Transplantation

Volume 41

BALTIMORE, MD.
1986

February 1986
Volume 41
Number 2

Transplantation

Official Journal of the Transplantation Society

Contents

OVERVIEW

Inducible expression of class II major histocompatibility complex antigens and the immunogenicity of vascular endothelium.
J.S. Pober, T. Collins, M.A. Gimbrone, Jr., P. Libby, and C.S. Reiss 144

EXPERIMENTAL TRANSPLANTATION

Cyclosporine and the ischemic rat kidney.
P. Jablonski, C. Harrison, B. Howden, D. Rae, G. Tavanlis, V.C. Marshall, and J.D. Tange . . . 147

Cyclosporine and experimental renal ischemic injury.
S.S. Chow, P. Thorner, R. Baumal, and D.R. Wilson 152

Local treatment of renal allografts—a promising way to reduce the dose of immunosuppressive drugs: Comparison of various ways of administering prednisolone.
T.J.M. Ruers, W.A. Buurman, J.F.M. Smits, C.J. van der Linden, J.J. van Dongen, H.A.J. Struyker-Boudier, and G. Kootstra 156

Evidence of free-radical-induced damage in rabbit kidneys after simple hypothermic preservation and autotransplantation.
C.J. Green, G. Healing, J. Lunec, B.J. Fuller, and S. Simpkin 161

The role of major and minor histocompatibility antigens in active enhancement of rat kidney allograft survival by blood transfusion.
I.V. Hutchinson and P.J. Morris 166

CLINICAL TRANSPLANTATION

Cyclosporine as an alternative to cyclophosphamide in the treatment of chronic graft-versus-host disease.
D. Bunjes, W. Heit, R. Arnold, T. Schmeiser, and H. Heimpel 170

Spontaneous anti-tubular-basement-membrane antibody production by lymphocytes isolated from a rejected allograft.
S.C. Jordan, S.C. Barkley, J.M. Lemire, R.S. Sakai, A. Cohen, and R.N. Fine 173

The effects of delayed function on recipients of cadaver renal allografts: A study of 158 patients randomized to cyclosporine or ALG-azathioprine.
D.M. Canafax, A. Torres, D.S. Fryd, J.E. Heil, M.H. Strand, N.L. Ascher, W.D. Payne, D.E.R. Sutherland, R.L. Simmons, and J.S. Najarian 177

The decreased incidence of aseptic necrosis in renal transplant recipients: A case control study.
P.S. Parfrey, D. Farge, N.A. Parfrey, J.A. Hanley, and R.D. Guttman 182

IMMUNOBIOLOGY

Protein kinase activation and the immunosuppressant cyclosporine.
R.K. Fidelus and A.H. Laughter 187

Hypersensitivity reactions in the small intestine: VII. Induction of the intestinal phase of the murine graft-versus-host reaction by Lyt 2^- T cells activated by I-A alloantigens.
A.M. Mowat, A. Borland, and D.M.V. Parrott 192

Difference in sensitivity to cyclosporine in vitro of human alloreactive lines and clones.
F. Manca, S. Carrozzi, A. Kunkl, S. Barocci, V. Dessi, U. Valente, I. Fontana, and F. Celada. 199

Altered patterns of organ distribution of autologous and grafted blood cells in mice treated with hydroxyurea.
M. Lévy 204

Allograft rejection and immune responses against allogeneic antigens in neonatally thymectomized mice.
K. Nomoto, H. Mayumi, K. Himeno, Y. Watanabe, M. Mitani, and N. Tokuda. 209

The migration of activated T lymphocytes in vitro: III. Paralysis and recovery of locomotor function during mitosis.
R.A. Hoffman, B.J. Hyland, N.L. Ascher, and R.L. Simmons. 214

Development of a simplified counterflow centrifugation elutriation procedure for depletion of lymphocytes from human bone marrow.
S.J. Noga, A.D. Donnenberg, C.L. Schwartz, L.C. Strauss, C.I. Civin, and G.W. Santos. ... 220

The relative immunogenicity of corneal epithelium, stroma, and endothelium: The role of major histocompatibility complex antigens.
P.A. Treseler, G.N. Foulks, and F. Sanfilippo. 229

Effect of storage on lymphocyte surface markers in whole blood units.
H.E. Prince and L. Arens. 235

The graft-versus-host reaction and immune function: III. Functional pre-T cells in the bone marrow of graft-versus-host-reactive mice displaying T cell immunodeficiency.
M. Seddik, T.A. Seemayer, and W.S. Lapp. 238

The graft-versus-host reaction and immune function: IV. B cell functional defect associated with a depletion of splenic colony-forming units in marrow of graft-versus-host-reactive mice.
M. Seddik, T.A. Seemayer, and W.S. Lapp. 242

IMMUNOGENETICS, HISTOCOMPATIBILITY AND TISSUE ANTIGENS

The expression of major histocompatibility complex and leukocyte antigens by cells in the rat cornea.
P.A. Treseler and F. Sanfilippo. 248

Public determinants of HLA indicated by pregnancy antibodies.
Y. Konoeda, P.I. Terasaki, A. Wakisaka, M.S. Park, and M.R. Mickey. 253

BRIEF COMMUNICATIONS

Severe immunosuppression in a renal transplant recipient with HTLV-III antibodies.
D.B.G. Oliveira, C.G. Winearls, J. Cohen, P.W. Ind, and G. Williams. 260

Late cellular rejection in renal transplant recipients.
L.R. Solomon, S. Martin, C.D. Short, W. Lawler, R. Gokal, R.W.G. Johnson, and N.P. Mallick. 262

Successful treatment with infrared contact coagulation of excessive fluid leakage after spontaneous decapsulation of a renal allograft.
R.G.W.L. Tiggeler, R.F. van der Sluis, T. Wobbes, R.A.P. Koene, and J.H.M. Berden. 265

In vivo interaction of cyclosporine and intralipid.
R. Wassef, Z. Cohen, and B. Langer. 266

Increased Leu-7-positive T lymphocytes during cytomegalovirus infection following allogeneic bone marrow transplantation for hematologic malignancies.
S.J. Forman, J.A. Zaia, C. Wright, M.T. Gallagher, and K.G. Blume. 268

Comparison of splenic and renal subcapsular islet autografting in dogs.
U.J. Hesse, D.E.R. Sutherland, P.F. Gores, A. Sitges-Serra, and J.S. Najarian. 271

Prolongation of skin graft survival in dogs treated with 8-aminoguanosine.
J.B. Benear, D. Frederick, L. Townsend, and R.B. Epstein. 274

Cyclosporine blood concentrations in the management of renal transplant recipients.
M.E. Rogerson, J.T. Marsden, K.E. Reid, M. Bewick, and D.W. Holt. 276

April 1986
Volume 41
Number 4

Transplantation

Official Journal of the Transplantation Society

Contents

OVERVIEW

The regulation of expression of major histocompatibility complex products.
P.F. Halloran, A. Wadgymar, and P. Autenried. 413

EXPERIMENTAL TRANSPLANTATION

Rejection of cultured thyroid allografts by the transfer of sensitized Lyt 2^+ T cells.
H.S. Warren and R.G. Pembrey. 421

Prolonged reversal of diabetes in the rat by transplantation of allogeneic islets from a single donor and cyclosporine treatment.
A. Dibelius, H. Königsberger, P. Walter, W. Permanetter, W. Brendel, and B.U. von Specht. 426

The influence of OKT8F treatment on allograft survival in Rhesus monkeys.
M. Jonker, F.J.M. Nooij, P. van Suylichem, P. Neuhaus, and G. Goldstein. 431

CLINICAL TRANSPLANTATION

Serologic methods for the early diagnosis of pneumocystis carinii infection in renal allograft recipients.
M. Jarowenko, L. Pifer, R. Kerman, and B.D. Kahan. 436

Comparison of monoclonal antibodies used for immunological monitoring of renal transplant recipients.
F.C. Henny, P.J. Oljans, H.J. Tanke, L.C. Paul, and L.A. van Es. 442

Serum antibody reactivity of broadly sensitized patients with HLA-matched peripheral blood T lymphocytes.
D.J. Cook and J.C. Scornik. 447

Assessment of plasma neopterin in clinical kidney transplantation.
A.J. Schäfer, V. Daniel, K. Dreikorn, and G. Opelz. 454

Demographic factors affecting the pharmokinetics of cyclosporine estimated by radioimmunoassay.
B.D. Kahan, W.G. Kramer, C. Wideman, S.M. Flechner, M.I. Lorber, and C.T. Van Buren. . . 459

An assessment of intrarenal hydrostatic pressure measurements in the diagnosis of acute renal allograft rejection.
C.P. Gibbons, C.B. Summerton, P.G. McNally, R. Kay, C.B. Brown, and A.T. Raftery. 464

Failure of platelet transfusion to improve human renal allograft survival.
J.R. Chapman, A. Ting, M. Fisher, N.P. Carter, and P.J. Morris. 468

The importance of the Lewis system in cadaver renal transplantation.
M.P. Posner, M.B. McGeorge, G. Mendez-Picon, T. Mohanakumar, and H.M. Lee. 474

Adaptation of adult bone marrow transplant recipient long-term survivors.
D.L. Wolcott, D.K. Wellisch, F.I. Fawzy, and J. Landsverk. 478

Psychological adjustment of adult bone marrow transplant donors whose recipient survives.
D.L. Wolcott, D.K. Wellisch, F.I. Fawzy, and J. Landsverk. 484

IMMUNOBIOLOGY

Immune reactivity in congenic mice after allogeneic or isogeneic transfusion.
M.L. Wood, R. Gottschalk, and A.P. Monaco. 489

Suppressive effect of mizoribine on humoral antibody production in DBA/2 mice.
M. Okubo, X. Chen, K. Kamata, Y. Masaki, and T. Uchiyama. 495

Detailed analysis and demonstration of differences in the kinetics of induction of class I and class II major histocompatibility complex antigens in rejecting cardiac and kidney allografts in the rat.
A.D. Milton, S.C. Spencer, and J.W. Fabre. 499

Relative contribution of major histocompatibility complex antigens to the immunogenicity of corneal allografts.
P.A. Treseler and F. Sanfilippo. 508

Second-set allograft responses in the earthworm *Lumbricus terrestris*: Kinetics and characteristics.
E.L. Cooper and P. Roch. 514

Specificity and precursor frequency of cytotoxic T cells in the response to minor H antigens.
L.M. Pilarski. 521

BRIEF COMMUNICATIONS

Lack of effect of splenectomy on the influence of pretransplant blood transfusions on cardiac allograft survival in histoincompatible rats.
R. Pollak, J.M. Blanchard, and M.R. Mozes. 527

Comparison of the immunogenicity of purified and unpurified murine islet allografts.
P.F. Gores, J. Mayoral, M.J. Field, and D.E.R. Sutherland. 529

Intrathecal allotransplantation of pancreatic endocrine cells in diabetic rats.
W.J. Tze and J. Tai. 531

The relationship between lymphokine responsiveness and HLA DR antigens as prognostic indicators of renal transplant survival.
J.M. MacSween, S.L. Eastwood, A.D. Cohen, and K. Rajaraman. 534

Asymptomatic extravasation of contrast material in the unused bladder.
W.K. O'Neal, A. Naimark, R.K. Babayan, and B.A. Idelson. 536

Cyclosporine for steroid-resistant acute rejection of renal cadaver grafts.
F.W. Ballardie, C.G. Winearls, D.J. Evans, A.J. Rees, and G. Williams 537

Doppler ultrasound as a screen for hepatic artery thrombosis after liver transplantation.
M.C. Segel, A.B. Zajko, A. Bowen, M.L. Skolnick, K.M. Bron, R.J. Penkrot, B.S. Slasky, and T.E. Starzl. 539

Cyclosporine-associated microangiopathy in renal transplantation: A severe but potentially reversible form of early graft injury.
J.A. Wolfe, R.L. McCann, and F. Sanfilippo. 541

Lethal graft-versus-host disease in a recipient of a pancreas-spleen transplant.
M.H. Deierhoi, H.W. Sollinger, M.J. Bozdech, and F.O. Belzer. 544

DIARY OF FORTHCOMING EVENTS 546

May 1986
Volume 41
Number 5

Transplantation

Official Journal of the Transplantation Society

Contents

OVERVIEW

Suppressor T cells in allogeneic models.
I.V. Hutchinson 547

EXPERIMENTAL TRANSPLANTATION

Lifelong reversal of the metabolic abnormalities of advanced diabetes in rats by whole-pancreas transplantation.
M.J. Orloff, G.E. Greenleaf, P. Urban, and B. Girard . . . . . 556 *

Monoclonal antibody analysis of canine hematopoietic cells: Role of Ia-like and Thy-1 antigens in bone marrow engraftment.
M.M. Prendergast, K.F. Bradstock, A.F. Broomhead, W.G. Hughes, A. Kabral, M.C. Berndt, and K. Tiver 565

CLINICAL TRANSPLANTATION

Monoclonal antibody therapy: Anti-idiotypic and non-anti-idiotypic antibodies to OKT3 arising despite intense immunosuppression.
G.J. Jaffers, T.C. Fuller, A.B. Cosimi, P.S. Russell, H.J. Winn, and R.B. Colvin 572

ALG treatment of steroid-resistant rejection in patients receiving cyclosporine.
A.J. Matas, V.A. Tellis, T. Quinn, D. Glichlick, R. Soberman, R. Weiss, G. Karwa, and F.J. Veith 579

Severe aplastic anemia associated with chronic mucocutaneous candidiasis: Immunologic and hematologic reconstitution after allogeneic bone marrow transplantation.
H.J. Deeg, L.G. Lum, J. Sanders, G.J. Levy, K.M. Sullivan, P. Beatty, E.D. Thomas, and R. Storb 583

Antigen-specific antibody responses of lymphocytes to tetanus toxoid after human marrow transplantation.
S. Shiobara, L.G. Lum, R.P. Witherspoon, and R. Storb 587

Diagnosis of tubular injury in renal transplant patients by a urinary assay for a proximal tubular antigen, the adenosine-deaminase-binding protein.
N.E. Tolkoff-Rubin, A.B. Cosimi, F.L. Delmonico, P.S. Russell, R.E. Thompson, D.J. Piper, W.P. Hansen, N.H. Bander, C.L. Finstad, C. Cordon-Cardo, L.H. Klotz, L.J. Old, and R.H. Rubin 593

A critical look at survival of diabetics with end-stage renal disease: Transplantation versus dialysis therapy.
R.B. Khauli, D.R. Steinmuller, A.C. Novick, C. Buszta, M. Goormastic, S. Nakamoto, D.G. Vidt, M. Magnusson, E. Paganini, and M.J. Schreiber. 598

Plasma exchange for platelet alloimmunization.
W.I. Bensinger, C.D. Buckner, R.A. Clift, S.J. Slichter, and E.D. Thomas. 602

Results of living-related kidney transplantation in Puerto Rico.
E.A. Santiago-Delpín, Z. González, E. Rivé-Mora, J.H. Amadeo, and R. Ramirez-González. 606

The effects of cyclosporine on *Toxoplasma gondii* in vivo and in vitro.
R.E. McCabe, B.J. Luft, and J.S. Remington. 611

Autonomic system dysfunction and polyneuropathy in nondiabetic uremia: A one year follow-up study after renal transplantation.
G. Solders, A. Persson, and H. Wilczek. 616

IMMUNOBIOLOGY

Allospecificity of activated T cells grown from endomyocardial biopsies from heart transplant patients.
A. Zeevi, J. Fung, T.R. Zerbe, C. Kaufman, B.S. Rabin, B.P. Griffith, R.L. Hardesty, and R.J. Duquesnoy. 620

Induction of transplantation tolerance in rats by spleen allografts: I. Evidence that rats tolerant of spleen allografts contain two phenotypically distinct T suppressor cells.
W.R. Duncan, S.M. Stepkowski, and H. Bitter-Suermann 626

Skin allograft rejection by both L3/T4$^+$ and Lyt-2$^+$ T cell subsets.
S. Cobbold and H. Waldmann 634

Improved renal allograft function and survival following nonspecific blood transfusions: I. Induction of soluble suppressor factors inhibiting the mitogenic response.
R. Roy, J. Lachance, R. Noel, J.H. Grose, and R. Beaudoin. 640

Treatment and prevention of acute graft-versus-host disease with thalidomide in a rat model.
G.B. Vogelsang, A.D. Hess, G. Gordon, and G.W. Santos. 644

BRIEF COMMUNICATIONS

Transfusion of donor class I MHC antigen prior to kidney transplantation in dogs.
P.F. Gores, A. Sitges-Serra, U.J. Hesse, J.S. Najarian, and D.E.R. Sutherland. 648

The influence of the transplantation technique on the duration of endocrine function of pancreas allografts in the rat model.
W. Timmermann, T. Schang, and A. Thiede. 650

The effect of exchange blood transfusions on the cytotoxic alloantibody response in AS strain rats.
N. Mistry, T. Horsburgh, P.S. Veitch, and P.R.F. Bell. 652

Optimization by timing of oral cyclosporine to prevent acute kidney allograft rejection in dogs.
M. Cavallini, F. Halberg, D.E.R. Sutherland, G. Cornélissen, J. Heils, and J.S. Najarian. 654

Determination of cyclosporine concentration in bile.
L. Scanlon, R. Baloh, B. Gridelli, K.M. Rao, B. Shaw, T. Starzl, and A. Sanghvi. 657

Encapsulation of cyclosporine by phosphatidylinositol-cholesterol liposomes.
L. Stuhne-Sekalec, J. Chudzik, and N.Z. Stanacev 659

Effect of cyclosporine and low-temperature culture on prevention of rejection of islet xenografts (rat-to-mouse).
R. Terasaka, P.E. Lacy, R.P. Bucy, and J.M. Davie 661

Positive direct antiglobulin tests associated with intravenous gamma globulin use in bone marrow transplant recipients.
C.F. Whitsett, J.A. Pierce, and L.E. Daffin. 663

Hematuria and hypercalciuria following renal transplantation.
J.E. Springate, R.D. Fildes, S.M. Mauer, and L.G. Feld. 664

Successful treatment of persistent post-transplant hyperparathyroidism with diphosphonate.
K.M.L. Leunissen, F-J.F.E. Vismans, R.J.M. van Leendert, and J.P. van Hooff 666

June 1986
Volume 41
Number 6

Transplantation

Official Journal of the Transplantation Society

Contents

EXPERIMENTAL TRANSPLANTATION

Functional preservation of the mammalian kidney: VII. Autologous transplantation of dog kidneys after treatment with dimethylsulfoxide.
A.M. Karow, Jr., M. McDonald, T. Dendle, and R. Rao. . . . 669

Amplification of the graft-versus-host reaction by partial body irradiation.
S. Lehnert, W.B. Rybka, and T.A. Seemayer. . . . 675

Functional clonal deletion vs. suppressor cell–induced transplantation tolerance in chimeras prepared with a short course of total-lymphoid irradiation.
S. Slavin, S. Morecki, M. Weigensberg, S. Bar, and L. Weiss. . . . 680

Early events in natural resistance to bone marrow transplantation: Use of radiolabeled bone marrow cells.
G.A. Carlson, S.T. Marshall, and A. Kiesche. . . . 688

Passive transfer of cytomegalovirus by cardiac and renal organ transplants in a rat model.
J.H. Bruning, C.A. Bruggeman, C.P.A. van Boven, and P.J.C. van Breda Vriesman. . . . 695

The effect of hyperglycemia on isolated rodent islets transplanted to the kidney capsule site.
D.W.R. Gray, P. McShane, and P.J. Morris. . . . 699

Bone marrow transplantation in the rat: V. Lymphoid cell subclasses in the target organs during acute graft-versus-host disease.
R. Renkonen. . . . 704

CLINICAL TRANSPLANTATION

The prognostic value of the eosinophil in acute renal allograft rejection.
M.R. Weir, M. Hall-Craggs, S.Y. Shen, J.N. Posner, S.V. Alongi, F.J. Dagher, and J.H. Sadler. . . . 709

Use of a prognostic index in evaluation of liver transplantation for primary biliary cirrhosis.
J. Neuberger, D.G. Altman, E. Christensen, N. Tygstrup, and R. Williams. . . . 713

Relationship of interferon-gamma and neopterin levels during stimulation with alloantigens in vivo and in vitro.
W. Woloszczuk, J. Troppmair, E. Leiter, R. Flener, M. Schwarz, J. Kovarik, E. Pohanka, R. Margreiter, and C. Huber. . . . 716

Cellular immunity to vaccinations and herpesvirus infections after bone marrow transplantation.
J.W. Gratama, L.F. Verdonck, J.A. van der Linden, J.G. van Heugten, H.A.J.G. Kreeft, J. D'Amaro, F.E. Zwaan, C.C. Gast. . . . 719

Infections in heart-lung transplant recipients.
J.S. Dummer, C.G. Montero, B.P. Griffith, R.L. Hardesty, I.L. Paradis, and M. Ho. . . . 725

Prophylactic use of OKT3 monoclonal antibody in cadaver kidney recipients: Utilization of OKT3 as the sole immunosuppressive agent.
P. Vigeral, N. Chkoff, L. Chatenoud, H. Campos, M. Lacombe, D. Droz, G. Goldstein, J.F. Bach, and H. Kreis. . . . 730

IMMUNOBIOLOGY

Inhibition of rat skin allograft rejection by cyclosporine: In situ characterization of the impaired local immune response.
F.J. Guillén, W.W. Hancock, E. Towpik, J.W. Kupiec-Weglinski, F.R. Rickles, N.L. Tilney, and G.F. Murphy. . . . 734

The specificity of nephritogenic antibodies: IV. Binding of monoclonal antithymocyte antibodies to rat kidney.
W.M. Bagchus, J. Donga, J. Rozing, P. Hoedemaeker, and W.W. Bakker 739

The entry of lymphocytes into stimulated lymph nodes: The site of selection of alloantigen-specific cells.
M.T. Drayson. 745

Alloantigen presentation by canine endothelial cells: Presentation of autologous alloantigens in vitro.
G. Groenewegen, W.A. Buurman, G.M.A.A. Jeunhomme. 751

Increased oxidative burst potential exhibited by macrophages during graft-versus-host reactions in mice.
H. Goldin and Y. Keisari 755

Functional characterization of prethymic T cells committed to alloreactivity.
M. Blank, C. Gronau, M. Sauer, H.-U. Wottge, and W. Müller-Ruchholtz. 759

Impaired rejection of minor-histocompatibility-antigen–disparate skin grafts and acquisition of tolerance to thymus donor antigens in allothymus-implanted thymectomized *Xenopus*.
J.C. Arnall and J.D. Horton. 766

IMMUNOGENETICS, HISTOCOMPATIBILITY AND TISSUE ANTIGENS

Expression of class I and class II major histocompatibility antigens in normal and transplanted human heart.
M.L. Rose, M.I. Coles, R.J. Griffin, A. Pomerance, and M.H. Yacoub. 776

BRIEF COMMUNICATIONS

The effects of donor pretreatment on the transmission of murine cytomegalovirus with cardiac transplants and explants.
E.J. Wilson, D.N. Medearis, L.V. Barrett, A. Bhan, and R.H. Rubin. 781

Effect of cyclosporine upon the function of ischemically damaged kidneys in the rat.
G. Kanazi, N. Stowe, D. Steinmuller, H. Ho-Hsieh, and A.C. Novick. 782

Accelerated development of spontaneous thymic lymphomas in male AKR mice receiving cyclosporine.
A. Hattori, M.I.R. Perera, L.A. Witkowski, H.W. Kunz, T.J. Gill, III, and H. Shinozuka. 784

Donor type MHC positive cells in the host spleen after rat organ transplantation: Differences between pancreas and heart allograft recipients.
B. Steiniger and J. Klempnauer. 787

The rationale for antimitotic treatment prior to bone marrow transplantation.
M. Lévy. 790

Cyclosporine and Familial Mediterranean Fever amyloidosis.
B. Siegal, D. Zemer, and M. Pras. 793

Superoxide dismutase decrease in cardiac transplants.
M. Kloc, K. Mailer, and S. Stepkowski. 794

Erythromycin and cyclosporine.
T.A. Gonwa, D.D. Nghiem, J.A. Schulak, and R.J. Corry. 797

LETTERS TO THE EDITOR 800

ERRATA 801

AUTHOR INDEX 802

SUBJECT INDEX 805

Transplantation

Official Journal of the Transplantation Society

Transplantation (ISSN 0041—1337) is published monthly by Williams & Wilkins, 428 E. Preston Street, Baltimore, MD 21202. Second class postage paid at Baltimore, MD, and at additional mailing offices. Postmaster, send address changes (form 3579) to Williams & Wilkins, 428 E. Preston Street, Baltimore, MD 21202. Subscription rates $105.00 ($120.00 foreign); institutions $130.00 ($145.00 foreign); single copy $12.00 ($15.00 foreign). (Prices subject to change) Indexed by *Current Contents* and *Index Medicus.*

Transplantation

INSTRUCTIONS FOR AUTHORS

Articles dealing with completed research, and brief or preliminary reports designated as *Brief Communication* will be considered for publication. The latter should present new ideas or techniques or findings of special timeliness and significance. *Brief Communications* should not be divided into sections; it is recommended that the last paragraph be a summary and the entire double-spaced typewritten manuscript *including* tables and figures should not exceed 10 pages. *Letters to the Editor*, whether in commentary on articles appearing in TRANSPLANTATION or about other pertinent matters will also be considered. *Overview* articles should cover a topic of special interest in the field of transplantation. The *overview* should not exceed 4000 words and should not be divided in sections. The references should be done according to the instructions below for *References.* If and when manuscripts are accepted for publication, it will be necessary for The Williams & Wilkins Company to receive in writing the assignment of copyright from all authors of all manuscripts. Forms for this purpose will be supplied. *Submit an original, 2 copies, and 3 sets of illustrations.* Avoid extensive handwritten alterations. Failure to observe the format requested may delay processing of the manuscript.

Typescript must be *double-spaced throughout.* Use bond paper for the original copy. Maintain a minimum left margin of approximately 4 cm and a right margin of 2.5 cm. Number the pages in sequence.

Title page should carry the title, author's name under the title, and institution and address under the author's name. Include postal zone or "zip code" in the address. To avoid confusion in bibliographic indexing, it is preferable for authors to state given names in full.

Title should be concise (preferably not more than 15 words).

Summary of not more than 250 words is to be typed on a separate sheet.

Footnotes for the text should be typed double-spaced on a separate page, but all footnotes may be typed on the same page. Footnotes should be designated by superscript Arabic numbers and numbered in sequence. Footnotes should include source of support (cited as footnote to the title), current address, correspondence address, and abbreviations.

Abbreviations used in the text and their meanings should be listed alphabetically and typed double-spaced on a separate sheet of paper or on the page with other footnotes.

References should be typed double-spaced on a separate sheet. References should be numbered in the order in which they are cited in the text. Six or fewer authors should be listed. If there are seven or more, only the first three and "et al." should be listed. The titles of articles are to be included, and the journal names are to be abbreviated according to the *Index Medicus* style. Text citations of the references are placed in parentheses. Only papers that have been accepted for publication should be listed in the references. Manuscripts in preparation, unpublished observations, and personal communications should be referred to as such in the text. Completed manuscripts that have been submitted for publication may be cited as footnotes to the text. If the manuscript is subsequently in press, appropriate changes can be made in the galleys. The following are examples of the reference style:

1. Winearls CJ, Fabre JW, Millard PR, Morris PJ. Use of cyclophosphamide and enhancing serum to suppress renal allograft rejection in the rat. Transplantation 1979; 28: 271.
2. Osler AG. Complement: mechanisms and functions. Englewood Cliffs: Prentice Hall, 1976.
3. National Center for Health Sciences. Acute conditions: incidence and associated disability, United States July 1968–June 1969. Rockville, Md.: National Center for Health Statistics, 1972. (DHEW publication no. (HSN) 72-1036).

Tables should be typed *double-spaced throughout* (including column heads, footnotes, and data), each table on a separate sheet. Number the tables in sequence with Arabic numerals. For each table supply a concise descriptive heading. Designate explanatory footnotes by superscript lowercase Latin letters. Type footnotes immediately below the table to which they refer. All columns must carry concise headings descriptive of the data in the column. Photographs of tables are not acceptable. All tables are cited in the text in numerical order.

Figures (i.e., photomicrographs, charts, and graphs) are to be supplied as unmounted glossy photographic prints. Lettering on graphs should be large enough so that when the figure is reduced to the width of a single column (8.8 cm), the lettering is still legible (1.5 mm high for an 8.8-cm-wide figure). Photomicrographs and other photographs should be no larger than 8.8 cm in width, if possible. Number the figures in sequence in Arabic numbers. Figures should be labeled on the back with the author's name, figure number, and the word "top." All figures are cited in the text in numerical order. Figure legends, numbered to correspond with the figures, typed double-spaced, and assembled on a separate sheet are to be supplied for all figures. These legends should explain all symbols used on the figures and should indicate staining and magnification for photomicrographs.

Page charges. Authors will be charged $40.00 for each printed page per article. Under exceptional circumstances, page charges will be waived by the editors.

Submit manuscripts to either editorial office:

A. P. Monaco, M.D.
TRANSPLANTATION
North American Editorial Office
New England Deaconess Hospital
185 Pilgrim Road
Boston, Massachusetts 02215

J. R. Batchelor, M.D.
TRANSPLANTATION
European Editorial Office
Department of Immunology
Royal Postgraduate Medical School
Hammersmith Hospital
Ducane Road
London W12, England

Information for Subscribers

Published monthly, two volumes a year, beginning January and July.

Annual Subscription Rates—U. S. A. AND POSSESSIONS: personal, $105.00; institutional, $130.00; single copies, $12.00. FOREIGN: personal, $120.00; institutional, $145.00; single copies, $15.00. Institutional (multiple reader) rate applies to libraries, schools, hospitals, clinics, group practices, and federal commercial, and private institutions and organizations. A special in-training rate of $60.00 ($85.00 foreign) is available to residents, fellows, interns and students. (Prices subject to change) In requesting this rate, which is limited to three years, please give training status and name of institution. Subscribers may request that their copies be sent by air mail; the extra charge entailed for air service will be billed to the subscriber.

New and renewal subscriptions are entered to begin with the January or July issue. Correspondence regarding subscriptions should be addressed to the publishers.

Change of address. Publisher must be notified 60 days in advance. Undeliverable journals will be destroyed. Duplicates (if available) can be ordered from the publishers at the regular price of single issues.

Reprints of individual articles are available *only* from authors.

Microfilm. For availability, inquire of Williams & Wilkins.

Japanese Yen price is available from our sole agent: USACO Corporation, 13-12 Shimbashi 1-Chome, Minato-Ku, Tokyo 105, Japan, telephone 03-502-6471.

WILLIAMS & WILKINS

Publishers of Books and Periodicals in Medicine and the Allied Sciences
428 East Preston Street, Baltimore, Md. 21202, U.S.A.

AUTHOR INDEX

Arens, L., 235
Arnold, R., 170
Ascher, N. L., 177, 214

Barkley, S. C., 173
Barocci, S., 199
Baumal, R., 152
Benear, J. B., 274
Berden, J. H. M., 264
Bewick, M., 276
Blume, K. G., 268
Borland, A., 192
Bunjes, D., 170
Buurman, W. A., 156

Canafax, D. M., 177
Carrozzi, S., 199
Celada, F., 199
Chow, S. S., 152
Civin, C. I., 220
Cohen, A., 173
Cohen, J., 260
Cohen, Z., 266
Collins, T., 141

Dessi, V., 199
Donnenberg, A. D., 220

Epstein, R. B., 274

Farge, D., 182
Fidelus, R. K., 187
Fine, R. N., 173
Fontana, I., 199
Forman, S. J., 268
Foulks, G. N., 229
Frederick, D., 274
Fryd, D. S., 177
Fuller, B. J., 161

Gallagher, M. T., 268
Gimbrone, M. A., Jr., 141
Gokal, R., 262
Gores, P. F., 271
Green, C. J., 161
Guttmann, R. D., 182

Hanley, J. A., 182
Harrison, C., 147
Healing, G., 161
Heil, J. E., 177
Heimpel, H., 170
Heit, W., 170
Hesse, U. J., 271
Himeno, K., 209
Hoffman, R. A., 214
Holt, D. W., 276
Howden, B., 147
Hutchinson, I. V., 166
Hyland, B. J., 214

Ind, P. W., 260

Jablonski, P., 147
Johnson, R. W. G., 262
Jordan, S. C., 173

Koene, R. A. P., 264
Konoeda, Y., 253
Kootstra, G., 156
Kunkl, A., 199

Langer, B., 266
Lapp, W. S., 238, 242
Laughter, A. H., 187
Lawler, W., 262
Lemire, J. M., 173
Lévy, M., 204
Libby, P., 141

Lunec, J., 161

Mallick, N. P., 262
Manca, F., 199
Marsden, J. T., 276
Marshall, V. C., 147
Martin, S., 262
Mayumi, H., 209
Mickey, M. R., 253
Mitani, M., 209
Morris, P. J., 166
Mowat, A. M., 192

Najarian, J. S., 177, 271
Noga, S. J., 220
Nomoto, K., 209

Oliveira, D. B. G., 260

Parfrey, N. A., 182
Parfrey, P. S., 182
Park, M. S., 253
Parrott, D. M. V., 192
Payne, W. D., 177
Pober, J. S., 141
Prince, H. E., 235

Rae, D., 147
Reid, K. E., 276
Reiss, C. S., 141
Rogerson, M. E., 276
Ruers, T. J. M., 156

Sakai, R. S., 173
Sanfilippo, F., 229, 248
Santos, G. W., 220
Schmeiser, T., 170
Schwartz, C. L., 220
Seddik, M., 238, 242
Seemayer, T. A., 238, 242
Short, C. D., 262
Simmons, R. L., 177, 214
Simpkin, S., 161
Sitges-Serra, A., 271
Smits, J. F. M., 156
Solomon, L. R., 262
Strand, M. H., 177
Strauss, L. C., 220
Struyker-Boudier, H. A. J., 156
Sutherland, D. E. R., 177, 271

Tange, J. D., 147
Tavanlis, G., 147
Terasaki, P. I., 253
Thorner, P., 152
Tiggeler, R. G. W. L., 264
Tokuda, N., 209
Torres, A., 177
Townsend, L., 274
Treseler, P. A., 229, 248

Valente, U., 199
Van der Linden, C. J., 156
Van der Sluis, R. F., 264
Van Dongen, J. J., 156

Wakisaka, A., 253
Wassef, R., 266
Watanabe, Y., 209
Williams, G., 260
Wilson, D. R., 152
Winearls, C. G., 260
Wobbes, T., 264
Wright, C., 268

Zaia, J. A., 268

0041-1337/86/4102-0141$02.00/0
TRANSPLANTATION

Vol. 41, No. 2
Printed in U.S.A.

Transplantation

OVERVIEW

INDUCIBLE EXPRESSION OF CLASS II MAJOR HISTOCOMPATIBILITY COMPLEX ANTIGENS AND THE IMMUNOGENICITY OF VASCULAR ENDOTHELIUM[1]

JORDAN S. POBER,[2,3,4,5] TUCKER COLLINS,[2,3] MICHAEL A. GIMBRONE, JR.,[2,3] PETER LIBBY,[6] AND CAROL S. REISS[2,7]

Departments of Pathology, Brigham and Women's Hospital and Harvard Medical School; Department of Medicine, Tufts University; and Division of Pediatric Oncology, Dana Farber Cancer Institute, Boston, Massachusetts

The vasculature is a major target of immune-mediated injury in the process of allogeneic transplant rejection (*1*). This is certainly related to the continual exposure of the endothelial lining to blood-borne immune effector cells and molecules; the endothelium must bear the first wave of attack. An additional explanation may lie in the intrinsic immunogenicity of vascular endothelium. In vivo, alloantibodies specific for endothelial cell surface molecules (*2*) are readily demonstrable in rejected organs (*3*). In vitro, endothelial cultures strongly stimulate allogeneic responses (*4*). In both regards, endothelial cells appear more immunostimulatory than other vascular and stromal cell types. How can this enhanced allogeneic immunogenicity of endothelial cells be explained?

Two central conclusions may be drawn from the general study of the allogeneic response to foreign cells and tissues. First, the major (although not necessarily the only) pathways involved in generating specific effector cells, including delayed-type hypersensitivity (DTH)[8] effector cells and allospecific cytolytic T lymphocytes (CTL), require the participation of allospecific activated T helper cells (T_H). Second, the activation of T_H in an antigen-specific manner requires recognition of a polymorphic determinant of a class II major histocompatibility complex (MHC) molecule upon the surface of a stimulator cell (*5, 6*). Clonal cell analyses of T_H have shown that the same T cell antigen receptor may be triggered by polymorphic self (autologous) class II determinants "modified" by combination with nominal antigen (which may include foreign class I MHC antigens) or by polymorphic foreign (allogeneic) class II determinants, with or without combination with nominal antigen (*7*). Therefore, in order to be immunogenic and stimulate specific T_H, a foreign cell must express a class II MHC antigen. However, while expression of class II antigens is necessary for a foreign cell to stimulate an allogeneic response, it may not be sufficient. For example, not all class-II-bearing cells can stimulate a primary allogeneic T cell proliferative response, a measure of T_H activation (*8*). In addition, there is evidence that the requirements for activation of T_H are not constant. Naive resting T_H may require different signals from previously stimulated T_H that may be different yet from activated T_H blasts (*9*). Furthermore, T_H subsets activated by different types of stimulatory cells may have different functional properties (*10*).

In the 1970s, many investigators felt that bone-marrow-derived "immunocytes" (lymphocytes, mononuclear phagocytes, and dendritic cells) were the only cells that functionally expressed class II molecules and thus could interact with T_H. Much debate has been generated over the issue of whether all class-II-expressing leukocytes are equivalent. For example, can all B cells or mononuclear phagocytes or only some subset of them effectively stimulate allogeneic T cell proliferation in vitro, or is the classic mixed leukocyte reaction (MLR) largely a response to a minor subpopulation of nonphagocytic, nonlymphocytic "dendritic" cells. (There are recent examples of this controversy [*11, 12*]). In vivo, the postulated restriction of immunogenicity to bone-marrow-derived cells that express class II antigens has been formulated as the "passenger leukocyte" hypothesis—that is, a graft is immunogenic only if it contains bone-marrow-derived, class-II-bearing cells of the mononuclear phagocyte or dendritic cell lineage (*13, 14*).

Recent observations concerning the cellular range and control of class II MHC expression have dramatically challenged and broadened these ideas. In 1980, it was discovered that murine macrophages in vitro could be induced to express more surface Ia antigens (murine class II MHC molecules) by T cell factors present in crude lymphokine (*15, 16*). Furthermore, the percentage of macrophages in a peritoneal exudate that express class II antigen depended upon the nature of the eliciting signal and could also be modulated by lymphokine (*17*). Subsequently, the Ia-inducing factor was identified as immune interferon

[1] This work was supported by grants from NIH and The Cancer Research Institute.

[2] Department of Pathology, Harvard Medical School.
[3] Brigham and Women's Hospital.
[4] Jordan S. Pober is a Searle Scholar.
[5] To whom correspondence should be addressed, at Department of Pathology, Brigham and Women's Hospital, 75 Francis St. Boston, MA 02115.
[6] Tufts University.
[7] Dana Farber Cancer Institute.

[8] Abbreviations used: CTL, cytolytic T lymphocytes; DTH, delayed-type hypersensitivity; EC, endothelial cells; HUVE, human umbilical vein endothelial cells; Ia, I-region-associated antigen (used to collectively describe class II MHC antigens; IFN, interferon; IL-1, interleukin 1; IL-2, interleukin 2; MHC major histocompatibility complex; MLR, mixed leukocyte reaction; PBL, peripheral blood lymphocyte; SMC, smooth muscle cell; T_H, T helper cells.

(IFN-γ) (*18, 19*). These observations were extended to human monocytes (*20–22*) and established that class II antigen expression was not immutable. It was also observed that several human tumor cell lines of non-bone-marrow origin could express class II antigens (notably melanoma cells) and that this expression could also be increased or induced by immune interferon (*20*). Our laboratory reported that normal cultured human vascular endothelial cells could be induced to express HLA-DR antigens (the immunodominant human class II molecule) (*23*) and that this effect could be mediated by activated T cells or by immune interferon (*24*). We subsequently found that large and small vessel endothelial cells express HLA-DR—and, much to our initial surprise, so do human dermal fibroblasts (*25*). Recent studies from several laboratories have demonstrated that cultured cells from virtually every organ and embryonic germ layer can be induced to express HLA-DR in response to immune interferon (*26, 27*). Interferons of the nonimmune type (leukocyte and fibroblast) usually increase surface expression of class I but not class II MHC antigens (*21, 22, 25*). In vivo experiments have shown similar induction of class II molecules on stromal and epithelial cell types in rodent and human tissues at sites of cellular immune inflammation (*28–36*). (It is worth noting that human microvascular endothelial cells in situ may basally express some class II molecules, as detected by immunocytochemistry [*37–39*], although the origin [i.e., adsorption vs. endogenous synthesis] and function of such molecules is unknown. Furthermore, immune inflammation appears to increase the level of expression on human vascular endothelium.) Collectively, these observations have established that class II MHC antigen expression is not, as previously thought, restricted to an "immunologic" subset of bone-marrow-derived cell types either in vitro or in vivo.

As an aside, immune interferon is not the only mediator reported capable of modulating the expression of class II MHC antigens (*41–50*). Significantly, keratinocyte Ia expression can be induced in vivo under circumstances in which immune interferon production is highly unlikely (*51*). However, most agents other than interferon appear to work on the cell type under study (eg., murine macrophages or resting B cells) but not necessarily on other cell types (*26*). Furthermore, we have failed to identify any other agent that will modulate class II expression on cultured vascular cells. Thus immune interferon remains of special interest as a mediator because it is generated in situ during immune reactions at the site of observable class II induction; and it is a broadly acting agent in vitro with readily demonstrable class II-inducing activity on vascular and stromal cell types, including endothelium.

The mechanism of immune interferon action on the MHC has recently been investigated. In general, immune interferon appears to increase mRNA levels for class II molecules (*52–55*). For example, we have found that untreated human endothelial cells or dermal fibroblasts have no detectable mRNA for class II antigens, whereas immune interferon causes a rapid appearance of specific mRNAs that precedes surface expression (*55*). A general role of mRNA levels in regulating class II expression is supported by B cell "regulatory mutants" that show intact class II genes and basally depressed mRNA levels that can be rescued by introduction of "trans acting" factors (*56, 57*) that increase both mRNA and surface expression. It is likely that the induction of class II mRNA by immune interferon will involve activation of transcription, as has been shown for the induction of class I mRNA by leukocyte interferon (*58*). It is also likely that class II genes will contain regulatory sequences that "respond" to an interferon-induced trans acting signal (*59*). However, direct evidence for these conclusions is as yet lacking.

Several observations suggest that mRNA levels are not the only regulatory factor controlling class II surface expression. For example, we have found that withdrawal of interferon leads to rapid disappearance of class II mRNA in fibroblasts but only slow decline in surface expression (*55*). There are also large quantitative discrepancies between the size of the change in class I or class II message levels and the size of the change in surface expression (*52, 55*). The mechanisms of such posttranscriptional regulatory effects are unknown. Much speculation has been focused upon the potential posttranscriptional regulatory role of the "invariant chain" of the class II molecules (*60*), a nonpolymorphic protein encoded outside the MHC that is associated with intracellular biosynthetic intermediates of the mature class II antigens. According to one model, limiting quantities of invariant chain, under separate regulatory control, could limit surface expression of interferon-induced class II polypeptides. We have found that mRNA for invariant chain is coordinately induced with class II mRNAs in fibroblasts and endothelial cells when treated with immune interferon (*55*), and others have found increased invariant chain polypeptide in interferon-treated cells (*61, 62*). Thus, the invariant chain is unlikely to be limiting in interferon-exposed cells. Furthermore, there is no direct evidence as yet that invariant chain levels do in fact regulate class II antigen surface expression, inducible or otherwise.

While interferon-mediated induction of class II MHC antigens upon non-bone-marrow–derived cell types is now well established, the functional consequences of this phenomenon are not yet known. We have proposed that endothelial cell HLA-DR expression could be used to recruit antigen-specific T_H into the site of a developing immune response, serving as an amplification mechanism. In our model, presentation of nominal antigen by endothelial cells in combination with induced HLA-DR or other class II products would be used as a signal to the antigen receptor on a circulating T_H cell, leading to migration into the tissues at the site of the foreign antigen (*63*). Our model is in accord with the observations that induction of expression of class II antigens on endothelial cells precedes large scale mononuclear cell infiltration in DTH (*35*); and that the initial T cell infiltrate in DTH responses is enriched for antigen-specific T cells (*64*). Burger and Vetto have postulated that nominal antigen presentation by vascular endothelium might actually be the initial mechanism of T_H activation (*65*). Their model was developed prior to the realization that class II antigens on endothelial cells are subject to modulation, and that in the absence of activated T cell products (e.g., immune interferon), endothelial cell class II molecules may be at insufficient (basal) levels to function in presentation of antigen to resting T_H cells. The key premise underlying both these models is that the serologically-detected class II molecules can serve to activate T_H. We reported that HLA-DR induced on human endothelial cells or dermal fibroblasts had the characteristic two-polypeptide chain structure of lymphocyte HLA-DR and could be recognized by allospecific cloned CTL (*25*). The CTL assay has the advantage that only the antigen on the surface of an individual target cell is relevant to killing; there is no bystander effect and minor contaminating cell populations in the culture cannot account for the observed result. Therefore, our data clearly establish that endothelial cell HLA-DR can be recognized by a T cell antigen receptor. However, they do not directly address whether the T_H antigen receptor can recognize these molecules. Nominal antigen presentation to T_H by endothelial cell cultures in an HLA-DR restricted manner has been reported by several investigators (*66–68*), although contamination of the cultures by antigen-presenting cells of bone marrow origin was not rigorously ruled out. Other workers have since reported nominal antigen presentation by isolated murine astrocytes (*69*) or by human thyroid cells (*70*); contamination of the cultures in these experiments was not addressed. We have found presentation of tetanus toxoid by long-term, multiply passaged cultures of dermal fibroblasts to T cell clones and resting T cells (*71*). Antigen presentation by fibroblasts required preinduction of class II antigens by immune interferon, could be blocked by antibody against HLA-DR, and was HLA-DR-restricted (*71*). Contamination of such long-term cultures by bone-marrow-derived accessory cells is highly unlikely, and we conclude that fibroblast cells are the actual antigen-presenting cell in the cultures. Perhaps most convincing has been the report of Burger and coworkers who found that cloned endothelial cells would present nominal antigen to HLA-DR-matched cloned T cells (*72*). The direct implication of these experiments is that T_H can recognize class II molecules on nontraditional accessory cells, and that this recognition results in T_H activation. This conclusion is reinforced by the demonstration of nominal antigen presentation by murine L cells transfected with class II genes (*73, 74*). (The cell of origin of the L cell is not known; they are not fibroblasts, as commonly stated, however, it is unlikely that they are of bone-marrow origin).

The nominal antigen responses in the above experiments are memory responses, involving resting or activated memory T_H cells. Primary allogeneic responses, such as those triggered by allografts, differ in that they may involve naive T cells. Hirschberg et al. found that human umbilical vein endothelial (HUVE) cells can stimulate primary allogeneic responses in vitro (*4*). We have confirmed this result and extended it with long-term, serially passaged HUVE cultures. Surprisingly, it does not matter whether or not the endothelial cells are pretreated with immune interferon to express HLA-DR. Presumably this is because normal peripheral blood T cells in coculture with allogeneic endothelial cells rapidly induce endothelial cells to become HLA-DR-positive (*24*), perhaps through lymphokine secretion by a previously activated T cell subpopulation. By contrast, dermal fibroblasts are markedly less stimulatory of allogeneic lymphocyte proliferation, whether or not HLA-DR is preinduced to equivalent levels, and whether or not purified IL-1 is added to supplement the cultures (*25*) (Fig. 1). Cyclooxygenase inhibitors did not augment the response to fibroblasts. Some, but not all, fibroblast strains actively inhibited lymphocyte responses, although fibroblast-conditioned medium was not inhibitory. These experiments suggest that endothelial cells are, in some way, "special" with regard to their interactions with T_H cells compared with "stromal" cells.

It is hard to compare quantitatively the endothelial and fibroblast response of the allogeneic T cells shown in Figure 1 because (A) the endothelial cells used were in primary culture whereas the fibroblasts were serially passaged (and thus presumptively less likely to be contaminated by cells of bone marrow origin); and (B) the endothelial cells and fibroblasts were derived from different donors (and thus coincidentally could differ in their immunogenicity for a particular responder). We have addressed these problems by using serially passaged endothelial cells and "smooth muscle" cells derived from explants of the tunica media of the same saphenous vein segments. (The smooth muscle cultures are less well characterized then the endothelial cells because immunochemical criteria for passaged vascular smooth muscle are not readily available. Nevertheless, the morphologic appearance of these cultures is consistent with their identity as vascular smooth muscle). Smooth muscle cells are readily induced to express HLA-DR by immune interferon, and comparable amounts of HLA-DR is present in interferon-treated endothelial and smooth muscle cultures (data not shown). (We were unable to compare the number or surface density of HLA-DR molecules per cell because of difficulties in producing viable single-cell suspensions of smooth muscle cells for flow cytometric analysis.) The clear result is that passaged endothelial cells appear markedly more stimulatory than vascular smooth muscle cells (Fig. 2).

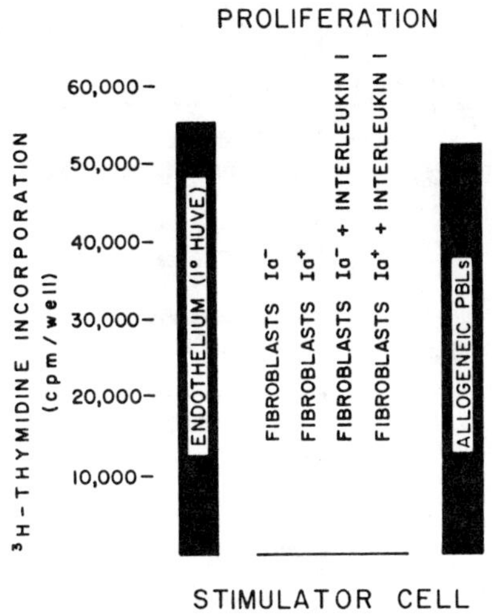

FIGURE 1. Proliferation of allogeneic lymphocytes to primary human umbilical vein endothelial cells (1° HUVE), human dermal fibroblasts, or allogeneic peripheral blood leukocytes (PBL). The cells were cultured and the assays performed as described previously (*24, 25*). In brief, endothelial cell or fibroblast stimulators were grown to confluence in flat-bottomed microtiter well plates (about 1×10^4 cells/well). Alternatively, allogeneic peripheral blood mononuclear leukocytes (1×10^5 cells/well) were used as stimulators in other wells. Stimulators were γ-irradiated prior to the assay. Responder cells (3×10^5 cells) were added to the wells on day 0, and proliferation was assessed on day 6 visually and by incorporation of ^{3}H-thymidine. Ia$^+$ refers to pretreatment of stimulator cells with recombinant immune interferon (200 U/ml) for 4 days prior to the proliferation assay to induce class II MHC antigen expression; and interleukin 1 refers to addition of affinity-purified, human monocyte-derived IL-1 (a generous gift of Dr. Charles Dinarello, Tufts Medical School, Boston, MA) at 10 U/ml to the proliferation assay on day 0.

Our experiments with vascular smooth muscle and dermal fibroblasts suggest that expression of HLA-DR is insufficient to generate an allogeneic response. Why are endothelial cells more immunogenic? One possibility is that class II MHC antigens other than HLA-DR may be important. This explanation seems unlikely because we have found that both endothelial cultures and dermal fibroblast cultures express DP and DQ (formerly SB and DC/DS/MB, respectively, the two other human class II antigens) upon immune interferon treatment

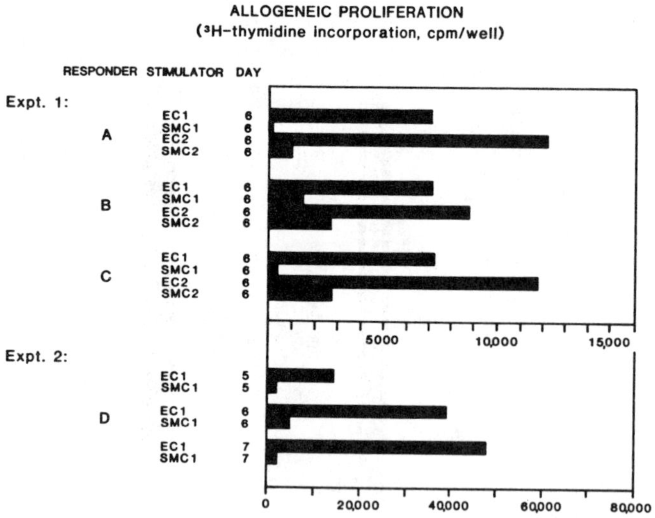

FIGURE 2. Proliferation of allogeneic lymphocytes to serially passaged saphenous vein endothelial cells (EC) or smooth muscle cells (SMC). Lymphocyte proliferation was measured as in Figure 1. Each pair of endothelial cells and smooth muscle cells was cultured from the same donor vascular segment according to methods described elsewhere (*75–77*). For the data shown, all of the stimulator cells were pretreated with immune interferon (200 U/ml) for four days prior to starting the proliferation assay; no consistent difference from untreated stimulator cells was noted.

(*55*). In both cases, DQ mRNA levels and surface expression is markedly less than for HLA-DR or DP. It has been suggested that resting murine B cells may express a posttranslationally altered (i.e., differently glycosylated) class II molecule that is less recognizable by T cells (*78*). Such diversity exists in humans as well. Human melanoma HLA-DR differs from B lymphoblastoid cell HLA-DR by glycosylation variations (*79*) and a monoclonal antibody has been described that can differentiate HLA-DR on human lymphoid cells from that on myeloid cells (*80*). There is as yet no biochemical data comparing endothelial cell HLA-DR with autologous smooth muscle or fibroblast HLA-DR. However, it seems unlikely that the class II molecules on fibroblasts are "structurally defective" because the same dermal fibroblast cultures that poorly stimulate primary allogeneic responses present nominal antigen to T cell clones or resting T cells and stimulate alloreactive T cell clones (*71*). It is possible that the surface density or surface display or lateral mobility of class II molecules may differ on endothelial cells compared with fibroblasts or smooth muscle cells in a way that is important for naive resting T_H activation. There are no data on these points. Alternatively, endothelial cells may secrete or display some second stimulatory molecule (e.g., IL-1) or fail to secrete or display an inhibitory molecule that modifies the response to class II determinants. We favor the hypothesis that some as-yet-to-be-identified factor, other than class II MHC expression or display, will account for enhanced allogeneic endothelial cell immunogenicity.

There are two final points. First the evaluation of endothelial cells as relatively more immunogenic than other vascular or stromal cells and uniquely capable of stimulating resting T_H is based entirely upon T cell thymidine incorporation experiments. This is an indirect analysis in that it measures a net sum of effects (e.g., IL-2 production, induction of IL-2 receptors, and other unspecified determinants of DNA replication) rather than component parts. Endothelial cells could be contributing stimulatory and inhibitory signals that integrate only slightly differently than those given by smooth muscle or fibroblasts, yet result in significantly more T cell proliferation under our in vitro experimental conditions. In vivo, the integration may be different. Second, T cell proliferation is only one measure of T_H function. The more relevant questions for transplantation may relate to the ability of endothelial cells to induce specific T_H subsets. For example, there is as yet no direct evidence that stimulation by foreign endothelial cells will lead to help for classic CTL development or for a delayed-type hypersensitivity response. It is the exploration of these questions that will establish the full functional significance of endothelial-cell-inducible class II MHC antigen expression for transplantation and normal immunity.

REFERENCES

1. McCluskey RT. Comments on targets in rejecting allografts. Transplant Proc 1980; 12 (suppl 1): 22.
2. Moraes, JR, Stastny P. A new antigen system expressed in human endothelial cells. J Clin Invest 1977; 60: 449.
3. Claas FHJ, Paul LC, van Es LA, van Rood JJ. Antibodies against donor antigens on endothelial cells and monocytes in eluates of rejected kidney allografts. Tissue antigens. 1980; 15: 19.
4. Hirschberg H, Evensen SA, Henriksen T, Thorsby E. The human mixed lymphocyte-endothelium culture interaction. Transplantation 1975; 19: 495.
5. Miller JFAP, Vadas MA, Whitelaw A, Gamble J. H-2 gene complex restricts transfer of delayed type hypersensitivity in mice. Proc Natl Acad Sci USA 1975; 72: 5095.
6. Weinberger O, Herrmann SH, Mescher MF, Benacerraf B, Burakoff SJ. Cellular interactions in the generation of cytolytic T lymphocyte responses: role of Ia-positive splenic adherent cells in presentation of H-2 antigen. Proc Natl Acad Sci USA 1980; 77: 609.
7. Sredni B, Schwartz R. Antigen-specific proliferating T lymphocyte clones: methodology, specificity, MHC restriction and alloreactivity. Immunol Rev 1981; 54: 187.
8. Glimcher LH, Kim KJ, Green I, Paul WE. Ia antigen-bearing B cell tumor lines can present protein antigen and alloantigen in a major histocompatibility complex-restricted fashion to antigen-reactive T cells. J Exp Med 1982; 155: 445.
9. Chu ET, Lareau M, Rosenwasser LJ, Dinarello CA, Geha RS. Antigen presentation by EBV-B cells to resting and activated T cells: role of interleukin 1. J Immunol 1985; 134; 1676.
10. Ramila G, Studer S, Mischler S, Erb P. Evaluation of Ia^+ tumor cell lines and peritoneal exudate macrophages as accessory cells: differential requirements for the activation of certain T cell functions. J Immunol 1983; 131: 2714.
11. van Voorhis WC, Valinsky J, Hoffman E, Luban J, Haor LS, Steinman RM. Relative efficiency of human monocytes and dendritic cells as accessory cells for T cell replication. J Exp Med 1983; 158: 174.
12. Gonwa TA, Picker LJ, Raff HV, Goyert SM, Silver J, Stobo JD. Antigen-presenting capabilities of human monocytes correlates with their expression of HLA-DS, an Ia determinant distinct from HLA-DR. J Immunol 1983; 130: 706.
13. Lafferty KJ, Prowse SJ, Silmeonovic CJ, Warren HS. Immunobiology of tissue transplantation: a return to the passenger leukocyte concept. Annu Rev Immunol 1983; 1: 143.
14. Faustman DL, Steinman RM, Gebel HM, Hauptfeld V, Davie JM, Lacy PE. Prevention of rejection of murine islet allografts by pretreatment with antidendritic cell antibody. Proc Natl Acad Sci USA 1984; 81: 3864.
15. Steinman RM, Nogueira N, Witmer MD, Tydings JD, Mellman IS. Lymphokine enhances the expression and synthesis of Ia

antigens on cultured mouse peritoneal macrophages. J Exp Med 1980; 152: 1248.
16. Steeg PS, Moore RN, Opperheim JJ. Regulation of murine macrophage Ia-antigen expression by products of activated spleen cells. J Exp Med 1980; 152: 1980.
17. Scher MG, Beller DI, Unanue ER. Demonstration of a soluble mediator that induces exudates rich in Ia-positive macrophages. J Exp Med 1980; 152: 1684.
18. Steeg PS, Moore RN, Johnson HM, Oppenheim JJ. Regulation of murine macrophage Ia antigen expression by a lymphokine with immune interferon activity. J Exp Med 1982; 156: 1780.
19. Sztein MB, Steeg PS, Johnson MM, Oppenheim JJ. Regulation of human peripheral blood monocyte antigen expression *in vitro* by lymphokines and recombinant interferons. J Clin Invest 1984; 73: 556.
20. Basham TY, Merigan TC. Recombinant interferon-γ increases HLA-DR synthesis and expression. J Immunol 1983; 130: 1492.
21. Kelley VE, Fiers W, Strom TB. Cloned human interferon-γ, but not interferon-α or -β, induces expression of HLA-DR determinants by fetal monocytes and myeloid leukemic cell lines. J Immunol 1984; 132: 240.
22. Becker S. Interferons as modulators of human monocyte-macrophage differentiation: I. Interferon-γ increases HLA-DR expression and inhibits phagocytosis of zymosan. J Immunol 1984; 132: 1249.
23. Pober JS, Gimbrone MA Jr. Expression of Ia-like antigens by human vascular endothelial cells is inducible *in vitro*: demonstration by monoclonal antibody binding and immunoprecipitation. Proc Natl Acad Sci USA 1982; 79: 6641.
24. Pober JS, Gimbrone MA Jr, Cotran RS, et al. Ia expression by vascular endothelium is inducible by activated T cells and by human γ interferon. J Exp Med 1983; 157: 1339.
25. Pober JS, Collins T, Gimbrone MA Jr., et al. Lymphocytes recognize human vascular endothelial and dermal fibroblast Ia antigens induced by recombinant immune interferon. Nature 1983; 305: 726.
26. Houghton AN, Thomson TM, Gross D, Oettgen HF, Old LJ. Surface antigens of melanoma and melanocytes: specificity of induction of Ia antigens by human γ-interferon. J Exp Med 1984; 160: 255.
27. Wong GHW, Bartlett PF, Clark-Lervis I, Battye F, Schrader JW. Inducible expression of H-2 and Ia antigens on brain cells. Nature 1984; 310: 688.
28. Lampert IA, Suitters AJ, Chisholm PM. Expression of IA antigens on epidermal keratinocytes in graft-versus-host disease. Nature 1981; 293: 149.
29. Mason DW, Dallman M, Barclay AN. Graft-versus-host disease induces expression of Ia antigen in rat epidermal cells and gut epithelium. Nature 1981; 293: 150.
30. Suitters AJ, Lampert IA. Expression of Ia antigen on epidermal keratinocytes is a consequence of cellular immunity. Br J Exp Pathol 1982; 63: 207.
31. Barclay AN, Mason DW. Induction of Ia antigen in rat epidermal cells and gut epithelium by immunological stimuli. J Exp Med 1982; 156: 1665.
32. de Waal RMW, Bogman MJJ, Maass CN, Cornelisson LMH, Tax WJM, Koene RAP. Variable expression of Ia antigens on the vascular endothelium of mouse skin allografts. Nature 1983; 303: 426.
33. Breathnach SM, Katz SI. Keratinocytes synthesize Ia antigen in acute cutaneous graft-versus-host disease. J Immunol 1983; 131: 2741.
34. Wadgymar A, Urmson J, Baumal R, Halloran PF. Changes in Ia expression in the kidney during acute graft-versus-host disease. J Immunol 1984; 132: 1826.
35. Sobel RA, Blanchette BW, Bhan AK, Colvin RB. The immunopathology of experimental allergic encephalomyelitis: II. Endothelial cell Ia increases prior to inflammatory cell infiltration. J Immunol 1984; 132: 2402.
36. Milton AD, Fabre JW. Massive induction of donor-type class I and class II major histocompatibility complex antigens in rejection cardiac allografts in the rat. J Exp Med 1985; 161: 98.
37. Benson EM, Coluin RB, Russell PS. Induction of IA antigens in murine renal transplants. J Immunol 1985; 134: 7.
38. Koyama K, Fukuwishi T, Barcos M, Tanigaki N, Pressman D. Human Ia-like antigens in non-lymphoid organs. Immunology 1979; 38: 333.
39. Baldwin WM III, Claas FHJ, van Es LA, van Rood JJ. Distribution of endothelial-monocyte and HLA antigens on renal vascular endothelium. Transplant Proc 1981; 13: 103.
40. Natali PG, Quaranta V, Nicotra MR, Apollonj C, Pellegrino MA, Ferrone S. Tissue distributions of Ia-like antigens in different species: analysis with monoclonal antibodies. Transplant Proc 1981; 13: 1026.
41. Snyder DS, Beller DI, Unanue ER. Prostaglandins modulate macrophage Ia expression. Nature 1982; 299: 164.
42. Snyder DS, Unanue ER. Corticosteroids inhibit murine macrophage Ia expression and interleukin 1 production. J Immunol 1982; 129: 1803.
43. Steeg PS, Johnson HM, Oppenheim JJ. Regulation of murine macrophage Ia antigen expression by an immune interferon-like lymphokine: inhibitory effect of endotoxin. J Immunol 1982; 129: 2402.
44. Yem AW, Parmley MJ. Modulation of Ia-like antigen expression and antigen-presenting activity of human monocytes by endotoxin and zymosan Am J Immunol 1981; 127: 2245.
45. Wong GHW, Clark-Lewis I, Hamilton JA, Schrader JW. P cell stimulating factor and glucocorticoids oppose the action of interferon-γ in inducing Ia antigens on T-dependent mast cells (P cells). J Immunol 1984; 133: 2043.
46. Acres RB, Lamb JR, Feldman M. Effects of PDGF and EGF on antigen-induced proliferation of human T-cell lines. Immunology 1985; 54: 9.
47. Walker EB, Maino V, Sanchez-Lanier M, Warner N, Stewart C. Murine gamma interferon activates the release of a macrophage-derived Ia-inducing factor that transfers Ia inductive capacity. J Exp Med 1984; 159: 1532.
48. Lu CY, Changelian PS, Unanue ER. α-fetoprotein inhibits macrophage expression of Ia antigens. J Immunol 1984; 132: 1722.
49. Roehm NW, Leibson HJ, Zlotnik A, Kappler J, Marrack P, Cambier JC. Interleukin-induced increase in Ia expression by normal mouse B cells. J Exp Med 1984; 160: 679.
50. Noelle R, Krammer PH, Ohara J, Uhr JW, Vitetta ES. Increased expression of Ia antigens on resting B cells: an additional role for B-cell growth factor. Proc Natl Acad Sci USA 1984; 81: 6149.
51. Daynes RA, Feman M, Krueger GG, Roberts LK. Expression of Ia antigens on epidermal keratinocytes after grafting of normal skin to nude mice. J Immunol 1983; 130: 1536.
52. Wallach D, Fellous M, Revel M. Preferential effect of γ interferon on the synthesis of HLA antigens and their mRNAs in human cells. Nature 1982; 299: 833.
53. Rosa F, Hatat D, Abadie A, Wallach D, Revel M, Fellous M. Human interferons enhance HLA-DR mRNA. EMBO J 1983; 2: 1585.
54. Nakamura M, Manser T, Pearso GDN, Daely M, Gefter ML. Effect of IFN-γ on the immune response *in vivo* and on gene expression *in vitro*. Nature 1984; 307: 381.
55. Collins T, Korman AJ, Wake CT, et al. Immune interferon activates multiple class II major histocompatability complex genes and the associated invariant chain gene in human endothelial cells and dermal fibroblasts. Proc Natl Acad Sci USA 1984; 81: 4917.
56. Long EO, Mach B, Accola RS. Ia-negative B cell variants reveal a coordinate regulation in the transcription of the HLA class II gene family. Immunogenetics 1984; 19: 349.
57. Levine F, Erlich HA, Mach B, Pious DS. Transcriptional regulation

of HLA class II and invariant chain genes. J Immunol 1985; 134: 637.
58. Friedman RL, Manly SP, McMahon M, Kerr IM, Stark GR. Transcriptional and post-transcriptional regulation of interferon-induced gene expression in human cells. Cell 1984; 38: 745.
59. Friedman RL, Stark GR. α-interferon-induced transcription of HLA and metallothionein genes containing homologous upstream sequences. Nature 1985; 314: 637.
60. Kvist S, Wiman K, Claesson L, Peterson PA, Dobberstein B. Membrane insertion and oligomeric assembly of HLA-DR histocompatibility antigens. Cell 1982; 29: 61.
61. McNicholas JM, King D, Jones PP. Biosynthesis and expression of Ia and H-2 antigens on a macrophage cell line are stimulated by products of activated T cells. J Immunol 1983; 130: 449.
62. Koch N, Wong GHW, Schrader JW. Ia antigens and associated invariant chain are induced simultaneously in lines of T-dependent mast cells by recombinant interferon-γ J Immunol 1984; 132: 1361.
63. Pober JS, Gimbrone MA, Jr. Collins T, et al. Interactions of T lymphocytes with human vascular endothelial cells: role of endothelial cell surface antigens. Immunobiol 1984; 168: 482.
64. Scheper RJ, van Dinther-Janssen CHM, Polak L. Specific accumulation of hapten-reactive T cells in contact sensitivity reaction sites. J Immunol 1985; 134: 1333.
65. Burger DR, Vetto RM. Vascular endothelium as a major participant in T-lymphocyte immunity. Cell Immunol 1982; 70: 357.
66. Hirschbert H, Bergh OH, Thorsby E. Antigen-presenting properties of human vascular endothelial cells. J Exp Med 1980; 152: 2495.
67. Burger DR, Vetto RM, Hamblin A, Goldstein A, Hubbard M, Dumonde DC. Endothelial cell presentation of antigen to human T cells. Hum Immunol 1981; 3: 209.
68. McCarron RM, Kempski O, Spatz M, McFarlin DE. Presentation of myelin basic protein by murine cerebral vascular endothelial cells.
69. Fontana A, Fierz W, Wekerle. Astrocytes present myelin basic protein to encephalitogenic T-cell lines. Nature 1984; 307: 273.
70. Londei M, Lamb JR, Bottazzo GF, Feldman M. Epithelial cells expressing aberrant MHC class II determinants can present antigen to cloned human T cells. Nature 1984; 312: 639.
71. Umetsu DT, Pober JS, Jabara HJ, et al. Human dermal fibroblasts present tetanus toxoid antigen to antigen specific T cell clones. J Clin Invest (in press).
72. Wagner CR, Vetto M, Burger DR. The mechanism of antigen presentation by endothelial cells. Immunobiol 1984; 168: 452.
73. Malissen B, Peele-Price M, Goverman JM, et al. Gene transfer of H-2 class II genes: antigen presentation by mouse fibroblast and hamster B cell lines. Cell 1984; 36: 39.
74. Norcross MA, Bertley DM, Margulies DH, Germain RN. Membrane Ia expression and antigen-presenting accessory cell function of L cells transfected with class II major histocompatibility complex genes. J Exp Med 1984; 160: 1316.
75. Watkins MT, Sharefkin JB, Zajtchuk R, et al. Adult human saphenous vein endothelial cells: assessment of their reproductive capacity for use in endothelial seeding of vascular prostheses. J Surg Res 1984; 36: 588.
76. Jarell B, Levine E, Shapiro S, et al. Human adult endothelial cell growth in culture. J Vasc Surg 1984; 1: 757.
77. Ross R, Kariya B. Morphogenesis of vascular smooth muscle in atherosclerosis and cell culture. In: Bohr DF, Somlyo AP, Sparks HY, eds. Handbook of Physiology: the cardiovascular System. vol. II. Baltimore: Williams & Wilkins, 1980: 69.
78. Cowing C, Chapdelaine JM. T cells discriminate between Ia antigens expressed on allogeneic accessory cells and B cells: a potential function for carbohydrate side chains on Ia molecules. Proc Natl Acad Sci USA 1983; 80: 6000.
79. Alexander S, Hubbard SC, Strominger JL. HLA-DR antigens of autologous melanoma and B lymphoblastoid cell lines: differences in glycosylation but not protein structure. J Immunol 1984; 133: 315.
80. Torok-Storb B, Nepom GT, Nepom BS, Hansen JA. HLA-DR antigens on lymphoid cells differ from those on myeloid cells. Nature 1983; 305: 541.

0041-1337/86/4102-0147$02.00/0
TRANSPLANTATION

Vol. 41, No. 2
Printed in U.S.A.

Transplantation

ARTICLES

CYCLOSPORINE AND THE ISCHEMIC RAT KIDNEY

P. JABLONSKI,[1] C. HARRISON, B. HOWDEN, D. RAE, G. TAVANLIS, V.C. MARSHALL, AND J.D. TANGE[2]

Monash University Department of Surgery, Prince Henry's Hospital, and University of Melbourne Department of Pathology

The effects of cyclosporine (CsA) on renal function and morphology have been studied in the rat after unilateral nephrectomy and warm renal ischemia. There is evidence of an enhanced CsA nephrotoxic effect after unilateral nephrectomy alone and of an additive or synergistic effect of CsA and renal ischemia upon renal function and morphology. These enhanced effects are most evident after longer periods of ischemia (60 min) and with higher doses of CsA (25 mg/kg/day). The findings may be relevant to clinical practice and suggest that the nephrotoxic effects of CsA upon the donor kidney may be greatest when there is coincident renal damage from other causes.

Cyclosporine (CsA) is a very effective immunosuppressive agent (*1*) that has been used in the transplantation of the kidney (*2, 3*), heart (*4*), bone marrow (*5*), and liver (*6*). However, there are indications that CsA may have adverse effects upon the kidney (*7*). Patients treated with the drug have increased serum concentrations of urea and creatinine (*5, 8*) and increased urinary excretion of N-acetyl-β-D-glucosaminidase (NAG)[3] (*9*), γ-glutamyl transferase (γ-GT) (*9*), and β_2-microglobulin (*9, 10*). These abnormalities all revert when treatment with the drug is stopped.

In contrast to these reversible changes with short-term treatment, long-term treatment in heart transplant recipients was associated with irreversible renal damage consisting of focal glomerular sclerosis and interstitial nephritis (*11*). These lesions are nonspecific and they may partly represent an indirect effect of long-term treatment with CsA even though the drug has been demonstrated within proximal convoluted tubule epithelium by immunofluorescence (*12*), and damage to these cells has been shown in the rat following very high doses of CsA (*13–15*). One possibility is that the adverse effect of the drug is accentuated by preexisting or associated renal damage. The Canadian Transplant Study Group (*16*) has reported that CsA-treated patients with initially nonfunctioning kidney grafts have a higher incidence of graft loss than those treated with azathioprine and steroids. A unit (*17*) transplanting donor kidneys with longer preservation times (>24 hr) found that CsA treatment reduced the proportion of kidneys with immediate function from 50% to 17%. In order to examine the possible interaction of CsA administration and renal damage we have induced unilateral warm renal ischemia in rats treated with CsA. We have used a rat model because (1) the effects of different periods of warm ischemia have been well-characterized (*18*); (2) the vulnerability of the kidney to stress can be increased by uninephrectomy (*19–21*); and (3) the rat kidney is relatively insensitive to the nephrotoxic effects of CsA (*13, 15*).

MATERIALS AND METHODS

Male Sprague-Dawley rats (250–300 g) were housed six to a cage and received standard rat pellets and water ad libitum. Rats were randomly assigned to three treatment groups:

1. Cyclosporine dissolved in olive oil, 1 ml/kg daily by gavage
2. Olive oil, 1 ml/kg daily by gavage
3. No treatment

Rats in each treatment group were subjected to 30 or 60 min warm renal ischemia and contralateral nephrectomy, or uninephrectomy alone (Table 1). Treatment commenced 2 days prior to the induction of warm renal ischemia and/or uninephrectomy, and continued for 14 days thereafter.

Cyclosporine A dosage. Doses of 5, 10, 25 mg/kg body weight were tested. The highest dose chosen was well below that (100 mg/kg/day) previously shown to produce tubular lesions in rats (*14, 15*). Dosage was recalculated daily on actual body weights. The lower doses (5, 10 mg/kg body weight) were given to rats subjected to 60 min warm renal ischemia only.

Warm renal ischemia. Animals were anesthetized with sodium pentobarbitone (21 mg, i.p.). The right renal artery was dissected near its aortic origin; heparin (50 IU, i.v.) was administered, and the artery was occluded for 30 or 60 min. At the end of the warm ischemic period, the left kidney was excised and the clip was removed from the right renal artery so that renal blood flow was reestablished. Control animals were subjected to left nephrectomy only.

Follow-up studies. Animals were examined and weighed daily. Serum creatinine and urea were determined prior to surgery and 2, 4, 6, 8, and 15 days after operation. Before the experiment all animals were placed in metabolic cages for 24 hr to assess renal function and food and water intake. Urine pH and osmolality and urinary excretion of sodium, potassium, creatinine, and protein were measured and creatinine clearance calculated. All these studies were repeated at weekly intervals

Received 3 March 1985.
Accepted 24 May 1985.

[1] Address correspondence to: P. Jablonski, Ph.D., M.Sc., Department of Surgery, Prince Henry's Hospital, St. Kilda Road, Melbourne, Vic., 3004, Australia.

[2] University of Melbourne.

[3] Abbreviations used: CsA, cyclosporine; γ-GT, γ-glutamyl transferase; NAG, N-acetyl-β-D-glucosaminidase; NT, nontreated.

TABLE 1. The effect of CsA on body weight after unilateral nephrectomy and warm renal ischemia

Duration of ischemia	No. rats	Maximum body wt. loss[a]	Final body wt.[a]
Nil:			
NT[b]	10	6±1	108±1
CsA (25 mg/kg/day)	5	12±2	92±4
30 min:			
NT[b]	14	8±2	110±1
CsA (25 mg/kg/day)	7	11±1	97±3
60 min:			
NT[b]	23	12±1	106±1
CsA (25 mg/kg/day)	6	17±1	88±22
CsA (10 mg/kg/day)	5	17±1	97±2
CsA (5 mg/kg/day)	4	11±1	105±2

[a] Expressed as % preoperative weight.
[b] NT: Combination of oil-treated and untreated animals.

after operation. Liver function was assessed before treatment and at the end of the experiment by the measurement of serum bilirubin, albumin, alkaline phosphatase, γ-glutamyl transferase, and aspartate transferase. Sodium and potassium were measured using a flame photometer with a LiCl internal standard. Creatinine (*22*), urea (*23*), total protein (*24*), albumin (*25*), bilirubin (*26*), alkaline phosphatase (*27*), γ-glutamyl transferase (*28*), and aspartate aminotransferase (*29*) were measured by standard methods using a Centrifichem (Roche Diagnostics).

At the end of the experiment the animals were killed, and the heart, liver and kidney were excised, weighed, and processed for light microscopy. The effects of the experimental procedures upon the kidney were assessed based on the amount of cortical damage present in a single longitudinal section. Hypertrophy of the remaining kidney was calculated by comparing its weight with that of the contralateral kidney removed at the beginning of the experiment.

All experimental functional and morphological data were recorded separately and analyzed on completion of the experiment. Results were analyzed statistically using a chi-square test or Wilcoxon's rank sum test.

RESULTS

All animals survived the experiment. Findings in the oil-treated and nontreated groups were not significantly different, and these have been combined into a single group (NT).

General. All rats lost weight postoperatively. Weight loss was influenced by two factors (Table 1): the duration of warm ischemia and treatment with CsA. Untreated rats started to regain weight 5 days postoperatively. CsA-treated animals continued to lose weight up to 12 days postoperative—consequently most were still below their initial weight at the end of the experiment. The effect of CsA was dose-related and not evident at 5 mg/kg/day.

After operation, food intake was significantly changed only in animals subjected to warm renal ischemia and treated with high-dose CsA (25 mg/kg). In such animals after 30 min ischemia there was significant ($P<0.01$) reduction in food intake one week postoperatively, but this returned to preoperative values after 15 days. After 60 min ischemia there was similar reduction in food intake (from 19±2 g/day to 14±1 g/day) and this persisted at 15 days. Lower doses of CsA had no significant effect on food intake. Water intake was affected only by warm ischemic damage. All rats subjected to 30 or 60 min warm renal ischemia and contralateral nephrectomy had significantly ($P<0.02$) increased water consumption that was not influenced by CsA at any dose level.

Renal function. Unilateral nephrectomy or 30 min warm ischemia, produced no significant changes in serum urea or creatinine (Figs. 1 and 2). The high dose of CsA (25 mg/kg) produced an appreciable rise in serum urea, but not in creatinine after unilateral nephrectomy alone, or combined with 30 min warm ischemia, and this rise was still apparent at the end of the experiment.

In contrast, 60 min warm ischemia resulted in large increases in serum urea (Fig. 1C) and creatinine (Fig. 2C) that returned towards, but not to, normal at 8 and 15 days. Furthermore both the CsA-25 and CsA-10 mg/kg/day groups had significantly higher serum urea (Fig. 1C) and creatinine (Fig. 2C) concentrations than untreated rats 4, 6, 8, and 15 days after 60 min ischemic damage. These changes were reflected in the creatinine clearance values (Table 2). Control animals with no warm ischemic damage showed no significant changes. Warm ischemia initially decreased creatinine clearance but values returned to normal in untreated rats and remained significantly ($P<0.05$) smaller in rats subjected to 30 min warm ischemia and treated with CsA 25 mg/kg; following 60 min warm ischemia the effect of CsA was more pronounced, being present with all 3 dosages.

After 60 min warm renal ischemia rats excreted large volumes of dilute urine and continued to do so until the end of the experiment (Table 3). Urine osmolality also fell significantly.

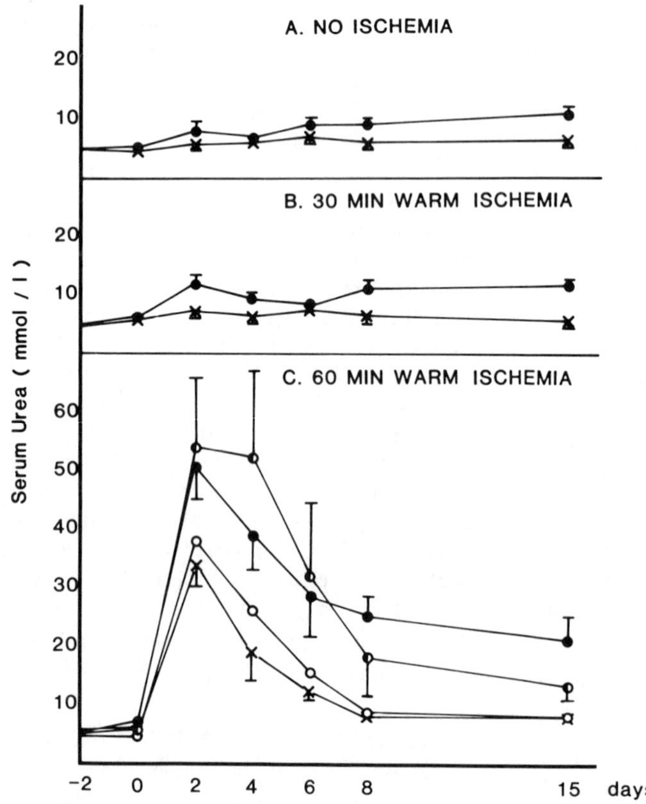

FIGURE 1. Serum urea after (A) contralateral nephrectomy alone or combined 30 min (B) and 60 min (C) warm renal ischemia. (●) CsA 25 mg/kg/day; (◐) CsA 10 mg/kg/day; (○) CsA 5 mg/kg/day; (×) NT.

Both these effects were enhanced by treatment with high-dose CsA.

Warm ischemia by itself did not significantly impair potassium excretion, (Table 4) but rats subject to 60 min warm ischemia and treated with CsA (10 or 25 mg/kg/day) had significantly diminished potassium excretion, and this persisted throughout the 15-day follow-up period. Transient impairment of potassium excretion (8 days only) was found in other experimental groups given CsA 25 mg/kg/day. Urinary sodium excretion was diminished in groups that received CsA (25 mg/kg/day) but these differences were not significant. CsA (25 mg/kg/day) treatment plus 60 min warm ischemia resulted in a significantly ($P<0.01$) diminished ratio of potassium:sodium excretion (preoperatively = 2.02±0.13; 8 days postischemia = 1.50±0.09; 15 days postischemia = 1.87±0.12). In contrast the ratio significantly ($P<0.05$) increased in untreated animals after 60 min warm ischemia (preoperatively = 1.96±0.08, 8 days postischemia = 2.21±0.15, 15 days postischemia = 2.23±0.16). These changes could not be related directly to diminished food intake in the animals that received CsA (25 mg/kg/day) and warm renal ischemia, although this may have been a contributing factor. Serum potassium and sodium remained unchanged in all treatment and control groups.

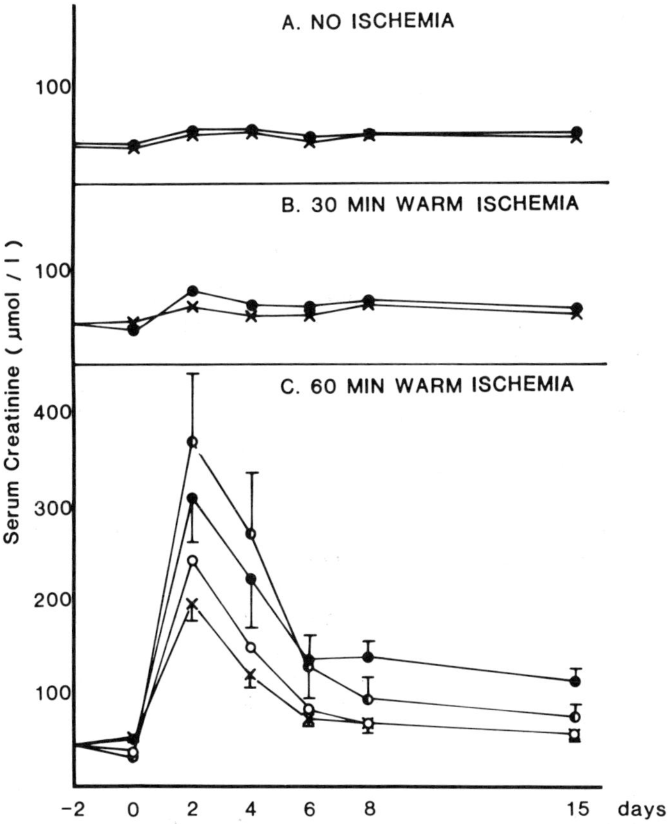

FIGURE 2. Serum creatinine after (A) unilateral nephrectomy alone or combined with 30 min (B) or 60 min (C) warm renal ischemia.

TABLE 2. The effect of CsA on creatinine clearance after unilateral nephrectomy and warm renal ischemia

Duration of ischemia	Creatinine clearance (ml/min) Preoperative	Postoperative 8 Days	Postoperative 15 Days
Nil:			
NT	1.51±0.05	1.53±0.08	1.65±0.05
CsA (25 mg/kg/day)	1.56±0.09	1.35±0.07	1.34±0.12
30 Min:			
NT	1.51±0.10	1.02±0.08	1.52±0.10
CsA (25 mg/kg/day)	1.56±0.12	0.92±0.07	1.18±0.10[a]
60 Min:			
NT	1.52±0.09	1.08±0.06	1.38±0.05
CsA (25 mg/kg/day)	1.68±0.18	0.49±0.07[b]	0.64±0.09[b]
CsA (10 mg/kg/day)	1.40±0.08	0.73±0.13[b]	0.93±0.14[b]
CsA (5 mg/kg/day)	1.37±0.18	0.96±0.13	0.91±0.13[b]

[a] $P<0.05$ compared with corresponding NT group.
[b] $P<0.01$ compared with corresponding NT group.

TABLE 3. The effect of CsA on urine volume and osmolality after unilateral nephrectomy and warm renal ischemia

Duration of ischemia	Urine output (g/24 hr) Preop.	Urine output (g/24 hr) Postop. (15 days)	Urine osmolality (mOsm/kg) Preop.	Urine osmolality (mOsm/kg) Postop. (15 days)
Nil:				
NT	5.9±0.8	7.6±0.4	2210±200	1880±100
CsA (25 mg/kg/day)	7.0±1.1	8.9±1.3	2090±260	1600±200
30 Min:				
NT	6.9±0.5	8.6±1.2	2010±170	1700±150
CsA (25 mg/kg/day)	6.8±0.7	10.6±2.5	2340±200	1730±190
60 Min:				
NT	7.1±0.7	12.5±0.8	2020±90	1440±60
CsA (25 mg/kg/day)	7.6±0.9	18.1±2.9[a]	2200±150	930±170[b]
CsA (10 mg/kg/day)	7.2±0.6	15.0±3.5	1680±280	1000±220
CsA (5 mg/kg/day)	6.8±1.1	15.2±3.5	2020±160	1100±150

[a] $P<0.05$ compared with NT 60 min.
[b] $P<0.02$ compared with NT 60 min.

Liver function. All CsA-25 mg/kg/day animals had significantly ($P<0.02$) reduced serum albumin (2.7±0.1 compared with 3.0±0 g/100 ml), elevated serum bilirubin (5±1 compared with 1±0 μmol/L), and alkaline phosphatase (460±40 compared with 380±30 U/L). Both γ-glutamyl transferase and aspartate aminotransferase were unaltered by treatment with CsA. Lower dosages of CsA (5 and 10 mg/kg/day) had a smaller effect on serum bilirubin (2±0 μmol/L) and no significant effect on serum albumin or alkaline phosphatase. These changes were independent of other experimental procedures.

Morphology. Uninephrectomy alone, or combined with warm renal ischemic damage resulted in significant hypertrophy and a variable degree of interstitial nephritis in the remaining kidney. Renal hypertrophy was characterized by increased kidney mass and increased diameter of proximal convoluted tubules; the height of tubular epithelial cells was increased, and there was increased numbers of cells around the circumference of the tubule. The degree of hypertrophy was related to the duration of warm renal ischemia. After 60 min warm ischemia the weight of the hypertrophied kidney in the NT group was 177±7% the original weight, compared with 154±8% after 30 min ischemia. Animals treated with CsA (25 mg/kg/day) did not have the same degree of renal hypertrophy (60 min ischemia = 149±8%, 30 min group = 126±5%). The degree of renal hypertrophy was not affected by treatment with lower doses of CsA.

The severity of the interstitial nephritis was principally determined by the duration of the warm renal ischemia. Untreated kidneys subjected to 30 min ischemia showed only minimal (<10% interstitial nephritis) damage, whereas 22% of the 60-min ischemia group showed severe damage (>30% interstitial nephritis). The administration of CsA appeared to exacerbate the extent but not the character of morphological damage following 60 min ischemia. All CsA (25 mg/kg/day)-treated animals showed moderate or severe damage (>20% interstitial nephritis) after 60 min ischemia, whereas only 60% of the CsA (10 mg/kg/day)-treated and 17% of the NT group showed such damage. Moreover 1 of 6 animals treated with CsA in high dosages and subjected to 30 min ischemia showed appreciable (10–20%) interstitial nephritis. Interstitial nephritis was also more severe in animals treated with 25 mg/kg CsA and subjected to uninephrectomy alone than in the NT group. In 2 of 6 animals interstitial nephritis was assessed at 10–20% and was accompanied by fine vacuolation and pyknosis in groups of proximal convoluted tubule epithelial cells (Fig. 3).

CsA (25 mg/kg/day)-treated animals had significantly ($P<0.01$) smaller hearts than untreated rats (0.88±0.3 g compared with 1.06±0.04 g), but without histological abnormalities. Liver weights and overall morphology were not affected by the treatment regimen, but 3 rats (2 treated with CsA 25 mg/kg/day) had granulomas in their liver. These were made up of variable combinations of necrosis and a mild chronic inflammatory reaction and were consistent with bacterial infection.

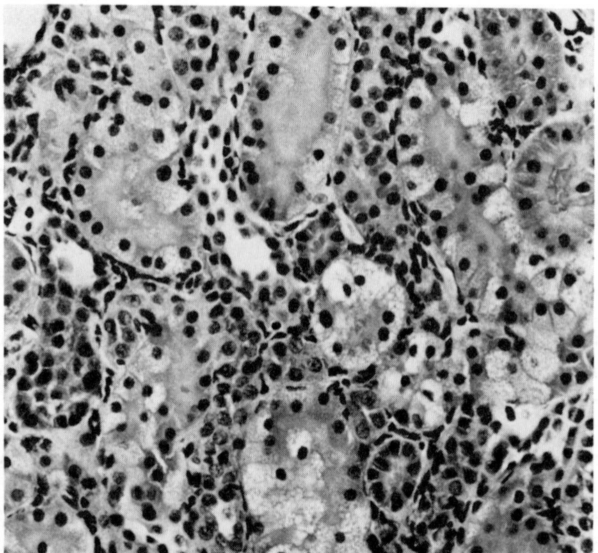

FIGURE 3. Photomicrograph of portion of rat kidney. Some proximal convoluted tubule epithelial cells show fine vesicular cytoplasm and pyknotic nuclei. These are surrounded by darker areas in which tubular cells are basophilic and in which interstitial connective tissue is increased; unilateral nephrectomy and CsA 25 mg/kg/day (H & E; ×160).

TABLE 4. The effect of CsA on urinary potassium excretion after unilateral nephrectomy and warm renal ischemia

Duration of ischemia	Urinary K excretion (μmol/24 hr)		
	Preoperative	Postoperative	
		8 Days	15 Days
Nil:			
NT	1910±90	1820±60	2090±100
CsA (25 mg/kg/day)	2020±60	1480±90[a]	1640±270
30 Min:			
NT	2070±110	2130±80	2390±150
CsA (25 mg/kg/day)	2300±120	1520±200[a]	2100±230
60 Min:			
NT	2180±90	2130±80	2470±60
CsA (25 mg/kg/day)	2460±100	1440±150[a]	1660±60[a]
CsA (10 mg/kg/day)	2420±130	1460±90[a]	2030±80[b]
CsA (5 mg/kg/day)	2150±210	1770±150	2010±320

[a] $P<0.01$ compared with the corresponding NT group.
[b] $P<0.05$ compared with the corresponding NT group.

DISCUSSION

These experiments have shown that the administration of CsA has adverse effects upon the repair and regeneration of the rat kidney after warm renal ischemia. Because the normal contralateral kidney was removed, the experimental model has some similarity to the clinical situation in which the donor kidney has sustained damage before or during preservation.

Renal function was depressed by CsA (25 mg/kg/day) during recovery from 60 min warm renal ischemia in a single kidney. Serum urea and creatinine were elevated; creatinine clearance and potassium excretion were reduced. Urine volume increased and urine osmolality decreased. These changes significantly exceeded those produced separately by CsA, warm renal ischemia, or unilateral nephrectomy. Following treatment with CsA, interstitial nephritis was more extensive, and increase in renal mass was less than after warm renal ischemia and unilateral nephrectomy.

Treated animals also showed significant weight loss and reduced food intake, and it is possible that these factors contributed to reduction in kidney weight. Significant loss of body weight did not occur in other toxicity studies (*15*) using higher doses of CsA in the absence of experimentally induced kidney damage. There was also marginal impairment of liver function in the absence of structural changes in the liver. In 3 animals, (NT [1]); CsA 25 mg/kg/day [1]; 60 min warm ischemia + CsA 25 mg/kg/day [1]) there were incidental focal inflammatory lesions in the liver having a pattern consistent with that produced by superimposed bacterial infection.

CsA is known to depress renal function in patients with heart transplants and these biochemical changes revert when the drug is stopped. When CsA was given for longer periods to patients receiving marrow transplants glomerular sclerosis and interstitial nephritis developed in the recipients kidneys (*11*). Glomerular lesions have not been reproduced in experimental animals. However, large doses of CsA (50–100 mg/kg/day) given to rats have produced morphological changes in proximal convoluted tubule epithelium (*14, 15*). Lower doses were deliberately chosen for our experiments—nonetheless similar fine vacuolation in tubular epithelium, together with obvious interstitial nephritis, was found in 2 of 6 rats given 25 mg/kg/day and subjected to unilateral nephrectomy only. This suggests that kidneys undergoing compensatory hypertrophy may be more susceptible to the toxic effects of CsA. A similar enhanced susceptibility has been demonstrated for other nephrotoxins, such as lead (*19*) and analgesics (*20, 21*). Except for a few very small foci in one animal after 30 min warm ischemia, this fine vacuolation of the tubular epithelium was not found in animals subjected to unilateral warm ischemia and treated with CsA; presumably the lesions are masked by the morphological changes produced by ischemia. There is other evidence of a synergistic effect between CsA and renal ischemia: acute experiments in the dog (*30*) have shown that CsA (5, 10, or 15 mg/kg) infused over 1 hr impaired urine output after 60 min occlusion of the left renal artery, and that the CsA-treated ischemic kidneys secreted larger quantities of γ-glutamyl transferase compared with untreated ischemic kidneys, indicating more severe proximal convoluted tubule damage.

Our observations suggest that besides its relatively minor functional and morphological effects upon normal kidneys, CsA has an additional deleterious effect upon a regenerating and repairing kidney. These experimental findings may be relevant to clinical practice, particularly after transplantation of donor kidneys with relatively long ischemic times (>24 hr) when preservation procedures have not been able to prevent some degree of renal damage.

Acknowledgments. We are grateful to Sandoz Ltd., Basle, for the cyclosporine used in these experiments.

REFERENCES

1. Borel JF. Cyclosporin-A: present experimental status. Transplant Proc 1981; 13: 344.
2. Calne RY, White DJG, Thiru S, et al. Cyclosporin A in patients receiving renal allografts from cadaver donors. Lancet 1978; 2: 1323.
3. Calne RY, Rolles K, White DJG, et al. Cyclosporin A as the only immunosuppressant in 34 recipients of cadaveric organs: 32 kidneys, 2 pancreases and 2 livers. Lancet 1979; 2: 1033.
4. Oyer PE, Stinson EB, Jamieson SW, et al. Cyclosporin-A in cardiac allografting: a preliminary experience. Transplant Proc 1983; 15: 1247.
5. Powles RL, Clink HM, Spence D, et al. Cyclosporin A to prevent graft-versus-host disease in man after allogeneic bone-marrow transplantation. Lancet 1980; 1: 327.
6. Starzl TE, Klintmalm GBG, Porter KA, Iwatsuki S, Schroter PJ. Liver transplantation with use of cyclosporin A and prednisone. N Engl J Med 1981; 305: 267.
7. Bennett WM, Pulliam JP. Cyclosporine nephrotoxicity. Ann Intern Med 1983; 99: 851.
8. Hows JM, Smith JM, Baughan A, Gordon-Smith EC. Nephrotoxicity in marrow graft recipients treated with cyclosporine. In: Kahan BD, ed. Cyclosporine. Orlando: Grune & Stratton, 1983: 492.
9. Devineni R, McKenzie FN, Kostuk WJ. Renal effects of cyclosporin. Heart Transplant 1983; 2: 219.
10. Marbet UA, Graf V, Mihatsch MJ, Gratwohl A, Muller W, Thiel G. Renale nebenwirkungen der therapie mit cyclosporin A bei chronischer polyarthritis und nach knochenmarktransplantation. Schweiz Med Wochenschr 1980; 110: 2017.
11. Myers BD, Ross J, Newton L, Leutscher J, Perlroth M. Cyclosporine-associated chronic nephropathy. N Engl J Med 1984; 311: 699.
12. von Willebrand E, Hayry P. Cyclosporin-A deposits in renal allografts. Lancet 1983; 2: 189.
13. Farthing MJG, Clark ML, Pendry A, Sloane J, Alexander P. Nature of the toxicity of Cyclosporin A in the Rat. Biochem Pharmacol 1981; 30: 3311.
14. Whiting PH, Thomson AW, Blair JT, Simpson JG. Experimental cyclosporin A nephrotoxicity. Br J Exp Pathol 1982; 63: 88.
15. Blair JT, Thomson AW, Whiting PH, Davidson RJL, Simpson JG. Toxicity of the immune suppressant Cyclosporin A in the rat. J Pathol 1982; 138: 163.
16. Stiller C. The Canadian trial of cyclosporine: cyclosporine therapy compared to standard immunosuppression in renal transplants: an exploration of nephrotoxicity. In: Kahan BD, ed. Cyclosporine. Orlando: Grune & Stratton, 1983: 263.
17. Shiel AGR, Hall BM, Tiller DJ, et al. Australian trial of cyclosporine (CsA) in cadavaric donor renal transplantation. In: Kahan BD, ed. Cyclosporine. Orlando: Grune & Stratton, 1983: 269.
18. Jablonski P, Howden BO, Rae DA, Birrell CS, Marshall VC, Tange J. An experimental model for assessment of renal recovery from warm ischemia. Transplantation 1983; 35: 198.
19. Tange JD, Hayward NJ, Bremner DA. Renal lesions in experimental plumbism and their clinical implications. Aust Ann Med 1965; 14: 49.
20. Molland EA. Aspirin damage in the rat kidney in the intact animal and after unilateral nephrectomy. J Pathol 1976; 120: 43.
21. Henry MA, Sweet RS, Tange JD. A new reproducible experimental model of analgesic nephropathy. J Pathol 1983; 139: 23.
22. Kovar KA, Schmid M. Die Bestimmung von Kreatin in serum mit einem neuentwickelten enzymatischen Farbtest. Arch Pharm (Weinheim) 1979; 312: 780.
23. Eisenwiener HG. Kinetische Bestimmung des Harnstoffes mit dem LKB-system. J Clin Chem Clin Biochem 1976; 14: 261.
24. Kingsley Gr. The determination of serum total protein, albumin, and globulin by the biuret reaction. J Biol Chem 1939; 131: 197.
25. Weichselbaum TE. An accurate and rapid method for the determination of proteins in small amounts of blood, serum and plasma. Am J Clin Pathol 1946; 16(tech suppl 10): 40.
26. Brechbuehler T, Eisenwiener HG. Comparative investigations on the total bilirubin determination with 2-4-dichloroaniline and sulfanilic acid. Chem Rundschr 1976; 29: 1.
27. Bessey OA, Lowry OH, Brock MJ. Method for rapid determination of alkaline phosphatase with 5 cubicmillimeters of serum. J Biol Chem 1946; 164: 321.
28. Szasz G. A kinetic photometric method for serum glutamyl transpeptidase. Clin Chem 1969; 15: 124.
29. German Society for Clinical Chemistry. Standardization of methods for the estimation of enzyme activities in biological fluids. Z Klin Chem Klin Biochem 1972; 10: 281.
30. Devineni R, McKenzie N, Duplan J, Keown P, Stiller C, Wallace AC. Renal effects of cyclosporine: clinical and experimental observations. In: Kahan BD, ed. Cyclosporine. Orlando: Grune & Stratton, 1983: 479.

0041-1337/86/4102-0152$02.00/0
TRANSPLANTATION
Vol. 41, No. 2
Printed in U.S.A.

CYCLOSPORINE AND EXPERIMENTAL RENAL ISCHEMIC INJURY[1]

STEPHEN S. CHOW, PAUL THORNER, REUBEN BAUMAL, AND DOUGLAS R. WILSON[2]

Department of Medicine and Department of Pathology, Faculty of Medicine, University of Toronto, Toronto, Ontario, Canada

To investigate the interaction of cyclosporine nephrotoxicity and renal ischemia, an animal model in rats with bilateral renal artery clamping was used. Rats given cyclosporine had a lower rate of recovery from ischemia. However, the percentages of reduction in glomerular filtration rate in vehicle and cyclosporine groups were the same in sham-operated or ischemically treated group. This suggests a superimposition of cyclosporine nephrotoxicity on the recovering kidneys rather than synergistic potentiation between ischemia and cyclosporine nephrotoxicity.

Cyclosporine (CsA) has been increasingly used in clinical transplantation in recent years but the drug is nephrotoxic. Patients on CsA have, as a group, higher serum creatinine levels and other manifestations of renal dysfunction including proteinuria, impaired concentrating ability, and elevated blood pressure (*1*, *2*). In addition, nephrotoxicity was potentiated when CsA was used with amphotericin B (*3*), ketconozole (*4*), or trimethoprim and cotrimoxazole (*5*). The potentiation of ischemic injury by CsA was suggested by the Canadian renal transplantation study (*1*). Poorer graft survival was seen in the CsA group if the graft was perfused for more than 24 hr or if the surgical anastomosis time was more than 45 min. The time taken for the graft to begin to function was about twice as long in the CsA group as in the standard treatment group. This delayed recovery from posttransplantation acute tubular necrosis during CsA therapy poses important questions concerning the optimal use of this drug in renal transplant recipients. To investigate the interaction between ischemic renal injury and CsA therapy we have used an experimental model in which CsA was given to rats after temporal bilateral renal artery clamping, and renal function and histology were followed for 1 week.

MATERIALS AND METHODS

Male Sprague-Dawley rats weighing 230–340 g were anesthetized with pentobarbital 50 mg/kg i.p. A midline abdominal incision was made. The right and left renal arteries were identified and separated from the renal vein, clamped, with tight vascular clips (stopping completely any blood flow to the kidney), and the incision was closed temporarily with staples. While the renal arteries were clamped, CsA (parenteral preparation) diluted in 1 ml 0.9% saline was injected s.c. Three dosages were given—5, 25, and 50 mg/kg. Another group was given parenteral vehicle (cremaphor and ethanol mixture), and an additional group 0.9% saline. The renal artery clips were removed at 30 or 40 min to produce different degrees of ischemia. Then 2 ml of 0.9% saline was injected into the peritoneal cavity to replace fluid loss, and the incision closed with surgical sutures. Sham-operated groups had an abdominal incision only, and they were also given various dosages of CsA, vehicle, or saline. The rats were kept in metabolic cages with fluids ad libitum, and fed with Purina rat chow. Body weight, fluid intake, and urinary outut were determined on days 2, 4, and 7. Injections of CsA, vehicle, or saline s.c. were continued daily until sacrifice. Blood was drawn or expressed from the tail for analysis for ureal nitrogen and creatinine. To document the recovery from ischemia at different intervals, inulin clearances were performed on groups of rats sacrificed on days 2, 4, and 7 after the ischemic injury. For clearance studies pentobarbital 50 mg/kg was injected i.p. and tracheostomy performed. An internal jugular vein, femoral artery, and the bladder were cannulated with PE 50 tubing for fluid infusion, blood sampling and blood pressure monitoring, and urine collection respectively. A priming dose of H^3 inulin 5 μC in 2 cc 0.9% saline was infused over 10 min followed by a maintenance dose of 5 μC/hr in 2.25 ml of saline. After an equilibration period of 30 min, three urine collections, each of 30 min duration were made, with blood sampling at the beginning and end of each period. 20 μl of blood and urine samples were counted in Acquasol solution. At the end of the study, the rats were sacrificed, exsanguinated, and a blood sample analyzed for urea nitrogen, creatinine, sodium, potassium and CsA level. Sections of kidneys were preserved in 1% glutaraldehyde for electron microscopy and in 10% formalin for light microscopy. To determine cortical tissue sodium, potassium, and calcium content, cortical slices were dried in an oven at 70°C. The dried tissue was then digested in 5 cc HCl and filtered. Sodium, potassium, and calcium concentration in the filtrate were measured, and from this measurement tissue content was calculated using wet and dry weight. Kidney CsA tissue level was determined using a double ether extraction method (*6*). Pieces of corticl renal tissue were homogenized in ether followed by centrifugation. The pellet was resuspended in ether and homogenized again. The supernatant was allowed to dry and 2 cc buffer solution was then added. The concentration of CsA in the buffer solution was measured using ratioimmunoassay, and the total amount of CsA in tissue consequently derived.

Sodium and potassium were measured by flame photometry. Calcium was measured by atomic absorption spectroscopy. Creatinine was measured with a Beckman creatinine analyzer, and urea nitrogen with diacetylmoxine method. The radioimmunoassay and buffer solution for CsA measurement were based on a kit from Sandoz. Results were analyzed using the

[1] This work was supported by a Grant from The Kidney Foundation of Canada, Ontario Branch.

[2] Address correspondence to: D. R. Wilson, M.D., Dean's office, Faculty of Medicine, University of Alberta, Edmonton, Alberta, Canada, T6M 2G3.

[3] Abbreviations used: BUN, blood urea nitrogen; CsA, cyclosporine; GFR, glomerular filtration rate.

unpaired student's t test and $P < 0.05$ was considered to be significant.

RESULTS

All groups of rats survived the operation, but in the groups given higher doses of CsA there was significant mortality by day 7. Among the eight animals with 30 min clamping that were given CsA 50 mg/kg/day, three died on day 4, two on day 5, and one on day 6. A similar mortality was seen in the sham animals given the same high doses of CsA with only one of six animals surviving on day 7. Seizures were seen in these animals prior to death. Renal failure did not appear to be the cause of death as serum creatinine remained normal or only mildly elevated in these animals.

TABLE 1. Weight loss (%) (mean ±SD [n])

	Day 4		Day 7	
Sham:				
Vehicle	11±5 (18)	> $P < 0.0002$	12±5 (11)	> $P < 0.05$
CsA 5 mg/kg	17±3 (14)		19±11 (7)	> $P < 0.01$
25 mg/kg	20±2 (6)		26±2 (6)	
50 mg/kg	17±3 (6)		—	
Ischemia 30′:				
Vehicle	13±6 (16)		12±8 (8)	
CsA 5 mg/kg	16±6 (13)		18±7 (8)	> $P < 0.02$
25 mg/kg	20±6 (8)		32±7 (7)	
50 mg/kg	17±4 (6)			
Ischemia 40′:				
Vehicle	13±6 (8)		20±9 (8)	
CsA 5 mg/kg	19±4 (8)		25±5 (8)	

Table 1 shows the weight changes. Weight loss occurred in all groups, but was greater in the higher-dosage CsA groups. There was no significant difference between the vehicle group and CsA 5 mg/kg/day group with 30-min or 40-min ischemia. More weight loss was seen, however, in the sham animals given CsA 5 mg/kg/day than in sham animals given vehicle. Urine output and fluid intake were similar in vehicle and CsA groups.

The BUN results are listed in Table 2. In the sham groups, there was about a two-fold rise in BUN in both CsA groups as compared with the vehicle group on day 7. No significant difference was seen between the CsA 5 mg/kg/day group and the 25 mg/kg/day group. In the 40-min ischemia groups, BUN in those given CsA 5 mg/kg/day was significantly higher on day 7 after partial recovery from the ischemic injury. Similarly in the 30-min ischemia groups, there were significant differences between CsA groups and vehicle groups on days 4 and day 7, with the higher-dosage group having higher BUN levels than the lower-dosage group.

Inulin clearances were performed on the vehicle and CsA 5 mg/kg/day group on days 2, 4, and 7, and results are shown in Table 3. With sham operation, the vehicle group showed no significant changes in inulin clearance on days 2, 4, and 7, but the CsA 5 mg/kg/day group had decreased clearance values, so that by day 7 it was about 50% that of the vehicle group. With 30-min ischemia the recovery from renal failure in the CsA group was prevented as compared with the vehicle group. Similarly, with 40-min ischemia, the clearance value of CsA 5 mg/kg/day group on day 7 was about 50% that of the vehicle group. Table 4 shows the corresponding serum creatinine on the day of inulin clearance as well as those of higher-dosage CsA groups

TABLE 2. Blood urea nitrogen (mg/dl) (mean ±SD [n])[a]

	Day 0	Day 2	Day 4		Day 7	
Sham:						
Normal saline	27±7 (6)	26±4 (6)	26±9 (6)		29±11 (6)	
Vehicle	32±16 (26)	27±13 (26)	28±12 (19)		26±8 (11)	> $P < 0.0001$
CsA 5 mg/kg	29±16 (21)	31±12 (21)	32±8 (12)		51±14 (7)	> P = NS
25 mg/kg	27±7 (6)	25±2 (6)	29±4 (6)		54±34 (6)	
50 mg/kg	22±4 (6)	28±4 (6)	39±25 (4)		—	
Ischemia 30′:						
Vehicle	25±9 (23)	55±32 (23)	33±11 (15)	$P < 0.02$	24±7 (8)	> $P < 0.03$
CsA 5 mg/kg	27±11 (23)	58±42 (23)	45±6 (15)	$P < 0.03$	45±16 (8)	
			72±49 (8)			
25 mg/kg	23±5 (8)	74±45 (8)	72±49 (8)		—	
50 mg/kg	27±11 (8)	53±23 (8)	62±40 (6)		—	
Ischemia 40′:						
Vehicle	41±9 (8)	53±23 (8)	42±13 (8)	> P = NS	43±12 (8)	> $P < 0.01$
CsA 5 mg/kg	45±13 (8)	66±43 (8)	52±16 (8)		65±17 (7)	

[a] n decreases on successive days because animals were sacrificed on successive days.

TABLE 3. Inulin clearance (ml/min/100 g BW) (mean ±SD [n])

	Day 2	Day 4	Day 7	
Sham:				
Normal saline	—	—	0.81±0.32 (6)	
Vehicle	0.83±0.31 (5)	0.75±0.18 (7)	0.89±0.31 (5)	> $P < 0.01$
CsA 5 mg/kg	0.79±0.22 (6)	0.68±0.27 (5)	0.44±0.14 (6)	
Ischemia 30′:				
Vehicle	0.35±0.16 (6)	0.63±0.29 (8)	0.72±0.27 (6)	> $P < 0.05$
CsA 5 mg/kg	0.29±0.19 (6)	0.49±0.19 (7)	0.43±0.29 (8)	
Ischemia 40′:				
Vehicle	—	—	0.55±0.12 (5)	> $P < 0.01$
CsA 5 mg/kg	—	—	0.27±0.13 (5)	

TABLE 4. Serum creatinine (mg/dl) (mean ±SD [n])

	Day 2	Day 4	Day 7
Sham:			
Vehicle	0.40±0.07 (5)	0.67±0.13 (8)	0.66±0.18 (11)
CsA 5 mg/kg	0.35±0.10 (6)	0.70±0.23 (8)	0.87±0.44 (7)
25 mg/kg	0.68±0.22 (5)	0.55±0.12 (5)	0.56±0.16 (5)
50 mg/kg	0.55±0.12 (6)	0.63±0.32 (4)	—
Ischemia 30′:			
Vehicle	1.46±1.2 (6)	0.64±0.19 (5)	0.63±0.15 (6)
CsA 5 mg/kg	1.54±1.6 (6)	0.75±0.20 (6)	0.72±0.19 (8)
25 mg/kg	1.27±0.71 (8)	0.93±0.39 (7)	0.56±0.11 (6)
50 mg/kg	0.87±0.18 (8)	0.65±0.26 (6)	—
Ischemia 40′:			
Vehicle	1.10±0.39 (8)	0.73±0.12 (8)	0.73±0.26 (8)
CsA 5 mg/kg	1.39±0.92 (8)	0.88±0.23 (8)	0.74±0.32 (7)

TABLE 5. CsA level in plasma (ng/ml) and kidney tissues (ng/g) (mean ±SD [n])

	Plasma	Tissue
Sham:		
CsA 5 mg/kg		
Day 2	287±101 (6)	[a]
Day 4	585±436 (8)	596±274 (8)
Day 7	507±205 (7)	543±376 (7)
CsA 25 mg/kg		
Day 7	3696±1934 (6)	[a]
Ischemia 30′:		
CsA 5 mg/kg		
Day 2	302±58 (8)	225±44 (3)
Day 4	468±443 (8)	749±284 (3)
Day 7	419±212 (8)	355±110 (7)
CsA 25 mg/kg		
Day 7	3397±1564 (7)	[a]
Ischemia 40′:		
CsA 5 mg/kg		
Day 7	647±72 (6)	484±96 (5)

[a] Results not available due to technical problems.

in which inulin clearances were not performed. In contrast to the BUN levels and inulin clearances there were no significant differences between the vehicle and CsA groups.

Table 5 shows the trough CsA plasma level 24 hr after the last injection and the kidney tissue CsA concentration. There appears to be no accumulation of CsA in kidney tissue despite renal failure.

Serum sodium, potassium, and renal cortical tissue content of sodium, potassium, and calcium were all similar in vehicle groups and CsA groups. There was no significant difference between vehicle and CsA groups in their fractional excretional rates of sodium on day 7, although inulin clearance indicated decreased glomerular filtration rate in the CsA group.

Kidneys of at least three rats in each group were examined by light microscopy. Rats that had had their renal arteries clamped showed tubular necrosis. Despite the difference in inulin clearance between the CsA and vehicle groups (Table 3), the degree of tubular necrosis was similar. No tubular necrosis was seen in sham-operated rats given CsA, although inulin clearance showed a decrease in GFR. Vacuolization of tubular epithelium was present in the CsA and vehicle groups, whether sham-operated or renal-artery-clamped (Fig. 1). Using a grid with 36 intersecting points (point counting), the percentage of tubular epithelial cells showing vacuolization was measured in three fields. Vacuolization was more extensive in the ischemic than in the sham-operated rats, and in the rats that were sacrificed on day 7 than at the earlier times. A sham-operated group given normal saline for seven days also showed vacuolization. Electron microscopy revealed that the vacuoles consisted of phagolyosomes containing granular and membranous debris (Fig. 2).

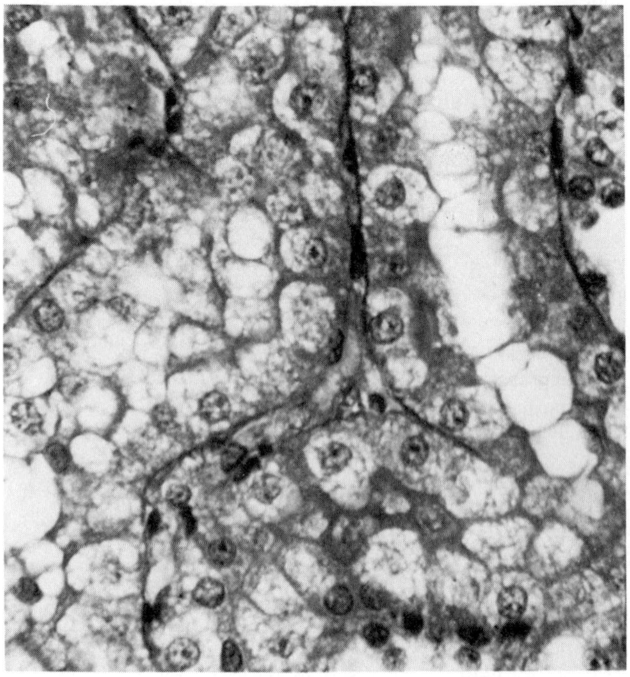

FIGURE 1. Light microscopy of an H & E-stained section from the kidney of a rat sham-operated and given CsA 5 mg/kg/day for 7 days. Vacuolization of the tubular epithelium is seen.

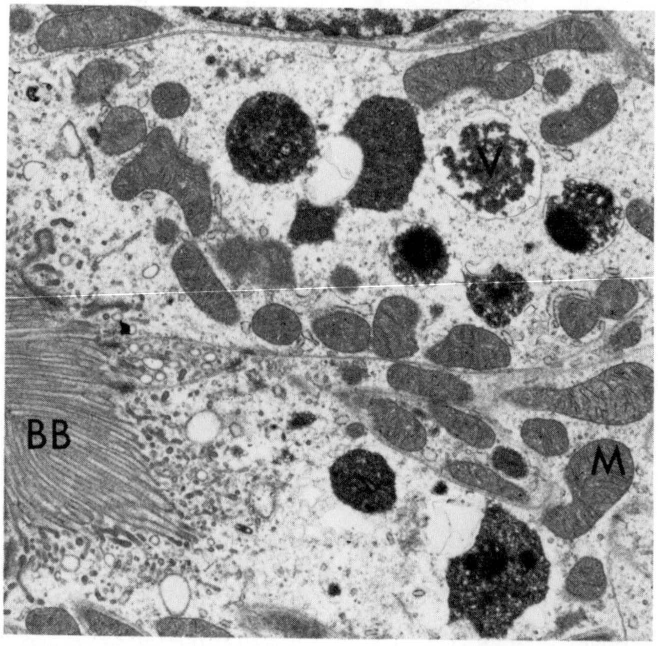

FIGURE 2. Electron micrograph of a proximal tubule showing normal brush border (BB), normal mitochondria (m), and vacuolar structure (V) with the appearance of phagolyosomes containing granular and membranous debris (×5100).

DISCUSSION

Previous studies investigating the interaction between ischemia and CsA have yielded varying results. Homan et al. (*7*) studied bilaterally nephrectomized dogs that received kidney autografts after 1 hr of warm ischemia. CsA 25 mg/kg was administered daily posttransplant to half the animals, and no difference was observed in the serum creatinine levels on subsequent days. After renal artery clamping for 45 min and contralateral nephrectomy, Dieperink et al. (*8*) also found no difference in serum creatinine and creatinine clearance values between rabbits given CsA 25 mg/kg/24 hr and those receiving no treatment. In contrast, Thiel et al. (*9*) observed delayed recovery from ischemia with CsA. They clamped the left renal artery in rats with previous right nephrectomy and administered CsA 20 mg or 50 mg/kg 1 hr before ischemia, followed by daily administration. The creatinine clearance on day 8 was decreased in the CsA group compared withe the vehicle group, but sham-operated animals given CsA had a similar decrease in creatinine clearance. In the present study a rat model of bilateral renal ischemia was used with a lower dosage of CsA more consistent with that used in humans. The lower dosage of CsA would also be expected to result in less nephrotoxicity, which might obscure the effect of interaction with ischemia. Different degrees of ischemia were used since interaction might be seen with a more severe degree of ischemia but not with a lesser one.

The results show that, with CsA administration, recovery from either 30 or 40 min ischemia appeared to be prevented, such that on day 7 inulin clearance in animals given CsA 5 mg/kg/day was about 50% of that in the vehicle group. Sham-operated animals given CsA 5 mg/kg/day, however, also had a decrease in renal function. Their inulin clearances on day 7 were also about 50% of those of the sham-operated group given vehicle. It is more likely, therefore, that the diminished degree of recovery from ischemia with CsA is a reflection of superimposition of CsA nephrotoxicity on the recovering kidneys. If there had been significant interaction between ischemia and CsA, one would have expected more than 50% reduction in clearance. Thus ischemia and CsA do not appear to have a synergistic effect on renal function in the rat, contrary to the impression from human renal transplant experience (*1*). Conceivably this is the result of species difference. The question remains, however, whether a lower dosage of CsA than was used in the present study might show an interaction because it might not have nephrotoxicity on its own. The trough plasma CsA levels in our rats given CsA 5 mg/kg/day were about 400–500 ng/ml, which is higher than the level (100–200) usually desired in human renal transplantation. In a recent study (*10*), however, a lower mean trough plasma level of 161 ng/ml in rats was also associated with significant diminution of inulin clearance after 13 days of therapy.

The mechanism of nephrotoxicity of CsA is unknown. Willibrand and Hayry (*11*), using fine-needle aspirate and indirect immunofluorescence, have demonstrated deposits of CsA in proximal tubular cells, the amount of which correlated with the degree of clinical nephrotoxicity in renal transplant recipients. The kidney tissue CsA content in our animals, however, was not increased with nephrotoxicity. Kahn et al. (*6*) found no selective renal disposition of CsA, unlike other body tissue, in a patient who manifested nephrotoxicity prior to death. Morphologic changes reported to be associated with acute nephrotoxicity in man have included arteriolar and glomerular capillary thrombosis, mesangial sclerosis, and tubulointerstitial changes with interstitial edema, vacuolization, and necrosis of tubular epithelium (*12*). Giant mitochondria with disoriented cristae and paracrystalline inclusion were seen on electron microscopy (*13*). Long-term therapy with CsA in cardiac transplant recipients has been found to be associated with extensive interstitial fibrosis, tubular atrophy, and focal global sclerosis of 10–20% of glomeruli (*14*). In our study, there was vacuolization of tubular epithelium—not only in CsA groups but also in vehicle groups. A group given normal saline had the same changes, although to a lesser extent. This finding suggests a technical artifact from the fixation technique. Similar difficulty was encountered by Dieperink et al. (*10*) in a study involving CsA on the same strain of rats. Other studies in rats have reported vacuolization in the proximal tubular epithelium with CsA and not with control (*15*, *16*). On electron microscopy, dilatation of endoplasmic reticulum, and an increased number of lysosomes, and myeloid bodies were seen and glomeruli were unaffected (*15*).

The fact that tubular changes predominated in morphology suggests that CsA is toxic to tubular epithelium. Urine N-acetylgluosamidase excretion, which reflects tubular damage, was elevated in rats receiving CsA (*15*) and also in two patients with CsA nephrotoxicity (*17*). The occurrence of impaired renal concentrating ability, metabolic acidosis, and hyperkalemia in transplant patients also indicates tubular damage (*2*, *18*). In our study, despite the reduced glomerular filtration rate, fractional excretion of sodium in the CsA groups was not significantly different from that in the vehicle groups. Others have found, in both human and animal studies, that fractional excretion of sodium decreases with CsA (*19*, *20*). Dieperink et al. (*10*), using lithium clearance methods, observed that in rats receiving CsA with resultant decrease in inulin clearance, proximal tubular fractional reabsorption of filtrate decreased. They concluded that nephrotoxicity was the result of glomerular effects, despite the absence of morphological changes. Hemodynamic alteration, with a reduction of renal blood flow and glomerular filtration rate, could be a possibility. The renin-angiotensin system has been found to be stimulated in rats given CsA and might contribute to a decreased glomerular filtration rate and decreased renal sodium excretion (*21*). CsA also reduces the prostaglandin stimulating plasma factor level, and the consequent disturbance in prostaglandin synthesis could potentiate hemodynamic alterations and affect the glomerular filtration rate (*22*).

In summary, using a model of ischemic injury induced by bilateral renal artery clamping, we have found no synergistic interaction between ischemia and CsA nephrotoxicity. Significant nephrotoxicity in rats was seen after 7 days of CsA administration at 5 mg/kg/day with the plasma CsA level around 400–500 ng/ml. The mechanism of CsA nephrotoxicity is unknown and evidence exists both for tubular and for glomerular mechanisms.

REFERENCES

1. The Canadian Multicentre Transplant Study Group. A randomized clinical trial of cyclosporine in cadaveric renal transplantation. N Engl J Med 1983; 309: 809.
2. Atkinson K, Biggs JC, Hayes J, et al. Cyclosporin A associated nephrotoxicity in the first 100 days after allogeneic bone marrow transplantation: three distinct syndromes. Br J Haematol 1983; 54: 59.
3. Kennedy MS, Deeg HJ, Siegel M, Crowley JJ, Storb R, Thomas

ED. Acute renal toxicity with combined use of amphotericin B and cyclosporine after marrow transplantation. Transplantation 1983; 35: 211.
4. Ferguson RM, Sutherland DER, Simmons RL, Najarian JS. Ketoconazole, cyclosporin metabolism, and renal transplantation. Lancet 1982; 2: 882.
5. Thompson JF, Chalmers DHK, Hunnisett AGW, Wood RFM, Morris PJ. Nephrotoxicity of trimethoprim and cotrimoxazole in renal allograft recipients treated with cyclosporine. Transplantation 1983; 36: 204.
6. Kahan BD, Van Buren CT, Boileau M, Ried M, Payne WD. Cyclosporin A tissue levels in a cadaveric renal allograft recipient. Transplantation 1983; 35: 96.
7. Homan WP, French ME, Morris PJ. Effect of cyclosporin A upon the function of ischemically damaged renal autografts in the dog. Transplantation 1980; 30: 228.
8. Dieperink H, Starklint H. Effect of cyclosporin A on ischemically damaged rabbit kidneys. Dan Med Bull 1983; 30: 278.
9. Thiel G, Torhorst J, Brunner FP. Renal toxicity of cyclosporin A in the rat. Proc Clin Dial Transplant Forum 1980; 62.
10. Dieperink H, Starklint H, Leyssac PP. Nephrotoxicity of cyclosporine—an animal model: study of the nephrotoxic effect of cyclosporine on overall renal and tubular function in conscious rats. Transplant Proc 1983; 15: 2736.
11. Willebrand EV, Hayry P. Cyclosporin A deposits in renal allografts. Lancet 1983; 2: 189.
12. Shulman H, Striker G, Deeg HJ, Kennedy M, Storb R, Thomas ED. Nephrotoxicity of cyclosporin A after allogeneic marrow transplantation. N Engl J Med 1981; 305: 1392.
13. Mihatsch MJ, Olivieri W, Marbet Y, Thiel G, Harder F, Zollinger HU. Giant mitochondria in renal tubular cells and cyclosporin A. Lancet 1981; 1: 1162.
14. Myers BD, Ross J, Newton L, Luetscher J, Perlroth M. Cyclosporine-associated chronic nephropathy. N Engl J Med 1984; 311: 699.
15. Blair JT, Thompson AW, Whiting PH, Davidson RJL, Simpson JC. Toxicity of the immune suppressant cyclosporin A in the rat. J Pathol 1982; 138: 163.
16. Whiting PH, Simpson JG, Davidson RJL, Thompson AW. Pathological changes in rats receiving cyclosporin A at immunotherapeutic dosage for 7 weeks. Br J Exp Pathol 1983; 64: 437.
17. Sweny P, Hopper J, Gross M, Varghese Z. Nephrotoxicity of cyclosporin A. Lancet 1981; 1: 663.
18. Hamilton DV, Evans DB, Henderson RG, et al. Nephrotoxicity and metabolic acidosis in transplant patients on cyclosporin A. Proc Eur Dial Transplant Assoc 1981; 18: 400.
19. Devineni R, McKenzie N, Duplan J, Keown P, Stiller C, Wallace AC. Renal effects of cyclosporine: clinical and experimental observations. Transplant Proc 1983; 15: 2695.
20. Tonnesen AS, Hamner RW, Weinmann EJ. Cyclosporine and sodium and potassium excretion in the rat. Transplant Proc 1983; 15: 2730.
21. Siegl H, Ryffel B, Petric R, et al. Cyclosporine, the renin-angiotensin-aldosterone system, and renal adverse reactions. Transplant Proc 1983; 15: 2719.
22. Neild GH, Rocchi G, Imberti L, et al. Effect of cyclosporin A on prostacyclin synthesis by vascular tissue. Thromb Res 1983; 32: 373.

Received 31 January 1985.
Accepted 23 May 1985.

0041-1337/86/4102-0156$02.00/0
TRANSPLANTATION
Vol. 41, No. 2
Printed in U.S.A.

LOCAL TREATMENT OF RENAL ALLOGRAFTS, A PROMISING WAY TO REDUCE THE DOSAGE OF IMMUNOSUPPRESSIVE DRUGS

COMPARISON OF VARIOUS WAYS OF ADMINISTERING PREDNISOLONE[1]

T. J. M. RUERS,[2] W. A. BUURMAN, J. F. M. SMITS,[3] C. J. VAN DER LINDEN, J. J. VAN DONGEN, H. A. J. STRUYKER-BOUDIER,[3] AND G. KOOTSTRA

The Department of Surgery and The Department of Pharmacology, Biomedical Center, University of Limburg, 6200 MD Maastricht, The Netherlands

A method is described for continuous administration of immunosuppressive drugs directly into rat renal allografts. The drug is given via a catheter, introduced into the suprarenal or testicular artery of the transplanted kidney. The cannula is connected to an implantable osmotic minipump that delivers an immunosuppressive drug with continuous flow for 13 days. It is demonstrated that the technique as such has no detrimental or enhancing effects on renal allograft survival. Depending upon the pharmacokinetic properties of the drug administered, this technique allows a more or less selective treatment of renal allograft rejection.

The method was used to test the effect of intrarenal administration of prednisolone on renal allograft survival. Intrarenal administration of this drug appeared to be superior to any other way of administration tested.

[1] This work was supported by the Dr. Saal van Zwanenberg Stichting.
[2] Address correspondence to: T.J.M. Ruers, Department of Surgery, University of Limburg, P.O. Box 616, 6200 MD Maastricht, The Netherlands.
[3] The Department of Pharmacology.

A low dose of 4 mg/kg body weight per day given by continuous intrarenal infusion results in significant prolongation of graft survival, whereas continuous systemic administration of this dose is not effective. To induce prolongation of graft survival by i.p. administration the prednisolone dose had at least to be doubled. The results prove that during graft rejection local events within the graft are vulnerable to prednisolone. It is concluded that local treatment of allograft rejection is possible and that this approach represents a potentially important way to manipulate the immune response.

In rats, a method was developed for local drug delivery into the renal artery of a transplanted kidney (further called intrarenal or local drug delivery). Thus it became possible to deliver immunosuppressive drugs directly to the renal allograft. The technique was derived from chronic local drug infusion into the renal artery of unrestrained rats as described earlier (*1*). Depending upon the pharmacokinetic properties of the drug used, this approach allows a more or less selective treatment of the transplanted kidney. More precisely, intrarenal drug delivery results in high renal exposure of the drug with low systemic exposure, if total body clearance of the drug is high or the extraction ratio by the kidney is high.

Local events within the kidney play an important role during the afferent, as well as during the efferent, phase of the immune response (*2–8*). When selective administration of immunosuppressive drugs to renal allografts can interfere with these processes, allograft rejection may be manipulated locally. This approach to immunosuppressive therapy offers interesting perspectives because reduced systemic drug levels lead to fewer systemic side effects of the immunosuppressive agents used. We have tested the effect of local administration of prednisolone on renal allograft survival since the plasma half-life of prednisolone in the rat is short (*9*). The results are compared with those obtained with prednisolone administered by other routes. It is demonstrated that local continuous infusion of prednisolone is an effective way to induce immunosuppression. It appears to be superior to any other way of administration tested.

MATERIALS AND METHODS

Animals. Inbred male Brown Norway (BN)[4] (RT^n) and Lewis rats (RT^1) were obtained from the department of experimental animal services of the University of Limburg. Rats of 250–300 g were used for all experiments. Rats were supplied with acidified water and rat chow ad libitum.

Kidney transplantation. Kidneys were transplanted from Brown Norway rats to Lewis rats. In BN rats the right renal artery branches from the suprarenal artery or the testicular artery. Both arteries can be used for catheter implantation. Therefore only right donor kidneys were used. Renal allografting was performed according to the technique of Lee (*10*) with the modifications of Lameyer (*11*) for the urether bladder anastomosis.

Both recipient kidneys were removed during the operation and graft survival was assessed by animal survival. Serum urea levels were determined on day 3, day 7, and at weekly intervals thereafter. Urea concentrations were measured using a urease colorimetric assay (Boehringer, Mannheim, FRG). Serum urea levels in normal animals were 50–55 mg/100 ml. Recipients were killed on the 50th day after transplantation if rejection had not occurred.

Technique of intrarenal and i.v. drug delivery. For intrarenal treatment a catheter was introduced in the suprarenal or testicular artery of the transplanted kidney in a way similar to that previously described in normal rats (*1*) (Fig. 1). The catheter was secured to the vessel, preventing the tip of the cannula from protruding into the arterial lumen. After patency of the infusion system was checked, the catheter was immediately connected to the pump.

Catheters were constructed of a 10-cm piece of polyethylene (PE)-10 tubing (Clay Adams, Parsippany, NJ). The tip of the catheter was stretched over a hot soldering iron to reduce its outer diameter to approximately 0.2 mm. An inner diameter of 0.1 mm was maintained by the previous introduction of a steel wire of that diameter. The catheter was extended by a 5-cm piece of PE-60 tubing (Clay Adams) that was heat-sealed to the PE-10 tubing (*1*).

For i.v. drug delivery a Silastic catheter (602–155 Silastic tubing Dow Corning, Midland, MI) was introduced into the jugular vein, guided to the abdominal cavity, and connected to the osmotic minipump.

Drug administration. Prednisolone was given by means of continuous infusion intrarenally, i.v., or i.p. Administration of prednisolone i.p. was also performed by bolus injection once daily.

Continuous delivery of prednisolone was performed with Alzet osmotic minipumps (model 2ML2, Alza, Palo Alto, CA). The pumps were implanted in the abdominal cavity immediately after transplantation. Pumps delivered prednisolone directly into the abdominal cavity or were connected to a catheter to deliver the drug intrarenally or i.v. In this way prednisolone was delivered i.p. intrarenally, or i.v. at a constant rate of approximately 6 μl/hr from day 0 till day 13. Prednisolone

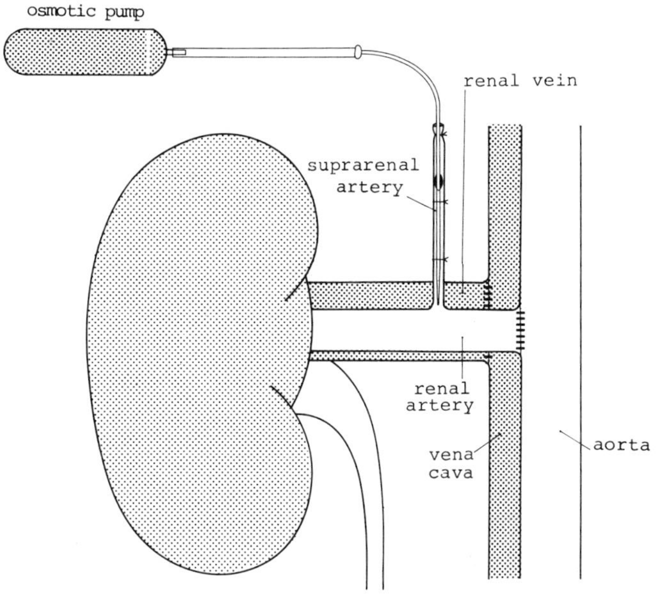

FIGURE 1. Schematic outline of the experimental model used for drug infusion into the renal artery of a transplanted kidney. A catheter is introduced into the suprarenal (or testicular) artery of the transplanted kidney and connected to an osmotic minipump implanted in the abdominal cavity. The osmotic minipump delivers the drug in a continuous fashion from day 0 until day 13.

[4] Abbreviations used: BN, Brown Norway; MST, median survival time; PE, polyethylene.

(Nogepha, Alkmaar, The Netherlands) was dissolved in pyrogen-free distilled water without heparin, and the dose of the drug was adjusted to the body weight of the recipient at day -1. In animals that received intrarenal or i.v. treatment correct position of the catheter was checked at autopsy.

Rats, treated with i.p. bolus injections were injected once daily. Solutions were prepared at day -1 and kept at 37°C in order to permit comparison of results with those obtained with continuous infusion. The dose of prednisolone was adjusted to the body weight of the recipient at day -1 and remained constant during the experiment. Drug administration started on day -1 and lasted till day 13.

Statistical analysis. Comparisons between groups were made using the Wilcoxon rank test. Differences were considered to be statistically significant if $P<0.05$ in a two-tailed test.

RESULTS

To test the effect of the intrarenal infusion technique on graft survival Lewis recipients were untreated or received continuous intrarenal infusion with saline. The results, shown in Table 1, demonstrate that the intrarenal infusion technique has no influence on renal allograft survival. Median survival time (MST) in animals treated with continuous intrarenal infusion was 7 days, which did not significantly differ from the MST observed in untreated rats. To evaluate the function of renal allografts during intrarenal infusion, early graft function was determined by estimating serum urea levels on day 3 posttransplant (Table 1). Untreated rats and saline-treated rats showed similar serum urea levels, which indicates that the technique of intrarenal infusion does not interfere with early graft function. From these observations it can be concluded that the intrarenal infusion technique has neither detrimental nor enhancing effects on renal allograft survival.

To study the effect of intrarenal prednisolone therapy on renal allograft survival various prednisolone treatments were tested. Prednisolone was administered in four ways and dose-response studies were performed to establish the optimal regimen of administration. The drug was given by continuous infusion (intrarenal, i.v., or i.p.) or by i.p. bolus injections. The results of these experiments are given in Table 2.

At a dose of 4 mg/kg body wt/day intrarenal prednisolone delivery resulted in significant ($P<0.01$) prolongation of graft survival (MST 26 days). As depicted in Figure 2, serum urea levels of these animals remained low. The histological appearance of kidneys of these animals is, apart from slight infiltration with mononuclear cells, essentially normal (Fig. 3a). In contrast, i.v. or i.p. administration of prednisolone at this dosage proved to be ineffective, and MST of these groups were not statistically different from controls. Kidneys of these animals showed a dense interstitial mononuclear cell infiltrate, fibrinoid deposits, and obstructions of arterioles (Fig. 3b).

A beneficial effect on graft survival by any route of administration other than intrarenal was only obtained if the dose of prednisolone was doubled. Continuous i.p. infusion of prednisolone at a dose of 8 mg/kg body wt/day resulted in a moderate improvement of graft survival (MST 16 days). Serum urea levels of these animals are depicted in Fig. 2. The peak on day 7 and the large SD on this day are caused by the heterogeneity of the group. Three animals died within 10 days after transplantation and showed a mean serum urea level on day 7 of 586 mg/100 ml. Five animals survived for 2 weeks or more, these animals showed a mean serum urea level of 280 mg/100 ml after one week.

Prednisolone (8 mg/kg body wt/day) given by i.p. bolus injections did not prolong allograft survival; MST was 8 days. If the dose was increased to 12 mg/kg body wt/day, i.p. bolus injections were still ineffective. Animals treated with 12 mg/kg body wt/day showed high serum urea levels on day 7 (Fig. 2), which demonstrates that these animals died from rejection and not from other causes.

The data show that intrarenal administration of prednisolone is a successful way to achieve immunosuppression. Prednisolone administered in this way is effective at a low dosage (4 mg/kg body wt/day), whereas a dose more than 2 times higher is necessary if the drug is delivered by continuous i.p. infusion.

TABLE 1. Effect of the intrarenal infusion technique upon the survival and the serum urea levels of Lewis rats receiving BN renal allografts

Treatment	Survival times (days)	MST[a]	Urea ± SD (day 3)[b]
—	7.7.8.8 8.9.9	8	111±50
Saline Intrarenal	6.7.7.7.7 7.8.12	7	127±47

[a] MST = median survival time.
[b] Mean serum urea levels ± SD (mg/100 ml).

TABLE 2. Effect of various prednisolone treatments upon the survival of Lewis rats receiving BN renal allografts

Prednisolone (mg/kg/day)	Daily i.p. injections: Survival times	Daily i.p. injections: MST[a]	Continuous infusion, Intraperitoneal: Survival times	Intraperitoneal: MST	Intravenous: Survival times	Intravenous: MST	Intrarenal: Survival times	Intrarenal: MST
4	7.7.7.7.7 8.8.10.11	7	9.9.9.9 9.10.10.11	9	7.7.7.8 9.15.18	8.5	17.17.18 26.26>50 >50	26[b]
8	7.7.7.8.8 8.8.32	8	9.9.10.14 18.20.41>50	16[c]				
12	7.7.7.8 8.10.10	8						

[a] MST = median survival time (days).
[b] Wilcoxon rank test for difference between animals treated with intrarenal prednisolone (4 mg/kg body wt/day) and animals treated with this dose by continuous infusion i.v. ($P<0.05$), continuous infusion i.p. ($P<0.01$), or i.p. bolus injections ($P<0.01$).
[c] Wilcoxon rank test for difference between animals treated with continuous infusion i.p. (8 mg/kg body wt/day) and animals treated with this dose by i.p. bolus injections ($P<0.01$).

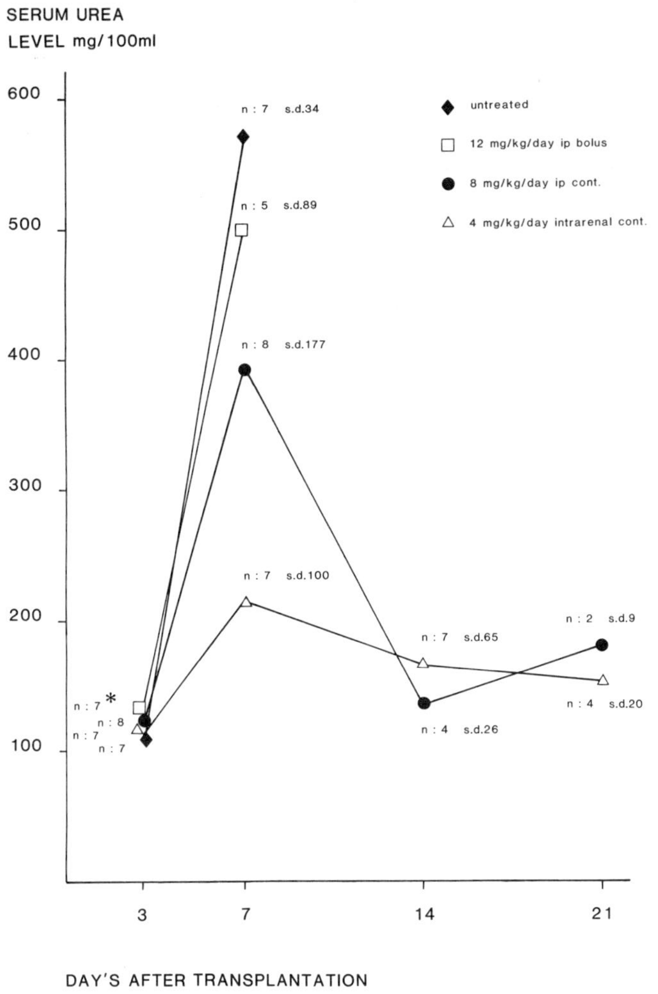

FIGURE 2. Mean serum urea levels in Lewis rats receiving BN renal allografts. Lewis recipients were untreated or received various prednisolone treatments. SD and the number of animals are indicated in the figure; (*) SD for all groups <55.

DISCUSSION

In this study we describe a technique for intrarenal drug delivery to kidney allografts in rats. It was shown that the method itself has no influence on renal allograft survival. This finding is in agreement with earlier observations that the technique did not interfere with kidney function in uninephrectomized rats (*1*). Depending upon the pharmacokinetic properties of the drug used the technique allows selective renal allograft treatment.

We demonstrated that the immunosuppressive effect of prednisolone administered by continuous intrarenal infusion is superior to the immunosuppressive effect obtained during continuous systemic infusion. This observation proves that local prevention and treatment of graft rejection is feasible. The data suggest that inhibition of local events within the graft, such as occur during the initiation phase and during the effector phase, can result in effective immunosuppression. In our model prednisolone may interact with both stages. In mice expression of Ia antigens on macrophages and Langerhans cells can be inhibited in vivo and in vitro by prednisolone (*12–13*). Local administration of prednisolone may likewise suppress the induction of the immune response by reducing the expression of Ia antigens. However, a wide range of other corticosteroid actions may also explain the immunosuppressive effect during local treatment. For example it was observed that corticosteroids inhibit interleukin 1 production (*12*) or render interleukin-2-producing T cells unresponsive to interleukin 1 (*14*). Moreover it was reported that dexamethasone inhibits the synthesis of interleukin 2 mRNA in human peripheral blood lymphocytes in vitro (*15*).

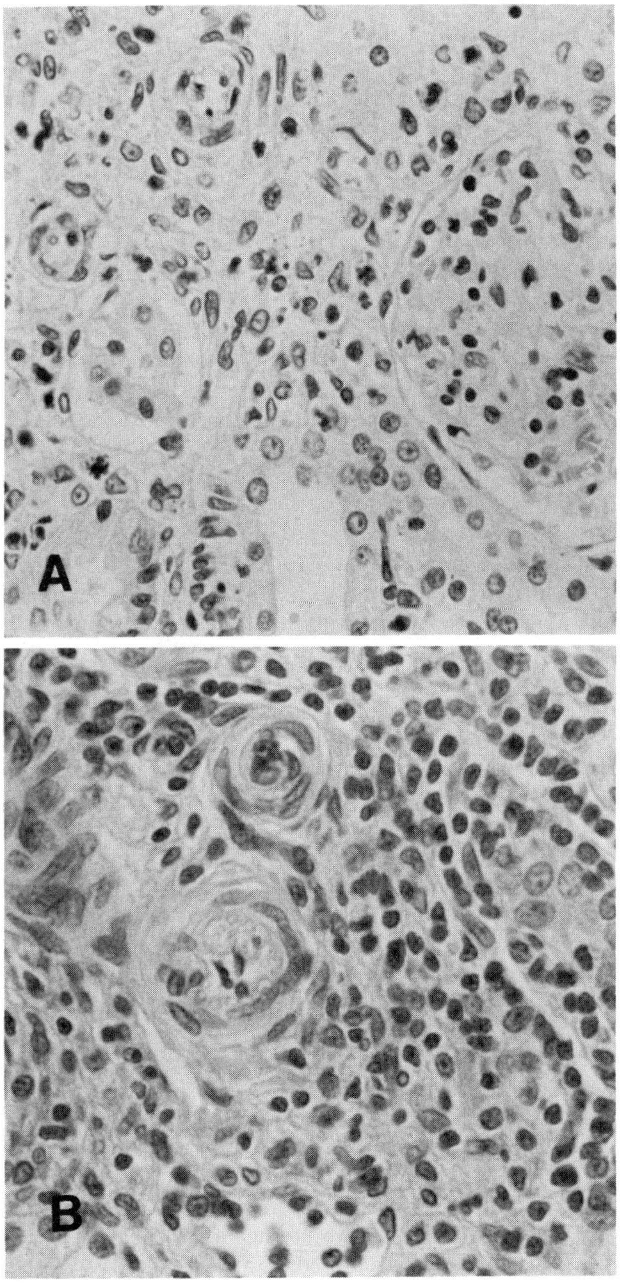

FIGURE 3. (A) Kidney of an animal treated with intrarenal prednisolone 4 mg/kg body wt/day. On day 8 the animal was killed while the graft was functioning well (serum urea level at day 8: 195 mg/100 ml). Apart from slight infiltration with mononuclear cells the histological picture is essentially normal (H & E; ×400). (B) BN kidney grafted in Lewis recipient, killed after 7 days of continuous i.p. prednisolone infusion (4 mg/kg body wt/day). A dense interstitial mononuclear cell infiltrate, fibrinoid deposits, and almost complete obstruction of an arteriole are clearly seen (H&E; ×500).

In man the effector mechanisms of the immune response are relatively insensitive to corticosteroids. Inhibition of cytotoxic T lymphocytes by corticosteroids, in vivo or in vitro, was described sporadically and was mostly achieved with extremely high concentrations or prolonged incubations (*16, 17*). Rats, in contrast to man, are corticosteroid sensitive—which, among other things, means that corticosteroid treatment results in leukocyte lysis. This property may interact with effector mechanisms during allograft rejection in rats.

Continuous infusion of prednisolone resulted in a better immunosuppressive effect than i.p. bolus injections. This finding is consistent with the results of Provoost (*18*), who demonstrated the superiority of continuous s.c. infusion of prednisolone over daily s.c. injections. These observations can be explained by the short half-life of the drug in rats, which is about 30 min (*9*). However, it was reported also that during continuous administration of prednisolone the side effects of the drug increase (*19–21*). A way to reduce systemic side effects is local administration, leading to a constant level of prednisolone in the target organ with low systemic levels. Intrarenal delivery of prednisolone is an example of this approach.

Our data show that the dosage of prednisolone may be reduced by at least 50% when given intrarenally, as compared with systemic administration. On the basis of theoretical considerations, the ratio between arterial blood levels during local intraarterial drug infusions (Cloc) and systemic infusions (Csys) is given by Cloc/Csys = (1+Ks/Qt) (*22*), where Ks represents systemic clearance of the drug and Qt is blood flow through the target tissue. In man, clearance of prednisolone is largely metabolic (*23*). In rats, prednisolone is also eliminated mostly by liver metabolism. Systemic clearance should be expected to be maximally equal to liver blood flow—i.e., 15 ml/min. Taken together with a value for renal blood flow of ≈ 15 ml/min through a single kidney in rats (*1*), this would result in a maximal ratio of Cloc/Csys ≈ 2. The advantage of intrarenal drug delivery can be much greater if Ks ≫ Qt—in other words, if the systemic clearance of the drug is much greater than the blood flow through the kidney. Experiments are currently in progress with this kind of high-clearance immunosuppressive drugs.

In 1969 Kountz and Cohn (*24*) had already shown excellent graft survival in renal transplant patients treated with intrarenal delivery of methylprednisolone over a short period. They also reported that patients treated this way did not develop systemic side effects of the drug, in contrast to patients who received systemic therapy. Our data strongly support their suggestion that local drug delivery is, in principle, an effective way to induce immunosuppression. The method of intrarenal drug delivery used by Kountz and Cohn, a catheter introduced into the renal artery via a small stabwound in the common iliac artery, has its drawbacks, however, in immunosuppressed patients. An attractive new way to achieve local drug delivery clinically is by means of prodrugs. These prodrugs are by themselves inactive, however within the organ (e.g., the kidney) they are converted into an active drug. This conversion may be an enzymatic reaction. Recently, renal prodrugs (which are activated within the kidney) were described (*25, 26*) and it would be a promising approach to immunosuppressive therapy if short-acting immunosuppressive drugs could be synthesized in this prodrug form. Our model of intrarenal drug delivery offers the possibility for selection among immunosuppressive drugs of candidates for transformation into such prodrug form.

Acknowledgments. We thank M. Havenith, M.D. of the Department of General Pathology, Annadal Hospital, Maastricht, for his advice, as well as Mrs. K. Spronck for her secretarial assistance.

REFERENCES

1. Smits JF, Kasbergen CM, van Essen H, Kleinjans JC, Struyker-Boudier HA. Chronic local infusion into the renal artery of unrestrained rats. Am J Physiol 1983; H: 304.
2. Lechler RI, Batchelor JR. Restoration of immunogenicity to passenger cell-depleted kidney allografts by the addition of donor strain dendritic cells. J Exp Med 1982; 155: 31.
3. Lafferty KJ. Immunogenicity of foreign tissue. Transplantation 1980; 29: 179.
4. Bach JF. Comment on Lafferty KJ. Immunogenicity of foreign tissue. Transplantation 1980; 29: 182.
5. Ascher NL, Chen S, Hoffman R, Simmons RL. Maturation of cytotoxic effector cells at the site of allograft rejection. Transplant Proc 1981; 13: 1105.
6. Nemlander A, Soots A, von Willebrand E, Husberg B, Häyry P. Redistribution of renal allograft-responding leucocytes during rejection. II. Kinetics and specificity. J Exp Med 1982; 156: 1087.
7. Häyry P. Intragraft events in allograft destruction. Transplantation 1984; 38: 1.
8. Ascher NL, Hoffman R, Hanto DW, Simmons RL. Cellular events within the rejecting allograft. Transplantation 1983; 35: 193.
9. Kort WJ, Weijma IM, Westbroek DL. Reductive effect of phenobarbital on graft survival in prednisolone treated rats. Eur Surg Res 1979; 11: 317.
10. Lee S. An improved technique of renal transplantation in the rat. Surgery 1967; 61: 771.
11. Lameyer LD, Smith J, Mowbray JF. Effect of kidney perfusion on renal allograft survival in azathioprine treated rats. Br J Exp Pathol 1972; 53: 130.
12. Snijder DS, Unanue ER. Corticosteroids inhibit murine macrophage Ia expression and interleukin 1 production. J Immunol 1982; 129: 1803.
13. Nordlund JJ, Ackles AE, Lerner AB. The effects of ultraviolet light and certain drugs on Ia-bearing Langerhans cells in murine epidermis. Cell Immunol 1981; 60: 50.
14. Palacios R, Sugawara I. Hydrocortisone abrogates proliferation of T cells in autologous mixed lymphocyte reaction by rendering the Il-2 producer T cells unresponsive to Il-1 and unable to synthesize the T cell growth factor. Scand J Immunol 1982; 15: 25.
15. Arya SK, Wong-Staal F, Gallo RC. Dexamethasone-mediated inhibition of human T cell growth factor and γ-interferon messenger RNA. J Immunol 1984; 133: 273.
16. Rosenberg JC, Lysz K. Suppression of human cytotoxic lymphocytes by methylprednisolone. Transplantation 1978; 25: 115.
17. Balow JE, Hunninghake GW, Fauci AS. Corticosteroids in human lymphocyte mediated cytotoxic reactions. Transplantation 1977; 23: 322.
18. Provoost AP, de Keyzer MH, Kort WJ, Wolff ED. Superiority of continuous infusion of prednisolone over daily injections in the prolongation of heart allograft survival in rats. Transplantation 1982; 34: 221.
19. Reed WP, Lucas ZJ, Cohn R. Alternate-day prednisone therapy after renal transplantation. Lancet 1970; 1: 747.
20. Sheagren JN, Jowsey J, Bird DC, Gurton ME, Jacobs JB. Effect on bone growth of daily versus alternate day corticosteroid administration: an experimental study. J Lab Clin Med 1977; 89: 120.
21. McEnery PT, Gonzalez LL, Martin LW, West CD. Growth and development of children with renal transplants: use of alternate-day steroid therapy. J Pediatr 1973; 83: 806.
22. Smits JF, Thijssen HH. Spatial control of drug action: theoretical considerations on the pharmacokinetics of target-aimed drug delivery. In: Struyker-Boudier HAJ, ed. Rate controlled drug

administration and action. Boca Raton (USA): CRC Press (in press).

23. Gambertoglio JG, Amend WJ, Benet LZ. Pharmacokinetics and bioavailability of prednisone and prednisolone in healthy volunteers and patients: a review. J Pharmacokinet Biopharm 1980; 8: 1.
24. Kountz SL, Cohn R. Initial treatment of renal allografts with large intrarenal doses of immunosuppressive drugs. Lancet 1969; 1: 338.
25. Orlowski M, Mizoguchi H, Sherwin W. N-acyl-γ-glutamyl derivatives of sulfamethoxazole as models of kidney selective prodrugs. J Pharmacol Exp Ther 1980; 212: 167.
26. Smits JF, Struyker-Boudier HAJ. Preferential renal vasodilator effects of CGP 22979A in conscious spontaneously hypertensive rats. J. Pharmacol Exp Ther 1985; 232: 845.

Received 26 February 1985.
Accepted 21 May 1985.

0041-1337/86/4102-0161$02.00/0
TRANSPLANTATION

Vol. 41, No. 2
Printed in U.S.A.

EVIDENCE OF FREE-RADICAL-INDUCED DAMAGE IN RABBIT KIDNEYS AFTER SIMPLE HYPOTHERMIC PRESERVATION AND AUTOTRANSPLANTATION

C. J. GREEN,[2] G. HEALING,[2] J. LUNEC,[3] B. J. FULLER,[4] AND S. SIMPKIN[1]

Surgical Research Group, M.R.C. Clinical Research Centre, Northwick Park Hospital, Harrow, Middlesex; Department of Biochemistry, Selly Oak Hospital, Raddlebarn Road, Birmingham, B29 6JD; and Academic Department of Surgery, Royal Free Hospital Medical School, Pond Street, London, NW3 2OG, England

Rabbit kidneys were stored for 24 or 48 hr at 0°C after single-passage vascular flush with 30 ml of cold hypertonic citrate solution or 0.9% isotonic sodium chloride solution. They were then subjected to in vitro biochemical assay for evidence of free-radical damage immediately after storage or after they had been orthotopically autotransplanted and reperfused with blood in vivo for 60 min. Kidney homogenates were incubated at 37°C and assayed for fluorescent conjugated Schiff bases as indicators of lipid peroxidation, as well as for superoxide dismutase activity and reduced and oxidized glutathione.

In kidneys flushed with hypertonic citrate, no evidence of peroxidation could be detected immediately after storage for 24 or 48 hr. However, after in vivo reperfusion significantly more peroxidation ($P<0.01$) was evident. Storage in isotonic saline solution produced still higher levels of peroxidation damage whether reperfused or not ($P<0.001$). Schiff base formation was inversely proportional to the reduced and oxidized glutathione levels measured. No changes in superoxide dismutase levels could be detected. It is concluded that lipid peroxidation is important during cold ischemia but most damage occurs during the 60-min of reperfusion in vivo immediately after transplantation.

The causes of deterioration and eventual loss of renal function in kidneys during prolonged periods of ex vivo storage for transplantation remain obscure. Several pathological events have been documented, including depletion of cellular stores of high-energy adenine nucleotides (*1*), accumulation of metabolites, especially H^+ ions (*2*), autolysis by release of lysosomal enzymes (*3*), damage to cellular membranes with loss of constituent phospholipids (*4*), and vascular injury that results in edema, loss of circulating proteins, and—in its most severe form—leakage of blood cells into the extravascular compartment (*5*). The diversity of these changes suggests that they are secondary or tertiary events and not symptomatic of the primary lesion. This view is strengthened by the observation that correction of one particular pathological change—e.g., stimulation of net synthesis of high-energy adenine nucleotides by using various substrates and inhibitors of degradation—does not, in fact, improve other components of the "storage-damage syndrome," such as renal mitochondrial function (*6*). The spectrum of preservation damage mirrors that seen in simple renal ischemia at normothermia, although in the latter instance the damage accumulates much more quickly.

In simple normothermic ischemia, many of the pathological changes only become evident after blood circulation has been restored. For example, several workers have shown that most myocardial damage occurs during the early phases of recirculation and reoxygenation after ischemia (*7, 8*). The microvascular changes occurring during reperfusion of organs after long periods of ischemia have been well described, and the end result is an outflow block after initial flow through the vascular bed (*9–11*), but what actually initiates the lesions has been the subject of speculation; hard evidence is not available. However, prevention or delay in the chain of events involving endothelial swelling, protein leaks to the extravascular space, escalating edema, and loss of erythrocyte deformability have been claimed in several systems to which free-radical scavengers, such as superoxide dismutase (*12*), α-tocopherol, and coenzyme Q_{10}

[1] This work was supported by a grant from The Peter Samuel Fund.
[2] Northwick Park Hospital.
[3] Selly Oak Hospital.
[4] Royal Free Hospital Medical School.

(13), glutathione peroxidase (14), ascorbic acid (15), selenium salts (16), or iron chelators (17) have been added. Hence, there is now sufficient circumstantial evidence to incriminate toxic free-radical products as the possible culprits in initiating this cascade, both because sudden reoxygenation produces an overload of such free radicals as superoxide, hydroxyl radicals, and lipid peroxides, and because the activity of endogenous scavengers has been saturated during ischemia. Before the role of free radicals during and after ischemia can be demonstrated with confidence, however, it is important that accurate measurements of free-radical activity, in particular the lipid peroxides generated, should be made in tissues where the clinical and histopathological outcome of warm and cold ischemia is already well known, so that valid correlations can be made.

The actual detection of lipid peroxides in ischemic kidneys has previously proved difficult. The traditional assay involves the detection of a colored product formed when lipid peroxides are heated in the presence of thiobarbituric acid (18). However, although this reaction has been used extensively in several biological systems, it does not provide an accurate index of free-radical reactions that have occurred in vivo (19). Tappel and his co-workers have developed an alternative assay that depends on the reactivity of lipid peroxides in vivo with all primary amino groups to form characteristically fluorescence-conjugated Schiff bases (20). Detection of these lipid-soluble Schiff bases, thought to result from the conjugation of peroxides and aldehydes with membrane phospholipids, appears to be a more sensitive and specific test for the presence of lipid peroxides in vivo (21). We have already shown that these assays do correlate well with warm ischemic damage in rabbit kidneys, both before and after restoration of circulation to the tissue (22).

The aims of the present studies were: (1) to look for evidence of lipid peroxidation in rabbit kidneys subjected to cold ischemia for periods already known to be or not to be compatible with subsequent viability, depending on the "storage" solution used; (2) to compare this with the generation of lipid peroxides after the stored organs had been autografted and reperfused with blood for 60 min; and (3) to assay superoxide dismutase activity and glutathione redox status to see whether these correlated with the degree of lipid peroxidation.

Kidneys were stored at 4°C for various periods after vascular flush with hypertonic citrate (HCA) (23) or isotonic sodium chloride solutions, and then were assayed with or without autotransplantation and recirculation of blood in vivo for 60 min. The HCA solution has previously proved an excellent preservation medium, whereas isotonic saline is damaging in the storage of rabbit kidneys (24, 25).

MATERIALS AND METHODS

Materials. All chemicals were Analar grade except chloroform and methanol, which were special spectral grade.

Surgical technique. Seven groups of adult New Zealand White rabbits each weighing 3 kg were anesthetized by i.m. injection of fentanyl-fluanisone (Hypnorm) at 0.2 ml/kg, followed 3 min later by slow i.v. injection of diazepam (1.0 mg/kg). They were then supplied via an open face mask with oxygen flowing at 2 L/min for the duration of the operations.

[5] Abbreviations used: GSH, reduced glutathione; GSSG, oxidized glutathione; HCA, hypertonic citrate.

The right kidney was exposed through a mid-line abdominal incision and removed after careful dissection and ligation of the vessels and ureter under magnification. The warm ischemic period was less than 2.0 min. The renal artery was then cannulated and the kidney was flushed with 30 ml of sterile HCA solution (23) or with sterile isotonic 0.9% sodium chloride solution, each previously cooled to 2°C. It was then placed in a sterile beaker containing 60 ml of the identical flush solution and surrounded by ice within a closed polystyrene container held in a refrigerator. The storage temperature was thus maintained at a steady 0°C for the duration of storage, which was either 24 or 48 hr.

In groups in which kidneys were to be assessed for free-radical production after autotransplantation and 60 min of reperfusion in vivo, the donor rabbit was again anesthetized and opened along the same mid-line incision. The left kidney was carefully skeletalized and removed after clamping the artery and vein proximally and then dividing these vessels and the ureter as close to the renal hilus as possible to leave the maximum length of free renal vessel. The stored right kidney was then autografted into the recently vacated left renal bursa. The renal vessels were both anastomosed by a simple cuff ligature technique (26) that is so rapid that additional ischemia can be minimized; it allows excellent flow to the kidneys immediately after vessel clamps are removed. The total anastomosis time was less than 15 min and the kidney was kept cool locally by cold isotonic saline on swabs to minimize additional warm ischemic damage. Blood was allowed to reflow through the kidney for 60 min, during which the abdominal viscera were returned to their normal position and the incision was closed temporarily with clips. The rabbits were maintained anesthetized on a heated pad to keep body temperature at 37°C, and were hydrated with 60 ml of isotonic sodium chloride solution by constant i.v. infusion over this period.

In the control groups, the kidneys were simply harvested by the same careful technique described above using an identical anesthetic management protocol, and the organs were assayed without flushing, storage, or autotransplantation.

Assay for Schiff base formation. All the kidney specimens were processed within 60 min of removal from the animal. Thin slices were taken, weighed, homogenized and incubated at 37°C in open vessels with mechanical shaking. Lipid extracts (20) were monitored for a fluorescence maximum between 400 and 450 nm.

Assay for superoxide dismutase. Incubated samples were assayed by spectrophotometry for superoxide dismutase activity by the method of McCord and Fridovich (27) using a xanthine and xanthine oxidase system for the generation of superoxide (O_2^-,) radicals and cytochrome c as an electron acceptor. The presence of superoxide dismutase activity is characterized by the percentage of inhibition of cytochrome c reduction. All results were corrected for variability in the protein concentration of homogenates using the method of Lowry (28).

Measurement of reduced glutathione (GSH) and oxidized glutathione (GSSG). Further incubated samples were examined for the status of glutathione redox activity. A direct assay was found to be unreliable, so an indirect method was used based on that described by Hissin and Hilf (29) in which the concentrations of GSH and of GSSG were measured. The ratio of GSH to GSSG was used as a relative index of redox activity present.

Experimental protocol. The experimental protocol was as follows:

Gp. 1: Control kidneys were neither flushed nor stored.
Gp. 2: Kidneys were flushed with 30 ml HCA and stored for 24 hr at 0°C.
Gp. 3: Kidneys were flushed with 30 ml HCA and stored for 48 hr at 0°C.
Gp. 4: Kidneys were flushed with 30 ml HCA, stored 24 hr at 0°C, autotransplanted, and assayed after 60 min of recirculation with blood.
Gp. 5: Kidneys were flushed with 30 ml HCA, stored 48 hr at 0°C, autotransplanted, and assayed for 60 min of recirculation with blood.
Gp. 6: Kidneys were flushed with 30 ml of 0.9% w/v NaCl solution and stored for 24 hr at 0°C.
Gp. 7: Kidneys were flushed with 30 ml of 0.9% NaCl solution, stored for 24 hr at 0°C, autotransplanted, and assayed after 60 min of recirculation with blood.

RESULTS

Schiff base formation. There was no significant difference in the mean rate of change in fluorescence intensity between control kidneys (gp. 1) and those stored, whether for 24 (gp. 2) or 48 hr (gp. 3) after initial vascular flush with HCA (Table 1). This suggests that there was little change in the susceptibility to lipid peroxidation in these kidneys attributable to cold ischemia alone. However, recirculation of blood for 60 min through the stored and autografted kidneys, flushed with HCA (gps. 4 and 5) produced a dramatic and highly significant increase in Schiff base formation ($P<0.01$) but it made little difference whether the organs had been stored for 24 or 48 hr.

In kidneys flushed with isotonic saline solution, however, the results were quite different. Now, the greatest change in susceptibility to lipid peroxidation occurred during the 24-hr storage period, and the difference between control kidneys (gp. 1) and those in gp. 6 was highly significant ($P<0.001$). Schiff base formation had increased still further when tested after 60 min of recirculation (gp. 7) but this difference failed to reach significance.

Levels of superoxide dismutase. There were no significant differences in the mean amount of superoxide dismutase (SOD) present in control kidneys compared with those in gps. 2, 5, 6, or 7 (Table 2). However, the differences from controls obtained after 48-hr storage only with HCA (gp. 3) and 24-hr storage with HCA plus 60 min reflow (gp. 4) were significant ($P<0.02$ and <0.001, respectively).

TABLE 1. Results of assays for Schiff base formation after storage for 24 or 48 hr with and without reperfusion in vivo with blood

Experimental group (n=12 in each)	Mean rate of change in fluorescence intensity/mg protein (FI/hr±SD)	Significant differences from controls (*t* test)
Gp.1	1.05 (±1.04)	—
Gp.2	1.89 (±2.01)	NS
Gp.3	1.99 (±1.93)	NS
Gp.4	3.89 (±2.44)	$P<0.01$
Gp.5	2.89 (±1.54)	$P<0.01$
Gp.6	4.72 (±2.58)	$P<0.001$
Gp.7	5.55 (±2.52)	$P<0.001$

TABLE 2. Results of assays measuring mean amounts of superoxide dismutase (SOD) after storage for 24 or 48 hr with and without reperfusion in vivo with blood

Experimental group (n=12 in each case)	Mean amount of superoxide dismutase in tissue mg SOD/mg protein ± SD)	Significant differences from controls
Gp.1	$2.88\times10^{-3}(\pm0.39\times10^{-3})$	—
Gp.2	$2.85\times10^{-3}(\pm0.95\times10^{-3})$	NS
Gp.3	$3.68\times10^{-3}(\pm0.95\times10^{-3})$	$P<0.02$
Gp.4	$4.19\times10^{-3}(\pm0.81\times10^{-3})$	$P<0.001$
Gp.5	$3.03\times10^{-3}(\pm0.77\times10^{-3})$	NS
Gp.6	$2.67\times10^{-3}(\pm0.49\times10^{-3})$	NS
Gp.7	$2.72\times10^{-3}(\pm0.49\times10^{-3})$	NS

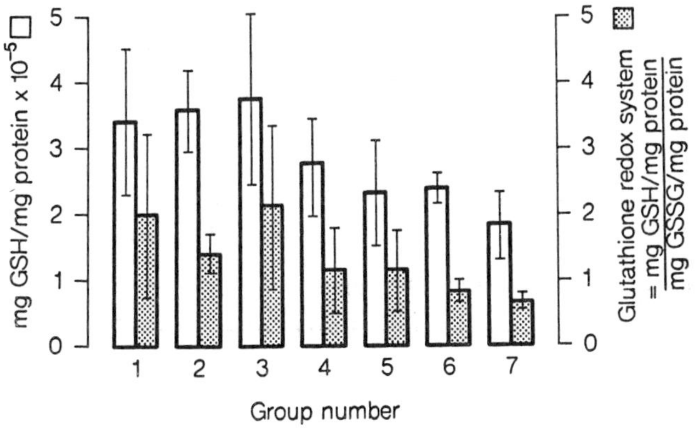

FIGURE 1. Mean levels of reduced glutathione (GSH) and the glutathione redox system.

Superoxide dismutase is an inducable enzyme, but within the time scale of these experiments the levels measured did not rise or fall in line with Schiff base indicators of lipid peroxidation. No correlation could be made in the case of the two groups that did experience a significant increase, and these data are difficult to interpret.

Glutathione redox system. The mean concentrations of GSH measured at the beginning and end of incubation, shown in Figure 1, correlate with the changes in Schiff base formation. Again there was no significant difference between control values and those in kidneys stored for 24 or 48 hr in HCA (gps. 2 and 3). However, there was a significant difference between controls and gp. 4 ($P<0.05$) and gp. 5 ($P<0.02$), although not between these two groups. The differences between control values and kidneys stored for 24 hr in isotonic saline (gp. 6) was highly significant ($P<0.01$), and there was a similar difference between gp. 6 and 7 ($P<0.01$).

From the mean concentrations of oxidized glutathione (GSSG) shown in Figure 2, in which storage in isotonic saline for 24 hr again showed the greatest changes (gp. 6 $P<0.001$ and gp. 7 $P<0.02$), the redox status of glutathione was obtained indirectly (Fig. 1). These results again correlate well and were inversely proportional to susceptibility to lipid peroxidation. There was no significant difference between control values and straight 24-hr or 48-hr storage in HCA, but there was a significant fall after recirculation for 60 min before assay (gps. 4 and 5), although there was no difference between these two groups. Similarly, there was a significant fall in gp. 6 from control values ($P<0.01$), and levels were still further depressed after recirculation for 60 min ($P<0.02$). The glutathione redox status expressed as a ratio of GSH to GSSG levels showed a clear difference between tissues subjected to cold ischemia alone and

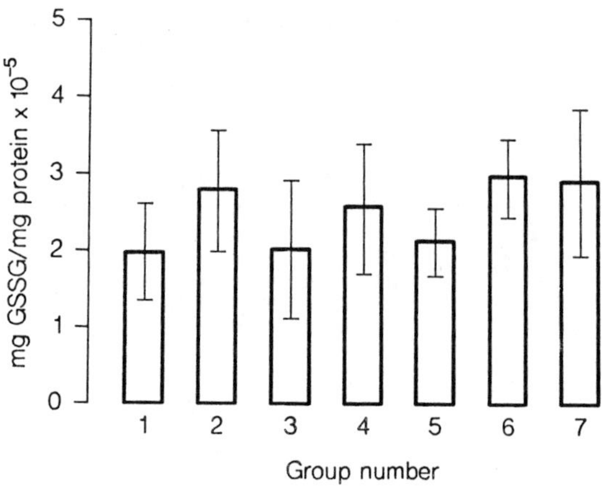

FIGURE 2. Mean activity of oxidized glutathione (GSSG).

kidneys reperfused with blood in vivo—as well as providing further evidence that initial flush with isotonic saline solution is itself damaging, with reperfusion playing a lesser role in the latter instance.

DISCUSSION

Rabbit kidneys autografted after an initial vascular flush with HCA and simple refrigeration for from 24 hr to a maximum of 48 hr have already been shown capable of supporting life in the unilaterally nephrectomized recipient, but they are universally damaged after storage for 72 hr (*24*). The results with isotonic sodium chloride solution flush, conversely, have been poor even after 16 hr of refrigeration (*25*). The present experiments were designed to test the hypothesis that lipid peroxidation is likely to be a major cause of damage during the period immediately after transplantation when the blood flow is reestablished; comparison of renal tissue was made after simple infusion storage using HCA as a good flush medium and isotonic saline as an unsuitable solution.

One undesirable consequence of tissue damage is the destabilization and destruction of cell membrane. Biological membranes contain polyunsaturated fatty acids that, because of their almost unique structure (methylene-interrupted double bonds) are highly susceptible to peroxidation (autoxidation). This chain reaction is perhaps the best piece of evidence for the occurrence of primary free-radical reactions. It is a chain reaction because the primary products of the reaction also act as initiators of further peroxidation. This propagation of the reaction is catalyzed by the presence of trace metal catalysts, such as iron and copper, that can become decompartmentalized, and thus potentially toxic during tissue injury.

Although we have not been able to detect lipid peroxidation immediately following ischemia of kidneys, we believe that the events that lead to peroxidation have occurred, and primary free-radical reactions have been induced. If our hypothesis is correct, the propensity for tissues to undergo peroxidation in vitro will be increased. From the data obtained in these experiments it is clear that susceptibility to lipid peroxidation, as measured by Schiff base formation, as well as by the redox activity of glutathione, behave as predicted and fit in well with the functional transplantation assessment of the two solutions. Most important, in kidneys flushed with HCA, the greatest damage seems to occur during reperfusion of the organ with blood.

The reason that the levels of GSH and the glutathione redox status are related to levels of lipid peroxidation is probably that glutathione peroxidase is a scavenging enzyme; in addition to being involved in the removal of superoxide anions converted to H_2O_2 by superoxide dismutase, it is also involved in the removal of lipid hydroperoxides formed as a result of lipid peroxidation. This reaction is related directly to the oxidation of glutathione:

$$\underset{\text{(H—OOH)}}{\text{Lipid—OOH}} + 2\ \text{GSH} \xrightarrow{\text{glutathione peroxidase}} \underset{\text{(H—OH)}}{\text{Lipid—OH}} + \text{GSSG} + H_2O$$

Hence, as lipid peroxidation proceeds, more hydroproxides are produced, so GSH is used up in the reaction and its level falls. Similarly, it can be seen that the ratio of GSH:GSSG, the indicator of redox activity, falls as oxidative stress increases.

The levels of GSSG and SOD do not fall into any pattern, and their role has not been established in these studies. It does seem strange that levels of GSSG should not rise corresponding to the fall in GSH levels as described above, but it is possible that reductase activity cannot cope with the production of peroxides, which are then oxidizing GSH.

Superoxide dismutase, although an inducible enzyme, showed no increased activity during the reperfusion period, so it must be concluded that this enzyme was not induced within the 60 min of reperfusion examined. Although raised levels were observed in two cases, these were not correlated with the Schiff base, GSH, or glutathione redox assays—so no definite conclusions can be reached.

It is likely that peroxidation damage to membrane lipids, occurring mostly during reflow after rabbit kidneys were stored in HCA and at a still higher level during reperfusion after storage in isotonic saline solution, resulted from the action of a free radical. From previous experiments in which antioxidants apparently protected tissues from warm ischemic damage, it seems likely that oxygen free radicals and lipid peroxidases do cause cell damage and, consequently, are responsible for—or at least contribute to—ischemic cell death (*13*).

Two probable reasons for damage occurring almost exclusively during reperfusion of the kidneys flushed with HCA can be advanced. Firstly, during ischemia, decreased oxygen ensures that available high energy nucleotide stores are rapidly used up. ATP has been shown to be catabolized in tissues during hypoxia to yield increased levels of hypoxanthine:

$$\text{ATP} \longrightarrow \text{AMP} \longrightarrow \text{inosine} \longrightarrow \text{hypoxanthine}$$

When an unstored kidney is transplanted and reperfused, xanthine oxidase acts quickly on the hypoxanthine, oxidizing it to xanthine, and finally to uric acid. However, under conditions of reduced oxygen availability during ischemia, the enzyme is converted to a form capable of producing superoxide (*30*), which then proceeds to peroxidize tissue membranes. Endogenous scavengers, which have been depleted during storage anyway, are then saturated by this abnormal overload. Second, during ischemia, the components of the electron transport chain accumulate in their reduced states—and, once oxygen becomes available, spontaneous oxidation occurs and free radicals are formed in large amounts. Hence, we conclude from our studies that the sudden delivery of oxygen to the kidney that has undergone ischemic changes cannot be utilized by the tissues and is reduced to toxic free radicals. These, in turn, initiate lipid peroxidation and almost certainly give rise to cell damage and cell death.

REFERENCES

1. Calman KC, Quinn RO, Bel PRF. Metabolic aspects of organ storage and the prediction of viability. In: Pegg DE, ed. Organ preservation. London: Churchill Livingstone, 1973: 225.
2. Chan L, Bohr P, Ross BD. Possible new approaches to organ preservation. In: Marberger M, Dreikorn K, eds. Renal preservation. Baltimore/London: Williams and Wilkins, 1983: 323.
3. Pavlock GS, Southard JH, Starling JR, Belzer FO. Lysosomal enzyme release in hypothermically perfused dog kidneys. Cryobiology 1984; 21: 521.
4. Southard JH, Ametani MS, Lutz MF, Belzer FO. Effects of hypothermic perfusion of kidneys on tissue and mitochondrial phospholipids. Cryobiology 1984; 21: 20.
5. Green CJ. [PhD Thesis.] London University, 1976.
6. Southard JH, Lutz MF, Ametani MS, Belzer FO. Stimulation of ATP synthesis in hypothermically perfused dog kidneys by adenosine and PO_4. Cryobiology 1984; 21: 13.
7. Hearse DJ, Humphrey SM, Nayler WG, Slade A, Border D. Ultrastructural damage associated with reoxygenation of the anoxic myocardium. J Mol Cell Cardiol 1975; 7: 315.
8. Buckberg GD. A proposed "solution" to the cardioplegic controversy. J Thorac Cardiovasc Surg 1979; 77: 803.
9. Summers WK, Jamison RL. The no reflow phenomenon in renal ischemia. Lab Invest 1971; 25: 635.
10. Majno G, Ames A, Chiang J, Wright RL. No reflow after cerebral ischemia. Lancet 1967; 2: 635.
11. Willerson JT, Powell WJ, Gruiney TE, Stark JI, Saunders CA, Leaf A. Improvement in myocardial function and coronary blood flow in ischemic mycardium after mannitol. J Clin Invest 1972; 51: 2989.
12. Granger DN, Rutili G, McCord JM. Suproxide radicals in intestinal ischemia. Gastroenterology 1981; 81, 22.
13. Takenaka M, Tatsukawa Y, Dohi K, Ezaki H, Matsukawa K, Kawasaki T. Protective effects of α-tocopherol and coenzyme Q_{10} on warm ischemic damage of the rat kidney. Transplantation 1981; 32: 137.
14. McCay PB, Gibson DB, Fong KL, Hornbrook KR. Effect of glutathione peroxidase activity on lipid peroxidation in biological membranes. Biochim Biophys Acta 1976; 431: 459.
15. Pryor WA. The role of free radical reactions in biological systems. In: Pryor WA, ed. Free radicals in biology, (vol 1). New York: Academic, 1976: 1.
16. Franconi F, Manghi N, Giotti A, Martini F, Dini M. Effect of selenium on the contractile force of isolated and perfused guinea-pig heart. Acta Pharmacol Toxicol (Copenh) 1980; 46: 98.
17. Blake DR, Hall ND, Bacon PA, Dieppe PA, Halliwell B, Gutteridge JMC. Effects of a specific iron chelating agent on animal models of inflammation. Ann Rheum Dis 1983; 42: 89.
18. Asakawa T, Matsushita S. Thiobarbituric acid test for detecting lipid peroxides. Lipids 1979; 14: 401.
19. Dillard CJ, Tappel AL. Fluorescent products of lipid peroxidation of mitochondria and microsomes. Lipids 1971; 6: 715.
20. Tappel AL. In: Trump BF, Arstila AV, eds. Pathobiology of Cell Membranes. New York: Academic, 1975: 145.
21. Bidlack WR, Tappel AL. Damage to microsomal membrane by lipid peroxidation. Lipids 1973; 8: 177.
22. Lunec J, Fuller B, Green CJ. Evidence of lipid peroxidation damage in rabbit kidneys during ischemia. Cryobiology 1983; 20: 731.
23. Ross H, Marshall VC, Escott ML. 72-hr canine kidney preservation without continuous perfusion. Transplantation 1976; 21: 498.
24. Green CJ, Pegg DE. The effect of variation in electrolyte composition and osmolality of solutions for infusion and hypothermic storage of kidneys. In: Pegg DE, Jacobsen IA, eds. Organ preservation II. London: Churchill Livingstone, 1979: 86.
25. Green CJ, Pegg DE. A comparison of nonperfusion and perfusion methods for preservation of rabbit kidneys. In: Pegg DE, ed. Preservation I. London: Churchill Livingstone, 1973: 16.
26. Green CJ. Rabbit renal autografts as an organ preservation model. Lab Anim 1973; 7: 1.
27. McCord JM, Fridovich I. The reduction of cytochrome c by milk xanthine oxidase. J Biol Chem 1968; 243: 5753.
28. Lowry OH, Rosebrough NJ, Farr AL, Randall RJ. Protein measurements with the Folin phenol reagent. J Biol Chem 1951; 193: 265.
29. Hissin PJ, Hilf R. A fluorometric method for determination of oxidised and reduced glutathione in tissues. Anal Biochem 1976; 74: 214.
30. McCord JM. Oxygen-derived free radicals in postischemic tissue injury. N Engl J Med 1985; 312: 159.

Received 14 February 1985.
Accepted 16 May 1985.

0041-1337/86/4102-0166$02.00/0
TRANSPLANTATION

Vol. 41, No. 2
Printed in U.S.A.

THE ROLE OF MAJOR AND MINOR HISTOCOMPATIBILITY ANTIGENS IN ACTIVE ENHANCEMENT OF RAT KIDNEY ALLOGRAFT SURVIVAL BY BLOOD TRANSFUSION[1]

IAN V. HUTCHINSON AND PETER J. MORRIS

The Nuffield Department of Surgery, University of Oxford, John Radcliffe Hospital, Oxford OX39DU, United Kingdom

Rats given a blood transfusion do not reject a subsequent kidney allograft from the same donor strain. This effect is strain-specific so that pretransplant blood transfusion from a LEW ($RT1^l$) rat will protect a LEW kidney in a DA ($RT1^a$) recipient but not a PVG/c ($RT1^c$) kidney. The same is true in other combinations. Using DA or PVG.$RT1^a$ congenic recipients we have shown that sharing of all or part of the MHC or of minor alloantigens by the blood transfusion and kidney transplant donors is sufficient to prolong allograft survival. Activation of suppression against minor alloantigens appears to require two signals: one is the minor alloantigen and the other may be a major histocompatibility complex alloantigen.

Pretreatment of recipients with donor-specific antigen can enhance the survival of subsequent rat renal allografts. This phenomenon, known as *active enhancement*, can be produced with whole blood (*1, 2*) or leukocytes from lymph nodes (*3*), spleen (*4, 5*) and bone marrow (*6, 7*), although crude antigen preparations such as sonicates (*8*) or papain digests (*9*) can be shown to enhance in some experiments. In addition, nonleukocyte antigen preparations such as erythrocytes (*10*) and platelets (*11, 12*) of donor origin were effective in some active enhancement protocols. In most studies a clear-cut immunological specificity was seen, such that only when the donors of the antigen used for pretreatment and the kidney graft were of the same strain was enhancement observed.

The active enhancement effect may have clinical significance. It has been recognized for some time that patients who are transfused before kidney transplantation have a better graft survival rate than nontransfused recipients (*13–15*). Not only are random transfusions effective, but a single random transfusion can have a beneficial effect in 20–25% of patients (*16*). Although donor-specific transfusions are effective in living-related kidney transplantation (*17*), they are perhaps little more effective than random blood transfusions (*18*). Thus the transfusion effect in clinical practice is apparently broadly specific or nonspecific, in contrast to the results of rodent studies.

A rational immunological explanation for the transfusion effect in clinical renal transplantation has not emerged, despite general acceptance of the phenomenon in clinical practice. How can the clinical and experimental data be reconciled? One possibility is that only minimal sharing of antigens between the blood transfusions and the kidney donors is necessary to achieve a positive effect, and that the antigens shared need not be those coded by genes of the major histocompatibility complex (MHC).[2] For this reason we have examined the role of MHC and minor alloantigens in the blood transfusion effect and have demonstrated that either or both can enhance the survival of kidney allografts transplanted across MHC barriers in the rat.

MATERIALS AND METHODS

Animals. Rats of the DA ($RT1^a$), LEW ($RT1^l$), PVG/c ($RT1^c$) PVG.$RT1^l$, PVG.$RT1^a$, and PVG.$RT1^{r1}$ ($RT1^{a/c}$) inbred lines were raised in the Animal House of the John Radcliffe Hospital, Oxford. The breeding stock of the PVG lines was obtained from Olac 1976 Ltd., Bicester, Oxon. BN ($RT1^n$) strain and (LEW×BN)F_1 hybrid rats were obtained from the Animal House of the Charing Cross Hospital, London. WAG ($RT1^u$) rats were supplied by Olac. The major and minor histocompatibility antigens of these rats are summarized in Table 1.

Blood transfusions. For this procedure 1 ml of blood, heparinized at 30 U/ml, was injected i.v. into recipient rats 7 days before transplantation.

Kidney transplantation. The left kidney of recipient rats was dissected and removed, and a similarly prepared kidney from a heparinized donor was transplanted in its place using end-to-end anastomoses of the renal artery, renal vein and ureter. This operation was performed under chloral/ether anesthesia, as previously described (*19*). Warm ischemia time was less than 25 min. The recipient's remaining (right) kidney was removed 7 days after the transplantation operation. Transplants were examined during the contralateral nephrectomy, and beyond this time survival of the recipient depended on the continued function of the transplant.

RESULTS

Strain specificity of the transfusion effect. DA rats that were not previously transfused acutely rejected their allografts (Table 2, groups 1 and 6). Blood transfusion of donor-specific origin prolonged indefinitely the survival of allografts from LEW or PVG donors (Table 2, groups 2 and 7). This effect was specific because blood from third-party donors did not cause enhancement (Table 2, groups 3, 4, 5, and 8).

Haplotype specificity of the blood transfusion effect. Transfusion of LEW blood into DA rats prolonged the survival of LEW, but not BN, kidney transplants (Table 3, groups 2 and 4, respectively). However, LEW transfusion protected (LEW×BN)F_1 transplants, despite the fact that the DA recipients had not been exposed previously to BN antigens (Table 3, group 6).

The role of MHC antigens in the blood transfusion effect. The

[1] This work was supported by grants from the Medical Research Council of the U.K. and the National Kidney Research Fund.

[2] Abbreviations used: CTL, cytotoxic T lymphocytes; DTH, delayed-type hypersensitivity; MHC, major histocompatibility complex; Ts, T; suppressor cells.

TABLE 1. Major and minor antigens of the inbred rat strains used

Strain	RT1 (MHC) antigens		Background (minor) antigens
	RT1A (class I)	RT1B (class II)	
DA	a	a	DA
LEW	l	l	LEW
PVG/c	c	c	PVG
PVG.RT1[a]	a	a	PVG
PVG.RT1[l]	l	l	PVG
PVG.RT1[c]	c	c	PVG
PVG.RT1[rl]	a	c	PVG
BN	n	n	BN
WAG	u	u	WAG

TABLE 2. Strain specificity of the transfusion effect in DA recipients

Group	Blood[a]	Kidney[b]	n[c]	Survival (days)[d]	MST[e]
1	—	LEW	8	10 (×6), 11 (×2)	10
2	LEW	LEW	5	>100 (×5)	>100
3	PVG/c	LEW	4	10, 10, 10, 10	10
4	BN	LEW	5	10, 10, 10, 11, 11	10
5	WAG	LEW	5	10, 10, 10, 10, 11	10
6	—	PVG/c	5	10, 10, 10, 10, 10	10
7	PVG/c	PVG/c	9	>100 (×9)	>100
8	LEW	PVG/c	5	10, 10, 10, 10, 10	10

[a] DA rats were given 1 ml allogeneic blood i.v. 7 days before transplantation.
[b] Kidneys were transplanted from LEW or PVG/c donors into DA recipients.
[c] Number in groups.
[d] Individual survival time (days) posttransplant.
[e] Median survival time.

TABLE 3. The effect of haplotype sharing between the blood transfusion and kidney donors on renal allograft survival in DA recipients

Group	Blood[a]	Kidney[b]	n[c]	Survival (days)[d]	MST[e]
1	—	LEW	8	10 (×5), 11 (×3)	10
2	LEW	LEW	5	>100 (×5)	>100
3	—	BN	5	10 (×5)	10
4	LEW	BN	4	10 (×4)	10
5	—	(LEW×BN)F_1	5	10 (×5)	10
6	LEW	(LEW×BN)F_1	5	>100 (×5)	>100

[a] DA recipients were given 1 ml LEW blood i.v. 7 days before transplantation.
[b] Kidneys were transplanted from LEW, BN, or (LEW×BN)F_1 donors into DA recipients.
[c] Number in group.
[d] Individual survival time (days) posttransplant.
[e] Median survival time.

rats in this experiment were recombinant animals that shared the same PVG background genes. Hence the strains used differed only at the MHC or at part of the MHC. In all groups the recipients were PVG.RT1[a] rats. Kidneys differing at class I and class II loci of the MHC were acutely rejected in 10 days (Table 4, groups 1 and 3), whereas when the difference was only at the B locus (class II) the rejection process was greatly attenuated (Table 4, group 2); two rats survived indefinitely although they showed clinical signs of a rejection crisis in the 2–3-week postoperative period.

Transfusion with donor-specific blood led to prolonged survival in all three cases tested (Table 4, groups 4, 8, and 12), while third-party blood was not effective (groups 6, 9, 10, and 11). When the transfusion and the kidney donors shared only the class II RT1.B locus and other telomeric genes, enhancement was still seen (groups 5 and 7) even if the kidney donor had class I antigens that were not present in the preoperative blood transfusion (group 7).

The role of minor alloantigens in the blood transfusion effect. Rats of the DA (RTl[a]) strain were given blood transfusions and kidneys from PVG congenic and LEW rats in these experiments to test the influence of pretransplant exposure to PVG minor antigens (alone or in association with MHC antigens) on kidney allograft survival. Kidney donors were PVG congenic rats (expressing PVG minor antigens) or LEW strain rats (having LEW minor background antigens [Table 5]). LEW, PVG.RT1[l] and PVG.RT1[c] kidneys were acutely rejected by untreated DA rats (Table 5, groups 1–3).

Blood transfusions with LEW blood protects LEW kidneys, which share both MHC and minor antigens with the blood transfusion (group 4), and PVG.RT1[l] kidneys, which share MHC but not minor antigens (group 5). PVG.RT1[c] kidneys, which share neither MHC nor minor antigens with the blood transfusion, were acutely rejected (group 6). When the blood transfusion donor was of the PVG.RT1[l] strain, LEW, PVG.RT1[l], and PVG.RT1[c] kidneys were all enhanced (groups 7, 8, and 9, respectively). The three kidney donors, respectively, share MHC, MHC plus minor, or minor antigens only with the PVG.RT1[l] blood donor.

When the blood transfusion donor was of the PVG.RT1[c] strain, PVG.RT1[c] grafts (sharing MHC plus minor antigens) and PVG.RT1[l] kidneys (sharing minor antigens only) were enhanced (groups 11 and 12), while LEW kidneys were rejected (group 10—compare with group 7). Hence sharing of major or minor alloantigens was sufficient to cause enhancement.

An unexpected finding was that PVG.RT1[a] blood did not cause active enhancement of PVG.RT1[l] or PVG.RT1[c] kidneys in DA (RT1[a]) recipients (groups 14 and 15). Thus it appears that a third-party allogeneic MHC difference is required to activate suppression against minor alloantigens (compare groups 14 and 15 with groups 9 and 11).

DISCUSSION

The clinical blood transfusion effect is either very broadly crossreactive or nonspecific since a few random blood transfusions can have dramatic effects on later kidney transplant survival (*13–16*). In general, chance sharing of HLA antigens does not account for the effect. If, however, sharing of some minor antigens between donors of the blood transfusion and the kidney graft were sufficient to induce a strong transfusion effect, this would account both for the beneficial effect of preoperative transfusion in recipients given few transfusions and for the apparent lack of HLA specificity. It is this possibility we addressed with our rat experiments in which strains sharing major and/or minor alloantigens were used.

The results show that not all antigens expressed on the graft need be present in the prior transfusion. This is true for sharing of a haplotype (MHC plus minor), MHC, or minor antigens only (Tables 3, 4, and 5, respectively). Activation of suppression to one set of antigens (e.g., minor antigens) can suppress rejection responses against another set (e.g., MHC antigens) to which there has been no previous exposure. This phenomenon

TABLE 4. The role of MHC antigens in the blood transfusion effect: recipients of blood transfusions and kidney allografts were always PVG.RT1[a] rats (RT1A[a]B[a])

Group	Blood[a]	Blood MHC antigens	Kidney[b]	Graft MHC antigens	Shared MHC antigens[c]	n[d]	Survival (days)[e]	MST[f]
1	None	—	PVG/c	A^c B^c	—	5	10, 10, 10, 10, 10	10
2	None	—	PVG.RT1[r1]	A^a B^c	—	5	20, 20, 28, >50 (×2)	28
3	None	—	PVG.RT1[l]	A^l B^l	—	5	10, 10, 10, 10, 11	10
4	PVG/c	A^c B^c	PVG/c	A^c B^c	A^c B^c	5	>50 (×5)	>50
5	PVG/c	A^c B^c	PVG.RT1[r1]	A^a B^c	B^c	5	>50 (×5)	>50
6	PVG/c	A^c B^c	PVG.RT1[l]	A^l B^l	None	5	10, 10, 11, 11, 12	11
7	PVG.RT1[r1]	A^a B^c	PVG/c	A^c B^c	B^c	5	>50 (×5)	>50
8	PVG.RT1[r1]	A^a B^c	PVG.RT1[r1]	A^a B^c	B^c	4	>50 (×4)	>50
9	PVG.RT1[r1]	A^a B^c	PVG.RT1[l]	A^l B^l	None	3	10, 10, 10	10
10	PVG.RT1[l]	A^l B^l	PVG/c	A^c B^c	None	4	10, 10, 11, 12	10.5
11	PVG.RT1[l]	A^l B^l	PVG.RT1[r1]	A^a B^c	None	4	9, 20, 23, 34	21.5
12	PVG.RT1[l]	A^l B^l	PVG.RT1[l]	A^l B^l	A^l B^l	5	>50 (×5)	>50

[a] PVT.RT1[a] recipients were given 1 ml allogeneic blood i.v. one week before kidney transplantation.
[b] Kidney donors were all PVG congenic rats.
[c] RT1 class I and class II antigens shared by the blood and kidney donor strains but absent from the recipient strain.
[d] Number in group.
[e] Individual survival time (days) posttransplant.
[f] Median survival time.

TABLE 5. The role of minor alloantigens in the blood transfusion effect: recipients of blood transfusions and kidney allografts were always DA (RT1[a]) rats

Group	Blood donor[a]			Kidney donor[b]			Antigens shared[c]	n[d]	Survival (days)[e]	MST[f]
	Strain	MHC	Minor	Strain	MHC	Minor				
1	None	—	—	LEW	l	LEW	—	8	10 (×6), 11 (×2)	10
2	None	—	—	PVG.RT1[l]	l	PVG	—	5	10 (×5)	10
3	None	—	—	PVG.RT1[c]	c	PVG	—	5	10 (×5)	10
4	LEW	l	LEW	LEW	l	LEW	MHC+minor	5	>100 (×5)	>100
5	LEW	l	LEW	PVG.RT1[l]	l	PVG	MHC only	5	>100 (×5)	>100
6	LEW	l	LEW	PVG.RT1[c]	c	PVG	None	5	10 (×5)	10
7	PVG.RT1[l]	l	PVG	LEW	l	LEW	MHC only	5	>100 (×5)	>100
8	PVG.RT1[l]	l	PVG	PVG.RT1[l]	l	PVG	MHC+minor	5	>100 (×5)	>100
9	PVG.RT1[l]	l	PVG	PVG.RT1[c]	c	PVG	Minor only	5	12, >100 (×4)	>100
10	PVG.RT1[c]	c	PVG	LEW	l	LEW	None	5	10 (×5)	10
11	PVG.RT1[c]	c	PVG	PVG.RT1[l]	l	PVG	Minor only	5	29, 35, >100 (×3)	>100
12	PVG.RT1[c]	c	PVG	PVG.RT1[c]	c	PVG	MHC+minor	5	>100 (×5)	>100
13	PVG.RT1[a]	a	PVG	LEW	l	LEW	None	5	10 (×5)	10
14	PVG.RT1[a]	a	PVG	PVG.RT1[l]	l	PVG	Minor only	5	10, 10, 11, 12, 13	11
15	PVG.RT1[a]	a	PVG	PVG.RT1[c]	c	PVG	Minor only	5	7, 10, 10, 11, 11	10

[a] DA rats were given 1 ml blood i.v. from the specified donor one week before transplantation. The MHC haplotype and the minor background antigens of these rats is indicated.
[b] The kidney donor strain, along with its MHC haplotype and minor background antigens is indicated.
[c] The MHC and minor antigens shared by the blood and kidney donors, but absent from the DA recipient strain, are shown.
[d–f] See footnotes *d–f* of Table 4.

could be due to specific-reactivation by the alloantigens of the subsequent kidney graft of blood-transfusion primed suppressor cells to release nonspecific suppressor factors (*20*), to the formation of immunosuppressive complexes between antibody (elicited by the transfusion) and kidney donor alloantigens (*20, 21*) or to idiotype-specific suppressor T cells that exert their effects via "antigen bridges" between the T suppressor (Ts) receptor and the receptor of the target cell (*20*). We have clear examples of each sort of suppression in other systems (Hutchinson IV, Morris PJ, manuscript in preparation). We know that suppressor cells appear rapidly after transplantation in blood-transfused rats (Hutchinson IV, Wood KJ, and Morris PJ, unpublished data), which favors the first or the last explanation.

Activation of suppression to minor alloantigens did not occur in DA rats unless the minor alloantigens were presented with a third-party MHC allogeneic stimulus (Table 5). This strongly suggests that the process of activation requires help provided by the recognized MHC alloantigen. This two-signal model of activation of suppressor T cells is closely analogous to the activation of cytotoxic T lymphocytes (*22*). There is, however, a clear difference between Ts and cytotoxic T lymphocyte (CTL) activation in that CTL specific for minor antigens are restricted by the MHC (*23*) while, in this case, Ts are evidently not.

A recent study of suppression of delayed-type hypersensitivity (DTH) to alloantigens in mice by pretreatment with minor alloantigens suggested that minor determinants could play a dominant role in the transfusion effect (*24*). In those experiments, i.v. injection of splenocytes from animals differing at

MHC or minor histocompatibility loci induced the appearance of Ly-2^+ Ts that could regulate the DTH response to fully allogeneic cells injected into the foot-pad of sensitized mice. In the present study we have shown that both MHC and minor antigens can induce unresponsiveness to kidney allografts. The possibility that different subregions of the MHC may have different enhancing potential (*25–27*) has not been addressed here. We can conclude from our data that sharing of RT1.A (class I) antigens by the blood and kidney donors is not essential (Table 4, group 7) and that prior exposure to class II antigens (plus other MHC antigens coded to the right of RT1.B) is sufficient to enhance the survival of kidneys expressing those class II antigens (plus other MHC antigens coded to the right of RT1.B) is sufficient to enhance the survival of kidneys expressing those class II antigens (Table 4, groups 5, 7, and 8). Recombinant rat strains are available to allow proper investigation of active enhancement by RT1-subregion antigens.

The concept of strain specificity in the blood transfusion effect (Table 2) appears to conflict with the finding that sharing of some MHC or minor alloantigens can lead to suppression because different strains certainly do share some antigens. Most rat strains were derived from a limited number of stocks, particularly those of the Wistar Institute (*28*). However, the sharing of minor antigens in our experiments was for the products of all the genes of the PVG background, not just a few random and coincident shared antigens. We do not know yet which are the most important. In addition, in our strain specificity experiments, we chose rat strain combinations that, in our experience, do not crossreact in enhancement assays. There are some known crossreactions—for instance, BUF ($RT1^b$) blood enhances the survival of $(LEW \times BN)F_1$ kidneys in LEW rats because the BUF and BN strains share the public class II specificity 15 (*29*). Sharing of public class I antigens is common (*30*) and active enhancement of rat cardiac allografts can be achieved by preimmunization with class I or class II antigens alone (*10, 11, 25–27*).

In summary, then sharing of MHC and/or minor histocompatibility antigens between the donors of preoperative blood transfusions and kidney transplants can lead to a positive blood transfusion effect with prolonged survival of renal allografts in the rat. These experiments finally provide a rational explanation for observations made in clinical renal transplantation—namely, not only that donor-specific transfusions in living-related transplantation improve graft survival, but also that random blood transfusions improve both living-related graft survival and cadaveric graft survival.

REFERENCES

1. Marquet RL, Heystek GA, Tinbergen WJ. Specific inhibition of organ allograft rejection by donor blood. Transplant Proc 1971; 3: 708.
2. Fabre JW, Morris PJ. The effect of donor strain blood pretreatment on renal allograft rejection in rats. Transplantation 1972; 14: 608.
3. Enomoto K, Lucas ZJ. Immunological enhancement of renal allografts in the rat. Transplantation 1973; 15: 8.
4. Stuart FP, Saitoh T, Fitch FW. Rejection of renal allografts: specific immunologic suppression. Science 1968; 160: 1463.
5. Stuart FP, Fitch FW, Rowley DA. Specific suppression of renal allograft rejection by treatment with antigen and antibody. Transplant Proc 1970; 2: 483.
6. Ockner SA, Guttmann RD, Lindquist RR. Renal transplantation in the inbred rat. XIII. Modification of rejection by active immunization with bone marrow cells. Transplantation 1970; 9: 30.
7. Ockner SA, Guttmann RD, Lindquist RR. Renal transplantation in the inbred rat. XIV. Mechanism of the modified rejection produced by bone marrow cell pretreatment. Transplantation 1970; 9: 39.
8. Zimmerman CE. Active enhancement of renal allografts. Transplant Proc 1971; 3: 701.
9. Von Haefen U, Wren SFG, Shaipanich T, Martins ACP, Busche GJ, Wilson RE. Active enhancement of rat renal allografts with papain-released specific antigens. Transplantation 1973; 16: 295.
10. Wood KJ, Evins J, Morris PJ. Suppression of renal allograft rejection in the rat by class I antigens on purified erythrocytes. Transplantation 1985; 39: 56.
11. Hibberd AD, Scott LJ. Allogeneic platelets increase the survival of rat renal allografts. Transplantation 1983; 35: 622.
12. Wood KJ, Morris PJ. The blood tranfusion effect: suppression of renal allograft rejection in the rat using purified blood components. Transplant Proc 1985; 17: 1135.
13. Opelz G, Terasaki PI. Poor kidney transplant survival in recipients with frozen-blood transfusions or no transfusions. Lancet 1974; 2: 696.
14. Opelz G, Mickey MR, Terasaki PI. Calculations on long-term graft and patient survival in human kidney transplantation. Transplant Proc 1977; 9: 27.
15. Van Es AA, Balner H. Effect of pretransplant and transfusions on kidney allograft survival. Transplant Proc 1979; 11: 127.
16. Persijn GG, van Leeuwen A, Parleviek J, Cohen B, Landsbergen Q, d'Amaro J, van Rood JJ. Two major factors influencing kidney graft survival in Eurotransplant: HLA-DR matching and blood transfusion(s). Transplant Proc 1981; 13: 150.
17. Salvatierra O, Vincenti F, Amend W, Potter D, Iwaki Y, Opelz G, Terasaki PI, Duca R, Cochrum K, Hawes D, Stoney RJ, Feduska NJ. Deliberate donor-specific blood transfusions prior to living related renal transplantation. A new approach. Ann Surg 1980; 192: 543.
18. Opelz G. Blood transfusions and renal transplantation. In: Morris PJ, ed. Kidney transplantation: principles and practice. 2nd ed. London, New York, Orlando: Grune & Stratton, 1984: 323.
19. Hutchinson IV, Zola H, Batchelor JR. Immunological enhancement of rat renal allografts using rabbit antisera with specificity for rat transplantation antigens. Transplantation 1976; 22: 273.
20. Hutchinson IV. Specific immunosuppression. In: Morris PJ, ed. Kidney transplantation: principles and practice. 2nd ed. London, New York, Orlando: Grune & Stratton, 1984: 301.
21. Barber WH, Hutchinson IV, Morris PJ. Enhancement of rat kidney allografts using haptenated alloantigens and anti-hapten antibody. Transplantation 1983; 36: 475.
22. Bach RF, Bach M, Sondel PM. Differential function of major histocompatibility antigens in T-lymphocyte activation. Nature 1976; 259: 273.
23. Bevan MJ. Minor H antigens introduced on H-2 different stimulating cells cross-react at the cytotoxic T cell level during in vivo priming. J Immunol 1976; 117: 2233.
24. Perry L, Williams IR, Dirusso S. Suppressor T cell recognition of major and minor histocompatibility antigens: selected suppression of MHC-directed responses by minor alloantigen Ts. J Immunol 1984; 133:16.
25. Guttmann RD, Forbes RDC, Cramer DV, Gell TJ. Cardiac allograft rejection and enhancement in natural recombinant rat strains. Transplantation 1980; 30: 216.
26. Soulillou JP, Blandin F, Günter E, Lemoine V. Genetics of the blood transfusion effect of heart allografts in rats. Transplantation 1984; 38: 63.
27. Soulillou JP, Blandin F, Günter E. Sharing of RT1.B region between organ donor and blood donor is required for optimal prolongation of heart allografts by blood transfusion. Transplant Proc 1985; 17: 1914.
28. Palm J, Black G. Interrelationships of inbred rat strains with

respect to Ag-B and non-Ag-B antigens. Transplantation 1971; 11: 184.

29. Lowry RP, Carpenter CB. Public B cell alloantigen determinants (Ia) and active enhancement of renal allografts in the rat. Transplantation 1980; 30: 347.

30. Günter E, Stark O. The major histocompatibility system of the rat. In: Götze D, ed. The major histocompatibility system in man and animals. Berlin, Heidelberg, New York: Springer-Verlag, 1977: 207.

Received 29 May 1985.
Accepted 11 June 1985.

0041-1337/86/4102-0170$02.00/0
TRANSPLANTATION

Vol. 41, No. 2
Printed in U.S.A.

CYCLOSPORINE AS AN ALTERNATIVE TO CYCLOPHOSPHAMIDE IN THE TREATMENT OF CHRONIC GRAFT-VERSUS-HOST DISEASE

D. BUNJES,[1] W. HEIT, R. ARNOLD, TH. SCHMEISER, AND H. HEIMPEL

Bone Marrow Transplantation Unit, Department of Internal Medicine III, Ulm University, Ulm, Federal Republic of Germany

Four patients with progressive extensive chronic graft-versus-host disease or dose-limiting toxicity on conventional therapy (cyclophosphamide + prednisolone) were treated with a regimen of cyclosporine + prednisolone as induction therapy and cyclosporine as maintenance therapy. All 4 showed clinical improvement and 3 of 4 are alive at 9 months. The incidence of infections was not affected by this regimen, but steroid requirements were reduced.

Chronic graft-versus-host disease (GVHD)[2] is a syndrome with features of several autoimmune diseases that occurs as a late complication in approximately 30% of bone marrow transplant patients (*1*). The disease is disabling and is associated with a high mortality if left untreated (*2*). The only effective treatment regimen reported to date consists of a combination of steroids and a cytotoxic drug (cyclophosphamide or azathioprine). Though undoubtedly effective with regard to response rate and survival, this regimen is associated with serious complications. The most important is a high incidence of recurrent and frequently fatal bacterial infections that is related to the underlying disease and to the drug-induced damage to nonspecific and specific host defense mechanisms (*2, 3*). Since these patients require prolonged, intensive immunosuppressive therapy we were also concerned about the long-term consequences of steroid and cytotoxic drug therapy, such as aseptic bone necrosis, glaucoma, cataract, and secondary malignancies. In the hope of reducing the incidence of serious infections and avoiding the prolonged use of steroids we have switched 4 patients with progressive extensive chronic GVHD or dose-limiting toxicity on conventional therapy to cyclosporine as maintenance therapy.

[1] To whom correspondence should be addressed.

[2] Abbreviations used: aGVHD, acute GVHD, AUL, acute undifferentiated leukemia; GVHD; graft-versus-host disease; SGOT, serum glutamic oxaloacetic transaminase; SGPT, serum glutamic pyruvic transaminase; TMP-SMX, trimethoprim sulfamethoxazol.

MATERIALS AND METHODS

Patients. The report deals with 4 male patients aged 19–21 who received an allogeneic bone marrow graft from an HLA-identical, MLC-negative sibling donor (2 patients with acute leukemia, 2 patients with aplastic anemia).

Transplant regimen. All patients were transplanted according to the Seattle protocol (*4*). In brief, conditioning regimens consisted of cyclophosphamide (50 mg/kg on four successive days) for aplastic anemia or cyclophosphamide (60 mg/kg for 2 days) followed by 10 Gy total-body irradiation (TBI) for patients with leukemia. GVHD prophylaxis consisted of methotrexate administered during the first 100 days posttransplant following the Seattle schedule. Prednisolone was used to treat grade I and grade II acute GVHD (aGVHD) and prednisolone + ATG was used for grades III and IV aGVHD not responsive to high-dose steroids.

Diagnosis of chronic GVHD. The diagnosis of chronic GVHD was established by clinical and histopathological criteria (*1*). Skin and lip biopsies plus a Schirmer test were performed on all patients for staging purposes and liver biopsies when indicated (*1*).

Treatment regimen and follow-up. All patients were initially treated with cyclophosphamide (1–2 mg/kg) and prednisolone (1–2 mg/kg). The dosage was adjusted according to the clinical response and the WBC. When allocated to the cyclosporine protocol patients initially received 5 mg/kg/d i.v. and prednisolone 2 mg/kg/day. After a stable, effective blood level of cyclosporine had been established (500–800 mg/ml whole blood) patients were switched to oral cyclosporine (12 mg/kg/day). Cyclosporine blood levels were determined daily during the i.v. phase and weekly thereafter. The cyclosporine dose was adjusted to maintain a blood level of 300–800 mg/ml and the steroid dose was adjusted according to the clinical response. In all patients an attempt to discontinue steroids was made. Supportive therapy consisted of prophylactic trimethoprim-sulfamethoxazole (TMP-SMX, 320 mg/1600 mg/day) and protective sunblocking creams.

All patients were initially treated as inpatients. They were examined daily and a laboratory check-up was performed 2–3 times per week (complete blood count, bilirubin, serum glutamic oxaloacetic transaminase (SGOT), (SGPT) serum glutamic pyruvic transaminase, alkaline phosphatase, cholinesterase, creatinine). Once significant clinical improvement had occurred, they were followed as outpatients at regular intervals (2–4 weeks). The follow-up consisted of a physical examination and a blood chemistry profile. Radiological investigations were performed if clinically indicated. After six months of treatment skin biopsies were obtained to monitor the histological response. The overall response to treatment was assessed by determining the Karnofsky performance score.

RESULTS

Case Histories

Patient No. 1. This patient initially had acute undifferentiated leukemia (AUL) at the age of 19. He was transplanted in second complete remission in November 1982. He developed grade IV aGVHD involving the skin, the liver and the gut. This was followed by extensive chronic GVHD (skin, liver, oral mucosa). There was an initial response to cyclophosphamide and prednisolone complicated by a *Pseudomonas aeruginosa* pneumonia that necessitated reduction of imunosuppressive therapy. Dose reduction resulted in a flare-up of chronic GVHD. This cycle of reactivation of GVHD followed by massive immunosuppression resulting in another life-threatening infection repeated itself several times and the patient required continuous hospitalization for a period of 7 months. Finally, in October 1983 we substituted cyclosporine for cyclophosphamide. The skin and mucosa responded rapidly with gradually decreasing steroid requirements. At a dose of 7.5 mg/day the disease flared up and the amount had to be raised again. Four months after the initiation of therapy the patient developed acute B-hepatitis and died in acute liver failure accompanied by a terminal *Listeria monocytogenes* septicemia.

Patient No. 2. AUL was diagnosed in this man at the age of 19. He was transplanted in first remission in March 1983. He suffered grade II aGVHD of the skin that merged into chronic GVHD of the skin and oral mucosa and possibly the liver (the liver biopsy was not definitive). After initially successful treatment with the standard regimen the patient was readmitted to hospital with progressive dyspnea unresponsive to antibiotic therapy and florid chronic GVHD of the skin and mucosa in March 1984. An open lung biopsy revealed no evidence of infection but showed a lymphoplasmacellular infiltrate with interstitial fibrosis interpreted as chronic GVHD of the lung. Lung function studies revealed a primarily restrictive defect, although airway resistance was raised as well. Disease of the skin, liver, mucosa, and lung responded rapidly to treatment with cyclosporine and prednisolone. Two months after being discharged the patient developed herpes encephalitis that responded to acyclovir. The patient has now been off steroid treatment for 3 months with no evidence of disease reactivation. The liver values are still raised but improving (SGOT <50 U/L, cholinesterase and bilirubin normal, alkaline phosphatase 500-700 U/L). Lung function has returned to normal and a control biopsy of the skin revealed no disease activity.

Patient No. 3. Severe aplastic anaemia was the indication for allogeneic bone marrow transplantation in this 20-year-old man. He had grade II aGVHD (skin) that developed into chronic GVHD (skin, mucosa, liver). He was initially treated with the standard regimen but was changed to cyclosporine and prednisolone because of progressive disease of the skin and mucosa. The skin and mucosa responded rapidly and there has been some improvement in the liver values. In September 1984 the patient developed a severe herpes zoster infection with bacterial superinfection which responded to acyclovir and antibiotics. The patient is a Turkish national with a limited knowledge of German. This caused compliance problems with large fluctuations in cyclosporine blood levels and a rise in serum creatinine. This forced us to return to a regimen of cyclophosphamide and steroids at a dose of 1 mg/kg.

Patient No. 4. This 21-year-old man was first seen with severe aplastic anemia in June 1982. Bone marrow transplantation was performed in July 1982. It was complicated by grade III aGVHD (skin and liver) that developed into chronic GVHD. During treatment with the standard regimen bilateral avascular necrosis of the femoral head occurred. Steroids were discontinued and an attempt was made to control the disease with 3 mg/kg cyclophosphamide alone, which proved unsuccessful. We changed the patient to cyclosporine with rapid improvement of skin and mucosa. SGOT and SGPT improved (<50 U/L) but alkaline phosphatase levels continued to rise. A liver biopsy revealed periductular fibrosis but no inflammatory infiltrate providing a diagnosis of residual bile duct damage as a result of preceding chronic GVHD. The patient is currently recovering from orthopaedic surgery to his femoral heads. A valid assessment of the Karnofsky index is currently impossible.

DISCUSSION

The results presented in this paper suggest that cyclosporine in combination with prednisolone is effective in treating extensive chronic GVHD. All 4 patients have shown clinical improvement and 3 of 4 are alive at 9 months. The relative ease with which disease of the skin, the mucosa, and lung can be treated and the less impressive results obtained in chronic liver GVHD raise several issues (Table 1). One aspect to be considered is the question of whether the response rates reported in this study might be due to patient selection. We consider patient selection an unlikely explanation since 3 of 4 patients were classified as having the prognostically unfavourable progressive type of chronic GVHD (direct progression of acute GVHD to

TABLE 1. Clinical features and response to therapy

Patient No.	Diagnosis	Type of onset	Organs affected	Organ response to therapy		Karnofsky index
1	AUL	Progressive GVHD	Skin Liver Mucosa	Skin Liver Mucosa	Good[a] Definite[b] Good	0%
2	AUL	Progressive GVHD	Skin Liver Mucosa Lung	Skin Liver Mucosa Lung	Good Definite Good Good	80%
3	AA	Progressive GVHD	Skin Liver Mucosa	Skin Liver Mucosa	Good Definite Definite	70%
4	AA	Progressive GVHD	Skin Liver Mucosa	Skin Liver Mucosa	Good Poor[c] Good	Not evaluable

[a] Good response: no clinical and/or histological disease activity.
[b] Definite response: definite improvement in all disease parameters (a) liver: transaminases <50 U/L, alkaline phosphatase <800 U/L, normal bilirubin, normal cholinesterase; (b) lung: no active disease, evidence of residual organ damage in lung function tests; (c) mucosa: residual lichenoid lesions.
[c] Poor response: improvement in some disease parameters.

chronic GVHD) (*2*). We do not believe that the effects we have observed are the result of fluctuations in disease activity, a well-known feature of several connective tissue to autoimmune diseases, because all the data on the natural history of extensive chronic GVHD show that it takes an unremitting course (*2*). Whether pretreatment with the standard regimen may have conditioned the response is hard to judge, but it is improbable considering the clinical course described in the case histories.

We believe that the effect of cyclosporine on the clinical course of chronic GVHD can be explained by its mechanism of action. Chronic GVHD is considered to be a T-lymphocyte-mediated disease and cyclosporine is a T-cell-specific immunosuppressive drug that inhibits the release of a variety of lymphokines required for the activation and proliferation of T lymphocyte clones (*5, 6*). Steroids have a synergistic effect on lymphokine secretion, affect lymphocyte distribution in the body, and have potent antiphlogistic effects (*7*). The combination of cyclosporine and steroids in the induction phase can be expected to inactivate and prevent the clonal expansion of host-reactive T cells, and the presence of cyclosporine in the maintenance phase should inhibit the reactivation of these cells. The clinical results confirm the predictions of this hypothesis. Since, in our experience, chronic GVHD requires continuous therapy with cyclosporine we have no evidence as yet that the drug induces a state of tolerance, as has been suggested by several authors (*8, 9*).

The reasons for the incomplete response of liver GVHD to cyclosporine are unclear. We have observed a typical response pattern in our patients consisting of a marked improvement or normalization of transaminase values, an improvement in cholestatic enzymes (with the exception of patient 4) and normal values for bilirubin and cholinesterase. Table 1 but raised serum levels of alkaline phosphatase persisted; these could be due to: (A) residual bile duct damage after a prolonged period of active GVHD; (B) a persistent viral infection such as chronic non-A–non-B hepatitis; or (C) drug toxicity.

The routine use of liver biopsies in treatment evaluation may resolve this problem, but our own experience with patient 4 and results reported by others (*10, 11*) raise some doubts about the value of liver biopsy in dealing with the difficult differential diagnosis of liver dysfunction after bone marrow transplantation.

The regimen of cyclosporine and steroids has not reduced the overall incidence of infections. Our data suggest, however, that the introduction of cyclosporine may reduce the steroid requirements in these patients. Two of the three surviving patients are off steroids at present with no evidence of disease reactivation.

The side effects of cyclosporine therapy have been minor and easily reversible by dose reduction. The three most frequent ones have been an asymptomatic rise in serum creatinine, nausea, and tremor.

Overall, these results are encouraging and suggest that cyclosporine is a valuable alternative to cyclophosphamide in the therapy of chronic GVHD. Obviously a larger number of patients and a longer period of observation are required to assess the long-term results and the long-term toxicity of this regimen.

REFERENCES

1. Shulman HM, Sullivan KM, Weiden PL, et al. Chronic graft-versus-host syndrome in man. A long-term clinopathological study of 20 Seattle patients. Am J Med 1980; 69: 204.
2. Sullivan KM, Shulman HM, Storb R, et al. Chronic graft-versus-host disease in 52 patients. Adverse natural course and successful treatment with combination immunosuppression. Blood 1981; 57: 267.
3. Atkinson K, Storb R, Prentice PL. Analysis of late infections in 89 long-term survivors of bone marrow transplantation. Blood 1979; 53: 720.
4. Thomas ED, Storb R, Buckner CD, et al. Bone marrow transplantation. N Engl J Med 1975; 292: 832.
5. Bunjes D, Hardt C, Deusch K, et al. Studies on the mechanism of action of cyclosporin A in the murine and human T cell response in vitro. In: White DJG, ed. Cyclosporin A. Amsterdam, New York, Oxford: Elsevier, 1982: 261.
6. Borel JF, Feurer C, Magnee C, et al. Effects of the new anti-lymphocytic peptide cyclosporin A in animals. Immunology 1977; 32: 1017.
7. Cupps JR, Fauci AS. Corticosteroid-mediated immunoregulation in man. Immunol Rev 1982; 65: 133.
8. Hess AD, Tutschka PJ, Santos GW. Effect of cyclosporin A on human lymphocyte responses in vitro. II. Induction of specific allogantigen unresponsiveness mediated by a nylon wool adherent suppressor cell. J Immunol 1981; 126: 961.
9. Wang BS, Heacock EH, Zheng CX, et al. Evidence for the presence of suppressor T cells in animals treated with cyclosporin A. J Immunol 1982; 128: 1382.
10. Snover DC, Weisdorf S, Ramsay NK, et al. Hepatitic graft-versus-host disease: a study of the predictive value of liver biopsy in diagnosis. Hepatology 1984; 4: 123.
11. Berman MD, Rabin L, O'Donnell J, et al. The liver in long-term survivors of marrow transplant chronic graft-versus-host disease. Clin Gastroenterol 1980; 2: 53.

Received 26 February 1985.
Accepted 23 May 1985.

0041-1337/86/4102-0173$02.00/0
TRANSPLANTATION
Vol. 41, No. 2
Printed in U.S.A.

SPONTANEOUS ANTI–TUBULAR-BASEMENT-MEMBRANE ANTIBODY PRODUCTION BY LYMPHOCYTES ISOLATED FROM A REJECTED ALLOGRAFT[1]

S. C. JORDAN,[2,3] S. C. BARKLEY, J. M. LEMIRE, R. S. SAKAI, A. COHEN,[4] AND R. N. FINE

Division of Pediatric Nephrology, Department of Pediatrics, University of California, Los Angeles, School of Medicine; and Department of Pathology, Harbor-UCLA School of Medicine, Torrance, California

The immunological events mediated by, and antigen specificity of, allograft-bound lymphocytes (ABLs) are poorly understood. To further define the role of antibody-mediated rejection, a rejected allograft from a patient with primary anti-TBM disease was sterilely minced and pressed through a microscreen. The ABLs were isolated by density gradient centrifugation. Using this technique, 8.5×10⁶ ABLs were isolated. Then 1×10⁶ washed ABLs/ml were suspended in RPMI 1640 with 20% fetal calf serum and cultured in microtiter plates with media only, or with pokeweed mitogen (PWM) (100 μg/culture). The cells were incubated for 7 days and supernatants were collected and assayed for total IgG and IgM by a solid-phase enzyme immunoassay (EIA) and reactivity with normal human kidney targets by indirect immunofluorescence (IF) and immunoperoxidase (IP) techniques. Total IgG production was 500 ng/ml for both spontaneous and PWM stimulated cells. No IgM production was detected. IF and IP studies demonstrated IgG-anti-TBM antibodies in the spontaneous supernatants only. IgG antibodies reactive with peritubular capillaries (anti-PTC) were also noted. IgG-anti-TBM anti-bodies and antibodies reactive with arterioles were subsequently demonstrated by direct immunofluorescence techniques in the rejected allograft. Analysis of serum samples obtained at the time of allograft rejection showed no IF or IP reactivity with the kidney targets. Subsequent analysis of anti-TBM production by the patient's peripheral blood mononuclear cells (PBMs) showed IgM-anti-TBM only. These studies suggest that the IgG-anti-TBM and IgG-anti-PTC antibodies reactive with the allograft resulted from in situ antibody production by ABLs; the role of anti-TBM antibodies in mediating the AR is unclear, but their presence suggests recurrence of the original disease in the allograft. Anti-PTC antibodies could be important in mediation of the vascular AR.

Renal allografts lost to rejection not only feature intense cellular infiltrates of lymphocytes, plasma cells, and monocytes, but also commonly feature profound degrees of vasculitis (*1*). Traditionally, vascular rejection is thought to be mediated by circulating antibodies reactive with vascular-endothelial (V-E)[5] antigens (primarily located on the peritubular capillaries [PTC]); however, consistent demonstration of serum antibodies to V-E antigens has been difficult (*2, 3*). Recent studies (*4*) have shown that B-lymphocytes and plasma cells isolated from allografts with vascular rejection were capable of secreting immunoglobulin (Ig). Although the antigen specificity of the secreted Ig was not determined, these investigators concluded that in situ antibody production by ABLs could be an important mechanism of humorally-mediated allograft injury (*4*). Antibodies reactive with tubular basement membrane (anti-TBM) have been described in association with immune-mediated glomerular injury (*5–7*), in patients with allergic interstitial nephritis (*8*), and as a primary disease (*9*). However, anti-TBM antibody production without anti-GBM production most frequently occurs after renal transplantation (*10, 11*).

The immunopathogenic capacity of these posttransplant anti-TBM antibodies is questionable (*11, 12*). Since anti-TBM antibodies can induce severe tubulointerstitial nephritis in experimental animals, their posttransplant pathogenic capacity must, however, be considered. This report describes a 14-year-old boy with well-documented and previously described (*9*) primary anti-TBM nephritis who received a renal allograft. The allograft functioned poorly and underwent severe rejection at 4 weeks posttransplant and was excised at 8 weeks posttransplant. Allograft-bound lymphocytes (ABLs) isolated from the allograft produced IgG-anti-TBM and IgG-anti-PTC antibodies detected on a panel of 5 human kidney targets. Immunofluorescence studies of the rejected allograft showed linear staining of the tubular basement membrane without anti-GBM antibody. Indirect immunofluorescence (IF) and immunoperoxidase (IP) analysis of serum obtained at the time of allograft nephrectomy showed no significant anti-TBM or anti-PTC reactivity with the kidney targets. In situ production of IgG-anti-TBM and IgG-anti-PTC may have been responsible for the allograft dysfunction and loss in this patient.

Case Presentation. A 14-year-old boy with end-stage renal disease secondary to anti-TBM nephritis was admitted to UCLA for a second cadaver renal transplant (donor antigens: HLA-AB 30,49,52—Dr 2,5); Patient: (HLA-AB 30, 11,49,52—Dr 2,63). The complement-dependent cytotoxicity assay was

[1] This work was supported by grants from the National Institute of Arthritis, Diabetes and Digestive and Kidney Diseases (1-R01-AM-32568), and by the Peter Boxenbaum Research Fund.

[2] Dr. Jordan is the recipient of a Research Career Development Award (1-KO4-AM 01183) from the National Institute of Arthritis, Diabetes and Digestive and Kidney Diseases.

[3] Please address reprint requests to: Stanley C. Jordan, M.D., Assistant Professor of Pediatrics, UCLA Medical Center, Division of Pediatric Nephrology, Room A2-331 MDCC, Los Angeles, CA 90024.

[4] Harbor-UCLA School of Medicine

[5] Abbreviations used: ABL, allograft-bound lymphocyte; CAPD, continuous ambulatory peritoneal dialysis; EIA, enzyme immunoassay; FBS, fetal bovine serum; HRP, horseradish peroxidase; IF, immunofluorescence; Ig, immunoglobulin; IP, immunoperoxidase; PBM, peripheral blood mononuclear cell; PBS, phosphate-buffered saline; PTC, peritubular capillaries; PWM, pokeweed mitogen; TBM, tubular basement membrane; V-E, vascular-endothelial.

negative (*13*). The allograft functioned well for 4 weeks, but the subsequent posttransplant course was stormy and was complicated by several severe rejection episodes unresponsive to Solu-Medrol therapy and antithymocyte globulin. At 4 weeks posttransplant an allograft biopsy was performed, and the patient was begun on continuous ambulatory peritoneal dialysis (CAPD). At 8 weeks posttransplant an allograft nephrectomy was performed due to hypertension and severe persistent rejection. Previously, in 1979, the patient had rejected a cadaver allograft over 6 months. Review of the pathology reports from the first transplant showed a severe vascular rejection without anti-TBM antibodies. Postnephrectomy, the signs and symptoms of rejection (fever, hypertension, abdominal tenderness, and edema) abated, and the patient is currently stable on CAPD.

MATERIALS AND METHODS

Immunopathologic studies. Histopathological studies of the patient's renal biopsy (light, immunofluorescence, and electron microscopy) were carried out as previously described (*9, 14*). After approval of the UCLA Human Subjects Protection Committee and informed consents were given, blood was obtained for assays for nephritogenic (antitubular basement membrane, antiglomerular basement membrane and anti-V-E antibodies) in the patient's and control sera, and from cell free culture supernatants of the patient's allograft-bound lymphocytes (ABLs). Peripheral blood mononuclear cells (PBMs) and PBMs from controls were developed in our laboratory using modifications of previously described indirect IF and IP techniques (*9, 14, 15*).

Briefly, cryostat sections of renal cortical tissue obtained from a panel of five normal human kidneys were incubated (30 min, 25°C) with serial dilution of the patient's and control sera and culture supernatants. The slides were washed in 0.01 M phosphate-buffered saline (PBS) pH 7.4 (×3), and counterstained with fluoresceinated goat antihuman IgG and IgM (Cappell Labs, Cochranville, PA) or with horseradish peroxidase (HRP)-labeled protein A (Sigma, St. Louis, MO.) and HRP-labeled anti-IgM (Cappell Labs, Cochranville, PA). The details of the IF techniques have been previously described (*9, 14*).

Preparation for IP staining was carried out as follows. Prior to incubation of renal cortical sections with test sera or culture supernatants, endogenous peroxidase activity was blocked by preincubating the sections with 0.3% H_2O_2 in methanol (60 min, 25°C). The slides were washed in PBS and 25 μl of appropriately diluted HRP-labeled antibody or protein A was added and incubated (45 min, 25°C). After washing in PBS, 25 μl of HRP-substrate (19 ml 0.1 m acetate with 100 μl 3% H_2O_2 and 1 ml 3-amino-9 ethyl carbazole) was added and incubated (5 min, 25°C). The slides were then washed in PBS, dried, cover slipped, and examined by light microscopy.

The amount of IF and IP staining was arbitrarily scored as negative, trace, 1^+, 2^+, and 3^+ in IF and IP analysis of test sera and supernatants. ABLs were isolated from the rejected allograft using a modification of previously described methods (*4, 16*). After a 4-hr soak in RPMI 1640 (to isolate non-ABLs), renal cortical tissue from the rejected allograft was minced and disrupted by forcing 40-g portions of renal cortex (total 500 g) through a stainless steel No. 115 mesh sieve into a receiving pan containing 50 ml complete RPMI-1640. The sieved material was suspended in the RPMI and centrifuged on Ficoll-Hypaque (Histopaque, Sigma, St. Louis, MO). The isolated lymphocyte fraction contained >95% mononuclear cells.

The cells were counted and cultured as follows. PBMs were obtained from the patient and controls by centrifugation of heparinized venous blood on Ficoll-Hypaque (Histopaque, Sigma, St. Louis, MO). The isolated fraction contained more than 95% mononuclear cells. Cells were cultured in medium RPMI-1640 supplemented with penicillin (50 U/ml), streptomycin (50 μg/ml), L-glutamine (0.29 mg/ml), and 20% heat-inactivated fetal bovine serum (FBS) in microtiter plates (all from Flow Laboratories, McLean, VA) at a concentration of 1×10^6 cells/ml. Cells were cultured in media alone or with PWM (2.5 μg/ml), and incubated at 37°C in an atmosphere of 5% CO_2, 95% humidified air. Ig production by ABLs, non-ABLs, and PBMs was determined by an enzyme immunoassay (EIA) system previously developed in our laboratory (*17*). After 7 days in culture, IgG and IgM were measured from culture supernatants on flat-bottomed microtiter plates (Linbro, Flow Laboratories, McLean, VA). Samples were analyzed on an automated spectrophotometer (Flow Laboratories) with each supernatant assayed in triplicate. The values were related to a standard concentration of IgG and IgM (Calbiochem-Behring, La Jolla, CA). The results were expressed in absolute values (ng/ml). Cell viability was checked at the end of the culture period by resuspending the cell pellets in RPMI-1640 and counting the cells in the presence of trypan blue. Viability was always >95%.

RESULTS

Light microscopic examination of the rejected allograft showed a moderate-to-marked degree of interstitial edema associated with accumulation of large numbers of mononuclear cells (mostly lymphocytes and plasma cells). Many lymphocytes and monocytes were located in the peritubular capillaries and in the walls of tubules. Direct immunofluorescence studies revealed linear staining of tubular basement membranes (TBMs) with antihuman IgG (3^+), C3-(3^+), and kappa and lambda light chains (2^+). The walls of arteries stained with antihuman IgG (2^+), C3-(2^+), and kappa and lambda light chains (2^+) (Fig. 1).

Briefly, 8.5×10^6 ABLs were isolated from the rejected allograft. The results of total, anti-TBM and anti-PTC (IgM/IgG) production by 1×10^6 cells/culture ABLs, non-ABLs, and PBMs, are depicted in Table 1. Spontaneous ABL supernatants (4 wells) contained 500 ng of IgG per well, which reacted strongly with target TBMs in an interrupted linear pattern and with PTCs (V-E antigens) (Fig. 2). PWM stimulated cells produced more total IgG (1000 ng/well), but anti-TBM and anti-PTC IgG production was abrogated by mitogen stimulation. Neither PWM nor spontaneous supernatants of non-ABL cultures contained significant amounts of Ig, anti-TBM, or anti-PTC. Interestingly, the PBMs produced anti-TBM and anti-PTC, but only IgM. No IgM-anti-TBM was noted in the patient's rejected allograft. Indirect IF and IP analysis of the patient's postnephrectomy serum failed to reveal significant anti-TBM or anti-PTC activity. Studies of PBM cell culture supernatants and serum from normal controls showed no activity with the kidney targets.

DISCUSSION

The pathogenic role of anti-TBM antibodies in producing tubulointerstitial nephritis in man is well established (*5–11*).

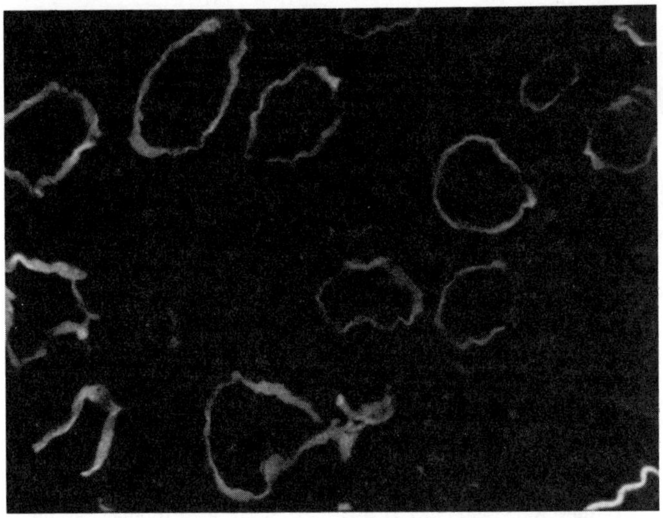

FIGURE 1. Allograft biopsy findings (Immunofluorescence Microscopy). All glomeruli (10–15/section) were completely negative. TBMs stained in a linear fashion with anti-human IgG (3^+), C3-(3^+) and kappa and lambda light chain (2^+). The walls of arterioles stained with anti-human IgG (2^+), C3-(2^+) and kappa and lambda light chains (2^+). (×250).

TABLE 1. The total anti-TBM and anti-PTC IgM and IgG produced by ABLs, non-ABLs, and PBMs

Cell type[a]	Culture conditions	Total Ig (IgM/IgG ng/well)	Anti-TBM (IF/IP) (IgM/IgG)	Anti-PTC (IF/IP) (IgM/IgG)
ABLs	Spontaneous	<50/500	Neg/3^+	Neg/3^+
ABLs	PWM-stimulated	100/1000	Neg/TR-neg	Neg/neg
Non-ABLs	Spontaneous	<50/50–100	Neg/neg	Neg/neg
Non-ABLs	PWM-stimulated	50–100/50–100	Neg/neg	Neg/neg
PBMs	Spontaneous	<50/126	3^+/Neg	1^+/Neg
PBMs	PWM-stimulated	500/900	3^+/TR	3^+/Neg

[a] Each determination represents the mean amount of Ig produced by 1×10^6 cells/well. Four wells were set up for each point.

However, the pathogenic role of posttransplant anti-TBM antibodies is questionable (*11, 12*). Since this patient's end-stage renal disease (ESRD) was secondary to anti-TBM disease (*9*), we designed a study to assess the contribution of recurrent anti-TBM disease to the allograft rejection process. Despite evidence for anti-TBM antibody in the allograft biopsy, no significant amount of circulating anti-TBM antibody was demonstrated in the patient's sera. Since infiltrating cells were successfully isolated from the rejected graft, their ability to produce specific antibody was assessed. Our data showed that ABLs secreted primarily IgG-anti-TBM and IgG-anti-PTC antibodies. The anti-TBM antibodies reacted in an interrupted linear pattern. This type of reactivity has been previously described (*18*), and it may represent denatured or immunologically inaccessable TBM antigens in certain areas of the target tissues. Mitogen stimulation of ABLs abrogated the specific antibody responses even though the total Ig production was increased. Mitogen stimulation of mature antigen-specific B cells most likely inhibits specific antibody production without affecting nonspecific Ig production by non-committed or less-mature B cells (*19, 20*). This could explain the abrogation of specific (IgG-anti-TBM and IgG-anti-PTC) antibody responses in mitogen-stimulated ABLs. The PBMs produced IgM-anti-TBM and IgM-anti-PTC but not IgG. As noted, no IgM-anti-TBM was found in the patient's allograft biopsy. It is known that antibody production by lymphocytes isolated from various lymphoid organs is extremely variable (*21*). The lack of pathogenic (IgG-anti-TBM) antibody production by PBMs suggest that the lymphoid cells from the circulation may be developmentally immature and less responsive to specific antigen (TBM or V-E than memory cells located in other lymphoid organs such as the spleen (*22*).

Allograft rejection is characterized by infiltration of cytotoxic lymphocytes and by generation of antibodies to transplant antigen (HLA and V-E antigens). Vascular rejection is often characterized by deposits of Ig in PTCs and other vascular structures similar to those in this patient (*1, 2*). This antibody-mediated vascular injury to renal allografts is thought to be mediated by circulating antibody to V-E antigens. This study suggests that alternative pathogenic mechanisms (i.e., in situ

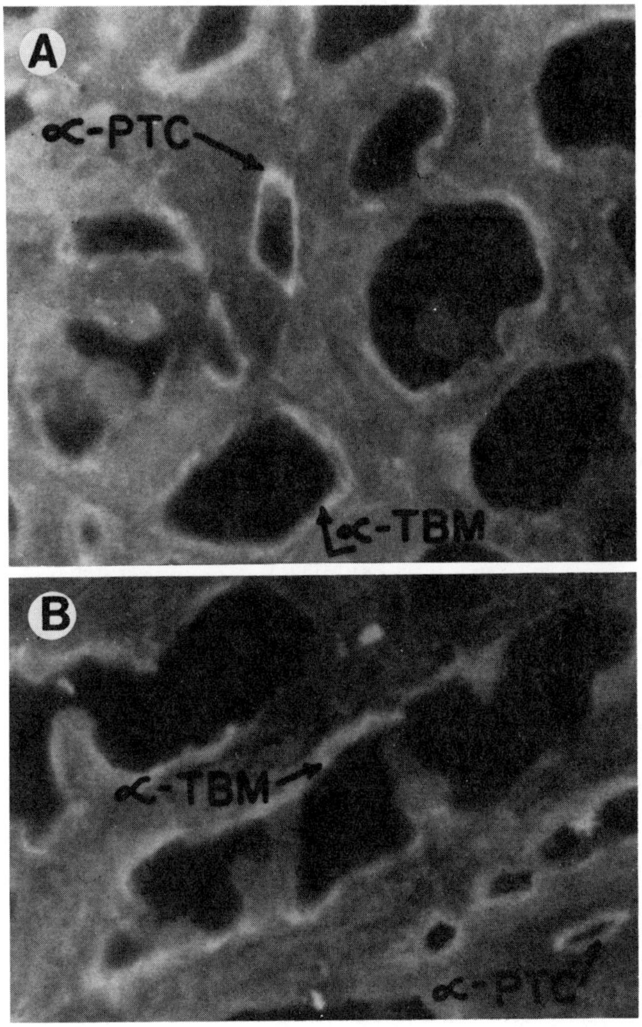

FIGURE 2. Indirect Immunofluorescence (IF) of cell culture supernatant on two normal human renal cortex targets (A and B). Supernatants of ABLs cultured in RPMI 1640 with 20% FCS (HI) showed IgG antibodies that reacted with TBMs (anti-TBM) of normal human renal cortex (5 targets). Reactivity was primarily in an interrupted linear pattern. Antibodies reactive with PTC were also noted (anti-PTC). The nephritogenic antibodies were of IgG class, were found only in the spontaneous cultures, and were only in ABLs. Analysis of serum samples obtained posttransplant revealed no significant antibody to TBM or to PTC. Analysis of samples by immunoperoxidase techniques revealed similar findings. PBMs produced IgM-anti-TBM and IgM-anti-PTC but no pathogenic IgG. (×250)

antibody production and injury) are responsible, since no circulating antibody reactive with V-E antigens could be demonstrated at the time of rejection and cell-free supernatant of PBMs did not contain the pathogenic IgG-anti-PTC antibody. However, ABLs isolated from the graft secreted significant amounts of IgG-anti-PTC while failing to secrete the IgM-anti-PTC.

This data adds a new dimension to the traditional concept of renal injury mediated by circulating nephritogenic antibody reacting with kidney-specific antigens (*18*). The renal allograft most likely expressed antigens (TBM and V-E) that acted as specific immunoabsorbents for circulating migratory memory cells (TBM-specific and V-E specific), which resulted in in situ localization, maturation, and nephritogenic antibody synthesis by these antigen-specific B cells. Experimental evidence for in situ pathogenic antibody production exists (*23*). Using a rabbit model of autoimmune thyroiditis, investigators have shown that antibody producing cells reactive with thyroglobulin first appeared in the spleens of immunized animals; however, significant thyroiditis did not appear until antibody-producing cells were isolated from the thyroid. The severity of the thyroiditis also correlated with the number of antibody producing cells isolated from the thyroid (*23*).

Our inability to demonstrate nephritogenic (IgG-anti-TBM and IgG-anti-PTC) antibody in the circulation at the time of rejection suggest in situ production and immunoabsorption of nephritogenic antibody to the allograft. If nephritogenic antibody were produced at extra-allograft sites, the absence of detectable serum levels could be explained by immunoabsorption of circulating antibody by the allograft (*23*). Another potential problem with indirect IF and IP analysis of serum and culture supernatants is the limited degree of ascertainment inherent in these methods. We have recently developed EIA methods to determine anti-TBM levels that we hope will resolve this problem. Future therapeutic protocols for treating humoral allograft rejection should take into account this study, since it suggests that the immunologic events resulting in allograft dysfunction and loss were mediated by in situ IgG-secreting ABLs and not by circulating nephritogenic antibody.

In summary, ABLs isolated from a rejected allograft in a patient with ESRD-secondary anti-TBM nephritis spontaneously produced IgG-anti-TBM and IgG-anti-PTC antibody reactive with a panel of normal human renal cortical tissues. Supernatants of non-ABLs isolated from the allograft "soak" and PBMs failed to show this reactivity. Serum samples obtained during the AR episodes failed to show significant reactivity with target kidney TBM and V-E antigens. The presence of IgG-anti-TBM probably represents recurrence of the original disease (*9*) in the allograft, while the IgG-anti-PTC most likely represents anti-V-E that can be implicated in the mediation of vascular rejection. The production of IgG-anti-TBM and IgG-anti-PTC by ABLs suggests that in situ nephritogenic antibody synthesis and deposition may be a significant pathogenic mechanism producing allograft dysfunction and loss.

Acknowledgments. We are grateful to Karen Varma and Amy Landsberg for preparing the manuscript.

REFERENCES

1. Busch GJ, Schamberg JF, Moretz RC, et al. Four patterns of human renal allograft rejection: a cytologic and in vitro analysis of the infiltrates in 24 irreversibly rejected kidneys. Transplant Proc 1977; 9: 37.
2. Paul LC, Claas FHJ, van Es LA, Kalff MW, de Graeff J. Accelerated rejection of a renal allograft associated with pre-transplant antibodies directed against donor antigens on endothelium and monocytes. N Engl J Med 1979; 300: 1258.
3. Paul LC, van Es LA, van Rood JJ, van Leeuwen A, Brutel de la Riviere G, de Graeff J. Antibodies directed against antigens on the endothelium of peritubular capillaries in patients with rejecting renal allografts. Transplantation 1979; 27: 175.
4. Garovoy MR, Reddish MA, Busch GJ, Tilney NL. Immunoglobulin secreting cells recovered from rejected human renal allografts. Transplantation 1982; 33: 109.
5. Wilson CB, Dixon FJ. Anti-glomerular basement membrane antibody induced glomerulonephritis. Kidney Int 1973; 3: 74.
6. McCluskey RT, Klassen J. Immunologically mediated glomerular, tubular and interstitial renal disease. N Engl J Med 1973; 288: 564.
7. Morel-Marogen L, Kourilsky O, Milgrom F, et al. Antitubular basement membrane antibodies in rapidly progressive post-streptococcal glomerulonephritis: report of a case. Clin Immunol Immunopathol 1974; 2: 185.
8. Border WA, Lehman DH, Egan JD, et al. Anti-tubular basement membrane antibodies in methicillin-associated interstitial nephritis. N Engl J Med 1974; 291: 381.
9. Bergstein J, Litman N. Interstitial nephritis with anti-tubular basement membrane antibody. N Engl J Med 1975; 292: 875.
10. Andres GA, McCluskey RT. Tubular and interstitial renal disease due to immunologic mechanisms. Kidney Int 1975; 7: 271.
11. Klassen J, Kano K, Milgrom F, et al. Tubular lesions produced by autoantibodies to tubular basement membrane in human renal allografts. Int Arch Allergy Immunol 1973; 45: 675.
12. Nocl LH, Rotellar C, Droz D, et al. Significances of antitubular basement membrane antibodies in renal transplant recipients [Abstract]. Los Angeles: 9th Int Congress of Nephrology, 1984; 485A.
13. Terasaki PI, McClelland JD. Microdroplet assay of human serum cytotoxins. Nature 1964; 204: 998.
14. Jordan SC, Buckingham B, Sakai R, Olson D. Studies of immune complex glomerulonephritis mediated by human thyroglobulin. N Engl J Med 1981; 304: 1212.
15. Farr AG, Nakane P. Immunohistochemistry with enzyme labelled antibodies: a brief review. J Immunol Methods 1981; 47: 129.
16. Spiro R. Studies on the renal glomerular basement membrane. J Biol Chem 1967; 242: 1915.
17. Lemire J, Adams J, Sakai R, Jordan SC. $1,25(OH)_2D_3$ suppresses proliferation and immunoglobulin production by normal human peripheral blood mononuclear cells. J Clin Invest 1984; 74: 657.
18. Wilson CB, Dixon FJ. Renal injury from immune reactions involving antigens in or of the kidney. In: Wilson CB, Brenner BM, Stein JH, eds. Immunologic mechanism of renal disease. New York: Churchill Livingstone, 1979: 35.
19. Stevens RH. Regulation of human B-lymphocyte function in secondary humoral immune responses. In Inglis JR, ed. B Lymphocytes Today. Amsterdam: Elsevier, 1982: 107.
20. Lawton AR, Lucivero G, Levitt D, Cooper M. Aspects of mitogen activation of human B-cells. In: Fauci AS, Ballieux RE. Human B-lymphocyte function, activation and immunoregulation. New York: Raven Press, 1982: 37.
21. Rynnel-Dagoo B, Kunor T, Ringden O, Moller E. Induction of antibody synthesis in human lymphocytes from different organs by different PBA substances. In: Fauci AS, Ballieux RE, eds. Antibody production in man. New York: Academic, 1979: 35.
22. Singal NH, Dosch HM. Parallel quantitation in individual microcultures of antigen-and class-specific immunoglobulins. In: Fauci AS, Ballieux RE, eds. Human B-lymphocyte function, activation and immunoregulation. New York: Raven Press, 1982: 103.
23. Clinton BA, Weigle WO. Cellular events during the induction of experimental thyroiditis in the rabbit. J Exp Med 1972; 136: 1605.

Received 26 March 1985.
Accepted 11 June 1985.

0041-1337/86/4102-0177$02.00/0
TRANSPLANTATION
Vol. 41, No. 2
Printed in U.S.A.

THE EFFECTS OF DELAYED FUNCTION ON RECIPIENTS OF CADAVER RENAL ALLOGRAFTS

A STUDY OF 158 PATIENTS RANDOMIZED TO CYCLOSPORINE OR ALG-AZATHIOPRINE[1]

DANIEL M. CANAFAX,[2] ARMANDO TORRES, DAVID S. FRYD, JOHN E. HEIL, MARILYN H. STRAND, NANCY L. ASCHER, WILLIAM D. PAYNE, DAVID E.R. SUTHERLAND, RICHARD L. SIMMONS, AND JOHN S. NAJARIAN

The Departments of Pharmacy and Surgery, University of Minnesota Hospitals, Minneapolis, Minnesota 55455

We randomized 158 recipients of cadaver renal allografts to cyclosporine-prednisone (*83*) or antilymphocyte globulin–azathioprine-prednisone (*75*) to evaluate: (1) the effects of immunosuppression and pretransplant risk factors on the incidence of delayed graft function, (2) the effects of immunosuppression on the resolution of delayed graft function, and (3) the effects of delayed graft function and pretransplanted risk factors on patient and graft survival. Cyclosporine did not increase the incidence of delayed graft function, compared with ALG-azathioprine–treated patients (33% versus 27%, *P*=0.550) but doubled the mean (±SD) duration of oliguria (11.8±11.0 versus 5.9±3.2 days, *P*=0.002) and the number of required dialyses (6.6±7.6 versus 3.2±1.3, *P*=0.031). Retransplanted patients had a higher incidence of delayed graft function that recipients of primary grafts in both the cyclosporine (82% versus 25%, *P*=0.001) and ALG-azathioprine (55% versus 22%, *P*=0.025) treatment groups. The presence of delayed function reduced one-year graft survival from 89% in all patients without delayed function to 72% (*P*=0.011) in all patients with delayed function. Cyclosporine-treated patients had a slightly, but not significantly better one-year graft survival rate than ALG-azathioprine treated patients both with (73% versus 68%, *P*=0.750) and without (92% versus 82%, *P*=0.069) delayed graft function. A preservation time longer than 24 hr did not increase the incidence of delayed graft function in cyclosporine-treated patients (34% versus 32%, *P*=0.811) or ALG-azathioprine-treated patients (27% versus 27%, *P*=0.902). Cyclosporine-treated patients given kidneys with greater than 24 hr of preservation time had reduced graft survival only when delayed graft function occurred (67% versus 92%, *P*=0.009). In conclusion, (1) cyclosporine did not increase the incidence of delayed graft function over ALG-azathioprine treatment; (2) cyclosporine did significantly slow recovery of kidneys with delayed function; (3) delayed graft function correlated with poorer graft survival rate in both treatment groups; but (4) prolonged preservation time did not increase the incidence of delayed graft function or reduce graft survival.

Cyclosporine is a potent immunosuppressive drug that selectively inhibits the T lymphocytes, possibly by preventing the cell from manufacturing, releasing, or binding interleukin-2 (*1–4*). The proved clinical efficacy of cyclosporine has lead to its wide use for organ transplant immunosuppression (*5–9*). An important limitation of transplanting cadaver renal allografts is the frequent occurrence of acute renal failure that, on histologic examination, appears to be tubular necrosis (*10*). This complication combined with cyclosporine's dose-related nephrotoxicity, raises the concern that cyclosporine increases the incidence of delayed graft function, prolongs periods of oliguria, and reduces graft survival rates (*11–13*). These concerns lead us to analyze the results of our randomized, prospective comparison of cyclosporine-prednisone versus antilymphocyte globulin–azathioprine-prednisone immunosuppression with respect to the impact of immunosuppressive therapy and delayed graft function on the clinical course, incidence of rejection, and patient and graft survival rates.

MATERIALS AND METHODS

A group of adult recipients of cadaver allografts were randomized into two groups who received either cyclosporine and prednisone (referred to as *cyclosporine*) or (b) azathioprine, antilymphocyte globulin (ALG), and prednisone (referred to as *ALG-azathioprine*) immunosuppression. The study was approved by the University of Minnesota Committee on Use of Human Subjects in Research. Reports have appeared concerning other aspects of this study (*8, 9*). Patients were prospectively stratified according to the presence or absence of diabetes mellitus, age, and number of previous transplants. All patients had their spleen removed before transplantation and were given at least five unrelated donor transfusions one or more months before transplant. Kidneys were preserved by hypothermic pulsatile perfusion or were stored in Collins' solution at 4°C. Entrance into the study ended June 8, 1984, and patients have been followed for a mean (±SD) of 28.4±13.4 months.

Four patients in the cyclosporine group and five in the azathioprine group, had immediate posttransplant technical complications or hyperacute rejection and no graft function. Of the remaining 149 patients evaluated, 79 had been randomized to cyclosporine treatment, which included 46 diabetics and 68 primary grafts. Seventy patients had been randomized to ALG-azathioprine: 42 diabetics and 59 primary grafts. The patients ranged in age from 18 to 55 years; the mean (±SD) age of cyclosporine patients was 38±8 years and that of ALG-azathioprine patients was 37±8 years.

Cyclosporine was given orally just prior to transplantation, and for one week thereafter at a dose of 14 mg/kg/day. The dose was then adjusted to 12 mg/kg/day or less based on serum creatinine concentration and trough whole-blood-cyclosporine concentration assayed by high-performance liquid chromatog-

[1] This work was supported in part by National Institutes of Health Grants AM 13083 and RR-400.

[2] To whom correspondence should be addressed.

raphy, to maintain the serum creatinine at less than 2 mg/dl and the cyclosporine concentration between 100 and 200 ng/ml. Prednisone was given initially at a dose of 2 mg/kg/day, rapidly tapered to 0.4 mg/kg/day by 30 days and to 0.2 mg/kg/day by one year posttransplant in the cyclosporine-treated patients. ALG-azathioprine–treated patients were given 5 mg/kg/day azathioprine before transplantation, and then doses were tapered to 2.5 mg/kg/day by one week posttransplant. The prednisone dose began at 2 mg/kg/day and was decreased to 0.5 mg/kg/day by 30 days and then to 0.3 mg/kg/day at one year posttransplant. ALG was given as a 30 mg/kg/day dose i.v. for 14 doses in the immediate posttransplant period. All patients were given prophylactic trimethoprim/sulfamethoxazole.

Delayed renal allograft function was defined as requiring dialysis during the first two weeks posttransplant. Oliguria was defined as posttransplant urine volumes less than 400 ml in 24 hr. Three patients in each group required dialysis but were not oliguric. Graft loss was defined by patient death, even if the graft still functioned, or by the institution of chronic dialysis. Acute rejection episodes were defined by a rise in serum creatinine concentration that subsequently decreased with supplemental prednisone administration. Almost all rejections were confirmed by histologic evidence (*14*). Cyclosporine nephrotoxicity was defined by increased creatinine concentration that subsequently decreased with lower cyclosporine doses and verified by renal biopsy evidence of cyclosporine effects, as described by Sibley et al. (*14*).

Statistical analysis employed the Student's *t* test, chi-square, and the Wilcoxon test for differences between groups of patients, as appropriate. Actuarial techniques were used to calculate patient and graft survival rates (*14a*). A generalized Wilcoxon test was used to determine *P* values over the entire period of analysis.

RESULTS

Effect of patient characteristics on posttransplant delayed graft function. Age and gender were evenly distributed in both the cyclosporine and ALG-azathioprine treatment groups and had no effect on the incidence of delayed graft function. The duration of preservation (>24 versus <24 hr) and type of preservation (machine versus Collins' solution) also did not affect the incidence of delayed graft function in the cyclosporine (P=0.729 and 0.524) or ALG-azathioprine–treated patients (P=0.590 and 0.540).

The incidence of delayed graft function was increased in retransplanted patients, when compared with recipients of primary allografts, in both the cyclosporine (82% versus 25%, P=0.001) and ALG-azathioprine–treated patients (55% versus 22%, P=0.025). Diabetics had a slightly lower incidence of delayed graft function than their nondiabetic counterparts in the cyclosporine (25% versus 42%, P=0.123) and ALG-azathioprine–treated patient groups (24% versus 32%, P=0.551), although the differences were not significant.

Effects of immunosuppression and delayed graft function on the clinical course. Cyclosporine did not increase the incidence of posttransplant delayed graft function, compared with ALG-azathioprine treatment (33% versus 27%, P=0.550) but did prolong the duration (Table 1). All grafts with delayed function eventually functioned, but cyclosporine-treated patients required twice the number of dialyses, and oliguria was present six days longer.

TABLE 1. The effects of immunosuppression and delayed graft function (ATN) on the posttransplant clinical course (N)[a]

ATN Patients	CsA	ALG-AZA	P
Incidence of delayed function:	33% (26/79)	27% (19/70)	0.550
Number of dialyses			
mean ± SD:	6.6±7.6	3.2±1.3	0.031
range:	1–39	1–6	
median:	4.5	3.0	
Days of oliguria			
mean ± SD:	11.8±11.0	5.9±3.2	0.002
range:	0–48	0–12	
median:	10.5	7.0	
Days to last dialysis			
mean ± SD:	15.7±18.4	7.7±3.0	0.026
range:	2–94	2–14	
median:	11.0	7.0	
Hospitalization (days)			
mean ± SD:	29±19	25±11	0.756
range:	9–101	13–58	
median:	21	23	

Cyclosporine-treated patients with delayed graft function tended to require slightly longer mean (±SD) posttransplant hospitalization than ALG-azathioprine–treated patients with delayed graft function (29±19 versus 25±11) but the differences were not statistically significant (P=0.756). In the absence of delayed graft function, hospitalization was reduced in the cyclosporine-treated patients compared with the ALG-azathioprine–treated patients (12±8 versus 16±4 days, P=0.001).

At the time of discharge from the hospital, the mean (±SD) serum creatinine concentrations in patients with delayed graft function were higher for cyclosporine-treated patients than ALG-azathioprine–treated patients (3.2±2.0 versus 1.9±0.8 mg/dl, P=0.001). This difference was lost over the follow-up period and the current mean (±SD) serum creatinine levels are equal in the two treatment groups (1.9±0.5 versus 1.9±1.1 mg/dl, P=0.905). Cyclosporine-treated patients without delayed graft function also had higher creatinine concentrations than ALG-azathioprine–treated patients (2.0±0.8 versus 1.4±0.5 mg/dl, P=0.001), and this difference was maintained over the follow-up period (2.0±0.6 versus 1.3±0.3 mg/dl, P=0.001).

Effect of delayed graft function and immunosuppression on patient and graft survival. The actuarial patient survival rates at three years for cyclosporine and ALG-azathioprine–treated patients were 87% versus 86%, P=0.948. The actuarial graft functional survival rates at one year for cyclosporine and ALG-azathioprine–treated patients were 82% versus 75%, P=0.301. Excluding the technical losses, the one-year graft survival rates were 87% versus 79%, P=0.262. All patients with delayed graft function had a decreased one-year graft survival compared with all patients without delayed graft function (72% versus 89%, P=0.011).

Figure 1 (A–D) shows the effects of delayed graft function on patient and graft survival rates. Cyclosporine-treated patients had a nonsignificant trend toward better graft survival than did ALG-azathioprine–treated patients, both with (73% versus 68%, P=0.749) and without (92% versus 82%, P=0.122) delayed graft function. Patient survival was not different for these same groupings, (81% versus 90%, P=0.226) and 94% versus 90%, P=0.130).

Within the cyclosporine treatment group, patient and graft

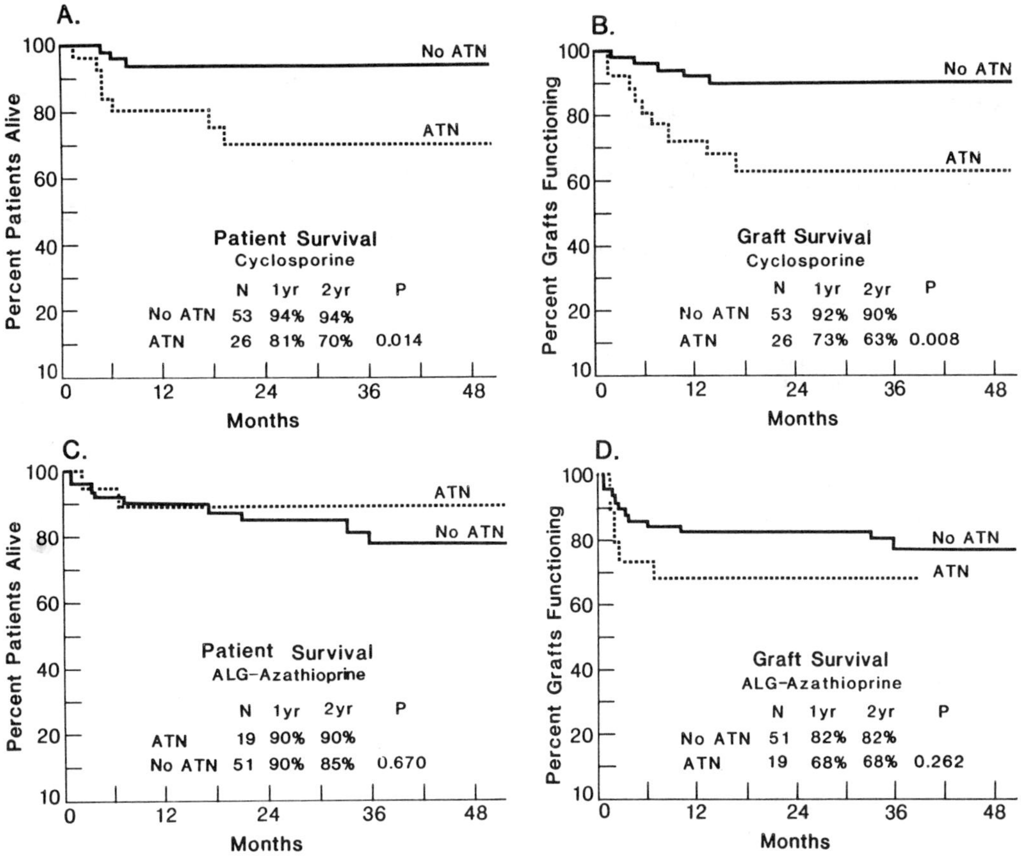

FIGURE 1. Patient (A,C) and renal allograft functional (B,D) survival rates are shown for cyclosporine-treated patients (A,B) and ALG-azathioprine-treated patients (C,D) with and without delayed graft function (ATN).

survival rates were both reduced by delayed graft function (Fig. 1 A,B) (94% versus 81%, P=0.014) and (92% versus 73%, P=0.008). Within the ALG-azathioprine treatment group patient survival was not altered (90% versus 90%, P=0.670) but delayed function tended to reduce graft survival (82% versus 68%, P=0.262) (Fig. 1 C,D).

The cyclosporine-treated diabetic patients had better graft survival than the ALG-azathioprine–treated diabetic patients (85% versus 66%, P=0.033). In the cyclosporine treatment group, diabetics with delayed graft function had reduced graft survival (Fig. 2 A). In the ALG-azathioprine treatment group, nondiabetic patients had better graft survival than diabetics (93% versus 69%, P=0.012) and delayed graft function was an important contributing factor (Fig. 2 B).

Effect of delayed graft function and immunosuppression on acute rejections. Cyclosporine-treated patients had fewer acute rejection episodes than did the ALG-azathioprine-treated patients by one-year posttransplant (32% versus 58%, P=0.001). Delayed graft function did not increase the incidence of acute rejection episodes in either immunosuppressive treatment group. The incidence of acute rejection in cyclosporine-treated patients with and without delayed graft function was 32% versus 33%, P=0.896, and in the ALG-azathioprine–treated patients it was 68% versus 53%, P=0.620.

Effect of preservation technique on posttransplant delayed graft function. The mean (±SD) duration (hours) of pretransplant kidney preservation did not differ for the cyclosporine and ALG-azathioprine treated patients with (34. 8±13.0, versus 33.6±12.1, P=0.901) or without (36.9±12.2 versus 35.8±13.2, P=0.875) delayed graft function. Kidneys preserved longer than 24 hr had similar incidence of delayed graft function in the cyclosporine (34%) and the ALG-azathioprine (27%) treatment group (P=0.803), as did those with less than 24 hr preservation time (32% versus 27%, P=0.845).

Table 2 shows the one-year graft survival as a function of preservation time. Cyclosporine-treated patients given kidneys with greater than 24 hr of preservation time had reduced graft survival when delayed function occurred (67% versus 92%, P=0.009)—thus the combination of prolonged cold ischemia and delayed graft function reduced the graft survival rate in cyclosporine-treated patients.

Cold storage in Collins' solution resulted in a slightly greater incidence of delayed graft function than machine perfusion in the cyclosporine-treated patients (40% versus 31%, P=0.524). ALG-azathioprine-treated patients had virtually identical results (36% versus 25%, P=0.540).

Figure 3 shows that machine preservation of the kidney, with subsequent delayed function, reduced graft survival when compared with patients without delayed function (P=0.023). This same trend occurred in the kidneys preserved with Collins' solution, and these patients had an overall reduction in graft survival when compared with machine preservation (73% versus 85%, P=0.152).

Patients who were oliguric for prolonged periods (9–48 days) did not have a reduced graft survival compared with patients with oliguria for 0–8 days (79% versus 65%, P=0.189).

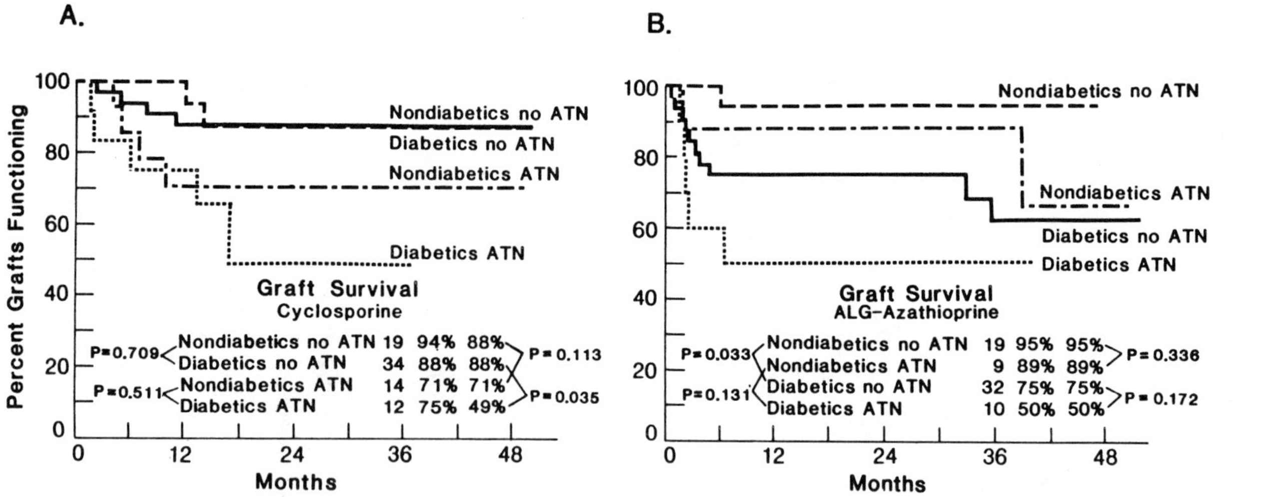

FIGURE 2. Renal allograft functional survival rates are shown for cyclosporine-treated patients (A) and ALG-azathioprine-treated patients (B) with and without diabetes and delayed graft function (ATN).

TABLE 2. The effect of cold preservation duration, type of immunosuppression, and presence of delayed graft function on one-year cadaver graft survival (N)[a]

	Preservation >24 hours			Preservation <24 hours		
	ATN % (N)	No ATN % (N)	P	ATN % (N)	No ATN % (N)	P
Cyclosporine:	67(10)	92(22)	0.009	83(12)	88(26)	0.125
ALG-Azathioprine:	70(10)	86(10)	0.197	67(9)	83(24)	0.149

	ATN Preservation			No ATN Preservation		
	>24 hrs	<24 hrs	P	>24 hrs	<24 hrs	P
Cyclosporine:	67(10)	83(12)	0.243	92(22)	88(26)	0.161
ALG-Azathioprine:	70(10)	67(9)	0.480	86(21)	83(24)	0.485

[a] Abbreviation: ATN = delayed graft function.

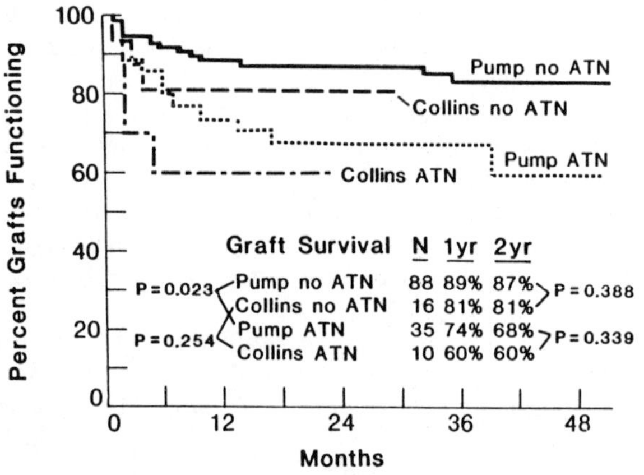

FIGURE 3. Renal allograft functional survival rates are shown for kidneys preserved pretransplant by pulsatile perfusion (pump) or cold storage in Collins' solution.

DISCUSSION

Cyclosporine is a potent immunosuppressant that prolongs renal allograft survival but has the undesirable potential of nephrotoxicity (*6–9*). Since recipients of cadaver renal allograft often have a delay in graft function (*10, 15*), the concern has arisen that cyclosporine might increase the number of kidneys with this problem, prolong the duration of delayed function, or decrease graft survival. Therefore, at some centers, cyclosporine therapy is given only to patients diuresing immediately after transplantation (*5*).

Our prospective, randomized and stratified trial has the advantage of directly comparing the incidence, severity, and long-term influence of early renal transplant malfunction using two immunosuppressive regimens with and without cyclosporine. There is the further advantage that we have found no effect on short-term or long-term graft survival with the two regimens (*8, 9*). The results are clear: the incidence of graft malfunction that required at least one episode of hemodialysis did not differ in patients given cyclosporine or ALG-azathioprine. The return of function, however, was significantly delayed in cyclosporine-treated patients, thereby making cyclosporine more costly therapy when delayed function did occur. Retransplanted patients receiving cyclosporine had a high incidence of delayed graft function, which suggests that cyclosporine should be withheld until oliguria resolves in this patient group. It is important to note, however, that no additional detrimental long-term effects of delayed graft function were found when cyclosporine was used, as compared with ALG-azathioprine. Therefore, although cyclosporine is inconvenient and expensive in the presence of delayed graft function, its long-term effects are as good as ALG-azathioprine. Unfortunately, ALG-azathioprine has the major disadvantage of an increased incidence of reversible rejection episodes and an increased incidence and severity of cytomegalovirus infection (*8, 9*).

Delayed graft function is, however, not an innocuous event. There is growing evidence that delayed graft function is associated with decreased one-year renal allograft survival (*16–19*). Our experience agrees, and we have previously reported that delayed function in some way reduces graft survival (*16*). The present randomized study confirms this finding both for cyclosporine and ALG-azathioprine–treated patients. A possible contributory factor is the difficulty in detecting acute rejection episodes during periods of oliguria, but our experience cannot clarify this issue.

We cannot find definitive evidence that cyclosporine should only be used with one or another type of preservation, or that only short-term preservation is safe. The same incidence of delayed function occurred in patients with short and long periods of preservation, confirming our previous report (16). Significantly lower graft survival rates for cyclosporine-treated patients with delayed function were found in patients who had received kidneys with prolonged preservation times, suggesting that this particular combination is detrimental to graft survival. Kidney preservation by machine perfusion, however, only slightly reduced the incidence of delayed graft function. However, machine preserved kidneys without delayed function did have the best graft survival, and Collins'-stored kidneys with delayed function the worst (P=0.001). Obviously, this will remain controversial, as it has in the past.

We have no explanation for the finding that delayed function reduced the graft survival rate in ALG-azathioprine–treated diabetic patients compared with cyclosporine-treated diabetics. This difference may have been due to fewer acute rejection episodes in the cyclosporine-treated patients and, on the surface, suggests that cyclosporine may be the preferred drug for diabetic recipients of cadaver allografts who might develop delayed function—but idiosyncratic findings even in large randomized studies frequently defy analysis.

We have previously reported that patients with delayed graft function who were converted from cyclosporine to azathioprine within the first two months posttransplant recovered renal function, but had a high risk of rejection and infections (*20*). This finding and the correlation between cyclosporine and longer periods of delayed function suggest that conversion is best considered within two to three weeks after transplantation. Our current practice is to reduce the cyclosporine dosage while adding azathioprine, and to continue with a regimen of azathioprine-cyclosporine-prednisone (*21, 22*). To avoid the problem entirely, our current cadaver graft protocol utilizes a short course of ALG with azathioprine-prednisone, then cyclosporine is added and the ALG terminated when creatinine clearance returns. This approach has decreased the duration of oliguria (*22*). With this approach we hope to avoid early nephrotoxicity while gaining the antirejection benefits of cyclosporine. Patients treated in this manner are then maintained on cyclosporine-azathioprine-prednisone indefinitely thereafter.

REFERENCES

1. Borel JF, Feurer C, Gubler H, Stahelin H. Biological effects of cyclosporine A: a new antilymphocytic agent. Agents Actions 1976; 6:468.
2. Andrus L, Lafferty KJ. Inhibition of T-cell activity by cyclosporine A. Scand J Immunol 1982; 14: 449.
3. Larsson EL. Cyclosporine A and dexamethasone suppress T-cell responses by selectively acting at distinct sites of trigering process. J Immunol 1980; 124: 2828.
4. Bunges D, Hardt C, Rollinghoff M, Wanger H. Cyclosporine A mediates immunosuppression of primary cytotoxic T-cell responses by impairing the release of Interleukin-1 and Interleukin-2. Eur J Immunol 1981; 8: 657.
5. Calne RY, White DJG, Evans DB. Cyclosporine A in cadaver transplantation. Br Med J 1981; 282: 934.
6. European Multicenter Trial. Cyclosporine A as sole immunosuppressive agent in recipients of kidney allografts from cadaver donors. Lancet 1982; 2: 57.
7. Canadian Multicentre Transplant Study Group. A randomized clinical trial of cyclosporine in cadaveric renal transplantation. N Engl J Med 1983; 309: 809.
8. Najarian JS, Strand M, Fryd DS, et al. A single institution randomized prospective trial of cyclosporine versus azathioprine-antilymphocyte globulin for immunosuppression in renal allograft recipients. Ann Surg 1985; 201: 142.
9. Sutherland DER, Fryd DS, Strand MH, et al. Results of the Minnesota randomized prospective trial of cyclosporine versus azathioprine-antilymphocyte globulin for immunosuppression in renal allograft recipients. Am J Kid Dis 1985; 5: 318.
10. Rao KV, Kjellstrand CM. Post-transplant acute renal failure: a review. Clin Exper Dial and Apleresis 1983; 7: 127.
11. Castro LA, Hillebrand G, Schneider LB, Gunther K, Gurland J. Cyclosporine in patients with oligioanuria after cadaveric kidney transplantation. Transplant Proc 1983; 15: 2699.
12. Flechner M, Payne WD, Van Buren C, Kerman R, Kahan BD. The effect of cyclosporine A on early graft function in human renal transplantation. Transplantation 1983; 36: 268.
13. Sheil AGR, Hall BM, et al. Australian trial of cyclosporine (CsA) in cadaveric donor renal transplantation. Transplant Proc 1983; 15: 2485.
14. Sibley RK, Ferguson RM, Sutherland DER, Simmons RL, Najarian JS. Morphology of cyclosporine nephrotoxicity and of acute rejection in cyclosporine-prednisone immunosuppressed renal allograft recipients. Transplant Proc 1983; 15: 2836.

14a. Merrell N, Schulman LE. Determination of prognosis in chronic disease. J Chron Dis 1955; 1: 12.

14b. Gehan E. A generalized Wilcoxon test comparing arbitrarily singly sensored samples. Biometrika 1965; 52: 203.

15. Brophy D, Najarian JS, Kjellstrand CM. Acute tubular necrosis after renal transplantation. Transplantation 1980; 29: 245.
16. Heil J, Sutherland DER, Fryd DS, Ascher NL, Simmons RL, Najarian JS. Acute tubular necrosis of cadaver renal allografts does not correlate with organ sharing or preservation time but portends a poorer prognosis for long-term graft survival. Transplant Proc 1984; 16:270.
17. Williams GM, White HJO, Hume DM. Factors influencing the long-term functional success rate of human renal allografts. Transplantation 1967; 5: 837.
18. Davison JM, Uldall PR, Ross-Taylor RM. Relation of immediate post-transplant renal function to long-term function in cadaver kidney recipients. Transplantation 1977; 23: 310.
19. McDonald JC, Vaughn W, Filo RS, et al. Cadaver donor renal transplantation by centers of the Southeastern Organ Procurement Foundation. Ann Surg 1981; 193: 1.
20. Canafax DM, Sutherland DER, Ascher NL, Simmons RL, Najarian JS. Cyclosporine nephrotoxicity in renal allograft recipients: conversion to azathioprine to improve renal function. Transplant Proc 1983; 15: 2874.
21. Canafax DM, Strand M, Ascher NL, Sutherland DER, Simmons RL, Najarian JS. Two methods of managing cyclosporine nephrotoxicity: conversion to azathioprine, prednisone, or cyclosporine, azathioprine and prednisone. Transplant Proc 1985; 17: 1176.
22. Simmons RL, Canafax DM, Strand MH, et al. Management and prevention of cyclosporine nephrotoxicity after renal transplantation: use of low doses of cyclosporine, azathioprine, and prednisone. Transplant Proc 1985; 17: (suppl 1) 266.

Received 26 October 1984.
Accepted 18 June 1985.

0041-1337/86/4102-0182$02.00/0
TRANSPLANTATION
Vol. 41, No. 2
Printed in U.S.A.

THE DECREASED INCIDENCE OF ASEPTIC NECROSIS IN RENAL TRANSPLANT RECIPIENTS—A CASE CONTROL STUDY

P. S. PARFREY,[1] D. FARGE, N. A. PARFREY, J. A. HANLEY, AND R. D. GUTTMAN

Transplant Service, Departments of Clinical Epidemiology and Pathology, Royal Victoria Hospital, McGill University, Montreal, Canada; and The Division of Nephrology, The Health Sciences Centre, St. John's, Newfoundland

Before 1971 the incidence of aseptic necrosis in renal transplant recipients was 29%, and after 1971 it was 5%. To investigate the reasons for this decreased incidence and to elucidate the causes of aseptic necrosis we studied all 26 transplant patients with aseptic necrosis and 42 controls matched for year of transplantation, age, and sex.

Development of aseptic necrosis was not related to duration of dialysis before transplant, severity of uremia at the time the patient started dialysis, adequacy of dialysis before transplantation, transplant dysfunction at the time aseptic necrosis was diagnosed, hyperparathyroidism before or after transplantation, lack of Vitamin D supplementation after transplantation, or fatty infiltration of liver. Total steroid dose 1 month after transplantation was actually lower in aseptic necrosis compared with the control group (2.47±0.3 g vs. 3.6±0.3 g SEM g) and was similar after 4 months (6.72±0.55 g vs. 7.14±0.6 g), as were total numbers of i.v. doses of methylprednisolone or hydrocortisone. However, blood urea nitrogen (BUN) during the dialysis period was significantly higher in the aseptic necrosis group. Of the aseptic necrosis group, 27% had a previous transplant compared with 5% of controls. Half the aseptic necrosis group (5/10) had parenchymal iron on liver biopsy one year after transplant compared with 15% (2/13) of those without aseptic necrosis. Patients transplanted before 1971 (with and without aseptic necrosis) received significantly more i.v. hydrocortisone and less i.v. methylprednisolone, had higher BUN levels at the time of starting dialysis, and had lower serum calcium and higher serum phosphate at transplantation compared with patients transplanted in or after 1971.

The incidence of aseptic necrosis following transplantation has decreased during the past 13 years for reasons that are unclear. Risk factors for aseptic necrosis may include previous transplantation, severe iron overload that may lead to marrow fibrosis and osteopenia, and increased protein catabolism/turnover during dialysis.

Aseptic necrosis of bone is a disabling complication of renal transplantation. We have recently reported (*1*) that the incidence of aseptic necrosis in renal transplant recipients has dramatically decreased in our population during the past decade from 29% before 1971 to 4% during or after 1971. A similar decrease in incidence has been ascribed to low-dose prednisolone (*2*) and also to vitamin D2 (*3*).

Despite numerous studies, the exact pathogenesis of aseptic necrosis remains unknown (*4–6*). Although most of the patients with aseptic necrosis unrelated to trauma or systemic disease have received steroids prior to the development of symptoms (*6–17*) many studies have failed to identify how steroids are pathogenic to the bone. Is the cumulative dose, the number of i.v. doses, or the duration of high oral steroid therapy the important risk factor? The time on dialysis before transplantation, the development of secondary hyperparathyroidism, hyperlipemia, fatty liver and fat embolization to bone, osteoporosis, abnormal blood viscosity, and coagulability have been suggested as possible risk factors (*5, 10, 16–25*). In view of these controversies we undertook a case control study in which all patients who developed aseptic necrosis of bone between 1958 and 1983 were matched with controls (who did not develop aseptic necrosis) by year of transplantation, age, and sex. We assessed the role of the following putative risk factors:

(1) Dose of steroid therapy and method of administration
(2) Duration and quality of dialysis before transplantation
(3) Secondary hyperparathyroidism
(4) Transplant dysfunction
(5) Liver disease, including iron overload, and fatty liver.

We compared patients with aseptic necrosis to the control group without aseptic necrosis, and we also compared patients transplanted before 1971 (with and without aseptic necrosis) with those transplanted in 1971 or after.

MATERIALS AND METHODS

All patients who had a functioning renal transplant for at least one year, from 1958 to 1983, from a living-related or a nonliving donor were studied. During that period, 231 renal transplant recipients had transplants that functioned for at least one year, and 216 (93%) had serial bone roentgenograms available for analysis. Aseptic necrosis was diagnosed by a history of joint pain and radiographic evidence of bone necrosis, using the criteria of Ficat et al. (*26*).

The 26 patients were matched with 2 control patients, when possible, according to year of transplantation ±2 years, age at time of transplantation ±15 years, and sex, when possible.

Two controls were available for 16 patients and 1 control for the remaining 10 patients. In the group transplanted before 1971, 18 patients developed aseptic necrosis and 26 matched controls were available. In the group transplanted in 1971 or after, 8 patients developed aseptic necrosis and 16 controls were available. In all 26 patients with aseptic necrosis and in the 42 matched controls, the following data were collected and analyzed.

(1) demographic data including age, sex, and nature of original disease that led to endstage renal failure
(2) Duration of dialysis before transplantation

[1] Address reprint requests to: P. S. Parfrey, M.D., Division of Nephrology, The Health Sciences Centre, St. John's, Newfoundland, Canada, A1B 3V6.

(3) Severity of uremia when patients started dialysis and adequacy of dialysis before transplantation, as assessed by blood urea nitrogen (BUN)[2], serum creatinine, serum uric acid, and hemoglobin values at the time patients and controls started dialysis, monthly predialysis values, (when available) during the 6 months on dialysis before transplantation, and levels on the day of transplantation
(4) The total dose of steroids received by each recipient at 1 month and 4 months after transplantation, and the cumulative dose when aseptic necrosis was diagnosed or the corresponding number of months in the matched control. The way steroids were administered was assessed by recording the total number of i.v. doses of methylprednisolone or hydrocortisone given to each recipient, as well as the number of days of oral prednisone >40 mg/day and the number of days of oral prednisone >100 mg/day.
(5) Nutritional status was evaluated by recording BUN, serum albumin, and blood glucose, when patients started dialysis, at the time of transplantation, and at the time aseptic necrosis was diagnosed (or 1 year after transplant in the control group—this being the assessment that we predicted before the study began would be closest to the time of diagnosis in these cases).
(6) Coexistence of secondary hyperparathyroidism was assessed by reviewing hand and skull roentgenograms obtained at one year after transplantation. Also serum calcium, phosphorus, and alkaline phosphatase was obtained at the time patients started dialysis, on the day of transplantation, and at time aseptic necrosis was diagnosed (or 1 year after transplant in the control group).
(7) Liver function was evaluated by serum glutamic oxaloacetic transaminase (SGOT) values when aseptic necrosis was diagnosed, or at one year posttransplantation for the controls. Liver biopsies performed one year after transplant were available from other prospective studies (*27, 28*). Ten biopsies in the group who developed aseptic necrosis and 13 in the control group were reviewed by a pathologist who was blind to the clinical state. Each biopsy was classified according to histological diagnosis (no hepatitis, acute reactive hepatitis, ground glass appearance of hepatitis B, chronic persistent hepatitis, chronic active hepatitis, or cirrhosis). The presence or absence of parenchymal iron deposits or fatty infiltration was also determined.

Immunosuppression. From 1971 onward a formal immunosuppressive protocol was introduced. This regimen consisted of high-dose prednisone immediately following transplantation but tapering quickly to 50 mg/day at 3 weeks, 30 mg/day at 9 weeks, 20 mg/day at 6 months, finally to a maintenance dose of 15 mg/day at 1 year (*29*). In addition 4 infusions of 750 mg of methylprednisolone were usually given in the first 14 days. Azathioprine 2 mg/kg/day was also prescribed. Patients who developed evidence of acute rejection during the follow-up were usually treated with i.v. methylprednisolone (750 mg) ±400 mg cyclophosphamide. Before 1971, prednisone therapy was less formalized. However, prednisone 40–60 mg/day was given for the first 6 weeks and acute rejection was usually treated by increasing oral prednisone for 4–7 days, sometimes up to 200 mg/day (*30*). Hydrocortisone i.v. was sometimes prescribed for rejection in doses varying from 100 to 200 mg/day.

[2] Abbreviations used: BUN, blood urea nitrogen; SGOT, Serum glutamic oxaloacetic transaminase.

Statistics. Comparisons were performed between all aseptic necrosis patients (n=26) and their controls (n= 42) using unpaired t tests for quantitative data, and chi-square tests for nonquantitative data. Also patients transplanted before 1971 (with and without aseptic necrosis) (n=44) were compared with those transplanted in or after 1971 (n=24), because new formalized immunosuppressive schedules were introduced in 1971. Results are presented as mean ± SE and $P< .05$ is considered significant.

RESULTS

Incidence of aseptic necrosis. Of 216 patients, 26 developed aseptic necrosis, having received a renal transplant between 1958 to 1983. Before 1971, 18 of 59 patients (29%) developed aseptic necrosis, compared with 8 of 157 (5%) patients who were transplanted in 1971 or after (X2 = 23.8, $P< .001$). Aseptic necrosis was diagnosed after a mean follow-up of 19.3±3.7 months.

Evolution of aseptic necrosis. Hip joints were affected in all but 1 patient. Number of affected joints varied from 1 to 7. Seven of the 26 patients (27%) had more than 2 joints involved, 12 (46%) patients had 2 joints involved, and 7 (27%) had 1 joint involved. An orthopedic operation was performed in 8 patients. Fifteen patients had symptomatic disease not requiring an operation, and 3 patients had spontaneous resolution of the observed radiological lesions.

Comparison of Patients Who Did and Did Not Develop Aseptic Necrosis

Demographic details concerning cases and controls are available in Table 1. The diseases that led to end-stage renal failure were not different in both groups of patients. The majority of cases and controls had glomerulonephritis (Table 1).

Duration and adequacy of dialysis. Duration of dialysis before transplantation was not significantly different in both groups (Table 1). There was no significant difference in serum creatinine values, uric acid, albumin, or hemoglobin between patients and controls when they started dialysis, before transplantation, or at the time of transplantation (Table 2). However, during the dialysis period the predialysis BUN levels were generally higher in the aseptic necrosis group. The mean predialysis

TABLE 1. Demographic data and original disease in patients with aseptic necrosis (n=26) and controls (n=42)

	Aseptic necrosis	No aseptic necrosis
Mean age (years ± SEM)	29±2	31±2
Number of male patients	19 (73%)	30 (71%)
Original disease:		
Glomerulonephritis	14 (54%)	24 (57%)
Chronic pyelonephritis/obstruction	4 (15%)	7 (17%)
Polycystic kidney disease	2 (8%)	8 (19%)
Other disorders	6 (21%)	3 (7%)
Time on dialysis before transplant (months ± SEM)	16.9±4.2	11.2±1.9
Months posttransplant when aseptic necrosis was diagnosed	19.3±3.7	70.6±7.6[a]

[a] Duration of follow-up after transplant in patients in the control group, who did not develop aseptic necrosis.

TABLE 2. Degree of uremia, nutritional status, and calcium/phosphorus status at the time dialysis began, at the time of transplant, and at the time aseptic necrosis was diagnosed in patients with (n=26) and without (n=42) aseptic necrosis

	When dialysis began		At transplantation		Diagnosis	
	Aseptic necrosis	Control	Aseptic necrosis	Control	Aseptic necrosis	Control
Serum creatinine (mg/dl)	16.6±1.0	15.6±0.6	13.5±0.8	12.8±0.5	2.8±0.8	2.0±0.2
Blood urea nitrogen (mg/dl)	121±9	107±6	98±10	83±5	28±2	32±6
Serum uric acid (mg/dl)	10.9±1.0	9.3±0.6	8.4±0.6	8.3±0.5	7.1±0.4	7.4±0.3
Hemoglobin (g/L)	84±5	77±3	84±5	83±3	120±6	127±4
Platelets (10^6/ml)	289±23	292±18	237±27	268±20	214±26	270±16
Serum albumin (g/dl)	3.3±0.3	3.3±0.2	3.4±0.2	3.4±0.1	3.7±0.2	3.9±0.2
Blood glucose (mg/dl)	119±10	114±5	141±9	149±9	115±7	105±5
Serum calcium (mg/dl)	8.2±1.6	8.1±1.6	8.5±0.3	8.5±0.2	9.5±0.1	9.4±0.1
Serum phosphorus (mg/dl)	8.2±1.1	8.5±3.3	6.7±0.9	8.9±1.8	3.2±0.2	3.6±0.2
Serum alkaline phosphatase (u/L)	24±6	40±8[a]	16±3	24±5	32±10	21±3

[a] Significant difference between aseptic necrosis group and control group.

BUN during the dialysis period in the aseptic necrosis group was 110±10 compared with 86±4 in the control group (P<.05), whereas the mean predialysis serum creatinine was 14.5±0.9 compared with 13.9±0.6 mg/dl (P-ns).

Hyperparathyroidism. No significant differences were observed for serum calcium, phosphorus, or alkaline phosphatase at the time of transplantation, or at the time aseptic necrosis was diagnosed. In fact serum alkaline phosphatase was higher in the control group at the time dialysis was started. No patient who developed aseptic necrosis had hyperparathyroidism on hand roentgenograms at the time aseptic necrosis was diagnosed, compared with 9% of the control group who had hyperparathyroidism on roentgenogram 1 year after transplant.

Steroid therapy. Table 3 summarizes the cumulative doses of steroids received by cases and controls, and the way they were administered. The total dose of steroids administered, whether by oral or i.v. routes, at 1 and 4 months after transplant and at the time aseptic necrosis was diagnosed was not higher in patients who developed aseptic necrosis. In fact the control group received significantly more steroids than the aseptic necrosis group in the first month after transplantation. The mean dose of steroids at the time aseptic necrosis was diagnosed was 16.9±0.6 g. In the control group the mean cumulative dose up to the last follow-up was 39.1±3.9 g. The mean number of i.v. methylprednisolone or hydrocortisone boluses received by patients with aseptic necrosis was less than or equal to the mean number received by the control group. Patients with aseptic necrosis received oral steroid doses >40 mg/day for 44.9 days ±7.7, but this was not significantly different from the control group, nor was the duration of therapy with >100 mg oral prednisone significantly different comparing both groups.

Seven (27%) patients with aseptic necrosis and 2 (5%) controls without aseptic necrosis had been transplanted previously. However, even when this was taken into account no significant differences in steroid doses were observed. The number of days of treatment with >100 mg/day oral prednisone now increased to 20.2±6.5 in the group with aseptic necrosis compared with 12.2±1.5 in the control group (P-ns) and the number of days of treatment with >40 mg/day oral prednisone was 50.3±8.8 compared with 38.9±4.2 (P-ns).

Hepatic disease. SGOT were usually normal in both groups of patients (26±3 U/L vs 33±7 U/l). Liver biopsies were available in 10 (42%) patients who developed aseptic necrosis and in 13 (31%) controls. No histological diagnosis was predominant in either group. Of the 10 patients with aseptic necrosis, 4 had marked parenchymal liver iron and 1 had mild parenchymal liver iron on a biopsy performed one year after transplant, compared with none and two (2/13) of the controls, respectively. Mild fatty infiltration was found in 3 of the 10 patients with aseptic necrosis and in 62% (8/13) of the controls.

TABLE 3. Cumulative dosages and way of administration of steroid therapy in patients with (n=26) and without (n=42) aseptic necrosis

Steroids administered	Aseptic necrosis (mean + SEM)	Control group (mean + SEM)	*P*
Total dose in first month posttransplant (g)	2.47±0.3	3.60±0.31	<.02
Total dose in first 4 months posttransplant (g)	6.72±0.55	7.14±0.60	NS
Number of i.v. doses of methylprednisolone	1.7±0.6	2.9±0.6	NS
Number of i.v. doses of hydrocortisone	2.5±0.8	2.5±0.4	NS
Number of days of oral prednisone >40 mg/day	44.9±7.7	37.3±3.8	NS
Number of days of oral prednisone >100 mg/day	18.3±6.3	11.9±1.5	NS

Comparison of Patients Transplanted Before and After 1971

Adequacy of dialysis: (Table 4) Serum creatinine values were similar at the time of starting dialysis, during the dialysis period, and at transplantation in patients transplanted before 1971 (whether or not they had aseptic necrosis) (n=44), compared with those treated in or after 1971 (n=24). However, BUN was significantly higher in the pre-1971 group at the time dialysis was first undertaken, although not subsequently. At the time of transplantation serum calcium was significantly lower in the pre-1971 group and serum phosphate was signifi-

TABLE 4. Steroid dosage, adequacy of dialysis, and calcium/phosphorus status in patients transplanted before 1971 (with and without aseptic necrosis) (n=44) compared with those transplanted in or after 1971 (n=24)

	Transplanted before 1971 (mean + SEM)	Transplanted in or after 1971 (mean + SEM)	P
Serum creatinine at time dialysis began (mg/dl)	16.2±0.8	15.5±0.9	NS
BUN at time dialysis began (mg/dl)	121.0±0.7	100.0±0.7	<.05
Mean predialysis serum creatinine (mg/dl)	14.6±0.6	13.2±0.7	NS
Mean predialysis BUN (mg/dl)	100.0±0.6	88.0±0.6	NS
Duration of dialysis (months)	14.8±2.9	11.0±2.2	NS
At transplant:			
Serum creatinine (mg/dl)	13.0±0.6	13.1±0.7	NS
BUN (mg/dl)	88.0±0.7	88.0±0.6	NS
Serum calcium (mg/dl)	8.2±0.3	8.9±0.2	<.05
Serum phosphorus (mg/dl)	8.2±0.7	5.6±0.5	<.02
Serum alkaline phosphatase (u/L)	22.1±5.8	18.7±2.2	NS
Serum albumin (g/L)	32.3±1.3	35.9±1.4	NS
Hemoglobin (g/L)	89.0±0.3	77.0±0.4	<.02
Steroid Dosage:			
Total dose in first month posttransplant (g)	2.02±0.16	4.46±0.33	<.001
Total dose in first 4 months posttransplant (g)	5.27±0.35	9.13±0.65	<.001
Number of i.v. doses of methylprednisolone	0.19±0.1	5.8±0.8	<.001
Number of i.v. doses of hydrocortisone	3.3±0.5	1.3±0.6	<.02
Number of days of oral prednisone >40 mg/day	39.8±4.7	41.7±6.1	NS
Number of days of oral prednisone >100 mg/day	11.3±2.0	19.3±5.1	NS

cantly higher. However, serum alkaline phosphatase levels were similar.

Prednisone schedules: Patients transplanted before 1971, compared with the patients transplanted in 1971 or thereafter, received i.v. methylprednisolone significantly less often and i.v. hydrocortisone more often (Table 2). Cumulative steroid doses were higher after 1970, but no significant differences were shown in the duration of high oral prednisone intake.

DISCUSSION

Corticosteroids probably play a central role in aseptic necrosis of bone in transplant recipients, but how they exert this effect is uncertain. Conflicting reports have been published of correlations between the total dose of prednisone administered and the development of aseptic necrosis, positive correlations being found by some investigators (*11, 14, 16*) but not by others (*5, 22*). In one study the incidence of avascular necrosis decreased when the total dose of prednisone was reduced during the first three weeks of transplantation (*13, 14*), an observation also made in a recent trial of low-vs.-high dose oral prednisolone (*2*). However, our results show that the development of aseptic necrosis after transplantation is not related to the maximal or cumulative dose of corticosteroid administered, or to the dosage received at one or four months after transplant. A similar observation was made in the initial report concerning aseptic necrosis from the Royal Victoria Hospital (*8*). Moreover, the reduced incidence observed in our center since 1971 corresponded with an increased absolute dose of steroids (*1*).

It is possible that the cumulative doses in the short term or the long term are not important risk factors for aseptic necrosis, but the way steroids are administered may be more important. Prolonged treatment with prednisone above 40 mg/day may be more damaging than intermittent infusions of 750 mg methylprednisolone. However, when we compared the dosage protocols in patients treated before 1971 (who had a high incidence of aseptic necrosis) with those treated in 1971 or later (who had a low incidence) there was no difference in the number of days of treatment with high oral doses. The difference was in the increased use of i.v. hydrocortisone before 1971 and the increased use of i.v. methylprednisolone after 1970. However when we compared the cases with aseptic necrosis with the control patients we could find no significant differences between the two groups in the number of boluses of hydrocortisone or methylprednisolone, or in the number of days treated with >100 mg/day or >40 mg/day oral prednisone. Therefore it appears that neither high cumulative doses of steroids nor the method of administration of steroids are related to the decreased incidence of aseptic necrosis observed during the past 13 years.

One hypothesis for the pathogenesis of aseptic necrosis is that increased bony resorption due to prior or continuing secondary hyperparathyroidism, combined with steroid induced osteoporosis and inhibition of new bone formation by steroid therapy and osteoporosis, could lead to trabecular collapse—which, in addition to weight bearing, could produce bony necrosis (*25, 31*). Chronic renal failure and time on hemodialysis before transplant could also modify the bone status of future transplant recipients. In the current study calcium/phosphorus status at the time of transplantation was significantly different comparing with pre-1971 group to the group transplanted later on. However, our results demonstrate that the development of aseptic necrosis was not related to the duration of dialysis before transplantation, or to transplant dysfunction after the graft, or to the presence of hyperparathyroidism one year after transplantation. There were no differences in serum calcium, phosphorus, or alkaline phosphatase between cases and controls at the time they started dialysis, at the time of transplantation, or at the time of diagnosis of aseptic necrosis—suggesting that secondary hyperparathyroidism before transplantation was not an important risk factor for aseptic necrosis. This latter result confirms the observation made in the initial report from the royal Victoria Hospital (*1*) and other reports (*5, 32*). It has recently been suggested that Vitamin D2 supplements may have been responsible for the decreased incidence of aseptic necrosis observed during the last decade (*3*). However our patients did not receive Vitamin D, and a similar decrease in the incidence nonetheless occurred.

Previous transplantation may be a risk factor for aseptic necrosis (*5*). In the current study 27% of aseptic necrosis patients had had a previous transplant compared with 5% of control patients. We were unable to implicate excess steroids as the explanation for this observation. However, it is possible that failed transplantation has an adverse catabolic effect on the skeletal structure, predisposing the bone to aseptic necrosis on retransplantation.

During the period in which aseptic necrosis decreased in incidence, the management of end-stage renal failure has improved in many respects. In addition to the use of vitamin D to prevent hyperparathyroidism, nutrition has improved and dialysis techniques have been modified. We attempted to document this suggested improvement in management by comparing patients transplanted before 1971 with those treated in or after 1971. Significant differences between these two groups were observed: higher BUN in the pre-1971 group at time they started dialysis, with lower hemoglobin, lower serum calcium, and higher serum phosphate at time of transplantation. However, when we tried to discover whether adequacy of dialysis and nutritional status, as reflected by biochemical tests, were worse in the group with aseptic necrosis compared with the control group, no significant differences were observed, except in mean predialysis BUN. The observation of similar pretransplantation serum creatinine, uric acid, and hemoglobin levels in aseptic necrosis patients and in controls suggests that adequacy of dialysis was comparable in both groups. However, the raised predialysis BUN levels observed during the dialysis period in the aseptic necrosis group may indicate that excess catabolism/protein turnover was occurring, which may have had an adverse effect on the skeletal structure. Other explanations are possible—such as increased dietary intake of protein, increased protein breakdown in the gut, or increased exercise producing increased protein turnover. This third suggestion may have pathogenetic relevance, because patients habituated to exercise may start exercise soon after transplantation. This may produce a disequilibrium between articular weight-bearing and the decreased mechanical resistance of the bone and muscle apparatus, leading to aseptic necrosis. This disequilibrium may be exacerbated by steroid-induced posttransplant weight gain, proximal muscle atrophy, and osteopenia (*31*).

Another hypothesis is that corticosteroid-induced hyperlipemia and fatty infiltration of the liver predispose to nontraumatic embolization from the fatty liver, with subchondral arteriolar fat embolization and occlusion, which subsequently leads to ischemic necrosis (*8, 9, 11, 15, 19, 31*). Analysis of liver biopsies in this study does not support this hypothesis. Fatty infiltration was very mild and occurred more frequently in the controls than in those who developed aseptic necrosis. In another study no significant differences were found in the amount or location of fat in the femoral heads of those with aseptic necrosis and other patients (*4*). Serum lipid abnormalities in renal transplant recipients who developed avascular necrosis have not been confirmed in some recent studies (*5, 32*).

An interesting observation in the liver biopsies available to us was that heavy, parenchymal liver iron was present in 40% of the patients with aseptic necrosis, and in none of the controls. This observation is in keeping with a report of aseptic necrosis in Bantu iron overload (*33*). It is conceivable that severe iron overload can lead to marrow fibrosis and osteopenia making the femoral head more vulnerable to the development of aseptic necrosis.

The key event that initiates the subchondral fracture in aseptic necrosis is the local weakness produced by the resorption of the peripheral portion of the lateral aspect of the subchondral plate and the overlying cartilage, that occurs during the repair process (*4*). Normally bone is being constantly remodeled throughout life, but in transplant patients corticosteroids may depress bone turnover and may prevent the bone from responding to abnormal loads (*32*). The local weakness that initiates the fracture may be exacerbated by the catabolic effects of previous transplantation, by increased protein turnover/catabolism during dialysis, and by the fibrotic effects of iron overload.

Although our detailed case control study has identified important differences between aseptic necrosis patients and their controls—higher predialysis BUN levels during the dialysis period, higher occurrence of iron overload, and higher number of patients with previous transplants—we were unable to demonstrate that high cumulative dosages of steroids in the short term or the long term, the way steroids were prescribed, duration of dialysis before transplantation, adequacy of dialysis, hyperparathyroidism before or after transplantation, lack of Vitamin D supplementation after transplant, transplant dysfunction, or fatty infiltration of the liver contributed to the development of aseptic necrosis.

REFERENCES

1. Farge D, Parfrey PS, St. André C, et al. Aseptic necrosis following renal transplantation: a 25 year experience. Transplant Proc 1985; 17: 1947.
2. Morris PJ, Chan L, French ME, Ting A. Low dose oral prednisolone in renal transplantation. Lancet 1982; 1: 525.7.
3. Scholz D, Mebel M, Topelmann I, et al. Prevention of osteonecrosis following renal transplantation by using vitamin D_2 (ergocalciferol) Proc Eur Dial Transplant Assoc 1983; 20: 331.
4. Glimcher MJ, Kenzora JE. The biology of osteonecrosis of the human femoral head and its clinical implications. III. Discussion of the etiology and genesis of the pathological sequelae: comments on treatment. Clin Orthop 1979; 140: 273.
5. Ibels LS, Alfrey AC, Muffer WE, Weil R. Aseptic necrosis of bone following renal transplantation. Experience in 194 transplant recipients and review of the literature. Medicine 1978; 57: 25.
6. Nixon JE. Early diagnosis and treatment of steroid induced avascular necrosis of bone. Br Med J 1984; 288: 741.
7. D'Aubigne RM. Idiopathic necrosis of the femoral head in adults. Ann R Coll Surg Engl 1964; 34: 143.
8. Cruess RL, Blennerhassett J, MacDonald FR, et al. Aseptic necrosis following renal transplantation. J Bone Joint Surg 1968; 50A: 1577.
9. Fisher DE, Bickel WH, Holley KE. Histological demonstration of fat emboli in aseptic necrosis associated with hypercortisonism. Mayo Clin Proc 1969; 44: 252.
10. Boettcher WG, Bonfiglio M, Hamilton H, et al. Non traumatic necrosis of the femoral head. I. Relation of altered hemostatis to etiology. J Bone Joint Surg 1970; 52A: 312.
11. Fisher DE, Bickel WH. Corticosteroid-induced avascular necrosis. A clinical study of 77 patients. J Bone Joint Surg 1971; 53A: 859.
12. Solomon L. Drug induced arthropathy and necrosis of the femoral head. J Bone Joint Surg 1973; 55B: 246.
13. Harrington KD, Murray WR, Kountz SL, Belzer FO. Avascular necrosis of bone after renal transplantation. J Bone Joint Surg 1971; 53A: 203.

14. Murray WR. Hip problems associated with organ transplants. Clin Orthop 1973; 90: 57.
15. Bewick M, Stewart PH, Rudge C, et al. Avascular necrosis of bone in patients undergoing renal allotransplantation. Clin Nephrol 1976; 5: 66.
16. Hawking KM, Van Den Bosch BF, Wilmink JM. Avascular necrosis of bone after renal transplantation. N Engl J Med 1976; 294: 397.
17. Fisher DE, Bickel WH, Holley KE, Ellefson RD. Corticosteroid induced avascular necrosis. II Experimental study. Clin Orthop 1972; 84: 200.
18. Jaffe WL, Epstein M, Heyman N, Mankin HJ. The effect of cortisone on femoral and humeral heads in rabbit. An Experimental Study. Clin Orthop 1972; 82: 221.
19. Jones JP, Engleman EP, Steinbach HL, et al. Fat embolization as a possible mechanism producing avascular necrosis. Arthritis Rheum 1965; 8: 449.
20. Jones JP, Engleman EP. Fat embolization complicating hypercortisonism. Arthritis Rheum 1965; 8: 448.
21. Fisher DE. The role of fat embolism in the etiology of corticosteroid induced avascular necrosis. Clinical and experimental results. Clin Orthop Rel Res 1978; 130: 68.
22. Pierides AM, Simpson W, Stainsby D, et al. Avascular necrosis of bone following renal transplantation. Q J Med 1975; 44: 459.
23. Kenzora JE, Steele RE, Yosipovitch ZH. Glimcher MJ. Experimental osteonecrosis of the femoral head in adult rabbits. Clin Orthop 1978; 130: 8.
24. Briggs WA, Hamper CL, Merrill JP, et al. Aseptic necrosis in the femur after renal transplantation. Ann Surg 1972; 195: 282.
25. Chatterjee SN, Massry SG, Friedler R, et al. The high incidence of persistent secondary hyperparathyroidism after renal transplantation. Surg Gynecol Obstet 1976; 143: 440.
26. Ficat P, Arlet J, Picci A, Fournial JC. Resultats therapeutiques du forage biopsie dans les osteonecroses femoro capitales primitive (100 cas). Rev Rheum Mal Osteoartic 1971; 38: 369.
27. Parfrey PS, Forbes RDC, Hutchinson TA, et al. The clinical and pathological course of hepatitis B liver disease in renal transplant recipients. Transplantation 1984; 37: 461.
28. Parfrey PS, Forbes RDC, Hutchinson TA, et al. The prevalence and progression of liver disease in renal transplant recipients: a histological study. Transplant Proc 1984; 16: 1103.
29. Lowry RP, Guttmann RD. Diagnosis and treatment of rejection. In: Levine, DZ, ed. Care of renal patient. Philadelphia: Saunders, 1983: 371.
30. Dossetor JB, Gault MH, Nephron failure: conservation, substitution, replacement. Springfield: CC Thomas, 1971; 371.
31. Slatapolsky E, Martin K. Glucocorticoids and renal transplant osteonecrosis. Adv Exp Med Biol 1984; 171: 353.
32. Feletti C, Di Felice A, Scolaxi MP, Bonomini V. Glucocorticoids and avascular bone necrosis in renal transplantation. Adv Exp Med Biol 1984; 171: 361.
33. Bothwell TH, Charlton RW. In: Schiff L. Diseases of the liver, 4th ed. Philadelphia: Lippincott, 1975; 990.

Received 17 April 1985.
Accepted 18 June 1985.

0041-1337/86/4102-0187$02.00/0
TRANSPLANTATION

Vol. 41, No. 2
Printed in U.S.A.

PROTEIN KINASE ACTIVATION AND THE IMMUNOSUPPRESSANT CYCLOSPORINE[1]

ROSANNE K. FIDELUS[2,3] AND ARLINE H. LAUGHTER[4]

Nuclear Hematology Research Laboratory, Veterans Administration Medical Center, Albany, New York 12208; and Immunohematology Research Laboratory, Veterans Administration Medical Center, Houston, Texas 77030

Cyclosporine (CsA), a potent immunosuppressant for the prevention of transplant rejection, modulates T lymphocyte activation by blocking antigen stimulation and the production of interleukin-2. The mode of action by which CsA generates this immunosuppressive effect is unknown. We have studied two early intracellular enzymes associated with mitogen activation. They include calcium/phospholipid-dependent protein kinase (C-kinase) and cAMP-dependent protein kinase (cAMPd PK). Changes in protein kinase activation were correlated with the immunosuppression of polyamine and DNA synthesis measured by ornithine decarboxylase (ODC) induction and 3_H-thymidine incorporation, respectively. These studies utilized murine T cell tumor lines sensitive to the effects of CsA.

Similar to the mitogen activation of human peripheral blood lymphocytes, CsA was capable of inhibiting the induction of ODC and ^{3}H-thymidine uptake of T cell tumor lines cultured with either fresh serum or mitogen. In contrast, C-kinase and cAMPd PK activation stimulated by the addition of fresh serum was not affected by CsA. Further, CsA did not inhibit the direct activation of C-kinase with phorbol esters or the activation of cAMPd PK with exogenous cAMP.

[1] This work was supported by U.S. PHS Grant AI 21995 and by the Veterans Administration.
[2] V.A. Medical Center, Albany.
[3] Address correspondence to: Rosanne K. Fidelus, Ph.D., Medical Research Service (151D), VA Medical Center, 113 Holland Avenue, Albany, New York 12208.
[4] V.A. Medical Center, Houston.
[5] Abbreviations used: cAMPd PK, cyclic-AMP-dependent protein kinase; C-kinase, calcium/phospholipid-dependent protein kinase; CsA, cyclosporine; ^{3}HTdr, ^{3}H-thymidine; IL-2, interleukin-2; IBMX, isobutyl-1-methyl-xanthine; ODC, ornithine decarboxylase; PMA, 4B-phorbol 12B-myristic 13α-acetate; PMSF, phenylmethylsulfonyl fluoride; SW49 k$^-$, kinase negative; SW49 wt, SW49 wild type.

We conculde that CsA does not affect the activation of either C-kinase or cAMPd PK in T cell tumor lines when activated by either fresh serum or when stimulated with chemical agents. The suppression of ODC induction and ^{3}H-thymidine incorporation associated with CsA treatment cannot be accounted for with changes in C-kinase and cAMPd PK activation.

The immunosuppressive agent CsA has made important contributions to our understanding of the immune system. CsA was first used clinically for the prevention of oxygen rejection in transplantation, following initial studies demonstrating that CsA blocked the mixed lymphocyte reaction and mitogen-induced T cell activation (*1, 2*). Recent studies have tried to identify the mode of action by which CsA blocks T cell, but not B cell, activation. These data have demonstrated that CsA inhibits antigen and mitogen responses of primed and unprimed T lymphocytes (*3, 4*); it does not block the activation of primed T cells stimulated with interleukin-2 (IL-2) (*4, 5*). There has been some evidence for a CsA receptor on T lymphocytes (*6*), while Palacios (*7*) has suggested that CsA may act by blocking the receptors for HLA-Dr. Although the actual events responsible for CsA's immunosuppressive activity continues to elude us, evidence does implicate very early responses in antigen-triggered T cell activation (*8*).

In hopes of determining the initial event responsibility for CsA's immunosuppressive ability, we began evaluating a series of intracellular events associated with lymphocyte activation. It was well established that CsA similarly blocks DNA synthesis in both mitogen-activated and peripheral blood lymphocytes (*1–4*). Similarly, the proliferation of T cell tumor lines is inhibited by CsA at concentrations comparable to those at which immunosuppression of mitogen activation of normal peripheral blood lymphocytes occurs (*6, 9*). We examined an enzymatic event preceding but associated with DNA synthesis—namely, polyamine synthesis using T lymphoblastic cell lines. We have previously reported that CsA blocks the induction of ornithine decarboxylase (*4*), the initial enzyme in the polyamine cascade, which is triggered by mitogen and antigen in human peripheral blood lymphocytes. We currently extend these observations by examining enzymatic events that precede and may be responsible for the induction of ODC. The data demonstrate that CsA does not affect the activation of two protein kinases, cAMP-dependent and calcium-phospholipid dependent protein kinase.

MATERIALS AND METHODS

Cells. EL4 is a thymic leukemia cell line of murine origin. The proliferation of these cells is blocked by CsA (*9*). They also respond to phorbol ester stimulation (*10*). SW49 wild-type (SW49 wt) and SW49 kinase-negative (SW49 k^-) are murine T cell lines, one of which contains cAMP-dependent protein kinase (SW49 wt), and one of which is cloned for its deficiency in cAMP-dependent protein kinase (SW49 k^-) (*11*). These cells were kindly provided by Dr. Phil Coffino, (University of California, San Francisco). Cells were cultured in RPMI-1640 containing 10% fetal calf serum, 25 mM Hepes (Gibco, Grand Island, NY) with 100 units/ml penicillin and 100 μg/ml streptomycin. Synchronization of these cell lines into a nondividing state was achieved by 24 hr of serum deprivation. The addition of serum-containing media stimulated DNA replication after a 6–8 hr lag.

Reagents. CsA (Sandoz, Basel, Switzerland) was dissolved in ethanol at a concentration of 40 mg/ml and diluted in media to the proper concentration in culture. Control concentrations of ethanol in media were used to assess its effect on lymphocytes. 4B-phorbol 12B-myristic 13α-acetate (PMA) (Sigma Chemical Co., St. Louis, MO) was dissolved in ethanol (1 mg/ml) and diluted with media to the appropriate concentration.

Calcium/phospholipid-dependent protein kinase (C-kinase). This enzyme was measured according to the methods of Kraft et al. (*12*). EL4 cells (2.0×10^6) were incubated in the presence or absence of PMA (20 ng/ml) for 2 hr in 5% CO_2 at 37°C. Cells were then harvested and sonicated in 0.1 ml of homogenizing buffer that contained 20 mM Tris (pH 7.5), 0.33 M sucrose, 2 mM EDTA, 015 mM EGTA, and 2 mM phenylmethylsulfonyl fluoride (PMSF). The sonicated mixture was spun at 15,000 rpm in an Eppendorf microfuge, and 0.01 ml of the supernate was incubated with 0.05 ml of the assay mixture and 0.01 ml of phospholipids (20 μg phosphotidylserine and 10 μg diolein) or 0.01 ml of homogenizing buffer. The assay mixture contained 800 μg/ml histone F_2b (Sigma Chemical Co.), 20 mM Tris pH 7.5, 5 mM $CaCl_2$, 75 mM Mg acetate, 10 μg/ml leupeptin and 5 μm ^{32}P-ATP (Amersham, Arlington Hts., IL). After incubation for 3 min at 30°C, 0.05 ml is spotted onto a 3MM Whatman filter and washed for 60 min in 10% trichloroacetic acid. The filter paper is then dried and counted in a liquid scintillation counter.

Ornithine decarboxylase (ODC). Induction of ODC was measured as previously described (*13*). Cells were suspended at 2.0×10^6/ml in 1 ml of RPMI-1640 in 16-mm cells (Cluster[24], Costar, Cambridge, MA). After incubation for 2 hr at 37°C in a 5% CO_2 atmosphere, cells were harvested and centrifuged for 2 min at 15,000 rpm in an Eppendorf microfuge. Cell pellets were sonicated in 50 mM Na_2HPO_4 (pH 7.2) containing 0.1 mM EDTA, 2.0 mM dithiothreitol, 5 mM NaF, 2 mM PMSF, and 60 μM pyridoxal phosphate. After centrifugation for 5 min at 15,000 rpm at 4°C, aliquots (0.18 ml) of supernate were incubated with 0.2 ml of L-(1-^{14}C)-ornithine (40–60 mCi/mmol) for 60 min at 37°C. Released $^{14}CO_2$ was collected on filter paper to which 0.02 ml of 2N NaOH was added. The reaction was terminated with 1M citric acid and the filter paper counted by standard liquid scintillation spectroscopy.

cAMP-dependent protein kinase (cAMPd PK). This enzyme was measured according to the methods of Klimpel et al. (*14*) and Haddox et al. (*15*) with some modification. cAMPd PK was determined by measuring the amount of ^{32}P-labeled histone that resulted from incubation of the sonicated lymphocyte preparation with ^{32}P-ATP and F_2b histone in the presence or absence of cAMP. The cAMPd PK activity is expressed as a ratio of total phosphorylating activity (+cAMP/−cAMP) in the lymphocyte preparation.

Cells were incubated with appropriate concentrations of stimulating agents at a density of 2×10^6 cells/ml in 16-mm wells. Following a 2-hr incubation (unless otherwise indicated) at 37°C in 5% CO_2, cells were scraped, pelleted, and sonicated in 100 μl of the homogenizing buffer. The homogenizing buffer contained 10 mM potassium phosphate buffer (pH 6.5), 2 mM EDTA, 0.05 mM isobutyl-1-methyl-xanthine (IBMX), 5 mM NaF, and 100 mM KCl. Following sonication, cells were spun at 15,000 rpm for 5 min. A 10-μl aliquot of the resulting supernate was then mixed with 50 μl of the reaction mixture that contained 20 mM potassium phosphate (ph 6.5), 6 mM Mg acetate, 0.5 mM IBMX, 5 mM NaF, 2.5 mg/ml F_2b histone, and 0.5 μCi of ^{32}P-ATP (10 Ci/mmole, Amersham, Arlington Heights, IL). The resulting reaction was carried out in the presence of cAMP (10^{-4}M) or an equal volume of homogenizing buffer in a final volume of 70 μl. After a 10-min incubation at 30°C, 50 μl was spotted onto 3MM filter paper and washed for 1 hr in 10% trichloroacetic acid. After drying, the filter paper was counted by liquid scintillation.

DNA synthesis. ^{3}H-thymidine (^{3}HTdr) (New England Nuclear) incorporation as a marker of DNA synthesis, was determined by incubating 1×10^5 cells in RMPI-1640 containing 10% fetal calf serum cultured in 96 well plates (Costar, microtiter plates, Cambridge, MA) for 24 hr with a 6-hr terminal pulse with 1 μCi of ^{3}HTdr. Cells were harvested and counted by standard liquid scintillation.

RESULTS

We have previously reported that T cell tumor lines, both human and murine, have sensitivities to the immunosuppressive action of CsA similar to those of helper T lymphocytes (*9*). Since many of the T cell tumor lines also respond to mitogens and product growth factors identical to stimulated helper T cells and are easily available in a larger number, the EL4 and SW49 cell lines were utilized in these studies. The EL4 cell line was used for its responsiveness to phorbol ester stimulation (*10*) and sensitivity to CsA (*9*) and SW49 for the availability of cAMPd PK deficient clone (SW49k$^-$) and the normal counterpart, SW49 wt.

To verify that CsA does inhibit the proliferation of these murine T cell lines similar to helper T lymphocytes, we examined the induction of ODC and the ^{3}HTdr incorporation as a response in cellular replication. Enzyme activation and DNA synthesis were determined in the presence and absence of various concentrations of CsA. In the representative experiment depicted in Figure 1, the effect of CsA on the induction of ODC and on ^{3}HTdr uptake was examined in the EL4 cell line. ODC activity was determined after 2 h of incubation in fresh media, while ^{3}HTdr uptake was determined after 24 hr of

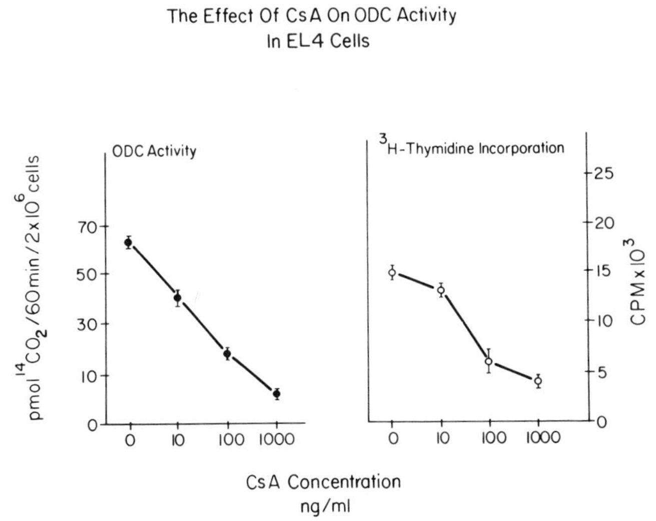

FIGURE 1. The effect of CsA on ODC activity in EL4 cells. ODC activity was determined after 2 hr of incubation and calculated as pmol $^{14}CO_2$ released/60 min/2×10 cell. ^{3}H-thymidine incorporation was determined after 24 hr of incubation and a 6-hr terminal pulse using 2×10^5 cells. The results are expressed as the mean ± SD in 3 experiments.

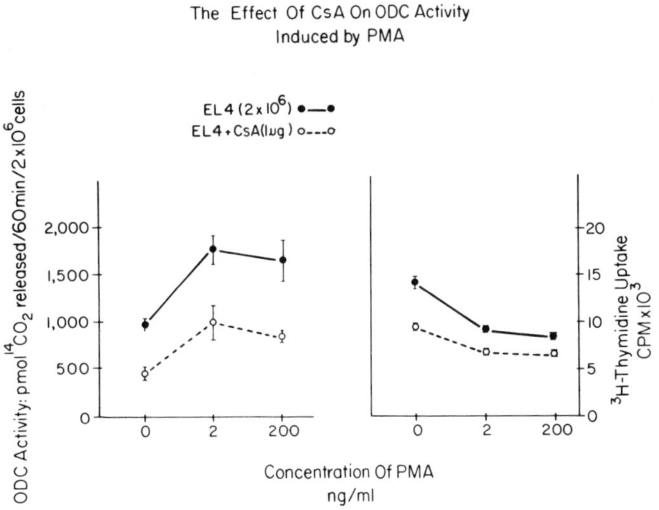

FIGURE 2. The effect of CsA on ODC activity and ^{3}H-thymidine uptake in PMA-stimulated EL4. ODC activity was determined after 2 hr of incubation and expressed as pmol of $^{14}CO_2$ released/60 min/2×10^6 cells. ^{3}H-thymidine incorporation was determined after 24 hr of incubation with a 6-hr terminal pulse using 2×10^5 cells. The results are expressed as the mean ± SD of 3 experiments.

culture. Although the level of ODC activity in EL4 cells was highly variable, a consistant dose-dependent inhibition in ODC activity and in ^{3}HTdr incorporation was noted that was maximal at 1 μg/ml. This level of sensitivity is comparable to that seen in helper T lymphocytes responding to mitogen stimulation (*5*).

Since EL4 cells are responsive to phorbol esters and the PMA receptor has been identified as C-kinase (*16–18*), we next tested the activation of EL4 cells by PMA as measured by the induction of ODC, ^{3}H-thymidine uptake, and as an activation of the C-kinase enzyme. These studies were performed in the absence and presence of CsA (1 μg/ml). Figure 2 is a representative experiment demonstrating the activation of ODC by various concentrations of PMA. The stimulation of ODC activity in PMA-treated EL4 cells was consistently suppressed by CsA, although enhanced activity over control levels in the absence of PMA was noted. In contrast to the increase in ODC activity, PMA suppresses ^{3}HTdr incorporation. The decrease in DNA synthesis with PMA stimulation has been reported by previous investigators (*10*, *18*), and has been associated with the ability of PMA to retard cells in late G_1—as opposed to the S—phase in which DNA synthesis occurs. CsA further suppresses the ^{3}HTdr uptake in both PMA-treated and nontreated cells.

We had established that CsA would partially suppress the level of ODC activity achieved with PMA stimulation, so we examined an earlier event associated with PMA-initiated lymphocyte activation, the activation of calcium/phospholipid dependent protein kinase. C-kinase is normally present in the cytosol—but, when activated, it leaves the cytosol and binds to the inner membrane of the cell through diacylglycerol (*16*, *17*). Therefore, changes in the level of enzyme activity are detected by increases or decreases in the cytosolic level of C-kinase activity. PNA can directly activate C-kinase by substituting the diacylglycerol causing a decrease in cytosolic enzyme activity. In Table 1, the levels of C-kinase activity were determined in the cytosol of PMA and/or CsA-treated EL4 cells. We could

TABLE 1. The effect of cyclosporine on C-kinase activity[a] in PMA-stimulated EL4 cells[b]

	Protein kinase activity		Ratio of activity[d]
	Without phospholipids[c]	With phospholipids[c]	
	cpm×10^3	cpm×10^3	
EL4 (2×10^6) cells	7.0±.45	8.7±.11	0.80
+CsA (1 μg/ml)	7.4±.31	9.0±.01	0.83
+PMA (20 ng/ml)	7.2±.38	7.0±.31	1.03
+PMA CsA	6.5±.20	6.8±.25	0.97

[a] C-Kinase activity was assayed in the presence of 5 mM $CaCl_2$ and phospholipids (20 μg phosphotydlserine and 10 μg diolein) and is the amount of acid-precipitable ^{32}P that has reacted with F_2b histone under standard conditions (see the *Materials and Methods* section).

[b] Mean ± SD of 4 independent experiments.

[c] This is the protein kinase activity determined in the absence and presence of phospholipids.

[d] The protein kinase activity ratio (−phopholipids/+phospholipids) is a measure of the activated fraction of the total CA^{++}-dependent protein activity.

not detect any statistically significant difference in the level of C-kinase activity between unactivated and CsA-treated EL4 cells. PMA did activate the enzyme, causing a loss in cytosolic enzyme level (+ phospholipids enzyme activity). CsA, however, could not block the PMA activation of C-kinase. These enzyme levels were determined after 2 hr of incubation with mitogen and/or CsA. The data suggest that, although CsA causes a slight suppression in the induction of ODC by PMA, it does not appreciably affect an event occurring earlier in the generation of lymphocyte activation, namely C-kinase activation.

To further examine the effect of CsA on C-kinase activation, we next examined cytosolic enzyme activity in synchronized EL4 cells cultured in the presence and absence of CsA. Cells were synchronized by serum-deprivation, as described in the *Materials and Methods* section, and were tested for C-kinase activity at various times over an 18-hr period following the addition of serum-containing media or serum-containing media plus CsA (1 μg/ml). The results are depicted in Figure 3. Time zero is enzyme activity in the absence of serum for 24 hr. There was no significant differences in the levels of enzyme activity determined in the presence or absence of CsA. Further, the level of enzyme activity showed little change with the addition of serum to the media suggesting that C-kinase may play an insignificant role in replication of EL4 cells.

We had determined that CsA could partially suppress the induction of ODC by PMA, but had no effect on the activation of C-kinase in the EL4 T cell tumor line. We therefore questioned whether CsA would affect other protein kinases associated with the induction of ODC and lymphocyte activation. It has been shown that cAMPd PK activity increases in mitogen-triggered lymphocyte activation and this activity is associated with increased ODC activity in lymphocytes (*14*), so we examined the activation of cAMPd PK in murine T cell lines—one of which contains the enzyme (SW49 wt) and one of which is a clone deficient in cAMPd PK (SW49 k^-).

To test whether the immunosuppressive effects of CsA are directed at cAMPd PK activation, we cultured the SW49 cell lines with various concentrations of CsA and determined the level of ODC activity and ^3H-thymidine uptake after 2 and 24 hr, respectively. The results are shown in Figure 4. Although the levels of ODC activity differ between the cell lines, CsA suppressed enzyme activity in SW49 wt and SW49 k^-, but only at the level of 1 μg/ml. A slight enhancement in ODC activity was seen at lower drug concentrations. ^3H-thymidine uptake was similarly depressed with higher doses of CsA. Of importance is that both cell lines responded comparably to the effects of CsA despite the absence of cAMPd PK in SW49 k^- cells. These data suggest that the immunosuppressive effects of CsA in the SW49 T cell lines is not manifested through the inhibition of cAMPd PK.

To further exemplify this fact, Figure 5 demonstrates the effect of CsA on cAMPd PK-activity in synchronized EL4 cells. CsA did not alter enzyme activity following the addition of serum-containing media to the cells.

Finally, we tested whether CsA could affect the activation of cAMPd PK by cAMP. Table 2 describes the level of cAMPd

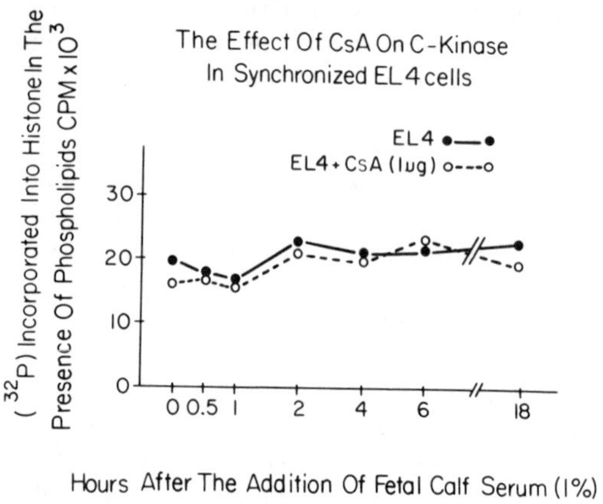

FIGURE 3. The effect of CsA on C-kinase activity in synchronized EL4 cells. C-kinase activity is expressed as cpm×10^3 of ^{32}P incorporated into F_2b histone in the presence of phospholipids. C-kinase activity was determined in EL4 cells (2×10^6) at various times following the addition of serum or serum plus CsA (1 μg/ml). These are results of a representative experiment. Similar results were obtained on 4 occasions.

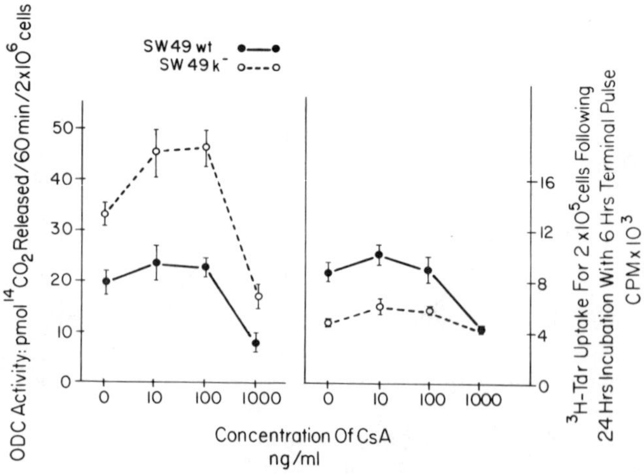

FIGURE 4. The effect of CsA on the ODC activity and ^3H-thymidine uptake in 2 SW49 cell lines. ODC activity was determined after 2 hr of incubation and calculated as pmol of $^{14}CO_2$ released/60 min/2×10^6 cells. ^3H-thymidine incorporation was determined after 24 hr incubation and a 6-hour terminal pulse using 2×10^5 cells. The results expressed are the mean ± SD of 4 experiments.

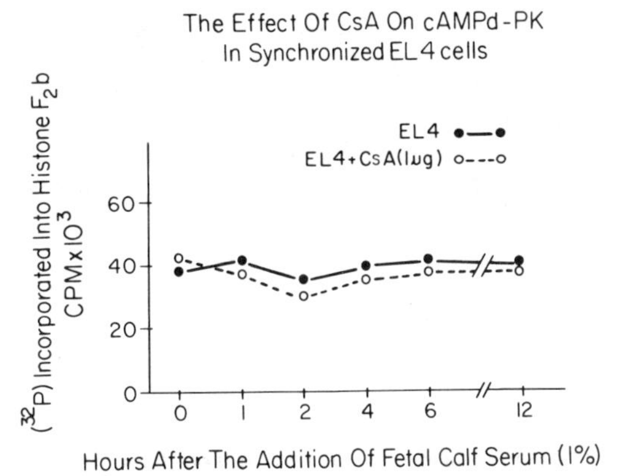

FIGURE 5. The effect of CsA on cAMPd PK activity in synchronized EL4 cells. cAMPd PK activity is expressed as cmpx10^3 of ^{32}P incorporated into F_2b histone in the presence of cAMP. cAMP PK activity was determined on EL4 cells (2×10^6) at various times following the addition of serum or serum plus CsA (1 μg/ml). These are results of a representative experiment, with similar findings noted in at least 2 experiments.

TABLE 2. The effect of cyclosporine on cAMP-dependent protein kinase activity

Control	Ratio of enzyme activity[a]	Change in ratio from control cells
SW49 wt (2×10^6 cells)	0.66±0.03	
+CsA (1 μg/ml)	0.70±0.02	+0.04
+cAMP (10^{-4} M)	0.94±0.02	+0.24
+cAMP +CsA	0.89±0.03	+0.19
SW49 k^- (2×10^6 cells)	0.98±0.01	
+CsA (1 μg/ml)	1.00±0.02	+.02
+cAMP (10^{-4} M)	1.00±0.02	+.02
+cAMP +CsA	0.97±0.03	−.01

[a] The cAMP-dependent protein kinase activity ratio (mean ± SD) was determined following 2 hr of incubation in 3 experiments, as described in the *Materials and Methods* section.

PK activity determined in SW49 cells cultured for 2 hr with cAMP (10^{-4}M) and/or CsA (1 μg/ml). There was no difference in the level of enzyme activity between CsA-treated and non-treated SW49 wt cells—and, more imortant, CsA did not affect enzyme activation when cells were cultured with exogenous cAMP. As a control, no cAMPd PK activity was detected in cultured SW49 k^- cells.

DISCUSSION

Lymphocyte activation at the intracellular level has been studied by many investigators over the years. The mechanisms examined have included calcium flux, phospholipid metabolism, phosphorylating activity, protein kinase activation, polyamine synthesis, and DNA and protein synthesis (*14–16, 19–21*). We still do not know which early events when activated can ultimately lead to cellular proliferation. Further, we have not determined how these events are coupled and which series of events is associated with antigen, mitogen, or lymphokine-triggered activation. CsA is more than immunosuppressive agent, it is a modern tool to help dissect events that are responsible for the proliferation of an immune response. Its specificity in blocking mitogen and antigen-triggered T cell activation, but not interleukin-2-stimulated proliferation, establishes a difference between cell response to each signal. These data also demonstrate that CsA does not merely coat the cell surface, preventing a cellular response, but rather inhibits a specific series of events. The data presented here further exemplify the fact that certain mitogenic and chemical stimuli can generate enzymatic responses at the intracellular level that are unaffected by CsA. What we can not address is whether these events are crucial to lymphocyte activation. CsA, when used as a probe in these studies of mitogen-stimulated T cell tumor lines, has defined specific nuclear events that are affected by the immunosuppression of CsA—i.e., polyamine synthesis and nucleic acid synthesis—demonstrable in both human peripheral blood lymphocytes and in T cell tumor lines. The fact that C-kinase and cAMPd PK activation are not affected by CsA suggests two possibilities: these pathways are not normally involved in lymphocyte proliferation or the immunosuppressive activity associated with CsA is at the nuclear level, prior to polyamine synthesis.

In these studies we have utilized T cell tumor lines to investigate the role of C-kinase and cAMPd PK in T lymphocyte activation for their accessibility when cells are needed in large number. These cells are not normal helper T lymphocytes, yet they can respond to mitogenic and chemical stimuli and are sensitive to the immunosuppressive action of CsA at concentrations causing similar effects in helper T lymphocytes. Since these are activated cells we cannot be sure that protein kinase activation is comparable in malignant cell lines and normal peripheral blood lymphocytes. Certainly some protein kinase activation is occurring to maintain continuous cell growth. There are, however, many interesting similarities between T lymphoblastoid cell lines and normal human T lymphocytes.

We conclude that CsA does not affect the activation of C-kinase or cAMPd PK in T lymphoblastoid cell lines when activated by normal growth factors or when stimulated with chemical agents. The suppression of ODC activity and ^{3}H-thymidine incorporation associated with CsA treatment cannot be accounted for with changes in C-kinase and cAMPd PK activation.

REFERENCES

1. Borel JF, Feurer C, Magnee C, Stahlin H. Effects of the new anti-lymphocyte peptide cyclosporin A in animals. Immunology 1975; 32: 1017.
2. Borel JF. Comparative study of in vitro and in vivo drug effects on cell mediated cytotoxicity. Immunology 1976; 31: 631.
3. Hess AD, Tutschka PJ, Zhang PV, Santos GW. Effect of cyclosporin on human lymphocyte responses in vitro. IV. Production of T cell stimulatory growth factors and development of responsiveness of these growth factors in CsA-treated primary MLR cultures. J Immunol 1982; 128: 360.
4. Hess AD, Tutschka PJ, Santos G. Effect of cyclosporin A on human lymphocyte responses in vitro. II. CsA inhibits the production of T lymphocyte growth factors in secondary mixed lymphocyte responses but does not inhibit the response of primed lymphocytes to TCGF. J Immunol 1982; 128: 355.
5. Fidelus RK, Widmer M, Wee S-L, Bach F, Ferguson RM, Orosz C. The effect of cyclosporin A on murine and human T helper cell clones. Transplantation 1982; 34: 308.
6. Handschumacher RE, Harding MW, Rice J, Drugge RJ. Cyclophilin: a specific binding protein for cyclosporin A. Science 1984; 226: 544.

7. Palacios R, Moller G. Cyclosporin A blocks receptors for HLA-Dr antigens on T cells. Nature 1981; 290: 792.
8. Lafferty KJ, Borel JF, Hodgkins P. Cyclosporine-A (CsA). In Models for the mechanism of action in cyclosporine: biological activity and clinical applications. New York: Grune & Stratton, 1984: 26.
9. Fidelus RK, Orosz C, Ferguson RM. The effect of cyclosporine A (CsA) on murine and human T and B cell tumor lines. Transplant Proc 1983; 15: 554.
10. Farrar JJ, Fuller-Farrar J, Simon PL, Hilfiker ML, Stadler BM, Farrar WL. Thymoma production of T cell factor (Interleukin 2). J Immunol 1980; 125: 2555.
11. Coffino P, Gray JW, Tomkins GM. Cyclic AMP, a non-essential regulator of the cell cycle. Proc Natl Acad Sci USA 1975; 72: 878.
12. Kraft AS, Anderson WB, Cooper HL, Sando JJ. Decrease in cytosolic calcium/phospholipid-dependent protein kinase activity following phorbol ester treatment of EL4 thymoma cells. J Biol Chem 1982; 257: 13193.
13. Haddox MK, Magun BE, Russell DH. Ornithine decarboxylase induction during G_1 progression of normal and Rous sarcoma virus-transformed cells. Cancer Res 1980; 40: 604.
14. Klimpel SG, Byus CV, Russell DH, Lucas DO. Cyclic AMP-dependent protein kinase activation and the induction of ornithine decarboxylase during lymphocyte mitogenesis. J Immunol 1979; 123: 817.
15. Haddox MK, Magun BE, Russell DH. Differential expression of type I and type II cAMP-dependent protein kinases during cell cycle and cAMP induced growth arrest. Proc Natl Acad Sci USA 1980; 77: 3445.
16. Kraft AS, Anderson WB. Phorbol esters increase the amount of Ca^{2+} phospholipid protein kinase associated with plasma membrane. Nature 1983; 301: 621.
17. Kolata G. Clues to cell growth and differentiation. Science 1983; 220: 291.
18. Sando JJ, Hilfiker ML, Piacentini MJ, Laufer TM. Identification of phorbol ester receptors in T cell growth factor producing and non-producing EL4 mouse thymoma cells. Cancer Res 1982; 42: 1676.
19. Tsein RY, Pozzan T, Rink TJ. T cell mitogens cause early changes in cytoplasmic free Ca^{2+} and membrane potential in lymphocytes. Nature 1982; 295: 68.
20. Maino VC, Hayman MJ, Crumpton MJ. Relationship between enhanced turnover of phosphatidylinositol in lymphocyte activation by mitogens. Biochem J 1975; 146: 247.
21. Sarkadi EA, Szasy I, Gardos G. Active calcium transport and calcium-dependent membrane phosphorylation in human peripheral blood lymphocytes. Cell Calcium 1982; 3: 163.

Received 1 April 1985.
Accepted 22 May 1985.

0041-1337/86/4102-0192$02.00/0
TRANSPLANTATION

Vol. 41, No. 2
Printed in U.S.A.

HYPERSENSITIVITY REACTIONS IN THE SMALL INTESTINE

VII. INDUCTION OF THE INTESTINAL PHASE OF MURINE GRAFT-VERSUS-HOST REACTION BY LYT 2⁻ T CELLS ACTIVATED BY I-A ALLOANTIGENS[1]

ALLAN McI. MOWAT, ANNETTE BORLAND, AND DELPHINE M. V. PARROTT

Department of Bacteriology and Immunology, Western Infirmary, Glasgow Gll 6NT, Scotland

This study has examined the nature of the T lymphocytes and the alloantigens that induce the intestinal phase of graft-versus-host reaction in unirradiated F_1 mice. Parental spleen cells were depleted of T cells subsets by treatment with anti-Lyt monoclonal antibodies and complement, and we show that Lyt 2^- cells alone induce the increased lymphocytic infiltration of the epithelium that characterizes the intestinal graft-versus-host reaction. Lyt 2^- cells are also required to induce some of the associated crypt hyperplasia, but the full crypt changes require both Lyt 2^- and Lyt 2^+ T cells. In intra-H-2 recombinant congenic F_1 mice with graft-versus-host reaction, a disparity at the I-A locus was alone sufficient and necessary for crypt hyperplasia and increased intraepithelial lymphocyte counts, while an I-J incompatibility led to suppression of both these indices. The results support the hypothesis that the intestinal pathology of acute GVHD is induced by class II MHC-restricted delayed-type hypersensitivity effector T cells.

Small intestinal damage is an important cause of morbidity and mortality in patients with acute graft-versus-host disease after allogeneic bone marrow transplantation, but the pathogeneic mechanisms are still unclear (*1, 2*). The pathological features of intestinal graft-versus-host disease (GVHD)[2] include villus atrophy, crypt necrosis, preceded by crypt hyperplasia, infiltration of the mucosa by lymphocytes, and—in severe cases—malabsorption and protein-losing enteropathy

[1]This work was supported by MRC Grants 8011059 and 8224559; Annette Borland was in receipt of a Vacational Scholarship from the Wellcome Trust.

[2] BMT, bone marrow transplant; B10, C57B1/10; CCPR, crypt cell production rate; CTL, cytotoxic T lymphocyte; DTH, delayed-type hypersensitivity; GVHD, graft-versus-host disease; GVHR, graft-versus-host reaction; H & E, hematoxylin and eosin; IEL, intraepithelial lymphocyte; MHC, major histocompatibility complex; T_{DTH}, effector T lymphocyte of delayed-type hypersensitivity; T_s, suppressor T lymphocyte.

(1–4). These features present severe clinical problems, thus it would be important to clarify the mechanisms involved. Furthermore, mucosal alterations similar to those of GVHD are found during parasitic infestations of the intestine (*5–7*) and in patients with enteropathy due to food hypersensitivity (*8*). Therefore, elucidation of the basis of intestinal GVHD should contribute to our understanding of these other important conditions.

The tissue damage during allograft reactions including GVHD is often considered to be due to cytotoxic T lymphocytes, but recent evidence indicates that cytotoxic T lymphocytes (CTL) are not essential for acute GVHD in rodents (*9, 10*). In previous studies of graft-versus-host reaction (GVHR) in unirradiated F_1 mice, we have shown that the principal mucosal alterations are increases in crypt cell mitotic activity and in numbers of intraepithelial lymphocytes. The changes occur in the absence of antihost cytotoxic T lymphocytes and are present as a "bystander phenomenon" in intestinal grafts that are syngeneic to the lymphocytes used to induce the GVHR (*11, 14*). As these mucosal changes also develop in parallel with the proliferative phase of the systemic GVHR, these results are strong, but indirect, evidence that delayed-type hypersensitivity is the principal effector mechanism. We have now attempted to define further the exact mechanisms of intestinal GVHR by examining directly the nature of the T-cell-mediated immune response. Thus, we have determined the phenotype of the T cells responsible for the intestinal phase of GVHR in unirradiated mice and have elucidated the alloantigenic stimulus that activates these T cells. Our results support the hypothesis that the mucosal pathology characteristic of this model of GVHR is due to Lyt 2^- T cells activated by antigens coded by the I-A region of the major histocompatibility complex.

MATERIALS AND METHODS

Mice. CBA, BALB/c, and C57BL/10 Sc Sn mice were obtained from departmental stocks, while original breeding pairs of B10.A, B10.A3R, B10.A4R, B10.AKM, B10.BR, B10.AQR, A.TH, and A.TL mice were obtained from Olac Ltd, Bicester, England. Thereafter, these were bred and maintained in the department, as were all F_1 hybrids. The H-2 haplotypes of these strains are shown in Table 1.

Preparation of cell suspensions. Spleens were trimmed of adherent tissues, gently minced through a fine wire-mesh filter, and washed three times in RPMI 1640 (Flow Labs). Viabilities were assessed by phase contrast microscopy and were normally >80%.

TABLE 1. H-2 haplotypes of strains used in GVHR experiments

Strain	H-2 Allele				
	K	*A*	*J*	*E/C*	*D*
CBA	k	k	k	k	k
BALB/c	d	d	d	d	d
B10.BR	k	k	k	k	k
B10	b	b	b	b	b
B10.A4R	k	k	b	b	b
B10.A5R	b	b	k	k	d
B10.A3R	b	b	b	k	d
B10.A	k	k	k	k	d
B10.AQR	q	k	k	k	d
B10.AKM	k	k	k	k	d
A.TH	s	s	s	s	d
A.TL	s	k	k	k	d

Induction of graft-versus-host reactions. Adult F_1 hybrid mice were injected with 6×10^7 viable parental spleen cells in 0.2 ml i.p., while neonatal F_1 mice received 2.5×10^7 viable parental spleen cells in 0.1 ml. Controls received RPMI 1640 only. The intensity of the GVHR was assessed by the spleen Index of Simonsen (*15*).

Elimination of T cell subsets. Spleen cell suspensions were depleted of Lyt subsets by incubation with 1:1000 monoclonal anti-Lyt 1.1 (NEN clone NEI003) or 1:500 anti-Lyt 2.1 (NEN clone NEI 004) for 40 min at 4°C followed by 30 min. at 37°C in 1:10 rabbit complement (Low Tox M, Cedarlane Ltd.). Cells were washed three times before use and used without adjustment for cell depletion. In our hands, depletion of Lyt 1^+ and Lyt 2^+ T cells in this way lyses 25–30% and 15–20% of mouse spleen cells, respectively, while Lyt 2^- cells are incapable of allospecific CTL activity in vitro.

Assessment of mucosal alterations. Villus length, crypt length, and crypt cell production rate were measured as described previously (*11, 12, 16*). Briefly, mice were injected with 7.5 mg/kg colchicine (Sigma) i.p. and killed at intervals from 20–120 min thereafter. Pieces of jejunum 10 cm from the pylorus were fixed in 75% ethanol/25% acetic acid and stained in bulk with Schiff Reagent (Difco Ltd.) by the modified Feulgen reaction. Villus and crypt lengths were measured using an eyepiece micrometer under a dissecting microscope and the number of metaphases per crypt were counted. The crypt cell production rate (CCPR) was then calculated by linear regression analysis of the accumulation of metaphases against time, and was expressed as the cell production per crypt per hour. For each specimen, values for 10 villi and crypts were obtained.

Intraepithelial lymphocyte (IEL) counts. Intraepithelial lymphocytes were counted in H & E-stained sections of jejunum by the method of Ferguson and Murrary (*17*) and expressed as the number of IEL/100 epithelial cells.

Statistics. Results were expressed as means + 1 SD and compared by Student's *t* tests. Crypt cell production rates were compared using covariance analysis to establish nonparallelism of lines obtained by linear regression analysis.

RESULTS

Role of T cell subsets in induction of intestinal GVHR. As delayed-type hypersensitivity (DTH) effector cells and CTL differ in Lyt phenotype, our first approach in assessing the role of T_{DTH} in intestinal GVHR was to examine the Lyt phenotype of the T cells responsible for intestinal pathology.

Unirradiated (CBA×BALB/C) F_1 mice were injected with 2.5×10^7 CBA spleen cells i.p. on the sixth day of life, the parental spleen cells having been treated previously either with anti-Lyt-1 or anti-Lyt 2 and complement, or with complement alone. As shown previously, this dose of spleen cells produced a moderately intense GVHR, that was maximal after 8–10 days, as assessed by the spleen index, but there were no clinical signs of GVHR (*12*). The mice were killed on day nine and the intestinal phase of the GVHR was assessed in the jejunum by measuring the intraepithelial lymphocyte count, crypt length, and crypt cell production role, as these parameters have been shown to be reliable indices of mucosal GVHR (*11, 12*). Mice receiving unseparated parental cells had a significantly higher IEL count than controls, and this increase was abolished by depletion of Lyt 1^+ T cells from the parental cell inoculum (Fig. 1). In view of the fact that all mouse T cells may carry the Lyt

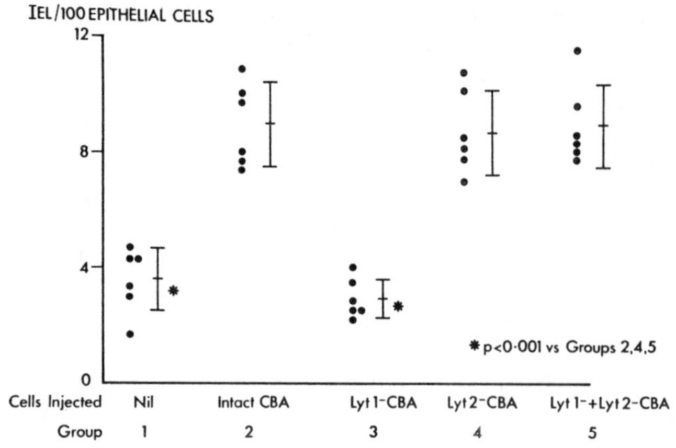

FIGURE 1. Phenotype of T lymphocytes mediating the intestinal phase of GVHR: intraepithelial lymphocyte counts in the jejunum of neonatal (CBA×BALB/c)F_1 mice nine days after induction of GVHR with normal, Lyt-1-depleted or Lyt-2-depleted CBA spleen cells. Results shown are means ± 1 SD.

1 marker (*18*) this result is not altogether surprising and may merely reflect depletion of all alloreactive donor T lymphocytes. However, the significant findings from this experiment were that depletion of Lyt 2^+ cells did not affect the increase in IEL count, and that addition of Lyt-2-depleted cells restored the ability of Lyt-1-depleted cells to induce the increased IEL count. As this last group of cells lacks Lyt 1^+2^+ T cells, we conclude that Lyt 2^- cells are alone sufficient to produce the increased lymphocytic infiltration of the jejunal epithelium in GVHR.

When alterations in mucosal architecture and epithelial cell kinetics were examined, a similar, but not identical, pattern emerged (Fig. 2). Recipients of unseparated spleen cells had significant increases in crypt length and CCPR compared with controls (134.2±8.9 μm and 12.4±2.5 vs. 85.4±4.0 μm and 3.4±0.7, $P<0.001$ and $P<0.005$, respectively) and once again these were eliminated by depleting T cells with anti-Lyt-1 and complement (88.9±3.4 μm and 3.5±0.6). In this case, recipients of Lyt-2-depleted cells also had significantly smaller crypts and a lower CCPR than recipients of intact cells (108.4±5.1 μm and 6.5±1.0, $P<0.001$ and $P<0.002$, respectively) although both indices were still significantly increased compared with those in control mice ($P<0.001$ and $P<0.002$). Addition of Lyt-2-depleted to Lyt-1-depleted cells did not restore the full increases in crypt length and CCPR, these values being identical to those found with Lyt-2-depleted cells alone. Villus atrophy was not observed in any group. We interpret these results as showing that Lyt 2^- T cells can alone induce significant alterations in mucosal architecture and cell proliferation but that these cells have to interact with an Lyt 2^+ T cell to produce their full effect.

Nature of the MHC alloantigens that stimulate intestinal GVHR. The predominant role of Lyt 2^- cells in inducing the intestinal phase of the GVHR is consistent with the hypothesis that conventional T_{DTH} are the effector cells involved, and also suggests that class II MHC alloantigens should provide the stimulus for activating these cells. We therefore examined this directly by studying the intestinal changes during a GVHR induced across specified MHC incompatibilities. Adult F_1 hybrid mice were bred from congenic parents differing at individual loci (Table 1), injected with 6×10^7 parental spleen cells i.p. and killed at the peak of the GVHR, on day ten.

Intensity of systemic GVHR. The ability of different MHC regions to induce a proliferative systemic GVHR was assessed in several individual experiments by the spleen index (Table 2). A GVHR across the whole H-2 complex (in [B10×B10.BR] F_1 mice) or involving H-2K+I-A only (B10→ [B10×B10.A4R]) produced marked splenomegaly that was identical in the two strain combinations. Significantly, incompatibility at H-2K alone did not induce significant splenomegaly (B10.A→ [B10.A×B10.AQR]), while an isolated I-region incompatibility did (ATH→ [A.TH×A.TL]). In addition, significant splenomegaly did not occur in a GVHR induced by H-2D (B10.BR→ [B10.BR×B10.AKM]) or J-D (B10→ [B10×B10.A5R]). These findings confirm that class II MHC antigens provide the major stimulus for a proliferative GVHR, and indicate that the I-A region is the single most important locus involved. Interestingly, mild splenomegaly was consist-

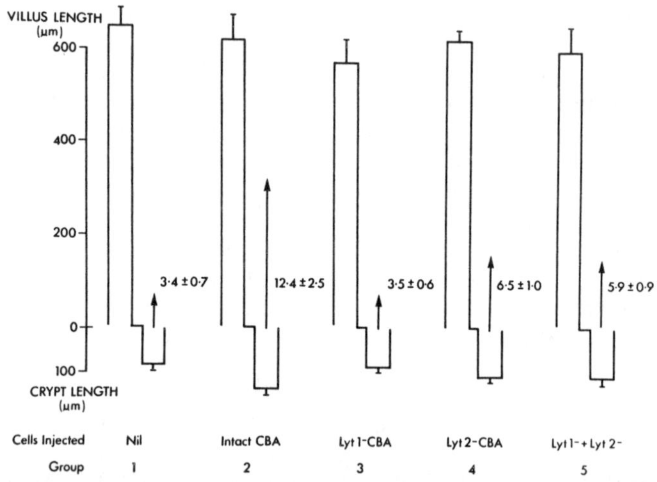

FIGURE 2. Phenotype of T lymphocytes mediating the intestinal phase of GVHR: mucosal architecture in jejunum of neonatal (CBA×BALB/c)F_1 mice nine days after induction of GVHR with normal, Lyt-1-depleted or Lyt-2-depleted CBA spleen cells. Bars represent villus length and crypt length and arrows represent CCPR. Results shown are the means + 1 standard deviation for six mice per group. Mice in groups 2, 4, and 5 had significantly longer crypts than control mice ($P<0.001$), while crypts in groups 4 and 5 were significantly smaller than after injection of untreated spleen cells (group 2: $P<0.001$). The CCPR of groups 2, 4, and 5 were significantly greater than controls ($P<0.005$; $P<0.005$; $P<0.02$, respectively), while those in groups 4 and 5 were lower than in recipients of untreated cells ($P<0.02$).

TABLE 2. Ability of H-2 loci to induce splenomegaly in unirradiated F_1 mice nine days after injection of 6×10^7 parental spleen cells[a]

Donor→host combination	H-2 disparity	Spleen index
B10→ (B10×B10.BR)F_1	H-2	2.23±0.71 (18)
B10→ (B10.×B10.A4R)F_1	K + A	2.40±0.77 (27)
B10.A→ (B10×B10.AQR)	K	1.07±0.11 (15)
B10→ (B10×B10.A5R)	J − D	1.05±0.19 (15)
B10.BR→ (B10.BR×B10.AKM)	D	1.18±0.20 (16)
A.TH→ (A.TH×A.TL)	I	1.64±0.39 (15)
B10→ (B10.A3R×B10A5R)	J	1.20±0.22 (10)

[a] Results shown are pooled from 2–4 experiments and are the mean spleen index ±1 SD for the number of mice shown in parentheses.

ently observed during a GVHR in (B10.A3R×B10.A5R) mice, which differ at I-J alone.

Intraepithelial lymphocyte counts. Intraepithelial lymphocytes were counted in the jejunum of the mice described above—and, as anticipated, a GVHR across a full H-2 incompatibility produced a significant increase in IEL count compared with controls (Fig. 3). Significantly increased IEL counts were also observed in mice with a GVHR induced across differences at the I region and at H-2K + I-A. In contrast, incompatibility at H-2K or for the H-2 complex to the right of I-A did not provoke an increased IEL count during GVHR. Indeed, mice with GVHR induced by class I MHC antigens frequently had lower IEL counts than controls, although this did not attain statistical significance. When the GVHR was stimulated only by the I-J region, however, IEL counts were significantly lower than in control mice.

Thus, incompatibility at the I-A region is alone sufficient and necessary for the increased lymphocytic infiltration of the intestinal epithelium in GVHR.

Mucosal architecture and epithelial cell kinetics. Villus and crypt lengths and crypt cell production rates were also measured in these mice. No significant alterations were found in villus length in any mice with GVHR, except for (A.TH×A.TL) mice, which had slight villus atrophy (Table 3). In contrast, mice with GVHR induced across the whole H-2 region, the I region, or only H-2K+IA had significantly increased crypt lengths and CCPR compared with controls (Fig. 4). No such increases were observed when the incompatibility involved only H-2K, H-2D,

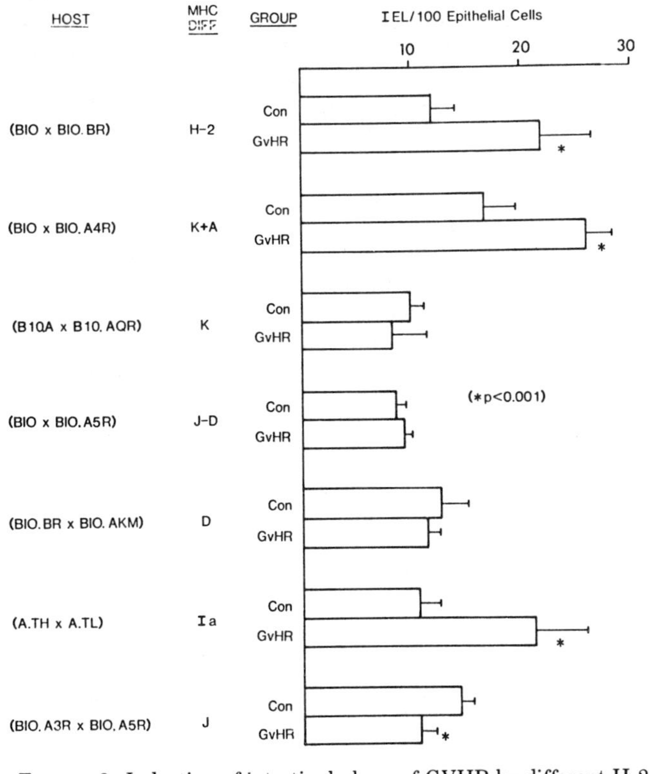

FIGURE 3. Induction of intestinal phase of GVHR by different H-2 incompatibilities: intraepithelial lymphocytes counts in the jejunum of adult F_1 mice nine days after injection 6×10^7 parental spleen cells. Results shown are the mean number of IEL/100 epithelial cells + 1 SD for 5–6 mice per group.

TABLE 3. Villus lengths during a GVHR induced across different H-2 loci

GVHR host	H-2 disparity	Villus length (μm) Control	GVHR
(B10×B10.BR)F_1	H-2	580±57.4	585.0±58.5
(B10×B10.A4R)F_1	K + A	674.1±36.4	690.0±37.0
(B10.A×B10.AQR)F_1	K	662.3±55.3	691.2±47.8
(B10×B10.A5R)F_1	J − D	625.8±35.2	634.1±32.4
(B10.BR×B10.AKM)F_1	D	682.5±56.1	687.8±59.5
(A.TH×A.TL)F_1	I	762.1±18.0	670.1±35.0[b]
(B.10A3R×B10.A5R)F_1	J	584.9±27.5	567.6±25.9

[a] Results shown are mean villus lengths ± 1 SD for 5–6 mice/group on day nine of GVHR.
[b] $P<0.005$.

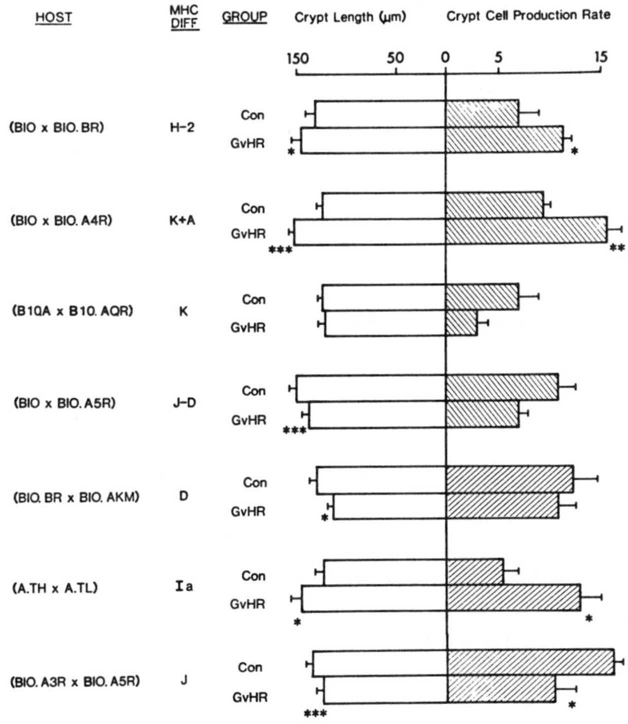

FIGURE 4. Induction of intestinal phase of GVHR by different H-2 incompatibilities: crypt lengths (open bars) and crypt cell production rate (hatched bars) in the jejunum of adult F_1 mice nine days after injection of 6×10^7 parental spleen cells. Results shown are means + 1 SD for 5–6 mice per group. (*) $P<0.05$; (**) $P<0.02$; (***) $P<0.005$).

or J-D—and, as with the IEL count, a GVHR across class I MHC antigens alone often produced shorter crypt lengths and lower CCPR than in controls. Similarly, an I-J region difference caused significant suppression of these parameters during a GVHR. Once again, the I-A region is the only stimulus for enhanced crypt cell proliferation and crypt hypertrophy during the GVHR, while I-J alloantigens may induce suppression of crypt cell mitosis.

DISCUSSION

This study demonstrates that Lyt 2^- T cells are responsible for inducing the intestinal phase of the GVHR in unirradiated mice and that class II MHC alloantigens provide the stimulus. Thus our results substantiate the concept the intestinal pathology in this model of GVHR is induced by class II MHC-restricted T_{DTH}.

The pathogenesis of immunologically mediated intestinal damage has not yet been studied in detail, not only because few experimental models are available but also because there has been a lack of reliable indices for measuring the immune pathology. In this study, we have used the IEL count and CCPR as parameters of the local immune response, as our previous experiments established these to be accurate measures of intestinal cell-mediated immunity (CMI). This is shown by the increases in both IEL count and CCPR that occur during allograft rejection of gut (*16, 19*), in T-cell-dependent responses to intestinal parasites (*5–7*), and in the intestines of mice with local DTH to fed protein antigens (*20*). Furthermore, in GVHR, increases in IEL count and CCPR occur in parallel with the proliferative phase of the systemic GVHR (*12*), and are directly related to the cell dose used to induce the GVHR.[3] For these reasons, we consider increases in IEL count and CCPR to be direct consequences of intestinal CMI in GVHR. Our finding that Lyt 1^+ cells are essential for inducing these intestinal alterations during the GVHR in unirradiated mice must be interpreted with caution in the light of the demonstration that virtually all murine T cells may be Lyt 1^+ (*18*). Thus, the elimination of intestinal GVHR by anti-Lyt-1^+ complement could merely reflect the removal of all T cells from the donor inoculum rather than a selective effect on one functional subpopulation. Nevertheless, our results using Lyt 2-depleted cells and mixed populations of Lyt 1^- and Lyt 2^- cells show clearly that Lyt 2^- T cells are essential for the intestinal phase of the GVHR in unirradiated F_1 mice, and that Lyt 1^+2^- cells are the single most important population. There are no similar studies of individual organ damage in GVHR, but our findings are supported by studies of systemic GVHR across MHC incompatibility. Thus, in rats, lethal GVHR can be induced by CTL-depleted helper/inducer T cells (*9*), while a local GVHR in the popliteal lymph node is due principally to cells with the phenotype of inducer T cells (*20*).

Lyt 2^- cells were alone able to induce an increased number of IEL in GVHR and produced a significant degree of crypt hyperplasia. However, as others have shown in systemic GVHD both for mortality (*22, 23*) and splenomegaly (*24, 25*), the full crypt alterations also required Lyt 2^+ cells—possibly indicating that more alloreactive T cells are necessary to stimulate major tissue alterations like crypt cell hyperplasia. We propose that this interaction reflects the cooperation of Lyt 2^- T_{DTH} and Lyt 2^+ precursor T_{DTH}, rather than CTL and their precursors, which are also Lyt 2^+ (*26*), for the following reasons. First, the intestinal alterations in (CBA×BALB/c)F_1 mice with GVHR occur in the absence of CTL (*14*) and in grafts of intestine that are syngeneic to the donor lymphocytes and therefore cannot present allogeneic targets for antihost CTL (*11, 13*). It is also known that systemic GVHR can be induced by CTL-depleted donor cells (*9, 22, 24, 27*) and does not correlate with the presence of CTL in the host (*10, 28, 29*). Second, alloreactive DTH precedes lethal GVHD in irradiated mice (*30, 31*) and correlates with allograft rejection by unprimed T cells (*32, 33*)—and both phenomena require interaction between Lyt 2^- and Lyt 2^+ T cells. It is believed that these cells are T_{DTH} and their precursors, and we suggest that the intestinal phase of GVHR induced by unprimed cells reflects a similar mechanism. Finally, the strongest evidence against a role of CTL and their precursors is our finding that I-A disparity is an absolute prerequisite for the intestinal changes of GVHR.

This result is entirely consistent with other studies showing that the I-A locus is the single most important stimulus for several different aspects of GVHR, including splenomegaly (*34*) mortality (*35*), macrophage activation (*36*), allohelper T cell induction (*37*) and antihost DTH (*38*). In addition, alloreactive T cells directed at I-A alone can induce a lethal GVHD in which CTL are not found (*10*). In contrast, we found that class I MHC alloantigens induced neither proliferative changes in the intestine nor splenomegaly. Class I antigens induce little antihost DTH in GVHR (*38, 39*) and so the genetic basis of intestinal GVHR supports our hypothesis that T_{DTH}, and not CTL, are the effector cells involved. Current studies are aimed at confirming the role of I-A-restricted T_{DTH} directly by investigating the presence of the L3T4 antigen on the cells responsible for intestinal GVHR.

Two other interesting features emerged from studying the intestinal GVHR across specified MHC differences. First, there was no synergy observed between class I and II MHC alloantigens, despite the fact that splenomegaly was greater across H-2K+I-A than across the I region itself. Synergy between class I and II antigens, which has been found previously for GVHR-induced mortality (*35, 37*), splenomegaly (*34*), and antihost DTH (*38, 39*), has usually been ascribed to the induction of different T cell populations. Our results, therefore, indicate that intestinal GVHR in unirradiated mice is induced by a single class of effector T cell. The second important finding was that suppressed IEL counts and crypt measurements were found during the GVHR across an I-J difference. This supports the ability of I-J alloantigens to induce suppressor T cells (*40*) and suppress macrophage activity (*36*) in vivo, despite the controversy over the genetic basis of the I-J region (*41*). Interestingly, as others have noted (*36*), an additional I-A disparity overcame the inhibitory effect of the I-J region. In addition to the I-J locus, certain class I differences also suppressed the intestinal indices. Although this requires confirmation in other combinations, it is entirely consistent with the ability of class I loci to activate allosuppressor T cells both in vivo and in vitro (*37, 42*). These findings, plus those using Lyt-depleted cells, indicate that the intestinal alterations in a GVHR across the entire MHC mainly reflect a proliferative phase due to I-A restricted T_{DTH}, but that this is also regulated by T_S activated by I-J and/or class I antigens. Furthermore, they raise the intriguing possibility that intestinal epithelial renewal is regulated by mucosal T cells under normal conditions, as well as pathological conditions such as GVHR and food-sensitive enteropathy. We are currently examining the role of T lymphocyte products in maintaining the homeostasis of normal epithelial cell turnover. This study did not identify the source of the stimulating I-A antigens but we believe that these are presented by bone-marrow-derived cells. Although intestinal epithelial cells express I-A antigens and this is enhanced during a GVHR (*43*), these cells have not been shown to activate T cells. In contrast, our more recent work suggests that I-A^+ bone-marrow-derived cells are necessary to stimulate intestinal GVHR (manuscript in preparation) and we propose that these cells migrate through the mucosa where they stimulate precursor T_{DTH}.

The results presented here are consistent with the hypothesis

[3] Ziegler K, Strobel S, Ferguson A. manuscript submitted for publication.

that T_{DTH} are the effector cells responsible for inducing the intestinal pathology of acute GVHD in man. Nevertheless, it is important to assess their relevance for these clinical disorders. In our experiments we examined an entirely proliferative GVHR in unirradiated hosts, whereas acute GVHD after BMT occurs in patients conditioned with lethal irradiation and/or chemotherapy and across non-MHC differences. Under these conditions in mice, lethal GVHD may occur, and it is due to class I MHC-restricted Lyt 2^+ T cells, suggesting a possible role for CTL rather than T_{DTH} (*45*). Furthermore, the tissue lesions of human GVHD are infiltrated by lymphocytes with a suppressor/cytotoxic phenotype (*46*). However, T_{DTH} can be class I MHC-restricted and these are frequently Lyt 2^+ cells (*47*). In addition, although the IEL infiltrating the gut of unirradiated mice with GVHR show the same preponderance of Lyt 2^+ cells as normal IEL (Mowat A, Micklem HS, unpublished observations) we have demonstrated that IEL from mice with GVHR have no CTL activity (*14*). These observations suggest that T_{DTH} may indeed be the effector cells in acute, lethal GVHD, but their phenotype and restriction elements may differ from those described here. The second issue to consider is that we have reproduced the crypt hyperplasia and lymphocytic infiltration but not the villus atrophy typical of acute GVHD (*1, 2*). The reasons for this are unclear, but we have suggested previously that crypt hyperplasia is a direct effect of enteropathic lymphokines released by mucosal T_{DTH} and represents an early stage of enteropathy, of which villus atrophy is the final and most severe manifestation (*48*). It is known that the villus damage found in rejecting allografts of gut and in irradiated mice with GVHD is preceded by a phase of crypt cell proliferation (*16*, and Mowat A, Felstein MV, manuscript in preparation). Villus atrophy may therefore reflect a severe DTH response that proceeds unchecked due to the continued presence of antigen or to the elimination of host regulation by irradiation. Alternatively, sequential activation of allosuppressor T cells by allohelper T cells can produce a lethal GVHD in some unirradiated mice (*37, 49*) and it is possible that the development of destructive enteropathy from an early proliferative response involves a similar sequence of T cell activation. We are, at present, studying the nature and regulation of the mucosal T cells that respond to alloantigens and food proteins with a view to resolving these issues.

Note added in proof. The I-A region has recently been shown to be the only stimulus for intestinal damage in irradiated mice with GVHR (Piguet P-F. GVHR elicited by products of class I or class II loci of the MHC: analysis of the response of mouse T lymphocytes to products of class I and class II loci of the MHC in correlation with GVHR-induced mortality, medullary aplasia and erteropathy. J Immunol 1985; 135: 1637.)

REFERENCES

1. Slavin RE, Santos GW. The graft-versus-host reaction in man after bone marrow transplantation. Pathology, pathogenesis, clinical features and implications. Clin Immunol Immunopathol 1973; 1: 472.
2. Woodruff JM, Hansen JA, Good RA, Santos GW, Slavin RE. The pathology of the GVHR in adults receiving BM. transplants. Transplant Proc 1976, 8: 675.
3. Hedberg CA, Reiser S, Reilly RW. Intestinal phase of the runting syndrome in mice. II. Observations on nutrient absorption and certain disaccharidase abnormalities. Transplantation 1968; 6: 104.
4. Weisdorf SA, Salati LM, Longsdorf JA, Ramsay NKC, Sharp HL. Graft-versus-host disease of the intestine: a protein-losing enteropathy characterized by fecal α-antitrypsin. Gastroenterology 1983; 85: 1076.
5. Ferguson A, Jarrett EEE. Hypersensitivity reactions in the small intestine. I Thymus dependence of experimental "partial villus atrophy." Gut 1975; 16: 114.
6. Manson-Smith DF, Bruce RG, Parrott DMV. Villus atrophy and expulsion of intestinal Trichinella spiralis are mediated by T cells. Cell Immunol 1979; 47: 285.
7. Ruitenberg EJ, Leenstra F, Elgersma A. Thymus dependence and independence of intestinal pathology in a Trichinella spiralis infection: a study in congenitally athymic (nude) mice. Br J Exp Pathol 1977; 58: 311.
8. Ferguson A, Mowat A.McI. Immunological mechanisms in the small intestine. In: Wright R, Ed. Recent advances in gastrointestinal Pathology. Philadelphia: Saunders, 1980: 93.
9. Mason DW. Subsets of T cells in the rat mediating lethal graft-versus-host disease. Transplantation 1981; 32: 222.
10. Jadus MR, Peck AB. Lethal murine graft-versus-host disease in the absence of detectable cytotoxic T lymphocytes. Transplantation 1983; 36: 281.
11. Mowat A.McI, Ferguson A. Hypersensitivity reactions in the small intestine. VI. Pathogenesis of the graft-versus-host reaction in the small intestinal mucosa of the mouse. Transplantation 1981; 32: 238.
12. Mowat A.McI, Ferguson A. Intraepithelial lymphocyte count and crypt hyperplasia measure the mucosal component of the graft-versus-host reaction in mouse small intestine. Gastroenterology 1982; 83: 417.
13. Elson CO, Reilly RW, Rosenberg IH. Small intestinal injury in the GVHR: an innocent bystander phenomenon. Gastroenterology 1977; 72: 886.
14. Borland A, Mowat A.McI, Parrott DMV. Augmentation of intestinal and peripheral natural killer activity during the graft-versus-host reaction in mice. Transplantation 1983; 36: 513.
15. Simonsen M. Graft versus host reactions: their natural history and applicability as tools of research. Prog Allergy 1962; 6: 349.
16. MacDonald TT, Ferguson A. Hypersensitivity reactions in the small intestine. III. The effects of allograft rejection and of GVHD on epithelial cell kinetics. Cell Tissue Kinet 1977; 10: 301.
17. Ferguson A, Murray D. Quantitation of intraepithelial lymphocytes in human jejunum. Gut 1971; 12: 988.
18. Ledbetter JA, Rouse RV, Micklem HS, Herzenberg LA. T cell subsets defined by expression of Ly-1,2,3 and Thy-1 antigens. Two parameter immunofluorescence and cytotoxicity analysis with monoclonal antibodies modifies current views. J Exp Med 1980; 152: 280.
19. MacDonald TT, Ferguson A. Hypersensitivity reactions in the small intestine II. Effects of allograft rejection on mucosal architecture and lymphoid cell infiltrate. Gut 1976; 17: 81.
20. Mowat, A.McI, Ferguson A. Hypersensitivity in the small intestinal mucosa. V. Induction of cell mediated immunity to a dietary antigen. Clin Exp Immunol 1981; 43: 574.
21. Spickett GP, Brandon MR, Mason DW, Williams AF, Woollett GR. MRC OX-22, a monoclonal antibody that labels a new subset of T lymphocytes and reacts with the high molecular weight form of the leucocyte-common antigen. J Exp Med 1983; 158: 795.
22. Vallera DA, Soderling CCB, Kersy JH. Bone marrow transplantation across major histocompatibility barriers in mice. III. Treatment of donor grafts with monoclonal antibodies directed against Lyt determinants. J Immunol 1982; 128: 871.
23. Rolink AG, Gleichmann E. Allosuppressor and allohelper-T cells in acute and chronic graft-versus-host (GVH) disease. III. Different Lyt subsets of donor T cells induce different pathological syndromes. J Exp Med 1983; 158: 546.
24. Kisielow P, Hirst JA, Shiku H, Beverley PCL, Hoffmann MK,

Boyce EA, Oettgen HF. Ly antigens as markers for funtionally distinct subpopulations of thymus derived lymphocytes of the mouse. Nature 1975; 253: 219.
25. Mage M, Mathieson B, Sharrow S, McHugh L, Hammer V, Kanellopoulos-Langevin C, Brideau D, Thomas CA. Preparative nonlytic separation of Lyt 2^+ and Lyt 2^- lymphocytes, functional analyses of the separated cells and demonstration of synergy in graft-versus-host reaction of Lyt 2^+ and Lyt 2^- cells. Eur J Immunol 1981; 11: 228.
26. Beverley PCL, Woody J, Dunkley M, Feldmann M, McKenzie IFC. Separation of suppressor and killer T cells by surface phenotype. Nature 1976; 262: 495.
27. Mage MG, McHugh LL. Retention of graft-versus-host activity in non-adherent spleen cells after depletion of cytotoxic activity by incubation on allogeneic target cells. J Immunol 1973; 111: 652.
28. Van Elven EH, Rolink AG, Van Der Veen F, Gleichmann E. Capacity of genetically different T lymphocytes to induce lethal graft-versus-host disease correlates with their capacity to generate anti-F_1 killer cells. A non-H-2 locus determines the inability to induce lethal graft-versus-host disease. J Exp Med 1981; 153: 1474.
29. Hamilton BL. Absence of correlation between cytolytic T lymphocytes and lethal murine graft-versus-host disease in response to minor histocompatibility antigens. Transplantation 1984; 38: 357.
30. Wolters EAJ, Benner R. Immunobiology of the graft-versus-host-disease. Symptoms of graft-versus-host disease in mice are preceded by delayed-type hypersensitivity to host histocompatibility antigens. Transplantation 1978; 26: 40.
31. Bril H, Molendijk-Lok BD, Hussaarts-Odijk LM, Benner R. Synergism of T lymphocyte subsets in the response to Ms-locus coded antigens during graft-versus-host reaction. Cell Immunol 1984; 83: 370.
32. Loveland BE, McKenzie IFC. Delayed-type hypersensitivity and allograft rejection in the mouse: correlation of effector cell phenotype. Immunology 1982; 46: 313.
33. Loveland BE, McKenzie IFC. Cells mediating graft rejection in the mouse. III. Ly-1^+ precursor T cells generate skin graft rejection. Transplantation 1982; 33: 407.
34. Klein J. Allograft rejection against H-2 region antigens. Transplant Proc 1977; 9: 847.
35. Klein J, Chiang CL. Ability of H-2 Regions to induce graft-versus-host disease. J Immunol 1976; 117: 736.
36. Rolink AG, Pals ST, Gleichmann E. Allosuppressor and allohelper T cells in acute and chronic graft-vs-host disease. II. F_1 recipients carrying mutations at H-2K and/or I-A. J Exp Med 1983; 157: 755.
37. Zinkernagel RM. Activation or suppression of bactericidal activity of macrophages during a graft-versus-host reaction against I-A and I-J region differences respectively. Immunogenetics 1980; 10: 373.
38. Wolters EAJ, Benner R. Functional separation in vivo of both antigens encoded by H-2 subregion and non H-2 loci. Nature 1979; 279: 642.
39. Wolters EAJ, Benner R. Different H-2 subregion-coded antigens as targets for T-cell subsets in graft-versus-host reaction. Cell Immunol 1981; 59: 115.
40. Liew FY. Regulation of delayed-type hypersensitivity. VII. The role of I-J subregion gene products of delayed-type hypersensitivity to major histo-compatibility antigens by specific suppressor T cells. Eur J Immunol 1981; 11: 883.
41. Klyczek KK, Carter H, Hayes CE. T-cell surface I-J glycoprotein: concerted action of chromosome -4 and -17 genes forms an epitope dependent on -D-mannosyl residues. J Exp Med 1984; 159: 1604.
42. Rolink AG, Van Der Meer W, Melief CJM, Gleichmann E. Intra H-2 and T cell requirements for the induction of maximal positive and negative allogeneic effects. Eur J Immunol 1981; 13: 191.
43. Mason DW, Dallman M, Barclay AN. Graft-versus-host disease induces expression of Ia antigen in rat epidermal cells and gut epithelium. Nature 1981; 293: 150.
44. Mowat A.McI. Ia^+ bone-marrow-derived cells are the stimulus for the intestinal phase of murine graft-versus-host reaction. Transplantation (in press).
45. Korngold R, Sprent J. Features of T cells causing H-2 restricted lethal graft-versus-host disease across minor histocompatibility barriers. J Exp Med 1982; 155: 872.
46. Janossy G, Montano L, Selby WS, Duke O, Panayi G, Lampert I, Thomas JA, Granger S, Bofill M, Tidman N, Thomas HC, Goldstein G. T cell subset abnormalities in tissue lesions developing during autoimmune disorders, viral infection and graft versus host disease. J Clin Immunol 1982; 2(suppl): 425.
47. Leung KN, Ada GL. Different functions of subsets of effector T cells in murine influenza virus infection. Cell Immunol 1982; 67: 312.
48. Ferguson A, MacDonald TT. Effects of local delayed hypersensitivity on the small intestine. Ciba Found Symp 1977; 46: 305.
49. Pals ST, Radaszkiewicz T, Gleichmann E. Allosuppressor and allohelper T cells in acute and chronic graft-versus-host disease. IV. Activation of donor allosuppressor cells is confined to acute GVHD. J Immunol 1984; 132: 1669.

Received 28 February 1985.
Accepted 14 May 1985.

0041-1337/86/4102-0199$02.00/0
TRANSPLANTATION

Vol. 41, No. 2
Printed in U.S.A.

DIFFERENCE IN SENSITIVITY TO CYCLOSPORINE IN VITRO OF HUMAN ALLOREACTIVE LINES AND CLONES[1]

FABRIZIO MANCA,[2,3] SILVIA CARROZZI,[4] ANNALISA KUNKL,[2] SERGIO BAROCCI,[2] VITALIA DESSI,[2] UMBERTO VALENTE,[5] IRIS FONTANA,[5] AND FRANCO CELADA[2]

Department of Immunology, XIII U.S.L., Department of Nephrology, XIII U.S.L., Department of Surgical Anatomy, University of Genoa, Genoa, Italy

The effectiveness of cyclosporine (CsA) as immunosuppressive agent in human kidney graft rejection is well established. However, in spite of efforts to maintain optimal plasma levels, a fraction of transplanted patients undergo rejection episodes and/or irreversible chronic rejection. This suggests that immunosuppression by CsA cannot control the alloreactive response if there is a high degree of histoincompatibility for HLA or non-HLA antigens, or it has little effect on the "high responder" patient. Both possibilities are difficult to test in the human system. A third hypothesis, the existence of individual CsA resistance, was tested by evaluating the in vitro inhibitory activity of CsA on alloreactive T cell lines from several individuals. A different degree of in vitro sensitivity to the drug was observed among alloreactive lines generated from different individuals and among clones obtained from the same bulk line. The variability at the individual level and at the clonal level may account for the onset of CsA-resistant rejection assuming that in vivo a positive selection in the presence of the drug occurs and allows for the resistant clones, if present, to dominate the sensitive ones.

The effect of cyclosporine (CsA)[6] in preventing graft rejection has been extensively demonstrated by a number of reports and in multicenter trials (*1, 2, 3*). Although CsA is presently the immunosuppressive drug of choice for kidney transplantation in the opinion of several authors (*4, 5, 6*), a fraction of CsA-treated patients undergo rejection episodes or irreversible rejection of the graft. The number of mismatches for HLA class I and class II antigens does not correlate with graft survival in CsA-treated patients (*7*), and previous blood transfusions do not improve graft outcome in some reports (*8, 9*). We can hypothesize that graft rejection in CsA-treated recipients depends on the particular antigenicity of some mismatched combinations, on mismatches for non-HLA antigens, or on a high or low immune responsiveness of the recipient. All these possibilities are difficult to test in the outbred human population. The possibility that differences in susceptibility to the drug may exist is supported by a previous report from our group in which the variability of individual sensitivity to CsA in mitogen-induced lymphocyte proliferation was described (*10*). Since the mitogen-induced stimulation may be unrelated to the immune events leading to the recognition of transplantation alloantigens, we generated alloreactive lines and clones from individuals as a more likely counterpart of graft recognition. These lines were characterized for their sensitivity to CsA when stimulated with allogeneic cells.

[1] This work was supported in part by Grant 84.01173.95 (PF Chimica Fine e Secondaria) from The National Research Council (C.N.R.), Rome, Italy.

[2] Department of Immunology.

[3] Address correspondence to: Fabrizio Manca, M.D., Servizio di Immunologia, XIII U.S.L., Viale Benedetto XV, 16132 Genova, Italy.

[4] Department of Nephrology.

[5] Department of Surgical Anatomy.

[6] Abbreviations used: CsA, cyclosporine; EBV, Epstein-Barr virus; FCS, fetal calf serum; ID50, dose of CsA inhibiting 50% of the response; MLR, mixed lymphocyte culture; PBL, peripheral blood lymphocytes; PHA, phytohemagglutinin.

MATERIALS AND METHODS

Media. RPMI 1640 (Flow Laboratories) was supplemented with penicillin 100 U/ml, streptomycin 100 μg/ml, L-glutamine 10 mM, Hepes 10 mM, 2-mercaptoethanol 5×10^{-5}M and 5% fetal calf serum (FCS, Sterile System, Logan, Utah; lot. 100360). CsA, kindly provided by Sandoz (Basel), was dissolved in ethanol-Tween 80 20% at 10 mg/ml and diluted to 1 mg/ml in RPMI to obtain a stock solution.

Lymphoblastoid lines. The lines were generated by transformation with Epstein-Barr Virus (EBV) as previously described (*11*). The cells were maintained in complete medium containing 10% FCS. When used as stimulators the cells were irradiated with 5000 rads from a ^{137}Cs source (Atomic Energy of Canada).

Preparation of human interleukin-2 (IL-2). IL-2-containing supernatant (IL-2) was generated by culturing human lymphocytes from normal spleens obtained at surgery in complete RPMI medium at 2×10^6/ml in the presence of PHA-P (Difco) at 10 μg/ml for 48 hr. The cells were spun down and the clear supernatant was stored at 4°C. After titration on the IL-2-dependent murine line CTLL and on human IL-2 dependent lines the supernatant was used at 10% final concentration.

Alloreactive lines. Peripheral blood lymphocytes (PBL) were obtained by Ficoll gradient centrifugation of heparanized blood samples from uremic patients and from normal individuals. Then 10^6 cells were cultured in 1.5 ml medium in 24-well plates (Costar) along with 4×10^5 irradiated stimulator cells. This is a simple procedure for the generation of T lines that recognize class II determinants (*12*). Eight days later each culture was split into four wells and IL-2-containing supernatant at 10% final concentration was added. Five to eight days later the cells showed a vigorous growth, and 2×10^5 viable cells were restimulated with an equal number of the same irradiated lymphoblastoid cells. The established lines were maintained by weekly restimulation in the absence of exogenous IL-2. The lines are designated with the first initial of the responder and the first initial of the stimulator.

Clones were obtained by limiting dilution at 1 or 0.5 cells/well, plus IL-2 and 10^4 unrelated irradiated PBL as the feeder in 96-well flat-bottomed microtiter plates. The positive wells

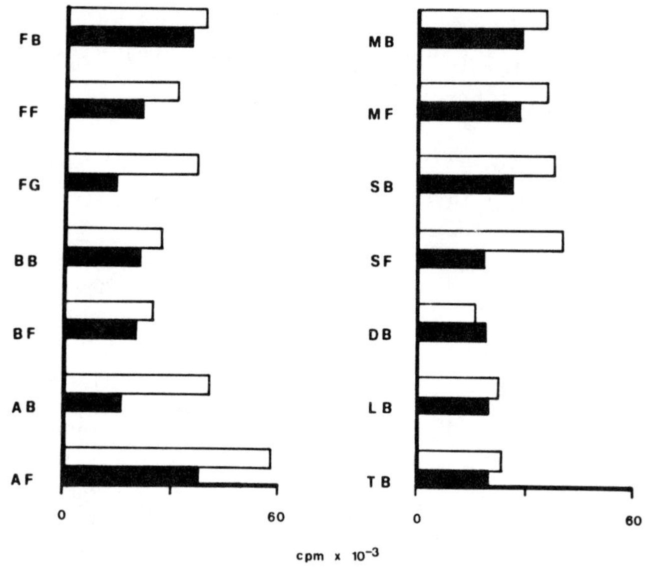

FIGURE 1. Proliferative response of alloreactive lines in the presence of the irradiated stimulator lymphoblastoid cells used for their generation (open bars) and in the presence of optimal amounts of IL-2 (full bars). The lines are indicated with the first initial of the responder and of the stimulator. F (HLA A2, x; B5, 7; DR2, x) and B are normal individuals; A (HLA A2, w19; Bw35, 12), M (HLA A2, 3; Bw21, w53), S, D (HLA A9, 11; Bw35, 27), L (HLA A2, 3; B12, 40; DR7, w6), and T are uremic patients. It can be seen that the specific stimulus is more effective than the lymphokine for most of the lines.

were expanded and subsequently grown in the absence of exogenous IL-2, as described for the bulk lines.

Proliferation assay. The responder cells (20×10^3) and an equal number of irradiated stimulator cells (the same lymphoblastoid line used for the generation and the maintenance of the alloreactive line) were cultured in flat-bottomed microtiter plates for 48 hr, pulsed with 0.5 μCi ^{3}H-thymidine (Amersham, 5 Ci/mmol) and harvested 12 hr later. Incorporated thymidine was measured in a liquid scintillation counter (LKB Wallac).

RESULTS

Proliferative response to alloreactive lines. Alloreactive lines were generated from normal individuals and uremic patients. Figure 1 depicts the proliferation of different lines in the presence of stimulator cells or IL-2. Responders F and B are normal individuals; A, M, S, D, L, and T are uremic patients. It is evident that optimal stimulation for most of the lines was achieved in the presence of the irradiated stimulator rather than in the presence of exogenous IL-2 and that alloreactive lines can be generated from uremic patients as well as from normal controls.

It should be noted that with both F and B as responders a vigorous proliferation is also obtained with autologous transformed cells as stimulators. This fact does not necessarily imply that the response to lymphoblastoid lines is not specific. It rather indicates that EBV-transformed cells are effective stimulators of alloreactive and autoreactive clones. Similar results, in fact, can be obtained by using T cell lines established and

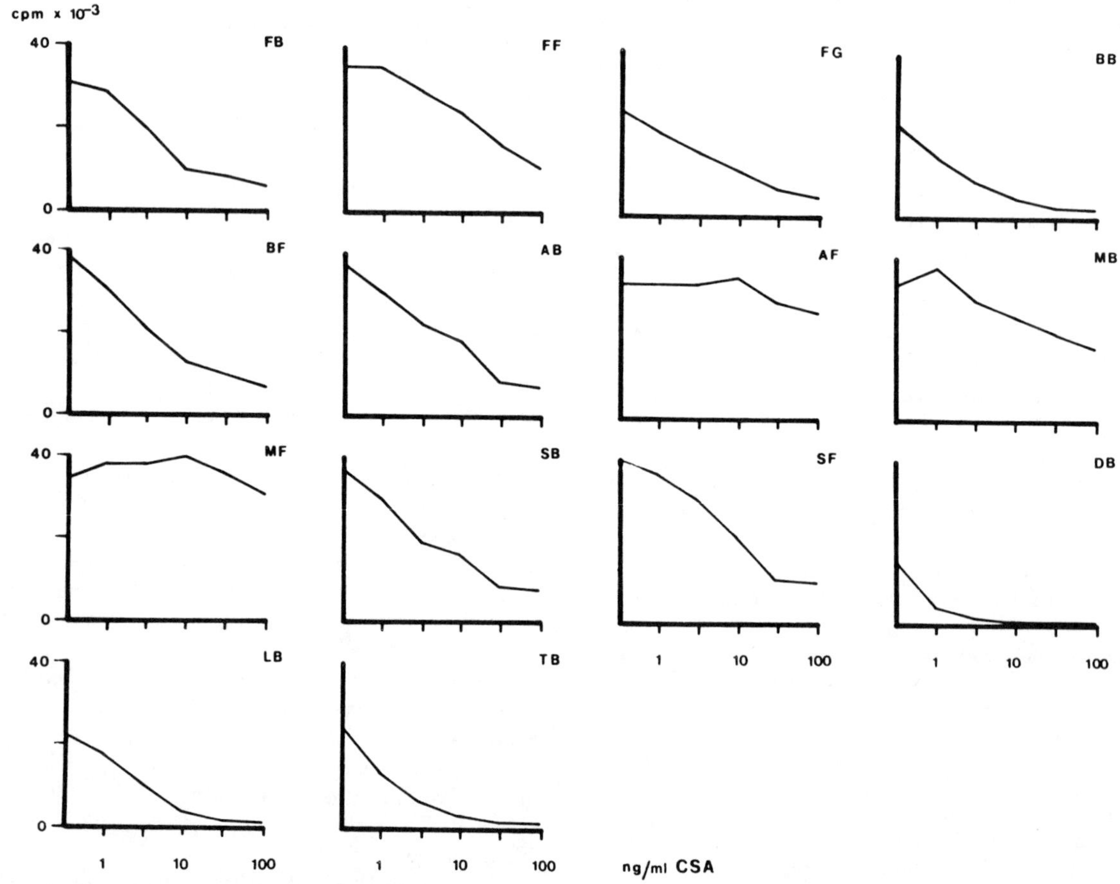

FIGURE 2. The alloreactive lines were stimulated with the corresponding irradiated lymphoblastoid lines in the presence of various amounts of CsA. Inhibition of thymidine uptake was measured. CsA concentration ranged from 0 to 100 ng/ml. Different inhibition curves were obtained. The dose of CsA yielding 50% inhibition (ID 50) is reported in Table 1.

maintained by using irradiated PBL as stimulators (Manca et al. manuscript in preparation).

CsA sensitivity of alloreactive lines. Figure 2 shows a titration of CsA on 14 alloreactive lines from 6 individuals. The lines show an impressive range of patterns of individual sensitivity. Table 1 summarizes the sensitivity of the different lines as the dose of CsA required to inhibit 50% of the maximal proliferative response (ID 50). ID 50 ranges from 0.6 to >100 ng/ml CsA. Maximal proliferation does not correlate with ID 50 (r=0.0825).

CsA sensitivity of alloreactive clones. We then asked the question whether the difference in sensitivity of the alloreactive lines was homogenously distributed among the clones or the resistant lines included only a fraction of clones with a markedly higher resistance.

Two lines generated from the same individual against two different lymphoblastoid lines, although extensively crossreactive, displayed a different sensitivity to the drug (lines FB and FP, Fig. 3). Both lines were subsequently cloned by limiting dilution, and the individual clones that could be expanded were tested for sensitivity to CsA. All of the clones from the FB line displayed a similar inhibition pattern in the presence of various concentrations of CsA (Table 2). On the contrary, whereas 18 of 20 clones from line FP showed an average sensitivity to CsA, 2 clones exhibited a higher resistance. The distribution analysis of the two families shows a mode of ID 50 equal to 2 ng/ml in the FB family, corresponding to the sensitivity of the bulk line, and a mode of 8 ng/ml in the FP family, which is not very different from the value of 10 for the FP bulk line. In the latter group, however, two outstanding clones are highly resistant with an ID 50 greater than 100 ng/ml.

Comparison of sensitive and resistant clones. We then compared the behavior of a "sensitive" (FP 12) and a "resistant" clone (FP 16) by measuring their proliferative response to IL-2 and to the allogeneic stimulus, as well as the CsA-induced inhibition of alloantigen-dependent proliferation and IL-2 production. It can be seen in Figure 4, panels a and b, that sensitivity to IL-2 and to different amounts of stimulator cells does not differ between the two clones. On the contrary the sensitivity to CsA of antigen-induced IL-2 production (panel c) and the proliferative response (panel d) differ between the two clones. A 50% inhibition of IL-2 production measured as thymidine incorporation by the CTLL lines is inducd by 3 ng/ml CsA on clone FP 12 and 0.5 ng/ml CsA on clone FP 16.

TABLE 1. ID 50 of CsA of different alloreactive lines[a]

Line	Maximal proliferation (cpm×10^{-3})	ID 50 (ng/ml CsA)
FB	31	5.5
FF	35	25
FG	26	6
BB	23	2
BF	39	3
AB	37	7
AF	33	>100
MB	33	65
MF	35	>100
SB	37	10
SF	40	10
DB	16	0.6
LB	23	2.4
TB	25	1

[a] The maximal proliferative response in the absence of CsA and the dose of CsA yielding 50% inhibition (ID 50) as obtained from the titration curves shown in Figure 2 are reported. No correlation was seen between the two parameters considered ($r = 0.0825$).

DISCUSSION

The results presented in this article can be summarized as follows:

(1) Alloreactive lines can be generated from uremic patients as well as from normal individuals.

(2) Differences in sensitivity to CsA were found in these lines irrespective of the individual from whom they were derived and of the stimulator line.

(3) Clones obtained from a "resistant" line also show heter-

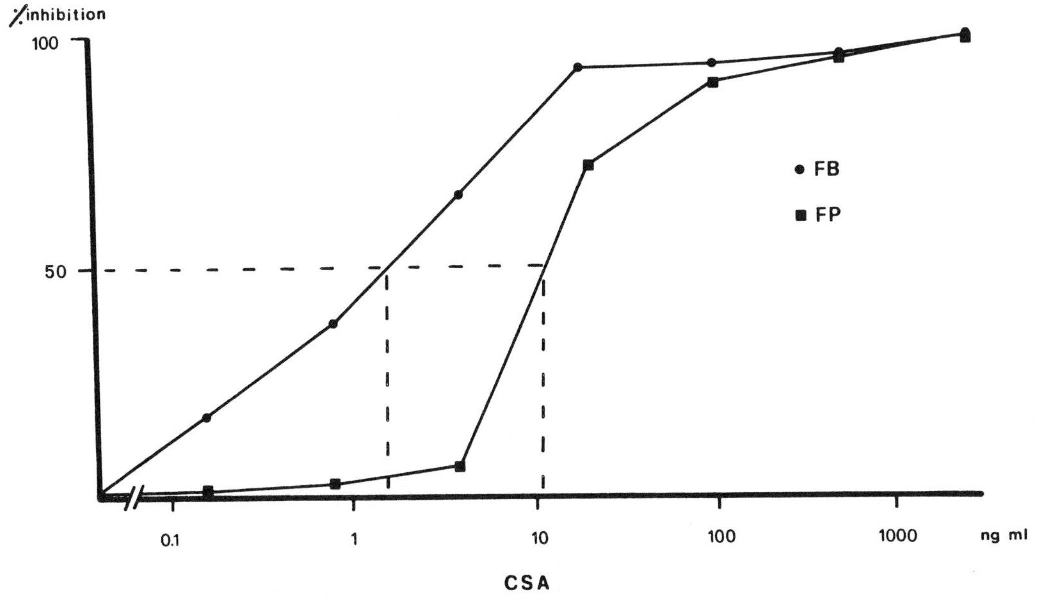

FIGURE 3. Two lines generated by stimulating responder F with lymphoblastoid lines B and P were selected for different sensitivity to CsA and cloned by limiting dilution. Fluctuations in ID 50 were seen in different experiments and thus comparison of different lines and clones was always done within the same experiment.

ogeneity: a minority are resistant to the drug while most are sensitive.

The first point suggests that the well-known condition of immunodepression of uremic patients can be overcome when the cells are maintained in vitro by repeated stimulation with allogeneic cells. The second and third observations indicate that the concept of CsA resistance cannot be applied at the individual level, but refers only to the family of clones capable of responding to a given antigen (in the case of organ transplantation the oligoclonal alloreactive response to the relevant donor). In this context, resistance and sensitivity to CsA could probably be best defined in terms of the proportion of resistant clones during the antiallograft response. The presence of CsA-resistant clones has already been recently reported in a murine system in which the development of cytotoxic clones from resting precursors is examined in vitro (*13*). A minority of the clones, in fact, is resistant to 100 ng/ml CsA chosen as the cut-off dose.

We should also consider that, as in the case of mutant bacteria resistant to a given antibiotic, in the presence of the immunosuppressive drug the few resistant clones may be selected for thanks to their selective advantage over the sensitive ones. Thus a CsA-resistant immune response may eventually result. An adaptation of the concept of phenotypic variations of bacteria stemming from random changes in the genetic material (*14*) to the area of cancer chemotherapy and drug resistance has been recently proposed (*15*). On the other hand we do not know whether the tempting similarity between drug resistance induced in bacteria and detected in immunocompetent clones indicates a comparable underlying genetic mechanism. This possibility will be tested in vitro by using increasing amounts of CsA in the culture medium of stimulated T lines to select for the resistant clones.

It is well known that CsA preferentially affects cell types with defined functions, such as helper and interleukin-producing cells. Thus we can expect that the clones differing in

TABLE 2. Clonal variability of CsA sensitivity[a]

Clones from line FB	ID 50	Clones from line FP	ID 50
1	2.5	1	6
3	4	2	>100
7	2	3	8
9	4	9	17
14	2.5	12	4
17	2	13	9
21	2	14	2.5
22	3	15	13
FB bulk	2	16	>100
		17	8
		18	15
		20	7
		21	11
		22	14
		23	8
		FP bulk	10

[a] The alloreactive lines FB and FP were cloned by limiting dilution and the clones that could be expanded were tested for CsA sensitivity. The different inhibition patterns obtained from the titration curves of CsA on each individual clone stimulated with the corresponding lymphoblastoid line are given as ID 50.

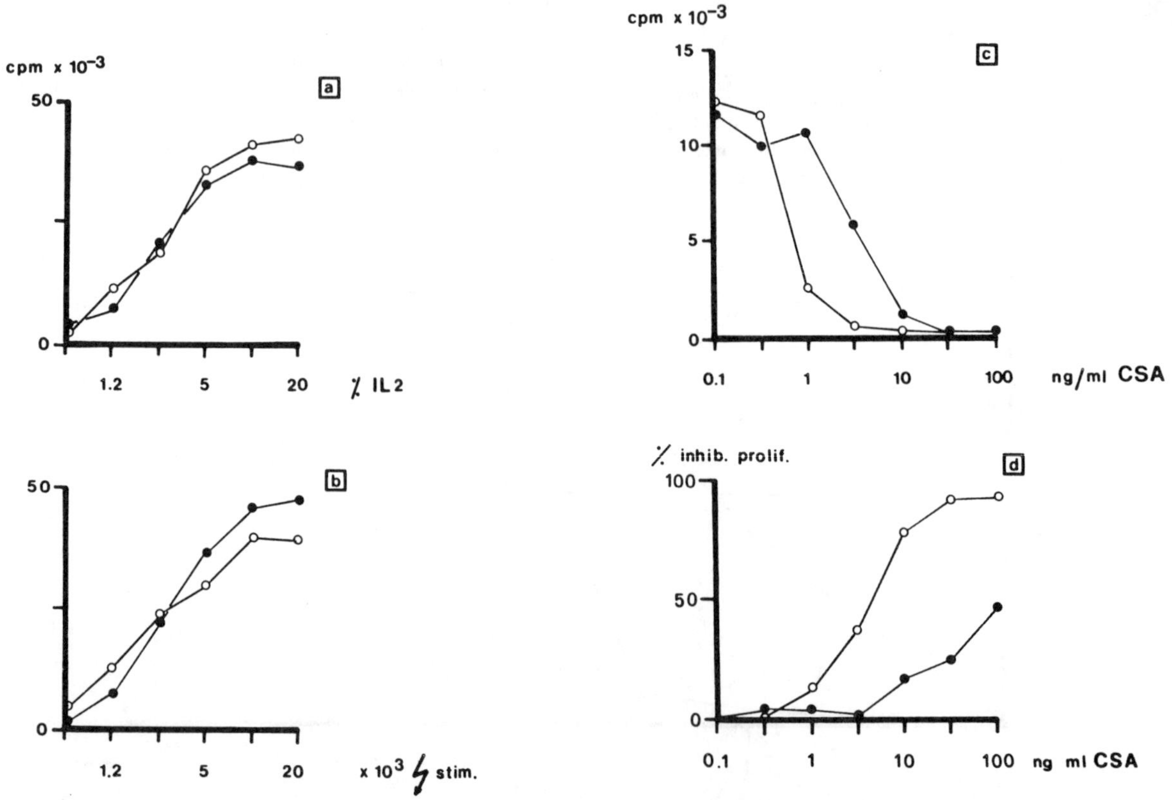

FIGURE 4. Two clones generated from line FP, representative of the sensitive (FP.12) (●——●) and of the resistant (FP.16) (○——○) families were further analyzed for sensitivity to IL-2 (panel a) and to the alloreactive stimulus (panel b), for inhibition of IL-2 production (panel c), and for proliferation following allostimulation (panel d) in the presence of different amounts of CsA. IL-2 production was measured by adding the 48-hr culture supernatants at 25% final concentration to 10^4 CTLL cells in flat-bottomed microtiter plates. Thymidine incorporation was measured 24 hr later after 4 hr of pulsing.

sensitivity also differ from a functional and phenotypic point of view. Work is in progress to ascertain whether this is the case. The demonstration that drug sensitivity can correlate with a given phenotype might account for the difference in sensitivity we observed both at the clonal and at the bulk line level. Clones differing in sensitivity to CsA also allow to test a possible correlation with T cell receptor avidity for antigen either for proliferating or for cytotoxic cells and drug sensitivity. A point that has both theoretical and practical implications is whether the clones resistant to a given drug are homogeneously distributed among the various oligoclonal alloreactive families of the same individual. If this were the case the analysis at the clonal level of a test alloreactive response in a prospective graft recipient could yield valuable information on possible postgraft behavior and help the clinicians to select the immunosuppressive treatment of choice. the long term follow-up of these lines in the absence of CsA will allow us to detect whether a drift in sensitivity to the drug spontaneously occurs or whether the selective pressure of the drug is required.

REFERENCES

1. White DJG, Calne RY. The use of Cyclosporin A immunosuppression in organ grafting. Immunol Rev 1982; 65: 115.
2. The Canadian Multicentre Transplant Study Group. A randomized clinical trial of Cyclosporine in cadaveric renal transplantation. N Engl J Med 1983; 309: 811.
3. European Multicentric Trial Group. Lancet 1983; 2: 986.
4. Thiel G, Harder F, Loertscher R, Brünisholz M, Landmann J, Brunner F, Follat F, Wenk M, Mihatsch M. Cyclosporine alone or in combination with prednisone in cadaveric renal transplantation. Transplant Proc 1984; 5: 1187.
5. Sells RA. A prospective randomized substitutive trial of Cyclosporine as a prophylactic agent in human renal transplant rejection. Transplant Proc 1983; 4: 2495.
6. Morris PJ, French ME, Dunnil MS, Hunnisett AGW, Ting A, Thompson JF, Wood RFM. A controlled trial of Cyclosporine in renal transplantation with conversion to azathioprine and prednisolone after three months. Transplantation 1983; 36: 273.
7. Kahan BD, Van Buren CT, Flechner SM, Payne WD, Boileau M, Kerman RH. Cyclosporine immunosuppression mitigates immunologic risk factors in renal allotransplantation. Transplant Proc 1983; 4(suppl 1): 2469.
8. Van Buren CT, Flechner SM, Kerman RH, Vaughn W, Kahan BD. Cyclosporine improves outcome in high-risk cadaveric renal allograft recipients. Transplant Proc 1984; 5: 1162.
9. Gardner B, Harris KR, Tate DG, Digard NJ, Gosling DC, Searle M, Slapak M. The effect of pretransplant blood transfusions on renal allograft survival in patients on Cyclosporine. Transplant Proc 1984; 5: 1172.
10. Manca F, Carozzi S, Kunkl A, Barocci S, Valante U, Fontana I, Celada F. Individual sensitivity to Cyclosporine in vitro can be detected in kidney failure patients. Transplant Proc 1985; 17: 1265.
11. Bird AG, McLachlan SM, Britton S. Cyclosporin A promotes spontaneous outgrow in vitro of Epstein-Barr virus-induced B cells lines. Nature 1981; 289: 300.
12. DeMars R, Chang CC, Shaw S, Reitnauer PJ, Sondel PM. Homozygous deletions that simultaneously eliminate expressions of class I and class II antigens of EBV-transformed B lymphoblastoid cells. I. Reduced proliferative responses of autologous and allogeneic T cells to mutant cells that have decreased expression of class II antigens. Hum Immunol 1984; 11: 77.
13. Heeg K, Deusch K, Solbach M, Bunjes D, Wagner H. Frequency analysis of Cyclosporine-sensitive cytotoxic lymphocyte precursors. Transplantation 1984; 38: 532.
14. Luria SE, Delbruck M. Mutations of bacteria from virus sensitivity to virus resistance. Genetics 1943; 28: 491.
15. Goldie JH, Coldman AJ, Gudauskas GA. Rationale for the use of alternating non-cross resistant chemotherapy. Cancer Treat Rep 1982; 66: 439.

Received 5 March 1985.
Accepted 23 May 1985.

0041-1337/86/4102-0204$02.00/0
TRANSPLANTATION

Vol. 41, No. 2
Printed in U.S.A.

ALTERED PATTERNS OF ORGAN DISTRIBUTION OF AUTOLOGOUS AND GRAFTED BLOOD CELLS IN MICE TREATED WITH HYDROXYUREA

MARTINE LÉVY[1]

Unité d'Immunobiologie, Institut Pasteur, 75724 Paris Cédex 15, France

Migration and distribution of lymphocytes and red blood cells were profoundly altered in C57BL/6 mice treated with the anti-mitotic drug hydroxyurea (HU). HU treatment given twice daily for four consecutive days, markedly reduced the population of nucleated cells in the spleen and bone marrow; the numbers of nucleated cells in spleen and bone marrow were reduced to 20% and 10% of normal values, respectively. Paradoxically, in the bone marrow of HU-treated mice, the numbers of mature erythrocytes were increased 8-fold, while in the spleen erythrocyte values were decreased. To explore this altered pattern of red blood cell partition, radiolabeled cells were injected and their migration traced in normal and HU-treated recipients. Both erythrocyte and leukocyte populations were observed to migrate preferentially to the bone marrow of HU-treated animals. The altered pattern of blood cell partition in the bone marrow could be explained by the induction of abnormal permeability of the bone marrow-blood barrier by the antimitotic drug. This point may be of importance when considering clinical bone marrow transplantation. It stresses the need for antimitotic treatment before grafting individuals with hemopoietic precursors.

It is generally accepted that hemopoiesis in adult mammals occurs in bone marrow, where pluripotent stem cells develop into committed stem cells that give rise to all types of terminally differentiated blood cells (*1*). All blood cells have limited life spans, consequently newly arising differentiated cells must be continuously produced throughout life to keep peripheral cell numbers in a steady state. It has, in fact, been established that very important renewal rates are observed in normal conditions, and in response to particular requirements of the organism (*2–4*). Entry of cells into the circulation requires transit through the marrow sinus wall (*5–8*). The factors controlling this transit of cells are incompletely understood, but it is likely that they involve specific interactions and properties of both the migrating cells themselves and the sinus wall (*9–11*).

I report here observations indicating that migration and distribution of lymphocytes and red blood cells are profoundly altered in mice treated with the antimitotic drug hydroxyurea. This finding may be of importance to consider when grafting hemopoietic precursors into individuals submitted to chemotherapy.

MATERIALS AND METHODS

Mice. Mice of the C57BL/6 strain bred at the Pasteur Institute were used between 10 and 14 weeks of age.

Drug treatment. Hydroxyurea (HU,[2] SIGMA, St Louis, MO) was dissolved in NaCl 0.9% and administered i.p. according to Hodgson et al. (*12*): two doses of 1 mg/g body weight of hydroxyurea were injected 7 hr apart. Mice received two doses of HU per day for 4 consecutive days.

Cell suspensions. Spleen cell suspensions were prepared by passing the spleen through a 200-mesh stainless steel screen. Bone marrow cells were collected by cutting the ends of the femurs and by flushing the marrow cavity with 5 ml of balanced salt solution (BSS) from a syringe equipped with a 26 G×0.45 needle. Cell clumps were dissociated by repeated pipetting with a 10-ml plastic pipette (Falcon, Division of Becton, Dickinson and Co., MD) 10 times, the cells were washed twice in BSS, and viability assessed by trypan blue exclusion.

Immunofluorescence. Immunofluorescence was performed using procedures previously described in detail (*13*). B cells were identified with a rhodamine-labeled rabbit antimouse μ antibody or a fluorescein-labeled polyvalent rabbit antimouse Ig. T cells were identified with a rat monoclonal antimouse Thy-1 (J1J: μ, κ, a kind gift from Dr. J. Sprent, University of Pennsylvania, Philadelphia, PA) followed by fluorescein-conjugated mouse monoclonal anti-rat κ antibody (MAR 18.5) (*14*). For each determination, at least 200 cells were scored.

Labeling. Mouse red blood cells: C57BL/6 mice were bled into Alsever solution and the blood washed three times in saline. Labeling was performed using ^{51}Cr (sodium chromate, Amersham, UK) at a concentration of 100 μCi/ml of packed red cells for 60 min at 37°C. The blood was then washed three times in BSS and a 25% suspension prepared. Mice were injected i.v. with 200 μl of this suspension (400,000 cpm), and 60 min later recipients were killed and the amount of radioactivity recovered in the spleen and femurs was measured in cell suspensions of these organs.

Lymphocytes: Spleen and bone marrow cell suspensions were labeled with ^{51}Cr after removal of erythrocytes (10 min at 4°C in 0.87% NH_4Cl). Labeling was performed using 50 μCi of ^{51}Cr/10^8 cells, as for red cells, but recipient mice received 100,000 cpm in 200 μl of the lymphocyte suspensions, which corresponds to a range of 1–5×10^6 cells injected per mouse.

RESULTS

Experimental protocol. HU is a drug that kills cells synthesizing DNA (*15, 16*) by inhibiting ribonucleoside phosphate reductase (*17, 18*); it also acts as a synchronizing agent by blocking the passage of G_1 cells into S phase (*19*). It follows that two doses of HU, 7 hr apart, kill all cycling cells in the animal (*12*). Thus, at the time of the first injection all cells in S phase degenerate, but proliferating cells in other phases of

[1]Address correspondence to: Dr. Martine Lévy, Unité d'Immunobiologie, Institut Pasteur, 25 rue du Docteur Roux, 75724 Paris Cédex 15, France.

[2] Abbreviations used: ASAA, acquired severe aplastic anemia; BSS, balanced salt solution; HU, hydroxyurea; Ig: immunoglobulin(s).

the cell cycle continue to accumulate at the G_1/S boundary (*20*). As HU concentrations rapidly drop to ineffective levels, these cells at the G_1/S boundary move into S phase and become vulnerable to the second injection of HU.

This treatment was applied to normal mice for four days, attempting to eliminate proliferating cells in experiments investigating half-lives of B lymphocytes. In the course of these experiments, I observed unusually high concentrations of red cells in bone marrow, so I have investigated cell turnover and migration into different lymphoid organs under these conditions.

Recovery of blood cells after four days of HU treatment in spleen and bone marrow. Mice were injected twice a day on four consecutive days with HU at 1 mg/g body weight, a dose previously established to kill all cycling cells when administered twice with a 7-hr interval (*12*). On the day following the last injection, mice were killed, and the numbers of both nucleated cells and erythrocytes in the spleen and two femurs were evaluated (Table 1). This antimitotic treatment kills over 75% of nucleated cells in spleen, and around 90% in the bone marrow. When the treatment was continued in time, the recovery of nucleated cells in spleen and bone marrow does not drop any further (data not shown).

The numbers of red blood cells recovered were somewhat surprising. In the spleen of HU-treated animals, they were decreased by a factor of 14, while being increased by a factor of 8 in the bone marrow (Table 1). If the bone marrow–spleen ratios of blood cells are compared in normal and HU-treated animals, nucleated cells are somewhat more depleted in marrow (3.9 versus 2.1 ratios for normal and HU-treated animals, respectively), while red cells are far more affected in spleen and actually increased in marrow (1.4 versus 167.0 ratios for normal and HU-treated animals, respectively) (Table 2). The relationship between such bone marrow/spleen ratios gives a striking quantitative demonstration of the differential HU effects in the two cell and organ compartments. Indeed, the ratio of HU/normal is less than one for nucleated cells and more than 100 for erythrocytes (Table 2).

^{51}Cr-labeled exogeneous syngeneic red blood cells showing the same abnormal distribution in HU-treated recipients. Chromium-labeled red blood cells were injected i.v. (400,000 cpm/mouse) to normal and HU-treated mice. Mice were killed 60 min later, and radioactivity in spleen and bone marrow suspensions was counted (Table 3). These results partially reproduce the above observations on the alterations in partition of red blood cells in spleen and bone marrow of normal versus HU-treated animals. If the bone-marrow–to–spleen ratios are again calculated, a value of HU/normal = 16.1 is obtained, showing that exogeneous red blood cells somehow follow the same pattern of partition observed in situ in normal and HU-treated animals. I conclude, therefore, that HU treatment during four consecutive days, leads to an alteration of the bone marrow–blood barrier with an enhanced permeability and abnormal passage of red cells from the blood to the marrow.

Migration of ^{51}-Cr-labeled leukocytes in normal and HU-treated mice. It has previously been shown that HU treatment does not alter lymphocyte migration (*22*). To evaluate the possibility that HU treatment alters bone marrow blood permeability, the same type of migration/homing experiments were performed with leukocytes taken from spleen or bone marrow. In this case, however, I compared the homing in normal or HU-treated recipients of leukocytes obtained from normal and HU-treated donors. The results obtained are presented in Table 4. The recovery of grafted normal spleen cells in the spleen of HU-treated recipients was roughly 10 times lower than that obtained in normal recipients. Lower spleen homing in HU-treated animals is also observed with spleen cells recovered from HU-treated donors. In contrast to spleen, bone marrow of HU-treated animals seems to be more "permeable" to the entrance of transfused cells, because 3–4 times more counts are recovered in the marrow of such recipients, whether the injected cells are spleen or bone marrow cells from normal or HU-treated donors. It appears, therefore, that HU treatment alters local conditions in bone marrow and allows for a higher migration and "homing" of circulating cells into this organ. This effect could explain the decrease in spleen "homing" observed in HU-treated animals as a secondary effect. On the other hand, HU does not appear to significantly alter the pattern of migration of cells recovered from treated donors. Thus, as shown in Table 4, both spleen and bone marrow cells from HU-treated donors follows the same pattern of migration into bone marrow as cells recovered from untreated donors, while their homing in spleen is only slightly decreased. Hemopoietic cell grafts are often performed in allogeneic combinations, so I have also assessed the influence of histocompatibility differences in localization of spleen cells in HU-treated versus normal recipients. No significant differences between the migration of syn-

TABLE 1. Blood cell concentrations in spleen and bone marrow of normal and HU-treated C57BL/6 mice[a]

Organ	HU treatment	Nucleated cells/organ	Red blood cells/organ
Spleen	−	77.4×10^6 (×/÷1.1)	8.2×10^6 (×/÷1.1)
	+	17.2×10^6 (×/÷1.0)	5.7×10^6 (×/÷1.5)
Bone marrow	−	19.2×10^6/femur (×/÷1.2) 304.7×10^6/total bone marrow	7.6×10^6/femur (×/÷1.3) 120.6×10^6/total bone marrow
	+	2.3×10^6/femur (×/÷1.2) 36.5×10^6/total bone marrow	60.0×10^6/femur (×/÷1.3) 952.2×10^6/total bone marrow

[a] C57BL/6 mice (14 weeks old) were injected twice a day for 4 consecutive days with HU (1 mg/g body weight per injection) or saline. The day following the last injection, viable nucleated cells were counted using the trypan blue exclusion method. Each value represents the geometric mean of results obtained in 5 mice. The standard deviations of the mean are given in brackets. The number of cells per total bone marrow has been calculated to be 15.87 times the number of cells in a single femur using a conversion factor according to Benner et al. (*21*).

TABLE 2. Bone marrow to spleen ratios of different blood cells in normal and HU-treated C57BL/6 mice[a]

	Nucleated cells	Red blood cells
Untreated mice	$\frac{304.7\times10^6}{77.4\times10^6} = 3.93$	$\frac{120.6\times10^6}{82.1\times10^6} = 1.46$
HU-treated mice	$\frac{36.5\times10^6}{17.1\times10^6} = 2.13$	$\frac{952.2\times10^6}{5.7\times10^6} = 167.05$
$\frac{HU}{N}$	0.54	114.41

[a] Bone marrow:spleen ratios were calculated using results given in Table 1. HU = treatment described in Table 1; N = normal untreated mice.

TABLE 3. Recovery of radioactivity in different lymphoid organs of normal and HU-treated C57BL/6 mice injected with ^{51}Cr-labeled syngeneic mouse red blood cells[a]

Organ	HU treatment	Counts recovered per organ (in cpm)	% Recovery of the injected radioactive dose	Bone marrow: spleen ratios
Spleen	−	10,975 ($\times\!\!/\!\div$ 1.2)	2.7	1.09
Bone marrow	−	12,019 ($\times\!\!/\!\div$ 1.1)	3.0	
Spleen	+	4034 ($\times\!\!/\!\div$ 2.9)	1.0	17.57
Bone marrow	+	70,872 ($\times\!\!/\!\div$ 1.1)	17.7	

[a] C57BL/6 mice (13 weeks old) were treated as in Table 1, and on the day following the last injection, they were injected i.v. with ^{51}Cr-labeled red blood cells (400,000 cpm per mouse); 60 min later, spleen and bone marrow cell suspensions were prepared and the amount of radioactivity in these suspensions was determined. Each value represents the geometric mean of results obtained in 5 mice. The standard deviations of the mean are given in brackets. Radioactivity recovered in total bone marrow is calculated from one femur using 15.87 as the conversion factor (see Table 1 and the *Materials and Methods* section for details).

TABLE 4. Recovery of radioactivity in spleen and bone marrow of normal and HU-treated C57BL/6 mice injected with different sources of ^{51}Cr-labeled leukocytes[a]

Origin of ^{51}Cr-labeled injected cells	HU treatment: Donor	HU treatment: C57BL/6 recipient	% Recovery of the injected radioactive dose: Spleen	% Recovery of the injected radioactive dose: Total bone marrow
C57BL/6 spleen	−	−	17.8	4.1
		+	2.6	12.2
	+	−	10.1	4.3
		+	2.1	7.7
C57BL/6 bone marrow	−	−	8.1	3.9
		+	1.0	12.4
	+	−	17.6	4.6
		+	3.0	18.4
BALB/c spleen	−	−	21.5	5.2
		+	2.2	19.5

[a] The protocol is the same as in Tables 1 and 3, except that mice were injected with ^{51}Cr-labeled erythrocyte-depleted spleen or bone marrow cells (100,000 cpm per mouse) obtained from different sources as indicated. The amount of radioactivity is expressed as the percentage of the total cellular radioactivity injected.

geneic and allogeneic cells into spleen and bone marrow could be detected (Table 4). Again, however, HU treatment of recipients does result in a sharp decrease in spleen recoveries and in augmentation in bone marrow migration.

Cellular composition of blood in normal and HU-treated animals. To determine whether these modifications in the distribution of blood cells in the various lymphoid organs were secondary to an altered representation of the different cell types in blood, blood cell counts were perfomed in normal and HU-treated animals. Table 5 shows results of T and B lymphocyte counts determined by immunofluorescence techniques, as well as the enumeration of red and white cells in circulation. The concentration of white cells in the blood of HU-treated mice was altered to the same extent as in the spleen (as shown in Table 5, 20% of normal white blood cell counts were recovered in treated animals). The proportion of B lymphocytes in the blood is not altered, and there is only a slight increase in the relative proportion of circulating T cells. Surprisingly, HU-treated mice do not show any significant difference in the concentration of red blood cells when compared with normal mice. Although these results may be the consequence of a modification in the plasma volume, they still indicate that the circulating compartment may be the most tightly regulated, and demonstrate that homing and cell distribution alterations are not the consequence of abnormal cell composition in blood.

TABLE 5. Enumeration of cell components in blood of normal and HU-treated C57BL/6 mice[a]

HU treatment	Blood counts: Red cells	White cells	Ig^+ cells[b]	IgM^+ cells[b]	Thy-1^+ cells[b]
−	$10.7\times10^6/mm^3$ (±0.29)	$7.43\times10^3/mm^3$ (±1.37)	30%	28%	48%
+	$9.9\times10^6/mm^3$ (±0.78)	$1.60\times10^3/mm^3$ (±0.14)	31%	ND	65%

[a] Five animals were used per group. Red cells were enumerated after dilution of blood in a Potin pipet, white cells after red cell lysis in 2% acetic acid. Percentages of Ig^+ or Thy-1^+ cells were determined using immunofluorescence methods (for details, see the *Materials* and *Methods* section). Arithmetic means were calculated, and standard deviations are given in brackets.

[b] Expressed as percentage of total white cell counts.

DISCUSSION

The experiments reported here describe the distribution and migration of blood cells after prolonged HU treatment. Two doses of HU, 7 hr apart, given four times to normal female C57BL/6 mice on consecutive days markedly reduced the population of nucleated cells in the blood, spleen, and bone marrow. Only 20–30% of blood or spleen cells and 10% of bone marrow cells were recovered after this protocol of in vivo treatment with HU. This depletion in the spleen reflects not only the killing of cells dividing in the organ, but primarily the absence of replenishment by newly formed cells arising from the precursor pool in the bone marrow that is necessary to substitute the rapidly decaying peripheral compartments (*22–24*).

The altered pattern of partition of red blood cells is not likely to result directly from the killing of erythrocyte progenitors, which are known to be actively proliferating in normal mice (*20*). As a matter of fact, the mean lifespan of mouse red cells was determined, using ^{14}C-labeled glycine as hemoglobin precursor or other methods, to be between 40 and 43 days (*25, 26*). Therefore, the killing of cycling precursor cells for 4–5 days should not affect the total number of red cells in the organism—consequently, alterations in their partition cannot be a side effect of red cell depletion. Indeed, mice treated with this protocol of HU injections do not show any significant differences in their red blood cell concentrations in the circulation (Table 5). This is in agreeement with the findings of Hodgson et al., who have previously reported that the packed red blood cell volume was not significantly affected by two doses of HU (*12*). It is, of course, very difficult to calculate from these data the total number of erythrocytes in the whole body of the animal. The difference in partition of red cells, particularly in the bone marrow, could be explained in one of several different ways, or by a combination of them.

Enhancement of erythropoiesis. Although dividing erythrocyte progenitors in the bone marrow were killed, some late precursors, at a stage of differentiation when no division is required, could actually be activated by this treatment. In fact, several authors have reported normal numbers of erythropoietin-sensitive cells on the first day after HU-treatment (*27*) and a rapid HU-dependent enhancement of preferential marrow differentiation into the erythroid line (*28–30*). This first possibility can be excluded because it cannot entirely explain the distribution pattern of exogeneously infused labeled red blood cells.

Infection. A major portion of the increase of red cells in the bone marrow may be due to abnormal migration of these cells from the vasculature to the marrow tissue. Infection of these animals as a consequence of the granulocytopenia (*12*) could be a factor contributing to this unexpected migration into the marrow. Again, this argument cannot explain the migration of labeled exogeneous red blood cells.

Free bone marrow space. In normal conditions, 85–95% of the available marrow space is occupied with hemopoietic cells, one-third of which are erythrocyte precursors, and two-thirds of which are white blood cell precursors (*31, 32*). The tremendous drop in numbers of nucleated cells in the bone marrow of HU-treated animals (10% of normal counts, compare with Table 1) leaves free the majority of extravascular space in the organ. It could then be argued that the higher blood cell concentration in the femoral shaft is due to an expansion of vascular sinuses in order to compensate for the relative "emptiness" of the extravascular space, with a consequent greater blood volume per shaft. By comparing the relative distributions of T and B lymphocytes in the circulating pool and in the femoral shaft, there is no doubt that this possibility alone cannot account for the present results. As a matter of fact, T cells go from 1% in normal marrow up to 40% in the bone marrow of HU-treated mice, which corresponds roughly to 1×10^6 T cells per femur in treated mice (manuscript submitted for publication). From Table 5 it can be calculated that around 1000 T cells are present in 1 μl of blood. As the femoral vascular volume has been evaluated to be 0.25 μl (Milon G, Marchal G, personal communication), the number of T cells due to the vasculature in the femoral shaft is consequently 250. It is most improbable, if not impossible, that an expansion of the femoral vasculature by itself could account for the present results, since it would require a $10^6/250 = 4000$-fold increase in the volume of the marrow sinusoids.

Alteration of the bone marrow-blood barrier. The wall of vascular sinuses forms an anatomical barrier between the hemopoietic compartment and the circulation. This barrier controls the migration of reticulocytes and other mature cells from the extravascular space into the sinusoids and ensures orderly traffic of newly formed cells in the response to particular requirements of the organism (*5, 6, 33*). The sinusoids of the bone marrow are lined by a simple flattened endothelium having the function of permitting the passage of cells into (or, rarely, out of) the circulation, leading to the assumption that the wall is a dynamic structure (*34*). Moreover, marrow-sinus endothelial cells are incompletely covered on their abluminal surface by adventitial reticular cells, which can be rearranged under certain conditions (*35, 36*). It follows that, in response to agression, blood cells may both enter and leave the marrow, and the relative sizes of the populations migrating in either direction are related to the particular requirement for these cells (*7*). In addition, macrophages abound in the vicinity of the sinus wall. They can phagocytose intact erythroblasts and other cells. Approximately 2% of erythroid cells are normally removed before reaching the circulation (*10*). According to the organism demand, they can form a barrier that modulates the rate of transinal passage of red cells. These perisinal macrophages could also be involved in the modulation of the partition of red cells in the bone marrow. In normal conditions, mature red blood cells live their entire life span in the circulatory space and do not go back to the extravascular space of the bone marrow. This whole process may show considerable variations that could explain the partition of cells observed in the organs of HU-treated mice. Most likely there is abnormal permeability of the bone marrow-blood barrier as a consequence of disappearance of endothelial and rearrangement of adventitial cells. Indeed, endothelial cells could be very active cycling cells—consequently, they would be killed by the HU-treatment, leading to drastic modifications of the traffic through the wall in both directions.

Altered patterns of migration were also observed with spleen and bone marrow cells injected into normal and HU-treated animals. Although these results were limited to a single time-window, the differences in the localization of transfused cells in normal and HU-treated animals are quite obvious.. Thus, whatever the ^{51}Cr-labeled injected cells are (syngeneic or allogeneic spleen cells, syngeneic marrow cells, both recovered from normal or HU-treated animals), the distribution/homing of these cells in HU-treated recipients is changed such that they migrate ten times less into the spleen. On the other hand, the recovery of cells in bone marrow of HU-treated animals is four times higher than that of normal animals (Table 4). This particular point is quite important in connection with clinical bone marrow transplantation. The fact that bone marrow cells localize far more efficiently to the recipient marrow after HU-treatment may be explained by the increased permeability of the blood to the marrow barrier, suggested here for all types of circulating cells, including erythrocytes. As argued above, this increased permeability is likely to be due to a combination of endothelial cell destruction and adventitial cell arrangement by the antimitotic treatment. These results could very well explain the findings of Appelbaum et al. (*37*), who have reported that patients with acquired severe aplastic anemia (ASAA) did not recover following transplantation of syngeneic bone marrow, while, when conditioned with cyclophosphamide, the grafts did readily "take" in the recipients. ASAA is actually the best available model to emphasize the importance of antimitotic treatment before bone marrow transplantation. Thus, because of the absence of underlying malignant or myeloproliferative process, and because of the complete "emptiness" of the marrow, ASAA would not theoretically need any particular immunosuppressive treatment before syngeneic bone marrow transplantation (*38*). This can eliminate the "bone marrow free space" argument in explaining abnormal migration of cells into this organ. The present demonstration of enhanced permeability of the bone marrow–blood barrier after antimitotic treatment most satisfactorily explains these clinical observations and stresses the crucial importance of an antimitotic treatment regimen prior to bone marrow transplantation. In fact, in most other situations where bone marrow transplantation is required, this is currently done, but for reasons other than that indicated here.

Acknowledgments. I thank Antonio Coutinho for helpful discussions and critical reading of the manuscript, Jacqueline Badella for excellent secretarial work, and Odile Burlen for expert technical assistance.

REFERENCES

1. Metcalf D, Moore MAS. Regulation of growth and differentiation in haemopoietic colonies growing in agar. In: Wolstenholme GEW, O'Connor M, eds. Haemopoietic stem cells, Ciba Foundation Symposium. Amsterdam: Elsevier, Associated Scientific Publishers, 1973: 157.
2. Osmond DG, Miller SC, Yoshida Y. Kinetic and haemopoietic properties of lymphoid cells in the bone marrow. In: Wolstenholme GEW, O'Connor M, eds. Haemopoietic stem cells, Ciba Foundation Symposium, Amsterdam: Elsevier, Associated Scientific Publishers, 1973: 131.
3. Osmond DG, Nossal GJV. Differentiation of lymphocytes in mouse bone marrow. II. Kinetics of maturation and renewal of antiglobulin-binding cells studied by double labelling. Cell Immunol 1974; 13: 132.
4. Osmond DG. Generation of B lymphocytes in the bone marrow. In: Cooper M, Mosier DE, Sher I, Vitteta ES, eds. B lymphocytes in the immune response. New York: Elsevier/North Holland, 1979: 63.
5. Weiss L. Transmural cellular passage in vascular sinuses of rat bone marrow. Blood 1970; 36: 189.
6. De Bruyn PPH, Michelson S, Thomas TB. The migration of blood cells of the bone marrow through the sinuosidal wall. J. Morphol 1971; 133: 417.
7. Chen LT, Weiss L. The role of the sinus wall in the passage of erythrocytes through the spleen. Blood 1973; 41: 529.
8. Leblond PF. Etude au microscope électronique à balayage de la migration des cellules sanguines à travers les parois des sinusoides spléniques et médullaires chez la rat. Nouv Rev Fr Hématol 1973; 13: 71.
9. Hudson G, Yoffey JM. The passage of lymphocytes through the sinusoidal endothelium of guinea-pig bone marrow. Proc R Soc Lond [Biol] 1966; 165: 486.
10. Tavassoli M. Bone marrow erythroclasia: the function of perisinal macrophages relative to the uptake of erythroid cells. J Reticuloendothel Soc 1974; 15: 163.
11. Chamberlain JK, Weiss L, Weed RI. Bone marrow sinus cell packing: a determinant of cell release. Blood 1975; 46: 91.
12. Hodgson GS, Bradley TR, Martin RF, Sumner M, Fry P. Recovery of proliferating haemopoietic progenitor cells after killing by hydroxyurea. Cell Tissue Kinet 1975; 8: 51.
13. Forni L. Reagents for immunofluorescence and their use for studying lymphoid cell products. In: Lefkovits I, Pernis B, eds. Immunological methods, vol 1. New York: Academic, 1979: 151.
14. Lanier LL, Gutman GA, Lewis DE, Griswold ST, Warner NL. Monoclonal antibodies against rat immunoglobulin Kappa chains. Hybridoma 1982; 1: 125.
15. Sinclair WK. Hydroxyurea: differential lethal effects on cultured mammalian cells during the cell cycle. Science 1965; 150: 1729.
16. Schwartz HS, Garofalo M, Steinberg SS, Philips FS. Hydroxyurea: inhibition of Deoxyribonucleic acid synthesis in regenerating liver of rats. Cancer Res 1965; 25: 1867.
17. Young CW, Hodas S. Hydroxyurea: inhibitory effect on DNA metabolism. Science 1964; 146: 1172.
18. Skoog L, Nordenskjöld B. Effects of hydroxyurea and 1- -D-arabinofuranosyl cytosine on deoxyribonucleotide pools in mouse embryo cells. Eur J Biochem 1971; 19: 81.
19. Sinclair WK. Hydroxyurea: effects of Chinese hamster cells grown in culture. Cancer Res 1967; 27: 297.
20. Hodgson G, Blackett W. In vivo synchronization of haemopoietic stem cells with hydroxyurea. Exp Hematol 1977; 5: 423.
21. Benner R, Van Oudenaren A, Koch G. Induction of antibody formation in mouse bone marrow. In: Pernis B, Lefkovits I, eds. Immunological methods, vol 2. New York: Academic, 1980: 247.
22. Freitas AA, Rocha B, Forni L, Coutinho A. Population dynamics of B lymphocytes and their precursors: demonstration of high turnover in the central and peripheral lymphoid organs. J Immunol 1982; 128: 54.
23. Freitas AA, Coutinho A. Very rapid decay of mature B lymphocytes in the spleen. J Exp Med 1981; 154: 994.
24. Rocha B, Freitas AA, Coutinho A. Population dynamics of T lymphocytes. Renewal rate and expansion in the peripheral lymphoid organs. J Immunol 1983; 131: 2158.
25. Von Ehrenstein G. The life span of the erythrocytes of normal and of tumour-bearing mice as determined by glycine-2-^{14}C. Acta Physiol Scand 1958; 44: 80.
26. Van Putten LM. The life span of red cells in the rat and the mouse as determined by labeling with DFP^{32} in vivo. Blood 1958; 13: 789.
27. Nečas E, Neuwirt J. Study of the effect of hydroxyurea on the erythropoietin-sensitive cells. Cell Tissue Kinet 1976; 9: 257.
28. Nečas E, Poňka P, Neuwirt J. Changes in stem cell compartments in mice after hydroxyurea. Cell Tissue Kinet 1978; 11: 119.
29. Rencricca NJ, Morse BS, Monette FC, Howard D, Stohlman Jr F. Hydroxyurea-induced erythroid differentiation. Proc Soc Exp Biol Med 1975; 149: 1052.
30. Ebert PS, Wars I, Buell DN. Erythroid differentiation in cultured friend luekemia cells treated with metabolic inhibitors. Cancer Res 1976; 36: 1809.
31. Endicott KM, Gump H. Hemograms and myelograms of healthy female mice of C-57 brown and CFW strains. Blood (special issue) 1947; 1: 61.
32. Brecher G, Endicott KM, Gump H, Brawner HP. Effects of X-ray on lymphoid and haemopoietic tissues of albino mice. Blood 1948; 3: 1259.
33. Campbell FR. Ultrastructural studies of transmural migration of blood cells in the bone marrow of rats, mice and guinea pigs. Am J Anat 1972; 135: 521.
34. Weiss L. The structure of bone marrow. Functional interrelationship of vascular and hematopoietic compartments in experimental hemolytic anemia: an electron-microscopic study. J Morphol 1965; 117: 467.
35. Tavassoli M. Adaptation of marrow sinus wall to fluctuation in the rate of cell delivery: studies in rabbits after blood-letting. Br J Haematol 1977; 35: 15.
36. Tavassoli M. Red cell delivery and the function of the marrow-blood barrier: a review. Exp Hematol 1978; 6: 257.
37. Appelbaum FR, Fefer A, Cheever MA, et al. Treatment of aplastic anemia by bone marrow transplantation in identical twins. Blood 1980; 55: 1033.
38. Lu DP. Syngeneic bone marrow transplantation for treatment of aplastic anaemia; report of a case and review of the literature. Exp Hematol 1981; 9: 257.

Received 4 April 1985.
Accepted 11 June 1985.

0041-1337/86/4102-0209$02.00/0
TRANSPLANTATION
Vol. 41, No. 2

Printed in U.S.A.

ALLOGRAFT REJECTION AND IMMUNE RESPONSES AGAINST ALLOGENEIC ANTIGENS IN NEONATALLY THYMECTOMIZED MICE[1]

KIKUO NOMOTO, HISANORI MAYUMI,[2] KUNISUKE HIMENO, YOSHITSUGU WATANABE, MASAMITSU MITANI, AND NORIAKI TOKUDA

Department of Immunology, Medical Institute of Bioregulation, Kyushu University, Fukuoka 812, Japan

Skin allograft survival and immune responses against allogeneic antigens homologous to skin grafts were observed in BALB/c Cr Slc (BALB)[3] mice (H-2^d) thymectomized at 1 day after birth and grafted with skin from major histocompatibility complex (MHC)-incompatible, fully allogeneic C3H/HeN (C3H) (H-2^k) or MHC-compatible allogeneic DBA/2 Cr Slc (DBA) mice (H-2^d), at 14 weeks of age. In neonatally thymectomized (NTx) BALB mice, survival of C3H skin grafts was not prolonged at all, but survival of DBA skin grafts was prolonged significantly, although the survival periods of DBA skin grafts were very different among individual recipients. In NTx recipients grafted with C3H skin, delayed foot-pad reaction (DFR) was not reduced, but cytotoxic lymphocyte (CTL) activity and cytotoxic antibody (CTAb) production were appreciably depressed. CTL and CTAb were reduced profoundly and consistently in all NTx mice grafted with DBA skin, while DFR was reduced to various degrees in each. The degrees of depression of DFR in these NTx mice correlated well with the prolongation of DBA skin survival, although the sample number was small. The rejection of skin allografts appears to be attributable largely to a T cell subset, the function of which can be expressed as DFR. Thymus dependency in the ontogenic development is low as compared with other T cell subsets.

Effects of neonatal thymectomy (NTx) on allograft rejection were first reported by Miller (*1*) and by Martinez et al. (*2*). They and other authors have reported that NTx animals show acceptance of skin xenografts (*3*), skin allografts (*1–7*), and tumor allografts (*6, 8*). Martinez et al. have shown that early thymectomy serves to depress immunological capacity sufficently to overcome a small histocompatibility difference, but its depressive effect is not enough to overcome the strong difference caused by different H-2 histocompatibility genes (*2*). Miller has also reported that the earlier in life a thymectomy is performed, the less competent is the mouse to reject skin grafts of increasing "foreignness" (*3*)—that is to say, prolongation of survival of skin allografts from MHC-compatible strains can be achieved by NTx more easily than with MHC incompatible strains. Moreover, several immunological parameters—including peripheral lymphocyte counts (*1–3*), sizes, and structures of lymphoid organs (*1, 3, 6*), delayed hypersensitivity (*4*), graft-versus-host reaction (*3, 6, 9*), and antibody production—(*1, 6, 7, 10*) are depressed in NTx animals.

To completely comprehend the immunological status of NTx mice, simultaneous evaluation of multiple parameters—especially for cell mediated immune responses—should be employed, as we have shown in a cyclophosphamide-induced tolerance system reported previously (*11–14*). Shimamoto et al. have compared DFR, CTL, and antibody production in response to chicken erythrocytes (*15*), and have shown that DFR production resists the effects of NTx most strongly. Therefore, we conducted the present study to confirm the effects of NTx on rejection of MHC-compatible and incompatible skin allografts, and to examine the degree of impairment of DFR, CTL, and CTAb against MHC-compatible and incompatible antigens in NTx mice.

In the present study, the prolongation of skin graft survival by NTx correlated well with the degree of impairment of DFR, for which a T cell subset showing a low degree of thymus dependency in its ontogenic development may be responsible.

MATERIALS AND METHODS

Animals. Newborn BALB/c Cr Slc (BALB) (H-2^d) mice bred in the Institute of Experimental Animals, Kyushu University, were operated on and maintained under specific-pathogen-free conditions; all were female. Inbred female mice of C3H/HeN (C3H) (H-2^k) and DBA/2 Cr Slc (DBA) (H-2^d) strains were obtained from the Institute of Experimental Animals, Kyushu University, and the Shizuoka Agricultural Association for Laboratory Animals (Hamamatsu, Japan), respectively. These 8–10-week-old mice were used as donors of skin grafts and spleen cells.

Thymectomy. The thymus of BALB mice was removed 1 day (24–48 h) after birth, as described by Sjodin et al. (*16*). Control mice were sham-operated (sternotomy alone) at the same time. At the beginning of the experiments, the thymectomized and sham-operated female mice were 14 weeks of age. All of the NTx mice were tagged, and the thymus-free state was ascertained macroscopically prior to CTL and CTAb assay. When the thymus was observed macroscopically in the mediastinum, the mice were excluded from all of the assays, including the DFR assay.

Antigenic cells. C3H or DBA spleen cells were used as antigens for elicitation of DFR assay and for i.p. boosting for the

[1] This work was supported by a Grant-in Aid for Scientific Research from Ministry of Education, Science and Culture, Japan.

[2] Address correspondence to: Hisanori Mayumi, M.D., Department of Immunology, Medical Institute of Bioregulation, Kyushu University 69, 3-1-1 Maidashi, Higashi-ku, Fukuoka City, 812, Japan.

[3] Abbreviations used: ANOVA, analysis of variance; BALB, BALB/c Cr Slc; Con A, concanavalin A; CTAb, cytotoxic antibody(ies); CTL, cytotoxic lymphocyte(s); C3H, C3H/HeN; DBA, DBA/2 Cr Slc; DFR, delayed foot-pad reaction; GNA-PEC, glass-nonadherent peritoneal exudate cells; HBSS, Hanks' balanced salt solution; MHC, major histocompatibility complex; MST, mean survival time; NTx, neonatal thymectomy(ized); PEC, peritoneal exudate cells; SD, standard deviation (SD_{n-1}).

CTL assay. DBA spleen cells were also used as s.c. immunizing antigens in some experiments. Spleens were disrupted by pressing them between two glass slides in cold Hanks' balanced salt solution (HBSS). The cell suspension was filtered through cotton gauze and washed twice. C3H or DBA skin grafts were used as immunizing antigens for DFR, CTL, and CTAb assays as described previously (*14*).

Skin grafting. Skin grafting was carried out as previously described (*11–14*). Briefly, full-thickness square grafts, 1 cm × 1 cm, were prepared from trunk skin. Graft beds, 1 cm × 1 cm, were prepared on the right lateral thoracic wall. Grafts were sutured to the graft beds by 8 interrupted sutures. The first inspection of skin grafts was done on the 7th day, followed by daily inspections. The end-point of rejection was judged according to criteria described previously (*14*). In brief, grafts were considered rejected in most cases when they formed a dry scab. In some mice, grafts were estimated to be rejected when all hair was gone from the grafts. Survival was expressed as mean survival time (MST) ±SD (days).

Assay of DFR. Elicitation of DFR was carried out by injecting 0.5 ml of HBSS containing 1×10^7 C3H or DBA spleen cells into the right hind foot-pad of BALB mice 16 days after grafting with C3H or DBA skin. In some experiments, however, BALB mice were immunized s.c. with 1×10^7 DBA spleen cells 51 days after grafting with DBA skin, followed by the elicitation 7 days later, because the end-points of rejection were scattered in a wide range (13–49 days) in the thymectomized group. Swelling was measured at 24 hr and expressed as the mean value of 4–6 mice ±SD (1/10 mm).

Assay of CTL. Boosting for the CTL assay was carried out concomittantly with elicitation for the DFR assay (16 days after skin grafting) in each mouse by injecting 0.2 ml of HBSS containing 1×10^7 C3H or DBA spleen cells into the peritoneal cavity of BALB mice.

In some experiments, BALB mice were immunized with DBA spleen cells, followed by boosting 7 days later. Peritoneal exudate cells (PEC) of 4–6 mice were obtained by washing the peritoneal cavity with 5 ml of HBSS 3 days after i.p. boosting with C3H or DBA spleen cells. Glass-nonadherent (GNA) PEC were obtained from the unfractionated PEC, as described previously (*11–14*), and used as effector cells for the CTL assay. RPMI-1640 (Gibco) supplemented with 5% heat-inactivated fetal calf serum was used as a standard medium for all assays.

C3H or DBA spleen cells incubated with concanavalin A (Con A) (type IV, Sigma Chemical Co., St. Louis, MO) were prepared (5 μg/ml Con A, 5×10^6 cells/ml for 48 hr) and used as target cells.

A standard ^{51}Cr-release assay was used (4 hr at 37°C in a humidified 5% CO_2 incubator) and the percentage of specific lysis was calculated as described elsewhere (*11–14*). Briefly, all assays were carried out in quadruplicate in round-bottomed microtiter plates in a total volume of 0.2 ml. Labeled target cells in 0.1 ml (1×10^4) were added to 0.1 ml (25×10^4 or 50×10^4) effector cells.

The percentage of specific release was calculated as follows:

$$\frac{\text{experimental release} - \text{spontaneous release}}{\text{maximal release} - \text{spontaneous release}} \times 100$$

Maximal release was obtained by adding 0.1 ml 1% Triton X-100 to 0.1 ml of target cells. *Spontaneous release* means the cpm released from target cells incubated with medium alone. All values represent the mean percentage of specific ^{51}Cr-release of quadruplicate samples ±SD.

Assay of CTAb. Sera were collected from 5 or 6 mice in the control groups and pooled when the mice were killed for CTL assay. In NTx groups, however, blood from each mouse was kept separately until confirmation that the mice were thymus-free. The trypan-blue dye exclusion method was employed as described (*11–14*). C3H or DBA Con A blast cells (1×10^6 in 0.1 ml of RPMI) were incubated with the sera (×1, 0.1 ml) and guinea pig complement (×1, 0.1 ml) (Miles Scientific, Naperville, IL) for 30 min at 37°C in a humidified 5% CO_2 incubator. Live Con A blasts were isolated by using Ficoll-Hypague separation (Litton Bionetics, Kensington, MD) before use for this assay.

The percentage of dead cells was calculated as follows:

$$\frac{\text{dead cell count} - \text{total cell count} \times \text{rate of spontaneous cell death}}{\text{total cell count} - \text{total cell count} \times \text{rate of spontaneous cell death}} \times 100$$

The rate of spontaneous cell death was the dead cell count divided by the total cell count in the target cells incubated with the medium (0.1 ml) and complement (×1, 0.1 ml). Usually 200–300 cells were counted as the total cell number. This procedure was repeated twice for each group and the percentage of dead cells was expressed as the mean value ±SD.

Statistics. Group data in each experiment were compared by the analysis of variance (ANOVA) and conventional Student's *t* test. A *P* value of less than 0.05 was taken as significant.

TABLE 1. Skin allograft survival in NTx BALB (H-2^d) mice

Group	NTx	Donor of skin graft	No. mice	Skin graft survival[a]	MST±SD (days)
1	−	C3H(H-2^k)	6	9, 9, 9, 10, 10, 11	9.7±0.8
2	+	C3H(H-2^k)	5	8, 9, 9, 10, 11	9.4±1.1[b]
3	−	DBA(H-2^d)	6	11, 11, 11, 11, 12, 12	11.3±0.5
4-a	+	DBA(H-2^d)	4	13, 14, 14, 16	14.3±1.3[c]
4-b	+	DBA(H-2^d)	4	18[e], 18[f], 26[g], 49[h]	27.8±14.7[i]

(Groups 1–4-a bracketed: [d]; groups 1–4-b bracketed: [j])

[a] Skin grafting was carried out on day 0.
[b] Not significant compared with group 1.
[c] *P*=0.0008 compared with group 3.
[d] In these groups, elicitation for DFR and boosting for CTL and CTAb assays were carried out on day 16 (Figs. 1 and 2, and Table 2).
[e,f,g,h] DBA skin graft survival varied in NTx BALB mice. Therefore, the mice that rejected the grafts by day 16 (group 4-a) were used for the assays mentioned above. The others (group 4-b) were called nl (e), n2 (f), n3 (g) and n4 (h), and were kept to observe the end-points of the skin graft rejection, followed by DFR, CTL, and CTAb assays (Table 3).
[i] *P*=0.0219 compared with group 3. Not significant compared with group 4-a.
[j] ANOVA; *P*=0.0006.

RESULTS

Skin allograft survival in NTx mice. NTx or sham-operated BALB (H-2[d]) mice were grafted with C3H (H-2[k]) or DBA (H-2[d]) skin (Table 1). Graft survival of MHC-incompatible C3H skin was not prolonged at all by NTx (group 1 versus group 2), but that of MHC-compatible DBA skin was prolonged significantly (group 3 versus groups 4a or 4b). NTx mice grafted with DBA skin were divided into two groups—the group in which grafted skin was rejected within 16 days after grafting (group 4a) and the group in which grafted skin survived more than 18 days (group 4b). The mice of groups 1, 2, 3, and 4a were used for DFR, CTL, and CTAb assays soon after the graft rejection, with groups 5 and 6 added as sham-operated, nongrafted controls (Figs. 1 and 2, Table 2). The mice of group 4b were kept to observe the end-points of the graft rejection. By 49 days after grafting, all the grafted DBA skin was rejected. These mice were further immunized with DBA spleen cells 51 days after grafting in order to synchronize the immunity, and were used for DFR, CTL and CTAb assays as described above (Table 3). In these late assays, groups 7 and 8 were added as sham-operated, nongrafted controls (Table 3).

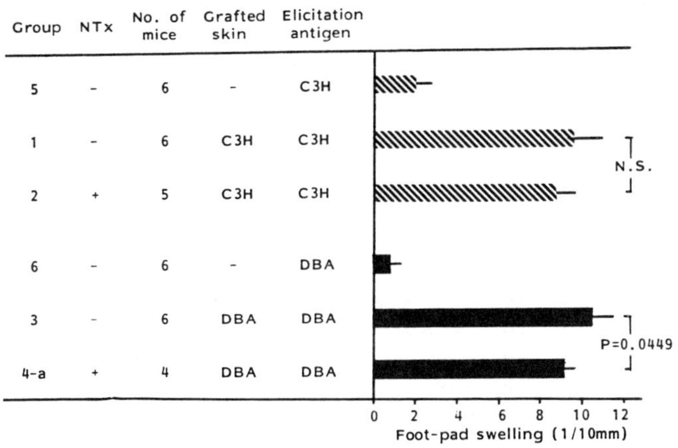

FIGURE 1. DFR in NTx BALB mice. The BALB mice represented as groups, 1, 2, 3, and 4a in Table 1 received the elicitation for DFR assay 16 days after skin grafting (the same groups). Sham-operated, nongrafted controls were set up as negative controls (groups 5 and 6) (thin bars = SD; ANOVA: $P < 0.0001$).

DFR in NTx mice. In both sham-operated and NTx mice grafted with skin (Fig. 1), high levels of DFR were detected against C3H (groups 1 and 2) and DBA (groups 3 and 4a) antigens compared with nongrafted controls (groups 5 and 6). However, DFR against DBA was slightly impaired in these NTx mice compared with sham-operated and grafted controls (group 3 versus group 4a), while that against C3H antigens was not impaired (group 1 versus group 2).

CTL activity in NTx mice. The experimental groups were the same as those described in the DFR assay (Table 2). Boosting for this assay was carried out concomitantly with the DFR assay by using the same mice.

The CTL activity against C3H was slightly impaired by NTx (group 1 versus group 2; E:T = 50:1)—although a high level of CTL activity was detected against C3H in sham-operated (group 1) and NTx mice (group 2) grafted with C3H skin, as compared with the nongrafted group (group 5).

In contrast, CTL activity against DBA was completely abrogated in NTx mice grafted with DBA skin (group 4a), while such an activity was considerably higher in mice sham-operated and grafted with DBA skin (group 3).

CTAb activity in NTx mice. Sera used in this assay were obtained when the mice were killed for the CTL assay (Fig. 2).

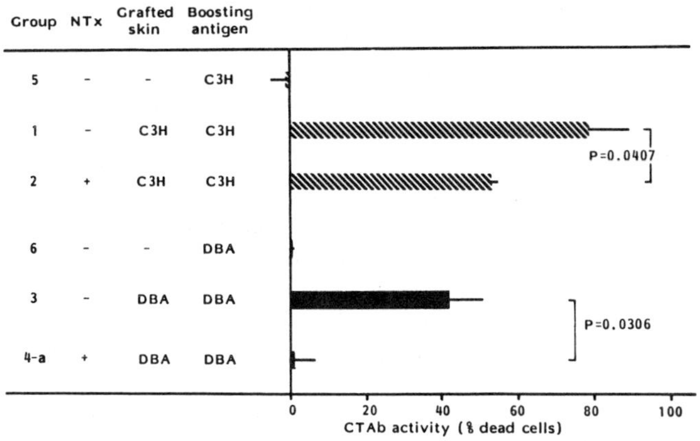

FIGURE 2. CTAb activity in NTx BALB mice. Sera were obtained when BALB mice were killed for the CTL assay. C3H or DBA Con A blasts were used as target cells (thin bars = SD; ANOVA: $P < 0.0001$).

TABLE 2. CTL activity in NTx BALB mice

Group	NTx	Donor of skin graft	Boosting antigen[a]	CTL activity (% lysis)	
				25:1	50:1[b]
5	−	—	C3H	−2.5±1.1	1.3±4.9 [e] [h]
1	−	C3H	C3H	59.9±2.8	78.2±3.8 [e] [h]
2	+	C3H	C3H	52.1±7.3[c]	64.3±5.0[d] [e] [h]
6	−	—	DBA	−3.8±3.4	1.9±4.2 [g] [h]
3	−	DBA	DBA	37.0±6.4	53.8±1.9 [g] [h]
4-a	+	DBA	DBA	−2.9±3.1[f]	3.9±5.3[f] [g] [h]

[a] BALB mice were boosted i.p. with C3H or DBA spleen cells 16 days after C3H or DBA skin grafting and were killed 3 days later to collect PEC.
[b] E:T.
[c] Not significant compared with group 1.
[d] P=0.0044 compared with group 1.
[e] Target cells were C3H Con A blasts.
[f] $P<0.0001$ compared with group 3. Not significant compared with group 6.
[g] Target cells were DBA Con A blasts.
[h] ANOVA; $P<0.0001$.

TABLE 3. DFR, CTL, and CTAb assays in NTx BALB mice with prolonged DBA skin graft survival of more than 18 days

Group	NTx	Skin grafting (on day 0)	No. mice	Code of mouse	Graft survival (days)[a]	Im (on day 51)[b]	E and B (on day 58)[c]	DFR (1/10 mm)[d]	CTL (% lysis)[e]		CTAb (% dead cells)[g]
									25:1	50:1[f]	
7	–	–	5	—	—	—	DBA	0.7±0.6	0.3±1.6	−1.4±2.1	−0.7±1.5
8	–	–	6	—	—	DBA	DBA	9.4±0.4	59.6±2.7	68.0±3.4	2.2±2.4
				n1	18			12.3			
				n2	18			11.5			
4-b	+	DBA	4	n3	26	DBA	DBA	3.8	11.2±1.7[h]	18.3±2.1[h]	−1.3±1.3[i]
				n4	49			0.3			

[a] Four NTx mice shown in Group 4-b of Table 1 were used for this experiment. Skin grafting was carried out on day 0.
[b] Sham-operated (group 8) and NTx mice (group 4-b) were immunized s.c. with 1×10^7 DBA spleen cells on day 51.
[c] Elicitation for DFR assay and boosting for CTL and CTAb assays were carried out on day 58.
[d] In group 4-b, foot-pad swelling of each mouse is presented.
[e] In group 4-b, PEC from the 4 mice (n1–n4) were pooled and used for the CTL assay; ANOVA for the CTL assay—$P<0.0001$.
[f] E:T.
[g] In group 4-b, sera from the 4 mice (n1–n4) were pooled and used for the CTAb assay; ANOVA for the CTAb assay—$P=0.2616$.
[h] $P<0.0001$ compared with groups 7 and 8.
[i] Not significant compared with groups 7 and 8.

Although CTAb activity against C3H was impaired by NTx (group 1 versus group 2), a high level of CTAb activity against C3H was still detected after grafting with C3H skin, not only in sham-operated mice (group 1) but also in NTx mice (group 2).

On the other hand, CTAb activity against DBA was completely abrogated in the sera obtained from NTx mice grafted with DBA skin (group 4a), while such an activity was considerably higher in those from mice sham-operated and grafted with DBA skin (group 3).

Assays of DFR, CTL, and CTAb in NTx BALB mice with prolonged DBA skin graft survival of more than 18 days. Group 4b (Table 1) was employed in this experiment, and nonimmune (group 7) and immune (group 8) sham-operated and nongrafted controls were added (Table 3).

In the DFR assay, a high level of the response was detected in immunized controls (group 8) and in n1 and n2 mice of group 4b, both of which showed 18 days' graft survival. In contrast, the response was low or absent in n3 or n4 mice showing 26 or 49 days' graft survival, respectively (group 4b). Thus, the level of DRF in group mice correlated inversely with the survival periods of skin grafts (group 4b), although the sample number was small. CTL activity was high in immunized controls (group 8), but it was very low in NTx mice (group 4b). CTAb activity was not detectable in NTx mice grafted with DBA skin (group 4b) or in sham-operated mice immunized with DBA spleen cells (group 8).

DISCUSSION

In our present study, survival of skin allografts from an MHC-compatible strain was prolonged, but that from an MHC-incompatible strain was not prolonged at all in 14-week-old BALB mice thymectomized at 1 day after birth. These results may be somewhat inconsistent with those reported by many authors (*1–7*), because permanent survival of the grafts was never achieved in our present experiments. However, as Miller (*3*), Martinez et al. (*2, 6*), and our colleagues (*15*) have shown, the degree of immunity in NTx mice depends on the time of the NTx operation (*2, 3, 6, 15*), the age of the NTx mice used in experiments (*3, 6*), and the combination of murine strains employed (*2, 3, 6*). Another possible reason for the difference is the performance of the NTx operation, although we have histologically excluded this possibility in our previous study (*17*).

As Loveland et al. have described previously (*18, 19*), rejection of skin grafts appears to be mediated by an Lyt-1^+2^- T lymphocyte population responsible for DFR in mice. However, Mason et al. have refuted this explanation because rejection of the allografts may be due to collaboration between the injected helper T cells and CTL precursors in the T-cell-deprived host, as well as to the existence of CTL precursors contained in the subset of T cells with helper phenotype that are able to specifically lyse class-II-incompatible targets (*20*). Our previous results support the results of the former authors, because skin allografts survival in a congenic murine combination disparate only at the MHC was markedly prolonged by tolerance induction with cyclophosphamide, accompanied by depletion of DFR, despite the significantly high activity of residual CTL (*21*). Moreover, in the present study MHC-compatible allogeneic skin grafts were rejected in the absence of CTL activity (Table 2). On the other hand, DFR correlated inversely with skin graft survival (Table 1 and Fig. 1). This inverse correlation between skin graft survival and DFR was evident in the late assays for DFR against the MHC-compatible antigens (Table 3). It may be hasty to draw a conclusion from only 4 mice—but, as shown in Table 3, NTx mice (n1-n4) showed skin graft survival of 12–49 days and foot-pad swelling of 12.3–0.3 units. In the n4 mouse, DFR was not detectable even after the mouse had rejected the graft by day 49 and received further immunization on day 51. This may be ascribed to our criteria of graft rejection—i.e., the graft was judged to be rejected on day 49 when no normal hair was found on it, as mentioned above. However, a small amount of scarlike graft tissue was still found in the graft bed at the time of the DFR assay (data not shown), suggesting that the skin grraft had not really been rejected yet.

The general immunological characteristics of NTx mice in the present study demonstrated that the degrees of immunological impairments by NTx were CTAb>CTL>DFR against both MHC-compatible and incompatible antigens, and that MHC-compatible were greater than MHC-incompatible systems for each immunological parameter. CTL and CTAb activities were reduced by NTx slightly against MHC-incompatible antigens and greatly against MHC-compatible ones. Moreover, all the immunological parameters were profoundly depressed against MHC-compatible antigens in some NTx mice (n3 and n4 mice in Table 3). These results may suggest that effector mechanisms responsible for DFR, CTL, and CTAb—as well as those reactive against MHC-incompatible antigens and MHC-compatible ones—develop ontogenically in those respective orders when the thymus is present. The ontogenic development of the immunological parameters is consistent with the results reported by Shimamoto et al. (*15*), and the ontogenic difference between the immunologically competent cell population reactive against MHC-incompatible antigens and that against MHC compatible ones is consistent with the results from Martinez et al. (*2*) and Miller (*3*).

As a whole, immunological activity in NTx mice is depressed compared with that in sham-operated mice, but the degree of the depression is more severe in immune responses against MHC-compatible allogeneic antigens than in those against MHC incompatible allogeneic antigens. Therefore, the lymphocyte population reactive against MHC-incompatible, fully allogeneic antigens appears to contain a higher proportion of lymphocytes that are less thymus-dependent in ontogenic development than those reactive against MHC-compatible allogeneic antigens.

REFERENCES

1. Miller JFAP. Immunological functions of the thymus. Lancet 1961; 2: 748.
2. Martinez C, Kersey J, Papermaster BW, Good RA. Skin homograft survival in thymectomized mice. Proc Soc Exp Biol Med 1962; 109: 193.
3. Miller JFAP. Role of the thymus in transplantation immunity. Ann NY Acad Sci 1962; 99: 340.
4. Arnason BG, Jankovic BD, Waksman BH. Effect of thymectomy on "delayed" hypersensitive reaction. Nature 1962; 144: 99.
5. Dalmasso AP, Martinez C, Good RA. Further studies of the homograft reaction by thymectomy in the mouse. Proc Soc Exp Bio Med 1962; 111: 143.
6. Martinez C, Dalmasso AP, Good RA. Effect of thymectomy on development of immunological competence in mice. Ann NY Acad Sci 1964; 113: 933.
7. Miller JFAP, Osoba D, Dukor P. A humoral thymus mechanism responsible for immunologic maturation. Ann NY Acad Sci 1965; 124: 95.
8. Martinez C, Dalmasso A, Good RA. Acceptance of tumour homografts by thymectomized mice. Nature 1962; 194: 1289.
9. Dalmasso AP, Martinez C, Good RA. Failure of spleen cells from thymectomized mice to induce graft vs. host reactions. Proc Soc Exp Biol Med 1962; 110: 205.
10. Papermaster BW, Dalmasso AP, Martinez C, Good RA. Suppression of antibody forming capacity with thymectomy in the mouse. Proc Soc Exp Biol Med 1962; 111: 41.
11. Shin T, Mayumi H, Himeno K, Sanui H, Nomoto K. Drug-induced tolerance to allografts in mice. I. Difference between tumor and skin grafts. Transplantation 1984; 37: 580.
12. Mayumi H, Shin T, Himeno K, Nomoto K. Drug-induced tolerance to allografts in mice. II. Tolerance to tumor allografts of large doses associated with rejection of skin allografts and tumor allografts of small doses. Immunobiology 1985; 147: 169.
13. Mayumi H, Himeno K, Shin T, Nomoto K. Drug-induced tolerance to allografts in mice. IV. Mechanisms and kinetics of cyclophosphamide-induced tolerance. Transplantation 1985; 39: 209.
14. Mayumi H, Himeno K, Shin T, Nomoto K. Drug-induced tolerance to allografts in mice. VI. Tolerance induction in H-2 haplotype-identical strain combinations in mice. Transplantation 1985; 40: 188.
15. Shimamoto Y, Taniguchi K, Kubo C, Nomoto K. Differences in thymus-dependency among various T-cell function. Immunology 1980; 41: 167.
16. Sjodin K, Dalmasso AP, Smith JM, Martinez C. Thymectomy in newborn and adult mice. Transplantation 1963; 1: 521.
17. Nomoto K, Shimamoto Y, Taniguchi K, et al. Development of immunity against Listeria monocytogens in athymic nude versus neonatally thymectomized mice. Cell Immunol 1983; 75: 134.
18. Loveland BE, Hogarth PM, Ceredig RH, McKenzie IFC. Cells mediating graft rejection in the mouse. I. Lyt-1 cells mediate skin graft rejection. J Exp Med 1981; 153: 1044.
19. Loveland BE, McKenzie IFC. Delayed type hypersensitivity and allograft rejection in the mouse: correlation of effector cell phenotype. Immunology 1982; 46: 313.
20. Mason DW, Dallman MJ, Arthur RP, Morris PJ. Mechanisms of allograft rejection: the roles of cytotoxic T-cells and delayed-type hypersensitivity. Immunol Rev 1984; 77: 167.
21. Shin T, Himeno K, Mayumi H, Nomoto K. Drug-induced tolerance to allografts in mice. III. Prolongation of skin graft surival by tolerance induction in congeneic mice disparate in the major H-2 antigens. Transplantation 1985; 39: 333.

Received 20 February 1985.
Accepted 21 May 1985.

0041-1337/86/4102-0214$02.00/0
TRANSPLANTATION
Vol. 41, No. 2
Printed in U.S.A.

THE MIGRATION OF ACTIVATED T LYMPHOCYTES IN VITRO

III. PARALYSIS AND RECOVERY OF LOCOMOTOR FUNCTION DURING MITOSIS[1]

ROSEMARY A. HOFFMAN,[2] BONNIE J. HYLAND, NANCY L. ASCHER, AND RICHARD L. SIMMONS

The Department of Surgery, University of Minnesota, Minneapolis, Minnesota 55455

Previous reports have stated that activated lymphocytes are more motile than unsensitized lymphocytes and that certain subpopulations of lymphocytes are more motile than others. In order to determine at what stage of activation lymphocytes become motile, we have examined lymphocyte motility as well as other functions at various times after mitogenic or allogeneic stimulation in culture. Lymphocytes cultured with concanavalin A (Con A)[3] or with alloantigen become most motile after peak thymidine incorporation has occurred. Allosensitized lymphocytes need not possess cytolytic capacity in order to become motile. Allosensitized lymphocytes retain the ability to locomote at near maximal rates for at least 2 weeks after stimulation. When these motile, allosensitized lymphocytes are recultured in the presence of fresh irradiated stimulator cells, they lose their ability to locomote during active thymidine incorporation and become motile again when thymidine incorporation has abated. Lymphocyte clones demonstrated motility cycles similar to cycles observed with bulk cultures (i.e., peak motility is observed only after peak thymidine incorporation has occurred in the subculture). All T lymphocyte clones tested are motile, regardless of Lyt phenotype or function, if tested for motility on the appropriate day of subculture. Studies of clone motility at intervals less than 24 hr after restimulation revealed that motility ceased before tritiated thymidine uptake occurred. The migratory potential of lymphocytes in vitro does not seem to depend on phenotype or the nature of the mitogenic stimulus. It seems instead to be part of the cyclic response of the cell to activation, with early inhibition of motility and subsequent recovery of locomotor function. Whether ability to locomote is intrinsic to the activated cell or depends on environmental factors requires further investigation.

Both directional and random lymphocyte motility must certainly influence two critical immunologic functions in vivo—the capacity of lymphocytes to emigrate from a lymphoid depot into the circulation—and, conversely, their capacity to migrate from a capillary into an inflammatory site or lymphoid depot. Reviews by Parrott and Wilkinson (*1*), Wilkinson et al (*2*), and deSousa (*3*) have summarized many of the findings on lymphocyte motility. Most investigators agree that activated lymphocytes are more motile than unstimulated lymphocytes (*4, 5*). We recently reported that the sensitized T lymphocytes recovered from a sponge matrix allograft are very motile and are not actively incorporating thymidine. Furthermore, within a bulk population of in vitro allosensitized lymphocytes, the cells that are most motile are not incorporating thymidine and bear Lyt-1 surface markers (*6*). The present studies were designed to determine the effect of cell cycle changes on lymphocyte motility in vitro. Both bulk cultures and lymphocyte clones of defined Lyt phenotype were utilized. No attempt was made here to study chemotaxis because substances governing directional lymphocyte motility have not yet been clearly defined.

[1] This work was supported by NIH Grants AI 16869 and CA 11605.

[2] To whom correspondence should be addressed, at Box 185 Mayo, University of Minnesota Hospitals, Minneapolis, MN 55455.

[3] Abbreviations used: CB, cytochalasin B; Con A, concanavalin A; DMEM, Dulbecco's modified Eagle's medium; FBS, fetal bovine serum; ^{3}H-TdR, tritiated thymidine; 2°MLC-SN, secondary mixed leukocyte culture supernatant; NMS, normal mouse serum; PHA-P, phytohemagglutinin.

MATERIALS AND METHODS

Female BALB/c AnNCrlBR and C57BL/6 NCrlBR mice were obtained from Charles River Breeding Laboratory (Wilmington, MA). DBA/2J mice were obtained from Jackson Laboratories (Bar Harbor, ME). Alpha 17 and Beta 16 mice (C57BL/6 congenic mice) were obtained from the mouse colony of the Immunobiological Research Center. (Minneapolis, MN). The mice were housed in plastic cages, provided with Purina Rodent Chow and tap water ad libitum, and used at 12–20 weeks of age.

Mitogenic stimulation. A single cell suspension was prepared from the inguinal, axillary, and brachial lymph nodes of BALB/c mice by gently compressing the nodes with a glass stopper. The suspension was washed 3× and counted using trypan blue. Viability ranged from 75–90%. The cells were cultured in Click's medium (Altick Associates, River Falls, WI) supplemented with 0.6% BALB/c normal mouse serum (NMS). Con A (Pharmacia, Piscataway, NJ) was added at a final concentration of 1 μg/ml. Then 30×10^6 cells were cultured in a final volume of 15 ml per flask (25-cm^2, Corning) and placed upright in a 37°C, humidified, 5% CO_2 atmosphere.

Mixed leukocyte cultures. A single cell suspension was prepared from spleens by gently compressing with a glass stopper. Cells were washed 3×, counted (85–95% viability), and 17.5×10^6 responder cells were cultured with 22×10^6 irradiated (2000 rads) stimulator cells (25-cm^2 Corning flasks, incubated upright) in a final volume of 10 ml. The cultures were supplemented with 0.6% or 1% NMS from the responding strain. For short-term (days 3–7) MLC, Click's medium was utilized. For long-term (days 4–14) MLC, Dulbecco's modified Eagle's medium (GIBCO, Grand Island, NY), supplemented with 1.5 mM L-glutamine, 1×10^5 units/L penicillin, 1×10^5 μg/L streptomycin, 6 mg/L folic acid, 36 mg/L L-asparagine, 116 mg/L L-arginine-HCL (all GIBCO), 1 mM sodium pyruvate (M.A. Bioproducts, Walkersville, MD) and 5×10^{-5} M 2-mercaptoethanol (Sigma, St. Louis, MO), as described by Cerrottini et al. (*7*), was used.

Preparation of secondary mixed leukocyte culture supernatant (2°MLC-SN). As described by Ryser et al. (*8*), fifty million C57BL/6 splenocytes were cultured with 100×10^6 irradiated (2000 rads) DBA/2 splenocytes in a final volume of 40 ml 2%

fetal bovine serum (FBS)-DMEM (as above, except with 2% FBS added) in 75-cm^2 Falcon flasks. The cultures were maintained at 37°C in humidified 10% CO_2 atmosphere for 11–14 days. Cells were then harvested and 30×10^6 were recultured with 120×10^6 irradiated (2000 rads) DBA/2 splenocytes in a final volume of 30 ml. (Syngeneic 2° MLC-SN was prepared by culturing primed C57BL/6 anti DBA/2 splenocytes with irradiated C57BL/6 splenocytes). After 18–24 hr the supernatant was harvested, aliquoted, and stored at −20°C. The 2° MLC-SN was sterilized by membrane filtration (0.22 μm).

Derivation of clones. Three T lymphocyte clones were derived by Derry Roopenian, Ph.D., and have been characterized (*9*). Eight other clones were derived by limiting-dilution analysis (0.25 cells/well) of cells from a C57BL/6 anti DBA/2 mixed lymphocyte culture (days 5–8 of culture). Cells from growth-positive wells were subcultured in 16-mm wells (COSTAR) with $6–8\times10^6$ irradiated stimulator cells and 20–30% 2° MLC-SN in a a final volume of 1.5 ml 2% FBS-DMEM. Weekly subculture of $1–5\times10^4$ cells/well was performed. Clones were analyzed for proliferative and cytolytic capacity and Lyt phenotype.

Assessment of proliferation of lymphocyte clones. For this purpose, 1×10^4 cells were cultured with 1×10^6 irradiated spleen cells in round-bottomed microtiter wells in 0.2 ml of 2% FBS-DMEM. On day 2 of culture 2 μCi of ^{3}H-TdR (5 Ci/mM, New England Nuclear, Boston, MA) was added per well. After 6.5 hr incubation the cultures were harvested with a multiple sample harvester and counted in a Beckman LS 2800 (Beckman Instruments, Fullerton, CA). Results are expressed as mean cpm ± SD of triplicate samples. For all the lymphocyte clone proliferation studies a positive control of 20% 2° MLC-SN was included to be sure of the viability of the cells (data not shown).

Phenotyping surface antigens on lymphocyte clones. Lymphocyte clones were incubated with monoclonal Thy 1.2, Lyt 1.2, or Lyt 2.2 antisera (New England Nuclear), washed, and incubated with fluorescein-conjugated IgG fraction of goat anti-mouse immunoglobulin (IgG + IgM + IgA) (Cappel Laboratories, Malvern, PA). The percentage of fluorescence was determined with a FACS IV (Becton Dickinson, Mountainview, CA). Fluorescence background was determined by treating cells with the fluorescein conjugate alone. Fluorescence levels below 10% were arbitrarily considered negative. Thymocytes from Alpha 16 and Beta 17 mice were used as positive and negative controls for the allele specificity of Lyt 1.2 and Lyt 2.2 antisera.

Cytotoxicity assay. Target cell blasts were generated by culturing spleen cells (2×10^6/ml) for 48 hr with 5 μg/ml Con A or 40 μg/ml lipopolysaccharide (LPS) (*Escherichia coli* 0111:B4, Difco, Detroit, MI) in Eagle's MEM supplemented with 1.0 mM sodium pyruvate, 0.1 mM nonessential amino acids (all M.A. Bioproducts) 2.0 mM L-glutamine, 1×10^5 units/L penicillin, 1×10^5 μg/L streptomycin, and 10% FBS (all GIBCO). The Con A blasts were washed with 0.3 mM alpha-methyl-D mannoside (Sigma) prior to being labeled with sodium chromate ^{51}Cr (New England Nuclear). EL4 and P815 tumor lines were maintained in vitro by twice-weekly subcultures. Spleen cell blasts (1×10^4) or 2×10^3 tumor cells were incubated with various numbers of effector cells in conical-bottomed microtiter wells (final volume 0.2 ml of 5% FBS-MEM). When necessary 0.5 μl/ml phytohemagglutinin (PHA-P) (Difco) was included in the cytotoxicity assay to detect lectin-mediated cytotoxicity. The microtiter plate was centrifuged at 20×g for 2 min, incubated at 37°C for 4 hr, and centrifuged at 700×g for 10 min, after which 0.1 ml of supernatant was removed and counted in a Bio-Gamma II (Beckman Instruments). The percentage of cytotoxicity of the mean of triplicate samples was calculated by using the formula:

$$\frac{\text{experimental cpm} - \text{spontaneous cpm}}{\text{total cpm} - \text{spontaneous cpm}} \times 100 = \%\ \text{cytotoxicity}$$

Assessment of lymphocyte locomotion. On various days of culture, cells were harvested (cells from at least 2 flasks or multiple wells were pooled) by washing 3× in protein-free RPMI-1640-25mM HEPES (GIBCO). Cells numbering 0.5×10^6 in a 0.1 ml volume of RPMI were added to blind well chemotaxis chambers (Neuroprobe, Bethesda, MD). A 5-μm pore-size membrane (Sartorius, Hayward, CA) was used. RPMI containing 10% BALB/c NMS or 1–2 mg/ml alpha-casein (Sigma) was placed in the well of the chamber. The chambers were incubated for 1 hr in a 37°C, humidified 5% CO_2 atmosphere. The filters were removed, stained, cleared, and mounted on glass slides. Migration was assessed by determining the leading front (distance in micrometers that the leading 2 cells had migrated in 4 different areas of triplicate filters). This assessment was determined by using an automated chemotaxis data acquisition system (ACDAS) (*10*) and is expressed as mean ± SD. We have previously utilized the mean aggregate number (MAN) as an additional technique of assessing locomotion (*6*). Because results using this technique did not differ in qualitative terms from the simpler leading front technique, the MAN method was not utilized in these experiments.

^{3}H-TdR incorporation. On each day of migration assessment the ^{3}H-TdR incorporation was also determined. For this procedure, 1 μCi ^{3}H-TdR was added to 1×10^5 cells per microtiter well in a final volume of 0.2 ml RPMI. After a 4-hr incubation in a 37°C, 5% CO_2, humidified atmosphere, the samples were harvested. The mean cpm ± SD of triplicate samples were determined.

Reagents for motility assay. Alpha-casein (Sigma) was diluted at 2 mg/ml in RPMI, aliquoted, and stored at −70°C. (Casein was used as an attractant in these assays because it has previously been used in neutrophil and monocyte motility assays). Pooled NMS was made by cardiac puncture of 10–15 BALB/c, allowing blood to clot, centrifuging to obtain serum, aliquoting, and storing at −70°C.

RESULTS

Time course of motility of lymph node lymphocytes after stimulation with Con A. On days 1–5 after stimulation of lymph node lymphocytes with Con A, the cells were harvested and motility, ^{3}H-TdR incorporation, and cell yield were determined (Fig. 1). ^{3}H-TdR incorporation peaked on day 2 of culture and declined on days 3–5. The random migration in protein-free media (media control) as well as the migration in response to casein began to increase after peak ^{3}H-TdR incorporation, and increased steadily on days 3–5 of culture. Proliferation was evidenced by the increasing numbers of cells recovered from the cultures.

Time course of lymphocyte locomotion after allogeneic stimulation. BALB/c splenocytes were cultured with C57BL/6 irradiated splenocytes (H-2 and background-disparate combination) and with DBA/2 irradiated splenic lymphocytes (H-2-identical, MLS-disparate combination) (Fig. 2). The cells were harvested on days 3–7 of culture. Motility, ^{3}H-TdR incorpora-

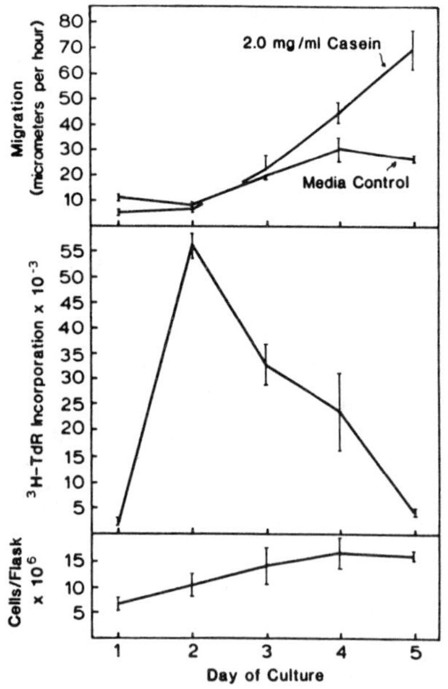

FIGURE 1. The motility, ^{3}H-TdR incorporation and cell yield per flask of BALB/c lymph node lymphocytes stimulated with Con A. On days 1–5 of culture, the migration in response to protein-free media (media control) and (2 mg/ml) casein was determined. The ^{3}H-TdR incorporation per 1×10^5 cells in 4 hr is expressed as cpm. The data represent the mean ± SE of pooled results from 3 experiments.

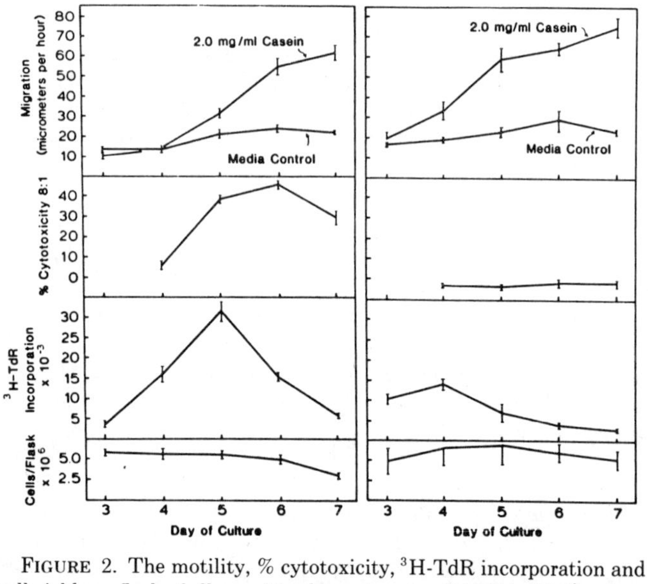

FIGURE 2. The motility, % cytotoxicity, ^{3}H-TdR incorporation and cell yield per flask of allosensitized lymphocytes. BALB/c (H-2^d) splenocytes were stimulated with C57BL/6 (H-2^b) irradiated spenocytes (left panel) or DBA/2 (H-2^d) irradiated splenocytes (right panel). On days 3–7 of culture, migration in response to protein-free media (media control) and casein (2 mg/ml) was assessed. The percentage of cytotoxicity against Con A blasts of the stimulator strain was determined at 8:1 effector:target ratio. The ^{3}H-TdR incorporation per 1×10^5 cells in 4 hr is expressed as cpm. The data represent the mean ± SE of results of 3 different experiments.

tion, % cytotoxicity, and cell yield per flask were determined. The random migration (media control), as well as the migration in response to casein, began to increase after the peak in ^{3}H-TdR incorporation occurred. Although the amount of ^{3}H-TdR incorporated per 1×10^5 cells were markedly different for the two combinations (30,000 cpm for the H-2 disparate and 15,000 cpm for the H-2-identical combination), the increase in motility in response to casein was comparable. In fact, migration was slightly better on days 4 and 5 of culture in the H-2-compatible combination in which proliferation was less. The cytotoxic potential of the cell population did not seem to be a factor in the increase in motility, since no cytotoxicity against DBA/2 was detected in the H-2-compatible combination.

Motility of lymphocytes on various days of primary and second-set allostimulation. On days 6, 8, 10, 12, and 14 of primary culture, the motility and ^{3}H-TdR incorporation of BALB/c splenocytes stimulated with C57BL/6 splenocytes was determined. On day 14 of primary culture the cells were harvested and restimulated with fresh C57BL/6 irradiated splenocytes. On days 2, 4, 6, 8, and 10 of second-set culture, motility and ^{3}H-TdR incorporation were assessed. The results of these studies are depicted in Fig. 3. On days 6, 8, 10, 12, and 14 of primary stimulation the lymphocytes remained motile and were incorporating a low level of ^{3}H-TdR. After restimulation with fresh alloantigen, the ^{3}H-TdR incorporation reached a maximum level (70,000 cpm/1×10^5 cells) on day 2, at which time the motility of the lymphocytes were severely impaired. As the ^{3}H-TdR incorporation began to wane (days 4, 6, 8, and 10 of second-set culture) the lymphocytes again became motile.

Motility of lymphocyte clones on various days of subculture. The eleven lymphocyte clones tested were characterized with respect to their proliferative responses (to allogeneic stimulation), cytotoxicity, and Lyt phenotype (Table 1). Clones 5M/B6-5, 5M/B6-6, and LPA-8 were isolated and characterized by Derry Roopenian, Ph.D., and their characteristics have been reported in detail (*9*). They have been characterized as helper-cell-independent cytolytic T cell clones. The remaining clones were derived in our laboratory. Some of the clones were able to proliferate in response to irradiated specific allogeneic spleen cells. Clones 123-6 and 123-20 were directly cytotoxic, while 170-19, 170-21, and 170-29 were cytotoxic only in the presence

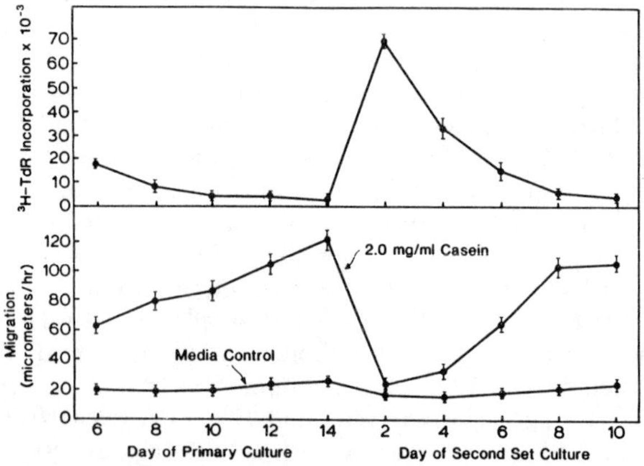

FIGURE 3. Motility and ^{3}H-TdR incorporation of allosensitized lymphocytes on various days of primary and second-set culture. BALB/c splenocytes were stimulated with C57BL/6 irradiated splenocytes and motility and ^{3}H-TdR uptake were determined on days 6–14 of primary culture and on days 2–10 of second-set culture (cells from day 14 primary culture were restimulated with irradiated C57BL/6 splenocytes). The migration (in micrometers per hour) in response to protein-free media (media control) and casein represents the mean ± SD of triplicate filters. ^{3}H-TdR incorporation per 1×10^5 cells in 4 hr is expressed as mean ± SD of triplicate wells.

TABLE 1. Functional characteristics of lymphocyte clones used in motility studies

Clone	Derived from mixed lymphocyte culture		Proliferation in reponse to irradiated splenocytes[a]		% Cytotoxicity of radiolabeled targets		Phenotype
	Responder	Stimulator			30:1	E:T ratio[b]	
			NONE	*C57BL/6*	*BALB/c*	*C57BL/6*	
5M/B6-5[c]	B10.129 (5M)	C57BL/6	526±597	7803±1503	4	44	Lyt 1^-2^+
5M/B6-6[c]	B10.129 (5M)	C57BL/6	798±48	12,596±1697	4	51	Lyt 1^-2^+
			B10.LP-H-3[b]	*C57BL/10*		*EL4*	
LPA-8[c]	B10.LP-H-3[b]	C57BL/10	164±57	19,038±815	ND	98	ND
			C57/BL/6	*DBA/2J*	*EL4*	*P815*	
58-5	C57BL/6	DBA/2J	2718±508	17,927±1431	0	0	ND
58-7	C57BL/6	DBA/2J	1972±314	23,328±170	0	0	ND
123-6	C57BL/6	DBA/2J	652±108	1514±157	0	86	Lyt 1^-2^+
123-20	C57BL/6	DBA/2J	363±30	879±179	0	80	Lyt 1^-2^+
170-7[d]	C57BL/6	DBA/2J	783±22	15,627±2301	0	0	Lyt 1^+2^-
170-19[d]	C57BL/6	DBA/2J	368±12	1557±12	0	0	Lyt 1^-2^+
170-21[d]	C57BL/6	DBA/2J	285±46	10,383±1595	0	0	Lyt 1^+2^+
170-29[d]	C57BL/6	DBA/2J	447±39	3449±620	0	0	Lyt 1^+2^+

[a] Proliferation was assessed by culturing 1×10^4 lymphocytes in the presence of 1×10^6 irradiated splenocytes in round-bottomed microtiter wells in a final volume of 0.2 ml 2% FBS-DMEM. On day 2, 2 μCi ^{3}H-TdR was added per well, and thymidine uptake was determined after a 6.5-hr incubation (mean ± SD of triplicate wells).

[b] 1×10^4 ^{51}Cr-labeled spleen cell LPS blasts or 2×10^3 tumor cells were incubated with various numbers of lymphocytes in conical bottom microtiter in a final volume of 0.2 ml 5% FBS-DMEM. After a 4-hr incubation % ^{51}Cr release was determined. Clones 58–5, 58–7, and 170–7 were not cytotoxic at E:T ratios up to 100:1 with and without PHA-P present. Clones 170–19, 170–21, and 170–29 were cytotoxic only in the presence of PHA-P.

[c] These clones were gifts from D. C. Roopenian, Ph.D., Department of Pathology, Harvard Medical School.

[d] Motility of these clones was similar to other clones depicted in Figure 5 (Data not shown).

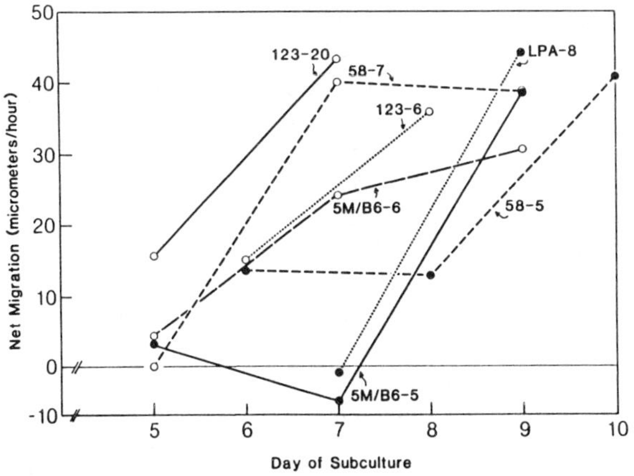

FIGURE 4. Motility of lymphocyte clones on various days of subculture. On each harvest day, cells from several wells were pooled, washed, and suspended at 5×10^6/ml in RPMI. After 1 hr incubation, the net migration in micrometers (micrometers migrated in response to 10% normal mouse serum minus micrometers migrated in presence of protein free media) was determined. (*See* Table 1 for functional characterization of clones and Table 2 for cell yields and thymidine incorporation.)

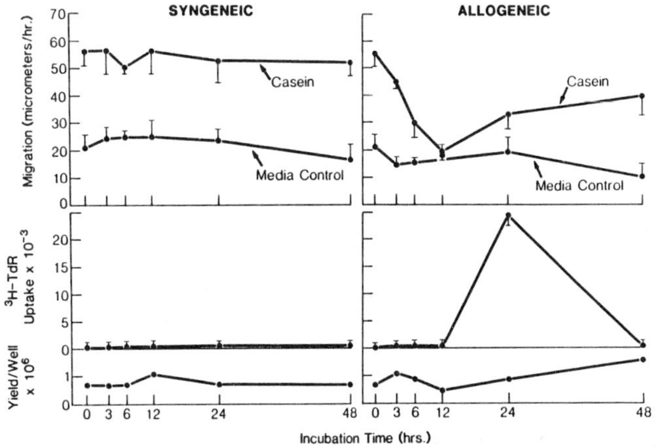

FIGURE 5. Motility of clone 123-6 after various incubation times in syngeneic or allogeneic secondary mixed lymphocyte culture supernatant. On day 7 of subculture, clone 123-6 was exposed to 50% (v/v) syngeneic or allogeneic 2°MLC-SN for various times. At each time point, the cells were harvested, (minimum of 6 wells pooled) washed, and motility, ^{3}H-TdR uptake, and cell yield were determined.

of lectin. Clones 58-5, 58-7, and 170-7 were not cytotoxic, even in the presence of lectin. Clones were either Lyt 1^+, 2^+, or both. The motility of Clones 170-7, 170-19, 170-21, and 170-29 was similar to the others depicted in Figure 4. (Data not shown). On various days of subculture, cells from multiple wells were harvested and the motility in response to normal mouse serum and casein was determined. Regardless of the function of the clone (Table 1) the lymphocytes were most motile when tested as late in the subculture period as possible (Fig. 4). As with bulk cultures, each clone was most motile after thymidine incorporation had abated. (Table 2).

Lymphocyte clone motility early after mitogenic stimulation. To determine at what point after mitogenic stimulation a lymphocyte becomes immotile, motile lymphocytes (Clone 123-6) on day 7 of subculture were incubated with 50% syngeneic (v/v) or allogeneic 2° MLC-SN. At 3, 6, 12, 24, and 48 hr time points, motility, thymidine uptake, and cell recovery were determined (Fig. 5). The syngeneic supernatant did not affect motility, thymidine uptake, or cell yield at any time examined. After exposure to allogeneic supernatant, lymphocyte motility was moderately inhibited at 6 hr and severely inhibited at 12 hr; it began to recover by 24 hr. Thymidine uptake had not begun at 12 hr when motility was severely impaired.

TABLE 2. Cell recovery and thymidine uptake of lymphocyte clones on various days of subculture[a]

Clone		Day 5	Day 6	Day 7	Day 8	Day 9	Day 10
5M/B6-5	Yield	0.9×10^6		0.6×10^6		0.4×10^6	
	^{3}H-TdR	102,310±4890	ND	10,710±1651	ND	4030±850	ND
5M/B6-6	Yield	0.6×10^6		0.8×10^6		0.4×10^6	
	^{3}H-TdR	100,270±1685	ND	7180±1492	ND	2870±195	ND
LPA-8	Yield			1.2×10^6		1.5×10^6	
	^{3}H-TdR	ND	ND	1516±404	ND	500±69	ND
58–5	Yield		0.7×10^6		0.9×10^6		0.7×10^6
	^{3}H-TdR	ND	81,870±2572	ND	4040±529	ND	5193±489
58–7	Yield	1.1×10^6		1.1×10^6		0.9×10^6	
	^{3}H-TdR	42,340±3409	ND	926±85	ND	899±1010	ND
123–6	Yield		0.3×10^6		0.2×10^6		
	^{3}H-TdR	ND	36,309±895	ND	3138±277	ND	ND
123–20	Yield	0.3×10^6		0.4×10^6			
	^{3}H-TdR	47,945±3182	ND	1410±77	ND	ND	ND

[a] Cloned lymphocytes (2×10^4) were subcultured in 16-mm wells in the presence of 2° MLC-SN and irradiated stimulator cells. On various days of subculture, cells from a minimum of 6 wells were pooled and motility (Fig. 4), cell yield/well, and ^{3}H-TdR uptake were determined. The ^{3}H-TdR uptake was determined after a 4-hr incubation of 1×10^5 cells with 1 μCi of ^{3}H-TdR, and is expressed as cpm ± SD.

DISCUSSION

Studies of lymphocyte motility in vitro are designed to provide information about factors governing in vivo lymphocyte passage from the lymph nodes to blood and migraton from blood to sites of inflammation. Until recently, efforts devoted to establishing a reproducible and quantifiable lymphocyte motility assay in vitro have been disheartening. Standardized techniques have not always provided data that is easily interpretable. In part this is because the standards used for neutrophil motility assays have been applied to studies of lymphocyte locomotion. It is becoming clear that different "rules" apply for lymphocyte motility than for neutrophil motility: (A) Neutrophils readily adhere to various surfaces but lymphocytes do not. Lymphocytes are, therefore, unable to locomote on a planar surface (*1*, *12*) and require a three-dimensional matrix, like micropore filters or collagen gels (*13*), on which to locomote. (B) Unlike neutrophils, lymphocytes can locomote in vitro in the total absence of an exogenous protein source. Lymphocyte locomotion is, however, facilitated in media containing protein. (C) True chemotaxis, as defined by the Zigmond checkerboard assay (*14*), has been difficult to demonstrate with bulk lymphocyte populations. The extreme heterogeneity of lymphocytes recovered from a lymphoid depot makes them unsuitable for the Zigmond assay, in which homogeneity of the test population is a requirement. Because of such observations, Wilkinson et al. (*2*) have suggested that lymphocytes may accumulate at inflammatory sites in vivo because of lack of attachment points (or other unknown mechanisms) rather than by chemotactic mechanisms that account for neutrophil accumulation.

For these reasons, our motility assays were carried out in the total absence of protein (media control), and in the presence of casein or 10% NMS placed on the side of the membrane distal to the cells. No attempt was made to study chemotaxis.

Many investigators have reported that lymphocytes activated in vitro or in vivo are more motile than unsensitized lymphocytes (*4*, *5*, *15*). We have confirmed these observations using lymphocytes activated in vivo and in vitro (*6*). All previously studied activated lymphocyte preparations have been composed of cells of various Lyt phenotypes, in various stages of the mitotic cycle, and with various immune capacities (i.e., helper, cytolytic, etc.). The present studies of the motility of lymphocytes on various days after stimulation with mitogen or alloantigen were prompted by our previous observation that the most motile lymphocytes within the allosensitized lymphocyte population were Lyt-1-positive, noncytolytic T lymphocytes that were not actively incorporating thymidine. These studies utilized allosensitized lymphocytes on day 5 of culture. The present studies extend these preliminary observations. Lymphocytes activated in vitro are most motile after thymidine incorporation has peaked and abated. This observation applies to heterogeneous populations of lymphocytes stimulated with mitogen or alloantigen, as well as to T lymphocyte clones with proliferative, cytolytic, or both proliferative and cytolytic functions. This general observation holds true for clones with various Lyt phenotypes (Table 1). These data are consistent with the idea that the state of activation rather than the function of a lymphocyte is the more important determinant of lymphocyte motility. We cannot exclude the possibility that some clones will move faster than others—although the data suggests that the kinetics of activation may have a greater influence on the relative motility of lymphocyte subpopulations than difference in lymphocyte phenotype. These observations are consistent with our previous work (*6*) in which within a bulk population the cells that are migratory are not actively incorporating thymidine.

Our previous observations that Lyt-1$^+$ and not Lyt-2$^+$ lymphocytes, within an allosensitized bulk culture, were motile might seem incongruous with the present results. However, in the previous study, motility was assayed only on day 5 of culture when active thymidine incorporation was occurring. Perhaps in a bulk culture Lyt-1$^+$ cells enter and complete the mitotic cycle before Lyt-2$^+$ cells do. If the analysis of the Lyt phenotype of the migrated cells had been carried out on various days of culture, the data would certainly have shown that Lyt-2$^+$ lymphocytes are also motile.

There have been several publications concerning the differential motility of lymphocyte subpopulations (*5*, *6*, *16–20*). Considering the present data demonstrating differential motility depending on the state of activation, day of subculture, etc., it seems important to test each lymphocyte subpopulation in question under various conditions (after culture, after activation, etc.) before definitive statements about ability to locomote in response to a particular stimulus can be made. Ideally, clonded lymphocytes with defined function and surface phenotype should be used before conclusions can be made about differential motility of lymphocyte subsets.

Our studies demonstrate that T lymphocyte functional maturity correlates with the ability to locomote. This observation is in accordance with other studies correlating maturity with migratory function. Stamper and Woodruff (*21*) have demonstrated that thymocytes do not adhere to high endothelial venules as do lymphocytes obtained from lymph node, spleen, and thoracic duct. Otteskog and Sundqvist (*22*) have reported a differential anchorage and spreading capacity of thymic cells and peripheral blood T cells in an in vitro assay. These authors concluded that the spreading capacity reflects the stage of maturation of T cells. Mouse thymocytes demonstrate virtually no motility in the micropore membrane motility assay (unpublished observations) compared with lymph node lymphocytes (*23*). Lymph node lymphocytes are much less motile (2–3 hr migration times) than activated lymphocytes (1 hr migration time). Thus, lymphocyte populations containing many activated lymphocytes (in vitro activated cells) are more motile than populations containing few activated cells (lymph node lymphocytes), which in turn are more motile than populations containing virtually no activated cells (thymocytes).

Two phenomena, in fact, have been observed in these experiments: functionally mature T lymphocytes are able to locomote; and upon mitogenic stimulation, locomotor activity is lost. Utilizing clone 123-6 it was determined that, upon mitogenic stimulation, loss of motility occurs many hours before thymidine incorporation (S-phase) occurs. Therefore, when a lymphocyte receives the signal to initiate mitosis, perhaps there is a coincident signal to stop moving. Alternatively, another substance (or substances) produced during activation may inhibit lymphocyte motility, and mitosis may not be the immediate cause of the inhibition of lymphocyte motility.

The possible in vivo correlates of these observations are speculative. The initial paralysis of antigen-stimulated lymphocytes may function to limit the escape of maturing lymphocytes from lymphoid depots. However, after division the sensitized cells may escape into the circulation by virtue of their increased motility. By similar reasoning, restimulation of the sensitized cells within the inflamed tissue may serve to trap the paralyzed, sensitized subpopulation.

The above scenario does not exclude other mechanisms controlling the migration of lymphocytes to sites of inflammation or antigeneic deposition. Such influences include adherence to specially adapted vascular endothelium, changes in endothelial permeability within lymphoid depots or inflammed tissues (*24–26*), the acquisition of specialized receptors on sensitized cells for specific or nonspecific components of the inflammatory response (*3*), the possible role of antigen as a chemotactic agent, and/or the elaboration of nonspecific lymphocyte chemotactic factors by immunological interactions. In the latter regard, using an in vivo recruitment model, we have demonstrated that sensitized lymphocytes (*27*), 2° MLC-SN supernatant, and purified IL-1 (unpublished observations), all can act to attract circulating lymphocytes in vivo. We have not shown preferential in vivo recruitment of recently sensitized cells. In fact, most in vivo data support the idea that proliferation and maturation of sensitized cells at the site of antigeneic deposition are more important for the local enrichment of the sensitized cell population than recruitment of mature sensitized cells from the circulating pool (*28*). The change in the inherent motility of a sensitized lymphocyte may, however, play an important role in allowing the first few sensitized cells to reach the reaction site and initiate the local response.

Acknowledgments. The editorial contributions of Ellen Debe are appreciated. The technical expertise of Michael Hupke on the FACS IV is also appreciated. We thank Michael B. Widmer, Ph.D., and Derry C. Roopenian, Ph.D., for their contributions in deriving and characterizing the lymphocyte clones used in these studies.

REFERENCES

1. Parrott DMV, Wilkinson PC. Lymphocyte locomotion and migration. Prog Allergy 1981; 28: 193.
2. Wilkinson PC, Haston WS, Shields JM. Some determinants of the locomotory behavior of phagocytes and lymphocytes in vitro. Clin Exp Immunol 1982; 50: 461.
3. De Sousa M. Lymphocyte circulation: experimental and clinical aspects. New York: Wiley, 1981.
4. Wilkinson PC, Parrott DMV, Russell RJ, Sless F. Antigen-induced locomotor responses in lymphocytes. J Exp Med 1977; 145: 1158.
5. O'Neill GJ, Parrott DMV. Locomotion of human lymphoid cells. I. Effect of culture and Con A on T and non-T lymphocytes. Cell Immunol 1977; 33: 257.
6. Hoffman RA, Ascher NL, Hanto DW, Simmons RL. The migration of activated murine T lymphocytes in vitro. II. Evidence for differential locomotion of T cell subsets. J Immunol 1983; 130: 1610.
7. Cerrottini J-C, Engers HD, MacDonald HR, Brunner KT. Generation of cytotoxic T lymphocytes in vitro. I. Response of normal and immune mouse spleen cells in mixed leukocyte cultures. J Exp Med 1974; 140: 703.
8. Ryser JE, Cerottini J-C, Brunner KT. Generation of cytolytic T lymphocytes in vitro. IX. Induction of secondary CTL responses in primary long-term MLC by supernatants from secondary MLC. J Immunol 1978; 120: 370.
9. Roopenian DC, Widmer MB, Orosz CG, Bach FH. Helper cell independent cytolytic T lymphocytes specific for a minor histocompatibility antigen. J Immunol 1983; 130: 542.
10. Turner SR. ACDAS: An automated chemotaxis data acquisition system. J Immunol Methods 1979; 28: 355.
11. Becker EL, Davis AT, Estensen RD, Quie PG. Cytochalasin B. IV. Inhibition and stimulation of chemotaxis of rabbit and human polymorphonuclear leukocytes. J Immunol 1972; 108: 396.
12. Haston WS, Shields JM, Wilkinson PC. Lymphocyte locomotion and attachment on two-dimensional surfaces and in three-dimensional matrices. J Cell Biol 1982; 92: 747.
13. Schor SL, Allen TD, Winn B. Lymphocyte migration into three-dimensional collagen matrices: a quantitative study. J Cell Biol 1983; 96: 1089.
14. Zigmond SH, Hirsch JG. Leukocyte locomotion and chemotaxis. New methods for evaluation and demonstration of a cell-derived chemotactic factor. J Exp Med 1973; 137: 387.
15. Russell RJ, Wilkinson PC, Sless F, Parrott DMV. Chemotaxis of lymphoblasts. Nature 1975; 256: 646.
16. Wilkinson PC, Roberts JA, Russell RJ, McLoughlin M. Chemotaxis of mitogen-activated human lymphocytes and the effects of membrane-active enzymes. Clin Exp Immunol 1976; 25: 280.
17. Parrott DMV, Good RA, O'Neill GJ, Gupta S. Heterogeneity of locomotion in human T cell subsets. Proc Natl Acad Sci USA. 1978; 75: 2392.
18. Gupta S, Miescher A, Good RA. Subpopulations of human T lymphocytes. VIII. Locomotion of lymphocyte subpopulations in patients with primary immunodeficiency disorders. Thymus 1979; 1: 109.
19. Gupta S. Selective migration of T-cell subset in pleural fluid from non-Hodgkin's lymphoma. Thymus 1981; 2: 277.
20. Van Epps DE, Durant DA, Potter JW. Migration of human helper/

inducer T cells in response to supernatants from Con A-stimulated suppressor/cytotoxic T cells. J Immunol 1983; 131: 697.
21. Stamper HB Jr, Woodruff JJ. Lymphocyte homing into lymph nodes: in vitro demonstration of the selective affinity of recirculating lymphocytes for high-endothelial venules. J Exp Med 1976; 144: 828.
22. Otteskog P, Sundqvist KG. Anchorage and lymphocyte function. Spreading capacity distinguishes common thymocytes and peripheral T lymphocytes. Immunology 1983; 48: 675.
23. Hoffman RA, Ascher NL, Nelson RD, Simmons RL. Migration of mouse lymphocytes in vitro. I. Normal lymph node lymphocytes. Transplantation 1981; 31: 195.
24. Rose ML, Parrott DMV, Bruce RG. The accumulation of immunoblasts in extravascular tissues including mammary gland, peritoneal cavity, gut and skin. Immunology 1978; 35: 415.
25. Jungi TW, McGregor DD. Activated lymphocytes trigger lymphoblast extravasation. Cell Immunol 1978; 38: 76.
26. Ottaway CA, Parrott DMV. Regional blood flow and its relationship to lymphocyte and lymphoblast traffic during a primary immune reaction. J Exp Med 1979; 150: 218.
27. Hanto DW, Hopt UT, Hoffman RA, Simmons RL. Lymphocyte recruitment, regional blood flow and vascular permeability at sites of allogeneic cellular interactions. J Immunol 1982; 129: 2437.
28. Ascher NL, Chen S, Hoffman RA, Simmons RL. Maturation of cytotoxic T cells within sponge matrix allografts. J Immunol 1983; 131: 617.

Received 22 March 1985.
Accepted 18 June 1985.

0041-1337/86/4102-0220$02.00/0
TRANSPLANTATION

Vol. 41, No. 2
Printed in U.S.A.

DEVELOPMENT OF A SIMPLIFIED COUNTERFLOW CENTRIFUGATION ELUTRIATION PROCEDURE FOR DEPLETION OF LYMPHOCYTES FROM HUMAN BONE MARROW[1]

STEPHEN J. NOGA[2], ALBERT D. DONNENBERG,[2,3] CINDY L. SCHWARTZ,[4] LEWIS C. STRAUSS,[4] CURT I. CIVIN,[4,5] AND GEORGE W. SANTOS[2]

Bone Marrow Transplant Unit, Johns Hopkins Oncology Center, Baltimore, Maryland 21205

Graft-versus-host disease (GVHD) remains a major complication of allogeneic bone marrow (BM) transplantation. Techniques that effectively purge BM of mature T lymphocytes should reduce the incidence of GVHD and improve survival. We have developed a simplified, two-flow rate, fixed rotor speed counterflow centrifugation-elutriation (CCE) procedure that reproducibly depletes 99% of lymphocytes from Ficoll-Hypaque(F/H)-separated BM or BM buffy-coat. Two predetermined flow rates (24 and 28 ml/min) were used to purge small and intermediate-to-large lymphocytes, respectively, whereas faster sedimenting cells were recovered at the termination of the run. Lymphocyte depletion was substantiated by pan-T monoclonal antibody analysis as well as by complete loss of responsiveness to alloantigens and mitogens. Despite the lack of mature T cells, the depleted marrow fraction retained lymphoid colony-forming ability. Lymphocyte-purged marrow was obtained in high yield (72%), and retained high viability (>97%) and hematopoietic colony-forming ability (>99%). The ratio of total myeloid/erythroid colony-forming cells to T lymphocytes was 73-fold higher in the lymphocyte-depleted fraction than in unseparated BM. We concluded that a two-step CCE procedure can be used to rapidly deplete lymphocytes from both F/H-separated and buffy-coat BM inocula without altering hematopoietic capacity as measured by the in vitro clonogenic assays. It may be possible to adapt this procedure to the separation of the large number of marrow cells required for human BM transplantation.

Allogenic bone marrow transplantation (BMT)[6] is the treatment of choice for severe aplastic anemia and severe combined

[1] This work was supported by Grants CA15396, CA31687, and CA3218 from the National Cancer Institute.

[2] Bone Marrow Transplant Unit.
[3] To whom correspondence should be addressed, at Bone Marrow Transplant Unit, Johns Hopkins Oncology Center, Rm. 3-127, 600 N. Wolfe Street, Baltimore, MD 21205.
[4] Pediatric Oncology Division.
[5] Dr. Civin is a Scholar of the Leukemia Society of America.

[6] Abbreviations Used: BFU-E, erythroid burst forming units; BM, bone marrow; BMT, bone marrow transplantation; CCE, counterflow centrifugation elutriation; CFU-GEM, granulocyte/erythroid/monocyte colony forming units; CFU-GM, granulocyte/monocyte colony forming units; CFU-L, lymphoid colony forming units; EDTA, ethylenediaminotetraacetic acid; F/H, Ficoll-Hypaque; FITC, fluorescein isothiocyanate; FMF, flow microfluorometric analysis; GVHD, graft-versus-host disease; HBSS, hanks balanced salt solution; I1-2, interleukin-2; MLR, mixed lymphocyte reaction; PBML, peripheral blood mononuclear leukocytes; PBS, phosphate-buffered saline; PHA, phytohemagglutinin; R/O, rotor-off—residual cells in elutriator chamber; SI, stimulation index; UNQ, unique transplantation number; V/V, volume/volume; W/V, weight/volume.

immune deficiency, and has become a viable therapeutic option for leukemia. It also shows great promise for the treatment of other neoplastic diseases and congenital disorders (*1–2*). One of the major factors currently limiting the success of this modality is the occurrence of GVHD , which is believed to be mediated by donor T lymphocytes present in the graft preparation. Accordingly, methods that remove the majority of T lymphocytes from the graft prior to transplantation may be expected to increase survival by reducing the incidence of GVHD and infectious complications associated with this process.

The use of lectin agglutination followed by T cell–sheep erythrocyte (E) rosette depletion has been successful in preventing GVHD in immune-deficient recipients of haplo-mismatched (parental) BM (*3–5*). This technique is also being evaluated for the treatment of acute leukemias. Although promising, this method is time consuming and may require multiple transplants to establish marrow engraftment. Recently, encouraging results were reported when monoclonal antibodies directed against T cell surface antigens were used to reduce the incidence of GVHD among allogeneic transplant recipients (*6–9*).

Counterflow centrifugation elutriation can be used to separate large numbers of cells on the basis of differing sedimentation characteristics without impairing cell function or yield (*10–14*). Several investigators have recently used CCE to deplete a substantial proportion of lymphocytes from canine (*15*), simian (*16*), and human BM (*17, 18*), while retaining in vitro clonogenic and reconstructive capacity. These techniques succeeded in removing the majority of T lymphocytes from the donor graft—but, in the case of human BM, elutriation required a complicated collection and monitoring system to ensure separation (*17, 18*). The aim of our present study was to determine if CCE could be used to provide a lymphocyte-depleted fraction with high lymphohematopoietic clonogenic capacity while employing minimal manipulation, time, and instrumentation. Characterization of the lymphocyte-depleted fraction was performed with special attention to: phenotypic and functional detection of residual lymphocytes, and retention of hematopoietic and lymphocyte colony-forming cells.

MATERIALS AND METHODS

Bone marrow preparation. A 5–15-ml aliquot of human BM harvested from normal donors for allogeneic transplantation was used for each set of experiments. Written informed consent was obtained from each donor under a protocol approved by The Johns Hopkins Joint Committee for Clinical Investigation. The *experiment number* used in the tables refers to the unique transplant number (UNQ) assigned to each patient. Mature erythrocytes, granulocytes, and platelets were moved by isopyknic centrifugation over an F/H gradient of specific gravity 1.079 (*19*). Before underlaying with F/H, the BM sample was diluted 1:1 with calcium and magnesium-free Hanks' balanced salt solution (HBSS) containing 0.3 mM ethylenediaminetetraacetic acid (EDTA). After centrifugation (400×g, 40 min, 18°C), mononuclear cells were removed from the gradient interface and washed once in HBSS. The cells were then resuspended in elutriation medium consisting of calcium-and-magnesium–free HBSS (pH 7.20) with 0.3 mM EDTA, and 0.5% (W/V) bovine serum albumin (osmolality 290 mosm/L). In addition to F/H separation, an alternative method of cell preparation was used for samples obtained from two ABO–incompatible donors. BM samples were first processed by a Haemonetics Model-30 Cell Separator (Haemonetics Corp., Braintree, MA), which removed the majority of mature erythrocytes and a variable percentage of neutrophils. Aliquots of 1 ml from each of the two erythrocyte-depleted buffy-coat preparations destined for recipient reinfusion were combined, washed once in elutriation medium, and counted. Total cell counts were made by hemocytometer and by Coulter Counter, Model ZBI (Coulter Electronics Inc., Hialeah, FL). Viability was determined by trypan blue dye exclusion.

CCE. The use of predetermined flow rates at fixed rotor speed for the separation of leukocyte populations having small modal volume differences has been reported (*20–21*). Briefly 25–400×10^6 nucleated cells suspended in 5–10 ml of elutriation medium were injected into the inlet stream leading into the Beckman J-21 centrifuge that was equipped with a JE-6B elutriator rotor and standard chamber (Beckman Instruments, Spinco Division, Palo Alto, CA). A Masterflex peristaltic pump (Cole-Parmer Instrument Co., Chicago, IL) equipped with a vernier potentiometer provided precisely metered flow. The cells were loaded into the chamber at a flow rate of 15 ml/min, rotor speed of 3000 RPM, and a temperature of 18°C. A 50-ml eluate was collected and counted to confirm that fewer than 5×10^5 cells were eluted during loading. Rotor speed was held constant, and the cells were eluted by changing the flow rate. The flow rate was then increased to 24 ml/min and cells were collected by eluting to exhaustion (400 ml). This process was repeated after raising the flow rate to 28 ml/min. Cells remaining in the elutriator chamber were collected by continuing medium flow after stopping the rotor. Each cell fraction was collected by centrifugation (300×g, 15 min), washed twice in RPMI 1640, and counted, after which viability was determined. Slides were prepared using a cytocentrifuge (Shandon Southern Instruments Inc., Sewickly, PA) at 5×10^4 cells per slide in 20% human AB serum. Cell differentials were done on 500 cells stained with Wright-Giemsa (Camco Quick Stain, American Scientific Products, Ocala, FL). A Zeiss-3 microscope and camera were used to photograph the stained slides.

Monoclonal antibody analysis. Ficoll-Hypaque-separated BM and CCE-separated fractions were analyzed for surface antigen expression using monoclonal antibodies directly conjugated to fluorescein isothiocyanate (FITC, Beckton Dickinson, Sunnyvale, CA). One million viable cells in 100 μl phosphate-buffered saline (PBS) with 0.1% sodium azide were incubated with 5–10 μl of direct-conjugated antibody for 30 min at room temperature in 12×75-mm polystyrene tubes (Falcon Plastics, Oxnard, CA). After three washes with PBS (0.1% azide), the cells were fixed with paraformaldehyde (1% in PBS) and kept in the dark at 4°C until analyzed. Flow microfluorometric (FMF) analysis of antibody binding (*22*) was performed using FACSII instrumentation (Beckton Dickinson).

Colony forming assays: CFU-GM, BFU-E, GEM, CFU-L. Day 14 multilineage colonies (*23–25*) were assayed in duplicate using a modification of a previously described method (*26*). Ficoll-Hypaque-separated or CCE-fractionated BM (1×10^5 cells) were cultured in Iscove's modified Dulbecco's medium (GIBCO, Grand Island, NY) containing 30% fetal bovine serum, 0.96% (W/V) methylcellulose, 5% (V/V) GCT-conditioned medium (GIBCO), 1.5 U/ml erythropoietin (Connaught, Toronto Canada), and 5×10^5M 2-mercaptoethenol (1 ml medium/35-mm well). Colonies were scored on day 14 as CFU-GM, BFU-E, or CFU-GEM with colony number being a linear function of total cells plated. PHA-dependent, IL-2-responsive CFU-L were assayed using a modification of the whole-blood techniques previously described (*27–30*). Briefly, 1×10^5 fractionated or F/H separated BM or peripheral blood mononuclear leukocytes (PBML) were cultured (1 ml/35-mm well) in the presence of autologous irradiated (1500 rads) whole peripheral blood (3% V/V) in RPMI 1640 medium containing 15% human AB serum, 0.5% agarose, and supplements as previously described (*30*). Replicate cultures were established in the absence or presence of PHA-M (250 μg/ml), Difco Laboratories, Detroit, MI) plus IL-2 (1.0 unit/ml). IL-2 was derived from culture supernatants of the MLA-144 gibbon ape lymphoma cell line, which constitutively secretes IL-2 but no other known lymphokine (*31*). In all colony assays, colonies were enumerated using an inverted phase microscope (200×). The morphology of lymphoid colonies was determined by oil-immersion light microscopy (1000×) on Wright-Giemsa-stained agarose layers mounted on glass slides.

Mixed lymphocyte response and phytohemagglutinin assays. The ability of lymphocytes in F/H-separated BM and in the postelutriation fractions to respond to allogeneic lymphocytes in a mixed lymphocyte reaction (MLR) or to phytohemagglutinin (PHA) was assayed using thymidine incorporation as previously described (*3, 32*). Briefly, MLR was assayed under optimal conditions by mixing 1×10^5 effector cells (A) with an equal number of irradiated (1500 rads) allogeneic (Bx) or autologous PBML (Ax, control) and culturing for 6 days in 96-well U-bottomed Linbro plates (Flow Laboratories, Inc. Mc Lean, VA) at 37°C and 5% CO_2. ^{3}H-thymidine (0.5 μCi/well) was added 16 hr before harvesting. An optimized concentration of PHA-M (250 μg/ml) was added to 1×10^5 cells in 96-well Linbro plates with thymidine incorporation (4-hr labeling time) measured at 72 hr (*3, 32*).

RESULTS

Elutriation characteristics of Ficoll-Hypaque-separated human bone marrow. In preliminary experiments, it was determined that the majority of lymphocytes contaminating human bone marrow grafts exit the elutriator at 24 ml/min when the rotor speed is held constant at 3000 RPM. Size variability among donor lymphocytes results in incomplete purging of all lymphocytes even after a 400 ml collection volume. Some investigators have used continuous cell volume analysis to adjust flow rates for individual cell size variations (*17, 33*). We found this unnecessary for lymphocyte depletion, but rather a second 400-ml fraction taken at 28 ml/min was effective in removing all detectable lymphocytes from the elutriator chamber. In preliminary experiments, more efficient lymphocyte depletion was obtained when the majority of lymphocytes were first purged from the chamber at 24 ml/min rather than starting at 28 ml/min. In addition, we have previously shown that a critical cell density ($1–2\times10^8$) is necessary when separating cells of small diameter differences to prevent the premature elution of intermediate-sized cells due to chamber turbulence (*21*). Therefore, we used the two-step procedure to collect fractions at fixed flow rates of 24 and 28 ml/min for all experiments. A third fraction consisting of all cells still residing in the chamber was collected by stopping the rotor but continuing medium flow (designated the "rotor off" (R/O) fraction). When available, optimal cell numbers were initially loaded into the chamber.

TABLE 1. Leukocyte separation characteristics of CCE-fractionated human bone marrow[a]

Fraction	Percentage of eluted cells	Leukocyte differential[b]										
		Lymphocytes	Blast	Promyelocyte	Myelocyte	Band forms & metamyelocyte	Polymorphonuclear	Monocyte	Eosinophil	Basophil	Plasmacyte	Megakaryocyte[c]
Unseparated bone marrow	100	17.4±1.7	6.0±1.7	4.7±1.0	11.0±2.3	41.3±4.7	6.3±1.3	7.5±1.5	1.7±0.6	0.7±0.2	0.8±0.2	2.8±0.7
24 ml/min	18.0±1.1	97.1±0.6	0	0	0.1±0.1	0.1±0.1	0.1±0.1	2.6±0.4	0	0	0	0.1±0.7
28 ml/min	5.2±1.1	67.1±6.6	1.0±0.4	0.8±0.2	1.0±0.3	3.7±1.9	1.3±0.6	19.6±3.8	0	4.4±1.7	0.1±0.1	1.3±0.4
R/O	72.4±2.1	0.2±0.1	7.3±1.6	5.9±2.4	10.9±2.2	55.0±5.4	8.6±2.1	6.4±1.3	1.8±0.4	0.6±0.2	0.9±0.2	3.0±0.9

[a] Data are reported as mean ± SE on 10 consecutive experiments. The unseparated bone marrow was prepared by Ficoll-Hypaque separation of bone marrow harvested for allogeneic BMT.

[b] Percentage determined by evaluation of 500 leukocytes on Wright-giemsa-stained cytocentrifuge preparations.

[c] Megakaryocytes included in leukocyte differential.

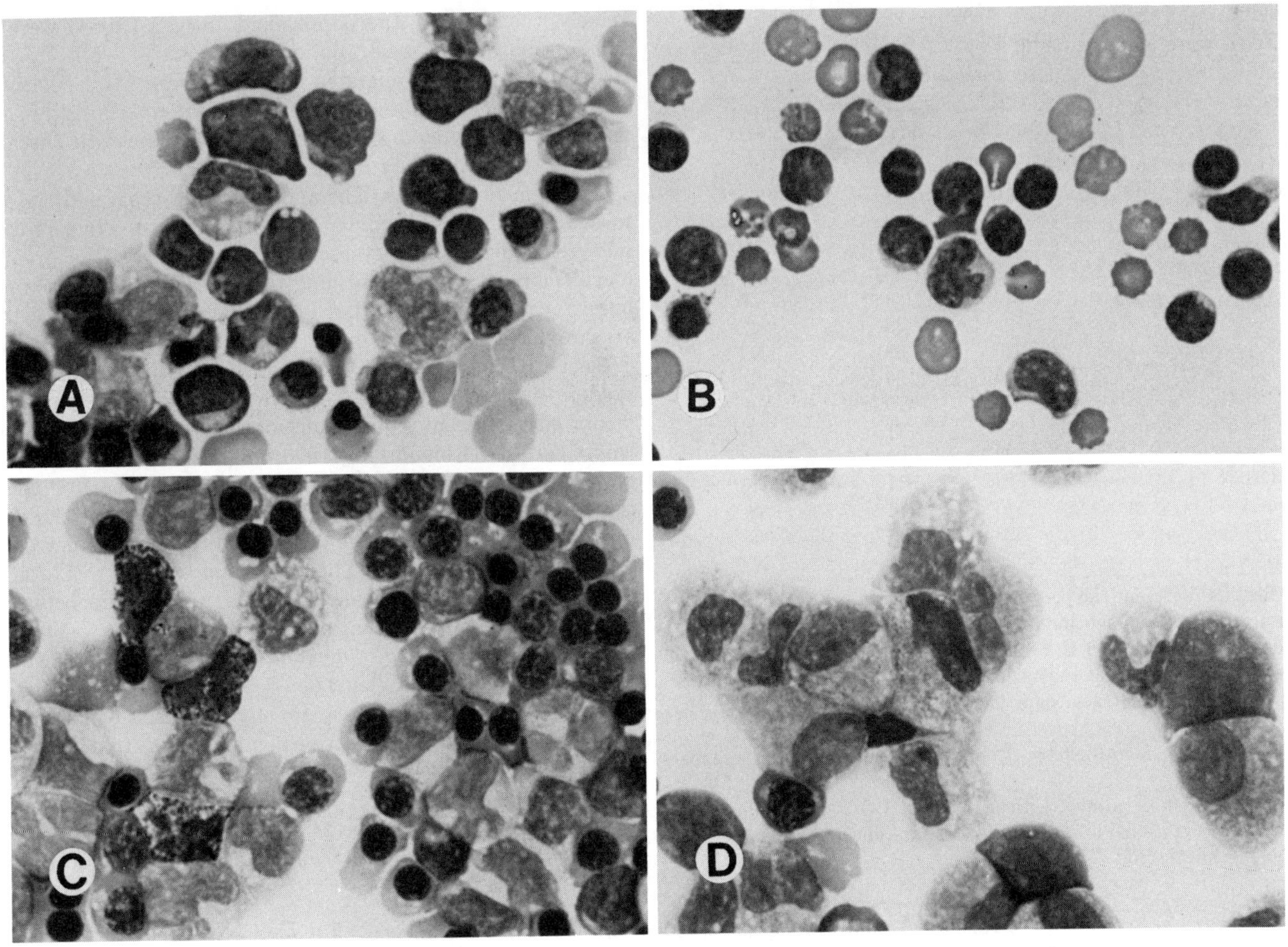

FIGURE 1. Morphology of human bone marrow fractions separated by CCE (Wright-Giemsa; ×1000). (A) Initial F/H-separated bone marrow preparation shows diverse cell populations including lymphocytes. (B) The 24 ml/min fraction is mainly composed of lymphocytes and mature erythrocytes. An occasional monocyte (off-center) can be identified. (C) The 28 ml/min fraction contains intermediate and large-sized lymphocytes, monocytes, basophils, and poly/orthochromotophilic normoblasts. (D) The R/O fraction contains 72% of the recovered cells; it lacks morphologically identifiable lymphocytes but possesses all the other leukocyte elements found in F/H-separated bone marrow.

Table 1 summarizes the elutriation characteristics of morphologically defined BM leukocytes. The leukocyte separation characteristics of BM from all 10 experiments are presented. Overall leukocyte recovery was 90% with greater than 97% viability in all fractions. Of total cells recovered, 18% were eluted at 24 ml/min. Morphologically, the leukocytes in this fraction were mostly lymphocytes and monocytes (97% and 3%, respectively) with mature erythrocytes making up the erythroid component (Fig. 1 B). Lymphocytes (67%) and monocytes (20%) were also the leukocytes most frequently found in the 28 ml/min fraction (Fig. 1C). Additionally, erythrocytes of various maturational states were present. A small percentage of cells in this fraction were identified as blasts (1.0%), promyelocytes (0.8%), and other myeloid precursors (5%). However, in 5 of 10 experiments in which greater cell numbers (75×10^6–400×10^6) were loaded into the elutriator, the 28 ml/min fraction was totally devoid of early myeloid elements. More importantly, irrespective of the loading cell number, this fraction was a small proportion of the eluted nucleated cells (range: 0.6–11%).

The third fraction, consisting of cells purged from the rotor at the completion of the run (R/O), retained all myeloid elements present in the unseparated BM (Fig. ID) but was essentially free of morphologically detectable lymphocytes (0.2%). The R/O fraction accounted for 72% of recovered cells. We concluded from these experiments that the two-step elutriation procedure provided a high-yield, simple rapid and reproducible means of depleting morphologically identifiable lymphocytes from human BM.

Monoclonal antibody analysis of CCE fractions. Ficoll-Hypaque-separated BM and elutriation fractions were analyzed using monoclonal antibodies to further characterize the cell populations, and to substantiate the observed morphologic depletion of lymphocytes in the R/O fraction. The fractions were profiled using leu-1 FITC (*34*), leu-4 FITC (*35*), and anti-My-1 FITC (*22*). A cocktail of leu-1 FITC and leu-4-FITC (pan-T) was used to detect the presence of mature T lymphocytes. Anti-My-1 FITC served as a pan-myeloid maker, since it binds to all cells of the granulocyte lineage beyond the myeloblast stage (*22*).

As shown in Table 2, <1% of R/O leukocytes displayed pan-T markers. In contrast, 5–12% of unseparated BM leukocytes were pan-T-positive. As expected, the lymphocyte-rich 24 and 28 ml/min fractions showed substantial pan-T binding. Con-

TABLE 2. Phenotypic analysis of human bone marrow leukocytes separated by CCE

Fraction	UNQ[b]	% leukocytes positive[a] For pan-T (FITC)	For My-1 (FITC)
F/H-separated bone marrow	506[c]	12	65
	510[c]	5	70
	523	8	63
	526	10	NT[d]
24 ml/min	506[c]	35	<1
	510[c]	38	<1
	523	59	<1
	526	58	NT
28 ml/min	506[c]	90	3
	510[c]	10	65
	523	71	1
	526	79	NT
R/O	506[c]	<1	75
	510[c]	<1	83
	523	<1	79
	526	<1	NT

[a] Results represent the percentage of total leukocytes that bind the directly conjugated monoclonal Leu 1/4 FITC (pan-T), and My-1 FITC, as determined by FACS II FMF analysis of 30,000 cells. IgG_1 FITC was used as control and subtracted from the respective experimental counterparts. Percentages below minimal level of FACS II sensitivity are listed as <1%.

[b] Subjects are identified by their unique transplantation number (UNQ).

[c] Experiments performed with fewer than 1×10^8 cells (suboptimal separation conditions) initially loaded into the elutriator chamber.

[d] NT = not tested.

versely, cells bearing the panmyeloid antigen (My-1) were a small proportion of 24 ml/min leukocytes (<1%), while 79% of R/O and 66% of unseparated BM cells were My-1-positive. Thus, differences in the phenotypic markers expressed on mature lymphocytes and myeloid cells correlate with characteristics permitting their resolution by CCE.

Colony-forming assays. The ability of CCE-separated BM to form myeloid and erythroid colonies was evaluated in a 14-day methylcellulose culture system by the enumeration of granulocyte/monocyte colony-forming units (CFU-GM), erythroid burst-forming units (BFU-E), and granulocyte/monocyte/erythroid colony-forming units (CFU-GEM). Additionally, the presence of lymphoid colony-forming units (CFU-L) was measured in a 6-day PHA, IL-2-dependent agarose system that displayed a stringent requirement for the presence of irradiated whole peripheral blood (3%, 1500 rads). Essentially all CFU-GM, BFU-E, and CFU-GEM were recovered in the R/O fraction (Table 3). In experiments performed with suboptimal cell numbers, a small percentage of colonies (3–7%) was detected in the 28 ml/min fraction. The 24 ml/min fraction was totally devoid of all 3 types of colonies. The relationship between hematopoietic colony retention and T lymphocyte depletion was expressed as a ratio of myeloid-plus-erythroid colonies to phenotypically defined (leu-1/leu-4-positive) T lymphocytes (Table 3). This parameter was greatly increased (73±23-fold, mean ± SEM) in the R/O fraction compared with that observed in F/H-separated BM.

In contrast, considerable CFU-L were detected in all elutriation fractions (Table 4). The 24 and 28 ml/min fractions grew colonies having the typical cellular morphologies of PHA-

TABLE 3. Colony-forming ability of human bone marrow separated by CCE

Fraction	UNQ[a]	CFU-GM Colony efficiency per 10^5[b]	CFU-GM Total colonies per fraction[c]	BFU-E Colony efficiency per 10^5	BFU-E Total colonies per fraction[c]	GEM Colony efficiency per 10^5	GEM Total colonies per fraction[c]	Myeloid & erythroid colonies: T cell ratio[d]
F/H-separated bone marrow	506[e]	159	120	103	78	0	0	0.02
	510[e]	91	14	372	57	0	0	0.09
	523	122	545	61	272	0	0	0.02
	526	192	299	210	327	2	3	0.04
	527[e]	352	153	162	70	2	1	NT[f]
24 ml/min	506[e]	0	0	0	0	0	0	0
	510[e]	0	0	0	0	0	0	0
	523	0	0	0	0	0	0	0
	526	0	0	0	0	0	0	0
	527[e]	0	0	0	0	0	0	NT
28 ml/min	506[e]	76	3	101	4	12	0.5	0.002
	510[e]	59	1	134	3	2	0	0.03
	523	0	0	0	0	0	0	0
	526	116	1	198	2	14	0	0
	527[e]	88	3	76	3	16	0.6	NT
R/O	506[e]	212	116	176	96	3	2	1.95
	510[e]	167	16	390	38	2	0.2	1.13
	523	168	551	83	272	3	10	1.27
	526	245	314	225	289	4	5	4.75
	527[e]	436	123	288	81	8	2	NT

[a] Data were obtained on five consecutive elutriations of normal donor marrow harvested for allogeneic transplantation. The subjects are identified by their unique transplant numbers (UNQ).

[b] Values represent the mean number of colonies per 10^5 viable cells plated in duplicate in a 14-day methylcellulose culture system. The number of F/H-separated bone marrow cells used for each experiment was variable, resulting in differences in total colonies found within the fractions.

[c] Total colony number expressed in thousands (efficiency × total nucleated cells in fraction).

[d] The ratio of total myeloid/erythroid colonies to cells bearing the mature T cell markers Leu 1 and/or Leu 4.

[e] Experiments performed with fewer than 1×10^8 cells initially loaded into the elutriator chamber.

[f] NT = not tested.

TABLE 4. Lymphoid colony-formation in human bone marrow fractions separated by CCE

Fraction	UNQ[a]	Colony-forming efficiency[b]	
		PHA + IL2	No PHA, No IL-2
Peripheral blood	523	260	0
	526	72	0
	527[c]	31	0
F/H-separated	523	99	26
	526	20	3
	527[c]	59	0
24 ml/min	523	120	0
	526	79	0
	527[c]	14	0
28 ml/min	523	100	5
	526	35	0
	527[c]	22	0
R/O	523	129	42
	526	29	0
	527[c]	61	2

[a] Subjects are identified by their unique transplantation number.

[b] Data are reported as colonies/10^5 cells (means of triplicate determinations).

[c] Experiments performed with fewer than 1×10^8 cells initially loaded into the elutriation chamber.

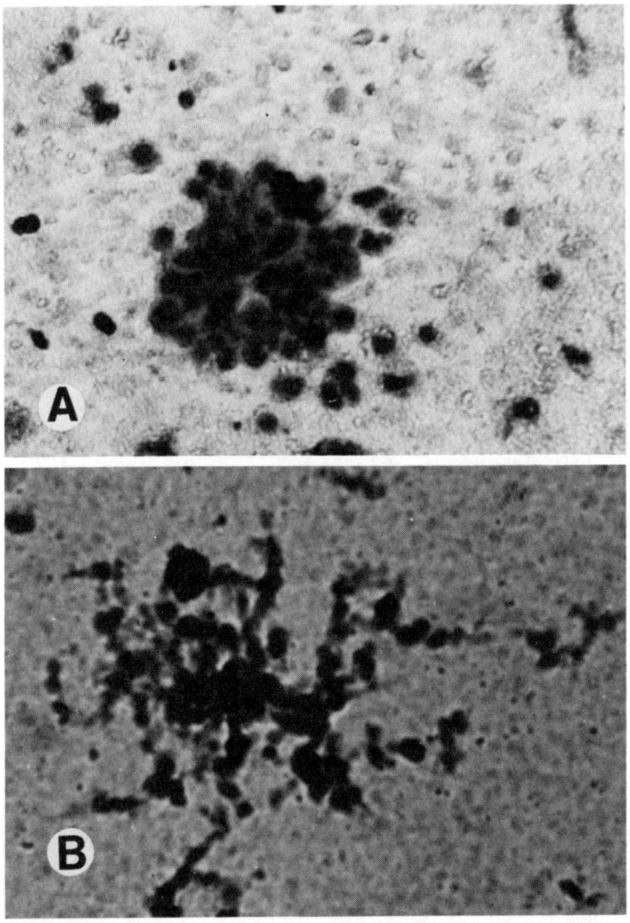

FIGURE 2. Morphology of human lymphoid colonies obtained before and after T lymphocyte depletion by CCE. (A) Typical discoid-shaped colony found in unseparated human BM. Individual cells possess a small dark-staining nucleus with scant cytoplasm. (B) Diffuse colony found within the lymphocyte-depleted R/O fraction. Individual cells possess increased cytoplasmic volume, large euchromatic nuclei, and one or more long pseudopodia.

stimulated peripheral blood T lymphocytes. Two principal colony types were detected. Surface colonies were discoid or spherical, with individual cells possessing a small dark staining nucleus and large amounts of heterochromatin (Fig. 2A). Diffuse colonies arising within the medium consisted of stellate cells with a higher cytoplasm-to-nucleus ratio than the surface colonies. Frequently these colonies contained a nidus of closely packed cells surrounded by a diffuse cellular halo. In contrast, the R/O fraction contained primarily diffuse colonies. Although some of these diffuse colonies closely resembled those found in peripheral blood, the majority were of different cellular morphology. Cells within these colonies were characterized by increased cytoplasmic volume, large euchromatic nuclei and one or more long pseudopodia (Fig. 2B). The number of cells per colony was variable, ranging from 50 to several thousand cells. All three colony types were detected in cultures derived from the initial F/H-separated BM. In the absence of PHA plus IL-2, no colonies were detected using PBML or the 24 ml/min fraction. Low numbers of colonies were detected sporadically in the 28 ml/min and R/O fractions, as well as in F/H-separated BM. The majority were clearly of myeloid morphology. Thus, aliquots of actual graft preparations used for allogeneic BMT were substantially depleted of mature T lymphocytes without appreciably reducing the number of myeloid, erythroid, or early lymphoid colonies, all of which may provide an index of the hematopoietic potential.

MLR and PHA response of elutriated bone marrow. Inability to respond to MLR has been used to substantiate the purging of mature alloreactive lymphocytes from the marrow preparation (*3, 4*). Additionally, response to mitogens such as PHA provides a sensitive means of detecting residual lymphocytes. Consequently, all elutriation fractions were analyzed for lymphocyte functional activity by contrasting the MLR and PHA response of CCE-separated BM with that of the original unelutriated preparation. Lymphocyte-containing fractions (24 and 28 ml/min had stimulation indices (SI) for both MLR and PHA comparable to those obtained for PBML (Table 5). Ficoll-Hypaque-separated BM showed moderate reactivity to allogeneic cells (SI 1.2–3.6) and PHA (SI 2.3–5.4), while minimal or depressed responses were obtained with R/O cells (SI 0.3–1.4 MLR, 0.7–1.5 PHA). It should be noted that the background incorporation of thymidine in unseparated BM and in the R/O fraction was considerably higher than that of the 24 ml/min, 28 ml/min, and PBML fractions. These results are consistent with the retention in the R/O fraction of a cell population having an inherently high proliferative component. The lack of thymidine incorporation in excess of background following allogeneic or PHA stimulation provides functional evidence for the substantial depletion of lymphocytes in the R/O fraction.

Elutriation of haemonetics-separated bone marrow buffy-coat. Large-volume blood cell processors, such as the Haemonetics-30, are in routine use for depleting BM of erythrocytes prior to infusion into ABO-incompatible recipients (*36*). The resulting buffy-coat provides a concentrated source of erythrocyte-depleted and granulocyte-depleted cells with in vitro reconstitutive properties indistinguishable from unseparated marrow. To determine whether this procedure could replace F/H separation as a means of reducing cell number prior to elutriation, we injected Haemonetics-separated BM (2 ml) directly into the inlet stream of the elutriator rotor without further manipulation. Samples from two ABO-incompatible transplants were processed. These samples contained a mean of 1.0×10^8 leukocytes and 2.1×10^9 erythrocytes. The R/O frac-

TABLE 5. Mixed lymphocyte reactivity and PHA response of CCE-fractionated human bone marrow

Fraction	UNQ[a]	Mixed lymphocyte response			PHA response		
		A + Bx (cpm×10³)	A + Ax Control (cpm×10³)	Stimulation index	PHA (cpm×10³)	Medium control	Stimulation index
Peripheral blood mononuclear cells	510	NT[c]	NT	NT	NT	NT	NT
	523	22.8±0.9	0.9±0.2	25.3	34.7±6.3	0.3±0.1	115.7
	526	28.2±3.8	0.5±0.2	56.4	25.0±1.3	0.2±0.1	125.0
	527	22.9±3.7	0.3±0.1	76.3	26.0±0.8	0.1±0.1	260.0
F/H-separated bone marrow	510[b]	6.6±0.3	5.8±0.4	1.2	NT	NT	NT
	523	21.1±3.1	5.9±0.5	3.6	21.0±1.5	9.1±0.8	2.3
	526	12.3±1.0	7.0±0.3	1.8	22.4±0.9	4.2±0.1	5.3
	527[b]	9.5±1.4	6.0±0.2	1.6	27.2±8.3	5.0±0.3	5.4
24 ml/min	510[b]	13.4±2.6	0.9±0.1	14.9	NT	NT	NT
	523	15.3±0.4	0.6±0.1	25.5	24.8±2.4	0.5±0.1	49.6
	526	24.7±2.3	0.8±0.1	30.9	25.0±2.1	0.7±0.1	35.7
	527[b]	16.4±5.3	0.2±0.1	82.0	20.7±0.1	0.1±0.1	207
28 ml/min	510[b]	3.8±0.6	1.9±0.2	2.0	NT	NT	NT
	523	25.7±5.9	1.0±0.1	25.7	22.3±0.7	0.6±0.2	37.2
	526	27.5±4.6	2.3±0.2	12.0	15.2±1.0	1.8±0.3	8.4
	527[b]	32.6±4.3	1.2±0.1	27.2	14.5±1.2	0.5±0.1	29.0
R/O	510[b]	2.7±1.0	8.5±0.5	0.3	NT	NT	NT
	523	5.7±1.0	4.2±0.4	1.4	7.9±1.2	12.0±0.7	0.7
	526	2.4±0.4	6.7±0.6	0.4	4.3±0.2	5.2±0.4	0.8
	527[b]	5.1±1.0	5.3±0.3	1.0	8.8±0.8	6.0±0.2	1.5

[a] Data are reported as mean ± SE on individual consecutive experiments identified by their unique transplant number (UNQ). Irradiated autologous (Ax, control) or allogeneic (Bx) lymphocytes were added to an equal number of cells (A) from the various fractions. The control (Ax) for experiment 510 was medium alone. Reactivity was determined at 6 days. PHA-M (250 μg/ml) was added to 1×10⁵ responder cells in a 3-day assay.

[b] Experiments performed with fewer than 1×10⁸ cells initially loaded into the elutriation chamber.

[c] NT = not tested.

TABLE 6. Lymphocyte depletion of Ficoll/Hypaque-separated BM versus BM buffy coat[a]

	Ficoll-Hypaque-separated BM	Bone marrow buffy coat	
		Exp 1	Exp 2
Nucleated cell recovery	72%±6	88%	92%
Lymphocyte depletion determined by:			
Morphology[b]	99.9%±0.1	99.8%	99.7%
Pan T-FMF analysis[b]	99%±0.1	99%	99%
Lymphocyte responsiveness (stimulation index):			
MLR	0.8±0.5	0.2	0.6
PHA	1.0±0.4	0.4	0.8
Colony recovery:			
CFU-GM	100±13	NT	NT
BFU-E	99±23	NT	NT
CFU-GEM	133±47	NT	NT
CFU-L	76±20	82	90

[a] Normal donor marrow harvested for allogenic transplantation was first separated on Ficoll-Hypaque (SG 1.079). Alternatively, BM buffy coat was prepared on a Haemonetics-30 cell separator. The data represent the mean of 4–5 experiments ± SEM on Ficoll-Hypaque-separated BM and two experiments using the Haemonetics-30 (UNQ 523, 526).

[b] Formula for calculating lymphocyte depletion:

$$\left[1 - \left(\frac{\text{R/O nucleated cells} \times \%\ \text{lymphs.}}{\text{Input nucleated cells} \times \%\ \text{lymphs.}}\right)\right] \times 100.$$

tion was similar in analysis to that of F/H-separated marrow (Table 6) but yielded even higher recovery in the R/O fraction (90%).

DISCUSSION

CCE has been used to separate and characterize BM from a variety of mammalian species (*12–14*). In particular, CCE fractionated marrow has recently been used to successfully reconstitute simians (*16*), canines (*15*), and humans (*37, 38*) receiving marrow lethal drugs and/or irradiation. The methodologies employed in these studies were dependent upon the collection of multiple fractions (*15–17*). In some cases, continuous cell size monitoring equipment was employed to ensure separation of mature lymphocytes from the remainder of the cells in the graft (*37–38*). For elutriation to be used effectively in the prevention of GVHD in allogeneic BMT recipients, the technique should meet three basic criteria: 1. It must be effective in the removal of mature T lymphocytes from the donor graft. 2. The methods of depletion should not cause an appreciable reduction in the hematopoietic capacity of the donor graft. 3. It must be highly reproducible from donor to donor. Additionally, the utility of such a separation procedure would be greatly increased if it were rapid, simple, and inexpensive.

Toward this end we performed pilot experiments using a simplified two-step, fixed rotor speed separation procedure. We found this method strikingly effective in the removal of morphologically, phenotypically, and functionally identifiable lymphocytes from human BM. The samples used were aliquots from actual preparations harvested for allogeneic BMT, and contained higher percentages of T lymphocytes than that found in "first-pull" marrow. Despite this considerable contamination with mature peripheral blood lymphocytes, leukocyte differentials showed that lymphocytes were >99% depleted from the residual chamber fraction (R/O) in the 10 patient marrows separated to date. We believe this to be a more thorough lymphocyte depletion than reported previously for CCE. Monroy et al. achieved a 95–97% reduction of lymphocytes in the monkey (*16*), Jemionek and coworkers a 46–81% depletion in the fraction reconstituting the dog (*15*), and DeWitte and colleagues reported a 95–98% depletion with human BM preparations (*17, 37, 38*). In the latter most recent series (20 patients), this degree of lymphocyte depletion appeared to be adequate to prevent GVHD when combined with chemoprophylaxis (*38*). None of 18 patients receiving CCE-separated BM plus chemophrophylaxis (methotrexate or cyclosporine) developed GVHD, whereas 2 subjects receiving CCE-separated BM alone developed significant disease. Morphologic and in vitro functional data reported for other methodologies that purge lymphocytes from BM were not demonstrably superior to our CCE procedure. Lectin binding coupled with E-rosette depletion (*3, 4*) or monoclonal antibody treatment (*8*) depleted 95.7% and >99%, respectively, of lymphocytes from human marrow. We documented T cell purging from the R/O fraction by FMF analysis with pan-T (Leu 1/4) markers. Less than 1% of leukocytes displayed these T cell markers. Other investigators, using sequential CCE fractionation, detected 1.8–4.6% OKT3 (Pan-T)-positive cells in the purged BM inocula (*17*). Monoclonal antibodies alone or with complement have also been reported to effectively kill or deplete the majority of cells identified by pan-T markers from human BM without interfering with engraftment—and in most cases reduced the incidence of GVHD (*8, 9, 39–42*).

Ablation of lymphocyte functions, particularly alloreactivity, is important in a BM fraction designed to reconstitute without mediating GVHD. We have shown that the R/O fraction had substantially lower MLR and PHA reactivity than the F/H-separated BM. These results compare favorably with those reported by Reissner and coworkers on lectin-treated, rosette-depleted, haploidentical marrow used to reconstitute patients with acute leukemia (*4*) or severe combined immunodeficiency syndrome (*5*). Reduction of PHA and MLR responses in our series was comparable to that reported by DeWitte et al. (*43*) for CCE preparations used in allogeneic BMT.

The desirability of rigorous lymphocyte depletion must be balanced against the reconstitutive capacity of the fractionated preparation. This criterion was evaluated indirectly by in vitro colony-forming assays. Colony assays showed that nearly all CFU-GM, BFU-E, and CFU-GEM were recovered in the R/O fraction. The total myeloid-plus-erythroid colony:T cell ratio of the R/O fraction increased 73-fold over that of unseparated BM (Table 3), indicating a marked enrichment of colony-forming cells relative to mature lymphocytes. Even when sub-optimal cell concentrations were used in the elutriator, only low numbers of CFU-GM, BFU-E, and CFU-GEM were eluted in the 28 ml/min fraction. Since this fraction constituted 5% of nucleated BM cells, the actual number of colony-forming units not recovered in the R/O fraction was minimal. DeWitte et al. (*17*) have reported a 90% CFU-GM and 98.6% BFU-E recovery following CCE of human BM, while Monroy and colleagues reported a 20–50% recovery of the original CFU-GM activity in the CCE fraction reconstituting the monkey (*16*). In their initial studies, Reissner and coworkers recovered 22.2% of the original CFU-C activity following lectin and rosette depletion of human BM, but were still able to achieve engraftment (*3–5*).

We have also assessed the ability of cells present in the R/O fraction to give rise to mature T lymphocytes using a PHA-dependent lymphoid colony assay (Table 4). The R/O fraction formed T cell colonies having morphology compatible with that described for BM radically depleted of mature T cells by treatment with monoclonal antibody and complement (*44–45*). In one experiment (UNQ 526) colonies were found to contain mature T cells by direct immunofluorescent staining with a cocktail of FITC-conjugated Leu-1/4 monoclonal antibodies (data not shown). The relatively high efficiency of colony formation suggests that the colonies detected in the R/O fraction were derived from immature precursors rather than from contaminating lymphocytes. It is not currently known whether these cells can mediate GVHD. However, similar colony-forming cells have also been observed in BM treated with anti-T-cell monoclonal antibody and complement (*44–46*), a regimen that has been successful in reducing GVHD (*9, 47*).

Although in vitro clonogenic assays do not necessarily predict in vivo reconstitution, the present data, taken together with previously reported results (*37, 38*), strongly suggest that the R/O fraction contains the cell population(s) necessary for complete hematopoietic reconstitution.

The third stipulation involves high reproducibility in the composition of the final fraction with respect to lymphocyte depletion and retention of clonogenic capacity. The results (Tables 1–5, summarized in Table 6), indicate that lymphocyte contamination (measured morphologically or phenotypically) never exceeded 1%. Although greater variability was encountered with respect to retention of clonogenic capacity, the CFU-GM and BFU-E recovery always exceeded 80% and 70%, respectively, and CFU-GEM recovery always exceeded 100%. The remaining colony-forming cells were recovered in the 28 ml/min fraction. Experiments in which the initial loading concentration of cells was suboptimal accounted for the greatest loss of colony-forming cells in this series.

We anticipate that the procedure described in this report will be of value in facilitating the study of lymphohematopoietic differentiation in the absence of contaminating mature T cells. Its ultimate clinical application as a rapid means of purging lymphocytes from human BM grafts will depend upon the success of scale-up experiments currently in progress. Marrow preparations harvested for allogeneic BMT contain on the order of $2\text{–}4 \times 10^{10}$ nucleated cells, and have hematocrits as high as 25%. The number of nucleated cells can be reduced by over 50% and the erythrocyte number lowered by 96% using centrifugation techniques currently employed for erythrocyte depletion in ABO mismatched BMT (*36*). The resulting preparation is well within the reported capacity of the newly developed Beckman JE-10X elutriator chamber, making possible the elutriation of an entire marrow preparation in a single run. Our small-scale pilot studies reported here indicate that erythrocyte-depleted BM buffy-coat can be loaded directly into the elutriation chamber without compromising the resolution of the separation (Table 6). Experiments are currently in progress to determine whether similar resolution can be achieved using the high capacity chamber and rotor.

Acknowledgments. Dr. Allan Hess was instrumental in establishing the initial MLR assays. Dr. Strauss is a fellow of the Leukemia Society of America. We wish to express our appreciation to Emilie Bright, Dr. Mona Lisa C. Banquerigo, Karen Dattilio, and Linda Norton for their exceptional technical assistance. We are grateful for the assistance of Connie Rutter and Lisa Alai in the careful preparation of the manuscript.

REFERENCES

1. O'Reilly RJ, Allogeneic bone marrow transplantation: current status and future directions. Blood 1983; 62(5): 941.
2. Santos GW, Kaizer H. Bone marrow transplantation in acute leukemia. Semin Hematol 1982; 19(3): 227.
3. Reisner Y, Kapoor N, O'Reilly RJ, Good RA. Allogeneic bone marrow transplantation using stem cells fractionated by lections. VI. In vitro analysis of human and monkey bone marrow cells fractionated by sheep red blood cells and soybean agglutinin. Lancet 1980; 2: 1320.
4. Reisner Y, Kapoor N, Kirkpatrick D, Pollack MS, Dupont B, Good RA, O'Reilly RJ. Transplantation for acute leukaemia with HLA-A and B nonidentical parental marrow cells fractionated with soybean agglutinin and sheep red blood cells. Lancet 1981; 2: 327.
5. O'Reilly RJ, Kapoor N, Kirkpatrick D, Cunningham-Rundles S, Pollack MS, Dupont B, Hodes MZ, Good RA, Reisner Y. Transplantation for severe combined immunodeficiency using histoincompatible parental marrow fractionated by soybean agglutinin and sheep red blood cells: experience in six consecutive cases. Transplant Proc 1983; 15(1): 1431.
6. Prentice HG, Blacklock HA, Janossy G, Bradstock KF, Skeggs D, Goldstein G, Hoffbrand AV. Use of anti-T-cell monoclonal antibody OKT3 to prevent acute graft-versus-host disease in allogeneic bone-marrow transplantation for acute leukemia. Lancet 1982; 1: 700.
7. Filipovich AH, McGlave PB, Ramsay NK, Goldstein G, Warkentin PI, Kersey JH. Pretreatment of donor bone marrow with monoclonal antibody OKT3 for prevention of acute graft-versus-host disease in allogeneic histocompatible bone-marrow transplantation. Lancet 1982; 1: 1266.
8. Filipovich AH, Vallera DA, Youle RJ, Quinones RR, Neville Jr DM, Kersey JH. Ex-vivo treatment of donor bone marrow with anti-T-cell immunotoxins for prevention of graft-versus-host disease. Lancet 1984; 1: 469.
9. Prentice HG, Blacklock HA, Janossy G, Gilmore MJML, Price-Jones L, Tidman N, Trejdosiewicz LK, Skeggs DBL, Panjwani D, Ball S, Graphakos S, Patterson J, Ivory K, Hoffbrand AV. Depletion of T lymphocytes in donor marrow prevents significant graft-versus-host disease in matched allogeneic leukaemic marrow transplant recipients. Lancet 1984; 1: 472.
10. Grabske RJ. Separating cell populations by elutriation. Fractions 1978; 1: 1.
11. Pretlow II TG, Pretlow TP. Centrifugal elutriation (counter streaming centrifugation) of cells. Cell Biophys 1979; 1: 195.
12. Meyskens Jr FL, Kiefer CA, Holmes DK, Gerner EW. Separation of normal human bone marrow cells by counterflow centrifugal elutriation. I. morphological analysis and subfractionation of neutrophilic granulocytes. Exp Hematol 1979; 7(8): 402.
13. Inque T, Carsten AL, Cronkite EP, Kelley JET. Separation and concentration of murine hematopoietic stem cells (CFU_s) using a combination of density gradient sedimentation and counterflow centrifugal elutriation. Exp Hematol 1981; 9(6): 563.
14. Jemionek JF, MacVittie TJ, Byrne PJ, Schein PS, Walden DA. Fractionation of mammalian bone marrow by counterflow centrifugation-elutriation using a continuous albumin gradient: analysis of granulocytemacrophage colony-forming units. Br J Haematol 1982; 50: 257.
15. Jemionek JF, Monroy RL, MacVittie TJ, Contreras TJ, Espy SB. Bone marrow reconstitution of lethally irradiated canines using autologous bone marrow fractions obtained by counterflow centrifugation elutriation. Br J Haematol 1982; 51: 585.
16. Monroy RL, Darden JH, MacVittie TJ, Patchen ML, Schwartz GN. Transplantation of a hematopoietic stem cell population isolated by counterflow centrifugation-elutriation from monkey bone marrow. Exp Hematol 1984; 12: 384.
17. De Witte T, Plas A, Koekman E, Blankenborg G, Salden M, Wessels J, Haanen C. Cell size monitored counterflow centrifugation of human bone marrow resulting in clonogenic cell fractions substantially depleted of small lymphocytes. J Immunol Methods 1983; 65: 171.
18. De Witte T, Plasa, Koekman E, Blankenborg G, Salden M, Wessels J, Haanen C. Separation of human bone marrow by counterflow centrifugation monitored by DNA-flowcytometry. Br J Hematol 1984; 58: 249.
19. Boyum A. Separation of leucocytes from blood and bone marrow with special reference to factors which influence and modify sedimentation properties of hematopoietic cells. Scand J of Clin Lab Invest 1968; 21(suppl 97): 9.
20. Noga SJ, Normann SJ, Weiner R. Separation and characterization of guinea pig monocyte subsets using counter-flow centrifugation elutriation (CCE). In: Norman SJ, Sorkin E, eds. Macrophages and natural killer cells. New York: Plenum, 1982: 221.
21. Noga SJ, Normann SJ, Weiner RS. Isolation of guinea pig monocytes and Kurloff cells: characterization of monocyte subsets by morphology, cytochemistry, and adherence. Lab Invest 1984; 51(2): 244.
22. Strauss LC, Stuart RK, Civin CI. Antigenic analysis of hematopoiesis. I. Expression of the My-1 granulocyte surface antigen on human marrow cells and leukemic cell lines. Blood 1983; 61(6): 1222.
23. Fauser AA, Messner HA. Identification of megakaryocytes macrophages, and eosinophils in colonies of human bone marrow containing neutrophilic granules and erythroblasts. Blood 1979; 53: 1023.
24. Nakahata T, Spicer SS, Ogawa M. Clonal origin of human erythroeosinophilic colonies in culture. Blood 1982; 59: 857.
25. Iscove N, Sieber F, Winterhalter E. Erythroid colony formation in cultures of mouse and human bone marrow: analysis of the requirement for erythropoietin by gel filtration and affinity chromatography in agarose conconavalin A. J Cell Physiol 1974; 83: 309.
26. Civin CI, Strauss LC, Brovall C, Fackler MJ, Schwartz JF, Shaper JH. Antigenic analysis of hematopoiesis. III. A hematopoietic progenitor cell surface antigen defined by a monoclonal antibody raised against KG-1a cells. J Immunol 1984; 133(1): 157.
27. Knox SJ, Shifrine M, Wilson FD, Rosenblatt LS. The selective growth of human T lymphocyte colonies from whole blood in a semisolid culture system. Exp Hematol 1981; 9(9): 926.
28. Donnenberg AD, Elfenbein GJ. Lymphocyte colony formation in human allogeneic bone marrow transplant recipients. Exp Hematol 1981; 9(9): 62.
29. Donnenberg AD, Elfenbein GJ, Santos GW. Cell-cell cooperation in lymphocyte colony formation: studies in human allogeneic marrow transplantation. J Immunol 1982; 129: 1080.
30. Hess AD, Donnenberg AD, Engel P, Tutschka PJ, Santos GW. Suppressor-cell amplification circuitry in cyclosporine-treated MLR cultures. Transplant Proc 1983; 15(4): 2343.
31. Henderson LE, Hewetson JF, Hopkins III RF, Sowder RC, Neubauer RH, Rabin H. A rapid large scale purification procedure for gibbon interleukin 2. J Immunol 1983; 131(2): 810.
32. Rotter V, Yakir Y, Trainin N. Role of L-alanine in the response of human lymphocytes to PHA and Con A. J Immunol 1979; 123: 1726.
33. Sanderson RJ, Shepperdson FT, Vatter AE, Talmage DW. Isolation and enumeration of peripheral blood monocytes. J Immunol 1977; 118(4): 1409.

34. Engleman EG, Warnke R, Fox RI, Levy R. Studies of a human T lymphocyte antigen recognized by a monoclonal antibody. Proc Natl Acad Sci USA 1981; 78: 1791.
35. Ledbetter JA, Evans RL, Lipinski M, Cunningham-Rundles C, Good RA, Herzenberg LA. Evolutionary conservation of surface molecules that distinguish T lymphocyte helper/inducer and T cytotoxic/suppressor subpopulations in mouse and man. J Exp Med 1981; 153: 310.
36. Braine HG, Sensenbrenner LL, Wright SK, Tutschka PJ, Saral R, Santos GW. Bone marrow transplantation with major ABO blood group incompatibility using erythrocyte depletion of marrow prior to infusion. Blood 1982; 60(2): 420.
37. De Witte T, Raymakers R, Plas S, Koekman E, Wessels H, Haanen C. Bone marrow repopulation capacity after transplantation of lymphocyte-depleted allogeneic bone marrow using counterflow centrifugation. Transplantation 1984; 37(2): 151.
38. DeWitte T, Raymakers R, Wessels J, Haanen C. Successful prevention of graft-vs-host disease after allogeneic bone marrow transplantation with marrow depleted of lymphocytes by counterflow centrifugation. Exp Hematol 1984; 12(6): 411.
39. Granger S, Janossy G, Francis G. Elimination of T lymphocytes from human bone marrow with monoclonal T antibodies and cytolytic complement. Br J Haematol 1982; 50: 367.
40. Thierfelder S, Hoffmann Fezer G, Rodt H. Anti lymphocytic antibodies and marrow transplantation. Transplantation 1983; 35: 249.
41. Trigg ME, Billing R, Sandel PM. Depletion of T-cells from human bone marrow with monoclonal antibody CT-2 and complement. J Biol Response Mod, 1984; 3: 406.
42. Reinherz EL, Ge Ha R, Rappeport JM. Reconstitution after transplantation with T lymphocyte depleted HLA haplotype-mismatched bone marrow for severe combined immunodeficiency. Proc Natl Acad Sci USA 1982; 79: 6047.
43. De Witte T, Koekman E, Geestman E, Plas A, Blaukeuborg G, Wessels J, Haanen C. Depletion of immunocompetent lymphocytes from human pluripotent progenitor cells (CFU-GEMM) by means of counterflow centrifugation. In: DeWitte T, ed. Physical elimination of lymphocytes from human bone marrow [Doctoral Dissertation]. The Netherlands: University of Nijmegen, 1983: 78.
44. Muraoka S, Miller RG. Cells in bone marrow and in T cell colonies grown from bone marrow can suppress generation of cytotoxic T lymphocytes directed against their self antigens. J Exp Med 1980; 152: 54.
45. Moreau JF, Miller RG. Growth at limiting dilution of human T cell colonies from T cell-depleted peripheral blood leukocytes. J Immunol 1983; 120(3): 1139.
46. Ching L, Muraoka S, Miller RG. Differentiation of T cells from immature precursors in murine T cell colonies. J Immunol 1981; 127(5): 2156.
47. Trigg ME, Billing R, Sandel PM, Exten R, Houg R, Bozdeck MJ, Horowitz SD, Finlay JL, Moen R, Lougo W, Erickson C, Peterson A. Clinical trial depleting T lymphocytes from donor marrow for matched and mismatched allogeneic bone marrow transplants. Cancer Treat Rep 1985; 69: 377.

Received 19 February 1985.
Accepted 18 June 1985.

0041-1337/86/4102-0229$02.00/0
TRANSPLANTATION
Vol. 41, No. 2
Printed in U.S.A.

THE RELATIVE IMMUNOGENICITY OF CORNEAL EPITHELIUM, STROMA, AND ENDOTHLIUM

The Role of Major Histocompatibility Complex Antigens

Patrick A. Treseler,[1] Gary N. Foulks, and Fred Sanfilippo[2]

Departments of Microbiology and Immunology, Ophthalmology, Pathology, and Surgery, Duke University and Durham V.A. Medical Centers, Durham, North Carolina 27710

Corneal allografts have been shown to give rise to immune responses, but the role and relative importance of individual corneal cell populations in evoking such responses remain unclear. We dissected ACI (RT1^a) rat corneas into separate epithelial, stromal, and endothelial components by a method that yields pure cell populations in tissue culture, and grafted these components separately to groups of fully allogeneic PVG (RT1^c) recipients). Grafts of corneal stroma elicited strong cellular cytotoxic immune responses in a cell-mediated lymphocytotoxic assay, but corneal epithelium failed to generate any detectable response. Grafts of corneal endothelium alone, however, evoked a potent cellular cytotoxic response.

Using congenic rats, it was found that grafts from PVG.1A (RT1^a) donors to PVG (RT1^c) recipients (which differ at both the RT1.A and B loci) yielded identical results. However, no corneal component graft from PVG.R1 (RT1^{r1}) donors to PVG recipients (which differ only at RT1.A) generated a detectable immune response. Use of target lymphoblasts from congenic strains established that at least part of all responses detected were directed against class I (RT1.A) major histocompatibility complex antigens.

These findings indicate that there is differential im-

[1] Supported by the Medical Scientist Training Program, NIH Grant 5-T32GM07171.

[2] Address reprint requests to Dr. Sanfilippo, at Box 3712, Duke University Medical Center, Durham, NC 27710.

munogenicity of specific corneal tissue components in the rat that may be further influenced by the degree of MHC disparity between donor and recipient.

Corneal allografts are known to give rise to humoral (*1*) and cellular (*2, 3*) immune responses, but the relative contribution of the three major corneal cell layers (i.e., epithelium, stroma, and endothelium) to graft immunogenicity remains largely unknown. It has been postulated that cells of the corneal endothelium may be responsible for sensitizing the host to orthotopic corneal grafts (*4*), yet except for one early report suggesting that all three layers of the rabbit cornea may be immunogenic (*5*), there is no evidence that the endothelium alone may sensitize a grafted individual, and little to suggest what the role of the other corneal layers may be in evoking an allograft response.

Using a microdissection technique, we have performed heterotopic allografts of individual corneal cell layers in inbred rats, and have found that isolated corneal stroma and endothelium both elicit a cellular immune response, while grafts of isolated corneal epithelium do not. Use of congenic animals has further allowed us to establish that antigens of the major histocompatibility complex (MHC)[3] alone may evoke these responses—which are, at least in part, directed against class I MHC antigens.

MATERIALS AND METHODS

PVG ($RT1^c$), PVG.1A ($RT1^a$), and PVG.R1 ($RT1^{r1}$) rats were obtained from Olac, Ltd. (Bicester, Oxon, UK). ACI ($RT1^a$) animals were obtained from M.A. Lab Animals (Walkersville, MD). The PVG.1A rat is a congenic animal, bearing the RT1 haplotype of the ACI rat on a PVG genetic background. The PVG.R1 animal is also congenic, bearing the RT1.A region of the ACI rat on a PVG background; it thus varies from PVG only at loci encoding class I MHC antigens (*6*). The RT1 haplotypes of these strains are summarized in Table 1.

Isolated donor corneal buttons free of limbal tissue were dissected into separate epithelial, stromal, and endothelial components following the method of Stocker and associates (*7*). By this procedure, corneal endothelial cells were removed in a continuous sheet along with the underlying Descemet's membrane. Corneal epithelium was dissected from the underlying Bowman's layer—occasionally in a continuous layer, but more commonly, in four or five large fragments. This procedure has been shown to yield pure cultures of corneal cell subpopulations in tissue culture of dissected human (*8, 9*) and rabbit (*7, 10*) corneas. Using similar tissue culture techniques (*11*) we have confirmed that similar dissection of rat corneas yields pure populations of corneal, epithelial, stromal, and endothelial cells (unpublished observations).

Recipients grafted with corneal components were given all of that component (i.e., epithelium, stroma, or endothelium) from two identical donor corneal buttons. The grafting techniques (*1*) and cell-mediated lymphocytotoxicity (CML) assays (*2*) were conducted as previously described. Briefly, groups of three recipient PVG rats were given grafts of skin, cornea, or corneal components from the appropriate donor strain to the chest wall. Ten days later, recipient splenocytes were put in mixed lymphocyte culture with irradiated ACI splenocytes and, after six days, the recipient splenocytes were removed from culture and tested for their ability to lyse ^{51}Cr-labeled Con A lymphoblasts at several effector-to-target ratios. All assays were performed in triplicate, and the percentage of specific ^{51}Cr release was calculated as previously described (*2*).

In order to compare quantitatively the levels of cytotoxicity obtained using different effector cell populations, a best-fit quadratic curve was obtained for each lysis plot (i.e., the plot of the percentage of specific ^{51}Cr release vs. effector-to-target ratio) using the GPLOT procedure (a non-linear least-squares fitting program) of the Statistical Analysis Systems (*12, 13*). The 99% and 95% confidence limits for these curves were then compared at an effector-to-target ratio of 7.5:1, which corresponds to the approximate midpoint of the linear, preplateau region of the lysis curves. All comparisons represent groups grafted and assayed on the same days with values calculated relative to the same controls. It should be noted that fully allogeneic ACI splenocytes were used as in vitro stimulators in the secondary CML assay for all PVG recipient splenocytes, regardless of the graft the animals received. Thus all recipient splenocytes were treated identically after being removed from the host, and any significant differences in the ability of the various effector cell populations to lyse target cells should be due entirely to differences in the grafts the animals received.

TABLE 1. Immunogenetic relationship of rat strains utilized

Strain[a]	RT1 haplotype[b]
PVG	A^c B^c
PVG.R1	A^a B^c
PVG.1A	A^a B^a
ACI	A^a B^a

[a] PVG, PVG.R1, and PVG.1A strains possess identical background (i.e., non-RT1) genes.

[b] Limited information exists concerning the genotype of these strains at the RT1.C, RT1.D, and RT1.E loci, so strains have been characterized only in terms of genotype at RT1.A and RT1.B.

RESULTS

In initial experiments, PVG recipients were grafted with isolated corneal epithelium, corneal stroma, or corneal endothelium from fully allogeneic ACI donors. PVG rats given grafts of intact syngeneic PVG cornea were used as negative controls, while PVG recipients of ACI skin grafts served as a positive control population (*2*). When effector splenocytes from these recipients were tested for their ability to lyse ACI target cells (Fig. 1), it was found that high levels of cytotoxicity were obtained using effector cells from recipients given ACI skin, ACI corneal stroma, and ACI corneal endothelium. Effector cells from recipients of ACI corneal epithelium or control PVG cornea grafts yielded substantially lower, and essentially equivalent, levels of target cell lysis. Quantitative comparison of the best-fit quadratic equations for these lysis plots (Table 2) confirmed that ACI target cell lysis by effectors from recipients of ACI skin, corneal stroma or corneal endothelium was significantly ($P<0.01$) above control levels, while target cell lysis using effector cells from animals grafted with ACI corneal epithelium did not differ significantly from controls. Identical results were obtained when these same PVG effector cells were used against congenic PVG.1A (RT1-disparate) or PVG.R1 (RT1.A-disparate) targets (Table 2); in each case, there were significant cytotoxic responses following grafts of ACI corneal stroma or ACI corneal endothelium, but not following ACI

[3] Abbreviations used: CML, cell-mediated lymphocytotoxicity; MHC, major histocompatibility complex.

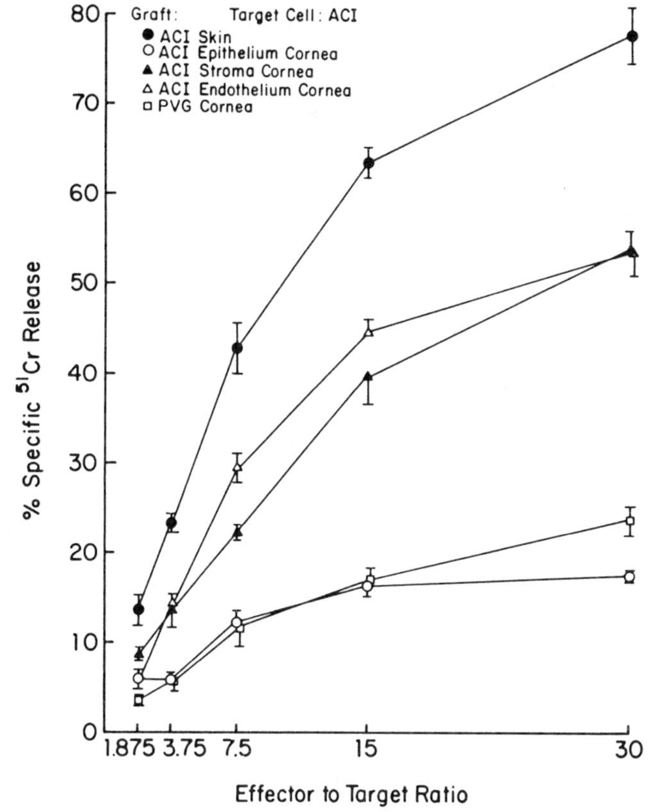

FIGURE 1. Lysis of ACI target lymphoblasts by effector cells from recipients of ACI corneal epithelial, stromal, and endothelial grafts.

corneal epithelial grafts. There was no significant lysis of syngeneic PVG targets by an effector cell population (Table 2).

These experiments were repeated using congenic PVG.1A rats as donors of corneal cell populations to PVG recipients. As with tissue from ACI donors, grafts of PVG.1A corneal stroma or endothelium were found to be immunogenic, yielding effector cells substantially more cytotoxic toward cells of donor strain than effector cells from syngeneically grafted controls (Fig. 2), whereas in separate experiments, grafts of PVG.1A corneal epithelium again yielded no cytotoxicity above control levels (Fig. 3). Statistical analysis confirmed that the levels of PVG.1A target cell lysis were significantly ($P<0.01$) above control levels following PVG.1A corneal stromal or endothelial grafts, but not following grafts of PVG.1A corneal epithelium (Table 3). Identical patterns of reactivity were seen when these same effector cell populations were used to lyse ACI and PVG.R1 targets—but, as before, there was no significant lysis of syngeneic PVG targets by any effector group (Table 3). When PVG.R1 rats were used as a source of corneal component grafts given to PVG hosts, however, no significant cytotoxicity was detectable regardless of the corneal component graft used (Fig. 4).

Because Descemet's membrane is dissected from the corneal stroma in our procedure of isolating corneal endothelium for grafting, it is possible that a few corneal stromal cells remained adherent. In order to exclude rigorously the possibility that such "passenger" stromal cells were responsible for the immune response to ACI and PVG.1A corneal endothelial grafts, ACI donor grafts of Descemet's membrane with corneal endothelium were compared with ACI Descemet's membrane stripped of

TABLE 2. Cytotoxicity using effector cells from PVG recipients of isolated ACI corneal cell populations

Target cell	Graft	Percentage of specific ^{51}Cr release at 7.5:1 E:T ratio[a]		
		Total	Above control	
ACI	ACI skin	42.8±2.8	31.3±3.4	($P<0.01$)[b]
	ACI epithelium	12.2±0.8	0.7±2.2	(NS)[c]
	ACI stroma	22.1±0.9	10.6±2.2	($P<0.01$)
	ACI endothelium	29.5±1.6	18.0±2.6	($P<0.01$)
	PVG cornea (control)	11.5±2.0		
PVG.1A	ACI skin	35.0±2.4	27.6±2.7	($P<0.01$)
	ACI epithelium	7.1±1.0	−0.3±1.6	(NS)
	ACI stroma	15.6±1.5	8.2±1.9	($P<0.01$)
	ACI endothelium	23.2±0.9	15.8±1.5	($P<0.01$)
	PVG cornea (control)	7.4±1.2		
PVG.R1	ACI skin	25.0±0.9	18.1±1.0	($P<0.01$)
	ACI epithelium	10.2±0.6	3.3±0.8	(NS)
	ACI stroma	14.1±1.0	7.2±1.1	($P<0.01$)
	ACI endothelium	14.8±1.2	7.9±1.3	($P<0.01$)
	PVG cornea (control)	6.9±0.5		
PVG	ACI skin	−1.9±0.8	0.5±1.4	(NS)
	ACI epithelium	−1.5±0.9	0.9±1.4	(NS)
	ACI stroma	−4.2±0.5	−1.8±1.2	(NS)
	ACI endothelium	−1.9±0.7	0.5±1.3	(NS)
	PVG cornea (control)	−2.4±1.1		

[a] 7.5:1 E:T ratio corresponds to approximate midpoint of linear, preplateau region of lysis curves.

[b] Significance assessed by comparing confidence limits of best-fit quadratic curves at 7.5:1 E:T ratio.

[c] Not significant.

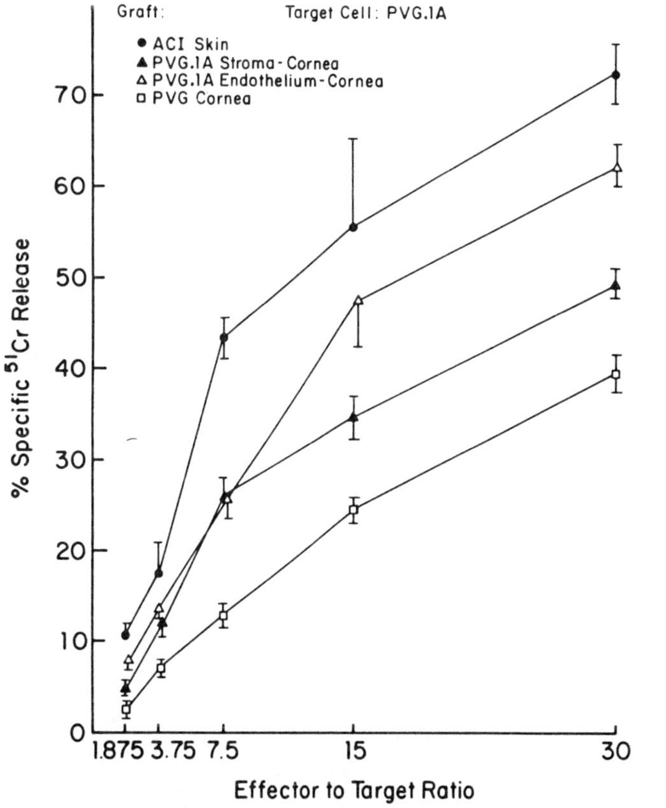

FIGURE 2. Lysis of PVG.1A target lymphoblasts by effector cells from recipients of PVG.1A corneal stromal and endothelial grafts.

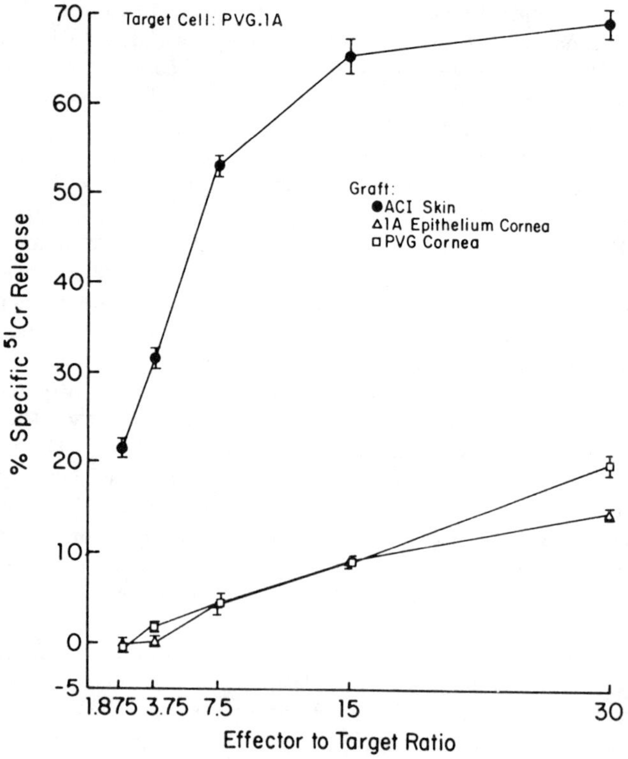

FIGURE 3. Lysis of PVG.1A target lymphoblasts by effector cells from recipients of PVG.1A corneal epithelial grafts.

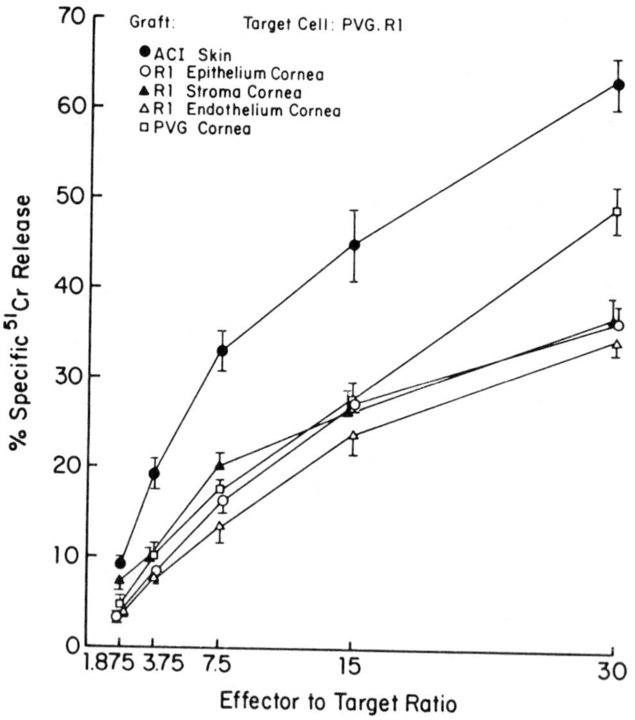

FIGURE 4. Lysis of PVG.R1 target lymphoblasts by effector cells from recipients of PVG.R1 corneal epithelial, stromal, and endothelial grafts.

TABLE 3. Cytotoxicity using effector cells from PVG recipients of isolated PVG.1A corneal cell populations

Target cell	Graft	Percentage of specific ^{51}Cr release at 7.5:1 E:T ratio[a]		
		Total	Above control	
A. Stroma and endothelium				
ACI	ACI skin	51.4±3.9	37.5±4.2	(P<0.01)[b]
	PVG.1A stroma	22.7±1.3	8.8±2.1	(P<0.01)
	PVG.1A endothelium	31.2±0.7	17.3±1.7	(P<0.01)
	PVG cornea (control)	13.9±1.6		
PVG.1A	ACI skin	43.4±2.2	30.5±2.5	(P<0.01)
	PVG.1A stroma	26.0±2.0	13.1±2.3	(P<0.01)
	PVG.1A endothelium	25.6±2.0	12.7±2.3	(P<0.01)
	PVG cornea (control)	12.9±1.2		
PVG.R1	ACI skin	32.9±2.2	15.5±2.5	(P<0.01)
	PVG.1A stroma	26.6±0.9	9.2±1.4	(P<0.01)
	PVG.1A endothelium	30.3±3.5	12.9±3.7	(P<0.01)
	PVG cornea (control)	17.4±1.1		
PVG	ACI skin	1.5±0.6	1.0±0.8	(NS)[c]
	PVG.1A stroma	1.7±0.7	1.2±0.9	(NS)
	PVG.1A endothelium	−0.8±1.3	−1.3±1.4	(NS)
	PVG cornea (control)	0.5±0.7		
B. Epithelium				
ACI	ACI skin	52.0±1.4	44.0±3.0	(P<0.01)
	PVG.1A epithelium	4.5±0.5	−3.5±2.7	(NS)
	PVG cornea (control)	8.0±2.7		
PVG.1A	ACI skin	53.0±1.1	48.6±1.4	(P<0.01)
	PVG.1A epithelium	1.8±0.3	−2.6±0.9	(NS)
	PVG cornea (control)	4.4±0.9		
PVG.R1	ACI skin	49.1±0.8	42.1±2.6	(P<0.01)
	PVG.1A epithelium	5.1±0.7	−1.9±2.6	(NS)
	PVG cornea (control)	7.0±2.5		
PVG	ACI skin	−0.6±0.3	1.4±0.7	(NS)
	PVG.1A epithelium	−0.7±0.8	1.3±1.0	(NS)
	PVG cornea (control)	−2.0±0.6		

[a] 7.5:1 E:T ratio corresponds to approximate midpoint of linear, preplateau region of lysis curves.
[b] Significance assessed by comparing confidence limits of best-fit quadratic curves at 7.5:1 E:T ratio.
[c] Not significant.

endothelial cells, which were removed by scraping with a surgical scalpel. PVG rats given grafts of ACI Descemet's membrane with endothelium yielded effector splenocytes which were significantly ($P<0.01$) more cytotoxic for ACI target cells than were control effectors from recipients of PVG isografts; grafts of Descemet's membrane without endothelium from ACI donors, on the other hand, yielded no lysis of ACI target cells above control levels (Table 4). The same result was seen with PVG.1A and PVG.R1 target cells as well (Table 4).

DISCUSSION

It is apparent from the results of these studies that, in the rat, both isolated corneal stroma and isolated corneal endothelium are capable of provoking a cytotoxic immune response in allogeneic recipients. With tissue from fully allogeneic ACI or MHC-disparate PVG.1A donors, PVG recipients of corneal stroma or corneal endothelial grafts generated effector splenocytes that were significantly more cytotoxic for donor-strain target cells than appropriate controls. Grafts of corneal epithelium, however, never yielded cytotoxic responses above control levels.

The potent responses to PVG.1A stromal and endothelial grafts indicate that MHC antigens alone are capable of evoking immune responses to these corneal components. Furthermore, the level of target cell lysis using effector cells raised to a particular PVG.1A graft met or exceeded that using the comparable anti-ACI effectors in all cases, suggesting that grafts from the two strains may be equally immunogenic. This suggests that MHC antigens alone may be responsible for evoking the immune responses to even fully allogeneic ACI grafts. MHC antigens are certainly involved as major targets of these responses since PVG.1A lymphoblasts were effectively lysed by anti-ACI effectors, and the finding that PVG.R1 cells were effective targets for both anti-ACI and anti-PVG.1A effectors further suggests that at least a proportion of these cytotoxic effector cells were directed against class I MHC antigens.

TABLE 4. Effect of endothelial cells on graft immunogenicity

Target cell	Graft	Percentage of specific ^{51}Cr release at 7.5:1 E:T ratio[a]	
		Total	Above control
ACI	ACI skin	43.4±2.2	34.8±2.3 ($P<0.01$)[b]
	ACI Descemet's membrane with endothelium	14.1±0.9	5.5±1.1 ($P<0.01$)
	ACI Descemet's membrane without endothelium	10.0±0.7	1.4±0.9 (NS)[c]
	PVG cornea (control)	8.6±0.6	
PVG.1A	ACI skin	46.4±1.3	35.7±1.5 ($P<0.01$)
	ACI Descemet's membrane with endothelium	14.6±0.8	3.9±1.1 ($P<0.01$)
	ACI Descemet's membrane without endothelium	9.1±0.7	−1.6±1.0 (NS)
	PVG cornea (control)	10.7±0.7	
PVG.R1	ACI skin	43.8±1.3	29.5±1.5 ($P<0.01$)
	ACI Descemet's membrane with endothelium	19.2±0.7	4.9±1.1 ($P<0.01$)
	ACI Descemet's membrane without endothelium	12.6±0.6	−1.7±1.0 (NS)
	PVG cornea (control)	14.3±0.8	
PVG	ACI skin	0.1±0.2	0.5±0.3 (NS)
	ACI Descemet's membrane with endothelium	1.0±0.5	1.4±0.5 (NS)
	ACI Descemet's membrane without endothelium	−0.2±0.2	0.2±0.3 (NS)
	PVG cornea (control)	−0.4±0.2	

[a] 7.5:1 E:T ratio corresponds to approximate midpoint of linear, preplateau region of lysis curves.

[b] Significance assessed by comparing confidence limits of best-fit quadratic curves at 7.5:1 E:T ratio.

[c] Not significant.

None of the corneal cell populations isolated from PVG.R1 donors provided an immunogenic stimulus to PVG recipients detectable by our methods. It is unlikely that all three corneal components from these donors are truly nonimmunogenic, since we have previously found that whole PVG.R1 corneal grafts induce a slight but significant cellular immune response in PVG hosts. (*14*) Most likely, either the grafting of only portions of PVG.R1 corneas has reduced the mass of immunogenic tissue below the threshold required to evoke a response, or the response generated is too slight to be detected by our assay system.

It was not unexpected that allogeneic corneal stroma should prove immunogenic. The stroma constitutes the bulk of the cornea and has been found to contain cells positive for class I and class II MHC antigens, both in the human (*15*) and the rat (*16*). Somewhat unexpected, however, was the finding that allogeneic corneal epithelium failed to provoke any detectable immune response. In the human, the corneal epithelium is rich in class I and class II MHC antigen-positive cells (*14*), and the removal of the donor epithelium prior to human corneal transplantation has been associated with reduced rates of graft rejection (*17*). In the rat, however, we have noted that the corneal epithelium, though containing many class I MHC antigen-positive cells, is almost devoid of cells bearing class II MHC antigen, especially compared with the human. Such class II antigen-bearing cells in the corneas of human, rat, and other species have been rigorously shown to be Langerhans cells (*18*), which are dendritic cells thought to make a major contribution to the immunogenicity of many allogeneic tissues (*19, 20*). Their relative absence from the rat corneal epithelium could explain that tissue's failure to provoke an allograft response.

Allogeneic corneal endothelium proved to be a surprisingly potent immunogenic stimulus considering its relatively meager contribution to the corneal mass: it generated levels of target cell lysis at least as great as the entire corneal stroma. This effect, however, was not entirely unpredictable in light of evidence that orthotopic corneal grafts, constructed such that the endothelium is the only foreign element, initiate host immune responses in both allogeneic (*5*) and xenogeneic (*21*) combinations. Furthermore, since desquamated corneal endothelial cells have been identified in the aqueous humor of orthotopic corneal allograft recipients (*4*), and no other corneal cell type has obvious access to the host immune system when a graft is made to an avascular corneal bed, it is possible that corneal endothelial cells play a dominant role in the elicitation of a typical corneal allograft rejection episode.

The possibility that the responses seen to grafts of corneal endothelium could be due to stromal cells accidentally removed along with Descemet's membrane during isolation of the endothelium was considered (though thought unlikely in view of the pure endothelial cell cultures thus obtained). This possibility was excluded, however, by experiments showing that mechanical removal of the endothelial cells prior to the isolation of Descemet's membrane from the underlying stroma abolished the immunogenicity of the graft.

It appears then, that the immune response to allogeneic corneal endothelium is due entirely to the endothelial cells themselves. Corneal endothelial cells, however, in the human (*14*) and in the rat (*16*) normally express only modest amounts of class I, and no detectable class II, MHC antigen. Based on this phenotype, they would not be predicted to be potent allostimulators. However, it is interesting to note that many vascular endothelial cells (which share some structural (*22*) and many functional (*23*) characteristics with endothelial cells of the cornea) also normally lack class II MHC antigens in rodents, but can be induced to express them by contact with alloreactive T lymphocytes (*24*) or other immunologic stimuli (*25*). Whether rejecting corneal endothelium is induced to express class II MHC antigens and what role this may play in corneal graft rejection is unknown. Nevertheless, these results clearly indicate that, in the rat, the corneal endothelium, along with the corneal stroma, provides the major contribution to corneal allograft immunogenicity.

Acknowledgments. We thank Beth Graybeal, Mary Digel, Teven Harmon, and Julie Fuller for expert technical assistance, and Nancy Hall for help in preparing the manuscript.

REFERENCES

1. Treseler PA, Sanfilippo F. Humoral immunity to heterotopic corneal allografts in the rat. Transplantation 1985; 39: 193.
2. Treseler PA, Treseler CB, Foulks GN, Sanfilippo F. Cellular immunity to heterotopic corneal allografts in the rat. Transplantation 1985; 39: 196.
3. MacDonald AL, Basu PK, Miller RG. The systemic production of cytotoxic lymphoid cells in corneal allograft reaction. 1. A quantitative study utilizing ^{51}chromium release assay. Transplantation 1977; 23: 431.
4. Silverstein AM, Khodadoust AA, Prendergast RA. Desquamation of corneal endothelial cells. Invest Ophthalmol Vis Sci 1982; 22: 351.
5. Khodadoust AA, Silverstein AM. Transplantation and rejection of individual cell layers of the cornea. Invest Ophthalmol 1969; 8: 180.
6. Howard JC. The major histocompatibility complex of the rat: a partial review. Metabolism 1983; 32(suppl 1): 41.
7. Stocker FW, Eiring A, Georgiade R, Georgiade N. A tissue culture technique for growing corneal epithelial, stromal, and endothelial tissues separately. Am J Ophthalmol 1958; 46: 294.
8. Newsome DA, Takasugi M, Kenyon KR, Stark WF, Opelz G. Human corneal cells in vitro: morphology and histocompatibility (HL-A) antigens of pure cell populations. Invest Ophthalmol 1974; 13: 23.
9. Baum JL, Niedra R, Davis C, Yue BYJT. Mass culture of human corneal endothelial cells. Arch Ophthalmol 1979; 97: 1136.
10. Perlman M, Baum JL. The mass culture of rabbit corneal endothelial cells. Arch Ophthalmol 1974; 92: 235.
11. Yue BYJT, Baum JL. Studies of corneas in vivo and in vitro. Vision Res 1981; 21: 41.
12. SAS User's Guide: Statistics, 1982 ed. Cary, North Carolina: SAS Institute.
13. SAS User's Guide: Basics, 1982 ed. Cary, North Carolina: SAS Institute.
14. Treseler PA, Sanfilippo F. Relative contribution of major histocompatibility complex antigens to the immunogenicity of corneal allografts. Transplantation (in press).
15. Treseler PA, Foulks GN, Sanfilippo F. The expression of HLA antigens by cells in the human cornea. Am J Ophthalmol 1984; 98: 763.
16. Treseler PA, Sanfilippo F. The expression of major histocompatibility complex and leukocyte antigens by cells in the rat cornea. Transplantation 1986; 41: 248.
17. Tuberville AW, Foster CS, Wood TO. The effect of donor cornea epithelium removal on the incidence of allograft rejection reactions. Ophthalmology Rochester 1983; 90: 1351.
18. Rodriques MM, Rowden G, Hackett J, Bakos I. Langerhans cells in the normal conjunctiva and peripheral cornea of selected species. Invest Ophthalmol Vis Sci 1981; 21: 759.
19. Lafferty KJ, Prowse SJ, Simeonovic CJ. Immunobiology of tissue transplantation: a return to the passenger leukocyte concept. Ann Rev Immunol 1983; 1: 143.
20. Hunter JAA. The Langerhans cell: from gold to glitter. Clin Exp Dermatol 1983; 8: 569.
21. Bahn CF, MacCallum DK, Lillie JH, Meyer RF, Martonyi CL. Complications associated with bovine corneal endothelial cell-lined homografts in the cat. Invest Ophthalmol Vis Sci 1982; 22: 73.
22. Treseler PA, Foulks GN, Sanfilippo F. The expression of ABO blood group, hematopoietic and other cell-specific antigens by cells in the human cornea. Cornea (in press).
23. Gospodarowicz D, Vlodavsky I, Greenburg G, Alvarado J, Johnson LK, Moran J. Studies on atherogenesis and corneal transplantation using cultured vascular and corneal endothelia. Recent Prog Horm Res 1979; 35: 375.
24. deWaal RMW, Bogman MJJ, Maass CN, Cornelissen LMH, Tax WJM, Koene RAP. Variable expression of Ia antigens on the vascular endothelium of mouse skin allografts. Nature 1983; 303: 426.
25. Pober JS, Gimbrone Jr MA, Cotran RS, Reiss CS, Burakoff SJ, Fiers W, Ault KA. Ia expression by vascular endothelium is inducible by activated T cells and by human gamma interferon. J Exp Med 1983; 157: 1339.

Received 13 March 1985.
Accepted 18 June 1985.

0041-1337/86/4102-0235$02.00/0
TRANSPLANTATION

Vol. 41, No. 2
Printed in U.S.A.

EFFECT OF STORAGE ON LYMPHOCYTE SURFACE MARKERS IN WHOLE BLOOD UNITS

HARRY E. PRINCE[1] AND LIINA ARENS

Cellular Immunology Laboratory, American Red Cross Blood Services, Los Angeles-Orange Counties Region, Los Angeles, California 90006

Pretransplant transfusions of stored donor-specific blood have been shown to improve renal allograft survival while reducing the frequency of lymphocytotoxic antibody production when compared with fresh blood. As part of studies to define the mechanism(s) of this phenomenon, we have monitored lymphocyte surface markers during storage of four units of whole blood. Both mononuclear cell preparations (obtained by density gradient centrifugation) and whole blood preparations were analyzed using monoclonal antibodies and a flow cytometer enabling lymphocytes to be distinguished from other white cells and nonviable cells. In both cell preparations, the percentage of viable lymphocytes expressing CD3 (all T cells), CD4 (T helper cells), CD8 (T suppressor cells,) HLA-class I (A,B,C), or HLA-DR antigens remained stable for at least 14 days, although median fluorescence intensity declined for the first three markers. After day 14, the number of viable lymphocytes recovered from a standard volume of whole blood was insufficient for further assessment of surface markers, even though the white cell count (determined by cell volume) remained near original levels. Thus the distribution of viable lymphocyte subpopulations defined by surface markers was stable for at least two weeks in stored blood; however, a nonspecific loss of lymphocyte viability began after 10 days of storage. These findings suggest that loss of cell viability, rather than loss of specific lymphocyte subpopulations, may be related to the mechanism by which pretransplant transfusion of stored blood improves renal allograft survival without inducing a high incidence of lymphocytotoxic antibody.

While pretransplant donor-specific blood transfusions significantly improve subsequent renal allograft survival (*1*), approximately 30% of recipients develop cytotoxic antibodies that recognize HLA antigens or donor lymphocytes (*2*). These sensitized patients thus become ineligible for transplantation of that donor's kidney. Recent studies (*3, 4*) have shown that transfusion of stored blood, rather than fresh blood, still produces the beneficial effect for graft survival, but decreases the sensitization rate to 5–10%.

The mechanism responsible for decreased sensitization rates after transfusion of stored blood remains unknown. Some workers have suggested that a selective loss of T lymphocytes during storage is associated with a lower incidence of lymphocytotoxic antibody production (*5, 6*). These workers, however, analyzed mononuclear cells obtained by density gradient centrifugation, rather than directly analyzing the lymphocyte component of the whole blood.

Accordingly, we have analyzed lymphocyte surface markers using whole blood as well as mononuclear cell preparations from stored blood. Our flow cytometric system enabled us to distinguish viable lymphocytes from monocytes, granulocytes, and nonviable cells, and thus to determine surface markers on viable lymphocytes only. We show that the percentages of viable lymphocytes expressing several markers remain stable over two weeks of storage, but lymphocyte viability nonspecifically decreases after 10 days.

MATERIALS AND METHODS

A unit of blood was collected (with CPD-A as anticoagulant) from each of four donors who met standard criteria for whole-blood donation. A 10-ml aliquot was removed from the bag with a needle and syringe following donation, and after 1, 2, 4, 6, 10, 14, and 21 days of storage at 4°C. Aliquots were brought to room temperature by incubation for 10 min in a 37°C water bath. White blood cell counts were determined using a Coulter Counter (Model M4-30, Hialeah, FL). Then 6 ml of each aliquot was mixed with an equal volume of phosphate-buffered saline (PBS),[2] layered over 6 ml of Ficoll-Paque (Pharmacia Fine Chemicals, Piscataway, NJ), and centrifuged at 2000 rpm (Sorvall GLC-2B centrifuge) for 25 min at room temperature (*7*). The resulting interface band was transferred to a 15-ml plastic tube and washed twice in PBS. The washed cells were resuspended in 1 ml of PBS containing 2% bovine albumin (cell concentration = $2–8\times10^6$ cells/ml), and constituted the mononuclear cell preparation.

Either 100 μl of whole blood or 100 μl of mononuclear cells was placed in each of seven tubes, followed by the addition of 100 μl of PBS. The tubes were then placed in a wet ice bath, and 5 μl of one of the following monoclonal antibodies (volume giving antibody excess) were added: Flourescein isothiocyanate (FITC)-OKT3 (CD3 [*8*], all T cells, Ortho Diagnostic Systems, Raritan, NJ), FITC-OKT4A (CD4, T helper cells, Ortho), FITC-OKT8 (CD8, T suppressor cells, Ortho), FITC-mouse IgG1 antibody (nonspecific control, Becton Dickinson, Mountain View, CA) OKIa (cells expressing HLA-DR, Ortho), anti-HLA-A,B,C (Cooper Diagnostics, Cochranville, PA), or mouse ascites fluid (nonspecific control, Cooper). After 20 min, red cells were lysed with ammonium chloride (lysing reagent, Ortho), and the remaining cells washed twice in cold PBS. Cells stained with FITC-labeled monoclonal antibodies were resuspended in 1 ml of cold PBS. Cells stained with unlabeled monoclonal antibodies were treated with 100 μl of FITC-goat antimouse immunoglobulin (1:100 dilution, Tago, Burlingame,

[1] Address correspondence to: Harry E. Prince, Ph.D., American Red Cross Blood Services, Los Angeles-Orange Counties Region, Cellular Immunology Laboratory, 1130 South Vermont Avenue, Los Angeles, CA 90006.

[2] Abbreviations used: PBMC, peripheral blood mononuclear cell; PBS, phosphate-buffered saline; VLTC, viable lymphocyte trigger region count.

CA) for an additional 20 min, and then washed in cold PBS, The cells were then resuspended in 1 ml cold PBS.

Lymphocyte fluorescence was analyzed using a Spectrum III flow cytometer (Ortho Diagnostic Systems, Westwood, MA). Nonviable cells were gated out electronically, and viable lymphocytes were distinguished from monocytes and granulocytes by correlated analysis of forward and right-angle scatter (*9*). A lymphocyte trigger region was thus established, and the percentage of cells within this trigger region that was positive for fluorescence was measured. Background fluorescence of the control mouse antibodies was substracted from the results. The mean value and standard deviation were determined for each marker at each time.

RESULTS

With whole blood preparations, the number of cells within the lymphocyte trigger region served as an indicator of the number of viable lymphocytes recoverable from a standard volume (100 μl) of whole blood. As shown in Figure 1, the viable lymphocyte trigger region count (VLTC) remained around 100% of original values (mean = 3000 cells) through day 6 of storage. By day 14, however, the number had markedly decreased, with only around 20% of original levels obtained. By day 21, the number of cells in this trigger region was too low (10% of original levels, less than 500 cells) to obtain reliable data. Thus, surface marker data are presented through day 14 of storage. In contrast, the white cell count was essentially unchanged after 21 days of storage (Fig. 1) (original mean WBC = 6000 cells/μl). White cell determinations, however, were based solely on cell volume (Coulter counter), and thus included nonviable as well as viable cells.

Figures 2 and 3 present a comparison of whole blood and mononuclear cell preparations with respect to the stability of three T cell markers (CD3, CD8, CD4) during storage. Whole blood and mononuclear cell values were comparable at essentially all times. The proportion of viable lymphocytes expressing these markers was stable in blood stored at 4°C for 14 days, regardless of the cell preparation used. A slight decrease in the percentage of $CD8^+$ lymphocytes was observed on day 14 (Fig. 2), but this change did not represent a drastic decrease from day 10 values, and may reflect the markedly reduced cell number in the viable lymphocyte trigger region (Fig. 1).

Similarly, the proportion of viable lymphocytes expressing HLA antigens remained stable over 14 days of storage (Fig. 4). As with other markers, values for whole blood and mononuclear cell preparations were comparable at all time points.

Figure 5 presents changes in median fluorescence intensity of positive cells during storage. For whole-blood samples (Fig. 5a), the median fluorescence intensity of HLA-DR and HLA-A,B,C markers on lymphocytes remained at 85–100% of original values during 14 days of storage. The T cell markers (CD3,

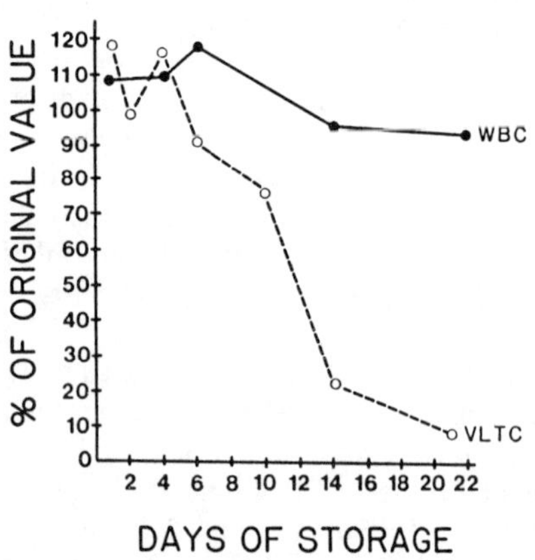

FIGURE 1. Changes in white blood cell count (WBC, ●——●) and viable lymphocyte trigger region count (VLTC, O- - -O) in stored whole blood. The white cell count was determined with a Coulter counter, and VLTC was determined by flow cytometry.

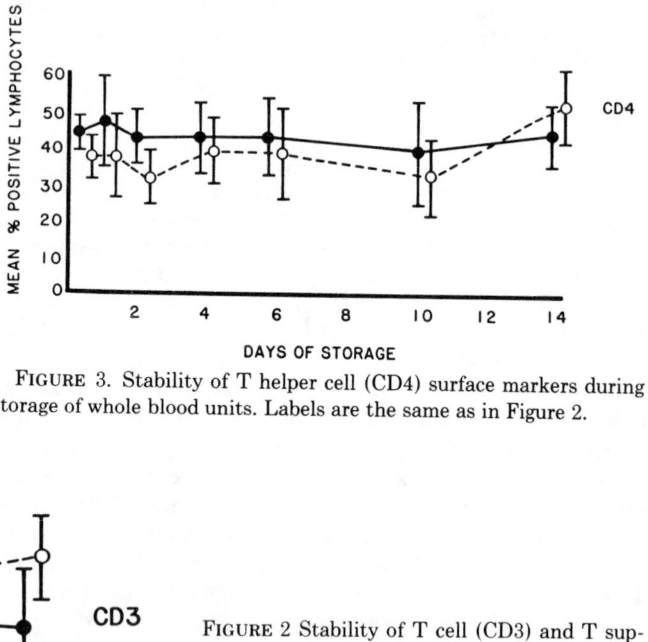

FIGURE 3. Stability of T helper cell (CD4) surface markers during storage of whole blood units. Labels are the same as in Figure 2.

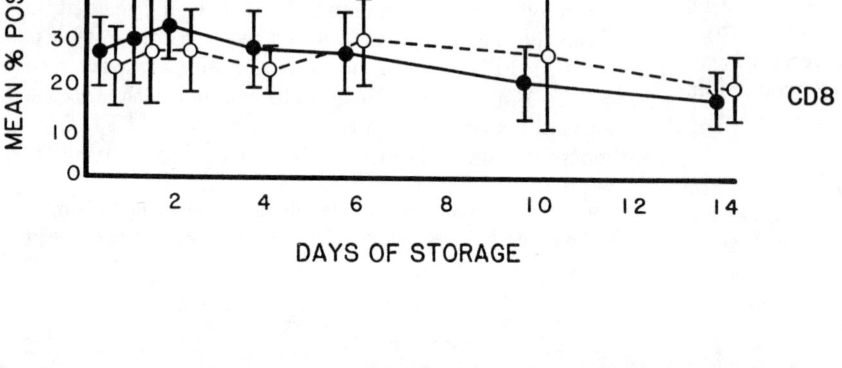

FIGURE 2 Stability of T cell (CD3) and T suppressor cell (CD8) surface markers during storage of whole blood units. Whole blood preparations (●——●) and mononuclear cell preparations (O- - -O) gave similar results. Bars represent standard deviation (n=4).

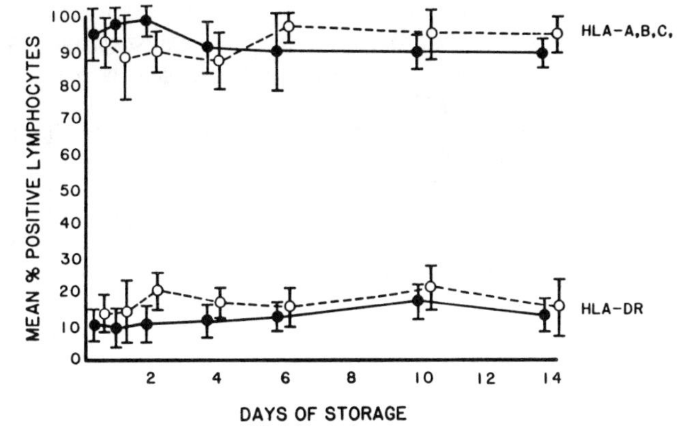

FIGURE 4. Stability of HLA antigen markers on lymphocytes during storage of whole blood units. Labels are the same as in Figure 2.

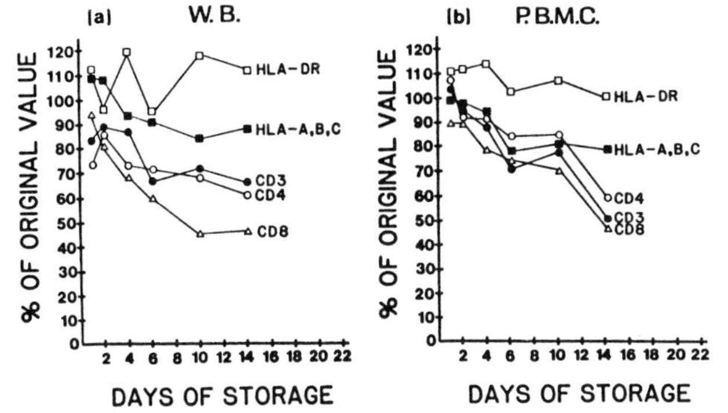

FIGURE 5. Changes in median fluorescence intensity for lymphocyte markers during storage: (a) whole blood (WB) preparations; (b) peripheral blood mononuclear cell (PBMC) preparations.

CD4, and CD8), however, exhibited reduced fluorescence intensity values (<80% of original values) within 4–6 days after storage, with continued reductions to 40–60% of original levels by day 14 of storage. Similar trends were observed using peripheral blood mononuclear cells (PBMC) (Fig. 5b).

DISCUSSION

Several workers have examined the effects of various storage conditions on lymphocyte surface markers detected by monoclonal antibodies. Kahan et al. (*10*) found that PBMC isolated from fresh blood and held overnight at 4°C express T cell markers at levels comparable to controls. Nicholson et al. (*11*) found that whole blood specimens held for four days at room temperature gave results comparable to original values, with PBMC giving similar but less consistent findings. These workers also found that granulocytes contaminate PBMC preparations from blood more than one day old, confirming previous findings (*12*). They further pointed out that by using a flow cytometer equipped with forward and right-angle scatter, lymphocyte markers could be measured, with no interference by the contaminating granulocytes.

Other groups (*5, 6, 13*) have found a 40–60% reduction in the percentage of T cells and T helper cells in PBMC obtained from whole blood stored for only one day at 4°C. These workers, however, did not use flow cytometers equipped with both forward and right-angle scatter, and thus did not analyze markers on lymphocytes only. Dzik et al. (*6*) corrected their findings for granulocyte contamination, but did not directly measure markers on only lymphocytes in PBMC preparations.

By using a flow cytometer equipped with forward and right-angle scatter, we therefore focused only on lymphocytes (i.e., cells with the scatter properties of lymphocytes) when measuring cell fluorescence. By this method, we found that the proportion of viable lymphocytes expressing a given cell surface marker was relatively stable over 14 days of storage at 4°C. Further, we found that percentages for a given marker at a given time were comparable when whole blood or mononuclear cell preparations were used. This observation indicates that differential recovery of lymphocyte subpopulations by density gradient centrifugation of stored blood is not a problem.

In addition to monitoring the percentage of cells positive for fluorescence, we also monitored median fluorescence intensity during storage. Since our assay system was in antibody excess, changes in fluorescence intensity reflected changes in antigen density (*14*). The T cell markers (CD3, CD4, CD8) showed reductions to roughly half (40–60%) of original values by day 14 of storage, while HLA markers remained near original values. This reduction in the density of T cell markers may have been interpreted by other workers as a change from "positive" to "negative" for expression of these markers, particularly if conditions of antibody excess were not used.

The most profound change we observed was not the loss of specific lymphocyte subpopulations, but a marked nonspecific reduction in the number of recoverable viable lymphocytes after 10 days of storage at 4°C. Concomitantly, the white cell count (determined by cell volume) after 10 days of storage remained essentially unchanged from initial values. These observations indirectly suggest that between 10 and 21 days of storage, many lymphocytes die but remain intact. Alternatively, the reduction in the number of cells in the viable lymphocyte trigger region may reflect changes in the forward and right-angle scatter properties of viable lymphocytes induced by long-term storage alone, and/or the effect of the erythrocyte lysing agent on stored lymphocytes. While our data cannot rule out this possibility, visual inspection of dot plots of forward and right-angle scatter for stored whole blood revealed an increased number of cells in the area characteristic of dead cells. Thus, we favor the hypothesis that reduced levels of viable lymphocytes reflect increased levels of intact, nonviable lymphocytes.

Assuming these intact but nonviable lymphocytes (and other white cells) pass through transfusion filters and enter the recipient's circulation, their fate in the recipient is unknown. They may be rapidly cleared by the reticuloendothelial system, and thus limited in their ability to serve as a source of HLA antigens for the induction of lymphocytotoxic antibodies. This reduction in antigenic load could therefore result in decreased sensitization rates in recipients of stored blood.

Acknowledgments. We thank Norman Morris for graphics, and Ann Sarkisian for preparing the manuscript.

REFERENCES

1. Salvatierra DJ, Vincenti F, Amend W Jr, et al. Four year experience with donor-specific blood transfusion. Transplant Proc 1983; 15: 924.
2. Fine RN, Terasaki PI, Ettenger RB, Danovitch B, Ehrlich RM. Renal transplantation update. Ann Intern Med 1984; 100: 246.
3. Whelchel JD, Shaw JF, Curtis JJ, Luke RG, Diethelm AG. Effect of pretransplant stored donor-specific blood transfusions on early renal allograft survival in one-haplotype living related transplants. Transplantation 1982; 34: 326.
4. Cheigh JS, Suthanthiran M, Kaplan M, et al. Induction of immune

alterations and successful renal transplantation with a simplified method of donor-specific blood transfusion. Transplantation 1984; 38: 501.
5. Light JA, Metz S, Oddenino K, et al. Donor-specific transfusion with diminished sensitization. Transplantation 1982; 34: 352.
6. Dzik WH, Neckers L. Mononuclear cell-surface antigens during storage of banked blood. Transplantation 1984; 38: 67.
7. Boyum A. Separation of lymphocytes from blood and bone marrow. Scand J Clin Lab Invest 1968; 21(suppl 97): 77.
8. Bernard A, Bernstein I, Boumsell L, et al. Differentiation human leukocyte antigens: a proposed nomenclature. Immunol Today 1984; 5: 158.
9. Reinherz EL, Schlossman SF. The differentiation and function of human T lymphocytes. Cell 1980; 19: 821.
10. Kahan A, Kahan A, Amor B. Lymphocyte subpopulations during blood storage. Arch Intern Med 1984; 144: 2101.
11. Nicholson JKA, Jones BM, Cross GD, McDougal JS. Comparison of T and B cell analyses on fresh and aged blood. J Immunol Methods 1984; 73: 29.
12. Dzik WH. Granulocytes in gradient separations of stored blood. Transfusion 1983; 23: 538.
13. Weiblen BJ, Debell K, Valeri CR. "Acquired immunodeficiency" of blood stored overnight. N Engl J Med 1983; 309: 793.
14. Holter W, Majdic O, Liszka K, Stockinger H, Knapp W. Kinetics of activation antigen expression by in vitro-stimulated human T lymphocytes. Cell Immunol 1985; 90: 322.

Received 9 April 1985.
Accepted 18 June 1985.

0041-1337/86/4102-0238$02.00/0
TRANSPLANTATION

Vol. 41, No. 2
Printed in U.S.A.

THE GRAFT-VERSUS-HOST REACTION AND IMMUNE FUNCTION

III. Functional Pre-T Cells in the Bone Marrow of Graft-Versus-Host–Reactive Mice Displaying T Cell Immunodeficiency[1]

Mona Seddik,[2] Thomas A. Seemayer,[3] and Wayne S. Lapp[4]

Department of Physiology, McGill University, Montreal, Quebec H3G 1Y6; and Department of Pathology, Montreal Children's Hospital and the McGill University-Montreal Children's Hospital Research Institute, Montreal, Quebec, Canada

Studies were performed to determine whether pre-T cells develop normally in the bone marrow of mice displaying thymic dysplasia and T cell immunodeficiency as a consequence of a graft-vervus-host (GVH) reaction. GVH reactions were induced in CBA×AF$_1$ mice by the injection of A strain lymphoid cells. To test for the presence of pre-T cells in GVH-reactive mice, bone marrow from GVH-reactive mice (GVHBM) was injected into irradiated syngeneic F$_1$ mice and 30–40 days later thymic morphology and function were studied. Morphology studies showed nearly normal thymic architectural restoration; moreover, such glands contained normal numbers of Thy-1-positive cells. Functional pre-T cells were evaluated by transferring thymocytes from the irradiated GVHBM-reconstituted mice into T-cell-deprived mice. These thymocytes reconstituted allograft reactivity, T helper cell function and Con A and PHA mitogen responses of T-cell-deprived mice. These results suggest that the pre-T cell population in the bone marrow is not affected by the GVH reaction. Therefore, the T cell immunodeficiency associated with the GVH reaction is not due to a deficiency of pre-T cells in the bone marrow but is more likely associated with GVH-induced thymic dysplasia.

It has been demonstrated that thymic epithelial injury associated with the graft-versus-host (GVH)[5] reaction results in a block of T cell differentiation into alloreactive (*1, 2*), helper, and mitogen-responsive cells (*3*). No suppressor cells were detected in thymuses of mice experiencing GVH reactions, thus excluding the possibility of active suppression (*3*). These studies showed that the state of immunosuppression that characterizes a chronic GVH reaction is, in part, the result of thymic epithelial injury and the concomitant block in T cell maturation. Subsequently, it was established that thymuses of late GVH mice (40 and more days after GVH induction) were able to recruit pre-T cells, and to impart the Thy-1 alloantigen onto parental and F$_1$ bone marrow cells (*4*). The latter study dem-

[1] This work was supported by grants from the Medical Research Council, the National Cancer Institute of Canada, and the McGill University-Montreal Children's Hospital Research Institute.
[2] MRC of Canada Fellow
[3] McPherson, Fraser, Monat University Associate.
[4] Reprint requests to W. S. Lapp, Department of Physiology, McIntyre Medical Center, McGill University, 3655 Drummond Street, Montreal, Quebec, H3G 1Y6, Canada.

[5] Abbreviations used: ATxBM, adult thymectomized, irradiated, bone-marrow-reconstituted; Con A, concanavalin A; GVH, graft-versus-host; GVHBM, bone marrow obtained from GVH-reactive mice; LPS, lipopolysaccharide; NBM, bone marrow obtained from normal mice; PFC, plaque-forming cell; PHA, phytohemagglutinin; SRBC, sheep erythrocytes.

onstrated that the acquisition of the Thy-1 marker was independent of differentiation into functional T lymphocytes. The failure of thymocytes, obtained from GVH mice, to reconstitute T cell function could also be due in part to a T cell precursor defect in the bone marrow. Such an event could possibly prevent the normal development of pre-T cells and their usual migration into a normal thymus. The following study was undertaken to investigate whether the GVH reaction caused a defect in the production of pre-T cells in the bone marrow.

The results demonstrate that the bone marrow of GVH-reactive mice continues to produce pre-T cells—and, furthermore, that the T cell immunodeficiency associated with the GVH reaction is not associated with defective pre-T cell genesis in the marrow.

MATERIALS AND METHODS

Animals. Mice of the inbred strains A ($H\text{-}2^a$), CBA ($H\text{-}2^k$), and Balb/c ($H\text{-}2^d$), as well as the (CBA×A) F_1 hybrid (BAF_1) were used. All mice were bred and maintained in our animal colony.

GVH reaction induction. Adult BAF_1 mice were injected i.v. with 75×10^6 A strain lymphoid cells as described elsewhere (*5*).

Preparation of T-cell-deprived mice (ATxBM). Adult BAF_1 mice were surgically thymectomized. Four days later, they were lethally irradiated (850–900 rads) and reconstituted (on the same day) by the i.v. injection of $15\text{–}20\times10^6$ bone marrow cells. ATxBM mice were used 15 days later. A small group of mice were not reconstituted with bone marrow after irradiation. The irradiated control group all died within two weeks.

Splenic mitogen responses. Splenic mitogen responses were measured using a technique previously described (*6, 7*). Briefly, for each 1 ml splenic cell suspension (containing 3×10^6 cells/ml), 0.1 ml of phytohemagglutin (PHA) (Wellcome Reagents, Beckenham, England), (2.5 μg/ml), concanavalin A (Con A) (Pharmacia, Uppsala, Sweden), (2.5 μg/ml), or lipopolysaccharide (LPS) (Difco, Detroit, MI) (10 μ/ml) were added. These mixtures were plated in microtiter plates and incubated (5% CO_2, 95% air, 37°C) for 48 hr. Thymidine methyl ^3H (New England Nuclear, Boston, MA) was added to the microtiter plates after they had been incubated for 48 hr in a final dilution of 1 μCi/well and the plates were incubated for 4–6 hr. The cells were then harvested using a multiple automated sample harvester on glass fiber filters. Filters were air dried and placed in scintillation vials, each containing 5 ml scintillation fluid, and were counted in a liquid scintillation counter.

Direct plaque-forming cell (PFC) assay. PFC assays were carried out as described previously (*8–10*). Mice were injected with 5×10^8 sheep red blood cells (SRBC) 4–5 days before being sacrificed for the PFC assay.

Skin grafting. Skin grafts were applied according to the technique of Bliss (*11*). Bandages were removed on the 9th postoperative day and grafts were visually inspected daily. The grafts were scored from 0 to 100 based on the amount of healthy epithelium. Grafts with 10% or less healthy epithelium were considered rejected.

Histology. Thymuses from representative groups of mice were prepared for light microscopy studies as described previously (*1, 12*).

TABLE 1. Summary of immunosuppression data and thymus histology of GVH-reactive BAF_1 mice used as bone marrow donors

Experimental groups	No. mice per group	PFC response to SRBC/spleen ($\bar{x}\pm SE\times10^{-3}$)	Thymic histology[a]	
			Hassall's corpuscles	Epithelial cell injury
Normal BAF_1	3	278.5±41.0	+	−
GVH days 10–12	4	0	+	−
GVH days 22–24	4	0	−	+
GVH days 40–45	4	0	−	++

[a] Thymic histology: For Hassall's corpuscles: + denotes their presence, − denotes their absence, For epithelial cell injury: − = absence of injury, + = presence of epithelial cell injury, ++ = severe epithelial cell injury.

RESULTS

Immunosuppression and thymic dysplasia. It was important first to establish the intensity of the GVH reaction of F_1 mice injected with parental strain cells and that the GVH reaction induced thymic medullary epithelial cell injury. The results presented in Table 1 confirmed earlier studies showing that the PFC response to SRBC was completely immunosuppressed by day 9 after GVH induction and remained so for the remainder of the experiment. Also, light microscopic studies demonstrated thymic medullary epithelial cell injury and the disappearance of Hassall's corpuscles by 38–40 days after GVH induction (Table 1). Thus, immunosuppression and thymic dysplasia were confirmed in a randomly selected group of GVH mice prior to their utilization in the following studies.

Repopulation of the lymphoid organs by bone marrow cells from normal (NBM) or GVH mice (GVHBM). The first study was designed to investigate the ability of GVHBM cells to repopulate the lymphoid organs of normal irradiated (800–900 rads) syngeneic BAF_1 mice. The results in Table 2 show that GVHBM was as effective as NBM in providing cells for repopulation of the spleen, thymus, and bone marrow of irradiated mice. The spleens of irradiated animals repopulated with

TABLE 2. The mean number of cells in the thymus, spleen, and bone marrow, and the percentage of Thy-1-positive cells in thymus of irradiated normal BAF_1 mice reconstituted with NBM or GVHBM cells

Experimental groups	BM cells used for reconstitution	No. mice per group	Mean number of cells per organ ±SE × 10^{-6}			% Thy-1^+ cells/thymus
			Thymus	Spleen	Bone marrow/2 femurs	
Normal	—	5	52.3±6.9	53.0±17.1	24.0±1.5	92
Irradiated[a]	NBM	6	105.3±4.4	86.8±5.1	21.2±1.2	92
Irradiated[a]	GVHBM[b]	12	94.9±3.1	186.0±6.4	25.5±1.2	94
GVH	—	6	7.0±2.0	33.8±3.6	ND[c]	90

[a] Normal BAF_1 mice were lethally irradiated (850–900 rads), injected with BM cells, and then sacrificed 35–40 days after bone marrow treatment.

[b] GVHBM cells were obtained from mice 45–50 days after GVH induction.

[c] ND = not done.

GVHBM contained significantly more cells than irradiated animals repopulated with NBM. The thymuses of mice reconstituted with NBM or GVHBM contained approximately twice as many cells as age-matched nonirradiated normal mice. In addition, the thymuses of mice reconstituted with either NBM or GVHBM contained 92 and 95% Thy-1-positive cells, respectively. Therefore, GVHBM was as efficient as NBM for restoring the cellularity of lymphoid organs—and, as well, GVHBM appeared to provide adequate numbers of pre-T cells for reconstituting the Thy-1 population in the thymus.

Representative thymuses from irradiated BAF_1 mice reconstituted with NBM demonstrated a thymocyte-rich cortex, sharp corticomedullary demarcation, and many Hassall's corpuscles. Thymuses from irradiated BAF_1 mice reconstituted with GVHBM demonstrated relatively sharp corticomedullary demarcation, occasional Hassall's corpuscles, and individual medullary epithelial cells.

Functional studies. These studies were undertaken to investigate the ability of normal and irradiated BAF_1 thymuses to process NBM and GVHBM cells into immunocompetent T lymphocytes. The degree of functional maturity of T cell subsets was measured following the transfer of 50×10^6 thymus cells into ATxBM mice. Thymus cells were obtained from BAF_1 mice, or from irradiated normal BAF_1 mice given NBM or GVHBM cells. The degree of reconstitution of cell-mediated immunity (allograft survival time); humoral immunity (PFC response to SRBC); and splenic PHA, Con A, and LPS responses was determined in ATxBM mice treated with the different thymus cells.

To measure the degree of reconstitution of cell-mediated immunity, ATxBM mice restored with thymus cells were grafted with an H-2-incompatible third-party skin graft (Balb/c skin graft). The results given in Table 3 show that BAF_1 mice had a mean graft survival time of 10.6 days. ATxBM mice reconstituted with thymus cells from irradiated BAF_1 mice given NBM or GVHBM cells had a median graft survival time of 15 days. However, thymocytes taken directly from a GVH-dysplastic thymus failed to restore T cell function when transferred to ATxBM mice. ATxBM mice not reconstituted with thymus cells failed to reject their skin allografts within 60 days. Therefore, it appeared that pre-T cells were present in GVHBM and became immunocompetent T cells, able to mediate allograft rejection, after residing in a host with a normal thymic architecture.

TABLE 3. Survival time of Balb/c skin allografts on ATxBM mice reconstituted with thymocytes from irradiated BAF_1 mice given NBM or GVHBM cells

Thymocyte donors	Thymocyte recipients	No. mice per group	Skin allograft survival time of thymocyte recipients (mean ± SE)
None	Normal BAF	3	10.6±0.8
BAF_1 irradiated + NBM[a]	ATxBM	4	14.7±1.2
BAF_1 irradiated + GVHBM[a]	ATxBM	5	15.0±0.5
None	ATxBM	4	>60
GVH BAF_1	ATxBM	10	>60

[a] Normal BAF mice were irradiated (850–900 rads), injected with normal bone marrow cells (NBM) or GVH bone marrow cells (GVHBM), and sacrificed 30–40 days later; their thymocytes were used to reconstitute T cell function in AT×BM mice. Each AT×BM animal received 50×10^6 thymocytes.

TABLE 4. The PFC responses to SRBC of ATxBM mice reconstituted with thymocytes obtained from irradiated normal BAF_1 mice injected With NBM or GVHBM cells

Thymocyte donors	Thymocyte recipients	No. mice per group	PFC response of thymocyte recipients: x̄ PFC±SE/ spleen × 10^{-3}	PFC response of thymocyte recipients: x̄ PFC±SE/ 10^6 cells
None	Normal BAF_1	6	183.0±6.3	1,860.7±246.0
BAF_1 irradiated + NBM[a]	ATxBM	6	205.3±34.3	3,840.2±296.0
BAF_1 irradiated + GVHBM[a]	ATxBM	9	51.6±2.3	1,029.0±7.0
GVH BAF_1	ATxBM	12	0.2±0.2	23.0±6.0
None	GVH	8	0	0
None	ATxBM	20	0.6±0.3	18.2±4.6

[a] Normal BAF_1 mice were irradiated (850–900 rads), injected with normal bone marrow cells (NBM) or GVH bone marrow cells (GVHBM), and sacrificed 30–40 days later; their thymocytes were used to reconstitute T cell function in ATxBM mice. Each ATxBM animal received 50×10^6 thymocytes.

To measure the reconstitution of the humoral immune response, ATxBM mice were restored with thymus cells and were immunized with SRBC. PFC responses to SRBC were measured 9–10 days later. The results included in Table 4 show that ATxBM mice reconstituted with thymocytes from irradiated BAF_1 mice given NBM cells responded somewhat better than normal mice. ATxBM mice reconstituted with thymocytes from irradiated BAF_1 mice given GVHBM demonstrated a mean splenic PFC response approximately 25% that of normal mice, however, the PFC response per 10^6 splenic cells was greater than 50% of normal. In contrast thymocytes from GVH mice failed to reconstitute the PFC response of ATxBM mice. These results demonstrated that GVHBM contained pre-T cells capable of maturing into competent T cells when processed by a normal thymus. In contrast cells processed by a GVH dysplastic thymus failed to mature into competent T cells.

The data in Table 5 indicate that BAF_1 mice had splenic PHA and Con A responses of 52×10^3 and 41×10^3 cpm, respectively. The ATxBM mice reconstituted with thymocytes taken from irradiated BAF_1 mice, treated either with NBM cells or GVHBM cells, displayed similar reconstituted splenic PHA and Con A responses, although the background response was higher in the latter group. The splenic PHA and Con A responses of GVH spleen cells were not significantly different from background values. Furthermore, the thymocytes derived from GVHBM did not suppress the LPS response. Therefore, pre-T cells in NBM and GVHBM developed into mitogen-responsive T cells when processed through a normal thymus.

DISCUSSION

The results suggest that pre-T cell production in the bone marrow is not significantly affected by the GVH reaction. There was very little difference between normal BM and GVHBM in their ability to repopulate thymus glands of irradiated mice. In both cases, cells in the repopulated thymus glands expressed Thy-1 antigen. In addition, thymocytes obtained from thymuses repopulated with GVHBM were nearly as effective as thymocytes obtained from thymuses repopulated with NBM in reconstituting allograft reactivity, T helper cell function, and T-mitogen responses. Conversely, it was shown—in this study and in previous studies from this laboratory—that thymocytes

TABLE 5. Splenic PHA, Con A, and LPS responses of ATxBM mice reconstituted with thymocytes obtained from irradiated normal BAF_1 mice injected with NBM or GVHBM cells

Thymocyte donors	Thymocyte recipients	Splenic mitogen response ($\bar{x}$ cpm±SE×10^{-3})[c]			
		No mitogen	PHA	Con A	LPS
None	Normal BAF_1	1.9±0.7	52.1±0.8	41.2±0.6	19.3±0.6
BAF_1 irradiated + NBM[a]	ATxBM	1.1±0.9	14.6±2.1	29.5±1.7	77.3±0.3
BAF_1 irradiated + GVHBM[b]	ATxBM	6.5±0.3	19.5±0.3	27.3±4.8	76.4±0.1
GVH BAF_1	ATxBM	14.3±0.3	10.6±0.2	17.6±0.3	46.0±0.8
None	ATxBM	4.1±0.1	5.5±0.4	4.8±0.4	39.1±3.5

[a] Normal BAF_1 mice were irradiated (850–900 rads), injected with normal bone marrow cells (NBM) or GVH bone marrow cells (GVHBM), and killed 30–40 days later; their thymocytes were used to reconstitute T cell function in ATxBM mice. Each animal received 50×10^6 thymocytes.

[b] GVH BAF_1 mice were used 43–46 days after GVH induction.

[c] The mean of triplicate cultures from pooled spleen cells from 3–5 mice. Two experiments were performed and both gave similar results. The result of one representative experiment is shown.

obtained either from a GVH-reactive mouse or from a GVH-reactive mouse that was irradiated and reconstituted with normal bone marrow cells, failed to restore T-cell function when injected into T-cell-deprived mice (*1–4*). Thus, the results presented in this report strongly suggest that the T cell immunodeficiency that is associated with the GVH reaction is not due to the absence of pre-T cells in the GVHBM, but rather to maturational defect(s) in the thymus of GVH-reactive mice as suggested by earlier studies (*1*, *2*).

Previous studies from this laboratory (*4*) and by others (*13*) strongly suggest that the cells in the thymus 35–40 days after irradiation and reconstitution are nearly all of donor origin. Kadisch and Basch (*13*) showed an early burst of radiation-resistant host cells during the first few days, but by day 5 after irradiation 25% of the cells were of donor origin, and by day 20 more than 90% of the cells were of donor origin. In the present study there was no significant difference between the number of cells in the thymus of irradiated mice that received NBM or GVHBM, and both contained nearly twice as many thymocytes as mice that had not been irradiated and reconstituted. In addition, histological examination showed a near-normal cortical and medullary demarcation in irradiated mice reconstituted with either NBM or GVHBM. Therefore, it appears that the GVHBM was as effective as NBM in providing pre-T cells for repopulation of the thymuses of irradiated mice.

There is evidence that pre-T cells undergo an early differentiation in the bone marrow, and that the bone marrow or fetal liver environment is essential to commit cells to the pre-T cell lineage. Kadish and Basch (*13*) showed few, if any, pre-T cells in the marrow of mice for at least the first 10 days following irradiation. Stutman (*14*) demonstrated that when bone marrow cells, fetal liver cells, and yolk sac cells were used to repopulate thymus grafts, no yolk sac cells were detected in the thymus during the first 10 days, whereas bone marrow and fetal liver cells were evident by day 10. However, 20–30 days later cells from all three sources were readily detected. When ^{89}Sr was used to abrogate the stromal cells in the marrow, yolk sac cells failed to migrate to the thymus for up to 75 days after injection (*15*). These studies suggest that the bone marrow environment is important in the commitment of undifferentiated cells to the pre-T cell lineage.

Since the GVHBM was as effective as NBM, it appears that the bone marrow stromal cells that are necessary for the early differentiation of pre-T cells are not affected by the GVH reaction. However, it is possible that those cells are injured and that the GVHBM received the early differentiation signal after it was transferred into the irradiated non-GVH-reactive mouse. The studies of Kadisch and Basch (*13*), however, tend to rule out production of pre-T cells by bone marrow of irradiated mice.

Some insight can be obtained into lymphoid cell differentiation in the bone marrow of GVH-reactive mice from these studies. All hemopoietic cells in the periphery are thought to originate from a common stem cell following progressively more specialized differentiation steps (*16*). The lymphoid cell lineage gives rise to both pre-T and B cells in the bone marrow (*17*). In previous studies we showed that B cell, as well as T cell, functions were suppressed during the GVH reaction. It has recently been shown that GVHBM does not reconstitute normal B cell function when employed to restore B-cell-deprived mice (*18*). Therefore, it appears that an arrest in B cell differentiation occurs in the bone marow after the pre-T cells have formed. The results from the present experiments suggest that the block in B cell differentiation is not due to a differentiation defect in the early lymphoid lineage. Rather, it appears that the B cell differentiation defect occurred after the T and B cell differentiation had diverged into their respective cell lines, since pre-T cells were not affected as severely as B cells. An early divergence of pre-T and pre-B cells has been demonstrated in other studies (*17*). Therefore, early lymphoid differentiation does not seem to be affected by the GVH reaction, whereas later maturational events of B cells in the marrow (*18*) and T cells in the thymus are affected (*1–3*).

Studies on bone marrow stromal cell injury during the GVH reaction may aid in identifying cells and/or products that play important roles in lymphoid differentiation in the bone marrow of normal animals.

Acknowledgments. We thank Ailsa Lee Loy and Rosmarie Siegrist-Johnstone for careful technical assistance, and Sandra James for typing the manuscript.

REFERENCES

1. Seddik M, Seemayer TA, Lapp WS. T cell functional defect associated with thymic epithelial cell injury induced by a graft-versus-host reaction. Transplantation 1980; 29: 61.
2. Seddik M, Seemayer TA, Kongshavn P, Lapp WS. Thymic epithelial functional deficit in chronic graft-versus-host reaction. Transplant Proc 1979; 11: 967.
3. Seddik M, Seemayer TA, Lapp WS. The graft-versus-host reaction and immune function: I. T-helper cell immunodeficiency associated with graft-versus-host induced thymic epithelial cell damage. Transplantation 1984; 37: 281.
4. Seddik M, Seemayer TA, Lapp WS. The graft-versus-host reaction and immune function: II. Recruitment of pre-T cells in vivo by graft-versus-host induced dysplastic thymuses following irradia-

tion and bone marrow treatment. Transplantation 1984; 37: 286.
5. Lapp WS, Wechsler A, Kongshavn PAL. Immune restoration of mice immunosuppressed by a graft-versus-host reaction. Cell Immunol 1974; 11: 419.
6. Seddik M, Seemayer TA, Lapp WS. In vitro study of the effects of the GVH reaction on T-cell immunocompetence. In: Kaplan JG, ed. The molecular basis of immune cell function. Amsterdam: Elsevier, 1979: 549.
7. Kirchner H, Muchmore AV, Chused TM, Holden HT, Heberman RB. Inhibition of proliferation of lymphoma cells and T lymphocytes by suppressor cells from spleens of tumor-bearing mice. J Immunol 1975; 114: 206.
8. Elie R, Lapp WS. Graft-versus-host induced immunosuppression: mechanism of depressed T-cell helper function in vitro. Cell Immunol 1977; 34: 38.
9. Treiber W, Lapp WS. Stimulation of humoral immune responses to a thymic-independent antigen in mice immunosuppressed by a graft-versus-host reaction. Cell Immunol 1978; 37: 118.
10. Parthenais E, Lapp WS. Evidence for two types of non-specific suppressor cells activated by the graft-versus-host reaction in mice. Scand J Immunol 1978; 7: 215.
11. Bliss JQ. The development of a congeneic pair from the A and CBA strains of mice. Transplantation 1965; 3: 730.
12. Seemayer TA, Lapp WS, Bolande RP. Thymic epithelial injury in graft-versus-host reactions following adrenalectomy. Am J Pathol 1978; 93: 325.
13. Kadish JL, Basch RS. Hematopoietic thymocyte precursors. I. Assay and kinetics of the appearance of progeny. J Exp Med 1976; 143: 1082.
14. Stutman O. Migration of yolk sac cells to thymus grafts: requirement of prior sojourn in bone marrow (or liver?). Ann Immunol (Inst Pasteur) 1976; 127C: 943.
15. Fried W, Gurney CW, Swatek M. The effect of Strontium-89 on the stem cell compartment of the spleen. Radiat Res 1966; 29: 50.
16. Micklem HS, Ford CE, Evans EP, Gray J. Interrelationships of myeloid and lymphoid cells: studies with chromosome marked cells transplanted into lethally irradiated mice. Proc Soc Lond [Biol] 1966; 165: 78.
17. Abramson S, Miller RG, Phillips RA. The identification in adult bone marrow of pluripotent and restricted stem cells of the myeloid and lymphoid systems. J Exp Med 1977; 145: 1567.
18. Seddik M, Seemayer TA, Lapp WS. The graft-versus-host reaction and immune function: IV. B-cell functional defect associated with a depletion of CFU-s in marrow of graft-versus-host reactive mice. Transplantation 1985; 41: 242).

Received 2 January 1985.
Accepted 6 June 1985.

0041-1337/86/4102-0242$02.00/0
TRANSPLANTATION Vol. 41, No. 2
Printed in U.S.A.

THE GRAFT-VERSUS-HOST REACTION AND IMMUNE FUNCTION

IV. B CELL FUNCTIONAL DEFECT ASSOCIATED WITH A DEPLETION OF SPLENIC COLONY-FORMING UNITS IN MARROW OF GRAFT-VERSUS-HOST-REACTIVE MICE[1]

MONA SEDDIK,[2] THOMAS A. SEEMAYER,[3] AND WAYNE S. LAPP[4]

Department of Physiology, McGill University, Montreal, Quebec H3G 1Y6; and Department of Pathology, Montreal Children's Hospital and the McGill University—Montreal Children's Hospital Research Institute, Montreal, Quebec, Canada

Studies were conducted to determine whether a functional B cell defect occurred in the bone marrow of mice experiencing a GVH reaction (GVHBM). GVH reactions were induced in AxCBA F_1 adult mice by an injection of A strain lymphoid cells. The GVH reaction was confirmed by immunosuppression and thymus histology. At various intervals after GVH induction, GVHBM was tested for its ability to restore B cell function in adult thymectomized irradiated mice reconstituted with normal thymocytes. GVHBM cells obtained seven days after GVH induction restored but slightly the plaque forming cell (PFC) response to sheep erythrocytes and the mitogen response to lipopolysaccharide (LPS). GVHBM cells obtained 10 days or later failed to reconstitute the PFC or LPS responses. GVHBM cells suppressed neither the T or B cell function of normal spleen cells nor the LPS mitogen response of normal bone marrow cells. In addition, the splenic colony-forming units (CFU-s) in GVHBM were slightly decreased by day 10 after GVH induction and markedly depressed by day 22 after GVH induction. These results suggest that the GVH reaction may affect two different events in B cell differentiation. The early decrease in functional B cells that occurs before there is any change in the CFU-s population suggests a direct effect on B cell production, whereas the later absence of functional B cells could be due to the marked decline in stem cell production (CFU-s).

[1] This work was supported by grants from the Medical Research Council, the National Cancer Institute of Canada, and the McGill University-Montreal Children's Hospital Research Institute.

[2] MRC of Canada Fellow.

[3] McPherson, Fraser, Monat Associate.

[4] Reprint requests to W.S. Lapp, Department of Physiology, McIntyre Medical Center, McGill University, 3655 Drummond Street, Montreal, Quebec, H3G 1Y6, Canada.

Experimental graft-versus-host (GVH)[5] reactions induce suppression of cell-mediated and humoral immune responses (*1–4*). In the course of investigating mechanisms responsible for this immunosuppression, a distinct lesion was observed in the thymus of F_1 mice experiencing a GVH reaction (*5*). The thymus of such animals incurred a form of injury to medullary epithelium and Hassall's corpuscles that resulted in a histological appearance indistinguishable from thymic dysplasia, the morphological hallmark of severe combined immunodeficiency.

The documentation of this thymic alteration led to a series of experiments demonstrating an associated block in T cell differentiation into alloreactive (*6*), helper, and mitogen-responsive cells (*7*). It was later shown that the thymic lesion was associated with an arrest in T cell maturation in the thymus, with the primary defect resulting in deficient IL-2 production (*9*) rather than abnormal pre-T cell production in the marrow (*10*).

Early studies showed that the B cell response to thymic independent antigens was depressed during the GVH reaction (*4, 11, 12*). In addition, the splenic mitogen response to LPS was also suppressed following the GVH reaction, and all animals remained permanently suppressed (*2, 13*). The early suppression of B cell function in experimental animals was, in part, attributed to suppressor cells (*10, 13*) and/or increased release of prostaglandin (PG) (*13*). The PG mediated suppression subsided within a short time, however, B cell function remained suppressed. It was not known whether the permanent B cell functional abnormality was the result of a central failure of B cell production in the bone marrow or whether it was due to some suppression or cytostatic activity in the peripheral lymphoid organs.

The purpose of the present study was to determine whether the GVH reaction caused a central defect in the production of functional B cells in the bone marrow of mice experiencing a chronic GVH reaction and, if so, to determine the time when functional B cell production ceased. Using a bone marrow transfer system, our experiments show that GVH bone marrow was not able to reconstitute B function in B-cell-deprived mice as early as 7 days after GVH induction and that GVHBM remained functionally B-cell-deficient during the entire course of a chronic GVH reaction. In addition, stem cell production was also depressed in GVH bone marrow. These results are consistent with the hypothesis that a GVH reaction causes a central failure in the production of functional B as well as T lymphocytes.

MATERIALS AND METHODS

Animals. Mice of inbred strains A(H-2^a), CBA (H-2^k), and the CBA×A F_1 hybrid (BAF_1) were used. All mice were bred and maintained in our animal colony. Donors and recipients were between 12 and 16 weeks of age.

GVH reaction induction. Single-cell suspensions were prepared from pooled spleens and lymph nodes of strain A animals as described previously (*14*). GVH reactions were induced in adult BAF_1 mice by the i.v. injection of 75×10^6 A strain lymphoid cells.

Direct plaque-forming cell (PFC) assay. Spleen cells were assayed for the total number of direct PFCs per spleen to sheep red blood cells (SRBC) using the technique of Cunningham and Szenberg (*15*) as modified in this laboratory (*16*). Mice were injected i.v. with 5×10^8 SRBC 4–5 days before being killed for the PFC assay.

Splenic mitogen responses. Splenic mitogen responses to PHA, Con A, and LPS were tested using the technique of Kirchner et al. (*17*) as described previously (*7, 13*).

Histology. Thymuses from representative control and GVH-reactive mice were obtained at various intervals after the induction of the GVH reaction and were studied by light microscopy as described previously (*5*).

Preparation of adult thymectomized, irradiated (ATx) mice. Normal BAF_1 mice were thymectomized at 8–10 weeks of age. Four days later, they were lethally irradiated with 850–900 rads and were reconstituted with bone marrow within 24 hr as described previously (*16*). At the end of each experiment all animals were autopsied. Any animal with macroscopic or microscopic thymic remnants was discarded from the experimental group.

Spleen and thymus cell suspensions. Spleen and thymus cell suspensions were prepared from normal BAF_1 mice in the same manner as the spleen and lymph node cell suspensions used to induce a GVH reaction.

Colony forming unit (CFUs) assay. The in-vivo colony forming ability of bone marrow cells was determined by counting the number of visible macroscopic colonies per spleen in adult thymectomized, lethally irradiated (850–900 rads) BAF_1 mice (ATx), 10–11 days after reconstitution with 8×10^4 bone marrow cells.

Bone marrow cell suspension. Single-cell suspensions were prepared from bone marrow aspirates from the femurs and tibia of normal (NBM) or GVH mice (GVHBM) as described previously (*6*).

RESULTS

Three experiments were performed utilizing bone marrow cells from mice experiencing a GVH reaction. To assure that a GVH reaction had been induced, a representative group of mice presumed to have incurred a GVH reaction was tested to satisfy two conditions prior to initiating the experiments. The first requisite was that the thymus reflect the histological features of GVH-induced thymic dysplasia. The second requirement was that the mice be immunosuppressed and remain so throughout the experiment, as determined by the PFC response to SRBCs and the splenic mitogen responses to PHA, Con A, and LPS. Both conditions were fulfilled (Table 1).

The first experiment was designed to test the ability of bone marrow from GVH-reactive mice (GVHBM) to reconstitute B cell function in B-cell-deprived mice. Adult thymectomized BAF_1 mice were lethally irradiated and were reconstituted with 15×10^6 bone marrow cells from GVH-reactive mice (ATx-GVHBM) or normal mice (ATxNBM) within 24 hr. Fifteen days later, 50×10^6 thymocytes from normal syngeneic BAF_1 mice (NTc) were administered. These animals were divided

[5] Abbreviations used in this article: ATx, adult thymectomized, irradiated; ATxGVHBM, adult thymectomized, irradiated, reconstituted with bone marrow obtained from GVH-reactive mice; ATxNBM, adult thymectomized, irradiated, reconstituted with bone marrow obtained from normal mice; CFU-s, splenic colony forming units; Con A, conconavalin A; GVH, graft-versus-host; GVHBM, bone marrow obtained from GVH-reactive mice; LPS, lipopolysaccharide; NBM, bone marrow obtained from normal mice; NSc, normal spleen cells; NTc, thymocytes obtained from normal mice; PFC, plaque-forming cell; PHA, phytohemagglutin; SRBC, sheep erythrocytes.

into two groups: the first received SRBC and the PFC response to SRBC was determined 9–10 days later; the second was used to measure the splenic mitogen response to LPS.

The results presented in Table 2 demonstrate that NBM plus NT restored the PFC response to SRBC of ATx mice to nearly 50% of the normal response based on the PFC response per 10^6 spleen cells. In contrast GVHBM, obtained as early as 7 days after GVH induction, plus NT, only slightly restored the PFC response (10% of normal per 10^6 spleen cells). GVHBM cells obtained 24–42 days after GVH induction failed to restore the PFC response of ATx mice that also received NT. The response of ATx mice that received both NT and 24–42-day GVHBM cells was not different from that of the ATx mice that received either NBM or GVHBM and no thymus cells. The results suggest that GVHBM is markedly deficient in B cell production as early as 10 days after induction and remains deficient for at least 42 days after GVH induction.

The data in Table 3 indicate that ATxNBM mice, with or without NTc reconstitution, had normal splenic LPS responses. In contrast, the splenic LPS responses were profoundly reduced in ATx mice reconstituted with GVHBM as early as 10 days after initiation of the GVH reaction. In addition, the results in Table 3 show that the addition of normal thymocytes to ATxGVHBM mice failed to restore the LPS response.

These experiments document a B cell functional deficiency in the marrow of GVH-reactive mice. Several mechanisms that might contribute to the observed results include the presence of suppressor cells in GVHBM, a lack of B cell functional maturation, or a marked deficiency of bone marrow stem cells capable of maturing into immunocompetent B cells. Experiments were then designed to test these possibilities.

The second series of experiments was designed to test whether GVHBM contained suppressor cells capable of suppressing the function of normal syngeneic spleen cells (NSc), and/or the function of normal syngeneic bone marrow cells (NBM).

To test the former possibility, ATx mice received a mixture of 60–80×10^6 NSc and 15×10^6 GVHBM cells (the latter provided by GVH-reactive mice 40–42 days after GVH induction) within 24 hr after x-irradiation. Subsequently, the splenic PFC response was determined. Table 4 illustrates that ATx mice given either NSc or NSc and NBM cells had a mean PFC response of 34.7 and 26.3×10^3/spleen respectively. ATx mice reconstituted with the mixture of NSc and GVHBM cells had a mean PFC response of 24.7×10^3/spleen. Thus, GVHBM cells did not suppress the ability of NSc to reconstitute the PFC response in ATx mice.

To test whether GVH bone marrow contained cells capable of suppressing normal syngeneic bone marrow cells, ATx mice received a mixture of 15×10^6 NBM cells and 15×10^6 GVHBM cells, the latter provided by GVH-reactive mice 42 days after GVH induction. Fifteen days later, 50×10^6 NTc were administered. The PFC response was measured 9–10 days following the administration of SRBC.

Table 4 shows that the PFC response was restored in ATx mice reconstituted with a mixture of NBM cells and late GVHBM cells followed by NTc. Thus, GVHBM cells did not suppress the PFC response in ATxr mice reconstituted with syngeneic normal bone marrow cells and thymocytes. Since the PFC response to SRBC represents a humoral response dependent upon T and B cell cooperation, one may conclude that GVHBM cells failed to suppress both T and B cells.

TABLE 1. Immune function and histology of thymuses of animals used as bone marrow cell donors

Experimental groups	No. of mice per group	Days after GVH induction	Immune function: PFC response to SRBC/spleen (x̄±SE × 10^{-3})	Mitogen response (% of normal responses)[a]: PHA	ConA	LPS	Histological observations[b]: Hassall's corpuscles	Epithelial cell injury
Normal BAF_1	3	—	278.5±41.0	100	100	100	+	−
GVH	4	10–12	0	87.2	131.4	104.8	+	−
GVH	4	22–24	0	22.6	111.7	21.9	−	+
GVH	4	40–45	0	2.2	2.2	8.2	−	++

[a] % of normal mitogen response was calculated using the following equation:

$$\frac{\text{GVH} - \text{background}}{\text{Control} - \text{background}} \times 100.$$

Normal BAF_1 mice were used as the control group. The background denotes the response when no mitogens were added.

[b] Hassall's corpuscles: + denotes their presence, − denotes their absence; Epithelial cell injury: − = no epithelial cell injury, + = evident epithelial cell injury, ++ = severe epithelial cell injury.

TABLE 2. The PFC response to SRBC of ATx mice reconstituted with NTc and GVHBM cells obtained on different days after GVH induction

Experimental group	Source of cells for reconstitution: Thymus cells	BM cells	Days after GVH induction	No. mice per group	PFC response of reconstituted mice: X̄PFC±SE/spleen×10^{-3}	X̄PFC±SE/10^6 spleen cells (% of normal)
Normal BAF_1	—	—	—	21	199.2±18.2	2600.1±265.4 (100)
ATx	—	Normal	—	17	0.5±0.2	15.4±2.5 (0.5)
ATx	normal BAF_1	Normal	—	20	30.0±2.9	1238.1±14.3 (47.6)
ATx	normal BAF_1	GVH	7	5	5.8±1.8	260.7±37.1 (10.0)
ATx	normal BAF_1	GVH	10	3	0.7±0.3	28.6±5.9 (1.1)
ATx	normal BAF_1	GVH	24	6	1.7±1.2	39.9±13.7 (1.5)
ATx	normal BAF_1	GVH	42	12	0.5±0.3	14.4±3.9 (0.5)
ATx	—	GVH	42	3	1.0±1.0	44.5±14.8 (1.7)

The splenic PHA, Con A, and LPS responses in ATx mice reconstituted with normal thymocytes and GVHBM are shown in Table 5. ATx mice given NTc had reconstituted splenic PHA, Con A, and LPS responses. ATx mice reconstituted with NBM but not NTC were able to respond to LPS. In addition, ATx mice reconstituted with a mixture of NBM and GVHBM displayed a normal LPS response. When this latter group was further reconstituted with NTc the responses to PHA, Con A and LPS were restored. These results further confirm that GVHBM did not exert a suppressive effect on either NBM cells or on normal T lymphocyte function.

The third experiment was designed to determine whether the GVH reaction induced a deficiency in the bone marrow stem cell population. For this study, the splenic colony-forming ability (CFU-s) of GVHBM cells was measured at different days after GVH induction by injection 8×10^4 GVHBM cells i.v. into x-irradiated mice and by counting the number of macroscopic CFU-s in the spleen of each animal 10–11 days later. The results show that mice reconstituted with NBM averaged 13.5 colonies per spleen (Table 6). In mice reconstituted with GVHBM cells 3–7 or 10–13 days after GVH induction, relatively normal numbers of splenic colonies were present. In contrast, mice that received GVHBM cells, obtained 22–66 days after GVH induction demonstrated a marked decrease in the number of CFU-s. Therefore, the GVH reaction appeared to markedly reduce the stem cell renewal potential of bone marrow obtained late during the GVH reaction, and as well caused a marked reduction in the total number of marrow cells.

TABLE 3. Splenic LPS response of ATx BAF_1 mice reconstituted with normal BAF_1 thymocytes and bone marrow obtained from BAF_1 mice on different days after GVH induction

Experimental groups	No. mice per group	Reconstituted with normal thymocytes	Source of bone marrow cells used for reconstitution: Donor	Days after GVH induction	LPS response (SI)[a]
Normal	5	–	—	—	28.07
ATx	5	–	Normal BAF_1	—	29.0
ATx	8	+	Normal BAF_1	—	31.92
ATx	8	+	GVH	10	1.53
ATx	5	+	GVH	24	0.92
ATx	6	+	GVH	42	1.44

[a] The stimulation index (SI) was calculated as follows:

$$\frac{\text{mean cpm mitogen stimulated culture}}{\text{mean cpm of control cultures}}.$$

DISCUSSION

These experiments demonstrate that GVH reactions in F_1 mice induce B cell functional defects that accompany the T cell functional deficiencies previously documented (*6, 7*). Bone marrow cells from GVH-reactive mice were unable to reconstitute the humoral immune (PFC) response to SRBCs and splenic LPS response in B-cell-deprived mice. The inability to effect these B cell functions does not appear to be the consequence of cells contained in GVH bone marrow capable of

TABLE 6. The splenic colony-forming ability of GVHBM cells obtained on different days after GVH induction

Source of BM cells injected	No. animals	Days after GVH induction	$\bar{X}$ number of bone marrow cells per animal[a]	$\bar{x}$ CFU-s/ spleen
Normal BAF_1	11	—	19.3	13.5±0.4
GVH	6	3–7	17.0	13.2±0.3
GVH	7	10–13	12.0	11.2±0.7
GVH	9	22–27	8.5	3.6±0.3
GVH	5	64–66	8.3	3.7±0.3

[a] The cells were collected from femurs and tibias of each mouse and were pooled.

TABLE 4. The PFC response to SRBC of ATx mice reconstituted with GVHBM cells, plus normal spleen cells or normal BM and normal thymus cells

Experimental groups[a]	Source of cells used for reconstitution: BM cells	Normal spleen cells	Normal BAF_1 thymocytes	Days after GVH induction	$\bar{X}$PFC/spleen ±SE×10^{-3}	XPFC±SE/10^6 spleen cells
ATx	—	NSC	—	—	34.7±3.5	1,796.1±166.2
ATx	NBM	NSC	—	—	26.3±2.0	1,052.1±122.3
ATx	GVHBM	NSC	—	40–42	24.7±1.9	882.5±441.3
ATx	NBM + GVHBM	—	NT	40–42	20.8±4.7	1,504.3±191.8
ATx	NBM	—	NT	—	30.0±2.9	1,238.1±14.3
ATx	GVHBM	—	NT	40–42	0.5±0.3	14.4±3.9

[a] A minimum of 5 animals was included in each experimental group.

TABLE 5. Splenic mitogen response of ATx BAF_1 mice reconstituted with normal BAF_1 thymus cells and bone marrow cells from normal BAF_1 and GVH-reactive mice

Experimental group[a]	No. mice per group	Reconstituted with normal thymocytes	Source of bone marrow cells used for reconstitution	Mitogen response (SI)[a]: PHA	Con A	LPS
Normal BAF_1	6	–	—	30.0	35.0	26.7
ATx	7	–	Normal BAF_1	1.3	1.4	40.2
ATx	8	+	Normal BAF_1	31.1	35.5	45.0
ATx	7	–	Normal + $GVHBAF_1$	1.3	1.5	39.7
ATx	7	+	Normal + $GVHBAF_1$	25.7	45.7	42.1
ATx	6	–	$GVHBAF_1$	1.1	1.2	1.2

[a] As for footnote [a], Table 3.

suppressing either normal spleen or bone marrow cells. An additional effect of GVH reactions on the marrow is a profound reduction in the number of stem cells, as measured by the number of CFU-s. Since the B cell functional deficiencies documented in this study antedated the decline in colony-forming ability of GVH bone marrow cells, the reduction in marrow stem cells cannot account solely for the observed functional consequences.

These results suggest that, in addition to the suppression of B cell function that has been observed in the spleen of mice experiencing a GVH reaction (*4, 11, 12*), there is also a marked absence of B cells and/or B cell precursors in the marrow of GVH-reactive mice. The absence of B cells in the marrow suggests a central failure in the production of functional B cells as early as 7 days after GVH induction (Table 2). The central failure of B cell production could be due either to the generalized destruction of myeloid and lymphoid elements in the marrow—including pre-B cells and, perhaps, pluripotent stem cells—or to some selective injury to the pre-B or stromal cells that may influence B cell production. The present results suggest that the B cell defect is not due to a generalized destruction of bone marrow but rather to some selective effect on B cell production. Evidence for this speculation is based on several observations by us and others.

First, the inability to transfer functional B cells in GVHBM occurs very early after the onset of the GVH reaction, at a time before marked hypoplasia or aplasia is seen in the marrow. Since the turnover of B cells is very high in the marrow and the half-life of pre-B and B cells is very short (*18*), any defect in B cell production in the marrow would be followed by a rapid decline in functional B cells within 2–3 days. In addition, the decrease in B cells preceded the decrease in CFU-s production by nearly one week. The generalized hypoplasia occurred in these animals at least 14 days after GVH induction. Therefore, extensive cell destruction cannot account for the early decline in B cells but bone marrow aplasia could contribute to the later absence of B cells in GVH bone marrow. Thus, it is quite possible that decreased B cell function following the GVH reaction could be due to two independent events. The initial suppression could stem from a selective effect on pre-B and B cells, whereas the long term depression of functional B cells may be associated with the decreased stem cell production.

Second, the marked decrease in B cell production occurred without a concommittant absence of erythroid and myeloid stem cells and pre-T cells. It is true that the number of CFU-s did decline during the GVH reaction and that CFU-s can consist of pluriopotent stem cells as well as myeloid restricted stem cells (*19, 20*). However, from other studies carried out in this laboratory and the present study we have demonstrated that bone marrow cells from GVH-reactive mice can reconstitute erythroid and myeloid production in lethally irradiated mice since ATxr mice reconstituted with GVH bone marrow cells survived, whereas ATxr mice not reconstituted died within the first week after irradiation (these controls are not shown in the results section). In addition, we have recently shown that GVH bone marrow that is devoid of functional B cells still contains near normal numbers of pre-T cells (*10*). Abramson et al. (*20*) have suggested that both the pre-T and myeloid cells in the bone marrow are each derived from their own restricted stem cell compartment. In contrast, the B cell line appears to be derived directly from the pluripotent stem cell compartment. Based on the model described by Abramson et al. (*20*) it appears quite possible that the B lymphocyte cell line could be selectively abolished with sparing of T or myeloid-restricted stem cell compartments. Our observations are compatible with this notion (*20*) and, in fact, support the concept that pre-T and pre-B cells diverge very early during ontogeny in the bone marrow. We therefore suggest that B cell production is selectively inhibited in the marrow of mice undergoing a chronic GVH reaction.

It is noteworthy that both hypoplasia and a reduced splenic colony-forming ability (*22*) of bone marrow have been demonstrated in F_1 mice experiencing a GVH reaction. It is plausible, but not yet established, that a GVH reaction may inflict injury, not only to established marrow cell lines, but to more primitive stromal cells, in a manner analogous to events in the thymus (*5–7*). Several types of stromal cells have been described in the bone marrow of rodents (*23*) and are believed to function either by cell-cell contact or through the elaboration of humoral factors. Injury to such stromal cells with alteration of the physical and/or molecular microenvironment of the marrow may contribute to the B cell functional deficiencies documented.

A complex assortment of immunodeficiencies and disorderd immune function, affecting both the cellular and humoral immune systems, has been documented as a consequence of GVH reactions in humans following bone marrow transplantation (*24–26*). Earlier studies showed that patients who had undergone bone marrow transplantation for a variety of disorders routinely developed a combined deficiency of cell-mediated and humoral immunity (*27, 28*). Ringden et al. (*29*) demonstrated that patients with chronic GVH disease displayed a significantly lower IgG, IgA, and IgM PFC response to S. aureus than normal patients for the first 101 days after grafting; as well, chronic GVH patients displayed a decreased IgM response for more than 1 year following transplantation. More recently, from a total of nine bone marrow transplant patients studied, Korsmeyer et al. (*24*) have shown that while for some patients the absence of normal B-cell function was due to suppressor cell activity, others, (four of the nine) possessed defective B-cells. Thus, both suppressor cell activity and defective B-cell production may contribute to the hypogammaglobulinemia that occurs in patients who develop chronic GVH disease following bone marrow transplantation. The mechanism responsible for the B-cell defect in man following bone marrow transplantation is not known, but from our experimental GVH studies it appears that the defect may occur in the B cell lineage in the bone marrow.

Acknowledgments. We thank Ailsa Lee Loy and Rosmarie Siegrist-Johnstone for careful technical assistance and Sandra James for typing the manuscript.

REFERENCES

1. Howard JG, Woodruff MFA. Effect of graft-versus-host reaction on the immunological responsiveness of the mouse. Proc R Soc Lond [Biol] 1961; 154: 532.
2. Blaese RM, Martinez C, Good RA. Immunologic incompetence of immunologically runted animals. J Exp Med 1964; 119: 211.
3. Lapp WS, Möller G. Prolonged survival of H-2 incompatible skin allografts in F_1 animals treated with parental lymphoid cells. Immunology 1969; 17: 339.
4. Möller G. Suppressive effect of graft-versus-host reaction on immune response to heterologous red cells. Immunology 1971; 20: 597.

5. Seemayer TA, Lapp WS, Bolande RP. Thymic involution in murine graft-versus-host reaction. Am J Pathol 1977; 88: 119.
6. Seddik M, Seemayer TA, Lapp WS. T cell functional defect associated with thymic epithelial cell injury induced by a graft-versus-host reaction. Transplantation 1980; 29: 61.
7. Seddik M, Seemayer TA, Lapp WS. The graft-versus-host reaction and immune function. I. T helper cell immunodeficiency associated with graft-versus-host induced thymic epithelial cell damage. Transplantation 1984; 37: 281.
8. Seddik M, Seemayer TA, Lapp WS. The graft-versus-host reaction and immune function. II. Recruitment of pre T cells in vivo by graft-versus-host induced dysplastic thymuses following irradiation and bone marrow treatment. Transplantation 1984; 37: 286.
9. Mendes ML, Rode H, Peres A, Kongshavn PAL, Lapp WS. Interleukin 1 and Interleukin 2 defects associated with murine graft-versus-host induced immunodeficiency. Transplantation 1985; 39: 418.
10. Seddik M, Seemayer TA, Lapp WS. The graft-versus-host reaction and immune function. III. Occurrence of pre-T cells in the bone marrow of graft-versus-host reactive mice manifesting a T-cell immunodeficiency. Transplantation 1986; 41: 238.
11. Byfield P, Christie GH, Howard JG. Alternative potentiating and inhibitory effects of GVH reaction on formation of antibodies against a thymus independent polysaccharide (SIII). J Immunol 1973; 111: 72.
12. Treiber W, Lapp WS. Stimulation of humoral immune responses to a thymic-independent antigen in mice immunosuppressed by a graft-versus-host reaction. Cell Immunol 1978; 37: 118.
13. Lapp WS, Mendes M, Kirchner H, Gemsa D. Prostaglandin synthesis by lymphoid tissue of mice experiencing a graft-versus-host reaction: relationship to immunosuppression. Cell Immunol 1980; 50: 271.
14. Lapp WS, Wechsler A, Kongshavn PAL. Immune restoration of mice immunosuppressed by a graft-versus-host reaction. Cell Immunol 1974; 11: 419.
15. Cunningham AJ, Szenberg A. Further improvements in the plaque technique for detecting single antibody-forming cells. Immunology 1968; 14: 599.
16. Elie R, Lapp WS. Graft-versus-host induced immunosuppression: mechanism of depressed T-cell helper function in vitro. Cell Immunol 1977; 34: 38.
17. Kirchner H, Muchmore AV, Chused TM, Holden HT, Herberman RB. Inhibition of proliferation of lymphoma cells and T lymphocytes by suppressor cells from spleens of tumor-bearing mice. J Immunol 1975; 114: 206.
18. Osmond DG. Production and differentiation of B lymphocytes in the bone marrow. In: Battisto JR, Knight KL, eds. Immunoglobulin genes and B cell differentiation. Amsterdam: Elsevier, 1980: 185.
19. Micklem HS, Ford EC, Evans EP, Gray J. Inter-relationships of myeloid and lymphoid cells: studies with chromosome-marked cells transfused into lethally irradiated mice. Proc R Soc Lond [Biol] 1966; 165: 78.
20. Abramson S, Miller RG, Phillips RA. The identification in adult bone marrow of pluripotent and restricted stem cells of the myeloid and lymphoid systems. J Exp Med 1977; 145: 1967.
21. Ishihara K, Shimamine T. Structural changes of the murine bone marrow in graft-versus-host reaction. Pathol Res Pract 1980; 169: 84.
22. Hirabayashi N. Studies on graft versus host (GVH) reactions. I. Impairment of hemopoietic stroma in mice suffering from GVH disease. Exp Hematol 1981; 9: 101.
23. Weiss L. The hematopoietic microenvironment of the bone marrow. An ultrastructural study of the stroma in rats. Anat Rec 1976; 186: 161.
24. Korsmeyer SJ, Elfenbein GJ, Goldman CK, Marshall SL, Santos GW, Waldmann TA. B cell, helper T cell, and suppressor T cell abnormalities contribute to disordered immunoglobulin synthesis in patients following bone marrow transplantation. Transplantation 1982; 33: 184.
25. Reinherz EL, Parkman R, Rappeport J, Rosen FS, Schlossman SF. Aberrations of suppressor T cells in human graft-versus-host disease. N Engl J Med 1979; 300: 1061.
26. Noel DR, Witherspoon RP, Storb R, et al. Does graft-versus-host disease influence the tempo of immunologic recovery after allogenic human marrow transplantation? An observation on 56 long-term survivors. Blood 1978; 51: 1087.
27. Elfenbein GJ, Anderson PN, Humphrey RL, et al. Immune system reconstitution following allogenic bone marrow transplantation in man: a multiparameter analysis. Transplant Proc 1976; 8: 641.
28. Thomas ED, Buckner CD, Bonaje M, et al. One hundred patients with acute leukemia treated by chemotherapy, total body irradiation, and allogenic marrow transplantation. Blood 1977; 49: 511.
29. Ringden O, Witherspoon RP, Storb R, Ekelud E, Thomas ED. Increased in vitro B-cell IgG secretion during acute graft-versus-host disease and infection. Observations in 50 human marrow transplant recipients. Blood 1980; 55: 179.

Received 2 January 1985.
Accepted 6 June 1985.

0041-1337/86/4102-0248$02.00/0
TRANSPLANTATION

Vol. 41, No. 2
Printed in U.S.A.

THE EXPRESSION OF MAJOR HISTOCOMPATIBILITY COMPLEX AND LEUKOCYTE ANTIGENS BY CELLS IN THE RAT CORNEA

PATRICK A. TRESELER[1] AND FRED SANFILIPPO[2]

Departments of Microbiology and Immunology, Pathology, and Surgery, Duke University Medical Center, Durham, North Carolina 27710

The well-characterized immunogenetic constitution of the rat has made it a valuable resource for the study of corneal transplantation. However, little is known about the expression of histocompatibility antigens in the rat cornea or about the populations of passenger leukocytes rat corneal grafts may contain. Thus the relevance of rat corneal transplantation to the human situation is unclear. We examined the expression of antigens of the histocompatibility complex (MHC) of the rat (RT1) and of antigens identifying rat leukocyte populations in corneas of selected rat strains using a sensitive immunoperoxidase technique. Class I MHC antigens were found in fairly uniform association with most cells of the rat corneal epithelium, endothelium, and stroma. In contrast, class II MHC antigens were not associated with most corneal parenchymal cells, but were clearly present on multiple isolated dendritic cells throughout the corneal stroma, especially near the limbus, and on very rare isolated cells in the limbal epithelium; these antigens were not detectable on the corneal endothelium. Cells expressing an antigen common to all rat leukocytes were present in a distribution similar to that of class II MHC antigen-bearing cells. There was no consistent expression of antigens associated with T lymphocytes, macrophages, neutrophils, or NK cells. It thus appears that the expression of MHC and leukocyte antigens by cells in the rat cornea is similar to that reported in the human, indicating that the rat may indeed provide a good model of human corneal transplantation.

The rat has become widely used as an experimental model for the study of corneal transplantation (*1–6*), and appears to be well suited for this role. Unlike the rabbit and cat, which have been extensively employed by earlier investigators, the rat has a well-characterized immunogenetic constitution (*7, 8*), and many inbred, congenic, and recombinant strains exist (*8*), permitting transplantation across well-defined histocompatibility barriers and examination of the role of individual transplantation antigens in allograft responses (*1, 5, 6*). However, unlike the mouse, which is also an immunogenetically well-characterized experimental animal, the rat is large enough to allow full-thickness orthotopic corneal transplantation, providing a closer analogy to the clinical situation in humans (*4*).

Despite the recent extensive use of the rat in experimental corneal transplantation, important questions concerning the antigenic composition of the rat cornea remain unanswered. Antigens of the major histocompatibility complex (MHC)[3] have been repeatedly implicated in the rejection of corneal allografts in both human (*9–16*) and animal (*16, 17*) systems. While sensitive techniques have recently permitted demonstration in the human of class I MHC antigens on virtually all corneal epithelial, stromal, and endothelial cells, as well as class II MHC antigens on dendritic cells in the human corneal epithelium and stroma (*18–20*), almost nothing is known about the expression of MHC antigens by cells in the rat cornea. Also, despite the apparent important contribution of passenger leukocytes to the immunogenicity of various allogeneic tissues (*21*) including cornea (*22*), the types and numbers of bone-marrow-derived cells in the rat cornea remain virtually unknown. Without such information, the relevance of the rat model to the transplantation of human cornea remains unclear.

In this report, we describe the immunoperoxidase staining of corneas from selected rats strains with monoclonal antibodies reactive with rat class I and class II MHC antigens as well as leukocyte markers. With only relatively minor exceptions, the antigenic composition of the rat cornea was found to be closely analogous to that of the human.

MATERIALS AND METHODS

PVG ($RT1^c$), PVG.R1 ($RT1^{r1}$), and PVG.1A ($RT1^a$) rats were obtained from Olac Ltd. (Bicester, Oxon, UK). ACI ($RT1^a$) animals were obtained from M.A. Lab Animals (Walkersville, MD). The PVG.1A rat is a congenic animal, bearing the RT1 haplotype of the ACI rat on a PVG genetic background. The PVG.R1 animal is also congenic, bearing the RT1.A region of the ACI rat on a PVG background; it thus varies from PVG only at loci encoding class I MHC antigens (*8*).

Monoclonal antibodies reactive with various rat MHC and leukocyte antigens were obtained from Sera-tec Ltd. (Bicester, Oxon, UK). Table 1 shows the specificity of each primary antibody used. These reagents are all mouse IgG_1 antibodies obtained in the ascites form. Biotinylated rabbit anti-mouse IgG_1 antibody was obtained from Zymed Labs.

Donor rats seven weeks old were killed by CO_2 exposure and enucleated. Corneas were then immediately dissected from the rest of the eye with a 2-mm. margin of limbal tissue left attached. Each cornea was stored in immunofixative transport medium, then washed, embedded, frozen, and sectioned as described elsewhere (*23*).

Immunoperoxidase staining of corneal sections was performed following the avidin-biotin complex technique (*24*) using the primary monoclonal antibodies at a 1:100 dilution and the biotinylated rabbit antimouse IgG_1 secondary antibody at a 1:50 dilution. Each mouse monoclonal antibody was tested for its ability to react with rat spleen sections and found to yield significant staining of appropriate cell populations (data not shown). At least three cornea sections from each donor rat strain were labeled with each antibody.

[1] Dr. Treseler was supported by the Medical Scientist Training Program, Grant 5-T32GM07171, from the National Institutes of Health.

[2] Address reprint requests to Fred Sanfilippo, M.D., Ph.D., Box 3712, Duke University Medical Center, Durham, NC 27710.

[3] Abbreviation used: MHC, major histocompatibility complex.

TABLE 1. Monoclonal antibodies used in labeling

Antibody	Specificity
OX-18	Rat class I MHC antigen, monomorphic determinant[a]
OX-6	Rat class II MHC antigen, monomorphic determinant
OX-1	Rat leukocyte-common antigen
OX-19	Rat T lymphocytes and thymocytes
W3/13	Rat T lymphocytes, thymocytes, neutrophils, and brain
W3/25	Rat helper/inducer T lymphocytes and macrophages
OX-8	Rat cytotoxic/suppressor T lymphocytes, thymocytes, and most NK cells

[a] Present on all MHC antigens of that class.

Each corneal structure (i.e., epithelium, stroma, and endothelium) in every stained tissue section was assigned a score having the form X/Y, as previously described (*18*)—where X represented the intensity of staining (using a subjective scale of 0–4, with 0 indicating no staining above background levels, 1 indicating minimal but significant staining above background, and 4 indicating maximally intense staining), and Y represented the proportion of cells staining in this manner (rare = <1%, occasional = 1–10%, 1 = 11–25%, 2 = 26–50%, 3 = 51–75%, and 4 = 76–100%). There was no significant variation of a given structure's staining score between tissue sections of the same triplicate. Background levels of staining were assessed using several control slides for each cornea in which the primary monoclonal antibody was replaced with phosphate-buffered saline or a mouse monoclonal IgG_1 antibody that did not stain corneal tissue but nonetheless gave significant staining of positive control tissue. The control slide giving the highest intensity staining for each cornea was used as the appropriate background reference slide for that tissue.

RESULTS

Table 2 shows the results of corneal staining with monoclonal antibodies reactive with monomorphic determinants (invariant components) of rat MHC antigens. Virtually all corneal epithelial cells from all rat strains tested showed expression of class I MHC antigens that was most intense in the superficial epithelium (Fig. 1). This pattern did not vary significantly from central to limbal epithelium. Most corneal endothelial cells showed specific staining for class I MHC antigens as well (Fig. 2). About half the apparent keratocyte cell nuclei present in the corneal stroma of all strains appeared to have class I MHC antigens present in close association, presumably at the cell surface, but about an equal proportion showed no significant staining (Figs. 1 and 2). Isolated strands of class I antigen could also be seen throughout the stroma of all corneas, possibly reflecting class I antigen-bearing keratocyte membranes present at some distance from the cell nucleus. The expression of class I MHC antigens by all corneal components was uniformly more intense in ACI, PVG.1A, and PVG.R1 corneas than in PVG corneas (Table 2).

Class II MHC antigens were present on a much more restricted population of corneal cells (Table 2). Isolated class II antigen-positive cells were most frequent in the limbal stroma (Fig. 3), but a few scattered positive cells were consistently found even in the central cornea of all strains (Fig. 4). These cells often had a dendritic morphology, with spindly cytoplasmic processes (Fig. 3 and 4). Class II MHC antigen-positive cells in the corneal epithelium were extremely rare, but could occasionally be found in the peripheral cornea of some strains.

TABLE 2. MHC antigen expression in the rat cornea

Antibody	Corneal structure	Rat strain			
		ACI	PVG.1A	PVG.R1	PVG
OX-18	Epithelium (central)	2/4[a]	1/4	2/4	1/3
	Epithelium (limbal)	2/4	1/4	2/4	1/3
	Stroma (central)	2/2	1/2	2/2	1/2
	Stroma (limbal)	2/2	1/2	2/2	1/2
	Endothelium	2/3	2/3	2/2	1/3
OX-6	Epithelium (central)	0[b]	0	0	0
	Epithelium (limbal)	4/rare	4/rare	0	0
	Stroma (central)	4/rare	4/rare	4/rare	4/rare
	Stroma (limbal)	4/1	4/occ.	4/occ.	4/rare
	Endothelium	0	0	0	0

[a] Scored as X/Y: X = intensity of staining (1 to 4: 1 = slightly but significantly above background levels, and 4 = maximal staining intensity); Y = proportion of cells stained (rare = <1%, occasional (occ.) = 1–10%, 1 = 11–25%, 2 = 26–50%, 3 = 51–75%, 4 = 76–100%).

[b] No significant staining above background levels.

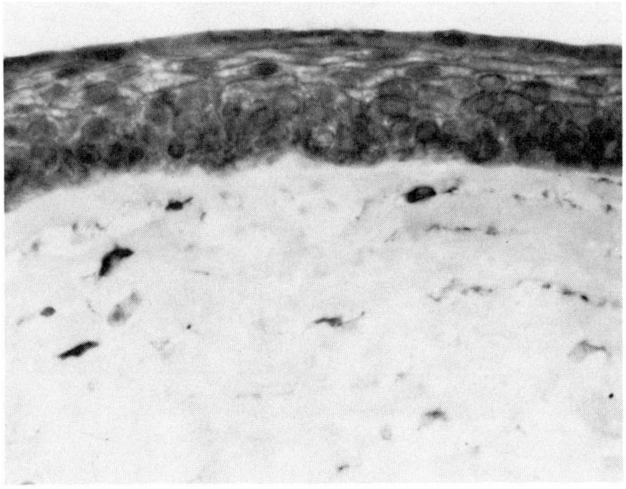

FIGURE 1. Class 1 MHC antigen expression in central ACI rat corneal epithelium and stroma (×400).

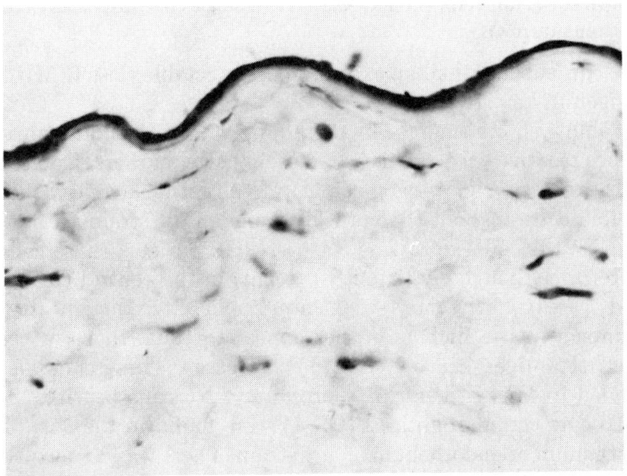

FIGURE 2. Class I MHC antigen expression in central PVG.1A rat corneal endothelium and stroma (×400).

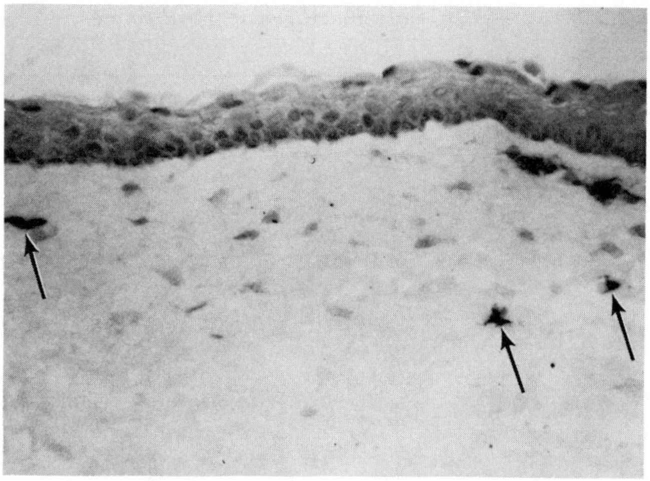

FIGURE 3. Class II MHC antigen expression in peripheral (left) and limbal (right) ACI rat cornea (×190). Frequency of class-II-positive stromal cells (arrows) is much higher near the limbus.

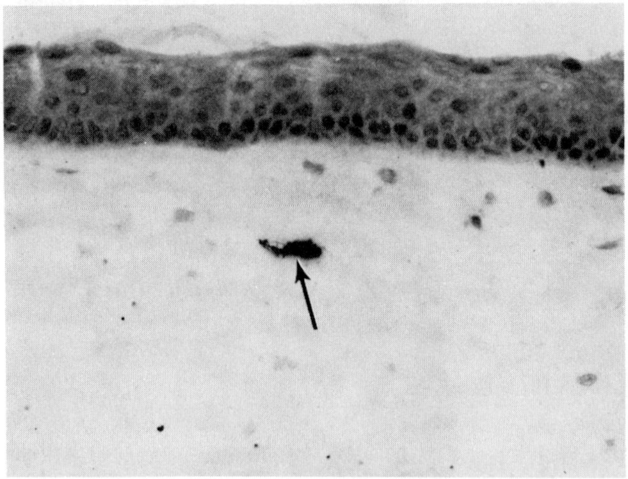

FIGURE 4. Class II MHC antigen expression in central ACI rat corneal epithelium and stroma (×250). Note single class-II-positive cell in stroma (arrow).

TABLE 3. Leukocyte antigen expression in the rat cornea

Antibody	Corneal structure	Rat strain			
		ACI	PVG.1A	PVG.R1	PVG
OX-1	Epithelium (central)	0[a]	0	0	0
	Epithelium (limbal)	0	0	0	0
	Stroma (central)	3/rare[b]	3/rare	3/rare	3/rare
	Stroma (limbal)	3/rare	3/occ.	3/rare	3/rare
	Endothelium	0	0	0	0
OX-19	Epithelium (central)	0	0	0	0
	Epithelium (limbal)	0	0	0	0
	Stroma (central)	4/rare	0	0	0
	Stroma (limbal)	0	0	0	0
	Endothelium	0	0	0	0
W3/13	Epithelium (central)	0	0	0	0
	Epithelium (limbal)	0	0	0	0
	Stroma (central)	0	0	0	0
	Stroma (limbal)	0	0	0	0
	Endothelium	0	0	0	0
W3/25	Epithelium (central)	4/rare	0	0	0
	Epithelium (limbal)	0	0	0	0
	Stroma (central)	0	0	0	0
	Stroma (limbal)	0	0	0	0
	Endothelium	0	0	0	0
OX-8	Epithelium (central)	0	3/rare	0	0
	Epithelium (limbal)	0	0	0	0
	Stroma (central)	0	0	0	0
	Stroma (limbal)	0	0	0	0
	Endothelium	0	0	0	0

[a] No significant staining above background levels.
[b] Scored as X/Y: X = intensity of staining (1 to 4: 1 = slightly but significantly above background levels, and 4 = maximal staining intensity); Y = proportion of cells stained (rare = <1%, occasional (occ.) = 1–10%, 1 = 11–25%, 2 = 26–50%, 3 = 51–75%, 4 = 76–100%).

The corneal endothelium expressed no detectable class II MHC antigen in any strain.

Table 3 shows the results of staining with monoclonal antibodies reactive with a variety of rat leukocyte markers. Isolated cells expressing an antigen common to all rat leukocytes could be found throughout the corneal stroma of all strains tested. As with the cells expressing class II MHC antigen, these cells were rare (though consistently present) in the central cornea, and were slightly more frequent peripherally, though their numbers in the limbus did not appear to equal those of the class II antigen-bearing cells in most cases. These cells also tended to have a dendritic morphology. No cells bearing the leukocyte-common antigen (OX-1) were found in the corneal epithelium or endothelium of any strain. There was no consistent expression of markers for rat T lymphocytes, thymocytes, neutrophils, macrophages, or natural killer cells (as detected by OX-19, W3/13, W3/25, and OX-8) by any cells in the cornea of any rat strain (Table 3).

DISCUSSION

In the rat, as in the human (*18*), it appears that class I MHC antigens are associated with most corneal epithelial, stromal, and endothelial cells. The quantitative expression of class I MHC antigens in the rat cornea appears appears to differ from the human only in the epithelium, where the human shows a marked increase in antigen expression from central to limbal cornea (*18*); the rat appears to express a low, uniform level of class I MHC antigen throughout the corneal epithelium. The class I MHC antigen associated with the rat corneal endothelium may constitute a crucial target antigen in corneal allograft rejection: irreversible rejection of corneal allografts appears to involve destruction of the endothelial layer (*25, 26*), and cellular and humoral immune responses to rat corneal allografts are primarily directed against class I MHC antigens (*5, 6, 27*). Consistent expression of class I MHC antigens in the human corneal endothelium has not been found by some groups using less sensitive techniques or limited serologic reagents (*19, 20*), whereas with the more sensitive (*24*) avidin-biotin complex method used in these studies we have also found uniform expression of class I antigens in the human cornea (*18*), paralleling our similar findings in the rat.

The expression of class II MHC antigens by the rat and human cornea appears to be similar in the corneal stroma, where both contain isolated, frequently dendritic, class II antigen-positive cells that are more common near the limbus (*22*). The human and rat cornea appear to differ somewhat in the frequency of cells expressing class II MHC antigen in the epithelium. In the human, isolated class II antigen-positive cells are quite common in the epithelium, especially near the limbus (*18*). In the rat cornea, however, epithelial cells expressing class II antigen were extremely rare, and were not found in the central cornea.

Previous investigators have documented by ultrastructural analysis that the cells bearing class II MHC antigen in the corneal epithelium of the human, rat, and other species are indeed Langerhans cells (*28*). Langerhans cells are bone-marrow-derived (*29*) dendritic cells increasingly implicated as important contributors to the immunogenicity of various allogeneic tissues (*21, 30*). We have found using congenic animals that the addition of a class II MHC antigen difference markedly augments the immunogenicity of class I MHC antigen disparate rat corneal allografts (*31*), indicating that these class II MHC antigen-positive Langerhans cells may play an important role in the rejection of corneal allografts as well. Others have shown that mouse corneas depleted of cells bearing class II MHC antigen by treatment with hyperbaric oxygen are much less immunogenic (*22, 32*). Preliminary results in our laboratory indicate that the same may also be true in the rat (*33*).

Dendritic cells such as the Langerhans cell, derived from bone marrow, frequently express "leukocyte-common antigens" used as markers for hematopoietically derived cells (*34*). It thus seems likely that the rat corneal cells that stained with the OX-1 monoclonal antibody may represent the same population of cells found by OX-6 staining to express class II MHC antigen, as is also suggested by their similar cell morphology and pattern of distribution. The frequency of OX-1-positive cells, however, appeared slightly less than that of OX-6-positive cells (i.e., fewer at the limbus, none in the epithelium). This could simply be due to simply a slight variation in Langerhans cell numbers in different sections of the same cornea, a failure of all Langerhans cells to express the OX-1 antigen, the presence of a separate OX-6-positive cell population not expressing the OX-1 antigen, or a combination of these factors.

It should be noted that one group of investigators has published multiple reports claiming that the cornea is devoid of class II MHC antigens and Langerhans cells, based in large part on their inability to demonstrate specific staining in corneal whole mounts (*35*), and their grafting experience with a single Ia antigen-disparate mouse strain combination (*36, 37*). Their conclusions have been widely cited as evidence that class II MHC antigens play no role in corneal grafting (*38–40*). In light of the repeated demonstration by our laboratory (*18*) and many others (*20, 28, 41–44*) of class II MHC antigen-bearing cells throughout the cornea of the human and mouse—and now the rat (including the report previously mentioned that used ultrastructural analysis to prove that these cells are Langerhans cells by all accepted criteria [*28*])—we believe that the general applicability of any claim that the cornea lacks class-II-positive Langerhans cells should be seriously questioned. The previously mentioned studies indicating a significant contribution of class II MHC antigens (*31*) and dendritic cells (*22, 32*) to corneal allograft immunogenicity further suggest that corneal Langerhans cells not only exist, but may also play an important role in corneal allograft rejection.

There appear to be no significant populations of T lymphocytes, natural killer cells, macrophages, and neutrophils in the normal rat cornea. This is consistent with an earlier report that macrophages and mast cells are absent from the normal rat cornea (*45*). These findings are also in general agreement with data from the human cornea, where no consistent expression of cells expressing leukocyte markers other than leukocyte-common antigens—and (in the adult) T lymphocytes (*46*) and occasionally B cells (*47*)—have been reported.

The cornea of the rat thus appears to show expression of MHC and leukocyte antigens in a pattern quite similar to that seen in the human, with the subtle differences of uniform epithelial class I MHC antigen density and reduced numbers of epithelial class II MHC antigen-positive cells. Rat models of corneal transplantation thus appear to represent an appropriate model for studying mechanisms that may also be involved in human corneal allograft rejection.

Acknowledgments. We thank Julie Fuller for expert technical assistance, and Marie Thomas for help in preparing the manuscript.

REFERENCES

1. Lang RF, Riekhof FT, Steinmuller D. Interlamellar corneal grafts in rats. Arch Ophthalmol 1975; 93: 349.
2. Gronemeyer U, Pulhorn G, Muller-Ruchholtz W. Histoincompatibility and allogeneic corneal grafting between inbred strains of rats. Mod Probl Ophthalmol 1976; 16: 161.
3. Gebhardt BM. Factors affecting corneal allograft rejection in inbred rats. Transplant Proc 1981; 13: 1091.
4. Williams KA, Coster DJ. Penetrating corneal transplantation in the inbred rat: a new model. Invest Ophthalmol Vis Sci 1985; 26: 23.
5. Treseler PA, Treseler CB, Foulks GN, Sanfilippo F. Cellular immunity to heterotopic corneal allografts in the rat. Transplantation 1985; 39: 196.
6. Treseler PA, Sanfilippo F. Humoral immunity to heterotopic corneal allografts in the rat. Transplantation 1985; 39: 193.
7. Gill III TJ, Cramer DV, Kunz HW, Misra DN. Structure and function of the major histocompatibility complex of the rat. J Immunogenet 1983; 10: 261.
8. Howard JC. The major histocompatibility complex of the rat: a partial review. Metabolism 1983; 32(suppl 1): 41.
9. Ehlers N, Ahrons S. Corneal transplantation and histocompatibility. Acta Ophthalmol (Copenh) 1971; 49: 513.
10. Gibbs DC, Batchelor JR, Casey TA. The influence of HL-A compatibility on the fate of corneal grafts. In: Porter R, Knight J, eds. Corneal graft failure, Ciba Foundation Symposium 15 (new series). Amsterdam: Elsevier, 1973: 293.
11. Vannas SK, Karjalainen K, Ruusuvaara P, Tiilikainen A. HLA-compatible donor cornea for the prevention of allograft rejection. Albrecht v. Grefe's. Arch Klin Exp Ophthalmol 1976; 198: 217.
12. Volker-Dieben JHM, Kok-Van Alphen CC, Oosterhuis JJ, Van Dorp G, Van Leeuwen A. First experiences with HLA-matched corneal grafts in high risk cases. Ophthalmol 1977; 44: 39.
13. Stark WJ, Taylor HR, Bias WB, Maumenee AE. Histocompatibility (HLA) antigens and keratoplasty. Am J Ophthalmol 1978; 86:595.
14. Ehlers N, Kissmeyer-Nielsen F. Corneal transplantation and HLA histocompatibility: a preliminary communication. Acta Ophthalmol (Copenh) 1979; 57: 738.
15. Foulks GN, Sanfilippo F. Beneficial effects of histocompatibility in high-risk corneal transplantation. Am J Ophthalmol 1982; 94: 622.
16. Bennet TO, Peyman GA, Tissot R, Cohen C. Histocompatibility matching in poor-prognosis penetrating keratoplasty. Acta Ophthalmol (Copenh) 1975; 53: 403.
17. Ehlers N, Ahrons S. The influence of histocompatibility upon the corneal immune reaction after interlamellar allotransplantation in rabbits. Tissue Antigens 1971; 1: 23.
18. Treseler PA, Foulks GN, Sanfilippo F. The expression of HLA antigens by cells in the human cornea. Am J Ophthalmol 1984; 98: 763.
19. Williams KA, Ash JK, Coster DJ. Histocompatibility antigen and passenger cell content of normal and diseased human cornea. Transplantation 1985; 39: 265.
20. Whitsett CP, Stutting RD. The distribution of HLA antigens in human corneal tissue. Invest Ophthalmol Vis Sci 1984; 25: 519.
21. Lafferty KJ, Prowse SJ, Simeonovic CJ. Immunobiology of tissue transplantation: a return to the passenger leukocyte concept. Annu Rev Immunol 1983; 1: 143.

22. Chandler JW, Ray-Kiel L, Gillette TE. Experimental corneal allograft rejection: description of murine model and a new hypothesis of immunopathologenesis. Curr Eye Res 1983; 2: 387.
23. Borowitz MJ, Croker BP, Burchette J. Immunocytochemical detection of lymphocyte surface antigens in fixed tissue sections. J Histochem Cytochem 1982; 30: 171.
24. Hsu S, Raine L, Fanger H. Use of avidin-biotin-peroxidase complex (ABC) in immunoperoxidase techniques: a comparison between ABC and unlabeled antibody (PAP) procedures. J Histochem Cytochem 1981; 29: 577.
25. Khodadoust AA, Silverstein AM. Transplantation and rejection of individual cell layers of the cornea. Invest Ophthalmol 1969; 8: 180.
26. Polack FM. Clinical and pathologic aspects of the corneal graft rejection. Trans Am Acad Ophthalmol Otolaryngol 1972; 77: 418.
27. Treseler PA, Foulks GN, Sanfilippo F. The relative immunogenicity of corneal epithelium, stroma, and endothelium: the role of major histocompatibility complex antigens. Transplantation 41: 229.
28. Rodrigues MM, Rowden G, Hackett J, Bakos I. Langerhans cells in the normal conjunctiva and peripheral cornea of selected species. Invest Ophthalmol Vis Sci 1981; 21: 759.
29. Katz SI, Tamaki K, Sachs DH. Epidermal Langerhans cells are derived from cells originating in bone marrow. Nature 1979; 282: 324.
30. Hunter JAA. The Langerhans cell: from gold to glitter. Clin Exp Dermatol 1983; 8: 569.
31. Treseler PA, Sanfilippo F. Relative contribution of major histocompatibility complex antigens to the immunogenicity of corneal allografts. Transplantation (in press).
32. Ray-Keil L, Chandler JW. Rejection of murine heterotopic corneal transplants. Transplantation 1985; 39: 473.
33. Geier SS, Fuller J, Sanfilippo F. The effect of hyperbaric oxygen on corneal allograft immunogenicity and mixed lymphocyte culture responsiveness. Hum Immunol 1985; 14: 171.
34. Nussenzweig MC, Steinman RM, Unkeless JC, Witmer MD, Gutchinov B, Cohn ZA. Studies of the cell surface of mouse dendritic cells and other leukocytes. J Exp Med 1981; 154: 168.
35. Bergstresser PR, Fletcher CR, Streilein JW. Surface densities of Langerhans cells in relation to rodent epidermal sites with special immunologic properties. J Invest Dermatol 1980; 74: 77.
36. Streilein JW, Towes GB, Bergstresser PR. Corneal allografts fail to express Ia antigens. Nature 1979; 282: 326.
37. Rubsamen PE, McCulley J, Bergstresser PR, Streilein JW. On the Ia immunogenicity of mouse corneal allografts infiltrated with Langerhans cells. Invest Ophthalmol Vis Sci 1984; 25: 513.
38. Steinman RM. Dendritic cells. Transplantation 1981; 31: 151.
39. Morris PJ, Ting A. Studies of HLA-DR with relevance to renal transplantation. Immunol Rev 1982; 66: 103.
40. Butcher GW, Howard JC. Genetic control of transplant rejection. Transplantation 1982; 34: 161.
41. Mayer DJ, Daar AS, Casey TA, Fabre JW. Localization of HLA-A, -B, -C and HLA-DR antigens in the human cornea: practical significance for grafting technique and HLA typing. Transplant Proc 1983; 15: 126.
42. Fujikawa LS, Colvin RB, Bhan AK, Fuller TC, Foster CS. Expression of HLA-A/B/C and -DR locus antigens on epithelial, stromal, and endothelial cells of the human cornea. Cornea 1982; 1: 213.
43. Gillette TE, Chandler JW, Greiner JV. Langerhans cells of the ocular surface. Ophthalmology 1982; 89: 700.
44. Chandler JW, Cummings M, Gilletter TE. Presence of Langerhans cells in the central corneas of normal human infants. Invest Ophthalmol Vis Sci 1985; 26: 113.
45. Allansmith MR, Baird RS, Bloch KJ. Macrophages in ocular tissues of rats: determination of their number after local anaphylaxis and other procedures. Arch Ophthalmol 1983; 101: 1930.
46. Treseler PA, Foulks GN, Sanfilippo F. The expression of ABO blood group, hematopoietic, and other cell-specific antigens by cells in the human cornea. Cornea (in press).
47. Vantrappen L, Geboes K, Missotten L, Maudgal PC, Desmet V. Lymphocytes and Langerhans cells in the normal human cornea. Invest Ophthalmol Vis Sci 1985; 26: 220.

Received 26 March 1985.
Accepted 11 June 1985.

0041-1337/86/4102-0253$02.00/0
TRANSPLANTATION
Vol. 41, No. 2
Printed in U.S.A.

PUBLIC DETERMINANTS OF HLA INDICATED BY PREGNANCY ANTIBODIES[1]

YOSHIKI KONOEDA, PAUL I. TERASAKI,[2] AKEMI WAKISAKA, M. S. PARK, AND M. R. MICKEY

Department of Surgery, UCLA School of Medicine, University of California, Los Angeles, California 90024

A tentative table of public specificities in the HLA-A and -B loci is provided. It is based on an all-inclusive survey of placenta extracts from 50,000 pregnancies. We postulate that most of the specificities found are directed against public epitopes. In support of this postulate are the facts that certain combinations occur very frequently, monoclonal antibodies have been made to some of the epitopes, and some have already been established by absorption experiments as being a single specificity.

The immunogenicity score for each private and public specificity was computed by taking into account the chance of immunization. It was shown that immunogenicity can vary by factors of more than ten between different specificities. Significantly, immunogenicity of the public epitopes was just as high as against the private ones. This indicates that the public epitopes should be considered as independent, separate antigens in transplantation. Establishment of a table of public specificities and the recognition of each by international nomenclature would be the first step in evaluating public epitopes for transplantation matching.

Tables of public specificities have been published for the mouse H-2 system (*1*). In man, there is abundant evidence that the HLA molecule is analogous to the H-2 of the mouse, and that in addition to the private specificities, which have been given international recognition by the WHO Nomenclature Committee, public specificities also exist in HLA. Legrand and Dausset suggested the sharing of determinants by two or more different allelic products (*2*). Schwartz et al. have verified this concept immunochemically (*3, 4*) and Oldfather et al. have performed extensive absorption tests to establish certain public specificities that are shared by the private specificities (*5*). Monoclonal antibodies to these shared public determinants have contributed evidence to their validity (*6, 7*).

We provide here a tentative working table of public specificities based on analysis of antibodies from 50,000 pregnancies. Although the table will have to be refined and corrected in the future, it is provided as the first step in recognition of these epitopes. These epitopes are shown to be just as immunogenic as the private determinants by the frequency with which antibodies are produced against them.

MATERIALS AND METHODS

The microlymphocytotoxicity test was used throughout the study (*8*). Oriental samples from approximately 12,000 Japanese and 20,000 Korean placentas were screened with a selected panel of 100 frozen cells. Approximately 18,000 Caucasian samples were screened against a panel of 60 well-defined frozen cells.

Clusters of reactivities were noted when more than three similar combinations occurred or when patterns previously encountered were found.

In order to calculate an immunogenicity score, the phenotype frequencies for the private specificities were utilized from the 8th International Histocompatibility Testing Workshop. The chance of immunization was (1 − P.F.) G.F., where P.F. = phenotype frequency and G.F. = gene frequency. The immunogenicity score was the number of samples found/(total samples × chance of immunization) × 100.

RESULTS

As shown in Table 1, approximately 5% of the placenta extracts from the 50,000 placentas were cytotoxic for both Orientals and Caucasians. Among the positive sera, 41% were directed against the B locus, 24% against the A locus, and 3% against the C locus. Thus, the immunogenicity of specificities in these three loci can be thought of as being highest for the B locus and lowest for the C locus. The immunogenicity of the A, B, and C loci products were almost exactly the same for Caucasians and Orientals.

The number of antisera found against various private determinants of the A locus is given in Table 2. HLA-A2 was by far the most frequent antibody found in both Caucasian and Oriental populations. As many as 66 sera against A2 were found in Caucasians and 54 in Orieintals. In 50,000 samples, antibodies against some of the specificities were not found at all. The phenotype frequency of each specificity, of course, determines the frequency with which immunization can be expected to take place. Upon accounting for the rate of immunization expected, the immunogenicity score was calculated as described in the *Materials and Methods* section. It can be noted that the immunogenicity for the various antigens varied from 2.55 to 0. Some variation was noted between the two races, though strong antigens tended to be similar in both racial groups.

Antibodies to the private B locus specificities found are listed in Table 3. As many as 43 antisera against B7 were found in Caucasians, and 32 antisera against B51 were found in Orientals. The immunogenicity, however, was strongest for B49 in the Caucasians and Bw65 in the Orientals. Antibodies against certain specificities occurred much more frequently than to others even after correction for the phenotype frequencies.

The antibodies encountered against public specificities of the A locus are given in Table 4. Arbitrary numbers were assigned for the specificities in the left hand column. Within the body of Table 4 are the component private specificities that made up each of the public specificities. For example, on the first line, the public specificity 84 was composed of A1, A3, A11, A24, and Aw36. Two such antisera were found in the Caucasian

[1] This work was supported by National Institute of Arthritis, Diabetes, Digestive, and Kidney Disease Grant AM 2375.

[2] Address reprint requests to: Paul I. Terasaki, 1000 Veteran Avenue, Los Angeles, CA 90024.

TABLE 1. Frequency of positive samples with lymphocytotoxic antibodies

Race	No. PF samples	Positive	A locus	B locus	C locus
Oriental	32,000	1628 (5.09%)	372 (22.85%) (0.618)[a]	663 (40.72%) (0.689)[a]	50 (3.07%)
Caucasian	18,000	965 (5.36%)	252 (26.11%) (0.739)[a]	398 (41.12%) (0.849)[a]	39 (4.01%)
Total	50,000	2593 (5.19%)	624 (24.06%)	1061 (40.91%)	89 (3.43%)

[a] Chance of immunizing.

TABLE 2. Number of samples with antibodies to HLA-A locus private antigens

HLA-A	Caucasian			Oriental		
	No. found	PF[a]	Immuno-genicity	No. found	PF	Immuno-genicity
A 1	15	0.257	0.813	4	0.019	1.352
A 2	66	0.466	2.550	54	0.487	1.159
A 3	7	0.260	0.376	2	0.029	0.444
A 11	10	0.125	0.983	28	0.161	1.239
A 23	9	0.050	2.079	0	0.000	0.000
A 24	7	0.128	0.674	13	0.496	0.278
A 25	7	0.042	1.913	0	0.000	0.000
A 26	8	0.072	1.306	13	0.147	0.621
A 29	1	0.081	0.146	3	0.012	1.514
A 30	1	0.051	0.227	2	0.019	0.676
A 31	1	0.062	0.188	1	0.147	0.048
A 32	3	0.071	0.496	0	0.000	0.000
Aw33	1	0.034	0.335	1	0.198	0.037
Aw34	0	0.005	0.000	0	0.000	0.000
Aw36	0	0.007	0.000	0	0.000	0.000
Aw43	0	0.002	0.000	0	0.000	0.000

[a] PF = phenotype frequency

TABLE 3. Number of samples with antibodies to HLA-B locus private antigens

HLA-B	Caucasian			Oriental		
	No. found	PF[a]	Immuno-genicity	No. found	PF	Immuno-genicity
B 7	43	0.187	2.988	21	0.097	1.454
B 8	14	0.171	1.048	4	0.006	4.019
B 13	10	0.053	2.184	18	0.049	2.396
B 18	1	0.097	0.124	0	0.000	0.000
B 27	9	0.075	1.414	2	0.025	0.510
B 35	10	0.156	0.810	3	0.151	0.140
B 37	0	0.032	0.000	1	0.038	0.172
B 38	0	0.062	0.000	0	0.012	0.000
B 39	2	0.036	0.635	3	0.033	0.592
Bw41	2	0.039	0.587	0	0.000	0.000
Bw42	0	0.006	0.000	0	0.000	0.000
B 44	10	0.261	0.536	5	0.151	0.234
B 45	3	0.014	2.406	0	0.000	0.000
Bw46	0	0.061	0.000	1	0.061	0.107
Bw47	0	0.004	0.000	0	0.000	0.000
Bw48	1	0.013	0.863	1	0.040	0.161
B 49	13	0.047	3.187	1	0.006	1.046
Bw50	2	0.026	0.872	1	0.006	1.005
B 51	11	0.093	1.414	32	0.169	1.365
Bw52	1	0.028	0.405	5	0.087	0.385
Bw53	0	0.009	0.000	0	0.000	0.000
Bw54	2	0.000	0.000	8	0.126	0.438
Bw55	1	0.043	0.267	4	0.058	0.454
Bw56	0	0.011	0.000	1	0.010	0.607
Bw57	2	0.072	0.326	3	0.000	uncalculated
Bw58	3	0.022	1.541	0	0.017	0.000
Bw59	0	0.008	0.000	3	0.029	0.664
Bw60	2	0.110	0.221	3	0.109	0.188
Bw61	0	0.020	0.000	0	0.151	0.000
Bw62	3	0.095	0.378	3	0.163	0.132
Bw63	0	0.019	0.000	0	0.000	0.000
Bw64	0	0.056	0.000	1	0.005	1.255
Bw65	0	0.017	0.000	1	0.001	6.255
Bw67	0	0.001	0.000	2	0.013	1.000

[a] PF = phenotype frequency.

population and three in the Orientals. The phenotype frequency and immunogenicity for the two races are also given.

The antibodies formed against public specificities of the B locus are listed in Tables 5 and 6. It can be noted that the arrangement is not random and that there is a clustering of antisera against certain specificities. Moreover, there is again a wide variation in the immunogenicity of the different specificities. Antibodies against certain public specificities were found very often, as compared with others.

DISCUSSION

The antibody specificities found upon testing 50,000 placental extracts were summarized and listed in tables. Interestingly the antibodies did not consist of random mixtures, but rather tended to have specificities that had been previously noted as "crossreactive groups." Tables of the specificities found are provided here with the suggestion that many of the combined specificities listed are not simply multispecific mixtures, but represent antibodies against a single determinant shared by different private specificities. The reasons for this belief are the following:

1. Antisera against certain combinations of specificities occur much too frequently to have been a chance occurrence. For example, A23-A24 occurred 26 times, anti-B7-B27 was found eight times, and anti-B35-B51 was noted seven times. Thus, these combinations are probably detecting single shared epitopes. As in the establishment of private HLA specificities, the frequent occurrence of strong antisera for a given specificity is a simple guide to validity of a specificity.
2. Some of the combinations in the table have already been encountered and shown to be monospecific by absorption tests. Specificity 89 containing A2, 28 [68, 69] and 9 [23, 24] is exactly the same combination shown by Oldfather et al. (*5*) to a public specificity. These authors also describe a public specificity A28, 33, 34, and 26, which excludes A25. The specificity 110 is quite like this specificity and reacts with 26 excluding 25, except that it also contains A30 and 31.

Several of the specificities of the B7 crossreacting group reported by Darke in pregnancy antisera are similar to these encountered here (*9*). If we exclude BW67 (which may not have been typed for by Darke), specificity 190 containing 54, 55, 56, 42, 27, and 7 was also noted in his series. Others that are in common are 121 [42, 27, 7]; 116

TABLE 4. Number of samples with antibodies to HLA-A locus public antigens

Number of determinant	1	2	3	11	23	24	25	26	29	30	31	32	33	34	36	43	66	68	69	B LOCUS	Caucasian No. found	Caucasian P.F.	Caucasian Immuno-genicity	Oriental No. found	Oriental P.F.	Oriental Immuno-genicity
84	1		3	11		24									36						2	0.654	0.078	3	0.651	0.066
85	1		3	11			25	26				32	33	34	36		66				0	0.708	0.000	4	0.511	0.085
86	1		3	11					29	30	31		33	34			66				0	0.709	0.000	3	0.536	0.063
82	1			11			25	26						34	36						3	0.462	0.116	6	0.322	0.157
83	1			11											36						3	0.370	0.128	0	0.186	0.000
81	1				23	24									36						0	0.412	0.000	3	0.519	0.064
80	1														36						12	0.263	0.639	0	0.022	0.000
92		2	3	11			25	26	29	30	31	32	33	34			66	68	69		0	0.901	0.000	3	0.892	0.129
93		2	3	11			25	26						34	36			68	69		0	0.786	0.000	3	0.715	0.071
89		2			23	24												68	69		1	0.591	0.038	3	0.823	0.092
87		2																68	69		12	0.466	0.464	30	0.488	0.644
88		2																	69		5	0.466	0.193	14	0.488	0.300
99			3	11	23	24	25	26				32	33	34							0	0.651	0.000	3	0.827	0.093
98			3	11																	0	0.367	0.000	3	0.195	0.113
100				11			25	26	29	30	31	32	33	34				68	69		1	0.477	0.038	7	0.603	0.149
101				11			25	26						34							2	0.234	0.116	6	0.303	0.163
9					23	24															26	0.175	1.912	43	0.503	0.917
106							25	26	29	30	31	32	33	34			66	68	69		0	0.380	0.000	3	0.486	0.064
105							25	26				32	33	34							1	0.214	0.062	3	0.338	0.076
107							25	26					33	34			66				0	0.149	0.000	3	0.338	0.076
10							25	26						34							2	0.117	0.208	4	0.151	0.187
104							25	26													4	0.112	0.432	6	0.151	0.281
103							25					32									0	0.111	0.000	1	0.000	0.000
110								26		30	31		33	34				68	69		0	0.214	0.000	3	0.477	0.065
109								26					33	34							0	0.109	0.000	3	0.338	0.076
108								26						34							0	0.077	0.000	2	0.151	0.094
19									29	30	31	32	33								2	0.281	0.102	6	0.367	0.145
111									29	30	31		33	34			66	68	69		0	0.223	0.000	3	0.367	0.072
113										30	31		33	34			66				0	0.148	0.000	3	0.357	0.074
112										30	31										0	0.171	0.000	0	0.164	0.000
102													33	34							1	0.039	0.294	5	0.204	0.182
28																		68	69		1	0.099	0.121	0	0.006	0.000
91		2																68	69	B17	0	0.534	0.000	3	0.501	0.064
90		2																		B17	6	0.466	0.232	4	0.488	0.086
97		2																		B 7	4	0.600	0.151	0	0.560	0.000
95		2																		B12	3	0.466	0.116	0	0.488	0.000
94		2																		B22	0	0.466	0.000	3	0.488	0.064
96		2																		B35, 53	3	0.584	0.113	0	0.600	0.000

TABLE 5. Number of samples with antibodies to HLA-B 5 complex public antigens

Number of determinants	49	50	52	51	53	35	57	58	63	79	62	71	72	46	18	64	65	8	59	44	45	37	Caucasian No. found	Caucasian PF	Caucasian Immuno-genicity	Oriental No. found	Oriental PF	Oriental Immuno-genicity
173	49	50	52	51	53	35	57	58	63	79	62	71	72										4	0.509	0.151	4	0.538	0.084
176	49	50	52	51	53	35			63	79	62	71	72		18	64	65						0	0.562	0.000	3	0.530	0.063
159	49	50	52	51																			1	0.187	0.069	2	0.258	0.061
21	49	50																					3	0.072	0.487	0	0.012	0.000
158	49		52	51	53				63														3	0.189	0.206	3	0.253	0.093
156	49		52	51	53																		0	0.172	0.000	7	0.253	0.216
132	49		52	51																			3	0.415	0.233	13	0.243	0.278
155	49		52																59				0	0.082	0.000	4	0.120	0.229
133	49		52																				2	0.074	0.317	4	0.093	0.290
172		50				35				79	62												4	0.266	0.212	0	0.312	0.000
139		50				35				79	62	71	72										1	0.280	0.051	2	0.321	0.052
134		50								79	62	71	72										1	0.136	0.092	2	0.179	0.081
142			52	51	53	35									18								0	0.356	0.000	4	0.384	0.094
138			52	51	53	35																	2	0.273	0.104	7	0.384	0.165
154			52	51	53																		0	0.128	0.000	19	0.248	0.595
5			52	51																			6	0.120	0.613	16	0.248	0.501
127				51	53	35																	2	0.249	0.111	3	0.312	0.080
135				51	53																		1	0.102	0.119	3	0.169	0.128
126				51		35																	7	0.241	0.398	0	0.312	0.000
175				51											18								3	0.185	0.210	0	0.169	0.000
171					53	35				79													2	0.164	0.155	0	0.158	0.000
128					53	35																	2	0.164	0.155	3	0.158	0.135
17							57	58															11	0.093	1.412	9	0.017	3.352
137							57		63	79	62												2	0.181	0.143	2	0.163	0.088
15									63	79	62												2	0.113	0.215	1	0.163	0.044
147										79	62												0	0.095	0.000	1	0.163	0.044
184															18	64	65						2	0.166	0.154	0	0.006	0.000
181																64	65	8	59				4	0.244	0.225	0	0.041	0.000
114																64	65	8					2	0.237	0.115	0	0.012	0.000
14																64	65						9	0.095	1.135	6	0.013	2.886
115																		8	59				2	0.178	0.145	3	0.035	0.550
12																				44	45		20	0.273	1.037	14	0.158	0.630
131	49	50																		44	45		5	0.335	0.227	0	0.170	0.000
130	49																			44	45		3	0.313	0.142	0	0.164	0.000
129	49																			44			3	0.301	0.145	0	0.164	0.000
4	49		52	51	53		57	58	63										59	44		37	1	0.648	0.039	3	0.524	0.064
180	49		52	51	53		57	58	63											44		37	0	0.593	0.000	4	0.484	0.086
6		50				35				79	62	71	72	46	18	64	65	8			45		5	0.819	0.267	4	0.794	0.111
177	49	50																					0	0.278	0.000	3	0.307	0.081
179	49	50				(see Table 6)																	0	0.292	0.000	4	0.343	0.101
157	49	50																					0	0.448	0.000	4	0.424	0.090

TABLE 6. Number of samples with antibodies to HLA-B 7 complex public antigens

Number of determinants	38	39	54	55	56	67	42	27	7	41	48	60	61	47	13	49	50	Caucasian No. found	Caucasian PF	Caucasian Immuno-genicity	Oriental No. found	Oriental PF	Oriental Immuno-genicity
190			54	55	56	67	42	27	7									0	0.307	0.000	3	0.314	0.080
189				55		67	42	27	7									0	0.297	0.000	2	0.192	0.077
122						67	42	27	7									2	0.261	0.107	0	0.138	0.000
121							42	27	7									1	0.260	0.054	2	0.127	0.109
188								27	7			60	61					4	0.365	0.172	0	0.360	0.000
187								27	7		48	60						1	0.360	0.043	3	0.266	0.089
116								27	7									8	0.254	0.437	2	0.127	0.109
186		39	54	55	56	67	42		7	41	48	60						0	0.423	0.000	3	0.553	0.063
185		39	54	55	56	67	42		7									0	0.273	0.000	3	0.319	0.079
123			54	55	56	67	42		7									4	0.242	0.227	2	0.291	0.056
118			54	55	56				7									2	0.235	0.116	0	0.280	0.000
151				55	56	67	42		7									5	0.242	0.283	0	0.176	0.000
183				55			42		7									0	0.231	0.000	4	0.155	0.183
182						67	42		7									0	0.193	0.000	5	0.113	0.303
120						67			7									1	0.188	0.069	1	0.113	0.061
117							42		7									4	0.192	0.272	8	0.101	0.538
124									7	41	48	60	61					3	0.346	0.133	3	0.373	0.072
191									7		48	60	61		13			1	0.357	0.044	4	0.415	0.091
125									7		48	60	61					4	0.314	0.189	8	0.373	0.192
144									7		48	60						1	0.297	0.049	9	0.242	0.287
143									7		48							1	0.199	0.066	6	0.142	0.297
193									7			60	61	47	13			0	0.350	0.000	3	0.381	0.071
119									7			60	61					2	0.303	0.097	3	0.338	0.076
174								27				60	61	47				0	0.202	0.000	4	0.275	0.116
148								27							13			2	0.126	0.195	0	0.079	0.000
170	38	39				67	42											0	0.104	0.000	1	0.060	0.110
16	38	39																2	0.097	0.248	1	0.047	0.137
169		39	54	55		67	42											0	0.085	0.000	2	0.222	0.068
168		39				67	42											3	0.043	0.804	0	0.046	0.000
167		39				67												0	0.037	0.000	4	0.046	0.563
140			54	55	56	67	42											1	0.061	0.192	9	0.201	0.332
22			54	55	56													1	0.054	0.215	5	0.189	0.193
141			54	55			42											2	0.050	0.463	10	0.191	0.383
136			54	55														4	0.043	1.068	16	0.180	0.645
153			54		56													0	0.011	0.000	2	0.136	0.103
164				55	56	67	42											0	0.061	0.000	4	0.080	0.333
152				55	56													0	0.054	0.000	2	0.068	0.195
163				55		67	42											0	0.050	0.000	6	0.070	0.567
162						67	42											1	0.007	1.596	2	0.013	1.000
150							42			41								1	0.045	0.256	0	0.000	0.000
178										41	48	60	61	47	13			0	0.229	0.000	4	0.333	0.102
166										41	48	60	61					1	0.177	0.073	3	0.289	0.084
165										41		60	61	47				0	0.169	0.000	3	0.251	0.093
192											48	60	61		13			1	0.190	0.069	0	0.333	0.000
146											48	60	61					0	0.141	0.000	10	0.289	0.281
160											48	60						0	0.122	0.000	6	0.149	0.284

TABLE 6. *Continued*

Number of determinants	38	39	54	55	56	67	42	27	7	41	48	60	61	47	13	49	50	Caucasian No. found	Caucasian PF	Caucasian Immuno-genicity	Oriental No. found	Oriental PF	Oriental Immuno-genicity
145												60	61	47	13			0	0.182	0.000	5	0.297	0.138
161												60	61	47				0	0.133	0.000	3	0.251	0.093
149												60	61		13			1	0.178	0.072	0	0.297	0.000
40												60	61					6	0.129	0.574	10	0.251	0.310
157									7	41	48	60	61	47	13	49	50	0	0.448	0.000	4	0.424	0.090
179										41	48	60	61	47	13	49	50	0	0.292	0.000	4	0.343	0.101
177										41		60	61		13	49	50	0	0.278	0.000	3	0.307	0.081
4	38							27						47	13	49		1	0.648	0.039	3	0.524	0.064
180	38														13	49		0	0.593	0.000	4	0.484	0.086
6		39	54	55	56	67	42		7	41	48	60	61				50	5	0.819	0.267	4	0.794	0.111

[27, 7]; 186 [39] 54, 55, 56, 42, 7, [41] 48, 60 61; 151 [55, 56, 42, 7]; 183 [55, 42, 7]; and 144 [7, 48, 60]. The appearance of the same combinations in the two studies could not have been a chance occurrence.

3. Monoclonal antibodies have been made to the same combinations of specificities as found in the extracts of the placenta, such as anti-A2-28 (*7*), B17, (*10*), A28-B7 (*11*), A25-A32 (*12*), and A3-11 (*13*). It is likely that monoclonal antibodies are not mixtures of antibodies but are detecting a single epitope shared by the specificities noted. Furthermore, allogeneic antibodies to determinants such as A2-B17 (specificity 91) have been reported (*14*).
4. If we assume that most pregnancies involve a single father, even with multiple pregnancies, only two specificities at the A locus and two specificities at the B locus could be the immunizing antigens. In pregnancies in which the father's immunizing haplotype is known, multiple specificities are often found (*9, 15, 16*). This indicates that antibodies are made to epitopes other than the private ones identified at the A and B loci.
5. Antibodies against specificities that are lacking in a given racial population are sometimes found. For example, many antisera that react to BW42 are produced in Orientals who do not have BW42 in the population. This phenomenon can be explained by BW42 molecules having a separate epitope that is shared, for example, with B7. Immunization against B7 results, then, in antibodies to the separate epitope—which, when tested in another population having BW42, would react with such cells.

   We have previously given examples of antibodies produced in a race in which the antigen does not occur (*17*). Caucasians produce BW54 and BW59 against Orientals and AW34, AW36, and BW42 against Negroes. Orientals produce AW30, AW34, BW45, BW38, and BW42, and Negroes produce BW38 and BW56. The antibodies are probably not against these specificities themselves, but rather against the public epitope. These sera having interracial reactions are probably a good source of antibodies to the public specificities.
6. Although it is generally agreed that the HLA system is quite analogous to the H-2 of mice, no table of public specificities, such as that accepted for the mouse H-2, has been published as yet for the HLA system. From the precedence of the mouse H-2, it is likely that the HLA molecules have several epitopes along its chain that are alloimmunogenic. Such epitopes probably result in alloimmunization in man as they do in mice.

An important reason for construction of the tables is the recognition that the public specificities have as much validity and significance as the private ones. That is, they represent polymorphic epitopes that function as alloantigens. They deserve equal footing and recognition by the International Nomenclature Committee. Eventually we can be confident that the public specificities will be identified as a determinant on the amino acid sequence as, for example, the identification of the HLA-A28-B7 shared determinant on asparagine residue 74 (*11*).

Although public specificities tend not to be as useful in disease association and paternity studies as the private specificities, they may be very important for transplantation studies. That is, in the past, public specificities have not been accounted for as a separate epitope that is immunogenic. In fact, public specificities have been invoked to reduce the number of mismatches given by the private specificities (*18–20*). In other words, by matching for the public specificities, there would be fewer mismatches than if one were to match for the private determinants. Contrary to this view, we suggest that public specificities should be counted as other epitopes in addition to the incompatibilities showed by the private specificities. There is no reason to expect that the public epitopes would be of lesser strength, since antibodies against them are elicited at about the same rate as to private epitopes. This means that the number of mismatches generated by the A and B loci would be considerably more than the conventional maximum two mismatches at each locus. Consequently, the number of mismatches can be quite high, particularly when we are considering unrelated cadaver donors. Analysis of transplant results based on this concept is the subject of a subsequent publication.

It is quite likely that different epitopes will have different relative immunogenicity strengths. This is evident from the computations of the immunogenicity score for each specificity. This score was calculated to take into account how often immunization would take place as compared with how often antibodies were produced against the given specificity. Two antigens that occur at almost the same phenotypic frequencies, such as HLA-B49 and HLA-BW55, are quite different in their immunogenicities, since antibodies are formed against B49 10 times more often than to BW55. In Orientals, B51 and BW62 are also of similar frequencies but antibodies against B51 are 10 times more frequent than against BW62. In a similar way, the public specificities differ from each other in their immunogenicity score. There does not, however, seem to be any clear difference in immunogenicity between the private and public specificities indicating that, in general, they would be of comparable antigenic strengths.

In crossmatching for transplantation, Delmonico et al. (*21*) have drawn attention to the possibility that antibodies to public specificities may be responsible for many of the positive crossmatches. Certainly it is difficult to account for all the reactions simply by the private HLA determinants. Taking the public specificites into account may aid in the selection of crossmatch-negative donor and recipient pairs.

It can be expected that not all specificities listed will be validated in the future. Combinations that occur more frequently have a greater likelihood of validity. Comparison with the combinations of specificities encountered within the B14-crossreactive group (*15*) and within the B12, B40 groups (*16*) indicate that many more combinations than those identified here may actually exist. Large-scale international exchange of antisera should be the best means of rapidly establishing the table of specificities, which eventually should attain recognition by the International Nomenclature Committee.

REFERENCES

1. Klein J, Flaherty L, Van de Berg JL, Shreffer DC. H-2 haplotypes, genes, regions, and antigens: first listing. Immunogenetics 1978; 6: 489.
2. Legrand L, Dausset J. Serological evidence of the existence of several antigen determinants (or factors) on the ML-A gene products. In: Dausset J, Colombani J, eds. Histocompatibility testing 1972. Copenhagen: Munksgaard, 1972: 441.
3. Schwartz BD, Luehrman LK, Rodey GE. Public antigenic determinant on a family of HLA-B molecules, basic for cross-reactivity and a possible link with disease predisposition. J Clin Invest 1979; 64: 938.
4. Schwartz BD, Luehrman LK, Lee J, Rodey GE. A public antigenic determinant in the HLA-B5 cross-reacting group—a basis for cross-reactivity and a possible link with Behcet's disease. Hum Immunol 1980; 1: 37.
5. Oldfather JW, Gebel HM, Holmes DJ, Rodney GE. Detection of two distinct public specificities on HLA-A28 bearing lymphocytes. Tissue Antigens 1983; 22: 16.
6. Parham P. Monoclonal antibodies against two separate alloantigenic sites of HLA-B40. Immunogenetics 1981; 13: 509.
7. Parham P, Brodsky FM. Partial purification and some properties of BB7. 2a cytotoxic monoclonal antibody with specificity for HLA-A2 and a variant of HLA-A28. Hum Immunol 1981; 3: 277.
8. Terasaki PI, Bernoco D, Park MS, Ozturk G, Iwaki Y. Microdroplet testing for HLA-A, -B, -C, and -D antigens. Am J Clin Pathol 1978; 69: 103.
9. Darke C. A reanalysis of the HLA-B7 cross-reactive group. Tissue Antigens 1983; 22: 326.
10. McMichael AJ, Parham P, Rust N, Brodsky F. A monoclonal antibody that recognizes an antigenic determinant shared by HLA-A2 and B17. Hum Immunol 1980; 1: 121.
11. Lopez de Castro JA, Strominger JL, Strong DM, Orr HT. Structure of crossreactive human histocompatibility antigens HLA-A28 and HLA-A2: possible implications for the generation of HLA polymorphism. Immunology 1982; 79: 3813.
12. Vilella R, Yague J, Vives J. Monoclonal antibody against HLA-AW32 A25. Is HLA-Aw32 an allele with no unique antigenic determinant? Hum Immunol 1983; 6: 53.
13. Billing R, Clark B, Lucero K, Shi BJ, Terasaki PI. A monoclonal antibody recognizing a determinant common to HLA-A3 and A11. Tissue Antigens 1982; 19: 121.
14. Class F, Castelli-Visser R, Schreuder I, Van Rood J. Allo-antibodies to an antigenic determinant shared by HLA-A2 and B17. Tissue Antigens 1982; 19: 388.
15. Darke C. The inclusion of HLA-BW42, BW54 and BW55 within the HLA-B14 crossreactive group. Tissue Antigens 1983; 21: 246.
16. Darke C. The HLA-B12 and -B40 cross-reactive groups and their serological relationships. Tissue Antigens 1983; 21: 281.
17. Nakata S, Terasaki PI, Omori K. Interracial crossreactivity. In: Terasaki PI, ed. Histocompatibility testing 1980. Los Angeles: UCLA Tissue Typing Laboratory, 1981, 590.
18. Roy R, Fradet Y, Lachance J. Influence of HLA-A and HLA-B cross-reactive antigen matching on kidney graft survival. Tissue Antigens 1981; 18: 101.
19. Grifford RRM, Schmidtke JR, Sutherland DER, Simmons RL, Najarian JS. Improved renal allograft survival with selected HLA antigen matching. Surgery 1979; 86: 316.
20. Sanfillippo F, Vaughn WK, Spees EK, Heise ER, LeFor WM. The effect of HLA-A, -B matching on cadaver renal allograft rejection using public versus private specificities. Transplantation 1984; 38: 483.
21. Delmonico FL, Fuller A, Cosmini AB, et al. New approaches to donor crossmatching and successful transplantation of highly sensitized patients. Transplantation 1983; 36: 629.

Received 17 April 1985.
Accepted 18 June 1985.

0041-1337/86/4102-0260$02.00/0
TRANSPLANTATION

Vol. 1, No. 2
Printed in U.S.A.

Transplantation

BRIEF COMMUNICATIONS

SEVERE IMMUNOSUPPRESSION IN A RENAL TRANSPLANT RECIPIENT WITH HTLV-III ANTIBODIES

The acquired immunodeficiency syndrome (AIDS)[1] was first recognized over three years ago (*1–3*) and the cause has recently been linked to a retrovirus, the human T cell lymphotropic virus (HTLV-III) (*4*). However, it seems likely that many patients with serological evidence of past exposure to HTLV-III do not develop overt AIDS (*5*) and that other factors are required for the expression of the syndrome. It has been suggested that AIDS may itself be an opportunistic disease and that the AIDS agent only causes disease in individuals who are already immunocompromised (*6*). This hypothesis predicted first, that evidence of previous exposure to the AIDS agent would be found in individuals who had had the immune capability to suppress its pathogenicity, and second, that AIDS would eventually be encountered in other exposed immunodeficient individuals.

We report here a patient with HTLV-III antibody who became disproportionately immunosuppressed following renal transplantation and developed a pattern of opportunistic infections suggestive of AIDS.

In October 1981 a 57-year-old British man, resident in the USA for more than ten years, was first seen in a hospital in Los Angeles with end-stage renal failure. There was a past history of accelerated hypertension and focal segmental glomerulosclerosis. He was a heterosexual and denied i.v. drug abuse. Regular hemodialysis treatment was started, and he received a number of blood transfusions because of anemia. In June 1982 he transferred to the Hammersmith Hospital, London, England to continue treatment. He remained well, on hemodialysis for the next 7 months. In January 1983 he received a cadaver renal transplant from a young male donor. The total lymphocyte count on the day of transplantation was 2.6×10^9/L. Immunosuppression was achieved with prednisolone (300 mg/day, halving every three days to 15 mg/day) and azathioprine (5 mg/kg i.v. preoperatively and 2.5 mg/kg/day thereafter). Nystatin mouthwashes (200,000 units 8-hourly) were given prophylactically. The early postoperative course was complicated by pancreatitis, multiple duodenal ulcers, and severe oral candidiasis. After an initial delay the transplant functioned well but an episode of rejection on day 14 was treated with high-dose oral steroids. From then on his course was marked by multiple opportunist infections. On day 34 he was readmitted with pyrexia, rapidly deteriorating renal function, and marked dysphagia due to severe oral candidiasis. He was treated with a total of 6 g of i.v. methylprednisolone, oral nystatin, and topical amphotericin B; hemodialysis was reinstituted. Azathioprine was reduced to 100 mg/day and then increased to 125 mg/day on day 53. Renal function recovered 16 days after the onset of the rejection episode. During this admission he developed a perianal vesicular eruption from which herpes simplex was grown. These lesions resolved after treatment with oral acyclovir. He lost seven kilograms in weight and had a continuing fever, attributed to a primary cytomegalovirus (CMV) infection. The CMV complement fixation test (CFT) was <1/8 at transplantation and >1/256 5 months later.

Over the next three months there were two further episodes of oral herpes simplex that resolved with topical idoxuridine and oral acyclovir. Prednisolone was reduced to 12.5 mg/day three and a half months after transplantation. He was readmitted one month later for investigation of dysphagia and dyspepsia and further weight loss of 2 kg. Gastroscopy revealed severe candidal esophagitis which was treated with amphotericin B lozenges and ketoconazole. Prednisolone was reduced to 10 mg/day and maintained at this level. Azathioprine was reduced to 100 mg/day. There was a further episode of oral candidiasis and herpes simplex infection but gastroscopy three weeks later showed a marked improvement. Six months following transplantation he became tachypneic and pyrexial. A chest roentgenogram showed a ground-glass appearance and his arterial pO_2 on room air was 56 mm Hg (7.45 kPa). *Pneumocystis carinii* pneumonia (PCP) was confirmed by transbronchial biopsy, and treatment with high-dose oral cotrimoxazole (trimethoprim 20 mg/kg/day, and sulfamethoxazole 100 mg/kg) was administered for three weeks. At this point his lymphocyte subpopulations were determined by immunofluorescence with the Leu series of monoclonal antibodies (Becton Dickinson). There was a marked lymphopenia and the helper:suppressor ratio was 2.2 (see Table 1). During the course of treatment the liver enzymes (alkaline phosphatase and aspartate transaminase) rose, and a liver biopsy showed nonspecific granulomata. A reaction to cotrimoxazole was thought to be the most likely cause, but in view of the known hepatotoxicity of azathioprine this drug was stopped. His fever settled and blood gases and chest roentgenographic findings became normal. A repeat bronchoscopy and biopsy one month after starting treatment showed no evidence of *Pneumocystis.*

Over the next three months his condition improved and his weight returned to normal. One and a half months after the episode of PCP azathioprine was restarted at 75 mg/kg and increased to 100 mg/day two weeks later. During this time he developed a nodule on the forearm that proved on excision biopsy to be a basal cell carcinoma. Three and a half months after the episode of PCP he developed a fever and became tachypneic. He was hypoxemic, had increased shadowing on the chest roentgenogram, and a transbronchial biopsy revealed large numbers of cysts of *Pneumocystis carinii.* A repeat lymphocyte subset count showed persistent lymphopenia and a helper:suppressor ratio of 3.3. He made an immediate clinical and radiological response to reinstitution of high-dose oral cotrimoxazole, and there was no disturbance of liver function on this occasion. During this admisson he complained of visual impairment and fundoscopy revealed features consistent with CMV retinitis.

[1] Abbreviations used: AIDS, acquired immunodeficiency syndrome; CDC, Center for Disease Control; CFT, complement fixation test; CMV, cytomegalovirus; HTLV-III, human T cell lymphotropic virus; PCP, *Pneumocystis Carinii* pneumonia.

TABLE 1. Lymphocyte counts and subsets (counts $\times 10^9$/L)[a]

Day	Total	Helper/ inducer	Suppressor/ cytotoxic	Helper/ suppressor ratio
0	2.60	—	—	—
180	0.35	0.23	0.1	2.2
285	0.13	0.07	0.02	3.3
700	0.28	—	—	—
Normal range	1.25–2.5	1.0–1.6	0.55–0.9	1–3

[a] Leu series (Becton-Dickinson).

Following this second episode of PCP, azathioprine was stopped, the dose of prednisolone reduced to 10 mg/day, and he received continuous oral cotrimoxazole as prophylaxis against *Pneumocystis*. There were no further episodes of PCP, but the CMV retinitis progressed so that he became blind and he continued to excrete CMV in the urine. Renal function remained unchanged despite the reduction in the immunosuppression. The lymphocyte count remained low at 0.28×10^9/L. His general condition deteriorated slowly and he died two years after transplantation. Because of the clinical similarities to AIDS, stored sera were tested by membrane immunofluorescence for HTLV-III antibody (PHLS Virus Reference Laboratory, Colindale, London, UK). These included specimens taken: at the time of starting hemodialysis in London seven months before transplantation; immediately posttransplant; and during the second episode of PCP. All these, and the last sample taken 18 months after transplantation, were positive. No sample was available from the renal donor but the recipient of the other kidney, who also developed a CMV infection, is well and without HTLV-III antibody (Dr. D. J. Jeffries, St. Marys Hospital, London). Attempts to trace the source of the blood transfusions in the USA have failed.

There are obvious difficulties, both semantic and clinical, in diagnosing AIDS in a renal transplant recipient who has received pharmacological immunosuppressive treatment (*7*). However the clinical pattern and the severity of this patient's infections were such that it was likely that some factor other than azathioprine and prednisolone treatment accounted for his immunodepressed state. Recurrent PCP in particular is exceedingly rare in renal transplant patients (we are aware of only one other well documented case [8]) but is frequently encountered in patients with AIDS (*9, 10*). That he remained profoundly immunosuppressed was suggested by the fact that, despite the reduction in immunosuppressive therapy, there was no sign of allograft rejection; the CMV retinitis progressed and he continued to excrete CMV in the urine two years after transplantation; and he remained lymphopenic.

The finding of HTLV-III antibodies in this patient raised the question of whether his immunodepressed state was accounted for by AIDS although this diagnosis would strictly be excluded by the Centers for Disease Control (CDC) definition (*7*).

He had a marked T cell lymphopenia, which is characteristic of AIDS, but his helper:suppressor ratio was normal, which is not. The primary abnormality in AIDS is depletion of helper T cells with the derangement in the helper:suppressor ratio occurring secondarily. This ratio may have been modified by his concurrent treatment with prednisolone and azathioprine (*11*). It can be argued that the past exposure to HTLV-III is irrelevant and that his posttransplant course can be explained simply by extreme sensitivity to azathioprine and prednisolone. An alternative is that he had AIDS, which by chance manifested after he had received a renal transplant. Assuming that exposure to the virus was via blood transfusion, the timing is compatible with what is known of the incubation period (*12–14*). However, the CDC definition of AIDS now seems out of date and we believe that this patient developed transplant-related AIDS. He was probably previously exposed to the virus by blood transfusion (*12, 14, 15*) and later developed AIDS as an opportunist disease when he received additional pharmacological immunosuppression.

As more patients are tested for HTLV-III infection it is probable that more affected transplant patients will be identified. Dialysis patients awaiting renal transplantation almost invariably receive blood transfusions and it is possible that such patients, particularly in the USA, may regularly be exposed to the virus. If additional immunosuppression is required for clinical expression, then they may be another population with a significant risk of developing AIDS. The implications for patient screening and hemodialysis practice are considerable.

David B. G. Oliveira
Christopher G. Winearls[2]
Jonathan Cohen
Philip W. Ind
Gordon Williams
The Departments of Medicine, Bacteriology, and Surgery
Hammersmith Hospital
London W12 OHS

[2] Address correspondence to: Dr. C.G. Winearls, Renal Unit, Hammersmith Hospital, Ducane Road, London W12 OHS, United Kingdom.

REFERENCES

1. Gottlieb MS, Schroff R, Schanker HM, et al. Pneumocystis carinii pneumonia and mucosal candidiasis in previously healthy homosexual men. Evidence of a new acquired cellular immunodeficiency. N Engl J Med 1981; 305: 1425.
2. Masur H, Michelis MA, Greene JB, et al. An outbreak of community-acquired Pneumocystis carinii pneumonia. Initial manifestation of cellular immune dysfunction. N Engl J Med 1981; 305: 1431.
3. Siegal FP, Lopez C, Hammer GS, et al. Severe acquired immunodeficiency in male homosexuals, manifested by chronic perianal ulcerative Herpes simplex lesions. N Engl J Med 1981; 305: 1439.
4. Broder S, Gallo RC. A pathogenic retrovirus (HTLV-III) linked to AIDS. N Engl J Med 1984; 311: 1292.
5. Cheinsong-Popov R, Weiss RA, Dalgleish A, et al. Presence of antibody to human T-lymphotropic virus type III in AIDS and AIDS-risk patients in Britain. Lancet 1984; 2: 477.
6. Levy JA, Ziegler JL. Acquired immunodeficiency syndrome is an opportunist infection and Keposi's sarcoma results from secondary immune stimulation. Lancet 1983; 2:78.
7. Update on acquired immunodeficiency syndrome (AIDS)-United States MMWR 1982; 31: 507.
8. Sirotzky L, Memoli V, Roberts JL, Lewis EJ. Recurrent pneumocystis pneumonia with normal roentgenograms. JAMA 1978; 240: 1513.
9. Mildvan D, Mathur U, Enlow RW, et al. Opportunistic infections and immune deficiency in homosexual men. Ann Intern Med 1982; 96: 700.
10. Follansbee SE, Busch DF, Wolfsy CB, et al. An outbreak of Pneumocystis carinii pneumonia in homosexual men. Ann Intern Med 1982; 96: 705.
11. Sweny P, Tidman N. The effect of cyclosporin A on peripheral

blood T cell subpopulations in renal allografts. Clin Exp Immunol 1982; 47: 445.
12. Ammann AJ, Cowan MJ, Wara DW, et al. Acquired immunodeficiency in an infant: possible transmission by means of blood products. Lancet 1983; 1: 956.
13. Special Report of the CDC Task Force: epidemiologic aspects of the current outbreak of Kaposi's sarcoma and opportunistic infections. N Engl J Med 1982; 306: 248.
14. Andreani T, Modigliani R, le Charpentier Y, et al. Acquired immunodeficiency with intestinal cryptosporidiosis: possible transmission by Haitian whole blood. Lancet 1983; 1: 1187.
15. Groopman JE, Salhuddin SZ, Sarngadharan MG, et al. Virologic studies in a case of transfusion-associated AIDS. N Engl J Med 1984; 311: 1419.

Received 3 May 1985.
Accepted 6 September 1985

LATE CELLULAR REJECTION IN RENAL TRANSPLANT RECIPIENTS

After the first three months, progressive failure of a renal graft is usually due to chronic vascular rejection, the histology of which shows fibro-obliterative lesions of the arterial intima; this rejection is not improved by increased immunosuppressive therapy (*1, 2*). However, patients with stable graft function may occasionally suffer rejection episodes many months or years after transplantation, when the main histological finding is an interstitial cellular infiltrate. We describe eight such patients, in whom treatment with increased doses of corticosteroids produced stabilization or improvement in renal function.

During a two-year period (January 1982 to December 1983) eight patients (aged 18–48, four men, four women) suffered an unexpected decline in renal function between 10 and 127 (mean 55) months posttransplantation (Table 1) and had renal biopsies (Fig. 1) showing preponderantly interstitial cellular rejection of a type usually associated with acute rejection (*3*). Patients 1, 2, 3, 4, and 6 had been receiving prednisolone and azathioprine, and patients 5, 7, and 8 cyclosporine alone. The dose of immunosuppressants had been unchanged for between 4 and 45 months. All patients were treated with 1 g methylprednisolone i.v. daily for five days. Oral prednisolone was increased to 20 mg per day in the patients taking prednisolone and azathioprine. Mean plasma creatinines were 140, 471, and 256 μmol/L three months before, at the time of, and four weeks after diagnosis and treatment, respectively (Wilcoxson matched pairs signed ranks: for each comparison tau = 0 $P < .01$). The fall in plasma creatinine occurred without a reduction in the dose of cyclosporine, which makes cyclosporin toxicity unlikely in patients 5, 6, and 8.

In addition to cellular rejection, each of our patients showed some degree of chronic rejection (Table 2). Since chronic vascular rejection does not respond to corticosteroids, this was probably the main determinant of long-term prognosis. Thus patient 7, who was the only patient with complete recovery of function, displayed the least chronic vascular change and interstitial fibrosis; and patients 2, 4, 5, and 6, who had the most severe vascular changes, had the highest plasma creatinines at follow-up.

Late interstitial cellular rejection occurs sporadically and at a time when follow-up is infrequent. There is, therefore, little information on underlying causes. We reviewed the clinical history to identify possible precipitating events. Infection, inadequate immunosuppression, and genetic disparity between donor and host are likely underlying factors.

Infections. Patients 2, 4, and 7 had suffered recent *Escherichia coli* urinary infections that had been treated with Cephradine, Cotrimoxazole, and Amoxycillin, respectively. However, urinary infections are common among renal transplant recipients and the association could have been fortuitious. The role of viral infection is also uncertain. Interferons, which are released during viral infection, induce the cellular expression of HLA class I and class II antigens—ands might, therefore, mediate rejection(*4*). Patients 5 and 6 gave a history of cough and aching limbs during the preceding two weeks, and a viral infection was suspected. Patient 4 had recently suffered a primary cytomegalovirus infection that was followed by the appearance of lymphocytotoxic antibodies. Patient 1, who initially had symptoms of fluid overload, and patients 3 and 8, who were asymptomatic, had no clinical evidence of infection. In all cases, an array of sera, which spanned the date of rejection, were investigated for the presence of viral antibodies using complement-fixation tests. Except for patient 4, no specific antibodies to cytomegalovirus, herpes simplex, influenza A and B, herpes varicella, measles and adenovirus, or to *Chlamideae* and *Coxsiella burnetti* were detected. Patient 4 became seropositive for cytomegalovirus.

Immunosuppression. Several reports suggest that complete cessation of immunosuppression is followed by rejection of the majority of cadaver grafts (*5, 6*). Among our patients it is difficult to relate the onset of rejection to the dosage of azathioprine, because this was similar in the control group and had not been changed since transplantation in patients 2, 3, and 6, and for 45 months in patient 1. Patient 4 had discontinued azathioprine for a five-week period for four months previously, during the CMV infection, but was again taking her original dose. However, the maintenance dosage of prednisolone could have been too low. In particular, patient 2 had not taken prednisolone for four months because she was concerned about side effects. In one study, mixed cellular and vascular rejection occurred in 5 of 10 renal allograft recipients who had been stable on 10 mg prednisolone/day for two years posttransplant, and in whom the dose of prednisolone was reduced below 7 mg/day (*6*). It was suggested that this may be the minimum "safe" dosage. However, 15 of our 19 controls were taking a lower dose, and among our patients with rejection the last dosage reduction had been 4–75 months previously. Thus, although a low corticosteroid dose may have predisposed to rejection, the considerable lag between dose reduction and rejection suggests other causes.

Genetics. Serum samples were collected from all patients prior to transplantation and at three monthly intervals thereafter. They were screened in the standard microlymphocytotoxicity assay against a panel of HLA-A, B, and DR-typed lymphocytes from 30 volunteers and 10 patients with chronic lymphocytic leukemia as a source of B cells. In addition, sera from five of the eight patients were crossmatched against spleen cells from their respective donors to test for the production of antidonor antibodies. Nineteen randomly selected primary graft recipients (aged 25–59, eight men and eleven women) who had received unchanged maintenance doses of prenisolone and

TABLE 1. Clinical and laboratory data

Patient No.	Age	Sex	Months post-transplant	Immunosuppressive dose			Plasma creatinine (μmol/L)			Follow-up (months)[b]
				Pred[a] mg/day	Aza[a] mg/day	CsA[a] mg/kg/day	Three months before diagnosis	Peak	One month after diagnosis	
1	26	F	127	5(75)	75(45)		97	187	163	188(25)
2	30	F	95	0(4)	100(95)		98	324	196	259(13)
3	30	M	68	5(21)	100(67)		151	247	234	212(7)
4	19	F	65	5(11)	100(64)		183	432	264	291(15)
5	22	M	33			7(16)	130	825	348	782(11)
6	46	M	27	10(7)	150(27)		202	1069	447	554(20)
7	20	F	17			7(12)	144	384	160	143(5)
8	18	M	10			7(4)	115	302	237	179(13)
Mean			55				140[c]	471[c]	256[c]	326
Controls (n=19) range										
Mean			84	5.6 (13–122)	104 (24–132)					112
Range			60–123	5–10	50–150					81–184

[a] Months since latest reduction of dose.
[b] Months after rejection episode in brackets.
[c] $P = .01$, Wilcoxon; all paired comparisons.

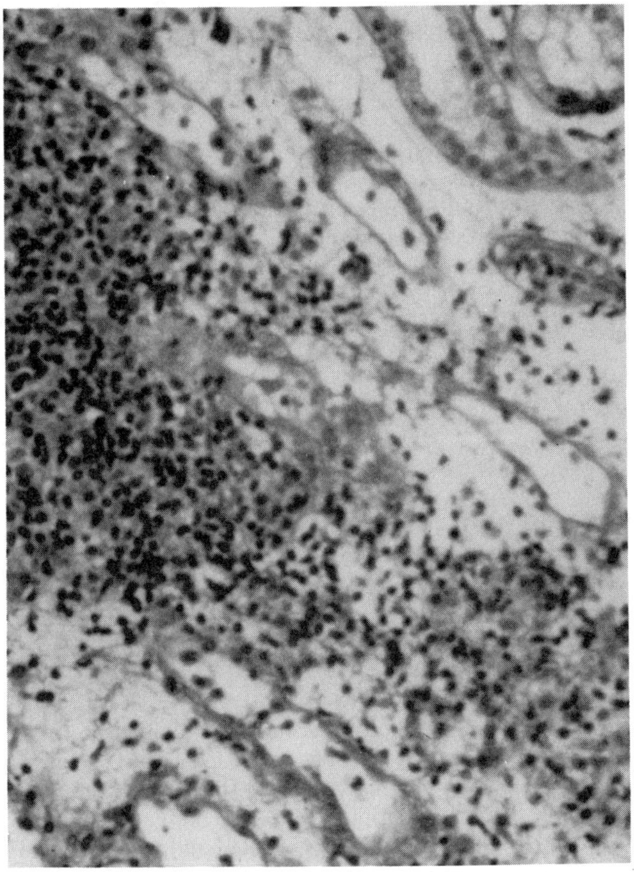

FIGURE 1. An edematous interstitium showing variable but fairly heavy infiltration by lymphocytes, immunoblasts, plasma cells, and macrophages.

azathioprine for between 13 and 122 months acted as controls for the immunogenetic studies.

All patients and controls had received a crossmatch-negative kidney. The mean number of HLA-A and -B matches and mismatches were 2.6 versus 1.25 and 2.0 versus 1.5 among patients and control subjects respectively (neither significant by Mann-Whitney U test).

None of the subjects had lymphocytotoxic antibodies before transplantation. Following transplantation, 4 of 19 (21%) controls and 6 of the 8 (75%) patients with late onset rejection developed lymphocytotoxic antibodies directed against panel cells (Table 3). (Fisher's exact test, P=0.014). Donor spleen

TABLE 2. Semiquantitative pathological assessment of biopsy changes[a]

Patient Number	Interstitial cellular infiltrate	Chronic vascular changes	Interstitial fibrosis	Glomerular changes
1	++	+	+/	+GP
2	++	+/++	++D	+GP;1
3	+/++	+	+/−	N
4	+/++	+/++	++F	+I
5	+/++	++/+++	+++D	++I
6	++/+++	+/++	+F	+GP
7	++	N	+F	N
8	+/++	+	+/−	N

[a] Key: (N) nil, (+/−) equivocal, (+) mild, (++) moderate, (+++) severe, (D) diffuse, (F) focal, (GP) transplant glomerulopathy, (I) focal ischemic changes.

TABLE 3. Posttransplant occurrence of lymphocytotoxic antibodies reactive with panel and donor cells for patients with late-onset acute rejection

Recipient	Nonabsorbed sera			Platelet-absorbed sera		
	PBL	CLL	Donor B cells	PBL	CLL	Donor B cells
1	−	−	ND[a]	−	−	ND
2	−	+	ND	−	+	ND
3	+	+	+	−	+	−
4	+	+	ND	−	−	ND
5	−	+	+	−	+	+
6	−	+	+	−	+	+
7	−	−	−	−	−	−
8	−	+	+	−	+	+

[a] ND = no donor cells available.

cells were available for five patients (Nos. 3, 5, 6, 7, and 8) and the lymphocytotoxic antibodies were reactive against these in four cases (Nos. 3, 5, 6, and 8). For patients 2, 3, 4, 5, and 8 antibodies were detectable for 4–60 days, and patient 6 had fluctuating levels for nine months prior to diagnosis. Platelet absorption removed all lymphocytotoxic antibody activity in patient 4, indicating that the antibodies were directed against HLA class I determinants. In the other five class cases anti-B-cell activity remained following absorption, suggesting that the antibodies were directed against HLA class II, as well as class I, antigens. The antibodies in cases 5 and 8 were specifically directed against a donor antigen (HLA DR4) that had been mismatched with the recipient. For the other three patients with B cell lymphocytotoxins it was not possible to assign a specificity. These antibodies could have been directed against Ia-like antigens other than DR or against non-Ia-related B cell antigens (*7*).

Finally, complacency among both doctors and patients may be the most important avoidable factor. After a long period of graft stability, it is tempting to reduce both the frequency of follow-up and the dose of medication. Rejection episodes no longer immediately follow reduction of immunosuppression, but typically occur after several months. Occasional lapses in compliance have no obvious adverse effect and may become common. Therefore, transplant recipients must be warned that it is always dangerous to stop immunosuppression (*5, 6*)—and, whenever the dosage of immunosuppressants is decreased, frequent (e.g., six-weekly) follow-up should continue for at least one year. Since cellular rejection may be first-observed with an acute symptomatic illness or an asymptomatic increase in plasma creatinine, we recommend that regular follow-up (e.g., three-monthly) be continued indefinitely, and that plasma creatinine be checked following all suspected infections. Prompt diagnosis of late interstitial cellular rejection is important because high-dose corticosteroid therapy improves renal function.

Laurence R. Solomon[1]

[1]Address correspondence to: Dr. L. R. Solomon, Renal Unit, Manchester Royal Infirmary, Oxford Road, Manchester M13 9WL, England.

Susan Martin[2]
Colin D. Short
William Lawler[3]
Ramanlal Gokal
Robert W. G. Johnson
Netar P. Mallick
Renal Unit
Manchester Royal Infirmary
Tissue Typing Laboratory
St Mary's Hospital
Department of Pathology
Manchester University
Manchester, England

[2] Tissue Typing Laboratory, St. Mary's Hospital.
[3] Deparment of Pathology, Manchester University.

REFERENCES

1. Morris PJ. Renal transplantation. In: Black DAK, Jones NF, eds. Renal disease. Oxford, London, Edinburgh, Melbourne: Blackwell, 1979: 549.
2. Strom TB, Tilney NL. Clinical management of the renal transplant recipient. In: Brenner BM, Stein JH, eds. Chronic renal failure. London: Churchill Livingstone, 1981: 255.
3. Zollinger HV, Mihatsch MJ. Renal pathology in biopsy. Berlin: Springer Verlag, 1978: 564.
4. Rosa F, Fellous M. The effect of gamma interferon on MHC antigens. Immunol Today 1984; 5(9): 261.
5. Zoller KM, Cho SI, Cohen JJ, Harrington JT. Cessation of immunosuppresive therapy after successful transplantation: a national survey. Kidney Int 1980; 18: 110.
6. Naik RB, Chakraborty J, English J, Marks V, Slapak M, Lee HA. Serious renal transplant rejection and adrenal hypofunction after gradual withdrawal of prednisolone two years after transplantation. Br Med J 1980; 1337.
7. Nunez G, McPhaul JJ, Statsny P. Characterization of B cell antibodies in kidney transplant recipients. Transplantation 1983; 35: 446.

Received 12 March 1985.
Accepted 4 June 1985.

SUCCESSFUL TREATMENT WITH INFRARED CONTACT COAGULATION OF EXCESSIVE FLUID LEAKAGE AFTER SPONTANEOUS DECAPSULATION OF A RENAL ALLOGRAFT

Spontaneous renal decapsulation with excessive fluid loss several years after transplantation is a rare complication. After our first description of two patients (*1*) three additional cases have been reported (*2, 3*). Despite several attempts to control the fluid leakage, the otherwise perfectly functioning graft had to be removed in 4 of these 5 patients, because of the excessive fluid loss. In one patient a marsupialization into the peritoneal cavity was successful (*2*). In the other four patients a spontaneously formed connection to the peritoneal cavity resulted in intractable ascites formation (*1, 3*). In our first patient we have tried to form a new capsule by painting with butylcyanoacrylate (Histoacryl) or by covering the kidney with lyophilized human dura (Lyodura), but both attempts failed. In two other patients, drainage of the perirenal fluid by a LeVeen shunt or a Denver shunt only led to temporary relief— and ultimately the grafts had to be removed (*1, 3*). Recently, we have seen another transplant patient with renal decapsulation with excessive fluid loss. This time we were successful in treating the problem by infrared contact coagulation of the entire kidney surface.

A woman born in 1950, with chronic renal failure caused by chronic pyelonephritis secondary to reflux nephropathy, underwent cadaveric kidney transplantation in October 1978 after 4 years of hemodialysis treatment. Except for a successfully treated rejection period immediately after transplantation, she did not have any problems until July 1984. Her graft function was excellent and stable (serum creatinine 88 μmol/L); and blood pressure was normal. From January 1981 there was a slight proteinuria of 1–1.5 g/24 hr without any signs of rejection. On July 25th she was admitted to our hospital because a large and painful swelling of the graft had developed suddenly, preceded by pain in the graft for three days. There was no history of trauma. The graft was tender and heavily swollen. On palpation there was fluctuation suggesting a large fluid collection. Blood pressure was normal and the serum creatinine had increased to 144 μmol/L. Ultrasound examination showed a perirenal fluid collection. A subsequent explorative laparotomy disclosed a completely decapsulated kidney, with a fluid collection of 410 ml inside the capsule. The fluid leaked profusely from the entire surface of the soft and swollen kidney. A drain was inserted into the cavity formed by the original capsule. Examination of the perirenal fluid showed a sodium concentration of 139 mmol/L, potassium 4.0 mmol/L, total protein content 1.5 g/L, and creatinine of 100 μmol/L. In the subsequent 9 days the fluid production remained unchanged (mean daily production 2440 ml, range 1540–3600 ml), while the serum creatinine gradually decreased to a normal value: 81 μmol/L. As expected on the basis of observations in the earlier described cases, the leakage did not subside. After nine days we performed a second operation, and attempted to control the leakage by infrared contact coagulation of the kidney surface. The graft was separated from the loose capsule surrounding it and, with the probe of the infrared sapphire coagulator ISC 81 (manufactured by G. Nath, Ph.D., Munich, F.R.G.) (*4*), the whole surface of the kidney was carefully coagulated, with maximal coagulation episodes of 2 sec. After the coagulation the fluid leakage of the surface was still visible, but it had evidently diminished. The kidney was then covered with a slip of omentum, and finally the original capsule was placed around the omentum-covered transplant and a drain was left behind. A biopsy taken during the procedure showed, on histological examination, severe interstitial edema with scattered, slight mononuclear cell infiltrates. Endothelial cells of small arteries showed some swelling. The result of immunofluorescence staining for immunoglobulins and complement components was negative. After the coagulation procedure the fluid production was 810 ml/24 hr, while the serum creatinine had increased to 158 μmol/L. During subsequent weeks fluid production gradually decreased without further treatment. On control echograms of the transplant at 1 and 6 days after the coagulation procedure some fluid collection was still visible around the graft, while at 14 days it had completely disappeared. Twenty-seven days after the procedure the patient was discharged from the hospital with a drain production of 310 ml and a serum creatinine of 116 μmol/L. Three weeks later the fluid production had completely stopped and the drain could be removed. At 9 months after the procedure the patient is doing well; her serum creatinine is 108 μmol/L, and she has normal blood pressure. The proteinuria has remained unchanged (1.7 g/24 hr). Ultrasound investigation of the graft reveals no abnormalities.

Until now only one patient has been reported in whom spontaneous decapsulation with excessive fluid leakage from the renal transplant did not lead to graft removal. In this patient marsupialization to the peritoneal cavity wsas successful—however, in the remaining four patients, a spontaneous connection to the peritoneal cavity did not solve the problem. Since earlier attempts to induce the generation of a new capsule had failed, we tried a new technique in this patient. Infrared contact coagulation has been successfully used in recent years for hemostasis of parenchymal bleeding from spleen or liver (*4–7*) and for the treatment of hemorrhoids (*8*). With this technique, in which infrared light is generated by a wolfram-halogen source and transmitted to the tissue by a sapphire crystal, coagulation areas of 20 mm^2 can be achieved that descend up to 4 mm into the underlying tissue depending on the probe used and the duration of coagulation. A capsule of fibrous tissue will form within 4–6 weeks after the procedure. This technique has been found to be superior to other techniques, such as laser coagulation or butylcyanoacrylate painting (*4*). In this patient we observed, immediately after the coagulation procedure, an abrupt decrease in fluid production of an average of 2440 ml per day to 810 ml per day; fluid production subsequently gradually diminished and ultimately disappeared after weeks. This gradual decrease in fluid leakage seems to parallel the formation of fibrous tissue at the coagulation site. Although we cannot completely rule out a spontaneous recovery of the fluid leakage, this seems very unlikely in view of other cases reported (*1–3*). The cause of this rare complication after kidney transplantation remains obscure. The successful treatment achieved in this patient supports our original hypothesis (*1*) that the fluid leakage is secondary to the decapsulation, since formation of a new capsule led to disappearance of the leakage.

ROLAND G. W. L. TIGGELER[1]
RIGTJE F. VAN DER SLUIS[2]
THEO WOBBES[2]
ROBERT A. P. KOENE[1]
J. H. M. BERDEN[1]
The Departments of Nephrology and Surgery
Sint Radboudziekenhuis
University of Nijmegen
Nijmegen, The Netherlands

[1] Department of Nephrology.
[2] Department of Surgery.

REFERENCES

1. Koene RAP, Skotnicki SH, Debruyne FM. Spontaneous renal decapsulation with excessive fluid leakage after transplantation. N Engl J Med 1979; 300: 1030.
2. Nghiem DD, Schulak JA, Corry RJ. Decapsulation of the renal transplant as a mechanism of lymphocele formation. Transplant Proc 1982; 14: 741.
3. Sollings HW, Starling JR, Oberley T, Glass NR, Belzer FO. Severe "weeping" kidney disease after transplantation: a case report. Transplant Proc 1983; 15: 2157.
4. Lauterjung KL, Nath G, Heberer G. Blutstillung mit einem neunen infrarot-Saphir-Coagulator (ISC-81). Chirurg 1982; 53: 88.
5. Guthy E. Die Behandlung der verletzten Milz. Langenbecks Arch Chir 1981; 354: 173.
6. Guthy E, Kiefhaber P, Nath G, Kreitmar A. Infrarot-Kontakt-Koagulation. Langenbecks Arch Chir 1979; 348: 105.
7. Guthy E, Brölsch C, Neuhaus P, Pichlmayr R. Infrarot-Kontaktcoagulation an der Leber: Technik, Taktik, Ergebnisse. Langenbecks Arch Chir 1984; 363: 129.
8. Templeton JL, Spence RAJ, Kennedy TL, Parks TG, McKenzie G, Hanna WA. Comparison of infrared coagulation and rubber band ligation for first and second degree hemorrhoids: a randomized prospective trial. Brit Med J 1983; 286: 1387.

Received 26 March 1985.
Accepted 6 August 1985.

IN VIVO INTERACTION OF CYCLOSPORINE AND INTRALIPID[1]

Cyclosporine (CsA) is a potent immunosuppressive agent that has been shown to inhibit humoral immunity to T-cell-dependent antigens and to strongly suppress cell-mediated immunity. Prolonged graft survival under CsA treatment has been achieved in a great variety of species using a great variety of organs, several of which have been grafted successfully for the first time (e.g., nerve and muscle cells, lung, and small bowel in experimental animals) (*1*).

In certain circumstances, successful organ transplantation may require nutritional support in the postoperative period. Although few well-controlled, well-designed, randomized clinical trials have documented conclusively the efficacy of perioperative nutritional support, there is sufficient data to justify this practice in selected cases (*2–4*), particularly following major abdominal procedures. The inclusion of fat (Intralipid) in parenteral nutritional regimens supplies a large portion of non-protein calories at a lower osmolarity than hypertonic glucose systems and prevents essential fatty acid deficiency. It thus allows peripheral venous administration of nutrients, with the added safety and convenience of this (*5*). Although some controversy remains as to the ability of fat to substitute for glucose as a caloric source under all circumstances (especially under severe stress), a growing number of studies have demonstrated the efficacy of fat in achieving nitrogen sparing in a variety of clinical or experimental settings (*6–9*).

Our interest in small intestinal transplantation has been rekindled by the advent of CsA (*10–12*). Because of the obvious essential role of (TPN) in such a possible clinical undertaking, it was imperative to look at possible interactions between these therapeutic modalities. CsA is an extremely lipophilic agent (*13*) with known tendencies to bind with lipoproteins (*13–15*) in plasma. Because of the rise in serum triglyceride level known to occur with the use of i.v. fat emulsions (*7*) such as Intralipid, the effects of the concomitant use of CsA and Intralipid were studied.

The purpose of this study was therefore to determine if the concomitant use of CsA and Intralipid produced an alteration in the plasma levels achieved after a standard IV dose of CsA; the clearance of CsA from the circulation, after a standard i.v. dose of CsA; and the in-vivo distribution of CsA in plasma.

Five adult mongrel dogs (3 male and 2 female) weighing 20–24 kg were used. In group 1, a single dose of CsA, 3 mg/kg, diluted in 300 ml of saline 0.9%, was infused over 1 hr. Blood samples were collected at 1, 2, 4, 6, 8, and 10 hr and CsA serum levels were determined by radioimmunoassay (RIA).[2] Biochemical analyses including blood urea nitrogen (BUN), creatinine, and triglycerides were performed on samples collected at the end of the infusion (hour 0) and at 10 hr.

In the second part of the experiment (group 2), an infusion of fat emulsion (Intralipid 10%) was started and maintained at a rate of 20 ml/hr (or approximately 2 g/kg/24/hr) for the duration of the experiment (14 hr). Four hours after starting the fat emulsion infusion, a single dose of CsA, prepared exactly as in part one, was infused through a different venous access route over 1 hr. Blood samples were collected according to the schedule above for CsA-RIA and biochemical analyses (Fig. 1).

To minimize in-vitro variations of CsA distribution, handling of all samples was standardized according to a process described by Smith et al. (*16*): Samples were collected in heparinized tubes and separated by centrifugation after two hours of equilibration at room temperature. CsA concentration was determined by RIA.

To study the distribution of CsA in plasma, KBr was added to each plasma sample to bring its density to 1.25 mg/ml. The resulting solution was then overlayered with a 1.25 mg/ml KBr solution (pH:7.4). Fractionation of plasma by ultracentrifugation at 45,000 rpm × 48 hr at 10°C was performed using a 50.3 rotor (Beckman Instruments). CsA concentration was then determined by RIA in the lipoprotein fraction, which was collected from the top of the tubes.

The total area under the CsA concentration-time curve (AUC) was computed for each dog, using the trapezoid rule, to obtain the area up to the last measured sample (10 hr). Slopes were computed on the log-transformed CsA concentrations by linear regression analysis. All comparative analyses were performed using the Student's *t* test.

Biochemical analysis demonstrated that triglycerides were elevated to twice their original level in group 2—fat emulsion infusion—(Table 1). The mean ± SE was raised from 0.62± 0.06 mmol/L in group 1, to 1.43±0.19 mmol/L in group 2. This difference was statistically significant ($P<0.01$ by paired Student's *t* test).

Although mean creatinine levels were slightly more elevated after the experiment (i.e., after two i.v. doses of CsA) than at the start of the experiment (153±46.7 μmol/L vs. 114.3±16.7 μmol/L—Table 1), this difference failed to achieve statistical significance.

CsA concentrations in unmodified plasma (Fig. 2) were slightly more elevated in group 2 (fat emulsion infusion), but this difference also failed to achieve statistical significance at any given time (Student's *t* test). In both groups, large variations in CsA concentration were noted in the early hours after i.v. infusion of the drug. There was a rapid decrease in plasma levels during the first 4 hr, followed by a slower decline up to 10 hr.

Determination of the total AUC (hr 2–10) by the trapezoidal rule for each group gave the following results: mean AUC for group 1: 2978.8±573 $\mu g \cdot hr \cdot l^{-1}$; for group 2: 3805.5±612 $\mu g \cdot hr \cdot l^{-1}$. This was not a statistically significant difference (Student's *t* test).

Linear regression on the log-transformed CsA levels (plotted

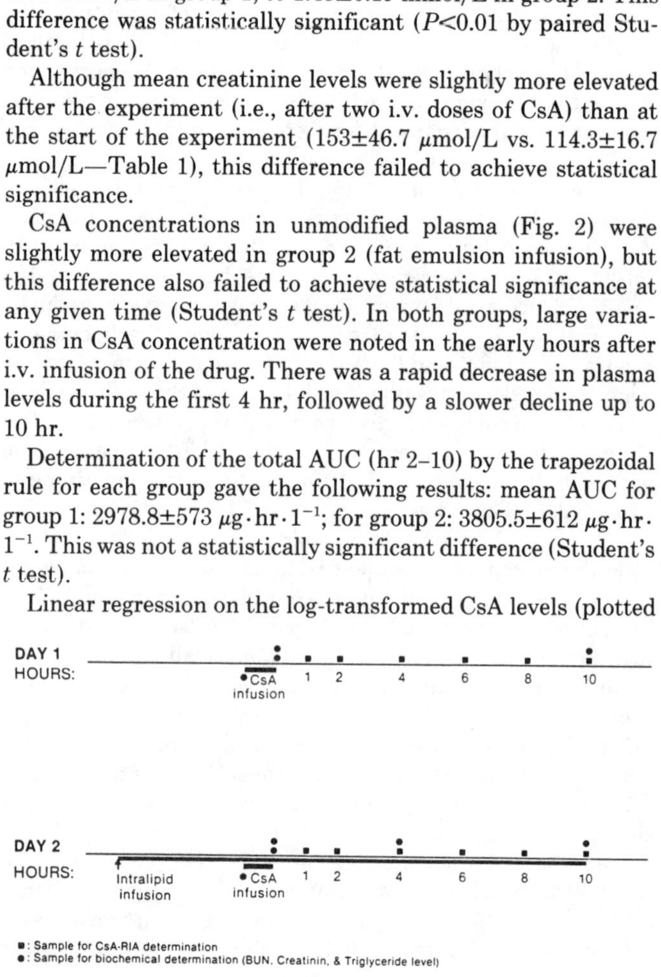

FIGURE 1. Experimental design.

[1] This work was supported by a grant from the Physicians Services Incorporated Foundation, Toronto, Ontario and by the Lawrence & Elsie Pifko Foundation.

[2] Abbreviations used: AUC, area under curve; BUN, blood urea nitrogen; RIA, radioimmunoassay.

TABLE 1. Summary of values in experimental groups 1 and 2

Measurement	Group 1	Group 2	P
Triglycerides (mmol/L)	0.62±0.06	1.43±0.19	<0.01
Creatinine (μmol/L)	153.0±46.7	114.3±16.7	0.08
AUC (Hr 2–10) (μg·hr·l^{-1})	2978.8±573	3805.5±612	0.82
SLOPE (log CsA) (hr^{-1})	−0.312±0.058	−0.263±0.065	0.15
Bound fraction (%)	88.0±3.2	86.4±9.4	0.76

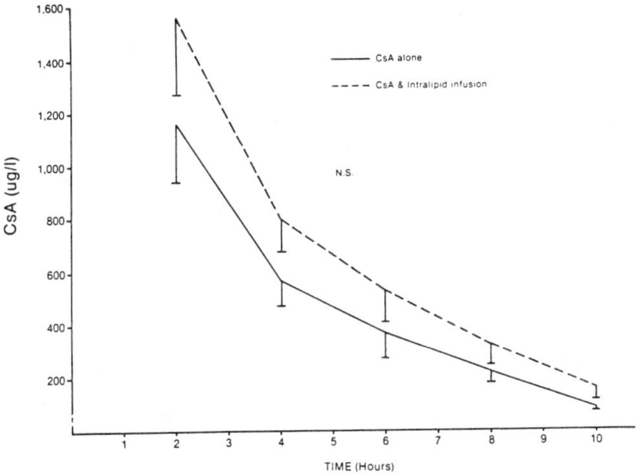

FIGURE 2. Cyclosporine plasma levels in dogs receiving cyclosporine alone (group 1) and in dogs receiving cyclosporine and intralipid (group 2).

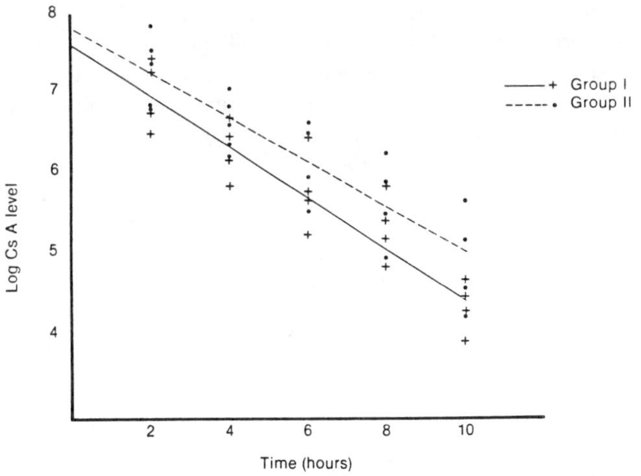

FIGURE 3. Scattergram of log-transformed cyclosporine plasma levels and linear regression equations in dogs receiving cyclosporine alone (group 1) and in dogs receiving cyclosporine and intralipid (group 2).

against time [Fig. 3]) was performed using the least squares method. The resulting equation for group 1, with an intercept of 7.63 and a slope of −0.31, demonstrated a correlation coefficient of −0.92. In group 2, a similar intercept of 7.83 and a similar slope of −0.28 characterized the resulting equation, with its correlation coefficient of −0.87. Again, the Student's t test failed to demonstrate a significant difference between the two groups.

Fractionation of plasma by ultracentrifugation revealed most of the CsA to be bound to lipoproteins. The fraction of CsA bound (Table 1) was (mean ± SE) 88.0±3.2% in group 1 and 86.4±9.4% in group 2 (no statistically significant difference).

CsA has become an important part of many immunosuppressive regimens for a variety of clinical and experimental organ transplantation protocols. Patients undergoing these major procedures often require adjuvant nutritional support, which may be provided in the form of parenteral solutions. Although TPN regimens using hypertonic glucose are widely used, fat emulsion solutions have also proved to be a valuable caloric source (*6–9*).

The binding of CsA to plasma lipoproteins has previously been described (*13–15*). These observations, however, did not address the possible interference of i.v. fat emulsion infusions (or the elevations of lipoproteins known to occur when using fat as a caloric source [*7, 17*]) with the pharmacokinetics of CsA, or even its distribution in plasma. Although a previously reported study (*13*) showed no correlation between the serum concentrations of total cholesterol, triglycerides, lipoproteins or erythrocytes, and plasma levels of CsA after administration of a standardized dose in renal transplant patients, the variations noted among patients could not reflect accurately the increase of lipoproteins (*7*) expected with the use of fat emulsion infusion.

All blood samples were allowed to separate for 2 hr, at room temperature, to ensure uniform equilibration of CsA (*16, 18*). It has been shown repeatedly that immediate separation, or a longer waiting period at room temperature, resulted in higher CsA serum levels (because of lack of CsA uptake by the erythrocytes—or, in the second case, because of back-diffusion of CsA from the red blood cells). A uniform handling technique thus minimizes in-vitro variations.

Determination of CsA levels in the plasma was performed by RIA. Controversy still exists over the accuracy of the RIA method for determination of CsA (*19–21*) as opposed to the method of high performance liquid chromatography (HPLC). RIA measures metabolites of CsA as well as the parent molecule, while HPLC measures only CsA itself. However, there is no evidence that the metabolites are any less nephrotoxic than CsA itself. In addition, the HPLC method is less available, and it requires a greater degree of technical expertise and higher initial and maintenance costs. The RIA remains widely used, which is thought by many authors to be justified (*18, 20–22*).

This in-vivo study of the interactions of the lipophilic oligopeptide CsA with fat emulsion solutions has helped to elucidate the following points. Even after raising the triglycerides levels to twice their original level, no significant modification in the CsA concentration was noted. The great variation of CsA concentration in the early hours after i.v. administration (noted in both groups) has previously been reported (*23*) and is thought to be due to variations among distribution and/or tissue binding. The curves depicting CsA plasma levels with and without fat emulsion infusion showed a very similar "two-slope" decline, with a rapid fall in plasma level during the first 4 hr, followed by a slower decline up to 10 hr, when only minimal levels could be detected. This has also been previously reported (*24*) and is suggestive of a two-compartment model of drug distribution. The log (CsA level) vs. time curves showed a very similar slope, without a statistically significant difference (Student's t test). This strongly suggests that tissue distribution of the drug is not affected.

Previous reports have shown that 70–90% of CsA is bound to lipoproteins (*13–15*) in plasma (this bond has, in fact, been shown to be temperature-dependent [*16*]). Although the exact nature of this binding remains to be determined, similar findings have been reported for different lipophilic drugs (*25*). The distribution of CsA among the different blood components was unaltered by the infusion of i.v. fat emulsion, even though this undoubtedly raised the major plasma pool of binding sites (lipoproteins).

These findings strongly suggest that the concomitant use of i.v. fat emulsion and CsA is safe, and does not require modifications in the drug dosage schedule, since no alterations in the pharmacokinetic profile of CsA could be demonstrated, using the RIA method for analysis.

In summary, we conclude that the concomitant use of fat emulsion as a caloric source and of CsA as an immunosuppressant does not seem to alter the normal pharmacokinetic profile of CsA, when measured by RIA. There does not appear to be a significant alteration in the plasma concentrations achieved, and clearance of the drug from the vascular pool is also unaffected. Therefore no changes in the drug schedule seem warranted when parenteral nutritional support with fat emulsions is used concomitantly with the immunosuppressant CsA. In addition, the distribution of the drug among the different blood components seems to be unaffected, with a similar proportion of the drug being bound to plasma lipoproteins.

Acknowledgments. We acknowledge P. Y. Wong, Ph.D., for CsA radioimmunoassays, and Monica Craig for technical assistance. Cyclosporine was generously provided by Sandoz Canada Ltd.

Ramses Wassef[3]
Zane Cohen[4]
Bernard Langer
The Division of General Surgery
Toronto General Hospital
The Department of Surgery
University of Toronto
Toronto, Canada

[3] Fellow of the Medical Research Council of Canada.

[4] Address correspondence and reprint requests to: Zane Cohen, M.D., F.R.C.S.(C), F.A.C.S., Division of General Surgery, Toronto General Hospital, 101 College Street, Eaton 9-211, Toronto, Ontario, Canada M5G 1L7.

REFERENCES

1. Borel J. Cyclosporine: historical perspectives. Transplant Proc 1983; 15: 2219.
2. Buzby G. Preoperative nutritional support: nutritional indications for delaying surgery. Clin Consult 1982; 2: 1.
3. Mullen J, Gertner M, Buzby G, et al. Implications of malnutrition in the surgical patient. Arch Surg 114: 121.
4. Mullen J, Buzby G, Waldman M, et al. Prediction of operative morbidity and mortality by preoperative nutritional assessment. Surg Forum 1979; 30: 80.
5. Jeejeebhoy K. Close M. Total parenteral nutrition by peripheral venous infusion. Clin Consult 1981; 1: 3.
6. Bark I, Holm I, Hakansson I, et al. Nitrogen sparing effect of fat emulsion compared with glucose in postoperative period. Acta Chir Scand 1976; 142: 423.
7. Jeejeebhoy K, Anderson G, Nakhooda K, et al. Metabolic studies in total parenteral nutrition lipid in man: comparison with glucose. J Clin Invest 1976; 57: 125.
8. Freund H, Fischer J. Is intravenous fat nitrogen sparing in the post injury state? Surg Forum 19 30: 83.
9. Souba W, Long J, Dudrick S. Energy intake and stress as determinants of nitrogen excretion in rats. Surg Forum 1978; 29: 76.
10. Craddock G, Nordgren S, Reznick R, et al. Small bowel transplantation in the dog using Cyclosporine. Transplantation 1983; 35: 284.
11. Reznick R, Craddock G, Langer B, et al. Structure and function of small bowel allografts in the dog: immunosuppression with Cyclosporine A. Can J Surg 1982; 25: 51.
12. Mackenzie R, Nordgren S, Lossing A, et al. Cyclosporin A absorption in canine small intestinal transplantation. Transplant Proc 1982; 14: 646.
13. Mraz W, Zink R, Graf A, et al. Distribution and transfer of Cyclosporine among the various human lipoprotein classes. Transplant Proc 1983; 15: 2426.
14. Niederberger W, Lemaire M, Maurer G, et al. Distribution and binding of Cyclosporine in blood and tissues. Transplant Proc 1983; 15: 2419.
15. Wood A, Maurer G, Niederberger W, et al. Cyclosporine: pharmacokinetics, metabolism, and drug interactions. Transplant Proc 1983; 15: 2409.
16. Smith J, Hows J, Gordon-Smith E. In vitro stability and storage of Cyclosporine in human serum and plasma. Transplant Proc 1983; 15: 2422.
17. Adamkin DH, Gelke KN, Andrews BF. Fat emulsions and hypertriglyceridemia. J Parenter Nutrition 1984; 8: 563.
18. Cohen DJ, Loertscher R, Rubin MF, et al. Cyclosporine: a new immunosuppressive agent for organ transplantation. Ann Intern Med 1984; 101: 667.
19. Varghese Z, Chan MK, Steele LV, et al. How to measure cyclosporine. Lancet 1984; 8391: 1407.
20. Holt DW, White DJ. How to measure Cyclosporine. Lancet 1984; 8396: 228.
21. Woloszczuk W, Schindler J, Hamilton G, et al. How to measure cyclosporine. Lancet 1984; 8403: 638.
22. Nelson PW. Cyclosporine. Collective review. Surg Gynecol Obstet 1984; 159: 297.
23. Lokiec F, Devergie A, Poirier O, et al. Pharmacologic monitoring in the clinical use of cyclosporine. Transplant Proc 1983; 15: 2442.
24. Newburger J, Kahan B. Cyclosporine pharmaco-kinetics in man. Transplant Proc 1983; 15: 2413.
25. Danon A, Chen Z. Clin Pharmacol Ther 1979; 25: 316.

Received 22 February 1985.
Accepted 18 June 1985.

INCREASED LEU-7-POSITIVE T LYMPHOCYTES DURING CYTOMEGALOVIRUS INFECTION FOLLOWING ALLOGENEIC BONE MARROW TRANSPLANTATION FOR HEMATOLOGIC MALIGNANCIES[1]

The months following allogeneic bone marrow transplantation are associated with profound immunosuppression despite normal numbers of leukocytes. Several studies have outlined the pattern and pace of immune reconstitution and have shown that the newly developing immune system acquires T cell and B cell immunocompetence within 2–12 months after the return of mononuclear cells to the peripheral blood (*1, 2*). In addition, previous work has shown that natural killer cell (NK)[2] activity

[1] This work was supported in part by Program Project Grant CA 30206 and Cancer Center Core Grant CA 33572 from the National Institutes of Health.

[2] Abbreviations used: CMV, cytomegalovirus; GVHD graft-versus-host disease; HCMV, human CMV; IL-2, interleukin 2; NK, natural killer; PBMC, peripheral blood mononuclear cells.

also returns within the first two months after grafting of the marrow (*3*). NK cells are thought to be primitive immune cells and have the characteristic of being able to react with tumor or viral target antigens without prior sensitization (*4*). Their function can be augmented by γ-interferon and interleukin-2 (IL-2) and suppressed by drugs such as cyclosporine (*5–8*). Despite this, the role of NK cells in the overall immune response to viral infections and graft-versus-host disease (GVHD) is uncertain. Previous reports have correlated NK activity and its augmentation by interferon with survival of patients with cytomegalovirus (CMV) infection following bone marrow allografting (*9*). In addition, some investigators have noted a fall in NK activity during overwhelming CMV infection after marrow transplantation (*3*).

As part of our ongoing studies involving immune reconstitution and the immune response to CMV after marrow transplantation, we studied markers of the NK cell population to determine the relationship between the appearance of these cells, which mediate NK activity, with the onset and course of CMV infection following marrow transplantation.

The monoclonal IgM antibody Leu7 reacts with approximately 15% of normal blood lymphocytes and is a marker for a homogeneous population of medium-sized lymphocytes with abundant neutrophilic cytoplasm containing azurophilic granules (*10, 11*). Depletion of Leu7-positive cells from the peripheral blood mononuclear cell (PBMC) population by complement-mediated lysis reduces NK activity against K-562 target cells. This antibody appears to detect a differentiation antigen that is expressed on human NK cells. We therefore used this antibody to follow the appearance of cells, after marrow grafting, bearing the antigen associated with NK activity.

Patients undergoing marrow transplantation were transplanted using high-dose chemotherapy and radiation therapy. The details of marrow transplantation, GVHD prophylaxis, and treatment are described as in previous publications from our center (*12, 13*).

Mononuclear cells from the blood of recipients of marrow allografts were studied for the appearance of Leu7-positive cells every two weeks following the return of 1000 white cells to the peripheral blood. NK activity against the K-562 cell line was measured every two weeks during the observation period as previously described (*14*). Granulocytes were cultured for cytomegalovirus on a weekly basis between day +35 and day +120 to detect CMV viremia as previously described (*15*). IgG antibody to CMV antigen was determined weekly between days +35 and +120 using an immunofluorescence assay. Cell surface marker studies on PBMC cells were performed every other week as previously described; these included the markers for OKT3 (T cells), OKT8 (suppressor/cytotoxic cells), OKT4 (helper/inducer), and Leu7 (NK cells) (*16*). Monocytes were depleted by adherence to plastic petri dishes prior to staining. The resulting cell population contained <5% esterase-positive cells.

Table 1 summarizes our observation on 18 patients who were treated with bone marrow transplantation for hematologic malignancies. Eleven of these patients were found to have evidence of CMV infection by both seroconversion and positive granulocyte cultures. Seven patients were followed who did not develop serologic and virologic evidence of human cytomegalovirus (HCMV) infection. The increased number of Leu7-positive cells was detected only in patients who had evidence of reactivated CMV infection. Normal individuals (n=15) in our laboratory showed a range of NK cells from 5–27% (median 14%). Patients with CMV infection (n=12) showed a range of 40–86% positive cells (median 66%). Patients without CMV infection (n=7) showed a range of positive cells between 12 and 43% (median 18%). The absolute number of Leu7-positive cells in the patients in the group with CMV viremia was statistically significant ($P<.001$ by Wilcoxon rank sum test) when compared with patients who did not develop CMV viremia. In general, the pattern of development of these Leu7-positive cells was typical of the group with the increase in the cell population

TABLE 1. Leu-7-positive cells (peak %) following allogeneic bone marrow transplantation (BMT):
I. Group 1—positive granulocyte culture for HCMV

UPN	Diagnosis[a]	Day after BMT	Day of 1st HCMV-positive culture	Leu 7	Acute GVHD	Interstitial pneumonia	NK activity[b]
166	CML	56	41	68	IV	Yes	18.2 (52)
168	ANLL	70	70	60	0	0	40 (100)
181	ANLL	62	41	86	0	0	32.9 (70)
186	LL	72	34	64	II	0	28.2 (51)
188	CML	90	42	86	0	0	70.9 (127)
202	ANLL	62	27	87	0	0	53.9 (103)
214	ALL	76	41	64	0	0	NT
220	CML	62	55	40	IV	Yes	NT
225	CML	90	41	53	0	0	31.3 (55)
237	ANLL	76	27	61	0	0	36.7 (72)
244	ANLL	90	41	66	II	0	36.2 (62)
II. Group II—negative granulocyte culture for HCMV							
163	ALL	83		12	0	0	47.2 (122)
187	ALL	83		16	0	0	42.3 (70)
212	CML	84		15	0	0	NT
215	ANLL	96		30	0	0	59.4 (200)
224	ANLL	90		18	0	0	33.1 (104)
229	ANLL	71		43	0	0	49.8 (194)
245	ANLL	84		24	0	0	NT

[a] CML = chronic myelocytic leukemia: ANLL = acute nonlymphoblastic leukemia; ALL = acute lymphoblastic leukemia, LL = lymphoblastic lymphoma; HCMV = human cytomegalovirus.

[b] Percentage of natural killer cell activity vs. K 562 at a 50:1 effector:target ratio; percentage of normal control in parentheses.

occurring after the onset of CMV viremia. Granulocyte cultures for HCMV became positive a median of 34 days prior to the peak of Leu7-positive cells in the blood. For reasons that are not clear, some patients with CMV viremia demonstrated these high numbers of Leu7-positive cells for up to a year after marrow transplantation, despite the resolution of CMV viremia by day +100.

Double labeling experiments were performed to further define the phenotype of these Leu7-positive cells. These experiments show that these cells are OKT3-positive, OKT8-positive and Leu7-positive. Despite the increase in the numbers of Leu7-positive cells, there was no increase in NK activity against the K-562 target. In addition, the appearance of these cells did not correlate with the presence or absence of acute GVHD, and it was not related to whether the patient received methotrexate/prednisone or cyclosporine/prednisone for GVHD prophylaxis.

CMV infection following marrow transplantation is a common virologic event that is sometimes associated with fatal interstitial pneumonitis (*17, 18*). However, many patients develop a benign viremia that may persist for weeks without the development of any significant clinical findings in the patient (*15*). It is known that in the marrow transplant patient there are several immune responses that occur in association with the occurrence of CMV infection. These include the development of IgG-specific antibody without a concomitant rise in IgM antibody, the development of a proliferative response to antigens associated with CMV, and the development of cytotoxic T cells (*17, 19, 20*). The last has been correlated with survival following marrow transplantation.

NK cell activity has also been studied following allogeneic marrow grafting. These reports have suggested that NK activity appears soon after the return of mononuclear cells following the grafting procedure (*3*). Some investigators correlated change in NK activity with the outcome of CMV infection (*3*). In this study we followed the appearance of a mononuclear cell population bearing the NK marker to determine the relationship between the appearance of Leu7-positive cells and CMV infection. The studies summarized above suggest that a cell population bearing a Leu7 antigen expands during CMV viremia and persists for some time.

Further studies with monoclonal antibodies made against NK cells have suggested that there are subpopulations of NK cells that can be delineated by antibodies directed against the Leu7 and Leu11 antigens (*21*). Although most of the NK activity on peripheral blood can be found in a $Leu7^{+}/Leu11^{+}$ cell population, this activity is highest in the population of cells that are $Leu7^{-}/Leu11^{+}$. We therefore determined the number of Leu11 cells in the blood at the time of the measurement of the Leu7 cells in patients who demonstrated high numbers of Leu7-positive cells up to 433 days after transplantation. These data are summarized in Table 2 and show that the number of Leu11 cells remained normal despite the increased number of Leu7 cells. The data presented here suggest that the expansion of this Leu7-bearing T cell population defined by double labeling techniques is an expanded T cell population that is reacting to the presence of CMV infection. Patients who do not have any CMV infection still maintain a predominantly OKT8 positive phenotype of T cells, but the cells do not express the antigen marked by the Leu7 antibody.

As noted above, NK activity against the K-562 target remained normal despite the increased numbers of Leu7-positive cells. Although there is an association with CMV infection, it is not clear what function these Leu7-positive T cells have in the immune reaction to the virus. In addition, it is also unknown why these cells persist for so long after viremia is no longer detectable (Table 2). It may be that these cells mediate the suppression of further reactivation of latent CMV infection. At present, we can conclude that the appearance of a Leu7-positive T cell correlates with the presence of CMV infection during the early phase of immune reconstitution following marrow transplantation. The function of these cells in an effective immune response to CMV following marrow transplantation remains to be determined.

TABLE 2. Relationship between Leu 7 and Leu-11-positive cells (%) after bone marrow transplantation (BMT)

UPN	Diagnosis[a]	Day after BMT	Leu 7	Leu 11
216	ALL	45	54	5
203	ANLL	62	87	15
214	ALL	76	64	13
208	ANLL	94	55	2
200	ANLL	175	72	4
188	CML	181	78	23
183	ANLL	262	82	29
174	ALL	272	63	17
152	ALL	385	52	9
172	ALL	433	61	17

[a] CML = chronic myelocytic leukemia; ANLL = acute nonlymphoblastic leukemia; ALL = acute lymphoblastic leukemia.

STEPHEN J. FORMAN[3]
JOHN A. ZAIA
CHRISTINE WRIGHT
MICHAEL T. GALLAGHER
KARL G. BLUME
City of Hope National Medical Center
Duarte, California

[3] Address correspondence to: Stephen J. Forman, M.D., Assistant Director, Department of Hematology and Bone Marrow Transplantation, City of Hope National Medical Center, 1500 E. Duarte Road, Duarte, CA 91010.

REFERENCES

1. Noel DR, Witherspoon RP, Storb R, et al. Does graft-versus-host disease influence the tempo of immunologic recovery after allogeneic human marrow transplantation? An observation on 56 long-term survivors. Blood 1978; 51: 1087.
2. Storb R, Ochs HD, Weiden PL, et al. Immunologic reactivity in marrow graft recipients. Transplant Proc 1976; 8: 637.
3. Dokhelar M-C, Wiels J, Lipinski M, et al. Natural killer cell activity in human bone marrow recipients. Early reappearance of peripheral natural killer activity in graft-versus-host disease. Transplantation 1981; 31: 61.
4. Herberman RB, Holden HT. Natural cell-mediated immunity. Adv Cancer Res 1978; 27: 305.
5. Henney CS, Kuribayashi K, Kern DE, Gillis S. Interleukin-2 augments natural killer cell activity. Nature 1981; 291: 335.
6. Herberman RB, Ortaldo JR, Rubinstein M, Pestka S. Augmentation of natural and antibody-dependent cell-mediated cytotoxicity by pure human leukocyte interferon. J Clin Immunol 1981; 1: 149.
7. Introna M, Allavena P, Spreafico F, Mantovani A. Inhibition of human natural killer activity by cyclosporin A. Transplantation 1981; 31: 113.
8. Svedersky LP, Shepard HM, Spencer SA, Shalaby MR, Palladino

MA. Augmentation of human natural cell-mediated cytotoxicity by recombinant human interleukin 2. J Immunol 1984; 133: 714.
9. Rook AH, Frederick WRJ, Burns WH, et al. Natural killer cell activity and interferon release predict survival from viral infection in bone marrow transplant recipients. Transplant Proc 1983; 15: 1773.
10. Abo T, Cooper MD, Balch CM. Characterization of HNK-1⁺ (Leu-7) human lymphocytes. I. Two distinct phenotypes of human NK cells with different cytotoxic capability. J Immunol 1982; 129: 1752.
11. Abo T, Balch CM. Characterization of HNK-1⁺ (Leu-7) human lymphocytes. II. Distinguishing phenotypic and functional properties of natural killer cells from activated NK-like cells. J Immunol 1982; 129: 1758.
12. Blume KG, Beutler E, Bross KJ, et al. Bone-marrow ablation and allogeneic marrow transplantation in acute leukemia. N Engl J Med 1980; 302: 1041.
13. Forman SJ, Spruce WE, Farbstein MJ, et al. Bone-marrow ablation followed by allogeneic marrow grafting during first complete remission of acute nonlymphocytic leukemia. Blood 1983; 61: 439.
14. Thong YH, Hensen SA, Vincent MM, et al. Use of cryopreserved virus-infected target cells in a lymphocytotoxicity ^{51}Cr release microassay for cell-mediated immunity to cytomegalovirus. Infect Immun 1976; 13: 643.
15. Zaia JA, Forman SJ, Gallagher MT, Vanderwal-Urbina E, Blume KG. Prolonged human cytomegalovirus viremia following bone marrow transplantation. Transplantation 1984; 37: 315.
16. Forman SJ, Nöcker P, Gallagher M, et al. Pattern of T cell reconstitution following allogeneic bone marrow transplantation for acute hematological malignancy. Transplantation 1982; 34: 96.
17. Neiman PE, Reeves W, Ray G, et al. A prospective analysis of interstitial pneumonia and opportunistic viral infection among recipients of allogeneic bone marrow grafts. J Infect Dis 1977; 136: 754.
18. Meyers JD, Spencer HC, Watts JC, et al. Cytomegalovirus pneumonia after human marrow transplantation. Ann Intern Med 1975; 82: 181.
19. Meyers JD, Flournoy N, Thomas ED. Cytomegalovirus infection and specific cell-mediated immunity after marrow transplant. J Infect Dis 1980; 142: 816.
20. Quinnan Jr. GV, Kirmani N, Rook AH, et al. Cytotoxic T cells in cytomegalovirus infection. HLA-restricted T-lymphocyte and non T-lymphocyte cytotoxic responses correlate with recovery from cytomegalovirus infection in bone-marrow transplant recipients. N Engl J Med 1982; 307: 7.
21. Lanier LL, Le AM, Phillips JH, Warner NL, Babcock GF. Subpopulations of human natural killer cells defined by expression of the Leu-7 (HNK-1) and Leu-11 (NK-15) antigens. J Immunol 1983; 131: 1789.

Received 13 March 1985.
Accepted 18 June 1985.

COMPARISON OF SPLENIC AND RENAL SUBCAPSULAR ISLET AUTOGRAFTING IN DOGS[1]

Diabetes has been ameliorated in pancreatectomized dogs by autotransplantation of dispersed pancreatic tissue prepared and engrafted by a variety of techniques (*1–5*). In a recent report Toledo-Pereyra et al. (*6*) presented data suggesting that the renal subcapsular space was an immunologically privileged site for pancreatic islet allografting in dogs; they used a collagenase-free method for tissue preparation, and the results of autotransplantation were not reported. Previous studies using a collagenase digestion technique in our laboratory indicated that intrasplenic injection was preferable to intraportal injection for islet autotransplantation in dogs (*2*), but we had not tested the renal subcapsular space as a site. In the experiments reported herein we compared the results of autotransplantation of collagenase-dispersed pancreatic islet tissue to the spleen or kidney in totally pancreatectomized dogs.

Forty mongrel dogs weighing between 13.2 and 24.4 kg (mean ± SD of 19.4±3.3 kg) were made diabetic by total pancreatectomy. Fifteen untreated pancreatectomized animals survived a mean (± SD) of 7.0±4.2 days with a mean (± SD) plasma glucose level of 402±19 mg/dl before death. The pancreases of 25 dogs were intraductally distended with Hanks' balanced salt solution (HBSS)[2] at 4°C for 10 min, followed by 20–40 min intraductal perfusion with collagenase (Sigma Type I 180 units/mg) at a concentration of 7200 units/dl at 37°C, a modification of the technique described by Horaguchi et al. (*3*). The digested pancreas was coarsely minced with a scissors and finely minced by machine (*7*), followed by shaking in a water bath in 3 steps of 10 min duration each. After each step, the suspension was filtered through a steel mesh of 400-μm pore size and washed three times with HBSS in a refrigerated centrifuge. The settled tissue volume was 10–15 ml. A double antibody radioimmunoassay method (8) was used to determine the insulin content in the washes and in the final tissue suspension on aliquots subjected to acid-alcohol extraction. Tissue insulin content roughly correlates with beta cell mass (*9*) and function (*10*) as previously described. The mean (± SD) total insulin content of the final tissue preparations (n=25) was 1067±657 μg, compared with a total pancreatic tissue insulin content (calculated from the sum of the final tissue preparation plus the insulin content of the washes and discarded tissue) of 3728±1318 μg, an average yield of 29%.

The prepared tissue was autotransplanted by injection through a 20-gauge needle. In 14 dogs injection was into the trabecular system of the spleen by reflux into the splenic venous tributaries. The mean (± SD) insulin content of the tissue injected into the spleen of 14 dogs was 1077±808 μg.

In 11 dogs the material was injected under the renal capsule of the left kidney. (In one dog both kidneys were used.) The capsule was carefully dissected from the cortex by a scoop prior to injection, and the site of injection was closed by a pursestring suture. The mean (± SD) insulin content of tissue injected under the kidney capsule of the 11 dogs was 1053±432 μg.

Between 7% and 56% of the original total pancreatic insulin content was contained in the final tissue preparations. The mean (± SD) yield was 29±12% in all 25 dogs, and the mean yields in the splenic injection group (n=14) and in the renal subcapsular injection group (n=11) were similar: 30±15% and 27±6%, respectively, ($P>.2$, Wilcoxon test).

After grafting the animals received a high protein diet containing Viokase as a substitute for the exocrine pancreatic enzymes. Daily fasting plasma glucose levels were measured by

[1] This work was supported by a grant from the Vegas Corporation and the Juvenile Diabetes Foundation, Inc.

[2] Abbreviations used: HBSS, Hanks' balanced salt solution; IVGTT, intravenous glucose tolerance test.

using a Beckman glucose analyzer Type II. The dogs were considered normoglycemic when plasma glucose levels were ≤ 150 mg/dl. Intravenous glucose tolerance tests (IVGTTs) (0.5 gm/kg in a bolus, with samples for plasma glucose obtained at 0, 1, 3, 5, 10, 20, 30, 60, 90, 120, and 180 min) were performed 14 days posttransplant in all surviving animals, and the results were compared with the pretransplant values obtained in 15 dogs one day prior to pancreatectomy. Five normoglycemic recipients of tissue into the spleen also had an additional IVGTT performed at six weeks posttransplant, followed by splenectomies to prove successful grafting. The organs were processed for histological examination using hematoxylin and eosin and aldehyde fuchsin staining, as well as immunoperoxidase staining for insulin.

None of the 11 recipients of tissue under the renal capsule became normoglycemic. They died at a mean (± SD) of 19.4±8.6 days posttransplant with a mean plasma glucose level at death of 413±138 mg/dl.

Of 14 spleen-injected dogs, 10 (72%) became normoglycemic between 1 and 5 days after transplantation. The 10 normoglycemic dogs were killed between 2 and 6 weeks after transplantation, and their mean (± SD) plasma glucose level at the time of sacrifice was 110±20 mg/dl. Four recipients of islets into the spleen did not return to normoglycemia and died at a mean (± SD) of 20.0±18.0 days posttransplant with a mean plasma glucose level of 310±95 mg/dl. The mean (± SD) tissue insulin content of the processed (transplanted) tissue was higher in the ten dogs that became normoglycemic (1238±915 μg) than in the four that did not (674±125 μg), as was the mean insulin content of the transplanted tissue as a percentage (yield) of the original total pancreatic tissue insulin content (32±17% vs. 25±2%), but the differences were not significant (P>.2).

Four animals in the renal subcapsular injection group died or were killed before IVGTTs could be performed. IVGTT results at 14 days were nearly normal in the spleen-injected normoglycemic dogs (group 1, n=10), although the mean K value was significantly lower than that obtained prior to pancreatectomy and autotransplantation (P<.05) (Fig. 1). In the diabetic spleen-injected dogs (group 2, n=4) and in the renal subcapsular-injected dogs (group 3, n=7), IVGTT curves were very abnormal (Fig. 1), and K values were significantly lower than in group 1 dogs (P<.01), but were not significantly different from each other (P>.2). However, there is some evidence of islet function in group 2 and group 3 dogs, since their mean (± SD) survival times of 20.5±7.8 days and 19.4±8.6 days were significantly longer than the mean survival (7.0±4.2 days) of the apancreatic nontransplanted dogs (P<.01).

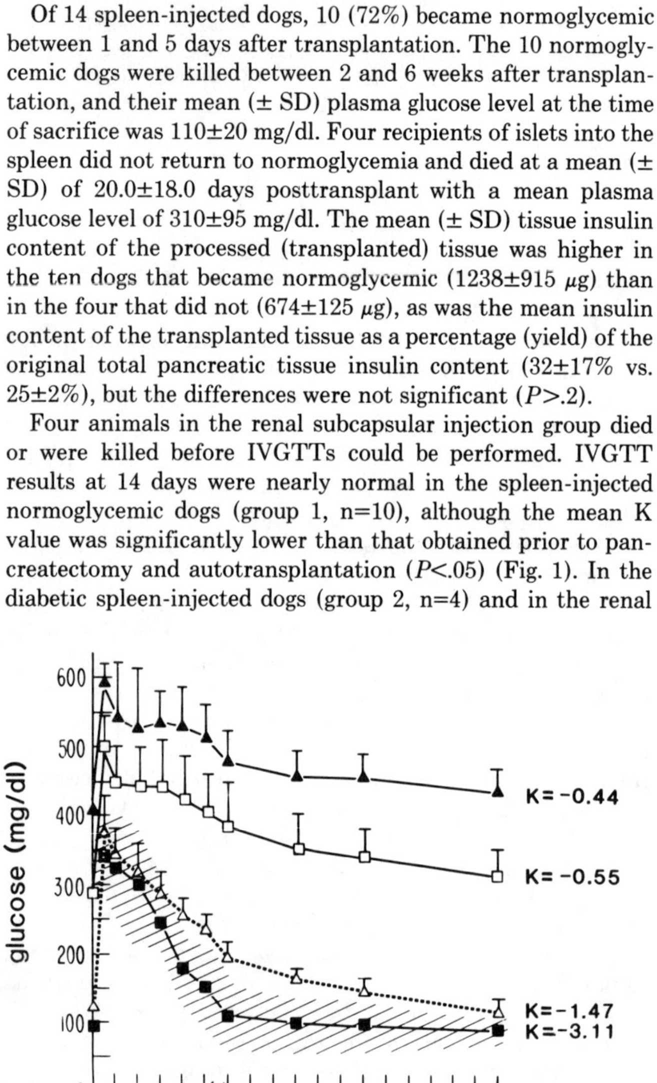

FIGURE 1. Intravenous glucose tolerance test results in normal dogs (■) (n=15) and at two weeks posttransplant in totally pancreatectomized recipients of collagenase-dispersed autologous pancreatic tissue into the spleen (10 normoglycemic dogs [△] and 4 diabetic dogs [□]) or under the kidney capsule (▲) (n=7).

In five normoglycemic animals of group 1, a second IVGTT was performed at six weeks after transplantation. The mean (± SD) K value was −1.7±0.70%—similar to the one obtained at 14 days posttransplant. After splenectomy all five animals became hyperglycemic and died within two or three days.

In animals of all groups tissue was seen at the site of transplantation, grossly and upon histological examination (Fig. 2). Insulin-containing cells were identified in the spleen (Fig. 2A) and under the renal capsule (Fig. 2B) in the appropriate groups by specific immunoperoxidase staining. The tissue under the renal capsule was situated near capillaries, but was surrounded by fibrous tissue (Fig. 2B), while that in the spleen was not enveloped by a fibrotic reaction (Fig. 2A).

The amount of islet tissue that became engrafted was estimated from total insulin content measurements in the spleens of 6 dogs (3 in group 1 and 3 in group 2) and in the kidneys of 5 dogs of group 3 at the time of killing (Table 1). The insulin content of the transplanted tissue was similar in all 3 groups, both in absolute amount and as a percentage of the preprocessing pancreatic tissue insulin content (yield). The mean insulin content of the spleens was higher in the dogs of group 1 than of group 2 (P<.05), as was the percentage of engraftment, but the latter difference was not significant (P>.2). The most significant observations were that the mean insulin content and the percentage of engraftment were lower in the kidneys of group 3 dogs than in the spleens of group 1 or group 2 dogs (P<.05).

Both the method of pancreatic islet preparation and the site of implantation appeared to influence the results of islet transplantation in dogs. Using a collagenase digestion technique, we found the renal subcapsular site to be unsatisfactory, while intrasplenic grafting was successful. In contrast, Toledo-Pereyra et al. (*6*) ameliorated diabetes in pancreatectomized dogs by allotransplantation under the kidney capsule of mechanically dispersed pancreatic tissue not subjected to collagenase digestion. Toledo-Pereyra et al. (*6*) did not evaluate the spleen as a site for transplantation of mechanically dispersed pancreatic tissue, nor did they give information on the success rate of their technique; rather, they gave information only on the successfully transplanted dogs. Furthermore, they did not transplant autologous tissue. It is possible that these differences in tissue preparation technique protocol could account for the difference in results between our experiments and those of Toledo-Pereyra et al., but we were unable to make a pancreatic tissue preparation that would fit under the kidney capsule by purely mechanical means.

However, the intraductal collagenase perfusion technique we used resulted in a mean recovery of 29% of the original insulin-containing tissue in the pancreas, a yield similar to that obtained by others using this technique (*3*, *4*). Furthermore, we had practically no warm ischemia time in our preparation. Therefore, we must conclude that the kidney capsule site is inferior to the spleen for islet autotransplantation in dogs. Various implantation sites have been used for islet transplantation in rodents, including the peritoneal cavity, portal vein,

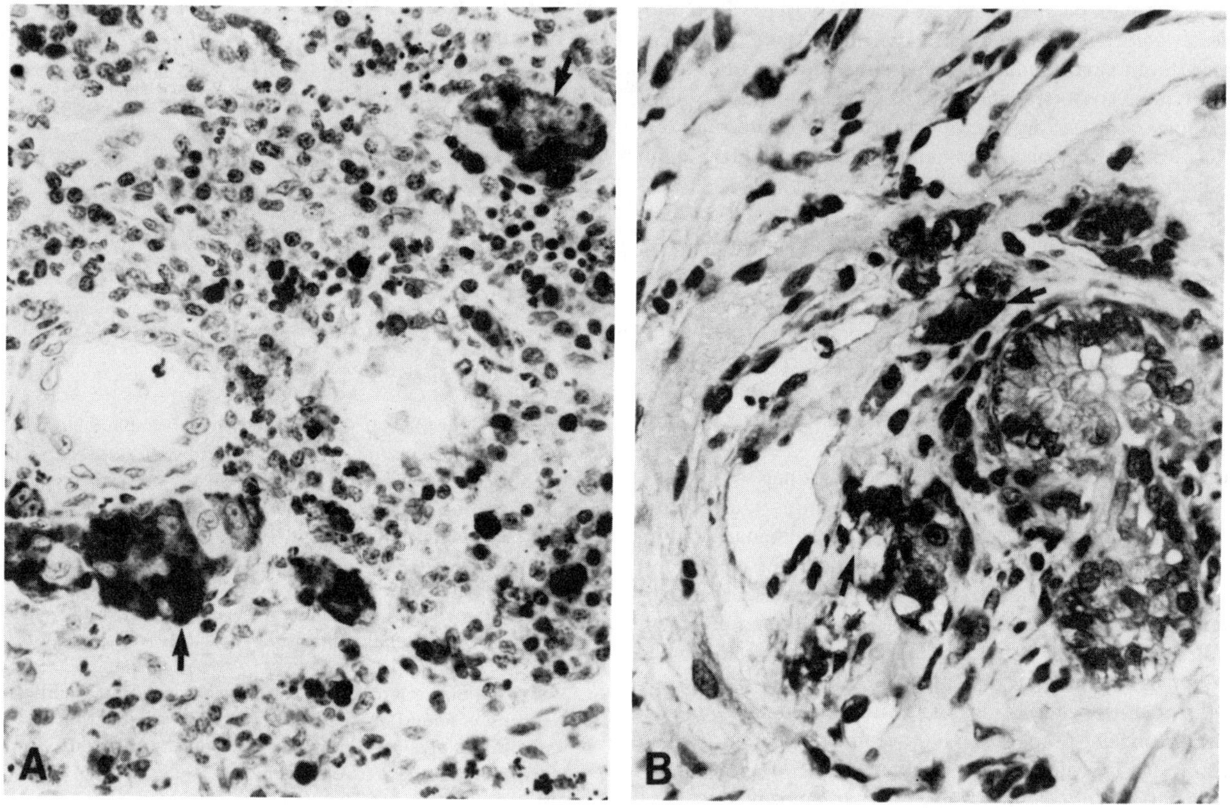

FIGURE 2. Photomicrograph of spleen (A) of one animal of group 1 at 6 weeks posttransplant and of the renal subcapsular site (B) of one animal of group 3 at 2 weeks posttransplant. Both sections were stained by immunoperoxidase technique for insulin and both were photographed at a magnification of 480×. Insulin staining cells (→) are seen in both the spleen and kidney, but the cells are enveloped in fibrous tissue in the latter.

TABLE 1. Mean (± SD) insulin content of injected tissue at the time of transplantation and insulin content of the recipient organ at death

Site of transplant	Insulin content (μg) of tissue transplanted[a]	Insulin content (μg) of organ at removal[b]	Percentage of recovery of insulin in recipient organ (engraftment)[c]
Spleen (n=6)	845±670	32.5±18.0	8.5±11.3
Group 1 (n=3)	866±611	47.6±9.1	12.9±15.8
Group 2 (n=3)	825±865	17.3±5.5	4.1±3.1
Kidney (group 3, n=5)	1159±361	2.1±0.7	.20±.09

[a] Mean ± SD insulin contents after processing as a percentage of the insulin contents of the pancreases prior to processing were : 25.0± 17.9% in the 6 spleen dogs (30.0±21.3% in group 1 and 20.0±16.7% in group 2) and 36.6±8.0% in the 5 kidney dogs, similar yields in all three groups ($P \geq .1$) based on preprocessing pancreas insulin contents of 3130±873 in the 6 spleen dogs (2751±735 in group 1 and 3510±967 in group 2) and 3355±1659 in the 5 kidney dogs (group 3).

[b] $P < .05$ for organ insulin content at removal in group 1 vs. group 2 and $P < .05$ for groups 1 and 2 vs. group 3.

[c] $P < .02$ for engraftment in group 3 vs. engraftment in both group 1 and group 2.

spleen, omentum, and kidney capsule (*5*). In large animals, except for the report of Toledo-Pereyra et al. (*6*), only intraportal and splenic injection sites have been associated with amelioration of diabetes (*1–5, 10–13*). Previous studies in dogs showed that when an impure islet preparation is used, the spleen is superior to the portal vein because of a high incidence of intraportal hypertension with the latter technique (*2*). The intraductal collagenase digestion method also gives an impure preparation (*3*). In our experiments, reflux of the material into the spleen via the splenic vein prevented diabetes in 10 of the 14 animals (72%). However, when the tissue was injected directly into the renal subcapsular space, the results were inferior. The recipients of tissue injected under the kidney capsule never became normoglycemic and IVGTTs were impaired.

Nevertheless, animal survival was prolonged and histological findings showed the presence of insulin-producing tissue. Presumably, the amount that became engrafted was insufficient to produce normoglycemia. These results are in high contrast to those of Toledo-Pereyra et al. (*6*) who used a collagenase-free islet preparation technique. He reported indefinite graft survival without or with only minimal immunosuppression and suggested that the renal capsule was a privileged site for islet transplantation. Toledo-Pereyra et al. (*6*) reported that K values were actually higher in transplanted than in normal dogs, which is remarkable since almost all other allotransplant and autotransplant studies have found that K values were significantly reduced compared with normal animals even when the recipients were otherwise normoglycemic (*2, 4, 12, 13*). Again, it should be noted that our tissue preparation technique was different from that of Toledo-Pereyra et al., so we cannot claim to refute these results.

Nevertheless, we conclude that the spleen is a superior injection site. In previous experiments in dogs, using a collagenase digestion technique that resulted in 50–90% loss of islet tissue, autotransplantation in the spleen still produced normoglycemia (*2*), as was the case in one of the dogs reported here, who received tissue containing only about 7% of the original insulin content of the pancreas. The spleen is richly vascularized and provides a favorable environment for engraftment and for function of even small quantities of tissue. A larger amount of tissue may have to be transplanted to the subcapsular region of the kidney, since a larger proportion of the islets may die before neovascularization occurs and a sufficient nutritional supply for the implanted tissue is provided. The lack of immediate blood supply and the narrowness of the subcapsular space limits engraftment to the cortex and capsule. We attempted to compensate for this limitation in one dog by splitting the tissue between both kidneys, but this maneuver did not improve the functional outcome. Thus, the usual collagenase technique for islet preparation in dogs will not result in amelioration of diabetes when the tissue is injected under the renal capsule as an autograft. In contrast, the splenic site has been repeatedly proved to be practical in the canine model.

In summary, the subcapsular space of the kidney was evaluated for pancreatic islet autografting in a canine model, and compared with the standard approach of intrasplenic injection. The intraductal collagenase perfusion technique for islet preparation after total pancreatectomy yielded a beta cell recovery (as judged by tissue insulin content) of 7–56% (mean ± SD of 29±12%). A total of 15 totally pancreatectomized animals became hyperglycemic and died at a mean (± SD) of 7.0±4.2 days after operation. Of 14 dogs that underwent intrasplenic injection of the islet preparation, 10 became permanently normoglycemic by 2–5 days posttransplant. None of 11 animals receiving islets under the renal capsule became normoglycemic, suggesting that the renal capsule is not an appropriate site for transplantation of dispersed pancreatic islet tissue prepared by collagenase digestion.

Acknowledgments. We appreciate John Heil, Michelle Dunning, Murray Richardson, Fred Gould, Jane Field, and Frances Rabe for their helpful assistance, as well as Tom Groppoli for histological immunoperoxidase staining. Janet Sanders and Jennifer May prepared the manuscript and Martin Finch produced the figures. Traysolol for islet preparation was generously provided by Mobay FBA Pharmaceuticals, 425 Park Avenue, New York, NY.

UWE J. HESSE
DAVID E. R. SUTHERLAND[3]
PAUL F. GORES
ANTONIO SITGES-SERRA
JOHN S. NAJARIAN
The Department of Surgery
University of Minnesota
Minneapolis, Minnesota

[3] Address correspondence to: Dr. Sutherland, Box 280, University of Minnesota Hospitals, 420 Delaware Street S.E., Minneapolis, MN 55455.

REFERENCES

1. Mirkovitch V, Campiche M. Successful intrasplenic autotransplantation of pancreatic tissue in totally pancreatectomized dogs. Transplantation 1976; 21: 265.
2. Kretschmer GJ, Sutherland DER, Matas AJ, Payne WD, Najarian JS. Autotransplantation of pancreatic fragments to the portal vein and spleen of totally pancreatectomized dogs. Ann Surg 1978; 187: 79.
3. Horaguchi A, Merrell RC. Preparation of viable islet cells from dogs by a new method. Diabetes 1981; 30: 455.
4. Warnock GL, Rajotte RV, Procyshyn AW. Normoglycemia after reflux of islet containing pancreatic fragments into the splenic vascular bed in dogs. Diabetes 1983; 32: 452.
5. Sutherland DER. Pancreas and islet transplantation. I. Experimental studies. Diabetologia 1981; 20: 161.
6. Toledo-Pereyra LH, Bandlien KO, Gordon DA, MacKenzie GH, Reyman TA. Renal subcapsular islet cell transplantation. Diabetes 1984; 33: 910.
7. Matas AJ, Sutherland DER, Steffes MW, Najarian JS. Short-term culture of adult pancreatic fragments for purification and transplantation of islets of Langerhans. Surgery 1976; 80: 183.
8. Morgan AR, Lazarow A: Immunoassay of insulin: two antibody system. Diabetes 1973; 12: 115.
9. Sutherland DER, Matas AJ, Steffes MW, Najarian JS. Infant human pancreas: a potential source of islet tissue for transplantation. Diabetes 1976; 25: 1123.
10. Ward SL, Sutherland DER, Najarian JS. Correlation of function and engraftment of canine intrasplenic islet autotransplants. Surg Forum 1984; 35: 374.
11. Hanson SL, Sutherland DER, Field MJ, Rabe F, Najarian JS. Comparison of techniques for pancreatic islet transplantation in dogs. Surg Forum 1981; 32: 365.
12. Alderson D, Farndon JR. The effects of transplant mass on insulin release by collagenase-dispersed pancreatic fragments in the diabetic dog. World J Surg 1984; 8: 598.
13. Williams MD, Walshaw R, Bull RW, Schall WD, Padgett GA, Gossain VV, Nachreiner RF. Effect of cyclosporine on allotransplanted pancreatic islets in DLA-MLC compatible dogs. Transplant Proc 1983; 15(suppl 1): 3004.

Received 5 March 1985.
Accepted 24 May 1985.

PROLONGATION OF SKIN GRAFT SURVIVAL IN DOGS TREATED WITH 8-AMINOGUANOSINE

Inherited deficiencies of the enzymes adenosine deaminase (ADA)[1] and purine nucleoside phosphorylase (PNP) result in severe immunodeficiency disease in man (*1, 2*). Specific inhibitors of ADA and PNP in normal man may therefore prove useful as immunosuppressive agents. Administration of 2-deoxycoformycin, a competitive inhibitor of ADA has been shown to prolong skin grafts in dogs and rodents (*3, 4*). While ADA deficiency results in depression of both cell-mediated and humoral immune responses, congenital deficiency of PNP results in impaired cellular immune responses with preservation of antibody production (*1, 2*). Children with this disorder have frequent infections, lymphopenia, and variable elevation of PNP substrates in urine and blood (*5*). Studies in murine and human lymphoid cell lines show that deoxyguanosine (dGuo), a substrate for PNP, is toxic to T lymphocytes—having, perhaps, subset specificity (*6–8*). Suppressor T cell activity in mice is completely depressed by daily i.p. administration of 0.1 mg dGuo. Effector T cells are not affected until the dose was increased to 10 mg/day (*9*). Rapid degradation of dGuo by PNP rich red cells is thought to prevent its toxicity in man (*10*). The guanosine analog, 8-aminoguanosine (8-AG), is an inhibitor of PNP activity with a K_i of 1.7×10^{-5}M (*11*). Studies in

[1] Abbreviations used: ADA, adenosine deaminase; 8-AG, 8-aminoguanosine; dGuo, deoxyguanosine; MLC, mixed lymphocyte culture; PNP, purine nucleoside phosphorylase.

TABLE 1. Clinical and laboratory observations following 8-aminoguanosine treatment

Dog No.	Skin graft survival (days)	No. treatments	Wt. loss	Emesis	Lethargy	Thrombo-cytopenia	Last treatment (% of initial lymphocyte count)
8438	20[a]	8	No	No	No	Yes	34.2
8456	24	12	Yes	Yes	No	No	65.5
8457	31[b]	12	Yes	Yes	Yes	No	54.5
8478	29	12	Yes	No	Yes	Yes	39.7
8479	28	12	Yes	No	No	Yes	27.5
8466	29	9	Yes	Yes	No	No	49.2
Controls	Mean ± 1 SD						
n=12	11.2±1.3						

[a] Died under general anesthesia day 20 with viable skin graft.
[b] Found dead day 31 with viable skin graft.

vitro using a combination of dGuo and 8-AG showed little effect on resting lymphoid cells but significant toxicity to stimulated lymphocytes (*11*). The present studies were carried out in canines to evaluate the in vivo immunosuppressive activity and toxicity of the PNP inhibitor 8-AG.

Random mongrel dogs weighing 5–13 kg were immunized against hepatitis, parvovirus, and distemper; they were treated for parasitic infestation and observed for at least 4 weeks prior to use.

The 8-aminoguanosine was synthesized by the method of Holmes and Robins (*12*). In preliminary studies 8 dogs were given 8-AG i.v. in solutions of hydrochloric or citric acid of pH 2.5–5.0, or an alkaline solution of 0.05N NaOH titrated with 0.05N HCl to pH 10–12. 8-AG could be solubilized at 8–10 mg/cc at pH 10.5–11 and administered over 10–20 min in doses of 10–100 mg/kg without acute toxic effects. Venous sclerosis resulted from multiple injections, but venous access could be maintained by rotating extremity injection sites.

Following preliminary studies, 6 dogs were treated with 8-AG 100 mg/kg i.v. 3 times weekly. At 24 hr following the fourth dose of drug, full-thickness fitted 2.5×2.5-cm skin grafts were performed under general anesthesia using mixed lymphocyte culture (MLC)-positive random donors. Four dogs received 8 subsequent doses of drug while 2 dogs received 4 and 5 doses, respectively. Graft rejection was considered complete when total induration of the transplanted skin occurred. In addition to skin graft monitoring, clinical assessment of weight loss and activity were made daily. Plasma samples, complete blood counts, and absolute lymphocyte counts were obtained on all dogs 3 times per week. Following sacrifice, gross and histologic examinations were performed. Selected dogs had serial plasma samples analyzed by high pressure liquid chromatography methods for levels of 8-AG, inosine, deoxyinosine, guanosine, and deoxyguanosine, adapted from the method of De Abreu, et al. (*13*). A C-18 column with 0.5M phosphate buffer, (pH 6.7):methanol (90:10), mobile phase was used on a high pressure liquid chromatograph (Hewlett Packard, Palo Alto, CA).

Table 1 summarizes skin graft survival and ancillary clinical and laboratory findings in the 6 dogs treated with 8-AG. Significant prolongation of skin graft survival as compared with controls occurred in treated animals (mean ± 1 SD, 26.8 ± 4.6 days versus 11.2 ± 1.3 days) $P<0.01$. In 5 of 6 dogs, as shown in Table 1, this regimen had significant toxicity. Five dogs had anorexia with a mean weight loss of 22%; 2 animals were lethargic during treatment but improved after the drug was discontinued. Of 6 dogs, 3 developed significant thrombocytopenia (nadirs of 4×10^3, 1.7×10^4, and $1.5\times10^4/mm^3$). Clinical bleeding did not occur and platelet counts returned to normal following drug discontinuation. Bone marrow examination during the thrombocytopenic episode revealed megakaryocytic hyperplasia. Lymphocyte counts declined during treatment by a mean of 53±14% compared with pretreatment level. During treatment 2 dogs died. One was found dead on day 31 postgrafting, two weeks following the last 8-AG administration. Autopsy did not reveal a specific cause of death, the skin graft was viable, and chemistries at the time of last treatment, 10 days before death, showed only elevation of blood urea nitrogen to 56 mg/dl. The other dog died while under general anesthesia for a bone marrow aspiration. The bone marrow showed megakaryocytic hyperplasia.

One animal had serial plasma samples analyzed at intervals following a bolus injection of 100 mg/kg 8-AG. Peak concentration of 8-AG were 88 micromolar immediately following injection and rapidly declined to less than 1 micromolar in 25 min. Inosine plasma concentrations were followed during 8-AG treatment in all dogs. Initial inosine concentrations were undetectable (less than 1 micromolar). All dogs had elevated inosine levels during treatment, with the highest level attained being 20.4 micromolar. No deoxyadenosine, guanosine, or deoxyguanosine were detected (detection limit = 1 micromolar) in plasma samples. In vitro studies on dog whole blood demonstrated 8-AG disappearance from plasma decreasing from 100 μmol/L to 1 μmol/L in 20 min.

In summary 8-AG in doses of 100 mg/kg body weight given i.v. on a 3-times-per-week schedule could be demonstrated to significantly prolong skin graft survival in dogs. Clinical toxicity was moderate-to-severe. Thrombocytopenia was noted in 50% of the treated dogs and was associated with megakaryocytic hyperplasia of the bone marrow. One dog died of unknown causes. PNP inhibition resulting in depressed cell-mediated immunity is suggested as the mechanism of action of 8-AG. Inhibitors of purine nucleotide metabolic pathways may provide a new class of immunosuppressive agents for further study.

JOHN B. BENEAR
DON FREDERICK
LEROY TOWNSEND[2]
ROBERT B. EPSTEIN[3]
Department of Medicine
University of Oklahoma Health Science Center

[2] University of Michigan.
[3] Reprint requests should be sent to: Robert B. Epstein, M.D., Chief, Section of Oncology, University of Oklahoma Health Science Ctr., P.O. Box 26901, Oklahoma City, OK 73190.

University of Michigan School of Pharmacy
Department of Medicinal Chemistry
Section of Oncology
Veterans Administration Center
Oklahoma City, Oklahoma

REFERENCES

1. Giblett ER, Amman AJ, Wara DW, Sandman R, Diamond LK. Nucleoside-phosphorylase deficiency in a child with severely defective T-cell immunity and normal B-cell immunity. Lancet 1975; 1: 1010.
2. Giblett ER, Anderson JE, Cohen F, Pollara B, Meuwissen HJ. Adenosine deaminase deficiency in two patients with severely impaired cellular immunity. Lancet 1972; 2: 1067.
3. Epstein RB, Fey T, Sarpel S. Prolongation of canine skin graft survival by deoxycoformycin. Transplantation 1982; 33; 208.
4. Ruers TJM, van der Linden CJ, Koostra G. 2 Deoxycoformycin: a new immunosuppressive drug with a potency comparable to Cyclosporin A. 10th Int Cong Transplant Soc 1984; S14.6(A).
5. Edwards LN, Gelfand EW, Biggar D, Fox IH. Partial deficiency of purine phosphorylase: studies of purine pyrimidine metabolism. J Lab Clin Med 1978; 91: 736.
6. Gelfand EW, Cohen A, How A, Dosch HM. Selectivity of nucleoside toxicity during T-cell ontogeny: implication for therapy. Clin Res 1980; 28: 346A.
7. Lelchuk R, Cooke A, Playfair JHL. Differential sensitivity to 2-deoxyguanosine of antigen specific and nonspecific suppressor T-cells in delayed hypersensitivity. Cell Immunol 1982; 72: 202.
8. Dosch HM, et al. Inhibition of suppressor T-cell development following deoxyguanosine administration. Nature 1980; 285: 494.
9. Bril H, van den Akker TW, Molendijik-Lok BD, Bianchi ATJ, Benner R. Influence of 2-deoxyguanosine upon the development of DTH effector T-cells and suppressor T-cells in vivo. J Immunol 1984; 132: 599.
10. Cohen A, Lee JW, Gelfand EW. Selective toxicity of deoxyguanosine and arabinosyl guanine for T-leukemic cells. Blood 1983; 61: 600.
11. Kazmers IS, Mitchell BS, Dadonna PE, Wotring LL, Townsend LB, Kelley WN. Inhibition of purine nucleoside phosphorylase by 8-aminoguanosine: selective toxicity for T lymphoblasts. Science 1981; 214: 1137.
12. Holmes RE, Robins RK. Purine nucleosides IX. The synthesis of 9-B-ribofuranosyl uric acid and other related 8-substituted purine ribonucleosides. J Am Chem Soc 1965; 87: 1772.
13. De Abreu RA, Van Baal JM, De Bruyn C, Bakkeren J, Schretlen E. High-performance liquid chromatographic determination of purine and pyrimidine bases, ribonucleosides, deoxyribonucleosides and cyclic ribonucleotides in biological fluids. J Chromatogr 1982; 229: 67.

Received 15 May 1985.
Accepted 24 May 1985.

CYCLOSPORINE BLOOD CONCENTRATIONS IN THE MANAGEMENT OF RENAL TRANSPLANT RECIPIENTS

A group of 58 renal allograft recipients received initial oral cyclosporine (CsA)[1] doses of 10 mg/kg for three days, together with a steroid supplement. Subsequently, dosage adjustment of CsA was made in the light of clinical signs of graft rejection and pre-dose whole-blood concentrations of CsA measured by a commercially available radioimmunoassay kit (Sandoz Products Ltd.). Retrospective analysis of the CsA concentrations measured during the two months following transplantation showed that, in 23 of 32 patients who had shown signs of graft rejection responding to therapy with methylprednisolone CsA, blood concentrations were below 200 μg/L close to the rejection episode; the association between graft rejection and this threshold value was statistically significant. Two months after transplantation there was a poor correlation between dosage and blood CsA concentrations. It is concluded that measurement of blood CsA concentrations is a useful guide to optimal dosage, being more helpful than knowledge of the daily dose.

CsA is a cyclic undecapeptide of fungal origin that is being used increasingly as an immunosuppressive drug following transplant surgery. There is no concensus on the value of measuring CsA concentrations in patients receiving the drug, a problem compounded by methodological variables, including the choice of analytical technique and sample matrix. (*1*, *2*). A recent review (*3*) suggested that access to drug monitoring facilities, though interesting, was not essential to clinical management. We present our experience of blood CsA measurements as a guide to dosage requirements following renal transplantation.

A group of 58 renal allograft recipients (47 M/11 F, age [mean±SD] 42±12years) were studied following transplantation (50 cadaveric, 8 living-related). There were 36 patients who had undergone their first graft; 22 had already had one or more failed transplants on a regimen of azathioprine and steroids. Five patients were diabetic, and a further five had been desensitized for 12–18 weeks prior to transplantation, using cyclophosphamide and prednisolone (with plasma exchange in one case), in an attempt to remove and suppress HLA antibodies (*4*). The clinical and laboratory data for the first two months of intensive monitoring following transplantation were reviewed retrospectively.

Prior to transplantation all patients were transfused with six units of blood. More recently each unit of blood contained 5 mg CsA (as the i.v. preparation). Preoperatively, immunosuppression was commenced with 1 g i.v. methylprednisolone and one oral dose of CsA, 5 mg/kg. Postoperatively, irrespective of graft function, patients received prednisolone 10 mg and CsA 5 mg/kg orally, at 12-hourly intervals, for three days. Subsequently, the CsA dose was reduced to a maintenance dose of 5 mg/kg/day, or less, depending on clinical signs and CsA blood concentrations. Following earlier experience in this unit, CsA doses were adjusted to maintain predose blood concentrations within a target range of 200–400 μg/L. The prednisolone dose was reduced to 10 mg daily after about one month, depending on graft function. Patients receiving a second graft, or whose cytotoxic antibody titer had been high preoperatively, also received antithymocyte globulin (2 mg/kg/day) for 10 days.

Cimetidine, 200 mg twice daily, was administered to 20 patients for the period under study. Other drug therapy comprised: phenobarbitone (1), phenytoin (2), depot phenothiazine (1), and antituberculous therapy (rifampicin and isoniazid [2], isoniazid [1]).

Graft function was assessed clinically and with the help of ultrasonography and thrice-weekly isotope renograms (*5*). The

[1] Abbreviations used: CsA, cyclosporine; CV, within-assay reproducibility; RIA, radioimmunoassay.

diagnosis of acute rejection was made clinically by evaluation of the following symptoms and signs: malaise, graft tenderness, oliguria, increasing blood pressure, and pyrexia (without other evidence of infection). The diagnosis was supported by a rising serum creatinine concentration and/or a deterioration in the renogram flow index. Graft rejection was treated with three daily 1 g i.v. boluses of methylprednisolone and changes in CsA dosage, where appropriate. Renal biopsy was performed when the diagnosis of an episode of poor transplant function was uncertain or the response to increased immunosuppression was unsatisfactory. CsA-induced nephrotoxicity was assumed only after excluding other causes of graft dysfunction.

Blood samples for renal function tests and CsA analysis were drawn before the morning dose of CsA and, when possible, before breakfast; samples were collected daily during in-patient care, and three times per week from out-patients. Whole-blood concentrations of CsA were measured using a radioimmunoassay kit (Sandoz Products Ltd.). The within-assay reproducibility (CV) of the method at 500 μl/L was 5% (n=10) while the between-assay value at this concentration was 8% (n=25); the limit of accurate measurement was 65 μg/L. Appropriate control samples, prepared from an independent stock solution of CsA hydrochloride, were included in each assay, and the laboratory was a participant in the UK Cyclosporin Quality Assessment Scheme. Results were usually available 2–3 days after sampling.

During the first two months after transplantation CsA concentrations averaged less than 200 μg/L for at least two consecutive measurements in 28 of the 58 patients. Of these 28 patients, 23 (82.1%) showed signs of rejection—which, in 22 cases, responded to the appropriate therapy; the remaining five patients had no documented evidence of rejection. The rejection episodes occured 5±3 days (range 1–15) after a period of low CsA concentrations; the mean CsA concentration during these periods was 160±96 μg/L (n=93 observations). The patient who failed to respond to treatment had her rejection episode 22 days posttransplant; her mean CsA concentration over this period was 174±158 μg/L (n=12), despite doses of up to 8.9 mg/kg/day.

In 18 patients CsA concentrations were consistently in the range of 200–1000 μg/L. Of these patients 13 suffered no rejection episodes—the mean CsA concentration during the two months following transplantation being 452±218 μg/L (n=309). Five patients showed symptoms and signs consistent with the diagnosis of rejection and responded to therapy. In these latter patients the mean CsA concentration in the five days preceding each rejection episode was 583±221 μg/L (n=25).

CsA concentrations greater than 1000 μg/L were recorded on at least two consecutive occasions in 12 patients. Of these, eight were free from graft rejection throughout the two-month period (mean CsA 560±427 μg/L [n=227]). However, four patients did have signs consistent with rejection. In two cases this followed a CsA dosage reduction that produced CsA concentrations in the range of 200–300 μg/L; for the five days preceding the diagnosis of rejection CsA concentrations were 237±143 μg/L. These rejection episodes responded to therapy with steroids and an increase in CsA dose. In the remaining two cases signs of rejection occurred in association with CsA concentrations in the range 155–1238 μg/L, following CsA dose reduction; the mean CsA concentration for the five days preceding rejection was 582±376 μg/L. In these cases the episodes were refractory to treatment, and one of the grafts was ultimately lost after two months; on biopsy the kidney showed signs of chronic rejection. The remaining patient showed slow improvement and continues with good renal function (serum creatinine 100 μmol/L at two months).

Thus, of 58 patients, 32 had signs of rejection during the first two months after transplantation; in 23 of these CsA concentrations below 200 μg/L had been noted. The association between rejection and this threshold value of 200 μg/L was significant, $\chi^2=13.9$, $P<0.001$.

Two months after transplantation the mean CsA concentration in our patients was 402±168 μg/L; the dose varied widely, 2.3–9.6 mg/kg/day, mean 5.1±1.9, and there was no significant correlation between daily dose and CsA concentration (r=0.06, $P=0.6$).

The effect of methylprednisolone therapy on CsA concentrations was noted in 22 of our patients who received three daily pulses of the drug without any alteration in CsA dosage. Mean pre-dose CsA concentration on the day methylprednisolone therapy started was 282±207 μg/L, compared with 359±213 μg/L on the third day of therapy ($P<0.01$, Wilcoxon test). No data relating the effect of other drug therapy on CsA concentrations could be collected systematically because of small patient numbers or concurrent changes in CsA dosage.

Cyclosporine has been used in the treatment of a variety of clinical conditions, but its principal indication is as an immunosuppressive agent following organ transplantation. In this latter situation it may be used as a single agent or with a low-dose steroid supplement, its efficacy in combination with prednisolone being as good or better than conventional regimens (*6*). In addition, its more selective action and steroid-sparing capacity, compared with alternative therapy, have led to a reduction in the incidence of posttransplant complications (*7*).

The use of cyclosporine may result in nephrotoxicity that, although well recognized, can be difficult to distinguish from acute (or chronic) rejection episodes following renal transplantation. Differential diagnosis of drug-induced renal toxicity or rejection may require the use of invasive techniques, such as renal biopsy, fine-needle aspiration for differential cell count, or intrarenal pressure monitoring (*3*)—and, even then, the results may not give a definitive answer.

We have used the radioimmunoassay (RIA) measurement of whole blood CsA concentrations as a guide to the dosage requirements of renal allograft recipients. Two months after transplantation the mean concentration achieved was 402 μg/L, but the dose necessary to achieve the observed concentrations varied widely, and knowledge of the daily dose alone would have been a poor indicator of the blood concentration.

During the first two months of intensive monitoring there was a clear association between graft rejection and pre-dose concentrations below 200 μg/L, while blood CsA concentrations in excess of 1000 μg/L appeared to confer no additional clinical benefit. Each episode of rejection responded to treatment, with the exception of one patient with a persistently low CsA concentration and two patients who had been noted to have comparatively high concentrations. Whether CsA-induced toxicity had contributed to the clinical signs in any of our cases is not clear, owing to our lack of a selective diagnostic test. However, in all but the two latter cases, the response to steroid therapy was sustained, despite an unaltered or increased CsA dose.

Several groups have already suggested a relationship between the clinical effects of CsA and its concentration in blood, plasma, or serum (*8–10*). The interpretation of these data is complicated by a number of methodological problems. First, CsA concentrations are substantially higher if measured by RIA, using the kit supplied by Sandoz Products, compared with the more selective technique of high-performance liquid chromatography (*11*). This finding is to be expected since the antibody supplied with the RIA kit crossreacts with several metabolites of CsA that are closely related to the parent compound (*12*). However, with the use of standardized times for sample collection, a relatively constant relationship between the two techniques has been shown (*13*). Second, whichever technique is used, the choice of sample matrix affects the result. The drug exhibits temperature-dependent binding to erythrocytes, resulting in lower plasma and serum CsA concentrations compared with whole-blood concentrations (*14*). Although it has been suggested that separation of plasma from whole blood under temperature-controlled conditions yields reproducible results (*15*), others have found such procedures unreliable (*16*). Finally, inter-center comparison of results is difficult since there has been no standardization of sample collection time or choice of sample.

Despite these problems there are some practical advantages to the use of the RIA and its crossreactivity with CsA metabolites does not preclude the possibility of it producing results that are clinically useful, since neither the immunosuppressive nor toxicological properties of these compounds have been clearly defined.

Whether a more selective measurement of cyclosporine, using high-performance liquid chromatography or a more specific antibody in the RIA, would prove more useful clinically has yet to be established (*17*). The results presented here indicate that, despite the inherent problems noted with the currently available RIA, the measurement of CsA in predose blood samples is of clinical value. The blood concentrations were a better guide to dosage requirements than standardized doses and may, therefore, be of help in selecting the optimum effective dose. While the findings of this study help to clarify the minimum effective concentrations of the drug needed during the early period after renal transplantation, they do not define the significance of the measurements on long-term graft function or their role during chronic maintenance therapy. Studies are in progress to address these areas.

M.E. ROGERSON[2,3]
J.T. MARSDEN[4]
K.E. REID[2]
M. BEWICK,[2]
D.W. HOLT[5,6]

[2] Dulwich Hospital.

[3] Present address: St. Mary's Hospital, Portsmouth, Hants. PO3 6AD.

[4] King's College Hospital.

[5] Guy's Hospital.

[6] To whom correspondence should be addressed.

Renal Unit, Dulwich Hospital, London SE 22
Chemical Pathology Department, King's College Hospital, London SE 5
Poisons Unit, Guy's Hospital, London SE 1

REFERENCES

1. Varghese Z, Chan MK, Steele LV, et al. How to measure cyclosporin. Lancet 1984; 1: 1407.
2. Dieperink H. Temperature dependency of CSP plasma levels. Lancet 1983; 1: 416
3. Salaman JR. Cyclosporin in renal transplantation: a guide to management. Lancet 1984; 2:269.
4. Taube DH, Williams DG, Cameron JS, et al. Renal transplantation after removal and prevention of resynthesis of HLA antibodies. Lancet 1984; 1: 824.
5. Hilson AJW, Maisey MN, Brown CB, Ogg CS, Bewick MS. Dynamic renal transplant imaging with Tc99M DTPA supplemented by a transplant perfusion index in the management of renal transplantation. J Nucl Med 1978; 19: 994.
6. Canadian Multicentre Transplant Study Group. A randomised clinical trial of cyclosporin in cadaveric renal transplantation. N Engl J Med 1983; 309: 809.
7. European Multicentre Trial Group. Cyclosporin in cadaveric renal transplantation: one year follow-up of a multicentre trial. Lancet 1983; 2: 986.
8. Keown PA, Ulan RA, Wall WJ, et al. Immunological and pharmacological monitoring in the clinical use of cyclosporin A. Lancet 1981; 1: 686.
9. Myers BD, Ross J, Newton L, Luetscher J, Perlroth M. Cyclosporine associated chronic nephropathy. N Engl J Med 1984; 311: 699.
10. Irschik E, Tilg H, Niederwieser D, et al. Cyclosporin blood levels do correlate with clinical complications. Lancet 1984; 2: 692.
11. Carruthers SG, Freeman DJ, Koegler JC, et al. Simplified liquid chromatographic analysis for cyclosporin A, and comparison with RIA. Clin Chem 1983; 29: 180.
12. Schran HF, Abisch E. Monitoring of cyclosporine: a status report. Ther Drug Monit 1984; 6: 371.
13. Robinson WT, Schran HF, Barry EP. Methods to measure cyclosporine levels: high pressure liquid chromatography, radioimmunoassay and correlation. Transplant Proc 1983; 15(suppl 1): 2403.
14. Wenk M, Follath F, Abisch E. Temperature dependency of apparent cyclosporin A concentrations in plasma. Clin Chem 1983; 29: 1865.
15. Yatscoff RW, Rush DN, Jeffery JR. Effects of sample preparation on concentrations of cyclosporin A measured in plasma. Clin Chem 1984; 30: 1812.
16. Bennett MJ, Carpenter KH, Worthy E, Lilleyman JS. Cyclosporin concentrations in whole blood and plasma. Clin Chem 1984; 30: 817.
17. Holt DW, White DJG. How to measure cyclosporin. Lancet 1984; 2: 228.

Received 19 March 1985.
Accepted 9 June 1985.

About to emerge...

a major advance in immunosuppressive therapy

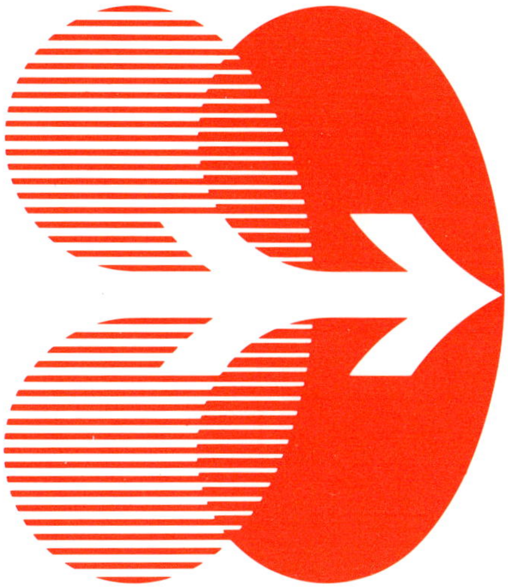

ORTHO

ORTHO PHARMACEUTICAL CORPORATION
Raritan, New Jersey 08869

OJ-374

Information for Subscribers

Published monthly, two volumes a year, beginning January and July.

Annual Subscription Rates—U. S. A. AND POSSESSIONS: personal, $105.00; institutional, $130.00; single copies, $12.00. FOREIGN: personal, $120.00; institutional, $145.00; single copies, $15.00. Institutional (multiple reader) rate applies to libraries, schools, hospitals, clinics, group practices, and federal commercial, and private institutions and organizations. A special in-training rate of $60.00 ($85.00 foreign) is available to residents, fellows, interns and students. (Prices subject to change) In requesting this rate, which is limited to three years, please give training status and name of institution. Subscribers may request that their copies be sent by air mail; the extra charge entailed for air service will be billed to the subscriber.

New and renewal subscriptions are entered to begin with the January or July issue. Correspondence regarding subscriptions should be addressed to the publishers.

Change of address. Publisher must be notified 60 days in advance. Undeliverable journals will be destroyed. Duplicates (if available) can be ordered from the publishers at the regular price of single issues.

Reprints of individual articles are available *only* from authors.

Microfilm. For availability, inquire of Williams & Wilkins.

Japanese Yen price is available from our sole agent: USACO Corporation, 13-12 Shimbashi 1-Chome, Minato-Ku, Tokyo 105, Japan, telephone 03-502-6471.

WILLIAMS & WILKINS

Publishers of Books and Periodicals in Medicine and the Allied Sciences
428 East Preston Street, Baltimore, Md. 21202, U.S.A.

AUTHOR INDEX

Autenried, P., 413

Babayan, R. K., 536
Ballardie, F. W., 537
Belzer, F. O., 544
Blanchard, J. M., 527
Bowen, A., 539
Bozdech, M. J., 544
Brendel, W., 426
Bron, K. M., 539
Brown, C. B., 464

Carter, N. P., 468
Chapman, J. R., 468
Chen, X., 495
Cohen, A. D., 534
Cook, D. J., 447
Cooper, E. L., 514

Daniel, V., 454
Deierhoi, M. H., 546
Dibelius, A., 426
Dreikorn, K., 454

Eastwood, S. L., 534
Evans, D. J., 537

Fabre, J. W., 499
Fawzy, F. I., 478, 484
Field, M. J., 529
Fisher, M., 468
Flechner, S. M., 459

Gibbons, C. P., 464
Goldstein, G., 431
Gores, P. F., 529
Gottschalk, R., 489

Halloran, P. F., 413
Henny, F. C., 442

Idelson, B. A., 536

Jarowenko, M., 436
Jonker, M., 431

Kahan, B. D., 436, 459
Kamata, K., 495
Kay, R., 464
Kerman, R., 436
Königsberger, H., 426
Kramer, W. G., 459

Landsverk, J., 478, 484
Lee, H. M., 474
Lorber, M. I., 459

MacSween, J. M., 534
Masaki, Y., 495
Mayoral, J., 529
McCann, R. L., 541
McGeorge, M. B., 474
McNally, P. G., 464
Mendez-Picon, G., 474
Milton, A. D., 499

Mohanakumar, T., 474
Monaco, A. P., 489
Morris, P. J., 468
Mozes, M. R., 527

Naimark, A., 536
Neuhaus, P., 431
Nooij, F. J. M., 431

Okubo, M., 495
Oljans, P. J., 442
O'Neal, W. K., 536
Opelz, G., 454

Paul, L. C., 442
Pembrey, R. G., 421
Penkrot, R. J., 539
Permanetter, W., 426
Pifer, L., 436
Pilarski, L. M., 521
Pollak, R., 527
Posner, M. P., 474

Raftery, A. T., 464
Rajaraman, K., 534
Rees, A. J., 537
Roch, P., 514

Sanfilippo, F., 508, 541
Schäfer, A. J., 454
Scornik, J. C., 447
Segal, M. C., 539
Skolnick, M. L., 539
Slasky, B. S., 539
Sollinger, H. W., 544
Spencer, S. C., 499
Starzl, T. E., 539
Summerton, C. B., 464
Sutherland, D. E. R., 529

Tai, J., 531
Tanke, H. J., 442
Ting, A., 468
Treseler, P. A., 508
Tze, W. J., 531

Uchiyama, T., 495

Van Buren, C. T., 459
Van Es, L. A., 442
Van Suylichem, P., 431
Von Specht, B. U., 426

Wadgymar, A., 413
Walter, P., 426
Warren, H. S., 421
Wellisch, D. K., 478, 484
Wideman, C., 459
Williams, G., 537
Winearls, C. G., 537
Wolcott, D. L., 478, 484
Wolfe, J. A., 541
Wood, M. L., 489

Zajko, A. B., 539

0041-1337/86/4104-0413$02.00/0
TRANSPLANTATION

Vol. 41, No. 4
Printed in U.S.A.

Transplantation
OVERVIEW

THE REGULATION OF EXPRESSION OF MAJOR HISTOCOMPATIBILITY COMPLEX PRODUCTS[1]

PHILIP F. HALLORAN,[2] ARTURO WADGYMAR, AND PETER AUTENRIED[3]

The Department of Research, Mount Sinai Hospital; and the Departments of Medicine and Immunology, University of Toronto, Toronto, Ontario, Canada

Recent overviews have summarized the state of knowledge concerning the alloantigens of vascular endothelium (*1*) and the changes that these antigens undergo with interferons (*2*). The purpose of the present discussion is to highlight some recent work concerning regulation of class I and class II antigens of the major histocompatibility complex (MHC),* especially in non-marrow-derived cells, emphasizing the observations relevant to the biology of transplantation. In particular, we discuss the evidence that MHC product expression can be modulated by many physiologic, pathologic, and pharmacologic influences, and that these changes may be crucial to the immune events in the tissue. Reference cannot be made to all relevant publications because of space limitations, and the reader is referred to some recent reviews (*3–7*). Class III genes and Qa-Tla genes will not be discussed.

Why study MHC regulation? The concept that class II antigen expression quantitatively influences immune responses is supported by certain studies of I-E expression in F_1 hybrid mice (*8, 9*). In these experiments, low responsiveness in the I-E-restricted response to a nominal antigen (pigeon cytochrome c) was found to be due to quantitative reduction in I-E product. Using antigen-presenting cells varying quantitatively in I-E product expression, these workers found that an 8-fold diminution in Ia antigen expression per cell rendered the antigen-presenting cells ineffective, unless much higher quantities of nominal antigen were used. Indeed, the responsiveness of cloned T cells to the nominal antigen on antigen-presenting cells was proportional to the product of the Ia antigen concentration and the nominal antigen concentration (*10*). Thus, in an I-E restricted response, with a fixed amount of nominal antigen, responsiveness of T cells varied directly with the density of the I-E product on the antigen-presenting cell. Certain results indicate that similar considerations hold for the I-A molecule (*5*), and that Ia density on B cells influences the interactions of B cells with T cells (*11*).

Parallel considerations point to the conclusion that class I MHC product expression is relevant to the function of cytotoxic T cells of the Lyt-2 or T8-positive phenotype. The amount of MHC product appears to determine target cell susceptibility to lysis: various viruses can alter MHC product expression on target cells either up or down, and the susceptibility of the target cells to lysis by cytotoxic T cells varies in the same direction (*12*). Oncogenicity of adenovirus type 12 may be related to its ability to depress MHC product expression on infected cells, whereas nononcogenic adenoviruses increase MHC product expression (*13, 14*). Similarly, increases in class I antigen expression on reticulocytes also may influence outcome of malarial infections (*15*).

These considerations also apply to alloimmunity: it is likely that alterations in MHC antigen density influence the alloimmune response in much the same manner as the MHC-restricted response. One of the reasons for the large number of clones responding to particular MHC alleles could be the relatively high density of allodeterminants when compared with the "modified self" type of determinant in MHC-restricted responses (*16*).

Another effect of MHC product modulation is that decreasing MHC expression may increase target cell sensitivity to natural killer (NK) cells (*17*). It is possible to visualize the NK system as preventing abnormal cells from eluding destruction by down-regulating their MHC product expression to avoid recognition by T cells. Finally, MHC antigen expression may affect non-immunologic phenomena, such as myelopoiesis (*18*), malignant transformation (*19*), and tumor metastatic behavior (*20*).

Regulatory sequences flanking MHC genes. The regulation of gene expression generally involves certain DNA sequences located upstream (5′) to the gene, in the area known as the *promoter.* Two common promoter region sequences are the TATA-box and the CCAAT box. The TATA box, for example, appears to influence the site of initiation of transcription. These and other promoter sequences govern the level of binding of regulatory proteins to DNA, which in turn regulate mRNA polymerase activity and therefore gene transcription (*21*). Promoters are located only at the 5′ end and are a limited distance from the start of the gene, usually 100–1000 bases. In contrast, another type of regulatory element is the *enhancer* sequence, which may be 1000 bases or more upstream or downstream from the gene, and can work in either orientation.

[1] This work was supported by Grant MT5739 from the Medical Research Council of Canada, and by a grant from the Kidney Foundation of Canada.

[2] Address correspondence to: Philip F. Halloran, M.D., Mount Sinai Hospital, Suite 435, 600 University Avenue, Toronto, Canada M5G 1X5.

[3] P.A. was supported by a fellowship from the Kidney Foundation of Canada.

* Abbreviations used: AIDS, acquired immunodeficiency syndrome; EM, electron microscopy; GVHD, graft-versus-host disease; IFN, interferon; LPS, lipopolysaccharide; MHC, major histocompatibility complex; mRNA, messenger RNA; NK, natural killer.

Some regulatory sequences flanking the MHC genes are beginning to be mapped. At least some MHC genes have TATA and CCAAT sequences 5′ to the gene. All murine class II genes have common upstream sequences (*22*) known as the class II box, which may be relevant to their expression. A region of approximately 30 base pairs has recently been described 5′ to two class I genes and one class II gene that is involved in the ability of interferon to induce increased MHC gene expression (*23*). In addition, an enhancer element specific for certain cell types has been reported in association with the class II gene E_B in mouse, which could influence the tissue distribution of class II molecules (*24*).

Some additional factors regulating gene expression could be anti-sense RNA (*25*); alterations in the extent of DNA methylation (*26*); and changes in DNA coiling or helix arrangement. In general, the impact of such types of factors on the expression of MHC products is unknown. Changes in chromatin structure within the MHC have been noted after activation of the DR alpha chain gene (*27*).

Although much of the control of gene expression in eukaryotes (nucleated cell forms) is at the level of transcription, other levels of control are known. Alternative messenger RNA (mRNA) processing has been shown for one MHC gene (*28*) and other mechanisms may also be operating at the translational or post-translational level (*7*). Thus increased mRNA may not necessarily be followed by increased product, and increased product in the whole cell may not be accompanied by increased product expressed on the membrane.

Membrane expression of MHC products in vivo. It is difficult to determine whether MHC products expressed in a cell or tissue in vivo are, in fact, exposed on the membrane of that cell, as they must be to have immunologic relevance. As a result, the in vivo insertion of class I or II molecules into the cell membrane is often assumed but seldom proved. One difficulty is that class I and II antigens in whole tissues are often undetectable after fixation, so that immunoperoxidase and immunofluorescent localization of membrane antigens in tissues is usually done on frozen unfixed sections, which lack definition. Electron microscopic localization is also a problem, since intact tissue may not give ready access to antibodies, and the antigens frequently do not survive the fixation steps necessary for electron microscopy (EM). More work needs to be done with EM localization, since it would also assist studies of the intracellular processing and localization of MHC products.

Ubiquitous and restricted expression of MHC products. It is often stated that class I antigens are ubiquitous, whereas class II antigens have a restricted tissue distribution. In fact, the class I antigens cannot be demonstrated in sections of certain tissues when allospecific antibodies are used: for example, rat (*29*) and mouse (*30*) renal tubules, and rat pancreatic acinar cells (*31*) are negative for class I antigens in tissue sections. The data for human kidney have been reviewed (*32*); again, epithelium of kidney is sometimes negative for class I when allospecific antibodies were used, although it does stain with antibody against monomorphic class I determinants, which stain all the A, B, and C products. In vitro, class I expression in normal cultured cells is the rule, even when no class I can be demonstrated in such cells in vivo. For example, mouse kidney epithelium is negative in vivo but kidney cell cultures are positive in vitro for class I antigens (*30*). Does this mean that class-I-negative cell types in vivo become positive in vitro, or that class I expression in vivo is underestimated by methods based on tissue sections? As a generalization, we can state that class I antigens are not detectable in all cells in vivo, although the possibility of low but undetectable levels remains. The level of class I expression tends to be higher in class-II-positive cells and lower in class-II-negative cells, suggesting that these products are regulated by similar mechanisms under some circumstances. Moreover, stimuli that induce or increase class II expression usually increase class I expression. Nevertheless, the distinctive ontogeny and tissue distribution of class I compared with class II products indicates that the regulation of the two must involve independent as well as common regulatory mechanisms. The relative expression of individual class I genes, or individual class II genes, can vary (see below)—suggesting that even among genes of the same class, some regulatory differences must exist. Thus the old generalizations such as "restricted" and "ubiquitous" should now be more appropriately expressed in quantitative terms based on observations of the expression of that gene in that tissue.

Regulation of transfected MHC genes. Two types of transfection have been instructive: introducing human or other xenogeneic MHC genes into mouse cells (*33–36*) and introducing allogeneic MHC genes into mouse cells (*37–39*). In either case the genes show evidence of being regulated by influences such as interferon (*33, 35–37*). Transfected human class I genes in mouse cells respond to mouse, but not human, interferon (*34*), indicating that either the receptor binding or some aspect of the postreceptor signalling is species-specific. In mouse embryonal carcinoma cells, the expression of a transfected mouse class I gene has been shown to be developmentally regulated—the same as the normal class I genes in these cells (*38*)—but a transfected rabbit MHC gene was not developmentally regulated in these cells, indicating some species specificity in the developmental regulatory mechanism.

Interferons and MHC expression in vitro. One of the principal modulating influences on MHC product expression in vitro and in vivo is probably interferon. The ability of interferon to induce MHC product expression was first shown by Lindahl, Gresser, and their colleagues (*40–44*), who showed that interferon induced increased histocompatibility antigen expression on mouse L1210 lymphoma cells in vitro and on lymphoid cells in vivo. The investigators showed that the effect in vitro was not due to the accumulation of cells in one phase of the cell cycle. Subsequently their observations have been confirmed and extended many times, using both marrow-derived and non-marrow-derived cells. The effect has been demonstrated with both natural and recombinant DNA-derived-interferons, both of type I (alpha and beta) and of type II (gamma). However, the most striking effects are demonstrable with gamma interferon induction of class II genes.

The marrow-derived cells that have been shown to respond to interferons with altered MHC product expression include macrophages (*45–47*), monocytes (*48, 49*), Langerhans cells (*49, 50*), and mast cells (*51*)—as well as many tumor cell lines derived from these cells (*52*). B cells are more variable in their responsiveness to interferons (*11, 53*), but mitogen-stimulated T cells do respond (*54*). A host of apparently normal non-marrow-derived cells also respond in tissue culture, including endothelial cells (*2, 55, 56*), fibroblasts (*2, 44, 55, 56*), thyroid epithelial cells (*57, 58*), renal tubule epithelial cells (*30, 59*), keratinocytes (*60, 61*), melanocytes (*59, 62, 63*), astrocytes, and other brain cells (*64, 65*), and gut epithelial cells (*66*). A wide variety of cell lines derived from non-marrow-derived cells or tumors respond to interferons in vitro with increased MHC product expression—including heart, kidney, colon, pancreas, bladder, lung, ovary, brain, and melanomas (*59, 63, 67*). Most of the above cells respond to gamma interferon with an increase in class I and class II antigens; among the exceptions were choriocarcinoma and teratocarcinoma, in which class I expression increased but class II antigens could not be induced.

In many studies (*7, 47, 56*) class I or class II mRNA was studied as well as MHC product expression. The mRNA is almost always increased when the MHC product is increased, indicating that transcription is probably a major site of control. It is less clear whether interferon itself is inducing a second mediator: in at least one system this appears to be the case (*68*).

The relative induction of DR versus other class II products in vitro has been studied in certain systems. In some systems DR is increased more than DQ or other class II products (*62, 69*) but the reverse has also been recorded (*49, 63*).

The effects of the interferons on virus replication, NK activity, cell growth, and induction of class I and II MHC antigens tend to differ, such that the NK, growth, and MHC effects differ from the antiviral affects. For example, interferon gamma generally has more effect on MHC gene expression per unit of antiviral activity than have type I interferons, at least in vitro. Some studies have suggested that MHC class II induction is an exclusive property of interferon gamma (*59, 60, 62*), but other studies have disputed this view (*63, 70*). The concensus is that type I interferons induce increased class I MHC product expression with variable class II expression, whereas gamma interferon induces both class I and class II very efficiently. One suggestion is that both beta and gamma interferons can increase class I and class II MHC in cells already transcribing them, but that only gamma can induce class II MHC gene expression de novo (*71*).

Individual I region alpha and beta chain genes may be regulated independently. For example, both the A beta 2 and the A beta 1 genes are transcribed in B cells, but only the A beta 1 gene is transcribed in macrophages, even after interferon (*72*). This observation is interpreted as suggesting that both cell-type-specific and gene-specific mechanisms regulate class II gene expression.

In at least one report (*73*) cultured cells regulated their own class I MHC expression by autocrine production of type I interferon. It will be important to determine how common autocrine interferon production is in the regulation of class I MHC expression in vivo. Similarly, autocrine gamma interferon production could alter T cell MHC expression.

Role of interferons in "normal" MHC product expression. Class I MHC products appear very early in embryonic life, whereas class II antigens appear later—in humans, between the 20th and 32nd weeks of gestation (*74*). The issue of whether class I and/or class II products in various sites are induced or constitutive has not been resolved. For example, in mouse, class I gene expression is detectable at the midsomite (10-day) stage but is induced earlier by interferons, prompting the suggestion that interferon is the physiologic inducer of MHC expression (*75*). This concept has some merit: type I interferon can be produced by many more cell types than type II interferon, and could regulate the more ubiquitous expression of class I antigens. On the other hand, type II interferon production would then await maturation of the T cell system, and then induce class II (as well as increased class I) antigens in a more selected distribution. A physiologic role for gamma interferon in the induction of class II MHC products has also been suggested by studies of the effects of cyclosporine, although such conclusions are debated (see below). It seems likely that some role for "physiologic" interferon levels (*76*) in regulation of normal MHC product expression will be found, but that this may be highly dependent on other variables, such as age, species, microbial flora, and baseline immunologic activity of the host.

The effect of prostaglandins and nonsteroidal antiinflammatory drugs on the expression of MHC genes. Snyder et al. (*77*) first showed that prostaglandins of the E series depress the expression of class II MHC products on macrophages. The nonsteroidal antiinflammatory drug indomethacin augmented MHC product expression on peritoneal macrophages in vivo. This has also been observed with Langerhans cells in vitro (*78*). The mechanism of action of prostaglandins on MHC expression is unknown.

In our studies of MHC product in mouse kidney, we have found moderate but highly variable effects of indomethacin (increased renal tubular class I and class II expression). Thus it is possible that interferons and prostaglandins have a tonic push-pull effect on MHC product expression. Indomethacin may act either to decrease prostaglandin, thereby producing an interferon-like effect, or to increase leukotrienes, actually releasing interferon.

A related phenomenon may be the effect of membrane vesicles, which are known to act through prostaglandin release to inhibit MHC product expression in vitro (*79*). Such vesicles could be relevant to the immunosuppressive effects of some tumors in vivo.

The prostaglandin-interferon link may explain an observation we made in mice given immune stimuli—namely, that when renal tubule class I or class II antigens increase, expression of the same antigens on interstitial cells usually declines (*30*). This could reflect the ability of immune stimuli to increase prostaglandins, which might then inhibit interstitial MHC product expression. The significance of such shifts is unknown.

The regulation of Ia expression by endotoxin or lipopolysaccharide. (LPS). Bacterial endotoxin consists of an aggregate of several LPS chains, plus the associated protein, of various gram-negative bacteria. The LPS is itself a complex lipid (lipid A, a complex of glycosamine sugars with fatty acid side chains) with a polysaccharide side chain consisting of an O region and an R region (*80*). The proliferative response in mouse cells to LPS is under genetic control (*81*).

LPS administration has complex effects on Ia induction, these influences being either positive (*82*) or negative (*83, 84*). The effects could be mediated by the known role of LPS in inducing both interferon (*85*) and prostaglandins in vivo. Curiously, although endotoxin induces interferon production in some cell types, it also induces hyporesponsiveness in many other cell types. The late interferon response is acid-stable but the early response is acid-labile (*86*). It is possible that LPS and endotoxin have no direct effect on MHC product expression, but may alter it by releasing prostaglandin or interferon from target cells, or by inducing an immune response that releases such mediators. The effects of LPS on Ia expression on macrophages and elsewhere may be relevant to the immunomodulatory effects of LPS.

MHC regulation in vivo in non-marrow-derived cells. In vivo the patterns of MHC expression alter in some tissues during local or systemic responses in which interferon is likely to be produced. Sensitivity of various cell types to MHC induction differs: for example, in mouse kidney proximal tubules are more readily induced to express Ia than distal tubules or other epithelial cells (*30*). Capillary endothelial cells remain unchanged or have reduced Ia in these kidneys (*30*). It is not clear whether such differences between various cell types reflect true differences in response, or differences in the amount of interferon or other mediators to which the cells are exposed in a tissue in vivo. Presumably a systemic interferon response in vivo will produce much higher exposure of some cells than others. For example, renal proximal tubule cells normally reabsorb filtered low-molecular-weight proteins such as light chains (molecular weight 25,000 Daltons). Since the molecular weight of interferons in vivo is believed (based on the size of the products of cloned genes) to be at least partially in this range (*87–89*), the filtration and tubular reabsorption mechanism may be responsible for catabolism of a certain amount of interferons (and other mediators) (*90*). The question in such a case is whether interferon that is absorbed from the lumen would be biologically active.

In vivo, increased class II antigen has been studied more frequently than increased class I antigen. Class II is increased in capillary endothelium in the rejection of mouse skin allografts (*91*), and possibly early in rejection of other organ grafts, such as pancreas (*31*). In kidney, MHC products may be induced on endothelium of arteries but remain unchanged in capillary endothelium. Epithelial Ia has been reported to be increased in many situations: in gut epithelium during systemic graft-versus-host disease (GVHD) (*92–94*) and during intraluminal parasitic infections (*93*); in skin epithelium during GVHD (*92–94*), but also after skin grafting (*95*) and during various skin diseases (*96*); in kidney during a wide variety of systemic challenges—including GVHD (*30, 97, 98*), rejection of ascites tumor allografts (*30*), rejection of skin allografts, and in response to interferon—inducing stimuli such as human influenza virus and poly I/poly C.[4] Renal tubule epithelium also becomes positive during kidney graft rejection (*99, 100*), as do parenchymal cells of pancreas (*31*) and myocardium (*101*) during local rejection processes. The relative importance of local versus systemically released lymphokines in each case needs to be determined. It is of interest to note that systemic interferon therapy can induce rejection in human renal transplants (*102*).

The effect of LPS on the expression of renal class I and II MHC antigens in vivo has recently been studied in our laboratory.[5] LPS administration induced an increase in renal tubule epithelial Ia and H-2K, occurring several days after administration of the LPS.

The many examples of altered class II antigen in disease models and human diseases in vivo have recently been reviewed (*3*). In local disease in various organs, particularly immunologic disease, certain parenchymal cells become class II antigen positive. In many other types of disease class II antigen induction has been reported, including autoimmune thyroiditis, various immunologic skin diseases, and certain local inflammatory processes, such as delayed-type hypersensitivity.

In the autoimmune nephritis of MRL-lpr/lpr mice, which have increased macrophage Ia expression (*103*), we have found that the renal lesions are accompanied by a marked increase in intrarenal MHC class II and class I expression. At least some of this is in the tubular epithelium (*104*). There are also extensive peritubular immunoglobulin deposits, and large mononuclear cell infiltrates.

The effect of immunosuppression on MHC product expression. A variety of recent observations have indicated that immunosuppressives may down-regulate normal MHC product expression, or prevent the increase in MHC products that occurs during immunologic stimulation. Cyclosporine has recently been shown to decrease normal MHC product expression in dogs, suggesting that normal MHC product expression is lymphokine-dependent rather than constitutive (*105, 106*). In our studies of mouse kidney, very high levels of cyclosporine result in a modest decrease in normal MHC product expression, although the usual blood levels of cyclosporine do not (*107*). Rose has also raised doubts about the effect of cyclosporine on normal levels of MHC product expression (*108*).

In contrast, cyclosporine is capable of totally inhibiting the induction of increased MHC product expression by immunologic stimuli, at least in mouse kidney (*107, 109*). We believe that, regardless of whether cyclosporine reduces normal MHC product expression, its ability to abrogate induction of increased MHC products may be a critical component of its immunosuppressive effect. Since cyclosporine is known to inhibit gamma interferon production, either directly or through the inhibition of IL-2 production, the suppression of in vivo MHC induction by cyclosporine is probably a reflection of its ability to block lymphokine production.

Other immunosuppressives may have similar effects. Corticosteroids are known to depress class II expression in macrophages (*110*), dendritic cells (*111*), and mast cells (*51*). Whole-body irradiation without reconstitution also decreases renal class I and II expression in mouse kidney (Halloran P.F., unpublished observations). Interestingly, young nude mice, which are very deficient in T cells, appear to have MHC expression similar to that of their normal (nu/+) littermates, casting doubt on the importance of T cell lymphokines in normal MHC product expression. Nude mice do not respond to immunologic challenges by increased renal MHC expression, however (*30*).

The expression of MHC products is abnormal in some human immunodeficiency diseases. In the acquired immunodeficiency syndrome (*AIDS*), class II antigens are reduced on epidermal Langerhans cells (*112*). This in turn could be either a consequence or a cause of the deficient production of IL-2 and gamma interferon in these patients. All MHC products are reduced on lymphocytes in one hereditary combined immunodeficiency syndrome, although the relationship between the immunodeficiency and the defective HLA antigen expression is unknown. The disease is probably a defect in MHC gene regulation, since the MHC genes can be detected in these patients by hybridization with specific DNA probes (*113*). In one variant, class-II-deficient severe combined immunodeficiency, evidence has been presented that the defect is in a transacting, non-MHC gene, which is necessary for class II gene expression and responses to gamma interferon (*114*).

In summary, immunosuppression and some types of immunodeficiency may be associated with reduced MHC product expression. The effect of immunosuppression on normal MHC expression seems variable, perhaps because normal MHC expression may have both constitutive and induced components (see above). It is more clear that immunosuppressives or T cell

[4] Halloran et al., manuscript submitted for publication.

[5] Jephtha-Ochola et al., manuscript submitted for publication.

deficiency can blunt or inhibit the induction of massive increases in MHC product expression during immune stimuli, which may be crucial to the pathogenesis of some local immune processes. If so, this could be a major effect of immunosuppressives or of immunodeficiency states such as AIDS. But pathways of induction via type I interferon and other factors from non-T cells may also exist: for example, we have recently demonstrated that poly I/C, a type I interferon inducer, induces increased Ia and H-2K expression in mouse kidney, even in nude mice and in mice on cyclosporine. Thus resistance of MHC expression to immunosuppressives should not necessarily imply that expression is constitutive: non-lymphokine-inducing factors such as type I interferons may also play a role in vivo.

Other influences. The influences on MHC gene expression can be summarized as follows:

Positive	Negative
1. Ontogeny and differentiation	1. Malignant transformation
2. Cell activation	2. Alpha fetoprotein
3. Interferons	3. Cyclosporine
4. Non-interferon interleukin	4. Glucocorticoids
5. Calcitriol	5. Chloramphenicol
6. Virus infection	6. Virus infection
7. Lipopolysaccharide	7. Lipopolysaccharide
8. Indomethacin	8. Prostaglandins
9. Sodium butyrate	9. Membrane vesicles from tumor cells
10. Lactogenic hormones	10. F_c-receptor binding
11. Non-MHC gene(s)	11. Beryllium

One of the initial demonstrations of induction of class II antigens was in breast epithelial cells in response to lactation and lactogenic hormones (*115*). Alpha fetoprotein has been reported to inhibit macrophage Ia expression in vitro (*116*), an action that could be relevant to the proposed immunoregulatory effect of this protein in pregnancy. Calcitriol (*117*) and sodium butyrate (*118*) induce class I antigen expression on certain tumor lines in vitro. Chloramphenicol moderately decreases lymphoid H-2 antigen expression in vivo (*119*), and F_c receptor binding downregulates gamma-interferon-induced Ia induction on macrophages (*120*). Beryllium and other adjuvants also increase macrophage Ia expression (*121*). Malignant transformation, on the other hand, may select for low expression of class I MHC antigens, as a strategy to escape from host immune responses (*122, 123*).

Some problems in MHC product regulation. From these considerations, we are left with many areas of uncertainty, such as:

(A) What DNA binding proteins alter MHC gene transcription? To what sites do they bind?

(B) How important are alternative mRNA processing, translational, posttranslational, and other levels of control of MHC product expression, compared with transcriptional control, in the regulating amount of biologically relevant MHC product on the cell membrane?

(C) How can we decide whether MHC products in tissue sections are inserted into the plasma membrane?

(D) Is normal MHC product expression, particularly in nonlymphoid cells, constitutive, or does it depend on interferons or other soluble inducers? How do interferons regulate MHC product expression and what "second messengers" or mediators are involved? How can normal MHC product expression be suppressed?

(E) MHC product expression is frequently altered in disease states in tissues. Is this a primary event, essential to the development of the disease state, or is it secondary to tissue injury? Which in vivo changes are relevant to immune mechanisms and which are irrelevant epiphenomena?

(F) Is induction of increased MHC products on parenchymal cells or on arterial endothelium necessary for graft rejection—either cell-mediated or humoral or both—to occur?

This information is thus essential to evaluate the key hypothesis: that MHC product expression is a major determinant of T cell activation, a common pathway through which many influences such as IL-2, prostaglandins, and interferons may act. A corollary is that many immunosuppressives may act at this level as well—e. g., corticosteroids and cyclosporine. If so, monitoring and manipulation of MHC product expression could prove to be useful in clinical management of immune processes.

REFERENCES

1. Paul LC, Baldwin WM, van Es LA. Vascular endothelial antigens in renal transplantation. Transplantation 1985; 40: 117.
2. Pober JS, Collins T, Gimbrone MA, Libby P, Reiss CS. Inducible expression of class II major histocompatibility complex antigens and the immunogenicity of vascular endothelium. Transplantation (in press).
3. Forsum U, Claesson K, Hjelm E, et al. Class II transplantation antigens: distribution in tissues and involvement in disease. Scand J Immunol 1985; 21: 389.
4. Mengle-Gaw L, McDevitt HO. Genetics and expression of mouse Ia antigens. Annu Rev Immunol 1985; 3: 367.
5. Janeway CA, Bottomly K, Babich J, et al. Quantitative variation in Ia antigen expression plays a central role in immune regulation. Immunol Today 1984; 5: 99.
6. Trinchieri G, Perussia B. Immune interferon: a pleiotropic lymphokine with multiple effects. Immunol Today 1985; 6: 131.
7. Rosa F, Hatat D, Abadie A, Fellous M. Regulation of histocompatibility antigens by interferon. Ann Inst Pasteur [Immunol] 1985; 136C: 103.
8. McNicholas JM, Murphy DB, Matis LA, et al. Immune response gene function correlates with the expression of an Ia antigen: I. Preferential association of certain A_e and E_a chains results in a quantitative deficiency in expression of an A_e:E_a complex. J Exp Med 1982; 155: 490.
9. Matis LA, Jones PP, Murphy DB, et al. Immune response gene function correlates with the expression of an Ia antigen: II. A quantitative deficiency in A_e:E_a complex expression causes a corresponding defect in antigen presenting cell function. J Exp Med 1982; 155: 508.
10. Matis LA, Glimcher LH, Paul WE, Schwartz RH. Magnitude of response of histocompatibility-restricted T-cell clones is a function of the product of the concentrations of antigen and Ia molecules. Proc Natl Acad Sci USA 1983; 80: 6019.
11. Kehrl JH, Muraguchi A, Fauci AS. The modulation of membrane Ia on human B lymphocytes. Cell Immunol 1985; 92: 391.
12. Flyer DC, Burakoff SJ, Faller DV. Retrovirus induced changes in major histocompatibility complex antigen expression influence susceptibility to lysis by cytotoxic T lymphocytes. J Immunol 1985; 135: 2287.
13. Schrier PI, Bernards R, Vaessen RTMJ, Houweling A, van der Eb AJ. Expression of class I major histocompatibility antigens switched off by highly oncogenic adenovirus 12 in transformed rat cells. Nature 1983; 305: 771.
14. Rosenthal A, Wright S, Quade K, Gallimore P, Cedar H. Grosvelld F. Increased MHC H-2K gene transcription in cultured mouse embryo cells after adenovirus infection. Nature 1985; 315: 579.
15. Jayawardena AN, Mogil R, Murphy DB, Burger D, Gershon RK.

Enhanced expression of H-2K and H-2D antigens on reticulocytes infected with *Plasmodium yoelii.* Nature 1983; 302: 621.
16. Bevan MJ. High determinant density may explain the phenomenon of alloreactivity. Immunol Today 1984; 5: 128.
17. Taniguchi K, Kaerre K, Klein G. Lung colonization and metastasis by disseminated B16 melanoma cells: H-2 associated control at the level of the host and the tumor cell. Intl J Cancer 1985; 36: 503.
18. Broxmeyer HE, Dupont B. A role for class II major histocompatibility complex antigens in the regulation of myelopoiesis. Prog Allergy 1985; 36: 203.
19. Brickell PM, Latchman DS, Murphy D, Wilson K, Rigby PWJ. The class I major histocompatibility antigen gene activated in a line of SV 40 transformed mouse cells is H-2D^d not Qa/Tla. Nature 1985; 316: 162.
20. Hammerling GJ, Wallich R, Bulbuc N, Katzav S, Segal S, Feldman M. Abrogation of metastatic properties of tumour cells by de novo expression of H-2K antigens following H-2 gene transfection. nature 1985; 315: 301.
21. Dynan WS, Tjian R. Control of eukaryotic messenger RNA synthesis by sequence-specific DNA binding proteins. Nature 1985; 316: 774.
22. Saito H, Makai RA, Clayton LK, Tonegawa S. Complete primary structures of the E beta chain and gene of the mouse major histocompatibility complex. Proc Natl Acad Sci USA 1983; 80: 5520.
23. Friedman RL, Stark GR. Alpha-interferon-induced transcription of HLA and metallothionein genes containing homologous upstream sequences. Nature 1985; 314: 637.
24. Gillies SD, Folsom V, Tonegawa S. Cell type specific enhancer element associated with a mouse MHC gene, E_B. Nature 1984; 310: 594.
25. Travers A. Regulation by anti-sense RNA. nature, 1984; 311: 410.
26. Bird AP. DNA methylation: how important in gene control? Nature 1984; 307: 503.
27. Peterlin BM, Hardy KJ. Changes in chromatin structure associated with HLA DR alpha gene activation. Fed Proc [abstract] 1985; 44: 2174.
28. Kress M, Glaros D, Khoury G, Jay G. Alternative RNA splicing of the H-2K gene. Nature 1983; 306: 602.
29. Mayrhofer G, Schon-Hegrad MA. Ia antigens in rat kidney, with special reference to expression in tubular epithelium. J Exp Med 1983; 157: 2097.
30. Halloran PH, Jephthah-Ochola J, Urmson J, Farkas S. Systemic immunologic stimuli increase class I and II antigen expression in mouse kidney. J Immunol 1985; 135: 1053.
31. Steiniger B, Klempnauer J, Wonigeit K. Altered distribution of class I and class II MHC antigens during acute pancreas allograft rejection in the rat. Transplantation 1985; 40: 234.
32. Paul LC, van Es LLA, Baldwin WM. Antigens in human renal allografts. Clin Immunol Immunopathol 1981; 19: 206.
33. Rosa F, Le Bouteiller PP, Abadie A, Mishal Z, Lemonnier FA, et al. HLA class I genes integrated into murine cells are inducible by interferon. Eur J Immunol 1983; 13: 495.
34. Rabourdin-Combe C, Mach B. Expression of HLA-DR antigens at the surface of mouse L cells co-transfected with cloned human genes. Nature 1983; 303: 670.
35. Satz ML, Singer DS. Effect of mouse interferon on the expression of a porcine major histocompatibility gene introduced into mouse L cells. J Immunol 1984; 132: 496.
36. Yoshie O, Schmidt H, Reddy ES, Weissma S, Lengyel P. Mouse interferons enhance the accumulation of a human HLA RNA and protein in transfected mouse and hamster cells. J Biol Chem 1982; 257: 13169.
37. Malissen B, Steinmetz M, McMillan M, Pierres M, Hood L. Expression of I-A^k class II genes in mouse L cells after DNA-mediated gene transfer. Nature 1983; 305: 440.
38. Rosenthal A, Wright S, Cedar H, Flavell R, Grosveld F. Regulated expression of an introduced MHC H-2K bml gene in murine embryonal carcinoma cells. Nature 1984; 310: 415.
39. Folsom V, Gold DP, White J, Marrach P, Kappler J, Tonegawa S. Functional and inducible expression of a transfected murine class II major histocompatibility complex gene. Proc Natl Acad Sci USA 1984; 81: 2045.
40. Lindahl P, Leary P, Gresser I. Enhancement by interferon of the expression of surface antigens on murine leukemia L 1210 cells. Proc Natl Acad Sci USA 1973; 70: 2785
41. Lindahl P, Gresser I, Leary P, Torey M. Interferon treatment of mice: enhanced expression of histocompatibility antigens on lymphoid cells. Proc Natl Acad Sci USA 1976; 73: 1284.
42. Vignaux F, Gresser I. Differential effects of interferon on the expression of H-2K, H-2D, and Ia antigens on mouse lymphocytes. J Immunol 1977; 118: 721.
43. Killander D, Lindahl P, Lundin L, Leary P, Gresser I. Relationship between the enhanced expression of histocompatibility antigens on interferon-treated L1210 cells and their position in the cell cycle. Eur J Immunol 1976; 6: 56.
44. Vignaux F, Gresser I. Enhanced expression of histocompatibility antigens on interferon-treated mouse embryonic fibroblasts. Proc Soc Exp Biol Med 1978; 157: 456.
45. Beller DI, Ho K. Regulation of macrophage populations: V. Evaluation of the control of macrophage Ia expression in vitro. J Immunol 1982; 129: 971.
46. Steeg PS, Moore RN, Johnson HM, Oppenheim JJ. Regulation of murine macrophage Ia antigen expression by a lymphokine with immune interferon activity. J Exp Med 1982; 156: 1780.
47. Nakamura M, Manser T, Pearson GDN, Daley MJ, Gefter ML. Effect of IFN-y on the immune response in vivo and on gene expression in vitro. Nature 1984; 307: 381.
48. Gonwa TA, Stoho JD. Differential expression of Ia molecules by human monocytes. J Clin Invest 1984; 74: 859.
49. Basham T, Smith W, Lanier L, Morhenn V, Merigan T. Regulation of expression of class II major histocompatibility antigens on human peripheral blood monocytes and Langerhans cells by interferon. Hum Immunol 1984; 10: 83.
50. Berman B, Duncan MR, Smith B, Ziboh VA, Palladino M. Interferon enhancement of HLA-DR antigen expression on epidermal Langerhans cells. J Invest Dermatol 1985; 1: 54.
51. Wong AHA, Clark-Lewis I, Hamilton JA, Schrader JW. P cell stimulating factor and glucocorticoids oppose the action of interferon-gamma in inducing Ia antigens on T-dependent mast cells (P cells). J Immunol 1984; 133: 50.
52. Wong GHW, Clark-Lewis I, McKimm-Bresshkin JL, Harris AW, Schrader JW. Interferon-induced enhanced expression of Ia and H-2 antigens on B lymphoid, macrophage, and myeloid cell lines. J Immunol 1983; 131: 788.
53. Roehm NW, Leibson HJ, Zlotnik A, Kappler J, Marrack P, Camier JC. Interleukin-induced increase in Ia expression by normal mouse B cells. J Exp Med 1984; 160: 679.
54. Miyawaki T, Seki H, Taga K, Taniguchi N. Interferon gamma can augment expression ability of HLA-DR antigens on pokeweed mitogen-stimulated human T lymphocytes. Cell Immunol 1984; 89: 300.
55. Pober JS, Collins T, Gimbrone MA Jr, et al. Lymphocytes recognize human vascular endothelial and dermal fibroblast Ia antigens induced by recombinant immune interferon. Nature 1983; 305: 726.
56. Collins T, Korman AJ, Wke CT, et al. Immune interferon activates multiple class II major histocompatibility complex genes and the associated invariant chain in human endothelial cells and dermal fibroblasts. Proc Natl Acad Sci USA 1984; 81: 4917.
57. Pujol-Borrell R, Hanafusa T, Chiovato L, Bottazzo GF. Lectin-induced expression of DR antigen on human cultured follicular thyroid cells. Nature 1983; 304: 71.
58. Londei M, Lamb JR, Bottazzo GF, Feldmann M. Epithelial cells expressing aberrant MHC class II determinants can present

antigen to cloned human T cells. Nature 1984; 312: 639.
59. Houghton AN, Thomson TM, Gross D, Oettgen HF, Old LJ. Surface antigens of melanoma and melanocytes: specificity of induction of Ia antigens by human y-Interferon. J Exp Med 1984; 160: 255.
60. Aubock J, Niederwieser D, Romani N, Fritsch P, Huber C. Human interferon-gamma induces expression of HLA-DR on keratinocytes and melanocytes. Arch Dermatol Res 1985; 277: 270.
61. Basham TY, Nickoloff BJ, Merigan TC, Morhenn VB. Recombinant gamma interferon induces HLA-DR expression on cultured human keratinocytes. J Invest Dermatol 1984; 83: 88.
62. Basham TY, Nickoloff BJ, Merigan TC, Morhenn VB. Recombinant gamma interferon differentially regulates class II antigen expression and biosynthesis on cultured normal human keratinocytes. J Interferon Res 1985; 5: 23.
63. Giacomini P, Aguzzi A, Pesstka S, Fisher PB, Ferrone S. Modulation by recombinant DNA leukocyte (alpha) and fibroblast (beta) interferons of the expression and shedding of HLA- and tumor-associated antigens by human melanoma cells. J Immunol 1984; 133: 1649.
64. Fierz W, Endler B, Reske K, Wekerle H, Fontano A. Astrocytes as antigen-presenting cells. I. Induction of Ia antigen expression on astrocytes by T cells via immune interferon and its effect on antigen presentation. J Immunol 1985; 134: 3785.
65. Wong GHW, Bartlett PF, Clark-Lewis I, Battye F, Schrader JW. Inducible expression of H-2 and Ia antigens on brain cells. Nature 1984; 310: 688.
66. Cerf-Bensussan N, Quaroni A, Kurnick JT, Bhan AK. Intraepithelial lymphocytes modulate Ia expression by intestinal epithelial cells. J Immunol 1984; 132: 2244.
67. Schwartz R, Momburg F, Moldenhaueer G, Dorken B, Schirrmacher V. Induction of HLA class II antigen expression on human carcinoma cell lines by IFN-Gamma. Int J Cancer 1985; 35: 245.
68. Walker EB, Maino V, Sanchez-Lanier M, Warner N, Stewart C. Murine gamma interferon activates the release of a macrophage-derived Ia-inducing factor that transfers Ia inductive capacity. J Exp Med 1984; 159: 1532.
69. Koeffler HP, Ranyard J, Yelton L, Billing R, Bohman R. Gamma interferon induces expression of the HLA-D antigens on normal and leukemic human myeloid cells. Proc Natl Acad Sci USA 1984; 81: 4080.
70. Capobianchi MR, Ameglio F, Tosi R, Dolei A. Differences in expression and release of DR, BR, and DQ molecules in human cells treated with interferon-gamma: comparison to other interferons. Hum Immunol 1985; 13: 1.
71. Shaw AR, Chan JK, Reid S, Seehafer J. HLA-DR synthesis induction and expression in HLA-DR negative carcinoma cell lines of diverse origins by interferon-gamma but not by interferon-beta. J Natl Cancer Inst 1985; 74: 1261.
72. Wake CT, Flavell RA. Multiple mechanisms regulate the expression of murine immune response genes. Cell 1985; 42: 623.
73. Yarden A, Shure-Gottlieb H, Chebath J, Revel M, Kimchi A. Autogenous production of interferon beta switches on HLA genes during differentiation of histiocytic lymphoma U937 cells. EMBO J 1984; 3: 969.
74. Natali PG, Russo C, Ng A-K, et al. Tissue distribution of human Ia-like antigens. In: Ferrone S, David CS, eds. Ia Antigens, vol II. Boca Raton, FL: CRC Press, 1982: 81.
75. Ozato K, Wan Y-J, Orrison BM. Mouse major histocompatibility class I gene expression begins at midsomite stage and is inducible in earlier-stage embryos by interferon. Proc Natl Acad Sci, USA 1985; 82: 2427.
76. Bocch V. The physiologic interferon response. Immunol Today 1985; 6: 7.
77. Snyder DS, Beller DI, Unanue ER. Prostaglandins modulate macrophage Ia expression. Nature 1982; 299: 163.
78. Berman B, Duncan MR, Smith B, Ziboh VA, Palladino M. Interferon enhancement of HLA-DR antigen expression on epidermal Langerhans cells. J Invest Dermatol 1985; 84: 54.
79. Taylor DD, Black PH. Inhibition of macrophage Ia antigen expression by shed plasma membrane vesicles from metastatic murine melanoma lines. J Natl Cancer Inst 1985; 74: 859.
80. Klein J. Immunology: the science of self-nonself discrimination. New York: Wiley, 1982: 367.
81. Watson J, Riblet R. Genetic control of responses to bacteria lipopolysaccharides in mice: I. evidence for a single gene that influences mitogenic and immunogenic responses to lipopolysaccharides. J Exp Med 1974; 140: 1147.
82. Ziegler HK, Staffileno KL, Wentworth P. Modulation of macrophage Ia expression by lipopolysaccharide: I. Induction of Ia expression in vivo. J Immunol 1984; 133: 1825.
83. Steeg PS, Johnson HM, Oppenheim JJ. Regulation of murine macrophage Ia antigen expression by an immune interferon-like lymphokine: inhibitory effect of endotoxin. J Immunol 1982; 129: 2402.
84. Yem AW, Parmely MJ. Modulation of Ia-like antigen expression and antigen-presenting activity of human monocytes by endotoxin and zymosan A. J Immunol 1981; 127: 245.
85. Ho M, Breinig MC, Maehara N. Cellular basis of interferon formation and hyporeactivity after exposure to bacterial lipopolysaccharide. J Infect Dis 1976; 133: 30.
86. Apt RN, Ascher D, Pluznik DH. Genetic analysis of generation of serum interferon by bacterial lipopolysaccharide. J Immunol 1977; 119: 1898.
87. Gray PW, Leung DW, Pennica D, et al. Expression of human immune interferon cDNA in *E Coli* and monkey cells. Nature 1982; 295: 503.
88. Gray PW, Goeddel DV. Cloning and expression of murine immune interferon cDNA. Proc Natl Acad Sci USA 1983; 80: 5842.
89. Rinderknecht E, O'Connor BH, Rodriguez H. Human natural interferon gamma: Complete amino acid sequence and determination of sites of glycosylation. J Biol Chem 1984; 259: 6790.
90. Bocci V, Pacini A, Muscettola M, et al. Renal filtration, absorption, and catabolism of human alpha interferon. J Interferon Res 1981; 1: 347.
91. de Waal RMW, Bogman MJJ, Maass CN, Cornelissen LMH, Tax WJM, Koene RAP. Variable expression of Ia on vascular endothelium of mouse skin grafts. Nature 1983; 303: 426.
92. Mason DW, Dallman M, Barclay AN. Graft-versus-host disease induces expression of Ia antigens in rat epidermal cells and gut epithelium. Nature 1981; 293: 150.
93. Barclay N, Mason D. Induction of Ia antigen in rat epidermal cells and gut epithelium by immunological stimuli. J Exp Med 1982; 156: 1665.
94. Lambert IA, Suitters AJ, Chisholm PM. Expression of Ia antigen on epidermal keratinocytes in graft vs. host disease. Nature 1981; 293: 149.
95. Daynes RA, Eman M, Krueger GG, Roberts LK. Expression of Ia on keratinocytes after the grafting of normal skin to nude mice. J Immunology 1983; 130: 1536.
96. Volc-Platzer B, Majdic O, Knapp W, et al. Evidence of HLA-DR antigen biosynthesis by human keratinocytes in disease. J Exp Med 1984; 159: 1784.
97. Wadgymar A, Urmson J, Baumal R, Halloran PF. Changes in Ia expression in mouse kidney during acute graft-vs-host disease. J Immunol 1984; 132: 1826.
98. Sinclair G, Wadgymar A, Halloran PF, Delovitch TL. Graft-vs-host reactions induce H-2 class II gene transcription in host kidney cells. Immunogenetics 1984; 20: 503.
99. Hall BM, Bishop GA, Duggin GG, Horvath JS, Philips J, Tiller DJ. Increased expression of HLA-DR antigens on renal tubular cells in renal transplants: relevance to the rejection response. Lancet 1984; 2: 247.
100. Benson EM, Colvin RB, Russell PS. Induction of Ia antigens in murine renal transplants. J Immunol 1985; 134: 7.

101. Milton AD, Fabre JW. Massive induction of donor-type class I and class II major histocompatibility complex antigens in rejecting cardiac allografts in the rat. J Exp Med 1985; 161: 98.
102. Kramer P, Ten Kate FWJ, Bijnen AB, Jeekel J, Weimar W. Recombinant leucocyte interferon A induces steroid-resistant acute vascular rejection episodes in renal transplant recipients. Lancet 1984; 1: 989.
103. Kelley VE, Roths JB. Increase in macrophage Ia expression in autoimmune mice: role of the lpr gene. J Immunol 1982; 129: 923.
104. Halloran PF, Autenried P. Mechanism and significance of the changes in renal MHC expression in the mouse. (abstract presented at the 17th Annual Meeting of the American Society of Nephrology, Washington, December, 1984).
105. Groeneweg G, Buurman WA, Jeunehomme, GMAA, van der Linden CJ. Effect of cyclosporine on MHC-class II expression on arterial and venous endothelium in vitro. Transplantation 1985; 40: 21.
106. Groenewegen G, Buurman WA, van der Linden CJ. Lymphokine dependence of *in vivo* expression of MHC class II antigens by endothelium. Nature 1985; 316: 361.
107. Autenried P, Halloran PF. Cyclosporine blocks the induction of class I and class II MHC products in mouse kidney by graft-vs-host disease. J Immunol 1985; 135: 3922.
108. Rose ML. Immunoregulation of MHC antigen expression. Immunol Today 1985; 6: 297.
109. Halloran PF, Wadgymar A, Autenried P. Inhibition of MHC product induction may contribute to the immunosuppressive action of cyclosporin. Prog Allergy (in press).
110. Warren MK, Vogel SN. Opposing effects of glucocorticoids on interferon-gamma-induced murine macrophage Fc receptor and Ia antigen expression. J Immunol 1985; 134: 2462.
111. Belsito DV, Flotte TJ, Lim HW, et al. Effect of glucocorticosteroids on epidermal Langerhans cells. J Exp Med 1982; 155: 291.
112. Hengy W, Kelley VE, Strom TB, et al. Decreased expression of human class II antigens on monocytes from patients with acquired immune deficiency syndrome. J Clin Invest 1984; 74: 2089.
113. Marcadet A, Cohen D, Dausset J, Fischer A, Durandy A, Griscelli C. Genotyping with DNA probes in combined immunodeficiency with defective expression of HLA. N Engl J Med 1985; 312: 1287.
114. dePreval C, Lisowska-Grospierre B, Loche M, Griscelli C, Mach B. A transacting class II regulatory gene unlinked to the MHC controls expression of HLA class II genes. Nature 1985; 318: 291.
115. Klareskog L, Forsum U, Peterson PA. Hormonal regulation of the expression of Ia antigens on mammary gland epithelium. Eur J Immunol 1980; 10: 958.
116. Lu CY, Changelian PS, Unanue ER. Alpha Fetoprotein inhibits macrophage expression of Ia antigens. J Immunol 1984; 132: 1722.
117. Ball ED, Guyre PM, Glynn JM, Rigby WF, Fanger MW. Modulation of class I HLA antigens on HL-60 promyelocytic leukemia cells by serum-free medium: re-induction by gamma-IFN and 1, 25 dihydroxy-vitamin D3 (calcitriol). J Immunol 1984; 132: 2424.
118. Sutherland J, Mannoni P, Rosa F, Huyat D, Turner AR, Fellous M. Induction of the expression of HLA class I antigens on K562 by interferons and sodium butyrate. Hum Immunol 1985; 12: 65.
119. Navarro J, El-Ansary M, Royo C, de Maeyer E, Touraine JL. Lymphocyte homing in mice: lack of significant alteration when H-2 antigen is moderately modulated. Immunobiology 1984; 167: 404.
120. Hanaumi K, Gray P, Suzuki K. F_c gamma-receptor mediated suppression of gamma-interferon-induced Ia antigen expression on a murine macrophage cell line (P338D1). J Immunol 1984; 133: 2852.
121. Behbehani K, Beller DI, Unanue ER. The effects of beryllium and other adjuvants on Ia expression by macrophages. J Immunol 1985; 134: 2047.
122. Klein G, Klein E. Evolution of tumours and the impact of molecular oncology. Nature 1985; 315: 190.
123. Sanderson AR, Beverley PE. Interferon, B-2-microglobulin and immunoselection in the pathway to malignancy: a blinkered view from Nag's Head Yard. Immunol Today 1983; 4: 211.

0041-1337/86/4104-0421$02.00/0
TRANSPLANTATION
Vol. 41, No. 4

Printed in U.S.A.

Transplantation

ARTICLES

REJECTION OF CULTURED THYROID ALLOGRAFTS BY THE TRANSFER OF SENSITIZED LYT 2+ T CELLS[1]

HILARY S. WARREN[2] AND RICHARD G. PEMBREY

Cancer Research Unit, Woden Valley Hospital, Woden, ACT 2606, Australia

Cultured BALB/c (H-2^d) thyroid allografts, which are accepted permanently in fully immunocompetent allogeneic CBA/H (H-2^k) recipients, are rejected following the transfer of immune spleen cells generated by immunization of recipient-strain mice with P815 (H-2^d) which, like the cultured thyroid, expresses only class I major histocompatibility (MHC) antigens. Depletion of Lyt 2$^+$ T cells from the transferred population abolished the capacity of immune spleen cells to trigger rejection, whereas depletion of L3T4$^+$ T cells was without effect. Transfer of in-vitro-activated H-2^d specific Lyt 2$^+$ T cells also triggered rejection of cultured thyroid allografts. The results are consistent with previous studies showing that sensitized Lyt 2$^+$ T cells are required for rejection of cultured pancreatic islet allografts, which also express only class I MHC antigens. These results are in accord with the notion that Lyt 2$^+$ T cells are activated by and are active against class I MHC antigens.

The T cell subclass triggering graft rejection has been investigated in a number of rodent systems. In the majority of cases (*1–6*), untreated grafts are transplanted and these survive for prolonged periods only when the recipients are rendered immunoincompetent by irradiation and T cell depletion. An alternative system is the cultured organ allograft model, in which the graft is depleted of passenger leukocytes by organ culture and this results in the indefinite survival of the graft following transplantation into allogeneic recipients (*7, 8*). The cultured organ allograft, therefore, provides a model for investigating the T cell subclass triggering rejection in which the recipient is fully immunocompetent.

Specifically sensitized Lyt 2$^+$ T cells have been shown to trigger rejection of cultured pancreatic islet allografts. We previously reported that transfer of H-2^d-specific immune spleen cells triggered the acute rejection of cultured BALB/c (H-2^d) pancreatic islet allografts in CBA/H (H-2^k) recipients (*9*), and that the capacity to trigger rejection was dependent upon sensitized Lyt 2$^+$ T cells in the inoculum. Recent studies by Hodgkin et al. (*10*) show that in-vitro-activated Lyt 2$^+$ T cells also trigger graft rejection when transplanted together with the pancreatic islets. The immune spleen cells and in-vitro-activated Lyt 2$^+$ T cells were generated using as immunogen P815 cells—which, like the cultured pancreatic islets, express only class I major histocompatibility (MHC)* antigens (*11, 12*). The results obtained are consistent with the notion that Lyt 2$^+$ T cells are class I MHC antigen reactive.

In contrast to these studies, Vesole et al. (*13*) concluded that sensitized Lyt 2$^-$ T cells may trigger the rejection of cultured thyroid allografts. In their studies cultured BALB/c (H-2^d) thyroid allografts in C57B1/6 (H-2^b) recipients were rejected in a protracted fashion by the transfer of P815 immune spleen cells, but the ability of the immune spleen cells to trigger rejection did not correlate with the cytotoxic activity of the inoculum. Lyt 2$^-$ T cells are considered to be class II MHC reactive (*14, 15*), but cultured thyroid expresses only class I MHC antigens (*11*). In this article we present data showing that sensitized Lyt 2$^+$ T cells do trigger rejection of cultured thyroid allografts. Some of these results have been presented in preliminary form (*16*).

MATERIALS AND METHODS

Mice. BALB/c An Bradley Wehi Can (H-2^d) and CBA/CaH Wehi Can (H-2^k) male mice were bred at the Animal Breeding Establishment, John Curtin School of Medical Research, Australian National University, Canberra, and were used at 9–12 weeks of age.

Preparation of grafted mice. BALB/c mice were treated with cyclophosphamide (300 mg/kg) at 4 and 2 days prior to removal of thyroids. The thyroids were cultured for 21 days in 95% O_2 and 5% CO_2 as described previously (*7*). Single thyroid lobes were transplanted under the kidney capsule of thyroidectomized CBA/H mice. Graft acceptance was assessed at 3 weeks posttransplantation by ^{125}I-uptake or by visual inspection of the graft at laparotomy. Accepted grafts were seen as clear follicular grafts. Occasionally grafts had evidence of a mononuclear cell infiltrate giving the graft a milky white appearance—these mice were discarded.

Assessment of graft rejection. Graft rejection was assessed by the absence of ^{125}I-uptake and/or by histological examination of the grafts. ^{125}I-uptake was measured 3 days following i.p. injection of 15 μCi Na^{125}I using a purpose-built scintillation probe (*7*). For fully functional grafts between 5000 and 16000 cpm was measured. Grafts were considered rejected when the cpm measured was below the mean +3 SD of cpm for uncultured thyroids 3 weeks posttransplantation (*7*). This value was 500 cpm. Rejection measured as absence of function requires that

[1] This work was supported by a grant from the National Health and Medical Research Council of Australia.

[2] Address correspondence to: Dr. H. S. Warren, Cancer Research Unit, Woden Valley Hospital, P.O. Box 11, Woden, A.C.T. 2606, Australia.

* Abbreviations used: CU, cytotoxic units; MHC, major histocompatibility complex; MNC, mononuclear cells.

the graft be totally destroyed, thus results are recorded as time taken for total tissue destruction. Histological assessment of rejection allows the degree of rejection to be assessed at a particular time after cell transfer. Histological assessment was made on 4-μ sections taken at 18 sections apart through the entire graft. Each section was scored on an arbitrary scale from 1 to 7, and the average of scores for the graft was recorded: score 1: focal point of mononuclear cells (MNC) at the edge of the graft; score 2: less than 25% MNC infiltration; score 3: 25–50% MNC infiltration; score 4: 50–75% MNC infiltration; score 5: 75–100% MNC infiltration; score 6: total graft destruction; score 7: scar tissue only.

Tumor cell lines. The tumor lines P815 (H-2^d) and EL-4 (H-2^b) were maintained by serial passage in tissue culture as described previously (*9*).

Immunization. CBA/H male mice were immunized by i.p. injection of 2.5×10^7 P815 or EL-4. Spleens were harvested at 10 days, and cell suspensions prepared.

Measurement of cytotoxic activity. Spleen cells and subpopulations were assayed for their cytotoxic activity on the appropriate tumor cell target by methods described previously (*9*). Cytotoxic activity on ^{51}Cr-labeled target cells is expressed as cytotoxic units (CU), which adjusts the percentage of specific lysis to a value linearly related to the number of effector cells (*17*). One CU is defined as the amount of activity that causes the specific lysis of one target cell during a 4-hr incubation period.

Subfractionation of immune spleen cells. Immune spleen cells were depleted of various subpopulations by panning (*18*). Monoclonal antibodies used were Lyt 2.1 (Australian Monoclonal Development, Sydney) and GK 1.5 (*19*) (obtained from a hybridoma cell line supplied by F. Fitch, M.D., Ph.D., Chicago, IL). Polyclonal antibodies, rabbit antimouse and rabbit antirat immunoglobulins (Z109 and Z147, Dako-Immunoglobulins A/S, Denmark) were ultracentrifuged to remove immune complexes. All antibodies were used at predetermined optimum concentrations. Immune spleen cells were left untreated or were incubated for 7 min at room temperature, at a concentration of 2×10^7/ml, with the monoclonal antibodies Lyt 2.1 or GK 1.5. After washing, the untreated and monoclonal antibody treated cells were plated at 3×10^7 cells/3 ml on 90-mm bacteriological petri dishes coated with rabbit antimouse immunoglobulin (to deplete Ig^+ cells and Lyt 2^+ cells) or a mixture of rabbit antimouse and rabbit antirat immunoglobulins (to deplete Ig^+ cells and L3T4$^+$ cells). Nonadherent cells were recovered after 70 min at 4°C, and were depleted further by incubation on a second antibody-coated plate. Then 5×10^7 immune spleen cells or subpopulations derived from the same number of cells were injected i.p. into thyroid-grafted mice on 3 occasions at 2 day intervals. Thyroid-grafted mice were used at between 35 and 100 days posttransplant (*20*).

Fluorescent analysis of subpopulations. Samples for fluorescent studies were stored in liquid nitrogen and thawed just prior to analysis. Immune spleen cells and subpopulations were treated with Lyt 2.1 or GK 1.5 monoclonal antibodies for 7 min at room temperature, washed, and incubated for 1 hr on ice with fluorescein-conjugated rabbit antimouse IgG, $F(ab')_2$ fragment (Cappel laboratories cat. no. 1311-0082) and fluorescein-conjugated rabbit antirat IgG (Cappel laboratories, cat. no. 1213-0082), respectively. Controls were cells incubated with the fluorescein-conjugated antibodies alone. Cells were enumerated by fluorescent microscopy.

Generation of in vitro activated Lyt 2^+ T cells. Spleen cells were prepared from mice immunized with P815 at least 2 months previously. Cultures contained 10^6 spleen cells and 1.6×10^5 UV-irradiated P815 per ml of Eagle's medium supplemented with 24 mM $NaHCO_3$, 0.1 mM 2-mercaptoethanol, antibiotics, 10% fetal calf serum, and an optimum amount of an interleukin-2-containing human tonsillar lymphokine (*21*) preparation. UV-irradiation of cells was as described previously (*22*). Cultures were incubated in a gas phase of 7% O_2, 10% CO_2, and 83% N_2 for 5 days at 37°C. The activated cells were harvested and subcultured into lymphokine-containing medium for a further 3–5 days. Activated cells specifically killed P815 and were greater than 95% Lyt 2^+ as assessed by fluorescent analysis. In-vitro-activated cells were injected i.p. in one dose. Grafts were taken for histological analysis at 3 weeks after cell transfer.

RESULTS

Immune and nonimmune cells. Cultured BALB/c thyroids survive indefinitely following transplantation into fully immunocompetent CBA/H recipients. As shown in Table 1, thyroid allograft rejection, as measured by total tissue destruction, does not occur following transfer of normal CBA/H spleen cells or CBA/H spleen cells sensitized to third-party (H-2^b) alloantigens, but does occur following transfer of CBA/H spleen cells specific for graft (H-2^d) alloantigens. All grafts are rejected by 10 weeks. This result confirms studies by Vesole et al. (*13*) who examined the requirements for rejection of BALB/c thyroid grafts in C57B1/6 (H-2^b) recipients following i.v. transfer of 5×10^7 immune spleen cells. In our studies, consistent rejection required that a total of 15×10^7 immune spleen cells be given i.p. in 3 doses at 2-day intervals.

Immune spleen cell subpopulations obtained by panning. Immune spleen cells were depleted of Ig^+ cells, or Lyt 2^+ and Ig^+ cells, or L3T4$^+$ and Ig^+ cells by "panning", as described in the *Materials and Methods* section. The depleted populations were analyzed by fluorescence and the total T cells of each subclass injected was calculated (Table 2). There were 8% residual Lyt 2^+ cells in the Lyt 2^+ and Ig^+-depleted populations and 11% residual L3T4$^+$ cells in the L3T4$^+$ and Ig^+-depleted population compared with the number of Lyt 2^+ and L3T4$^+$ cells in the control Ig^+-depleted population. Measurement of cytotoxic activities showed that Lyt 2^+ depletion reduced the cytotoxic activity to less than 7% of that in the untreated immune spleen cell populations (Tables 2 and 3).

Immune spleen cell subpopulations and thyroid graft rejection. Immune spleen cells and subpopulations were compared for their capacity to trigger thyroid allograft rejection (Tables 2 and 3). Results in Table 3 record graft rejection as the time

TABLE 1. Rejection of thyroid allografts following the transfer of specifically sensitized cells

Spleen cells transferred[a]	Cytotoxic activity ($CU\times10^{-4}$)[b]	Graft rejection (rejected/total)[c]		
		Weeks 2–3	Weeks 5–6	Weeks 9–10
Normal CBA/H		0/9	0/8	0/8
CBA/H anti-EL-4	213	0/5	0/4	0/4
CBA/H anti-P815	87	5/9	7/8	8/8

[a] A total of 15×10^7 cells were given in 3 i.p. doses at 2-day intervals.
[b] Total cytotoxic activity injected measured on the relevant target.
[c] Grafts were considered rejected when ^{125}I incorporated was <500 cpm.

TABLE 2. Immune spleen cell subpopulations and thyroid allograft rejection: histological studies

Spleen cells	Total T cells transferred ($\times 10^{-5}$)[a]		Cytotoxic activity ($CU\times 10^{-4}$)[b]	Average histological score[c]		Rejected/total[d]
	Lyt 2^+	L3T4$^+$		For each graft	For all grafts	
None	NT	NT	—	1.8, 1.1, 1.0 0.7, 0.4, 0.2	0.9	0/6
Normal CBA/H	NT	NT	—	2.3, 1.9, 0.2 0.0, 0.0	0.9	0/5
Immune						
Total	NT	NT	150	6.5, 5.4, 4.8 4.8, 4.6, 4.3	5.0	6/6
Ig$^+$-depleted	198	258	122	5.1, 5.0, 4.4 3.0, 2.9	4.1	4/5
Lyt 2^+ and Ig$^+$-depleted	17	246	10	2.9, 1.8, 1.6 0.8	1.8	0/4
L3T4$^+$ and Ig$^+$-depleted	222	29	147	5.7, 5.0, 4.8 4.1, 3.8, 3.0	4.4	6/6

[a] T cell subpopulations derived from 15×10^7 immune spleen cells are the total injected i.p. in 3 doses at 2-day intervals.
[b] Total cytotoxic activity injected.
[c] Histological scores are on a scale from 1 to 7: 1 = focal MNC, 2 = 25% MNC, 3 = 25–50% MNC, 4 = 50–75% MNC, 5 = 75–100% MNC, 6 = total graft destruction, 7 = scar tissue.
[d] Rejection was arbitrarily designated as occurring when the average histological scores across a graft exceeded 3.0.

TABLE 3. Immune spleen cell subpopulations and thyroid allograft rejection: functional studies

Immune spleen cells transferred[a]	Cytotoxic activity ($CU\times 10^{-4}$)[b]	Graft rejection (rejection/total)[c]				
		Weeks 2–3	Weeks 5–6	Weeks 9–10	Week 15	Week 20
Total	162	2/10	6/9	8/9	9/9	
Ig$^+$-depleted	144	0/10	0/10	2/9	6/9	8/9
Lyt 2^+ and Ig$^+$-depleted	7.5	0/9	0/9	0/8	0/7	0/7

[a] A total of 15×10^7 immune spleen cells or subpopulations derived from this number were given in 3 i.p. doses at 2-day intervals.
[b] Total cytotoxic activity transferred for each subpopulation.
[c] See Table 1 footnote.

taken for total tissue destruction as assessed by the absence of ^{125}I-uptake. Results in Table 2 show graft rejection assessed histologically at 4 weeks after cell transfer using an arbitrary scale from 1 to 7 to denote increasing graft destruction (Fig. 1). The histological scores recorded are an average of sections cut at 72-μ intervals across the entire graft. Grafts with average histological scores exceeding 3.0 (greater than 25% of the graft showing mononuclear cell infiltration) were considered rejected. Histological analysis of grafts from untreated mice revealed that there was a low level of MNC infiltration. The mean histological score was 0.9 (range 0.2–1.8). This observation is in agreement with studies by La Rosa and Talmage (*23*) who also reported that mononuclear cells are observed to varying degrees at the graft site. All 5 grafts from mice receiving normal CBA/H spleen cells had a histological score below 3.0. The mean histological score for all grafts was 0.9 (range 0–2.3).

Results in Tables 2 and 3 show that Ig$^+$-depleted immune spleen cells retained the capacity to trigger graft rejection. However, compared with total immune spleen cells, rejection triggered by Ig$^+$-depleted cells was slower. Thus total tissue destruction (Table 3) was recorded for 20% of grafts at 3 weeks and 100% of grafts at 15 weeks for mice receiving total immune spleen cells. In comparison, it was 10 weeks following transfer of Ig$^+$-depleted immune spleen cells when 20% of the grafts were totally destroyed, and 20 weeks before most of the grafts were destroyed. The slower rejection of grafts following transfer of Ig$^+$-depleted immune spleen cells was confirmed by histological assessment of the grafts at 4 weeks after cell transfer (Table 2). The degree of tissue destruction was less for grafts from mice receiving Ig$^+$-depleted immune spleen cells (mean histological score 4.1, range 2.9–5.1) compared with total immune spleen cells (mean histological score 5.0, range 4.3–6.5), and 1 of 5 grafts had a histological score below 3.0. We do not know if the slower rejection by Ig$^+$-depleted immune spleen cells reflects a requirement for Ig$^+$ cells in the rejection process, or whether it reflects a nonspecific effect of the cell handling required in the panning procedure.

Lyt 2^+ and Ig$^+$-depleted immune spleen cells were examined for their capacity to trigger thyroid allograft rejection. All 7 grafts showed no functional impairment over the observation period of 20 weeks (Table 3). Histological analysis at 4 weeks after cell transfer showed that 4 of 4 grafts had a histological score below 3.0. The mean histological score for grafts from mice receiving Lyt 2^+ and Ig$^+$-depleted immune spleen cells was 1.8 (range 0.8–2.9)—which was only slightly greater than for grafts from control mice (mean 0.9, range 0.2–1.8) (Table 2).

L3T4$^+$ and Ig$^+$-depleted immune spleen cells triggered thyroid allograft rejection in 6 of 6 cases. Results in Table 2 show that grafts from mice receiving L3T4$^+$ and Ig$^+$-depleted immune spleen cells had a mean histological score of 4.4 (range 3.0–5.7), which was not different from the mean score of 4.1 (range 2.9–5.1) for mice receiving Ig$^+$-depleted immune spleen cells.

In-vitro-activated Lyt 2^+ T cells and thyroid graft rejection. The results in Table 4 show that the i.p. transfer of in-vitro-

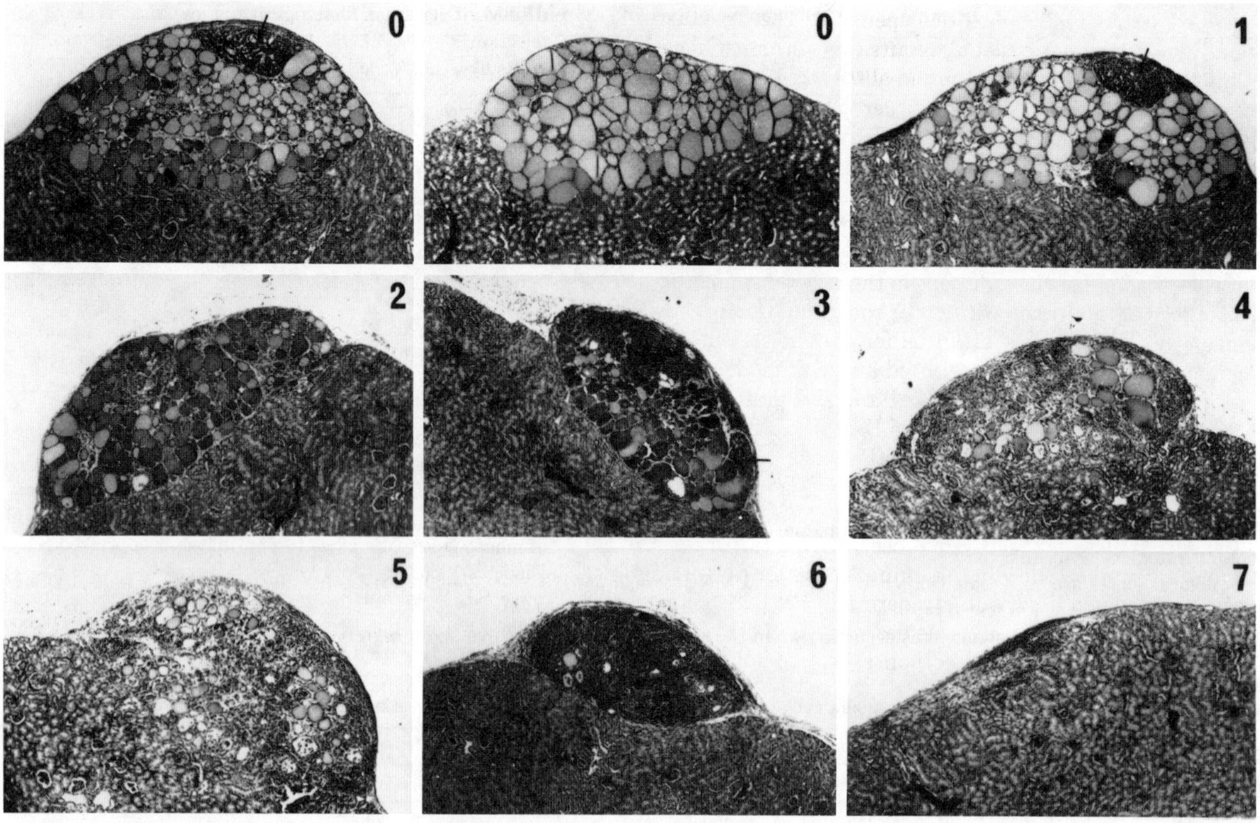

FIGURE 1. Histological analysis of rejecting thyroid grafts. Grafts were scored according to the degree of mononuclear cell infiltration and tissue destruction. The scores are indicated in the top right hand corner and are as follows: 0: intact graft; 1: focal point of MNC; 2: <25% MNC; 3: 25–50% MNC; 4: 50–75% MNC; 5: 75–100% MNC; 6: total graft destruction; 7: scar tissue. The parathyroid, where present, is indicated by an arrow.

TABLE 4. In-vitro-activated Lyt 2^+ T cells triggering thyroid allograft rejection

No. cells transferred ($\times10^{-6}$)[a]	Cytotoxic[b] activity (CU$\times10^{-6}$)[b]	Average histological score[c]		Rejected/total[d]
		For each graft	For all grafts	
5	6–10	3.4, 2.5, 2.5 2.2, 2.1, 2.0 1.7, 1.1, 0.1	2.0	1/9
12.5	30	5.9, 4.8, 3.0	4.6	3/3
25	60	6.6, 5.0	5.8	2/2
50	120–820	7.0, 6.7, 6.5 6.5, 6.0, 5.4 5.1, 4.7	6.0	8/8
50 (UV-killed)		1.0, 0.0, 0.0	0.3	0/3

[a] Cells were injected in one i.p. dose.
[b] Range is indicated for different preparations.
[c] At 3 weeks after cell transfer.
[d] See Table 2.

activated H-2^d-specific Lyt 2^+ T cells triggers thyroid allograft rejection. Rejection is dependent upon Lyt 2^+ cells and is not mediated by any contaminating P815 antigen in the inoculum, since rejection is not triggered when the cells are UV-irradiated prior to transfer. On a per-cytotoxic-unit basis, in-vitro-activated Lyt 2^+ T cells are less effective in triggering thyroid allograft rejection than in-vivo-activated cells (compare Tables 2 and 3 with Table 4). This may reflect an impaired migration of in-vitro-activated cells due to their larger size (*24*), or it may indicate that the capacity of cells to trigger rejection is not related to their cytotoxic activity.

DISCUSSION

The data presented show clearly that cultured thyroid allograft rejection is triggered by specifically sensitized Lyt 2^+ T cells. Graft rejection was triggered by transfer of the total immune spleen cell population and by Ig^+-depleted or L3T4$^+$ and Ig^+-depleted populations, but not by Lyt 2^+ and Ig^+-depleted populations. Transfer of in-vitro-activated Lyt 2^+ T cells triggered thyroid allograft rejection. The results obtained are in accord with the notion that Lyt 2^+ T cells are class I MHC reactive (hereafter referred to as *class I T cells*), since the cultured thyroid (*11*) and P815 used as immunogen (*12*) express only class I MHC antigens. The L3T4$^+$ T cell subclass, identified by the monoclonal antibody GK1.5 (*19*) and activated by class II MHC antigens (class II T cells) (*14, 15*), is either not activated using P815 as immunogen or is unable to trigger rejection of cultured allografts. As argued by Lafferty et al. (*12*), if T cells are activated against graft-strain class I MHC antigens in association with recipient-strain class II MHC antigens, the T cells so activated would not be graft-specific. The results presented here are consistent with earlier studies showing that rejection of cultured pancreatic islet allografts is triggered by P815-sensitized Lyt 2^+ T cells (*9, 10*).

The mechanism by which sensitized class I T cells trigger rejection of the two cultured grafts may involve a direct cytotoxic mechanism and/or lymphokine-dependent reactions (*25, 26*). In the case of pancreatic islet allograft rejection triggered by transferred sensitized T cells the rejection process is lymphokine-dependent (*10*). These studies do not rule out a role for a cytotoxic mechanism since the maintenance of sensitized

T cells in vivo may be lymphokine-dependent. The time taken for rejection of pancreatic islet allografts (days) compared with the time taken for rejection of thyroid allografts (weeks) might suggest that the rejection process triggered by sensitized class I T cells differs in the two cases. Alternatively, the difference might be explained by differences in the amount of grafted tissue—and/or, in the case of pancreatic islet allografts, the amount of tissue below which normal blood glucose levels cannot be maintained.

The essential role of class I T cells in the rejection of cultured murine allografts contrasts with other rodent allograft models in which class II T cells are essential for graft rejection (*1–6*). These models differ from the cultured allograft model in that the recipients are immunosuppressed and the grafts contain cells expressing both class I and class II MHC antigens. How sensitized class II T cells trigger rejection of skin, heart, and renal allografts is not known, but this triggering may involve an associated sensitization of host-derived class I T cells (*3, 27*). Sensitized class I T cells have been shown to trigger an inflammatory response leading to skin destruction in semiallogeneic hosts when injected intradermally (*28*). Sensitized class II T cells can also cause tissue destruction in the absence of a measurable class I T cell response in a tumor allograft model (*29*).

The T cell subclass triggering rejection may simply reflect the class of MHC antigen expressed by the graft or by cells essential for graft survival. In the case of cultured allografts the vascular endothelium is of host, not donor, origin (*30*). Thus the graft epithelial cells, which express only class I MHC antigens, must be the target for graft rejection. In the case of skin, heart, and renal allografts, the vascular endothelium is of donor origin. Since murine vascular endothelium can express class II MHC antigens during an immune response (*31*), destruction of the vascular endothelium by sensitized class II T cells would lead to graft rejection. Whether sensitized class I or class II T cells trigger graft rejection, the mechanism of graft destruction in both cases most likely involves a cascade of inflammatory reactions triggered by lymphokine release from the activated cells.

Note added in proof. Recent studies (Warren HS, Simeonovic CJ, Allan W, and Hume DA, unpublished data) have shown that thyroid grafts, which are negative for class II MHC antigens, strongly express class II MHC antigens within 3 days of transfer of sensitized Lyt 2^+ T cells. In contrast, under identical conditions, pancreatic islet allografts do not show induced expression of class II MHC antigens. Thus, although both cultured grafts are rejected following the transfer of sensitized Lyt 2^+ T cells, the pathways to tissue destruction probably differ.

Acknowledgments. The expert technical assistance of Ms. Tania Kwesius is gratefully acknowledged. We thank Ms. Jane Dixon for preparing the GK1.5 monoclonal antibody concentrate from the hybridoma cell line supplied by F. Fitch, M.D. Ph.D., and J Allan Ph.D. for supplying the fluorescein-conjugated antirat immunoglobulin.

REFERENCES

1. Loveland BE, Hogarth PM, Ceredig Rh, McKenzie IFC. Cells mediating graft rejection in the mouse I. Lyt-1 cells mediate skin graft rejection. J Exp Med 1981; 153: 1044.
2. Dallman MJ, Mason DW, Webb M. The roles of host and donor cells in the rejection of skin by T cell-deprived rats injected with syngeneic T cells. Eur J Immunol 1982; 12: 511.
3. Hall BM, deSaxe I, Dorsch SE. The cellular basis of allograft rejection in vivo III. Restoration of first-set rejection of heart grafts by T helper cells in irradiated rats. Transplantation 1983; 36: 700.
4. Lowry RP, Gurley KE, Clarke Forbes RD. Immune mechanisms in organ allograft rejection. I. Delayed-type hypersensitivity and lymphocytotoxicity in heart graft rejection. Transplantation 1983; 36: 391.
5. Gurley KE, Lowry RP, Clarke Forbes RD. Immune mechanisms in organ allograft rejection. II. T helper cells, delayed-type hypersensitivity, and rejection of renal allografts. Transplantation 1983; 36: 401.
6. Lowry RP, Gurley KE. Immune mechanisms in organ allograft rejection. III. Cellular and humoral immunity in rejection of organ allografts transplanted across MHC subregion disparity RT1.B(RT1.D). Transplantation 1983; 36: 405.
7. Lafferty KJ, Bootes A, Dart G, Talmage DW. Effect of organ culture on the survival of thyroid allografts in mice. Transplantation 1976; 22: 138.
8. Bowen KM, Andrus L, Lafferty KJ. Successful allotransplantation of mouse pancreatic islets to non-immunosuppressed recipients. Diabetes 1980; 29 (suppl 1): 98.
9. Prowse SJ, Warren HS, Agostino M, Lafferty KJ. Transfer of sensitized Lyt 2^+ cells triggers acute rejection of pancreatic islets. Aust J Exp Biol Med Sci 1983; 61: 181.
10. Hodgkin PD, Agostino M, Sellins K, Prowse SJ, Bellgrau D, Lafferty KJ. T lymphocyte function in vivo: ambivalence of the Class I MHC antigen reactive subset. Transplantation 1985; 40: 288.
11. Parr EL, Lafferty KJ, Bowen KM, McKenzie IFC. H-2 complex and Ia antigens on cells dissociated from mouse thyroid glands and islets of Langerhans. Transplantation 1980; 30: 142.
12. Lafferty KJ, Prowse SJ, Simeonovic CJ, Warren HS. Immunobiology of tissue transplantation: a return to the passenger leucocyte concept. Annu Rev Immunol 1983; 1: 143.
13. Vesole DH, Dart GA, Talmage DW. Rejection of stable cultured allografts by active or passive (adoptive) immunization. Proc Natl Acad Sci USA 1982; 79: 1626.
14. Swain SL, Dennert G, Wormsley S, Dutton RW. The Lyt phenotype of a long-term allospecific T cell line. Both helper and killer activities to IA are mediated by Ly-1 cells. Eur J Immunol 1981; 11: 175.
15. Meuer SC, Schlossman SF, Reinherz EL. Clonal analysis of human cytotoxic T lymphocytes: $T4^+$ and $T8^+$ effector cells recognize products of different major histocompatibility complex regions. Proc Natl Acad Sci USA 1982; 79: 4395.
16. Warren HS, Pembrey RG. Thyroid allograft rejection is triggered by the transfer of sensitized Lyt 2^+ cells. Transplant Proc 1985; XVII: 1641.
17. Davidson WF. Cellular requirements for the induction of cytotoxic T cells in vitro. Immunol Rev 1977; 35: 263.
18. Wysocki LJ, Sato VL. Panning for lymphocytes: a method for cell selection. Proc Natl Acad Sci USA 1978; 75: 2844.
19. Dialynas DP. Quan ZS, Wall KA, Pierres A, Quintans J, Loken MR, Pierres M, Fitch FW. Characterization of the murine T cell surface molecule, designated L3T4, identified by monoclonal antibody GK1.5: similarity of L3T4 to the human Leu-3/T4 molecule. J Immunol 1983; 131: 2445.
20. Donohoe JA, Andrus L, Bowen KM, Simeonovic C, Prowse SJ, Lafferty KJ. Cultured thyroid allografts induce a state of partial tolerance in adult recipient mice. Transplantation 1983; 35: 62.
21. Warren HS, Pembrey RG. A method for the production and quantitative assay of human lymphokine preparations. J Immunol Methods 1981; 41: 9.
22. Lafferty KJ, Warren HS, Woolnough JA, Talmage DW. Immunological induction of T lymphocytes: role of antigen and the lymphocyte costimulator. Blood Cells 1978; 4: 395.
23. La Rosa FG, Talmage DW. The failure of a major histocompatibility antigen to stimulate a thyroid allograft reaction after

culture in oxygen. J Exp Med 1983; 157: 898.
24. Kimura AK, Wigzell H. Development and function of cytotoxic T lymphocytes (CTL). I. In vivo maturation of CTL precursors in the absence of detectable proliferation results as a normal consequence of alloimmunisation. J Immunol 1983; 130: 2056.
25. Andrus L, Prowse SJ, Lafferty KJ. Interleukin 2 production by both Ly2$^+$ and Ly2$^-$ T cell subsets. Scand J Immunol 1981; 13: 297.
26. Geurne P-A, Piguet P-F, Vassalli P. Production of interleukin 2, interleukin 3, and interferon by mouse T lymphocyte clones of Lyt-2$^+$ and -2$^-$ phenotype. J Immunol 1984; 132: 1869.
27. LeFrancois L, Bevan MJ. A re-examination of the role of Lyt-2-positive T cells in murine skin graft rejection. J Exp Med 1984; 159: 57.
28. Tyler JD, Galli SJ, Snider ME, Dvorak AM, Steinmuller D. Cloned Lyt-2$^+$ cytolytic T lymphocytes destroy allogeneic tissue in vivo. J Exp Med 1984; 159: 234.
29. Fujiwara H, Fukuzawa M, Yoshioka T, Nakajima H, Hamaoka T. The role of tumor-specific Lyt-1$^+$2$^-$ T cells in eradicating tumor cells in vivo. I. Lyt-1$^+$2$^-$ T cells do not necessarily require recruitment of host's cytotoxic T cell precursors for implementation of in vivo immunity. J Immunol 1984; 133: 1671.
30. Parr EL, Bowen KM, Lafferty KJ. Cellular changes in cultured mouse thyroid glands and islets of Langerhans. Transplantation 1980; 30: 135.
31. De Waal RMW, Bogman MJJ, Maass CN, Cornelissen LMH, Tax WJM, Koene RAP. Variable expression of Ia antigens on the vascular endothelium of mouse skin allografts. Nature 1983; 303: 426.

Received 23 April 1985.
Accepted 1 August 1985.

0041-1337/86/4104-0426$02.00/0
TRANSPLANTATION
Vol. 41, No. 4

Printed in U.S.A.

PROLONGED REVERSAL OF DIABETES IN THE RAT BY TRANSPLANTATION OF ALLOGENEIC ISLETS FROM A SINGLE DONOR AND CYCLOSPORINE TREATMENT

A. DIBELIUS,[1] H. KÖNIGSBERGER,[1] P. WALTER,[3] W. PERMANETTER,[2] W. BRENDEL, AND B. U. VON SPECHT[1,4]

Institute for Surgical Research and Department of Pathology, University of Munich; and Department of Surgery, University of Homburg/Saar, Federal Republic of Germany.

Islets were isolated using neutral red as a dye to exclude lymphatic and acinar impurities in the transplant preparation. In a one donor–one recipient model, intraportally transplanted isogeneic islets survived indefinitely. Mean graft survival could be prolonged from 5 to 90 days, using a 3-dose rejection prophylaxis with CsA in allografts of (DA [RT1a] → Lew (RT 1l). Histological examination revealed intact islets in the grafted normoglycemic animals. Immunohistochemical staining of these islets showed B cells with insulin-rich cytoplasma. Blood glucose levels and the results of i.v. glucose tolerance tests 50 days after transplantation are presented. The different outcomes of our experiments are discussed.

Total endocrine replacement therapy for experimental diabetes mellitus can be achieved either by segmental pancreas grafting or by transplantation of isolated islets of Langerhans.

To date segmental pancreatic allografts combined with immunosuppressive agents like cyclosporine (CsA), showed considerably longer survival times than comparable islet allografts (*1–3*). The surgical technique, however, is more complex and the problems associated with exocrine portion of the organ have not been solved satisfactorily. Duct occlusion techniques give problems of islet atrophy due to whole organ fibrosis—and open duct procedures, although working in some animal models, may cause problems in patients.

Although pancreatic islet transplantation is a promising approach to avoid the problems of segmental grafting, there are several difficulties to overcome. First relatively low yields of islets, as described by several investigators (*4, 5*), limit a one donor–one recipient application. Furthermore, the considerably higher amounts of acinar and lymphatic impurities that may be transplanted together with the islets, can influence the rejection process (*5–10*). Finally, it is striking that CsA, while providing a significant prolongation of allograft survivals in segmental pancreatic transplants, seems to be less effective for islet grafts, especially those transplanted across a major histocompatibility barrier (*1, 3*).

We have investigated in an allogeneic rat model whether one donor–one recipient transplants using neutral red islet isolation (which provides lower amounts of impurities), show improved graft survival times using CsA as immunosuppression.

MATERIALS AND METHODS

Animals. DA donor rats (RT1a) (11), male or female, between 150–250 g and male Lewis (RT1l) (11) or DA recipients, of

[1] Institute for Surgical Research, University of Munich, FRG.
[2] Department of Pathology, University of Munich.
[3] Department of Surgery, University of Homburg/Saar, FRG.
[4] Address correspondence to: B. U. von Specht, M.D., Ph.D., Institute for Surgical Research, Klinikum Grosshadern, Marchioninistr. 15, D-8000 München 70, FRG.

about 300 g, were obtained from Zentralinstitut für Versuchstierkunde, Hannover, FRG.

Chemicals. Streptozotocin, Neutral Red (3-amino-m-dimethylamino-2-methylphenazinhydrochlorid) and DNAse were obtained from Sigma, Taufkirchen, FRG. Collagenase from clostridium histolyticum (0.2–0.8 U/mg) was obtained from Serva, Heidelberg, FRG; Trasylol from Bayer AG, Leverkusen, FRG; di-ethyl-ether from Hachst AG, Frankfurt, FRG; and CsA from Sandoz (Basel, Switzerland). All other chemicals were obtained from Merck, Darmstadt, FRG, and were of the highest purity available.

Induction of diabetes. Male DA or Lewis rats of about 300 g bodyweight were injected with 65 mg/kg bodyweight streptozotocin in 1 ml of phosphate-buffered saline (PBS) i.v. by the penile vein. Blood samples were taken from the tail vein every 2–4 days. Serum glucose levels were determined by the glucose dehydrogenase method using an autoanalyzer (Eppendorf ACP 50/40, Eppendorf AG, Hamburg, FRG). Body weight was determined at one-day or two-day intervals.

Diabetes. Animals were considered diabetic if the glucose levels remained over 16.5 mMol/L in four sequential determinations made 1–3 weeks postinjection (*12*). Only rats with a concurrent weight loss of at least 50 g were taken for transplantation.

Isolation of pancreatic islets. DA rats were anesthetized by diethyl-ether, shaved, and the skin was disinfected with isopropanol. All steps were performed under sterile conditions. The abdomen was opened by midline incision. Both kidney arteries were electrocoagulated. The abdominal aorta was cannulated near the bifurcation with a teflon catheter (65–12, 18G Becton, Dickinson GmbH, Heidelberg, FRG). The mesenteric arteries were clamped below the coeliac axis. Perfusion of the pancreas was then performed through the cannulated aorta with 40 ml of ice-cold neutral red solution (0.08 mg/ml neutral red dissolved in Hank's solution) (*13*). Successful perfusion was correlated with homogenous red staining of the pancreas. Immediately after perfusion the pancreas was removed and placed in a petri dish on ice. For isolation of islets each pancreas was chopped using two pairs of scissors in tandem into pieces about 1–3 mm in diameter. The fragments were placed in a cell stirrer (Wheaton, Millville, NJ) equipped with a thermojacket and connected to a 37° water bath.

Collagenase solution was prepared immediately before use by dissolving 12 IU collagenase per pancreas in 4 ml Hank's buffer and added to the minced pancreas. The mixture was stirred at 1000 rpm for 5–10 min. The degree of digestion was controlled by microscopic observations of samples taken at 1-min intervals. Optimal digestion was obtained when the red-stained islets were liberated from connective acinar tissue.

The digestion was terminated by adding 50 ml ice-cold Hank's buffer containing 400 U/ml Trasylol, and the mixture centrifugated (190 g) at 4°C in aliquots of 10 ml. The supernatant was discarded and the pellet washed twice with ice-cold Hank's solution. To prevent agglutination, a pinch of DNAse was added. The washed and resuspended islets were stored on ice. For isolation the islets were transferred into petri dishes 6 cm in diameter (Falcon; Becton, Dickinson GmbH, Heidelberg, FRG) and picked under a dissection microscope using siliconized glass capillaries. To improve purification, the picking procedure was repeated at least twice. The number of islets was determined by counting during the last picking step. All purification steps were performed under sterile conditions (*5, 14, 15*).

In vitro glucose stimulation test. To determine the viability and function of the isolated islets, in vitro glucose stimulation tests were performed. For this purpose 150 freshly isolated islets were placed in glucose-free medium. After transfer into a medium (RPMI 1640 supplemented with 10% fetal calf serum, GIBCO Europe) containing 25 mMol/L glucose, insulin levels were determined at 5-min intervals for 35 min, at 60 min, and at 90 min. Insulin RIA (Amersham & Buchler, Braunschweig, FRG) was used.

Islet transplantation. Recipient Lewis or DA rats were operated under ether anaesthesia. The abdomen was opened by midline incision under sterile conditions. The portal vein was prepared and 800 freshly isolated islets, suspended in 0.2 ml of RPMI 1640 were injected through a 27 G needle (5/8, 0.4×16 Becton, Dickinson GmbH, Heidelberg FRG) into the portal vein. The abdomen was closed by running suture. Antibiotic protection with Totocillin (Bayer, Leverkusen, FRG) (2.5 mg/kg) was given i.v. for two days.

Three groups were studied:

(1) An isogenic group with 1 DA donor and 1 DA recipient, to determine whether the number of islets isolated from one donor with a neutral red technique would be sufficient to reverse streptozotocin-induced diabetes.

(2) An allogenic group with 1 DA donor and 1 Lewis recipient, to characterize the pattern of rejection.

(3) An allogeneic group, as above, but with the recipient receiving CsA (30 mg/kg bodyweight) as immunosuppression.

The latter groups were compared to reveal effects of CsA.

Rejection. Grafts were considered clinically rejected when glucose levels of transplanted animals rose above 16 mmol/L.

Intravenous glucose tolerance test. For this purpose, 1 g glucose/kg bodyweight was given i.v. by the penile vein. Blood samples were collected at various intervals from the tail vein, and glucose levels were determined. In parallel, blood insulin levels were determined with the insulin RIA, as described before.

Mixed lymphocyte culture. The spleen was removed aseptically and single-cell suspensions were prepared in Dulbecco's modified Eagle's medium by pressing the spleen through a wire mesh. Triplicates of cell suspensions (1×10^5 cells/01. ml) were plated in microtiter plates (Nunc GmbH, Wiesbaden, FRG).

Stimulator cells were irradiated with 2000 rads, and 0.1 ml of stimulator cells (1×10^5 cells) was added to the responder cells. The cells were kept for 6 days in a humidified incubator (5% CO_2). During the last 72 hr cells were pulsed with ^3H-thymidine (2 μCi/well). The cells were harvested with a Mash II cell harvester on Whatman glass fiber filters (934 AH), and the radioactivity was counted in a Packard liquid scintillation counter.

Histological methods. For histological examination, the formalin-fixed whole livers of transplanted rats were divided into thin slices, which were embedded in paraffin; 5-μm sections of these tissue blocks were examined in series by H&E staining and with antiinsulin serum, which demonstrates insulin by the indirect immunoperoxidase method (*16*). From the isogenic group, two animals 200 and 240 days posttransplantation were sacrificed to examine the function in grafts. Four allotransplanted animals receiving no immunosuppression were sacrificed for histological examination after rejection. Three animals of the allotransplanted group receiving CsA were examined at 110, 129, and 150 days, respectively.

RESULTS

Using the neutral red procedure 800–1000 islets could be isolated from one donor, and there islets showed normal function using an in vitro glucose tolerance test. The number of islets was sufficient to decrease diabetic glucose levels to normal immediately following transplantation (Figures 1–3). The isogeneic transplanted animals remained normoglycemic for the observation period up to 240 days (Fig. 4). The glucose tolerance test excluded a latent diabetic status (Fig. 5). There were no striking differences between normal rats (group A) and isotransplanted rats (group D). Allogeneic islet grafts without immunosuppression were rejected between 3 and 9 days after transplantation (Fig. 4). Once rejected, glucose levels never returned to prerejection values and the animals survived only in poor condition up to 35 days after rejection (Fig. 2). If recipients were treated with CsA, a prolongation of graft survival could be observed. The glucose levels remained normal for 28–150 days (Figs. 3 and 4), with 3 animals having normoglycemic survival beyond this period. The mean graft survival was 90 days (Fig. 4). The weight gain was similar to that observed in successfully transplanted rats of the isogeneic group. Glucose tolerance tests performed 50 days posttransplantation showed normal values and were not significantly different from nondiabetic controls (Fig. 5, groups B and E). Both the diabetic controls and transplanted rats tested 10 days after rejection had the same pathologic glucose tolerance (Fig. 5, groups G and F). Lymphocytes from CsA-treated, normoglycemic recipients, when compared with lymphocytes of recipients that had rejected their islet grafts, did not reveal significant differences in stimulation indices. No definite conclusion could

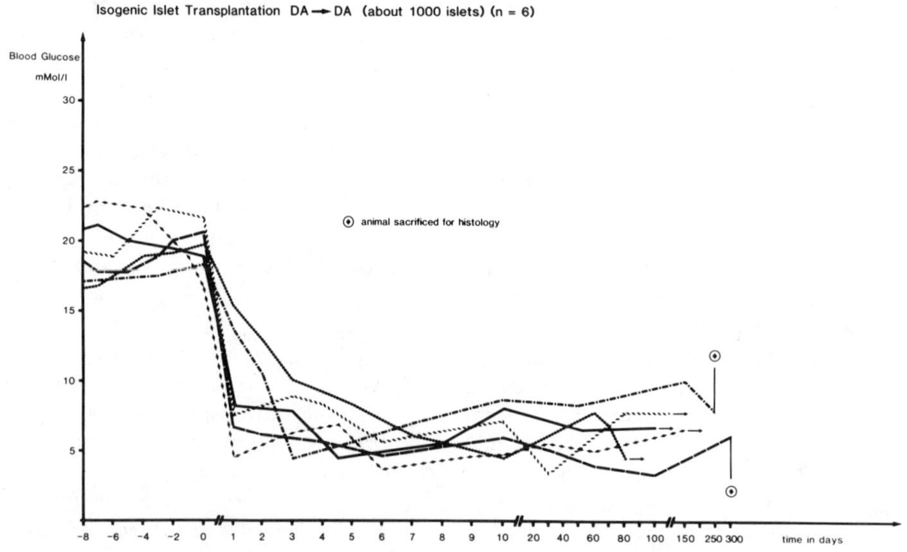

FIGURE 1. Isogeneic (DA→DA) islet transplantation (n = 6): nonfasting glucose levels before and after intraportal transplantation of about 1000 islets.

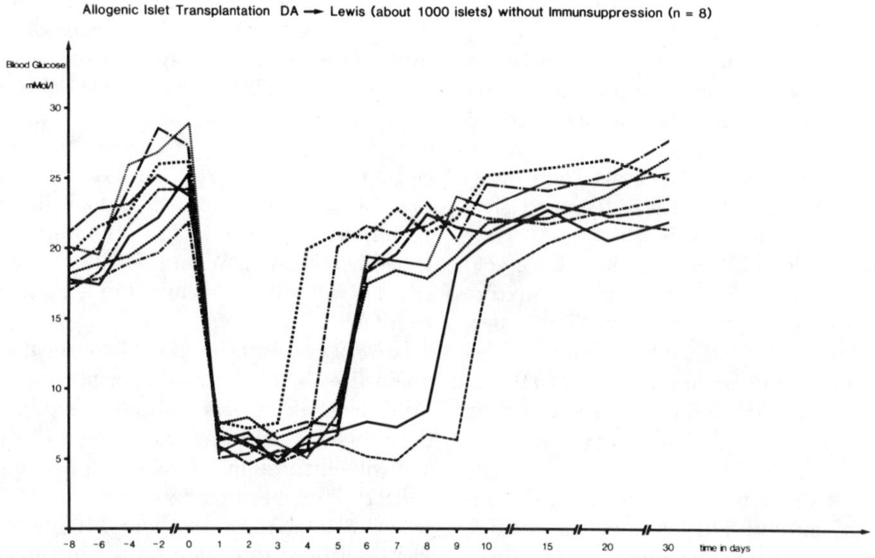

FIGURE 2. Allogeneic (DA→LEW) islet transplantation without immunosuppression (n = 8). Nonfasting glucose levels before and after intraportal transplantation of about 1000 islets. Observation period 30 days.

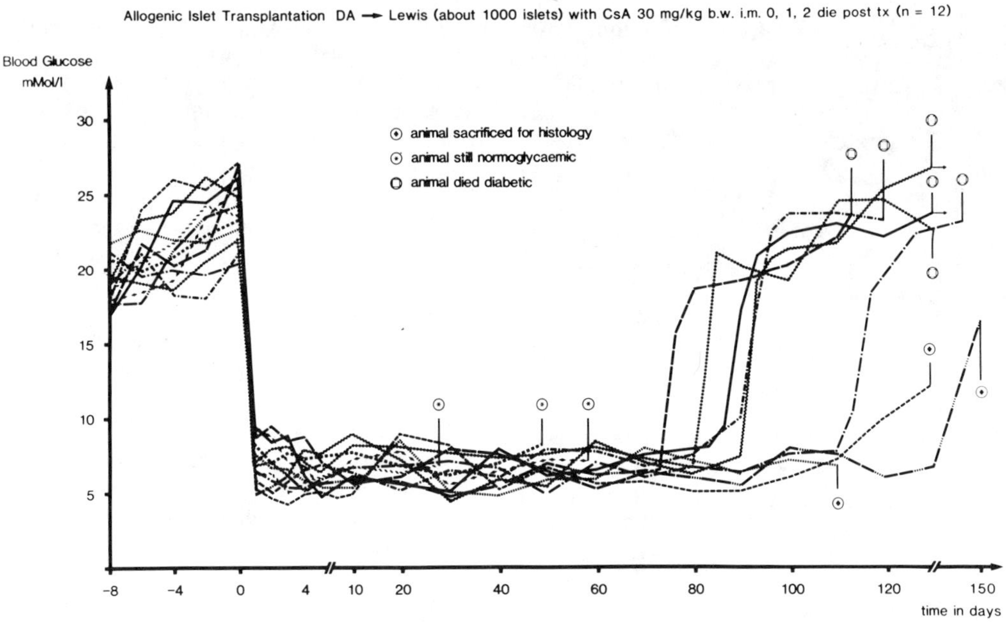

FIGURE 3. Allogeneic (DA→LEW) islet transplantation with CsA (30 mg/kg b.w. i.m. at days 0, 1, and 2 posttransplantation) (n = 12). Nonfasting glucose levels before and after intraportal transplantation of about 1000 islets.

Survival of Islet Grafts

	n	graft survival (days)	mean survival (days)
isogenic DA → DA	6	>53·, >63·, >68·, 124, 200•, 240•	124,6 ± 78,9
allogenic DA → Lew	8	3, 4, 5, 5, 5, 5, 8, 9	5,5 ± 2,0
allogenic DA → Lew + 3x CsA 30 mg/kg b.w. 0, 1, 2 die p.tx	12	>28·, >49•, >59·, 73, 82, 88, 94, 110•, 111, 117, 129•, 150•	90,8 ± 35,1

• – animal sacrificed for histology
· – animal still normoglycaemic

FIGURE 4. Islet graft survival times in three groups. (1) isogeneic transplantation DA→DA; (2) allografts without immunosuppression DA→LEW; (3) allografts with CsA 30 mg/kg b.w. i.m. at days 0, 1, and 2 posttransplantationem (DA→LEW). About 1000 islets were isolated using a neutral red isolation method and transplanted intraportally.

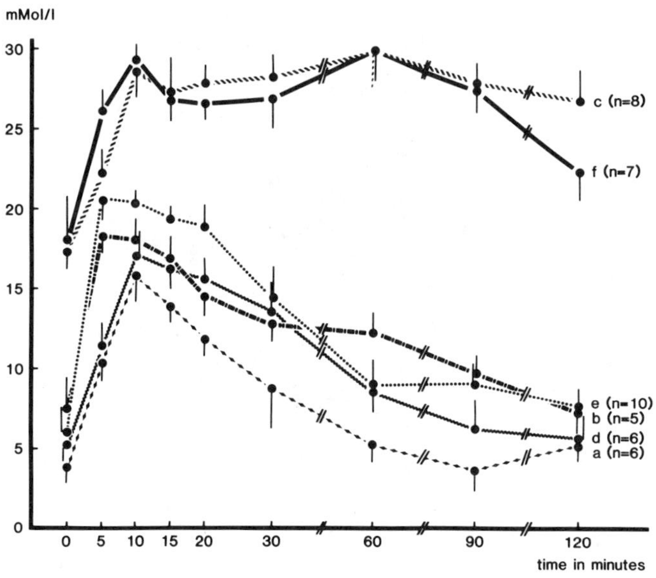

FIGURE 5. Glucose tolerance of different groups with 1 g glucose/kg b.w. i.v. Blood samples were taken at 0, 5, 10, 15, 20, 30, 60, 90 and 120 min.

be drawn as to whether or not a donor-specific tolerance was induced by the CsA treatment.

Histological findings. In the first week after isogeneic and allogeneic transplantation under normoglycemic conditions, embolic islets with normal morphology could be demonstrated within the portal veins. Later, up to 200 days after isogenic transplantation, organization of the thromboembolic material in portal veins could be seen. Aggregates of insulin-positive islets cells were covered with a newly formed intima. In other cases, the whole lumen of one portal vein branch was filled with islet cell complexes.

After clinical rejection of allografts and a reversion to hyperglycemic conditions, small thrombotic plaques with a dense infiltration of lymphatic cells could be seen in portal veins. Islet tissue could not be demonstrated by routine staining or by immunohistochemical reaction with antiinsulin serum. Three rats of the allografted and CsA-treated group were sacrificed for histological examination; two were normoglycemic at 150 and 110 days postallotransplantation, and one showed a slightly increased blood glucose level 129 days posttransplantation. The livers of all animals showed many portal fields containing transplanted islets. The islets were positive on insulin staining. Rudiments of surrounding portal veins could be seen only with difficulty. The islet cells showed strikingly broad and sometimes vacuolated cytoplasm (Fig. 6 A and B). In the rat with increasing glucose levels (which we examined in order to see what happened histologically during the phase of rejection) a greater number of islet cells were negative to insulin

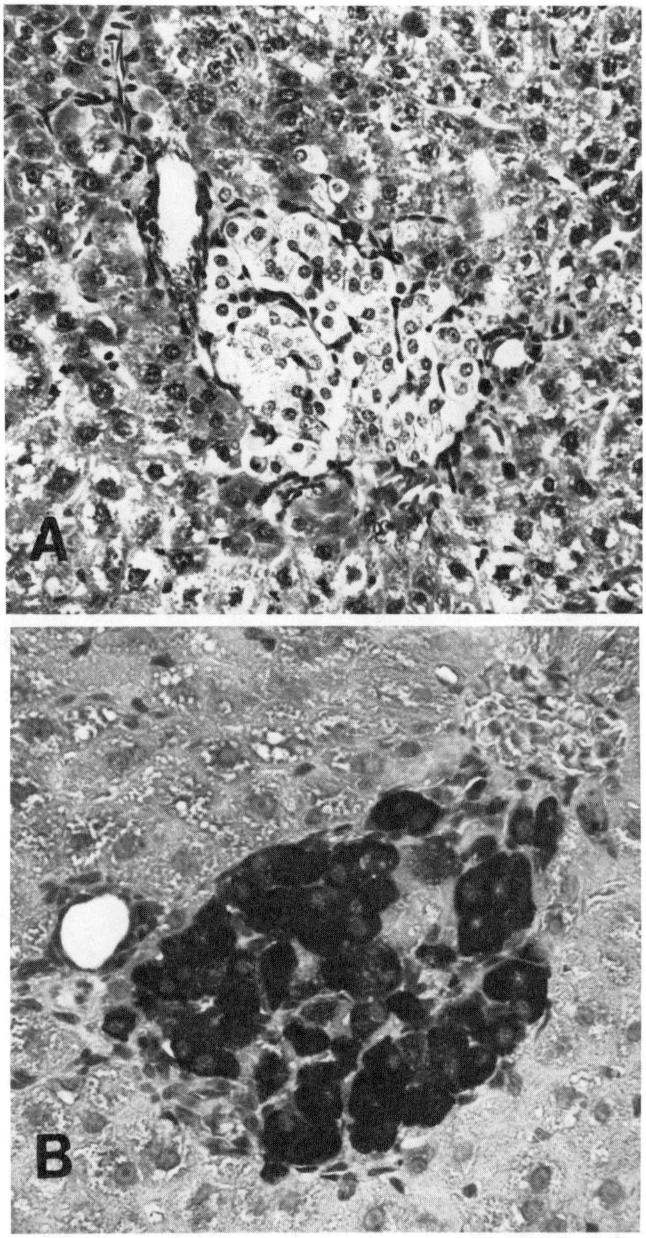

FIGURE 6. (A) Transplanted islet within a portal field under CsA therapy with normal blood glucose level 150 days posttransplantation. Only a minimal lymphatic infiltrate can be seen around the islet. (H&E; 100×). (B) Immunohistochemical demonstration of insulin in a transplanted islet of the same animal.

staining. It is noteworthy that in this animal the lymphatic infiltrate was more intensive than in a rat with normoglycemic glucose levels.

DISCUSSION

In contrast to previous reports (*17–20*) we found that CsA prolongs the survival of allogeneic transplanted islets across the MHC barrier (*11*). Three i.m. injections of 30 mg/kg bodyweight CsA were sufficient to prolong graft survival up to more than 150 days, as proved by histological examination, serum glucose levels, and glucose tolerance tests. The results of Selawry et al. (*21*) showed that islet graft acceptance was independent of the degree of histocompatibility between different rat strains. On the other hand, it was reported that CsA may prolong islet graft survival in transplantation across minor histoincompatibility barriers (*1*). These two facts may indicate that CsA principally interferes with the complex reaction involved in graft rejection in our DA → Lewis model. The reason for the previously disappointing results must be something else—especially, if one supports the hypothesis that endocrine tissue is less immunogenic than other tissues, such as heart or kidney, in which survival can be prolonged by CsA treatment (*22*). It seems possible that during the isolation process the immunogenicity of the transplant preparation is altered in such a way that the immunosuppressive effect of CsA is not strong enough to guarantee long term graft survival. We present two possible explanations:

(1) Recently several authors have emphasized the importance of the purity of the transplant preparation (*23*). We performed islet isolations using the Ficoll method (*14, 15*) and found lower yields of islets and higher amounts of non-islet contamination of the transplant preparation, compared with the neutral red technique. Histological examination of the contamination showed mainly lymphatic cells. These cells may stimulate the rejection process and prevent the beneficial effect of CsA in islet transplantation. Tissue culture, under certain conditions may guarantee an even higher degree of purity, but this requires manipulations that may alter islet function and viability—and, therefore, may make a one donor–one recipient model impractical. Nevertheless, we think that the combination of tissue culture methods and the use of CsA may lead to a further prolongation of graft survival.

(2) Ficoll itself may affect the immunogenicity by altering islet cell surface antigens. Further investigation of the ultrastructure of islets and islet cells isolated under different conditions should provide more information.

Pharmacokinetic studies (*24*) have shown that CsA blood levels vary according to the form of administration of the drug. In contrast to other authors (*1*), we gave CsA i.m. This may lead to a prolonged effect of CsA—through a depot effect, for example. This proposal is supported by the fact that we could still measure CsA blood levels of about 90 ng/ml 70 days after transplantation. On the other hand, long-term graft survival of heart and kidney transplants in small animals (*22*) after initial CsA immunosuppression was shown to be independent of a depot effect.

Islet transplantation must deal with two major problems: obtaining sufficient yields from one donor pancreas and preventing graft rejection. Our results show that by modifying the isolation technique, a one donor–one recipient model in the rat can be achieved. Furthermore an immunosuppressive effect of CsA could be demonstrated in our experiments, and seems to enable more successful islet transplantation.

Acknowledgments. We thank PD DR. R. Teichmann for preparing the insulin RIAs, Professor Vogt for determining the blood glucose levels, and Dr. K. Geisen for helping us to deal with the neutral red method.

REFERENCES

1. Rynasiewicz JJ, Sutherland DER, Kawahara K, Gorecki P. Najaran JS. Cyclosporin A prolongation of segmental pancreatic and islet allograft function in rats. Transplant Proc 1980; 12: 270.
2. Sutherland DER. Pancreas and islet transplantation. Diabetologia 1981; 20: 161.

3. Gray DWR, Morris PJ. Cyclosporine and pancreas transplantation. World J Surg 1984; 8: 230.
4. Kemp CB, Knight MJ, Sharp DW, Ballinger WF, lay PE. Effect of transplantation site on the results of pancreatic islets isografts in diabetic rats. Diabetologia 1973; 9: 486.
5. Kemp CB, Knight MB, Sharp DW, Lacy PE, Ballinger WF. Transplantation of isolated pancreatic islets into the portal vein of diabetic rats. Nature 1973; 244: 447.
6. Griffith RC, Sharp DW, Hartmann BK, Ballinger WF, Lacy PE. A morphologic study of intrahepatic portal vein isografts. Diabetes 1977; 26: 201.
7. Rabinovitch A, Alejandro R, Neol J, Brunschwig JP, Ryan US. Tissue culture reduces Ia antigen-bearing cells in rats and prolongs islets allograft survival diabetes. Diabetes 1982; 31(suppl 4): 48.
8. Lafferty KJ, Prose SJ. Theory and practice of immunoregulation by tissue treatment prior to transplantation. World J Surg 1984; 8: 187.
9. Lacy PE. Experimental immunoalteration. World J Surg 1984; 8: 198.
10. Hevely MA, Lan HT, Weber C, Reemtsma K. lsBS Pancreatic islets transplantation: immunoalteration with UV-irradiation. World J Surg 1984; 8: 207.
11. Günther B, Stark O. The major histocompatibility system of the rat. In: Göke D, ed. The MHS in man and animals. Berlin: Springer Verlag, 1977:
12. Junod A, Lambert AE, Stauffacher W, Renold AE. Diabetic action of streptozotocin, relationship of dose to metabolic response. J Clin Invest 1969; 48: 1969.
13. Bensley RR. Studies on the pancreas of the guinea pig. Am J Anat 1912; 3: 297.
14. Lacy PE, Kostianovsky M. Method for the isolation of intact islets of Langerhans from the rat pancreas. Diabetes 1967; 16: 35.
15. Sharp WD. Isolation and transplantation of islet tissue. World J Surg 1984; 8: 143.
16. Nathrath WBJ, Wilson PD, Trejdosiewicz LK. Immunohistochemical demonstration of epithelial and urothelial antigens at light- and electronmicroscope levels. Acta Histochem 1982; 25(suppl): 73.
17. Bell PRF, Wood RFM, Peters M, Nash JR. Comparison of various methods of chemical immunosuppression in islet cell transplantation. Transplant Proc 1980; 12: 291.
18. Reece-Smith H, Du toit DF, McShane P, Morris P. Effect of CyA on rejection of pancreatic islets transplanted under the renal capsule. Transplantation 1981; 32: 333d.
19. Vialettes B, Simon MC, Lassmann V, et al. Prolonged survival in allotransplanted islets of Langerhans after CyA treatment in rats. Transplantation 1979; 25: 180.
20. Garvey JFW, Morris PJ, Finch DRA, et al. Experimental pancreas transplantation. Lancet 1979; 1: 971.
21. Selawry HP, Mui MM, Paul RD, Distasio JA. Improved allograft survival using highly enriched populations of rat islets. World J Surg 1984; 8: 198. Transplantation 1984, 2: 202.
22. White DJG, NAgao T, Davies HS. Immunoalteration with UV-irradiation. Experimental Transplantation in small animals. In: White DJG, ed. Cyclosporin A. Amsterdam, New York, Oxford: Elsevier Biomedical Press, 1982: 89.
23. Hegre OD, Hichly GE, Marshall S, Serie JR. Modification of allograft immunogenicity in perinatal islets isolated and purified in vitro. Transplantation 1984; 3: 227.
24. Beveridge T. Pharmacakinetics and metabolism of Cyclosporine A. In: White DJG, ed. Cyclosporine A. Amsterdam, New York, Oxford: Elsevier Biomedical Press, 1982: 35.

Received 12 December 1984.
Accepted 31 July 1985.

0041-1337/86/4104-0431$02.00/0
TRANSPLANTATION

Vol. 41, No. 4
Printed in U.S.A.

THE INFLUENCE OF OKT8F TREATMENT ON ALLOGRAFT SURVIVAL IN RHESUS MONKEYS[1]

M. JONKER,[2] F. J. M. NOOIJ,[2] P. VAN SUYLICHEM,[3] P. NEUHAUS,[4] AND G. GOLDSTEIN[5]

Primate Center TNO, Dept. of Surgery, State University Leiden, The Netherlands; Medizinische Hochschule, Hannover, Federal Republic of Germany; Ortho Pharmaceutical Company, Raritan, NJ

The immunosuppressive effect of a monoclonal antibody specific for the cytotoxic/suppressor T cells (CD8) was investigated in rhesus monkeys. This antibody (OKT8F) removed the CD8-positive T cells from the circulation and prolonged skin allograft survival. Since most patients awaiting a kidney allograft are transfused prior to transplantation, the immunosuppressive potency of OKT8F was subsequently investigated in transfused recipients. No significant prolongation of the mean survival time was observed when OKT8F was given prophylactically. However, no early rejections were observed, while 30% of the control animals rejected their kidneys within 2 weeks. This might indicate that OKT8F prevents early rejection of a kidney allograft in transfused recipients.

It has previously been shown that monoclonal antibodies specific for helper (CD4) as well as cytotoxic/suppressor (CD8) T cell subsets can suppress skin and renal allograft rejection in monkeys (*1–4*). However, when kidney graft recipients received blood transfusions before transplantation, no additional favorable effect of treatment with CD4 antibodies (OKT4+4A) was

[1] This work was supported in part by FUNGO and Nierstichting Nederland.
[2] Primate Center TNO.
[3] Department of Surgery, State University Leiden.
[4] Medizinische Hochschule, Hannover.
[5] Ortho Pharmaceutical Company, Raritan, NJ.

seen (2). It was suggested that pretransplant blood transfusions may have generated highly reactive effector cells in some recipients that could not be blocked by CD4 antibodies. Since most patients awaiting a kidney allograft are transfused, it is important to know whether other monoclonal antibodies, which might be useful in suppressing the rejection of an allograft, are immunosuppressive in unprimed as well as in transfused recipients. This study reports the immunosuppressive effects of a CD8 antibody (OKT8F) in unprimed and transfused monkeys.

MATERIALS AND METHODS

Animals. Young unrelated male and female rhesus monkeys (*Macaca mulatta*) weighing 2–4 kg were used. About 50% of these were imported from China; the others were born at the Rijswijk Primate Center. The animals were not alloimmunized prior to these experiments. Donor recipient pairs were unrelated and mismatched for the RhLA-A, B, and DR antigens.

Skin grafting. Skin grafts were exchanged between nonimmunized monkeys. These animals were unrelated and differed for one RhL-A or -B antigen only. Because no influence of DR matching on skin graft survival has been found in rhesus monkeys, DR disparities were not taken into account (5). Such combinations have a mean skin graft survival time of 10.23 days (SE = 0.27, n = 42; range 8.5–13 days), which is slightly longer than when completely mismatched combinations are used (5).

The skin grafting technique has been described previously (6). Grafts of about 2-cm diameter (two grafts per donor) were taken from the donors abdominal skin and, after removing the subcutaneous tissue, they were transplanted onto the back of the recipient. The grafts were fixed with sutures and a special dressing was used to immobilize the area and exert pressure on the grafts. From day 5 on, the skin grafts were inspected on alternate days by briefly opening and closing the dressing. About 10 days after transplantation, the dressing was permanently removed. After that time, grafts were examined twice a day and their condition was recorded until total rejection was observed. Major hemorrhages and crust formation over virtually the entire graft were taken as the endpoint of graft survival. Monoclonal antibody treatment was started at one or two days before skin grafting and continued for as long as the skin grafts were not rejected, up to a maximum of 16 days. The antibody dose, 5 mg in saline per day, was given i.v. in a single injection of 5 ml.

Kidney transplantation. Kidney grafting was performed as described previously (7). Renal vessels were anastomosed end-to-side with the aorta and vena cava. In order to accurately determine the end-stage failure of the renal grafts, recipients were bilaterally nephrectomized immediately after transplantation. Death attributable to graft failure was considered the endpoint of graft survival. After transplantation, blood creatinine and urea levels were regularly determined. Autopsies and histopathological examinations of the recipients were done routinely. All animals received 1 mg of prednisolone and 2 mg of azathioprine daily for 45 days posttransplantation.

Monoclonal antibodies and subset analysis. Monoclonal antibodies (MCAs)* were produced at Ortho Pharmaceutical Co. (8), the Primate Center TNO (9), or in Munich (Rieber, E. P. personal communication). The MCAs used in this study were: MT910, specific for CD2 (IgG1; Rieber, E. P. personal communication); OKT4 (IgG2b) (8), OKT4A (IgG2a) (10) specific for CD4 cells; OKT8F (IgG2a) (11), and GM9 (IgG1) specific for CD8 cells; and GM11 (IgG2b) (9) specific for B cells.

The distribution of various lymphocyte subsets was determined by using monoclonal antibodies and an indirect immunofluorescence technique. Subset analysis was carried out before antibody administration, at two days after the first injection, once on days 5–7 after the first injection, once on days 9–11 after the first injection, and subsequently at weekly intervals. In approximately 50% of the animals, subset analysis was carried out more frequently in the first two weeks after injection. The stained cell samples were analyzed by means of a FACS II (Becton Dickinson, Mountain View, CA). Fluorescence of viable lymphocytes only was measured by setting the appropriate electronic windows around this population on the basis of forward and perpendicular light-scatter characteristics. Absolute numbers of the various subsets were calculated from differential blood counts. Determination of antimouse Ig antibodies was performed with an ELISA technique as described previously (1).

RESULTS

OKT8F crossreacted well with rhesus monkey lymphocytes and stained the same proportion of cells as other CD8-like antibodies in this species (12).

When OKT8F was injected i.v., the CD8 positive cells promptly disappeared from the circulation. This could be observed as soon as 10 minutes after injection and lasted for at least 9 days when daily injections were given. This was accompanied by a decrease of the lymphocyte number by 50% (range 19%–77%) in two-thirds of the animals. Table 1 shows the relative numbers of lymphocyte subsets. The relative number of CD4-positive cells increased in all animals while the absolute number of CD4 cells remained the same in two animals, increased in four animals, and decreased in six animals—more or less depending on the change in total lymphocyte numbers. The relative number of B cells did not change very much in all animals but the absolute number decreased in ten of the twelve monkeys. The relative number of null cells (cells that did not stain with T-cell or B-cell-specific antibodies) increased in 75% of the animals, usually accompanied by an increase in absolute numbers of null cells. The number of cells stained by a pan-T-

TABLE 1. Relative numbers of lymphocyte subsets before, and 7 days after, the first OKT8F injection

Monkey	Relative number of lymphocytes							
	CD4		CD8		B		Null	
	Day 0	Day 7	Day 0	Day 7	Day 0	Day 7	Day 0	Day 7
1 K[a]	29	53	29	1	36	37	6	9
2 K	29	46	31	2	34	34	6	18
3 K	30	48	27	2	29	20	14	30
4 K	28	36	30	2	34	35	8	27
5 K	24	49	34	2	33	26	9	23
6 K	41	45	21	2	30	31	8	22
7 K	29	46	28	2	27	25	16	27
8 K	21	45	35	1	34	33	10	21
9 S	45	53	25	0	12	13	18	34
10 S	48	55	20	1	12	11	20	33
11 S	39	57	30	1	17	24	14	18
20 S	42	61	29	1	13	24	16	14

[a] K: kidney graft recipient; S: skin graft recipient.

* Abbreviation used: MCAs, monoclonal antibodies.

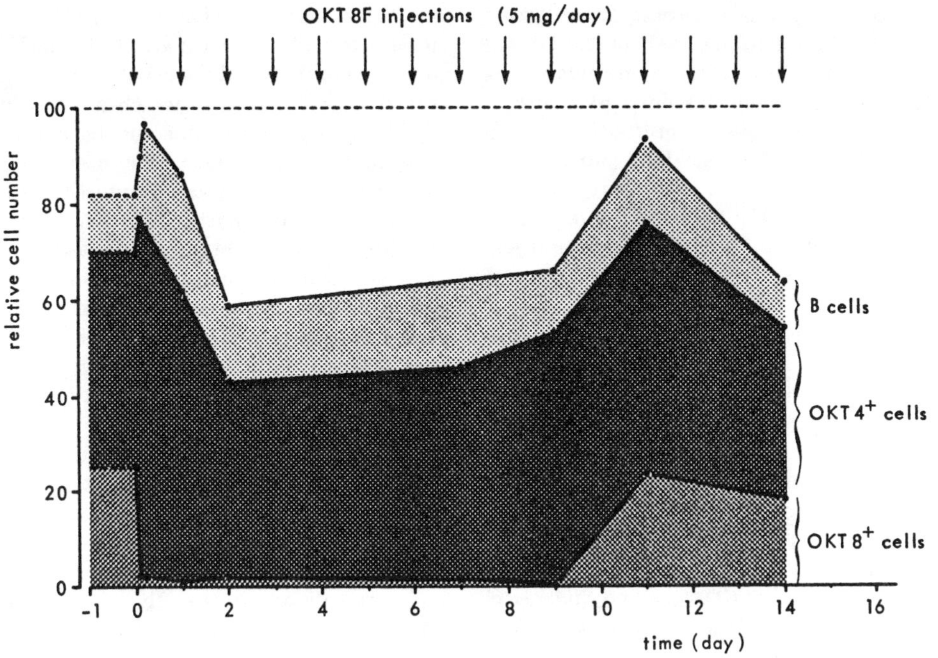

FIGURE 1. Effect of daily OKT8F injections on rhesus monkey peripheral blood lymphocyte subsets: representative example (monkey 9S). The intermediate shaded area represents the relative number of OKT8F+ cells. The dark shaded area represents the relative number of OKT4+ cells, and the top line of this area represents the sum of OKT8F+ and OKT4+ cells. The lightly shaded area represents the relative number of B cells, and the top line of this area represents the sum of OKT8F+, OKT4+ and B cells. The white area between the upper line and the 100% line represents the relative number of unstained "null" cells.

cell antibody (MT910) was approximately the same as the sum of the number of cells stained by CD4 and CD8 antibodies. Figure 1 shows the changes in the relative numbers of lymphocytes of monkey 9S as a typical example.

Skin graft experiments. The immunosuppressive potential of OKT8F was first assessed in skin graft experiments. Forty-four animals served as a control group. These animals were skin grafted for the production of alloantisera during the past ten years (*5*). The mean skin graft survival was 10.41±0.17 days (Table 2). Four animals were given OKT8F treatment, started at two days before trnsplantation, and received a skin graft. The mean skin graft survival time was 13.88±1.13 days (Table 2). This was significantly longer than the mean survival time of the control animals ($P<0.001$, Mann-Whitney U test).

Kidney graft experiments. Eight monkeys received three pretransplant blood transfusions from random donors at two-week intervals. The last transfusion was given at three weeks before transplantation. The blood donors shared no RhLA-A or -B locus antigens with the prospective kidney donors. Therefore there was no sensitization against these antigens. The animals were transplanted with an allogeneic MHC-mismatched kidney. One animal died on day 17 due to urine leakage from the bladder without signs of graft rejection. The other seven animals survived 20–56 days (MST = 40.6±4.9 days) (Table 3). The results are compared with a nontransfused control group and a transfused control group. These same groups of animals served as control groups in previous studies (*2, 13*). Nontransfused rhesus monkeys were transplanted with MHC-mismatched kidneys. All these monkeys rejected their kidneys within 22 days: mean graft survival 12.8±1.2 days (Table 3). The transfused control animals also received blood transfusions from random donors at two-week intervals. Again, the blood donors shared no RhLA-A or -B locus antigens with the prospective kidney donors. The mean graft survival time was 33.6 days, which is significantly longer than that of untransfused animals ($P = <0.01$, Mann-Whitney U test) (Table 3). Thus, the additional treatment of transfused animals with OKT8F did not give an additional graft-prolonging effect. It should be noted that none of the OKT8F-treated animals died before day

TABLE 2. Immunosuppressive effect of OKT8F (skin graft experiments)

Treatment	Skin graft survival times	
None	8.5 8.5 8.5 8.5	
	9 9 9	
	9.5 9.5 9.5 9.5 9.5	
	10 10 10 10 10 10 10 10 10	
	10.5 10.5 10.5 10.5 10.5 10.5 10.5	
	11 11 11 11	
	11.5 11.5 11.5 11.5 11.5 11.5 11.5	
	12 12 12	
	12.5 13	
	Mean: 10.41; SE: 0.17	
OKT8F	12 12.5 14 17	$P<0.001$
	Mean: 13.88; SE: 1.13	

TABLE 3. The effect of OKT8F on kidney graft survival times in transfused monkeys

Pretreatment of recipient	OKT8F	Graft survival times (MST±SE)		
None	No	9 9 10 10 11 12 12 14		
		14 17 22	(12.8±1.2)	
3 Blood transfusions	No	9 10 11 12 12 13 13 19		$P<0.001$
		22 29 32 32 34 41 43 43 44		
		53 53 56 56 61 75	(33.6±4.1)	
3 Blood transfusions	Yes	20 35 35 35 48 55 56	(40.6±4.9)	NS

20, while 30% of the control animals rejected their kidneys within two weeks. The serum creatinine levels of the OKT8F treated animals did not differ from those of the transfused control animals, which were matched for kidney graft survival times. No correlation was found between graft survival time and degree of lymphopenia due to OKT8F treatment.

DISCUSSION

OKT8F is a monoclonal antibody reactive with the cytotoxic-suppressor T cell population. It has been shown to be a potent inhibitor of MHC-class-I–specific CTL responses in man (*14*). To assess whether OKT8F could be immunosuppressive in vivo, it was first tested in a skin graft experiment. When a potential immunosuppressive agent can prolong the survival time of an allogeneic skin graft, this will be highly predictive of its immunosuppressive potencies for kidney allografts (*15*) and is then considered for further studies. Injection of OKT8F resulted in a prompt disappearance of CD8-positive cells. This was a true disappearance and not a modulation of the CD8 antigen, since the remaining T cells as defined by a CD2-specific antibody were virtually all CD4-positive. Nearly all animals showed similar changes in the relative numbers of lymphocyte subsets: an increase of the proportion of CD4 cells and null cells, and no change in the proportion of B cells. Thus, the OKT8F treatment had a predictable effect on the subset proportions. The effect on the total lymphocyte count varied, but this may be due to influences other than the OKT8F treatment. Daily sedation and animal handling carried out for the transplantation experiments may have caused a nonspecific reduction or increase of peripheral blood lymphocytes.

The administration of OKT8F to rhesus monkeys receiving the MHC mismatched skin allograft resulted in a significant prolongation of the survival times of these grafts. Thus, it can be concluded that OKT8F is immunosuppressive and that OKT8F-positive cells do play a role in the allograft rejection. This is in contrast to earlier findings that CD8 antibodies did not prolong skin allograft survival in rhesus monkeys (1, 16). This cannot be explained by the immunoglobulin isotype of the antibodies employed, since the other two antibodies tested—OKT8A (*1*) and B9.8 (*16*)—were, like OKT8F, IgG2a. It could be that the effect the antibody has on the CD8-positive T cells is important. OKT8F administration resulted in a prompt disappearance of CD8-positive cells, while B9.8 only coated the cells and OKT8A reduced the number of CD8 cells not completely, with the effect starting only after a few days of administration. It is, however, not clear whether CD8 cells should be removed in order to achieve immunosuppression. In another experiment a pool of six CD8-specific monoclonal antibodies (B9 pool) was used; this resulted in prolongation of skin graft survival times while the CD8 cells were coated by the antibody in vivo (Jonker M, unpublished results). Since CD8 antibodies can recognize many different epitopes of the CD8 molecule (*17*) it could be that, by using this pool of CD8 antibodies, the immunoactive site of the molecule was coated and could not carry out its function effectively. Thus, either elmination of the CD8 cells, or coating of the active site of the CD8 molecule can result in immunosuppression. We have previously shown also that CD4-positive cells play a role in skin allograft rejection (*1*), and from these results it appears that both cell types are needed for the rejection of a class-I and class-II–mismatched skin allograft.

Experiments carried out by Cosimi et al. (*4*) have shown that a CD8-like antibody (Leu2a) can also be immunosuppressive in monkeys when a mismatched kidney is transplanted in an unprimed recipient. In view of our previous experience with transfused recipients, in which no additional favorable effect of OKT4+4A treatment could be observed, and because in clinical situations most kidney graft recipients have received blood transfusions, we chose to test OKT8F only in transfused recipients. It was postulated that blood transfusions could condition the recipients in one of two ways; either they become nonresponsive to antigens of the kidney donor and show a prolonged graft survival time, or they become sensitized and have high-affinity effector cells of the CD4 and/or the CD8 type. These CD4-positive effector cells could apparently not be blocked by coating the cells with OKT4+4A antibodies (*2*). This study showed that no significant additional favorable effect of OKT8F and blood transfusions was found. However, no acute rejections occurred (graft survival time of <14 days) in the OKT8F-treated group, although it was observed in 30% of the untreated group of recipients and also in recipients receiving OKT4+4A treatment (*2*). Since the number of animals transplanted in the OKT8F treated group is small, this difference is not significant. From the results reported here it might be an indication that removal of CD8-positive cells by OKT8F antibody eliminated effector cells in those recipients that otherwise would have rejected their kidneys early. This would indicate that in primed (blood-transfusion-primed) recipients one needs to eliminate the effector cells in order to prevent early rejection while coating the cells with antibody is sufficient in unprimed recipients.

Our experiments have shown that a primary response can be suppressed by OKT4+4A (*2*) and by OKT8F antibodies (shown in this study) in nontransfused recipients. This could mean that a primary response directed against antigens expressed on the transplanted kidney is already suppressed or does not occur in blood-transfusion-primed recipients. It seems unlikely that CD8 positive suppressor cells play a significant role in prolonging kidney graft survival since OKT8F certainly does not shorten the graft survival in transfused animals.

Taken together, the findings with OKT8F and our previous results with OKT4+4A (*2*) suggest that it is unlikely that these types of subset-specific monoclonal antibodies will eventually be useful in clinical immunosuppression when applied singly. When using monoclonal anti-T-cell antibodies as immunosuppressive agents two approaches are possible: elimination (or inactivation) of all mature T cells or elimination of cells that are directly responsible for allograft rejection. The first approach is not essentially different from antithymocyte globulin treatment, and success has been achieved with OKT3. This antibody proved to be immunosuppressive in man when used prophylactically (*18*) as well as when used as rejection treatment (*19*, *20*). Also another pan-T-cell antibody (T12, [*21*]) proved to be immunosuppressive, but other pan-T-cell antibodies failed to reverse a rejection episode effectively (Hulyml, ref. 22 and WT1; Tax W, personal communication). Using a combination of CD4 and CD8 antibodies could be an alternative to pan-T-cell antibodies, again aiming at elimination or inactivation of all mature T cells. The second approach—elimination of only those cells that are responsible for rejection—has successfully been used by Takahashi et al. (*23*). However, the CBL1 antibody crossreacts with tissues other than activated T cells (*24*), and a further search for useful antibodies that react only with activated T cells is needed.

Since many antihuman T cell monoclonal antibodies crossreact with subhuman primates (*11*) the rhesus monkey is a useful animal model in which to test the immunosuppressive efficacy of these reagents.

Acknowledgments. We thank A. Kok, Z. de By-Aghai, G. van Meurs, H. D. Wiersema, and A. Arkesteijn for their excellent technical assistance and D. de Keizer and E. J. v. d. Reyden for their help in preparing the manuscript. We thank Prof. E. P. Rieber for the donation of the MT910 antibody.

REFERENCES

1. Jonker M, Goldstein G, Balner H. Effects of in vivo administration of monoclonal antibodies specific for human T cell subpopulations on the immune system in a rhesus monkey model. Transplantation 1983; 35: 521.
2. Jonker M, Neuhaus P, Zurcher C, Fucello A, Goldstein G. OKT4 and OKT4A antibody treatment as immunosuppression for kidney transplantation in rhesus monkeys. Transplantation 1985; 39: 247.
3. Cosimi AB, Burton RC, Kung RC, et al. Evaluation in primate renal allograft recipients of monoclonal antibody to human T-cell subclasses. Transplant Proc 1981; 13: 499.
4. Cosimi AB. Anti T cell monoclonal antibodies in transplantation therapy. Transplant Proc 1983; 15: 1889.
5. Vreeswijk W, Balner H. MHC-matching and other factors influencing skin allograft survival in related and unrelated rhesus monkeys. Transplantation 1980; 30: 196.
6. Balner H. Transplantation 1969; 8: 281.
7. Neuhaus P, Neuhaus R, Wiersema HD, et al. The technique of kidney transplantation in rhesus monkeys. J Med Primatol 1982; 11: 155.
8. Kung PC, Goldstein G, Reinherz EL, Schlossman SF. Monoclonal antibodies defining distinctive human T cell surface antigens. Science 1979; 206: 347.
9. Jonker M, Meurs G van. Monoclonal antibodies specific for B cells, cytotoxic/suppressor T cells and a subset of cytotoxic/suppressor T cells in the rhesus monkey. In: Bernard A, et al, eds. Leucocyte typing. Berlin: Springer, 1984: 328.
10. Bach MA, Phan-Dinh-Tuy F, Bach JF, et al. Unusual phenotypes of human inducer T cells as measured by OKT4 and related monoclonal antibodies. J Immunol 1981; 127: 980.
11. Reinherz EL, Kung PC, Goldstein G, et al. Discrete stages of human intrathymic differentiation: analysis of normal thymocytes and leukemic lymphoblasts of T-cell lineage. Proc Natl Acad Sci USA 1980; 77: 1588.
12. Jonker M, Nooij FJM. The phylogeny of T cell antigens. In: Leucocyte Typing II. (in press).
13. Borleffs JCC. Kidney transplantation in rhesus monkeys [Thesis]. Leiden, 1982.
14. Biddison WE, Rao PE, Talle MA, et al. Distinct epitopes on the T8 moleculare are differentially involved in cytotoxic T cell function. Hum Immunol 1984; 9: 711.
15. Ceppellini R, Bigliani S, Curtoni ES, Leigheb G. Experimental allotransplantation in man. Transplant Proc 1969; 1: 390.
16. Jonker M, Malissen M, Mawas C. The effect of in vivo application of monoclonal antibodies specific for human cytotoxic T cells in rhesus monkeys. Transplantation 1983; 35: 374.
17. Hansen JA, Martin PJ, Beatty PG, et al. In: Bernard, et al, eds. Leukocyte typing. Berlin: Springer, 1984: 195.
18. Kreis H, Chkoff H, Vigeral P, et al. Prophylactic treatment of allograft recipients with a monoclonal anti-$T3^+$ cell antibody. Transplant proc 1985; 17: 1315.
19. Cosimi AB, Burton RC, Colvin RB, et al. Treatment of acute renal allograft rejection with OKT3 monoclonal antibody. Transplantation 1981; 32: 535.
20. Goldstein G, Schindler J, Sheahan M, et al., Orthoclone OKT3 treatments of acute renal allograft rejection. Transplant Proc 1985; 17: 129.
21. Kirkman RL, Araujo JL, Busch GJ, et al. Treatment of acute renal allograft rejection with monoclonal anti-T12 antibody. Transplantation 1983; 36: 620.
22. Thurlow PJ, Lovering E, D'Apice AJF, McKenzi IFC. A monclonal anti-pan T-cell antibody. In vitro and in vivo studies. Transplantation 1983; 36: 293.
23. Takahashi H, Terasaki PI, Kinukawa T, et al. Reversal of transplant rejection by monoclonal antiblast antibody. Lancet 1983; 2: 1155.
24. Terasaki P, Cats S, Cicciarelli J, et al. Use of monoclonal antibodies for kidney transplant patients. Transplant Proc 1985; 17: 1521.

Received 22 March 1985.
Accepted 17 July 1985.

0041-1337/86/4104-0436$02.00/0
TRANSPLANTATION
Vol. 41, No. 4

Printed in U.S.A.

SEROLOGIC METHODS FOR THE EARLY DIAGNOSIS OF *PNEUMOCYSTIS CARINII* INFECTION IN RENAL ALLOGRAFT RECIPIENTS[1,2]

MARK JAROWENKO, LINDA PIFER,[3] RONALD KERMAN, AND BARRY D. KAHAN

The Division of Immunology and Organ Transplantation, Department of Surgery, The University of Texas Medical School at Houston, Texas 77030

Because of the nephrotoxic action of trimethoprim-sulfamethoxazole (TMP-SMX) in cyclosporine (CsA)-treated patients, combined with the possibility of selecting resistant gram-negative or *Nocardia* asteroides organisms, a monitoring tool to detect early *Pneumocystis carinii* (PC) infection permitting a selective treatment approach is highly desirable. A review of 401 consecutive renal transplants revealed 26 cases (18 suspected and 8 histologically proved) of PC infection in 21 cadaver and 5 living-related renal recipients. The diagnosis was confirmed in 8/18 patients who were invasively studied by open-lung biopsy (1/2), bronchoscopy with transbronchial biopsy (4/9), bronchoscopy with brushing (1/2), bronchoscopy with bronchoalveolar lavage (2/5), and transpleural needle biopsy (0/1)—yielding a confirmed incidence of 2% (8/401). All positive invasive studies had been performed prior to or within 24 hr of the inception of TMP-SMX therapy. Nine of ten negative invasive studies were performed after more than 24 hr of treatment. The mean time from transplantation to the onset of clinical symptoms was 2.5±1.5 months. The infection rate would be 6.5%, assuming all 18 suspected cases would be PC-positive if studied pretreatment. In order to assess the efficacy of a variety of serologic methods of PC detection, qualitative counterimmunoelectrophoresis (CIE) for *P carinii* antigen (PC-Ag), IgG antibody reactive with PC (enzyme-linked immunosorbent assay [ELISA]), and a latex particle agglutination test (LPA) were performed on 279 sera; 85 sera from the 26 suspected or proved cases, 100 sera from normal age-matched controls, and 94 sera from 78 asymptomatic allograft recipients followed as outpatients. In the eight histologically proven cases, CIE was positive in only 3/8 and turned positive late in the clinical course. LPA was positive in all histologically proved cases; however, it was also positive in 60% of asymptomatic renal recipients. In cases that developed clinical disease, LPA increased in titer weeks to months prior to the onset of symptoms. Additionally, LPA titers decreased or stabilized during successful TMP-SMX therapy, providing an early therapeutic index. Measurement of anti-PC IgG was not useful per se, as it was elevated in both controls and documented PC infection. The combination of very low antibody titer (≤1:16) with a positive or increasing LPA PC-Ag titer appeared to be disease-predictive. Both histologic and serologic criteria appeared to indicate an increase in *P carinii* pneumonia (PCP) incidence in this transplant population. Serial studies of LPA PC-Ag and ELISA PC antibody titers will aid in the development of monitoring tools to improve the care of transplant recipients at high risk for PC infection.

Pneumocystis carinii (PC)* was originally identified by the Delanos at the Pasteur Institute in Paris (*1*). This probable protozoan has at least a two-phase life cycle. In the cyst phase, a 4–6-μ organism contains up to eight smaller units called sporozoites, which mature into trophozoites, extracystic forms that attach to the host cell until they encyst (*2*). Even when this ubiquitous organism causes fulminant infections, as it does in hosts immunocompromised by virtue of chemotherapeutic or immunosuppressive drug therapy, of congenital or acquired immune deficiency, or of severe malnutrition, it generally remains restricted to the lungs. The incidence of *P carinii* pneumonia (PCP) in allograft recipients is generally between and 0 and 4% (*3, 4*). A recent report suggests an increased incidence from 3.4 to 9.0% since the introduction of the T-cell-selective immunosuppressive drug cyclosporine (CsA[*5*]). Other workers believe the change in disease incidence is unrelated to the advent of CsA (*3*).

The increased incidence of PCP demands new therapeutic approaches. The response of instituting routine trimethoprim-sulfamethoxazole (TMP-SMX) prophylaxis appeared to result in at least temporary eradication of the problem (*5*). However, concerns regarding this approach are two-fold: first, mass TMP-SMX prophylaxis may lead to the selection of resistant strains not only of PC, but also of other, currently, susceptible bacteria. Therapeutic failures have been already noted in cases of PCP, in spite of adequate TMP-SMX serum levels (*6*). Since the mortality rate in untreated patients is 95–100%, drug resistance has ominous implications (*7*). The second difficulty is the synergistic nephrotoxicity of TMP-SMX with CsA. Significant declines in creatinine clearance have been noted in TMP-SMX–treated renal allograft recipients immunosuppressed with azathioprine (*9*)—or particularly with CsA (*8*). Thus although the prophylactic approach may superficially appear advantageous, there may be potential both for the emergence of resistant organisms and for significant nephrotoxicity.

A clearly preferable alternative would be the development of

[1] Presented at the 11th Annual Meeting of The American Society of Transplant Surgeons, May 1985, Chicago, IL.

[2] This work was supported by National Institutes of Health National Cancer Institute Grant IU01 CA 34987-01.

[3] *Pneumocystis carinii* Serologic Reference Laboratory, Department of Pediatrics, University of Tennessee Center for the Health Sciences, and Le Bonheur Children's Medical Center, Memphis, TN 38163.

* Abbreviations used: CEL, chick epithelial lung; CIE, counterimmunoelectrophoresis; CsA, cyclosporine; ELISA, enzyme-linked immunosorbent assay; LPA, latex particle agglutination; PC, *Pneumocystis carinii;* Pc-Ag, *Pneumocystis carinii* antigen; PCP, *Pneumocystis carinii* pneumonia; TMP-SMX, trimethoprim-sulfamethoxazole.

a rapid, noninvasive diagnostic test for PCP, which would discern allograft recipients requiring therapy prior to the onset of fulminant disease. At the present time, a variety of invasive approaches are necessary to obtain samples to identify the organism by the Gomori methenamine silver and the Giemsa stains, which each discern individual phases of the organism's life cycle (*14*). Open-lung biopsy is considered the most precise diagnostic tool, since it has almost 100% accuracy with a 10% morbidity rate and a reported mortality range of 3–10% (*10, 11*). Bronchoscopy with bronchial brushing, a less invasive alternative, may be 80% accurate, but may incur a 25% incidence of pneumothorax (*12*). Bronchoalveolar lavage and transbronchial biopsy have yielded a positive diagnosis in greater than 80% of cases in some reports (*13*).

The advent of methods to cultivate PC in embryonic chick epithelial lung cells (CEL) in vitro has permitted extraction and purification of *P carinii* antigen (Pc-Ag) and production of specific antisera to titer Pc-Ag content, using counterimmunoelectrophoresis (CIE), latex particle agglutination (LPA [*15*]), or enzyme-linked immunosorbent assay (ELISA [*16, 17*]) tests. This communication presents a preliminary evaluation of a combined approach utilizing clinical and serologic approaches to diagnose PCP in 401 renal allograft recipients, including 26 patients suspected of harboring, or proved to suffer, from the disease.

TABLE 1. Summary of invasive pulmonary studies for the diagnosis of PCP in the 18 suspected cases studied invasively

Patient	Method	Result	<24 hr[b]	>24 hr[c]	>48 hr[d]
307	Open biopsy	+	x		
409	Closed (transbronchial) biopsy	+	x		
	Open biopsy[a]	−		x	
185	Closed biopsy	−		x	
234	Closed biopsy	−			x
298	Closed biopsy	−	x		
371	Closed biopsy	+	x		
389	Closed biopsy	−		x	
525	Closed biopsy	−			x
529	Closed biopsy	+	x		
548	Closed biopsy	+	x		
534	Brush biopsy	+	x		
543	Brush biopsy	−		x	
474	Wash	+	x		
515	Wash	+	x		
547	Wash	−		x	
550	Wash	−		x	
559	Wash	−		x	
275	Transpleural biopsy	−			x

[a] Open lung biopsy was performed because preliminary stains were negative on closed lung biopsy.

[b,c,d] Time of invasive study in relation to start of TMP-SMX therapy.

MATERIALS AND METHODS

Clinical material. The clinical courses of 401 consecutive renal allografts performed between February 1981 and March 1985 were reviewed, including 82 living-related donor kidneys and 319 transplants from cadaver donors. All patients were immunosuppressed with the CsA-prednisone regimen previously described in detail (*18*). There were 26 cases (18 suspected and 8 histologically proved) of PCP based upon standard invasive and histologic techniques. Cases evoking suspicion of the diagnosis displayed (1) an acute presentation with dyspnea and fever to greater than 101°F; (2) PaO_2 <60 mmHg with no previous pulmonary disease or evidence of cardiac failure; (3) infiltrate on chest roentgenogram; and (4) absence of a definite pathogen by routine gram stain and/or culture of sputum. The 26 cases of clinically suspected or proved PCP were analyzed for the following characteristics: (1) method of diagnosis, including staining techniques and serologic correlation; (2) time from transplantation to onset of clinical illness; (3) correlations of serologic data with diagnostic and prognostic factors; and (4) impact of anti-PC therapy on clinical outcome and serologic data.

Clinical management. Table 1 summarizes the results and timing of invasive studies using standard methods—namely, open lung biopsy, closed lung biopsy, brush biopsy, bronchoalveolar lavage, and needle transpleural biopsy. Noteworthy is the fact that none of the invasive studies was performed prior to the initiation of TMP-SMX therapy. All patients in the series of 26 were treated with a minimum of one week of TMP-SMX therapy, at least five days of which were delivered i.v. (20 mg trimethoprim/kg/24 hr). Oxygen and mechanical ventilatory support were provided as required. In cases documented invasively or when the clinical course was consistent with the diagnosis of PCP, i.v. therapy was continued until substantial improvement occurred, namely ventilation was no longer needed and the chest roentgenogram significantly improved. All patients were subsequently continued on oral TMP-SMX therapy for at least six months.

Serologic material. The 279 samples submitted for analysis included 85 sera from the 26 suspected or proved cases, 100 sera from normal age-matched controls, and 94 sera from 78 asymptomatic allograft recipients being followed as outpatients. All serum specimens were frozen immediately following separation from the clot by centrifugation, coded, and shipped on dry ice directly to the laboratory of Dr. L. Pifer. Each patient's serum was tested in triplicate by LPA and CIE methods for PC antigenemia and by ELISA method for patient IgG antibody to PC. Due to serologic laboratory time constraints and the availability of ELISA PC antibody control data from other series, the ELISA was performed on only 20 of the 100 normals in this series. Control samples included normal human sera and samples from nontransplant patients with tissue-documented PC.

Latex particle agglutination test (LPA). Rabbit antibody (*15, 19*) raised against in-vitro-cultured PC organisms, which were originally derived from cortisone-acetate-treated Sprague-Dawley rats, was bonded to latex beads and mixed on a ring slide with doubling dilutions of either patient serum (1:2, 1:4, 1:8, etc.), or positive and negative controls. After the slides were rotated until agglutination appeared complete, the Pc-Ag titer was recorded as the highest serum dilution displaying flocculation or agglutination visible to the unaided eye. Tests failing to show agglutination were recorded as negative for the presence of antigen.

Counterimmunoelectrophoresis test (CIE). Counterimmunoelectrophoresis was performed on 75×50-mm glass slides precoated with 10 ml 0.75% agarose (Marine Colloids, Inc., Rockland, ME) in 0.05 M barbital buffer, pH 8.2 (Spectra Biologicals, Oxnard, CA). After 3-mm-diameter wells were cut 2 mm apart in the agarose, undiluted rabbit antibody and antigen-containing sera were placed in the anodal and cathodal wells, respectively. Electrophoresis was carried out for 45 min at 50 V, 10 mamp at room temperature. The appearance of a discrete precipitin band between the wells signified a specific antigen-antibody reaction (*19*).

Enzyme-linked immunosorbent assay (ELISA). Patient IgG antibody toward PC was titered in serum by a micro-ELISA technique (*17*). Pc-Ag suspended in carbonate buffer was bound to microtiter plates (Dynatech Laboratories, Inc.) by incubation at 40°C. The plates were rinsed with phosphate-buffered saline containing Tween 20 (PBST) and dried. Diluted serum specimens were added to the wells, incubated for 1 hr at room temperature and then drained prior to washing the plates with PBST. Peroxidase-tagged, heavy and light chain-specific, goat antihuman IgG (Kirkegaard and Perry Laboratories, Inc.) was added to each well, incubated for 2 hr at room temperature, and then rinsed with PBST. Then 50 μl of substrate, consisting of ABTS (2.2 azina-di-[3-ethyl-benz-thiazoline sulfonate 6]) in cacodylic acid buffer combined with equal parts of H_2O_2, was added prior to the plates being incubated in the dark for 30 min at room temperature, and then analyzed at 405 nm on an Abbott EIA micro-ELISA plate reader. Serum IgG antibody to PC was also semiquantitated by an indirect immunofluorescence (IFF) method (*19*) in parallel testing with the ELISA technique. The ELISA results were highly consistent with the IIF, although ELISA titers tended to be proportionately higher, reflecting a greater sensitivity of the procedure.

RESULTS

The 401 renal allograft recipients included 26 suspected or proved cases of PCP. If all suspected cases of PCP had been histologically proved, the overall incidence would be 6.5% (26/401), including 21/320 cadaver recipients (6.6%) and 5.82 living-related recipients (6.1%). Table 1 summarizes the invasive studies for the presence of PCP in 18/26 cases: Open lung biopsy was positive in 1/2 cases; bronchoscopy with transbronchial biopsy in 4/9 cases; bronchoscopy with brushing in 1/2 cases; bronchoscopy with bronchoalveolar lavage in 2/5 cases; and transpleural needle biopsy in 0/1 cases. All invasive studies that were positive for PC organisms by histologic techniques had been peformed prior to or within 24 hr of the inception of TMP-SMX therapy. Of the ten invasive studies that did not yield PC organisms, only one (case No. 298) was performed within 24 hr of the initiation of therapy; the remainder occurred later in the treatment course. The mean time from transplantation to clinical presentation was 2.5±1.5 months. Finally, a review of CMV titers revealed a similar distribution of infection with CMV in the histologically proved group A (4/8), histologically negative group B (6/10), and group C, not studied histologically (4/8).

The cases were divided into five categories in order to evaluate the serologic results: group A, the 8 biopsy-proved PCP cases; group B, the 10 histologically negative cases of suspected PCP; group C, the 8 suspected cases of PCP not invasively studied; group D, the 78 asymptomatic outpatient allograft recipients; and group E, the 100 normal control persons (of whom antibody determinations were performed on 20 random subjects).

CIE. Table 2 shows that all normal individuals were negative by CIE for Pc-Ag. Among 78 asymptomatic outpatient renal allograft recipients (group D), only one was positive for antigen. Indeed, this patient was convalescing from invasively documented PCP, had been previously antigen 4^+ positive, and now was antigen 1^+ positive. Five of the invasively documented cases failed to show antigenemia. Three cases with negative invasive studies had a positive CIE, but all had been treated for greater than 24 hr prior to the study. In general, CIE determinations became positive late in the clinical course, rendering them not useful diagnostic tools. However, the one case showing a decreased antigen level in convalescent sera did display a benign clinical course, whereas the two patients who succumbed showed a persistent antigen 4^+ positive result without a decrease accompanying therapy.

LPA. Table 3 summarizes the results of Pc-Ag levels detected by the LPA test. Among the group E normal persons, 5% of sera were positive undiluted, consistent with the occasional histological finding of incidental PCP at autopsy. Group A, patients with proved PCP, showed only one patient with an antigen titer of 1:2; all biopsy-proved cases were antigen-positive. The mean titer in the PCP-proved group was 1:4.28±1.67, significantly greater than the mean titer of 1:1.82±2.21 in the outpatient population ($P<0.05$, Wilcoxon rank sum). Groups B and C showed serum antigen titers of 1:2 or greater with the exception of three cases, who, on review of their clinical courses and treatment responses, were independently judged to represent misdiagnoses of PCP. Not only were their antigen titers negative throughout the clinical course, but also cytomegalovirus titers subsequently increased, suggesting that this agent was the cause of pneumonia. The LPA was positive in five cases in which invasive studies were negative; however, in all cases treatment had been underway for more than 24 hr prior to the invasive study. Finally, among group D outpatient recipients, 62% displayed positive antigen determinations at undi-

TABLE 2. Summary of Pc-Ag determinations using CIE

Group	n	CIE[b] result				
		4+	3+	2+	1+	Negative
A	7[a]	2	0	0	0	5
B	6[a]	1	1	0	1	3
C	6[a]	1	1	0	0	4
D	78	0	0	0	1	77
E	100	0	0	0	0	100
Total	197	4	2	0	2	189

[a] The values recorded reflect samples collected during the clinical illness.

[b] CIE scored by a subjective assessment was made. The degree of reaction scaled 1–4+ antigen-positive in relation to the size of the discrete precipitin band between the wells.

TABLE 3. Summary of Pc-Ag titer determined by LPA

Group[a]	n	Negative	Maximum antigen titer[b]					
			Undiluted	1:2	1:4	1:8	1:16	Mean
A	7	0	0	1	5	1	0	4.28
B	6	2	0	2	0	2	1	5.14
C	6	1	0	0	3	0	1	5.60
D	78	30	10	22	10	6	0	1.82
E	100	95	5	0	0	0	0	0.05

[a] Groups A–D values represent maximum titers; n has been reduced in A–C if no titer was available during clinical illness. In the outpatient group n has been reduced by dropping the convalescent titers, and repeat values on the same patient on subsequent visits.

[b] Titer was recorded as the highest serum dilution displaying flocculation or agglutination visible to the unaided eye.

luted or greater titer: 8% at 1:8, 13% at 1:4, 28% at 1:2, 13% undiluted, and 38% negative. These antigen levels were significantly different from the normal controls ($P<0.01$, Wilcoxon rank sum).

Although a given titer of Pc-Ag did not predict disease, the entire group of allografted patients showed 20/36 (56%) patients reaching a Pc-Ag titer of at least 1:4 and 9/35 (26%) recipients at 1:2 developed clinical disease. The few cases in which serial sera were available demonstrated a progressive increase in Pc-Ag titer prior to clinical onset. Figures 1–3 depict the serologic time courses in patients with proved or suspected PCP, in whom there were sera available for analysis during, before, and after the clinical illness. Figure 1 illustrates seven cases of invasively documented PCP (from group A). Figure 2 provides similar data on four of six histologically negative cases meeting the sera availability criterion. Figure 3 provides similar data on three suspected PCP cases (group C) that were not invasively studied. All nine cases (A, 1–4; B, 1–3; C, 1 and 3) with serial sera preceding the onset of clinical illness displayed at least a doubling of antigen titer as long as two months prior to the onset of clinical illness. All antigen-positive cases that survived their illness showed a plateau or decline in antigenemia during therapy. Among the 13 evaluable cases, 9 patients

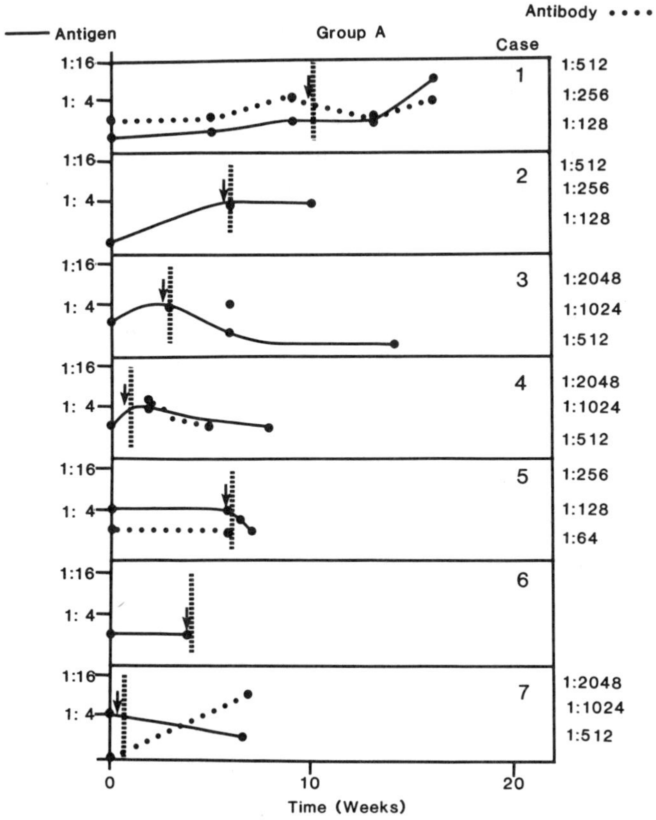

FIGURE 1. Group A: serial serologic studies in seven cases of histologically documented PCP. Case eight did not have serial studies. The point of clinical disease onset is marked by the black vertical arrow. Initiation of TMP-SMX therapy is indicated by the vertical line. Case 1 was open-lung-biopsy–negative and closed-lung-biopsy–positive for PCP. Cases 2, 3, and 7 were closed-lung-biopsy–positive. Case 4 is brush-biopsy–positive. Cases 5 and 6 are bronchoalveolar-lavage–positive. The solid line indicates PC antigen detected by latex particle agglutination assay. The dotted line represents IgG antibody to PC antigen detected by ELISA.

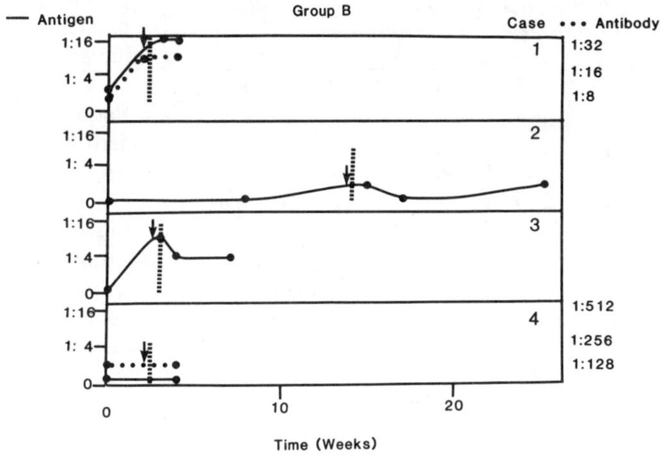

FIGURE 2. Group B: serial serologic studies in histologically negative cases. Four cases histologically negative for PC that had serial serology available are illustrated serologically here. Cases without data during clinical illness are also excluded. Coded as in Figure 1.

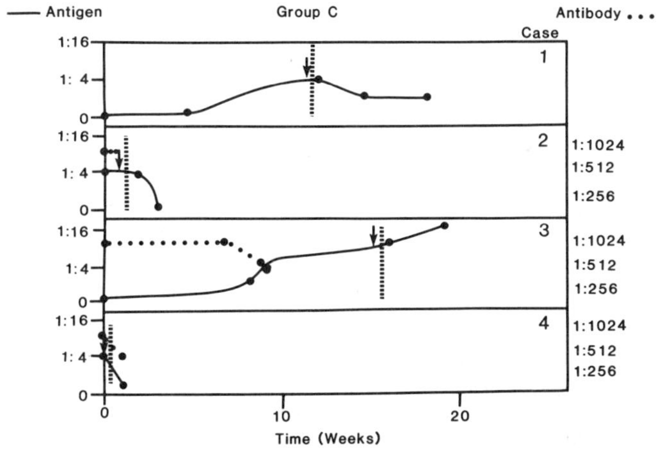

FIGURE 3. Group C: serial serologic studies in suspected PCP cases. Four cases suspected of PCP, but not invasively documented, are illustrated herein. Cases in this group without serial data or data during clinical illness are excluded. Coded as in Figure 1.

(A-3, 4, 5, 7; B-2, 3; C-1, 2, 4) showed a decline in antigenemia, 2 recipients displayed stable antigen levels (A-2; B-1), and the 2 individuals (A-1; C-3) showing an increase both died of progressive disease.

ELISA P carinii *antibody*. The overall distribution of IgG antibody specific for PC is illustrated in Table 4. Noteworthy is that an antibody titer of 1:16 or less, in the presence of an antigen titer (by LPA) of 1:2 or more, consistently predicted the subsequent development of clinical pneumonia in four cases. Supporting the probable impact of serial ELISA tests was the observation that a fall in antibody titer accompanied a rise in LPA antigen titer in one of the deaths. In the suspected or proved PCP cases, the antibody levels were erratic, but generally higher toward completion of the clinical course in recovered patients. Five of the six sera in group D outpatients showing greater than 1:512 titer were actually from convalescent patients, who had been treated for invasively documented PCP. Similar to normal adults, all of whom were antibody-positive, outpatient allograft recipients uniformly had detectable antibody. None of the outpatients who remained healthy

TABLE 4. Summary of ELISA PC antibody distribution

Group	n[b]	Antibody titer[a]									
		0	1:8	1:16	1:32	1:64	1:128	1:256	1:152	1:1024	1:2048
A	3	0	0	0	0	1	1	1	0	0	0
B	5	0	3	1	0	0	0	1	0	0	0
C	4	0	0	0	0	0	0	0	2	2	0
D[c]	62	0	0	0	4	11	11	18	12	4	2
E[d]	20	0	0	0	0	1	7	2	8	0	2

[a] Maximum titers attained in the clinically ill patients (A–C).

[b] Number of patients examined was reduced due to limitations in serologic laboratory time and amount of stored sera.

[c] The outpatient sera were biased, since the ELISA was run preferentially on those patients exhibiting LPA Pc-Ag positive results, which also reduced n in this group.

[d] ELISA was only performed on 20 normal controls.

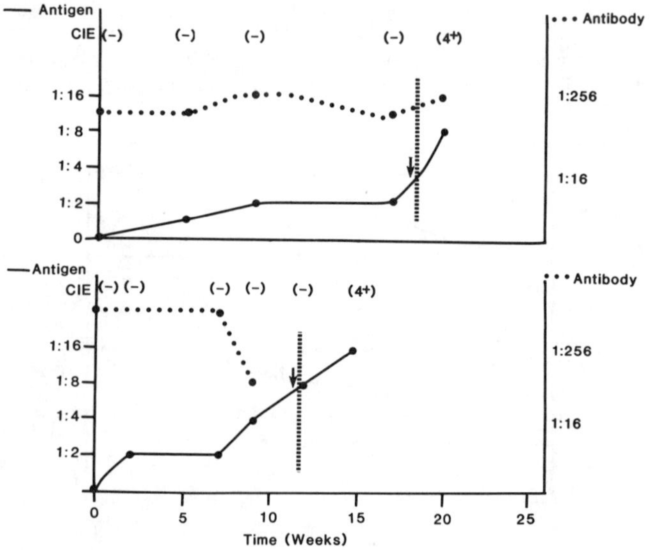

FIGURE 4. Seroanalysis of two deaths. Illustrated here is the serologic analysis of two PC pretransplant-seronegative recipients. Coded as in Figure 1.

displayed antibody titers <1:32 in the presence of antigen detected by LPA.

Combined clinical and serologic analysis. Four deaths occurred in the series of 26 patients. One patient was histologically (closed-lung biopsy) and serologically (LPA-0, CIE-0) negative for PCP. A second case was histologically negative, but serologic evaluation preceding clinical disease showed a low IgG antibody titer to Pc-Ag in the presence of a positive LPA Pc-Ag test. The LPA titer immediately preceding the illness decreased, but in the absence of sera during the course of the illness the case is indeterminate. The serological courses of the remaining two deaths are illustrated in Figure 4. These pretransplant PC-seronegative patients are believed to have PCP; one documented by open-lung biopsy and the other not studied invasively, but showing increasing Pc-Ag titer with stable or decreasing antibody titer.

Combining the clinical and serological data, it appears that the incidence of PCP may be lower than originally suspected (Table 5). The LPA antigen test was positive in seven cases documented to have disease by invasive means, excluding one case where no serum was available during the period of clinical illness. Among ten histologically negative cases, six recipients

TABLE 5. Combined clinical and serological data

Histology	Pc-Ag	Conclusion	Number
(+)	(+)	PCP	8[a]
(−)	(−)	Not PCP	3[b]
(−)	No change	Not PCP	1[c]
(−)	(+)	PCP	4[d]
(−)	1:2	PCP	1[e]
(−)	(−)	Not PCP	1
NA	(+)	PCP	4[f]
NA	(−)	Not PCP	4[g]
Total: 17 likely PCP cases			

[a] Eight invasively documented PCP cases.

[b] Three cases seronegative prior to illness onset; sera not available (NA) during illness.

[c] This case was Pc-Ag positive undiluted with no titer change prior to clinical onset.

[d] Four cases, all Pc-Ag positive with increasing titers preceding illness.

[e] Very low (<1:8) ELISA antibody titer in the presence of positive (1:2) LPA.

[f] Findings as in [d].

[g] Four cases seronegative prior to or during illness.

were evaluable. However, the sera preceding the onset of clinical illness in the four excluded cases was clearly Pg-Ag-negative in three cases and positive undiluted with no titer change just prior to clinical illness in the fourth case. Thus the serologic results were consistent with the biopsy data in at least three cases without PCP. Four of the remaining six cases had antigen detectable by LPA. A fifth case had a single value of 1:2 positive, which combined with a low antibody titer is suggestive of PCP. The sixth case not only had repeatedly negative LPA preceding and during his clinical illness, but also had negative histology, making the diagnosis of PCP unlikely. Of the remaining group of suspected PCP cases who were not studied invasively, four were LPA Pc-Ag positive, two were LPA Pc-Ag negative, and two nonevaluable, although their sera preceding the onset of clinical illness was negative. Therefore combining clinical and serologic data, the number of suspected or proved PCP cases is more likely to be 17, excluding the patients who are nonevaluable from a serologic standpoint, as well as the obviously seronegative recipients, but including all biopsy-proved cases. This incidence of 17/401 (4.2%) includes 14 cadaver and 3 living-related kidney recipients.

DISCUSSION

In contradistinction to individuals with acquired immune deficiency syndrome in whom PCP infection is often first seen as a 2–3-week prodrome of fever, malaise, and weight loss preceding the onset of pneumonia, transplant recipients suffer a rapid 24–36-hr onset of pulmonary distress, hypoxia, and fever (*20*), demanding rapid and accurate diagnosis. The presently available definitive diagnostic modalities not only are invasive—e.g., open-lung biopsy, bronchoscopy with biopsy brushing, or lavage, and/or direct needle biopsy—but also carry significant attendant morbidity and occasional mortality, particularly in this markedly immunocompromised population. While combinations of gallium scans, chest roentgenograms, and arterial blood gases may suggest the diagnosis, they do not afford definitive confirmation (*21*).

In vitro propagation of PC from human sources has yielded a source of Pc-Ag for the development of serologic tests to detect circulating antigen and specific antibody levels (*14*). In initial studies, polyclonal rabbit antisera raised against CEL-derived Pc-Ag was utilized in CIE: 95% of children undergoing chemotherapy were antigenemic, 15% of children without pneumonitis were reactive, and all normal children were negative (*19*). In contrast, the data presented herein on renal transplant recipients demonstrated antigenemia detected by CIE in only 7/26 suspected PCP cases. Five cases proved to have PCP by invasive means were negative. Thus the CIE test does not appear to have diagnostic utility. It only turned positive late in the clinical course of cases studied with serial sera. However, the test may have prognostic utility, since decreasing antigen titers during TMP-SMX therapy appeared to correlate with eventual clinical resolution.

The LPA, a second-generation test for Pc-Ag, showed 62% of asymptomatic immunosuppressed transplant recipients, but only 5% of normal persons, to be antigenemic. In addition to the histologically documented cases, five histologically negative cases of PCP were antigen-positive by LPA. The failure of biopsies to reveal organisms in the latter group of cases may be due to the invasive maneuvers being performed at least 24 hr after TMP-SMX therapy. Since it has been reported that PC can be cultured from histologically negative lung sections (*19*), and that antigenemia may resolve within 24 hr of treatment in some cases (*14*), the seropositive cases were probably not false positives. Finally, the limitation of the pure histologic approach is illustrated by one of the cases wherein transbronchial biopsy was PCP-positive, while open-lung biopsy performed several hours later was negative.

The CsA-prednisone regimen may be particularly vulnerable to the complication of PCP. On the one hand, 2–3 months of corticosteroid administration to antibiotic-treated rats results in uniformly fatal PCP (*22, 23*). On the other hand, administration of CsA alone yields PCP at approximately half the rate observed in the steroid model, in a dose-dependent fashion (*24*). Therefore the combined CsA-prednisone immunosuppressive regimen may predispose to significant PCP incidence at 2–3 months posttransplant, a time in agreement with the 2.5 month mean interval to clinical presentation observed herein. Thus the serologic result of 60% (48/78) Pc-Ag-positive allograft recipients is not unlikely. The challenge will be to discern among these PC-Ag-positive cases patients who require TMP-SMX therapy.

The LPA test is consistently positive in the presence of documented disease. When serial sera were tested, titer changes indicated impending disease weeks to several months prior to clinical presentation. Additionally, stabilization or decreasing antigen titers during therapy indicated a favorable clinical outcome, whereas persistently increasing titers in spite of therapy appeared to be an ominous sign since both patients died of PCP. The LPA may therefore provide an index for unresponsiveness to therapy. Preliminary observations utilizing the ELISA to measure IgG antibody to PC indicate that low antibody levels in the presence of positive or increasing LPA Pc-Ag titers strongly suggests impending clinical disease. The presence of antibody without changes in antigen levels may indicate previous exposure, but as previously reported (*25*), does not appear to be clinically useful per se. The presence of positive antibody titers in normal adult controls is consistent with the fact that most (75–100%) normal persons are reactive by age four (*21, 26*). Serial peritransplant studies will have to be obtained, in order to assess whether serologic monitoring of LPA Pc-Ag and ELISA PC antibody titers can predict impending PCP disease, thereby obviating mass prophylaxis and/or invasive testing. The development of clinically useful serologic monitoring tools will be expected to markedly improve the care of transplant recipients at high risk for PC infection.

Acknowledgments. We are grateful to Rebecca E. Joyner and Carol C. Edward of the University of Tennessee, and to Dianne Houston-Hawkins of the University of Texas Medical School at Houston, for their expert technical assistance.

REFERENCES

1. Delano P, Delano M. Sur les rapports des lcystes de carinii du poumon des rats avec le Trypanosoma lewisic. C R Seances Acad Sci 1918; 155: 658.
2. Hughes WT. Pneumocystis carinii pneumonitis. Chest 1984; 85: 810.
3. Ballardie FW, Wineads CG, Williams G. Cyclosporine and steroids in renal transplantation: risk of Pneumocystis carinii pneumonia? Lancet 1984; 2: 638.
4. Kuller J, First MR, D'Achiandi R, Munda R. Pneumocystis carinii pneumonia in renal transplant recipients. Am J Nephrol 1982; 2: 312.
5. Hardy AM, Wajszczuk CP, Suffredini AF, Hakala TR, Ho M. Pneumocystis carinii pneumonia in renal transplant recipients treated with cyclosporine and steroids. J Infect Dis 1984; 149: 143.
6. Mitsayasu RT, Corwin HL, Harris AA, Trenholme GH, Levin S, Karakusis PH. Failure of trimethoprim-sulfamethoxazole in the therapy of Pneumocystis carinii pneumonia. Am Rev Respir Dis 1982; 125: 762.
7. Ettinger LJ, Torrisi J, Wood BP, Anderson VM. Spontaneous improvement of Pneumocystis carinii pneumonia in childhood acute lymphocytic leukemia. Med Pediatr Oncol 1982; 10: 477.
8. Thompson JF, Chalmers DHK, Hunnisett AG, Wood RFM, Morris PJ. Nephrotoxicity of trimethoprim and cotrimoxazole in renal allograft recipients treated with cyclosporine. Transplantation 1983; 36: 204.
9. Nyberg G, Gabel H, Althoff P, Biork S, Herlitz H, Brynger H. Adverse effect of trimethoprim on kidney function in renal transplant patients. Lancet 1984; 1: 394.
10. Mason WH, Siegel SE, Tucker BL. Diagnostic open lung biopsy for diffuse pulmonary disease in immunocompromised pediatric patients. Am J Pediatr Hematol Oncol 1982; 4: 355.
11. Kelley J. Alveolar lavage, bronchial irrigation and the diagnosis of pneumoncystis. Am Rev Respir Dis 1984; 129: 649.
12. Prat JJ, Besson-Leaud M, Lavaud J, Cloup M, Nezelof C. Diagnosis of Pneumocystis carinii pneumonia using an endobronchial brushing technique. Eur J Pediatr 1980; 133: 41.
13. Ognebene FP, Shelhamer J, Gill V, Mocher AM, Loew D, Parker MM, et al. The diagnosis of Pneumocystis carinii pneumonia in patients with the acquired immune deficiency syndrome using subsegmental bronchoalveolar lavage. Am Rev Respir Dis 1984: 129: 929.
14. Pifer LL. Pneumocystis carinii: a diagnostic dilemma. Pediatr Infect Dis 1983; 2: 177.
15. Pifer LL, Hughes WT, Murphy MJ. Propagation of Pneumocystis carinii in vitro. Pediatr Res 1977; 11: 305.
16. Maddison SE, Hayes GV, Slemenda SB, Norman LG, Ivey MH. Detection of specific antibody by enzyme-linked immunosorbent assay and antigenemia by counterimmunoelectrophoresis in humans infected with Pneumocystis carinii. J Clin Microbiol 1982; 15: 1036.
17. Pifer LL, Niell H, Langdon S, Neely C, Woods D, Edwards C, et al. Pneumocystis carinii antigen and antibody profiles in AIDS patients with P. carinii pneumonia. In: Proceedings of the 24th Interscience Conference on Antimicroagents and Chemotherapy, 1984: 230.

18. Flechner SM, Kerman RH, Van Buren C, Payne W, Kahan BD. The use of cyclosporine and prednisone for high MLC haploidentical living related renal transplants. Transplant Proc 1983; 15: 442.
19. Pifer LL, Hughes WT, Stagno S, Woods DR. Pneumocystis carinii infection: evidence for high prevalence in normal and immunosuppressed children. Pediatrics 1978; 61: 35.
20. Sterling RP, Bradley BB, Khalil KG, Kerman RH, Conklin RH. Comparison of biopsy proven Pneumocystis carinii pneumonia in acquired immune deficiency syndrome patients and renal allograft recipients. Ann Surg 1984; 38: 494.
21. Goodman JL, Tashin DA. Pneumocystis with normal CXR film and arterial oxygen tension. Arch Intern Med 1983; 143: 1981.
22. Wolzer PD, Powell RD Jr, Yoneda K, Rutledge ME, Milder JE. Growth characteristics and pathogenesis of Pneumocystis carinii pneumonia. Infect Immun 1980; 27: 928.
23. Hendley JO, Weller TH. Activation and transmission in rats of infection with pneumocystis. Proc Soc Exp Biol Med 1971; 137: 1401.
24. Hughes WT, Smith B. Provocation of infection due to Pneumocystis carinii by cyclosporine. J Infect Dis 1982; 145: 767.
25. Meyers JD, Pifer LL, Sale GE, Thomas ED. The value of Pneumocystis carinii antibody and antigen detection for diagnosis of Pneumocystis carinii pneumonia after marrow transplantation. Am Rev Respir Dis 1979; 120: 1283.
26. Meuwissen JHET, Taber I, Leeuwenberg ADEM, Beckers PJA, Sieben M. Parasitologic and serologic observations of infection with pneumocystis in humans. J Infect Dis 1977; 136: 43.

Received 6 June 1985.
Accepted 23 August 1985.

0041-1337/86/4104-0442$02.00/0
TRANSPLANTATION
Vol. 41, No. 4
Printed in U.S.A.

COMPARISON OF MONOCLONAL ANTIBODIES USED FOR IMMUNOLOGICAL MONITORING OF RENAL TRANSPLANT RECIPIENTS[1]

F. C. Henny,[2] P. J. Oljans,[3] H. J. Tanke,[3] L. C. Paul[2] and L. A. van Es[2]

Department of Nephrology and Department of Histochemistry and Cytochemistry, University Hospital, Leiden, The Netherlands

To investigate the comparability of the OKT and Leu monoclonal antibodies (mAbs) used for immunological monitoring, T cell subpopulations in 360 blood samples from 35 renal allograft recipients were studied by flow cytometry using both series of mAbs. To identify the activated cells in the different subpopulations, those labeled with the Leu mAbs were double-labeled with an anti-HLA-DR mAb. The percentages of T cells that stained with the Leu3a and Leu2a mAb using a direct immunofluorescence technique were significantly lower than the percentages of cells that stained with the OKT4 and OKT8 mAb using an indirect immunofluorescence technique (47.6±12.8% and 14.5±9.1% [mean ± SD] versus 50.5±11.2% and 18.3±8.0%, respectively; $P<0.0001$). Since the difference between the Leu2a$^+$ and OKT8$^+$ cells was relatively greater (21%) than that between the Leu3a$^+$ and OKT4$^+$ cells (6%), the mean Leu3a/2a ratio was significantly higher than the mean OKT4/8 ratio (6.64±9.7 versus 3.60±2.82; $P<0.0001$). The differences between the Leu2a$^+$ and OKT8$^+$ cells were not attributable to a difference in the sensitivity of the direct and indirect immunofluorescence technique. A large difference between the Leu2a$^+$ and OKT8$^+$ cells correlated with a high percentage of DR$^+$ cells within the Leu2a population ($P<0.001$). No correlation was found for the difference between the OKT4$^+$ and Leu3a$^+$ cells and the DR expression in the Leu3a$^+$ cell population. These observations suggest that activation of some T cells of the "cytotoxic-suppressor" phenotype leads to antigen modulation in which the OKT8 epitope is not affected but the Leu2a epitope disappears or cannot be detected with the present method.

Since the description of two functional subsets of T cells in man, defined by antisera against heterologous membrane determinants (*1*), both the development and production of mAbs* against these determinants have progressed rapidly (*2, 3*). The application of these mAbs for the monitoring and treatment of renal transplant patients may provide new insights into the mechanisms of the immune response (*4*). Furthermore, the ratio of T cell subsets that express the "helper-inducer" to those expressing the "cytotoxic-suppressor" phenotypes can be of prognostic value for recipients of renal allografts (*5*) or of diagnostic value for patients with the acquired immunodeficiency syndrome (AIDS) (*6*).

An increasing number of mouse anti-human mAbs that appear to react with the same T cell subsets as the OKT4 or OKT8 reagents are at present commercially available (*2*). It is

[1] This work was supported by the Dutch Kidney Foundation (grant C81.308).
[2] Department of Nephrology.
[3] Department of Histochemistry and Cytochemistry.

* Abbreviations used: AIDS, acquired immunodeficiency syndrome; BSA, bovine serum albumin; FACS, fluorescence-activated cell sorter; FITC, fluorescein isothiocyanate; mAbs, monoclonal antibodies; PBS, phosphate-buffered saline; PE, phycoerythrin.

known that the Leu and OKT mAbs react with the same molecule, which has been found to be a glycoprotein with a molecular weight of 62,000 daltons on T cells expressing the helper-inducer phenotype and a glycoprotein of 34,000 daltons on T cells expressing the cytotoxic-suppressor phenotype (*7*). However, the Leu reagents apparently recognize other epitopes than the OKT reagents, as indicated by competitive blocking assays and immunoprecipitation studies (*8–10*).

To evaluate the practical significance of this finding for immunological monitoring, we used both the OKT and the Leu mAbs for sequential monitoring of T cell subsets in renal allograft recipients and compared the results obtained with the two antibodies.

MATERIALS AND METHODS

Patients. Cells were collected within the first 6 months of transplantation from 35 adult patients who had received a cadaveric renal allograft. Samples were taken three times a week during hospitalization and once a week during the follow-up period in the out-patient clinic. The number of determinations varied from 5 to 25 per patient. Immunosuppressive therapy consisted of azathioprine or cyclosporine in combination with low doses of prednisone. Rejection episodes were diagnosed independent of the monitoring results and were treated with rabbit antithymocyte globulin (RATG), high doses of prednisone, or bolus injections of methylprednisolone. For control purposes, cells were also collected from 10 normal controls and 20 renal transplant recipients with a stable renal function more than 6 months after transplantation.

Monoclonal antibodies. The mAbs used are listed in Table 1. The OKT mAbs were purchased from Ortho Pharmaceutical Corporation, Beerse, Belgium, and the Leu mAbs from Becton Dickinson Laboratory Systems, Mechelen, Belgium. The Leu mAbs were conjugated directly with fluorescein isothiocyanate (FITC); the binding of the OKT mAbs to cells was visualized by an indirect fluorescence technique using a goat antimouse IgG conjugated with FITC (Nordic Immunological Laboratories, Tilburg, The Netherlands), which gave a background labeling on the lymphocytes of a maximum of 3%, as described previously (*5*). To identify the percentage of activated T cells, a phycoerythrin (PE) labeled mAb against the nonpolymorphic structure of HLA-DR was used (Becton Dickinson). The mAbs and the FITC-conjugated goat antimouse IgG were diluted in phosphate-buffered-saline, pH 7.8, containing bovine serum albumin (PBS/BSA; 5 g/l) to a concentration to obtain optimal staining.

Cell isolation and incubation. Mononuclear cells were isolated from 10 ml of citrated blood by Ficoll-Isopaque density gradient centrifugation. Preincubation of the cells with ferrocarbonylic particles (0.5 mg/ml blood) at 37°C for 30 min substantially reduced the number of monocytes. After isolation the cells were washed twice in PBS/BSA. Subsequently 5–10×10^5 lymphocytes were centrifuged (5 min at 200 g) and incubated at 4°C for 30 min with 30 μl unlabeled OKT (1 μg/ml) or the FITC-conjugated Leu mAb (10 μg/ml). The cells were washed and centrifuged (5 min at 200 g); the OKT-labeled cells were then incubated with 30 μl goat antimouse FITC (50 μg/ml). The cells labeled with the FITC-conjugated Leu mAbs were double-labeled by incubating them with 30 μl PE-conjugated anti-HLA-DR mAb (10 μg/ml). Finally, the cells were washed once more, resuspended in 0.25 ml PBS/BSA, and analyzed by flow cytometry within 2 hr of staining.

To confirm the observation that different epitopes are recognized by the different mAbs, competitive blocking experiments were performed in 4 cases; after preincubation with OKT mAbs, the cells were incubated with the FITC-conjugated Leu mAbs directed against the corresponding T cell subsets. For control purposes the Leu-FITC-labeled cells were also blocked with unlabeled Leu mAbs.

Flow cytometry. Flow cytometric analysis was performed using a fluorescence-activated cell sorter (FACS IV, Becton Dickinson, Sunnyvale, CA). An argon ion laser tuned at 488 nm with an intensity of 300 mW was used as light source. Cell debris, red blood cells, nonviable lymphocytes, and the majority of the monocytes that remained after lymphocyte isolation were eliminated electronically on the basis of their forward-angle light scatter signal. Fluorescence histograms were recorded using logarithmic amplification. Histograms of the fluorescence values of approximately 10,000 viable lymphocytes were analyzed. The number of positive cells was expressed as the percentage of the total number of cells analyzed. Most of the fluorescence histograms of the OKT8 and Leu2a-labeled cells showed two distinct subgroups including a discrete population of bright-stained cells and a smaller population of dull-stained cells. In accordance with previous observations from this laboratory (*5*) the bright-stained $OKT8^+$ and $Leu2a^+$ cells were considered positive. A three-parameter analysis was performed to determine the percentage of $Leu3a^+$ or $Leu2a^+$ cells that coexpress HLA-DR antigens. The $Leu3a^+$ or $Leu2a^+$ cells were identified on the basis of their forward light scatter and their green FITC-fluorescence and the cells coexpressing HLA-DR by the simultaneous red fluorescence of the PE-conjugated anti-HLA-DR. Green (FITC) and red (PE) fluorescence were separated using a 560 nm dichroic beam splitter. Green fluorescence was measured through a short-pass 550 nm interference filter and the red fluorescence through a long-pass 580 nm glass filter. The PE emission did not pass through the 550 nm interference filter, and therefore did not disturb the measurements in the green channel. The FITC emission passed through the 580 filter and caused a background fluorescence in the red channel that was indicated by a dull peak in the histogram that was distinct from the bright peak of the PE fluorescent-positive population. We did not try to compensate for this "cross-talk"

TABLE 1. Serologic specificities and immunoglobulin isotypes of the different mAbs

Name	Specificity	Immunoglobulin isotype	Reference
OKT4	helper/inducer T cells	IgG_{2b}	*2,11*
OKT8	suppressor/cytotoxic T cells	IgG_{2a}	*2,12*
Leu3a	helper/inducer T cells	IgG_1	*3,13*
Leu2a	suppressor/cytotoxic T cells	IgG_1	*3,13*
anti–HLA-DR	B lymphocytes, monocytes, macrophages, activated T lymphocytes	IgG_{2a}	*14,15*

phenomenon electronically, since the separation of the two populations was very clear (Fig. 1).

Results were statistically analyzed by Fisher's test on a 2×2 table and the Student's t test for paired observations.

RESULTS

The percentages of the T cells that expressed the helper-inducer phenotype as well as those expressing the cytotoxic-suppressor phenotype, determined in 360 blood samples with either the OKT4 or Leu3a mAbs or the OKT8 or Leu2a mAbs, respectively, are listed in Table 2. The percentages of the two T cell subpopulations found with the Leu mAbs are significantly lower than the percentages obtained with the OKT reagents. The relative difference between the percentages of $Leu2a^+$ and $OKT8^+$ cells is 21% versus 6% between the $Leu3a^+$ and $OKT4^+$ cells. The mean Leu 3a/2a ratio (6.64±9.17) is therefore significantly higher than the mean OKT 4/8 ratio (3.60±2.82 [$P<0.0001$]). As is shown in Figure 2, the difference between the $OKT8^+$ and $Leu2a^+$ populations is highly variable; this variability is also illustrated by the OKT8/Leu2a ratio, which varies from 0.6 to 13.0. Samples with a very low percentage of $Leu2a^+$ cells in particular are responsible for the very high mean Leu3a/2a ratio.

The cells of 353 patient samples were incubated with both the Leu and the anti HLA-DR mAbs. The percentage of $Leu2a^+$ cells that coexpressed the DR antigen varied from 1% to 56%; the maximum percentage of $Leu3a^+$ cells that were DR-positive was 40%. The correlation between the percentage of DR^+ cells in the $Leu2a^+$ and the $Leu3a^+$ cell populations was low (r=0.58).

In 10 normal controls and 20 renal allograft recipients with a stable renal function more than 6 months after transplantation, a maximum of 6% of the $Leu2a^+$ cells was found to be HLA-DR-positive. The percentage of $Leu3a^+$ cells that expressed the DR antigen varied considerably among the various individuals; the maximum was 19%. No difference between the $OKT4^+$ and $Leu3a^+$ or the $OKT8^+$ and $Leu2a^+$ cells was found (51.0±10.4% vs. 51.2±11.3% and 20.4±9.6% vs. 20.5±11.6%, respectively). The OKT8/Leu2a ratio varied from 0.7 to 1.4. We therefore consider an OKT8/Leu2a ratio <1.5 and a percentage of $Leu2a^+$ cells that coexpress the DR antigen ≦6% as normal.

For the experimental patient group a correlation between an increase in DR expression by $Leu2a^+$ cells and the difference between the percentage of $OKT8^+$ and $Leu2a^+$ cells was found. The number of determinations showing that the OKT8/Leu2a ratio was less than 1.5, together with ≦6% DR^+ cells, or that the OKT8/Leu2a ratio was ≧1.5, together with >6% DR^+ cells, was significantly higher than the number of samples with either

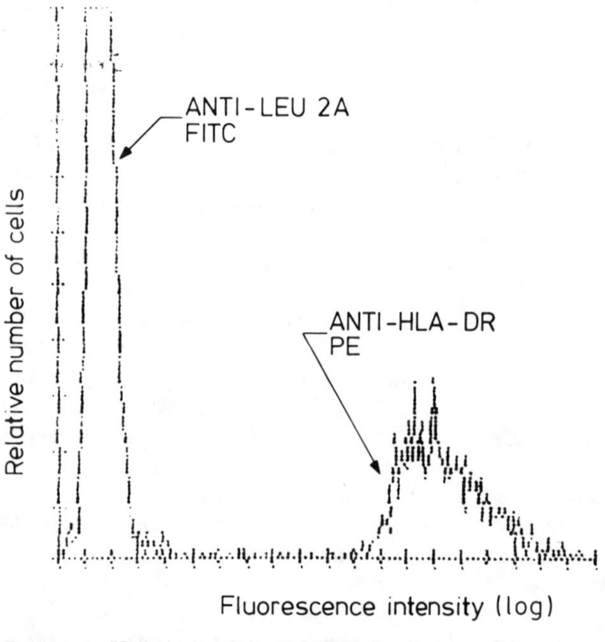

FIGURE 1. Histogram of the red (PE) fluorescence of lymphocytes that are double-labeled with Leu 2a-FITC and anti-HLA-DR-PE.

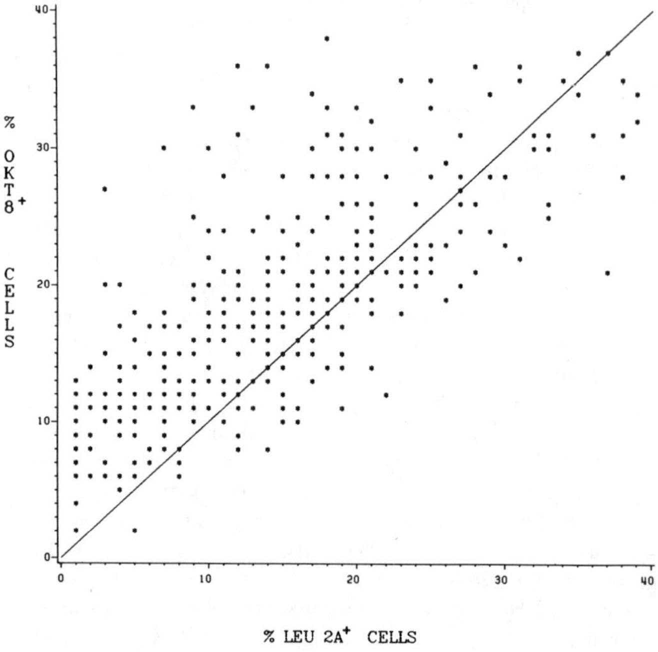

FIGURE 2. Relation of the percentages of T cells expressing the cytotoxic-suppressor phenotype when stained with either the OKT8 or the Leu2a mAbs.

TABLE 2. Percentage of cells belonging to the different T subsets and their ratios in 360 blood samples from 35 renal allograft recipients, as assessed with different mAbs

Antibody	Percentage (mean ± SD)	Correlation coefficient	Difference (mean ± SD)
OKT4	50.5±11.2	0.837	2.9±7.0[a]
Leu3a	47.6±12.8		
OKT8	18.3±8.0	0.752	3.8±6.1[a]
Leu2a	14.5±9.1		
OKT4/8 ratio	3.60±2.82	0.55	3.04±7.97[a]
Leu 3a/2a ratio	6.64±9.17		

[a] $P<0.0001$.

an OKT8/Leu2a ratio ≧1.5 or a percentage of DR^+ cells >6% alone (P<0.001) (Table 3).

When the data were analyzed per patient rather than as single determinations (Table 4), 11 of the 35 patients never showed an OKT8/Leu2a ratio ≧1.5 and more than 6% $Leu2a^+$ DR^+ cells; in 6 of these 11 cases more than 8 samples per patient were analyzed. Twenty patients had an OKT8/Leu2a ratio ≧1.5 and more than 6% DR^+ cells in the $Leu2a^+$ population; in this group of patients at least one sample showed both characteristics. Occasionally, in some samples obtained from these patients at other times, only the OKT8/Leu2a ratio was ≧1.5 or the percentage of DR^+ cells was >6%. During follow-up three patients exhibited only an OKT8/Leu2a ratio ≧1.5 without an increase in DR^+ $Leu2a^+$ cells, whereas only one patient had more than 6% DR^+ cells without an increase in the OKT8/Leu2a ratio (in 2 of 5 samples). Neither the OKT8/Leu2a ratio nor the percentage of DR^+ cells was constant per patient. Whenever the OKT8/Leu2a ratio exceeded 1.5 it was always due to a decrease in the percentage of $Leu2a^+$ cells rather than an increase in the percentage of $OKT8^+$ cells. There was no correlation between the type of immunosuppressive therapy given and the difference between the percentages of $OKT8^+$ and $Leu2a^+$ cells or the percentage of DR^+ cells.

TABLE 3. Difference between the percentage of $OKT8^+$ and $Leu2a^+$ cells in relation to the percentage of $Leu2a^+$ cells that express DR antigens

	DR^+ cells ≦6%	DR^+ cells >6%	Total
OKT8/Leu 2a <1.5	170	41	211
OKT8/Leu 2a ≧1.5	68	74	142
Total	238	115	353
P<0.001.			

TABLE 4. Patients grouped on the basis of the difference between the percentage of $OKT8^+$ and $Leu2a^+$ cells and the percentage of $Leu2a^+$ cells expressing DR, as observed during the follow-up period

	DR^+ cells ≦6%	DR^+ cells >6%	Total
OKT8/Leu 2a <1.5	11	1	12
OKT8/Leu 2a ≧1.5	3	20	23
Total	14	21	35
P<0.001.			

To investigate whether the discrepancies between the $OKT8^+$ and $Leu2a^+$ cells were due to the different labeling techniques (indirect fluorescence versus direct fluorescence technique, respectively) 25 cell suspensions in which a discrepancy between the $OKT8^+$ and $Leu2a^+$ percentages was found were incubated with an unconjugated Leu2a antibody followed by staining using the FITC-conjugated goat antimouse antibody. As is shown in Table 5 the percentage of $Leu2a^+$ cells detected with the indirect fluorescence technique was significantly lower than the percentage of $OKT8^+$ cells, but was not different from the numbers of $Leu2a^+$ cells detected using the direct immunofluorescence technique.

Furthermore, to exclude the possibility that the double-labeling technique somehow caused the difference between the percentages of $OKT8^+$ and $Leu2a^+$ cells, 60 additional cell suspensions were incubated with either FITC-conjugated Leu2a mAb alone or FITC-conjugated Leu2a mAb together with PE-conjugated mAb against HLA-DR. The number of $Leu2a^+$ cells was not significantly influenced by double-labeling (Table 5).

The wide variation in the percentage of $Leu3a^+$ cells, which are also DR^+, found for the 30 controls was also exhibited by the experimental patient group. No correlation between the OKT4-Leu3a difference and the percentage of $Leu3a^+$ cells that are also DR^+ was found.

The results of the competitive binding experiments are listed in Table 6. It can be seen that the OKT4 mAb could not reduce the percentage of $Leu3a^+$ cells, whereas the OKT8 mAb partially inhibited the binding of Leu2a-FITC. Furthermore it was shown that, after incubation of the cells with the unlabeled Leu mAbs only, between 0 and 2% of the cells stained after additional incubation with FITC-labeled Leu mAb—which illustrates that the concentration of Leu mAbs used was a saturating concentration.

DISCUSSION

This report describes a comparison of mAbs of the OKT and Leu series used for immunological monitoring of renal allograft recipients. Although it has been shown with immunoprecipitation techniques that these mAbs react with the same cell-surface glycoprotein (*9*), the results of sequential monitoring with OKT and Leu antisera have never been compared. We have shown that, shortly after transplantation, highly variable

TABLE 5. Percentages of $Leu2a^+$ cells detected with different labeling techniques compared with the percentage of $OKT8^+$ cells

Labeling technique	Number of samples	Percentage	P value
OKT8 indirect	25	19.7±9.0	<0.001
Leu2a indirect	25	13.9±7.8	>0.05
Leu2a direct	25	14.8±8.4	
Leu2a direct without αHLA-DR	60	14.3±9.9	>0.05
Leu2a direct together with αHLA-DR	60	14.9±10	

TABLE 6. Competitive binding inhibition experiments using the FITC-conjugated Leu monoclonals (Leu-FITC) together with the unlabeled OKT and Leu mAbs

Patients	Percentage of Leu 3a–FITC-positive cells			Percentage of Leu2a–FITC-positive cells		
	Not preincubated	Preincubated with unlabeled Leu3a	Preincubated with unlabeled OKT4	Not preincubated	Preincubated with unlabeled Leu2a	Preincubated with unlabeled OKT8
1	36	2	31	17	0	9
2	43	1	39	39	1	24
3	43	0	49	25	0	15
4	52	2	48	12	0	7

results—especially with respect to the percentages of T cells expressing the cytotoxic-suppressor phenotype and therefore the ratio's between the T cell subsets—can be obtained with different mAbs against the same cell-surface glycoprotein. The very high mean Leu3a/2a ratio was due to a relatively large number of samples with a very low percentage (<10%) of Leu2a$^+$ cells (Fig. 2). Compared with other published studies (*4, 16*) the mean OKT4/8 ratio in our patient population was high. This is probably because only the bright fluorescent OKT8 population was considered positive, in accordance with previous studies from this laboratory (*5*). Although both subpopulations determined by the Leu mAbs were smaller than those assessed with the OKT reagents, it is not clear whether the total number of T cells measured by the mAbs from the Leu series (anti-Leu1) differs from the total number of T cells found with OKT mAbs (anti-OKT3), since we did not use these mAbs in the present experiments. The difference observed between the percentage of cells belonging to the different T cell subsets is probably attributable to the fact that the Leu and OKT mAbs react with different epitopes of the same cell-surface glycoprotein (*8, 9*). The results of the competitive blocking experiments, also found by others (*8, 10*), support this possibility. Since the OKT4 mAb could not block the binding of the Leu3a mAb, the Leu3a epitope appears to be distinct from the OKT4 epitope. The OKT8 antibody, however, partially inhibited the binding of the Leu2a mAb, which suggests that the two epitopes are sterically close to one another. The possibility that a difference in the affinities of the two mAbs is responsible for the observed differences and blocking results has not been excluded. However, the fact that differences between the Leu2a$^+$ and OKT8$^+$ cells differ in time in the same patient suggests that antigen modulation may occur. Other authors have suggested that in vivo modulation of membrane antigens can occur after treatment with mAbs (*17*) and that reduced staining with Leu mAbs could be caused by drugs that affect the expression of antigen density (*18*). However, in our study the differences between the OKT8$^+$ and Leu2a$^+$ populations were not related to the type of immunosuppressive therapy. From our data it appears that there is a relation between the degree of HLA-DR expression in the Leu2a$^+$ T cell subpopulation and the difference between the percentages of OKT8$^+$ and Leu2a$^+$ cells. This finding may suggest that in vivo activation of some of the T cells expressing the cytotoxic-suppressor phenotype results in a modulation of the cell membrane structure in which the Leu2a epitope cannot be recognized or has disappeared, but the OKT8 epitope is maintained. Clinically there seemed to be a correlation between this phenomenon and rejection episodes. None of the 11 patients listed in Table 4 with a percentage of DR$^+$ cells $\leqq$6% and an OKT8/Leu 2a ratio <1.5 underwent a rejection episode during the study period. In contrast 11 of the 20 patients exhibiting an increase in both DR expression (>6%) and OKT8/Leu 2a ratio ($\geqq$1.5) during follow-up received an antirejection treatment within 10 days of this observation. Proliferation of OKT8$^+$ Leu2a$^-$ cells or crossreactivity of the goat antimouse FITC antibody with OKT8$^+$ DR$^+$ cells, cannot be excluded, but the finding of a decrease in the percentage of Leu2a$^+$ cells rather than an increase in the percentage of OKT8$^+$ cells makes these possibilities unlikely.

The wide variation in DR expression in the Leu3a population found for the 10 normal controls and 20 renal allograft recipients with a stable graft function probably was due to the fact that anti Leu3a mAbs also react with cytoplasmic structures of the monocytes which remain behind in variable amounts and can be DR-positive (*19*).

In conclusion, our study shows that different percentages of T cells belonging to the different T cell subsets, and therefore also different T cell subset ratios, can be obtained when different mAbs against the same T subsets are used. Since the percentage of Leu2a$^+$ cells decreases in patients with an increased DR expression in the cytotoxic-suppressor subpopulation—whereas the percentage of OKT8$^+$ cells remains unchanged—the results of this study suggest that in vivo activation of cells expressing the cytotoxic-suppressor phenotype is associated with membrane modulation in which the Leu2a epitope becomes undetectable and the OKT8 epitope remains unchanged.

Acknowledgments. We are indebted to Dr. J. Hermans for his comments on the statistical aspects of this study.

Note added in proof. In 20 additional blood samples in which differences between percentages of OKT8$^+$ and Leu2a$^+$ cells were found (21±6% vs. 14±5%, respectively), no significant differences were found between the percentages of OKT8$^+$ cells and percentages of cells stained with the Leu2b mAb (21±6% vs. 20±5%, respectively). In 14 of these 20 samples >6% HLA-DR$^+$ cells were found within the Leu2a population. The Leu2b mAb, which has the same immunoglobulin isotypes as the OKT8 mAb has (IgG2a), was kindly provided by Dr. N. Warner from Becton Dickinson Co., Mountain View, CA.

REFERENCES

1. Evans RL, Lazarus H, Penta AC, Schlossman SF. Two functionally distinct subpopulations of human T cells that collaborate in the generation of cytotoxic cells responsible for cell-mediated lympholysis. J Immunol 1978; 120: 1423.
2. Reinherz EL, Kung PC, Goldstein G, Schlossman SF. Separation of functional subsets of human T cells by a mAb. Proc Natl Acad Sci USA 1979; 76: 4061.
3. Engleman EG, Benike CJ, Glickman E, Evans RL. Antibodies to membrane structures that distinguish suppressor/cytotoxic and helper T lymphocyte subpopulations block the mixed leucocyte reaction in man. J Exp Med 1981; 154: 193.
4. Cosimi AB, Colvin RB, Burton RC, et al. Monoclonal antibodies for immunologic monitoring and treatment in recipients of renal allografts. N Engl J Med 1981; 305: 308.
5. Van Es A, Tanke HJ, Baldwin WM III, Oljans PJ, Ploem JS, Van Es LA. Ratios of T lymphocyte subpopulations predict survival of cadaveric renal allografts in adult patients on low-dose corticosteroid therapy. Clin Exp Immunol 1983; 52: 13.
6. Lane MC, Masur H, Edgar LC, Whalen G, Rook AH, Fauci AS. Abnormalities of B-cell activation and immunoregulation in patients with the acquired immunodeficiency syndrome. N Engl J Med 1983; 309: 453.
7. Terhorst C, Van Agthoven A, Reinherz EL, Schlossman SF. Biochemical analysis of human T lymphocyte differentiation antigens T4 and T5. Science 1980; 209: 520.
8. Fuller TC, Trevithick JE, Fuller AA, Colvin RB, Cosimi AB, Kung PC. Antigenic polymorphism of the T4 differentiation antigen expressed on human T helper/inducer lymphocytes. Hum Immunol 1984; 9: 89.
9. Snow P, Spits H, De Vries J, Terhorst C. Comparison of target antigens of monoclonal reagents OKT5, OKT8 and Leu2a, which inhibit effector function of human cytotoxic T lymphocytes. Hybridoma 1983; 2: 187.
10. Martin PJ, Ledbetter JA, Clark EA, Beatty PG, Hansen JA. Epitope mapping of the human surface suppressor/cytotoxic T cell molecule Tp32. J Immunol 1984; 132: 759.

11. Reinherz EL, Kung PC, Goldstein G, Schlossman SF. Further characterization of the human inducer T cell subset defined by a mAb. J Immunol 1979; 123: 2894.
12. Reinherz EL, Kung PC, Goldstein G, Schlossman SF. A mAb reactive with the human cytotoxic/suppressor T cell subset previously defined by a hetero antiserum termed TH-2. J Immunol 1980; 124: 1301.
13. Evans RL, Wall DW, Platsoucas CD, et al. Thymus-dependent membrane antigens in man: inhibition of cell-mediated lympholysis by mAbs to T_{H2} antigen. Proc Natl Acad Sci USA 1981; 78: 544.
14. Warnke R, Miller R, Grogan R, Pederson M, Dilley J, Levy R. Immunological phenotype in 30 patients with diffuse large-cell lymphoma. N Engl J Med 1980; 303: 293.
15. Warnke R, Levy R. Detection of T- and B cell antigens with hybridoma mAbs: a biotin-avidin horse radish peroxidase method. J Histochem Cytochem 1980; 28: 771.
16. Carter NP, Cullen PR, Thompson JF, Bewick ALT, Wood RFM, Morris PJ. Monitoring lymphocyte subpopulations in renal allograft recipients. Transplant Proc 1983; 15: 1157.
17. Chatenoud L, Baudrikaye MF, Kreis H, Goldstein G, Schindler J, Bach JF. Human in vivo antigenic modulation induced by the anti-T cell OKT3 mAb. Eur J Immunol 1982; 12: 979.
18. Guttmann RD, Poulsen RS. FACS analysis of lymphocyte subsets after renal transplantation: clinical correlates and evidence for reduced expression of antigen density associated with chronic immunosuppression. Transplant Proc 1983; 15: 1962.
19. Wood GS, Warner NL, Warnke RA. Anti-Leu3/T4 antibodies react with cells of monocyte/macrophage and Langerhans lineage. J Immunol 1983; 131: 212.

Received 9 May 1985.
Accepted 8 August 1985.

0041-1337/86/4104-0447$02.00/0
TRANSPLANTATION

Vol. 41, No. 4
Printed in U.S.A.

SERUM ANTIBODY REACTIVITY OF BROADLY SENSITIZED PATIENTS WITH HLA-MATCHED PERIPHERAL BLOOD T LYMPHOCYTES[1]

DANIEL J. COOK[2] AND JUAN C. SCORNIK[3]

Department of Pathology, University of Florida College of Medicine, Gainesville, Florida

The sera of 45 hypersensitized patients with more than 90% panel reactive antibodies were tested for reactivity against peripheral blood T lymphocytes from 7 donors matched for HLA-A,B antigens. The target cells were phenotypically homozygous HLA-A1,B8 or A2,B44. Tests for lymphocytotoxic antibodies were essentially negative except for one target cell in which 10 of 25 sera were positive. More positive reactions were detected by flow cytometry, and the proportion of positive specimens ranged from 15% to 48% with the different target cells. Most positive reactions involved the HLA-A2 and B44 antigens, in which heterogeneity within the serologically defined specificities has been described. The positive reactions were further evaluated by testing the effect of purified soluble HLA molecules on the binding of antibodies to the HLA-marched targets. Purified HLA produced a detectable inhibition of antibody binding in the majority of the serum-target combinations studied. These results document that anti-HLA antibodies can still react with HLA-matched lymphocytes, which may be due to the recognition of subtypes of the known serologically defined specificities.

[1] This work was supported Grant AM-31959 from the National Institutes of Health.

[2] Present address: Tissue Typing Laboratory, University of California at Los Angeles, CA 90024.

[3] Address correspondence to: Juan C. Scornik, M.D., Department of Pathology, Box J-275, University of Florida College of Medicine, Gainesville, FL 32610.

Allogeneic cells, in the form of transplants or transfusions, are being used with increasing frequency for therapeutic purposes. As a consequence, a growing number of patients develop anti-HLA class I antibodies that may react with cells from a high proportion of donors. HLA hypersensitization is a major problem for renal transplantation (*1*) platelet transfusions (*2*), and perhaps also for heart transplantation (*3*).

The use of HLA-matched donors in HLA-sensitized patients has made it possible to perform successful renal transplants (*4*) and platelet transfusions (*2*). Since fully HLA-matched donors can be found only on rare occasions, the concept of HLA matching has been extended to include absence of detectable mismatch or mismatch with crossreactive class I antigens (*5*). The full impact of these practices, however, has been difficult to document (*6*). Obviously, the basic assumption for the use of HLA-matched donors is that patients will not have (or make) antibodies to molecules that are identical to self. Since crossreactive antigens are not identical, and even serologically defined antigens are known to be heterogeneous (*7, 8*) the question arises as to whether hypersensitized patients may have antibodies reacting with epitopes in HLA molecules that otherwise are very similar to self.

In the present study we systemically evaluated sera containing broadly reactive antibodies for their reactivity with HLA-matched T lymphocytes. Although lymphocytotoxic reactions were rare, binding measured by flow cytometry was frequently detected and shown to be due to HLA reactivity by specific inhibition by purified HLA molecules.

MATERIALS AND METHODS

Sera. Normal human sera (NHS)* were obtained from normal, nontransfused male individuals. Sera from highly sensitized patients whose HLA phenotypes included the antigens HLA-A1 and B8 or HLA-A2 and B44 were obtained from our own and from the following institutions: New England Organ Bank, Boston, MA; Mayo Clinic, Rochester, MN; Jewish Hospital (University of Louisville), Louisville, KY; Johns Hopkins University, Baltimore, MD; University of Pittsburgh, Pittsburgh, PA; New York Hospital, New York, NY; and Blood Center of Southeastern Wisconsin, Milwaukee, WI. All the sera had lymphocytotoxic antibodies reacting with more than 90% of panel cells and were from end-stage renal disease patients on cadaveric donor renal transplant waiting lists.

Microcytotoxicity. HLA typing (*9*) was performed with antisera procured locally and from commercial sources (University of California at Los Angeles, CA). Alloantibody reactivity was determined by the Amos modified technique (*10*) and the antiglobulin technique (*11*).

Target cells and immunofluorescence staining. Peripheral blood lymphocytes (PBL) were isolated from leukocyte concentrates of blood units from donors phenotypically homozygous for HLA-A1,B8 or HLA-A2,B44. Blood from such donors was provided by the Civitan Regional Blood Center (Gainesville, FL) or the South Florida Blood Service (Miami, FL). Mononuclear cells were cryopreserved (*12*) using a controlled-rate freezing apparatus (Planer LTD, Sunbury-on Thames, UK). T lymphocytes were identified in two-color immunofluorescence analysis using a phycoerythrin-conjugated anti-Leu 1 monoclonal antibody (Becton-Dickinson, Mountain View, CA). For single-color fluorescence using the patient's sera 2–4×10^6 PBL were incubated with 30 μl of a 1:3 serum dilution for 20 min at 37°C, and washed twice with phosphate-buffered saline (PBS) with 0.1% sodium azide. The pellets were resuspended in 50 μl of a 1:20 dilution of fluorescein-conjugated goat antihuman IgG $F(ab')_2$ (Kallestad, Austin, TX), incubated 20 min at 4°C, washed twice with PBS, resuspended in 0.5 ml PBS, and kept on ice. For two-color studies, the cells were further incubated with 5 μl of the anti-Leu-1 reagent for 20 min at 4°C.

Flow cytometric analysis. Samples were analyzed using a FACS II (Becton Dickinson, Sunnyvale, CA). Fluorescence was excited using the 488 nm line of a 4-watt argon ion laser, and the forward light scatter, green fluorescence (515–530 nm), and right-angle light scatter (for single-color analyses) or red (>580 nm) fluorescence signals of 10^4 cells/sample were acquired. For single-color studies, electronic gating of forward and right-angle light scatter signals was employed to select viable lymphoid cells for analysis (*13*), and green fluorescence data were transferred to and stored in a Hewlett Packard 9845T microcomputer (Palo Alto, CA) for later analysis. For two-color analyses, electronic compensation was used to correct for green-into-red and red-into-green fluorescence spill-over (*14*), and electronic gating of forward light scatter and red fluorescence was used to select viable T lymphocytes for analysis.

IgG alloantibody binding measured by flow cytometry was quantitated by comparing the fluorescence intensity produced by the test serum with a normal serum control (*15*) and expressing the results as a percentage of positive cells according to the Kolmogorov-Smirnov (K-S) test (*16*). This way of expressing the results is very useful when the concentration of antibodies is low (*15*). At high antibody concentrations the fluorescence peaks produced by the normal serum and experimental serum do not overlap, and the K-S analysis would not distinguish different antibody levels. In these cases quantitation was accomplished by calculating the mean channel number (MCN) of fluorescence intensity (*17*).

Purification of HLA-A,B,C molecules. HLA class I molecules were purified from pooled platelets from 200 donors (Scantibodies, Lakeside, CA) by affinity chromatography using the W6/32 monoclonal antibody (*18*). Gel electrophoresis of the purified material showed only the two subunits (44,000 and 12,000 m.w.) of the HLA molecules (*19*). The preparation contained 0.1% Nonidet P40 (NP40) used to solubilize the platelets, so that when 10 μl of a 0.2 mg/ml solution of purified HLA was used, 10 μl of 30% bovine serum albumin was also added to minimize the effect of the detergent on the target cells (*20*). Controls in the absence of purified HLA contained equivalent amounts of NP40 and bovine albumin. Patient serum (10 μl) was incubated for 1 hr at room temperature with either 10 μl of the HLA or the control preparation, and 10 μl of albumin. After that target cells were added and the fluorescence staining procedure was continued without other changes. Purified HLA inhibited the binding of the W6/32 antibody to lymphocytes or lymphoblastoid cells in a dose-dependent fashion, with 0.2 μg producing complete inhibition. This amount did not interfere with the binding of monoclonal antibodies to the T4 antigen or to HLA-DR antigens. Details of the effects of purified HLA are described elsewhere (*19*).

RESULTS

Quantitation of antibody binding by flow cytometry. The first experiments were performed to compare the binding of broadly-reactive antibodies to HLA-matched and unmatched lymphocytes using flow cytometry. Figure 1 shows binding of antibodies from a broadly sensitized patient to target cells of different degrees of HLA matching. In the top panel the results are expressed in MCN; illustrating that the differences in antibody binding are very apparent at high antibody concentrations but become gradually undetectable with increasing serum dilutions. In contrast, when the results are expressed using the K-S test (Fig. 1, bottom panel) minor differences from the normal serum control are made very evident and the curves of antibody binding activity remain separated even at high serum dilutions. The K-S test, as expected, did not quantitate antibody binding accurately at high antibody concentrations. The results shown in Figure 1 indicate that there is more antibody binding to lymphocytes having a 3-HLA antigen mismatch with the patient than to lymphocytes mismatched for ony 1 HLA antigen. In addition, when there were no HLA antigens mismatched the binding was very weak in 2 cases and undetectable in 2 other cases. We next performed a systematic evaluation of sera from 45 broadly sensitized patients with lymphocytes from 7 HLA-matched individuals.

* Abbreviations used: K-S, Kolmogorov-Smirnov; MCN, mean channel number, NHS: normal human serum, PBL: peripheral blood lymphocytes, PBS: phosphate-buffered saline.

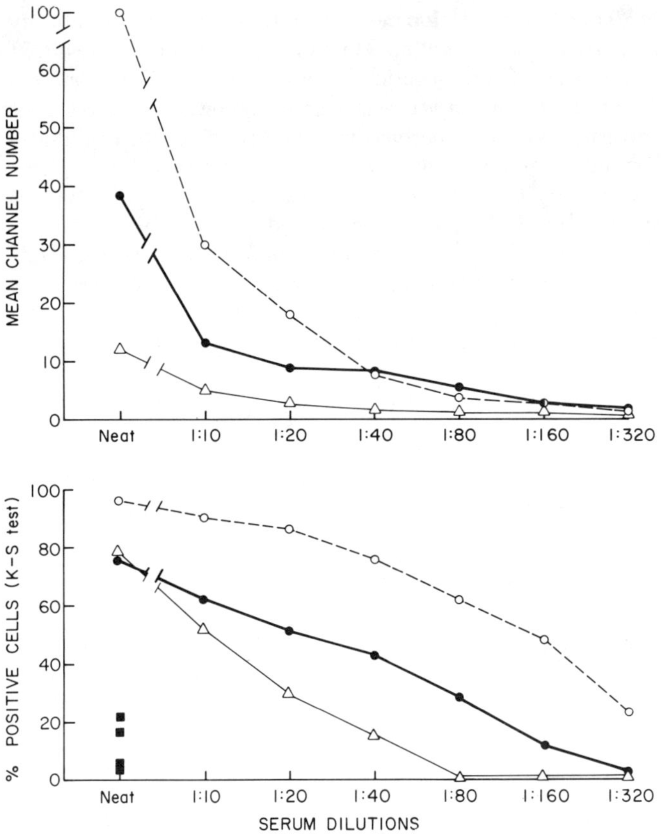

FIGURE 1. Antibody binding activity of serum from patient A1B8-10 (HLA-A1,A3,B8,B35) to HLA-matched and mismatched lymphocytes. Top panel: flow cytometry results expressed as MCN; bottom panel: same results expressed as percentage of positive cells (K-S test). The heavy line is a 3-antigen mismatch target (HLA-A2,A26,B8,B16); the fine line is a 1-antigen mismatch target (HLA-A1,A3,B7,B8); and the squares represent lymphocytes from different individuals who are a 0-antigen mismatch (HLA-A1,B8). The dotted line is serum from another broadly sensitized patient against mismatched target cells. Since variability not due to antibodies can account for up to 15 per cent of the binding measured by the K-S test (*15*), the top two curves in the bottom panel appear significantly different at all points, whereas the middle and bottom curves appear different only at the 1:20, 1:40, and 1:80 dilutions.

Reactions against HLA-matched targets detected by microcytotoxicity. First, reactivity against HLA-matched targets was studied by conventional cytotoxicity (Table 1). When sera from 20 broadly sensitized patients who were positive for HLA-A1 and B8 were tested against 4 A1,B8 homozygous cells, 17 of them were negative. Of the 3 specimens giving positive reactions, 2 (A1B8-19 and 20) were negative by flow cytometry (see below) suggesting that these antibodies may have been IgM and possibly directed to autologous antigens. Sera from 25 HLA-A2,B44 positive broadly sensitized patients were tested against 3 HLA-A2,B44 homozygous cells. Again, the reactions were mostly negative, although one target cell (No. 3) appeared to be more susceptible to cytotoxicity than the others (Table 1). The results were essentially the same using the antiglobulin technique.

Reactions against HLA-matched targets detected by flow cytometry. All 45 specimens were also evaluated against their respective HLA-matched targets using flow cytometry. We have previously established (*15*) that normal ulntransfused male

TABLE 1. HLA-matched microcytotoxicity reactions against HLA-A1,B8 or HLA-A2,B44[a] target cells

A. A1,B8 targets

Serum (n = 20)	Target No. 1	Target No. 2	Target No. 3	Target No. 4
ATS[b]	8/8[c]	8/8	8/8	8/8
NHS[d]	1/1	1/1	1/1	1/1
RM[e]	8/8	8/8	8/8	8/8
DB[e]	8/8	8/8	8/8	8/8
A1B8-11	2/4	0/0	6/6	6/6
A1B8-19	4/1	4/6	4/4	1/1
A1B8-20	4/6	4/4	6/6	1/1
All others (n = 17)	1/1	1/1	1/1	1/1
% Positive[f]	15%	10%	15%	5%

B. A2,B44 targets

Serum (n = 25)	Target No. 1	Target No. 2	Target No. 3
ATS[b]	8/8[c]	8/8	8/8
NHS[d]	1/1	1/1	1/1
RM[e]	8/8	8/8	8/8
BC[e]	8/8	8/8	8/8
A2B44-9	1/1	1/1	1/4
A2B44-10	1/1	1/1	4/2
A2B44-11	1/1	1/1	4/4
A2B44-12	1/2	1/1	6/4
A2B44-13	1/1	1/1	6/6
A2B44-14	1/1	1/2	4/2
A2B44-15	2/2	1/1	2/4
A2B44-20	1/1	1/1	1/4
A2B44-24	1/1	1/1	6/6
A2B44-25	1/1	2/2	6/6
All others (n = 15)	1/1	1/1	1/1
% Positive[f]	0%	0%	40%

[a] Target cells were phenotypically HLA-A,B homozygous.
[b] Antithymocyte serum (positive control).
[c] Cytotoxicity score (*9*); 1 is all cells alive; 8 is all cells dead; 2, 4, and 6 are increasing proportions of dead cells; 0 is unreadable wells. Results shown are of duplicate wells.
[d] Normal human serum.
[e] Unmatched sensitized patient's serum.
[f] Cytotoxicity score of 4 or more.

serum give K-S values of 15% of less, and we used 15% as the cut-off point to distinguish positive from negative reactions. Once positive reactions were identified, results were expressed as MCN for a more quantitative comparison with reactions with unmatched targets. Table 2 shows the patients' sera that were positive in any of the HLA-A1,B8 combinations (8 sera out of 20). All the reactions were very low when compared with unmatched patients' sera and 3 sera were positive with only one target cell. The tests were repeated using 2-color flow cytometry measuring antibody binding only in T cells identified by phycoerythin-conjugated anti-Leu 1 antibody. Only 2 of the 4 targets were available for these tests, and the results were similar with the exception of serum A1B8-12, which was negative with target No. 1, and serum A1B8-16, which remained positive with target No. 1 but negative with target No. 2. Similar experiments were performed with the HLA-A2,B44 combinations, and since all 3 targets were available for 2-color flow cytometry, the results shown in Table 3 are on Leu-1-positive cells. In general, more positive reactions were detected in the HLA-A2,B44 combinations than in the HLA-A1,B8 combinations.

Specificity of HLA-matched positive reactions. The next experiments focused on the positive reactions in order to gain further understanding of the specificities involved. Since antigenically active soluble HLA molecules can be purified by affinity chromatography using monoclonal antibodies (*18*) such HLA preparation was produced and tested in the HLA-matched combinations in which antibody binding was detected. Table 4 shows that purified HLA, at the concentrations used, produced an almost complete inhibition of the antibody binding in an unmatched combination (RM) but it did not affect the binding of the OKT4 monoclonal antibody. When tested with 5 sera and 2 targets of the HLA-A1,B8 combinations, purified HLA significantly inhibited antibody binding in 3 patients (in one only with one target) and produced little or no inhibition in the remaining 2 patients (Table 4). The inhibition studies performed in the HLA-A2,B44 combinations are detailed in Table 5. If we arbitrarily consider significant inhibition a value of 20 per cent inhibition or more, purified HLA was inhibitory in all patients except 2 (A2B44-14 and 17). It is of interest that similar degrees of inhibition were seen for the same patients with the different target cells. Figure 2 shows the fluorescence patterns seen in 2 examples in which purified HLA produced significant inhibition or no inhibition of antibody binding.

Summary of HLA-matched reactions. Table 6 summarizes the results of the studies performed in all combinations by cytotoxicity, flow cytometry and inhibition by purified HLA. In the HLA-A1, B8 group there were 5 out of 20 sera with clear-cut T cell reactivities detected by flow cytometry, and 3 of them (15%) were inhibited by purified HLA. In contrast, 13 of 25 sera were positive in the HLA-A2, B44 group, 11 of them (44%) inhibited by HLA ($P<0.05$).

TABLE 2. Mean fluorescence intensity of HLA-matched reactions against HLA-A1,B8 lymphocytes

Serum	Target No. 1	Target No. 2	Target No. 3	Target No. 4
NHS[a]	7.0[b]	10.0	8.4	13.7
RM[c]	69.0	83.8	94.1	62.9
DB[c]	168.0	145.8	181.9	111.6
A1B8-3	16.0	21.7	19.9	–[e]
A1B8-4	–	–	–	15.2
A1B8-8	19.0	26.2	33.5	15.6
A1B8-10	17.4	–	22.1	–
A1B8-11	12.5	24.7	30.6	39.9
A1B8-12	18.6[d]	–	–	–
A1B8-15	–	14.2	–	–
A1B8-16	24.4[d]	27.4	–	–
% Positive[f]	30%	25%	20%	15%

[a] Normal human serum.
[b] Mean channel number of green fluorescence.
[c] Unmatched sensitized patient's serum.
[d] NHS control MCN was 17.2.
[e] The dash (–) indicates a value of less than 15% by the K-S test.
[f] Percentage positive of all HLA-matched sera.

TABLE 3. Mean fluorescence intensity of HLA-matched reactions against HLA-A2,B44 T lymphocytes

Serum	Target No. 1	Target No. 2	Target No. 3
NHS[a]	4.9[b]	11.0	7.5
RM[c]	182.2	172.2	113.1
A2B44-1	–[d]	40.6	–
A2B44-2	–	26.0	25.8
A2B44-3	–	17.7	36.6
A2B44-4	43.0	103.1	31.2
A2B44-5	28.8	52.2	65.4
A2B44-6	–	14.3	15.3
A2B44-7	–	–	41.4
A2B44-8	–	17.1	14.4
A2B44-10	–	22.0	28.3
A2B44-14	–	40.0	45.0
A2B44-16	–	19.1	–
A2B44-17	42.0	52.6	50.6
A2B44-20	–	15.2	–
% Positive[e]	12%	48%	40%

[a] Normal human serum.
[b] Mean channel number of green fluorescence.
[c] Unmatched sensitized patient's serum.
[d] The dash (–) indicates a value of less than 15% by the K-S test.
[e] Percentage positive of all HLA-matched sera.

TABLE 4. Inhibition of HLA-A1,B8-matched reactions on T cells by purified HLA antigens

Serum	Target No. 1			Target No. 3		
	PBS[a]	HLA[b]	Inhibition (%)[c]	PBS	HLA	Inhibition (%)
OKT4	63.0	75.6	(−22)	60.1	61.9	(−2)
RM[d]	79.5	6.2	98	73.0	6.3	97
A1B8-3	12.1	11.3	10	9.9	10.2	(−6)
A1B8-8	34.5	6.4	93	20.5	7.8	79
A1B8-10	13.1	8.3	54	8.8	5.6	75
A1B8-11	10.4	10.5	(−2)	8.9	6.9	46
A1B8-16	12.9	13.1	(−3)	–[e]	–	–
NHS[f]	4.3			4.5		

[a] Serum preincubated with 10 μl PBS–0.1% NP40, MCN of green fluorescence signal.
[b] Serum preincubated with 2 μg affinity-purified HLA-A,B,C in 10 μl PBS–0.1% NP40. MCN of green fluorescence signal.
[c] Using 100-([MCN-HLA]-[MCN-NHS])/([MCN-PBS]-[MCN-NHS]) × 100.
[d] Unmatched sensitized patient.
[e] The dash (–) indicates a value of less than 15% by the K-S test.
[f] Normal human serum.

TABLE 5. Inhibition of HLA-A2,B44-matched reactions on T cells by purified HLA antigens

Serum	Target No. 1			Target No. 2			Target No. 3		
	PBS[a]	HLA[b]	Inhibition (%)[c]	PBS	HLA	Inhibition (%)	PBS	HLA	Inhibition (%)
OKT4	55.7	55.7	(0)	85.1	88.3	(−4)	87.6	88.6	(−1)
RM[d]	182.2	17.0	93	172.2	55.3	72	113.1	43.3	66
A2B44-1	–[e]	–	–	40.6	30.3	35	–	–	–
A2B44-2	–	–	–	26.0	15.8	68	25.8	21.9	21
A2B44-3	–	–	–	17.7	13.1	69	36.6	16.8	68
A2B44-4	43.0	24.8	48	103.1	66.9	39	31.2	21.4	41
A2B44-5	28.8	16.7	50	52.2	40.2	29	65.4	41.3	42
A2B44-6	–	–	–	14.3	12.8	46	15.3	12.3	38
A2B44-7	–	–	–	–	–	–	41.4	12.8	84
A2B44-8	–	–	–	17.1	12.8	71	14.4	12.1	33
A2B44-10	–	–	–	22.0	19.3	24	28.3	16.8	55
A2B44-14	–	–	–	40.0	37.2	10	45.0	40.9	11
A2B44-16	–	–	–	19.1	14.8	53	–	–	–
A2B44-17	42.0	42.8	(−2)	52.6	50.5	5	50.6	51.0	(−1)
A2B44-20	–	–	–	15.2	10.9	100	–	–	–
NHS[f]	4.9			11.0			7.5		

[a] Serum preincubated with 10 μl PBS–0.1% NP40. MCN of green fluorescence signal.
[b] Serum preincubated with 2 μg affinity-purified HLA-A,B,C in 10 μl PBS–0.1% NP40. MCN of green fluorescence signal.
[c] Using 100-([MCN-HLA]-[MCN-NHS])/([MCN-PBS]-[MCN-NHS]) × 100.
[d] Unmatched sensitized patient.
[e] The dash (–) indicates a value of less than 15% by the K-S test.
[f] Normal human serum.

TABLE 6. Summary of HLA-matched reactions

Number of cases	HLA-A1,B8		HLA-A2,B44		Total	
	Sera[a]	Combin.[b]	Sera	Combin.	Sera	Combin.
Total	20	80	25	75	45	155
Positive by cytotoxicity	3	9	10	10	13	19
Positive by flow cytometry	8	18	16	32	24	50
Positive T cells only	5	9[c]	13	25	18	34
Inhibited by HLA	3	5[c]	11	20	14	25
Not inhibited by HLA	2	4[c]	2	5	4	9
Total reactions HLA specific[d]	18	76	23	70	41	146
% Reactions HLA specific[d]	90	90	92	93	91	94

[a] HLA-matched sera from highly sensitized patients.
[b] Serum:target combinations.
[c] Only two HLA-A1,B8 targets were available for these analyses.
[d] Includes the broadly reactive sera that were negative with the HLA-matched targets plus positive ones that were inhibited by purified HLA.

DISCUSSION

The approach in this study has been to use sera from highly sensitized patients as an experimental situation in which the capacity of each patient to respond to different HLA epitopes is expressed as broadly reactive antibodies. Such a repertoire is known to involve determinants defining the known serological specificities, crossreactive or supertypic specificities (*4*)—and, conceivably, other crossreactive determinants not yet defined. Since the HLA molecules of a single specificity may not be identical in unrelated individuals (*8*), it is possible that the differences may elicit antibody responses, either directly or through crossreactivity with epitopes in other HLA molecules to which the patient has been exposed. By testing sera from many highly sensitized patients with HLA-matched targets using conventional (microcytotoxicity) and highly sensitive (flow cytometry) techniques we addressed the questions of how often positive reactions would be found, how strong they would be and whether HLA or non-HLA specificities would be involved.

The target cells chosen for these studies were HLA typed as being homozygous for HLA-A1,B8,CW7 or HLA-A2,B44,CW5 (possible CW4 with target No. 3). The HLA-A1,B8 (*21*) and A2,B44 (*22*) haplotypes are very frequent and in linkage desequilibrium, increasing the possibilities that the cells were truly homozygous. In addition, it allowed us to study a larger number of patients matching with one of the 2 types of targets. The sera of these patients produced strong reactions with unmatched targets, even when there was only a 1-antigen mismatch (Fig. 1). Even though family members of the target cell donors were not available for confirmatory genotyping, the fact that most of the sera reacted weakly or not at all with the matched target cells provided convincing evidence for homozygocity of the target cells.

The microcytotoxicity reactions were essentially negative with few exceptions. In 2 of the 3 positive cases with the HLA-A1B8 targets such positivity was not confirmed by flow cytometry, in which antibodies are detected with a fluorescein-conjugated anti-IgG reagent. This suggests that the antibodies were possibly IgM and perhaps autoantibodies (*23*) (cells from the patients could not be procured for testing). With the HLA-A2,B44 targets there were no positive reactions with cells from 2 donors and several with cells from the remaining donor—a fact that, as discussed below, may be due to polymorphism within the serologically defined antigens. The use of flow cytometry revealed a considerable number of reactions that were

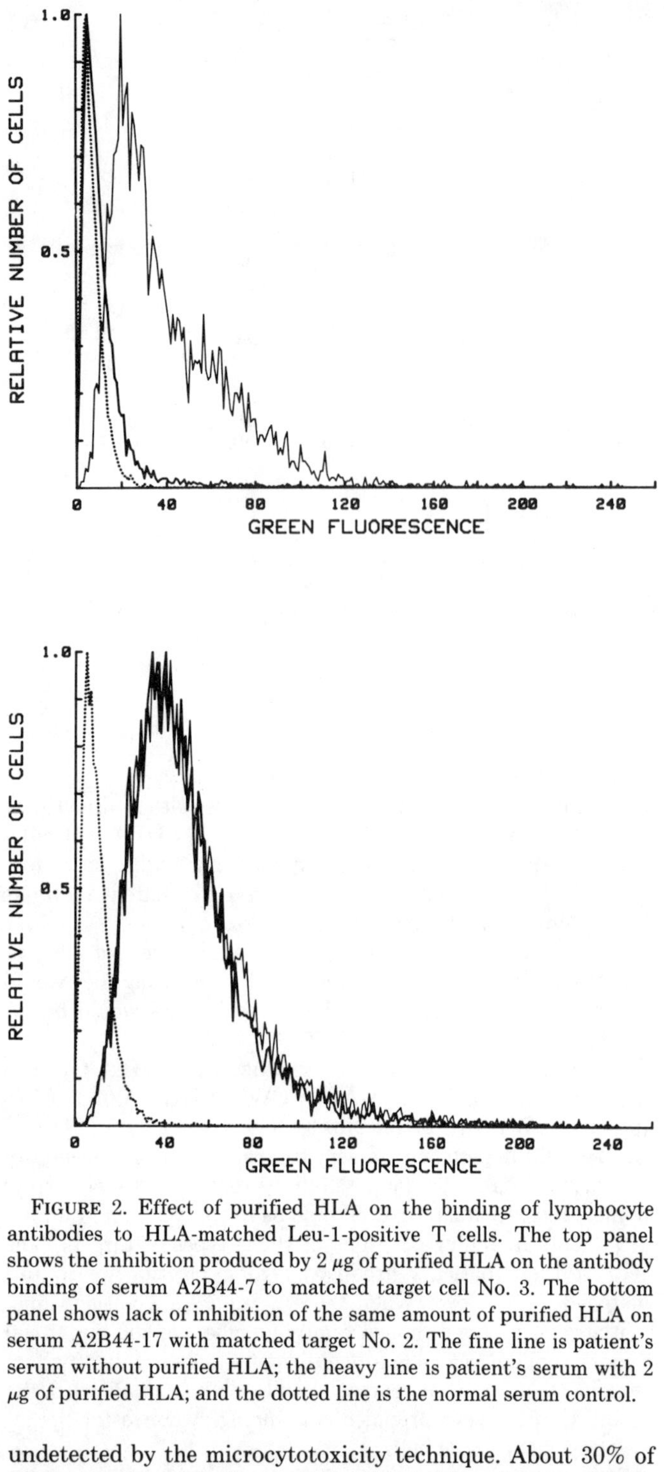

FIGURE 2. Effect of purified HLA on the binding of lymphocyte antibodies to HLA-matched Leu-1-positive T cells. The top panel shows the inhibition produced by 2 μg of purified HLA on the antibody binding of serum A2B44-7 to matched target cell No. 3. The bottom panel shows lack of inhibition of the same amount of purified HLA on serum A2B44-17 with matched target No. 2. The fine line is patient's serum without purified HLA; the heavy line is patient's serum with 2 μg of purified HLA; and the dotted line is the normal serum control.

undetected by the microcytotoxicity technique. About 30% of the matched combinations were positive, although most of these reactions involved relatively little antibody binding as judged by the MCNs of the green fluorescence. While non-HLA antibody reactions could be responsible for these findings, there are alternative explanations. Positive reactions were found more frequently with the HLA-A2,B44 targets than with HLA-A1,B8 targets. The HLA-B44 antigen is a subtype of HLA-B12 (*24*), and it has been shown that the B44 antigen itself can be further subdivided serologically (*7*). Thus, patient and target cell donor may belong to different subtypes of HLA-B44, and the positive reactions may in fact have involved HLA specificities. Subtypes have also been described for HLA-A2 (*8*). In contrast, the recognition of HLA-A1 is straightforward using serology, and it seems that the HLA-B8 specificity may be the result of a single epitope (*25*). Thus, the increased reactions seen with the HLA-A2,B44 target cells could be the result of the relative complexity in serologically defining the HLA-A2 and B44 antigens. The HLA-C antigens of many of the patients were unknown, and some of the positive reactions could conceivably have involved HLA-C specificity.

Experimental support for HLA specificity was given by the inhibition seen with purified HLA. The production of purified HLA antigens using cells from one or a few individuals would not be effective because of the limited number of individual specificities that would be present in such preparation. The use of platelets from a large pool of individuals provided a means of obtaining a preparation that included many different antigens. Using this preparation, the majority of the reactions seen in the matched combinations could be inhibited to some degree. Given the complexity of this polymorphic antigen system, along with the differences in specificities, affinities, and titers that would be expected in the different sera studied, the inhibition produced by the HLA preparation strongly suggests that most of these reactions were due to antibodies reacting with HLA class I antigens, particularly HLA-A and B, as HLA-C is only weakly expressed on platelets (*26*). In some of the reactions that were not inhibited by the HLA preparation, increasing the amount of HLA antigen did result in a slight decrease in the fluorescence intensity of the reaction (not shown). This suggests that epitopes possibly involved in this particular reactions are present in relatively small amounts in the HLA preparation, so that even in the few cases in which purified HLA was not inhibitory HLA specificity could not be definitively ruled out.

The results presented here allowed us to draw some conclusions relevant to histocompatibility and transplantation. First, we could not confirm previous reports (*27*) that T cell non-HLA antibodies were significantly involved in the renal transplant patient population. Antibodies to non-HLA antigens accounted for little or none of the antibody reactivity in the broadly sensitized renal patients that we studied. Second, antibodies to HLA-matched unrelated lymphocytes were detected in a significant proportion (about 30%) of our patients. However, the antibodies were infrequently cytotoxic and were present in rather low concentrations. These weakly reactive antibodies may still be significant in renal transplantation although they do not appear to produce hyperacute rejections (*17*). Third, the reactivity against HLA-matched targets was still largely due to anti-HLA antibodies, probably involving the recognition of distinct epitopes in the otherwise serologically HLA-matched molecules, especially in the A2,B44 targets. Of course, further work is necessary to confirm or rule out this possibility. These results reinforce the importance of HLA-A, B matching in sensitized patients and suggest that when positive crossmatches do occur, even with well-matched donors it would not be safe to dismiss them as due to non-HLA specificities.

Finally, the weak or absent reactivity with HLA-matched targets defines an experimental model in which the immunogenicity of similar antigens (e.g., HLA-A2 vs. A28) could be tested in the future. Such information will undoubtedly be very useful in the selection of donors for renal transplantation and platelet transfusions.

Acknowledgments. We are very grateful to the laboratory personnel of other institutions who kindly provided sera and cells from HLA-typed patients and blood donors. The skillful technical assistance of Theodor Teimer and Joan Ireland is deeply appreciated.

REFERENCES

1. Terasaki PI. Presidential address: Transplantation Society. Transplant Proc 1983; 15: 14.
2. Mittal KK, Ruder EA, Green D. Matching for histocompatibility (HL-A) antigens for platelet transfusion. Blood 1976; 47: 31.
3. Singh G, Thompson M, Griffith B, Berstein R, Rabin BS, Hardesty R, Nalesuik M, Bahnson HT. Histocompatibility in cardiac transplantation with particular reference to immunopathology of positive serologic crossmatch. Clin Immunol Immunopathol 1983; 28: 56.
4. Delmonico FL, Fuller A, Cosimi AB, Tolkoff-Rubin N, Russell PS, Rodey GE, Fuller TC. New approaches to donor crossmatching and successful transplantation of highly sensitized patients. Transplantation 1983; 36: 629.
5. Duquesnoy RJ, Filip DJ, Rodey GE, Rimm AA, Aster RH. Successful transfusion of platelets "mismatched" for HLA antigens to alloimmunized thrombocytopenic patients. Am J Hematol 1977; 2: 219.
6. Schiffer CA, Keller C, Dutcher JP, Aisner J, Hogge D, Wiernik PH. Potential HLA-matched platelet donor availability for alloimmunized patients. Transfusion 1983; 23: 286.
7. Heise ER, Tekolf WA, Hampton JP. Serologic recognition of a HLA-B44 (12) subgroup associated with the 44.2 specificity defined by CML. Hum Immunol 1984; 11: 163.
8. Biddison WE, Kostyu DD, Strominger JL, Krangel MS. Delineation of immunologically and biochemically distinct HLA-A2 antigens. J Immunol 1982; 129: 730.
9. Terasaki PI, Bernoco D, Park MS, et al. Microdroplet testing for HLA-A,-B,-C and -D antigens. Am J Clin Pathol 1978; 69: 103.
10. Amos DB. Cytotoxicity testing. In: Ray JG Jr, Hare DB, Pedersen PD, Mullally DI, eds. NIAID manual of tissue typing techniques. Publication No. (NIH) 77-545. Washington, DC: US Department of Health, Education and Welfare 1976: 25.
11. Johnson AH. Antiglobulin cross-match for transplantation. In: Rose NR, Friedman H, eds. Manual of clinical immunology. 32nd ed. Washington, DC: American Society for Microbiology, 1980: 1000.
12. Jewett MAS, Hansen JA, DuPont B. Cryopreservation of lymphocytes. In: Rose NR, Friedman H, eds. Manual of clinical immunology. Washington, DC: American Society for Microbiology 1980; 1026.
13. Hoffman RA, Kung PC, Hansen WP, Goldstein G. Simple and rapid measurement of human T lymphocytes and their subclasses in peripheral blood. Proc Natl Acad Sci 1980; 77: 4914.
14. Loken MR, Parks DR, Herzenberg LA. Two-color immunofluorescence using a fluorescence activated cell sorter. J Histochem Cytochem 1977; 25: 899.
15. Scornik JC, Ireland JE, Howard RJ, Pfaff WW. Assessment of the risk of broad sensitization by blood transfusions. Transplantation 1984; 37: 249.
16. Young IT. Proof without prejudice: use of the Kolmogorov-Smirnov test for the analysis of histograms from flow systems and other sources. J Histochem Cytochem 1977; 25: 935.
17. Garovoy MR, Rheinschmidt MA, Bigos M, Perkins H, Colombe B, Salvatierra O. Flow cytometry analysis: the ultimate crossmatch technique? Transplant Proc 1983; 15: 1939.
18. Parham P, Barnstable CJ, Bodmer WF. Use of a monoclonal antibody (W6/32) in structural studies of HLA-A,B,C antigens. J Immunol 1979; 123: 342.
19. Cook DJ, Scornik JC. Purified HLA antigens to probe human alloantibody specificity. Hum Immunol 1985; 14: 234.
20. Dawson JR, Shasby SS, Amos DB. Serologic assay of HL-A antigens in the presence of detergents. J Immunol 1973; 111: 281.
21. Ivaskova E. AI. In: Terasaki PI, ed. Histocompatibility testing 1980. UCLA Tissue Typing Laboratory, Los Angeles, CA, 1980: 292.
22. Marshall WH, Barnard JM. A2. In: Terasaki PI, ed. Histocompatibility testing 1980. UCLA Tissue Typing Laboratory, Los Angeles, CA, 1980: 295.
23. Ting A. The lymphocyte crossmatch test in clinical renal transplantation. Transplantation 1983; 35: 403.
24. Mittal KK. BW44. In: Terasaki PI, ed. Histocompatibility testing 1980. UCLA Tissue Typing Laboratory, Los Angeles, CA, 1980: 398.
25. Antonelli P, Nisperos B, Braun M, Hansen JA. Recognition by a murine monoclonal antibody of a unique epitope specific for the human alloantigen HLA-B8. Hum Immunol 1984; 11: 11.
26. Mueller-Eckhard G, Hauck M, Kayser W, Mueller-Eckhard C. HLA-C antigens on platelets. Tissue Antigens 1980; 16: 91.
27. Reed E. Suciu-Foca N, Hardy M, Lattes C, McCabe R, Brensilver J, Reemtsma K. Alloantibodies to a non-HLA system and their relevance to transplantation. Transplant Proc 1983; 15: 245.

Received 19 June 1985.
Accepted 13 August 1985.

0041-1337/86/4104-0454$02.00/0
TRANSPLANTATION
Vol. 41, No. 4

Printed in U.S.A.

ASSESSMENT OF PLASMA NEOPTERIN IN CLINICAL KIDNEY TRANSPLANTATION

A. J. SCHÄFER, V. DANIEL, K. DREIKORN,[1] AND G. OPELZ[2]

Department of Transplantation Immunology, Institute of Immunology, and Department of Urology, Surgical Center, University of Heidelberg, Heidelberg, Federal Republic of Germany

Serial plasma samples of 172 kidney transplant recipients and 42 chronic dialysis patients were evaluated retrospectively in a radioimmunoassay to determine the clinical relevance of plasma neopterin levels. Dialysis patients had a higher neopterin level 196±82 nmol/L (mean±SD) than 70 healthy controls (7±4 nmol/L). In 45 patients with a completely uneventful postoperative course, elevated pretransplant neopterin levels dropped rapidly within a week to a mean of 30 nmol/L and remained stable thereafter. In 22 outpatients with stable graft function there was a highly significant correlation between 170 paired serum creatinine and plasma neopterin values (r = 0.94). A group of 13 patients had experienced delayed graft function (ATN) without rejection. Their one-week mean neopterin level was 100 nmol/L and continued to drop in parallel with the serum creatinine. Another 15 patients rejected their kidneys irreversibly within 3 weeks—6 of them had extremely high neopterin levels during the rejection process (range 500–1000 nmol/L) that were not seen in other patients. A total of 169 rejection episodes in 43 patients were treated with bolus-dose cortisone. On the day of bolus therapy, both serum creatinine ($P<0.002$) and neopterin ($P<0.005$) were elevated. At 24 hours prior to bolus cortisone therapy, creatinine levels were not significantly elevated, whereas there was a significant rise in plasma neopterin ($P<0.01$). The overall sensitivity of neopterin increase was 86% with a 17% probability of false positives, and the sensitivity was 95% in biopsy-proved rejections. Plasma neopterin appears to be a useful marker for early detection of rejection and for identifying severe rejections that are not responsive to treatment.

Early diagnosis of rejection is essential for successful rejection treatment. Ideally, one would like to diagnose rejection prior to the induction of significant cellular damage and the subsequent rise in serum creatinine. In spite of many attempts to devise immunological tests for the diagnosis of rejection, few have gained wide clinical acceptance.

Complex events associated with the allograft response lead to an activation of specific effector T lymphocytes mediating allograft rejection. Activated T lymphocytes release interferon gamma that is capable of activating in macrophages a guanosine triphosphate-specific cyclohydrolase leading to increased synthesis and excretion of neopterin (*1*). Neopterin can be utilized as a marker for the clinical assessment of cell-mediated immune responses (*2*). Elevated urinary and serum neopterin levels have been demonstrated in patients with various viral and malignant diseases (*3*). Furthermore, increased urinary neopterin levels determined by high-performance liquid chromatography have been reported to precede rejection in human allograft recipients (*4–7*).

We report here our experience with radioimmunoassay plasma neopterin determinations. Serially collected and frozen-stored plasma samples of 172 kidney transplant recipients were assayed retrospectively and correlated with the transplants' clinical course.

MATERIALS AND METHODS

Patients. From June 1982, through March 1985, 172 consecutive renal allografts were performed in 166 patients at the Department of Urology, University of Heidelberg: 13 grafts were from living-related donors and 153 from cadaveric donors. There were 146 first and 25 second transplants, and 1 fourth transplant.

Plasma samples. Upon admission to the hospital and thrice weekly thereafter until discharge, heparinized blood was obtained and plasma samples were kept frozen at −20°C until use in the neopterin assay. Serum creatinine was monitored and recorded daily, in addition to body temperature, morning weight, urine excretion, blood pressure, creatinine-clearance, urea, dialysis treatments, acute rejection treatments, biopsies, urinary and serum electrolytes.

Clinical chemistry. Creatinine: Serum creatinine was determined by an automated Jaffe-picrate reaction on an SMA 12/60 (Technicon Instruments Corp.).

Neopterin (Neopterin RIAcid, Henning, Berlin): Each standard curve concentration was determined in triplicate: 50 μl plasma was pipetted into Radioimmuno-Special Vials (Sarstedt, Numbrecht, F.R.G.) and 100 μl of 125-iodine neopterin tracer and 100 μl of preprecipitated antibody complex (rabbit anti-neopterin and goat antirabbit IgG) was added. The suspension was incubated overnight at 22°C, resuspended with 0.3 ml polyethylene glycol (PEG)* solution (6% in water) and centrifuged twice for 10 min at 2500 g. The supernatant was removed and pellet radioactivity was counted in a gamma counter (LKB, Munich). Neopterin plasma levels were computed using lin/log transformation and cubic spline interpolation.

The neopterin level in plasma of 70 healthy individuals was 7±4 nmol/L (mean±SD). We defined the upper limit of normal (mean±2 SD) with 95% confidence as 15 nmol/L.

Diagnosis of acute rejection. For the purpose of this study, rejection was defined as occurring when the composite clinical

[1] Department of Urology.

[2] Address correspondence to: Gerhard Opelz, M.D., Institute of Immunology, University of Heidelberg, Im Neuenheimer Feld 305, D-6900 Heidelberg, F R. Germany.

* Abbreviations used: ATN, acute tubular necrosis; CMV, cytomegalovirus; EBV, Epstein-Barr virus; ELISA, enzyme-linked immunosorbent assay; HSV, herpes-simplex virus; HPLC, high-performance liquid chromatography; PEG, polyethylene glycol.

decision to initiate antirejection therapy was made. The diagnosis of acute rejection was based on clinical symptoms (diminished urinary output, fever, increase in blood pressure, increased bodyweight, graft tenderness, graft swelling) clinical chemistry of blood and urine (decreased creatinine clearance, increase of serum creatinine and urea, increased β-2-microglobulin), renal scanning (functional and sequence scintigraphy with 131-iodine-hippuran and 99 m-technetium-nuclide), renal biopsy, and immunological and virological tests (lymphocyte subpopulations, virus antibody titers).

Diagnosis of actue tubular necrosis (ATN). ATN was defined as persistent postoperative renal disfunction during which the scintigram showed good transplant perfusion, without urine production, serum creatinine levels of >3 mg/100 ml, dialysis requirement but no evidence of acute rejection, and subsequent normalization of function without therapy for rejection.

Virology. From January 1982, through June 1984, virus-antibody titers against cytomegalovirus (CMV), Epstein-Barr virus (EBV) and Herpes-simplex virus (HSV) were determined weekly by a complement-fixation reaction using commercial antigens (Behring, Marburg). Since June 1984, enzyme-linked immunosorbent assays (ELISA) for anti-CMV-IgG and CMV-IgM antibodies were performed routinely (Enzygnost, Behring), because from that time all patients were immunized with CMV-hyperimmunoglobulin (Behring, Marburg). Patients with a positive titer were excluded from second and third immunization with CMV-hyperimmunoglobulin.

Statistical analysis. Arithmetic means±SD are given unless otherwise stated. Significance was determined by Student's t test. Sensitivity was calculated as true-positive / (true positive + false negative) and the probability of false positive was calculated as false positive / (true positive + false positive).

RESULTS

Figure 1 shows the distribution of neopterin levels in healthy controls and hemodialysis patients. The 70 healthy controls showed a narrow range of plasma neopterin concentrations with a mean of 7±4 nmol/L, whereas there was a wide range in 42 chronically dialyzed patients with a mean of 196±82 nmol/L (Fig. 1). The mean neopterin value in 45 transplanted patients with uncomplicated posttransplant course was 29±21 nmol/L from day 9 posttransplantation until discharge (Fig. 2). In 22 transplant patients with stable graft function seen in the outpatient clinic, the relationship between neopterin and creatinine is drawn as the best fit of a regression line for 170 sets of parallel tests (Fig. 3). Even with well-functioning grafts, patients do not reach the low point of neopterin and creatinine values in healthy controls, however, the regression line cuts that point (Fig. 3). The excellent correlation (r = 0.94) between creatinine and neopterin demonstrates the dependence of both substances on glomerular clearance. We can conclude that there is a biological relationship between renal function and neopterin levels. Consequently, neopterin should be useful in estimating renal function. The fluctuations of creatinine, urea, and plasma neopterin concentrations in patients on dialysis treatment show a similar pattern (Fig. 4), whereas the molar ratio of neopterin to creatinine is constant. The parallel time course of creatinine and neopterin in 13 patients with delayed function without rejection is obvious and documented by a nearly constant molar ratio (Fig. 5).

Having established these baseline characteristics of plasma neopterin, we next analyzed its utility to predict immunological

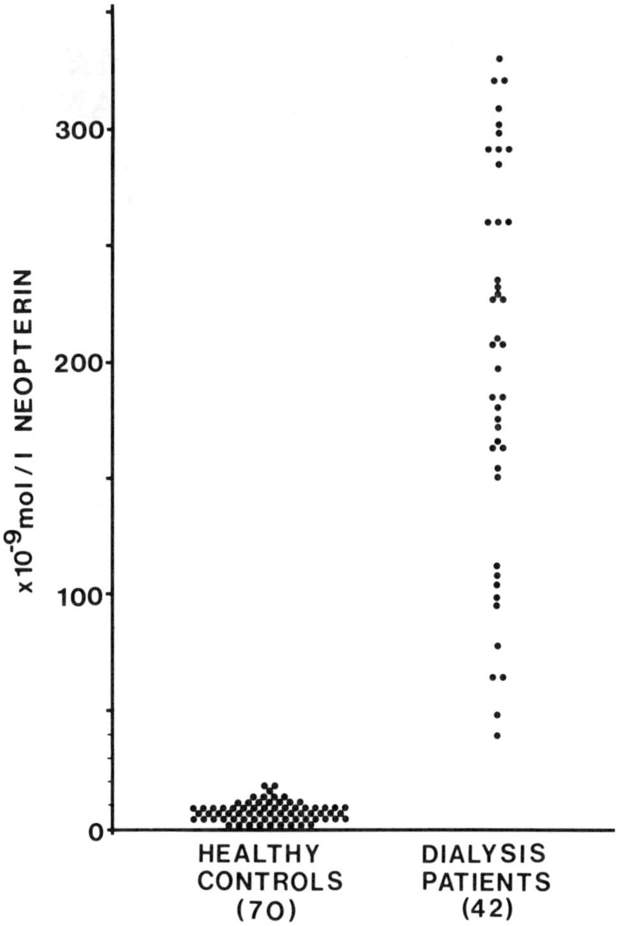

FIGURE 1. Plasma neopterin in healthy controls and dialysis patients. Numbers of patients studied are given in parentheses.

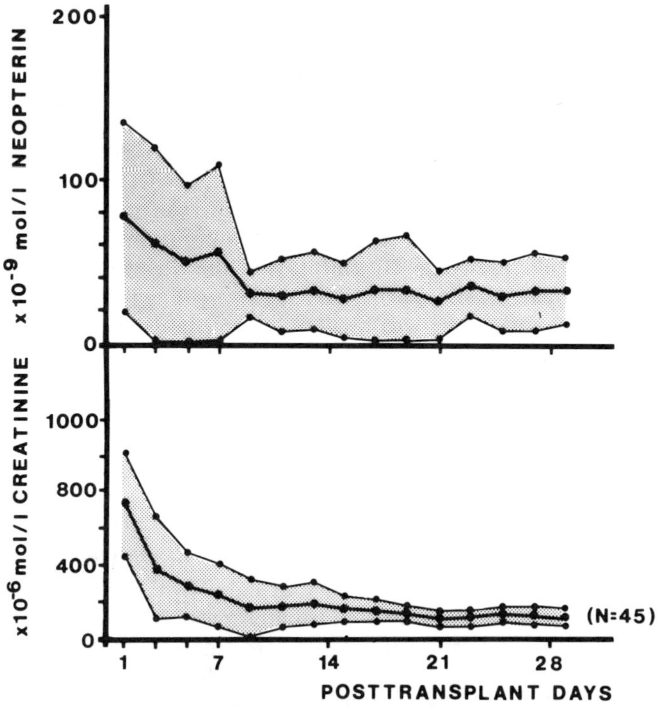

FIGURE 2. Posttransplant course in 45 patients with good graft function. Serial levels of plasma creatinine and neopterin are given as curves of mean level±SD.

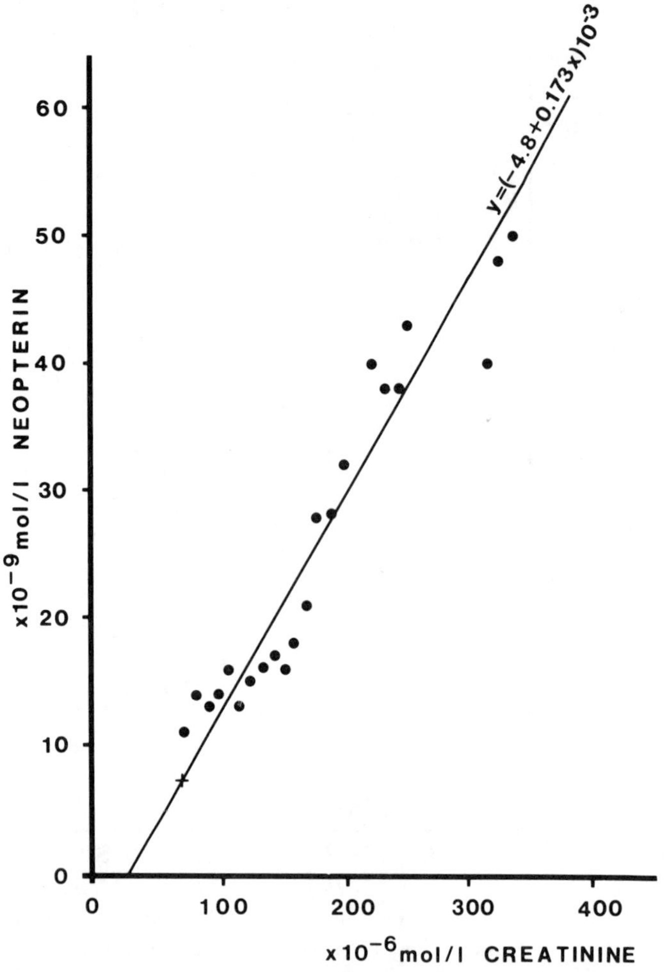

FIGURE 3. Relationship between plasma neopterin and plasma creatinine in transplant recipients. Regression line is drawn as best fit through mean neopterin and corresponding creatinine values. A total of 170 paired values determined in 22 outpatients with stable graft function were analyzed (correlation coefficient r = 0.94)

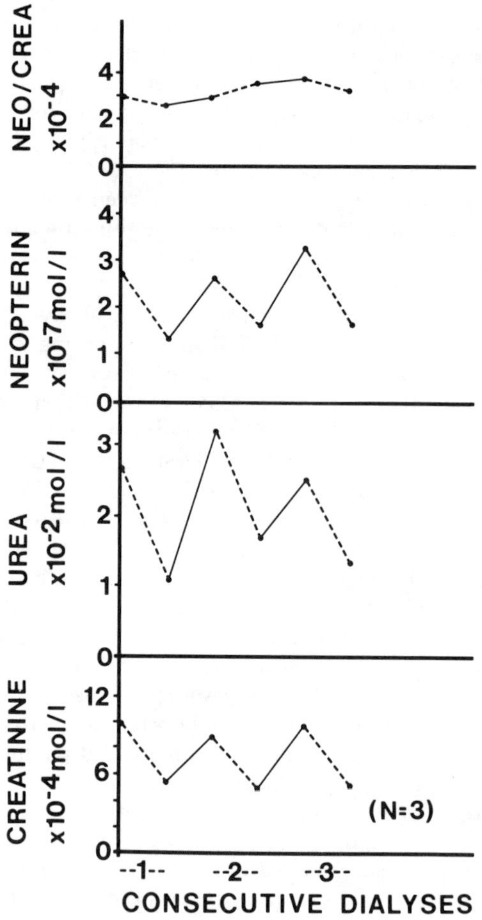

FIGURE 4. Variation of creatinine, urea, and plasma neopterin concentrations in 3 uremic patients during three consecutive hemodialyses. Neo/crea (top) represents molar ratio of neopterin over creatinine.

rejection. Of 15 irreversible rejections, 6 had extremely high neopterin levels that were not seen in any other of our 172 patients. Mean neopterin levels increased even though these patients showed stable creatinine levels during hemodialysis and plasma exchange treatment (Fig. 6). In other words, whereas dialysis and plasma exchange were able to normalize creatinine, neopterin was produced in such vast excess that normalization did not occur. Thus, extreme increases in plasma neopterin may be helpful in identifying rejections that are refractory to immunosuppressive treatment. However, 9 of the 15 patients with irreversible rejection showed only moderately increased neopterin levels indistinguishable from increases observed in patients with reversible rejection episodes. In 43 measurements during rejection episodes without dialysis, mean levels of neopterin ($P<0.005$) and creatinine ($P<0.02$) were elevated significantly on the day of bolus cortisone therapy. Importantly, the mean level of neopterin was elevated significantly 24 hr prior to an elevation of creatinine (Fig. 7).

Increased neopterin values in the urine have been described previously in connection with viral diseases (*1*, *3*). In immunosuppressed allograft recipients, reactivation of latent virus infection plays an important role. We analyzed mean neopterin levels for 10 days before and after detection of a significant rise in virus titer. Of 24 titer increases, neopterin was increased in 10 (42%). Neopterin increase per rise of different virus titers was 7/11 (64%) for CMV, 3/5 (60%) for EBV, and 0/8 (0%) for HSV.

Table 1 shows the sensitivity of neopterin elevations with respect to three stages of clinical decision for antirejection therapy. To define increased neopterin we used the 29±21 nmol/L observed in patients with an uncomplicated posttransplant course at the time of discharge (Fig. 2). For transplanted patients, the upper limit of normal was defined as a mean of 50 nmol/L—and, to exclude daily variations, increases of neopterin had to be higher than 2SD (42 nmol/L) above the patients' mean base line level. We arrive at a sensitivity of neopterin at bolus cortisone therapy of 86%, and in the biopsy-proved rejection group of 95% (Table 1). Table 2 shows an analysis of all 169 neopterin elevations with respect to clinical findings. They are distributed over 141 bolus cortisone therapies, 10 virus infections, and 18 others. The probability of a false positive elevation on bolus cortisone therapy is only 17%. The reasons for false positives were virus infection (6%), unknown reasons (5%), bacteriuria (2%), unspecified fever (2%), pneumonia, cyclosporine nephrotoxicity, blood transfusion, and possibly atypical rejection (2%).

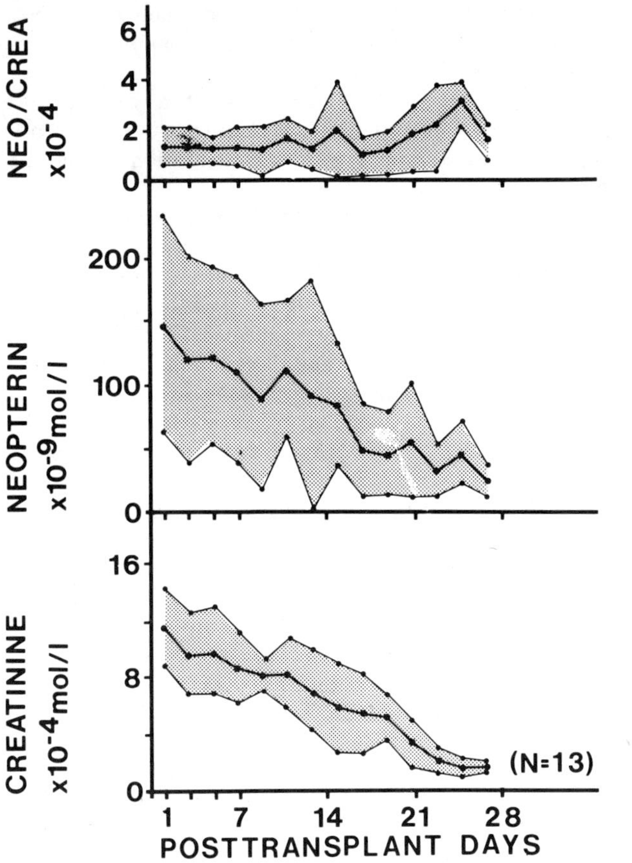

FIGURE 5. Posttransplant course in 13 patients who experienced delayed function (ATN) without rejection. Means±SD are plotted.

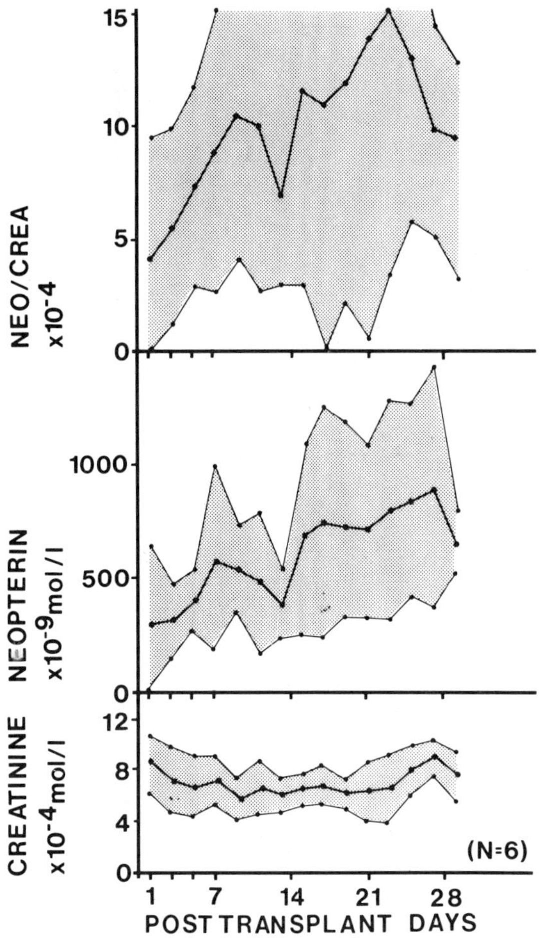

FIGURE 6. Posttransplant course in 6 patients with extremely high neopterin levels during acute irreversible rejection. Note relatively stable creatinine values in contrast to high neopterin values despite hemodialysis treatment.

DISCUSSION

Previous studies have shown an association of urinary neopterin increase with rejection episodes or viral infections (*5*). It can be assumed that neopterin is preferentially released at the site of allogeneic stimulation and penetrates through the tissue into the blood compartment. It is then filtered via the glomeruli and excreted. Blood plasma or serum appear to be most suitable for neopterin determination, especially when no urine is produced during impaired graft function because of acute tubular necrosis. ATN occurred in 23% of the transplants monitored by us. Thus there is an advantage of the plasma neopterin RIA assay as compared with neopterin determination by reversed-phase high-performance chromatography (HPLC) in urine (*8*). To use the HPLC method for plasma is time-consuming, and requires different precolumns, columns, and deproteinization—so that the method becomes impractical. Another disadvantage of measuring neopterin in the urine is that, because of the physiological variation in urine volume and concentration (e.g., the measurement would give different values in the morning or the evening), it is necessary to relate urinary neopterin to creatinine. The neopterin/creatinine ratio eliminates these disturbing effects to some extent. Plasma RIA neopterin determination provides the advantage of technical simplicity. There is no requirement for sample pretreatment, it can be performed from as little as 0.5 ml blood, hundreds of samples can be processed simultaneously, and instrumentation is readily available. The accuracy of neopterin determination by HPLC or RIA is comparable, with similar variation coefficients (*11*).

Our analysis of the neopterin assay's accuracy in predicting rejection depends on correct rejection diagnosis. Therefore, we distinguished three rejection categories. The accuracy of rejection prediction was 95% (60/63) in the group with clinical rejection symptoms proved by biopsy, 88% (80/91) in the group with strong clinical and diagnostical evidence of rejection (without biopsy), and 10% (1/10) in the group with fever and creatinine increase only. Thus, in this retrospective analysis, we found a good correlation between plasma neopterin increase and rejection. With urinary neopterin, an accurate prediction of rejection was made in 95% (16 patients) when rejections were diagnosed on the basis of clinical symptoms, blood chemistry, renal scanning, and fine-needle aspiration cytology (*5*). Thus, it appears that urine and plasma neopterin elevations have essentially the same accuracy in predicting rejection.

Analysis of rejection episodes in 43 patients without dialysis treatment showed a significant increase in plasma neopterin 24 hr prior to a significant rise in creatinine and clinical diagnosis of rejection. These results are concordant with reported urinary neopterin elevations 1–2 days (*7*), 1.6 days (*4*), and 1.9 days (*5*) prior to rejection therapy. Among 15 patients with fulmi-

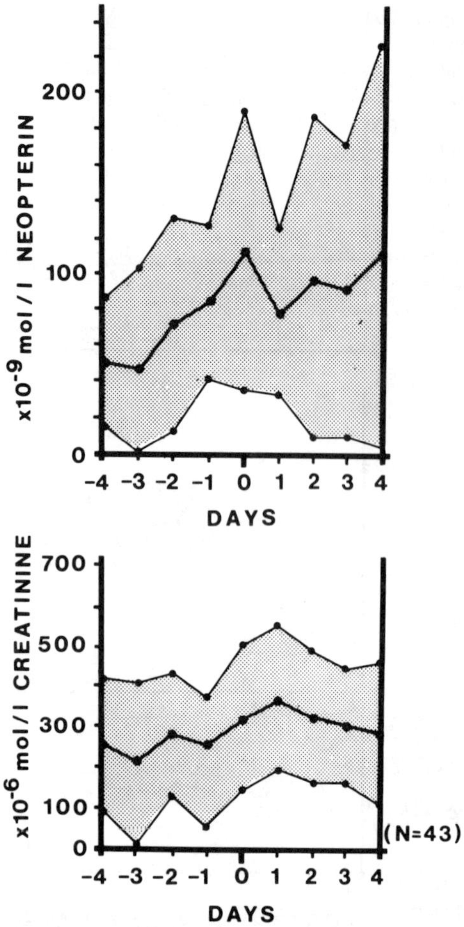

FIGURE 7. Changes in neopterin and creatinine levels in 43 patients before and after bolus cortisone therapy. On the day of bolus therapy (day 0) both plasma creatinine ($P<0.02$) and neopterin ($P<0.005$) were elevated significantly. At 24 hr prior to bolus cortisone therapy only neopterin was significantly increased ($P<0.01$). Means±SD are plotted; day 0 = day of first cortisone bolus.

nant irreversible rejections, 6 showed extremely high neopterin levels not seen in other patients. The remaining 9 patients showed moderate neopterin elevations. It is conceivable, although we cannot provide evidence, that the types of rejection in these two groups of patients were different. With respect to the parameters examined by us, differentiation was not possible.

One complicating factor in the interpretation of increased plasma neopterin is that virus infections can cause changes similar to those of graft rejection. In our patients, a significant rise in virus titer was accompanied by a rise in plasma neopterin in 64% (7/11) of CMV infections, 60% (3/5) of EBV infections, and 0% (0/8) of HSV infections. These numbers are too small to be conclusive. Among our patients with viral infection, 42% (10/24) had elevated plasma neopterin levels as compared with a reported 100% (23/23) with elevated urinary neopterin (5). Our criterion of viral infections was based on a rise of virus titers tested by complement fixation or ELISA, and not additionally or alternatively by evidence of clinical symptoms, which may explain this difference.

In this series of 172 transplants, low and stable plasma neopterin values were associated with an immunologically uncomplicated posttransplant course, whereas neopterin increases were associated with rejection. Our data indicate that plasma neopterin determination may be a useful and practical method of posttransplant immunological monitoring.

Acknowledgments. We acknowledge the excellent technical assistance of Elke Kairies and Clara Hofmann, and the assistance of Ulrike Mülker in preparing the manuscript.

REFERENCES

1. Huber Ch, Batchelor R, Fuchs Ch, et al. Immune response-associated production of neopterin. J Exp Med 1984; 160: 310.
2. Huber Ch, Fuchs D, Hausen A, et al. Pteridines as a new marker to detect human T cells activated by allogeneic or modified self major histocompatibility complex (MHC) determinants. J Immunol 1983; 130: 1047.

TABLE 1. Sensitivity of neopterin elevation in relation to method of rejection diagnosis

Clinical decision for antirejection therapy	Increased neopterin/total: Elevation range neopterin (nmol/L)			False-negative/total:
	50–80	81–150	>150	
Clinical + laboratory diagnostics + biopsy	10/63 (16%)	7/63 (11%)	43/63 (68%)	3/63 (5%)
Clinical + laboratory diagnostics	21/91 (23%)	24/91 (26%)	35/91 (38%)	11/91 (12%)
Fever + creatinine increase	—	1/10 (10%)	—	9/10 (90%)
		141/164 (86%)		23/164 (14%)

TABLE 2. Analysis of 169 neopterin elevations in relation to clinical status

Clinical status	Increased neopterin/total. Elevation range in Neopterin (nmol/L)			
	50–80	81–150	>150	>50 (SUM)
Bolus cortisone	31/169 (18%)	32/169 (19%)	78/169 (46%)	141/169 (83%)
Rejection therapy				
Virus infection	1/169 (1%)	2/169 (1%)	7/169 (4%)	10/169 (6%)
Others:	4/169 (2%)	9/169 (5%)	5/169 (3%)	18/169 (11%)
8 Unknown				
3 Bacteriuria				
3 Fever				
1 Pneumonia				
1 Cyclosporine nephrotoxicity				
1 Blood transfusions				
1 Atypical rejection?				

3. Wachter H, Hausen A, Grassmayr K. Increased urinary excretion of neopterin in patients with malignant tumors and with virus diseases. Hoppe-Seyler's Z. Physiol Chem Phys 1979; 360: 1957.
4. Fuchs D, Hausen A, Huber Ch, et al. Pteridine secretion as a marker for the proliferation of alloantigen-induced lymphocytes. Hoppe-Seyler's Z. Physiol Chem Phys 1982; 363: 661.
5. Margreiter R, Fuchs D, Hausen A, et al. Neopterin as a new biological marker for diagnosis of allograft rejection. Transplantation 1983; 36: 650.
6. König P, Margreiter R, Huber Ch, et al. Neopterin levels in long-term renal allograft recipients. Immunobiology 1985; 169: 208.
7. Fuchs D, Hausen A. Reibnegger G, et al. Assessment of urinary neopterin in the early diagnosis of human allograft rejection. In: Blair JA, ed. Chemistry and biology of pteridines. Berlin: Walter de Gruyter, 1983: 885.
8. Hausen A, Fuchs D, König K, Wachter H. Determination of neopterin in human urine by reversed-phase high performance liquid chromatography. J. Chromatogr 1982; 227: 61.
9. Dhondt JL, Bellahsene Z, Vanhille Ph, Noel C. Tetrahydrobiopterin metabolism in chronic uraemia: possible explanation of dialysis encephalopathy. Lancet 1982; 1: 491.
10. Dhondt JL, Vanhille Ph. Serum pteridines in patients on chronic hemodialysis. In: Wachter H, Curtius Ch, Pfleiderer W, eds. Biochemical and clinical aspects of pteridines. Berlin: Walter de Gruyter, 1982: 229.
11. Rokos H, Rokos K. A radioimmunoassay for determination of D-erythro-neopterin. In: Blair JA, ed. Chemistry and biology of pteridines. Berlin: Walter de Gruyter, 1983: 815.

Received 14 June 1985.
Accepted 8 August 1985.

0041-1337/86/4104-0459$02.00/0
TRANSPLANTATION
Vol. 41, No. 4
Printed in U.S.A.

DEMOGRAPHIC FACTORS AFFECTING THE PHARMACOKINETICS OF CYCLOSPORINE ESTIMATED BY RADIOIMMUNOASSAY

BARRY D. KAHAN,[1] WILLIAM G. KRAMER,[2] CAROL WIDEMAN, STUART M. FLECHNER, MARC I. LORBER, AND CHARLES T. VAN BUREN

The Division of Immunology and Organ Transplantation, Department of Surgery, The University of Texas Medical School at Houston; and the Department of Pharmaceutics, College of Pharmacy, University of Houston, Houston, Texas 77030

In order to assess the impact of demographic factors on serum levels of cyclosporine (CsA) estimated by radioimmunoassay (RIA) in renal allograft recipients, 493 pharmacokinetic studies were performed in 212 patients. Neither the presence of diabetes mellitus nor the CsA dosing frequency affected the measured pharmacokinetic parameters. Age over 45 years led to slower CsA clearance with resultant increase in maximum serum concentration (Cmax) per administered milligram, and increased volume of distribution. Female patients showed more rapid drug clearance, but greater volume of distribution. Concomitant hepatic impairment reduced drug clearance, increasing the area under the curve (AUC) per administered milligram of drug, and the Cmax. Patients treated with a rapid steroid taper showed a shorter half-life and lower Cmax than those receiving a slow steroid taper. Nephrotoxicity was associated with increased AUC per administered mg, while patients with acute tubular necrosis requiring dialysis showed poorer drug absorption, lower Cmax, and longer time to peak. The only effect of cimetidine administration was a slightly shortened time to peak. Serial analyses posttransplant in 17 patients suggested a tendency toward improved drug absorption with no effect on other parameters. These studies demonstrating the significant impact of demographic factors thus afford a basis on which to predict the trend of anticipated CsA levels as measured by RIA in renal allograft recipients.

Despite the widespread use of cyclosporine (CsA),* a fungal endecapeptide of novel chemical structure, as an immunosuppressive agent both for clinical organ transplantation (*1–3*) and for disorders of putative autoimmune mechanisms (*4*), there is little information stipulating drug dosing regimens. At the present time, clinicians assess drug bioavailability by symptom review for complaints of nausea, vomiting, and diarrhea, which may be associated with poor absorption from the gastrointestinal tract, and by inquiry about concomitant drug administration that could alter CsA metabolism (*5*). Because of significant differences in dosing regimens, various renal transplant centers report widely disparate drug efficacy with variable incidence of allograft rejection episodes (*6, 7*), drug toxicity (*8, 9*), and lymphoproliferative disorders (*9, 10*). Because of its simplicity, flexibility, and consistency, the radioimmunoassay (RIA) has

[1] Address correspondence to: Dr. Kahan, Department of Surgery, The University of Texas Medical School, 6431 Fannin, Suite 6240 MSMB, Houston, TX 77030.
[2] Department of Pharmaceutics, College of Pharmacy, University of Houston, Houston, TX 77030.

* Abbreviations used: AUC, area under the curve; CAD, cadaver donor; Cmax, maximum serum concentration; CsA, cyclosporine; LRD, living-related donor; RIA, radioimmunoassay.

become the most widely applied, convenient technique for therapeutic drug monitoring of transplant recipients. Although it measures both parent compound (CsA) and a narrow array of metabolites, Robinson et al. (*11*) showed that these metabolites display similar pharmacokinetic behavior to the parent compound. Serum rather than whole blood determinations have been widely utilized, since under carefully controlled conditions trough serum levels correlate well with clinical conditions. In general, low or exceedingly high levels of CsA as measured by RIA (*12*) correlate with the overall clinical course (*13–15*). Furthermore, Wood (*16*) agrees that estimates of bioavailability and drug clearance by this technique afford useful information to predict therapeutic effects.

The overall purpose of the studies presented herein was to improve therapeutic management by identifying the potential contributions of a variety of demographic factors to CsA pharmacokinetics and bioavailability. Demographic factors have been shown to be important in the management of patients undergoing therapy with theophylline, aminoglycosides, and digoxin (*17*). The present studies demonstrate that acute tubular necrosis causing impaired renal function requiring dialysis reduces CsA absorption, that age, male sex, hepatic impairment, and higher prednisone dosages reduce CsA clearance, and that there is a greater volume of drug distribution in female patients.

METHODS

Patients. The present studies were conducted upon 212 recipients of cadaver (CAD) or living-related donor (LRD) renal allografts. CsA was administered at 14 mg/kg preoperatively and for seven days postoperatively (12 mg/kg on days 7–14; 10 mg/kg on days 14–28). Dosages were adjusted to maintain serum trough levels at 100–250 ng/ml (*13*). By day 60, patients received an average of 7±0.5 mg/kg and by one year an average of 5.5±0.5 mg/kg. Two steroid regimens were employed: the high-dose regimen, which had been the usual regimen with azathioprine, tapered patients from 1.7 mg/kg to 0.6 mg/kg prednisone by daily decrements of 10 mg. After an additional 20 days, they were decreased gradually to 0.4 mg/kg prednisone until day 60, when they were reduced to 0.2 mg/kg by six months. The low-dose regimen tapered the prednisone from 1.7 mg/kg to 0.6 mg/kg by 20 mg decrements, reaching 0.4 mg/kg at day 6, the level at which the patient was maintained until day 30, whence he was gradually tapered to 0.2 mg/kg by three months. Nephrotoxicity was assumed to be the case if the serum creatinine had risen by 25% above a 2.0 mg/dl baseline with no signs of rejection. Hepatic toxicity was evidenced by a bilirubin rise above a level of 1.0 mg/dl or a rise in either transaminase above a level of 100 IU/L without other cause. The diagnosis was routinely confirmed by greater than 50% improvement upon dose reduction.

Pharmacokinetic analysis. Pharmacokinetic analysis was performed with 493 studies in 212 patients as follows: oral studies included samples drawn at trough (0 hour), every hour for 14 hr, then every 2 hr from 14 to 24 hr. Intravenous studies included samples at trough (0 hour), then every 15 min during drug infusion over 1 hr, every half hour postinfusion for 2 hr, every hour from 2 hr to 14 hr, then finally every 2 hr from 18 to 24 hr. After each 2–2½ cc whole-blood sample was clotted at 4°C for at least 2 hr, the serum was separated and analyzed using the RIA kit provided by Sandoz (Basle, Switzerland [*17*]). The competition assay, including tritiated CsA, polyclonal sheep antibody, and patient serum sample, was incubated at room temperature for 2 hr. Labeled antigen-antibody complexes were detected by liquid scintillation counting. The assay was sensitive to 40 ng/ml; concentrations above 250 ng/ml were estimated by further dilution of the sample. A computer program was used for logit-log transformation of data to yield a standard curve from which the coefficient of variation of duplicates of each sample was checked to ensure quality control (*12*).

Semilogarithmic plots of serum CsA concentration against time are shown in Figures 1 and 2 for representative i.v. and p.o. studies, respectively. Data points in the terminal portion of the dosing interval that appeared to fall in a nearly straight line were used to calculate the elimination rate constant, k, equal to the negative of the slope of the line. All slopes were calculated using linear regression of the natural logrithm of concentration against time; rate constants were expressed in terms of elimination half-life, $t\,½$, according to equation 1:

$$t\,½ = 0.693/k \qquad (1)$$

The area under the serum CsA concentration time curve for the dosing interval was calculated using the linear trapezoidal method. For patients in whom samples had been collected for only a portion of the dosing interval, the area was extrapolated to the end of the interval using equation 2:

$$AUC_{O\rightarrow\tau} = AUC_{O\rightarrow t^*} + \frac{C^*}{k}\left(e^{-kt^*} - c^{-k\tau}\right) \qquad (2)$$

where C^* is the last measured concentration, taken at time t^*,

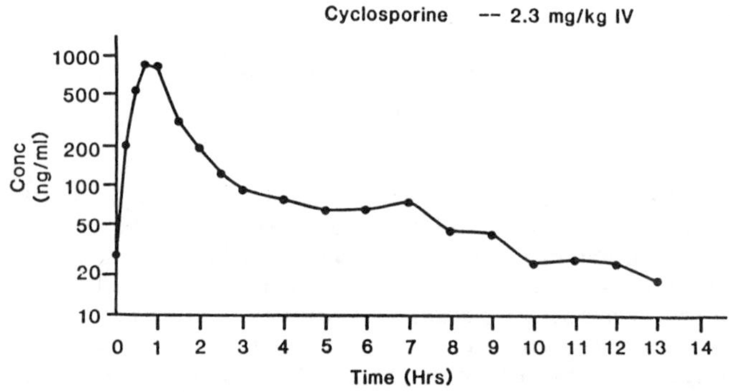

FIGURE 1. Semilogarithmic plot of serum CsA concentration determined by RIA against time after administration of 2.3 mg/kg i.v. over 1 hr.

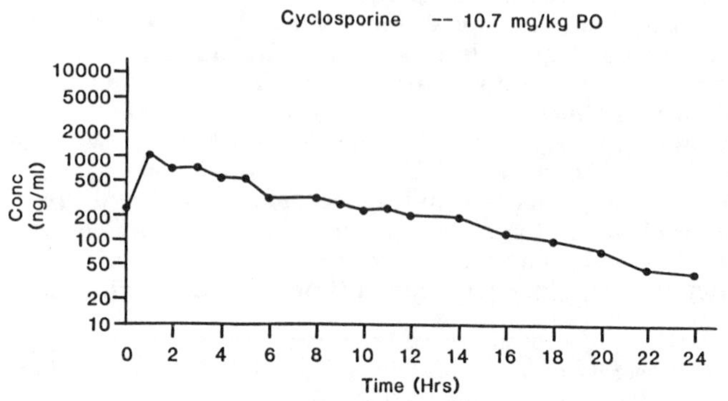

FIGURE 2. Semilogarithmic plot of serum CsA concentration determined by RIA against time after administration of 10.7 mg/kg orally.

τ is the dosing interval, and AUC the area under the curve, appropriately subscripted. For both i.v. and p.o. administration, AUC was normalized to the milligram per kilogram administered dose. Following i.v. delivery of CsA, total plasma clearance (CL) and volume of distribution (V) were calculated according to equations 3 and 4:

$$CL = \text{Dose}/\text{AUC} \tag{3}$$

$$V = CL/k \tag{4}$$

Both parameters were normalized to the patient's body weight. In addition, the maximum plasma concentration, Cmax, and time to reach the maximum concentration, t_p, were obtained directly from the data after p.o. drug administration.

For patients in whom i.v. and p.o. studies were performed on successive days, the percentage absorbed (F) was calculated according to equation 5:

$$F = \frac{(\text{AUC}/\text{dose})_{\text{p.o.}}}{(\text{AUC}/\text{dose})_{\text{i.v.}}} \times 100\% \tag{5}$$

Mean parameter values were compared as appropriate by analysis of variance using patients and the effect to be tested as the classification variables. For effects with three or more groups, individual means were compared using Duncan's multiple range test. Differences were considered to be significant if $P<0.05$.

RESULTS

The pharmacokinetic parameters of CsA absorption and disposition are summarized in Table 1. The frequency distribution of clearance and volume of distribution are shown in Figures 3 and 4. While CsA pharmacokinetics and bioavailability were unaffected by diabetes mellitus or dosing frequency (Table 2), they were significantly altered by age, sex, hepatic impairment, nephrotoxicity and the rapidity of the steroid taper (Tables 2 and 3). Patients over the age of 45 years appeared to have a lower CsA clearance, 9.45 ml/min/kg, compared with 13.3±8.97 in younger patients. This approximately 30% decreased clearance corresponded to an approximate 50% increase in AUC, as would be expected from the relationship shown in equation 1. The change may also account for the increased maximum concentration seen in older patients. This decreased drug clearance has been documented for many drugs and is presumably due to decreased organ function and/or perfusion associated with aging. CsA volume of distribution decreased with age by approximately the same percentage as the clearance (Table 3). However, since half-life (t ½) is a function of both of these parameters ($t_{1/2} = 0.693 \cdot V/Cl$), it was not different in the two age groups (8.74±4.44 hr versus 7.79±3.23 hr and <45 years versus ≥45 years, respectively).

Male and female patients differed significantly in their ability to clear and distribute CsA. Male clearance averaged 11.4±5.93 ml/min/kg compared with 14.8±12.0 ml/min/kg female clearance. The volume of distribution of 10.3±6.92 L/kg in female patients was larger than in male patients (7.85±4.89 L/kg).

TABLE 1. Summary of CsA pharmacokinetic parameters for absorption and disposition[a]

Parameter	i.v.	p.o.
AUC (ng/ml/hr)/(mg/kg)	1938±1337	765±593
t ½ (hr)	8.6±4.6	9.6±5.8
CL (ml/min/kg)	12.3±8.2	—
V (l/kg)	8.7±6.2	—
Cmax (ng/ml)	—	1087±744
t_p (hr)	—	3.8±2.6
F (%)	—	29±24

[a] Values reported as mean ± SD.

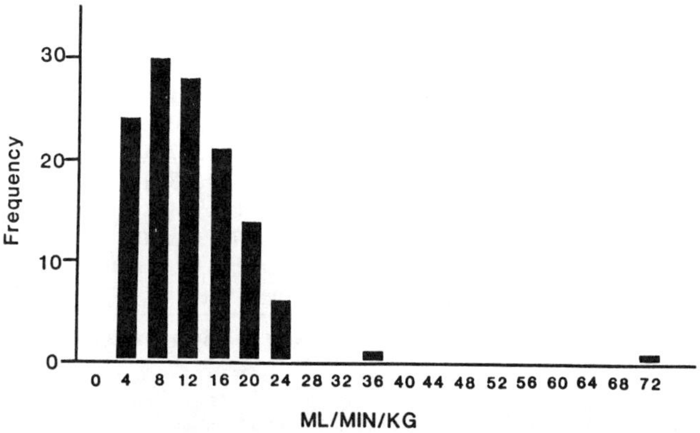

FIGURE 3. Frequency distribution among 212 renal allograft recipients of CsA clearance (in ml/min/kg).

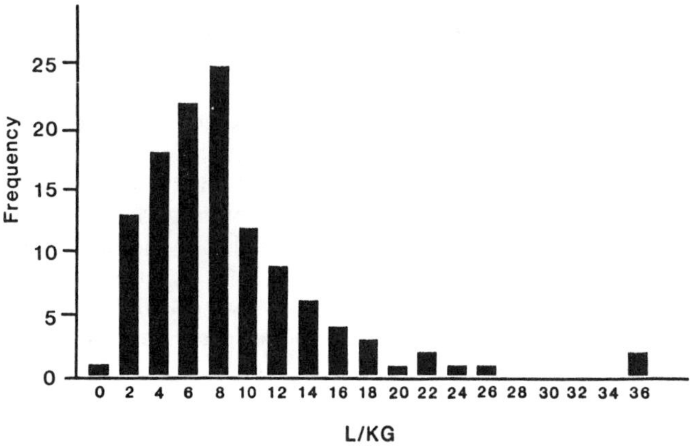

FIGURE 4. Frequency distribution among 212 renal allograft recipients of CsA volume of distribution (in L/kg).

TABLE 2. The effect of demographic variables on CsA pharmacokinetics

Parameter	Number of pharmacokinetic studies[a]		Effect[b]
	Positive	Negative	
Age[c]	350	95	Yes
Sex[c]	323	170	Yes
Diabetes mellitus	131	362	No
Hepatotoxicity	63	388	Yes
Nephrotoxicity	84	367	Yes
Dosing frequency[c]	460	31	No
Steroid taper[c]	167	300	Yes

[a] Repetitive studies in the same patient were considered as separate cases. There were 283 repeat studies.

[b] Variables with a positive effect are detailed in Table 3.

[c] Positive = <45 years, male sex, once-daily dosing, and fast steroid taper; negative = ≥45 years, female sex, twice-daily regimen, and slow steroid taper.

Both groups displayed similar ratios of the volume to clearance, yielding the same elimination half-life.

CsA is cleared from the body primarily by hepatic metabolism. Consequently, patients exhibiting altered liver function should be expected to clear the drug more slowly, and subsequently have higher plasma levels. Patients with hepatic impairment cleared the drug at an average of 8.75±5.43 ml/min/kg, a one-third decrease compared with nonhepatotoxic patients (13.1±8.72 ml/min/kg). This change may be responsible for the 30–50% increase in AUC (equation 1) following i.v. and p.o. dosing and in Cmax following p.o. dosing (Table 3).

Patients suffering from CsA-induced nephrotoxicity showed an increased AUC/dose following oral administration. Since there was no apparent effect of nephrotoxicity on the disposition parameters of CsA, the exact mechanism of this effect cannot be determined from our data. It may be related to changes in the extent of absorption, as patients with nephrotoxicity had a trend toward a higher percentage absorbed (37.8±35.1 for nephrotoxic patients versus 26.4±18.2 for those with normal kidney function), although the difference was not statistically significant, due to the small number of cases in which *F* could be calculated and the consequent higher variation. Patients showing signs of acute tubular necrosis or requiring dialysis showed a decreased extent of absorption, as indicated by a lower AUC/dose. Absorption also appeared to occur more slowly, as evidenced by a longer time to reach peak concentrations. The combination of these factors significantly reduced the peak concentration.

Patients administered the slow steroid taper tended to have a longer CsA half-life following i.v. administration and to reach a higher peak concentration following oral administration than those receiving a fast taper. Finally, patients receiving cimetidine concurrently with CsA tended to absorb the drug more rapidly, as evidenced by a shorter average time to reach the peak concentration (Table 3).

The length of time between transplant and the pharmacokinetic study had no apparent effect on the i.v. disposition parameters of CsA (Table 4); although there was variation, it was not statistically significant. This may be due, in part, to the majority of cases falling within the 0–14-day period (76 per cent of the total i.v. cases). Among oral parameters for which the number of cases is somewhat more evenly distributed, there were significant effects of posttransplant time on AUC/dose and Cmax. For AUC/dose, the mean value for pretransplant studies was significantly less than for the posttransplant cases; all posttransplant cases, however, were not different from the pre-transplant value. Cmax showed the most variation, and the group means are compared in Table 5. It appears from Table 5 that Cmax increases through the first 90 days posttransplant and then begins to decrease again; however, more cases in the post-90-day period are needed to confirm this observation.

DISCUSSION

Since CsA elimination and bioavailability exhibit large interpatient variability, therapeutic efficacy might be improved by measuring pharmacokinetic parameters in individual patients. Since the RIA is the most widely utilized method to estimate serum levels, it was employed in the studies presented herein, recognizing that the conclusions reflect both CsA and cross-reactive metabolites. Certain demographic characteristics affecting CsA disposition were apparent from the data, and may serve as guides not only for the initial dosing, but also for interpretation of serially measured CsA serum concentrations.

Patients over the age of 45 years clear the drug more slowly. Thus, to maintain a given range of serum concentrations, patients in this age group should require about one-third less

TABLE 3. Comparison of CsA pharmacokinetic parameters for classification variables with significant effects[a, b]

Parameter	Classification variable	Response[c]	
		Negative	Positive
Intravenous			
AUC/dose (ng/ml/hr)/(mg/kg)	Age	1750±1094 (90)	2371±1526 (23)
	Hepatic impairment	1726±987 (98)	2864±1951 (15)
Clearance (ml/min/kg)	Age	13.3±8.97 (90)	9.45±5.20 (23)
	Sex	11.4±5.93 (77)	14.8±12.0 (36)
	Hepatic impairment	13.1±8.72 (98)	8.75±5.43 (15)
Volume (L/kg)	Age	9.33±6.06 (87)	6.04±3.02 (22)
	Sex	7.85±4.89 (73)	10.3±6.92 (36)
Half-life (hr)	Steroid taper	9.27±4.18 (44)	7.78±3.55 (63)
Oral			
AUC/dose (ng/ml/hr)/(mg/kg)	Nephrotoxicity	733±580 (264)	1011±685 (68)
	Hepatic impairment	755±601 (284)	997±644 (48)
	ATN/dialysis	818±623 (295)	562±468 (37)
Maximum concentration (ng/ml)	Hepatic impairment	1033±726 (284)	1409±872 (48)
	Steroid taper	1138±767 (235)	970±736 (94)
	Age	1037±756 (260)	1270±747 (72)
	ATN/dialysis	1134±772 (295)	715±511 (37)
Peak time (hr)	Cimetidine administration	3.84±2.69 (312)	2.66±1.33 (19)
	ATN/dialysis	3.62±2.37 (295)	5.00±4.06 (37)

[a] Significance based upon unpaired Student's *t* test, repetitive studies in the same patient considered as separate cases, no pretransplant cases used, and $P<0.05$.

[b] Values reported as mean ± SD, number of cases in parentheses.

[c] Negative = <45 years of age, male sex, no for hepatic impairment, nephrotoxicity, ATN/dialysis, and cimetidine administration; = slow for steroid taper. Positive = ≥45 years of age, female sex, yes for hepatic impairment, nephrotoxicity, ATN/dialysis and cimetidine administration; = fast for steroid taper.

TABLE 4. Parameters at various times after transplantation

A. Group	Time (days)	n	Intravenous			
			AUC/dose	CL	V	t ½
1	Pretransplant	12	2511±2182	10.3±5.56	9.27±10.2	8.83±7.33
2	0–14	95	1788±1204	13.1±8.80	8.64±5.93	8.03±3.79
3	14–28	6	2194±750	8.67±4.00	8.81±3.75	13.2±7.62
4	28–90	4	2785±1723	7.80±4.41	7.54±1.07	10.1±2.98
5	90–180	4	2633±1349	9.99±9.73	7.37±2.14	10.7±5.49
6	180–365	3	1284±314	13.6±3.65	12.6±8.88	10.0±4.30

B. Group	Time (days)	n	Oral				
			AUC/dose	t ½	Cmax	t peak	F
1	Pretransplant	36	537±279	8.16±4.34	1089±595	3.94±1.79	25.9±19.4
2	0–14	170	628±524	9.39±5.57	1004±737	4.34±3.21	24.2±18.1
3	14–28	63	900±588	9.14±5.00	1328±730	3.29±1.52	51.4±43.0
4	28–90	37	1172±865	10.2±5.69	1437±827	2.64±1.23	35.1±27.4
5	90–180	29	912±473	11.4±7.78	1026±744	3.28±1.60	48.5±48.6
6	180–365	15	956±693	11.9±5.61	771±331	3.13±1.46	50.2±7.85
7	>365	18	816±529	9.93±8.65	674±771	3.72±2.87	27.2

TABLE 5. Effect of time posttransplant on maximum plasma concentration after oral administration of CsA

Group	Time	Cmax	Comparison[a]
1	Pretransplant	1089	A B C
2	0–14	1004	B C D
3	14–28	1328	A B
4	28–90	1437	A
5	90–180	1026	B C D
6	180–265	771	C D
7	>365	674	D

[a] Means with the same letter are not significantly different, Duncan's multiple range test, $P<0.05$.

drug per dosing interval than younger persons. The attainment of steady-state conditions should occur at about the same rate in all patients, since the decreased clearance in the older age group is offset by a similar decrease in distribution volume, giving the same elimination half-life as in younger patients. Similarly, male patients may require slightly less drug than female patients because of their lower clearance. Again because of differences in the volume of distribution, both groups display the same half-life and should reach steady-state levels at the same rate. The most dramatic effect appears to be hepatotoxicity, since it affects the primary organ responsible for CsA elimination. Patients with signs of hepatotoxicity may require substantially less drug than those with normal hepatic function to maintain equivalent serum CsA levels due to their decreased clearance, a conclusion similar to that reached by analysis of 41 pharmacokinetic profiles using the RIA in bone marrow transplant recipients (*18*). While the present data agree that there is no change in the volume of distribution and time to peak concentration, they do demonstrate a higher maximum serum concentration in hepatotoxic patients.

An insufficient amount of data are available from our study to make positive conclusions regarding the role of nephrotoxicity. However, the association of that condition with increased drug absorption may represent the cause of the disordered renal function or an unexplained result of this condition. Failure to observe a change in drug elimination in nephrotoxic patients confirms the previous findings of Follath et al. (*19*), who noted unchanged CsA kinetics after i.v. drug administration to four renal failure patients. In addition to these demographic factors, there appear to be effects of the rate of steroid taper, concomitant cimetidine administration, and length of therapy that are less prominent, but yet significant, determinants of pharmacokinetic parameters. Thus consideration of demographic factors may assist the clinician in drug dosing in order to avert suboptimal or alternatively toxic levels of CsA.

REFERENCES

1. Calne RY, Thiru S, McMaster P, et al. Cyclosporin A in patients receiving renal allografts from cadaver donors. Lancet 1978; 2: 1323.
2. The Canadian Multicentre Transplant Study Group. A randomized clinical trial of cyclosporine in cadaveric renal transplantation. N Engl J Med 1983; 309: 809.
3. Kahan BD, Van Buren C, Flechner S, Payne WD, Boileau M, Kerman R. Cyclosporine immunosuppression mitigates immunologic risk factors in renal allotransplantation. Transplant Proc 1983; 15(4): 2469.
4. Stiller CR, Dupre J, Gent M, et al. Effects of cyclosporine immunosuppression in insulin-dependent diabetes mellitus of recent onset. Science 1984; 223: 1362.
5. Salaman JR. Cyclosporin in renal transplantation: a guide to management. Lancet 1984; 1: 269.
6. Starzl TE, Hakala TR, Rosenthal JT, Iwatsuki S, Shaw BW. Variable convalescence and therapy after cadaveric renal transplantation under cyclosporin-A and steroids. Surg Gynecol Obstet 1982; 154(6): 819.
7. Kahan BD, Kerman RH. Allograft rejection in renal allograft recipients under cyclosporine-prednisone immunosuppressive therapy. In: Williams GM, Burdick JF, Solez K, eds. Kidney transplant rejection: diagnosis and treatment. New York: M. Dekker, in press.
8. Laupacis A. Complications of cyclosporine therapy—a comparison to azathioprine. Transplant Proc 1983; 15(4): 2748.
9. Kahan BD, Van Buren CT, Flechner S, et al. Clinical and experimental studies using cyclosporine in renal transplantation. Surgery 1985; 97: 125.
10. Starzl TE, Nalesnik MA, Porter KA, et al. Reversibility of lymphomas and lymphoproliferative lesions developing under cyclosporin-steroid therapy. Lancet 1984; 1: 583.

11. Robinson WT, Schran HR, Barry EP. Methods to measure cyclosporine levels—high pressure liquid chromatography, radioimmunoassay, and correlation. Transplant Proc 1983; 15(4): 2403.
12. Donatsch P, Abisch E, Homberger M, Traber R, Trapp M, Voges R. A radioimmunoassay to measure cyclosporin A in plasma and serum samples. J Immunoassay 1981; 2: 19.
13. Kahan BD, Van Buren CT, Lin SN, et al. Immunopharmacological monitoring of cyclosporin A-treated recipients of cadaveric kidney allografts. Transplantation 1982; 34: 36.
14. Kahan BD, Wideman C, Ried M, Gibbons S, Jarowenko M, Flechner S, Van Buren CT. The value of serial serum trough cyclosporine levels in human renal transplantation. Transplant Proc 1984; 16: 1195.
15. Keown PA, Stiller CR, Sinclair NR, et al. The clinical relevance of cyclosporine blood levels as measured by radioimmunoassay. Transplant Proc 1983; 15(4): 2438.
16. Wood AJ. In the discussion of pharmacologic aspects of cyclosporine therapy: pharmacokinetics. Transplant Proc 1985; 17: 37.
17. Burton ME, Vasko MR, Brater DC. Comparison of drug dosing methods. Clin Pharmacokinet 1985; 10: 1.
18. Yee, GC, Kennedy MS, Storb R, Thomas ED. Effect of hepatic dysfunction on cyclosporine pharmacokinetics in marrow transplant patients. Blood 1984; 64: 1277.
19. Follath F, Wenk M, Vozeh S, et al. Intravenous cyclosporine kinetics in renal failure. Clin Pharmacol Ther 1983; 34: 638.

Received 23 May 1985.
Accepted 12 August 1985.

0041-1337/86/4104-0000$02.00/0
TRANSPLANTATION

Vol. 41, No. 4
Printed in U.S.A.

AN ASSESSMENT OF INTRARENAL HYDROSTATIC PRESSURE MEASUREMENTS IN THE DIAGNOSIS OF ACUTE RENAL ALLOGRAFT REJECTION

CHRISTOPHER PETER GIBBONS,[1,2] CHRISTOPHER BARRY SUMMERTON,[1] PAUL GERARD MCNALLY,[1] RICHARD KAY,[3] COLIN BERTRAM BROWN,[1] AND ANDREW THOMAS RAFTERY[1]

Department of Nephrology and Transplantation, Royal Hallamshire Hospital, Sheffield S10 2JF; and Department of Probability and Statistics, University of Sheffield, Sheffield S10 2TN, England

Postoperative intrarenal pressure measurements may be an aid to the diagnosis of acute renal transplant rejection, especially in patients treated with cyclosporine. Serial measurements of intrarenal pressure were made in 38 recipients using a fine-needle technique. Thirty-two intraoperative and 207 postoperative measurements were made, and 39 clinical rejection episodes (23 confirmed by biopsy) monitored. Intraoperative pressures in grafts with immediate function (37.4±4.0 mmHg, mean±SEM) were not significantly different from those with delayed function (30.9±4.8 mmHg), whereas postoperative pressures were greater (*P*<0.01) in kidneys with acute tubular necrosis (29.4±1.9 mmHg) than in functioning grafts (20.4±0.9 mmHg). Pressures recorded during clinical rejection episodes (44.3±2.3 mmHg) exceeded (*P*<0.001) those during quiescent periods (23.6±1.0 mmHg). During rejection episodes, higher pressures (*P*<0.01) were recorded from tender or palpably enlarged grafts (52.5±3.0 mmHg) than in the absence of these signs (36.3±3.1 mmHg), and patients whose transplants biopsies showed cellular rejection tended to have greater pressures (50.1±4.1 mmHg) than those with concomitant vasculopathy (36.4±3.9 mmHg), but the latter did not reach statistical significance. In 7 cases of cyclosporine toxicity the intrarenal pressure was 17.8±4.2 mmHg. Using a diagnostic cut off point of 40 mmHg, the investigation failed to recognize 26% of acute rejection episodes—and, in the presence of acute tubular necrosis, it wrongly categorized 21% of nonrejectors. While its predictive capacity was limited, the test may occasionally be helpful in the differentiation of cyclosporine toxicity and rejection in functioning kidneys.

Graft swelling is a major feature of acute rejection in renal transplants. This is accompanied by a rise in hydrostatic pressure measured in the subcapsular space (*1, 2*) and renal parenchyma (*3*). It has been proposed that such measurements offer a useful means for monitoring the progress of renal transplant recipients, by aiding the early diagnosis of acute rejection and by differentiating rejection from cyclosporine nephrotoxicity (*3, 4*). A modification of these techniques has been used routinely for intraoperative and postoperative monitoring of renal transplant recipients over a period of one year in this center. The results of this investigation have been analyzed with a particular emphasis on the predictive value and accuracy of this technique in the diagnosis of acute rejection.

MATERIALS AND METHODS

Intrarenal pressure was measured by a fine-needle injection technique with strict asepsis using disposable equipment. The apparatus consisted of a 25-gauge spinal needle connected by

[1] Royal Hallamshire Hospital.
[2] Address correspondence to: Mr. C. P. Gibbons, Singleton Hospital, Sketty, Swansea SA2 8QA, England.
[3] University of Sheffield.

rigid plastic tubing (Lectrocath; Vygon, Ecouers, France) to a Bentley Trantec Arterial 800 pressure transducer (American Hospital Supplies, Didcot, England) fitted with a plastic dome with Linden seal (Cobe Laboratories Inc., CO) and two 3-way taps (Vygon, Ecouers, France), the whole system being filled with sterile saline from a 20-ml syringe. The transducer was connected to an Alpha 9 amplifier and display system (Spacelabs, Chatsworth, CA) calibrated to read zero pressure with the needle at the level of the anterior superior iliac spine. For postoperative readings the needle was introduced into the s.c. tissue without anaesthetic, flushed with 0.5 ml sterile saline, and advanced toward the kidney, keeping laterally to remain extraperitoneal. Resistance was usually felt as the capsule was breached and the needle was advanced a further 2–3 cm into the renal parenchyma. For intraoperative measurements, the needle was introduced directly into the exposed kidney to a depth of 2–3 cm. 50 μl of sterile saline was then injected into the kidney from the 1-ml syringe, and the three way taps rotated to exclude both syringes. Recorded pressure decayed toward a plateau with a variable time course. Gentle rotation of the needle was found to aid this process and prevent blockage. The plateau pressure was recorded as the intrarenal pressure. On withdrawal of the needle, a step in pressure was usually observed as the tip passed out through the kidney capsule. In most cases duplicate readings were taken from different areas of the kidney.

Intraoperative intrarenal pressure was measured in 32 cadaver renal transplants immediately prior to abdominal closure. A total of 207 postoperative intrarenal pressure measurements were made in one living-related donor and 37 cadaver renal transplants at intervals of approximately 3–4 days until renal function was regarded as stable. The investigation was well tolerated and the only complication was a single transient episode of hematuria.

The initial immunosuppression was cyclosporine-plus-prednisolone in 24 patients (11 converted to azathioprine within 3 weeks, in most cases because of continuing acute tubular necrosis at a time when facilities for measuring cyclosporine were lacking) and azathioprine-plus-prednisolone in 14 patients (4 converted to cyclosporine within 3 weeks). 39 rejection episodes were monitored, of which 23 were confirmed by biopsy. Clinically identified rejection episodes were treated conventionally by pulsing with from three to a maximum of six daily injections of 1 g methylprednisolone.

Carefully recorded clinical data, including graft tenderness and swelling, urine output, temperature, blood pressure, laboratory data, (including serum creatinine and urea and DTPA perfusion index [5]—and, when appropriate, the response to steroid pulsing were used to identify periods of rejection or acute tubular necrosis. In addition, when a biopsy was performed during a rejection episode, the intrarenal pressure readings within that period were classified according to whether the biopsy showed significant cellular or vascular rejection, or both. The pressures for each group were expressed as mean±SEM. Group comparisons were made using a two-factor analysis of variance (*6*), one factor corresponding to patients and the other to the particular two-group comparison. Calculations were performed using the statistical package MINITAB (MINITAB data analysis software, MINITAB Inc., PA) implemented on the PRIME computer. Predictive probabilities were obtained by fitting a logistic regression model (*7*) with rejection or nonrejection as the response and intrarenal pressure as the regressor variable. The logistic model was fitted using the statistical package GLIM (1977 Royal Statistical Society, London) implemented on the PRIME computer.

RESULTS

Intraoperative measurements. Intrarenal pressures were recorded immediately prior to abdominal closure in 32 transplants. The variability of these readings was high (mean±SEM of difference between duplicates 9.1±1.6 mmHg)—widely disparate values often being obtained from different areas of the same kidney. The mean pressure recorded was 34.0±3.2 mmHg. Analysis of variance failed to reveal any significant difference in pressure between 15 kidneys with immediate function (37.4±4.0 mmHg) and 17 with delayed function (30.9±4.0 mmHg) due to acute tubular necrosis (ATN)* (requiring dialysis in the postoperative period).

Postoperative measurements. Postoperative pressures were less variable ($P<0.001$ [Student's t test]) than intraoperative values (mean±SEM of difference between duplicates 4.5±0.3 mmHg).

In kidneys with immediate function, the first postoperative pressure, taken 3–4 days after transplantation, was significantly reduced when compared with intraoperative values (Table 1). Subsequent pressures tended to be lower, but this failed to reach significance. In contrast, kidneys with ATN maintained a relatively high postoperative pressure at 3–4 days after grafting, which fell significantly after resumption of function. An analysis of variance of all postoperative results (Table 2) confirmed a significantly increased pressure in kidneys with ATN in comparison with functioning kidneys in the absence of rejection. In one patient whose graft had suffered an initial warm ischemia of 1 hr with partial function returning only after 6 weeks, intrarenal pressure was initially very high (94 mmHg in the operating theater), reducing gradually to normal levels (20 mmHg) over 2–3 weeks. In this patient, as in several others, the DTPA perfusion index paralleled intrarenal pressure. In most patients with ATN, the rise in intrarenal pressure was much less marked.

Acute rejection caused a much greater rise in intrarenal pressure than ATN (Table 2). This pressure rise usually appeared simultaneously with graft swelling and tenderness, although in some cases local signs were evident earlier. The mean of all pressures obtained during clinically diagnosed rejection episodes was similar to those during biopsy-confirmed rejection, but was significantly greater than the mean pressure recorded during quiescent periods. The mean pressure recorded during rejection episodes in functioning kidneys (44.2±3.3 mmHg) did not differ significantly from that during rejection episodes in kidneys with acute tubular necrosis (44.1±3.4 mmHg). Rejecting kidneys which were tender or palpably enlarged had significantly higher pressures than those without local signs, but the latter were still significantly elevated in comparison with quiescent phase values.

Kidneys with cellular rejection tended to have higher pressures than those with concomitant vasculopathy, but this failed to reach significance. In one patient who had three severe cellular rejection episodes, each with increasing vasculopathy on biopsy, culminating in graft failure at 11 weeks after transplantation, the maximum intrarenal pressure was lower with each succeeding episode (78, 51, and 11 mmHg, respectively).

* Abbreviation used: ATN, acute tubular necrosis.

TABLE 1. The effect of acute tubular necrosis on intraoperative and postoperative intrarenal pressures[a]

Transplant function	No. patients	Intrarenal pressure (mmHg)[b]		
		Intraoperative	First postoperative	Last postoperative
Delayed	10	32.6±7.8	34.3±5.6[c]	21.9±2.5[d]
Immediate	10	37.5±5.1	24.4±4.0[d]	18.8±3.4[c]

[a] All patients having both intraoperative and postoperative readings performed were included, unless rejection was diagnosed at the first or last postoperative reading.

[b] Mean±SEM.

[c] No significant difference from reading in preceding column (paired *t* test).

[d] *P* for difference from reading in preceding column <0.05 (paired *t* test).

TABLE 2. Postoperative intrarenal pressure in 38 renal transplant recipients

Condition	No. observations	Intrarenal pressure (mmHg)[a]	
Overall:			
Not rejecting	130	23.6±1.0	
Rejecting	77	44.3±2.3	$P<0.001$[b]
Biopsy-proved rejection	43	42.5±3.0	$P<0.001$[b]
Nonrejectors:			
Functioning kidneys	83	20.4±0.9	
Acute tubular necrosis	47	29.4±1.9	$P<0.01$[b]
Rejectors:			
Tenderness and/or swelling	38	52.5±3.0	
No tenderness or swelling	39	36.3±3.1	$P<0.01$[b]
Biopsy-proved rejectors:			
Cellular rejection	19	50.1±4.1	
Vascular ± cellular rejection	24	36.4±3.9	N.S.[b,c]

[a] Mean±SEM.

[b] Analysis of variance.

[c] Low power comparison based on 1 patient with rejection episodes of both types.

Seven episodes of unequivocal cyclosporine toxicity were monitored, although some degree of cyclosporine-induced renal impairment may have occurred in several other patients. These episodes were diagnosed by a rising serum creatinine and a rising whole-blood cyclosporine level, followed by a fall in both these parameters when cyclosporin dosage was reduced. (In the early part of this study cyclosporine monitoring was not available and suspected cyclosporine toxicity occurring during this period was regarded as unconfirmed.) The intrarenal pressure in these seven cases of known cyclosporine toxicity was 17.8± 4.2 mmHg.

Despite the highly significantly rise in intrarenal pressure with rejection, the predictive value of the test was disappointing due to the large scatter in the results. The fitted logistic model gave the relationship $\ln 1-P/P = 3.092-0.0798y$ (where P is the probability of rejection and y is the intrarenal pressure), so that the predicted probability of rejection was:

$$P = \frac{1}{1 + e^{3.092-0.0798y}} \text{ (Fig. 1)}$$

From this, the probability of rejection was calculated to exceed 0.5 when the intrarenal pressure was greater than 38.7 mmHg.

Taking 40 mmHg as the threshold for rejection, as suggested by others (*2, 3*), 74% of all rejection episodes were diagnosed correctly (Table 3). This figure rose to 90% for clinically tender or swollen kidneys or for kidneys with biopsy-proved cellular rejection, but fell to 56% for nontender kidneys and 54% for kidneys with concomitant vasculopathy. There were also 11 false positives in 130 quiescent-phase measurements (8.5%) of which 10/47 (21.3%) occurred during ATN and 1/83 (1.2%) during normal function. All false positives were recorded in the first 12 days and 5 were obtained 3 or 4 days after transplantation. Five out of 16 (31%) of readings taken at 3–4 days during ATN were falsely positive.

DISCUSSION

The present technique, like that of Salaman and Griffin (*3*) used a 25-gauge spinal needle, but this has been combined with an electrical recording system similar to that described by Wagner (*2, 4*). Fine-needle techniques obviate the need for retaining a catheter for long periods in the subcapsular space, with the attendant risk of infection, and allow measurements to be made at any time, even after discharge from hospital. However, positioning of the needle is imprecise and pressure measurement via a subcapsular catheter placed at operation may give less variable results (*2, 4*).

Baseline intrarenal pressures in the absence of rejection or acute tubular necrosis were found to be slightly lower than those reported by Salaman and Griffin (*3*) but similar in magnitude to the subcapsular hydrostatic pressures of Wagner et al. (*2, 4*). The tissue pressure of normal human kidneys is

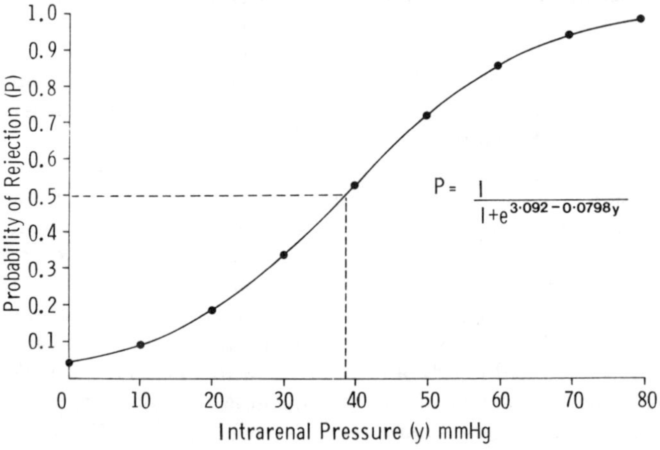

FIGURE 1. Predicted probability of rejection in relation to intrarenal pressure.

TABLE 3. Number of rejection episodes with peak intrarenal pressure exceeding 40 mmHg[a]

Condition	Total No.	No. at 40 mmHg	%
All clinical rejection episodes	39	29	74
Rejection with tenderness/swelling	21	19	90
Rejection without tenderness/swelling	18	10	56
Cellular rejection	10	9	90
Cellular + vascular rejection	13	7	54

[a] *P* for association between graft tenderness/swelling and pressure 40 mmHg = 0.01 (Fisher exact test); *P* for association between absence of vascular rejection and pressure 40 mmHg = 0.07 (Fisher exact test).

not known, but needle pressures in the kidneys of experimental animals (10 to 26 mmHg) are similar to those reported here (*10, 11, 14*). A tendency toward lower pressures was seen with increasing time after transplantation, even in kidneys with immediate function.

The relatively high intrarenal pressures found in transplanted kidneys when measured 45–60 min after reestablishing the circulation is a new finding. The pressure at this time, however, is of no predictive significance and intraoperative measurements have now been abandoned. By the first postoperative measurement the pressure in functioning kidneys had fallen to baseline levels, whereas those in kidneys with ATN remained elevated, reducing later after regaining function. This extends the findings of Wagner et al. (*2*) using subcapsular hydrostatic pressure, although Salaman and Griffin (*3*) failed to find any significant change in fine-needle pressure in acute tubular necrosis.

The increase in intrarenal pressure with acute rejection confirms the results of previous workers (*2–4*). They have emphasized the value of this parameter as a diagnostic test that may be particularly useful for the differentiation of rejection and cyclosporine toxicity. In the latter the pressure remains unchanged and the results of the seven patients with cyclosporine toxicity in this series are consistent with this. Severe cyclosporine toxicity was uncommon in this series, and this may have been a result of the close monitoring of whole-blood cyclosporine levels introduced during the course of this study.

Whereas find-needle pressure may not necessarily be a true measure of interstitial pressure (*8*), it is likely to have similar determinants. Thus the increased pressures recorded in rejection and ATN may result from the interstitial edema accompanying immune and ischemic damage, respectively. The physical swelling of the graft within its relatively inelastic capsule is less likely to contribute to the pressure rise because removal of the capsule has little effect on needle pressure in the dog (*9*). The relatively high pressures found intraoperatively may also be due to edema and reactive hyperemia after ischemic insult—but in this case an increased level of hydration and the infusion of mannitol may have contributed, since these are known to increase intrarenal pressure in experimental animals (*9, 10*). Experiments in dogs have also shown that intrarenal pressure is dependent upon arterial perfusion pressure (*9*) but the effect may only become significant during severe hypotension (*11*). Arterial and arteriolar constriction produced by catecholamine infusion reduces intrarenal pressure in experimental animals (*9*) and this may be analagous to the effect of vascular rejection, which narrows the lumen of arteries and arterioles within the graft. Thus vasculopathy may be expected to counter the rise in intrarenal pressure produced by cellular rejection. Similarly an increase in arterial resistance is likely to contribute to the reduced perfusion seen during acute rejection (12–14), and this might explain some of the lower pressures recorded during rejection episodes.

Animal studies have also demonstrated a rise in intrarenal pressure or subcapsular hydrostatic pressure with venous or ureteric obstruction (*8, 9, 11*). In clinical studies, Salaman and Griffin (*3*) found a high intrarenal pressure in a transplant recipient with renal vein thrombosis but not in a case of ureteric obstruction. Pyelonephritis may also be expected to cause renal edema and thereby increase intrarenal pressure, but in two patients of the present series with biopsy evidence of pyelonephritis (in one case associated with cellular rejection) the pressures were only 18 mmHg and 19 mmHg, respectively.

The present study confirms that a cut-off point in the region of 40 mmHg is appropriate for the diagnosis of rejection. However, using this figure, 26% of clinical rejection episodes would have been missed and the majority (8–10) of these were kidneys without the local signs of tenderness and swelling. False-positive results were rare in functioning kidneys (1.2%) but rose to 21.3% in acute tubular necrosis, and were especially frequent (31%) during ATN within 4 days of transplantation when local signs are more difficult to interpret. Thus the test was of least value in patients in whom extra diagnostic information would have been most helpful.

It is concluded that intrarenal manometry is a well tolerated investigation that may be safely used for postoperative transplant monitoring. While marked pressure changes may be found during acute rejection, its value as a diagnostic test is limited by wide variability and low power of discrimination, especially when ATN is present. The investigation must, therefore, be regarded as an adjunct to conventional diagnostic methods that may be helpful in occasional cases, particularly when cyclosporine toxicity is being considered in functioning kidneys.

REFERENCES

1. Wagner E, Schweitzer J. Effect of administering a high dosage glucocorticoid bolus on the survival and subcapsular hydrostatic pressure of rat kidney allografts. Eur Surg Res 1980; 12: 179.
2. Wagner E, Pichlmayr R, Wonigeit K, Hecker H. The subcapsular hydrostatic pressure of allogeneic kidney grafts. A new clinical method for postoperative transplant monitoring. Transplant Proc 1983; 15: 1707.
3. Salaman JR, Griffin PJA. Fine needle intrarenal manometry: a new test for rejection in cyclosporin-treated recipients of kidney transplants. Lancet 1983; 2: 709.
4. Wagner E, Pichlmayr R, Wonigeit K, Klempnauer J, Bunzendahl H, Lauchart W. Differentiation between rejection and cyclosporin A nephrotoxicity by monitoring interstitial pressure in human renal allografts. Transplant Proc 1983; 15: 489.
5. Hilson AJW, Maisey MN, Brown CB, Ogg CS, Bewick MS. Dynamic renal transplant imaging with Tc ⁻99M DTPA (Sn) supplemented by a transplant perfusion index in the management of renal transplants. J Nucl Med 1978; 19: 994.
6. Armitage P. Statistical methods in medical research. 1st ed. Oxford, Eng: Blackwell, 1974: 217.
7. Cox DR. The analysis of binary data. 1st ed. London: Methuen, 1970.
8. Wunderlich P, Persson E, Schnermann J, Ulfendahl H, Wolgast M. Hydrostatic pressure in the subscapular interstitial space of rat and dog kidneys. Pflügers Arch 1971; 328: 302.
9. Miles BE, De Wardener HE. Intrarenal pressure. J Physiol (Lond) 1954; 123: 131.
10. Herbert LA, Arbus GS. Renal subcapsular pressure—a new intrarenal pressure measurement. Am J Physiol 1971; 220: 1129.
11. Gottschalk CW. A comparative study of renal interstitial pressure. Am J Physiol 1952; 169: 180.
12. Cohn R, Kountz SL. Relationship of blood flow in the kidney to the homograft reaction. Am J Surg 1964; 108: 245.
13. Kountz SL, Truex G, Earley LE, Belzer FO. Serial haemodynamics after renal allotransplantation in man. Circulation 1970; 41: 217.
14. Jackson BT, Mannick JA. Serial blood flow in first set renal homotransplants undergoing rejection. Surg Gynecol Obstet 1964; 119: 1265.

Received 2 May 1985.
Accepted 25 July 1985.

0041-1337/86/4104-0468$02.00/0
TRANSPLANTATION
Vol. 41, No. 4
Printed in U.S.A.

FAILURE OF PLATELET TRANSFUSION TO IMPROVE HUMAN RENAL ALLOGRAFT SURVIVAL[1]

J. R. CHAPMAN,[2] A. TING, M. FISHER, N. P. CARTER, AND P. J. MORRIS

Nuffield Department of Surgery, University of Oxford, and Regional Transfusion Centre, John Radcliffe Hospital, Headington, Oxford, England OX3 9DU

Platelets, expressing only class I antigens on their surface, have been shown to improve renal allograft survival in some experimental models but do not lead to humoral sensitization. In this pilot study, 24 previously untransfused patients were given 3 platelet transfusions at 2-week intervals before renal transplantation. Twelve patients (group 1) received 200×10^8 platelets contaminated by 15×10^6 leukocytes in each transfusion, and 42% developed cytotoxic antibodies; 12 further patients (group 2) received a purified preparation containing 200×10^8 platelets and <5×10^6 leukocytes, and no cytotoxic antibodies were detected. Using a more sensitive flow cytometry technique, 83% of group 1 but only 17% of group 2 ($P<0.004$) responded to their platelet donors. From each group 9 patients have been transplanted. Four grafts in group 1 and 6 in group 2 have failed, yielding a 1-year graft survival rate of 44%, compared with 69% in blood-transfused patients ($P = 0.03$). Pure platelet transfusions, using our protocol, do not appear to improve renal allograft survival, and minimal contamination by leukocytes can lead to humoral sensitization.

Transfusion of whole blood can induce antibodies directed at HLA class I antigens. Since these antibodies lead to a positive lymphocytotoxic crossmatch and thus prevent renal transplantation, it was thought to be important to avoid blood transfusion in potential renal allograft recipients. When the first paper (*1*) was published suggesting improved graft survival in patients transfused with blood, it was viewed with some scepticism (*2*). But it subsequently became apparent both from individual centers (*3, 4*) and from multicenter data (*5*) that transfusion did indeed improve the results of renal transplantation. Because the problem of humoral sensitization due to whole-blood transfusions was thought to be significant, a number of studies were directed at finding a blood preparation that reduced the rate of antibody formation. Frozen-thawed blood (*5*) and depletion of leukocytes by filtration (*6*) decreased the sensitization rate but also appeared to abrogate or abolish the beneficial effect on transplant outcome.

The concept that transfusion of platelets, expressing only class I antigens, would not lead to humoral sensitization and would modify subsequent immune responses was espoused by Batchelor and Welsh (*7, 8*). Support for this view has come from experimental work in rats (*7–10*), mice (*11, 12*), monkeys (*13–17*), and mongrel (*18*), though not Beagle, dogs (*19, 20*). Considerable interest was generated by the first report (*13*) of platelet transfusion in the rhesus monkey, which showed a low sensitization rate and improved renal allograft survival.

Our pilot study of the effect of platelet transfusion in the clinical situation started in 1982. The trial was designed to assess the humoral response to 3 platelet transfusions and measure the outcome of allografts in patients who had only received platelets before renal transplantation.

MATERIALS AND METHODS

A group of 24 previously untransfused patients, with a mean age of 37.8 years, awaiting their first cadaver transplant were selected: 11 were women and 4 of these had previously been pregnant. Informed consent was obtained and a careful search of their previous medical histories undertaken to confirm that there had been no prior blood transfusions.

Platelet transfusions. Platelet transfusions were prepared as previously described in detail (*21, 22*). The first 12 patients (group 1) received platelets separated from blood group O volunteers by use of a V50 Cell Separator (Haemonetics Corporation, Braintree, MA). The remaining 12 patients (group 2) were given a highly purified preparation of platelets using an IG500 Filter (*23*) (Terumo Corporation, Tokyo) that allowed leukocytes to be filtered from the platelet suspensions. The mean leukocyte contamination was measured by an electronic particle counter (S Plus, Coultern Electronics, Luton, England) and the results for each group are shown in Table 1. All patients received 3 platelet transfusions from different donors at 2-week intervals, serum samples being taken before each transfusion and 2 and 4 weeks after the last.

Antibody status. A standard eosin dye exclusion, complement-dependent cytotoxicity (CDC) assay * with 2-hr postcomplement incubation was used to detect sensitization. The 5 serum samples were tested against the patients' 3 platelet donors; panels of 20 PBLs, and the separated T and B cells, from normal volunteers; and a panel of cells from 20 patients with chronic lymphatic leukemia (CLL). The decision to transplant was taken on the basis of a negative CDC crossmatch against separated donor T and B cells, with 3 exceptions. Two patients had positive crossmatches due to autoantibodies and one had a peak serum that was positive with donor B cells that was not attributable to autoantibody, but was negative with serum taken at the time of the transplant.

Sensitization to the respective platelet and kidney donors was also measured by flow cytometry using a method similar to that reported by Garavoy and his colleagues (*24*) that detects binding antibodies. Platelet and kidney donor lymphocytes were prepared at a concentration of 5×10^6/ml and 50-μl aliquots

[1] This work was supported in part by the Medical Research Council of the United Kingdom.

[2] JRC is an MRC Training Research Fellow.

* Abbreviations used: CDC, complement-dependent cytotoxicity; CsA, cyclosporine; PBL, peripheral blood lymphocyte; CLL, chronic lymphatic leukemia; FC, flow cytometry; FITC, fluorescein isothiocyanate.

were incubated with 50 μl of each sample of the patients' serum for 30 min at 22°C. Following two washes, the cells were incubated with an FITC F(ab')$_2$ goat antihuman immunoglobulin (Tago, Burlingame, CA) for 30 min at 4°C. After two further washes the cells were suspended at a final concentration of 1×10^6 ml in 1% formaldehyde. Analysis of the bound fluorescein was performed using a Cytofluorograf System 50L coupled to a 2150 Data Handler (Ortho, Westwood, MA). Comparison of the experimental mean of the T cell peak, with that of a control antibody-negative serum produced the "T cell peak shift." A shift of greater than 20 channels (+20) was considered a positive result.

Blood transfusion. Five patients were transfused with blood after their platelets and before their transplants. One received 3 transfusions from a potential living-related donor to whom he became sensitized. He subsequently was transplanted with a crossmatch-negative cadaver kidney. Another patient required blood for urgent clinical reasons. When the poor graft outcome from platelet transfusion became apparent, the 3 patients still awaiting kidneys who had not developed cytotoxic antibodies were transfused deliberately with 3 units of random 10-day-old whole blood. But it was thought unwise to stimulate, still further, patients who had already developed antibodies.

Renal transplantation. Of the 24 patients, 18 have been transplanted with cadaver donor kidneys—9 from each group. The patients were entered into the ongoing second Oxford Cyclosporine Trial which involved all cadaver grafts performed between November 1981 and November 1984 (*25*). This trial compared two immunosuppressive regimens so 10 of the platelet patients were randomly allocated to conventional azathioprine and low-dose prednisolone, while 8 were randomized to receive cyclosporine alone for the first 90 days followed by conversion to azathioprine and prednisolone for maintenance therapy. Acute rejection episodes in both groups were treated with i.v. boluses of 0.5 g methylprednisolone for 3–5 days.

Statistical analysis. Comparison of the humoral sensitization rates was performed by Fisher's exact test. Actuarial graft survival curves were calculated by the method of Peto et al., and tests for the significance of differences performed by the Mantel-Cox test (*26*).

RESULTS

Sensitization. Screening of the patients by CDC before transfusion revealed 5 patients in group 1 and 3 patients in group 2 with antibodies. One untransfused male patient had a monospecific anti-DR4; 3 patients had autoreactive B cell and 2 autoreactive T and B cell antibodies; 2 female patients, neither of whom had been pregnant, had broadly reactive antibody without definable HLA specificity. No change in the antibody status of these patients was detected after the platelet transfusions.

Five patients in group 1, who did not have antibodies and were transfused with the impure platelet preparation, developed cytotoxic antibodies after the transfusions (Table 1). Two multiparous female patients developed anti-HLA B8 and A2 antibodies respectively. Two nulliparous female recipients developed anti-HLA A2 and broad reactivity. One male patient developed autoreactive B cell antibodies that had been weakly detectable 1 and 2 years previously. CDC thus demonstrated a sensitization rate of 42% in group 1—i.e. those who received platelets contaminated with just 15×10^6 leukocytes, this degree of contamination being equivalent to the number of leukocytes in 2–3 ml of whole blood. In group 2, when leukocyte contamination was below the particle counter background of 5×10^6 cells per transfusion, no antibodies were detected in patients who did not have antibodies before transfusion.

TABLE 1. Platelet transfusion details

	Group 1	Group 2	
Number of patients	12	12	
Transfusions:			
Number of platelets per transfusion	200×10^8	200×10^8	
Number of leukocytes per transfusion	15×10^6	$<5\times10^6$	
Antibody status:			
Cytotoxic antibodies			
Number with antibodies before platelets	5	3	
Number with antibodies after platelets	10	3	
Sensitization rate	42%	0%	($P<0.04$)
Flow cytometry:			
Number responding to platelet donors	10	2	
Sensitization rate	83%	17%	($P<0.004$)
Transplantation:			
Number of patients transplanted	9	9	
Number who also received blood	2	1	
One-year graft survival	56%	33%	

Flow cytometry (FC) represents a more sensitive technique than CDC for detecting antibody bound to the surface of lymphocytes and was thus used as an adjunct to CDC screening. The patients' sera were tested against lymphocytes from their 3 platelet donors and, when transplanted, also their kidney donor. 10 patients in group 1 responded to their platelet transfusions as judged by development of a positive FC result against one of their platelet donors' T cells following transfusion, 3 patients actually responded to 2 donors (Fig. 1). By contrast ony 2 patients in group 2 responded to the transfusions (Fig. 2) and these were much weaker than the majority of group 1 responses. Thus the sensitization rates assessed by FC were significantly different at 83% and 17% for groups 1 and 2, respectively ($P<0.004$).

The renal donor CDC crossmatch was also compared with the FC crossmatch result. The individual T cell peak shifts in all of the sera were negative except for 3 patients who had a positive FC crossmatch judged by the most reactive serum. However all patients were negative when serum from the time of the transplant was used. Two of the 3 peak-positive transplants were successful and 1 failed. The 9 other patients with rejected grafts had negative peak and current FC crossmatches.

Blood transfusion after platelets. Of the 5 patients who received subsequent blood transfusions, 2 developed cytotoxic antibodies after the blood that were not present after the platelets (Table 2). One of these patients had fresh blood on 3 occasions from his father who was intended to be a single-haplotype-matched living-related kidney donor. After developing donor-specific T cell antibodies the patient was given a cadaver graft that is functioning at 18 months. The other patient to respond to the blood transfusions produced anti-HLA A1 and weak B8 specificities, but has not yet been transplanted.

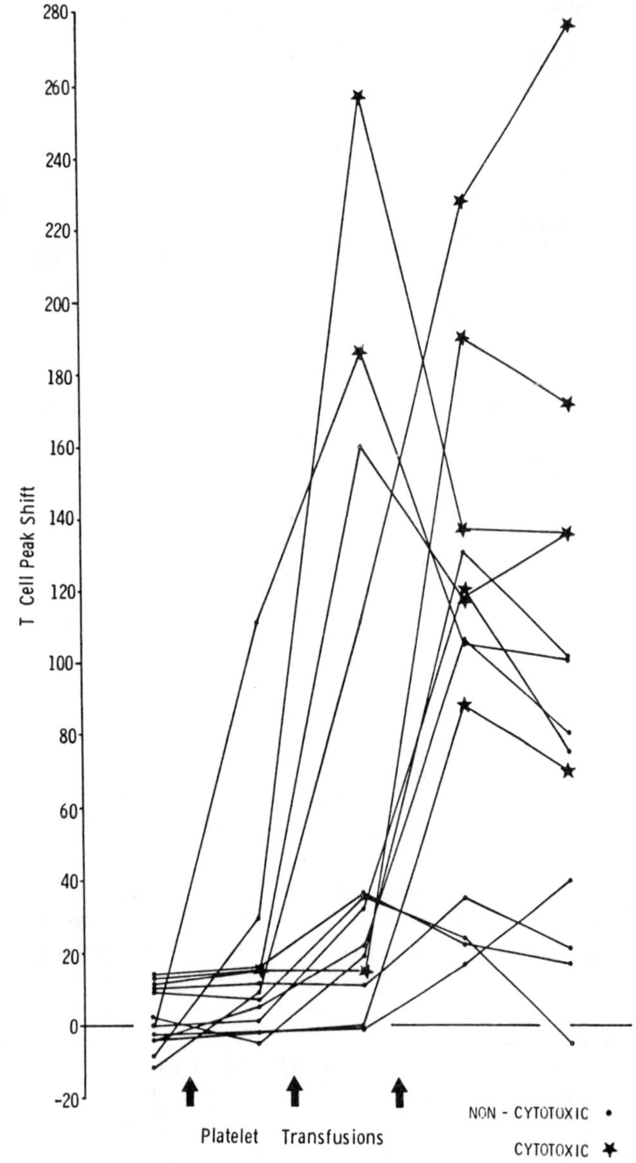

FIGURE 1. Flow cytometer crossmatch results of sera from patients in group 1 against the patients' platelet donors, showing the results for responders only.

Transplant outcome. Details of the transplanted patients are shown in Table 3 (group 1) and Table 4 (group 2), 9 patients from each group received cadaver renal allografts. In group 1 (those transfused with impure platelets) 4 patients rejected their grafts rapidly and 5 have functioning grafts 14–23 months after transplantation. Two of those with surviving grafts (numbers 5 and 7) received blood transfusions after their platelets and before their transplants. All patients with surviving grafts were demonstrated, by FC, to have mounted a humoral response to their platelet donors. In group 2, those given pure platelets only, with the exception of patient 17 who was given deliberate blood transfusions, the results of transplantation were poor. Three patients rejected their grafts rapidly and 3 others died. Patient 16 died from cytomegalovirus infection and *Pseudomonas* septicemia, with a functioning graft. Patient 17 died from cytomegalovirus infection and respiratory complications after emergency surgery for a perforated duodenal ulcer, during which time her graft failed. Patient 18 had multiple acute rejection episodes and renal artery stenosis requiring correction. He died from septicemia, and his graft showed histological evidence of severe rejection. Patients 18 and 19 were the only patients in group 2 to mount a humoral response to their platelet donors. There was no correlation between the graft

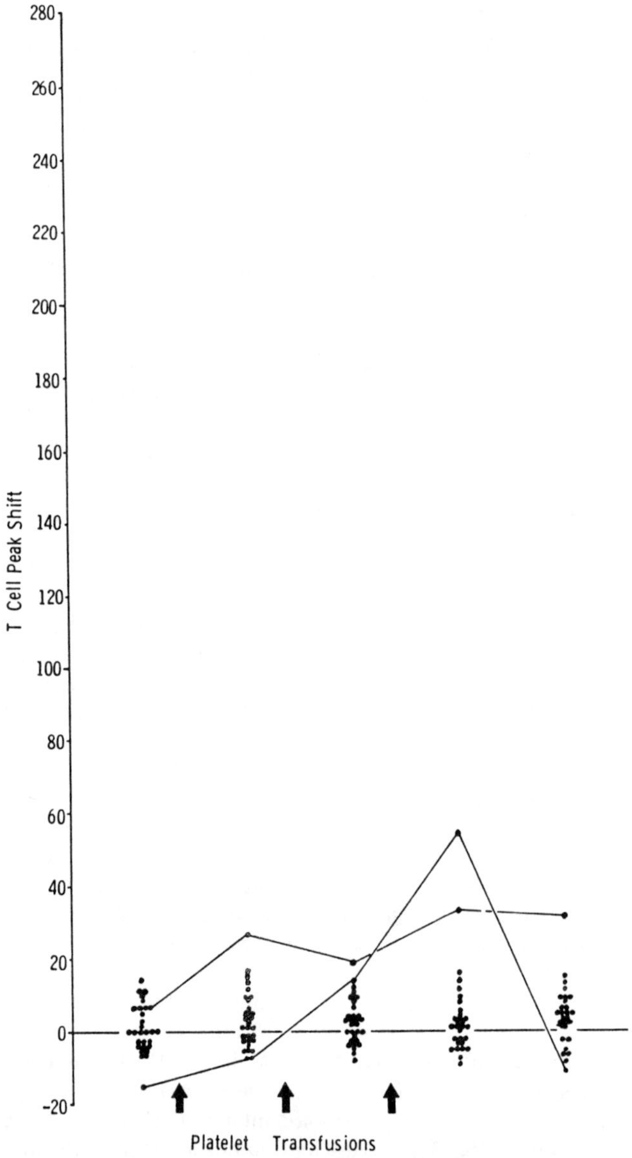

FIGURE 2. Flow cytometer crossmatch results of sera from patients in group 2 against the patients' platelet donors, showing the results for all patients, and demonstrating that only 2 patients produced any response (the connected points).

TABLE 2. Blood transfusion after platelets

Patient	Blood	Sensitization	Transplant outcome
Group 1			
MJ	2 × Random	No change	Success
TL	3 × Single donor	Sensitized to blood donor	Success
Group 2			
DH	3 × Random	No change	Died[a]
MP	3 × Random	Anti-A1, weak B8	Not transplanted
JC	3 × Random	No change	Not transplanted

[a] Patient No. 17.

TABLE 3. Group 1 results

Patient	Ab response[a] CDC	Ab response[a] FC	Immuno suppression	CDC Xm	Graft survival	Current creatinine µmol/L
1.	+	+	Aza	—	0 Days	Rejection
2.	−	+	CsA	—	3 Days	Rejection
3.	−	+	CsA	B non-auto	6 Days	Rejection
4.	−	+	Aza	—	43 Days	Rejection
5.	−	+	Aza (B1)	B Auto	14 Months	157
6.	+	+	CsA	—	15 Months	205
7.	+	+	Aza (B1)	—	18 Months	169
8.	−	+	Aza	—	23 Months	80
9.	+	+	Aza	—	23 Months	111
10.	+	+	Awaiting transplantation.			
11.	−	−				
12.	−	−				

[a] Aza = azathioprine and low-dose prednisolone; CsA = Cyclosporine; Ab response = response to platelet transfusion; CDC = assessed by CDC; FC = assessed by FC, B = B cell positive crossmatch; (B1) = pretransplant blood transfusions; CDC Xm = Cytotoxic crossmatch.

TABLE 4. Group 2 results

Patient	Ab response[a] CDC	Ab response[a] FC	Immuno suppression	CDC Xm	Graft survival	Current creatinine µmol/L
13.	−	−	Aza	—	0 Days	Rejection
14.	−	−	Aza	—	13 Days	Rejection
15.	−	−	Aza	—	29 Days	Rejection
16.	−	−	CsA	—	66 Days	Died Functioning
17.	−	−	Aza (B1)	TB Auto	71 Days	Died
18.	−	+	CsA	—	5 Months	Died
19.	−	+	CsA	—	14 Months	144
20.	−	−	CsA	—	16 Months	124
21.	−	−	Aza	—	22 Months	82
22.	−	−	Awaiting transplantation.			
23.	−	−				
24.	−	−				

[a] Abbreviations as for Table 3.

outcome and the interval between the last platelet transfusion and the day of transplantation. Similarly no clear pattern could be discerned relating outcome to HLA matching, mismatching, or the sharing of class I antigens between the platelet donors and the kidney donors.

The actuarial graft survival for the 18 platelet-transfused patients is demonstrated in Figure 3 and compared with the graft survival of first cadaver grafts in 52 blood transfused patients transplanted during the same period. The difference between the two curves is significant ($P = 0.03$), suggesting that platelet and blood transfusion do not lead to similar graft survival rates. The 1-year graft survival for all the platelet-transfused patients is 44%, but for those who received pure platelets only, the figure is 38% (though the number of patients is small). The 1-year graft survival of 128 untransfused patients receiving first cadaver grafts in Oxford up to 1982 was 56%, suggesting that platelet-transfused patients may have fared even worse than if they had not been transfused at all. Further evidence suggesting that those transfused with pure platelets did not behave as if they were naive untransfused recipients was the speed with which acute rejection occurred: 4 patients had their first acute rejection episode diagnosed before day 4, and a further 2 patients by day 7.

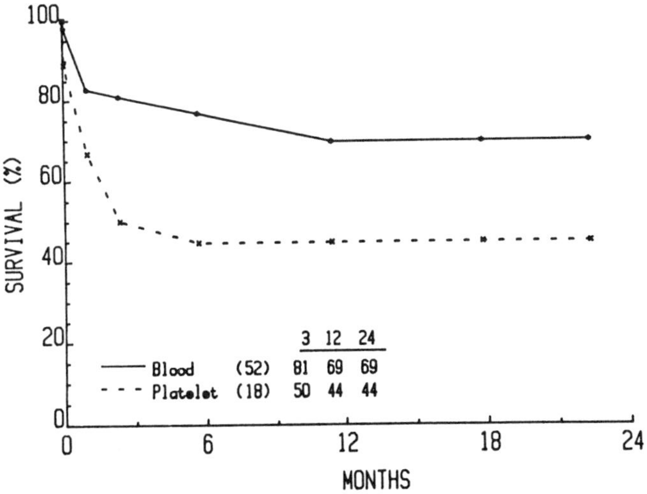

FIGURE 3. Actuarial renal allograft survival rates of platelet transfused patients compared with blood-transfused patients receiving first cadaver grafts over the same period. The tabular material on the figure shows the percentage of survival in the two groups at 3, 12, and 24 months. The difference between the two curves is significant, $P = 0.03$ (*26*).

DISCUSSION

This small pilot study of platelet transfusions in patients awaiting a renal transplant has produced results that were unexpected on the basis of previous experience in animal models. These models would have suggested that sensitization would be low, and that subsequent graft survival might be at least comparable to that produced by blood transfusions.

In the rat neither platelets nor red blood cells (both of which express class I antigen only) induce a primary lymphocytotoxic response, but platelets will induce a secondary response to class I antigens if the animal has been primed with lymphoid cells. Transfusion of platelets (*8*) or red blood cells (*28*) enhances rat renal allograft survival. A number of experiments have confirmed that donor, but not third-party, strain platelets enhance survival of rat renal allografts (*9, 10*), mouse skin allografts (*11*), and mouse islet allografts (*12*). In the rhesus monkey, random platelet transfusion produced improved renal allograft survival comparable to blood transfusions, and little humoral sensitization (*13, 14*). It has also been shown that platelet transfusions not only lead to low rates of humoral sensitization in the rhesus monkey but they also alter humoral responses to subsequent transfusion with whole blood (*15–17*). In Oxford, mongrel dog renal allografts were chosen as a model to assess the effect of platelet transfusions (*18*). This study demonstrated similar and improved graft survival times after whole-blood and purified platelets, but 2 of the 5 platelet transfused dogs developed antibodies. On the other hand, Marquet and his colleagues showed that random platelet transfusions in Beagle dogs resulted in a high incidence of humoral sensitization, and renal allograft survival was not prolonged (*19, 20*).

The degree of contamination of the platelet preparations by leukocytes was variable in the animal studies. In man, deliberate immunization of volunteers for the production of HLA antibodies suggested that a minimum of 15 ml on several occasions would be required to induce a response (*27*). The leukocyte contamination of our first platelet preparations (group 1) was small, in that the equivalent of 2–3 ml of whole blood was given on 3 occasions, and so we did not anticipate a humoral response. However, using the cytotoxicity assay we detected 42% sensitization, and by the more sensitive FC assay 83% were sensitized. Purification of the platelets (group 2), such that leukocyte contamination was below the ability to measure it accurately, markedly reduced the sensitization rate, although 2 patients were sensitized as detected by FC, thus showing that very small numbers of contaminating leukocytes can produce a weak humoral response. However in general, pure platelets did not produce any response, tending to confirm in the clinical situation the experimental observations that primary exposure to i.v. class I antigen alone does not induce a humoral response.

This was a phase-one study and was not expected to produce poor graft survival. There were thus no randomized blood transfused or untransfused groups for comparison. Nevertheless, despite the small number of transplanted patients, some useful comparisons can be made. Blood-transfused recipients of first cadaver grafts transplanted during the same period as the platelet recipients, fared significantly better. Therefore this study does not show that random platelet transfusions, using our protocol, improve renal allograft survival in the same way as blood. Indeed it would even seem that patients given platelet transfusions did worse than untransfused patients. There were no untransfused patients transplanted over the period of the study for comparison, because those patients all entered the platelet trial. Oxford had a relatively high proportion of untransfused recipients before 1982 and their 1-year survival was considerably higher than that achieved by the whole platelet group, and much higher than the dismal results in the few who received only pure platelets. Certainly the clinical course of many of the subsequent renal allografts in platelet-transfused patients suggested that these patients were sensitized against the renal donor, for there was a high number of very early acute rejections in this group, well before any primary response to the graft would have been mounted. There is thus reason to believe that the platelet-transfused patients may not have acted as if they were unsensitized untransfused recipients of renal allografts. Although there was little evidence of donor-specific sensitization in the patients given a renal transplant, as determined by the donor-recipient crossmatch, it is possible that donor-specific sensitization was present at a cellular level.

Three other studies of platelet transfusion in the clinical situation have been undertaken. Land, using a donor-specific protocol, harvested platelets from 1000 ml of cadaver-donor blood and transfused them 24 hr before performing the kidney transplant (*29*). The results in a limited number of patients showed that this protocol conferred no advantage over random blood and the procedure has been abandoned. Pallardo et al. (*30*) undertook a similar study to our own, giving fresh platelets on 5 occasions at 4-week intervals. Their preparation contained three times as many platelets and was also contaminated with more leukocytes than our suspensions. They concluded that the sensitization rate was comparable with that from 5 blood transfusions, and that graft survival was poor—50% of the grafts being acutely rejected. Betuel and Traeger (*31*) have recently reported early results from their trial of platelet transfusion in which 4 times the number of pure platelets was given from a larger number of donors than in our trial, and on 5 occasions instead of 3. They did not experience humoral sensitization from this protocol and the early results of renal transplantation, using prophylactic antilymphocyte globulin, are encouraging.

When faced with these poor graft survival rates we, like Pallardo, decided to blood-transfuse the remaining patients in the hope that we might confer some benefit. Data from rats (*8*) and monkeys (*16, 17*) suggest that sensitization to blood would be less likely when given after platelets. We decided, however, not to transfuse patients who had already developed cytotoxic antibodies, for fear of inducing high sensitization. A total of 5 patients thus received blood—and, of these, 2 produced cytotoxic antibodies and 1 produced a response detectable by FC analysis; 3 of these patients have been transplanted and 1 graft has failed.

This study of 3 transfusions of random platelets in nontransfused recipients did not produce the expected results. First, a small contamination with leukocytes did result in sensitization, as judged by the development of both lymphocytotoxic antibodies and binding antibodies detected by flow cytometry. Second, highly purified platelets did not sensitize the recipients. Finally, graft survival was poor in both groups regardless of the immunosuppression used.

REFERENCES

1. Opelz G, Sengar DPS, Mickey MR, Terasaki PI. Effect of blood transfusions on subsequent kidney transplants. Transplant Proc 1973; 5: 253.
2. Opelz G, Terasaki PI. Dominant effect of transfusions on kidney graft survival. Transplantation 1980; 29: 153.
3. Van Es AA, Balner H. Effect of pretransplant transfusions on kidney allograft survival. Transplant Proc 1979; 11: 127.
4. Spees EK, Vaughn WK, Williams GM, Filo RS, McDonald JC, Mendez-Picon G, Niblack G. Effects of blood transfusion on

cadaver renal transplantation. The Southeastern Organ Procurement Foundation Prospective Study (1977–1979). Transplantation 1980; 30: 455.
5. Opelz G, Terasaki PI. International study of histocompatibility in renal transplantation. Transplantation 1982; 33: 87.
6. Madsen M, Graugaard B, Fjeldborg O, Hansen HE, Posborg V, Kissmeyer-Nielsen F. HLA-DR antigen matching in cadaveric renal transplantation: an analysis of 201 consecutive transplants performed in Aarhus from 1978 to 1983. Transplant Proc 1985; 17: 47.
7. Batchelor JR, Welsh KI, Burgos H. Immunological enhancement. Transplant Proc 1977; 9: 931.
8. Welsh KI, Burgos H, Batchelor JR. The immune response to allogeneic rat platelets; Ag-B antigens in matrix form lacking Ia. Eur J Immunol 1977; 7: 267.
9. Martin DC, Hewitt CW, Osbourne JG, Dowdy SF, Fristoe TL, Russell LA, Cote J. Enhanced kidney graft survival in rats by single or multiple blood transfusions and various blood products. Transplant Proc 1982; 14: 407.
10. Hibberd AD, Scott LJ. Allogeneic platelets increase the survival of rat renal allografts. Transplantation 1983; 35: 622.
11. Kapnick SJ, Monaco AP. Induction of unresponsiveness to skin allografts with donor strain platelets in antilymphocyte-serum-treated mice. Transplant Proc 1979; 11: 982.
12. Weber CJ, Pemis B, Reemtsma K. Donor specific platelet transfusion prolongs mouse islet allograft survival. Transplant Proc 1985; 17: 1116.
13. Borleffs JCC, Neuhaus P, Van Rood JJ, Balner H. Platelet transfusions improve kidney allograft survival in rhesus monkeys without inducing cytotoxic antibodies. Lancet 1982; 1: 1117.
14. Borleffs JCC, Neuhaus P, Van Rood JJ, Balner H. Platelet transfusions have a positive effect on kidney allograft survival in rhesus monkeys and induce virtually no cytotoxic antibodies. Transplant Proc 1983; 15: 985.
15. Oh JH, McClure HM. Lymphocytotoxic antibodies induced by fresh blood, stored blood, and platelets in rhesus monkeys. Transplant Proc 1982; 14: 410.
16. Oh JH, McClure HM, Tuttle EP. Immunological unresponsiveness induced by platelet transfusion in rhesus monkeys. Transplantation 1983; 36: 727.
17. Oh JH, McClure HM. Platelet induced immunosuppression in rhesus monkeys. Transplant Proc 1985; 17: 1113.
18. Errett LE, Allen N, Deierhoi MH, Denton TG, Wood RFM, Morris PJ. The effect of platelet transfusions on renal allograft survival and sensitization in dogs. Tissue Antigens 1985; 25: 28.
19. Marquet RL, Tank B, Heineman E, et al. Pre-transplant platelet transfusions do not improve kidney graft survival in beagle dogs. Lancet 1983; 1: 774.
20. Bijnen AB, Heineman E, Marquet RL, Niessen GJCM, Obertop H, Tank B, Jeekel J. Lack of beneficial effect of thrombocyte transfusions on kidney graft survival in dogs. Transplantation 1984; 37: 213.
21. Fisher M, Chapman JR, Ting A, Morris PJ. Alloimmunization to HLA antigens following transfusion with leukocyte poor and purified platelet suspensions. Vox Sang 1985; 49: 331.
22. Chapman JR, Fisher M, Ting A, Morris PJ. Platelet transfusion before renal transplantation in humans. Transplant Proc 1985; 17: 1038.
23. Lichtiger B, Del Valle L, Arminto M, Trujillo JM. Use of Imugard Ig500 filters for preparation of leukocyte-poor blood for cancer patients. Vox Sang 1984; 46: 136.
24. Garovoy MR, Rheinschmidt MA, Bigos M, Perkins H, Colombe B, Feduska N, Salvatierra O. Flow cytometry analysis: a high technology crossmatch technique facilitating transplantation. Transplant Proc 1983; 15: 1939.
25. Wood RFM, Thompson JF, Ting A, Benjamin IS, Allen NH, Morris PJ. A randomized controlled trial of short term cyclosporine therapy in renal transplantation (Trial II). Transplant Proc 1985; 17: 1164.
26. Peto R, Pike MC, Armitage P, et al. Design and analysis of randomized clinical trials requiring prolonged observation of each patient. II. Analysis and examples. Br J Cancer 1977; 35: 1.
27. Ferrara GB, Tosi RM, Azzolina G, Carminati G, Kissmeyer-Nielsen F. The production of anti-HL-A cytotoxic antisera through planned immunization by intravenous injection of small aliquots of whole blood. I. Immunization of unrelated recipients. Tissue Antigens 1972; 2: 359.
28. Wood KJ, Evins J, Morris PJ. Suppression of renal allograft rejection in the rat by class I antigens on purified erythrocytes. Transplantation 1985; 39: 56.
29. Land W, Mempel W, Scholz S, Illner WD. Cadaveric donor specific platelets transfusion prior to renal transplantation. Netherlands J Med 1985; 28: 262.
30. Pallardo LM, Moll JL, Montoro J, et al. Las transfusiones de plaquetas no mejoran la supervivencia del trasplante renal de cadaver. Nefrologia 1984; 4: 111.
31. Betuel H, Traeger J. Platelet transfusion. 17th International Course on Transplantation and Clinical Immunology, Lyon, May 1985.

Received 14 June 1985.
Accepted 23 July 1985.

0041-1337/86/4104-0474$02.00/0
TRANSPLANTATION
Vol. 41, No. 4

Printed in U.S.A.

THE IMPORTANCE OF THE LEWIS SYSTEM IN CADAVER RENAL TRANSPLANTATION[1]

M.P. POSNER, M.B. MCGEORGE, G. MENDEZ-PICON, T. MOHANAKUMAR,[2] AND H.M. LEE

The Division of Vascular and Transplantation Surgery and the Tissue Typing Laboratory, Department of Surgery, Medical College of Virginia, Virginia Commonwealth University, Richmond, Virginia

Previous reports have suggested that Lewis (Le) antigens may exert a significant effect on cadaver renal allograft (CRA) survival, especially in black recipients in whom there is a higher frequency of Le-negative phenotypes. We review our experience with this problem in 70 donor-recipient pairs of CRA who underwent prospective Le typing and received conventional immunosuppression between 1980 and 1983.

Recipient typing alone yielded the following graft survival (GS) and patient survival (PS) at 2 years by life table analysis: (a^+,b;$^-$) (n = 12) 51% GS, 93% PS; (a^-,b^+) (n = 44) 57% GS, 88% PS; and (a^-,b^-) (n = 14) 51% GS, 93% PS(*P*-ns for GS, PS). Recipient racial characteristics did not effect ultimate graft survival, as whites and blacks had similar two-year GS in all phenotypic groups. When Le matching was considered, no significant differences in one-year graft survivals could be ascertained between Le-matched and Le-mismatched donor-recipient pairs, and this effect persisted despite stratification for race and HLA-A,B and DR histoincompatibilities.

In light of these results, we do not recommend using Lewis compatibility as a criterion for donor selection in cadaver renal allografting, as this substantially increases the difficulty in finding suitable matches, especially in the (a^-,b^-) recipient group.

The Lewis (Le)* system is considered by some to be influential in allograft survival. Lewis system products are very closely related in structure to the gene products of the ABO system; they arise from a common precursor molecule. Additionally, antibodies directed against Lewis a and b substances are among the most common naturally occurring blood group antibodies, second only to the antibodies to major blood group antigens in frequency.

The significance of Lewis phenotype in cadaveric renal allografts has been supported by the observations of Oriol (*1*), Pfaff (*2*) and others (*3*), who noted decreased survival in recipients lacking the Lewis gene (thus expressing the [a^-,b^-] phenotype). Moreover, Williams et al. (*4*) reported rejection of a renal allograft of an HLA-compatible kidney in a Lewis mismatched recipient who demonstrated Lewis antibody at the time of graft loss. It has been suggested that the higher frequency of the (a^-,b^-) phenotype in the black population may contribute, at least in part, to the poorer graft survival rate that has been reported in blacks (*1*).

Most of the reported literature regarding the relevance of the Lewis system in transplantation has been based on retrospective analysis and has included only recipient—not donor—phenotyping. Thus, the presence of a Lewis match or mismatch in a donor-recipient combination can be assessed only by statistical presumption, based on the relative frequencies of the three recipient phenotypes. In addition to the retrospective nature of these studies, other factors may have played a role in determining ultimate results—to wit, patient selection processes and multicenter effects. Notwithstanding these facts, retrospective data have been confirmed by the results of at least one prospective study (*5*), wherein Lewis-"identical" donor-recipient pairs were found to have improved graft survivals when compared with Lewis "nonidentical" pairs, and this effect was augmented by increasing MHC disparity. In order to more accurately reflect the effect of Lewis matching on our recipient population, we conducted a single-center prospective study, involving both recipient and donor Lewis typing.

MATERIALS AND METHODS

Seventy-five consecutive recipients of cadaveric renal allografts (CRA) performed between 1980–1983 were screened for Lewis substances on red blood cells to form the basis of this report. Five patients were excluded from the study due to primary nonfunction of the kidney, leaving 70 patients in the study group. These kidneys were presumably lost to causes other than Lewis incompatibility, since all five patients were matched with their donors in terms of Lewis phenotyping. Patients were statistically similar with regard to sex, age, number of transplants, donor characteristics, preservation methods and times, preoperative and perioperative blood transfusion history, and HLA and DR matching among the phenotypic groups. The race distribution, as expected, was not similar—with 12/14 (86%) of the Lewis negative (a^-,b^-) group being black. Recipient Lewis typing was performed at the time of initial HLA typing and the donor was typed just prior to transplant. The mean MHC incompatibility consisted of a 2-HLA-A,B-matched kidney during the entire study period, and Lewis typing was used prospectively during the period from 1980 to 1982, such that no recipient received a Lewis incompatible kidney within that time.

The techniques of transplantation and conventional immunosuppression have been described elsewhere (*6*), and have included the routine use of prophylactic ATG. As noted (Table 1), it was decided that donor kidneys of phenotype (a^-,b^+) transplanted into (a^+,b^-) recipients would also be considered a mismatch, based on reports of the presence of anti-b antibody in Lewis (a^+,b^-) individuals (*7*). This was the case in 6/18 (33%) of mismatched patients.

Graft survival was calculated using actuarial methods described by Kaplan-Meier (*8*). The *P* values were generated by the methods of Breslow (which give greater weight to earlier observations) and Mantel-Cox (*9, 10*). A failed graft was con-

[1] This work was supported by NIH Grant AM 32253.

[2] T. Mohanakumar is a recipient of ACS FRA No. 246.

* Abbreviations used: CRA, cadaver renal allograft; GS, graft survival; Le, Lewis; PS, patient survival.

sidered to have occurred if the patient was returned to a normal dialysis schedule, regardless of the cause of organ failure. However, in order to more accurately reflect graft loss secondary to immunological injury, death with a functioning graft was not considered a failed graft, but rather was censored.

RESULTS

From 1980 to 1983, it was the policy of our center to only transplant Lewis-matched patients. Subsequently, after preliminary assessment of the data, Lewis typing was continued, but matching was not considered in the decision to transplant—thus, as will become apparent, Lewis-mismatched recipients were few.

The relative phenotypic frequencies in the study group were as follows: (a^+,b^-): (n = 12) 17%; (a^-,b^+): (n = 44) 63%; and (a^-,b^-): (n = 14) 20%. Comparative graft survival curves of these three recipient groups are illustrated in Figure 1. These patients were grouped on the basis of recipient phenotype only, and as noted, no one group held a significant survival advantage over a two-year period. Two-year graft survival for the (a^+,b^-) group was 51%, 57% for the (a^-,b^+) group, and 51% for the (a^-,b^-) group (*P* = ns).

In order to determine whether race affected overall graft survival, patients were further grouped according to race. Figures 2 and 3 represent graft survival of the three phenotypes in white and black populations. Whites had 2-year graft survival rates of 31% in the (a^+,b^-) group, 61% in the (a^-,b^+) group, and 50% in the (a^-,b^-) group (*P* = ns). Blacks had 2-year graft survivals of 75% for (a^+,b^-) patients, 47% for (a^-,b^+), and 49% for (a^-,b^-) individuals (*P* = ns). The overall 2-year graft survival rates for blacks versus whites at our center over the last 12 years in recipients of cadaver renal allografts were statistically equivalent at about 55%—and, specifically, the 2-year graft survival (regardless of Lewis type or match) for 42 white recipients in this series was 48%, versus 63% for 28 black recipients ($P<0.44$).

TABLE 1. The criteria for match and mismatch Lewis antigens

Recipient phenotype	Donor phenotype	
a^-,b^+	a^+,b^-	Match
	a^-,b^+	Match
	a^-,b^-	Match
a^+,b^-	a^+,b^-	Match
	a^-,b^-	Match
	a^-,b^+	Mismatch
a^-,b^-	a^+,b^-	Mismatch
	a^-,b^+	Mismatch
	a^-,b^-	Match

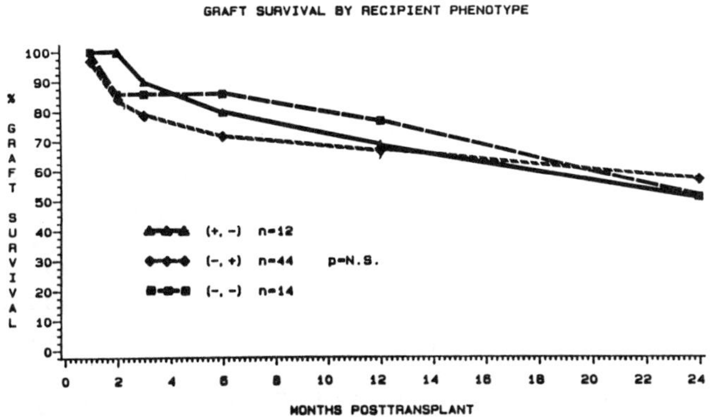

FIGURE 1. Actuarial renal allograft survival related to Lewis phenotype in all recipients.

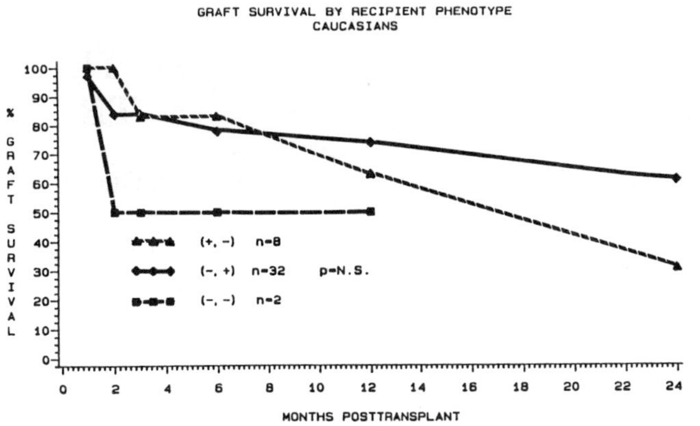

FIGURE 2. Actuarial renal allograft survival related to recipient Lewis phenotype and race (whites).

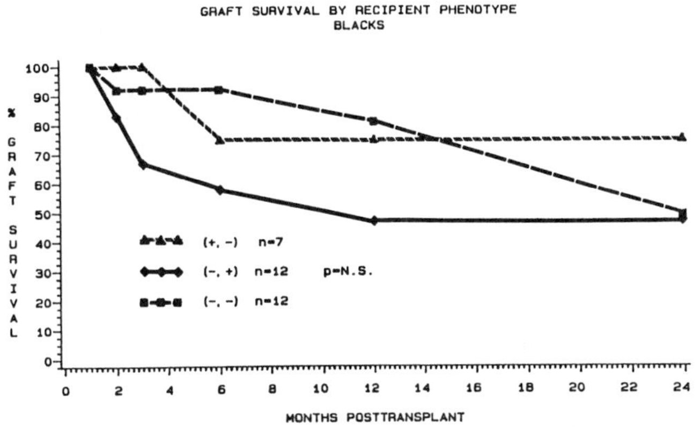

FIGURE 3. Actuarial renal allograft survival related to recipient Lewis phenotype and race (blacks).

Patients were subsequently grouped according to Lewis match or Lewis mismatch, which was not based solely on the presence or absence of the Lewis gene, but rather the specific phenotypes, as described in methods. Figure 4 illustrates the graft survivals of patients who were matched and mismatched for Lewis. No significant differences were noted in the two groups with 1-year survival rates for matched and mismatched patients at 70% and 69%, respectively. At two years survival looked quite different among the two groups. This was most likely due to the fact that the majority of the mismatched patients were censored by the two-year period, since mismatching has only been accepted in our protocol since 1982. Hence, there were very few mismatched patients at the two-year survival period; thus, no firm conclusions can be made with respect to the two-year survival interval. Overall, however, the survival rates were not significantly different.

Furthermore, when these patients were stratified for race, no remarkable differences were noted (Figs. 5 and 6), with Lewis-matched white patients having a 1-year graft survival of 74% versus 63% in the mismatched group. Likewise, blacks had 1-year graft survivals of 61% in the matched, versus 72% in the mismatched, group.

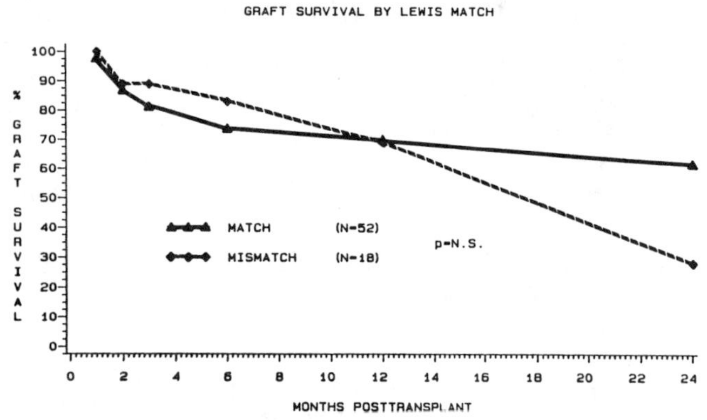

FIGURE 4. Actuarial renal allograft survival in all recipients according to donor-recipient pair Lewis matching.

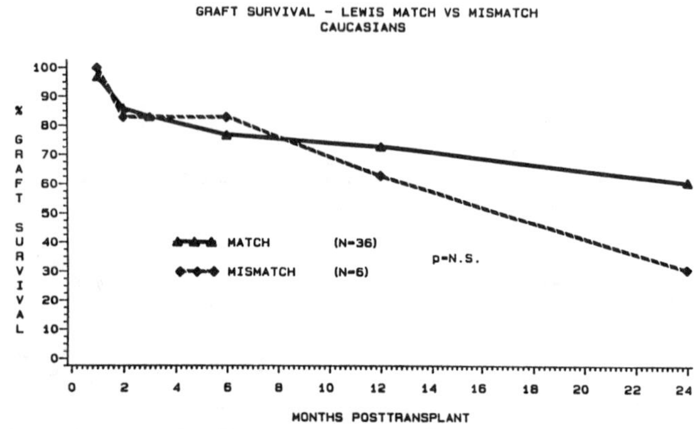

FIGURE 5. Actuarial renal allograft survival in donor-recipient pairs according to Lewis matching: white recipients only.

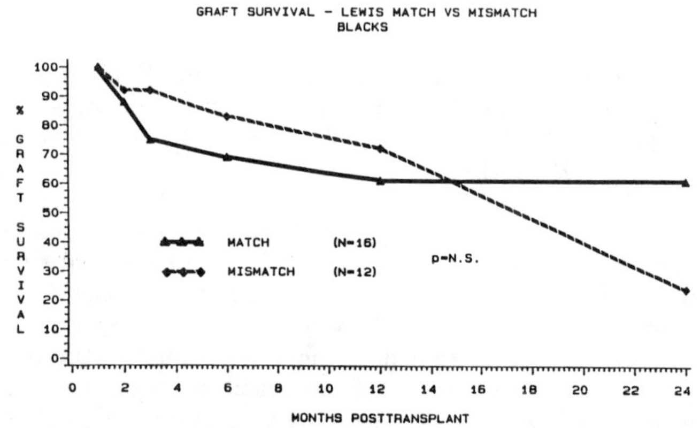

FIGURE 6. Actuarial renal allograft survival in donor-recipient pairs according to Lewis matching: black recipients only.

DISCUSSION

The Lewis system is among the most complex of the blood group systems, the phenotypic expression of which is influenced by more than one gene. While the Lewis system shares many similarities with the ABO system, there are several factors distinguishing the two. Unlike major blood group antigens, Lewis substances are soluble antigens present in saliva and plasma that are merely passively adsorbed onto cell surfaces. Blood transfusions can result in an inaccurate Lewis test result, which is particularly relevant in the case of multiply transfused dialysis patients awaiting transplant, as well as cadaver donors, who often have been transfused prior to donor nephrectomy. There are three commonly expressed Lewis phenotypes. The phenotypes (a^+,b^-) and (a^-,b^+) indicate the presence of the Lewis gene. The phenotype (a^-,b^+) indicates that an additional gene is present that allows the conversion of the "a" substance to the "b" substance—which those of phenotype (a^+,b^-) lack. On the other hand, the phenotype (a^-,b^-) is indicative of a patient who lacks the Lewis gene altogether. Based on reports of others (*1–3*) concerning the frequency distribution of the three Lewis phenotypes, our results are consistent; therefore, we assumed that our test results were accurate, notwithstanding the above limitations.

Most of the previous reports regarding the importance of the Lewis system and transplantation have involved retrospective analysis and considered only recipient phenotype (*1, 2*). Lewis-negative (a^-,b^-) recipients have been reported to have a graft survival ranging from 8% to 100% lower at one year when compared with Lewis-positive patients (*1, 2*). When considering only recipient phenotype, however, Lewis negative patients receiving Lewis-negative kidneys were grouped with Lewis-negative patients receiving Lewis-positive kidneys. Admittedly, this represents a comparatively small portion of the donor-recipient combinations; however, typing of both donor and recipient eliminates this problem and seems to more accurately reflect the role of Lewis compatibility in allograft rejection.

Another advantage of typing both donor and recipient is that one can determine which of the Lewis (a^+,b^-) recipients received (a^-,b^+) kidneys. Lewis (a^+,b^-) individuals lack the Lewis b substance altogether; therefore, they should have the ability to form anti-b antibody (*7*), and for this reason they were considered as mismatches in our study. Of the six donor-recipient combinations who were of these phenotypes, three rejected, two currently have functioning grafts, and one patient died with a functioning graft.

The relationship between Lewis antibody and allograft rejection has thus far been difficult to assess. Although anti-Lewis antibodies have been shown to be hemolytic and cytotoxic, titers of this naturally occurring antibody vary substantially among individuals (*7*), and this may be true even in recipients of identical Lewis phenotypes. Antibodies to Lewis antigens can also result from an immune response—and, perhaps, be augmented by blood transfusion. This may be, at least in part, the explanation for the lack of effect of Lewis incompatibility in our patients, since we were not using a routine pretransplant transfusion protocol in our cadaveric recipients at that time—in spite of the fact that, statistically, transfusion histories were similar among recipients in all phenotypic groups.

The observations of Spitalnik et al. (based on highly sensitive k-ELISA antibody assay) (*11*) have suggested a temporal relationship between Lewis antibody and renal allograft rejection. Anti-Lewis antibody was detected in eight Lewis negative recipients who received Lewis-incompatible grafts, all of whom rejected their renal allografts. A more detailed analysis of the kinetics of the response to Lewis antigens and the onset of allograft rejection may provide even further insight into the significance of these antigens in the transplant setting; this is something we are presently looking into in our Lewis-incompatible donor-recipient pairs.

Since we did not establish Lewis "identity" as a criterion for Lewis "compatibility," our results are not strictly comparable to those of Lenhard et al. (*5*) who found in their prospective series a 14% graft survival advantage at one year in recipients of Lewis-identical (compatible) renal allografts. Moreover, this methodological difference between the two studies may also account for the fact that even when we stratified Lewis match and HLA-A,B, and DR incompatibility, we could find no significant survival differences (data not shown). We cannot truly comment on this latter important difference between our results and those of Lenhard et al. (*5*) who found the influence of Lewis matching to be that much greater in recipients of HLA-incompatible renal allografts, because the small group size in our data makes it difficult to obtain statistically meaningful results. However, it is clear that there is no apparent influence of the Lewis system overriding the major histocompatibility complex.

In conclusion, our experience with prospective Lewis typing has indicated that matching for Lewis antigens does not appear to be a useful criterion in improving graft survival. In contrast to the large multicenter study reported by Oriol et al., neither race nor Lewis status has been a significant risk factor in our patient population. The black population, which represents approximately 40% of our recipient pool has, over the last 12 years, had survival rates equivalent to those of whites (unpublished observations), and when stratified for Lewis phenotype, there have been no remarkable differences noted. In light of these results, we do not recommend using Lewis compatibility as a criterion for donor selection, since this substantially increases the difficulty in finding suitable matches, specifically in the (a^-,b^-) recipient group.

REFERENCES

1. Oriol R, Cartron J, Yvart J, et al. The Lewis system: new histocompatibility antigens in renal transplantation. Lancet 1978; 1: 574.
2. Pfaff WW, Howard RJ, Ireland J, Scornik J. The effect of Lewis antigen and race on kidney graft survival. Transplant Proc 1983; 15(1): 1139.
3. Fischer E, Lennard V, Rosner W, Dreikorn K, Scharer K, Roelcke D. The Lewis antigen system and its relevance for clinical transplantation. Z Immun-Forsch 1979; 155: 420.
4. Williams G, Pegrum GD, Evans CA. Lewis antigens in renal transplantation. Lancet 1978; 1978: 878.
5. Lenhard V, Roelcke D, Dreikorn K, et al. Significance of Lewis and HLA system in kidney transplantation: a multicenter study in Germany. Transplant Proc 1981; 13(1): 930.
6. Lee HM. Surgical techniques of renal transplantation. In: Morris PJ, ed. Kidney transplantation, 1979; 145.
7. Mollison PL. Blood transfusion in clinical medicine. 6th ed. Oxford: Blackwell, 1972; 255.
8. Kaplan EL, Meier P. Nonparametric estimation from incomplete observations. J Am Stat Assoc 1958; 53: 457.
9. Breslow N. A generalized Kruskal-Wallis test for comparing K samples subject to unequal patterns of censorship. Biometrika 1970; 57: 579.
10. Mantel N. Evaluation of survival data and two new rank order statistics arising in its consideration. Cancer Chemother Rep 1966; 50: 163.
11. Spitalnick S, Pfaff W, Cowles J, Ireland JE, Scornik J, Blumberg N. Correlation of humoral immunity to Lewis blood group antigens with renal transplant rejection. Transplantation 1984; 37: 265.
12. Oriol R, Cartron JP, Cartron J, Mulet C. Biosynthesis of ABH and Lewis antigens in normal and transplanted kidneys. Transplantation 1980; 29: 184.

Received 13 May 1985.
Accepted 1 August 1985.

0041-1337/86/4104-0478$02.00/0
TRANSPLANTATION
Vol. 41, No. 4
Printed in U.S.A.

ADAPTATION OF ADULT BONE MARROW TRANSPLANT RECIPIENT LONG-TERM SURVIVORS

DEANE L. WOLCOTT,[1] DAVID K. WELLISCH, FAWZY I. FAWZY, AND JOHN LANDSVERK

Department of Psychiatry, School of Medicine, Neuropsychiatric Institute, and Liaison Psychiatric Service, University of California at Los Angeles

Although there is a small literature on psychosocial and psychiatric aspects of bone marrow transplants (BMT) in adult recipients during the BMT hospitalization phase, adaptation of long-term adult BMT recipient survivors has received little study.

This study surveyed the adaptation of BMT recipient survivors over age 17 who were an average of 42 months posttransplant. Study variables included the recipients' current self-reported health status, mood state, social role function, self esteem, life satisfaction, and relationships with their BMT donors and other family members. A companion study of those who donated BMT to the recipients eligible for this study was also performed.

The study participants were preponderantly young adults who currently were in an intimate relationship and vocationally active. About ¼ of the subjects reported ongoing medical problems. Also, 15–25% reported significant emotional distress, low self-esteem, and less-than-optimal life satisfaction. The subjects' current quality of relationship with their donors was highly correlated with many measures of their psychosocial status.

The findings indicate that about 75% of BMT recipient long-term survivors are doing well from a psychosocial as well as a medical standpoint, that the recipient-donor relationship may be sensitive to any changes in the recipient's status, and that 15–20% of BMT recipient survivors report a degree of psychological distress that might benefit from specific psychological/psychiatric intervention.

Bone marrow transplantation (BMT)* is an alternative to conventional treatment, for which the primary established indications in adults include severe aplastic anemia and leukemia (*1*). BMT requires a histocompatible donor (usually a sibling). BMT is an arduous procedure associated with significant early morbidity and mortality. Individuals who survive for more than one year posttransplant free of their original disease have a good prognosis for long-term survival.

The estimated number of BMTs performed in the United States in individuals over the age of 18 increased from 125 in 1979 to 550 in 1984 (Bortin M, personal communication). The one-year post-BMT recipient survival rate is about 50–60% (*2*), so there is a small, but increasing, number of adult BMT recipient long-term survivors in the United States.

Ware has indicated that comprehensive assessment of adaptation in individuals who are medically ill should consider biological, personal (self-care, daily activities, mobility), psychological distress/well being, general health perceptions, and social/role function variables (*3*). Multiple previous investigations have indicated that cancer and its treatment can have serious adverse effects on individual functioning in each of the areas Ware has outlined (*4–13*). Holland has advocated that psychosocial research in cancer document the psychosocial adaptation and quality of life of long-term survivors (*14*).

There exists a small body of literature concerning psychiatric aspects of BMT for recipients, donors, family members, and BMT staff during the BMT hospitalization (*15*). An earlier cost-benefit analysis of BMT has included a health professional global estimate of the quality of life of BMT recipient survivors (*16*). However, the authors are aware of no previously published studies concerning the adaptation of adult BMT recipient long-term survivors. Clinically, some BMT recipient survivors report an excellent quality of life, while others have significant medical and psychosocial morbidity. Furthermore, a significant minority of donor-recipient pairs have new or exacerbated interpersonal conflicts after BMT. This is in contrast with living-related kidney transplantation, in which donor psychosocial outcome, and donor-recipient relationship outcome appear to be almost uniformly positive (*17*).

This study focused on adult BMT recipients who had survived at least one year after undergoing BMT. Our major purpose was to document the health status and psychosocial adjustment of BMT recipient survivors who had a good long-term medical prognosis.

This was a cross-sectional study using self-report instruments that assessed demographic, mood state, self-esteem, social adjustment, health status, general health perception, recipient-donor relationship, and recipient attitude about BMT variables. A parallel study was performed simultaneously with BMT donors whose recipient was eligible for this study. The variables studied in these two BMT groups were identical except that health status and social adjustment were not studied in donors. This research strategy allowed for comparison of BMT donors' and recipients' psychosocial status, their perceptions about their relationships, and their attitudes toward bone marrow donation.

MATERIALS AND METHODS

All UCLA BMT recipient survivors who were more than one year post-BMT as of December 1981, who were fluent in English, who lived in the United States, and who were born prior to July 1964, were eligible to participate. The donors to these eligible recipients were eligible for the comparison donor study. Recruitment letters explaining the purposes and procedures of the study were sent to eligible recipients and to their

[1]Address correspondence to: Deane L. Wolcott, M.D., UCLA-NPI, 760 Westwood Plaza, Los Angeles, CA 90024.

* Abbreviations used: BMT, bone marrow transplantation; GVHD, graft-versus-host disease; POMS, profile of mood states; (SAS-SR), Social Adjustment Scale–Self-Report; TMD, total mood disturbance.

donors. When replies to the recruitment letter were not received, and no information was obtained that the recipient was deceased, attempts were made to contact the recipient and/or donor through family members. Subjects who agreed to participate in the study were then sent the research packet containing a further description of the study, two copies of the informed consent form, and the self-report instruments and questionnaires.

From the UCLA BMT records, thirty-six potential recipient subjects who met entrance criteria were identified. Twenty-six subjects (72%) actually returned completed research packets. Of the 10 originally identified potential recipient subjects who did not participate, we were unable to locate 5 (14%), two (6%) agreed to participate but never returned completed packets, and three (8%) did not wish to participate. Eighteen of 36 (50%) potential donors, and 12/36 (33%) of potentially eligible recipient-donor pairs, participated.

The research instruments for the recipients consisted of a demographic questionnaire, a current medical status form, an investigator-constructed recipient questionnaire, the Profile of Mood States (POMS), the Simmons Scale, and the Social Adjustment Scale–Self Report (SAS-SR).

The investigator-constructed current medical status form consisted of multiple-choice questions regarding the recipient's frequency of current systemic symptoms related to the BMT conditioning regimen and/or graft-versus-host disease (GVHD), vegetative functions, infections and medical care utilization in the previous 12 months, and his/her global self-perceived current health status.

The recipient questionnaire was a 63-item multiple-choice instrument that asked recipients about their current positive mood, the degree of current approval they felt from family members, their current life satisfaction in five areas, and the intensity, (positive) quality, and degree of conflict in their relationship with their donors, both prior to the BMT and in the previous three months. It also asked about recipients' general attitudes about BMT and bone marrow donation.

The POMS is a 65-question self-report adjective checklist with six subscales including tension/anxiety, depression, anger, fatigue, vigor, and confusion/bewilderment. The POMS measures mood disturbance in the previous week and has college student and psychiatric outpatient reference group data (*18*). It has previously been used in studying cancer patients (*19*).

The Simmons Scale is a 9-item self-report measure of self-esteem adapted from the Rosenberg Self-Esteem Scale (*20*). Simmons has documented improvement in the self-esteem of chronic dialysis patients after successful kidney transplantation using this scale, as well as reliability and validity data (*12, 21*).

The Weissman SAS-SR is a 54-item questionnaire with seven subscales in the expressive or role-function areas of work, social/leisure activities, marital, parental, economic, family, and extended-family relationships. Weissman has reported reliability and validity data on the SAS-SR, and reference group data for psychiatric patient groups as well as for a community sample (*22–24*). The SAS-SR has been used in psychosocial studies of chronic hemodialysis patients (*25*).

BMT donor subjects were asked to complete a shorter packet consisting of the same demographic questionnaire, the POMS, The Simmons Scale, and a donor questionnaire. The donor questionnaire asked identical (but reciprocally worded) questions about the donor's perceptions of the donor-recipient relationship pretransplant and in the past three months, as well as his/her experience of, and attitudes about, BMT. Both donors and recipients were encouraged to make written comments about their reactions to the BMT and its effects on their lives.

Data Analysis

The recipients' age, sex, marital status, educational history, religious preference, and current vocational status were assessed. Recipients' original disease diagnoses and the interval in months from BMT to study participation were also documented.

The subjects' POMS responses were coded, and scores were calculated for each of the six subscales. A total mood disturbance (TMD) score was also calculated for each recipient using standard techniques (*18*). Higher POMS subscale and TMD scores indicate greater mood disturbance.

The Simmons Scale was scored for each subject according to Simmons' method. The potential range of scores on the Simmons scale is 0–9, with higher scores indicating greater self-esteem (*21*).

A current *family approval* score was determined for each subject based on responses to two recipient questionnaire questions about the general degree of approval the subject felt from parents and siblings, as well as response to a question about any experiences of major family disapproval.

A *Positive Mood* score was obtained from each subject's responses to 5 questions about happiness and cheerfulness "today" and "in general," and his/her endorsement of the statement "I get a lot of fun out of life." Current life satisfaction was assessed by single-item replies in the five areas of work/school, leisure, family life, friendships, and health and physical condition.

Recipient-donor relationship characteristics were assessed for two time dimensions (prior to BMT, and the previous 3 months), and for three relationship characteristics. The relationship characteristics assessed were intensity (3 questions of interactional frequency), positive quality (5 questions indicating positive emotional support from the other person), and conflict (one question each about anger, arguments, and avoidance).

The recipient's current global illness variable score was based on the subject's reply to one question self-rating his/her overall health in the last 3 months as excellent, good, fair, or poor. Subjects' responses were scored 1–4, with a higher score indicating poorer health.

Individual SAS-SR subscale mean scores were calculated for each subject using Weissman's method (*24*). The potential range of subscale mean scores in each area is 1–5. A higher individual mean subscale score indicates increased self-rated impairment in that role area in the previous two weeks.

Comparisons between groups were analyzed by means of t tests. Tests for equality of variance determined the specific P value. Comparisons of perceived relationship characteristics before BMT and currently were analyzed by constructing change scores (current–before BMT) and comparing the recipient and donor change scores by means of t tests. Throughout, the significance level was set at .05.

Intercorrelations of the global health, interval in months, POMS-TMD, Simmons Scale, SAS-SR subscale scores, and recipient-donor relationship variables were assessed by calculating Pearson product-moment correlation coefficients.

The BMT donor group scores for mood state (POMS-TMD), self-esteem (Simmons Scale), donor-recipient relationship characteristics, and current life satisfaction were scored using the same methods, and are reported for comparison.

RESULTS

Demographic. Table 1 shows the demographic characteristics of the recipient participants. Sixteen females and ten males participated, with an average age of 27.9 (range 17–51). Of the 26 subjects, 15 (58%) were married, and 2 others (8%) were living with a sexual partner. Their average level of education was two years of college. At the time of the study 84% were actively participating in work, school, or household activities. Their original disease diagnoses were exactly split between severe aplastic anemia (50%) and leukemia (50%). The average interval between the BMT and completion of the research packet was 42 months. Thus, this was a preponderantly young adult population, most of whom were well educated, currently vocationally active, living with a sexual partner, and—on average—3½ years post-BMT.

TABLE 1. Demographic and disease characteristics of BMT recipients

Characteristic				n (26)	%
Original diagnosis	Aplastic anemia			13	50.0%
	Acute myelogenous leukemia			7	26.9%
	Acute lymphocytic leukemia			3	11.5%
	Chronic myelogenous leukemia			3	11.5%
Sex	Female			16	61.5%
	Male			10	38.5%
Marital status	Single			9	34.6%
	Married			15	57.7%
	Living with sexual partner			2	7.7%
Employment status	Employed full-time			9	34.6%
	Maintaining household			6	23.1%
	In school full-time or part-time			7	26.9%
	Unemployed/retired			4	15.4%
Ethnicity	Caucasian			18	69.2%
	Hispanic			6	23.1%
	Asian-American			2	7.7%
Age (years)	Mean = 27.9	SD = 8.3	Range = 17–51		
Education (years)	Mean = 14.6	SD = 3.9	Range = 8–20		
Interval between BMT and study (months)	Mean = 42	SD = 21.7	Range = 19–91		

TABLE 2. Current frequency of selected symptoms for BMT recipients

Symptom	Never/rarely		Frequently/always	
	n	%	n	%
Dry mouth	18	72.0%	7	28.0%
Mouth soreness	19	73.1%	7	26.9%
Trouble swallowing	24	92.3%	2	7.7%
Nausea	24	92.3%	2	7.7%
Vomiting	24	92.3%	2	7.7%
Abdominal cramps/pain	21	80.8%	5	19.2%
Diarrhea	19	73.1%	7	26.9%
Skin rash	23	88.5%	3	11.5%
Skin itching	19	73.1%	7	26.9%

Current health status. Table 2 shows the subjects' responses to selected questions from the author-constructed current medical status questionnaire. Between 8–28% of the recipient respondents indicated they currently had each symptom *frequently* or *always*, and 15% (n = 4) rated their current symptoms of graft-versus-host disease as being *moderate* or *severe*.

A total of 80% of participants indicated that they were usually at least moderately well rested on awakening, 84% that food had regained its usual taste, 88% that their appetite was at least as good as usual, and 76% that their current weight was at least 85% of their ideal weight.

About one-third of the recipients (Table 3) reported a high number of infections (colds, pneumonia, or other major infections) and a significant number of visits to a physician in the year prior to study participation. Emergency room visits were reported by 35% (n = 9), and 15% (n = 4) reported one or more hospitalizations within the previous 12 months. Of the 25 recipients who responded to the question about their current health, 4 (16%) rated it *excellent*, 13 (52%) rated their health *good*, 7 (28%) rated it *fair*, and 1 (4%) rated her health *poor*.

Mood states. Figure 1 shows the scores of four groups on the POMS. These include two BMT recipient groups categorized by sex (males n = 10, females n = 16), and two BMT donor groups (males n = 12, females n = 6). Group mean POMS subscale *t* scores for each group are shown with reference to a historical healthy college student sample (*18*). A *t* score of 50 is equal to the reference group mean score, with each 10-point score interval greater or less than 50 equalling 1 SD from the mean. The POMS-TMD scores shown are group mean raw scores.

The male and female BMT recipient subjects did not have significantly different group mean POMS subscale or total mood disturbance scores. Female BMT recipients had higher group mean POMS scores than female BMT donors on the tension/anxiety (12.1 vs. 5.2, *P* = .03), depression (10.6 vs. 4.0,

TABLE 3. Illness episodes and use of medical services last 12 months

Illness episode/use of service		n	%
Colds	Less than two	14	56.0%
	Two-to-four	7	28.0%
	Five or more	4	16.0%
Pneumonia	None	22	88.0%
	One	2	8.0%
	Two or more	1	4.0%
Other major infections	None	18	69.2%
	One	4	15.4%
	Two or more	4	15.4%
Physician/clinic visits	Less than three	13	54.2%
	Three-to-ten	7	29.2%
	Eleven to twenty	2	8.3%
	Twenty-one or more	2	8.3%
Emergency room visits	None	15	62.5%
	One	5	20.3%
	Two	4	16.7%
Hospitalizations	None	22	84.6%
	One	2	7.7%
	Two or more	2	7.7%

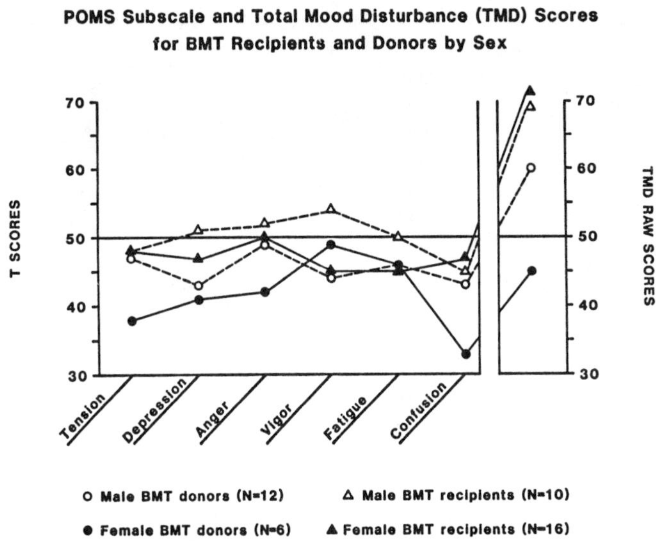

FIGURE 1. Group mean POMS subscale *t* scores and raw total mood disturbance (TMD) scores for 4 post-BMT groups: male and female recipients, male and female donors. The *t* scores are with reference to a historical heterosexual group of healthy college students (n = 856). For each subscale a *t* 50 score equals the reference group mean score with each 10-point score interval above or below 50 equalling 1 SD from the mean. The TMD group mean raw scores were calculated—using standard techniques—adding the five negative subscale scores plus the negative vigor (32-vigor) subscale score. The significance of group subscale and TMD score differences are reported in the text of the papers.

$P = .10$), anger (9.7 vs. 4.0, $P = .07$), and confusion (9.6 vs. 3.0, $P = .02$) subscales, as well as on the POMS total mood disturbance score (71.4 vs. 45, $P = .04$).

The male BMT recipients had nonsignificantly higher group mean scores than the male BMT donor group on the POMS depression (14.0 vs. 6.1), anger (11.0 vs. 8.5), and fatigue (10.4 vs. 7.6) subscales, and on the POMS-TMD (69.8 vs. 60.0). Thus male and female BMT recipients reported higher levels of anxiety, depression, anger, and total mood disturbance than did sex-matched BMT donors. Of 25 BMT recipients, 5 had POMS-TMD scores greater than 100, and higher scores than any of the BMT donors studied.

For the twelve matched pairs of BMT donors and recipients who participated in this study, the recipient group had almost significantly higher mean POMS-TMD scores than the donor group (82.4 vs. 56.8, $P = .07$). All POMS subscale scores in the recipient groups were highly intercorrelated with each other and with the POMS-TMD score.

Self-esteem. The recipients' group mean Simmons score was nonsignificantly lower than the BMT donor group's mean Simmons score (4.6 vs. 5.1), indicating slightly lower self-esteem in the recipient group. The BMT recipients' group mean Simmon's score was moderately lower than the group mean scores of 117 previously studied nondiabetic kidney transplant recipients with a functioning kidney transplant (4.6 vs. 5.3) (Simmons R, personal communication).

Recipient donor self-ratings of current life satisfaction areas. Table 4 compares the BMT recipient and donor groups' self-ratings of their current life satisfaction. Subjects' replies were divided into those who reported being at least "quite a bit" satisfied with each life area, and those who reported lesser degrees of current life satisfaction. Although the donor group had a higher percentage of highly satisfied ratings in 4/5 of these life areas, about ¾ of the recipients indicated a high level of current satisfaction with relationships and activities.

Social adjustment scale–self report. Table 5 indicates the mean scores in each role performance area for BMT recipients by sex compared with a historical healthy community sample (*24*). The BMT recipient groups' mean SAS-SR subscale scores tended to be higher than the community sample groups' mean scores, but these differences did not reach statistical significance. The relatively small absolute differences in group mean SAS-SR subscale scores between the BMT recipient and community sample groups suggests that the BMT recipients' current level of social role function was very similar to that of the healthy general population. The SAS-SR results are consistent

TABLE 4. Percentage of BMT recipients and donors expressing life satisfaction[a]

Area of satisfaction	Recipients (n = 25)	Donors (n = 18)
Work/school	68.0%	82.4%
Leisure	68.0%	88.9%
Family life	72.0%	88.9%
Friendships	84.0%	83.3%
Health and physical condition	64.0%	72.2%

[a] Life satisfaction was indicated by subject choosing the response category "quite a bit" or more for each particular life area.

TABLE 5. Social adjustment scale–self report scores for BMT recipients and community respondents by sex

Role areas	Sample	Males			Females		
		(n)	Mean[a]	(SD)	(n)	mean	(SD)
Work	BMT	(8)	1.48	(0.42)	(11)	1.76	(0.75)
	Community	(127)	1.26	(0.31)	(272)	1.46	(0.50)
Social/leisure	BMT	(10)	2.24	(0.57)	(16)	1.95	(0.64)
	Community	(205)	1.83	(0.51)	(277)	1.83	(0.53)
Extended family	BMT	(10)	1.65	(0.52)	(16)	1.71	(0.75)
	Community	(201)	1.33	(0.31)	(274)	1.34	(0.35)
Marital	BMT	(8)	1.63	(0.33)	(9)	1.91	(0.61)
	Community	(170)	1.72	(0.46)	(191)	1.77	(0.49)
Parenting	BMT	(5)	1.60	(0.29)	(8)	1.47	(0.36)
	Community	(101)	1.35	(0.41)	(175)	1.43	(0.43)
Family unit	BMT	(7)	1.86	(0.26)	(9)	1.78	(0.82)
	Community	(194)	1.35	(0.51)	(270)	1.54	(0.62)
Economics	BMT	(10)	2.10	(1.45)	(15)	1.87	(1.46)

[a] High scores in each role area indicate more self-reported role impairment.

with the demographic information that most BMT recipients were vocationally active, and 65% of recipients were involved in intimate relationships. No statistically significant differences were found on any group mean SAS-SR subscale scores between male and female BMT recipients.

Recipient-donor relationship and attitudes toward donation. Table 6 shows the group mean scores for the recipient-donor relationship variables for the recipient and donor groups, prior to the BMT and currently. In general the results indicate remarkably congruent perceptions between the recipient and donor groups about their relationships at both intervals. Recipients reported nonsignificantly less conflict in their relationships with their donors for both periods than the BMT donors reported. Recipients perceived little change in the intensity and quality of their relationship with their donors from prior to the BMT to the present. These findings were mirrored in the reports of the 12 matched recipient-donor pairs.

There were no significant differences between the recipient and donor groups on the current *positive mood* and *family approval* variable scores constructed from the recipient (and donor) questionnaires. Recipients who reported less work-role impairment on the SAS-SR also tended to have high family approval scores ($r = -.72$, $P = .002$).

A total of 96% of recipients agreed that a BM donor is "almost a hero," 78% felt that BM donation is "a sacrifice out of the ordinary," and 76% indicated that they had felt a special obligation to the donor since the BMT.

Intercorrelations of study variables. Table 7 presents the intercorrelations of the adaptation variables studied. Recipients' self-esteem scores (Simmons Scale) were strongly negatively correlated with the POMS-TMD, global health, and 6/7 SAS-SR subscale scores. Thus, health status, social role function, mood state, and self-esteem tend to improve or deteriorate together in BMT recipients.

The interval in months from BMT to study participation variable negatively correlated with the *global current illness* score, indicating that self-rated health status improved with time after BMT. The interval-in-months variable was not significantly correlated with any of the psychosocial variables measured.

TABLE 6. Reported recipient-donor relationship characteristics before BMT and currently by recipients and donors

Relationship characteristic	Sample	Before BMT Mean	Before BMT (SD)	Current Mean	Current (SD)
Total study group:					
Intensity[a]	Recipients (n = 26)	13.6	(4.4)	13.0	(3.5)
	Donors (n = 18)	13.1	(3.8)	14.3	(2.9)
Quality[b]	Recipients	17.3	(4.0)	17.4	(4.7)
	Donors	16.3	(4.4)	17.7	(4.3)
Conflict[c]	Recipients	4.6	(1.8)	4.0	(1.8)
	Donors	5.7	(2.3)	5.2	(1.7)
Matched recipient-donor pairs:					
Intensity[a]	Recipients (n = 12)	12.9	(4.8)	12.6	(4.4)
	Donors (n = 12)	11.6	(5.4)	12.8	(3.4)
Quality[b]	Recipients	15.4	(4.4)	16.5	(5.5)
	Donors	15.6	(6.3)	17.4	(6.0)
Conflict[a]	Recipients	4.8	(2.1)	3.3	(0.6)
	Donors	5.8	(3.5)	5.0	(2.3)

[a] High intensity indicates greater frequency of interaction.
[b] High quality indicates greater emotional support from the other person.
[c] High conflict indicates greater conflict in the relationship.

TABLE 7. Selected intercorrelations among recipient adaptation variables

	BMT study interval	Global illness	POMS-TMD	Self-esteem	Recipient-donor relationship quality
Global illness[a]	−.41[b]		−.50[b]	−.60[c]	−.27
POMS-TMD[d]	−.22	.50[b]		−.57[c]	−.40
Self-esteem[e]	.40	−.60[c]	−.57[c]		.66[c]
Relationship quality[f]	.17	−.27	−.40	.66[c]	
SAS-SR work[g]	−.10	.58[c]	.85[c]	−.64[c]	−.57[c]
SAS-SR social/leisure	−.14	.10	.28	−.47[b]	−.57[c]
SAS-SR extended family	−.23	.50[c]	.70[c]	−.65[c]	−.61[c]
SAS-SR marital	−.30	.46	.34	−.60[c]	−.66[c]
SAS-SR parenting	−.05	.29	.02	−.14	−.23
SAS-SR family	.13	.59[b]	.74[c]	−.69[c]	−.55[b]
SAS-SR economics	−.10	.18	.34	−.44[b]	−.30

[a] High current global illness scores indicates poor health.
[b] $P<.05$.
[c] $P<.01$.
[d] POMS-TMD high score indicates more total mood disturbance.
[e] High score indicates high self-esteem.
[f] High recipient-donor relationship quality score indicates more current positive emotional support received from the donor, as perceived by the recipient.
[g] High SAS-SR subscale scores indicate more role impairment.

The current recipient-donor relationship quality variable (as perceived by the recipient) was significantly positively correlated with recipient self-esteem and with decreased recipient social role impairment.

Comparison of BMT recipients by original disease diagnosis. There were no significant demographic, health status, mood state, self-esteem, social role function, or recipient-donor relationship differences between the two recipient groups categorized by the original disease diagnosis of severe aplastic anemia (n = 13), or by a form of leukemia (n = 13).

DISCUSSION

It is highly probable that most, if not all, of these subjects would not have been alive at the time of this study if they had not undergone BMT. The fact of their survival represents a triumph of medical technology. A potential problem in societal/medical ethics arises when one considers the quantity of resources expended to achieve the survival of even one BMT recipient, balanced against the limits in the resources available to the health care system. In the face of this dilemma documentation of the adaptation of long-term survivors takes on increased significance. This study was an attempt to provide a relatively comprehensive view of adult BMT long-term survivors with assessment of current health, psychological state, social/role function, and recipient-donor relationship variables.

The high study participation rate of eligible subjects (72%), and of those actually contacted (84%), indicates the gratitude these individuals felt towards the BMT team for saving their lives. This participation rate reflects a high likelihood of having obtained a reasonably unbiased sample of the population of then-current UCLA adult BMT recipient long-term survivors.

A major finding in this study was the frequency of chronic physical symptoms in these BMT recipients: about ¼ of these subjects reported significant physical symptoms, high rates of infections, and high medical care utilization—on the other hand, about 70% reported current good health.

Although the recipient' mood disturbance (POMS-TMD) scores were not remarkably higher than a reference group of college students, they do indicate that the recipient group has more current emotional distress than was present in the group of bone marrow donors. The recipients' relatively low TMD scores support the tenet that cancer patients do not manifest high levels of psychological symptoms when they are not in extraordinarily stressful circumstances (*26*). The other measures of the recipients' current subjective state also indicated that they had a mildly less-positive emotional balance than BM donors, which may represent a residual adverse psychological effect of their original illness, and its treatment, on their lives. Their self-rated current role functioning indicated somewhat more impairment than reported by a historical healthy community sample (*24*). Thus, on a number of measures of functional status and subjective state most BMT recipients compared quite favorably with healthy control or reference groups. The lack of correlation between the interval since BMT and the psychosocial variables indicates that a recipient's level of adaptation will not necessarily improve with time alone. Health status is clearly related to psychosocial measures of adaptation in BMT recipients, so that poor health status in recipients may be an indicator of poor psychosocial adaptation.

The recipients and donors had very similar views of the impact of BMT on their relationship. We predicted the data would show that BMT had exerted a strong effect on the recipient-donor relationship, either positively or negatively. This hypothesis was not borne out by the data.

The highly significant correlations between the recipient-donor current relationship quality variable, self-esteem, current global health, POMS-TMD, and 5/7 social adjustment subscale scores in the recipient group was not expected. The donor's reported current donor-recipient relationship quality variable was also highly correlated with 5/7 recipient social adjustment subscale scores (*27*). The quality of the donor-recipient relationship, as perceived by both recipient and donor, may be highly sensitive to changes in the recipient's health and psychosocial status. A recipient's deterioration might have significant adverse psychological consequences for his/her donor, and on their relationship.

The study design allows comparison of the adaptation of BMT recipients with historical reference population groups only, and not with the most relevant comparison group, which would be long-term conventionally treated survivors with the same disease. The design also does not allow discrimination among premorbid adaptation, illness effects, and modality-specific effects on recipients' current level of adaptation.

Potential limits to the generalization of these findings arise because all participants were from only one BMT center, the design was cross-sectional, and the sample size was small. Current patient selection criteria also differ in many centers from the late 1970s, when many of these subjects received transplants. BMT recipients from programs providing routine psychosocial support services in the posttransplant period might have an even more favorable experience.

The results do indicate that the majority of BMT recipient long-term survivors have an objectively and subjectively acceptable level of functioning. A number of aspects of psychosocial status appear to be highly intercorrelated with each other, and with health status, in these individuals.

Although the findings of this study are generally quite positive, about 15–25% of long-term BMT recipient survivors may have significant psychological distress and poor adaptation. This finding suggests that clinicians treating this special group of patients should be alert to evidence of psychological distress, particularly in recipients who are having continuing health problems.

Determining whether routine use of a brief psychological-state screening instrument such as the POMS can effectively and accurately identify the highly distressed BMT recipient—and whether psychiatric intervention can effectively relieve the distress of such identified individuals—should be a high priority of research on BMT recipient outcome.

The present study is only a start in investigation of the adaptation of long-term BMT survivors. Clearly, prospective longitudinal research is needed to more accurately document the acute and chronic psychosocial consequences of undergoing BMT.

The existence of posthospitalization psychosocial phases of BMT (such as have been described in cancer patients [*28*]); the incidence, severity, duration and reversibility of cognitive dysfunction (*15*); and the predictors (if any) of poor psychosocial outcome and need for psychosocial intervention in BMT recipient survivors can only be adequately studied by such prospective longitudinal research.

REFERENCES

1. Gale RP (ed). Recent advances in bone marrow transplantation. New York: AR Liss, 1983.
2. Gale RP. Progress in bone marrow transplantation in man. Surv Immunol Res 1982; 1: 40.
3. Ware JE, Jr. Conceptualizing disease impact and treatment outcomes cancer 1984; 53(suppl): 2316.
4. Petty F, Noyes R Jr. Depression secondary to cancer. Biol Psychiatry 1981; 16: 1203.
5. Derogatis LR, Morrow GR, Fetting J, et al. The prevalence of psychiatric disorders among cancer patients. JAMA 1983; 249: 751.
6. Meyerowtiz BE, Heinrich RL, Schag CC. A competency-based approach to coping with cancer. In: Burish TG, Bradley LA, eds. Coping with chronic disease: research and applications. New York: Academic Press, 1983: 137.
7. Singer JE. Some issues in the study of coping. Cancer 1984; 53(suppl): 2303.
8. Silberfarb PM, Maurer LH, Crouthamel CS. Psychosocial aspects of neoplastic disease. I. Functional status of breast cancer patients during different treatment regimens. Am J Psychiatry 1980; 137: 450.
9. Sanders JB. Adaptive coping mechanisms in adult leukemia patients in remission. JAMA 1977; 238: 952.
10. Silberfarb PM, Greer S. Psychological concomitants of cancer: clinical aspects. Am J Psychother 1982; 36: 470.
11. Wellisch DK. Work, social recreation, family, and physical status. Cancer 1984; 53(suppl): 2290.
12. Feldman FL. Work and cancer health histories. In: Cohen J, Cullen JW, Martin LR, eds. Psychosocial aspects of cancer. New York: Raven Press, 1982: 199.
13. Wortman CB. Social support and the cancer patient: conceptual and methodologic issues. Cancer 1984; 53(suppl): 2339.
14. Holland JCB. Need for improved psychosocial research methodology: goals and potentials. Cancer 1984; 53(suppl): 2218.
15. Wolcott DL, Fawzy FI, Wellisch DK. Psychiatric aspects of bone marrow transplantation: a review and current issues. Psychiatr Medicine (in press).
16. Schweitzer SO, Scalzi CC, Keating MV. Social cost versus effectiveness of bone marrow transplant therapy. UCLA Cancer Center Bulletin 1979; 6(1): 3.

17. Simmons RG. Long-term reactions of renal recipients and donors. In: Levy NB ed. Psychonephrology, vol 2. New York: Plenum, 1983: 275.
18. McNair DM, Lorr M, Droppleman LF. Manual for the profile of mood states. San Diego: Education and Industrial Testing Service, 1981.
19. Weisman AD, Worden JW, Sobel HJ. Psychosocial screening and intervention with cancer patients. National Cancer Institute 1980; CA 19797.
20. Rosenberg M. Society and the adolescent self image. Princeton, NJ: Princeton University Press, 1965.
21. Simmons RG, Klein SD, Simmons RL. Gift of life: the social and psychological impact of organ transplantation. New York: Wiley, 1977.
22. Weissman MM, Sholomskas D, John K. The assessment of social adjustment: an update. Arch Gen Psychiatry 1981; 38: 1250.
23. Weissman MD, Bothwell S. Assessment of social adjustment by patient self-report. Arch Gen Psychiatry 1976; 33: 1111.
24. Weissman MD, Prusoff B, Thompson WD, Harding PS, Myers JK. Social adjustment by self-report in a community sample and in psychiatric outpatients. J Nerv Ment Dis 1978; 166: 317.
25. Maher BA, Lamping DL, Dickinson CA, et al. Psychosocial aspects of chronic hemodialysis: the national cooperative dialysis study. Kidney Int 1983; 23(suppl 13): S-50.
26. Bloom JR, Ross RD. Measurement of the psychosocial aspects of cancer: sources of bias. In: Cohen J, Cullen JW, Morton LR, eds. Psychosocial aspects of cancer. New York: Raven Press, 1982: 255.
27. Wolcott DL, Wellisch DK, Fawzy FI, Landsverk J. Psychological adjustment of adult bone marrow transplant donors whose recipient survives. Transplantation 1986; 41: 484.
28. Weisman AD. A model for psychosocial phasing in cancer. Gen Hosp Psychiatry 1979; 1: 187.

Received 5 March 1985.
Accepted 24 July 1985.

0041-1337/86/4104-0484$02.00/0
TRANSPLANTATION
Vol. 41, No. 4
Printed in U.S.A.

PSYCHOLOGICAL ADJUSTMENT OF ADULT BONE MARROW TRANSPLANT DONORS WHOSE RECIPIENT SURVIVES

DEANE L. WOLCOTT,[1] DAVID K. WELLISCH, FAWZY I. FAWZY, AND JOHN LANDSVERK

Department of Psychiatry, School of Medicine, Neuropsychiatric Institute, and Liaison Psychiatric Service, University of California at Los Angeles

The psychosocial and psychiatric impact of donating bone marrow (BM) has received little study. This mail questionnaire study of bone marrow donors whose recipient had survived more than one year post-BMT was undertaken to document the psychosocial consequences of donation on "successful" BM donors.

Demographic, mood state, self-esteem, current life satisfaction, and donor-recipient relationship characteristics, donor-perceived approval from family members, and donor attitudes about BM donation were studied.

A companion study of BM recipients was also performed to provide comparative data on the psychosocial status of donors and recipients.

As a group BM donors manifested little emotional distress, high self-esteem, and a high degree of current life satisfaction. Donors reported little change in their relationships with their recipients since the BMT. However the current quality of their relationships with their recipients was highly correlated with several recipient health status and psychosocial variables, suggesting that recipient deterioration might significantly adversely impact donor psychosocial status. From 10% to 20% of donors indicated at least some negative consequences of donating.

[1]Address correspondence to: Deane L. Wolcott, M.D., UCLA-NPI, 760 Westwood Plaza, Los Angeles, CA 90024.

Bone marrow (BM) transplantation in adults is primarily performed in recipients who have severe aplastic anemia or certain forms of leukemia. The number of bone marrow transplants has been increasing rapidly in the last 6–8 years, in adults and children. The Statistical Center of the International Bone Marrow Transplant Registry has estimated that 1000 bone marrow transplants (BMT) were performed in the United States in 1984, approximately 55% (550) of them in individuals over age 18 (*1*). Although BMT recipient survival figures vary according to the patient's age, underlying disease process, and other variables, approximately 50–60% of BMT recipients survive at least one year posttransplant (*2*).

The long-term psychological effects of donating bone marrow have received little attention in the literature. Two major factors probably account for this: the donation of bone marrow is a minor surgical procedure that ordinarily has no associated significant physical morbidity; and the literature concerning kidney donation indicates that the long-term psychological adjustment of living-related kidney donors is very positive, even if the transplant fails (*3*).

However a number of psychologically important differences exist between bone marrow and living-related kidney donation. The BMT recipient candidate has a life-threatening illness for which there is no alternative curative or chronically life-sustaining procedure. Living-related kidney transplant recipient candidates have access to other life-sustaining treatment alternatives, including cadaveric transplantation. Thus, the potential living-related kidney donor is never in the position of being the only possible rescuer of his/her family member. The timing of the living-related kidney transplant is essentially elective, whereas the timing of BMT is usually more urgent. Kidney donation is widely recognized as being an extraordinary altruistic act, while donating bone marrow (which rapidly regenerates) usually brings much less praise for the donor.

Additionally, a major cause of BMT recipient morbidity and mortality is graft-versus-host disease, in which the donor's transplanted BM immunologically attacks the recipient's skin and internal organs. Thus, the BM donor is at risk of feeling that the donated tissue caused the recipient's morbidity or death.

Previous reports have anecdotally described BMT donor psychological problems mainly in terms of donor guilt, in the early postdonation period (*4–8*). These reports have led to suggestions that postdonation adverse psychological responses in donors are frequent and severe enough that routine predonation psychiatric evaluation might be indicated (*6, 7*).

One might assume that when the BMT recipient does well medically the psychological effect on the donor, and the course of the donor-recipient relationship, would be uniformly positive. However, our clinical experience at UCLA has been that some donor-recipient relationships have become estranged even though the recipient became a long-term disease-free survivor.

This study was undertaken to obtain information about selected aspects of the psychosocial adjustment of adult BMT donors including their mood state, self-esteem, and psychological reactions to BM donation. Another focus concerned the donor's perceptions of changes in the donor-recipient relationship from the predonation period to the present. This was a companion study of a study of adult BMT recipient long-term survivors. The study of BMT recipients examined the same variables and used the same instruments as the BMT donor study, and additionally included measures of current health status and social role function (*9*). Attempts were made to study as many donor-recipient pairs as possible in parallel.

MATERIALS AND METHODS

Many of the BMT donors (and recipients) eligible to participate in this study lived at a great distance from UCLA, and no longer received medical care at UCLA, so it was decided to use mailed self-report investigator-constructed questionnaires and standardized research instruments. UCLA BMT recipients transplanted from the inception of the BMT program until December 1980 who were still alive in December 1981, fluent in English, lived in the United States, and born prior to July 1964 were eligible for the study. All donors whose recipient met these criteria were eligible to participate in the donor study. These criteria were chosen to obtain information about the long-term psychosocial effects of donating on successful donors, whose recipient had a good prognosis for long-term disease-free survival.

Eighteen of 36 eligible donors (50%) returned completed research packets. We were unable to locate 10 (28%) of the eligible donor subjects. Seven (19%) of the eligible donors indicated interest but never returned completed packets, and 1 (3%) refused. Twenty-six of 36 eligible recipients (72%) returned completed packets. Twelve matched donor-recipient pairs participated (33%). We have no information about the characteristics of eligible BMT donors who did not participate.

Procedures. Donors were contacted by letter. Donors who indicated their willingness to participate were sent a study packet that included two copies of the informed consent form, a demographic questionnaire, the Profile of Mood States (POMS), an investigator-constructed donor questionnaire, and the Simmons Scale. The Profile of Mood States is a 65-question adjective self-report checklist, with six subscales measuring mood state within the last seven days; it has reference group norms (*10*). The Simmons Scale is a 9-item self-report measure of self-esteem previously used in her studies of adaptation of living-related kidney donors and recipients (*11*). The donor questionnaire is a 63-item investigator-constructed multiple-choice questionnaire that measures aspects of the donor's experience of, and attitudes about, BM donation, as well as the donor's perceptions of his/her relationship with the recipient before the donation and currently. A reciprocally worded recipient questionnaire with otherwise-identical questions was used in the parallel study of BMT recipients.

Data Analysis

Demographics. Demographic characteristics of the donor group were compiled, as well as their recipients' original disease diagnoses, and the interval in months between donation and study participation.

Profile of mood states and Simmons scale. The Profile of Mood States responses were coded, and individual scores were calculated for each of the six subscales of tension/anxiety, depression, anger, fatigue, confusion, and vigor. A *total mood disturbance* (TMD) score was also calculated for each subject using standard techniques (*10*). Higher POMS subscale and TMD scores indicate more psychological distress.

The Simmons self-esteem score was determined for each subject using Simmons' scoring procedures (*11*). The range of scores on the Simmons Scale is 0–9, with higher scores indicating higher self-esteem.

Donor questionnaire. Variable scores constructed from donor questionnaire items included current *family approval, positive mood*, and donor-recipient relationship scores. The donor-recipient relationship variables were intensity, positive quality, and conflict, as reported for two periods—prior to the BMT and in the previous three months. The details of the variable construction scoring are reported in the companion report on BMT recipient adaptation (*9*). Additionally, multiple questions were asked of the donors concerning their predonation decision-making process and feelings and their postdonation positive and negative reactions to being a BM donor.

The recipient variables studied included all donor variables studied, as well as measures of recipients' current global health status and social role function. Recipient's social role function was measured by the Weissman Social Adjustment Scale-Self Report (SAS-SR), which measures self-assessed instrumental or expressive role performance in the previous two weeks in the role areas of work, social/leisure, extended family, marital, parental, family, and economic function (*12, 13*). Higher recipient SAS-SR scores indicate more self-rated social role impairment.

The recipient *current global illness* score was calculated from a self-rated current health status question, with response options from *excellent* (scored 1) to *poor* (scored 4).

Intercorrelations between variables. Pearson product-moment correlations of the interval (time in months since donation), mood disturbance (POMS-TMD), self-esteem (Simmons Scale), donor-recipient relationship (intensity, quality, conflict both pre-BMT and currently), donor family approval, and donor positive mood variable scores were then determined. Correlations between the donor variable and recipient variable scores were also determined for the subgroup of 12 matched donor-recipient pairs. Intergroup comparisons were analyzed by means of paired *t* tests.

RESULTS

Table 1 shows the demographic characteristics of the donor subjects. On average they had donated about 3½ years before participating in the study (range 18–89 months). They were mostly young adults.

Figure 1 of the companion report (*9*) shows group mean Profile of Mood States (POMS) subscale scores comparing male donors (n = 12), female donors (n = 6), male recipients (n = 10), and female recipients (n = 16). The POMS group mean subscale scores are shown as *t* scores in comparison with a healthy college reference group (n = 856) (*10*). Male donors had significantly higher POMS tension/anxiety (P = .03), confusion (P = .007), and TMD (P = .03) scores than female donors. However almost all individual donor POMS subscale scores were well within 1 SD of the mean scores of the college reference group. The donor group's mean POMS depression, anger, confusion, and TMD scores were nonsignificantly lower than the comparable scores of the BMT recipient group; 20% (5/25) of the recipients had POMS TMD scores that were higher than those of any BMT donor, another indicator that the BMT donors were less distressed than BMT recipients.

On the current *family approval* and *positive mood* variables, the BMT donor and recipient groups had similar mean scores. The donor group's mean Simmons Scale score (5.1) indicated very positive self-esteem in the donor group and was comparable to scores of a previously studied group of living-related kidney donors 5–9 years after donation (mean score = 5.3, n = 84) (Simmons R, personal communication). The BMT donor group's mean Simmons Scale score was nonsignificantly higher than the BMT recipient group's mean score (5.1 vs. 4.6).

TABLE 1. Demographic characteristics of BMT donors

Characteristic		n (18)	%
Sex	Female	12	66.7%
	Male	6	33.3%
Marital status	Single	6	33.3%
	Married	11	61.1%
	Divorced	1	5.6%
Employment status	Employed full-time	12	66.7%
	Employed part-time	2	11.1%
	Maintaining household	1	5.6%
	In school full-time or part-time	3	16.7%
Ethnicity	Caucasian	13	72.2%
	Hispanic	4	22.2%
	Asian-American	1	5.6%
Original diagnosis of recipient	Aplastic anemia	11	61.1%
	Acute myelogenous leukemia	5	27.8%
	Acute lymphocytic leukemia	1	5.6%
	Chronic myelogenous leukemia	1	5.6%
Age (years)	Mean = 28.8 SD = 7.5	Range = 17–49	
Education (years)	Mean = 13.7 SD = 2.1	Range = 11–18	
Interval between BMT and study (months)	Mean = 42.9 SD = 19.9	Range = 18–89	

Donor's responses to the *current life satisfaction* question are shown in Table 4 of the accompanying report (*9*). As compared with recipients' responses, a higher percentage of donors indicated high current satisfaction in 4/5 life areas.

Table 6 of the companion BMT recipient study report (*9*) shows the donors' ratings of the intensity, quality, and conflict in their relationships with their recipients. The donors as a group reported little change in their relationships with their recipients from before the BMT to the present. Donors and recipients were generally congruent in their perceptions of their relationships at both times. The donors reported nonsignificantly more donor-recipient relationship conflict than the recipients reported for both intervals studied. The relationship variable scores of intensity, positive quality, and conflict were based on author-constructed items for this population; data from other populations for comparison purposes is not available.

The majority of donors (14/18) reported having experienced no ambivalence about donating, while 4/18 (22%) reported some predonation doubts. All of the donors (n = 18) indicated that they would donate again if asked. Several questions asked about any negative emotional or somatic consequences subsequent to the donation. Three of 18 (16%) donors agreed with the statement "I have given something that is part of me for nothing in return." Four of 18 (22%) donors reported having had physical problems they attributed to donating BM. Three reported minor transient back pain, while one reported chronic erectile dysfunction that he attributed to the BMT donation. Two of 18 donors (11%) reported feelings of self-blame when their recipient had medical complications.

Further analysis revealed that the donor's mood disturbance (POMS TMD), self-esteem (Simmons Scale), and donor-recipient relationship variable scores were not significantly correlated. The donors' perception of the current quality of the donor-recipient relationship variable score was very highly correlated with donors' current *family approval* scores (r = .66, P = .0098).

Twelve matched donor-recipient pairs participated in this study. Table 2 shows correlations between the donors' perceptions of the current quality of their relationships with their recipients and a number of recipient status variables for the matched sibling pairs. Current perceptions of the quality of the relationship were highly positively correlated with two recipient psychosocial variables: recipients' perceived current *family approval* (r = .967, P = .0001), and *positive mood* scores (r = .65, P = .023), but were negatively correlated with four of seven recipient social role impairment (SAS-SR) subscale scores, and with the recipients' global illness scores.

The current quality of the relationship between the donor and recipient is, therefore, linked, in the donor's mind, to the degree of esteem each is accorded by the larger family unit, and to the recipient's health and social function status—of note is the finding that it was not correlated with the interval in months between the donors' BMT donation and study participation.

DISCUSSION

This study documents the psychosocial consequences of BM donation on a group of late adolescent/young adult donors whose recipients have become long-term survivors. Data from a companion study of BMT recipients using several identical instruments allowed for comparison of the psychosocial status

TABLE 2. Correlations between donor-perceived quality of donor-recipient relationship and selected donor and recipient adaptation variables (for matched donor-recipient pairs, N=12)

	Donor-perceived quality of donor-recipient relationship
Donor family approval	.66[a]
Recipient family approval	.97[a]
Recipient global illness[b]	−.56
Recipient POMS-TMD[c]	−.51
Recipient positive mood	.65[d]
Recipient SAS-SR work[e]	−.96[a]
Recipient SAS-SR social/leisure	−.53
Recipient SAS-SR extended family	−.86[a]
Recipient SAS-SR marital	−.76[b]
Recipient SAS-SR parental	.13
Recipient SAS-SR family	−.94[a]
Recipient SAS-SR economics	.33
Interval between BMT and study (months)	.09

[a] $P<.01$.
[b] High current global illness scores indicates poor health.
[c] POMS-TMD high score indicates more total mood disturbance.
[d] $P<.05$.
[e] High SAS-SR subscale scores indicate more role impairment.

of BMT donors and recipients. The relatively lengthy mean BMT donation–study participation interval (42.9±19.9 months) provides a cross-sectional view of the long-term—and presumably relatively stable—psychosocial status of BMT donors, and of their relationships with their recipients. This study does not present information about the psychosocial status of donors during the presumably more stressful BMT hospitalization and early posthospitalization periods. Nor does it provide information about the status of BMT donors whose recipients have died, probably a much more stressed donor group.

The donor participation rate (18/36, 50%), was acceptable for mail questionnaire research. However the matched-pair participation rate of 33% (12/36) was somewhat disappointing. The demographic and psychosocial characteristics of the matched-pair donors and of the donor group as a whole were quite similar.

The bone marrow donors in this study strongly tended to be well educated, married, and engaged in work and other productive activities. They reported little current mood disturbance, high self-esteem, and a high degree of satisfaction with current life activities. They reported an overall perception of stability in their relationships with their recipients from the pre-BMT period to the present, with no dramatic positive or negative changes. They minimized the stresses in the predonation period and any heroic aspects of their donating. They endorsed very positive statements about the effects on their lives of donating bone marrow, and indicated that donating was a "high point." All said they would donate to a family member again, and several spontaneously wrote that they would also gladly donate to an unrelated recipient. Several commented that the opportunity to do something that might save the life of their sibling was especially gratifying.

The donors were sharply differentiated from other family members at the time of the BMT, who could only passively hope that treatment would be successful. This element of active participation in the BMT may place donors in a double-bind. As compared with other family members, the donors' sense of contributing by being an active participant during the BMT procedure can give donors a greatly enlarged sense of guilt if the transplant fails. If the recipient deteriorates or dies, the donor often feels that it is not his or her body that failed—but "my body failed my sibling". Thus, donor guilt is potentially very great.

We have seen several situations in which the donor-recipient relationship was fraught with preillness sibling rivalry and competition. Family members may also value siblings differently. As one mother remarked openly to us recently, "Isn't it strange that it ends up our black sheep (son) is the donor to our favorite (daughter)." The staff aptly questioned, "What will these parents do to this donor son psychologically if she dies?"

Although the numbers are small, approximately 10–20% of donors indicated that they had negative experiences or feelings subsequent to donating. Several recipients and donors who have become estranged, and who were eligible to participate in the present study, did not. This clinical observation suggests a "tip-of-the-iceberg" phenomenon, such that the true incidence of adverse psychological consequences in donors whose recipients survive may be significantly higher than reflected by the current study sample. Even the finding of adverse psychosocial consequences in 10–20% of successful donors, if replicated, would indicate a higher incidence of postdonation psychosocial problems in BMT donors than has been reported in studies of living-related kidney transplant donors (*3*).

Turning to the 12 donor-recipient participant pairs, several issues are noteworthy. The donors' perception of the current quality of the donor-recipient relationship was highly correlated with recipients' self-reported current health, mood state, social role functioning, and family approval status. This finding suggests that physical or psychosocial deterioration in BMT recipients may result in significant psychological distress in the donor.

The suggested relationship in our study between recipient medical decline and donor distress could lead to clinical programs to assess and support BMT donors especially carefully when the recipient is medically and/or psychosocially deteriorating. Time since donation was not correlated with measures of the donors' current psychosocial status, or with measures of the donor-recipient relationship. The dynamic factors bearing upon the donor's current quality of relationship with his/her recipient appear not so much time-dependent as recipient-state-dependent.

Several methodological issues, in addition to the small simple size and moderate return rate, limit the data and the conclusions that may be drawn from these results. The design of this study was retrospective and cross-sectional. This limits its ability to document the psychological stresses of donating BM. However, we were primarily interested in the current status of BMT donors, and therefore the potential retrospective distortion problem is less serious.

The use of an unvalidated author-constructed questionnaire to measure reactions to donation, as well as the donor-recipient relationship, is a second methodological limitation. This was necessitated by the novel nature of BMT and the previous lack of systematic research in this area. A third methodological concern is the development of BMT technology over time. The donors in this study were from a pool who donated bone marrow over several years in the mid-to-late 1970s. In the 1970s many aspects of BMT procedures and selection criteria were not as well standardized as they are today. The findings may not necessarily be as applicable to current adolescent/young adult BMT donors.

A final methodological limitation is that all subjects came from one BMT center. Other BMT centers may draw patients from populations with different family relationship patterns who have different demographic and recipient primary disease characteristics. Different BMT centers may also provide different predonation and postdonation psychosocial services to donors and recipients, which could affect donor psychological outcome.

Prospective longitudinal research is needed to more definitively characterize the psychosocial impact on donors of BM. Prospective longitudinal psychosocial research with BMT donors would also help us begin to understand the psychological consequences for donors whose recipients do not survive. Clinical experience indicates that donors to BMT recipient nonsurvivors have a relatively high incidence of pathological grief reactions, but more systematic evidence is needed to verify or refute this clinical impression.

This study suggests that most bone marrow donors whose recipient becomes a long-term survivor do well from a psychosocial standpoint. However, a minority—possibly 10–20%—have at least some adverse psychological sequelae. These findings provide arguable support for previous recommendations in the literature that prospective BM donors should be routinely psychiatrically assessed prior to donation, although there is currently no evidence that such assessment would result in accurately identifying psychologically "high-risk" donors, or in preventing adverse psychological sequelae in these individuals. The study also suggests that the perception of the quality of the donor-recipient relationship may be heavily dependent on the health status and social role function of the recipient. Decline in these recipient functions may be especially stressful to the psychological equanimity of the donors. Our findings suggest that particular psychological attention should be given to donors in this circumstance.

REFERENCES

1. Personal communication. Mortimor Bortin, MD. Director, International BMT Registry, Milwaukee, Wisconsin.
2. Gale RP, ed. Recent advances in bone marrow transplantation. New York, AR Liss, 1983.
3. Simmons RG. Long-term reactions of renal recipients and donors. In: Levy NB, ed. Psychonephrology 2. New York: Plenum, 1983: 275.
4. Gardner CG, August CS, Githens J. Psychological issues in bone marrow transplantation. Pediatrics 1977; 60(4): 625.
5. Pinegger-O'Connor G, Bender-Gotze CH. Betreuung minderjahriger Knochenmarksspender Psychologsche aspekte. MMW 1980; 122(16): 597.
6. Brown HN, Kelly MJ. Stages of bone marrow transplantation: a psychiatric perspective. Psychosom Med 1976; 38: 439.
7. Fawzy FI, Wellisch DK, Yager J. Psychiatric liaison to the bone marrow transplant project. In: Hollingsworth C, Pasnau RO, eds. The family in mourning. New York: Grune and Stratton, 1977: 181.
8. Wolcott DL, Fawzy FI, Wellisch DK. Psychiatric aspects of bone marrow transplantation: a review and current issues. Psychiatric Med (in press).
9. Wolcott DL, Wellisch DK, Fawzy FI, Landsverk J. Adaptation of adult bone marrow transplant recipient long-term survivors. Transplantation 1986; 41: 478.
10. McNair DM, Lorr M, Droppleman LF. Manual for the profile of mood states. San Diego, Educational and Industrial Testing Service, 1981.
11. Simmons RG, Klein SD, Simmons RL. Gift of life: the social and psychological impact of organ transplantation. New York: Wiley, 1977.
12. Weissman MM, Bothwell S. Assessment of social adjustment by patient self-report. Arch Gen Psychiatry 1976; 33: 1111.
13. Weissman MM, Prusoff B, Thompson WD, et al. Social adjustment by self-report in a community sample and in psychiatric outpatients. J Nerv Ment Dis 1978; 166: 317.

Received 5 March 1985.
Accepted 24 July 1985.

0041-1337/86/4104-0489$02.00/0
TRANSPLANTATION
Vol. 41, No. 4

Printed in U.S.A.

IMMUNE REACTIVITY IN CONGENIC MICE AFTER ALLOGENEIC OR ISOGENEIC TRANSFUSION[1]

MARY L. WOOD,[2] RITA GOTTSCHALK, AND ANTHONY P. MONACO

Department of Surgery, Harvard Medical School, New England Deaconess Hospital, Boston, MA 02215

Pretransplant donor-specific blood transfusion has a beneficial effect on subsequent skin graft survival in B10 congenic mice when donor and recipient differ at both the K and I regions of the H-2 complex, but has no effect on graft survival in donor-recipient combinations differing at the K region alone. Immune reactivity was studied in B10.A recipients after a single allogeneic transfusion from B10 donors differing either at both K and I regions or at K alone, or after a transfusion of isogeneic B10.A blood. Spleen cells were assayed for the ability to respond in mixed lymphocyte culture (MLC) and cell mediated lymphocytotoxicity (CML) assays against blood donor and third-party at 2, 9, 16, and 30 days after transfusion. MLC and CML responses were nonspecifically suppressed in recipients transfused with allogeneic blood from K or K and I region disparate donors. The responses of mice receiving K region disparate blood were partially recovered by 9 days posttransfusion and had returned to normal 16 days posttransfusion. Responses of mice receiving K and I region disparate blood remained suppressed 30 days post transfusion. Isogeneic transfusion induced a suppression of the MLC response. Two days posttransfusion, the MLC response was suppressed to a variety of stimulators representing disparity at K alone; K and I; or K, I, and D. The response to K region disparate stimulators had recovered 9 days after isogeneic transfusion, but the response to K and I or K, I, and D region disparate stimulators remained suppressed 30 days after transfusion. The suppression observed after allogeneic or isogeneic transfusion was not due to a shift in the day of peak response in the transfused mice. Kinetic studies showed that the day of peak MLC and CML responses in the transfused mice corresponded to that of normal controls, but the level of response was significantly lower in the transfused mice.

The beneficial effect of donor-specific transfusions (DST)* on the survival of subsequent allografts has been demonstrated in clinical transplanation and in various animal models (*1–3*). The mechanism that induces the posttransfusion unresponsive state is unclear, but evidence both in man and in animals suggests that the recipient's immune responses to the blood donor are impaired, as shown by a suppression of the mixed lymphocyte culture (MLC) response and the ability to generate antidonor cytotoxic effector cells (*3, 4*). Some of the mechanisms proposed for the induction of unresponsiveness after blood transfusions are activation of suppressor cells and/or the production of antiidiotypic antibodies (*5, 6*). The influence of the major histocompatibility complex (MHC) on the transfusion effect has not been precisely defined, although it has been proposed that both non-MHC-restricted and MHC-restricted mechanisms play a role (*7*). There is evidence from experiments in mice that transfusion is more effective if donor and recipient differ at both the K region (encoding class I antigens) and the I region (encoding class II antigens) of the major H-2 complex. We have reported previously that DST was more effective in prolonging DBA/2 skin allografts in $B6AF_1$ mice, in which donor and recipient differ in both K and I regions, than in prolonging C3H/He skin grafts in $B6AF_1$ mice, in which donor and recipient differ at the D region and IC subregion only (*8*). In experiments studying the effect of nonspecific transfusions on graft survival, transfusions were more beneficial if the blood donor and recipient differed at both K and I regions, regardless of the genetic relationship between the skin and blood donor and the recipient (*9*). To examine the role of the MHC in the transfusion effect further, congenic mice were used to study the effect of DST on skin allograft survival. This made it possible to have donor-recipient combinations that differed from each other at defined regions of the H-2 complex and minimized the effect of minor histocompatibility antigens. Donor-recipient combinations of B10 congenic mice were used that differed at both K and I regions of the H-2 complex or at K alone. DST significantly prolonged subsequent skin allograft survival when donor and recipient differed at both the K and I regions (*10*). In contrast, DST had no effect on graft survival when donor and recipient differed at the K region alone (*10*). In the present studies, in vitro antidonor immune reactivity has been studied in congenic mice that have received donor-specific transfusion alone without subsequent skin grafting. Mice received a single transfusion from a donor differing either at K and I or at K alone, and their spleen cells were assayed at various intervals posttransfusion for the ability to respond in MLC and cell-mediated lymphocytotoxicity (CML) assays to the specific blood donor and third party. In addition, immune reactivity was studied in recipients after transfusion with isogeneic blood.

MATERIALS AND METHODS

Mice. Adult male congenic and recombinant mice developed on the B10 background were used. B10.A and B10.D2 mice were obtained from Jackson Laboratory, Bar Harbor, ME. B10.AQR mice were obtained from J. Wayne Streilein, M.D., University of Texas Health Science Center, Dallas, TX. A.Sw($H-2^s$) mice, used as third-party donors, were obtained from Jackson Laboratory.

Blood transfusion. Blood was obtained from the tail veins of donor mice, collected in heparin-coated tubes, pooled, and

[1] This work was supported by USPHS Grant AI 14551-07.

[2] Address correspondence to: Mary L. Wood, New England Deaconess Hospital, 185 Pilgrim Road, Boston, MA 02215.

* Abbreviations used: Con A, concanavalin A; CML, cell-mediated lymphocytotoxicity; DST, donor-specific transfusion; E:T, effector:target; MHC, major histocompatibility complex; MLC, mixed lymphocyte culture; MLR, mixed lymphocyte response; SI, stimulation index.

transfused within 1 hr. Recipient mice received 0.25 ml whole blood i.v.

Preparation of spleen cell suspensions. Spleens were removed by sterile technique and single-cell suspensions were prepared in Click's medium (Altick Associates, River Falls, WI) supplemented with 0.5% normal mouse serum. Spleens were removed from at least three mice in treated or control groups, and cells were pooled within a group for assay. Each experiment was repeated on at least two occasions.

Mixed lymphocyte culture. MLC were done in 16-mm flat-bottomed culture wells. Responder spleen cells from normal or transfused recipients were cultured with x-irradiated stimulator cells from the blood donor or third-party in a volume of 2 ml. In the case of B10.A stimulated by B10.D2, 7.5×10^6 responder and 5×10^6 stimulator cells were used. In the case of B10.A stimulated by B10.AQR 5×10^6 responder and 5×10^6 stimulator cells were used. Cultures were incubated at 37°C in a humid atmosphere of 5% CO_2. B10.A cells stimulated with B10.D2 were incubated for 3 days and B10.A cells stimulated with B10.AQR were incubated for 4 days, as it had been determined previously that these were the days of peak MLC response for normal mice in these strain combinations. After incubation, each well was mixed with a Pasteur pipette and 0.25 ml of the cell suspension was transferred to a microtiter well. Triplicate cultures were pulsed for 12 hr with 2 μCi (^{3}H) thymidine. The cultures were harvested on filter paper and counted in a scintillation counter.

Cell-mediated cytotoxicity. For determination of CML, MLC were prepared as described above and cultured for 5 days. The ^{51}Cr release assay for CML was performed according to the technique of Brunner et al. (*11*). Target cells consisted of P815 (H-2^d) tumor cells or concanavalin A (Con-A)-induced spleen cell blasts. Con A blasts were prepared by incubating 100×10^6 spleen cells in 50 ml RPMI 1640 supplemented with 5 ml fetal calf serum, 2 ME, and 250 μg Con A. The cells were incubated for 48 hr at 37°C and washed with 0.3 mM D-(d-methyl)-mannoside before labeling with ^{51}Cr. For assay, ^{51}Cr-labeled target cells (2×10^4) were placed in microtiter plates, and varying numbers of effector cells were added. Each effector to target (E:T) ratio was plated in triplicate. The final volume of the wells was adjusted to 0.2 ml. The plates were centrifuged for 2 min at 200×G and incubated for 4 hr at 37°C. After incubation, the plates were centrifuged for 10 min at 2000×G, and 0.1 ml supernatant was removed from each well and counted for ^{51}Cr release. Total counts on the target cells were determined by direct counting of 2×10^4 cells. Spontaneous release was determined by counting 0.1 ml supernatant from 2×10^4 target cells incubated in medium alone. Spontaneous release of ^{51}Cr never exceeded 15% of the total cpm in any experiment. Cytotoxicity was expressed as a percentage according to the formula:

$$\frac{\text{Experimental cpm} - \text{spontaneous cpm}}{\text{total cpm} - \text{spontaneous cpm}} \times 100$$

RESULTS

Table 1 shows the H-2 haplotypes of the congenic mice.

Effect of transfusion in mice disparate at the K region alone. The effect of transfusion in K region disparate mice was studied in B10.A mice transfused with B10.AQR blood. Spleen cells from B10.A mice were assayed 2, 9, and 16 days after B10.AQR transfusion for the ability to respond in MLC and CML to the blood donor and to third-party A.Sw cells. Both MLC and CML responses to the blood donor and third party were significantly suppressed 2 days posttransfusion, as shown in Figures 1 and 2. Nine days posttransfusion, there was variation in the pattern of MLC and CML responses among 4 groups of transfused mice tested. Three of the four groups still showed supressed MLC and CML responses to the blood donor, as illustrated in Figures 1 and 2. In these groups, the MLC response to third party had returned to normal while the CML response was still suppressed (Figs. 1 and 2). In the fourth group assayed, MLC and CML responses to both donor and third party had returned to normal. Sixteen days posttransfusion, all B10.A mice transfused with B10.AQR blood showed normal MLC and CML responses to blood donor and third party. MLC and CML responses were also assayed 16 days posttransfusion in the reverse K disparate combination—i.e., B10.AQR transfused with B10.A blood. As shown in Table 2, MLC and CML responses were elevated in the transfused mice to blood donor and third party.

TABLE 1. H-2 typing of B10 congenic mice

	K	I ABJEC	D
B10.A	k	kkkkd	d
B10.AQR	q	kkkkd	d
B10.D2	d	ddddd	d

Effect of transfusion in mice disparate at the K and I region. The effect of transfusion in K and I region disparate mice was assayed in B10.A mice transfused with B10.D2 blood. Spleen cells of B10.A recipients were assayed 2, 9, 16, and 30 days after B10.D2 transfusion for the ability to respond in MLC and CML to the blood donor and to third-party A.Sw cells. The MLC and CML responses of transfused mice were significantly suppressed to both blood donor and third party 2, 9, and 16 days after transfusion, as shown in Figures 3 and 4. Thirty days after transfusion, the MLC and CML responses were still suppressed. B10.A mice transfused with B10.D2 blood had a stimulation index (SI) of 12.2 when stimulated in MLC with B10.D2 stimulators 30 days post B10.D2 transfusion, compared with a normal SI of 21.4. The net cpm in the normal controls was 25943±356 compared with 14654±212 in the transfused group. The CML response of transfused mice at an E:T ratio of 20:1 was 24% compared with 48% in the normal controls.

The effect of transfusion was also assayed in two other K and I region disparate combinations, B10.D2 transfused with B10.AQR and B10.D2 transfused with B10.A. Spleen cells from transfused recipients were assayed 16 days posttransfusion for the ability to respond in MLC and CML against the blood donor and third party. As shown in Table 3, MLC and CML responses were suppressed to blood donor and third party after transfusion in both strain combinations.

Effect of transfusion with isogeneic blood. The effect of isogeneic transfusion was assayed in B10.A mice transfused with B10.A blood. Spleen cells of B10.A recipients were assayed 2, 9, 16, and 30 days posttransfusion for the ability to respond in MLC and CML to B10.AQR (K region disparate), B10.D2 (K and I region disparate), and A.Sw (K, I, and D region disparate). Two days posttransfusion, the MLC response to all three stimulators was significantly suppressed in the transfused mice compared with normal B10.A, as shown in Figure 5. Nine days

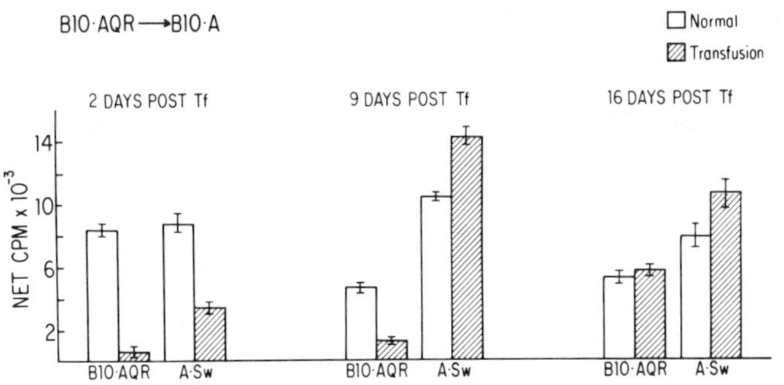

FIGURE 1. MLC response of B10.A mice to blood donor and third party 2, 9, and 16 days after B10.AQR blood transfusion (K region disparity).

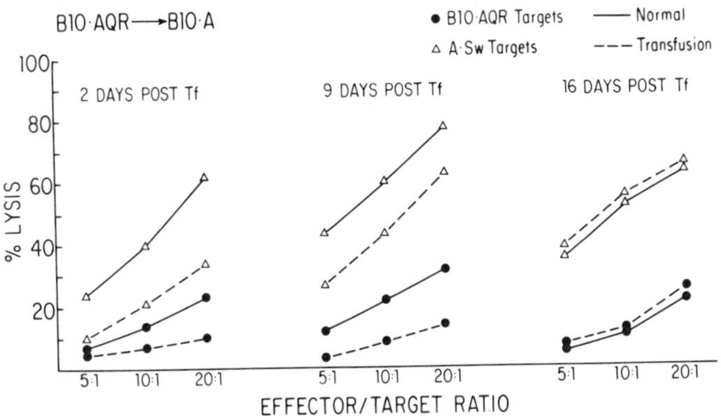

FIGURE 2. CML response of B10.A mice to blood donor and third party 2, 9, and 16 days after B10.AQR blood transfusion.

TABLE 2. MLC and CML responses 16 days posttransfusion with K-region-disparate blood

Responder[a]	Stimulator	MLC cpm[b]	MLC (SI)[c]	CML 20:1	CML 10:1	CML 5:1[d]
B10.AQR vs. B10.A:						
Norm. B10.AQR	B10.A	5933±232	(3.4)	31	21	13
	A.Sw	8313±378	(4.7)	56	40	27
Tf B10.AQR	B10.A	11876±238	(5.7)	40	27	18
	A.Sw	43721±3477	(21)	79	74	70

[a] Spleen cells from three mice were pooled in each group for testing.
[b] Mean counts (minus background) per minute of ^{3}H thymidine uptake ± SD.
[c] Stimulation index.
[d] Effector/target ratios. CML results are expressed as percentage of lysis, as shown by ^{51}Cr release.

after isogeneic transfusion, the MLC response to K region disparate stimulators had returned to normal in the transfused mice, while the response to K and I or K, I, and D region disparate stimulators was still suppressed 16 days posttransfusion (Figure 5). Thirty days posttransfusion, the MLC response remained suppressed, as shown by the SI of 12.4 in isogeneically transfused B10.A stimulated by B10.D2, compared with an index of 21.4 in normals. The net cpm in the transfused mice was 14958±398 compared with a net count of 25943±356 in the controls. The response of isogeneically transfused mice in CML was not consistent. In 3 of 8 assays of the CML response 2–16 days posttransfusion in isogeneically transfused mice, the CML response was suppressed compared with normal controls, but not to the extent of allogeneically transfused mice. For example, in an assay 16 days after transfusion comparing B10.A mice transfused with B10.D2 blood or B10.A blood in their response to B10.D2 stimulators at E:T ratios of

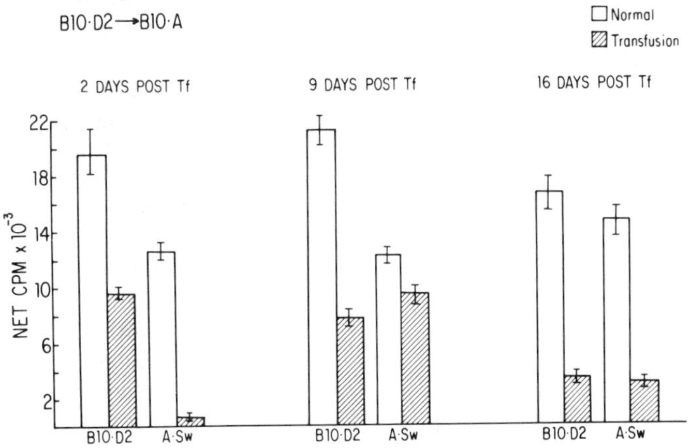

FIGURE 3. MLC response of B10.A mice to blood donor and third party 2, 9, and 16 days after B10.D2 blood transfusion (K and I region disparity).

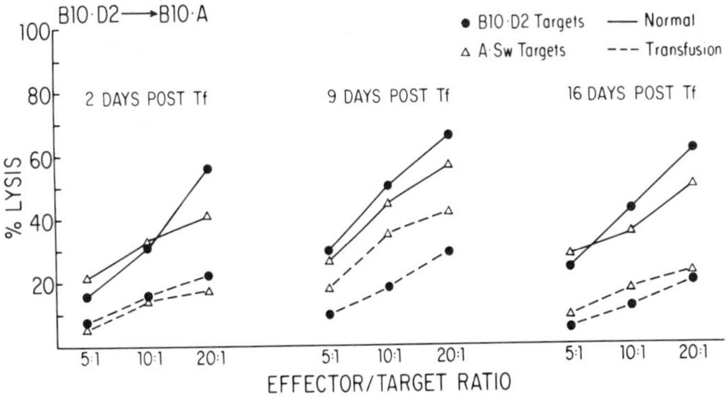

FIGURE 4. CML response of B10.A mice to blood donor and third party 2, 9, and 16 days after B10.D2 blood transfusion.

TABLE 3. MLC and CML responses 16 days posttransfusion with K and I-region-disparate blood

Responder[a]	Stimulator	MLC cpm[b]	MLC (SI)[c]	CML 20:1	CML 10:1	CML 5:1[d]
B10.D2 vs. B10.AQR:						
Norm. B10.D2	B10.AQR	27571±1269	(5.5)	82	76	57
	A.Sw	33637±1227	(6.7)	77	71	59
Tf B10.D2	B10.AQR	9989±226	(3.9)	47	32	19
	A.Sw	9115±369	(3.6)	53	41	25
B10.D2 vs. B10.A:						
Norm. B10.D2	B10.A	33106±1985	(6.6)	73	68	51
	A.Sw	33637±1227	(6.7)	77	71	59
Tf B10.D2	B10.A	4205±317	(1.2)	33	17	10
	A.Sw	6749±698	(1.9)	63	52	37

[a] Spleen cells from three mice were pooled in each group for testing.
[b] Mean counts (minus background) per minute of ^{3}H thymidine uptake ± SD.
[c] Stimulation index.
[d] Effector/target ratios. CML results are expressed as percentage of lysis, as shown by ^{51}Cr release.

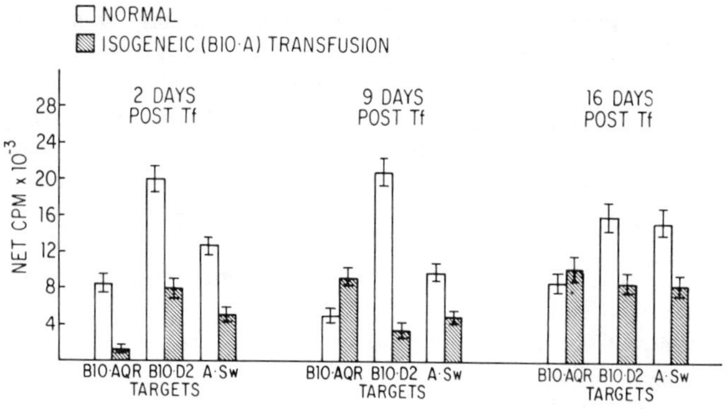

FIGURE 5. MLC response of B10.A mice to B10.AQR, B10.D2 and A.Sw 2, 9, and 16 days after isogeneic B10.A blood transfusion.

20:1, 10:1, and 5:1, the normals showed 75%, 61%, and 42% lysis; the B10.D2-transfused 20%, 11%, and 5% lysis; and the B10.A-transfused 58%, 38%, and 20% lysis. In other assays, the CML response after isogeneic transfusion was normal, as shown in Table 4 (see kinetic studies below).

Kinetics of MLC and CML Responses in Transfused Mice

K region disparate transfusion. The kinetics of the MLC response to the blood donor in B10.A mice transfused with B10.AQR blood was assayed 9 days posttransfusion to determine whether the suppressed response observed in transfused mice was due to a shift in the day of peak MLC response compared with the normal controls. Responder spleen cells from normal B10.A or B10.A transfused with B10.AQR blood 9 days previously were cultured with x-irradiated B10.AQR stimulator cells, as described above. Cultures of normal and transfused responders were incubated for 3, 4, or 5 days before pulsing with (^{3}H) thymidine and counting. The MLC response of transfused mice was significantly suppressed on all 3 days of culture compared with normal (data not shown) and the small peak in the response of transfused mice occurred on day 4 of culture, corresponding to the peak response in normal controls.

K and I region disparate transfusion. The kinetics of the MLC response to the blood donor in B10.A mice transfused with B10.D2 blood was assayed 2, 9, and 16 days posttransfusion, and the kinetics of the CML response was assayed 2 and 16 days posttransfusion. Responder cells from normal B10.A or B10.A transfused with B10.D2 blood 2, 9, or 16 days previously were cultured with x-irradiated B10.D2 stimulators, as described above. MLC cultures of normal and transfused responders were incubated for 2, 3, 4, or 5 days before pulsing with (^{3}H) thymidine and counting. Cultures of normal and transfused mice were assayed for CML 4, 5, 6, or 7 days after initiation of culture. The peak MLC response in normal mice occurred on day 3, as shown in Figure 6. The assays 2 days posttransfusion and 9 and 16 days posttransfusion were performed on different days, so that the normal control curves are different, but the normal peak in both assays is on day 3. Figure 6 shows that the peak response in transfused mice assayed 2 days after allogeneic transfusion occurred one day later than in the normal controls. However, a comparison of the peak response in the normal controls (day 3) and in the transfused mice (day 4) showed that the MLC response was significantly suppressed in the transfused mice, with a peak SI of 20 in the controls and 11.9 in the transfused mice ($P<0.02$). The MLC response of transfused mice 9 and 16 days posttransfusion was significantly suppressed, but the small peak that occurred was on day 3.

The peak CML response in normal mice occurred on day 5 and the response remained at peak on days 6 and 7, as shown in Table 4. In mice assayed 2 days posttransfusion, the peak response also occurred on day 5, but was significantly lower than that of normal mice (Table 4). The response remained at peak level on days 6 and 7. The peak CML response in mice assayed 16 days posttransfusion occurred on day 5, as in normal controls, but was significantly lower than the normal response. There was a significant drop in the CML response from peak level in this group of transfused mice on day 6 of culture.

Isogeneic transfusion. The kinetics of the MLC response to B10.D2 stimulators (K and I region disparate) in B10.A mice transfused with B10.A blood was assayed 2, 9, and 16 days posttransfusion, and the CML response was assayed 2 and 16 days posttransfusion. Responder cells from normal B10.A or

TABLE 4. Kinetics of CML response in B10.A mice 2 and 16 days after B10.D2 or B10.A transfusion

Day of culture	Responder	CML 2 days post Tf			CML 16 days post Tf		
		20:1	10:1	5:1[a]	20:1	10:1	5:1
4	Norm B10.A	26	13	8	21	12	8
	B10.D2 Tf	10	5	3	14	8	5
	B10.A Tf	28	16	10	23	14	9
5	Norm B10.A	61	45	23	61	42	20
	B10.D2 Tf	26	14	6	45	28	15
	B10.A Tf	67	53	32	61	45	25
6	Norm B10.A	68	52	30	65	48	27
	B10.D2 Tf	21	13	5	27	15	7
	B10.A Tf	82	64	44	70	52	32
7	Norm B10.A	66	46	30	63	46	27
	B10.D2 Tf	25	13	6	25	14	4
	B10.A Tf	69	46	27	65	43	29

[a] Effector/target ratios. CML results are expressed as percentage of lysis of B10.D2 targets, as shown by ^{51}Cr release.

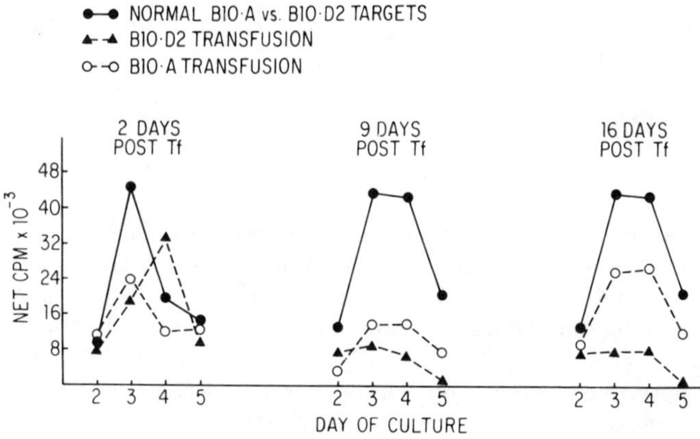

FIGURE 6. Kinetics of the MLC response of B10.A mice to B10.D2 2, 9, and 16 days after transfusion with allogeneic B10.D2 or isogeneic B10.A blood. Response was assayed 2, 3, 4, and 5 days after initiation of MLC.

B10.A transfused with B10.A blood 2, 9, or 16 days previously were cultured with x-irradiated B10.D2 stimulators, as described above. MLC cultures of normal and transfused responders were incubated for 2, 3, 4, or 5 days before pulsing with (^{3}H) thymidine and counting. Cultures of normal and transfused responders were assayed for CML 4, 5, 6, or 7 days after initiation of culture. The peak MLC response of isogeneically transfused mice occurred on day 3, as in the normal controls (Fig. 6), when assayed 2, 9, or 16 days posttransfusion, but the peak response was always significantly suppressed compared with normals. The CML response in the isogeneically transfused mice was as high as the normals on day 5 and peaked even higher on day 6 (Table 4).

DISCUSSION

These results indicate that isogeneic as well as allogeneic transfusion can induce a state of suppressed immune reactivity. The degree and duration of suppression appears to depend on the degree of genetic disparity in the H-2 complex between donor and recipient. B10.A mice receiving a transfusion from a K (B10.AQR) or a K and I (B10.D2) region disparate donor exhibited suppressed MLC and CML responses as early as 2 days posttransfusion. The suppression was nonspecific, as responses to both blood donor and third party were suppressed. The responses of mice receiving K region disparate blood showed some evidence of recovery by 9 days after transfusion and their responses had returned to normal 16 days posttransfusion. In contrast, MLC and CML response of mice transfused with K and I region disparate blood remained suppressed as long as 30 days after transfusion. These results correlate with the prolongation of skin graft survival that can be achieved by DST in these strain combinations. B10.D2 skin can be prolonged on B10.A after DST, but DST has no effect on prolonging B10.AQR skin on B10.A (*10*). The suppression of both MLC and CML responses was not due to an earlier peak response in transfused recipients, as kinetic studies showed that the peak response in transfused mice occurred on the same day or 1 day later than in the normal controls, and the peak responses of transfused mice were significantly lower than those of the normals.

Isogeneic transfusion induced a significant suppression of the MLC response. Two days posttransfusion, the MLC response was suppressed to a variety of stimulators, representing disparity in the H-2 complex at the K region alone; at K and I; and at K, I, and D. The MLC response of the transfused mice to a K region disparity had recovered by day 9 posttransfusion, but the MLC response to mice differing at K and I or at K, I, and D remained suppressed for 30 days after transfusion. A study of the kinetics of the response in isogeneically transfused mice showed that the time of peak response in MLC in the transfused mice was identical to that of normal controls, but that the response was significantly lower than normal. In some CML assays, the CML response appeared to be suppressed after isogeneic transfusion, but the response in these assays may not have represented the peak. The 3 assays showing suppression were performed after 5 days in culture. However, the study of the kinetics of the CML response in isogeneically transfused mice showed that the CML response reached its peak on day 6.

Studies are in progress to compare the mechanism underlying the suppression observed after allogeneic and isogeneic transfusion in congenic mice. Previous experiments in our laboratory studying the effect of DST in noncongenic mice showed that cells from transfused mice could suppress the normal MLC in coculture (*12*). There is substantial evidence that allogeneic stimulation not only induces cytotoxic effector cells, but also cells that suppress and regulate the immune response. Lymphocytes obtained from mice after i.v. injection of antigen or injection of antigen into the foot-pads have been shown to suppress the immune response when restimulated by the sensitizing antigen in vitro (*13, 14*). In addition, spleen cells harvested from MLC or cultured in the presence of Con A can suppress both MLC and CML responses (*15, 16*). The cells responsible for suppression can be antigen-specific or nonspecific Thy-1$^+$ lymphocytes or Thy-1$^-$ plastic-adherent activated macrophages. Suppressor T lymphocytes have been shown to develop after antigenic stimulation through a series of complex cellular events that involves several subpopulations. Determinants coded by the IJ subregion are thought to be present on suppressor cells and on the suppressor factors produced by these cells (*17, 18*). Macrophages can be activated by a factor produced by Con-A-stimulated lymphocytes to produce a second factor that nonspecifically suppresses the proliferative responses of T and B lymphocytes (*19*). It is possible that the suppression observed 2 days after allogeneic transfusion is mediated by a pathway different from that of the suppression observed two weeks after transfusion, and the target of suppression at various times may be different subpopulations of lymphocytes in the recipient. The fact that the responses remained suppressed for a longer period when donor and recipient differed at both K and I regions may indicate the importance of disparity at the IJ subregion in inducing suppressor cells. Alternatively, the greater degree of suppression in I region disparate combinations may reflect a feedback inhibition of helper cell activation that may not be present in mice disparate at the K region alone.

The significant suppression of the MLC response after isogeneic transfusion was unexpected. It has been demonstrated in animals and man that T cells can proliferate in MLC in response to syngeneic non-T cells without antigen being present (*20, 21*). This syngeneic or autologous mixed lymphocyte response (MLR) is thought to have an important role in immunoregulation, as the cells that proliferate have been shown to have a suppressive effect on the proliferative and cytotoxic responses of fresh syngeneic cells (*22, 23*). It is possible that transfusion with isogeneic blood induces a syngeneic MLR in vivo that, in turn, generates a population of suppressor cells. The primary target of suppression after isogeneic transfusion appears to be the proliferative response, in contrast to the effect of allogeneic transfusion on both MLC and CML responses. The response to stimulation by K and I region disparate stimulators remained suppressed for a longer period after isogeneic transfusion than the response to stimulation by mice disparate to the K region alone, suggesting that isogeneic transfusion affected the helper cell response. Experiments are being done to examine the effect of isogeneic transfusion on allograft prolongation.

A comparison of the similarities and/or differences in the cell populations responsible for suppression of the immune response after allogeneic and isogeneic transfusion may help define the requirements for activation of suppressor cells that are important in inducing allograft prolongation, and it may lead to an understanding of the mechanism of pretransplant transfusion.

REFERENCES

1. Salvatierra O, Vincenti F, Amend W, et al. Deliberate donor specific transfusions prior to living related renal transplantation. Am Surg 1980; 192: 543.
2. Borleffs JC, Marquet RL, Balner H. Pretransplant blood transfusions have an additive positive effect on kidney graft prognosis in D/Dr matched rhesus monkeys. Transplantation 1981; 32: 48.
3. Marquet RL, Heystek GA, Borleffs JC. Suppressor cells in rats with actively induced unresponsiveness to allogeneic heart grafts. Transplant Proc 1981; 13: 48.
4. Klatzmann D, Gluckman JC, Foucault C, et al. Modification of mixed lymphocyte reactivity after blood transfusions in man. Transplant Proc 1983; 15: 1016.
5. Maki T, Okazaki H, Wood ML, Monaco AP. Suppressor cells in mice bearing intact skin allografts after blood transfusions. Transplantation 1981; 32: 463.
6. Nagarkatti PS, Joseph S, Singal DP. Induction of antibodies by blood transfusions capable of inhibiting responses in MLC. Transplantation 1983; 36: 695.
7. van Rood JJ. Pretransplant blood transfusions. Sure! But how and why? Transplant Proc 1983; 15: 915.
8. Okazaki H, Maki T, Wood ML, Monaco AP. Effect of a single transfusion of donor specific and nonspecific blood on skin allograft survival in mice. Transplantation 1980; 30: 421.
9. Okazaki H, Maki T, Wood ML, Jones S, Monaco AP. Prolongation of skin allograft survival in H-2 K and I region-incompatible mice by pretransplant blood transfusion. Transplantation 1981; 32: 111.
10. Wood ML, Monaco AP. Induction of unresponsiveness to skin allografts in adult mice disparate at defined regions of the H-2 complex. II. Effect of pre-graft donor specific blood transfusions in ALS-treated mice. Transplantation 1984; 37: 39.
11. Brunner KT, Engers HD, Cerotinni JC. The ^{51}Cr release assay as used for the quantitative measurement of cell-mediated cytolysis in vitro. In: Bloom BR, David JR, eds. In vitro methods in cell-mediated immunity. NY: Academic Press, 1976: 423.
12. Wood ML, Gottschalk R, Monaco AP. Comparison of immune responsiveness in mice after single or multiple donor specific transfusions. J Immunol 1984; 132: 651.
13. Miller RG, Phillips RA. Reduction of the in vitro cytolytic lymphocyte response produced after in vivo exposure to semiallogeneic cells: recruitment or active suppression? J Immunol 1976; 117: 1913.
14. Truitt GA, Rich RR, Rich SS. Regulation of cytotoxic lymphocyte responses in vitro by alloantigen-activated spleen cells. J Immunol 1977; 119: 31.
15. Hirano T, Nordin AA. Cell-mediated immune response in vitro. The development of suppressor cells and cytotoxic lymphocytes in mixed lymphocyte culture. J Immunol 1976; 116: 1115.
16. Peavy DL, Pierce CW. Cell-mediated immune responses in vitro. I. Suppression of the generation of cytotoxic lymphocytes by concanavalin A and concanvalin A-activated spleen cells. J Exp Med 1974; 140: 356.
17. Tada T, Taniguchi M, David CS. Properties of the antigen-specific suppressive T-cell factor in the regulation of antibody responses in the mouse. IV. Special subregion assignment of the gene(s) that codes for the suppressive T-cell factor in the H-2 histocompatibility complex. J Exp Med 1976; 144: 173.
18. Usui M, Aoki I, Sunshine GH, Dorf ME. Requirements for suppressor T cell activation. J Immunol 1984; 133: 1137.
19. Aune T, Pierce CW. Mechanism of action of macrophage derived suppressor factor produced by soluble immune response suppressor-treated macrophages. J Immunol 1981; 127: 368.
20. Smith JB, Pasternak RD. Syngeneic mixed lymphocyte reaction in mice: strain distribution, kinetics, participating cells and absence in NZB mice. J Immunol 1978; 121: 1889.
21. Sakane T, Green I. Specificity and suppressor function of human T cells responsive to autologous non-T cells. J Immunol 1979; 123: 584.
22. Smith JB, Knowlton RP. Activation of suppressor T cells in human autologous mixed lymphocyte culture. J Immunol 1979; 123: 419.
23. Yamashita U, Ono S, Nakamura H. The syngeneic mixed leukocyte reaction in mice. I. The cellular and genetic mechanism of the syngeneic mixed leukocyte reaction. J Immunol 1982; 128: 1003.

Received 24 June 1985.
Accepted 26 July 1985.

0041-1337/86/4104-0495$02.00/0
TRANSPLANTATION
Vol. 41, No. 4
Printed in U.S.A.

SUPPRESSIVE EFFECT OF MIZORIBINE ON HUMORAL ANTIBODY PRODUCTION IN DBA/2 MICE[1]

MICHIHITO OKUBO,[2] XING-MEI CHEN, KOUJU KAMATA, YOSHIHIKO MASAKI, AND TAKEHIKO UCHIYAMA

Departments of Medicine and Experimental Animals, Kitasato University School of Medicine, Sagamihara 228; and Department of Microbiology, Tokyo Women's Medical College, Tokyo 162, Japan

The mode of action of mizoribine (MZR) as a B cell inhibitor was studied using DBA/2 mice. Its in vitro administration significantly delayed the primary response in hemagglutinin production against sheep erythrocytes by suppressing the IgM antibody formation. In vitro plaque-forming cell (PFC) response against both T-dependent and T-independent antigens, such as TNP-SRBC and TNP-*Brucella abortus*, was dose-dependently suppressed by MZR. Since PFC formation by the T-depleted fraction of splenocytes was likewise suppressed, MZR may inhibit humoral antibody response by directly affecting the B cells (and/or macrophages) as well as by modulating the regulatory T cells. MZR may only act on a certain stage of the cell cycle of B lymphocytes following antigenic stimulation. It may not interfere with the initial antigen recognition or with mature B cells.

Mizoribine (MZR* [Bredinin]), an imidazole nucleoside isolated from *Eupenicillium brefeldianum* M-2166, was originally developed as a T cell inhibitor (*1, 2*). It is currently in clinical use in Japan as an immunosuppressant for posttransplant patients (*3*) because of lesser side effects but potency comparable to that of azathioprine (*1*). In the meantime, we found that its long-term administration in vivo produced prolonged survival of New Zealand black/white F_1 hybrid mice (NZB/W F_1), and a delay in the development of glomerulonephritis that spontaneously occurs in this murine model (*4*). Using DBA/2 mice sharing the same H-2 antigen system with NZB/W F_1 mice, the present study was designed to clarify the mode of action of MZR as a B cell inhibitor. It was found that MZR suppresses antibody generation by directly acting on B cells (and/or by affecting macrophages [Mø]), as well as by indirect action through the modulation of T cells. Moreover, MZR was shown only to act on a certain stage of the B cell cycle, without interfering with the antigen recognition or with mature B cells.

[1] This work was supported in part by the Toyo Jozo Fund and the Life Science Laboratories Fund.

[2] Address correspondence to: Michihito Okubo, Department of Medicine, Kitasato University School of Medicine, 1-15-1 Kitasato, Sagamihara-228, Japan.

* Abbreviations used: Con A, concanavalin A; HBSS, Hanks' balanced salt solution; Ig, immunoglobulin; Il, interleukin; Mø, macrophage; 2-ME, 2-mercaptoethanol; MZR, mizoribine; NZB/W F_1, New Zealand black/white F_1 hybrid mice; PBS, phosphate-buffered saline; PFC, plaque forming cell; RRBC, rabbit erythrocytes; SRBC, sheep red blood cells; TD, T-cell-dependent antigen; TI, T-cell-independent antigen; TNP-Ba, trinitrophenyl-*Brucella abortus*; TRF, T-cell-replacing factor.

MATERIALS AND METHODS

Animals. Weanling female DBA/2 mice were purchased from Shizuoka Experimental Animals (Shizuoka, Japan), and kept at our mouse unit until used at 10 weeks of age.

In vivo studies. To study the effect of MZR on the primary phase of antisheep erythrocytes (SRBC) hemagglutinin production, each group of 10 animals was given 0, 20, or 40 mg of MZR per kg body weight s.c. every day for 16 days starting 2 days prior to the i.p. injection of 0.2 ml of 20% SRBC. Animals were consecutively bled through the tail vein as indicated (Fig. 1), and 200 μl of blood was collected into capillary tubes. Serum anti-SRBC hemagglutinin was measured as routine. An aliquot of each serum was preincubated with an equal amount of 0.1 M 2-mercaptoethanol (2-ME, Wako Chemicals, Tokyo) at 37°C for 1 hr prior to the measurement of the anti-SRBC antibodies.

In Vitro Studies

Preparation of spleen cells. DBA/2 mouse spleens were aseptically taken immediately following the sacrifice of the animals by cervical dislocation. Whole spleen cells were obtained by pressing the spleens with forceps and passing them through stainless steel mesh. Contaminating erythrocytes were lyzed with 0.83% tris ammonium chloride. After washing the cells 3 times with Hanks' balanced salt solution (HBSS), they were suspended at the concentration of 1×10^7 cells/ml in complete Click's medium (*5*) with 10% fetal calf serum (lot No. 404, Flow Laboratories, Stanmore, N.S.W., Australia), 2 mM l-glutamine, 5×10^{-5} M 2-ME, 0.18% $NaHCO_3$, 100 units/ml penicillin, and 100 μg/ml streptomycin.

Cell culture. The spleen cells were incubated in 35×10-mm plastic Petri dishes (Nunc, Roskilde, Denmark) in duplicate. They were stimulated with varying doses of MZR at 37°C in 5% CO_2 in air for 4 days. Trinitrophenyl-*Brucella abortus* (TNP-Ba, 10^{11} organisms/ml), (which was prepared by the method of Mond et al. [*6*], and generously provided by Dr. Tadakuma, Keio University School of Medicine, Department of Microbiology, Tokyo), was used as the T-independent antigen (TI). TNP-SRBC, (prepared by a slight modification of the Rittenberg and Pratt [7] method), was used as the T-dependent antigen (TD). Using the trypan blue exclusion test, the viability of splenocytes cultured for 96 hr with TNP-Ba and MZR at 0.5–10 μg/ml was found to be more than 90%. The number of harvested cells was always comparable to that of the control cells cultured without MZR.

Plaque-forming cell (PFC) assay. Details have been described previously (*8*). Briefly, 0.2 ml of recovered cells were mixed with 0.05 ml of 50% TNP-SRBC or TNP-horse erythrocytes (when TNP-SRBC was used as antigen) and 2 ml soft agar in a 47°C water bath. The mixture was immediately poured into a 10-cm plastic dish covered with base agar. After 1 hr of incubation at 37°C, 2 ml fresh guinea pig serum diluted to 1/20 in HBSS, which had been twice absorbed with TNP-SRBC at 0°C, was added as a complement source, and incubated for an additional 1 hr. After the plate was counted for direct anti-TNP PFC, 2 ml antimouse immunoglobulin (Ig) rabbit serum, which was diluted to 1/100 in HBSS, was added after aspirating off the guinea pig serum using a Pasteur pipette. Following an additional 2-hour incubation, anti-mouse Ig was again replaced by complement prior to another 1-hour incubation and subsequent enumeration of indirect anti-TNP PFC.

Depletion of T cells. T cells were depleted by incubating 2×10^7 whole spleen cells at 0°C for 30 min in 1 ml of monoclonal anti-thy-1 antibody, HO-13 (*9*), a generous gift from Dr. Ishikawa, Keio University School of Medicine, Department of Microbiology, Tokyo, which was finally diluted to 1/50 in HBSS, and then by incubating them in 1 ml of fresh guinea pig serum, which was diluted to 1/10, for another 30 min at 37°C. After washing 3 times with HBSS, the cells were suspended at 1×10^7/ml in complete Click's medium. The loss of functioning T cells in the fraction obtained was confirmed by the absence of response to T cell mitogens such as concanavalin A (Con A, Sigma Chemical, St Louis, MO) and phytohemagglutinin P (Difco Laboratories, Detroit, MI), although the response to B cell mitogens, such as purified protein derivatives of tuberculin (preservative-free, Parke-Davis, Detroit, MI), and lipopolysaccharide (from *Escherichia coli* 055: B5, Difco Laboratories) remained unchanged compared with the response of the whole spleen cells.

Production of T cell replacing factor (TRF). Following the Watson, Aarden, and Lefkovits (*10*) method, 1×10^7 whole spleen cells were cultured with 3 μg Con A for 2 days at 37°C. The culture supernatant was harvested and stored at −20°C until use.

Development of TNP-specific memory B cells. DBA/2 mice were sensitized every 2 weeks with 2 i.p. injections of 0.2 ml 20% TNP-rabbit erythrocytes (RRBC). Two weeks after the second injection, the animals were sacrificed, and the T-cell-depleted fraction of spleen cells was prepared as described above. The cells were stimulated in vitro with TNP-SRBC in the presence of various concentrations of MZR. Then, 48 hr after the start of the culture, various amounts of TRF were added. The culture was continued for another 48 hr prior to measuring the anti-TNP PFC generated.

Statistics. Statistical analyses were performed using Student's unpaired *t* test. Data are expressed as mean ± 1 SE.

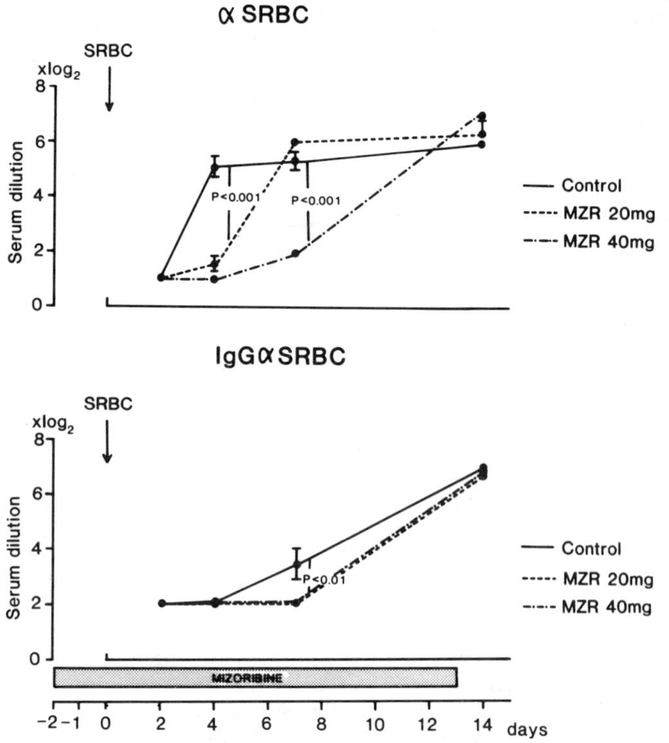

FIGURE 1. Effect of MZR on primary antihemagglutinin response in vivo. Three groups of 10 mice were studied. On day 0, 0.2 ml 20% SRBC was injected, i.p., into all of the animals; on days −2 through 13, each of the 3 groups daily received, s.c., 100 μl of PBS only, or 20 or 40 mg/kg body weight of MZR dissolved in the same amount of PBS. Animals were bled on days 2, 4, 7, and 14. On the upper panel is the hemagglutinin level of untreated sera; on the lower panel, that of 2-ME-pretreated sera (see the *Materials and Methods* section). The mean ± 1 SE of 10 animals is shown.

RESULTS

In vivo studies. The serum anti-SRBC hemagglutinin level on day 4 in the group of mice given 20 mg MZR/kg body weight daily, and on days 4 and 7 in another group given 40 mg, was significantly lower compared with the control group, which was given 100 μl of phosphate-buffered saline (PBS, used as carrier) only ($P<0.001$; Fig. 1, upper panel). Pretreatment of sera with 2-ME abolished the early antibody response seen on days 4 and 7 in the control group and on day 7 in the group given 20 mg of MZR. No difference in the IgG antibody level was detected between the control and the experimental groups on day 4, while on day 7 the difference was significant ($P<0.01$; Fig. 1, lower panel).

In vitro studies. To confirm the differential degree of T cell dependency of TNP-SRBC and TNP-Ba, the whole spleen cells and their T-cell-depleted fraction were stimulated with these antigens (Table 1). Anti-TNP PFC production by the T-depleted fraction, which was stimulated with TNP-SRBC, was much lower compared with the whole spleen cells stimulated with the same antigen. On the other hand, both the whole spleen cells and their T-depleted fraction produced a comparable level of PFC when stimulated with TNP-Ba, suggesting the T-independency of this antigen.

MZR caused dose-dependent suppression in in vitro anti-TNP PFC production induced by both TD and TI antigens, such as TNP-SRBC and TNP-Ba (Fig. 2). Response to TNP-SRBC was inhibited by a lower dose, 250 ng/ml, compared with TNP-Ba.

The T-cell-depleted fraction of splenocytes, which was stimulated with either TNP-Ba or with TNP-SRBC plus 100 μl of Con-A-induced TRF, likewise showed significantly decreased response in the presence of MZR at 1 μg/ml (Fig. 3).

Direct PFC generation by TNP-specific memory B cells, which were stimulated in vitro with TNP-SRBC in the presence of TRF, was significantly suppressed by MZR at 0.5–1 μg/ml (Fig. 4). In contrast, indirect PFC response was not significantly lower in the presence of MZR up to 1 μg/ml.

To specify the timing of action during the course of 4-day culture, MZR was added at various intervals following the start of culture. At 24 hr after adding MZR, the cultured cells were

TABLE 1. Anti-TNP PFC production by the whole spleen cells and their T-cell-depleted fraction stimulated with TD or TI antigen

Cell source	Antigen	Anti-TNP PFC/ 10^6 cells	
		Exp. 1	Exp. 2
Whole splenocytes[a]	—	86	97
	TNP-SRBC	1710	3038
	TNP-Ba	1341	1540
T-cell-depleted fraction	—	82	143
	TNP-SRBC	379	406
	TNP-Ba	1216	1696

[a] 1×10^7 whole spleen cells or their T-cell-depleted fraction were cultured in vitro at 37°C in 5% CO_2 in air for 96 hr with either 5×10^5 TNP-SRBC or TNP-Ba diluted to $1/10^4$.

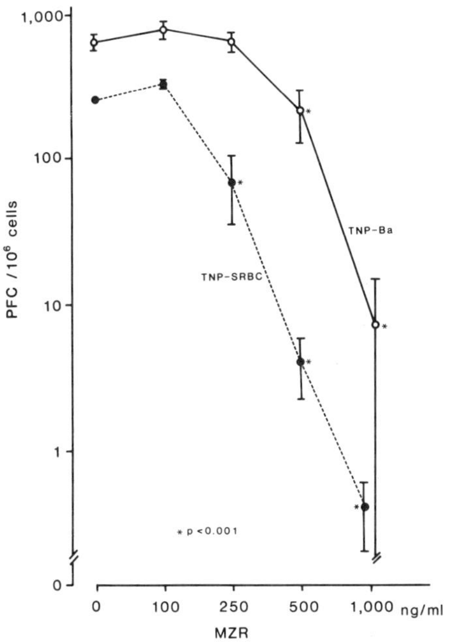

FIGURE 2. In vitro effect of MZR on anti-TNP PFC generation by spleen cells stimulated with TNP-SRBC or TNP-Ba: 1×10^7 spleen cells were cultured with 5×10^5 TNP-SRBC or TNP-Ba diluted to $1/10^4$ in the absence or presence of various doses of MZR for 96 hr prior to measuring the direct anti-TNP PFC produced. The mean ± 1 SE of 5 experiments is shown; $P<0.001$ versus control.

extensively washed. The culture then continued in a fresh media for the remainder of the time. The 24-hr MZR pulse on days 1–2 at 1 μg/ml caused marked reduction in PFC production against TNP-Ba, which was as few as 8±3.2% of the control (Fig. 5; $P<0.005$ vs. control). In contrast, 1000 ng MZR pulses on days 0–1, days 2–3, or days 3–4 caused no significant decrease in PFC generation compared with their respective controls without MZR treatment.

DISCUSSION

Although MZR has been used mainly as a T cell inhibitor for posttransplant patients (*3*), there is some experimental evidence that it may also modulate humoral immune responses. Kobayashi, Shigematsu, and Masaki (*11*) reported that early treatment in crescentic glomerulonephritis with MZR suppressed the production of humoral antibody and prevented progression of the glomerular lesions. Our therapeutic trials with MZR on experimental lupus nephropathy of NZB/W F_1 mice (*4*) resulted in a prolonged survival of the animals and a delay in the development of the glomerulopathy.

The present study was designed to provide a basis to explain the mode of action of MZR in suppressing the humoral antibody production in NZB/W F_1 mice. The result of the in vivo study suggested that MZR may inhibit IgM class antibody production.

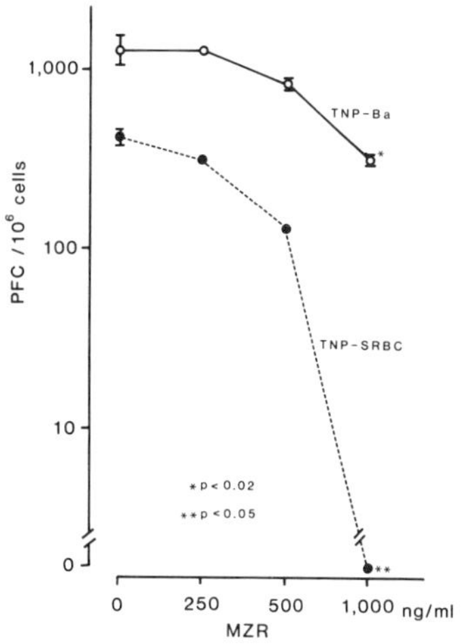

FIGURE 3. In vitro effect of MZR on anti-TNP PFC produced by T-cell-depleted fraction of spleen cells stimulated with TNP-SRBC or TNP-Ba: 1×10^7 T-depleted spleen cells were cultured with 5×10^5 TNP-SRBC or TNP-Ba diluted to $1/10^4$ with or without MZR for 96 hr. 100 μl of Con-A-induced TRF was added to the cells stimulated with TNP-SRBC 48 hr after the start of the incubation. In the absence of the TRF, the TNP-SRBC-stimulated cells generated no appreciable level of anti-TNP PFC. The mean ± 1 SE of 3 experiments is shown.

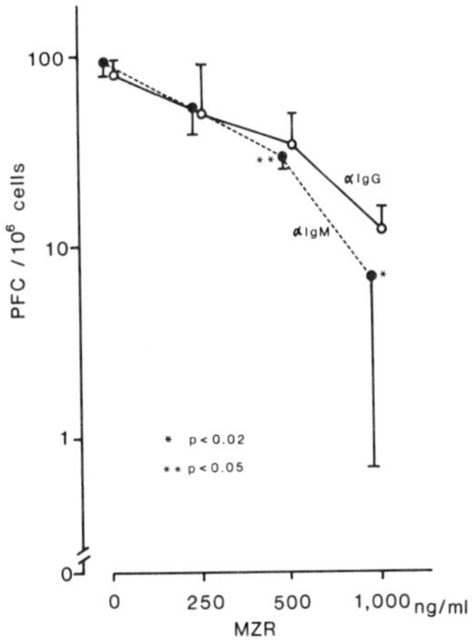

FIGURE 4. In vitro effect of MZR on direct and indirect anti-TNP PFC production by T-depleted fraction of spleen cells obtained from mice presensitized with TNP-RRBC that was stimulated in vitro with TNP-SRBC: 1×10^7 T-depleted spleen cells obtained from mice twice presensitized with TNP-RRBC were cultured with 5×10^5 TNP-SRBC with or without MZR. At 48 hr after the start of the incubation, 100 μl of TRF was added. At 96 hr, both direct and indirect anti-TNP PFC production were measured. The cells obtained from the animals injected with PBS only showed no appreciable level of indirect PFC generation when similarly stimulated in vitro with TNP-SRBC. The mean ± 1 SE of 2 experiments is shown.

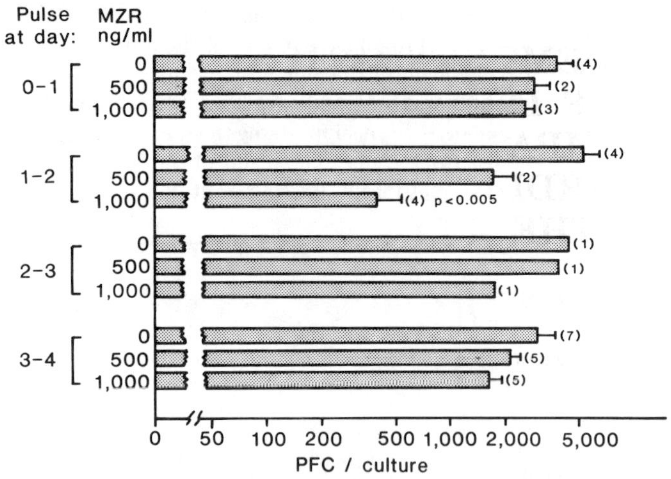

FIGURE 5. In vitro effect of intermittent 24-hr MZR pulse on anti-TNP PFC generation by spleen cells stimulated with TNP-Ba. Aliquots of 1×10^7 spleen cells were cultured with TNP-Ba diluted to $1/10^4$. They were pulse-treated with PBS only, or 500 or 1000 ng/ml of MZR at various intervals after the start of the culture. Then they were extensively washed 24 hr after the pulse treatment, the cells reconstituted to 1×10^7/ml in fresh medium without antigen, and the culture continued for the remainder of the experiment. At 96 hr, anti-TNP PFC production was measured. The number of experiments is shown in the parentheses to the right of bars. The mean ± 1 SE is shown.

Although its effect on IgG antibody has not been shown for sure in the present study, our recent analysis by ELISA showed that IgG anti-double-stranded-DNA antibody generation in NZB/W F_1 mice was significantly suppressed by MZR treatment (10 mg/kg body weight every other day [unpublished data]).

MZR suppressed antibody generation in vitro against TI (TNP-Ba), as well as TD (TNP-SRBC), antigens. In contrast, cyclosporine, which we used at a concentration of 25–100 ng/ml, did not show an inhibitory effect in vitro on antibody production induced by TNP-Ba (TI-1), in agreeement with earlier data (*12–14*), although it blocked the TNP-SRBC stimulus as effectively as MZR (*15*). It is most likely that MZR suppresses antibody production by modulating the function of the regulatory T cells (*1, 2, 16*), although Ichikawa et al. (*17*) recently reported that MZR had no inhibitory action on interleukin 2 (Il 2) production. On the other hand, the results of the present study suggest that MZR may directly act on B cells or indirectly by affecting the Mø function. No data is available at present to discriminate between the latter two possibilities.

Results of the 24-hr MZR pulse suggested that it may only be active on B cells stimulated by an antigen for at least 24 hr. MZR may not affect the initial antigen recognition or mature B cells. This reminds us of the report by Ichikawa et al. (*18*) on mixed lymphocyte reaction, which showed that MZR suppressed lymphoproliferation, but had no effect on the recognition phase or effector phase of cytotoxic lymphocytes. As an alternative explanation, MZR may indirectly act on B cells by modulating Mø function, since T independent B cell responses are known to be enhanced by Mø-produced Il-1, at least in cultures at limiting dilution, and the stimulation and induction of Il-1 by antigen has an 18-hr lag (*19*). Further characterization of the timing of action in reference to the antigen stimulation is clearly indicated.

Acknowledgments. The technical assistance provided by Miss Kazumi Nakazato is greatly appreciated. Mizoribine was a generous gift from the Toyo Jozo Co. Ltd.

REFERENCES

1. Uchida H, Yokota K, Akiyama N, et al. Effectiveness of a new drug, Bredinin, on canine kidney allotransplant survival. Transplant Proc 1979; 11: 865.
2. Okubo M, Kamata K, Yokota K, et al. Effect of Bredinin on cellular and humoral immune responses and on canine kidney allograft survival. Transplant Proc 1980; 12: 515.
3. Inou T. Immunosuppressive effects of Bredinin on renal transplantation. Summarized by Bredinin Research Committee. Japan J Transplant 1982; 17(suppl): 547. (In Japanese).
4. Kamata K, Okubo M, Uchiyama T, Masaki Y, Kobayashi Y, Tanaka T. Effect of mizoribine on lupus nephropathy of New Zealand Black/White F_1 hybrid mice. Clin Immunol Immunopathol 1984; 33: 31.
5. Click RE, Enck L, Alter BJ. Immune response in vitro. I. Culture conditions for antibody synthesis. Cell Immunol 1972; 3: 246.
6. Mond JJI, Scher DE, Mosier DE, Baese M, Paul PE. T-independent response in B cell-defective CBA/N mice to Brucella abortus. Eur J Immunol 1978; 8: 459.
7. Rittenberg MP, Pratt KL. Anti-trinitrophenyl (TNP) plaque assay. Primary response of Balb/c mice to soluble and particulate immunogens. Proc Soc Exp Biol Med 1969; 132: 575.
8. Okubo M, Kamata K, Uchiyama T. Pseudoplaque formation by cytophilic immunoglobulin in the sera of lupus patients as measured using reverse haemolytic plaque assay. Clin Exp Immunol 1982; 48: 499.
9. Kubota E, Ishikawa H, Saito K. Evidence for a cloned hybridoma (HO-13-4-9) producing 2 kinds of antibody molecules different in specificity, one directed to thy 1.2 gene products and the other to antigen on a subpopulation of thy 1.1 thymocytes. J Immunol 1981; 127: 1498.
10. Watson J, Aarden LA, Lefkovits IL. The purification and quantitation of helper T cell-replacing factors secreted by murine spleen cells activated by concanavalin A. J Immunol 1979; 122: 209.
11. Kobayashi Y, Shigematsu H, Masaki Y. Modification of crescentic masugi nephritis in the rabbit by bredinin, a new immunosuppressant. Virchows Arch (Cell Pathol) 1983; 43: 103.
12. Borel JF, Feurer C, Magnee C, Stähelin H. Effects of a new antilymphocytic peptide cyclosporin A in animals. Immunology 1977; 32: 1017.
13. Kunkl A, Klaus GGB. Selective effects of cyclosporin A on functional B cell subsets in the mouse. J Immunol 1980; 125: 2526.
14. Shidani B, Colle J-H, Motta I, Truffa-Bachi P. Effect of cyclosporin A on the induction and activation of B memory cells by thymus-independent antigens in mice. Eur J Immunol 1983; 13: 359.
15. Okubo M, Chen X-M, Kamata K, Masaki Y, Uchiyama T. Immunosuppressive effect and mode of action of cyclosporin A (CyA) and mizoribine (MZR) on humoral immune response in mice. Japan J Nephrol (in press).
16. Kamata K, Okubo M, Ishigamori E, et al. Immunosuppressive effect of Bredinin on cell-mediated and humoral immune reactions in experimental animals. Transplantation 1983; 35: 144.
17. Ichikawa Y, Ihara H, Takada K, Ishibashi M, Sagawa S. Effect of mizoribine on interleukin 2 synthesis. Transplant Proc 1984; 16: 322.
18. Ichikawa Y, Ihara H, Takahara S, et al. The immunosuppressive mode of action of mizoribine. Transplantation 1984; 38: 262.
19. Endres RO, Kushnir E, Kappler JW, Marrack P, Kinsky SC. A requirement for nonspecific T cell factors in antibody responses to "T cell independent" antigens. J Immunol 1983; 130: 781.

Received 23 May 1985.
Accepted 31 July 1985.

0041-1337/86/4104-0499$02.00/0
TRANSPLANTATION
Vol. 41, No. 4

Printed in U.S.A.

DETAILED ANALYSIS AND DEMONSTRATION OF DIFFERENCES IN THE KINETICS OF INDUCTION OF CLASS I AND CLASS II MAJOR HISTOCOMPATIBILITY COMPLEX ANTIGENS IN REJECTING CARDIAC AND KIDNEY ALLOGRAFTS IN THE RAT[1]

ANDREW D. MILTON, SARAH C. SPENCER,[2] AND JOHN W. FABRE

Blond McIndoe Centre, Queen Victoria Hospital, East Grinstead, Sussex RH19 3DZ, England

In this paper, we analyze in detail donor class I and class II major histocompatibility complex (MHC) antigen induction in heart and kidney allografts in the DA-to-PVG rat strain combination. The immunohistological techniques and quantitative absorption analyses utilize monoclonal antibodies and assay systems specific for donor class I and class II MHC antigens, to enable precise interpretation of the results in terms of the MHC antigens of the graft. Quantitative absorption analyses were performed on homogenates comprising 4–6 allografts pooled at each interval examined (days 1–5 for kidneys, days 3–7 for hearts). In the heart allografts, donor class I antigen induction begins at day 3 after transplantation and proceeds rapidly on the 4th and 5th postoperative days. The maximum level (a 10-fold increase in comparison with normal heart) occurs at day 6, and thereafter the level declines. Donor class II antigen induction in the heart allografts follows a similar pattern. In kidney allografts, it was of particular interest that donor class I induction occurred much more rapidly, being already evident on the first postoperative day, and reaching levels 20-fold greater than normal kidney by day 3. Maximum levels (approximately 30-fold that of normal kidney) of donor class I antigens were reached on days 4 and 5. Donor class II induction, by contrast, developed in kidney grafts with kinetics similar to that seen for class II induction in heart grafts (beginning at day 3 and reaching a maximum of 7-fold over normal kidney at day 5). Immunohistological studies were performed at days 1, 3, 5, and 7 after transplantation. These confirmed the early induction of donor class I antigen in the kidney allografts. In kidney, by the fifth postoperative day, all tubules in the cortex and medulla, and the arteriolar vascular endothelium, were strongly positive for class II antigens. However, the glomerulus, including the glomerular capillary endothelium, remained donor-class-II–negative, except for induction of class II antigens on Bowman's capsule. The endothelium of interstitial capillaries also probably remained class-II-negative. These results have potentially important implications for understanding the development of the rejection response.

The immune effector mechanisms involved in allograft rejection have not been clearly defined, but it seems likely that T cell-mediated cytotoxic (Tc)* and delayed-type hypersensitivity (DTH) responses both play an important role (*1–3*). These effector mechanisms show a class preference in the major histocompatibility complex (MHC) antigens to which they respond, with Tc reactions being directed predominantly at Class I MHC antigens (*4*), and DTH responses predominantly at class II MHC antigens (*5*). Moreover, although additional factors, such as lymphokine production, are essential for accessory cell function, recent studies suggest that the expression of class II MHC antigens on virtually any cell type is likely to confer on that cell the capacity to present antigens to T lymphocytes. Of particular relevance are elegant transfection experiments, in which the transfer of mouse class II MHC genes into mouse fibroblasts and the subsequent expression of class II antigens confer antigen-presenting capacity on the fibroblasts (*6*).

It follows that the presence or absence, the amount, and the location of class I and class II MHC antigens within the tissues of a graft are likely to be of primary importance in determining the mechanisms whereby a graft induces a rejection response and the effector mechanisms involved in the rejection process. At the time of grafting, the commonly transplanted organs (kidney, heart, and liver) show marked differences in their distribution and content of class I and class II MHC antigens (*7–9*)—and, in addition, human but not rat vascular endothelial cells normally express class II MHC antigens (*10*). These differences might be important in relation to the ability of the graft to initiate rejection responses (*11*). Once initiated, however, the cellular infiltrate of the rejection response will release a wide variety of lymphokines into the interstitial connective tissue of the graft. Among these lymphokines will be γ interferon from activated T lymphocytes, α interferons from a wide variety of other leukocytes, and perhaps also β interferon from fibroblasts and other cell constituents of the graft itself (*12*), α and β interferons have been shown to induce class I MHC antigens in a wide variety of different cell types in vitro (*13, 14*) while γ interferon is a potent inducer of both class I and class II MHC antigens (*15*).

In a previous report (*16*), we demonstrated that myocardial cells, which normally express little or no class I MHC antigens, and no class II MHC antigens, become strongly positive for both class I and class II MHC antigens by day 5 of the rejection process. Class II MHC antigens were also strongly induced on

[1] This work was supported by the British Heart Foundation.

[2] Rank Foundation Scholar.

* Abbreviations used: BSA, bovine serum albumin; DTH, delayed-type hypersensitivity; MHC, major histocompatibility complex; PBS, phosphate-buffered saline; PVC, polyvinylchloride; RAM, immunoadsorbent-purified rabbit F(ab′)$_2$ antimouse F(ab′)$_2$; RBC, red blood cell; Tc, cytotoxic T lymphocyte.

the vascular endothelial cells of the graft. The earliest studies demonstrating class II MHC antigen induction on the vascular endothelial (*17*) and epidermal (*18*) cells of skin allografts in rodents have also more recently been extended by other groups, using immunohistological techniques. Thus, class II antigen induction has been reported in transplanted kidneys in man, and this appears to correlate with rejection (*19*). In addition, mouse kidney allografts examined at day 6 after transplantation, showed induction of class II antigens of proximal convoluted tubules and the parietal layer of Bowman's capsule (*20*). Both class I and class II induction has been reported in pancreatic allografts in the rat (*21*).

In this report, we extend the data on cardiac allografts with a detailed, quantitative analysis of the kinetics of donor class I and class II MHC expression from the time of grafting to the time of rejection. In addition, we report similar detailed immunohistological and quantitative kinetic analyses on kidney grafts, for two reasons. First, the kidney is the most commonly transplanted organ and therefore of widespread clinical interest. Second, in contrast to heart, kidneys normally express large amounts of class I MHC antigens (*7*)—and, also in contrast to heart, kidneys express class II antigens on some of the parenchymal cells (*7, 8*). We felt that these differences might result in different patterns of MHC induction in heart and kidney allografts during rejection. Indeed, among a number of findings, we report that class I MHC induction occurs much more rapidly in kidneys than in hearts, and reaches an astonishing 30-fold increase over resting levels by the fifth postoperative day.

MATERIALS AND METHODS

Animals. Inbred DA ($RT1^a$), and PVG ($RT1^c$), and PVG $RT1^a$ male rats were obtained from OLAC 1976 Ltd., Bicester, Oxon., England, and were used between 3 and 6 months of age for organ transplantation.

Heart transplantation. Heterotopic heart allografts were performed using microsurgical techniques. After the left kidney was removed, donor hearts were anastomosed to the recipient using end-to-end anastomoses between the renal and left common carotid arteries, and between the left branch of the pulmonary artery and the renal vein. Ischemia times were in the range of 40–50 min. Heartbeat was checked daily by palpation through the abdominal wall.

Kidney transplantation. Orthotopic left kidney grafts were performed using microsurgical techniques, with end-to-end anastomoses of the renal artery and vein, and end-to-end anastomosis of the ureter. Ischemia times were in the range of 30–40 min. The recipient's right kidney was not removed.

Tissue homogenates. Homogenates were prepared from normal DA hearts and kidneys, and DA-to-PVG allografted hearts and kidneys. Organs were removed and frozen immediately at −40°C until used. On thawing, the tissues were minced with scissors in Tris-buffered saline containing proteolytic inhibitors (2.5 mM iodoacetamide, 5 mM ethylenediaminotetraacetate and 2 mM phenylmethylsulfonyl fluoride). The tissue was forced through a metal sieve and then mechanically homogenized with a Teflon pestle. The homogenate was washed twice in Tris-buffered saline by centrifuging at 30,000 g for 20 min. The pellet of the second wash was resuspended in an equal volume of Tris-buffered saline and frozen at −40°C until used. All procedures were carried out at 4°C or on ice.

Cell suspensions. Spleen cell suspensions were prepared fresh, immediately before use. Spleens were removed and rinsed in phosphate-buffered saline (PBS) to remove excess blood. They were then minced with scissors in PBS and forced through a metal sieve. The resulting cell suspension was washed twice in 0.5% bovine serum albumin (BSA) in PBS by centrifuging at 500 g for 10 min.

Red blood cell (RBC) suspensions were prepared by exsanguinating a rat into a syringe containing 200 units of heparin. The blood was washed four times by centrifuging at 500 g for 10 min and removing the buffy coat and upper layer of RBC after each wash. All cell preparations were done at 4°C or on ice.

Antibodies. Immunoadsorbent-purified rabbit $F(ab')_2$ anti-mouse $F(ab')_2$ (RAM) was prepared as described previously (*22*), and iodinated using the chloramine T method.

The F17-23-2 (*23*), MN4-91-6 (*16*), and F16-4-4 (*8*) monoclonal antibodies have previously been described in detail. All are BALB/c spleen/NS-1 hybridomas. F17-23-2 reacts with I/A homologue of rat class II MHC antigens. It is polymorphic in that it reacts with the DA, LEW, and BN strains, but not the PVG or WAG strains. MN4-91-6 reacts with RT1-A class I MHC antigens of the DA strain, and appears to be highly specific for the DA ($RT1^a$ haplotype. It does not react with other strains tested to date, including PVG, WAG, and LEW. F16-4-4 reacts with a monomorphic determinant of rat class I MHC antigens.

The MRC OX6 and MRC OX17 monoclonal antibodies react with monomorphic determinants of the rat I/A and I/E class II homologues, respectively (*24*). These two cell lines were a kind gift of Dr. A. F. Williams, MRC Cellular Immunology Unit, Oxford. The MRC OX1 antibody (*25*) against the rat leukocyte common antigen was also a gift of Dr. Williams. All monoclonal antibodies were used as immune ascites partially purified by ion-exchange chromatography.

PVG anti DA spleen alloserum was prepared by immunizing 5 PVG rats each with approximately 5×10^7 DA nucleated spleen cells in complete Freund's adjuvant in the hind foot-pads. The rats were boosted twice with approximately 5×10^7 DA spleen cells in incomplete Freund's adjuvant at weeks 4 and 7, and bled out 1 week after the last injection. The sera from the 5 rats were pooled.

Immunohistology. Tissue samples for immunohistology were frozen in liquid nitrogen immediately after harvesting. Cryostat sections of 5 μm were cut and air-dried on gelatinized slides, fixed in acetone, and stored at −20°C until used. To stain the sections, the slides were thawed and the appropriate mouse monoclonal antibody was put on the sections at saturating concentrations. This was incubated at room temperature for 30 min and washed twice in Tris-buffered saline. Horseradish-peroxidase–coupled rabbit antimouse immunoglobulin (Dako, Copenhagen, Denmark) was used at a 1:7 dilution in 20% normal rat serum to block antibodies crossreacting with rat immunoglobulins. This second incubation was also at room temperature for 30 min, after which the slides were washed twice as above. The coloration was developed at 37°C with diaminobenzidine (Sigma Chemical Co., London) at 6 mg/10 ml containing 3 μl of 100 vol. hydrogen peroxide. Sections were counterstained with Harris's hematoxylin.

Quantitative absorption analyses for donor class I MHC antigens. Initial titration of MN4-91-6 immune ascites was performed using the binding assay (described in the next paragraph) to choose a dilution that represented conditions of target antigen excess in the assay system. Absorptions were performed at this dilution, by incubating equal volumes (80 μl) of MN4-91-6 antibody at the chosen dilution in 0.5% BSA/PBS with tripling dilutions of homogenates or cell suspensions in 0.5% BSA/PBS. For the absorptions, homogenates were used at starting concentrations as prepared above—i.e., 50% solid tissue; spleen cell suspensions were used at starting concentrations of 5×10^8 nucleated cells/ml; and RBC suspensions at 3×10^9/ml. After absorption for 1 hr, the absorbing tissue was removed by centrifugation and the supernatants assayed in a binding assay, essentially as described by Morris and Williams (*26*).

Duplicate 25 μl samples to be assayed were transferred to LP3 tubes (Luckham Ltd., Burgess Hill, Sussex). DA RBC (25 μl) at 10^9/ml in 0.5% BSA/PBS were added as targets and incubated for 1 hr. The cells were then washed twice in 0.1% BSA/PBS, and to the pellet of the second wash was added 100 μl of ^{125}I-labeled RAM in 0.5% BSA/PBS (approximately 300,000 cpm/tube). The target cells were resuspended, incubated for a further 1 hr, and washed twice as above. The pellet of the second wash was resuspended in 0.5 ml of PBS, transferred to fresh LP3 tubes, and the target cell bound radioactivity was measured in a gamma counter (LKB Produkter, Bromma, Sweden). All of the above procedures were performed at 4°C or on ice.

Quantitative absorption analyses for donor class II MHC antigens. As explained in the *Results* section, the polymorphic mouse monoclonal antibodies to rat class II MHC antigens were unsuitable for absorption analysis. The following assay was therefore devised.

The target in this assay was purified I/A type class II MHC antigen noncovalently bound to 96-well polyvinylchloride (PVC) microtiter plates (Dynatech, Billingshurst, Sussex). Details of the class II antigen purification will be given elsewhere. Briefly, the antigen was purified from detergent solubilized DA spleen homogenates using a combination of MRC OX6 monoclonal antibody affinity and Sepharose CL6B (Pharmacia, Uppsala, Sweden) gel permeation chromatography. The purified antigen gave the classic 28,000/33,000 Mr heterodimer when analyzed on nonreducing sodium dodecyl sulfate gels, with no contaminants seen when approximately 5 μg of antigen was loaded on to the gel, and the gel stained with silver (Bio-Rad, Watford, Hertfordshire, England).

Twenty-five μl of the pure antigen at approximately 10 μg/ml was incubated overnight in each well of the PVC plates. The antigen was then removed, and the remaining protein-binding sites were blocked by incubating the wells with 200 μl of 5% BSA/PBS for 30 min. This was removed, and the wells washed three times in 0.1% BSA/PBS. The antigen-coated plates were then ready for use.

The polyspecific PVG anti-DA spleen serum was the source of anti–class-II antibodies. The specificity of the assay derives from the fact that a pure antigen preparation was used as the target. For the initial titration, 25 μl of doubling dilutions of the PVG anti DA antiserum was added to the class-II-antigen–coated wells, and incubated for 1 hr. The antiserum was then removed, the wells washed 3 times in 0.1% BSA/PBS, and 50 μl of ^{125}I-labeled RAM containing 300,000 cpm was added. After a further 1 hr incubation, the wells were washed 3 times as above. The individual wells were then cut out and the bound radioactivity measured in a gamma counter (LKB Produkter, Bromma, Sweden). All steps were performed at 4°C.

Although the PVG anti-DA serum is of rat origin, the RAM was used as the second antibody because of the substantial (≥ 80%) crossreactivity of the antimouse $(Fab')_2$ antibodies for rat $F(ab')_2$. The absorption and subsequent assays on the class II plates were, in principle, identical to that described for MN4-91-6.

RESULTS

A critical factor for unequivocal interpretation of studies on donor MHC antigen induction in transplantation is the development of antibodies and assay systems specific for *donor* class I and class II MHC antigens. In this way, the MHC antigens present on the infiltrating recipient leukocytes do not obscure or interfere with the interpretation or quantitation of the induction.

In a previous report (*16*), we demonstrated that the MN4-91-6 mouse monoclonal antibody (antirat class I MHC antigen) was specific for DA in both immunohistological and quantitative absorption analyses, DA tissues being strongly positive and PVG tissues completely negative. The F17-23-2 antibody (antirat class II MHC antigen) was also specific for DA and functioned well in immunohistological studies. However, the F17-23-2 proved unsuitable for absorption analyses over a wide range of dilutions, probably because low affinity of the antibody results in high free antibody concentrations even in conditions of antigen excess in the absorption (*16*).

We have therefore developed an assay specific for DA class II MHC antigens by using polyspecific PVG anti-DA spleen alloserum and assaying this on pure DA class II MHC antigens immobilized on PVC plates, as detailed in the *Materials and Methods* section. The specificity of this assay for class II antigens is inherent in the molecular purity of the target antigen used, but further proof is given in Figure 1, where it can be seen the PVG RT1^a spleen cells absorb well, but PVG

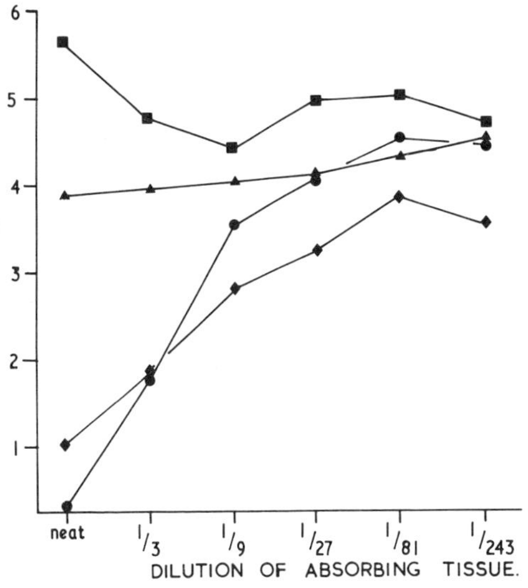

FIGURE 1. Specificity of anti DA class II assay. PVG anti-DA alloserum at a 1:15 dilution was absorbed with equal volumes of tripling dilutions of various cell suspensions. The absorbed serum was assayed for residual antibody by adding it to PVC microtiter plates to which DA class II MHC antigens had been noncovalently bound. Binding of the alloserum to the plates was detected with ^{125}I-labeled RAM. The absorbing cells were: (▲) PVG spleen; (●) DA spleen; (◆) PVG RT1^a spleen; and (■) DA RBC. The starting concentration for the spleen cell suspension was 5×10^8/ml—and for the RBC, 3×10^9/ml.

spleen cells and DA RBC do not give any absorption. Proof of strain specificity of this assay is also given in Figure 1, where it can be seen that DA spleen absorbs well, but PVG spleen is negative. With this assay, we could proceed with quantitative studies on class II MHC antigen induction in the DA-to-PVG allograft model.

Heart Allografts

In the previous study (*16*) immunohistological studies demonstrated focal induction of class I and class II MHC antigens in the myocardium at day 3. By day 5, there was strong induction of both class I and class II antigens throughout the myocardium, including class II induction on the vascular endothelial cells of arterioles. Quantitation of donor class I induction at day 5 showed a remarkable 5–10-fold increase in class I expression in comparison with the normal DA heart. Here, we report more detailed kinetic studies.

Quantitation of donor class I MHC antigen induction in heart allografts. DA cardiac allografts were removed on days 3, 4, 5, 6, and 7 after transplantation into PVG recipients, and immediately frozen. Between 4 and 6 allografts were pooled for each interval, and the pooled allografts homogenized for the absorption studies. The results are given in Figure 2. At day 3 there is a relatively modest increase of only 50% in class I expression, which is consistent with the weak, focal induction seen on immunohistology. However, once donor class I MHC antigen expression has begun it proceeds rapidly. At day 4, there is a 4-fold increase over normal heart (approximately 3-fold over the day 3 rejecting heart). At day 5 the increase is 7-fold over normal heart (approximately 2-fold over day 4 heart), and at day 6 there is a 10-fold increase over normal heart (approximately 50% increase over day 5 heart). Whether the decrease in the pace of induction at day 6 is a reflection of physiological control mechanisms, or represents damage to the myocardial cells as a result of the rejection process, cannot be distinguished. Certainly, at day 7, when there is obvious and widespread myocardial necrosis, the amount of donor class I in the rejecting heart is reduced to half the level seen at day 6, although this still represents 5 times the amount of class I antigen in normal DA heart.

Quantitation of class donor II MHC antigen induction in heart allografts. Quantitations here were done at days 3, 5, and 7 after grafting, using the cardiac allograft homogenates described in the preceding section. The results are given in Figure 3. The class II MHC antigen content of normal heart is low and it gives weak absorption curves, as previously described (*7*). This is because the only class II positive structure in normal heart is the interstitial dendritic cell, which is the presumed immunogenic passenger leukocyte (*9*). By day 3, (at which time one can see focal induction on immunohistology), there is probably a detectable increase in the quantity of class II MHC antigen expression by absorption analysis, but the absorption curve is not much different from that of normal heart. By day 5, however, there is a clear and substantial increase in the level of donor class II antigen expression in the rejecting graft. Precise quantitation is obviously not possible given the shallow slope of the absorption curve for normal DA heart. However, a comparison of the absorption curves for the day 5 allograft with the day 3 allograft suggests an approximately 5-fold increase in class II antigen content. By day 7, the donor class II MHC antigen content drops to about 50% of that seen at day 5 (approximately 2–3 times the amount in normal heart).

The kinetics of donor class II MHC antigen induction in the cardiac allografts is very similar to that for donor class I antigen induction.

Kidney Allografts

It was mentioned in the *Introduction* that class II MHC antigen induction has been reported in the tubular cells of transplanted kidneys in man (*19*), and in proximal convoluted tubules and the parietal layer of Bowman's capsule at one time (day 6) in mouse kidney allografts (*20*). Here we present a detailed immunohistological and quantitative analyses for both

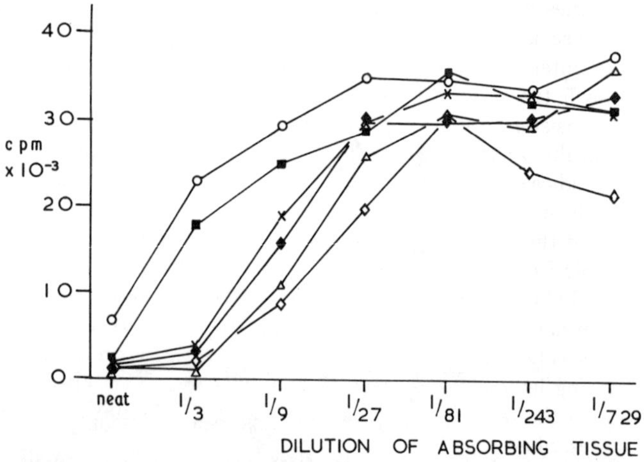

FIGURE 2. Kinetics of donor class I MHC antigen induction in cardiac allografts. The MN4-91-6 antibody was absorbed with tripling dilutions of homogenates of normal DA heart and DA-to-PVG allografted hearts. Residual antibody was assayed by incubating with DA RBC and detecting binding with ^{125}I-labeled RAM. The absorbing tissues were: (○) normal DA heart; (■) day 3 allografts; (×) day 4 allografts; (△) day 5 allografts; (◇) day 6 allografts; and (◆) day 7 allografts.

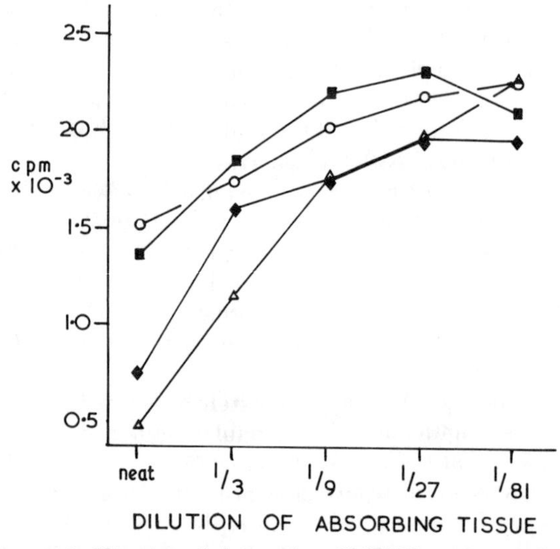

FIGURE 3. Kinetics of donor class II MHC antigen induction in cardiac allografts. The PVG anti-DA serum at a 1:15 dilution was absorbed with homogenates of normal DA heart and DA-to-PVG allografted hearts. Residual antibody was assayed on DA class II antigen-coated plates, as indicated in the legend to Figure 1. The absorbing tissues were: (○) normal DA heart; ■, day 3 allografts; (△) day 5 allografts; and (◆) day 7 allografts.

class I and class II donor MHC induction at various times after grafting in the DA-to-PVG rat kidney allograft model.

Immunohistological studies of donor class I MHC antigen induction. Three kidney allografts at each of the intervals 1, 3, 5, and 7 days after grafting were examined by the immunoperoxidase technique on frozen sections.

In normal DA kidney, all tubular cells in the cortex and medulla are definitely but relatively weakly positive for class I MHC antigens, with the medullary tubules staining more weakly than cortical tubules. As previously noted (*8*), this staining tends to be confined to the basal half of the cell. Interstitial structures, presumably mainly capillary endothelial and interstitial dendritic cells, stain more intensely than the tubular epithelial cells. Glomeruli also stand out as more intensely stained than the tubular cells, but Bowman's capsules are not stained (Fig. 4a). It should be noted that this picture in kidney is qualitatively different from that which exists in heart. In heart, only interstitial structures and intercalated discs are positive—and the major component, the myocardial cell, appears negative for class I MHC antigens.

On the first postoperative day we were surprised to note a weak but definite increase in the level of tubular staining in both cortex and medulla in all 3 kidney grafts examined. In fact, in one kidney, in addition to the generalized weak increase in staining, there were foci of very strong staining. These foci occurred both in the cortex and medulla, were approximately 5 tubules wide, and covered about one-tenth of the area of the slide (Fig. 4b). Within these foci, staining of the tubular cells was no longer confined to the base of the cells, but occurred throughout the cell.

On day 3, in marked contrast to the weak and patchy induction seen in cardiac allografts (*16*) all 3 kidney allografts showed strong induction of class I MHC antigens. Two of the three kidneys showed strong staining of all tubules in the cortex and medulla. In the third kidney, the strong staining was focal and covered about half the area of the kidney, the strong foci being approximately 10 tubules wide. Outside these foci, induction was present but less intense. At this stage, in spite of the obvious class I MHC induction in the tubules, glomeruli were no more intensely stained than in normal kidneys.

By day 5 there was an intense leukocyte infiltrate, such that all tubules, arterioles, and glomeruli were completely surrounded by several layers of leukocytes (Fig. 4d). Interestingly, as can be seen in Figure 4d, this extensive infiltrate did not extend at all into the glomerulus. At this stage, all tubules on the cortex and medulla were staining extremely intensely for donor class I MHC antigens (Fig. 4c). The glomeruli now were also staining more intensely than normal, but not as intensely as the tubules. Bowman's capsules were now clearly stained in most glomeruli.

By day 7, the grafts had become extensively damaged, and in two cases were infarcted, so meaningful immunohistology could not be done at this stage.

All of the above immunohistological studies with the polymorphic MN4-91-6 antibody were repeated with the F16-4-4 monoclonal antibody. F16-4-4 reacts with a monomorphic determinant of rat class I MHC antigens, so it stained class I antigens on recipient infiltrating leukocytes as well as donor tissues. This obscured some of the details, but the results were very similar to those just described with MN4-91-6.

Immunohistological studies of donor class II MHC antigen induction. In the normal DA kidney (Fig. 4e) epithelial cells of the proximal convoluted tubules are positive for class II MHC antigens, the staining being restricted to the basal half of the epithelial cells (*23*). Occasional, isolated tubules in the medulla are also class II positive, but weakly so. Scattered, strongly class II positive cells are seen in the interstitial connective tissues, and are more prominent in the medulla than in the cortex. These probably mainly represent interstitial dendritic cells as described in detail in the rat heart (*9*).

In contrast to the rapid induction of donor class I MHC antigens, the pace of donor class II MHC antigen induction more closely resembled that seen in cardiac allografts (*16*). Within the tubular cells, class I induction was well advanced before class II induction was observed.

On the first postoperative day, no noticeable change in donor class II MHC antigen expression had occurred in the kidney grafts.

By day 3, staining for class II antigens in the kidney cortex was noticeably stronger than normal. There appeared to be a normal number of class II negative tubules, and it is possible that the induction had occurred mainly in the already class-II–positive proximal convoluted tubules. In some instances, half a tubule was class II positive, and the other half of the same tubule was class II negative or only weakly positive (Fig. 4f). At this stage, in the kidney medulla, focal induction of class II antigens had occurred in areas approximately 5–10 tubules wide in two kidneys, while in the third kidney the induction was seen throughout the medulla. At day 3 there was essentially no induction of class II antigens in the glomerulus or the arteriolar vascular endothelium, but very occasionally one could see a glomerulus with class-II–positive Bowman's capsule and an arteriole with weak staining of the endothelium.

At day 5 all the tubules in the cortex and medulla were strongly positive for donor class II MHC antigens, the cortical tubules being more strongly stained than medullary tubules. The vascular endothelium of arterioles was now clearly and consistently class-II–positive (Fig. 4h) but it is interesting to note that the glomerular vascular endothelium was class-II–negative (Fig. 4g). The vascular endothelium of the peritubular capillaries was also probably class-II–negative, as one would otherwise have expected to see donor class II positive structures in the interstitial tissues, but these were rarely seen (Fig. 4g). At day 5, the epithelial cells of Bowman's capsules were clearly and consistently class-II–positive (Fig. 4g) but the rest of the glomerulus was completely donor-class-II–negative.

As indicated above, immunohistological assessment was not possible at day 7.

All of the above immunohistological studies with the polymorphic F17-23-2 antibody were repeated with the MRC OX6 and MRC OX17 antibodies. These reacted with monomorphic determinants of rat I/A and I/E type class II MHC antigens, respectively, and therefore stained class II antigens on recipient filtrating leukocytes as well as donor tissues. This obscured some of the details, but the results were very similar to those just described with F17-23-2.

Quantitation of donor class I MHC antigen induction in kidney allografts. DA kidney allografts were removed at 1,2, 3, 4, and 5 days after transplantation into PVG recipients, and immediately frozen. Between 4 and 6 allografts were pooled for each interval, and the pooled allografts homogenized for the absorption studies.

The immunohistological studies had suggested a rapid induction of donor class I MHC antigens and this was clearly

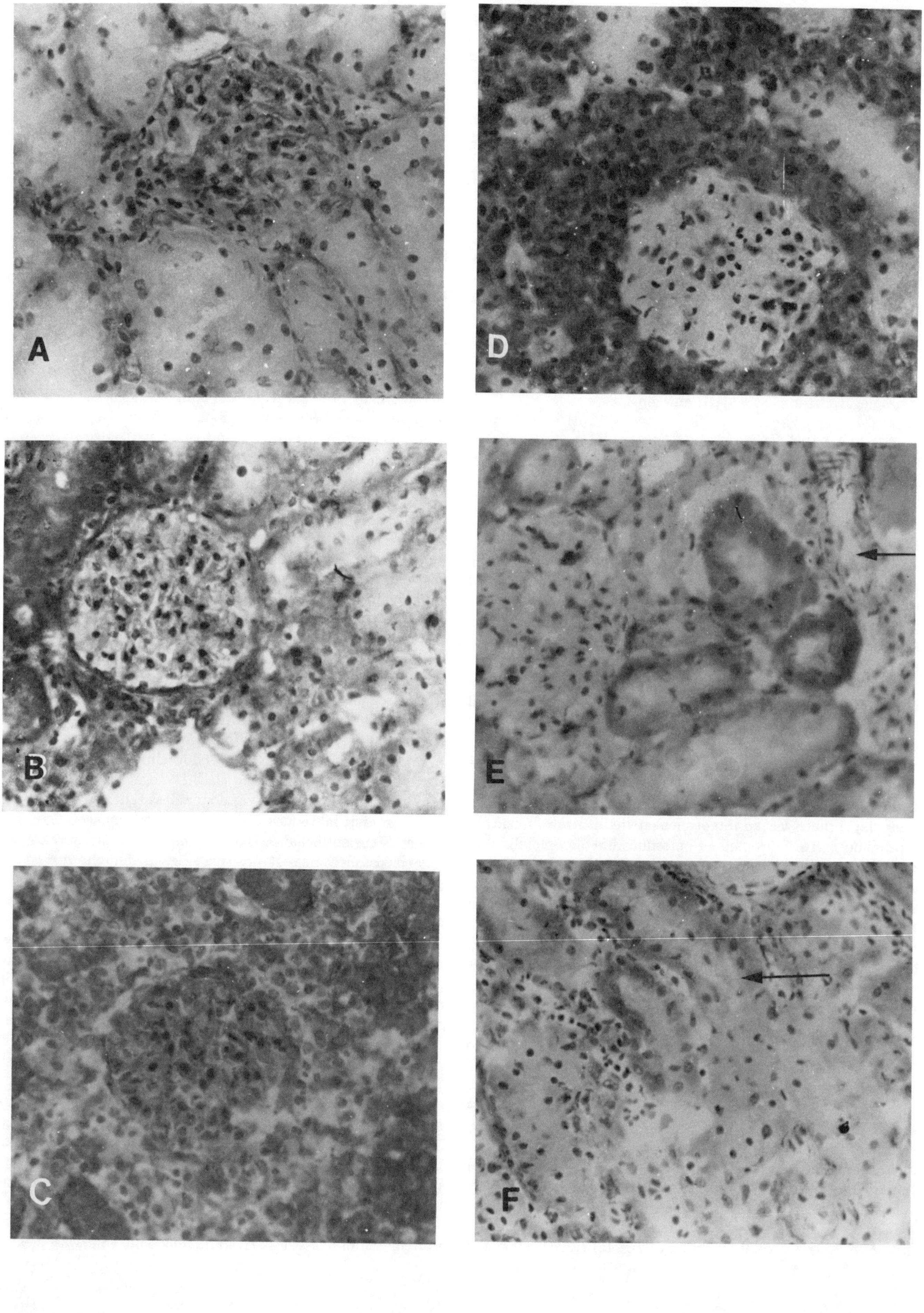
A
D
B
E
C
F

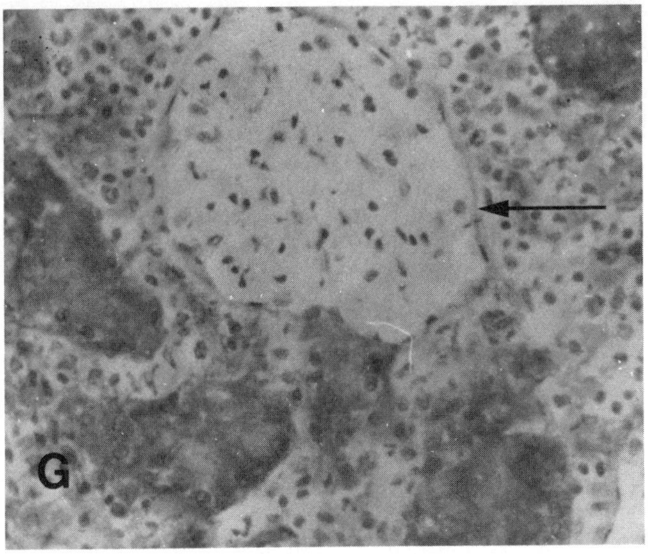

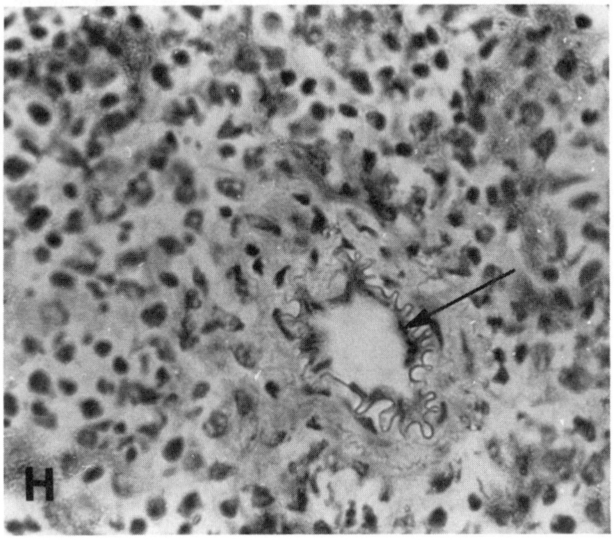

confirmed by the quantitative absorption analysis shown in Figure 5. Even at day 1, one can see that donor class I expression had approximately doubled when compared with normal DA kidney. By day 2 there had been a 5-fold increase, and by day 3 this had become a 20-fold increase in comparison to normal DA kidney.

Maximum induction of donor class I antigens in the kidney occurred at days 4 and 5, when there was a 25–30-fold increase when compared with normal DA kidney. It is important to note that the rate of increase of donor class I expression in kidney slowed markedly beyond day 3, there being only a 50% increase at day 5 as compared with day 3.

Quantitation of donor class II MHC induction in kidney allografts. Quantitations were done at day 1, 2, 3, 4, and 5 after grafting, using the same kidney graft homogenates described in the preceding section. The results are given in Figure 6.

In contrast to heart, normal kidney gives a good absorption for class II antigens, because of the expression of class II antigens on the proximal convoluted tubules. At days 1 and 2 after transplantation, one can see that the amount of class II expression actually seemed to be reduced 2–3-fold. This is a surprising result, and is presumably a consequence of the ischemia to which the kidney was subjected at the time of grafting. One should remember, however, that there had been a 5-fold increase in class I expression by day 2.

By day 3 after grafting, at which time one could see focal induction by immunohistology, there was a 2–3-fold increase in donor class II expression in the kidney. By day 4 this increase had become 7-fold over normal kidney, with no further increase at day 5.

The kinetics of class II MHC antigen induction in kidney are clearly much slower than that for class I induction, and resemble more closely class I and class II MHC antigen induction in the heart allografts.

MHC Induction in Recipient Tissues

It was possible that the allograft response produced sufficient quantities of lymphokines to raise blood levels beyond the threshold necessary for induction of MHC antigens in the tissues of the recipient. The recipient's own heart and kidney were removed for immunohistological studies from several PVG rats at day 7 after they had received DA cardiac or kidney allografts, but there was no evidence at all for MHC induction in recipient tissues.

DISCUSSION

This study establishes the massive scale on which increase in MHC expression occurs during rejection of heart and kidney grafts. We demonstrate increases measured not in terms of 20% or 30% but of up to 30-fold in the space of 5 days. Moreover, we show a clear and very interesting difference in the kinetics of class I antigen induction in kidney grafts as compared with class II antigen induction in kidney grafts, and also as compared with class I and class II antigen induction in

FIGURE 4. Immunohistological studies of donor class I and class II antigen induction in DA-to-PVG kidney grafts. DA kidneys were grafted to PVG recipients and removed at various times after grafting for immunohistology. Frozen sections were stained for class I MHC antigens (A-C), the leucocyte common antigen (D), and class II MHC antigens (E-H). (A) normal DA kidney, MN4-91-6 antibody: Note that the glomerulus stands out as more strongly staining than the weak, basal staining of the tubules. (B) kidney allograft, day 1, F16-4-4 antibody: Note the strong staining in the left half of the section—and, in contrast to normal kidney in (A), the stronger staining of the tubules in comparison with the glomerulus. (C) kidney allograft, day 5, MN4 91-6 antibody: Note strong staining of tubules and glomerulus. (D) kidney allograft, day 5, MRC OX1 antibody: Note the intense leucocyte infiltrate and the complete absence of leukocytes in the glomerulus. (E) normal kidney, F17-23-2 antibody: Note negative glomerulus and arteriole (arrow), and positive and negative tubules. (F) kidney allograft, day 3, F17-23-2 antibody: Note positive and negative tubules with some tubules (e.g. arrow) having strongly and weakly positive areas. (G) kidney allograft, day 5, F17-23-2 antibody: Note strongly positive tubules and negative glomerulus, except for positive Bowman's capsule (arrow). Note also the demonstration of donor specificity of antibody, as infiltrating leukocytes do not stain. (H) kidney allograft, day 5, F17-23-2 antibody: Note positive arteriolar endothelium (arrow). All ×250.

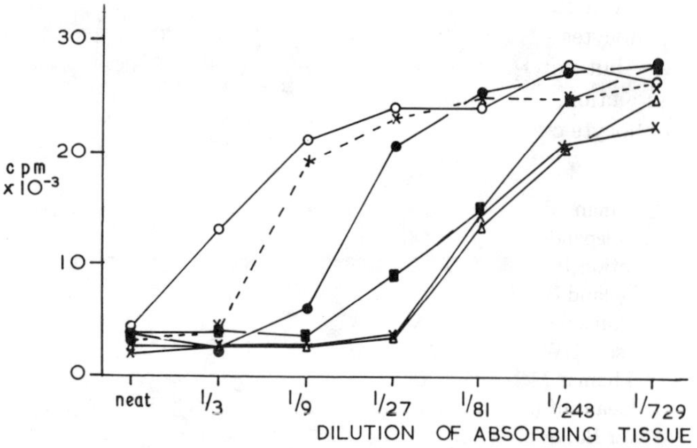

FIGURE 5. Kinetics of donor class I MHC antigen induction in kidney allografts. The MN4-91-6 antibody was absorbed with tripling dilutions of homogenates of normal DA kidney and DA-to-PVG allografted kidneys. Residual antibody was assayed by incubating with DA RBC and detecting binding with ^{125}I-labeled RAM. The absorbing tissues were : (○) normal DA kidney; (×- - - - -×) day 1 allografts; (●) day 2 allografts; (■) day 3 allografts; (×———×) day 4 allografts; and (△) day 5 allografts.

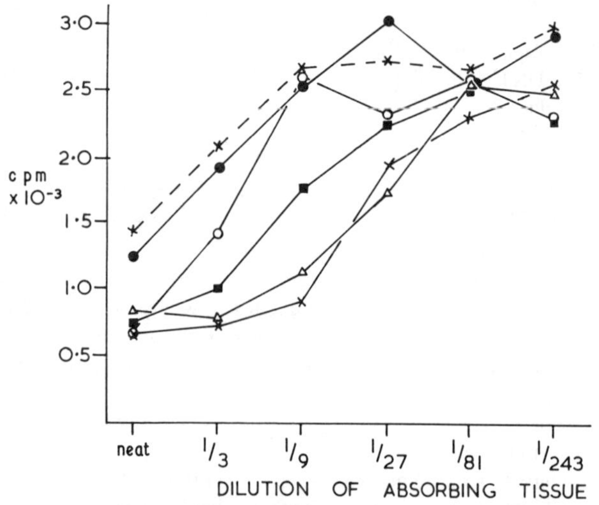

FIGURE 6. Kinetics of donor class II MHC antigen induction in kidney allografts. The PVG anti-DA serum at a 1:15 dilution was absorbed with homogenates of normal DA kidney and DA-to-PVG allografted kidneys. Residual antibody was assayed on DA class-II-antigen–coated plates, as indicated in the legend to Figure 1. The absorbing tissues were : (○) normal DA kidney; (×- - - - -×) day 1 allografts; (●) day 2 allografts; (■) day 3 allografts; (×———×) day 4 allografts; and (△) day 5 allografts.

heart grafts. These quantitative aspects of the induction kinetics are illustrated in Fig. 7.

The early and rapid increase in class I expression in kidney is of particular interest for two reasons. First, it suggests that, in kidney at least, class I and class II antigen induction is probably occurring by different mechanisms. Small foci of infiltrating leukocytes are seen at day 1 after kidney grafting, and it is possible that lymphokines released from these foci diffuse widely and are primarily responsible for the early class I induction. However, it is also possible that the inducing stimulus comes from the graft itself as a response to the ischemia at the time of transplantation. The biochemical basis for the difference in class I induction kinetics between heart and kidney are obviously unknown, but it could be related to the fact that the kidney tubules already express class I antigen in the resting state (*8*), whereas myocardial cells express little or no class I antigen (*7–9*).

Class II induction in kidney, as in heart, is most likely a result of γ interferon release from activated T lymphocytes, and therefore reflects the degree of leukocytic infiltration into the graft. It would seem that, by the time γ interferon is released in sufficient concentration into the connective tissue of the kidney graft, class I induction is already approaching maximal levels. The fact that class I induction in kidney approaches its maximum plateau at the time when γ-interferon-induced class II expression is occurring also suggests that the observed class I induction represents the maximum induction possible, and that the plateau is the result of biological constraints rather than cell destruction consequent on the rejection process. In heart allografts, γ interferon might well be the major inducing agent for both class I and class II MHC antigens.

The early induction of class I antigens in kidney grafts also represents a potentially important immunological difference between heart and kidney grafts. As previously discussed (*16*), the induction of class I MHC antigens will almost certainly increase the susceptibility of the kidney tissue to class I–specific alloreactive cytotoxic T cells, and probably also improve its capacity to induce the maturation of cytotoxic T cell precursors. The massive amount of class I antigens present by day 3 of the rejection process raises the possibility that cytotoxic T cell responses might be playing an important part in initiating kidney graft destruction at an early stage of the rejection process. It is possible that the cytotoxic T cell arm of the rejection response might occur earlier and play a greater role in the destruction of kidney grafts as compared with heart grafts. Certainly, in the grafts we studied, the cellular infiltrate was much greater in the kidneys, and the kidneys were destroyed earlier.

We have previously mentioned (*16*) that class II induction

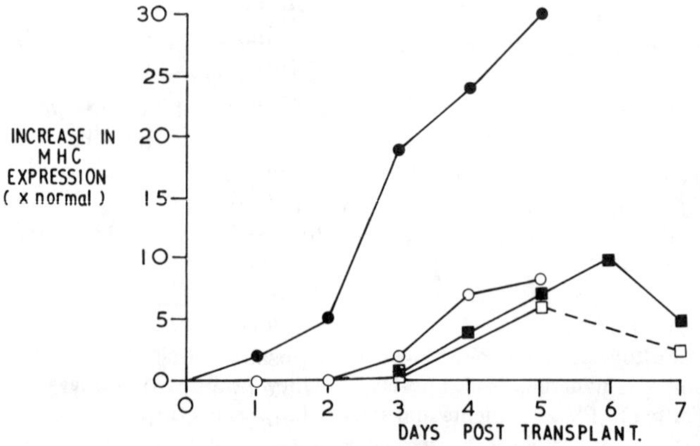

FIGURE 7. Quantitative kinetics of donor class I and class II MHC antigen induction in heart and kidney allografts. At each interval after grafting, the increase in MHC expression is plotted as the factor by which it is increased over levels in the normal organ. Calculations are based on the quantitative absorption analyses given in Figures 2, 3, 5, and 6. (●) class I antigens in kidney grafts; (○) class II antigens in kidney grafts; (■) class I antigens in heart grafts; and (□) class II antigens in heart grafts.

might play an important role in establishing and enhancing DTH type reactions in the rejecting graft. In addition, it probably enables parenchymal cells (such as myocardial and tubular cells) to present class I and minor histocompatibility antigens to the infiltrating lymphocytes (*16*). Although a variety of lymphokines are required, in addition to class II expression, for effective antigen presentation, the interstitial tissues of a rejecting graft will be bathed in many lymphokines, and therefore very likely provide an ideal milieu for class II positive epithelial and myocardial cells to act as effective antigen-presenting cells.

We feel that MHC induction probably plays an important role in the development of the rejection response. Not only does the de novo expression or the massive increase in MHC expression increase the vulnerability of the cellular components to cytotoxic and DTH type responses—but, in addition, it places the rejection response on an amplification loop similar to an expanding chain reaction. Once a focus of response has developed sufficiently for local interferon production to induce class I and (perhaps more important) class II antigens, this will make further development of the immune response progress more easily, which in turn generates more γ interferon, and so on, in an expanding and self-regenerating cycle that terminates with the destruction of the graft. Indeed, this might well explain why a brief course of therapy frequently reverses rejection episodes. If the graft can be removed from the influence of the host's immune system for even a few days, it might allow the foci of MHC induction to abate. In this way, the self-regenerating cycle is broken, and whatever coalescence of favorable local circumstances is needed to restart the process must begin once more from scratch.

One interesting observation we made was that, although there was induction of class II antigens on arteriolar endothelium, there was never any induction of class II antigen on the capillaries of the glomerulus, into which the arterioles drain. Since blood levels of lymphokines were not sufficiently high to induce MHC antigens on the recipient's own tissue, it is likely that the inducing agent had to diffuse across the arteriolar wall to the endothelial cells. The interposition of Bowman's space between the glomerular tuft and the interstitial spaces of the kidney probably shielded the glomerulus from inducing lymphokines. The other important and most interesting factor protecting the glomerulus from MHC induction was, of course, the virtually complete absence of infiltrating leukocytes in the glomeruli, in spite of massive leukocyte infiltrates throughout the rest of the graft.

Although it is difficult to make absolute statements about the endothelium of capillaries, a careful examination of the interstitial tissues for donor class II expression made it likely that class II induction was not occurring on capillary endothelium. In the published studies of de Waal et al. (*17*) on mouse skin allografts, we could see clear endothelial staining only on the major vessels. We think it is possible that the arteriolar endothelium is particularly susceptible to class II induction. If so, this might explain why leukocyte infiltration occurs, as described from the earliest days of transplantation, as periarteriolar cuffs. One would think, on general grounds, that any inducing stimulus would be far more effective at causing leukocyte infiltration across capillaries, since the diffusion of the inducing agent would be more effective across the much thinner capillary wall—and, moreover, the leukocytes would pass more slowly and be in constant contact with the endothelial cell surface during passage through the capillary bed. However, if class II induction facilitates the attachment of alloreactive lymphocytes to endothelium, and if the arteriolar endothelium—but not the capillary endothelium—demonstrates class II induction, this might explain the enigmatic periarteriolar lymphocyte cuff.

REFERENCES

1. Dallman MJ, Mason DW. Role of thymus derived and thymus independent cells in murine skin allograft rejection. Transplantation 1980; 33: 221.
2. Loveland BE, McKenzie IFC. Which T cells cause graft rejection? Transplantation 1982; 33: 217.
3. Mason DW, Arthur RP, Dallman MJ, Green JR, Spickett GP, Thomas ML. Functions of rat T lymphocyte subsets isolated by means of monoclonal antibodies. Immunol Rev 1984; 14: 57.
4. Alter BJ, Schendel DJ, Bach ML, Bach FH, Klein J, Stimpfling J. Cell-mediated lympholysis. Importance of serologically defined H-2 regions. J Exp Med 1973; 137: 1303.
5. Engleman EG, Benike CJ, Grumet FC, Evans RL. Activation of human T lymphocyte subsets; helper and suppressor/cytotoxic T cells recognize and respond to distinct histocompatibility antigens. J Immunol 1981, 127: 2124.
6. Malissen B, Price MP, Goverman JM, McMillan M, White J, Kappler J, Marrack P, Pierres A, Pierres M, Hood L. Gene transfer of H12 class II genes: antigen presentation by mouse fibroblast and hamster B cell lines. Cell 1984, 36: 319.
7. Hart DNJ, Fabre JW. Quantitative studies on the tissue distribution of Ia and SD antigens in the DA and Lewis rat strains. Transplantation 1979; 27: 110.
8. Hart DNJ, Fabre JW. MHC antigens in rat kidney, ureter and bladder: localization with monoclonal antibodies and demonstration of Ia positive dendritic cells. Transplantation 1981; 31: 318.
9. Hart DNJ, Fabre JW. Demonstration and characterisation of Ia positive dendritic cells in the interstitial connective tissues of rat heart and other tissues, but not brain. J Exp Med 1981; 154: 347.
10. Daar AS, Fuggle SV, Fabre JW, Ting A, Morris PJ. The detailed distribution of MHC class II antigens in normal human organs. Transplantation 1984; 38: 293.
11. Fabre JW. The rat kidney allograft model: was it all too good to be true? Transplantation 1982; 34: 223.
12. Clemens MJ, McNurlan MA. Regulation of cell proliferation and differentiation by interferons. Biochem J 1985; 226: 345.
13. Fellous M, Nir U, Wallach D, Merlin G, Rubinstein M, Ravel M. Interferon dependent induction of mRNA for the major histocompatibility antigens in human fibroblasts and lymphoblastoid cell lines. Proc Natl Acad Sci USA 1982; 79: 3082.
14. Wong GHW, Clark-Lewis I, Harris AW, Schrader JW. Effect of cloned interferon-γ-on expression of H-2 and Ia antigens on cell lines of hemopoetic, lymphoid, epithelial, fibroblastic and neuronal origin. Eur J Immunol 1984; 14: 52.
15. Morhen V, Merigan TC. Regulation of expression of class II major histocompatibility antigens on human peripheral blood monocytes and langerhans cells by interferon. Hum Immunol 1984; 10: 83.
16. Milton AD, Fabre JW. Massive induction of donor type class I and class II MHC antigens in rejecting cardiac allografts in the rat. J Exp Med 1985; 161: 98.
17. de Waal RMW, Bogman MJJ, Mass CN, Cornelissen LMH, Tax WJM, Koene RAP. Variable expression of Ia antigens on the vascular endothelium of mouse skin allografts. Nature 1983; 303: 426.
18. Dallman MJ, Mason DW. Induction of Ia antigens on murine epidermal cells during the rejection of skin allografts. Transplantation 1984; 36: 222.
19. Hall BM, Duggin CG, Philips J, Bishop GA, Horvarth JS, Tiller DJ. Increased expression of HLA-DR antigens on renal tubular cells in renal transplants: relevance to the rejection response. Lancet 1984; 2: 247.

20. Benson EM, Colvin RB, Russell PS. Induction of IA antigens in murine renal transplants. J Immunol 1985; 134: 7.
21. Steiniger B, Klempnauer J, Wonigeit K. Effect of the rejection process on class I and class II major histocompatibility complex antigen expression in the rat pancreas. Transplant Proc 1985; 17: 407.
22. Dalchau R, Fabre JW. Identification and unusual tissue distribution of the canine and human homologues of Thy-1 (Θ). J Exp Med 1979; 149: 576.
23. Hart DNJ, Fabre JW. Endogenously produced Ia antigens within cells of convoluted tubules of rat kidney. J Immunol 1981; 126: 2109.
24. Fukumoto T, McMaster WR, Williams AF. Mouse monoclonal antibodies against rat major histocompatibility antigens. Two Ia antigens and expression of Ia antigens and class I antigens in thymus. Eur J Immunol 1982; 12: 237.
25. Sunderland CA, McMaster WR, Williams AF. Purification with monoclonal antibody of a predominant leucocyte-common antigen and glycoprotein from rat thymocytes. Eur J Immunol 1979; 9: 155.
26. Morris RJ, Williams AF. Antigens on mouse and rat lymphocytes recognized by rabbit antiserum to rat brain; the quantitative analysis of a xenogeneic antiserum. Eur J Immunol 1975; 5: 274.

Received 2 July 1985.
Accepted 6 August 1985.

0041-1337/86/4104-0508$02.00/0
TRANSPLANTATION

Vol. 41, No. 4
Printed in U.S.A.

RELATIVE CONTRIBUTION OF MAJOR HISTOCOMPATIBILITY COMPLEX ANTIGENS TO THE IMMUNOGENICITY OF CORNEAL ALLOGRAFTS

PATRICK A. TRESELER[1] AND FRED SANFILIPPO[2]

The Departments of Microbiology and Immunology, Pathology, and Surgery, Duke University Medical Center, Durham, NC 27710

The relative contributions made by the major class I (RT1.A) and class II (RT1.B) antigens of the rat major histocompatibility complex (MHC) to the immunogenicity of corneal and skin allografts were investigated using congenic animals. PVG (RT1[c]) recipients were given skin or heterotopic cornea grafts from congenic PVG.1A (RT1[a]) or PVG.R1 (RT1[r1]) donors, which respectively share the entire RT1 complex or only the RT1.A (major class I MHC antigen) region with fully allogeneic ACI (RT1[a]) rats. Recipient splenocytes were tested at ten days posttransplant for their ability to lyse ACI, PVG.1A, PVG.R1, and PVG target cells in a secondary CML following 6 days in vitro stimulation with irradiated ACI spleen cells. Effector cells from PVG recipients of both RT1.A and B disparate (PVG.1A donor) and RT1.A disparate (PVG.R1) skin or cornea grafts lysed ACI, PVG.1A, and PVG.R1 (but not PVG) targets at levels significantly above controls given syngeneic grafts. However, the level of cytotoxicity against PVG.R1 as well as ACI and PVG.1A allogeneic targets was always significantly higher following PVG.1A grafts than following PVG.R1 grafts, indicating that the addition of a class II MHC antigen difference markedly augmented the immunogenicity of class I MHC antigen disparate cornea and skin grafts. Taken together with other recent evidence confirming the presence of Langerhans cells in the normal rat (and human) cornea, these results suggest that class II MHC-bearing cells make an important contribution to the immunogenicity of corneal allografts.

Corneal allografts have been shown to give rise to both humoral (*1*) and cellular (*2–4*) immune resposes. Antigens of the major histocompatibility complex (MHC)*, have been widely implicated in the process of corneal allograft rejection, and have been documented to act as target antigens for immune responses to allogeneic cornea (*1*, *2*). However, the role and relative importance of the various MHC antigens in evoking such responses remains unclear. In the mouse, in which the MHC has been especially well characterized (*5*, *6*), skin grafts disparate for only class I as well as skin grafts disparate for only class II MHC antigens both appear to be immunogenic. However, the immunogenicity of slowly rejected class I disparate skin may be increased by the addition of a class II antigen difference, which consistently induces more prompt rejection (*7*). However, with other tissue grafts, the presence of allogeneic class I MHC antigens alone may fail to provoke an immune response (*8*, *9*).

In this study, rats congenic for antigens of the MHC were utilized in order to determine the contribution of these various antigens to the immunogenicity of corneal allografts. Using a cellular cytotoxicity assay, it was found that class I MHC antigen disparate corneal (or skin) grafts were immunogenic, but that immunogenicity could be greatly increased by the

[1] P. A. Treseler was supported by the Medical Scientist Training Program, Grant 5-T32GM07171, from the National Institutes of Health.
[2] Address correspondence to: Dr. Fred Sanfilippo, Box 3712, Duke University Medical Center, Durham, NC 27710.

* Abbreviations used: CML, cell-mediated lymphocytotoxicity; MHC, major histocompatibility complex.

addition of a class II MHC antigen difference. Recent findings by ourselves (*10*) and others (*11–16*) indicating that class II MHC antigen-bearing Langerhans cells are present in normal corneal epithelium and stroma support the concept that disparity for class II MHC antigens is important in corneal allograft immunogenicity.

MATERIALS AND METHODS

Animals. PVT ($RT1^c$), PVG.1A ($RT1^a$), and PVG.R1 ($RT1^{r1}$) rats were obtained from Olac, Ltd. (Bicester, Oxon, UK). ACI ($RT1^a$) animals were obtained from M. A. Lab Animals (Walkersville, MD). The PVG.1A rat is a congenic animal bearing the RT1 haplotype of the ACI rat on a PVG genetic background. The PVG.R1 animal is also congenic, bearing the RT1.A region of the ACI rat on a PVG background; it thus appears to vary from PVG only at loci encoding class I MHC antigens (*17*). The RT1 haplotypes of these strains are summarized in Table 1 for the A and B loci; the C, D, and E locus haplotypes have not been reported.

Grafting and cytotoxicity assays. The grafting techniques (*1*) and cell-mediated lymphocytotoxicity (CML) assays (*2*) used have been previously described. Briefly, groups of at least 3 recipient PVG rats were each given skin or heterotopic corneal grafts from the appropriate donor strain to the chest wall. Ten days later, recipient splenocytes were put in mixed lymphocyte culture with irradiated ACI splenocytes, and after six days the recipient splenocytes were removed from culture and tested for their ability to lyse ^{51}Cr-labeled target concanavalin-A-treated lymphoblasts at several effector-to-target ratios. All assays were performed in triplicate, and the percentage of specific ^{51}Cr release was calculated as previously described (*2*).

Statistical analysis. In order to compare quantitatively the levels of cytotoxicity obtained using different effector cell populations, a best-fit quadratic curve was obtained for each lysis plot (i.e., the plot of the percentage of specific ^{51}Cr release vs. effector-to-target ratio) using the GPLOT procedure (a nonlinear least-squares fitting program) of the Statistical Analysis Systems (*18, 19*). The 99% and 95% confidence limits for these curves were then compared at an effector-to-target ratio of 7.5:1, which corresponds to the approximate midpoint of the linear, preplateau region of the lysis curves. All comparisons involved groups that were grafted and assayed on the same days with values calculated relative to the same controls.

RESULTS

RT1-disparate grafts. PVG strain rats were grafted with skin or cornea from RT1-disparate (PVG.1A) or RT1.A-disparate (PVG.R1) congenic donors. PVG recipients of syngeneic PVG cornea grafts served as negative controls. Figure 1 shows that, when ACI targets were used, high levels of cytotoxicity were obtained with effector cells from PVG rats grafted with either

TABLE 1. RT1 haplotypes of rat strains utilized

Rat strain[a]	RT1 haplotype A	RT1 haplotype B
PVG	c	c
PVG.R1	a	c
PVG.1A	a	a
ACI	a	a

[a] PVG, PVG.R1, and PVG.1A strains possess identical background (i.e., non-RT1) genes.

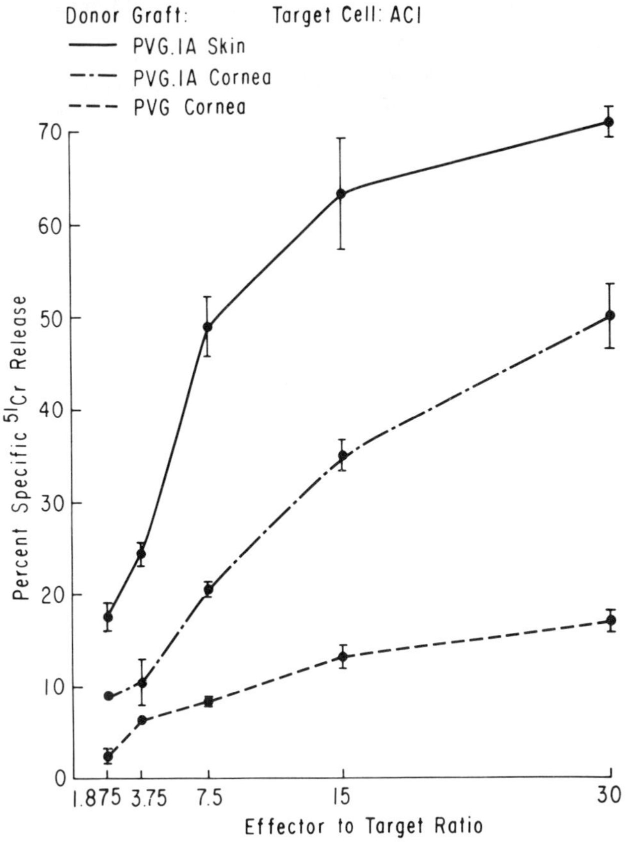

FIGURE 1. Lysis of ACI target lymphoblasts by PVG anti-PVG.1A effector cells.

PVG.1A skin or PVG.1A cornea. Effector cells from recipients of syngeneic PVG cornea yielded substantially lower levels of target cell lysis. Similar results were obtained when PVG.1A or PVG.R1 target cells were used in place of ACI cells (Figs. 2 and 3), but there was no significant lysis of syngeneic PVG targets by any effector cell population at any effector-to-target ratio (data not shown). Quantitative comparison of the best-fit quadratic equations for these lysis plots confirmed that, for all allogeneic target cells used (i.e., ACI, PVG.1A, and PVG.R1 lymphoblasts), cytotoxicity using effector cells from PVG rats grafted with either PVG.1A skin or PVG.1A cornea was significantly higher ($P<0.01$) than cytotoxicity obtained with effectors from syngeneically grafted animals.

RT1.A-disparate grafts. Figures 4, 5, and 6 show the results obtained when the same allogeneic targets (i.e., ACI, PVG.1A, and PVG.R1, respectively) were exposed to effector cells from PVG rats grated from PVG.R1 skin, PVG.R1 cornea or syngeneic PVG cornea. As with PVG.1A donor tissue, grafts of PVG.R1 skin or cornea to PVG recipients yielded effector cells that were substantially more cytotoxic toward ACI (Fig. 4), PVG.1A (Fig. 5), and PVG.R1 (Fig. 6) targets than were control effector cells from PVG recipients of syngeneic cornea grafts. These differences were again found to be significant by quantitative comparison of the cytotoxicity curves. As before, there was no significant reactivity of any of these effector cell populations with syngeneic PVG targets (data not shown).

Relative graft immunogenicity. By comparing the best-fit quadratic equations for the lysis plots generated using anti-PVG.1A and anti-PVG.R1 effector cells, PVG.1A grafts ap-

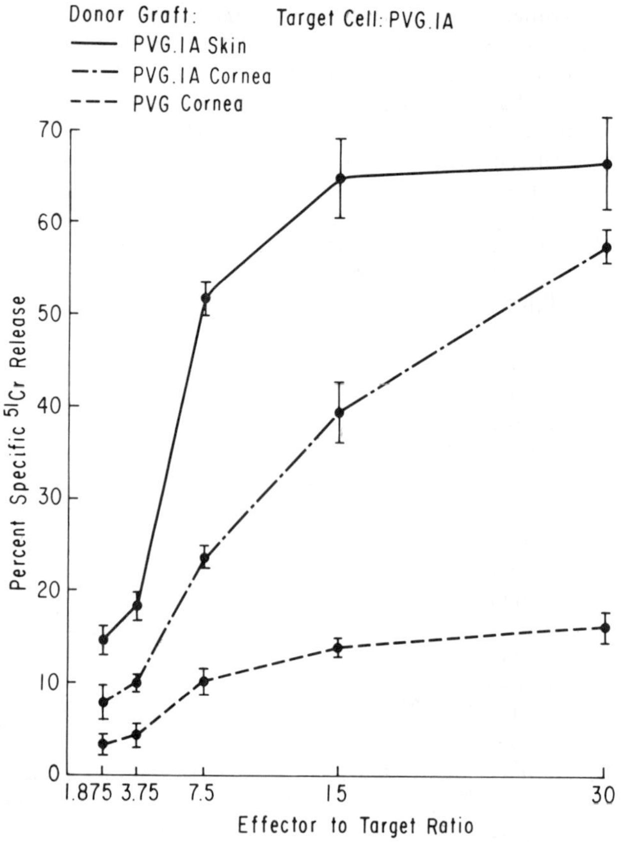

FIGURE 2. Lysis of PVG.1A target lymphoblasts by PVG anti-PVG.1A effector cells.

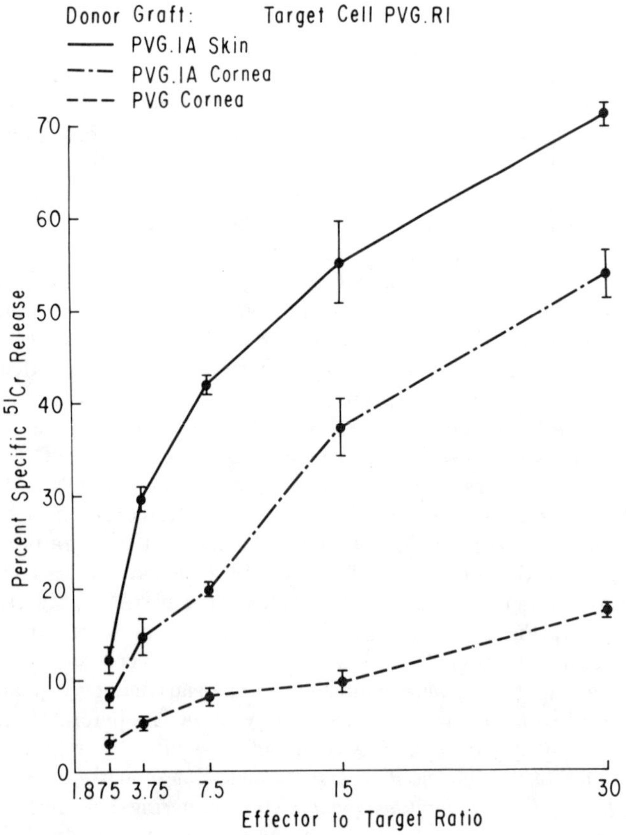

FIGURE 3. Lysis of PVG.R1 target lymphoblasts by PVG anti-PVG.1A effector cells.

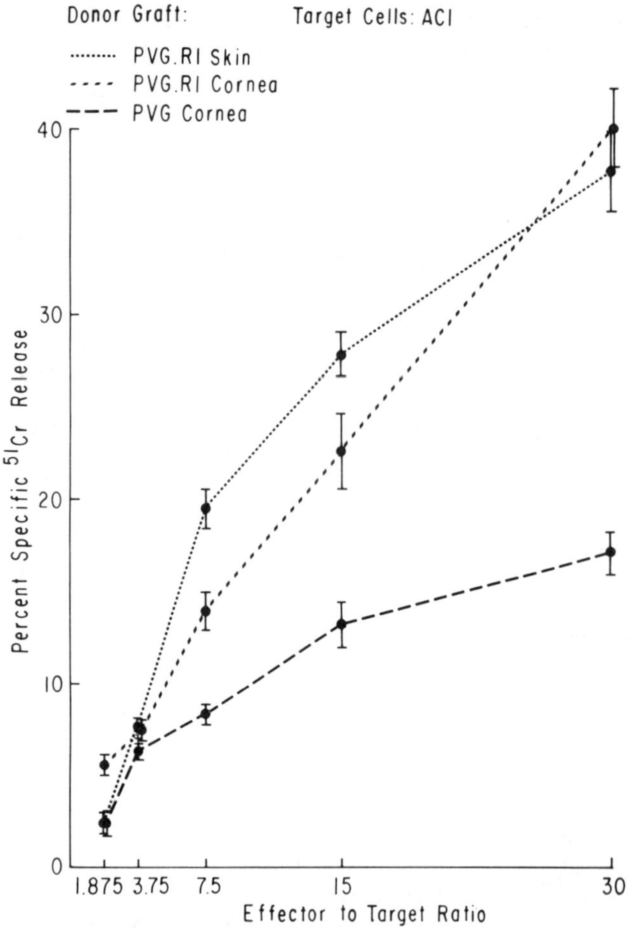

FIGURE 4. Lysis of ACI target lymphoblasts by PVG anti-PVG.R1 effector cells.

peared to be significantly more immunogenic for PVG hosts that PVG.R1 grafts. Table 2 shows the level of cytotoxicity of the two anticornea effector cell populations relative to controls and each other. For each allogeneic target cell used, cytotoxicity resulting from PVG.1A and PVG.R1 corneal grafts was significantly above controls, but the level of target cell lysis was always significantly higher ($P<0.01$) with PVG.1A grafts than with PVG.R1 grafts. Precisely the same result was obtained when PVG.1A and PVG.R1 skin grafts were compared (Table 3).

DISCUSSION

It is apparent from the results of these and our previous studies that MHC-disparate corneas are capable of evoking a cellular immune response. Splenic effector cells from PVG animals receiving RT1 disparate corneal grafts were always significantly more cytotoxic toward allogeneic target cells than were splenocytes from PVG rats given control syngeneic corneal grafts. We have previously demonstrated that the low levels of cytotoxicity yielded by effector cells from recipients of syngeneic corneas are due entirely to the in vitro stimulation that all effectors receive in this secondary CML assay (*2*). These levels of target cell lysis following PVG.1A corneal grafting are roughly equivalent to those seen when PVG rats were grafted with fully allogeneic ACI cornea (*2*), suggesting that MHC antigens alone may be responsible for the immunogenicity of corneal grafts. Indeed, other work from our labora-

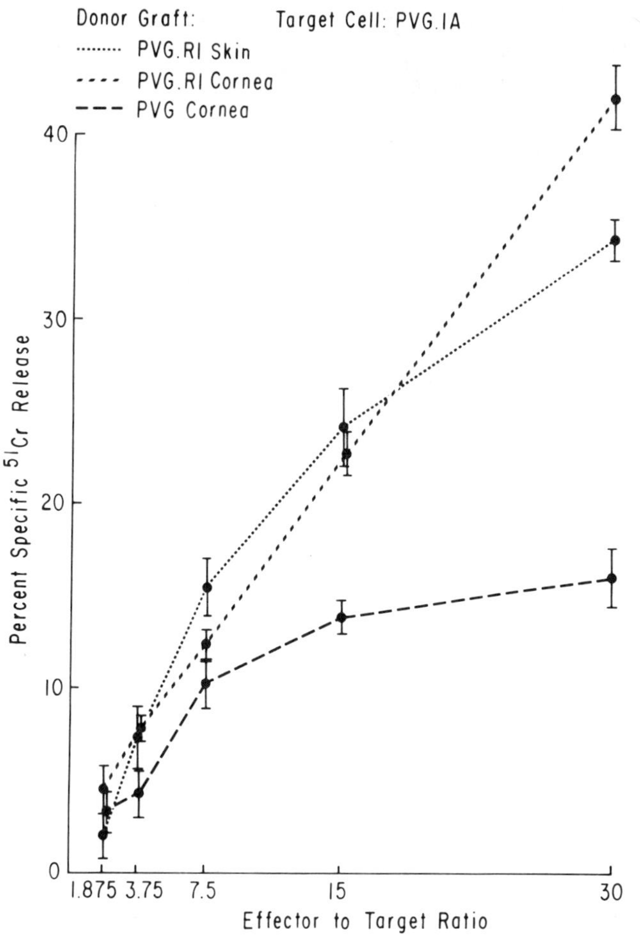

FIGURE 5. Lysis of PVG.1A target lymphoblasts by PVG anti-PVG.R1 effector cells.

tory, designed to examine the role played by non-RT1 antigens in these corneal immune responses, has shown no detectable contribution by such antigens.[3] That MHC-disparate cornea should be highly immunogenic is, in large part, predictable from the many studies linking corneal allograft failure with donor-recipient MHC disparity in animals (*20, 21*) and in humans (*21–30*). Since PVG.R1 rats vary from PVG animals only at the RT1.A region, which is only known to encode a class I MHC antigen (*31*) or antigens (*32*), the finding that PVG.R1 cells were lysed efficiently by effector cells from PVG.1A-grafted PVG rats suggests that class I MHC antigens serve as major target antigens in cell-mediated cytotoxicity against MHC-disparate corneal grafts. A similar result was previously noted for fully allogeneic grafts (*2*).

It also appears from our results that corneal grafts mismatched for only class I MHC antigens are capable of giving rise to cellular immune responses. As discussed above, PVG.R1 and PVG rats appear to differ by only a short stretch of chromosome encoding class I MHC antigens. Yet, when PVG.R1 cornea (or skin) was grafted onto PVG recipients, the recipient splenocytes were significantly more cytotoxic for allogeneic targets than were controls. This also is not entirely unexpected, since grafts of other class I MHC antigen disparate tissue have been shown to be rejected by congenic hosts in other model systems (*33–35*). Indeed, even H-2 mutant mouse skin (which in many cases may differ from the strain from which it was derived by only a few amino acids in a single class I MHC antigen [*36*]) may be briskly rejected by an otherwise identical host (*34*). Since our results deal with the in vitro measurement of cellular responses following heterotopic corneal grafts, it is unclear whether orthotopic corneal grafts would provide the same stimulus, or accessible targets for immune mediated rejection in vivo. However, a recent report clearly demonstrates that orthotopic corneal grafts are easily rejected when transplanted between different strains of inbred rats (*37*).

In addition to documenting the immunogenicity of completely MHC-disparate as well as class I MHC antigen disparate cornea grafts, our results indicate that the former is more immunogenic than the latter. In all cases, cytotoxicity following PVG.1A corneal or skin grafting was significantly higher than following PVG.R1 grafting. This marked increase in the immunogenicity of class I MHC antigen-disparate grafts by the addition of a class II MHC antigen difference suggests the possible important contribution by Langerhans cells to the immunogenicity of MHC-disparate corneal allografts.

Langerhans cells are bone-marrow-derived (*38*) dendritic cells present in many tissues (*39*), including human and rat cornea (*11*). In the cornea (*11*), as elsewhere (*40, 41*), they have been shown to express class II MHC antigens, and are known to be potent stimulators of alloreactive T lymphocytes (*42, 43*). Marked allostimulation is seen only if the Langerhans cell and T cell are class II MHC antigen disparate (*42*), and

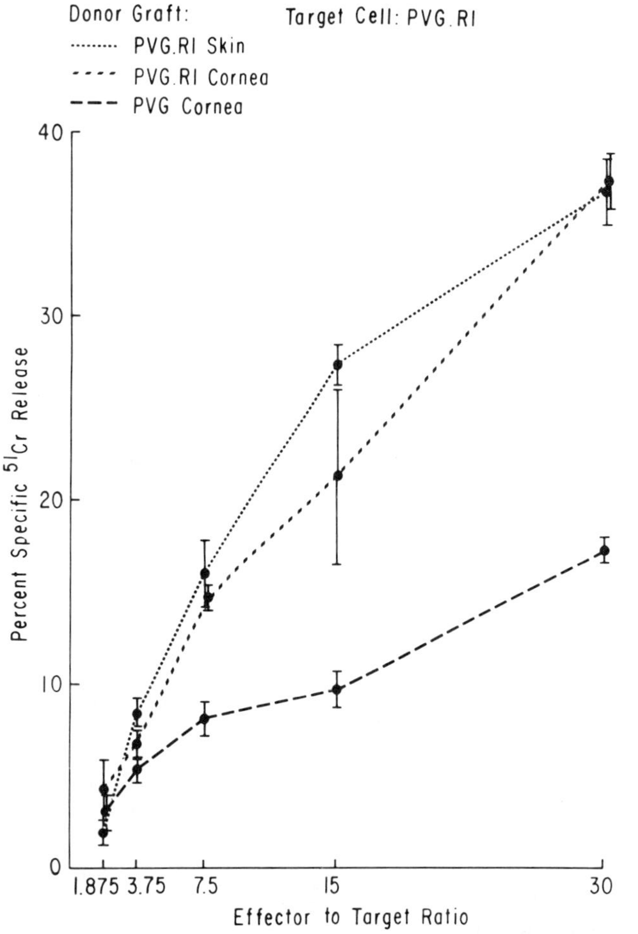

FIGURE 6. Lysis of PVG.R1 target lymphoblasts by PVG anti-PVG.R1 effector cells.

[3] Treseler et al., manuscript in preparation.

TABLE 2. Cytotoxicity using PVG anticornea effector cells

Target cell	Graft	Percentage of specific ^{51}Cr release at 7.5:1 E:T ratio[a]		
		Total	Above control	Above PVG.R1
ACI	PVG.1A cornea	20.6±0.7	12.3±0.9 ($P<0.01$)[b]	6.7±1.2 ($P<0.01$)
	PVG.R1 cornea	13.9±1.0	5.6±1.1 ($P<0.01$)[b]	
	PVG cornea (control)	8.3±0.5		
PVG.1A	PVG.1A cornea	23.6±1.2	13.4±1.8 ($P<0.01$)	11.2±1.4 ($P<0.01$)
	PVG.R1 cornea	12.4±0.8	2.2±1.5 ($P<0.05$)	
	PVG cornea (control)	10.2±1.3		
PVG.R1	PVG.1A cornea	19.8±0.7	11.7±1.1 ($P<0.01$)	5.1±1.0 ($P<0.01$)
	PVG.R1 cornea	14.7±0.7	6.6±1.1 ($P<0.05$)	
	PVG cornea (control)	8.1±0.9		
PVG	PVG.1A cornea	−1.7±0.5	0.4±0.9 (NS)[c]	−0.4±1.5 (NS)
	PVG.R1 cornea	−1.3±1.4	0.8±1.6 (NS)	
	PVG cornea (control)	−2.1±0.7		

[a] 7.5:1 Effector:target ratio corresponds to approximate midpoint of linear preplateau region of lysis curves.
[b] Significance assessed by comparing confidence limits of best-fit quadratic curve at 7.5:1 E:T ratio.
[c] Not significant.

TABLE 3. Cytotoxicity using PVG antiskin effector cells

Target cell	Graft	Percentage of specific ^{51}Cr release at 7.5:1 E:T ratio[a]		
		Total	Above control	Above PVG.R1
ACI	PVG.1A skin	49.0±3.2	40.7±3.2 ($P<0.01$)[b]	29.5±3.4 ($P<0.01$)
	PVG.R1 skin	19.5±1.0	11.2±1.1 ($P<0.01$)	
	PVG cornea (control)	8.3±0.5		
PVG.1A	PVG.1A skin	51.7±1.8	41.5±2.2 ($P<0.01$)	36.3±2.3 ($P<0.01$)
	PVG.R1 skin	15.4±1.5	5.2±2.0 ($P<0.05$)	
	PVG cornea (control)	10.2±1.3		
PVG.R1	PVG.1A skin	42.0±1.0	33.9±1.3 ($P<0.01$)	26.0±2.1 ($P<0.01$)
	PVG.R1 skin	16.0±1.8	7.9±2.0 ($P<0.01$)	
	PVG cornea (control)	8.1±0.9		
PVG	PVG.1A skin	−0.4±0.8	1.7±1.1 (NS)[c]	1.6±1.4 (NS)
	PVG.R1 skin	−2.0±1.1	0.1±1.3 (NS)	
	PVG cornea (control)	−2.1±0.7		

[a] 7.5:1 Effector:target ratio corresponds to approximate midpoint of linear, preplateau region of lysis curves.
[b] Significance assessed by comparing confidence limits of best-fit quadratic curve at 7.5:1 E:T ratio.
[c] Not significant.

may be blocked by preincubating the Langerhans cell with monoclonal antibodies reactive with its class II MHC antigens (*43*). Such dendritic cells have increasingly been implicated as important "passanger leukocytes" that contribute greatly to allograft immunogenicity (*44*). Many reports suggest that the immunogenicity of allogeneic endocrine tissue may be greatly reduced, or even eliminated if it is purged of such cells (*45–48*); such findings have recently been extended to the cornea as well (*45*).

This concept of Langerhans cell allostimulation is consistent with our results concerning relative graft immunogenicity. Fully MHC disparate corneal grafts (i.e., PVG.1A-to-PVG) would be expected to yield a potent immune response since they would contain Langerhans cells bearing foreign class II MHC antigens. Recent studies also suggest that class II MHC antigen expression can be induced on the corneal endothelium by in vivo inflammation or in vitro (*50*) manipulation. With grafts differing for only class I MHC antigens (i.e., PVG.R1 to PVG), any Langerhans cells present would bear the same class II antigen as the host, and would thus lack this strong immunogenic potential. Such grafts could still provoke an immune response by other presumably less efficient routes, such as the processing of foreign class I MHC antigens by host antigen-presenting cells (*51*), resulting in the lower level of host sensitization seen with these grafts.

While possible, it is unlikely that the greater immunogenicity of PVG.1A (compared with PVG.R1) grafts is due to differences in class-I-like MHC alloantigens encoded at the RT1.E and RT1.C loci. The PVG.1A congenic rat is known to bear the $RT1^a$ genotype at the RT1.A and RT1.B loci; its genotype at the other loci has not been formally established, but it likely shares the ACI ($RT1^a$) haplotype at some or all of these sites as well. Likewise, unless the PVG.R1 is a triple recombinant, it probably expresses the PVG ($RT1^c$) haplotype at these loci. Since we have found that PVG.R1 (as well as ACI and PVG.1A) target cells were lysed more effectively by effector cells from PVG recipients grafted with corneas from PVG.1A donors versus PVG.R1 donors, the possibility of this difference reflecting contributions from class I-like antigens at the RT1.C or E loci is effectively excluded. This is true regardless of the genotype of these strains at these class I loci: if, indeed, the PVG.R1 expresses $RT1^c$ at the C or E locus and the PVG.1A expresses $RT1^a$, the RT1.C and RT1.E class I antigens of target PVG.R1 cells would be identical to those of the PVG graft recipient ($RT1^c$), and reactivity to $RT1.C^a$ or $RT1.E^a$ could not be detected. Conversely, if PVG.R1 is $RT1^a$ and PVG.1A is $RT1^c$ at these loci, there would be no difference between the PVG.1A donor and PVG recipient at these loci—and, therefore, no expected contribution to immunogenicity. Differences between these strains at other class II loci (e.g., RT1.D) may also exist, however, and these would only provide additional class II contributions to the increased immunogenicity associated with the known RT1.B class II disparity.

It should be noted that there have been reports that in certain animal strains corneal tissue may be devoid of Langerhans cells and class II MHC antigens (*52–54*). These results have been cited as evidence that class II MHC antigens play no role in corneal allograft rejections (*55–58*). We and others have repeatedly identified cells bearing class II MHC antigens in corneal epithelium and stroma of human, rat, and other species (*10–16, 59*). Using elegant immunolabeling and ultrastructural analyses one group has proven conclusively that these corneal class II MHC antigen-positive cells are indeed Langerhans cells by all accepted criteria (*11*). We believe that these studies clearly indicate that Langerhans cells are present in the cornea and, based on the results described in this report, they appear to provide an important contribution to the immunogenicity of corneal allografts.

Acknowledgments. We thank Gregory Ness, Teven Harmon, and Beth Graybeal for expert technical assistance, and Beth Barnhill for help in manuscript preparation.

REFERENCES

1. Treseler PA, Sanfilippo F. Humoral immunity to heterotopic corneal allografts in the rat. Transplantation 1985; 39: 193.
2. Treseler, PA, Treseler CB, Foulks GN, Sanfilippo F. Cellular immunity to heterotopic corneal allografts in the rat. Transplantation 1985; 39: 196.
3. Gronemeyer U, Pulhorn G, Muller-Ruchholtz W. Histocompatibility and allogeneic corneal grafting between inbred strains of rats. Mod Probl Ophthalmology 1976; 16: 161.
4. MacDonald AL, Basu PK, Miller RG. The systemic production of cytotoxic lymphoid cells in corneal allograft reaction. I. A quantitative study utilizing ^{51}chromium release assay. Transplantation 1977; 23: 431.
5. Klein J, Kiretoc A, Baxevanis CN, Nagy ZA. The traditional and a new version of the mouse H-2 complex. Nature 1981; 291: 455.
6. Klein J, Figueroa F, David CS. H-2 haplotypes, genes antigens: second listing. II. The H-2 complex. Immunogenetics 1983; 17: 553.
7. McKenzie IFC, Henning MM, Morgan GM. Skin graft enhancement studies with antigenic differences arising from the H-2K, H-2D, and H-2L loci. Transplantation 1980; 29: 439.
8. Lafferty KJ, Bootes A, Killby VAA, Burch W. Mechanisms of thyroid allograft rejection. Aust J Exp Biol Med Sci 1976; 54: 573.
9. Parr EL, Lafferty KJ, Bowen KM, McKenzie IFC. H-2 Complex and Ia antigens on cells dissociated from mouse thyroid gland and islets of Langerhans. Transplantation 1980; 30: 142.
10. Treseler PA, Foulks GN, Sanfilippo F. The expression of HLA antigens by cells in the human cornea. Am J Ophthalmol 1984; 98: 763.
11. Rodrigues MM, Rowden G, Hackett J, Bakos I. Langerhans cells in the normal conjunctiva and peripheral cornea of selected species. Invest Ophthalmol Vis Sci 1981; 21: 759.
12. Mayer DJ, Daar AS, Casey TA, Fabre JW. Localization of HLA-A,-B,-C and HLA-DR antigens in the human cornea: practical significance for grafting technique and HLA typing. Transplant Proc 1983; 15: 126.
13. Fujikawa LS, Colvin RB, Bhan AK, Fuller TC, Foster CS. Expression of HLA-A/B/C and -DR locus antigens on epithelial, stromal, and endothelial cells of the human cornea. Cornea 1982; 1: 213.
14. Whitsett CF, Stulting RD. The distribution of HLA antigens on human corneal tissue. Invest Ophthalmol Vis Sci 1984; 25: 519.
15. Gillette TE, Chandler JW, Greiner JV. Langerhans cells of the ocular surface. Ophthalmology 1982; 89: 700.
16. Chandler JW, Cummings M, Gillette TE. Presence of Langerhans cells in the central corneas of normal human infants. Invest Ophthalmol Vis Sci 1985; 26: 113.
17. Howard JC. The major histocompatibility complex of the rat: a partial review. Metabolism 1983; 32(suppl 1): 41.
18. SAS user's guide: basics, 1982 ed. Cary, North Carolina: SAS Institute.
19. SAS user's guide: statistics, 1982 ed. Cary, North Carolina: SAS Institute.
20. Ehlers N, Ahrons S. The influence of histocompatibility upon the corneal immune reaction after interlamellar allotransplantation in rabbits. Tissue Antigens 1971; 1: 23.
21. Bennett TO, Peyman GA, Tissot R, Cohen C. Histocompatibility matching in poor-prognosis penetrating keratoplasty. Acta Ophthalmol 1975; 53: 403.
22. Ehlers N, Ahrons S. Corneal transplantation and histocompatibility. Acta Ophthalmol 1971; 49: 513.
23. Ehlers N, Kissmeyer-Nielsen F. Influence of histocompatibility on the fate of the corneal transplant. In: Porter R, Knight J, eds. Corneal graft failure, Ciba Foundation Symposium 15 (new series). Amsterdam: Elsevier, 1973: 307.
24. Gibbs DC, Batchelor JR, Casey TA. The influence of HLA compatibility on the fate of corneal grafts. In: Porter R, Knight J, eds. Corneal graft failure, Ciba Foundation Symposium 15 (new series). Amsterdam: Elsevier, 1973: 293.
25. Gibbs, DC, Batchelor JR, Werb A, Schlesinger W, Casey TA. The influence of tissue-type compatibility on the fate of full thickness corneal grafts. Trans Ophthalmol Soc UK 1974; 94: 101.
26. Vannas S, Karjalainen K, Ruusuvaara P, Tiilikainen A. HLA-compatible donor cornea for the prevention of allograft rejection. Albrecht v. Graefe's Arch Klin Exp Ophthalmol 1976; 198: 217.
27. Volker-Dieben JHM, Kok-Van Alphen CC, Oosterhuis JJ, Van Dorp G, Van Leeuwen A. First experiences with HLA-matched corneal grafts in high risk cases. Documenta Ophthalmol 1977; 44: 39.
28. Stark WJ, Taylor HR, Bias WB, Maumenee AE. Histocompatibility (HLA) antigens and keratoplasty. Am J Ophthalmol 1978; 86: 595.
29. Ehlers N, Kissmeyer-Nielsen F. Corneal transplantation and HLA histocompatibility: a preliminary communication. Acta Ophthalmol 1979; 57: 738.
30. Foulks GN, Sanfilippo F. Beneficial effects of histocompatibility in high-risk corneal transplantation. Am J Ophthalmol 1982; 94: 622.
31. Gill TJ III, Cramer DJ, Kunz HW, Misra DN. Structure and function of the major histocompatibility complex of the rat. J Immunogenet 1983; 10: 261.
32. Blankenhorn EP, Cecka JM, Gotze D, Hood L. Partial N-terminal amino acid sequence of rat transplantation antigens. Nature 1978; 274: 90.
33. McKenzie IFC, Henning MM. The H-2 complex: immunogenicity and enhancement studies of the H-2K region alloantigens. J Immunogenet 1977; 4: 249.
34. McKenzie IFC, Henning MM, Morgan GM. Skin graft enhancement studies with antigenic differences arising from the H-2K, H-2D and H-2L loci. Transplantation 1980; 29: 439.
35. Isakov N, Bach FH. High frequency of splenic anti-class I cytotoxic T lymphocyte precursors correlates with in vivo rejection of K/D region disparate thyroid and islet grafts in mice. J Immunol 1984; 132: 50.
36. Nairn R, Yamaga K, Nathenson SG. Biochemistry of the gene

products from murine MHC mutants. Annu Rev Genet 1980; 14: 241.
37. Williams KA, Coster DJ. Penetrating corneal transplantation in the inbred rat: a new model. Invest Ophthalmol Vis Sci 1985; 26: 23.
38. Katz SI, Tamaki K, Sachs DH. Epidermal Langerhans cells are derived from cells originating in bone marrow. Nature 1979; 282: 324.
39. Hunter JAA. The Langerhans cell: from gold to glitter. Clin Exp Dermatol 1983; 8: 569.
40. Rowden G, Lewis MG, Sullivan AK. Ia antigen expression on human epidermal Langerhans cells. Nature 1977; 268: 247.
41. Tamaki K, Stingl G, Gullino M, Sachs DH, Katz SI. Ia antigens in mouse skin are predominantly expressed on Langerhans cells. J Immunol 1979; 123: 784.
42. Braathen LR, Thorsby E. Studies on human epidermal Langerhans cells. I. Allo-activating and antigen-presenting capacity. Scand J Immunol 1980; 11: 401.
43. Faure M, Frappaz A, Schmitt D, Dezutter-Dambuyant C, Thivolet J. Role of HLA-DR bearing Langerhans and epidermal indeterminate cells in the in vitro generation of alloreactive cytotoxic T cells in man. Cell Immunol 1984; 83: 271.
44. Lafferty KJ, Prowse SJ, Simeonovic CJ. Immunobiology of tissue transplantation: a return to the passenger leukocyte concept. Annu Rev Immunol 1983; 1: 143.
45. Chandler JW, Ray-Keil L, Gillette TE. Experimental corneal allograft rejection: description of murine model and a new hypothesis of immunopathogenesis. Curr Eye Res 1983; 2: 387.
46. Leuker DC, Sharpton TR. Survival of Ovarian allografts following maintenance in organ culture. Transplantation 1974; 18: 457.
47. Lafferty KJ, Bootes A, Dart G, Talmage DW. Effect of organ culture on the survival of thyroid allografts in mice. Transplantation 1976; 22: 138.
48. Talmage DW, Dart GA. Effect of oxygen pressure during culture on survival of mouse thyroid allografts. Science 1978; 200: 1066.
49. Bowen KM, Andrus L, Lafferty KJ. Successful allotransplantation of mouse pancreatic islets to nonimmunosuppressed recipients. Diabetes 1980; 29(suppl): 98.
50. Donnelly JJ, Li W, Rockey JH, Prendergast RA. Class II (Ia) alloantigens induced on corneal endothelium in vivo and in vitro. Invest Ophthalmol Vis Sci 1985; 26(suppl): 316.
51. Lechler RI, Batchelor JR. Restoration of immunogenicity to passenger cell-depleted kidney allografts by the addition of donor strain dendritic cells. J Exp Med 1982; 155: 31.
52. Rubsamen PE, McCulley J, Bergstresser PR, Streilein JW. On the Ia immunogenicity of mouse corneal allografts infiltrated with Langerhans cells. Invest Ophthalmol Vis Sci 1984; 25: 513.
53. Bergstresser PR, Fletcher CR, Streilein JW. Surface densities of Langerhans cells in relation to rodent epidermal sites with special immunologic properties. J Invest Dermatol 1980; 74: 77.
54. Streilein JW, Toews GB, Bergstresser PR. Corneal allografts fail to express Ia antigens. Nature 1979; 282: 326.
55. Steinman RM. Dendritic cells. Transplantation 1981; 31: 151.
56. Wolff K, Stingl G. The Langerhans cell. J Invest Dermatol 1983; 80(suppl): 17s.
57. Morris PJ, Ting A. Studies of HLA-DR with relevance to renal transplantation. Immunol Rev 1982; 66: 103.
58. Butcher GW, Howard JC. Genetic control of transplant rejection. Transplantation 1982; 34: 161.
59. Treseler PA, Sanfilippo F. The expression of MHC and leukocyte antigens by cells in the rat cornea. Transplantation (accepted).

Received 10 June 1985.
Accepted 26 July 1985.

0041-1337/86/4104-0514$02.00/0
TRANSPLANTATION
Vol. 41, No. 4
Printed in U.S.A.

SECOND-SET ALLOGRAFT RESPONSES IN THE EARTHWORM *LUMBRICUS TERRESTRIS*

KINETICS AND CHARACTERISTICS[1]

EDWIN L. COOPER, AND PHILIPPE ROCH[2]

Department of Anatomy, School of Medicine, University of California Los Angeles, CA 90024

Second-set *Lumbricus terrestris* allografts from the same donor to the same recipient undergo accelerated rejection if transplanted less than 10 days after first-set allografts. In contrast, second-set allografts, transplanted at longer intervals (20–90 days) show no accelerated rejection. Accelerated rejection of allotransplants under these kinetic conditions agrees with earlier intrafamilial xenotransplant results obtained in earthworms affirming an essential experimental variable: the time of second-set transplantation. Accelerated rejection, weak specificity, and short-term "memory" are three characteristics of the earthworm's allogeneic cellular defense/immune system. These reactions probably result from intense responses (although of short duration) of coelomocytes activated by first transplants that are still present at the time of second-set grafting but absent or inactive at later periods.

[1] This work was supported in part by Grants BRSG, AI 15976-03, and HD 09333-06 (E.L.C.) and by a postdoctoral fellowship from NATO and from The Philippe Foundation (P.R.).

[2] Present address: UA CNRS 1136, Institut de Biologie Animale, Avenue des Facultes, 33405 Talence Cedex, France.

The "memory" component associated with invertebrate graft responses, first investigated in earthworms (*1–3*) has been recently analyzed in the more primitive noncoelomate protostomes, including nemertines (*4*), sponges (*5, 6*) and corals (*7*), and in the advanced deuterostomes, such as starfish and sea urchins (*8, 9*). In earthworms (family Lumbricidae), three criteria have been used for assessing immunological memory: (1) rejection time of a second transplant; (2) adoptive transfer by coelomocytes, and (3) specificity of the second-set response. Since these first studies, the importance of coelomocytes has been stressed because they play a prominent role in earthworm graft rejection (*10–13*). With regard to specific coelomocyte types, the small undifferentiated leukocytes recognize foreign antigens, show evidence of proliferation, and then differentiate into cells that attack the grafted tissues (*14–16*).

Although only single first-set allografts were previously exchanged in the earthworms *Lumbricus* (*17*) and *Eisenia* (*2, 18, 19*), a specific second-set graft reaction was first shown in *Eisenia fetida* hosts, in allocombinations (*2, 16*) as well as in xenocombinations using other earthworms (family Lumbricidae) as donors (*1, 20, 21*). In more detail, specificity and short-term "memory" have been analyzed by three criteria. First, in both these intrafamilial transplantation experiments, heightened coelomocyte responses occurred only when the second graft was transplanted no later than a week after first-set transplantation (*22, 23*). Second, adoptive transfer of this accelerated response has been achieved by passively transferring coelomocytes from a primed earthworm to a naive one, shortening the second host's response to the new transplant (*11, 23*). Third, regarding specificity, using xenografts, accelerated reactions have been observed against a second graft performed at the same time as "third"-party grafts; these third-party test grafts showed an independent first-set rejection time (*23, 24*).

To complete the numerous transplantations devoted to gross assessment of earthworm first-set and second-set graft rejection responses begun 20 years ago, this report describes the results after second-set allografts transplanted onto *Lumbricus* hosts at 4, 7, 10, 20, 30, and 90 days after first allotransplantation. Essential controls consist of intrapopulation and interpopulation allografts transplanted in combination with autografts at various times.

MATERIALS AND METHODS

Earthworms: Outbred (mixed Canada and Idaho), sexually mature *Lumbricus terrestris* were obtained from Sure-Live Meal Worm Co., Torrance, California, and those from Bordeaux (France) came from local pasture land. Their maintenance in the laboratory in darkness at 15°C constant temperature has been described previously (*20*). Donors and recipients were always maintained individually in separate boxes.

Grafts: After 1-hr anesthesia in 5% alcohol, body-wall grafts 4-mm^2 were transplanted onto hosts 10 segments posterior to the clitellum and allowed to heal without suturing. Although not suturing increases technical losses, allowing grafts to heal normally decreases trauma and shortens grafting time. Routinely, 100 transplants are easily performed in 1 hr by this procedure. A second-set graft, always from the same donor to the same recipient, was grafted 10 segments posterior to the primary site at 4, 7, 10, 20, 30, or 90 days after the first allotransplantation, except when the second and third transplants were either autogeneic or interpopulation-allogeneic controls.

Criteria for assessing intensity of incompatibility and allograft rejection: Any transplant not well healed on all four sides 24 hr after grafting, assessed by gross observation and palpation, was eliminated from the experiment as a technical loss. We routinely obtained 80% well-healed grafts without suturing. After healing, to assess beginning allograft incompatibility leading to rejection, transplants were scored first after 24 hr, then every two days using gross criteria as revealed by a dissecting microscope. We defined a gradual scale of incompatibility and rejection responses, and arbitrarily assigned to these gross criteria increasing numerical values, so that responses could be quantified (Table 1). For example, a well-healed graft (GH)* was assigned the number 0. The presence of discrete patches of destroyed pigment cells in the graft epidermis indicated a rejection beginning (RB); this stage was assigned the number 10. Finally, a "white graft"—all pigment cells destroyed, edema, and swelling, indicating graft rejection (GR) was assigned the number 18. The results are expressed as the arithmetic means of no less than 25 worms ± SE.

Histological observations: In order to assess the veracity of the gross criteria and the commercial values assigned to them, some of the grafted earthworms were anesthetized, the transplants removed, then fixed for 48 hr in Bouin-Holland fixative. Sections (5-μm) of grafted tissue and normal host tissue surrounding the entire graft were stained with Masson-trichrome.

RESULTS

Number of transplants: Our experiments involved 608 first-set allografts, 300 autografts and 410 second-set allografts within random and nonrandom Canada-Idaho populations, and one population from Bordeaux. Among these 1318 body-wall transplants, we observed 23% technical losses and 3% deaths on day 1, mainly due to anesthetic intolerance. The reaction curves reported herein represent ranges of responses observed in 97% of grafted earthworms. Meanwhile, 1% of first-set and second-set allografts, showed acute pigment cell destruction (scored as 18) in less than 10 days. In contrast, 2% of the grafts showed no true rejection, except for slight graft resorption (scored as 4) without pigment cell destruction (Table 1).

Fate of single autograft control: Control autografts (100 transplants) showed no evidence of rejection (score 0), except for early swellings in some instances during the first 11 days (Fig. 1). The maximum mean value of "rejection intensity" (1.85± 1.03) was obtained 5 days after grafting and corresponded to a distended graft area without any visible sign of true graft rejection. This swelling effect disappeared rapidly.

First-set allograft response in random interpopulation from Canada and Idaho: Incompatibility leading to allograft rejection responses developed gradually over a 45-day observation period, as expressed kinetically in Figure 1. The mean maximum rejection intensity (14.25±2) was calculated on the basis of 409 scored transplants and reached 33 days after grafting. At this time, most of the grafts showed various gross signs of incompatibility including breakdown of pigment cells, swelling, and edema (Fig. 2). Because the grafts were never sloughed—i.e., there was gradual resorption and replacement by host tissue—it was necessary to perform histopathologic observations as confirmatory evidence of destruction and to correlate it with the correct score.

Fate of a first-set interpopulation allograft derived from a

* Abbreviations used: GH, well-healed graft; GR, graft rejection; RB, rejection beginning.

TABLE 1. Definition of gross graft conditions, numerical values, morphological features and endpoint reaction criteria for first-set allografts

Symbols	Numerical values	Morphological features
GH (graft healed)	0	All 4 sides of the graft totally and strongly healed (mechanical test)
GS (graft swollen)	2	Graft area distended by coelomic fluid accumulation
R25 (25% graft resorption)	4	
R50 (50% graft resportion)	6	Graft progressively replaced by cicatricial tissue starting from the edges
R75 (75% graft resorption)	8	
RB (rejection beginning)	10	Discrete patches of pigment in graft epidermis
R25 (25% graft rejection)	12	Pigment patches in 1/4 of graft surface epidermis with progressive depigmentation
R50 (50% graft rejection)	14	Pigment patches in half the graft surface epidermis
R75 (75% graft rejection)	16	Pigment patches in 3/4 of graft surface epidermis
GR (100% graft rejected)	18	"White graft" totally without pigmentation

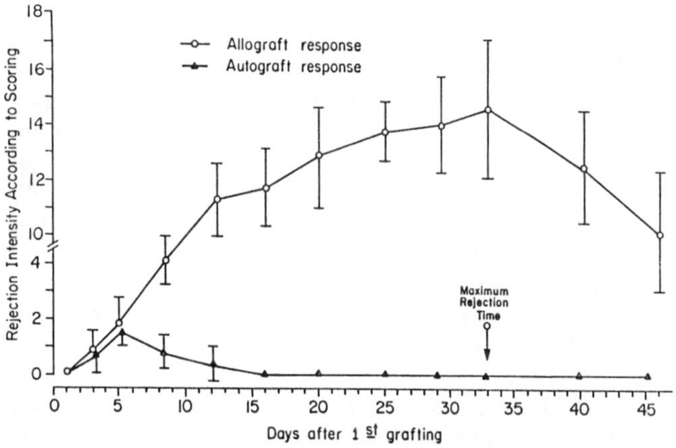

FIGURE 1. Kinetic curve of *L. terrestris* first allograft response between the 2 populations from Canada and Idaho compared with the first autograft response. Rejection intensity defined according to Table 1. Each point represents the arithmetic mean of at least 25 earthworms ±SE.

single donor on multiple nonrandom interpopulation hosts: Instead of using random mutual donors and recipients from a single population, we used one donor from each of three populations of *Lumbricus* collected from Canada, Idaho, and Bordeaux, as a source of multiple grafts onto 50 recipients per group. The results are presented for days 1 and 7 in the Idaho/Canada combinations and for the days 1, 7, and 14 in the Bordeaux/Idaho combination.

Idaho → Canada. On day 1, 100% of the transplants were well healed, corresponding to a rejection score of 0. By day 7, 58% of the transplants were still scored as 0, whereas 42% of the transplants received a score of 8, evidence of weak alloincompatibility (Fig. 3a).

Canada → Idaho. In the opposite combination—i.e., a single Canadian donor on multiple Idaho recipients—the results were somewhat different, even on day 1 when three diverse reactions were observed: 37% of the transplants were well healed (score 0), 17% showed varying degrees of swelling (score 2), and 46% showed strong alloincompatibility reactions (score 14). By day 7, the distribution had changed only slightly with 51% (score 0), 7% (score 2), and 42% showing strong alloincompatibility reactions (score 14) (Fig. 3b).

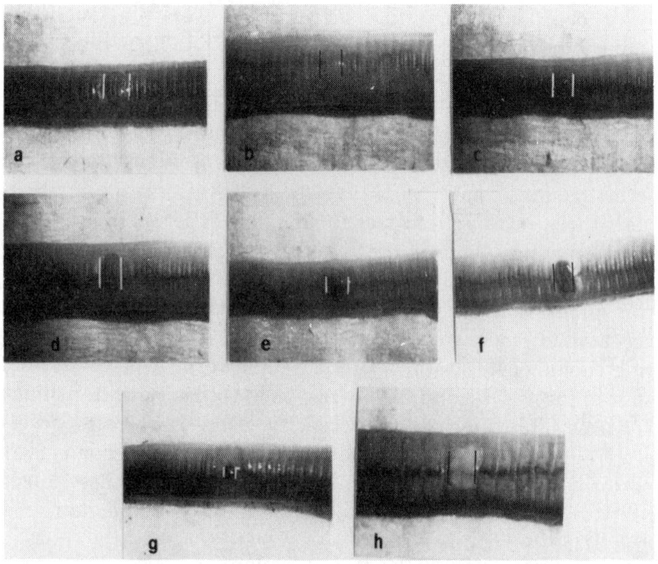

FIGURE 2. Gross features of allograft rejection in *L. terrestris*. Autograft observed 1 day (a), 10 days (b), and 30 days (c) postgrafting (note the difficulty in distinguishing the graft area after 30 days). Some typical stages of allograft incompatibility and rejection observed 1 day (d) and 5 days (e) postgrafting. Allograft rejection equivalent to score 12, observed at 12 days (f), score 16 at 20 days (g), and allograft considered as rejected (score 18) at 33 days (h). (Masson-trichrome; ×4).

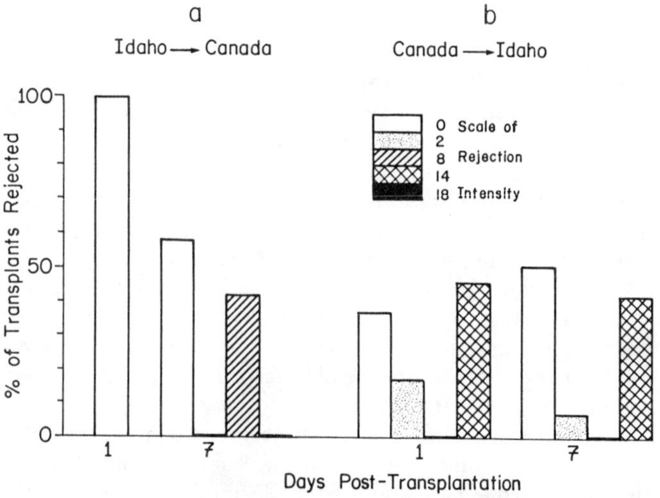

FIGURE 3. Fate of first-set interpopulation allografts derived from single donors on multiple nonrandom interpopulation hosts from Canada and Idaho. Note that a greater number of allografts were well healed in Canadian *L. terrestris*, in contrast to strong reactions in hosts from Idaho.

Bordeaux → Idaho. Allografts from a single Bordeaux donor to 50 different Idaho recipients developed several reaction patterns (Fig. 4). On day 1, 49% of the transplants were well healed (score 0), when 51% were swollen (score 2). Later, ranges of incompatibility varied so that on days 7 and 14 four distinct patterns were observed. On day 7, 48% of the transplants were still scored 0 and no rejection reactions occurred for them. All other transplants were involved in gradual rejection responses with 7% (score 8), 38% (score 14), and 7% (score 18) indicating a graft totally rejected. By day 14, the incompatibility reaction developed leading to 29% (score 0), 3% (score 8), 45% (score 14), and 23% total rejection (score 18).

Fate of first allografts exchanged between Idaho and Canadian hosts and an autograft transplanted simultaneously: On day 1 after transplantation, 24% of the autografts and 28% of the allografts showed no evidence of incompatibility (score 0). By day 3 only 8% of the autografts were scored 0 when 16% were swollen (score 2). At that time, 8% of the allografts were swollen (score 2) and 8% showed strong alloreactivity (score 8). At 7 days, 8% of the autografts were still scored 0 when 8% of the allografts were swollen (score 2) and 4% involved in graft rejection (score 14). At the end of the observations, 21 days after grafting, the response changed little except for persistent swelling (score 2) in 8% of the autografts (data not shown).

Second-set allograft response in a random population from Canada and Idaho: Second-set allografts (210 transplants) were performed at 4, 7, 10, 20, 30, and 90 days after first-set allografting from the same donor to the same recipient. Among the four curves reflecting the intensity of second-set reactions, three were essentially similar, indicating a maximum rejection time of 12–14 days (Fig. 5). The fourth curve that reflects rejection of the second allograft transplanted 20, 30, or 90 days after the first one, resembles the kinetics of first-set allograft reactions (Fig. 1). As revealed by histology, cellular responses involved in rejection of second-set allografts were identical to those described for first-set allografts (see Fig. 7). However, the sequence developed more rapidly.

Influence of a second-set allograft on the behavior of first-set allograft and autograft: Groups of 50 worms from Idaho were transplanted with an autograft and an intrapopulation allograft simultaneously. At day 7, 60% of the grafted worms showed no evidence of incompatibility (score 0). On day 7, we performed second-set allografts from the same donors to the same recipients. No change was observed even after 21 days in the first autograft and allograft behavior after transplanting the second allograft (data not shown).

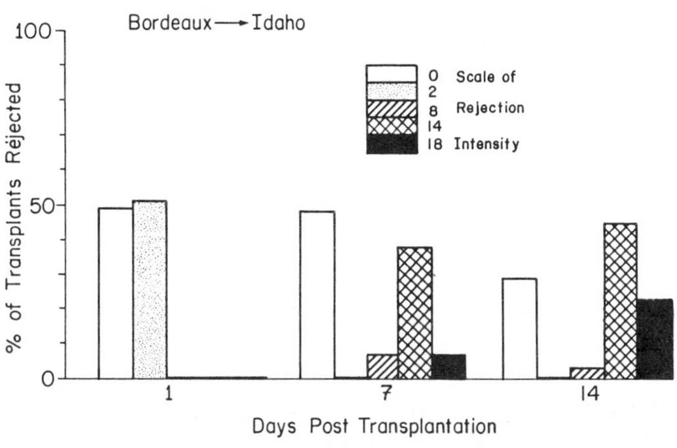

FIGURE 4. Fate of first-set allografts derived from one Bordeaux donor onto Idaho recipients. Note the stronger and faster reactions in this combination with 7% of complete rejection by day 7.

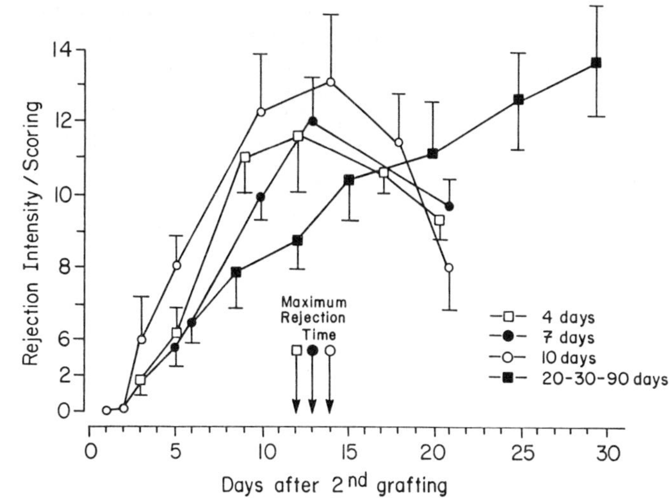

FIGURE 5. Second-set allograft responses from the same donor to the same recipient in *L. terrestris* performed 4, 7, and 10, and 20, 30, and 90 days after the first allograft. No accelerated rejections occurred after second-sets grafted at 10 days. Symbols as in Figure 1.

Condition of first-set autograft and first-set allograft exchanged between Canada and Idaho followed 11 days later by a second-set autograft: At the end of the first day, all (60) autografts and allografts were well healed (score 0), but by day 4, only 50% of allografts were still scored 0 (Table 2); the other 50% showed various degrees of incompatibility (score 4–8). Of the autografts, 80% were scored 0, and 20% scored 2. By 10 days, the scoring did not change significantly except for 2% of autoreactivity (score 4) and some increased alloreactivity (18% of score 8). At 11 days, 41 second-set autografts were transplanted—revealing, on day one, no evidence of incompatible reactions. Although by day 3, autograft patterns had changed, most of the first and second sets were well healed, despite various degrees of resorption of 8% first sets (Table 2). The first-set allografts showed the following reactions on day 14: 30% revealed no incompatible responses (score 0), whereas 70% revealed incompatibilities ranging from scores 8 to 18. At 21 days when the experiment was terminated, we observed little change from the earlier conditions (Table 2). It must be noted that the two worms showing autoreactivity (score 6 on day 14) did not react against the second autograft, suggesting some nonspecific mechanism(s) involved in reactions against the first autograft.

Fate of a first-set allograft exchanged between Canada and Idaho, grafted 15 days later with a second-set allograft from the same donor and a first-set autograft: To demonstrate specificity of recognition and differential response to autogeneic and allogeneic grafts, we grafted between two populations of *Lumbricus* from Canada and Idaho. At 15 days later, second-set allografts were exchanged between original donors and recipients and a single autograft transplanted. One week after the first transplantation 75% of the Canadian worms showed no response to Idaho allografts, whereas the remaining 25% showed destructive reactions varying from score 2 to 8. In the Idaho hosts, by contrast, only 20% showed evidence of incompatibility that ranged from score 6 to 10, whereas the remaining 80% showed no evidence of incompatibility (score 0).

TABLE 2. Condition of first-set autografts and allografts exchanged between Canada and Idaho earthworms, and the influence of a second autograft transplanted 11 days later (expressed as % of total [60] transplants)

Days after first-set transplantation	Days after second-set transplantation	First autografts %	First autografts Score	First allografts %	First allografts Score	Second allografts %	Second allografts Score
1		100	0	100	0		
4		80	0	50	0		
		20	2	50	4 to 8		
10		78	0	64	0		
		20	2	78	2		
		2	4	18	8		
12	1	—		—		100	0
14	3	78	0	30	0	70	0
		14	2	4	8	30	2
		6	4	23	10		
		2	6	15	12		
				11	14		
				12	16		
				5	18		
21	10	74	0	53	0	100	0
		14	2	5	10		
		4	4	13	12		
		5	6	26	14		
		3	8	3	18		

Three days after second-set autografting, the results changed somewhat. In recipients from both Canada and Idaho, 90% of the first allografts were still well healed (score 0) without any visible sign of incompatibility when only 10% (score 2) of the grafts were swollen (Table 3). In the Idaho recipients, reactions of the first-set allograft indicated development of rejection phenomena with 38% of the grafts (score 12 to 16). In contrast, among the Canada hosts, the rejection reaction developed more rapidly with 63% of the grafts showing rejection (score 14 to 18). At this time, 100% (for Idaho hosts) and 80% (for Canada hosts) of the second allografts (grafted 3 days before) were scored 0. One week after second allografting, the behavior of first autografts and allografts did not change. The second allograft developed a rejection reaction more rapidly in Canada hosts, with 14% (score 14), than in Idaho hosts, 14% (but score 10).

Influence of second allografts on acceleration of first-set allograft rejection times: When the rejection intensities in first-set allografts and in first-set allografts on worms bearing a second allograft exchanged randomly between Canada and Idaho populations are compared, there is acceleration of the first-set rejection (Fig. 6). The maximum rejection intensity of these grafts occurred at 20 days instead of 33 when only first-set allografts were present.

Histopathology of graft rejection: As the rejection reaction developed, the graft was progressively infiltrated by numerous leukocytes (coelomocytes) that caused complete destruction of the graft's morphological structure, best evidenced by loss of muscle integrity, death of epithelial cells, and disappearance of the basement membrane (Fig. 7). On the host side or in autografts, the muscle was always in excellent condition (Fig. 7A). Between the healthy host tissue and the graft there was a well-formed cicatrix characterized by the presence of connective tissue. In some instances, there was a fine line of demarcation between elements of the cicatrix and penetrating coelomocytes from the coelomic cavity (Fig. 7B). Coelomocytes were arranged

TABLE 3. Fate of a first-set allograft exchanged between Canada and Idaho followed 15 days later by a second allograft from the same donor and a first-set autograft

	Days after second-set transplantation	First autografts %	First autografts Score	First allografts %	First allografts Score	Second allograft %	Second allograft Score
Idaho:							
	3	90	0	39	0		
		10	2	23	10	100	0
				23	12		
				8	14		
				7	16		
Canada:							
		90	0	10	0	80	0
		10	2	9	2	2	2
				18	10	1	14
				45	14		
				9	16		
				9	18		
Idaho:							
	7	88	0	33	0	72	0
		12	2	9	2	14	2
				25	10	14	10
				17	12		
				8	14		
				8	16		
Canada:							
		77	0	10	0	14	0
		23	2	10	2	72	2
				20	10	14	14
				50	14		
				10	16		

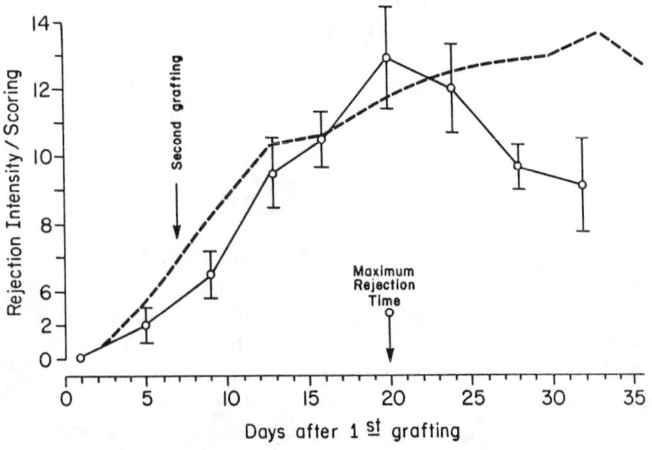

FIGURE 6. Kinetics of the first-set allograft rejection when a second allograft from the same donor is grafted 7 days after the first one. There is an accelerated rejection of the first allograft. First-set allograft reference curve (Fig. 1) is indicated as a dashed line. Symbols as in Figure 1.

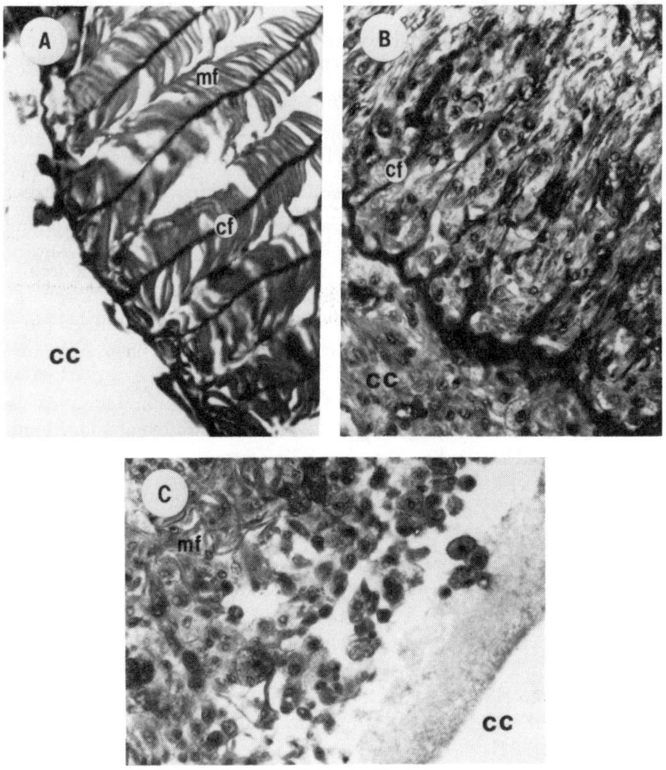

FIGURE 7. Histological aspects of allograft rejection in *L. terrestris.* Longitudinal muscle structure in a 25-day-old autograft (A) compared with a 25-day-old allograft (B–C). Note the complete destruction of muscle fibers (B), the persistence of a connective tissue stroma filled with leukocytes (B–C), the accumulation of leukocytes beneath the graft (B–C) and the presence of edema caused by swelling (C). Magnification, ×100. (cc): coelomic cavity; (mf): muscle fiber; (cf): connective tissue framework. (Masson-trichrome; ×240).

in a palisading manner, moving from the coelomic cavity into the graft matrix. Those coelomocytes which ultimately penetrated the remaining muscle just beneath the epithelium appeared to be granular, whereas those nearest the coelomic cavity were less granular and lighter staining. Beneath the graft, there was clear evidence of strong inflammatory reactions, such as the presence of patches of edema or fluid-filled spaces (Fig. 7C). In some instances blood vessels were quite prominent in the graft/host interface.

DISCUSSION

The present investigation shows evidence of a second-set response to allografts in *Lumbricus terrestris*, in 97% of the worms receiving first- and second-set allografts from the same donor to the same recipient. Other control experiments using different donor-host combinations confirm these results. This is in marked contrast to autografts, which in a few instances showed swelling 3–8 days postautografting, a response probably due to inflammatory reactions induced by wounding and healing (*25*).

Our results on second-set allograft responses in *Lumbricus terrestris* agree with previous investigations in *Eisenia fetida* where it was also clearly shown that in allograft (*2*) as well as in xenograft (*1*) rejection reactions, a second transplant is destroyed in an acute, specific fashion, demonstrating an immune reaction against foreign tissue antigens. Dealing with xenografts, accelerated rejections occurred if second-set grafts were transplanted 5–7 days after primary grafting. In addition, not only was there an accelerated rejection of the second xenograft, but the rejection time of the first xenograft was also shortened.

Coelomocytes are free cells found in the coelomic fluid of earthworms. In *Lumbricus*, the total number of coelomocytes increased after a first-set xenograft, with a peak at 3–5 days postgrafting, whereas a second-set xenograft induced an early proliferation (*24*). During the first few days postgrafting, coelomocyte multiplication may represent nonspecific phenomena, induced by any perturbations of the coelomic cavity (*25*). In *Eisenia*, a special group of small undifferentiated leukocytes has been shown to play a prominent role in graft rejection (*14*). These undifferentiated leukocytes are stimulated by the grafts, with a peak 4 days postgrafting (*19*)—when, by contrast, they did not react after a wound. Large leukocytes resembling macrophages were stimulated by inflammatory reactions (*16*). In *Lumbricus* the two mechanisms of stimulation, grafts and inflammation, have been thought to be due to recruitment or proliferation of stimulated cells; coelomocyte sub-types have not yet been defined (*26*).

To begin to assess the specificity of accelerated responses, it was necessary to challenge a host, previously sensitized by an allograft, with an autograft and an allograft, operating on the assumption that coelomocytes will only respond strongly to the allograft. We wished to confront the hosts (Idaho-Canada) with self autografts along with nonself allografts simultaneously. We predicted that the initial events occurring after transplantation—i.e., inflammation followed by cicatrization, would be relatively equal, but that the host, in the ensuing days, would make distinctions between autografts and allografts. Distinction between self and nonself was exactly what we observed, since the condition of both sets of grafts was essentially the same during the first 2 days. However, host antiallograft reactions began to become obvious on day 3 and were increasingly more pronounced by day 7; by day 21 some of the allografts were rejected.

There is some cause, however, to question the sharpness of this distinction since we did observe some persistent swelling in some of the autografts. At least with respect to allografts, the host did make sharper distinctions between first-set and second-set allografts provided the second-set grafts were transplanted at varying intervals, at least 4, 7, or 10 days. Since 4 days represents the earliest time for transplanting second-set allografts, there is no relevant information on the behavior of two allografts transplanted simultaneously to compare with the condition following the simultaneous transplantation of an autograft and allograft (Fig. 5 and Table 3). Given the existence of sharp specificity, one would predict unequivocal host responses against two allografts derived from the same donor and grafted simultaneously.

Since hosts were shown to make distinctions between autografts and allografts if performed simultaneously, and between two allografts if the second is transplanted as early as 4 days but not more than 10 days after first-set transplantation, we designed another experiment to further test for specificity. Although we had observed earlier that Idaho-Canada hosts were able to distinguish between first-set autografts and allografts if transplanted simultaneously, the same experiment failed to show distinctions if the hosts were challenged at day

7 with a second-set allograft (data not shown). We offer the following possible explanations for these results.

The first result—i.e., autografts and allografts transplanted simultaneously, provoking little or no response—is probably due to an inherently weak response, as borne out by the fact that a second-set allograft performed at 7 days evoked no reaction—perhaps the 4-day interval is the maximum challenge time. Moreover, in this experiment, we exchanged interpopulation (Idaho) allografts—which, at least in the case of other intrapopulation allografts, stimulate weaker host reactions than in interpopulation allografts (*24*). The first variable influencing the rejection is the source of the allograft. If interpopulation allografts are exchanged simultaneously with autografts and followed later by a "challenging" second-set autograft at 11 days, there is no reaction against either the two autografts except for some persistent swelling in a few of the autografts, but there is rejection of certain allografts (Table 2). Although 11 days is longer than the 7-day maximum effective time, the fact that the challenging autograft did not change the reaction, supports the existence of a specific component in the rejection process.

Up to now, specificity is shown by distinctions made by the host: (1) between autografts and allografts; (2) between sources of allografts, and (3) between challenge times after first-set transplantation. Thus, the maximum rejection intensity of second-set allografts occurred at 20 days, whereas that of first sets was at 33 days. These reactions and our conclusions are based upon the results of experiments involving first-set and second-set interpopulation and intrapopulation allografts using Canada and Idaho donors and recipients.

In earthworms, "graft memory" lasts for no longer than about 10 days. Such accelerated responses may result from the presence of large numbers of competent leukocytes induced by the first-set graft. These stimulated leukocytes are thus ready to rapidly attack the newly grafted tissues. As this "memory" disappeared long before the first graft was destroyed (at least 45 days), these activated leukocytes may not reflect the presence of a separate population of long-lived memory cells such as those found in most vertebrates.

REFERENCES

1. Valembois P. Recherches sur la nature de la réaction antigreffe chez le lombricien Eisenia fetida Savigny. CR Acad Sci Paris Ser D 1963; 257: 3489.
2. Duprat P. Mise en évidence de réaction immunitaire dans les homogreffes de paroi du corps chez le lombricien Eisenia fetida typica. CR Acad Sci Paris Ser 3 1964; 259: 4177.
3. Cooper EL. Rejection of body-wall xenograft exchanged between Lumbricus terrestris and Eisenia fetida. *Am Zool* 1965; 5: 665.
4. Langlet C, Bierne J. Immunologie des invertébrés. Recherches sur l'immunité de greffe chez les némertiens du genre Lineus. Rejet accéléré des secondes greffes hétérospécifiques incompatibles. CR Acad Sci Paris Ser D 1975; 281: 595.
5. Hildemann WH. Immunocompetence and allogenic polymorphism among invertebrates. Transplantation 1979; 27: 1.
6. Bigger CH, Hildemann WH, Jokiel PL, Johnson IS. Afferent sensitization and efferent cytotoxicity in allogeneic tissue responses of the marine sponge Callyspongia diffusa. Transplantation 1981; 31: 461.
7. Hildemann WH, Raison RL, Cheung G, Hull CJ, Akaka L, Okumoto J. Immunological specificity and memory in a scleractinian coral. Nature 1977; 270: 219.
8. Karp RD. Specific immunoreactivity in echinoderms. In: Wright RK, Cooper EL, eds. Phylogeny of thymus and bone-marrow-bursa cells. Amsterdam: Elsevier North Holland, 1976: 37.
9. Coffaro KA, Hinegardner RT. Immune response in the sea urchin, Lytechinus pictus. Science 1977; 197: 1389.
10. Duprat P. Etude de la prise et du maintien d'un greffon de paroi du corps chez le lombricien Eisenia fetida typica. Ann Inst Pasteur 1967; 113: 867.
11. Bailey S, Miller BJ, Cooper EL. Transplantation immunity in annelids. II. Adoptive transfer of the xenograft reaction. Immunology 1971; 21: 81.
12. Valembois P. Rôle des leucocytes dans l'aquisition d'une immunité spécifique chez les lombriciens. Arch Zool Exp Gen 1971; 112: 97.
13. Hostetter RK, Cooper EL Coelomocytes as effector cells in earthworm immunity. Immunol Commun 1972; 1: 155.
14. Roch Ph, Valembois P, Du Pasquier L. Response of earthworm leukocytes to Con A and transplantation antigens. Adv Exp Med Biol 1975; 64: 45.
15. Linthicum DS, Marks DH, Stein EA, Cooper EL. Graft rejection in earthworms: an electron microscopic study. Eur J Immunol 1977; 7: 871.
16. Valembois P, Roch Ph. Identification par autoradiographie des leucocytes stimulés à la suite de plaies ou de greffes chez un ver de terre. Biol Cell 1977; 28: 81.
17. Cooper EL. Chronic allograft rejection in Lumbricus terrestris. J Exp Zool 1969; 171: 69.
18. Cooper EL, Rubilotta LM. Allograft rejection in Eisenia fetida, Transplantation 1969; 8: 220.
19. Roch Ph. Leukocyte DNA synthesis in grafted lumbricids: an approach to study histcompatibility in invertebrates. Dev Comp Immunol 1979; 3: 417.
20. Cooper EL. Transplantation immunity in annelids. I. Rejection of xenografts exchanged between Lumbricus terrestris and Eisenia fetida. Transplantation 1968; 6: 322.
21. Hostetter RK, Cooper EL. Cellular anamnesis in earthworms. Cell Immunol 1973; 9: 384.
22. Cooper EL. 1985. Leukocyte activity during earthworm inflammatory reactions. Tissue Reactions (in press).
23. Roch Ph. Contribution à l'étude du transfert de l'immunité antigreffe chez le lombricien Eisenia fetida sav. CR Acad Sci Paris Ser D 1973; 276: 1369.
24. Cooper EL, Specific tissue graft rejection in earthworms. Science 1969; 166: 1414.
25. Cooper EL, Roch P. Earthworm leukocyte interactions during early stages of graft rejection. J Exp Zool 1984; 232: 67.
26. Lemmi CAE, Cooper EL. Induction of coelomocyte proliferation by xenografts in the earthworm Lumbricus terrestris. Dev Comp Immunol 1981; 5 (suppl 1): 73.

Received 13 February 1985.
Accepted 24 July 1985.

0041-1337/86/4104-0521$02.00/0
TRANSPLANTATION
Vol. 41, No. 4
Printed in U.S.A.

SPECIFICITY AND PRECURSOR FREQUENCY OF CYTOTOXIC T CELLS IN THE RESPONSE TO MINOR H ANTIGENS[1]

LINDA M. PILARSKI

Department of Immunology, University of Alberta, Edmonton, Alberta T6G2H7 Canada

The cytotoxic T cell response to minor histocompatibility antigens (MIHA) has been characterized in terms of the specificity repertoire, Lyt phenotype and precursor frequency. In the response of primed BALB/c spleen cells to B10.D2 or DBA/2 MIHA, the cytotoxic T lymphocyte (CTL) generated bear Thy-1.2, and are Lyt-1^+2^+.

In the response to intact stimulator cells we have been able to distinguish at least three different specificities of anti-MIHA CTL in the response of primed BALB/c T cells to DBA/2 MIHA. These subsets exhibit differential inductive requirements and are derived from CTL precursors (CTLp) present at different frequencies in primed spleen. As reported by others, at high responder cell numbers (10^7) the CTL generated see MIHA shared between DBA/2 and B10.D2 in H-2-restricted fashion. However, at lower numbers (3×10^5), the CTL generated are only weakly crossreactive between DBA/2 and B10.D2 as defined by cold target competition. These CTL show a higher activity for DBA/2 than for B10.D2 regardless of the hot target used in the competition assay. CTLp are depleted by absorption on DBA/2 but not B10.D2 monolayers. These CTLp are present at higher frequency than are the CTLp responsive to shared MIHA—yet are undetectable at high responder cell numbers, suggesting strong clonal dominance effects. At low cell numbers (3×10^4) in the response to intact stimulators, the CTL are specific for MIHA unique to DBA/2, and crossreactive CTL able to lyse B10.D2 are no longer detectable. Addition of growth factors to cultures restores the crossreactive CTL, suggesting a requirement for higher levels of help and indicating that these two subsets derive from different CTLp.

Finally the frequency of CTLp responsive to MIHA on intact cells was found to be 40-fold higher than the frequency of CTLp responsive to MIHA on membrane fragments. These data are discussed in terms of strong immunodominance mechanisms that appear to operate in the response to MIHA.

The cytotoxic T cell (CTL)* response to minor histocompatibility antigens (MIHA) differs in a number of important properties from CTL responses to major histocompatibility (MHC) antigens. CTL specific for MIHA are, in most cases, stringently H-2-restricted both in the induction of CTL precursor (CTLp) cells and in the ability of CTL effectors to bind to target cells (*1–7*). The frequency of CTLp specific for MIHA appears to be sufficiently low that priming in vivo is required in order to obtain CTL responses in vitro (*1, 2*), and suppressive effects predominate in unprimed populations of responder cells (*8–11*). Like the response to MHC antigens (*12–14*), the secondary response to MIHA is regulated by both helper and suppressor T cells (*15, 16*). Perhaps as a result of these regulatory cells it exhibits dramatic shifts in immunodominance patterns (*17, 18*).

Although regulatory cells appear to exert a strong influence on the CTL induced in response to MIHA (*9, 11, 15, 19–21*), the nature of the antigen plays a major role. We have shown that while H-2-restricted CTL are induced in response to intact adherent cells bearing intrinsically expressed MIHA, apparently unrestricted CTL are induced when challenged with membrane fragments bearing MIHA and presented by syngeneic adherent cells (*17*). In bulk cultures the magnitude of these two types of response appears to be equal, suggesting that challenge with subcellular MIHA inhibits CTLp specific for MIHA in association with H-2 while stimulating those that recognize MIHA in unrestricted fashion. The reverse pattern appears when the challenge is with intact cells bearing intrinsic MIHA (*17*).

In this work, we show that the specificity repertoire of the H-2-restricted CTL is considerably more exclusive in its recognition of target cell determinants than was previously thought. We describe three different specificity subsets of MIHA-specific CTL that appear to have quite different inductive requirements. Finally, the precursor frequencies of the restricted and unrestricted CTL are shown to be of very different magnitude.

MATERIALS AND METHODS

Mice: BALB/cCr, DBA/2, C57BL10/J (B10), and B10.D2 mice were bred at the Medical Sciences Animal Breeding Center at the University of Alberta. Unless otherwise indicated, BALB/cCr mice were primed in vivo with 2×10^7 irradiated DBA/2 spleen cells at approximately 6–7 weeks of age. Spleen cells were removed for in vitro culture at least 4 weeks postpriming.

Generation of CTL in vitro: Two types of culture conditions were employed. For Lyt typing the CTL, 10^7 nylon-wool-passed (*17*) responder T cells were cocultured with the irradiated adherent cells from 10^7 B10.D2 spleen cells, or the membrane fragments derived from 10^7 B10.D2 spleen presented by the irradiated adherent cells from 10^7 BALB/c spleen cells. Membrane fragments, referred to as *freeze-thaw antigen* (FTA), were prepared by freezing and thawing of spleen cells followed by centrifugation to remove any intact cells, as previously described (*17*). Culture was in 24-well Linbro plates (Linbro Chemical Co., Hamden, CT) containing 2 ml of minimal essential medium (F-15, Gibco, Grand Island, NY) supplemented with 10^{-4} M beta-mercaptoethanol, 10% fetal calf serum

[1] This work was supported by the Medical Research Council of Canada.

* Abbreviations used: B10, C57BL10/J; CTL, cytotoxic T lymphocyte; CTLp, cytotoxic T lymphocyte precursor; FTA, freeze-thaw antigen; MIHA, minor histocompatibility antigens; MHC, major histocompatibility complex antigens; TCGF, T cell growth factors.

(Gibco) and antibiotics. Cultures were incubated for 5 days at 37°C in 10% CO_2. Groups included at least 3 replicate cultures that were pooled prior to treatment with antibodies and assay. Each group was assayed at 1/10, 1/20, and 1/40 of a culture.

All other experiments were done using microculture conditions as previously described (*14, 22*). Media and culture conditions were as above. Unfractionated or nylon-wool-passed responder cells were cocultured with the adherent cells derived from 3×10^5 intact irradiated stimulator cells, or with the FTA derived from 3×10^5 spleen cells presented on the adherent cells derived from 3×10^5 BALB/c spleen. Culture was in 96-well microtiter trays (Linbro, Flow Laboratories, Mississaugua, Ontario, Canada). All groups included 6–12 replicate cultures assayed individually. For competition assays the wells in a group were pooled prior to assay at several dilutions of effectors.

For limiting dilution experiments to determine precursor frequencies, culture of nylon-wool-passed primed T cells was in 96-well microtiter trays as above with the addition of an optimal concentration of a partially purified IL-2-containing T cell growth factor preparation (fraction III, [22]), and with or without irradiated primed responder cells to provide any necessary helper or other function for the CTLp. Each cell concentration of the series included 48 wells. To confirm the H-2 restriction properties of the CTL in these cultures, the CTL generated in cultures with 1×10^4 responders were tested in a competition assay after pooling a separate set of 48 wells.

Assay for cytotoxicity: CTL activity was assayed in situ or by pooling of cultures in a group as described, using ^{51}Cr-labeled B10.D2 or DBA/2 Con A blast cells as targets and using Con A blast cells as cold competitors (*17*). Killer to target ratios were in the range of 0.05–2:1. Spontaneous release was 25–30% of detergent release. The percentage of specific lysis was calculated as follows:

$$\frac{\text{sample cpm} - \text{spontaneous cpm}}{\text{detergent cpm} - \text{spontaneous cpm}} \times 100$$

Antibodies and treatment: Anti-Thy-1.2, anti-Ly-1.2, and anti-Lyt-2.2 were monoclonal antibodies purchased from New England Nuclear (Quebec, Canada). Viable cells after 5 days of culture were suspended at no more than 10^7 cells/ml in the indicated antibody, incubated at room temperature for 20 min, washed, and resuspended in a 1/5 dilution of absorbed rabbit complement and incubated at 37°C for 45 min (*14*). Treated cells were washed, counted for viable cells and used at numbers equivalent to the controls treated with complement alone to avoid enrichment of the remaining cell types (*14*).

RESULTS

Preferential recognition of DBA/2-specific antigens by CTL derived from low numbers of primed responder cells. There are reports in the literature that anti-MIHA CTL are able to kill essentially any H-2-matched target cell due, presumably, to the overlap in MIHA expressed by different strain backgrounds (*1, 2*). As a prelude to limiting dilution studies, anti-MIHA CTL derived from different numbers of responder cells that had been cultured with intact DBA/2 stimulator cells were assayed on DBA/2 and B10.D2 target cells (Fig. 1). In cultures containing 3×10^5 or more responder cells we were able to repeat the results of others and detected the same quality of killing on both types of target cell. However as the responder cell number was decreased, the specificity of the CTL began to change until at 3×10^4 or fewer responders per culture, the ability to kill B10.D2 targets was completely lost. These data suggest a population of CTLp present at high frequency but not induced at high numbers of responder cells. It appears to be specific for antigens expressed exclusively on DBA/2 and not on B10.D2 (Fig. 1) or on (BALB/c×B10)F_1 target cells (data not shown). Control experiments with other populations of CTL indicated that these two targets were as susceptible to lysis as were DBA/2 targets (data not shown).

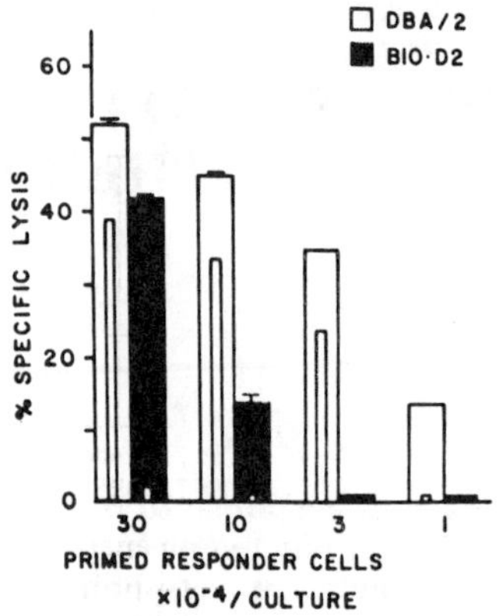

FIGURE 1. CTL generated in response to DBA/2 preferentially recognize MIHA unique to DBA/2 at low responder cell numbers. The indicated number of unfractionated spleen cells from primed BALB/c mice were cocultured with DBA/2 irradiated stimulator cells for 5 days in microtiter wells. All wells in a group were pooled and diluted, and aliquots were assayed on ^{51}Cr-labeled DBA/2 or B10.D2 blast cells. Columns represent the percentage of specific lysis by the equivalent of 1/2 a culture per assay well. The inner columns represent the lysis by 1/4 of a culture per assay well. Each group was assayed in triplicate at 1/2, 1/4, and 1/8 dilution on each target. No lysis of B10 targets was detectable. Effector-to-target ratios ranged from 2:1 for cells from cultures of 3×10^5 responders down to 0.05:1 for cells from cultures containing 1×10^4 responders. Values represent the mean ±SD. This experiment has been repeated 13 times with the same pattern of results. However, in some experiments the killing of B10.D2 target cells was minimal even at a dose of 3×10^5 responder cells.

Preferential recognition of DBA/2-specific antigens is confirmed by cold target inhibition studies. To determine whether the preference of anti-DBA/2 CTL for unique DBA/2 MIHA existed even at 3×10^5 responder cell numbers, we performed cold target competition assays on the CTL induced (Fig. 2). Aliquots of the same population of CTL that was able to kill DBA/2 (20% specific lysis) and B10.D2 (32% specific lysis) were subjected to cold target competition with DBA/2 and B10.D2 blast cells. When the CTL were assayed on hot DBA/2 targets, only DBA/2 cold blasts showed specific inhibition of the CTL response with no specific competition by B10.D2 blasts, indicating higher avidity for DBA/2 than for B10.D2 MIHA. Unexpectedly based on the literature, but as might be expected from the data in Figure 1, a similar pattern was observed for competition for the CTL able to kill B10.D2 targets. Specific competition for the anti-B10.D2 killers was seen with B10.D2 cold targets only at a ratio of 40:1 (Fig. 2b). DBA/2 cold targets competed more successfully for the anti-B10.D2 killers. This confirms the higher avidity of the CTL induced by DBA/2 for DBA/2 MIHA even in cultures in which comparable killing of both targets is observed.

When similar experiments were done using mice primed to

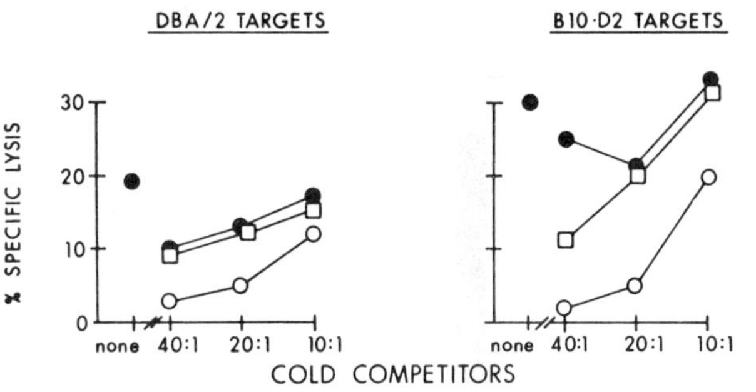

FIGURE 2. For cold target competition analysis of CTL able to lyse DBA/2 or B10.D2 3×10^5 unfractionated primed BALB/c responder cells were cultured with DBA/2 stimulator cells. At day 5, cultures were pooled and aliquots tested for their ability to lyse ^{51}Cr-labeled DBA/2 or B10.D2 blasts with or without the presence of a 10–40-fold excess of cold blast cell competitors of the indicated types. In other similar experiments B10 cold competitors were tested and competed at the same level as the BALB/c blasts did. (○) = DBA/2 cold competitors; (●) = BALB/c cold competitors; (□) = B10.D2 cold competitors; (●) = Killing in the absence of competitors; These experimental results have been reproduced 3 times.

B10.D2 in vivo, and challenged with B10.D2 in vitro, comparable killing was observed on DBA/2 and B10.D2 targets at all responder cell numbers (data not shown). Thus this phenomenon may be most easily detected using BALB/c anti- DBA/2 CTL.

Preferential binding of CTLp to DBA/2-specific antigens. To determine whether or not the preferential lysis of DBA/2 targets existed at the precursor as well as at the CTL effector cell level, we performed adsorption experiments with responder cells. Spleen cells from primed mice were allowed to adsorb to monolayers of peritoneal exudate cells of various strain origins and the nonadherent population was assayed for its ability to generate CTL effectors in response to DBA/2 stimulator cells (Table 1). As a control, aliquots of the same populations were stimulated with allogeneic B10 cells. The response to DBA/2 MIHA was eliminated almost completely by adsorption of the CTLp on DBA/2 but not on B10.D2, B10, or syngeneic BALB/c monolayers. This suggests preferential recognition of MIHA unique to DBA/2 by the majority of CTLp responding to DBA/2. The CTL response to B10 was removed by adsorption on B10, but not on DBA/2, B10.D2, or BALB/c monolayers, confirming the specificity of the adsorption method. As might be expected based on reports in the literature (*1, 2*) CTL generated by culture of 10^7 responder cells with DBA/2 stimulator cells were able to kill B10.D2 as well as DBA/2 target cells and were adsorbed with equal efficiency by both DBA/2 and B10.D2 monolayers (data not shown).

Revelation of CTL crossreactive with both DBA/2 and B10.D2 by culture with helper-replacing factors. In order to characterize the conditions for determining precursor frequency, a limiting dilution experiment was set up with or without addition of a semipurified population of T cell growth factors (TCGF) able to replace helper function (*16, 22*) (Table 2). This experiment shows that helper function was a limiting factor in the response to intact DBA/2 stimulator cells.

The subset of CTL able to kill both DBA/2 and B10.D2 target cells, shown in Figure 1 to be absent from the population of CTL generated from low numbers of responders, was restored by the addition of TCGF (Table 2, columns 5 and 6). This crossreactive subset of CTLp was induced by intact cells and appeared to be present at a frequency comparable to that of the DBA/2-specific subset. The properties of this subset are most easily explained by the assumption that its induction requires considerably higher levels of help than does the DBA/2-specific subset of CTLp.

Previous work has demonstrated the existence of an otherwise undetectable subset of CTL generated in the response to MIHA expressed on membrane fragments of freeze-thaw ruptured spleen cells (FTA) (*17*). This subset is able to kill both DBA/2 and B10.D2 target cells in an H-2-unrestricted fashion (*17*), and is present at a considerably lower frequency than are the H-2-restricted CTL subsets (Table 2, columns 3, 4, and 6).

Frequency of H-2-restricted and H-2-unrestricted CTLp responsive to MIHA. Since the limiting dilution analysis shown in Table 3 did not allow precise quantitation of precursor frequency in the response to intact DBA/2 cells, a more comprehensive limiting dilution series was done to compare the frequency of H-2-restricted CTLp that are responsive to intact cells with the frequency of H-2-unrestricted CTLp that are responsive to FTA (Fig. 3). Limiting numbers of T cells were cultured with antigen, with TCGF, and with or without additional irradiated unfractionated primed spleen cells to provide any necessary helper or differentiative factors. In the case of the response to MIHA on intact cells, the addition of these "fillers" gave a marginal increase in the frequency of CTLp from 1/158 to 1/112 T cells (Fig. 3). However in the case of the response to MIHA on FTA presented by BALB/c adherent cells, the generation of CTL was severely decreased by the addition of fillers such that a frequency of CTLp could not be calculated (data not shown). These calculations based on Poisson analysis (*23*) indicate that, within a population of primed spleen cells, the H-2-restricted CTLp (89/10^4 T cells) able to respond to MIHA on intact adherent cells are 40-fold more frequent than the H-2-unrestricted CTLp responsive to MIHA on FTA (2.0/10^4 T cells).

Lyt phenotype of CTL generated in response to cellular versus subcellular antigen. Wettstein and Frelinger (*18*) have reported that shifts in the Lyt phenotype of CTL specific for MIHA correlated with shifts in the immunodominant determinants. Experiments were designed to determine whether the CTL specific for H-2 restricted MIHA, and induced by intact stim-

TABLE 1. Preferential binding of CTLp to MIHA unique to DBA/2

Treatment of responder cells	% Specific lysis	
	DBA/2 stimulators: DBA/2 targets	B10 stimulators: B10 targets
Untreated	42.2±2	47.7±1
Adsorbed on DBA/2	5.6±3	43.7±4
Adsorbed on B10.D2	28.9±4	47.5±4
Adsorbed on B10	35.6±2	0.4±6
Adsorbed on BALB/c	24.7±4	20.2±4

Spleen cells from primed BALB/c mice were adsorbed on monolayers of thioglycollate-induced peritoneal exudate cells of the indicated origin as previously described (17). Recovery of responder cells after adsorption was 53%. 1.6×10^5 of the spleen cells nonadherent to the monolayer were cultured with the indicated stimulator cells for 5 days. Assay was on the indicated type of Con A blast cells. Each group included 4 replicate cultures assayed individually. Values represent the mean ± S.E. This experiment has been repeated 3 times with comparable results.

TABLE 2. Requirement for TCGF in the generation of anti-DBA/2 CTL crossreactive with B10.D2 induced by both cellular and subcellular forms of MIHA[a]

Responders × 10^{-3}	% Specific lysis of DBA/2: stimulator Ag				% Specific lysis of B10.D2: stimulator Ag	
	Intact DBA/2: TCGF		DBA/2 FTA: TCGF		Intact DBA/2: + TCGF	DBA/2 FTA: + TCGF
	−	+	−	+		
300	92±4	91±7	53±4	37±4	86±2	31±4
100	53±3	88±7	23±1	42±5	81±2	23±3
30	18±1	88±7	21±2	27±3	83±2	31±6
10	15±1	75±6	7±2	10±1	75±3	33±5
3	13±1	62±4	6±1	14±2	66±3	17±4
Precursor frequency/10^4 nylon-wool-passed T cells (No. containing 1 CTLp)	3.98 (1/2511)	>10 (>1/1000)	1.2 (1/7943)	6.9 (1/1445)	>10 (>1/1000)	3.5 (1/2819)

[a] Nylon-wool-nonadherent spleen cells primed to DBA/2 were cultured at the indicated number with intact DBA/2 irradiated adherent cells or with DBA/2 FTA presented by BALB/c irradiated adherent cells, with or without an optimal concentration of TCGF as indicated. Each group included 12–24 cultures assayed individually. A positive well was defined as one with ^{51}Cr release that was >3 SD of the mean spontaneous release. Frequency was calculated from a plot of the percentage of negative wells, as shown in Figure 3. There was a strong correlation between the percentage of negative wells and the number of responder cells per well (r ≃ 1 for the analyses of columns 1, 3, 4, and 6).

TABLE 3. Lyt phenotype of CTL specific for MIHA[a]

	% Specific lysis			
	Hot B10.D2	Cold competitors		
		B10.D2	B10	BALB/c
Response to B10.D2 adherent cells:				
Complement control	51.4±1	0	40.8±1	51.8±3
Anti-Lyt-1.2 + C′	17.5±2	0	7.5±2	20.7±2
Anti-Lyt-2.2 + C′	5.6±2	0	0	13.7±3
Anti-Thy-1.2	0	0	0	0
Predominant phenotype:	Lyt-1^+2^+, Thy-1^+, H-2-restricted			
Response to B10.D2 FTA:				
Complement control	44.0±3	0	15.9±1	57.4±2
Anti-Lyt-1.2 + C′	15.9±3	0	0	12.3±1
Anti-Lyt-2.2 + C′	4.5±1	0	0	7.1±2
Anti-Thy-1.2	0	0	0	0
Predominant phenotype:	Lyt-1^+2^+, Thy-1^+, H-2-unrestricted			

[a] Nylon-wool-passed responder spleen cells were from BALB/c mice primed in vivo with B10.D2. Cultures were as described in the *Materials and Methods* section. At day 5 of culture all wells in a group were harvested and pooled. Aliquots of each group were treated as indicated with complement alone, anti-Lyt-1.2 or 2.2, or anti-Thy-1.2. Each aliquot was then assayed in a cold target competition assay in triplicate at dilutions of 1/10, 1/20, 1/40 of a culture per assay well. Values in the table are from the 1/40 assay point. Cold competitors were added at a 30-fold excess. This experiment was repeated 3 times with results as shown. Values are the mean ± SD.

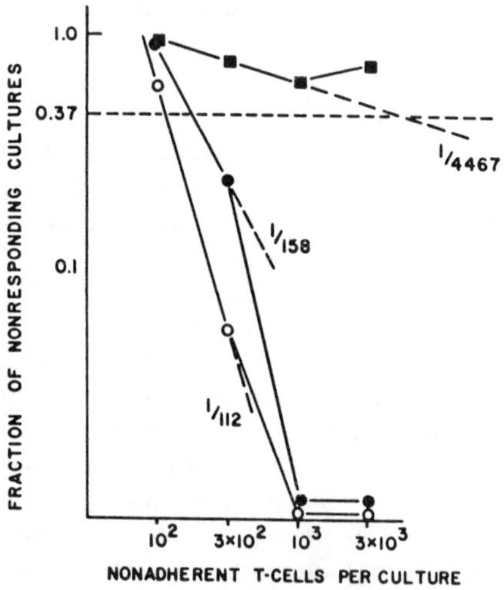

FIGURE 3. Limiting dilution analysis of the CTLp responsive to MIHA on intact cells or subcellular MIHA (FTA). The indicated number of nylon-wool-passed primed responder T cells was cultured with TCGF, with or without 1×10^5 irradiated unfractionated primed cells as "fillers," and with DBA/2 adherent cells or DBA/2 FTA as antigen. (■) = response to DBA/2 FTA; (●) = response to DBA/2 adherent cells without fillers; (○) = response to DBA/2 adherent cells with fillers; A well was considered to be positive if the ^{51}Cr released exceeded the mean of the spontaneous release by >3 SD. Each point was derived from assay of 48 individual cultures. The frequency of responding units was taken as the number of cells which, when cultured, would give rise to 37% negative wells (*23*) as calculated from the plot of the percentage of negative wells versus the responder cell number. Limiting dilution experiments such as this and the one in Table 3 have been repeated 6 times with comparable results.

ulator cells were of a different Lyt phenotype from the CTL recognizing apparently unrestricted MIHA and induced by FTA presented on adherent cells (Table 3).

CTL generated after 5 days of culture were pooled within each group and divided into aliquots to be treated with complement, anti-Lyt-1.2, anti-Lyt-2.2, or anti-Thy-1.2. After treatment the remaining CTL were tested for specificity in a cold target competition assay. CTL generated in response to intact cells bearing MIHA were H-2-restricted, Lyt-1^+2^+, and Thy-1^+ (Table 3, lines 1–4). CTL generated in response to FTA on antigen presenting cells were also Lyt-1^+2^+, Thy 1^+ cells but they were, as reported (*17*), not H-2-restricted (lines 5–8). A pattern of results identical to those in Table 3 was seen when DBA/2 rather than B10.D2 was the stimulating antigen (data not shown). Although we reported previously that anti-DBA/2 H-2-restricted CTL were of the Lyt-1^-2^+ phenotype (*16*), we have been unable to detect such CTL in this series of experiments performed 2 years later. The anti-Lyt-1.2 antiserum used previously was equally efficient as the monoclonal anti-Lyt-1.2 used here, indicating the sensitivity of the assay systems was comparable. The observation may reflect differences in the specificity of the antibodies, as has been reported in another system (*14*), or it could reflect environmental changes in the mouse colony.

DISCUSSION

The experiments reported here document the existence of at least three distinct subsets of CTL that can be generated in the response to MIHA. These subsets cannot be distinguished by Lyt phenotype because all three are Lyt-1^+2^+—however, they have different receptor specificity, are present at different frequencies in a population of primed spleen cells, and appear to have different inductive requirements. The most frequent subset is H-2-restricted in its recognition of MIHA, preferentially recognizes MIHA uniquely expressed on DBA/2, is induced in response to MIHA on intact stimulator cells, and is very frequent ($1/112$ T cells). A second subset is also H-2-restricted and induced in response to MIHA on intact cells; it is able to recognize target MIHA expressed on both DBA/2 and B10.D2 and, although exhibiting a requirement for higher levels of help, it appears to be present at comparable frequency. This set appears to consist of two specificities of CTL: those that have equal avidity for both DBA/2 and B10.D2 as reported by Bevan (*1, 2*), and those that kill both targets but have detectably higher avidity for DBA/2 MIHA. The third subset is apparently H-2-unrestricted, is induced only in response to subcellular MIHA on FTA, and is present at a 40-fold lower frequency of CTLp ($1/4467$ T cells).

The existence in populations of primed BALB/c T cells of a high-frequency CTLp subset responsive to MIHA uniquely expressed by DBA/2 has not been previously reported and appears to be an unexpected immunodominance pattern in the response to multideterminant MIHA antigens. In cultures containing 3×10^5 or more responder cells, the CTL response generated appears to lyse target cells from any strain background with equal efficiency as long as they bear the appropriate H-2 class I antigens (Fig. 1, and [*1*]). Since different strains share many MIHA alleles it seemed likely that shared MIHA were the immunodominant determinants. In the present work, however, we have analyzed the ability of CTL to lyse both DBA/2 (the challenge antigen) and B10.D2 target cells. Suprisingly, at low numbers of responder cells the CTL generated were fully able to lyse DBA/2 cells but had lost the capacity to recognize B10.D2. These CTL were, however, fully H-2-restricted as defined by their inability to kill DBA/1 (H-2^q) (data not shown). The nature of the antigen apparently uniquely expressed on DBA/2 is unknown.

Cold target competition experiments were designed to further analyze the CTL generated at higher responder numbers. At very high numbers of responder cells (10^7), the CTL were able to lyse DBA/2 and B10.D2 targets, and blast cells from both strains were equally good competitors ([*1*], and Pilarski L, unpublished data) suggesting that the predominant CTL subset recognized MIHA shared between the two strains. This category of response is analogous to that described by Bevan (*1*). However, when the responder number was reduced to 3×10^5, the character of the response altered. Although the CTL were able to lyse both targets, the pattern of cold target competition indicated that the avidity of the CTL was considerably greater for DBA/2 than for B10.D2. This suggested a population of CTL weakly crossreactive with B10.D2 but with preferential recognition of DBA/2-specific MIHA.

Analysis of the specificity of CTLp using the technique of monolayer adsorption can be interpreted to indicate preferential binding to DBA/2 confirming the existence of this subset at the precursor as well as the effector level. However, an alternative explanation is that the adsorption preferentially removes helper cells. Since our results suggest that the level of help has a profound influence on the specificity of CTLp induced, it is possible that the crossreactive CTLp were still present in the adsorbed population but were silent due to an inadequate amount of help. More sophisticated experiments are needed to dissect the relationship between CTLp specificity and help.

Thus, as a result of changes in the responder cell number, a shift in specificity occurs that results in a loss of CTL responsive to shared MIHA, suggesting that these CTLp must have been present at only a low frequency. At high responder cell numbers (10^7) this relatively infrequent population appeared to exert clonal dominance over the more frequent, but unexpressed, DBA/2-specific CTLp. A similar phenomenon, involving different specificities of CTL has been reported by Matzinger and Mirkwood (*24*). The mechanism(s) responsible for the various patterns of immunodominance are far from clear. Based on the observation that the DBA/2/B10.D2 crossreactive subset of CTLp appears to require higher levels of help than the DBA/2-specific set of CTLp does, one might postulate that regulatory events play a key role. However to explain the dominance of infrequent CTLp subsets over frequent CTLp subsets, one must invoke quite selective inhibitory effects. Selectivity could be due to the receptor specificity of the inhibitory cells, or to differential suceptibility of various CTLp subsets to the negative signalling mechanism. Further experiments will be required to resolve this complex problem.

We previously reported the generation of apparently H-2-unrestricted CTL in response to a subcellular form of MIHA (*17*). The characteristics of that response were paradoxical in that, although the magnitude of the CTL response was the same whether the immunogen was MIHA on intact cells or MIHA on membrane fragments (FTA), only H-2-restricted CTL were detected in the former and only H-2-unrestricted CTL in the latter response. In this study we have shown that the frequency of apparently unrestricted CTLp is 40-fold less than the frequency of H-2-restricted CTLp. This could provide an explanation for the inability to detect unrestricted CTL in conditions favoring the generation of H-2-restricted CTL. However, it appears that the presentation of MIHA on FTA either allows maximal clonal dominance by the infrequent H-2-unrestricted CTLp, or the antigen recognized by H-2-restricted CTLp no longer exists on the FTA. Further work is required to answer these questions.

In conclusion, we have demonstrated the existence of three specificity subsets of CTL whose generation in culture is dependent upon the number of responder cells, the availability of help, and the form in which the antigen is presented. In agreement with the work of others (*18*), we find strong immunodominance effects operating in the response to MIHA, and we suggest that, at least in the case of BALB/c mice primed to DBA/2 MIHA, the predominant CTL subset is one that is specific for MIHA unique to DBA/2 rather than MIHA shared between DBA/2 and B10.D2.

Acknowledgments. We are grateful to Ms. Zarina Mohamed and Ms. Mary Tretiak for their excellent technical assistance, and thank Dr. Arun Fotedar for his critical reading of the manuscript.

REFERENCES

1. Bevan MJ. Interaction antigens detected by cytotoxic T cells with the major histocompatibility complex as modifier. Nature 1975; 256: 419.

2. Bevan MJ. The major histocompatibility complex determines susceptibility to cytotoxic T cells directed against minor histocompatibility antigens. J Exp Med 1975; 142: 1349.
3. Bevan MJ. H-2 restriction of cytolysis after immunization of minor H congenic pairs of mice. Immunogenetics 1976; 3: 177.
4. Gorden RD, Simpson E, Samelson LE. In vitro cell-mediated immune responses to the male-specific (H-Y) antigen in mice. J Exp Med 1975; 142: 1108.
5. Matzinger P, Bevan MJ. Induction of H-2 restricted cytotoxic T cells: in vivo induction has the appearance of being unrestricted. Cell Immunol 1977; 33: 92.
6. Wettstein PJ, Frelinger JA. H-2 effects on cell-cell interactions in the response to single non-H-2 alloantigens. II. H-2D region control of H-7.1-specific stimulator function in mixed lymphocyte culture and susceptibility to lysis by H-7.1-specific cytotoxic cells. J Exp Med 1977; 146: 1356.
7. Wettstein PJ, Frelinger JA. H-2 effects on cell-cell interactions in the response to single non H-2 alloantigens. III. Evidence for a second Ir-gene system mapping in the H-2K and H-2D regions. Immunogenetics 1980; 10: 211.
8. Hayes CE, Macphail S, Bach FH. Generation of primary cytotoxic lymphocytes against non-major histocompatibility complex antigens by anti-Ia serum plus complement-treated lymphocytes. J Exp Med 1980; 151: 1305.
9. Macphail S, Stutman O. Suppressor T cells activated in a primary in vitro response to non-major histocompatibility alloantigens. J Exp Med 1982; 156: 1398.
10. Macphail S, Yron I, Stutman O. Primary in vitro cytotoxic T cell response to non-major histocompatibility complex alloantigens in normal mice. J Exp Med 1982; 156: 610.
11. Gasgoine NRJ. Suppression of the cytotoxic T cell response to minor alloantigens in vivo. II. Fine specificity of suppressor cells and lack of restriction by immunoglobulin heavy chain-linked gene products. Eur J Immunol 1984; 14: 677.
12. Pilarski LM. A requirement for antigen-specific helper T cells in the generation of alloantigen-specific cytotoxic T cells from thymocyte precursors. J Exp Med 1977; 145: 709
13. Al Adra AR, Pilarski LM, Antigen-specific suppression of cytotoxic T cell responses. I. Suppressor cells are not cytotoxic T cells. Eur J Immunol 1978; 8: 504.
14. Al-Adra AR, Pilarski LM, McKenzie IFC. Surface markers on the T cells that regulate cytotoxic T-cell responses I. The Ly phenotype of suppressor T cells changes as a function of time and is distinct from that of helper or cytotoxic T cells. Immunogenetics 1980; 10: 521.
15. Pilarski LM. Regulation of the cytotoxic T cell response to minor histocompatibility antigens. Transplantation 1981; 32: 188.
16. Pilarski LM, McKenzie IFC. Lyt antigens on the T cells specific for minor histocompatibility antigens. Suppression by a Lyt 1+2- regulator. Transplantation 1981; 32: 363.
17. Pilarski LM, Vergidis D. Cytotoxic T cell response to minor histocompatibility antigens: apparent lack of H-2 restriction in killers stimulated by membrane fragments. J Exp Med 1982; 156: 217.
18. Wettstein PJ, Frelinger JA. T lymphocyte responses to non H-2 histocompatibility antigens. I. Role of Ly-1+2+ T cells as cytotoxic effectors and requirement for Ly-1+2+ T cells for optimal generation of cytotoxic effectors. J Immunol 1981; 127: 43.
19. Rammensee H-G, Nagy ZA, Klein J. Suppression of cell-mediated lymphocytotoxicity against minor histocompatibility antigens mediated by Lyt-1+ Lyt-2+ T cells of stimulator-strain origin. Eur J Immunol 1982; 12: 930.
20. Rammensee H-G, Juretic A, Nagy ZA, Klein J. Class I restricted interaction between suppressor and cytolytic cells in the response to minor histocompatibility antigens. J Immunol 1984; 132: 668.
21. Baum LL, Pilarski LM. In vitro generation of antigen-specific helper T cells that collaborate with cytotoxic T cell precursors. J Exp Med 1978; 148: 1579.
22. Shaw J, Caplan B, Paetkau V, Pilarski LM, Delovitch TL, McKenzie IFC. Cellular origins of co-stimulator (IL-2) and its activity in cytotoxic T lymphocyte responses. J Immunol 1980; 124: 2231.
23. Lefkovits I, Waldmann H. Limiting dilution analysis of the cells of immune system. I. The clonal basis of the immune response. Immunol Today 1984; 5: 265.
24. Matzinger P, Mirkwood G. In a fully H-2 incompatible chimera, T cells of donor origin can respond to minor histocompatibility antigens in association with either donor or host H-2 type. J Exp Med 1978; 148: 84.

Received 25 April 1985.
Accepted 23 July 1985.

0041-1337/86/4104-0527$02.00/0
TRANSPLANTATION

Vol. 41, No. 4
Printed in U.S.A.

Transplantation

BRIEF COMMUNICATIONS

LACK OF EFFECT OF SPLENECTOMY ON THE INFLUENCE OF PRETRANSPLANT BLOOD TRANSFUSIONS ON CARDIAC ALLOGRAFT SURVIVAL IN HISTOINCOMPATIBLE RATS

The beneficial effect of pretransplant blood transfusions on allograft survival has been firmly established both experimentally and in the clinical setting (*1–3*). Splenectomy has been shown to facilitate allograft survival in some animal models but not in others (*4–8*). In the clinical setting the role of splenectomy has been controversial, with beneficial effects either not demonstrable (*9*) or restricted to certain subgroups of patients (*10*). The role of the spleen in the blood transfusion effect has not been adequately studied. Elucidation of the role of splenectomy on the enhancing effect of donor-specific blood transfusion is of special interest both in terms of gaining further insight into mechanisms of enhancement and because of its clinical implications. We performed a series of experiments in a histoincompatible rat model to study the consequences of splenectomy on the donor-specific transfusion effect.

Retired breeder male Brown Norway (BN,* $RT1^n$) and Lewis (Lew, $RT1^l$) rats from the same supplier were used as a histoincompatible donor-recipient pair. Lew rats acted as recipients of BN blood and cardiac allografts. Wistar-Furth (WF, $RT1^u$) and Lew rats provided third-party hearts or syngeneic blood transfusions, respectively. One milliliter of heparinized fresh donor blood was injected into the tail vein of the recipient rat 7 days prior to cardiac allograft placement, as described by Martin et al. (*1*). Heterotopic cardiac allotransplantation was then performed after the method of Ono and Lindsay (*11*), and function assessed by daily palpation of the recipient abdomen for cardiac activity. The endpoint of rejection was established by the absence of a palpable heartbeat, and confirmed by electrocardiogram when necessary. Subsequent histological examination of the resected allograft was also done in some instances to confirm allograft rejection. The timing of splenectomy varied with relation to the blood transfusion, as well as to the timing of the cardiac transplant procedure. The spleen was removed through an upper midline incision after ligation of its vascular pedicle. Sham splenectomies were performed by using the same incision, and consisted of atraumatic clamping of the splenic vascular pedicle for one minute. The clamp was then removed and the organ allowed to recover in its anatomical position. The results were analyzed for significance using the Student's *t* test.

Preoperative transfusion of BN blood significantly prolonged the survival of BN hearts in Lew recipients. This effect was donor-specific because third-party hearts (WF) were rejected significantly earlier (Table 1). Splenectomy in unconditioned Lew recipients of BN hearts also prolonged cardiac allograft survival over sham-splenectomized controls. The timing of the splenectomy did not significantly influence the outcome (Table 2). The prolongation of allograft survival associated with splenectomy was less than that achieved with pretransplant blood transfusions. In experiments in which blood transfusions and splenectomy were combined, splenectomy—regardless of its relative timing—did not have an effect on the prolongation of cardiac allograft survival over that seen with transfusion alone (Table 3).

The prolongation of BN cardiac allograft survival in Lew recipients by preconditioning of the recipient with donor-specific blood transfusions is in agreement with other studies in which similar prolongation has been observed with other organ allografts performed in this donor-recipient strain combination (*1*). The mechanisms underlying the effects of pretransplant immunization with donor spleen cells or blood and the resulting prolongation in allograft survival are speculative and have been variously attributed to the induction of antiidiotypic antibodies (*12, 13*), phagocytic cell depression (*14*), suppressor cell activation (*15*), or, in the clinical setting, a selection bias by elimination of strong responders who produce antileukocyte antibodies (*2*). Current experimental evidence favors the theory that conditioning by donor alloantigen or hyperimmune serum administered pretransplant induces a specific suppressor cell network that maintains a state of immune unresponsiveness in the posttransplant period (*16, 17*). This is especially true of donor-recipient pairs in which the histocompatibility barriers are considerably weaker than in the present study (*18*). The induction of these suppressor cells in rats may be restricted by the major histocompatibility complex in that recent evidence suggests that the RT1.B region (coding for Ia-like antigens) must be shared by the blood and graft donor to mediate significant graft prolongation (*19*).

TABLE 1. Influence of blood transfusions on cardiac allograft survival in Lew rats transfused 7 days prior to allograft placement with 1 ml of blood

	Recipient	Blood donor	Heart donor	MST (days) ± SD[a]	P
n=9	Lew	Lew	BN	6.9±0.8	—
n=12	Lew	BN	BN	14.1±2.8	<0.01
n=11	Lew	BN	WF	7.8±0.9	0.03

[a] MST = mean survival time.

TABLE 2. Effect of splenectomy performed in the pretransplant or posttransplant period on unconditioned Lew recipients of BN cardiac allografts

Splenectomy	MST (days) ± SD[a]	P
Before (day −3) (n=4)	8.75±1.5	
		0.04
Sham (n=4)	6.0±0	
After (day +3) (n=4)	9.75±1.0	
		0.01
Sham (n=4)	7±0	

[a] MST = mean survival time.

* Abbreviations used: BN, Brown Norway; Lew, Lewis, WF, Wistar-Furth.

TABLE 3. The combined effect of donor-specific BN blood transfusions and splenectomy on cardiac allograft survival

Splenectomy[a]	Lew recipients[b]	MST (days) ± SD[c]	P
Day −14	Yes (n=6)	13.0±1.5	NS
	No (n=4)	11.5±1.3	
Day −0	Yes (n=4)	12.5±0.53	0.05
	No (n=4)	14.25±1.3	
Day +3	Yes (n=4)	13.75±1.5	NS
	No (n=4)	13.33±1.2	

[a] Splenectomy (Yes) or sham splenectomy (No) was performed at various times relative to transplantation.

[b] All recipients received 1 ml blood at 7 days pretransplant (day −7).

[c] MST = mean survival time.

There is still controversy as to whether presence of the spleen is a requirement for the effects of passive or active enhancement of organ allografts in suitable recipients. This requirement is influenced by the strain combinations used and the experimental model system employed. Our data suggest that in the BN to Lew donor-recipient pair, preconditioning of the Lew recipient by BN donor blood was effective regardless of the presence of the spleen. Furthermore, the timing of splenectomy also had no effect on graft outcome. These results are in contrast to the findings in a similar experiment utilizing B10/J mice as recipients and 129/J mice as donors. In this experiment the transfusion effect appeared dependent on the presence of the spleen (*20*). B10/J(H-2^b) mice and 129/J(H-2^b) mice are compatible at the H-2 locus and only differ by multiple minor non-H-2 antigen differences. Thus the requirement for the spleen to be present to achieve significant enhancement by blood transfusion is in agreement with the experimental evidence cited earlier relating to the induction of specific suppressor cell networks in weakly histoincompatible strain combinations (*4*). Similarly, we have shown that these enhancing suppressor cells do exist in the spleens of Lew rats bearing long-term surviving BN heart allografts by adoptive transfer of these spleen cells. This transfer is associated with prolonged BN heart allograft survival in irradiated naive Lew recipients when compared with control irradiated Lew rats (unpublished data). Suppressor cells are not only found in the spleen but also have been harvested from the thymus 6 days after allograft implantation (*21*). Thus—at least in some situations and especially when there is a strong histocompatibility barrier—the spleen may not be a necessary requirement for the blood transfusion effect.

The effect of splenectomy on allograft survival and on the blood transfusion effect in man has also generated considerable controversy. The controlled clinical trials of the effect of splenectomy on graft outcome were carried out in a transfused recipient population. These studies showed no effect or a relatively short-term beneficial effect of splenectomy (*9, 24, 25*). Therefore it is not unreasonable to assume that splenectomy is not a requirement for the blood transfusion effect in man. When subgroups of patients are examined in greater detail, it appears that splenectomy is beneficial in patients with leukopenia (*22*) or those treated with antilymphocyte globulin (*23*). The splenectomy in these individuals allowed larger doses of immunosuppressive therapy to be administered, this being the probable mechanism for the improved allograft survival observed.

Thus, in conclusion, our data has demonstrated that pretransplant blood transfusions prolong cardiac allograft survival in histoincompatible rats. In this particular strain combination of BN-to-Lew, the presence of the spleen is not a requirement for the blood transfusion effect to be manifested, and splenectomy does not enhance this effect regardless of its timing. Based on these findings and observations by others it appears unlikely that splenectomy will significantly influence the blood transfusion effect in the outbred or strongly incompatible experimental model or in the clinical setting.

Acknowledgments. We thank Suzanne M. Renfroe for her careful and attentive work in the preparation of this manuscript.

RAYMOND POLLAK[1]
JACQUELINE M. BLANCHARD
MARTIN F. MOZES
Department of Surgery
Division of Transplantation
University of Illinois College of Medicine at Chicago
Chicago, Illinois 60680

[1] Address reprint requests to: Dr. Raymond Pollak, University of Illinois College of Medicine at Chicago Department of Surgery, Division of Transplantation, Box 6998 (m/c 958), Chicago, IL 60680.

REFERENCES

1. Martin DC, Hewitt CW, Osborne JG, et al. Enhanced kidney graft survival in rats by single or multiple blood transfusions and various blood products. Transplant Proc 1982; 14: 407.
2. Salvatierra O, Vincenti F, Amend W, et al. Deliberate donor-specific blood transfusions prior to living related renal transplantation: a new approach. Ann Surg 1980; 192: 543.
3. Glass NR, Miller DT, Sollinger HW, Belzer FO. A four-year experience with donor blood transfusion protocols for living donor renal transplantation. Transplantation 1985; 39: 615.
4. Fabre JW, Batchelor JR. The role of the spleen in the rejection and enhancement of renal allografts in the rat. Transplantation 1975; 20: 219.
5. Souther SG, Norris RE, Vistres LM. Prolongation of rat cardiac allograft survival by splenectomy following transplantation. Transplantation 1974; 17: 317.
6. Tilney NL, Bell PRF. Studies on enhancement of cardiac and renal allografts in the rat. Transplantation 1974; 18: 31.
7. Kountz SL, Cohn R. Prolonged survival of a renal homograft by simultaneous splenectomy and splenic homotransplantation. Surg Forum 1962; 13: 59.
8. Birinyi LK, Baldwin WM III, Tilney NL. Influence of selective splenectomy on survival of cardiac and skin allografts in enhanced rats. Transplantation 1980; 30: 59.
9. Sutherland DER, Fryd DS, So SKS, et al. The long term effect of splenectomy versus no splenectomy on renal allograft survival: reanalysis of a randomized prospective study. Transplant Proc 1985; 17: 136.
10. Rohrer R, Meller J, Reckard CR, et al. Splenectomy revisited: more restricted indications for pretransplant splenectomy. Transplant Proc 1985; 17: 132.
11. Ono K, Lindsey ES. Improved technique of heart transplantation in rats. J Thorac Cardiovasc Surg 1969; 57: 225.

12. Singal DP, Joseph S. Role of blood transfusions on the induction of antibodies against recognition sites on T-lymphocytes in renal transplant patients. Hum Immunol 1982; 4: 93.
13. Stuart FP, Fitch FW, McKearn TJ. Enhancement of rat renal allografts with idiotypic and antiidiotypic monoclonal alloantibodies. Transplant Proc 1982; 14: 313.
14. Keown PA, Descamps B. Improved renal allograft survival after blood transfusion: a nonspecific erythrocyte mediated immunoregulatory process. Lancet 1979; 1: 20.
15. Lenhard V, Massen G, Seifert P, Johannsen R, Grosse-Wilde H. Characterization of transfusion-induced suppressor cells in prospective kidney allograft recipients. Transplant Proc 1982; 14: 329.
16. Marquet RL, Heystek GM, Niessen GJCM, Jeekel J. Induction of suppressor cells by a single blood transfusion in rats. Transplant Proc 1982; 14: 397.
17. Hall BM. Mechanisms maintaining enhancement of allografts. I. Demonstration of a specific suppressor cell. J Exp Med 1985; 161: 123.
18. Batchelor JR, Phillips BE, Grennah D. Suppressor cells and their role in the survival of immunologically enhanced rat kidney allografts. Transplantation 1984; 37: 43.
19. Soulillou JP, Blandin F, Gunther E, Lemoine E. Genetics of the blood transfusion effect on heart allografts in rats. Transplantation 1984; 38: 63.
20. Shelby J, Wakely E, Corry RJ. Suppressor cell induction in donor-specific transfused mouse heart recipients. Surgery 1984; 96: 296.
21. Tilney NL, Graves MJ, Strone TB. Prolongation of organ allograft survival by syngeneic lymphoid cells. J Immunol 1978; 121: 1980.
22. Pollak R, Nishikawa RA, Mozes MF, Jonasson O. Azathioprine induced leukopenia: clinical significance in renal transplantation. J Surg Res 1980; 29: 258.
23. Mozes MF, Spigos DG, Thomas PA, Nishikawa RA, Cohen C, Jonasson O. Antilymphocyte globulin and splenectomy or partial splenic embolization: evidence for a synergistic beneficial effect on cadaver renal allograft survival. Transplant Proc 1983; 15: 613.
24. Alexander JW, First MR, Majeski JA, et al. The late adverse effect of splenectomy on patient survival following cadaveric renal transplantation. Transplantation 1984; 37: 467.
25. Peters TG, Williams JW, Harman HC, Britt LG. Splenectomy and death in renal transplant patients. Arch Surg 1983; 118: 795.

COMPARISON OF THE IMMUNOGENICITY OF PURIFIED AND UNPURIFIED MURINE ISLET ALLOGRAFTS[1]

Some of the earliest islet allograft experiments that were reported seemed to show that islets transplanted as free grafts across a major histocompatibility barrier were either highly immunogenic or very susceptible to rejection effector mechanisms. Islets appeared to be rejected earlier than skin (*1–3*), heart (*3–5*), or kidney allografts (*3*)—and immunosuppressive regimens that prolonged the survival of skin, heart, or kidney allografts were shown to be less effective in promoting the survival of islet allografts (*1, 3, 4, 6, 7*). In addition, islet allografts were more susceptible to immune destruction than islets transplanted as part of an immediately vascularized intact pancreatic graft (*5, 7–9*). However, all of these experiments were performed in rats and all utilized islet grafts that had been prepared solely by mechanical separation techniques and thus were contaminated with a relatively large amount of acinar and endothelial tissue. Therefore it has not been possible to determine whether the endocrine portion of the allograft or the contaminating exocrine and vascular debris, or both, are responsible for the apparent heightened immunogenicity.

More recent studies using congenic mice seem to indicate that meticulously handpicked islet preparations are actually of low immunogenicity in many strain combinations (*10, 11*). Even when an entire H-2 disparity is involved, the frequency of islet allograft rejection has ranged from 10–100% depending on the strain combination used (*11*). It has been unclear how much of this phenomenon is attributable to the use of relatively pure islet preparations and how much is due to the immunogenetics of histocompatibility in this model.

Nevertheless, it has generally been assumed that clean handpicked islet preparations containing only a few associated endothelial and acinar cells are less immunogenic than preparations contaminated with a significant amount of exocrine tissue (*12, 13*). However, no controlled experiment testing this hypothesis has yet been reported. We sought to answer this question by performing a series of islet allografts with the only variable being the amount of exocrine tissue transplanted along with the islets.

C57B1/6 (H-2^b) and B10.BR (H-2^k) mice were obtained from Jackson Laboratory, Bar Harbor, ME and from the mouse colony at the University of Minnesota. Six-to-eight-week-old male C57B1/6 mice were donors, and 12-to-16-week-old male B10.BR mice were recipients. This strain combination was chosen because it had been shown earlier that the incidence of rejection of clean handpicked islets is low (*11*). Therefore if unpurified islets are in fact more immunogenic a clear difference should be seen. Recipient mice were made diabetic by the i.p. injection of streptozotocin (200 mg/kg body wt.) a gift from Upjohn Laboratories, Kalamazoo, MI. Plasma glucose was determined by the glucose oxidase procedure of the Sigma Chemical Co., St. Louis, MO, on samples obtained from the retroorbital venous plexus. Only mice with plasma glucose levels >400 mg/dl were used as recipients.

Both dirty (contaminated with exocrine tissue) and clean (only a few endothelial and acinar cells present) islet preparations were obtained by a sequential collagenase-digestion technique (*14*). Fourteen donor mice were fasted overnight prior to each isolation. Following cervical dislocation the pancreases were rapidly excised and cut into three pieces. The fragments were placed in six vials with 8 ml of a 1 mg/ml collagenase (Type I, Sigma Chemical Co., St. Louis, MO) solution. After vigorous shaking (200 cycles/min) in a 37°C water bath for 11 min the partially digested tissue was transferred to four vials with 6 ml of 0.5 mg/ml collagenase solution for sequential 5-min digestions. After each digestion the liberated tissue in suspension was washed once with Hanks' solution and free islets were handpicked under a dissecting microscope.

When a dirty preparation was the goal the islets were only handpicked once after the digestion process was stopped. Pure preparations were obtained after several sequential cleanings by means of handpicking.

Three tissue preparations containing 500–800 islets were used for transplantation: purified islets with only a few contam-

[1] National Institutes of Health Grant AM34360-02.

inating endothelial and acinar cells present; unpurified islets such that approximately 40% of the tissue present was acinar and 60% was endocrine; and unpurified islets as described, but further contaminated with the addition of 10–20×10^6 donor-strain splenocytes. In each case the tissue was placed beneath the left renal capsule by injection through a 21-gauge butterfly needle. A technical success was defined as a reversion to normoglycemia (<200 mg/dl) on at least two separate occasions. Rejection was defined as the permanent return of plasma glucose to >200 mg/dl.

In order to quantitate the degree of exocrine contamination present the insulin and amylase content of clean and dirty islet preparations was determined and compared with that of the intact gland.

The tissue was homogenized in a ground-glass homogenizer and extracted with acid-alcohol. Insulin content was measured by the double-antibody radioimmunoassay technique of Morgan and Lazarow (*15*). Amylase was quantitated by the colorimetric technique of Jamieson et al (*16*).

The mean insulin content of the whole pancreases was 35.3 μg ±8.7 μg gland (Table 1). This corresponds closely to the amount of insulin present in the preparations used for transplantation. For example, 400 purified islets contain 24.9 μg of insulin. Therefore 500–800 purified islets contain 31.1 to 49.8 μg of insulin. The mean insulin content of an islet was approximately 62 ng, which is in agreement with previously published figures for a variety of species (*17, 18*).

The amylase content of the dispersed tissue not subjected to rigorous islet isolation was more than two times that of purified islets, and the difference was statistically significant ($P<.01$). However, even the unpurified preparations were considerably enriched in insulin producing tissue when compared with whole pancreases. The insulin/amylase ratio of the unpurified islets was increased nearly 300-fold over the ratio of the whole pancreases, and that of pure islets was increased nearly 1000-fold.

Islet allograft survival times in the three different groups are given in Table 2. Rejection was observed in three of fourteen recipients of purified islets at a mean (±SD) of 19±13 days, and in four of sixteen recipients of unpurified islets at a mean of 17±19 days ($P>.8$). When islets were further contaminated with 10–20×10^6 donor splenocytes, five of five recipients rejected their grafts at a mean of 12±5 days.

Four animals that received purified allogenic islets and did not spontaneously reject the grafts were challenged with 5.0×10^7 donor-strain splenocytes i.v. at >100 days posttransplantation. All four mice rejected their established islet allografts at a mean of 9 days.

TABLE 1. Mean (±SD) insulin and amylase content of islet preparations[a]

	No. of preparations	Insulin content (μg)[b]	Amylase content (IU)[c]	Insulin/amylase
Purified islets	4	24.9±6.7	3.3×10^{-3} ±1.5×10^{-3}	7500
Unpurified islets	4	23.0±7.8	10×10^{-3} ±3.2×10^{-3}	2300
Whole pancreas	5	35.3±8.7	4.4×1.4	8.0

[a] Insulin and amylase content normalized to 400 islets per preparation; Two-tailed student's *t* test used for statistical analysis.

[b] $P>.7$ for purified vs. unpurified islets.

[c] $P<.01$ for purified vs. unpurified islets.

TABLE 2. Functional survival of islet allografts according to degree of purification

Group	Tissue transplanted	No.	Functional survival	% rejection[a]
1	Purified islets	14	7, 19, 32, >100×11	21%
2	Unpurified islets	16	10, 10, 20, 28, >100×12	25%
3	Unpurified islets plus donor splenocytes	5	6, 9, 12, 13, 20	100%

[a] $P>.8$ for groups 1 vs. 2 and $<.02$ for groups 3 vs. 1 and 2; Chi-square test used for statistical analysis.

Thus the present study fails to demonstrate any difference in immunogenicity between clean and dirty islet preparations in one mouse donor-recipient strain combination. However, when the islets were further contaminated with donor splenocytes, the resulting preparation was highly immunogenic, with 100% of recipients acutely rejecting their grafts.

Current theories of allograft rejection propose that two signals are required for lymphocyte activation (*19*). Signal one is provided by alloantigen binding to the T cell receptor. Signal two is postulated to be provided by an inductive molecule elaborated by an accessory lymphoid cell—the most likely candidate being the Ia-rich dendritic cell (*20*).

With this theoretical background in mind, it follows that allograft immunogenicity might be reduced by eliminating Ia-positive cells from the tissue prior to transplantation. Several different approaches along this line have proved successful, including pretransplant culture (*21, 22*), incubation with anti-Ia alloantisera and complement (*23*), incubation with anti-dendritic-cell monoclonal antibody and complement (*24*), and ultraviolet irradiation followed by 24-hr culture (*25*). Because it seemed logical to expect that pure islets would be less immunogenic than islet preparations contaminated with exocrine elements all of these experiments utilized clean hand-picked islets.

However this study failed to reveal an advantage of purified over unpurified islets. Murine islets as well as exocrine tissue are both apparently of low immunogenicity. Since purified islet preparations are difficult to obtain and result in a diminished islet yield per donor pancreas it would be advantageous if unpurified preparations could be used. Our data suggest that this may be the case.

It remains to be determined whether the methods that have recently been reported to decrease the immunogenicity of purified islet allografts will exert a similar effect on unpurified islets. Such experiments would be important to perform since it may be impossible to obtain purified islets from large animal or human pancreases.

In summary, we compared the ability of C57BI/6 mice to reject B10.BR islet allografts contaminated with varying degrees of exocrine tissue. Purified islet preparations containing only a few associated endothelial and acinar cells were rejected by 21% of recipients. Unpurified islet preparations consisting of approximately 40% exocrine tissue and 60% endocrine cells were rejected by only 25% of recipients. When donor strain splenocytes were added to the preparation, 100% of the grafts were rejected. We conclude that there is no difference in immunogenicity between purified and unpurified islet allograft preparations in this model.

Paul F. Gores[2]
Jaime Mayoral
M. Jane Field
David E. R. Sutherland
The Department of Surgery
University of Minnesota Hospitals
Minneapolis, Minnesota 55455

[2] Recipient of National Research Service Award AM07187.

REFERENCES

1. Reckard CR, Zeigler MM, Barker CF. Physiological and immunological consequences of transplanting isolated pancreatic islets. Surgery 1973; 74: 91.
2. Reckard CR, Stuart FP, Schulak JA. Immunologic comparison of isolated pancreatic islets and whole-organ allografts. Transplant Proc 1979; 11: 563.
3. Nash JR, Peters M, Bell PRF. Comparative survival of pancreatic islets, heart, kidney, and skin allografts in rats with and without enhancement. Transplantation 1977; 24: 70.
4. Rynasiewicz, JJ, Sutherland DER, Ferguson RM, Squifflet JP, Morrow CE, Goetz FC, Najarian JS. Cyclosporine A for immunosuppression: observations in rat heart, pancreas and islet allograft models and in human renal and pancreas transplantation. Diabetes 1982; 31: 92.
5. Perloff LH, Naji A, Barker CF. Vascularized pancreas versus isolated islet allografts: an immunological comparison. Surgery 1980; 88: 222.
6. Squifflet JP, Sutherland DER, Rynasiewicz JJ, Field J, Heil J, Najarian JS. Combined immunosuppressive therapy with Cyclosporin A and Azathioprine: a synergistic effect in three of four experimental models. Transplantation 1982; 34: 315.
7. Reckard CR, Stuart FG, Clayman JL, Buckingham F, Schulak JA. Differential susceptibility of segmental and isolated islet allografts of rat pancreas to rejection and enhancement. Transplant Proc 1981; 13(1): 819.
8. Sutherland DER, Rynasiewicz JJ, Kawahara K, Gorecki P, Najarian JS. Rejection of islets versus immediately vascularized pancreatic allografts: a quantitative comparison. J Surg Res 1980; 29: 240.
9. Squifflet JP, Sutherland DER, Morrow CE, Florack G, Field J, Najarian JS. Comparison of rejection of intraportal islet versus immediately vascularized segmental pancreatic allografts in rats in relations to beta cell mass engrafted. Transplant Proc 1983; 15(1): 1344.
10. Morrow CE, Sutherland DER, Steffes MW, Najarian JS, Bach FH. Rejection of established mouse pancreatic islet allografts by active immunization requires Class I (H-2 K, D) antigen disparities. J Surg Res 1984; 36: 332.
11. Zhu XY, Sutherland DER, Steffes MW, Morrow CE, Gores PF, Najarian JS, Bach FH. Rejection of mouse islet allografts according to donor and recipient genotypes. Transplant Proc 1985; 17: 425.
12. Lacy PE, Davie JM, Finke EH. Transplantation of insulin producing tissue. Am J Med 1981; 70: 589.
13. Downing R. Historical review of pancreatic islet transplantation. World J Surg 1984; 8: 137.
14. Steffes MW, Nielsen O, Dyrberg T, Baekkeskov S, Scott J, Lernmark A. Islet transplantation in mice differing in the I and S subregion of the H-2 complex. Transplantation 1981; 31: 476.
15. Morgan AR, Lazarow A. Immunoassay of insulin: two-antibody system. Diabetes 1973; 12: 115.
16. Jamieson AD, Pruitt KM, Caldwell RC. An improved amylase assay. J Dent Res 1969; 48: 483.
17. Rabinovitch A, Cuendet GS, Sharp GWG, Renold AE, Mintz DM. Relation of insulin release to cyclic AMP content in rat pancreatic islets maintained in tissue culture. Diabetes 1978; 27: 766.
18. Trimble ER, Renold AE. Ventral and dorsal areas of rat pancreas: islet hormone content and secretion. Am J Physiol 1981; 240: E422.
19. Lafferty KJ, Prowse SJ, Simeonovic CJ. Immunobiology of tissue transplantation: a return to the passenger leukocyte concept. Ann Rev Immunol 1983; 1: 143.
20. Lechlen RI, Batchelor JR. Restoration of immunogenicity to passenger cell-depleted kidney allografts by the addition of donor strain dendritic cells. J Exp Med 1982; 155: 31.
21. Lacy PE, Davie JM, Finke EM. Prolongation of islet allograft survival following in vitro culture (24°C) and a single injection of ALS. Science 1979; 204: 312.
22. Bowen KM, Lafferty KJ. Reversal of diabetes by allogeneic islet transplantation without immunosuppression. Aust J Exp Biol Med Sci 1980; 58: 441.
23. Faustman D, Hauptfeld V, Lacy P, Davie J. Prolongation of murine islet allograft survival by pretreatment of islets with antibody directed to Ia determinants. Proc Natl Acad Sci USA 1981; 78: 5156.
24. Faustman D, Steinman R, Gebel H, Hauptfeld V, Davie J, Lacy P. Prevention of rejection of murine islet allografts by pretreatment with anti-dendritic cell antibody. Proc Natl Acad Sci USA 1984; 81: 3864.
25. Hardy MA, Lau HT, Weber C, Reemstma K. Pancreatic islet transplantation: immuno-alteration with ultraviolet irradiation. World J Surg 1984; 8: 207.

Received 6 May 1985.
Accepted 24 July 1985.

INTRATHECAL ALLOTRANSPLANTATION OF PANCREATIC ENDOCRINE CELLS IN DIABETIC RATS[1]

It has been repeatedly demonstrated that the diabetic state in rodents and in larger animals can be ameliorated by pancreatic islet transplantation (*1*). However graft rejection invariably occurs in allotransplantation if steps for the induction of permanent graft survival are not taken (*2*). Recently brain tissue has been demonstrated to be able to provide a suitable environment for the survival of transplanted allograft and xenograft of neural and endocrine tissues including pancreatic islet cells (*3–6*). The present study examines the immunological status of the subarachnoid space and the feasibility of using it as a site for allotransplantation by the injection of pancreatic islet cells into the cisterna magna of streptozotocin-induced diabetic rats.

Male rats of outbred Wistar (Wi)* strain, with body weights of 350–500 g were used as donors of pancreatic tissue, and rats of the ACI (AgB 4/4) strain were used as streptozotocin-induced (55 mg/kg i.v.) diabetic recipients. Pancreatic tissue was di-

[1] This work was supported by the Medical Research Council of Canada; by Funds For Medical Research from the Royal Canadian Legion (Branch 177, Vancouver, British Columbia); and by the Canadian Diabetes Association.

* Abbreviations used: BG, blood glucose; BW, body weight; EDTA, ethylenediaminotetraacetate; HBSS, Hanks' balanced salt solution; H–F, Hypaque-Ficoll; i.c., intracerebral; PEC, pancreatic endocrine cells.

gested with collagenase, and the islets were hand-picked under a dissection microscope. Contaminating acinar tissues and blood vessels were removed from the islets by the single-layer Hypaque-Ficoll (H–F) separation technique (7). Clean islets collected at the interface were used for transplantation study or immediately dissociated into single-cell suspensions (8). Every minute 1000 islets were suspended and resuspended in 3 ml of 0.04% ethylenediaminotetraacetate (EDTA) in Ca^{2+}-Mg^{2+}-free Hanks' balanced salt solution (HBSS), pH 7.2, at 25°C for 5 min followed by treatment with 3 ml of 0.02% VMF trypsin solution (Worthington, Freehold, NJ) in HBSS at 37°C. Cells from a quantity of 1500 islets were suspended in 15 ml of culture medium (M199 containing 15% fetal calf serum), dispensed into a 100×20-mm plastic Petri dish, and cultured in a humidified 5% CO_2 incubator at 26°C overnight. To rid them of dead cells, the cultured cells were suspended in a single layer H–F gradient solution and centrifuged at 800 G for 8 min. Viable PEC collected at the interface of the H–F gradient was used for transplantation study.

PEC or whole islets from 5–6 donor rats were suspended in a 40-μl volume in a ½-cc U-100 Monoject syringe (Sherwood Medical, St. Louis, MO) for intraportal, intracerebral, or intrathecal transplantation. Streptozotocin-induced diabetic ACI rats were used as recipients. Intracerebral transplantation of PEC or whole islets was achieved with a stereotactic instrument (5). For intrathecal implantation, the recipient was anesthetized with ether and the nape was shaved. The neck of the animal was flexed ventrally, using the occipital protuberance as the landmark, and the needle was inserted through the muscle layers between the occipital protuberance and atlas vertebra directly into the cisterna magna to a depth of approximately 3–4 mm. Gentle aspiration was applied, and after the appearance of clear CSF, the PEC or whole islets were slowly injected.

Random blood glucose (BG), body weight (BW), 24-hr urine volume, and water intake for each recipient were assessed daily prior to, and for 2 weeks following transplantation, as well as at regular intervals thereafter. In addition 24-hr serial BG tests were performed on these rats at around 13 weeks following transplantation. Rejection was considered to have occurred when the BG level exceeded 200 mg/dl for 2 successive days following transplantation. BG levels were measured with a Beckman glucose analyzer.

To further confirm the existence of a functioning endocrine pancreatic allograft in diabetic ACI recipients rendered normoglycemic by the Wi allograft, Wi skin grafts were implanted in 6 of these animals for the purpose of inducing graft rejection (9).

To determine the distribution of intrathecally transplanted cells, normal rats were injected intrathecally with PEC stained with 1% crystal violet in 20% ethanol for 10 min or with 1% trypan blue in Puck's saline for 30 min following 1 hr fixation in 1% buffered formalin. The stained cells were washed repeatedly with Puck's saline to remove excess dye and subsequently suspended to 40 μl in Puck's saline for intrathecal injection. At 10 min, 2 hr and 24 hr following intrathecal injection, rat recipients were killed by exsanguination. The whole animal was fixed with 300 ml of 10% phosphate-buffered formalin by perfusion through the left ventricle, and then the skull and dura were carefully removed to allow gross examination of the brain.

For morphological study of the intrathecal transplants, rat recipients were exsanguinated by cardiac puncture. The brain

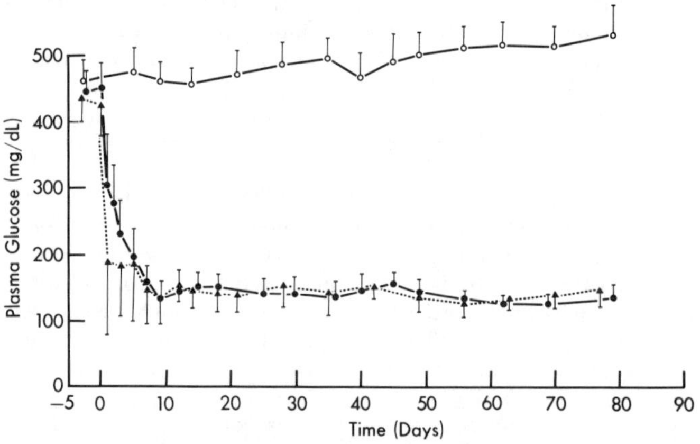

FIGURE 1. Plasma glucose (mg/dl; mean ± SD) of sham-operated diabetic ACI (O– – –O, n = 6); of diabetic recipients of intracerebral PEC (●– – –●, n = 8); and of intrathecal PEC (▲—▲, n = 13).

TABLE 1. Survival of allogeneic Wistar pancreatic endocrine cells (PEC)/whole islets in streptozotocin-induced diabetic ACI rats

Donor tissue	Transplant route	Transplant site	Individual survival (days)
PEC	Intrathecal	Subarachnoid space	7, 67,[a] 77,[b] 78,[b] 94,[a] 96,[a] 98,[a] 99,[a] >227, >269, >274, >349, >394, >398
Islets	Intrathecal	Subarachnoid space	7, 10, 10, 20,[b] 54,[b] 184,[a] >353, >354
PEC	Intracerebral	Brain	118,[b] >204, >205, >208, >209, >211, >215, >215
Islets	Intracerebral	Brain	6, 6, 8, 9, 17, 21, 60, >206, >210
PEC	Intraportal	Liver	4, 6, 6, 6, 8, 8
Islets	Intraportal	Liver	5, 6, 6, 6, 7, 7, 8

[a] Received skin graft.

[b] Killed for histological examination.

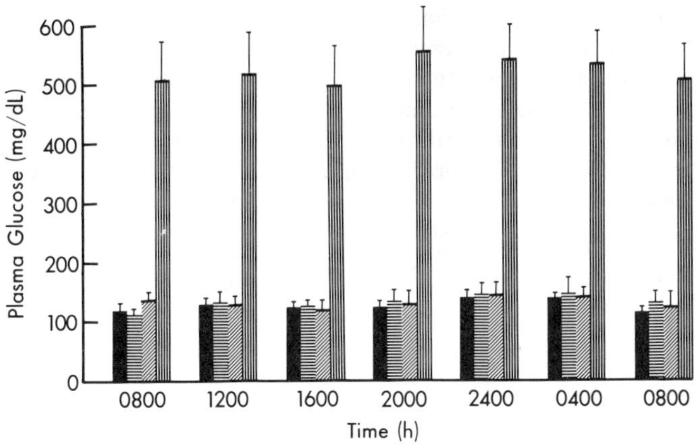

FIGURE 2. The 24 hr serial plasma glucose (mg/dl; mean ± SD) at around 90 days following transplantation of PEC in 4 experimental animal groups. Normal controls (■, n = 6); ACI recipients of Wi PEC intrathecally (▤, n = 8); ACI recipients of Wi PEC intracerebrally (▨, n = 7); ACI diabetic controls (▥, n = 6).

tissue was fixed in situ with 10% phosphate-buffered formalin and processed for microscopic examination.

Table 1 shows the allograft survival time in ACI diabetic recipients of intraportal, intracerebral, and intrathecal PEC or whole-islet transplants from Wi donors. The transplanted PEC normalized the BG levels in all the diabetic recipients within 1 week following the intracerebral or intrathecal transplantation (Fig. 1). 13/14 of the intrathecal transplants of PEC remained functional for the entire observation period, but only 5/8 of the whole-islet grafts had achieved prolonged survival time. These results were very similar to that of intracerebral transplantation, as 8/8 of the PEC grafts and 5/9 of the whole-islets grafts had maintained long-term function. By comparison, intraportal transplants of PEC or whole islets were rejected within 7 days.

There was an initial decrease in BW in some of the recipients of both PEC and whole-islet grafts. However most of them regained their BW within 1 week, with further steady BW gain over the observation period. All successfully transplanted diabetic recipients showed a marked reduction of water intake and urine output. The volumes were comparable to normal control animals.

Figure 2 shows the normal pattern of 24-hr serial BG in ACI recipients with successful long-term intracerebral or intrathecal PEC allografts.

A recurrence of hyperglycemic state as evidence of rejection of the functional islet allograft was observed in 11.5±2.0 (mean ± SD) days in all 6 diabetic ACI recipients with a permanent PEC allograft challenged with Wi skin grafts. Also, within a 2-week period all skin grafts were rejected.

Intrathecal transplantation with stained PEC revealed that they were found mainly in the cisterna magna and subarachnoid space on the dorsal and lateral aspects of the cerebellum and ventral surface of the brain. A small number of cells were also

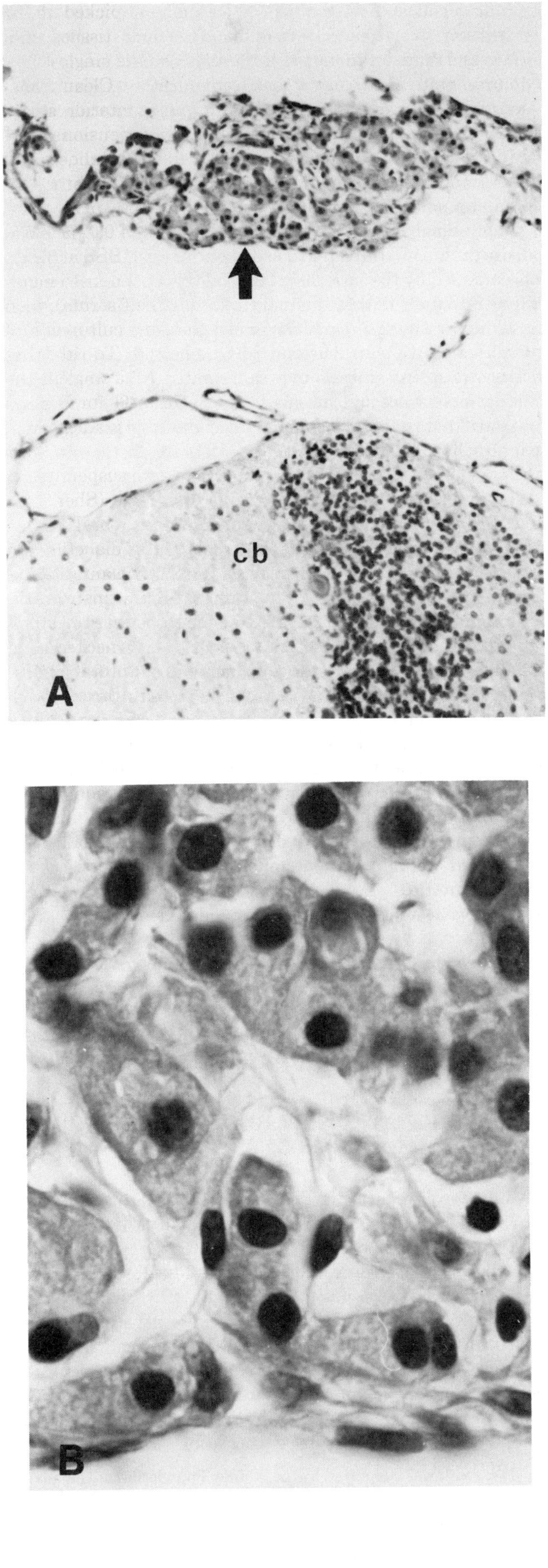

FIGURE 3. Morphology of grafted pancreatic endocrine cells following intrathecal transplantation. (A) Coronal section of brain showing transplanted pancreatic endocrine cells, well vascularized, in the subarachnoid space above the cerebellum (Cb). (B) Higher magnification of a designated area in (A) (arrow) showing cords of normal-looking pancreatic endocrine cells and no evidence of lymphocytic infiltration and inflammatory reaction around the grafted cells. Magnification: (A)×185; (B)×1500.

seen on dorsal and ventral aspects of the spinal cord at the cervical level. Very few cells were found on the dorsal cerebral surface and none was detected in the ventricular system.

Representative histology of successful intrathecal PEC transplants for 10 weeks is shown in Figure 3. Islet cell aggregates with normal appearance, permeated with capillaries, were present in the subarachnoid space above the cerebellum. There was no evidence of lymphocytic infiltration and inflammatory reaction around the grafted cells.

Longitudinal follow up of the BG, BW, and 24-hr blood glucose profile indicated that the diabetic state of the recipients was corrected by the intrathecal PEC allograft. The recurrence of hyperglycemia in these animals following the challenge with the donor strain skin graft confirmed the functional state of intrathecal transplants. Histological examination revealed that in these recipient animals the transplanted PEC were in the subarachnoid space and appeared to be healthy. These findings suggested that the cerebrospinal fluid–containing subarachnoid space is a hospitable site for the survival of the PEC and whole-islet transplants.

The following observations from the present study indicate that the subarachnoid space is an immunologically privileged site: (1) The allogeneic PEC and whole islet have achieved long-term survival when transplanted intrathecally in the diabetic recipients across a major histocompatibility barrier without immunosuppression. (2) There was no evidence of lymphocytic infiltration around the grafted cells. (3) The outcome of intrathecal transplants to the subarachnoid space was almost identical to that of intracerebral transplants to the brain, which is a known immunologically privileged site. However, immunological protection provided by the site is incomplete and delicate. The type of donor tissue preparation used for transplantation is an important factor influencing the outcome of the allograft survival. This is evidenced by 3 of 8 whole-islet grafts being rejected by the recipients, compared with 1 of 14 PEC grafts—devoid of contaminating cells—being rejected. Furthermore PEC graft in the subarachnoid space is shown to be susceptible to immune rejection induced by donor strain skin graft.

Transplantation of cells into the cisterna magna is a benign and simple procedure that involves no surgery. Rat recipients following serial cisterna magna puncture for CSF collection did not suffer detectable ill effects. The combination of the discovery of the subarachnoid space as an immunologically privileged site and the simplicity of the intrathecal transplantation procedure offers an opportunity to carry out further transplantation studies. Since only a small mass of PEC is required to correct the hyperglycemia in a diabetic recipient, and the biological characteristics of PEC have a long life span, the intrathecal approach to transplantation of PEC has potential for application in the treatment of human diabetes.

Acknowledgments. We thank S. Ng, D. Mallory, C. Graves, D. Tze, N. Bassida, B. Kotzte, R. Mah, and J. E. van den Broek for their technical assistance; Dr. F. Durity for his advice; and R. Bogyo for secretarial help.

WAH JUN TZE,[2]
JOSEPH TAI
Departments of Paediatrics and Pathology
University of British Columbia
Vancouver, British Columbia, Canada

[2] Address correspondence to: Dr. W. J. Tze, Children's Hospital, 4480 Oak Street, Vancouver, B.C., Canada V6H 3V4.

REFERENCES

1. Sutherland DER. Pancreas and islet transplantation. I. Experimental studies. Diabetologia 1981; 20: 161.
2. Lafferty KJ, Prowse SJ, Simeonovic CJ, Hegre O, Chase HP. Current status of experimental islet transplantation. Transplant Proc 1984; 16: 813.
3. Marx JL. Transplants as guides to brain development. Science 1982; 217: 340.
4. Kolata G. Grafts correct brain damage. Science 1982; 217: 342.
5. Tze WJ, Tai J. Successful intracerebral allotransplantation of purified pancreatic endocrine cells in diabetic rat. Diabetes 1983; 32: 1185.
6. Tze WJ, Tai J. Intracerebral allotransplantation of purified pancreatic endocrine cells and pancreatic islets in diabetic rats. Transplantation 1984; 38: 107.
7. Tze WJ, Wong FC, Tingle AJ. The use of Hypaque-Ficoll in the isolation of pancreatic islets in rats. Transplantation 1976; 22: 201.
8. Tze WJ, Tai J. Preparation of pseudoislets for morphological and functional studies. Transplantation 1982; 34: 228.
9. Billingham RE, Medawar PB. The technique of free skin grafting in mammals. J Exp Biol 1951; 28: 385.

Received 11 July 1985.
Accepted 5 August 1985.

THE RELATIONSHIP BETWEEN LYMPHOKINE RESPONSIVENESS AND HLA DR ANTIGENS AS PROGNOSTIC INDICATORS OF RENAL TRANSPLANT SURVIVAL[1]

A number of reports support the concept that patients who exhibit vigorous immunological responses to a variety of stimuli have a poorer prognosis for successful renal transplantation than those with weaker responses (*1–4*). The observation that individuals who were positive for HLA DRw6 had a higher incidence of rejection than those who were negative (*5*) supported the concept of high and low immunological responders and suggested that nonspecific responsiveness might be genetically determined in humans. We have observed a polymorphism in the human population in that some individuals consistently produce macrophage migration inhibition factor (MIF)* when their cells are stimulated by concanavalin A (Con A) while others produce migration stimulation factor (MStF) (*6*). MIF responders had a higher incidence of rejection of renal transplants than MStF responders and MIF responses were associated with HLA DR7 while MStF responses were associated with HLA DR1. We therefore reviewed our data to determine if the outcome of renal transplantation related more closely to the lymphokine responses or to the DR antigens of the recipients.

[1] This work was supported by the Kidney Foundation of Canada.

* Abbreviations used: AET, 2-aminoethyl isothiouronium; BSS, balanced salt solution; Con A, concanavalin A; MIF, migration inhibition factor; MStF, migration stimulation factor.

Heparinized peripheral blood was obtained by venepuncture from healthy volunteers, blood donors, and patients with renal failure prior to transplantation. Mononuclear cells were obtained by centrifugation on Ficoll-Isopaque (Pharmacia, Montreal) and suspended in endotoxin-free RPMI 1640 medium (Microbiological Associates, Walkersville, MD) without serum in a concentration of 5 million cells/ml. Stimulated cells were obtained by pulsing the cells for 2 hr with 10 μg/ml Con A while control cells were incubated for the same period without Con A. The cells were washed three times and one or two stage migration assays carried out in duplicate as described previously (*7, 8*). The results were expressed as migration indices obtained by multiplying the ratio of test to control migration areas by 100. Indices of 90 or less were identified as MIF responses and those of 110 or more as MStF responses.

Peripheral blood mononuclear cells were also used for the identification of HLA DR antigens. T lymphocytes were removed by rosetting with sheep erythrocytes (Woodland Laboratories, Quelph, Ontario) which were treated with 2-aminoethyl isothiouronium (AET) bromide hydrobromide, (Sigma, St. Louis). The sheep cells were prepared by washing five times in saline and were suspended in 200 mg AET dissolved in 10 ml distilled water with the pH adjusted to 8.0 with sodium hydroxide. After 15 min at 37°C the cells were washed five times in Hanks' balanced salt solution (BSS) and added in a 1% V-V suspension to Hanks, BSS containing 40% heat inactivated fetal calf serum. Three ml of the mononuclear cells at a concentration of 5×10^6 ml in Hanks' BSS were added to 3 ml of the sheep erythrocyte suspension, centrifuged for 5 min at 240 g and resuspended gently with a pipette. The cells were layered over 3 ml ficoll-isopaque and centrifuged for 20 min at 400 g. The T-cell-depleted cells at the interface were then recovered and washed in Hanks' BSS.

DR typing was performed using trays from the laboratory of P. Terasaki, Los Angeles (originally), and (for the last two years) from the Canadian Red Cross National Reference Laboratory, Toronto. Hanks' BSS, 1 μl, containing approximately 2000 cells was added to each well and the trays were kept at room temperature for 1 hr. Then 5 μl of rabbit complement was added to each well, the trays were kept at room temperature for a further 2 hr, and viability was estimated by eosin exclusion.

The transplant recipients reported here all received kidneys from cadaver donors. DR antigens were determined in 243 transplants involving 230 patients. Forty-one patients were treated with prednisone and azathioprine and the remainder received prednisone and cyclosporine. Virtually all the patients received at least two blood transfusions prior to transplantation. Successful transplants were identified on the basis of functioning kidneys 100 days after transplantation.

Lymphokine responses were evaluated in 288 individuals who had also been typed for HLA DR antigens. Eighty-seven of these were patients with renal failure while the rest were healthy individuals. The correlations between lymphokine responses and DR antigens were the same in the two groups as reported earlier (*6*). The cumulative data are summarized in Table 1. A total of 112 (38.9%) were MIF responders, 111 (38.5%) were negative, and 65 (22.6%) were MStF responders. Sixty-eight individuals were positive for HLA DR 1 and, of these, 11 (16.2%) were MIF responders while 27 (39.7%) were MStF responders. There were 220 individuals who were negative for HLA DR1, 101 (45.9%) being MIF responders and 38 (17.3%) MStF responders. These differences were highly significant ($\chi^2 = 24$, $P<0.0001$). Seventy-three individuals were positive for DR7 and, of these, 42 (57.5%) were MIF responders while 7 (9.6%) were MStF responders. Seventy of 215 (32.6%) individuals who were negative for DR7 were MIF responders, while 56 (26%) were MStF responders. These differences were also significant ($\chi^2 = 16.5$, $P<0.0005$) and were still highly significant when correlated for the 6 DR types that were analyzed ($P<0.0006$ and $P<0.003$). Other DR antigens were not associated with differences in lymphokine responses. Thirty-seven individuals were found to be positive for HLA DRw6 in all the groups studied, including transplanted patients. Eleven were MIF responders, 16 were negative, and 10 were MStF responders.

TABLE 1. Correlation of lymphokine responses with HLA DR antigens

HLA DR phenotype	Total number	Lymphokine responses to Con A (% of total)		
		MIF	Negative	MStF
DR1-positive	68	16.2	44.1	39.7
DR1-negative	220	45.9	36.8	17.3
DR2-positive	108	45.4	38.9	15.7
DR2-negative	180	35.0	39.4	25.6
DR3-positive	72	45.8	40.3	13.9
DR3-negative	216	36.6	38.4	25.0
DR4-positive	103	39.8	39.8	20.4
DR4-negative	185	38.4	38.4	23.2
DR5-positive	50	26.0	46.0	28.0
DR5-negative	238	41.6	37.8	20.6
DR7-positive	73	57.5	32.9	9.6
DR7-negative	215	32.6	41.4	26.0

The outcome of 243 renal transplants in relation to the presence of DR antigens in the recipients is shown in Table 2. The success rate was similar for all the antigens except DRw6 that was associated with a success rate decreased to 50%. Although only 20 individuals were identified as positive for DRw6, there was a significant difference between the success rate of these and all others transplanted ($\chi^2_c = 6.1$, $P<0.02$). The DRw6-positive individuals who had successful transplants had immunosuppressive protocols similar to those with failed transplants. There were 3 MIF responders and 3 MStF responders to Con A in the DRw6-positive successful group, and 6 MIF responders and 1 MStF responder in the failed group. Lymphokine responses to extracts of donor cells (*9*) were determined after transplantation in 5 of the successful group, and all 5 demonstrated MStF responses, while the only one tested in the failed group gave an MIF response.

We have reported previously that the mean migration index resulting from Con A stimulation was significantly higher in individuals who were positive for HLA DR1 than in those who were negative, and was significantly lower in those who were positive for HLA DR7 (*6*). Since individuals tend to have similar lymphokine responses when tested repeatedly (*6*), we reviewed our results from the standpoint of identifying MIF responders and MStF responders on the basis of individual migration indices. There were almost twice as many MIF responders as MStF responders in the general population. Individuals who were positive for HLA DR1 had a highly significant increase in the proportion who were MStF responders, while those positive for HLA DR7 had an increased proportion of MIF responders. There was no significant association between the lymphokine responses and other DR antigens. Since both positivity for HLA DRw6 (*5*) and MIF responses to Con A (*8, 9*) have been associated with an increased incidence of renal transplant rejection we wished to determine if DRw6 was associated with MIF responsiveness. We identified 37 individuals who were positive for DRw6 among the healthy groups, patients with renal failure, and transplant recipients. There were similar numbers of MIF and MStF responders in the DRw6-positive group so that we have no evidence of such an association. While this suggests that MIF responsiveness and DRw6 may influence transplant survival through independent mechanisms, 6 of 7 DRw6 positive patients who rejected their transplants exhibited MIF responses to Con A prior to transplantation. Five DRw6-positive recipients who had successful transplants had lymphokine responses to extracts of donor cells evaluated during the first two weeks after transplantation. All five exhibited MStF responses, suggesting that a "favorable" donor-recipient combination is important for success in this group.

When we examined the relationships between the HLA DR antigens of the recipients and the clinical outcome of transplantation (Table 2), patients positive for DR1 had a slightly higher success rate (83%) than those who were positive for DR7 (76%), but the difference was not significant. On the other hand, we have found significantly decreased graft survival in MIF responders tested prior to transplantation than in MStF responders (*8*).

It therefore seems apparent that the lymphokine responses, rather than positivity for DR1 or 7, were the more important parameters relating to transplant survival. It is of interest that 20 recipients who were positive for HLA DRw6 had significantly reduced graft survival (50%) at 100 days. While the numbers are small, this supports the observation of a poorer prognosis for DRw6 recipients in Europe (*5*). While this association was not supported by a study in the United States (*10*), our results suggest that DRw6 may also relate to a poorer prognosis for graft survival in a North American population.

TABLE 2. Correlation of HLA DR phenotype of renal transplant recipients with clinical outcome

Positive antigens	Successes	Failures	Percentage of success
DR1	44	9	83
DR2	53	15	78
DR3	55	15	79
DR4	69	25	73
DR5	31	12	72
DR6	10	10	50
DR7	45	14	76
DR8	15	4	79

Acknowledgments. We thank Marie DeCoste for technical assistance and Pat Godin for secretarial assistance.

JOSEPH MICHAEL MACSWEEN
STUART LESLIE EASTWOOD
ALLAN DAVID COHEN
KAUSALYA RAJARAMAN
Department of Medicine
Dalhousie University
Camp Hill Hospital and Transplantation Unit
Victoria General Hospital
Halifax, Nova Scotia, Canada, B3H 3G2

REFERENCES

1. Opelz G, Mickey MR, Terasaki PI. Identification of unresponsive kidney transplant recipients. Lancet 1972; 1: 868.
2. Morris PJ, Dumble LJ. Use of lymphoblastoid cell-lines to determine responsiveness in cadaveric renal transplantation. Lancet 1973; 2: 16.
3. Jones AR, Vaughan RW, Bewick M, Batchelor JR. Transformation of lymphocytes from patients awaiting cadaver renal transplants. Lancet 1976; 2: 529.
4. Watson MA, Briggs JD, Diamondopoulos AA, Hamilton DNH, Dick HM. Endogenous cell-mediated immunity, blood transfusion, and outcome of renal transplantation. Lancet 1979; 2: 1323.
5. Hendricks GFJ, Schreuder GMTH, Class FHJ, et al. HLA-DRw6 and renal allograft rejection. Br Med J 1983; 286: 85.
6. MacSween JM, Eastwood SL, Cohen AD, Rajaraman K, Fox RA. Lymphokine responses to Concanavalin A stimulation: association with HLA DR antigens. Clin Immunol Immunopathol 1984; 32: 368.
7. MacSween JM, Rajaraman K, Rajaraman R, Fox RA. Macrophage migration inhibition factor (MIF): reducing the variables. J Immunol Methods 1982; 52: 127.
8. MacSween JM, Cohen AD, Rajaraman K. Donor-specific cellular responses and pre-existing non-specific responsiveness as interrelated determinants of renal transplant survival. Transplant Proc 1984; 16: 1410.
9. MacSween JM, Cohen AD, Rajaraman K, Fox RA. Lymphokine responses to mitogenic and antigenic stimulation. Predictive value in renal transplantation. Transplantation 1982; 34: 196.
10. Kerman RH, Flechner SM, VanBuren CT, Kahan BD. DRw6 phenotype, immune responder status, and renal allograft outcome. Transplant Proc 1985; 17: 44.

Received 19 June 1985.
Accepted 21 August 1985.

ASYMPTOMATIC EXTRAVASATION OF CONTRAST MATERIAL IN THE UNUSED BLADDER

Patients who are potential renal transplant recipients often undergo retrograde cystography as part of their pretransplant evaluation. These patients usually have been on long-term hemodialysis, and consequently have virtually unused urinary bladders. Day (*1*) and Caroline (*2*) have recently reported the phenomenon of self-limited extravasation of contrast material during retrograde cystography in patients with unused urinary bladders. Caroline (*2*) reports that the extravasation begins at the lateral border of the trigone near the ureteral orifices, never extends much further, and never is massive. We report a case in which there was considerable extravasation of contrast without symptoms or sequelae.

Our patient, a 57-year-old man with end-stage renal disease secondary to accelerated hypertension, underwent a retrograde cystogram as part of his pre-renal-transplant work-up. The patient had been on hemodialysis for approximately two years prior to this examination and was virtually anuric at this time (less than 30 cc per day). A gravity drip infusion technique was used. The total volume infused was 300 cc. Extravasation of contrast material was first noted during the late filling phase of the exam while performing fluoroscopy. Filling was immediately terminated. Films demonstrated marked bilateral extravasation of contrast material into the perivesicular soft tissues (Fig. 1). The patient was totally asymptomatic and was able to immediately resume his normal activities. Cystoscopy revealed mild chronic inflammatory changes, but no lacerations. There were no sequelae.

Extravasation from the urinary bladder is usually caused by severe trauma and requires surgical management. The situation we are describing is quite different. Chronic renal failure patients are a unique clinical population. These patients are

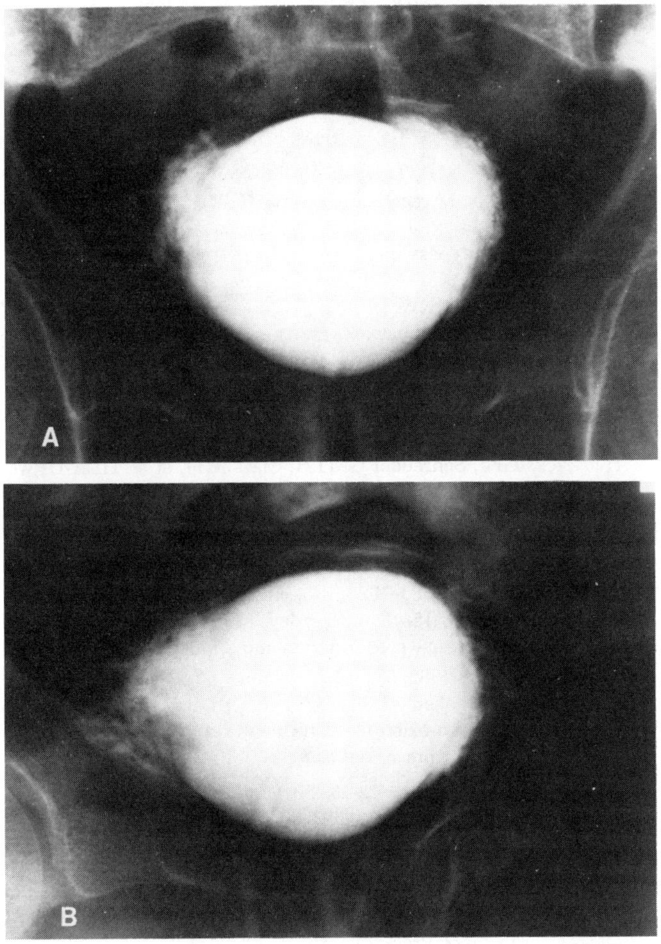

FIGURE 1. Anteroposterior (A) and oblique (B) views of the bladder during the retrograde cystogram demonstrate extensive extravasation of contrast into the wall and surrounding tissues of the bladder circumferentially.

frequently anuric but have urinary bladders which are intrinsically normal. Since this phenomenon has been observed only in this group of patients, Caroline (*1*) has inferred that failure of the bladder to distend and empty regularly somehow compromises its status as a water-tight viscus. At cystoscopy, the bladders of these patients are found to be grossly normal without evidence of laceration. Histologically, they may be normal or show mild inflammatory changes. Also, following renal transplantation, these patients show normal bladder function.

To explain this phenomenon, it has been postulated (*1, 2*) that changes must occur in the mucosa of unused bladders that somehow render them more friable or vulnerable to injury. When these bladders are acutely distended during retrograde cystography, small rents or tears may occur in the bladder mucosa that allow contrast material to escape and dissect through the fascial planes into the perivesical soft tissues.

Our patient demonstrates that this asymptomatic extravasation can be pronounced. It is important for both the radiologist and clinician to recognize this as an innocuous phenomenon that does not indicate irreversible nondistensibility of the unused bladder.

In summary, our experience indicates that even when extravasation from the bladder during retrograde cystography on pre-renal-transplant patients is extensive, conservative management suffices to be guided by the clinical course.

WILLIAM K. O'NEAL[1]
ALLAN NAIMARK[1,2]
RICHARD K. BABAYAN[3]
BELDON A. IDELSON[4]
Departments of Radiology, Urology, and Renal Medicine
University Hospital
Boston University School of Medicine
Boston, Massachusetts

[1] Department of Radiology.

[2] Address reprint requests to Dr. A. Naimark, Department of Radiology, University Hospital, 75 East Newton Street, Boston, MA 02118.

[3] Department of Urology.

[4] Department of Renal Medicine.

REFERENCES

1. Day DL. Extravasation of contrast material from unused bladders during voiding cystourethrography. Radiology 1985; 155: 105.
2. Caroline DF, Pollack HM, Banner MP, Schneck C. Self-limited extravasation in the unused urinary bladder. Radiology 1985; 155: 311.

Received 6 August 1985.
Accepted 21 August 1985.

CYCLOSPORINE FOR STEROID-RESISTANT ACUTE REJECTION OF RENAL CADAVER GRAFTS

Cyclosporine has been shown to improve the survival of cadaveric renal allografts in controlled trials comparing it with conventional immunosuppression with azathioprine and prednisolone (*1, 2*). However there is concern about its long-term effects on the kidney (*3*) and the difficulty in differentiating nephrotoxicity from allograft rejection (*4*). These have contributed to the less-than-universal acceptance of cyclosporine as a primary immunosuppressant.

Patients treated with conventional immunosuppression present a major therapeutic dilemma when repeated courses of high-dose steroids fail to control rejection. The options include: stopping high-dose prednisolone to minimize morbidity and mortality, usually at the expense of the graft, or administering further steroids, or other immunosuppressants such as antilymphocyte globulin, thereby increasing the risk of infection. The use of cyclosporine is rarely considered in these circumstances, partly because it is ineffective for established acute renal allograft rejection in the rat (*5*), but also because of present understanding of its mechanism of action (*6*), which suggests that effector T lymphocytes are insensitive to the drug. Nevertheless, there are reports that cyclosporine can reverse acute rejection in dogs (*7*) and abrogate second-set rejection in presensitized rats (*8*). There are also tentative suggestions that cyclosporine can reverse acute renal allograft rejection in man, but these have not included a morphological assessment of the rejection process (*9, 10*). We have observed recovery from histologically proved acute rejection with interstitial and vascular components, apparently resistant to high-dose steroids, when cyclosporine has been introduced as a secondary immunosuppressant.

In the period from January 1982 to August 1984, 55 cadaver renal allograft recipients were treated with a standard immunosuppressive protocol to suppress rejection. All recipients had received third-party blood transfusions and were treated initially with prednisolone 300 mg per day, reducing to 20 mg daily by the twelfth day after transplantation. Azathioprine 2–5 to 3 mg/kg/day was given throughout. Rejection episodes were treated either with i.v. methylprednisolone, 1 g daily for 3 or 4 days, or high-dose oral prednisolone for twelve days, in a total dose of 2.2 g. Of the 55 grafts, seven were excluded from the study for the following reasons: primary non function, not treated for rejection (4); technical failure (1); sepsis (1); and late acute rejection found with nonfunctioning graft (*1*). Throughout this period, no more than two courses of high-dose steroids were given for treatment of a rejection episode. Thereafter, rejection was considered resistant. Twenty patients bearing 22 grafts had "resistant" rejection so defined. All had, in total, at least two courses of high-dose steroids for treatment of rejection, and further courses were considered inadvisable. Function in these 22 grafts had continued to deteriorate for a further 7–16 days (mean 12 days) after commencing the last course of bolus steroids.

Until mid-1983, the recipients of 14 grafts with resistant rejection received no additional immunosuppression after treatment with a mean of 6.9 g of bolus prednisolone. Eleven failed, and 3 recovered (Fig. 1a). Since then, cyclosporine at 15–17 mg/kg/day, orally, was given to recipients of 8 grafts with rejection that did not respond to more than 7 g of bolus corticosteroids. Azathioprine was stopped when cyclosporine was introduced and prednisolone maintained at basal dose. There has been no other alteration in management of recipients. Six grafts treated in this way recovered and 2 failed (Fig. 1b). Levels of cyclosporine measured 5–11 days after starting the drug were within or above our therapeutic range (equilibrated plasma, trough levels of 100–300 ng/ml). At follow up, at a mean of 13±6.4 months later, recipients of the 6 grafts that recovered had a mean plasma creatinine of 202 μmol/L; one had suffered a further acute rejection that was treated successfully with prednisolone. The survival of grafts with resistant rejection is significantly greater in patients with cyclosporine, (6 of 8 with cyclosporine compared with 3 of 14; $P<0.05$, Fisher's exact 2-tailed test). One patient who was not treated with cyclosporine died from primary cytomegalovirus infection. The patient characteristics are shown in Table 1 and do not provide an alternative explanation for the improved graft survival in the patients treated with cyclosporine.

Percutaneous needle biopsies were performed on 17 of the 22 grafts with resistant rejection. These were assessed blind for severity of rejection by the criteria of Herbertson (*11*), prognostic scores were calculated, and results for patients treated with and without cyclosporine compared. The 10 biopsies from patients not treated with cyclosporine were taken at a time comparable to that of the 7 who received cyclosporine (mean 13±12 days and 6±9 days, respectively, from diagnosis of resistant rejection). All biopsies from patients receiving cyclosporine showed evidence of vascular rejection of moderate severity, as did 9 of 10 of the grafts from the earlier series. They all had evidence of moderate-to-severe mononuclear cell interstitial

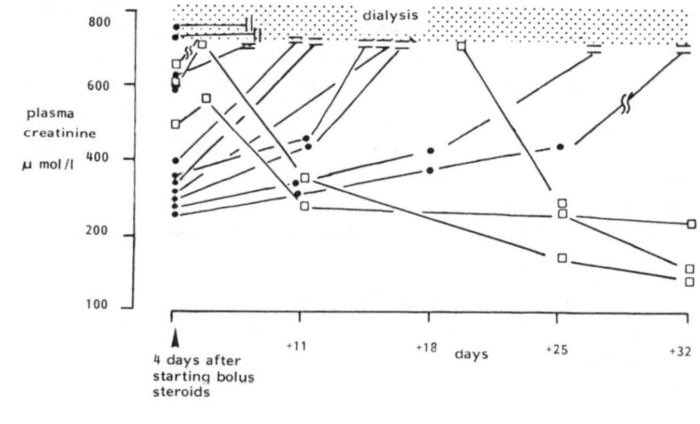

(a)

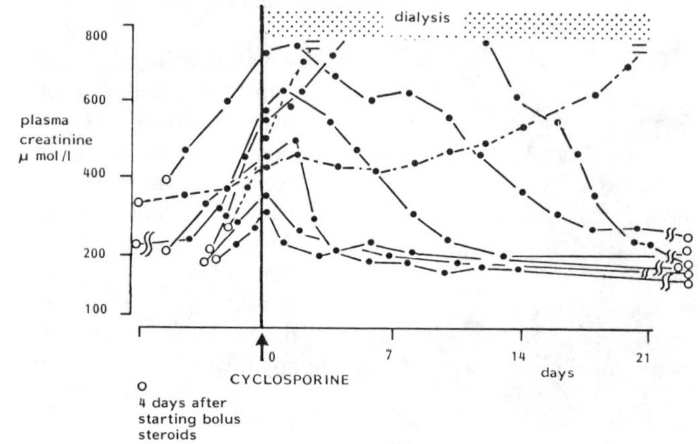

(b)

FIGURE 1. Graft function of kidneys with resistant acute rejection from 4 days after starting the final course of high dose corticosteroids: (a) 1982–1983, in recipients of 14 transplants: 3 grafts recovered function and 11 failed. (b) 1983–1984, in recipients of 8 transplants, converted to cyclosporine, 15–17 mg/kg/day, orally, after discontinuing azathioprine: 6 grafts recovered function and 2 failed.

TABLE 1. Patient characteristics of recipients of grafts with resistant rejection

	1982–1982 (14 grafts)	1983–1984 (8 grafts [+ cyclosporine])
Patients	13	7
Age	44±12	48±7
Second grafts	3	1
HLA mismatches:		
A, B	2.8	2.5
DR	0.9	0.4
Rejection episodes	1.7	2.1
Bolus steroids	6.9 g	8.5 g

TABLE 2. Mean scores for prognostic indices (range 0–2 [11] in 17 biopsies of 22 grafts with resistant rejection

	Mean score (±SD)	
	1982–83: (10)	1983–84: (+ cyclosporine [7])
Arteries:		
Mononuclear infiltrate	1.6±0.7	1.4±0.8
Medial necrosis	0.4±0.7	0.3±0.5
Glomeruli:		
Thrombosis	0.2±0.5	0
Endothelial swelling	1.1±0.6	0.9±0.7
Interstitial hemorrhage	0.7±0.3	0.8
Tubules:necrosis	0.1	0

infiltrate, and there was no difference between the prognostic scores (Table 2).

These findings suggest that acute vascular rejection not controlled by conventional immunosuppression may respond, in some cadaver graft recipients, to introduction of cyclosporine. Vascular rejection has not previously been shown to improve with cyclosporine used as a secondary immunosuppressant. Other studies supporting its efficacy have shown variable benefit, without assessment of graft histology (*9, 10, 12, 13*). This suggests that some of the advantages of cyclosporine may be achieved by those preferring to use azathioprine and prednisolone as initial immunosuppression. Cyclosporine may complement the role of conventional therapy for treatment of acute vascular rejection.

F. W. BALLARDIE
C. G. WINEARLS
D. J. EVANS
A. J. REES
G. WILLIAMS
Departments of Medicine, Pathology, and Surgery
Royal Postgraduate Medical School
Hammersmith Hospital
London W12 OHS, England

REFERENCES

1. European Multicentre Trial Group. Cyclosporine in cadaveric renal transplantation: one year follow-up of a multicentre trial. Lancet 1983; 2: 986.
2. The Canadian Multicentre Transplant Study Group. A randomized clinical trial of cyclosporine in cadaveric renal transplantation. N Engl J Med 1983; 309: 809.
3. Farnsworth A, Hall BM, Kerican P. Pathology in renal transplant patients treated with cyclosporine A. Transplant Proc 1983; 15: 2852.
4. Salaman JR. Cyclosporin in renal transplantation: a guide to management. Lancet 1984; 2: 269.
5. Homan WP, Fabre JW, French ME, Millard PR, Denton TG, Morris PJ. Studies on the immunosuppressive properties of cyclosporine A in rats receiving renal allografts. Transplantation 1980; 29: 361.
6. Borel JF. Cyclosporine A—present experimental status. Transplant Proc 1981; 13: 344.
7. Homan WP, Fabre JW, French ME, Millard PR, Denton TG, Morris PJ. Reversal of acute rejection episodes by cyclosporine A in dogs receiving renal allografts. Transplantation 1980; 29: 262.
8. Schulak JA, Manson D, Shelby J, Corry RJ. Abrogation of second-set rejection with Cyclosporine A. Transplantation 1983; 36: 289.
9. Margreiter R, Huber C, Spielberger M, Koenig P. Cyclosporine in the treatment of acute cadaveric kidney graft rejection refractory to high dose methylprednisolone. Transplantation 1983; 36: 203.
10. MacDonald AS, Belitsky P, Cohen A. Cyclosporine for steroid resistant rejection in azathioprine treated renal graft recipients. Transplant Proc 1983; 15(suppl 4,1): 2535.
11. Herbertson BM, Evans DB, Calne RY, Banergee AK. Percutaneous needle biopsies of renal allografts: relationship between morphological changes present in biopsies and subsequent allograft function. Histopathology 1977; 1: 161.
12. Margreiter R, Lang A, Koenig P. Cyclosporine in the treatment of acute allograft rejection refractory to high dose methylprednisolone: results of a prospectively randomised trial. Transplant Proc 1984; 16: 1202.
13. Pettersson E, Ahonin J, Edkaldn K. Treatment of acute rejection with cyclosporine. Transplant Proc 1984; 16: 1205.

Received 19 March 1985.
Accepted 30 July 1985.

DOPPLER ULTRASOUND AS A SCREEN FOR HEPATIC ARTERY THROMBOSIS AFTER LIVER TRANSPLANTATION

Doppler ultrasound combined with real-time ultrasound allows evaluation of both the hepatic artery and hepatic parenchyma after liver transplantation. Hepatic artery thrombosis following liver transplantation is a devastating event that may require emergency retransplantation. Unfortunately, clinical signs are often nonspecific. Results of angiographic evaluation for clinically suspected hepatic artery thrombosis have been normal in 76% of patients at our institution.

In a prospective study utilizing pulsed Doppler and real-time ultrasound, 29 transplant patients were examined. Six transplants had no hepatic artery Doppler pulse. All six had abnormal angiograms: four had hepatic artery thrombosis, one had a significant anastomotic stenosis, and one had slow flow with biopsy-proved ischemia. Of 23 patients with a Doppler pulse, two had surgically proved hepatic artery thrombosis. However, both had a focal abscess in the liver by real-time ultrasound. There were no cases of hepatic artery thrombosis in 21 patients with both a normal Doppler hepatic artery pulse and normal liver parenchyma.

Our data demonstrate that a combination of hepatic artery Doppler ultrasound and anatomical imaging of the liver currently is the optimal screening test for selecting which patients need hepatic angiography following liver transplantation.

Doppler ultrasound (pulsed Doppler imaging combined with real-time ultrasound) is an exciting new radiographic imaging modality available to physicians involved in liver and renal transplantation (*1–3*). This duplex imaging device detects blood flow via the Doppler shift from a single selected vessel localized by real-time ultrasound. Thus, noninvasive detection of arterial and venous blood flow to and from the allograft organ is now possible.

Hepatic artery thrombosis following liver transplantation usually occurs within the first three postoperative months and is a devastating event that, in the majority of patients, requires

TABLE 1. Comparison of Doppler and real-time ultrasound (RTU) findings with the incidence of hepatic artery thrombosis after liver transplantation

Ultrasound findings	Number of transplants	Hepatic artery thrombosis
Normal Doppler, normal RTU	21	None[c]
Normal Doppler, abnormal RTU[a]	2	2
Abnormal Doppler,[b] normal RTU	3	1[d]
Abnormal Doppler,[b] abnormal RTU[a]	3	3

[a] Abnormal RTU = focal hepatic abscess or infarct.

[b] Abnormal Doppler = absent hepatic artery flow.

[c] Three by angiography, eighteen by clinical follow-up.

[d] In the other two patients, both had patent but abnormal hepatic arteries. In one, a severe anastomotic stenosis was present, and the other showed markedly reduced flow with biopsy-proved ischemia.

immediate therapeutic intervention. The patient may develop fever and elevated liver enzymes, especially serum transaminases. If hepatic infarction develops, infection often supervenes. Finally, toxic septicemia results from septic hepatic gangrene (*4, 5*). Emergency hepatic retransplantation is the patient's only hope for survival (*6*).

Angiography, an invasive examination, has been the definitive procedure to evaluate patency of the hepatic artery following liver transplantation (*7*). On the basis of clinical criteria alone, one cannot effectively predict which transplant patient needs an arteriogram.

From January 1981 to October 1984, prior to the availability of Doppler ultrasound, 33 angiographic studies (18 children, 15 adults) were performed at the University Health Center of Pittsburgh for the clinical suspicion of hepatic artery thrombosis after liver transplantation. Of these, 61% (11/18) of the children and 93% (14/15) of the adults had patent hepatic arteries.

Currently, we use three noninvasive imaging modalities to evaluate the liver after transplantation: computed tomography (CT),* real-time ultrasound, and Doppler ultrasound. CT and real-time ultrasound are useful for evaluating the liver parenchyma to detect focal areas of infarction and/or abscess. However, only Doppler ultrasound can detect flow within the allograft hepatic artery.

The purpose of this communication is to demonstrate the immense value of noninvasive imaging as a screen for angiography in liver transplant patients with suspected hepatic artery thrombosis. In our institution, the allograft liver parenchyma is imaged with real-time ultrasound when the patency of hepatic artery is evaluated with pulsed Doppler ultrasound. If ultrasonic visualization of the liver parenchyma is unsatisfactory or equivocal then CT of the liver may be performed without and with intravenous contrast material.

During the 51 month period from January 1981 to April 1985, 330 patients (147 children, 183 adults) received 435 orthotopic liver transplants at the University Health Center of Pittsburgh. Seventy-seven patients received two transplants each and 14 patients received three transplants each. There were 150 male and 180 female patients with an age range from 4 months to 57 years.

During this time 42 angiographic studies (25 in children, 17 in adults) were performed for evaluation of hepatic artery patency after liver transplantation. This includes the initial 33 patients evaluated prior to Doppler and 9 additional patients

* Abbreviation used: CT, computed tomography.

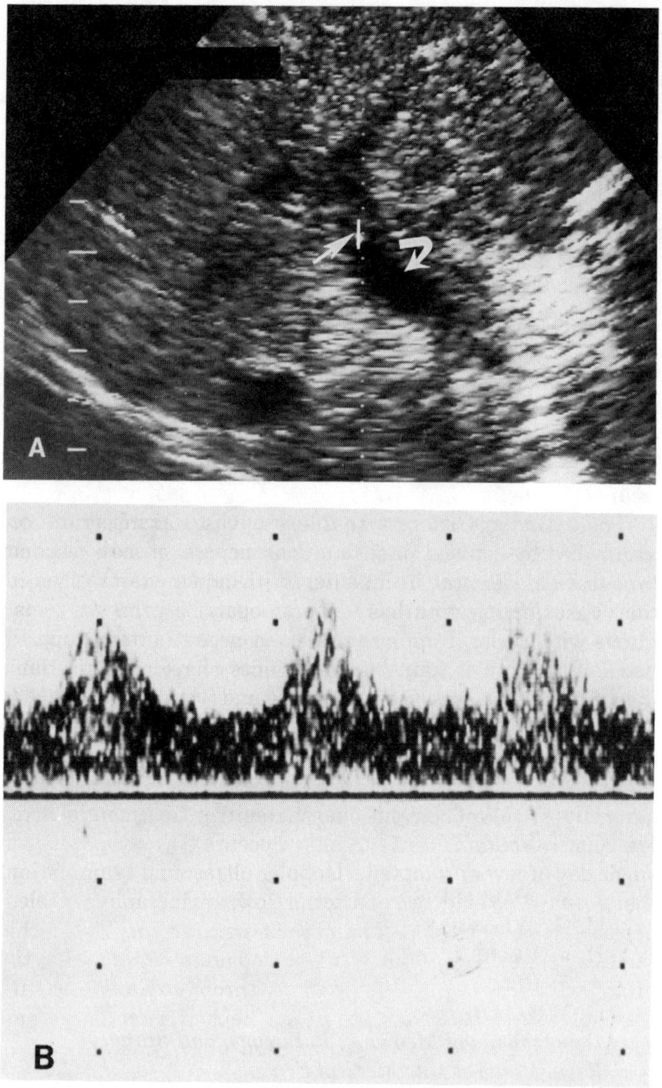

FIGURE 1. Normal Doppler ultrasound findings. (A) position of cursor line through hepatic artery (straight arrow) on sagittal view for Doppler waveform shown in (B). Portal vein (curved arrow); (B) normal Doppler hepatic artery waveform.

studied since Doppler ultrasound became available. In all cases, angiography was performed within the first two months following liver transplantation.

Between October 1984 and April 1985, pulsed Doppler and real-time ultrasound examinations have been performed on 29 liver transplants to evaluate hepatic artery patency and the liver parenchyma. Eighteen have been followed clinically without angiography. Nine transplants underwent angiography and two had emergency surgery without angiography.

Doppler and real-time ultrasound imaging were performed on 29 transplanted livers. A comparison of the Doppler and real-time ultrasound findings with the incidence of hepatic artery thrombosis is shown in Table 1. In 23 transplants, Doppler ultrasound demonstrated arterial flow to the liver (Fig. 1). Three patients underwent angiography that demonstrated patent hepatic arteries in each case. In twenty transplants, angiography was not performed, based on the normal Doppler study. In two of the twenty transplants, a focal abscess was identified in the liver by real-time ultrasound. Because of clinical deterioration, both patients required emergency retransplantation. Both had hepatic artery thrombosis. Of the remaining eighteen, none have developed hepatic artery thrombosis. Four have required retransplantation for reasons other than hepatic artery thrombosis. Two patients died, one of graft failure and one of cardiac arrest.

In six transplants, no evidence of hepatic arterial flow was identified in the liver hilum by Doppler imaging. Angiography was abnormal in all six cases. Four had hepatic artery thrombosis. In one of the four, angiography also revealed arterial collaterals to the transplanted liver while a small infarct was seen on ultrasound. In the fifth transplant, a severe stenosis was found at the hepatic artery anastomosis. In the sixth transplant, the hepatic arterial tree was narrowed with markedly reduced washout of contrast within the liver, suggesting slow flow. Liver biopsy showed changes consistent with ischemia.

Hepatic artery thrombosis following liver transplantation should be suspected if there is a focal hepatic abscess/infarct, or if there is absence of blood flow by Doppler examination in the hepatic artery within the porta hepatis. In the six transplants with absent Doppler findings of hepatic artery flow, all had abnormal angiograms. Of 14 patients with focal alterations (abscess/infarct) in the liver by CT and/or ultrasound from 1982 to 1985, 86% (12/14) have had hepatic artery thrombosis (*3*).

Doppler ultrasound imaging of the hepatic artery is the only currently available noninvasive method for detecting hepatic artery thrombosis before infarction occurs. In one patient, a single day of fever prompted a Doppler ultrasound examination that detected no evidence of arterial flow; angiography revealed hepatic artery occlusion. The patient was retransplanted the same day. Pathology of the liver revealed no evidence of hepatic infarction, even though hepatic artery thrombosis was present.

Doppler ultrasound imaging of the hepatic artery, together with real-time ultrasound examination of liver parenchyma, should be the initial test in patients suspected of having hepatic artery thrombosis after liver transplantation. CT may give complimentary information in difficult or equivocal cases. In experienced hands, Doppler confirmation of hepatic arterial flow with normal liver parenchyma on real-time ultrasound obviates angiography. Absence of hepatic artery flow in the porta hepatis by Doppler imaging or the presence of a focal hepatic abscess or infarct by real-time ultrasound or CT warrants immediate angiography.

Acknowledgment. We thank Donna Scahill for manuscript preparation.

Mark C. Segel[1]
Albert B. Zajko[1,2]
A'Delbert Bowen[3]
M. Leon Skolnick[1]
Klaus M. Bron[1]
Ronald J. Penkrot[1]
B. Simon Slasky[1]
Thomas E. Starzl[4]
Department of Radiology, Presbyterian-University Hospital
Department of Radiology, Children's Hospital of Pittsburgh
Department of Surgery, University Health Center of Pittsburgh, Pittsburgh, Pennsylvania

REFERENCES

1. Taylor KJW, Burns PN. Doppler ultrasound: continuous and pulsed superficial and deep. In: Goldberg BB, ed. Chapter in syllabus—categorical course in ultrasound. Presented at the annual meeting of the Radiological Society of North America. Washington, D.C., November, 1984: 139–169.
2. Taylor KJW, Burns PN, Weltin G, Rigsby C. Pulsed Doppler in the evaluation of vascular integrity of the transplanted kidney. Presented at the annual meeting of the American Roentgen Ray Society Meeting. Boston, MA. April, 1985.
3. Segel MC, Zajko AB, Bowen A, Skolnick ML, Penkrot RJ, Starzl TE. Hepatic artery thrombosis after liver transplantation: radiologic evaluation. AJR 1986; 146: 137.
4. Starzl TE (with the assistance of Putman CW). Intra- and postoperative complications and care. In: Experience in hepatic transplantation. Philadelphia: Saunders, 1969: 144.
5. Starzl TE (with the assistance of Putman CW). Acute rejection and hepatic gangrene. In: Experience in hepatic transplantation. Philadelphia: Saunders, 1969: 308.
6. Shaw BW Jr, Gordon RD, Iwatsuki S, Starzl TE. Hepatic retransplantation. Transplant Proc 1985; 17: 264.
7. Zajko AB, Bron KM, Starzl TE, et al. Angiography of liver transplantation patients. Radiology 1985; 157: 305.

Received 11 July 1985.
Accepted 15 August 1985.

[1] Presbyterian-University Hospital.
[2] Address correspondence and requests for reprints to: Albert B. Zajko, M.D., Department of Radiology, Presbyterian-University Hospital, DeSoto at O'Hara Streets, Pittsburgh, PA 15213.
[3] Childrens Hospital of Pittsburgh.
[4] University Health Center of Pittsburgh.

CYCLOSPORINE-ASSOCIATED MICROANGIOPATHY IN RENAL TRANSPLANTATION: A SEVERE BUT POTENTIALLY REVERSIBLE FORM OF EARLY GRAFT INJURY

Cyclosporine (CsA)* is a fungal metabolite that has been shown to have immunosuppressive properties, presumably through modulation of T lymphocyte activity (*1–3*). These properties have made CsA a clinically useful drug in suppressing rejection of transplanted bone marrow (*4*), kidney (*5–7*), liver (*7, 8*), and heart/lung (*9*). However, several important side-effects of CsA such as renal toxicity (*10*), hepatic injury (*10–12*), and hypertension (*13, 14*) have been found to interfere with the drug's usefulness. One complication that has been well documented in bone marrow transplant recipients given CsA is a condition similar to hemolytic-uremic syndrome (HUS), manifested by azotemia, anemia with red blood cell fragmentation, hypertension, thrombocytopenia, and glomerular capillary thromboses (*15–17*). This complication of CsA has not yet been reported as arising de novo in renal transplant recipients, perhaps because of the clinical and histopathological similarities to acute humoral-vascular rejection. We here describe a case of thrombotic microangiopathy and glomerulopathy in a renal allograft associated with CsA use, with rapid resolution upon withdrawal of the drug. This is a particularly important

* Abbreviations used: CsA, Cyclosporine; DVAH, Durham Veterans' Administration Hospital; HUS, hemolytic-uremic syndrome; PRA, percentage of panel-reactive antibody.

condition to differentiate from allograft rejection in renal transplant patients because of the entirely different treatment indicated.

The patient was a 30 year old man who was first seen at an outside hospital with headaches in May 1982. He was found to have significant hypertension (180/150 mm Hg), as well as heavy proteinuria and a serum creatinine of 4.2 mg/dl. He was referred to the Durham Veterans' Administration Hospital (DVAH) for further evaluation. A renal biopsy was performed, showing focal segmental glomerulosclerosis. An arteriovenous fistula was placed in February 1983, and hemodialysis was begun in June 1983 and continued until February 1984, during which time routine pretransplant blood transfusions were given without complications. In March 1984 the patient was admitted to the DVAH for cadaveric renal transplantation. Histocompatibility testing showed a three-antigen HLA-A, B match (O mismatch) and O antigen HLA-DR match (1 mismatch) with the donor. The patient had no detectable presensitization to leukocyte HLA antigens (percentage of panel reactive antibody, PRA, = 0) and a negative lymphocyte crossmatch with all sera available. The cadaveric donor kidney was transplanted into the patient's left iliac fossa on 3/2/84 without complications. Azathioprine and 500 mg of methylprednisolone were given on the day of surgery. Prednisone (80 mg/day) was begun preoperatively and tapered to 40 mg/day by posttransplant day 27. Postoperatively the patient never received high-dose steroid bolus therapy. During the first postoperative week, the serum creatinine fell progressively from 20.3 to 13.5 mg/dl. CsA (15 mg/kg p.o. q.d.) was started on 3/6/84 (postoperative day 4), and the azathioprine was rapidly tapered and stopped. Hemodialysis was performed on 3/6/84, bringing the serum creatinine to 11 mg/dl. An ultrasound examination of the renal allograft showed no perirenal fluid collection and no hydronephrosis. However, the patient complained of pain around the graft site, his urine output fell significantly, and blood began draining from his penis around the urethral catheter. A repeat ultrasound study on 3/8/84 revealed hydronephrosis of the transplant kidney. A percutaneous nephrostomy tube was placed. On 3/9/84, left flank and left thigh swelling was noted, and the patient was taken to the operating room where a left pelvic hematoma was evacuated and an open renal biopsy was performed. After this procedure, urine output improved, but he continued to have gross hematuria and his serum creatinine rose to 15 mg/dl in spite of hemodialysis. The patient's platelet count also fell as low as 44,000, his hemoglobin dropped from 11 to 6 mg/dl despite multiple transfusions, and serum bilirubin rose from 0.6 to 5.7 mg/dl. CsA trough levels were 1100 ng/ml on 3/8/84 and 650 ng/ml on 3/12/84. The biopsy findings were not typical of acute vascular-humoral or cellular-interstitial rejection, or obstruction, but they were consistent with the CsA-associated microangiopathy and glomerulopathy previously reported in bone marrow allograft recipients (*15–17*). Based on the clinical course and pathologic findings, the CsA was stopped on 3/13/84 and immunosuppression with azathioprine resumed. Subsequently the gross hematuria resolved after one day—and, over the next several days, the serum creatinine fell to the 6–9 mg/dl range, the serum bilirubin decreased back to 0.7 mg/dl, and the platelet count increased to the 75,000–120,000/ml range. The patient's course continued to improve, and he was discharged on 3/29/84 with a serum creatinine of 7.0 mg/dl. Follow-up serum creatinine on 4/9/84 was 2.7 mg/dl. The allograft has continued to function well with stable serum creatinine levels in the 3.0–3.5 mg/dl range.

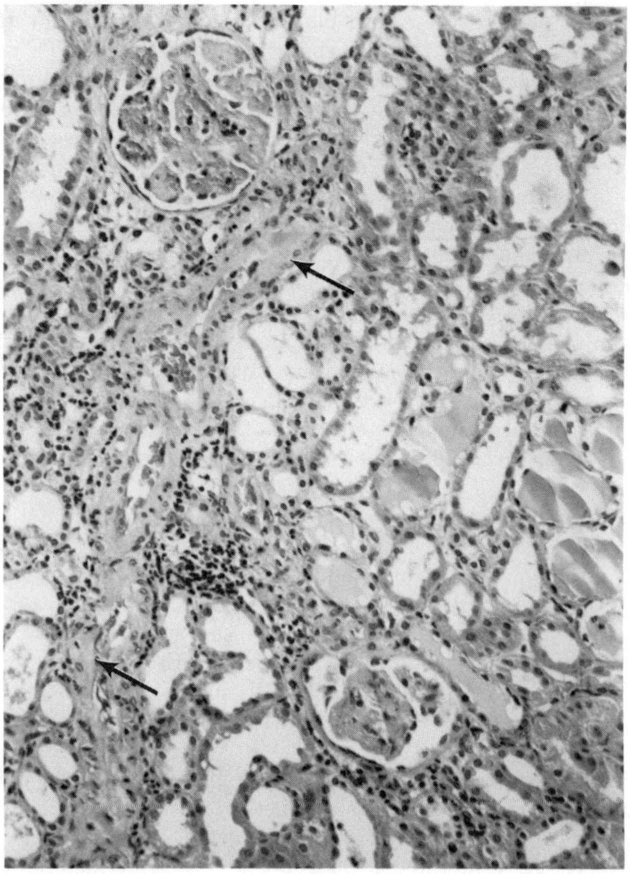

FIGURE 1. Focal dilatation of renal tubules with cast formation. Note glomerular thrombosis and acellular hyaline material (arrows) within wall of interlobular artery (H&E; 170×).

Paraffin-embedded sections of the renal allograft biopsy showed two fragments of renal cortex with approximately 30 glomeruli per section for evaluation. No vessels larger than interlobular arteries were present in the sections. The overall cortical architecture was mildly disrupted by interstitial fibrosis. Occasional small subcapsular foci of mononuclear inflammatory cells were seen that were composed of lymphocytes, but there was no other significant interstitial inflammation. Numerous tubules were mildly dilated; some contained proteinaceous casts, red blood cells, or a few polymorphonuclear neutrophils; some proximal tubular epithelial cells were flattened while others were swollen and vacuolated (Fig. 1). The arterioles and small interlobular arteries had thickened walls with acellular amorphous proteinaceous material between the swollen and reactive smooth muscle cells (Fig. 1). Many of the endothelial cells also appeared swollen and reactive in these arterioles. No inflammation was present within these blood vessel walls. Most of the glomeruli showed various degrees of capillary loop thickening with fibrin deposition along the capillary endothelial surfaces. Other glomerular capillary loops were dilated. Many of the glomeruli showed fibrin thrombi within capillaries and segmental necrosis with occasional polymorphonuclear neutrophils within these areas (Fig. 2). No glomerular proliferative changes or crescents were present. Direct immunofluorescence studies demonstrated extensive fibrin deposition within the glomeruli, including multiple dilated capillary loops filled with fibrin. There was no significant immunoglobulin or complement staining except for focal hya-

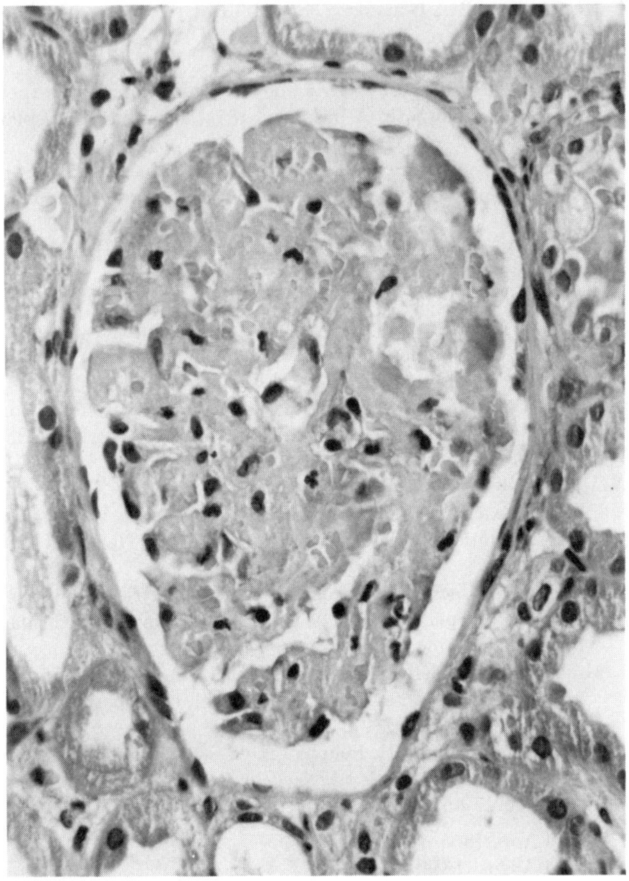

FIGURE 2. Prominent accumulations of fibrin within glomerular capillaries with partial glomerular necrosis (H&E; 400×).

line IgM and C3 within arterioles and occasional glomeruli. Renal cortical tissue was removed from the paraffin block for transmission electron microscopy with a moderate amount of fixation artifact present. No immune-complex type deposits were seen within glomeruli, but fibrin was present within glomeruli and tubular lumens. Arterioles and small muscular arteries contained large collections of electron-dense hyaline-like material within their walls located both between smooth muscle cells and just beneath the endothelial basement membrane, and platelet clumps were noted within peritubular capillaries.

This case manifests many of the clinical features reported in previous cases of CsA-induced microthrombotic disease in bone marrow allograft recipients (*15–17*). These features include progressive or unresolving azotemia, anemia, thrombocytopenia, and hypertension. These clinical signs may, of course, be manifestations of other problems that more commonly arise in the early post-renal-transplantation period, such as allograft rejection or severe (malignant) hypertension. Renal biopsy can be an extremely useful tool in making this distinction. The allograft biopsy in this patient showed little interstitial inflammation to suggest acute interstitial graft rejection. Also, there was no inflammation or necrosis within blood vessel walls to indicate acute humoral-vascular rejection. Kohler and Tilney (*18*) have described a patient with hyperacute renal allograft rejection who had findings similar to HUS in the renal biopsy and who was not on CsA—but they saw diffuse interstitial mononuclear cell infiltration as well as arteritis on the biopsy, two features not present in this case.

Interestingly, one patient (case No. 3) mentioned in a report of the early clinical trials of CsA in England (*10*) was found to have fibrin deposited in the walls of small arteries and in a glomerulus. This case was thought to be vascular rejection, but to the authors' surprise, the patient subsequently did well with good allograft function. In retrospect, this case may actually have represented CsA-induced microangiopathy rather than rejection, thus accounting for the patient's excellent course.

Mihatsch et al. (*19*) have seen a CsA-associated arteriolopathy (severe hyaline change involving arterioles and small arteries without significant vascular wall inflammatory infiltrate) in many of their renal allograft recipients on CsA. However, since this type of arteriolar hyaline deposition is also a feature of hypertension, differentiation between these processes may be difficult. The patient in the case we report here did have severe hypertension, but this was present before, during, and after his stormy postoperative period, and there was no apparent correlation between the degree of hypertension and the dramatic changes seen in his clinical course following CsA withdrawal.

The pelvic hematoma obstructing the allograft ureter in this case raises the possibility that much of this patient's postoperative renal failure was a result of obstruction. However, the biopsy finding of glomerular and vascular thrombosis is normally not seen with obstructive disease alone. Furthermore, surgical evacuation of the obstructing hematoma did not significantly alter his declining renal function or clinical course. Clearly, one of the most convincing bits of evidence that CsA was largely responsible for this patient's postoperative renal problems was that discontinuance of the drug resulted in rapid and marked improvement in function.

CsA-associated recurrence of HUS has also been reported (*20*), but our patient had no history of HUS or any other type of coagulopathy. The importance of this case report lies in the recognition that this type of CsA-associated toxicity may occur in renal transplant patients independent of a prior history of HUS. Both clinicians and pathologists should be aware of this entity—and, in appropriate circumstances, attempt to differentiate it from acute allograft rejection, which it may simulate. Microangiopathic hemolytic anemia (with fragmented erythrocytes on peripheral blood smear and increased plasma free hemoglobin, serum lactic dehydrogenase, and serum bilirubin) and marked thrombocytopenia in patients receiving CsA with progressive posttransplantation azotemia should alert clinicians to this possibility. Pathologically, glomerular thrombosis and necrosis with arteriolopathy in the absence of vasculitic changes, larger vessel involvement, and other features of acute humoral rejection help lead to the diagnosis. Distinguishing this condition from acute humoral-vascular rejection is critical to prevent needless aggressive immunosuppressive therapy or allograft nephrectomy for this disorder, which is potentially reversible by reduction or withdrawal of CsA treatment.

Acknowledgments. We thank M. Horsley for manuscript preparation; J. Burchette and M. Hale for expert technical assistance; and S. Embry, T. Sprinkle, and S. Conlon for photomicrograph preparation.

JOHN A. WOLFE[1]
RICHARD L. MCCANN
FRED SANFILIPPO

[1] Address correspondence and reprint requests to Dr. Wolfe, Department of Pathology, Box 3712, Duke University Medical Center, Durham, NC 27710.

Departments of Pathology and Surgery
Duke University and Durham Veterans Administration Medical Centers
Durham, North Carolina 27710

REFERENCES

1. Borel JF, Feurer C, Gubler HU, Stahelin H. Biologic effects of cyclosporin A: a new antilymphocyte agent. Agents Actions 1976; 6: 468.
2. Wagner H. Cyclosporin A: mechanism of action. Transplant Proc 1983; 15: 523.
3. Borel JF, Lafferty KJ. Cyclosporin: speculation about its mechanism of action. Transplant Proc 1983; 15: 1881.
4. Powles RL, Clink HM, Spence D, et al. Cyclosporin A to prevent graft-versus-host disease in man after allogeneic bone marrow transplantation. Lancet 1980; 1: 327.
5. Ferguson RM, Rynasiewicz JJ, Sutherland DER, Simmons RL, Najarian JS. Cyclosporin A in renal transplantation: a prospective randomized trial. Surgery 1982; 92: 175.
6. Merion RM, White DJG, Thiru S, Evan DB, Calne RY. Cyclosporin: five years' experience in cadaveric renal transplantation. N Engl J Med 1984; 310: 148.
7. Calne RY, Rolles K, White DJG, et al. Cyclosporin A initially as the only immunosuppressant in 34 recipients of cadaveric organs: 32 kidneys, 2 pancreases, and 2 livers. Lancet 1979; 2: 1033.
8. Starzl TE, Iwatsuki S, Shaw BW, et al. Analysis of liver transplantation. Hepatology 1984; 4: 47S.
9. Reitz BA, Wallwork JL, Hunt SA, et al. Heart-lung transplantation: successful therapy for patients with pulmonary vascular disease. N Engl J Med 1982; 306: 557.
10. Calne RY, White DJG, Thiru S, et al. Cyclosporin A in patients receiving renal allografts from cadaver donors. Lancet 1978; 2: 1323.
11. Klintmalm GBG, Iwatsuki S, Starzl TE. Cyclosporin A hepatotoxicity in 66 renal allograft recipients. Transplantation 1981; 32: 488.
12. Fernando ON, Sweny P, Farrington K, et al. Preliminary experience with cyclosporin A in human renal allografts. Transplant Proc 1980; 12: 244.
13. Hamilton DV, Charmichael DJS, Evans DB, Calne RY. Hypertension in renal transplant recipients on cyclosporin A and corticosteroids and azathioprine. Transplant Proc 1982; 14: 597.
14. Joss DV, Barrett AJ, Kendra JR, Lucas CF, Desai S. Hypertension and convulsions in children receiving cyclosporin A [letter]. Lancet 1982; 1: 906.
15. Shulman H, Striker G, Deeg HJ, et al. Nephrotoxicity of cyclosporin A after allogeneic marrow transplantation: glomerular thromboses and tubular injury. N Engl J Med 1981; 305: 1392.
16. Hows JM, Chipping PM, Fairhead S, et al. Nephrotoxicity in bone marrow transplant recipients treated with cyclosporin A. Br J Haematol 1983; 54: 69.
17. Atkinson K, Biggs JC, Hayes J, et al. Cyclosporin A associated nephrotoxicity in the first 100 days after allogeneic bone marrow transplantation: three distinct syndromes. Br J Haematol 1983; 54: 59.
18. Kohler TR, Tilney NL. Microangiopathic hemolytic anemia associated with hyperacute rejection of a kidney allograft. Transplant Proc 1982; 14: 444.
19. Mihatsch MJ, Thiel G, Spichtin HP, et al. Morphologic findings in kidney transplants after treatment with cyclosporine. Transplant Proc 1983; 15: 2821.
20. Leithner C, Sinzinger H, Pohanka E, et al. Recurrence of haemolytic uraemic syndrome triggered by cyclosporin A after renal transplantation [letter]. Lancet 1982; 2: 1470.

Received 4 April 1985.
Accepted 1 August 1985.

LETHAL GRAFT-VERSUS-HOST DISEASE IN A RECIPIENT OF A PANCREAS-SPLEEN TRANSPLANT

Acute graft-versus-host disease (GVHD)* is a frequent complication of bone marrow transplantation and has been reported in immunodeficient patients receiving nonirradiated blood transfusions. Acute GVHD is a potential problem in any transplant involving immunocompetent tissue. We report here a case of fatal acute GVHD following a combined pancreaticosplenic transplant for insulin-dependent diabetes mellitus.

A 35-year-old man was admitted to the University of Wisconsin Hospital on 9/4/84 for a pancreas transplant. Past medical history was significant for insulin-dependent diabetes mellitus since age 5 with associated complications of retinopathy, neuropathy, and end-stage renal failure. One year prior to admission the patient had received a living-related renal transplant. Current immunosuppression consisted of azathioprine 150 mg/day and prednisone 15 mg/day, and renal function on admission was excellent with serum creatinine of 1.3 mg/dl (130 μmol/L).

A pancreaticosplenic transplant was performed on 9/5/84 using our standard technique as previously described (*1*). Donor and recipient were complete HLA mismatches with the exception of a shared A2. Posttransplant immunosuppression consisted of cyclosporine 5 mg/kg i.v. daily, prednisone in a tapering dose schedule beginning at 120 mg daily, and azathioprine 25 mg daily. The graft functioned immediately and the patient required no further insulin administration. The early postoperative course was uneventful. A pancreaticosplenic scan revealed good perfusion of both organs.

Approximately one week postoperatively the patient developed progressively worsening leukopenia, the total white cell count falling to less than 1000 cells/mm^3. Azathioprine was stopped along with other drugs that could cause leukopenia. Serial viral antibody titers demonstrated no evidence of cytomegalovirus, Epstein-Barr virus, or herpesvirus infection, and multiple blood cultures were negative. A bone marrow biopsy revealed normal cellularity and normal precursors for all three lines of formed blood elements. Although a labeled white cell scan did not demonstrate any localized white cell collections, it was suspected that splenic sequestration was occurring and splenic irradiation was performed, with a total of 1000 rads administered over 3 days. Despite this treatment severe leukopenia persisted with total white cell levels as low as 200 cells/mm^3. Transplant splenectomy was performed on 9/24/84, but leukopenia persisted and the patient was placed in reverse isolation. Histology of the spleen revealed a normal pattern of reactive hyperplasia.

Over the next two weeks the patient developed a severe bullous epidermolysis of the head, trunk, and upper extremities. This was accompanied by progressive edema of the head and neck with slowly increasing upper airway obstruction. Sinus films demonstrated maxillary sinusitis and the patient was placed on antibiotics. At this point the patient's general condition deteriorated rapidly with multiple organ system involvement. Intubation was required for progressive airway obstruc-

* Abbreviations used: CT, computerized tomography; GVHD, graft-versus-host disease.

tion, and the patient developed respiratory insufficiency and diffuse interstitial infiltrates on chest roentgenograms. Bronchoscopy and bronchoalveolar lavage were performed and demonstrated no definite pathogen. Simultaneously, impairment of liver function developed with a steadily rising bilirubin which reached a level of 25 mg/dl associated with an elevation of alkaline phosphotase and normal transaminase levels. Low grade gastrointestinal tract bleeding developed. Abdominal computerized tomography (CT) scans did not reveal abscesses or biliary tract obstruction. Upper and lower endoscopy revealed diffuse gastritis and mild colitis. Pancytopenia developed with platelet counts falling to 20–40,000/mm^3 and hemoglobin levels requiring almost daily transfusions to maintain a level of 10 gm/dl. A skin biopsy revealed toxic epidermal necrolysis consistent with GVHD. Cyclosporine was stopped and in consultation with the Bone Marrow Transplant service the patient was started on high-dose steroid therapy, initially receiving 3 g methylprednisilone i.v. daily. One week later, as no clinical response was noted, a course of CBL-1, an anti-T-lymphoblast monoclonal antibody was given after the patient's family gave informed consent, following a protocol approved by the Human Subjects Committee. Bone marrow biopsy on 10/30/84 revealed severe hypocellularity, and HLA typing of peripheral blood lymphocytes revealed 80–100% donor-type cells. Cultures from multiple sites became positive for *Candida albicans*, and shortly thereafter the patient succumbed to progressive respiratory failure on 11/4/84.

An autopsy revealed consolidation of both lungs with multiple fungal granulomas; hypocellular bone marrow, lymph nodes, and spleen; and toxic epidermal necrolysis. These findings were consistent with acute GVHD, adult respiratory distress syndrome, and diffuse fungal sepsis.

Acute GVHD is a clinical entity that most commonly involves the skin, liver, and GI tract—causing rash, hyperbilirubinemia, and profuse diarrhea. It occurs frequently in HLA-matched bone marrow transplant recipients, in whom it is thought to be due to mismatched minor histocompatibility antigens between donor and recipient. It has also been reported as a result of transfusions of nonirradiated blood products into immunodeficient patients or maternofetal cell transfers in severely immunodeficient infants (*2–4*).

Acute GVHD has been described in several animal models of splenic transplants including dog and rat (*5, 6*). Extensive studies by Bitter-Suermann in rats demonstrated frequent occurrence of fatal acute GVHD, particularly when the donor had been pretreated with recipient antigen in the form of lymphocytes or when the recipient had been irradiated prior to transplantation (*7*).

A limited number of spleen transplants have been performed in the clinical setting. Isolated spleen transplants have been performed in attempts to boost tumor-specific immunity—in a single patient with Gaucher's disease, and in one patient with classic hemophilia (*8–10*). All failed in short periods with no evidence of immunologic complications. More recently, splenic transplants have been performed by several groups, including our own, to increase total blood flow in pancreaticosplenic transplants and thereby prevent graft loss due to venous thrombosis. We have thus far performed 8 combined transplants, and Starzl et al. have reported on 4 others (*11*). This is the first case of acute GVHD reported in a patient who received a splenic transplant. Although the presentation was somewhat atypical with leukopenia being the initial sign, the classic symptoms of GVHD rapidly developed, with skin, liver, and GI tract involvement. Despite vigorous treatment with steroids and monoclonal antibody, the patient succumbed to severe GVHD complicated by overwhelming fungal infection.

In our own series and in the cases reported by Starzl, several other less severe immunologic problems have occurred. We have had one patient who developed isolated thrombocytopenia that responded to splenic irradiation. A second patient developed a skin rash that was not acute GVHD by skin biopsy; nevertheless this patient also had circulating lymphocytes of donor HLA type. Starzl has also reported two similar patients—as well as another patient whose blood was type A and who developed hemolytic anemia after receiving a type O pancreaticosplenic transplant (*11*). The donor spleen produced anti-A antibodies resulting in hemolytic anemia. Both of these problems resolved following splenectomy. Corry recently reported a case of nonfatal GVHD following a pancreaticosplenic transplant (personal communication).

The spleen contains a variety of immunocompetent cells capable of several types of immune responses following transplantation, the most serious being acute GVHD. The type of response seen with splenic transplantation likely depends on the balance between a number of factors in both the donor and host immune systems. The prior immunosuppression of our recipient for a renal transplant may account for the development of GVHD in this situation in a manner similar to the rat model, in which irradiation of the recipient promoted acute GVHD. It is also possible that the donor had somehow been primed to the recipient, perhaps by previous transfusions.

The risk of GVHD following transplantation of the spleen is unknown. Nevertheless, due to the serious nature of this complication and the difficulty in treating established GVHD, it would seem prudent to approach further splenic transplantation with caution until it has been better studied in animal models. Because of this risk of GVHD occurring in future patients we are no longer including the spleen in our whole-organ pancreas transplants.

M. H. Deierhoi
H. W. Sollinger
M. J. Bozdech
F. O. Belzer
Departments of Surgery and Medicine
University of Wisconsin Hospital
Madison, Wisconsin

REFERENCES

1. Sollinger HW, Kalayoglu M, Hoffmann RM, Belzer FO. Results of segmental and pancreatico-splenic transplantation with pancreatico-cystostomy. Transplant Proc 1985; 17(1): 360.
2. James WD, Odom RB. Graft-v-host disease. Arch Dermatol 1983; 119: 683.
3. Rosen RC, Huestis DW, Corrigan JJ. Acute leukemia and granulocyte transfusions: fatal graft-v-host reaction following transfusion of cells obtained from normal donors. J Pediatr 1978; 93: 268.
4. Morhann VB, Maibach HI. Graft-v-host reactions in a newborn. Acta Derm Venereol Stockh 1974; 54: 133.
5. Simonsen M. Biological incompatibility in kidney transplantation in dogs. II. Serological investigations. Acta Pathol Microbiol Scand 1953; 32: 36.

6. Bitter-Suermann H, Herbertson BM. Morphologic features of splenic allografts in rats. Am J Pathol 1975; 81: 283.
7. Bitter-Suermann H. Different ways of using graft-versus-host reactivities to achieve acceptance of rat spleen allografts in the same donor-recipient pairing. Transplantation 1974; 18: 515.
8. Marchioro TL, Fudenberg H, Rowlands DT, Rifkind D. Splenic homotransplantation. Ann NY Acad Sci 1964; 120: 626.
9. Groth CG, Blomstrand R, Dreborg S, et al. Splenic transplantation in Gaucher's disease. In: Bergsma D, Desnick RJ, Bernbohr RW, Krivil W, eds. Enzyme therapy in genetic diseases, birth defects: original article series. New York: The National Foundation, 1973; 10: 102.
10. Hathaway WE, Mull MM, Githens JH, et al. Attempted spleen transplantation in classical hemophilia. Transplantation 1969; 7: 73.
11. Starzl TE, Iwatsuki S, Shaw BW, et al. Pancreaticoduodenal transplantation in humans. Surg Gynecol Obstet 1984; 159: 265.

Received 25 June 1985.
Accepted 1 August 1985.

DIARY OF FORTHCOMING EVENTS

Anyone organizing a meeting likely to be of interest to the readers of *Transplantation* may submit essential information about the meeting to any editorial office, which will consider its inclusion in the Diary of Events. This information should be received by the North American Editorial Office at least six months before the event. The Diary appears four times annually.

DATE	PLACE	SUBJECT	SECRETARIAT
June 1–6	Dubrovnik, Yugoslvaia	Second International Workshop on Neuroimmunomodulation	Dr. B.D. Jankovic Immunology Research Center Vojvode Stepe 458 11221 Belgrade, Yugoslavia
June 29–July 3	Budapest, Hungary	23rd Congress of the EDTA	Congress Bureau Motesz EDTA—EDTNA H-1361 Budapest P.O.B. 32 Hungary
June 29–July 3	Denver, Colorado	Annual Meeting of the North American Transplant Coordinators Organization	NATCO 5000 Van Nuys Blvd. Suite 400 Sherman Oaks, CA 91403
July 1–5	Toronto, Canada	3rd International Congress of Reproductive Immunology	Dr. David Clark 3V39 McMaster Univ. 1200 Main St., West Hamilton, Ontario, Canada
July 14–17	Buffalo, N.Y.	Vaccines: New Concepts and Developments	Dr. James Mohn 210 Sherman Hall SUNY Buffalo, N.Y. 14214
July 21–25	Kona, Hawaii	5th Annual Meeting of the North American Symposium on Dialysis and Transplantation	Dr. Robert Mendez 1893 Wilshire Blvd. Los Angeles, CA 90057
July 30–Aug. 1	Amsterdam, The Netherlands	6th International Workshop on Alloantigenic Systems in the Rat	Dr. L.C. Paul Academisch Ziekenhuis Leiden Rijnsburgerweg 10 2333 AA Leiden, The Netherlands
August 3–8	Helsinki, Finland	XIth International Congress of the Transplantation Society	Dr. Pekka Hayry Transplantation Laboratory Univ. of Helsinki Haartmaninkatu 3 Helsinki, Finland

Information for Subscribers

Published monthly, two volumes a year, beginning January and July.

Annual Subscription Rates—U. S. A. AND POSSESSIONS: personal, $105.00; institutional, $130.00; single copies, $12.00. FOREIGN: personal, $120.00; institutional, $145.00; single copies, $15.00. Institutional (multiple reader) rate applies to libraries, schools, hospitals, clinics, group practices, and federal commercial, and private institutions and organizations. A special in-training rate of $60.00 ($85.00 foreign) is available to residents, fellows, interns and students. (Prices subject to change) In requesting this rate, which is limited to three years, please give training status and name of institution. Subscribers may request that their copies be sent by air mail; the extra charge entailed for air service will be billed to the subscriber.

New and renewal subscriptions are entered to begin with the January or July issue. Correspondence regarding subscriptions should be addressed to the publishers.

Change of address. Publisher must be notified 60 days in advance. Undeliverable journals will be destroyed. Duplicates (if available) can be ordered from the publishers at the regular price of single issues.

Reprints of individual articles are available *only* from authors.

Microfilm. For availability, inquire of Williams & Wilkins.

Japanese Yen price is available from our sole agent: USACO Corporation, 13-12 Shimbashi 1-Chome, Minato-Ku, Tokyo 105, Japan, telephone 03-502-6471.

WILLIAMS & WILKINS

Publishers of Books and Periodicals in Medicine and the Allied Sciences
428 East Preston Street, Baltimore, Md. 21202, U.S.A.

AUTHOR INDEX

Amadeo, J. H., 606

Baloh, R., 657
Bander, N. H., 593
Beatty, P., 583
Beaudoin, R., 640
Bell, P. R. F., 652
Bensinger, W. I., 602
Berndt, M. C., 565
Bitter-Suermann, H., 626
Bradstock, K. F., 565
Broomhead, A. F., 565
Buckner, C. D., 602
Bucy, R. P., 661
Buszta, C., 598

Cavallini, M., 654
Chudzik, J., 659
Clift, R. A., 602
Cobbold, S., 634
Colvin, R. B., 572
Cordon-Cardo, C., 593
Cornélissen, G., 654
Cosimi, A. B., 572, 593

Daffin, L. E., 663
Davie, J. M., 661
Deeg, H. J., 583
Delmonico, F. L., 593
Duncan, W. R., 626
Duquesnoy, R. J., 620

Feld, L. G., 664
Fildes, R. D., 664
Finstad, C. L., 593
Fuller, T. C., 572
Fung, J., 620

Girard, B., 556
Glichlick, D., 579
González, Z., 606
Goormastic, M., 598
Gordon, G., 644
Gores, P. F., 648
Greenleaf, G. E., 556
Gridelli, B., 657
Griffith, B. P., 620
Grose, J. H., 640

Halberg, F., 654
Hansen, W. P., 593
Hardesty, R. L., 620
Heils, J., 654
Hess, A. D., 644
Hesse, U. J., 648
Horsburgh, T., 652
Hughes, W. G., 565
Hutchinson, I. V., 547

Jaffers, G. J., 572

Kabral, A., 565
Karwa, G., 579
Kaufman, C., 620
Khauli, R. B., 598
Klotz, L. H., 593

Lachance, J., 640
Lacy, P. E., 661
Leunissen, K. M. L., 666
Levy, G. J., 583
Luft, B. J., 611
Lum, L. G., 583, 587

Magnusson, M., 598
Matas, A. J., 579
Mauer, S. M., 664
McCabe, R. E., 611
Mistry, N., 652

Najarian, J. S., 648, 654
Nakamoto, S., 598
Noel, R., 640
Novick, A. C., 598

Old, L. J., 593
Orloff, M. J., 556

Paganini, E., 598
Persson, A., 616
Pierce, J. A., 663
Piper, D. J., 593
Prendergast, M. M., 565

Quinn, T., 579

Rabin, B. S., 620
Ramirez-González, R., 606
Rao, K. M., 657
Remington, J. S., 611
Rivé-Mora, E., 606
Roy, R., 640
Rubin, R. H., 593
Russell, P. S., 572, 593

Sanders, J., 583
Sanghvi, A., 657
Santiago-Delpín, E. A., 606
Santos, G. W., 644
Scanlon, L., 657
Schang, T., 650
Schreiber, M. J., 598
Shaw, B., 657
Shiobara, S., 587
Sitges-Serra, A., 648
Slichter, S. J., 602
Soberman, R., 579
Solders, G., 616
Springate, J. E., 664
Stanacev, N. Z., 659
Starzl, T., 657
Steinmuller, D. R., 598
Stepkowski, S. M., 626
Storb, R., 583, 587
Stuhne-Sekalec, L., 659
Sullivan, K. M., 583
Sutherland, D. E. R., 648, 654

Tellis, V. A., 579
Terasaka, R., 661
Thiede, A., 650
Thomas, E. D., 583, 602
Thompson, R. E., 593
Timmermann, W., 650
Tiver, K., 565
Tolkoff-Rubin, N. E., 593

Urban, P., 556

Van Hooff, J. P., 666
Van Leendert, R. J. M., 666
Veitch, P. S., 652
Veith, F. J., 579
Vidt, D. G., 598
Vismans, F-J. F. E., 666
Vogelsang, G. B., 644

Waldmann, H., 634
Weiss, R., 579
Whitsett, C. F., 663
Wilczek, H., 616
Winn, H. J., 572
Witherspoon, R. P., 587

Zeevi, A., 620
Zerbe, T. R., 620

0041-1337/86/4105-0547$02.00/0
TRANSPLANTATION
Copyright © 1986 by The Williams & Wilkins Co.

Vol. 41, No. 5
Printed in U.S.A.

Transplantation
OVERVIEW

SUPPRESSOR T CELLS IN ALLOGENEIC MODELS[1]

IAN V. HUTCHINSON

Nuffield Department of Surgery, University of Oxford, John Radcliffe Hospital, Oxford, OX3 9DU, England

Acceptance of a tissue allograft is quite readily achieved in some experimental systems using donor-specific antibodies (*1–4*), antigen pretreatment (*1, 5, 6*), or certain agents such as cyclosporine (*7, 8*) or antilymphocyte serum (*9*). In many instances the state of long-term unresponsiveness induced is specific for the donor even in cases in which ostensibly nonspecific immunosuppression was used for the induction (*9–11*). The immunological mechanisms that operate in the induction and maintenance of this donor-specific unresponsiveness have obvious relevance to clinical transplantation.

Possible mechanisms of allograft acceptance by immunocompetent recipients include alteration of the antigenicity or immunogenicity of the graft (*12, 13*), depletion (*14, 15*) or clonal deletion (*16*) of alloreactive lymphocytes, blocking of effector cells by alloantibody and/or alloantigen (*17–19*) and, the subject of this overview, suppressor cells. The literature considered here will be mainly confined to studies in rodents.

The phenotype, specificity, interactions and mode of action of suppressor cells and their role in regulation of allograft rejection have been extensively studied, but no clear consensus has been reached. Some cells suppress nonspecifically. For instance, immature bone-marrow-derived lymphocytes may have nonspecific suppressive activity in vitro and in vivo (see below). However, specific cell-mediated suppression is a function of T lymphocytes (*20–22*) or macrophages armed by specific T cell factors (*23, 24*).

Specific T suppressor cells (Ts)* were first demonstrated by Gershon and Kondo (*25*) in a model in which mice injected with large doses of sheep red blood cells (SRBC) had a depressed humoral response to a subsequent challenge with SRBC. Many subsequent studies have detected Ts in various models, including suppression of humoral or delayed type hypersensitivity (DTH) responses to such antigens as haptens (*20, 26, 27*), xenogeneic erythrocytes (*28*), avian lysozymes (*29*), marine hemocyanins (*30*) and synthetic polypeptides (*31, 32*).

Alloreactive suppressor cells were first described by Jirsch et al. (*33*) who showed their presence in the lymph nodes of mice that had been lethally irradiated, reconstituted with syngeneic bone marrow, and given a heart allograft. Ts were found, too, in the lymphoid tissues of skin-grafted mice given liver extracts (*34*) pretreated with donor antigens and ALS or with various other agents (*35–41*). Suppressor cells have since been shown to be present in many allogeneic systems (see below), but studies in which their exact nature—(lymphocyte or macrophage), "suppressor" or "helper" phenotype, specificity (nonspecific, antigen-specific or antiidiotypic) and sensitivity to irradiation and various drugs—was examined have lead to conflicting reports.

For the sake of clarity and ease of crossreference the markers on T cell subsets will be referred by the recently agreed nomenclature for human lymphocytes, namely CD4 (the assumed analogues being OKT4 or Leu-3, L3T4, and W3/25 in the human, mouse and rat, respectively) and CD8 (OKT8 or Leu-2, Lyt-2, OX8). The currently used epithets "T helper cell" for $CD4^+$ T cells and "T cytotoxic/suppressor cell" for T cells with the $CD8^+$ phenotype wrongly imply an absolute relationship between these markers and cell function. In this overview the term Ts refers directly to function and not to cell surface antigens.

It is now clear that there is not a single entity that can be described as "the specific suppressor T lymphocyte." Indeed, both macrophages and T lymphocytes (of both $CD4^+$ and $CD8^+$ phenotype) can exert specific or nonspecific effects in allogeneic models. These cells apparently interact to give rise to the state we recognize as specific unresponsiveness—mediated, at least in part, by T suppressor cells.

Detection of Alloreactive Suppressor Cells

Alloreactive suppressor cells are detected either in vitro by their ability to suppress mixed lymphocyte reactions (MLR) and generation of cell-mediated lymphocytotoxicity (CML) or in vivo by their capacity to adoptively transfer unresponsiveness to a syngeneic recipient. There are problems with interpretation in both systems.

Culture conditions in vitro have to be carefully controlled to ensure that the addition of "regulator" cells to an MLR does not interfere with, say, responder:stimulator cell-to-cell contact or deplete essential nutrients too rapidly. In some cases activated cells expressing interleukin-2 (IL-2) receptors have been shown to absorb IL-2 and produce artifactual nonspecific "suppression," an effect reversed by addition of exogenous IL-2 (*42*). Addition of excess helper cells may accelerate the MLR response so that the peak is dramatically advanced, while addition of cytotoxic cells may cause suppression by destroying stimulator cells. Interpretation is complicated, especially when suppression measured at a single time point is in the 20–50% range or when the magnitude of the response is unchanged but the kinetics of the response is merely advanced or delayed. However, for human studies, suppression of responses in MLR/CML cultures is the only available method.

* Abbreviations used: ALS, antilymphocyte serum; CML, cell-mediated lymphocytotoxicity; CsA, cyclosporine; Cy, cyclophosphamide; Cy^R, cyclophosphamide-resistant; Cy^S, cyclophosphamide-sensitive; DTH, delayed-type hypersensitivity; IL-2, interleukin-2; LTS, long-term-surviving; MHC, major histocompatibility complex; MLR, mixed lymphocyte reaction; SRBC, sheep red blood cells; TNP, trinitrophenyl; Ts, T suppressor cells.

[1] Work from this department discussed in this overview was supported by grants from The Medical Research Council of the UK and The National Kidney Research Fund.

Adoptive transfer studies are seemingly more straightforward: cells from a suppressed animal thought to possess suppressor cell activity are injected into a syngeneic recipient, which is then challenged with an allograft. If graft survival is prolonged the conclusion is drawn that the cell inoculum contained functional suppressor cells. However, some form of partial immunosuppression of the recipient is often required to reveal suppressor cell activity. Thus irradiation in the sublethal 200–500 rad range (*43–45*) or a course of antilymphocyte serum (ALS) therapy is used (*37, 38, 41, 46*). In a similar system animals are lethally irradiated and then reconstituted with just sufficient normal cells to cause acute rejection. The addition of putative suppressor cells to the normal reconstituting cells then provides a semiquantitative estimate of suppressor activity (*47–49*).

An alternative to attenuating the rejection response by treating the recipient is to weaken the vigor of the reaction by using challenge grafts depleted of passenger leukocytes by a period of residence in an immunosuppressed intermediary host (*50, 51*). This approach works but is complicated by the presence of suppressor cells within the retransplanted graft (see below).

Neither partial immunosuppression nor the use of retransplanted grafts are unreasonable approaches if one considers that the number of cells adoptively transferred (typically 10^6–10^8 cells) is only a fraction of the lymphoid population of the donor animal and that, in the maintenance phase in long-term survivor animals, the graft being protected by suppressor mechanisms is reduced in immunogenicity by loss of passenger leukocytes.

A major question is whether these assays are measuring the function of the same cells. In our studies (see below) Ts in rats that accept renal allografts are exclusively $CD8^+$ ($OX8^+$). By contrast, in the experiments of Hall (*48, 49*), who uses a rat heart allograft model, only $CD4^+$ ($W3/25^+$) Ts can be demonstrated. However, we use sublethal irradiation (200 rads) and a kidney allograft challenge (*9, 45, 52, 53*). For kidney transplant rejection cytotoxic mechanisms mediated by $CD8^+$ ($OX8^+$) T cells are thought to be crucial (*54*). By contrast, Hall uses a lethal irradiation and reconstitution system with a heart graft challenge, a situation in which reconstitution with $CD4^+$ ($W3/25^+$) T cells restores acute rejection (*49*). It is, therefore, a possibility that $CD4^+$ Ts effector cells suppress rejection by $CD4^+$ T-cell-mediated mechanisms and, likewise, that $CD8^+$ Ts effector cells regulate $CD8^+$ cytotoxic cells. Hence, the assay system, in vivo or in vitro, may dictate the results obtained.

Suppressor Cells in Allogeneic Models

Neonatally induced tolerance. The allospecific unresponsiveness of neonatally tolerized animals cannot be attributed solely to deletion or irreversible inactivation of alloreactive clones of lymphocytes (*55*). Neonatal rodents are immunologically incompetent (*55, 56*), and there appears to be a population of relatively immature lymphoid cells—possibly of the $Lyt\text{-}1^+2^-$ phenotype—that have nonspecific suppressor activity (*57, 58*). Antigen exposure in the presence of these nonspecific suppressor cells is permissive of induction of specific suppressor cells (*59*).

However, although specific suppressor cells have been demonstrated in the neonatally tolerized adult after grafting (*47, 60, 62*), their generation is dependent on the genetic disparity between the host and the tolerogen (*63*). Thus Class II disparities, especially at the putative I-J subregion are associated with activation of suppressor cells that act in the afferent phase of the immune response, while Class I differences lead to tolerance via a different pathway involving clonal deletion (*64*) or Ts that act in the efferent phase of the generation of cytotoxic T cells (*65*). Some studies have suggested two populations of suppressor T cells in neonatally tolerized mice: one regulates generation of cytotoxic T cell precursors from bone marrow while the other prevents the activation of those that do arise (*66*). It is probably the latter that is detected in MLR/CML suppression and adoptive transfer assays (see below) and that might act on the T helper cells. The former suppressor cells could account for the deficiency of cytotoxic precursor cells in tolerized mice (*67*). Hence, although suppressor cells may not have an exclusive role in neonatal tolerance, they could have important functions in the induction and maintenance of the unresponsive state, a subject reviewed very recently by Streilein (*68*).

Immunological reversion in the adult. In many respects the immunological status of recipients in which lethal radiation and bone marrow reconstitution (*33, 69*) or fractionated total-lymphoid irradiation (*70*) are used closely resembles neonatal tolerance in rodents. These techniques operate by eliminating mature lymphocytes and cause immunological reversion to an immunoincompetent (neonatal-like) state. The cells that arise from the inoculated or residual bone marrow contain nonspecific suppressor cells of the CD4/Lyt-1 phenotype), and exposure to antigen during their presence tends to activate the regenerating specific suppressor cells rather than helper or cytotoxic elements (*71*). Hence, an allogeneic organ or hematopoietic graft engenders the appearance of specific suppressor cell activity that protects the graft in the face of a recovering population of immunocompetent lymphocytes.

Any agent that has a selective effect on mature lymphocytes rather than bone marrow cells may cause temporary immunological reversion, at least in some parts of the immune system. ALS, cyclosporine (CsA), or high-dose steroids may act in this way—and giving the agent alone may elicit nonspecific cell-mediated suppression as a primary event, an effect most clearly demonstrated in the experiments of Maki et al. (*72*).

Suppressor cells in immunocompetent adults. Suppression of alloreactivity can be achieved in the immunocompetent adult by a variety of methods. These include treatment with antigen (*5, 6, 73–75*), antibody (*1–4, 76, 77*) or both (*1, 4, 74*), with or without the use of drugs (*78–81*) or other agents (*82, 83*). There are three principle models: suppression of allogeneic DTH reactions in rats (*84*) and mice (*85–87*), suppression of skin graft rejection in mice (*33–41, 80, 81*), and prevention of rejection of a vascularized allograft in rats (*48, 49, 52, 53, 88, 89*).

An i.v. preimmunization of mice or rats with donor antigen before sensitization and challenge for a DTH response will lead to a specific suppression of the reaction (*84–87*). The suppression is transferable by T cells from the preimmunized animal to normal syngeneic recipients (*90, 91*). Strong suppression is induced by preimmunization with donor cells differing from the recipient at Class II major histocompatibility complex (MHC) loci (*87*), although suppression to associated Class I (*85*) and minor alloantigens (*86*) is observed, too. These studies emphasize the importance of Class II antigens in the induction of suppressor T cells. This subject will be discussed again later.

Treatment with antigens i.v., including blood transfusions, can prolong the survival of subsequent skin allografts in mice

(*33–41, 80, 81*). In most cases this is donor-specific—although, depending on the histocompatibility barrier between the graft and the host and the dose of antigen used, nonspecific suppression can be observed (*92*). Specific suppressor cells, probably T cells, have been detected by in vitro and in vivo assays in the spleens and lymph nodes of mice that have accepted skin allografts after treatment with donor blood and ALS (*93*).

Suppressor cells in rats bearing kidney or heart allografts were elusive for some time. Attempts to transfer suppression with spleen cells from rats with actively enhanced kidneys into normal recipients (*94*) or from passively treated cell donors into partially immunosuppressed (ALS-treated) recipients (*46*) were unsuccessful. A transient appearance of suppressor cells in the thymuses of rats pretreated 10–11 days before grafting with antigen and antibody was demonstrated when cells were transferred to unmodified recipients (*89*).

Since these equivocal experiments it has been clearly shown that there are suppressor cells in rats bearing long-term surviving (>50 days) vascularized kidney or heart (*48, 50, 52, 53, 88, 89*) allografts treated with passive antidonor enhancing serum (*50, 52*) or active enhancement with donor-specific antigens (*88, 95*). In addition, the maintenance of graft survival induced by treatment with drugs such as CsA (*49, 53, 96, 97*) or cyclophosphamide (Cy) (*51*) may be due to suppressor T cells.

Suppressor T Cells in a Rat Renal Allograft Model

Techniques used for fractionation of Ts. The first step is to remove B lymphocytes. We use panning of populations on plates coated with anti-rat Ig antibody (*98*) or rosetting with the monoclonal mouse antirat B cell antibody, OX12, and anti-mouse Ig-coated sheep red blood cells (*99*). $CD4^+$ cells are depleted by rosetting with the monoclonal antibody W3/25, while $CD8^+$ cells are removed by rosetting with the OX8 monoclonal antibody (*99*). Antigen binding (idiotype-positive, [id^+]) cells are depleted by panning on monolayers of allogeneic spleen leukocytes formed in plates using poly-L-lysine (*100*). Anti-idiotypic (anti-id^+) cells are specifically inactivated by incubation in antidonor alloantibody and rabbit complement (see later). Finally, susceptibility of cells to Cy is tested by treatment of cell donors with 50 mg/kg Cy i.p. 2 days before cell transfer. These techniques will be detailed in future publications.

Suppressor T cells in acutely rejecting allograft recipients. When DA rats are grafted with a LEW kidney, suppressor cells can be detected in their spleens within 3 days. These cells persist in the spleen until day 14 after transplant but disappear by day 28. Suppressor cells are present, too, in the graft itself at day 5 but their activity wanes (or is overwhelmed) by day 7 during the rejection response (Hutchinson IV, Wood KJ, Morris PJ, manuscript in preparation). The phenotype of the suppressor cells found in the spleen at day 5 is Ig^- W3/25^+ $OX8^-$. These cells are Cy-sensitive (Cy^S) and specifically bind to LEW donor antigen monolayers. They are specifically suppressive in syngeneic rats but are effective only if transferred before grafting the adoptive recipient, suggesting an afferent mode of action (Hutchinson IV, Morris PJ, manuscript in preparation).

We have sonicated day 5 rejecting spleen T cells and have studied the properties of the soluble supernate (after 100,000 G centrifugation). This material suppresses graft rejection when given in place of the cells themselves (Hutchinson IV, unpublished results). The suppression is specific for LEW antigens and the active principle is absorbed out by LEW lymphocytes. Activity is removed, too, by absorption with unfractionated syngeneic DA spleen cells, but not by DA spleen cells passed through a column of G-10 Sephadex to remove adherent cells. The suppressive activity of this sonicate is not MHC-restricted: sonicates of cells from PVG·$RT1^a$ rats grafted with LEW kidneys are active in PVG·$RT1^c$ congenic recipients (in which the $RT1^a$ and $RT1^c$ rats differ only at the MHC complex). Conversely, PVG·$RT1^c$ anti-LEW sonicate is active in PVG·$RT1^a$ rats. However, there does appear to be a genetic restriction for minor alloantigens since DA ($RT1^a$) anti-LEW sonicate does not suppress LEW renal allograft rejection in PVG·$RT1^a$ recipients, and PVG·$RT1^a$ anti-LEW sonicate does not work in DA rats. (DA and PVG·$RT1^a$ rats share the same MHC complex but differ for minor background genes.) Allotype restriction has been reported in mouse suppressor cell systems (*101*), a possibility we have been unable to test directly without allotype congenic strains.

Treatment of normal DA rats with DA anti-LEW T cell sonicate induces in their spleens specific suppressor cell activity present in the $CD8^+$ (W3/25^- $OX8^+$) T cell fraction 7 days after injection of sonicate.

These results are interpreted in the following way. Challenge of the recipient with alloantigens on the graft induces, in addition to the rejection response, the appearance of $CD4^+$ (W3/25^+ $OX8^-$) Ts inducer cells. These cells elaborate an antigen-specific factor that is taken up by adherent cells and activates $CD8^+$ (W3/25^- $OX8^+$) T suppressor cells (i.e., of the classic phenotype). These afferent $CD4^+$ Ts inducer cells fail to prevent the rejection response, perhaps because the induction of $CD8^+$ Ts effector cells is a time-dependent process (*101*). One can speculate that application of a form of immunosuppression that delays rejection without interfering with the induction of $CD8^+$ Ts could lead to long-term acceptance of the allograft. We are currently investigating the action of CsA in this regard, since this agent is thought to have a selective Ts-sparing effect (*96*).

We are also engaged in a parallel study looking at the appearance of Ts in blood-transfused recipients (Hutchinson IV, Wood KJ, Morris PJ, unpublished results). Pretreatment alone with blood or spleen leukocytes does not elicit transferrable suppressor cells, these appearing only after grafting. Suppressor cells in these animals appear by days 3–5, as in untreated animals, but are nonspecific at this time. Suppressor cells in treated animals persist for the life-time of the animal both in the spleen and in the graft itself—and, in the long-term survivors, their action is specific (Hutchinson IV, Morris PJ, manuscript submitted for publication).

Suppressor T cells in long-term-surviving allograft recipients. The suppressor cell activity in the spleens of long-term surviving (LTS) LEW-to-DA kidney allograft recipients is confined to the $CD8^+$ (W3/25^- $OX8^+$) fraction in animals in which allograft acceptance was induced by blood transfusion or with trinitrophenyl (TNP) haptenated LEW donor alloantigen and TNP-specific suppressor cells (*45, 102*, and see below). There are two subpopulations of $CD8^+$ Ts (Hutchinson IV, Morris PJ, manuscript in preparation). One is cyclophosphamide-resistent (Cy^R) Ig^- W3/25^- $OX8^+$ id^- anti-id^+, while the other is Cy^S Ig^- W3/25^- $OX8^+$ id^+ anti-id^-. Both are effective if transferred four days after grafting in the adoptive transfer assay, suggesting an efferent mode of action. Both are strain-specific and prevent rejection of a LEW but not of a third-party graft. However, if the Cy^S $OX8^+$ id^+ cells are transferred with LEW antigen they act nonspecifically to suppress rejection of third-party transplants. This activation of nonspecific suppression is specific since unrelated antigens from BN, WAG, or PVG/c rats fail to activate third-party suppression. Specific activation of nonspecific suppression will be discussed below.

Another feature distinguishing the Cy^S and Cy^R $OX8^+$ Ts in LTS rats is that Cy^R Ts do not suppress in Cy-treated adoptive cell recipients. This suggests that they are not directly suppressive but need to act on a Cy^S element in the recipient rat. The coexistence of Cy^R and Cy^S Ts in LTS rats might indicate a mutual requirement for both cells to maintain effective long-term unresponsiveness.

The Cy^R $OX8^+$ Ts is thought to be antiidiotypic because it is inactivated by donor alloantibody and complement. In the strain combination used here, LEW-to-DA, the idiotype-positive receptors are DA anti-LEW and the antiidiotypic receptors DA anti-(DA anti-LEW). In our experiments, anti-id^+ cells are inactivated by cytotoxic DA anti-LEW antibody but not by DA anti-WAG antibody or by DA anti-LEW antibody absorbed with LEW spleen cells. By this criterion the antiidiotypic receptor has the internal image of antigen.

If the Cy^R $OX8^+$ Ts is really antiidiotypic one might expect allotype restriction of its interactions (see above). We tested for restriction for minor antigens by transferring DA ($RT1^a$) Cy^R $OX8^+$ Ts across a minor histocompatibility barrier into PVG·$RT1^a$ recipients and, likewise, PVG·$RT1^a$ Cy^R $OX8^+$ Ts into DA rats. By contrast to their effectiveness in syngeneic recipients, Cy^R $OX8^+$ Ts adoptively transferred across minor barriers were not effective. This result was probably not due to rejection because Cy^S $OX8^+$ Ts could be shown to suppress across these minor barriers. Assuming the restriction is due to allotype genes, these observations are compatible with the notion of antiidiotypic specificity of at least a subpopulation of $OX8^+$ Ts. Recent in vitro studies (*103*) in which spleen cells from LTS rats were shown to respond specifically to antidonor blasts are further evidence of an antiidiotypic cell population in specifically unresponsive rats.

Mechanisms of Suppression Mediated by T Cells

How do the "suppressor T cells" identified in our experiments really regulate the immune response to an allograft? The first cell, which has the $CD4^+$ ($W3/25^+$) "T helper" phenotype, could help or accelerate the production of enhancing antibodies by B cells in the adoptive recipient. A preliminary experiment suggests that the titer of cytotoxic antibody in such recipients is not increased. However the change may be more subtle (e.g., an increase in a noncytotoxic antibody subclass) than can be detected in our assay. The observation that the sonicate of $CD4^+$ ($W3/25^+$) T cells still "suppresses" in our assay does not answer the question, since this material could contain specific helper factors (the factors would have to be specific rather than nonspecific—e.g. IL-2—to account for the specificity of suppression). Arguing against the hypothesis of help is the observation that the sonicate induces in normal syngeneic rats suppressive activity in the $CD8^+$ ($OX8^+$) T cell fraction of their spleens. Hence, assuming the $CD4^+$ ($W3/25^+$) T cells in the spleen elaborated the factor in the sonicate, it would appear that the $CD4^+$ T cell is a T suppressor inducer cell. However, further cell fractionation studies are required to substantiate this interpretation.

Do $CD8^+$ ($OX8^+$) suppressor T cells act by a cytotoxic mechanism? This is another question which is difficult to answer directly. Cytotoxic T cells in the rat are $OX8^+$ and there are no rat markers equivalent to the mouse MHC I-J antigens, supposedly present on all suppressor cells, that could be used to distinguish cytotoxic and suppressor functions.

A cytotoxic antiidiotypic cell could conceivably kill all alloreactive cells expressing the appropriate receptor. This elimination would be exquisitely spcific. There are some reasons for suggesting that this does not occur. In the first place, an idiotype-anti-idiotype interaction between two killer cells could lead to their mutual destruction, but this phenomenon is not seen with alloreactive killer T cells (*104*) or in an allorestricted killer cell system (*105*). Second, we have tested $OX8^+$ Ts for cytotoxic activity on ^{51}Cr-labeled MLR-activated T cell blasts, with negative results in all assays. The difficulty here is establishing a proper positive control (especially because, as suggested above, the phenomenon might not exist anyway). The third reason is that, in our experiments, Cy^R antiidiotypic $OX8^+$ T cells do not suppress in a Cy-treated recipient, a result that cannot be explained by a cytotoxic mechanism of action of antiidiotypic Ts on alloreactive cells.

The idiotype-positive $OX8^+$ T cell could operate by killing certain stimulator cells, such as dendritic cells, in the graft. The early infiltrate into kidneys transplanted to blood-transfused recipients is consistent with such a hypothesis, even when the donors of the blood transfusion and the kidney need share only some antigens (*106*). Again, there are some reasons for discarding this hypothesis. Although cell populations from long-surviving allografted rats containing suppressor cells can respond to donor antigens in MLR (*107*) and graft-versus-host (*108, 109*) assays, they are not cytotoxic to donor antigens when freshly isolated from the LTS rats after culture with donor-strain stimulator cells. Here, a positive control is no problem. Furthermore, the antigen-binding cells from LTS DA rats bearing LEW grafts can protect a third-party graft when restimulated with LEW antigens. Unless there is massive bystander killing, a cytotoxic mechanism of suppression is not a plausible explanation.

Suppression, if it is not due to help or cytotoxicity, must be a distinct function. How this is achieved, by the interaction of T cells and ultimately the arming of cells for nonspecific suppression, is discussed in the next section. Whether the function of suppression is mediated by a distinct subclass of T cells will be discussed later.

Idiotype-Antiidiotype Networks and Pathways in Suppressor T Cell Function

The network concept has long been accepted and substantiated for antibody-producing cells. It is not unreasonable to assume that T cells can interact in the same way.

It has been proposed that Ts in the mouse DTH model interact in pathways (*101, 110, 111*). Accordingly, an antigen-reactive cell with T helper (CD4, Lyt-1) phenotype acts as a Ts inducer (or Ts1) cell and produces a factor (TsF1) that activates antiidiotypic Ts2 cells carrying CD8 (Lyt-2) antigens. The factor, TsF2, from this second cell induces a third cell, Ts3, which is again antigen binding. The TsF3 from this last cell apparently specifically arms macrophages for nonspecific suppression. Hence, it is thought that there is an idiotype–anti-idiotype–idiotype network (alternatively referred to as an inducer-transducer-effector pathway) that is an amplifier system for antigen-driven suppression leading to nonspecific unresponsiveness.

The results obtained in our rat experiments are largely compatible with the mouse work. The T cell from the spleens of untreated rats 5 days after a renal transplant have the Cy^S Ig^- $W3/25^+$ $OX8^-$ id^+ properties that make it analogous to the mouse Ts1 (Ts inducer) cell. Both our rat Ts1 cells and those in the mouse DTH system produce an antigen-specific factor that is absorbed by syngeneic spleen cells and induces a further set of $CD8^+$ ($OX8^+$, $Lyt\text{-}2^+$) suppressor cells in a manner restricted by minor but not MHC antigens. In the mouse, minor restriction is due to IgH allotype genes, reflecting a direct interaction between two receptor molecules—for instance, in idiotype-anti-idiotype recognition.

The $OX8^+$ suppressor cells we have characterized so far are not those induced by "rat TsF1." They were obtained from LTS rats. The two populations found, Cy^R Ig^- $W3/25^-$ $OX8^+$ anti-id^+ and Cy^S Ig^- $W3/25^-$ $OX8^+$ id^+, correspond directly to the mouse Ts2 (transducer) and Ts3 (effector) cells. The action of both mouse Ts2 and rat Cy^R anti-id^+ cells is restricted by minor alloantigens (we have not tested for MHC restriction in the rat). There is one difference between mouse DTH Ts3 cells and our rat Cy^S id^+ alloreactive T cells in that the rat cells are not minor-restricted at this stage. However, an unrestriction action of TsF3 in B cell suppression has been reported (*101*).

The pathway or cascade concept is attractively simple and can account for both specific and nonspecific effects and for the potency of minimal numbers of transferred cells. The proposed sequential and time-dependent activation of afferent Ts1 (inducer), efferent Ts2 (transducer), and Ts3 (effector) cells or their rat analogues could explain many of our observations. However, one difficulty remains: MHC restriction phenomena. How can a $CD4^+$ (class-II-restricted) idiotypic Ts1 (inducer) cell activate a $CD8^+$ (class-I-restricted) antiidiotypic Ts2 (transducer) cell, which then turns around and switches on a $CD8^+$ Ts3 (effector) cell? By definition, the antiidiotypic receptor of the Ts transducer cell interacts with both the class-II-restricted receptor on the Ts inducer cell and the class-I-restricted receptor on the Ts effector cell. How? Either the receptors of Ts cells (or perhaps of anti-idiotypic Ts) are not MHC restricted—a possibility that is difficult to countenance—or only the idiotype and not the MHC restricting element of the T cell receptor is seen as "antigen" by the antiidiotypic cell. In this way, a $CD8^+$ Ts2 cell would see idiotype in association with class I MHC molecules on the surface of the Ts1 cell, while a $CD4^+$ Ts2 cell would recognize the idiotype with class II MHC antigens. If this is so, the CD phenotype of the Ts inducer cell is immaterial, and one could envisage activation of suppressor cell pathways by class-II-restricted receptors on $CD4^+$ (T helper/inducer) cells or by class-I-restricted receptors on $CD8^+$ (T cytotoxic/suppressor) cells.

Do T suppressor cells exist as a distinct T cell subclass?

The number of different antigen-specific T cells reported in the literature is large: there are helpers for B cells, helpers for cytotoxic cells, mediators of DTH, cytotoxic effectors, T contrasuppressor inducers, T contrasuppressor transducers, T contrasuppressors, various Ts and so on. The list continues to grow—T cell proliferation, indeed. Are there truly so many distinct cells each with an individual function? My current view is that there are only two mature T cell subsets, one being $CD4^+$ (OKT4, T3T4, W3/25), the other $CD8^+$ (OKT8, Ly-2, OX8), and that their phenotype is a reflection of their restriction specificity ($CD4^+$ cells restricted by class II MHC); their function (along with secondary markers) is dictated by their activation environment. The reasoning behind this is deductive, and there is not room for a discussion here. Suffice it to say we can allow for $CD4^+$ or $CD8^+$ T cells with positive (helper or effector) or negative (suppressor or regulator) functions. Whether a cell can have more than one function at the same time, sequentially or at all, is not clear. Cloned cells in vitro can produce lymphokines and can help or suppress, depending on the assay system (*112, 113*). The relevance of these observations on cloned lines to the in vivo situation is not known.

Specificity of Ts-Mediated Suppression

In our rat renal allograft model, transfusion of DA rats with LEW blood one week before transplantation specifically induces acceptance of LEW kidneys, but not grafts from unrelated WAG, BN, or PVG/c rats. However, $(LEW\times BN)F_1$ kidneys are accepted despite the fact that the recipients have not been preexposed to BN antigens (*106*). We (*6, 106*) and others (*95, 114*) can show that sharing of only some MHC antigens (either class I or class II) can elicit a "transfusion" effect. Further analysis in our system shows that sharing of only minor antigens by the donors of the blood transfusion and the kidney allograft is sufficient to induce acceptance of grafts expressing disparate MHC antigens (*106*). The explanation we favor is that Ts specific for minor alloantigens on allogeneic cells can regulate the response to MHC antigens on the same cell surface. This interpretation is supported by the finding that DA rats treated with TNP-haptenated LEW antigen and given $CD8^+$ ($OX8^+$) TNP-specific Ts accept LEW but not third-party kidney grafts (*45, 102*). In simple terms, the TNP-LEW antigen forms a "bridge" between TNP-specific Ts and LEW-specific donor-reactive cells. What actually happens is rather more complicated: TNP-specific Ts elaborate a soluble "factor" that is active in vivo in place of the Ts cells (Hutchinson IV, unpublished data). The TNP-specific Ts are Cy^S Ig^- $W3/25^-$ $OX8^+$, and are thus similar to the Ts3-like effector cells described above, except that they do not suppress nonspecifically when restimulated with TNP (*45*). Furthermore, TNP-specific rat-rat suppressor T cell hybridomas created by fusion of TNP-tolerant spleen cells with a lymphoma line are all $CD4^+$ ($W3/25^+$) and express only low levels of the CD8 (OX8) antigen (Curling EMA, Hutchinson IV, Griffiths AJ, Morris PJ, manuscript in preparation). These hybridomas therefore have the antigens associated with Ts1 (inducer) cells rather than Ts3 (effector) cells. In the TNP system, then, there is probably more than one active cell, and the further possibility exists that Ts3-like cells can suppress specifically or nonspecifically, depending on the assay conditions.

The nonspecific action of Ts3-like effector cells can be restimulated by MHC or minor alloantigens in our adoptive transfer assay (Hutchinson IV, unpublished data). This may account for a peroperative transfusion effect we have recently discovered. DA rats given a transfusion from a LEW rat 7 days before transplantation will accept a LEW, but not a third-party, WAG kidney allograft. However, if the DA rat pretreated with LEW blood is peroperatively retransfused with LEW blood, a third-party WAG transplant is accepted. The restimulation is specific so that only peroperative LEW blood and not PVG/c or BN blood will do. By using different strain combinations we can show that major or minor histocompatibility antigens can restimulate nonspecific suppression. Thus, it appears that a second exposure to an antigen (and in our most recent experiments we have used sheep erythrocytes as the antigen) at the time of operation will lead to graft acceptance (Hutchinson IV, Wood KJ, Morris PJ, manuscript in preparation). In the case of donor-specific transfusion the second antigenic stimulus is the graft itself.

Genetic Requirements for Activation of Suppression

Many studies have suggested that class II differences are important in establishing unresponsiveness in neonatally-induced tolerance (*63–65*) or active enhancement/blood transfusion (*81, 95, 106, 114, 115*) models, although there are exceptions (*6*). We have only limited data on this point. To establish unresponsiveness to minor alloantigens in the blood transfusion experiments described above there must be an MHC difference between the blood donor and recipient (*106*). For instance, transfusion of a DA ($RT1^a$) rat with PVG·$RT1^l$ blood ($RT1^l$ MHC antigens on a PVG background) will induce acceptance of a PVG·$RT1^c$ kidney graft. By contrast, pretreatment with PVG·$RT1^a$ blood does not lead to enhancement of PVG·$RT1^c$ allograft survival in DA ($RT1^a$) rats, in which the blood donor and the recipient strains share the same MHC (*106*). A mixture of LEW ($RT1^l$) and PVG·$RT1^a$ blood induces acceptance of PVG·$RT1^c$ grafts (while LEW blood alone does not)—showing, in this case, that the MHC and minor alloantigens do not have to be physically linked to elicit induction of suppression. A similar mixing procedure is required for the first immunization in the induction of the peroperative transfusion effect elicited by SRBC—i.e., LEW blood + SRBC on day −7 and SRBC on day 0 will cause acceptance of a WAG allograft. The same is true for the peroperative transfusion effect mediated by minor alloantigens (Hutchinson IV, Wood KJ, Morris PJ, manuscript in preparation).

Our experiments confirm the importance of MHC antigens in inducing the unresponsive state—and, where we have looked, class II MHC antigens can act in this situation. Class I antigens may be able to provide an appropriate allogeneic stimulis, since erythrocytes can cause active enhancement (*6*). We interpret these results in terms of a requirement for a "second signal," in addition to antigen, for Ts activation, although further studies are required to confirm this. Once established, suppression is independent of MHC antigens, at least in our acute experiments.

Are Ts Responsible for Allograft Survival?

Several mechanisms of specific unresponsiveness can operate in animals bearing long-term accepted allografts. We have recently demonstrated four levels of unresponsiveness in DA animals that have accepted LEW kidney transplants.[2] The graft is less immunogeneic, having lost its complement of passenger leukocytes (*12, 13*).[2] There are suppressor T cells in the central lymphoid tissue (at least in the spleen) that can regulate antidonor MLR in vitro and graft rejection in adoptive recipients (*101*). Any lymphocytes that do respond are likely to be removed from the circulation and not home to the allograft (*14, 15*).[2] Finally, any activated cell that does reach the transplant meets a population of efferent suppressor cells present in the graft organ.[2] Simple experiments like adoptive transfer of activated antidonor cells or treatment with cyclophosphamide do not abrogate unresponsiveness,[2] although combined manipulations may lead to rejection in some strain combinations. On this basis it is difficult to ascribe a necessary role to the Ts cells. Streilein has argued forcefully for a critical role for Ts in neonatally tolerized adult mice (*68*), and supports his conclusions with the demonstration that anti-IJ antibody can abrogate the unresponsive state. The ubiquitous presence of Ts in the maintenance phase of rat renal allograft survival, regardless of the method of induction, strongly suggests that they are there for a reason. However, they may be just one mechanism of unresponsiveness, the importance of which may vary with the tissue transplanted and the histocompatibility barrier.

Conclusions

Experiments in the rat have shown that there are several cells with suppressor function. They can be of the CD4 (OKT4, L3T4, W3/25) phenotype or of the CD8 (OKT8, Lyt-2, OX8) phenotype, and these markers probably reflect their MHC restriction specificity rather than their function. There is, at present, no good reason to suppose that T cell cells with suppressor function constitute a distinct subset with receptors that are not MHC-restricted. As a consequence, simple analysis of the phenotype of cellular infiltrates into grafts or of CD4:CD8 ratios is unlikely to be informative. However, secondary markers (such as I-J antigens in the mouse) may indicate functional activity.

Suppressor T cells are difficult to assay in vitro or in vivo. Although helper or cytotoxic cells could, under certain circumstances, cause artifactual suppression, this is apparently not how they operate in the experiments described here. Rather, Ts seem to operate in pathways or networks involving idiotype-anti-idiotype interactions. There is a striking similarity between the cells identified in our experiments and those described in the mouse DTH pathway. These pathways can culminate in nonspecific suppression such that, depending on the level at which the analysis is made, suppression may or may not appear to be specific. Thus, specificity, like beauty, is in the eye of the beholder.

The action of suppressor cells can explain various aspects of the blood transfusion effect and of long-term allograft acceptance, but it is not possible to attribute an absolute or exclusive role in specific unresponsiveness. Indeed, this is quite unlikely. However, it is clear that Ts could play a critical role in graft survival. The better understanding of the identity, activation, interactions and mode of action of Ts and their factors that is emerging from experimental studies may point the way to the clinical application of this knowledge.

[2] Hutchinson IV, Barber WH, Morris PJ. Mechanisms maintaining long-term survival of rat kidney allografts (manuscript submitted for publication).

LITERATURE CITED

1. Stuart FP, Saitoh T, Fitch FW. Rejection of renal allografts: specific immunologic suppression. Science 1968; 160: 1463.
2. French ME, Batchelor JR. Enhancement of renal allografts in rats and man. Transplant Rev 1972; 13: 115.
3. Morris PJ. Suppression of rejection of organ allografts by alloantibody. Immunol Rev 1980; 49: 93.
4. Stuart FP, McKearn TJ, Weiss A, Fitch FW. Suppression of rat renal allograft rejection by antigen and antibody. Immunol Rev 1980; 49: 127.

5. Enomoto K, Lucas ZJ. Immunological enhancement of renal allografts in the rat. Transplantation 1973; 15: 8.
6. Wood KJ, Evins J, Morris PJ. Suppression of renal allograft rejection in the rat by class I antigens on purified erythrocytes. Transplantation 1985; 39: 56.
7. Homan WP, Fabre JW, Williams KA. Studies on the immunosuppressive properties of cyclosporin A in rats receiving renal allografts. Transplantation 1980; 29: 361.
8. White DJG, Rolles K, Ottawa T, Turell O. Cyclosporin A-induced long-term survival of fully incompatible skin and heart grafts. Transplant Proc 1980; 12: 261.
9. Al Mahdi N, Hutchinson IV, Brent L. Specific unresponsiveness to fully allogeneic kidney allografts in rats induced by procarbazine hydrochloride and antilymphocyte serum. Transplantation 1983; 36: 480.
10. Homan WP, Fabre JW, Morris PJ. Nature of the unresponsiveness induced by cyclosporin A in rats bearing renal allografts. Transplantation 1979; 28: 439.
11. Winearls CG, Fabre JW, Millard PR, Morris PJ. Use of cyclophosphamide and enhancing serum to suppress renal allograft rejection in the rat. Transplantation 1979; 28: 271.
12. Hart DNJ, Winearls CG, Fabre JW. Graft adaptation: studies on possible mechanisms in long-surviving rat renal allografts. Transplantation 1980; 30: 73.
13. Lechler RI, Batchelor JR. Mechanisms of reduced immunogenicity of retransplanted rat kidney allografts. Transplant Proc 1983; 15: 316.
14. Hutchinson IV, Zola H. Antigen-reactive cell opsonization (ARCO): a mechanism of immunological enhancement. Transplantation 1977; 23: 464.
15. Hutchinson IV. Antigen-reactive cell opsonization (ARCO) and its role in antibody-mediated immune suppression. Immunol Rev 1980; 49: 167.
16. Billingham RE, Brent L, Medawar PB. Quantitative studies on tissue transplantation: III Actively acquired tolerance. Phil Trans R Soc Lond (Biol) 1956; 239: 357.
17. Stuart FP, Fitch FW, Rowley DA, Biesecker JL, Hellstrom KE, Hellstrom I. Presence of cell-mediated immunity and serum blocking factors in rat renal allografts enhanced by passive immunization. Transplantation 1971; 12: 331.
18. Strom TB, Carpenter CB, Garavoy M, Abbas AK, Corson JM, Soullilou JP. Modification of the rat alloimmune response by enhancing antibodies and the role of blocking antibodies in the survival of renal grafts. Transplantation 1975; 20: 368.
19. Stuart FP, Scollard DM, McKearn TJ, Fitch FW. Cellular and humoral immunity after allogeneic transplantation in the rat: V. Appearance of anti-idiotypic antibody and its relationship to cellular immunity after treatment with donor spleen cells and alloantibody. Transplantation 1976; 22: 455.
20. Bach BA, Sherman L, Benacerraf B, Green MI. Mechanisms of regulation of cell-mediated immunity. J Immunology 1979; 122: 1899.
21. Finberg R, Burakoff SJ, Benacerraf B, Green MI. The cytolytic T lymphocyte response to trinitrophenyl-modified syngeneic cells: II. Evidence for antigen-specific suppressor T cells. J Immunol 1979; 123: 1210.
22. Braley-Mullen H. Direct demonstration of specific suppressor T cells in mice tolerant to type III pneumococcal polysaccharide. J Immunol 1980; 125: 1849.
23. Tada T, Okumura K. The role of antigen-specific T cell factors in the immune response. Adv Immunol 1980; 28: 1.
24. Ptak W, Zembala M, Asherson GL, Marcinkieicz J. Inhibition of contact sensitivity by macrophages. Int Arch Allergy Appl Immunol 1981; 65: 121.
25. Gershon RK, Kondo K. Cell interactions in the induction of tolerance. Immunology 1970; 18: 723.
26. Asherson GL, Zembala M. Suppression of contact sensitivity by T cells in the mouse: I. Demonstration that suppressor cells act on the effector phase of contact sensitivity. Proc R Soc Lond (Biol). 1974; 187: 329.
27. Weinberger JA, Germain RN, Ju ST, Green MI, Benacerraf B, Dorf ME. Hapten specific T cell responses to 4-hydroxy-3-nitrophenyl acetyl: II. Demonstration of idiotypic determinants on suppressor T cells. J Exp Med 1979; 150: 761.
28. Liew FY. Regulation of delayed-type hypersensitivity: I. T suppressor cells for delayed-type hypersensitivity to sheep erythrocytes in mice. Eur J Immunol 1977; 7: 714.
29. Sercarz EE, Yowell RL, Turkin D, Miller A, Araneo B, Adorini L. Different functional specificity repertoires for suppressor and helper T cells. Immunol Rev 1978; 39: 108.
30. Herzenberg LA, Tokuhisa T. Epitope-specific regulation: I. Carrier-specific induction of suppression for IgG anti-hapten antibody responses. J Exp Med 1982; 155: 1730.
31. Kapp JA, Pierce CW, Schlossman S, Benacerraf B. Genetic control of the immune response *in vitro*: V. Stimulation of suppressor T cells in non-responder mice by the terpolymer L-glutamic acid-L-alanine-L-tyrosine (GAT). J Exp Med 1974; 140: 648.
32. Debre P, Kapp JA, Dorf ME, Benacerraf B. Genetic control of specific immune suppression: II. H-2 linked dominant genetic control of the immune response by the random copolymer L-glutamic acid-L-tyrosine (GT). J Exp Med 1975; 142: 1447.
33. Jirsch DW, Kraft N, Diener E. Tolerance induction to a heterotopic cardiac allograft in the irradiated reconstituted mouse. Transplantation 1974; 18: 155.
34. Hilgert I. The involvement of activated specific suppressor T cells in maintenance of transplantation tolerance. Immunol Rev 1979; 46: 27.
35. Brent L, Hansen JA, Kilshaw PJ, Thomas AV. Specific unresponsiveness to skin allografts in mice: I. Properties of tissue extracts and their synergistic effect with antilymphocyte serum. Transplantation 1973; 15: 160.
36. Pinto M, Brent L, Thomas AV. Specific unresponsiveness to skin grafts in mice: III. Synergistic effects of tissue extracts, *Bordetella pertussis* and antilymphocyte serum. Transplantation 1974; 17: 477.
37. Kilshaw PJ, Brent L, Pinto M. Suppressor T cells in mice made unresponsive to H-2 incompatible skin grafts. Nature 1975; 255: 489.
38. Kilshaw PJ, Brent L. Further studies on suppressor T cells in mice made unresponsive to H-2 incompatible skin grafts. Transplant Proc 1977; 9: 717.
39. Rieger M, Gunther J, Kristofova H, Hilgert I. Evidence of a suppressor cell mechanism of allograft tolerance induced by spleen extract and hydrocortisone. Folia Biol (Praha) 1978; 24: 145.
40. Brent L, Opara SC. Specific unresponsiveness to skin allografts in mice: V. Synergy between donor tissue extract, procarbazine hydrochloride and antilymphocyte serum in creating a long-lasting unresponsiveness mediated by suppressor T cells. Transplantation 1979; 27: 120.
41. Horsburgh T, Wood PJ, Brent L. *In vivo* induction of specific suppressor lymphocytes to histocompatibility antigens. Transplant Proc 1981; 13: 637.
42. Palacious R, Moller G. T cell growth factor abrogates Con-A-induced suppressor cell function. J Exp Med 1981; 153: 1360.
43. Steinmuller D. Suppressor cells and transplantation tolerance. Transplantation 1978; 26: 2.
44. Stuart FP, McKearn TJ, Fitch FW. Immunological enhancement of renal allografts by antireceptor antibody. Surgery 1976; 80: 130.
45. Hutchinson IV, Barber WH, Morris PJ. Specific suppression of allograft rejection by TNP-induced suppressor cells in recipients treated with TNP-haptenated donor alloantigens. J Exp Med 1985; 162: 1409.
46. Batchelor JR, Brent L, Kilshaw PJ. Absence of suppressor cells

from rats bearing passively enhanced kidney allografts. Nature 1977; 270: 552.

47. Dorsch S, Roser R. Recirculating, suppressor T cells in transplantation tolerance. J Exp Med 1977; 145: 1144.
48. Hall BM. The cellular basis of the maintenance of passive enhancement. Transplant Proc 1981; 13: 640.
49. Hall BM, Jelbart ME, Gurley KE, Dorsch SE. Specific unresponsiveness in rats with prolonged cardiac allograft survival after treatment with cyclosporine: mediation of specific suppression by T helper/inducer cells. J Exp Med 1985; 162: 1683.
50. Batchelor JR, Phillips BE, Greenan D. Suppressor cells and their role in the survival of immunologically enhanced rat kidney allografts. Transplantation 1984; 37: 43.
51. Chui YL, Batchelor JR. Mechanisms underlying continued survival of rat kidney allografts after a short period of chemical immunosuppression. Transplantation 1985; 40: 150.
52. Barber WH, Hutchinson IV, Morris PJ. The role of suppressor cells in maintaining passively enhanced rat kidney allografts. Transplantation 1984; 38: 548.
53. Barber WH, Hutchinson IV, Morris PJ. Mechanisms of kidney allograft maintenance in rats treated with cyclosporine. Transplant Proc 1985; 17: 1391.
54. Bradley JA, Mason DW, Morris PJ. Evidence that renal allografts are rejected by cytotoxic T cells and not by non-specific effectors. Transplantation 1985; 39: 169.
55. Brent L, Brooks CG, Medawar PB. Transplantation tolerance. Br Med Bull 1976; 32: 101.
56. Billingham RE, Brent L, Medawar PB. "Actively acquired tolerance" of foreign cells. Nature 1953; 172: 603.
57. Ptak W, Skowron-Cendrzak A. Fetal suppressor cells: their influence on the cell-mediated immune responses. Transplantation 1977; 24: 45.
58. Argyris BF. Nature of the neonatal splenic suppressor cells in the mouse. Cell Immunol 1982; 66: 352.
59. Okada S, Strober S. Spleen cells from adult mice given total lymphoid irradiation or from newborn mice have similar regulatory effects in the mixed lymphocyte reaction: II. Generation of antigen specific suppressor cells in the MLR after the addition of spleen cells from newborn mice. J Immunol 1982; 129: 1892.
60. Argyris BF. Adoptive tolerance: transfer of the tolerant state. J Immunol 1963; 90: 29.
61. Argyris BF. Role of the thymus in adoptive tolerance. J Immunol 1968; 100: 1255.
62. Holan V, Chutna J, Hasek M. Specific suppressor cells in rats with neonatally induced transplantation tolerance. Folia Biol (Praha) 1977; 26: 66.
63. Streilein JW. Neonatal tolerance: towards an immunogenetic definition of self. Immunol Rev 1979; 46: 125.
64. Streilein JW, Gruchalla RS. Analysis of neonatally induced tolerance to transplantation antigens: I. Adoptive transfer indicated that tolerance of class I and class II antigens is maintained by distinct mechanisms. Immunogenetics 1981; 12: 161.
65. Streilein JW, Gruchalla RS, Strome P. Neonatal transplantation tolerance results from two types of suppression acting during induction and at the effector stage. Transplant Proc 1981; 13: 578.
66. Gorczynski RM, MacRae S. Suppression of cytotoxic response to histoincompatible cells: II. Analysis of the role of two independent T suppressor pools in maintenance of neonatally induced allograft tolerance in mice. J Immunol 1979; 122: 747.
67. Wood PJ, Strome P, Streilein JW. Clonal frequency of alloreactive cells in mice tolerant of H-2. Transplant Proc 1985; 17: 1137.
68. Streilein JW. Suppressor cells are necessary for tolerance. Transplant Proc 1985; 17: 1558.
69. Rapaport FT, Bachvaroff RJ, Akiyama N, Sato T, Ferrebee JW. Specific allogeneic unresponsiveness in irradiated dogs reconstituted with autologous bone marrow. Transplantation 1980; 30: 23.
70. Strober S. Natural suppressor (NS) cells, neonatal tolerance and total lymphoid irradiation: exploring obscure relationships. Ann Rev Immunol 1984; 2: 219.
71. Okada S, Strober S. Spleen cells from adult mice given total lymphoid irradiation or from newborn mice have similar regulatory effects in the mixed leukocyte reaction: I. Generation of antigen-specific suppressor cells in the mixed leukocyte reaction after the addition of spleen cells from adult mice given total lymphoid irradiation. J Exp Med 1982; 156: 522.
72. Maki T, Simpson M, Monaco AP. Development of suppressor T cells by antilymphocyte serum treatment in mice. Transplantation 1982; 34: 376.
73. Marquet RL, Heystek GA, Tinbergen WJ. Specific inhibition of organ allograft rejection by donor blood. Transplant Proc 1971; 3: 708.
74. Fabre JW, Morris PJ. The effect of donor strain blood pretreatment on renal allograft rejection in rats. Transplantation 1972; 14: 608.
75. Stuart FP, Weiss A, Fitch FW. Induction and maintenance of immunological enhancement. In: Stuart FP, Fitch FW, eds. Immunological tolerance and enhancement. Lancaster, England: MTP Press 1979: 29.
76. Hutchinson IV, Zola H, Batchelor JR. Immunological enhancement of rat renal allografts using rabbit antisera with specificity for rat transplantation antigens. Transplantation 1976; 22: 273.
77. Morris PJ. Suppression of rejection of organ allografts by alloantibody. Immunol Rev 1980; 49: 93.
78. Chutna J. The mechanism of immunological enhancement of H-2 incompatible skin grafts in mice. Transplantation 1971; 12: 28.
79. Winearls CG, Millard PR, Morris PJ. Effect of azathioprine and prednisolone on passive enhancement of rat renal allografts. Transplantation 1978; 25: 229.
80. Okazaki H, Maki T, Wood ML, Monaco AP. Effect of a single transfusion of donor-specific and non-specific blood on skin allograft survival in mice. Transplantation 1980; 30: 421.
81. Wood ML, Monaco AP. Induction of unresponsiveness to skin allografts in adult mice disparate at defined regions of the H-2 complex: II. Effect of pre-graft donor-specific blood transfusions in ALS-treated mice. Transplantation 1984; 37: 39.
82. Batchelor JR, Fabre JW, Morris PJ. Passive enhancement of kidney allografts: potentiation with antithymocyte serum. Transplantation 1972; 13: 610.
83. Medawar PB. The use of antigenic extracts to weaken the immune reaction against skin homografts in mice. Transplantation 1963; 1: 21.
84. Prop J, Hutchinson IV, Morris PJ. Persistent suppression against bystander haptens and alloantigens. Cell Immunol (in press).
85. Van der Kwast TH, Bianchi ATJ, Bril H, Benner R. Suppression of anti-graft immunity by preimmunization: I. Kinetic aspects and specificity. Transplantation 1981; 31: 79.
86. Perry LL, Williams IR, DiRusso S. Suppressor T cell recognition of major and minor histocompatibility alloantigens: selected suppression of MHC-directed responses by minor alloantigen Ts. J Immunol 1982; 33: 69.
87. Liew FY. Regulation of delayed-type hypersensitivity to histocompatibility antigens. Transplantation 1982; 33: 69.
88. Marquet RL, Heystek GA. Induction of suppressor cells by donor-specific blood transfusions and heart transplantation in the rat. Transplantation 1981; 31: 272.
89. Hendry WS, Tilney NL, Baldwin WM. Transfer of specific unresponsiveness to organ allografts by thymocytes: specific unresponsiveness by thymocyte transfer. J Exp Med 1979; 149: 1042.
90. Polak L, Ruick C. Persistent activity of suppressor cells in T cell-

mediated immune responses. J Immunol 1978; 121: 762.
91. Bril H, De Ruiter H, Hussaarts-Odijk LM, Bianchi ATJ, Benner R. Suppression of antigraft immunity by preimmunization: IV. Persistence of long-lived recirculating suppressor T cells. Transplantation 1985; 40: 417.
92. Okazaki H, Maki T, Wood ML, Monaco AP. Effect of blood transfusion on skin allograft survival in immunosuppressed mice. Transplant Proc 1981; 13: 515.
93. Maki T, Okazaki H, Wood ML, Monaco AP. Suppressor cells in mice bearing intact skin allografts after blood transfusions. Transplantation 1981; 32: 463.
94. Fabre JW, Morris PJ. The mechanism of specific immunosuppression of renal allograft rejection by donor strain blood. Transplantation 1972; 14: 634.
95. Nagata M, Ochiai T, Asano T, et al. Role of I-A positive cells in the beneficial effect of donor blood transfusion and induction of suppressor cells in cardiac allotransplantation in rats. Transplantation 1984; 38: 522.
96. Hutchinson IF, Shadur CA, Duarte JSA, et al. Cyclosporin A spares selectively lymphocytes with donor-specific suppressor characteristics. Transplantation 1981; 32: 210.
97. Kupiec-Wglinski JW, Lear PA, Bordes-Aznar J, Tilney NL, Strom TB. Acute rejection in cyclosporin A-treated graft recipients occurs following abrogation of suppressor cells. Transplant Proc 1983; 15: 531.
98. Mage MG, McHugh LL, Rothstein TL. Mouse lymphocytes with or without surface immunoglobulin: preparative scale separation on polystyrene culture dishes coated with specifically purified anti-immunoglobulin. J Immunol Methods 1977; 15: 47.
99. Mason DW. Subsets of T cells in the rat mediating lethal graft versus host disease. Transplantation 1981; 32: 222.
100. Kedar E, Ortiz de Landazuri M, Bonavida B, Fahey JL. Cellular immunoadsorbents: an improved technique for specific depletion of cytotoxic T lymphoid cells. J Immunol Methods 1974; 5: 97.
101. Dorf ME, Benacerraf B. Suppressor cells and immunoregulation. Annu Rev Immunol 1984; 2: 127.
102. Hutchinson IV, Barber WH, Morris PJ. Specific prolongation of rat renal allograft survival mediated by TNP-hapten induced suppressor T cells and TNP-modified donor alloantigens. Transplant Proc 1985; 17: 1922.
103. Lancaster F, Chui YL, Batchelor JR. Anti-idiotypic T cells suppress rejection of renal allografts in rats. Nature 1985; 315: 336.
104. Kuppers RC, Henney CS. Studies on the mechanism of lymphocyte-mediated cytolysis: X. Relationships between antigen recognition and lytic expression in killer T cells. J Immunol 1977; 118: 71.
105. von Boehmer, Haas W. H-2 restricted cytolytic and noncytolytic T cell clones: isolation, specificity and functional analysis. Immunol Rev 1981; 54: 27.
106. Hutchinson IV, Morris PJ. The role of major and minor histocompatibility antigens in active enhancement of rat kidney allograft survival by blood transfusion. Transplantation 1986; 41: 166.
107. Weiss A, Stuart FP, Fitch FW. Immune reactivity of cells from long-term rat renal allograft survivors. Transplantation 1978; 26: 346.
108. French ME, Batchelor JR, Watts HG. The capacity of lymphocytes from rats bearing enhanced kidneys to mount graft-versus-host reactions. Transplantation 1971; 12: 45.
109. Hutchinson IV, Brent L. Depressed graft-versus-host reactivity of blood leukocytes from rats bearing passively enhanced long-surviving renal allografts. Transplantation 1982; 34: 305.
110. Germain RN, Benacerraf B. A single major pathway of T lymphocyte interactions in antigen-specific immune suppression. Scand J Immunol 1981; 13: 1.
111. Green DR, Flood PM, Gershon RK. Immunoregulatory T cell pathways. Annu Rev Immunol 1983; 1: 439.
112. Dennert G, Weiss S, Warner JF. T cells may express multiple activities: specific allohelp, cytolysis, and delayed-type hypersensitivity are expressed by a cloned T cell line. Proc Natl Acad Sci USA 1981; 78: 4540.
113. Lukacher AE, Morrison LA, Braciale VL, Malissen B, Braciale TJ. Expression of specific cytolytic activity by H-2I region-restricted, influenza virus-specific T lymphocyte clones. J Exp Med 1985; 162: 171.
114. Soullilou JP, Blandin F, Gunter E, Lemoine V. Genetics of the blood transfusion effect on heart allografts in rats. Transplantation 1984; 38: 63.
115. Wood ML, Gootschalk R, Monaco AP. Immune responses in mice transfused with blood from donors differing at defined regions of the H-2 complex. Transplant Proc 1985; 17: 1108.

0041-1337/86/4105-0556$02.00/0
TRANSPLANTATION
Vol. 41, No. 5
Printed in U.S.A.

Transplantation

ARTICLES

LIFELONG REVERSAL OF THE METABOLIC ABNORMALITIES OF ADVANCED DIABETES IN RATS BY WHOLE-PANCREAS TRANSPLANTATION[1]

MARSHALL J. ORLOFF,[2] GLENN E. GREENLEAF, PAUL URBAN, AND BARBARA GIRARD

Department of Surgery, School of Medicine, University of California, San Diego; University of California Medical Center, San Diego, California 92103

Evidence suggests that metabolic abnormalities are responsible for the widespread microvascular complications of insulin-dependent diabetes mellitus (IDDM). Interest in endocrine pancreas replacement therapy, including pancreas transplantation, is based on the hope that such treatment will reverse the complications of IDDM by providing more precise metabolic control than conventional therapy. To determine if whole pancreas transplantation is capable of reversing well-established metabolic abnormalities of diabetes mellitus (DM) and maintaining strict metabolic control for life, we performed monthly metabolic studies for 2 years in 141 nondiabetic control rats, 273 diabetic control rats with alloxan-induced DM, and 267 diabetic rats that received syngeneic whole pancreaticoduodenal transplants 6, 9, 12, 15, 18, and 21 months after induction of DM with alloxan. Whole-pancreas transplantation in rats with long-standing DM permanently reversed the metabolic disorders. Elevated plasma glucose concentrations were permanently reduced to normal, depressed plasma insulin levels were permanently increased to normal, elevations of BUN and serum creatinine were permanently normalized, and there was a striking gain in body weight. Hyperglycemia during glucose tolerance tests was of lesser magnitude and shorter duration than normal, as a result of greater-than-normal plasma insulin levels. The only abnormality that persisted was hyperglucagonemia, but it did not interfere with control of hyperglycemia and is of unknown significance. These results indicate that whole-pancreas transplantation produces the most complete and sustained correction of the metabolic abnormalities of experimental DM of any available therapeutic modality.

It is well established that insulin-dependent diabetes mellitus (IDDM)* results from destruction of the beta cells of the islets of Langerhans in the pancreas of a genetically predisposed subject (*1–7*). Although not yet proved, substantial evidence suggests that the widespread microangiopathic complications in IDDM are due to beta cell insufficiency and the resultant metabolic disorders. Conventional treatment of IDDM with insulin injections and diet has not prevented the development or progression of these secondary complications, presumably because of failure to correct the metabolic abnormalities of the disease (*8–10*). For this reason, there is considerable interest in various forms of endocrine pancreas replacement therapy, based on the premise that such treatment will provide close-to-physiologic beta cell function and precise metabolic control. It is not yet known if endocrine pancreas replacement therapy is capable of preventing, stabilizing, or reversing diabetic microangiopathy.

Research studies have focused on three types of endocrine pancreas replacement therapy: (1) artificial insulin delivery devices; (2) transplantation of isolated islets of Langerhans; and (3) transplantation of all or a segment of the pancreas as a vascularized graft. The first two of these therapeutic modalities—artificial insulin delivery devices and isolated islet transplants—have been unsuccessful in preventing or reversing diabetic nephropathy or retinopathy in the few studies that have been done to date, perhaps because they have not produced precise metabolic control (*11–25*). It has been demonstrated clearly that both insulin pump therapy and isolated islet transplantation, while lowering blood glucose levels and correcting other metabolic and hormonal abnormalities (*19–31*), have failed to normalize the disturbed carbohydrate and lipid metabolism in IDDM (*32–41*). No investigations have been reported of the effect of the third form of endocrine pancreas replacement therapy—whole-pancreas transplantation—on established complications of IDDM.

Studies that we have reported previously have shown that whole-pancreas transplants performed shortly after diabetes mellitus (DM) is induced with alloxan in rats produce prolonged normalization of the metabolic abnormalities of diabetes (*42*). However, potential clinical use of pancreas transplantation is unlikely to occur immediately after onset of DM, but will be used in patients with long-established DM and serious complications. Therefore, the present investigation was undertaken to determine if whole-pancreas transplantation is capable of reversing well-established metabolic abnormalities of DM and providing strict metabolic control for life. To this end, we performed serial metabolic studies for 2 years in highly inbred

[1] This work was supported by NIH Grant AM30825 and by a grant from the Weingart Foundation.

[2] Address reprint requests to: Marshall J. Orloff, M.D., Department of Surgery, H-899, UCSD Medical Center, 225 Dickinson Street, San Diego CA 92103.

* Abbreviations used: BUN, blood urea nitrogen; DM, diabetes mellitus; IDDM, insulin-dependent diabetes mellitus.

rats that received whole pancreas transplants 6, 9, 12, 15, 18, and 21 months after induction of DM with alloxan.

MATERIALS AND METHODS

Experimental groups. The animals used in this study were 6-month-old, highly inbred Lewis strain rats (Simonsen Laboratories, Gilroy, CA), which uniformly accept tissue transplants from each other without rejection. The rats were housed 2–5 to a cage and fed standard rat chow and water ad libitum during the entire study. The animals were distributed among 3 groups as follows:

Group NC (nondiabetic controls) contained 141 unaltered rats.

Group DC (diabetic controls) contained 273 untreated diabetic rats in which DM was induced by i.v. injection of alloxan monohydrate (Sigma Chemical Co., St. Louis, MO) in a dose of 42–44 mg/kg. Only rats with plasma glucose levels that were at least above 200 mg/dl on both the third and seventh days after alloxan injection were accepted into the study. Many rats had plasma glucose levels above 300 mg/dl. Approximately 10% of the rats had a decrease in severity of hyperglycemia with time, but no rats in this group were eliminated from the study after DM was established in the first week.

Group DT (diabetic transplant) contained 267 diabetic rats that received syngeneic whole pancreaticoduodenal transplants from age-matched donor rats 6, 9, 12, 15, 18, and 21 months after DM was induced by the same method used in group DC; 94% of the rats had plasma glucose concentrations above 300 mg/dl at the start. All rats accepted for transplantation had continuous DM documented by serial plasma glucose measurements above 300 mg/dl. Eighty-eight animals underwent successful whole-pancreas transplantation after 6 months, 62 after 9 months, 65 after 12 months, 39 after 15 months, 6 after 18 months, and 7 after 21 months of continuous DM.

In the control groups, 2 rats were sacrificed every month, and in the transplant subgroups, 2–4 rats were sacrificed every month following transplantation for 24 months after the onset of DM in order to perform quantitative morphologic studies that are the subject of a separate report.

Technique of whole pancreas transplantation. The microvascular surgical technique of heterotopic pancreaticoduodenal transplantation in the rat originated in our laboratory in 1971 (*43, 44*). The pancreaticoduodenal graft was harvested from an age-matched donor rat with a segment of aorta containing the celiac and superior mesenteric arteries supplying the graft, and with a segment of portal vein containing the venous drainage from the graft. The pancreaticoduodenal graft was transplanted into the recipient rat by performing end-to-side vascular anastomoses with continuous 9–0 nylon sutures between the graft aortic segment and the host aorta, and between the graft portal vein and the host inferior vena cava. The proximal end of the graft duodenum was closed and the distal end was anastomosed end-to-side to the third portion of the host duodenum using a continuous 7–0 silk suture. The graft ischemia time was 25±5 minutes.

Metabolic studies. Monthly measurements were made of body weight and concentrations of glucose, insulin, glucagon, creatinine, and urea nitrogen in the blood. All blood studies were performed on specimens of blood obtained from the tail vein of the rat between 9:00 A.M. and 10:00 A.M. Plasma glucose was measured by a modification of the O-toluidine method, which involves the spectrophotometric detection of N-glucosylamine formed from the reaction of glucose with O-toluidine in glacial acetic acid in the presence of heat. Plasma insulin was measured by a double antibody radioimmunoassay, according to the principle of Yalow and Berson (*45*). Plasma glucagon was measured by the radioimmunoassay of Faloona and Unger using an antiserum that was highly specific for pancreatic glucagon (*46*). Blood urea nitrogen (BUN) was measured by urease and the Berthelot reaction, and serum creatinine was determined with Lloyd's reagent. Glucose tolerance tests were performed monthly and consisted of measurements of plasma glucose and insulin concentrations before and 40, 70, and 130 minutes after intraperitoneal injection of a 30% glucose solution in an amount required to provide a glucose load of 3 g/kg.

Since the normal life span of the Lewis rat in our laboratory usually ranges from 24 to 30 months, and the metabolic studies spanned the period from age 6 months to age 30 months, metabolic data were obtained over almost the entire life span of the animals.

Statistical analysis. A two-tailed Student's *t* test was used to examine differences between mean values.

RESULTS

Body weight. Table 1 and Figure 1 show the effect of pancreas transplantation on body weight in diabetic rats. Nondiabetic control rats (group NC) reached their peak weight 15 months after entry into the study, by which time they had sustained a 65% weight gain. Diabetic control rats (group DC) failed to gain weight; after 24 months of DM they weighed essentially

TABLE 1. Effect of pancreas transplantation on body weight in rats with DM

GROUP	Weight (g) on day of entry into study		Weight (g) immediately pretransplant		Peak weight (g)			Weight (g) after 24 months	
	Mean ± SEM	n	Mean ± SEM	n	Mean ± SEM	n	Mo.	Mean ± SEM	n
Nondiabetic control (NC)	337±2.7	141	—		556±2.5	77	15	517±3.0	47
Diabetic control (DC)	327±2.6	273	—		341±4.8	20	21	330±5.4	10
Diabetic transplant (DT):									
6-Month transplant	338±2.6	88	354±5.6	88	510±5.4	9	21	472±6.9	4
9-Month transplant	329±2.7	61	345±7.6	62	486±13.0	2	24	486±13.0	2
12-Month transplant	336±3.0	64	336±5.9	63	468±13.8	19	21	436±26.9	8
15-Month transplant	343±4.9	39	339±7.8	33	446±13.3	23	21	385±22.4	9
18-Month transplant	331±11.6	6	327±22.3	6	437±12.3	9	21	424±36.2	5
21-Month transplant	322±6.9	7	341±23.5	4	396±24.0	3	24	396±24.0	3

the same as on the day of entry into the study (330 g vs. 327 g). Similarly, diabetic rats in group DT failed to gain weight prior to pancreas transplantation. However, there was a striking gain in body weight following pancreas transplantation, even when it was performed 15, 18, or 21 months after induction of DM. Rats that received pancreas transplants after 6 months of DM had a 51% peak weight gain, after 9 months had a 48% peak weight gain, after 12 months had a 39% peak weight gain, after 15 months had a 30% peak weight gain, after 18 months had a 32% peak weight gain, and after 21 months had a 23% peak weight gain.

Blood glucose. Table 2 shows the mean results of serial plasma glucose determinations in the 3 groups of rats, and Figure 2 shows the mean plasma glucose levels in group DT before and after pancreas transplantation. Blood samples were obtained between 9:00 A.M. and 10:00 A.M. The rats were not fasted. Diabetic control rats had marked hyperglycemia throughout life, with plasma glucose levels that were 3–4 times those observed in the nondiabetic controls. Similarly, until the time of pancreas transplantation, the rats in group DT had plasma glucose concentrations that were more than 3 times those found in the nondiabetic controls. Following pancreas transplantation performed at any time from 6 to 21 months after induction of DM, plasma glucose levels were reduced to normal and maintained below 100 mg/dl. Plasma glucose levels in group DT were not significantly different from those in group NC at any time after transplantation.

Plasma insulin. Table 3 shows the mean plasma insulin concentrations in the 3 groups of rats, and Figure 3 shows the mean insulin levels before and after pancreas transplantation in group DT. Diabetic controls had markedly depressed plasma insulin concentrations that ranged from 18% to 24% of the

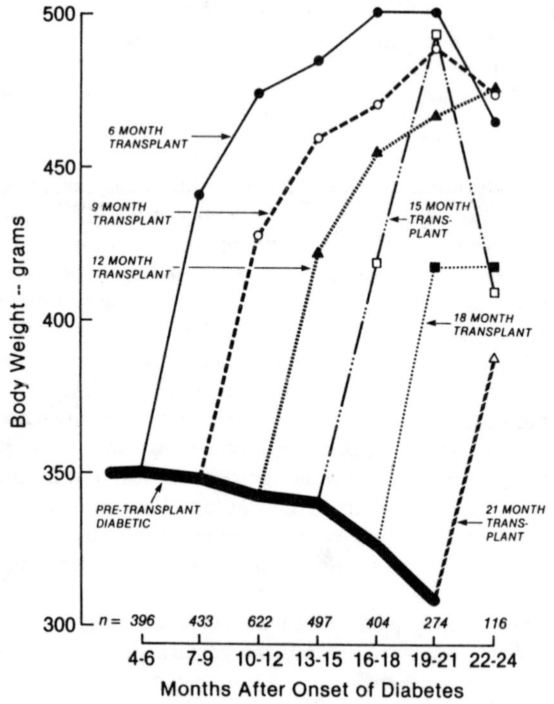

FIGURE 1. Changes in mean body weight following whole-pancreas transplantation performed 6–21 months after induction of DM.

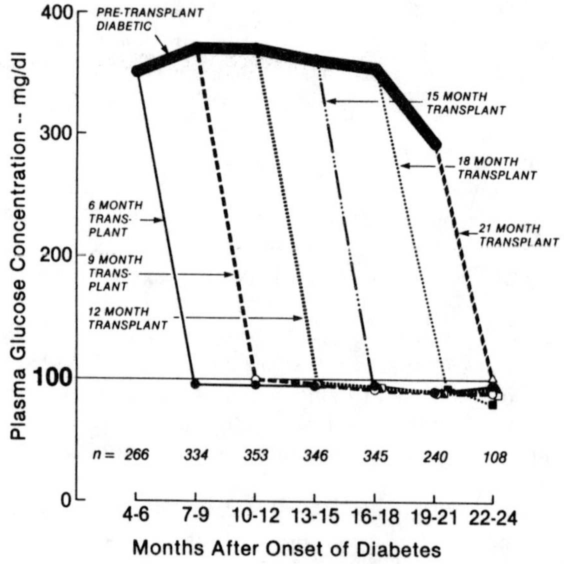

FIGURE 2. Changes in mean plasma glucose concentration following whole-pancreas transplantation performed 6–21 months after induction of DM.

TABLE 2. Plasma glucose concentrations (mg/dl) in nondiabetic controls, diabetic controls, and diabetic transplanted rats before and after pancreas transplantation (mean ± SEM)

GROUP	Months after entry into study															
	1–3		4–6		7–9		10–12		13–15		16–18		19–21		22–24	
	n	X̄ ± SEM	n	X̄ ± SEM	n	X̄ ± SEM	n	X̄ ± SEM	n	X̄ ± SEM	n	X̄ ± SEM	n	X̄ ± SEM	n	X̄ ± SEM
Nondiabetic control	116	87±1.6	105	119±2.2	98	87±1.1	113	82±0.7	106	85±1.3	91	83±1.1	76	85±1.2	42	98±1.6
Diabetic control	272	288±6.0[b]	245	305±5.9[b]	198	297±4.6[b]	156	303±5.1[b]	134	296±5.3[b]	84	270±8.6[b]	43	299±14.9[b]	28	264±6.3[b]
Diabetic transplant:[a]																
6-Month transplant	87	328±5.8[b]	88	338±4.9[b]	158	*95±0.6*	102	*95±0.7*	65	*93±1.0*	34	*94±1.3*	22	*89±1.3*	10	*95±1.9*
9-Month transplant	62	334±5.6[b]	61	343±5.5[b]	61	375±7.7[b]	136	*99±2.2*	79	*94±0.9*	61	*91±0.7*	36	*89±1.0*	10	*88±2.9*
12-Month transplant	65	349±6.7[b]	65	354±5.4[b]	64	371±5.8[b]	63	370±8.2[b]	156	*96±0.8*	110	*92±1.2*	68	*90±0.9*	27	*93±1.2*
15-Month transplant	39	352±8.3[b]	39	362±8.7[b]	38	355±7.7[b]	39	365±5.7[b]	33	359±13.2[b]	129	*93±0.8*	79	*89±2.8*	37	*87±1.5*
18-Month transplant	6	321±10.3[b]	6	337±14.9[b]	6	361±11.0[b]	6	374±17.2[b]	6	374±25.9[b]	6	353±16.9[b]	31	*92±2.3*	15	*80±3.1*
21-Month transplant	7	320±16.1[b]	7	372±19.9[b]	7	373±8.9[b]	7	380±15.2[b]	7	358±12.7[b]	5	353±17.6[b]	4	292±26.0[b]	9	*102±17.2*

[a] Plasma glucose levels obtained after pancreas transplantation are in italics.
[b] $P<0.001$ compared with nondiabetic controls.

TABLE 3. Plasma insulin concentrations (pg/ml) in nondiabetic controls, diabetic controls, and diabetic transplanted rats before and after pancreas transplantation (mean ± SEM)

GROUP	Months after entry into study: 1–3		4–6		7–9		10–12		13–15		16–18		19–21		22–24	
	n	$\bar{X}$ ± SEM	n	$\bar{X}$ ± SEM	n	$\bar{X}$ ± SEM	n	$\bar{X}$ ± SEM	n	$\bar{X}$ ± SEM	n	$\bar{X}$ ± SEM	n	$\bar{X}$ ± SEM	n	$\bar{X}$ ± SEM
Nondiabetic control	337	523±1.4	196	540±1.1	258	492±1.0	208	479±1.1	74	440±1.2	116	417±1.1	113	394±0.9	68	389±1.6
Diabetic control	448	94±1.4[b]	277	100±1.2[b]	259	104±1.2[b]	241	86±1.3[b]	228	106±0.6[b]	130	102±1.1[b]	56	83±1.4[b]	12	110±2.3[b]
Diabetic transplant:[a]																
6-Month transplant	88	134±1.2[b]	88	112±0.90[b]	157	*566±1.2*	101	*588±3.9*	64	*508±1.4*	24	*564±3.3*	7	*464±4.9*		—
9-Month transplant	62	145±1.7[b]	62	103±0.9[b]	62	152±5.3[b]	129	*973±0.5*[b]	67	*477±1.4*	44	*467±2.1*	7	*510±6.7*		—
12-Month transplant	65	115±1.4[b]	64	115±0.9[b]	61	80±0.6[b]	62	101±1.2[b]	148	*474±1.2*	87	*487±1.3*	24	*560±6.2*[b]		—
15-Month transplant	39	125±1.2[b]	39	95±1.0[b]	36	77±0.7[b]	38	93±0.9[b]	31	142±1.7[b]	104	*419±1.0*	21	*413±2.7*		—
18-Month transplant	6	130±2.8[b]	6	66±1.8[b]	5	70±1.9[b]	6	89±2.4[b]	6	91±1.7[b]	4	185±5.9[b]	10	*385±2.3*		—
21-Month transplant	7	103±2.8[b]	7	78±2.4[b]	7	70±1.3[b]	7	88±3.5[b]	5	50±0.6[b]	5	212±2.9[b]	3	193±4.9[b]	6	*400±2.4*

[a] Plasma insulin levels obtained after transplantation are in italics.
[b] $P<0.001$ compared with nondiabetic controls.

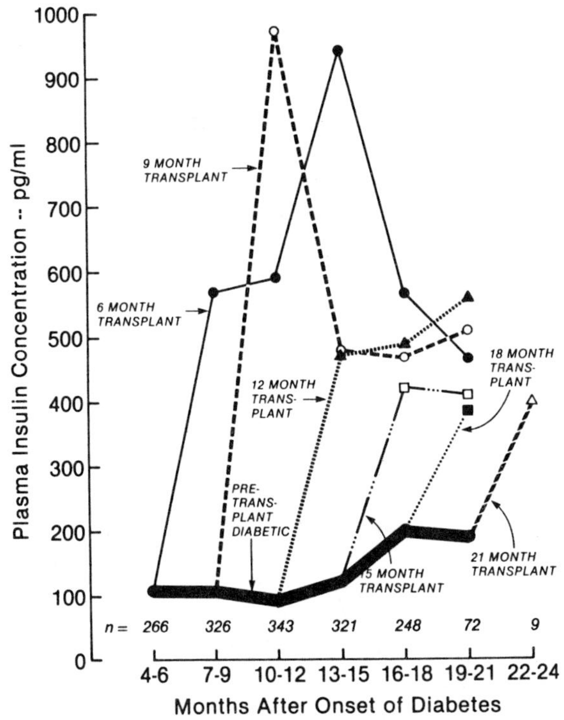

FIGURE 3. Changes in mean plasma insulin concentration following whole-pancreas transplantation performed 6–21 months after induction of DM.

levels observed in the nondiabetic controls. Similarly, plasma insulin concentrations in group DT were markedly depressed up until the time of pancreas transplantation. Following pancreas transplantation at any time from 6-21 months after onset of DM, plasma insulin rose to levels that were higher than those in the nondiabetic controls, although in only 2 instances were they significantly elevated above normal.

Glucose tolerance tests. Table 4 shows mean plasma glucose and insulin concentrations during serial glucose tolerance tests throughout the study in the 3 groups of rats, and Figures 4 and 5 show typical mean results of glucose tolerance tests performed 13–15 months after the start of the study in group NC, group DC, group DT before transplantation, and group DT rats that received pancreas transplants 6 months and 12 months after induction of DM. Nondiabetic control rats developed peak plasma glucose and insulin levels that were approximately 2–2.5 times the baseline levels 40 min after a glucose load. After 130 min, plasma glucose concentrations were still 50–102% above the baseline level, and plasma insulin was still 41–66% above basal. In the diabetic control rats and the diabetic transplant rats before pancreas transplantation, all 4 blood glucose and insulin levels during the glucose tolerance test, at all intervals throughout life, were significantly different from those in the nondiabetic controls ($P<0.001$). The diabetic glucose tolerance curve started at a much higher level than the normal curve, did not show as large a percentage increase above the baseline, peaked at 70 min rather than at 40 min, and remained markedly elevated at 130 min. Basal insulin secretion in the diabetic rats was very low and the peak increase was only 12–40% above basal. Whole-pancreas transplantation at all intervals almost normalized the glucose tolerance curve. Peak plasma glucose levels were shifted back to 40 min after administration of the glucose load and were approximately twice the baseline level. However, there was a greater-than-normal decline of plasma glucose concentration after 130 min. Secretion of insulin in the transplanted rats was significantly greater than normal, with plasma concentrations at 40 min often exceeding 2.5 times the basal level.

Plasma glucagon. Table 5 shows the mean plasma glucagon concentrations in the 3 groups of rats. DM was associated with a persistent increase in plasma glucagon. Whole-pancreas transplantation resulted in a further significant increase in plasma glucagon compared with the levels found in diabetic rats before transplantation and in the diabetic controls.

Blood urea nitrogen and serum creatinine. Table 6 and Figures 6 and 7 show the mean concentrations of BUN and serum creatinine in Group DT before and after pancreas transplantation. DM resulted in significant increases in BUN and serum creatinine early in the course of the disease. Whole-pancreas transplantation produced significant reductions of BUN and serum creatinine to the levels found before induction of DM, even when the transplants were performed 15 months after the onset of DM.

TABLE 4. Glucose tolerance tests after i.p. injection of glucose in a dose of 3 g/kg in nondiabetic controls, diabetic controls, and diabetic transplant (DT) rats before and after pancreas transplantation, showing mean plasma concentration of glucose in mg/dl and insulin in pg/ml[a]

GROUP	1–3 Months GTT (min) 0	40	70	130	No. rats	4–6 Months GTT (min) 0	40	70	130	No. rats	7–9 Months GTT (min) 0	40	70	130	No. rats	10–12 Months GT (min) 0	40	70	130	No. rats
NC:																				
Glu	101	202	176	146	25	123	269	230	224	25	92	200	178	162	26	84	199	186	170	48
Ins	518	1080	972	729	25	542	1204	1079	819	25	490	1067	935	701	26	482	996	851	681	48
DC:																				
Glu	311	419	446	431	58	350	464	487	488	52	308	413	444	436	35	304	410	430	414	29
Ins	102	132	125	110	58	101	136	129	112	52	105	145	134	114	35	96	127	121	108	29
DT-6 Mo.:[b]																				
Glu	328	432	475	464	44	338	440	486	468	44	*95*	*192*	*160*	*125*	44	*95*	*202*	*168*	*135*	35
Ins	122	159	151	133	44	101	130	124	108	44	*560*	*1402*	*1050*	*735*	44	*572*	*1483*	*1097*	*768*	35
DT-9 Mo.:[b]																				
Glu	334	440	489	472	30	343	460	497	486	30	375	472	504	493	30	*99*	*200*	*172*	*134*	30
Ins	118	153	145	128	30	100	132	122	106	30	104	141	134	118	30	*774*	*1703*	*1192*	*834*	30
DT-12 Mo.:[b]																				
Glu	349	467	492	488	32	354	470	498	482	31	371	474	521	502	30	371	470	512	498	28
Ins	120	157	149	130	32	103	135	125	110	31	102	136	129	111	30	96	128	121	105	28
DT-15 Mo.:[b]																				
Glu	352	468	492	487	20	362	483	516	504	20	355	479	509	499	19	365	483	520	506	18
Ins	116	151	142	125	20	99	137	130	114	20	98	131	122	107	19	98	129	121	104	18
DT-18 Mo.:[b]																				
Glu	320	430	467	460	3	337	442	483	471	3	361	482	517	503	3	374	476	522	511	3
Ins	128	166	157	138	3	104	141	133	117	3	103	133	125	108	3	99	130	122	107	3
DT-21 Mo.:[b]																				
Glu	320	436	463	442	3	372	471	512	498	3	373	478	518	506	3	308	482	532	523	3
Ins	129	173	164	143	3	105	137	127	112	3	106	141	132		3	100	129	121	117	3

[a] (NC) nondiabetic controls; (DC) diabetic controls; (DT) diabetic transplanted; (GLU) glucose; (dns) insulin.
[b] Plasma glucose and insulin levels obtained after transplantation are in italics.

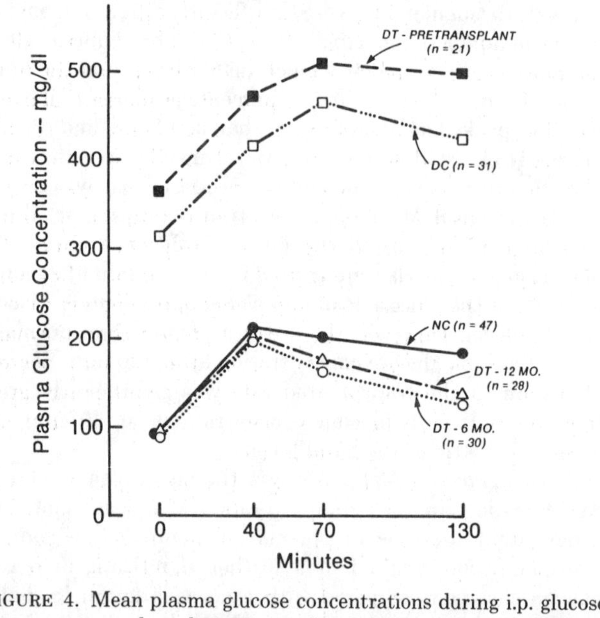

FIGURE 4. Mean plasma glucose concentrations during i.p. glucose tolerance tests conducted 13–15 months after the start of the study in nondiabetic control rats (NC), diabetic control rats (DC), and diabetic transplant rats (DT) before and after whole-pancreas transplantation performed 6 months and 12 months after induction of DM.

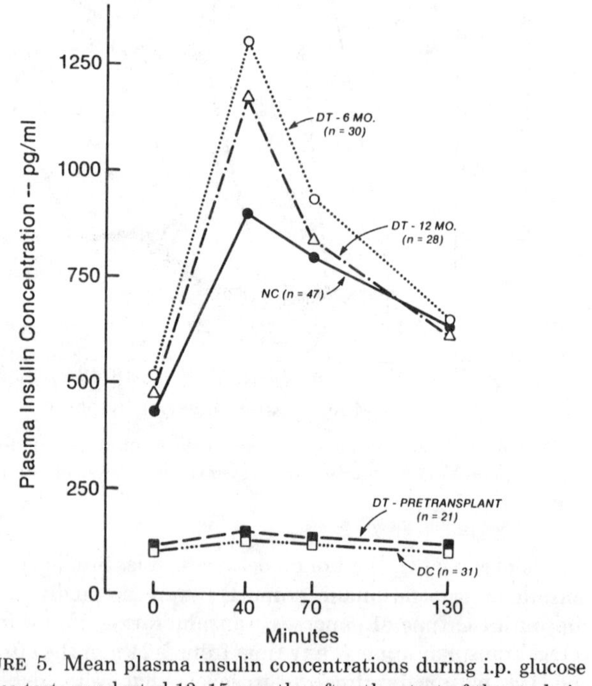

FIGURE 5. Mean plasma insulin concentrations during i.p. glucose tolerance tests conducted 13–15 months after the start of the study in nondiabetic control rats (NC), diabetic control rats (DC), and diabetic transplant rats (DT) before and after whole-pancreas transplantation performed 6 months and 12 months after induction of DM.

DISCUSSION

The relationship between metabolic control of IDDM and the development of microvascular complications is a controversial issue, particularly because it has not been proved that precise, even physiologic metabolic control can prevent, stabilize, or reverse diabetic lesions in the kidney, eye, nerves, and other organs. If, indeed, the metabolic abnormalities of IDDM cause microangiopathy, as the weight of evidence suggests, an important question is: how strictly must metabolic control be

13–15 Months					16–18 Months					19–21 Months					22–24 Months				
GTT (min)				No. rats	GTT (min)				No. rats	GTT (min)				No. rats	GTT (min)				No. rats
0	40	70	130		0	40	70	130		0	40	70	130		0	40	70	130	
93	213	200	185	47	86	206	178	171	42	89	224	183	168	40	87	207	189	176	21
438	902	801	643	47	408	950	873	655	42	391	880	796	616	40	390	904	817	647	21
316	417	460	427	31	303	436	468	455	16	254	535	541	520	5	—	—	—	—	—
100	128	120	104	31	97	120	110	101	16	88	118	112	95	5	—	—	—	—	—
93	*198*	*162*	*126*	30	*94*	*206*	*170*	*142*	17	*89*	*190*	*158*	*132*	10	*95*	*203*	*166*	*136*	5
514	*1307*	*941*	*640*	30	*552*	*1401*	*1037*	*830*	17	*462*	*1247*	*935*	*655*	10	*457*	*1051*	*757*	*568*	5
94	*192*	*160*	*132*	25	*91*	*188*	*158*	*133*	20	*89*	*185*	*156*	*128*	16	*88*	*192*	*160*	*131*	4
498	*1245*	*934*	*700*	25	*464*	*1206*	*892*	*642*	20	*490*	*1323*	*953*	*667*	16	*476*	*1095*	*799*	*599*	4
96	*203*	*175*	*136*	28	*92*	*190*	*169*	*138*	28	*90*	*187*	*170*	*130*	16	*93*	*189*	*166*	*128*	6
471	*1178*	*884*	*619*	28	*483*	*1207*	*905*	*652*	28	*548*	*1260*	*945*	*661*	16	*492*	*1132*	*815*	*611*	6
359	471	504	497	15	*93*	*202*	*171*	*141*	15	*89*	*190*	*162*	*136*	15	*87*	*189*	*165*	*130*	8
115	150	141	124	15	*420*	*1051*	*788*	*583*	15	*412*	*1071*	*803*	*562*	15	*423*	*973*	*730*	*547*	8
374	472	528	509	3	353	469	508	496	3	*92*	*193*	*163*	*131*	3	*80*	*184*	*161*	*132*	3
118	156	148	130	3	172	201	189	175	3	*392*	*1019*	*754*	*528*	3	*411*	*1028*	*761*	*571*	3
358	467	512	495	3	352	473	506	489	3	300	428	457	438	2	*99*	*198*	*158*	*129*	2
120	147	139	124	3	180	212	198	181	3	190	214	201	192	2	*406*	*1015*	*741*	*556*	2

TABLE 5. Plasma glucagon concentrations (pg/ml) in nondiabetic controls, diabetic controls, and diabetic transplant rats before and after pancreas transplantation (mean ± SEM)

GROUP	Months after entry into study									
	1–3		4–6		7–9		10–12		13–15	
	n	$\bar{X}$ ± SEM	n	$\bar{X}$ ± SEM	n	$\bar{X}$ ± SEM	n	$\bar{X}$ ± SEM	n	$\bar{X}$ ± SEM
Nondiabetic control	233	275±11.4	197	228±14.0	199	228±12.1	179	404±21.3	72	258±17.4
Diabetic control	456	613±19.0[b]	368	774±27.2[b]	340	716±30.5[b]	237	884±32.1[b]	156	848±31.4[b]
Diabetic Transplant:[a]										
6-Month	85	239±20.3	87	459±17.9[b]	151	*894*±30.3[b]	63	*1007*±35.8[b,c]	10	*1375*±422.4[b,c]
9-Month	62	210±19.7	61	413±20.7[b]	61	533±23.1[b]	61	*912*±58.0[b,c]	1	*1160*[b,c]
12-Month	64	344±23.3	64	489±19.5[b]	58	483±21.5[b]	31	584±30.6[b]	26	*1154*±52.0[b,c]

[a] Plasma glucagon levels obtained after pancreas transplantation are in italics.
[b] $P < 0.01$ compared with nondiabetic control.
[c] $P < 0.01$ compared with diabetic control and diabetic pretransplant.

maintained in order to influence the pathologic manifestations? Since conventional therapy with insulin injections and diet has failed to prevent or reverse secondary complications (*8–10*), it appears that conventional treatment does not achieve sufficiently strict metabolic control to affect microangiopathy. The same may be true of insulin pump therapy and of transplantation of isolated pancreatic islets.

Although there have been anecdotal reports of improvement of diabetic complications in patients treated by s.c. insulin infusion with a portable pump in conjunction with home glucose monitoring, a number of recent studies have demonstrated progression of retinopathy (*11, 13–16*) and nepnropathy (*12, 17, 18*) during insulin pump therapy. Artificial insulin delivery devices have been shown to substantially lower levels of blood glucose and glycosylated hemoglobin (*26–29*), and to correct abnormalities of amino acids, lipids, catecholamines, and growth hormone (*30, 31*) in patients with IDDM, but they have not maintained normal blood glucose concentrations over a prolonged period (*32, 33*). Presumably, insulin pump therapy has not achieved sufficiently precise metabolic control to stabilize or reverse diabetic lesions in the eye and kidney.

Prevention and reversal of diabetic nephropathy and eye lesions by isolated islet transplants have been examined in a number of studies in rodents with chemical DM, but all of

TABLE 6. BUN and serum creatinine (Cr) concentrations in diabetic transplant rats (Group DT) before and after pancreas transplantation

Group DT (time of transplant)	Before DM		Months after onset of DM: 3		6		7–9		10–12		13–15		16–18		19–21	
	n	X̄ ± SEM	n	X̄ ± SEM	n	X̄ ± SEM	n	X̄ ± SEM	n	X̄ ± SEM	n	X̄ ± SEM	n	X̄ ± SEM	n	X̄ ± SEM
6-month[a]																
BUN-mg/dl	22	18.7±0.5	87	28.9±0.6	88	27.3±0.6	141	*22.4±0.6*[b]	54	*21.9±1.2*[b]	10	*19.5±0.5*[b]	9	*22.1±0.6*[b]		—
Cr-mg/dl	32	0.27±.05	77	0.80±.18	88	0.58±.04	141	*0.57±.03*	54	*0.52±.03*	11	*0.23±.02*[b]	9	*0.23±.05*[b]		—
9-Month[a]																
BUN-mg/dl	15	16.5±0.7	62	26.7±0.5	62	26.7±0.5	61	31.1±0.7	42	*23.5±0.6*[b]	18	*22.2±0.7*[b]	2	*23.0±0*[b]		—
Cr-mg/dl	22	0.23±.07	60	0.60±.04	62	0.66±.03	61	0.69±.03	43	*0.43±.04*[b]	19	*0.40±.07*[b]	2	*0.25±.01*[b]		—
12-Month[a]																
BUN-mg/dl	22	19.3±0.8	65	29.7±1.1	65	28.6±0.5	55	30.2±0.8	24	29.0±1.1	20	*21.7±1.0*[b]	13	*21.8±0.7*[b]	3	*23.7±1.8*[b]
Cr-mg/dl	18	0.25±.03	50	0.61±.05	65	0.61±.04	55	0.65±.03	24	0.65±.03	16	*0.46±.05*[b]	13	*0.46±.08*[b]	3	*0.13±.03*[b]
15-Month[a]																
BUN-mg/dl	5	17.6±1.1	39	28.2±0.8	39	28.0±0.8	20	28.7±0.9	5	28.8±0.7	8	28.9±2.9	17	*25.0±0.9*[b]	5	*21.2±0.9*[b]
Cr-mg/dl	17	0.26±.06	32	0.58±.07	39	0.48±.05	20	0.64±.07	5	0.64±.09	8	0.65±.05	18	*0.26±.04*[b]	5	*0.25±.09*[b]

[a] BUN and serum creatinine levels obtained after pancreas transplantation are in italics.
[b] $P<0.01$ compared with pretransplant values.

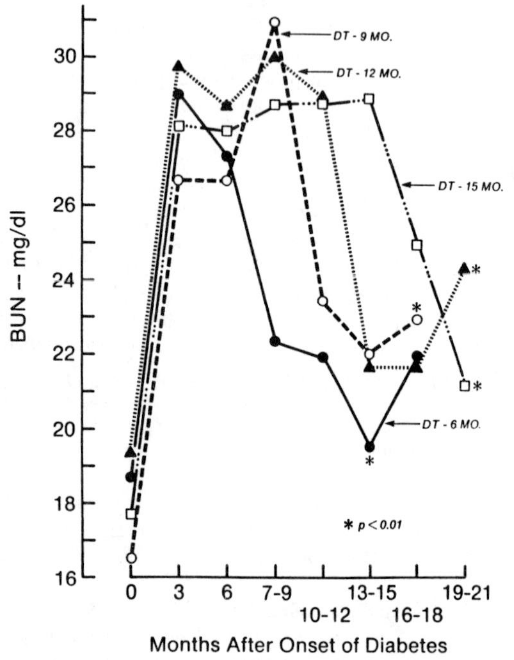

FIGURE 6. Changes in mean BUN concentration following whole-pancreas transplantation performed 6, 9, 12, and 15 months after induction of DM.

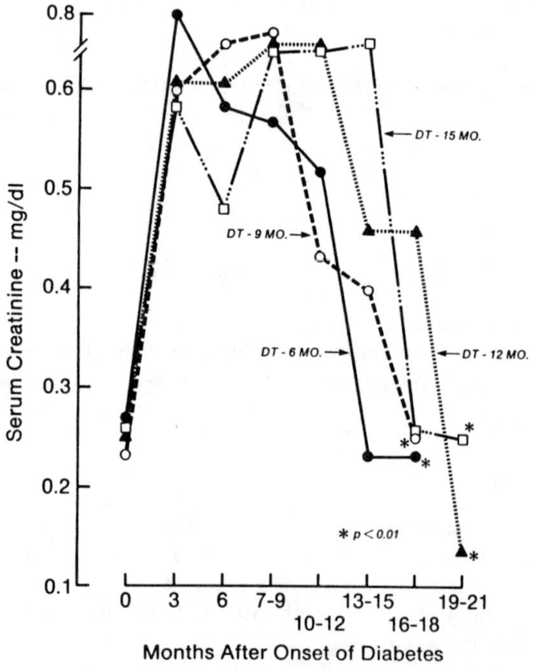

FIGURE 7. Changes in mean serum creatinine concentration following whole-pancreas transplantation performed 6, 9, 12, and 15 months after induction of DM.

these have been short-term investigations performed in a small number of animals, and most have not involved quantitative morphologic methods or a "blind" protocol. Of the 6 quantitative studies that have been reported (*19–21, 23–25*), 5 have shown failure to reverse diabetic lesions in the kidney (*20, 21, 23, 25*) or the eye (*19*). Metabolic studies in diabetic animals with isolated islet transplants have all been of short duration and conducted in a few animals, and most have involved transplantation shortly after induction of DM (*19, 22, 23, 25, 34–41*). These studies have shown considerable improvement in metabolic control, but persistence of significant abnormalities of glucose and lipid metabolism. In particular, a substantial percentage of animals with isolated islet transplants have not become normoglycemic; in those with normal blood glucose levels, hyperglycemia has often recurred within 6–12 months; plasma insulin concentrations have been lower than normal; and oral and i.v. glucose tolerance test results have remained abnormal. In one study, plasma triglyceride and cholesterol levels remained elevated (*38*). Thus isolated islet transplants have not achieved precise metabolic control, even in short-term trials, and this may account for their failure to reverse diabetic kidney and eye lesions.

Regarding whole-pancreas transplantation, studies that we have reported previously showed that whole pancreas isografts transplanted shortly after induction of DM in rats produced precise metabolic control for life (*42*). Furthermore, quantitative morphologic studies in these alloxan-diabetic rats demonstrated that whole pancreas transplants prevented glomerular basement membrane thickening (*47*) and mesangial enlargement (*48*) in the kidney for the full natural life span of the animals. Finally, in recent studies, we found that whole-pancreas transplantation was capable of reversing well-established mesangial enlargement in long-standing DM (*49*). Other than our investigations, there have been no reports of detailed long-term metabolic studies or quantitative morphologic studies of the effectiveness of whole-pancreas transplants. Ongoing metabolic studies are being carried out in humans with whole-pancreas transplants (*50*), but they are difficult to interpret at this early point because of the small number of patients and short periods of follow-up.

The results of the present study provide convincing evidence that whole-pancreas transplantation in an animal model of DM is capable of reversing long-established metabolic abnormalities and maintaining very tight metabolic control for life. Pancreas transplants performed 6–21 months after induction of DM invariably reduced plasma glucose concentrations to normal and maintained them below 100 mg/dl. Depressed plasma insulin concentrations were restored by pancreas transplantation to levels that were higher than normal, although not significantly higher. Glucose tolerance tests i.p. after whole-pancreas transplantation produced hyperglycemia of lesser magnitude and shorter duration than normal, as a result of greater-than-normal insulin secretion. Elevations of BUN and serum creatinine were reduced to normal by pancreas transplants. Correction of the metabolic disturbances of DM by pancreas transplantation resulted in marked growth and gain in body weight. Precise metabolic control was associated with striking reversal of mesangial enlargement in these same rats (*49*).

The only abnormality that was not improved by whole-pancreas transplantation was hyperglucagonemia. As others have reported (*41, 51–54*), plasma glucagon concentration was elevated in the diabetic rats, and as others have found (*40, 54*), heterotopic pancreas transplantation was associated with a further increase in the plasma glucagon level. The cause and significance of this abnormality are not known, but it clearly did not interfere with elimination of hyperglycemia by pancreas transplantation.

The results of the present study indicate that, of the various methods of treating DM, whole-pancreas transplantation produces the strictest metabolic control and is the most effective means of correcting the metabolic abnormalities. It appears that precise metabolic control is required to influence diabetic microangiopathy, since to date only whole-pancreas transplants have been successful in preventing and reversing the kidney lesions of experimental DM.

Acknowledgments. We thank Hazel J. Sayers and Sun Lee for technical assistance with the transplantation operations.

REFERENCES

1. Gepts W, Lecompte P. The pancreatic islets in diabetes. Am J Med 1981; 70: 105.
2. Nerup J, Lernmark A. Autoimmunity in insulin-dependent diabetes mellitus. Am J Med 1981; 70: 135.
3. Cahill GF Jr, McDevitt HO. Insulin-dependent diabetes mellitus: the initial lesion. N Engl J Med 1981; 304: 1454.
4. Cudworth AG, Wolf E. The genetics of type I (insulin-dependent) diabetes. Curr Probl Clin Biochem 1983; 12: 45.
5. Yoon Y-W. Viruses in the pathogenesis of type I diabetes. Curr Probl Clin Biochem 1983; 12: 11.
6. Brogren CH, Baekkeskov S, Dryberg T, Lernmark A, Marner B, Nerup J, Papadopoulos GK. Role of islet cell antibodies in the pathogenesis of type I diabetes. Curr Probl Clin Biochem 1983; 12: 65.
7. Doniach D, Bottazzo GF, Cudworth AG. Etiology of type I diabetes mellitus: heterogeneity and immunological events leading to clinical onset. Ann Rev Med 1983; 34: 13.
8. Tchobroutsky G. Relation of diabetic control to development of microvascular complications. Diabetologia 1978; 15: 143.
9. Cahill CF Jr. Diabetes mellitus: a brief overview. Johns Hopkins Med J 1978; 143: 155.
10. Siperstein MD. Diabetic microangiopathy and the control of blood glucose. N Engl J Med 1983; 309: 1577.
11. Puklin JE, Tamborlane WV, Felig P, Genel M, Sherwin RS. Influence of long-term insulin infusion pump treatment of type I diabetes on diabetic retinopathy. Ophthalmology (Rochester) 1982; 89: 735.
12. Tamborlane WV, Press CM. Insulin infusion pump treatment of type I diabetes. Pediatr Clin North Am 1984; 31: 721.
13. Lauritzen T, and the Steno Study Group. Effect of one year of near-normal blood glucose levels on retinopathy in insulin-dependent diabetes. Lancet 1983; 1: 200.
14. Kroc Collaborative Study Group. Near-normal glycemia control does not slow progression of mild diabetic retinopathy. Diabetes 1983; 32(suppl 1): 10A.
15. Hooymans JMM, Ballegoole EV, Schweitzer NMJ, Doorenbos H, Reitsma WP, Sluiter WJ. Worsening of diabetic retinopathy with strict control of blood sugar. Lancet 1982; 2: 438.
16. Lawson PM, Champion MC, Canny C, Kingsley R, White MC, Dupre J, Kohner DM. Continuous subcutaneous insulin infusion (CSII) does not prevent progression of proliferative and preproliferative retinopathy. Br J Opthalmol 1982; 66: 762.
17. Tamborlane WV, Puklin JE, Bergman M, Verdon KC, Rudolf MC, Felig P, Genel M, Sherwin R. Long-term improvement of metabolic control with the insulin pump does not reverse diabetic microangiopathy. Diabetes Care 1982; 5(suppl 1): 58.
18. Viberti GC, Bilous RW, Mackintosh D, Bending JJ, Keen H. Long-term correction of hyperglycemia and progression of renal failure in insulin-dependent diabetes. Br Med J 1983; 286: 598.
19. Naeser P, Andersson A. Effects of pancreatic islet implantation on the morphology of retinal capillaries in alloxan diabetic mice. Acta Ophthalmol 1983; 63: 38.
20. Weber CJ, Silva FG, Hardy MA, Lirani CL, Reemtsma K. Effect of islet transplantation on renal function and morphology of short- and long-term diabetic rats. Transplant Proc 1979; 11: 549.
21. Gotzsche O, Gundersen HJG, Osterby R. Irreversibility of glomerular basement membrane accumulation despite reversibility of renal hypertrophy with islet transplantation in early diabetes. Diabetes 1981; 30: 481.
22. Mauer SM, Sutherland DER, Steffes MW, Leonard RJ, Najarian JS, Michael AF, Brown DM. Pancreatic islet transplantation effects on the glomerular lesions of experimental diabetes in the rat. Diabetes 1974; 23: 748.
23. Steffes MW, Brown DM, Basgen JM, Matas AJ, Mauer SM. Glomerular basement membrane thickness following islet transplantation in the diabetic rat. Lab Invest 1979; 41: 116.
24. Steffes MW, Brown DM, Basgen J, Mauer SM. Amelioration of mesangial volume and surface alterations following islet transplantation in diabetic rats. Diabetes 1980; 29: 509.
25. Steffes MW, Vernier RL, Brown DM, Basgen J, Mauer SM. Diabetic glomerulopathy in the uninephrectomized rat resists amelioration following islet transplantation. Diabetologia 1982; 23: 347.
26. Pickup J, White M, Keen H, Parsons J, Alberti K. Long-term continuous subcutaneous insulin infusion in diabetics at home. Lancet 1979; 2: 870.
27. Tamborlane MV, Sherwin RS, Genel M, Felig P. Reduction to normal of plasma glucose in juvenile diabetics by subcutaneous administration of insulin with a portable infusion pump. N Engl J Med 1979; 300: 573.
28. Tamborlane WV, Sherwin RS, Genel M, Felig P. Outpatient treatment of juvenile-onset diabetes with a preprogrammed portable subcutaneous insulin infusion system. Am J Med 1980; 68: 190.
29. Champion MC, Shephard GAA, Rodger NW, Dupre J. Continuous

subcutaneous infusion of insulin in the management of diabetes mellitus. Diabetes 1980; 29: 206.
30. Tamborlane WV, Sherwin RS, Genel M, Felig P. Restoration of normal lipid and amino-acid metabolism in diabetic patients treated with a portable insulin-infusion pump. Lancet 1979; 1: 1258.
31. Tamborlane WV, Sherwin RS, Koivisto V, Handler R, Genel M, Felig P. Normalization of the growth hormone and catecholamine response to exercise in juvenile onset diabetics treated with a portable insulin infusion pump. Diabetes 1979; 28: 785.
32. Lauritzen T, Pramming S. Insulin pumps—still a research tool? Ann Clin Res 1984; 16: 98.
33. Mecklenburg RS, Benson JW Jr, Becker NM, Brazel PL, Fredlund PN, Metz RJ, Nielsen RL, Sannar CA, Steenrod WJ Jr. Clinical use of the insulin infusion pump in 100 patients with type I diabetes. N Engl J Med 1982; 307: 513.
34. Ballinger WF, Lacy PE. Transplantation of intact pancreatic islets in rats. Surgery 1972; 72: 175.
35. Ziegler MM, Reckard CR, Barker CF. Long-term metabolic and immunological considerations in transplantation of pancreatic islets. J Surg Res 1974; 16: 575.
36. Gray BN, Watkins E. Prolonged relief from diabetes after syngeneic or allogeneic transplantation of isolated pancreatic islets in rats. Surg Forum 1974; 25: 382.
37. Steffes MW, Sutherland DER, Mauer SM, Leonard RJ, Najarian JS, Brown DM. Plasma insulin and glucose levels in diabetic rats prior to and following islet transplantation. J Lab Clin Med 1975; 85: 75.
38. Vialettes B, Sutherland DER, Matas AJ, Payne WD, Najarian JS. Amelioration of streptozotocin-induced diabetes in rats: effect of islet isografts on plasma lipids and other metabolic abnormalities. Metabolism 1979; 28: 489.
39. Pipeleers D, Pipeleers-Marichal MA, Kipnis D. Metabolic and morphologic studies in long-term islet transplanted rats. Diabetes 1975; 24(suppl 1): 420.
40. Weber CJ, Hardy MA, Lerner RL, Felig P, Reemtsma K. Hyperinsulinemia and hyperglucagonemia following pancreatic islet transplantation in diabetic rats. Diabetes 1976; 25: 944.
41. Trimble ER, Karakash C, Malaisse-Lagal F, Vassutine I, Orce L, Renold E. Effects of intraportal islet transplantation on the transplanted tissue and the recipient pancreas. I. Functional studies. Diabetes 1980; 29: 341.
42. Orloff MJ, Lee S, Charters AC, Grambort DE, Storck LG, Knox D. Long-term studies of pancreas transplantation in experimental diabetes mellitus. Ann Surg 1975; 182: 198.
43. Orloff MJ, Lee S, Chandler JG, Krubel R, Rosen H. Heterotopic transplantation of the whole pancreas in inbred rats. Gastroenterology 1971; 61: 704.
44. Lee S, Tung SK, Koopmans H, Chandler JG, Orloff MJ. Pancreaticoduodenal transplantation in the rat. Transplantation 1972; 13: 421.
45. Yalow RS, Berson SA. Immunoassay of endogenous insulin in man. J Clin Invest 1960; 39: 1157.
46. Faloona GR, Unger RH. Glucagon. In: Jaffe BM, Behrman HR, eds. Methods of hormone radioimmunoassay. New York: Academic Press, 1974: 317.
47. Bell RH Jr, Fernandez-Cruz L, Brimm JE, Sayers HJ, Lee S, Orloff MJ. Prevention by whole pancreas transplantation of glomerular basement membrane thickening in alloxan diabetes. Surgery 1980; 88; 31.
48. Orloff MJ, Bell RH Jr, Greenleaf GE, Yamanaka N, Girard B. Lifelong prevention of mesangial enlargement by whole pancreas transplantation in rats with insulin-dependent diabetes mellitus. Diabetologia in press.
49. Orloff MJ, Yamanaka N, Greenleaf GE, Huang Y-t, Hung D-g, Leng X-s. Reversal of mesangial enlargement in rats with long-standing diabetes by whole pancreas transplantation. Diabetes 1986; 35: 347.
50. Sutherland DER, Goetz FC, Najarian JS. One hundred pancreas transplants at a single institution. Ann Surg 1984; 200; 414.
51. Buchanan KD, McCarrol AM. Abnormalities of glucagon metabolism in untreated diabetes mellitus. Lancet 1972; 2: 1394.
52. Muller WA, Faloona GR, Unger RH. The effect of experimental insulin deficiency on glucagon secretion. J Clin Invest 1971; 50: 1992.
53. Unger RH, Orci L. Glucagon and the A cell. Physiology and pathophysiology. N Engl J Med 1981; 304: 1518.
54. Brekke IB, Oyasaeter S, Vidnes J. Long-term effect of pancreas transplantation on diabetic hyperglucagonemia. Eur Surg Res 1982; 14: 211.

Received 17 July 1985.
Accepted 17 September 1985.

0041-1337/86/4105-0565$02.00/0
TRANSPLANTATION
Copyright © 1986 by The Williams & Wilkins Co.

Vol. 41, No. 5
Printed in U.S.A.

MONOCLONAL ANTIBODY ANALYSIS OF CANINE HEMOPOIETIC CELLS

ROLE OF IA-LIKE AND THY-1 ANTIGENS IN BONE MARROW ENGRAFTMENT[1]

MARGARET M. PRENDERGAST[2], KENNETH F. BRADSTOCK, ALAN F. BROOMHEAD, WILBUR G. HUGHES, ARNOLD KABRAL, MICHAEL C. BERNDT AND KENNETH TIVER

Department of Haematology, Institute of Clinical Pathology and Medical Research, and Departments of Medicine and Radiation Oncology, Westmead Centre, Westmead, N.S.W. Australia

The expression of Ia-like (class II MHC) antigens on canine hemopoietic cells was investigated using a cytotoxic murine monoclonal antibody, WM-2, reactive with dog Ia-like antigens. Another monoclonal antibody, WMD-1, reactive with canine Thy-1 antigen, was used as a positive control. Depletion of Ia$^+$ cells from dog bone marrow by complement-mediated lysis with WM-2 antibody failed to inhibit growth of granulocyte-macrophage progenitors (CFU_{GM}) in vitro, while WMD-1 produced complete inhibition of CFU_{GM}. Lethally irradiated dogs receiving bone marrow autografts depleted of Ia-positive cells ex vivo showed initial engraftment, followed by prolonged pancytopenia, and eventual complete recovery of marrow function in the majority of animals. In contrast, dogs receiving autografts treated with WMD-1 and complement all died of marrow failure. We interpret these results as indicating: (1) that Thy-1 antigen is present on hemopoietic stem cells essential for marrow engraftment; and (2) that the expression of Ia antigens on hemopoietic cells is heterogeneous and related to the level of stem cell maturation. While Ia appears to be present on a stem cell population at an earlier stage than CFU_{GM}, as evidenced by the transient phase of graft failure seen in dogs receiving Ia-depleted marrow, the most primitive stem cell, responsible for long-term engraftment, is effectively Ia-negative.

Ia-like (class II) antigens of the major histocompatibility complex are widely distributed on lymphohemopoietic cells, and play a prominent role in the regulation of the immune response (*1, 2*). The presence of Ia antigens on bone marrow myeloid progenitor cells has also suggested a regulatory function in myelopoiesis. Ia antigens have been demonstrated on bone marrow progenitors assayable in semisolid media, including cells committed to the granulocyte-macrophage lineage (CFU_{GM}),* (*3–6*), and to erythropoiesis (BFU_E and CFU_E) (*7–10*). More recently, the more primitive multi-lineage myeloid progenitor cells (CFU_{GEMM}) have also been reported to express Ia antigens (*10–12*). However, evidence has accumulated that the true pluripotential stem cell, giving rise to both lymphoid and myeloid lineages, and representing the essential cell for restoration of hemopoiesis after marrow transplantation, is Ia-negative. In the mouse, depletion of Ia-positive hemopoietic cells with cytolytic heteroantiserum failed to inhibit the growth of spleen colony forming cells (CFUs), thought to represent the mouse pluripotential stem cell (*13*). Similarly, Hetherington and coworkers showed that pretreatment of marmoset bone marrow with 2 monoclonal anti-Ia antibodies and complement had no inhibitory effect on bone marrow engraftment (*14*). In addition, Moore et al., using a long-term human bone marrow culture system, failed to inhibit the growth of marrow inoculum by pretreatment with anti-Ia antibody (*15*); results of this study have been recently confirmed by Keating and coworkers (*16*). We have further investigated the expression of Ia-like antigens on hemopoietic progenitor cells, using canine bone marrow and murine monoclonal antibodies reactive with dog cells. The in vitro growth of hemopoietic colonies after depletion of Ia$^+$ cells was compared with the regeneration pattern of Ia-depleted autologous marrow in lethally irradiated dogs. We report that, although a complex short-term pattern of inhibition of bone marrow regeneration was seen, long-term engraftment of marrow occurred despite ex vivo treatment of marrow cells with cytolytic anti-Ia antibody and complement.

MATERIALS AND METHODS

Monoclonal antibodies. Murine monoclonal antibodies were prepared according to published methods (*17, 18*). BALB-C mice were immunized with the human B cell line Daudi, or with canine thymocytes, and splenic lymphocytes fused with NS1 myeloma cells. Antibody secretory clones were injected i.p. into mice, and high-titer ascitic fluid harvested under sterile conditions.

For evaluation of efficiency of removal of Ia-positive bone marrow cells, 3 further monoclonal antibodies reactive with canine p28,33 antigens were used for immunofluorescence studies; these consisted of 7.2 (New England Nuclear) (*19, 20*), CA-135 (*21*), and ISCR-3 (*22*).

Immunofluorescence. Indirect immunofluorescence was carried out as previously described (*23*). Briefly, 1×10^6 mononuclear cells were incubated with saturating concentrations of monoclonal antibody, or with negative control antibody WM-21 (*24*) (antihuman CALLA; unreactive with canine cells), washed with phosphate-buffered saline containing 1% bovine

[1] This work was supported by a grant from the National Health and Medical Research Council of Australia.

[2] Address correspondence to: M. Prendergast, Department of Haematology, Institute of Clinical Pathology and Medical Research, Westmead Centre, Westmead N.S.W. 2145 Australia.

* Abbreviations used: BFU_E, burst-forming unit, erythroid; BSA, bovine serum albumin; CFU_E, colony-forming unit, erythroid; CFU_{GEMU}, progenitor cells forming mixed colonies containing granulocytes erthrocytes, macrophages, and megakaryocytes. CFU_{GM}, granulocyte-macrophage progenitors; CFUs, spleen colony-forming cells; DMEM, Dulbecco's minimal essential medium; GAM-FITC, goat antimouse immunoglobulin conjugated with fluorescein isothiocyanate; PBSA, phosphate-buffered saline containing 1% bovine serum albumin and 0.1% sodium azide; TBI, total-body irradiation.

albumin and 0.1% sodium azide (PBSA), and reacted with goat antimouse immunoglobulin conjugated with fluorescein isothiocyanate (GAM-FITC). After 2 further washes with bovine serum albumin (BSA), cells were examined under a Zeiss fluorescence microscope. A minimum of 200 cells was scored for each antibody assay.

Complement. Fresh blood from 6-week-old New Zealand White rabbits was collected under sterile conditions and allowed to clot. Serum was tested for background toxicity and lytic ability with monoclonal antibodies by Trypan blue exclusion. Sera selected on the basis of high lytic activity were pooled and stored at −70°C for further use.

Canine CFU_{GM} assay. A modification of the method of Pike and Robinson was used to evaluate CFU_{GM} in canine marrow (*25*). Briefly, 10^5 washed bone marrow mononuclear cells in McCoy 5A medium were plated in 0.3% agar, with 10% fetal calf serum (Flow Laboratories), penicillin/streptomycin, supplemental vitamins, and 0.1 ml of giant cell tumor conditioned medium (Flow Laboratories) as the source of colony-stimulating factor. Petri dishes were incubated at 37°C in 5% CO_2 in air. In some experiments, cells were preincubated with rabbit serum with or without monoclonal antibody, washed, and plated as above. Plates were evaluated at 7 and 10 days, with colonies being scored as groups of more than 40 cells. Preliminary studies, using combined esterase stains of fixed colony preparations from plates, had established that cells growing under these conditions were granulocytic and/or monocytic in type.

Immunoprecipitation. Immunoprecipitation experiments were performed according to published methods (*26*). WM-18, reactive with human platelet glycoprotein IIb/IIIa and FMC18 directed against *Toxoplasma*, were used as negative controls. The cells used were the Ia-positive cell lines Daudi (human) and CT45-S (canine) (*20*). Washed cells were incubated in sodium iodide (^{125}I) at 1mCi/ml and 13.4 micromolar lactoperoxidase, prior to addition of hydrogen peroxide. Labeled cells were mixed with leupeptin and DFP, and solubilized in 11% Triton X-100. Centrifuged lysates were precleared with protein-A-coated *S Aureus*, and incubated with monoclonal antibody. Goat antimouse IgG was added, and immunoprecipitation performed with fixed *S Aureus* cells (Pansorbin). Immunoprecipitates were electrophoresed in exponential 5–20% sodium dodecyl sulfate polyacrylamide gels, as previously described (*26*), and Coomassie-brilliant-blue–stained gels subjected to autoradiography against Kodak X-Omat x-ray film.

Animals. Adult mongrel dogs (15–20 kg body weight) were observed for at least 2 weeks prior to transplantation, and vaccinated against distemper, parvovirus, and canine hepatitis.

Bone marrow transplantation. Bone marrow was aspirated under general anesthesia from the humerus, femur, and iliac crest of heparinized animals. Marrow was collected in acid-citrate-dextrose and heparin, diluted with Dulbecco's minimal essential medium (DMEM), and centrifuged over Ficoll-Isopaque in 50-ml tubes at 500g for 30 min. Interface mononuclear cells were washed twice in DMEM containing 25 units/ml deoxyribonuclease (Sigma) and 1% bovine albumin, and adjusted to a concentration of 2×10^7 ml. Cells were then incubated with monoclonal antibody (10 μg/ml) at 20°C for 15 min, followed by freshly thawed rabbit serum (40% v:v) at 37°C for 45 min, or with rabbit serum alone. Cells were then centrifuged and resuspended in DMEM. In some experiments, a second treatment with antibody and complement was carried out as above. Washed cells in DMEM were then injected i.v. into the same dogs within 6 h of irradiation.

Total-body irradiation. All dogs received brief general anesthesia for total-body irradiation (TBI). Radiotherapy was delivered using a 6 meV linear accelerator (Therac, Atomic Energy Canada Limited) via parallel opposed lateral fields at a dose rate of 0.55 Gy/min. The dose was prescribed to the midplane on the central axis of the beam. Bolus therapy was used to improve the uniformity of dose distribution to the limbs, and a 1-cm perspex sheet suspended 15–20 cm above the dog ensured delivery of the full radiation dose to the skin. Dosimetric measurements in test animals suggested that a dose uniformity of ±5% at the midplane was achieved by this technique. Total received doses are detailed below.

Posttransplantation care. Dogs were housed in isolation, and given parenteral penicillin/streptomycin for fever (rectal temperature >39.7°C) during periods of neutropenia. Daily full blood counts were performed for the first month, and 1–2 times weekly thereafter. Fresh whole blood transfusions, irradiated with 20 Gy, were given as required to maintain the hemoglobin above 10g/dl and the platelet count above 10×10^9 L. Intravenous fluids were given as clinically indicated as replacement for TBI-induced vomiting and diarrhea. Postmortem examinations were conducted on dogs that died after transplantation.

RESULTS

Reactivity of monoclonal antibodies with canine cells (Table 1). Two murine monoclonal antibodies reactive with canine cells were used for this study. WM-2, raised against the human B cell line Daudi, immunoprecipitated two chains with molecular weights of 28 and 33 kilodaltons (Fig. 1). This antibody crossreacted with canine cells—and, in parallel immunoprecipitation studies using the dog CT45-S line, bound to canine p28,33 antigens (Fig. 1). WM-2 reacted with 43% of normal canine peripheral blood mononuclear cells, a high proportion of thoracic duct and splenic lymphocytes, and a minor subpopulation of dog bone marrow cells (Table 1). It is a cytolytic antibody of IgG_{2a} subclass.

WMD-1, produced using canine thymocytes as immunogen, reacted with the majority of peripheral blood mononuclear cells, thymocytes, and thoracic duct lymphocytes, as well as a proportion of spleen cells (Table 1). In addition, it labeled a subpopulation of bone marrow mononuclear cells. WMD-1 is an IgM complement-fixing antibody. Pretreatment of canine peripheral blood lymphoid cells with WMD-1 and complement abolished the proliferative response of these cells to phytohemagglutinin and allogeneic stimulation in mixed lymphocyte culture (data not shown). Recently, competitive binding studies and immunoprecipitation experiments have confirmed that WMD-1 reacts with the canine Thy-1 molecule (*27*).

Effect of monoclonal antibodies on CFU_{GM} growth. Although both WM-2 and WMD-1 reacted with minor subpopulations of marrow cells, differing patterns of reactivity with CFU_{GM} were seen (Table 2). Elimination of WM-2-positive cells by complement lysis did not inhibit CFU_{GM} growth, whereas WMD-1 abolished colony formation in parallel cultures.

Bone marrow transplantation studies. The effect of various ex vivo bone marrow manipulations on hemopoietic regeneration was evaluated in five experimental groups of irradiated dogs. Regeneration patterns of neutrophils and platelets are given in Figures 2 and 3. Group A (n=5) received 5 Gy TBI

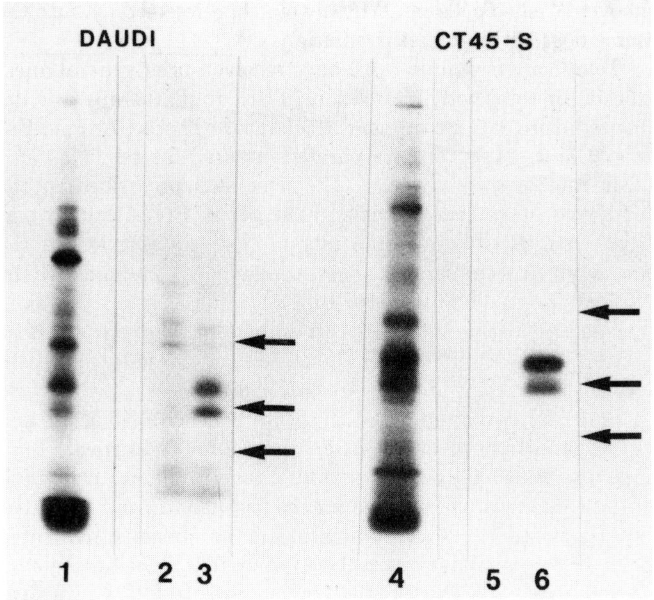

FIGURE 1. Autoradiography of exponential 5%–20% SDS-polyacrylamide gels run under reducing conditions of the WM-2 immunoprecipitates derived from lactoperoxidase-labeled, Triton-X-100-solubilized Daudi or CT45-S cells. Lane 1: 1-in-10 dilution of Daudi lysate; lanes 2 and 3: WM-18 (negative control) and WM-2 immunoprecipitates, respectively, derived from the cell lysate shown in lane 1; lane 4: 1-in-10 dilution of CT45-S lysate; lanes 5 and 6: FMC-18 (negative control) and WM-2 immunoprecipitates, respectively, derived from the cell lysate shown in lane 4. Molecular weight markers in decreasing order of molecular weight are ovalbumin (43,000), carbonic anhydrase (29,000), and soybean trypsin inhibitor (21,000).

TABLE 1. Reactivity of monoclonal antibodies with normal canine leukocytes

Cell type	Antibody[a]	
	WM-2	WMD-1
Peripheral blood mononuclear cells	40 (24–67; n = 6)	66 (58–72; n = 7)
Thoracic duct lymphocytes	60 (n = 1)	75 (72–80; n = 3)
Thymocytes	<1 (n = 2)	90 (n = 2)
Splenic lymphocytes	50 (n = 1)	33 (23–56; n = 5)
Bone marrow mononuclear cells	13 (2–23; n = 8)	26 (18–33; n = 6)

[a] Percentage of cells reactive with WM-2 and WMD-1 by indirect immunofluorescence. Figures in parentheses indicate range of results and number of samples tested.

and no bone marrow rescue (Fig. 2). All dogs in this control group died of bone marrow failure by a mean of day 11 (range 10–13 days). Histological examination of postmortem bone marrow sections showed no evidence of hemopoietic recovery. Group B (n=4) also received 5 Gy TBI, followed by bone marrow cells incubated with complement alone (mean cell dose 8.6×10^7/kg; range $7–12\times10^7$/kg) (Fig. 2). After a nadir in the neutrophil count at day 7 after TBI (mean count 0.06×10^9/L) and in the platelet count at days 9–12 (mean count 13×10^9/L), all animals showed prompt and complete hematological recov-

TABLE 2. Reactivity of monoclonal antibodies with canine CFU_{GM}[a]

Treatment of cells	Experiment No.	CFU_{GM} per 10^5 cells	
		Day 7	Day 10
Complement alone	1	137	153
	2	91	91
	3	144	175
	4	64	99
WM-2 plus complement	1	126	134
	2	70	73
	3	108	172
	4	55	96
WMD-1 plus complement	1	0.5	1
	2	0	0.5
	3	1	0
	4	0	0

[a] Growth of canine granulocyte-macrophage progenitor colonies in agar. Results indicate the number of colonies greater than 40 cells and represent the mean of triplicate plates.

ery (mean neutrophil count 2.0×10^9/L by day 14, mean platelet count 40×10^9/L by day 15), and required no blood product or antibiotic support therapy.

Dogs in group C (n=2) received 5 Gy TBI, and bone marrow cells treated with WMD-1 and complement (Fig. 2). Dogs were given cell doses of 19×10^7/kg and 24×10^7/kg respectively, but died on days 12 and 14 with severe pancytopenia and no evidence of neutrophil recovery. Histological examination of postmortem marrow revealed gross hypocellularity, but with one small focus of hemopoietic regeneration seen in each animal. One further dog received bone marrow tested with two cycles of WMD-1 and complement after 7.5 Gy TBI; this animal died on day 19 with pancytopenia and a completely aplastic marrow.

Dogs in group D (n=8) were irradiated with 5 Gy TBI, followed by infusion of bone marrow treated with a single incubation with WM-2 and complement (Fig. 3). Immunofluorescence analysis of bone marrow cells before and after antibody-complement treatment showed complete removal of Ia-positive cells in 3 of 4 dogs analyzed (Table 3). In one experiment, 3% weakly staining residual cells were seen after treatment. Following the neutrophil nadir at day 7 (mean neutrophils 0.2×10^9/L), there was evidence of initial engraftment at days 9–12 (mean count 1.2×10^9/L). Subsequently, a second nadir occurred at days 16–20 (mean count 0.3×10^9/L), after which gradual but complete regeneration was seen in 5 dogs (mean neutrophils 2.0×10^9/L by day 36). All dogs in this group required multiple transfusions for prolonged anemia and thrombocytopenia, and antibiotic therapy for febrile episodes. The five surviving dogs were given a mean cell dose of 9.4×10^7/kg (range $5–20\times10^7$/kg). Three dogs receiving a mean cell dose of 3.5×10^7/kg (range $2–4.3\times10^7$/kg) showed evidence of initial neutrophil recovery, but subsequently died by mean day 16 with severe pancytopenia.

In order to investigate the possibility that the long-term bone marrow recovery seen in the 5 group D dogs was due to ineffective removal of Ia-positive cells from the marrow inoculum, or to an insufficient radiation dose, a further group of dogs was studied (Fig. 3). Group E (n=3) received either 5 Gy TBI (one dog) or 7.5 Gy TBI (2 dogs), followed by bone marrow treated with 2 incubation cycles of WM-2 and complement.

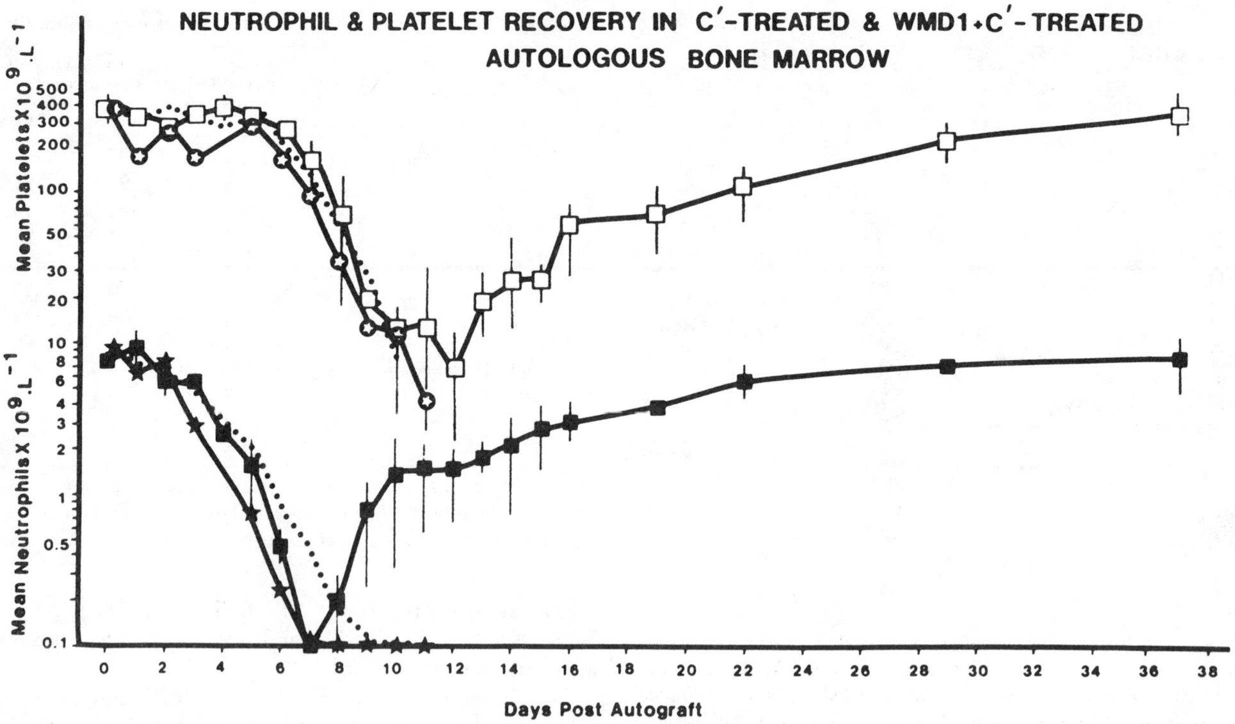

FIGURE 2. Neutrophil and platelet counts in irradiated dogs (5 Gy) given no bone marrow rescue (. . . . [group A]), bone marrow cells treated with complement alone (□) platelets, (■) neutrophils [groupB]), or bone marrow cells treated with WMD-1 plus complement. (✪) platelets, (★) neutrophils [group C]). Symbols represent mean of absolute counts; vertical bars indicate range of values in group B (not given for groups A and C).

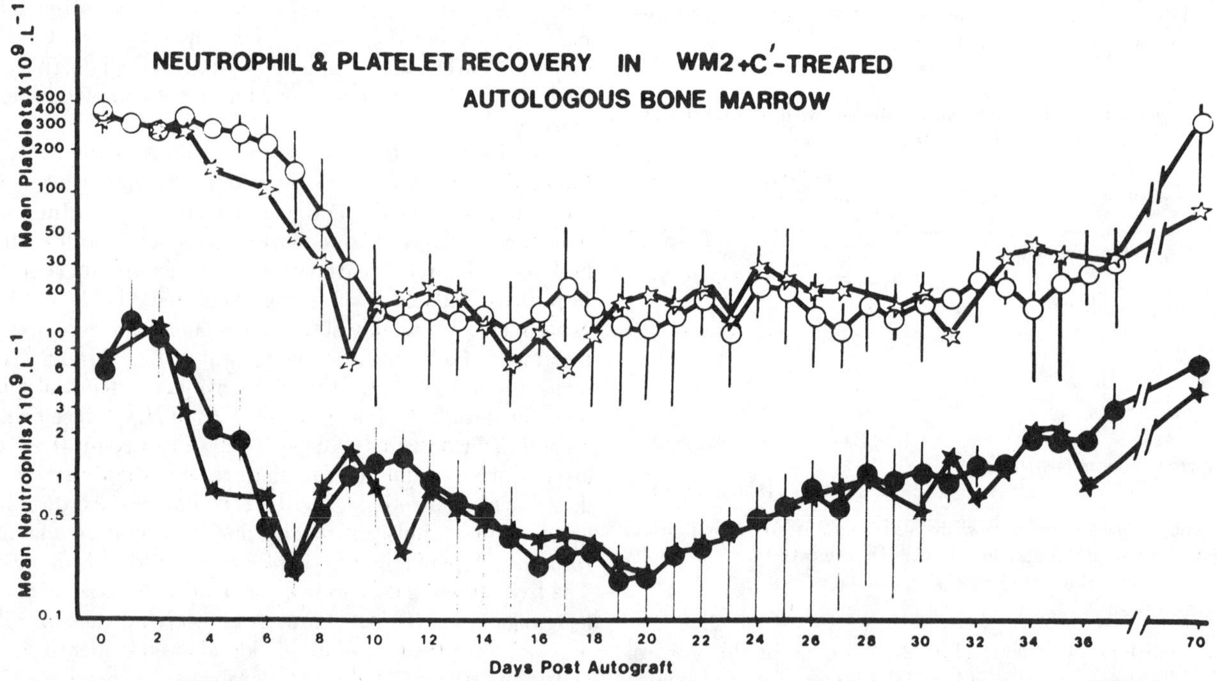

FIGURE 3. Neutrophil and platelet counts following total-body irradiation and marrow transplantation with WM-2-plus-complement–treated cells. Dogs were treated with 5 Gy TBI and one treatment of cells (○) platelets, (●) neutrophils (group D), or with 7.5 Gy TBI or 2 cell treatments (☆) platelets, (★) neutrophils (group E). Symbols represent mean of absolute counts; vertical bars indicate range of values.

The dog given 5 Gy and 4×10^7 cells/kg. showed early neutrophil recovery at day 10, but died with only partial engraftment at day 27 (data not shown). The 2 dogs treated with 7.5 Gy and cell doses of 22×10^7/kg and 12×10^7/kg showed similar recovery patterns to group D dogs, and both became long-term survivors.

Immunofluorescence studies carried out to evaluate the efficiency of Ia depletion in group E dogs demonstrated complete removal of WM-2^+ cells after 2 antibody-complement treatment (Table 3). In 2 further experiments, marrow was incubated with two treatment cycles of WM-2 plus complement,

TABLE 3. Analysis of Ia-positive marrow cells before and after WM-2-complement treatment

Dog No.	Radiation dose (Gy)	No. of treatment cycles[a]	Percentage of Ia-pos. cells[b]	
			Pretreatment	Posttreatment
1	5.0	1	ND[c]	ND
2	5.0	1	21	3
3	5.0	1	ND	ND
4	5.0	1	ND	ND
5	5.0	1	11	0
6	5.0	1	ND	ND
7	5.0	1	2	0
8	5.0	1	7	0
9	5.0	2	4	0
10	7.5	2	9	0
11	7.5	2	10	0

[a] Number of marrow treatments with monoclonal antibody and complement.

[b] Percentage of cells reactive with antibody WM-2, determined by indirect immunofluorescence before and after antibody-complement treatment.

[c] (ND) not done.

TABLE 4. Analysis of efficiency of removal of bone marrow Ia positive cells

Antibody	Percentage of Ia-positive bone marrow cells[a]			
	Pretreatment[b]		Posttreatment[b]	
	Dog 1	Dog 2	Dog 1	Dog 2
WM-21[c]	<1	<1	<1	<1
WM-2	6	4	<1	<1
CA-135	8	3	<1	<1
7.2	7	8	<1	<1
ISCR-3	26	26	<1	<1

[a] Canine mononuclear bone marrow cells in each case washed, incubated with monoclonal antibody, washed, and incubated with GAM-FITC, prior to analysis by fluorescence microscopy.

[b] Bone marrow cells stained by indirect immunofluorescence with one of the panel of antibodies, before or after 2 incubation cycles ex-vivo with WM-2 and complement.

[c] Control antibody WM-21, reactive with human CALLA, but unreactive with canine cells.

and re-stained with one of a panel of antibodies plus GAM-FITC (Table 4). Before treatment, the percentages of marrow cells labeled by WM-2, CA-135, and 7.2 were similar for both marrows; ISCR-3 antibody, however, labeled a greater proportion of cells at higher fluorescence intensity. However, after two cycles of WM-2 plus complement, no residual p28,33-positive cells could be detected using any of the above 4 antibodies.

DISCUSSION

This study documents the effect of two cytolytic monoclonal antibodies on the engraftment potential of canine bone marrow cells, as judged by in vitro clonal assays and by in vivo hemopoietic regeneration in irradiated animals. Monoclonal antibody WM-2, reactive with human p28,33 antigens, crossreacts with canine Ia-like antigens, as has been demonstrated with antibodies 7.2 and ISCR-3 (*20, 21*). Unlike the CFU_{GM} of the marmoset (*14*) and man (*3–6*), we have shown that the canine CFU_{GM} is not inhibited by cytolytic anti-Ia antibody. It is unlikely that this is a technical artefact related to the conditions of antibody-mediated cytotoxicity. WM-2 markedly inhibits the growth of human CFU_{GM} using similar culture conditions (data not shown), while WMD-1 similarly abolishes canine CFU_{GM} growth. The relative mature progenitor cells committed to the granulocyte-macrophage lineage in the dog are therefore predominantly Ia-negative. We have been unable to perform clonal assays for the canine equivalent of human CFU_{GEMM} to determine the Ia status of earlier multipotential myeloid stem cells.

Autologous transplantation experiments using Ia-depleted bone marrow showed a complex pattern of hemopoietic regeneration, with three components based on the peripheral blood neutrophil counts. After the initial nadir, a prompt rise in neutrophils was seen in all animals receiving Ia-treated marrow, similar to that seen in complement-only controls. It is tempting to equate this early, self-limited engraftment peak with the Ia-negative status of the canine CFU_{GM}. It is recognized that CFU_{GM} is a stem cell relatively late in maturation, capable of only a limited number of divisions before maturing into functional end-stage leukocytes, and having only limited self-replication capacity (*28*). It is pertinent that this initial peak was not observed in irradiated animals given no marrow rescue or marrow treated with the CFU_{GM}-reactive monoclonal antibody WMD-1. It has been demonstrated that the Thy-1 antigen is present on rat pluripotential stem cells (CFU_S) (*29*). Since the tissue distribution of canine Thy-1 is very similar to that seen in the rat (*30*) the failure of engraftment of WMD-1-treated marrow may be due to the expression of Thy-1 on canine hemopoietic stem cells as well as CFU_{GM}.

An alternative explanation for the failure of engraftment of WMD-1-treated marrow might be removal of an accessory T lymphocyte population, rather than a direct effect on stem cells. It should be noted, however, that Vriesendorp and coworkers have shown prompt marrow reconstitution following autologous transplantation of marrow enriched for CFU_{GM} and depleted of T cells by gradient separation, implying that T cells are not essential for engraftment (*31*). Final resolution of the question must await development of antibodies fully specific for dog T cells.

The second phase, seen in all dogs receiving Ia-treated marrow, was a second nadir in neutrophil counts in the second and third weeks, accompanied by persistent thrombocytopenia. It is clear that this was due to removal of a stem cell or accessory population expressing Ia antigens, as this second nadir phenomenon was not observed in the complement control group. As noted above, we were unable to further investigate this effect in vitro by analysis of pre-CFU_{GM} progenitor cells.

The final phase seen in the groups of dogs receiving Ia-treated marrow was slow but complete bone marrow recovery. This phenomenon was cell-dose-dependent, as all dogs receiving Ia-depleted marrow inocula with cell counts less than 5×10^7/kg died in the second nadir phase with minimal evidence of engraftment. The origin of the stem cells responsible for the final marrow regeneration cannot, of course, be finally determined in autografting experiments. It is possible that these stem cells either escaped the ex vivo antibody-complement treatment, or survived the effects of radiotherapy. However, for the reasons discussed below, we think that it is probable that regeneration occurred from true Ia-negative stem cells.

It is unlikely that the long-term marrow recovery in these dogs receiving Ia-depleted marrow was due to a suboptimal dose of TBI. The LD_{50} for the bone marrow syndrome in dogs has been previously established to be between 2.7 and 3.7 Gy using dose rates lower than those employed in this study (*31, 32*). Animals irradiated with 5.0 Gy without marrow rescue all died of bone marrow failure (*31, 33*). In this study, all 4 dogs irradiated with 5 Gy and given no rescue died. It is possible, of course, that if these dogs had survived longer, some reconstitution of hemopoiesis might have occurred, but this hypothesis is untestable with existing supportive measures. A 50% increase in TBI to 7.5 Gy did not alter the pattern of engraftment seen in dogs receiving Ia-treated marrow. We cannot completely exclude the possibility that some undefined factor present in these Ia-depleted marrows may have stimulated the regrowth of stem cells surviving the radiotherapy, but note that this effect could not have occurred with WMD-1-treated marrows. In other experiments, we have found that a further increase in dose to 9 Gy given at a dose rate of 0.55 Gy/min resulted in death due to lethal gastrointestinal syndrome (data not shown), despite supportive measures, precluding further testing at this dose level. Taken together, these data indicate that the 5.0 Gy and 7.5 Gy TBI doses used in our study lie between the LD_{100} for bone marrow and gastrointestinal syndromes, and are capable of ablating hemopoiesis in all animals.

An alternative explanation for permanent engraftment of dogs receiving Ia-treated marrow is inadequate antibody-complement lysis ex vivo. However, our results suggest that this is unlikely. First, one lytic cycle of WM-2 was sufficient to remove all detectable Ia^+ cells in 3 of 4 animals. Second, marrow engraftment was effectively abolished in dogs given marrow treated with one cycle of WMD-1 antibody, and completely inhibited after two WMD-1 cycles. Third, engraftment occurred in 2 dogs receiving cells treated with 2 lytic cyles of WM-2 and complement. Under these conditions, Ia-positive cells were undetectable by immunofluorescence using a panel of independent anti-Ia antibodies, including ISCR-3, which shows significantly higher binding affinity to dog cells than the other antibodies used. The term *Ia-negative* is, of course, an operational one, and may not indicate a complete absence of Ia antigens. It is possible that some cells may still express low levels of Ia, but below the detection limits of immunofluorescence and complement-mediated lysis. Our results imply that the vast majority of Ia-positive cells was removed by WM-2 cytolytic treatment. Finally, using complement of high lytic activity in adequate concentrations, other investigators have shown that 2 lytic treatment cycles are sufficient to eradicate detectable antibody-coated cells from marrow suspensions (*34*).

We therefore favor the explanation that a subpopulation of primitive stem cells in the dog is Ia-negative, and capable of repopulating the marrow in irradiated dogs after ex vivo depletion by anti-Ia antibody. Our findings are in agreement with previous related studies in mice (*13*) and the common marmoset (*14*). In the latter study, bone marrow treated with two cytolytic anti-Ia antibodies promptly engrafted in all recipients, with 2 of 4 animals becoming long-term survivors. Although no differences in regeneration patterns between control and Ia-treated animals were seen, blood counts were done at relatively infrequent intervals, and transient nadirs may not have been detected.

In our group of dogs receiving Ia-depleted marrow, we believe that the second phase of pancytopenia seen in the third and fourth weeks posttransplant was due to depletion of an Ia-positive stem cell population. The delay in peripheral blood recovery presumably reflected the time taken for regeneration of the depleted stem cell compartment by surviving Ia-negative cells. This delay may have been simply a dosage effect related to the gross depletion of Ia-positive stem cells. Alternatively, it is possible that stem cells at various levels of maturation differ in Ia expression, with Ia being absent on the most primitive resting cells, and acquired as stem cells are recruited into active proliferation and maturation.

In support of the latter hypothesis, Broxmeyer and coworkers have reported on further characteristics of human myeloid progenitor cells (*35, 36*). The majority of human CFU_{GM} and CFU_{GEMM} were demonstrated to be Ia-positive, engaged in active DNA synthesis, and sensitive to inhibition by acidic isoferritins. However, a subpopulation of both CFU_{GM} and CFU_{GEMM} were noted to be Ia-negative, not in active cell cycle, and insensitive to isoferritins. Hemopoietic stem cells are therefore heterogeneous with respect to a number of properties, including proliferative activity and self-renewal capacity, and Ia antigen may function as a receptor for inhibitory feedback mechanisms on proliferating cells. We therefore hypothesize that the stem cells escaping cytolytic treatment with anti-Ia antibody in our study were the resting, nonproliferative fraction of progenitor cells not expressing Ia antigens; when transplanted into irradiated animals, however, these resting cells were induced into a state of self-replication and subsequent differentiation. Further studies of Ia depletion of allogeneic cells bearing a chromosomal marker will be required to confirm this hypothesis.

Acknowledgments. We are indebted to Dr. G. Stewart for this critical review of the manuscript, and to Mrs. C. Dorrington for expert secretarial assistance.

REFERENCES

1. Thomas DW, Yamashita U, Shevach EM. The role of Ia antigens in T cell activation. Immunol Rev 1977; 35: 97.
2. Winchester RJ, Kunkel HG. The human Ia system. Adv Immunol 1979; 28: 221.
3. Kaplan J, Inoue S, Ottenbreit MJ. Myeloid colony-forming cells express human B lymphocyte antigens. Nature 1978; 271: 458.
4. Fitchen JH, Ferrone S, Quaranta V, et al. Monoclonal antibodies to HLA-A,B and Ia-like antigens inhibit colony formation by human myeloid progenitor cells. J Immunol 1980; 125: 2004.
5. Levine MN, Fay JW, Jones NH, et al. Phenotypic characterization of human bone marrow granulocyte-macrophage forming progenitor cells. Blood 1981; 58: 1047.
6. Goldman JM, Hibbin J, Kearney L, et al. HLA-DR monoclonal antibodies inhibit the proliferation of normal and chronic granulocytic leukaemia myeloid progenitor cells. Br J Haematol 1982; 52: 411.
7. Robinson J, Sieff C, Delia D, et al. Expression of cell-surface HLA-DR, HLA-ABC and glycophorin during erythroid differentiation. Nature 1981; 289: 68.
8. Torok-Storb B, Hansen JA. Modulation of in vitro BFU-e growth by normal Ia positive T cells is restricted by HLA-DR. Nature 1982; 298: 473.
9. Belzer MB, Fitchen JH, Ferrone S, et al. Expression of Ia-like antigen on human erythroid progenitor cells as determined by monoclonal antibodies and heteroantiserum to Ia-like antigens. Clin Immunol Immunopathol 1981; 20: 111.
10. Falkenberg JHF, Jansen J, van der Vaart-Duinkerken N, et al. Polymorphic and monomorphic HLA-DR determinants on human hematopoietic progenitor cells. Blood 1984; 63: 1125.
11. Fitchen JH, Le Fevre C, Ferrone S, Cline MJ. Expression of Ia-like and HLA-A,B antigens on human multipotential hematopoietic progenitor cells. Blood 1982; 59: 188.
12. Bodger MP, Izaguirre CA, Blacklock HA, et al. Surface antigenic

determinants on human pluripotent and unipotent hematopoietic progenitor cells. Blood 1983; 61: 1006.
13. Basch RS, Janossy G, Greaves MF. Murine pluripotential stem cells lack Ia antigen. Nature 1977; 270: 520.
14. Hetherington CM, Crawford DH, Blacklock HA, et al. Successful bone marrow transplantation with whole marrow and CFU[c] depleted marrow in the marmoset (Callithrix jacchus). In: Touraine JL, Gluckman E, Griscelli C, eds. Bone marrow transplantation in Europe II. Excerpta Medica 1981; 274.
15. Moore MA, Broxmeyer HE, Sheridan AP, et al. Continuous human bone marrow culture: Ia antigen characterization of probable pluripotential stem cells. Blood 1980; 55: 682.
16. Keating A, Powell J, Takahashi M, Singer JW. The generation of long-term marrow cultures from marrow depleted of Ia (HLA-DR) positive cells. Blood 1984; 64: 1159.
17. Kohler G, Milstein C. Continuous cultures of fused cells secreting antibody of predefined specificity. Nature 1975; 256: 495.
18. Fazekas de St Groth S, Scheidegger D. Production of monoclonal antibodies: strategy and tactics. J Immunol Methods 1980; 35: 1.
19. Hansen JA, Martin PJ, Nowinski RC. Monoclonal antibodies identifying a novel T-cell antigen and Ia antigens of human lymphocytes. Immunogenetics 1980; 10: 247.
20. Deeg HJ, Wulff JC, De Rose S, et al. Unusual distribution of Ia-like antigens on canine lymphocytes. Immunogenetics 1982; 16: 445.
21. Charron DJ, McDevitt HO. Characterization of HLA-D region antigens by two-dimensional gel electrophoresis. J Exp Med 1980; 152: 18.
22. Watanabe M, Suzuki T, Taniguchi M, Shinohara N. Monoclonal anti-Ia murine alloantibodies cross-reactive with the Ia-homologues of other mammalian species including humans. Transplantation 1983; 36: 712.
23. Janossy G, Bollum FJ, Bradstock KF, et al. Terminal transferase positive human bone marrow cells exhibit the antigenic phenotype of common acute lymphoblastic leukaemia. J Immunol 1979; 123: 1525.
24. Bradstock KF, Favaloro EJ, Kabral A, et al. Standardization of monoclonal antibodies for use in autologous bone marrow transplantation for common acute lymphoblastic leukemia. Pathology, in press.
25. Pike BL, Robinson A. Human bone marrow colony growth in agar-gel. J Cell Physiol 1970; 76: 77.
26. Berndt MC, Gregory C, Chong BH, et al. Additional glycoprotein defects in Bernard-Soulier syndrome: confirmation of genetic basis by parental analysis. Blood 1983; 62: 800.
27. Prendergast MM, Bradstock KF, Grimsley P, et al. Membrane antigens of canine lymphocytes and haemopoietic cells defined by monoclonal antibodies. Manuscript in preparation.
28. Quesenberg P, Levitt L. Hematopoietic stem cells. N Engl J Med 1979; 301: 755.
29. Goldschneider I, Metalf D, Battye F, Mandel T. Analysis of rat haemopoietic cells on the fluorescence-activated cell sorter. I. Isolation of pluipotent haemopoietic stem cells and granulocyte-macrophage progenitor cells. J Exp Med 1980: 182: 419.
30. McKenzie SL, Fabre JW. Studies with a monoclonal antibody on the distribution of Thy-1 in the lymphoid and extracellular connective tissues of the dog. Transplantation 1981; 31: 275.
31. Vriesendorp HM, Klapwyk WM, Heidt PJ, et al. Factors controlling the engraftment of transplanted dog bone marrow cells. Tissue Antigens 1982; 20: 63.
32. Morris WP, Fritz TE, Rehfeld CE, Poole CM. The response of the beagle dog to Cobalt-60 gamma radiation: determination of the LD50 and description of associated changes. Radiat Res 1968; 35: 681.
33. Thomas ED, Le Blond R, Graham T, et al. Marrow infusions in dogs given midlethal or lethal irradiation. Radiat Res 1970; 41: 113.
34. Prentice HG, Blacklock HA, Janossy G, et al. Depletion of T lymphocytes in donor marrow prevents significant graft-versus-host disease in matched allogeneic leukaemic marrow transplant recipients. Lancet 1984; 1: 472.
35. Broxmeyer HE. Relationship of cell-cycle expression of Ia-like antigenic determination on normal and leukaemia human granulocyte-macrophage progenitor cells to regulation in vitro by acidic isoferritins. J Clin Invest 1982; 69: 632.
36. Lu L, Broxymeyer ME, Meyers PA, et al. Association of cell cycle expression of Ia-like antigenic determinants on normal human multipotential (CFU^{GEMM}) and erythroid (BFU^{E}) progenitor cells with regulation in vitro by acidic isoferritins. Blood 1983; 61: 250.

Received 14 May 1985.
Accepted 10 August 1985.

0041-1337/86/4105-0572$02.00/0
TRANSPLANTATION

Vol. 41, No. 5
Printed in U.S.A.

MONOCLONAL ANTIBODY THERAPY

ANTI-IDIOTYPIC AND NON-ANTI-IDIOTYPIC ANTIBODIES TO OKT3 ARISING DESPITE INTENSE IMMUNOSUPPRESSION[1]

GREGORY J. JAFFERS, THOMAS C. FULLER, A. BENEDICT COSIMI, PAUL S. RUSSELL, HENRY J. WINN, AND ROBERT B. COLVIN[2]

Transplantation-Immunology and Immunopathology Units, Departments of Surgery and Pathology, Massachusetts General Hospital and Harvard Medical School, Boston, Massachusetts 02114

The frequency, timing, and specificity of the humoral antibody response to a murine monoclonal antibody (OKT3, IgG_{2a}) were measured in 21 consecutive renal allograft recipients. These patients received i.v. OKT3, 1–5 mg/day for 10–20 days as treatment for acute graft rejection. Maintenance immunosuppression consisted of azathioprine and corticosteroids. Using three different assays, an antibody response was detected in 75% of the 20 patients with adequate samples. The ELISA assay of the overall IgM and IgG reactivity to OKT3 revealed that IgM anti-OKT3 appeared in 65% and IgG anti-OKT3 in 50% of the patients, reaching a peak 20–33 days after the last dose of OKT3. The IgM preceeded the IgG in most cases ($P<0.02$) and in 8 cases was detected during therapy. One patient had high levels of IgM anti-OKT3 before therapy, yet responded normally to OKT3. Interference with the therapeutic effectiveness was evident in one patient who developed IgG antibodies during therapy. His serum blocked the binding of F-OKT3 to normal lymphocytes in the presence of normal BALB/c serum. The blocking assay, done by flow cytometry, measured anti-idiotypic (Id) reactivity since the sera did not affect the binding of OKT8 (another IgG_{2a}) or anti-Leu4 (another anti-T3), and the blocking activity remained after affinity absorption with normal mouse IgG. Using this assay, 60% of the pateints made an anti-Id response. One made only anti-Id, and several had anti-Id at times when other reactivities were undetectable. Antibodies to non-idiotypic, presumably isotypic, determinants represented on OKT8 occurred in only 44%, while other reactivity (OKT4; $IgG_{2b}\kappa$) was less common (12%) and weaker.

While no adverse allergic reactions occurred in this group of patients, the anit-Id antibodies, which are a prominent feature of the immune response to this and probably other monoclonal antibodies, can block their therapeutic effectiveness and can arise despite intense immunosuppression. This response may require the use of different idiotypes for prolonged or repeated courses of therapy and may be the major obstacle to the use of human monoclonal antibodies.

The parenteral administration of foreign serum proteins has been known since the early days of serotherapy to stimulate an immune response. The typical allergic manifestations include fever, skin rash, anaphylaxis, and serum sickness. This phenomenon has acquired new relevance with the application of murine hybridoma-derived antibodies to clinical medicine. Despite some initial optimism, the injection of these murine proteins into man, as expected, regularly provokes an immune response by the host (*1–11*).

We have had extensive experience with the use of one monoclonal antibody, OKT3 ($IgG_{2a}\kappa$, BALB/c), used as an adjuvant to azathioprine and prednisone for treatment of acute renal allograft rejection (*1, 2, 11*). This antibody, reactive with an invariant component (T3)* of the T cell antigen receptor complex (*12*), has proved to be dramatically effective in reversing acute cellular rejection when administered at doses of 1–5 mg/day over 10–20 days. This report describes in detail the specificity of the antibody response to OKT3 in 21 renal allograft recipients, and the implications for therapy. A preliminary report of the first 11 patients has been presented (*6, 7*).

MATERIALS AND METHODS

Patients. The 21 consecutive OKT3-treated patients studied were initially treated with prednisone and azathioprine after receiving a cadaver donor renal allograft (*1, 2*). They were given OKT3 (Ortho Pharmaceuticals, Raritan, NJ) when they had their first episode of renal allograft rejection. The antibody was given once daily as a 1–5-mg i.v. bolus. No patient manifested a skin reaction to intradermal OKT3 (0.1 μg) prior to treatment. In an attempt to modify the immune response to OKT3, 6 patients also received cyclophosphamide (patients Nos. 10 and 17–21).

Serum samples. Blood samples were collected in acid-citrate-dextrose (ACD) at least twice weekly beginning at the time of transplantation and continuing for up to ten months after OKT3 therapy. An average of 19 samples per patient were analyzed in 20 patients (range 12–24). One patient (No. 3) had only 3 posttreatment samples (all negative) and therefore was not included in further analysis. The samples were centrifuged at 1500 rpm and the plasma was stored at −20°C. Peripheral blood lymphocytes from these samples were used for immunologic monitoring as described previously (*1*).

Enzyme-linked immunosorbent assay (ELISA). This assay, performed by a slight modification of published methods (*13*), was used to detect both anti-Id and non-anti-Id anti-OKT3 antibodies. Polyvinyl vinyl plastic microtiter plates (Imulon I,

[1] This work was supported by USPHS Grant HL-18646 and by funds provided by the Ortho Pharmaceutical Corporation.

[2] Reprint requests should be addressed to R.B. Colvin, M.D., Immunopathology Unit, Department of Pathology, Massachusetts General Hospital, Boston, MA 02114.

* Abbreviations used: ACD, acid citrate dextrose; CAF_1, (BALB/c×A/J)F_1; ELISA, enzyme-linked immunosorbent assay; F-, fluorescein-conjugated (e.g., F-OKT3); Id, idiotype; MFC, median fluorescence channel; PBS, phosphate-buffered saline; PHA, phytohemagglutinin; T3, the 20–25 kilodalton surface antigen of mature T cells.

Dynatech, Alexandria, VA) were coated with 1 μg/ml of purified parenteral grade OKT3, 0.05 M $NaHCO_3$ buffer (pH 9.6). The plates were incubated overnight at 4°C then washed with phosphate-buffered saline containing .05% (v/v) Tween-20 (0.01 Na phosphate, 0.14 M NaCl, (pH 7.4) (PBS-Tween). Each serum sample was diluted 1:240 in PBS-Tween (5 μl/1.2 ml buffer). 200 μl of this mixture was added to the wells. The plates were incubated for 2 hr at room temperature, washed with PBS-Tween, and 200 μl of a 1:500 dilution of alkaline-phosphatase-conjugated goat antihuman IgG (Kirkegaard-Perry, Gaithersberg, MD)—or goat antihuman IgM (both heavy chain specific) was added at a similar concentration. Anti-IgG with light chain reactivity was used in early studies as a screening test. These solutions were incubated for 2 hr at room temperature and washed again using PBS-Tween. Finally, 200 μl of 1 mg/ml p-nitrophenyl phosphate in 10% diethanolamine was added. The resultant color change of substrate was read on an ELISA plate spectrophotometer (Bio-Tek Instruments) at 405 nM. Sera from 15 healthy volunteers and assays without OKT3, serum, or anti-Ig were used as controls. All assays were done in triplicate. Each daily run was standardized by running aliquots of a known postive control. This serum had a net OD_{405} (test-blank) of about 650 and 70 for the IgG and IgM assays, respectively. Standardized values for IgG were obtained by multiplying the net OD_{405} of the test sample by 650/(OD_{405} of standard) on that day (or 70/OD_{405} of standard for IgM). A sample was considered positive if the corrected OD_{405} was 2 SD above the mean of the controls (95th percentile) in the case of the pretreatment samples, or if the OD_{405} was more than double the pretreatment OD_{405} in the case of subsequent samples (provided the OD_{405} was >100).

PHA blast preparation. The preparation of phytohemagglutinin (PHA)-stimulated T cell blasts was accomplished by methods previously described (*14*). Briefly, normal peripheral mononuclear cells were isolated on Ficoll-Hypaque gradients and stimulated with 1 μg of PHA per 10^6 lymphocytes in 1 ml of RPMI 1640 medium containing 5% normal human serum, antibiotics, and 5 μM mercaptoethanol. Cells were maintained by dilution to 10^5/ml in T cell growth factor medium containing interleukin-2 about every third day.

Enhancing assay for non-Anti-Id antibodies. Using flow cytometry, non-anti-Id human antibodies that included isotype-specific reactivity to murine IgG_{2a} were detected by the binding to OKT8-coated ($IgG_{2a}\kappa$,CAF_1) PHA blasts. Antibodies not specific for Id or isotype were similarly measured with OKT4-coated ($IgG_{2b}\kappa$,CAF_1) targets. OKT3-coated targets were used as a positive control. PHA blasts (which contained both $T3^+T4^+$ and $T3^+T8^+$ cells) were suspended at a concentration of 10^6/ml in RPMI 1640. Nonfluoresceinated OKT8, OKT4, or OKT3 (0.5 μg) or PBS was added to each tube containing 50 μl of PHA blasts. The suspensions were incubated at 4°C for 30 min and washed twice with PBS. 50 μl of test or normal serum was added and the mixture incubated and washed as before. Fluoresceinated goat antihuman IgG (heavy and light chain reactive) was then added and the tubes were incubated and washed as before. The median intensity of the positive staining was evaluated using the Spectrum III flow cytometer (Ortho Diagnostics System, Westwood, MA) (*15*). The percentage of increase in the median fluorescence channel (MFC, linear units) above uncoated blasts (no monoclonal antibody) for each sample was calculated. This corrects for any contribution by anti-T-cell antibodies that may be present in the patient's serum, e.g., anti-HLA. Positive values were defined as 2 SD units above the mean of 21 normals.

Affinity columns. OKT3 and normal mouse IgG (Miles) were coupled to CNBr-activated Sepharose 4B (Pharmacia) by standard techniques, with approximately 10 mg of protein/ml swollen gel. Columns were 12×0.9 cm (mouse IgG) and 4.5×0.9 cm (OKT3). Fractions were eluted in PBS and then 3M KSCN, dialyzed, and reconcentrated to the starting volume by positive pressure filtration (Amicon XM-50).

Anti-idiotype (Id) assay. The basis of this assay is that certain anti-Id block the binding of the Id-bearing antibody with antigen. The test was done by flow cytometry using fluoresceinated OKT3 (F-OKT3) as the Id and $T3^+$ T cell blasts (or normal peripheral blood lymphocytes) as the antigen in the presence of the test serum. Normal BALB/c mouse serum was added to block non-anti-Id antibodies. The controls included normal human serum and fluoresceinated OKT8 (F-OKT8). The amount of F-OKT3 required to saturate PHA blasts or peripheral lymphocytes was determined by titration with a constant number of cells, plotting the MFC-vs.-concentration of F-OKT3 used (Fig. 1). Saturation was achieved at 8 μg/ml of F-OKT3; beyond this point no further shift in the MFC was achieved. A point of about 30% saturation was selected (2.5 μg/ml) for use in the assays to maximize sensitivity. A similar point was determined for F-OKT8.

The assay was performed by adding 25 μl of test or normal serum to 20 μl of BALB/c serum and incubating for 30 min at room temperature. Subsaturating amounts of F-OKT3 or F-OKT8 were added and these were incubated for 30 min on ice. Normal buffy coat peripheral blood lymphocytes (25 μl), previously prepared from ACD blood, were added to each tube with further incubation for 30 min at 4°C. Residual erythrocytes were lysed with NH_4Cl and the cells were washed twice in PBS. Samples were analyzed using the Spectrum III flow cytometer gated on the lymphocyte or lymphoblast cluster. The MFC of the positive cells above the positive threshold channel was taken as the index of staining intensity. Pretreatment samples had inhibition of 7±7%. Therefore a decrease in the MFC of greater than 20% of the normal serum control, provided there was not a concommitant inhibition of F-OKT8, was taken as evidence for the presence of anti-Id antibody. Samples

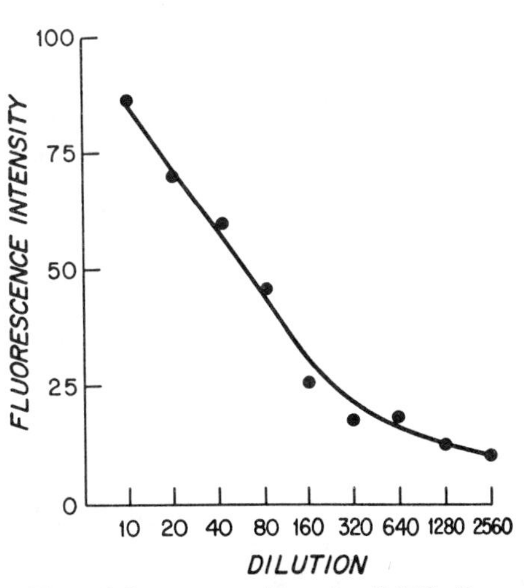

FIGURE 1. Plot of fluorescence intensity (MFC, linear units) vs. dilution of F-OKT3 on PHA lymphoblasts. A point of about 30% saturation was selected for the anti-Id inhibition assay.

containing no BALB/c serum were analyzed in parallel. F-anti-Leu 4 (Becton Dickinson Monoclonal Center, Mountain View, CA) was used for comparison.

Statistical analysis. Values given are mean ± SD unless otherwise noted. Student's *t* and Fisher's exact tests were used for evaluating statistical significance. An antibody response was considered positive if two or more sample values were above the defined threshold, either a doubling of the pretreatment value or above the 95th percentile of normal controls.

RESULTS

ELISA: total Anti-OKT3 response. Using the ELISA with OKT3 as the antigen, the IgG and IgM antibodies of all specificities to OKT3 were determined. Except for patient No. 18, the ELISA reactivity of the patient's pretreatment serum was similar to that of the 15 controls, both for IgG and for IgM (Table 1) and the anti-Ig with light chain reactivity gave essentially the same result as anti-γ chain.

Patient No. 18 had the highest pretreatment reactivity, which was exclusively IgM. This binding could be completely eliminated by preincubation of the test serum with BALB/c serum, and partially blocked with preincubation in normal goat serum. A rheumatoid factor assay with human IgG was within normal limits (<60 I.U.). The level of the IgM antimouse IgG antibody did not change by more than 5% during treatment, and the patient responded normally to the OKT3 therapy (Table 2).

An anti-OKT3 antibody response, defined as doubling of the pretreatment OD_{405}, was detectable at various times posttreatment in 14 (70%) of those individuals (Tables 2 and 3). Four had only IgM and one had only IgG. The IgG was detected significantly later than the IgM by an average of 10 days, although the time of the peak level was the same (20–23 days) (Tables 2–4). Antibodies were detected during OKT3 administration in 8 patients. All 8 had IgM antibodies and 2 also had IgG. Only one patient (No. 4), who had IgG as well as IgM anti-OKT3, showed resistance to the pharmacologic effects of OKT3. The other 7 cleared their T cells normally despite the presence of IgM anti-OKT3. Only 10% (IgG) and 33% (IgM) of the responders had persistent antibodies when checked 6 weeks or longer after the last dose. Two had detectable levels 14 weeks posttherapy (Nos. 7, 15).

Enhancing assay. This assay was used to detect isotype and light chain reactivity by assaying $T8^+$ and $T4^+$ PHA blasts coated with OKT8, OKT4, or OKT3 antibodies. Three patients (Nos. 10, 12, and 14) had pretreatment reactivity above the 95th percentile (Tables 1 and 2). Of the 16 tested, 7 (44%) showed a two-fold or greater increase in reactivity to OKT8 ($IgG_{2a}\kappa$)-coated cells. Only two (12%) bound (both weakly) to OKT4 ($IgG_{2b}\kappa$)-coated cells, suggesting that the reactivity detected was primarily to isotype specificities on the heavy chain. The timing of the anti-isotype was closer to that of the IgM than the IgG (Table 4).

OKT8 and OKT3 enhancing reactivity were disparate in 2 patients. The serum from patient No. 1 reacted with OKT8 coated, but not OKT3 coated cells. She had blocking anti-Id antibodies and it is possible that these displaced the OKT3 from the target cell, giving a false negative. A similar phenomenon may explain the negative OKT3-enhancing results in patients Nos. 2 and 17 who also had blocking anti-Id. A second patient (No. 14) had the opposite pattern, reacting with OKT3-coated, but not OKT8-coated cells. The restricted reactivity in this case may have been due to anti-Id of the nonblocking type.

Blocking anti-Id assay. None of the pretreatment sera specifically blocked the binding of F-OKT3 or F-OKT8 to normal lymphocytes (Table 1). However, after the course of OKT3 therapy, 12 patients (60%) developed antibodies that selectively blocked the antigen-binding of F-OKT3. The sera blocked F-OKT3 in the presence of normal BALB/c serum and did not block F-OKT8 or F-anti-Leu 4, arguing that the specificity was restricted to idiotypic—and not allotypic or isotypic—determinants on OKT3 (Fig. 2).

TABLE 2. Onset of anti-OKT3 antibodies and effect on OKT3 response[a]

Patient	ELISA-OKT3		Blocking	Enhancing			Response to OKT3 (cells/mm³)[d]	
	IgG	IgM	Anti-Id	OKT3	OKT8	OKT4	T3	T4+T8
1	19	4	8	–[c]	8	–	3	153
2	15	−4	25	–	–	–	15	276
3[b]	–	–	–	–	–	–	7	402
4	0	−2	0	1	1	–	477	524
5	11	7	2	2	7	–	0	41
6	–	8	5	1	1	–	0	153
7	–	–	–	–	–	–	1	118
8	5	−3	2	2	2	–	3	191
9	6	−8	10	4	4	–	0	130
10	–	–	–	p–	p–	p–	5	56
11	1	28	–	–	–	45	5	80
12	–	–	–	p–	p–	–	0	34
13	–	2	2	2	2	72	1	392
14	31	−10	8	p3	p–	p–	16	379
15	−1	−5	–	–	–	–	23	242
16	–	–	–	–	–	–	4	129
17	–	–	14	–	–	–	17	436
18	10	p–	8				17	274
19	–	−10	–				30	231
20	–	−6	45				24	598
21	–	–	–				1	105

[a] The day when antibody was first detected (0 = last day of OKT3 therapy; negative numbers-days before therapy ended).

[b] Only 3 posttreatment samples.

[c] Abbreviations: p = pretreatment sample positive, >95th percentile of normal controls; – = negative; blank = not done.

[d] Last blood values on OKT3.

TABLE 1. Pretreatment reactivity

	ELISA (OD_{405})[a]			Enhancing assay (% increase)			Blocking assay (% inhibition)	
	Ig	IgG	IgM	OKT3	OKT8	OKT4	OKT3	OKT8
Patients	369±219	339±147	60±92	59±76	144±297	38±80	7±7	8±11
Controls	322±125		198±151	29±30	27±34	16±21		

[a] Excludes patient No. 18 whose values were 1384 (Ig), 118 (IgG), and 1718 (IgM) on the 3 ELISA assays. Ig was a screening test using goat antihuman immunoglobulin reactive to γ heavy chain and both light chains, while IgG and IgM were detected by heavy-chain-specific antisera.

TABLE 3. Maximum antibody level[a]

Patient	ELISA-OKT3: OD_{405}		Blocking:	Enhancing (% increase MFC)		
	IgG	IgM	Anti-Id (% Inhibition)	OKT3	OKT8	OKT4
1	634(19)	*596(59)*[b]	75(8)	–	1122(19)	–
2	1761(15)	142(75)	*89(25)*	–	–	–
3	–	–	–	–	–	–
4	1314(14)	460(5)	83(14)	358(1)	569(2)	–
5	1723(15)	226(10)	*91(12)*	489(7)	178(7)	–
6	–	*292(8)*	*92(14)*	1116(14)	1183(19)	–
7	–	–	–	–	–	–
8	1971(12)	5583(12)	*94(8)*	*640(22)*	200(22)	–
9	*782(10)*	881(10)	33(10)	*400(13)*	*263(13)*	–
10	–	–	–	–	–	–
11	599(39)	*608(45)*	–	–	–	94(52)
12	–	–	–	–	–	–
13	–	869(13)	89(2)	*1200(76)*	*1500(76)*	67(76)
14	900(55)	538(29)	55(14)	1067(3)	–	–
15	655(−1)	*385(−1)*	–	–	–	–
16	–	–	–	–	–	–
17	–	–	88(22)	–	–	–
18	865(30)	–	92(16)			
19	–	*597(0)*	–			
20		*199(45)*	58(45)			
21	–	–	–			

[a] Day of maximum (after OKT3 therapy ended) in parentheses.
[b] Assays in italics were positive in the last sample tested (more than 6 weeks from the last OKT3 dose).

TABLE 4. Summary of time course of antibody response

	Number	Onset[a]	Peak[a]
IgM	13	0±3[b]	23±7
IgG	10	10±3	20±5
Idiotype	12	11±4	16±3
Isotype	7	4±1	23±9

[a] Day after last OKT3 dose, mean ± SE.
[b] Preceeds IgG, $P<.02$.

Further experiments were performed to document whether the effect was indeed due to anti-Id antibodies. The presence of residual free OKT3 in the serum was ruled out by the lack of detectable mouse Ig on normal lymphocytes after incubation in the blocking serum. In all patients OKT3 antibody was undetectable in the serum by 2 days after therapy had ended (data not shown). For this reason only sera taken at least 48 hr after the end of therapy were analyzed (except for patient No. 4 who was demonstrated to clear the OKT3 within 7 hr). Serum that blocked OKT3 did not block F-anti-Leu 4, an IgG_1 antibody to a different epitope on the same molecule (Fig. 2). This argues strongly against free or complexed T3 antigen itself as a significant source of antigenic competition in the blocking assay.

Sera from two of the patients were analyzed by affinity chromatography using columns with immobilized OKT3 or normal mouse IgG. The sera from patients Nos. 4 (Fig. 2 and 3) and 8 (Figs. 4 and 5) were absorbed with mouse IgG on Sepharose. The effluent and the dialyzed 3M KSCN eluate were tested for blocking activity. The eluate from normal mouse IgG (patient No. 8, day 5) showed equivalent blocking of F-OKT3 and F-OKT8 of 88% and 83%, respectively, in the absence of BALB/c serum. The analogous eluate from patient No. 4 had no blocking activity. In contrast, the effluent blocked F-OKT3 completely but had little activity against F-OKT8, even in the absence of added BALB/c serum (Fig. 4). The effluent (patient No. 4) and the starting serum were then absorbed on an OKT3 column. This removed the blocking activity, which was undetectable even after reconcentration. Taken together, these data indicate that the blocking activity was due to antibodies that reacted selectively with OKT3 and not to other mouse immunoglobulins, satisfying the criteria for anti-Id specificity.

The time course of the anti-Id antibody production was variable, but generally paralleled that of the IgG (Table 4). The anti-Id antibodies first became detectable at an average of 11 days (range 0–45) after therapy had ended. The most rapid antibody response was manifested at 12 days after the start of therapy in patient No. 4 (Fig. 3). At this time he became refractory to the T lymphopenic effect of OKT3. The only clinical signs of an allergic reaction were an eosinophilia of 12% and a fever upon administration of the OKT3. No serum sickness lesions (glomerulonephritis, vasculitis, mouse Ig deposits by immunofluorescence) were seen in renal biopsy taken during the OKT3 treatment. The patient suffered no adverse systemic effects from this response, although the rejection process became reactivated and the allograft was eventually rejected. This was the only patient whose therapy was stopped because of anti-OKT3 antibodies. Three other patients had anti-Id antibody in the first sample analyzed, 2 days after therapy ended. Anti-Id antibody persisted in 33% of patients after 6 weeks; the longest documented was 6 months (No. 8).

Of the 12 patients that made a blocking anti-Id antibody, 3 (25%) had no IgG and 2 (17%) had no IgM reactivity detectable by ELISA. Similarly, 30% of those with blocking anti-Id had no isotype/light chain reactivity detectable by the enhancing assay. Patient No. 17 made exclusively an anti-Id response, detectable only in the blocking assay. Furthermore, the anti-Id assay detected antibody on one or more occasions in 7 other patients when the other assays were negative. This can be seen, for example, in the time course of the antibody response in patient No. 8 (Fig 4), in which the anti-Id response was persistently positive when the ELISA and enhancing assays were negative. Two patients (Nos. 11 and 15) made anti-OKT3 antibody detected on ELISA that did not block antigen binding or have reactivity to OKT8. These antibodies may include nonblocking anti-Id.

To estimate the portion of the antibody response that was anti-Id, serum from patient No. 8 at the peak of the antibody response (day 12, Fig. 4) was analyzed by ELISA using normal BALB/c serum as a competitive inhibitor for non-anti-Id antibodies. Normal mouse serum (100 μl) was able to block 69% of the IgG binding to OKT3, while 100% could be blocked by 10 μg OKT3, so that anti-Id constituted about 31% of the reactivity.

Correlations with clinical course. With the exception of the one patient (No. 4) who developed anti-Id antibodies that neutralized the in vivo effectiveness of OKT3, no adverse effects were associated with the antimouse Ig or anti-OKT3 idiotype response. The response to therapy and outcome of the graft were not correlated with the presence or absence of an antibody response. However, of the 6 patients who received cyclophosphamide (Nos. 10 and 17–21) only 17% made an IgG anti-OKT3 response detectable in ELISA, whereas 9 of 14 of

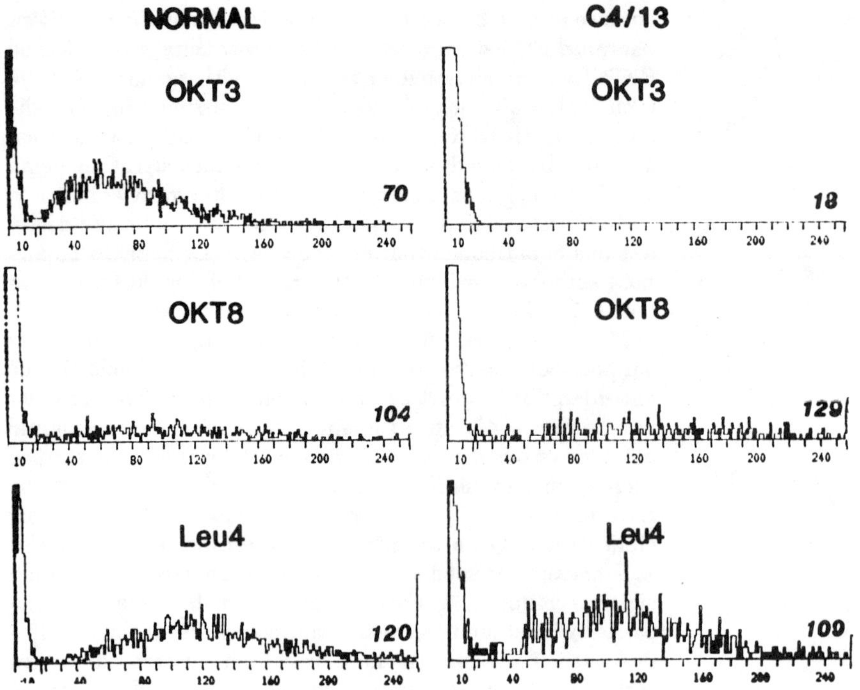

FIGURE 2. Fluorescence histograms of blocking anti-Id assay. Normal lymphocytes stained with fluoresceinated monoclonal antibodies in the presence of normal BALB/c serum and either normal human serum (left column) or serum from patient No. 4 (right column). The patient's serum blocks F-OKT3, but not F-OKT8 (both are IgG_{2a}) or F-anti-Leu 4 (IgGl, reactive to the T3 antigen). Cell number is on the y-axis and fluorescence intensity is on the x-axis. The number in the lower right of each histogram is the median fluorescence channel of the positive cells.

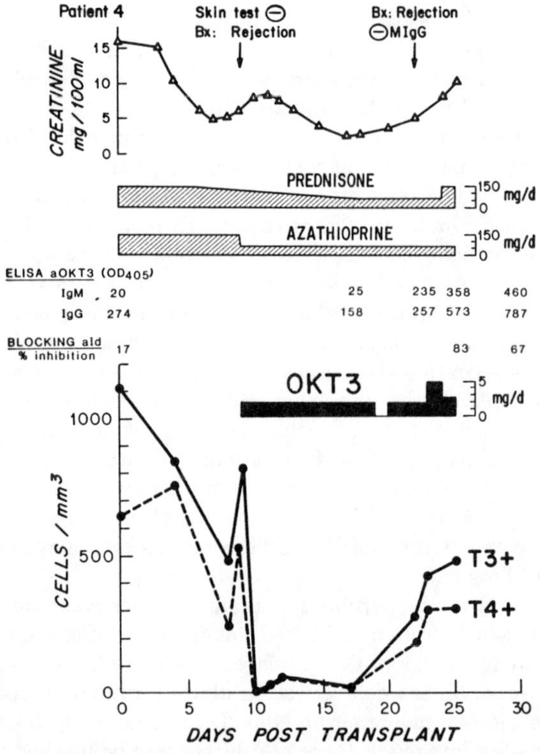

FIGURE 3. Clinical course of patient No. 4, who developed blocking anti-Id during therapy and became resistent to the T lymphopenic effects of OKT3. IgG and IgM anti-OKT3 was detected during therapy. Blocking anti-Id appearance was accompanied by resistance to the T lymphopenic response to OKT3 (day 22).

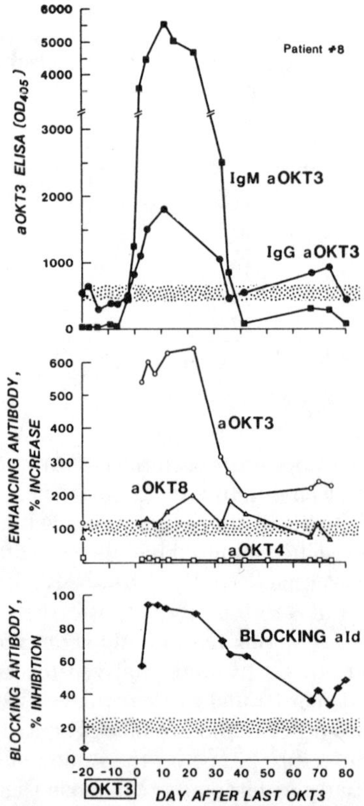

FIGURE 4. Time course of antibody response in patient No. 8, as detected by each assay in this study. The horizontal bar is the threshhold of positivity (2 SD above the mean of normals). Note the early rise of IgM and the presence of both blocking anti-Id and anti-isotype (OKT8 enhancing assay). No antibodies to OKT4 were detectable.

the non-cyclophosphamide group made such antibodies ($P<0.076$). Cyclophosphamide had little effect on the blocking anti-Id response, which still occurred in 50% of patients—although somewhat later than the others, peaking at 16–45 days. No correlation with the recipient's HLA phenotype and the antibody response was found.

DISCUSSION

In this series 60% of the patients treated with OKT3 developed anti-Id antibodies and 44% anti-isotypic antibodies, despite intense immunosuppressive treatment (Table 5). The

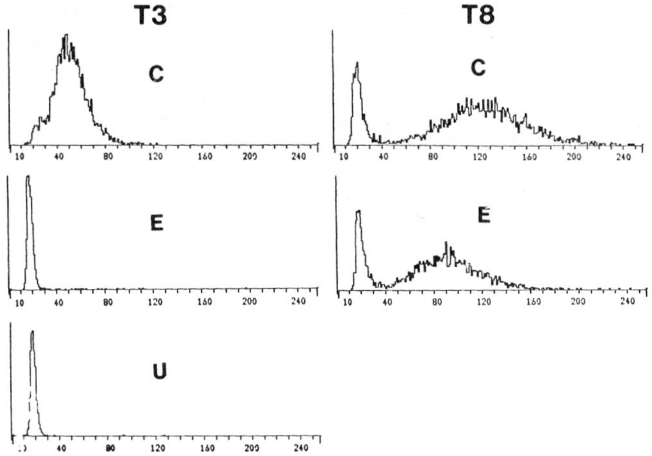

FIGURE 5. Blocking assay of the mouse IgG absorbed serum from patient No. 8, day 5. Fluorescence histograms of T cell blasts stained with F-OKT3 (T3) or F-OKT8 (T8) in the presence of the effluent (E) that passed through the mouse IgG column or the control (C) which was the ultrafiltrate of the effluent (passed through XM-50). (U) unstained cells. No BALB/c serum was added. The effluent completely blocks F-OKT3, in contrast to its slight inhibitory effect on F-OKT8.

TABLE 5. Summary of response pattern

N	Anti-OKT3 by ELISA	Blocking anti-Id	Antiisotype[a]
7	+	+	+
4	+	+	–
3	+	–	–
1	–	+	–
5	–	–	–

[a] Four patients were not tested for antiisotype.

response was transient and, with one exception, did not affect therapeutic outcome even though IgM antibodies frequently appeared before the completion of therapy.

A number of experiments indicated that these patients did make antibody with anti-Id specificity. The patient's serum blocked the antigen binding of OKT3, but not OKT8, a monoclonal of the same isotype, and the blocking occured even in the presence of BALB/c serum and after absorption with mouse immunoglobulin. These data indicate that the activity is specific for OKT3 and not due to reactivity with other mouse immunoglobulin. Three other possibilities for this blocking activity were considered: free OKT3 antibody, free T3 antigen, and autologous anti-T3 antibody (anti-anti-Id). Residual free OKT3, able to bind T3 antigen, was ruled out by the inability to detect mouse Ig binding to normal T cells by flow cytometry and the ability of OKT3 affinity columns to remove the activity. The presence of free T3 antigen was rendered unlikely by the inability of the test sera to block the binding of anti-Leu 4, a monoclonal antibody to a different epitope on the same antigen complex. Similarly, no inhibition was obtained with 12F6, another IgG_{2a} monoclonal antibody to T3 (unpublished data). One would have to postulate blocking by a fragment or altered T3 molecule. Finally, an anti-anti-Id response with human anti-T3 activity was considered, as has been described in patients treated with an antitumor monoclonal antibody (*9*). This was unlikely because of the inability of the test serum to bind normal T lymphocytes (the control for the enhancing assay) and the ability of an OKT3 affinity column to remove the blocking activity.

The nonidiotypic reactivity detected by the binding of OKT8 was probably isotypic, because little reactivity was found to OKT4. We cannot exclude the possibility that a portion of the OKT8 reactivity may be to allotypic determinants not expressed on OKT4. OKT3 was derived from a BALB/c mouse, and both OKT8 and OKT4 were obtained from (BALB/c×A/J) F_1 mice (*16*). The strains of origin of the heavy chains in OKT4 and OKT8 are unknown. Several IgG_{2a} allotypic determinants of BALB/c are expressed by A/J but none are apparently expressed on IgG_{2b} (*17*). Anti-isotype specificities have been detected in other patients treated with OKT3 (*10*).

The presence of some degree of reactivity to mouse immunoglobulin in the pretreatment sera and in normal controls was expected. Antibodies to equine ATG have been detected by passive hemagglutination in up to 50% of patients awaiting renal transplantation with no previous exposure to ATG (*18*). These antihorse immunoglobulin antibodies were found to crossreact with goat and rabbit immunoglobulin. The specificity of these antibodies has not been established. They may be crossreactive antibodies to immunoglobulin antigens absorbed orally (beef, pork, etc.) or rheumatoid factors. We found no correlation between preexisting antibodies and the severity of side effects from monoclonal therapy. The one patient with a high titer prior to treatment responded fully to OKT3 therapy for rejection. A further analysis of these antibody crossreactivities will be necessary to determine the importance of these interactions.

Although early studies were optimistic that monoclonal antibodies might have low immunogenicity (*1, 3, 19*), following our initial report (*6*), several other studies have documented the presence of both non-anti-Id and anti-Id responses (*4, 5, 7, 9, 10, 14, 15*). The production of such antibodies may be influenced by the particular monoclonal antibody used and the immune reactivity of the individuals treated. More than half the patients treated for lymphoreticular malignancies with a nonmitogenic antibody (anti-Leu 1) produce antimouse antibody, similar to that of our transplant recipients. Although these antibodies do not cause immune complex disease, the response effectively neutralized the monoclonal antibody, as in our patients (*15*).

OKT3 does not seem particularly more or less immunogenic than other anti-T-cell or antitumor antibodies, despite its known mitogenic activity. The one distinctive feature of the immune response to OKT3 may be the predominance of the anti-Id response. Only 5% of the antibodies to the murine immunoglobulin have been to idiotypic determinants in lymphoma patients treated with anti-Leu 1 (*20*), whereas in one of our patients only anti-Id antibodies were detected, and in another they accounted for 31% of the antibody response. Overall, 75% of our patients who had any antibody response made anti-Id that was able to block antigen binding. Why OKT3 should be particularly effective at promoting an anti-Id response is unknown, but one could speculate that this might be related to the target molecule, a part of the T cell antigen receptor complex. However, the strong anti-Id response is not unique to OKT3, as anti-Id constituted about one-third of the antibody response of goats immunized with myeloma proteins (*21*). Furthermore, we have observed blocking anti-Id in monkeys treated with anti-Leu 2a (Cosimi et al., manuscript in preparation).

That the recipients of murine monoclonal antibodies should develop an immune response to these foreign proteins is, of course, expected. Such responses have been described in recipients of antithymocyte (or lymphocyte) globulin (ATG) made in horses or rabbits (*22, 23*). However, with more recent preparations of ATG that have been deaggregated and administered i.v., the antibody response is typically inconsequential and does not preclude repeated use of ATG (*24, 25*).

Two likely possibilities exist for the differences between the intensity of the response to monoclonal and polyclonal antibodies. The broadly reactive ATG may be more effective at destroying the T cells and/or B cells needed to make an antibody response. If this is the case, a monoclonal antibody—or drug, such as cyclophosphamide—might be added that would interfere with B cell function. A second possibility is that the substantial amount of nonreactive immunoglobulin in the polyclonal preparations acts to promote tolerance in the recipients. It is likely that more intense deaggregation of the monoclonal antibody will be ineffective, since essentially all of the soluble monoclonal antibody becomes "aggregated" when it binds to the target cell surface. Indeed, some years ago, Lance and Dresser demonstrated that rabbit ATG was more immunogenic in mice than normal, nonimmune, rabbit IgG (*21*). Based on this observation, a possible solution is to give a loading dose of nonreactive monoclonal antibody of the same isotype.

At this time, anti-immunoglobulin and anti-Id antibodies represent barriers to the prolonged or repeated application of murine monoclonal antibodies. The anti-Id barrier will likely also exist for human monoclonal antibodies: the magic "bullets" are stopped by equally magic "shields." Although monoclonal antibodies have exceptional promise for specific modulation of immune responses, the antibody response will need to be eliminated to permit their widest therapeutic and diagnostic application.

Acknowledgments. We are grateful for the excellent technical assistance of Helen Goldsman, Carol Struzziero, Amy Luttinger, and Victoria Hull. James T. Kurnick, M.D., kindly provided the PHA blast lines.

REFERENCES

1. Cosimi AB, Colvin RB, Burton RC, et al. Use of monoclonal antibodies to T-cell subsets for immunologic monitoring and treatment in recipients of renal allografts. N Eng J Med 1981; 305: 308.
2. Cosimi AB, Burton RC, Colvin RB, et al. Treatment of acute renal allograft rejection with OKT3 monoclonal antibody. Transplantation 1981; 32: 535.
3. Miller RA, Maloney DG, McKillop J, Levy R. In vitro effects of murine hybridoma monoclonal antibody in a patient with T-cell leukemia. Blood 1981; 58: 78.
4. Sears HG, Atkinson B, Mattis J, et al. Phase-I clinical trial of monoclonal antibody in treatment of gastrointestinal tumors. Lancet 1982; 2: 762.
5. Dillman RO, Shawler DL, Sobol RE, et al. Murine monoclonal antibody therapy in two patients with chronic lymphocytic leukemia. Blood 1981; 59: 1036.
6. Colvin RB, Cosimi AB, Burton RC, Kurnick JT, Struzziero C. Anti-idiotype antibodies in patients treated with murine monoclonal OKT3 [Abstract] Fed Proc 1982; 41: 363.
7. Jaffers GJ, Colvin RB, Cosimi AB, et al. The human immune response to murine OKT3 monoclonal antibody. Transplant Proc 1983; 15: 646.
8. Chatenoud L, Baudrihaye MF, Chkoff N, Kreis H, Bach JF. Immunologic follow-up of renal allograft recipients treated prophylactically by OKT3 alone. Transplant Proc 1983; 15: 643.
9. Koprowski H, Herlyn D, Lubeck M, DeFreitay E, Sears HF. Human anti-idiotype antibodies in cancer patients: is the modulation of the immune response beneficial to the patient. Proc Natl Acad Sci USA 1984; 81:216.
10. Baudrihuye MF, Chatenoud L, Kreis M, Goldstein G, Bach JP. Unusually restricted anti-isotype human immune response to OKT3 monoclonal antibody. Eur J Immunol 1984; 8: 686.
11. Thistlethwaite JR, Cosimi AB, Delmonico FL, et al. Evolving use of OKT3 monoclonal antibody for treatment of renal allograft rejection. Transplantation 1984; 38: 695.
12. van der Elsen P, Sheplen B-A, Borst J, et al. Isolation of cDNA clones encoding the 20K T3 glycoprotein of human T-cell receptor complex. Nature 1984; 312: 413.
13. Voller A. Heterogenous enzyme-immunoassays and their applications. In: Maggio ET, ed. Enzyme-immunoassay. Boca Raton, FL: CRC Press, 1980: 181.
14. Kurnick JT, Warren AR, Moscicki RA, Leary CP. T-cell subsets in human lymphocytes maintained in IL-2 medium after PHA or mixed lymphocyte reaction activation. Clin Immunol Immunopathol 1984; 27: 444.
15. Moscicki RA, Luttinger AL, Colvin RB. Analysis of human T cells in blood with monoclonal antibodies and flow cytometry. In: Yoshida T, ed. Investigation of cell-mediated immunity. London: Churchill Livingston 1985: 6.
16. Kung PC, Talle MA, DeMaria M, Butler M, Lifter J, Goldstein G. Strategies for generating monoclonal antibodies defining human T lymphocyte differentiation antigens. Transplant Proc 1980; 12(suppl 1): 141.
17. Altman PL, Katz DD, eds. Inbred and genetically defined strains of laboratory animals. Part I: mouse and rat. Bethesda, MD: Fed Amer Soc Exp Biol, 1979: 108.
18. Amemiya H, Kashiwagi N, Putnam CW, Starzl TE. Cross-reactivity studies of horse, goat and rabbit anti-lymphocyte globulin. Clin Exp Immunol 1970; 6: 279.
19. Kirkman RL, Araunjo JL, Busch GJ, et al. Treatment of acute renal allograft rejection with monoclonal anti-T12 antibody. Transplantation 1984; 36: 620.
20. Levy R, Miller RA. Tumor therapy with monoclonal antibodies. Fed Proc 1983; 42: 2650.
21. Haber J, Winn JH. An isotopic antiglobulin test for quantitation of anti-sheep red blood cell antibodies of individual Ig classes in the mouse. J Immunol Methods 1982; 48: 61.
22. Martin WJ II, Blumenthal M, Roitman MS, Condie R, Simmons R, Najarian J. Antilymphoblast globulin in renal transplant patients: no allergic reactions. JAMA 1976; 236: 1729.
23. Satoh P, Elberg A, Davis J, Uittenbogaart C, Fine R, Hardy MA. Effects of different ATG (ATGAM) regimens on the levels of rosette-forming cells (RFC), serum horse IgG (HoI), and anti-horse antibodies in kidney transplant recipients. Transplant Proc 1979; 11: 1427.
24. Vincent C, Revillard JP. Antibody response to horse γ-globulin in recipients of renal allografts. Transplantation 1977; 24: 141.
25. Hiotsma AJ, Reekers P, Kreeftenberg JG, VanLier HJJ, Capel PJA, Koene RAP. Treatment of acute rejection of cadaveric renal allografts with rabbit antilymphocyte globulin. Transplantation 1982; 33: 12.
26. Lance EM, Dresser DW. Antigenicity in mice of antilymphocyte gamma globulin. Nature 1967; 215: 488.

Received 26 June 1985.
Accepted 4 September 1985.

0041-1337/86/4105-0579$02.00/0
TRANSPLANTATION
Copyright © 1986 by The Williams & Wilkins Co.

Vol. 41, No. 5
Printed in U.S.A.

ALG TREATMENT OF STEROID-RESISTANT REJECTION IN PATIENTS RECEIVING CYCLOSPORINE

ARTHUR J. MATAS,[1] VIVIAN A. TELLIS, THERESA QUINN, DAN GLICHLICK, ROBERT SOBERMAN, ROBERT WEISS, GATTU KARWA, AND FRANK J. VEITH

The Department of Surgery, Montefiore Medical Center, New York, New York 10467

Thirty-one episodes of biopsy-proved acute rejection (R) in 28 patients maintained on cyclosporine did not respond to high-dose steroids and were treated with antilymphocyte globulin (ALG). Cyclosporine was discontinued in all but three during ALG administration. (A) Twenty-four patients received 26 courses of ALG within 90 days of transplant (11 1st R, 15 2nd or 3rd). Seven treatment courses were cut short due to infection (4), ongoing R (2) and a combination of infection and rejection (1). Only 1 of 7 has a functioning graft. Of the remaining 19 full ALG courses (17 patients) (8 1st R, 11 2nd or 3rd), 13 (11 patients) responded (7 1st R, 6 >1st). The remaining 6 patients lost their grafts to ongoing acute rejection. (B) Five patients were treated after 6 months posttransplant; two responded but no grafts currently function. (C) Overall 7 patients developed systemic infection (7 viruses, 1 *Candida*) with 1 death, and 2 additional patients developed severe thrombocytopenia and leukopenia. Patients responding to their ALG course were restarted on cyclosporine. We conclude that ALG is not as effective in reversing steroid-resistant rejection in patients maintained on cyclosporine as it has been in patients maintained on azathioprine. However, more than 50% of steroid-resistant rejection episodes are reversed.

Reported advantages of cyclosporine immunosuppression in renal transplantation have included an increase in patient and graft survival (*1–6*), with a decrease in infection episodes (*7, 8*), a reduction in the need for steroids (*6–9*), and a shortened hospital stay (*5, 7*). Importantly, cyclosporine has been reported to significantly reduce the frequency and severity of posttransplant rejection episodes (*3, 5, 7, 9, 10*). In some studies, as few as 10%–30% of cadaver transplant recipients are reported to experience an acute rejection episode (*3, 7*). However, rejection remains the major cause of graft loss in transplant recipients maintained on cyclosporine.

Our experience has differed from that reported in many studies in the literature. Although graft survival in cyclosporine recipients has been excellent, 80% of our patients have had one or more rejection episodes, many which have not responded to increased steroid doses. Since steroid-resistant rejections in patients maintained on prednisone and azathioprine frequently respond to antilymphocyte globulin (ALG) (*11–13*), we studied whether or not steroid resistant rejections in cyclosporine treated patients would similarly respond to ALG.

MATERIALS AND METHODS

Between March 1983 and March 1985 ninety-one recipients of cadaveric kidneys at the Albert Einstein College of Medicine/Montefiore Medical Center and were immunosuppressed with cyclosporine and prednisone. Prior to transplantation, all patients received a minimum of five blood transfusions. All patients received ABO-compatible kidneys that were crossmatch-negative by the Amos modified NIH lymphocytotoxicity assay (*14*). During this period, we were attempting to determine whether kidneys could be successfully transplanted to patients with a past positive crossmatch. Initially, transplants were done only if sera from the preceding eighteen months were crossmatch-negative (*15*). This period has been progressively reduced to 12 months, 9 months—and, currently, to the 6 months preceding the transplant. No attempt was made to select recipients on the basis of HLA or Dr matching.

Following transplantation, prednisone was started at 40 mg/day and was tapered to 30 mg/day on the fifth postoperative day and to 25 mg/day on the fourteenth postoperative day. The first fifteen cadaver recipients received cyclosporine according to a fixed protocol without measurement of cyclosporine blood levels. The first three patients received a starting dose of 14 mg/kg/day orally, whereas the subsequent twelve received 17 mg/kg/day. If there was concern about gastrointestinal function, the first dose was given i.v. (1/3 of the oral dose). The cyclosporine dose in all 15 patients was tapered to 10 mg/kg at one month, and then by 1 mg/kg/month until patients were receiving 5–6 mg/kg/day.

The subsequent 76 recipients received cyclosoprine according to a consistent protocol. If possible, cyclosporine was given preoperatively (14 mg/kg orally). If no preoperative dose was given, the drug was started in the recovery room (5 mg/kg i.v., administered over 6–8 hr). Postoperatively, oral cyclosporine (14 mg/kg/day) was initiated. Patients with functioning kidneys and those with oliguria were managed similarly. Cyclosporine levels were measured and the dose was adjusted for the first three months to maintain serum trough levels at 100–200 ng% by radioimmunoassay. Subsequently, the dose was adjusted to maintain trough levels above 50 ng%. In addition, pharmokinetic studies were done on all patients, and when indicated the drug was given in two divided daily doses. The cyclosporine radioimmunoassay was done according to the technique of Donatsch et al. (*16*).

Rejection episodes were diagnosed by clinical and laboratory criteria, by deterioration of I^{131} iodohippuran scan, and by percutaneous allograft biopsy. Alternate causes of serum creatinine elevation were excluded (*17*). In cases in which the diagnosis was in doubt, the cyclosporine dose was lowered as a therapeutic trial. If serum creatinine levels continued to rise, antirejection therapy was instituted. Rejection episodes were initially treated with i.v. methylprednisolone (1 g×3). If there was no response to the steroids within five days of treatment (increase in urine output, fall in serum creatinine level) the patient underwent biopsy of the transplant. Rejection was

[1] Address reprint requests to Arthur J. Matas, M.D.

* Abbreviations used: ALG, antilymphocyte globulin; CMV, cytomegalovirus; SSR, steroid-resistant rejection.

diagnosed and differentiated from cyclosporine-induced changes using the histopathologic criteria outlined by Sibley et al. (*18*). If the biopsy demonstrated acute rejection, the patient received another course of i.v. methylprednisolone or was started on ALG (Minnesota) (20 mg/kg/day) with a planned treatment course of 14 days. The ALG dose was decreased if there was a fall in the platelet or leukocyte count. Cyclosporine was continued during ALG administration for the first two patients. Both developed serious systemic infections—therefore in subsequent patients cyclosporine was discontinued during ALG administration and was restarted at the termination of the ALG course.

We evaluated the incidence of rejection in our cadaver kidney recipients maintained on cyclosporine, and the percentage and timing of rejection episodes that did not respond to increased steroid doses. In addition, we studied whether ALG treatment of steroid resistant rejections in patients maintained on cyclosporine was efficacious and was associated with significant morbidity and mortality.

Case report. The clinical course of our second cyclosporine-treated patient is shown in Figure 1. The patient required dialysis until the sixth postoperative day. He was treated with cyclosporine 17 mg/kg/day and prednisone 40 mg/day. Five days posttransplant he developed fever, graft tenderness, and decreased urine output. He received 3 g of methylprednisolone and responded with disappearance of symptoms, increased urine output, and fall in creatinine level. On the seventeenth postoperative day, he again developed fever, graft tenderness, decreased urine output and a rise in serum creatinine from 3.3 to 4.8 mg%. A second steroid treatment was followed by a temporary increase in urine output and fall in serum creatinine level. However, shortly after completion of the steroid course, urine output again began to fall and creatinine level to rise. Percutaneous allograft biopsy done at this time revealed edema and a mononuclear interstitial cell infiltrate consistent with moderate-to-severe rejection. Antilymphocyte globulin was started with a dramatic response. Urine output increased, and serum creatinine level fell to 2.5 mg% and was stable for 12 months.

RESULTS

Between March 1983 and March 1985 ninety-one recipients of cadaver kidney transplants were immunosuppressed with prednisone and cyclosporine. Patient demographics for this group are shown in Table 1. The mean HLA and Dr antigen matches were 0.8 and 0.5, respectively. A total of 34% of the patients had antibodies to over 50% of a panel of lymphocytes, and one-quarter had antibodies to more than 70% of the panel (Table 1). For the entire group, one year actuarial patient and graft survival were 98% and 73%, respectively (17 patients at risk one year). Seventy-three patients (80%) had one or more rejection episodes and were treated with i.v. methylprednisolone. Thirty-one episodes of biopsy-proved rejection in twenty-eight patients did not respond to high dose steroids and were treated with antilymphocyte globulin. ALG-treated patients were divided into two groups based on the interval from transplant to ALG treatment.

ALG within 90 days of transplant. Twenty-four patients received 26 courses of ALG within 90 days of transplantation to treat eleven first and fifteen second or third rejections (Fig. 2). Seven of these patients received an incomplete ALG course. ALG was discontinued in three because of the development of systemic infection (3 virus, 1 *Candida*). Two of these three patients had not had their cyclosporine discontinued during ALG administration. Two patients had ALG terminated because of ongoing severe symptomatic rejection (fever, oliguria, and graft tenderness), and both underwent transplant nephrectomy. One patient had both herpes virus infection and ongoing rejection; ALG was discontinued and the graft was removed.

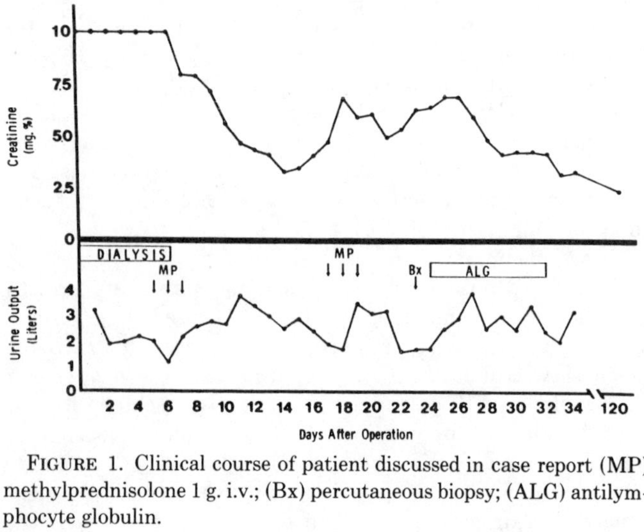

FIGURE 1. Clinical course of patient discussed in case report (MP) methylprednisolone 1 g. i.v.; (Bx) percutaneous biopsy; (ALG) antilymphocyte globulin.

TABLE 1. Characteristics of 91 cadaver transplant recipients receiving cyclosporine

Characteristic	
Mean age±SE (range):	37±2 (4–58)
Sex	
%Male	57
%Female	34
Race:	
%Caucasian	41
%Black	29
%Hispanic	19
%Asian	2
Multiple transplant:	
#:Second	13
#:Third	3
#:Fourth	2
Mean HLA match (±SE):	0.8±0.2
Dr match (±SE):	0.5±0.3
Highest PRA:	
#:≥70%	23
#:50–70%	8
#:30–50%	18
#:≤30%	42

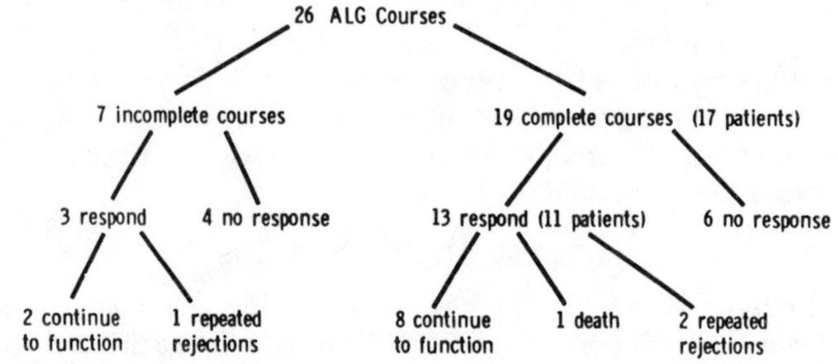

FIGURE 2. Outcome following 26 courses of ALG in 24 patients within 90 days of transplantation.

One patient with a healing herpetic lip lesion had an excellent early response to ALG and was given an abbreviated course because of concern about reactivating and disseminating the virus. Three of the seven patients responded to ALG with an improvement in graft function. Two kidneys continue to function three months after their ALG course and the third was lost secondary to chronic rejection at fourteen months.

Seventeen patients treated within the first 90 days received nineteen full ALG courses (eight first rejections, eleven second or third rejections) (Fig. 2). Thirteen rejection episodes in eleven patients responded with an increased urine output and a fall in serum creatinine level (seven first, six second or third rejections). The remaining six patients lost their grafts to ongoing acute rejection. Eight patients (Fig. 2) have functioning grafts 4–13 months posttransplant, 3–12 months post ALG treatment. Two grafts in the eleven patients having an initial response were lost to additional repeated rejection episodes. Five of these 17 patients developed viral infection after ALG treatment. There was one localized herpes simplex infection and two mild cytomegalovirus (CMV) infections. Two patients had severe disseminated cytomegalovirus. One had leukopenia (100/mm^3) and thrombocytopenia (10,000/mm^3) and was hospitalized for six weeks after completion of the ALG course. The second patient with disseminated CMV had two courses of ALG—the first immediately posttransplant and the second two months posttransplant. She developed CMV after the second treatment and died of disseminated infection after a protracted course.

ALG more than six months after transplant. No patients received ALG between 90 days and 6 months posttransplant. Five patients were treated after 6 months with a full two-week ALG course (one first, four second or third rejections). Two patients (both third rejection episodes) responded with a fall in serum creatinine level. However, both patients had additional rejection episodes and both returned to dialysis ten months posttransplant and three months post ALG. The three patients not responding to ALG all returned to dialysis. There were no infections in this group as a result of ALG administration. However, one patient developed a severe aplastic anemia requiring hospitalization for an additional month before platelet, white blood cell, and red cell counts returned to normal.

DISCUSSION

When cyclosporine was approved by the Food and Drug Administration, we were completing an evaluation of antirejection therapy in patients receiving prednisone and azathioprine for maintenance immunosuppression (*13*). Patients were randomized at the onset of their first rejection episode to receive for antirejection treatment either high-dose steroids plus ALG or steroids alone with ALG reserved for steroid-resistant rejections. Graft survival and patient morbidity and mortality were equivalent for both groups. We demonstrated that in patients maintained on prednisone and azathioprine, 60% of first and 50% of second rejection episodes responded to steroids alone. The majority of the remainder responded to a delayed course of ALG. Thus it appeared to be effective to treat rejection episodes initially with steroids, saving ALG for steroid resistant rejections.

Many of the initial reports on the use of cyclosporine for maintenance immunosuppression stressed the low incidence of rejection episodes (*3, 5, 7, 9, 10*). In addition, when rejection did occur, it was reported to be relatively easy to reverse with high doses of steroids. Our experience has been considerably different. Despite using cyclosporine doses similar to those described in the literature, and adjusting the cyclosporine dose with the aid of trough levels, we have had a high incidence of acute rejection episodes. In contrast to the findings in many other reports, these episodes were frequently associated with symptoms (fever, graft tenderness). Many of these rejections did not rapidly reverse with i.v. pulses of methylprednisolone. Given our success in using ALG to treat steroid-resistant rejection (SRR) in patients maintained on prednisone and azathioprine, we attempted to use ALG to treat SRR in patients maintained on cyclosporine. In contrast to our previous experience (*13*), 30% of first and 50% of second or third rejection episodes that were steroid-resistant were also resistant to ALG. In addition, three cyclosporine-treated patients had ongoing severe symptomatic rejection while receiving ALG and underwent transplant nephrectomy before completion of their ALG course.

The frequency of acute rejection episodes in our cadaver transplant recipients (80%) is higher than that reported in many other studies. The reason for this difference is not entirely clear. All our patients were transfused. Although recently we have done transplants when historical sera were positive (*15*), the majority of recipients in this study had crossmatch-negative historical and current sera. We made no attempt at HL and Dr matching, but others have demonstrated that there is little significance to matching in patients maintained on cyclosporine (*3, 19–22*). One-third of the patients were highly sensitized and had a percentage of radioactive antibody (PRA) of over 50%. Our rate of acute tubular necrosis (ATN) (50%) is higher than many other centers reporting a decreased rejection incidence. The diagnosis of rejection in patients who have posttransplant ATN and are receiving cyclosporine can be exceedingly difficult. As discussed above, we have seen symptomatic rejections in the immediate posttransplant period. On other occasions, however, rejection has been diagnosed by percutaneous allograft biopsy. The cyclosporine regimen used in our patients, although not identical, was similar to that used in the aforementioined studies, and the majority of our rejection episodes occurred in patients whose cyclosporine levels were in the therapeutic range. One major difference in our protocol was the low dose of steroids used. A relationship between initial steroid dose at a number of centers and the percentage of cyclosporine treated patients who are rejection-free can be seen in Table 2.

This is the first report of the use of ALG for treatment of steroid-resistant rejection episodes in renal transplant recipients maintained on cyclosporine. Oyer et al. (*23*) and Halloran et al. (*24*) report using ALG for prevention as well as treatment of rejection in cardiac and renal transplant recipients maintained on cyclosporine. When ALG was used in this manner, there was a high incidence of tumors and infection. Sommer and Ferguson (*25*) have used a five-day course of ALG for rejection prophylaxis. All patients were switched to cyclosporine on the sixth postoperative day. There was no increase in the incidence of infection in their patients. Tilney et al. (*5*) have used anti T12 monoclonal antibody to treat rejection in cyclosporine-treated patients. In an attempt to limit steroids, the monoclonal antibody was used as primary antirejection treatment in thirteen patients (12 early rejections, 1 late). Seven required the addition of high-dose steroids in order to reverse the rejection episode.

TABLE 2. Percentage of cyclosporine-treated cadaver kidney recipients who are rejection free

Institution	Initial cyclosporine, dose (mg/kg)	Daily initial prednisone dose	% Rejection-free	Reference No.
U. of Texas	14	120 mg	90	(*3*)
U. of Minnesota	14	2 mg/kg	66	(*7*)
Medizinishe Hochschule, Hanover	14	2 mg/kg	63	(*10*)
Brigham and Woman's	17	30 mg	47	(*5*)
U. of Louvain, Brussels	14	0.4 mg/kg	45	(*9*)
Huddinge Hospital, Karolinska Institute	17	100 or 60 mg	44	(*27*)
U. of Cambridge	17	0	39	(*6*)
Queen Elizabeth Hospital, Birmingham	15	20	33	(*28*)
Canadian Study Group	15	Alternate day	25	(*29*)
		0	33	
U. of Sydney, Royal Prince Albert Hospital	17	0	17	(*30*)
Montefiore Medical Center	14	40	20	

An alternative approach to antirejection treatment in our patients could have been an additional course of high-dose methylprednisolone. However, this would negate a major advantage of cyclosporine, namely a reduction in complications because of its steroid-sparing effect. We had reduced the steroid dosage that our patients received even before the introduction of cyclosporine and had already seen a marked decrease in steroid-related complications.

In using ALG in patients maintained on cyclosporine, we were concerned about the potential development of tumors and/or severe infection. To date, with a follow-up of three months to two years, we have not seen a malignancy in our ALG treated patients. However, we have had two patients develop severe aplastic anemia—both required over a month of hospitalization before reversal. One of these two also had severe disseminated cytomegaloviris infection. Two other patients also had severe cytomegalovirus infection, resulting in death in one patient. We had not seen either aplastic anemia or CMV of this degree of severity in our patients maintained on prednisone and azathioprine who had received ALG for steroid-resistant rejection. It may be that a shorter course of ALG would decrease the risk of these problems.

Because of similar concerns, we debated whether to resume cyclosporine in patients responding to ALG or to start azathioprine. By definition, these patients had severe rejection on cyclosporine therapy. However, graft survival rates are reported to be lower in patients switched from cyclosporine to azathioprine (*7*). In addition, as originally reported by Calne et al. (*26*), when cyclosporine was used in conjunction with multiple other immunosuppressive agents, there was a high incidence of both tumors and fatal infection. As a result, we are currently restarting cyclosporine at the end of the ALG course.

Although ALG is not as efficacious in reversing SRR in patients maintained on cyclosporine as compared with SRR in those maintained on prednisone and azathioprine, over 50% of rejection episodes are reversed. We believe that cyclosporine should be stopped during ALG administration.

REFERENCES

1. Canadian Multicenter Transplant Study Group. A randomized trial of cyclosporine in cadaveric renal transplantation. N Engl J Med 1983; 309: 809.
2. European Multicenter Trial Group. Cyclosporine in cadaveric renal transplantation: one year follow up of a multicenter trial. Lancet 1983; 2: 986.
3. Kahan BD, Van Buren CT, Flechner SM, Payne WD, Boileau M, Kerman RH. Cyclosporine immunosuppression mitigates immunologic risk factors in renal allotransplantation. Transplant Proc 1983; 15: 2469.
4. Starzl TE, Hakala TR, Rosenthal JT, Iwatsuki S, Shaw BW Jr. The Colorado-Pittsburgh cadaveric renal transplantation study with cyclosporine. Transplant Proc 1983; 15: 2459.
5. Tilney NL, Milford EL, Araujo JL, Strom TB, Carpenter CB, Kirkman RL. Experience with cyclosporine and steroids in clinical renal transplantation. Ann Surg 1984; 20: 605.
6. Merion RM, White DJG, Thiru S, Evans DB, Calne RY. Cyclosporine: five years' experience in cadaveric renal transplantation. N Engl J Med 1984; 310: 148.
7. Najarian JS, Fryd DS, Strand M, et al. A single institution, randomized, prospective trial of cyclosporine versus azathioprine-antilymphocyte globulin for immunosuppression in renal allograft recipients. Ann Surg 1985; 201: 142.
8. Hakala TR, Starzl TE, Rosenthal JT, Shaw B, Iwatsuki S. Cadaveric renal transplantation with cyclosporine-A and steroids. Transplant Proc 1985; 15: 465.
9. Squifflet JP, Pirson Y, Jamart J, Wallemacq P, Westelinck K, Alexandre GPJ. Cyclosporine in cadaver renal transplantation at a center with good results using conventional treatment. Transplant Proc 1985; 1212.
10. Bunzendahl H, Wonigeit K, Klempnauer J, Brolsch C, Pichlmayr R. Cyclosporine and steroids: effects on the clinical course after renal allotransplantation. Transplant Proc 1983; 15: 2531.
11. Hardy MA, Nowygrod R, Elberg A, Appel G. Use of ATG in treatment of steroid-resistant rejections. Transplantation 1980; 29: 162.
12. Light JA, Alijani MR, Bigger JA, Oddenino K, Reinmuth B. Antilymphocyte globulin (ALG) reverses "irreversible" allograft rejection. Transplant Proc 1981; 13: 475.
13. Matas AJ, Tellis VA, Quinn T, et al. Treatment of renal transplant rejection episodes in patients receiving prednisone and azathioprine: a cost effective approach. Transplantation 1985; 40: 35.
14. Amos PB. Cytotoxicity testing. NIAID manual of tissue typing techniques 1979–80. NIH publication No. 80, 545: 42.
15. Matas AJ, Nehlsen-Cannarella S, Tellis VA, Kuemmel P, Soberman R, Veith F. Successful kidney transplantation with current-sera-negative/historical-sera-positive T cell crossmatch. Transplantation 1984; 37: 111.
16. Donatsch P, Abisch E, Hornberger M, et al. A radioimmunoassay

to measure cyclosporine A in plasma and serum samples. J Immunoassay 1981; 2: 18.
17. Matas AJ, Simmons RL, Kjellstrand CM, Najarian JS. Pseudorejection; factors mimicking rejection in renal allograft recipients. Ann Surg 1977; 186: 51.
18. Sibley RK, Rynasiewicz J, Ferguson RM, et al. Morphology of cyclosporine nephrotoxicity and acute rejection in patients immunosuppressed with cyclosporine and prednisone. Surgery 1983; 94: 225.
19. Rosenthal JT, Hakala TR, Iwatsuki S, Shaw BW, Jr, Starzl TE. Cadaveric renal transplantation under cyclosporine-steroid therapy. Surg Gyn Obstet 1983; 157: 309.
20. Harris KR, Digard NJ, Gosling DC, et al. HLA-dr matching in renal transplant patients on cyclosporine. Transplant Proc 1985; 17: 42.
21. Klintmalm G, Brynger H, Flatmark A, et al. The blood transfusion, dr matching, and mixed lymphocyte culture effects are not seen in cyclosporine-treated renal transplant recipients. Transplant Proc 1985; 17: 1026.
22. Taylor RJ, Andrews W, Rosenthal JT, Carpenter B, Hakala TR. Dr matching in cadaveric renal transplantation with cyclosporine. Transplant Proc 1985; 17: 1194.
23. Oyer PE, Stinson EB, Jamieson SW, et al. Heart and lung transplantation. Transplant Proc 1983; 15: 2546.
24. Halloran P, Ludwin D, Aprile M, and the Canadian Multicentre Transplant Study Group. Comparison of antilymphocyte globulin-imuran, cyclosporine, and antilymphocyte globulin-cyclosporine therapy for cadaver renal transplantation. Transplant Proc 1985; 17: 1201.
25. Sommer BG, Ferguson RM. Immediate post-renal transplant immunotherapy: comparison of three adjunct protocols combined with maintenance cyclosporine [Abstract]. Presented at the 10th meeting of the Amer Soc Transplant Surgeons, June 1984.
26. Calne RY, Rolles K, White DJG, et al. Cyclosporin A initially as the only immunosuppressant in 34 recipients of cadaveric organs: 32 kidneys, 2 pancreases, and 2 livers. Lancet 1979; 2: 1033.
27. Ringden O, Ost L, Klintmalm G, et al. Improved outcome in renal transplantation recipients above 55 years of age treated with cyclosporine and low doses of steroids. Transplant Proc 1983; 15: 2507.
28. McMaster P, Haynes IG, Michael J, et al. Cyclosporine in cadaveric renal transplantation: a prospective randomized trial. Transplant Proc 1983; 15: 2523.
29. Stiller C, for the Canadian Transplant Study Group. The requirements for maintenance steroids in cyclosporine-treated renal transplant recipients. Transplant Proc 1983; 15: 2450.
30. Sheil AGR, Hall BM, Tiller DJ, et al. Australian trial of cyclosporine (CsA) in cadaveric donor renal transplantation. Transplant Proc 1983; 15: 2485.

Received 6 June 1985.
Accepted 17 September 1985.

0041-1337/86/4105-0583$02.00/0
TRANSPLANTATION
Vol. 41, No. 5
Printed in U.S.A.

SEVERE APLASTIC ANEMIA ASSOCIATED WITH CHRONIC MUCOCUTANEOUS CANDIDIASIS

IMMUNOLOGIC AND HEMATOLOGIC RECONSTITUTION AFTER ALLOGENEIC BONE MARROW TRANSPLANTATION[1]

H. JOACHIM DEEG,[2] LAWRENCE G. LUM, JEAN SANDERS, GARY J. LEVY, KEITH M. SULLIVAN, PATRICK BEATTY, E. DONNALL THOMAS,[3] AND RAINER STORB

The Fred Hutchinson Cancer Research Center and the Departments of Medicine and Pediatrics, the University of Washington School of Medicine, Seattle, Washington; and the Louisiana State University School of Medicine, Shreveport, Louisiana

Chronic mucocutaneous candidiasis (CMC) is typically associated with the inability of T lymphocytes to proliferate and produce lymphokines in response to *Candida* antigen. A 7-year-old girl with CMC developed severe aplastic anemia and, after conditioning with cyclophosphamide, 200 mg/kg, underwent bone marrow transplantation from her HLA-identical sister. Engraftment was prompt and complete. The patient is surviving more than 3 years after transplantation with normal donor-derived hemopoiesis and immune function. Manifestations of CMC have resolved completely and she has not received antifungal therapy for more than 2 years.

Chronic mucocutaneous candidiasis (CMC)* comprises a symptom complex including chronic superficial candidiasis involving the mucous membranes and extending onto adjacent

Received 1 August 1985.
Accepted 11 September 1985.
[1] This work was supported in part by Grants CA 30924, CA 18221, CA 18029, and CA 15704 awarded by the National Cancer Institute, DHHS.
[2] Address correspondence to: H. J. Deeg, M.D., Fred Hutchinson Cancer Research Center, 1124 Columbia Street, Seattle, WA 98104.
[3] Dr. Thomas is the recipient of a Research Career Award AI 02425 from the National Institute of Allergies and Infectious Disease.

* Abbreviations used: Con A, concanavalin A; CMC, chronic mucocutaneous candidiasis; HLA, human leukocyte antigen (major histocompatibility complex); MLC, mixed leukocyte culture; PWM, pokeweed mitogen; TT, tetanus toxoid.

skin. Satellite patches may occur on the trunk, extremities, and nail beds (*1–3*). Clinical findings often develop during the first year of life. In some patients CMC may be associated with endocrinopathies such as hypoparathyroidism or hypoadrenalism (*4*). Most patients demonstrate defects of cellular immunity with an inability of T lymphocytes to proliferate or produce lymphokines in response to *Candida* antigen (*2, 5–7*). The responses to other antigens are usually normal. Patients can have hemolytic anemia or anemia related to iron-, B12-, folic acid-, biotin, or pyridoxin deficiency (*2, 8*). Pure red cell aplasia (*9*) or aplastic anemia (*10*) have also been described but usually have been associated with the presence of thymoma (*11*). We report here a patient with juvenile-onset CMC who developed severe aplastic anemia. Allogencic marrow transplantation carried out for the treatment of aplastic anemia also corrected the patient's immunological defect and apparently cured her CMC.

Case Report

The patient (unique patient number 1604), is a girl born in 1974 as the product of a normal full-term pregnancy and delivery. She was first seen at 10 months of age with a severe *Candida albicans* infection of pharynx, larynx, and esophagus. Laboratory investigations (summarized in Tables 1 and 2) showed a depressed lymphocyte proliferation response to *C albicans*. Specific IgA antibody titers to *Candida* were low (effective titer <1:4 as compared with 1:52 in a normal human pool), IgG and IgM titers were in the normal range. Skin tests to *Candida* were nonreactive. Subsequent studies intermittently revealed defects of neutrophil and monocyte chemotaxis in Boyden chambers and agarose. Beginning at the age of 1½ years, the patient had recurrent febrile episodes associated with maxillary and ethmoid sinusitis and pulmonary atelectases of undetermined cause. At the age of 2 years, she was found to have marked hepatosplenomegaly and mildly elevated serum alkaline phosphatase. Serum bilirubin, transaminases, and alphaantitrypsin were normal. A liver biopsy showed 15% glycogen by weight. Electronmicroscopic studies suggested hepatic phosphatidyl kinase deficiency but no enzymatic defect could be demonstrated. There was no histological evidence of acute or chronic hepatitis. On one occasion hormone studies suggested adrenal hyporesponsiveness but an unequivocal defect could not be demonstrated.

The patient was treated with i.v. amphotericin B, mycostatin in various preparations, and gentian violet, with only partial and transient responses. There was transient improvement with the addition of 5-fluorocytosine but the administration of this drug resulted in drug resistance. There was no response to prolonged treatment with transfer factor. Her candidiasis was finally controlled when she was placed on ketoconazole in July 1981.

At that time the patient presented with bruising, a platelet count of 1×10^9/L, a hematocrit of 0.20, a reticulocyte count of 7.4% and megaloblastic changes (MCV 116.5 fl). A total leukocyte count was 3.6×10^9/L with normal differential. A marrow aspirate showed megaloblastoid changes. A two-stage Schilling test was interpreted as consistent with pernicious anemia. The folic acid level was normal. She was treated with parenteral vitamin B12 without response. A repeat marrow aspirate in November 1981 revealed severe hypoplasia. The hematocrit was 0.18 with <1% reticulocytes. The white blood cell count was 2.7×10^9/liter with 3% neutrophils and a platelet count 3×10^9/L. The diagnosis of severe aplastic anemia was made.

TABLE 1. Patient characteristics before and after transplantation

Datum	1975 (age 10 mo.)	11/81	1/29/82 (=d. −12)[a]	2/24/82 (=d. 14)	3/3/82 (=d. 22)	5/12/82 (=d. 91)	8/20/82 (=d. 191)	8/12/83 (=d. 548)	5/2/84 (=d. 812)	1/14/85 (=d. 1069)
Lymphocytes ($\times10^9$/L)	3.1		0.8	0.5	0.5	1.1	2.5	3.9	2.3	1.9
E-rosette⁺ % (patient/control)[b]	61/54			58/76				38/70		
T4+ % (patient/control)[b]				21/62				45/44		
T8+ % (patient/control)[b]				75/21				27/30		
Granulocytes ($\times10^9$/L)	6.1	0.9	0.01	0.04	0.08	2.7	5.4	9.5	5.5	6.3
Platelets ($\times10^9$/L)	Normal	3	6	30	9	26	95	152	235	290
Hematocrit	0.37	0.18	0.25	0.30	0.30	0.30	0.43	0.46	0	0.45
Bone Marrow		Severely hypoplastic	15% cellular[c] no megs M:E = 8:1	5% cellular M+E graft	15% cellular Trilineage graft	50% cellular M:E = 2:1				
Serum IgG (mg/dl)	1,150		495 (564–1765)[d]					913		853
IgA (mg/dl)	165		58 (85–385)					35		96
IgM (mg/dl)	155		47 (45–250)					74		76
IgE (units/ml)	25		ND					160 (<200)[d]		
Complement: C3 (mg/dl)	60							118 (100–200)		189
C4 (mg/dl)	36							32 (14–51)		40

[a] Abbreviations: megs = megakaryocytes; M = myeloid; E = erythroid; ND = not done; d = days relative to marrow transplantation.
[b] Cells from the marrow donor served as control.
[c] Cellularity in % of normal.
[d] Values in parentheses show normal range; no normal brackets were available for the determinations carried out in 1975.

TABLE 2. In vitro lymphocyte proliferation[a]

Datum	1975 (age 10 mo.)	1/29/82 (=d. −12)	2/24/82 (=d. 14)	6/30/83 (=d. 505)	8/12/83 (=d. 548)
Lymphocyte stimulation (% of control)[c]					
Candida	[574/1.1][b]	9.8	176	52	168
Con A		135	ND	32	145
PWM					
TT		552	40	ND	65
MLC		ND	74	7	9
		127	31	ND	93

[a] Abbreviations: ConA = concanavalin A; PWM = pokeweed mitogen; TT = tetanus toxoid; MLC = mixed leukocyte culture; ND = not done; d = days relative to marrow transplantation.
[b] No control value available; median cmp/stimulation index is given.
[c] Results obtained with lymphocytes from the bone marrow donor, tested on the same days as cells from the patient, served as control values.

While thrombocytopenic she had an intracranial right occipital hemorrhage and generalized convulsions. She was treated with diphenylhydantoin and transfusions of platelets and washed red blood cells. Prednisone, 60 mg/m^2/day was initiated on December 26, 1981 without effect. She then developed a myositis manifested by pain, elevated serum creatine phosphokinase and aldolase, nerve conduction abnormalities, and a muscle biopsy consistent with polymyositis. Tissue typing of her siblings revealed that she had an 11-year-old sister who was HLA-identical as determined by serologic typing and mixed leukocyte culture nonreactivity. The patient was referred for marrow transplantation.

MATERIALS AND METHODS

Marrow Transplantation

The procedures used for conditioning the patient for marrow transplantation and the postgrafting care have been described (*12*). Briefly, the patient was given cyclophosphamide, 50 mg/kg i.v. for 4 consecutive days, followed 2 days later by the infusion of 12.2×10^9 (5.3×10^8/kg) marrow cells from her HLA-identical sister. On days 1–5 following marrow transplantation, 44×10^9 unirradiated donor buffy coat cells (19.1×10^8/kg) were infused (*13*). Methotrexate as prophylaxis for graft-versus-host disease was given on days 1, 3, 6, and 11 and at weekly intervals thereafter, as described (*12*). Sustained marrow engraftment was assessed by monitoring peripheral blood granulocyte counts and by the demonstration of erythrocytes of the donor phenotype. Criteria for diagnosis and management of acute and chronic graft-versus-host disease have been described (*14*).

Immunologic Studies

Purification of lymphocytes. Peripheral blood mononuclear cells from patient, marrow donor, and unrelated control individuals were obtained by standard ficoll-hypaque gradient centrifugation. T and non-T (B) cells were separated by E-rosetting as described (*15*).

Lymphocyte proliferation studies. The proportions of total T (determined by rosetting with AET-modified sheep erythrocytes), OKT4, and OKT8-positive cells were determined as described (*15*). In vitro lymphocyte proliferative responses to optimal concentrations of concanavalin A (Calbiochem, San Diego, CA), pokeweed mitogen (Gibco, Grand Island, NY), *Candida*, and tetanus toxoid (Massachusetts Health Department, Boston, MA) were assessed using standard flat-bottomed microwells and ^{3}H-thymidine incorporation after 3 or 6 days of culture as described (*16*).

Delayed cutaneous hypersensitivity. The skin test antigens used included *Candida* (Dermatophytin 1:100, Hollister-Stier, Spokane, WA), mumps (Eli Lilly, Indianapolis, IN), trichophytin (1:10; Hollister-Stier, Spokane, WA), and tetanus toxoid (Massachusetts Health Department, Boston, MA).

Humoral immunity. Serum immunoglobulin and complement levels were determined using standard assays.

RESULTS

Hemopoietic reconstitution. Hematologic parameters before and following transplantation are summarized in Table 1. Analyses of red blood cell antigen and enzyme phenotypes 6, 12, and 24 months after transplantation showed 100% of the patient's erythrocytes to be of donor origin.

The postgrafting course was complicated by graft-versus-host disease developing on day 23 and involving skin, liver, and intestinal tract. She improved on treatment with methylprednisolone, 2 mg/kg/day. She returned home on day 98, on treatment with prednisone, gradually being reduced to 1 mg/kg every other day. Upon further dose reduction there was a flare-up of graft-versus-host disease of the skin, and prednisone was increased to 2 mg/kg on alternate days.

One year after transplantation the patient was well except for mild chronic graft-versus-host disease of the skin—and prednisone, 15–20 mg every other day, was continued. All other medications had been discontinued. Hematologic parameters are shown in Table 1. Three years after transplantation the patient is hematologically normal. She still has chronic GVHD, and is being treated with prednisone and azathioprine (*17*).

Immunologic reconstitution. To control CMC, treatment with ketoconazole, 100 mg/day, was given in the pretransplant period. Although there was no evidence of CMC, prophylactic ketoconazole was continued until day 247 after transplantation. In addition, prophylactic amphotericin B, 20 mg every other day, was administered from day 6 before until day 31 after transplantation. Because of the serious clinical condition no detailed immunologic studies could be carried out before transplantation. Her myositis resolved within a week of marrow transplantation. There has been no evidence of *Candida* or any other fungal infection since transplantation. Skin tests for *Candida*, mumps, trichophytin, and tetanus toxoid one year after transplantation were nonreactive. Three years after transplantation skin tests for mumps, trichophytin and tetanus toxoid remained negative; however, the test for *Candida* had converted to positive.

The results of in vitro immune function studies are summarized in Table 2. Pretransplant lymphocyte proliferative responses to mitogens and alloantigens (mixed leukocyte culture) were normal. The response to *Candida*, however, was depressed to 9.8% of donor control. By 18 months after transplantation proliferative responses, except to tetanus toxoid, were intact.

DISCUSSION

Both CMC and severe aplastic anemia are rare disorders (*2, 18*). Although multiple hematologic abnormalities have been recognized in association with CMC (*2*), only one case of aplastic anemia coexistent with chronic candidiasis has been reported (*10*). That patient, however, had chronic candidiasis of adult onset in the presence of a thymoma. The cause of this patient's aplastic anemia could not be determined. In some patients cells or serum factors capable of suppressing erythropoiesis in vitro have been described (*2, 9*), but no such studies were carried out in our patient. There was no evidence of autoantibodies. It appears unlikely that this patient's aplastic anemia was related to 5-fluorocytosine since there was an interval of more than 3 years from the last administration of this drug to diagnosis. Nevertheless, since aplastic anemia can be treated successfully by allogeneic marrow transplantation (*12, 13, 18*), the present case provided the opportunity of investigating the effect of marrow transplantation—not only on hemopoietic reconstitution but also on the immunological deficiencies associated with CMC.

Our results show that both hematologic and immunologic defects could be corrected, and the child is surviving 3 years after transplantation, off antifungal therapy, and without evidence of CMC. This is remarkable in view of the fact that the patient is receiving prednisone for the treatment of chronic graft-versus-host disease (*17*). In vitro responses of the patient's lymphocytes to *Candida* and skin tests for delayed type hypersensitivity to *Candida* are normal.

The etiology of CMC is not clear, and it is likely that different mechanisms are involved in the various symptom complexes that have been described. The severe forms may be reminiscent of thymic aplasia (DiGeorge syndrome) (*19*). Most patients are committed to continuous antifungal therapy. Many attempts at treating CMC have aimed at correcting T cell defects. Inconsistent and only transient responses to transfer factor (*20, 21*), transplantation of cultured thymus fragments (*22, 23*), or the H_2-blocker cimetidine (*24*) have been observed. One patient was given transfusions of leukocytes from an HLA-identical healthy brother and had prolonged improvement of CMC (*25*). Similarly, Buckley et al. (*26*) observed striking clinical improvement in one patient following the infusion of paternal marrow cells. However, in neither case was sustained engraftment of the transfused cells demonstrated. The patient reported here is the first in whom CMC was corrected by allogeneic marrow transplantation.

In summary, we have shown that the immunological defects of CMC of juvenile onset can be corrected by allogeneic marrow transplantation replacing abnormal effector cells with a normal T cell repertoire derived from marrow cells from the normal donor.

Acknowledgments. We thank Drs. Frank Schmalstieg and Hans Ochs for referring this patient to us, the physicians and nurses involved in the patient's care for their support, and Margaret Seigneuret for expert technical assistance.

REFERENCES

1. Dwyer JM. Chronic mucocutaneous candidiasis. Ann Rev Med 1981; 32: 491.
2. Kirkpatrick CHH, Sohnle PG. Chronic mucocutaneous candidiasis. In: Safai B, Good RA, eds. Comprehensive immunology, immunodermatology. New York: Plenum, 1981; 7: 495.
3. Jorizzo JL. Chronic mucocutaneous candidosis. Arch Dermatol 1982; 118: 963.
4. Digeorge AM, Paschkis K. The syndrome of Addison's disease, hypoparathyroidism and superficial moniliasis. Am J Dis Child 1957; 94: 476.
5. Lehner T, Wilton JMA, Ivanyi L. Immunodeficiencies in chronic mucocutaneous candidosis. Immunology 1972; 22: 775.
6. Gupta S, Kirkpatrick CH, Good RA. Subpopulations of human T lymphocytes. XI. T cells with receptors for IgM or IgG and locomotion of T and non-T cells in peripheral blood from patients with chronic mucocutaneous candidiasis. Clin Immunol Immunopathol 1979; 14: 86.
7. Sams WM Jr, Jorizzo JL, Snyderman R, et al. Chronic mucocutaneous candidiasis. Immunologic studies of three generations of a single family. Am J Med 1979; 67: 948.
8. Higgs JM, Wells RS. Chronic mucocutaneous candidiasis: associated abnormalities of iron metabolism. Br J Dermatol 1972; 86(suppl): 88.
9. Krantz SB. Pure red-cell aplasia. N Engl J Med 1974; 291: 345.
10. Twomey JJ, Waddell CC, Krantz S, et al. Chronic mucocutaneous candidiasis with macrophage dysfunction, a plasma inhibitor, and co-existent aplastic anemia. J Lab Clin Med 1975; 85: 968.
11. Schmid JR, Kiely JM, Harrison EG Jr, Bayrd ED, Pease GL. Thymoma associated with pure red-cell agenesis. Review of literature and report of 4 cases. Cancer 1964; 18: 216.
12. Storb R, Thomas ED, Buckner CD, et al. Marrow transplantation for aplastic anemia. Semin Hematol 1984; 21: 27.
13. Storb R, Doney KC, Thomas ED, et al. Marrow transplantation with or without donor buffy coat cells for 65 transfused aplastic anemia patients. Blood 1982; 59: 236.
14. Deeg HJ, Storb R. Graft-versus-host disease: pathophysiological and clinical aspects. Ann Rev Med 1984; 35: 11.
15. Lum LG, Orcutt-Thordarson N, Seigneuret MC, Storb R. The regulation of Ig synthesis after marrow transplantation. IV. T4 and T8 subset function in patients with chronic graft-versus-host disease. J Immunol 1982; 129: 113.
16. Lum LG, Benveniste E, Blaese RM. Functional aspects of T-cells bearing Fc-receptors for IgA. I. Mitogen responsiveness, mixed lymphocyte culture reactivity and helper activity of T_A cells as compared to T_G and T_M cells. J Immunol 1980; 124: 702.
17. Sullivan KM, Shulman HM, Storb R, et al. Chronic graft-versus-host disease in 52 patients: adverse natural course and successful treatment with combination immunosuppression. Blood 1981; 57: 267.
18. Camitta BM, Storb R, Thomas ED. Aplastic anemia. Pathogenesis, diagnosis, treatment, and prognosis. N Engl J Med 1982; 306: 645.
19. Rosen FS, Wedgwood RJ, co-chairmen. Primary immunodeficiency diseases [Meeting report]. Prepared for the WHO by a scientific group on immunodeficiency. Clin Immunol Immunopathol 1983; 28: 450.
20. Spitler LE, Levin AS, Fudenberg HH. Transfer factor. In: Bach FH, Good RA, eds. Clinical immunobiology. New York: Academic Press, 1974: 153.
21. Griscelli C, Revillard JP, Betuel H, Herzog C, Touraine JL. Transfer factor therapy in immuno-deficiencies. Biomedicine 1973; 18: 220.
22. Levy RL, Bach ML, Huang S-W, et al. Thymic transplantation in a case of chronic mucocutaneous candidiasis. Lancet 1971; 2: 898.
23. Hong R, Dibbell DG. Cultured thymus fragment transplant in chronic candidiasis complicated by oral carcinoma. Lancet 1981; 1: 773.
24. Jorizzo JL, Sams WM Jr, Jegasothy BV, Olansky AJ. Cimetidine as an immunomodulator: chronic mucocutaneous candidiasis as a model. Ann Intern Med 1980; 92: 192.
25. Valdimarrson H, Holt PJL, Moss PD, Hobbs JR. Treatment of chronic mucocutaneous candidiasis with leucocytes from HL-A compatible sibling. Lancet 1972; 1: 469.
26. Buckley RH, Lucas ZJ, Hattler BG Jr, Zmijewski CM, Amos DB. Defective cellular immunity associated with chronic mucocutaneous moniliasis and recurrent staphylococcal botryomycosis: immunological reconstitution by allogeneic bone marrow. Clin Exp Immunol 1968; 3: 153.

0041-1337/86/4105-0587$02.00/0
TRANSPLANTATION
Copyright © 1986 by The Williams & Wilkins Co.

Vol. 41, No. 5
Printed in U.S.A.

ANTIGEN-SPECIFIC ANTIBODY RESPONSES OF LYMPHOCYTES TO TETANUS TOXOID AFTER HUMAN MARROW TRANSPLANTATION[1]

SHINTARO SHIOBARA,[2] LAWRENCE G. LUM,[3] ROBERT P. WITHERSPOON, AND RAINER STORB

The Fred Hutchinson Cancer Research Center and the Division of Oncology, Departments of Medicine and Pediatrics, University of Washington School of Medicine, Seattle, Washington

In vitro IgG anti–tetanus toxoid (IgG anti-TT) antibody produced by peripheral blood lymphocytes (PBL) from 16 normal subjects (9 marrow donors and 7 random healthy subjects) and 17 marrow graft recipients from 45–1058 days postgrafting was measured with an enzyme-linked immunosorbent assay (ELISA). PBL from 11 of 13 seropositive (anti-TT ≥1:1024) normal subjects produced IgG anti-TT in vitro, whereas the PBL from the 3 seronegative (IgG anti-TT <1:1024) normal subjects did not. In our normal subjects, there was a high correlation between seropositivity and in vitro IgG anti-TT production (P=.0048, χ^2, two-tailed). PBL from only one of 13 seropositive marrow graft recipients produced in vitro IgG anti-TT antibody.

B and T cell functions of 8 marrow graft recipients were assessed by coculturing their T and B cells with those from their HLA-identical marrow donors. One short-term patient and 7 long-term patients (4 with and 3 without chronic graft-versus-host disease) were studied. Recipient B cells failed to produce antibody in the presence of donor T cells in 7 of these 8 cases. However, T cells from long-term survivors provided helper activity to immune donor B cells in 7 of 9 evaluable cases.

TT-specific helper T cell activity was present in most seropositive long-term recipients, and B cells from marrow recipients failed to produce specific antibody in the presence of normal donor TT-specific helper T cells. These results, TT-specific T cell helper activity, and normal circulating serum IgG anti-TT antibody levels in marrow graft recipients without postgrafting TT boosters suggest that specific immunity had been transferred from the marrow donor to the marrow recipient.

Human marrow graft recipients have humoral and cellular immune deficiencies that resolve over time, except in recipients with chronic graft-versus-host disease (GVHD) (*1–9*).* Previous studies using pokeweed mitogen (PWM) showed defects in B and T cell functions in nearly all patients within the first 3 months postgrafting, and these defects tended to persist in patients with chronic GVHD (*2, 3, 6, 7*). However, there have been few attempts to probe the immunodeficiency after marrow grafting using in vitro antigen-specific antibody production systems (*10, 11*).

Recently, we developed a new approach using a microculture system for eliciting and detecting IgG anti–tetanus toxoid (IgG anti-TT) antibody from peripheral blood lymphocytes (PBL) stimulated in vitro with tetanus toxoid (TT) (*12*). Responses were T-cell-dependent and antigen-specific. It is possible to induce in vitro IgG anti-TT antibody production in over 85% of immune normal subjects without recent booster immunizations.

This new approach uses high concentrations of lymphocytes in multiple replicate cultures, washout of the TT after 4 days of culture, replacement of culture medium, and assaying the supernatants for specific antibody synthesis after an additional 8 days of culture (*12*). The approach does not require recent in vivo booster immunizations or selection of immune subjects with high TT titers.

This investigation was undertaken to study the in vitro antigen-specific T and B cell functions in assays of specific IgG anti-TT antibody synthesis in marrow graft recipients, and to determine if cells capable of mediating antigen-specific antibody responses were transferred from marrow donors to marrow recipients.

MATERIALS AND METHODS

Patients. Sixteen of 17 patients with leukemia, lymphoma, or severe aplastic anemia ranging in age from 13 to 45 years, received marrow grafts from HLA-identical siblings. One recipient (UPN 2078) with lymphoma received a marrow graft from the HLA-haploidentical father and another (UPN 2141) with leukemia received a cryopreserved autologous marrow graft. Six patients were studied during the first 3 months after marrow grafting ("short-term" patients). Six patients with chronic GVHD and five without chronic GVHD were studied at intervals of 348–1058 days postgrafting ("long-term" patients).

The pertinent clinical data including clinical characteristics, time of study posttransplant, treatment regimens, and immunization histories are presented in Table 1. Patients with leukemia were conditioned for marrow transplantation with cyclophosphamide and total-body irradiation (*13–16*). Patients with aplastic anemia were conditioned for marrow transplantation with cyclophosphamide alone (*16*). Six patients received cyclosporine (*17*), and 8 patients received methotrexate (MTX) weekly for 3 months for GVHD prophylaxis. Two patients (UPNs 2158 and 1835) received MTX through day 11 after marrow infusion and cyclosporine from days -1 to 180. To

* Abbreviations used: ELISA, enzyme-linked immunosorbent assay; GVHD, graft-versus-host disease; Ig, immunoglobulin; IgG anti-TT, IgG anti-tetanus toxoid; MTX, methotrexate; PBL, peripheral blood lymphocytes; TT, tetanus toxoid; PWM, pokeweed mitogen.

[1] This work was supported by Grants CA 18221, HL36444 (formerly CA 30924), CA 25139, CA 15704, CA 18029, and CA 09319 awarded by the National Cancer Institute, DHHS.

[2] Shintaro Shiobara was supported in part by a Fellowship from Kanazawa University while a visiting scientist from the Third Department of Internal Medicine, 13-1 Takara-machi, Kanazawa University School of Medicine, Kanazawa, P.C. 920, Japan.

[3] Address correspondence to: Lawrence G. Lum, M.D., Fred Hutchinson Cancer Research Center, 1124 Columbia Street, Seattle, WA 98104.

TABLE 1. Patient characteristics, treatments, and immunizations

UPN[a] Diagnosis		Age (years) sex	Day of Study p̄ BMT	Acute GVHD > grade 2	Rx of acute or chronic GVHD	Day of last transfusion[b]
Short-term patients:						
2207	ALL	23/M	45	−	−	15
2196	CML	45/M	63	−	−	50
2141	ALL[au]	15/F	66	−	−	38
2201	AMML	13/M	76	+	−	6
2158	CML	22/M	88	+	CsA	63
2078	Lymph[m]	17/M	91	+	CsA + ATG	24
Long-term patients with chronic GVHD:						
1835	AA	39/F	348	−	−	190
1808	CML	20/M	431	−	−	No
1884	AMML	41/M	460	+	−	No
1693	AMOL	15/F	486	+	P11	No
1434	AA	37/F	930	+	−	No
1353	CML	39/F	1058	+	P	No
Long-term patients without chronic GVHD:						
1962	CML	26/F	383	+	−	No
1827	ALL	20/F	391	+	−	No
1857	AMML	29/F	395	−	−	No
1476	AMML[TT]	24/F	649	−	−	No
1523	AML	23/F	756	−	−	No

[a] UPN = unique patient number; BMT = bone marrow transplant; au = autologous; m = mismatched; ALL = acute lymphocytic leukemia; AML = acute myelogenous leukemia; CML = chronic myelogenous leukemia; AMOL = acute monocytic leukemia; AMML = acute myelomonocytic leukemia; AA = aplastic anemia; Lymph = lymphoma; CsA = cyclosporine; ATG = antithymocyte globulin; P11 = prednisone + study drugs; P = prednisone; TT = boosted with tetanus toxoid 5 days before study.

[b] No = no transfusions given after 100 days posttransplant.

prevent recurrent leukemia, an autologous transplant recipient (UPN 2141) received i.v. MTX weekly for 3 months (*18*).

PBL from the marrow donors were used as normal controls whenever possible. Otherwise, PBL from healthy random subjects were used as controls. Only donor T and B lymphocytes were used in coculture with recipient T and B lymphocytes.

History of TT immunizations. One recipient (UPN 1476) received a TT immunization 5 days before our study. The other recipients had no TT immunizations after marrow grafting. All normal subjects, including 9 marrow donors, had not been boosted in the 1-year interval prior to study. Two of three seronegative normal subjects were Japanese persons who had no history of TT immunizations.

Purification of mononuclear cells. PBL were obtained from whole heparinized blood by density gradient centrifugation with Ficoll-Hypaque and were separated into T (E^+) and non-T (E^-) cells by rosetting with sheep red blood cells (*19–21*). The T cell fraction consistently contained more than 95% E^+ cells and the non-T cell fraction (designated as B cells) contained less than 3% E^+ cells (*3, 4*).

Culture conditions. In vitro anti-TT antibody biosynthesis was induced using a new antigen-specific system employing high numbers of lymphocytes, high numbers of replicate cultures, and antigen washout after 4 days of culture. The specific details of the microculture system for the optimal induction of IgG anti-TT antibody have been described (*12*). In brief, 6×10^5 to 8×10^5 PBL/microculture or 6×10^5 T cells and 2×10^5 B cells/microculture from marrow graft recipients or normals were cocultured in the presence or absence of TT antigen (25 ng/ml). B cells were not limiting at a dose of 2×10^5 B cells/microculture, as determined by previous studies (*12*). The TT was purchased from the Commonwealth of Massachusetts Department of Public Health, Division of Biologic Laboratories. All cultures were performed in round-bottomed microwells (NUNC, Denmark) containing 250 μl of RPMI 1640 (GIBCO) supplemented with heat-inactivated fetal calf serum, antibiotics, and glutamine.

All experiments had a time zero supernatant defined as the supernatant from 4×10^6/ml PBL incubated for at least 1 hr at 37°C. These consistently measured zero. Supernatants were collected after 4 days of culture to rule out spontaneous specific antibody production and stored at −20°C until the assays were performed. All of the cultures were washed free of soluble antigen at day 4 to optimize antibody production (*12*). Eight days after washing, culture supernatants were collected and stored at −20°C until they were assessed for IgG anti-TT antibody by ELISA. The majority of the antibody produced in this in vitro system is directed at tetanus toxoid when stimulated by doses of TT less than 250 ng/ml. Higher doses of TT (>250 ng/ml) used to stimulate in vitro IgG anti-TT antibody production tend to elicit polyclonal IgG responses.

Preparation of IgG anti-TT antibody standard. IgG anti-TT antibody standard was prepared from hyperimmune serum from boosted normal subjects 1–2 weeks postimmunization with TT as described (*12*). The affinity-purified IgG anti-TT was acid eluted from a TT-linked Sepharose 4B column (Pharmacia, Piscataway, NJ). The affinity purified standard was calibrated against commercial IgG standard (TAGO, Burlingame, CA) assuming all of the IgG antibody present to be specific for TT.

Quantitation of IgG anti–tetanus toxoid antibody. Culture supernatants were assayed by a modification of an ELISA technique described elsewhere (*12, 22*).

Samples or known amounts of affinity-purified IgG anti-TT antibody standard were added to the wells and incubated for 2 hr at 37°C. After three washes with phosphate-buffered saline with 0.05 Tween 20, 100 μl of 1:1500 dilution of peroxidase-conjugated goat antibody directed at human IgG (TAGO, Burlingame, CA) was added to microwells.

After a 1hr incubation at 37°C, the plates were washed and 100 μl of a solution of ABTS (2,2′-azinodi-[3-ethylbenzthiazoline sulfonic acid], Sigma, St. Louis) at 1 mg/ml in 0.1 M citrate buffer, pH 4, with 0.03% H_2O_2 was added to each well, and the optical density at 414 nm was measured with a Titertek Multiscan Unit (Flow, McLean, VA).

The amount of IgG anti-TT antibody in samples was estimated by direct comparison to best-fit linear regression line determined by the standard samples (affinity-purified IgG anti-TT at 6 concentrations ranging from 7.3 to 55 ng/ml). The lower limit of sensitivity for detectable IgG anti-TT antibody varied between 2 and 8 ng/ml from assay to assay.

Tetanus toxoid antibody titers on a normal population. Over 110 normal immune subjects ranging in age from 3 to 50 years served as controls to determine a normal interval that included 95% of all determinations. Anti-TT antibody titers ≥1:1024 were considered positive. Since ELISA assays are more sensitive than hemagglutination methods, the negative cutoff titer using ELISA methodology was nearly two logs higher than the hemagglutination methodology. Agammaglobulinemic serum had IgG anti-TT antibody titers <1:128. Titers 1:512 or less were considered background in the ELISA. The mean serum antibody titer of the normal population to TT was 1:27,394 with a range from 1:1024 to 1:131,072. All antibody titer determinations were done by ELISA.

Statistics. Results were compared using χ^2, two-tailed test.

Informed consent. The studies described herein were performed using protocols approved by the Investigational Review Board of The Fred Hutchinson Cancer Research Center.

RESULTS

Correlation between in vivo and in vitro IgG anti-TT antibody production in marrow recipients. Table 2 shows the lack of correlation between in vivo seropositivity and in vitro IgG anti-TT production by lymphocytes from marrow recipients. Five of 6 short-term recipients, 3 of the 6 long-term recipients with chronic GVHD, and all 5 long-term recipients without chronic GVHD had serum antibody titers to TT. However, this in vitro study shows that PBL from all but one recipient failed to produce IgG anti-TT antibody. The PBL that produced IgG anti-TT antibody were from a female recipient (UPN 1827) who received bone marrow from a male donor. Cytogenetics showed peripheral blood lymphoid chimerism (12 with 46.XY; 8 with 46.XX) 391 days posttransplant (an unusual finding). Cytogenetics in the other marrow graft recipients revealed lymphocytes of donor type exclusively when there were evaluable cytogenetic markers at or before the time of study.

Cocultures using donor and recipient T and B cells. Figure 1 illustrates the type of experiments used to assess T and B cell functions. A long-term recipient (UPN 1523) without chronic GVHD 756 days after marrow transplantation was studied. Cultures containing recipient T and donor B cells and cultures containing donor T and recipient B cells were compared with control cultures of donor T and B cells to assess TT-specific helper activity and B cell function. Six of 12 cultures containing donor T and donor B cells produced 7, 13, 31, 42, 47, and 60 ng IgG anti-TT antibody/ml (mean = 16.7 ng/ml). In contrast, none of 12 cultures containing recipient T and B cells responded. Eight of 12 cultures containing recipient T and donor B cells produced 9, 12, 18, 21, 39, 52, 55, and 61 ng IgG anti-TT antibody/ml (mean = 22.0 ng/ml), while none of the cultures containing donor T and patient B cells produced IgG anti-TT antibody.

Failure of B cells to produce IgG anti-TT antibody. Table 3 summarizes the results of cultures on 9 cases studied using recombinations of donor and patient lymphocytes after TT stimulation to assess T and B cell functions. Autologous cul-

TABLE 2. In vivo and in vitro IgG anti-TT antibody production in marrow transplant recipients

UPN	Day after BMT[a]	In vivo IgG anti-TT titer[b]	In vitro IgG anti-TT production[c]		
			With TT (day 4)	With TT (day 12)	With medium (day 12)
Short-term patients:					
2207	45	1:1024[d]	0/12	0/10	ND[g]
2196	63	1:1024	1/12 (7)[e]	0/24	0/24
2141	66	1:131072	0/12	0/12	0/12
2201	76	1:128	0/12	0/24	0/24
2158	88	1:131072	0/4	0/8	ND
2078	91	1:16384	0/8	0/8	0/4
Long-term patients with chronic GVHD;					
1835	348	1:1024	0/4	0/4	0/4
1808	431	1:1024	0/12	0/12	0/12
1884	460	1:16384	0/12	0/18	ND
1693	486	1:128	ND	0/11	ND
1434	930	1:128	ND	0/24	ND
1353	1058	1:128	0/18	0/20	ND
Long-term patients without chronic GVHD;					
1962	383	1:131072	0/12	0/16	ND
1827	391	>1:131072	0/12	11/12 (16, 36, 28, >55, >55, >55, >55, >55, >55, >55, >55)[f]	0/12
1857	395	1:1024	0/12	0/12	0/12
1476	649	1:16384	ND	0/18	0/8
1523	756	1:1024	0/18	0/18	0/12

[a] Days postgrafting when the recipients were studied.

[b] The serum Ab titers were performed and reported as 2-fold dilutions of serum. Titers <1:1024 were defined as seronegative, and titers ≥1:1024 were defined as seropositive, see the *Materials and Methods* section.

[c] Positive wells/total wells.

[d] The last positive serum dilution expressed as $\log_2$.

[e] Numbers in parentheses show amount of IgG anti-TT antibody (ng/ml).

[f] > symbol indicates ELISA determinations that were greater than the highest standard point.

[g] ND = not done.

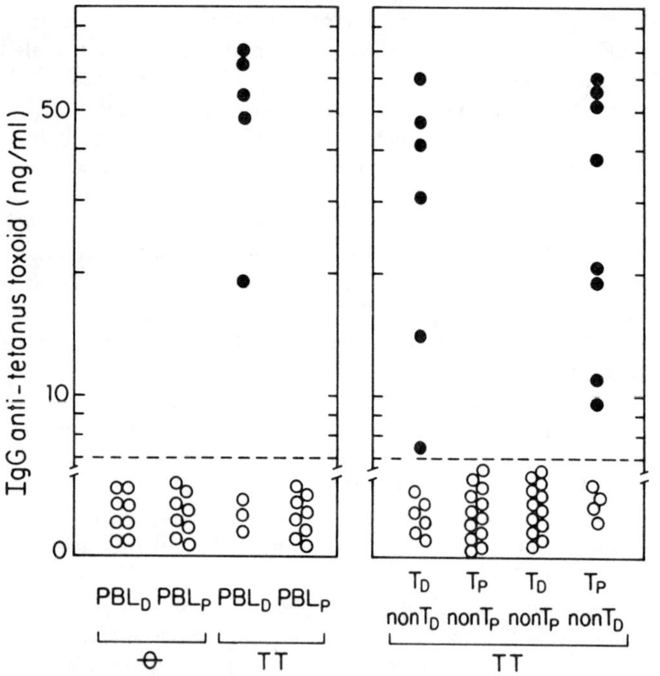

FIGURE 1. Patient non-T cells fail to produce IgG anti-TT antibody in the presence of donor T cells. The amounts of IgG anti-TT antibody production per well at 12 days stimulated by TT antigen are shown on the vertical axis; the various cocultures used to identify the cells responsible for in vitro failure are shown on the horizontal axis; (PBL) peripheral blood lymphocytes, (T) T cells, (non T) non-T cells (D) donor, (P) patient, (-⊖-) medium only, and (TT) tetanus toxoid. The PBL cultures contained 8×10^5 cells and the (T + non-T) cultures contained 6×10^5 T cells and 2×10^5 non-T cells.

tures of donor T and B cells produce IgG anti-TT antibody in 6 of 9 cases tested. Only one of 8 recipients had autologous T and B cells that produced IgG anti-TT antibody; and this patient (UPN 1827) was a lymphoid chimera.

Recipient T and donor B cells could produce IgG anti-TT antibody in 7 of 9 evaluable cases, while donor T and patient B cells from only one (UPN 1827) of 9 cases produced IgG anti-TT antibody. No IgG anti-TT antibody was detected in the 12 day supernatants from unstimulated PBL from the marrow recipients. These results demonstrate evidence for the presence of antigen-specific helper T cell activity and impaired specific antibody synthesis by recipient B cells.

DISCUSSION

The long-term marrow recipients had T cells that provided TT-specific T cell helper activity to donor B cells in 6 of 7 marrow recipients. On the other hand, B cells from marrow recipients failed to produce IgG anti–tetanus toxoid antibody in the presence of TT-specific donor helper T cells. These findings contrast with findings in PBL from normal individuals where the presence of a serum IgG anti–tetanus toxoid titer correlates with the ability to produce in vitro antibody.

A few studies show that specific humoral immunity may be transferred from immune marrow donors to marrow recipients. Early studies in dogs showed marrow graft recipients developed distemper titers without postgrafting immunizations (*23*). Another investigation using IgG anti–keyhole-limpet-hemocyanin (KLH) as an immunologic marker showed transfer of anti-KLH antibody activity from an immunized identical twin donor to an unimmunized recipient who received a marrow transplant for treatment of leukemia (*24*). Recently, one study showed transfer of anti-acetylcholine-receptor immunity from the donor to a recipient who developed myasthenia gravis postgrafting (*25*). A recent study of ours demonstrated levels of IgG anti–tetanus toxoid antibody in a group of long-term marrow recipients who had not received tetanus toxoid immunizations postgrafting (*26*).

The origin of the serum IgG anti-TT is likely different between marrow graft recipients in the first 100 days after marrow grafting and the recipients at intervals greater than 1–3 years postgrafting. Immunoglobulin allotype studies show that host-type immunoglobulins are no longer detectable in 97% of the recipients by 120 days postgrafting (*27*). Furthermore, studies of the long-term survivors are not confounded by passive antibody received through blood products. On the other hand, the short-term survivors may have a mixture of cells and antibodies of donor and host origin. Postgrafting cytogenetic analyses have shown PBL to be of donor origin as early as 14 days after marrow transplantation (*13, 28*) and peripheral blood monocytes and tissue macrophages in lung and liver to be of donor type by day 80 (*21, 29–31*).

Our findings suggest that infused donor B cells are producing specific IgG anti-TT antibody in the recipient without booster immunization. However, we were unable to stimulate PBL with TT to produce in vitro IgG anti-TT antibody and our results show that B cells were likely responsible for the in vitro failure since in vitro monocyte accessory cell function of long-term marrow recipients in pokeweed-mitogen-driven immunoglobulin production has been shown to be generally intact in the majority (10/12) of cases (*21*). The frequency of monocyte mediated suppression of polyclonal antibody synthesis in the pokeweed mitogen system was low (2/12) cases. The possibility of monocyte mediated TT-specific suppression needs to be further investigated but was not within the scope of this study.

Antigen-specific B cells exist in sufficient numbers in the marrow recipients to produce circulating levels of IgG anti-TT but do not circulate in great enough numbers for detection under the current conditions of our assay system. In vitro B cell failure may be due to low precursor frequency of antigen-specific B cells, sequestration of antibody producing B cells, insensitivity of the recipient B cells to antigenic stimulation, and/or a lack of in vivo and/or in vitro B cell growth and differentiation factors. Culturing higher than usual ($>8.0\times10^5$/culture) numbers of PBL from marrow graft recipients tends to enhance IgG anti-TT antibody production (Lum et al, unpublished data). Although we expected less-than-normal antigen-specific T cell helper activity we did not observe impaired antigen-specific helper activity or excessive antigen-specific suppressor T cell activity. Since marrow recipients have polyclonal suppressor T cells (*2–4, 26*), it would not be surprising to find T cells from marrow recipients that suppress in this assay system. The role of suppressor T cells is not clear since cell numbers did not permit us to screen the T cell subpopulations for suppressor activity. Additional studies are necessary to determine whether antigen-specific suppressor T cells play a role in the marrow recipients.

Our results suggest that donor T cells may carry specific memory to tetanus toxoid and can communicate in an antigen-specific fashion with donor B cells. These findings contrast with those of Dosch et al. who described communication failure between T cells and B cells in the production of specific antibody in their patient with chronic GVHD (*10*). Although controversial, the presence of circulating IgG anti-TT titers

TABLE 3. The non-T-cell fraction is responsible for in vitro failure of IgG anti-TT antibody production

UPN	anti-TT antibody titers[a]		Td + non-Td[c]	Recombination of donor and patient cells[b]		
	Donor	Patient		Tp + non-Tp	Td + non-Tp	Tp + non-Td
Short-term patients:						
2078	1:16384	1:16384	2/8 (53, 49)[d]	0/8	0/8	0/8
Long-term patients with chronic GVHD:						
1835	1:16384	1:1024	3/7 (32, 45, >55)	0/4	0/4	3/7 (14, 16, >55)
1808	1:16384	1:1024	12/24 (7, 7, 8, 10, 10, 12, 31, 41, 49, 54, >55, >55)	0/12	0/12	3/18(12, 24, >55)
1693	1:16384	1:128	4/12 (20, >55, >55, 11)	0/11	0/11	0/11
1353	1:1024	1:128	0/9	0/9	0/9	1/9 (+)
Long-term patients without chronic GVHD:						
1827	1:131072	>1:131072	0/6	11/12 (16, 28, 36, >55, >55, >55, >55, >55, >55, >55, >55)	1/6 (34)	1/12 (35)
1476	1:16384	1:16384	9/12 (18, 30, 39, 35, +, +, +, +, +)	0/12	0/12	10/12 (8, 25, 19, 40, 49, >55, +, +, +, +)
1523	1:131072	1:1024	6/12 (7, 13, 47, 31, >55, 42)	0/12	0/12	8/12 (12, 9, 21, 18, 39, 52, 55, >55)

[a] <1:1024 means seronegative and ≥1:1024 means seropositive.
[b] Positive wells/total wells.
[c] "T + non-T" indicates coculture of 6×10^5 T cells and 2×10^5B cells per well; d = donor, p = patient.
[d] Numbers in parentheses show amount of IgG anti-TT antibody (ng/ml). + = ELISA wells positive for IgG anti-TT antibody, but the amount of antibody not determined.

(*26*) and the presence and antigen-specific helper T cells suggest that antigen-specific T cell memory may be transferred from the donor to the recipient.

Saxon et al. and Ringden et al. reported increased spontaneous Ig production associated with GVHD, hypergammaglobulinemia and infection (*6, 32*), and decreased polyclonal immunoglobulin production responses to in vitro stimulation with *Staphylococcus aureus* bacteria (*32*). Only one marrow graft recipient in the first 100-day interval postgrafting had spontaneous IgG anti-TT production after in vitro stimulation with TT. The differences between the studies that showed increased spontaneous Ig production and this study may be due to differences in the study populations and differenes in polyclonal and antigen-specific assay systems.

This study demonstrates that the immunodeficiency observed after marrow grafting can be examined using an antigen-specific culture system. Future studies will explore the antigen-specific B cell failure using limiting dilution techniques. We hypothesize that B cells from some of the marrow graft recipients will produce antibody if the number of T and B cells/microculture is increased. If our hypothesis is correct, then we will have been able to establish a basis for in vivo/in vitro correlative studies using the tetanus toxoid–specific system.

Acknowledgments. We acknowledge the assistance of Jan Noges, Deborah Gayle, and Lori Ausburn in the preparation of the manuscript.

REFERENCES

1. Noel DR, Witherspoon RP, Storb R, et al. Does graft-versus-host disease influence the tempo of immunologic recovery after allogeneic human marrow transplantation? An observation on 56 long-term survivors. Blood 1978; 51: 1087.
2. Witherspoon RP, Lum LG, Storb R, Thomas ED. In vitro regulation of immunoglobulin synthesis after human marrow transplantation. II. Deficient T and non-T lymphocyte function within 3–4 months of allogeneic, syngeneic, or autologous marrow grafting for hematologic malignancy. Blood 1982; 59: 844.
3. Lum LG, Seigneuret MC, Storb RF, Witherspoon RP, Thomas ED. In vitro regulation of immunoglobulin synthesis after marrow transplantation. I. T-cell and B-cell deficiencies in patients with and without chronic graft-versus-host disease. Blood 1981; 58: 431.
4. Lum LG, Orcutt-Thordarson N, Seigneuret MC, Storb R. The regulation of Ig synthesis after marrow transplantation. IV. T4 and T8 subset function in patients with chronic graft-versus-host disease. J Immunol 1982; 129: 113.
5. Tsoi MS, Storb R, Dobbs S, et al. Nonspecific suppressor cells in patients with chronic graft-vs-host disease after marrow grafting. J Immunol 1979; 123: 1970.
6. Saxon A, McIntyre RE, Stevens RH, Gale RP. Lymphocyte dysfunction in chronic graft-versus-host disease. Blood 1981; 58: 746.
7. Witherspoon RP, Storb R, Ochs HD, et al. Recovery of antibody production in human allogeneic marrow graft recipients. Influence of time post-transplantation, the presence or absence of

chronic graft-versus-host disease, and antithymocyte globulin treatment. Blood 1981; 58: 360.

8. Mori T, Tsoi M-S, Gillis S, Santos E, Thomas ED, Storb R. Cellular interactions in marrow-grafted patients. I. Impairment of cell-mediated lympholysis associated with graft-vs-host disease and the effect of interleukin 2. J Immunol 1983; 130: 712.
9. Witherspoon RP, Kopecky K, Storb R, et al. Immunologic recovery in 48 patients following syngeneic marrow transplantation for hematological malignancy. Transplantation 1982; 33: 143.,
10. Dosch H-M, Gelfand EW. Failure of T and B cell cooperation during graft-versus-host disease. Transplantation 1981; 31: 48.
11. Pahwa SG, Pahwa RN, Friedrich W, O'Reilly RJ, Good RA. Abnormal humoral immune responses in peripheral blood lymphocyte cultures of bone marrow transplant recipients. Proc Natl Acad Sci (USA) 1982; 79: 2663.
12. Lum LG, Culbertson NJ. The induction and suppression of in vitro IgG anti-tetanus toxoid antibody synthesis by human lymphocytes stimulated with tetanus toxoid in the absence of in vivo booster immunizations. J Immunol 1985; 135: 185.
13. Thomas ED, Buckner CD, Banaji M, et al. One hundred patients with acute leukemia treated by chemotherapy, total body irradiation, and allogeneic marrow transplantation. Blood 1977; 49: 511.
14. Thomas ED, Clift RA, Hersman J, et al. Marrow transplantation for acute nonlymphoblastic leukemia in first remission using fractionated or single-dose irradiation. Int J Radiat Oncol Biol Phys 1982; 8: 817.
15. Clift RA, Buckner CD, Thomas ED, et al. Allogeneic marrow transplantation using fractionated total body irradiation in patients with acute lymphoblastic leukemia in relapse. Leuk Res 1982; 6: 401.
16. Storb R, Thomas ED, Buckner CD, et al. Allogeneic marrow grafting for treatment of aplastic anemia. Blood 1974; 43: 157.
17. Deeg HJ, Storb R, Thomas ED, et al. Marrow transplantation for acute nonlymphoblastic leukemia in first remission: preliminary results of a randomized trial comparing cyclosporine and methotrexate for the prophylaxis of graft-versus-host disease. Transplant Proc 1983; 15: 1385.
18. Stewart P, Buckner CD, Bensinger W, et al. Autologous marrow transplantation in patients with acute nonlymphocytic leukemia in first remission. Exp Hematol 1985; 13: 267.
19. Pellegrino MA, Ferrone S, Dierich MP, Reisfeld RA. Enhancement of sheep red blood cell human lymphocyte rosette formation by the sulfhydryl compound 2-aminoethylisothiouronium bromide. Clin Innumol Immunopathol 1975; 3: 324.
20. Lum LG, Benveniste E, Blaese RM. Functional properties of human T cells bearing Fc receptors for IgA. I. Mitogen responsiveness, mixed lymphocyte culture reactivity, and helper activity for B cell immunoglobulin production. J Immunol 1980; 124: 702.
21. Shiobara S, Witherspoon RP, Lum LG, Storb R. Immunoglobulin synthesis after HLA-identical marrow grafting. V. The role of peripheral blood monocytes in the regulation of in vitro immunoglobulin secretion stimulated by PW mitogen. J Immunol 1984; 132: 2850.
22. Engvall E, Perlmann P. Enzyme-linked immunosorbent assay, ELISA. III. Quantification of specific antibodies by enzyme-labeled anti-immunoglobulin in antigen-coated tubes. J Immunol 1972; 109: 129.
23. Ochs HD, Storb R, Thomas ED, et al. Immunological reactivity in canine marrow graft recipients. J Immunol 1974; 113: 1039.
24. Starling KA, Faletta JM, Fernbach DJ. Immunologic chimerism as evidence of bone marrow graft acceptance in an identical twin with acute lymphocytic leukemia. Exp Hematol 1975; 3: 244.
25. Smith CIE, Aarli JA, Biberfeld P, et al. Myasthenia gravis after bone marrow transplantation; evidence for a donor origin; N Engl J Med 1983; 309: 1565.
26. Lum LG, Seigneuret MC, Orcutt-Thordarson N, Noges JE, Storb R. The regulation of immunoglobulin synthesis after HLA-identical bone marrow transplantation. VI. Differential rates of maturation of distinct functional groups within lymphoid subpopulations in patients after human marrow grafting. Blood 1985; 65: 1422.
27. Witherspoon RP, Schanfield MS, Storb R, Thomas ED, Giblett ER. Immunoglobulin production of donor origin after marrow transplantation for acute leukemia or aplastic anemia. Transplantation 1978; 26: 407.
28. Storb R, Thomas ED, Weiden PO, et al. Aplastic anemia treated by allogeneic bone marrow transplantation; a report on 49 new cases from Seattle. Blood 1976; 48: 817.
29. Tsoi M-S, Dobbs S, Brkic S, Ramberg R, Thomas ED, Storb R. Cellular interactions in marrow-grafting patients. II. Normal monocyte antigen-presenting and defective T-cell proliferative functions early after grafting and during chronic graft-versus-host disease. Transplantation 1984; 37: 556.
30. Thomas ED, Ramberg RE, Sale GE, Sparkes RS, Golde DW. Direct evidence for a bone marrow origin of the alveolar macrophage in man. Science 1976; 192: 1016.
31. Gale RP, Sparkes RS, Golde DW. Bone marrow origin of hepatic macrophages (Kupffer cells) in humans. Science 1978; 201: 937.
32. Ringden O, Witherspoon R, Storb R, Ekelund E, Thomas ED. B cell function in human marrow transplant recipients assessed by direct and indirect hemolysis-in-gel assays. J Immunol 1979; 123: 2729.

Received 20 May 1985.
Accepted 5 September 1985.

0041-1337/86/4105-0593$02.00/0
TRANSPLANTATION
Vol. 41, No. 5

Printed in U.S.A.

DIAGNOSIS OF TUBULAR INJURY IN RENAL TRANSPLANT PATIENTS BY A URINARY ASSAY FOR A PROXIMAL TUBULAR ANTIGEN, THE ADENOSINE-DEAMINASE-BINDING PROTEIN[1]

N. E. TOLKOFF-RUBIN,[2] A. B. COSIMI, F. L. DELMONICO, P. S. RUSSELL, R. E. THOMPSON, D. J. PIPER, W. P. HANSEN, N. H. BANDER, C. L. FINSTAD, C. CORDON-CARDO, L. H. KLOTZ, L. J. OLD, AND R. H. RUBIN

The Dialysis-Transplantation Unit of the Medical and Surgical Services of the Massachusetts General Hospital, and the Department of Medicine and Surgery of Harvard Medical School, Boston, Massachusetts; the Cambridge Research Laboratory, Cambridge, Massachusetts; and the Laboratory of Human Cancer Serology of The Memorial-Sloan Kettering Cancer Center, New York, New York

Two murine monoclonal antibodies (URO-4 and URO-4a)—which detect different epitopes of a proximal tubular cell glycoprotein antigen, the adenosine-deaminase-binding protein (ABP)—have been formatted into a sandwich enzyme immunoassay for detection of ABP in the urine. Serial urine samples from 34 renal transplant patients during the first six months posttransplant were analyzed to determine the correlation of this test with clinical rejection and cyclosporin (CsA) nephrotoxicity.

In 29/29 acute rejection episodes the ABP level was elevated, beginning 1–7 days prior to treatment of rejection. Eighteen patients were treated for rejection with courses of OKT3 or antithymocyte globulin: 0/6 whose ABP level fell to normal during therapy had rerejection; 10/12 whose ABP level remained elevated had rerejection within 7 days of therapy completion. Of 15 patients treated with CsA, 7 had no rejection or drug toxicity; all 7 had normal ABP levels. The remaining 8 had CsA nephrotoxicity, all in association with elevated ABP levels that rapidly fell to normal with decreased CsA dose. An additional 7 patients with creatinine elevations more than 6 months posttransplant were studied: 5 had chronic vascular changes on biopsy, no response to increased immunosuppression, and normal ABP levels; 2 had a cellular infiltrate on biopsy, response to increased immunosuppression, and elevated ABP levels. We conclude that the urinary ABP assay provides information useful in the management of renal transplant patients with acute and chronic rejection and CsA toxicity.

A basic tenet of kidney transplantation is that allograft rejection is better prevented than treated, and that the earlier a rejection episode is recognized and treatment initiated, the greater the chance of reversing the rejection episode with the least amount of permanent renal damage. Unfortunately, short of renal biopsy, there is no definitive diagnostic test for the presence of acute allograft rejection. Usually, the diagnosis is based upon the recognition of one or more of the cardinal clinical signs of rejection—weight gain, falling urine output, increasing serum creatinine, hypertension, fever, and graft enlargement and tenderness. Pediatric transplant recipients, who have small muscle masses—and, frequently, adult-sized kidneys in place—present an even more difficult diagnostic dilemma, with fever often being the only early indication of rejection. Unfortunately, the same signs and symptoms can result from a variety of types of allograft injury—including the tubulointerstitial injury of classic cellular rejection, but also technical complications of the transplant procedure, acute tubular necrosis, drug toxicity (such as that caused by cyclosporine or gentamicin), vascular rejection associated with humoral factors, a glomerulopathy associated with cytomegalovirus infection, pyelonephritis, and recurrent disease. Only the first of these, classic cellular rejection, is likely to respond to increases in immunosuppressive therapy.

There remains, therefore, a compelling need for specific and sensitive noninvasive tests that might provide an early warning of allograft rejection. Ideally, such a test should help to distinguish among the various forms of allograft injury and be useful for assessing the response to a given therapeutic regimen. A variety of approaches attempting to fulfill these needs has been taken, ranging from immunologic monitoring (*1–4*) to the measurement of the release of a various serum proteins and renal enzymes into the urine with renal injury (*5–13*). All of these approaches have provided useful information, but none has proved sufficiently specific to permit clinical management decisions to be made on the basis of its results alone.

We have evaluated a new approach to this problem. A series of monoclonal antibodies (Mabs) has been generated that recognize surface glycoproteins on cells restricted to specific regions of the nephron (*14–16*). Since the nephron is bathed in urine, a body fluid easily sampled, we postulated that if we could develop assays using Mabs for one or more of these glycoproteins, we would have a quantitative means of assessing both the site and extent of nephron injury. In addition, since serial samples of urine could be obtained easily, we could monitor the activity of the disease process and its responsiveness to therapy. To test this hypothesis, we have developed a sandwich ELISA assay for a 120,000 dalton glycoprotein (*17*),

* Abbreviations used: ABP, adenosine-deaminase-binding; ATG, antithymocyte globulin; CsA, cyclosporine; EDTA, ethylenediaminotetraacetate; ELISA, enzyme-linked immunosorbent assay; Mabs, monoclonal antibodies.

[1] Presented in part at the 17th Annual Meeting of The American Society of Nephrology, Washington, D.C., December, 1984.

[2] Reprint requests should be addressed to: Nina E. Tolkoff-Rubin, M.D., Hemodialysis Unit; Massachusetts General Hospital; Boston, MA 02114.

the adenosine-deaminase-binding protein (ABP), which is found on the brush border of the proximal tubular epithelial cell (*18*). This test has been shown to be an excellent marker for proximal tubular injury, and to distinguish reliably between glomerular and tubular injury in patients with native kidney disease (*19*). This report summarizes our experience with this assay in patients undergoing renal transplantation.

MATERIALS AND METHODS

Assay. URO-4 and URO-4a, two commercially available murine Mabs (Cambridge Research Laboratory, Cambridge, MA) which recognize different epitopes of the soluble forms of ABP were formatted into a sandwich enzyme-linked immunosorbent assay (ELISA) assay as previously described (*17*) In brief, the two Mabs were obtained as ascites fluid and then purified on Protein A–Sepharose according to the methods of Ey et al. (*20*). URO-4a was conjugated to horseradish peroxidase by the method of Wilson and Nakane (*21*). Purified URO-4 was passively absorbed onto the surfaces of Immulon 2 microtiter plates (Dynatech Laboratory, Inc., Alexandria, VA) by leaving 125 μl of URO-4 solution (10 μg/ml, in $Na_2CO_3/NaHCO_3$ buffer, 50 mmol/L, pH 9.6) in each well to adsorb overnight at 4°C. The plates were then washed with phosphate-buffered saline solution containing Tween 20 polyoxyethylene sorbitan monolaurate (0.5 ml/L). Any remaining binding sites were blocked by the addition of a 10 g/L solution of bovine serum albumin in phosphate-buffered saline for 1 hr at 25°C. The plates were then kept stored at 4°C until use, at which time they were washed three additional times with the Tween-containing phosphate-buffered saline.

To perform the assay, duplicate 100-μl portions of patients' urine, assay controls, and known assay standards (prepared from pooled positive urine samples) were inoculated onto the previously prepared URO-4-coated microtiter plates, and incubated for 1 hr at 25°C. The plates were then washed three times with the Tween-containing phosphate-buffered saline to remove unbound antigen and other materials. To each well was then added 100 μl of URO-4a-horseradish-peroxidase conjugate (0.4 mg/L), which was allowed to incubate for 1 hr at 25°C. The unbound conjugate was then aspirated, and the wells washed three more times with Tween-containing phosphate-buffered saline. At this point, 100 μl of the chromogen solution, which contained, per liter, 2 g of o-phenylenediamine and 500 μl of 30% H_2O_2 in citrate (19 mmol/L)-Na_2HPO_4 (62 mmol/L) buffer, pH 5.0. After incubating for 1 hr at 25°C, the enzymic activity was halted by the addition of 100 μl of 4.5 mol/L sulfuric acid. An MR600 microtiter plate reader (Dynatech) was used to quantify the enzyme activity by measuring at 490 nm the absorbance of the color that had developed. A standard curve was established with each assay, using the prepared standard, and based on arbitrary units of reactivity, with 1 A.U. being defined as the amount of ABP in 100 μl of sample that increased the absorbance at 490 nm by one absorbance unit in the assay. Patients' urinary concentrations of ABP were calculated by comparison with the standard curve.

Patient selection and urine collection. A total of 34 consecutive renal transplant recipients, including 23 recipients of kidneys from cadaveric donors and 11 recipients of kidneys from living-related donors, were entered into this study beginning on the day following transplantation. Of these 34 patients, 19 were treated with azathioprine and prednisone from the time of transplantation according to our usual protocol (*22*). The remaining 15 patients were treated with CsA and prednisone as follows: CsA, at a dosage of 15 mg/kg/day, orally, is started on the day of transplant, then gradually tapered to maintain a plasma level of 100–400 ng/ml (by radioimmunoassay [23]), reaching a maintenance dosage of 4–6 mg/kg/day by about eight weeks posttransplant. Prednisone therapy is initiated at a dose of 200 mg/day on the day of transplant, with a daily decrease in dose of 40 mg/day, until a daily maintenance dose of 20 mg/day is reached on the fifth posttransplant day. Untimed urine specimens from each of these patients were obtained daily while they were in the hospital and at each follow-up outpatient visit during the first six months posttransplant. On average, in the uncomplicated patient, daily urine specimens were obtained for the first three weeks posttransplant, twice a week for six weeks, once a week for four weeks, and then once or twice a month for the rest of the six-month period when the patient remained in the study. Patients with complicated courses—e.g., those with rejection or CsA toxicity—were studied more frequently (usually daily during the course of the complication). These urine specimens had preservatives added to give the following final concentrations: Tris 20 mmol/L, benzamidine 1 mmol/L, and ethylenediaminotetraacetate (EDTA) 10 mmol/L. The pH of the specimens then ranged from 6.0 to 7.5. All debris and insoluble material were removed by centrifugation (1500 ×g, 10 min), and then the specimens were stored at 4°C until assayed.

Acute transplant rejection was diagnosed on the basis of a 50% or greater increase in serum creatinine level over a period of less than three days that was not explained by some other cause. Such episodes were treated with 1–3-pulse doses (250–500 mg) of i.v. methylprednisolone at a dose of 10 mg/kg. If rejection activity still continued, these patients were then treated with antithymocyte globulin (ATG) (*24*) of the anti-T-cell monoclonal antibody OKT3 (*25*), as previously reported.

For purposes of this study, CsA nephrotoxicity was defined as episodes of creatinine elevation in which the serum creatinine levels fell ≥0.4 mg/dl within 72 hr of decreasing the CsA dose.

An additional seven patients with chronic allograft rejection were entered into this study and met the following criteria: they were found more than six months posttransplant to have a greater than 50% increase in serum creatinine level over a period of more than seven days, and were then subjected to renal biospy and increased immunosuppressive therapy. Such patients had serial urine samples assayed during the course of this evaluation and treatment. Such urine specimens were handled in a fashion identical to that described previously.

RESULTS

Eleven of the 34 prospectively studied patients (32.4%) had neither acute allograft rejection nor evidence of CsA toxicity in the first six months posttransplant. Of these, seven had been treated with the CsA and prednisone protocol, the remaining four with azathioprine and prednisone. As delineated in Figure 1 and 2, in such patients the urinary ABP levels fell to a level of <0.35 A.U. during the first week following transplantation, and remained at that level. Such a pattern occurred in all 11 patients with an uncomplicated clinical course, without regard to the form of immunosuppression being administered.

In contrast, 29 of 29 episodes of acute allograft rejection, that occurred in 23 individuals (in 15 of these episodes the clinical diagnosis was confirmed by renal biopsy that revealed the

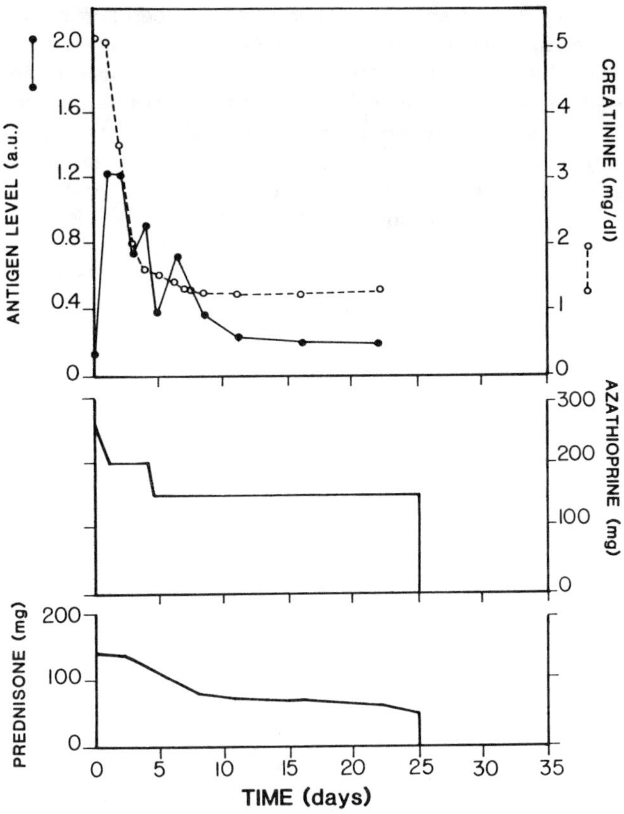

FIGURE 1. Results of urinary proximal tubular antigen (the adenosine-deaminase-binding protein) assays and serum creatinine determinations in a cadaveric renal allograft recipient immunosuppressed with azathioprine and prednisone who had an uncomplicated posttransplant course.

typical tubulointerstitial inflammatory changes of acute cellular rejection) were associated with urinary ABP levels >0.6 A.U. (P<.01), beginning 1–7 days prior to the clinical diagnosis of rejection. Particularly noteworthy was the experience with the pediatric transplant recipient whose course is outlined in Figure 3. In this patient, intermittent fevers of unknown cause and increased urinary ABP levels that were unresponsive to two pulse doses of methylprednisolone both began more than five days prior to the point when the definitive diagnosis of acute allograft rejection could be made and full antirejection treatment instituted. Such therapy was ineffective, the kidney was lost, and the patient returned to chronic dialysis.

A total of 18 patients with acute rejection were treated with either OKT3 or ATG and had a "successful reversal" of their acute rejection process. Of these 18, six (33%) had their urinary ABP levels fall to a level <0.35 A.U. by the completion of the course of antirejection therapy. None of these six rerejected over the next three months. In contrast, 12 patients (67%) had increased levels of urinary ABP (>0.6 A.U.) at the completion of the antirejection therapy, with 10 of these (83%) having a repeat episode of rejection within seven days of discontinuing the ATG or OKT3 regimen (P<.05). The patient whose course is outlined in Figure 4 is representative of this phenomenon. The acute rejection episode initially responded to treatment with OKT3 and cyclophosphamide, with the serum creatinine falling from a peak of 5 mg/dl to 2.4 mg/dl, but with only partial and temporary improvement in the urinary ABP level. Rerejection ensued within two days of discontinuing the OKT3 regimen, resulting in further therapy with ATG. On this occasion, not only the patient's creatinine level but his ABP level fell, and he remained free of further rejection activity.

Fifteen patients in this study were immunosuppressed with

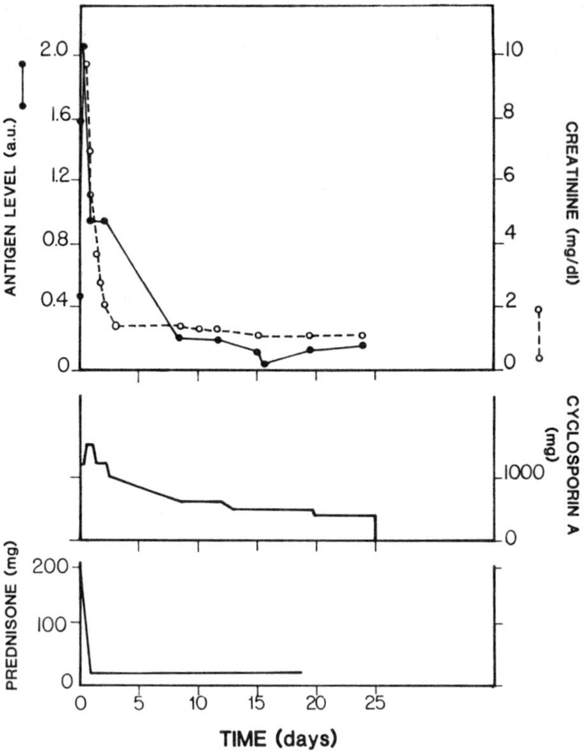

FIGURE 2. Results of urinary proximal tubular antigen (the adenosine-deaminase-binding protein) assays and serum creatinine determinations in a cadaveric renal allograft recipient given CsA and prednisone who had an uncomplicated posttransplant course.

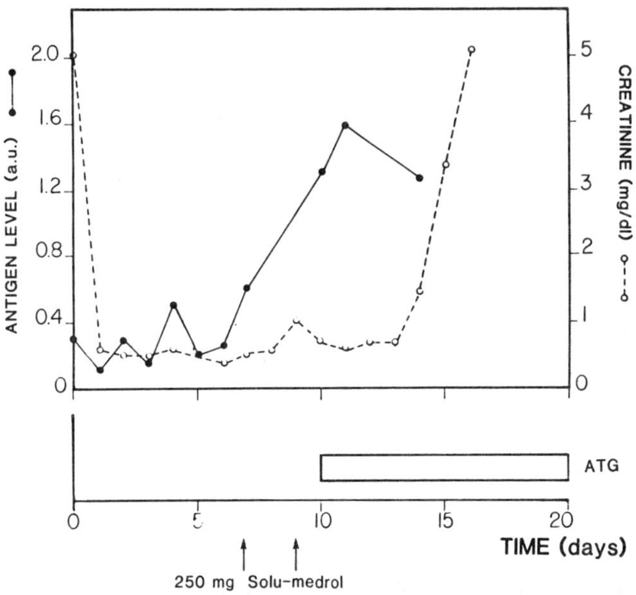

FIGURE 3. Results of urinary proximal tubular antigen (the adenosine-deaminase-binding protein) assays and serum creatinine determinations in a pediatric patient who had received an HLA-identical kidney from a sibling. Particular attention is called to the fact that the assay became abnormal approximately five days before a definitive diagnosis of rejection was made and ATG therapy instituted, and seven days before the serum creatinine level began to rise.

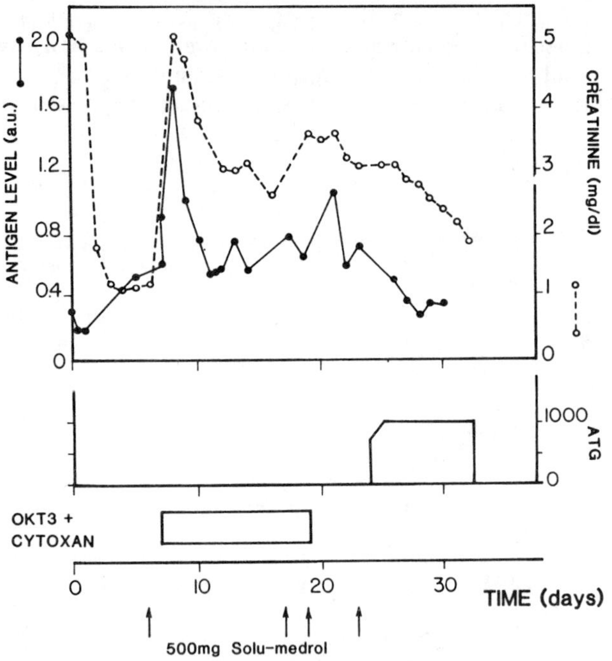

FIGURE 4. Results of urinary proximal tubular antigen (the adenosine-deaminase-binding protein) assays in a cadaveric renal allograft recipient who underwent two episodes of acute rejection, the first treated with OKT3, cyclophosphamide, and two pulse doses of methylprednisolone, the second with one pulse dose of methylprednisolone and ATG. Particular attention is called to the fact that, at the completion of the first course of therapy, the antigen level was still elevated and rerejection quickly ensued. In contrast, at the end of the second course of therapy the antigen level was normal and no further rejection developed.

CsA and prednisone following transplantation. Of these, seven had no clinical evidence of allograft rejection or CsA toxicity—all had urinary ABP levels <0.35 A.U. In contrast, eight patients had evidence of CsA toxicity, with all eight manifesting urinary ABP levels >0.6 A.U. that fell to normal within 36 hr of decreasing the CsA dose. In six of these eight patients CsA blood levels were greater than 400 ng/ml by radioimmunoassay at the time clinical toxocity was diagnosed.

Seven patients with chronic allograft rejection were studied at the time of presentation. Of these, five had chronic vascular changes on biopsy, with minimal evidence of tubulointerstial inflammation, and had no clinical response to increased immunosuppression therapy. All five had urinary ABP values of <0.35 A.U. In contrast, two patients had at least moderate amounts of tubulointerstitial inflammation on biopsy, and both responded to increases in their immunosuppressive regimen with significant falls in their serum creatinine levels. The urinary ABP levels prior to therapy were 0.79 and 0.96 A.U., falling to 0.27 and 0.18 A.U. posttherapy in the two patients.

DISCUSSION

We believe that there is a compelling need in clinical renal transplantation for a noninvasive, diagnostic test that would accomplish the following tasks:

1. Provide an early warning of allograft rejection and a measure of the activity and reversability of the process
2. Provide a mechanism for monitoring the effectiveness of antirejection therapy
3. Provide a means of distinguishing between acute cellular rejection, which is treatable with increased immunosuppressive therapy, from other forms of allograft injury that do not respond to such treatment

The data presented here suggest that serial, urinary ABP measurements may accomplish at least some of these objectives. There is a clear distinction between patients with a clinical course uncomplicated by either drug toxicity or rejection (urinary ABP levels <0.35) from those with acute allograft injury caused by acute rejection or CsA toxicity (urinary ABP levels >0.6 A.U., $P < .01$). Particularly in pediatric patients, as illustrated by the patient whose course is outlined in Figure 3, in whom the early diagnosis of rejection can be especially challenging, this assay appears to provide an early warning of significant rejection before serum creatinine levels begin to rise. Since it is believed that transplant rejection is easier to treat the earlier it is diagnosed, it is interesting to speculate about the possible outcome if this patient had been intensively treated at the time when the ABP level rose, rather than five days later when the serum creatinine level began to rise.

Particularly convincing in this study was the correlation between the risk of rerejection and urinary ABP levels at the completion of therapy for acute rejection with ATG or OKT3. Patients whose urinary ABP levels were <0.35 A.U. at the completion of the course of antirejection therapy were free of further rejection; in contrast, 10 of 12 patients (83.3%) with elevated urinary ABP levels at the completion of such a treatment rerejected quite promptly ($P < .05$), even if their serum creatinine levels had fallen to baseline at the completion of this course of treatment. It is not unreasonable to propose that if treatment had been continued or intensified during the first course of therapy until the ABP level returned to normal, the second rejection episode might have been prevented. Moderate prolongation or intensification of a primary course of antirejection therapy is likely to be associated with lesser total amounts of immunosuppression and immunosuppression-related side effects—and, perhaps, better long-term renal function—than if repeat rejection injury ensues and a new intensive course of therapy is required.

In this same vein, the experience of stratifying patients with chronic rejection according to which might be responsive to increased immunosuppression appears to be quite promising. While salvage of kidney function in such patients is obviously quite desirable, this is just the group of patients with the highest risk of life-threatening infection associated with added immunosuppression (*26*). Therefore a predictor of success of such added immunosuppression would be quite useful. In this study, all five patients who failed to respond to increased immunosuppression had normal urinary ABP levels, as opposed to elevated levels in the two patients who did respond to such therapy.

It must be emphazised that the urinary ABP assay is not specific for allograft rejection or CsA toxicity. Rather, it is a sensitive Mab-based assay for a glycoprotein found on the brush border of the renal proximal tubule and initial portion of the loop of Henle. Unlike previous urinary tests of renal injury, such as the beta-2-microglobulin and N-acetyl-beta-D-gluosaminidase assays (*27*), this test appears to be specific for tubular injury and to be unaffected by changes in urinary pH (*17, 19*). What it cannot do, however, is distinguish among different forms of proximal tubular injury. Thus, acute tubular necrosis, acute cellular rejection, CsA and gentamicin toxicity, myoglobinuria, etc., all produce similar changes in the urinary ABP level (19). Despite this overlap, useful information can be gained by correlating the assay results with the clinical situation and by serial performance of this assay. Thus, acute tubular necrosis or drug toxicity would be unlikely in the absence of nephrotoxic drugs or hypotension. In addition, the urinary ABP level appears to be quite responsive to manipulations in the immunosuppressive regimen. Thus patients with CsA toxicity and increased urinary ABP levels manifest a fall in ABP levels within 36 hr of decreasing the dose—frequently before a fall in serum creatinine level has occurred. Similarly, patients with acute rejection treated with increased immunosuppression usually lower their ABP levels prior to any fall in the serum creatinine levels.

We believe, however, that the ultimate answer lies in the development of other urinary Mab-based assays of renal injury. The urinary ABP assay appears clinically useful by itself. Equally important, in our opinion, is to view this antigen and this Mab-based assay as a model system. This model has shown that renal injury damaging a specific site on the nephron is associated with the quantitative release into the urine of an antigen specific for this nephrone site that can be correlated with the activity of the disease process, its responsiveness to therapy, and the adequecy of a given therapeutic regimen (*19*). Although CsA toxicity and acute allograft rejection both produce injury to the proximal tubule, they probably have divergent effects on the rest of the nephron. Therefore, Mab-based assays for antigens specific to these other nephron sites should allow one to distinguish among these different forms of renal injury. Thus a battery of such noninvasive tests should allow the clinician to make an earlier specific diagnosis and permit more precise therapy. Such an application of Mab technology should result in more individualized and improved care for the renal transplant patient.

REFERENCES

1. Cosimi AB, Colvin RB, Burton RC, Rubin RH, Goldstein G, Kung PC, Hansen WP, Delmonico FL, Russell PS. Use of monoclonal antibodies to T-cell subsets for immunologic monitoring and treatment in recipients of renal allografts. N Engl J Med 1981: 305: 308.
2. Colvin RB, Cosimi AB, Burton RC, Delmonico FL, Jaffers G, Rubin RH, Tolkoff-Rubin NE, Giorgi JV, McCluskey RT, Russell PS. Circulating T-cell subsets in 72 human renal allograft recipients: the $OKT4^+/OKT8^+$ cell ratio correlates with reversibility of graft injury and glomerulopathy. Transplant Proc 1983; 15: 1166.
3. Thomas J, Thomas F, Mendez-Picon M, Lee HM. Immunologic monitoring of long-surviving renal transplant recipients. Surgery 1977; 81: 125.
4. Kerman R, Floyd M, Van Buren C, McConnell B, McConnell R, Kahan B. Correlation of non-specific immune monitoring with rejection or impaired function of renal allografts. Transplantation 1981; 32: 16.
5. Koo GCG, Moroghan ED, Gault MH, Maclean LD. Comparative value of lymphocyturia, serum and urinary enzymes in the diagnosis of renal homograft rejection. Surg Forum 1965; 16: 256.
6. Ward JP. Urinary gamma-glutamyl transpeptidase an indicator of renal ischaemic injury and homograft rejection. Br J Urol 1976; 47: 765.
7. Wellwood JM, Ellis BG, Hall J, Robinson DR, Thomson AE. Early warning of rejection? Br Med J 1973; 2: 261.
8. Whiting PH, Nicholls AJ, Catto GRD, Edward N, Engeset J. Pattern of N-acetyl-β-D-glucosaminidase excretion after renal transplantation. Clin Chem Acta 1980; 108: 1.
9. Whiting PH, Petersen J, Power DA, Stewart RDM, Catto GRD, Edward N. Diagnostic value of urinary N-acetyl-β-D-glucosaminidase, its isoenzymes and the fractional excretion of sodium following renal transplantation. Clin Chim Acta 1983; 130: 369.
10. Hart CA, Alexander LC, Steen S. Immunological evaluation of renal transplant patients: changes in levels of beta-2-micromicroglobulin, immunoglobulins and complement components during graft rejection. J Clin Lab Immunol 1983; 12: 17.
11. Edward LC, Halderman JH, Hamm LL, Ludwin D, Gailiunas P Jr., Hull AR. Noninvasive monitoring of renal transplant function by analysis of beta-2-microglobulin. Kidney Int 1983; 23: 767.
12. Woo J, Floyd M, Cannon DC. Albumin and beta-2-microglobulin radioimmunoassays applied to monitoring of renal-allograft function and in differentiating glomerular and tubular diseases. Clin Chem 1981; 27: 709.
13. Dyck RF, Cardella CJ, Sacks MA. Urinary lysosomal enzyme excretion after renal allotransplantation. Clin Chem Acta 1979; 91: 111.
14. Ueda R, Ogata SI, Morrissey DM, Szkudlarek J, Whitmore WF, Ooettgen HF, Lloyd KO, Old LJ. Cell surface antigens of human renal cancer defined by mouse monoclonal antibodies: identification of tissue-specific kidney glycoproteins. Proc Natl Acad Sci USA 1981; 78: 5122.
15. Cordon-Cardo C, Bander NH, Fradet Y, Finstad CL, Whitmore WF Jr, Lloyd KO, Oettgen HF, Melamed MR, Old LL. Immunoanatomic dissection of the human urinary tract by monoclonal antibodies. J Histochem Cytochem 1984; 32: 1035.
16. Bander NH, Cordon-Cardo C, Finstad CL, Whitmore WF Jr, Vaughan ED Jr, Oettgen HG, Melamed M, Old LJ. Immunohistologic dissection of the human kidney using monoclonal antibodies. J Urol 1985; 133: 502.
17. Thompson RE, Piper DJ, Galberg C, Chan TH, Tolkoff-Rubin NE, Rubin RH. Adenosine diaminase binding protein, a new diagnostic marker for kidney disease. Clin Chem 1985; 31: 679.
18. Andy RJ, Finstad CL, Old LJ, Lloyd KO, Kornfeld R. The antigen identified by a mouse monoclonal antibody raised against human renal cancer cells in the adenosine deaminase binding protein. J Biol Chem 1984; 259: 12844.
19. Tolkoff-Rubin NE. Monoclonal antibodies in the diagnosis of renal disease: a preliminary report. Kidney Int 1986; 29: 142.
20. Ey PL, Prowse SJ, Jenkin CR. Isolation of pure IgG_1, IgG2b immunoglobulins from mouse serum using Protein A-sepharose. Immunochemistry 1978; 15: 429.
21. Wilson MB, Nakane PK. Recent development in the periodate method of conjugating horseradish peroxidase (HRPO) to antibodies. In: Knapp W, Holubar K, Wick G, eds. Immunofluorescence and related staining technique. Amsterdam; Elsevier/North-Holland, 1978: 215.
22. Cosimi AB, Wortis HH, Delmonico FL, Russell PS. Randomized clinical trials of antithymocyte globulin in cadaver renal allograft recipients: importance of T cell monitoring. Surgery 1976; 80: 155.
23. Donatsch P, Abisch E, Homburger M, et al. A radioimmunoassay to measure cyclosporin A in plasma and serum samples. J Immunoassay 1981; 2: 19.
24. Nelson PW, Cosimi AB, Delmonico FL, Rubin RH, Tolkoff-Rubin NE, Fang L, Russell PS. Antithymocyte globulin as the primary treatment of renal allograft rejection. Transplantation 1983; 36: 587.
25. Thisthlewaite JR Jr, Cosimi AB, Delmonico FL, Rubin RH, Tolkoff-Rubin NE, Nelson PW, Fang L, Russell PS. Evolving use of OKT3 monoclonal antibody for treatment of renal allograft rejection. Transplantation 1984; 38: 695.
26. Rubin RH. Infection in the renal transplant patient. In: Rubin RH, Young LS, eds. Clinical approach to infection in the compromised host. New York: Plenum, 1981: 553.
27. Sherman RL, Drayer DL, Leyland-Jones BR, Reidenberg MM. N-acetyl-beta-glucosaminidase and beta-2-microglobulin, their urinary excretion in patients with renal parenchymal disease. Arch Int Med 1983; 143: 1183.

Received 15 May 1985.
Accepted 5 September 1985.

0041-1337/86/4105-0598$02.00/0
TRANSPLANTATION
Copyright © 1986 by The Williams & Wilkins Co.

Vol. 41, No. 5
Printed in U.S.A.

A CRITICAL LOOK AT SURVIVAL OF DIABETICS WITH END-STAGE RENAL DISEASE

TRANSPLANTATION VERSUS DIALYSIS THERAPY

RAJA B. KHAULI, DONALD R. STEINMULLER, ANDREW C. NOVICK,[1] CAROLINE BUSZTA, MARLENE GOORMASTIC, SATORU NAKAMOTO, DONALD G. VIDT, MAGNUS MAGNUSSON, EMIL PAGANINI, AND MARTIN J. SCHREIBER

The Section of Renal Transplantation The Cleveland Clinic Foundation Cleveland, Ohio 44106

The survival of 100 consecutive patients with diabetic nephropathy after treatment with hemodialysis, peritoneal dialysis, or renal transplantation was reviewed at our institution from 1976 to 1982. Standard actuarial survival analysis revealed an overall survival of 83% and 61% at one and two years, respectively. Coronary angiography was used as a screening procedure for renal transplantation. In the dialysis group, 27 patients were considered acceptable transplant candidates on the basis of the coronary angiography but were not transplanted for other reasons. When the survival analysis was limited to those "transplant candidates" the survival rates were 78%, 51%, and 8% at 1, 2, and 5 years, respectively. In comparison, survival after transplantation was 81%, 67%, and 45%, at 1, 2, and 5 years, respectively. In order to eliminate bias, survival comparisons were subsequently made using the Cox Proportional Hazard Model to take into account the time the transplant patients spent on dialysis prior to renal transplantation. When this analysis was performed, there was no significant difference in survival between transplantation and dialysis for the first two years, but overall survival after five years was significantly better after renal transplantation even when the comparison was limited to acceptable transplant candidates who remained on dialysis (*P*=.04). Survival for patients with significant coronary disease (>70% stenosis of a coronary vessel or moderate to severe left ventricular dysfunction) was analyzed according to therapeutic modality. Although overall prognosis was poor in this group as a whole (1, 2, and 5 year survivals were 76%, 45%, and 19%, respectively), the cardiac patients had a trend to better survival after renal transplantation than when maintained on dialysis (*P*=.22). In addition to other factors such as quality of life, rehabilitation, and progression of other diabetic complications, the benefit of renal transplantation on patient survival must be considered when deciding between renal transplantation and maintenance dialysis therapy for diabetic patients with renal failure.

Patients with long-standing diabetes who develop diabetic nephropathy and end-stage renal disease (ESRD)* remain some of the most difficult patients for whom to care for all physicians involved with dialysis and transplantation. Diabetic complications in other organ systems, atherosclerotic disease involving the heart, cerebrovascular system or peripheral vessels, and infectious complications all result in diminished patient survival after the onset of dialysis or after renal transplantation. Initial results with kidney transplantation were not as good as those for nondiabetics (*1*), but the survival rates of diabetics receiving renal allografts have been reported to exceed those of diabetic patients maintained on chronic dialysis (*1, 2*). More recently there have been some reports of improved survival in diabetics following renal transplantation along with better overall rehabilitation when compared with dialysis therapy (*3–9*). Concomitantly, the past few years have witnessed an overall improvement of results with dialysis therapy with the advent of better techniques for hemodialysis (*10*) and the development of continuous ambulatory peritoneal dialysis (CAPD) (*11*). The results of dialysis at these centers have recently matched those of transplantation, with one-year survival of 80–90%. Despite this better short-term outlook for diabetics with ESRD, there still are questions regarding long-term survival with different therapeutic modalities. Moreover, comparison between these therapeutic modalities have, in general, been poorly controlled and have encountered biases with regard to the selection of patient populations and the statistical methods utilized.

This report reviews the experience with 100 patients with diabetic nephropathy and ESRD at one institution and specifically addresses the question of early and late survival of these patients with different therapeutic modalities.

MATERIALS AND METHODS

From January 1976 to July 1982, 100 insulin-dependent diabetic patients with ESRD secondary to diabetic nephropathy were evaluated for renal transplantation at the Cleveland Clinic. All of the patients were felt to have diabetic nephropathy on the basis of long-standing diabetes, typical clinical features of hypertension and proteinuria, the presence of other diabetic complications—and, in some patients, on the basis of renal morphology. The policies regarding the pretransplant evaluation have been previously described (*12*), and in diabetics include the performance of coronary angiography (*13*). Fifty-two patients received renal transplants, 12 from a living-related donor (LRD) and 46 from a cadaver (six patients received two transplants). Prior to transplantation, 33 patients were maintained on hemodialysis alone, seven were maintained on peritoneal dialysis alone (intermittent [IPD] CAPD), and nine patients were maintained sequentially on a combination of peritoneal and hemodialysis. Three patients were transplanted

[1] Address reprint requests to: Andrew C. Novick, M.D., Head, Section of Renal Transplantation, The Cleveland Clinic Foundation, 9500 Euclid Avenue, Cleveland, Ohio 44106.

* Abbreviations used: ALG, antilymphoblast globulin; CAPD, continuous ambulatory peritoneal dialysis; ESRD, end-stage renal disease; IPD, intermittent peritoneal dialysis; LRD, living-related donor.

prior to initiation of dialysis. During this period, 48 patients were treated with dialysis alone; 27 were maintained on hemodialysis, 16 were maintained on peritoneal dialysis (ten IPD and six CAPD), and five were maintained sequentially on a combination of hemodialysis and peritoneal dialysis. Of the 48 patients maintained exclusively on dialysis, 25 were not considered suitable as transplant candidates because of other serious medical problems and therefore were recommended for maintenance dialysis therapy. Of these, 17 patients had extensive cardiovascular disease on the basis of coronary angiography and transplantation was not recommended due to their poor overall prognosis. Because of other medical problems, eight patients never stabilized adequately to be considered as serious transplant candidates. Thus, 23 of the 48 patients maintained exclusively on dialysis were considered acceptable "transplant candidates," based on their overall medical condition including the results of coronary angiography. These "transplant candidates" were not transplanted due to the unavailability of a cadaver or living related donor kidney or because of patient choice.

Transplant patients received standard immunosuppression consisting of azathioprine and prednisone. In 20 cadaver recipients, adjunctive prophylactic immunosuppression was administered in the form of Minnesota antilymphoblast globulin (ALG) 15–30 mg/kg/day for the first 14 days posttransplantation. Prophylactic ALG was not administered to 22 cadaveric recipients, nor to any LRD recipients. In most patients, episodes of acute rejection were treated with 1 g/day of i.v. methylprednisolone in four divided doses. For statistical analysis, a change of the mode of dialysis for a period of less than three months was regarded as no change in treatment. Eighteen patients on chronic peritoneal dialysis were started on IPD in-hospital, then switched to home CAPD (n=8) or maintained on IPD (n=10). Because of the small number of patients in each of these subgroups, the peritoneal dialysis group has been considered one single entity in terms of therapy.

For descriptive purposes, the Kaplan-Meier (*14*) method was used to calculate survival curves by patient group and by treatment modality. The three patient groups were transplantation, dialysis, and the subgroup of dialysis patients who were acceptable transplant candidates. In considering the survival for the treatment modality of dialysis, the survival time on dialysis for the transplant patients (100% survival) prior to the transplant procedure was incorporated with the survival of dialysis patients.

Since transplantation is usually a change in treatment modality rather than the initial treatment and graft rejection often forces a switch back to dialysis, patients usually belong in both treatment groups at different times. Comparisons of the usual survival curves cannot take these treatment switches into account and can give biased and misleading results. To adequately handle this situation, an analysis using the Cox proportional hazards model (*15*) was done. In the models used, treatment modality was dependent on time. Previous to their transplant operation all but three of the transplant patients were classified as dialysis patients.

Patient survival was also compared with respect to cardiac status as determined by angiography, using the Cox Proportional Hazards Model.

Transplant patients were considerd to remain in their treatment modality (transplantation) for varying times after returning to dialysis. This was done based on the assumption that complications related to transplantation and immunosuppressive therapy often occur long after graft failure. Analyses were performed switching from the transplant treatment modality to dialysis at 0, 6, and 12 months after a failed transplant and return to dialysis. To address the question of biases introduced by the selection process for renal transplantation, the analysis includes only dialysis patients who were considered acceptable transplant candidates but for various reasons were never transplanted. Follow-up interval for the whole group range from two to eight years.

RESULTS

The causes of death for patients in each of the three groups (transplant, transplant candidates, and transplant exclusions) are shown in Table 1. Cardiovascular and cerebrovascular disease accounted for 60% of patient deaths in the transplant exclusions. The causes of death in the transplant patients and transplant candidates were more variable. The age and duration of diabetes are shown in Table 2 for the three groups—dialysis patients as a whole, transplant candidates, and transplant patients.

Table 3 shows the differences in patient survival at 1, 2, and 5 years for the dialysis group as a whole, first row, and the transplant candidates, row two. Also shown in rows three and four is the effect of considering survival for the treatment modality of dialysis; in other words, incorporating the time on dialysis (with 100% survival) for the transplant patients prior to the transplant procedure. Row three considers only trans-

TABLE 1. Cause of death for diabetic ESRD patients

	Transplant (n = 52)	Dialysis (n = 48)	
		Transplant candidates (n = 23)	Transplant exclusions (n = 25)
Cardiac event	5 (10%)	6 (26%)	15 (60%)
CVA		2 (9%)	2 (8%)
Sepsis	7 (14%)	2 (9%)	2 (8%)
Hyperkalemia	2 (4%)	2 (9%)	1 (4%)
Hypoglycemia	1 (2%)		1 (4%)
GI bleeding	1 (2%)	1 (4%)	
Hepatic failure	1 (2%)		
Pulmonary embolism	2 (4%)		1 (4%)
Unknown	2 (4%)	4 (17%)	2 (8%)
Total mortalities (%)	21/52 (40%)	17/23 (74%)	24/25 (96%)

TABLE 2. Description of age and duration of diabetes

A. Age

Age (years)[a]	N	Mean ± SD	Min-max
Overall	100	38±10	18–61
Dialysis patients	48	42±10	24–61
Transplant candidates	23	39±8	24–55
Transplant patients	52	34±9	4–40

[a] at onset of treatment

B. Duration of diabetes

Diabetes (years)	N	Mean ± SD	Min-Max
Overall	100	20±6	5–40
Dialysis patients	48	19±6	5–40
Transplant candidates	23	18±6	5–31
Transplant patients	52	21±67–38	

plant candidates and transplant patients and represents the survival for the treatment modality of dialysis as outlined above. Row four considers all dialysis patients including the transplant exclusions and shows the survival for the treatment modality of dialysis for those patients.

As can be seen, the one-year survival for the treatment modality of dialysis, excluding patients with severe cardiac disease or other medical problems that excluded them from consideration of transplantation, is 89%. The five-year dialysis survival, however, is only 12%. Table 4 compares the same dialysis survival (again excluding patients not acceptable for transplantation) with survival after renal transplantation. For this analysis, a patient was considered to have returned to the treatment modality of dialysis 12 months after the date of his or her failed transplant. As can be seen, early survival (one and two years) is comparable for the dialysis and transplant treatment modalities (89% versus 81% at one year and 74% versus 67% at two years)—a slight but statistically insignificant advantage for the treatment modality of dialysis. The five-year survival, however is 45% for the transplantation modality compared with only 12% for dialysis (P=.04).

Table 5 illustrates the effect of using different intervals for switching patients from the transplantation treatment modality to the dialysis treatment modality after a failed graft. This was performed at 0, 6, and 12 months after a failed allograft. The relative risk of dying for transplantation as a modality of therapy compared with dialysis varies from .2 to .49; with P values ranging from P<.0001 to P=.04. Twelve months is a figure probably biased slightly in favor of dialysis since some mortality, unrelated to a failed transplant, may occur prior to 12 months after a failed graft. Thus, the relative risk of dying after transplantation is at least one-half or less that of dying on dialysis for patients with ESRD secondary to diabetic nephropathy (P=.04).

Of the 100 total patients, 87 underwent coronary angiography, as a part of their transplant evaluation. Thirty-eight had ≥70% stenosis of one or more vessels and/or moderate to severe left ventricular dysfunction. This group was designated the *cardiac* group. Four of these patients underwent coronary bypass procedures. Forty-nine had neither 70% stenosis of any coronary vessel, nor moderate left ventricular dysfunction. This group was designated the *noncardiac group.* As previously stated, 17 of the 38 cardiac patients were not recommended for transplantation primarily on the basis of their cardiac disease. Twelve of the 52 transplant recipients had significant heart disease (70% stenosis of one or more coronary vessels and/or moderate to severe left ventricular dysfunction). Nevertheless, they were all transplanted because of a strong preference for transplantation despite the risk, or after successful coronary bypass (four patients). It is interesting to note that 50% (19 patients) of the cardiac group were asymptomatic despite the positive angiographic findings and 22% (9 patients) of the noncardiac group were symptomatic (chronic congestive heart failure (CHF), angina, or electrocardiogram changes) despite the absence of disease on angiography.

TABLE 3. Cumulative percentage of survival

	1 Yr	2 Yr	5 Yr
1. Dialysis (48)	65%	35%	6%
2. Transplant candidates (23)	78%	51%	8%
3. Dialysis survival (transplant and transplant candidates) (75)[a]	89%	74%	12%
4. Dialysis survival (all patients) (100)[a]	80%	53%	11%

[a] Patients are censored at the time of first transplant.

TABLE 4. Cumulative percentage of survival

	1 Yr	2 Yr	5 Yr	
Dialysis survival (transplant and transplant candidates) (75%)[a]	89%	74%	12%	p = .04
Transplant Patients (censored if return to dialysis 12 months) (52)	81%	67%	45%	

* Patients are censored at the time of first transplant.

TABLE 5. COX model with time-dependent covariates—multiple treatment switches: transplant candidates vs. transplant recipients

Time of switch	P value	Relative risk
Treatment switch	$P<0.0001$	0.20
>6 For dialysis after transplant	$P = 0.0002$	0.24
>12 For dialysis after transplant	$P = 0.04$	0.49

TABLE 6. Cumulative percentage of survival

	1 Yr	2 Yr	5 Yr	P
Cardiac status (87)[a]				
No (49)	94%	75%	40%	$P = 0.0002$
Yes (38)	76%	45%	19%	
Cardiac patients (38)[a]				
Transplant (12)	100%	67%	40%	$P = 0.05$
Transplant candidates (9)	67%	44%	15%	
Nontransplant candidates (17)	65%	29%	6%	

[a] From onset of first ESRD treatment.

Table 6 (row one) shows the patient survival for cardiac and noncardiac groups without considering treatment modality. The survival of the cadiac group is much worse: two-year survival of 45% versus 75% for the noncardiac group (P=0.0006). Row two of Table 6 shows survival by treatment group for the cadiac patients only. As can be seen, survival after transplantation is better than survival on dialysis, with a two-year survival of 67% for the former. This represents a relative risk of dying of .68 for the treatment modality of transplantation, but does not reach statistical significance (P=.22).

DISCUSSION

Comparison of patient survival for various modalities of therapy for end-stage renal disease is frought with a number of problems. The primary bias, favoring patients who undergo renal transplantation, is the selection process prior to the transplantation surgery (*16*). The second bias relates to the fact that most patients who undergo transplantation survive for some time on dialysis prior to the transplant (*17*). This survival time on dialysis for transplant recipients should be included as survival for the treatment modality of dialysis. Patients who reject a renal transplant create another problem in comparing survival between modalities of therapy. Using the preceding argument, dialysis time or death after the failure of the graft could be considered as survival or death for the treatment modality of dialysis. However, it is clear that significant mortality directly or indirectly related to transplantation and its immunosuppression still occurs for an indeterminate period after failure of an allograft. Thus it is very difficult to know whether to label a death after a failed transplant as a dialysis-related or transplant-related event. Even detailed analysis of specific cases may leave considerable doubt, and often death is due to a combination of dialysis and transplantation-related problems or complications.

Other analyses comparing survival on dialysis with survival after transplantation for all renal failure patients (*3, 18*) or diabetics (*5*), have shown a significant advantage for transplantation. These studies have generally not addressed the above problems and biases. Two analyses comparing survival for age-matched dialysis patients and cadaver transplant recipients found no signficiant difference when the dialysis survival time of the transplant recipients was incorporated into dialysis survival (*16, 19*) These studies included all end-stage renal failure patients, not exclusively diabetic patients as in this study.

This review has tried to address all biases as well as possible. All patients were seen at a single center. The patients in the transplant candidate group were well-matched to the transplant patients with respect to the extent of cardiac disease—the major cause of death in diabetic patients with ESRD. Although the transplant recipients were younger than the transplant candidates, age was not found to be a significant covariate overall, and it does not account for the difference in survival. The dialysis survival for the transplant patients prior to transplantation was incorporated into dialysis survival, avoiding that particular bias.

It might be argued that transplant recipients should not be switched back to dialysis in performing the analysis of survival after a failed transplant. The use of an interval of 12 months before switching back to dialysis is probably biased in favor of dialysis since almost all complications related to transplantation and its immunosuppression do not necessarily affect survival for a period of 12 months after a failed graft.

Despite this careful analysis to avoid any bias in favor of transplantation, there was significantly better survival beyond two years after renal transplantation when compared with dialysis. Early survival (from zero to two years), however, as shown in other studies (*9, 16, 19*) was similar for both modalities of treatment. This is not unexpected since it may take time for improved survival after transplantation to make up for early mortality related to surgery, rejection, and the more aggressive immunosuppressive therapy in the early posttransplant period.

We included 12 living-related donor transplant recipients in our transplant group, a subgroup that is recognized to have a better survival (*19*) compared with those receiving dialysis or cadaver transplantation. However, the small number of patients, and the similar survival for this subgroup (*8*) (80% at one year), compared with the cadaver transplant recipients (79% at one year) makes this unlikely to be the reason for the better survival after transplantation.

Rehabilitation, stabilization of other diabetic complications, and overall improvement in well-being are other advantages of transplantation compared with dialysis that we have previously documented in this group of patients (*9*). These factors are of primary importance early after transplantation, with improved survival being a more prominent factor over the long run (greater than two years).

Although severe cardiac disease was considered a relative contraindication to transplantation, these results suggest that survival after transplantation may be better for diabetic patients despite significant cardiac disease than for those remaining on dialysis. The reason for considering cardiac disease a relative contraindication to transplantation was the poor overall prognosis in this group of patients (*13*). This poor prognosis for the cardiac diabetic patients was documented in this study. However, it may be best to individualize therapy since overall survival may still be better if a more aggressive approach to transplantation is undertaken.

In conclusion, early survival (zero to two years) for patients with diabetic nephropathy and ESRD is similar for all modalities of therapy. The apparent benefit of transplantation, based on standard Kaplan-Meier survival curves, is due primarily to patient selection and the bias present when dialysis intervals prior to transplantation are not taken into consideration. Late survival (two to five years) for patients with diabetic nephropathy and ESRD is better after transplantation, with a five-year survival rate of 45% versus a five-year survival rate of 12% for similar patients on dialysis (P=.04). The survival of diabetic ESRD patients with coronary disease is poor (two-year survival of 45%) but may be better after transplantation. These survival data must be considered along with other factors (such as quality of life, rehabilitation, and progression of other diabetic complications) when deciding between various therapeutic modalities for diabetic renal failure patients.

REFERENCES

1. Najarian JS, Sutherland DER, Simmons RL, et al. Kidney transplantation for the uremic diabetic patient. Surg Gynecol Obstet 1977; 144: 682.
2. Totten MA, Izenstein B, Glaeson RE, Kassissieh SD, Libertino JA, D'Elia JA. Chronic renal failure in diabetes: survival with hemodialysis versus transplantation. Kidney Int 1977; 12: 492.
3. Kjellstrand CM. Cadaver transplantation versus hemodialysis. Trans Am Soc Artif Intern Organs 1980; 26: 611.
4. Najarian JS, Sutherland DER, Simmons RL, et al. Ten years' experience with renal transplantation in juvenile onset diabetics. Ann Surgery 1979; 190: 487.
5. Sutherland DER, Morrow CE, Fryd DS, Ferguson R, Simmons RL, Najarian JS. Improved patient and primary renal allograft survival in uremic diabetic recipients. Transplantation 1982; 34: 319.
6. Okiye SE, Engen DE, Sterioff SS, et al. Primary and secondary renal transplantation in diabetic patients. JAMA 1983; 249: 492.
7. Libetino JA, Zinman L, Salerno R, D'elia J, Kaladny A, Weinrauch LA. Diabetic renal transplantation. J Urol 1980; 124: 593.
8. Khauli RB, Novick AC, Braun WE, Steinmuller D, Buszta C. Goormastic M. Improved results of cadaver renal transplantation in the diabetic patient. J Urol 1983; 130: 867.
9. Khauli RB, Novick AC, Steinmuller DR, et al. Patient survival and rehabilitation of diabetics with end-stage renal disease: comparison of therapeutic modalities. Trans Proc 1985; 17: 178.
10. Shapiro FL, Conty CM. Hemodialysis in diabetics: 1981 update. In: Friedman EA, L'Esperance FA, eds. Diabetic renal retinal syndrome. New York: Grune and Stratton, 1981: 309.
11. Amair P, Khanna R, et al. Continuous ambulatory peritoneal dialysis in diabetic with end-stage renal disease. In: Friedman EA, L'Esperance FA, eds. Diabetic renal retinal syndrome. New York: Grune and Stratton, 1981: 331.
12. Novick AC, Braun WE, Magnusson M, Stowe N. Current status of

renal transplantation at the Cleveland Clinic. J Urol 1979; 122: 433.
13. Braun WE, Phillips D, Vidt DG, et al. The course of coronary artery disease in diabetics with and without renal allografts. Transplant Proc 1983; 15: 1114.
14. Kaplan EL, Meier P. Non-parametric estimation from incomplete observations. J Am Stat Assoc 1958; 53: 457.
15. Cox DR. Regression model in life table. J R Statisticians Soc 1972; 34(B): 187.
16. Hutchinson TA, Thomas DC, Lemieux JC, Harvey CE. Prognostically controlled comparison of dialysis and renal transplantation. Kidney Int 1984; 26: 44.
17. Weller JM, Port FK, Swartz RD, Ferguson CW, Williams GW, Jacobs JF. Analysis of survival of end-stage renal disease patients. Kidney Int 1982; 21: 78.
18. Krakauer H, Grauman JS, McMullan MR, Creede CC. The recent US experience in the treatment of end-stage renal disease by dialysis and transplantation. N Engl J Med 1983; 308(26): 1558.
19. Vollmer WM, Wahl PW, Blagg CR. Survival with dialysis and transplantation in patients with end-stage renal disease. 1983; 308(26): 1553.

Received 13 June 1985.
Accepted 14 August 1985.

0041-1337/86/4105-0602$02.00/0
TRANSPLANTATION
Vol. 41, No. 5

PLASMA EXCHANGE FOR PLATELET ALLOIMMUNIZATION[1]

WILLIAM I. BENSINGER,[2] C. DEAN BUCKNER, REGINALD A. CLIFT, SHERRILL J. SLICHTER, AND E. DONNALL THOMAS[3]

The Department of Medicine, Fred Hutchinson Cancer Research Center, University of Washington School of Medicine, Seattle, Washington, 98104

We studied the effectiveness of plasma exchange for reversing antiplatelet alloimmunization in 18 patients undergoing marrow transplantation. Patients received one-to-three daily exchanges. Most exchanges occurred during the pretransplant conditioning phase. Overall, eleven of 18 patients had a beneficial response to plasma exchange, defined as an improvement in post-platelet-transfusion increments. More patients responded who had received two or more exchanges. Patients who had lymphocytotoxic antibodies pretransplant were more likely to benefit from the exchange. Our results show that plasma exchange may improve the posttransfusion platelet increments in alloimmunized patients undergoing marrow transplant.

The morbidity and mortality associated with iatrogenic thrombocytopenia has been significantly decreased by the availability of platelet transfusions. This has allowed physicians to use more intensive chemotherapy and radiotherapy for the treatment of malignancies. Pooled platelets from random donors are the most commonly used and least costly source. However, approximately 38%–50% of patients become refractory to platelets from random donors within a relatively short time (*1, 2*).

In immunized, refractory patients matching for HLA antigens is the most widely used method of selecting compatible platelet donors (*3, 4*). Unfortunately this selection process has variable and unpredictable success. A poor transfusion response from HLA-matched platelets may indicate that other antigenic systems, autoimmunity, or other complicating clinical conditions are involved.

Efforts to improve selection of donors have centered on platelet crossmatch tests, which suffer from lack of sensitivity and reproducibility (*5, 6*). Suitable donors cannot be found for many alloimmunized, thrombocytopenic patients. These patients might benefit from measures that remove platelet reactive antibodies, especially if the thrombocytopenia is likely to be of limited duration, as is the case in marrow transplant recipients or patients with leukemia and lymphoma undergoing chemotherapy. Plasma exchange has been successfully used to manage autoimmune thrombocytopenia (*7*), has reduced the titers of HLA antibodies in patients actively rejecting renal allografts (*8*), and has been suggested for the management of alloimmunization (*14*). It thus seemed rational to try this approach in alloimmunized thrombocytopenic patients. This report presents our preliminary experience with plasma exchange in marrow transplant recipients who were alloimmunized.

MATERIALS AND METHODS

Between 1978 and 1983 eighteen patients with aplastic anemia or leukemia who were refractory to random donor platelets underwent plasma exchange. Patients were considered to be refractory when the 1-hr posttransfusion platelet increment was less than $500/\mu l$ per unit (approximately 5.5×10^{10} platelets/unit) of transfused platelets on two successive occasions. Some

* Abbreviations used: CY, cyclophosphamide; TBI, total-body irradiation.

[1] This work was supported by PHS Grants CA 18579, CA 30924, and CA 18029 awarded by the National Cancer Institute, DHHS.

[2] Address reprint requests to: William I. Bensinger, M.D., Fred Hutchinson Cancer Research Center, 1124 Columbia Street, Seattle, WA 98104.

[3] Dr. Thomas is a recipient of a Research Career Award AI 02425 from the National Institute of Allergy and Infectious Diseases.

of these patients were also refractory to platelets from selected community plateletpheresis donors, matched for two-to-four HLA antigens or family members HLA matched or mismatched for one-to-four HLA antigens, including the intended marrow donor.

The plasma exchange procedure was usually performed during the pretransplant conditioning phase of treatment before or during the chemoradiotherapy. In some patients the exchange was performed during the posttransplant period. Patients received pregrafting chemotherapy consisting of cyclophosphamide (CY) 60 mg/kg on each of two consecutive days or 50 mg/kg on each of four consecutive days. In addition patients with leukemia received total-body irradiation (TBI) as a single dose or in daily fractionated doses (*9*). Some patients received additional conditioning with antithymocyte globulin.

Ten patients received transplants from HLA-identical siblings, nine of whom were additionally used as platelet donors. Five patients received transplants from relatives mismatched for one or two antigens. One patient (a child) received a transplant from her identical twin. Another patient received a transplant from his aunt who was phenotypically HLA-identical. One patient received an autologous transplant using cryopreserved marrow.

Patient characteristics are shown in Table 1. Eighteen patients received one or more plasma exchanges. Eight patients were transplanted for aplastic anemia and received only CY in preparation for transplant. The other 10 patients had leukemia and received pretransplant TBI in addition to CY. Six patients had major ABO incompatibility (the presence of anti-A or anti-B antibodies against donor red cells) with their donors, and the plasma exchanges were performed both to remove anti-red-cell antibodies and to improve responsiveness to platelets (*10*).

Plasma exchanges were performed using a continuous-flow blood cell separator for plasma separation (IBM 2997, AMINCO Celltrifuge I, or Fenwal Celltrifuge II). Blood access was obtained through the use of Scribner-type arteriovenous shunts or Hickman-type double-lumen central venous catheters (*11*). Exchange fluid consisted of pooled, cryoprecipitate-depleted, fresh-frozen plasma. Each patient underwent a series of one-to-three daily exchanges. One patient (UPN 1236) received multiple exchanges over 6 weeks.

Following plasma exchange, patients received platelet transfusions from family members including the marrow donor ("related"), HLA-selected community plateletpheresis donors, or pooled random donors. Blood samples for platelet counts were drawn 1 hr after transfusion. Platelet transfusion increments were calculated by subtracting the pretransfusion count from the posttransfusion count and dividing by the number of units of platelets transfused. To minimize day-to-day variability in platelet increments we averaged the increments for all transfusions received for 30 days after the plasma exchanges.

Tests for lymphocytotoxic antibodies were performed using a panel of lymphocytes derived from fifty random donors. Tests for the presence of antibodies against B lymphocytes utilized a modified microcytotoxicity assay against purified B cells derived from unrelated donors (*12*).

RESULTS

Two patients received a single plasma exchange. Eight patients were treated with two plasma exchanges performed over 2 days. Seven patients had a series of three plasma exchanges. A single patient received eight exchanges over a 6-week period because of definite, yet transient, benefit from the exchange procedure. Patient information, the exchange volume, and the timing of the exchange in relation to the marrow transplant are presented in Table 1.

Fourteen patients had cytotoxic antibodies to various members of a panel of unfractionated lymphocytes. Details of the lymphocytotoxic antibody tests are presented in Table 2. Six

TABLE 1. The timing of plasma exchanges and the total volume of plasma exchanged

UPN	Diagnosis	Age	Sex	ABO-INC[a]	Days of Exchange[c]	Volume of plasma per series (L)
813	AA[b]	14	F	No	−2, −1, 0	30
861	AA	18	M	Yes	−4, −3	20
948	AA	44	M	Yes	−3, −2, −1	30
1236	AML	33	F	No	33, 34	20
					48	10
					54	10
					71	10
					74	10
					78	10
					81	10
1362	AML	35	F	No	75	10
1395	AA	18	M	No	−2, −1	20
1407	CGL	6	F	No	30, 31	10
1425	AML	33	M	No	50	10
1465	CGL	29	M	No	−4, −3, −2	30
1486	CGL	31	M	No	−2, −1, 0	30
1525	AA	20	M	Yes	−2, −1	20
1588	AML	9	M	Yes	−1, 0	20
1690	AML	40	F	No	−6, −5, −4	30
1730	AA	19	M	No	−6, −5, −4	30
1816	AML	40	F	No	−6, −5	20
1835	AA	38	F	Yes	−1, 0	20
1859	AA	11	M	No	−6, −5, −4	30
1886	ALL	7	M	Yes	−2, −1	8

[a] Major ABO incompatibility; recipient vs. donor.

[b] AA = aplastic anemia; AML = acute myelogenous leukemia; ALL = acute lymphocytic leukemia; CGL = chronic granulocytic leukemia.

[c] Day of transplantation = day 0.

TABLE 2. Antibody screening data

UPN	Lymphocytotoxicity[a]	
	Unfractionated	B cells
813	27/50	17/19
861	50/50	19/19
948	49/50	19/19
1236	44/50	0/20
1362	9/50	0/20
1395	44/50	0/20
1407	0/50	0/20
1425	0/50	0/20
1465	45/50	0/20
1486	15/50	0/20
1525	0/50	0/20
1588	34/50	0/20
1690	29/50	0/20
1730	1/50	0/20
1816	46/50	20/20
1835	18/18	0/20
1859	44/50	20/20
1886	37/50	20/20

[a] Ratio represents the number of cell donors with a positive cytotoxicity test (numerator) over the number of donors tested (denominator).

of these 14 patients additionally had demonstrable cytotoxic antibodies to a panel of B cells from unrelated donors.

Averages of the preexchange and postexchange platelet transfusion increments from HLA-selected community, random, and related donor platelets are presented in Table 3. Six of 18 patients who initially had average transfusion increments of <500/μl/unit from random donor platelets achieved posttransfusion increments >2000/μl/unit after plasma exchange. Two additional patients achieved posttransfusion increments of >2000/μl/unit from random donor platelets, but this effect lasted for only 10 days (UPNs 1690 and 1730). Another patient (UPN 1236) showed transient increments >2000/μl/unit to related, random, and community donor platelets following multiple plasma exchanges.

Thirteen of the 18 patients received platelets from related donors preexchange. Eight of these 13 patients were evaluable for the effect of plasma exchange on response to related platelet transfusions. Six patients had preexchange related transfusion increments of <500/μl/unit, and five of them achieved postexchange transfusion increments of >2000/μl/unit to the same donors, while one was unchanged. Two patients who had average pretreatment transfusion increments of 625 and 1666/μl/unit had posttreatment increments of 2934 and 1989/μl/unit. Five other patients had preexchange increments >2000/μl/unit and could not be evaluated for the effect of plasma exchange on related platelet transfusions.

TABLE 3. Increments for transfusions from community donors, random pooled donors, or relatives.[a]

UPN	Preexchange: Platelet donor			Postexchange: Platelet donor		
	COM	RAN	REL	COM	RAN	REL
813	–	278	0	–	3972	6138
861	–	0	0	–	166	2547
948	–	0	1666	–	3750	1989
1236	3531	246	0	2933	851	3300
	3555	138	1500	687	1583	5187
	687	1583	5187	2485	1417	7375
	700	603	8000	666	2624	–
	666[b]	2624	–	0	1721	–
	0[b]	1721	–	125	2625	–
	125[b]	2625	–	3488	1434	–
1362	0	0	–	222	94	–
1395	–	159	250	–	416	9400
1407	–	0	0	–	166	0
1425	–	0	625	–	1472	2934
1465	–	0	4795	–	469	1343
1486	–	400	10250	4031	150	10729
1525	11500	500	–	5500	3600	6952
1588	6476	0	–	19277	10447	–
1690	800	0	0	8256	1861	8140
1730	5250	313	–	2434	966	5750
1816	13500	187	–	1100	240	5900
1835	0	0	6875	–	1000	7400
1859	9083	175	18750	5950	2591	11518
1886	–	0	12500	–	3819	18714

[a] Increments are expressed in counts/μl/unit transfused from blood samples drawn 1 hr after tranfusion and are averages for all transfusions received. Preexchange data were calculated from all transfusions received for 7 days prior to the exchange. Postexchange data were calculated for all transfusions received for 30 days after the exchange or until death.

[b] Preexchange increments based on days between exchanges.

We further examined the role of full HLA matching by analyzing the results of transfusions from HLA-identical siblings. Seven of the 18 patients received preexchange transfusions from HLA-identical siblings. Three of the seven had preexchange increments of <500/μl/unit, and all three averaged increments of >2000/μl/unit postexchange. A single patient who had preexchange increments averaging 750/μl/unit achieved postexchange increments averaging 2835/μl/unit. The other three patients had pretreatment increments to platelets from HLA-identical siblings of >2000/μl/unit. Two other patients received HLA-identical platelets but only beginning after the plasma exchanges.

Nine patients received platelets from community donors who were partially HLA-matched prior to plasma exchange. Of two patients who had an average transfusion increment <500/μl/unit, one was unchanged postexchange and another did not receive community donor platelets. A single patient with a preexchange increment of 800/μl/unit had a postexchange increment averaging 8256/μl/unit. The other six patients were all responsive to community donor platelets preexchange and thus unevaluable for the effect of exchange.

If one defines *response* as a patient whose preexchange transfusion increment averaged <500/μl/unit and who averaged >2000/μl/unit postexchange it is possible to make the following conclusions. Neither of the two patients who received a single plasma exchange had a response. Five of the eight patients receiving two plasma exchanges responded to either related or random donor platelets. Similarly, five of eight patients given three or more plasma exchanges responded.

Overall, 11 of the 18 patients plasma exchanged for platelet refractoriness became responsive to platelets from random or related donors. Six of the responding patients had aplastic anemia, while five responders had leukemia. Fourteen patients received plasma exchanges during the conditioning phase of bone marrow transplantation. Nine of these patients derived benefit. Only four patients were treated with plasma exchange after marrow transplantation and one of these had benefit.

There was the suggestion of a correlation between a beneficial effect of plasma exchange and the pretreatment presence of lymphocytotoxic antibodies. Eight of 13 patients positive for antibody became responsive compared with one of five patients who were negative for antibody pretreatment (P not significant).

DISCUSSION

In this article we have reviewed our experience in the use of plasma exchange for the management of alloimmunized patients undergoing marrow transplantation. Our results indicate that a significant proportion of patients who are refractory to platelet transfusions can benefit from this procedure. None of the 18 patients experienced major bleeding episodes during the procedures. Nine of 14 patients had responses when plasma-exchanged before transplant, while only one of four patients benefited when the exchange procedure was performed during the posttransplant phase, but these numbers are too small to indicate whether plasma exchange performed during the conditioning phase of transplant is more efficacious.

It is interesting to note that six of eight patients who had aplastic anemia responded to plasma exchange while five of 10 patients with leukemia responded. Since patients with leukemia received TBI and CY while patients with aplastic anemia received only CY this could indicate that TBI had no additional effect on the suppression of alloantibodies. Small numbers limit the validity of this conclusion.

However, the possible lack of an immunosuppresive effect of TBI could also be due to a stronger sensitization prior to transplant, as most of the patients with leukemia received numerous platelet and red cell transfusions during induction chemotherapy. Although all the patients with AA had received some transfusions prior to transplant, only four of eight received more than four transfusions. The two patients with AA who did not benefit from plasma exchange had only recently acquired their disease—1 week and 1 month previously, and were immunized after receiving only one and two transfusions, respectively.

The proportion of patients responding to plasma exchange performed once was lower than the proportion of patients responding who were treated with two or three exchanges (neither of two versus 10 of 16). Thus there was a suggestion of a dose effect with plasma exchange, but again the number of patients treated was too small to permit definite conclusions.

The failure of some patients to benefit from plasma exchange could be due to several mechanisms, including (1) refractoriness caused by nonimmunologic (consumptive) causes; (2) transient removal of alloantibodies but rapid resynthesis by host cells, and (3) new synthesis of alloantibodies by the emerging donor lymphoid cells.

The first possibility includes factors other than alloimmunization, such as infection, active bleeding or the primary disease itself. We have observed variable posttransfusion increments from the same single donor (to related or unrelated community donors). Although a higher proportion of lymphocytotoxic antibody-positive patients responded to exchange than those who were antibody-negative, we were not able to monitor antibody levels serially postexchange. This might have provided evidence of a role for the other two mechanisms. Our data on the return of anti-red-cell alloantibodies after plasma exchange suggest that one-third of such patients continue to synthesize antibody for up to 3–4 months, presumably from residual host plasma cells (*10*).

Because of these problems it may be difficult to judge the effect of measures designed to reverse alloimmunization. We chose to average the posttreatment platelet transfusion increments over a 30-day period when possible to minimize the day-to-day variability. This method of analysis does have limitations, as evidenced by two patients who initially responded to random platelets after plasma exchange, but by 2 weeks were reimmunized. Although their initial average increments for 10 days postexchange were greater than 2000/μl/unit, transfused their 30 day average was less than 2000/μl/unit.

Other investigators have noted the relationship between the presence of lymphocytotoxic antibodies and refractoriness to random donor platelet transfusions (*13*). It is of interest that there was a suggestion of a correlation between the presence of pretreatment antibodies and a response to therapy (eight of 13 with antibody responded versus one of five without). This positive correlation would tend to add weight to the theory that lymphocytotoxic or other alloantibodies mediate alloimmunization. The availability of an improved system for measuring platelet-specific antibodies may shed more light on this issue. In any case, our findings suggest that plasma exchange as adjunctive therapy in the management of alloimmunized, platelet-refractory patients undergoing bone marrow transplant deserves further investigation, preferably in a randomized, controlled study. We are currently studying methods of improving plasma exchange by specific immunoadsorption of alloantibodies.

REFERENCES

1. Dutcher JP, Schiffer CA, Aisner J, Wiernik PH. Alloimmunization following platelet transfusion: the absence of a dose-response relationship. Blood 1981; 57: 395.
2. McFarland JG, Slichter SJ, Appelbaum F. Alloimmune vs consumptive platelet "refractoriness" in AML. Blood 1982; 60(supple 1): 180a.
3. Yankee RA, Graff KS, Dowling R, Henderson ES. Selection of unrelated compatible platelet donors by lymphocyte HL-A matching. N Engl J Med 1973; 288: 760.
4. Mittal KK, Ruder EA, Green D. Matching of histocompatibility (HL-A) antigens for platelet transfusion. Blood 1976; 47: 31.
5. Freedman J, Hooi C, Garvey MB. Prospective platelet crossmatching for selection of compatible random donors. Br J Haematol 1984; 56: 9.
6. Hecht T, Wolf JL, Mraz L, Scott EP, Petz LD. Platelet transfusion therapy in an alloimmunized patient. JAMA 1982; 248: 2301.
7. Branda RF, Tate DY, McCullough JJ, Jacob HS. Plasma exchange in the treatment of fulminant idiopathic (autoimmune) thrombocytopenic purpura. Lancet 1978; 1: 688.
8. Rifle G, Chalopin JM, Turc JM, et al. Plasmapheresis in the treatment of renal allograft rejections. Transplant Proc 1979; 11: 20.
9. Thomas ED. Bone marrow failure and bone marrow transplantation. In: Petersdorf RG, Adams RD, Braunwald E, Isselbacher KJ, Martin JB, Wilson JD, eds. Harrison's principles of internal medicine. New York: McGraw-Hill, 1983: 1885.
10. Bensinger WI, Buckner CD, Thomas ED, Clift RA. ABO-incompatible marrow transplants. Transplantation 1982; 33: 427.
11. Buckner CD, Clift RA, Sanders JE, et al. ABO-incompatible marrow transplants. Transplantation 1978; 26: 233.
12. Mittal KK, Mickey MR, Singal DP, Terasaki PI. Serotyping for homotransplantation. XVIII. Refinement of microdroplet lymphocyte cytotoxicity test. Transplantation 1968; 6: 913.
13. Hogge DE, Dutcher JP, Aisner J, Schiffer CA. Lymphocytotoxic antibody is a predictor of response to random donor platelet transfusion. Am J Hematol 1983; 14: 363.
14. Klein CA, Blajchman MA. Alloantibodies and platelet destruction. Semin Thromb Hemostas 1982; 8: 105.

Received 26 June 1985.
Accepted 11 September 1985.

0041-1337/86/4105-0606$02.00/0
TRANSPLANTATION
Vol. 41, No. 5
Printed in U.S.A.

RESULTS OF LIVING-RELATED KIDNEY TRANSPLANTATION IN PUERTO RICO

EDUARDO A. SANTIAGO-DELPÍN,[1] ZULMA GONZÁLEZ, ERNESTO RIVÉ-MORA, JOSÉ H. AMADEO, AND RAFAEL RAMÍREZ-GONZÁLEZ

The Transplant Program, Surgical and Medical Services, San Juan Veterans Administration Hospital, San Juan, Puerto Rico 00936

A total of 103 kidney transplantations from living-related donors were performed in the Puerto Rico Kidney Transplant Program between January 1977 and June 1984. The majority of these patients were male, 76% were between 21 and 50 years of age, 33% were indigent, and 38% were either black or of mixed race. Rigid exclusion criteria were established in the selection of kidney donors. All donor operations were at least 2-antigen-compatible. Surgical technique and posttransplant management were standard, except that in 1980 the immunosuppressive policy was changed as follows: posttransplant prednisone was very rapidly tapered to 20 mg/day at two weeks after transplantation and antilymphocyte globulin was used to treat all rejections. The overall 3-year patient survival for the 7½ years is 91.6%, but after 1980 it increased to 98% perhaps a reflection of the changes in immunosuppressive policy. Eight of ten deaths were due to sepsis, most of them related to rejection treatment. The 3-year kidney survival was 77%. All kidney losses were due to rejection. A low incidence of urological complications is reported. There were no technical losses. A relatively low incidence of cancer is reported. Cutaneous mycosis is highly prevalent in our patients, but systemic fungi are virtually absent.

The incidence of end-stage renal disease in Puerto Rico has changed from the initial projection of 44 new cases per million per year, to the most recent appraisal of 119.2 new cases per million per year (*1*). This is perhaps a reflection of improved diagnosis, enhanced communications, an active outreach program to the community, and increased facilities for renal care. There are currently 8 in-hospital hemodialysis centers, 8 satellite dialysis units, 8 continuous ambulatory peritoneal dialysis (CAPD)* programs, 8 chronic continuous peritoneal dialysis (CCPD) programs, one kidney transplant program, two nephrology training programs, one transplant surgery training program, one histocompatibility laboratory, an End-Stage Renal Disease Network (No. 29), several professional and patient organizations, and a Puerto Rico Kidney Foundation to serve a population of 3.2 million inhabitants.

The Puerto Rico Kidney Transplant Program was started in January 1977 based at the San Juan Veterans Administration Hospital but serving both veteran and community patients. The lack of appropriate legislation to permit cadaver organ retrieval made it difficult to develop an effective cadaver organ procurement program. In 1983 the 1974 Organ Donations Law was amended to incorporate a definition of death including a brain death clause, but for many years the program was skewed to living-related donor transplantation. A total of 103 kidney transplantations from living related donors performed between January 1977 and June of 1984 form the basis of this report.

MATERIALS AND METHODS

Patient population. The transplant histories of 103 recipients of organs from living-related donors were analyzed for patient and kidney survival and for immunological, technical, and nontechnical complications.

Sixty-six patients were male and 37 female. Ages ranged from 5 to 61 years; there were 6 children and 13 adolescents; 76% of the patients fell within the age limits of 21–50 years. Fourteen patients were veterans and 89 were nonveterans from the community. Thirty-three patients were considered indigent using family income and dwelling site criteria (*2*), 62 were middle class, and 8 were upper middle class. The Puerto Rican population consists of a mixture of African black and European white elements (*3*). It is usually difficult to define in a given person the color or race. In our identification of race we used color as well as facial features. We considered 19 presumably black, 63 presumably white, and 21 mixed.

Exclusion criteria were the presence of cancer, major cardiac or cerebrovascular disease not amenable to operation, liver disease or alcoholism, severe pulmonary disease, and a positive crossmatch. The causes of the primary renal failure of our patient population are listed in Table 1. The vast majority of patients with end-stage renal disease had a diagnosis of chronic glomerulonephritis, usually established clinically by the referring nephrologist.

Donors. Every effort was made to evaluate as many prospective donors as possible from the usually large Puerto Rican families, with the hope of encountering HLA-identical relatives. Donor distribution by family relationship was as follows:

Mother (15)
Father (13)
Brother (33)
Sister (33)
Son (4)
Daughter (2)
Nephew (2)
Cousin (1)

Very rigid donor acceptance criteria were used and the compatible donor rejection rate was 33%. The reasons for rejection

[1] Please address all correspondence and reprint requests to: E.A. Santiago-Delpín, Professor of Surgery and Pathology, Surgical Service, San Juan VA Hospital, San Juan, P.R. 00936.

* Abbreviations used: ALG, antilymphocyte globulin; CAPD, continuous ambulatory peritoneal dialysis; CCPD, chronic continuous peritoneal dialysis; MLC, mixed lymphocyte culture; PHA, phytohemagglutinin.

TABLE 1. Etiology of primary renal failure

Cause	No. patients
Chronic glomerulonephritis	53
End stage renal disease—unspecified	18
Chronic pyelonephritis/interstitial nephritis	8
Structural, obstructive or reflux: either congenital or acquired	8
Hypertension	7
Hereditary nephritis	2
Diabetic nephropathy	2
Schoenlein-Henoch	2
IgA nephropathy	1
Lupus	1

included obesity, mild hypertension, urinary tract infection, kidney stones, metabolic disease, and peptic ulcer disease.

Histocompatibility. Histocompatibility determinations included typing for HLA-A, B, and C loci using the NIH microtoxicity assay, plus mixed lymphocyte culture (MLC). The histocompatibility profile of donor and recipients is shown in Table 2 and is compared with that of the Puerto Rican population.

The latter is abstracted from the results of 847 independent cases obtained from a total of 1500 tissue types on file from the paternity section of our histocompatibility laboratory. When available, predicted haplotype was used in the selection of the most compatible donor. On the basis of a previous study (*4*), MLC stimulation index was used to assess cellular reactivity. A high stimulation index (over 3) was an indication for donor-specific blood transfusions—a total of 3 under temporary azathioprine coverage. Tests measuring transformation induced by phytohemagglutination (PHA) and skin reactivity to injected recall antigens were dropped from our protocol because of their lack of correlation with morbidity and mortality (*5*), or the eventual posttransplant course (*4*).

Splenectomy. Pretransplant splenectomy has been intermittently practiced in our program. Splenectomy was routinely performed between 1977 and 1979. In 1979, the operation was discontinued and a pilot study started, since mounting evidence of postsplenectomy sepsis placed the procedure under critical scrutiny. An increased severity of rejection was found, which prompted us to reinstitute the practice (*6*) as part of the conventional immunosuppressive protocol reported here. More recently however, we dropped it again from our routine protocol after adopting cyclosporine immunosuppression in all our cases.

Surgical technique. Donor nephrectomies were performed using a flank approach. The donors were maximally hydrated, and mannitol was usually given within 30 min of vascular occlusion (*7*). Although the transplant operation in the recipient was frequently performed by junior staff or supervised fellows or residents, only senior staff were involved in the donor operation. There was minimal manipulation of the donor kidney during the dissection, and removal occurred only under generous diuresis.

After flushing, the kidney was transplanted into the right iliac fossa of the recipient using standard vascular technique. The vein was always anastomosed end-to-side to the external or common iliac vein, and the artery was anastomosed either end-to-side to the external or common iliac artery or end-to-end to the internal iliac artery (*8*). In children, anastomosis was carried out to the inferior vena cava and aorta. From 1977 to 1981, a standard Politano-Leadbetter ureteroneocystostomy was used for ureteral implantation into the bladder, but for the last three years we have used a modified Lich-Gregoir operation. The technique, including the use of nonabsorbable polypropylene sutures in the muscular bladder wall, is described elsewhere (*8*). In children with bladder anomalies we used an ileal conduit, an iliocecal pouch, or transplantation into a mature end ureterostomy (*9*). Infrequently, Hemovac drains were placed lateral to the kidney and removed within 48 hr. Wound irrigation with antibiotic-containing saline was very frequently done during the operation.

Posttransplant management. All recipients were well hydrated and routine massive posttransplant diuresis was the rule. The bladder catheter was usually removed within 48 hr unless this was prevented by excessive diuresis or a small bladder capacity. Prednisone, azathioprine, and Minnesota an-

TABLE 2 (A). Histocompatibility profile (gene frequency [%])

Antigen	Recipients	Donors	Puerto Rican population
HLA A-1	4.9	5.8	6.1
2	23.8	24.8	21
3	9.7	8.3	9.8
9	14.7	14.7	14.8
(23)	( )[a]	( )	(4.9)
(24)	( )	( )	(9.9)
10	5.4	3	6.7
(25)	( )	( )	(1.3)
(26)	( )	( )	(5.4)
11	5.4	4.4	4.2
28	4.9	4.4	6.3
29	7.3	7.3	6.2
30	5.9	5.4	6.6
31	3.4	3.9	3.3
32	2.9	3.0	3.3
33	2.5	2.0	3.7
Blanks	8.8	12.5	7.6

[a] Data unavailable for early cases.

TABLE 2 (B). Histocompatibility profile (gene frequency [%])

Antigen	Recipents	Donors	Puerto Rican population
HLA B-5	9.2	10.2	9.7
7	5.4	4.9	5.7
8	3.9	1.0	3.5
12	13.6	17.0	16
(44)	( )[a]	( )	(12.2)
(45)	( )	( )	(3.8)
13	2	3	1.2
14	4.4	4.4	5.3
15	4.9	4.9	6.4
16	3.4	4.4	5
(38)	( )	( )	(3.7)
(39)	( )	( )	(1.3)
17	10.2	10.2	9.0
18	5.3	5.3	3.4
21	4.9	4.4	4.7
22	2	0	2.2
27	2.4	3	1.8
35	11.2	13.1	11.6
40	6.8	6.8	7.1
42	1.0	1.0	1.6
Blanks	9.2	4.9	4.0

[a] Data unavailable for early cases.

tilymphoblast globulin (ALG) were the mainstay of immunosuppression.

However, in 1980 two major changes in the immunosuppression protocol were established. The first concerned prednisone. The drug was tapered much more rapidly, the recipients usually being discharged home two weeks after the transplant on only 20 mg/day of prednisone. Azathioprine toxicity was monitored by liver function and white blood cell counts, and the dosage altered if signs of toxicity appeared (*10*). Minnesota antilymphocyte globulin was given prophylactically at 20 mg/kg for a total of 14 doses.

The second change in policy concerned the management of rejection. Prior to 1980, rejection was treated with three 1-g pulses of methylprednisolone and, if no response was detected, recycling of steroids was instituted. This consisted of increasing the dose of prednisone to 2 mg/kg and very slowly tapering it down to baseline levels again. Starting in 1980, all rejections were treated with antilymphocyte globulin and a fast recycling of the steroids was only used if response was not detected. Three or more rejections were not treated with increased immunosuppression. Minor elevations of creatinine that could have been secondary to a minor third or fourth rejection were treated with a single methylprednisolone pulse—and, if no response was noted, no further immunosuppressive treatment was given. Ten patients received more than one ALG course for rejection.

Posttransplant follow-up includes hematologic, hepatic, and renal function, urinalysis, and weight and blood pressure measurements at close intervals: three times a week for a month, twice a week for two months, and weekly thereafter until six months. A careful urinalysis of a fresh specimen is particularly important since persistent leukocyturia appears to be of prognostic value (*11*). Sonographic and radionuclide functional and anatomical evaluations are routinely performed in the posttransplant period and in cases of renal dysfunction (*12*). All patients with fever are admitted to the hospital. All infections, especially pulmonary infections, are managed very aggressively. Viral serology is routinely performed.

RESULTS

Survival. Table 3 shows our patient and kidney survival calculated using the life table method. There were only 22 recipients of HLA-identical, MLC-negative kidneys, and such a small number would not be strong enough for independent statistical analysis. Therefore, the 100% patient survival and the 84% graft survival of this subgroup at 3 years was added to the whole population, and these were analyzed together. The overall 3-year patient survival for the 7½ years reported here is 91.6%. When only the last four years were analyzed, as an index of the effect of the changes in prophylactic immunosuppression and the management of rejection, the 3-year patient survival increased to 98%. This increase was achieved with only minimal drop in 3-year graft survival to 77%.

Most of the deaths (70%) were related to the management of rejection: they occurred during the treatment for rejection or immediately thereafter; 80% of the deaths were due to bacterial sepsis (Table 4), although one case of disseminated *Strongyloides stercoralis* resulted in the death of one of our recipients (*13*). After institution of the use of ALG for rejection, the rejection-related death rate dropped to zero.

With the exception of 3 cases of late kidney loss due to recurrence of the disease, all other losses were due to acute rejection (9 cases), accelerated rejection (1 case), chronic rejection (6 cases), or chronic rejection with superimposed acute rejection (4 cases). In general, kidneys removed within the first six months showed chronic rejection with superimposed acute rejection ($P<0.01$, chi-square).

Mortality was not related to socioeconomic status or race. On the other hand, race appeared to have an independent impact on loss by rejection. Thirty-five percent of black or mixed recipients lost their kidneys to rejection, versus 13% in whites (chi-square=7.24; $P=0.007$). This was not accounted for by socioeconomic status, location of dwelling, or a higher incidence of infection or hypertension. Also, direct questioning failed to disclose differences in compliance. HLA match was similar in blacks and whites.

Infectious complications. Table 5 describes our infectious complications. We commonly encountered urinary tract infections and prostatitis, usually symptomatic and responding rapidly to antibiotic treatment. Tuberculosis is still seen in Puerto Rico, and most of our cases rapidly responded to antituberculous medications. Upper respiratory infections, pneumonia, and viruses are also frequently found, usually of mild-to-moderate severity and responding to appropriate antimicrobial therapy.

Cutaneous mycoses are highly prevalent in Puerto Rico. In one study (in preparation) we found that 60% of our patients had evidence of epidermophytosis, 10% of which were symptomatic and severe. This did not appear to be related to socioeconomic status, but patients with the more severe forms of infection were receiving higher doses of azathioprine and prednisone, and this was statistically significant ($P<.05$). Con-

TABLE 4. Deaths

Cause	No. patients
Sepsis	
Mycotic aortic aneurysm (*Salmonella*)	1[a]
Acute bacterial endocarditis (*S aureus*)	1[a]
Overwhelming sepsis (*E coli*)	1[a]
Pneumonia, necrotizing (*K pneumonia*)	2[a]
Pneumonia (*P carinii*)	1[a]
Pneumonia and respiratory failure	1[a]
Disseminated *S stercoralis*	1
Pulmonary embolus	1
Pancreatitis, obesity, fractures	1

[a] Associated with management of rejection.

TABLE 3. LRD % survival[a]

Survival	1 Mo.	6 Mo.	1 Yr.	2 Yr.	3 Yr.
Patient survival					
1977–1984	100±0 (103)	96±0.95 (102)	94±1.7 (98)	93±2.0 (81)	91.6±2.4 (68)
1980–1984 only	100±0 (50)	98±0(50)	98±0 (46)	98±0 (27)	98±0 (14)
Kidney survival					
1977–1984	97.1±1.7 (103)	91±2.0 (99)	89±2.4 (92)	84.6±7.4 (75)	81.7±9.3 (60)
1980–1984 only	96±2.8 (50)	94±2.7 (49)	89.9±3.9 (45)	83±15.3 (26)	77±15.3 (13)

[a] Percentage of survival ± SE. The number in parentheses is the size of the group at risk at the beginning of the interval.

versely, systemic fungi were absent from our population with the exception of one case of cryptococcal meningitis in a patient who had traveled extensively abroad.

"Rare" infections were all-too-present in our program too. An active diagnostic effort and very aggressive treatment has resulted in excellent survival of the rare infections described in Table 5. Of particular interest are the *Mycobacterium Kansasii* pneumonia (*14*) and a patient with cutaneous chromoblastomycosis (*15*). Appendicitis is very rare in the transplant patient (review submitted for publication) but in 1984 we had two patients admitted almost simultaneously, both with perforated appendicitis and intraabdominal abscesses. Both patients survived after aggressive surgical and antimicrobial therapy.

Technical complications. These are described in Table 6. A relatively low rate of urological complications is reported, the most dramatic of which was a patient with acute tubular necrosis so severe that it resulted in total necrosis of the ureter and pelvis. All complications, including this necrosis, were cured by appropriate surgical intervention. Lymphoceles were treated by repeated aspiration—and, if recurrent, by internal marsupialization. No arterial or venous thromboses were reported. There were no deep infections, and no patients or kidneys were lost to technical complications (*8*).

Nontechnical complications are listed in Table 7. Although our program is located in a tropical country, we have only seen one case of basal cell carcinoma on the dorsum of the hand; one lip leukoplakia, in a 58-year old recipient; and no other patient with cutaneous cancer. An adenocarcinoma of the rectum was successfully treated with abdominoperineal resection. One microinvasive carcinoma of the vulva was treated by wide excision and vulval reconstruction. A "lymphoid lung tumor" responded to segmental resection of the lung.

TABLE 5. Infectious complications

Common	Rare
Urinary tract infection	*M kansasii* pneumonia
Prostatitis	*L monocytogenes* sepsis
Tuberculosis	*Salmonella* sepsis
Pneumonia	*P carinii* pneumonia
Upper respiratory infections	*M morgagni* pneumonia
	Necrotizing staphylococcal pneumonia
Virus	*S stercoralis* sepsis
Skin fungi	Chromoblastomycosis
Intestinal parasites	Herpes encephalitis
	Toxoplasma hepatitis
	Disseminated Herpes zoster
	Perforated appendicitis with abscess
	Mycotic aortic aneurysm

TABLE 6. Technical complications

Complication		Number(percentage)
Urological complications		10 (9.7%)
Early ureteral stenosis	4 (3.9%)	
Late ureteral stenosis	2 (1.9%)	
Stones	2 (1.9%)	
Extravasation	1 (0.9%)	
Total ureteral necrosis	1 (0.9%)	
Lymphocele		7 (6.7%)
Acute renal failure with dialysis		6 (5.9%)
Bleeding		4 (3.9%)
Infection		
Superficial	3 (2.9%)	3 (2.9%)
Deep	0 (0)	
Anastomoses	0 (0)	
Early renal artery stenosis		1 (0.9%)
Hernia		0 (0)
Venous complications		0 (0)
Technical losses		0 (0)
Deaths due to technical complications		0 (0)

TABLE 7. Nontechnical complications

Complication	No. patients (%)
Hypertension	32 (31%)
Steroid-induced diabetes mellitus	9 (8.7%)
Aseptic necrosis of the hip	5 (4.9%)[a]
Late renal artery stenosis	4 (3.9%)
Deep thrombophlebitis	3 (2.9%)
Cataracts with severe visual impairment	2 (1.9%)
Cancer	4 (3.9%)
"Lymphoid lung tumor"	1 (.9%)
Adeno carcinoma of rectum	1 (.9%)
Carcinoma in situ of vulva	1 (.9%)[b]
Basal cell carcinoma of skin	1. (.9%)
Dysplasia cervix uteri	1 (.9%)[b]

[a] 3 bilateral.
[b] Same patient.

DISCUSSION

Kidney transplantation has become routine in the treatment of end-stage renal disease. The behavior of our end-stage renal disease patients and our transplant patient population is similar to that reported in other centers of the United States. However, there are several salient points in our experience. Patient survival improved significantly coincident with the change in immunosuppression protocol. The liberal use of ALG for rejection, together with more conservative use of prednisone, resulted in an important increase in patient survival (*16*) while only minimally decreasing the kidney survival. Rejection is being treated earlier and more aggressively with antilymphocyte globulin, while the acute overdose with steroids and the chronic use of moderately high steroid doses were eliminated from our practice. A combination of these factors had a salutary effect on the results.

We have no explanation for the very low incidence of systemic fungi. *Histoplasma*, *Sporotrix*, *Candida*, and *Aspergillus* all occur in Puerto Rico, and have been seen in cancer patients undergoing chemotherapy as well as in immunosuppressed patients on hyperalimentation. Conversely, we report an unusually high incidence of cutaneous mycoses, probably a reflection of humidity and temperature. A significant correlation exists between level of immunosuppression and severity of infection.

There is also a relatively low incidence of tumors as compared with the national average (*17*). Of particular significance is the low incidence of skin tumors, especially since Puerto Rico is a tropical country with a high ultraviolet index. Sheil (*18*) reports that 19% of all Australian transplant patients develop skin cancer, and the Swedish report a similar 19.9% premalignant or malignant skin lesions. Our low incidence could be a reflection of a relatively short follow-up or of our racial admixture.

The low incidence of wound infection may be the result of the use of prophylactic antibiotics during and immediately postoperatively, the use of antibiotic solutions for all wound lavages during surgery, and the low incidence of urological complications, confirming the experience of other centers.

A very aggressive approach to all fevers has been continuously in operation since the inception of the program. This permits early diagnosis of common or rare infections and early institution of antimicrobial therapy. In the case of pulmonary infections, identification of the offending organism is a priority, and if tissue or secretions for diagnosis cannot be obtained actively by expectoration, then bronchoscopy and washings or biopsy are immediately performed, with negligible complication rate.

Acknowledgment. We recognize the selfless, dedicated involvement of our coordinators and consultants in the management of the patients.

REFERENCES

1. Statistics, ESRD Kidney Network Council #29. San Juan, PR, 1984.
2. Matos D, Rodríguez N, Santiago R, Torres M, Zayas A. La Rehabilitación del Paciente Después de un Trasplante Renal, [Master Thesis]. Puerto Rico: University of Puerto Rico, 1978.
3. Nettleship E, Santiago-Delpín EA. The HLA profile of the Puerto Rican population. Fed Proc 1983; 42: 940.
4. Santiago-Delpín EA, Nettleship E, Ruiz ML. Pretransplant predictors in renal transplantation. Amer J Surg 1983; 146: 586.
5. Santiago-Delpín EA, Ruiz ML, Echegaray S, Cancio M, Ramírez-González R. A high incidence of failed delayed hypersensitivity in hemodialysis patients does not correlate with increased morbidity & mortality. Dial Transplant 1983; 12: 708.
6. González Z, Santiago-Delpín EA. Massive irreversible rejection in kidney transplantation in man. Puerto Rico Health Sci J 1982; 1: 5.
7. Najarian JS, Gulyassy PP, Stoney RJ, Duffy G, Braunstein P. Protection of the donor kidney during homotransplantation. Ann Surg 1966; 164: 398.
8. Santiago-Delpín EA, Baquero A, González Z, Low incidence of urological complications in kidney transplantation. Amer J Surg (in press).
9. Santiago-Delpín EA, Acosta-Otero A, Vázquez-Lugo A. Ureteral implantation in kidney transplantation: the use of a mature end-ureterostomy. J Urol 1980; 124: 513.
10. Santiago-Delpín EA. Principles of clinical immunosuppression. Surg Clin North Am 1979; 59: 283.
11. Baquero A, Santiago-Delpín EA. The prognostic significance of sterile leukocyturia after kidney transplantation. Dial Transplant 1984; 13: 758.
12. Rivera JV, Santiago-Delpín EA. Radionucleide studies in the evaluation of renal transplants. Bol Asoc Med P Rico 1980; 72: 71.
13. Santiago-Delpín EA, Rodríguez-Campos B, Ramírez-González R, Miranda JL. Strongyloidiasis in the immunosuppressed host. Bol Assoc Med P Rico 1982; 74: 134.
14. Cruz N, Ramírez-Muxó O, Bermúdez RH, Santiago-Delpín EA. Pulmonary infection with *M kansasii* in a renal transplant patient. Nephron 1980; 26: 187.
15. Morales L, González Z, Santiago-Delpín EA. Chromoblastomycosis in renal transplantation. Nephron 1985; 40: 238.
16. Krakauer H, Grauman JS, McMullan MR, Creede CC. The recent US experience in the treatment of end stage renal disease by dialysis & transplantation. N Engl J Med 1983; 308: 1558.
17. Penn I, Lymphomas complicating organ transplantation. Transplant Proc 1983; 15: 2790.
18. Sheil AGR, Mahoney JF, Horwath JS, et al. Cancer following successful cadaveric donor renal transplantation. Transplant Proc 1981; 13: 733.

Received 23 May 1985.
Accepted 12 September 1985.

0041-1337/86/4105-0611$02.00/0
TRANSPLANTATION
Vol. 41, No. 5

Printed in U.S.A.

THE EFFECTS OF CYCLOSPORINE ON *TOXOPLASMA GONDII* IN VIVO AND IN VITRO[1]

ROBERT E. MCCABE,[2] BENJAMIN J. LUFT,[3,4] AND JACK S. REMINGTON,[5]

Department of Immunology and Infectious Diseases, Research Institute, Palo Alto Medical Foundation, Palo Alto, California 94301; and Department of Medicine, Stanford University, Stanford, California 94305

We examined the effect of cyclosporine on *Toxoplasma* infection in vivo and in vitro. Administration to mice of 150 mg/kg/day cyclosporine variably affected mortality in four separate experiments. IgG (Sabin-Feldman dye test) and IgM enzyme-linked immunosorbent assay antibody titers were significantly depressed in mice treated with cyclosporine. These results suggested the possibility that cyclosporine possesses anti-*Toxoplasma* activity. Thus, macrophages were incubated with cyclosporine before and after infection with *Toxoplasma*. Treatment with 0.5, 1, and 5 μg cyclosporine/ml during or after challenge of macrophage monolayers with *Toxoplasma* inhibited replication of *Toxoplasma* (and resulted in killing of *Toxoplasma*). The effect of cyclosporine on development of activated macrophages was studied. Cyclosporine administered to mice at a dose of 150 mg/kg/day neither accelerated nor delayed activation of macrophages (assessed by inhibition of *Toxoplasma* replication in vitro) by i.v. injection of either *Corynebacterium parvum* or *Toxoplasma*. Cyclosporine affects mortality variably in murine toxoplasmosis, depresses synthesis of IgG and IgM *Toxoplasma* antibody in vivo, does not prevent activation of macrophages in vivo, and possesses anti-*Toxoplasma* activity in vitro and perhaps in vivo. Cyclosporine may be the preferred immunosuppressive agent for recipients of an organ transplant who are at high risk for toxoplasmosis (e.g., seronegative recipients who have received organ from seropositive donors).

Disseminated toxoplasmosis is a major cause of morbidity and mortality in patients with organ transplants (*1–3*). Primary rather than recrudescent infection probably causes most cases of toxoplasmosis in transplant recipients (*1–3*), and approximately 17% of heart transplant recipients seronegative for *Toxoplasma* antibody receive a heart from a seropositive donor (*2*). The use of cyclosporine has significantly ($P<0.05$) reduced the incidence of significant changes of *Toxoplasma* serologies in comparison with other immunosuppressive regimens in heart transplant recipients (*1*), although the incidence of clinical toxoplasmosis is not known to be lower. Reduction of infectious complications due to other organisms has been reported for cyclosporine-treated recipients of transplant organs other than hearts (*4–6*). Cyclosporine selectively suppresses T lymphocytes, particularly T helper cells (*7–9*). It is noteworthy that patients with acquired immunodeficiency syndrome (AIDS)* who are afflicted with a remarkably high incidence of central nervous system toxoplasmosis (*10, 11*) are lymphopenic, with a relative decrease in T helper cells (*12, 13*).

We considered it important to study the effect of cyclosporine on *Toxoplasma* infection in vitro and in a murine model because of the aforementioned observations. The studies in vitro were performed to determine if cyclosporine has intrinsic anti-*Toxoplasma* activity, whether this activity is directed against intracellular or extracellular organisms, and whether cyclosporine affects activation of macrophages that constitute the major host defense mechanism against *Toxoplasma* and other intracellular pathogens (*14*). The murine model of *Toxoplasma* infection was studied to determine if the anti-*Toxoplasma* activity of cyclosporine is significant in vivo when immunosuppressive doses of cyclosporine are used.

MATERIALS AND METHODS

Mice. Swiss-Webster female mice, weighing 20–22 g (Simonsen Laboratories, Gilroy, CA) were used.

Infection of mice with Toxoplasma. Tachyzoites of the C56 strain (*14*) were obtained from peritoneal fluid of mice as previously described (*15*). Mice were infected i.v. via the tail vein.

Macrophage cultures. Mouse peritoneal cells were harvested and monolayers established in 8-chamber tissue culture slides (Lab-Tek, Miles Laboratories, Naperville, IL) (*15*). In some experiments, macrophages were activated by i.v. injection of 1400 μg of killed *Corynebacterium parvum* (Wellcome Laboratories, Research Triangle Park, NC) or by i.v. injection of 2×10^3 tachyzoites of the C56 strain (*14*).

Challenge of macrophages with Toxoplasma. Tachyzoites of the highly virulent RH strain were used to infect macrophage monolayers as previously described (*14*). Macrophage monolayers were washed and incubated with medium containing *Toxoplasma* for 1 hr. Extracellular *Toxoplasma* then were washed from the monolayers. This is considered the zero time point, and monolayers were fixed and stained routinely at this time to determine the number of organisms phagocytosed. Separate monolayers were incubated for 18 hr, which is sufficient for approximately three doublings of a single *Toxoplasma* in a

[1] This work was supported by Grant AI04717 from the National Institutes of Health.

[2] Robert E. McCabe is the recipient of an Edith J. Milo Memorial Fellowship and Fellowship Grant AI06723 from the National Institutes of Health.

[3] Benjamin J. Luft is the recipient of an Edith J. Milo Memorial Fellowship, an Upjohn Fellowship, and BRSG No. S07 RRO 5513.

[4] Benjamin J. Luft is currently located at the Division of Infectious Diseases, Department of Medicine, State University of New York, Stony Brook, NY 11794.

[5] Please address all communications and reprint requests to Jack S. Remington, M.D., Research Institute, Palo Alto Medical Foundation, 860 Bryant Street, Palo Alto, CA 94301.

* Abbreviations used: AIDS, acquired immunodeficiency syndrome; ELISA, enzyme-linked immunosorbent assay.

normal mouse macrophage. The size of the *Toxoplasma* challenge was calculated to infect approximately 20–40% of the macrophages, as determined by counting 500 cells stained with Giemsa stain. The number of *Toxoplasma* per vacuole was determined by counting 50 infected cells. A rosette is defined here as *eight or more* Toxoplasma *within a single vacuole*. Each data point is the mean for duplicate monolayers. According to the particular experimental protocol, cyclosporine was present in the medium of the macrophage cultures: (1) before challenge of the macrophages with *Toxoplasma*; (2) during incubation of extracellular *Toxoplasma* with macrophages for the 1 hr before the zero time point; (3) for the 18 hr of incubation after the extracellular *Toxoplasma* had been washed from the cultures (after the zero time point); or (4) a combination of these.

Toxoplasma *serology*. The Sabin-Feldman dye test was performed as previously described (*16*). This test measures complement-dependent neutralizing IgG antibody. Measurement of serum IgM antibody specific for *Toxoplasma* was done by the double sandwich enzyme-linked immunosorbent assay (ELISA)* method (*17*).

Reagents. Cyclosporine was kindly supplied by Drs. E. Wiskott and M. Hugener, Sandoz Ltd., Basel, Switzerland. Tissue culture medium was RPMI 1640 (Gibco Laboratories, Grand Island, NY) supplemented with 10% inactivated fetal calf serum (Gibco) and 100 U/ml of penicillin and 100 μg/ml of streptomycin. For in vivo experiments, cyclosporine was solubilized in olive oil and administered by s.c. injection at a dose of 150 mg/kg/day (*18*). We had previously established that a single injection of this dose produces a peak serum level in mice of 630 ng/ml 2 hr after injection and a level of 155 ng/ml 24 hr after injection (*19*). We and others had previously demonstrated that this dose of cyclosporine is immunosuppressive for mice infected with *Listeria monocytogenes* (*18*) and *Trypanosoma cruzi* (*20–22*). Control animals received only olive oil. In preliminary experiments, this dose of cyclosporine administered to mice for three weeks did not affect the mice adversely as assessed by inspection and weight gain compared with controls. For in vitro experiments, cyclosporine was solubilized in 100% ethanol and then diluted to the desired concentration in medium such that the final concentration of ethanol was 0.01% (v/v) for all concentrations of cyclosporine and for controls.

RESULTS

Effect of cyclosporine on time to death. Mice were treated with 150 mg/kg/day for 48 hr before infection with 2×10^4 tachyzoites of the C56 strain. Of four separate experiments (Fig. 1) of similar design, one (Fig. 1A) showed that cyclosporine treated mice had a significantly earlier time to death than controls ($P<.05$). No significant differences in time to death were observed in the other three experiments. One of these experiments showed a slight deleterious effect and two showed a slight protective effect of cydclosporine. In the experiments in which administration of cyclosporine produced a protective effect, control animals died earlier than in the experiments in which cyclosporine produced an apparent immunosuppressive effect despite use of comparable inocula of *Toxoplasma*.

Effect of cyclosporine on serum antibody titers. For the experiment depicted in Figure 1A, in which a statistically significant earlier time to death was produced by cyclosporine, five treated and five control mice were bled on days five and fifteen for dye test and IgM antibody determination (Table 1). Mice treated with cyclosporine had lower dye test and IgM serum antibody

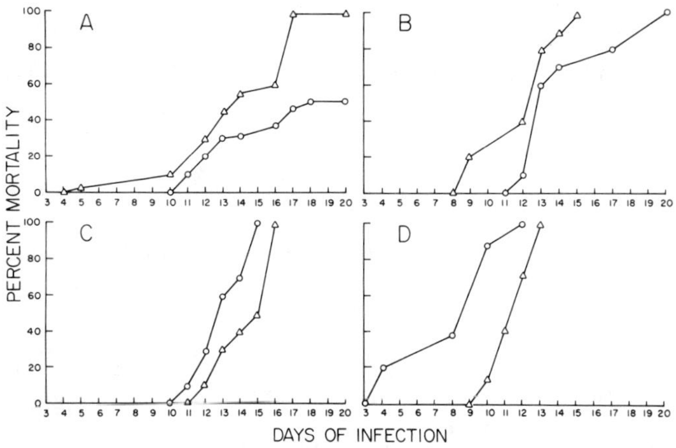

FIGURE 1. Effect of cyclosporine on *Toxoplasma* infection in vivo: Mice were infected i.v. with 2×10^4 tachyzoites of the C56 strain on day 0, except for experiment C in which 5×10^4 tachyzoites were administered. Mice were treated with cyclosporine (△) (150 mg/kg/day s.c.) or olive oil (○) started 48 hr before infection. The number of cyclosporine-treated and untreated mice were (22, 21), (10, 10), (9, 10), and (7, 8) in A, B, C, and D, respectively. In experiment A, cyclosporine-treated mice had significantly greater mortality than controls ($P<0.05$, Fisher exact test).

TABLE 1. Effect of cyclosporine on serum IgG and IgM antibody titers

Group[a]	IgG: day of infection		IgM: day of infection	
	5	15	5	15
Controls	37±26[b]	538±223	29±16	717±210
Cyclosporine	Neg. (<4)	39±12[c]	3±4	10±4[c]

[a] Five mice in each group were infected with 2×10^4 C56 i.v. Starting 48 hr before infection, mice were treated with 150 mg/kg/day of cyclosporine or olive oil. Mice were bled from the retroorbital venous plexus on days 5 and 15 of infection for serum for antibody testing.
[b] Reciprocal titer ± SE.
[c] $P<0.05$ (Student's t test) compared with control.

titers on days 5 and 15 of infection. These differences were statistically significant on day 15 ($P<.05$). Dye test levels were also performed in an experiment in which a slight protective effect of cyclosporine was observed on time to death. Dye test titers were significantly reduced in the cyclosporine-treated mice on day 9 of infection ($P<.05$).

Effect of cyclosporine on Toxoplasma *in vitro*. Experiments were performed with the use of two protocols to determine if the presence of cyclosporine during either the *Toxoplasma* infection incubation period (i.e., during the 1 hr challenge period before the zero time point when extracellular *Toxoplasma* are washed from the monolayers) or after extracellular *Toxoplasma* had been washed from the monolayers affected replication of *Toxoplasma*. Results of a representative experiment are shown in Table 2. When extracellular *Toxoplasma* and cyclosporine at concentrations of 1 and 5 μg/ml were incubated with the macrophage cultures for 1 hr and then washed to remove both *Toxoplasma* and drug, both the number of infected macrophages and the number of rosettes were markedly reduced compared with controls. Similar results were obtained when cyclosporine was added to the monolayers after extracellular *Toxoplasma* had been washed from the monolayers (Table 2). In separate but similar experiments, 0.5 μg cyclosporine/ml was tested for its effect on *Toxoplasma* replication.

TABLE 2. Effect of cyclosporine on *Toxoplasma* replication in vitro

Concentration of cyclosporine (μg/ml)	Cyclosporine present during infection[a]			Cyclosporine present after infection[b]		
	Percentage of MØ infected	Tv[c]	Percentage of rosettes[d]	Percentage of MØ infected	Tv	Percentage of rosettes
0	40	6.0	55	33.3	6.6	41
0.1	40	6.2	58	28.2	5.6	40
1.0	28	6.5	42	14.1	4.3	17[e]
5	14[e]	5.2	33	10.3	4.0	14[e]

[a] Macrophage monolayers were challenged for one hour with *Toxoplasma* in medium containing cyclosporine. Cyclosporine and extracellular *Toxoplasma* were then washed from the monolayers. Monolayers were incubated for 18 hr more; data is presented for monolayers at this time.

[b] Cyclosporine was present only during the 18 hr after extracellular *Toxoplasma* had been removed from the monolayers.

[c] *Toxoplasma* per vacuole.

[d] Percentage of infected vacuoles that contained at least eight *Toxoplasma*.

[e] $P<0.05$ (Student's *t* test).

For both protocols, this concentration of drug markedly decreased the number of infected cells compared with controls but had little effect on the development of rosettes by surviving *Toxoplasma* (data not shown).

The foregoing experiments suggest that cyclosporine may have a direct effect on extracellular *Toxoplasma*. To further test this possibility, *Toxoplasma* were incubated with cyclosporine for 30 min at 37°C, washed with medium that did not contain cyclosporine, and then used to challenge macrophage monolayers. In a second protocol, cyclosporine was added to macrophage monolayers 1 hr after extracellular *Toxoplasma* had been washed from monolayers to minimize the possibility of contact of cyclosporine with *Toxoplasma* that may have adhered to the cell membrane of the macrophage but had not yet been internalized at the zero time point. *Toxoplasma* incubated with 1 or 5 μg cyclosporine/ml prior to infection of monolayers produced slightly decreased numbers of infected cells, *Toxoplasma* per vacuole, and rosettes by 18 hr of infection when compared with controls. For macrophages incubated with cyclosporine starting 1 hr after extracellular *Toxoplasma* had been washed from the monolayers, 5 μg cyclosporine/ml caused significant decreases in numbers of infected cells, *Toxoplasma* per vacuole, and rosettes. One μg cyclosporine/ml produced significant decreases of rosettes only, with lesser decreases in the other two parameters.

In none of the foregoing experiments did treatment with cyclosporine affect the number of macrophages infected or the number of *Toxoplasma* per infected macrophage at the zero time point.

To determine if preincubation of macrophages with cyclosporine would enable macrophages to kill *Toxoplasma*, macrophage monolayers were incubated with cyclosporine at concentrations of 0.1, 1, and 5 μg/ml. After extensive washing, the monolayers were infected with *Toxoplasma* and incubated in medium that did not contain cyclosporine. No effect on replication was observed (data not shown).

Effect of cyclosporine on macrophage activation. Activated macrophages are important for defense against *Toxoplasma* infection in vivo (*15*). Thus we considered it important to determine if administration of cyclosporine to mice affected activation of macrophages. Two methods were used to activate mouse peritoneal macrophages—i.v. injection of 2×10^3 tachyzoites of the C56 strain or i.v. injection of 1400 μg of heat-killed *C parvum* (*14, 15, 23*). Both of these methods for macrophage activation confer resistance to challenge with *Toxoplasma* or *Listeria* (*14*), and treatment of mice with *C parvum* confers resistance to infection with *T cruzi* (*24*). Mice were treated with cyclosporine at a dose of 150 mg/kg/day or olive oil for 48 hr before injection with C56 tachyzoites or *C parvum*. Peritoneal cells were harvested from groups of four mice at varying times thereafter, and macrophage monolayers established with these cells were challenged with *Toxoplasma* of the RH strain. Macrophage activation was assessed by inhibition of replication of RH *Toxoplasma* by macrophages (*14*).

Results of an experiment that utilized macrophages harvested 6 days after infection with *Toxoplasma* are shown in Figure 2. Macrophages from infected mice treated with cyclosporine or olive oil were activated since they markedly inhibited *Toxoplasma* replication when compared with macrophages from

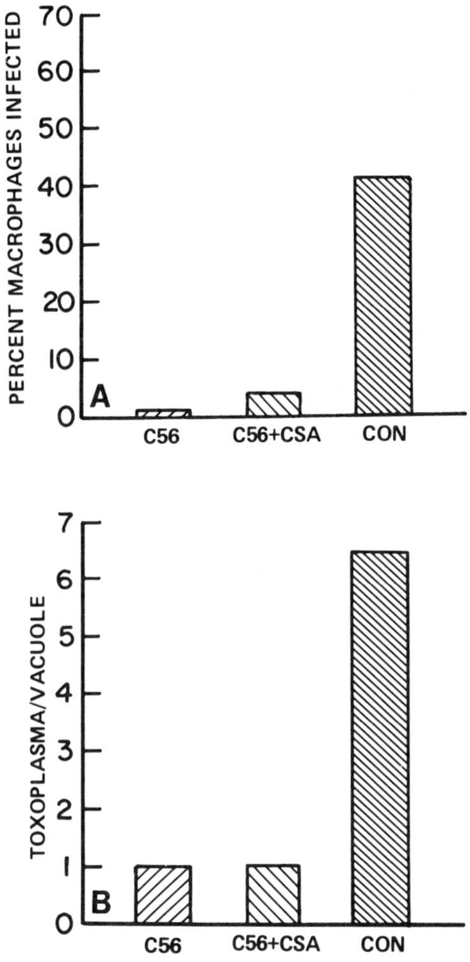

FIGURE 2. Effect of cyclosporine on activation of macrophages: Mice were infected i.v. with 2×10^3 tachyzoites of the C56 strain and treated with cyclosporine (CsA+C56, with daily s.c. injections at 150 mg/kg) or olive oil (C56). Six days after infection, peritoneal macrophages were harvested and challenged with *Toxoplasma* of the RH strain in vitro. The number of *Toxoplasma* per vacuole (A) and percentage of macrophages infected (B) were determined after 18 hr of incubation. The number of macrophages infected at the zero hour time point (see the *Materials and Methods* section) was approximately 27% for all experimental groups. (Con) = uninfected and untreated mice. Treatment of uninfected mice with cyclosporine or olive oil did not affect the number of infected macrophages or replication of *Toxoplasma*.

uninfected mice ($P<.05$, Student's t test) (Fig. 2A). These activated macrophages killed *Toxoplasma*; this was evidenced by a greater than fourfold decrease in the percentage of infected macrophages from *Toxoplasma*-infected mice as compared with macrophages from uninfected mice ($P<.05$) (Fig. 2B). In contrast, macrophages obtained from mice three days after infection with *Toxoplasma* did not inhibit replication of *Toxoplasma*, regardless of whether the macrophages were obtained from mice treated with cyclosporine (data not shown). In addition, administration of cyclosporine to mice infected with *Toxoplasma* did not affect the ability of macrophages to phagocytose *Toxoplasma* in vitro, as assessed by inspection of monolayers fixed and stained at the zero time point. Controls for these experiments consisted of macrophages from uninfected mice treated with cyclosporine, olive oil, or nothing. There was no difference among the controls with respect to either phagocytosis or replication of *Toxoplasma*.

Similar experiments were performed with macrophages from mice injected with *C parvum* and treated or not treated with cyclosporine. Administration of cyclosporine did not appear to affect development of activated macrophages. Macrophages obtained from cyclosporine-treated or untreated mice seven days after injection with *C parvum* inhibited replication of *Toxoplasma* as in controls. For *C parvum*-activated macrophages obtained from mice treated with cyclosporine or olive oil, infected vacuoles contained a mean of 2.2±0.3 (SEM) and 2.4±0.1 *Toxoplasma* ($P>.05$, Student's t test), whereas infected vacuoles from nonactivated macrophages contained a mean of 5.0±0.2 *Toxoplasma* ($P<.025$ when compared with *C parvum*-activated macrophages from mice treated or untreated with cyclosporine). Macrophages were not activated by five days after injection of *C parvum* (data not shown) in mice either treated with cyclosporine or untreated.

DISCUSSION

The cyclosporine treated mice in this study were clearly immunosuppressed. Administration of doses of cyclosporine to mice infected with *Toxoplasma* that achieved serum levels within the range observed in humans (*25*) produced significant depression of the IgG and IgM *Toxoplasma*-specific antibody responses. In studies by ourselves and other investigators, similar dosages of cyclosporine administered to mice infected with either of the intracellular pathogens *L monocytogenes* (*18*) or *T cruzi* (*20–22*) were clearly immunosuppressive via their effects on T lymphocytes. In our study reported here, cyclosporine treatment of mice infected with *Toxoplasma* produced a variable response with respect to mortality in four separate experiments. Our in vitro studies confirm a previous report that cyclosporine has intrinsic anti-*Toxoplasma* activity (*26*) and demonstrate that the drug is effective against both intracellular and extracellular forms of the organism.

The variability in mortality may be related to a balance between the anti-*Toxoplasma* activity of cyclosporine and its immunosuppressive properties. The anti-*Toxoplasma* activity may be most evident in experiments with quickly lethal inocula (e.g., experiment D, Figure 1), while immunosuppressive activity may be more prominent with prolonged infections that allow development of immunity. It is very difficult to formally test these possibilities in an experiment with many inocula of *Toxoplasma* that are chosen to span LD_0 to LD_{100}, due to the experimental constraints of i.v. injection of large numbers of mice with tachyzoites of the C56 strain that are in limited supply and have limited life span in vitro before injection.

Cyclosporine has been shown to suppress the responsiveness of murine B cells to thymus-independent-2 antigens (*27, 28*), to inhibit the help provided by T helper cells for antibody production in the mouse (*9*), and to inhibit an early step in human B cell activation (*29*). The role of specific antibody in host resistance to acute infection with *Toxoplasma* is not clear; some data support a role for antibody in resistance (*30–32*), while others do not (*33–35*). Our studies demonstrated a significant suppression of *Toxoplasma*-specific IgG and IgM antibody. However, our studies cannot distinguish between the relative importance of humoral and cellular effector mechanisms.

A considerable amount of evidence suggests that the activated macrophage is an imortant effector cell for resistance to *Toxoplasma* (*15, 23, 36, 37*). For this reason, we examined the effect of cyclosporine on activation of macrophages to kill *Toxoplasma* with use of two different activation stimuli, *Toxoplasma* of the C56 strain and killed *C parvum*, with use of an in vitro ex vivo approach. Administration of cyclosporine did not retard development of macrophage activation in this system. Cyclosporine has been shown to decrease production of human and murine interferon gamma from human leukocytes (*38, 39*), human thymocytes (*40*), and murine spleen cells (*39*) in vitro. Interferon gamma activates human monocytes and murine macrophages to kill *Toxoplasma* (*41, 42*). Under the conditions of our studies, cyclosporine may not have suppressed the production of interferon gamma sufficiently to prevent activation of macrophages; or lymphokines other than interferon gamma involved in macrophage activation were relatively unaffected by cyclosporine.

The anti-*Toxoplasma* effect of cyclosporine in vitro was observed at concentrations (0.5–1.0 μg/ml) that can be achieved in serum of humans and mice (*21, 25*). While our experiments were in progress, Mack and McLeod reported that cyclosporine at a concentration of 2 μg/ml, inhibited replication of *Toxoplasma gondii* within macrophages when assayed by uptake of radiolabeled uracil (*26*). Mack and McLeod speculated that compounds related to cyclosporine may prove useful for treatment of toxoplasmosis. Borel (*43*) has reviewed the accumulated data and suggested that the antiparasitic activity of cyclosporine that has been demonstrated in murine models of schistosomiasis and malaria (*44–47*) does not result from immunosuppression and is not related to the portion of the cyclosporine molecule that affects T cell functions. Therapy of *Toxoplasma* infection in humans, particularly for immunosuppressed patients, is unsatisfactory at present, and congeners of cyclosporine that are not immunosuppressive may be useful for treatment of *Toxoplasma* infections.

Toxoplasmosis is a frequent opportunistic pathogen in recipients of cardiac transplants, particularly for seronegative recipients of a heart from a seropositive donor (*1, 2*). The foregoing data suggest that cyclosporine is the immunosuppressive agent of choice for these heart transplant patients, and perhaps for other organ transplant recipients as well if they are at risk of developing toxoplasmosis.

Acknowledgments. We greatly appreciate the technical assistance of Michael Gallo and Dorothy Gibbons.

REFERENCES

1. Luft BJ, Naot Y, Araujo FG, Stinson EB, Remington JS. Primary and reactivated Toxoplasma infection in patients with cardiac transplants: clinical spectrum and problems in diagnosis in a defined population. Ann Intern Med 1983; 99: 27.
2. Nagington J, Martin AL. Toxoplasmosis and heart transplantation.

Lancet 1983; 2: 679.
3. Ryning FW, McLeod R, Maddox JC, Hunt S, Remington JS. Probable transmission of Toxoplasma gondii by organ transplantation. Ann Intern Med 1979; 90: 47.
4. Preiksaitis JK, Rosno S, Grumet C, Merigan TC. Infections due to herpes viruses in cardiac transplant recipients: role of the donor heart and immunosuppressive therapy. J Infect Dis 1983; 147: 974.
5. Dummer JS, Hardy A, Poorsattar A, Ho M. Early infections in kidney, heart, and liver transplant recipients on cyclosporine. Transplantation 1983; 36: 259.
6. Najarian JS, Ferguson RM, Sutherland DER, Rynasiewicz JJ, Simmons RL. A prospective trial of the efficacy of cyclosporine in renal transplantation at the University of Minnesota. Transplant Proc 1983; 15: 438.
7. White DJG. Cyclosporine A: clinical applications and immunology. Clin Immunol All 1983; 3: 287.
8. Morris PJ. Cyclosporin A. Transplantation 1981; 32: 349.
9. Klaus GGB, Kunkl A. Effects of cyclosporine on the immune system of the mouse II. Cyclosporine inhibits the effector function of primary T helper cells, but not helper cell priming. Transplantation 1983; 36: 80.
10. Luft BJ, Brooks RG, Conley F, McCabe RE, Remington JS. Toxoplasmic encephalitis in patients with AIDS. JAMA 1984; 252: 913.
11. Wong B, Gold JWM, Brown AE, et al. Central-nervous-system toxoplasmosis in homosexual and parenteral drug abusers. Ann Intern Med 1984; 100: 36.
12. Gottlieb MS, Groopman JE, Weinstein WM, Fahey JL, Detels R. The acquired immunodeficiency syndrome. Ann Intern Med 1983; 99: 208.
13. Rogers MF, Morens DN, Stewart JA, Kaminski RM, Spira TJ, Feorino PM, Larsen SA, Francis DP, Wilson M, Kautman L. The Task Force on Acquired Immune Deficiency Syndrome. National case control study of Kaposi's sarcoma and Pneumocystis carinii pneumonia in homosexual men: part 2, laboratory results. Ann Intern Med 1983; 99: 151.
14. Swartzberg JE, Krahenbuhl JL, Remington JS. Dichotomy between macrophage activation and degree of protection against Listeria monocytogenes and Toxoplasma gondii in mice stimulated with Corynebacterium parvum. Infect Immun 1975; 12: 1037.
15. McLeod R, Remington JS. Studies on the specificity of killing of intracellular pathogens by macrophages. Cell Immunol 1977; 34: 156.
16. Sabin AB, Feldman HA. Dyes as microchemical indicators of a new immunity phenomenon attending a protozoon parasite (Toxoplasma). Sience 1948; 108: 660.
17. Siegel JP, Remington JS. Comparison of methods for quantitating antigen-specific immunoglobulin M antibody with a reverse enzyme-linked immunosorbent assay. J Clin Microbiol 1983; 18: 63.
18. Schaffner A, Douglas H, Davis CE. Models of T cell deficiency in listeriosis: the effects of cortisone and cyclosporin A on normal and nude Balb/c mice. J Immunol 1983; 131: 450.
19. Donatsch P, Abisch E, Homberger M, Traber R, Trapp M, Voges R. A radioimmunoassay to measure cyclosporin A in plasma and serum samples. J Immunoassay 1981; 2: 19.
20. Kierszenbaum F, Gottlieb CA, Budzko DB. Exacerbation of Trypanosoma cruzi infection in mice treated with the immunoregulatory agent cyclosporin A. Tropenmed Parasitol 1983; 34: 4.
21. McCabe RE, Remington JS, Araujo FG. Effect of cyclosporin A on T. cruzi. Fed Proc 1984; 43: 31.
22. McCabe RE, Remington JS, Araujo FG. In vivo and in vitro effects of cyclosporin A on Trypanosoma cruzi. Am J Trop Med Hyg 1985; 34: 861.
23. Remington JS, Krahenbuhl JL, Mendenhall JW. A role for activated macrophages in resistance to infection with Toxoplasma. Infect Immun 1972; 6: 829.
24. Brener Z, Cardoso JE. Nonspecific resistance against Trypanosoma cruzi enhanced by Corynebacterium parvum. J Parasitol 1976; 62: 645.
25. Kahan BD, Ried M, Newburger J. Pharmacokinetics of cyclosporine in human renal transplantation. Transplant Proc 1983; 15: 446.
26. Mack DG, McLeod R. New micromethod to study the effect of antimicrobial agents on Toxoplasma gondii: comparison of sulfadoxine and sulfadiazine individually and in combination with pyrimethamine and study of clindamycin, metronidazole, and cyclosporin A. Antimicrob Agents Chemother 1984; 26: 31.
27. Kunkl A, Klaus GGB. Selective effects of cyclosporin A on functional B cell subsets in the mouse. J Immunol 1980; 125: 2526.
28. Dongworth DW, Klaus GGB. Effects of cyclosporin A on the immune system of the mouse. I. Evidence for a direct selective effect of cyclosporin A on B cells responding to anti-immunoglobulin antibodies. Eur J Immunol 1982; 12: 1018.
29. Muraguchi A, Butler JL, Kehrl JH, Falkoff RJM, Fauci AS. Selective suppression of an early step in human B cell activation by cyclosporin A. J Exp Med 1983; 158: 690.
30. Nakayama I. Effects of immunization procedures in experimental toxoplasmosis. Keio J Med 1965; 14: 63.
31. Krahenbuhl JL, Ruskin J, Remington JS. The use of killed vaccines in immunization against an intracellular parasite: Toxoplasma gondii. J Immunol 1972; 108: 425.
32. Hafizi A, Modabber FZ. Effect of cyclophosphamide on Toxoplasma gondii infection: reversal of the effect by passive immunization. Clin Exp Immunol 1978; 33: 389.
33. Huldt G. Experimental toxoplasmosis. Effect of inoculation of Toxoplasma in seropositive rabbits. Acta Pathol Microbiol Scand 1966; 68: 592.
34. Eichenwald HF. Experimental toxoplasmosis. II. Effect of sulfadiazine and antiserum on congenital toxoplasmosis in mice. Proc Soc Exp Biol Med 1949; 71: 45.
35. Gill HS, Prakash O. Chemotherapy of experimental Toxoplasma gondii (RH strain) infection. Indian J Med Res 1970; 58: 1197.
36. Mackaness GB. Resistance to intracellular infection. J Infect Dis 1971; 123: 439.
37. Jones TC, Yeh S, Hirsch JG. Assessment in vitro of immunity against Toxoplasma gondii. J Exp Med 1975; 141: 466.
38. Abb J, Abb H. Effect of cyclosporine on human leukocyte interferon production: selective inhibition of IFN-gamma synthesis. Transplant Proc 1983; 15: 2380.
39. Kalman VK, Klimpel GR. Effects of cyclosporine on the production of various interferons. Transplant Proc 1983; 15: 2383.
40. Reem GH, Cook LA, Palladino MA. Cyclosporine inhibits interleukin-2 and interferon gamma synthesis by human thymocytes. Transplant Proc 1983; 15: 2387.
41. Nathan CF, Murray HW, Wiebe M, Rubin BY. Identification of interferon-γ as the lymphokine that activates human macrophage oxidative metabolism and antimicrobial activity. J Exp Med 1983; 158: 670.
42. McCabe RE, Luft BJ, Remington JS. Effect of murine interferon gamma on murine toxoplasmosis. J Infect Dis 1984; 150: 961.
43. Borel JF. Cyclosporine: historical perspectives. Transplant Proc 1983; 15: 2219.
44. Bueding BE, Hawkins J, Cha YN. Antischistosomal effects of cyclosporin A. Agents Actions 1981; 11: 380.
45. Thommen-Scott K. Antimalarial activity of cyclosporin A. Agents Actions 1981; 11: 770.
46. Bout D, Deslee D, Capron A. Protection against mouse schistosomiasis by a non-schistosomicide drug, cyclosporine A. Research for an immune mechanism. Fed Proc 1983; 42: 1246.
47. Nickel SP, Scheibel LW, Cole GA. Inhibition by cyclosporin A of rodent malaria in vivo and human malaria in vitro. Infect Immun 1982; 37: 1093.

Received 11 July 1985.
Accepted 17 September 1985.

0041-1337/86/4105-0616$02.00/0
TRANSPLANTATION
Vol. 41, No. 5
Printed in U.S.A.

AUTONOMIC SYSTEM DYSFUNCTION AND POLYNEUROPATHY IN NONDIABETIC UREMIA[1]

A ONE-YEAR FOLLOW-UP STUDY AFTER RENAL TRANSPLANTATION

GÖRAN SOLDERS,[2,3] ANDERS PERSSON,[2] AND HENRYK WILCZEK[4]

Departments of Clinical Neurophysiology, Neurology, and Transplantation Surgery, Huddinge University Hospital, S-141 86 Huddinge, Sweden

Polyneuropathy and autonomic dysfunction were studied in 15 patients with nondiabetic terminal uremia before renal transplantation and again at 6 and 12 months after the transplantation. Beat-to-beat variation of the electrocardiogram (ECG) relative to mean beat interval was used as an observation of the function of the parasympathetic vagal reflex arc. Marked autonomic dysfunction—i.e., reduced beat-to-beat variation and a mild diffuse polyneuropathy—was found. The neuropathy was mainly of axonal type, but a slowing of conduction velocities was also found. The latter was markedly improved after transplantation and is suggested to be caused by a toxic metabolic factor, possibly causing nodal dysfunction. Action potential amplitudes and autonomic function did not improve during the study. This implies a structural damage that is not repaired in 12 months. Neurological examination should be included in the care of patients with uremia, and the results should be one of the factors considered when transplantation is discussed.

Symptoms of autonomic systemic dysfunction and polyneuropathy are common findings in patients with uremia (*1–3*). The polyneuropathy is easy to document by showing reduced nerve conductivity. To establish autonomic dysfunction many tests have been used, for example beat-to-beat variation of the electrocardiogram (the R-R test) (*3–8*), valsalva test (*4–7, 9–13*), forced handgrip test (*4, 7, 10, 12–13*), cold pressure test (*5–7, 9, 13*), sweat test (*14, 15*), baroreflex studies (*16–18*) and atropine test (*7*). In most cases pathological findings have been reported.

In earlier reports we have used the R-R test to study the relative beat-to-beat variability in the electrocardiogram (ECG)* and have shown that reduced variability may be a sign of parasympathetic dysfunction (*19*). A profound impairment was found in uremic patients and no acute improvement occurred by hemodialysis (HD) (*3*). The aim of the present study was to observe the short-term and long-term effects of renal transplantation on autonomic dysfunction compared with its effects on motor and sensory neuropathy.

* Abbreviations used: CV, conduction velocity; DL, distal latencies; ECG, electrocardiogram; ENeGIx, electroneurography index; HD, hemodialysis; MCV, motor conducting velocity; SCV, sensory conducting velocity; SNAP, sensory nerve action potential.

[1] This work was supported by funds from the Karolinska Institute.

[2] Department of Clinical Neurophysiology.

[3] Department of Neurology.

[4] Department of Transplantation Surgery.

MATERIALS AND METHODS

Patients and controls. 15 nondiabetic patients with terminal uremia were examined before (−5.9 months ±4.4) renal transplantation and again at about 6 months (7.7 months ±3.3) and about 12-months (14.2 months ±3.8) after the transplantation. The patients were compared with age-matched normal values used in the laboratory. The patient group consisted of 6 male and 9 female patients aged 16–64 ($\bar{x}$ = 43.5±12.0).

The underlying renal disease was chronic glomerulonephritis in eight patients; two patients had chronic pyelonephritis; and the remaining five patients suffered from papillary necrosis, nephrosclerosis, oxalosis, nephronopthisis and SLE-nephritis.

Before transplantation all but two patients had been treated by regular dialysis. Twelve patients were treated by regular HD and one patient by peritoneal dialysis. The time on pretransplant dialysis ranged from 2 to 82 months ($\bar{x}$ = 18). Following transplantation none of the patients required further treatment by regular dialysis. Some relevant laboratory data are given in Table 1.

Six patients were normotensive without the use of antihypertensive medication, while nine patients had well controlled blood pressure with β-receptor blockers, alone or in combination with hydralazine. All except one patient used small doses of diuretics (furosemide). Eleven patients received transplants from cadaveric donors and four patients from living-related donors.

Informed consent was obtained and the study was approved by the Ethical Committee at Huddinge University Hospital.

Immunosuppressive regimen. All patients were immunosuppressed with cylcosporine and prednisolone. Cyclosporine was given in an initial dose of 15 mg/kg b. wt./day, which was then reduced by 2 mg/kg b. wt./day after 14, 30, and 60 days to reach a maintenance dose of 9 mg/kg b. wt./day. For all patients additional dose adjustments were made when toxic side effects occurred. Prednisolone was given in a dose of 100 mg/day from the day of operation, which was then tapered off so that 20 mg/day was reached after 3 months. All patients also received 0.5 g of hydrocortisone i.v. intraoperatively. In all patients rejection episodes were treated with pulses of methylprednisolone, 0.5 g i.v. on the first day, followed by 0.25 g/day for another 3 days.

Due to severe nephrotoxicity in one patient, cyclosporine was replaced by azathioprine after 1 month. Two more patients also were switched to azathioprine, one after 4 and one after 9 months, due to impaired renal function. Azathioprine and prednisolone were given according to regimens previously described (*20*).

Recording procedure. The beat-to-beat variation of the ECG

TABLE 1. Laboratory data of the patients

Laboratory data	Months after transplantation		
	0	6	12
Hemoglobin	81.6±13.9	126.5±18.9	138.6±17.9
Ref. value (115–165)			
Creatinine	956.5±270.7	211.2±83.7	212.4±95
Ref. value (0–115 μmol/L)			
Urea	26.1±8.3	14.7±6.4	13.9±6.9
Ref. value (3.0–7.5)			
S-Ca	2.44±0.30	2.50±0.16	2.48±0.15
Ref. value (2.07–2.55 mmol/L)			
S-PO_4	1.99±0.48	1.21±0.27	1.16±0.20
Ref. value (0.6–1.6 mmol/L)			

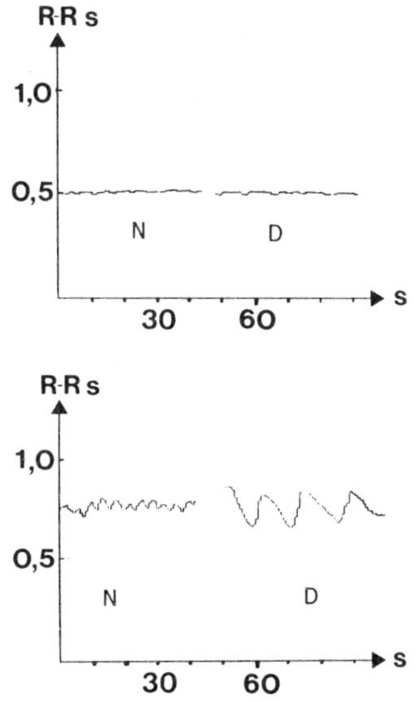

FIGURE 1. R-R variations during normal breathing (N) and during deep breathing (D). Top recording: uremic patient on HD; bottom recording: healthy control subject.

(R-R variation) was recorded with the patients resting in supine position using a Rate Display unit (Neurolog) and plotted against time using an X-Y recorder (Fig. 1). The R-R variation relative to mean R-R interval was calculated during 1 min of normal breathing (N%) and during 1 min of deep breathing (D%). Recording procedure and calculations have been described in detail earlier (*19*).

Motor conduction velocity (MCV) and distal latencies (DL) in the median and peroneal nerves, sensory conduction velocity (SCV), and the amplitude of the sensory nerve action potential (SNAP) in the median and sural nerves were recorded with conventional neurophysiological techniques. Recordings were made at room temperature. Skin temperature was controlled and care was taken that all recordings were made at normal skin temperatures.

Statistical methods. The degree of polyneuropathy was expressed by the electroneurography index (ENeG-Ix) as described by Hillbom and Wennberg (*21*). This consists of the mean deviation of MCV, DL, SCV and SNAP from normal values of age-matched controls expressed in standard deviations. The normal limit for individuals (i.e., for $P<0.05$) of the ENeG-Ix is $\pm 2/\sqrt{\text{number of examined parameters}}$. In this study (10 parameters) the individual normal limit is ±0.63.

Values are given as mean ±SD. For N% and D%, the patients were compared with the laboratory control values for their age, and the mean deviation from normal was tested by the *t* test or, when the variances differed significantly, the approximative *t'*-test. Intraindividual variations at 0, 6, and 12 months were tested by the *t* test of differences. The level of significance was set at P<0.05. (*22*).

RESULTS

Before transplantation, the uremic patients as a group showed impaired R-R variations (N% = 6.0±1.4, D% = 16.4±10.5) as compared with age-matched laboratory normal values (N% = 19.4±4.1, D% = 29.5±6.0). The differences are significant (Table 2, Fig. 2). The ENeG-Ix in the uremic group before transplantation was −1.17±0.41, which was significantly ($P<0.001$) below normal (0±0.63). This indicated that the patients had a clear but mild diffuse polyneuropathy (Table 3).

After the transplantation there was a rapid improvement of the ENeG-Ix. At about 6 months the index was −0.49 ($P<0.01$) and at about 12 months the index was −0.35 ($P<0.05$). The improvement compared with the pretransplantation index is significant at $P<0.01$ and $P<0.001$ for 6 and 12 months, respectively. Compared with the normal values, an improvement was found in several individual parameters, especially in the conduction velocities. The amplitudes of the action potentials remained low (Table 3).

TABLE 2. N%, D%, and ENeG-Ix before transplantation

	Patients (n = 15)	Age-matched normal (n = 80)	Statistical analysis	
N%	6.00±1.41	19.40±4.12	$\sigma_1^2 \neq \sigma_2^2$ f' = 20	t' = 11.92 $P<0.001$
D%	16.36±10.54	29.50±5.99	$\sigma_1^2 \neq \sigma_2^2$ f' = 22	t' = 4.20 $P<0.001$
ENeG-Ix	−1.17±0.41	0±0.63	f = 14	t = 11.05 $P<0.001$

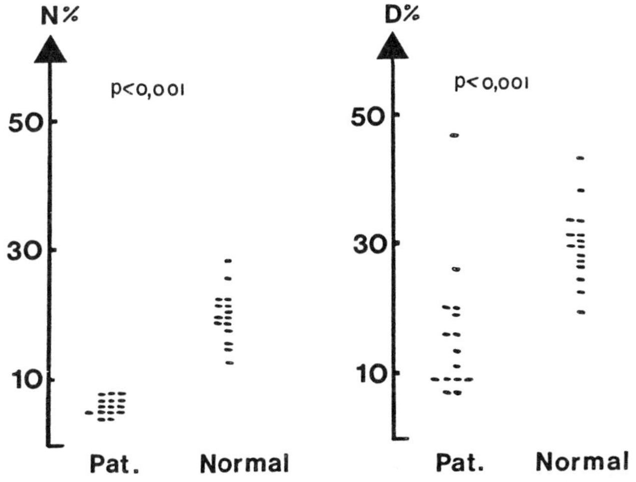

FIGURE 2. N% (left) and D% (right). Uremic patients before renal transplantation compared with age-matched normal values used in the laboratory.

TABLE 3. Neuropathy status of the patients, significance tested vs. laboratory normal

	Age-matched laboratory normal (n=80)	Patients before transplantation (n=15)		Patients at half year after transplantation		Patients at one year after transplantation	
Median nerve							
MCV m/s	55.9	50.5±6.4	$P<0.01$	52.6±5.2	$P<0.05$	52.6±6.8	ns
Distal SCV m/s	54.3	51.3±6.1	ns	58.8±7.6	ns	54.8±6.5	ns
Distal SNAP μV	17.3	14.9±10.2	ns	14.2±7.7	ns	16.6±11.2	ns
Prox. SCV m/s	63.7	58.5±5.2	$P<0.01$	60.4±6.0	$P<0.05$	63.1±7.1	ns
Prox. SNAP μV	30.9	13.5±7.3	$P<0.001$	15.4±10.7	$P<0.001$	16.3±9.5	$P<0.001$
Peroneal nerve							
MCV m/s	47.9	42.1±6.9	$P<0.01$	43.8±5.1	$P<0.01$	43.3±6.6	$P<0.05$
Sural nerve							
SCV m/s	43.1	37.8±5.5	$P<0.01$	41.1±7.8	ns	41.1±6.0	ns
SNAP μV	11.9	4.5±2.7	$P<0.001$	6.7±3.6	$P<0.001$	7.7±5.4	$P<0.01$
ENeG-Ix	0.00±0.63	−1.17±0.41	$P<0.001$	−0.49±0.64	$P<0.01$	−0.35±0.46	$P<0.05$

TABLE 4. N%, D%, and ENeG-Ix: intraindividual changes after transplantation[a]

	Intraindividual changes		Statistical analysis	
0–6 Months	N%	$\bar{d}$= 0.43±2.98	t = 0.56	ns
	D%	$\bar{d}$ = 4.23±11.53	t = 1.42	ns
	ENeG-Ix	$\bar{d}$ = 0.68±0.86	t = 3.08	$P<0.01$
6–12 Months	N%	$\bar{d}$ = 1.07±2.34	t = 1.76	ns
	D%	$\bar{d}$ = 2.93±8.90	t = 1.28	ns
	ENeG-Ix	$\bar{d}$ = 0.13±0.50	t = 1.02	ns
0–12 Months	N%	$\bar{d}$ = 0.71±2.05	t = 1.35	ns
	D%	$\bar{d}$ = 0.57±10.63	t = 0.26	ns
	ENeG-Ix	$\bar{d}$ = 0.82±0.71	t = 4.44	$P<0.001$

[a] $\bar{d}$ = mean difference.

Contrary to the improvement of the polyneuropathy after transplantation, we could not demonstrate any recovery of the autonomic dysfunction. At about 6 months the N% and D% were 6.5±2.6 and 20.9±9.1 and at about 12 months the N% and D% were 5.4±1.8 and 17.2±5.7, respectively. There was no significant intraindividual change in N% or D% during the 12-month follow-up period (Table 4).

DISCUSSION

The results of the present investigation show that autonomic dysfunction was common in nondiabetic uremia patients and that it did not improve after renal transplantation. A high frequency of autonomic dysfunction associated with uremia has been reported in several other studies that have used similar or other methods to demonstrate autonomic neuropathy.

In our previous study of autonomic dysfunction in uremia no acute improvement was seen in the R-R test by HD. Neither could we now demonstrate any effect on the autonomic neuropathy by renal transplantation. The effect of renal transplantation on autonomic dysfunction has not been extensively studied. Röckel et al. (*23*), however, found an improvement of autonomic dysfunction (pupillary reaction to tyramine, valsalva, and postural tolerance test) after renal transplantation, but not after HD.

Before transplantation the patients as a group showed signs of a mild diffuse neuropathy. The most significant changes were found in the low amplitudes of the action potentials, indicating a primarily axonal neuropathy. This is in agreement with other reports of polyneuropathy in chronic uremia (*24*), including four reports of sural nerve biopsies (*25–28*) in which axonal degeneration dominated and demyelination was seen only as a secondary finding. It is worth noting that in our study potential amplitudes did not improve much during the 12-month follow-up after transplantation—i.e., the axonal dysfunction remained.

The conduction velocities (CV) before transplantation were low in all nerves examined, indicating a dysfunction of the myelin sheet also. The CV had recovered to normal values in all nerves except the peroneal at one year after transplantation. Most of the improvement was seen during the first half-year, as can be seen by the change in the ENeG-Ix. Many studies have reported similar rapid improvement of conduction velocities after transplantation (*28–31*), in some cases even within a few days (*32*). The rapid change has, as in our study, been followed by a long period of further normalization of the CV.

All our patients had chronic terminal uremia and had been on HD before transplantation. In acute experimental uremia in the rat a slowing of MCV can be seen within 48 hr (*33*); it is probably caused by dysfunction of the nodal membrane with decreased sodium permeability (*34*). A toxic factor has been suggested as a cause of this slowing of CV, a factor that is not altered by HD but is eliminated by renal transplantation. This factor is thought to cause a reversible impairment of the membrane of the node of Ranvier (*34*).

The slow second phase of the improvement of the CV, and the persisting low action potential amplitudes may, on the other hand, be explained by structural damage to the nerve that is not repaired for a long time.

In contrast to the peripheral neuropathy, the autonomic dysfunction did not improve after transplantation. The tests used to study autonomic function give information about the parasympathetic vagal reflex arc. The nerves in this system consist mainly of thin myelinated and unmyelinated fibers. The damage to this reflex in chronic uremia seems to be structural—possibly axonal—and is not reversed within a year after transplantation. This is in contrast to the acute demyelinative neuropathies, in which a profound, but reversible, impairment of the N% and D% can be seen (*35–37*). The possibility that the persistence of the autonomic neuropathy may be caused by cyclosporine cannot be excluded by this study. We have, however, found no earlier report of neuropathy caused by cyclosporine. Only further studies in neurologically healthy patients taking cyclosporine can answer this question.

In conclusion, nondiabetic patients with terminal uremia showed signs of a mild polyneuropathy and of autonomic dysfunction. The neuropathy was mainly axonal but a slowing of the conduction velocities was also seen. This slowing was not altered by HD but was quickly (at least partially) restored by renal transplantation—and may, therefore, be caused by a toxic metabolic factor. The autonomic dysfunction, reduced heart frequency variability, was not improved within a year after transplantation, which implies structural nerve damage with a long time for repair.

REFERENCES

1. Thomas PK, Uraemic neuropathy. Proc Eur Dial Transplant Assoc 1976; 13: 109.
2. Arieff AI. Neurological complications of uremia. In: Brenner BM, Rector FC, eds. The kidney. Philadelphia: WB Saunders, 1981: 2306.
3. Solders G, Persson A, Gutierrez A. Autonomic dysfunction in non-diabetic terminal uraemia. Acta Neurol Scand 1985; 71: 321.
4. Ewing DJ, Winney R. Autonomic function in patients with chronic renal failure on intermittent haemodialysis. Nephron 1975; 15: 424.
5. Zuccala A, Esposti EP, Sturani A, et al. Autonomic function in haemodialyzed patients. Int J Artif Organs 1978; 1: 76.
6. Bach C, Iaina A, Eliahou HE. Autonomic nervous system disturbance in patients on chronic hemodialyses. Isr J Med Sci 1979; 9: 761.
7. Zoccali C, Ciccarelli M, Maggiore Q. Defective reflex control of heart rate in dialysis patients: evidence for an afferent autonomic lesion. Clin Sci 1982; 63: 285.
8. Burgess ED. Cardiac vagal denervation in hemodialysis patients. Nephron 1982; 30: 228.
9. Nies AS, Robertson D, Stone WI. Hemodialysis hypotension is not the result of uremic peripheral autonomic neuropathy. J Lab Clin Med 1979; 94: 395.
10. Campese VM, Romoff MS, Levitan D, Lane K, Massry SG. Mechanisms of autonomic nervous system dysfunction in uremia. Kidney Int 1981; 20: 246.
11. Naik RB, Mathias CJ, Wilson CA, Reid JL, Warren DJ. Cardiovascular and autonomic reflexes in haemodialysis patients. Clin Sci 1981; 60: 165.
12. Levitan D, Massry SG, Romoff MS, Campese VM. Autonomic nervous system dysfunction in patients with acute renal failure. Am J Nephrol 1982; 2: 213.
13. Yashpal LC, Issar U. Autonomic failure of circulation in chronic uremia. Indian J Med Sci 1982; 36: 69.
14. Hennessy WJ, Siemens AW. Autonomic neuropathy in chronic renal failure. Clin Res 1968; 16: 385.
15. Doerr HO, Follette W, Scribner BH, Elisdorfer C. Electrodermal response dysfunction in patients on maintenance renal dialysis. Psychophysiology 1980; 17: 83.
16. Levy SB, Lilley JJ, Stone RA. Baroreflex function in uraemic and hypertensive man. Am J Med Sci 1978; 276: 57.
17. Tomiyama O, Shiigai T, Ideura T, et al. Baroreflex function in uraemic and hypertensive man. Am J Med Sci 1978; 276: 57.
18. Wehle B, Bevegård S, Castenfors J, Davidsson S, Lindblad LE. Carotid baroreflexes during hemodialysis. Clin Nephrol 1983; 19: 236.
19. Persson A, Solders G. R-R variations, a test of autonomic dysfunction. Acta Neurol Scand 1983; 67: 285.
20. Wilczek H, Gunnarsson R, Lundgren G, Öst L. Improved results of renal transplantation in diabetic neuropathy. Transplant Proc 1984; 16: 623.
21. Hillbom M, Wennberg A. Prognosis of alcoholic peripheral neuropathy. J Neurol Neurosurg Psychiatry 1984; 47: 699.
22. Snedecor GW, Cochran WG. Statistical methods. 6th ed. Ames, Iowa: Iowa State University Press, 1967.
23. Röckel A, Hennemann H, Sternagel-Haase A, Heidland A. Uraemic sympathetic neuropathy after haemodialysis and transplantation. Eur J Clin Invest 1979; 9: 23.
24. Caccia MR, Mangili A, Mecca G, Ubiali E, Zanoni P. Effects of hemodialytic treatment on uremic polyneuropathy. J Neurol 1977; 217: 123.
25. Dayan AD, Gardner-Thorpe C, Down PF, Gleadle RI. Peripheral neuropathy in uremia, pathological studies on peripheral nerves from 6 patients. Neurology 1970; 20: 649.
26. Dyck PJ, Johnson WJ, Lambert EH, O'Brien PC. Segmental demyelination secondary to axonal degeneration in uremic neuropathy. Mayo Clin Proc 1971; 46: 400.
27. Thomas PK, Hullinrake K, Lascelles RG, O'Sullivan DJ, Baillod RA, Moorhead JF. The polyneuropathy of chronic renal failure. Brain 1971; 94: 761.
28. Ahonen RE. Peripheral neuropathy in uremic patients and in renal transplant recipients. Acta Neuropathol (Berl) 1981; 54: 43.
29. Ibrahim M, Crosland J, Honigsberger L, Barnes A, Dawson-Edwards P, Newman C. Effect of renal transplantation on uraemic neuropathy. Lancet 1974; 2: 739.
30. Nielsen K. The peripheral nerve function in chronic renal failure. Recovery after renal transplantation. Electro-physiological aspects (sensory and motor nerve conduction). Acta Med Scand 1974; 195: 171.
31. Bolton C. Electrophysiologic changes in uremic neuropathy after successful renal transplantation. Neurology (Minneap) 1976; 26: 152.
32. Oh SJ, Clements RS, Lee YW, Diethelm AG. Rapid improvement in nerve conduction velocity following renal tranplantation. Ann Neurol 1978; 4: 369.
33. Tegnér R, Brismar T. Experimental uremic neuropathy. Part 1. Decreased nerve conduction velocity in rats. J Neurol Sci 1984; 65: 29.
34. Brismar T, Tegnér R. Experimental uremic neuropathy. Part 2. Sodium permeability decrease and inactivation in potential clamped nerve fibers. J Neurol Sci 1984; 65: 37.
35. Edmonds ME, Sturrock RD. Autonomic neuropathy in the Guillain-Barré syndrome. Br Med J 1979; 2: 668.
36. Frisón JC, Sanchez L, Garnacho A, Bofill J, Oliveró R, Miquel C. Heart rate variations in the Guillain-Barré syndrome. Br Med J 1980; 281: 649.
37. Persson A, Solders G. R-R variations in Guillain-Barré syndrome: a test of autonomic dysfunction. Acta Neurol Scand 1983; 67: 294.

Received 16 July 1985.
Accepted 9 September 1985.

00078

0041-1337/86/4105-0620$02.00/0
TRANSPLANTATION

Vol. 41, No. 5
Printed in U.S.A.

ALLOSPECIFICITY OF ACTIVATED T CELLS GROWN FROM ENDOMYOCARDIAL BIOPSIES FROM HEART TRANSPLANT PATIENTS[1]

ADRIANA ZEEVI,[2] JOHN FUNG, TONY R. ZERBE, CHRISTINA KAUFMAN, BRUCE S. RABIN, BARTLEY P. GRIFFITH, ROBERT L. HARDESTY, AND RENE J. DUQUESNOY

Departments of Pathology and Surgery, University of Pittsburgh and Central Blood Bank of Pittsburgh, Pennsylvania

Studies were conducted to determine the functional characteristics of lymphocytes infiltrating human heart allografts. We have developed methodologies to generate lymphocyte cultures from endomyocardial biopsies. Thirteen biopsies from four heart transplant recipients, obtained at different days during a posttransplant period of less than two months, were cultured in interleukin-2 (IL-2)-containing medium supplemented with irradiated autologous peripheral blood lymphocytes as feeder cells. Lymphocyte cultures were obtained from all 13 biopsies and they exhibited a proliferative response to IL-2, suggesting the presence of activated T cells that express IL-2 receptors. Several cultures consisted of Leu 3 (helper/inducer) T cells, whereas others were primarily Leu 2 (cytotoxic/suppressor) T cells or a mixture of both types of cells. Cultured lymphocytes were also shown to be able to undergo secondary proliferation to donor-specific leukocytes as measured by primed lymphocyte testing (PLT). The PLT specificity of these cells was frequently toward class II HLA antigens of the donor, but certain cultures had PLT specificity associated with class I HLA antigens.

These results demonstrate the feasibility of growing functionally active T cells from heart transplant biopsies. An analysis of the phenotypes and allospecificity, as well as a functional characterization of these cells, should generate useful information about the types of T cells involved in cardiac transplant rejection.

The diagnosis of cardiac allograft rejection depends largely on the histological evaluation of endomyocardial biopsies. Rejection is manifested by perivascular and endocardial infiltrates of mononuclear cells—which, during later phases, extends to the interstitium and causes myocyte necrosis (*1*). Severe rejection is evidenced by additional hemorrhage and infiltration of neutrophils. Resolving rejection is characterized by scars, iron pigment, and scant residual mononuclear cells.

Although T lymphocytes are well known to mediate transplant rejection, little is understood about the functional characteristics of these cells infiltrating the cardiac allograft. The use of monoclonal antibodies in immunohistological staining of leukocyte subsets has provided opportunities to define the types of T cells infiltrating cardiac allografts. Reported studies have primarily focused on the detection of OKT-4 or Leu-3 (helper/inducer) and OKT8 or Leu-2 (cytotoxic/suppressor) T cell subsets in endomyocardial biopsies in relation to transplant rejection (*2–5*). It has been reported that OKT4 cells are primarily found during early stages of rejection, whereas OKT8 cells reach maximal levels during late stages of rejection (*4*).

Although these studies provide information about different types of infiltrating T cells, little is known about the functional characteristics and their specificity of allorecognition. To learn more about T cells involved in cardiac allograft responses, we have developed methodologies of generating in vitro cultures of activated T cells grown from endomyocardial biopsies. The technique is based on the concept that transplant biopsies undergoing an allograft response would be infiltrated by activated T cells capable of responding to interleukin-2 (Il-2)* in vitro. We describe here a method of growing activated T cells from heart transplant biopsies. These activated cells exhibit alloreactivity toward donor specific HLA antigens.

MATERIALS AND METHODS

Biopsy specimens. Serial endomyocardial biopsies were taken from heart transplant recipients one week after transplantation and thereafter, generally at two-week intervals during a two-month period. Thereafter, biopsies were obtained when rejection was suspected.

Under fluoroscopic guidance, right heart ventricular catheterization was accomplished utilizing an internal jugular vein approach. Four biopsy samples were obtained with a bioptome. Three were placed in 10% buffered formalin for histological evaluation, and one was suspended in sterile saline for tissue culture.

Histology. Four sections were prepared from each biopsy; three were stained with hematoxylin and eosin and one was stained with marron trichrome. All biopsy slides were evaluated in a blind manner by one of us (T.Z.) using Billingham's criteria for heart rejection (*1*).

Generation of lymphocyte cultures from heart biopsies. Each biopsy was divided into 2 or 3 fragments and placed in 100 μl tissue culture medium (TCM) supplemented with 100 μl Il-2 and 10^5 irradiated autologous feeder cells. TCM consisted of RPMI-1640 (Medastat) supplemented with 10% normal human serum, 4 mM L-glutamine, 24 mM Hepes buffer, and 60 mg/ml gentamycin. Sources of Il-2 were lectin-depleted supernatants of two-day phytohemagglutinin (PHA-M) cultures of normal peripheral blood leukocytes (PBL) as previously de-

[1] This work was supported by Grants AI-12410 and from the National Institute of Allergy and Infectious Diseases, Grant IM-373 from the American Cancer Society, and Grant AA93 from the United Way, Health Research and Services Foundation.

[2] Dr. Zeevi is a recipient of New Investigator Award AI-18923 from the National Institute of Allergy and Infectious Diseases.

* Abbreviations used: EBV, Epstein-Barr virus; IL-2, interleukin 2; HB, heart biopsy; HLA, human leukocyte antigen; LCL, lymphoblastoid cell lines; MLR, mixed leukocyte reaction; PBL, peripheral blood leukocytes; PHA-M, Phytohemagglutinin; PLT, primed lymphocyte test; TCM, tissue culture medium.

scribed (*6*). Irradiated autologous feeder cells were prepared from PBL from the recipient by Ficoll Hypaque gradient centrifugation and x-irradiation with 6000 rads as previously described (*7*).

Biopsy cultures were grown at 37°C in a humidified 5% CO_2 atmosphere. After 3–4 days, the culture supernatants were replenished with fresh TCM supplemented with 50% Il-2. The cultures were observed daily on an inverted stage microscope for cellular outgrowth. When growth ws observed, the contents of each well were transferred to another well on a 48-well culture plate (Costar 3548) and TCM supplemented with 50% Il-2 was added. Thereafter, the cultures were expanded with 50% IL2 until sufficient cells were obtained for functional studies.

PLT assay. The PLT activity of lymphocyte cultures grown from heart biopsies was measured in 3-day assays as previously described for alloreactive T cell clones (*7*). Prior to testing, the lymphocyte cultures had not received Il-2 for 3 days. In each PLT assay, 5×10^3 cells were incubated for 72 hr with 5×10^4 irradiated (2000 rads for PBL and spleen cells and 14000 rads for lymphoblastoid cell lines) stimulators in 96-well round-bottomed microplate wells. During the final 20 hr of incubation, each culture was labeled with 1 μCi of ^{3}H-thymidine (specific activity, 20 mCi/mmol, New England Nuclear Products). The cultures were harvested with a multiple sample harvester (Skatron, Inc.) and radioactivity was determined by liquid scintillation counting.

T cell phenotyping. Lymphocytes grown from heart biopsies were tested for T cell differentiation antigens. The tests were performed in the laboratory of Bruce S. Rabin M.D., Ph.D., (University of Pittsburgh). The monoclonal antibodies used were Leu 4 (pan/mature T cells), Leu 3a (helper T cells) and Leu 2a (suppressor/cytotoxic T cells); they were purchased from Becton Dickenson (Sunnyvale, CA). Cytocentrifuge smears for lymphocyte immunostaining were prepared and fixed in acetone immediately after preparation. The cytocentrifuge smears were stained using an avidin-biotin-peroxidase procedure as previously described (*8*). For each antibody, 2.5×10^4 cells were stained and 200–300 cells were analyzed per stain.

HLA phenotyping. Peripheral blood lymphocytes, donor spleen cells, and lymphoblastoid cell lines (LCL) were typed for HLA-A, B, C antigens by the standard NIH microlymphocytotoxicity technique. Serological typing for HLA-D region markers, HLA-DR, and DQ was done by the prolonged incubation microlymphocytotoxicity test using enriched B cell preparations made by carbonyl-iron treatment and by sedimentation following rosetting of PBL with neuraminidase-treated sheep erythrocytes. LCL were obtained from the human Genetic Mutant Cell Repository (Camden, NJ) or were generated in our laboratory by transforming PBL and spleen cells with Epstein-Barr virus (EBV) in the presence of cyclosporine according to previously described methodologies (*9, 10*).

RESULTS

Generation of lymphocyte cultures from heart biopsies. Lymphocyte cultures were generated from thirteen biopsies from four adult patients with heart transplants. Although each patient experienced one or more rejection episodes, all are currently alive 72–122 days posttransplant. From each patient three or four biopsies were obtained at different days during a posttransplant period of less than two months. These biopsies were grown in Il-2-containing medium supplemented with irradiated autologous PBL as feeder cells. After 6–8 days in culture it was possible to observe outgrowths of mononuclear cells from the biopsy tissue (Fig. 1). In many instances, distinct clusters of proliferating cells appeared at the periphery of these biopsies.

Secondary proliferation of cultured lymphocytes. The cultures were expanded by restimulation with Il-2 and transferred to additional wells until sufficient numbers of cells were obtained to conduct various assays. For these biopsies, the culture periods varied from 12 to 27 days (Table 1). Generally, a longer culture period was necessary to generate sufficient numbers of lymphocytes from biopsies obtained during the first week following transplantation.

Prior to PLT testing, the cells were cultured without exogenous Il-2 for 3 days. This was necessary to reduce the degree of background proliferation in the secondary stimulation assays. Table 1 shows the proliferative responses of biopsy-cultured lymphocytes to irradiated spleen cells from the transplant donor and to Il-2. Each patient had received a heart transplant from a donor with several HLA incompatibilities. In this article, each heart biopsy (HB) culture is referred to by a unique number that identifies the patient and the posttransplant period when the biopsy was obtained. For instance, HB 1.4 was obtained from patient 1 on day 4 posttransplant and HB 2.13 was obtained from patient 2 on day 13 posttransplant. The PLT responses of HB cells were measured in three-day assays. In many cases, the proliferation (expressed as cpm) was strong—and, in our experience, in the same range as that observed with cloned alloreactive lymphocytes generated from in vitro MLR cultures (*7*). However, cultured lymphocytes from one early biopsy, namely HB 1.4, did not exhibit PLT reactivity against the original donor cells. Also, HB 3.8 showed a weak PLT response. Each HB culture exhibited a proliferative response to Il-2 suggesting the presence of activated cells expressing Il-2 receptors. It may be seen in Table 1 that the magnitudes of PLT and Il-2 responses varied between the HB cultures. The variations seemed unrelated to the histological rejection grade observed in the transplant biopsies.

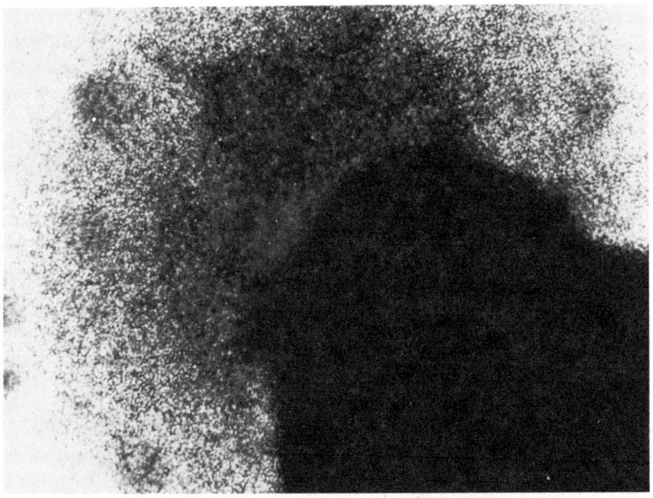

FIGURE 1. In vitro propagation of lymphocytes from a heart biopsy culture. This is a 400× magnification (moderately reduced) taken with an inverted stage microscope 8 days after expansion in tissue culture medium supplemented with IL-2. The dark area in the right corner is the heart biopsy tissue.

TABLE 1. Donor-specific PLT and exogenous Il-2 responses of lymphocyte cultures grown from heart transplant biopsies

HLA Phenotype			Heart biopsy	Histological rejection grade	Days in culture	Background (cpm±SD)	Donor-specific PLT activity (cpm±SD)	Exogenous Il-2 response (cpm±SD)
A	B	DR						
R: 2, –	44, 60	2, 5	1.4	0	27	275±40	315±110	2441±220
D: 2, –	35, 57	1, –	1.17	1	14	444±177	8586±788	5418±775
			1.43	2[a]	14	1399±316	46971±2276	28190±4020
			1.62	1	23	394±248	6966±179	3724±757
R: 3, 28	7, 18	2, 6						
D; 11, 23	44, 51	1, 4	2.13	3	14	298±329	183696±15351	24341±7878
			2.22	3[a]	18	234±137	8104±2701	21365±327
			2.29	1	13	94±22	11810±468	1211±3
R: 3, 26	7, 14	–, –	3.8	4	22	332±122	3231±2759	16197±46
D: 2, 11	8, 62	3, 4	3.14	0	20	113±3	37141±2052	8765±468
			3.22	1	12	876±704	14447±157	16548±234
R: 2, 3	27, 44	7, –	4.9	0	20	269±290	15679±4728	6740±704
D: 3, 26	14, 51	1, 5	4.25	1	13	965±907	33751±1621	12318±2071
			4.38	3	12	389±121	41958±668	11980±157

[a] Resolving.

Donor-specific HLA allospecificity of biopsy/cultured lymphocytes. For each HB lymphocyte culture, we determined the PLT responses against a small panel of unrelated stimulators selected to share HLA antigens with the original transplant donor. The results of these PLT assays are shown in Figures 2 through 5.

Patient 1. Four biopsies were cultured from patient 1 who had received a heart transplant from a donor who typed as A2, –; Bw35, w57; DR1, w6. The first biopsy (HB 1.4), obtained four days posttransplant, showed very minimal mononuclear cell aggregation in the endocardium and a rare pericapillary mononuclear aggregate. The histological pattern was interpreted as not being clinically significant rejection. Activated lymphocytes were generated from this biopsy and tested after 27 days in culture. No PLT activity was demonstrated for HB 1.4 cells against the original donor or to any stimulator from a selected panel of 6 unrelated donors (data not shown). The second biopsy (HB 1.17), obtained 17 days posttransplant, showed grade 1 rejection with minimal perivascular cellular infiltrates histologically. Lymphocytes grown from HB 1.17 exhibited PLT responses against 2 of 10 panel cells (Fig. 2). One stimulator shared Bw35 and DR1, and the other stimulator did not share any HLA antigens with the transplant donor. From these data it was not possible to determine the PLT specificity of HB 1.17 cells. A preliminary cell-mediated lympholysis assay showed significant cytolytic activity against 2 of 4 target cells; both were positive for Bw35 (data not shown).

Shortly thereafter, the patient received steroids (Solumedrol 1 gm/day for 5 days) and rabbit antithymocyte globulin (ATG) (5 cc/day for 3 days) as treatment of a rejection episode. A biopsy on day 43 showed some perivascular and endocardial cellular infiltrates consistent with resolving rejection. Lymphocytes grown from HB 1.43 showed strong PLT responses against 2 of 7 unrelated stimulators, both of which shared DR1 with the original transplant donor (Fig. 2). Two Bw35 panel cells induced very weak PLT responses of HB 1.43 cells. Nineteen days later biopsy HB 1.62 showed histologically normal endomyocardium with a few focal pericapillary infiltrates of small mononuclear cells. Lymphocytes grown from this biopsy exhibited a strong DR1-associated PLT reactivity. The results of these assays on HB cells from patient 1 demonstrate a

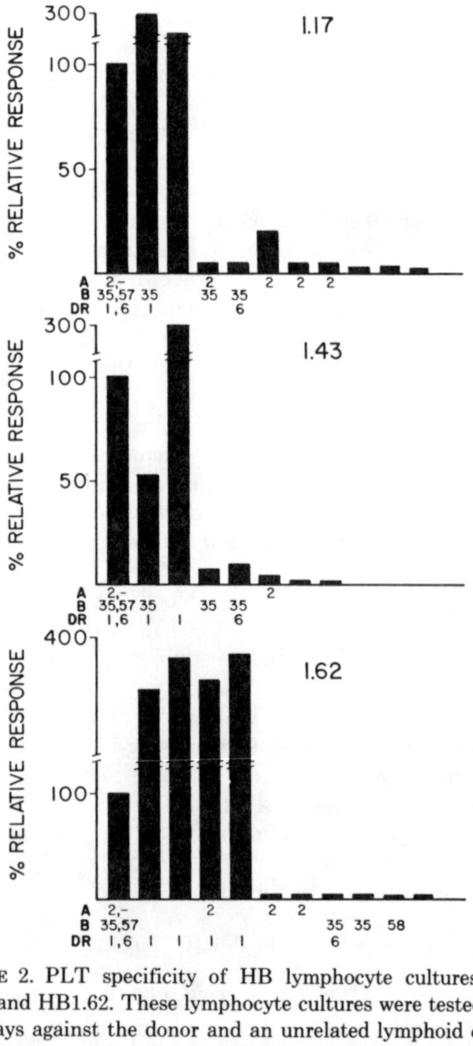

FIGURE 2. PLT specificity of HB lymphocyte cultures HB1.17, HB1.43, and HB1.62. These lymphocyte cultures were tested in 3-day PLT assays against the donor and an unrelated lymphoid cell panel. The HLA antigens shared with the donor are listed below each unrelated panel cell. Data are expressed as percentage of relative response to donor lymphocytes and calculated using the following formula:

$$\% \text{ RR} = \frac{\text{cpm unrelated cell}}{\text{cpm donor}} \times 100$$

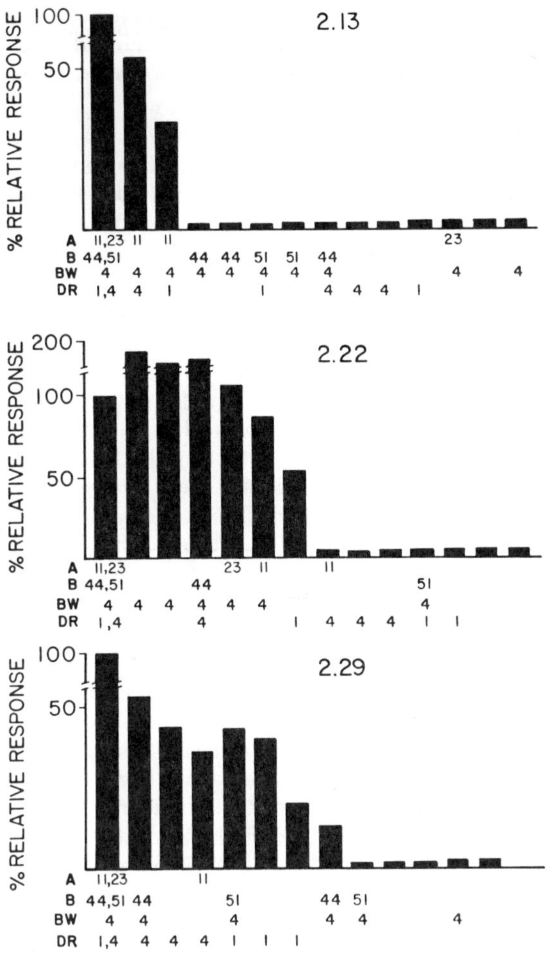

FIGURE 3. PLT specificity of HB lymphocytes HB2.13, HB2.22, and HB2.29. The data are expressed as percentage of relative response (see legend to Figure 2).

persistence of DR1-associated alloreactive T cells in three subsequent transplant biopsies.

Patient 2. Three biopsies were cultured from patient 2, who had received a transplant from a donor who typed as A11,23;B44,51;DR1,4. The first biopsy obtained 13 days posttransplant showed histological evidence of moderate rejection (grade 3). Lymphocytes grown from HB 2.13 showed strong PLT activity toward the donor and also 2 of 13 stimulators, both of which shared A11 with the transplant donor (Fig. 3). Eleven cells failed to induce a PLT response of HB 2.13, including several cells that shared one or more HLA antigens with the original donor. Since none of these cells typed for A11, it seems likely that the PLT specificity of HB 2.13 lymphocytes was associated with A11. These data also suggeted that no PLT specificity was demonstrable associated with B44, B51, DR1, and DR4 determinants found on the transplant donor. The rejection episode was treated with Solumedrol for 3 days and ATG for 3 days. A biopsy on day 22 showed a histological pattern consistent with resolving rejection. Cells grown from HB 2.22 showed PLT response to 6 of 13 panel cells (Fig. 3). Their PLT specificity appeared to be associated with Bw4 because 5 of 6 Bw4-positive cells induced strong stimulation, whereas 6 of 8 Bw4-negative cells did not stimulate. The Bw4 associated PLT specificity of HB 2.22 is concordant with the fact that the transplant donor was homozygous for Bw4, while the patient was homozygous for Bw6. The PLT results on HB 2.22 also demonstrated an absence of alloreactivity toward DR1 and DR4 antigens shared with the transplant donor.

A biopsy obtained 29 days posttransplant showed minimal focal cellular infiltrates (grade 1). Lymphocytes grown from HB 2.29 showed PLT reactivity with seven panel cells, six of which shared DR1 or DR4 with a transplant donor. None of the five panel cells which failed to induce a PLT response of HB 2.29 was positive for these DR antigens. These data suggested that the PLT specificity of HB 2.29 cells was primarily associated with DR1 and DR4. Another possibility is that HB 2.29 cells recognized the recently described MC1 determinant associated with DR1 and DR4 (*11*). With this cell panel it was

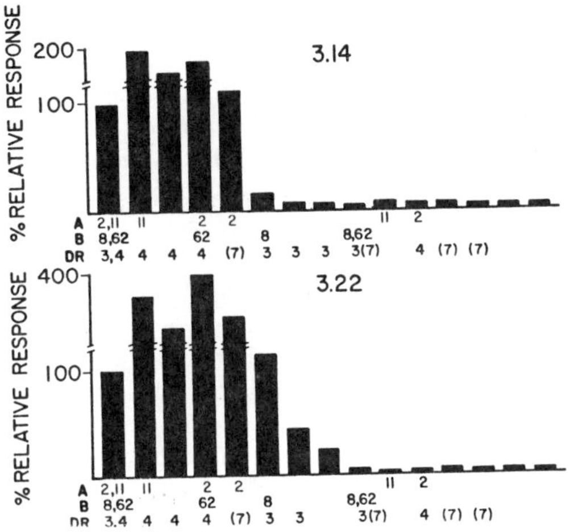

FIGURE 4. PLT specificity of HB lymphocyte cultures HB3.14 and HB3.22. The HLA-DR7 antigen listed in parentheses is crossreactive with donor HLA-DR4. The data are expressed as percentage of relative response (see legend to Figure 2).

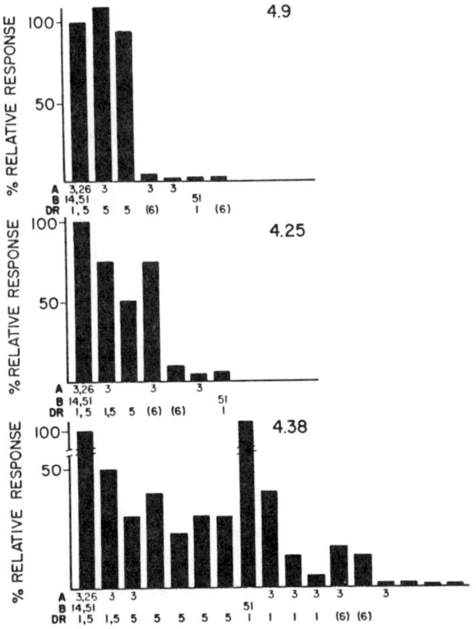

FIGURE 5. PLT specificity of HB lymphocyte cultures HB4.9, HB4.25, and HB4.38. HLA-DR6 antigen listed in parenthesis is crossreactive with donor HLA-DR5 (see legend to Figure 2).

not possible to demonstrate a significant association between the PLT specificity of HB 2.29 with Bw4.

These results in patient 2 suggested that the PLT specificity of cells grown from early biopsies was initially associated with class I antigens (A11, Bw4) and later switched to class II antigens—namely, DR1 and DR4.

Patient 3. Three biopsies were cultured from patient 3 who had received a heart transplant from an A2,11;B8,62;DR3,4 donor. The first biopsy obtained 8 days posttransplant showed histological signs of grade 4 rejection. Cells grown from this HB3.8 showed weak PLT activity against the original donor (Table 2) and 6 of 13 unrelated cells (data not shown). The specificity of the weak PLT reactions of HB 3.8 cells could not be defined. The rejection episode was treated with Solumedrol and ATG. A second biopsy on day 14 showed no or minimal mononuclear cell infiltrate and the endocardial myocardial and interstitial structures appeared normal. Cells grown from HB 3.14 showed strong PLT reactivity against the original donor plus three DR4 cells and one DR7 cell. This suggested that the PLT specificity of HB 3.14 might be toward DR4 or related to DRw53, which is associated with DR4 and DR7 (Fig. 4).

Another biopsy obtained eight days later was relatively normal and showed very minimal focal mononuclear cell infiltrate in the pericapillary area. Lymphocytes grown from HB 3.27 exhibited DR4 (or DRw53)-associated PLT specificity and additional reactivity toward DR3 cells.

These data on patient 3 showed that an early biopsy undergoing severe rejection generated activated T cells with weak PLT reactivity for which no specificity could be defined. After reversal of the rejection episode, lymphocytes from two subsequent biopsies showed PLT specificity associated with donor-specific class II HLA antigens. Both biopsies showed almost no evidence of rejection histologically.

Patient 4. Three biopsies were cultured from patient 4 who had received a transplant from an A3, 26; B14, 51; DR1, 5 donor. A biopsy on day 9 posttransplant showed no histological evidence of rejection. Cells grown from HB 4.9 exhibited PLT activity against the donor and 2 of 6 panel cells (Fig. 5). Both panel cells shared DR5 with the transplant donor. A biopsy on day 25 showed minimal focal infiltration of mononuclear cells in the interstitial pericapillary spaces. HB 4.25 cells showed PLT activity toward 3 of 6 unrelated cells, two of which were DR5, and one of which expressed the crossreacting DRw6 specificity (Fig. 5). A biopsy on day 38 posttransplant showed histological evidence of mild rejection, as indicated on several focal aggregates of mononuclear cells around blood vessels and subendothelial cellular infiltrates.

The PLT reactivity of HB 4.38 cells was associated with donor DR5 and DR1 antigens. The extra reactivity with DRw6 cells was probably due to crossreactivity between DRw6 and DR5. The findings on patient 4 showed that lymphocytes from biopsies had PLT specificity associated with DR5 of the transplant donor. The biopsy on day 38 posttransplant also contained DR1-associated PLT cells.

Relation of T cell phenotype and PLT specificity of cultured T lymphocytes to biopsy histology. Table 2 summarizes the PLT results of biopsy-grown lymphocytes in relation to donor-recipient HLA incompatibility, and their T cell phenotypes. It may be seen that the PLT specificity of cultured lymphocytes was always toward HLA antigens found on the transplant donor. This suggested that alloactivated T cells grown from these biopsies were donor-specific. For three patients, the PLT specificity of biopsy lymphocytes was associated with class II HLA antigens. Early biopsies from patient 2 grew activated T cells specific for class I HLA antigens, while a later biopsy produced class-II-specific PLT cells. Table 2 also shows that there was no evidence of a correlation between the Leu 2/Leu 3 cell composition and the PLT specificity toward class I or class II HLA antigens. Several reports have demonstrated that class-I-specific alloreactive T cells are primarily Leu 2 (or OKT8)-positive while class-II-specific alloreactive T cells express Leu 3 (or OKT4) (*12, 13*). In this group of patients, the two class-I-specific cells from HB 2.13 and HB 2.22 contained a mixture of Leu 2 and Leu-3-positive cells, whereas class II specific PLT reactivity was observed with other biopsy cells that were primarily Leu-2-positive (eg., HB 1.43, HB 4.38) or Leu-3-positive (eg., HB 1.17, HB 3.22). However, it should be noted that the biopsy-cultured cells may contain mixtures of activated cells and that the detected PLT specificity may be expressed by a small subset of T cells in such mixtures. Cloning procedures are necessary to further evaluate the relation between PLT specificity and T cell phenotype expression. Nevertheless, the reversal of Leu 3/Leu 2 cell composition from HB 1.17 to HB 1.43 is intriguing because both biopsy cultures showed the same DR1-associated specificity. This change in cell composition may be related to the immunosuppressive bolus of steroids and ATG used to treat a rejection episode during the period between these biopsies.

TABLE 2. Relation of T cell phenotype and PLT specificity of cultured lymphocytes to biopsy histology

HLA phenotype			HB	T cell phenotype			PLT specificity
A	B	DR		Leu4	Leu3	Leu2	
R: 2, –	44, 60	2, 5	1.4	98	93	4	No activity
D: 2, –	35, 57	1, –	1.17	96	80	15	DR1
			1.43	—	13	70	DR1
			1.62	—	—	—	DR1
R: 3, 23	7, 18	2, 6	2.13	—	37	49	A11
D: 11, 23	44, 51	1, 4	2.22	96	55	25	Bw4
			2.29	—	—	—	DR1, DR4
R: 3, 26	7, 14	–, –	3.8	98	10	77	Weak activity
D: 2, 11	8, 62	3, 4	3.14	—	—	—	DR4 (DRw53)
			3.22	95	89	1	DR4 (DRw53), DR3
R: 2. 3	27, 44	7, –	4.9	—	—	—	DR5
D: 3. 26	14, 51	1, 5	4.25	—	—	—	DR5 (+w6)
			4.38	97	6	93	DR5 (+w6), DR1

DISCUSSION

The results of this study demonstrate the feasibility of growing activated lymphocytes from endomyocardial biopsies from heart transplant patients. These cells were cultured directly from the heart biopsy in the presence of Il-2, which was necessary to induce proliferation of activated cells. As feeder cells we used irradiated autologous cells rather than donor cells to avoid de novo alloactivation of biopsy lymphocytes. Under these culture conditions it was possible to grow activated T lymphocytes that expressed T cell differentiation markers, exhibited Il-2 responsiveness, and—in most instances—showed PLT reactivity against donor lymphoid cells. Our studies also demonstrated that biopsy grown cells contained activated lymphocytes capable of responding to donor-specific HLA antigens. These findings are analogous to recent observations by Kurnick and coworkers, who propagated allospecific T lymphocytes from human renal allografts undergoing rejection (*14, 15*).

For each patient, we cultured cells from biopsies obtained on different days during the immediate posttransplant period of up to 6 weeks. These serial biopsy cultures provided an opportunity of studying the sequential appearance of different types of T cells infiltrating the transplant. Using this approach it was possible to study the types of cells involved during the early phases of allograft response even before any histological evidence of graft rejection. In several instances, it was possible to grow alloactivated T cells from heart biopsies that had been judged histologically to contain no mononuclear cellular infiltrates (e.g., HB 3.14 and HB 4.9).

Another advantage of studying cells from serial biopsies is that it is possible to learn about the types of cells mediating allograft responses during the early and late posttransplant periods. In this regard, most informative were the data on patient 2 from whom class-I-specific PLT cells were grown from early biopsies, whereas a later biopsy propagated class-II-specific PLT cells.

The recognition of PLT specificity of biopsy-grown lymphocytes toward HLA-A and HLA-B antigens further strengthens the concept that class I HLA antigens can directly stimulate alloactivated T cells. This concept, based on our previous observations (*16*) and confirmed by others (*17, 18*), is that certain alloreactive T cell clones generated from mixed leukocyte cultures have class I HLA-antigen-specific PLT reactivity that can be inhibited by class-I-specific monoclonal antibodies. Of special interest is the Bw4-associated specificity of HB 2.22 cells. Bw4 is a serologicaly defined public antigen encoded by HLA-B and belonging to the diallelic Bw4/Bw6 system (*19*). This antigen represents a distinct epitope (*20*) shared between a group of HLA-B molecules expressing private specificities, including B5, B13, B17, and B27 (*19*). Our data agree with the observations by Mayer et al. (*14*) that certain alloactivated T cells grown from rejecting allografts may recognize public HLA determinants.

Each patient in this study was on cyclosporine immunosuppression while rejection episodes were treated with an immunosuppressive bolus of prednisone (Solumedrol) and ATG. In spite of frequently high doses of immunosuppressive drugs, alloactivated T cells can frequently be grown from endomyocardial biopsies, even when such biopsies showed minimal cellular infiltrates.

These results demonstrate the feasibility of growing functionally active T cells from heart transplant biopsies. An analysis of the phenotypes and allospecificity, as well as a functional characterization of these cells, should generate useful information about the types of T cells involved in cardiac transplant rejection.

Acknowledgments. The authors thank Ms. Ellen Hamill, Ms. Loretta DiVechia, and Mr. David Bockstoce for excellent technical assistance. We also thank Ms. Kathy Hess and Ms. Laura Dillman for preparation of the manuscript.

REFERENCES

1. Weintraub D, Masek M, Billingham ME. The lymphocyte subpopulations in cyclosporine treated human heart rejection. Heart Transplant 1985; 4: 213.
2. Singh G, Rabin B, Griffith B, Thompson M, Nalesnik M, Hardesty R. Post-transplant monitoring in cardiac allografts. Transplant Proc 1983; 15: 1802.
3. Yacoub MH, Gracie JA, Rose ML, Cox J, Fraser AK, Chisolm PM. T-cell characterization in human cardiac allografts. Heart Transplantation 1983; 2: 259.
4. Hoshinaga K, Mohanakumar T, Goldman MH, Wilfgang TC, Szentpetery S, Lee HM, Lower RR. Characterization of mononuclear cell infiltrates in human cardiac allografts. Transplantation 1984; 38: 634.
5. Marboe CC, Schierman SW, Rose E, Reemtsma K, Fenoglio JJ Jr. Characterization of mononuclear cell infiltrates in human cardiac allografts. Transplant Proc 1984; 16: 1598.
6. Zeevi A, Chiu KM, Duquesnoy RJ. Functional differences between cells from MLR colonies grown in soft agar cultures. J Immunol 1980; 125: 1130.
7. Zeevi A, Scheffel C, Annen K, Bass G, Marrari M, Duquesnoy RJ. Association of the PLT specificity of alloreactive lymphocyte clones with HLA-DR, MB, and MT determinants. Immunogenetics 1982; 16: 209.
8. Paradis IL, Merrall EJ, Krell JM, Dauber HJ, Rogers MR, Rabin BS. Lymphocyte enumeration a comparison between modified avidin-biotin-immunoperoxidase system and flow cytometry. Histochem Cytochem 1984; 32: 358.
9. Thorley-Lawson DA, Chess L, Strominger JL. Suppression of in vitro Epstein-Barr virus infection. A new role for human T lymphocytes. J Exp Med 1977; 146: 495.
10. Zeevi A, Duquesnoy RJ. Specificity of alloactivated human T lymphocyte clones in secondary proliferation, cell-mediated lympholysis and interleukin-2 release. Immunogenetics 1985; 12: 17.
11. Duquesnoy RJ, Marrari M, Hackbarth S, Zeevi A. Serological and cellular definition of a new HLA-D determinant MC1, and its association with rheumatoid arthritis. Hum Immunol 1984; 10: 165.
12. Meuer SC, Schlossman SF, Reinherz EL. Clonal analysis of human cytotoxic T lymphocyte T4+ and T8+ effector T cells recognize products of different major histocompatibility complex region. Proc Natl Acad Sci USA 1982; 79: 4395.
13. Flomenberg N, Duffy E, Naito K. Two distinct phenotypes of HLA-DR specific cytotoxic T cell lines. Immunogenetics 1983; 17: 317.
14. Mayer TG, Lazarovits AI, Boyle LA, Sullivan ER, Leary CP, Fuller AA, Fuller TC, Bhan AK, Colvin RB, Collins AB, Kurnick JT. Functional allospecific T lymphocytes isolated from human renal allograft biopsies. Transplant Proc 1985; 17: 816.
15. Mayer TG, Fuller AA, Fuller TC, Lazarovits AI, Boyle LA, Kurnick JT. Characterization of in vivo activated allospecific T lymphocytes propagated from human renal allograft biopsies undergoing rejection. J Immunol 1985; 134: 258.

16. Zeevi A, Scheffel C, Annen K, Duquesnoy RJ. Primed lymphocyte testing specificity of alloreactive lymphocyte clones for HLA-B locus determinants. Proc Natl Acad Sci USA 1983; 80: 1440.
17. Reinsmoen N, Anichini A, Bach FH. Clonal analysis of T lymphocyte response to an isolated class I disparity. Hum Immunol 1983; 8: 195.
18. Flomenberg N, Russo C, Ferrone S, Dupont B. HLA class I-specific T lymphocyte clones with dual alloreactive functions. Immunogenetics 1984; 19: 39.
19. Schreuder I, D'Amaro J, Hackbarth S, Duquesnoy RJ. Histocompatibility testing 1980, UCLA tissue typing, Los Angeles, CA.
20. Ayres J, Cresswell, P. HLA-B specificities and w4, w6 specificities are on the same polypeptide. Eur J Immunol 1976; 6: 794.

Received 6 June 1985.
Accepted 12 September 1985.

0041-1337/86/4105-0626$02.00/0
TRANSPLANTATION
Vol. 41, No. 5

Printed in U.S.A.

INDUCTION OF TRANSPLANTATION TOLERANCE IN RATS BY SPLEEN ALLOGRAFTS

I. EVIDENCE THAT RATS TOLERANT OF SPLEEN ALLOGRAFTS CONTAIN TWO PHENOTYPICALLY DISTINCT T SUPPRESSOR CELLS[1]

WILLIAM R. DUNCAN,[2,3] STANISLAW M. STEPKOWSKI, AND HINRICH BITTER-SUERMANN

Laboratory of Transplantation Biology, Department of Surgery, Dalhousie University, Halifax, Nova Scotia, B3H 4H7, Canada

We have examined suppressor cell activity in transplantation tolerant (TT) rats bearing vascularized spleen allografts in several different donor-recipient combinations. More than 60% of WAG (RT-1^u) and 65% of AGUS (RT-1^l) spleen allografts were permanently accepted when transplanted to AGUS and PVG (RT-1^c) rats, respectively. All (WAG×AGUS)F$_1$ to AGUS and (AGUS×PVG)F$_1$ to PVG spleen allografts survived indefinitely. Unseparated LNC, TDL, and whole T cell or W3/25$^+$, OX8$^-$ T cell populations obtained from AGUS rats bearing (WAG×AGUS)F$_1$ spleens exhibited reduced mixed lymphocyte reaction (MLR) responses to the spleen donor, and to some extent to BN(RT1^n) third-party stimulators, but responded normally to PVG.A(RT1^a) stimulators. Coculture experiments demonstrated that lymph node cells (LNC) and thoracic duct lymphocytes (TDL) of TT rats contain RT1 specific suppressor cells. Furthermore, T cells isolated from all donor-recipient combinations contained two phenotypically distinct suppressor cell populations: a radiosensitive W3/25$^+$, OX8$^-$ (T$_{h/i}$) and a relatively radioresistant W3/25$^-$, OX8$^+$ (T$_{s/c}$). These Ts may be responsible for the maintenance of TT.

We have previously shown that the spontaneous acceptance of vascularized spleen allografts between RT-1 incompatible strains of rats (*1*) and guinea pigs incompatible at the class II region of the major histocompatibility complex (MHC)* (*2*) induces specific transplantation tolerance (TT). Recipients bearing long-term allografts subsequently accepted donor-type skin and pancreas grafts in rats (*3, 4*) and skin grafts in guinea pigs (*2*). The i.v. injection of spleen cells instead of transplantation of a spleen graft, did not induce TT (*3*).

In vitro experiments with LNC and TDL from tolerant rats (*5, 6*), and LNC from spleen-grafted tolerant guinea pigs (*7*) demonstrated reduced mixed lymphocyte reaction (MLR) responses to the spleen donor stimulators. MLR coculture experiments using lymph node cells (LNC) or thoracic duct lymphocytes (TDL) of tolerant rats (*5, 8*) and LNC of tolerant guinea pigs (*7*) indicated that the tolerant state might be due to the active involvement of suppressor cells.

In the present study, we utilized different spleen donor-recipient combinations to characterize the phenotype and genotype of the suppressor cells present in rats that spontaneously accepted fully allogeneic or F$_1$ spleen grafts. Our results demonstrate the presence of two phenotypically different Ts populations of host origin: a radiosensitive W3/25$^+$, OX8$^-$ T helper/inducer (T$_{h/i}$) and relatively radioresistant W3/25$^-$, OX8$^+$ T suppressor/cytotoxic (T$_{s/c}$).

MATERIALS AND METHODS

Animals. Inbred 6–8 week old WAG (RT-1^u), AGUS (RT-1^l), PVG (RT-1^c), PVG.A(RT1^a), (WAG×AGUS)F$_1$, and (AGUS×PVG)F$_1$ rats were obtained from OLAC (Bicester,

[1] This work was supported by grant MA-9108 from the Medical Research Council of Canada.

[2] W. R. Duncan is a Scholar of the Medical Research Council of Canada.

[3] Correspondence and reprint requests should be addressed to: William R. Duncan, Ph.D., Department of Surgery, Laboratory of Transplantation Biology, Dalhousie University, CRC Building, Halifax, Nova Scotia, B3H 4H7, Canada.

* Abbreviations used: BSS, balanced salt solution; C, complement; FCS, fetal calf serum; GVH, graft-vs-host; GVHD, graft-versus-host disease; Ig, immunoglobulin; MHC, major histocompatibility complex; MLR, mixed lymphocyte reaction; LNC, lymph node cells; TDL, thoracic duct lymphocytes; T$_{h/i}$, T helper/inducer; T$_{s/c}$, T suppressor/cytotoxic; TT, transplantation tolerance.

Oxfordshire, England). BN (RT-1^n) rats were purchased from Harlan Sprague-Dawley, Walkersville, MD.

Spleen grafting and thoracic duct cannulation. The techniques of splenic transplantation and thoracic duct cannulation have been described (*9, 10*).

Preparation of responder and stimulator cells for MLR studies. Responder cell populations were prepared by gently teasing biopsied mesenteric, cervical, and axillary lymph nodes and recipient spleens. Erythrocytes were removed by treatment with Tris-buffered ammonium chloride. Stimulator cells were obtained from the thymus of appropriate strains and irradiated with 2000 rads (^{60}Co source, Atomic Energy of Canada, at a rate of 100 rads/min). All populations of cells were suspended in medium consisting of balanced salt solution (BSS) supplemented with 1% fetal calf serum (FCS).

Separation of T cell populations on Degalan bead columns. To isolate the Ig^- (T cell) population, single-cell suspensions of LNC and recipient spleen cells from TT or normal rats were passed over rabbit anti-rat IgG (heavy and light-chain specific, Cappel Laboratories Cochranville, PA) coated Degalan bead (V26 polymethylmethacrylate beads, Degussa Corporation, Teterboro, NJ) columns, as described by Duarte et al. (*11*). The outflow rate was adjusted to approximately 0.7 ml/min and the Ig^- population was collected by flushing 30 ml medium through the column. The effluent cells (≥95% Ig^- T cells) were tested in vitro or coated with mouse antirat W3/25 or MRC OX8 monoclonal antibodies (Cedar Lane labs, Hornby, Ontario, Canada). After incubation for 1 hr, lymphocytes were further fractionated on goat antimouse IgG (heavy and light-chain specific, Cappel Laboratories Inc., Cochranville, PA) coated Degalan bead columns into two phenotypically distinct populations: $T_{h/i}$ W3/25^+, $OX8^-$ and $T_{s/c}$ W3/25^-, $OX8^+$ populations. Purity of separated populations was enumerated by immunofluorescent microscopy.

Briefly, the effluent cells from the rabbit antirat IgG columns were stained with fluoresceinated rabbit antirat IgG (heavy and light-chain specific, Cappell Laboratories, Cochranville, PA) to determine the percentage of Ig^+ cells. In all experiments, ≤5% Ig^+ cells were detected.

The effluent cells from the goat antimouse IgG columns were mixed with the monoclonal antibodies W3/25 and MRC OX8. Following 30 min incubation at 4°C, the cells were washed and stained with fluoresceinated goat antimouse IgG (heavy and light-chain sp., Microbiological Associates, Bethesda, MD). In all experiments when Ig^- (T cells) were coated with W3/25 and passed over goat antimouse IgG columns, the effluent cells contained ≤5% W3/25^+ cells and ≥95% $OX8^+$ cells. In all experiments, when Ig^- (T cells) were coated with MRC OX8 and passed over goat antimouse IgG columns, the effluent cells contained ≤5% MRC $OX8^+$ cells and ≥95% W3/25^+ cells.

Mixed lymphocyte reaction (MLR). LNC, TDL, or purified T cells, W3/25^+, and $OX8^+$ T cells obtained from tolerant or syngeneic normal control rats were used as responders. Stimulator cells were prepared from the thymus of appropriate strains and were irradiated with 2000 rads. All cell populations were suspended in complete medium consisting of RPMI 1640, supplemented with 25 mmol/L HEPES, 2 mmol/L glutamine, 100 μg/ml gentamycin, 5% rat serum, and 1% FCS. Triplicate cultures of 2×10^5 responders and 4×10^5 stimulators were set up in round-bottomed microtiter plates in a volume of 200 μl and incubated for 4 or 5 days at 37°C in a humidified atmosphere containing 5% CO_2. During the last 18 hr of culture, each well was pulsed with 1 μCi tritiated thymidine (^{3}H-TdR, 6.7 Ci/mM, sp. act., New England Nuclear, Boston, MA) and later harvested onto glass fiber filter discs. The results of triplicate cultures are expressed as total cpm per culture. The SEM of triplicate samples was never ≥10% of the mean, and for simplicity, only the mean of triplicate samples is reported.

In some experiments, Δ cpm was calculated as follows: Δ cpm = (cpm responder + irradiated stimulator) − (cpm responder + irradiated responder)

MLR coculture experiments. Populations of purified T cells isolated from normal AGUS or PVG rats or normal AGUS TDL were used as responders. LNC, TDL, or purified populations of whole T cells, W3/25^+, and $OX8^+$ T cells isolated from tolerant or normal control rats were tested for their ability to suppress syngeneic normal T-responders in the MLR. For some experiments cocultured populations were irradiated with 1500 rads. In coculture, tolerant and normal cells were mixed in a ratio of 1:1 with syngeneic responders in the presence of appropriate stimulators in a volume of 250 μL. In some experiments we utilized 1:1, 1:2, 1:4, and 1:8 ratios of cocultured cells to responders. Suppression of the MLR was calculated in the following fashion: % suppression = 1 − (cpm with cocultured cells from tolerant rats ÷ cpm with cocultured cells from normal rats) × 100.

Antibody depletion of lymphocytes. Complement-mediated depletion of lymphocytes was performed according to the method of Klein et al. (*12*). Briefly, 15×10^6 cells were incubated with 200 μL alloantiserum for 30 min at 4°C. After two washes the cells were incubated for 30 min at 37°C with baby rabbit complement (C) (1/10) (Pel Freeze, Rogers, Arkansas), and then washed twice with medium, recounted, and then tested.

RESULTS

MLR responses of AGUS rats tolerant of WAG spleen grafts. More than 60% of AGUS rats accepted WAG spleen allografts without any signs of graft-versus-host disease (GVHD). Some animals developed clinical signs of GVHD and eventually died within 3 weeks after transplantation. For the in vitro experiments, we utilized animals that had well-preserved spleen allografts and were at least 8 weeks posttransplantation. LNC from tolerant AGUS rats demonstrated reduced MLR responses to donor-type stimulators (Fig. 1B). Similarly, TDL collected from tolerant AGUS recipients overnight and tested in MLR exhibited diminished proliferative responses to donor antigen (Fig. 1A) that frequently approached 90%. However, half the tested animals also had reduced responses to BN stimulators. Unseparated T cells and the W3/25^+, $OX8^-$ T cell population isolated from AGUS recipients exhibited reduced MLR responses to WAG and moderately reduced responses to BN stimulators (Fig. 1C, 3A). These results indicate that AGUS rats that accepted WAG spleen grafts have an altered T cell alloreactivity, primarly to donor-type RT-1^u antigens.

MLR responses of PVG rats tolerant of AGUS spleen grafts. In this strain combination 65% of AGUS spleen allografts were accepted and the remainder were rejected. LNC from PVG recipients displayed distinctly reduced proliferative responses to donor stimulators (Fig. 2A). Purified T cells and W3/25^+, $OX8^-$ T cells fractionated from tolerant PVG rats were nonresponsive to spleen donor-type stimulators (Figs. 2B, 3B). Reduction of the T cell MLR response was, in most cases, RT-1^l alloantigen-specific, suggesting the presence of a specific immunoregulatory mechanism.

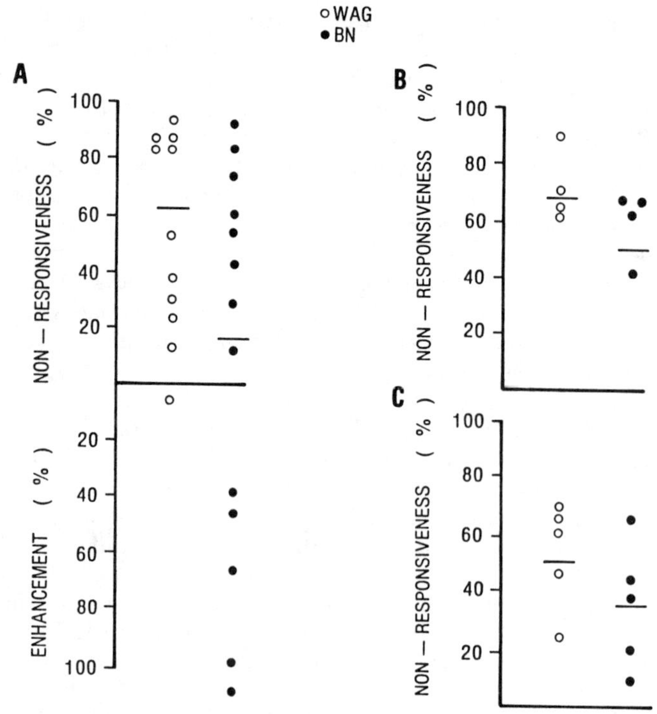

FIGURE 1. MLR responses of TDL(A), LNC(B) and purified T cells(C) isolated from AGUS rats bearing WAG spleens. Each point represents the MLR response of tolerant rats to WAG (o) or BN (●) stimulators in comparison with normal controls studied on the same day. Each bar represents the mean percentage of nonresponsiveness. The percentage of nonresponsiveness represents the decreased proliferative response of tolerant rats in comparison with normal syngeneic controls. The percentage of enhancement represents the increased proliferative response of tolerant rats in comparison with normal syngeneic controls. Percentage of nonresponsiveness (% enhancement) =

$$1 - \frac{\text{cpm tolerant spleen grafted rat}}{\text{cpm normal control rat}} \times 100$$

2×10^5 responder cells were cultured with 4×10^5 irradiated (2000 rads) WAG, AGUS, or BN stimulators. Control values (cpm responder + cpm irradiated syngeneic stimulators) varied from 800 to 5000 cpm and never exceeded 5% of alloresponse.

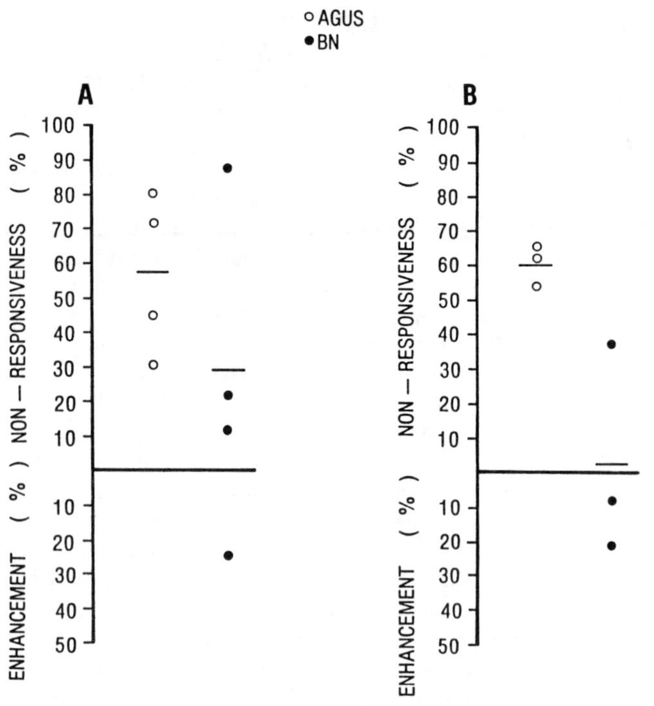

FIGURE 2. MLR responses of LNC(A) or purified T cells(B) isolated from PVG rats bearing AGUS spleens. Each point represents the MLR response of tolerant rats to AGUS (o) or BN (●) stimulators in comparison with normal controls studied on the same day. Each bar represents the mean percentage of nonresponsiveness (% enhancement) as calculated in Figure 1.

MLR responses of AGUS rats tolerant of (WAG×AGUS)F$_1$ spleen grafts. Since it is possible that the altered T cell reactivity, following the transplantation of allogeneic spleens, could be due to an ongoing chronic graft-vs-host (GVH) reaction, we examined the T cell responses of AGUS recipients of (WAG×AGUS)F$_1$ spleen grafts, in which no classic GVH reaction could ensue.

T cell populations obtained from AGUS recipient spleens and lymph nodes, (Fig. 3C), had reduced MLR responses to both donor (mean 72.5%) and BN (mean 69.5%) stimulators. W3/25$^+$, OX8$^-$ T$_{h/i}$ populations had reduced responses to donor (mean 66.6%) and slightly reduced responses to BN stimulators (mean 26.6%).

Therefore, AGUS recipients bearing F$_1$ spleen grafts similar to those bearing WAG spleen grafts also exhibit reduced MLR responsiveness, indicating that chronic GVH reaction alone, cannot account for reduced T cell reactivity.

Presence of W3/25$^-$ OX8$^+$ Ts in AGUS rats tolerant of WAG spleen grafts. In order to further evaluate the reduced anti-WAG MLR responses, MLR coculture experiments were performed. Tolerant TDL, irradiated with 1500 rads, suppressed the normal TDL response to WAG stimulators (Fig. 4A), but half the tested animals also suppressed the response to BN stimulators. Unseparated LNC from tolerant AGUS rats specifically suppressed the normal MLR response (27%) (Fig. 4B). Purified tolerant AGUS T cells also specifically suppressed (21%) normal T cell proliferation. Furthermore, the tolerant W3/25$^-$, OX8$^+$ T$_{s/c}$ population suppressed the normal MLR response to donor and BN stimulators (Fig. 5). In contrast, the irradiated tolerant W3/25$^+$, OX8$^-$ T$_{h/i}$ population enhanced normal T cell MLR responses by 45% to WAG but not to BN stimulators. These results clearly indicate that tolerant AGUS rats contain radioresistant W3/25$^-$, OX8$^+$ Ts and also radioresistant W3/25$^+$, OX8$^-$ T helper cells (Th), which in contrast to the former are able to enhance the MLR proliferative response.

Presence of two Ts populations in AGUS recipients of (WAG×AGUS)F$_1$ spleen grafts. T cells isolated from tolerant AGUS recipients bearing F$_1$ spleen grafts demonstrated reduced alloreactivity in MLR to donor (WAG) as well as BN antigens. The unseparated T cell population and the separated W3/25$^-$, OX8$^+$ T cell subpopulation markedly suppressed the normal MLR response (Fig. 6) and this suppressive activity was not radiosensitive. When the irradiated W3/25$^+$, OX8$^-$ T cell subpopulation was tested, no suppression was detectable (Fig. 6), while nonirradiated W3/25$^+$, OX8$^-$ T cells exhibited potent suppressor activity to WAG (61.2%) and BN (29.6%) stimulators (Fig. 7). Similar results (data not shown) were also obtained using nonirradiated W3/25$^+$, OX8$^-$ T cells isolated from AGUS recipients of WAG, as well as PVG recipients of AGUS spleen

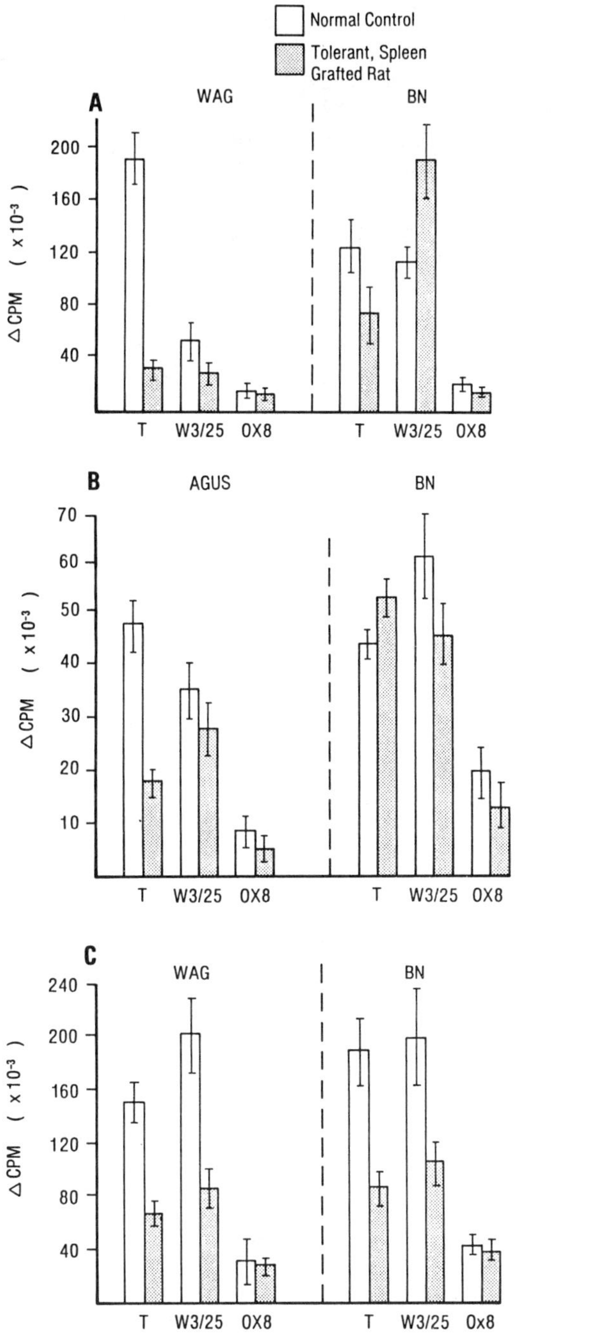

FIGURE 3. MLR responses of T, W3/25$^+$, OX8$^-$ T, and W3/25$^-$, OX8$^+$ T cell populations isolated from an AGUS rat tolerant of WAG spleen (A), a PVG rat tolerant of AGUS spleen (B), and an AGUS rat tolerant of (WAG×AGUS)F_1 spleen(C). Each bar represents the Δ cpm ± SEM. Δ cpm was calculated as follows; (cpm responder + irradiated stimulator) − (cpm responder + irradiated responder); control values (cpm responder + irradiated responder) varied from 2000 to 10000 cpm and never exceeded 5% of alloresponse (cpm responder + irradiated responder).

grafts. These data indicate that AGUS rats bearing F_1 spleens, contain at least two distinct Ts populations, one requiring cell division and with the surface phenotype W3/25$^+$, OX8$^-$ $T_{h/i}$ and the other being relatively radioresistant, W3/25$^-$ OX8$^+$, $T_{s/c}$.

Specificity of Ts in AGUS rats tolerant of (WAG×AGUS)F_1 spleen grafts. To further examine the specificity of altered T cell reactivity, AGUS rats bearing long-term (WAG×AGUS)F_1 spleen grafts were tested in MLR and coculture studies against WAG, BN, PVG, and PVG.A stimulators. As seen in Table 1, tolerant T cells exhibited reduced reactivity to WAG, as well as BN, stimulators, but responded normally to PVG and PVG.A stimulators. In coculture experiments, tolerant T cells suppressed normal T cell responses to both WAG and BN, but failed to inhibit the response to PVG or PVG.A. These results clearly indicate that spleen-graft-induced Ts cells are alloantigen-specific but may also recognize some determinants shared between the WAG and BN strains.

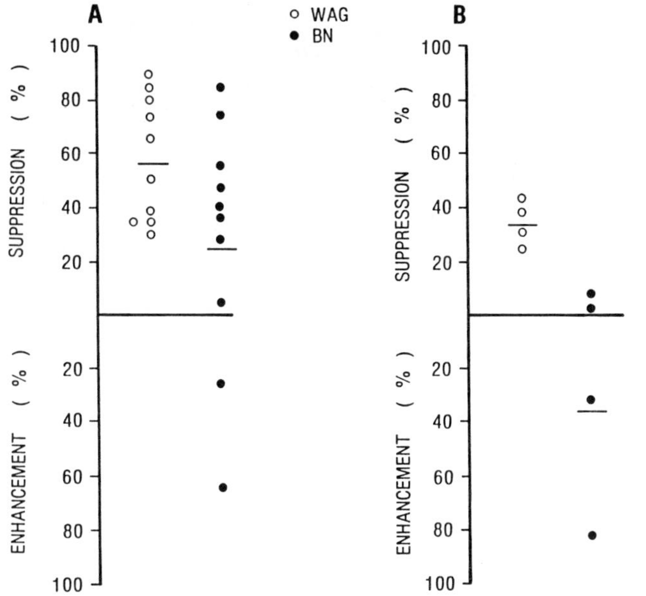

FIGURE 4. Presence of radioresistant TDL(A) and LNC(B) suppressor cells isolated in AGUS rats tolerant of WAG spleens. Each point represents the suppression or enhancement of the normal MLR response by irradiated tolerant cells to WAG (o) or BN (●) stimulators as compared with normal cocultures studied on the same day; 2×10^5 responder cells were cocultured with irradiated (1500 rads) 2×10^5 normal or tolerant cells and irradiated (2000 rads) 4×10^5 allogeneic, syngeneic, or third-party stimulators. Control values (responder + irradiated syngeneic stimulators) never exceeded 5% of alloresponsiveness. The percentage of suppression represents the decreased proliferative response of normal T cells when cocultured with tolerant T cells. The percentage of enhancement represents the increased proliferative response of normal T cells when cocultured with tolerant T cells. Each bar represents the mean percentage of suppression or enhancement. Percentage of suppression (enhancement) =

$$1 - \frac{\text{cpm coculture with tolerant cells}}{\text{cpm coculture with normal control cells}} \times 100$$

Genotype of Ts present in AGUS recipients of (WAG×AGUS)F_1 spleen grafts. The results of antibody depletion experiments are presented in Table 2. C-treated tolerant T cells suppressed the AGUS MLR response to WAG (56.5%)—and, to some extent, to BN stimulators (33%). Anti-WAG-plus-C-treated tolerant T cells similarly suppressed the normal AGUS proliferative response to WAG (62.4%), indicating that the Ts are of host origin.

DISCUSSION

Vascularized spleen allografts were spontaneously accepted when transplanted among several different strains of rats and

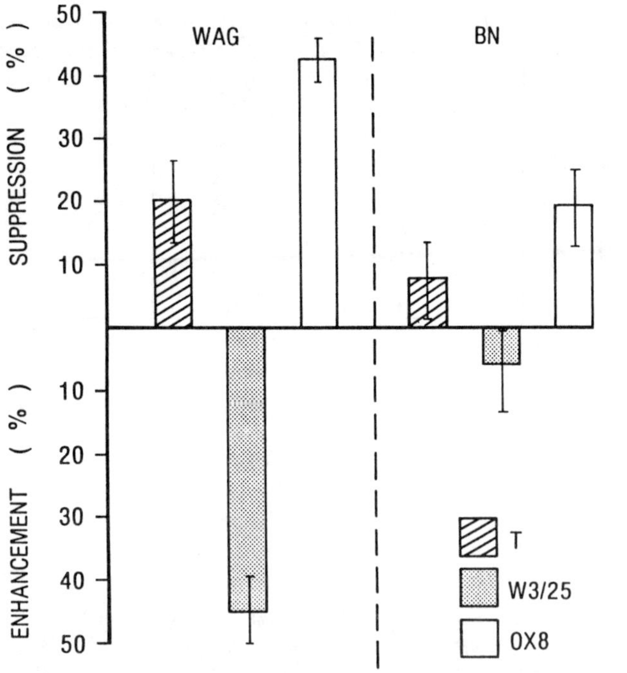

FIGURE 5. Presence of radioresistant W3/25$^+$, OX8$^-$ Th and W3/25$^-$, OX8$^+$ Ts in AGUS rats tolerant of WAG spleens; 2×10^5 normal AGUS responders were cocultured with 2×10^5 irradiated (1500 rads) tolerant or normal T, W3/25$^+$, OX8$^-$ T, or W3/25$^-$, OX8$^+$ T cell populations in response to 4×10^5 irradiated (2000 rads) WAG, AGUS, or BN stimulators. Control values (AGUS stimulators) never exceeded 5% of alloresponse. Each bar represents the mean ± SEM from four experiments. The percentage suppression or percentage of enhancement was calculated as indicated in Figure 4.

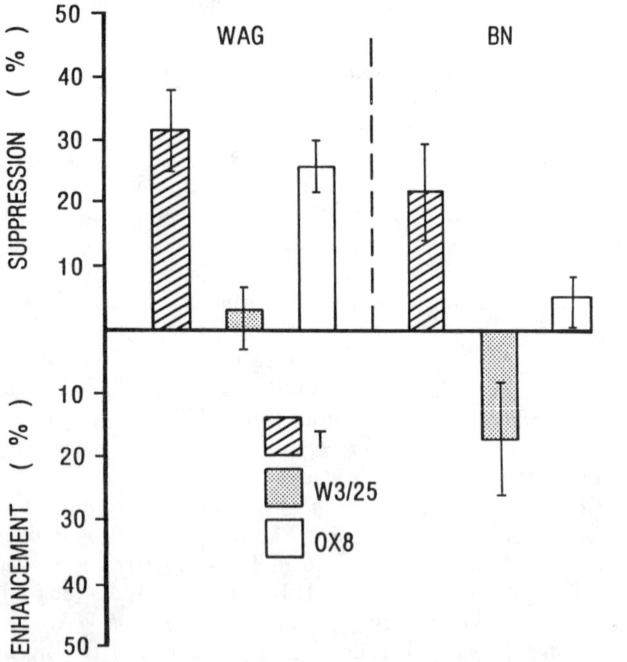

FIGURE 6. Presence of radioresistant W3/25$^-$, OX8$^+$ Ts in AGUS rats tolerant of (WAG×AGUS)F$_1$ spleens; 2×10^5 normal AGUS T responders were cocultured with 2×10^5 irradiated (1500 rads) tolerant or normal T, W3/25$^+$, OX8$^-$ T, or W3/25$^-$, OX8$^+$ T cell populations in response to 4×10^5 irradiated (2000 rads) WAG, AGUS, or BN stimulators. Each bar represents the mean ± SEM from four experiments. The percentage of suppression or percentage of enhancement was calculated as indicated in Figure 4.

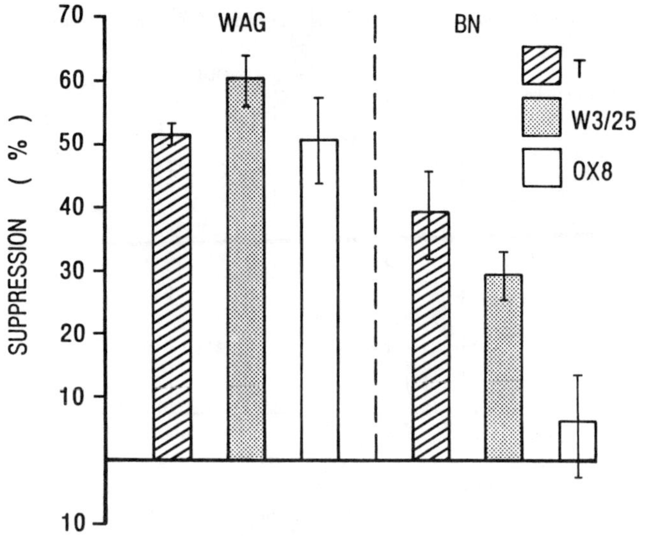

FIGURE 7. Presence of two Ts populations in AGUS rats tolerant of (WAG×AGUS)F$_1$ spleens; 2×10^5 AGUS T responders were cocultured with 2×10^5 nonirradiated tolerant or normal T, W3/25$^+$, OX8$^-$ T or W3/25$^-$, OX8$^+$ T cell populations in response to 4×10^5 irradiated (2000 rads) WAG, AGUS, or BN stimulators. Each bar represents the mean ± SEM from four experiments. Control values (AGUS-T responders + irradiated AGUS stimulators) never exceeded 5% of experimental values (AGUS-T responders + irradiated WAG or BN stimulators). Percentage suppression was calculated as indicated in Figure 4.

TABLE 1. Specificity of nonresponsiveness and suppression of tolerant AGUS rats bearing F$_1$ (WAG×AGUS) spleens

A. AGUS Tol (WAG×AGUS) F$_1$ responder[a]: % Nonresponsiveness			
WAG	BN	PVG	PVG.A
54.8±6.3	46.7±3.3	12.2±5	5.9±1.7
B. N-AGUS T & AGUS Tol F$_1$ responder[b]: % Suppression			
WAG	BN	PVG	PVG.A
49.1±5.8	47.8±0.7	17.3±8.1	6.1±3.2

[a] Nonresponsiveness represents the response of tolerant AGUS-T in comparison with normal AGUS-T studied on the same day. 2×10^5 tolerant or normal AGUS-T were cultured with 4×10^5 irradiated WAG(RT-1^u), BN(RT-1^n), PVG(RT-1^c) and PVG.A(RT-1^a) stimulators; % nonresponsiveness = 1 − (cpm tolerant AGUS-T/cpm normal AGUS-T) × 100.

[b] Suppression of 2×10^5 normal AGUS-T cells by 2×10^5 tolerant or normal AGUS-T cells in response to 4×10^4 irradiated WAG, BN, PVG, or PVG.A stimulators, % suppression = 1 − (cpm cocultured cells from tolerant rats/cpm cocultured cells from normal rats) × 100. Control values (responders + irradiated syngeneic AGUS stimulator) varied from 2000 to 8000 and never exceeded 5% of alloresponse. Each number represents the means ± SEM from three experiments.

induced alloantigen-specific transplantation tolerance (*1, 3*). The studies reported here demonstrate that rats bearing long-term allogeneic or semiallogeneic spleen grafts exhibited reduced T cell proliferative responses to donor alloantigens. At the same time, the acceptance of RT1-disparate spleen grafts, in all strain combinations studied, correlated with the presence of two phenotypically distinct populations of Ts, a radiosensitive W3/25$^+$, OX8$^-$ and a relatively radioresistant W3/25$^-$, OX8$^+$ population.

Both allogeneic and F$_1$ spleen grafts induced suppressor cells, although F$_1$ spleens appeared to be more efficient. In the two strain combinations studied, (AGUS → PVG and WAG →

TABLE 2. Presence of host Ts in tolerant AGUS rats bearing F_1 (WAG×AGUS) spleens[a]

Responder cells	Coculture cells	Antiserum treatment	Stimulators (cpm)	
			WAG	BN
AGUS-T[b]	AGUS-T	—	142627	115800
AGUS-T	563-T[c]	—	62145 (56.5)[d]	77679 (33)
AGUS-T	AGUS-T	C	156188	95015
AGUS-T	563-T	C	67668 (56.7)	108005 (−13)
AGUS-T	AGUS-T	Anti-WAG + C[e]	135540	98010
AGUS-T	563-T	Anti-WAG + C[f]	51042 (62.4)	97868 (0)

[a] These data are representative of four independent experiments. Control values (AGUS stimulators) varied but never exceeded 5% of alloresponse.

[b] Isolated from normal AGUS rats; 2×10^5 normal AGUS responder cells were cocultured with 2×10^5 normal or tolerant T cells before or after treatment with anti-WAG serum and C.

[c] Isolated from an AGUS recipient bearing a (WAG×AGUS)F_1 spleen graft.

[d] Percentage of suppression.

[e] Treatment with anti AGUS+C killed 100% of cells; treatment with anti-WAG+C killed 12% of cells.

[f] Treatment with anti AGUS+C killed 97% of cells; treatment with anti-WAG+C killed 20% of cells.

AGUS) approximately 60–70% of the recipients accepted spleen allografts permanently, but some of the recipients apparently developed acute GVHD and eventually died two to three weeks posttransplantation. Recipients surviving beyond three weeks continued to gain weight and displayed no signs of GVH reaction or increased susceptibility to infection. This suggests that in the allogeneic combination, there is a delicate balance between GVH responses and host-vs-graft responses resulting in acceptance of the allograft or development of acute GVHD. In contrast, practically 100% of F_1 spleens survived when transplanted in the two combinations studied, (WAG×AGUS)$F_1 \rightarrow$ AGUS and (AGUS×PVG)$F_1 \rightarrow$ PVG, and no F_1 spleen graft recipients developed clinical signs of GVH reaction, as would be expected. These data clearly suggest that F_1 spleens induce potent immunosuppression that prevents rejection of the spleen. Since both allogeneic and F_1 spleens induce Ts cells, it is unlikely that GVH alone is the sole mechanism responsible for the observed alteration in T cell reactivity. However it is possible that acute or chronic GVH responses could play a role in the induction of Ts following allogeneic spleen transplantation.

The observation that spleen allografts induce acute GVHD in normal, nonimmunosuppressed recipients suggests that some form of immunoregulation develops. It is likely that, in response to the splenic allograft, the host antidonor immune response is suppressed, allowing donor T cells, present in the graft, to mount a lethal GVH response. Similarly, Shevach et al. have reported that strain 13 spleen grafts induce lethal GVHD in strain 2 recipients, indicating that in guinea pigs, as well as in rats, spleen allografts may induce immunosuppression resulting in the development of GVHD in normal adult hosts (*7*). In contrast, transplantation of irradiated spleens or other allogeneic tissues— i.e., heart or skin—fails to induce GVHD or TT ([*1*] and unpublished results), suggesting that the lymphoid nature of the splenic graft is crucial for the induction of immunosuppression, resulting in GVHD or TT.

Analysis of the cells responsible for suppression of MLRs revealed that Ts could be isolated from AGUS rats bearing allogeneic (WAG) spleen grafts, and that two distinct populations were present. The Ig^-, whole T cell population, and the W3/25$^+$, OX8$^-$ (nonirradiated) population strongly suppressed the normal MLR response to donor alloantigens as well as BN stimulators, however the W3/25$^-$, OX8$^+$ Ts population primarily suppressed the donor response and only minimally altered the response to BN. These results indicate either that the suppressor cells present in the whole T cell population, as well as the W3/25$^+$, OX8$^-$ population, are antigen-nonspecific or that they may recognize alloantigenic determinants shared between the WAG and BN strains. In other experimental models in which chronic or acute GVHD occur, suppressor T cells can be identified that are alloantigen-nonspecific (*13–15*)—and it is possible, even though no clinical signs of chronic GVHD exist, that Ts present in animals bearing long-term allogeneic spleens are similar to the Ts present in hosts undergoing chronic GVHD.

Evidence against the argument that the GVH reaction is required for the induction of TT and Ts generation was obtained by analyzing AGUS rats bearing long-term (WAG×AGUS)F_1 spleen grafts. The Ig^- and W3/25$^+$, OX8$^-$ (nonirradiated) populations suppressed MLR responses to both WAG and BN stimulators, but the W3/25$^-$, OX8$^+$ populations specifically suppressed the response to WAG. Therefore the suppression of the response to BN (RT1^n) stimulators most likely represents the recognition of determinants shared between WAG and BN by a subpopulation of T suppressor cells. At the same time, these data suggest that the W3/25$^+$, OX8$^-$ and W3/25$^-$, OX8$^+$ Ts cells may recognize different MHC determinants. Further evidence that a subpopulation of Ts may recognize determinants shared between WAG and BN was obtained by analyzing the response of AGUS rats bearing F_1 spleens to stimulators expressing different RT1 haplotypes. Both in the MLR and suppressor assays, the Ts could recognize determinants expressed by both the RT1^u and RT1^n haplotypes, but failed to recognize determinants expressed by the RT1^c or RT1^a haplotypes. In an elegant study, Wettstein (*16*) has shown that RT1^u and RT1^n haplotypes do share class II determinants that could be recognized by RT1^l (AGUS) responders. Since the majority of the crossreactivity in our model was seen when class-II-reactive W3/25$^+$ T cells were present, it is quite possible that class II antigens may induce W3/25$^+$ T suppressor-effector or suppressor-inducer cells.

A number of different mechanisms have been proposed to explain the induction and maintenance of TT: clonal deletion of antigen reactive cells (*17, 18*), antigen-specific suppressor cell activity (*19, 20*), or blocking alloantibodies of undefined or antiidiotypic specificity (*21, 22*). In our model of spleen-graft-induced TT we have demonstrated that Ts are present in long-term, tolerant recipients. In addition, the sera of AGUS rats bearing WAG or (WAG×AGUS)F_1 spleen grafts do not contain cytotoxic antibodies ([*5*] and Duncan et al., unpublished observations), however they may contain blocking or antiidiotypic antibodies, and we are currently analyzing tolerant sera for such activity. Evidence that the Ts activity detected in vitro plays a role in vivo in the maintenance of the tolerant state was obtained utilizing adoptive transfer studies. Previously, we have demonstrated that LNC, TDL, and spleen cells from AGUS rats bearing viable WAG spleens specifically prolonged the survival of WAG hearts when transferred to normal, nonirradiated AGUS recipients (*23*). Further, T cells isolated from

F_1 spleen-grafted AGUS rats, when transferred to irradiated syngeneic recipients, indefinitely prolonged the survival of WAG but not PVG.A heart allografts (Duncan et al., manuscript in preparation). These results substantiate the role of Ts in maintaining the tolerant state, however it is possible that antibodies (i.e., antiidiotypic) may be involved in the induction as well as maintenance phase of spleen graft induced TT.

It is interesting to note that clonal deletion of donor alloantigen-specific T cells does not occur in this model of TT, in which the MLR response to donor alloantigens was reduced only 50–80% in tolerant animals. However in mice rendered tolerant by neonatal injection of F_1 bone marrow cells, no detectable MLR response to donor alloantigens could be detected (*24*). In the neonatal tolerance model there is also ample evidence for some form of clonal deletion that may involve either prethymic or postthymic Ts cells (*19, 25*). Interestingly, in the neonatal TT model, it is difficult to detect Ts in vitro (*24*), and this method of inducing tolerance most likely resembles the induction of self tolerance, in which foreign antigen is introduced prior to the complete development of immunocompetence by the host. However, in most other models of TT in which tolerance is induced in adult hosts, there is no compelling evidence for clonal deletion (*26, 27*). Thus spleen-graft-induced tolerance resembles enhancement, and cyclosporine-induced models of tolerance, in that donor-specific Ts are involved and no significant clonal deletion occurs (*28–32*). However, there are some unique differences between the spleen graft model and enhancement, in that the in vitro MLR responses are significantly reduced in spleen-graft-tolerant rats although they remain relatively normal in enhanced animals (*27*).

Our present results suggest that spleen-graft-tolerant rats contain two distinct populations of Ts: a radiosensitive $W3/25^+$, $OX8^-$ and a radioresistant $W3/25^-$, $OX8^+$. Previous studies in the rat by others have indicated that suppression is primarily mediated by the $W3/25^-$, $OX8^+$ T cell subpopulation and T cell help is mediated by the $W3/25^+$, $OX8^-$ subpopulation (*33–35*). However, recently Hall et al. (*36*) have suggested that specific suppression in cyclosporine-treated rats bearing long-term heart allografts may require interaction of both the $W3/25^+$, $OX8^-$ $T_{h/i}$ and the $W3/25^-$, $OX8^+$ $T_{s/c}$ subpopulation. In other systems in which suppressor cells have been thoroughly analyzed, it has been clearly shown that the typical helper subpopulation, $Lyt1^+$ in the mouse and the $T4^+$ subpopulation in man, contains Ts effector or Ts inducer cells (*37–40*). Therefore it would not be so unusual for two distinct Ts populations to exist in the rat and for the $W3/25^+$, $OX8^-$ subpopulation to contain a T suppressor-inducer population. Presently we have no evidence that the $W3/25^+$, $OX8^-$ Ts is an inducer cell—however, in light of preliminary results it appears that this T cell subpopulation can directly suppress the proliferative response of purified normal $W3/25^+$, $OX8^-$ T cells to donor alloantigens, indicating that this subpopulation may contain a suppressor-effector cell (Duncan et al., unpublished observations). The $W3/25^-$, $OX8^+$ Ts subpopulation resembles the classic Ts effector cell described by other laboratories (*35*). Further, it is likely that either Ts subpopulation may recognize class I or class II MHC determinants or recognize the idiotype of the responding T cells. Studies are currently underway to examine the specificity of these two subpopulations of Ts.

We also investigated the genotypic identity of Ts in our model of TT. Since TT was induced using an allograft containing large numbers of viable lymphoid cells, recipient and/or donor Ts may be present. Our data indicate that AGUS recipients bearing long-term F_1 spleen allografts contain recipient Ts, because treatment with AGUS anti-WAG alloantisera and C failed to remove Ts activity. However, these results do not rule out the possibility that donor (F_1) Ts also exist. Recent studies by Kimura and Wilson (*41*) indicate that F_1 antiparent (antiidiotypic) cytotoxic T cells are responsible for GVH resistance in rats. Similar cells could be generated when F_1 spleens are transplanted to normal parental recipients, and they may play a role in the induction and maintenance of TT.

These experiments demonstrate that rats that spontaneously accept allogeneic or semiallogeneic spleen grafts develop specific TT and contain donor-specific Ts cells. Two distinct subpopulations of Ts have been identified that apparently are involved in the maintenance of the in vivo tolerant state.

Acknowledgments. The excellent technical assistance of Mr. John Smith, Ms. Debby Currie, and Ms. Jane Hutchinson, and preparation of the manuscript by Ms. Debbie Brown are greatly appreciated. Helpful discussion and criticism of the manuscript was obtained from Richard M. O'Hara, Jr, Ph.D.

REFERENCES

1. Bitter-Suermann H. Survival of unmodified spleen allografts in rats. Nature 1974; 247: 465.
2. Bitter-Suermann H, Shevach EM. Induction of transplantation tolerance in guinea pigs by spleen allografts. I. Operative techniques and clinical results. Transplantation 1982; 33: 45.
3. Bitter-Suermann H. Prolonged survival of auxilliary spleen allografts in rats inducing acceptance of skin allografts. Transplantation 1974; 17: 75.
4. Bitter-Suermann H, Save-Soderbergh J. The course of pancreas allografts in rats conditioned by spleen allografts. Transplantation 1978; 26: 28.
5. Pennline KJ, Smith JP, Bitter-Suermann H. The cellular basis of transplantation tolerance in spleen-grafted rats. Transplant Proc 1983; 15: 704.
6. Stepkowski SM, Duncan WR, Smith JP, Bitter-Suermann H. Suppressor cells in the thoracic duct lymph of tolerant spleen-grafted rats. Can J Surg 1984; 27: 22.
7. Shevach EM, Chan C, Bitter-Suermann H. Induction of transplantation tolerance in guinea pigs by spleen allografts. II. Responses in the mixed leukocyte reaction correlate with the tolerant state. J Immunol 1982; 129: 710.
8. Stepkowski SM, Duncan WR, Smith JP, Bitter-Suermann H. Mixed lymphocyte reaction responses of thoracic duct lymphocytes from tolerant spleen-grafted rats. Transplant Proc 1984; 16: 1138.
9. Bitter-Suermann H. Surgical aspects of spleen grafting in rats. Eur Surg Res 1974; 7: 34.
10. Gowans JL. The recirculation of lymphocytes from blood to lymph in the rat. J Physiol (Lond) 1959; 146: 54.
11. Duarte AJS, Carpenter CB, Strom TB. Expression of T cell differentiation antigens and Ia on rat cytotoxic T lymphocytes. J Immunol 1982; 128: 580.
12. Klein J, Hauptfeld V, Hauptfeld M. Evidence for a fifth (G) region in the H-2 complex of the mouse. Immunogenetics 1975; 2: 141.
13. Shand FL. Ly and Ia phenotype of suppressor T cells induced by graft-vs-host reaction. Eur J Immunol 1977; 7: 746.
14. Elkins WL. Cellular immunology and pathogenesis of graft-vs-host reactions. Prog Allergy 1971; 15: 78.
15. Pickel K, Hoffmann MK. Suppressor T cells in mice undergoing a graft-vs-host response. J Immunol 1977; 118: 653.
16. Wettstein PJ. Serological characterization of rat class II (RT1.B) alloantigens. Analysis of $RT1^l$, $RT1^u$ and $RT1^n$ haplotypes. Immunogenetics 1981; 14: 541.
17. Billingham RE, Silvers WK, Wilson DB. Further studies on adop-

tive transfer of sensitivity to skin homografts. J Exp Med 1963; 118: 397.

18. Nossal GJV, Pike BL. Functional clonal deletion in immunological tolerance to major histocompatibility complex antigens. Proc Natl Acad Sci USA. 1981; 78: 3844.
19. Wood PJ, Streilein JW. Immunogenetic basis of acquired transplantation tolerance. Transplantation 1984; 37: 223.
20. Dorsch S, Roser B. Suppressor cells in transplantation tolerance. I. Analysis of the suppressor status of neonatally and adoptively tolerized rats. Transplantation 1982; 33: 518.
21. Hellstrom I, Hellstrom KE, Allison AC. Neonatally induced allograft tolerance may be mediated by serum-borne factors. Nature 1971; 230: 49.
22. Binz H, Wigzell H. Specific transplantation tolerance by autoimmunization against the individual's own, naturally occurring idiotypic, antigen binding receptors. J Exp Med 1976; 144: 1438.
23. Smith JP, Duncan WR, Stepkowski SM, Bitter-Suermann H. Transfer of spleen graft-induced transplantation tolerance in rats. Transplant Proc 1984; 16: 1136.
24. Gruchalla RS, Strelein JW. Analysis of neonatally induced tolerance of H-2 alloantigens. II. Failure to detect alloantigen specific T lymphocyte precursors and suppressors. Immunogenetics 1982; 15: 111.
25. Wood PJ, Streilein JW. Ontogeny of acquired immunological tolerance to H-2 alloantigens. Eur J Immunol 1982; 12: 188.
26. Kupiec-Weglinski JW, Araujo JL, Heidecke CD, Filho MA, Tilney NL. Does cyclosporin inhibit T helper or spare T suppressor lymphocytes in the maintenance phase of allograft survival? Transplant Proc 1985; 17: 1339.
27. Stuart FP, McKearn TJ, Weiss A, Fitch FW. Suppression of rat renal allograft rejection by antigen and antibody. Immunol Rev 1980; 49: 127.
28. Hall BM, Jelbart ME, Dorsch SE. Suppressor T cells in rats with prolonged cardiac allograft survival after treatment with cyclosporin. Transplantation 1984; 37: 595.
29. Hall BM. Mechanisms maintaining enhancement of allografts. I. Demonstration of a specific suppressor cell. J Exp Med 1985; 161: 123.
30. Batchelor JR, Phillips BE, Grennah D. Suppressor cells and their role in the survival of immunologically enhanced rat kidney allografts. Transplantation. 1984; 37: 43.
31. Bordes-Aznar J, Kupiec-Weglinski JW, Duarte AJS, Milford EL, Strom TB, Tilney NL. Function and migration of suppressor lymphocytes from cyclosporin-treated heart graft recipient. Transplantation 1983; 35: 185.
32. Kupiec-Weglinski JW, Filho MA, Strom TB, Tilney NL. Sparing of suppressor cells: a critical action of cyclosporin. Transplantation 1984: 97.
33. White RAH, Mason DW, Williams AF, Galfre G, Milstein C. T-lymphocyte heterogeneity in the rat: separation of functional subpopulations using a monoclonal antibody. J Exp Med 1978; 148: 664.
34. Brideau RJ, Carter PB, McMaster WR, Mason DW, Williams AF. Two subsets of rat T lymphocytes defined with monoclonal antibodies. Eur J Immunol 1980; 10: 609.
35. Mason DW, Arthur RP, Dallman MJ, Green JR, Spickett GP, Thomas ML. Function of rat T-lymphocyte subsets isolated by means of monoclonal antibodies. Immunol Rev 1983; 74: 57.
36. Hall BM, Jelbart ME, Dorsch SE. Function of $W3/25^+$ Th cells in rats with prolonged cardiac allograft survival after treatment with cyclosporin. Transplant Proc 1985; 17: 1372.
37. Thomas Y, Rogozinski L, Irigoyen OH, Friedman SM, Kung PC, Goldstein G, Chess L. Functional analysis of human T cell subsets defined by monoclonal antibodies. IV. Induction of suppressor cells within the $OKT4^+$ population. J Exp Med 1981; 154: 453.
38. Thomas Y, Rogozinski L, Irigoyen DH, Shen H, Talle MA, Goldstein G, Chess L. Functional analysis of human T cell subsets defined by monoclonal antibodies. V. Suppressor cells within the activated $OKT4^+$ population belong to a distinct subset. J Immunol 1982; 128: 1386.
39. Dorf ME, Benacerraf B. Suppressor cells and immune regulation. Ann Rev Immunol 1984; 2: 127.
40. Green DR, Flood PM, Gershon RK. Immunoregulatory T cell pathways. Ann Rev Immunol 1983; 1: 439.
41. Kimura H, Wilson DB. Anti-idiotypic cytotoxic T cells in rats with graft-vs-host disease. Nature 1984; 308: 463.

Received 3 December 1984.
Accepted 5 September 1985.

0041-1337/86/4105-0634$02.00/0
TRANSPLANTATION
Vol. 41, No. 5

Printed in U.S.A.

SKIN ALLOGRAFT REJECTION BY L3/T4+ AND LYT-2+ T CELL SUBSETS[1]

STEVE COBBOLD[2] AND HERMAN WALDMANN

Division of Immunology, Department of Pathology, University of Cambridge, Cambridge CB2 1QP, United Kingdom

The L3/T4+ and Lyt-2+ T-cell subsets can be depleted from mice, using selected monoclonal antibodies in vivo, at different times during rejection of, or priming to, allogeneic skin grafts. Although L3/T4+ cells are sufficient to reject skin grafts in naive Lyt-2-depleted mice, we show that Lyt-2+ cells can become involved, after an initial delay, in intact mice. Furthermore, these Lyt-2+ cells are primed to dominate the accelerated rejection of a normal secondary response. Mice depleted of L3/T4+ cells cannot be primed in this way, suggesting that priming of Lyt-2+ cells is dependent on help from L3/T4+ cells. However, in mice depleted of Lyt-2+ cells, priming for rapid rejection can be achieved, presumably via the L3/T4+ population. This suggests that the rejection of skin allografts in a given situation reflects different contributions of multiple effector mechanisms.

It has long been recognized that graft rejection is dependent on thymus-derived T cells (*1–3*). Attempts to suppress this process after organ transplantation have often focussed on reducing T cell activity—by using, for example, serotherapy with antithymocyte globulin (*4*). More recently it has been possible to define subsets of T cells according to their function in vitro (*5*) and the presence of specific surface antigens defined by monoclonal antibodies (*6–8*). The helper/inducer T cells recognize antigens presented with class II major histocompatibility complex (MHC)* molecules (*9*)—and, in the mouse, express the L3/T4 surface antigen (*10*), while the cytotoxic/suppressor T cells are generally restricted to antigens in the context of class I MHC molecules (*11*) and express the Lyt-2 antigen (*12*). The possibility of manipulating T cell subsets in vivo with monoclonal antibodies (*13*)—or with other reagents, such as cyclosporine (*14*)—to achieve more refined immunosuppression in therapeutic organ grafting requires the definition of the relative contributions of different T cells to the rejection process.

The immune system has a large repertoire of effector systems, including alloantibody, cytotoxic T lymphocytes (CTL), activated macrophages, natural killer (NK) cells, antibody-dependent cell cytotoxicity (ADCC), and delayed-type hypersensitivity (DTH). All of these have been implicated in the rejection of allografts (*15–19*) and most are thought to be regulated by, or dependent on, the presence of T cells. There has been considerable debate over which effector system is responsible for destruction of the graft, so that a number of models have been developed that involve adding back individual components (cellular or humoral) to skin grafted, immunocompromised animals. The thymectomized and irradiated, bone-marrow-reconstituted (ATXBM) model (*20*) is just one example in which different interpretations have implicated either the helper/DTH subset (*18*) or the cytotoxic T cells (*21, 22*).

Here we use a completely different approach by actively depleting T cell subsets either before or during the rejection of a skin graft. This is performed by the administration to adult mice of rat IgG2b monoclonal antibodies to one or more of the T cell antigens, leading to a substantial depletion of the target T cells, which in the case of adult thymectomized mice can be permanent (*13*). This method has the unique advantage that the importance of each T cell subset can be questioned at different phases of the response to the graft. We demonstrate that the normal rejection process in naive mice, and the ability to prime the Lyt-2+ cells, which we show normally dominate the secondary response, are dependent on the presence of L3/T4+ T cells. However, in the absence of Lyt-2+ cells the L3/T4+ T cells are able to reject and can also be primed in their own right. This suggests that skin graft rejection may occur through more than one effector mechanism, with these mechanisms operating together and perhaps competing for destruction and removal of the antigenic stimulus.

MATERIALS AND METHODS

Mice. CBA/CaH (H-2^k), BALB/c (H-2^d), and C57B10.BR (H-2^k) mice, and (LOU×DA)F_1 rats, were bred and maintained in the animal facility of Department of Pathology, Cambridge.

Monoclonal antibodies (MAbs). The monoclonal antibodies used for in vivo depletion were all rat IgG2b and were against the following mouse T cell antigens: Thy-1 (YTS 154.7), Lyt-1 (YTS 121.5), L3/T4 (YTS 191.1), and Lyt-2 (YTS 169.4) (*13*). These were produced from ascitic fluid by growing the hybridomas, which had been derived from fusion with the Y3/Ag1.2.3 myeloma (*23*), in pristane-primed (LOU×DA)F_1 rats. The antibody was partially purified by precipitation with 50% $(NH_4)_2SO_4$, followed by dialysis against phosphate-buffered saline (PBS). Each batch was tested in an in vitro, competitive enzyme-linked binding assay (*24*) using a monoclonal mouse anti-rat IgG2b (NORIG 7.16.2; [*25*]) coupled to β-galactosidase to check specificity and titer against batches with known activity. Specific titers were in the range 1:2×10^4 to 1:2×10^5 for 50 μl binding to 5×10^5 CBA thymocytes. Antibody was stored frozen below −20°C at 5–10 mg protein/ml (equivalent to approx. 1–2 mg/ml of active antibody). All preparations were microfuged at 14,000 rpm for 10 min before use.

Depletion of T cell subsets in vivo. Two methods were used for depeleting T cell subsets from mice: either repeated injec-

[1] This work was supported by the Medical Research Council, UK.

[2] Address correspondence to: S. P. Cobbold MA., PhD., Division of Immunology, Level 3, Laboratories Block, New Addenbrooke's Hospital, Hills Road, Cambridge CB2 2QQ. UK.

* Abbreviations used: ADCC, antibody-dependent cell-mediated cytotoxicity; ATX, adult thymectomized; ATXBM, adult thymectomized and bone-marrow-reconstituted; CTL, cytotoxic T lymphocyte; DTH, delayed-type hypersensitivity; MAb, monoclonal antibody; MGS, mean graft survival (in days); MHC, major histocompatibility complex; NK, natural killer.

tions for short-term depletion during the first two-to-three weeks after skin grafting, or two injections only to adult thymectomized mice in which longer-term depletion was required. In all cases each injection was of 0.2 ml of the monoclonal antibody preparation at 5–10 mg protein/ml (approx. 200–400 μg active antibody) given i.v. (tail vein)—or, in the case of any injection more than 10 days after the first, i.p. to avoid lethal anaphylaxis in the YTS 169.4 (anti-Lyt-2)-treated groups. All mice were given antibiotics (oxytetracycline, 50 mg/L) in the drinking water (Terramycin; Pfizer, UK), but were otherwise healthy and free from obvious infections.

Confirmation that the monoclonal antibodies had depleted the appropriate T cells in vivo was obtained for representative members of each group by the immunoperoxidase method on frozen sections of spleens removed on the day following rejection of the skin graft (*26*).

Thymectomy. Male CBA mice 5 to 6 weeks of age were thymectomized by the method of Monaco et al. (*27*). These were allowed to recover for at least 10 days before administration of monoclonal antibodies. Skin grafting or priming of these mice was not initiated until a minimum of a further three weeks after the last injection of antibody.

Priming to alloantigens. Irradiated (1500 rads), allogeneic (BALB/c or B10.BR) spleen cells (10^7) were injected into CBA mice i.p. 4–8 weeks prior to skin grafting.

Skin grafts. Allogeneic tail skin in pieces about 10 mm square was grafted onto the lateral thoracic wall of recipient mice by the method of Billingham et al. (*2*). The grafts were covered with paraffin-impregnated gauze, lint, and plaster bandage, which were removed on day 10 after grafting (day 8 in primed animals). The grafts were observed daily for rejection, which was considered complete when no viable graft was visible.

The arithmetic mean of graft survival in days (MGS) was calculated for each group, and the level of statistical significance between groups of interest estimated by values of P derived from the chi-square at 1 degree of freedom obtained by the Logrank (nonparametric) method (*28*).

RESULTS

Graft rejection in depleted athymic mice. Adult thymectomized (ATX) mice treated with appropriate monoclonal antibodies remain substantially depleted of either T cell subset for periods in excess of 12 months (*13*). In vivo depletion was shown to confirm the results obtained in ATXBM models in which animals lacking L3/T4$^+$ cells (or their equivalents) were substantially reduced in their capacity to reject skin allografts (*18, 21*). However, the grafts still rejected more rapidly in L3/T4-depleted mice when compared with pan-T-cell (Thy-1 + Lyt-1) depletion. There are two likely interpretations of these results—first, that there were residual L3/T4$^+$ cells that escaped the antibody treatment; and second, that L3/T4-negative cells were responsible for this slower rejection. We therefore aimed to confirm and extend our original observations in adult thymectomized subset-depleted mice with particular reference to these points.

Adult thymectomized CBA mice were depleted of T cell subsets by using monoclonal antibodies in vivo 4–8 weeks prior to grafting allogeneic (BALB/c) tail skin. The results shown in Figure 1 confirmed our previous observations (*13*) that Lyt-2 depletion did not delay rejection, while L3/T4 depletion prolonged survival of the skin grafts by approximately 5 days (controls MGS=13.6; L3/T4-depleted MGS=19.0: $P \leq 0.0001$).

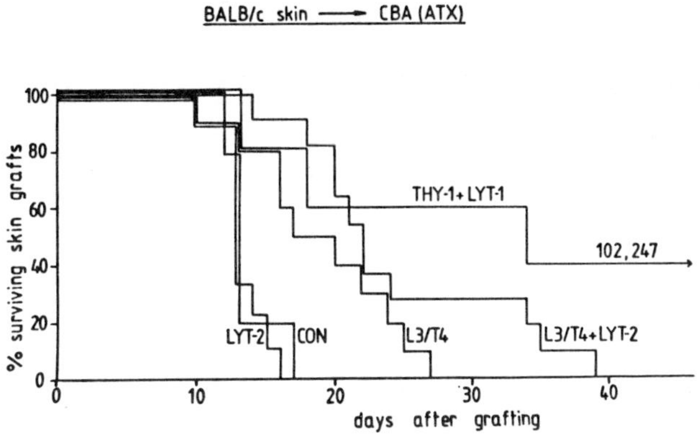

FIGURE 1. Graft rejection in adult thymectomized, T-cell-subset-depleted mice. Adult thymectomized CBA mice were depleted of different T cells by two i.v. injections of monoclonal antibodies to L3/T4 (YTS 191.1, n=10), Lyt-2 (YTS 169.4, n=10), both L3/T4 and Lyt-2 (1:1, n=11), or both Thy-1 and Lyt-1 (YTS 154.7 + YTS 121.5, 1:1, n=5). Control adult thymectomized mice received no antibody (CON, n=5). BALB/c tail skin was grafted to these mice 8 weeks after the last injection of monoclonal antibody. Mice rejecting grafts beyond day +100 are indicated by the figures in parentheses.

However, the combination of anti-L3/T4 and anti-Lyt-2 was unable to prolong the survival of any graft beyond 40 days, and was not significantly different from the delay obtained with anti-L3/T4 alone (L3/T4+Lyt-2-depleted MGS=24.5; L3/T4-depleted MGS=19.0: $P \leq 0.139$). This suggests that Lyt-2$^+$ cells were probably not the primary cause of the late rejection seen in these circumstances. Depletion with anti-Thy-1 plus anti-Lyt-1 was more effective with 2 of 5 grafts intact beyond day +100 (L3/T4+Lyt-2-depleted and L3/T4-depleted combined MGS=21.9; Thy-1+Lyt-1-depleted MGS=83.0: $P \leq 0.063$). This may reflect a residual capacity to reject by a cell that is negative for both L3/T4 and Lyt-2 at the time of depletion, or there could be insufficient depletion by the monoclonal anti-L3/T4 in vivo.

In order to investigate the level of depletion, ATX mice depleted of L3/T4$^+$ cells were given various numbers of syngeneic spleen cells i.v. in the presence of excess anti-Lyt-2 (Fig. 2). It was found that as few as 2×10^5 L3/T4$^+$ cells began to reconstitute the normal rejection of allogeneic skin grafts (group receiving no spleen cells MGS=26.3; group receiving 2×10^5 L3/T4$^+$ spleen cells MGS=17.8: $P \leq 0.003$). This implies that L3/T4-depleted mice have fewer than 2×10^5 residual L3/T4$^+$ cells—probably equivalent to 99–99.9% depletion. However, as the frequency of cells able to respond to alloantigens is disproportionately high (*29*), it cannot be ruled out that residual cells were expanded by the antigenic stimulus to eventually reach sufficient numbers to reject. This objection can be answered, in part, by administering antibody continuously over the rejection period—thereby reducing any tendency of cells to expand in response to the antigen. The direct administration of antibody during rejection also has two other advantages—first, there is no need to thymectomize, which makes the results more applicable to serotherapy during clinical organ grafting; and second, the antibodies can be used to deplete cells at different times during rejection. This helps to solve a major problem in interpreting results obtained in depleted (or ATXBM) animals in which the observed response may have been biased by the experimental manipulations before exposure to the graft. We therefore investigated graft rejection in eu-

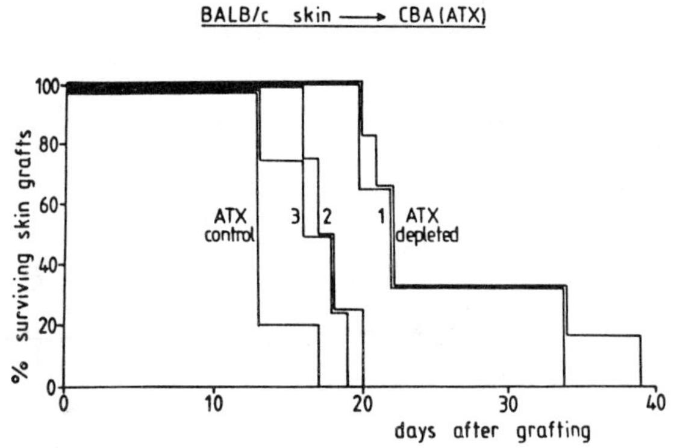

FIGURE 2. Reconstitution of L3/T4-dependent rejection in depleted mice. Adult thymectomized CBA mice were depleted of L3/T4$^+$ cells as described in the *Materials and Methods* section, with the exception of ATX controls. After 8 weeks, randomly selected groups of depleted mice received different numbers of syngeneic spleen cells (equivalent to 2×10^4 in group 1, 2×10^5 in group 2, and 2×10^6 in group 3 L3/T4$^+$ cells, assuming these to be 20% of normal spleen lymphocytes) i.v. plus 0.2 ml of YTS 169.4 to deplete Lyt-2$^+$ cells in both the inoculum and the recipient. One group (n=6) received only the antibody and no spleen cells (ATX depleted). All the mice were grafted with BALB/c tail skin after three more weeks.

thymic mice given antibodies to T cell subsets both early and late in the response to the graft.

Graft rejection in euthymic, intact mice involving participation of both T cell subsets. Fully allogeneic (H-2 and minor-antigen-mismatched) BALB/c skin was grafted onto euthymic CBA mice. These were given three i.v. injections of monoclonal antibodies to L3/T4, Lyt-2, or no antibody (controls). When these injections were given early in the course of grafting (days −1, +2, +5) it was found that depletion of the Lyt-2$^+$ cells caused no delay compared with controls receiving no antibody (controls MGS=13.4, Lyt-2-depleted MGS=13.6), while anti-L3/T4 treatment lead to considerable prolongation (L3/T4-depleted MGS=26.1; controls + Lyt-2-depleted combined MGS=13.5: $P\leq0.001$) of the skin grafts (Fig. 3). This confirmed previous observations that L3/T4$^+$ cells were sufficient to promote rapid rejection in this model (*13, 26*). However, if the injections were delayed until days +7, +10, +12, it was found that either L3/T4 or Lyt-2 depletion delayed rejection (compared with controls; anti-L3/T4 late MGS=19.7, $P\leq0.009$; anti-Lyt-2 late MGS=18.0, $P\leq0.023$; [Fig. 3]). Under these conditions, either antibody given alone was less effective than giving anti-L3/T4 from day -1 (anti-L3/T4 early compared with late, $P\leq0.069$) or both antibodies together from day -1 (MGS=25.4 [not shown]). The delay caused by giving anti-Lyt-2 late was not a nonspecific inhibition, because similar results could be obtained in adult thymectomized mice only if the Lyt-2$^+$ cells were present prior to antibody administration (ATX-Lyt-2-predepleted MGS=13.3; ATX-Lyt-2-depleted late (day+7) MGS=17.6; ATX Lyt-2-predepleted as well as anti-Lyt-2 late MGS=13.0: $P\leq0.035$). This suggests that, in the intact mouse, both L3/T4$^+$ and Lyt-2$^+$ cells participate in a response to the graft—but the Lyt-2$^+$ population seems to be dependent on the L3/T4$^+$ cells and is active only after an initial delay. This is consistent with the interpretation that Lyt-2$^+$ cells are primed during the course of rejection, and predicts that these cells should become more important in secondary responses.

Responsibility of Lyt-2$^+$ T cells for accelerated rejection after priming. In order to investigate graft rejection after priming, CBA mice were given irradiated BALB/c spleen cells six weeks before grafting BALB/c skin on day 0. Monoclonal antibodies were then injected i.v. to groups of randomly selected, primed mice on days −1, +3, +7 and i.p. on day +11. Control primed mice given no antibody rejected more rapidly (Fig. 4, MGS=8.5) than when unprimed (MGS=13.2; $P\leq0.0001$), demonstrating the effect of previous challenge with antigen. In marked contrast to the unprimed mice, depletion of the L3/T4$^+$ cells gave only a slight delay in rejection (MGS=11.2 vs. controls MGS=8.5; $P\leq0.089$), while anti-Lyt-2 was now more effective (Fig. 4, MGS=15.6 vs. controls MGS=8.5; $P\leq0.003$). Neither antibody alone prolonged graft survival as effectively as depletion of all T cells with the combinations of either anti-L3/T4 plus anti-Lyt-2 or anti-Thy-1 plus anti-Lyt-1, in which rejection was not different in tempo from that obtained by pan-T or L3/T4$^+$ cell depletion in unprimed mice (naive pan-T-depleted MGS=26.1; primed pan-T-depleted MGS=27.8; $P\leq0.606$). This suggests that the increased rejection rate of primed mice is mainly due to Lyt-2$^+$ cells, but removal of these then allows slower (MGS=15.6) "unprimed" rejection, probably via the L3/T4$^+$ cells.

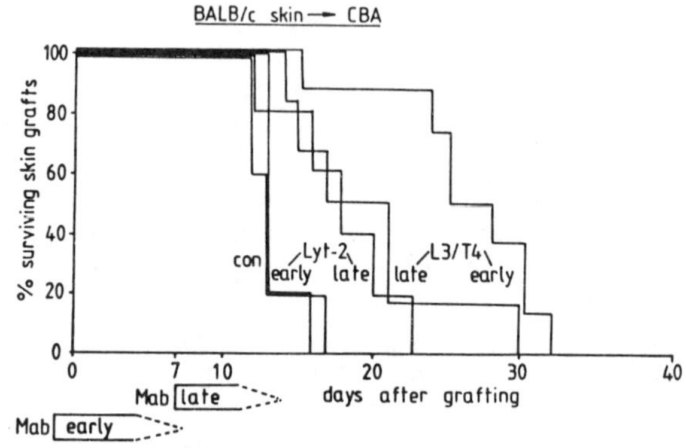

FIGURE 3. Both L3/T4$^+$ and Lyt-2$^+$ T cells reject allogeneic skin in naive mice. Euthymic CBA mice (6–10 per group) were grafted with BALB/c tail skin on day 0. Monoclonal antibodies to L3/T4 (YTS 191.1), or Lyt-2 (YTS 169.4) were administered as described in the *Materials and Methods* section. These were either given early (i.v. on days −1, +2, +5) or late (i.v. on days +7, +10, +12) during the course of rejection. Control mice received no antibody (CON).

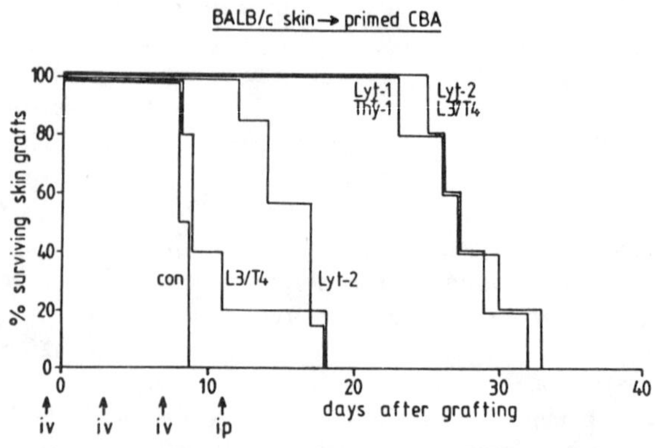

FIGURE 4. Lyt-2$^+$ cells are responsible for accelerated rejection after priming. Euthymic CBA mice (5–7 per group) were primed with irradiated BALB/c spleen cells 6 weeks prior to grafting BALB/c tail skin on day 0. Monoclonal antibodies to L3/T4, Lyt-2, both L3/T4 and Lyt-2 (1:1), or both Thy-1 (YTS 154.7) and Lyt-1 (YTS 121.5), were administered i.v. on days −1, +3, +7 and i.p. on day +11. Control mice received no antibody (CON).

Dependence of priming of Lyt-2⁺ cells on the L3/T4⁺ population. All the above experiments suggest that $Lyt\text{-}2^+$ cells only reject rapidly in the presence of $L3/T4^+$ cells. This would predict that the accelerated rejection, shown above to be due to $Lyt\text{-}2^+$ cells, would also depend on $L3/T4^+$ cells at the time of priming. This was tested by attempting to prime ATX subset-depleted mice with allogeneic spleen cells before grafting. It can be seen in Figure 5 that the pattern of results was essentially the same as in unprimed ATX depleted mice (Fig. 1), except that rejection was accelerated in all groups. Lyt-2-depleted mice were not different from undepleted controls (Fig. 5, MGS=8.4), while anti-L3/T4 delayed rejection (MGS=15.9: $P \leq 0.003$), demonstrating that $L3/T4^+$ cells are required for priming of the $Lyt\text{-}2^+$ cells normally responsible for acclerated rejection. However, both undepleted and Lyt-2-depleted primed mice rejected faster (MGS=8.7) than the similarly treated unprimed group (MGS=13.8; $P \leq 0.0051$), suggesting that it is also possible to prime in the absence of $Lyt\text{-}2^+$ cells.

The role of T cell subsets in rejection of minor-antigen-mismatched grafts. The experiments described above define the major roles of both $L3/T4^+$ and $Lyt\text{-}2^+$ cells in the rejection of, and priming to, fully allogeneic (MHC-mismatched) skin grafts. It is also important to determine whether MHC-matched, but minor-antigen-mismatched, grafts behave similarly, because this is often the situation in clinical organ transplantation. Many patients will also have been primed to minor antigens after receiving blood transfusions, so it is of particular interest to compare naive and primed responses to minor antigens.

B10.BR tail skin was grafted onto euthymic CBA mice. This is matched ($H\text{-}2^k$) for the MHC but differs at a number of minor histocompatibility loci (minor antigens). Monoclonal antibodies were given i.v. on days 0 and +7, and i.p.on day 12. In control mice given no antibody, or mice given anti-Lyt-2, it can be seen (Fig. 6) that the multiple-minor-antigen–mismatched graft was rejected after 13.3 and 14.5 days, respectively. Depletion of $L3/T4^+$ or all T cells lead to a substantial delay in rejection that lasted long past the time when repopulating T cells could be demonstrated in the spleen by immunoperoxidase staining of sections, or by the recovery of a response to sheep red blood cells (days 30–40, results not shown). All of the grafts were eventually rejected in these euthymic mice.

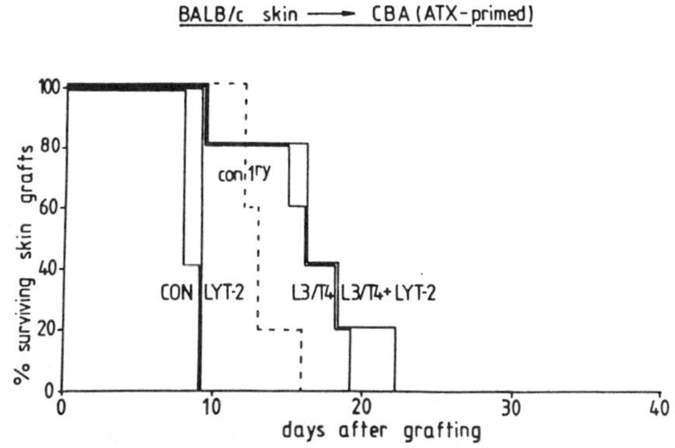

FIGURE 5. Graft rejection after priming in adult thymectomized, T-cell-subset–depleted mice. Adult thymectomized CBA mice (5 per group) were depleted with monoclonal antibodies to L3/T4, Lyt-2, or both L3/T4 and Lyt-2 (1:1). Control thymectomized animals received no antibody (CON). At 3 weeks after depletion the mice were primed with irradiated BALB/c spleen cells. After 6 more weeks the mice were grafted with BALB/c tail skin on day 0. Rejection of unprimed adult thymectomized mice is shown for comparison (CON 1ʳʸ).

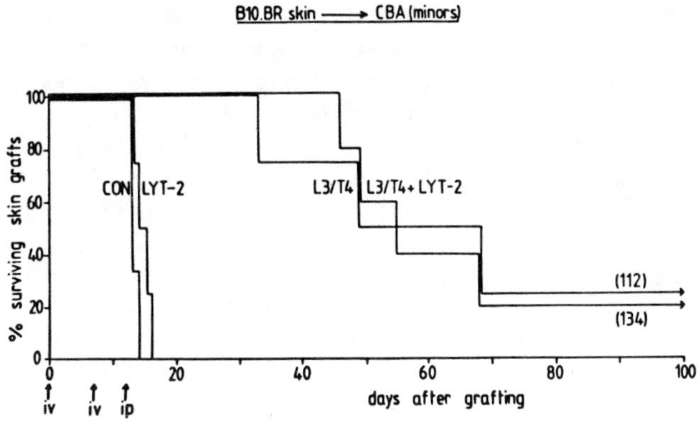

FIGURE 6. Rejection of H-2-matched, minor-antigen-mismatched, skin grafts in naive mice. Euthymic CBA ($H\text{-}2^k$, CBA minors) mice (5–8 per group) were grafted with B10.BR ($H\text{-}2^k$, C57B10 minors) tail skin on day 0. Monoclonal antibodies to Lyt-2, L3/T4, or both L3/T4 and Lyt-2 (1:1) were given i.v. on days 0 and +7, and i.p. on day +12. Control mice received no antibody (CON). Mice rejecting beyond day +100 are indicated by the figures in parentheses.

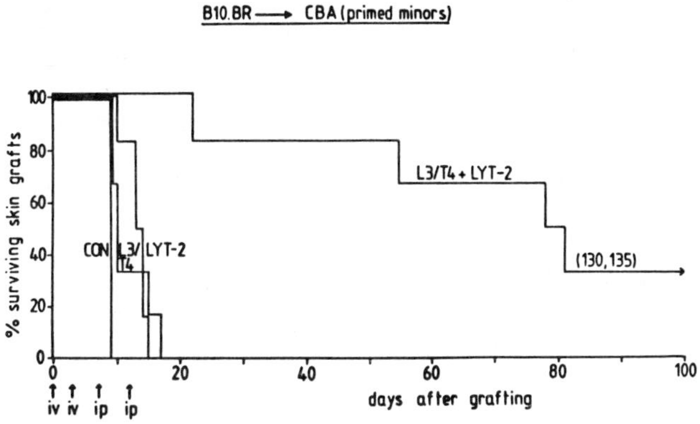

FIGURE 7. Rejection of H-2-matched, minor-antigen-mismatched skin grafts in primed mice. Euthymic CBA mice (6 per group) were primed with irradiated B10.BR spleen cells 8 weeks before grafting with B10.BR tail skin on day 0. Monoclonal antibodies to L3/T4, Lyt-2, or both L3/T4 and Lyt-2 (1:1) were given i.v. on days 0 and +3, and i.p. on days +8 and +12. Control mice were given no antibody (CON). Two mice in the L3/T4+Lyt-2 group rejected beyond day +100, as shown by the figures in parentheses.

When the recipient CBA mice had been previously primed to the B10.BR minor antigens, the grafts were lost more rapidly, and depletion of the $L3/T4^+$ subset was no longer effective at prolonging graft survival (Fig. 7). Depletion of both $L3/T4^+$ and $Lyt\text{-}2^+$ T cells, however, delayed rejection (MGS=83.5) in a manner similar to that observed in the unprimed mice after $L3/T4^+$ or pan-T-cell depletion (MGS=68.1; $P \leq 0.948$). Therefore, in both minor antigen and fully MHC mismatched skin grafts, $L3/T4^+$ cells are primarily responsible for rejection in naive mice, but $Lyt\text{-}2^+$ cells are primed in the presence of $L3/T4^+$ cells to accelerate rejection in the secondary response.

DISCUSSION

The development of monoclonal antibodies (*30*) lead to the discovery of a number of cell surface molecules defining different functional subpopulations of T cells in man (*8*) and rodents (*6, 7*). Combined with the ability of selected MAbs to eliminate their target cells in vivo (*13*), it has now become possible to manipulate different compartments of the immune system. This has lead to a hope that serotherapy for organ grafting might be directed specifically at T cells responsible for rejection, rather than the generalized immunosuppression obtained with antilymphocyte globulins—or, more recently, monoclonal anti–pan-T-cell reagents such as OKT3 (*31*). This has in turn stimulated the search for some global mechanism by which T cells control allograft rejection, concentrating logically on the major division into the so called helper/inducer and cytotoxic/suppressor subsets defined by the L3/T4 and Lyt-2 mouse antigens or their equivalents in rats (W3/25 and OX8, [*6*]) or man (OKT4:CD4 and OKT8:CD8 [*32*]). The results described here suggest that both these subsets are intimately involved in the rejection process. Therefore, there would be little advantage in directing immunosuppression at only one of these subsets unless individual circumstances can be defined—in particular, with regard to previous exposure to graft antigens.

Our results show that L3/T4$^+$ cells respond early in the first reaction to an allograft, and, in the absence of Lyt-2$^+$ cells, continue to reject the graft at the normal rate. However, in intact mice, this early L3/T4$^+$ response allows Lyt-2$^+$ cells to participate later in the rejection process. Late depletion of L3/T4$^+$ or Lyt-2$^+$ cells was found to be less immunosuppressive than removing L3/T4$^+$ cells early, implying that the L3/T4$^+$ cells are not as active when Lyt-2$^+$ cells are present from the beginning. This suggests that the activity of the two subsets is regulated, perhaps by competing for the graft antigens. The Lyt-2$^+$ cells activated during normal priming seem to be the major cause of accelerated rejection in a secondary response, with little participation of L3/T4$^+$ cells. However, if these primed Lyt-2$^+$ cells are eliminated, they no longer compete without the L3/T4$^+$ cells, which can then reject at a slower "primary" rate. If no Lyt-2$^+$ cells are present during priming, then it seems that L3/T4$^+$ cells can themselves mediate a more rapid rejection.

The above interpretation of our results assumes that the monoclonal antibodies are delaying rejection by a specific elimination of the L3/T4$^+$ or Lyt-2$^+$ cells. It is unlikely that any of the observed delays in rejection are nonspecific for four reasons: first, a number of irrelevant antibodies have been shown to have no effect on graft rejection (*33*); second, in most circumstances either the anti-Lyt-2 (primary response) or the anti-L3/T4 (secondary response) treated group was not markedly different from controls given no antibody; third, ATX subset-depleted mice were given time to clear the antibody and to reestablish any hypothetical thymus-independent cells that might have been affected by antibody treatment; and fourth, anti-Lyt-2 given late to ATX mice only delayed rejection when Lyt-2$^+$ cells had not already been eliminated. We are, therefore, confident that the delays obtained with monoclonal antibodies in vivo demonstrate that both T cell subsets are involved in the rejection process.

The ATXBM rodent models had previously implicated some participation of both T cell subsets in skin graft rejection, and it had been suggested that in the case of major histocompatibility differences the W3/25$^+$ T cells (in the rat) were most important—while in the case of minor antigens restriction was assumed to be by class I MHC antigens, so that the OX8$^+$ cells would be more prominent (*15*). Our results in the mouse clearly show that major and minor histocompatibility differences elicit similar responses for skin graft rejection: the L3/T4$^+$ cells are dominant in the primary response, while Lyt-2$^+$ cells become more important after priming. This stresses how model systems using primed cells cannot be compared with naive responses, and explains, for example, why cloned (primed) cytolytic T cells can destroy allogeneic skin in vivo (*19*) when adoptive transfer of OX8$^+$ or Lyt-2$^+$ naive cells is ineffective (*18, 21*). Weaker responses to minor antigens often need priming before observing a clear effect— for example, in anti-minor graft-versus-host reactions (*34*). It is possible that the apparent Lyt-2$^+$ cell involvement and class I MHC restriction of minor antigens are, in part, a consequence of this need to prime, although other factors, such as the nature of the grafted tissue, may also influence the T cells involved.

Priming for graft rejection was found to be dependent on the L3/T4$^+$ population, and one interpretation of this result would be that L3/T4$^+$ cells are supplying "help" for the generation of Lyt-2$^+$ cytotoxic T lymphocytes (CTL). However, although L3/T4 depleted mice do not generate allospecific CTL in vitro (*13*), it should be noted that such mice are able to generate H-2-restricted Lyt-2$^+$ cytotoxic T cells in vivo to allogeneic cells (unpublished data) and to herpes simplex virus (A. Nash, personal comunication). It should be borne in mind, however, that L3/T4$^+$ cells are necessary for antibody production in vivo (*13*), and complement or cell-mediated, antibody-dependent cytotoxicity would be mechanisms equally consistent with our results.

Adult thymectomized and T cell depleted mice eventually rejected all the skin grafts, even though athymic nude mice and rats or ATXBM animals are able to accept allogeneic, or even xenogeneic grafts, indefinitely. This might suggest that elimination of T cells by the monoclonal antibodies was incomplete, allowing expansion of the remaining cells upon antigenic challenge. However, as few as 2×10^5 L3/T4$^+$ cells given i.v. three weeks before grafting were observed to reconstitute rejection of allogeneic skin in depleted mice. This suggests that the number of active residual L3/T4$^+$ cells after depletion was less than 2×10^5—probably equivalent to a 99–99.9% reduction. It is likely that any residual cells could eventually be expanded sufficiently to reject, as long as a different mechanism, perhaps less important in intact mice, did not take over and reject the graft first. It is of interest to note that mice depleted with anti-Thy-1 maintained grafts for a longer period than those depleted with anti-L3/T4 plus anti-Lyt-2. This suggests that there might be a further mechanism of rejection that was Thy-1$^+$ L3/T4$^-$ Lyt-2$^-$ at the time of depletion. The difference in long-term graft survival between ATXBM or nude mice and the adult depleted thymectomized animals may also relate to other factors such as irradiation, genetic defects, the presence or absence of normal T cell function early in life, and the general state of health of the animals. For example, exposure to environmental antigens before depletion may have primed a variety of T and non-T-cell functions that could later influence responses in T-cell-subset–depleted mice.

The consensus about immunoregulation that has emerged in recent years is that it involves an organized set of T cell dependent mechanisms, each effector system controlled by interacting circuits of helper and suppressor cells. Our results suggest that the immune system is rather more plastic and adaptable than this. There may be a wide range of effector systems which are "opportunistic" and competitive in the destruction of the graft and removal of the antigenic stimulus. Some aspects of regulation by suppressive Lyt-2$^+$ cells observed in vitro could then be explained by competition of effector cells inappropriate to particular assay systems. For example, it has been suggested that cytotoxic T cells might inhibit help for antibody production by eliminating antigen on presenting cells (*35*).

This alternative, flexible immune system allows us to hold an ecumenical view of graft rejection. In the intact mouse, the L3/T4$^+$ cells start with an advantage, but as they help prime the Lyt-2$^+$ cells this advantage is lost. However, in animals that have been grossly manipulated, for example by irradiation and reconstitution, whichever mechanism is most capable in the circumstances will "assume responsibility" for rejecting the graft. Therefore, cloned cytotoxic T cells will reject if given appropriately (*19*)—and, in ATXBM models, L3/T4$^+$ cells (or their equivalents) will be sufficient to reject (*21*), but they may also help any residual cells of the cytotoxic lineage (*22*). Alloantibody, killer cell and NK cell activity, and class II restricted CTL may also play their part in appropriate circumstances. It will be interesting to see whether this view of the immune system is more widely applicable as we broaden our investigation of T-cell-subset–depleted mice to responses in viral, bacterial, and autoimmune diseases.

Acknowledgments. We thank Gill Martin and Penny Lovat for expert technical assistance.

REFERENCES

1. Mitchinson NA. Studies on the immunological response to foreign tumour transplants in the mouse. I. The role of lymph-node cells in conferring immunity by adoptive transfer. J Exp Med 1955; 102: 157.
2. Billingham RE, Brent L, Medawar PB. Quantitative studies on tissue transplantation immunity. II. The origin, strength and duration of actively and adoptively aquired immunity. Proc R Soc Lond [Biol] 1954; 143: 58.
3. Miller JFA. Effect of neonatal thymectomy on the immunological responsiveness of the mouse. Proc R Soc Lond [Biol] 1962; 156: 415.
4. Monaco AP, Wood ML, Gray JG, Russell PS. Studies on heterologous anti-lymphocyte serum in mice II. Effect on the immune response. J Immunol 1966; 96: 229.
5. Cantor H, Boyse EA. Functional subclasses of T lymphocytes bearing different Ly antigens. I. The generation of functionally distinct T cell subclasses in a differentiation process independent of antigen. J Exp Med 1975; 141: 1376.
6. Brideau RJ, Carter PB, McMaster WR, Mason DW, Williams AF. Two subsets of rat T lymphocytes defined with monoclonal antibodies. Eur J Immunol 1980; 10: 609.
7. Ledbetter JA, Herzenberg LA. Xenogeneic monoclonal antibodies to mouse lymphoid differentiation antigens. Immunol Rev 1979; 47: 63.
8. Reinherz EL, Meuer SC, Schlossman SF. The delineation of antigen receptors on human T lymphocytes. Immunol Today 1983; 4: 5.
9. Katz DH, Hamoaka T, Benacerraf B. Cell interactions between histoincompatible T and B lymphocytes. II. Failure of physiologic cooperative interactions between T and B lymphocytes from allogeneic donor strains in humoral responses to hapten-protein conjugates. J Exp Med 1973; 137: 1405.
10. Dialynas DP, Wilde DB, et al. Characterization of the murine antigenic determinant designated L3T4a recognised by a monoclonal antibody GK1.5: expression of L3T4a by functional T cell clones appears to correlate primarily with Class II MHC antigen reactivity. Immunol Rev 1983; 74: 29.
11. Zinkernagel RM, Doherty PC. Immunological surveillance against altered self components by sensitized T lymphocytes in lymphocytic choriomeningitis. Nature 1974; 251: 547.
12. MacDonald HR, Thiernesse N, Cerottini JC. Inhibition of T cell mediated cytolysis by monoclonal antibodies against Lyt-2: heterogeneity of inhibition at the clonal level. J Immunol 1981; 126: 1671.
13. Cobbold SP, Jayasuriya A, Nash A, Prospero TD, Waldmann H. Therapy with monoclonal antibodies by elimination of T-cell subsets in vivo. Nature 1984; 312, 548.
14. Palacios R, Moller G. Cyclosporin A blocks receptors for HLA-DR antigens on T cells. Nature 1981; 290: 792.
15. Mason DW, Dallman MJ, Arthur RP, Morris PJ. Mechanisms of allograft rejection: the roles of cytotoxic T-cells and delayed-type hypersensitivity. Immunol Rev 1984; 77: 167.
16. Hall BC, Dorsch SE. Cells mediating allograft rejection. Immunol Rev 1984; 77: 31.
17. Strom TB, Kupiec-Weglinski JW, Heidecke CD, Tilney NL. The cellular and molecular basis of allograft rejecton: fact and fancy. Transplant Proc 1985; 17: 801.
18. Loveland BE, Hogarth PM, Ceredig RH, McKenzie IFC. Cells mediating graft rejection on the mouse I. Lyt-1 cells mediate skin graft rejection. J Exp Med 1981; 153: 1044.
19. Tyler JD, Galli SJ, Snider ME, Dvorak AM, Steinmuller D. Cloned Lyt-2+ cytotoxic T lymphocytes destroy allogeneic tissue in vivo. J Exp Med 1984; 159: 234.
20. Huber BH, Cantor H, Shen FW, Boyse EA. Independent differentiation pathways of Ly-1 and Ly-23 subclasses of T cells. Experimental production of mice deprived of selected T cell subclasses. J Exp Med 1976; 144: 1128.
21. Dallman MJ, Mason DW, Webb M. The roles of host and donor cells in the rejection of skin allografts by T cell deprived rats injected with syngeneic T cells. Eur J Immunol 1982; 12: 511.
22. LeFrancois L, Bevan MJ. A re-examination of the role of Lyt-2 positive T cells in murine skin graft rejection. J Exp Med 1984; 159: 57.
23. Galfre G, Milstein C, Wright B. Rat x rat hybrid myelomas and a monoclonal anti-Fd portion of mouse IgG. Nature 1979; 277: 131.
24. Cobbold SP, Waldmann H. A rapid solid-phase enzyme-linked binding assay for screening monoclonal antibodies to cell surface antigens. J Immunol Methods 1981; 44: 125.
25. Aqel NM, Clark M, Cobbold SP, Waldmann H. Immunological screening in the selection of monoclonal antibodies: the use of isotype-specific antiglobulins. J Immunol Methods 1984; 69: 207.
26. Cobbold SP, Waldmann H. Immunosuppression with monoclonal antibodies—rules for effective serotherapy.
27. Monaco AP, Wood ML, Russel PS. Studies on heterologous anti-lymphocyte serum in mice. III. Immunologic tolerance and chimerism produced across the H-2 locus with adult thymectomy and anti-lymphocyte serum. Ann NY Acad Sci 1966; 129: 190.
28. Peto R, Pike MC, Armitage P, et al. Design and analysis of randomized clinical trials requiring prolonged observation of each patient. II. Analysis and examples. Br J Cancer 1977; 35: 1.
29. Lindahl KF, Wilson DB. Histocompatibility antigen-activated cytotoxic T lymphocytes. II. Estimates of the frequency and specificity of precursors. J Exp Med 1977; 145: 508.
30. Kohler G, Milstein C. Continuous cultures of fused cells secreting antibody of predefined specificity. Nature 1975; 256: 495.
31. Cosimi AB, Burton RC, et al. Treatment of acute renal allograft rejection with OKT3 monoclonal antibody. Transplantation 1981; 32: 535.
32. Bernard A, Boumsell L, Hill C. Leucocyte typing. In: Bernard A, Boumsell L, Dausset J, Milstein C, Schlossman SF, eds. Human leucocyte differentiation antigens detected by monoclonal antibodies- specification- classification- nomenclature. New York: Springer, 1984: 9.
33. Cobbold SP, Thierfelder S, Waldmann H. Immunosuppression with monoclonal antibodies: a model to determine the rules for effective serotherapy. Mol Biol Med 1983; 1: 285.
34. Korngold R, Sprent J. Lethal graft-versus-host disease after bone marrow transplantation across minor histocompatibility barriers in mice: prevention by removing mature T cells from marrow. J Exp Med 1978; 148: 1687.
35. Zamoyska R, Waldmann H. Allosuppression: evidence for the involvement of both "noncytotoxic" and cytotoxic T cells. Eur J Immunol 1984; 14: 645.

Received 16 July 1985.
Accepted 13 August, 1985.

0041-1337/86/4105-0640$02.00/0
TRANSPLANTATION
Vol. 41, No. 5

Printed in U.S.A.

IMPROVED RENAL ALLOGRAFT FUNCTION AND SURVIVAL FOLLOWING NONSPECIFIC BLOOD TRANSFUSIONS

I. INDUCTION OF SOLUBLE SUPPRESSOR FACTORS INHIBITING THE MITOGENIC RESPONSE[1]

RAYNALD ROY,[2] JEAN-GUY LACHANCE,[3] RÉAL NOEL,[3] JOHN H. GROSE,[3] AND ROGER BEAUDOIN

Unité de Recherche en Immunologie et Rhumatoloqie Centre Hospitalier de l'Université Laval, Ste-Foy Québec, Canada GIV 4G2

A small number of blood transfusions (1–3) seems sufficient to improve the cadaveric renal allograft outcome, probably via induction of some nonspecific suppressive activity. This activity was assessed by the concanavalin A (Con A) enhancement method; when present, the response of freshly isolated patients' cells to a submitogenic dose of Con A was lowered, leading to a Con A ratio >5, significantly (P<0.0001) higher than the one observed in normal controls or untransfused uremic patients. The correlation between this suppressive activity and graft outcome was determined. Thirty-five patients were studied over a 12-month period for graft function (creatinine level) and survival. Both parameters were significantly improved in the group of patients whose Con A ratio was >5 after transfusions. A soluble suppressor factor, or factors, released into the supernatant of patients' lymphocytes cultured for 48 hr, seems responsible for this suppressive activity. Moreover this process is nonspecific, since it suppresses mitogenic response of cells isolated from normal untransfused volunteers, and could be observed when peripheral blood mononuclear cells were used, but not with purified adherent or nonadherent cells. Addition of indomethacin to the cells during the elaboration of the supernatant abolished this activity. However, amounts of PGE_2 secreted into the supernatant during the 48 hr of culture could not be correlated with this suppressive activity. These findings suggest that induction of nonspecific immunosuppression by a few blood transfusions could predict a better kidney graft outcome.

The beneficial effect of pretransplant blood transfusions (BT)* on kidney graft survival is now well recognized. The role of recipient selection is still controversial (*1, 2*) but immunological mechanisms are certainly important. Many hypotheses such as suppressor cells (*3*), soluble suppressor factors (*4*), and antiidiotypic (*5*) or other enhancing antibodies (*6*) have been proposed to explain the effect of BT, which could be a multistep process as proposed by Van Rood (*7*). Many studies have shown that the response of lymphocytes to mitogenic or allogenic stimulation was lower in dialyzed patients following BT. Using the concanavalin A (Con A)-enhancement method we and others have reported recently such a suppressive effect after as few as 1–5 BT (*8, 9*). Some authors (*10*) using the same approach, have suggested that BT could induce a nonspecific immunosuppression mediated through activation of suppressor T cells, while others (*11*) have proposed that monocytes/macrophages were the cells implicated in this phenomenon. It has been suggested also that the suppression of mitogenic response observed with this method could be due to prostaglandins, an important bioactive secretion product of monocytes (*12*).

The aim of the study presented here was to try to correlate the presence of this suppressive activity (determined by the Con A enhancement method) observed following BT, with kidney graft function and survival, and to define the immune mechanism(s) involved in the acquisition of the beneficial effect of BT. We were particularly interested in learning whether this suppressive activity could be related to the presence of one or more soluble suppressor factors secreted by patients' cells, acting nonspecifically on the mitogenic response of normal controls.

MATERIALS AND METHODS

Patients. Thirty-five hemodialysis patients were selected for this study because they had never received blood transfusions previously. The 29 men and 6 women were aged 19–60 years (mean 38 years). After informed consents were obtained, each patient received up to five units of packed blood. Blood samples were obtained by venipuncture immediately before each transfusion, given every 4–8 weeks. All patients received a first cadaver kidney allograft (ABO compatible). HLA-A, B, C and Dr tissue typing was performed using the microlymphocytotoxicity technique with our own and Terasaki tissue-typing trays. Transplants were performed following a negative crossmatch reaction. Patients received conventional immunosuppressive therapy as previously described (*6*).

Isolation of cells and culture procedure. Peripheral blood lymphocytes (PBL) were isolated and cultured exactly as previously described (*8*). Cells suspended in RPMI 1640 with 10% fetal calf serum were incubated at 37°C in culture flasks (25 cm^2, Lux 5350) for 45 min. The nonadherent cells were harvested by washing with a Pasteur pipet, and subjected to a second incubation period to completely eliminate adherent cells. Adherent cells were obtained by gently scraping and vigorously washing the plates after the first incubation. The percentage of monocytes, determined by nonspecific esterase staining (*13*) and the immunofluorescence technique with Anti-Leu-M3 (Becton-Dickinson) monoclonal antibody, was >80% in adherent and <5% in nonadherent cell populations. Viability, as assessed by the trypan blue dye exclusion test, was always higher than 95%.

[1] This work was supported by a grant from the Kidney Foundation of Canada.

[2] Address reprint requests to: R. Roy, Unité de Recherche en Immunologie et Rhumatologie, Centre Hospitalier de l'Université Laval, 2705 Boulevard Laurier, Ste-Foy, Québec, Canada, G1V 4G2.

[3] Department of Nephrology, Hôpital Hôtel-Dieu de Québec, Québec, Canada.

* Abbreviations used: BT, blood transfusions; Con A, concanavalin A; PBL, peripheral blood lymphocyte; PGE, prostaglandin E.

Suppressive activity by the Con A enhancement method. This procedure was followed as previously described (*8*). Briefly, cells were incubated at 37°C, unstimulated (control) or stimulated with a suboptimal dose (3 μg/ml) of Con A (Sigma). Stimulation was performed in two parallel cultures. In the first, mitogen was added at the beginning of the culture (t0) while the second set of cells were incubated for 48 hr, washed, and resuspended in fresh medium to which Con A was added (t48). Both sets of cultures were cultured for 72 hr and pulsed with 0.2 μCi/well ^{3}H-thymidine for 16 hr before harvesting. The net cpm of triplicate cultures was calculated as the cpm of cells with mitogen minus the cpm of cells without mitogen. The Con A enhancement ratio was calculated by dividing the cpm obtained for t48 cultures by that for t0 cultures.

Suppressive activity in supernatants of cultured cells. The suppressive activity in the supernatant of nonpurified cells (PBL), adherent cells, and nonadherent cells was measured after cells were cultured at 37°C for 48 hr with or without indomethacin (Sigma, 1 μg/ml). This activity was defined as the capacity of the supernatant, used undiluted or diluted 1:2, to inhibit the response to a submitogenic dose of Con A (3 μg/ml) of freshly isolated lymphocytes from normal controls. Briefly, these cells were isolated and resuspended in medium or supernatant for the test (1×10^6/ml). Con A was then added and cells were cultured for 72 hr, harvested, and counted as described elsewhere (*8*).

Identification of monocytes/macrophages. Cells from the monocyte/macrophage lineage were identified by two methods. First, a direct immunofluorescence technique with Anti-Leu-M3 monoclonal antibody (Becton-Dickinson) and a fluorescence-activated cell sorter analyzer (Becton-Dickinson) were used as previously described (*8*). Monocytes were also identified by nonspecific esterase staining (*13*).

Quantification of PGE$_2$. Prostaglandin E$_2$ (PGE$_2$) was measured in the supernatant of cells after a 48-hr incubation using a direct specific radioimmunoassay as previously described (*14*). In this radioimmunoassay a specific antibody prepared and tested locally was used. Concentrations are expressed as pg/ml of cells, each milliliter containing 1×10^6 cells.

Statistical analysis. Results were compared using the nonpaired Student's *t* test. Transplant survival was analyzed using the chi square test with Yates' correction.

RESULTS

Con A enhancement ratio and graft outcome. Graft function and outcome at one year have been studied in 35 cadaveric renal allograft recipients who were subjected to a low number of blood transfusions during the dialysis period (Table 1). Patients were divided into two groups; sixteen of them had a post-BT Con A enhancement ratio (3.0±1.2) not significantly different from the one observed with untransfused normal controls (3.8±1.4), while 19/35 (54%) had a post-BT ratio (10.3±3.5) significantly higher ($P<0.0001$) than normal controls or the former group of 16 patients. Both groups had received an equal number of transfusions (3.4 vs. 4.0; not significant). The degree of donor HLA-matching was also comparable (data not shown) for both groups, while the interval between the last BT and transplantation was slightly longer in the group with a high ratio. The appearance of suppressive activity (Con A ratio >5) after BT could be related to significantly ($P<0.05$) improved survival (84% vs. 56% at one year) and to significantly better renal function, as evaluated by the serum creatinine level, measured at 1, 3, 6, and 12 month postgrafting ($0.0005<P<0.025$).

Suppressive activity in supernatants. Supernatants obtained from purified (adherent or nonadherent cells) and nonpurified patients' cells were then studied. Five of the 10 patients studied had a Con A ratio <5 (3.1±1.2), while the other 5 had a ratio >5 (9.4±2.3). The capacity of these supernatants to suppress the mitogenic proliferative response of normal cells was studied, and results are presented in Figure 1. In these experiments, the controls consisted of cells from normal donors incubated with supernatants obtained from unpurified normal cells cultured for 48 hr. In the group of patients with a Con A ratio <5, no significant inhibition of the mitogenic response could be observed no matter what the cell source (unpurified, adherent, or nonadherent) of the supernatant was. In other words, supernatants from any of these patients' cells had no effect on the proliferative response of normal cells. No effect was seen when supernatants were obtained from purified (adherent or nonadherent) cells from patients with a ratio of >5. However, a significant ($P<0.0005$) inhibition of the mitogenic response was observed when the supernatant was obtained from unpurified cells of these patients with a high ratio. This inhibitory capacity was gradually lost if the supernatant was diluted with culture medium before being added to the cells (data not shown) and this effect could no longer be observed if indomethacin was added during the 48 hr of elaboration of the supernatant. On the other hand, indomethacin had no effect when added to cells (purified or not) from patients with a low Con A ratio (Fig. 1) or from normal controls (data not shown).

The appearance of suppressive activity after BT could not be related to the number of circulating monocytes/macrophages as determined by nonspecific esterase staining or by direct

TABLE 1. Correlation between the Con A ratio observed after 1–5 blood transfusions (BT) and the kidney graft function and outcome up to one year posttransplantation (TX)

Con A ratio (t48/t0)	Number of patients	Interval between last BT and TX (mean No. of months)	Serum creatinine (mg%)				Survival for 12 Mo.
			1 Mo.[a]	3 Mo.	6 Mo.	12 Mo.	
3.0±1.2[b]	16	1.6±1.8	2.3±0.8 (16)[c]	2.2±1.0 (15)	2.5±1.9 (11)	1.7±0.3 (9)	56%
10.3±3.5	19	2.7±1.4	1.5±0.4[d] (19)	1.6±0.7[d] (17)	1.5±0.4[d] (16)	1.4±0.4[d] (16)	84%[e]

[a] Months postgrafting.
[b] Mean ± SD.
[c] Number of patients.
[d] $0.0005<P<0.025$.
[e] $P<0.05$.

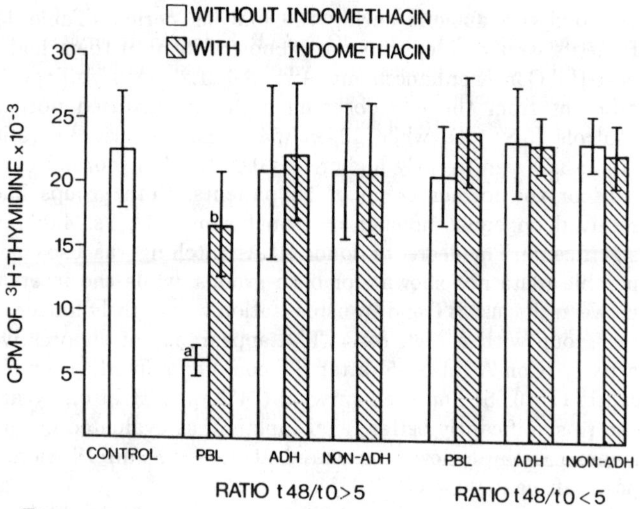

FIGURE 1. Suppression of ^{3}H-thymidine incorporation in normal cells by supernatants obtained with cells from normal volunteers (control) or with different preparations from transfused patients ([PBL] peripheral blood lymphocytes; [ADH] purified adherent cells; [NON-ADH] purified nonadherent cells). These cells were used untreated (empty bars) or treated with indomethacin (hatched bars). In the left panel, results from 5 patients with a high Con A ratio are shown (mean cpm ± SD) and in the right panel they are representative of 5 patients with a low Con A ratio post-BT. (a) $P<0.0005$; (b) not significant.

TABLE 2. Correlation between the percentage of monocytes/macrophages and the number of transfusions administered

Method used	Number of transfusions 0	1	2	3	4	Normal controls (33 exp.)
Esterase (17 patients)	16±12[a]	16±7	15±7	18±9	16±6	15±6
ANTI-Leu-M3 (17 patients)	15±6	15±8	15±6	18±8	15±5	15±5

[a] Mean % ± SD.

TABLE 3. Absence of correlation between Con A ratio and quantity of PGE2 secreted in vitro: results for 5 representative patients

Patient #	Transfusion No.	Con A ratio (t48/t0)	PGE2 secretion (pg/ml) −Indo.	+Indo.
1	0	2.9	826	34
	1	1.2	223	26
	2	5.8	235	31
	3	12.0	189	19
2	0	2.3	5,034	54
	1	2.2	4,519	35
	2	18.5	2,640	41
	3	5.3	2,532	23
3	0	1.2	124	26
	1	1.0	2,252	48
	2	5.8	2,100	43
	3	7.0	5,068	53
4	0	6.0	11,000	49
	1	11.8	552	32
	2	5.7	130	26
	3	7.0	76	33
5	0	8.5	24,813	57
	1	3.9	1,431	42
	2	1.3	1,263	35
	3	7.1	1,530	30

immunofluorescence using anti-Leu-M3 monoclonal antibody (Table 2).

Suppressive activity and PGE_2 secretion. We were also able to demonstrate (Table 3) that the increase in the Con A ratio during the transfusion protocol was not accompanied by a similar increase in in vitro PGE_2 secretion into the culture medium during the 48 hr of incubation of the cells—i.e., a high ratio did not imply that a higher quantity of PGE_2 was secreted into the supernatant. All patients whose results are shown in Figure 1 had a low level of PGE_2 secretion in vitro (1230±836 pg/ml). On the other hand, a very high level of PGE_2 secreted in vitro could perhaps explain the high Con A ratio observed in patients Nos. 4 (11,000 pg/ml and 6.0) and 5 (24,813 pg/ml and 8.5) before transfusion (Table 3). Indeed, addition of 10,000 pg/ml of commercial PGE_2 resulted in 50% and more inhibition of the mitogenic response of normal cells to Con A (data not shown).

DISCUSSION

In this study we were able to show that the alterations of immune response, revealed by the Con A enhancement method, that follow administration of a few donor nonspecific blood transfusions could be related to a better kidney graft outcome. This altered response was particularly associated with better renal function that was reflected by a lower serum creatinine level and improved graft survival. This phenomenon, when present, seems to last for some weeks since these patients received a kidney graft 2.7±1.4 months after their last BT. This is in accord with the findings of others who, using the same technique, reported that such an effect was lost by 20 weeks posttransfusion (*10*).

This effect of BT on immune response was reflected in vitro by a lower mitogenic proliferative response of patients' freshly isolated lymphocytes versus the same cells preincubated for 48 hr, leading to an increased Con A ratio (t48/t0) as previously shown by us (*8*). This increase in the Con A ratio has been reported to depend on elimination during the 48-hr period of "short-lived" suppressor cells (*15*). Moreover, it has been shown (*16*) that monocytes/macrophages can activate short-lived suppressor cells through secretion of PGE_2, and that such activation is prevented by indomethacin treatment.

As shown in Figure 1, this suppressive activity could be related to the release into the supernatant of a soluble suppressor factor by transfused patients' PBL with a high Con A ratio. Indeed, the addition of supernatant obtained after 48 hr of culture of such cells significantly inhibited the response of freshly isolated cells from normal donors. This effect was not observed if indomethacin was added for the 48 hr of elaboration of the supernatant indicating that prostaglandins or other substances sensitive to indomethacin could play a role in the induction of this factor.

Prostaglandins of the E series—more specifically PGE_2—were thus studied. Indeed, the effect of prostaglandins on inhibition of mitogen-stimulated T cell proliferation has been described (*17*). The suppressive activity observed in transfused patients (1–3 BT) does not seem, in fact, directly related to the amount of PGE_2 secreted in vitro by patients' cells, as shown by the absence of correlation between increase in Con A ratio and level of PGE_2 found in the supernatant after 48 hr of culture of the cells in vitro (Table 3). In a few untransfused patients, however, a low response at day t0 was observed, along with a very high level of PGE_2 (>10,000 pg/ml). Similar concentrations of PGE_2 added in vitro have already been shown to inhibit the mitogenic response of freshly isolated cells (*17*).

When we tried to generate this suppressor factor using purified adherent or nonadherent cells from the same patients, no effect was seen. It thus seems plausible that interaction between both cell populations could be necessary for the elaboration of this suppressor factor. The prostaglandins or related products could also play a role in this collaboration since addition of indomethacin inhibits the production of this suppressor factor. Moreover, in animals it has been suggested that prostaglandins produced by adherent cells could induce a suppressor T cell to elaborate a soluble suppressor factor (*18*).

Our data thus suggest that a better kidney graft outcome can be expected following the appearance of suppressive activity, defined by the Con A enhancement method, after a few nonspecific blood transfusions. We think, as Klatzmann et al. (*19*) do, that secretion products released by suppressor cells could play an important role in the elaboration of this state of suppression after BT. This phenomenon could be a major step in the process leading to the beneficial effect of blood transfusions on graft outcome.

Acknowledgments. We thank Lilliane Bérubé, Simone Lille, and Michèle Paré for their expert technical assistance. We are grateful to Patrice Poubelle, M.D., for a critical reading of the manuscript.

REFERENCES

1. Mickey MR, Cats S, Graves B, Perdue S, Terasaki PI. Transfusion and selection in cadaveric donor kidney grafts. Transplant Proc 1983; 15: 965.
2. Fehrman I, Ringden O, Moller E. Blood transfusions as pretreatment for kidney transplantation: immunization rate and effect on cellular immune response in vitro. Transplantation 1983; 35: 339.
3. Fisher E, Lenhard V, Seifert P, Kluge A, Johannsen R. Blood transfusion-induced suppression of cellular immunity in man. Hum Immunol 1980; 1: 187.
4. Sasporte M, Wollman E, Cohen D, Carosella E, Bensussan A, Fradelizi D, Dausset J. Suppression of the human allogeneic response in vitro with primed lymphocytes and suppressive supernatants. J Exp Med 1980; 152: 270s.
5. Singal DP, Joseph S. Role of blood transfusions on the induction of antibodies against recognition sites on T lymphocytes in renal transplant patients. Hum Immunol 1982; 4: 93.
6. Fradet Y, Roy R, Lachance JG, Noel R. Kidney graft survival: role of blood transfusions and lymphocytotoxic antibodies. Clin Nephrol 1982; 18: 69.
7. Van Rood JJ. Pretransplant blood transfusion: sure! but how and why? Transplant Proc 1983; 15: 915.
8. Roy R, Beaudoin R, Roberge F, Lachance JG, Pelletier G. Blood transfusions in renal dialysis patients. Effect on cellular immune response. Tissue Antigens 1984; 23: 203.
9. Smith MD, Williams JD, Coles GA, Salaman JR. The effect of blood transfusion on T-suppressor cells in renal dialysis patients. Transplant Proc 1981; 13: 181.
10. Smith MD, Williams, JD, Coles GA, Salaman JR. Blood transfusion, suppressor T cells, and renal transplant survival. Transplantation 1983; 36: 647.
11. Lenhard V, Massen G, Seifert P, Johannsen R, Grosse-Wilde H. Characterization of transfusion-induced suppressor cells in prospective kidney allograft recipients. Transplant Proc 1982; 14: 329.
12. Kalmar L, Gergely P. Enhancement of mitogen-induced lymphocyte proliferation after preincubation is due to altered sensitivity to prostaglandins. Immunol Lett 1982; 4: 179.
13. Yam LT, Li CY, Crosby WH. Cytochemical identification of monocytes and granulocytes. Am J Clin Pathol 1971; 55: 283.
14. Fradet Y, Simard J, Grose JH, Lebel M. Enhanced urinary prostaglandin E2 in postobstructive diuresis in humans. Prostaglandins Med 1980; 5: 29.
15. Bresnihan B, Jasin HE. Suppressor function of peripheral blood mononuclear cells in normal individuals and patients with systemic lupus erythematosus. J Clin Invest 1977; 59: 106.
16. Fischer A, Durandy A, Griscelli C. Role of prostaglandin E2 in the induction of nonspecific T lymphocyte suppressor activity. J Immunol 1981; 126: 1452.
17. Goodwin JS, Bankhurst AD, Messner RP. Suppression of human T-cell mitogenesis by prostaglandin: existence of a prostaglandin producing suppressor cell. J Exp Med 1977; 146: 1719.
18. Roger TJ, Campbell K, Calhoun I, Nowowiejski I, Webb DR. Suppression of B-cell and T-cell responses by the prostaglandin-induced T-cell-derived suppressor (PITS). I. Analysis of the PITS factor. Cell Immunol 1982; 66: 269.
19. Klatzmann D, Bensussan A, Gluckman JC, Foucault C, Dausset J, Sasportes M. Blood transfusions suppress lymphocyte reactivity in uremic patients. II. Evidence for soluble suppressor factors. Transplantation 1983; 36: 337.

Received 1 April 1985.
Accepted 15 August 1985.

0041-1337/86/4105-0644$02.00/0
TRANSPLANTATION
Copyright © 1986 by The Williams & Wilkins Co.

Vol. 41, No. 5
Printed in U.S.A.

TREATMENT AND PREVENTION OF ACUTE GRAFT-VERSUS-HOST DISEASE WITH THALIDOMIDE IN A RAT MODEL[1]

GEORGIA B. VOGELSANG, ALLAN D. HESS,[2] GARY GORDON, AND GEORGE W. SANTOS

The Bone Marrow Transplant Unit, The Johns Hopkins Oncology Center Baltimore, Maryland 21205

We have investigated the immunosuppressive effects of thalidomide (Thal) in a bone marrow transplant (BMT) model for graft-versus-host disease (GVHD). Lewis rats received RT1-incompatible marrow transplants from ACI rats after total-body irradiation. Twenty-two of twenty-three rats with established severe acute GVHD were successfully treated with Thal. Thal was given for therapy by gavage at 50 mg/kg/day or 100 mg/kg/day for 40 days after GVHD was clinically and histologically present. Fourteen of twenty-two received prophylaxis successfully with Thal at a dose of 50 mg/kg/day or 100 mg/kg/day. Acute GVHD did not develop after the drug was stopped. Three animals treated for severe GVHD later developed chronic GVHD. Chimerism was shown by permanent acceptance of ACI skin grafts and rejection of third-party skin grafts. Lymphocytes from Thal-treated animals likewise did not respond to Lewis or ACI cells in mixed lymphocyte culture but responded to third-party BN lymphocytes. Thal appears to be a potent new agent for therapy and prophylaxis of GVHD.

Thalidomide (Thal),* which achieved world wide notoriety for its unsuspected teratogenicity, was marketed originally as a sedative. Several early reports hinted that Thal had immunosuppressive activity. Sheskin first noted that the drug could rapidly alleviate the symptoms of reactional lepromatous leprosy (*1*). After this initial report, many case reports and two randomized studies showed that Thal could be effective in a number of inflammatory and autoimmune diseases (*2*). These data suggest that Thal is an immunosuppressive agent—but, unfortunately, these leads have not been extensively pursued. Although teratogenic drugs are widely used today, the failure to identify this major problem before marketing and the attendant tragedy of "thalidomide babies" has greatly inhibited any work with this compound.

Intrigued by the reports of the immunosuppressive effects of Thal, we examined this drug for its efficacy to prevent and/or treat graft-versus-host disease (GVHD) in a bone marrow transplant (BMT) model. To date there is only one early report in the literature of using Thal to partially alleviate GVHD in an animal model using spleen weight as an index of GVHD (*3*). The lack of toxicity other than teratogenicity made it an appealing choice to study, since all effective drugs to date used for GVHD have potentially life-threatening toxicities. Moreover, teratogenicity in patients post-BMT is not an issue, as these patients are sterile after their preparative regimen.

[1] This work was supported by Grant CA15396 from The National Cancer Institute, The National Institutes of Health.

[2] Scholar of the Leukemia Society.

* Abbreviations used: BMT, bone marrow transplant, GVHD, graft-versus-host disease, Thal, thalidomide, CsA, cyclosporine.

MATERIALS AND METHODS

Animals. Female Lewis ($RT1^l$), ACI ($RT1^a$), and BN ($RT1^b$) rats 12 weeks old were obtained from Sprague Dawley, Inc., Indianapolis, IN.

Drugs and irradiation. Thal (supplied by D. Blake, M.D., Johns Hopkins University) was prepared as a suspension in vegetable oil and given via gavage to animals in a volume of 0.25 ml. Cyclosporine (CsA), generously supplied by Sandoz, Ltd., Basle, Switzerland, was dissolved in 95% ethanol and added to a 4% Tween 20 solution in deionized water. The total dose of CsA per day per rat was 15 mg/kg and was given s.c. Total-body irradiation (TBI) was delivered using a dual source ^{137}Cs small animal irradiator at 116 rad/minute.

Bone marrow transplant. Recipient animals were given TBI at 1050 rads and 60×10^6 donor marrow cells were infused 24 h later. Donor animals were killed by asphyxiation with CO_2. The marrow from femurs, tibias, and humeruses were collected in RPMI tissue culture media (Flow Laboratory, McLean, VA) and 60×10^6 marrow cells were given by tail vein injection in 1 ml. The rats received medicated, acidified water containing Bactrim (generously supplied by Hoffman La Roche, Nutley, NJ), polymyxin, and neomycin. For the first 10 days after transplant, the rats also received gentamycin s.c. Radiation control (untransplanted) rats served to ensure that ablative therapy was given.

The clinical course was documented by biweekly weights and daily observation. GVHD was documented by its clinical appearance (erythema of the skin, ears, and foot-pads) and by skin biopsy. Previously described criteria were used for documenting histologic changes of GVHD in the rat (*4*).

Skin grafting was performed as previously described (*5*). Briefly, donor animals were killed with asphyxiation with CO_2. The animals were shaved, and an average of four 2.5-cm skin grafts were removed per animal and the excess fat removed. Recipient animals were anesthetized and shaved. A corresponding area of skin was removed from the dorsum and the graft was clipped into place using surgical staples. Ten days later the staples were removed and the graft observed for rejection.

Mixed lymphocyte cultures. Iron filing depletion of spleen cells was performed using previously described methods (*6, 7*). Spleens were harvested from animals and single-cell suspensions were made. Then 2×10^8 spleen cells were placed in RPMI and incubated with 50 mg of sterile carbonyl iron in 75-cm^2 culture flasks for 40 min at 37°C. The iron-containing cells (macrophages) were then removed by a magnet. The procedure was repeated once. Macrophage-depleted spleen cells were suspended in complete medium (RPMI supplemented with glutamine 0.25 μg/ml, amphotericin 2.5 μg/ml, penicillin 50 units/ml, streptomycin 50 μg/ml, and 10% heat-inactivated serum from DA strain rats).

Responder cells at 4×10^6 cells/well were cocultured at 37°C in microtiter plates with 6×10^6 irradiated (1500 rads from a ^{137}Cs source) stimulator cells for 5 days; 2 μCi of ^{3}H-thymidine was added and the cells were harvested after 18 h. The samples were then counted in a scintillation counter (Packard TriCarb liquid scintillation spectrometer model 3255).

RESULTS

Skin transplants. Serial trials of prolonging skin graft survival in normal Lewis rats given Thal after ACI skin transplants were uniformly unsuccessful. Animals were treated once a day with escalating doses of 5 mg/kg, 25 mg/kg, 50 mg/kg, and 100 mg/kg per day starting on the day of transplant until graft rejection, as shown in Table 1. All Thal-treated animals and all untreated controls had rejected their grafts by day 10 when the surgical clips were removed. Animals treated with twice-a-day Thal at 50 mg/kg/day had prolongation of their skin grafts to day 21. The effectiveness of Thal was compared with Lewis rats grafted with ACI skin grafts and treated with CsA. All CsA controls (treated at 15 mg/kg/day) had viable skin grafts while the drug was continued but were rejected within 10–14 days after stopping the drug.

Allogeneic BMT treatment of established GVHD. To ascertain whether Thal is effective in the therapy of established GVHD, RT1-mismatched transplants were performed and therapy started once GVHD was present (day 12±2). Lewis rats were transplanted with ACI bone marrow following TBI, as shown in Table 2. Radiation control rats received no marrow and died of aplasia. GVHD control rats received antibiotics only following BMT and died of GVHD within 21 days. Twenty-three rats were allowed to develop severe, blistering acute GVHD. The animals had liver disease as evident by bilirubinuria. Seventeen of these animals were treated with 100 mg/kg/day and 6 animals with 50 mg/kg/day of Thal for 40 days. Twenty-two of the 23 animals had resolution of their GVHD. One animal died of GVHD. After stopping the Thal there was no flare-up of GVHD. However, 3 animals that had severe GVHD did develop biopsy-proved chronic GVHD 3 weeks after Thal was stopped. Chimerism was shown by permanent (>100 days) acceptance of ACI skin grafts placed on the animals after completion of their therapy. In contrast, third-party BN skin grafts were rejected within 10 days.

Allogeneic BMT prophylaxis of GVHD. After showing that Thal could be used to treat GVHD, we tried to prevent GVHD by using Thal prophylactically and compared it with prophylaxis of animals with CsA. Lewis rats were transplanted with ACI bone marrow following TBI, as shown in Table 3. The 6 rats treated with 15 mg/kg/day of CsA remained free of GVHD while on CsA. All developed GVHD within 2 weeks of completing CsA therapy. Tutschka et al. (*8*) had reported permanent tolerance after CsA therapy in the same rat model. The occurrence of GVHD in these rats may be related to a different vehicle and/or a lower dosage regimen than used in the earlier report. Twenty-two rats were treated with Thal starting on the day of BMT, as shown in Table 3. Seventeen rats received 50 mg/kg/day and 5 rats received 100 mg/kg/day. Prophylaxis was successful in all rats that remained free of virus. Eight rats (all treated at 50 mg/kg) developed a clinical infection with rat corona virus characterized by weight loss and parotic swelling. These animals developed mild GVHD as shown by mild erythema of the ears and positive biopsies. All animals responded to continued therapy. Chimerism was shown by acceptance of ACI skin grafts for greater than 100 days and rejection within 10 days of a third-party BN skin graft. No GVHD was seen once the drug was stopped.

Mixed lymphocyte cultures. These were done 100 days after BMT using iron-filing-depleted spleen cells. There was no stimulation of the Thal-treated chimera by Lewis or ACI spleen

TABLE 1. Skin graft survival (in days)

Number of Animals	THAL therapy[a]	CsA Therapy[b]	Mean skin graft survival
8	—	—	≤10
8	—	15 mg/kg/day	52±2
4	5 mg/kg/day	—	≤10
4	25 mg/kg/day	—	≤10
4	50 mg/kg/day	—	±10
4	100 mg/kg/day	—	≤10
4	50 mg/kg/ BID	—	21±0.5

[a] Drug continued until graft rejection.
[b] Drug continued for 40 days.

TABLE 2. Treatment of established GVHD

Evaluable animals	Marrow	Thalidomide therapy[a]	Survival[b]		
			14 Days	40 Days	100 Days
3	None	0	0	0	0
3	ACI	0	3	0	0
6	ACI	50 mg/kg/day	6	6	6
17	ACI	100 mg/kg/day	17	16	15[c]

[a] Thalidomide therapy started when GVHD was clinically and histologically present.
[b] Survival measured from transplantation.
[c] One death from chronic GVHD.

TABLE 3. Prophylaxis for GVHD

Evaluable animals	Marrow	CsA Prophylaxis[a]	Thalidomide prophylaxis[a]	No GVHD		
				14 Days	40 Days	100 Days
3	None	0	0	0[b]	0	0
3	ACI	0	0	0	0	0
6	ACI	15 mg/kg/day	0	6	6	0
17	ACI	0	50 mg/kg/day	9[c]	9	9
5	ACI	0	100 mg/kg/day	5	5	5

[a] All drugs given for 40 days starting the day of transplant.
[b] Dead of aplasia.
[c] Animals developed GVHD following viral infection. GVHD resolved on continued therapy.

TABLE 4. Mixed lymphocyte cultures[a]

Responder	Stimulator	Counts per minute[b]
Thal-chimera	Lewis	767±95
Thal-chimera	ACI	261±32
Thal-chimera	BN	4547±1268
Thal-chimera	Thal-chimera	439±253
Lewis	Thal-chimera	9120±1737
ACI	Thal-chimera	479±210
ACI	ACI	348±52
Lewis	BN	11659±2094
ACI	BN	11137±2880

[a] Representative results from eight experiments.
[b] CPM±SD.

cells in 8 tested chimeric animals. Typical results are shown in Table 4. However, thalidomide chimeras did respond to third-party (BN) allogeneic strain cells.

DISCUSSION

Thal was first synthesized by Kunz et al. in 1956 and was marketed as a sedative (*9*). In 1961 it was withdrawn because of teratogenic effects, and interest in the drug diminished. However, Sheskin made interesting observations on the possible immunologic effects of Thal (*1*). Marked improvement in patients with reactional lepromatous leprosy (also called erythema nodusum leprosum) who were taking Thal as a sedative was observed. As recently reviewed by Barnhill et al. (*2*), Thal has been reported to be beneficial in a number of disorders with a probable immunologic basis including discoid lupus erythematosus, apthous ulcers, Behcet's syndrome, ulcerative colitis, pyoderma gangrenosum, actinic prurigo, and prurigo nedulari (*2*). Most of these reports deal with small numbers of patients in whom conventional therapy failed. Only in reactional lepromatous leprosy and actinic prurigo have larger trials been conducted showing the efficacy of Thal above placebo or conventional therapy (*10, 11*). These data imply the effect of Thal on immune function.

Investigation into the mechanism of Thal's action is scant. Hellmann et al. (*12*) first reported that Thal prolonged skin graft survival in mice with strong and weak H-2 histocompatibility differences. Skin graft survival was longest when the graft was incubated with Thal prior to transplant and the recipient received Thal posttransplant. The longest graft survival was 15 days, with controls lasting 10.9 days. The draining lymph nodes of the grafted animals were examined and found to contain fewer immunoblasts than control animals (*13*). Since no statistical analysis was provided in either study, these results must be viewed as marginal at best. Significant prolongation of skin graft survival after Thal therapy was not consistently found by other investigators (*14–19*).

The present studies examined the immunosuppressive activity of Thal in the prolongation of skin grafts and in the prevention and/or treatment of GVHD. In serial experiments Thal was unable to prolong skin graft survival when given once a day; these data are not in agreement with the observations of Hellman et al. (*12*). Dosage escalation from 5 mg/kg/day to 100 mg/kg/day doubled the survival of the skin grafts. These data indicate that prolonged and repeated treatment is necessary to achieve skin graft prolongation.

The present study also demonstrated the efficacy of Thal in treating established acute GVHD in the rat allogeneic BMT model. Of 23 animals with severe, blistering acute GVHD treated with Thal, 22 animals resolved their disease. The animals appeared to also have hepatic diseases as evidenced by bilirubinuria. Clinical signs, such as hair growth, weight, and erythema improved after about 1 week of therapy. Of importance, there was no clinical flare-up after stopping the drug. However, 3 of 22 surviving rats did develop clinical and biopsy-proved chronic GVHD.

When Thal was started in the recipients on the day of BMT and continued for 40 days post-BMT, no animal that remained free of apparent viral infection developed GVHD. The virally infected animals had mild GVHD that resolved on continued therapy. The etiologic role of viral infection in GVHD in this animal model remains unknown. Several studies have suggested a role of viral infections in triggering GVHD (*20*).

When Thal was used as a prophylactic agent or to treat GVHD, chimerism was established as evidence by acceptance of a skin graft from the marrow donor, but rejection of third-party skin grafts. Furthermore, spleen cells from the chimeric animals did not respond in mixed lymphocyte culture to recipient or donor lymphocytes but responded to third-party stimulator cells. The mechanism accounting for nonreactivity to original recipient lymphocytes in mixed lymphocyte culture and abatement or prevention of GVHD remains unknown. Preliminary studies in mixed lymphocyte culture implicate the presence of regulatory lymphocytes, in the spleens of these animals, that dampen immune responsiveness to host antigens. Previous studies in the Lewis-ACI bone marrow transplant model have demonstrated a critical role of suppressor T cells in the establishment of transplantation tolerance (*21*). Further studies are underway attempting to document suppressor T cells in Thal treated animals.

Thal in this setting was extremely well tolerated. There was more rapid weight gain following BMT in the Thal-treated animals than in the CsA controls (data not shown). There was no clinical evidence of significant toxicity from the Thal treatment. All animals have been kept for at least 3 months following completion of therapy without obvious sequelae except chronic GVHD in the allogeneic transplant group in which the rats had severe GVHD before starting therapy. Clinical studies using Thal to treat such disorders as reactional lepromatous leprosy have likewise shown no long-term sequelae in over 20 years of use (*2*).

Thus, Thal has shown impressive activity in treating and preventing GVHD. The drug was used successfully to treat animals with advanced disease. In animals remaining free of clinical viral infection, Thal prevented GVHD. Even in animals breaking through prophylaxis, GVHD was mild and resolved on further therapy. The drug was well tolerated by the animals, as it was in clinical studies before its withdrawal. Thal may represent an important immunosuppressive agent for use in BMT. The use of Thal in solid organ transplants needs to be further explored. Work on the mechanism of action of Thal has been hampered by its insolubility. New techniques are now being employed that should help clarify its mechanism of action.

REFERENCES

1. Sheskin J. Thalidomide in treatment of lepra reactions. Clin Pharmacol Ther 1965; 6: 303.
2. Barnhill RL, McDougall AC. Thalidomide: use and possible mode of action in reactional lepromatous leprosy and in various other conditions. J Am Acad Dermatol 1982; 7: 317.

3. Field EO, Gibbs JE, Tucker DF, Hellmann K. Effect of thalidomide on the graft versus host reaction. Nature 1966; 211: 1308.
4. Beschorner WE, Tutschka PJ, Santos GW. Sequential morphology of graft versus host disease in the rat radiation chimera. Clin Immunol Immunopathol 1982; 22: 203.
5. Santos GW, Owens AH. A comparison of the effects of selected cytotoxic agents on allogeneic skin graft survival in rats. Bull Hopkins Hosp 1965; 116: 327.
6. Weiss A, Fitch FW. Macrophages suppress CTL generation in rat mixed leukocyte cultures. J Immunol 1977; 119: 510.
7. Hirano T, Nordin AA. The development of suppressor cells and cytotoxic lymphocytes in mixed lymphocyte cultures. J Immunol 1976; 116: 1115.
8. Tutschka PJ, Beschorner WE, Allisom AC, Burns WH, Santos GW. Use of cyclosporine A in allogeneic bone marrow transplant (BMT) in the rat. Nature 1979; 280: 148.
9. Kunz W, Keller H, Mueckter H. N-Phthalyl-glutaminsaure-imid: experimentelle Untersuchungen an einem neuen synthetischen Product mit sedativen Eigenschaften. Arzneimittelforsch 1956; 6: 426.
10. Iyer CS, Languillon J, Ramunujam K, et al. WHO coordinated short term double blind trial with thalidomide in the treatment of acute lepra reaction in male lepromatous patients. Bull WHO 1971; 45: 719.
11. Tamayo L, Ruiz-Maldonado R. Dermatitis solar. Estudio doble clego cruzado Talidomida, Hidoxicina, Placeba. Proc Int Derm Congr Mex 1978; 219.
12. Hellmann K, Duke DI, Tucker DF. Prolongation of skin homograft survival by thalidomide. Br Med J 1965; 2: 687.
13. Hellmann K. Effect of thalidomide on the immunological response in local lymph nodes after a skin homograft. Lancet 1966; 1: 1134.
14. Playfair JHC, Leuchars E, Davies AJS. Effect of thalidomide on skin graft survival. Lancet 1963; 1: 1003.
15. Bore PJ, Scothorne RJ. Effect of thalidomide on survival of skin homografts in rabbits. Lancet 1966; 1: 1240.
16. Floersheim GL. Another chance for thalidomide? Lancet 1966; 1: 207.
17. Dukor P, Dietrich FM. Immunosuppression by thalidomide? Lancet 1967; 1: 569.
18. Mouzas GL, Gershon RK. The effect of thalidomide on skin allografts in mice: survival of the grafts. Transplantation 1968; 6: 476.
19. Murphy GP, Brede HD, Weber HW. Groenwald JH, Williams PD. Thalidomide immunosupression in canine renal transplantation. J Med Exp Clin 1970; 1: 66.
20. Pollard M, Truitt RL. Allogeneic bone marrow chimerism in free mice. I. Prevention of spontaneous leukemia in AKR mice. Proc Soc Exp Biol Med 1973; 144: 659.
21. Tutschka PJ, Hess AD, Beschorner WE, Santos GW. Suppressor cells in transplantation tolerance I. Suppressor cells in the mechanism of tolerance in radiation chimeras. Transplantation 1981; 32: 203.

Received 20 June 1985.
Accepted 15 August 1985.

0041-1337/86/4105-0648$02.00/0
TRANSPLANTATION

Vol. 41, No. 5
Printed in U.S.A.

TRANSFUSION OF DONOR CLASS I MHC ANTIGEN PRIOR TO KIDNEY TRANSPLANTATION IN DOGS[1]

Studies in rodent islet allograft models have supported the concept that the elimination of viable class II major histcompatibility (MHC)*-antigen-positive cells from an allograft prior to transplantation results in prolonged graft survival (*1, 2*). It has been postulated that the presentation of class I MHC antigens in this context conveys a tolerogenic signal to the recipient (*3*). This concept was further strengthened by the demonstration that pretransplant transfusion of donor strain blood depleted of viable class II MHC-positive cells leads to prolonged survival of fresh, untreated islet allografts in the congenic mouse and inbred rat models (*4, 5*). Similarly, renal allograft survival in the rat has been indefinitely prolonged by the pretransplant administration of donor cells expressing only class I antigen (*6*). We sought to determine whether this concept could be extended to the canine renal allograft model.

Rodent red blood cells express class I but not class II MHC antigens. These antigens are absent from the red blood cells of larger animals such as dogs and man, but class I MHC molecules are expressed on canine platelets while class II molecules are not (*7, 8*). Thus, a purified population of platelets seems to be the ideal preparation to use for pretransplant transfusion in large animal models.

Several investigators have examined the immune effects of platelet transfusions in large animals with conflicting results (*9–13*). In all of these studies the platelets were purified solely by mechanical means, with a resulting contamination of approximately one leukocyte per 5×10^4 platelets. Since between 4×10^9 (*11*) and 2×10^{10} (*12, 13*) platelets were used for transfusion, the number of leukocytes included in the transfusates varied from 8×10^4 to 4×10^5. Most canine peripheral blood lymphocytes express class II MHC antigens (*14*). Therefore, in the previous canine studies, approximately 2×10^5 viable class-II-antigen–positive lymphocytes were included in these transfusions, and their presence may have significantly influenced the results. Likewise immunosuppression was employed in these studies, and it has been demonstrated that immunosuppression may be detrimental to the induction and expression of tolerance (*15, 16*).

In this study we eliminated contaminating class-II-MHC-antigen–positive cells from the mechanically purified platelet suspension by treatment with a monoclonal antibody specific for canine class II antigens and complement. No pharmacologic immunosuppression was employed.

Mongrel dogs weighing between 17 and 22 kg were randomly assigned to pairs. Each member of a pair acted as the donor of both platelets and kidney for its partner. Platelets were isolated from 30 cc of ethylenediaminotetraacetate (EDTA) blood by repeated centrifugations and washings in a manner similar to that described by Claas (*17*). The resultant platelet suspension contained less than one leukocyte per 5×10^4 platelets.

Platelet preparations that were to be depleted of class-II-MHC–positive cells were treated with the murine monoclonal antibody B1F6 (IgG2a) (kindly supplied by Rodolfo Alejandro, M.D. and Daniel H. Mintz, M.D., of the University of Miami School of Medicine) followed by rabbit complement. This antibody recognizes a monomorphic determinant of canine Ia-like molecules (*7*). Microcytotoxicity testing demonstrated that incubation of canine lymphocytes with B1F6 for 60 min at 4°C followed by rabbit complement for 30 min at 37°C resulted in 70–80% cell killing, a figure that is consistent with the distribution of Ia-like antigens on canine lymphocytes reported by Deeg (*14*).

Recipients were divided into groups according to their transfusion status prior to transplantation. Group 1 served as a control group and was not transfused. A second control group received 1.3×10^9–1.7×10^9 donor platelets i.v. three weeks, two weeks, and one week prior to renal allografting. Group 3 received three transfusions at identical times pretransplant of 0.8×10^9–1.3×10^9 donor platelets that had been depleted of contaminating Class-II-positive lymphoid cells by incubation with B1F6 and rabbit complement. These preparations contained less than one leukocyte per 3×10^5 platelets.

To determine whether the presence of significant numbers of Class-II-MHC-antigen–negative lymphocytes influences tolerance induction, a fourth group of dogs received three transfusions of donor lymphocytes that had been depleted of Class-II-antigen–expressing cells by incubation with B1F6 and complement. To prepare these lymphocytes 30 cc of EDTA blood was centrifuged for 15 min at 500 g. The plasma and buffy coat were taken off and diluted 1:2 with Waymouth's media and layered over a Ficoll-hypaque gradient, specific gravity 1.077, in a 7 cc buffy coat:3 cc Ficoll-hypaque ratio and centrifuged for 30 min at 500 g. The lymphocyte layer was removed and incubated with B1F6 for 60 min at 4°C, washed once, and incubated for 30 min at 37°C with rabbit complement. The remaining cells were washed three times prior to transfusion. Each transfusate consisted of 2×10^6 to 4×10^6 cells.

The renal allografts were implanted into the right iliac fossa, and a bilateral nephrectomy was done at the time of transplantation. Serological crossmatches were not performed, and no pharmacologic immunosuppression was administered. Serum creatinine concentration was determined daily and the day when the serum creatinine equalled or exceeded 3.0 mg/dl was taken as the day of graft failure.

The results are depicted in Table 1. Donor-specific platelet transfusions were ineffective in prolonging graft survival. Furthermore, transfusions with donor platelets treated with anti-Class-II MHC monoclonal antibody and complement had no effect on renal allograft survival. Because the transfusions in

[1] This work was supported in part by a grant from the National Kidney Foundation of the Upper Midwest.

* Abbreviations used: EDTA, ethylenediaminotetraacetate, MHC, major histocompatibility complex.

Table 1. Renal allograft functional survival times according to pretransplant recipient treatment

Group	n	Pretransplant transfusion	Day when creatinine was ≥3.0	Mean ± SD
I	8	None	3, 5, 5, 5, 5, 6, 6, 7	5.3±1.2
II	7	Donor platelets	1, 1, 2, 3, 4, 4, 6	3.0±1.8
III	10	Donor platelets treated with $B1F_6$ + C′	2, 5, 5, 5, 5, 6, 7, 8, 11, 15	6.9±3.7
IV	4	Donor lymphocytes treated with $B1F_6$ + C′	1, 3, 4, 5	3.3±1.7

the rodent models included viable Class-II-MHC-antigen–negative lymphocytes that may have been important in the induction of the tolerant state we included a group of dogs that received a preparation of donor lymphocytes that had been treated with B1F6 monoclonal antibody and complement to remove the Class-II-MHC-antigen–positive cells. No prolongation of allograft survival was observed in these dogs.

Thus we have no evidence that the presentation of Class I major histocompatibility system antigens in the absence of Class II antigens leads to prolonged graft survival in a large animal model. This is not to argue, however, that different protocols of pretransplant platelet transfusions might not have a salutatory effect on allograft survival.

It has been argued that the inconsistent results, in terms of allograft survival, observed after the pretransplant administration of various blood products to recipients are due to the fact that the blood product preparations were contaminated with variable numbers of viable Ia-positive lymphoid cells and the fact that immunosuppressive drugs were employed (*4*). According to this line of reasoning the selective administration of donor Class I MHC antigen in the absence of generalized immunosuppression results in the preferential activation of suppressor cell networks. Our results do not support this concept.

In large animal models a beneficial effect of blood transfusions has been seen only in conjunction with the administration of immunosuppression (*18*). It has been hypothesized that blood transfusions immunize the recipient to donor histocompatibility antigens but the responding clones are eliminated by the high-dose immunosuppression employed postoperatively (*19*).

Bijnen et al. (*12, 13*) employed immunosuppression in conjunction with both third-party and donor-specific platelet transfusions and failed to observe a beneficial effect (*11, 12*). Likewise, the only reported clinical trial utilizing platelet transfusions failed to demonstrate a beneficial effect (*20*). Therefore, it appears that pretransplant platelet transfusions are ineffective in prolonging allograft survival whether or not generalized immunosuppression is employed.

In summary, prior to transplantation we administered donor-specific Class I MHC antigens to canine recipients of renal allografts in a model that did not employ immunosuppressive drugs. No prolongation of allograft function was observed. It did not matter whether the donor Class I antigen was presented to the recipient on the surface of donor platelets or donor lymphocytes. Our results do not support the argument that the selective administration of donor Class I MHC antigen in the absence of immunosuppression results in preferential activation of suppressor cell networks.

Paul F. Gores[2]
Antonio Sitges-Serra
Uwe J. Hesse
John S. Najarian
David E.R. Sutherland
The Department of Surgery
University of Minnesota Hospital
Minneapolis, Minnesota.

[2] Dr. Gores is a recipient of a NRSA Fellowship AM07187 from the National Institutes of Health.

REFERENCES

1. Faustman D, Hauptfeld V, Lacy P, Davie J. Prolongation of murine islet allograft survival by pretreatment of islets with antibody directed to Ia determinants. Proc Natl Acad Sci USA 1981; 78: 5156.
2. Lau H, Reemtsma K, Hardy MA. Prolongation of rat islet allograft survival by direct ultraviolet irradiation of the graft. Science 1984; 223: 607.
3. Lafferty KJ, Prowse SJ, Simeonovic CJ, Warren HS. Immunobiology of tissue transplantation: a return to the passenger leukocytes concept. Ann Rev Immunol 1983; 1: 143.
4. Faustman D, Lacy P, Davie J, Hauptfeld V. Prevention of allograft rejection by immunization with donor blood depleted of Ia-bearing. Science 1982; 217: 157.
5. Lau H, Reemtsma K, Hardy MA. Pancreatic islet allograft prolongation by donor-specific blood transfusions treated with ultraviolet irradiation. Science 1983; 221: 754.
6. Wood KJ, Evins J, Morris PJ. Suppression of renal allograft rejection in the rat by Class I antigens on purified erythrocytes. Transplantation 1985; 39: 56.
7. Alejandro R, Shienvold FL, Latif Z, Esquenazi V, Miller J, Mintz DH. Monoclonal antibodies recognizing canine and human Ia-like antigens. Transplantation 1984; 38: 542.
8. Deeg HJ. Personal communication.
9. Rowinski W, Ryffa T, Ruke M, Wasowska B, Tilney NL, Olszewski WL. Platelet-induced donor-specific unresponsiveness to kidney allografts in mongrel dogs treated with ALG. Transplant Proc 1981; 13: 586.
10. Oh JH, McClure HM, Tuttle EP. Immunological unresponsiveness induced by platelet transfusion in rhesus monkeys. Transplantation 1983; 36: 727.
11. Borleffs JCC, Neuhaus P, van Rood JJ, Bahner H. Platelet transfusions have a positive effect on kidney allograft survival in rhesus monkeys and induce virtually no cytotoxic antibodies. Transplant Proc 1983; 15: 985.
12. Bijnen AB, Heineman E, Marquet RL, et al. Lack of beneficial effect of thrombocyte transfusions on kidney graft survival in dogs. Transplantation 1984; 37: 213.
13. Bijnen AB, Marquet RL, Obertop H, Heineman E, Niessen GJCM, Jeekel J. Donor-specific transfusions of whole blood and thrombocytes prior to kidney transplantation in dogs. Transplant Proc 1985; 17: 1091.
14. Deeg HJ, Wulff JC, DeRose S. Unusual distribution of Ia-like antigens on canine lymphocytes. Immunogenetics 1982; 16: 445.
15. Kibshaw P, Brent L, Brooks CG, New RRC, Pinto M. Studies on the mechanism of specific unresponsiveness to skin allografts in mice. Transplant Proc 1975; 7: 385.
16. Wood ML, Monaco AP. Differential effect of cyclophosphamide on states of specific allograft unresponsiveness in immunosuppressed mice. Transplantation 1979; 27: 186.
17. Claas FHJ, Smeenk RJT, Schmidt R, van Steenbrugge GJ, Eernisse JG. Alloimmunization against the MHC antigens after

platelet transfusions is due to contaminating leukocytes in the platelet suspension. Exp Hematol 1981; 9: 84.
18. Niessen GJCM, Obertop H, Bijnen AB, Marquet TL, Jeekel J. Expression of beneficial blood transfusion effect in dogs is dependent upon immunosuppressants used. Transplant Proc 1982; 14: 400.
19. Terasaki PI. The beneficial transfusion effect on kidney graft survival attributed to clonal deletion. Transplantation 1984; 37: 119.
20. Chapman JR, Fisher M, Ting A, Morris PJ. Platelet transfusion before renal transplantation in humans. Transplant Proc 1985; 17: 1038.

Received 6 September 1985.
Accepted 18 September 1985.

THE INFLUENCE OF THE TRANSPLANTATION TECHNIQUE ON THE DURATION OF ENDOCRINE FUNCTION OF PANCREAS ALLOGRAFTS IN THE RAT MODEL

In experiments investigating the influence of the transplantation technique on the morphology and function of syngeneic pancreas grafts in the rat model, one of the important variables turned out to be the management of exocrine drainage. The techniques that are used can be divided into two types. The first type provides drainage of the exocrine secretion, leaving the appearance of the organ under the light microscope unchanged. The second type prevents the drainage of the exocrine secretion, leading, to a lesser or greater degree, to morphological and functional alterations in the graft (*1, 2*).

Comparatively little attention has been paid thus far to the significance of the amount of tissue being grafted—i.e., whether only a segment of the organ or the whole pancreas was grafted (*3*). The objective of the present experiments was to investigate the influence of these two variables—the management of exocrine drainage and the number of grafted islets—on the ability of allografts to maintain their endocrine function under a defined immunological attack. We therefore chose a strain combination that shows a very constant rejection reaction with few interindividual differences.

Initially we compared a group of animals with grafts with a reduced mass of islets and unphysiological management of the exocrine secretion (duct-ligated segmental grafts) with animals with grafts with physiological secretion drainage and the maximum mass of islets obtainable from one donor (pancreaticoduodenal grafts). In additional experiments the rejection reaction was delayed by short-term immunosuppression with cyclosporine. The rationale behind this measure was to allow alterations related to the technique, particularly to the ligation of the duct system, time to develop. A third group included in this series of experiments was recipients of duct-ligated whole organ grafts. With this we hoped to achieve a more detailed analysis of the influence of the islet cell mass and the secretion drainage on graft function.

LEW ($RT1^{l}$) rats, rendered diabetic by 55 mg/kg streptozotocin, were always used as recipients. Allograft donors were DA rats ($RT1^{av1}$), which are major histocompatibility complex and non-major-histocompatibility-complex-different from LEW rats. A rat was defined as being hyperglycemic and was used for transplantation after the induction of diabetes when the blood sugar level exceeded 20 mmol/L at least three days after the injection of streptozotocin. After transplantation, however, beginning of hyperglycemia or loss of graft function was defined as the first day of persisting hyperglycemia above 11 mmol/L.

For immunosuppression, cyclosporine was dissolved in olive oil and given via a gastric tube at a dose of 15 mg/kg/day. A group of diabetic animals (C_1, n=10) and a group of recipients of syngeneic grafts (C_2, n=10) served as controls. All pancreas grafts were transplanted heterotopically into the abdomen. Vascular supply was provided by a segment of the donor's aorta bearing the celiac axis and by the portal vein. Both vessels were anastomosed end-to-side to the recipient's infrarenal aorta and vena cava. The pancreaticoduodenal graft (n=20) consisted of the entire pancreas with the attached duodenum. The oral end of the duodenum was closed; the aboral end was anastomosed to the recipient's jejunum. In the case of the duct-ligated whole-organ grafts (n=23) the duodenum was also dissected from the pancreas, but the bile duct was ligated. The segmental graft (n=19) consisted of a left hemipancreas with ligated duct system (Fig. 1).

For statistical comparison of the different groups the Wilcoxon test was used. A difference was considered significant if $P<0.01$.

The animals in the untreated diabetic control group C_1 remained hyperglycemic, with blood sugar levels up to 30 mmol/L, constant polyuria, and weight loss over an observation period of 150 days. Diabetic recipients of pancreaticoduodenal isografts (group C_2) had a serum glucose level lower than 11 mmol/L on the first postoperative day and remained thus for more than 200 days. All animals in the experimental groups became hyperglycemic after rejection of their grafts. Duct-ligated segmental grafts discontinued their endocrine function between days 7 and 8 postoperatively—i.e., the serum glucose level of the recipients exceeded 11 mmol/L. Pancreaticoduodenal grafts ceased to function between 7 and 9 days postoperatively (Table 1). After 14 days of treatment with cyclosporine, duct-ligated segmental grafts functioned for a period of 18–24 days. Duct-ligated whole-organ grafts kept the recipient normoglycemic for 22–25 days, and pancreaticoduodenal grafts—i.e., whole-organ grafts with secretory drainage—for 25–27 days (Table 2).

From a merely statistical point of view, these results show that duct-ligated segmental grafts always function for a shorter period than whole-organ grafts with secretory drainage do. Following short-term immunosuppression, duct-ligated whole-organ grafts function longer than duct-ligated segmental grafts do, and whole organ grafts with secretory drainage function longer than duct ligated whole-organ grafts do.

The possible cause and the biological relevance of these findings need to be discussed. The MHC and non-MHC-different strain combination DA-LEW that we used is a combination that reacts particularly strongly. This is shown clearly by the very short rejection times for other organs (*4, 5*). In addition, the rejection reaction of the animals in the individual groups is quite uniform. This was established in previous investigations of the histological course of the rejection reaction (*6*) and is confirmed by the slight deviations from the mean in the experimental groups used in the present experiments. Thus we consider this model to be useful for investigating variables with only a slight absolute effect on the graft function.

How are the differences in the duration of endocrine function

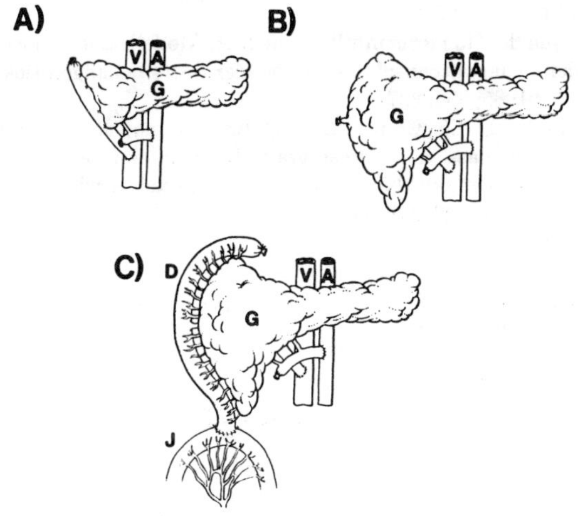

FIGURE 1. Techniques for pancreatic transplantation in the rat: (A) duct-ligated segmental graft; (B) duct-ligated whole organ; (C) pancreaticoduodenal graft (A = aorta, D = donor duodenum, G = graft, J = jejunum, V = vena cava inf.)

TABLE 1. Duration of endocrine function of pancreatic allografts (DA [$RT1^{av1}$] → LEW [$RT1^{l}$]) transplanted with two techniques

Technique	n	Days	Mean
Duct-ligated segment	10	7, 7, 7, 7, 7, 7, 7, 7, 7, 8	7.1
Pancreaticoduodenal graft (drained whole organ)	10	7, 8, 8, 8, 8, 8, 8, 9, 9, 9	8.2

TABLE 2. Duration of endocrine function of pancreatic allografts (DA [$RT1^{av1}$] → LEW [$RT1^{l}$]) transplanted with three different techniques after treatment of the recipient with 15 mg/kg/day cyclosporine orally for 14 days postoperatively

Technique	n	Days	Mean
Duct-ligated segment	9	18, 20, 21, 21, 21, 22, 22, 23, 24	21.3
Duct-ligated whole organ	13	22, 22, 23, 23, 23, 23, 23, 24, 24, 24, 24, 24, 25	23.4
Pancreaticoduodenal graft (drained whole organ)	10	25, 25, 25, 26, 26, 26, 26, 26, 26, 27	25.8

that we observed to be explained? One explanation is that a defined amount of insulin is necessary to achieve a defined blood sugar level (here 11 mmol/L was chosen), and the amount of insulin released depends on the quality and the quantity of islets available. During the course of these experiments the number of initially transplanted islets is affected not only by the rejection reaction but also by the results of the management of exocrine drainage—i.e., occlusion of the duct system or drainage. It is known from histological investigations that if the exocrine secretion is successfully drained, both the islets and the exocrine tissue remain intact. However, in the rat the differences between duct ligation and various forms of occlusion are only slight, and duct occlusion leads to the loss of exocrine tissue and to structural alterations in the islets, such as disintegration and connective tissue infiltration (*2, 7*).

With a normal, unmanipulated rejection reaction, the differences in the duration of exocrine function between the theoretically most favorable model (whole-organ graft with secretory drainage) and the least favorable model (duct-ligated segmental graft) were slight and presumably not relevant. Therefore we did not investigate further models along this line.

After the rejection reaction has been delayed with cyclosporine, the differences in the duration of exocrine function become more evident. For this reason we decided that it would be interesting to graft duct-ligated whole organs also. This made it possible to compare duct-ligated grafts with a reduced mass of islets and with a maximum mass of islets. It also made it possible to compare grafts with a maximum mass of islets with different methods of managing exocrine drainage.

Why does the effect of the transplantation technique on the function of the organs increase after immunosuppression? In our opinion, the reason is that during the administration of cyclosporine the destruction of the graft is prevented (*6*), whereas the processes induced by duct ligation are progressive (*2*). After immunosuppression is discontinued, the rejection reaction occurs in increasingly altered organs. These alterations evidently reduce the ability of the organs to withstand rejection. If a reduced mass of islets is grafted a priori, an even more rapid loss of function occurs. The changes following duct occlusion in the rat pancreas continue to progress for up to 300 days (*2*). Thus, it is possible that if the rejection reaction were delayed for an even longer period the differences in the duration of exocrine function between the transplantation models would be more evident.

We conclude from these results that, at least in the rat, the rejection of pancreas grafts, which is normally defined as the recurrence of hyperglycemia, is not only dependent on the immunogenetically defined rejection reaction, but also influenced, to a certain extent, by the transplantation technique. The best functional results are achieved with whole-organ grafts with secretory drainage. Thus the transplantation technique has a modifying influence on the course of the rejection reaction. The biological relevance of these findings is, in our view, that when an optimum transplantation technique is used, more functional reserves are evidently available. This is possibly advantageous for the treatment of acute rejection reactions and for overcoming rejection crises.

These results can be seen as experimental support for the view that to achieve optimum long-term function in human pancreas transplantation, it is important both to graft as large a number of islets as possible and to use a transplantation technique providing secretory drainage, to avoid unnecessary damage to the islets (*8*).

WOLFGANG TIMMERMANN
THOMAS SCHANG
ARNULF THIEDE
Chirurgische Universitätsklinik der Christian-Albrechts-Universität
D-2300 Kiel 1
Bundesrepublik Deutschland

REFERENCES

1. Steiniger B, Klempnauer J, Brüsch U, Wonigeit K. Histology of rejection in rat pancreas allografts with suppressed or preserved exocrine function. Transplant Proc 1984; 16: 783.
2. Nolan MS, Lindsey NJ, Savas CP, et al. Pancreatic transplantation in the rat. Long-term study following different methods of management of exocrine drainage. Transplantation 1983; 36: 26.
3. Squifflet JP, Sutherland DER, Morrow CE, Florack G, Field J, Najarian JS. Comparison of rejection of intraportal islet versus

immediately vascularized segmental pancreatic allografts in rats in relation to beta cell mass engrafted. Transplant Proc 1983; 15: 1344.
4. Engemann R, Ulrichs K, Thiede A, Müller-Ruchholtz W, Hamelmann H. Induction of liver graft tolerance in a primarily non-tolerant rat strain combination with temporary treatment of cyclosporine. Transplant Proc 1983; 15: 2986.
5. Homan WP, Fabre JW, Williams KA, Millard PR, Morris PJ. Studies on the immunosuppressive properties of cyclosporin A in rats receiving renal allografts. Transplantation 1980; 29: 261.
6. Timmermann W, Schang T, Thiede A. Modelle und Perspektiven der Pankreastransplantation bei der Ratte II. Langenbecks Arch Chir 1985; 363: 235.
7. Schang T, Timmermann W, Thiede A. Modelle und Perspektiven der Pankreastransplantation bei der Ratte I. Langenbecks Arch Chir 1985; 363: 227.
8. Sutherland DER, Chinn PL, Elick BA, Najarian JS. Maximization of islet mass in pancreas grafts by near or total whole organ excision without the duodenum from the cadaver donor's. Transplant Proc 1984; 16: 115.

Received 16 April 1985.
Accepted 9 September 1985.

THE EFFECT OF EXCHANGE BLOOD TRANSFUSIONS ON THE CYTOTOXIC ALLOANTIBODY RESPONSE IN AS STRAIN RATS

Plasmapheresis has been extensively used to treat a number of antibody-mediated diseases (*1–3*). Recently it has been used to reduce cytotoxic alloantibody levels in potential renal transplant patients (*4*). There have been several studies using purified protein antigens showing that plasmapheresis (*5*) or exchange transfusions (*6, 7*) can modify antibody responses producing "rebound" phenomena. However, the kinetics of alloantibody responses following modification of circulating immunoglobulin levels, such as by plasma exchange, has not been established. Because repeated intensive plasmapheresis in rats is impracticable, we have used whole-blood exchanges to mimic the effect of plasma exchange and its effects on cytotoxic alloantibody responses in AS ($RT1^l$) strain rats.

A whole-blood exchange was achieved by cardiac puncture that removed approximately half the circulating blood volume. This volume was immediately restored by nonheparinized syngeneic blood into a lateral tail vein. Four such exchanges within 24 hr was found to remove greater than 90% of the circulating blood volume as determined by the distribution of ^{51}chromium (^{51}Cr)-labeled syngeneic red cells administered i.v.

Cytotoxic antibody was determined using the modified technique of Gailiunas et al. (*8*) Briefly, 2×10^7 August ($RT1^c$, $RT2^a$, $RT3^a$) or LOU ($RT1^u$, $RT2^b$) strain spleen lymphocytes were labeled with ^{51}Cr (18 Mbq) in 100 μl of Hanks' balanced salt solution for 1 hr at 37°C. The cells were washed three times with Hanks' balanced salt solution and resuspended at 10^6 ml. Equal volumes of ^{51}Cr-labeled target cells (25 μl) and serially diluted rat sera were incubated for 30 min at room temperature. Guinea pig complement (25 μl; diluted 1:4 with Hanks' balanced salt solution) was added, and the mixture incubated for a further 1 hr. Additional Hanks' balanced salt solution was then added to give a final volume of 200 μl, the plates were spun at 800 g for 5 min, and half the supernatant removed for ^{51}Cr counting. Cytotoxicity was calculated by the following formula:

$$\%^{51}\text{Cr released} = \frac{\text{experimental cpm released—background cpm}}{\text{maximum cpm released—background cpm}} \times 100$$

The effect of four exchange blood transfusions within 24 hr of 1 ml August strain blood (i.v.) on the development of anti-August antibody response is shown in Figure 1.

Normally, the anti-August antibody response reached peak values five days after antigen administration, and these levels were sustained for at least a further 15 days. In the exchanged-transfused rats, the antibody response showed a similar time course, but the cytotoxic activity was enhanced on days 5 and 10 (significant to P=0.01 and P=0.05, respectively, Wilcoxon rank-sum test).

This elevation of antibody response was only observed when exchange transfusions were performed immediately after antigen administration but not at intervals of 10, 20, or even 50 days after injecting August blood (Table 1). This enhanced antibody response after exchange blood transfusions was not diminished upon several dilutions of the sera (Figure 2), and

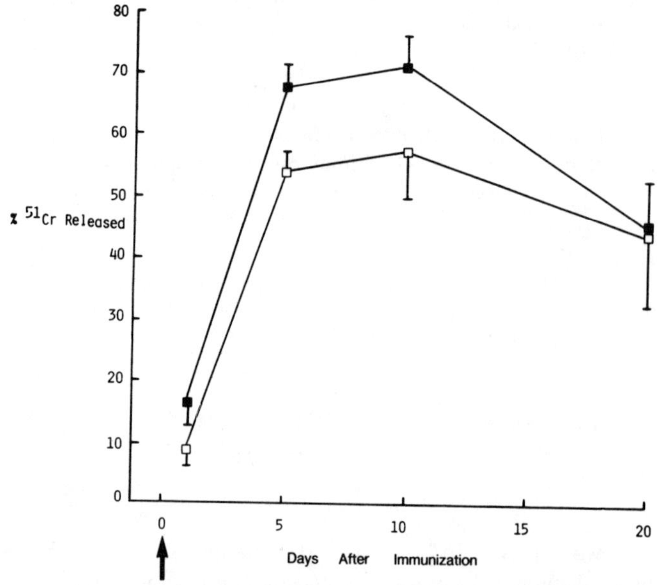

FIGURE 1. Anti-August antibody responses of AS rats given 1 ml August blood (i.v.) followed by 4 whole-blood exchanges within 24 hr. Five rats in each group; vertical bars represent standard deviations. (□) August blood only; (■) August blood and 4 whole-blood exchanges; (↑) Administration of 1 ml August blood (i.v.).

TABLE 1. Anti-August antibody responses in AS rats exchange-transfused at different times after 1 ml of August blood i.v.[a]

Groups	Time of exchange transfusions after August blood (days)			
	0	10	20	50
Controls	54.0±4.7[b]	60.6±6.8	43.3±8.6	12.7±1.0
Exchange-transfused	67.6±3.9	57.9±8.4	40.2±7.2	15.0±3.1

[a] Sera were taken five days after exchange transfusions and tested at 1:20 dilution. Five rats in each group except the day 50 groups which contained 3 rats.

[b] Mean % ^{51}Cr released±SD.

had greater cytolytic activity than an AS anti-August hyperimmune serum. This effect was antibody-mediated and specific, as indicated by controls omitting complement and assays using third-party LOU lymphocyte targets. Whole-blood exchange alone did not cause any increase in background ^{51}Cr release.

The effect of whole blood exchange on the secondary alloantibody response was also assessed. AS rats were primed with 1 ml August blood and then rechallenged 52 days later with a similar volume of blood, (by this time the primary antibody response had declined to background level) followed by four whole-blood exchanges within 24 hr. The anti-August antibody response is shown in Figure 3. As expected, the secondary anti-August antibody response was boosted by the additional August blood, with sustained antibody levels achieved five days after the second injection. However, whole-blood exchange had no detectable effect on development of anti-August antibody or its cytolytic activity (Figure 3).

Our data demonstrate that in rats only immediate intensive exchange transfusions following antigen administration stimulated the primary antibody response to alloantigens. Exchange transfusions failed to cause a rebound of an established primary antibody response and had no effect on the development of secondary antibody response.

These results partly agree with the studies of Brada et al. (5) and Bystryn et al. (7) who showed that delayed plasma exchange or exchange transfusions can modify a primary response to protein antigens. However, they conflict with the report of Brada in which the secondary response to bovine serum albumin was permanently depressed after plasma exchange. This may be because in our study whole blood was removed, rather than plasma alone. This would remove the current circulating lymphocyte population, which may disturb antigen dissemination, alter mononuclear cell homing, or remove suppressor cells. This may account for the effect of whole-blood exchange only being detected soon after administration of antigen. The secondary response is so vigorous that a similar increase in antibody response due to exchange transfusions could easily be obscured.

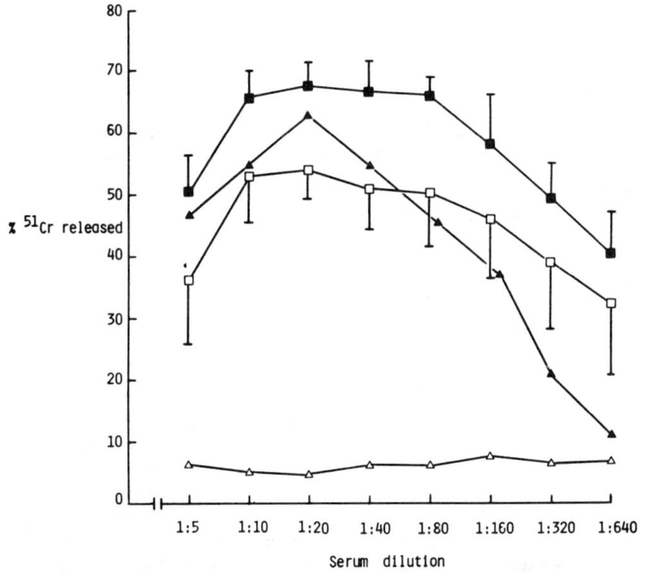

FIGURE 2. Titration of anti-August antibody responses from AS rats given 1 ml August blood (i.v.) followed by 4 whole-blood exchanges within 24 hr. Sera taken five days after treatment. Five rats in each group; vertical bars represent standard deviations. (□) August blood only; (■) August blood and 4 whole-blood exchanges; (▲) Hyperimmune AS-anti-August antiserum; (Δ) Pooled AS serum control.

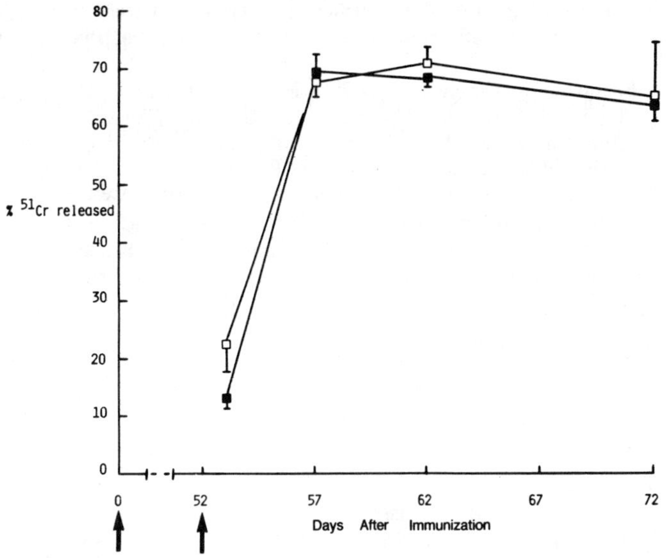

FIGURE 3. Anti-August antibody responses of AS rats given 1 ml August blood (i.v.) followed by a further 1 ml August blood 52 days later and 4 whole-blood exchanges within 24 hr. Five rats in each group; vertical bars represent standard deviations. (□) August blood days 0 and 52; (■) August blood day 0 and August blood plus 4 whole-blood exchanges on day 52; (↑) Administration of 1 ml August blood (i.v.).

In summary, we have shown that whole-blood exchanges in rats can modify their antibody response to alloantigeneic blood. This antibody response was only changed when the whole-blood exchanges were performed immediately after the primary challenge, but not if delayed or after secondary challenge. It appears that the timing and the type of immunogen may be important in the regulation of the feedback mechanism responsible for antibody synthesis and its modification by plasmapheresis.

N. MISTRY
T. HORSBURGH
P. S. VEITCH
P. R. F. BELL
Department of Surgery
Leicester General Hospital
Leicester LE5 4PW, England

REFERENCES

1. Pinching AJ. Recent advances in immunological therapy. Br J Anaesth 1979; 51: 21.
2. Wenz B, Barland P. Therapeutic intensive plasmapheresis. Semin Hematol 1981; 18: 147.
3. Dau PC. Plasmapheresis. Arch Neurol 1984: 647.
4. Taube DH, Cameron JS, Ogg CS, et al. Renal transplantation after removal and prevention of resynthesis of HLA antibodies. Lancet 1984; 14: 824.
5. Brada RF, Moldow CF, McCullough JJ, Jacob HS. Plasma exchange in the treatment of immune disease. Transfusion 1975; 15: 570.
6. Bystryn J, Graf MW, Uhr JW. Regulation of antibody formation by serum antibody. J Exp Med 1970; 132: 1279.
7. Bystryn J, Schenken I, Uhr JW. A model for regulation of antibody synthesis by serum antibody. Prog Immunol 1971: 627.
8. Gailiunas P, Suthanthiran M, Person A, Carpenter CB, Garovoy MR. Immunologic monitoring in the diagnosis of renal allograft rejection. Transplant Proc 1977; 9: 1823.

Received 11 July 1985.
Accepted 9 September 1985.

OPTIMIZATION BY TIMING OF ORAL CYCLOSPORINE TO PREVENT ACUTE KIDNEY ALLOGRAFT REJECTION IN DOGS[1]

Cyclosporine (CsA)* is a powerful immunosuppressive drug able to prevent or greatly delay the onset of acute allograft rejection both in experimental (*1*) and in clinical transplantation (*2*). Its utilization, however, has been correlated with a high incidence of nephrotoxicity already evident in therapeutic doses (*2, 3*). Since CsA nephrotoxicity is dose-related, the optimization of this drug's immunosuppressive properties could lower the dosage needed to prevent acute graft rejection and thus reduce nephrotoxicity. Earlier studies in rats have shown that the immunosuppressive properties of CsA can be enhanced by treatment timing. More specifically, male inbred Lewis rats kept in light (L) and darkness (D) alternating at 12-hr intervals (LD12:12) were studied for both CsA toxicity and immunosuppression (*4, 5*). Treatment during the dark span (the animals' active span) was associated with a higher susceptibility to lethal pulmonary infection of intact rats given high single daily doses of CsA i.p. (20 mg/kg body weight/day). Moreover, a rejection of a heart allografted across a major histocompatibility barrier was delayed with low single i.p. daily doses of CsA (1.25 mg/kg bw) given during the daily dark span. Two subsequent studies with segmental pancreas allografts from ACI rats into diabetic Lewis inbred rats extended the scope of the previous results. CsA circadian timing again determined the extent of prolongation of graft function (*6, 7*).

Against this background, we tested potential benefit from the circadian timing of CsA in a medium-sized animal, the dog, with a kidney allograft, kept on an LD12:12 regimen. CsA was administered i.v. via an implanted, externally programmable pump (Medtronic Inc., Minneapolis, MN). A circadian sinusoidal schedule of CsA peaking in the middle of the dark span was associated with a gain factor of nearly 2 (100% increase) in graft survival (when the duration of graft function associated with CsA delivery peaking in the middle of the light span was equated to 100%) (*8*). Accordingly, we tested and validated, in the experimental model of kidney-allografted dogs, the possibility that the results obtained with a pump could be exploited for the much more practical oral administration of the drug.

In August 1984, a total of 26 mongrel dogs of both sexes weighing between 13 and 29 kg, were utilized in this study. All animals were maintained in separate cages under standardized conditions of temperature (~24°C) and relative humidity (~50%) in LD12:12 with light-on at 06^{00}. Water and food were freely available. A two-team approach was utilized[2] and the kidneys exchanged between pairs of dogs; the remaining kidney of each dog was discarded. The allografts were heterotopically transplanted in the recipient's right iliac fossa. The renal vessels were anastomosed end-to-side to the iliac vein and end-to-end to the iliac artery. A ureterocystotomy completed the surgical procedure. Postoperative daily measurements of serum creatinine and weekly complete blood counts were obtained.

A graft was considered to be functional if the serum creatinine was <7 mg/dl and to have failed when the serum creatinine rose to >7 mg/dl (*9*). We refrained from biopsy of the kidney grafts in living dogs, in the face of a temporary functional impairment. In the latter case, reversibility was ascertained by a creatinine value that was acceptable, after a prior transient elevation or transient plateau. The reliance upon serial serum creatinines indeed allowed discrimination between an irreversible positive slope and a transient increase, by defining a failure of the kidney function ascertained by values larger than 7 mg/dl, which were invariably associated with subsequent death. This procedure is in keeping with an earlier choice of a creatinine value associated with irreversible kidney failure of 7 mg/dl by Canafax et al. (*9*).

Quasi-randomization was used to assign 20 dogs to two treatment groups, receiving CsA orally (single dose of 12.5 mg/kg body weight/day) at 1 of 2 circadian stages, 08^{30} or 20^{30}. Dogs arrived in pairs in the operating room; one animal, picked randomly, was to receive CsA daily at 08^{30} and the other at 20^{30}. The first dose of the drug was given on the day of the operation. Animals to be treated at 08^{30} received the entire first CsA dose preoperatively. Animals to be treated at 20^{30} received the first CsA dose in 2 fractions, the first half administered preoperatively and the second half at 20^{30} on the day of surgery. Thus, two experimental groups, each of 10 animals, were considered, and pairs of dogs received oral CsA at one of two circadian stages—at 08^{30} or at 20^{30}. Six dogs received no treatment (control group). In the long-term follow-up, CsA treatment was discontinued after 60 days from transplantation. At the end of the study, no statistically significant difference was seen between the two treated groups in terms of female/male ratio (2/10 vs 3/10) and mean (±SD) body weight (21.6±5.1 vs. 21.4±4.8 kg). At death, rejection (rather than nephrotoxicity) was confirmed by laparotomy and graft histology.

CsA was measured in whole-blood samples by high-pressure liquid chromatography (HPLC) (*10*). Blood was analyzed from each animal for CsA trough-concentration on the 5th postoperative day. In 4 dogs (2 dogs for each treatment schedule), a 24-hr blood CsA profile was performed between the 5th and 6th postoperative days. Blood samples were obtained at 7 times, 4 hr apart, from the time of the anticipated trough-concentration sample up to the anticipated trough-concentration sample on the following day.

Cosinor methods, used for data analysis (*11*), are specially designed for the analysis of rhythmic variations in short and sparse series of data. The single cosinor method tests the assumption of "no-rhythm" or zero-amplitude of the cosine function fitted by least-squares to the data. The result of this test is shown as a P value. Moreover, the following parameters are derived to describe the rhythm: the MESOR, a rhythm-adjusted mean; the amplitude, a measure of extent of predictable change around the MESOR; and the acrophase, a measure of timing of overall high values in the rhythm. Life tables were also calculated and compared in the 2 treated groups (*12*).

A statistically significant circadian variation was found to

[1] This work was supported by U.S. National Institutes of General Medical Sciences (GM-13981) and of Arthritis, Diabetes, Digestive and Kidney Diseases (AM-13083).

* Abbreviations used: ACTH, adrenocorticotropic hormone; bw, body weight; CsA, cyclosporine; HPLC, high-pressure liquid chromatography; LD12:12, light for 12 hr followed by darkness for 12 hr. ns: not significant (P>.05).

[2] Surgery was done in the morning between 8:30 and 11:30. The two-team approach allowed a similar surgical procedure in the 2 groups, especially in terms of cold ischemia and warm ischemia times. Each animal was assigned randomly to each team. The 8% technical failure is low; the teams worked in not-too-dissimilar a fashion since they each had one technical failure.

characterize CsA blood concentrations obtained from the 2 dogs treated at 08^{30} ($P<.001$) as well as those from the 2 dogs treated at 20^{30} ($P = .027$) (Fig. 1). In particular, the acrophases of the 24-hr cosine curve were at $15^{42}\pm00^{41}$ for the dogs treated at 08^{30} and at $03^{22}\pm01^{13}$ for those treated at 20^{30}. This figure clearly shows that the two curves are roughly in antiphase. The lack of a statistically significant difference, seen between the calculated areas under these curves (8719 ng/ml×h vs. 7740 ng/ml×h for the 08^{30} and 20^{30} schedules, respectively; ns.) would not suffice in itself to discuss pharmacokinetics, were it not that a lack of a statistically significant difference was also seen between the 2 groups in mean CsA trough concentration (± SE), now documented on the basis of a total of 18 dogs. For the 08^{30} treatment schedule, it was 191±60 ng/ml and for the 20^{30} treatment schedule 141±49 ng/ml (t = .65; ns.).

Two dogs (8% of all dogs entering the protocol), both receiving CsA at 20^{30}, became uremic within the 5th postoperative day because of technical failure (a renal artery thrombosis and an iatrogenous ureteral obstruction with hydronephrosis) and were not included in the statistical analysis. All 6 animals of the control group acutely rejected their graft within 7 days (mean graft survival ± SE 5.8±.2 days).

Eight of the dogs receiving CsA at 08^{30} acutely rejected their graft after 6, 6, 7, 7, 8, 10, 17, and 20 days. One dog with a functioning graft died from a bowel obstruction on the 9th postoperative day. Another dog (10%) had a functioning graft up to the 60th postoperative day. Median graft survival for this group was 8 days. Two dogs receiving CsA at 20^{30} acutely rejected their graft after 12 and 15 days. On the 28th postoperative day, 6 dogs of this treatment group (75%) were alive with a functioning graft, as apparent from both an acceptable serum creatinine and from histologic study of the graft. Subsequently, 2 animals were killed on the 28th and 31st postoperative days, and another died on the 38th postoperative day, all because of infection and malnutrition but with a functioning graft. The remaining 3 dogs (37.5%) were alive with a functioning graft at 60 days after transplantation. The mean and SE of graft survival times were 38.0±7.1 days for the treatment at 20^{30} and 15.0±5.2 days for the treatment at 08^{30}. The difference in graft function dependent upon CsA treatment timing is significant at the 1% level in a life-table analysis (Fig. 2). This analysis was done with the inclusion and exclusion of the dogs in the group treated at 20^{30}, dying within 5 days after operation. In both cases, the intergroup difference in mean survival time was significant ($P = .01$). This study validates the results of previous reports that have documented, in rodents (*5–7*) as well as in dogs, a gain in delaying graft rejection by circadian timing of CsA.

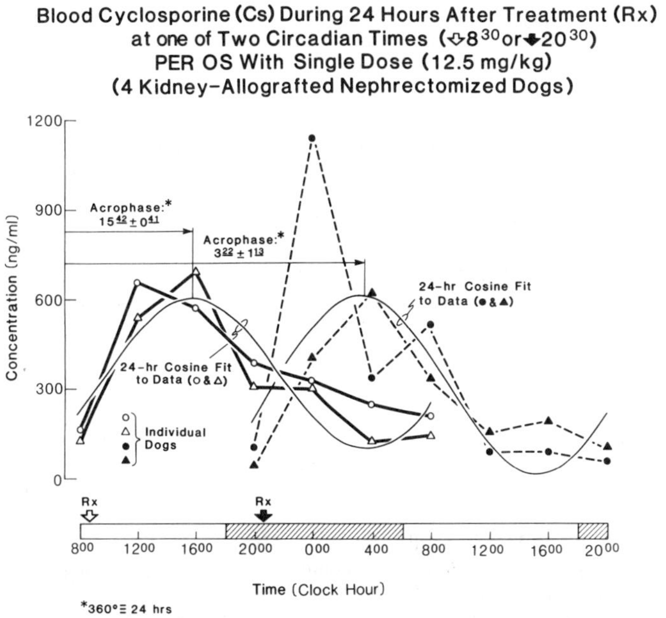

FIGURE 1. Circadian rhythm in CsA blood concentrations from 2 dogs treated at 08^{30} (○ & △) and from 2 dogs treated at 20^{30} (● and ▲) (dogs kept in light from 06^{00} to 18^{00} daily). Note difference in acrophase (measure of timing of high CsA concentration) in the absence of any difference in chronopharmacologic endpoints.

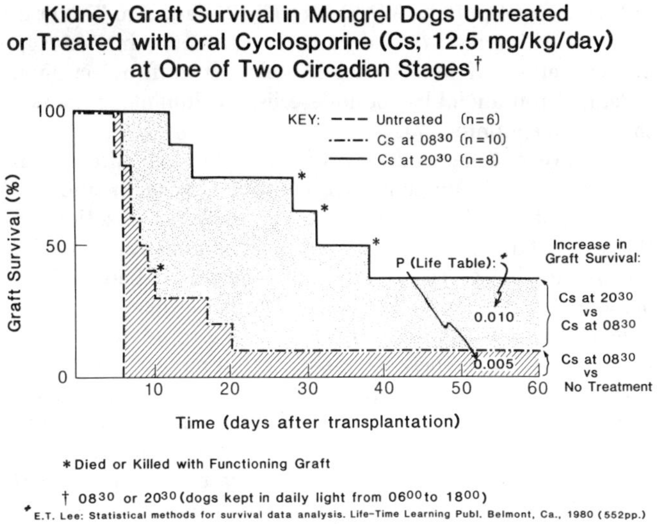

FIGURE 2. Kidney graft survival in untreated dogs and in dogs receiving oral cyclosporine at 08^{30} or at 20^{30} (dogs kept in light from 06^{00} to 18^{00} daily).

Like other drug responses, immunopharmacologic effects depend upon a spectrum of rhythms that constitutes part of an organismic time structure. Treatment timing is particularly promising in immunopharmacology, since it has been documented to account for the difference between immunosuppression and immunostimulation (*13*). Among other variables, a circadian bioperiodicity has been shown for T and B cell counts in human peripheral blood (*14–16*) and for in vitro lymphocyte response to mitogen (*17, 18*).

The mechanism of action of CsA is not well understood. The drug depresses humoral and cellular immunity, with a preferential and reversible action against T lymphocytes (*19, 20*). These effects are not accompanied by the bone marrow depression frequently found during treatment with azathioprine. The presence of CsA in patient plasma can block in vitro cell-mediated responses of peripheral blood lymphocytes in transplanted patients and healthy individuals (*21*). In that study, a circadian behavior of plasma inhibitory activity has been demonstrated in vitro in the circulation of transplanted patients given an oral dose of CsA.

The timing of the best schedule with CsA given during the dark span for diurnally active dogs is surprising in view of a similar timing found for the optimal CsA effect in nocturnally active rats bearing heart or pancreas allografts. Despite the difference in their activity-rest bioperiodicity, dogs share with human beings a similar circadian rhythm for melatonin, a hormone synthesized by the pineal gland during the dark span

(*22–24*). The reports of Womble et al. (*25*) and Liu Tao et al. (*26*) are of interest: they document a potential immunosuppressive effect of propranolol in delaying graft rejection in rodents. Propranolol has been described as inhibiting the synthesis of melatonin (*27*).

Whatever the mechanisms involved in the large difference in duration of graft function with respect to circadian timing of oral CsA, it is of interest that this circadian optimization was the result of a study with a modern drug administration device, the implantable, externally programmable pump. Thus, a result of modern technology, described in detail elsewhere (*8*), served to guide the timing of conventional (oral) drug administration. At the same time, these results confirm one of the merits of using the pump: circadian optimization. The pump remains highly desirable for a more refined drug administration patterned to account for rhythms with several frequencies. Benefit from timing treatment according to a circaseptan pattern (with a period of ~7 days) as well as according to circadian rhythms is documented in the rat (*7*).

The results herein must be interpreted in light of the practice of administering equal doses of CsA in the morning and in the evening. The extent to which the morning dose may be reduced remains a topic for future clinical studies. In the future, one might also consider interactions with the CsA effect of endogenous immunomodulators. Melatonin, ACTH, and corticosteroids come to mind, since their time-dependent effects are being found increasingly (*28–30*). Adjunctive corticosteroid treatment is advocated in reduced doses in CsA-treated patients in view of interactions between exogenous corticosteroid and CsA (*31*). The CsA dose at 20^{30} is likely to interact with less endogenous corticosteroid than the dose given at 08^{30}. Moreover, Öst (*32*) indicates that corticosteroids are metabolized in the liver, and that CsA may decrease metabolism by a hepatotoxic effect—by reducing the amount of hepatic cytochrome P-450, an effect recorded in the rat (*33*)—or there might be competitive inhibition since both CsA and corticosteroid utilize cytochrome P-450 in their metabolism (*32*).

Finally, the question may be raised as to whether the number of dogs suffices for the purpose on hand. Actually, already at the completion of work on 5 pairs of animals, the intertreatment difference between dogs receiving 12.5 mg/kg/day CsA in the morning or in the evening was significant below the 5% level. Nonetheless, the study was continued so that any reasonable criticism of the small number of dogs might not hold. After 10 pairs, the *P* value continued to rule out the effect of chance (*P* = .01). In the face of such consistent differences, the study of added dogs was judged neither humane nor financially responsible, the more so that these results already constitute a follow-up corroborating those obtained previously with an implanted, externally programmable pump.

Marco Cavallini[3,4]
Franz Halberg[5]
David E. R. Sutherland[6]
Germaine Cornélissen[5]
John Heil[6]
John S. Najarian[6]

[3] University of Rome Medical School.

[4] Marco Cavallini is a recipient of a fellowship from Istituto Pasteur, Fondazione Cenci-Bolognetti.

[5] Chronobiology Laboratories, University of Minnesota.

[6] Department of Surgery, University of Minnesota.

University of Rome Medical School, 1 Istituto di Clinica Chirurgia, Policlinico Umberto I, Rome, Italy
Chronobiology Laboratories, University of Minnesota, Minneapolis, Minnesota 55455
Department of Surgery, University of Minnesota, Minneapolis, Minnesota 55455

REFERENCES

1. Morris PJ. Cyclosporin A overview. Transplantation 1981; 32: 349.
2. Ferguson RM, Rynasiewicz JJ, Sutherland DER, Simmons RS, Najarian JS. Cyclosporin A in renal transplantation. A prospective randomized trial. Surgery 1982; 92: 175.
3. Klintmalm GBG, Iwatsuki S, Starzl TE. Nephrotoxicity of cyclosporin A in liver and kidney transplant patients. Lancet 1981; 1: 470.
4. Magnus G, Cavallini M, Halberg F, et al. Circadian toxicology of cyclosporine. Toxicol Appl Pharmacol 1985; 77: 181.
5. Cavallini M, Magnus G, Halberg F, et al. Benefit from circadian timing of cyclosporine revealed by delay of rejection of murine heart allograft. 1st Int Cong Cyclosporine, Houston, TX, May 16–19, 1983. Transplant Proc 1983; 15 (No. 4, Suppl 1): 2960.
6. Cavallini M, Halberg F, Liu T, Magnus G, Sutherland DER, Stipa S. Circadian stage-dependent prolongation by cyclosporine of segmental pancreatic allograft function in the rat. International Congress Immunology in Diabetes 1984, March 15–17, Rome, Italy, 1984, 22.
7. Liu T, Cavallini M, Halberg F, Cornélissen G, Field J, Sutherland DER. Multifrequency chronotherapy with circaseptan and eventually circannual optimization may follow early circadian-sinusoidal pump-implemented infusions of cyclosporine. In: Reinberg A, Smolensky M, Labrecque G, eds. Annual review of chronopharmacology. Proc 1st Int Montreux Conf of Biological Rhythms and Medications. Montreux, Switzerland, March 26–30, 1984. Oxford: Pergamon Press, 1984, 133.
8. Cavallini M, Halberg F, Cornélissen G, Enrichens F, Margarit C. Organ transplantation and broader chronotherapy with implantable pump and computer programs for marker rhythm assessment. J Contr Rel 1986; 3: 3.
9. Canafax DM, Sutherland DER, Ascher NL, Simmons RL, Najarian JS. Cyclosporine nephrotoxicity in renal allograft recipients: conversion to azathioprine to improve renal function. 1st Int Cong Cyclosporine. Houston, TX, May 16–19, 1983. Transplant Proc 1983; 15 (No. 4, suppl 1): 2874.
10. Sawchuk PS, Cartier LL. Liquid-chromatographic determination of cyclosporin A in blood and plasma. Clin Chem 1981; 27: 1368.
11. Bingham C, Arbogast B, Cornélissen Guillaume G, Lee JK, Halberg F. Inferential statistical methods for estimating and comparing cosinor parameters. Chronobiologia 1982; 9: 397.
12. Lee ET. Statistical methods for survival data analysis. Belmont, CA; Life-Time Learning Publ, 1980; 552.
13. Halberg F. Chronopharmacology and chronotherapy. In: Carpenter DO, ed. Cellular pacemakers. New York; Wiley, 1982; 261.
14. Elmadjian F, Pincus G. A study of the diurnal variations in circulating lymphocytes in normal and psychotic subjects. J Clin Endocrinol 1946; 6: 287.
15. Halberg F. Circadian temporal organization and experimental pathology. 7th Conf Internazionale della Società per lo Studio dei Ritmi Biologici. Siena; Edizioni Panminerva Medica, Sept 1960; 1.
16. Ritchie AWS, Oswald I, Spedding Micklem I, et al. Circadian variation of lymphocyte subpopulations: a study with monoclonal antibodies. Br Med J 1983; 286: 1773.
17. Haus E, Halberg F, Kühl JFW, Lakatua DJ. Chronopharmacology in animals. Chronobiologia 1974; 1 (suppl 1): 122.
18. Tavadia HB, Fleming KA, Hume PD, Simpson HW. Circadian rhythmicity of human plasma cortisol and pha-induced lymphocyte transformation. Clin Exp Immunol 1975; 22: 190.
19. Kunkl A, Klaus GGB. Selective effects of cyclosporin A on func-

tional B-cell subsets in the mouse. J Immunol 1980; 125: 2526.
20. Hess AD, Tutschka PJ. Effect of cyclosporin A on human lymphocyte responses in vitro. Cs-A allows for the expression of alloantigen-activated suppressor cells while preferentially inhibiting the induction of cytolytic effector lymphocytes in MLR. J Immunol 1980; 124: 2601.
21. Ferguson RM, Fidelus-Gort R. The immunosuppressive action of cyclosporine in man. 1st Int Cong of Cyclosporine. Houston, TX, May 16–19, 1983. Transplant Proc 1983; 15 (suppl 1): 2350.
22. Pelham RW, Vaughan GM, Sandock KL, Vaughan MK. Twenty-four-hour cycle of a melatonin-like substance in the plasma of human males. J Clin Endocrinol Metab 1973; 37: 341.
23. Lynch HJ, Wurtman RJ, Moskowitz MA, Archer MC, Ho MH. Daily rhythm in human urinary melatonin. Science 1975; 187: 169.
24. Ozaki Y, Lynch HJ, Wurtman RJ. Melatonin in rat pineal, plasma and urine: 24-hour rhythmicity and effect of chlorpromazine. Endocrinology 1976; 98: 1418.
25. Womble JR, Larson DF, Copeland JG, Russell DH. An effective immunosuppressive agent in rat heart-lung transplantation. Transplantation 1983; 35: 417.
26. Liu T, Sutherland DER, Field J, Najarian JS. Paradoxical effects of propranolol given with azathioprine on cyclosporine A in rat heart and islet allograft. Transplant Proc 1985; 17: 240.
27. Minneman KP, Wurtman RJ. the pharmacology of the pineal gland. Ann Rev Pharmacol Toxicol 1976; 16: 33.
28. Sánchez de la Peña S, Halberg E, Halberg F, Cornélissen G, Sothern RB, Yunis E. Circadian modulation of the anti-tumor effect of cyclosporine. Proc 1st Int. Workshop on Neuroimmunomodulation. Bethesda, MD, Nov 27–30, 1984 (in press).
29. Wrba H, Halberg F, Dutter A. Melatonin circadian-stage-dependently delays breast cancer development in mice injected daily for several months. Proc 1st Int Workshop on Neuroimmunomodulation. Bethesda, MD, Nov 27–30, 1984 (in press).
30. Sànchez de la Peña S, Halberg F, Halberg E, et al. Pineal modulation of ACTH 1–17 effect upon murine corticosterone production. Brain Res Bull 1983; 11: 117.
31. Langhoff E, Madsen S, Flachs H, Olgaard K, Ladefoged J, Hvidberg EF. Inhibition of prednisolone metabolism by cyclosporine in kidney-transplanted patients. Transplantation 1985; 39: 107.
32. Öst L. Effects of cyclosporine on prednisolone metabolism. Lancet 1984; 1: 451.
33. Cunningham C, Burke MD, Whiting PH, Simpson JG, Wheatley DN. Ketoconazole, cyclosporine and the kidney. Lancet 1982; 2: 1464.

Received 12 July 1985.
Accepted 17 September 1985.

DETERMINATION OF CYCLOSPORINE CONCENTRATION IN BILE

Cyclosporine (CsA),* a cyclic undecapeptide of fungal origin, is a potent immunosuppressive drug used to prevent the rejection of transplanted kidneys, livers, and hearts in man. Elimination of the drug is primarily biliary; only about 6% of the dose appears in the urine.

The disposition and metabolism of CsA remains poorly understood. Absorption from the gastrointestinal tract is incomplete and variable, and it is possible that the drug undergoes enterohepatic recirculation. Venkataramanan et al. observed increases in CsA blood levels following T tube clamping in liver transplant patients (*1*), and Kahan and coworkers noted the appearance of the drug in the ileostomy drainage of a patient (*2*).

CsA blood levels of transplant patients are routinely monitored in our laboratory by radioimmunoassay (RIA) or high-performance liquid chromatography (HPLC) of whole blood. The RIA measures CsA and many of its metabolites, whereas HPLC specifically measures the parent compound. A modification of both methods for determination of CsA in bile samples has been developed in our laboratory, and it has proved to be reliable in terms of accuracy, precision, and sensitivity. The determination of CsA concentration in bile is of potential value in the research setting as a tool for CsA disposition studies.

Bile samples were collected from a T tube in the common bile duct of five patients who had recently undergone orthotopic liver transplantation. Blank bile for preparation of assay standards and controls was from a patient not receiving CsA. Samples were obtained at various times after a dose of CsA and were stored at −20°C. CsA was administered as an oral dose (800–1200 mg; n = 3) or as a combination of i.v. infusion and oral dose (100–140 mg i.v., 450–1200 mg p.o.; n = 2).

For RIA, CsA standards and controls were prepared using a stock solution of 2.5 mg CsA in 25 ml of HPLC-grade methanol. The flask was wrapped in foil and stored upright at −20°C. Two sets of standards, 10, 20, 40, 69, and 100 μg/ml and 15, 40, 50, and 80 μg/ml, were prepared by pipetting the appropriate volumes of stock solution into glass flasks, evaporating the methanol under a stream of dry nitrogen, and adding 1.0 ml of blank bile. The flasks were covered with foil and stirred at room temperature for 1.5 hr. Each set of standards was diluted 50-fold to the final concentration with assay buffer A (0.05 M TRIZMA, pH 8.5), aliquoted into capped plastic tubes, and frozen until needed. Patient samples were diluted 50-fold with buffer A before analysis. One set of standards was used to obtain a standard curve and the other set to assess the accuracy of the measurement. The Sandoz RIA kit was used to measure CsA in samples according to the manufacturer's instructions.

HPLC bile standards and controls were prepared as above, but directly from the stock solution to yield the desired concentrations; no further dilution with buffer was performed. Patient samples were analyzed without dilution. HPLC determination of CsA was performed on a C18 reverse-phase Bondapack column, using a modification of the method of Sawchuk and Cartier (*3*). The column temperature was maintained at 70°C. Flow rate of the mobile phase, acetonitrile/methanol/distilled water (49/22/29 by volume), was 1.0 ml/min. Column effluent was monitored at 214 nm. Peak heights were measured electronically, and the ratio of CsA to the internal standard CsD was used to calculate drug concentration.

An index of CsA metabolite production was calculated using the concentrations obtained by RIA and HPLC by the following equation:

$$\text{CsA metabolite index (CMI)} = \frac{(\text{RIA} - \text{HPLC})}{(\text{RIA})}$$

A typical linear/log RIA standard curve of CsA in bile is shown in Figure 1. The assay is linear between bile CsA concentrations of 0.2 and 2.0 μg/ml. Patient samples were assayed in duplicate, and the coefficient of variation for duplicates within the run was less than 10%. Precision of the assay in routine use was determined by analyzing 12 bile samples

* Abbreviations used: CMI, cyclosporine metabolite index; CsA, cyclosporine; HPLC, high-performance liquid chromatography; RIA, radioimmunoassay.

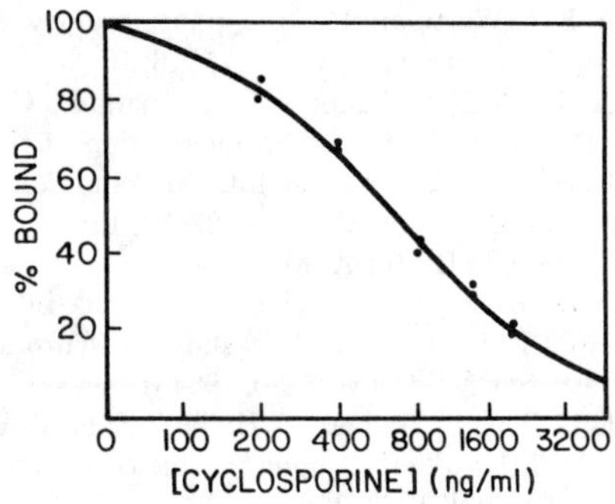

FIGURE 1. Linear/log RIA standard curve for determination of cyclosporine concentration in bile.

from five patients in duplicate daily for 10 days. The standard deviation of the difference of duplicate values was obtained for each set of determination, and from this data a coefficient of variation was calculated using standard statistical methods. Thus, the average between run variation was 11% with a range of 7%–14%. The highest variation was observed in a bile sample that contained pulpy debris. Four bile controls loaded with different concentrations of CsA were assayed in duplicate with each run of patient samples, and recovery of added CsA was 104±5.5% (Table 1).

When CsA concentration was determined in bile using HPLC, the limit of sensitivity was 0.1 μg/ml, and recovery of CsA in bile controls at all levels of CsA averaged 95%. The coefficient of variation for bile standards assayed on consecutive days was approximately 10%. The volumes of patient bile samples received in the laboratory for assay were insufficient for repeat analyses by HPLC.

Ten bile samples from four patients were assayed by RIA and HPLC for CsA concentration, and the results are shown in Table 2. Considerably higher values were obtained using RIA because of the high level of CsA metabolites present in bile. The actual metabolite concentration may be much higher than these values indicate, since CsA metabolites only partially crossreact with the antibody used in this assay. In contrast, HPLC, which specifically measures the parent drug only, yielded values 8–48-fold lower than those obtained by RIA.

Table 2 also includes a CMI that appeared to be relatively constant in any given patient and fluctuated within a narrow range for all patients studied. The CMI was 0.98 for all three samples from patient C, even though the samples were collected at different times during the dosing interval. Similarly, patient B had an average CMI value of 0.93.

The introduction of CsA for immunosuppression has been recognized as one of the major breakthroughs in organ transplantation in recent years. A greater understanding of CsA disposition and metabolism in the human body may further enhance its usefulness. The question of relative amount of parent drug and metabolites at various dosages is an important one, especially if there is a saturation level above which the liver is unable to metabolize more drug in a single pass.

A previous publication from this laboratory presented data on CsA levels in human bile (*1*). The analytical methods have since been modified to further increase precision, sensitivity, and CsA recovery. The most significant improvement has been the use of dry CsA for preparation of the stock standard solution instead of the standard included in the Sandoz RIA kit, which had limited solubility in the blank bile such that CsA recovery from standards and controls was variable and unacceptably low. This, in turn, led to a variable underestimation of CsA concentration in bile. The present bile CsA method has a high degree of precision, and recoveries are essentially 100%.

The present study shows that the levels of parent CsA in bile are quite low, and it is unlikely that bile CsA undergoes any significant enterohepatic recirculation. This is in general agreement with the results of Venkataramanan et al. (*1*), who found that less than 1% of the administered dose of CsA was excreted in bile. The question remains, however, whether CsA metabolites, which are present in bile in very high concentrations, are recycled to any significant extent. This is important because if any of these metabolites possess immunosuppressive properties, recycling may prolong the pharmacologic action of the drug. If, on the other hand, products of CsA metabolism are found to be toxic, their prolonged presence in the body could be harmful.

In this connection, the CMI could be a useful estimate of the level of CsA metabolites present in a sample. In blood, RIA determinations of CsA are two to three times higher than by HPLC (*1*), and the calculated CMI is found to be between 0.5 and 0.7. In contrast, the CMI for bile samples is considerably higher, around 0.93, consistent with the results of Venkataramanan and coworkers (*1*), from whose data a CMI value of approximately 0.97 may be calculated. This may be expected, as the metabolism of CsA is primarily hepatic. Unexpected was the finding that the CMI values were virtually identical in a given patient, regardless of the time elapsed since the last dose of CsA (Table 2). These data imply that the hepatic breakdown of the drug is fairly constant throughout the dosing interval for the patients in this study.

TABLE 1. Recovery of CsA added to control bile

CsA added (μg/ml)	CsA measured (μg/ml)	
	RIA	HPLC[a]
0.3	0.29±0.048	0.29±0.019
0.8	0.85±0.079	0.81±0.075
1.0	1.1±0.15	0.96±0.082
1.6	1.7±0.13	1.7±0.13

[a] n = 10 and 4, respectively, for RIA and HPLC for each concentration of CsA added to blank or control bile.

TABLE 2. RIA and HPLC determinations of cyclosporine concentration in bile samples at various times after a dose

Patient	Time after dose (hr)	Cyclosporine (μg/ml)		CMI[b]
		RIA[a]	HPLC	
A	4	97.7±12.8	6.69	0.93
B	1	36.8±5.50	2.64	0.93
	4	47.9±7.95	4.63	0.90
	9	46.7±6.25	3.08	0.93
	11	39.9±5.10	2.55	0.94
	12	44.8±6.70	3.12	0.93
C	5	29.6±3.85	0.714	0.98
	7	28.5±3.50	0.708	0.98
	12	21.5±3.15	0.451	0.98
D	2	15.6±3.15	1.85	0.88

[a] Mean (n = 10) and standard deviation are shown for RIA results. Insufficient sample volume prevented more than one HPLC determination for each sample.

[b] CMI-CsA metabolite index.

This method can be of value in the research setting for studies involving the disposition and metabolism of CsA. The results of RIA and HPLC CsA determinations in bile can be compared to estimate the fraction of total dose being excreted through the bile, as well as the amount of parent drug that is leaving the body unmetabolized.

Acknowledgments. We thank Linda Markivich, Diane Phillips, and Toni Campbell for their excellent technical assistance.

LENIA SCANLON[1]
ROSE BALOH[1]
BRUNO GRIDELLI[2]
K. MURALI RAO[1]
BYERS SHAW[2]
THOMAS STARZL[2]
AJIT SANGHVI[1]

[1] Department of Pathology.
[2] Department of Surgery.

Departments of Pathology and Surgery, University of Pittsburgh, School of Medicine, Pittsburgh, Pennsylvania 15261

REFERENCES

1. Venkataramanan R, Starzl TE, Yang S, Burckart GJ, Ptachcinski RJ, Shaw BW, Iwatsuki S, Van Thiel DH, Sanghvi A, Seltman H. Biliary excretion of cyclosporine in liver transplant patients. Transplant Proc (in press).
2. Kahan BD, Ried M, Newburger J. Pharmacokinetics of cyclosporine in human renal transplantation. Transplant Proc 1983; 15: 446.
3. Sawchuck RJ, Cartier LL. Liquid chromatographic determination of cyclosporine A in blood and plasma. Clin Chem 1981; 27: 1368.

Received 26 June 1985.
Accepted 12 September 1985.

ENCAPSULATION OF CYCLOSPORINE BY PHOSPHATIDYLINOSITOL-CHOLESTEROL LIPOSOMES[1]

Phospholipid vesicles (liposomes) are widely recognized as potential carriers of drugs (*1*) and other biologically active materials (*2*). Studies from our laboratory have demonstrated that they are appropriate for the reconstitution of cytochrome c oxidase (*3, 4*) and high density lipoproteins (*5, 6*), and may potentiate the immunogenicity of weak antigens (*7*). We have also shown that phosphatidylinositol-cholesterol liposomes are cytotoxic to tumor cell cultures (*8*).

Cyclosporine, a cyclic peptide that comprises 11 amino acids (*9*), has recently been recognized to be a very potent immunosuppressant; however, it is associated with undesirable side effects—e.g., nephrotoxicity (*10*). Because cyclosporine is hydrophobic it may become entrapped within the phospholipid bilayer of liposomes when it interacts with them; the resulting complex may be advantageous for the delivery and targeting of cyclosporine. A preliminary report on liposome-encapsulated cyclosporine used in a rat model has recently appeared, but the composition of phospholipids and the preparation of liposomes were not disclosed (*11*).

In this communication we report the preparation of phosphatidylinositol-cholesterol liposomes containing cyclosporine, and describe the centrifugation and the Sepharose-4B gel filtration of the liposome-cyclosporine complex. Our results clearly show that phosphatidylinositol, cholesterol, and cyclosporine form liposomes in a molar ratio of 2:1:0.22, establishing cyclosporine encapsulation by liposomes.

Liposomes were prepared as described elsewhere (*7*), with the following modifications: 2.4 μmol of soya bean phosphatidylinositol (Serdary Research Lab. Inc., London, Ontario), 4×10^5 cpm of 1-palmitoyl-2-[1-^{14}C]-linoleoyl-*sn*-3-phosphatidylinositol (specific activity 58 mCi/mmol (Amersham, Toronto, Ontario), 1.2 μmol of cholesterol (Sigma, St. Louis, MO), and 0.8 μmol of cyclosporine (a gift from Sandoz A.G., Basel, Switzerland) were dissolved in 1 ml of chloroform and evaporated to dryness. The residue was hydrated at 37°C for 2 hr with 1.5 ml of 0.15 M NaCl and then sonicated for 2 min. In the control experiment cyclosporine was omitted and liposomes yielded a clear solution that was applied to a Sepharose-4B (Pharmacia, Uppsala, Sweden) column.

Liposomes containing cyclosporine were milky and were subjected to centrifugation at 12,000 ×g for 10 min. The pellet containing 10.8 and 82.5% of starting [^{14}C]-phosphatidylinositol and cyclosporine, respectively, was not further investigated. The clear supernatant containing 1517 nmol of [^{14}C]-phosphatidylinositol and 170 nmol of cyclosporine was applied to the Sepharose-4B column and eluted with 0.15 M NaCl. Fractions

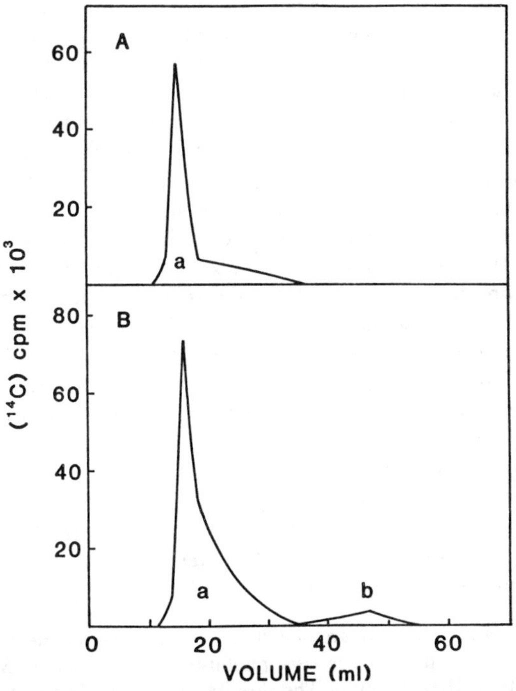

FIGURE 1. Sepharose-4B gel filtration. Elution pattern of A) phosphatidylinositol:cholesterol liposomes and B) phosphatidylinositol:cholesterol:cyclosporine liposomes, prepared as described in methods.

[1] This work was supported by a grant from the Medical Research Council of Canada.

TABLE 1. Sepharose-4B gel filtration of [^{14}C]-phosphatidylinositol-cholesterol-cyclosporine liposomes

Liposomes	Sepharose-4B					
	Applied		Recovered (nmol)			
			Peak a		Peak b	
	[^{14}C] PI	CsA	[^{14}C] PI	CsA	[^{14}C] PI	CsA
[^{14}C]-phosphatidylinositol-cholesterol (control)	2400 (100.0%)	–	2122 (88.4%)	–	–	–
[^{14}C]-phosphatidylinositol-cholesterol-cyclosporine (12,000 ×g supernatant)	1517 (100.0%)	170 (100.0%)	1071 (70.6%)	124 (72.8%)	99.6 (6.6%)	18.0 (10.6%)

Abbreviations: PI = phosphatidylinositol and CsA = cyclosporine.

of 2 ml were collected and assayed for radioactivity in standard fashion (Philips PW 4700 scintillation spectrometer). Cyclosporine in liposomes was determined spectrophotometrically at 240 nm in chloroform/methanol/water (2:1:0.8 v/v/v) against liposomes without cyclosporine in the same solvent.

When [^{14}C]-phosphatidylinositol-cholesterol (2:1) was hydrated, a clear solution of liposomes was obtained; this emerged from the Sepharose-4B column as a single sharp peak with the void volume and contained 88.4% of applied [^{14}C]-phosphatidylinositol (Fig. 1A and Table 1A). We therefore concluded that these liposomes were small and unilamellar, in agreement with the findings of Huang (*12*) and Hauser and Gains (*13*).

Hydration of the same phosphatidylinositol-cholesterol mixture in the presence of cyclosporine gave a heavy milky suspension. After centrifugation as described above it yielded a supernatant that was subjected to Sepharose-4B gel filtration. The elution pattern is shown in Fig. 1B and the recovery of [^{14}C]-phosphatidylinositol and cyclosporine is given in Table 1B. The major peak (a) eluted with the void volume was transparent, with negligible absorption at 410 nm, and contained both [^{14}C]-phosphatidylinositol and cyclosporine in a molar ratio of 1:0.12. The second, minor peak (b) eluted from Sepharose-4B contained only 6.6 and 10.6% of applied [^{14}C]-phosphatidylinositol and cyclosporine, respectively, and was not further examined. Since the elution volumes of the major peaks of the liposomes with and without cyclosporine were identical (Fig. 1), it is justifiable to suggest that the phosphatidylinositol-cholesterol-cyclosporine liposomes are identical with respect to size (small) and structure (unilamellar).

Because of its hydrophobic nature, the cyclosporine associated with these liposomes is, in all likelihood, entrapped within the hydrophobic regions of the phospholipid bilayer, but the experimental assessment of this distribution must be determined. Although cholesterol recovery was not determined in the experiments described here, we assumed that it was better than 90% on the basis of our previous experiments with cholesterol-containing liposomes (*7*).

The present experiments clearly show that cyclosporine can be associated with phosphatidylinositol-cholesterol liposomes that have high entrapment efficiency; the resulting carrier may prove useful in the administration, delivery, and targeting of cyclosporine.

Acknowledgments. We are grateful to Sandoz A.G. for the generous gift of cyclosporine. We are also grateful to Miss E. Shapter, Medical Publications Department of The Hospital for Sick Children, Toronto, for help in the preparation of the manuscript.

LIDIJA STUHNE-SEKALEC
JERZY CHUDZIK
NIKOLA Z. STANACEV[2]
The Department of Clinical Biochemistry
Banting Institute
University of Toronto and The Hospital for Sick Children
Toronto, Canada

[2] Address correspondence to: Dr. N.Z. Stanacev. The Banting Institute, Department of Clinical Biochemistry, University of Toronto, 100 College Street, Toronto, Ontario, Canada M5G 1L5.

REFERENCES

1. Gregoriadis G. Drug carriers in biology and medicine. New York: Academic, 1983: 363.
2. Knight CG, ed. Liposomes: from physical structure to therapeutic applications. Amsterdam: Elsevier/North Holland, 1981: 497.
3. Denes AS, Stanacev NZ. Spin-label study of the relation between enzymatic activity and lipid-protein organization in reconstituted cytochrome c oxidase. Can J Biochem 1978; 56: 905.
4. Denes AS, Stanacev NZ. Thermally induced changes in reconstituted and membranous cytochrome c oxidase. Can J Biochem 1979; 57: 238.
5. Vaughan DJ, Breckenridge WC, Stanacev NZ. Reconstitution of lipoproteins. I. Lipid-protein interaction of high density apoproteins, purified apoA-I and apoA-II with dimyristoyl-lecithin and dimyristoyl-lecithin: cholesterol vesicles studied by isomeric spin labelled lecithins. Can J Biochem 1980; 58:581.
6. Vaughan DJ, Stanacev NZ. Reconstitution of lipoproteins. II. Lipid-protein interaction between dimyristoyl-lecithin and dimyristoyl-lecithin: cholesterol vesicles and purified apolipoprotein C-I and $CIII_2$ studied by isomeric spin-labelled lecithins. Can J Biochem 1980; 58: 592.
7. Shek PN, Yung BYK, Stanacev NZ. Comparison between multilamellar and unilamellar liposomes in enhancing antibody formation. Immunology 1983; 49: 37.
8. Jett M, Chudzik J, Alving CR, Stanacev NZ. Metabolic fate of liposomal phosphatidylinositol in murine tumor cells: implications for the mechanism of tumor cell cytotoxicity. Cancer Res 1985; 45: 4810.
9. Wenger RM. Synthesis of cyclosporin and analogues: structural requirements for immunosuppressive activity. Angew Chemie Internatl 1985; 24: 77.
10. White DJG, ed. Cyclosporin A. Amsterdam: Elsevier, 1983: 573.
11. Hsieh HH, Schreiber M, Stowe N, et al. Preliminary report: the use of liposome-encapsulated cyclosporine in a rat model. Transplant Proc 1985; 17: 1397.
12. Huang C. Studies on phosphatidylcholine vesicles: formation and physical characteristics. Biochemistry 1969; 8: 344.
13. Hauser H, Gains N. Spontaneous vesiculation of phospholipids: a simple and quick method of forming unilamellar vesicles. Proc Natl Acad Sci 1982; 79:1683.

Received 12 August 1985.
Accepted 4 September 1985.

EFFECT OF CYCLOSPORINE AND LOW-TEMPERATURE CULTURE ON PREVENTION OF REJECTION OF ISLET XENOGRAFTS (RAT-TO-MOUSE)[1]

Cyclosporine (CsA) has been reported either to have no effect (*1*) or to produce a moderate prolongation of islet allograft survival in rats (*2*). If a short course of CsA therapy is combined with procedures that alter or destroy antigen-presenting cells in the donor islets, such as ultraviolet irradiation (*1*), low temperature culture or incubation with Ia antibodies and complement (*3*), rejection of islet allografts in rats is prevented. CsA has been shown to have only a marginal effect on prolongation of cardiac xenografts between rats and mice (*4*).

Marked prolongation of islet xenograft survival (rat-to-mouse) has been achieved in our laboratory by the combined use of low-temperature culture of the donor islets for seven days and a single injection of rat antilymphocyte serum (*5*), and by incubation of aggregates of donor islets in the presence of 95% O_2 for seven days prior to transplantation (*6*). The purpose of the present study was to determine the effect of CsA alone or in combination with low-temperature culture of donor islets on the survival of rat islets transplanted into diabetic mice.

CsA (25 mg/kg/day) injected at −1 and 0 days produced a mean survival time (MST) of 8.5±0.8 days, which was not significantly different from the controls (MST 8.2±0.5 days; groups 1 and 2, Table 1). The duration of treatment with CsA (25 mg/kg/day) was increased to −1, 0, +1, +3, +5, and +7 days, with day 0 as the time of islet transplantation. Increasing the duration of treatment with CsA (25 mg/kg/day) again had no effect on prolonging islet xenograft survival (MST 9.6±0.9 days, group 3). We next examined the effect of a higher dose of CsA on the survival of the islet xenografts. CsA (50 mg/kg/day) was injected at 0, +1, and +2 days after transplantation, and the effect of this regimen on islet xenograft survival was determined. This three-day course of CsA therapy produced a modest but significant prolongation of islet xenograft survival (MST 21.0±5.4 days; $P<0.05$).

In previous studies of rat islet allografts, we have found that a three-day course of CsA therapy beginning at the time of transplantation, in conjunction with culture of the donor islets at 24°C for seven days, produced 100% survival of rat islet allografts at 60 days after transplantation (*3*). In contrast, CsA therapy alone produced only a moderate prolongation of islet allograft survival, and low-temperature culture alone had no effect in prolonging survival (*11*). Thus we attempted to obtain further prolongation of islet xenograft survival by culturing the donor islets at 24°C for seven days before transplantation in addition to the three-day course of CsA (50 mg/kg/day). This regimen produced a marked prolongation of islet xenograft survival (MST >56.2±9.7 days, group 5) and three of the recipients had not rejected the islet xenografts at 100 days after transplantation.

TABLE 1. Effect of cyclosporine and low-temperature culture on the prevention of rejection of islet xenografts (rat-to-mouse)

Group	Islet treatment	CsA treatment	Transplant survival		
			Individual survival (days)	Mean±SEM	Survival 100 days
1.	—	—	7, 7, 7, 9, 9, 10	8.2±0.5	0%
2.	—	25 mg/kg/day −1 +0 days	7, 7, 7, 9, 9, 12	8.5±0.8	0%
3.	—	25 mg/kg/day −1 +0 +3 +5 +7 days	8, 8, 9, 10, 13	9.6±0.9	0%
4.	—	50 mg/kg/day 0 +1 +2 days	13, 14, 15, 21, 42	21.0±5.4[a]	0%
5.	Culture (24°C 7 days)	50 mg/kg/day 0 +1 +2 days	11, 11, 12, 24, 43, 47, 48, 69, 79, 87, >100×3	>56.2±9.7[b]	23%

[a] $P=<0.05$ compared with group 1.
[b] $P=<0.025$ compard with group 1.

Islets were isolated from male Wistar Furth rats by the collagenase technique (*7, 8*), separated on a Ficoll gradient (*9*), and hand-picked with the aid of a dissecting microscope. C57BL/6 mice were made diabetic by the i.v. injection of streptozotocin (160 mg/kg) and 400–500 islets were transplanted into the liver of the diabetic mice via the portal vein (*10*). The islets were cultured overnight at 37°C prior to transplantation or incubated at 24°C for seven days in CMRL-1066 tissue-culture medium containing fetal calf serum (10%), penicillin (100 units/ml), streptomycin sulfate (100 μg/ml), and D-glucose (1.5 mg/ml). CsA (a gift from the Sandoz Company) was dissolved in olive oil (10 mg/ml) and injected s.c. into recipient mice. Nonfasting plasma glucose levels were monitored three times weekly on blood from the orbital sinus, and rejection was considered to have occurred when the glucose levels exceeded 200 mg/dl on two consecutive determinations.

The livers were examined histologically in all the recipients that rejected the islet xenografts. In the controls and in recipients receiving only a low dose of CsA (groups 1, 2, and 3), only foci of lymphocytes were observed but no islet cells were present. In the group receiving the higher level of CsA (50 mg/kg/day, group 4), islets were found in the liver of the one recipient with an islet xenograft survival time of 42 days. Islets were also found in the livers of five of six recipients that had received low-temperature, cultured islets and the three-day course of CsA (group 5) and had rejected the xenografts beyond 40 days

[1] This work was supported in part by USPHS Grant AM-01226, by an ADA Feasibility grant, and by the United States Tobacco Company, Philip Morris Incorporated, and Brown and Williamson Tobacco Corporation.

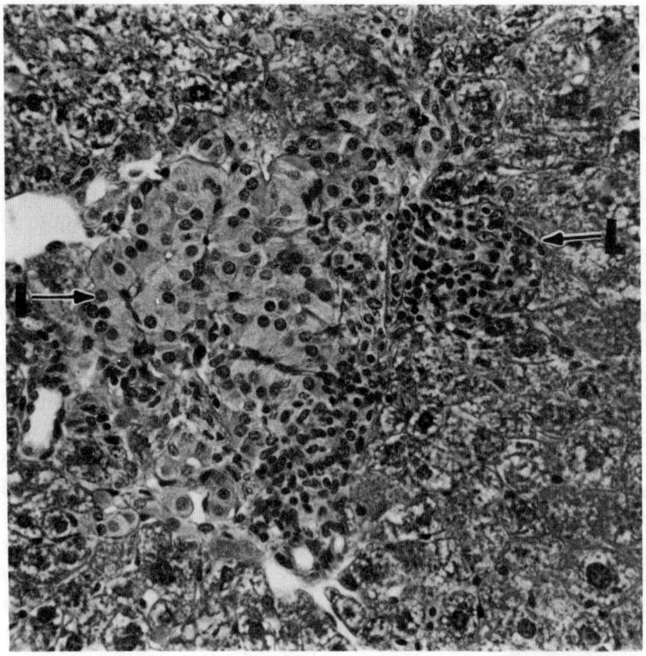

FIGURE 1. Photomicrograph of a rat islet xenograft in the liver of a normoglycemic mouse 154 days after transplantation. The donor rat islets had been cultured at 24°C for 7 days prior to transplantation and transplanted into the liver via the portal vein; the diabetic mouse recipient received CsA (50 mg/kg/day) for 3 days. The recipient became normoglycemic following transplantation and was normoglycemic at 154 days. Lymphocytes (L) are present only at the border of the rat islet (I) and are not infiltrating the islet (hematoxylin & eosin; ×320.

after transplantation. The beta cells in all of these islets were degranulated, indicating that they were responding to the return of hyperglycemia in these recipients. These findings indicate that, if the islet xenografts survived for several weeks, rejection was probably a gradual process resulting in the destruction of individual islets until the mass of islets remaining was insufficient to maintain normoglycemia in the recipients.

One of the recipients with a surviving islet xenograft at 100 days was killed at 154 days after transplantation and the liver was examined histologically. This animal was still normoglycemic, and islets containing beta cells with a normal degree of granulation were present in the liver. As shown in Figure 1, lymphocytes were present around the islets but not infiltrating them. In previous studies we had observed similar periinsular accumulations of lymphocytes in normoglycemic recipients with rat islet xenografts established by low-temperature culture and a single injection of antilymphocyte serum (*12*) or by in vitro culture of islet aggregates in the presence of 95% O_2 (*13*). Characterization of the periinsular infiltrate had shown that the infiltrate was composed of 80% T lymphocytes with a marked preponderance of $Ly2^+$ lymphocytes. It will be important to determine whether the periinsular infiltrate in established rat islet xenografts may be local accumulations of suppressor lymphocytes.

The findings in the present study indicate that a three-day course of CsA therapy and culture of the donor islets at 24°C for seven days will produce a marked prolongation of rat islet xenograft survival in diabetic mice, whereas a short course of CsA therapy alone produces only a modest prolongation of survival.

REIJI TERASAKA[2]
PAUL E. LACY[2]
R. PAT BUCY[2]
JOSEPH M. DAVIE[3]
Departments of Pathology and Microbiology and Immunology
Washington University School of Medicine
St. Louis, Missouri 63110

[2] Department of Pathology.
[3] Department of Microbiology and Immunology.

REFERENCES

1. Lau H, Reemtsma K, Hardy MA. The use of direct ultraviolet irradiation and cyclosporine in facilitating indefinite pancreatic islet allograft acceptance. Transplantation 1984; 38: 566.
2. Reece-Smith H, DuToit DF, McShane P, Morris PJ. Effect of cyclosporin A on rejection of pancreatic islets transplanted under the renal capsule. Transplantation 1981; 32: 333.
3. Terasaka R, Lacy PE, Hauptfeld V, Bucy RP, Davie JM. The effect of cyclosporine A, low-temperature culture and anti-Ia antibodies on prevention of rejection of rat islet allografts (submitted for publication).
4. Sugimoto K, Shelby J, Corry RJ. The effect of cyclosporine on cardiac xenograft survival. Transplantation 1985; 39: 218.
5. Lacy PE, Davie JM, Finke EH. Prolongation of islet xenograft survival without continuous immunosuppression. Science 1980; 209: 283.
6. Lacy PE, Finke EH, Janney CG, Davie JM. Prolongation of islet xenograft survival by in vitro culture of rat megaislets in 95% O_2. Transplantation 1982; 33: 588.
7. Lacy PE, Kostianovsky M. A method for the isolation of intact islets of Langerhans from the rat pancreas. Diabetes 1967; 16: 35.
8. Lacy PE, Walker MM, Fink CJ. Perfusion of isolated rat islets in vitro. The participation of the microtubular system in the biphasic release of insulin. Diabetes 1972; 21: 987.
9. Lindall A, Steffes M, Sorenson R. Immunoassayable insulin content of subcellular fractions of rat islets. Endocrinology 1969; 85: 218.
10. Kemp CB, Knight MJ, Scharp DW, Ballinger WF, Lacy PE. Effect of transplantation site on the results of pancreatic islet isografts in diabetic rats. Diabetologia 1973; 9: 486.
11. Lacy PE, Davie JM, Finke EH. Induction of rejection of successful allografts of rat islets by donor peritoneal exudate cells. Transplantation 1979; 28: 415.
12. Lacy PE, Davie JM, Finke EH. Prolongation of islet xenograft survival (rat to mouse). Diabetes 1981; 30: 285.
13. Janney CG, Davie JM, Lacy PE, Finke EH. Characterization of lymphocytes from rejected and nonrejected islet xenografts. Transplantation 1982; 33: 585.

Received 31 July 1985.
Accepted 15 August 1985.

POSITIVE DIRECT ANTIGLOBULIN TESTS ASSOCIATED WITH INTRAVENOUS GAMMA GLOBULIN USE IN BONE MARROW TRANSPLANT RECIPIENTS

Approximately 40% of bone marrow transplant recipients develop interstitial pneumonia following allogeneic transplantation (*1*). Cytomegalovirus (CMV)* is the pathogen most frequently isolated (*1, 2*). Both CMV immune plasma and CMV hyperimmune globulin favorably modify CMV infection and prevent interstitial pneumonia in these patients (*3, 4*). Since antibody titers to CMV in some lots of commercial i.v. immune globulin (IVIG)* are comparable to those found in CMV immune plasma (*5, 6*) CMV-negative bone marrow transplant recipients at our center are given IVIG. Here, we report on two patients who developed positive direct antiglobulin tests while receiving this therapy.

Case 1. L.D. was a 15-year old boy with acute myelogenous leukemia. Prior to transplantation his blood group was A Rh-positive. The direct antiglobulin test was negative and red cell alloantibodies were not detected in his serum. He received a bone marrow graft from an HLA-identical sibling who was group B Rh-positive. Red cell alloantibodies were not detected in the serum of his donor. On the day prior to transplantation Gamimune (i.v. immune globulin 5% in 10% maltose, Cutter Biological, Emeryville, CA) 1.15 gm/kg of body weight was begun and repeated at weekly intervals. Two units of washed irradiated red cells were transfused every four to five days to maintain the hemoglobin above 8 gm/dl. Fifteen days after transplantation the blood transfusion requirement increased to two units of washed red cells every two days. There was no clinical evidence of bleeding, and occult blood was not detected in the stool. Nineteen days after transplantation L.D.'s autocontrol was positive when routine crossmatching was performed. Direct antiglobulin testing revealed that his cells were weakly coated with IgG and C3d. When an acid eluate was performed, antibodies with anti-D specificity were recovered. Anti-D was not detected in his serum. The blood products he had received were from Rh-positive donors. Red cell alloantibodies were not detected in the sera of these individuals.

The lot of IVIG being administered was examined for red cell antibodies. Antibodies with anti-A, anti-B, and anti-D specificities were detected only in the undiluted product using the antiglobulin test and an anti-IgG reagent.

Since another lot of IVIG was not available, therapy was continued with the lot containing anti-D. The patient continued to have a positive direct antiglobulin test and antibodies with anti-D specificity were recovered in subsequent eluates. Although the direct antiglobulin test continued to be positive, the patient's transfusion requirement decreased. L.D. received the last dose of IVIG 34 days after transplantation. Twenty one days later, the direct antiglobulin test was negative with an anti-IgG reagent but remained positive with anti-C3d. An eluate prepared from that sample was unreactive.

Although anti-D present in the infused IVIG was clearly the cause of the positive direct antiglobulin test in this patient, the relationship of the positive direct antiglobulin test to the patient's increased transfusion requirement is unclear. If there were a causal relationship, one would expect the increased transfusion requirement to continue as long as therapy with IVIG was continued, but this did not occur. It has been demonstrated that high-dose IVIG decreases the clearance rate of Rh-positive cells sensitized with anti-D (*7*), presumably because of reticuloendothelial blockade. Therefore, continued therapy with IVIG may have prevented removal of sensitized red cells, causing the patient's transfusion requirements to return to the previous level.

Case 2. S.G. was a 39-year old woman with chronic myelogenous leukemia. Her blood group was A Rh-positive and her serum contained antibodies with anti-S and anti-JK^a specificites. She received a bone marrow graft from an HLA-identical sibling who was A Rh-positive. Gamimune 1.0 g/km of body weight was begun seven days after transplantation and repeated weekly. Eight days after the initial dose, the patient developed a positive direct antiglobulin test. Her cells were weakly coated with IgG and complement. Antibodies with anti-A_1, specificity were recovered in an acid eluate prepared from her cells. Anti-A_1 was not detected in her serum. All platelet and granulocyte products transfused were from A Rh-positive donors, none of whom had detectable anti-A_1 in their serum. The IVIG administered to this patient contained anti-A_1 detectable only in the antiglobulin test. As a precaution the patient was subsequently transfused with O Rh-positive blood. She had active gastrointestinal bleeding during most of her hospitalization. On several occasions the serum haptoglobin level was measured and was normal or elevated. These test results suggest that there was no significant intravascular red cell destruction. The direct antiglobulin test remained positive during the eight weeks that IVIG therapy was continued. One week after the last dose of IVIG her direct antiglobulin test was negative. The clinical importance of the positive direct antiglobulin test in this patient is also unclear.

Gamma globulin is prepared from plasma pools of 1000–2000 donors. It contains red cell isoagglutinins (anti-A, anti-B, anti-A,B) as well as protective antibodies to pathogens occurring in the donor population. Some lots of gamma globulin also contain anti-D and other red cell alloantibodies (*8, 9*). Dilutional effects are expected to reduce red cell antibodies to clinically insignificant levels; thus, federal regulations do not address the concentration of red cell antibodies in gamma globulin prepared for i.m. or i.v. administration. Isoagglutinin titers vary from lot to lot. When studying anti-A and anti-B gamma globulin products prepared for i.m. and i.v. use, one investigator observed that the titer of agglutinating anti-A_1 varied from undetectable to 64 (*8*). Anti-D reactive in the antiglobulin test was also detected in four products prepared for i.m. administration and in one product prepared for i.v. use.

Intravenous gamma globulin is used in the treatment of primary humoral immunodeficiency diseases and in the treatment of selected cases of idiopathic thrombocytopenic purpura (ITP). In humoral immunodeficiency diseases the dosage used is 150–300 mg/kg of body weight every two-to-three weeks (*10, 11*). The increase in serum IgG levels observed when immune globulin is given i.v. is much greater than that observed with i.m. administration (*10*). Although higher serum IgG levels are obtained with i.v. gamma globulin, problems have not been encountered with contaminating red cell antibodies at the dosage level used for humoral immune deficiency.

The dosage of i.v. gamma globulin used in the treatment of ITP is 0.4–1.5 g/kg of body weight for 4–5 days (*7, 12–15*). In

* Abbreviations used: CMV, cytomegalovirus; ITP, idiopathic thrombocytopenic purpura; IVIG, intravenous immune globulin.

most studies, the direct antiglobulin tests have been negative or not reported (*6, 7, 12–14*). However, a study of Warrier and Lusher (*15*) reported transiently positive direct antiglobulin tests in five of six pediatric patients with ITP treated with IVIG. They did not indicate whether the red cells were sensitized with IgG or complement.

The dose of IVIG used to ameliorate CMV infection in bone marrow transplant recipients is similar to that used in ITP. One would expect undesirable antibodies to become diluted when the product is administered. Because the half-life of IVIG is approximately 22 days, the serum concentration of these undesirable antibodies increases when large doses are given on a daily or weekly schedule. The development of a positive direct antiglobulin test in our two patients receiving such therapy indicates that low titer red cell antibodies present in IVIG may cause serologic problems.

CAROLYN F. WHITSETT
JULIA ANN PIERCE
LUNA E. DAFFIN
Department of Pathology and Laboratory Medicine
Emory University School of Medicine
Atlanta, Georgia 30322

[1] Address correspondence to: Carolyn F. Whitsett, M.D., Blood Bank, Emory University Hospital, 1364 Clifton Road, NE, Atlanta, Georgia 30322.

REFERENCES

1. Myers JD, Flournoy N, Thomas ED. Nonbacterial pneumonia after allogeneic marrow transplantation: a review of ten years' experience. Rev Infect Dis 1982; 4: 1119.
2. Neiman PE, Reeves W, Ray G, et al. A prospective analysis of interstitial pneumonia and opportunistic viral infection among recipients of allogeneic bone marrow grafts. J Infect Dis 1977; 136: 754.
3. Winston DJ, Pollard RB, Ho WG, et al. Cytomegalovirus immune plasma in bone marrow transplant recipients. Ann Intern Med 1982; 97: 11.
4. Condie RM, O'Reilly RJ. Prevention of cytomegalovirus infection by prophylaxis with an intravenous, hyperimmune, native unmodified cytomegalovirus globulin. Am J Med 1984; 76: 134.
5. Winston DJ, Ho WG, Rasmussen LE, et al. Use of intravenous immune globulin in patients receiving bone marrow transplants. J Clin Immunol 1982; 2(suppl): 42S.
6. Winston DJ, Ho WG, Lin CH, Budinger MD, Champlin RE, Gale RP. Intravenous immunoglobulin for modification of cytomegalovirus infections associated with bone marrow transplantation. Am J Med 1984; 76: 128.
7. Fehr J, Hofmann V, Kappeler U. Transient reversal of thrombocytopenia in idiopathic thrombocytopenic purpura by high-dose intravenous gamma globulin. N Engl J Med 1982; 306: 1254.
8. Hoppe I. Antibody screening of commercial immunoglobulin preparations, erythrocytes, HLA and autoantibodies. Blut 1979; 39: 9.
9. Romer J, Morgenthaler JJ, Scherz R, Skvaril F. Characterization of various immunoglobulin preparations for intravenous application. I. Protein composition and antibody content. Vox Sang 1982; 42: 62.
10. Cunningham-Rundles C, Siegal FP, Smithwick EM, et al. Efficacy of intravenous immunoglobulin in primary humoral immunodeficiency disease. Ann Intern Med 1984; 101: 435.
11. Pirofsky B. Intravenous immune globulin therapy in hypogammaglobulinemia: a review. Am J Med 1984; 76: 53.
12. Imbach P, Barandun S, Hirt A, Wagner HP. Intravenous immunoglobulin for idiopathic thrombocytopenic purpura (ITP) in childhood. Am J Pediatr Hematol Oncol 1984; 6: 171.
13. Carroll RR, Noyes WD, Rosse WF, Kitchens CS. Intravenous immunoglobulin administration in the treatment of severe chronic immune thrombocytopenic purpura. Am J Med 1984; 76: 181.
14. Bussel JB, Kimberly RP, Inman RD, et al. Intravenous gammaglobulin treatment of chronic idiopathic thrombocytopenic purpura. Blood 1983; 62: 480.
15. Warrier I, Lusher JM. Intravenous gamma globulin treatment for chronic idiopathic thrombocytopenic purpura in children. Am J Med 1984; 76: 193.

Received 28 May 1985.
Accepted 4 September 1985.

HEMATURIA AND HYPERCALCIURIA FOLLOWING RENAL TRANSPLANTATION

Isolated hematuria in children has recently been associated with hypercalciuria (*1*). We report a case of hematuria developing in a pediatric renal transplant patient with hypercalciuria.

This four-year-old boy developed end-stage renal disease in association with congenital nephrotic syndrome. Following bilateral nephrectomy and splenectomy, he received a renal transplant at age 2½ years. Hematuria was first noted one month after transplantation coincident with a urinary tract infection. A voiding cystourethrogram demonstrated reflux, and chronic suppressive antibiotic therapy was instituted. Subsequently, at least 5 separate episodes of painless gross or microscopic hematuria occurred, all resolving spontaneously. On each occasion, history and physical examination were unremarkable, urinalysis showed numerous red blood cells without cellular casts, and urine cultures were sterile. His medications included azathioprine, prednisone, penicillin, and trimethoprim-sulfamethoxazole.

Laboratory evaluation consistently documented normal transplant function with serum creatinines of 0.4 mg/dl, creatinine clearences of 105–116 ml/min/1.73 m^2, and total urinary protein excretions of less than 4 mg/m^2/day. Urine acidification, concentrating ability, and sodium handling appeared intact, as demonstrated by urine pHs less than 5, specific gravities greater than 1.025, and fractional excretions of sodium less than 1% during periods of fasting and mild dehydration. No glycosuria was detected. Complete blood counts, coagulation studies, serum complement levels, electrolytes, calcium, phosphate, and bicarbonate concentrations were all normal. Serial sonograms revealed normal renal architecture without evidence of nephrocalcinosis, urolithiasis, collecting system dilatation, or loss of corticomedullary differentiation.

A random "spot" urine calcium-to-creatinine ratio was elevated to 0.6 (normal: less than 0.18) (*2*). Two timed urine collections obtained on his usual diet containing approximately 700 mg of calcium/day confirmed the presence of hypercalciuria (greater than 4 mg/kg/day) (*2*). After one week on a low-calcium diet (less than 200 mg calcium/day), an oral calcium loading test was performed as described by Stapleton et al. (*1*). A fasting 2-hr urine collection and a blood sample were first obtained, followed by oral administration of 1 g elemental calcium/1.73 m^2 of body surface area. After the calcium dose, a 4-hr urine collection was obtained, together with a blood sample, at the end of the test period. Results are shown in Table 1.

TABLE 1. Results of oral calcium loading test[a]

Laboratory study	Fasting	Loading
Urine calcium/creatinine ratio	0.22(<0.21)	0.41(<0.27)
Urine cyclic-AMP (nmol/dl GFR) (1.8–4.6)	2.8	3.1
Urine phosphate (mg/dl)	11.3	
Serum calcium (mg/dl)	10.2	10.2
Serum phosphate (mg/dl)	4.5	5.2
TMP/GFR (5.0±0.6)[b]	5.17	
Serum intact N-terminal PTH (pg/ml) (11–24)	14	13

[a] Normal values are given in parentheses.

[b] TMP (tubular maximum phosphate reabsorption)/GFR was calculated using the nomogram of Walton and Byjvoet (15).

In addition, a 24-hr urinary calcium excretion from this patient's living-related donor, a 30-year-old woman was 137 mg (normal: less than 250 mg/day).

Hematuria following renal transplantation can result from a variety of causes, including rejection. Because of the child's consistently normal kidney function, idiopathic or benign hematuria appeared to be the most likely diagnosis. Harrison and Harrison were the first to suggest an association between unexplained hematuria and hypercalciuria (*3*). Subsequently, Kalia et al. (*4*) and Roy et al. (*5*) confirmed their impression in 11 children. Most recently, Stapleton et al. (*1*) documented the presence of hypercalciuria in 23 of 83 children with unexplained isolated hematuria.

Hypercalciuria can be idiopathic or secondary to a number of conditions (*2*). These include vitamin D intoxication, excessive calcium ingestion, hyperparathyroidism, sarcoidosis, malignancy, prolonged immobilization, furosemide therapy, and renal tubular disorders. Corticosteroid use is also associated with hypercalciuria (*2*). Although this association has not been specifically examined in renal transplant recipients, a review of the literature suggests that hypercalciuria is not common in transplanted patients (*6, 7*). When it occurs, posttransplantation hypercalciuria may be secondary to hypercalcemia, parathyroid hormone disorders, renal tubular acidosis, or phosphate depletion from chronic hyperphosphaturia (*8–10*). Our patient had no evidence of any of these secondary conditions.

The mechanisms responsible for idiopathic hypercalciuria remain unclear. Pak has suggested that idiopathic hypercalciuria constitutes two entities—intestinal hyperabsorption of calcium (absorptive hypercalciuria) and defective renal tubular calcium reabsorption (renal hypercalciuria) (*11*). He devised an oral calcium loading test similar to the one used for our patient to differentiate between the two types. Absorptive hypercalciuria is defined by normal urine-calcium–to–creatinine ratios during fasting and elevated ratios after an oral calcium load, while renal hypercalciuria is defined by excessive calcium excretion while fasting. Based on the results shown in Table 1, our patient appeared to have renal hypercalciuria.

A primary renal "leak" of calcium should induce elevations in serum parathyroid hormone levels and urinary cyclic adenosine monophosphate, particularly during fasting. No such elevations were found in our patient. Although this discrepancy may represent dietary "cheating" or delayed calcium hyperabsorption, others have noted similar discrepancies and proposed that idiopathic hypercalciuria may be caused by a single abnormality with varying degrees of expression (*12, 13*). This abnormality has yet to be specifically identified but may involve abnormal 1,25 dihydroxyvitamin D regulation (*14*). Interestingly, our patient's living-related donor did not have excessive urinary calcium excretion. This finding suggests that an extrarenal process was responsible for hypercalciuria in this case.

Regardless of its etiology, hypercalciuria should be considered during the evaluation of isolated hematuria following renal transplantation.

JAMES E. SPRINGATE
ROBERT D. FILDES
S. MICHAEL MAUER
LEONARD G. FELD[1]
The Division of Pediatric Nephrology and the Children's Kidney Center
Department of Pediatrics
Children's Hospital of Buffalo, New York
The Department of Pediatrics
University of Minnesota School of Medicine
Minneapolis, Minnesota

[1] Address correspondence to: Leonard G. Feld, M.D., Ph.D., Chief, Division of Pediatric Nephrology, Children's Hospital, 219 Bryant Street, Buffalo, NY 14222.

REFERENCES

1. Stapleton FB, Roy S, Noe N, Jerkins G. Hypercalciuria in children with hematuria. N Engl J Med 1984; 310: 1345.
2. Langman CB, Moore ES. Hypercalciuria in clinical pediatrics. Clin Pediatr 1984; 23: 135.
3. Harrison HE, Harrison HC. Disorders of calcium and phosphate metabolism in childhood and adolescence. Philadelphia: Saunders, 1979: 277.
4. Kalia A, Travis LB, Brouhard BH. The association of idiopathic hypercalciuria and asymptomatic gross hematuria in children. J Pediatr 1981; 99: 716.
5. Roy S, Stapleton FB, Noe NH, Jerkins G. Hematuria preceding renal calculus formation in children with hypercalciuria. J Pediatr 1981; 99: 712.
6. Rosenbaum RW, Hruska KA, Korkor A, Anderson C. Decreased phosphate reabsorption after renal transplantation: evidence for a mechanism independent of calcium and parathyroid hormone. Kidney Int 1981; 19: 568.
7. Garabedian M, Silve C, Levy-Bentolila D, Bourdeau A. Changes in plasma 1,25 and 24,25-dihydroxyvitamin D after renal transplantation in children. Kidney Int 1981; 20: 403.
8. Brien G, Scholz D, Oesterwitz H, Schubert G, Bick C. Urolithiasis after kidney transplantation-clinical and mineralogical aspects. Urol Research 1980; 8: 211.
9. Boyce NW, Holdsworth SR, Scott D, Atkins RC. Acute renal transplant failure resulting from obstruction with a calculus. Transplant Proc 1984; 16: 1364.
10. Green J, Better OS. Endocrine and metabolic dysfunctions following kidney transplantations. In: Robinson RR, ed. Nephrology. New York: Springer-Verlag, 1984: 1644.
11. Pak CYC. Physiological basis for absorptive and renal hypercalciurias. Am J Physiol 1979; 237: F415.
12. Coe FL, Favus MJ, Crockett T, Parks JH. Effects of low-calcium diet on urine calcium excretion, parathyroid function and serum 1,25 $(OH)_2$ D_3 levels in patients with idiopathic hypercalciuria and in normal subjects. Am J Med 1982; 72: 25.
13. Hymes LC, Warshaw BL. Idiopathic hypercalciuria. Am J Dis Child 1984; 138: 176.
14. Coe FL. Treatment of hypercalciuria. N Engl J Med 1984; 311: 116.
15. Walton RJ, Bijvoet OLM: Nomogram for derivation of renal threshold phosphate concentration. Lancet 1975; 2: 309.

Received 10 June 1985.
Accepted 4 September 1985.

SUCCESSFUL TREATMENT OF PERSISTENT POSTTRANSPLANT HYPERPARATHYROIDISM WITH DIPHOSPHONATE[1]

Progressive posttransplant hyperparathyroidism is always treated surgically by almost complete removal of the parathyroid glands (*1*). Until now no beneficial effect of drug treatment has been described. We report here the successful treatment of two patients with persistent posttransplant hyperparathyroidism with 3-amino-hydroxypropylidene-1, 1-disphosphonate (APD).* The first patient, a 58-year-old man, complained of persistent bone pain eight months after cadaveric renal transplantation. Corneal calcifications were seen. Bone biopsy, scintigraphy, and biochemical investigations were compatible with hyperparathyroidism. The serum calcium level was 2.95 mmol/L (2.1<n<2.6); alkaline phosphatase 550 U/L (30<n<120); and PTH 5.61 pmol P_2/L (n<0.75). Vitamin D levels were normal.

Because of worsening cardiac state, parathyroidectomy was thought to be contraindicated; therefore, after informed consent, APD 150 mg t.d.s. 30 min before meals was given. His usual drug regimen was continued: cyclosporine 250 mg b.d., prednisolone 2.5 mg daily, digoxine 0.125 mg daily, cimetidine 200 mg b.d., nifedipine 10 mg t.d.s. and isosorbidedinitrate 20 mg t.d.s. Serum calcium, phosphate, alkaline phosphatase, and PTH levels were measured at regular intervals. PTH (1–84) was measured according to the radioimmunoassy (RIA) method. In addition, 24-hr urine samples were collected to determine calcium, hydroxyproline, and creatinine.

The second patient, a 52-year-old woman, was treated with APD following the favorable results obtained in the first patient. Eleven months after a cadaveric renal transplantation she still complained of severe bone pain. Corneal calcifications were seen. Bone biopsy, scintigraphy, and biochemical investigations were compatible with hyperparathyroidism. The serum calcium level was 2.93 mmol/L, alkaline phosphatase 250 U/L, PTH 1.56 pmol P_2/l. Vitamin D levels were normal. The same APD regimen as in the first patient was followed. Her usual drug regimen was continued: cyclosporine 250 mg b.d., propranolol 40 mg t.d.s., and furosemide 40 mg daily. The same blood and urine measurements as in the first patient were performed.

Bone pain disappeared in both patients completely within the first week of treatment with APD. In both patients serum calcium decreased gradually to near normal levels during 26 weeks of treatment (Table 1). Serum phosphate remained unchanged. The alkaline phosphatase showed an initial increase but afterward there was a decrease in the alkaline phosphatase level. The PTH as well as hydroxyproline excretion decreased in both patients to normal levels. The urinary calcium:creatinine ratio remained unchanged. Vitamin D levels were stable during treatment. The bone biopsies after 12 weeks of treatment did not show any progression of renal osteodystrophy.

TABLE 1. The effect of APD on laboratory parameters of bone metabolism

	Patient 1			Patient 2		
	Baseline±SEM	After 12 weeks' treatment	After 26 weeks' treatment	Baseline±SEM	After 12 weeks' treatment	After 26 weeks' treatment
Clearance (ml/min)	45	45	45	50	50	60
Calcium (mmol/L; n: 2.10–2.65)	2.95±0.05	2.62	2.61	2.93±0.05	2.70	2.70
Parathyroid hormone (pmol p_2 L Ca ↑: [n<0.75])	5.61	2.00	0.41	1.56	0.92	0.65
Urinary hydroxy-proline excretion μmol/mmol creatinine	62	22	20	47	19	13
Alkaline phosphatase (n: 30–125)	550±40	561	251	250±40	294	184

The fall in serum calcium and hydroxyproline excretion are results of the inhibitive properties of APD on bone resorption (*2–4*). It is well known that APD, after inhibiting osteoclastic activity, also inhibits osteoblastic activity (*5–7*). This might explain the decrease in alkaline phosphatase after 3–4 months of treatment. PTH release is not autonomous in persistent posttransplant hyperparathyroidism; gland responsiveness to Ca^{2+} change is retained (*8*). The decrease of the PTH level in our patients, despite the decrease in serum calcium level, is therefore unexpected, and it might be due to inhibition of PTH release by APD. A spontaneous decrease in PTH release seems to be unlikely because in both patients clinical and biochemical parameters of hyperparathyroidism had been increasing in the pretreatment period. Moreover, the natural history of persistent posttransplant hyperparathyroidism shows a more gradual normalization of the various parameters over at least one year (*9*). Recently Mann observed a decrease in PTH during treatment with APD in a patient suffering from a parathyroid carcinoma (*10*). He suggested that the fall in PTH was a result of a direct cytotoxic effect of APD on the carcinoma cells. Our observations are in accordance with the findings of Mann with respect to the decrease of PTH during APD treatment.

In summary, the effects of the disphosphonate, APD, on two patients with persistent posttransplant hyperparathyroidism are described. The following observations were made: complete disappearance of bone pain within one week, the gradual decrease of serum calcium to near normal levels, and a decrease of serum PTH.

Acknowledgments. We thank Dr. W.H.L. Hackeng from the laboratory of endocrinology Bergwegziekenhuis Rotterdam for the determination of PTH, and Mrs. A. Wijnands for her excellent secretarial work.

* Abbreviations used: APD, 3-aminohydroxypropylidene-1, 1-diphosphophonate; RIA, radioimmunoassay.

[1] This work was supported by the Dutch Kidney Foundation.

K.M.L. Leunissen[2,3]
F-J.F.E. Vismans[4]
R.J.M. van Leendert[5]
J.P. van Hooff[2]
The Departments of Nephrology, Gastroenterology, and Endocrinology
Academic Hospital
Maastricht, The Netherlands

[2] Department of Nephrology.
[3]Address correspondence to: K.M.L. Leunissen, Academic Hospital, University of Limburg, P.O. Box 1918, NL-6201 BX Maastricht, The Netherlands.
[4] Department of Gastroenterology.
[5] Department of Endocrinology.

REFERENCES

1. Morris PJ. Kidney transplantation. Principles and practices. 2nd ed. New York: Grune & Stratton, 1984.
2. Bijvoet OLM, Frijlink WB, Jie K, et al. APD in Paget's disease of bone. Arthritis Rheum 1980; 23: 1193.
3. Frijlink WB, Bijvoet OLM, te Velde J, et al. Treatment of Paget's disease with 3-amino-1-hydroxypropilidene)-1, 1-disphosphonate (APD). Lancet 1979; 1: 788.
4. Breukelen van FJM, Bijvoet OLM, van Oosterom AT. Inhibition of osteolytic bone lesions by (3-amino-1-hydroxypropilidene)-1, 1-disphosphonate (APD). Lancet 1979; 1: 803.
5. Vismans F-JFE. APD, parathyreoidhormoon en osteoporose. 1984 Thesis Leiden.
6. Marks SC Jr, Walker DG. In: Bourne GH, ed. The biochemistry and physiology of bone. 2nd ed. New York: Academic Press, 1976; 4: 227.
7. Johson LC: Morphologic analysis of pathology: the kinetics of disease and general biology of bone. In: Frost HM, ed. Bone biodynamics. London: J&A Churchill, 1964: 543.
8. McCarron DA, Muther RS, Plant SB, Barry JM, Bennett WM, Krutzik S. Regulation of parathyroid hormone (PTH) secretion in post transplant hyperparathyroidism (Tx-HPTH): in vivo response to changes (A) in ionized calcium (Ca^{++}). [Abstract.] Amer Soc Nephrol 1984; 946.
9. de Graaf P, van Hooff JP, Boekhout M, et al. Hyperparathyroidism and vascular necrosis of bone after renal transplantation. Neth J Med 1982; 7: 237.
10. Mann K. Oral bisphosphonate therapy in metastatic parathyroid carcinoma. Lancet 1985; 1: 101.

Received 2 July 1985.
Accepted 9 September 1985.

ERRATUM

In the article entitled "Joint report of the Third International Workshop on Canine Immunogenetics: I. Analysis of homozygous typing cells" by Deeg et al., which appeared in the January 1986 issue of *Transplantation*, there is a mistake in Table 2 on page 114. The workshop assignment Dw8 was placed in the wrong column. Cells with the workshop numbers 7, 8 and 74 have the workshop specificity Dw7, and cells with the workshop numbers 25, 26, 42, 11, and 75 have the workshop specificity Dw8. We apologize for any inconvenience that this may have caused.

0041-1337/86/4106-0669$02.00/0
TRANSPLANTATION

Vol. 41, No. 6
Printed in U.S.A.

Transplantation
ARTICLES

FUNCTIONAL PRESERVATION OF THE MAMMALIAN KIDNEY

VII. AUTOLOGOUS TRANSPLANTATION OF DOG KIDNEYS AFTER TREATMENT WITH DIMETHYLSULFOXIDE (2.8 AND 4.2 *M*)[1]

ARMAND M. KAROW, JR.,[2,3] MALCOLM MCDONALD,[3] TRACY DENDLE,[3] AND RAGHUNATHA RAO[4]

Departments of Pharmacology and Toxicology and Pathology, Medical College of Georgia, Augusta, Georgia

This research demonstrates that dog kidneys perfused with dimethylsulfoxide (Me_2SO) in likely cryoprotective concentrations (2.8 *M*) can survive as the sole source of renal support when autologously transplanted. Kidneys were perfused in vitro with Me_2SO in one of two vehicles: solution A (K^+-Mg^{2+}-rich) or RPS-2 (K^+-glucose-rich). Me_2SO concentration in the vehicle was gradually increased to maximum (2.8 or 4.2 *M*) over a period of 28 to 35 min, held for 5–10 min, then decreased over 55–65 min. All groups except one consisted of 5 kidneys perfused at 25°C. *Survivors* were dogs living 21 days postoperatively. The first group received kidneys perfused with solution A; 5 dogs survived, serum creatinine on day 21 [Cr], [mean±SE] = 1.3±0.1. The second group received RPS-2 kidneys; 4 survived, Cr=1.4±0.1. The third group received solution A kidneys with 2.8 *M* Me_2SO; 3 survived, Cr=2.7±1.3. The fourth group received RPS-2 kidneys with 2.8 *M* Me_2SO; 5 survived, Cr=1.2±0.2. The fifth group received RPS-2 kidneys with 4.2 *M* Me_2SO; 2 survived, Cr=1.7±0.3. One group of 6 dogs received kidneys perfused at 10°C with 4.2 *M* Me_2SO in RPS-2; one survived, Cr=1.4. Results demonstrate beneficial interaction of vehicle with Me_2SO and the efficacy of 25°C perfusion.

Mammalian kidneys must be perfused with a cryoprotectant prior to long-term cryostorage. In recent screening studies cryoprotectant dimethylsulfoxide (Me_2SO) was found to be more effective against cryoinjury (*1*), and less toxic (*2–4*) to renal tissues, than ethylene glycol or glycerol. The screening studies used the rabbit divided kidney model that independently evaluates parenchymal and vascular renal components.

Here we present a confirmation of the utility of the rabbit divided kidney model in predicting preservation efficacy of dog kidneys tested by autologous transplantation. We also demonstrate that a large proportion of dog kidneys can serve as the sole source of renal support after being perfused with 2.8 *M* Me_2SO. The vehicle for Me_2SO perfusion and its temperature are shown to be important determinants in successful Me_2SO renal perfusion.

[1] This work was supported in part by a grant from USPHS National Institutes of Health (AM 31613) and by the American Heart Association Georgia Affiliate.

[2] To whom all correspondence should be addressed.

[3] Department of Pharmacology and Toxicology.

[4] Department of Pathology.

MATERIALS AND METHODS

Kidney extirpation. Female mongrel dogs (17.5±0.8 kg; [mean±SE]) were quarantined for 2 weeks prior to being placed in this study. Baseline laboratory studies indicated all dogs to have normal renal function and to be free of obvious infection. Baseline laboratory studies included hematocrit (47±0.8), serum glucose (93±7 mg/dl), serum creatinine ([Cr]*; 0.7±0.02 mg/dl), blood urea nitrogen ([BUN]; 42±0.7 mg/dl), and urinalysis by microscopy and chemistry. Anesthesia was induced with thiamyl sodium and maintained with nitrous oxide, methoxyflurane, and oxygen. During the operation each dog was supported with i.v. fluids, mannitol (0.5 g/kg body weight), methylprednisolone (250 mg) and penicillin (1 million units). Papaverine was infused around the renal artery of the kidney selected for perfusion, and a ureteral cannula was inserted. The kidney, freed of fat and connective tissue, was flushed with sterile perfusate (130±10 ml), either solution A or RPS-2 (Table 1) at room temperature (22°C), then placed in the perfusion circuit (Fig. 1). Extirpation required 1 min, and the period of renal anoxia prior to in vitro perfusion was 4.2±0.2 min. During external perfusion the contralateral common iliac artery and external iliac vein were prepared to receive the transplanted kidney. From the contralateral kidney a biopsy was taken, then the kidney was extirpated and discarded.

Perfusion circuit and solutions. The sterilized nonrecirculating perfusion circuit was assembled (Fig. 1) while the kidney was being prepared for extirpation. Perfusate pressure (at the bubble trap) and flow rate were monitored. The pressure was held at 60 mm Hg. Effluent from the ureter was collected.

The perfusates were sterilized by autoclave. During initial preparation Me_2SO in appropriate concentrations (Tables 2 and 3) was substituted for water in order to maintain the concentration of all other components at the values listed in Table 1. Separate solutions of sodium bicarbonate and hydrochloric acid were autoclaved and used to adjust the pH of solution A and of RPS-2 following autoclaving. (Precipitates tend to form in those solutions in which pH adjustment preceded autoclaving.) Oxygen that had been filtered (Bacterial Air Vent, Gelman Sciences) was passed continuously into these stock solutions prior to pouring them into the reservoir of the perfusion apparatus.

* Abbreviations used: BUN, blood urea nitrogen; Cr, serum creatinine.

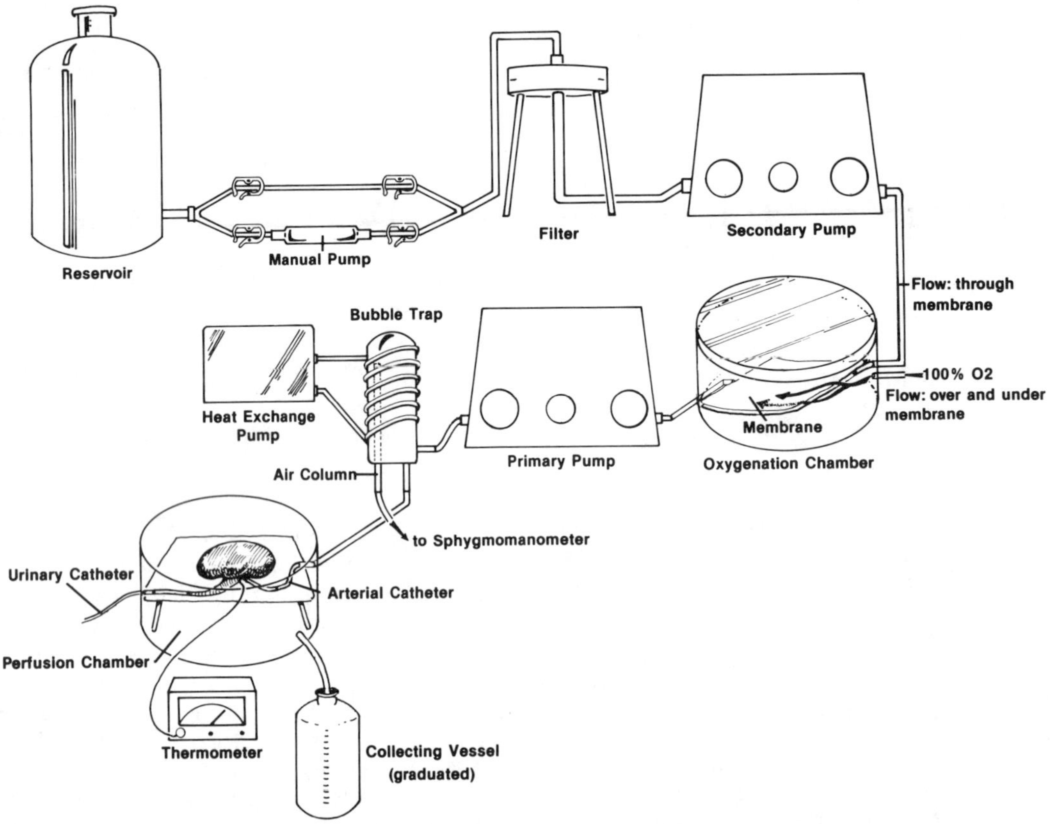

FIGURE 1. Perfusion Circuit. All surfaces in contact with perfusate are made of Silastic except as noted. Oxygenated perfusate (Table 1) is placed in the glass reservoir. As the reservoir is depleted, perfusates are added in sequence according to the schedules shown in Tables 2 and 3. The polyvinylchloride manual pump is used only to prime the circuit initially with Me_2SO-free perfusate. When the circuit is primed, the alternate path around the manual pump is used. The filter, 90-mm cellulose-acetate with 1.2 μ pores (RA-type, Millipore), is held in a stainless steel case. The secondary pump (Harvard Apparatus) has metal rods that sigmoidially compress Silastic tubing. The glass oxygenation chamber contains a Silastic membrane oxygenator (MOX, Waters Instrument) through which the perfusate flows. The primary pump is similar to the secondary pump. The glass bubble trap also serves as a heat exchanger, and as a port for measuring perfusion pressure by means of a sphygmomanometer. The external heat exchange pump can warm or cool the perfusate inside the bubble trap. To cool kidneys (10°C) an auxillary glass heat exchanger (not shown) is inserted between the bubble trap and the perfusion chamber. The glass perfusion chamber has a Teflon screen upon which the kidney rests. The catheters are made of polyethylene. The thermometer detects the temperature of the venous effluent, which is maintained at 25°C or 10°C as appropriate for the schedule (Tables 2 and 3). Perfusate flow and urine flow are determined by timed collections into graduated vessels, only one of which is shown.

TABLE 1. Composition of Solutions[a]

Components	Krebs-Henseleit	Sol. A	RPS-2	Collins'
NaCl	118	96.2	–	10
KCl	4.6	40.3	28.5	15
$CaCl_2$	2.5	1.7	1.0	–
$MgSO_4 \cdot 7H_2O$	1.2	12.5	–	30
$MgCl_2 \cdot 6H_2O$	–	–	2.0	–
$NaHCO_3$	24.9	11.9	10.0	10
KH_2PO_4	1.2	–	7.2	15
K_2HPO_4	–	–	–	4.2
Glucose	5.6	11.1	180	140
Glutathione	–	–	5.0	–
Adenine	–	–	1.0	–

[a] All concentrations expressed as m*M*; the solvent is water. Solution A and RPS-2 were used in the described experiments. The composition of Krebs-Henseleit and of Collins' solution are given for reference.

Experimental groups. Experimental groups of dogs receiving autologous kidney transplants were designated according to the in vitro renal perfusion regimen. The first group of dogs received kidneys perfused with solution A (no Me_2SO). The second group received RPS-2 kidneys. The third group received kidneys perfused with 2.8 *M* Me_2SO in solution A. The fourth group received kidneys perfused with 2.8 *M* Me_2SO in RPS-2. The fifth group received kidneys perfused with 4.2 *M* Me_2SO in RPS-2. Kidneys for groups 1-5 (5 dogs each) were perfused at 25°C. The sixth group (6 dogs) received kidneys perfused with 4.2 *M* Me_2SO in RPS-2 at 10°C (as explained in Table 3). In kidneys receiving Me_2SO, the concentration was increased step-wise over a period of 28–35 min, held at the maximum concentration of Me_2SO for 5–10 min, then decreased step-wise (with the help of 600 m*M* mannitol added to the vehicle) over the following 55–65 min. Details of concentration changes are given in Tables 2 and 3. All kidneys were perfused in vitro for 100 min.

Transplantation and postoperative evaluation. After perfusion the kidney was placed in the previously prepared inplantation fossa. Vascular anastomosis required 54.7 ± 1.7 min. The vesicle-ureteral anastomosis was accomplished by creating a submucosal tunnel (approx. 2.5 cm long) and then penetrating the muscularis and serosa of the bladder. Postoperatively dogs were supported with fluids, antibiotics, and appropriate food.

TABLE 2. Schedule of solutions to add and remove 2.8 *M* dimethylsulfoxide (Me_2SO)[a]

Time of addition (min)	Solution	Volume (ml)
0	Vehicle (without Me_2SO)	200
7	Vehicle with 0.7 *M* Me_2SO	200
14	Vehicle with 1.4 *M* Me_2SO	200
21	Vehicle with 2.1 *M* Me_2SO	200
28	Vehicle with 2.8 *M* Me_2SO	200
35	Vehicle with 2.1 *M* Me_2SO	200
42	Vehicle with 1.4 *M* Me_2SO and 600 m*M* mannitol	200
49	Vehicle with 0.7 *M* Me_2SO and 600 m*M* mannitol	200
56	Vehicle with 600 m*M* mannitol	650
78	Vehicle	>650
100	Discontinue; remove kidney	–0–

[a] Vehicle solution was solution A or RPS-2 (see Table 1 for composition). Solutions were placed in empty reservoir of perfusion circuit (see Figure 1). Unavoidable mixing of solutions occurred throughout the volume (dead space) of the apparatus. Perfusion was at 60 mm Hg and 25°C.

TABLE 3. Schedule of solutions to add and remove 4.2 *M* dimethylsulfoxide (Me_2SO)[a]

Time of addition (min)		Solution	Volume (ml)
Group 5	Group 6		
0	0	Vehicle (without Me_2SO)	200
5	5	Vehicle with 0.7 *M* Me_2SO	200
10	10	Vehicle with 1.4 *M* Me_2SO	200
15	15	Vehicle with 2.1 *M* Me_2SO	200
20	20	Vehicle with 2.8 *M* Me_2SO	200
25	25[b]	Vehicle with 3.5 *M* Me_2SO	300
30	35[b]	Vehicle with 4.2 *M* Me_2SO	300
35	45[b]	Vehicle with 3.5 *M* Me_2SO	300
40	55	Vehicle with 2.8 *M* Me_2SO	200
45	60	Vehicle with 2.1 *M* Me_2SO and 600 m*M* mannitol	200
50	65	Vehicle with 1.4 *M* Me_2SO and 600 m*M* mannitol	200
55	70	Vehicle with 0.7 *M* Me_2SO and 600 m*M* mannitol	200
60	75	Vehicle with 600 m*M* mannitol	500
80	80	Vehicle	700
100	100	Discontinue; remove kidney	–0–

[a] Vehicle solution was RPS-2 (see Table 1). Process of adding and removing given in footnote of Table 2 with exception of temperature. Group five was perfused at 25°C throughout the entire schedule.

[b] Group six was perfused at 25°C, except for these intervals on the schedule during which the temperature was 10°C.

Dogs were maintained individually in metabolism cages for 14 days so that 24-hr urine volumes could be measured periodically. Venous blood samples were taken daily through day 6, then on alternate days through day 14, and finally on day 21.

Dogs were killed by euthanasia (pentobarbital and phenytoin i.v.) upon advice of a veterinarian, when the Cr exceeded 8 mg/dl or blood urea nitrogen BUN exceeded 170 mg/dl or upon the twenty-first postoperative day. All dogs that lived three weeks postoperatively were considered to be survivors. An autopsy was done on all dogs.

Three general conditions represented reasons for excluding from the experiment some animals subjected to surgery. The first condition was severe problems not detected in presurgical evaluation, such as multiple renal arteries or disseminated afebrile abcesses. The second condition was severe difficulties encountered with perfusion, such as failure of a component of the perfusion apparatus. The third condition was surgical or postoperative complications, such as anastomotic failure, intussusception, pancreatitis, or septic peritonitis.

Quantitative data were subjected to Student's *t* test. Differences in experimental values were considered to be statistically significant if *t* values corresponded to *P* values of 0.05 or less.

Renal tissue was evaluated pathologically. This tissue consisted of wedge biopsies taken prior to perfusion, postperfusion wedge biopsies, wedge biopsies of contralateral kidneys, and excised kidneys at the end of the experiment. Phosphate-buffered 10% formalin was the primary fixative employed, but samples of the excised kidneys were also fixed in Bouin's fixative. All sections were paraffin-embedded. Hematoxylin-eosin stains were routinely performed. In selected cases of periodic-acid-Schiff, a modified picro-Mallory stain, and Jones' methenamine silver stains were used. Tissue from two kidneys was processed for epon embedding in glutaraldehyde; of these, one was also examined by transmission electron microscopy. Each tissue was evaluated without the benefit of the clinical history of the animal.

RESULTS

Postoperative changes in Cr and BUN were qualitatively identical, and therefore only Cr data are presented (Table 4). In our series a Cr value of 0.7±0.1 was typical of dogs with two functioning kidneys. In our experience with a group of ten dogs receiving nontreated autologous renal transplants with immediate contralateral nephrectomy, the Cr rose to 2.0 on the first postoperative day, fell to 1.3–1.6 by day 3, then declined over a one-week period to 0.8 to 1.2 for the remainder of the dog's life. In the experimental groups we consider in this report, Cr of surviving dogs rose to a peak value of 2.3–5.3 by day 4, then declined over a two-week period to a constant value of about 1.4 for the remainder of the dog's life. The kidney contralateral to the transplanted kidney was grossly and histologically normal in all dogs included in this study.

Perfusion without Me_2SO. Although considerations for aseptic technique precluded measurements of renal weight during perfusion, the development of edema was obvious in each kidney and its ureter. Perfusate flow for both vehicle perfusates was similar (Table 5), but urine flow was negligible for RPS-2 vehicle (Table 6).

The postoperative course of dogs perfused with either vehicle without Me_2SO was rather similar with regard to Cr. All of the solution A dogs survived, and all but one of the RPS-2 dogs survived.

The glomeruli from kidneys perfused with solution A or RPS-2 were hypercellular, and the tubular epithelium was swollen. Additionally, the tubular epithelium from solution A kidneys had markedly eosinophilic cytoplasm; the glomerular hypercellularity was very severe in one. No thrombosis in glomeruli or tubules, or necrosis, was evident.

An RPS-2 dog died on postoperative day 18; grossly the kidney had small scattered infarcts and the medulla was congested and microscopically tubular necrosis was evident. Infarcts were present in another RPS-2 kidney.

Perfusion with 2.8 M Me_2SO. The quality of survival of dogs receiving kidneys perfused with 2.8 *M* Me_2SO in RPS-2 was

TABLE 4. Postoperative serum creatinine in dogs receiving an autologous renal transplant

Kidney perfusate	Survivors			Serum creatinine,[c] survivors, preoperative and postoperative days (mg/dl)					
	N[a]	n[b]	$\frac{n}{N} \times 100$	Presurgery	3	6	10	14	21
RPS-2	5	4	80	0.7±0.07	4.9±0.8	3.8±0.9	2.4±0.3	2.4±0.4	1.4±0.1
Solution A	5	5	100	0.6±0.04	4.1±1.0	3.9±1.3	2.5±0.9	1.8±0.5	1.3±0.1
Solution A + 2.8 *M* Me_2SO	5	3	60	0.7±0.06	4.3±0.6	3.7±0.4	2.3±0.4	1.9±0.2	2.7±1.3
RPS-2 + 2.8 *M* Me_2SO	5	5	100	0.7±0.04	2.3±0.3	2.6±0.6	1.5±0.1	1.2±0.1	1.2±0.2
RPS-2 + 4.2 *M* Me_2SO (25°C)	5	2	40	0.70±0.00	5.2±0.9	3.8±0.2	2.4±0.5	2.0±0.3	1.7±0.3
RPS-2 + 4.2 *M* Me_2SO (10°C)	6	1	17	0.70	2.7	2.4	1.7	1.5	1.4

[a] N, total number of dogs included in group designated by kidney perfusate.

[b] n, number dogs in group that survived to day 21.

[c] Values = mean ±SE.

TABLE 5. Perfusate flow dynamics

	Kidney weight[a] (g)	Initial flow rate (ml/g/min)	Change in flow from initial (%)[a,b]					
			Me_2SO 2.8 *M* (25°C)		Me_2SO 4.2 *M* (25°C)		Me_2SO 4.2 *M* (10°C)	
			Peak	Washout	Peak	Washout	Peak	Washout
Solution A	51.2±4.3	0.82±0.2	−34.0[c]	−41.6[c]	Not applicable		Not applicable	
RPS-2	46.5±2.4	1.12±0.1	−39.6[c]	+38.7	−60.4[c]	−41.3[c]	−41.7[c]	−52.5[c]

[a] Values = mean ± SE.

[b] Kidneys were perfused with solution A or with RPS-2. Me_2SO concentration in these two vehicle perfusates was increaed to a peak value of 2.8 *M*–or, in the case of RPS-2, to 4.2 *M*. Then the Me_2SO was removed from the kidneys by washout. All kidneys were maintained at 25°C throughout perfusion except for a group that was cooled at 10°C during the time the Me_2SO concentration was in the range of 2.8–4.2 *M*. Change (%) in flow (ml/min) calculated as ([flow at experimental interval] − [flow at initial time without Me_2SO]) × 100 ÷ (flow at initial time without Me_2SO).

[c] Statistically significant from flow at initial time.

significantly better than in any other group. All dogs receiving kidneys perfused with 2.8 *M* Me_2SO in RPS-2 survived; 60% of dogs receiving kidneys perfused with Me_2SO in solution A survived (Table 4). The RPS-2/Me_2SO survivors had significantly lower Cr than the comparable solution A/Me_2SO dogs. The RPS-2/Me_2SO survivors had Cr that was lower but statistically similar to that of the two groups perfused only with vehicle.

During in vitro perfusion the administration of Me_2SO caused vascular resistance to rise (Table 5). During the washout period (decreasing Me_2SO concentration) vascular resistance remained elevated in all Me_2SO groups except RPS-2 with 2.8 *M* Me_2SO. In that group during washout renal vascular resistance typically decreased precipitously resulting in an increase in flow to an extent that maintenance of pressure became difficult. Immediately after the mannitol phase of washout all kidneys and ureters became extremely edematous, but the edema vanished almost immediately upon the resumption of blood flow.

Urine flow (Table 6) was sustained during in vitro perfusion when Me_2SO was used; for the RPS-2/Me_2SO group urine flow was significantly greater than solution A/Me_2SO.

Three kidneys perfused with 2.8 *M* Me_2SO in solution A showed fibrin thrombi in glomerular capillaries and interlobular arteries, necrosis of glomeruli and tubules, and focal infarcts. One kidney showed thrombi in only a few glomeruli.

All five kidneys perfused with 2.8 *M* Me_2SO in RPS-2 showed slight glomerular hypercellularity. However, the tubular epithelium was only slightly swollen because of osmotic nephropathy. No glomerular or vascular thrombi were noted in any of the animals in this group.

Perfusion with 4.2 M Me_2SO. Dogs receiving kidneys perfused with 4.2 *M* Me_2SO in RPS-2 had a significantly poorer prospect of survival than dogs in the other experimental groups (Table 4). Of the dogs perfused at 25°C that did not survive, all but one was killed by postoperative day 2 because of symptomatic renal failure; the exception was killed on day 4. Of the dogs perfused at 10°C that did not survive, 2 were killed by postoperative day 2, and the other 3 were killed on day 4.

Eight kidneys were studied microscopically in these groups. Severe glomerular and arterial thrombi were present with scattered infarcts of varying severity in seven. One kidney showed only slight glomerular hypercellularity.

TABLE 6. Urine flow during in vitro perfusion of dog kidneys

Kidney perfusate	N[a]	Urine volume[b] perfusion intervals		
		30 min	60 min	100 min
Solution A	5	33±11	23±11	49±13
RPS-2	5	4.3±3.9	0.04±0.04	0.09±0.04
Solution A + 2.8 *M* Me_2SO	5	50±18	78±27	62±14
RPS-2 + 2.8 *M* Me_2SO	5	7.8±3.0	27±10	84±17
RPS-2 + 4.2 *M* Me_2SO (25°C)	5	14±7.4	19±18	52±15
RPS-2 + 4.2 *M* Me_2SO (10°C)	6	29±7.8	a 33±9.8	53±14

[a] N, total number of dogs included in group designated by kidney perfusate.

[b] Urine (ml) accumulated during first 30 min, during second 30 min, and during final 40 min. Values = mean ± SE.

DISCUSSION

This is the first comprehensive report demonstrating dog kidney survival after perfusion with a high (cryoprotective) concentration of Me_2SO. The validity of the results should be considered in the context of the experimental process. Surgical experience in transplantation increased throughout the course of the experiment. Randomization of experimental groups was nonsystematic; a preponderance of animals in groups 1 and 2 were done early in the course of the experiment and animals in groups 5 and 6 were done late. In fact randomization by double-blind protocol of Me_2SO and non-Me_2SO groups is virtually impossible because Me_2SO is readily detected, even at concentrations less than half that used, by odor of solutions and breath of experimental animals that persists for at least 24 hr postoperatively. We believe our concern for these potential sources of interpretive error has helped mitigate their incursion.

Two general topics for discussion develop from the results of these experiments. The first is the possible consequences of findings relative to organ perfusion for cryopreservation. The second is the validation these results give to a rapid and inexpensive means of viability testing relative to the laborious and expensive process of transplanting canine kidneys.

Perfusion for Cryopreservation. We have focused on Me_2SO for many reasons. Relative to the other agents it is nontoxic (*2, 3*) in concentrations expected to be cryoprotective (*1, 5, 6*). Me_2SO diffuses across cell membranes much quicker than glycerol (*2, 7*) or ethylene glycol (*2*), and therefore has fewer adverse osmotic effects. Our group (*8*) and others (*9*) have demonstrated the tissue distribution and time course for Me_2SO perfused in mammalian kidneys at 37°C, 25°C, and 10°C; complete permeation is expected under the conditions of the experiment we report here. Electron microscopy by us (*10*) demonstrates good retention of vascular ultrastructure in kidneys perfused with 2.8 *M* Me_2SO in solution A without the benefit of gradual changes in concentration. Finally, Me_2SO has a facilitating effect when frozen tissue is thawed with electromagnetic radiation (*11–13*).

Cryoprotectant pharmacology has meaning only in the context of the vehicle solution. Relative to contemporary organ preservation, continuous perfusion with a potassium-rich solution is unusual. Keeler and associates (*14*) first demonstrated that a potassium-rich perfusate was important to the survival of kidneys perfused with Me_2SO. We (*8, 10, 15–18*) modeled solution A after Keeler's original solution. RPS-2, a relatively new vehicle solution developed by Fahy (*2, 20, 21*), is rich in potassium and glucose and also contains glutathione and adenine. Our previous work (*2–4*) and that reported here demonstrates that solution A without Me_2SO is less damaging to kidneys than is RPS-2 without Me_2SO. The damaging effects of RPS-2 and of Me_2SO seem to counteract each other. Glucose in high concentrations seems to inhibit the binding of Me_2SO to proteins (*3*); this benefit is not obtained when sucrose or mannitol is substituted for glucose in RPS-2. We (*19*) have found that glutathione, important in the economy of renal parenchyma, is depleted from kidneys perfused with vehicles deficient in this metabolite. Adenine, diffusable across cell membranes, is converted by cells to adenylate (adenosine monophosphate) and subsequently to other purine ribonucleotides by a well-known salvage reaction catalysed by adenine phosphoribosyl transferase (*23*). Evidence from several laboratories (*24–28*) suggests that nucleotide replenishment is effective in organ preservation. The absence of albumin from perfusate does not appreciably compromise the function of transplanted organs; this observation is amply confirmed by others who have transplanted canine kidneys (*29*) and canine hearts (*30*). Finally, in the washout perfusate, mannitol is incorporated to facilitate osmotically the removal of Me_2SO from cells (*3, 5, 22, 31, 32*).

The benefits of warm perfusion are numerous. Warm temperatures enhance the diffusion of Me_2SO across biological barriers (*7, 8, 33*). The use of warm temperatures obviates the admonition to change cryoprotectant concentrations gradually in order to minimize osmotic stress on cells (*32, 34*). Evidence from renal cortical slice studies (*3*) suggests that concentrations of Me_2SO up to 2.8 *M* may actually be less injurious at 25°C than at 10°C. Our earlier work (*8*) with solution A indicates that dog kidneys tested by transplantation might be safely perfused at 37°C with Me_2SO at concentrations of 1.4 *M*. The results of our present experiment demonstrate that dogs function quite well when their sole renal support is a kidney that has been perfused for 100 min at 25°C with solutions containing as much as 2.8 *M* Me_2SO. In the same study similar perfusion of dog kidneys with 4.2 *M* Me_2SO in RPS-2, whether at 25°C or 10°C, impairs renal function when tested in vitro and by transplantation. These results confirm an earlier report on cold perfusion of canine kidneys with 4 *M* Me_2SO (*6*). Thus we believe warm perfusion with Me_2SO is proper and we can find no argument to support the administration of Me_2SO at 10°C. Cold perfusion will only retard the tissue distribution of Me_2SO and exacerbate osmotic stress on cells.

Viability testing. We believe that this report validates the divided kidney model (*1*) as a suitable screening technique for organ preservation studies. This screening protocol divides the rabbit kidney into two independent components, the parenchymal and the vascular. The parenchymal component is biochemically evaluated in vitro using cortical slices. They are treated (e.g., with a cryoprotectant) then assayed with special emphasis on the potassium/sodium ratio (*35*). The vascular component is physiologically evaluated by ex vivo perfusion of treated whole kidneys—i.e. an allogeneic perfusor animal circulates blood through the kidney for a short time, perhaps 2 hr (*4, 36, 37*). By combining the results of both kinds of studies one gains, we believe, a clear indication of what to expect from organ transplantation. This is illustrated by a summary of our previous work (*2, 3, 4*).

Studies of cortical slices indicated to us (*2, 3*) that for the parenchymal component, RPS-2 was superior to either solution A or Krebs-Henseleit solutions as a vehicle for three cryoprotectants (ethylene glycol, glycerol, Me_2SO) and that Me_2SO was the least toxic of these cryoprotectants. Critical metabolic activities were maintained by cortical slices soaked in 2.8 *M* Me_2SO in RPS-2 for 40–60 min during a 2-hr total exposure period at 25°C. Slice metabolism deteriorated at higher concentrations of Me_2SO. Ex vivo perfusion (*4*) indicated that, for the vascular component, there was no significant difference between solution A and RPS-2 perfused for 2 hr—but, when 2.8 *M* Me_2SO was added at 25°C, the RPS-2 mixture depressed hemodynamics somewhat relative to Me_2SO in solution A. Higher concentrations (3.5 *M*) of Me_2SO accentuated this vascular depression. When the strongly favorable parenchymal effect and marginally unfavorable vascular effect were considered together, we concluded that RPS-2 was probably preferable to solution A as a vehicle for Me_2SO. The results of the present experiment confirms that judgement and enhances our confidence in the reliability of the divided kidney to reflect reality tested against the transplanted dog kidney.

Acknowledgments. The experimental surgery suite was kindly provided by Arlie R. Mansberger, Jr., M.D. We greatly appreciate training in canine renal transplantation provided by Arthur L. Humphries, Jr., M.D. Invaluable technical assistance was provided by Debbie Cribb,

Ricky Dent, William Hamilton, Maria Richard, and Robert Shimp, D.V.M. Excellent secretarial assistance was provided by Jennie Doby.

REFERENCES

1. Hawkins HE, Clark P, Karow AM. The influence of cooling rate and warming rate on the response of renal cortical slices frozen to −40°C in the presence of 2.1 M cryoprotectant (ethylene glycol, glycerol, or dimethyl sulfoxide). Cryobiology 1985; 22: 378.
2. Clark P, Fahy GM, Karow AM Jr. Factors influencing renal cryopreservation. I. Effects of three vehicle solutions and the permeation kinetics of three cryoprotectants assessed with rabbit cortical slices. Cryobiology 1984; 21: 260.
3. Clark P, Fahy GM, Karow AM Jr. Factors influencing renal cryopreservation. II. Toxic effects of three cryoprotectants in combination with three vehicle solutions in nonfrozen rabbit cortical slices. Cryobiology 1984; 21: 274.
4. Hawkins HE, Clark P, Lippert EC, Karow AM Jr. Functional preservation of the mammalian kidney. VI. Viability assessment of rabbit kidneys perfused at 25°C with dimethyl sulfoxide in RPS-2. J Surg Res 1985; 38: 281.
5. Segal NB, Guttman FM. Function of rabbit kidneys in vitro at normothermia following equilibration with 3.0 M Me_2SO and removal by hypertonic washout at 10°C. Cryobiology 1982; 19: 50.
6. Holst HI, Ketterer F, Lehr HB. Perfusate and microwave radiation effects on nonfrozen canine kidneys. Cryobiology 1970; 6: 590.
7. Bickis IJ, Kazaks K, Finn JJ, Henderson IWD. Permeation kinetics of glycerol and dimethyl sulfoxide in Novikoff hepatoma ascites cells. Cryobiology 1967; 4: 1.
8. Karow AM Jr, Wiggins S, Carrier GO, Brown R, Matheny JL. Functional preservation of the mammalian kidney. V. Pharmacokinetics of dimethyl sulfoxide (1.4 M) in kidneys (rabbit and dog) perfused at 37, 25, 10°C followed by transplantation (dog). J Surg Res 1979; 27: 93.
9. Segal NB, Guttman FM. Kinetics of permeation and intracellular events associated with Me_2SO permeation of rabbit kidneys during perfusion at 10°C. Cryobiology 1982; 19: 41.
10. Jeske AH, Fonteles MC, Karow AM Jr. Functional preservation of the mammalian kidney. III. Ultrastructural effects of perfusion with dimethylsulfoxide (DMSO). Cryobiology 1974; 11: 170.
11. Macklis JD, Ketterer FD. Microwave properties of cryoprotectants. Cryobiology 1978; 15: 627.
12. Karow AM Jr, Burdette EC. Design, development and performance of an electromagnetic illumination system for thawing canine kidneys. In: Freezing, frozen storage and freeze-drying. Paris: Institute International du Froid, 1977: 109.
13. Burdette EC. Engineering considerations in hypothermic an cryogenic preservation. In: Karow AM, Pegg DE, eds. Organ preservation for transplantation, 2nd ed. New York: Marcel Dekker, 1981: 213.
14. Keeler R, Swinney MC, Taylor RMR, Uldall PR. The problems of renal preservation. Br J Urol 1966; 38: 653.
15. Fonteles MC, Jeske AH, Karow AM Jr. Functional preservation of the mammalian kidney. I. Low flow and normothermia. J Surg Res 1973; 14: 15.
16. Jeske AH, Fonteles MC, Karow AM Jr. Functional preservation of the mammalian kidney. II. Ultrastructure with low flow perfusion at normothermia. J Surg Res 1973; 15: 4.
17. Karow AM Jr, Jeske AH. Functional preservation of the mammalian kidney. IV. Functional effects of perfusion with dimethylsulfoxide (DMSO) at normothermia. Cryobiology 1976; 13: 448.
18. Karow AM, Wiggins S, Carrier GO, Brown R, Matheny JL. Functional preservation of the mammalian kidney. V. Pharmacokinetics of dimethyl sulfoxide (1.4 M) in kidneys (rabbit and dog) perfused at 37, 25 or 10°C followed by transplantation (dog). J Surg Res 1979; 27: 93.
19. Leibach FH, Fonteles MC, Pillion D, Karow AM Jr. Glutathione in the isolated perfused rabbit kidney. J Surg Res 1974; 17: 228.
20. Fahy GM, Hornblower M, Williams H. An improved perfusate for hypothermic renal preservation. I. Initial in vitro optimization based on tissue electrolyte transport. Cryobiology 1979; 16: 618.
21. Collins GM, Fahy GM, Carter JM, Halasz NA. New flush solutions studied with a small animal preservation model. Cryobiology 1980; 17: 603.
22. Carruthers RK, Clark PB, Anderson CK, Parsons FM. Prevention of weight gain and protein loss during perfusion of the rat kidney for storage at −79°C. Br J Urol 1969; 44: 179.
23. Buhl MR, Jensen MH. Metabolic inhibition. In: Karow AM, Pegg DE, eds. Organ preservation for transplantation, 2nd ed. New York: Marcel Dekker, 1981: 497.
24. Garwin PJ, Castaneda M, Niehoff M, Jellinek M, Codd JE. An experimental evaluation of nucleotide enhancement techniques for kidney transplantation. J Surg Res 1985; 38: 29.
25. Fernando AR, Griffiths JR, O'Donoghue EP, Ward JP, Armstrong DMG, Hendry WF, Perrett D, Wickham JEA. Enhanced preservation of the ischemic kidney with inosine. Lancet 1976; 1: 555.
26. Nau T, Toledo-Pereyra LH, Simmons RL, Najarian JS. The effect of adenosine and allopurinol on the tolerance of the collapsed lung to warm ischemia. Surgery 1978; 83: 406.
27. Foker JE, Einzig S, Wang T, Anderson RW. Adenosine metabolism and myocardial preservation. J Thorac Cardiovasc Surg 1980; 80: 506.
28. Southard JH, Lutz MF, Ametani MS, Belzer FO. Simulation of ATP synthesis in hypothermically perfused dog kidneys by adenosine and PO_4. Cryobiology 1984; 21: 13.
29. Humphries AL JR, Russell R, Stoddard LD, Moretz WH. Perfusion of dog kidneys with cooled medium 199 followed by auto or allotransplantation. In: Norman JC, ed. Organ perfusion and preservation. New York: Appleton-Century-Crofts, 1968: 13.
30. Copeland JG, Jones M, Spragg R, Stinson EB. Successful orthotopic transplantation of canine hearts after in vitro preservation for 24 to 28 hours. Surg Forum 1972; 23: 202.
31. Pegg DE, Wusteman MC. Perfusion of rabbit kidneys with glycerol solutions at 5°C. Cryobiology 1977; 14: 168.
32. Jacobsen IA, Pegg DE, Wusteman MC, Robinson SM. Transplantation of rabbit kidneys perfused with glycerol at 10°C. Cryobiology 1978; 15: 18.
33. Karow AM Jr, Webb WR. Toxicity of various solute moderators used in hypothermia. Cryobiology 1965; 1: 270.
34. Carroll PM, Lin JH. The protection of frozen-thawed rat uterus by glycerol and dimethyl sulfoxide. Cryobiology 1968; 5: 226.
35. Fahy GM. Viability assessment. In: Karow AM, Pegg DE, eds. Organ preservation for transplantation, 2nd ed. New York: Marcel Dekker, 1981: 53.
36. Carter JN, Green RD, Halasz NA, Collins GM. Ex vivo perfusion. A renal preservation model. J Surg Res 1981; 31: 55.
37. Carruthers RK, Clark PB, Anderson CK, Parsons FM. Tubular function demonstrated in rat kidneys after storage at −79°C. Br J Urol 1969; 44: 186.

Received 12 August 1985.
Accepted 7 October 1985.

0041-1337/86/4106-0675$02.00/0
TRANSPLANTATION
Vol. 41, No. 6

Printed in U.S.A.

AMPLIFICATION OF THE GRAFT-VERSUS-HOST REACTION BY PARTIAL BODY IRRADIATION[1]

SHIRLEY LEHNERT,[2,3] WITOLD B. RYBKA,[4,5] AND THOMAS A. SEEMAYER[6]

Departments of Radiation Oncology and Medicine, The Montreal General Hospital Research Institute; and Department of Pathology, The McGill University-Montreal Children's Hospital Research Institute, Montreal, Quebec, Canada

An experimental model has been developed for the study of combined effects of partial body irradiation (PBI) and graft-versus-host disease (GVHD) in which irradiation is delivered to the thorax 24 hr prior to induction of GVHD in hybrid mice by the injection of parental lymphoid cells.

In mice irradiated to 1000 cGy or exposed to low doses of allogeneic lymphoid cells (20×10^6), survival was 100% at 250 days. In contrast, combination of the two treatments, GVHD and PBI, resulted in a mortality of 83% and a mean survival time of 29 days, indicating synergy between GVHD and PBI. From histological studies of the lung it appeared that about 40% of the deaths occurring after combined GVHD/PBR treatment might be attributable to pneumonia. The cause of death in the remaining mice receiving combined treatment is not known. Mice receiving combined PBI/lymphoid cell treatment develop a characteristic skin lesion that is not seen in nonirradiated mice and is confined to the irradiated area.

The effect of preinduction PBR on the timing and severity of GVHD is similar to that which would be produced by an increase in the number of effector cells.

Allogeneic bone marrow transplantation is a useful modality for the treatment of lethal marrow diseases such as acute leukemia and aplastic anemia (*1–3*). A complication of bone marrow transplantation that limits the fraction of recipients who derive long-term benefit from the procedure is acute respiratory failure caused by interstitial pneumonia (*4, 5*).

The pathophysiology of interstitial pneumonia is poorly understood, but a number of causative factors have been implicated including radiation, cytotoxic drugs, and graft-versus-host disease (GVHD). *A study in progress in this laboratory is focused on the elucidation of factors, separately or in combination, that might influence the incidence of interstitial pneumonia following bone marrow transplantation. In an initial phase of this investigation, factors influencing the response of the lung to a single modality, radiation, were studied (*6*). Subsequent studies have addressed the role of GVHD, which occurs frequently in recipients of allogeneic grafts (*7, 8*)—even though, for the majority, the donors are siblings matched at the major histocompatibility locus. Clinical studies have shown GVHD to be significantly associated with an increase in the incidence and the severity of interstitial pneumonia. Neiman (*9*), for instance, reported the incidence of pneumonia to be 2.4-fold greater in patients with GVHD than in non-GVHD patients.

An animal model system designed for the study of the interaction of GVHD with radiation damage to the lung is described below. In this model, radiation to the thorax is given prior to the induction of GVHD in F_1 hybrid mice by injection of parental cells. During the course of experiments using this system, it became apparent that GVHD and the response to thoracic irradiation probably involved lesions expressed both inside and outside the radiation field and had fatal consequences not directly associated with lung damage. These findings, which may have wide implications for the management of patients undergoing bone marrow and other forms of transplantation, are described below.

MATERIALS AND METHODS

Mice of the inbred strains A (haplotype H-2^a), C57L (haplotype H-2^b) and LAF$_1$, the F_1 hybrid A×C57L, were used.

Lymphoid cells used for inducing the graft-versus-host (GVH) reaction were prepared as described by Treiber and Lapp (*10*). Viable lymphoid cells, prepared from spleens and lymph nodes, were counted on the basis of trypan blue exclusion, and the required number was injected in a single inoculum via the lateral tail vein in a volume of 0.3 ml.

For the spleen weight assay, mice were killed 14 days after injection of lymphoid cells. Spleens were removed, weighed, and the relative spleen weight was expressed as milligrams of spleen weight/10 g body weight. The spleen index (*11*) of the injected mice was expressed as:

$$\frac{\text{mean relative spleen weight GVHD mice}}{\text{mean relative spleen weight controls.}}$$

For assay of plaque-forming cells (PFC), 5×10^8 sheep red blood cells (SRBC) were injected i.v. in a volume of 0.3 ml. Four days later, the mice were sacrificed, and the number of direct spleen PFCs to SRBC were assayed by the method of Cunningham and Szenberg (*12*).

For irradiation with ^{60}Coγ rays, groups of up to 8 unanesthetized mice were confined in adjustable holders of the type described by Travis et al. (*13*). Contoured lead blocks (5 cm) were arranged to shield the body above the clavicle and below

* Abbreviations used: GVH, graft-versus host; GVHR, GVH reaction; PBI, partial body irradiation; PFC, plaque-forming cells; SRBC, sheep red blood cells; TBI, total-body irradiation.

[1]This work was supported by the National Cancer Institute of Canada.

[2] Department of Radiation Oncology, The Montreal General Hospital Research Institute.

[3]Address correspondence to: Dr. Shirley Lehnert, Department of Radiation Oncology, The Montreal General Hospital, 1650 Cedar Ave., Montreal, Quebec, Canada, H3G 1A4.

[4] Department of Medicine, The Montreal General Hospital Research Institute.

[5] W.B. Rybka was supported, in part, by the T.H.P. Molson Award of the Montreal General Hospital Research Institute.

[6] The McGill University-Montreal Children's Hospital Research Institute.

the xiphisternum, leaving a treatment field approximately 2.5 cm wide. For irradiation of one lung, one side of the thorax up to the midline was shielded by an additional contoured lead block. Mice were irradiated to the dorsal surface through a build-up layer of 0.5 cm plastic. Dose rates were measured using an ionization chamber inserted in a mouse holder.

For histology, tissues from complete autopsies were fixed in 10% buffered formalin. Paraffin embedded sections were stained with hematoxylin-phloxine-saffron and examined as coded specimens.

RESULTS

Induction of Graft versus Host Disease in LAF_1 mice

Injection of F_1 hybrids with parental spleen or lymph node cells has been shown to lead to activation of parental lymphocytes that recognize major histocompatibility antigens of the other parental haplotype expressed by the F_1 host (*14*). Such recognition can lead to GVH reactions. Experiments were already in progress on radiation-induced lung damage using an F_1 hybrid mouse strain, LAF_1, so GVHD was induced in this strain by injection of lymphoid cells from either parental donor. The ability of the injected cells to induce GVHD in the recipient was assessed on the basis of spleen weight assay and immunosuppression as measured by the PFC response.

Spleen weight assay. LAF_1 mice were injected with 60×10^6 lymphoid cells from LAF_1, A, or C57L donors. The results are shown in Table 1. The high relative spleen weight produced in LAF_1 recipients by injection of A strain cells indicated a significant GVH reaction in these mice. Cells from C57L donors were less effective, confirming the occurrence of a natural resistance of the F_1 host to GVHD induction by lymphocytes of haplotype H-2^b, which has been reported previously (*15*).

Immunosuppression. GVHD has been observed to have an immunosuppressive effect, under appropriate conditions, for both cell-mediated and humoral immune responses (*16, 17*). The effect of an inoculum of A strain lymphoctyes on the humoral response of LAF_1 was studied by measuring the number of PFC in the spleen induced by challenge with SRBC in LAF_1 mice that had been injected with 75×10^6 syngeneic (LAF_1) or allogeneic (A) lymphoid cells. The results are shown in Table 2. Injection of A lymphoid cells reduced the level of PFCs in the spleen to undetectable levels. No significant effect was observed following the injection of LAF_1 cells. Also included in Table 2 are the results of a similar experiment using mice exposed only to 1400 cGy thoracic irradiation 14 days before injection of SRBC. The number of PFC/10^6 spleen cells in these irradiated mice was 83% of the number observed in controls, indicating only a slight suppression of the humoral immune response.

Results of the spleen weight assay and PFC response indicate that a GVHD reaction is induced in LAF_1 mice by injection of A strain lymphocytes. In subsequent experiments, the effect of partial body (thoracic) irradiation (PBI) on the incidence and severity of GVHD was investigated.

Gross Manifestations of GvHD

In mice given A strain parental lymphoid cells only, gross manifestation of GVHD were confined to hunched posture and wasting. Diarrhea was rarely seen and skin lesions were observed only in mice treated with lymphoid cells plus PBI. Weight changes in mice given lymphoid cells and/or PBI are shown in Figure 1. Following injection of 75×10^6 A strain lymphoid cells, weight loss commenced approximately 18 days after treatment and continued until the time of death at approximately 45 days. Mice exposed to PBI only showed a transient fall in weight that was greatest 4–5 days after treatment. Mice treated with lymphoid cells plus PBI showed an initial weight loss similar to that occurring after PBI only, which proved to be irreversible, continuing until the animals died at 12–16 days after combined treatment.

A skin lesion, characterized by hair loss and erythematous and scaly skin, was observed in mice surviving 30 or more days after treatment with lymphoid cells and PBI. In the experimental group given 42×10^6 lymphoid cells and 1400 cGy PBR, for example, the longest-lived survivors (4/12) died at 30–34 days after treatment, and all showed signs of cutaneous involvement. In contrast, 12 mice given 42×10^6 lymphoid cells but no irradiation died 32–62 days after treatment without skin lesions. Skin lesions were also seen in other experimental groups in which prolonged survival was seen following injection of reduced numbers of lymphoid cells and/or lower radiation doses. In GVHD models involving total-body irradiation, the skin lesion is frequently observed to start at the nape of the

TABLE 1. Body and spleen weights (mean ± SD) in LAF_1 mice injected with LAF_1 or parental spleen cells

Spleen cells injected	Mean body wt. (g)	Spleen wt. (mg)	Spleen index (mg/10 g body wt.)	Ratio
LAF_1	29.5	105±20	35	1.0
A	28.7	440±50	153	4.4
C57L	27.4	200±30	74	2.1

TABLE 2. PFC response to SRBC of spleen cells from control mice and from mice 13 days after injection of syngeneic or allogeneic lymphoid cells

Treatment	PFC/10^6 spleen cells
None	655±95
1400 cGy radiation to the thorax	545±53
75×10^6 LAF_1 lymphoid cells	882±198
75×10^6 A lymphoid cells	0±0

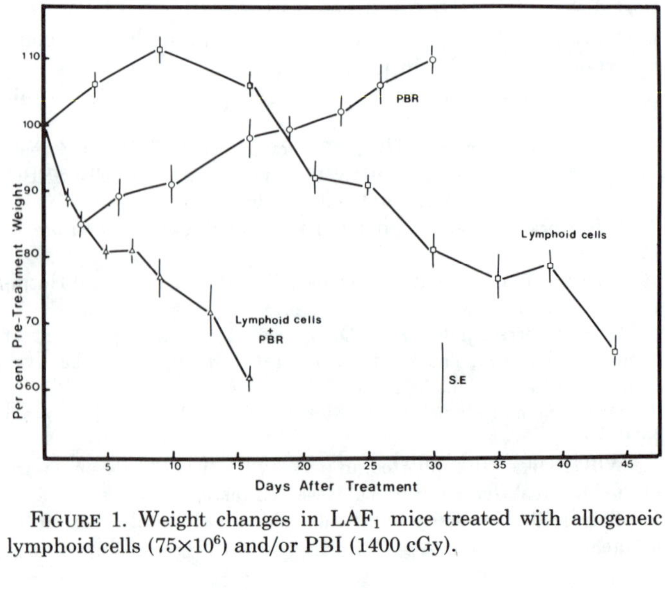

FIGURE 1. Weight changes in LAF_1 mice treated with allogeneic lymphoid cells (75×10^6) and/or PBI (1400 cGy).

neck and to progress across the dorsal and ventral surfaces of the thorax. This type of progression was also seen following PBI. However, the extent of the lesion was demarcated posteriorly and anteriorly by a sharp line corresponding to the edge of the radiation field. Macroscopic and histological skin changes were not seen beyond this line.

Histological Changes

Tissues were studied in four experimental groups:

1400 cGy to the thorax (PBI). The lungs showed only minor changes up to 45 days after irradiation. At 15 days postirradiation, small foci of inflammatory cells were present, and by 40 days small pneumonialike lesions were seen in some sections. Major changes, characteristic of radiation pneumonitis, did not become apparent until longer times after irradiation. Tissues outside the radiation field—including spleen, liver, and pancreas—showed normal histology.

Induction of GVHD by injection of 75×10⁶ parental lymphoid cells (GVHD). Lung sections showed moderate perivenular edema associated with variable degrees of perivenular mononuclear cell infiltration. In other organs, notable changes were seen in the pancreas where there was extensive periductular, perivenular, and acinar mononuclear infiltration. The spleen was the site of multifocal hemorrhage and fibrin deposition, intense megakaryocyte hyperplasia, and multifocal histiocytic replacement of red and white pulp.

PBR (1400 cGy) prior to induction of the GVH reaction(GVHD/PBR). Because of the short survival time of mice in this group, tissues were only available up to 20 days after treatment. Sections of lungs again showed variable degrees of perivenular edema with associated mononuclear cell infiltration between days 10 and 20 after GVH induction. In addition, 5 of 13 mice demonstrated multiple foci of acute pneumonia. The spleen showed extensive hemorrhagic, fibrinous necrosis and mild megakaryocytic hyperplasia. The pancreas featured lesser changes than in the GVHD only group with only slight mononuclear infiltration being noted.

Irradiation of half the thorax prior to GVHD induction. Changes observed in both lungs of these mice resembled those seen in the lungs of the GVHD only group. It was not possible to distinguish the irradiated from the nonirradiated lung in coded samples.

Mortality

Figure 2 shows survival patterns for mice given various doses of lympoid cells and/or PBI. No mice in the PBI only or PBI plus syngeneic (LAF_1) lymphoid cell groups died within 100 days of treatment. Of these, 50% died subsequently from radiation pneumonitis with a mean survival time of 163 days (*6*).

All mice given 75×10^6 and 42×10^6 A strain lymphoid cells died. The mean survival times were 40 and 45 days, respectively. Mortality was not observed in mice given 21×10^6 or fewer allogeneic cells.

Combined treatment with allogeneic cells and PBI reduced survival time in the 75×10^6 and 42×10^6 cell recipient groups to 13 and 23 days, respectively. Mortality was 100% in each case. Lower doses of allogeneic cells were also lethal when combined with PBI. Thus, for mice given 20×10^6, 10×10^6, and 5×10^6 allogeneic cells and 1400 cGY PBI, mortality was 100%, 83%, and 33% and mean survival times were 22, 25, and 41 days, respectively.

Not shown in Figure 2 is the response to irradiation of half the thorax prior to induction of GVHD by injection of 75×10^6 lymphoid cells. The mean survival time of these mice was 31± 5.7 days, intermediate between that of mice receiving irradiation to the whole thorax (13±4.7 days) and that of unirradiated mice (45±10 days).

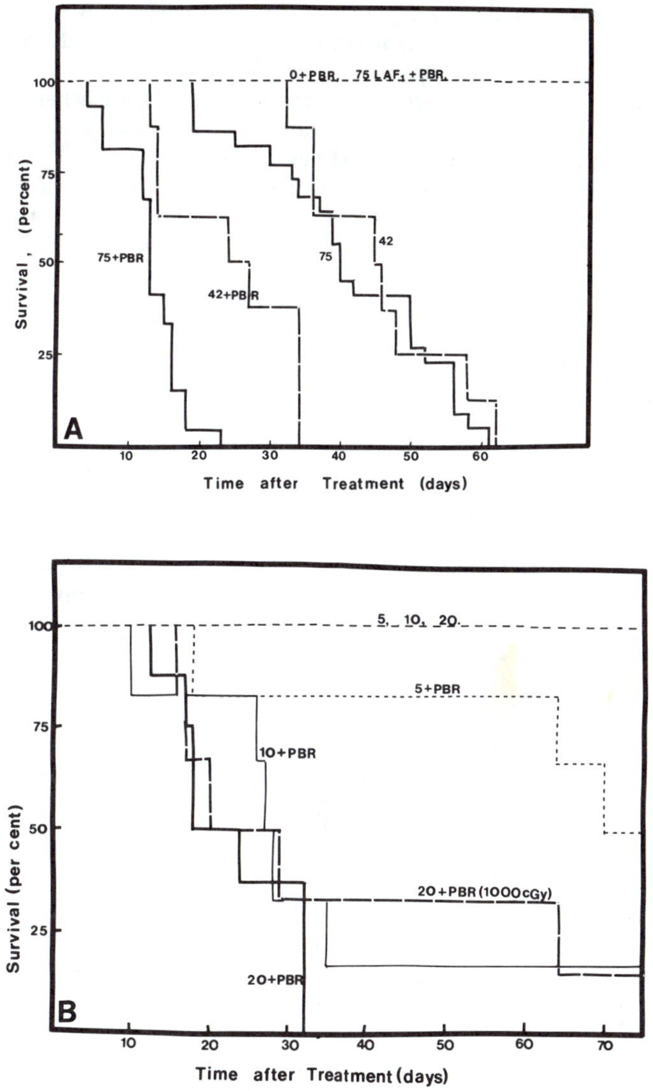

FIGURE 2. Survival as a function of time after injection of allogeneic lymphoid cells and/or PBI. Labels beside each line represent experimental groups. Numbers indicate number of cells injected $\times10^{-6}$. PBI indicates that the radiation dose was 1400 cGy unless otherwise indicated.

Also shown in Figure 2b is the response, in terms of early mortality, that is observed when a sublethal dose of PBI is combined with an inoculum of allogeneic lymphoid cells—which alone causes no reduction in life span. Survival after treatment with either 1000 cGy or 20×10^6 allogenic cells is 100% at 250 days. However, after combining these two treatments, mortality is 83% and mean survival time 29 days. This response indicates that synergism occurs when the two treatments interact.

DISCUSSION

Previous studies of the influence of radiation on the development of the GVH reaction have involved total-body irradiation (TBI). One of the earliest reports is that of Cole and Ellis

(*18*) who found that injection of spleen cells from A strain donors causes delayed death of LAF_1 recipients, survival time being related to the number of cells injected. The survival time was reduced if mice were exposed to 500 cGy TBI shortly before injection of spleen cells. A similar observation was made by Hilgard (*19*), who found that the extent to which survival time was reduced by radiation prior to induction of the GVH reaction was dependent on the size of the radiation dose. In another study involving TBI Claman and Jaffee (*20*) showed that minor histocompatibility differences could be demonstrated in vivo if the recipients were pretreated with TBI (600 cGy) although such incompatibilities were difficult to detect by mixed lymphocyte reactions in vitro. Thus, the potency of GVH effector cells in vivo appeared to be amplified by irradiation of the recipient.

In our studies, we found that a fatal reaction could be induced in LAF_1 mice by partial body irradiation prior to induction of the GVH reaction. This suggested that the intensity of the GVH reaction was enhanced by the effects of radiation. Lungs of 40% of the mice, sacrificed or autopsied 16–20 days after receiving combined GVHD/PBI treatment, showed multiple foci of acute pneumonia—while, within the same period, there was no sign of pneumonia in the groups receiving radiation alone or GVHD alone. It may be assumed from this that a proportion of the deaths that occur after combined treatment result from pulmonary injury culminating in an acute pneumonia. The sequence of events leading to this endpoint has yet to be elucidated, but the observation does suggest that the nonbacterial pneumonia observed in a proportion of bone marrow transplant patients is related to a combined effect of GVHD and radiation.

The occurrence of pneumonia was peculiar to mice receiving the highest does of parental lymphoid cells combined with thoracic radiation, all of whom died within 22 days of treatment. More than half the mice sacrificed or autopsied during this period, however, showed only minor lung lesions, so that death in these animals was unlikely to have been of pulmonary origin. Localization of the reaction to the site of radiation was also not apparent in animals receiving radiation to one side of the thorax only. Lungs from the irradiated and nonirradiated sides could not be distinguished from each other, although mice given irradiation to half the thorax did show a reduction in survival time. These observations prompted investigation of the possibility that some mice receiving combined treatment died as a result of an enhanced response occurring in unexposed organs as a result of a radiation-induced abscopal or systemic response. One mechanism by which this might be brought about is amplification of the GVH reaction in mice immunosuppressed by irradiation prior to GVHD induction. However, PBI alone was found to have only a mild immunosuppressive effect, manifest as a reduction in the number of PFCs to SRBC in irradiated mice to 83% of control values (Table 2). The problem was also investigated by examining histological changes occurring in organs outside the radiation field, comparing the mice in the GVHD group with those in the GVHD/PBI group. Results obtained were equivocal. While changes observed in the pancreas of mice in the GVHD/PBR group were less severe than those seen in the GVHD group, the reverse observation was made for the spleen, in which extensive hemorrhagic necrosis was seen in the GVHD/PBI group but not in the GVHD group. For other tissues such as liver, there was no difference between the two groups.

Localized interaction between radiation damage and the GVH reaction was noted in the skin. Whereas the skin lesion associated with GVHD could not be detected histologically or as a gross reaction in mice given parental lymphoid cells only, parental cells combined with PBI produced a skin lesion that was confined to the area exposed to radiation. In a study of skin biopsies from patients given cytotoxic drugs and/or radiation in conjunction with syngeneic or allogeneic bone marrow transplantation (*21*). Sale and coworkers concluded that, in terms of the skin lesion induced, the effects of GVHD in allograft recipients and of cytotoxic insult were almost identical, and that the effect of the two injuries was additive. In the murine system described here, a skin lesion was seen following combined treatment that was not apparent following radiation or allogeneic cell injection alone, suggesting that the effects of the two forms of insult are synergistic rather than additive.

A number of investigators have reported that in mouse models in which GVHD is induced by injection of allogeneic lymphoid cells, the survival time of the mice is a function of the number of lymphoid cells injected (*22, 23*). Okunewick et al (*24*) demonstrated that the survival time of the recipient was inversely related to the natural logarithm of the number of cells injected, implying that proliferation of GVH effector cells is required before a fatal GVH reaction occurs. Results described here also show correlation between recipient survival time and the number of GVH effector cells injected. This is shown in Figure 3, where the natural logarithm of the number of lymphoid cells injected is plotted against mean survival time of the recipients in groups in which early mortality was observed. Mean survival time for mice given PBI prior to GVHD induction is displaced from the line for unirradiated mice by a distance equivalent to a factor of 12. Thus, the effect of PBI on the recipient is an amplification of the response similar to that which would be produced by an increase in the number of lymphoid cells injected. As noted above, Claman and Jaffee

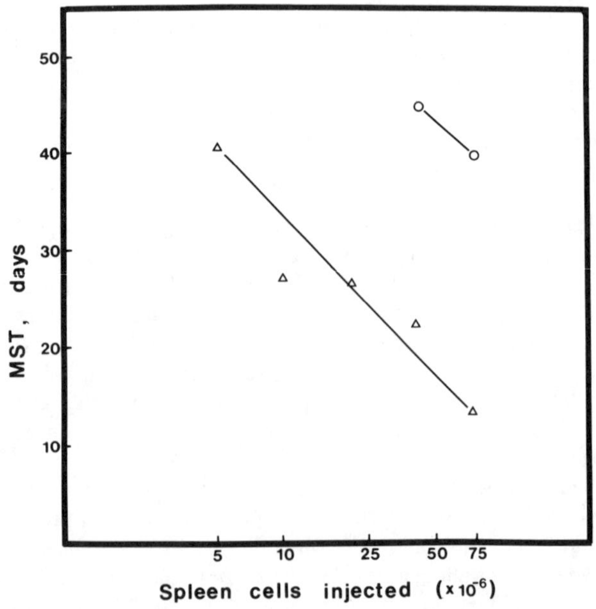

FIGURE 3. Mean Survival Time (MST) in days for LAF_1 mice as a function of the number of allogeneic lymphoid cells injected. (●——●) lymphoid cells only; (△——△) PBI (1400 cGy) prior to lymphoid cell inoculation.

(*20*) reported that the potential of GVH effector cells in vivo was amplified by TBI of the host.

The results described here are the first demonstration that partial body irradiation acts to amplify the GVH reaction. While the findings are preliminary, they suggest means by which the phenomenom of amplification of the GVH reaction by cytotoxic agents may be further investigated, and the possibility that the incidence and severity of GVHD occurring in recipients of allogeneic transplants could be modulated by manipulation of the cytotoxic preparatory regimen.

Acknowledgments. We are indebted to Wayne Lapp, Ph.D., for helpful discussions and to David Ivancic for expert technical assistance.

REFERENCES

1. O'Reilly RJ. Allogeneic bone marrow transplantation: current status and future directions. Blood 1983; 62: 941.
2. Dinsmore R, Kirkpatrick D, Flornenberg N, et al. Allogeneic bone marrow transplantation for patients with acute lymphoblastic leukemia. Blood 1983; 62: 381.
3. Thomas ED, Clift RA, Hersman J, et al. Marrow transplantation for acute nonlymphoblastic leukemia in first remission using fractionated or single dose irradiation. Int J Radiat Oncol Biol Phys 1982; 8: 817.
4. Barret A, Depledge MH, Powles RL. Interstitial pneumonitis following bone marrow transplantation after low dose total body irradiation. Int J Radiat Oncol Biol Phys 1983; 9: 1029.
5. Bortin MM, Kay HEM, Gale RP, Rimm AA. Factors associated with interstitial pneumonitis after bone marrow transplantation for acute leukemia. Lancet 1982; 1: 1137.
6. Lehnert S, Rybka WB. Dose rate dependence of response of mouse lung to irradiation. Br J Radiol 1985; 58: 74.
7. Thomas ED, Buckner CD, Banaji M, et al. One hundred patients with acute leukemia treated by chemotherapy, total body irradiation and allogeneic bone marrow transplantation. Blood 1977; 49: 511.
8. Bortin MM, Gale RP, Rimm AA. Allogeneic bone marrow transplantation for 144 patients with severe aplastic anemia. JAMA 1981; 245: 1132.
9. Neiman PE, Reeves W, Ray G, et al. A prospective analysis of interstitial pneumonia and opportunistic viral infection among recipients of allogenic bone marrow grafts. J Infect Dis 1977; 136: 754.
10. Treiber W, Lapp WS. Stimulation of humoral immune responses to thymic independent antigen in mice immunosuppressed by a graft versus host reaction. Cell Immunol 1978; 37: 118.
11. Mowat AM, Ferguson A. Hypersensitivity reaction in the small intestinal mucosa of the mouse. Transplantation 1981; 32: 238.
12. Cunningham AJ, Szenberg A. Further improvements in the plaque technique for detecting single antibody forming cells. Immunology 1968; 14: 599.
13. Travis EL, Parkins CS, Holmes SJ, Down JD. Effect of misonidazole on radiation injury to mouse spinal cord. Br J Cancer 1982; 45: 469.
14. Gleichmann E, Gleichmann H, Witke W. Auto-immunization and lymphomagnesis in parent-F_1 combinations differing at the major histocompatibility complex: model for spontaneous disease caused by self-antigens. Transplant Rev 1976; 31: 156.
15. Shearer GM, Polisson RP. Mutual recognition of parental and F_1 lymphocytes. IV. Parental determinants recognized by F_1 host mice in resistance to graft versus host associated immunosuppression to H-2D^2. J Immunol 1981; 126: 545.
16. Lapp WS, Moller G. Prolonged survival of H-2 incompatible skin allografts of F_1 animals treated with parental lymphoid cells. Immunology 1969; 17: 339.
17. Lapp WS. Synergistic effect of antilymphocyte serum and the graft versus host reaction on murine skin allograft suppression. Transplantation 1973; 15: 469.
18. Cole LJ, Ellis ME. Delayed deaths in sublethally X-rayed F_1 hybrid mice injected with parental strain spleen cells. Science 1958; 128: 32.
19. Hilgard HR. Dissociation of splenomegaly from graft versus host disease by host irradiation. Transplantation 1970; 10: 396.
20. Claman HN, Jaffee BD. Minor antigen versus host reactions revealed in irradiated spleen and popliteal lymph node assays. Transplantation 1984; 38: 392.
21. Sale GE, Lerner KG, Barker EA, Shulman HM, Thomas ED. The skin biopsy in the diagnosis of acute graft versus host disease in man. Am J Pathol 1977; 89: 621.
22. Korngold R, Sprent J. Lethal graft versus host disease following bone marrow transplantation across minor histocompatibility barriers in mice: prevention by removing mature T-cells from marrow. J Exp Med 1978; 148: 1687.
23. Gruska M, Lapp WS. Effect of lymphoid tissue transplants on the intensity of an existing graft versus host reaction. Transplantation 1974; 17: 157.
24. Okunewick JP, Meredith RF, Brozovich BJ, Seeman PR, Magliere K. Exponential relationship between spleen cell concentration and fatal graft versus host response after transplantation of allogeneic spleen-marrow cell mixtures. Transplantation 1980; 29: 507.

Received 23 July 1984.
Accepted 25 September 1985.

0041-1337/86/4106-0680$02.00/0
TRANSPLANTATION
Copyright © 1986 by The Williams & Wilkins Co.

Vol. 41, No. 6
Printed in U.S.A.

FUNCTIONAL CLONAL DELETION VERSUS SUPPRESSOR CELL–INDUCED TRANSPLANTATION TOLERANCE IN CHIMERAS PREPARED WITH A SHORT COURSE OF TOTAL-LYMPHOID IRRADIATION[1]

SHIMON SLAVIN, SHOSHANA MORECKI, MARILYN WEIGENSBERG, SARAH BAR, AND LOLA WEISS

Department of Bone Marrow Transplantation and Immunobiology Research, Hadassah University Medical Center, Jerusalem, Israel

Allogeneic bone marrow (BM) chimeras induced by infusion of BM cells into recipients conditioned with total lymphoid irradiation (TLI) were shown to develop humoral and cell-mediated tolerance to host and donor-type alloantigens by a number of in vitro and in vivo assays. Spleen cells of tolerant chimeras exhibited suppressive activity of mixed lymphocyte reaction (MLR). MLR suppression was not abrogated by depletion of Lyt-2 cells, and neither could Lyt-2-positive cells sorted from the spleens of tolerant chimeras suppress MLR or attenuate graft-versus-host reactivity in vivo. Likewise, specifically unresponsive spleen cells obtained from chimeras could not be induced to respond in MLR against tolerizing host-type cells following depletion of Lyt-2 or passage through a nylon-wool column. Tolerance of chimera spleen cells to host alloantigens, best documented by permanent survival of donor-type skin allografts, could be adoptively transferred into syngeneic recipients treated by heavy irradiation but not into untreated or mildly irradiated recipients. Adoptive transfer of tolerance seemed to be associated with experimental conditions favoring engraftment of tolerant cells rather than suppression of host reactivity. We speculate that although host and/or donor-derived suppressor cells may be operating in reducing the pool of specific alloreactive clones by blocking cell proliferation in response to allogeneic challenge, the final outcome in tolerant chimeras is actual or functional deletion of alloreactive clones.

Transplantation tolerance can be acquired during fetal stages and within the first few days after birth (*1*, *2*). Induction of transplantation tolerance can also be accomplished experimentally in adult animals by transplanting histoincompatible bone marrow (BM)* cells into properly conditioned recipients (*3*). In order to avoid the graft-versus-host disease (GVHD), which may result from introduction of immunocompetent cells into adequately immunosuppressed recipients, BM cells can be treated prior to transplantation by anti-T-cell antibodies (*4–6*) or lectins (*7*) for removal of alloreactive, mature T cells. Another approach that has been used to establish stable chimerism and specific tolerance to alloantigens without prior deletion of marrow T lymphocytes involves treatment of recipients with fractionated, high-dose total-lymphoid irradiation (TLI) prior to inoculation of BM cells (*8–10*). The transplantation tolerance that ultimately develops in the chimeras is defined as a state in which both alloantigen-specific host-versus-graft and graft-versus-host unresponsiveness result, whereas third-party alloantigens are still recognised as non-self. Specific unresponsiveness in chimeras can be documented in vivo by specific tolerance to skin allografts, and lack of GVHD against related strains by adoptive transfer experiments, and in vitro by mixed lymphocyte reactions (MLR) and cell-mediated lymphocytotoxicity (CML) assays. The mechanisms involved in establishing such specific unresponsiveness are not well understood. Antigen-specific, as well as antigen-nonspecific host-type suppressor cells were previously documented in nonreconstituted TLI-treated mice that were made tolerant to protein antigens or alloantigens (*9–14*). The key issue addressed here is whether tolerance of donor cells to host alloantigens in TLI-induced adult BM chimeras is maintained by regulatory suppressor cells or through functional deletion of alloantigen-specific clones.

MATERIALS AND METHODS

Animals. Inbred BALB/c (H-2^d) (BALB), C57BL/6 (H-2^b) (C57), (BALB/c×C57 BL/6)F_1 (H-$2^{d,b}$) (F_1), C3H/He(H-2^k) (C3H), ATH(H-2^{t2}) and A/Crgl(H-2^a) mice were used in all experiments. Male and female mice were used as tissue donors, or as recipients in cell transfer experiments. TLI recipients were 3–5 months old. Mice were kept in conventional animal facilities.

Total-lymphoid and whole-body irradiation. BALB and F_1 mice were anesthetized with pentobarbital for proper positioning in an apparatus designed to expose the major lymph nodes, thymus, and spleen—while most of the skull, ribs, lungs, hind legs, and tail were shielded with lead, as previously described in detail (*8*). TLI consisted of eight exposures of 200 rads/day, six times per week, to a total dose of 1600 rads delivered from a Phillips x-ray unit (250 kV, 20 mA) at a rate of 52 rads/min. The source to skin distance was 40 cm, and a 0.2-mm Cu filter was used. Whole-body irradiation (WBI) was delivered using the same source with a single exposure to 200 or 400 rads, as indicated, upon completion of TLI. Adoptive recipients of spleen cells were conditioned with a sublethal exposure of WBI consisting of 550 rads unless otherwise specified.

BM transplantation. BM cells were obtained by flushing minimal essential medium (MEM) without sodium bicarbonate (Grand Island Biological Co., Grand Island, NY) through the shafts of the femurs and tibias of donor mice. Cells were washed once and resuspended in MEM. Aliquots of 0.25 ml medium containing 30×10^6 nucleated cells were injected i.v. into the recipient mice, one day following termination of TLI.

[1] This work was supported by National Institutes of Health Grants 30313 and 15387; the Chief Scientist's Office, Israel Ministry of Health; Basic Research Foundation; The Israel Academy of Sciences; and The Lady Tata Memorial Trust.

* Abbreviations used: BM, bone marrow; CFU-GM, granuloid-macrophage colony-forming units; CFU-S, multipotential spleen colony-forming units; CML, cell-mediated lympholysis; FCS, fetal calf serum; FITC, fluorescein isothiocyanate; GVHD, graft-versus-host disease; LN, lymph node; MEM, minimal essential medium; MLR; mixed lymphocyte reaction; PBS, phosphate-buffered saline; TLI total-lymphoid irradiation; WBI, whole-body irradiation.

Skin grafting. A full-thickness skin graft was transplanted to the flank of several groups of irradiated and control mice as previously described (*15*). The grafts were followed by daily inspection and palpation. Rejection was taken as the time of complete sloughing, or when a dry scab was formed.

Assay for chimerism. Chimerism of the BM cell recipients was assayed by complement-dependent microtoxicity assays using antisera raised by immunizing mice with a donor-type skin allograft, followed by two injections of spleen cells i.p. Mice were bled after 2 weeks and the antisera were kept frozen after determination of dose response curves. The details of the microtoxicity assay were described elsewhere (*16*).

Detection of anti-H-2 antibodies in the serum. Mice were immunized with four i.p. injections of 50×10^6 spleen cells in 0.5 ml phosphate-buffered saline (PBS) at 2-week intervals, and they were bled 2 weeks after the last immunization. Sera were frozen until used at −70°C. Complement (rabbit)-dependent cytotoxic activity of antisera was determined using a microcytotoxic technique as previously described (*16*).

Antibodies. Monoclonal anti-Lyt-2 antibodies (NEI 006) used for cytotoxicity were a gift from New England Nuclear, Boston MA. The following reagents were obtained from E.S. Vitetta, Ph.D., University of Texas at Dallas, and were used for analysis and sorting by a fluorescence-activated cell sorter (FACS): rat hybridomas secreting IgG monoclonal antibodies against Lyt-2 (53.6.72) were prepared as previously described (*17*). Since rat chain is recognized by rabbit anti-mouse-γ (RAMγ), F(ab′)^2 fragments of RAMγ were prepared and coupled to fluorescein isothiocyanate (FITC) (*18*). FITC-F(ab′)^2 RAMγ antibodies were used to detect and sort spleen cells treated by monoclonal rat antibodies. The FITC-F(ab′)^2 RAMγ antibodies did not stain any significant amount of mouse B lymphocytes, the background being 2.6–4.0% of normal mouse spleen cells (similar to a negative stain control).

Indirect immunofluorescence analysis and sorting by FACS. Analysis of cells by FACS was performed as follows: Cells were suspended in PBS containing 10 mM sodium azide (PBS-azide) and incubated with optimal concentrations anti-Lyt-2 as the primary antibody at 4°C for 30 min. Cells were then washed, resuspended in PBS-azide, and incubated with optimal concentrations of the appropriate secondary antibody FITC-F (ab′)^2 RAMγ at 4°C for 15 min. Cells were washed and fixed at 4°C for at least 30 min. in 4% buffered paraformaldehyde (Eastman Kodak, Rochester, NY), resuspended in PBS-azide, and analyzed on the FACS III (B-D FACS system, Becton-Dickinson and Co., Sunnyvale, CA). Values for controls were subtracted as background. Spleen cells were also sorted sterilely in the FACS III using indirect immunofluorescence as described above. Sterile PBS was used instead of PBS-azide.

Elimination of Lyt-2$^+$ cells by cytotoxicity. Spleen cells (5×10^6/ml) were incubated with anti-Lyt-2 antibody (NEI-006) at 1/1000 dilution for 45 min at 37°C. Cells were washed once with RPMI-1640 and resuspended in 20% rabbit serum (complement) adsorbed on mouse splenocytes and thymocytes, for 45 min, at 37°C. Cells were then washed three times before resuspension in MLR culture medium.

Separation of nylon-wool-nonadherent spleen cells. Nylon wool obtained from a Leukapak leukocytic filter (Fenwal Laboratories, Division of Travenol Laboratories, Inc., Deerfield, IL) was pretreated by boiling in 0.2 N HCl for 60 min and washing in distilled water at 37°C for five days with two changes of water per day. Nylon wool was then dried for three days in a dry 37°C incubator and was shredded to a homogeneous fluff; 10 ml syringes were packed with 1.2 g nylon wool autoclaved and subsequently stored at room temperature until needed (*15*). Immediately before use, columns were washed with 100 ml warmed, serum-free medium followed by repeated washings with RPMI-1640 containing 20% fetal calf serum (FCS) in order to saturate the columns with protein. Then $75–100\times10^6$ spleen cells in 1.5–2.0 ml RPMI containing 10% FCS were loaded onto each column and incubated for a total of 45 min at 37°C in a humidified 5% CO_2-air incubator. At 15-min intervals, one-third of the suspension was eluted and collected from the bottom of the syringe, and fresh medium was added to the top. At the end of the incubation period the remaining nonadherent cells were eluted from the columns with 20 ml medium. Cells were spun down and resuspended at 10×10^6/ml in culture media. The cell yield was approximately 30%.

MLR assays. 1×10^6 responding cells were cultured in 0.25-ml flat-bottomed microculture wells (Sterilin, Cat. No. M29ARTL, Teddington, Middlesex, UK) with 1×10^6 stimulator lymphocytes, both isolated from peripheral lymph nodes. Stimulator cells were inactivated by a single in vitro exposure to 3000 rads from a radioactive cesium-137 source. Unless otherwise specified, 1×10^6 spleen cells from experimental chimeras, and an equal number from untreated mice, were cocultured in a one-way MLR to check for the presence of suppressor cells. Viability of cells was routinely checked by trypan blue exclusion. Cocultured cells were inactivated by irradiation prior to culturing, unless otherwise indicated, to eliminate proliferative responses to the responding or stimulating cells. The culture medium contained RPMI-1640 medium supplemented with human AB serum or newborn calf serum (Sera Lab. Ltd., Crawley Downs West Sussex, UK) (10%), glutamine (2 mM), mercaptoethanol (5×10^{-5} M), penicillin (100 U/ml) and streptomycin (100 μg/ml). Tissue culture media and reagents were purchased from Grand Island Biological Co., Grand Island, NY. Cells were incubated at 37°C in a humidified 5% CO_2/air incubator for 72 hr, and then pulsed for 16–18 hr with 1 μCi of ^{3}H-thymidine (5.0 Ci/mmol; Nuclear Research Center, Negev, Israel) per culture. Cells were subsequently collected on paper filters using a multiple sample harvester (Titertek, Skatron, Lierbyen, Norway) and counted in a Beckman liquid scintillation counter (Beckman Instruments, Inc., Fullerton, CA). Background proliferation was assessed in each experiment by adding irradiated lymph node (LN) cells syngeneic to responding cells. Background cpm were subtracted from MLR cpm and the resultant net cpm was used in all subsequent calculations. Suppressive activity was calculated according to the following formula: 100 − ([net cpm of tested cocultured cells/net cpm of normal cocultured cells] × 100).

Adoptive transfer experiments. Adoptive recipients were irradiated by WBI at the doses indicated 24 hr before i.v. inoculation of cells. Skin grafting of adoptive recipients was performed one day following cell transfer. Adoptive recipients were examined daily for skin graft survival and for clinical signs of GVHD including hunched back, ruffled skin, skin lesions, diarrhea, severe weight loss and death.

RESULTS

Evidence for Transplantation Tolerance in TLI-Induced BM Chimeras

Stable allogeneic chimerism, and specific unresponsiveness to donor-type alloantigens. Stable allogeneic chimerism was induced by infusing C57, A and BALB BM into BALB, F_1 and

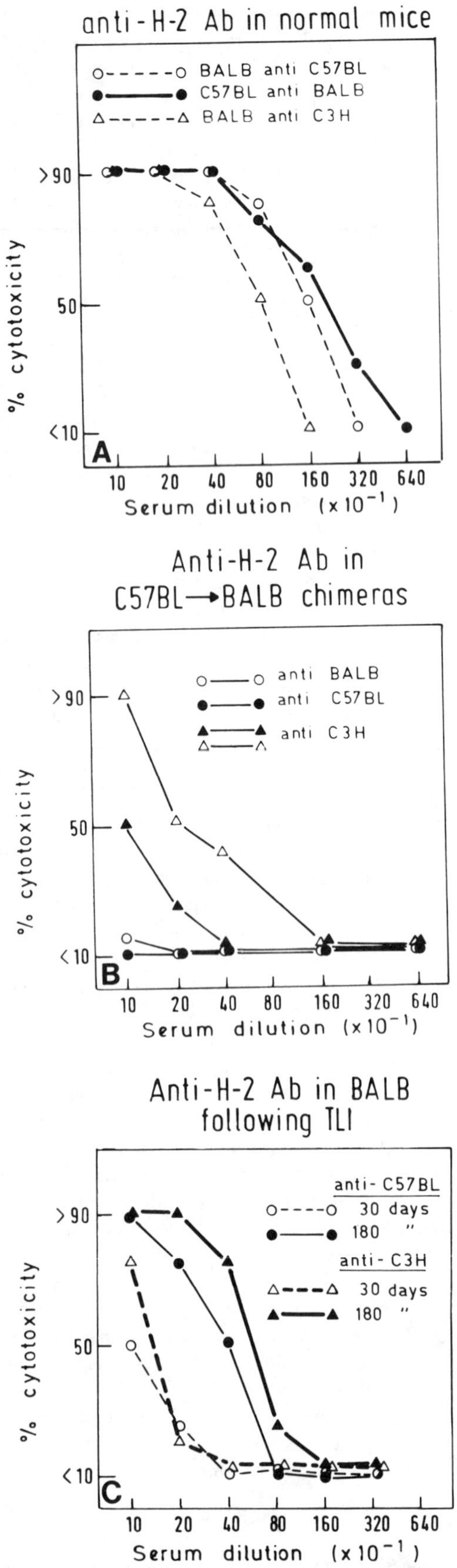

FIGURE 1. (A) Production of alloantisera in normal mice by complement-dependent microcytotoxic assay; (B) production of anti-BALB/c and anti-C57BL/6 as compared with anti-C3H/He alloantisera by C57BL/6→BALB/c chimeras immunized at 90 days (dark circles and triangles) and 180 days following induction of chimerism (open circles and triangles). (C) recovery of the capacity to produce anti-C57BL/6 and anti C3H/He alloantisera in TLI-treated BALB/c mice at different intervals following radiotherapy.

C3H recipients, respectively, conditioned with TLI consisting of 8 fractions of 200 rads (total dose of 1600 rads), followed by 400 rads WBI. Chimerism with semiallogeneic BM cells (C57→F_1 and BALB→F_1) was established following pretreatment of F_1 mice with TLI 1600 rads and 200 rads WBI. The percentage of donor-type cells ranged between 79±5 and 92±5 in the spleen of chimeras; C57→BALB, A→F_1, and BALB→C3H allogeneic chimeras maintained intact donor-type skin allografts (>180 days) while rejecting third-party skin grafts (12±2 days). No overt signs of GVHD were apparent in chimeras that were maintained in standard unprotected animal facilities.

Specific humoral unresponsiveness to alloantigens. As shown in Figure 1A, normal BALB as well as C57 mice produced good cytotoxic antisera against allogeneic C57, C3H, and BALB lymphocytes, respectively. In contrast, stable C57→BALB chimeras (at 90–180 days following BM transplantation) failed to produce cytotoxic antibodies against either of the parental strains (BALB, C57), although a significant antibody response was generated against unrelated C3H lymphocytes (Fig. 1B). In contrast, TLI-treated age-matched BALB mice recovered their ability to produce cytotoxic antibodies against C57, as well as C3H, alloantigens by day 180 following TLI alone (Fig. 1C).

Specific cell-mediated unresponsiveness to alloantigens in vitro. Tolerance to alloantigens was also documented in vitro. Spleen cells obtained from C57→BALB chimeras were unresponsive in one way MLR to both C57 and BALB LN cells. Similarly, spleen cells obtained from A→F_1 chimeras failed to respond to A and F_1 LN cells, but responded against unrelated ATH LN cells (data not shown). These results are similar to those described in chimeras prepared with heavier TLI doses (3400 rads) (*11*).

Specific unresponsiveness of spleen cells obtained from allogeneic chimeras to host alloantigens in vivo. Alloantigen-specific unresponsiveness of spleen cells obtained from stable C57→BALB chimeras was further documented in vivo by adoptive transfer experiments. Spleen cells (25×10^6) of chimeras with intact C57 skin grafts, containing 97% C57-type cells, were adoptively transferred into sublethally irradiated (550 rads) BALB or C3H mice. A similar number of normal C57 spleen cells was transferred into sublethally irradiated BALB or C3H mice serving as controls. None of the BALB recipients of C57→BALB spleen cells died of GVHD (>180 days observation), whereas all C3H mice receiving a similar inoculum died of GVHD within 12–16 days. Similarly, all BALB and C3H mice receiving normal C57 spleen cells died of GVHD within 9–13 and 8–14 days, respectively. The data suggest that C57 cells present in C57→BALB lack the ability to respond against BALB alloantigens in vivo.

Evidence for Suppressor Cells of MLR in Allogeneic Chimeras

Coculturing spleen cells isolated from well-established chimeras in MLR resulted in significant suppression of MLR. MLR suppressor cells were radioresistant to 750 rads; this dose of irradiation was administered to putative suppressor cells prior to culturing to avoid two-way MLR. The specificity of the inhibitory effects of the suppressor cells isolated from chimeras was variable. Spleen cells of C57→BALB chimeras blocked 60% of C57 vs. BALB MLR, as compared with 49% of BALB vs. C57, and 57% of C3H vs. BALB MLR. Spleen cells obtained from A→F_1 chimeras blocked 30% of A vs. F_1 MLR, as compared with 4% of A vs. unrelated ATH, and 0% of ATH vs. C57 MLR (Table 1).

Role of LyT-2⁺ cells in MLR suppression. The nature of MLR suppressor cells isolated from the spleen of chimeras was analyzed by positive and negative selection experiments using FACS analysis and sorting. Spleen cells isolated from A→F_1 and C57→F_1 chimeras revealed lower proportions of Lyt-2^+ cells than normal controls (9% as compared with 12–15% in A; 9% as compared with 12.5–14% in C57, respectively). In order to further analyze the possible role of Lyt-2^+ cells in inhibition of MLR, A→F_1 chimeric spleen cells were sorted sterilely by FACS into LyT-2^+ and LyT-2^- subpopulations. As shown in Table 1, coculturing of the LyT-2^+ cell fraction, containing 89% LyT-2^+ cells in an A vs. F_1 MLR, using even more than adequate numbers of Lyt-2^+ cells (0.25×10^6 as compared with an estimate of about 0.1×10^6 present in 1×10^6 unfractionated A→F_1 spleen cells), did not result in any suppression of MLR (0% vs. 30% by unfractionated spleen cells). In contrast, the Lyt-2^- cell fraction containing only 1.4% LyT-2^+ cells, retained the MLR suppressive capacity (52% vs. 30% suppression by the original spleen cells).

Role of Lyt-2^+ cells in unresponsiveness to alloantigens in chimeric spleen cells in vitro. Unfractionated spleen cells obtained from A→F_1 chimeras failed to respond in MLR against related (C57 or F_1) alloantigens (Table 2). Lyt-2-depleted spleen cells obtained from tolerant A→F_1 chimeras were used as responders in MLR in order to test whether specific unresponsiveness to recipient alloantigens is maintained by active Lyt-2-mediated suppression rather than deletion of alloreactive clones. As can be seen in Table 2, proliferative responsiveness of Lyt-2-depleted A→F_1 spleen cells against unrelated ATH cells was maintained, whereas no responsiveness could be recovered against host alloantigens (C57 or F_1). This experiment indicates that alloreactivity in MLR cannot be restored by depletion of Lyt-2^+ suppressor cells.

Similar experiments were carried out by studying the responsiveness of spleen cells obtained from BALB→F_1 and BALB→C3H chimeras against host-type lymphocytes in MLR before and after depletion by cytotoxic anti-Lyt-2 antibodies and rabbit complement. As shown in Table 3, Lyt-2-depleted BALB→F_1 and BALB→C3H spleen cells tolerant of host-type alloantigens failed to recover alloreactivity against tolerizing C57 and C3H cells, respectively.

Role of Lyt-2^+ cells in the maintenance and induction of unresponsiveness of the graft-versus-host reaction in chimeras. In order to test the possible role of Lyt-2^+ suppressor cells in maintaining unresponsiveness of the graft against the host, spleen cells obtained from C57→F_1 chimeras were incubated with anti-Lyt-2 antibodies, stained with FITC-RAMγ F(ab′)^2 and sorted sterilely by FACS. The proportion of Lyt-2^+ cells detectable in the negatively sorted population was 1.4%, whereas the positively sorted cell population contained 89% Lyt-2^+ cells. The first experiment was designed to investigate whether Lyt-2-depleted C57 spleen cells obtained from C57→F_1 chimeras regain their capacity to evoke GVHD against sublethally irradiated BALB recipients. The second experiment was designed to study the capacity of Lyt-2^+ cells isolated from

TABLE 2. The role of Lyt-2^+ cells in maintenance of specific unresponsiveness in MLR of spleen cells obtained from A→(BALB×C57)F_1 chimeras[a]

Responding spleen cells (1×10^6)	Stimulating LN cells (1×10^6)[b]	^{3}H-TdR uptake (mean cpm ± SD)
A	A	4465±484
A	F_1	38,575±9420
A	ATH	36,194±7446
A→F_1	A→F_1	3619±1804
A→F_1	F_1	3915±733
A→F_1	C57	3389±423
A→F_1	ATH	19,828±2748
Lyt-2-depleted A→F_1[c]	F_1	4757±554
Lyt-2-depleted A→F_1	C57	5765±594
Lyt-2-depleted A→F_1	ATH	12,674±2600

[a] Day ±180 A→F_1 chimeras; >90% A-type cells.
[b] LN: Lymph node cells irradiated with 3000 rads.
[c] Lyt-2 cells were depleted by sterile FACS sorting.

TABLE 1. The role of LyT-2^+ spleen cells of A→(BALB×C57)F_1 chimeras (A→F_1) in MLR suppression

Responding LN cells (1×10^6)[a]	Stimulating LN cells (1×10^6)	Cocultured spleen cells	^{3}H-TdR uptake (mean cpm ± SD)	% suppression[b]
A	F_1	1×10^6 normal A	18,544±1255	30%
A	F_1	1×10^6 A→F_1	13,239±1160	
A	ATH	1×10^6 normal A	17,072±9167	4%
A	ATH	1×10^6 A→F_1	16,440±2774	
A	F_1	0.25×10^6 normal A	14,723±2436	0%
A	F_1	0.25×10^6 LyT-2^{+c} A→F_1	22,760±3580	
A	ATH	0.25×10^6 normal A	16,146±3377	0%
A	ATH	0.25×10^6 LyT-2^+ A→F_1	22,971±1409	
A	F_1	1×10^6 LyT-2^{-d} A→F_1[4]	8947±1656	52%
ATH	C57	1×10^6 F_1	12,835±1061	0%
ATH	C57	1×10^6A→F_1	23,426±3272	

[a] LN: Lymph node.
[b] Suppression was calculated by comparing cpm of cocultured A cells obtained from A→F_1 chimera to CPM of cocultured normal A cells.
[c] Proportion of Lyt-2^+ in the positively sorted cells was 89%.
[d] Proportion of Lyt-2^+ in the negatively sorted cells was 1.4%.

stable C57→F_1 chimeras to suppress GVHD by coinjecting a challenge of 5×10^6 normal C57 spleen cells mixed with 1×10^6 Lyt-2^+ cells isolated from the spleens of stable C57→F_1 chimeras into sublethally irradiated BALB hosts. As can be seen in Table 4, 5×10^6 C57 spleen cells obtained from a C57→F_1 chimera did not result in GVHD upon inoculation into sublethally (550 rads) irradiated BALB mice, whereas a similar number of normal C57 spleen cells resulted in lethal GVHD within 12 days in all recipients. An identical number of Lyt-2-depleted spleen cells obtained from a C57→F_1 chimera failed to produce GVHD. Similarly, GVHD could not be prevented or even ameliorated by coinjecting a mixture of 5×10^6 normal C57 spleen cells with 1×10^6 Lyt-2^+ spleen cells isolated from a chimera (a final concentration of 17% Lyt-2^+ cells, as compared with 9% Lyt-2^+ cells present in the original spleen of the chimera). Thus these experiments imply that the lack of alloreactivity of the graft against the histoincompatible host in stable semiallogeneic chimeras cannot be attributed to Lyt-2^+ inhibitory cells alone.

TABLE 3. Responsiveness of spleen cells obtained from tolerant chimeras against host-type and unrelated alloantigens before and after depletion of Lyt-2^+ cells by anti-Lyt-2 antibody and complement

Responding spleen cells: Origin (1×10^6)	Treatment anti-Lyt-2+C′[a]	Stimulating LN cells (1×10^6)[b]	^{3}H-TdR uptake (mean cpm ± SD)
BALB	–	BALB	2451±207
BALB	–	C57	50,628±6002
BALB	–	C3H	73,700±7079
BALB→F_1[c]	–	BALB	1378±144
BALB→F_1	–	C57	4213±878
BALB→F_1	–	C3H	48,231±3828
BALB→F_1	+	BALB	661±29
BALB→F_1	+	C57	1476±293
BALB→F_1	+	C3H	47,192±2745
BALB	–	BALB	4851±650
BALB	–	C57	135,716±7161
BALB	–	C3H	113,477±85
BALB→C3H[d]	–	BALB	1042±85
BALB→C3H	–	C3H	3516±247
BALB→C3H	–	C57	7947±873
BALB→C3H	+	BALB	1507±401
BALB→C3H	+	C3H	4704±914
BALB→C3H	+	C57	9158±1189

[a] C′: complement.
[b] LN: Lymph node cells irradiated with 3000 rads.
[c] Day +73 chimeras; 100% donor-type cells in the peripheral blood.
[d] Day +154 chimeras; 100% donor-type cells in the peripheral blood.

TABLE 4. The in vivo role of Lyt-2^+ cells in the maintenance of unresponsiveness of the graft against the host in stable C57→(BALB×C57)F_1 (C57→F_1) chimeras[a]

Spleen cells used for GVHD challenge (i.v.)	No. BALB recipients[b]	Evidence of GVHD	Survival (days): median	(range)
5×10^6 normal C57	12	Yes	9	(7–12)
5×10^6 C57→F_1	4	None	>60	(>60)
25×10^6 C57→F_1	6	None	>60	(>60)
5×10^6 Lyt-2-depleted C57→F_1	4	None	>60	(>60)
5×10^6 normal C57 cells mixed with 1×10^6 Lyt-2^+ C57→F_1	4	Yes	12	(12–15)
None	6	None	>60	(>60)

[a] A pool of spleen cells obtained from day +220 C57→(BALB/c×C57BL/6)F_1 chimeras containing >90% C57-type cells with 9% Lyt-2^+ cells used in these experiments.
[b] All BALB recipients were conditioned with WBI 550 rads one day prior to cell transfer.

TABLE 5. Alloreactivity of spleen cells obtained from stable chimeras against related and third-party alloantigens before and after passage through nylon wool

Responding cells (1×10^6)	Stimulating lymph node cells (1×10^6): BALB	C57	C3H
BALB	6680±372[a]	174,278±7452	78,438±6414
BALB→F_1[b]	2252±312	2913±478	29,280±672
BALB (nylon-wool passed)	187±26	189,658±6179	34,905±7738
BALB→F_1 (nylon-wool passed)	146±16	431±148	34,613±2975

[a] ^{3}H-TdR uptake, cpm (mean ± SD).
[b] 166 days old BALB→F_1 chimeras >95% donor-type BALB cells in peripheral blood.

Attempts to recover alloreactivity of tolerant spleen cells against tolerizing alloantigens by passage through nylon wool. Alloreactivity against tolerizing host-type (C57) cells could not be restored by spleen cells obtained from BALB→F_1 chimeras after their passage over nylon wool. As can be seen in Table 5, nylon-wool-passed chimeric cells retained their alloreactivity in MLR against third-party stimulating lymph node cells but failed to respond against host-type cells.

Transfer of tolerance to skin allografts by spleen cells of chimeras. Spleen cells of chimeras were adoptively transferred into irradiated and nonirradiated naive recipients in order to ascertain whether specific unresponsiveness could be transferred by tolerant cells and/or antigen-specific suppressor cells. Sublethally irradiated BALB recipients infused with 25×10^6 C57→BALB spleen cells and cotransplanted with both C57 and C3H skin grafts accepted the former (>180) while rejecting the latter (unrelated) skin allografts (Table 6). These C57-tolerant adoptive recipients were proved to be chimeras themselves, since all spleen cells were found to be of C57 origin. All recipients of normal C57 spleen cells, on the other hand, died of GVHD within 4–34 (median 8) days. When an equal number (25×10^6) of C57→BALB spleen cells were irradiated in vitro (750 rads) prior to innoculation into sublethally irradiated BALB recipients, tolerance to C57 skin was not established (Table 6). The data suggest that the secondary BALB recipients acquired specific tolerance to C57 skin by being reconstituted with tolerant C57 cells rather than via active suppression by the suppressor cells found to be radioresistant in vitro. The latter conclusion is further supported by experiments summarized in Table 6. Tolerance to C57 skin allografts in naive recipients of 25×10^6 tolerant C57 cells obtained from C57→F_1 chimeras was established only in heavily irradiated BALB hosts (550 rads), whereas both unirradiated and suboptimally irradiated recipients (250 rads) promptly rejected C57 skin grafted one day following cell transfer. None of the adoptive recipients conditioned with 250 rads showed evidence of persisting C57 cells. In the mirror image experiment in which spleen cells obtained from C57→BALB chimeras were transferred into sublethally irradiated (550 rads) C57 recipients, none of the secondary C57 recipients accepted either BALB or C3H skin allografts (Table 6). The data indicate that although suppressor cells could be

TABLE 6. Transfer of specific unresponsiveness to allogeneic skin grafts by spleen cells obtained from C57→BALB and C57→(BALB×C57)F_1 chimeras

Adoptive recipients[a]	Spleen cell transfer (25×10⁶)	Skin allograft[b]	No. mice	Skin allograft survival in days
BALB WBI[c] 550 rads	C57→BALB[d]	C57	12	<180[e]
BALB WBI 550 rads	C57→BALB	C3H	12	12–16[e]
BALB WBI 550 rads	C57→F_1	C57	6	>180[e]
BALB WBI 550 rads	C57→BALB (750 rads)	C57	4	9–16
BALB WBI 550 rads	BALB	C57	10	9–15
BALB WBI 550 rads	BALB	C3H	10	9–14
BALB WBI 550 rads	none	C57	12	11–18
BALB WBI 550 rads	none	C3H	12	10–16
BALB WBI 250 rads	C57	C57	8	8–14
BALB WBI 250 rads	C57→BALB	C57	6	8–15[f]
BALB WBI 250 rads	C57→F_1	C57	3	23–26[f]
BALB unirradiated	C57	C57	6	9–12[f]
BALB unirradiated	C57→BALB	C57	4	11–16[f]
BALB unirradiated	C57→F_1	C57	4	12–15[f]
C57 WBI 550 rads	C57→BALB	BALB	6	13–18
C57 WBI 550 rads	C57→BALB	C3H	6	14–18
C57 WBI 550 rads	C57→F_1	BALB	4	9–16
C57 WBI 550 rads	C57	BALB	6	8–13
C57 WBI 550 rads	C57	C3H	6	10–12

[a] Adoptive recipients were conditioned by WBI at doses indicated 1 day prior to cell transfer.
[b] Skin allografts were transplanted one day after cell transfer.
[c] WBI: whole-body irradiation.
[d] >95% C57-type cells in the spleen.
[e] Chimerism was documented in all recipients; C57-type cells in the spleen >90%.
[f] Chimerism was not established in adoptive recipients.

documented in vitro in stable C57→BALB chimeras, abrogation of even attenuated C57 anti-BALB alloreactivity of sublethally irradiated C57 recipients could not be accomplished in vivo by suppressor cells known to be present in the spleen of chimeras.

Attempts to transfer suppression of graft-versus-host reactivity in vivo. Spleen cells obtained from stable C57→F_1 and A→F_1 chimeras were coinjected into irradiated BALB or F_1 recipients, respectively, together with normal donor-type spleen or BM cells as GVHD-inducing inocula. From 6 to 12 mice were used for each experimental or control group. Spleen cells (30×10⁶) obtained from stable chimeras (known to contain suppressive activity in vitro) failed to abrogate lethal GVHD induced by 5–10×10⁶ normal donor-type spleen cells (ratio of chimeric suppressor cell to effector cells of 6:1). Survival of recipients of chimeric spleen cells was only mildly prolonged in 3 of 4 experiments as compared with mice that received equal numbers of normal F_1 spleen cells (median survival 30 vs. 14 days, 49 vs. 15 days, 49 vs. 14 days, and 9 vs. 9 days, respectively). Lethal GVHD induced by normal BM cells was prevented by coinjecting chimeric spleen cells in only 1 of 3 experiments, while no significant inhibitory effects could be observed in the other 2 sets of experiments (median survivals >300 vs. 13 days, 37 vs. 13 days, and 20 vs. 25 days, respectively).

DISCUSSION

Experiments documented here were designed to elucidate the mechanism of specific unresponsiveness to alloantigens in TLI-induced BM chimeras by studying the nature and function of regulatory cells in tolerant chimeras with particular attention to the possible role of Lyt-2⁺ suppressor cells. The studies of transplantation tolerance induced by TLI extend previous observations in which the tolerogenic effects of TLI were exploited for induction of specific unresponsiveness across MHC in BM chimeras (*8–14*). In the present experiments tolerance was documented in several strain combinations by permanent survival of skin allografts, as well as by failure to generate anti-H-2 antibodies and proliferative responses in MLR against host-type or donor-type alloantigens. Since the specific unresponsiveness of donor-type cells against host alloantigens was associated with the presence of suppressor cells experiments were designed to investigate the possible role of Lyt-2 suppressor cells in the induction and/or maintenance of the specific unresponsive state.

Our studies indicate that Lyt-2⁺ cells are definitely not the sole mechanism for maintaining donor antihost unresponsiveness in long-term BM chimeras, mainly because effective elimination of these cells did not result in reconstitution of alloreactivity of spleen T cells against host alloantigens in vitro or in vivo. Also, Lyt-2⁺ cells isolated from tolerant chimeras failed to inhibit alloreactivity of mature T lymphocytes in vitro or in vivo. In general, it was not possible to document that tolerance to skin allografts could be transferred by suppressor cells of tolerant chimeras, but could be accomplished by reconstituting adoptive recipients with clonally inactive cells. On the other hand, certain experiments suggest that suppressor cells may play a role in down-regulation of the degree of clonal expansion of antihost-reacting cells, particularly of the small number of uncommitted T cell precursors present in the marrow, as may be inferred from the experiments presented in Table 6.

The failure to reconstitute alloreactivity of tolerant spleen cells in vitro in MLR assays and in vivo by GVHD assays following depletion of Lyt-2⁺ cells supports the concept that functional clonal depletion is the mechanism underlying maintenance of unresponsiveness in tolerant chimeras. Nevertheless, the possibility that specific suppressor cells other than Lyt-2⁺ may play a role cannot be ruled out, especially since the finding that suppressor cells belonging to the helper/delayed-type hypersensitivity subpopulation of cells was recently documented in neonatal tolerance (*9*). In that study, the degree of chimerism was minimal, as opposed to the BM chimeras induced by TLI in which virtually all the immunohematopoietic cells are of the donor type. Likewise, the specific unresponsiveness studied in the neonatal tolerance model was in the direction of the host against the graft, whereas the direction of tolerance studied in BM chimeras described here is in the direction of donor vs. host. This difference is particularly relevant since few, if any, residual host-type cells can be documented in such chimeras. Interestingly, the mechanism of tolerance to protein antigens (bovine serum albumin and bovine gamma globulin) that can be readily induced in TLI-treated mice not reconstituted with BM cells has been previously shown to be mediated by T lymphocytes (*12*)—which, by definition, are of host origin since no foreign cells were introduced. Other common immunological features of the post-TLI period and the neonatal state were recently reported (*20*).

Another approach used in the past to document the presence of alloreactive cells in tolerant chimeras was based on recovery of alloreactivity of tolerant cells against the tolerizing cells by removal of specific suppressor cells through passage over nylon wool (*21–24*). In TLI-induced BM chimeras, donor-type spleen cells tolerant to the host did not recover alloreactivity against host cells (Table 5) following passage through nylon-wool columns. Thus, specific unresponsiveness of donor vs. host in TLI-induced BM chimeras is not maintained by nylon-wool-adherent cells as has been suggested as evidence for the role of suppressor cells in transplantation tolerance by investigators working in neonatal tolerance (*21–23*) and radiation chimeras (*24*).

The mechanism by which TLI facilitates tolerance induction is not fully understood. We have recently documented that the TLI procedure results in potent immunosuppressive state that is probably due to a combination of both depletion of lymphocytes (*8*) as well as generation of massive antigen-nonspecific suppressor cells (*11–14, 25–27*) found among the large, nonlymphoid mononuclear cells that probably represent a population of immature cells likely to be more susceptible to tolerance induction (*26–28*). These nonspecific suppressor cells lack cell surface determinants characteristic of lymphocytes—including Thy-1, Lyt-1, Lyt-2, TL, assialo GM-1 and cell-surface immunoglobin, and cannot be depleted by adherence to nylon wool and plastic surfaces or passage through G-10 Sephadex for removal of monocytes (*25–27*). A large proportion of these cells, which are present within the first few weeks post TLI, have the ability to form colonies in vitro (CFU-GM) and in vivo (CFU-S) (*28*), and hence must represent a regeneration phase of the depleted immunohematopoietic system from the stem cell reservoir present in shielded marrow spaces of the peripheral bones and the tail. The large cells, shown to be capable of suppressing T cell mediated proliferative responses in vitro, can be agglutinated by soybean and peanut agglutinins (*27*) as BM stem cells can (*7*).

The biological role of the suppressor cells, which is readily demonstrable by various in vitro techniques either in TLI-treated, autoreconstituted mice (host-type), or in tolerant BM chimeras (donor-type), as well as the exact characterization and distinction between the two subsets of suppressor cells, is not clear. Although suppression of in vitro T-cell-mediated proliferative responses is radioresistant, irradiated spleen cells obtained from C57→BALB chimeras failed to block BALB anti-C57 or C57 anti-BALB alloreactivity in vivo (Table 6), suggesting that radioresistant suppressor cells may not play a role in blocking alloreactivity in vivo. On the other hand, tolerance to skin allografts could be adoptively transferred by nonirradiated chimeric spleen cells (Table 6). We designed several experiments to critically evaluate whether the adoptive transfer of transplantation tolerance is mediated by active antigen-specific cell-mediated suppression of the adoptive recipient's alloreactivity, or by reconstitution of adoptive recipients with tolerant cells. Transfer of 25×10^6 viable C57→BALB or C57→F_1 spleen cells into naive BALB recipients or BALB recipients irradiated by a suboptimal dose of WBI (250 rads) failed to prevent C57 skin allograft rejection. Tolerance of C57 skin could be established only in BALB recipients prepared with 550 rads WBI, which resulted in reconstitution of adoptive recipients with tolerant, C57-derived cells, most likely deleted of BALB-responding cells. On the other hand, a similar transfer of 25×10^6 donor-type spleen cells obtained from C57→BALB or C57→F_1 chimeras into syngeneic C57 recipients prepared with WBI 550 rads did not result in tolerance to BALB skin graft, suggesting that suppressor cells of C57 origin failed to abrogate anti-BALB reactivity of even attentuated, sublethally irradiated recipients by active suppressor cell mechanisms.

To explain these results on the basis of a clonal deletion theory, one must assume that 550 rads, shown to be sufficient for conditioning of BALB recipients, is insufficient to enable similar immunopoietic reconstitution in naive C57 recipients by BALB-tolerant C57→BALB or C57→F_1 spleen cells. This strain difference may be expected, since it is well known that C57 mice are substantially more resistant to irradiation than BALB mice.

In attempting to understand the complexity of the bilateral transplantation tolerance of the host vs. graft reaction, as well as the graft vs. host reaction, induced in TLI-treated recipients reconstituted with allogeneic BM cells, one must always bear in mind that two different regulatory events may function in concert. First, host-type suppressor cells regulating host immune reactivity may very likely be involved in induction of tolerance to alloantigens, as in their role in tolerance to protein antigens (*12*). Indeed, tolerance to perfused organ allografts can also be induced in TLI-treated rats, dogs, and primates in the absence of chimerism (*29–32*). Second, suppressor cells of the donor type present in recipients fully reconstituted with allogeneic BM cells may play some role in reducing the degree of alloreactivity to an allogeneic stimulus, as suggested by some studies in vitro and in vivo (*33*).

Nevertheless, data presented in this article suggest that the unresponsiveness of donor-type cells against the host is probably not induced, and certainly not maintained, by Lyt-2 suppressor cells. Taken together, failure to document the presence of alloreactive cells in tolerant chimeras, failure to completely abrogate GVHD alloreactivity induced by mature immunocompetent T cells by cotransferring normal and tolerant spleen cells obtained from stable chimeras, and lack of any evidence for a suppressive role of Lyt-2^+ cells obtained from tolerant chimeras using positive and negative selection experiments, do not support a major role for suppressor cells in actively preventing alloreactivity induced by mature donor-type T cells against the host. Since the possible role of serum factors in target receptor or effector cell blockade was also previously ruled out (*32*), functional clonal deletion is very likely to be the most adequate explanation for the lack of GVHD in tolerant chimeras. It is possible that Lyt-2-negative inhibitory cells—not necessarily alloantigen-specific—may still play an important role too by inhibiting alloantigen-induced cell proliferation as documented in vitro, thus reducing the pool of alloreactive cells or their precursors. Functional clonal deletion may therefore be established through ongoing inhibition and down-regulation of clonal expansion via inactivation or actual elimination of alloactivated clones, and resulting in abrogation of antigen-specific T cell functions.

Whatever the in vivo role of suppressor cells induced by the TLI conditioning may be in the induction of the unresponsive state, functional clonal deletion is likely to represent the final common pathway.

Acknowledgments. We thank Dr ES Vitetta, Department of Microbiology, the University of Texas Health Science Center at Dallas, for a generous supply of reagents and useful advice in operating the FACS.

REFERENCES

1. Billingham RE, Brent L. Quantitative studies on tissue transplantation immunity. IV. Induction of tolerance in newborn mice and studies on the phenomenon of runt disease. Philos Trans R Soc Lond [Biol] 154; 242: 439.
2. Billingham RE, Silvers WK. Quantitative studies on the ability of

cells of different origins to induce tolerance of skin homografts and cause runt disease in neonatal mice. J Exp Zool 1961; 146: 113.
3. Slavin S, Weiss L, Morecki S, Weigensberg M, Fuks Z. Immunosuppression and induction of transplantation tolerance by fractionated total lymphoid irradiation. In: Slavin S, ed. Tolerance in bone marrow and organ transplantation. Amsterdam: Elsevier, 1985; 105.
4. Korngold R, Sprent J. Surface markers of T cells causing lethal graft versus host disease in mice. In: Gale RP, ed. Recent advances in bone marrow transplantation. New York: Alan R Liss, 1983: 199.
5. Rodt HV, Thierfelder S, Eulitz M. Anti-lymphocytic antibodies and marrow transplantation. III. Effect of heterologous antibrain antibodies on acute secondary disease in mice. Eur J Immunol 1974; 4: 25.
6. Vallera DA, Filipovich AH, Soderling CCB, Kersey JH. Bone marrow transplantation across major histocompatability barriers in mice. Clin Immunol Immunopathol 1982; 23: 437.
7. Reisner Y, Itzicovitch L, Meshorer A, Sharon N. Hemopoietic stem cell transplantation using mouse bone marrow and spleen cells fractionated by lectins. Pro Natl Acad Sci USA 1978; 75: 2933.
8. Slavin S, Strober S, Fuks Z, Kaplan HS. Induction of specific tissue transplantation tolerance using fractionated total lymphoid irradiation in adult mice: long-term survival of allogeneic bone marrow and skin grafts. J Exp Med 1977; 146: 34.
9. Strober S, Slavin S, Gottlieb M, et al. Allograft tolerance after total lymphoid irradiation (TLI). Immunol Rev 1979; 46: 87.
10. Slavin S, Yatziv S. Correction of enzyme deficiency by allogeneic bone marrow transplantation in mice using total lymphoid irradiation. Science 1980; 210: 1150.
11. Slavin S, Strober S. Induction of allograft tolerance after total lymphoid irradiation (TLI). Development of suppressor cells of the mixed leukocyte reaction MLR. J Immunol 1979; 123: 942.
12. Zan-Bar I, Slavin S, Strober S. Induction and mechanism of tolerance to bovine serum albumin after total lymphoid irradiation. J Immunol 1978; 121: 1400.
13. King DP, Strober S, Kaplan HS. Suppression of the mixed leukocyte response and graft vs host disease by spleen cells following total lymphoid irradiation (TLI). J Immunol 1981; 126: 1140.
14. Okada S, Strober S. Spleen cells from adult mice given total lymphoid irradiation (TLI) or from newborn mice having similar regulatory effects in the mixed leukocyte reaction (MLR). I. Generation of antigen specific suppressor cells in the MLR after addition of spleen cells from adult mice given TLI. J Exp Med 1982; 156: 522.
15. Billingham RE, Medawar PB. The technique of free skin grafting in mammals. J Exp Biol 1951; 28: 385.
16. Slavin S, Fuks Z, Kaplan HS, Strober S. Transplantation of allogeneic bone marrow without graft vs host disease using total lymphoid irradiation (TLI). J Exp Med 1978; 147: 963.
17. Ledbetter JA, Herzenberg LA. Xenogeneic monoclonal antibodies to mouse differentiation antigens. Immunol Rev 1979; 47: 63.
18. Ligler F, Vitetta ES, Uhr JW. Cell surface immunoglobulin. XXII. Reappearance of surface IgM and IgD on murine splenocytes after removal by capping. J Immunol 1977; 119: 1545.
19. Stephenson P, Dorsch S, Roser B, Godden U, Herbert J. The identity of suppressor cells in neonatal tolerance. Transplant Proc 1983; 15: 850.
20. Okada S, Strober S. Spleen cells from adult mice given total lymphoid irradiation (TLI) or from newborn mice having similar regulatory effects in the mixed leukocyte reaction (MLR). II. Generation of antigen-specific suppressor cells in the MLR after addition of spleen cells from newborn mice. J Immunol 1982; 129: 1892.
21. Holan V, Chutna J, Hasek M. Specific suppression of antigen-reactive cells in neonatal transplantation tolerance. Nature 1978; 274: 895.
22. Hasek M, Chutna J. Complexity of the state of immunological tolerance. Immunol Rev 1979; 46: 3.
23. Roser BJ, Herbert J, Godden U. The role of suppressor cells in transplantation. Transplant Proc 1983; 15: 698.
24. Tutschka PJ, Hess AD, Beschorner WE, Santos GW. Suppressor cells in transplantation tolerance. I. Suppressor cells in the mechanism of tolerance in radiation chimeras. Transplantation 1981; 32: 203.
25. May RD, Slavin S, Vitetta ES. A partial characterization of suppressor cells in the spleens of mice conditioned with fractionated total lymphoid irradiation (TLI). J Immunol 1983; 131: 1108.
26. Weigensberg M, Morecki S, Weiss L, Fuks Z, Slavin S. Suppression of cell mediated immune responses following total lymphoid irradiation (TLI). I. Characterization of suppressor cell of the mixed lymphocyte reaction. J Immunol 1984; 132: 971.
27. Morecki S, Weigensberg M, Slavin S. Lectin separation of non-lymphoid suppressor cells induced by total lymphoid irradiation. European J Immunol (in press).
28. Slavin S, Seidel HJ. Hematopoietic activity in bone marrow chimeras prepared with total lymphoid irradiation (TLI). Exp Hematol 1982; 10: 206.
29. Slavin S, Reitz B, Bieber CP, Kaplan HS, Strober S. Transplantation tolerance in adult rats using total lymphoid irradiation (TLI): permanent survival of skin, heart and marrow allografts. J Exp Med 1978; 147: 700.
30. Howard RJ, Sutherland DER, Lum CT, et al. Kidney allograft survival in dogs treated with total lymphoid irradiation. Ann Surg 1981; 193: 196.
31. Myburgh JA, Smit JA, Browde S, Stark JH. Current status of total lymphoid irradiation. Transplant Proc 1983; 15: 659.
32. Slavin S, Fuks Z, Weiss L, Morecki S. Mechanisms of tolerance in chimeric mice prepared with total lymphoid irradiation (TLI). In: Gale R, Fox C, eds. Biology of bone marrow transplantation. ICN-UCLA Symposia on Molecular and Cellular Biology, vol 17. New York: Academic Press, 1980; 383.
33. Okada S, Palathumpat V, Strober S. Identification of donor-derived Ay-specific suppressor cells in murene bone marrow chimeras prepared with TLI. Transplantation 1983; 36: 417.

Received 23 April 1985.
Accepted 19 September 1985.

0041-1337/86/4106-0688$02.00/0
TRANSPLANTATION
Vol. 41, No. 1

Printed in U.S.A.

EARLY EVENTS IN NATURAL RESISTANCE TO BONE MARROW TRANSPLANTATION

USE OF RADIOLABELED BONE MARROW CELLS[1]

GEORGE A. CARLSON,[2] SUSAN T. MARSHALL, AND AMY KIESCHE[3]

The Jackson Laboratory Bar Harbor, Maine

Natural resistance against the proliferation of splenic colony-forming units (CFU-S) is seen in certain combinations of bone marrow donors and irradiated hosts. In order to examine the early events following bone marrow transplantaion and to determine whether genetically determined CFU-S repression is due to elimination of the transplanted cells from the spleen or to inhibition of their proliferation, we labeled proliferating cells in freshly isolated bone marrow or long-term bone marrow cultures (LTBMC) with radioactive I-iododeoxyuridine prior to injection. A heterogeneous mixture of cells was labeled in both freshly isolated marrow and LTBMC; CFU-S precursors were among the cells labeled as indicated by reduction of CFU-S numbers in the radiolabeled cell population.

Radiolabeled cells from C57BL/6J, DBA/2J, and B6D2F$_1$ mice were injected into syngeneic, semisyngeneic, and allogeneic irradiated mice that were killed at various times after injection to determine the amount of radioactivity remaining and the organ distribution of the labeled cells; additional mice were killed 7–8 days later to count CFU-S. Retention of label in the spleen was predictive of subsequent CFU-S numbers, suggesting that killing or elimination of the transplanted cells from the spleen is the cause of CFU-S depression in resistant animals. Further genetic analysis of the survival of the radiolabeled cells in the spleen indicated that mismatching of *H-2* homozygous donor cells with the host at *H-2D* was a prerequisite for resistance and that *H-2* heterozygous cells were not resisted in spite of *H-2* mismatching. Although natural killer (NK) cell-deficient beige mice were able to resist *H-2*-nonidentical bone marrow cells, pretreatment of the host with anti-asialo GM-1 antibodies completely abrogated natural resistance as assessed by splenic survival or radiolabeled cells. The findings that splenic survival of radiolabeled bone marrow cells reflects the immunogenetic specificity of CFU-S repression and that abrogation of CFU-S repression increases the splenic survival of the labeled cells strengthen the postulate that repression of CFU-S proliferation involves events occurring within the first 24 hr after injection.

[1] This work was supported by Grant CA28231 from the National Cancer Institute, U.S. Public Health Service.

[2] Address correspondence to: George A. Carlson, The Jackson Laboratory, Bar Harbor, ME 04609.

[3] Amy Kiesche was a participant in the Jackson Laboratory Summer Student Program and received financial assistance from the George I. Alden Trust, the Charles Ulrick and Josephine Bay Foundation, the Clark Foundation, General Funds of the Jackson Laboratory, and The Burroughs Wellcome Fund.

In apparent violation of the laws of transplantation, certain F$_1$ hybrid mice resist grafts of parental strain bone marrow cells (*1, 2*). This hybrid resistance, as well as resistance to allogeneic bone marrow, is quantitated by counting the numbers of colony-forming units (CFU-S)* in the spleens of irradiated hosts 7–10 days after transplantation (*3*). Using repression of CFU-S proliferation as the indicator of resistance, Cudkowicz and coworkers demonstrated that this resistance was nonadaptive and was controlled both *H-2* and *non-H-2* genes (*1, 2*). The *H-2*-linked genes appear to act by controlling a "recessive" antigen or a specific recognition event, with the *non-H-2* genes serving an "*Ir*-like" function or controlling the ability of the irradiated host to reject the *H-2*-nonidentical cells.

In previous studies we used leukemia cells prelabeled with ^{131}I-iododeoxyuridine (IdUrd) as a model for natural resistance against transplanted bone marrow cells (*4–6*). When the radiolabeled cells were injected into mice, more tumor cell death occurred in mice that were not identical with the transplanted cells at the major histocompatibility complex. In addition, the tumor cells were eliminated rapidly from the spleens of *H-2*-nonidentical mice, with differences apparent as soon as 4 hr postinjection. The genetic control of natural resistance to leukemia transplantation was remarkably similar to that for bone marrow transplantation; for example, after lethal doses of gamma irradiation only strains of mice that were capable of resisting bone marrow transplants retained the ability to resist *H-2*-nonidentical leukemia cells. In irradiated mice of the C57BL family, resistance to both bone marrow and leukemia transplantation is restricted to cases of *H-2D* nonidentity between the host and the graft (*1, 2, 5*). Resistance to both the normal and the malignant transplants is thymus-independent and involves members of the natural killer (NK) family of effector cells (*5, 7*). Based on these similarities we have inferred that resistance to bone marrow and to leukemia transplantation are manifestations of the same host response against nonsyngeneic cells.

However, given that CFU-S performance is assessed 7–10 days after injection, the possibility remains that natural resistance is due to inhibition or delay of stem cell proliferation (*8, 9*). The fact that resistant mice may be eventually repopulated by transplanted nonsyngeneic bone marrow has been cited as evidence for this interpretation (*10*). In contrast, retransplantation studies support the hypothesis that the transplanted

* Abbreviations used: ANOVA, analysis of variance; *bg*, beige; CFU-S, splenic colony-forming units; LTBMC, long-term bone marrow culture; NK, natural killer; PMN, polymorphonuclear leukocytes.

cells are rapidly eliminated from the spleens of resistant mice (*1, 2*). The ability to directly follow the survival and distribution of transplanted bone marrow cells shortly after injection, as we have done previously with leukemia cells, would prove useful in evaluating the mechanism of resistance to CFU-S proliferation. Recent studies by Orbach-Arbouys and coworkers (*11*) have indicated the feasibility of this approach. Using ^{125}I-IdUrd to label freshly isolated syngeneic bone marrow cells, these authors directly confirmed the assumption that lethal irradiation of the host allows a higher proportion of the injected bone marrow cells to survive in the spleen. Another study utilized radiolabeled marrow cells to analyze the role of NK cells in natural resistance, concluding that survival of the transplanted cells was reduced in high NK strains of mice (*12*). However, no effort was made to determine whether retention or elimination of the radiolabeled cells was predictive of their subsequent CFU-S performance.

The use of long-term bone marrow cultures (LTBMC) offers several advantages over freshly isolated marrow as a source of cells to be radiolabeled for use in following their survival in vivo. First, there is a small enrichment of CFU-S precursors (*13*)—but, more importantly, higher levels of labeling can be obtained in the LTBMC's than in freshly isolated marrow. CFU-S precursors are among the cells labeled, and it has been shown that nearly half these precursors are dividing after feeding or agitating the cultures (*14*). In this study we report results directly comparing the survival of labeled bone marrow cells with their subsequent CFU-S potential. Our emphasis in these studies is on the genetic control of natural resistance to marrow transplantation, and on the involvement of NK cells.

MATERIALS AND METHODS

Mice. All mice were obtained from Animal Resources or from our own research colony at the Jackson Laboratory, Bar Harbor, Maine, which is fully accredited by the American Association for the Accreditation of Laboratory Animal Care. The strains used are indicated in the *Results* section.

CFU-S assay. Numbers of CFU-S were counted essentially as originally reported (*3*). Recipients of labeled or unlabeled bone marrow cells obtained fresh or from LTBMC were given 900 rads of gamma irradiation 2–18 hr prior to injection. Irradiation was performed using a Shepherd Mark I, Model 68 Cesium Irradiator attentuated with lead shielding to give a dose rate of approximately 150 rads/min. The mice were killed 7 or 8 days after injection and their spleens were removed into Bouin's fixation for visualization of CFU-S. The spleen weight was also recorded in some experiments; it has been shown previously that spleen weight correlates with CFU-S proliferation (*15*).

Long-term bone marrow cultures. Cultures from mouse bone marrow were established using previously described methodology (*13*). Briefly, bone marrow cells were flushed from femurs and pooled, with small clumps left intact. Fisher's Medium (F-15, Grand Island Biological Company) supplemented with 10^{-7} M hydrocortisone, 20% preselected horse serum (Sterile Systems, Inc., Logan, UT), and penicillin-streptomycin were used throughout. Cultures were established in 25-cm^2 Corning tissue culture flasks each containing cells from approximately 1.5 femurs in 10 ml; the flasks were gassed with 5% CO_2 in air, closed, and incubated at 33°C. Cultures were fed weekly by gently shaking the flasks, removing 5 ml of the spent medium containing nonadherent cells, and adding 5 ml of fresh medium. Cultures were used for experiments between 7 and 16 weeks after their establishment.

Radiolabeling. Cells in LTBMC were labeled by adding 10–20 μCi of ^{131}I-IdUrd or ^{125}I-IdUrd (New England Nuclear) to each flask at the time of feeding. The cultures were then incubated at 33°C for 18–24 hr, shaken gently to remove loosely adherent cells, and all the cell-containing culture medium removed. The cells were then washed to remove unincorporated isotope, counted, and their concentration adjusted for injection. We generally obtained between 30,000 and 100,000 cpm per 10^6 cells when labeling by this procedure.

Freshly isolated bone marrow cells were washed and incubated at 10^6 cells/ml in RPMI-1640 (Grand Island Biological Laboratories) supplemented with 10% heat-inactivated fetal bovine serum and 5×10^{-5} M 2-mercaptoethanol in the presence of 1 μCi/ml of radioactive IdUrd. Labeling was allowed to proceed for 4–6 hr before harvesting. The degree of labeling was generally half to two-thirds that obtained in LTBMC.

Monitoring cell survival in vivo. After i.v. injection of radiolabeled bone marrow cells the mice were whole-body gamma counted to determine the initial radioactivity per animal using a Beckman Gamma 8000 scintillation counter as previously described (*4*). The animals were recounted before they were killed, and their spleens, livers, and lungs removed to determine the amount of isotope remaining in these organs. Previous studies have indicated that reutilization of released isotope is minimal and that this method provides an accurate indication of cell survival in vivo (*5, 16*). While intranuclear ^{125}I is approximately six-fold more radiotoxic than ^{131}I, either isotope is suitable for monitoring short-term survival and distribution of labeled cells because radiation-induced cell death does not occur within the first 48 hr after injection (*17, 18*).

Autoradiography. Bone marrow cells labeled with ^{125}I-IdUrd were prepared for autoradiography by cytocentrifugation using a Shannon cytocentrifuge. The methanol-fixed cells were then dipped in emulsion, exposed for 1–4 days, and developed by the Jackson Laboratory Histology Service. The slides were then stained with Giemsa and scored while still wet to preserve cell morphology.

Statistics. In addition to Student's t test for analysis of the significance of differences between groups, we also utilized the BMDP 1V statistical package (BMDP Statistical Software, Inc., 1983 version) to perform one-way analysis of variance and the planned contrast test on the Jackson Laboratory VAX-11 computer. The BMDP7D package was used for Levine test for equal variances and for the Bonferroni test. The value given for the Bonferroni test is the simultaneous significant P value of comparisons of all pairs of means—for example, after adjustment for the multiple comparison of all pairs of means, to be significant at the .01 level the P value must be less than 0.000667.

RESULTS

Cells labeled in freshly isolated marrow and in long-term bone marrow culture. LTBMCs established from C57BL/6J bone marrow 7 weeks previously were labeled for 24 hr at 33° with ^{125}I-IdUrd as described in the *Materials and Methods* section. Autoradiographs were prepared and differential counts were performed. Labeling in LTBMC was compared with that obtained with freshly isolated marrow cells incubated at 37° with isotope for 4 or 24 hr. Only minimal labeling of LTBMC cells was obtained after 4 hr. Representative results are shown in Table 1. The proportions of morphologically distinguishable cell types in LTBMC were similar to those previously published (*13*). Undifferentiated "blasts" made up approximately 60% of the cells labeled, while being less than 20% of the total cell population; as would be expected, more immature polymorphonuclear leukocyte (PMNs) were labeled than mature PMNs.

The most striking difference between the labeling obtained with freshly isolated marrow and that in LTBMC was in the lack of lymphocytes. LTBMC, though maintaining lymphoid precursors, do not normally contain mature lymphocytes; with freshly isolated marrow, over 40% of the cells labeled in 4 hr were lymphocytes. Increasing the time of labeling to 24 hr for fresh marrow led to a decrease in the percentage of cells labeled. It is important to note that in freshly isolated marrow and in LTBMC a heterogeneous mixture of cells was labeled, even without taking into account the fact that the morphologically homogeneous "blasts" are composed of a variety of functional types.

Survival and distribution of radiolabeled cells in vivo. Radiolabeled bone marrow cells were injected i.v. to determine the survival and distribution of the cells within the first 24 hr after injection. The same basic experimental design was used throughout. Cells from LTBMC or freshly isolated bone marrow cells were radiolabeled with IdUrd as described in the *Materials and Methods* section and 10^6 cells were injected into each mouse. The mice were whole-body gamma counted shortly after injection, and recounted prior to being killed 18–24 hr later when spleens, livers, and lungs were taken to determine the distribution of the surviving cells. These organs also were taken from groups of mice killed 2.5–4 hr after injection. Additional mice were injected with 10^6 unlabeled marrow cells from the same pools used for labeling to determine CFU-S numbers 8 days later. The results of representative experiments using C57BL/6J, DBA/2J, AND B6D2F$_1$ mice as marrow donors and as recipients are summarized in Table 2. The retention of radioisotope in the spleens of recipient mice 18–24 hr after injection paralleled CFU-S numbers in the same host-donor combination. For example, as reported previously (*1, 2*) and confirmed in this study (Table 2), B6D2F$_1$ mice strongly resisted parental C57BL/6J CFU-S proliferation, while allogeneic DBA/2J mice showed less resistance; the same pattern was seen in the retention of radiolabeled bone marrow cells. C57BL/6J mice retained 2.1±0.16% of labeled syngeneic bone marrow cells in their spleens 24 hr after injection, while DBA/2J and B6D2F$_1$ mice retained 1.1±0.08% and 0.62±0.01% of the ^{125}I-C57BL/6 cells. It is significant to note that the same pattern of resistance was observed with freshly labeled bone marrow cells and with labeled cells from LTBMC in spite of the fact that different cell populations were labeled as shown in Table 1.

Retention of labeled cells in the spleen 18–24 hr after injection paralleled subsequent CFU-S performance in all host-donor combinations tested. As shown in Table 2, the strong repression of DBA/2J CFU-S proliferation by C57BL/6J mice and the weaker resistance of B6D2F$_1$ mice is reflected by 0.44±0.04% and 1.1±0.1% retention of radiolabeled DBA/2J LTBMC cells, compared with 2.8±0.04% retention in syngeneic mice. Bennett (*19*) reported that *H-2* heterozygous bone marrow cells were not rejected by parental mice; the results in Table 2 confirm that B6D2F$_1$ cells were not strongly resisted by either parental strain, and also indicate no significant differences in retention of labeled cells in the spleens.

These results are in contrast to those of Riccardi and coworkers (*12*) who reported that survival of radiolabeled bone marrow cells in the spleens and lungs 4 hr after injection reflected the hosts' NK cell activity levels. C57BL/6J and B6D2F$_1$ mice have high levels of NK cell activity while DBA/2J is a low NK strain; rather than reflecting host NK levels, the results in Table 2 indicate that the survival of radiolabeled cells in the spleen 18–24 hr after injection is indicative of CFU-S potential in each host-donor combination. We found no indication that survival of the labeled cells in the lungs at either 4 or 24 hr after injection reflected the natural resistance of the host to bone marrow transplantation (data not shown). Significant differences in the survival of the total bone marrow cell inoculum as assessed by whole-body gamma counting were seen in most (9 out of 13), but not all, experiments. It is possible that CFU-S repression involves killing of the transplanted cells by the host, but the sensitivity of whole-body gamma counting mice that had received labeled bone marrow cells lacks the sensitivity to prove this point.

The differential between syngeneic mice and resistant mice is much greater using the CFU-S assay than indicated by splenic retention of radiolabeled cells. However, retention of radioactivity in the spleens of mice injected with prekilled cells were only slightly less than that with live cells in resistant mice. The results of one such experiment are illustrated in Figure 1. Groups of irradiated (1000 rads) C57BL/6J and B6D2F$_1$ mice were injected with 10^6 ^{125}I-labeled, freshly isolated C57BL/6J bone marrow cells that had been untreated or ex-

TABLE 1. Cells labeled with ^{125}I-IdUrd in fresh and long-term bone marrow culture

	Marrow cells	Hr labeled	Percentage labeled	Percentage[a]							
				Blasts	Lymph.	Mono.	PMN		Mega.	Mph.	PC
							Imm.	Mat.			
Total	Fresh	4	—	12	26	13	36	7	4	0	2
Labeled	Fresh	4	23	41	44	7	6	2	0	0	0
Total	Fresh	24	—	6	30	12	31	17	3	0	1
Labeled	Fresh	24	15	49	18	8	25	0	0	0	0
Total	LTBMC	24	—	17	0	10	19	35	1	18	0
Labeled	LTBMC	24	26	59	0	7	24	10	0	0	0

[a] Differential counts: *Blasts*, undifferentiated cells; *Lymph*, lymphocytes; *Mono*, monocytes; *PMN*, polymorphonuclear leukocytes; *Imm*, immature PMNs; *Mat*, mature PMNs; *Mega*, megakaryocytes; *Mph*, macrophages; *PC*, plasma cells.

TABLE 2. Splenic survival of radiolabeled bone marrow cells *in vivo*

Marrow source	Hours after injection	Percentage of injected ^{131}I-cells in spleen ± SE (whole-body retention of ^{131}I-cells [CFU-S day 8])		
		C57BL/6J	DBA/2J	B6D2F$_1$
C57BL/6J	4	6.2±0.37	5.2±0.21	5.5±0.31
Fresh	24	2.1±0.16	1.1±0.08[b]	0.62±0.01[b]
		(27.7±3.6)	(16.2±0.6)[b]	(16.6±1.3)[b]
		[TNTC][a]	[20±4]	[0]
			(Very small)	
C57BL/6J	2.5	8.0, 10.4[c]	11.0, 11.5	7.7, 7.0
LTBMC	22	1.5±0.17	0.6±0.06[b]	0.24±0.02[b]
		(33.2±1.0)	(29.0±2.5)	(29.0±1.2)
		[TNTC]	[0, 4, 1, 0]	[1, 1, 0]
DBA/2J	3.5	7.5±0.35[b]	12.5±0.9	8.0±0.7[b]
LTBMC	18	0.44±0.04[b]	2.8±0.04	1.1±0.1[b]
		(20.5±1.4)[b]	(36.6±2.0)	(35.1±2.9)
		[0]	[TNTC]	[~40 small]
B6D2F$_1$	4	4.7±0.31	4.0±0.18	4.4±0.3
LTBMC	24	1.1±0.04	0.81±0.13	0.78±0.08
		(23.2±2.7)	(23.5±3.8)	(20.8±1.1)
		[12.5±4.1]	[35.5±2.2]	[25±4.1]

[a] Too numerous to count.
[b] Significantly less than retention in syngeneic host to at least $P < 0.01$.
[c] Two mice per group, all other retention values are the means of 4–5 mice per group.

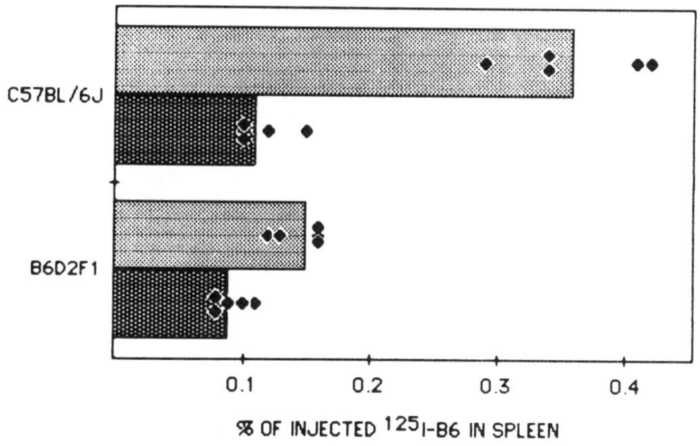

FIGURE 1. Splenic retention of label in syngeneic and F$_1$ hybrid mice receiving live or dead ^{125}I-IdUrd labeled C57BL/6 bone marrow cells. Each point represents one mouse with the lighter bars indicating the means for groups receiving live cells and the darker bars representing the means for groups injected with ultraviolet-radiation-prekilled cells.

posed to ultraviolet (UV) light (~15 cm from a General Electric 30W germicidal lamp for 45 min). The viability, as assessed by eosin dye exclusion, was >95% for the untreated cells and <15% for the UV-treated sample. In contrast to cells killed by gamma irradiation, which show survival identical to that of unirradiated cells for the first 48 hr after injection, UV-irradiated cells are rapidly eliminated from the host (*18*). The radioactivity remaining in the spleens was determined 18 hr after injection and retention of label in resistant B6D2F$_1$ mice given live cells was ony marginally greater than that in mice given prekilled cells. F$_1$ mice injected with live cells had significantly less label in their spleens than did the comparable parental group ($P<10^{-4}$), and retained only slightly more label than did F$_1$ mice injected with dead cells ($P<10^{-3}$). Similar results were obtained with cells killed by treatment with anti-H-2 antibody and complement prior to injection. In every experiment in which dead cell controls were incorporated, retention of radioactivity by resistant mice was similar or identical to that in mice receiving prekilled cells, suggesting that the transplanted cells are nearly totally eliminated from the spleens of resistant mice.

Given that CFU-S precursors form a small minority subpopulation of the labeled cells, we should emphasize that the distribution of labeled bone marrow cells is not a direct indication of CFU-S survival. However, as reported previously (*14*) and confirmed here, CFU-S precursors are among the cells labeled. Cells labeled with ^{131}I show a dramatic reduction in CFU-S numbers, and labeling with ^{125}I, which is approximately six-fold more radiotoxic, almost completely abolishes colony formation (data not shown).

Immunogenetic specificity. Natural resistance in mice of the C57BL family depends on mismatching at the *H-2D* region—that is, cells that are *H-2D*-identical with the host are not resisted in spite of mismatching at other *H-2* loci. LTBMCs from C57BL/6J mice established 8 weeks previously were labeled with ^{125}I-IdUrd, and 10^6 cells were injected i.v. into C57BL/6J (*H-2^b*), DBA/2J (*H-2^d*), B6D2F$_1$ (*H-2^b/H-2^d*), B10.BR/SgSn (*H-2^k*), B10.A(2R)/SgSn, and B10.A(5R)/SgSn mice. The mice were killed 24 hr later and the amount of label remaining in the spleens was determined. The alleles at the *K* A_β A_α E_β E_α S D L loci of the *H-2* complex for the intra-*H-2* recombinant strains are *kkkkkdbb* for B10.A(2R) and *bbbbkddd* for B10.A(5R). Mice of the same strains were also injected with unlabeled cells from culture to determine CFU-S performance. The results are illustrated in Figure 2. By one-way analysis of variance (ANOVA) differences between groups were highly significant (DF=5,30; F=21.93; P<<10^{-4}). The difference between D^b and non-D^b strains by the planned comparison test was significant (DF=30, T=11.06, $P<<10^{-4}$) and the Bonferroni test classified the strains into these two groups independent of a preformed hypothesis ($P<10^{-3}$). All allogeneic mice except B10.A(2R) retained significantly fewer of the labeled H-2^b cells than syngeneic mice; the same pattern was seen with CFU-S performance. As indicated above, B10.A(2R) is matched with the marrow donor at the *D* end of the *H-2* complex but mismatched at the *K* and *I* regions.

A similar experiment was performed using ^{131}I-labeled cells from DBA/2J LTBMC, and the results are illustrated in Figure 3. CFU-S were observed only in strains that shared the *D* end of the *H-2* complex with the H-2^d DBA/2J donor (B10.A/SgSn is *kkkkkddd*). Again, differences between groups of strains were highly significant(ANOVA-DF=5,22; F=27.62; $P<<10^{-4}$; planned comparison test comparing D^d and non-D^d strains, $P<<10^{-4}$). Retention of label in B10.A(5R) was significantly less than that in other D^d strains (Bonferroni test, $P<.01$); CFU-S numbers and spleen weights also were less in B10.A(5R) mice than in the three other H-$2D^d$ strains that allowed stem cell proliferation.

Involvement of natural killer cells. The beige (*bg*) mutation causes a deficiency in NK cell activity and *bg/bg* mice have been used to demonstrate a role for NK cells in vivo (*15, 20, 21*). Bone marrow cells from C57BL/6J mice were labeled with ^{131}I-IdUrd and 10^6 cells were injected i.v. into +/*bg* and *bg/bg* C57BL/6J and B6D2F$_1$ mice. Beige B6D2F$_1$ mice were produced by crossing C57BL/6J female mice (+/bg^J or bg^J/bg^J) with DBA/2JCo (bg^{8J}/bg^{8J} or +/bg^{8J}) (*22*). The percentages of the injected radiolabel found in the spleens 24 hr later are illustrated in Figure 4. There were no significant differences between +/*bg* and *bg/bg* animals. We reported previously (*15*) that beige mice retain much of the ability to repress allogeneic CFU-S proliferation.

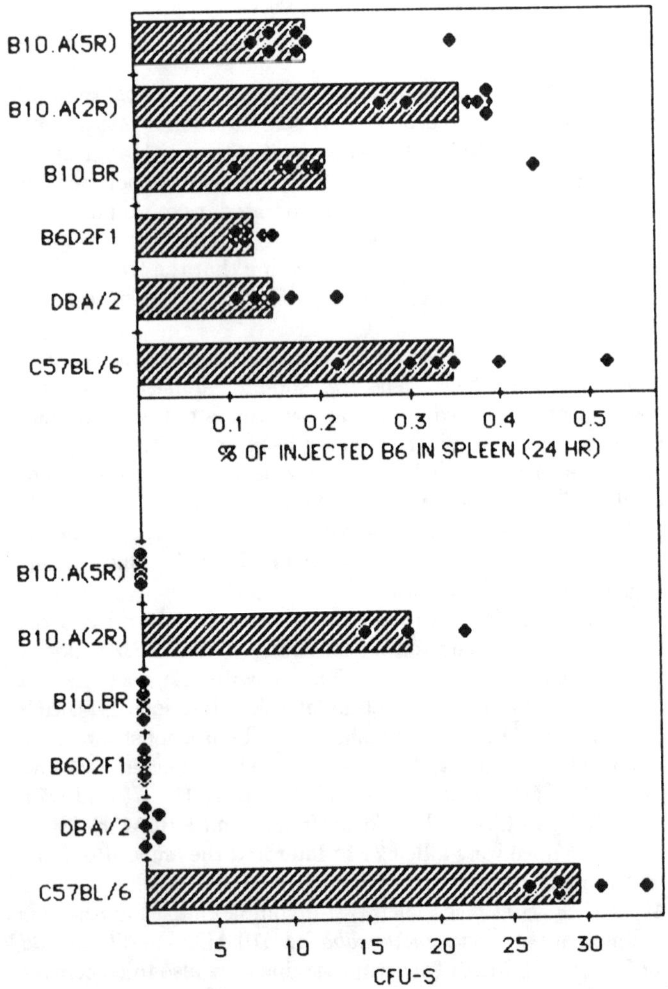

FIGURE 2. Immunogenetic specificity of natural resistance to C57BL/6 bone marrow transplantation as assessed by use of prelabeled LTBMC cells and by CFU-S activity.

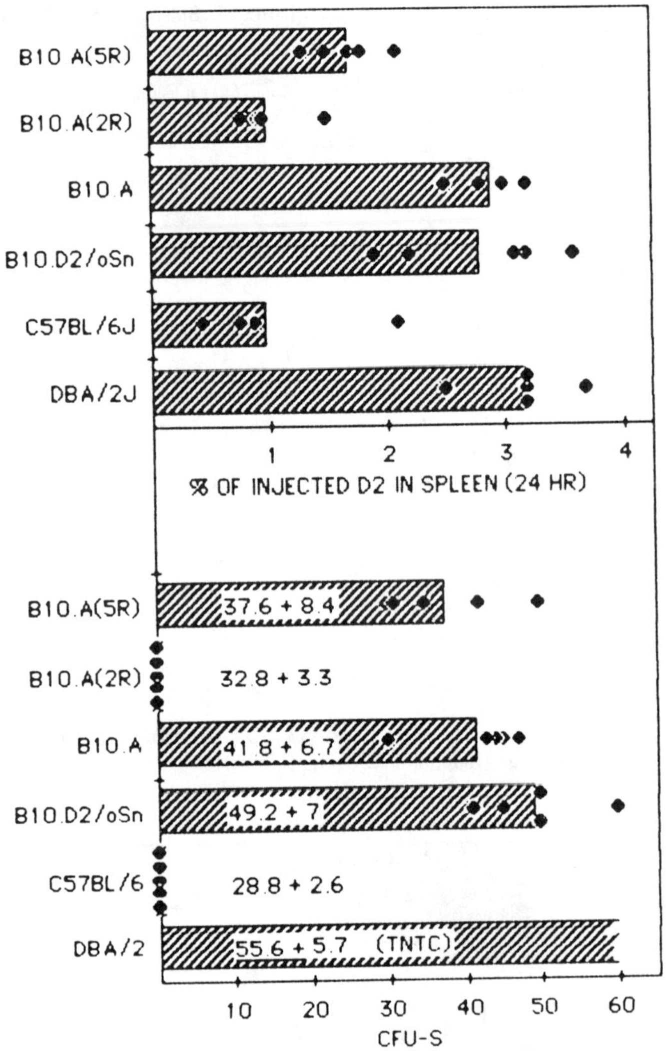

FIGURE 3. Immunogenetic specificity of natural resistance to DBA/2 bone marrow transplantation as assessed by the use of prelabeled TBMC cells and by CFU-S activity. The numbers superimposed on the CFU-S data are the means ± SD of the spleen weights for each group.

In contrast, treatment with rabbit anti-asialo GM 1, which abolishes both NK cell activity and natural resistance against bone marrow tranplantation (*23*), abolishes the ability of C57BL/6J mice to eliminate radiolabeled DBA/2J bone marrow cells from their spleens. DBA/2J and C57BL/6J mice were injected with 0.2 ml of a 1/10 dilution of normal rabbit serum or rabbit anti-asialo GM 1 (Wako Chemicals, Dallas, TX) 24 hr prior to injection of ^{131}I-IdUrd labeled freshly isolated DBA/2J bone marrow cells. The label remaining in the spleens was determined 18 hr after injection, and the results are illustrated in Figure 5. Treatment with ^{89}Sr caused similar reductions in resistance, as assessed by retention of labeled cells in the spleen (data not shown); ^{89}Sr-treated mice are also deficient in NK cell activity and in their ability to repress allogeneic CFU-S proliferation (*7*).

DISCUSSION

The results presented here strengthen the postulate that repression of *H-2* homozygous CFU-S proliferation by allogeneic or F_1 hybrid mice involves events occurring within the first 24 hr after injection. The retention of radiolabeled bone marrow cells in the spleen reflected the immunogenetic specificity of resistance to marrow grafts and abrogation of natural resistance to marrow transplantation with anti-asialo GM-1 or ^{89}Sr increased the early survival of the injected cells in the spleen. It is of interest that the survival of labeled cells from long-term culture or freshly labeled bone marrow was predictive of their subsequent CFU-S potential even though CFU-S precursors comprise only a small minority subpopulation of the

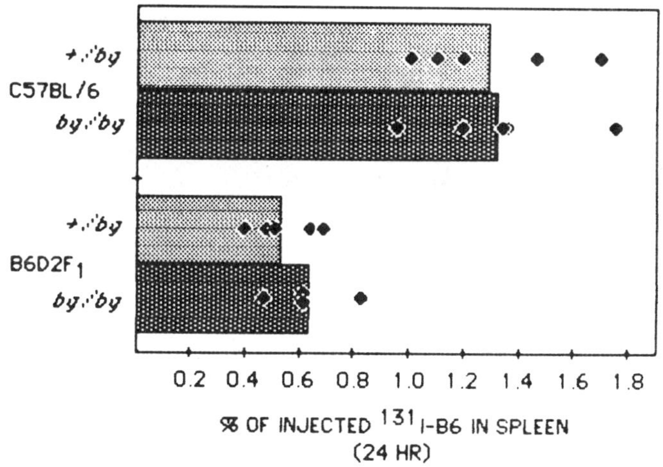

FIGURE 4. The ability to eliminate injected parental marrow cells from the spleen is intact in NK-deficient F_1 beige mice.

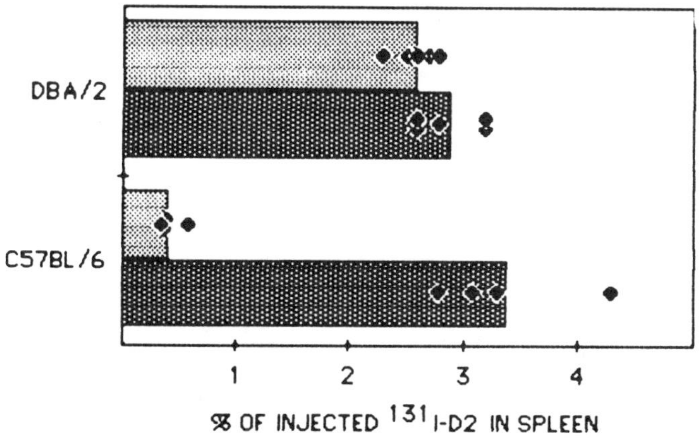

FIGURE 5. Treatment with anti-asialo GM 1 antibody abrogates the ability to eliminate allogeneic bone marrow cells from the spleen. Mice were injected with either normal rabbit serum (lighter bars) or rabbit anti-asialo GM 1 24 hr prior to injection of ^{131}I-IdUrd-labeled DBA/2 bone marrow cells. The label remaining in the spleens was determined 18 hr after injection.

labeled cells. This indicates that *H-2* associated natural resistance is expressed with the same immunogenetic specificity against other cell populations in the heterogeneous mixture. Our previous studies on the genetic control of natural resistance to leukemia and lymphoma cells is in accord with this interpretation (*4–6*).

The sensitivity of using radiolabeled bone marrow cells to assess natural resistance is less than that of the clonal CFU-S assay, but the results are informative as to the early events in CFU-S repression. Using leukemia cells as a model for natural resistance the same early elimination of the labeled cells from the spleens was observed but the differences between *H-2*-identical and nonidentical mice were much more pronounced. In comparison with malignant cells a much smaller fraction of radiolabeled bone marrow cells survive injection even in syngeneic mice, thus decreasing the sensitivity of the assay. Given the immunogenetic, mechanistic—and, based on this study, kinetic—similarities between natural resistance to leukemia cells and to bone marrow cells, labeled tumor cells remain preferable to labeled bone marrow for analysis of the early events of natural resistance.

While whole-body counting of mice injected with prelabeled cells suggests that cells may be killed during the course of resistance, reduced survival of the cells in the spleens of resistant mice is not sufficient evidence tht the spleen is the site of cytotoxicity against the *H-2*-nonidentical cells. Given the data from this study it is also possible that the failure of the cells to survive in the spleen is due to impaired interaction with the nonsyngeneic microenvironment leading to recirculation. Although reduced early survival of transplanted cells in the spleen was predictive of their subsequent colony forming ability, the possibility remains that other factors also can influence the proliferation potential of nonsyngeneic cells. For example, in Table 2 the partial resistance of $B6D2F_1$ mice against DBA/2J marrow cells was reflected as reduced survival of labeled cells in the spleen as well as reduction in size and a slight reduction in numbers of spleen colonies. Without further experimentation, several interpretations are possible, including a direct inhibitory effect on proliferation, a delay in seeding and effective interaction with the nonsyngeneic microenvironment due to recirculation of the transplanted cells, or lower susceptibility to resistance of CFU-S precursors with a reduced proliferative capacity.

The target "antigens," recognition structures, and effector mechanisms responsible for natural resistance against nonsyngeneic cells have yet to be elucidated, and it is highly probable that multiple host and donor influences are involved. For example, natural anti-H-2 antibodies can act in concert with NK cells against transplanted allogeneic bone marrow cells in irradiated mice (*24*) and provide an explanation for the greater strength of allogeneic resistance than hybrid resistance. It appears unlikely, however, that antibodies can fully account for natural resistance because of the absence of natural anti-self H-2 antibodies in *H-2* heterozygous mice (*25*). Based on this and previous studies (*6, 15*) the subset of NK cell affected by the beige mutation is not directly responsible for resistance, but NK-related cells are clearly involved in both hybrid and allogeneic resistance (*7*). Recognition of tumor cells by known subsets of NK cells is not dependent on *H-2* mismatching between the effector and target and host levels of NK activity are not predictive of natural resistance against nonsyngeneic cells. This implies that there is either a new subset of NK cells capable of recognizing *H-2* encoded target structures on hemopoietic cells or that an *H-2*-dependent recognition event precedes or induces lysis of the transplanted cells by *H-2* independent NK-related effectors. These possibilities were discussed more fully in an earlier publication (*6*).

Acknowledgments. We wish to thank Dr. Elaine Spooncer for helping us in establishing long-term marrow culture methodology, Dr. Robert Collins for assisting us with the statistical analyses, and Drs. David Harrison and Robert Evans for their critical reading of the manuscript and for helpful suggestions.

REFERENCES

1. Cudkowicz, G, Bennett M. Peculiar immunobiology of bone marrow allografts. I. Graft rejection by irradiated responder mice. J Exp Med 1971; 134: 83.
2. Cudkowicz G, Bennett, M. Peculiar immunobiology of bone marrow allografts. II. Rejection of parental grafts by resistant F_1 hybrid mice. J Exp Med 1971; 134: 1513.
3. McCulloch EA, Till JE. Proliferation of hemopoietic colony-forming cells transplanted into irradiated mice. Radiat Res 1964; 22: 383.
4. Carlson GA, Wegmann TG. Rapid in vivo destruction of semi-syngeneic and allogeneic cells by non-immunized mice as a consequence of nonidentity at H-2. J Immunol 1977; 118: 2130.
5. Carlson GA, Melnychuk D, Meeker MJ. H-2 associated resistance to leukemia transplantation: Natural killing in vivo. Int J Cancer 1980; 25: 111.
6. Carlson GA, Taylor BA, Marshall ST, Greenberg AH. A genetic analysis of natural resistance to nonsyngeneic cells: the role of H-2. Immunogenetics 1984; 20: 287.
7. Kiessling R, Hochman PS, Haller O, Shearer GM, Wigzell H, Cudkowicz G. Evidence for a similar or common mechanism for natural killer cell activity and resistance to hemopoietic grafts. Eur J Immunol 1977; 7: 655.
8. Goodman JW, Martin FB, Congdon CC. Histology of poor growth of parental marrow cells in F_1 hybrid mice. Absence of cellular immune response. Arch Pathol Lab Med 1970; 89: 226.
9. Buurman WA, van Bruggen I, Vos O. The influence of genetic resistance of CFU growth kinetics in spleen and femur. Cell Tissue Kinet 1975; 8: 111.
10. Chertkov JL, Gelfand IM, Gurevitch OA, Lemeneva LN, Udalov GA. Hybrid resistance to parental bone marrow transplantation: adaptive modification of hemopoietic stem cells in a nonsyngeneic environment. Proc Nat Acad Sci USA 1979; 76: 2955.
11. Orbach-Arbouys S, Ghazal I, Berdardet M. Direct measure of the destruction of bone marrow cells, after their injection into variously pretreated syngeneic hosts. Transplantation 1982; 34: 205.
12. Riccardi C, Santoni A, Barcozzari T, Herberman RB. In vivo reactivity of mouse natural killer (NK) cells against normal bone marrow cells. Cell Immunol 1981; 60: 136.
13. Dexter TM. Haemopoiesis in long-term bone marrow cultures. Acta Haematol 1979; 62: 299.
14. Toksöz D, Dexter TM, Lord BI, Wright EG, Lajtha LG. The regulation of hemopoiesis in long-term bone marrow cultures. II. Stimulation and inhibition of stem cell proliferation. Blood 1980; 55: 931.
15. Harrison DE, Carlson GA. Effects of the beige mutation and irradiation on natural resistance to marrow grafts. J Immunol 1983; 130: 484.
16. Forman J, Ketchell MM, Hofer KG. Tumor immunity in vivo. Use of the ^{125}IUdR prelabeling technique to monitor cell death in immune animals. Transplantation 1972; 14: 166.
17. Hofer KG, Hughes WL. Radiotoxicity of intranuclear tritium, ^{125}Iodine and ^{131}Iodine. Radiat Res 1971; 47: 94.
18. Mills GB, Carlson GA, Paetkau V. Generation of cytotoxic lymphocytes to syngeneic tumors by using co-stimulator (interleukin 2): in vivo activity. J Immunol 1980; 125: 1904.
19. Bennett M. Rejection of marrow allografts. Importance of H-2 homozygosity of donor cells. Transplantation 1972; 14: 289.
20. Talmadge JE, Meyers KM, Prieur DJ, Starkey JR. Role of NK cells in tumor growth and metastasis in beige mice. Nature 1980; 284: 622.
21. Kärre K, Klein GO, Kiessling R, Klein G, Roder JC. Low natural in vivo resistance to syngeneic leukemias in natural killer-deficient mice. Nature 1980; 284: 624.
22. Carlson GA, Marshall ST, Truesdale AT. Adaptive immune defects and delayed rejection of allogeneic tumor cells in beige mice. Cell Immunol 1984; 87: 348.
23. Okumura K, Habu S, Shimamura K. The role of asialo GM 1^+ cells in the resistance of tranplants of bone marrow or other tissues. In: Herberman RB, (ed). NK cells and other natural effector cells. New York: Academic, 1982: 1527.
24. Warner J, Dennert G. Bone marrow graft rejection as a function of antibody-directed natural killer cells. J Exp Med 1985; 161: 563.
25. Chow DA, Wolosin LB, Greenberg AH. Genetics, regulation, and specificity of murine natural anti-tumor antibodies and natural killer cells. J Natl Cancer Inst 1981; 67: 445.

Received 17 April 1985.
Accepted 27 September 1985.

0041-1337/86/4106-0695$02.00/0
TRANSPLANTATION
Vol. 41, No. 6

Printed in U.S.A.

PASSIVE TRANSFER OF CYTOMEGALOVIRUS BY CARDIAC AND RENAL ORGAN TRANSPLANTS IN A RAT MODEL[1]

JOHAN HENDRIK BRUNING,[2] CATHERINA ALBERTA BRUGGEMAN,[2] CORNELIS PIETER ANTON VAN BOVEN,[2] PETER JACOBUS CORNELIS VAN BREDA VRIESMAN[3,4]

Departments of Medical Microbiology and Immunology, University of Limburg, 6200 MD Maastricht, The Netherlands

Passive transfer of latent rat cytomegalovirus (R-CMV) infection by means of vascularized organ transplants was examined in inbred rat strains. LEWIS (LEW) rats 4–5 weeks old were infected with RCMV and used as donors at 5 months of age when the infection had become latent. Well-perfused LEW hearts and kidneys were transplanted into unmodified or 500-rad x-irradiated syngeneic or allogeneic Brown Norway (BN) recipients; recipients were sacrificed 3 weeks after transplantation, and RCMV virus from various organs was quantitated by means of a plaque assay. Passive transfer of latent infection could be accomplished with renal allografts (60%) and renal isografts (40%). When BN hosts were x-irradiated LEW renal allografts invariably transferred the latent infection (100%); cardiac allografts rarely did so (8%). X-irradiation of syngeneic hosts did not enhance the capacity of LEW kidneys to transfer the latent infection. The latent infection could not be transferred with thoracic duct lymphocytes. Results show the passive transfer of latent infection with well-perfused vascularized organ allografts to be a relative organ-specific phenomenon.

With the introduction of new effective immunosuppressive agents to control rejection, transplantations of a wide variety of tissues and organs can be used for the treatment of various diseases. These immunosuppressive agents, however, control rejection in a nonspecific manner, suppressing general immune responses rather than reactions to donor-specific antigens. This greatly enhances patient's susceptibility to microbial infections. Among these, herpes virus infections, especially cytomegalovirus (CMV)* infections play a dominant role, and have ever more frequently been associated with graft rejection (*1, 2*). Prospective studies have shown that CMV infection occurs in 50–90% of renal allograft recipients who are maintained on immunosuppressive drugs (*3–6*). Although primary infections occur in recipients of organ grafts from seronegative donors, reactivation of latent virus from the recipient or from the donated allograft accounts for most infections. In most instances primary infection is derived from the donated kidney allograft (*6–8*), but sometimes blood transfusions administered around the time of transplantation account for the infection. Probably the leukocytes within the blood transfused accounts for the transmission of CMV infection, because with non-leukocyte-containing blood derivates or frozen blood practically no primary infection occurs (*9, 10*). Recently we were able to isolate and characterize a CMV of the rat (RCMV) that closely resembles the human cytomegalovirus (HCMV) (*11–13*). This enabled us to investigate in a rat model the possibility that vascularized organ transplants taken from latently infected donors are capable of transferring CMV infection. In this study we compared heart and kidney organ grafts for their potential of transferring latent RCMV. The effect of an allogeneic barrier and immunosuppression of the recipient on the infection transfer rate was studied.

MATERIALS AND METHODS

Animals. Inbred Brown Norway (BN) and Lewis (Lew) rats from our own colonies were used. These rats were bred under specific-pathogen-free (SPF) conditions at the Department of Experimental Animal Services of the University of Limburg, Biomedical Center, Maastricht, The Netherlands.

Virus. In our studies we used an isolate of a wild rat cytomegalovirus (RCMV) strain recently isolated and characterized by our Department of Medical Microbiology (*11–13*). The virus stock consists of homogenates of salivary glands of four-week-old rats inoculated i.p. with 10^5 plaque-forming units (PFU) of virus. Virus was harvested four weeks after inoculation by homogenizing the salivary glands in a Ten Broeke grinder in PBS with 25% sorbitol, and subsequent sonication in a Branson B12 cell disrupter for 30 sec. After clarification by centrifugation (5 min, 400 xg) the supernatant was stored in small aliquots at −70°C until use, after quantification with plaque assay.

Infection. Experimental (acute) infections were established by inoculating 4–5-week-old rats i.p. with 10^4–10^5 PFU of RCMV. In previous work we defined rats to be chronically infected when only the salivary glands appeared to be RCMV-positive upon culture, with all the other organs being RCMV-negative. If all the organs of infected rats were found to be RCMV-negative upon culture, including the salivary glands, we defined them as latent. At 5 months after infection all organs of infected animals appeared to be RCMV-negative on culture except the salivary glands in some instances (*11, 12*). In this study we differentiated between latently and chronically infected animals merely by the absence or presence of RCMV in the salivary glands. For that purpose we took a surgical biopsy of the salivary glands and cultured their homogenates.

Virus assays. Quantitative assays for infectious virus were performed by plaque assays, a modification of the method described by Wentworth et al. (*14*), and Bruggeman et al. (*11*). In short, organ biopsies were homogenized in a Ten Broeke

[1]This work was supported by the Netherlands Kidney Foundation (NSN).

[2] Department of Medical Microbiology.
[3] Department of Immunology.
[4] To whom correspondence should be addressed, at Dept. of Immunology, University of Limburg, P.O. Box 616, 6200 MD Maastricht, The Netherlands.

* Abbreviations used: CMV, cytomegalovirus; HCMV, human cytomegalovirus; RCMV, rat cytomegalovirus; BN, Brown Norway; Lew, Lewis; MEM, minimal essential medium; PFU, plaque-forming units; REF, rat embryonic fibroblasts; SPF, specific-pathogen free.

grinder in minimal essential medium (MEM) (Gibco) supplemented with 10% newborn calf serum. This suspension (10% weight/volume) was further diluted ten times (volume/volume) and cultured on a monolayer of rat embryonic fibroblasts (REF) in a CO_2 incubator under a final concentration of 0.25% agarose. The plaques were counted by microscopic observations at 7 days postinfection after staining with methylene blue and are expressed in 10 log PFU/1 ml of 10% (v/v) diluted organ suspensions.

Immunosuppression. Immunosuppression of the rats that received an organ transplant was achieved by x-irradiation with 500 rads. X-rays were generated by a Philips-Müller MG 300 apparatus, and additionally filtered through 1.0-mm Cu. filter. The thickness of this filter was adapted to correct for field homogeneity. Rats to be irradiated were placed on a layer of 11 cm hardboard to obtain maximal backscatter. The x-ray dose was measured during irradiation using a 0.6-cc ionization chamber, connected to a digital dose/rate meter (Ionex 2500-3, Nuclear Enterprises, Beenham, England). Up to three rats were placed in a well-aerated round perspex box and irradiated at a source-to-subject distance of 42.5 cm. The x-rays were generated at 250 kV, 10 mA.

Transplantation. Orthotopic renal and cardiac transplantations were performed as described previously (*15*). In order to avoid an effect of uremia (*16*) on the reactivation of passively transferred virus, hearts and kidneys were transplanted into unilaterally nephrectomized recipients. LEW renal allografts inserted into unmodified BN recipients were removed 8 days postoperatively when they were invariably irreversible rejected. LEW kidneys transplanted into 500-rad x-irradiated BN hosts were not rejected histologically three weeks postoperatively when the hosts were sacrificed. The function of heart transplants was assessed by means of palpation; when grafts contracted vigorously (3+ on a scale of 1 to 3+) they were accepted as successful (*17*). Kidney transplants were considered successful when normal renal tissue was found at the time of sacrifice of isogeneic LEW, or x-irradiated BN hosts, or when classic hemorrhagic rejection was seen at 8 days postoperatively in LEW kidneys residing in unmodified BN hosts. In addition, the function of LEW kidneys residing in x-irradiated BN and LEW hosts was tested at 14 days postoperatively by means of ^{131}I hippuran nuclear imaging (*18*). In all instances a clearcut uptake of hippuran was seen in the transplant; no attempt was made to quantitate effective renal plasma flow. Thoracic duct cells were harvested as described previously (*17*).

Peripheral blood T cells and thoracic duct cells. Thoracic duct cells were harvested as described by van Schilfgaarde et al. (*17*). Peripheral blood T cells were obtained from heparinized blood. The buffy coat was further purified by lysing the erythrocytes with an ammonium chloride shock. The T cells were isolated from it as described by Julius et al. (*19*) on a nylon-wool column. These cells were 98% T cells, as was shown by positive staining with the monoclonal antibody W3/13 (Pan T, Sero-Tek).

RESULTS

Natural history. With plaque assays we were able to demonstrate virus in most organs only during the first week of an infection, as is shown in Table 1 (only kidney and heart in these experiments). After this first week no virus was detectable in any of the organs mentioned. The salivary glands, the organs in which the highest virus concentrations were reached, did not become rat cytomegalovirus (RCMV)-positive on culture before the end of the second week. In immunosuppressed animals, upon experimental infection, higher virus concentrations were measured in most organs. In the kidneys, for example, $2.5\times10_{log}$PFU/ml was measured in the immunosuppressed rats versus $1.2\times10_{log}$ PFU/ml in the untreated rats; and in the salivary glands $4.8\times10_{log}$ PFU/ml versus $3.5\times10_{log}$ PFU/ml in the untreated rats, at two weeks after infection. The spleen remained virus-positive upon culture up to more than four weeks in the immunosuppressed animals versus only a few days in the untreated rats (Table 1).

Transplantation: We used the salivary glands to detect the passive transfer of RCMV with organ grafts in our transplantation experiments, because in experimental infection with RCMV the highest concentration of virus was found in the salivary glands three to four weeks after inoculation. The homogenized suspension of a surgical biopsy of the recipients' salivary glands were used for plaque assay on REF-cells as described. It appeared that the latent RCMV-infection can readily be transferred by well-perfused renal transplants inserted into syngeneic and allogeneic recipients. When renal allografts were used, amplification of RCMV was observed in comparison to renal isografts, yielding a transfer rate of 67% versus 43% in the syngeneic model (Table 2). Apart from an allogeneic barrier, immunosuppression of the recipient appeared to enhance the reactivation of latent virus in the renal grafts, but only in the allogeneic model (100% in the immunosuppressed allogeneic recipients versus 67% in the untreated allogeneic recipients). In the syngeneic model transfer of RCMV infection with the renal grafts occurred even less frequently in the immunosuppressed recipients than in untreated rats (29% in the immunosuppressed versus 43% in the untreated recipients) (Table 2).

Well perfused heart allografts were far less effective than renal allografts in the transfer of RCMV infection. Only in 25% of the untreated recipient rats did we succeed in establishing an infection. When the recipient rats were immunosuppressed by total-body irradiation, this infection rate further decreased

TABLE 1. Natural history of RCMV-infection in unmodified and x-irradiated BN rats[a]

Days after infection	Unmodified rats					x-Irradiated rats				
	No. rats tested	Salivary glands	Spleen	Kidney	Heart	No. rats tested	Salivary glands	Spleen	Kidney	Heart
7	5	0	0	2	1	4	0	4	3	2
14	4	4	0	0	0	3	3	3	0	0
21	4	4	0	0	0	n.d.	—	—	—	—
28	4	4	0	0	0	3	3	3	0	0

[a] BN rats, 4 weeks of age, were given 10^4 PFU of RCMV i.p. on day 0. When desired, rats received 500 rads total-body irradiation at the time of infection. The presence of RCMV in various organs mentioned was determined by plaque assays at various instances after infection.

to only 8%. Another marked difference between cardiac and renal transplantations was the observed virus titers in the recipient organs 3 weeks after transplantation (data not shown). In the immunosuppressed recipients in which the highest titers were measured when transfer of infection had succeeded, 10^4–10^6 $10_{\log}$ PFU/ml was measured in the salivary glands of recipients of renal allografts versus 2.5–10^3 PFU/ml in the recipients of cardiac allografts. Surprisingly the spleen of the recipients of cardiac allografts remained virus-negative, even if they were immunosuppressed, whereas the spleens of the recipients of renal allografts reached virus titers of 10^2 PFU/ml when the recipients were immunosuppressed. In the untreated recipients no virus was measured in the spleens upon culture, nor in the spleens of recipients of renal isografts, whether or not they were immunosuppressed. When kidneys or hearts were transplanted into unmodified allogeneic recipients, the organ grafts were removed one week after transplantation.

Since the difference between heart and kidney might reside in latent virus carried in recirculating lymphocytes, buffy coat cells and thoracic duct cells of acutely infected and latent infected LEW hosts were passively transferred into x-irradiated BN recipients (Table 3). Only during acute infection—but not thereafter—was passive transfer with lymphocytes accomplished.

DISCUSSION

There were two main findings in this study. First, in the passive transfer of RCMV infection, kidney transplants are far more effective than heart transplants. This is particularly evident when allografts are inserted into immunosuppressed hosts. Second, passive transfer of latent infection cannot be accomplished by means of transfusion of peripheral blood cells or thoracic duct cells into syngeneic or allogeneic hosts.

In theory, passenger leukocytes are attractive candidates for passive transfer of CMV since clinical evidence supports a role for leukocytes in the transfer of human cytomegalovirus (HCMV) infections. Some authors have shown that blood transfusions of seropositive donors administered around the time of transplantation were frequently associated with active CMV infection—but, when leukocyte-deprived blood derivates of frozen blood were used, practically no primary infection occurred (*9, 10*). Human lymphocytes and monocytes can be infected with HCMV (*20, 21*). Thus passenger leukocytes residing in the kidney and heart transplants are potential candidates for the transfer of RCMV-infections.

These passenger leukocytes include bone-marrow-derived interstitially located dendritic cells (*22, 23*), T lymphocytes (*24*) and probably monocytes (*25*), and B lymphocytes (*26*). Compared with the heart, however, the rat kidney contains at least four times the number of recirculating lymphocytes (*17, 24*), part of which are mobile and capable of migrating out of the renal allograft into the spleen of the recipient (*24*).

Since we failed to transfer latent RCMV-infection with 10^7 thoracic duct cells (Table 3), which include all of the passenger leukocytes mentioned except significant numbers of dendritic-like cells, it is unlikely that the passive transfer of latent RCMV infection with allogeneic renal transplants is caused by any of these passenger leukocytes. The number of the thoracic duct cells used is far above the number of leukocytes thought to reside in one kidney (*17, 24*)—on the order of 2×10^6 cells. Although these experiments do not exclude passive transfer of RCMV via interstitial dendritic cells, these cells are unlikely candidates because both heart and kidney possess large numbers of these cells on the basis of immunohistochemical staining (*22, 23*). Thus, the observed "organ specificity" of transfer of infection with vascularized allograft cannot be easily explained in this way.

Alternatively, the latent virus is present in organ-specific cells—e.g., the renal tubular epithelial cells or (glomerular) vascular endothelium. This is supported by the findings in

TABLE 2. Passive transfer of RCMV by vascularized organ transplants taken from latently infected donors

Combinations of donor and recipient	Number of rats tested	Immunosuppression of recipient	Organ transplant	Organs tested for the presence of virus: Salivary gland	Spleen	Other organs[a]
Lew & Lew	14	—	kidney	6/14	0/14	0/14
Lew & Lew	7	500 rads	kidney	2/7	0/7	0/7
Lew & BN	3	—	kidney	2/3	0/3	ND
Lew & BN	11	500 rads	kidney	11/11	7/11	0/11
Lew & BN	4	—	heart	1/4	0/4	ND
Lew & BN	12	500 rads	heart	1/12	0/12	0/12

[a] Other organs tested included kidney and heart and were all negative. Recipients were 9–11 weeks old male rats. Donor rats were latently infected Lew rats, infected at the age of approximately 4 weeks. Latency was determined by plaque assays of a biopsy taken from the salivary gland at the age of about 4 months. The presence of RCMV in various organs as mentioned was determined by plaque assays at three weeks after transplantation.

TABLE 3. Evidence that RCMV infection cannot be transferred with blood or thoracic duct cells from chronically infected rats

Infectious state[a] donor	Donor and receptor	Transmitted cells injected i.p.	Immunosuppression of recipient	No. recipients virus + / No. recipients tested[c]
Ac	Lew×BN	whole blood (3 ml)	400 rads	6/6[c]
Ac	Lew×Lew	peripheral blood T lymphocytes	400 rads	3/3
Chr	Lew×BN	whole blood (3 ml)	500 rads	0/4
Chr	Lew×BN	thoracic duct cells[b]	500 rads	0/5

[a] (Ac) acutely infected; (Chr) chronically infected.

[b] Thoracic duct cells, washed 2× in buffered saline; 10^7 cells per recipient were infused i.v.

[c] Recipients tested for RCMV 3 weeks after i.p. injection by plaque assay of homogenates of salivary glands.

human kidneys, in which virus has been isolated from allografted kidneys sampled by needle biopsy and at autopsy (*1, 4, 5, 28, 29*). More pertinent is the observation that, in glomerular endothelial cells and renal tubular cells of human allografts, characteristic inclusion bodies have been observed histologically (*29, 30*) and the viral genome has been demonstrated by DNA in situ hybridization (*31, 32*). Preliminary data from our rat model support these findings (data not published). In this view latent RCMV infections are transferred more effectively with renal than with cardiac allografts because the kidney contains a greater number of infected cells.

Acknowledgments. We thank Ilse Heuts for doing the organ transplantations, Mieke Henfling for doing thoracic duct cannulation, and Wiel Debie and Gert Grauls for their valuable assistance in the virological assays. We also thank Fia Claus and Francine Teng for their secretarial expertise.

REFERENCES

1. Fiala M, Payne JE, Bern TV, Moore TC, Henle W, Montgomerie JZ, Chaterjee SN, Guze, LB. Epidemology of cytomegalovirus infection after transplantation and immunosuppression. J Infect Dis 1975; 132: 421.
2. Lopez C, Simmons RL, Mauer SM, Najarian JS, Good RA, Centry S. Association of renal allograft rejection with virus infections. Am J Med 1974; 56: 280.
3. Armstrong JR, Evans AS, RAO N, Ho M. Viral infections in renal transplant recipients. Infect Immun 1976; 14: 970.
4. Craighead JE, Hanshaw JB, Carpenter CB. Cytomegalovirus infection after renal allo transplantation. JAMA 1967; 201: 725.
5. Simmons RL, Lopez H, Balfour JR, et al. Cytomegalovirus: clinical virological correlations in renal transplant recipients. Ann Surg 1974; 180: 623.
6. Ho M, Suwansirikul S, Dowling JN, Youngblood LA, Armstrong JA. The transplanted kidney as a source of cytomegalovirus infection. N Engl J Med 1975; 292: 1109.
7. Betts RF, Freeman RB, Douglas RG Jr. Transmission of cytomegalovirus infection with renal allograft. Kidney Int. 1975; 8, 385.
8. Pass RF, Long WK, Whitley RJ, Soong SJ, Diethelm AG, Reynolds DW, Alford CA Jr. Productive infection with cytomegalovirus and herpes simplex virus in renal transplant recipients: role of source of kidney. J Infect Dis 1978; 137: 556.
9. Betts RF, Freeman RB, Douglas RG Jr, Talley TE. Clinical manifestations of renal allograft derived primary cytomegalovirus infection. Am J Dis Child 1977; 131: 759.
10. Thomas F, Lee HM, Wolf JS, Mendez-Picon G, Thomas J. Monitoring and modulation of immune reactivity in human transplant recipients. Surgery 1976; 79: 408.
11. Bruggeman CA, Meijer H, Dormans PHJ, Debie WMH, Grauls GELM and van Boven CPA. Isolation of a cytomegalovirus-like agent from wild rats. Arch Virol 1982; 73: 231.
12. Bruggeman CA, Debie WMH, Grauls GELM, Majoor F, van Boven CPA. Arch Virol 1982; 76: 189.
13. Meijer H, Dormans PHJ, Geelen JLML, van Boven CPA. Rat cytomegalovirus: studies on the viral genome and the proteins of vivious an nucleocapsids. J Gen Virol 1984; 65: 681.
14. Wentworth B, French L. Plaque assay of CMV strains of human origin. Proc Soc Exp Biol Med 1970; 135: 253.
15. van Breda Vriesman PJC, Swanen-Surag L, Vlek LFM. Cytotoxic and enhancing properties of early gamma-M alloantibodies elicited by first set renal allografts. Transplantation 1975; 20: 385.
16. Souhami RL, et al. The effect of uraemia on organ graft survival in the rat. Br J Exp Pathol 1973; 54: 183.
17. van Schilfgaarde R, et al. Role of mobile passenger lymphocytes in the rejection of renal and cardiac allografts in the rat. Transplantation 1980; 29: 209.
16. Souhami RL, et al. The effect of uraemia on organ graft survival in the rat. Br J Exp Pathol 1973; 54: 183.
18. Egleston TA, et al. ^{131}I-Hippuran in the evaluation of transplanted kidneys. Radiology 1969; 93: 1145.
19. Julius MH, et al. A rapid method for the isolation of functional thymus-derived mutine lymphocytes. Eur J Immunol 1973; 3: 645.
20. Rice GPA, et al. Cytomegalovirus infects human lymphocytes and monocytes: virus expression is restricted to immediate-early gene products. Proc Natl Acad Sci USA 1984; 81: 6134
21. Garnett HM, et al. Isolation of human cytomegalovirus from peripheral blood T-cells of renal transplant patients. J Lab Clin Med 1982; 99: 92.
22. Hart DNJ, et al. Demonstration and characterization of Ia-positive dendritic cells in the interstitial connective tissues of rat heart and other tissues, but not brain. J Exp Med 1981; 153: 347.
23. Hart DNJ, et al. Major histocompatibility complex antigens in rat kidney, ureter and bladder. Transplantation 1981; 31: 318.
24. v Schilfgaarde R, et al. Influence of recirculating lymphocytes in the rejection of renal and cardial allografts in the rat. Transplant Proc 1979; 11: 1485.
25. MacPherson GC, et al. The traffic of mononuclear phagocytes through renal allografts in sheep. Transplantation 1977; 24: 16.
26. MacDermott M, et al. Evidence for a common mucosal immunological system. J Immunol 1979; 122: 1892.
27. Spencer ES. Clinical aspects of CMV in kidney graft recipients. Scand J Infect Dis 1974; 6: 315.
28. Naraqi S, Jackson GG, Jonasson OM, et al. Prevalence, incidence and source of infections with herpes viruses in patients with renal allografts. J Infect Dis 1977; 136: 531.
29. Rifkind D, Goodman N, Hill Jr RB. The clinical significance of CMV infection in renal transplant recipients. Ann Intern Med 1967; 66: 1116.
30. Fetterman GH, Sherman FE, Fabrizio NS, et al. Generalized cytomegalic inclusion disease. Arch Pathol 1968; 86: 86.
31. Pagano JS. Diseases and mechanisms of persistent DNA virus infections: latency and cellular transformation. J Infect Dis 1975; 32: 209.
32. Myerson MD, et al. Widespread presence of histologically occult cytomegalovirus. Hum Pathol 1984; 15: 43.

Received 27 June 1985.
Accepted 25 September 1985.

0041-1337/86/4106-0729$02.00/0
TRANSPLANTATION
Copyright © 1986 by The Williams & Wilkins Co.

Vol. 41, No. 6
Printed in U.S.A.

THE EFFECT OF HYPERGLYCEMIA ON ISOLATED RODENT ISLETS TRANSPLANTED TO THE KIDNEY CAPSULE SITE[1]

DEREK W. R. GRAY, PHILIP MCSHANE, AND PETER J. MORRIS

Nuffield Department of Surgery, University of Oxford, John Radcliffe Hospital, Headington, Oxford OX3 9DU

The effect of hyperglycemia on transplanted rat pancreatic islets was studied using a new technique for transplanting a defined number of islets in a blood clot. Normal or streptozotocin-diabetic DA rats were given 400 DA islets under the left kidney capsule (a number shown to be insufficient to reverse diabetes). After 2 weeks the diabetic rats were given a further 1000 islets under the right kidney capsule to reverse diabetes. Kidneys from both groups were examined at 2 weeks after the initial islet implant and at 3 months for both gross and histological appearance and for insulin content. After 2 weeks left kidneys from nondiabetic rats showed abundant islet tissue, with an insulin content of 116 (± 14 SEM) milliunits, compared to 1±0.5 milliunits in the right kidney. Kidneys from diabetic rats showed no islets recognizable grossly. Histological examination showed vacuolated tissue scarcely recognizable as islet tissue, and the insulin content of the left kidney was reduced to 18±5 milliunits. However, 3 months after reversal of diabetes by transplantation of 1000 islets to the right kidney, histologically "normal" islet tissue was again visible on the left kidney, and the insulin content was 160±36 milliunits. Islets left in normal animals for 3 months contained 195±50 milliunits.

These experiments show that islets implanted beneath the kidney capsule in diabetic rats are not destroyed by two weeks hyperglycemia. This suggests that protection of islets after implantation by insulin treatment is unnecessary, even in the presence of a persistently raised blood sugar.

Successful isolation and transplantation of adult pancreatic islets to reverse diabetes was first demonstrated in the rat more than 13 years ago (*1*), and has been confirmed in numerous reports since then. However, the yield of islets obtained using the generally accepted method for islet isolation—namely, collagenase digestion and separation on a ficoll density gradient—has not usually been sufficient to allow reversal of diabetes by islets from a single-donor pancreas. The number of donors required varies with the site of implantation, the most efficient sites being those that allow portal venous drainage (*2*), but several pancreases are still required (*3*), 6 being the usual number. Despite this limitation many useful experiments have been performed in rodents, this being made possible by the availability of inbred strains as donors. This has allowed the potential of islet transplantation as a way of treating diabetes to be demonstrated.

The use of multiple donors for clinical transplantation, although theoretically possible, presents formidable practical obstacles. Furthermore, the use of islets from a single donor would be mandatory to allow avoidance of rejection by transplantation of islets into a host made tolerant of a renal allograft, a method for overcoming rejection that has been demonstrated to be very effective in the rodent model (*4–6*). However, attempts to produce a single donor model of purified islet transplantation in animals larger than rodents (usually as an autograft model) have, in general, been unsuccessful (*3*), as have attempts at clinical islet transplantation using single donors (*7*).

The problem of the multiple-donor requirement is not confined to isolated adult islet transplantation. Fetal pancreas transplantation is another method of transplanting insulin-secreting tissue, and initial studies in rodents again showed that multiple donors were necessary to produce normoglycemia (*8*). The fetal pancreas takes time to mature after transplantation, and thus normoglycemia is never achieved immediately. If the recipient is allowed to remain hyperglycemic during this maturation phase normoglycemia is eventually achieved, but multiple donors (usually 4–6) are needed (*9, 10*). However, if normoglycemia can be achieved during this maturation period, either by insulin treatment in vivo (*8, 11, 12*) or in vitro culture in normoglycemic medium (*13*), then it is possible to regularly reverse diabetes by a single-donor fetal pancreas transplant.

Thus it is possible that isolated adult islets may require a protective normoglycemic environment after implantation—i.e., islet implantation in the presence of persistent hyperglycemia may be impaired. The success of multiple-donor islet transplants does not exclude this possibility, since enough tissue is transplanted to allow rapid attainment of normoglycemia, possibly by initial nonspecific release of insulin. If islet implantation is impaired by persistent hyperglycemia, there is a rationale for insulin therapy after islet transplantation, in the hope that this would give better implantation and function of the tissue and allow islet transplantation from a single donor. In this study we have examined the ability of isolated rat islets to be implanted under the kidney capsule of syngeneic rats in the presence or absence of hyperglycemia, using a technique for transplanting islets that allows quantitative assessment of the success of islet implantation.

MATERIALS AND METHODS

Dark Agouti (DA, RT1[a]) rats supplied from our own colony were used throughout the study. Diabetes was induced by i.v. injection of streptozotocin (65 mg/kg), diabetes being confirmed if the serum glucose was above 22 mmol/L on 2 occasions at least 2 weeks after injection of streptozotocin. Islets were isolated from six donors by the collagenase digestion/ficoll separation technique (*1*), and then hand-picked under a dissecting microscope to remove impurities. Using a siliconized glass micropipette, islets were then carefully hand-picked into cone-shaped plastic receivers (constructed by cutting off the bottom of a plastic Universal container, Sterilin plastics). The islets were counted in groups of 40, taking care to allow an even

[1] This work was supported by grants from the Medical Research Council of the U.K. and the British Diabetic Association.

distribution of large and small islets and placing the islets in each receiver in rotation, until 420 islets had been deposited in each receiver. It was usually possible to fill 4 receivers with islets from 6 donors. The receivers were then allocated at random to the recipients.

For transplantation the islets were accumulated in the bottom of the conical receiver by aspirating the fluid under direct vision (taking care not to lose any islets) until the islets were tightly packed in the bottom of the cone, and as much of the fluid as possible was removed. A small drop of blood, obtained from the tail of the recipient, was then dropped on the islets and gently mixed using curved microforceps. The blood was left for 2 min to clot, then a drop of saline was layered above and clotting was confirmed. Under ether anesthesia the kidney of the recipient was exposed, an incision made in the capsule, and the capsule gently elevated by blunt dissection with curved forceps. The clot of blood containing the islets was then picked up using microforceps and deposited under the kidney capsule, which was allowed to fall over the clot, firmly pressing it to the kidney surface. The capsulotomy was left unsutured. Preliminary investigations showed that an average of 20 islets (±10) were lost in the procedure, leaving 400 islets in each transplant.

Islet transplants were performed in the following groups:

1. Normal rats given 400 islets under the left kidney capsule (n=9): Both kidneys were removed after 2 weeks and processed for histological examination (n=4) or extracted for insulin content (n=5).
2. Diabetic rats given 400 islets under the left kidney capsule (n=8): Both kidneys were removed after 2 weeks and processed for histological examination (n=4) or extracted for insulin content (n=4).
3. Normal rats given 400 islets under the left kidney capsule (n=2): Both kidneys were removed after 3 months and extracted for insulin.
4. Diabetic rats given 400 islets under the left kidney capsule (n=8): After 2 weeks diabetes was reversed by giving a full islet transplant (>1000 islets from 6 donors) placed under the right kidney capsule; 3 months later both kidneys were removed and processed for histological examination (n=4) or extracted for insulin (n=4).

Following transplantation all diabetic rats underwent regular blood glucose estimation. Blood glucose estimation was also performed before removing the kidneys from nondiabetic rats and normoglycemia confirmed in every case. Histological examination of formalin-fixed, paraffin-embedded sections of kidneys bearing islets was performed using hematoxylin-eosin and aldehyde fuchsin stains.

The insulin content of kidneys (some bearing transplanted islets) was measured by cooling the removed kidney in cold saline, chopping it into 1-mm particles in a cold mortar, then grinding the tissue with a pestle to ăn homogenate in 1 ml of acetone and a slush of solid CO_2. The homogenate was then carefully washed into a graduated 25 ml centrifuge tube using acid alcohol, and extracted overnight at 4°C in a volume of 25 ml. After centrifugation a 5 ml sample was taken and stored at −40°C. before insulin assay. The insulin content was assayed after neutralization by radioimmunoassay (*14*), and multiplied by the dilution factor to give the total insulin content of the kidney/islet tissue.

RESULTS

Normal DA rats given transplants of 400 DA islets under the left kidney capsule and examined at 2 weeks (group 1) showed a discrete patch of pearly white tissue with visible vessels at the site of implantation, all evidence of the transplanted blood clot having disappeared. Histological examination showed the presence of obvious and abundant endocrine tissue under the kidney capsule (Fig. 1A), with striking staining of B cells using aldehyde fuchsin stain (Fig. 1B). These features are typical of islet isografts transplanted under the kidney capsule.

Diabetic DA rats given 400 DA islets under the left kidney capsule (group 2) failed to reverse their diabetes (Fig. 2). Examination at 2 weeks showed an appearance different from

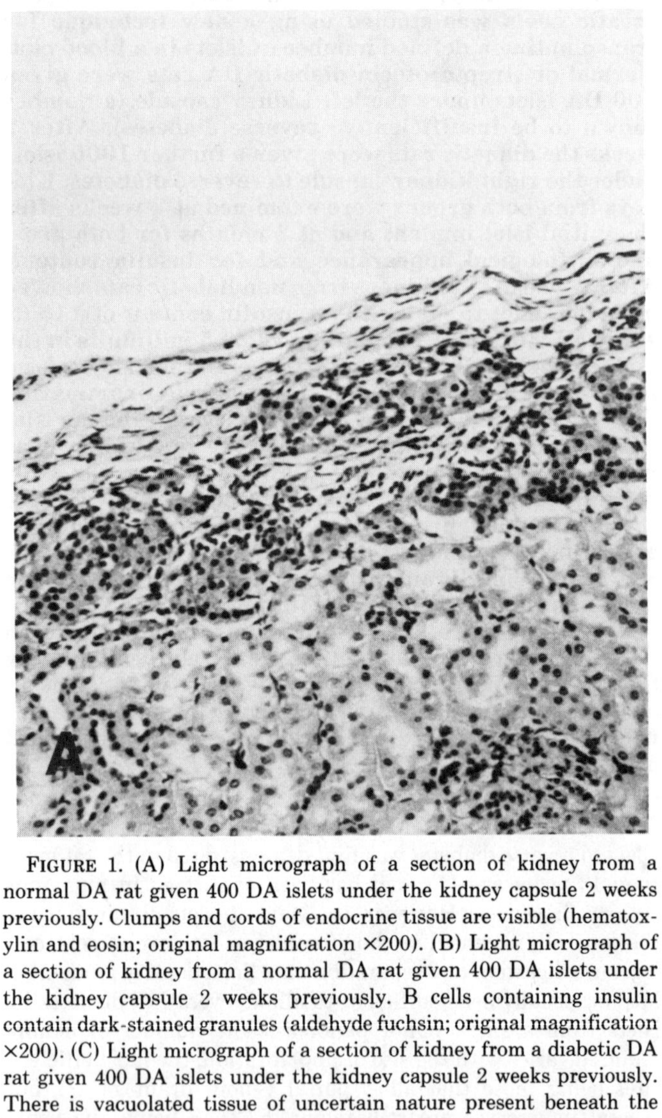

FIGURE 1. (A) Light micrograph of a section of kidney from a normal DA rat given 400 DA islets under the kidney capsule 2 weeks previously. Clumps and cords of endocrine tissue are visible (hematoxylin and eosin; original magnification ×200). (B) Light micrograph of a section of kidney from a normal DA rat given 400 DA islets under the kidney capsule 2 weeks previously. B cells containing insulin contain dark-stained granules (aldehyde fuchsin; original magnification ×200). (C) Light micrograph of a section of kidney from a diabetic DA rat given 400 DA islets under the kidney capsule 2 weeks previously. There is vacuolated tissue of uncertain nature present beneath the kidney capsule (haematoxylin and eosin; original magnification ×200). (D) Light micrograph of a section of kidney from a diabetic DA rat given 400 DA islets under the kidney capsule 2 weeks previously. In contrast to (B), there are no cells containing dark-stained granules (aldehyde fuchsin; original magnification ×200). (E) Light micrograph of a section of the left kidney from a diabetic DA rat given 400 DA islets under the left kidney capsule, then 2 weeks later given >1000 islets under the right kidney capsule and allowed to survive for a further 3 months before sacrifice. The tissue has reverted to an identifiably endocrine appearance (original magnification ×200). (F) Light micrograph of a section of the left kidney from a diabetic DA rat given 400 DA islets under the left kidney capsule, then 2 weeks later given >1000 islets under the right kidney capsule and allowed to survive for a further 3 months before sacrifice. B cells containing dark-stained granules are once again visible (aldehyde fuchsin; original magnification ×200).

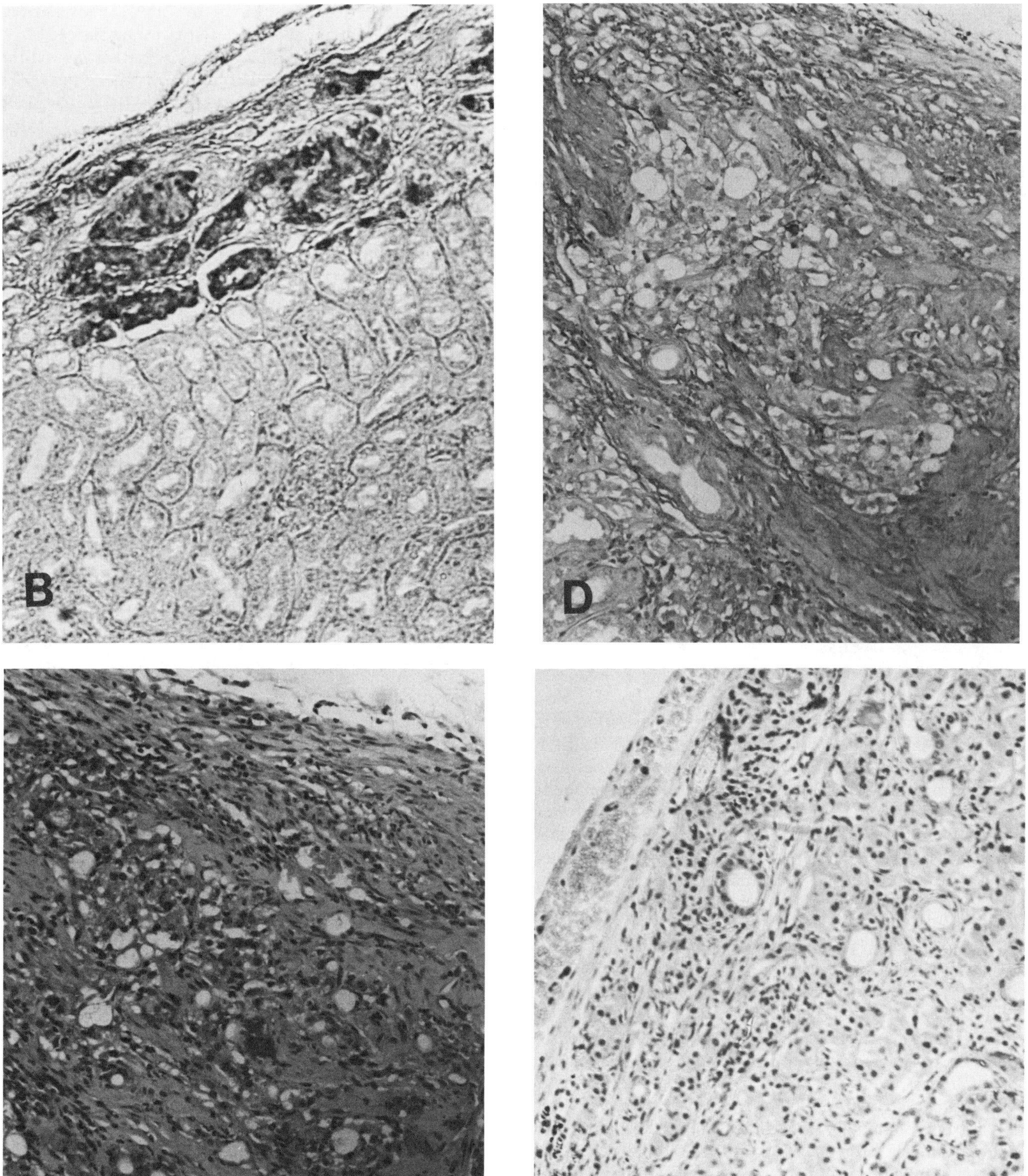

FIGURE 1 (continued)

that of group 1. The blood clot had not entirely disappeared from the site of implantation in some cases, and there was no obvious islet tissue to be seen, although careful inspection revealed the presence of almost translucent tissue beneath the kidney capsule, to which one or two fine vessels could be seen to course. Histological examination showed grossly vacuolated tissue at the site of inplantation that was difficult to recognize as endocrine tissue on hematoxylin/eosin stain (Fig. 1C), and

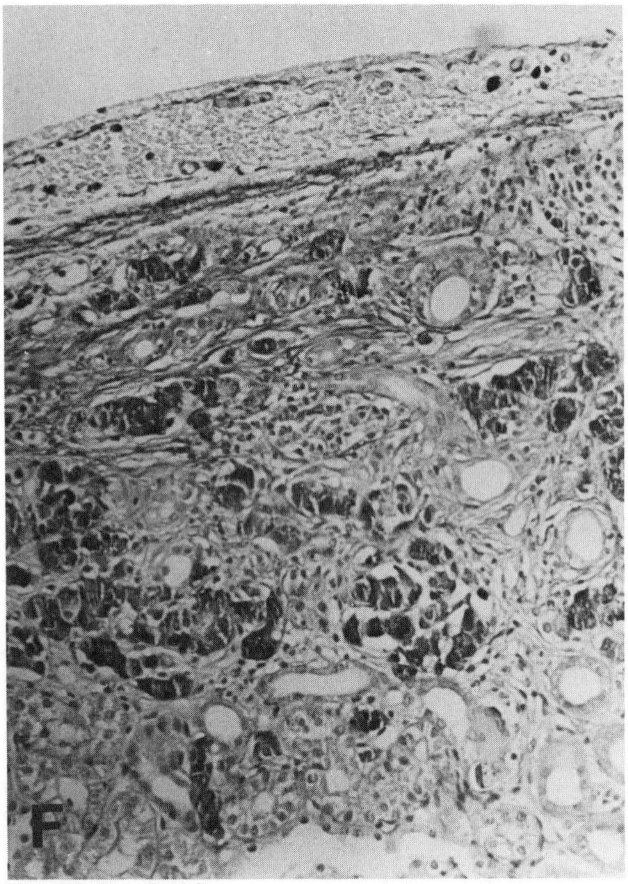

FIGURE 1 (continued)

there was no specific staining with aldehyde fuchsin (Fig. 1D).

Diabetic rats in group 3 were given 400 islets under the left kidney capsule, and also failed to reverse their diabetes (Fig. 3). Laparotomy at 2 weeks showed gross features similar to those described for group 2. These animals were then given a full transplant of DA islets (>1000 islets) under the right kidney capsule, which resulted in normoglycemia that was maintained for the next 3 months (Fig. 3). Examination of the left kidney at this time showed the return of apparent islet tissue at the original implantation site and a mass of islet tissue under the right kidney capsule. Histological examination confirmed the presence of identifiable endocrine tissue under the left kidney capsule (Fig. 1E), with specific staining by aldehyde fuchsin (Fig. 1F).

Normal animals given 400 DA islets and left for 3 months (group 4) showed gross and microscopic features similar to those of group 1.

The insulin content of kidneys removed from similarly treated groups of animals is shown in Table 1. The left kidney of normal animals given 400 islets (group 1) contained 116±14 (SEM) milliunits of insulin at 2 weeks, compared with 1±0.5 milliunits in the right kidney. The left kidney of diabetic animals given 400 islets (insufficient to reverse diabetes, group 2) contained 18±5 milliunits of insulin at 2 weeks, the right kidney containing 0.5±0.1 milliunits. Diabetic animals given 400 islets to the left kidney then a full transplant to the right kidney at 2 weeks (group 3) had an insulin content of 160±36 milliunits in the left kidney and 557±109 milliunits in the right kidney when the insulin content was measured 3 months later. Normal animals given 400 islets under the left kidney and left for 3 months had an insulin content of 195±50 milliunits on the left, compared with 0.06 milliunits on the right.

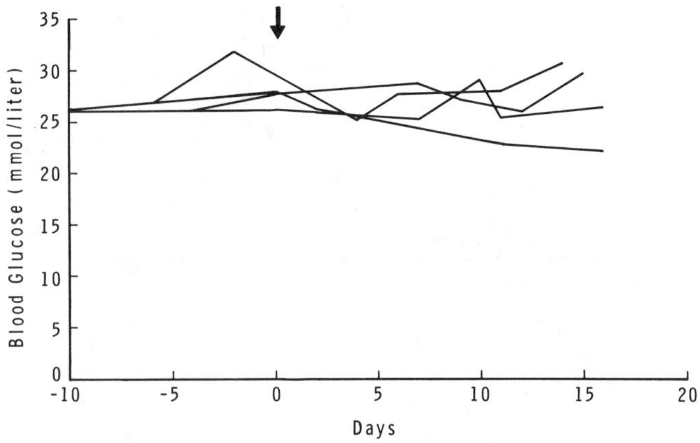

FIGURE 2. Serum glucose of diabetic DA rats given 400 DA islets under the left kidney capsule on day 0 (arrow).

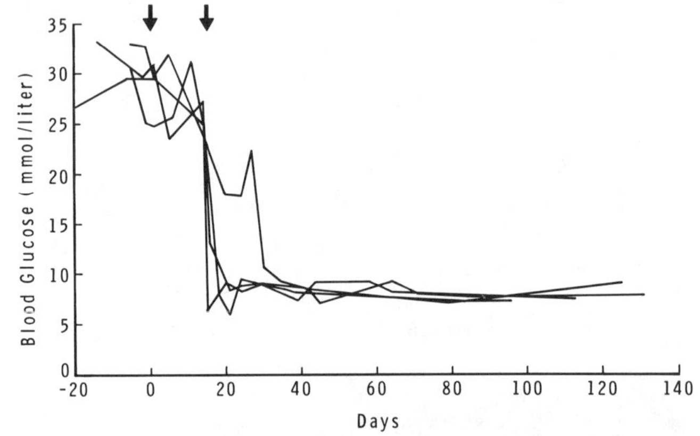

FIGURE 3. Serum glucose of diabetic DA rats given 400 DA islets under the left kidney capsule on day 0 (first arrow), and two weeks later given >1000 islets under the right kidney capsule (second arrow).

TABLE 1. The insulin content of kidneys bearing islets

Group No.	Islet Transplant	Insulin content (milliunits ± SEM)		
		(n)	Left kidney	Right kidney
1.	400 islets under left kidney capsule of normal animal for 2 weeks	5	116±14	1±0.5
2.	400 islets under left kidney capsule of diabetic animal for 2 weeks	4	18±5[a]	0.5±0.1
3.	400 islets under left kidney capsule of diabetic animal for 2 weeks and then a full islet transplant under the right kidney capsule and sacrifice at 3 months	4	160±36	557±109
4.	400 islets under left kidney capsule of normal animal for 3 months	2	195±50[b]	0.06

[a] Significantly different from left kidney, group 1.

[b] Not significantly different from left kidney, group 1 (Wilcoxon sign-rank test).

DISCUSSION

These results demonstrate that normoglycemia is not necessary for the successful implantation of adult islets under the kidney capsule of the rat. The gross and histological appearances of islets transplanted to the kidney capsule site have been described before (*15*), and the islets transplanted into normal rats (groups 1 and 4) showed typical features, with a white disc of tissue identifiable under the kidney capsule with the naked eye, and the histological features of endocrine tissue, the presence of islet tissue being easily confirmed by aldehyde fuchsin staining. In the present experiments (group 2) 400 islets were transplanted under the kidney capsule of syngeneic diabetic rats, this number having been chosen in preliminary experiments which showed that this was less than the number required to reverse diabetes. As predicted by these preliminary experiments the blood glucose did not fall, and examination at 2 weeks showed naked eye appearances suggesting failure of the islets to implant. Histological examination demonstrated that vacuolated tissue was present at the implantation site, although staining for insulin containing tissue with aldehyde fuchsin failed to provide positive confirmation that this was islet tissue. Reversal of diabetes by transplantation of a full islet transplant to the right kidney resulted in a "return" of the islet tissue, both grossly and by histological examination. This showed that the apparent absence of islet tissue in diabetic animals was not due to a failure of the isleted islets, but was due to the altered appearance of the tissue, presumably brought about by persistent exposure to hyperglycemia.

The measurement of the insulin content of standardized "packets" of islets implanted beneath the kidney capsule allows these changes to be quantitated. The insulin content of islets exposed to 2 weeks persistent hyperglycemia is a sixth that of islets implanted in a normoglycemic recipient, but the insulin content returns to "normal" after reversal of the diabetes by a full islet transplant to the opposite kidney. These findings confirm that hyperglycemia does not prevent islet implantation, and suggest that the abnormal gross and histological appearances are due to degranulation of the tissue, presumably in response to the persistent secretory stimulus provided by the hyperglycemia. This difficulty in identifying islet tissue in the presence of persistent hyperglycemia may have implications for studies of islet morphology and numbers in diabetic pancreases, and may be particularly relevent to reports of regeneration of native islets within the pancreas of streptozotocin-diabetic rodents following islet transplantation (*16*).

These findings suggest that, not only can islets successfully implant in the presence of hyperglycemia, but they can survive 2 weeks persistent hyperglycemic stimulus apparently unharmed. In a clinical setting these results might imply that the maintenance of strict normoglycemia by insulin therapy after islet transplantation would not be necessary, other than for normal patient management.

The effect of a persistent hyperglycemic stimulus on islets of Langerhans is of interest to diabetologists, since the demonstration of a harmful effect may have implications for the use of insulin pumps, etc., in newly diagnosed diabetics to prevent further loss of residual function. It is arguable whether transplanted islets correspond in any way to islets in the pancreas of a recent-onset insulin-dependent diabetic, but for what they are worth these results do not suggest that there is a striking detrimental effect of short term hyperglycemic exposure. However, this does not exclude the possibility of a long-term harmful effect and experiments are now being undertaken to investigate long term effects of hyperglycemia, using the quantitative model described above.

REFERENCES

1. Ballinger WF, Lacy PE. Transplantation of intact pancreatic islets in rats. Surgery 1972; 72: 175.
2. Kemp CB, Knight MJ, Scharp DW, Ballinger WF, Lacy PE. Effect of transplantation site on the results of pancreatic islet isografts in diabetic rats. Diabetologia 1973; 9: 486.
3. Sutherland DE. Pancreas and islet transplantation. I. Experimental studies. Diabetologia 1981; 20: 161.
4. Reece-Smith H, Homan WP, McShane P, Morris PJ. Indefinite survival of isolated pancreatic islets in rats rendered immunologically unresponsive to renal allografts. Transplantation 1982; 33: 452.
5. Gray DW, Reece-Smith H, Fairbrother B, McShane P, Morris PJ. Isolated pancreatic islet allografts in rats rendered immunologically unresponsive to renal allografts: the effect of the site of transplantation. Transplantation 1984; 37: 434.
6. Gray DW, Hibberd AD, McShane P, Morris PJ. Islet allografts in rats made tolerant of renal allografts by whole blood transfusion compared to islet allografts following blood transfusion alone. Transplant Proc 1984; 16: 863.
7. Sutherland DE. Pancreas and islet transplantation. II. Clinical trials. Diabetologia 1981; 20: 435.
8. Brown J, Molna IG, Clark W, Mullen Y. Control of experimental diabetes mellitus in rats by transplantation of fetal pancreases. Science 1974; 184: 1377.
9. Brown J, Clark WR, Molnar IG, Mullen YS. Fetal pancreas transplantation for reversal of streptozotocin-induced diabetes in rats. Diabetes 1976; 25: 56.
10. Garvey JF, Morris PJ, Millard PR. Early rejection of allogeneic foetal rat pancreas. Transplantation 1979; 27: 342.
11. McEvoy RC, Hegre OD. Syngeneic transplantation of fetal rat pancreas. III. Effect of insulin treatment on the growth and differentiation of the pancreatic implants after reversal of diabetes. Diabetes 1979; 28: 141.
12. Mullen YS, Clark WR, Molnar IG, Brown J. Complete reversal of experimental diabetes mellitus in rats by a single fetal pancreas. Science 1977; 195: 68.
13. Collier SA, Mandel TE, Carter WM. Detrimental effect of high medium glucose concentration on subsequent endocrine function of transplanted organ-cultured foetal mouse pancreas. Aust J Exp Biol Med Sci 1982; 60: 437.
14. Albano JD, Ekins RP, Maritz G, Turner RC. A sensitive, precise radioimmunoassay of serum insulin relying on charcoal separation of bound and free hormone moieties. Acta Endocrinol (Copenh) 1972; 70: 487.
15. Reece-Smith H, DuToit DF, McShane P, Morris PJ. Prolonged survival of pancreatic islet allografts transplanted beneath the renal capsule. Transplantation 1981; 31: 305.
16. Richardt M, Menden A, Bretzel RG, Federlin K. Islet tranplantation in experimental diabetes of the rat. VIII. B-cell restoration following islet transplantation. Preliminary results. Horm Metab Res 1984; 16: 551.

Received 27 June 1985.
Accepted 3 October 1985.

0041-1337/86/4106-0704$02.00/0
TRANSPLANTATION
Vol. 41, No. 6
Printed in U.S.A.

BONE MARROW TRANSPLANTATION IN THE RAT

V. LYMPHOID CELL SUBCLASSES IN THE TARGET ORGANS DURING ACUTE GRAFT-VERSUS-HOST DISEASE[1]

RISTO RENKONEN[2]

Transplantation Laboratory, University of Helsinki, Helsinki Finland

The distribution of white cell subclasses in different lymphoid (bone marrow, spleen, and blood) and parenchymal (liver, skin, lungs, and gut) target organs was studied after bone marrow transplantation in the rat. BN rats were irradiated and transplanted with 60–80×10^6 Lew (allogeneic) or BN (syngeneic) bone marrow cells. The recovery of lymphocytes was somewhat elevated in the bone marrow and spleen, slightly decreased in the blood, and markedly higher in the liver and skin in the allograft compared with the syngeneic graft recipient. A mild lymphocytic bronchitis was present in the lungs of the allografted animal, and the gut was hypocellular throughout the observation period. The total recovery of different lymphocyte subclasses; pan T, T helper, T suppressor-killer, class-II-positive cells, and surface-Ig-positive B cells in the different lymphoid organs—i.e., bone marrow, spleen, and blood—was similar in allogeneic compared with syngeneic graft recipients. In the liver and skin, which are the major target organs of acute graft-versus-host disease (aGVHD) in the rat, there was a massive infiltration of different T cell subclasses; high numbers of B cells were also seen in the liver. There was no difference in the T helper/T suppressor-killer ratio in the lymphoid organs or the liver of allograft compared with syngeneic graft recipients; in the skin and lungs the ratio was reduced more in the allograft compared with syngeneic graft recipient, whereas in the gut the situation was the opposite. These observations emphasize regional differences in the structure of inflammation in the different parenchymal target organs of aGVHD in the rat.

T lymphocytes have been recognized to be the initiators of the acute graft-versus-host disease (aGVHD)* (*1–5*), but other immunological mechanisms—e.g., B lymphocytes (*6, 7*)— are also involved, and the final structure of inflammation is extremely complex (*8, 9*).

For the first weeks after total-body irradiation and bone marrow transplantation in the human, the number of lymphocytes in the blood is very low. The reconstitution occurs within one month, but imbalances between different T cell subpopulations remain for many years. The major alterations are the decreased number of T helper (Th) cells and the increased number of T suppressor-killer (Tsk) cells, which lead together to a pathologically low Th/Tsk ratio in the blood (*10–13*).

[1] This work was supported by the Cancer Foundation of Finland, Helsinki, Finland.

[2] Address reprint requests to: Risto Renkonen, Transplantation Laboratory, Haartmaninkatu 3, SF 00290 Helsinki, Finland.

* Abbreviations used: aGVHD, acute graft-versus-host disease; Ia, class II; MGG, May-Grunwald-Giemsa; pan T, all T cells; PFC, plaque-forming cell; sIg, surface-immunoglobulin-positive B cell; Th, helper T cell; Tsk, suppressor-killer T cell.

The major histological manifestation of aGVHD in human and animal parenchymal target organs (liver, skin, and lungs) is the invasion of lymphocytes into the tissue, and later necrotic changes take place (*14–16*). There is preliminary data in humans showing that lymphocytes invading the skin during aGVHD are exclusively T suppressor/killer cells (*17*), but only few similar experiments have been reported from other target organs of aGVHD (*18, 19*).

In this work I have analyzed the structure of inflammation in the lymphoid and nonlymphoid (parenchymal) target organs of aGVHD in the rat using monoclonal antibodies.

MATERIALS AND METHODS

Rats. The nuclei for the Lewis (Lew;RT1 l) and Brown Norway (BN;RT1 n) strains were received through the courtesy of Dr. J. Howard from the Agriculture Research Council, Institute of Animal Physiology, Babraham, Cambridge and through the courtesy of Dr. I. Heron, University of Arhus, Arhus, Denmark. Male rats 12–16 weeks old and weighing 200 g were used.

Bone marrow transplantation. The BN rats were irradiated (Siemens Stabilipan) with 960 rads at a dose rate of 92 rads/min by rotating the recipients during irradiation in both horizontal and vertical plains. Before irradiation the rats were anesthetized with chloral hydrate (60 mg i.p.). Then 24 hr later the rats were given 60–80×10^6 nucleated Lew bone marrow cells. After transplantation the recipients received antibiotics for ten days (Bactrim 1.2 mg i.p.; Roche, Basel, Switzerland, and gentamycin 0.1 mg s.c.; Neofarma, Espoo, Finland). The control BN rats were irradiated and received 60–80×10^6 BN bone marrow cells or were left nontransplantated. The antibiotic scheme for these rats was the same as for the allotransplanted animals.

Isolation and quantitation of (inflammatory) white cells. The BN rats were killed at day −2 (normal control), or at days 0, 6, 10, 14, 20, and 25 after transplantation, and the bone marrow, spleen, blood, liver, ears (skin), lungs, and small intestine (gut) were removed. Parts of solid organs were embedded in Tissue Tek II (Lab-Tek Products, Division Miles Laboratories Inc., Naperville) and immediately frozen with liquid nitrogen; the remaining specimens were used for isolation of the inflammatory cells.

Bone marrow cells were recovered from one femur by opening the bone at both ends and flushing out the cell with RPMI tissue culture medium (Gibco Bio-Cult, Glasgow, Scotland). The blood specimen was drawn by cardiac puncture into a heparinized (0.1 mg, 5000 U/ml; Medica Pharmaceutical, Helsinki, Finland) syringe. Single-cell suspensions were made from the liver and spleen via mechanical disaggregation, clumps were removed by sedimentation, and the cells were washed twice with RPMI 1640. The ears were mechanically disaggregated, treated with collagen for 30 min at 37°C, filtered through cotton gauze, and washed with RPMI twice.

The total recovery of nucleated cells from each organ was determined in a hemocytometer. Then cytocentrifuge (Shandon Scintrefic Co. London, England) smears were made, stained in May-Grunwald-Giemsa (MGG), and the percentage of lymphocytes was counted. The total recovery of lymphocytes from each organ was calculated on the basis of total cell recovery and the percentage of lymphocytes.

Antisera. The following monoclonal antibodies directed against different rat white cell subclasses were used: W3/13 (MAS 010, Sera-Lab., Crawley Down, Sussex, England) reactive with rat T cells (pan T), W3/25 (MAS 1131) reactive with the T helper (Th) subset, MRC OX8 (MAS 041) reactive with the T suppressor/killer (Ts/k) subset, and MRC OX4 (MAS 029) reactive with the class II determinant of rat major histocompatibility complex (MHC). The specificity of these antibodies has been described (*20*). Polyclonal rabbit anti-rat Ig (Miles-Yeda Ltd, Rehovot, Israel) was also used.

Staphylococcus aureus *rosette assay for white cell subsets.* A method of Ranki et al. (*21*) was used. Approximately 1×10 cells deriving from the cell suspensions from different organs were suspended in 100 μl of RPMI containing a 1/20 dilution of the indicated antiserum and incubated for 30 min on ice. After two washes with RPMI, 100 μl heat-killed, formalin-fixed *Staphylococcus aureus* Cowan I bacteria (a gift from Professor H. Wigzell, Uppsala University, Uppsala, Sweden) was added so that the final concentration was 20 bacteria/cell. The suspension was centrifuged (100 g) for 3 min and left on ice for 30 min. The supernatant was discarded (with most of the nonattached bacteria), after which the cells were washed twice with RPMI, resuspended in fresh medium, cytocentrifuged onto microscopic slides, and stained with May-Grunwald-Giemsa (MGG). From the stained cell smears it is possible to differentiate a rosette-forming and a non-rosette-forming cell and concomitantly identifying the cellular morphology.

Immunoperoxidase staining. The frozen sections (5 μm) were fixed in chloroform for 30 min at room temperature. The specimens were then exposed for 30 min to MAS antibodies in humidified atmosphere, washed three times in PBS, exposed under the abovementioned conditions to peroxidase-conjugated rabbit antimouse Ig antibody, washed again three times in PBS, and exposed under the same conditions to peroxidase-conjugated goat antirabbit Ig antibody. The cells were washed three times in PBS and exposed under the humidified conditions to a mixture of ACE (3-amino-9-ethyl carbatzole), N'N'-dimethylformamide and H_2O_2 in 0.05 M acetate buffer, pH 5.0; washed in PBS; counterstained for 1 min in Mayer's hemalum; and mounted in Aquamount (BDH Chemicals Ltd., Poole, England).

Immunofluorescence stainings. For double direct immunofluorescence frozen sections were air-dried, fixed in acetone for 10 min at room temperature, covered with a mixture of MAS 029 and rabbit antirat Ig for 30 min, washed three times with phosphate-buffered saline (PBS), covered with a mixture of FITC-coupled goat antimouse Ig and TRITC-coupled goat antirabbit Ig for 30 min, washed three times with PBS, and finally mounted with PBS glycerol.

Identification of mononuclear phagocytes. To identify the mononuclear phagocytes and rule out their crossreaction with lymphoid antibodies, the rats were injected i.v. 2 hr before killing with a mixture of 0.2 ml of India ink and 0.3 ml of PBS. In the tissue sections the phagocytic cells were easily identified by ingested ink particles.

Definitions. The cells were considered positive according to the *Staphylococcus* rosette method if five or more bacteria were attached to the lymphocyte; crossreactive monocytes and granulocytes were ruled out by cell morphology. Normal mouse Ig control stainings were always made together with monoclonal antibody stainings.

The positive cells were counted from the tissue sections with a mesh (area 0.55255 mm^2) and a magnification of 400. From 10 to 20 fields were included in the analyses from each tissue (*19*).

RESULTS

Total recovery of lymphocytes. For the first few days after irradiation and transplantation the recovery of lymphocytes was very low in all organs (Fig. 1). Rapid reconstitution began in all compartments at day 6. When comparing allogeneic with syngeneic recipients a marginally higher lymphocyte recovery was obtained in the bone marrow and spleen for the first three weeks after transplantation; later a clear lymphopenia was present in the aGVHD-affected animal. In the blood there was a slight lymphopenia. Concomitantly there was a significant 5–10-fold increase of lymphocytes in the liver and skin associated with aGVHD. In the allogeneic transplanted animals' lungs there was a slight lymphocytic bronchitis, and the gut was hypocellular throughout the observation time. All the allograft recipients died of aGVHD between days 23–26 posttransplantation—meanwhile none of the syngeneic recipients showed any signs of aGVHD. No reconstitution was seen in the irradiated but nontransplanted animals at day 10, and approximately two-thirds of these animals survived more than one month.

Total recovery of different lymphoid cell subclasses. The subclasses in the different target organs of aGVHD were studied with monoclonal antibodies. The lymphoid organs and the liver were studied with the *Staphylococcus* rosette method, the lungs and gut with the immunoperoxidase method, and the skin with both the *Staphylococcus* rosettes and immunoperoxidase. In the control stainings with normal mouse Ig, no more than 1% of the cells were positive.

Immediately after irradiation and bone marrow transplantation the number of T and B cells was decreased in the bone marrow, but both cell subclasses were rapidly recovered during reconstitution (Fig. 2). At day 25 there were significantly ($P<0.05$) fewer Ia-positive cells in the allogeneic compared with the syngeneic recipients. The Th/Tsk-ratio remained approximately 1.0 throughout the observation period in both groups.

In the spleen the amount of pan-T-positive cells was significantly ($P<0.05$) lower in allogeneic compared with syngeneic graft recipients at day 25, whereas in the blood there were no differences. The T helper/suppressor ratio declined below 1 in both groups.

In the liver the number of pan-T, T helper, T suppressor-killer, class II (Ia), and surface-Ig-positive cells increased significantly, but the Th/Tsk-ratio was similar in the allograft recipients compared with the syngeneic recipients.

The skin was studied with the *Staphylococcus* rosette method and with frozen section immunoperoxidase stainings. In the frozen sections there was a clear dominance of T helper cells during the first 10 days after transplantation (Fig. 3), after

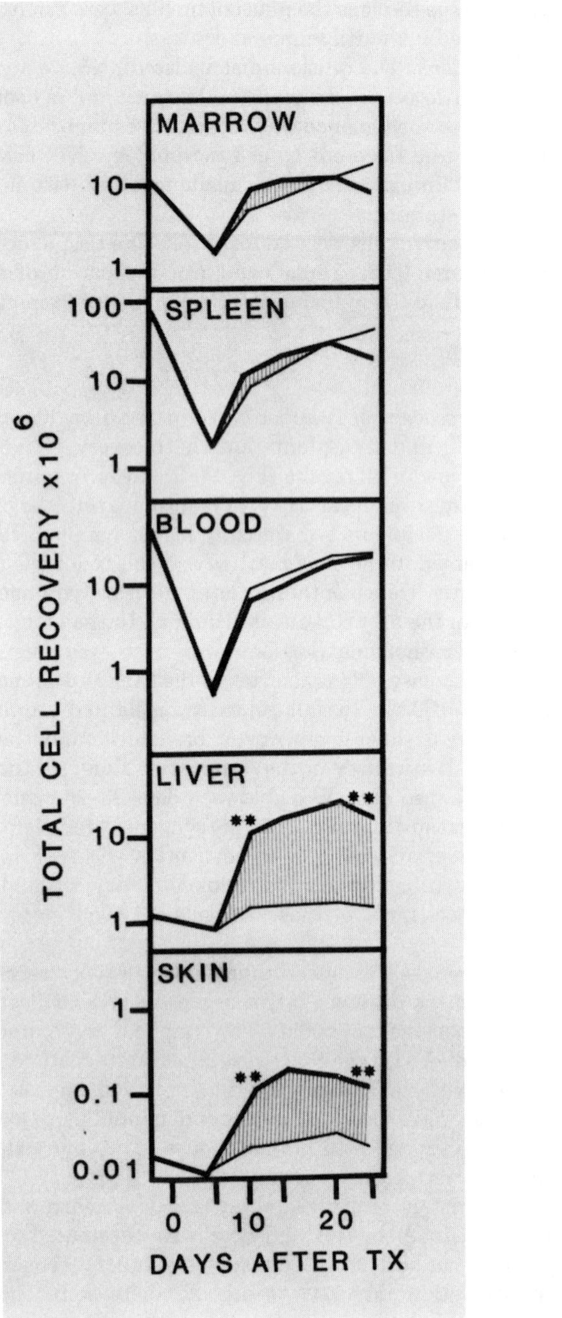

FIGURE 1. Total recovery of lymphocytes from different organs after bone marrow transplantation. Thick line: allograft recipients; thin line: syngeneic graft recipients. *P* values were calculated according to the Student's *t* test. (+) = $P<0.05$; (++) = $P<0.01$; (+++) = $P<0.001$. Values >0.05 were considered nonsignificant and left unmarked. The shaded area represents a positive increment between allograft and syngeneic graft recipients. The negative increment was left unmarked.

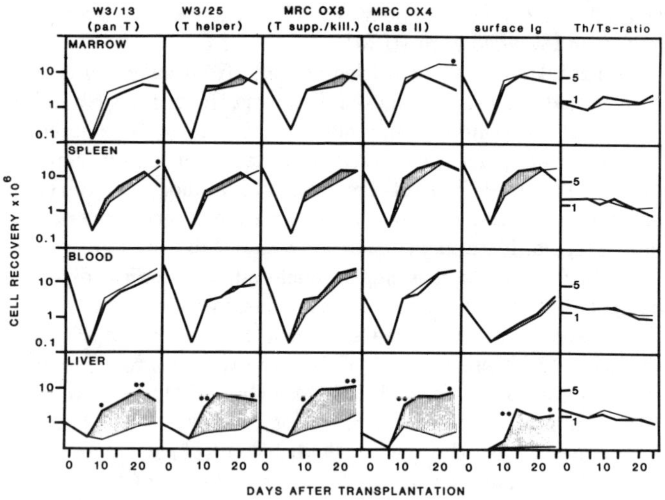

FIGURE 2. Total recovery of different lymphoid cell subclasses analyzed with the *Staphylococcus* rosette method. Thick line: allograft recipients; thin line: syngeneic graft recipients. For *P* values and shaded areas see the legend to Figure 1.

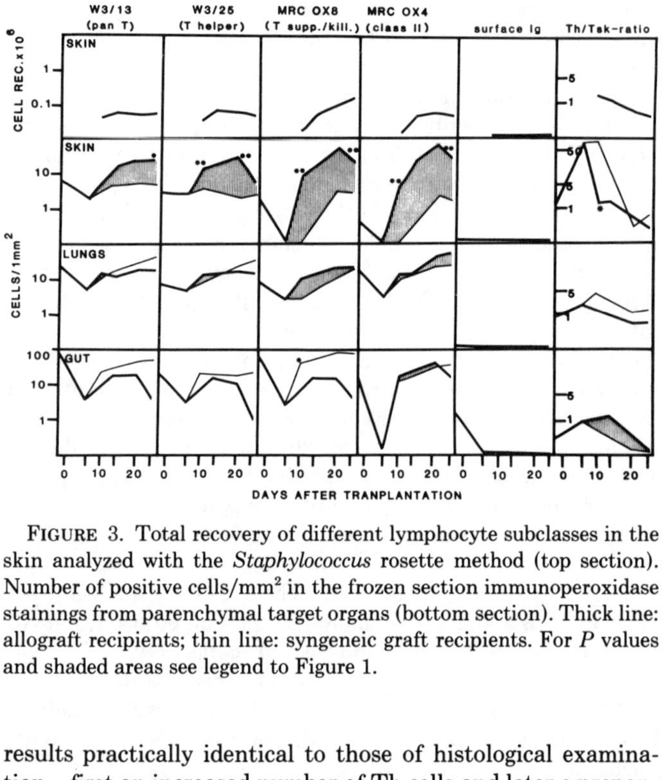

FIGURE 3. Total recovery of different lymphocyte subclasses in the skin analyzed with the *Staphylococcus* rosette method (top section). Number of positive cells/mm^2 in the frozen section immunoperoxidase stainings from parenchymal target organs (bottom section). Thick line: allograft recipients; thin line: syngeneic graft recipients. For *P* values and shaded areas see legend to Figure 1.

which the T suppressor/killer cells took over, leading to a significantly ($P<0.05$) decreased Th/Tsk-ratio in allograft compared with syngeneic graft recipients. The number of Ia-positive cells was significantly ($P<0.01$) higher in the allogeneic versus syngeneic graft recipients. No surface-Ig-positive cells were seen on any occasion in the skin. The *Staphylococcus* rosette assay of lymphoid subclasses (Fig. 3, top section) gave results practically identical to those of histological examination—first an increased number of Th cells and later a preponderance of Tsk cells.

The lungs appeared to be very similar in the two transplantation groups. In the gut there was a significantly ($P<0.01$) lower number of T suppressor/killer cells in the allograft versus the syngeneic graft recipients. No surface-Ig-positive cells were seen in the lungs or gut after bone marrow transplantation.

Percentage distribution of white cell subclasses. If the distribution of lymphoid subclasses in different organs were expressed in percentages rather than actual cell recoveries there would be practically no difference between allogeneic and syngeneic graft recipients (data not shown).

DISCUSSION

In normal bone marrow 25% of lymphocytes are T cells; the rest are B cells. The Th/Tsk ratio has been reported to be under 1 in normal conditions (*22*), and after bone marrow transplantation the ratio has been reported to be approximately 1 (*17*), which is in accordance with my results.

Approximately half the lymphocytes in the normal spleen are T cells and half are B cells. The T cell subclass distribution in the normal spleen closely resembles that in the blood—i.e., the Th/Tsk-ratio is approximately 1.4. After irradiation and bone marrow transplantation, the T helper/T suppressor-killer ratio declines and remains below 1 in the spleen and blood of both allogeneic and syngeneic recipients. To my knowledge there are no previous analyses of the white cell subpopulations of regenerating and/or GVHD-affected spleen.

The T cells are supposed to have an important role in the pathogenesis of aGVHD, and this may be one reason why white cell subclasses in the blood have been studied intensively after transplantation (*10–13*). The only consistent finding has been the reversal of Th/Tsk ratio in allografted, autografted, or syngeneically grafted patients (*12*). Recently Gratama et al. (*23*) demonstrated that the early monitoring of blood could give some predictive value to aGVHD. He showed that Th lymphocytes dominate in the blood for the first few weeks after transplantation and that the rate of Tsk cell regeneration is faster in patients who will develop aGVHD. On the other hand, my results do not show any difference in the blood Th/Tsk-ratio in rats with a poor prognosis (allogeneic) and with a good prognosis (syngeneic).

There are several double-staining analyses showing that the Tsk (OKT8 or Leu2-positive) cells dominating in the blood are concomitantly HLA-DR (class II) and HNK-1 (anti-natural-killer-cell) positive (*17, 24*). In these studies it was also shown that the proportion of class-II-positive Th is elevated in the early posttransplant period, which is thought to be due to activation of T cells during rapid regeneration. The distribution of T lymphocytes in the blood remains abnormal for 1–2 years after transplantation (*25*). It has recently been suggested that the OKT 8 or Leu 2 dominance seen in the blood after bone marrow transplantation could be related to the extremely high amounts of natural killer cells (*26*) and not to Tsk cells, as stated before. I made no double stainings because of the lack of a good rat natural killer cell antibody.

Liver is one of the major parenchymal target organs of aGVHD; the lymphocytes invade the portal area especially, and later piecemeal necrosis is seen. Leszczynski et al. (*19*) demonstrated that, in the normal liver, T helper cells dominated in the portal area, whereas there are equal numbers of Th and Tsk cells in the central vein area. During aGVHD there was a significantly high increase in the number of lymphocytes in the portal area representing mainly the T helper phenotype, whereas the few lymphocytes in the central vein area were exclusively T suppressor-killer cells. It must be noted that, concomitantly, there was a T suppressor/killer dominance in the blood.

An explanation of the discrepancy between these results and the results presented here, showing a reversal of the Th/Tsk ratio in the liver, is that there are approximately ten times more lymphocytes in the portal area, but its volume is only 1/10 of the central vein area—so finally the total number of lymphocytes in these two different areas are equal.

The skin infiltrate was distributed so that one-third of the cells were in the epidermis and two-thirds in the dermis. No differences in the subclass distribution in these two compartments was noted. The similarity between the results obtained from the histologic immunoperoxidase stainings and single-cell analyses with *Staphylococcus* rosettes in the skin confirms that there was no specific area of distribution of different subclasses in the skin, as reported earlier from the liver (*19*).

There are some reports from the skin showing that the infiltrating lymphocytes during aGVHD are exclusively of T suppressor-killer phenotype (*27, 28*), however contradictory results exist (*29*). Favrot et al. (*17*) showed also that these cells are class II (HLA-DR)-negative, which can be due to a later stage of differentiation of these cells (*17*) or to prednisone therapy given to aGVDH-affected patients. I, however, found class-II (Ia)-positive lymphocytes in the skin also, as did Muller et al. (*30*).

Bronchoalveolar lavation (BAL) has been used for diagnosis of different immunological lung processes (*31*). Preliminary results show that, in normal situations, the Th/Tsk ratio is approximately 1 and that after bone marrow transplantation and/or during aGVHD it is below 1 ([*18*] and E. Taskinen, personal communication).

Gut is a major aGVHD target organ in human bone marrow transplant recipients, but not in the Lew-to-BN rat model (*16*). In the rats there is no diarrhea and only few mild focal lymphocyte infiltrations are found in the lamina propria; on the contrary there is a severe hypocellularity in the epithelium. In the normal gut the intraepithelial lymphocytes are mainly T cells (over 90%) and most of them are of the T suppressor/killer subtype (*32*). In this analysis the aGVHD-affected rat gut showed pancytopenia and a low Th/Tsk ratio that was slightly higher than the ratio of the syngeneic animals. In the syngeneic recipient at day 26 the number of different T subpopulations was almost equal to normal.

Throughout this study it was observed that the sum of Th and Tsk was bigger than the number of pan-T-positive cells. This supports the suggestion that lymphocytes are immature after transplantation (*33*). There is also an increased number of Ia-positive cells in all compartments, both in allogeneic and syngeneic animals. This is interpreted to be a sign of activation in the T lymphocyte and/or mononuclear phagocyte population—in many places no B cells were present—due to regeneration, and it had little if any value in predicting aGVHD.

In the lymphohematopoietic tissue (bone marrow, spleen, and blood) and in the liver, there are surface-immunoglobulin-positive B cells throughout the observation period, which is also confirmed by analyzing PFC (*34*). On the contrary, the aGVHD lesions in the skin, lungs, and gut include neither surface-Ig-positive cells nor PFC (*34*), even though lymphoid blasts were present in the skin and lungs during aGVHD (*35*). These findings suggest the structure of inflammation is different in different parenchymal target organs.

There are no actual differences in lymphocyte subclass distributions in allogeneic and syngeneic transplanted rats if these distributions are expressed as percentages. However the total recovery of certain subclasses was significantly elevated in the parenchymal, but not the lymphoid, target organs. These results suggest the T and B cells are crucial in the development of graft-versus-host disease, but functional analyses must be done to understand their final role in the reaction. These analyses are underway.

Acknowledgments. I thank Professor Pekka Häyry for reading the manuscript.

REFERENCES

1. Dicke KA, van Hooft JIM, van Bekkum DW. The selective elimination of immunologically competent cells from bone marrow and lymphatic cell mixtures. Clin Immunol Immunopathol 1973; 1: 472.
2. Kornkold R, Sprent J. Lethal graft-versus-host disease after bone marrow transplantation across minor histocompatibility barriers in mice. J Exp Med 1978; 148: 1687.
3. Hamilton BL, Bevan MJ, Parkman R. Anti-recipient cytotoxic T lymphocyte precursors are present in the spleen of mice with acute graft-versus-host disease due to minor histocompatibility antigens. J Immunol 1981; 126: 621.
4. Prentice HG, Janossy G, Prince-Jones L, Trejdosiewicz LK, Panjwani D, Graphakos D, et al. Depletion of T lymphocytes in donor marrow prevents significant graft-versus-host disease in matched allogeneic leukemia marrow treated patients. Lancet 1984; 1: 472.
5. Filipovich AH, Youle RJ, Neville DM, Vallera DA, Quinones RR, Kersey JH. Ex-vivo treatment of donor bone marrow with anti-T-cell immunotoxins for prevention of graft-versus-host disease. Lancet 1984; 1: 469.
6. Ringden O, Persson U, Johansson SGO. Are increased IgE-levels a signal of an acute graft-versus-host reaction? Immunol Rev 1983; 71: 57.
7. Ringden O, Witherspoon RP, Storb R, Ekelund E, Thomas ED. Increased in vitro B-cell IgG secretion during acute graft-versus-host disease and infection. Observation in 50 human marrow transplant recipients. Blood 1980; 55: 179.
8. Tsoi MS. Immunological mechanisms of graft-versus-host disease in man. Transplantation 1982; 33: 459.
9. Seemayer TA, Gartner JG, Lapp WS. The graft-versus-host reaction. Hum Pathol 1983; 14: 3.
10. Hansen JA, Atkinson K, Martin PJ, Storb R, Longton G, Thomas ED. Human T lymphocyte phenotypes after bone marrow transplantation. T cells expressing Ia-like antigen. Transplantation 1983; 36: 277.
11. Fox R, McMillan R, Spruce W, Tani P, Mason D. Analysis of T lymphocytes after bone marrow transplantation using monoclonal antibodies. Blood 1982; 60: 578.
12. Atkinson K, Hansen JA, Storb R, Goehle S, Goldstein G, Thomas ED. T cell subpopulations identified by monoclonal antibodies after human marrow transplantation. I. Helper-inducer and cytotoxic-suppressor subsets. Blood 1982; 59: 1292.
13. Ekblom M, Ruutu T, Volin L, Leskinen R, Renkonen R, Hayry P. Immunological monitoring of bone marrow transplant recipients. I. Major leucocyte subclasses in the blood. Scand J Hematol 1984; 33: 113.
14. Woodruff JM, Hansen JA, Good RA, Santos GW, Slavin RE. The pathology of the graft-versus-host disease in adults receiving bone marrow tranplants. Transplant Proc 1976; 8: 675.
15. Beschorner WE, Tutschka PJ, Santos GW. Sequential morphology of graft-versus-host disease in the rat radiation chimera. Clin Immunol Immunopathol 1982; 22: 203.
16. Renkonen R, Hayry P. Bone marrow transplantation in the rat. I. Histologic correlations and quantitation of cellular infiltrates in acute graft-versus-host disease. Am J Pathol 1984; 117: 462.
17. Favrot M, Janossy G, Tidman N, Blacklock N, Lopez E, Bofill M, et al. T cell regeneration after allogeneic bone marrow transplantation. Clin Exp Immunol 1983; 54: 59.
18. Leskinen R, Tukiainen P, Taskinen E, Volin L, Renkonen R, Ruutu T, Hayry P. Bronchoalveolar lavage in the diagnosis of pulmonary complications in bone marrow transplant recipients. Exp Hematol 1984; 12(suppl 15): 24.
19. Leszczynski D, Renkonen R, Hayry P. Bone marrow transplantation in the rat. III. Structure of the liver inflammatory lesion in acute graft-versus-host disease. Am J Pathol 1985; 120: 316.
20. Williams AF, Galfre G, Milstein C. Analysis of cell surfaces by xenogeneic myeloma-hybrid antibodies. Differentiation antigens of rat lymphocytes. Cell 1977; 12: 632.
21. Ranki A, Totterman TH, Hayry P. Identification of mouse T and B lymphocytes from cytocentrifuged cell smears. Clin Exp Immunol 1976; 126: 632.
22. Janossy G, Montando L, Sleby S, Duke O, Panai G, Lampert I, et al. T cell subset abnormalities in tissue lesions developing during autoimmuno disorders, viral infection, and graft-versus-host disease. J Clin Immunol 1982; 2: 42S.
23. Gratama JW, Naipal A, Ojlans P, Zwaan FE, Vernoneck LF, Witte T, et al. T lymphocyte repopulation and differentiation after bone marrow transplantation. Early shifts in the ratio between T4+ and T8+ T lymphocytes correlate with the occurence of acute graft-versus-host disease. Blood 1984; 63: 1416.
24. Farrell C, Atkinson K, Chapman G, Renny R, Biggs J. Subsets of T lymphocyte subpopulations after human marrow transplantation defined by monoclonal antibodies and two-color fluorescence. Transplant Proc 1985; 17: 1704.
25. Ueda M, Harada M, Shiobara S, Nakoa S, Kondo K, Odaka K, et al. T lymphocyte reconstitution in long-term survivors after allogeneic and autologous marrow transplantation. Transplantation 1984; 37: 552.
26. Ault KA, Antin JH, Ginsburg D, Orkin SH, Rappeport JM, Koehan ML, et al. Phenotype of recovering lymphoid cell populations after marrow transplantation. J Exp Med 1985; 161: 1483.
27. Lampert IA, Suitters AJ, Janossy G, Thomas JA, Palmer S, Gordon-Smith E. Lymphoid infiltrates in skin in graft-versus-host disease. Lancet 1981; 2: 1352.
28. Lampert IA, Janossy G, Suitters AJ, Bofill M, Palmer S, Gordon-Smith E, et al. Immunological analysis of the skin in graft-versus-host disease. Clin Exp Immunol 1982; 50: 123.
29. Vasak E, Atkinson K, Munro V, Biggs J. Lymphoid cell subpopulations in the skin after bone marrow transplantation: definition with monoclonal antibodies. Transplant Proc 1984; 16: 1029.
30. Muller C, Schuch K, Pawelec G, Wilms K, Wernet P. Immunohistology of graft-versus-host disease mediated skin lesions and its correlation to a large granular lymphocyte surface phenotype. Blut 1982; 44: 89.
31. Hunninghake GW, Gadek JE, Kawanami O, Ferrans VJ, Crystal RG. Inflammatory and immune processes in the human lung in health and disease: evaluation by bronchoalveolar lavage. Am J Pathol 1981; 97: 149.
32. Taylor KB, Thomas HC. In: Stites DP, Stobo JD, Fudenberg HH, Wells JV, eds. Basic and clinical immunology. 5th ed. California: Lange, 1984: 520.
33. Rappeport JM, Dunn MJ, Parkman R. Immature T lymphocytes in the peripheral blood of bone marrow transplant recipients. Transplantation 1983; 36: 674.
34. Renkonen R, Wangel A, Hayry P. Bone marrow transplantation in the rat. IV. B cell activation during acute graft-versus-host disease. Transplantation 1986; 41: 290.
35. Renkonen R, Hayry P. Bone marrow transplantation in the rat. II. Quantitation of cellular infiltrates in parenchymal target organs in acute graft-versus-host disease. Submitted for publication. Scand J Immunol 1986; 23: 351.

Received 1 August 1985.
Accepted 1 October 1985.

0041-1337/86/4106-0709$02.00/0
TRANSPLANTATION
Vol. 41, No. 6

Printed in U.S.A.

THE PROGNOSTIC VALUE OF THE EOSINOPHIL IN ACUTE RENAL ALLOGRAFT REJECTION

MATTHEW R. WEIR,[1] MARY HALL-CRAGGS, STEVE Y. SHEN, JEFFREY N. POSNER, SHEILA V. ALONGI, FUAD J. DAGHER, AND JOHN H. SADLER

Renal Division and Transplantation Service, Departments of Medicine, Pathology, and Surgery, University of Maryland Hospital, Baltimore, Maryland

A case report of marked peripheral blood eosinophilia and eosinophilic infiltration of a rejected renal allograft in a transplant recipient stimulated our review of the clinical course of 132 consecutive renal transplant recipients. A total of 187 acute rejections occurred in 112 patients. Diagnosis was made by renal biopsy in 124 cases. The percentage of eosinophils in the leukocyte differential of patients with irreversible rejection was 5.2±5.7 (mean±SD) versus that seen in patients with reversible rejection, 2.9±3.5 (P<.05). The difference in the total eosinophil counts in each group was not statistically significant. Patients with peripheral blood eosinophil percentages greater than or equal to 4% had a 37.9% irreversible rejection rate, whereas those who had less than 4%, had a 22.4% loss rate (P<.01). Six of seven patients with greater than or equal to 2% eosinophils in the inflammatory infiltrate of their renal allograft lost their kidney, whereas grafts with less than 2% eosinophils had a 36.8% loss rate (P<.02). We conclude that the increased presence of eosinophils in the peripheral blood and/or renal allograft biopsy specimen is an adverse prognostic factor for acute rejection outcome.

The role of the eosinophil in the immune response remains controversial. There is evidence that it may function as a killer cell, especially when exposed to pathogenic parasites (*1, 2*). But, there is also evidence that it may have antiinflammatory actions, and thus have a restraining effect on the immune response (*1, 2*).

The role of the eosinophil in clinical transplantation has been neglected. Only one case report exists revealing peripheral blood eosinophilia associated with an acute rejection of a renal allograft (*3*). In the pathology literature, eosinophils are occasionally noted in the cellular infiltrate of an acutely rejecting kidney (*4, 5*). No systematic evaluation of the frequency, prevalence, or prognostic significance of eosinophils in either peripheral blood or renal biopsy specimens during a rejection has been performed.

Recently, we hospitalized a hemodialysis patient who experienced fever, severe peripheral eosinophilia, and pain over his renal transplant many months after his chronically rejected kidney had ceased to function. Subsequent to the transplant nephrectomy, his fever and eosinophilia disappeared. Histologic evaluation of the nephrectomy specimen revealed intense, interstitial inflammation consisting, in certain areas, of up to 80% eosinophils. These interesting observations prompted us to investigate the incidence and prognostic significance of eosinophilia in our transplant population during rejection episodes.

MATERIALS AND METHODS

Study group. A total of 132 consecutive cadaveric and living-related donor renal transplants were performed between January 1, 1977 and June 30, 1983 at the University of Maryland Hospital, and these formed the study group for investigation.

Clinical data. The transplant clinic and hospital charts were reviewed for each patient, and the dates of rejection episodes noted. The age, sex, race, and type of transplant for each patient was recorded. Patients who underwent percutaneous renal allograft biopsies were identified. None of these patients received antirejection treatment prior to having their biopsies performed or peripheral blood tested. All biopsies were performed within 24 hr of the clinical diagnosis of acute rejection.

Immunosuppressive regimen. All patients were treated with azathioprine, starting at 4 mg/kg/day, which was tapered to approximately 2 mg/kg/day within 1–2 weeks. This dose was maintained unless a significant depression of the white blood cell count or elevation of hepatocellular enzymes necessitated reduction. All patients also received corticosteroids. Haploidentical and cadaveric recipients started with a dose of 500 mg methylprednisolone each day, being tapered to 40 mg of prednisone by the end of 3 weeks. By one year the average dose was 20 mg/day of prednisone. HLA-identical recipients were initially treated with 250 mg of methylprednisolone daily, which was similiarly tapered. All acute rejections were treated with 500 mg of methylprednisolone on each of 4 consecutive days. If symptoms of rejection persisted after treatment with methylprednisolone pulse therapy, the patient was treated with 15 mg/kg/day of antithymocyte globulin (Upjohn) on each of 14 consecutive days, with the dose being reduced for thrombocytopenia, or neutropenia, or serum sickness.

Renal biopsy interpretation. The biopsy reports of all patients were reviewed. If the presence of eosinophils in the intersitial inflammatory infiltrate was noted, then the hematoxylin-and-eosin–stained slides of the renal biopsy were reexamined and the section with the most severe interstitial inflammation was used for quantitation of the presence of eosinophils. This was accomplished by performing a differential count of 20 random high-power fields. Further, a subjective assessment of the severity of total inflammation, degree of fibrosis, and vascular change, was made on each pathologic specimen.

Definitions and statistics. Acute rejection was defined clinically by the evidence of fever, allograft tenderness, and decreased urine output, in conjunction with a serum creatinine greater than 25% of baseline.

Reversible rejection was defined clinically by the eventual decrease and stabilization of serum creatinine to within 25% of

[1] Correspondence and requests for reprints should be addressed to M.R. Weir, Renal Division, University of Maryland Hospital, 22 S. Greene Street, Baltimore, MD 21201.

baseline levels after antirejection therapy. Irreversible rejection was defined as a continued rise in serum creatinine in spite of antirejection therapy ultimately necessitating reinstitution of dialysis.

Statistical analysis was performed using the *t* test for comparing the means of two independent samples. Additional groups were compared using a chi-square analysis.

RESULTS

Rejection episodes. A total of 187 acute renal allograft rejections occurred in 112 patients. Diagnosis of rejection was made by renal biopsy in 124 cases and by the clinical picture in 63 cases. There were no acute rejection episodes in 20 patients, and 134 rejections (71.7%) were successfully reversed, whereas 53 patients had irreversible loss of renal function (28.3%).

Peripheral blood analysis. The highest total eosinophil count and highest percentage of eosinophils in the peripheral blood leukocyte differential within seven days of the clinical diagnosis of rejection was recorded. The 20 patients with no rejection had fewer eosinophils both in total count and in percentage, compared with either groups with reversible or irreversible rejection (Table 1). The difference in total eosinophil counts did not reach statistical significance among any of these groups. However, the percentage of eosinophils in the differential of both the no-rejection group and the reversible-rejection group was significantly less than that seen in the irreversible-rejection group ($P<.05$).

As seen in Table 1, 66 patients had 4% or more eosinophils in peripheral blood leukocyte differential count at the time of rejection. Of these, 25 rejections were irreversible (37.9%). However, for the 125 patients suffering an acute rejection with fewer than 4% eosinophils in their peripheral leukocyte differential, only 28 irreversible rejections occurred (22.4%). This nearly two-fold difference in irreversible rejection rate is statistically significant ($P=.01$). The segregation of the two groups on the basis of peripheral blood eosinophil percentage was based on the finding (Table 1) that patients with reversible rejection had a mean of 2.9% eosinophils in their peripheral blood leukocyte differential.

Renal biopsy analysis. A total of 124 renal allograft biopsies were performed at the time of acute rejection. Of these, 26 were repeat biopsies in the same patient for recurrent rejection. Only one of seven patients with a biopsy eosinophil differential greater than or equal to 2% had a reversible rejection (Table 2)—whereas the majority (63.2%) of patients with biopsy eosinophil differentials less than 2% had reversible rejections ($P<.02$). Five patients had 4% or greater peripheral blood eosinophils, as well as 2% or greater eosinophils in the inflammatory infiltrate of their renal biopsy. All lost their allografts to irreversible rejection. The segregation of the two groups on the basis of percentage of eosinophils in the leukocyte infiltrate was based on the finding (Table 2) that patients with reversible rejection had a mean of 1.6% eosinophils in the inflammatory infiltrate. The subjective degrees of interstitial inflammation, fibrosis, and edema in the biopsy specimens were indistinguishable among groups.

DISCUSSION

The information derived from our retrospective review of the clinical course of our 132 renal transplant recipients suggests that the presence of increased numbers of eosinophils in the peripheral blood and/or renal biopsy predicts a poor outcome from an acute renal allograft rejection episode.

The purpose of the eosinophil in the immune response is still poorly understood. The cell bears a number of similarities to the neutrophil in its role as a defensive killer, as well as similarities in structure. Both eosinophils and neutrophils share similar chemotactic responses, phagocytic ability, and lysosomal enzymes (*1, 2*). Although the eosinophil has an oxidative metabolic response to membrane stimuli like the neutrophil, the eosinophil is clearly less efficient than a neutrophil at killing bacteria (*1, 2*).

Eosinophils and neutrophils respond quite differently to immunoregulatory mechanisms. Neutrophils, in contrast to eosinophils, appear to respond more effectively to antigenic stimuli independent of lymphocytes (*1, 2*). The responses of neutrophils and eosinophils to acute inflammation or corticosteroid administration are also quite different. A marked depression in the eosinophil count follows steroid administration or acute inflammation, whereas a marked increase in the neutrophil

TABLE 1. Relationship of the peripheral blood eosinophil count and percentage of eosinophils in the leukocyte differential to rejection outcome[a]

	No rejection (n=20)	Reversible rejection (n=134)	Irreversible rejection (n=53)
Peripheral blood eosinophil count	162±170	227±272	237±252
% Eosinophils in peripheral blood leukocyte differential	2.5±2.8	2.9±3.5	5.2±5.7
>4% Eosinophils in peripheral blood leukocyte differential	4	37	25
<4% Eosinophils in peripheral blood leukocyte differential	16	97	28

[a] All means expressed as ±SD.

TABLE 2. Relationship of the percentage of eosinophils in the leukocyte infiltrate of renal allografts to rejection outcome[a]

	Number	Reversible rejection	Irreversible rejection
>2% Eosinophils in leukocyte infiltrate	7	1	6
<2% Eosinophils in leukocyte infiltrate	117	74	43
% Eosinophils in leukocyte infiltrate in biopsies that noted eosinophils	17	1.6±2.0 (n=8)	3.9±2.9 (n=9)

[a] All means expressed as ±SD.

count occurs in these similar situations (*1, 2, 6, 7*). The eosinophil response is more closely related to T-lymphocyte-mediated immune responses (*1, 2, 8–10*).

The major distinguishing feature of eosinophils are their granules, which preferentially contain a variety of unique proteins. The granules contain high amounts of peroxidase, but no lysozyme or phagocytin as seen in neutrophils (*11*). The granules also contain arylsulfatase B, phospholipase D, eosinophil lysophospholipase, and eosinophil phospholipid exchange protein, the function of which is probably protective detoxification (*12*). The largest amount of protein by weight in the granules is the major basic protein that has been shown to be damaging to the schistosomules of *Schistosoma mansoni* (*13*), larvae of *Trichinella spiralis* (*14*), and many mammalian tissues (*15, 16*).

The eosinophilis' relationship with T lymphocytes and other aspects of cell-mediated immunity has been better defined recently, although many questions still remain. Speirs et al. have demonstrated that primed clones of lymphocytes in the presence of specific antigens are capable of enhancing eosinopoiesis and producing a local or systemic eosinophilia (*9*). Rechallenge with the same provoking stimulus can lead to a "secondary" or augmented response with increasing numbers of eosinophils. Rechallenge with a new stimulus provokes only a "primary" or a less-augmented response. This suggests an element of immunologic memory. Elegant studies have demonstrated the need of intact T cell function for eosinophilic response to such antigens as *Trichinella Spiralis* (*17*) or tetanus toxoid (*18*). Cohen and Ward have demonstrated that antigen-activated lymphocytes can release a factor that can combine with immune complexes to aid in generating an eosinophil chemotactic factor (*8*).

Experimental studies have suggested that eosinophilia generally results when antigens are introduced into the body as components that are too large to pass through the capillary bed. The same antigens as smaller particles do not cause a similar reaction (*19*). Some authors have speculated that the processing of antigens in the tissues, where inflammatory cells must migrate to meet the antigen, will more likely cause eosinophilia than the same material processed in the body's fixed macrophage system (*19–21*). This situation would be analagous to that occurring in an allograft transplant.

In general, the inflammatory reaction associated with involvement of eosinophils is a granulomatous one, with predominant mononuclear cellular infiltration with minimal evidence of neutrophils (*21, 22*). Pyogenic infiltration has been reported to produce factors that cause eosinopenia and suppress lymphocyte mediated stimuli for eosinophil production (*6*).

Only occasional studies report finding eosinophils in typical cell-mediated inflammatory reactions such as delayed-type hypersensitivity skin testing, and contact dermatitis (*23, 24*). Perhaps eosinophilic infiltration and/or eosinophilia represents only unusual cell-mediated reactions. Unfortunately, routine examination of tissues for eosinophils is not always performed.

It is interesting that the percentage of eosinophils in the peripheral blood, rather than the total eosinophil count, is a more reliable predictor of irreversible rejection. Perhaps this reflects the effects of both high-dose corticosteroids and azathioprine which tend to depress the number of peripheral blood eosinophils, thus making the total count more difficult to interpret. On the other hand, one might expect the percentage of eosinophils in the peripheral blood leukocyte differential to be decreased because corticosteroids do not depress neutrophil counts—and, if anything, tend to increase them (*7*). However, steroid-induced neutrophilia is balanced by the neutropenic effect of azathioprine. For these reasons, we were not suprised that the total eosinophil count was not as useful as the eosinophil percentage in the peripheral blood leukocyte differential in predicting rejection outcome.

The predictive value of the percentage of eosinophils in the peripheral blood was corroborated by the information we obtained from the percentage of eosinophils in the leukocyte infiltrate in the renal allograft biopsy. This reinforced the impression that the presence of eosinophils is an adverse prognostic factor in predicting the outcome of acute renal allograft rejection.

The purpose of the eosinophil in the rejecting leukocytic infiltrate remains open to speculation. Eosinophils could be accumulating locally in the graft to aid in the containment of a severe mononuclear inflammatory response associated with rejection, or they could be directly involved in tissue damage through release of their major basic protein. Eosinophils could also be transiently accumulating in the allograft during the healing phase of the local inflammatory insult from the acute rejection.

Another hypothesis is that the acute inflammation associated with renal allograft rejection stimulates IgE antibody production similar to that seen in allergic causes of anaphylaxis, thus leading to activation of mast cells in tissue, and basophils in the peripheral blood, the substances of which are chemoattractants for eosinophils. Thus, the acute rejection could produce local accumulation of eosinophils not only within the graft, but also within the peripheral blood, the purpose of which would be to suppress the hypersensitivity response of the rejecting kidney.

A third possibility is that the eosinophil may just be a nonspecific indicator of significant lymphocyte activation and a signal that an allograft rejection is occurring. Because of the poor prognosis associated with the presence of eosinophils, one might speculate that only the most severe rejections, associated with the most profound lymphocyte activation, would liberate enough eosinopoietic factors to cause an increase in peripheral blood eosinophils.

The case we described in the introduction clearly demonstrates the involvement of the eosinophil in the acute rejection process of a chronically rejected renal allograft, since the removal of the antigenic stimulus resulted in complete resolution of the patient's fever and peripheral blood eosinophilia. In addition, histologic examination of the allograft revealed an intense lymphocytic and eosinophilic infiltrate.

The eosinophil is somehow involved in the immunoregulatory response of the human body to acute allograft rejection. Whether the eosinophil is only a signal of an inflammatory insult, and thus an innocent bystander, or whether it has some role in modulating the immune response, remains controversial.

Acknowledgments. We thank Jean Marx and Linda Davis for their expert secretarial assistance in the preparation of the manuscript.

REFERENCES

1. Bass DA. The functions of eosinophils. Ann Intern Med 1979; 91: 120.
2. Beeson PB, Bass DA. The eosinophil (Major problems in internal medicine series) vol 14. Philadelphia: Saunders, 1977.
3. Shalev O, Rubinger D, Barlatzky Y, Kopolovic J, Drukker A.

Eosinophilia associated with allograft kidney rejection. Nephron 1982; 31: 182.
4. Antonovych TT, Mostofi FK. Renal transplantation. In: Atlas of kidney biopsies. Washington, DC: AFIP, 1980: chap 13.
5. Starzl TE, Klintmalm GBG, Weil R, et al. Cyclosporin A and steroid therapy in 66 cadaver kidney recipients. Surg Gyn Obstet 1981; 153: 486.
6. Bass DA, Gonwa TA, Szejda P, et al. Eosinopenia of acute infection: production of eosinopenia by the chemotactic factors of acute inflammation. J Clin Invest 1980; 65: 1265.
7. Hills AG, Forsham PH, Finch CA. Changes in circulating leukocytes induced by the administration of pituitary adrenocorticotrophic hormone in man. Blood 1948; 3: 755.
8. Cohen S, Ward PA. In vitro and in vivo activity of a lymphocyte and immune complex dependent chemotactic factor for eosinophils. J Exp Med 1973; 137: 133.
9. Speirs RS, Gallagher MT, Rauchwerger J, Heim LR, Trentin JJ. Lymphoid cell dependence of eosinophil response to antigen. II. Location of memory cells and their dependence on thymic influence. Exp Hematol 1973; 1: 150.
10. McGarry MP, Speirs RS, Jenkins VK, Trentin JJ. Lymphoid cell dependence of eosinophil response to antigen. J Exp Med 1971; 134: 801.
11. Archer GT, Hirsch JG. Isolation of granules from eosinophil leukocytes and study of their enzyme content. J Exp Med 1963; 118: 277.
12. Weller PF, Wasserman SI, Austin FF. Selected enzymes preferentially present in the eosinophil. In: Mahmoud AAF, Austen KF, Simon AS, eds. The eosinophil in health and disease. New York: Grune & Stratton, 1980: 115.
13. Butterworth AE, Wassom DL, Gleich GJ, et al. Damage to schistosomules of schistosoma mansoni induced directly by eosinophil major basic protein. J Immunol 1979; 122: 221.
14. Wassom DL, Gleich GJ. Damage to Trichinella spiralis newborn larvae by eosinophil major basic protein. Am J Trop Med Hyg 1979; 28: 860.
15. Gleich GJ, Frigas E, Loegering DA, et al. Cytotoxic properties of the eosinophil major basic protein. J Immunol 1979; 123: 2925.
16. Gleich GJ, Loegering DA, Frigas E, et al. The major basic protein of the eosinophil granule: physiochemical properties, localization and function. In: Mahmoud AAF, Austen KF, Simon AS, eds., The eosinophil in health and disease. New York: Grune & Stratton, 1980: 79.
17. Grove DI, Mahmoud AAF, Warren KS. Eosinophils and resistance to Trichinella spiralis. J Exp Med 1977; 145: 755.
18. Ponzio NM, Speirs RS, Lymphoid cell dependence of eosinophil response to antigen. VI. The effect of selective removal of T or B lymphocytes on the capacity of primed spleen cells to adoptively transferred immunity to tetanus toxoid. Immunology 1975; 28(2): 243.
19. Schriber RA Zucker-Franklin D. Induction of blood eosinophilia by pulmonary embolization of antigen-coated particles: the relationship to cell-mediated immunity. J Immunol 1975; 114: 1348.
20. Steele ASV, Rack JH. Cellular reaction to polystyrene-protein conjugates. J Path Bacteriol 1965; 89: 703.
21. Colley DG. Lymphocyte products. In: Mahmoud AAF, Austen KF, Simon AS, eds. The eosinophil in health and disease. New York: Grune & Stratton, 1980: 293.
22. Colley DG. Lymphokine-related eosinophil responses. Lymphokine Rep 1980; 1: 133.
23. Leber PD, Milgram M, Cohen S. Eosinophils in delayed hypersensitivity skin reaction sites. Immunol Commun 1973; 2: 615.
24. Hiroshima M, Hayashi H. The mediation of tissue eosinophilic in hypersensitivity reactions. I. Isolation of two different chemotactic factors from DNP-ascaris extract-induced skin lesions in guinea pig. Immunology 1976; 30: 203.

Received 11 July 1985.
Accepted 4 October 1985.

0041-1337/86/4106-0713$02.00/0
TRANSPLANTATION
Vol. 41, No. 6
Printed in U.S.A.

USE OF A PROGNOSTIC INDEX IN EVALUATION OF LIVER TRANSPLANTATION FOR PRIMARY BILIARY CIRRHOSIS

JAMES NEUBERGER,[1] DOUGLAS G. ALTMAN,[2] ERIK CHRISTENSEN,[3] NIELS TYGSTRUP,[4] AND ROGER WILLIAMS[1]

The Liver Unit, King's College Hospital and School of Medicine and Dentistry, Denmark Hill, London SE5 9RS; Division of Medical Statistics, Clinical Research Centre, Harrow, Middlesex, England; Department of Hepatology, Hvidovre Hospital, Copenhagen; and Medical Department A, Rigshospitalet, Copenhagen, Denmark

In the Cambridge/King's College Hospital program, one of the main criteria for recommendation of a liver transplant for a patient with primary biliary cirrhosis (PBC), as in other types of end-stage liver disease, has been the overall assessment that survival was likely to be less than one year. In the present study, a recently developed prognostic model, based on six variables, was used retrospectively to estimate the likely survival without transplantation of the first 29 patients receiving a transplant for PBC. Median estimated survival time for the complete group of patients was five months and in only four patients was survival in the absence of transplantation estimated to be more than one year. Comparison of actual survival curves after transplantation with the estimated survival in the absence of such a procedure shows that, despite an initial higher mortality related to surgery and the immediate postoperative period, grafting was associated with a statistically significant improvement in overall survival. No correlation between the outcome after transplantation and the severity of preexisting liver disease, (as assessed by the expected survival) could be determined, but further assessment of preoperative variables is warranted.

Primary Biliary Cirrhosis (PBC)* constitutes one of the major patient groups in the Cambridge/King's College Hospital series, as well as in those of other centers (*1–3*). There are two reasons for this: the degree of symptomatic improvement following a successful graft, and the apparent ability of these patients to withstand the considerable trauma of operation better than those with end-stage parenchymal liver disease from other causes. Nevertheless, there are difficulties in determining when liver transplantation should be carried out—with the prognosis for the individual case being sufficiently poor and yet with the patient not too ill to survive the operation and postoperative period. In our series the patients have been admitted to the program only when it appeared that the prognosis was less than one year, this estimate being based on the overall assessment by the physician concerned. It is known that of the various biochemical abnormalities, the extent of elevation in serum bilirubin level is an important prognostic guide (*4*). Thus Schaffner's group has shown that the expected survival is 17 months once the serum bilirubin exceeds 170 μmol/L on two successive occasions six months apart (*5*). In another study survival was likely to be less than two years once the serum bilirubin had reached 102 μmol/L (*6*). We have recently developed a statistical model to predict survival, based on six variables, including the serum bilirubin, that were found to imply a poor prognosis (*7*); and in the present study, we have used the model retrospectively to estimate the likely survival time without transplantation of the first 29 patients operated upon in the Cambridge/King's College Hospital series.

[1] King's College Hospital and School of Medicine and Dentistry.
[2] Clinical Research Centre.
[3] Hvidovre Hospital.
[4] Rigshospitalet.
* Abbreviations used: PBC, primary biliary cirrhosis; PI, prognostic index.

MATERIALS AND METHODS

The 29 patients underwent liver grafting (Prof. R. Y. Calne) between 1968 and April 1984 and comprised 26 women, aged 33 to 59 years and three men (Table 1). All the patients had complained of severe pruritus only partially controlled by cholestyramine; 15 had evidence of ascites and ten of these also had encephalopathy, with recurrent variceal hemorrhage a prominent feature in nine patients. At the time of transplantation, the serum bilirubin was above 100 μmol/L in all but one and exceeded 300 μmol/L in 18 and 500 μmol/L in seven. Serum albumin was below 30 g/L in 17 and prothrombin time was more than three seconds prolonged in ten patients. Liver biopsy showed that cirrhosis was present in all but three cases who were at histological stage 11/111 (*8*). Central cholestasis was present in 23 of the 29 patients. Seven of the patients had been on azathioprine 1 mg/kg/day and four others on d-penicillamine 250–1200 mg/day, for periods of one to three years.

Prognostic index (PI). The statistical model to predict survival was derived from data collected in an international controlled trial of azathioprine therapy versus placebo involving 216 patients, and validated in another group of patients receiving placebo as part of another controlled study (*9*). The six independent variables, identified by Cox regression analysis, are combined in the formula below to give a prognostic index (PI):

PI = 2.52 × $\log_{10}$ serum bilirubin μmol/1 + 0.0069 × exp. ([age yrs − 20]/10) − 0.05 × serum albumin g/l + 0.88 (if cirrhosis present) + 0.68 (if central cholestasis present) + 0.52 (if not treated with azathioprine).

and for any value of the index, the estimated survival function (S[t]) is obtained from the formula:

$$(\hat{S}[t]) = \exp.\ [-\hat{\Lambda}_0(t)\ \exp.\ (PI)]$$

where $\hat{\Lambda}_0$ (t) is the estimated cumulative underlying hazard function from the Cox regression analysis. The expected survival time for an individual was taken as the estimated median survival time, which was derived from $\hat{S}(t)$. The estimated survival function for a group of patients was taken as that

TABLE 1. Characteristics, prognostic index, and outcome of the 29 patients grafted for PBC

Patient	Age	Sex	Serum bilirubin (μmol/L)	PI	Survival (months) Estimated	Actual	Outcome
OL 5	48	F	120	5.91	11.2	1.6	Died, pneumonia
23	52	F	210	6.66	5.8	1.6	Died, bile leak
24	50	F	552	6.98	4.9	0.0	Died, cardiac arrest
56	51	M	90	5.12	20.7	59	Died, myocardial infarct
64	52	F	182	6.67	5.8	94	Alive
72	56	F	500	7.33	1.6	1.6	Died, pneumonia
74	56	M	780	7.94	0.6	84	Alive
76	50	F	410	7.18	3.2	21	Died, cholangitis
83	51	F	510	6.65	6.3	0.8	Died, pneumonia
84	56	F	390	7.14	3.2	0.7	Died, sepsis
93	40	F	386	5.82	13.8	2.2	Died, rejection
98	42	F	458	7.20	3.2	5.9	Died, rejection
101	36	F	590	7.72	1.3	49	Alive
103	36	F	354	7.16	3.2	1.4	Died, hepatic vein thrombosis
105	42	F	359	5.78	13.8	0.6	Died, sepsis
108	50	F	350	6.02	10.2	45	Alive
111	49	F	385	6.46	6.6	0.7	Died, sepsis
112	53	M	230	7.35	1.6	0.1	Died, hemorrhage
114	59	F	204	6.10	8.4	9.9	Died, pneumonia
122	42	F	317	7.07	4.7	32	Alive
125	33	F	552	7.59	1.3	1.0	Died, septicemia
128	55	F	122	6.10	8.4	1.8	Died, sepsis
129	42	F	384	7.33	1.6	5.4	Died, influenza
130	49	F	266	6.96	4.9	0.6	Died, respiratory failure
136	58	F	110	5.76	13.9	0.7	Died, sepsis
137	53	F	556	8.36	0.3	0.6	Died, *Candida*
138	36	F	380	7.19	3.2	0.7	Died, sepsis
140	36	F	271	6.30	8.0	0.6	Died, liver/kidney failure
145	48	F	166	6.04	9.0	0.3	Died, renal failure

corresponding to the average value of the PI of the patients ($\overline{S}[t]$).

Comparison of the observed outcome after transplantation with the expected survival using censored survival data was by a χ^2 test based on the calculation of $(O-E)^2/E$ where O is the observed number of deaths and E the expected number of deaths in the absence of grafting. Following Breslow (*10*), E was calculated as:

$$E = \sum_{i=1}^{29} -\log \overline{S}(t_i)$$

where ti is the observed survival of the "i" patient.

The observed survival curves after grafting were calculated using Kaplan-Meier statistics. The relation between the estimated (in the absence of grafting) and observed survival times was assessed by an index of concordance as described by Harrell et al. (*11, 12*). All pairings of the patients are considered in turn. For each pair, their observed and expected survival times are concordant if the patient with the longer expected survival time lived longer. If both patients are still alive or if only one is still alive but has not yet survived as long as the one who died, that pair is excluded. The index c is the proportion of concordant pairs among those that could be evaluated. Pairs with identical observed or expected survival time contributed ½ to the numerator of c. The index c must lie between 0 and 1. It was converted to a Kendall-type rank correlation by calculating 2 (c−½).

RESULTS

Nineteen of the 29 patients died within three months of transplantation as a consequence of complications directly related to surgery or to early postoperative problems (Table 1). A further three died between 3 and 12 months after surgery, one (OL 129) from a respiratory infection, a second (OL 98) from chronic rejection, and the third (OL 114) following a paraplegia induced by dislocation of an osteoporotic cervical spine. Of the seven patients who lived for more than one year, one (OL 76) succumbed to septicemia and cholangitis consequent upon biliary stricture at 21 months and one (OL 56) died from a myocardial infarct nearly five years after grafting. Of the remainder, who are all in good health, four are alive more than three years after grafting and the longest survivor is currently over nine years (as of December 31, 1984).

Calculation of values for the prognostic index gave a relatively narrow range of values, from 5.12 to 8.36 (median 6.96)—which, when related to expected survival, gave values of less than one year for 25 of the 29 patients, (3 months in 7, 3–6 months in 10, and 6–12 months in 8). In the four patients with an expected survival of greater than one year, this was 14 months in three (OPL 93, 105, and 106) and 21 months in the other (OL 56). Recurrent variceal hemorrhage was the indication for grafting in three of these patients (OL 56, 93, 136), severe fatigue and pruritus for the fourth.

Comparison of the actual survival after grafting and the expected survival in the absence of such a procedure shows that in 11 of the patients actual survival was greater than would be expected, although in 3 of these survival was prolonged by less than 3 months. However, comparison of the actual survival curves after grafting and the expected survival curve in the absence of grafting derived from the prognostic model shows that the two curves are of different shapes (Fig. 1). After an initial high perioperative mortality of 73% within 6 months,

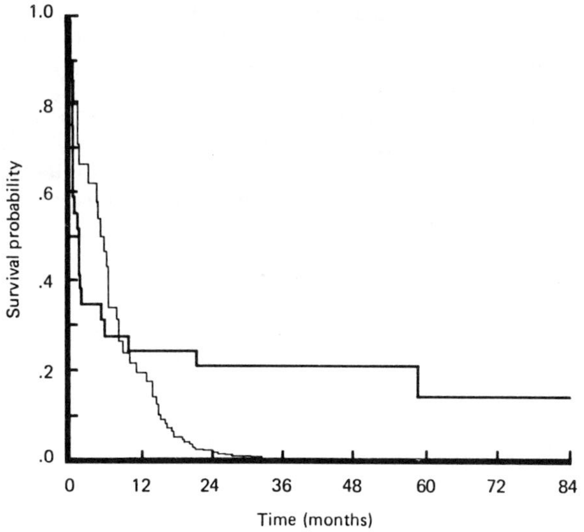

FIGURE 1. Actual (-----) and predicted (-----) survival of 29 patients following liver transplantation.

there were few deaths. Statistical analysis shows that the two curves were significantly different, with a better overall survival after transplantation (O=24, E=182, χ^2=137 with one degree of freedom, P<0.0001), although most of the difference is due to the three longest survivors.

Actual survival for the patients divided above and below the median PI of 6.96—which corresponds to an estimated survival of five months—was not significantly different (Fig. 2). Furthermore, the mean PI in the seven patients who survived for more than one year after grafting (6.82) was little different from that of those dying within one year (6.74). For the group with the worst prognosis there was little crossover of the observed and expected survival curves (Fig. 2, B).

Comparison of actual and expected survival in the absence of transplantation by means of a concordance statistic gave a value of c=0.492, which converts to a rank correlation coefficient of −0.02.

DISCUSSION

The reasonably close agreement between the doctors' estimate of survival and the results obtained using the statistical model is perhaps not surprising—for, in both cases, the serum bilirubin is a major component. The doctor's assessment is also likely to take into account other factors, such as pruritus and lethargy, that make the patient's life intolerable. Clinical features, such as ascites or variceal hemorrhage, although they may have an adverse effect on prognosis, were found not to constitute independent variables (*7*).

Comparison of the actual survival after transplantation with the expected survival shows that, despite an initial higher mortality related to the transplant procedure, survival overall was improved by grafting. Furthermore it is to be hoped that the high initial mortality of the procedure will be reduced, and indeed there is evidence from our 1984 results that this is occurring (*13*).

Statistical methods are most reliable for prediction taken near the center of observed data; predictions away from the mean of independent variables have wider confidence limits. Of the 216 patients in the trial from which the model was derived, only 5% had a PI greater than 7.0, whereas in the present group studied 45% did. In practice, such considerations are unlikely to be of great importance since the expected

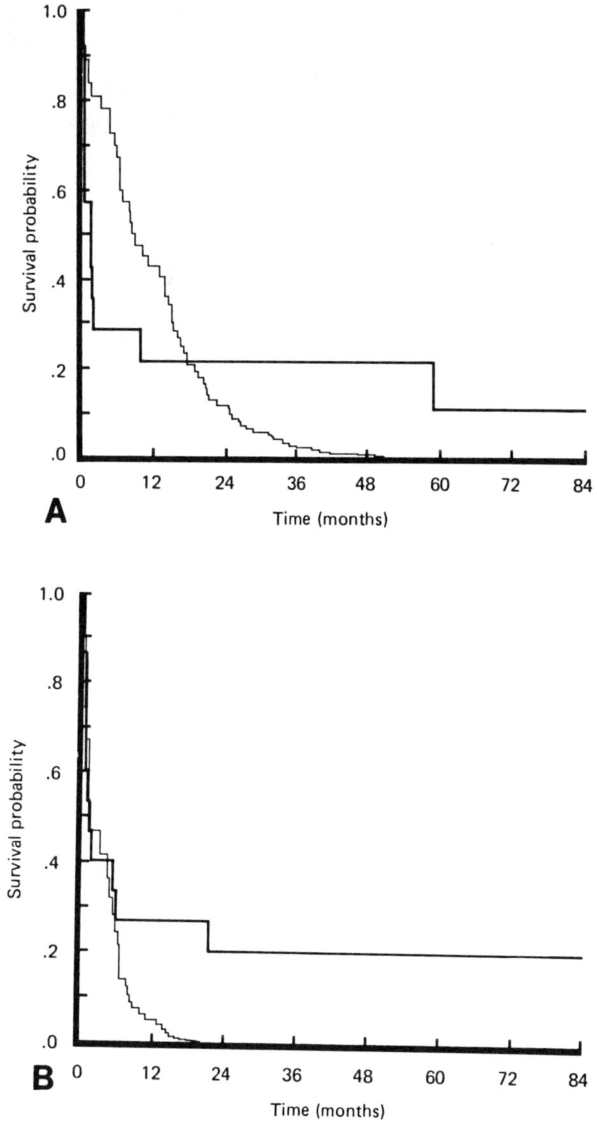

FIGURE 2. Actual (-----) and predicted (-----) survival of 16 patients (A) and 13 patients (B) with a prognostic index less than and greater than 6.96, respectively. The expected survival functions were based on the mean PI in each group.

survival times of patients with a PI greater than 7.0 is so short. In the total group studied, expected and actual survival curves cross, making interpretation of the benefits of transplantation difficult. However, among patients with the worst prognosis, the lines did not cross, and thus there was a clearer indication of the benefit of transplantation (Fig. 2, B). The outcome was no worse in those with a prognosis of less than three months than in those with a prognosis of greater than one year. The lack of correlation of PI with the outcome of the operation suggests that early postoperative death, at least in this sense, could not be directly related to the poor overall clinical state of the patient and that the patients are being operated on too late. Other factors, less closely related to the degree of hepatic impairment, may have important prognostic value in determining outcome of the operation—for example, the degree of malnutrition and closely related host defenses against infections.

REFERENCES

1. Rolles K, Williams R, Neuberger J, Caine RY. The Cambridge and King's College Hospital experience of liver transplantation. Hepatology 1983; 4: 50S.

2. Starzl TE, Iwatsuki I, Van Thiel D, et al. Evolution of liver transplantation. Hepatology 1982; 2: 614.
3. Krom RAF, Gips CH, Newton D, et al. A successful start of a liver transplant program. Transplant Proc 1983; 15: 1276.
4. Roll J, Boyer JL, Barry D, Klatskin G. The prognostic importance of clinical and histological factors in asymptomatic and symptomatic primary biliary cirrhosis. N Engl J Med 1983; 308: 1.
5. Shapiro JM, Smith H, Schaffner F. Serum bilirubin: a prognostic factor in primary biliary cirrhosis. Gut 1979; 20: 137.
6. Epstein O, Fraga EG, Keynan A, Sherlock S. When should patients with primary biliary cirrhosis be referred for liver transplantation? Liver 1984; 4: 82.
7. Christensen E, Neuberger J, Crowe J, et al. Beneficial effect of azathioprine and prediction of prognosis in primary biliary cirrhosis. Gastroenterology (in press).
8. Ludwig J, Dickson ER, McDonald GSA. Staging of chronic nonsuppurative cholangitis (syndrome of primary biliary cirrhosis). Virchows Arch [Pathol Anat] 1978; 379: 103.
9. Neuberger J, Christensen E, Portmann B, et al. Double-blind controlled trial of d-penicillamine in patients with primary biliary cirrhosis. Gut 1985; 26: 114.
10. Breslow NE. Analysis of survival data under the proportional hazard model. Int Stat Rev 1975; 1: 45.
11. Harrell FE, Lee KL, Califf RM, Pryor DB, Rosati RA. Regression modelling strategies for improved prognostic prediction. Stat Med 1984; 3: 143.
12. Harrell FE, Califf RM, Pryor DB, Lee KL, Rosati RA. Evaluating the yield of medical tests. JAMA 1982; 247: 2543.
13. Williams R, Calne RY, Rolles K, Polson R. Current results in orthotopic liver grafting in the Cambridge/King's College Hospital series. Br Med J [Clin Res] 1985; 49.

Received 2 July 1985.
Accepted 19 September 1985.

0041-1337/86/4106-0716$02.00/0
TRANSPLANTATION

Vol. 41, No. 6
Printed in U.S.A.

RELATIONSHIP OF INTERFERON-GAMMA AND NEOPTERIN LEVELS DURING STIMULATION WITH ALLOANTIGENS IN VIVO AND IN VITRO[1]

W. Woloszczuk,[2] J. Troppmair,[3,4] E. Leiter,[3] R. Flener,[5] M. Schwarz,[6] J. Kovarik,[6] E. Pohanka,[6] R. Margreiter,[7] and C. Huber[3]

Ludwig Boltzmann Institut für Klinische Endokrinologie, Vienna; Division of Clinical Immunobiology, Department of Internal Medicine, School of Medicine, University of Innsbruck; Second Department of Internal Medicine, University of Vienna; Boehringer Institut für Arzneimittelforschung, Vienna; and Division of Transplantation Surgery, Department of Surgery I, School of Medicine, University of Innsbruck, Innsbruck, Austria

We have recently shown that interferon-gamma is capable of activating the key enzyme of pterin biosynthesis in macrophages. This leads to excretion of the stable degradation product neopterin (*3*). In this article we present experimental evidence suggesting that stimulation of T cells by alloantigens is associated with release of interferon-gamma—which, in the case of rejection, is locally restricted and not always detectable in the bloodstream. Neopterin induced by this lymphokine, however, readily penetrates tissue barriers and is detectable in the serum. This conclusion is based on two different sets of observations:

(1) If supernatants of MLCs are compared with sera from patients with documented acute rejection episodes for their interferon-gamma and neopterin levels, a marked gradient is observed to exist between interferon levels measured in vitro and in vivo; this is not the case for neopterin for which comparable levels were seen.

(2) Detection of interferon-gamma in sera of allograft recipients invariably precedes an increase of neopterin; on the other hand, increasing neopterin counts are also seen in the absence of detectable interferon-gamma levels in the serum.

It thus appears that although interferon-gamma release during allograft rejection is primarily restricted to the tissue, evaluation of certain metabolites of interferon-dependent metabolic pathways enables definition of its endogenous release. Whereas interferon gamma represents a less reliable marker in the monitoring of rejection episodes, it might offer an additional means to differentiate rejection from systemic infections. Such a discrimination can not be achieved with the neopterin marker.

Despite the progress made during recent years in the field of prophylactic immunosuppression and prospective matching of organ grafts, acute cellular rejection still represents a major problem. Immunological monitoring that gains relevant and

[1] This work was supported by the Austrian research funds Zur Förderung der wissenschaftlichen Forschung, Project No. 5288.

[2] Ludwig Baltzmann Institut für Klinische Endokrinologie.
[3] Department of Internal Medicine, University of Innsbruck.
[4] Address correspondence to: J. Troppmair, Ph.D., Division of Clinical Immunobiology, Dept. of Internal Medicine, University of Innsbruck, Anichstr. 35, A-6020 Innsbruck, Austria.
[5] Boehringer Institut für Arzneimittelforschung.
[6] University of Vienna.
[7] Department of Surgery, University of Innsbruck.

early information with respect to ongoing allograft rejection would certainly facilitate clinical decisions. It is now well established that lymphokine release represents one of the earliest events after stimulation of T cells by alloantigens. Both IL-2 and interferon-gamma, however, are locally produced in peripheral tissues, and only detected with difficulty in the circulation (*1, 2*). We have recently obtained evidence that interferon-gamma activates the key enzyme of the pterin biosynthesis in macrophages, and that this leads to massive excretion of the degradation product neopterin (*3, 4*). Neopterin, in contrast to interferon-gamma, is a small and quite stable molecule that should easily penetrate tissue compartments and can be readily excreted. One thus might conclude that it represents a marker molecule reflecting endogenous production of interferons. We summarize here in vitro and in vivo evidence suggesting that interferon-gamma subsequent to alloantigenic stimulation in vivo only rarely enters the bloodstream; neopterin locally produced after induction by interferon-gamma can be easily detected in the circulation; and systemic infections are regularly accompanied by detectable levels of interferon-gamma. Our conclusion derived from these findings is that, under conditions in which lymphokines are not detected in the blood, stable metabolites produced under their control in peripheral tissues might be used to assess endogenous production of these molecules.

MATERIALS AND METHODS

Patients. In 36 consecutive patients receiving cadaveric kidney allografts interferon-gamma and neopterin serum levels were determined daily. Immunosuppressive therapy included cyclosporine and prednisolone with doses according to standard protocols (*5*). Additional therapy of rejection episodes consisted of a steroid bolus (250–500 mg methylprednisolone daily for at least three days) and, in cases of biopsy-proved steroid-resistant rejections, antithymocyteglobulin. Diagnosis of rejection in each case was based upon clinical parameters and biopsy.

Laboratory investigations. Peripheral blood mononuclear cells (PBMNC)* were isolated from heparinized venous blood of healthy volunteers by gradient centrifugation on Lymphoprep (Nygaard, Oslo, Norway). Stimulation of these cells was carried out by using an optimal concentration of phytohemagglutinin (PHA, Difco, Detroit, Michigan) or by cocultivation with cells of an Epstein-Barr virus (EBV)-transformed lymphoblastoid cell line in RPMI 1640 (Gibco, Grand Island, NY) supplemented with 20 mM Hepes buffer (Gibco, Grand Island, NY), antibiotics, and 15% heat-inactivated male pooled serum for the time indicated. The number of cells used in all experiments was 1×10^6/ml of tissue culture medium. Incubation was carried out at 37°C in 5% CO_2/95% air. Neopterin levels in culture supernatants and human sera were assessed by using a radioimmunoassay (*6*) (Henning, Berlin, FRG). Interferon-gamma concentrations were determined by immunoradiometry (Centocor, Malvern, PA). For the measurement of interferon-gamma in human serum this method was adapted for greater sensitivity as previously described (*7*).

RESULTS

Release of interferon-gamma and of neopterin from PBMNC stimulated in vitro with allogeneic cells or with mitogenic lectins.

* Abbreviations used: EBV, Epstein-Barr virus; FITC, fluorescein isothiocyanate; PBMNC, peripheral blood mononuclear cells; PHA, phytohemagglutinin.

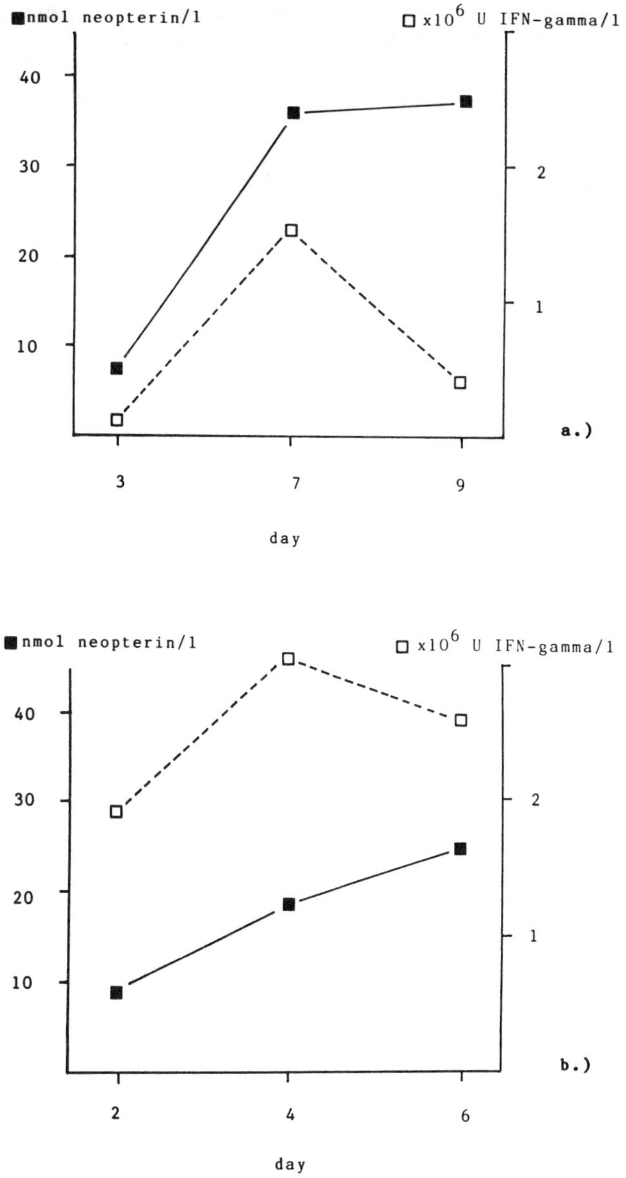

FIGURE 1. Levels of neopterin and IFN-gamma in supernatants from PBMNC-stimulated with allogeneic cells (a) or PHA (b).

Levels of interferon-gamma and of neopterin were simultaneously assessed in culture supernatants derived from PBMNC stimulated with allogeneic cells or with PHA. Results of a typical experiment are shown in Figure 1. In both culture systems rapidly increasing concentrations of interferon-gamma with peaks on day 4 or day 7, respectively, were observed. Neopterin values also increased and continued to rise until the end of the cultivation period. A compilation of all experiments performed is given in Table 1.

Levels of interferon-gamma and of neopterin in sera from patients with acute graft rejection or infection. Levels of interferon-gamma and of neopterin were also simultaneously assessed in sera of patients subsequent to transplantation. A total of 26 documented acute rejection episodes not accompanied by infection was observed in these cases during the time of observation. Also recorded were 9 serious infectious complications (7 bacterial, 2 viral infections) not associated with clinically detectable rejection.

TABLE 1. Comparison of interferon-gamma and neopterin peak levels subsequent to alloantigenic stimulation in vitro and in vivo[a]

	Interferon-gamma (U/L)		Neopterin (nmol/L)
Supernatants from MLC (day 7)	690500 (434200–1534800)	n = 3	36 (24–42.2)
Supernatants from PHA (day 2)	517700 (270400–1934700	n = 4	7.2 (7.0–8.4)
Patient sera during acute rejection[c]	140 (nd–260)[b]	n = 26	131 (42–385)
Patient sera during infections[c]	480 (120–1220)	n = 9	58 (25–116)

[a] Values given are median and range.
[b] n.d. = non detectable (<20 U/L).
[c] Day of diagnosis.

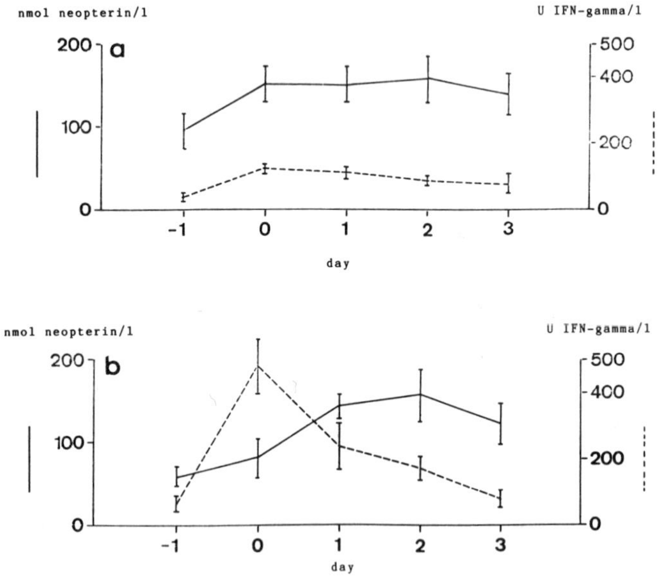

FIGURE 2. Levels of neopterin (solid line) and IFN-gamma (dotted line) during acute allograft rejections (a, 26 observations) or during infectious complications (b, 9 observations).

The levels in serum obtained during in vivo stimulation of immune cells by allografts or by infectious pathogens were compared with those determined after immune stimulation in vitro. Results are compiled in Table 1. As shown, neopterin serum levels obtained during allograft rejection or infection were somewhat higher than those measured in culture supernatants of antigenically activated mononuclear cells. In contrast the serum contained only 0.1% or even less of the amounts of interferon-gamma found in supernatants of activated immune cells. It thus appears that, although T cells subsequent to antigenic stimulation locally release large quantities of interferon-gamma, this molecule is only detectable simultaneously in trace amounts in the circulation. Also addressed was the question of whether acute rejections and infectious complications differ in their interferon-gamma and neopterin patterns. Levels of both markers at various times before, during, and after these clinical events are demonstrated in Figure 2. As shown, both interferon-gamma and neopterin levels peaked at the time of diagnosis of acute rejection; interferon-gamma levels, however, were very low and below the limit of detection in 5 of 26 sera tested. During infections interferon-gamma levels, in contrast, peaked 2 days earlier than neopterin and reached higher values than in the case of acute rejections.

DISCUSSION

This study aimed to answer the question of whether neopterin excretion subsequent to alloantigenic stimulation reflects endogenous production of interferon-gamma. Previous studies had shown that an intact hemolymphatic system is required to enable immune response-associated release of neopterin (*8*); in vitro macrophages can be stimulated by interferon-gamma to release neopterin (*4*) and that this is due to interferon-mediated enhancement of the activity of the key enzyme of this pathway (*3*); and interferon stimulates neopterin excretion in vivo also (*9*). The findings presented in this study indicate that: (1) the appearance of small amounts of interferon-gamma in sera of allograft recipients was invariably followed by increasing neopterin levels. Rejection episodes associated with increasing neopterin levels in the absence of detectable amounts of interferon-gamma were, however, also observed; and (2) after in vitro stimulation of PBMNC, neopterin is released in quantities ranging from 24–42 nmol, and interferon-gamma in quantities ranging from 0.4–1.5×10^6U/L at day 7. After allogeneic stimulation in vivo during the course of acute graft rejection episodes, comparable neopterin levels were observed in the serum—but much lower, interferon-gamma levels, invariably below 260 U/L, were detected.

Taken together, these findings strongly suggest that the increasing neopterin levels during the course of acute rejection episodes in fact reflect increased production of interferon-gamma in peripheral tissues. Whereas the mediator, due to its physicochemical properties and/or rapid removal and degradation, only rarely enters the bloodstream, neopterin with its small size and its chemical stability easily enters the circulation. There are several practical implications of this conclusion. Neopterin under these conditions seems to primarily reflect release of certain lymphokines by activated T cells. In addition, a systemic search for other biochemical markers, which are released under control of individual lymphokines, should be started to further enable assessment of their endogenous production. Lastly, the relative increases of interferon-gamma might be of diagnostic value for differentiation between the locally occurring rejection process and systemic immune challenge induced by infectious pathogens.

Acknowledgments. We are indebted to Mrs. M. Horzemsky and Mrs. T. Kössler for excellent technical assistance, and to Mrs. J. Gschnitzer and Mrs. M. Price-Placzek for competent secretarial help.

REFERENCES

1. Woloszczuk W, Schwarz M, Pohanka E, Kovarik J. Relation of neopterin to gamma interferon serum levels in patients with kidney transplants. In: Wachter H, Curtius HC, Pfleiderer W (eds). Biochemical and clinical aspects of pteridines, vol 4. New York: Walter de Gruyter, 1985: 489.
2. Bocci V. The physiological interferon response. Immunol Today 1985; 6: 7.
3. Troppmair J, Lang A, Huber C, Schoedon G, Niederwieser A, Adolf G. Intracellular changes in pterin releasing peripheral blood mononuclear cells after stimulation with interferon-gamma. In: Wachter H, Curtius HC, Pfleiderer W (eds). Biochemical and clinical aspects of pteridines, vol 4. Walter de Gruyter, 1985: 363.
4. Huber C, Batchelor JR, Fuchs D, et al. Immune response-associated production of neopterin. Release from macrophages primarily under control of interferon-gamma. J Exp Med 1984; 160: 310.
5. European Multicenter Trial Group. Cyclosporin in cadaveric renal transplantation: one-year follow-up of a multicentre trial. Lancet 1983; 2: 986.

6. Rokos K, Rokos H, Frisius H. Pteridines as tumor markers? Attempt of evaluation by HPLC and a radioimmunoassay for neopterin. In Wachter H, Curtius HC, Pfleiderer W, eds. Biochemical and clinical aspects of pteridines, vol 1. New York: Walter de Gruyter, 1982: 117.
7. Woloszczuk W. A sensitive immunoradiometric assay for gamma interferon, suitable for its measurement in serum. Clin Chem 1985; 31: 1090.
8. Niederwieser D, Huber Ch, Gratwohl A, et al. Neopterin as a new biochemical marker in the clinical monitoring of bone marrow transplant recipients. Transplantation 1984; 38: 497.
9. Lang A, Niederwieser D, Huber C, et al. Treatment with human recombinant interferon-alpha-2 induces increase of in vivo neopterin excretion. In: Pfleiderer W, Wachter H, Curtius H (eds.) Biochemical and clinical aspects of pteridines, vol 3, 1984: 249.

Received 11 July 1985.
Accepted 8 October 1985.

0041-1337/86/4106-0719$02.00/0
TRANSPLANTATION

Vol. 41, No. 6
Printed in U.S.A.

CELLULAR IMMUNITY TO VACCINATIONS AND HERPES-VIRUS INFECTIONS AFTER BONE MARROW TRANSPLANTATION[1]

J. W. GRATAMA,[2,4] L. F. VERDONCK,[3] J. A. VAN DER LINDEN,[3] J. G. VAN HEUGTEN,[3] H. A. J. G. KREEFT,[3] J. D'AMARO[4,5] F. E. ZWAAN,[5] AND G. C. DE GAST[3]

Departments of Immunohematology and Blood Bank and Hematology, University Hospital, Leiden; and Department of Hematology, University Hospital, Utrecht, the Netherlands

The cellular immune response to herpesviruses was studied in 46 recipients of marrow grafts (23 autologous, 23 allogeneic). That study was performed in vitro by evaluating the degree of lymphocyte proliferative responses to herpes simplex virus (HSV), cytomegalovirus (CMV), and varicella zoster virus (VZV).

No primary infections with any of those viruses were noted after bone marrow transplantation (BMT). The incidence of active infection in seropositive patients was significantly lower after autologous BMT than after allogeneic BMT (HSV, 2/22 vs. 11/22 patients, respectively, $P = 0.007$; CMV, 4/12 vs. 9/10 patients, respectively, $P = 0.02$; VZV, 3/23 vs. 11/23 patients, respectively, $P = 0.02$). After autologous BMT, the restoration of cellular immunity to the three viruses occurred at a clearly faster rate than after allogeneic BMT. That pattern may have contributed to the low incidence of active infections with those viruses after autologous BMT.

Recipients of allogeneic marrow from donors with a positive lymphocyte proliferation test to HSV had a significantly increased incidence of active HSV infection post-BMT (8/9 patients) than those who received marrow from donors with a negative test (3/13 patients; $P = 0.008$). Acute or chronic graft-versus-host disease (GVHD) decreased the cellular immune response to the three herpes viruses, but not significantly.

Our program of vaccinations with diptheria and tetanus toxoids started in the fourth month post BMT. Chronic GVHD patients who were vaccinated had a clearly impaired cellular immune response to both toxoids as compared with those without chronic GVHD.

Active infections with herpes simplex virus (HSV),* cytomegalovirus (CMV) and varicella zoster virus (VZV) are common after allogeneic bone marrow transplantation (BMT) (*1, 2*) but tend to occur less frequently following autologous BMT (*3*). Usually, the viruses are present in latent form at the time of BMT and subsequently become reactivated (*1*). Active HSV infection occurs mainly in the first month post-BMT, active CMV infection mainly in the second to fourth, and active VZV infection mainly in the fifth to ninth month post-BMT. The depression of cellular immunity after the cytoreductive therapy prior to grafting, which persists particularly after allogeneic BMT, may be the cause of the enhanced incidence and severity of those infections (*4, 5*). Graft-versus-host disease (GVHD) and its associated immunosuppressive therapy further delay the immunologic recovery following allogeneic BMT—and, consequently, also lead to an increased incidence of infections.

Serious and sometimes fatal infections with *Streptococcus pneumoniae* constitute a relatively late complication and usually occur six months or more after allogeneic BMT (*6*). Therefore, a vaccination protocol is used in our allogeneic BMT program, consisting of initial immunization with diphtheria

[1]This work was supported by the Queen Wilhelmina Fund (the Dutch Cancer League) (Grant UUKC-Haem '81) and by the J. A. Cohen Institute for Radiopathology and Radiation Protection (IRS).

[2]Address correspondence to: J. W. Gratama, M.D., Isolation Ward, Bldg. 16, University Medical Center. P.O. Box 9600, 2300 RC Leiden, The Netherlands.
[3] Department of Hematology, University Hospital, Utrecht.
[4] Department of Immunohematology and Blood Bank.
[5] Department of Hematology.

* Abbreviations used: BMT, bone marrow transplantation; CMV, cytomegalovirus; DT, diphtheria toxoid; DTP, diphtheria toxoid, tetanus toxoid, and killed poliomyelitis virus; GVHD, graft-versus-host disease; HSV, herpes simplex virus; PMNC, peripheral blood mononuclear cells; TT, tetanus toxoid; SI, stimulation index; VZV, varicella zoster virus.

toxoid, tetanus toxoid, and killed poliomyelitis virus (DTP)—followed, in the event of a positive antibody response to the initial vaccinations, by immunization with a polyvalent pneumococcal vaccine (Pneumovac).

We studied the recovery of cellular immunity against HSV, CMV, and VZV following autologous and allogeneic BMT, the influence of the cellular immunity of the marrow donors to those viruses on the occurrence of active infections post-BMT, and the immune response following vaccination with DTP. Particular attention was paid to the question of whether or not acute or chronic GVHD influenced those immune responses.

MATERIALS AND METHODS

Patients. Twenty-three recipients of autologous marrow grafts and 23 recipients of allogeneic marrow grafts and their HLA-A, B, C, DR-identical, MLR-nonreactive sibling donors were studied. Only patients with a follow-up of longer than 100 days were included in the study.

All recipients of autologous marrow grafts were acute leukemia patients in their first complete remission (n = 9) or patients with non-Hodgkin's lymphoma of high-grade malignancy, either in complete or partial remission or nonresponsive to chemotherapy (n = 14). All recipients of allogeneic marrow grafts had severe aplastic anemia (n = 3), acute leukemia in first or second complete remission (n = 19), or chronic myelogenous leukemia in its first chronic phase (n = 1).

All marrow graft recipients with leukemia or non-Hodgkin's lymphoma were prepared for transplantation using cyclophosphamide (60 mg/kg/day ×2) and total-body irradiation (8 Gy ×1, with lung shielding after 6 Gy). The three patients with severe aplastic anemia were prepared with cyclophosphamide (50 mg/kg/day ×4) and total-lymphoid irradiation (7.5 Gy ×1, n = 2; 2.0 Gy ×10, n = 1). The patients received a median of 1.8×10^8/kg (range $1.2–2.8\times10^8$) cryopreserved autologous nucleated bone marrow cells or a median of 2.1×10^8/kg (range $1.6–2.5\times10^8$) allogeneic nucleated bone marrow cells.

After allogeneic BMT, all patients received methotrexate as prophylaxis for acute GVHD (*7*). That complication was diagnosed and staged on the basis of the clinical criteria (*8*); in most patients, the diagnosis was confirmd histologically (*9*). Fourteen of the 23 patients developed acute GVHD: grade I in three, grade II, in nine and grade III in two patients. Therapy for acute GVHD consisted of one or more of the following modalities: high-dose methylprednisolone (20 mg/kg/12 hr for 2 days, followed by a rapid taper to zero in most patients [n = 9]), intermediate-dose prednisone (1–2 mg/kg/day for 10–14 days followed by a gradual taper to zero [n = 2]), and monoclonal antibody OKT3.PAN (Ortho Pharmaceutical Co., Raritan, NJ) (5 mg/day for 14 days [n = 4]). Chronic GVHD developed in 11 of the 23 patients; the complication was limited in four patients and extensive in seven. Therapy for chronic GVHD consisted of prednisone (0.3–1.0 mg/kg/day) and azathioprine (1–2 mg/kg/day). Two patients received a 7-day course of OKT3.PAN (5 mg/day).

The diagnosis of active HSV infection was based on clinical symptoms, in most cases confirmed by positive viral cultures. IgG-class antibodies to HSV were determined using an indirect immunofluorescence assay as previously reported (*10*). Active CMV infection was diagnosed on the basis of a four-fold or greater rise in IgG-class antibody titer and/or the occurrence of IgM-class antibodies, in combination with positive viral cultures in some patients. IgM- and IgG-class antibodies against CMV-late antigen were detected using an enzyme-linked immunosorbent assay (*11*). In the allogeneic marrow graft recipients, the interpretation of clinical signs of CMV infection was often hampered by the simultaneous presence of acute GVHD involving the gut and/or liver. The diagnosis of active VZV infection was always made on the basis of clinical symptoms and confirmed by serologic studies in most patients. For the detection of IgG-class VZV antibodies, an indirect immunofluorescence assay was used (*10*).

The DTP vaccinations were carried out as described previously (*1*). Antibodies against DTP were determined before immunization and 14 days after using an in-vivo toxin neutralization technique (*12*). In the event of a negative antibody response, the same procedure was repeated 45–90 days later. When a negative response was obtained again, the procedure was repeated once more. Patients were vaccinated with Pneumovac only when a positive antibody response to DTP was obtained. Prophylactic oral penicillin was given to all patients who had not yet been vaccinated with Pneumovac.

Isolation, preservation, and processing of mononuclear cells. Peripheral-blood mononuclear cells (PMNC) were obtained from heparinized venous blood, from the patients and their marrow donors 14–6 days prior to BMT. PMNC from the patients were also obtained at various times post-BMT. The PMNC of the autologous marrow graft recipients were isolated by Ficoll-Isopaque density gradient centrifugation and tested on the same day. For practical reasons, the PMNC of the allogeneic marrow graft recipients were frozen in RPMI-1640 medium containing 10% dimethylsulphoxide, stored in liquid nitrogen, and thawed prior to use, as described elsewhere (*13*). The cell viability was assessed by staining with trypan blue and was usually greater than 80%. Although the degree of lymphocyte proliferation to virus-infected and noninfected fibroblasts was generally higher in fresh samples than in frozen/thawed ones, their stimulation indices were similar (data not shown).

Lymphocyte stimulation by virus-infected fibroblasts. Cellular immunity to HSV, CMV, and VZV was tested by culturing PMNC with RIV-2 foreskin fibroblasts infected with HSV (type 1 strain MS), CMV (strain AD 169), or VZV (strain ZI 63-1444). The virus-infected fibroblasts were kindly supplied by Dr. A. Hekker (National Institute of Public Health and Environmental Hygiene, Bilthoven, the Netherlands) (*17*). In each experiment, fresh PMNC from a healthy volunteer with immunity to HSV, CMV and/or VZV were used as control. The culture medium consisted of RPMI-1640 medium containing penicillin and streptomycin, 2% glutamine, and 20% pooled human serum. Quadruplicate cultures were set up with 1×10^5 PMNC in round-bottomed microtiter plates in two ratios of PMNC to fibroblasts (1×10^4 and 5×10^3). Low-level control cultures and good stimulation were generally observed with 1×10^5 PMNC and 1×10^4 fibroblasts, and only the results of that ratio were analyzed. On the sixth day of culture, 1 μCi of ^{3}H-thymidine (Radiochemical Centre, Amersham, UK) was added, and the cultures were harvested 8 hr later. For the expression of the results the stimulation index (SI) was used, which is defined as follows:

$$SI = \frac{\text{mean cpm in cultures with virus-infected fibroblasts}}{\text{mean cpm in cultures with non-infected fibroblasts}}$$

An SI of >3 with an increment of at least 1000 cpm was considered positive.

Antigen-induced proliferation. Diphtheria toxoid (DT, 10 LF/

ml) and tetanus toxoid (TT, 10 LF/ml) (National Institute of Public Health and Environmental Hygiene, Bilthoven, the Netherlands) were used in cultures containing 1×10^5 PMNC and incubated for six days. The culture medium consisted of RPMI-1640 medium containing penicillin and streptomycin, 2% glutamine, and 20% pooled human serum. In each experiment, fresh PMNC from a healthy volunteer were used as control. On the last day of culture, 1 μCi of ^{3}H-thymidine was added and the cultures were harvested 8 hr later. For the expression of the the results the SI was used, which is defined as follows:

$$SI = \frac{\text{mean cpm in cultures with DT or TT}}{\text{mean cpm in cultures with culture medium only}}$$

An SI of >3 with an increment of at least 1000 cpm was considered positive.

Statistical analysis. Analysis of the data was performed using Wilcoxon's two-sample test (2-sided) and Fisher's exact test (2-sided).

RESULTS

Herpes simplex virus. Twenty-two of the 23 autologous and 22 of the 23 allogeneic marrow graft recipients had antibodies to HSV prior to BMT. The two seronegative patients did not develop HSV infection. The results of the seropositive patients were analyzed and are set out in Figure 1.

There was a significantly lower incidence of active HSV infection after autologous (2 of 22 patients) than after allogeneic BMT (11 of 22 patients, $P = 0.007$; Fisher's exact test). Prior to BMT, 14 autologous and 11 allogeneic marrow graft recipients had a positive lymphocyte stimulation test to HSV.

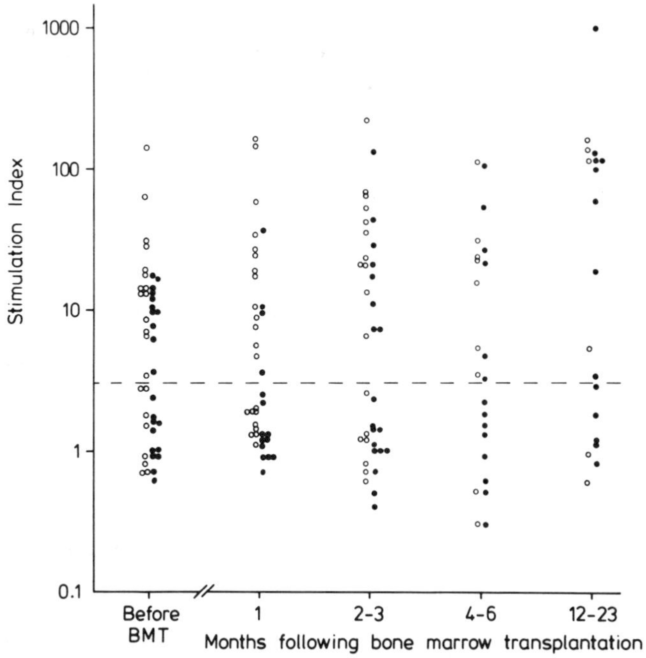

FIGURE 1. Lymphocyte proliferation to HSV-infected fibroblasts. Open circles indicate autologous marrow graft recipients (n = 22); closed circles, allogeneic marrow graft recipients (n = 22). Not all patients were monitored at every time point. A logarithmic scale has been used for the vertical axis in order to compress the figure. The dashed line indicates the cut-off level for positivity. The differences between both patient groups were significant at 1 month post-BMT ($P = 0.008$; Wilcoxon's 2 sample test).

At one month post-BMT, 13 of 22 autologous, but only four of 15 allogeneic marrow graft recipients, had a positive test. Consequently, the degree of lymphocyte proliferation after stimulation with HSV at that time was significantly higher in the autologous (median SI 6.6; range 1.1–157.5) than in the allogeneic (median SI 1.3; range 0.9–38.4) marrow graft recipients ($P = 0.008$; Wilcoxon's 2-sample test). Afterwards, the degree of lymphocyte proliferation to HSV of the allogeneic marrow graft recipients increased to a level that was not significantly different from that of the autologous marrow graft recipients.

The occurrence of GVHD decreased the magnitude of the cellular immune response to HSV in actively infected patients, but not significantly. When monitored at 2–3 months post-BMT, four patients with grades 0-I acute GVHD had a median SI of 17.9 (range 1.0–128.7) and six with grades II-IV had a median SI of 9.5 (range 1.4–43.6). Between 12 and 23 months post-BMT, four patients without chronic GVHD had a median SI of 119.1 (range 97.5–978.0) and four with chronic GVHD had a median SI of 38.4 (range 2.9–113.4).

A positive lymphocyte proliferation test to HSV in BMT recipients or in their marrow donors prior to allogeneic marrow grafting was significantly correlated with the occurrence of active HSV infection in the recipients (Table 1). Of the 11 recipients with active HSV infection post BMT, eight had prior to BMT a positive lymphocyte proliferation test after stimulation with HSV, whereas only two of the 11 without active HSV infection had a positive test ($P = 0.03$, Fisher's exact test). Eight of the 11 patients with active HSV infection received marrow from donors with a positive test, whereas only one of the 11 patients without active HSV infection had a donor with a positive test ($P = 0.008$, Fisher's exact test).

Cytomegalovirus. Twelve of the 23 autologous and 10 of the 23 allogeneic marrow graft recipients had antibodies to CMV prior to BMT. None of the seronegative patients developed CMV infection. The results of the seropositive patients were analyzed and are set out in Figure 2.

There was a significantly lower incidence of active CMV infection after autologous (4 of 12 patients) than after allogeneic BMT (9 of 10 patients, $P = 0.02$; Fisher's exact test). Prior to BMT, seven autologous and five allogeneic marrow graft recipients had a positive lymphocyte proliferation test after

TABLE 1. Pretransplant cellular immunity and posttransplant active infection in allogeneic marrow graft recipients

Virus	Pretransplant cellular immunity[a]		Posttransplant active infection[b]	
	Recipient	Donor	No	Yes
HSV	−	−	9	1
	−	+	0	2
	+	−	1	2
	+	+	1	6
CMV	−	−	1	2
	−	+	0	2
	+	−	0	4
	+	+	0	1
VZV	−	−	4	5
	−	+	4	1
	+	−	1	2
	+	+	3	3

[a] (− or +) negative or positive lymphocyte proliferation test.
[b] Number of patients.

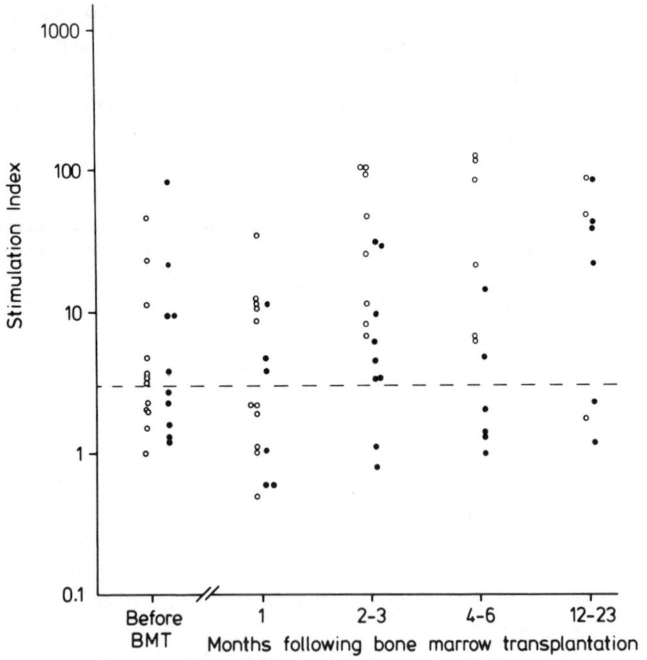

FIGURE 2. Lymphocyte proliferation to CMV-infected fibroblasts. Open circles indicate autologous marrow graft recipients (n = 12); closed circles, allogeneic marrow graft recipients (n = 10). For further details, see the legend for Figure 1. The differences between both patient groups were significant at 2–3 and 4–6 months post-BMT (P = 0.01 on both occasions; Wilcoxon's 2-sample test).

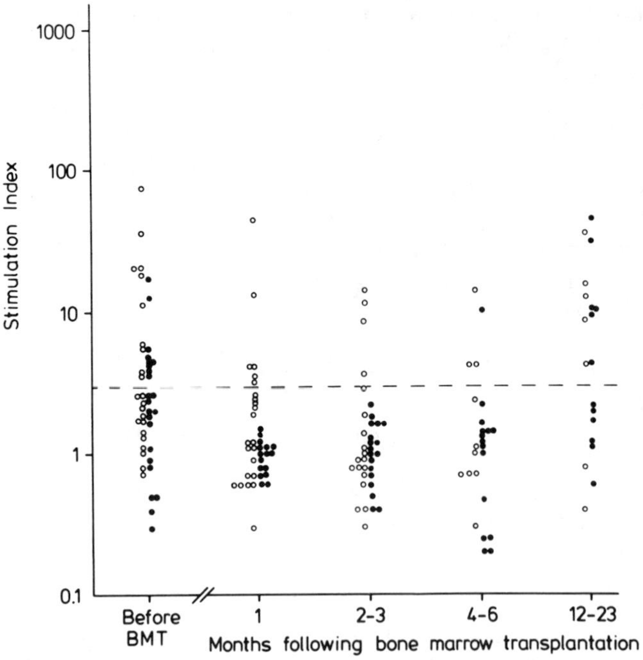

FIGURE 3. Lymphocyte proliferation to VZV-infected fibroblasts. Open circles indicate autologous marrow graft recipients (n = 23); closed circles, allogeneic marrow graft recipients (n = 23). For further details, see the legend for Figure 1. The differences between both patient groups were not significant.

stimulation with CMV. During the first six months following BMT, the degree of lymphocyte proliferation after stimulation with CMV increased at a faster rate and to higher levels in the autologous than in the allogeneic marrow graft recipients. The difference between both groups reached significance between two and six months post-BMT ($P = 0.01$, Wilcoxon's 2-sample test). The level of cellular immune responsiveness to CMV was similar in the actively infected patients with grades 0-I and those with grades II-IV acute GVHD; chronic GVHD caused a nonsignificant decrease (data not shown).

The presence of a positive lymphocyte proliferation test after stimulation with CMV prior to autologous BMT did not significantly correlate with the occurrence of active CMV infection post BMT: two of the four patients with active CMV infection and five of the eight patients without had a positive test prior to BMT. The influence of a positive test prior to allogeneic BMT could not be analyzed due to the low number of patients, in particular those without active CMV infection (Table 1).

Varicella zoster virus. All 23 autologous and all 23 allogeneic marrow graft recipients had antibodies to VZV prior to BMT, and their results are set out in Figure 3.

There was a significantly lower incidence of active VZV infection after autologous (3 of 23 patients) than after allogeneic BMT (11 of 23 patients, $P = 0.02$; Fisher's exact test). Prior to BMT, 10 autologous and 19 allogeneic marrow graft recipients had a positive lymphocyte proliferation test after stimulation with VZV. During the first six months following BMT positive reactions were observed in six autologous marrow graft recipients and in only one allogeneic marrow graft recipient. Between 12 and 23 months post-BMT, five of the seven autologous and six of the 12 allogeneic marrow graft recipients had developed a positive test. Because of the relatively late occurrence of active VZV infections, acute GVHD is not relevant. Chronic GVHD caused a nonsignificant decrease of the cellular response to VZV, just as it did for CMV (data not shown).

The presence of a positive lymphocyte proliferation test after stimulation with VZV prior to autologous BMT did not correlate significantly with the occurrence of active VZV infection post BMT: two of the three patients with active VZV infection and eight of the 20 patients without had a positive test prior to BMT. There was also no significant correlation between a positive test prior to allogeneic BMT, in the recipients or in the donors, and the occurrence of active VZV infection post-BMT (Table 1).

Immunity to DT and TT. Before BMT, the lymphocyte proliferation tests with DT were positive for 10 donors and six recipients, and the tests with TT were positive for 18 donors and 13 recipients. During the first three months after BMT, all DT and TT tests were negative. Seven of the 23 patients received no vaccinations because of their poor clinical condition. Their main clinical problem was severe chronic GVHD. For two patients, the immunologic follow-up studies were too brief to allow proper analysis. The remaining 14 patients could be evaluated with respect to their immune response against vaccination with DTP.

Seven patients showed a cellular response to DT, and in six of them the SIs ultimately exceeded 5.0. The same seven patients also showed a humoral response. Two of the seven patients who did not show a cellular response to DT had an increase in diphtheria antibodies (Table 2). Ten patients showed a cellular response to TT with all SIs ultimately exceeding 5.0. All 10 patients also had a humoral response to TT. Only one of the three patients who did not show a cellular response to TT had an increase in tetanus antibodies. The

TABLE 2. Immune reactivity to diphtheria toxoid and tetanus toxoid

Chronic GVHD	Number[b]	Diphtheria toxoid[a]				Tetanus toxoid[a]			
		Cellular		Humoral		Cellular		Humoral	
		+	−	+	−	+	−	+	−
−	9	6	3	6	3	9	0	8	1
+	5	1	4	3	2	1	4	3	2
Fisher's exact P		0.27				0.01			

[a] Number of patients with a positive or negative response to DT or TT after vaccination with DTP.
[b] Number of patients.

absence of a cellular response to TT was significantly associated with chronic GVHD (Table 2) ($P = 0.01$, Fisher's exact test).

DISCUSSION

Opportunistic infections, such as those caused by herpesviruses, are a major cause of morbidity and mortality after BMT. These infections seem to result mainly from the profound immune deficiency that develops after the cytoreductive therapy prior to BMT. Although such infections are more common in allogeneic than in autologous BMT recipients, in vivo and in vitro studies of that immune deficiency yielded similar results independent of the type of graft (*14–17*).

Our results in allogeneic marrow graft recipients are similar to those reported previously (*18–20*): recovery of lymphocyte proliferation to herpesviruses post-BMT is related to the occurrence of active infection. However, in autologous marrow graft recipients, such lymphocyte proliferation could often be demonstrated in the absence of active infection. In addition, the degree of lymphocyte proliferation in the autologous marrow graft recipients was generally higher than in the allogeneic recipients. There may be some reactivation of herpesviruses following autologous BMT, leading to increases in lymphocyte proliferation. That degree of reactivation does not meet our criteria for *active* infection—i.e., the demonstration of virus by culture, the presence of clinical signs, a four-fold or greater rise in IgG-class antibody titer, and/or the occurrence of IgM-class antibodies. We suggest that a rapid restoration of cellular immunity to HSV and CMV (and, to a lesser extent, VZV) may have contributed to the prevention of active infections. Such a phenomenon has recently been reported for CMV infection following renal allografting (*21*). However, the recovery of lymphocyte proliferation to CMV in allogeneic marrow graft recipients is not significantly correlated with a favorable outcome of active CMV infection (*5, 19*), but the presence of cytotoxic T lymphocytes specific for CMV has been shown to be (*5*).

Immunity to herpesviruses transmitted with the bone marrow graft may prevent reactivation of those viruses. That mechanism may be responsible for the low incidence of herpes virus reactivations after autologous BMT, since the regeneration of T cells in those patients is mainly due to proliferation of mature T cells in the graft (*22*). In patients who are seropositive for a given virus, those T cells confer immunity to that virus. Therefore, we also studied the cellular immunity of the donors of allogeneic marrow grafts, but we did not observe such phenomenon. In contrast, the presence of cellular immunity to HSV in the marrow donors was significantly associated with an increased incidence of active infection in their recipients. We suggest that a combination of the cytoreductive therapy prior to grafting (*23*) and an allogeneic effect (i.e., the recognition by mature donor T lymphocytes of minor histocompatibility antigenic differences [*24*]) are capable of inducing HSV reactivation. That phenomenon may be amplified when donor T lymphocytes immune for HSV recognize HSV-associated membrane determinants on infected cells.

The reactivity against fibroblasts infected with HSV, CMV, or VZV was not significantly affected by the occurrence of acute and chronic GVHD in patients with active infection. However, we emphasize that only patients who survived longer than 100 days were included in this study; patients who died before that time—e.g., from severe GVHD—may well have had impaired reactivity against these viruses. The occurrence of chronic GVHD had no significant influence on humoral responsiveness, but negatively influenced cellular reactivity against DT and TT.

The discrepancy between reactivity to HSV, CMV, and VZV and that to DT and TT may be explained by the hypothesis that those reactivating viruses present a much stronger antigenic challenge than DT or TT, with respect to amount and time of exposure. Noel et al. (*25*) reported that the ability to induce sensibilization to dinitrochlorobenzene was delayed in patients with chronic GVHD. Winston et al. (*26*) found a significant association between a poor antibody response to streptococcal vaccine and corticosteroid therapy for GVHD. Most of our patients with chronic GVHD were treated with corticosteroids and azathioprine.

In conclusion, the results of this study suggest that the cellular immunity against herpesviruses recovers at the fastest rate following autologous BMT, and at a slower rate following allogeneic BMT. The rate of recovery may be further affected by the occurrence of acute and chronic GVHD. Chronic GVHD particularly affects cellular immune reactivity against antigens with a limited presentation to the immune system, such as in vaccinations, as compared with those that are present for a prolonged period, such as reactivated herpesviruses.

Acknowledgments. We thank Ms. J. Blom and Ms. B. van Strijen for technical assistance, and Ms. M. L. Stokman and Ms. I. Curiël for secretarial help.

REFERENCES

1. Van der Meer JWM, Guiot HFL, Van den Broek PJ, Van Furth R. Infections in bone marrow transplant recipients. Sem Hematol 1984; 21: 123.
2. Meyers JD, Atkinson K. Infection in bone marrow transplantation. Clin Hematol 1983; 12: 791.
3. Verdonck LF, Dekker AW, Van Kempen L, et al. Intensive cytotoxic therapy followed by autologous bone marrow transplantation for non-Hodgkin lymphoma of high grade malignancy. Blood 1985; 65: 984.
4. Hirsch MS. Pathogenesis of viral infections. In: Galasso GJ, et al, eds. Antiviral agents and viral diseases of man, 2nd ed. New York: Raven Press, 1985: 35.
5. Quinnan GV Jr, Kirmani N, Rook AH, et al. Cytotoxic T cells in cytomegalovirus infection. HLA-restricted T-lymphocyte and non-T-lymphocyte cytotoxic responses correlate with recovery from cytomegalovirus infection in bone marrow transplant recipients. N Engl J Med 1982; 307: 7.
6. Winston DJ, Schiffman G, Wang DC, et al. Pneumococcal infections after human bone marrow transplantation. Ann Intern Med 1979; 91: 835.
7. Thomas ED, Buckner CD, Rudolph RH, et al. Allogeneic marrow

grafting for hematologic malignancy using HL-A matched donor-recipient sibling pairs. Blood 1971; 38: 267.
8. Thomas ED, Storb R, Clift RA, et al. Bone marrow transplantation. N Engl J Med 1975; 292: 832.
9. Glucksberg H, Storb R, Fefer A, et al. Clinical manifestations of graft-versus-host disease in human recipients of marrow from HLA-matched sibling donors. Transplantation 1974; 18: 295.
10. Hekker AC, Brand-Saathof B, Meijers RC. Indirect immunofluorescence test for detection of IgM antibodies to cytomegalovirus. J Infect Dis 1979; 140: 596.
11. Middeldorp JM, Jongsma J, Ter Haar A, Schirm J, The TH. Conditions for the detection of IgM and IgG antibodies against cytomegalovirus early and late antigens by ELISA. J Clin Microbiol 1984; 20: 763.
12. Van Ramshorst JD. Titration of diphtheria and tetanus antitoxins in sera of low titers. Bull WHO 1971; 45: 213.
13. Gratama JW, Lipovich-Oosterveer MA, Ronteltap C, et al. Natural immunity and graft-versus-host disease. Transplantation 1985; 40: 256.
14. Witherspoon RP, Storb R, Ochs HD, et al. Recovery of antibody production in human allogeneic marrow graft recipients: influence of time posttransplantation, the presence or absence of chronic graft-versus-host disease and antithymocyte globulin treatment. Blood 1981; 58: 360.
15. Witherspoon RP, Lum LF, Storb R, Thomas ED. In vitro regulation of immunoglobulin synthesis after human marrow transplantation. II. Deficient T and non-T lymphocyte function within 3–4 months of allogeneic, syngeneic or autologous marrow grafting for hematologic malignancy. Blood 1982; 59: 844.
16. Atkinson K, Hansen JA, Storb R, Goehle S, Goldstein G, Thomas ED. T-cell subpopulations identified by monoclonal antibodies after human marrow transplantation. I. Helper-inducer and cytotoxic-suppressor subsets. Blood 1982; 59: 1292.
17. Witherspoon RP, Matthews D, Storb R, et al. Recovery of in vivo cellular immunity after human marrow grafting: influence of time postgrafting and acute graft-versus-host disease. Transplantation 1984; 37: 145.
18. Meyers JD, Flournoy N, Thomas ED. Infection with herpes simplex virus and cell-mediated immunity after marrow transplant. J Infect Dis 1980; 142: 338.
19. Meyers JD, Flournoy N, Thomas ED. Cytomegalovirus infection and specific cell-mediated immunity after marrow transplant. J Infect Dis 1980; 142: 816.
20. Meyers JD, Flournoy N, Thomas ED. Cell-mediated immunity to varicella-zoster virus after allogeneic marrow transplant. J Infect Dis 1980; 141: 479.
21. Roenhorst HW, Middeldorp JM, Beelen JM, Schirm J, Tegzess AM, The TH. Maintenance of cytomegalovirus (CMV) latency and host immune responses of long-term renal allograft survivors. I. Prolonged suppression of in vitro lymphocyte responses against CMV-infected fibroblasts related to previous secondary CMV infection. Clin Exp Immunol 1985; 59: 709.
22. De Gast GC, Verdonck LF. Middeldorp JM, et al. Recovery of T cell subsets after autologous bone marrow transplantation is mainly due to proliferation of mature T cells in the graft. Blood 1985; 66: 428.
23. Lam MT, Pazin GJ, Armstrong JA, Ho M. Herpes simplex infection in acute myelogenous leukemia and other hematologic malignancies: a prospective study. Cancer 1981; 48: 2168.
24. Goulmy, E, Gratama JW, Blokland E, Zwaan FE, Van Rood JJ. A minor transplantation antigen detected by MHC-restricted cytotoxic T lymphocytes during graft-versus-host disease. Nature 1983; 302: 159.
25. Noel DR, Witherspoon RP, Storb R, et al. Does graft-versus-host disease influence the tempo of immunologic recovery after allogeneic human marrow transplantation? An observation on 56 long-term survivors. Blood 1978; 51: 1087.
26. Winston DJ, Ho WG, Schiffman G, Champlin RE, Feig SA, Gale RP. Pneumococcal vaccination of recipients of bone marrow transplants. Arch Intern Med 1984; 143: 1735.

Received 14 June 1985.
Accepted 8 October 1985.

0041-1337/86/4106-0725$02.00/0
TRANSPLANTATION
Vol. 41, No. 6

Printed in U.S.A.

INFECTIONS IN HEART-LUNG TRANSPLANT RECIPIENTS[1]

J. STEPHEN DUMMER,[2] CARLOS G. MONTERO, BARTLEY P. GRIFFITH, ROBERT L. HARDESTY, IRVIN L. PARADIS, AND MONTO HO

The Department of Infectious Diseases and Microbiology, Graduate School of Public Health, and the Departments of Surgery and Medicine, University of Pittsburgh School of Medicine, Pittsburgh, Pennsylvania

Infectious episodes were analyzed in 14 heart-lung transplant recipients who survived more than one week after transplantation. These patients had higher rates of infection than heart transplant recipients at our institution ($P<0.01$) and greater than 90% of all infections were potentially life-threatening. A total of 67% of all infections involved the lung or thoracic cavity as a primary site, and most of the rest were disseminated viral or fungal infections. *Pneumocystis carinii* infections occurred in six patients and were more common in this group than in patients who received heart transplants in the same period ($P<0.005$). Two patients followed more than one year developed a syndrome of chronic sputum production and bronchial colonization with *Pseudomonas aeruginosa*, which required recurrent treatment with i.v. antibiotics for symptomatic relief. The high rate of pulmonary infections in these patients presents a challenge to clinical management, and suggests that intensive and invasive monitoring for pulmonary infection is desirable.

Clinical heart-lung transplantation was first performed in 1968 (*1*), but early results were discouraging and the operation was abandoned until 1981. It was reintroduced in 1981 as part of the heart transplant program at Stanford University with cyclosporine (CsA)* as the main immunosuppressive drug (*2*). Early clinical results were encouraging, and long-term survival has been achieved (*3*). Our own heart-lung transplant program commenced in 1981 and 18 patients have now received 19 heart-lung allografts. We have a growing experience in the postoperative management of these patients and have found that the diagnosis and treatment of their infectious complications is a major challenge, even for clinicians experienced with transplant patients. A number of new problems have emerged, including a syndrome unique to transplant patients, chronic *Pseudomonas* bronchitis.

This article describes our early experience with the infectious complications of these heart-lung recipients, compares these complications with those of heart transplant patients at our institution, and makes recommendations for future modes of management and treatment.

[1]This work was supported in part by N.I.H. Grant 1 R01 AI 19377.

[2]Requests for reprints should be addressed to J. Stephen Dummer, M.D., A428 Crabtree Hall, Graduate School of Public Health, University of Pittsburgh, Pittsburgh, PA 15261.

* Abbreviations used: BAL, bronchoalveolar lavage; CMV, cytomegalovirus; CsA, cyclosporine; EBV, Epstein-Barr virus; EBV-VCA, Epstein-Barr viral capsid antigen; ELISA, enzyme-linked immunosorbent assay; HSV, herpes simplex virus; HTLV III, human T cell leukemia virus III; PCP, *Pneumocystis carinii* pneumonia; RATG, rabbit antithymocyte globulin; RIA, radioimmunoassay.

MATERIALS AND METHODS

Recipients. Of 18 patients transplanted, six transplant recipients had primary pulmonary hypertension (1°PH), six had secondary pulmonary hypertension (2°PH), and six had diffuse parenchymal disease. The latter diagnosis encompassed ailments such as emphysema (3), cystic fibrosis (1), pulmonary sarcoidosis (1), and eosinophilic granuloma (1). All patients were in end-stage cardiopulmonary failure, and three required some form of ionotropic support preoperatively.

Donors. Donors were matched by body size and ABO blood type. Thirteen allografts were harvested in an adjacent room. Six allografts were harvested at distant sites, one with cold saline flush for preservation, and the other five via a self-perfusing heart-lung graft. The experimental technique for the latter has been previously described (*4*).

Immunosuppression. All patients received CsA preoperatively (17 mg/kg) and 1 g methylprednisolone before weaning off bypass. Postoperatively, cyclosporine was tapered according to clinical criteria, and more recently by targeting whole blood levels of cyclosporine of 800–1000 ng/ml (radioimmunoassay (RIA) Sandoz kit). Methylprednisolone (125 mg) was given postoperatively every 8 hr for 3 doses. Steroids were withheld during the first two postoperative weeks, after which prednisone was introduced at maintenance doses (20 mg/day). During the first two weeks the patients received a 3–5-day course of rabbit antithymocyte globulin (RATG), 100 mg i.m./day. Azathioprine was also used for the first five patients in this series at 2–3 mg/kg/day during their first two postoperative weeks. Rejection episodes of the heart or lung were treated with three daily doses of methylprednisolone—or, if they were severe or persistent, with RATG 100 mg/day for three days.

Infections. Each episode of infection required the isolation of one or more pathogens in association with clinical abnormalities suggesting infection, such as fever, purulent drainage, or roentgenographic abnormalities. Recovery of multiple bacterial species from the same site—if present in large numbers—was listed as mixed infection. Isolations of different classes of organisms (i.e., bacteria and fungi) were always counted as separate episodes, even if obtained from the same site.

Thrush, minor afebrile upper respiratory infections, and catheter-associated bacteruria and candiduria were not counted. Two patients developed chronic bronchopulmonary infections with *Pseudomonas aeruginosa.* These were recorded as single infections, even though their treatment required multiple hospitalizations. Surveillance cultures were routinely performed on urine, throat washes, and buffy coat samples for herpes simplex virus (HSV) and cytomegalovirus (CMV) every two weeks during the first 8 postoperative weeks, then every 1–2 months for the next 6–10 months. Serum samples were obtained, when possible, from recipients and donors prior to the transplant operation and from recipients at monthly intervals after transplantation. CMV serologies on pretransplant and donor sera were initially performed by anti-complement immunofluorescence as previously described (5); more recently the presence or absence of CMV antibody was determined with a solid-phase immunoassay for IgG antibody to CMV (FIAX, International Diagnostic Technology, Santa Clara, CA). Titers of IgG antibodies to Epstein-Barr viral capsid antigen (EBV-VCA) were determined for pretransplant and posttransplant sera by immunofluorescence (*6*). Titers of IgG antibody to Human T cell leukemia virus III (HTLV III) were determined on sera from one patient by enzyme-linked immunosorbent assay (Litton Bionetics, Charleston, SC).

Viral syndromes caused by CMV were defined as the occurrence of fever over 38.0°C constantly or intermittently for at least one week in association with positive CMV cultures, and at least one other manifestation of CMV illness, including atypical lymphocytes greater than 3%, hepatitis with SGOT serum glutamic oxaloacetic transaminase greater than 40 IU, leukopenia less than 4000 WBC, or thrombocytopenia less than 100,000 platelets. Viral syndromes resulting from EBV were diagnosed if CMV cultures were negative and there was also a significant (≥4-fold) rise in antibody to EBV-VCA in a symptomatic patient. The finding of EBV nuclear antigen staining by immunofluorescence or EBV nucleic acid by nucleic acid hybridization in lymphoid tissue was taken as strong independent evidence of EBV infection.

RESULTS

Of the 18 patients transplanted, four died during the first week after transplantation and none of these four patients had an infection. Fourteen patients survived more than 30 days and were analyzed for infectious complications. These patients are listed in Table 1 with their sex, age, preoperative diagnosis, number of infections of each pathogen type, clinical follow-up, and number of episodes of biopsy-proved cardiac rejection. The average follow-up in these patients was 265 days (range: 33–874 days) and the mean age, 31 years (range: 19–45). The male:female ratio was 1:1.

Of these patients, 50% (7/14) had one or more episodes of biopsy-proved rejection. There was no significant difference in infection rate related to diagnosis, age, or incidence of cardiac rejection. There was a higher number of infections in male patients but this was thought to be related to longer follow-up in male patients.

Overall, 42 infections were recorded in the fourteen patients, for a mean incidence of 3.0 infections/pt. This was almost double the frequency of infections reported by us in 33 heart transplant patients with a similar mean follow-up time (277 days) (*7*). Statistical analysis of the two series shows the heart-lung recipient infection rate to be significantly higher ($P<0.02$; *t* test). Only two patients remained free of infection in the follow-up period (pts. 8, 14). All 12 infected patients had at least one infection that was potentially life-threatening, and all but three infections were life-threatening. Indeed, all seven deaths were associated with infection, although bleeding, severe lung rejection and neurological injury played a significant role in three patients (pts. 4, 5, 13). The pathogens causing infection are listed in Table 2. Bacterial isolates accounted for 50% of all infections and most isolates were enterobacteriaceae, *Pseudomonas*, or staphylococcal species. A sternal wound infection (pt. 13) was caused by a microaerophilic *Mycoplasma* species. The organism was isolated in pure culture from multiple operative cultures, as well as from chest tubes postoperatively. The infection was successfully treated with antibiotics, extensive debridement, and interposition of a pectoral muscle flap, but the muscle graft became superinfected with *Staphylococcus aureus* three weeks later in the context of intense immunosuppression for persistent severe heart and lung rejection. This unusual infection is being presented in greater detail elsewhere.[3]

Symptomatic viral infections were a significant cause of morbidity in the early part of the series, but were not seen in the last seven patients. CMV infections documented by culture occurred in nine of the 14 patients (64%) and included four primary infections, four reactivation infections, and one infection in which no pretransplant serum was available. Of these nine patients, five (55%) were symptomatic and four (44%) had histological or cultural evidence of CMV in lung tissue.

Seven of 13 patients had significant EBV antibody rises to VCA, and definite symptomatic EBV infection occurred in two patients with primary EBV infections and lymphoproliferative lesions. Both had evidence of EBV in tumor tissue by nucleic acid hybridization. These cases have been reported as part of a series of EBV lymphomas at our center (*8*). Symptomatic mucocutaneous HSV infection occurred in one patient. Adenovirus was isolated from a bronchoalveolar lavage (BAL) of a patient with *Pneumocystis* and staphylococcal pneumonia, but definite evidence of viral infection of the lung was lacking.

The higher incidence of symptomatic viral infection in the early patients appeared to be related to the large number of patients with primary viral infections (5/7) in this group. Only one of the second seven patients transplanted had a primary viral infection (EBV). She died 123 days after transplantation with other infections that may have obscured a viral syndrome. The additional use of azathioprine in the first five patients may have also contributed to the high rate of symptomatic viral illness in the early patients. The impact of receiving an allograft from a donor with serological evidence of past CMV infection could not be adequately evaluated because of the small number of such patients. There were six seronegative patients with available donor sera, and CMV infection occurred in two of three patients with seropositive donors and in one of three patients with seronegative donors.

Five fungal infections occurred in four patients, and included three cases of invasive *Candida* infection. These *Candida* infections occurred in critically ill patients who had received broad spectrum antibiotics in the intensive care unit. One of the patients with candida infections also had small foci of pulmonary aspergillosis discovered at autopsy. Another patient had disseminated cryptococcosis 144 days posttransplant. All four patients died. The rate of fungal infections in the heart-lung recipients (4/18; 22%) was higher than the rate of fungal infections in 92 adults who received heart transplants during the same period (1982–1984) (5/92; 5%), but the comparison was of borderline significance ($0.05<P<0.1$, χ^2-Yates).

Protozoal infections were found in seven patients (50%). Six patients had seven episodes of *Pneumocystis carinii* pneumonia (PCP), and one had reactivated toxoplasmosis discovered at autopsy. The diagnosis of PCP was made from lung tissue

[3]This work was supported by Steffensen DO, Dummer JS, Granick MS, Pasculle AW, Griffith BP, Cassell GH. Mycoplasma hominis median sternotomy infections. (Submitted for publication).

TABLE 1. Infections and rejection episodes in heart-lung transplant patients

Patient	Sex/age	Dx[a]	Infections				Rejection episodes[b]	Follow-up (days)	Outcome[c]
			Bacterial	Viral	Fungal	Protozoal			
1	M/28	1PH	2[d]	1	0	0	2	874	a/w
2	F/41	DPD	1	0	2	1	0	33	+
3	M/19	1PH	2	2	1	0	0	144	+
4	F/44	DPD	1	1	0	0	5	72	+
5	M/21	2PH	3[d]	2	0	1	4	575	+
6	M/24	DPD	1	1	1	0	2	52	+
7	M/26	DPD	2	1	0	1	0	442	a/w
8	F/40	2PH	0	0	0	0	0	343	a/w
9	M/30	2PH	2	0	0	2	2	245	+
10	F/22	1PH	1	0	0	1	0	272	a/w
11	F/36	2PH	2	0	0	1	0	271	a/w
12	M/45	1PH	1	0	0	1	0	200	a/w
13	F/30	1PH	3	0	1	0	3	71	+
14	F/28	2PH	0	0	0	0	0	123	a/w

[a] Diagnosis: 1PH (primary pulmonary hypertension); 2PH (secondary pulmonary hypertension), DPD (diffuse parenchymal disease).
[b] By endomyocardial biopsy, moderate or severe rejection.
[c] a/w (alive and well); + (death).
[d] These patients had chronic *Pseudomonas* bronchitis.

TABLE 2. Pathogens in heart/lung transplant infections

Pathogen	Number	% Infections
Bacterial:	21	50%
Gram+		
Staphylococcus sp.	6	
Gram−		
Pseudomonas sp.	4	
Escherichia coli	2	
Enterobacter	1	
Acinetobacter	1	
H influenzae	1	
Mixed flora	5	
Mycoplasma	1	
Viral:[a]	8	19%
HSV	1	
CMV	5	
EBV	2	
Protozoal:	8	19%
P carinii	7	
Toxoplasma	1	
Fungal:	5	12%
Candida	3	
Cryptococcus	1	
Aspergillus	1	
Total	42	100%

[a] HSV (herpes simplex virus); CMV (cytomegalovirus); EBV (Epstein-Barr virus).

samples in two cases and by BAL in five cases. The episodes occurred between three and 19 months after transplantation. The severity of illness varied considerably from fatal disease in one patient to minimally symptomatic disease in two. The latter patients had normal chest roentgenograms, and the diagnoses were made unexpectedly by routine BAL. The death due to *Pneumocystis* occurred in a patient who had been treated successfully for *Pneumocystis* pneumonia five months after transplantation but relapsed three months later and did not then respond to i.v. sulfamethoxazole-trimethoprim or pentamadine. We had not previously seen a relapse of *Pneumocystis* pneumonia after successful treatment in a transplant patient, although relapses are common in patients with the acquired immunodeficiency syndrome (*9*). IgG antibody to HTLV III was not found in this patient's sera taken 4 and 8 months after transplantation.

A comparison between *Pneumocystis* infection rates in heart and heart-lung transplant patients in 1982–1984 illustrates a high susceptibility to this pathogen in the latter group. Six (33%) of 18 heart-lung transplant recipients developed *Pneumocystis* pneumonia during this period, while the diagnosis was made in only 5 (5%) of 92 heart recipients ($P<0.005$; χ^2-Yates). The comparison remained significant even when four heart recipients who received high-dose sulfamethoxazole-trimethoprim for possible but not proved *Pneumocystis* infection were included in the analysis.

The diagnosis of pulmonary infection was problematic in the early posttransplant period. In the first 1–2 weeks after transplantation neutrophils were regularly found in tracheal secretions, often in association with bacteria. The differentiation among bronchitis, pneumonia, rejection, and a postimplantation response in the lung was therefore difficult. Our policy was to administer specific antibiotics to all patients who had had an infiltrate seen on chest roentgenogram and/or lack of steady improvement in arterial blood oxygen saturation.

Figure 1 gives the infection rates in the heart-lung recipients in relation to the time after transplant. The rates are corrected for the number of patients followed in each interval and normalized to one-year rates. The figure shows high infection rates in both the first and second three-month intervals after transplantation with a rapid decline to much lower, but still significant, infection rates thereafter. Viral and fungal infections were only seen in the first six months and only one case of protozoal infection (toxoplasmosis) occurred in the first three-month interval.

Infections after 360 days were seen in two patients (of three followed). Both patients developed bronchial colonization with *P aeruginosa* (mucoid and nonmucoid strains) that led to chronic sputum production and dyspnea. Both patients had multiple exacerbations, usually afebrile, requiring hospitalization for antibiotic therapy. A response to antipseudomonal antibiotics was seen, but the patients never became completely

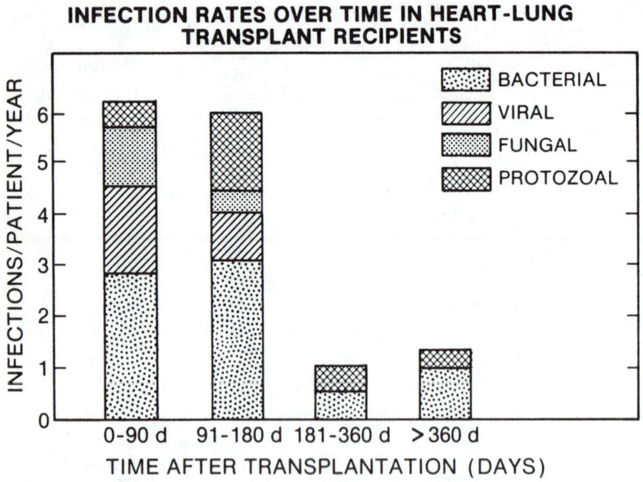

FIGURE 1. Infection rates over time in heart-lung transplant recipients. The infection rates are normalized to one-year rates for each interval.

asymptomatic between treatments. This syndrome, clinically similar to pulmonary cystic fibrosis or chronic bronchiectasis, caused mild-to-moderate disability in one patient and severe disability in the other. Chest roentgenograms in both patients showed an increase in lung markings that was stable over many months. There was no definite radiographic evidence of bronchiectasis, and bronchograms were not performed.

The site of infection was also investigated in these heart-lung recipients. A total of 67% of all infections occurred in the transplanted lung as a primary site, and 24% (all viral or fungal infections) were disseminated. Three infections (7%) involved the skin or mucocutaneous regions, and one patient developed an abdominal abscess at the site of a small bowel perforation during regression of a lymphoproliferative lesion involving the bowel wall. The relative frequency of lung infection in this group exceeds that in the other solid organ transplant groups at our institution (*10*).

DISCUSSION

Although a small number of heart-lung transplants have been done at our center, these represent a substantial portion of the world-wide experience. This and our intensive monitoring for infections allow us to make a preliminary statement about the infectious complications attendant upon this operation.

The sheer number of infections in this group presents a formidable problem in postoperative management. The average patient had three infections in the first six months after transplantation, and these were (in over 90% of the cases) potentially life-threatening. The finding that all seven patients who died after the early postoperative period had associated infections testifies to the severity of these infections. In contrast, infection accounts for only about half of all deaths in heart transplant patients (*7, 11*).

A total of 67% of all infections occurred primarily in the chest. Although we documented three pleural space infections and one case of mediastinitis, most cases were pneumonia caused by a broad range of pathogens. The chest was also an important site of involvement in seven of the ten cases of disseminated infection. Thus, the transplanted lung appears to be uniquely susceptible to infection. The reasons for this are likely to be multiple and include denervation (suppressing cough), early ischemia, lymphatic interruption, injury resulting from acute and chronic rejection, and, possibly, transmission of infectious agents such as CMV with the lung transplant, followed by reactivation in situ.

A brief report appearing from Stanford suggests that they have encountered similar infectious problems in their heart-lung transplant series and have also documented the primacy of the lung as a site of infection (*12*). However, not enough information is available to make a thorough comparison.

Serial bronchoalveolar lavages were introduced in July 1984 as part of a routine monitoring system for these patients. They have provided detailed microbiological information from the tracheobronchial tree—and, as noted by others, have been particularly useful in making a rapid, and at times early, diagnosis of *P carinii* pneumonia (*13*). Gryzan et al. note that cell counts and differentials of the pulmonary lavage fluid in heart-lung recipients were able to distinguish patients with rejection or infection in the lung from patients without either process, but they were less useful in distinguishing rejection from infection (*14*). Fortunately, microbiological stains and cultures, together with heart biopsies and attention to the clinical course of the patients and their chest radiographs, usually helped make that distinction. In difficult cases lung biopsies were performed (seven biopsies in five patients). In five of these cases, the biopsy was helpful or diagnostic, in one case it was not helpful, and in one case it was misleading. The latter patient had a lymphocytic interstitial infiltrate that was initially thought to represent rejection but was later found to represent CMV infection.

Viral infections were a significant source of morbidity in six patients, and included two cases of EBV-induced lymphoproliferative syndrome and five cases of symptomatic CMV infection, four of them involving the lung. We previously found that rates of symptomatic CMV infection and CMV pneumonia in heart-lung recipients were significantly higher than those in heart transplant recipients at our institution (*15*). This was ascribed to a high rate of primary CMV infection in the early heart-lung recipients. Follow-up of more heart-lung recipients should show whether they have a unique predisposition to viral infections.

Fungal infections were seen in four patients, always in the context of other serious illness, especially bacterial infections requiring broad-spectrum antibiotics. All patients with fungal infection died, but the fungal infection was not the sole cause of death in any patient. Although the rates of fungal infection were higher than in our heart transplant patients, the comparison was of borderline significance.

P carinii infection occurred in six patients; it was minimally symptomatic in two patients, but three patients were seriously ill, and one patient had recurrent disease that was fatal. The rates of disease were higher than in heart transplant patients who underwent transplant operations in the same period. This suggests an enhanced vulnerability to *Pneumocystis* infection in heart-lung recipients. The reasons for this are obscure, and little is known about the epidemiology and immunology of *Pneumocystis* infection in humans. We think all heart-lung recipients should receive sulfamethoxazole-trimethoprim as prophylaxis for *Pneumocystis* infection until better means are found to identify patients at risk for the infection.

The most interesting and the most worrisome infectious complication was chronic relapsing *Pseudomonas* bronchitis seen in two patients. Both cases had their onset more than a year after the transplant operation, and since we have only followed one other patient one year or more, it is not clear how frequent this condition will be and what its antecedents are. Both patients had symptomatic CMV syndromes, both had bacterial pneumonias, and both had episodes of rejection of at least moderate severity. Thus there were a number of preceding clinical processes that may have led to this syndrome via a mechanism of infectious or immunopathological lung injury.

The transplant group at Stanford have commented on the occurrence of obliterative bronchiolitis in seven of their heart-lung recipients (*16*). This was associated clinically with a productive cough and progressive airflow obstruction on pulmonary function testing. No comment was made on the bacteriology of the sputum. Lung tissue from five of their patients showed obliterative bronchiolitis; some patients also had pulmonary vascular disease or obliterative coronary arteriosclerosis. One of our patients with chronic bronchitis was retransplanted and the surgical lung specimen showed acute and chronic bronchitis with mild bronchiectasis but no definite obliterative bronchiolitis or vascular changes. Although the histology of Stanford's cases and our case do not match precisely, it seems likely that they are part of a spectrum of bronchial injury that results from rejection or infection, or a combination of both. With time these insults to the transplanted lung may irreversibly alter its function and lead to chronic airway disease. Clearly, further studies will have to be done to define the frequency of this syndrome, its important risk factors and ultimately its preventability.

Given the serious problems in management of these patients both in the immediate and extended postoperative period, it seems wise at present to restrict the use of heart-lung transplantation to a few centers with extensive experience in the management of transplant patients and a commitment to the science of transplantation. Our early observations of infections in these patients suggest that serial monitoring of these patients by means such as bronchial lavage, the use of antibiotic therapy and prophylaxis, as well as new approaches to the prevention and management of systemic viral infections are areas to explore in the struggle to improve the outcome of heart-lung transplantation.

Addendum. We recently did retrospective methenamine-silver staining of all heart-lung recipient bronchoalveolar lavage smears that had not previously been investigated for *P carinii.* Two additional patients (pts. 8, 14) were shown to have *Pneumocystis* infection. Patient 14 had a few *Pneumocystis* organisms detected on a bronchoalveolar lavage 94 days after transplant. She was placed on oral sulfamethoxazole-trimethoprim prophylaxis immediately thereafter. This was continued for two months and follow-up smears were negative. The other patient (pt. 8) had a few organisms detected 132 days after transplant. She also received oral sulfamethoxazole-trimethoprim prophylaxis, but not until 175 days later. Interim bronchoalveolar lavages were negative for *Pneumocystis.* Both patients were asymptomatic at the time the organism was detected. These findings show that *Pneumocystis* organisms may be found at an asymptomatic stage in these patients, and that, on occasion, the organism may disappear without specific treatment.

Acknowledgments. We thank Judy Fossati and Linda White for technical assistance, and Charles Rinaldo, Jr., Ph.D., for performing the HTLV-III assays.

REFERENCES

1. Cooley DA, Bloodwell RD, Hallman GL, Nora JJ, Harrison GM, Leachman RD. Organ transplantation for advanced cardiopulmonary disease. Ann Thor Surg 1979; 8: 30.
2. Reitz BA, Wallwork JL, Hunt SA, et al. Successful therapy for patients with pulmonary vascular disease. N Eng J Med 1982; 306: 557.
3. Jamieson SW, Baldwin J, Reitz BA, et al. Combined heart and lung transplantation. Lancet 1983; 1: 1130.
4. Ladowski JS, Kapelanski DP, Teodori MF, Stevenson WC, Hardesty RL, Griffith BP. Experimental use of an autoperfusing heart-lung block for organ preservation prior to heart-lung transplantation. J Heart Trans 1985; 4(2S): 128.
5. Dummer JS, Hardy A, Poorsattar A, Ho M. Early infections in kidney, heart, and liver transplant recipients on cyclosporine. Transplantation 1983; 36: 259.
6. Henle W, Henle GE. Epstein-Barr virus specific diagnostic tests in infectious mononucleosis. Hum Pathol 1979; 5: 551.
7. Dummer JS, Bahnson HT, Griffith BP, Hardesty RL, Thompson ME, Ho M. Infections in patients on cyclosporine and prednisone following cardiac transplantation. Transplant Proc 1983; 4: 2779.
8. Starzl TE, Nalesnik MA, Porter KA, et al. Reversibility of lymphomas and lymphoproliferative lesions developing under cyclosporin-steroid therapy. Lancet 1984; 1: 583.
9. Engelberg LA, Lerner CW, Tapper ML. Clinical features of pneumocystis pneumonia in the acquired immune deficiency syndrome. Am Rev Resp Dis 1984; 130: 689.
10. Ho M, Wajszczuk CP, Hardy A, et al. Infections in kidney, heart, and liver transplant recipients on cyclosporine. Transplant Proc 1983; 4: 2768.
11. Copeland JG, Stinson EB. Human heart transplantation. Curr Probl Cardiol 1980; 3: 4.
12. Brooks RG, Hofflin JM, Jamieson SW, Stinson EB, Remington JS. Infections in heart-lung transplant patients. Presented at the 24th Interscience Conference on Antimicrobial Agents and Chemotherapy, 8–10 Oct 1984, Washington DC
13. Stover DE, Zaman MB, Hajdu SI, Lange M, Gold J, Armstrong D. Bronchoalveolar lavage in the diagnosis of diffuse pulmonary infiltrates in the immunosuppressed host. Ann Intern Med 1984; 101: 1.
14. Gryzan S, Paradis IR, Dauber JH, Hardesty RL, Griffith BP. The role of bronchoalveolar lavage in monitoring patients after heart-lung transplantation. J Heart Trans 1985; 4: 134.
15. Dummer JS, White LT, Ho M, Griffith BP, Hardesty RL, Bahnson HT. Morbidity of cytomegalovirus infection in heart and heart-lung transplant patients on cyclosporine. J Infect Dis 1985; 152: 1182.
16. Burke CM, Morris AJ, Dawkins KD, et al. Obliterative bronchiolitis and chronic pulmonary rejection. J Heart Trans 1985; 4: 144.

Received 29 July 1985.
Accepted 25 September 1985.

0041-1337/86/4106-0730$02.00/0
TRANSPLANTATION
Vol. 41, No. 6
Printed in U.S.A.

PROPHYLACTIC USE OF OKT3 MONOCLONAL ANTIBODY IN CADAVER KIDNEY RECIPIENTS

UTILIZATION OF OKT3 AS THE SOLE IMMUNOSUPPRESSIVE AGENT

P. VIGERAL,[1] N. CHKOFF,[1] L. CHATENOUD,[2] H. CAMPOS,[1] M. LACOMBE[1] D. DROZ,[1] G. GOLDSTEIN,[3] J. F. BACH,[2] AND H. KREIS[1,4]

Unité de Transplantation, Hopital Necker, 75015 Paris; INSERM U25, Hopital Necker, 75015 Paris, France; Immunobiology Division, Ortho Pharmaceutical Corporation, Raritan, New Jersey

We describe the first clinical trial of OKT3, a monoclonal anti-T-cell antibody, for prevention of kidney transplant rejection. 13 patients receiving a first cadaveric kidney transplant were randomly assigned to conventional treatment with azathioprine and high-dose steroids (7 patients) or to treatment with daily injection of OKT3 alone (6 patients). The first OKT3 injection resulted in a dramatic decrease in T3$^+$, T4$^+$, and T8$^+$ cells, while patients simultaneously experienced fever, chills, and diarrhea. These symptoms did not recur with subsequent injections. All six OKT3-treated patients had a rejection necessitating introduction of steroids 12.8±2.9 days after surgery. Rejection was related to appearance of anti-OKT3 antibodies leading to disappearance of detectable OKT3 in the serum. Modulating (T3$^-$, T4$^+$ or T3$^-$, T8$^+$) cells were observed in all patients but were functionally inactive.

As no rejection was observed before day 9 posttransplant, despite the lack of additional immunosuppressive agents, we conclude that OKT3 is a powerful, well-tolerated immunosuppressive agent. However, it is highly immunogenic and anti-OKT3 antibodies lead to loss of clinical effectiveness in this protocol. The use of OKT3 alone for prevention of kidney graft rejection cannot be recommended until a method for reducing the effects of anti-OKT3 immunization is developed.

Antithymocyte globulins (ATG)* have been extensively used therapeutically in patients undergoing kidney transplant rejection and prophylactically (*1*, *2*). Inconsistent results have been reported, however, probably because of lot-to-lot variations and reactivity with other blood components, such as human erythrocytes and/or platelets (*3*). In vitro studies have shown that most of the functional properties of T lymphocytes are linked to the cell surface antigen T3 (*4*). OKT3 monoclonal antibody inhibits the function of this essential structure (*5*) Thus, this anti-T-cell monoclonal immunoglobulin may be suitable for administration to kidney transplant recipients. After the first reports of the successful use of OKT3 for the treatment of established allograft rejection (*6*, *7*), randomized trials were conducted to assess the efficiency of OKT3 (*8*) and other monoclonal antibodies (*9*, *10*) to treat first rejection episodes or as a rescue treatment for steroid and ATG-resistant rejection (*8*, *10*). Preliminary results showed reversibility in up to 90% of cases, but rerejection episodes necessitating the reintroduction of conventional treatment frequently occurred (*6*, *8*). Prophylactic use of OKT3 or other monoclonal antibodies in renal transplantation has never been reported. The first study was designed to compare the efficacy and safety of OKT3 given as the sole immunosuppressive agent with conventional immunosuppressive treatment for prevention of acute rejection after first cadaveric renal transplantation. The primary objective was to evaluate the capacity of OKT3 given before exposure of the patient to the transplant to induce tolerance.

[1]Unité de Transplantation, Hopital Necker.

[2]INSERM U25, Hopital Necker.

[3]Ortho Pharmaceutical Corporation.

[4]Requests for reprints should be addressed to H. Kreis, Unité de Transplantation Rénale, Département de Néphrologie, Hopital Necker, 161 rue de Sèvres, 75015 Paris, France.

* Abbreviations used: ATG, antithymocyte globulins; ELISA; enzyme-linked immunosorbent assay.

MATERIALS AND METHODS

Patients. Thirteen consecutive patients receiving a first cadaver kidney transplantation were enrolled in the study. Preimmunized recipients received an HLA-identical kidney (0 or 1 HLA mismatch) whereas HLA compatibility was not a prerequisite for nonresponder patients. Patients were randomly assigned to conventional treatment with azathioprine and steroids or to experimental treatment with OKT3 monoclonal antibody (Ortho Pharmaceutical Corp., Raritan NJ) without steroids or azathioprine. This study was approved by the local Institutional Review Board, and all patients gave written informed consent.

Monoclonal antibody. OKT3 is a monoclonal mouse IgG2a antibody directed against a 20,000-dalton glycoprotein present on the surface of all mature human T cells (*11*). The immunoglobulin is purified from mouse ascites and supplied by Ortho Pharmaceutical Corporation after testing for purity and safety as a sterile pyrogen-free solution suitable for i.v. use.

Treatment protocol. Six patients were assigned to the OKT3 group. A pretreatment skin test with OKT3 (0.1 ml of a 1/1000 solution) was performed to verify the absence of immunization against mouse immunoglobulin in each case. OKT3, 5 mg/day, was administered by i.v. push from the day before transplantation through day 13, without associated immunosuppressive drugs or steroids. Azathioprine alone, 3 mg/kg/day, was introduced at day 14 and continued thereafter. In case of acute rejection, OKT3 was stopped and conventional treatment with steroids and azathioprine was introduced. Seven patients constituted the control group. They received azathioprine and high-dose steroids according to the protocol employed in the transplantation center of Hopital Necker and detailed elsewhere (*12*). Azathioprine, 3 mg/kg/day, was given from the day before transplantation and thereafter; prednisolone, 5 mg/kg/day, was given for the first 5 days, then tapered to 0.25 mg/kg/day in 11 weeks.

Rejection. The patient was considered to be undergoing acute rejection when renal function progressively deteriorated for more than two days; other possible causes of renal dysfunction were excluded by appropriate tests. Percutaneous needle biopsy was performed in most instances.

Tolerance. Tolerance of OKT3 was studied by careful observation of any clinical evidence of serum sickness and daily monitoring of blood count, blood urea, serum creatinine, and urine protein excretion and by weekly assessment of hepatic function.

Immunological monitoring. Monitoring of peripheral lymphocyte subsets was begun before transplantation (before and 1 hr after the first OKT3 injection in the OKT3-treated patients). Blood was then collected two or three times weekly for four weeks. The number of $T3^+$ (total), $T4^+$ (mainly helper-inducer), and $T8^+$ (mainly cytotoxic/suppressor) T lymphocytes was determined by testing with OKT3, OKT4, and OKT8 monoclonal antibodies (kindly provided by Ortho Pharmaceutical Corp., Raritan, NJ). Peripheral mononuclear cells were obtained by gradient centrifugation of heparinized blood. $T3^+$, $T4^+$, and $T8^+$ cells were quantified by indirect immunofluorescence using goat antimouse isotype-specific antibodies conjugated with fluorescein (Nordic, Tilburg, the Netherlands) as previously described (*13*). The mononuclear cell suspension under study was analyzed under a Leitz Orthoplan microscope; an average of 200 cells per slide were counted. The proportions of $T3^+$, $T4^+$, and $T8^+$ cells were expressed as the percentages of labeled cells in relation to the total number of mononuclear cells. Strongly fluorescent cells only were considered labeled cells. When present, weakly fluorescent cells were noted as *faintly labeled cells* and were not taken into account for determination of percentages. Reappearance of $T3^+$ cells was defined as a percentage over 30% on two consecutive samples. Serum concentrations of OKT3 and circulating anti-OKT3 antibodies of the IgG or IgM type were evaluated by means of an enzyme-linked immunosorbent assay (ELISA) as previously reported (*14*).

RESULTS

The first administration of OKT3 was always followed by a systemic reaction consisting of fever, chills, anxiety, and diarrhea. These symptoms resolved within a few hours and did not recur with subsequent injections. Overall tolerance was therefore good. Three patients reported migratory arthralgias and two had mild and transient skin rashes, the relation of which to OKT3 could not be ascertained. Severe symptoms suggesting serum sickness were not observed. No serious infection occurred while patients received OKT3. After OKT3 was stopped and conventional immunosuppressive therapy begun, one patient in the OKT3 group has a severe bacterial infection that responded well to antibiotics. No OKT3-treated patient had severe viral infection. Two patients in the control group had a severe bacterial infection (one of whom died) and one had a severe cytomegalovirus infection.

Results of lymphocyte monitoring in OKT3-treated patients are shown in Table 1. Mean $T3^+$ cell level was $58.7\pm9.5\%$ (SEM) before treatment. The first monoclonal antibody injection resulted in a dramatic and concomitant decrease in $T3^+$, $T4^+$, and $T8^+$ cells. The $T3^+$ cell level was only 1–3% 1 hr after this injection. $T4^+$ and $T8^+$ cell levels were higher than the $T3^+$ cell level in patients 1 and 3, indicating the presence of $T3^-$, $T4^+$ and $T3^-$, $T8^+$ cells. This finding was similarly clear in all six OKT3-treated patients from the second day posttransplant. The $T3^+$ cell level remained close to zero for 10–17 days when it suddenly rose, rapidly followed by acute rejection (Fig. 1). In patients 2, 3, and 4 the detection of labeled cells were preceded by the appearance of faintly labeled cells.

Anti-OKT3 IgG were detected in all 6 OKT3-treated patients. The first positive sera were drawn between days 9 and 21 after the first OKT3 injection (Fig. 1). Anti-OKT3 IgM antibodies appeared in four patients; they were not detected in patients 2 and 4, suggesting that they were not of major importance in the reappearance of $T3^+$ cells. Serum concentrations of free OKT3 were determined in the six OKT3-treated patients. The 5 mg daily dosage used in this study induced plasma levels of 1730 ± 920 (SEM) ng/ml. When anti-OKT3 antibodies appeared, the serum concentration of free OKT3 quickly fell to undetectable levels.

There was no significant difference between the experimental and the control groups in patients' age, sex, duration of hemodialysis, total ischemia of the graft, and HLA compatibility (Table 2). All of the six OKT3-treated patients experienced an acute rejection episode early in the posttransplantation course (Fig. 1). Clinical diagnosis of acute rejection was confirmed by percutaneous renal biopsy in five patients. Patient 2 did not undergo renal biopsy. Introduction of conventional treatment with high-dose steroids and azathioprine promptly resulted in normalization of graft function in all six patients. Because of this early rejection, only patients 1 and 5 in the experimental

TABLE 1. Lymphocyte populations in six OKT3-treated patients[a]

	Patient 1			Patient 2			Patient 3			Patient 4			Patient 5			Patient 6		
	T3	T4	T8	T3	T4	T8	T3	T4	T8	T3	T4	T8	T3	T4	T8	T3	T4	T8
Before OKT3	72	48	21	50	31	18	56	36	22	61	50	15	45	22	25	68	60	10
One hour after first OKT3 injection	1	4	8	2	2	2	2	4	4	3	1	1	1	1	1	1	0	0
Day 2 PT[b]	1	11	15	0	2	1	0	4	6	1	1	4	0	6	6	2	5	2
Day 5 PT	1	18	20	0	16	13	0	7	2	0	30	13	0	7	5	1	7	15
Day 9 PT[c]	1	9	9	0	15	12	0	13	11	0	20	10	0	8	3	38	19	13
Day 13 PT	22	18	6	(38)	32	15	(16)	15	8	0	25	11	20	14	17	35	26	8
Day 14 PT	43	40	11	56	16	15	30	36	8	(4)	13	6	30	15	17	50	38	15
Day 17 PT	54	40	7	—	—	—	62	40	21	43	30	12	33	17	18	25	12	5

[a] Data are expressed as percentages of mononuclear cells. Numbers in parentheses represent faintly labeled cells.

[b] (PT) posttransplant.

[c] This determination was made on day 10 PT in patient 6.

group received the entire course of fourteen OKT3 injections. The mean time between surgery and rejection in this group was 12.8 days±2.9 (SEM). Two patients in the control group experienced an acute rejection episode during the first month posttransplant, on days 10 and 28 respectively. Both rejection episodes were successfully treated by an increase in steroid dosage. One patient in the control group died from sepsis on day 83. The remaining four patients in this group experienced acute rejection during the second or the third month posttransplant. The mean time between surgery and rejection (or death) in the control group was 51 days ±23.3 (SEM). This interval was significantly longer than that observed in the experimental group ($P<.01$, Student's t test).

DISCUSSION

OKT3 monoclonal antibody has proved to be effective in the treatment of established kidney transplant rejection (*6, 8*), but its usefulness in prophylaxis of graft rejection has never been tested. This first study demonstrated that OKT3 given alone daily from the day before transplantation does not induce tolerance to the transplant. On the contrary, each of the six OKT3-treated patients developed an acute rejection episode between days 9 and 18 posttransplantation. However, OKT3 was highly effective in preventing graft rejection during the initial posttransplantation course. Rapid normalization of serum creatinine was observed in all six patients. Since allogeneic kidney transplantation invariably results in acute rejection within the first 4 days in the absence of immunosuppression (*15*), the initially good kidney function in OKT3-treated patients confirms the strong clinical immunosuppressive action of OKT3 (*6, 8*). The first injection resulted in almost complete disappearance of circulating T cells. Cosimi and coworkers observed a similar dramatic decrease in peripheral T cells after administration of OKT3 for established acute rejection episodes (*6, 7*). Although OKT3 is a complement-fixing IgG 2a (*11*) that exhibits a lympholytic action in vitro (*16*), the mechanism of in vivo disappearance of T lymphocytes probably is not related to complement-mediated lympholysis, but rather to T cell opsonization followed by removal by the reticuloendothelial phagocytic system (*7, 17*). The rapid disappearance of circulating T lymphocytes that followed the first OKT3 injection in the six OKT3-treated patients occurred simultaneously with clinical manifestations consisting of fever, chills, and diarrhea. These reactions were probably related to release of endogenous pyrogens following the abrupt T cell removal and breakdown that occurs after the first initial injection of OKT3 (*7*). Similar reactions were not reported with other anti-T-cell monoclonal antibodies, such as the anti-T12 antibody (*9*), which probably do not induce lymphocyte destruction. These symptoms did not recur with subsequent injections; neither bronchospasm nor pulmonary edema were observed. Therefore, overall tolerance of OKT3 was quite good.

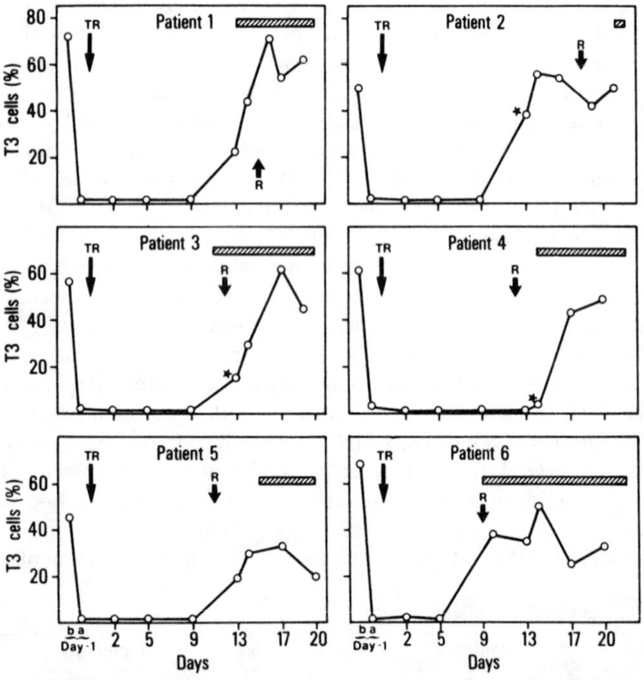

FIGURE 1. Monitoring of $T3^+$ lymphocytes (open circle) and anti-OKT3 IgG antibodies (shaded bar) in 6 prophylactically OKT3-treated kidney graft recipients. T cell counts were done twice on the day before transplantation (TR), before (b) and one hour after (a) the first OKT3 injection (*) indicates faintly labeled cells and (R) represents kidney graft rejection.

The presence of peripheral cells bearing T4 or T8 antigen, but not T3 antigen, was documented as early as 1 hr after the first OKT3 injection in patients 1 and 3, and from the second posttransplantation day in the four remaining patients. We (*14*) and others (*18*) have previously reported that the appearance of $T3^-$, $T4^+$ and $T3^-$, $T8^+$ peripheral lymphocytes after administration of OKT3 is related to the phenomenon of antigenic modulation whereby the expression of a membrane antigen is specifically inhibited by its antibody (*19, 20*). The same phenomenon was recently described during the treatment of leukemic patients with antilymphoblast monoclonal antibodies (*21*). Two mechanisms have been described: antigenic redistribution (or capping) with internalization of the molecule (*20*) and vertical movement (or shedding) with liberation of the molecule from the cell. Reappearance of peripheral T cells bearing T4 or T8 antigens, but not the T3 antigen, did not result in rejection. This finding emphasizes the vital importance of the T3 molecule in T lymphocyte function (*4*) and the fact that T3-modulated lymphocytes are functionally inactive.

Anti-OKT3 immunization appeared to be a major problem in the utilization of OKT3. The six OKT3-treated patients developed anti-OKT3 IgG antibodies. It can be assumed that anti-OKT3 antibodies led to the observed disappearance of effective free OKT3 plasma levels, resulting in the reappearance of $T3^+$ cells and the occurrence of rejection. In three patients, faintly labeled $T3^+$ cells reappeared a few days before

TABLE 2. Comparison of groups[a]

Group	No. Patients	Age	Sex (M/F)	Hemodialysis period (years)	Total ischemia (min)	HLA-compatible recipients
OKT3	6	34.3±9.2	3/3	3.9±1.6	1444±346	3
Steroids+ azathioprine	7	35.7±11.2	4/3	2.8±0.6	1408.3±299	2

[a] Data are reported as mean ± SEM. Differences are not statistically significant.

strongly labeled T3$^+$ cells, but our definition of reappearance did not include these faintly labeled cells. Anti-OKT3 antibodies have also been detected in patients treated with OKT3 for established acute rejection (*7, 22*). Precise characterization of antibodies following OKT3 therapy showed not only anti-mouse IgG antibodies but also antiidiotypic antibodies (*22*). Antixenogenic immunization is a well-known consequence of ATG treatment (*23*) that may clinically result in serum sickness (*24*). In our study, three patients had migratory arthralgias and two patients had transient mild skin rashes; however, severe symptoms suggesting serum sickness never occurred.

In summary, OKT3 monoclonal antibody is a well-tolerated and powerful immunosuppressive agent. However, in the present protocol it was highly immunogenic and anti-OKT3 antibodies consistently led to loss of clinical effectiveness. Therefore, since rapid graft tolerance was not established, the use of OKT3 alone cannot be recommended for prevention of kidney graft rejection. Whether the association of OKT3 with steroids or other immunosuppression agents will reduce the rate of anti-OKT3 immunization remains to be determined.

REFERENCES

1. Shield CF, Cosimi AB, Tolkoff-Rubin N, Rubin RH, Herrin J, Russel PS. Use of antithymocyte globulin for reversal of acute allograft rejection. Transplantation 1979; 28: 461.
2. Kreis H, Mansouri R, Descamps JM, et al. Antithymocyte globulin in cadaver kidney transplantation: a randomized trial based on T-cell monitoring. Kidney Int 1981; 19: 438.
3. Wechter WJ, Brodie JA, Morrel RM, Rafi M, Schulz JR. Antithymocyte globulin (ATGAM) in renal allograft recipients: multicenter trials using a 14-dose regimen. Transplantation 1979; 28: 294.
4. Reinherz EL, Meuer S, Fitzgerald KA, Hussey RE, Levine H, Schlossman SF. Antigen recognition by human T lymphocyte is linked to surface expression of the T3 molecular complex. Cell 1982; 30: 735.
5. Chang TW, Kung PC, Gingras SP, Goldstein G. Does OKT3 monoclonal antibody react with an antigen-recognition structure on human T cells? Proc Natl Acad Sci USA 1981; 78: 1805.
6. Cosimi AB, Colvin RB, Burton RC, et al. Use of monoclonal antibodies to T-cell subsets for immunologic monitoring and treatment in recipients of renal allografts. N Engl J Med 1981; 305: 308.
7. Cosimi AB, Burton RC, Colvin RB, et al. Treatment of acute renal allograft rejection with OKT3 monoclonal antibody. Transplantation 1981; 32: 535.
8. Norman DJ, Barry JM, Henell K, Funnel MB, Goldstein G, Bohannon L. Reversal of acute allograft rejection with monoclonal antibody. Transplant Proc 1985; 17: 39.
9. Kirkman RL, Araujo JL, Brusch GJ, et al. Treatment of acute renal allograft rejection with monoclonal anti-T12 antibody. Transplantation 1983; 36: 620.
10. Takahashi H, Okazaki H, Terasaki PI, et al. Reversal of transplant rejection by monoclonal antiblast antibody. Lancet 1983; 2: 1155.
11. Kung PC, Golstein G, Reinherz EL, Schlossman SF. Monoclonal antibodies defining distinctive human T-cell surface antigens. Science 1979; 206: 347.
12. Kreis H. Procedure for performing renal transplantation. In: Hamburger J, Crosnier J, Grunfeld JP, eds. Nephrology. New York: Wiley-Flammarion, 1979: 1311.
13. Chatenoud L, Bach MA. Abnormalities of T-cell subsets in glomerulonephritis and systemic lupus erythematosus. Kidney Int 1981; 20: 267.
14. Chatenoud L, Baudrihaye MF, Kreis H, Goldstein G, Schindler J, Bach JF. Human in vivo antigenic modulation induced by the anti T-cell OKT3 monoclonal antibody. Eur J Immunol 1982; 12: 979.
15. Kreis H, Lacombe M, Noel LH, Descamps JM, Chailley J, Crosnier J. Kidney graft rejection: has the need for steroid to be reevaluated? Lancet 1978; 2: 1169.
16. Van Wauve J, Goossens J. Monoclonal anti-human T-lymphocyte antibodies: enumeration and characterization of T-cell subsets. Immunology 1981; 42: 157.
17. Goldstein G, Schindler J, Lifter J. Towards immunomanipulation with monoclonal antibodies. In: Kuss R, Legrain M, eds. Semin Uro-Nephrol, Paris: Masson, 1983: 146.
18. Estabrook A, Berger CL, Mittler R, Logerfo P, Hardy M, Edelson RL. Antigenic modulation of human T-lymphocytes by monoclonal antibodies. Transplant Proc 1983; 15: 651.
19. Old LJ, Stockert E, Boyse EA, Kim JH. Antigenic modulation: loss of TL antigen from cells exposed to TL antibody. Study of the phenomenon in vitro. J Exp Med 1968; 127: 523.
20. Taylor RB, Duffus WPH, Raff MC, De Petris S. Redistribution and pinocytosis of lymphocyte surface immunoglobulin molecules induced by anti-immunoglobulin antibody. Nature New Biol. 1971; 223: 225.
21. Ritz J, Pesando JM, Sallan SE, et al. Serotherapy of acute lymphoblastic leukemia with monoclonal antibody. Blood 1981; 58: 141.
22. Jaffers GJ, Colvin RB, Cosimi AB. The human immune response to murine OKT3 monoclonal antibody. Transplant Proc 1983; 15: 646.
23. Kashiwagi N, Brantigan CO, Brettschneider L, Groth CG, Starzl TE. Clinical reactions and serologic changes after the administration of heterologous antilymphocyte globulin to human recipients of renal homografts. Ann Intern Med 1968; 68: 275.
24. Lawley TJ, Bielory L, Gascon P, Yancey KB, Young NS, Franck MM. Prospective clinical and immunologic analysis of patients with serum sickness. N Engl J Med 1984; 311: 1407.

Received 4 June 1985.
Accepted 14 September 1985.

0041-1337/86/4106-0734$02.00/0
TRANSPLANTATION
Vol. 41, No. 6

Printed in U.S.A.

INHIBITION OF RAT SKIN ALLOGRAFT REJECTION BY CYCLOSPORINE

IN SITU CHARACTERIZATION OF THE IMPAIRED LOCAL IMMUNE RESPONSE[1]

FRANCISCO J. GUILLÉN[2,3,5] WAYNE W. HANCOCK,[2,4,5] EDWARD TOWPIK,[6] JERZY W. KUPIEC-WEGLINSKI,[6] FREDERICK R. RICKLES,[7] NICHOLAS L. TILNEY,[6] AND GEORGE F. MURPHY[5]

Departments of Pathology and Surgery, Brigham and Women's Hospital and Harvard Medical School, Boston, Massachusetts 02115; and Division of Hematology-Oncology, Department of Medicine, University of Connecticut Health Center, Farmington, Connecticut 06032, and the Veterans Administration Center, Newington, Connecticut

Cyclosporine (CsA) is known to induce long-term survival of skin allografts, although the cellular mechanisms responsible for this effect are not well understood. To further define the effects of CsA-induced immunosuppression, we performed a morphological and immunohistological study of acute skin allograft rejection in the rat, comparing untreated and CsA-treated animals. Three significant differences were found between grafts in CsA-treated and untreated rats. First, CsA-allografts contained fewer MRC OX-8$^+$ cytotoxic T cells than untreated allografts. Second, although the presence and numbers of infiltrating macrophages (W3/25$^+$, W3/13$^-$ cells) was not influenced by CsA treatment, CsA treatment blocked expression of a macrophage membrane activation antigen, defined by the monoclonal antibody A1-3, which has previously been linked with development of macrophage procoagulant activity (PCA). Third, diminution in MRC OX-8$^+$ lymphocytes and A1-3$^+$ macrophages in CsA allografts was associated with an absence of the widespread thrombotic and necrotizing microvascular injury typical of acute rejection in untreated rats. We conclude that prolongation of skin allograft survival by CsA is related to its ability to prevent cell mediated injury to the endothelium of graft vessels, and possibly also to inhibition of macrophage PCA with consequent reduced thrombus formation.

[1] This work was supported by Grants AI 19071, CA 40358, and CA 22202 from the DHHS; and by grants from the American Heart Association and its Connecticut affiliate (83-957), the American Cancer Society (CH-39881), and the Research Service of the Veterans Administration (RDS-7446).

[2] Address correspondence and reprint requests to: Wayne Hancock, MD, PhD, Department of Pathology, Brigham and Women's Hospital, 75 Francis St., Boston, MA 02115.

[3] Visiting Fulbright Scholar; current address: Dept. of Pathology, University of Alicante Medical School, Alicante, Spain.

[4] Recipient of a Neil Hamilton-Fairley Fellowship from the National Health and Medical Research Council of Australia.

[5] Department of Pathology, Brigham and Women's Hospital and Harvard Medical School.

[6] Department of Surgery, Brigham and Women's Hospital and Harvard Medical School.

[7] University of Connecticut Health Center and The Veterans Administration Center.

* Abbreviations used: CsA, Cyclosporine; γ-IFN, gamma interferon; IL-1, interleukin-1; IL-2, interleukin-2; LPS, lipopolysaccharide; PCA, procoagulant activity; Tc, cytotoxic T cell; Th, helper T cell; Ts, suppressor T cell.

The fungal metabolite cyclosporine (CsA)* has remarkable immunosuppressive properties in both clinical and experimental settings (*1–11*). Although its mechanism of action is uncertain, CsA is thought to selectively inhibit particular lymphocyte functions by restricting clonal expansion and/or functional activation of immunocompetent cells (*12*). CsA interferes specifically with the induction of helper T cells (Th) and the generation of cytotoxic T cells (Tc), hampers release of both interleukins 1 and 2 (IL-1 and IL-2) (*13*, *14*), and selectively impairs secretion of gamma interferon (γ-IFN) (*15*). Moreover, in some experimental models, CsA appears to prevent the generation of Tc, while sparing or even amplifying the activity of suppressor T cells (Ts) (*16*).

In the rat, indefinite survival (>150 days) of skin allografts is possible using small maintenance doses of CsA (*17*). The basis for this effect may relate to the effect of CsA on the cellular interactions central to graft rejection. Recent morphological studies by Dvorak et al. (*18*) have shown that microvascular endothelium, and not the epidermal cell, is a critical target of the immune response in the rejection of first-set human skin allografts. These authors observed equal damage to donor vessels of the allograft, as well as to host vessels of the graft bed, and suggested that the final events in the acute rejection process were not entirely immunologically specific. The identity of mononuclear cells responsible for the effector limb of this response is controversial, although studies in rats (*19*, *20*), mice (*21*), and humans (*22*) have implicated Tc, Th, macrophages, and NK cells in the rejection phenomenon.

The observation of long-term skin allograft survival induced by CsA (CsA allografts) prompted us to compare acute allograft rejection with isografts and CsA allografts using light and electron microscopy and immunohistological techniques.

MATERIALS AND METHODS

Animals. Inbred male rats (Microbiological Associates, Walkersville, MD) weighing 250–300 g were used. Lewis (LEW, $RT1^l$) rats served as recipients of Brown-Norway (BN, $RT1^n$) skin grafts. For control isograft studies, skin grafts were exchanged between LEW rats.

Skin grafting. Full-thickness donor skin grafts measuring 4 × 4 cm were harvested, cleaned of subcutaneous fat, and sutured into comparable defects made in the recipient flanks. Dressings were removed on day 5, the sutures on day 7. The grafts were inspected daily and the time of clinical acute rejection was defined by the presence of necrosis of 50% of the graft surface.

Immunosuppressive therapy. CsA (Sandoz Inc, Basel, Switzerland) was dissolved in olive oil at 70°C, and administered daily s.c. at a dose of 15 mg/kg for the first 14 days, followed by a maintenance dose of 15 mg/kg every fourth day.

Graft biopsy and tissue processing for morphologic studies. Biopsies of the isografts (n = 21) and CsA allografts (n = 21) were obtained on days 4, 6, 8, 10, 14, 30, and 60. Biopsies from the allografts of nontreated animals (n = 12) were examined on days 4, 6, 8, and 10. For light microscopy, subdivided tissue was fixed in 10% neutral buffered formalin, processed routinely by embedding in paraffin, and stained with hematoxylin and eosin, or fixed in Karnovsky's II solution and prepared for 1 μm-thick plastic-embedded sections and for electron microscopy, as previously described (*23*).

Monoclonal antibodies. The specificities and tissue reactivities of the mouse anti-rat monoclonal antibodies used in this study, which were obtained from Sera-Lab, London, UK, are detailed elsewhere (*24–28*). Antibodies were directed against the leukocyte-common antigen (MRC OX-1) (*24*); Ia antigens (MRC OX-4) (*25*); rat T cells (W3/13), and cytotoxic/suppressor (MRC OX-8) or helper/inducer (W3/25) T cell subsets (*26–28*). In addition, we used the murine monoclonal antibody A1-3 (also known as HTF-1) which is directed against an activation antigen of mononuclear phagocytes (*29, 30*), and which neutralizes the PCA (*29*) characteristic of lipopolysaccharide (LPS) or lymphokine-treated monocytes and macrophages (*31*). We have previously shown that A1-3$^+$ macrophages are intimately associated with fibrin deposition in human renal allograft rejection (*32*), human glomerulonephritis (*33*), and pulmonary sarcoidosis (*30*). Parallel studies in our laboratory involving rat macrophages, to be published separately, have shown blood monocytes and pulmonary and peritoneal macrophages harvested from pathogen-free rats do not bind A1-3 but, like their human counterparts, become A1-3$^+$ after stimulation with LPS or lymphokine-rich conditioned media.

Immunohistological studies. Serially cut cryostat sections were incubated with optimally diluted monoclonal antibodies, followed by biotin-conjugated horse antimouse Ig, and avidin-biotin-horseradish peroxidase complex (Vector Laboratories Inc, Burlingame, CA). All sections were then incubated for 10 min with 3,3′-diaminobenzidine (Sigma, St. Louis, MO) in 0.1M Tris buffer containing 1M imidazole, rinsed in water, and counterstained lightly with hematoxylin. This technique was previously described in detail (*34*). Tissues were also stained with isotype-matched control monoclonal antibodies (IgG1, IgG2 and IgM). Labeled cells were enumerated in representative high power fields (40×) with the aid of an ocular grid micrometer. Statistical analysis of the numbers of labeled cells within each group was performed using the Student's *t* test.

RESULTS

Macroscopic Graft Appearance

Mean survival time of skin allografts (MST ± SD) was established as 9 ± 1 days; CsA allografts and isografts survived for the duration of the experiment. Both isografts and allografts healed in a similar pattern, with revascularization detectable from day 5. On day 8, however, abrupt changes in the appearance of allografts from animals not receiving CsA were observed, consisting of induration and localized epidermal sloughing, with necrosis of 50 to 100% of the graft surface by day 9.

Microscopic Description of the Grafts

Light microscopy. CsA allografts and isografts: The histologic changes observed in these groups were similar and are summarized in Table 1. During the first week, vessels of CsA allografts showed occasional endothelial degeneration, although vessel necrosis or thrombosis was not observed (Fig. 1). By 2–4 weeks, CsA allografts were similar to normal host skin and isografts, except for the presence of occasional and isolated mononuclear inflammatory cells.

Allografts: Early changes (day 4) in the epidermis and microvasculature were indistinguishable from those seen in the revascularization phase of isografts and CsA allografts (Table 1). By day 6, however, endothelial cells lining the microvasculature of the allografts exhibited focal degeneration and hypertrophy that resulted in occasional luminal obliteration, similar to that previously described during human skin allograft rejection (*18*). An inflammatory infiltrate, though present through all levels of the grafts, was particularly prominent around affected vessels, and in 1-μm sections these cells were seen to consist of lymphocytes and macrophages. Hypogranulated mast cells were also frequently encountered. In contrast to isografts and CsA allografts, a marked increase in the numbers of these inflammatory cells was observed by days 8–10. At this juncture, vascular lesions were most prominent, with marked hypertrophy and necrosis of endothelium and associated occlusive thrombosis (Fig. 1). By day 10, all allografts showed widespread signs of rejection, characterized by coagulation necrosis of the epidermis and cellular elements of the dermis. Vascular thrombosis and extracellular edema was extensive within the rejecting dermis, and numerous lymphocytes and macrophages were observed in association with the remaining intact vessels of the graft bed.

Immunohistology. The affected dermal vessels of allografts were surrounded by MRC OX-1$^+$ and MRC OX-4$^+$ (Ia$^+$) lymphocytes and macrophages (Fig. 2). Lymphoid cells were MRC OX-8$^+$, and most (>90%), but not all, reacted with W3/13. Macrophages were W3/25$^+$ and also A1-3$^+$ (Fig. 2), but were unreactive with the pan-T marker W3/13. This cellular infiltrate was seen by day 4, but was more pronounced by days 6–10.

The characteristics of the mononuclear cells infiltrating isografts and CsA allografts were similar in to those encountered in allografts (Table 1), though markedly diminished numbers

TABLE 1. Summary of morphological and immunohistological findings in skin allografts at days 8–10

Feature	Allografts	CsA allografts	Isografts
Endothelial damage	+++[a]	±	−
Thrombosis	++/+++	−	−
OX-8$^+$ cells	+++	+/++	+/++
W3/25$^+$, W3/13-cells	+++	+/++	+/++
A1-3$^+$ macrophages	+++	±	+/++
Ia$^+$ endothelial cells	++	−	−
Ia$^+$ epidermal cells	+++	+	+
Mast cell degranulation	++	−	−
Extracellular fibrin deposition	++	−	−

[a] Graded semiquantitatively, such that the feature indicated is either absent (−), or present to a trace (±), minor (+), moderate (++) or marked (+++) extent.

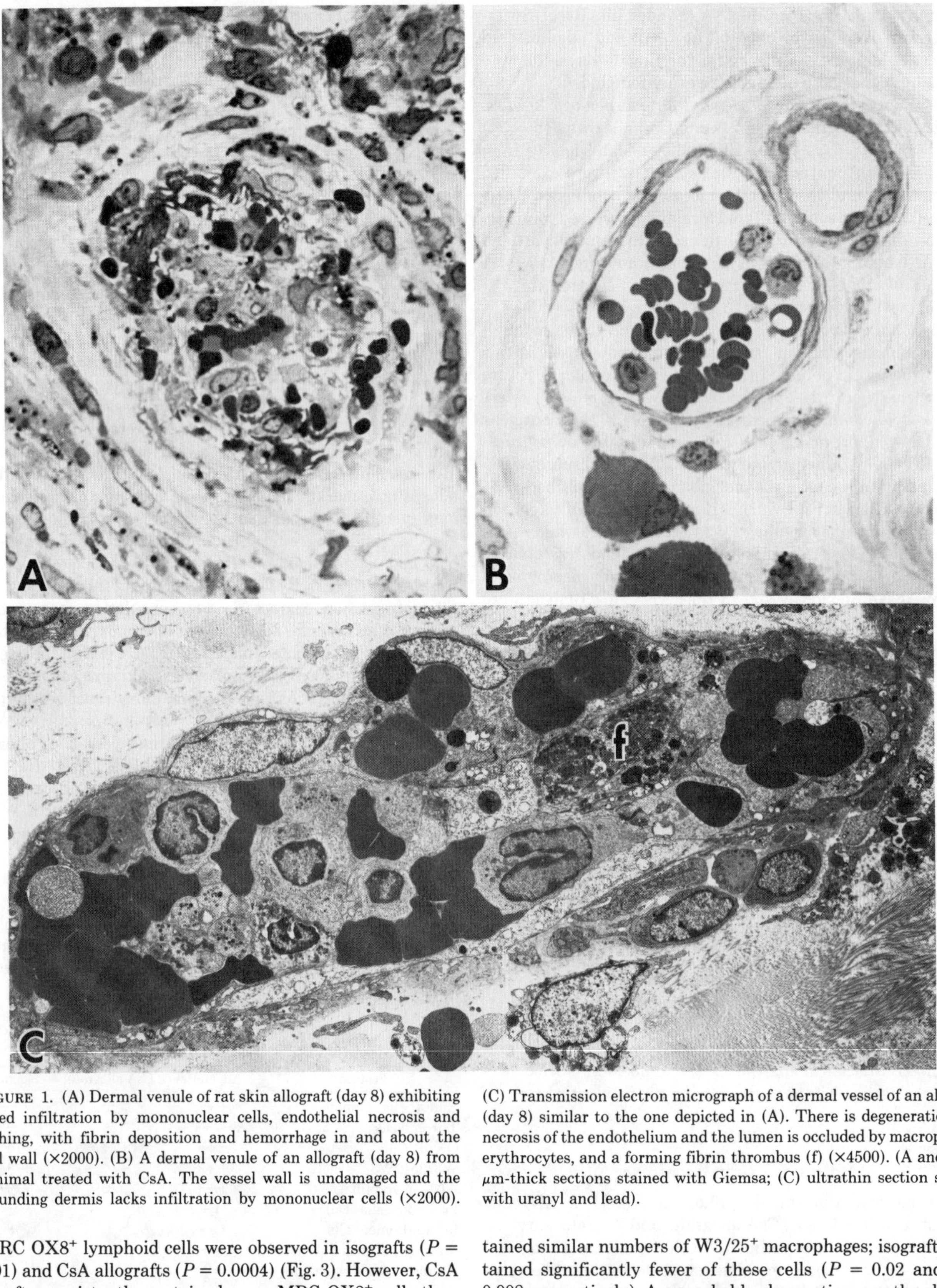

FIGURE 1. (A) Dermal venule of rat skin allograft (day 8) exhibiting marked infiltration by mononuclear cells, endothelial necrosis and sloughing, with fibrin deposition and hemorrhage in and about the vessel wall (×2000). (B) A dermal venule of an allograft (day 8) from an animal treated with CsA. The vessel wall is undamaged and the surrounding dermis lacks infiltration by mononuclear cells (×2000). (C) Transmission electron micrograph of a dermal vessel of an allograft (day 8) similar to the one depicted in (A). There is degeneration and necrosis of the endothelium and the lumen is occluded by macrophages, erythrocytes, and a forming fibrin thrombus (f) (×4500). (A and B) 1-μm-thick sections stained with Giemsa; (C) ultrathin section stained with uranyl and lead).

of MRC OX8$^+$ lymphoid cells were observed in isografts (P = 0.0001) and CsA allografts (P = 0.0004) (Fig. 3). However, CsA allografts consistently contained more MRC OX8$^+$ cells than control isografts (P = 0.001). Less than 35% of these MRC OX8$^+$ cells were W3/13$^+$, suggesting that the majority were non-Tc, NK cells (*19, 20*). Allografts and CsA allografts contained similar numbers of W3/25$^+$ macrophages; isografts contained significantly fewer of these cells (P = 0.02 and P = 0.008, respectively). A remarkable observation was the absence of reactivity for the antibody A1-3 in macrophages of CsA allografts ($P < 0.0001$) (Fig. 2). This was in sharp contrast to macrophages within allografts and in isografts, which were

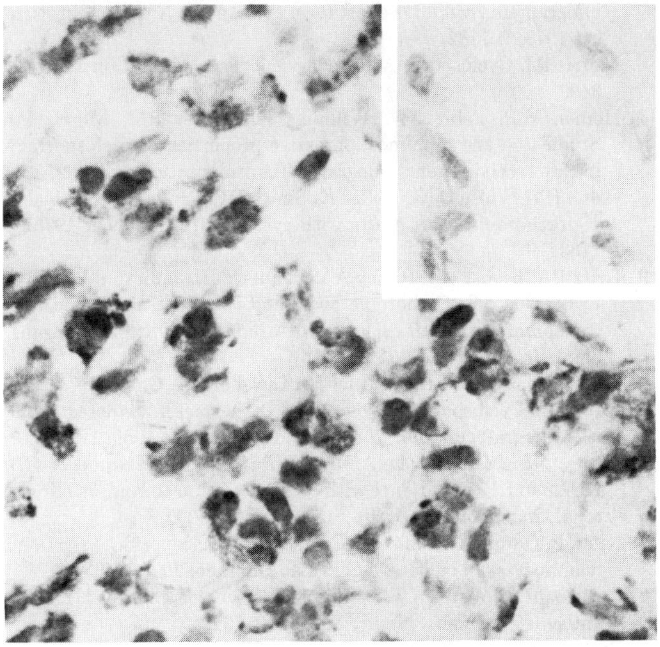

FIGURE 2. The dermal macrophages in rejecting allografts showed reactivity with the macrophage activation marker A1-3, whereas the majority of macrophages in allografts of CsA-treated animals were unreactive (inset) (immunoperoxidase; ×1500).

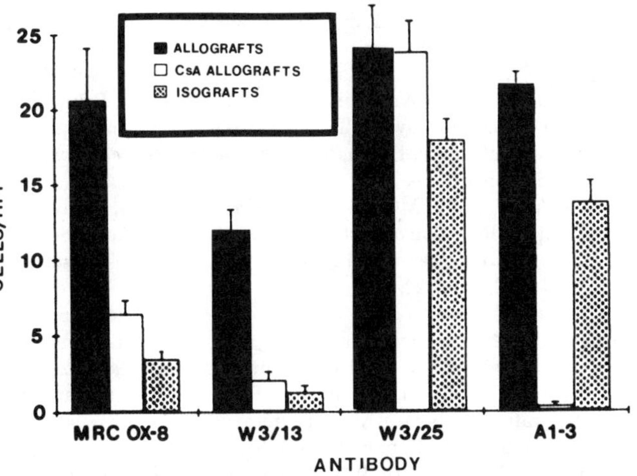

FIGURE 3. Numbers of dermal mononuclear cells from allografts, CsA allografts, and isografts (day 10), enumerated per high-power field (HPF), showing reactivity for the antibodies MRC OX-8, W3/13, W3/25, and A1-3. Note the marked reduction in the number of lymphocytes with phenotypes of cytotoxic cells (MRC OX-8$^+$) in CsA allografts compared with allografts ($P = 0.0004$). In addition, although allografts, CsA allografts, and isografts all contained W3/25$^+$ macrophages, expression of the macrophage activation marker A1-3 was significantly reduced only in animals receiving CsA ($P < 0.0001$).

almost all A1-3$^+$, though the total numbers of A1-3$^+$ macrophages in isografts were themselves decreased compared with allografts ($P = 0.0003$).

Dermal endothelial cells were stained variably by anti-Ia antibodies in all rejecting grafts, but not in CsA allografts and isografts. The epidermis and hair follicles of allografts, CsA allografts, and isografts showed reactivity for Ia antigen. The staining was focal and considerably weaker in CsA allografts and isografts, eventually disappearing by days 8–10.

Electron microscopy. The extent of microvascular injury observed in allografts was confirmed by transmission electron microscopy (Fig. 1). The venules and arterioles of the grafts prior to graft necrosis (days 6–8) exhibited endothelial alterations characterized by swelling and vacuolization of the endothelial cell cytoplasm, disruption of the cell membranes, nuclear pyknosis, focal areas of sloughing of endothelial cells, and luminal thrombosis. Vascular lesions were invariably accompanied by vasocentric infiltrates of mononuclear cells and fibrin deposition. Focal endothelial swelling was seen in vessels of CsA allografts, but necrosis and thrombosis were never observed. Endothelial alterations did not appear in isografts.

Ultrastructural examination confirmed that the large mononuclear cells in the dermal inflammatory infiltrates were macrophages, containing variable numbers of primary and secondary lysosomes. The accompanying lymphoid cells were of two types: most were compatible with conventional lymphocytes, while a minority exhibited indented nuclei and more abundant cytoplasm, and contained variable numbers of membrane-bound cytoplasmic granules. These latter cells had characteristics of large granular lymphocytes (*35*).

DISCUSSION

In this study we have established in a rodent model the importance of microvascular injury as an early and critical event in the pathogenesis of skin allograft rejection. Specific new findings to emerge are: that CsA-induced graft acceptance and survival are associated with ablation of necrotizing and occlusive microvascular lesions; that this ablation is associated with diminished numbers of mononuclear cells in the graft dermis with phenotypic characteristics of Tc and, to a lesser extent, macrophages; and that the absence of thrombotic vascular changes in CsA allografts is associated with markedly diminished expression of a macrophage activation antigen thought to be associated with PCA.

The use of monoclonal antibodies against antigens characteristic of different lymphoid cell subpopulations has aided in the in situ identification of mononuclear cells participating in skin allograft rejection (*19, 20, 22*). Our results are in keeping with previous observations that the cells infiltrating allografts are mostly activated (Ia$^+$) mononuclear cells with phenotypes of cytotoxic (MRC OX-8$^+$) lymphocytes (*19, 36*) and macrophages (W3/25$^+$, W3/13$^-$, A1-3$^+$). The fact that MRC OX-8$^+$ cells outnumber W3/13$^+$ cells has led to the speculation that some of these lymphoid cells represented NK cells (*19*); indeed we demonstrated occasional cells in rejecting allografts with the ultrastructural morphology of large granular lymphocytes. How these various mononuclear cell types affect endothelium, singly or in concert, could not be determined in this study, although isografts and CsA allografts did show markedly fewer infiltrating Tc, and lacked significant vascular injury, when compared with allografts. These observations suggest participation of Tc in the production of specific endothelial lesions.

Previous studies have failed to show a clear-cut role for macrophages in skin allograft rejection. Macrophages were found in large numbers in the infiltrates of healthy and rejecting grafts—and, in both cases these cells expressed Ia antigen, one marker of macrophage activation (*19*). In our study, the use of the monoclonal antibody A1-3, a new and additional marker of macrophage activation, provided findings that may contribute to understanding the role of macrophages in rejection. This novel antibody was shown recently to be a specific and sensitive marker for activated human monocytes and macrophages, and is capable of inhibiting the PCA of these cells (*29*). Furthermore, its membrane expression by tissue macrophages has been correlated with the formation and deposition of fibrin in rejecting human renal allografts (*30, 32*). In the current study, we observed reactivity for this antibody by macrophages infiltrating skin allografts and isografts, but not in CsA allografts. In allografts demonstrating endothelial cell injury, A1-3^+ macrophages were found in close proximity to occlusive thromboses within the affected vessels. In contrast, in isografts, in which no endothelial cell damage was present, A1-3^+ macrophages were not associated with thromboses. This result in isografts may reflect localization and activation of limited numbers of macrophages in response to nonspecific tissue injury, but without significant fibrinogen leakage from damaged vessels. Alternately, it should be noted that A1-3 antigen expression has in some cases been demonstrated in cells lacking PCA; e.g., following prolonged culture in vitro, activated A1-3^+ macrophages lose their PCA. Hence its expression by isograft macrophages may represent an example of dissociation of A1-3 antigen and expression of macrophage PCA.

The mechanism(s) for CsA inhibition of allograft related thrombogenesis is unknown. While some authors have suggested that CsA can inhibit the generation of macrophage PCA in vitro, in the setting of allogeneic stimulation (*37*), others have presented evidence that CsA can enhance modestly the capacity of macrophages to generate PCA in response to phorbol esters or mitogens (*38*). The inhibitory effect of CsA on development of macrophage PCA appears to be indirect, through inhibition of lymphokine production by helper T cells (*37, 39*). It is not possible to extrapolate from these isolated in vitro effects to the net effect of CsA in vivo. However, in skin graft rejection, CsA may prevent thrombotic vascular lesions by at least two mechanisms. The first mechanism may involve inhibition of activation and clonal expansion of those Tc cells that are important for the mediation of initial endothelial cell damage. The second mechanism, also due to an effect of CsA on T cells, may involve inhibition of production of the lymphokines responsible for induction of macrophage PCA, and thus inhibition of fibrin thrombus formation in and around already damaged vessels. Our results suggest that CsA can prevent vascular damage, and subsequent ischemic injury to an allograft, by both of these mechanisms.

Acknowledgments. We thank Ms. Eileen Fonferko for expert technical assistance.

REFERENCES

1. Borel JF, Feurer C, Gubler HU, Stähelin H. Biological effects of cyclosporin A: a new antilymphocytic agent. Agents Actions 1976; 6: 468.
2. Morris PJ. The impact of cyclosporine on transplantation. Adv Surg 1984; 17: 99.
3. Kostakis AJ, White DJG, Calne RY. Prolongation of rat heart allograft survival by cyclosporin A. Ir J Med Sci 1977; 5: 280.
4. Calne RY, White JG. Cyclosporine A—a powerful immunosuppressant in dogs with renal allografts. Ir J Med Sci 1977; 5: 595.
5. Green CJ, Allison AC. Extensive prolongation of rabbit kidney allograft survival after short term cyclosporin A treatment. Lancet 1978; 1: 1182.
6. Morris PJ. Cyclosporin A: an overview. Transplantation 1981; 32: 349.
7. Homan WP, Fabre JW, Williams KA, Peter RM, Morris PJ. Studies on the immunosuppressive properties of cyclosporin A in rats receiving renal allografts. Transplantation 1980; 29: 361.
8. Calne RY, White DJG, Rolles K, Smith DP. Prolonged survival of pig orthotopic heart grafts with cyclosporin A. Lancet 1978; 1: 1183.
9. Reitz BA, Bieber CB, Raney AA, Pennock JL, Janieson SW, Oyer P, Stinson EB. Orthotopic heart and combined heart and lung transplantation with cyclosporin-A immunosuppression. Transplant Proc 1981; 13: 393.
10. Rynasiewicz JJ, Sutherland DER, Kawahara K, Gorecki P, Najarian JS. Cyclosporin A prolongation of segmental pancreatic and islet allograft function in rats. Transplant Proc 1980; 12: 270.
11. Tilney NL, Milford EL, Araujo JL, Strom TB, Carpenter CB, Kirkman RL. Experience with cyclosporin and steroids in clinical renal transplantation. Ann Surg 1984; 200: 605.
12. Leoni P, Garcia RC, Allison AC. Effects of cyclosporin A on human lymphocytes in culture. J Clin Lab Immunol 1978; 1: 67.
13. Palacios R, Moller G. Cyclosporin A blocks receptors for HLA-DR antigens on T cells. Nature 1981; 290: 792.
14. Bunjes D, Hardt C, Röllinghoff M, Wagner H. Cyclosporin A mediates immunosuppression of primary cytotoxic T cell responses by impairing the release of interleukin 1 and interleukin 2. Eur J Immunol 1981; 11: 657.
15. Kalman VK, Klimpel GR. Effects of cyclosporin on the production of various interferons. Transplant Proc 1983; 15: 2383.
16. Kupiec-Weglinski JW, Filho MA, Strom TB, Tilney NL. Sparing of suppressor cells: a critical action of Cyclosporine. Transplantation 1984; 38: 97.
17. Towpik E, Kupiec-Weglinski J, Tyler D, Araujo J, Schneider T, Araneda D, Murphy GF, Tilney N. Cyclosporine and experimental skin allografts. I. Longterm survival in rats treated with low maintenance doses. Plast Reconstr Surg 1985; 76: 312.
18. Dvorak HF, Mihm MC Jr, Dvorak AM, Barnes BA, Manseau EJ, Galli SJ. Rejection of first-set skin allografts in man. The microvasculature is the critical target of the immune response. J Exp Med 1979; 150: 322.
19. Dallman MJ, Mason DW, Webb M. The roles of host and donor cells in the rejection of skin allografts by T cell-deprived rats injected with syngeneic T cells. Eur J Immunol 1982; 12: 511.
20. Mason DW, Dallman MJ, Arthur RP, Morris PJ. Mechanisms of allograft rejection: the roles of cytotoxic T-cells and delayed-type hypersensitivity. Immunol Rev 1984; 77: 167.
21. Loveland BE, Hogarth PM, Ceredig Rh, McKenzie IFC. Cells mediating graft rejection in the mouse. I. Lyt-1 cells mediate skin graft rejection. J Exp Med 1981; 153: 1044.
22. Bhan AK, Mihm MC, Jr, Dvorak HF. T cell subsets in allograft rejection. In situ characterization of T cell subsets in human skin allografts by the use of monoclonal antibodies. J Immunol 1982; 129: 1578.
23. Karnovsky MJ. The ultrastructural basis of capillary permeability studied with peroxidase as a tracer. J Cell Biol 1967; 35: 213.
24. Sunderland CA, McMaster WR, Williams AF. Purification with monoclonal antibody of a predominant leukocyte-common antigen and glycoprotein from rat thymocytes. Eur J Immunol 1979; 9: 155.
25. McMaster WR, Williams AF. Identification of Ia glycoproteins in rat thymus and purification from rat spleen. Eur J Immunol 1979; 9: 426.
26. Gilman SC, Rosenberg JS, Feldman JD. Membrane phenotype of the rat cytotoxic T lymphocyte. J Immunol 1982; 129: 1012.
27. Cantrell DA, Robins RA, Brooks CG, Baldwin RW. Phenotype of rat natural killer cells defined by monoclonal antibodies marking

rat lymphocyte subsets. Immunology 1982; 45: 97.
28. Barclay AN. The localization of populations of lymphocytes defined by monoclonal antibodies marking rat lymphocyte subsets. Immunology 1981; 42: 593.
29. Ewan VA, Cieplinski W, Hancock WW, Goldschneider I, Boyd AW, Rickles FR. Production and characterization of a monoclonal antibody (A1-3) that binds to activated monocytes and inhibits monocyte procoagulant activity. J Immunol 1986; 136: 2408.
30. Hancock WW, Rickles FR, Ewan VA, Atkins RC. Immunohistological studies with A1-3, a monoclonal antibody to activated human monocytes. J Immunol 1986; 136: 2416.
31. Edwards RL, Rickles FR. Macrophage procoagulants. Progr Hem Thromb 1984; 7: 183.
32. Hancock WW, Gee D, De Moerloose P, Rickles FR, Ewan VA, Atkins RC. Immunohistological analysis of serial biopsies taken during human renal allograft rejection. Changing profile of infiltrating cells and activation of the coagulation system. Transplantation 1985; 39: 430.
33. Hancock WW, Atkins RC. Activation of the coagulation pathways and fibrin deposition in human glomerulonephritis. Semin Nephrol 1985; 5: 69.
34. Hancock WW, Atkins RC. Immunohistological studies with monoclonal antibodies. In: di Sabato G, Langone JJ, van Vunakis, eds. Immunochemical techniques. Orlando: Academic Press, 1986: 2408.
35. Grossi CE, Cadoni A, Zicci A, Leprini A, Ferrarini M. Large granular lymphocytes in human peripheral blood: ultrastructural and cytochemical characterization of the granules. Blood 1982; 59: 277.
36. Bradley JA, Mason DW, Morris PJ. Evidence that rat renal allografts are rejected by cytotoxic T cells and not by nonspecific effectors. Transplantation 1985; 39: 169.
37. Helin HJ, Edgington TS. Cyclosporin A regulates monocyte/macrophage procoagulant response to allogeneic stimulation. J Immunol 1984; 132: 1074.
38. Carlsen E, Mallet AC, Prydz H. Effect of cyclosporine A on procoagulant activity in mononuclear blood cells and monocytes in vitro. Clin Exp Immunol 1985; 60: 416.
39. Thompson RW, Moon DK, Geczy CL, Nelson DS. Cyclosporin A inhibits lymphokine production but not the responses of macrophages to lymphokines. Immunology 1983; 48: 291.

Received 15 August 1985.
Accepted 9 October 1985.

0041-1337/86/4106-0739$02.00/0
TRANSPLANTATION
Vol. 41, No. 6
Printed in U.S.A.

THE SPECIFICITY OF NEPHRITOGENIC ANTIBODIES

IV. BINDING OF MONOCLONAL ANTITHYMOCYTE ANTIBODIES TO RAT KIDNEY[1]

W. M. BAGCHUS,[2] J. DONGA, J. ROZING,[3] PH. J. HOEDEMAEKER,[4] AND W. W. BAKKER

Department of Pathology, University of Groningen, 9713 EZ Groningen; Department of Internal Medicine, Erasmus University, Rotterdam; and Department of Pathology, University of Leiden, Leiden, The Netherlands

Polyclonal rabbit antirat thymocyte serum (ATS) has been shown to form in situ glomerular immune aggregates following perfusion into normal rat kidney ex vivo. This may be due to the presence of T-cell-like epitopes in the rat kidney, or it may be a result of contaminating anti-connective-tissue antibodies in ATS. To exclude the latter possibility we investigated binding to the rat kidney of three different (mouse) monoclonal antirat thymocyte antibodies (anti-T-cell MoAbs), directed to Thy 1.1 antigen, as well as (control) anti-B-cell MoAbs. The MoAbs were incubated in vitro with kidney sections or perfused into the blood-free rat kidney ex vivo. It was shown using immunofluorescence (IF) and immunoelectron microscopy (IEM) (peroxidase technique) that the anti-T-cell MoAbs used, in contrast to anti-B-cell MoAbs, are able to bind with glomerular capillary walls, and with mesangial structures after incubation in vitro or perfusion ex vivo. Although staining patterns are not completely identical, the reaction product is clearly demonstrated throughout the glomerular basement membrane (GBM) and along the plasma membranes of endothelial and epithelial cells, after contact with either of the three anti-T-cell MoAbs used. It is concluded that the presence of T-cell-like epitopes in the rat kidney may lead to immune complex formation following contact with anti-T-cell MoAbs. The nephritogenicity of rabbit ATS, as well as of some batches of clinically used ATS, may also be explained by this mechanism rather than by the usually assumed presence of contaminating antibodies in these polyclonal antisera.

Anti-human-thymocyte serum (a-human ATS)* is used as an immunosuppressive agent in transplantation (*1*, *2*). The

[1] This work was supported by a grant from the Dutch Kidney Foundation.

[2] Address correspondence to: W. M. Bagchus, University of Groningen, Oostersingel 63, 9713 EZ Groningen, The Netherlands.
[3] Erasmus University.
[4] University of Leiden.

* Abbreviations used: a-human ATS, anti-human-thymocyte serum; ATS, rabbit antirat thymocyte serum; DAB, diaminobenzidine; FITC, fluorescein isothiocyanate; GAM, goat antimouse IgG, GBM, glomerular basement membrane; IEM, immunoelectron microscopy; IF, immunofluorescence; LRE, lamina rara externa; MoAb, monoclonal antibody; PBS, phosphate-buffered saline; Tris MA, tris hydroxymethyl aminomethane maleic acid.

presence of nephritogenic antibodies in batches of this antiserum has been reported (*1, 2*). Contaminating stromal elements in the inoculum used for immunization are thought to be responsible for the presence of these undesired antibodies (*3*).

Rabbits immunized with thoroughly washed rat thymus cell suspensions also produce nephritogenic antibodies (ATS) (*4*). Administration of these antibodies into rats i.v. causes a transient glomerulopathy, characterized by immune aggregates localized in the kidney—mostly in the mesangium, and also along the glomerular basement membrane (GBM) (*5*). The possibility exists that the nephritogenicity of ATS is due to epitopes shared among T cell membranes and kidney structures, such as the Thy 1.1 antigen, which is present on rat thymocyte membranes and mesangium cells of the rat kidney (*6–9*).

Interestingly, rabbit antibodies directed to brushborder antigens—which, after injection into rats, induce heterologous immune complex glomerulopathy—also contain anti-T-cell specificity (*4, 10, 11*). In earlier studies we were able to demonstrate that this anti-T-cell activity is crucial for localization along the GBM after perfusion ex vivo (*12, 13*).

In order to characterize the epitopes presumably shared between thymocytes and kidney, we studied the renal binding of (mouse) monoclonal antibodies directed to thymocytes using immunofluorescence (IF) and immunoelectron microscopy (IEM). The binding was studied following incubation of kidney sections with the antibodies as well as after perfusion of these MoAbs in the normal rat kidney ex vivo.

The results show that monoclonal anti-T-cell antibodies, in contrast to monoclonal antibodies directed to rat B cells, are able to bind in mesangial matrix as well as in the GBM after ex vivo perfusion or incubation in vitro with rat kidney tissue. It is concluded that in glomerular mesangium as well as in GBM, epitopes occur that are recognized by anti-T-cell paratopes. It is likely, therefore, that the nephritogenicity of polyclonal ATS observed previously (*5*)—as well as that of some batches of a-human ATS prepared for clinical use—is due to the presence of T cell epitopes in the glomerulus rather than to antikidney antibodies induced by contaminating connective tissue in the inoculum used for preparation of these antisera.

MATERIALS AND METHODS

Animals. Female outbred Wistar rats of three months of age were used throughout the study. The rats were fed with RMBH (Woerden, The Netherlands) and received water ad libitum.

Monoclonal antibodies (MoAbs). Three mouse MoAbs against rat thymocytes and one against rat B cells were used in this study. Ascites-derived MoAbs were prepared using 50% saturated ammonium sulfate precipitation, according to standard techniques. After dialysis against phosphate-buffered saline (PBS), pH 7.3, for 72 hr, optical density was measured at 280 nM by spectrophotometry, and the antibodies were stored at −20°C at a concentration of 1 mg/ml. Some characteristics of these antibodies are summarized in Table 1.

Ex vivo perfusion of normal rat kidney with monoclonal antibodies. Ex vivo perfusion of normal female Wistar rats was done according to Van Damme (*10*) with minor modifications as described elsewhere (*5*). After kidney perfusion with PBS, pH 7.2, 37°C (2 ml/min), 10 ml MoAb containing 100 μg IgG/ml PBS was perfused. After perfusion of MoAb, subsequently 5 ml PBS was perfused to remove nonfixed antibodies and/or complexes. A small piece of kidney tissue was removed from the lower pole of the kidney, snap-frozen in freon 12, and stored at −80°C for IF microscopy. Kidneys were subsequently perfused for IEM with 20 ml of 0.2% freshly prepared glutaraldehyde, followed by perfusion with 5 ml Tris (hydroxymethyl) aminomethane (Tris) maleic acid, pH 7.3 (Tris MA). The kidney was taken out, and small pieces of kidney were rinsed in Tris MA for 2 hr at 4°C, snap frozen in freon 12 at −80°C, and processed as described below.

TABLE 1. Monoclonal antibodies used for in vitro incubation and ex vivo perfusion of normal rat kidney

Code[a]	Subclass	Antigenic determinant[b]	Distribution[c]
ER 14	IgG 1	25 kD	96% Thymocytes
			3% Spleen cells
			0% Peripheral lymphocytes
			31% Bone marrow cells
ER 4	IgG 2a	25 kD	98% Thymocytes
			1% Spleen cells
			5% Peripheral T lymphocytes
			20% Bone marrow
ER 5	IgG 3	25 kD	97% Thymocytes
			15% Spleen cells
			27% Bone marrow cells
HIS 11	IgG 1	—	B cell areas of the rat spleen

[a] The ER-coded antibodies were prepared by Dr. J. Rozing, Erasmus University, Rotterdam; MoAb HIS 11 was a gift from Prof. Dr. P. Nieuwenhuis, Department of Histology, Groningen.

[b] Molecular weight of antigenic determinants, as detected by immunoprecipitation is indicated in kilodaltons (kD) (*14*).

[c] Tissue distribution of the antibodies was determined by FACS analysis with fluorescein-isothiocyanate (FITC)-conjugated IgG (*14*). The FACS data were confirmed with immunohistology. The tissue distribution of HIS 11 (*15*) was detected by immunohistology (peroxidase method).

Immunofluorescence (IF) microscopy. To study binding of MoAb with normal rat kidney, in vitro cryostat sections (4-μm) of normal kidney tissue were washed twice in PBS followed by incubation with 0.05 ml MoAb (50 μg/ml) for 30 min, washed twice, and subsequently incubated with 0.05 ml fluorescein isothiocyanate (FITC)-conjugated goat antimouse IgG (GAM) (1/40, Nordic, Tilburg, The Netherlands) for 30 min. After two washings in PBS the sections were embedded in mounting medium (Gurr, pH 8.0) and examined under a Leitz Orthoplan fluorescence microscope with Ploemopak illumination. Localization of mouse IgG, after perfusion of MoAb into normal rat kidney, was studied by staining of 4-μm cryostat sections with FITC-conjugated GAM, as described above.

Immunoelectron microscopy (IEM). Binding of MoAbs to normal rat kidney at the ultrastructural level was studied using small pieces of 0.2% glutaraldehyde-perfused kidney cortex. Cryostat sections of 16 μm were washed 5 times with PBS, followed by incubation with 0.5 ml MoAb (350 μg/ml) for 3 hr. Subsequently they were washed 5 times with PBS and incubated with 0.5 ml peroxidase-conjugated rabbit antimouse IgG (1/20, Dakopatts, Denmark) for 3 hr, followed by 5 washings in PBS. Then 3.3 diaminobenzidine (DAB) tetra-hydrochloride (0.1%) was added containing 0.01% H_2O_2; after 25 min incubation with DAB, the sections were washed with PBS (5×). All incubation steps so far were performed at room temperature. Postfixation in 0.1 M phosphate buffered O_sO_4 for 45 min was done at 4°C. The sections were embedded in Epon and processed according to standard methods (*5*). Identical procedures were used for the detection of mouse IgG in kidneys that had been perfused with MoAbs.

RESULTS

Immunofluorescence microscopy. After incubation of cryostat sections of normal kidneys with anti-Thy 1.1 (ER 14) and FITC-GAM, mesangial staining, as well as a fine granular staining along the capillary walls, can be seen (Fig. 1A). In contrast, incubation with MoAb directed to B cells (HIS 11) did not result in staining of glomerular structures (Fig. 1B). Incubation with ER 4 (Fig. 1C) and ER 5 (Fig. 1 D) showed staining patterns similar to those seen using ER 14. Identical staining patterns (not shown here) occurred after perfusion into the rat kidney ex vivo of the MoAbs used in this study—i.e., positive staining after perfusion of ER 4, 5, and 14 and no detectable staining after perfusion of HIS 11.

Immunoelectron microscopy. Incubation of normal rat kidney tissue with anti-Thy-1.1 (ER 14) showed reaction product in the mesangial matrix and along mesangial cell membranes, in particular in areas where the mesangial cell borders the endothelial cell membrane (Fig. 2A). Reaction product can also be observed through the glomerular filtration barrier, including GBM and plasma membranes of endothelial and epithelial cells (Fig. 2B). After incubation with anti-B-cell MoAb (HIS 11) no reaction product was observed in the mesangium (Fig. 2C) or along the capillary walls (Fig. 2D).

Perfusion of ER 14 into the kidney resulted in localization of reaction product in the mesangium similar to that observed after in vitro incubation (Fig. 3A). Reaction product was also detected in the capillary wall—i.e., through the GBM in partic-

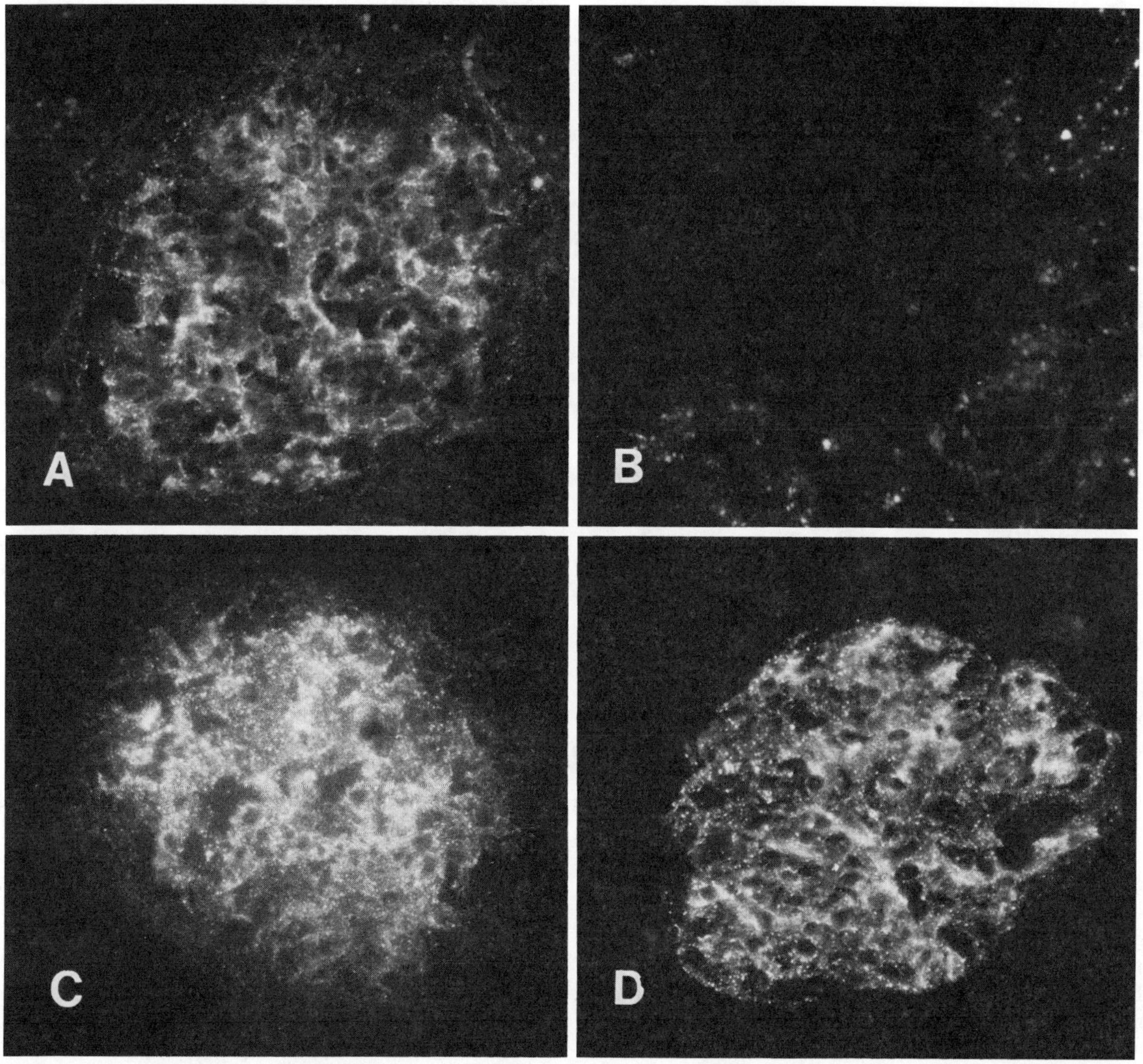

FIGURE 1. In vitro incubation of cryostat sections of normal rat kidney with 50 μg/ml of ER 14 (A), HIS 11 (B), ER 4 (C), or ER 5 (D), and FITC-conjugated goat anti-mouse IgG (1/40). All ER antibodies show confluent mesangial staining as well as fine granular staining along the capillary walls (A, C, and D: ×400). (In addition, some granular staining along Bowman's capsule is seen using ER 14 (A). Incubation with HIS 11 and FITC-conjugated goat antimouse IgG did not stain glomerular structures (B). Some autofluorescence of lysozomes in tubular structures can be seen (B: ×400).

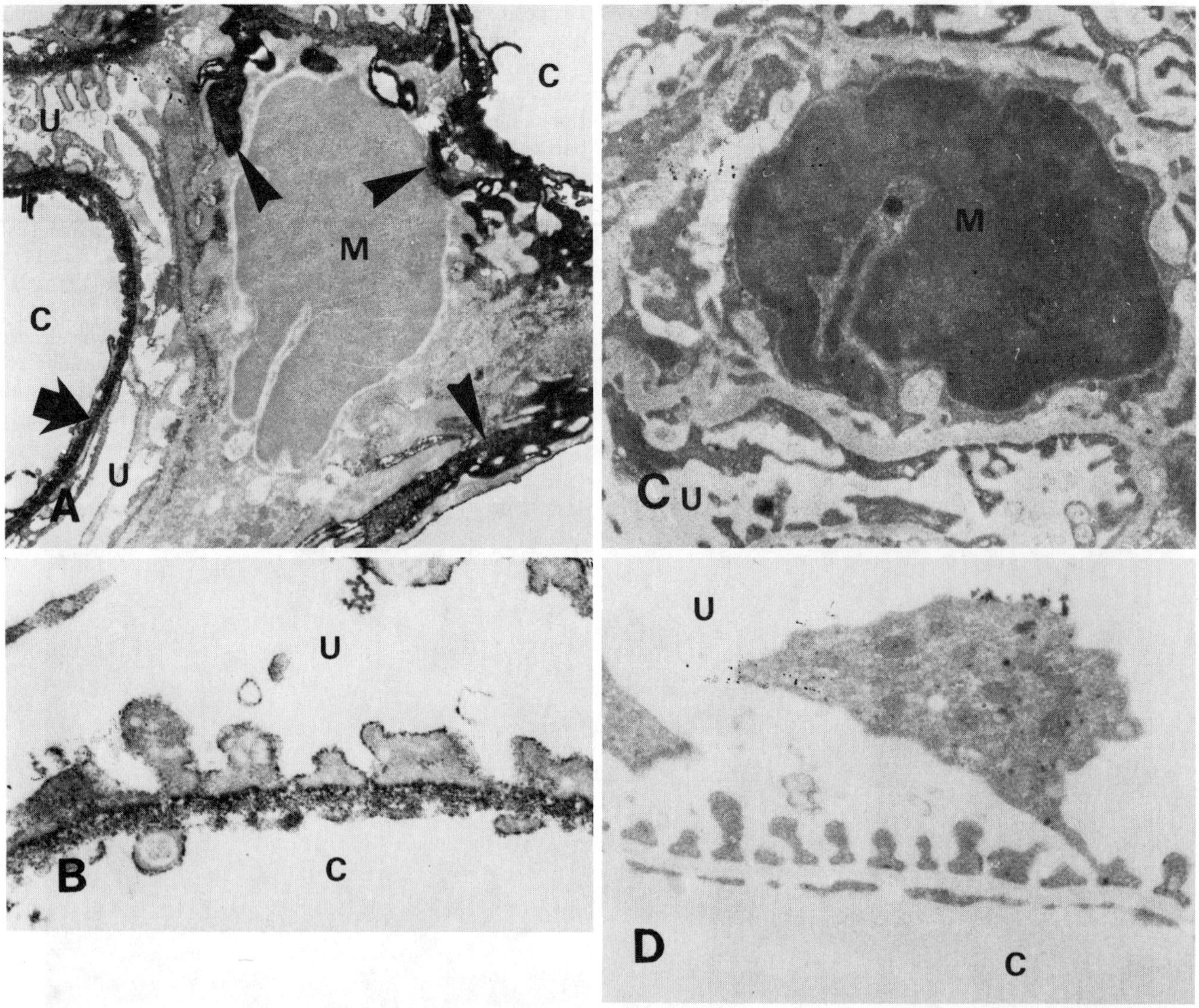

FIGURE 2. IEM of a normal rat kidney incubated with 0.5 ml containing 350 μg/ml ER 14 (A and B) or HIS 11 (C and D). Note the dark reaction product (arrowheads) present in the matrix of the mesangial cell (A: ×10,413). Staining of the GBM and endothelial cell membranes is also observed (arrow). (B) (×27,637) shows a peripheral part of the GBM. Reaction product is present throughout the GBM and along the membranes of the epithelial and endothelial cells. After incubation with HIS 11 no reaction product is detected (C: ×11,900 and D: ×26,780). (C: capillary lumen, M: mesangial cell, U: urinary space).

ular in the lamina rara externa (LRE) and along the membranes of epithelial and endothelial cells (Fig. 3B). No reaction product could be detected after perfusion of anti-B-cell MoAb (HIS 11) (results not shown). Following perfusion with ER 4 (Fig. 4A, B) or ER 5 (Fig. 5A, B) into the rat kidney ex vivo, reaction product along the mesangial matrix (Fig. 4A, 5A), as well as throughout the GBM (Fig. 4B, 5B), could be detected. After perfusion of ER 4, equal distribution of reaction product throughout the GBM can be detected (Fig. 4B), while after perfusion of ER 5 reaction product can be seen in particular at the LRE of the GBM (Fig. 5B). Both antibodies also stained membranes of endothelial and epithelial cells. Identical staining patterns were seen after in vitro incubation of rat sections with ER 4 or ER 5 (results not shown).

DISCUSSION

In the present study monoclonal anti-Thy 1.1 IgG 1 (ER 14) was compared with an anti-B-cell MoAb of identical IgG 1 subclass (HIS 11) with respect to its binding properties to the rat kidney in vitro and after perfusion ex vivo. In addition, two more anti-T-cell MoAbs of different IgG subclass (ER 4 and ER 5) were studied for their binding properties in the rat kidney, as well as MoAbs of the IgG 2a subclass directed to rat leukemic cells (pre-B-cell leukemia *16*), kindly provided by Prof. Dr. P. Nieuwenhuis, Groningen. The latter anti-B MoAbs did not show staining in vitro or after perfusion ex vivo using IF (data not shown).

The results show binding of anti-T-cell MoAbs to mesangium as well as GBM and plasma membranes of endothelial and epithelial cells, in contrast to anti-B cell MoAb HIS 11, which is negative in this respect (Fig. 1B; Fig. 2, C and D). It is concluded that the subclass of the anti-T-cell MoAb is not important for the observed binding to the rat kidney. Whether the pronounced accumulation of reaction product after perfusion of ER 14 (Fig. 3B) and ER 5 (Fig. 5B), in contrast to ER 4 (Fig. 4B), in the LRE of the GBM reflects differences in

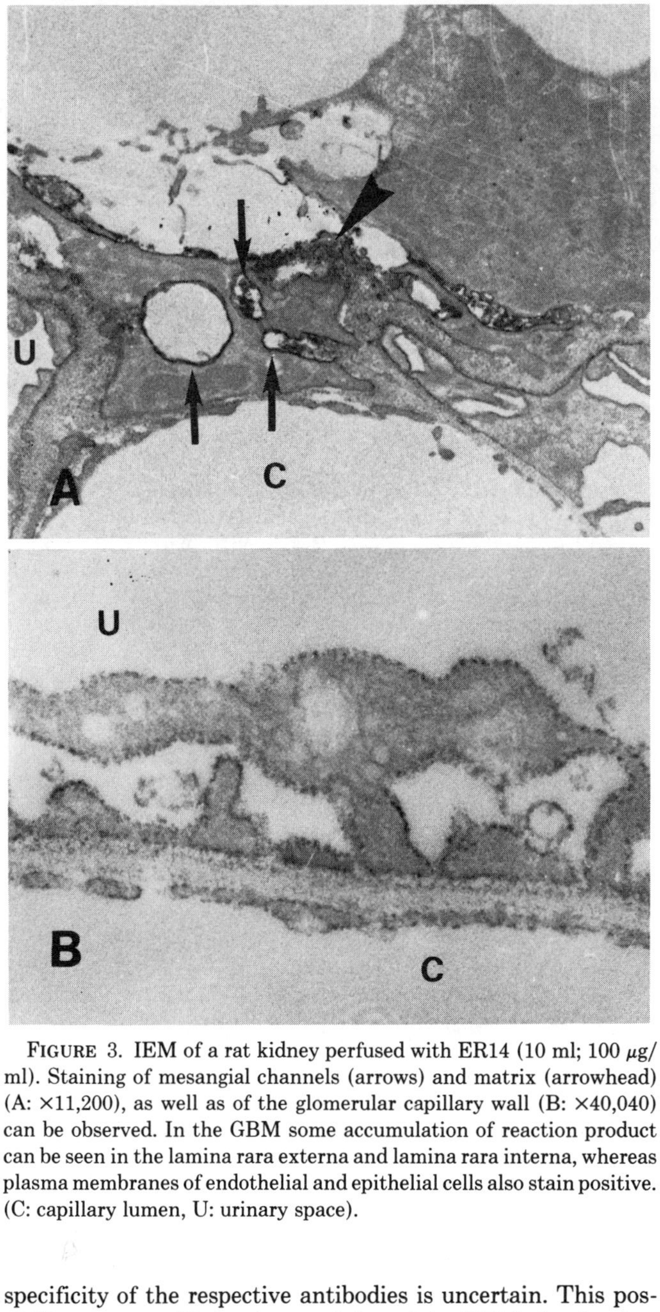

FIGURE 3. IEM of a rat kidney perfused with ER14 (10 ml; 100 μg/ml). Staining of mesangial channels (arrows) and matrix (arrowhead) (A: ×11,200), as well as of the glomerular capillary wall (B: ×40,040) can be observed. In the GBM some accumulation of reaction product can be seen in the lamina rara externa and lamina rara interna, whereas plasma membranes of endothelial and epithelial cells also stain positive. (C: capillary lumen, U: urinary space).

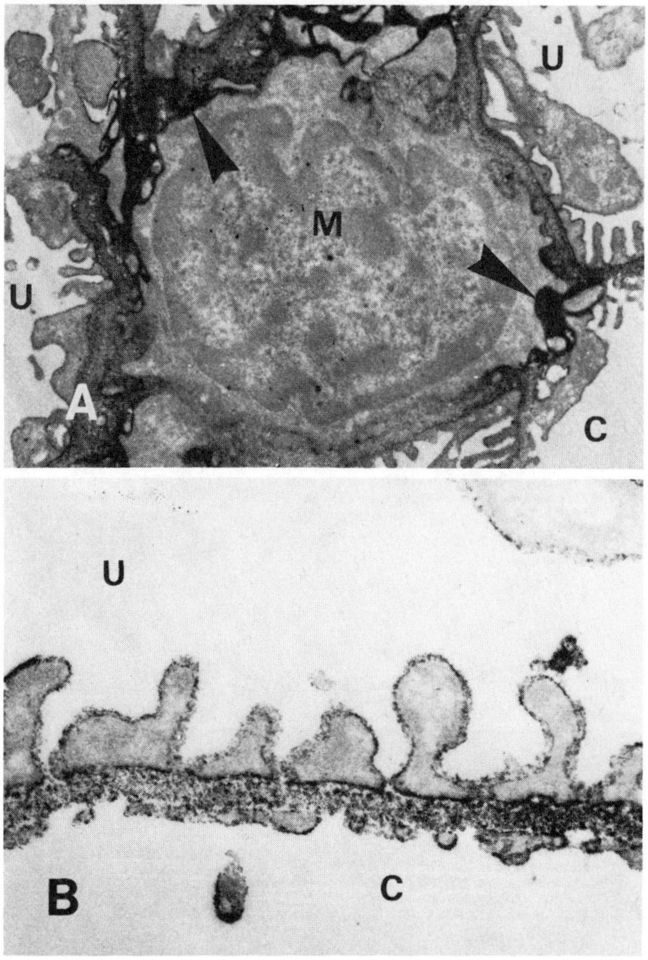

FIGURE 4. IEM of rat kidney after perfusion with ER 4. Prominent staining of the matrix of the mesangial cell (arrowheads) (A: ×10,080) is observed. Perfusion of ER 4 results in even distribution of reaction product in the GBM and staining of cell membranes of epithelial and endothelial cells (B: ×31,850). (C: capillary lumen, M: mesangial cell, U: urinary space).

specificity of the respective antibodies is uncertain. This possibility seems unlikely, since staining of the GBM after in vitro incubation of kidney sections with these anti-T-cell MoAbs resulted in identical staining patterns throughout the GBM (Fig. 2B).

The anti-T-cell MoAbs used in this study are directed to the Thy 1.1 antigens, since absorption with purified Thy 1.1 abolishes their anti-T-cell activity (*14*). The tissue distribution of the antigen recognized by ER 14 is indeed identical to the distribution of MoAb OX 7 against purified rat Thy 1.1 (*17*). However, since the Thy 1.1 molecule is characterized by a heterogenous glycosylation pattern (*18*), the three anti-T-cell MoAbs used may recognize different epitopes of this molecule. This is probably also reflected by the fact that the anti-T-cell MoAbs do not stain identical subsets of lymphoid cells (Table 1).

Whether differences in epitope recognition by these anti-T-cell antibodies are also reflected in different distribution of reaction product in the GBM, as stated above (Figs. 3B, 4B, and 5B) cannot be deduced from the present data; moreover it cannot be excluded completely, using these peroxidase techniques, that some diffusion of oxidized DAB plays a role.

Whatever the exact localization of the glomerular epitopes recognized by the anti-T-cell antibodies may be, from the IF data, as well as from the IEM results, it is clear that binding of anti-T-cell MoAb occurs in situ in mesangium, as well as within the GBM after contact with these MoAbs.

Since other glomerular constituents—i.e., type IV collagen, laminin, or entactin—are also present in the tubular basement membrane (*19–22*), which does not stain with the anti-T-cell MoAbs used, it is unlikely that our anti-T-cell MoAbs crossreact with these molecules. Similarly, crossreaction with actin (*23–25*) or fibronectin (*26*)seems unlikely, whereas these anti-T-cell MoAbs were not able to react with purified heparan sulfate using an in vitro assay (unpublished data).

In summary, the results of this study show that the GBM of the rat kidney contains T-cell-like epitopes, and they confirm the presence of Thy 1.1 antigen in the mesangium of the rat kidney, as demonstrated by other authors (*6–9*). This implicates that immune complex formation in situ after in vivo

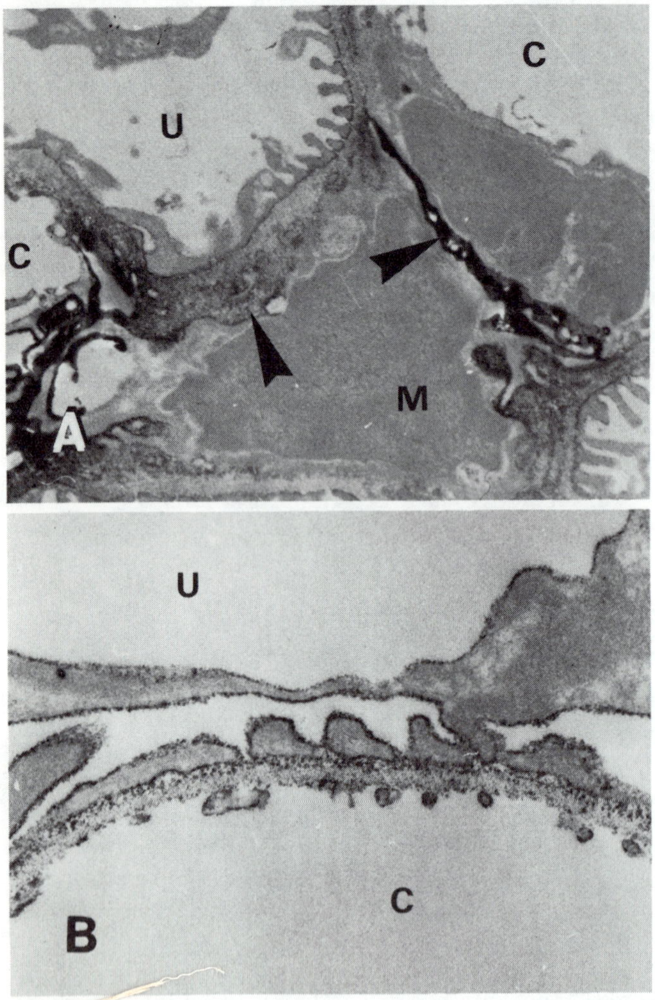

FIGURE 5. IEM of rat kidney perfused with ER 5. Staining of the matrix of the mesangial cell (A: ×10,515) is observed (arrowheads). Epithelial and endothelial cell membranes are also stained, and reaction product can be seen accumulated in the lamina rara externa (B: ×31,850), in the GBM, in particular (C: capillary lumen, M: mesangial cell, U: urinary space).

injection with polyclonal ATS, as shown previously (*5*), may be due to these T cell epitopes rather than to contaminating anti-connective-tissue antibodies, a mechanism generally assumed to explain the nephritogenicity in some batches of ATS prepared for clinical use (*2, 3*). The potential significance of T cell epitopes in the rat kidney is illustrated by massive proteinuria observed after a single injection of ER 4 (to be reported separately).

Acknowledgments. We thank Mr. H. Ferwerda and Mr. J. T. W. M. Vos for excellent technical assistance.

REFERENCES

1. Busch GJ, Birtch AG, Lukl P, Kobayashi K, Galvanek EG, Carpenter CB. Human renal allografts: glomerular deposits of horse immunoglobulin F and nephritis following administration of anti-lymphocyte globulin. Human Pathol 1971; 2: 299.
2. Strom B, Tilney NL, Merrill JP. Renal transplantation: clinical management of the transplant recipient. In: Brenner BM, Rector FC, eds. The kidney. Philadelphia: Saunders, 1981: 2618.
3. Monaco AP, Campion J-P, Kapnick SJ. Anti-lymphocyte globulins: clinical use of anti-lymphocyte globulin. Transplant Proc 1977; 9: 1007.
4. Bakker WW, Bagchus WM, Vos JTWM, Kooistra K, Hoedemaeker PhJ. The specificity of nephritogenic antibodies. I. Evidence on anti T-cell specificity in nephritogenic antibodies detected by cytotoxicity and MIF assays. Immunobiol 1981; 159: 235.
5. Bagchus WM, Donga J, Hoedemaeker PhJ, Bakker WW. The specificity of nephritogenic antibodies. II. Immune complex glomerulopathy in rats induced by heterologous antithymocyte serum. Transplantation 1984; 38: 165.
6. Ishizaki M, Sato S, Sano J, Fukuda Y, Sugisaki Y, Masugi Y. The presence of Thy-1.1 antigen in rat glomerular mesangial cells. Biomed Res 1980; 1: 438.
7. Harada K, Yamamoto T, Hara M, Kihara I. Antigenic association between kidney and thymocyte. Acta Pathol Jpn 1982; 32: 483.
8. Morris RJ, Ritter MA. Association of Thy 1 cell surface differentiation antigen with certain connective tissues in vivo. Cell Tissue Res 1980; 206: 459.
9. Paul LC, Rennke HG, Milford EL, Carpenter CB. Thy-1.1 in glomeruli of rat kidneys. Kidney Int 1984; 25: 771.
10. van Damme BJC, Fleuren GJ, Bakker WW, Vernier RL, Hoedemaeker PhJ. Experimental glomerulonephritis in the rat induced by antibodies directed against tubular antigens. V. Fixed glomerular antigens in the pathogenesis of heterologous immune complex glomerulonephritis. Lab Invest 1978; 38: 502.
11. Bakker WW, Bagchus WM, Hoedemaeker PhJ. Antithymus cell activity of nephritogenic antibodies. Transplantation 1979; 27: 217.
12. Bagchus WM, Vos JTWM, Bakker WW. Anti-T-cell specificity and localization of heterologous nephritogenic antibodies in the rat [Abstract]. Kidney Int 1984; 25: 732.
13. Bagchus WM, Vos JTWM, Hoedemaeker PhJ, Bakker WW. The specificity of nephritogenic antibodies. III. Binding of anti-FxiA antibodies in glomeruli is dependent on dual specificity. Clin exp Immunol 1986; 63: 639.
14. Rozing J, Joling P, Vaessen LMB. Determinants on the Thy-1 molecule expressed differentially during lympho-hematopoietic differentiation. Abstract book of the Fifth Int Workshop of Alloantigenic Systems in the Rat. Montreal, 1984.
15. Kroese FGM, Opstelten D, Wubbena AS, Deenen GJ, Aten J, Schwander EH, Leij L de, Nieuwenhuis P. Monoclonal antibodies to rat B-lymphocyte (sub-)populations. Proceedings of the 8th Int Conf on Lymphatic Tissues and Germinal Centres in Immune Reactions. Cambridge, 1984.
16. Rozing J, Vaessen LMB, Faber L, van Oven M, de Vries-Box L, de Jong B, Nieuwenhuis P. Pre B cell leukaemia in the rat. In: Nieuwenhuis P, van den Broek AA, Hanna Jr Mg, eds. Advances in experimental medicine and biology, vol 149: In vivo immunology. New York: Plenum Press, 1982: 111.
17. Mason DW, Williams AF. The kinetics of antibody binding to membrane antigens in solution and at the cell surface. Biochem J 1980; 187: 1.
18. Carlsson SR, Stigbrand T. Partial characterization of the oligosaccharides of mouse thymocyte Thy-1 glycoprotein. Biochem J 1984; 221: 379.
19. Hancock WH, Kraft N, Clarke F, Atkins RC. Production of monoclonal antibodies to fibronectin, type IV collagen and other antigens of the human glomerulus. Pathology 1984; 16: 197.
20. Abrahamson DR, Caulfield JP. Proteinuria and structural alterations in rat glomerular basement membranes induced by intravenously injected anti-laminin immunoglobulin G. J Exp Med 1982; 156: 128.
21. Jaffe R, Bender BL, Santamaria M, Chung AE. Segmental staining of the murine nephron by monoclonal antibodies directed against the GP-2 subunit of laminin. Lab Invest 1984; 51: 88.
22. Bender BL, Jaffe R, Carlin B, Chung AE. Immunolocalization of entactin, a sulfated basement membrane component, in rodent

tissues, and comparison with GP-2 (laminin). Am J Pathol 1981; 103: 419.
23. Scheinman JI, Fish AJ, Brown DM, Michael AJ. Human glomerular smooth muscle (mesangial) cells in culture. Lab Invest 1976; 34: 150.
24. Mendrick DL, Rennke HG, Cotran RS, Springer TA, Abbas AK. Monoclonal antibodies against rat glomerular antigens: production and specificity. Lab Invest 1983; 49: 107.
25. Dales S, Fujinami RS, Oldstone MBA. Serologic relatedness between Thy-1.2 and actin revealed by monoclonal antibody. J Immunol 1983; 131: 1332.
26. Courtoy PJ, Kanwar YS, Hynes RO, Farquhar MG. Fibronectin localization in the rat glomerulus. J Cell Biol 1980; 87: 691.

Received 20 August 1985.
Accepted 8 October 1985.

0041-1337/86/4106-0745$02.00/0
TRANSPLANTATION
Vol. 41, No. 6

THE ENTRY OF LYMPHOCYTES INTO STIMULATED LYMPH NODES

THE SITE OF SELECTION OF ALLOANTIGEN-SPECIFIC CELLS[1]

MARK T. DRAYSON[2]

Department of Immunology, Manchester University Medical School, Manchester M13 9PL, England

During a primary response to antigen, lymph nodes (LN) receive antigen-specific lymphocytes (ASL) from the recirculatory pool via specialized postcapillary venules (SPCV). Preliminary experiments demonstrated a three-fold increase in entry of ^{51}Cr-labeled thoracic duct lymphocytes (TDL) into the rat popliteal LN 3–4 days after alloantigenic stimulation. This increased entry was accounted for by an associated 4–5-fold increase in LN blood flow. It was unclear whether recruitment of ASL occurred within the SPCV lumen leading to selective entry of ASL—or, more conventionally, that entry of lymphocytes was a random process and that recruitment of ASL occurred in the extravascular space by selective retention. Thus a double-labeling technique was used to study the migratory characteristics of two populations of thoracic duct lymphocytes (TDL) that had been passaged from blood to lymph. The first population, passaged through a semiallogeneic animal, was negatively selected, and thus 99% depleted of ASL; the second population, passaged through a syngeneic animal, contained a normal complement of naive ASL. The two populations were combined before i.v. injection into syngeneic recipients. At 24 hr the right popliteal LN, which had previously been stimulated with the specific antigen, showed a preferential localization of the TDL containing ASL compared with the left (unstimulated) popliteal LN. This preferential localization was not present at 1 hr after injection. In the light of background data on the kinetics of lymphocyte traffic it is concluded that ASL were selected not at the luminal surface of SPCV but in the LN after they had left the bloodstream.

[1]This work was supported by an MRC research fellowship and by MRC Programme Grant G972/455B.

[2]Address correspondence to: Mark T. Drayson, Stopford Building, Oxford Road, Manchester M13 9PL, England.

The lymph node (LN),* although anatomically isolated, potentially provides a site for the presentation of antigen to the entire recirculating pool of lymphocytes (*1–4*). The major entry of lymphocytes into an LN occurs from the blood across the walls of specialized postcapillary venules (SPCV) (*5*). Following primary antigenic stimulation lymphocyte traffic is substantially increased by the combined effects of a greater blood flow to the LN and the expansion of the SPCV network—and possibly because of a more efficient extraction of lymphocytes from the blood (*6–10*). It is through this traffic of lymphocytes that antigen-specific lymphocytes (ASL) are delivered to the LN (*3, 4*).

It is generally held that lymphocytes cross SPCV irrespective of their antigenic specificity; it is only the encounter with antigen in the extravascular space that halts the migration of ASL while the majority of lymphocytes return to the blood via the efferent lymphatic (*3, 5*). A contrary conclusion was drawn from experiments in sheep suggesting that entry of lymphocytes into LN was not random (*11–13*) and that entry of ASL was selectively enhanced by the presentation of antigen on the luminal surface of SPCV (*12, 13*). This heterodox view was proposed as an explanation of the observation that the whole animal became specifically unresponsive if the sheep was deprived of the efferent lymph (removed by chronic drainage) emerging from a popliteal LN undergoing repeated antigenic stimulation. The plausibility of this notion (i.e., antigen selection within SPCVs) was strengthened by the finding that

* Abbreviations used: ASL, antigen-specific lymphocytes; dpm disintegrations per minute; Isl, index of selective localization; LN, lymph node; NSL, non-antigen-specific lymphocytes; PBS, phosphate-buffered saline; SPCV, specialized postcapillary venule; TDL, thoracic duct lymphocytes.

endothelial cells were shown to present histocompatibility antigens in vitro (*14, 15*).

The aim of the present study was to pinpoint the site of ASL selection relative to the blood vessel wall in antigenically stimulated LN. The experimental approach depended on measuring the localization of a *negatively selected* population of lymphocytes—i.e., lacking ASL, relative to the localization of a normal population that included ASL. The rationale depended heavily on a background of data on the kinetics of lymphocyte traffic through LN published by Smith and Ford (*16, 17*) as well as on preliminary experiments reported in the first section of the results.

MATERIALS AND METHODS

Experimental design. The experimental design is shown in Figure 1. The right popliteal LN was stimulated by a foot-pad injection of semiallogeneic LN cells. Syngeneic LN cells were injected into the left foot-pad and the left popliteal LN used as an internal control. Between 12 hr and 3 days later the rat was given an i.v. injection of syngeneic thoracic duct lymphocytes (TDL) containing a mixture of two marked populations. The first population was labeled with ^{3}H-uridine; having been passaged from blood to lymph in a syngeneic intermediate rat it contained a normal proportion of ASL, previously estimated to be between 2% and 12% of the total (*18–21*). The second population was labeled with ^{14}C-uridine; having been passaged from blood to lymph in a semiallogeneic intermediate rat, it was negatively selected and devoid of ASL (*22*). At either 1 hr or 24 hr after injection of labeled cells the animal was sacrificed and the ^{3}H/^{14}C ratios measured in the popliteal LN. Comparison of these ratios between the stimulated and internal control LN provided an index of selective localization–which, if greater than unity, indicated selective localization of ASL.

The interval between i.v. injection of labeled cells and sacrifice was critical to the analysis. It was shown by Smith and Ford (*15, 17*) that by 1 hr after i.v. injection the blood levels of labeled cells fell to 4% of the injected dose—a figure that remained constant over the next 23 hr. By contrast LN localization rose to maximum values by 1 hr after injection and remained relatively constant over the following 23 hr. In addition, labeled cells having entered an LN from the blood take a minimum of 2 hr and a modal time of 12 hr to traverse the LN space and reenter the blood via the lymphatic system. Thus any selective localization of ASL detected 1 hr after injection must have been due to selective entry across the SPCV. By 24 hr sufficient time would have elapsed to allow between one and two passages of labeled lymphocytes through the LN. Any selective localization of ASL would then be due to selective entry across SPCV and/or selective retention within the LN space.

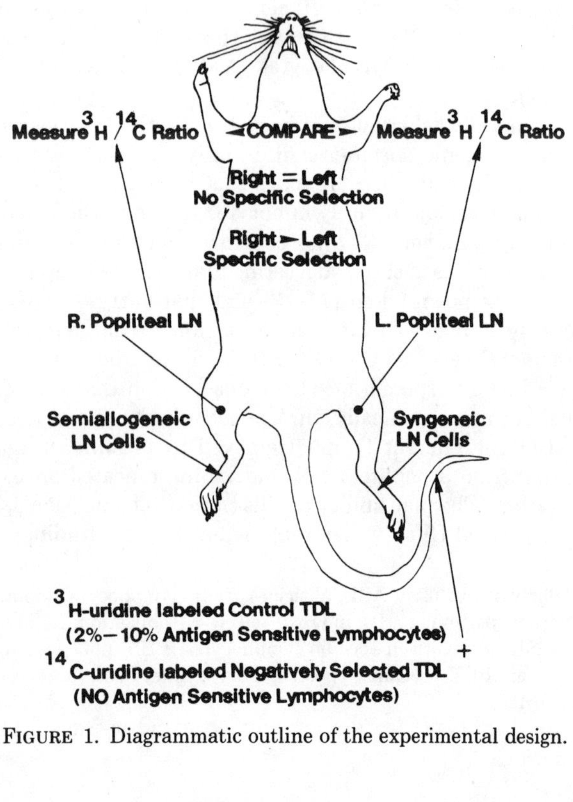

FIGURE 1. Diagrammatic outline of the experimental design.

Rats and major histocompatibility types. Two-to-three–months–old rats of the highly inbred AO strain (RT1^{u}) were used as donors of TDL, as intermediates for the passage of those TDL and as final recipients. Semiallogeneic rats for the passage of TDL or the provision of LN cells for foot-pad injection were (AO×DA)F_1 hybrids (RT1^{u}×RT1^{a}) or (AO×PVG) F_1 hybrids (RT1^{u}×RT1^{c}). Foot-pad injections s.c. consisted of 5×10^{6} mesenteric LN cells in phosphate-buffered saline (PBS) in a total volume of 100 μl.

Labeling and passage of TDL. Rats were cannulated by Gowans' method (*23*), and the first night collections of TDL on ice were pooled and divided into two. Half was labeled with [5-^{3}H] uridine at 6 μCi/ml, the other was labeled with [^{14}C] uridine at 1 μCi/ml (Radiochemical Centre, Amersham, UK TRA-178 and CFA-315, respectivley) (*23*). ^{3}H-uridine-labeled and ^{14}C-uridine-labeled cells were injected into syngeneic and semiallogeneic irradiated intermediate recipients, respectively, at a dose of 1–2×10^{9} cells per animal. Intermediates were irradiated with 400 rads over a 15-min period from a Cobalt 60 source 72 hr before cell transfer. Blood-to-lymph passage ensures that cells transferred to the final recipient are accredited recirculating lymphocytes; damaged and large lymphocytes are removed, and most of the radioactive uridine has entered the acid-insoluble fraction (*20*). Collection of passaged lymphocytes was made 0–36 hr after transfer to ensure that cells from semiallogeneic intermediates were negatively selected (*22*). Collection periods were limited to 4–6 hr at room temperature, and cells were subjected to a minimum of in vitro handling before i.v. injection into the final recipients to ensure rapid entry into LN (*16, 17*).

Five experiments were performed, the details of which are presented in Table 1. In experiment 2 the passage of ^{3}H and ^{14}C labeled cells was reversed such that ^{3}H-uridine labeled cells were passaged through the semiallogeneic intermediates. This reverse labeling procedure is normally a check against different elution rates of ^{3}H and ^{14}C. However this procedure was not essential to our present experimental design because the ^{3}H/^{14}C ratio in the stimulated LN was compared directly with that in the contralateral node, which provided an internal control. The validity of this will be demonstrated both by the lack of difference in the results of experiments 1 and 2 and also by the consistent lack of difference in the ^{3}H/^{14}C ratios of right and left unstimulated inguinal LN.

Final recipients and measurement of radioacativity. Final recipients were injected with a mixture of ^{3}H and ^{14}C-uridine-labeled TDL containing 3–10×10^{7} cells of each population adjusted to contain comparable cell numbers and similar levels

TABLE 1. Experimental details

Experiment number and group	Number of rats	Intermediates through which donor TLD were passaged		Final AO recipients-cells used to stimulate popliteal lymph nodes		Time of foot-pad injections before transfer of labeled cells	Time of sacrifice of final recipients after transfer of labeled cells
		^3H-labeled TDL	^{14}C-labeled TDL	Left foot-pad injection	Right foot-pad injection		
1A	7	AO	AO×DA	AO	AO×DA	3 days	1 Hr
2A	4	AO×PVG	AO	AO	AO×PVG	12 Hr	1 Hr
2B	6	AO×PVG	AO	AO	AO×PVG	3 Days	1 Hr
3A	5	AO	AO×PVG	AO	AO×PVG	16 Hr	24 Hr
3B	6	AO	AO×PVG	AO	AO×PVG	3 Days	24 Hr
4A	4	AO	AO×DA	AO	AO×DA	36 Hr	24 Hr
4B	7	AO	AO×DA	AO	AO×DA	3 Days	24 Hr
5A	6	AO×PVG	AO×DA	AO×PVG	AO×DA	3 Days	1 Hr
5B	6	AO×PVG	AO×DA	AO×PVG	AO×DA	3 Days	24 Hr

of detectable radioactivity. At 1 hr or 24 hr after injection the rats were killed by cervical dislocation under ether anesthesia. The popliteal, inguinal, cervical, and mesenteric LN, as well as the spleen, liver, and lung were removed and prepared for liquid scintillation counting (*23*). $^3H/^{14}C$ activity was measured in a Packard 460C Automatic Scintillation System programmed to count ^3H and ^{14}C activity separately and to convert cpm to dpm. $^3H/^{14}C$ ratios were calculated for individual tissues.

Simultaneous measurement of weight, blood flow, and lymphocyte influx. This was carried out by a method described previously (*10*). In brief lymphocyte influx was measured by i.v. injection of ^{51}Cr-labeled syngeneic TDL 1 hr before sacrifice. Blood flow was measured by Sapirsteins method of fractional distribution of indicators (*24*), which involved injecting a bolus of $^{86}RbCl$, 45 sec before the animal was killed by injection of saturated potassium chloride.

RESULTS

Changes in weight, blood flow, and lymphocyte influx after alloantigenic stimulation. The sequence of changes in popliteal LN weight, blood flow, and lymphocyte influx in 38 rats given semiallogeneic LN cells into their right feet and syngeneic LN cells into their left feet are depicted in Figure 2. The results were expressed as a ratio of the values of right to left popliteal LN on a log scale. The left popliteal LN controls did not show any significant change in any of the measurements. In alloantigen-stimulated LN, all three parameters increased to a peak at 4–5 days after foot-pad injection.

Note that the increase in blood flow in the stimulated LN preceded, and was at all intervals greater than, the increase in lymphocyte influx–peak values being approximately 5 times and 3 times control values, respectively. Thus the increase in lymphocyte influx could be entirely attributed to the increased blood flow. In consideration of ASL it was clear that there must have been a 3-fold increase in influx of ASL into the LN, even in the absence of enhanced entry across SPCV. In order to assess the role, if any, of SPCV in selective recruitment it was necessary to measure the entry of ASL during the inductive phase of the immune response. Therefore in the following experiments intervals between LN stimulation and measurement of selective localization of ASL were between 12 hr and 3 days.

Migratory characteristics after alloantigenic stimulation. Both ^3H and ^{14}C activities were distributed between the different lymphoid and nonlymphoid tissues in a pattern that was con-

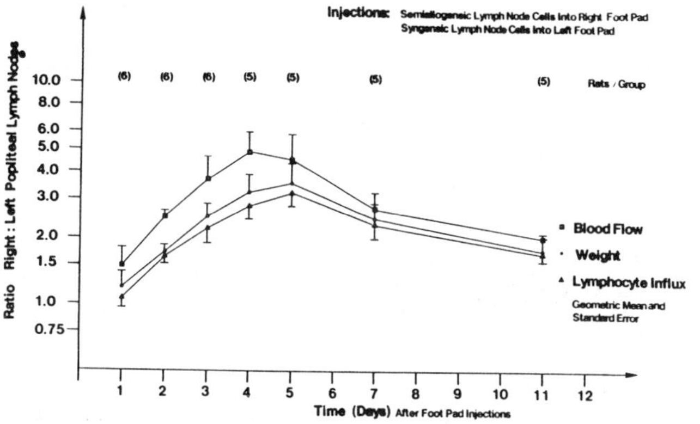

FIGURE 2. Sequential changes in weight, blood flow, and lymphocyte influx in the right popliteal LN following foot-pad injection of semiallogeneic LN cells at time 0. Note that the changes are depicted on a log scale and that the increase in blood flow is always greater than the increase in lymphocyte influx.

sistent with previous more detailed studies (*16, 17*). At 1 hr after injection, radioactivity in popliteal, inguinal, and cervical LN was approximately 50% of injected dose per gram of tissue; the percentage increased slightly by 24 hr. Mesenteric LN radioactivity was about 45% of injected dose per gram at 1 hr and rose to 100% by 24 hr. Conversely splenic radioactivity was 100% and 40% at 1 hr and 24 hr, respectively. There were differences between localization as assessed by ^3H and ^{14}C, particularly at 24 hr after i.v. injection: 2–5% less of ^3H activity at 1 hr as compared with ^{14}C, and 5–15% less of ^3H activity at 24 hr. These results were in accordance with previous studies (*16, 17, 20*) and there was no significant difference between the $^3H/^{14}C$ ratio of spleen and inguinal cervical and left popliteal LN of individual animals. Sequential changes in weight and lymphocyte influx in right popliteal LN at different intervals after foot-pad injection closely paralleled changes seen in the $^{51}Cr/^{86}Rb$ experiments.

Determination of selective localization. The results are expressed as an index of selective localization (Isl) according to the formula:

$$\text{Isl} = \left(\frac{\text{Ls}}{\text{Ln}}\right) \text{stimulated LN} \div \left(\frac{\text{Ls}}{\text{Ln}}\right) \text{control LN}$$

Where Ls = localization of syngeneic passaged TDL population, and Ln = localization of semiallogeneic passaged TDL population

Operationally this becomes:

$$\text{Isl} = \frac{{}^{3}\text{H dpm (stimulated LN)} \times {}^{14}\text{C dpm (control LN)}}{{}^{3}\text{H dpm (control LN)} \times {}^{14}\text{C dpm (stimulated LN)}}$$

Any selective localization of ASL in the stimulated right popliteal LN is signified by an Isl greater than 1.0. The geometric mean and standard errors of these indices are presented for individual groups of rats. Alternatively within any group the ^{3}H/^{14}C values of the stimulated LN were compared directly with those values in the internal control LN by means of a one-tailed Student's t test.

Possible differences between the migratory behavior of the two TDL populations through the alloantigen stimulated LN can be predicted by methods discussed in detail later. Prediction of differences in entry depends upon the proportion of cells in the syngeneic passaged TDL that are ASL (5–10%) and the degree of enhanced entry of ASL over that of NSL (2–4-fold). In the event of enhanced entry of ASL, the Isl would be in the range of 1.05–1.12. Prediction of differences in retention depends upon the proportion of cells in the syngeneic passaged TDL which are ASL (5–10%) and the number of passages of labeled cells through LN by 24 hr (1–2). The predicted range of Isl is thus 1.05–1.24.

Selective localization of ASL in stimulated LN 24 hr after injection. Figure 3 gives the results of experiments in which the 22 final recipients were killed 24 hr after i.v. injection of labeled cells. In experiment 3 (AO×PVG)F_1 hybrids were used as intermediates for passage of TDL and as donors for stimulation of the right popliteal LN. (AO×DA)F_1 hybrids were used in experiment 4 (See Table 1). In groups 4B and 3B studied 3 days after alloantigen stimulation, the mean Isl were 1.05 and 1.16, respectively. Group 4A studied 36 hr after alloantigen stimulation had a mean Isl of 1.10. Thus all these groups had significantly positive deviations from unity that were consistent with the predicted range (1.05–1.24). In group 3A studied only 16 hr after stimulation the mean Isl was 1.05, but not significantly different from unity. All inguinal LN pairs studied produced Isl that were not significantly different from unity.

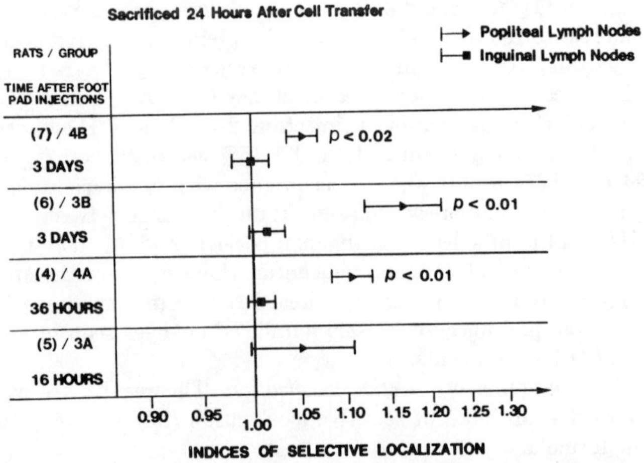

FIGURE 3. Indices of selective localization in alloantigen-stimulated LN 24 hr after injection of labeled cells. Indices greater than unity indicate selective localization of ASL. Geometric means and standard errors of groups of indices are displayed with the results of a one-tailed Student's t test of analyze significance of positive deviation from unity. Note positive deviations in groups studied 36 hr and 3 days after antigen stimulation, and that indices for inguinal LN pairs did not deviate from unity.

Thus at 24 hr after injection of labeled cells these experiments demonstrated a selective localization of ASL in LN at 36 hr and 3 days after alloantigen stimulation. However they did not elucidate whether selective localization was due to selective entry across SPCV or selective retention within the LN extravascular space.

Selective localization of ASL in stimulated LN 1 hr after injection. Figure 4 depicts the results of 17 rats killed 1 hr after cell transfer and 3 days or 12 hr after antigenic stimulation of the right popliteal LN. In all three groups the indices of selective localization both for popliteal and unstimulated inguinal LN pairs were not significantly different from unity. This demonstrates that there was no selective entry of ASL across SPCV, indicating that the selective localization of ASL found at 24 hr (Fig. 3) was due to selective retention of ASL within the LN extravascular space after random entry of TDL across SPCV.

In the next experiment both populations of labeled TDL were negatively selected but against different alloantigens (see Table 1). The ^{3}H-uridine-labeled population was negatively selected against the alloantigen used to stimulate the left popliteal LN, whereas the ^{14}C-uridine labeled population was negatively selected against the alloantigen used to stimulate the right popliteal LN. In the event of selective localization of both populations of ASL, one would expect the Isl to be approximately double that found in the previous experiments, assuming no significant crossreactivity between the two alloantigens used. Figure 5 depicts the results of 12 rats studied 3 days after foot-pad injection. In both groups indices for unstimulated inguinal LN pairs were not significantly deviated from unity. In group 5B killed 24 hr after injection of labeled cells, the mean index of selective localization (1.07) was highly significant. By contrast, in group 5A sacrificed 1 hr after injection of labeled cells, the mean Isl was 0.99—confirming again that ASL are selectively retained in the LN extravascular space after random entry across the SPCV.

DISCUSSION

The results reproducibly showed a selective localization of antigen-specific lymphocytes in the stimulated LN by 24 hr

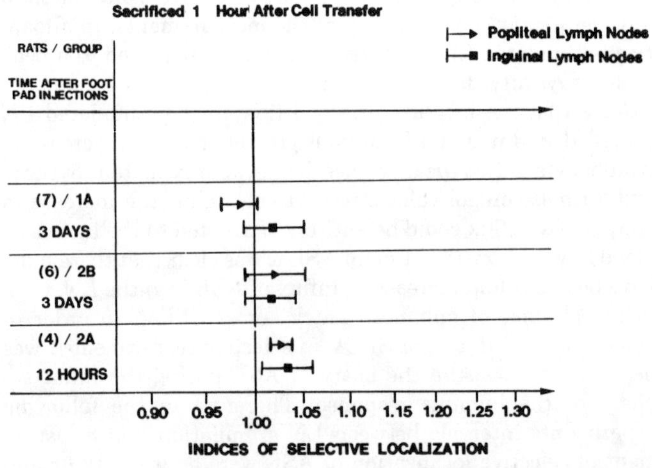

FIGURE 4. Indices of selective localization in alloantigen-stimulated LN 1 hr after injection of labeled cells. Indices greater than unity indicate selective localization of ASL. Geometric means and standard errors of groups of indices are displayed. Note that lack of significant deviation from unity in both popliteal and inguinal LN pairs, which was confirmed in a one-tailed Student's t test.

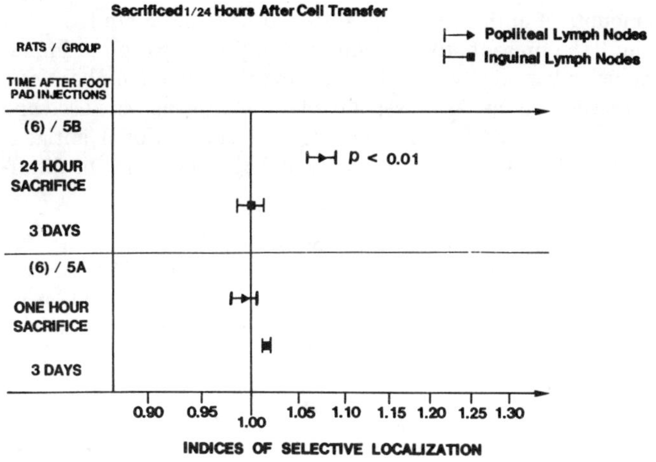

FIGURE 5. Indices of selective localization in alloantigen-stimulated LN 24 hr and 1 hr after injection of labeled cells. Indices greater than unity indicate selective localization of ASL. Note the statistically significant positive deviation from unity in the popliteal LN of animals sacrificed at 24 hr, but the lack of deviation in those sacrificed at 1 hr—as well as the lack of deviation in unstimulated inguinal LN pairs.

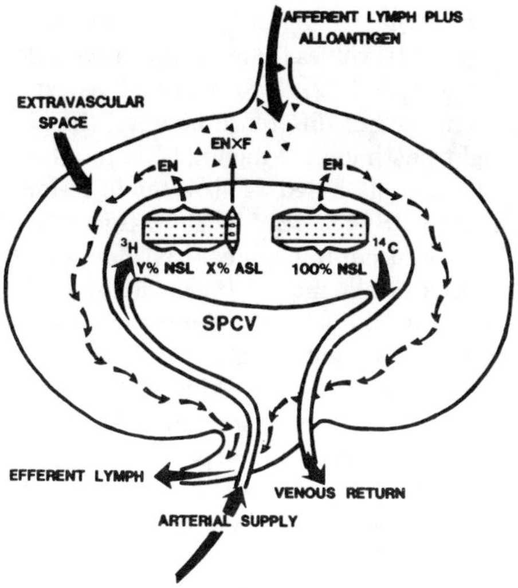

FIGURE 6. Topographical representation of alloantigen-stimulated LN demonstrating the theoretical basis of the experimental design. Two populations of TDL are shown passing through an SPCV—^{3}H-labeled syngeneic passaged population containing X% ASL and Y% NSL and a ^{14}C labeled semiallogeneic passaged population containing 100% NSL. EN is the proportion of NSL passing through SPCV that enter the extravascular space. F is the factor by which EN must be multiplied to derive the proportion of ASL that enter the extravascular space.

after injection. This selective localization may have been due to enhanced entry of ASL AND/OR selective retention of ASL. However the consistent lack of selective localization at 1 hr after injection indicated that selective entry of ASL across SPCV did not occur. The validity of this negative finding against the background of a positive demonstration of selective retention depends upon an analysis of predicted results versus actual results.

The basic concept of the experiments is illustrated in Figure 6, which shows the two TDL populations being delivered to the LN via the blood, the migration of ASL and NSL across the SPCV wall, and their subsequent movement in the extravascular space. The tempo of migration was eluciated by Smith and Ford (*16*, *17*)—and, as already discussed, provides the foundation for the present experimental design.

In consideration of entry of ASL and NSL, the relative localization of the normal and negatively selected TDL populations at 1 hr after injection can be predicted on the basis that the ^{3}H/^{14}C localization is determined by the equation (Fig. 6).

$$\frac{^{3}H}{^{14}C} = \frac{(EN \times Y) + (EN \times F \times X)}{(EN \times 100)} \qquad (1)$$

Since (EN×Y) represents entry of ^{3}H labeled NSL, (EN×F×X) represents entry of ^{3}H labeled ASL and (E×100) represents entry of ^{14}C labeled NSL. Because Y + X = 100 and in the left unstimulated LN F equals 1, we can substitute for ^{3}H/^{14}C ratios in the equation for the Index of selective localization presented in the results section to derive:

$$Isl = 1 + \frac{X(F-1)}{100} \qquad (2)$$

and x% is the proportion of lymphocytes in the normal syngenic passaged population of TDL sensitive to the antigen in question. In responses to sheep erythrocytes and flagellin the proportion has been estimated as being 1 in 10^5 and 1 in 10^6, respectively (*25*, *26*). In the case of alloantigens the proportion is very much higher. Various estimates have been made—at least 1–2% (*19*), 2–6% (*18*), and 30% (*27*)–but have not been fully satisfactory. Probably the most relevant estimates to these experiments were those produced by Ford, Atkins, and Simmonds who estimated that on passage from blood to lymph through an F_1 hybrid rat 5%–12% of donor lymphocytes were selectively retained because of antigen recognition (*20*, *21*), and thus these two figures have been used in predicting values for the Isl. F is the factor by which entry of ASL is enhanced over entry of NSL. If enhanced entry of ASL were to be of physiological significance one would expect F to be at least 2, and possibly a value of 4. Substitution of assumed values (X = 5–12%, F = 2–4) into equation 2 provides a predicted range of 1.05–1.12 for the index of selective localization at 1 hr after injection.

Let us now consider retention of ASL in the extravascular space of the stimulated LN. By 24 hr after injection of labeled cells there have been up to 2 passages of cells through the LN. Consequently one is considering 3 sets of cells of roughly equal numbers: cells that (1) entered LN as a bolus in the first 1 hr and have left by 12–13 hr; (2) entered LN 1–12 hr and left by 24 hr; and (3) entered LN 12–24 hr and were still present at 24 hr. In the absence of selective entry the ^{3}H/^{14}C ratio in the stimulated LN will be the same as that in the internal control LN if one only considers the contribution of the last set of cells. However, if retention of ASL occurs, ASL in the first 2 sets of cells will still be present at 24 hr and will thus alter the ^{3}H/^{14}C ratio according to the following equation:

$$\frac{^{3}H}{^{14}C}\ \text{stimulated LN} = \frac{100 + PX}{100} \qquad (3)$$

Where P is the number of cell passages through the LN (assumed to be between 1 and 2), and X is the percentage of ASL in syngeneic passaged TDL (assumed to be 5–12%)

Substitution into the equation for Isl produces:

$$Isl = 1 + \frac{PX}{100} \qquad (4)$$

with a predicted range of Isl values of 1.05–1.24.

In considering the validity of the results, note that the predicted ranges of Isl values for retention (1.05–1.24) is similar to that for entry (1.05–1.12). Note also that, as expected, there was a consistent lack of difference between the $^3H/^{14}C$ ratios of left and right unstimulated inguinal LN in all experiments. Results for 23 animals killed 24 hr after injection of labeled cells (experiments 3B, 4A, 4B, 5B) show that selection localization of ASL does occur in popliteal LN 36 hr and 3 days after foot-pad injection of alloantigen (mean Isl of 1.16, 1.10, 1.05, 1.07). These statistically highly significant results contrast sharply with the consistent inability to demonstrate selective localization of ASL in 23 animals killed 1 hr after injection of labeled cells. Mean Isl from experiments 1A, 2A, 2B and 5A were 0.99, 1.02, 1.02, and 0.99, respectively. Clearly selective localization of ASL in stimulated LN demonstrated 24 hr after injection must have been due to retention within the extravascular space after random entry across the SPCV.

Variation between the Isl in the groups killed at 24 hr may be due to experimental variation, but other factors are probably relevant: the different intervals after antigen stimulation of the LN, and the different combinations of MHC antigens used. In experiment 5 crossreactivity between the two alloantigens used may, in part, have been responsible for the index of selective localization being lower than expected. If one assumes that ASL represent 5% of the total population of syngeneic passaged TDL, the results are consistent with the selective retention of all ASL within the extravascular space. This is evident both at 36 hr and 3 days after antigen stimulation, but probably not at 16 hr—perhaps reflecting the time period required for alloantigen to be processed and presented by accessory cells.

With regard to the absence of enhanced entry of ASL, one should consider what proportion of recirculating lymphocytes delivered to a LN in the arterial blood actually leave the bloodstream. Two studies in sheep (*28, 29*) have utilized knowledge of LN blood flow, blood lymphocyte counts, and number of lymphocytes in efferent lymph to calculate that the proportion of lymphocytes entering a LN is about 25%. A more direct method (*30*) utilizing localization of ^{51}Cr-labeled TDL in an isolated chain of perfused mesenteric LN indicated a figure of about 11%. The latter estimate is probably an underestimate because less than optimal conditions for TDL migration were used (16 hr collections of TDL on ice, unpassaged after labeling); subsequently it was shown that TDL labeled, passaged from blood to lymph, and collected over 4-hr intervals at room temperature enter LN far more readily (*16, 17*). Furthermore not all blood entering an LN necessarily passes through an SPCV. Since all blood-borne lymphocytes enter LN via SPCV, the extraction of blood lymphocytes across the SPCV wall is probably greater than either of the above estimates and may approach 25–50%. Thus he maximum potential for enhanced entry of ASL could not be more than 2–4 times that of NSL. We have reliably shown that a 2-fold enhancement does not occur; any less of an enhancement would be of questionable physiological significance, particularly in the light of a 3-fold increase in total lymphocyte entry to the stimulated LN associated with increased blood flow.

The studies in sheep (*12, 13*) that suggested an enhanced entry of ASL into stimulated LN did not provide direct evidence for this putative phenomenon, but produced the hypothesis as an explanation of their findings. Other hypotheses might apply, such as the induction of tolerance by the leakage of small amounts of antigen into the system of the sheep. On the other hand, the present study is confined to the migration of immunologically naive lymphocytes during the inductive phase of a primary immune response; only two alloantigens were used and the physiology of a response against conventional antigens (particularly where the frequency of ASL is low) may be different.

Acknowledgments. I am deeply indebted to the late Professor Bill Ford whose encouragement and advice were essential. My thanks to Dr. Eric Bell for help in preparing the manuscript, Dr. S. Lucas for assistance with the statistical analysis, Mrs. J. Crosby for photographic work, and Mrs. S. John for secretarial work.

REFERENCES

1. Gowans, JL, McGregor DD. The immunological activities of lymphocytes. Prog Allergy 1965; 9: 1.
2. Ford WL, Gowans JL. The role of lymphocytes in antibody formation. II. The influence of lymphocyte migration on antibody formation in the isolated, perfused spleen. Proc R Soc B 1967; 168: 244.
3. Ford WL. Lymphocyte migration and immune responses. Prog Allergy 1975; 19: 1.
4. Hall JG, Morris B. The effect of X-irradiation of the popliteal lymph node on its output of lymphocytes and immunological unresponsiveness. Lancet 1964; 2: 1077.
5. Gowans JL, Knight EJ. The route of recirculation of lymphocytes in the rat. Proc R Soc B 1964; 159: 257.
6. Hay JB, et al. Relationships between changes in blood flow and lymphocyte migration induced by antigen. In: Essays on the anatomy and physiology of lymphoid tissue. Monogr Allergy 1980; 16: 112.
7. Herman PG. Microcirculation of organized lymphoid tissues. In: Essays on the anatomy and physiology of the lymphoid system. Monogr Allergy 1980; 16: 126.
8. Cahill RNP, Frost H, Trnka Z. The effects of antigen on the migration of recirculating lymphocytes through single lymph nodes. J Exp Med 1976; 143: 870.
9. Ottaway CA, Parrott DMV. Regional blood flow and its relationship to lymphocyte and lymphoblast traffic during a primary immune response. J Exp Med 1979; 150: 218.
10. Drayson MT, Smith ME, Ford WL. The sequence of changes in blood flow and lymphocyte influx to stimulated rat lymph nodes. Immunology 1981; 44: 125.
11. Cahill RNP, Hay JB, Frost H, Trnka Z. Changes in lymphocyte circulation after administration of antigen. Haematologia 1974; 8: 321.
12. McConnell I, Lachmann PJ, Hobart MJ. The restoration of specific immunological virginity. Nature 1974; 250: 113.
13. Hopkins J, McConnell I, Lachmann PJ. Specific selection of antigen reactive lymphocytes into antigenically stimulated lymph nodes in sheep. J Exp Med 1981; 153: 706.
14. Wagner C, Burger DR, McCall E. Antigen presentation and IL-1 production by HLA-DR compatible endothelial cells. Fed Proc 1983; 42(4): 835.
15. Pober JS, Gimbrone MA Jr, Cotran RS, et al. Ia expression by vascular endothelium is inducible by activated T cells and by human interferon. J Exp Med 1983; 157: 1339.
16. Smith ME, Ford WL. The recirculating lymphocyte pool of the rat: a systematic description of the migratory behaviour of recirculating lymphocytes. Immunology 1983; 49: 83.
17. Smith ME, Ford WL. The migration of lymphocytes across specialized vascular endothelium. VI. The migratory behaviour of thoracic duct lymphocytes retransfered from the lymph nodes, spleen, blood, or lymph of a primary recipient. Cell Immunol 1983; 78: 161.

18. Wilson DB, Blyth JL, Nowell PC. Quantitative studies on the mixed lymphocyte interaction in rats. III. Kinetics of the response. J Exp Med 1968; 135: 200.
19. Nisbet NW, Simonsen M, Zaleski M. The frequency of antigen sensitive cells in tissue transplantation. A commentary on clonal section. J Exp Med 1969; 129: 459.
20. Atkins RC, Ford WL. Early cellular events in a systemic graft-versus-host reaction. I. The migration of donor lymphocytes after intravenous injection. J Exp Med 1975; 141: 664.
21. Ford WL, Simmonds SJ, Atkins RC. Early cellular events in a systemic graft-versus-host reaction. II. Autoradiographic estimates of the frequency of donor lymphocytes which respond to each Ag-B-determined antigenic complex. J Exp Med 1975; 141: 681.
22. Ford WL, Atkins RC. Specific unresponsiveness of recirculating lymphocytes after exposure to histocompatibility antigen in F_1 hybrid rats. Nature 1971; 234: 178.
23. Ford WL. The preparation and labelling of lymphocytes. In: Weir DM, ed. Handbook of experimental immunology, 3rd ed. Oxford: Blackwell, 1977:
24. Sapirstein LA. Regional blood flow by fractional distribution of indicators. J Appl Physiol 1958; 193: 161.
25. Kennedy JC, Till JE, Siminovitch L, McCulloch EA. The proliferative capacity of antigen-sensitive precursors of haemolytic plague-forming cells. J Immunol 1966; 96: 973.
26. Armstrong WD, Diener E. A new method for the enumeration of antigen reactive cells responsive to a purified protein antigen. J Exp Med 1968; 129: 371.
27. Porter KA, Cooper EM. Transformation of adult allogeneic small lymphocytes after transfusion into newborn rats. J Exp Med 1962; 115: 997.
28. Hall JG. Quantitative aspects of the recirculation of lymphocytes. An analysis of data from experiments on sheep. QJ Exp Physiol Cogn Med Sci 1967; 52: 76.
29. Hay JB, Hobbs BB. The flow of blood to lymph nodes and its relation to lymphocyte traffic and the immune response. J Exp Med 1977; 145: 31.
30. Sedgley M, Ford WL, The migration of lymphocytes across specialized vascular endothelium. I. The entry of lymphocytes into the isolated mesenteric LN of the rat. Cell Tissue Kinet 1976; 231.

Received 14 June 1985.
Accepted 19 September 1985.

0041-1337/86/4106-0751$02.00/0
TRANSPLANTATION

Vol. 41, No. 6
Printed in U.S.A.

ALLOANTIGEN PRESENTATION BY CANINE ENDOTHELIAL CELLS

PRESENTATION OF AUTOLOGOUS ALLOANTIGENS IN VITRO[1]

G. GROENEWEGEN,[2] W. A. BUURMAN, AND G. M. A. A. JEUNHOMME

Department of Surgery, Biomedical Center, University of Limburg, 6200 MD Maastricht, The Netherlands

Presentation of autologous alloantigen by certain cells in an allograft can result in allograft rejection. The precise type of cell in a graft responsible for this aspect of allograft rejection remains to be established. Here we report the capacity of canine venous endothelial cells to activate, in vitro, allogeneic lymphocytes for proliferation and differentiation by presentation of alloantigen.

Antigen-presenting cell (APC)-depleted lymphocyte populations, prepared in a multistep procedure and tested for absence of APC, were cocultured with allogeneic venous endothelial cells. Proliferation and differentiation into cytotoxic T lymphocytes were measured. While mixed lymphocyte culture of APC-depleted lymphocytes did not result in proliferation and differentiation, coculture of allogeneic APC-depleted lymphocytes with venous endothelial cells resulted in proliferation and generation of cell-mediated cytotoxicity in these cultures. It is concluded that canine venous endothelial cells in vitro have the capacity to present alloantigen. The data suggest an essential role for endothelium in the initial phase of allograft rejection.

The presentation of antigens by specialized cells is an initial event in the immune response (*1*). Two types of antigen presentation can be distinguished. The first type, which occurs in immune responses against, e.g., viruses, is the presentation of antigens by accesory cells, which take up and express on the cell membrane the antigens involved, to activate lymphocytes; this is the accessory cell type. The second type of antigen presentation occurs in the artificial situation of allografting. In the graft certain donor cells present their autologous alloantigen to lymphocytes of the recipient, which are then triggered to proliferate and differentiate. The first type of antigen-presenting cells (accessory cell type) are macrophages (*1*), dendritic cells (*2*), B lymphocytes (*3*), epidermal Langerhans cells (*4*), and endothelial cells (*5–8*). For alloantigen presentation

[1] This work was supported Nier Stichting Nederland (Dutch Kidney Foundation) Grant C81.297, and by Fungo Grant 29.57.10.

[2] Address correspondence to: G. Groenewegen, Department of Surgery, Biomedical Center, University of Limburg, P.O. Box 616, 6200 MD Maastricht, The Netherlands.

monocytes (*9*), dendritic cells (10–12), and epidermal Langerhans cells (*13, 14*) have been suggested. These cells have the capacity to activate allogeneic T lymphocytes, independently of accessory cells of the responder. In the allograft situation the accessory-cell-type antigen-presenting cell would be a cell of recipient origin that presents donor-alloantigens shed from the graft to recipient lymphocytes. The cell presenting autologous alloantigen would be a cell of donor origin, which presents alloantigens to lymphocytes of the recipient to result in activation of recipient lymphocytes.

Endothelial cells are known to activate lymphocytes in vitro (*15–17*), but the dependence of this phenomenon on accessory cells is unknown. We have tested the capacity of endothelial cells to activate lymphocytes without the need for additional accessory cells.

MATERIALS AND METHODS

Animals. Dogs used in the experiments were kept in the kennels of the University of Limburg. They had not been immunized with alloantigen.

Endothelial cells. Canine venous endothelial cells were obtained by collagenase digestion of femoral veins and cultured as described before (*18*). The cultured cells were identified as a pure population of endothelial cells because of their oligoclonal origin, their growth pattern, their homogeneous reactivity with antibodies against angiotensin-converting enzyme and canine FVIII-related antigen, and the absence during culture of cells reactive with monoclonal antibodies against major histocompatibility (MHC)* class II antigens (*8, 18, 19*).

Preparation of lymphocyte suspensions. Lymphocytes were isolated from heparinized blood. Untreated lymphocytes were prepared by density centrifugation of blood on Lymphoprep (Nyegaard, Oslo, Norway). Lymphocytes depleted of antigen-presenting cells were prepared in a multistep procedure (*8*). In brief, diluted blood was incubated 45 min at 38°C with 12 mg/ml carbonyl iron to remove phagocytic cells. Leukocytes were separated by density centrifugation. After washing the cells, plastic adherent cells were removed by a 1-hr incubation at 38°C of the cells on plastic in RPMI 1640 containing 20% fetal calf serum. The plastic-nonadherent cells were decanted, washed once, and resuspended in RPMI 1640 containing 10% canine serum. The cells were then incubated for 45 min at 38°C in nylon-wool columns to remove canine dendritic cells (*20*). The cells obtained in this multistep procedure are nonphagocytic, not adherent to plastic, and not adherent to nylon-wool. The procedure resulted in enrichment of lymphocytes in the cell population because of depletion of other cells, such as monocytes and granulocytes. The cells consisted of >99% lymphocytes in morphological criteria and are referred to as APC-depleted lymphocytes (*8*).

Mixed cultures. APC-depleted lymphocytes or untreated lymphocytes were suspended in RPMI 1640, supplemented with 10% heat-inactivated canine serum and antibiotics (100 IU penicillin and 100 μg/ml streptomycin) at 10^6 cell/ml. The lymphocytes were cocultured with similarly prepared stimulator lymphocytes (4000 rads x-irradiated) at a responder-stimulator cell ratio of 2:1, or they were cocultured with endothelial cells (4000 rads x-irradiated) at a responder-stimulator cell ratio of 10:1. Mixed cultures were performed in triplicate in culture flasks and placed in a water-saturated atmosphere of air containing 5% CO_2 at 38°C.

Proliferation and differentiation assays. Proliferation of lymphocytes in mixed cultures was determined by measurement of ^{3}H-TdR incorporation. On day 8 of culture, 0.1 ml of the resuspended culture was pipetted into microtiter wells, to which 0.5 μCi ^{3}H-TdR (specific activity 5 Ci/mMol) (Amersham, England) was added during the final 4-hr of incubation (*17*). Proliferation in each culture flask was assayed in quadruplicate. Proliferation is expressed in counts per minute. Differentiation was determined by measurement of cell-mediated cytotoxicity in a ^{51}Cr-release assay, as described earlier (*18*). For detection of nonspecific lysis, third-party or responder-type lymphoblasts were used. Cell-mediated cytotoxicity was assayed in quadruplicate. Specific lysis of a target cell was calculated from:

$$\frac{\text{experimental release} - \text{spontaneous release}}{\text{maximum release} - \text{spontaneous release}} \times 100\% \quad (17).$$

Spontaneous release did not exceed 20% of ^{51}Cr-uptake of the target cells, whereas maximum release did exceed 85% of uptake. In syngeneic combinations of responder and stimulator cells, neither proliferation nor cell-mediated cytotoxicity could be detected (results not shown).

RESULTS

The capacity of endothelial cells to stimulate allogeneic lymphocytes in mixed lymphocyte endothelial cell cultures (MLEC) without the presence of antigen presenting cells (APC) in the lymphocyte population was studied. Contamination of the endothelial cells with nonendothelial cells was excluded on the basis of homogeneous positive reactivity, with two markers used for identification of endothelium in vitro.

Table 1 shows the proliferative response of untreated and APC-depleted lymphocytes in mixed cultures. Four representative experiments from a series of experiments are shown. Mixed lymphocyte culture (MLC) of untreated lymphocytes results in proliferation of lymphocytes, whereas proliferation in MLC of APC-depleted lymphocytes is negligible. Lack of response cannot be caused by depletion of stimulating antigen since, in an identical system, addition of responder-type endothelial cells could restore the response (*8*). It can therefore be concluded that APC are removed from the lymphocyte population by the depletion procedure employed. Proliferation in MLEC is not affected by the depletion of antigen-presenting cells from the lymphocyte population since, in MLEC of both untreated lymphocytes and APC-depleted lymphocytes, significant ^{3}H-TdR incorporation is observed. Incorporation of ^{3}H-TdR in MLEC with APC-depleted lymphocytes was 4–40 times higher than incorporation in MLC of APC-depleted lymphocytes. The increase in proliferative response in MLEC after depletion of APC from the responder cell population may be caused by depletion of cells that are able to inhibit the response—e.g., monocytes via production of PGE_2 (*21*) or by an increase in absolute number of reactive lymphocytes resulting from depletion of other cells. The experiments indicate that venous endothelial cells are capable of induction of a proliferative response in cultures of APC-depleted lymphocytes, and therefore have the capacity to present alloantigen.

* Abbreviations used: APC: antigen-presenting cell; CMC: cell-mediated cytotoxicity; MHC: major histocompatibility complex; MLC: mixed lymphocyte culture; MLEC: mixed lymphocyte endothelial cell culture; VEC: venous endothelial cell.

TABLE 1. Proliferation in mixed cultures of untreated and APC-depleted lymphocytes[a]

		Experiment			
		1	2	3	4
Untreated lymphocytes	MLC A/B^x	2831±1034	10333±1028	nt[b]	10895±311
	MLEC A/VEC B^x	2134±651	12891±636	8182±349	4990±253
APC-depleted lymphocytes	MLC A/B^x	705±351	560±343	776±470	1101±731
	MLEC A/VEC B^x	3022±477	25088±1661	12109±453	19295±2756

[a] Proliferation is expressed in cpm ^{3}H-TdR incorporation. Uptake by stimulator lymphocytes and stimulator VEC did not exceed respectively, 250 and 300 cpm. Mean cpm ± SD of ^{3}H-TdR incorporation in proliferation assay in quadruplicate is given.
[b] nt: not tested.

Differentiation of lymphocytes in mixed cultures was studied by measurement of cell-mediated cytotoxicity (CMC). The results of four experiments from a series of eight are given in Table 2. Three target cells have been used: lymphoblasts and endothelial cells of the stimulator and lymphoblasts of a third party or the responder. These target cells have been included for analysis of specificity of lysis. The effector cells from MLC of untreated lymphocytes lysed lymphoblasts and endothelial cells of the stimulator, without lysis of nonspecific lymphoblasts. An identical pattern of lysis was found for effector cells from MLEC of untreated lymphocytes. The cells from MLC with APC-depleted lymphocytes were not cytotoxic, even at effector-target ratios higher than 20:1 (data not given). In MLEC with APC-depleted lymphocytes high specific cytotoxicity was obtained. The cells of these cultures that were shown to proliferate appeared also to differentiate into cytotoxic T lymphocytes. It can be concluded that endothelial cells are capable of stimulating lymphocytes to proliferation and differentiation in the absence of APC in the lymphocyte population, and therefore function as cells presenting autologous alloantigen.

TABLE 2. Cell-mediated cytotoxicity generated in mixed cultures of lymphocytes[a]

Experiment		Target cell		
		Stimulator VEC	Stimulator lymphoblast	Nonspecific lymphoblast
Experiment 1: (responder 3284;[b] stimulator 126)				
Untreated lymphocytes	MLC	25±3.6	14±4.5	−23±7.2
	MLEC	83±18.8	74±10.5	−24±4.6
APC-depleted lymphocytes	MLC	−5±4.8	−2±1.8	−7±5.3
	MLEC	82±24.9	87±7.7	−14±5.0
Experiment 2: (responder 774; stimulator 132)				
Untreated lymphocytes	MLC	26±7.1	22±2.1	−13±7.6
	MLEC	29±5.2	40±7.0	−17±9.6
APC-depleted lymphocytes	MLC	0±1.7	1±3.0	nt[c]
	MLEC	13±2.7	32±6.1	−6±9.3
Experiment 3: (responder 787; stimulator 126)				
Untreated lymphocytes	MLEC	21±8.8	42±3.7	−1±3.1
APC-depleted lymphocytes	MLEC	66±10.1	63±7.0	1±3.6
Experiment 4: (responder 823; stimulator 3284)				
Untreated lymphocytes	MLEC	28±2.4	15±7.0	nt
APC-depleted lymphocytes	MLEC	32±8.2	68±4.9	nt

[a] Percentage of mean specific lysis ± SD of three cultures determined in quadruplicate is given. Effector:target cell ratio used was 20:1. Nonspecific lymphoblasts of responder or third-party origin were included for control of specificity of lysis.
[b] Responder and stimulator numbers in parentheses are identification numbers of individual dogs.
[c] nt: not tested.

DISCUSSION

The precise cell in an allograft that induces rejection of the allograft by the immune system of the recipient remains to be determined. The *passenger leukocyte* of donor origin, later identified as the *dendritic cell*, has been suggested to be responsible for the induction of rejection. However, it has been reported that, in the canine and murine model, skin allografts of a bone-marrow chimera were rejected by the marrow donor (*22*, *23*). Similar findings were observed for kidney allografts in the dog (Storb R, personal communication). These findings cast doubt on the exclusive role of bone-marrow-derived cells in induction of allograft rejection. The cell type responsible for induction of allograft rejection must, however, be within reach of the host's immune system and must express MHC-class II antigens, which have an essential role in the rejection process.

Recently we described the capacity of canine arterial and venous endothelial cells to function as antigen-presenting cells for alloantigens to syngeneic lymphocytes in mixed lymphocyte cultures (*8*). These experiments demonstrate, in the situation of an allograft, the capacity of recipient endothelial cells to present donor alloantigens to recipient lymphocytes. Here we studied the capacity of canine venous endothelial cells to stimulate allogeneic lymphocytes, without the need for additional antigen-presenting cells. For this purpose a system in which APC were removed from the lymphocyte population in a multistep procedure was used (*8*). It appeared that APC-depleted lymphocytes could be stimulated to proliferation and differentiation into cytotoxic T cells by venous endothelial cells. The expression of MHC class II antigens on the endothelial cells in the cultures is most likely induced by the lymphokines produced by the responder T lymphocyte population, since we could show that supernatants of unstimulated lymphocytes can induce MHC-class II antigens on endothelial cells (*19*).

Since the endothelial cells are capable of lymphocyte stimulation in the absence of APC in the lymphocyte population we conclude that venous endothelial cells function as cells presenting autologous alloantigen. The capacity of venous endothelial cells to present alloantigen allows donor endothelial cells in a vascularized allograft to present donor antigens to recipient lymphocytes in the initial events of an immune reaction leading to allograft rejection. Preliminary experiments demonstrate that arterial endothelial cells also have this capacity (unpublished observations).

Essential differences in cells expressing MHC-class II antigens in renal tissue between man and rat were described by Fabre (*24*). In the rat kidney MHC class II antigens are only present on dendritic cells and not on endothelium, whereas in the human kidney MHC class II antigens are present on capillary endothelium (*25*). Also canine endothelial cells have been reported to have the capacity to express MHC class II antigens (*19, 26*). Though cultured cells do not express the antigens, antigen expression could be induced in vitro by lymphokine-containing supernatants of both resting and stimulated lymphocytes (*19*). In vivo the antigens are expressed on capillary endothelium in skin and kidney, and the in vivo expression of MHC-class II antigens appears to be lymphokine dependent (*26*). Since dendritic cells are passenger cells, the rat renal allograft will be devoid of MHC class-II-antigen–positive cells a few days after transplantation. However, in the human renal allograft the endothelial cells still express the MHC class II antigens. The capacity of endothelial cells to present alloantigens, as demonstrated here, explains the observed difference in results in survival of renal allografts between man and rat described by Fabre (*24*).

The reported humoral reactions during rejection against non-MHC antigens on endothelium (*27, 28*) can be explained by the alloantigen-presenting capacity of endothelial cells. These antigens may be presented to lymphocytes by the endothelial cells in association with the immunogenic MHC-class II antigens, resulting in a reaction against these non-MHC antigens. The detrimental effect on allograft survival of such antigens has been demonstrated (*29*).

Acknowledgments. We thank Mrs.A. J. J. M. Daemen and Mrs. E. E. M. Spronken for their technical assistance, and Mrs. C. M. P. Spronck for her excellent secretarial assistance.

REFERENCES

1. Unanue ER, Beller DJ, Lu CY, Allen PM. Antigen presentation: comments on its regulation and mechanism. J Immunol 1984; 132: 1.
2. Sunshine GH, Katz DR, Feldmann M. Dendritic cells induce T cell proliferation to synthetic antigens under Ir-gene control. J Exp Med 1980; 152: 1817.
3. Chesnut RW, Grey HM. Studies on the capacity of B cells to serve as antigen presenting cells. J Immunol 1981; 126: 1075.
4. Braathen CR, Thorsby E. Studies on human epidermal Langerhans cells. I. Alloactivating and antigen-presenting capacity. Scand J Immunol 1980; 11: 401.
5. Hirscherg H, Bergh OJ, Thorsby E. Antigen-presenting properties of human vascular endothelial cells. J Exp Med 1980; 152: 249S.
6. Burger DR, Ford D, Vetto RM, Hamblin A, Goldstein A, Hubbard M, Dumonde DC. Endothelial cell presentation of antigen to human T cells. Human Immunol 1981; 3: 209.
7. Nunez G, Ball EJ, Stastny P. Accessory cell function of human endothelial cells. I. A. subpopulation of Ia positive cells is required for antigen presentation. J Immunol 1983; 131: 666.
8. Groenewegen G, Buurman WA. Vascular endothelial cells present alloantigens to unprimed lymphocytes. Scand J Immunol 1984; 19: 269.
9. Gonwa TA, Picker LJ, Raff HV, Gayert SM, Silver J, Stobo JD. Antigen presenting capabilities of human monocytes correlates with their expression of HLA-DS, an Ia-determinant distinct from HLA-DR. J Immunol 1983; 130: 706.
10. Steinman RM, Witmer MD. Lymphoid dendritic cells are potent stimulators of the primary mixed leukocyte reaction in mice. Proc Natl Acad Sci USA 1978; 75: 5132.
11. Klinkert WEF, LaBadie JH, Bowers WE. Accessory and stimulating properties of dendritic cells and macrophages isolated from various rat tissues. J Exp Med 1982; 156: 1.
12. Van Voorhis WC, Valinsky J, Hoffman E, Luban J, Hair LS, Steinman RM. Relative efficacy of human monocytes and dendritic cells as accessory cells for T cell replication. J Exp Med 1983; 158: 174.
13. Pollack MS, Goldenhersh M, Chin-Louie J, Safai B. The functional study of DR-positive human epidermal Langerhans cells in mixed cell cultures with allogeneic lymphocytes. Clin Immunol Immunopathol 1982; 24: 15.
14. Tscuhida T, Iijima M, Fugiwara H, Pehamberger H, Shearer GM, Katz SJ. Epidermal Langerhans cells can function as stimulatory cells but not as accessory cells in CTL induction. J Immunol 1984; 132: 1163.
15. Vetto RM, Burger DR. Endothelial cell stimulation of allogeneic lymphocytes. Transplantation 1972; 14: 652.
16. Hirschberg H, Evensen SA, Hendriksen T, Thorsby E. Stimulation of human lymphocytes by allogeneic endothelial cells in vitro. Tissue Antigens 1974; 4: 257.
17. Groenewegen G, Buurman WA, Jeunhomme GMAA, van der Linden CJ, Vegt PA, Kootstra G. In vitro stimulation of lymphocytes by vascular endothelial cells. A study with canine arterial and venous endothelial cells. Transplantation 1984; 37: 206.
18. Groenewegen G, Buurman WA, van der Linden CJ, Jeunhomme GMAA, Kootstra G. Cellular cytotoxicity against canine endothelial cells. Analysis of determinants recognized by CTL. Tissue Antigens 1983; 21: 114.
19. Groenewegen G, Buurman WA, Jeunhomme GMAA, van der Linden CJ. Cyclosporin A affects MHC-class II antigen expression by arterial and venous endothelial in vitro. Transplantation, 1985; 40: 214.
20. Goodell EM, Struckle MA, Blumenstock DA, Bowers WE. Canine dendritic cells as accessory cells in the canine lymphocyte activation [Abstract] . Immunobiology 1982; 163: 117.
21. Rappaport RS, Doge GR. Prostaglandin E inhibits the production of human interleukin 2. J Exp Med 1982; 155: 943.
22. Schroeder M-L, Storb R, Graham TC, Weiden PL. Canine radiation chimeras: an attempt to demonstrate serum blocking factors by an in vivo approach. J Immunol 1975; 14: 540.
23. Stuart PM, Bech-Maier B, Melvold RW. Provocation of skin graft rejection across murine class II differences by non bone-marrow-derived cells. Transplantation 1984; 37: 393.
24. Fabre JW. Rat kidney allograft model: was it all too good to be true? Transplantation 1982; 34: 223.
25. Natali PG, de Martino C, Marcellini M, Quaranta V, Ferrone S. Expression of Ia-like antigens on the vasculature of human kidney. Clinical Immunol Immunopathol 1981; 20: 11.
26. Groenewegen G, Buurman WA, van der Linden CJ. Lymphokine dependence of in vivo expression of MHC class II antigens by endothelium. Nature 1985; 316: 361.
27. Moreas JR, Stastny P. A new antigen system expressed in human endothelial cells. J Clin Invest 1977; 60: 449.
28. Paul LC, van Es LA, van Rood JJ, van Leeuwen A, Brutel de la Rivière G, de Graeff J. Antibodies directed against antigens on the endothelium of peritubular capillaries in patients with rejecting renal allografts. Transplantation 1979; 27: 175.
29. Cerilli J, Brasile L, Clarke J, Galouzis J. The vascular endothelial cell (VEC) specific antigen system: three years' experience in monocyte crossmatching. Transplant Proc 1985; 17: 567.

Received 19 March 1985.
Accepted 19 September 1985.

0041-1337/86/4106-0755$02.00/0
TRANSPLANTATION
Vol. 41, No. 6

Printed in U.S.A.

INCREASED OXIDATIVE BURST POTENTIAL EXHIBITED BY MACROPHAGES DURING GRAFT-VERSUS-HOST REACTIONS IN MICE[1]

HEDVA GOLDIN[2] AND YONA KEISARI[3]

Department of Human Microbiology, Sackler Faculty of Medicine, Tel-Aviv University, Tel-Aviv 69978, Israel

Graft versus host reactions (GVHR) in mice are accompanied by macrophage activation. Since macrophage oxidative burst (OB) was found to increase in activated macrophages (MPs), we examined the OB of peritoneal and spleen MPs from mice during GVHR. Parental spleen lymphocytes, were injected i.p. into F_1 hybrids (BALB/c×C57Bl/6) and at different intervals following injection we monitored the number of peritoneal exudate cells (PEC), spleen enlargement, and the OB of both peritoneal and spleen adherent MPs. Macrophage OB was assessed by measuring O_2^- and H_2O_2 production, following stimulation with the phorbol ester TPA. The spleen-to-body weight ratio increased by 40–70% in mice with GVHR during the period of 6–20 days postinjection and decreased to almost normal levels after 27 days. In such mice with GVHR the number of PEC returned to normal (≃6×10^6 cells/animal) after 20 days compared with 5 days in control mice (injected with F_1 spleen cells). Adherent peritoneal MPs from control mice and mice with GVHR exhibited increased OB activity 3 days following treatment. However, in the control mice the OB response returned to normal within 6 days, while in the experimental mice it showed a slight decrease after 6 days, increased again within 9–17 days, and finally decreased 20–27 days after treatment. Adherent spleen MPs from mice with GVHR generated a high response 6 days posttreatment, which gradually returned to the basal level after 17 days. These findings suggest that during GVHR in mice, macrophage OB was potentiated, giving rise to cytotoxic products such as O_2^- and H_2O_2, which may contribute to tissue damage during GVHR.

During the graft-versus-host reaction (GVHR),* macrophages that are mainly of host origin proliferate and infiltrate parenchymous organs (*1, 2*). The role of macrophages in the pathological changes occurring during the process is not entirely clear. Yet several studies reported that GVHR macrophages exhibit increased cytotoxic activity (*3–7*). In several studies it was reported that macrophage activation was associated with an increased capacity to produce and generate oxidative burst (OB) products such as superoxide ions O_2^- and hydrogen peroxide (H_2O_2) (*8, 9*). Such OB-derived products were reported to play a major role in the microbicidal and antiparasitic activity of macrophages (*8–11*), and were also reported to serve as lytic mediators in the destruction of erythrocytes (*12–14*) and tumor cells (*15–17*) by macrophages. In the present study we attempted to find out whether or not GVHR macrophages showed an activated OB response.

MATERIALS AND METHODS

Reagents. The phorbol ester derivative 12-*O*-tetradecanoyl-phorbol-13-acetate (TPA) was obtained from Sigma Chemical Co. (St. Louis, MO), dissolved in dimethylsulfoxide at 2 mM, and stored in the dark at −20°C. Cytochrome c (type III), horseradish peroxidase (HRP, type II, 165 purpurogallin units/mg protein), and phenol red (phenolsulfonphthalein sodium salt) were purchased from Sigma Chemical Co.

Animals. Male (BALB/c×C57Bl/6)F_1 (BCF_1) hybrid and BALB/c mice (Tel-Aviv University Animal House), 6 weeks old, were used in this study.

Peritoneal MPs. Adherent peritoneal macrophages (APM) were obtained from BCF_1 mice by peritoneal lavage, washed three times in Earle's balanced salt solution (BSS) and finally suspended in RPMI-1640 supplemented with 100 μg/ml streptomycin, 100 U/ml penicillin, 300 μg/ml glutamine, and 2.5% fetal calf serum (FCS) (RPMI-1640+FCS) (Biological Industries, Bet-Haemek, Israel). Cells were cultured in wells 16 mm in diameter (Cluster 24, Costar, Cambridge, MA), 1.5–2×10^6 cells in 0.5 ml/well, incubated for 1 hr a 37°C and 7.5% CO_2, and nonadherent cells were removed at the end of the incubation. PEC from mice with GVHR were plated at 1.5×10^6 cells/well with an efficiency of plating of 17.9±3.8%, and the resulting monolayer contained only 5±2.4% polymorphonuclear (PMN) cells. PEC from control mice were plated at 2×10^6 cells/well with an efficiency of plating of 12.6±2.9%, and the monolayers contained only 4.3±2.0% PMN.

Spleen cells. Spleen lymphocytes for injection were obtained from BALB/c and BCF_1 mice. Spleens were thoroughly disrupted in RPMI-1640 + FCS until a fine single-cell suspension was achieved), and fianlly resuspended in Earle's BSS (10^8/ml). Each mouse was injected with 10^8 cells i.p.

Spleen MPs. Adherent spleen macrophages (ASM) were obtained from spleen cell suspensions of GVHR and control animals in RPMI-1640 + FCS. The cells were plated in dishes 3 cm in diameter at 30×10^6, and 15×10^6 cells/3 ml, for control and mice with GVHR, respectively. The cultures were incubated for 1 hr at 37°C and 7.5% CO_2, and nonadherent cells were subsequently removed. The efficiency of plating was 4.8±1.8% and 2.8±0.7% for mice with GVHR and control mice, respectively. The ASM monolayers contained 6.0±1.7% (GVHR) and 5.6±1.9% (control) PMN cells out of the total number of cells.

[1] This work was supported by grants from the Vladimir Schrieber Memorial Fund and the Moise and Frida Eskenazy Institute for Cancer Research.

[2] This study is part of the M.Sc. studies of Ms. H. Goldin.

[3] To whom correspondence should be addressed.

* Abbreviations used: APM, adherent peritoneal macrophages; ASM, adherent spleen macrophages; FCS, fetal calf serum; GVHR, graft-versus-host reaction; HRP, horseradish peroxidase; MPs, macrophages; OB, oxidative burst; PEC, peritoneal exudate cells; PMN, polymorphonuclears; TPA, 12-O-tetradecanoyl-phorbol-13-acetate.

Adherent cell monolayers were stained with Camco Quik Stain (Cambridge Chemical Products, Inc., Fort Lauderdale, FL) for determination of the percentage of PMN cells.

Assay for O_2^- production. Production and release of O_2^- was assayed by the ferricytochrome c reduction method, as described by Babior et al. (*18*). APM monolayers in 16-mm wells and ASM in 3-cm dishes, were stimulated with TPA for 60 min in the presence of 80 μM ferricytochrome c as described (*19*).

Assay for H_2O_2 production. H_2O_2 production was quantitated according to Pick and Keisari (*20*) with a method based on the H_2O_2-mediated and horseradish-peroxidase (HRP)-dependent oxidation of phenol red to a product the absorbance of which is read at 610 nm. The assay was carried out with macrophage monolayers in 1.6-cm wells and 3-cm dishes as described (*19*). O_2^- and H_2O_2 production was expressed as nanomoles per 10^6 adherent cells. The number of adherent macrophages was determined following initial plating and removal of nonadherent cells. The adherent cells were scraped, resuspended in 1 ml Earle's BSS, and counted in an hemocytometer. All cell counts were performed in triplicate.

RESULTS

Parameters of GVHR. BCF_1 mice were injected i.p. with 10^8 spleen cells from BALB/c or BCF_1 mice. At different intervals following injection the animals were sacrificed and the number of peritoneal exudate cells (PEC), and the spleen-to-body weight ratio were determined. The results presented in Table 1 show that, compared with control mice spleen enlargement was evident in mice with GVHR 6 days following treatment (40–70% increase), remained stable for about 17 days, and declined to normal after 27 days. The number of PEC measured postinjection was found to decrease drastically in control mice from $18.7\pm2\times10^6$ per mouse at the 3rd day to $6.0\pm1.4\times10^6$ by the 6th day, while in mice with GVHR their number decreased gradually and reached the basal level ($\simeq6\times10^6$/mouse) after 20 days (Fig. 1).

The oxidative burst of adherent peritoneal macrophages (APM). APM monolayers were obtained as described in the *Materials and Methods* section by culturing 1.5×10^6 to 2×10^6 PEC from experimental and control mice, respectively. Such APM monolayers were prepared from PEC obtained from mice

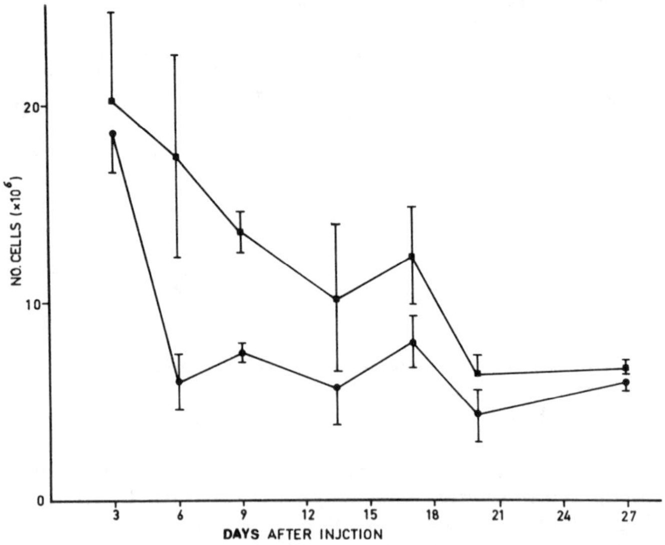

FIGURE 1. Number of peritoneal exudate cells (PEC) at different days following spleen cell injection. PEC from GVHR (■) and control (●) mice were collected from groups of 4–5 mice per experiment. The results represent mean ± SD from 3 experiments for days 3, 6, 9, 17, 20, and 27, and 12 experiments for day 13.

at different days after spleen cell injection, and were examined for their ability to generate H_2O_2 and O_2^- in response to TPA at various concentrations.

Superoxide generation by APM from control mice was high when tested 3 days following spleen cell injection, and drastically receded after 6 days, along with the drop observed in the amount of PEC (Fig. 2). APM from mice with GVHR also exhibited high O_2^- production 3 days following injection—but, unlike the control APM, their activity started to decrease only after 20 days, showing a transient fall in activity after 6 days (Fig. 2). The OB response to TPA was dose-dependent and followed the pattern observed with paraffin-oil-elicited macrophages (*19*). The generation of O_2^- was paralled by H_2O_2 production triggered with 20 nM TPA, and measured under the same conditions (Table 2).

APM monolayers from mice with GVHR were treated with BALB/c anti-C57B1/6 antibodies and guinea pig complement, and were subsequently tested for O_2^- generating capacity. The treatment reduced the O_2^- producing capacity of the cells from 35.8 ± 2.4 to 5.4 ± 6.6 nmol $O_2^-/10^6$ cells in 60 min, indicating that the responding cells were of host origin.

The OB of adherent spleen macrophages (ASM). ASM from mice at different periods following spleen cell injection were prepared as described previously, and tested for their O_2^- and H_2O_2 generating capacity in response to TPA (0–200 nM). ASM from mice with GVHR 6 days following treatment exhibited a profound O_2^--generating capacity (up to 32 nmol/10^6 cells/60 min), a capacity that was gradually diminished to almost zero on the 17th day posttreatment. ASM from control mice exhibited a marginal effect on the 6th day; this slightly increased on the 9th day—an increase that was not followed by a similar increase in H_2O_2—and disappeared later on (Fig. 3). Measurement of H_2O_2 production by ASM revealed a similar pattern of activity in response to 200 nM TPA (Table 3).

TABLE 1. Spleen enlargement in GVHR mice compared with control mice on different days following lymphocyte injection

Days after injection	Spleen/body weight ratio ($\times10^{-3}$) ± SD[a]		
	Control[b]	GVHR[c]	P[d]
3	5.0±0.5 (11)	5.4±0.9 (12)	ns
6	5.0±0.7 (10)	7.3±2.0 (15)	<0.05
9	5.0±0.7 (11)	9.0±1.5 (10)	<0.05
13	5.0±0.9 (40)	7.3±3.0 (49)	<0.01
17	5.0±0.7 (17)	8.0±3.1 (17)	<0.05
20	4.3±0.5 (8)	6.5±1.9 (8)	ns
27	4.8±0.4 (11)	5.7±0.8 (14)	ns

[a] The results are expressed as mean ± SD of spleen-to-body-weight ratio ($\times10^{-3}$), of control and GVHR mice at different days following GVH induction. Number in parentheses is the total number of mice tested.

[b] CBF_1 mice were injected with 10^8/mouse CBF_1 spleen cells.

[c] CBF_1 mice were injected with 10^8/mouse BALB/c spleen cells.

[d] The significance (P) of the difference between mean values of control and GVHR mice was calculated using the one-tailed Student's t test, (ns: not significant).

DISCUSSION

It has been implied in various studies that oxidative burst products, such as O_2^- and H_2O_2, are part of the cytotoxic arsenal

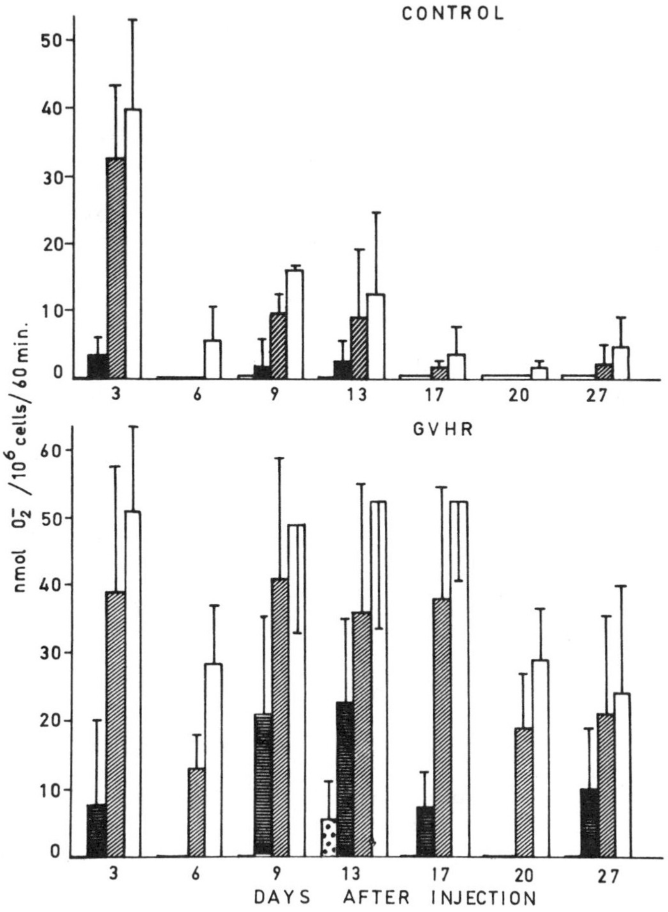

FIGURE 2. Superoxide (O_2^-) production by adherent peritoneal macrophages (APM) from mice with GVHR and control mice. Measurements were performed on APM monolayers containing 2.5–2.6×10^5 cells triggered with various concentrations of TPA (0-⊞; 2-▤; 20-▨; 200-□; nM). The results represent mean ± SD from 3 experiments for days 3, 6, 9, 17, 20, and 27 and 12 experiments for day 13, all done in duplicate.

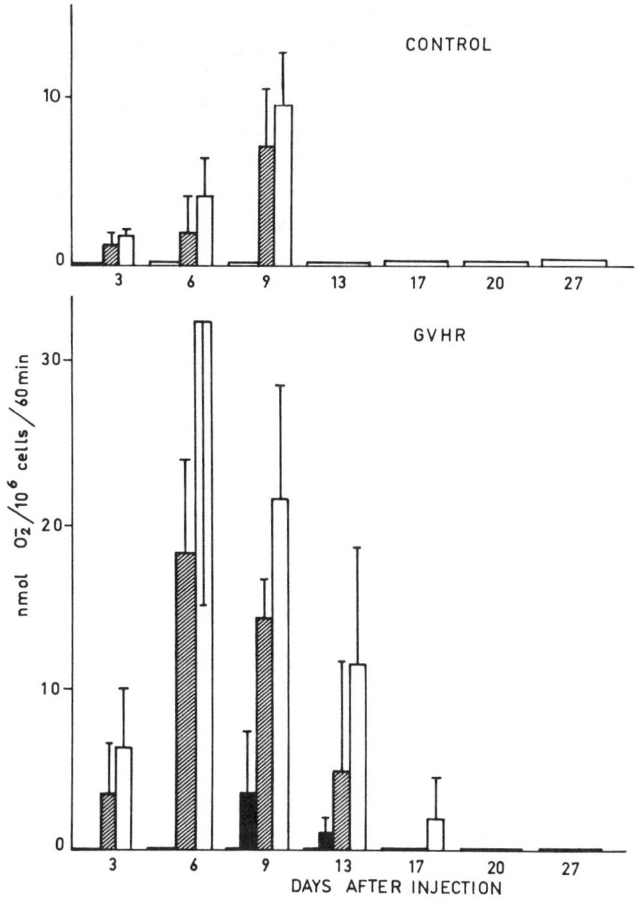

FIGURE 3. Superoxide (O_2^-) production by adherent spleen macrophages (ASM) from mice with GVHR and control mice. Measurements were performed on ASM monolayers containing ≃7.8×10^5 cells triggered with various TPA concentratons (0-⊞; 2-▤; 20-▨; 200-□; nM). The results represent mean ± SD from three experiments all done in duplicate.

TABLE 2. Hydrogen peroxide (H_2O_2) produced by oxidative-burst-stimulated adherent peritoneal macrophages from GVHR and control mice

Days after injection	No. expts.	H_2O_2 (nmol/60 min/10^6 cells ± SD)[a]		P[d]
		GVHR[b]	Control[c]	
3	3	22.5±9.0	17.2±5.9	ns
6	6	14.5±2.0	0	<0.001
13	12	21.0±5.4	2.6±3.2	<0.001
27	3	11.0±5.4	0	<.05

[a] Macrophages (≃2.6×10^5 cells/1.6-cm well) were incubated with 20 nM TPA for 60 min at 37°C in phenol red solution (140 mM NaCl, 10 mM potassium phosphate buffer, pH 7.0, 5.5 mM dextrose, and 0.28 mM phenol red) and 10 U/ml HRP.

[b] CBF_1 mice were injected i.p. with 10^8/mouse BALB/c spleen cells.

[c] CBF_1 mice were injected i.p. with 10^8/mouse CBF_1 spleen cells.

[d] The significance (P) of the difference between GVHR and control mice was calculated using the one-tailed Student's t test, (ns: not significant).

TABLE 3. Hydrogen peroxide (H_2O_2) produced by oxidative-burst-stimulated adherent spleen macrophages from GVHR and control mice

Days after injection	No. expts.	H_2O_2 (nmol/60 min/10^6 cells ± SD)[a]		P[d]
		GVHR[b]	Control[c]	
3	3	0	0	ns
6	3	25.9±8.7	7.0±3.9	<0.05
9	3	12.3±7.0	4.0±3.6	ns
13	3	14.2±3.8	5.3±1.4	<0.02
17	3	2.0±1.3	2.6±2.3	ns

[a] Macrophages (≃7.8×10^5 cells/3.0-cm plate) were incubated with 200 nM TPA for 60 min at 37°C in phenol red solution (140 mM NaCl, 10 mM potassium phosphate buffer, pH 7.0, 5.5 mM dextrose, and 0.28 mM phenol red) and 10 U/ml HRP.

[b] CBF_1 mice were injected i.p. with 10^8/mouse BALB/c spleen cells.

[c] CBF_1 mice were injected i.p. with 10^8/mouse CBF_1 spleen cells.

[d] The significance of the difference between GVHR and control mice was calculated using the one-tailed Student's t test, (ns: not significant).

of activated macrophages. In the present study, we measured the generation and release of OB products by peritoneal and spleen adherent macrophages from mice with GVHR and control mice, and correlated it with the state of the GVH response in these mice.

The results indicated that macrophages harvested from mice with GVHR were activated and exhibited an elevated OB potential compared with control mice. Such an elevated OB response was shown by macrophages following chemical elicitation or immunological activation, but not by resident peritoneal cells (*19, 21–24*).

The increased OB activity of peritoneal macrophages from mice with GVHR was observed during the period when spleen enlargement was also evident—namely, 6–20 days following GVHR induction. A similar pattern of macrophage activation was observed in other studies with different criteria for macrophage function. Macrophage-mediated destruction of target cells was at its peak within 7–14 days following induction of GVHR (*5,6*), and the phagocytic activity of resident macrophages was increased after 2 weeks (*25*). In another study spleen weight increased 18 days after GVHR induction, and was paralled by a higher resistance to *Listeria monocytogenes* infection, and an augmented capacity of peritoneal macrophages to kill bacteria in vitro (*3*). The above data and the presented results indicate that GVHR induction is accompanied by macrophage activation of both peritoneal and splenic origin.

The enhanced OB of macrophage from mice with GVHR probably reflects the activation of these cells by lymphokines that are presumably released by the injected parental T cells. Lymphokines were reported to enhance the capacity of macrophages to release OB products (*26, 27*), and to trigger H_2O_2 production by macrophages (*28*).

The role of macrophages in the pathophysiology of GVHR is yet to be elucidated. Indication of a possible role was given by the studies, which showed that antimacrophage serum reduced spleen enlargement and prolonged survival of mice in which GVHR had been induced (*29*). In view of the toxic nature of OB-derived reagents generated by macrophages, we suggest the involvement of such reagents in the damage inflicted upon host tissue. The possible effect of antioxidants in the reduction of tissue damage during GVHR is under investigation.

REFERENCES

1. Howard JG, Michie D, Simonsen M. Splenomegaly as a host response in graft-versus-host disease. Br J Exp Pathol 1961; 42: 478.
2. Zeiss IM, Fox M. Donor and host contribution to splenomegaly in homologous mouse chimaeras. Nature 1963; 197: 673.
3. Blanden RV. Increased antibacterial resistance and immunodepression during graft-versus-host reactions in mice. Transplantation 1969; 7: 484.
4. Stuart AE, Regunathan P. The allergic macrophage of graft versus host disease. Experientia 1971; 27: 197.
5. Ptak W, Hanczakowska M, Skowron-Cendrzak A. Cytotoxic macrophages in graft versus host reaction. Transplantation 1975; 19: 12.
6. Fung KY, Sabbadini E. Cytotoxicity in graft versus host reaction. II. Lysis of target cells of parental genotype by F_1 hybrid macrophages. Transplantation 1976; 22: 449.
7. Rhodes JM, Bennedsen J, Larsen D, Riisgaard S, Sparck JV. Correlation between in vivo and in vitro functional tests for activated macrophages. Infect Immun 1979; 23: 34.
8. Johnston RB Jr. Enhancement of phagocytosis-associated oxidative metabolism as a manifestation of macrophage activation. In: Pick E, ed. Lymphokines, vol 3. New York, London: Academic, 1981: 33.
9. Nathan CF. Secretion of oxygen intermediates—role in effector functions of activated macrophages. Fed Proc 1982; 41: 2206.
10. Johnston RB Jr. Oxygen metabolism and the microbicidal activity of macrophages. Fed Proc 1978; 37: 2759.
11. Murray HW, Cohn ZA. Mononuclear phagocyte antimicrobial and antitumor activity: the role of oxygen intermediates. J Invest Dermatol 1980; 74: 285.
12. Nathan CF, Brukner LH, Silberstein SC, Cohn ZA. Extracellular cytolysis by activated macrophages and granulocytes. I. Pharmacologic triggering of effector cells and the release of hydrogen peroxide. J Exp Med 1979; 149: 84.
13. Keisari Y, Pick E. Macrophage-mediated cytolysis of erythrocytes in the guinea pig. I. Activation by stimulators of the oxidative burst. Cell Immunol 1981; 62: 172.
14. Keisari Y. Macrophage-mediated cytolysis of erythrocytes in the guinea pig. II. Role of oxidative burst products in macrophage cytotoxicity activated by lectins and phorbol ester derivatives. Cell Immunol 1982; 67: 60.
15. Nathan CF, Silverstein SC, Brukner LH, Cohn ZA. Extracellular cytolysis by activated macrophages and granulocytes. II. Hydrogen peroxide as a mediator of cytotoxicity. J Exp Med 1979; 149: 100.
16. Flescher E, Gonen P, Keisari Y. Oxidative burst-dependent tumoricidal and tumorostatic activities of paraffin oil-elicited mouse macrophages. J Nat Cancer Inst 1984; 72: 1341.
17. Mavier P, Edgington TS. Human monocyte-mediated tumor cytotoxicity. I. Demonstration of an oxygen-dependent myeloperoxidase-independent mechanism. J Immunol 1984; 132: 1980.
18. Babior BM, Kipnes R, Curnette JT. Biological defense mechanisms: the production by leukocytes of superoxide, a potential bactericidial agent. J Clin Invest 1973; 52: 741.
19. Keisari Y, Braun L, Flescher E. The oxidative burst and related phenomena in mouse macrophages elicited by different sterile inflammatory stimuli. Immunobiol 1983; 165: 78.
20. Pick E, Keisari Y. A simple colorimetric method for the measurement of hydrogen peroxide produced by cells in culture. J Immunol Methods 1980; 38: 161.
21. Nathan CF, Root RK. Hydrogen peroxide release from mouse peritoneal macrophages. J Exp Med 1980; 146: 1648.
22. Johnston RB, Godzik CA, Cohn ZA. Increased superoxide anion production by immunologically activated and chemically elicited macrophages. J Exp Med 1978; 148: 115.
23. Murray HW, Cohn ZA. Macrophage oxygen-dependent antimicrobial activity. III. Enhanced oxidative metabolism as an expression of macrophage activation. J Exp Med 1980; 152: 1596.
24. Tomioka H, Saito H. Hydrogen peroxide-releasing function of chemically elicited and immunologically activated macrophages: differential response to wheat germ lectin and concanavalin A. Infect Immun 1980; 29: 469.
25. Anthony LSD, Stevenson MM, Lapp WS, Kongshavn PAL. Macrophage activity in mice undergoing chronic graft-versus-host reactions. Transplantation 1984; 38: 536.
26. Nathan CF, Nogueira N, Juangbhanich C, Ellis J, Cohn Z. Activation of macrophages in vivo and in vitro. Correlation between hydrogen peroxide release and killing of Trypanosoma cruzi. J Exp Med 1979; 149: 1056.
27. Nakagawara A, de Santis NM, Nogueira N, Nathan CF. Lymphokines enhance the capacity of human monocytes to secrete reactive oxygen intermediates. J Clin Invest 1982; 70: 1042.
28. Freund M, Pick E. The mechanism of action of lymphokines. VIII. Lymphokine-enhanced spontaneous hydrogen peroxide production by macrophages. Immunology 1985; 54: 35.
29. Ptak W, Skowron-Cendrzak A. A study of the immunosuppressive potency of antimacrophage serum. Ann Immunol 1972; 4: 205.

Received 25 June 1985.
Accepted 19 September 1985.

0041-1337/86/4106-0759$02.00/0
TRANSPLANTATION
Vol. 41, No. 6
Printed in U.S.A.

FUNCTIONAL CHARACTERIZATION OF PRETHYMIC T CELLS COMMITTED TO ALLOREACTIVITY[1]

MARION BLANK, CHRISTA GRONAU, MONIKA SAUER, HANS-ULRICH WOTTGE, AND WOLFGANG MÜLLER-RUCHHOLTZ[2]

Department of Immunology, University of Kiel, D-2300 Kiel, Federal Republic of Germany

The results of previous experiments on MHC fully allogeneic bone marrow transplantation (BMT) in nonthymectomizd recipients indicated that anti-MHC alloreactivity starts to become irreversibly committed at the prethymic level. This is a matter of some controversy. Since it is possible that conflicting results depend on the methods chosen, we reexamined our previous results by applying two new approaches. Adult thymectomized (ATX) Balb/c mice received a syngeneic fetal thymus either 3 weeks before or 3 weeks after lethal irradiation and reconstitution with C57BL/6 BM incubated in antiserum. Since monoclonal antibodies such as anti-Thy 1 are of limited value for investigations of the above type (Thy 1 antigen crosses the prethymic/thymic border), we used two highly selective, excessively cytotoxic xenoantisera for incubation of the donor BM—either a specific anti-T cell serum (SAT) that eliminated only mature T cells, or a specific antilymphocyte serum (SAL) that reacted additionally with a subset of prethymic T cells (PTC). In both experimental approaches the results were similar: (1) Recipients of SAT-BM developed antihost reactivity, in contrast to recipients of SAL-BM. (2) SAT-BM recipients became immunodeficient, whereas SAL-BM chimeras were immunocompetent. (3) Late mortality was observed only following SAT treatment. (4) Preliminary morphological findings in the lymphoid tissue of BM recipients agree fully with the functional observations. We conclude that the data confirm our previous results in nonthymectomized BM recipients—i.e., PTCs initiate antihost reactivity in MHC fully allogeneic BMT—and PTC commitment is thymus/thymus factor independent. These conclusions are discussed with regard to the problems of MHC allogeneic clinical BMT.

For successful bone marrow transplantation (BMT),* particularly in major histocompatibility complex (MHC) allogeneic systems it is of basic importance to avoid graft-versus-host reactions (GVHR), which are known to be induced by T cells of the grafted donor BM once these have become committed to alloreactivity (*1–3*). Hence the question arises at what stage of T cell differentiation this antiMHC alloreactivity becomes irreversibly determined. Contrary to the prevalent opinion that this stage is not reached prior to the differentiation processes occuring in the thymus, our previous findings have suggested that commitment to MHC alloreactivity begins at the prethymic level.

We have shown in a number of different experiments with rats and mice that to prevent not only acute but also delayed GVHR in MHC fully allogeneic BMT, both mature T cells and a subset of prethymic T cells (PTC) must be eliminated from the grafted BM (*4*). These data appear to conflict with the generalized hypothesis that prethymic cells have the capacity to become immunotolerant (*5–9*).

The different views, however, are not necessarily mutually incompatible, since they are based on different experimental approaches. It is difficult to compare our previous experiments directly with most of those reported in the literature for various reasons—one being that most other authors have worked with thymectomized or nude mice. The present study gives new results of experiments involving thymectomy and thymic reconstitution under varying conditions. They comfirm our former results. Nevertheless they can and will be discussed in terms of a unifying concept. The conclusions to be drawn are of clinical importance for adequate T cell depletion approaches in MHC allogeneic bone marrow transplantation.

General experimental approach. As demonstrated in Figure 1, two experimental approaches were used:

(A) Balb/c mice aged 6 weeks were thymectomized and reconstituted one week later with a syngeneic fetal thymus. After a further 3 weeks they received lethal irradiation and C57BL/6 (B6) BM incubated in SAT or in SAL.
(B) Balb/c mice aged 10 weeks and thymectomized 1 week previously were lethally irradiated and reconstituted with B6 BM incubated in SAT or in SAL. They received a syngeneic fetal thymus 3 weeks after BMT.

MATERIALS AND METHODS

Animals. Mice of the inbred strains Balb/c (H-2^d), C57BL/6 (B6; H-2^b), and C3H (H-2^k) were maintained conventionally.

Antisera. Two polyclonal xenogeneic antisera were prepared, rendered specific by absorptions, and tested as described in detail previously (*10*). In brief: A selective antilymphocyte serum (SAL) was prepared by absorbing a rabbit antirat thymocyte serum sequentially with rat erythrocytes, adherent peritoneal exudate cells, and fetal liver cells. The established term SAL originated from the finding that in the rat SAL was selectively specific for all lymphocytes—both T and B cells. Advantage was taken of its crossreactivity in the mouse, which is limited to thymocytes, peripheral T cells, and 25% of nylon-wool-passed spleen cells of nude mice. A selective anti-T-cell

[1]This work was supported by the Deutsche Forschungsgemeinschaft (SFB 111/A1).

[2] Address offprint requests to: W. Müller-Ruccholtz, Department of Immunology, University of Kiel, Brunswikerstr. 2-6, D-2300 Kiel, F.R.G.

* Abbreviations used: ATX, adult thymectomized; BM, bone marrow; BMT, bone marrow transplantation; CTL, cytotoxic T lymphocytes; FCS, fetal calf serum; GVHR, graft-versus-host reaction; MHC, major histocompatibility complex; MLC, mixed lymphocyte culture; PTC, prethymic T cell; SAL, specific antilymphocyte serum; SAT, specific anti–T cell serum.

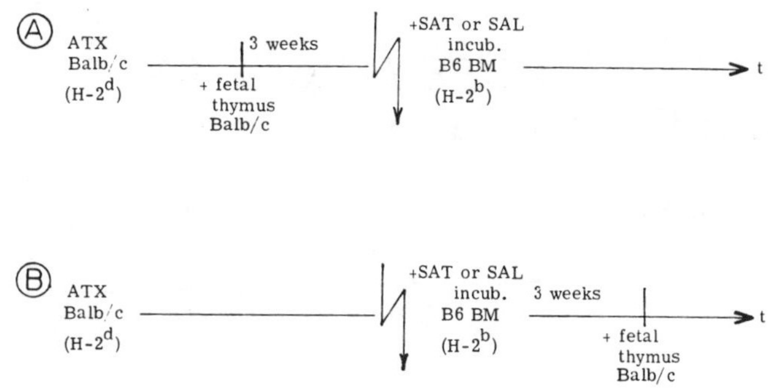

FIGURE 1. Schematic representation of experimental approaches A and B.

serum (SAT) was prepared by absorbing SAL additionally with lymphocytes from *B* rats (adult thymectomized, lethally irradiated and reconstituted with syngeneic bone marrow). SAT was cytotoxic to all mouse thymocytes and peripheral T cells, but did not react with 96–98% of nylon-wool-passed spleen cells of nude mice. All absorptions were proved to be serologically exhaustive, and both antisera were used strictly at equally, excessively cytotoxic titers. The most important difference between these two highly specific antisera is that SAT reacts with thymocytes and mature T cells only, while SAL has the additional capacity to eliminate a defined fraction of prethymic T cells.

Thymectomy. After anesthesia with Ketanest (Parke-Davis, Munich, F.R.G.) the thorax of 6–9-week-old female Balb/c mice was opened, and the thymus tissue was aspirated with a glass pipette.

Thymus transplantation. Adult thymectomized (ATX) Balb/c mice were engrafted with a syngeneic thymus from a 17–20-day-old fetus. The fetal thymus was placed under the right kidney capsule 3 weeks before or 3 weeks after BMT.

Irradiation and BMT. Balb/c mice aged 10 weeks were lethally irradiated (10.0 Gy from a ^{60}Co source, distance 60 cm, 2.1 Gy/min) and reconstituted with bone marrow from B6 mice aged 10–12 weeks (5×10^7 cells, i.v., 2–3 and 24 hr after irradiation) following incubation in SAT or SAL.

Treatment of the donor BM. 2×10^8/ml BM cells (B6) were mixed with an equal volume of antiserum (SAT or SAL at equicytotoxic titers four times as high as the 100% cytotoxicity end-point titer) and incubated for 15 min at 4°C. After four volumes of fresh rat serum were added as the source of complement, the cells were incubated for 30 min at 37°C, pelleted, and resuspended in normal mouse serum for injection into recipients (Balb/c).

Mixed lymphocyte cultures (MLC). Conventional MLC were performed. In brief, 1×10^5 responder spleen cells were cultured with 5×10^5 mitomycin-C-treated stimulator spleen cells in 200/μl RPMI 1640 medium containing 10% fetal calf serum (FCS) for 96 hr in microtiter plates. 24 hr before harvesting 1μ Ci ^{3}H-thymidine was added to each well. All experiments were done in quadruplicate.

Skin grafting. At 6–7 weeks after reconstitution the chimeras received full-thickness skin grafts from a third-party strain (C3H, H-2^k).

RESULTS

Failure of SAL⁺/SAT⁻ prethymic T cells (PTCs) to become tolerant of host alloantigens in MHC allogeneic ATX mice independent of the time of thymus implantation. Spleen cells from allogeneic BM chimeras produced by the two different experimental protocols (cf. Fig. 1) were tested in mixed lymphocyte cultures (MLC) 6–22 weeks after BMT in the first model and 5–20 weeks after thymus implantation in the second model. As shown in Figure 2A, ATX Balb/c mice that received a syngeneic fetal thymus 3 weeks before lethal irradiation and reconstitution with SAT-incubated B6 BM developed antihost reactivity in 9 of 11 cases. This contrasts markedly with recipients of SAL-treated B6 BM—i.e., bone marrow from which the SAL^+/SAT^- PTCs had been eliminated. Here chimera spleen cells were specifically tolerant of host alloantigens. They did not respond with increased ^{3}H-thymidine uptake following stimulation with host alloantigens, but reacted with third-party alloantigens.

A similar pattern of reactivity was obtained in ATX mice given a syngeneic thymus 3 weeks after BMT (Fig. 2B). Here the PTCs present in SAT-treated B6 BM were confronted with host alloantigens for 3 weeks before they had the chance to mature. Nevertheless, they developed antihost reactivity in 6 of 6 experiments. Again, B6 BM incubated with SAL resulted in specific unresponsiveness to host alloantigens, indicating

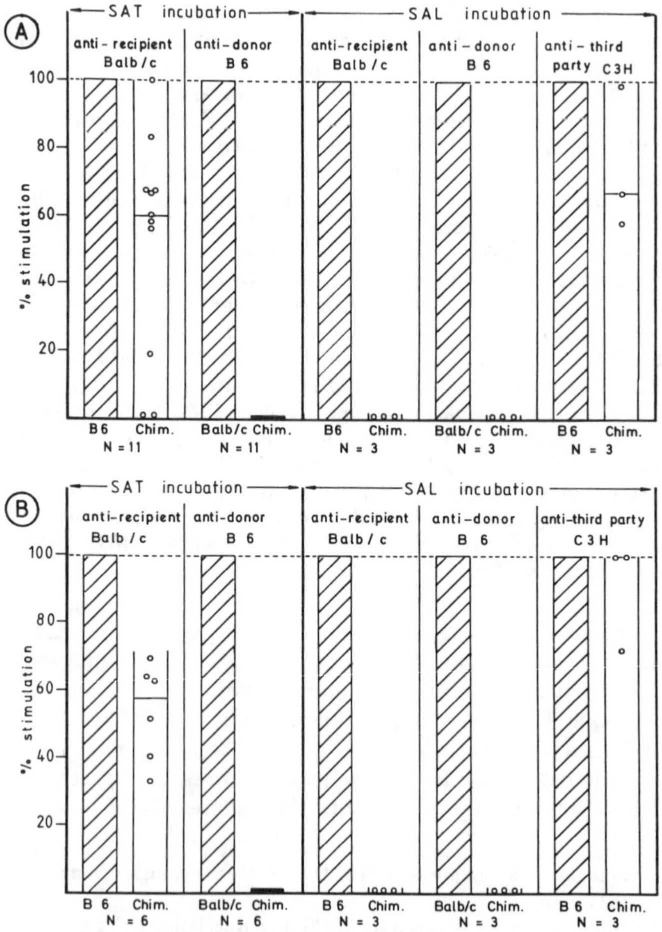

FIGURE 2. MLC reactivity of spleen cells from ATX, lethally irradiated Balb/c mice (Chim.) that received B6 BM incubated in SAT or SAL and a syngeneic fetal thymus 3 weeks before BMT (A) or 3 weeks after BMT (B). The results are expressed as percentage of stimulation of the alloreactivity of the corresponding untreated BM donor or recipient strain cells. (In previous experiments no differences in alloreactivity were found between normal mice and ATX mice reconstituted with syngeneic BM and fetal thymus.)

that SAL⁻/SAT⁻ PTCs achieved tolerance, in contrast to SAL⁺/SAT⁻ PTCs.

In both experimental models chimera spleen cells did not respond to BM donor (B6) alloantigens following incubation in SAT or SAL—i.e., no autoreactivity was found.

Immunodeficiency of chimeras reconstituted with MHC allogeneic BM containing SAL⁺/SAT⁻ PTCs. To demonstrate the restoration of immunocompetence of the chimeras, an in vivo test system was used, rather than an in vitro one, because in our experience it proved to be more sensitive. The chimeras were tested for their ability to reject third-party (C3H) skin grafts. In experimental approach A (cf. Fig. 1) the mice received full-thickness third-party skin grafts 6–7 weeks after BMT. The chimeras obtained by approach B were engrafted with third-party skin 6–7 weeks after thymus implantation. Thus in both cases PTCs were under the influence of a thymus during the same period before skin grafting.

The survival times of C3H skin grafts are shown in Figure 3. The majority (60–70%) of the ATX Balb/c mice that were reconstituted with SAT-incubated B6 BM rejected third-party (C3H) skin grafts between days 10 and 22, regardless of whether these chimeras had received a fetal thymus 3 weeks before or 3 weeks after BMT. That this skin graft rejection pattern indicated immunodeficiency in more than half the animals tested was confirmed by the results of control experiments with recipients of SAL-treated B6 BM. Here chimeras produced by transferring hematopoietic cells freed of SAL⁺/SAT⁻ PTCs rejected third-party skin grafts within 8 days, as normal untreated B6 mice do. There were no exceptions in this group, independent of the time of thymus implantation.

Late mortality caused by SAL⁺/SAT⁻ PTCs in MHC-allogeneic BMT chimeras. Because of the biological significance of long-term observation following MHC allogeneic BMT after different preconditioning regimens, the BMT recipients were observed for more than 120 days after BMT. This period was considered sufficient, since a mortality plateau was reached after 80–90 days.

In Figure 4A these rates are shown for chimeras that received a fetal thymus 3 weeks before BMT. Control animals, which received lethal irradiation only, all died within 15 days. No recipient of untreated allogeneic BM survived the first 30 days. Although nearly all (22–23) recipients of SAT-treated BM survived this period, 52% of them (12–23) died later between the 32nd and 77th day. In contrast, when the donor BM had been incubated with SAL, 7/8 of the chimeras survived for longer than 120 days.

The survival data of ATX mice that received a thymus graft 3 weeks after BMT (Fig. 4B) followed a pattern very similar to that of the group described above. Again, lethally irradiated control animals died within 15 days. Only 2 of 9 animals that had received untreated BM survived until thymus implantation at 21 days, and their physical condition was so poor that an implantation was not practicable. They died within the next week. Nearly all (19/20) recipients of SAT-treated BM, however, survived for 41 days after BMT—or, respectively, 20 days after thymus implantation. Nevertheless, within the next 50 days 55% of the animals in this group (11/20) died. In contrast,

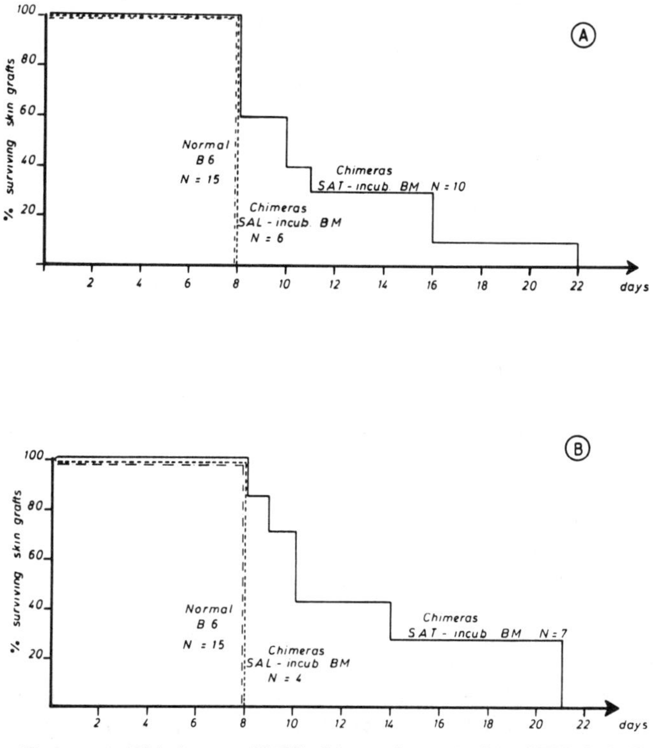

FIGURE 3. Third-party (C3H) skin graft survival in ATX, lethally irradiated Balb/c mice that received B6 BM incubated in SAT (——) or SAL (- - -) and a syngeneic fetal thymus 3 weeks before BMT (A) or 3 weeks after BMT (B), in comparison with normal mice of BM donor strain (–·–).

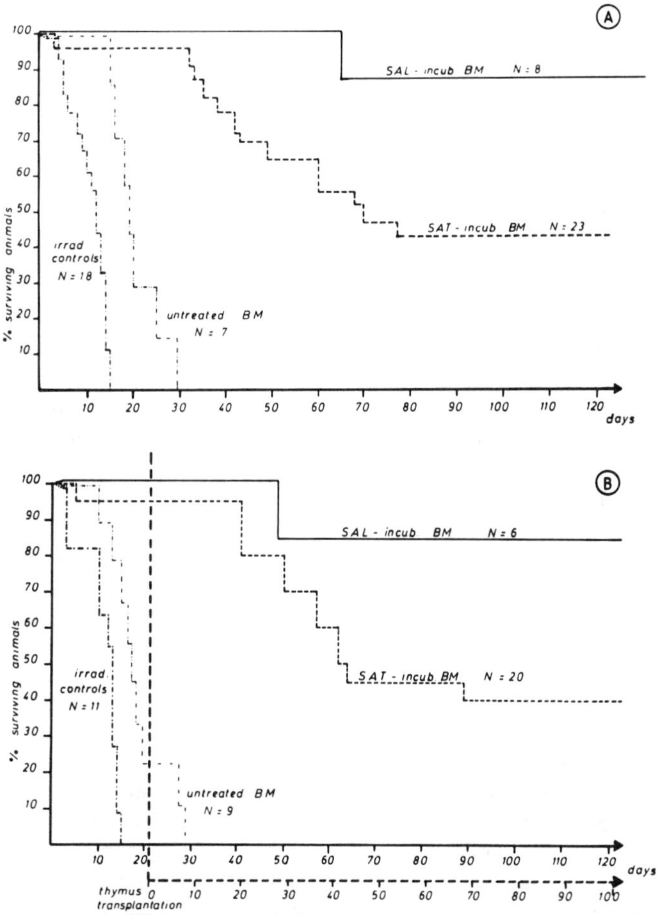

FIGURE 4. Survival rates of ATX, lethally irradiated Balb/c mice that received differently treated B6 BM and a syngeneic fetal thymus 3 weeks before BMT (A) or 3 weeks after BMT (B).

5/6 of the recipients of SAL-preconditioned BM survived for more than 120 days.

Taken together these survival data suggest that SAL⁺/SAT⁻ PTCs are responsible for late mortality in MHC allogeneic BMT, independent of the time of thymus implantation.

Confirmation of the functional findings by preliminary morphological data. In chimeras with both experimental approaches that were reconstituted with SAT-treated BM and died (mainly 4.5–11 weeks after BMT and 3–9.5 weeks after thymus implantation) the thymus implants were found to be atrophied and incompletely restored (Fig. 5, a and b). This limited thymus restitution was most apparent in chimeras that had received a syngeneic fetal thymus 3 weeks after BMT (experimental approach B). The appearance was similar to that observed in the control group given untreated BM, which showed signs of acute GVHR at death (2–4 weeks after BMT, as indicated in Fig. 4).

In contrast, elimination of SAL⁺/SAT⁻ PTCs from the grafted BM resulted in reconstitution of thymus tissue, with the cortex and medulla having their normal structure regardless of whether chimeras had received a fetal thymus 3 weeks before BMT or 3 weeks after BMT. For comparison with the above-described data, the thymus transplant histology of a chimera produced by SAL treatment of BM in the experimental approach B is shown in Figure 5, c and d. A complete evaluation of the histology of thymus and peripheral lymphatic tissue at various times following MHC allogeneic BMT in the different experimental approaches will be published by our pathologists. (Müller-Hermelink et al., manuscript in preparation).

DISCUSSION

The results of this study are summarized in Table 1, parts A and B. The different effects of SAL and SAT are shown in eight sets of experiments. The serological differences between these two antisera allowed us to test the extent to which GVHR can be prevented in MHC fully allogeneic BMT by eliminating only postthymic cells with SAT, or by simultaneously removing an additional portion of cells (25% of the nylon-wool-passed fraction of nude mouse spleen cells—tentatively termed *late* pre-T cells [*4*]) with SAL.

It should be recalled that comparisons of SAL and SAT were always made using equicytotoxic antiserum concentrations that had been shown in previous studies to lie well above the 100% thymocytotoxicity titer and even further above a T cell function inhibition titer (in the Simonsen assay).

In approach A, bone marrow chimeras (Table 1, A) received a syngeneic fetal thymus 3 weeks prior to irradiation and reconstitution with antiserum-treated BM. Thus they are immunobiologically identical with the animals used in our previous experiments (*4*) and correspond to the situation in clinical BMT to the extent that prethymic T cells contained in the grafted BM come into contact with both the alloantigen (irradiated recipient) and a functional thymus. Recipients of SAT-treated BM developed antihost reactivity and became immunoincompetent, which may explain their later mortality. In contrast, recipients of SAL-treated BM did not develop antihost reactivity or immunoincompetence and survived long-term in good general condition. Thus these results confirm the results of our earlier experiments (*4*) with nonthymectomized mice and rats (Table 1, parts C and D). The suggestion that the effects we have been studying were really effects of prethymic T cells rather than of other subpopulations, such as NK cells, is derived from the observation that the pertinent cells exert their effects with a significant delay (Table 1: A3; B3; C4) and become capable of mounting specific alloreactions, such as CTL or MLR, which are generally known to be T cell reactions (Table 1: A1; B1; C1, 2, 3; D1, 2). Taken together we have demonstrated with a total of 18 different experiments that in the MHC fully allogeneic model SAL anti-PTC reactivity is necessary to completely prevent GVHR.

This recognition is the result of a comparison of the effects of two highly specific but polyclonal antisera, SAL and SAT. Exhaustive absorption with prethymic T cells removes antibodies from SAL that are reactive against common antigens of PTCs and T cells. Since the resulting SAT does not react any longer with PTCs, but still shows reactivity against T cells, it must contain specific antibodies against antigens expressed solely on T cells—i.e., not on PTCs. In contrast, monoclonal antibodies, such as anti-Thy 1, have so far been of limited value for these studies, because differentiation antigens such as Thy 1 occur not only on mature T cells, but also—to a lesser degree—on prethymic T cells (*11–14*). Therefore, the most reasonable explanation of the varying results achieved with anti-Thy 1 antibodies in MHC fully allogeneic BMT (*7, 15–18*) appears to be that the antibody incubation was successful with regard to GVHR prevention when the antibody titer was sufficient to eliminate not only mature T cells, but also prethymic T cells (*7, 15, 16*). The same holds for polyclonal rabbit antimouse brain sera, which are presumably comparable to our SAL with regard to serological specificity (*19*) and the results obtained in MHC allogeneic BMT (*8, 20, 21*).

Our results following SAT incubation are in complete agreement with other studies showing that prethymic T cells can react specifically with alloantigens in vitro (*22–26*) and in vivo (*27, 28*). They appear, however, to contradict results obtained with nude mice or adult thymectomized mice, in which specific tolerance to the alloantigen of implanted fetal thymuses (*5, 7, 8, 20, 29*) or fetal thymus epithelial cells (*9, 30*) has been demonstrated. Therefore, we hypothesized (*4*) that SAL⁺/SAT⁻ PTCs can still become tolerant if, as in the above-mentioned experiments, they are not confronted with a normally functioning thymus or its products immediately after contact with the alloantigen. Our approach *B* was designed to test this hypothesis by exposing the PTCs only to the alloantigen (irradiated recipient) without thymus influence for 3 weeks.

Contrary to our hypothesis, ATX mice that did not receive a syngeneic fetal thymus until 3 weeks after irradiation and reconstitution with SAT-treated allogeneic BM developed antihost reactivity and became immunoincompetent (Table 1, B). Tolerance to the recipient was achieved only when the donor BM was treated with SAL, thus a subset of the PTCs was eliminated. Why did the SAL⁺/SAT⁻ cells not become tolerant in these experiments? An explanation may be that adult alloantigen (the irradiated recipient in our case) is much more immunogenic than fetal alloantigen (the fetal thymus in the other cases), which tends to be tolerogenic. This assumption is supported by experiments of Zinkernagel et al. (*29*). They achieved tolerance in nude mice following the implantation of a fetal thymus, but specific reactivity against nonshared alloantigens of the graft after implantation of an adult irradiated semiallogeneic thymus.

Taken together the results of our experiments allow the following conclusions: First, a portion of prethymic T cells is capable of inducing delayed and specific reactivity in MHC

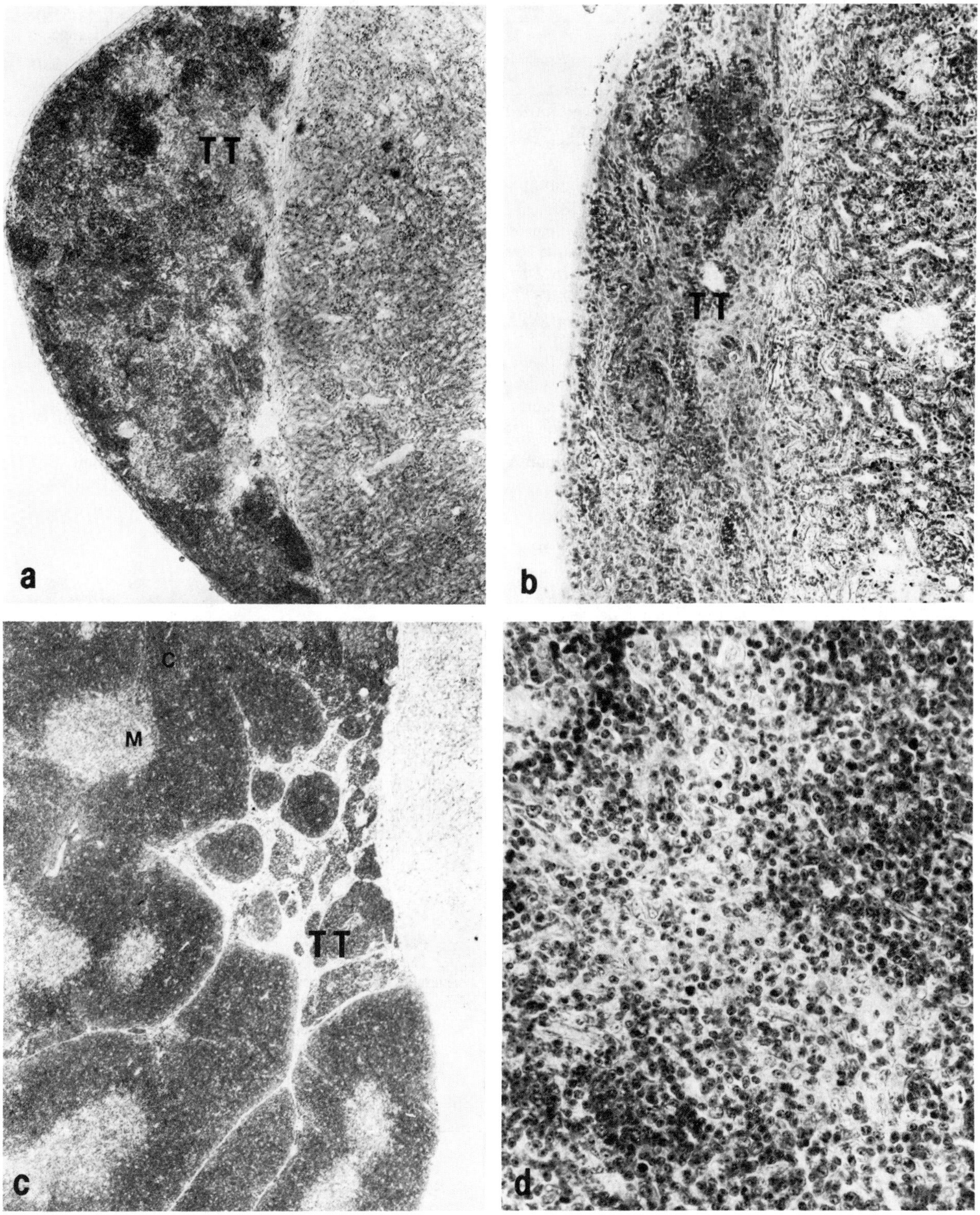

FIGURE 5. Thymus transplant (TT) histology of chimeras: (a) ATX Balb/c mouse that received a syngeneic fetal thymus 3 weeks before lethal irradiation and reconstitution with B6 BM incubated in *SAT*, 5 weeks after BMT (Giemsa, 70×); (b) ATX Balb/c mouse that received a syngeneic fetal thymus 3 weeks after lethal irradiation and reconstitution with B6 BM incubated in *SAT*, 5 weeks after thymus implantation (Giemsa, 170×) (Both thymus transplants [a and b] show incomplete restitution—most of the lymphoid cells are localized in the connective tissue surrounding thymus epithelial sheets with larger lymphoid cells); (c) ATX Balb/c mouse that received a syngeneic fetal thymus 3 weeks after lethal irradiation and reconstitution with B6 BM incubated in *SAL*, 4½ weeks after thymus implantation (Giemsa, 70×); (d) higher magnification of the thymus transplant in (c) showing the corticomedullary junction (Giemsa, 430×). Thymus transplant shows normal structure with cortex (C) and medulla (M).

TABLE 1. Summary of results showing that SAL anti-PTC reactivity is required for prevention of delayed GVHR in MHC fully allogeneic combinations

Exp. group	Experiment	Effects following application	
		SAL	SAT
A.	BM recipients: adult thymectomized and thymus-prereconstituted		
	Chimera: mouse (B6) $\xrightarrow{BM}$ ϟATX Balb/c+fet. Balb/c thymus 3 weeks before BMT		
	1. Prevention of MLC α-Balb/c	+	−
	2. Prevention of delayed third-party skin graft rejection	+	−
	3. Prevention of delayed mortality	+	−
	4. Normal lymphatic tissue histology	+	−
B.	BM recipients: adult thymectomized and thymus-postreconstituted		
	Chimera: mouse (B6) $\xrightarrow{BM}$ ϟATX Balb/c+fet. Balb/c thymus 3 weeks after BMT		
	1. Prevention of MLC α-Balb/c	+	−
	2. Prevention of delayed third-party skin graft rejection	+	−
	3. Prevention of delayed mortality	+	−
	4. Normal lymphatic tissue histology	+	−
C.	BM recipients: adult normal (non-ATX)		
	Chimera: mouse (C3H) $\xrightarrow{BM}$ ϟBalb/c		
	1. Prevention of CTL α-Balb/c	+	nt
	Chimera: mouse (B6) $\xrightarrow{BM}$ ϟBalb/c		
	2. Prevention of CTL α-Balb/c	+	−
	3. Prevention of MLC α-Balb/c	+	−
	4. Prevention of delayed mortality	+	−
	5. Normal lymphatic tissue histology	+	−
	Chimera: rat (CAP) $\xrightarrow{BM}$ ϟLEW		
	6. Thymus restitution	+	−
	7. Healthy permanent chimerism	+	−
D.	BM donors: thymusless		
	Chimera: nude mouse (B6) $\xrightarrow[spleen]{BM}$ ϟBalb/c		
	1. Prevention of CTL α-Balb/c	+	
	2. Prevention of MLC α-Balb/c	+	
	Chimera: B rat (LEW) $\xrightarrow{spleen}$ neonatal CAP		
	3. Prevention of delayed GVHR[a]	+	

[a] Splenomegaly, recognizable only on day 40, but not on days 10 or 20.

fully allogeneic BMT, which does not imply that the same must hold for non-MHC antigenic structures; and second, SAL^+/SAT^- PTCs did not become tolerant during the 3 weeks between BMT and thymus implantation during which they were in contact with MHC alloantigens. This shows that the commitment of prethymic T cells to anti-MHC alloreactivity is independent of the thymus or thymus factors.

Thus the success of GVHR prevention in MHC fully allogeneic BMT appears to depend on the extent to which not only mature T cells but also irreversibly determined prethymic T cells are eliminated. This recognition should help to overcome the MHC allogeneic barrier in clinical BMT and thus give us access to a much larger number of potential donors.

The aim of ongoing investigations is to characterize the SAL^+/SAT^- PTCs using cell biological markers. Preliminary data show that these cells are Thy 1^+, Lyt 1^-, Lyt 2^-, which further supports the possibility that they are prethymic.

Acknowledgments. We thank Mrs. H. Steffen for help in producing specific antisera; Mr. J. M. Jensen of the Department of Radiology, University of Kiel, for irradiation of animals; and Mrs. K. Dege for help in preparing and Mrs. U. Schwarz for typing the manuscript.

REFERENCES

1. Grebe SC, Streilein JW. Graft-verus-host reactions: a review. Adv Immunol 1976; 22: 119.
2. Elkins WL. Tolerance and the fate of the allogeneic bone marrow chimera. In: Stuart FP, Fitch FW, eds. Immunological tolerance and enhancement. Lancester: MTP Press Limited, 1979: 1.
3. Rolink AG, Radaszkiewicz T, Pals ST, van der Meer WGJ, Gleichmann E. Allosuppressor and allohelper T cells in acute and chronic graft-versus-host disease. I. Alloreactive suppressor cells rather than killer T cells appear to be the decisive effector cells in lethal graft-vs-host disease. J Exp Med 1982; 155: 1501.
4. Müller-Ruchholtz W, Blank M, Wottge H-U, Ulrichs K, Müller-Hermelink HK. Relevance of prethymic precursor cells for GVHR prevention in rat and mouse fully allogeneic combinations. Transplant Proc 1983; 15: 1463.
5. Kindred B. Lymphocytes which differentiate in an allogeneic thymus. I. Response to MLC determinants and skin grafts from the thymus donor strain. Cell Immunol 1976; 25: 189.

6. Besedovsky HO, Del Rey A, Sorkin E. Role of prethymic cells in aquisition of self-tolerance. J Exp Med 1979; 150: 1351.
7. Rayfield LS, Brent L. Tolerance, immunocompetence, and secondary disease in fully allogeneic radiation chimeras. Transplantation 1983; 36: 183.
8. Morrissey PJ, Singer A. Role of prethymic and intrathymic elements in the induction of T cell tolerance to allogeneic determinants: the thymus is not sufficient to prevent autoreactivity. In: Haynes BF, Eisenbarth GS, eds. Monoclonal antibodies. Probes for the study of autoimmunity and immunodeficiency. New York: Academic, 1983: 67.
9. Jordan RK, Robinson JH, Hopkinson NA, House KC, Bentley AL.Thymic epithelium and the induction of transplantation tolerance in nude mice. Nature 1985; 314: 454.
10. Müller-Ruchholtz W, Wottge H-U, Müller-Hermelink HK. Restitution potentials of allogeneically or xenogeneically grafted lymphocyte-free hemopoietic stem cells. In: Thierfelder S, Rodt H, Kolb J, eds. Immunobiology of bone marrow transplantation. Berlin, Heidelberg, New York: Springer, 1980: 153.
11. Raff MC. θ bearing lymphocytes in nude mice. Nature 1973; 246: 350.
12. Cantor H, Simpson E, Sato VL, Fathman CG, Herzenberg LA. Characterization of sub-populations of T lymphocytes. I. Separation and functional studies of peripheral T cells binding different amounts of fluorescent anti-thy 1.2 (theta) antibody using a flourescence activated cell sorter (FACS). Cell Immunol 1975; 15: 180.
13. Roelants GE, Loor F, von Boehmer H, Sprent J, Hägg L-B, Major KS, Rydén A. Five types of lymphocytes (Ig^-e^-, $Ig^-\ \theta^{+weak}$, $Ig^-\ \theta^{+strong}$, $Ig^+\ \theta^-$ and $Ig^+\ \theta^+$) characterized by double immunofluorescence and electrophoretic mobility. Organ distribution in normal and nude mice. Eur J Immunol 1975; 5: 127.
14. Basch RS, Berman JW. Thy-1 determinants are present on many murine hematopoietic cells other than T cells. Eur J Immunol 1982; 12: 359.
15. Matzinger P, Mirkwood G. In a fully H-2 incompatible chimera, T cells of donor origin can respond to minor histocompatibility antigens in association with either donor or host H-2 type. J Exp Med 1978; 148: 84.
16. Onoé K, Fernandes G, Good RA. Humoral and cell-mediated immune response in fully allogeneic bone marrow chimera in mice. J Exp Med 1980; 151: 115.
17. Zinkernagel RM, Althage A, Callahan G, Welsh RM. On the immunocompetence of H-2 incompatible irradiation bone marrow chimeras. J Immunol 1980; 124: 2356.
18. Rodt H, Thierfelder S, Kummer U. Effect of monoclonal antibodies on GVHR in minor and MHC-incompatible mouse models. Transplant Proc 1983; 15(1): 1472.
19. Sato VL, Waksal SD, Herzenberg LA. Identification and separation of pre T-cells from nu/nu mice: differentiation by preculture with thymic reticuloepithelial cells. Cell Immunol 1976; 24: 173.
20. Bradley SM, Morrissey PJ, Sharrow SO, Singer A. Tolerance of thymocytes to allogeneic I region determinants encountered prethymically: evidence for expression of anti-Ia receptors by T cell precursors before their entry into the thymus. J Exp Med 1982; 155: 1638.
21. Morrissey PJ, Kruisbeek AM, Sharrow SO. Tolerance of thymic cytotoxic T lymphocytes to allogeneic H-2 determinants encountered prethymically: evidence for expression of anti-H-2 receptors prior to entry into the thymus. Proc Natl Acad Sci USA 1982; 79: 2003.
22. Gillis S, Union NA, Baker PE, Smith MK. The in vitro generation and sustained culture of nude mouse cytolytic T lymphocytes. J Exp Med 1979; 149: 1460.
23. Hünig T, Bevan M. Specificity of cytotoxic T cells from athymic mice. J Exp Med 1980; 152: 688.
24. Fenneck MM, Letarte M, Osoba D. Responsiveness in the mixed leukocyte reaction by nu/nu cells bearing Thy-1 antigen and lacking Fc receptors. Cell Immunol 1981; 57: 339.
25. Waksal SD, Parkinson DR. Prothymocyte development: the role of specific microenviroments in normal and leukemia differentiation. Behring Inst Mitt 1982; 70: 14.
26. Ikehara S, Pahwa RN, Fernandes G, Hansen CT, Good RA. Functional T cells in athymic nude mice. Proc Natl Acad Sci USA 1984; 81: 886.
27. Wagner H, Hardt C, Heeg K, Röllinghoff M, Pfizenmaier K. T-cell-derived helper factor allows in vivo induction of cytotoxic T cells in nu/nu mice. Nature 1980; 284: 278.
28. O'Kunewick JP, Meredith RF, Raikow RB, Buffo MJ, Jones D. Possibility of three distinct and separable components to fatal graft-vs-host reaction. Exp Hematol 1982; 10(3): 277.
29. Zinkernagel RM, Althage A, Waterfield E, Kindred B, Welsh RM, Callahan G, Pincetl P. Restriction specificities, alloreactivity and allotolerance expressed by T cells from nude mice reconstituted with H-2-compatible or -incompatible thymus grafts. J Exp Med 1980; 151: 376.
30. Boehmer H von, Schubiger K. Thymocytes appear to ignore class I major histocompatibility complex antigens expressed on thymus epithelial cells. Eur J Immunol 1984; 14: 1048.

Received 18 July 1985.
Accepted 19 September 1985.

0041-1337/86/4106-0766$02.00/0
TRANSPLANTATION
Vol. 41, No. 6
Printed in U.S.A.

IMPAIRED REJECTION OF MINOR-HISTOCOMPATIBILITY-ANTIGEN–DISPARATE SKIN GRAFTS AND ACQUISITION OF TOLERANCE TO THYMUS DONOR ANTIGENS IN ALLOTHYMUS-IMPLANTED, THYMECTOMIZED *XENOPUS*[1]

JANE C. ARNALL[2] AND JOHN D. HORTON[3]

Department of Zoology, University of Durham, Durham, United Kingdom

We examine whether J strain *Xenopus laevis* and *X laevis/gilli* (LG) isogeneic hybrids, thymectomized (Tx) at 7 days and implanted with larval or postmetamorphic thymus (either normal or irradiated) in late larval life, can be used to explore the role of the developing thymus in the education of minor histocompatibility (H) antigen-reactive T cells and in the acquisition of tolerance to MHC (major histocompatibility complex) antigens.

Tx LG *Xenopus* implanted with isogeneic thymus display fully restored ability to reject both MHC-incompatible and minor H-disparate grafts. Allothymuses (both MHC- and minor-H-disparate) restore normal rejection of skin grafts with MHC incompatibility to thymus donor and Tx (J or LG) host, but reactivity to grafts with putative minor H disparity is impaired. Defective minor-H-disparate skin graft rejection occurs even when the Tx host has received a thymus of the "correct" MHC haplotype (i.e., the same MHC as the assay skin graft). This defect may be attributable to inadequate establishment of minor-H-reactive T lymphocytes, to sharing of minor antigens, or to"nonspecificity" of tolerance induction to minor antigens, since such tolerance is demonstrated here following perimetamorphic grafting of skin to control LG clones.

Skin grafts from *Xenopus* isogeneic to the donors of the MHC-incompatible larval and adult thymus implants are always tolerated by Tx hosts. In contrast, in vitro one-way MLC (mixed leukocyte culture) reactivity of splenocytes to thymus donor MHC antigens occurs when certain donor/host combinations are used but not when others are tested. Postmetamorphic thymus implants appear to promote in vitro MLC tolerance more effectively than larval thymus implants.

The South African clawed "toad," *Xenopus*, which belongs to the frog family Pipidae (*1*), is a useful comparative model for investigating development of the immune system (*2*). Many features of the mammalian immune system appear to be present in this anuran—for example, thymus (T)*-dependent and T-independent immune responses, T and B cell populations (against which monoclonal antibodies are now beginning to be prepared), a major histocompatibility complex (MHC),* genetically restricted T-B collaboration in vitro, IgM and low molecular weight IgY (IgG-like) (reviewed by Flajnik et al. [*3*]). However, in contrast to mammals, *Xenopus* can be surgically manipulated very early in life. This advantage is currently being put to use in several laboratories to assess the extent to which the thymus, at various stages of development, is involved in establishing tolerance of T-lineage lymphocytes to self- and alloantigens (*4*) and in restricting the MHC antigen specificities with which helper and effector T cell populations preferentially interact during recognition and/or destruction of non-MHC antigens (*3, 5–8*). These amphibian studies offer new approaches to investigate the role of the thymus in T cell education, which is still unresolved in mammals—despite, for example, many experiments on thymus/bone-marrow-reconstituted, irradiated mice and on thymus-implanted, nude mice (*9–12*).

Experiments involving thymus implantation into late larval and adult *Xenopus* that have been early-thymectomized (Tx) when only 4–7 days old (*5–7, 13*) suggest that host-derived stem cells, even when educated within a completely foreign (2-MHC-haplotype–disparate) thymus, can repopulate the periphery and collaborate effectively with host-derived antigen-presenting cells and B lymphocytes in in vivo IgM and IgY antibody responses to soluble and cellular T-dependent antigens. The thymectomy/thymus implant model has, therefore, not revealed a central role of the anuran thymus in establishing MHC restriction of helper T cells during late larval and early postmetamorphic life.

Recently Flajnik et al. (*3, 8*), using a different microsurgical approach, have presented data suggesting that during early development the *Xenopus* thymus is involved, to a limited extent, in establishing the MHC type with which T helper cells preferentially interact. They studied chimeric *Xenopus* made by joining the anterior portion of one 24-hour embryo (containing the thymic anlagen—i.e., thymus epithelium) to the posterior portion of an MHC-incompatible embryo (from which the hemopoietic stem cells, including lymphocytes, arise). When assayed for antibody production against dinitrophenylated keyhole limpet hemocyanin, such chimeric animals generally displayed normal IgM reactivity but kinetically delayed, or low, IgY antibody titers. Furthermore, the MHC haplotype of the thymus anlagen may also govern the MHC interaction antigen preference (*14*) of minor histocompatibility (H) antigen-reactive cells. This was implied by recent experiments (*3*) on allogeneically established chimeras that revealed minor H-disparate skin graft rejection of normal kinetics only when the

[1] This work was supported by grants from the Medical Research Council (G80/0720/2CB) and the North of England Cancer Research Campaign (to J. D. H.).

[2] A Durham University Research Studentship to J. C. A. is acknowledged.

[3] To whom correspondence should be addressed, at: Department of Zoology, University of Durham, South Road, Durham DH1 3LE, U.K.

* Abbreviations used: H, histocompatibility; J, J strain *Xenopus laevis*; LG, *Xenopus laevis/gilli* isogeneic hybrids; MHC, major histocompatibility complex; MLC, mixed leukocyte culture; T, thymus; Tx, early-thymectomized (at 7 days of age).

chimera had been constructed with its anterior region (i.e., thymus epithelium) MHC-compatible to the skin donor. Embryos created with their lymphocytes MHC-compatible to the skin donor, but with their thymic anlagen MHC-incompatible, were able to reject the minor antigens on display only in delayed fashion.

The major consideration of this article is whether the thymectomy/thymus implantation model can be used to demonstrate a role of the thymus during late larval and early adult life in educating minor-H-antigen reactive T cells. We examine, in a variety of donor/host combinations, whether alloimmunity (in particular to skin bearing only minor H differences to thymus donor and/or Tx host) is fully restored in Tx *Xenopus* implanted with isogeneic or allogeneic thymus in late larval life. The extent to which Tx animals are rendered tolerant to MHC antigens of the thymus donor and the specificity of this tolerance are also explored through in vivo skin grafting and by *in vitro* mixed leucocyte culture (MLC). In particular, we wished to know whether our experimental protocol achieves complete tolerance to thymus donor MHC antigens, since others have revealed split tolerance (tolerance in vivo but usually not in MLC) following thymus implantation to Tx frogs in adult life (*6*) and in chimeric *Xenopus* (*3*). Finally, to investigate the role that perimetamorphic tolerance (*2, 15, 16*) plays in our studies on minor H antigen graft rejection in Tx animals following thymus implantation, we have also briefly examined the range of in vivo alloimmune responses exhibited by control *Xenopus* bearing, as a consequence of late larval transplantation, a permanently surviving skin graft.

MATERIALS AND METHODS

Animals. Inbred J strain *X laevis* adults used for breeding were a gift from C. Katagiri (Hokkaido University, Sapporo, Japan). J strain *Xenopus* (originally called G-line by Katagiri (*17*) but subsequently rechristened J (*16*) to reflect their *J*apanese "origin") are MHC-identical (haplotype jj) and were initially thought not to reject skin and other tissues from one another (*17, 18*). However, that these clawed frogs display minor H antigen disparities was subsequently suggested by DiMarzo and Cohen (*16*), who revealed chronic intra-J skin graft destruction. A more detailed investigation of the alloimmune capabilities of our J strain colony is presented here. The adult *X laevis*/*X gilli* (LG) isogeneic hybrids used for breeding, originated from Basel (gift from L. DuPasquier, Basel Institute for Immunology, Switzerland) or were the F_1 offspring of these female frogs. The gynognetic clones used were LG17 (MHC haplotypes [ac]), LG15 (also ac but possessiong minor H antigenic differences to LG17), LG5 (ad), and LG3 (bd). Animals within a clone are identical to one another (*19*). Wild *X laevis* were purchased from Xenopus Ltd. (Surrey, UK). J strain *Xenopus*, wild *X laevis*, and the LG hybrids used in this study were bred and reared in the laboratory at 23°C as previously described (*19, 20*).

To prevent the possibility of back stimulation (*21*) in some of the one-way MLC experiments, hybrid JxLG5 and JxLM3 (*laevis*/*muelleri* isogeneic clonal *Xenopus*) were produced by fertilizing the endoreduplicated (2N) eggs that LG and LM *Xenopus* lay, with J sperm. The hybrids were checked for their triploidy by silver staining of blood cells (*22*). We have shown (Horton TL unpublished data) that J animals reject JLG5 and JLM3 skin within 3 weeks, whereas the hybrids fail to respond acutely to J strain skin grafts and fail to display MLC reactivity to J stimulators.

Thymectomy. Thymectomy was carried out using the microcautery technique of Horton and Manning (*20*). Thymuses were removed when the larvae were 7 days old (stage 47 of Nieuwkoop and Faber [*23*]). Tx larvae were checked for absence of thymus regeneration before metamorphosis and also postmortem.

Thymus implantation. Single thymus implants were subcutaneously transplanted to Tx larvae when 4–6 weeks old (stages 56–58; hind-limbs are well developed and fore-limbs erupt during stage 57—i.e., metamorphosis is beginning at this time) as described elsewhere (*7*). Donor thymuses were from larvae of similar age and stage to the host, or from 4–6-month-old froglets (these froglet thymuses are referred to as *adult* here; sometimes such thymuses required halving to allow implantation to proceed). Adult thymuses were used since it is only after metamorphosis that class I MHC antigens become detectable on *Xenopus* cells; class II MHC antigens have been recorded in larvae (*24*). Some thymuses were in vitro-irradiated prior to implantation to reduce the number of donor lymphocytes and thereby minimize their contribution in establishing allorestoration. Lack of involvement of donor implant T-lineage cells in restoration is suggested by our observations that nonirradiated larval spleen alloimplants (which contain T lymphocytes able to display MLC reactivity) fail to reconstitute the response of Tx *Xenopus* to MHC-disparate skin grafts. Irradiation of thymus was performed with a cobalt-60 source at a dose of 1000 rads (200 rads/min) or 3000 rads (600 rads/min). Previous histologic studies (*7*) have shown that nonirradiated allothymus implants develop normally. In contrast, irradiated thymuses observed within a few days of implantation consist mostly of stromal elements, although lymphocytes are still found scattered in the organ. Within one month of irradiation these thymuses display cortical/medullary differentiation and abundant lymphocytes; however, compared with nonirradiated implants, they remain extremely small and often become undetectable morphologically during early adult life. Extensive repopulation of both normal and irradiated larval and adult thymuses with host lymphocytes has been revealed by ploidy-labeling experiments in our laboratory ([*7*] and Russ JH [this laboratory], personal communication).

Skin grafting. Larvae were implanted with a single skin graft (approx. 2 mm^2) from 4–6-month-old froglets, when 4–6 weeks old (stages 56–58) as previously described (*25*); ventral (white) skin was used to aid long-term monitoring of these grafts (*26*). Adults (5–9 months old) were grafted with one or more 2–3-mm^2 dorsal, adult skin grafts (*20*). Grafted animals were kept at an elevated temperature of 25–26°C (so as to mimic the temperature used for in vitro MLC experiments). Rejection was monitored continually until at least 100 days (irregular observations were also made at later postgrafting periods). Rejection was considered complete at the time of total pigment cell destruction; histologically only collagen pad of the skin remains at the rejection end-point chosen here (*27*).

Mixed leukocyte culture. Splenocytes from 6–9-month-old froglets were used throughout these experiments and were suspended in fully supplemented L15 culture medium (Flow Laboratories) using a formula described elsewhere (*28*). Cells were incubated at 26°C in a water-saturated atmosphere of 5% CO_2 in air. Spleen cells were suspended at 1×10^6 viable leukocytes/ml in 1% decomplemented fetal calf serum (Flow)-supplemented medium and placed in triplicate (1×10^5 each of responder cells and stimulator cells) in 96-well, conical-bottomed tissue culture plates (M25 ARTL, Sterilin). Proliferative responses were measured in 1-way MLC using 5000-rad-irradiated stimulator cells. Cultures were pulsed at 72 hr with 1 μCi of ^{3}HTdR (tritiated thymidine)/well and harvested at 96 hr. Stimulation indices (SIs) were equal to the DPM of experimental cultures (i.e., responder cells from one animal cocultured with irradiated allogeneic stimulators) divided by the DPM of the same responder cells cocultured with irradiated autologous cells. The Student's t test was used to check the significance between experimental and control DPM.

RESULTS

Characterization of Histocompatibility Reactions Within J Strain Xenopus

Table 1 reveals the fate of first-set and second-set J strain allografts applied to J strain froglets. None of the first-set grafts was fully rejected by 30 days (the time within which first-set MHC-disparate skin grafts are usually rejected), but 63% were fully rejected by 100 days. Indeed, by the latter time, only 2/63 grafts remained in perfect condition; the other 21 nonrejected grafts displayed chronic rejection phenomena. Autografts, placed alongside allografts, always survived in perfect condition (Table 1).

Eighteen J froglets that had rejected, or were in the process of rejecting first-set allografts, were subsequently grafted wtih second-set (same donor as first-set) and third-party J skin to probe the immunological basis of intra-J graft rejection. A total of 77% of second-set grafts were now rejected *acutely* (here defined as within 30 days). Considerable minor H antigen sharing between animals in our colony was shown by the fact that this accelerated graft rejection was not specific to the original donor—thus 44% of third-party grafts were now also completely destroyed by 30 days. However, a certain degree of minor antigen polymorphism is indicated, since the proportion of secondary grafts not fully rejected by 100 days was higher when the grafts were third-party (50%, 9/18) than when from the original donor (17%, 3/18).

Figure 1 illustrates the chronology of graft rejection phases in the 18 regrafted J animals. Six hosts (Nos. 1, 4, 6, 7, 28, and 33) revealed accelerated (acute) rejection specific to the second-set transplant only. In contrast, 8 J hosts (Nos. 2, 3, 5, 19, 21, 27, 31, and 32) displayed acute rejection of both second-set and third-party grafts. A final group of 4 hosts (Nos. 8, 22, 29, and 30) failed to show acute destruction of second-set or third-party skin grafts. However, in all 4 hosts, such grafts reached phases 1 and 2 of rejection much earlier than did the first-set transplants.

J strain control animals failed to respond to J stimulator cells when tested in one-way MLC (see below).

Effect of Implantation of MHC- or Minor H Antigen-Disparate Thymus in Larval Life on Alloimmune Reactivity of Tx Animals

Skin graft experiments with J strain recipients. The results are illustrated in Figure 2. The data with J strain skin grafts applied to controls is taken from Table 1. In contrast to the subacute (30–50 days) or chronic rejection (>50 days) seen with minor-H-disparate skin, MHC-disparate grafts are rejected acutely (within 30 days). Early thymectomy generally abrogated the ability to destroy MHC-disparate grafts, although 3 LG17 transplants were rejected in subacute or chronic fashion. The finding that early-thymectomized *Xenopus* can ultimately reject MHC-disparate skin (when certain donor/host combinations are used) is discussed fully elsewhere (*26, 29, 30, 31*)), although the cellular mechanisms involved remain unresolved.

Implantation of minor-H-disparate J thymus, be it larval or adult, normal or irradiated, restores the allograft response of Tx J animals to MHC antigens; most grafts from LG or wild *X laevis* donors were now rejected in acute fashion, although a few transplants were rejected subacutely. In contrast, 24/26 J grafts (placed alongside the recognized MHC-disparate grafts) remained perfect for >100 days, only 2 being rejected in subacute fashion.

Implantation of MHC-disparate (LG) adult thymus (normal or irradiated) also restored the ability of Tx J animals to reject skin acutely or subacutely from donors MHC-disparate to host or thymus donor. Tolerance specific to thymus donor histocompatibility antigens is induced, since skin grafts from the thymus donor LG strain in 20/21 cases remained in perfect condition for >100 days, while neighboring unrelated transplants were being rejected. J transplants also remained in excellent health in this group of animals.

Skin graft experiments with LG recipients. The results are

TABLE 1. Fate of first-set and second-set J skin grafts applied to J strain *Xenopus laevis*

Donor skin type	No. of grafts	Graft rejection times (days)						Condition of grafts not fully rejected at 100+ days[a]			% Grafts fully rejected	
		0–15	16–30	31–45	46–60	61–75	76–100	Chronic rejection: Phase 2	Chronic rejection: Phase 1	Perfect	100 days	30 days
J strain *X laevis* 1st-set grafts[b]	63	—	—	24	11	5	—	19	2	2	63	0
J strain *X laevis* 2nd-set grafts[c]	18	—	14	1	—	—	—	3	—	—	83	77
J strain *X laevis* 3rd-party grafts[d]	18	—	8	1	—	—	—	9	—	—	50	44

[a] Phase 1: vascular disturbances and slight pigmentary defects; phase 2: pigment destruction modest to severe, glandular appearance of grafts; Rejected: complete pigment and skin gland destruction.

[b] 1st-set grafts: animals received 1 or 2 skin grafts from separate J individuals when 5 months old. (Those toadlets (N=11) given only 1 allograft were also given a control autograft; the latter was always in perfect condition >100 days).

[c] 2nd-set grafts: applied 100–120 days following 1st-set grafting. Animals received a single second-set graft (same donor as 1st-set).

[d] 3rd-party grafts: a single 3rd-party graft (from a new J donor) was applied alongside the 2nd-set graft.

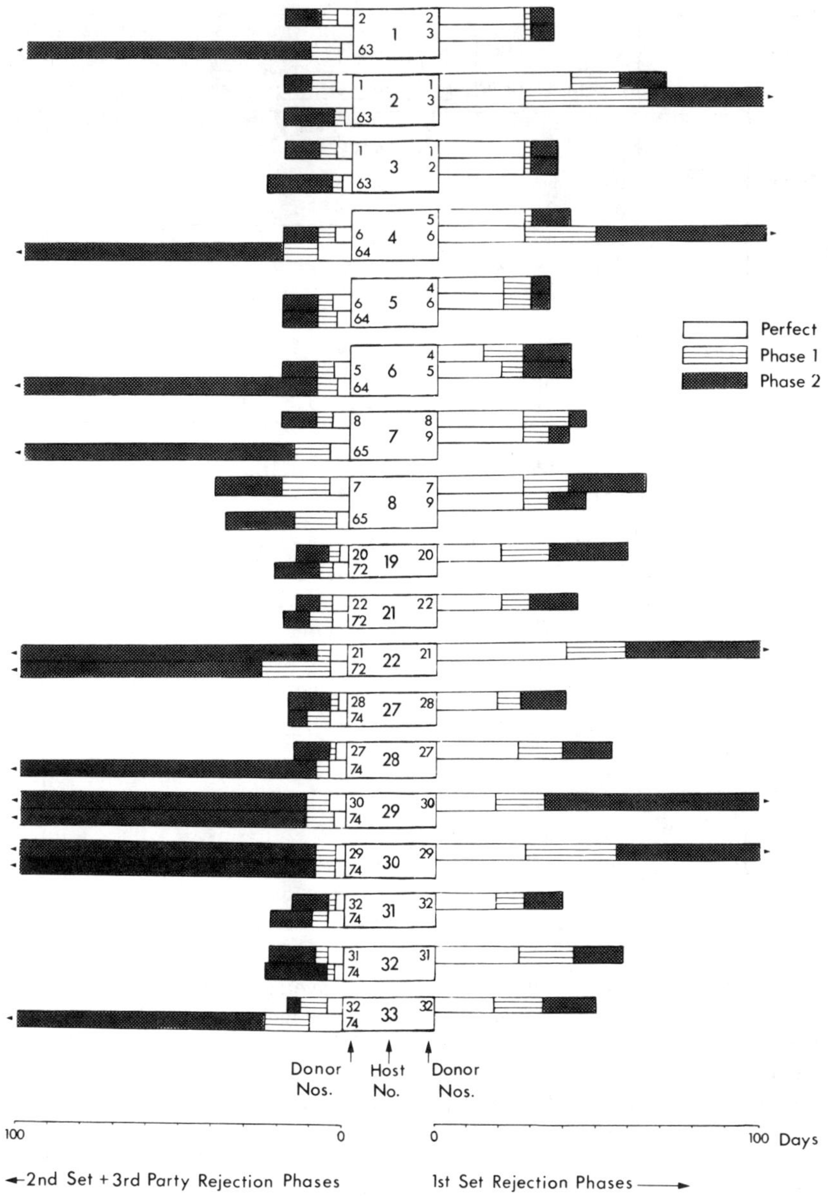

FIGURE 1. Chronology of graft rejection phases in J strain *X laevis*. Eighteen J Strain *Xenopus* hosts were given second-set and third-party J skin allografts 100–120 days following first-set grafting. For other experimental details, see legend to Table 1.

illustrated in Figure 3. MHC-disparate skin applied to LG17 and LG15 controls is rejected acutely, whereas minor graft destruction is generally subacute (30–50 days). Tx impairs (to varying extent depending on donor/host combination) rejection of MHC-incompatible grafts, but abrogates minor-H-incompatible graft rejection. As with the experiments on J strain *Xenopus*, MHC-incompatible larval and adult thymuses restore the ability of Tx animals to reject third-party, MHC-incompatible skin, but achieve tolerance to thymus donor strain skin grafts.

Implantation of an isogeneic larval thymus into Tx LG17 froglets fully restores both MHC- and minor-H-disparate graft rejection, revealing that absence of a thymus for a few weeks of larval life is not, in itself, the cause of the disturbed recognition of minor antigens that often occurs following allogeneic thymus implantation. LG17 and LG15 Tx animals implanted with one- or two-MHC-haplotype–incompatible thymus displayed (in all cases but one) impaired (when compared with controls) rejection of skin from donors bearing only minor H differences that can be recognized as foreign. It appears that impaired rejection of skin on which minor antigens were expected to be "on view" occurs both when the thymus is of completely different MHC to test skin graft donor, and even when the thymus shares one haplotype with the test skin graft (e.g., LG17 [ac] Tx implanted with LG3 [bd] thymus and grafted with LG5 [ad] skin). Furthermore, when the thymus implant was of identical MHC to the test skin graft (e.g., LG3 Tx implanted with LG15 thymus and assayed with LG17 skin) only 1/6 frogs completed rejection prior to 100 days.

MLC reactivity of splenocytes to thymus donor–strain MHC antigens. The MLC response is known to be an in vitro correlate of MHC-disparate graft rejection in *Xenopus* and is thymus-dependent (*29, 30*). We therefore wished to know whether the tolerance to thymus-strain skin allografts induced by allothymus implantation extended to MLC reactivity. (MLC reactivity is poor or nonexistent when cells expressing only minor H antigens are freshly cultured and mixed in vitro [*31*]).

Our initial experiments with LG responder cells are given in

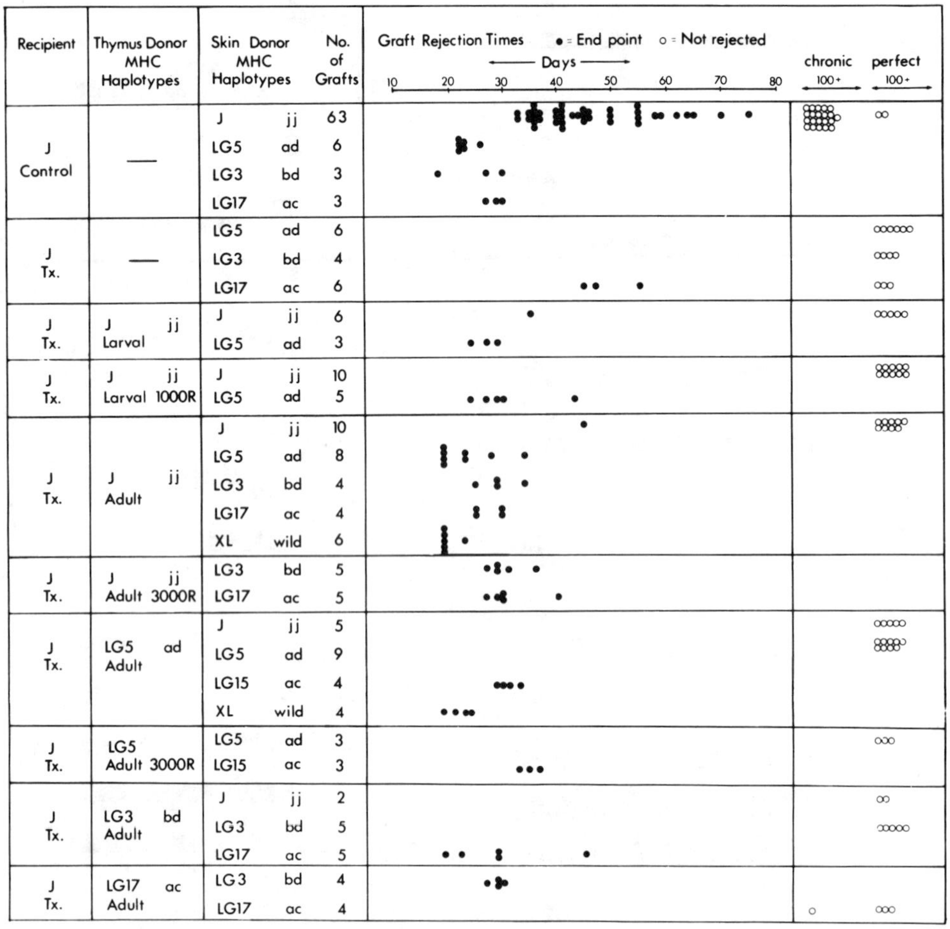

FIGURE 2. Effect of implantation of MHC-disparate or minor-H-antigen-disparate thymus on skin allograft responses of Tx J strain *X laevis*: Thymectomy at 7 days; thymus implants at 4–6 weeks (stage 56–58). Skin grafts were applied at 5–9 months. Each recipient usually received a total of 2 skin grafts that were from donors that were MHC-disparate to one another; exceptions to this included some controls, which were grafted with skin from 2 different J individuals only (Table 1), and some J-thymus-implanted animals that received a total of 3 grafts—2 from different J individuals as well as one MHC-disparate graft. For the thymus-implanted animals, individual J donors supplied maximally 2 skin grafts. J skin donor individuals were always different from J thymus donors.

Table 2. These reveal that all LG17 Tx animals given an MHC-incompatible LG3 larval thymus (normal or irradiated), still contain spleen lymphocytes capable of proliferating against thymus-type, irradiated stimulator cells. In contrast, LG15 Tx implanted with one-MHC-haplotype-disparate (LG5) adult thymus uniformly failed to display MLC reactivitiy against LG5 stimulators, while responding well to third-party cells. The very high SIs recorded with some LG15 splenocytes seem to be due to the particularly low background DPM seen with these cells (Table 2).

Subsequent experiments involved J strain responder cells (Table 3). In these studies we made use of hybrid stimulator cells (e.g., JLG5) to prevent the possibility of back stimulation in the MLC assay. Control J strain lymphocytes failed to respond in MLC to J stimulators, but recognized stimulators from MHC-disparate strains in normal fashion. Tx J strain *Xenopus* generally failed to respond to MHC-disparate cells; the small number of positive cultures appeared not to be the result of defective thymectomies, since these lymphocytes failed to respond to optimal mitogenic doses of the T-dependent mitogen phytohemagglutinin, in contrast to the excellent SIs (>10) recorded from control animals (data not shown). (MLC reactivity of alloimmunized, Tx animals in the absence of concomitant T cell mitogenicity has been recorded by others (*29*), although the nature of the cells involved remains to be elucidated.) Tx J strain *Xenopus* implanted with normal or irradiated adult J thymus generaly displayed significant MLC SIs to both JLG5 (6/7 cases) and JLM3 (5/7) stimulators. In contrast, animals implanted with adult LG5 thymus consistently (7/8 cases) responded well in vitro only to JLM3 stimulators; only 3/9 MLCs versus JLG5 stimulators were positive in this experimental group (2 of the 3 positive cultures contained responding cells from recipients implanted with irradiated thymus glands).

Alloimmune Responses of Control Xenopus *Following Larval Implantation of* MHC- *or Minor-H-Antigen-disparate Skin.*

Skin grafting assays. Table 4 illustrates how the fate of adult skin grafts implanted into stage 56–58 larvae is dependent on the genetic relatedness of donor and host: 100% of the isografts and minor-H-disparate grafts (J-to-J) remained in perfect condition for >100 days. In contrast, 89% of skin grafts bearing one MHC haplotype disparity (e.g., LG5-to-LG15) were tolerated, whereas only 57% (LG3-to-LG15), 40% (LG15-to-LG3), or 38% (LG5-to-J) of fully allogeneic grafts survived. That these larvally applied, surviving allografts induce in vivo tolerance to donor MHC antigens is indicated by the permanent survival of subsequent skin grafts from the same donor strain (Fig. 4). LG15 recipients tolerant of a perimetamorphic skin graft from LG3 or LG5 are still able to reject third-party (J) MHC-disparate grafts in acute fashion and their ability to visualize (LG17) minor antigens displayed in the context of host type MHC appears relatively normal. Thus, 4/6 animals implanted with LG3 skin rejected LG17 skin subacutely and 6/6 LG15 *Xenopus* bearing intact LG5 skin rejected LG17 skin in under 50 days.

The ability of skin-implanted control recipients to visualize minor H antigens displayed in the context of the skin implant

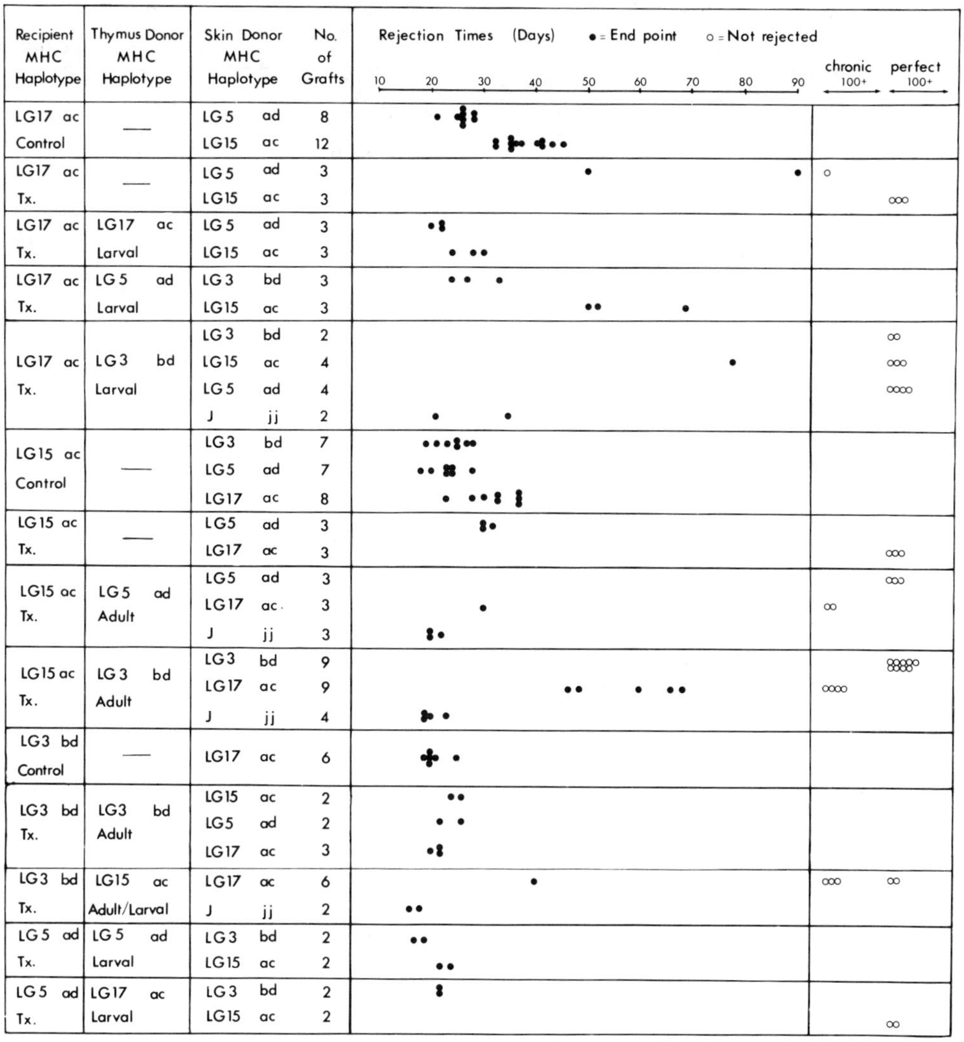

FIGURE 3. Effect of implantation of isogeneic or MHC-disparate thymus on skin allograft responses of Tx LG *Xenopus*. Experimental details mostly as in Figure 2. Here, each recipient usually received a total of 2 skin grafts from donors that were MHC-disparate to one another. A few animals receivd only a single skin allograft.

TABLE 2. MLC reactivity of splenocytes from thymectomized LG *Xenopus* following implantation of larval or adult thymus[a]

Recipients (MHC haplotypes)	Thymus donor (MHC haplotypes)	6000-rad stimulators: J (jj)	LG3 (bd)	LG5 (ad)	JLM3 (jwy)
LG17 control (ac)	—	3.43	1.55, 2.01, 2.07 2.50, 3.0	2.75, 3.54	ND[c]
LG17 Tx (ac)	LG17 larva (ac)	2.08, 2.04	2.44, 1.92, 2.03	2.53	ND
LG17 Tx (ac)	LG3 larva (bd)	2.18, 2.49 2.01, 3.34 3.04,[b] 2.70[b]	2.36, 3.51, 2.03 2.88, 2.82,[b] 2.57[b]	ND	ND
LG15 control (ac)	—	ND	ND	9.92, 11.40 8.49	12.96, 15.86 9.17
LG15 Tx (ac)	—	ND	ND	0.84[d]	1.42[d]
LG15 Tx (ac)	LG5 adult (ad)	ND	ND	0.94,[d] 0.76[d] 0.83,[d] 1.19[d]	17.98, 9.76 3.30, 3.17

[a] Thymectomy at 7 days. Thymus implants at 4–6 weeks. Assays at 6–8 months. Splenocytes from each implanted animal were tested against stimulator cells of thymus donor strain and of third-party origin. MLC results expressed as stimulation index (see the *Materials and Methods* section). Mean (±SE) ^{3}HTdR incorporation in autologous cultures (responder x irrad. autologous stimulators) = 5709±1671 (LG17 controls), 4000±1056 (LG17 Tx←LG17 Th.), 3069±563 (LG17 Tx←LG3 Th.), 381±83 (LG15 controls), 549 (LG15 Tx) and 1110±200 (LG15 Tx←LG5 Th.).

[b] Thymus implant 3000 rads–irradiated prior to implantation.

[c] (ND) not done.

[d] All SIs significant by *t* test ($P < 0.05$) except these.

TABLE 3. MLC reactivity of splenocytes from thymectomized J strain *Xenopus* following implantation of adult thymus[a, b]

Recipients (MHC haplotypes)	Thymus donor (MHC haplotypes)	6000-rad stimulators			
		J (jj)	LG17 (ac)	JxLG5 (jad)	JxLM3 (jwy)
J Control (jj)	—	1.08,[c] 0.91[c] 0.48,[c] 0.95[c] 0.89,[c] 0.35[c] 0.33,[c] 0.32[c]	1.98, 2.36 4.04	3.28, 6.93 2.60, 1.70	3.26, 8.73 1.70
JTx (jj)	—	ND[d]	0.88,[c] 1.91[c] 1.03,[c] 0.91[c] 2.81, 2.0	0.53,[c] 1.50[c] 1.00,[c] 1.00[c] 1.32,[c] 2.60	0.68,[c], 1.19[c] 1.0,[c] 2.1
J Tx (jj)	J adult (jj)	ND	ND	4.15, 4.59 5.40, 2.50 1.87,[e] 2.61[e] 1.85[c,e]	4.80, 6.62 13.6, 5.8[e] 2.52,[e] 1.72[ce] 2.13[c,e]
J Tx (jj)	LG5 adult (ad)	ND	ND	0.94,[c] 2.19[c] 1.30,[c] 0.80[c] 1.88,[c] 0.97[c,e] 2.3, 3.82[e] 3.99[e]	2.36, 2.27 5.0, 2.9 2.82, 8.97[e] 2.11,[e] 1.68

[a] Thymectomy, thymus implants, assays, and splenocyte testing as in Table 2.

[b] Mean (±SE) ^{3}HTdR incorporation in autologous cultures = 1268±262 (J controls); 2333±432 (J Tx); 2209±498 (J Tx←J Th.); 1615±268 (J Tx←LG5 Th.).

[c] All SIs significant by *t* test ($P<0.05$) except these.

[d] (ND) not done.

[e] Thymus implant 3000 rads–irradiated prior to implantation.

TABLE 4. Fate of adult skin grafts applied to larvae at stage 56–8 (i.e., during perimetamorphosis)

Recipients (MHC haplotype)	Skin donor (MHC haplotype)	No. animals	No. tolerant[a]	% tolerant
LG15 (ac)	LG3 (bd)	14	8	57%
LG15 (ac)	LG5 (ad)	9	8	89%
LG15 (ac)	LG15 (ac)	5	5	100%
LG3 (bd)	LG15 (ac)	10	4	40%
LG3 (bd)	LG3 (bd)	5	5	100%
LG5 (ad)	LG15 (ac)	9	8	89%
J (jj)	J (jjj) 3N	5	5	100%
J (jj)	LG5 (ad)	8	3	38%

[a] Tolerance = grafts in perfect condition >100 days.

donor MHC (rather than host MHC type) is also illustrated in Figure 4. Here, one of two LG3*Xenopus* and 6/6 LG5 recipients given LG15 skin as perimetamorphic larvae failed to reject LG17 grafts within 100 days. In contrast, when J controls were given jjj skin grafts at stage 56–58 and then asked to reject a subsequent graft from a new jj donor, rejection of these new minor-disparate grafts was effected in 9/10 cases within 100 days (7 in subacute manner, 2 in chronic fashion).

MLC studies. One MLC experiment with splenocytes from 9-month-old LG15 controls bearing permanently surviving grafts donated by LG15 or LG5 adults in late larval life was set up. One-way MLC SIs of splenocytes from two animals (bearing LG15 skin implants) to 5000-rad-irradiated LG5 stimulators were 4.0 and 2.0. Three LG15 animals carrying perfect LG5 skin also responded to LG5 stimulators with SIs of 3.4, 3.9, and 5.4. The MLC SIs of these latter animals to LG3 stimulators were 3.1, 5.2, and 4.3. All experimental DPM were significantly different from autologous cultures. Tolerance in vivo, but not in vitro to MHC antigens of the donor of the larvally-applied skin implant is suggested.

DISCUSSION

Our experiments on a variety of donor/host strain combinations reveal that an allothymus implanted a few weeks after early thymectomy will fully restore the ability of *Xenopus* to reject third-party, MHC-disparate skin grafts. The main aim of the present study, however, was not simply to confirm previous findings from this and other laboratories (*6, 13, 32, 33*), but to probe the ability of Tx/thymus implanted animals to display immune reactivity to minor H-disparate skin grafts and to begin to characterize the allotolerance that is acquired (*6, 32*) to thymus-donor-strain antigens.

Our planned restoration experiments with J strain *Xenopus* necessitated determination of the extent of histoincompatibility among individuals of our J colony. The in vivo (skin grafting) and in vitro (MLC reactivity) experiments extend the observations of others (*16*) that these animals are MHC-compatible but carry minor H antigenic differences, although the extent of polymorphism within the strain appears to be limited, as revealed by second-set and third-party grafting data. When J strain Tx individuals were implanted with MHC-disparate thymus, it was not surprising to find that J skin grafts failed

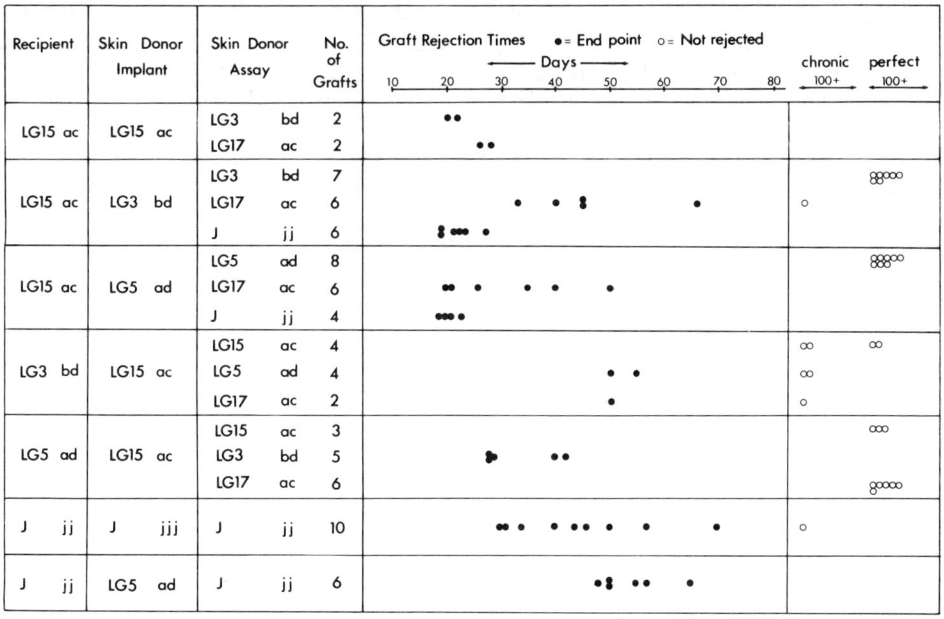

FIGURE 4. Effect of implantation of MHC-disparate or minor-H-antigen–disparate skin on subsequent allograft responses of control LG and J strain *Xenopus*. The initial skin implant was applied at 4–6 weeks (stage 56–58), and then the subsequent skin grafts were applied at 5–9 months. Implanted LG hosts were given 2 or 3 assay skin grafts from disparate donor strains. J recipients received 2 J assay grafts from separate J donors only. Only recipients bearing tolerated, larvally applied, skin implants are listed in this figure.

to be rejected—if one postulates that the T lymphocytes (developing from J stem cells) effecting rejection are attempting to visualize minor antigens following education in an MHC-disparate thymic environment. On the other hand, even when the thymus was of identical MHC to the TX recipient (i.e., J thymus–to–Tx J), subsequent J skin grafts were also (in 24/26 cases) tolerated. The limited minor H antigen polymorphism suspected within the J group could, it seemed, account for a proportion (but certainly not all) of the tolerant situations with thymus-restored Tx animals, since many of the skin graft donors would not present any new minor antigens to those already expressed in the host and thymus donor. It is possible that the only two J skin grafts to be rejected were on Tx animals that had received thymuses from donors that happened to be identical to the recipients in terms of minor H antigens (n.b. only 2/63 skin grafts exchanged between J strain controls remained perfect at >100 days). To gain a better understanding of this poor restoration of minor H antigen rejection, we decided to turn our attention to using clonal *Xenopus* as recipients and donors, since H differences between these hybrid animals are better defined (*19*). Frogs within an LG family have identical (major and minor) H antigens and, among the LG families available to us, some share the same MHC but differ routinely from each other by minor H antigens (e.g., LG17 and LG15 families).

The outcome of the allothymus restoration experiments with LG Tx recipients essentially backed up the findings with the J strain recipients, since they also revealed impaired rejection of skin expressing only minor antigenic differences. When the experimental combination was LG17 Tx (ac) implanted with LG3 (bd) thymus and then tested with LG15 (ac) skin, it seemed possible that the deficiency in rejecting the latter could be related to the recipients bearing the "wrong" MHC type of thymus—i.e., the T cells in these Tx LG17 animals learn to recognize minor antigens in the context of the MHC antigens expressed on cells within the implanted LG3 thymus, and therefore are inefficient at dealing with LG15 minor antigens expressed on ac cells. However, such a straightforward interpretation is not possible in view of the experiments on Tx LG3 recipients given an LG15 thymus (Fig. 3). Even with the 'right' thymus MHC type, these animals still dealt with LG17 skin (minor antigen-disparate to LG15) extremely poorly. Only when thymuses isogeneic to the host were implanted, was the Tx animal restored in its ability to visualize minor antigens.

One possible problem with our thymectomy/thymus implant model, in assessing the role of the thymus in educating minor H antigen-reactive cells, is that the age when the thymus is transferred marks the beginning of a temporary, perimetamorphic period when it is readily possible to achieve allotolerance to (skin) grafts (*2, 4, 15, 16, 25, 34*). This tolerance, which may be necessary to allow the animal to differentiate and not reject new adult-specific antigens (*35*), is thought not to be entirely specific in terms of minor H antigens. Thus DuPasquier (*2*) has noted that LG17 made tolerant at perimetamorphosis to LG15 skin, although able to reject subsequent MHC-disparate (LG3) skin grafts, were unable to reject LG7 skin of only minor H disparity to both LG17 and LG15. Whether this poor specificity in perimetamorphic tolerance is an indication of crossreaction between various minor antigens or represents a nonspecific blockade of effector mechanisms remains unclear. Although it is unknown how many minor H loci *Xenopus* minimally possess, both our own experiments with J strain *Xenopus* and other skin grafting studies (*36*) on gynogenetic *X laevis* reveal considerable sharing of minor H antigens and suggest limited polymorphism with respect to minor H loci at this level of evolution. Apparent nonspecific perimetamorphic tolerance could be influencing our skin graft experiments on allothymus-implanted animals. For example, LG3 Tx animals given an LG15 thymus may be unresponsive to LG17 skin because of this phenomenon. We have addressed this issue here by examining the alloimmune responses of control *Xenopus* (i.e., having their own thymus type) made tolerant to alloantigens by perimetamorphic implantation of skin. The outcome of the experiments with LG recipients indicates that perimetamorphic application of MHC-disparate skin can induce subsequent poor reactivity to skin of strains expected to display minor H antigens additional to those found in implant donor and host. Such impaired alloreactivity appears to occur routinely (see Fig. 4) when skin implant donor and assay skin donor are of the same MHC type (e.g., LG5 [ad] hosts implanted with LG15 [ac] skin and assayed with LG17 [ac] skin), but is seldom seen when assay and skin implant donors are MHC-disparate (e.g., LG15 hosts implanted with LG5 skin generally respond well to LG17 skin grafts). Poor alloreactivity to LG17 skin by LG5 recipients that had been implanted in late larval life with a skin graft from LG15 could be related to the fact that these LG5 hosts have a population of T cells preferentially restricted to recognize minor antigens in the context of their own (ad) thymus MHC type, rather than the skin donor assay type (ac). (This is the explanation given by Flajnik et al. [*3*] to explain the failure of LG3 *Xenopus*, which had been made tolerant to ac antigens by embryonic implantation of an LG15 eye, to reject LG6 [ac, but with minor H differences to LG15] skin.) In contrast, LG15 hosts implanted with LG5 skin are able to respond to LG17 skin, since they have the correct MHC (ac) thymus type.

The ability of J controls made tolerant to J skin by perimetamorphic grafting to reject skin from third-party J donors reveals that a specific allotolerance to the original donor can also ensue in *Xenopus* if recipient and skin implant donor are only minor-H-antigen–disparate. Therefore the reason for the impaired rejection of J skin by J Tx animals given a J thymus is unlikely to be due to minor H antigen sharing, unless the thymus differs from skin implant in its ability to present minor antigens and secure tolerance. The differences in outcome between skin and thymus implantation are not related to the fact that the skin implant donors were 3N (Fig. 4), whereas the thymus donors were 2N (Fig. 2), since 5/6 J Tx recipients given a 3N J thymus have recently been shown to carry intact third-party J grafts 100 days posttransplantation. For the moment, we must conclude that defective rejection of minor-H-disparate skin by Tx animals may, at least in some cases, relate primarily to defective restoration due to the use of allogeneic (even minor-H-disparate) thymus implants, rather than being merely effected by allothymus-induced tolerance. Minor-H-disparate thymuses implanted in late larval life may have a compromised ability to receive and/or educate sufficient numbers of host stem cells, because such histoincompatibility is reflected on cell membranes and affects cell-cell interactions. Interestingly, the migratory activity of triploid lymphoid cells through diploid tissue (e.g., thymus) seems to be impaired when compared with the activity of diploid cells (*6, 37*). Compromised interactions between stem cells and thymic stromal cells might result in failure of T lymphocytes involved in minor graft rejection to become established in sufficient number. In *Xenopus* the nature of minor-H-reactive cells is still uncertain; cytotoxic cells may (*38*) or may not (*31*) be involved.

The timing of thymus implantation in our experiments was chosen to allow sufficient time for the recipient to recover from the thymectomy operation, but not to allow too long for the animal to develop (abnormally?) in the absence of a thymic environment. Furthermore, we required the animal to be of sufficient size to receive "adult" thymus implants (expressing the full range of MHC antigens) and for the organ to be implanted before the period when a rapid growth of in situ thymus takes place at the end of metamorphosis (*39*). In retrospect, our findings of (A) defective minor-H-disparate graft destruction, even when the allothymus implant and the skin donor are both of the same MHC type as the Tx host, and (B) "nonspecific" (at the level of minor H antigens) perimetamorphic tolerance induction in some experiments, render our model system unsuitable for studying the possible role of the thymus in the restriction of minor-H-reactive T cells. The embryonic chimera model of Flajnik et al. (*3*) may be more appropriate for this sort of study, although this model system also presents some difficulties, such as the likelihood that host-derived restricting elements will migrate into the thymic epithelium (as they appear to do in mammals [*9*]) along with lymphoid stem cells— and, therefore, mask the educating role of the organ.

The suitability of amphibian embryos and larvae to study self- and allotolerance have been stressed by others before (*4*). In this paper we have shown that implantation of MHC-disparate larval or adult thymus to Tx *Xenopus* routinely induces a state of unresponsiveness to subsequent allografts of skin from the thymus strain donor. That the in vivo, thymus-induced tolerance extends to thymus donor strain tissues other than skin is suggested by our preliminary observations (unpublished data) on liver implants. These remain healthy when implanted s.c. *only* if isogeneic to the Tx host or isogeneic to the thymus donor.

Splenocytes taken from Tx animals rendered in vivo tolerant to thymus implant strain skin grafts display variable in vitro reactivity to thymus donor strain lymphocytes when tested in one-way MLC. Others have previously reported split tolerance (in vivo, but not in vitro) following allothymus implantation in Tx *Xenopus* in adult life (*6*) and in embryonic (histoincompatible) anterior/posterior chimeras (*3, 8*). Lymphoid cells from mice or rats bearing tolerated skin grafts after neonatal tolerance induction, also display MLC tolerance to donor cells in some cases, but not in others (*40*). In contrast to the split tolerance seen in some Tx/restored *Xenopus*, lymphocytes from nude mice implanted with allogeneic thymus, routinely display MLC tolerance to thymus donor strain cells, whereas in vivo reactivity to thymus strain skin grafts can occur (*41*).

Dimarzo and Cohen (*16*) have shown that following perimetamorphic skin allografting and the acquisition of in vivo nonreactivity to subsequent grafts from the same donor, the extent of in vitro MLR tolerance of splenocytes to cells of the skin donor is variable. We stress here that this is also true following thymus implantation to Tx animals. Moreover, our experiments suggest that the nature of the thymus implanted is a critical factor in the immunological outcome. Thus splenocytes from the majority of Tx *Xenopus* given adult thymus implants failed to respond in MLC against thymus strain stimulators, whereas those implanted with a larval thymus could proliferate to thymus-type MHC antigens. Whether the immunologic outcome relates to lymphocyte numbers within the thymus implant or is associated with qualitative changes (MHC antigen expression?) on thymic cells during ontogeny remains an open question. Interestingly, 2/3 J animals given irradiated LG5 adult thymus implants (i.e., reduced numbers of donor thymocytes) were able to display MLC reactivity to JLG5 stimulators. The phenomenon of in vivo tolerance but variable in vitro reactivity to thymus donor warrants further investigation. In particular, whether split tolerance represents tolerance to MHC determinants (possibly class 1 MHC antigens) centrally involved in skin allograft rejection, but not to molecules (class II antigens) known to effect MLC reactivity in *Xenopus* (Kaufman JF et al., unpublished data; quoted in

[3]) awaits clarification. The role of thymus-dependent suppressor cells (35, 42, 43) in maintaining the in vivo and in vitro states of nonreactivity are currently being investigated in our laboratory by adoptive-transfer experiments. The nature of the thymic cells effecting tolerance induction of immigrating T-lineage lymphocytes to allogeneic MHC antigens (which has recently come under scrutiny in mammals [44]) can now also begin to be examined within amphibian model systems, with the advent of reagents specific for class I and II MHC antigens (24) and the development of better cell makers (e.g., the *Xenopus borealis* fluorescent cell marker [45]) to trace the origins of cells within chimeric thymuses. We hope that *Xenopus* will continue to provide us with a developmental model that can give unique insight into the role that the thymus plays in the initial development of T lymphocyte reactivity.

Acknowledgments. We thank Miss P. Aitchison for technical assistance and to Mrs. T.L. Horton for typing the manuscript.

REFERENCES

1. Deuchar EM. The South African clawed frog. London: Wiley, 1975.
2. DuPasquier L. Ontogeny of immunological functions in amphibians. In: Cohen N, Sigel MM, eds. The reticulo-endothelial system: phylogeny and ontogeny. New York: Plenum, 1982: 633.
3. Flajnik MF, DuPasquier L, Cohen N. Immune responses of thymus/lymphocyte embryonic chimeras: studies on tolerance and major histocompatibility complex restriction in Xenopus. Eur J Immunol 1985; 15: 540.
4. Cohen N, DiMarzo S, Rollins-Smith L, Barlow E, Vanderschmidt-Parsons S. The ontogeny of allo-tolerance and self-tolerance in larval Xenopus laevis. In: Balls M, Bownes ME, eds. Metamorphosis. Oxford: (in press).
5. DuPasquier L, Horton JD. Restoration of antibody responsiveness in early thymectomized Xenopus by implantation of major histocompatibility complex-mismatched larval thymus. Eur. J Immunol 1982; 12: 546.
6. Nagata S, Cohen N. Induction of T cell differentiation in early-thymectomized Xenopus by grafting adult thymuses from either MHC-matched or from partially or totally MHC-mismatched donors. Thymus 1984; 6: 89.
7. Gearing AJH, Cribbin FA, Horton JD. Restoration of the antibody response to sheep erythrocytes in thymectomized Xenopus implanted with MHC-compatible or MHC-incompatible thymus. J Embryol Exp Morphol 1984; 84:287.
8. Flajnik MF, DuPasquier L, Cohen N. The ontogeny and phylogeny of MHC restriction and thymic education: studies with the frog, Xenopus. In: Cooper EL, Wright RK, eds. Proceedings 2nd ISDCI Congress. Dev Comp Immunol 1984; (suppl 3) 35.
9. Longo DL, Schwartz RH. T Cell specificity for H-2 and Ir gene phenotype correlates with the phenotype of thymic antigen presenting cells. Nature 1980; 287: 44.
10. Kindred B. A comparison of H-2 restriction of helper function using T cells from radiation chimeras and nude mice bearing thymus grafts. Cell Immunol 1981; 63: 228.
11. Zinkernagel RM. Selection of restriction specificities of virus-specific cytotoxic T cells in the thymus: no evidence for a crucial role of antigen-presenting cells. J Exp Med 1982; 156: 1842.
12. Kruisbeek AM, Sharrow SO, Singer A. Differences in the MHC-restricted self-recognition repertoire of intra-thymic and extra-thymic cytotoxic T lymphocyte precursors. J Immunol 1983; 130: 1027.
13. Horton JD, Arnall JC, Cribbin FA, Lallone RL, Gearing AJH. Reconstitution of T cell-dependent responses in thymectomized Xenopus: in vivo and in vitro studies on T cell education. In: Balls M, Clothier RH, eds. Second International Congress on Pathology of Amphibians and Reptiles. J Herpetopathology 1986; in press.
14. Bevan MJ. The major histocompatibility complex determines susceptibility to cytotoxic T cells directed against minor histocompatibility antigens. J Exp Med 1975; 142: 1349.
15. Barlow EH, DiMarzo SJ, Cohen N. Prolonged survival of major histocompatibility complex-disparate skin allografts transplanted to the metamorphosing frog, Xenopus laevis. Transplantation 1981; 32: 51.
16. DiMarzo SJ, Cohen N. Immunogenetic aspects of in vivo allotolerance induction during the ontogeny of Xenopus laevis. Immunogenetics 1982; 16: 103.
17. Katagiri C. Xenopus laevis as a model for the study of immunology. Dev Comp Immunol 1978; 2: 5.
18. Tochinai S, Katagiri C. Complete abrogation of immune response to skin allografts and rabbit erythrocytes in the early thymectomized Xenopus. Dev Growth Differentiation 1975; 17: 383.
19. Kobel HR, DuPasquier L. Production of large clones of histocompatible fully identical clawed toads (Xenopus). Immunogenetics 1975; 2: 87.
20. Horton JD, Manning MJ. Response to skin allografts in Xenopus laevis following thymectomy at early stages of lymphoid organ maturation. Transplantation 1972; 14: 141.
21. von Boehmer H. Separation of B and T lymphocytes and their role in the mixed lymphocyte reaction. J Immunol 1974; 112: 70.
22. Olert J. Interphase studies with a simplified method of silver staining of nucleoli. Experientia 1979; 35: 283.
23. Nieuwkoop PD, Faber J. Normal table of Xenopus laevis (Daudin). Amsterdam: North Holland, 1956.
24. Flajnik MFI, Kaufman J, DuPasquier L. Studies on the ontogeny of MHC expression in Xenopus. In: Basel Institute for Immunology Annual Report, 1983: 67.
25. Chardonnens X, DuPasquier L. Induction of skin allograft tolerance during metamorphosis of the toad Xenopus laevis: a possible model for studying generation of self tolerance to histocompatibility antigens. Eur J Immunol 1973; 3: 569.
26. Rimmer JJ, Horton JD. Allograft rejection in larval and adult Xenopus following early thymectomy. Transplantation 1977; 23: 142.
27. Horton JD. Ontogeny of the immune response to skin allografts in relation to lymphoid organ development in the amphibian, Xenopus laevis Daudin. J Exp Zool 1969; 170: 449.
28. Lallone RL. Histocompatibility recognition in effector and helper T cell responses of Xenopus [PhD Thesis]. UK: University of Durham, 1984.
29. Nagata S, Cohen N. Specific in vivo and nonspecific in vitro alloreactivities of adult frogs (Xenopus laevis) that were thymectomized during early life. Eur J Immunol 1983; 13: 541.
30. DuPasquier L, Horton JD. The effect of thymectomy on the mixed leukocyte reaction and phytohaemagglutinin responsiveness in the clawed toad, Xenopus laevis. Immunogenetics 1976; 3: 105.
31. Lallone RL, Horton JD. In vitro correlates of in vivo skin graft rejection in Xenopus. Transplantation 1985; 39: 223.
32. Horton JD, Horton TL. Development of transplantation immunity and restoration experiments in the thymectomized amphibian. Am Zool 1975; 15: 73.
33. Tochinai S, Nagata S, Katagiri C. Restoration of immune responsiveness in early thymectomized Xenopus by implantation of histocompatible adult thymus. Eur J Immunol 1976; 6: 711.
34. Bernardini N, Chardonnens X, Simon D. Tolérance des allogreffes cutanées chez Xenopus laevis: influence de la taille et de l'âge du greffon. C R Acad Sci 1970; 270: 2351.
35. DuPasquier L, Bernard CCA. Active suppression of the allogeneic histocompatibility reactions during the metamorphosis of the clawed toad Xenopus. Differentiation 1980; 16: 1.
36. Obara N, Kawahara H, Katagiri C. Response to skin grafts exchanged among siblings of larval and adult gynogenetic diploids

in Xenopus laevis. Transplantation 1983; 36: 91.
37. Turpen JB, Volpe EP, Cohen N. Stem cell influx following the heterotopic transplantation of the thymic primordia between frog embryos. Dev Comp Immunol 1977; 1: 255.
38. Watkins D. T cell function in Xenopus [PhD Thesis]. NY: University of Rochester, 1985.
39. DuPasquier L, Weiss N. The thymus during the ontogeny of the toad Xenopus laevis: growth, membrane-bound immunoglobulins and mixed lymphocyte reaction. Eur J Immunol 1973; 3: 773.
40. Hǎsek M, Chutná J. Complexity of the state of immunological tolerance. Immunol Rev 1979; 46: 3.
41. Kindred B. Lymphocytes which differentiate in an allogeneic thymus. I. Response to MLC determinants and skin grafts from the thymus donor strain. Cell Immunol 1976; 25: 189.
42. Barlow EH, Cohen N. The thymus dependency of transplantation allotolerance in the metamorphosing frog Xenopus laevis. Transplantation 1983; 35: 612.
43. Ruben LN, Buenafe A, Oliver S, Malley A, Barr K, Lukas D. Suppression in Xenopus laevis: thymus inducer, spleen effector cells. Immunology 1985; 54: 65.
44. Jordan RK, Robinson JH, Hopkinson NA, House KC, Bentley AL. Thymic epithelium and the induction of transplantation tolerance in nude mice. Nature 1985; 314: 454.
45. Thiébaud CH. A reliable new cell marker in Xenopus. Dev Biol 1983; 98: 245.

Received 1 August 1985.
Accepted 26 September 1985.

0041-1337/86/4106-0776$02.00/0
TRANSPLANTATION
Vol. 41, No. 6
Printed in U.S.A.

EXPRESSION OF CLASS I AND CLASS II MAJOR HISTOCOMPATABILITY ANTIGENS IN NORMAL AND TRANSPLANTED HUMAN HEART[1]

MARLENE L. ROSE, MARION I. COLES, ROBERT J. GRIFFIN, ARIELA POMERANCE, AND MAGDI H. YACOUB[2]

Cardiothoracic Unit, Harefield Hospital, Harefield, Middlesex UB9 6JH United Kingdom

The expression of monomorphic determinants of class I and class II histocompatability antigens in human heart before and after cardiac transplantation was examined using monoclonal antibodies and an immunoperoxidase technique. Thirty-five biopsy specimens were examined. Seven were from nontransplanted hearts and 28 were from patients who had received orthotopic cardiac transplantation 5–270 days previously. In normal hearts no class I was found on the surface of the myocardium, but intercalated discs were occasionally stained and interstitial structures (blood vessels and discrete mononuclear cells) strongly expressed the antigen. In contrast, of the 28 specimens from transplanted patients, 24 expressed class I antigen strongly on the outer surface and intercalated discs of the myocardium as well as on the interstitial structures. Class II antigen was not found on the myocardium of normal heart. It was present on small capillaries, the endothelia of some large capillaries, and discrete mononuclear cells. In 20 of 25 samples from transplant patients there was increased expression of class II antigen on interstitial structures but not on myocardium.

The increased expression of class I antigen on the myocardium following transplantation may make it a potential target for cytotoxic T cells. The relevance of increased expression of class I and class II antigens in response to transplantation is discussed.

Class I (HLA-ABC) and class II (HLA-DP, DQ, and DR) antigens are highly polymorphic glycoproteins encoded by the genes of the major histocompatibility complex found on chromosome 6 in man (*1*). Class I antigens are necessary for recognition of antigens by cytotoxic T cells (*2*), and class II antigens are necessary for antigen presentation to helper T cells (*3*). Class II antigens have a restricted tissue distribution—as well as being present on certain lymphoid cells (B cells, activated T cells, macrophages, and dendritic cells), they are also found on some human endothelia and epithelia (*4*, *5*). In addition there has been a detailed study of the distribution of class II antigens in human kidney (*6*). The distribution of class I antigens in all tissues and organs has not been as extensively documented. Until recently, it was thought that all nucleated cells expressed class I antigens (*7*). Such studies were based on the use of cell suspensions and hetero- or alloantisera as cytotoxic reagents. However, studies using frozen tissue sections, monoclonal antibodies (mabs),* and fluorosceinated (*8*) or enzyme-linked secondary antibodies (*9*) have demonstrated that class I distribution is not ubiquitous as was previously thought. We have investigated the distribution of the nonpolymorphic determinants of class I and class II antigens

[1] This work was supported in part by a grant from the British Heart Foundation.

[2] Address correspondence to: Mr. M. H. Yacoub, Cardiothoracic Unit, Harefield Hospital, Harefield, Middlesex, U.K.

* Abbreviations used: mabs, monoclonal antibodies; PBS, phosphate-buffered saline.

on normal, nontransplanted heart and have examined the effect of allotransplantation on expression of these determinants.

MATERIALS AND METHODS

Thirty-five specimens of myocardium have been examined. Seven of these were from nontransplanted "normal" hearts taken from the left atrium of the donor heart at the time of a cardiac transplant operation. The age of the donors varied from 12 to 29 years (mean 16.9, SD±5.9). Twenty eight specimens were cardiac biopsies from 12 patients who had received orthotopic cardiac transplantation from 5 days to 7 months previously (age range 33–56 years, mean 46.5, SD±7.2) Eight patients were receiving cyclosporine, azathioprine, and low-dose steroid immunosuppression, 4 were receiving cyclosporine and azathioprine only.

Transvenous endomyocardial biopsy is performed routinely on all cardiac transplant patients. At each session 4 pieces of right ventricular myocardium are removed, 3 pieces are fixed in formal saline and processed for paraffin wax embedding and conventional histological assessment of rejection, and 1 piece is snap-frozen for use with monoclonal antibodies (see below). The time between removal of the biopsy and snap-freezing is 1–2 min. Each biopsy specimen is 4–9 mm^2

Staining with Monoclonal Antibodies

Preparation of tissue specimens. Cardiac biopsies, covered in embedding medium (OCT compound, Tissue-Tek II) on cork slices were snap-frozen in precooled isopentane that was suspended over liquid nitrogen. The frozen tissue was stored in liquid nitrogen until use. Frozen sections (6-μm thick) were prepared, air-dried for 1 hr, and fixed in acetone at room temperature for 10 min. They were then covered in aluminium foil and stored (for not more than 7 days) at −40°C until use.

Immunoperoxidase technique. W6/32, a mouse mab (class IgG2a) with specificity against a human nonpolymorphic determinant common to all class I antigens (*10*), was used as a neat tissue culture supernatant and was kindly donated by Dr. C. Navarette and Professor H. Festenstein (The London Hospital, London, UK). NFK-1, a mouse mab with specificity against determinants common to class II antigens DP, DQ and DR (*6*), was kindly supplied by Dr. S. Fuggle (Radcliffe Infirmary, Oxford, UK). It was diluted 1:100 in phosphate-buffered saline (PBS). Frozen sections were warmed to room temperature, rehydrated in PBS and overlaid with W6/32 or NFK-1 for 30 min in a humid box at room temperature. This step was followed by washing in PBS, and 45 min incubation with affinity-purified biotinylated goat antimouse IgG and IgM (TAGO Products, from Tissue Culture Services). This second antibody was followed by 60 min incubation in avidin–biotin–horeseradish-peroxidase complexes (Vectastain, from Sera-Lab). Control slides were treated in the same way as the experimental slides, but the primary mab was omitted. No nonspecific staining was detected on cardiac biopsies by this procedure. The sites of peroxidase fixation were identified using diaminobenzidene tetrahydrochloride (0.3 mg/ml in PBS) and hydrogen peroxide (0.01%). The slides were counterstained in Harris's hematoxylin.

Histological grading of biopsies. For this study paraffin embedded sections of biopsies were graded on a scale of 1–4 according to the degree of cellular infiltration which occurs after transplantation (Table 1). Patients whose biopsies show changes corresponding to grades 3 and 4 were treated for acute rejection.

RESULTS

Class I antigens. In normal hearts, the outer surface of the myocardium did not bind W6/32; the intercalated discs were occasionally lightly stained, but all interstitial structures showed heavy staining (Fig. 1). The interstitial structures could be identified as small blood vessels and discrete mononuclear cells. In contrast, of the 28 biopsies from transplanted hearts, 24 contained areas of myocardium that strongly expressed class I antigens on the outer surface and intercalated discs (Fig. 2). In these biopsies the interstitial structures bound W6/32 as in the nontransplanted hearts. The correlation between histological grading of biopsies and the occurrence of class I positive myocardium is shown in Table 2. Of the biopsies showing no histological signs of rejection, 6 of 9 biopsies with no cellular infiltrate and 4 of 5 biopsies graded as 2 contained class-I-positive myocardium. However, all of the 14 biopsies showing minimal (grade 3) or mild (grade 4) rejection contained myocardium that stained heavily with W6/32 mab.

TABLE 1. Criteria for the four grades of cellular changes used in this study

Grade	Microscopic features
1	No cellular infiltration
2	Endocardial or interstitial cellular infiltration—not pyroninophilic
3	A few interstitial pyroninophilic cells, present in only a few adjacent fields
4	Scattered foci of interstitial, perivascular, or endocardial pyroninophilic mononuclear cells in many fields. Interstitial edema

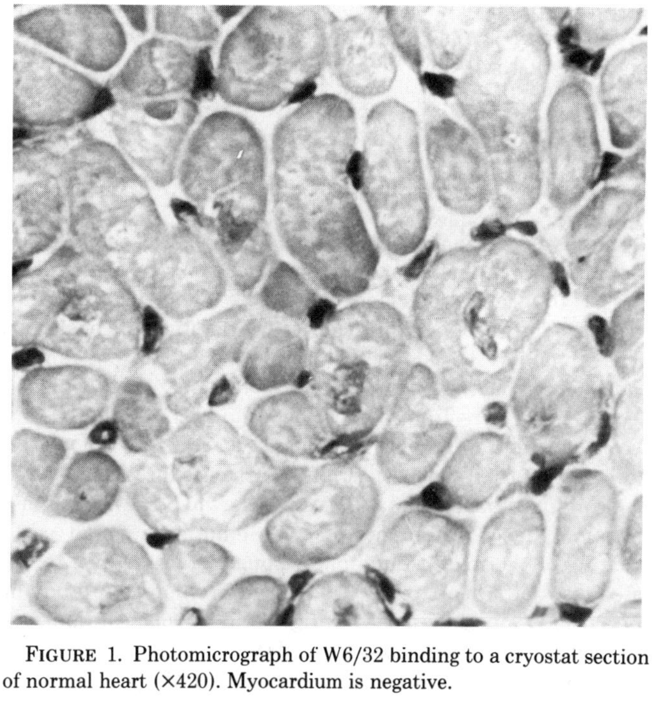

FIGURE 1. Photomicrograph of W6/32 binding to a cryostat section of normal heart (×420). Myocardium is negative.

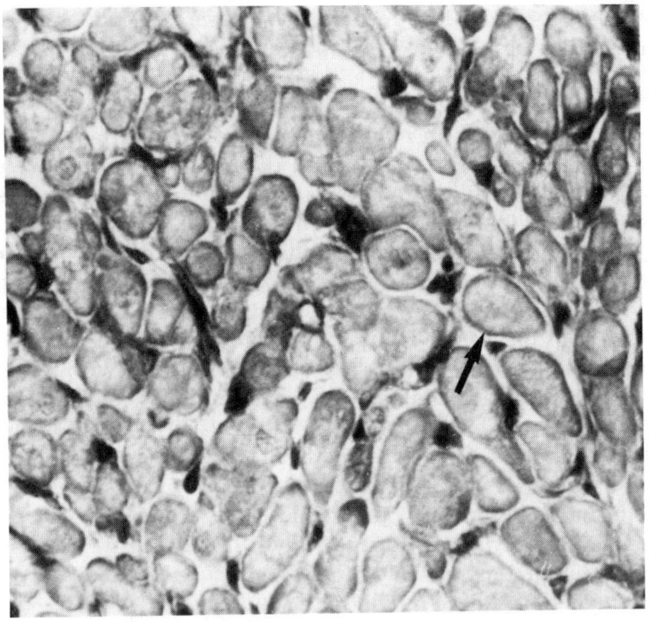

FIGURE 2. Photomicrograph of W6/32 binding to a cryostat section of a cardiac biopsy from a transplant patient (×420). Biopsy shows histological signs of mild rejection (grade 4). Arrow indicates an example of myocardium binding W6/32.

TABLE 2. Expression of class I and class II antigens and histological assessment of cardiac biopsies

Patient no.[a]	Biopsy no.	Days after transplantation	Histology grade	Class I[b]	Class II[c]
1	1	10	2	+++	ND
	2	21	3	++	+
	3	36	4	++	+
	4	45	1	+++	+
	5	74	1	+++	+
2	6	33	1	+++	+
	7	40	1	+++	+
	8	52	4	+	+
3	9	5	Severe rejection[d]	+++	+
4	10	20	4	++	+
5	11	26	3	++	+
	12	53	1	++	+
6	13	33	3	+	+
7	14	14	3	+	+
	15	20	4	+	+
	16	31	4	++	+
8	17	210	1	−	−
	18	270	1	−	−
9	19	31	2	+−	−
	20	45	2	−	+
	21	54	1	−	−
10	22	8	3	+	ND
	23	98	2	+−	+
	24	101	1	+−	−
11	25	21	4	+++	+
	26	200	4	+++	ND
12	27	12	2	++	+
	28	22	4	+++	+

[a] Patients 1, 2, 5, and 12 receiving cyclosporine and azathioprine immunosuppression.

[b] Expressed semiquantiatively: (+++) all myocardium of biopsy positive; (++) approximately ⅔ of myocardium positive; (+) approximately ⅓ of myocardium positive; (+−) 1 or 2 fibers only positive; (−) no positive myocardium.

[c] (+) increased expression compared with normal (includes interstitial leucocytes); (−) no increased expression. ND not determined.

[d] Postmortem specimen taken 5 days after rejection of second heart.

Class II antigens. NFK-1 bound to many interstitial structures in normal heart (Fig. 3), but not to myocardium. Some of the interstitial structures were identified as small capillaries and others as discrete nucleated cells (possibly dendritic cells). The endothelium of larger capillaries showed a heterogeneity within biopsies—some bound NFK-1 while others did not. Of the 25 biopsies from transplanted heart, 20 had an increase in the intensity and quantity of staining by NFK-1 (Table 2, Fig. 4). Much of this increase was due to interstitial infiltrating mononuclear cells that were strongly NFK-1-positive. Capillary endothelial cells remained class-II-positive, and some appeared to be staining more intensely with NFK-1 than in normal hearts. As in normal heart, not all large capillaries were NFK-1-positive and the myocardium remained negative for class II antigens. Of the 12 biopsies not showing histological signs of rejection, 8 had increased staining of interstitial structures. All 13 biopsies showing histological signs of rejection had increased expression of class II antigens on interstitial structures.

DISCUSSION

This study has demonstrated that the surface of the myocardium of normal nontransplanted hearts appears not to express class I antigens as detected by W6/32. The possibility that there is a low level of expression below the limit of sensitivity of the immunodetection method cannot be excluded. The nontransplanted hearts used in this study were not strictly normal, because they were from donors who had been ventilated and received various drugs over a number of days. There is however, no evidence that such drugs alter antigen expression by the myocardium. Daar et al. (*9*) using the mab PA2.6 against monomorphic determinants of class I antigens found weak staining of the myocardium and stronger staining of intercalated discs of a heart from a single cadaver donor. A study of the rat (*11*) found no class I antigens on the myocardium but intercalated discs were class-I-positive.

This study has shown induction of class I antigens on myocardium of transplanted heart. The significance of this finding is unclear. It could have important implications with regard to the process of acute rejection. Biopsies showing histological signs of rejection contain T cells of both suppressor/cytotoxic and helper/inducer phenotype (*12*). It is known that class I expression is necessary for cytotoxic T cells to recognize and lyse virally infected cells (*13*) or tissues bearing alloantigens (*2*). The induction of class I antigens on tissue that was previously class-I-negative may be an important prerequisite for T cell cytotoxicity and thus be an event preceeding cardiac myocyte damage during the rejection of cardiac allografts. Although we have found that all the biopsies showing histological signs of rejection contained class-I-positive myocardium, we also found 6 biopsies containing class-I-positive myocardium in the absence of a cellular infiltrate. All these biopsies were preceded or followed by rejection episodes. It may be, therefore, that the appearance of class I antigen is not directly related to the presence of the cellular infiltrate that is diagnostic of rejection. A recent study of cardiac transplantation in the rat has demonstrated induction of class I antigens on the myocardium during rejection (*11*). However, the same study reports that isografts also become class-I-positive, though to a

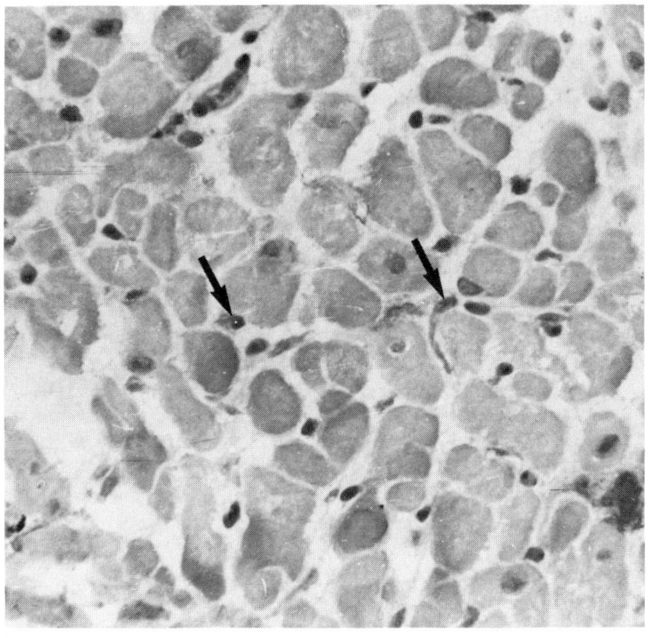

FIGURE 3. Photomicrograph of NFK-1 binding to a cryostat of normal heart (×420). Arrows indicate interstitial structures, possibly dendritic or endothelial cells, that are NFK-1-positive.

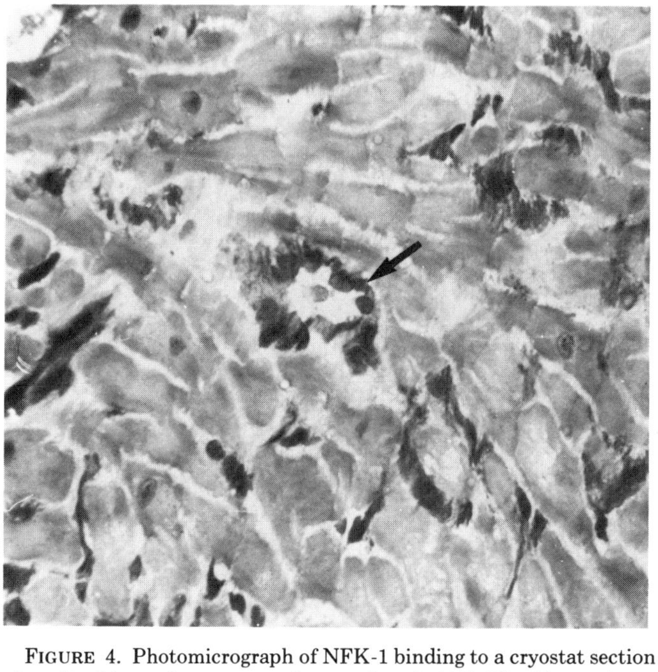

FIGURE 4. Photomicrograph of NFK-1 binding to a cryostat section of cardiac biopsy from a transplant patient (×420). The biopsy shows histological signs of mild rejection (grade 4). Arrow indicates a blood vessel that is NFK-1-positive.

lesser extent than allografts. This observation, taken together with the fact that class I antigens can be induced in vitro on human lymphoid cells by gamma interferon (*14*) and the recent report of increased class I antigen expression on skeletal muscle in a variety of muscle disorders (*15*), may indicate a more general role for class I antigens in pathogenic processes.

This study has shown that the distribution of class II antigens on normal heart is similar to that described in the rat (*16*), with the important exception that in the human the endothelium of small capillaries and some of the larger capillaries are class II positive. It confirms the original finding of Daar et al. (*17*) who studied the distribution of NFK-1 on a variety of human tissues and organs. Further studies are needed to characterize the interstitial nucleated cells that bind NFK-1 in particular to establish whether they are dendritic cells. In transplanted heart there was found to be increased expression of class II antigens on interstitial structures. Whereas much of this increase was due to infiltrating mononuclear cells, it also appeared that some vascular endothelial cells were staining more strongly with NFK-1 than in normal heart. It can be difficult to distinguish capillary endothelial cells from leukocytes using morphological criteria, and in the absence of an independent marker for endothelial cells, it cannot be stated for certain that there was induction of class II antigens on endothelial cells. Further studies are necessary to clarify this point. The induction of donor-specific class II antigens in transplanted heart could play a major role in acute graft rejection. When expressed on dendritic cells, class II antigens have been shown to be potent stimulators of the antiallograft response (*18*). Less certain is whether class II antigens can function as transplantation antigens when present on vascular endothelium, as some studies have suggested (*19*). There are experimental precedents for induction of class II antigens on allografted tissue, thus class II was induced on vascular endothelium (*20*) and epithelial cells (*21*) of rejecting skin, and a recent clinical study has shown an increase in HLA-DR expression on the tubular cells during rejection of renal allografts (*22*). The expression of class II antigens on transplanted heart in the present study was confined to capillaries and infiltrating mononuclear cells. Myocardium remained class-II-negative, unlike the rat heart allograft in which class II antigen was induced on the myocardium during rejection (*11*). Although in the present study increased class II expression was always found in biopsies showing histological signs of rejection (grades 3 and 4), 8 biopsies were found to contain increased class II expression in the absence of the cellular infiltrate that is diagnostic of rejection. The observation that gamma-interferon produced by activated T cells can induce class II antigens on human vascular endothelium (*23*) suggests that viral infections as well as rejection episodes could cause class II induction in clinical transplantation. Further studies are needed to clarify the exact role of class I and class II antigen expression in acute cardiac allograft rejection.

Acknowledgments. We thank Dr. C. Navarette and Professor H. Festenstein for their generous gift of W6/32 antibody, and Dr. S. Fuggle for her kind gift of NFK-1.

REFERENCES

1. Jongsma A, Someven H, Westerwald A, Hagemeijer A, Pearson P. Localization of human chromosomes by studies of human–Chinese hamster somatic cell hybrids. Hum Genet 1973; 20: 195.
2. Zinkernagel RM, Doherty PC. MHC cytotoxic T cells: studies on the biological role of polymorphic major transplantation antigens determining T cell restriction—specificity, function and responsiveness. Adv Immunol 1979; 27: 51.
3. Klein J, Hauptfeld V. Ia antigens: their serology, moleculr relationships and their role in allografted rejection. Transplant Rev 1980; 30: 83.
4. Natalie PG, Martino C, Quaranta V, et al. Expression of Ia-like antigens in normal human non-lymphoid tissues. Transplantation 1981; 31: 75.

5. Morris PJ, Ting A. Studies of HLA-DR with relevance to renal transplantation. Immunol Rev 1982; 66: 103.
6. Fuggle SV, Errasti P, Daar AS, Fabre JW, Ting A, Morris PJ. Localization of major histocompatibility complex (HLA-ABC and DR) antigens in 46 kidneys. Transplantation 1983; 35: 385.
7. Berah M, Hors J, Dausset J. A study of the HLA antigens in human organs. Transplantation 1970; 9: 185.
8. Fleming KA, McMichael A, Morton JA, Woods, J, McGee JO'D. Distribution of HLA class I antigens in normal human tissue and in mammary cancer. J Clin Pathol 1981; 34: 779.
9. Daar AD, Fuggle SV, Fabre JW, Ting A, Morris PJ. The detailed distribution of HLA-ABC antigens in normal human organs. Transplantation 1984; 38: 287.
10. Barnstable CJ, Bodmer WF, Brown G, et al. Production of monoclonal antibodies to group A erythrocytes, HLA and other human cell surface antigens—new tools for genetic analysis. Cell 1978; 14: 9.
11. Milton AD, Fabre JW. Massive induction of donor-type class I and class II major histocompatibility complex antigens in rejecting cardiac allografts in the rat. J Exp Med 1985; 161: 98.
12. Rose ML, Gracie JA, Fraser A, Chisholm PB, Yacoub MH. Use of monoclonal antibodies to quantitate T lymphocyte subpopulations in human cardiac allografts. Transplantation 1984; 38: 230.
13. McMichael AJ, Ting A, Zweevink HF, Askonas BA. HLA restriction of cell mediated lysis of influenza virus infected human cells. Nature 1977; 270: 524.
14. Fellows M, Kamoun M, Gresser I, Bono R. Enhanced expression of HLA antigens and B2-microglobulin on interferon-treated lymphoid cells. Eur J Immunol 1979; 9: 446.
15. Appleyard ST, Dunn MJ, Dubowitz V, Rose ML. Increased expression of HLA ABC class I antigens by muscle fibres in Duchenne muscular dystrophy, inflammatory myopathy, and other neuromuscular disorders. Lancet 1985; 1: 361.
16. Hart DNJ, Fabre JW. Demonstration of Ia-positive dendritic cells in the interstitial connective tissue of rat heart and other tissues, but not brain. J Exp Med 1981; 154: 347.
17. Daar AS, Fuggle SV, Fabre JW, Ting A, Morris PJ. The detailed distribution of MHC class II antigens in normal human organs. Transplantation 1984; 38: 293.
18. Lechler RJ, Batchelor JR. Restoration of immunogenecity to passenger cell depleted kidney allografts by the addition of donor strain dendritic cells. J Exp Med 1982; 155: 31.
19. Hirschberg H, Evensen SA, Henricksen T, Thorsby E. The mixed lymphocyte-endothelium culture interaction. Transplantation 1975; 19: 495.
20. de Waal RMW, Bogman MJJ, Mass CN, Cornelissen LMH, Tax WJM, Koene RAP. Variable expression of Ia antigens on the vascular endothelium of mouse skin allografts. Nature (Lond) 1983; 303: 426.
21. Dallman MJ, Mason DW. Induction of Ia antigens on murine epidermal cells during the rejection of skin allografts. Transplantation 1983; 36: 222.
22. Hall BM, Bishop GA, Duggin GG, Howath JS, Phelips J, Tillen DJ. Increased expression of HLA-DR antigens on renal tubular cells in renal transplantation: relevance to the rejection process. Lancet 1984; 1: 247.
23. Pober JS, Gimbrone MA, Cotran RS, et al. Ia expression by vascular endothelius is inducible by activated T cells and by human gamma interferon. J Exp Med 1983; 157: 1339.

Received 25 June 1985.
Accepted 16 September 1985.

0041-1337//86/4106-0781$02.00/0
TRANSPLANTATION
Vol. 41, No. 6

Printed in U.S.A.

Transplantation

BRIEF COMMUNICATIONS

THE EFFECTS OF DONOR PRETREATMENT ON THE TRANSMISSION OF MURINE CYTOMEGALOVIRUS WITH CARDIAC TRANSPLANTS AND EXPLANTS[1]

Cytomegalovirus (CMV)* is the most important single infectious agent that complicates the clinical course of cardiac transplant patients. It has been demonstrated by direct studies in a murine system (*1–3*) and by indirect, epidemiologic studies in humans (*4*) that the cardiac allograft itself is the major source of primary CMV infection in cardiac transplant recipients. Hearts removed from CMV-seropositive donors harbor latent CMV that is capable of being reactivated following the initiation of immunosuppression posttransplantation. With such reactivation, the seronegative recipient develops potentially lethal disseminated primary infection (*1, 3*).

Although it is now quite clear that the heart itself is the major source of primary CMV infection, the anatomic site within the heart that harbors the latent CMV remains unclear. The important question is whether the latent CMV lies primarily within passenger leukocytes that are not structural constituents of the heart, or within myocardial cells, vascular endothelial cells, or fibroblasts that are integral to cardiac structure. This is an important issue, since, if the passenger leukocytes are the major source of CMV reactivation, pretreatment of the heart donor aimed at destroying the passenger leukocytes would have the potential for eradicating primary CMV infection. In contrast, if the heart virus lies within integral cardiac structures, then all efforts for controlling CMV infection posttransplant will have to be directed at the organ recipient.

In this study two potential strategies for eliminating passenger leukocytes—high-dose cyclophosphamide pretreatment of the donor and total-body irradiation of the donor—are evaluated as to their effects on the reactivation of CMV infection from hearts harvested from donors latently infected with the virus.

Female BALB/C mice, purchased from Cumberland View Farm (Clinton, TN) were employed in all these experiments. Latent infection was produced in 5-week-old mice by the i.p. inoculation of 10^4 plaque-forming units (PFU) of virulent Smith-strain murine CMV (MCMV) maintained in this laboratory as previously described (*1, 5*). Control mice were injected with uninfected salivary gland homogenates (NSG) prepared in similar fashion (*1*). These mice were then maintained in our animal facility for 4–6 months, at which time they were subjected to the experimental protocol to be described. At this time, the latently infected animals were shown to have an antibody titer by indirect immunofluorescence assay (*1*) of 1:128 and to have no detectable virus on culture of their salivary glands. Control animals were shown to have an antibody titer <1:16. and virus was never recovered from their salivary glands.

* Abbreviations used: ATS, antithymocyte serum; CMV, cytomegalovirus; NSG, normal salivary gland; PFU, plaque-forming units.

[1] This work was supported in part by Grant HL18646 from the United States Public Health Service.

Latently infected animals, at the end of 4–6 months in the animal facility, were then treated with 0.35 mg/g of cyclophosphamide, i.p. or 1000 rads of total-body irradiation, administered as a single dose. Both treatments caused 100% mortality in 5–7 days. Four to five days after treatment, shortly before the expected demise of these animals, blood was obtained for white blood cell counts, the animals were anesthetized with a single i.p. injection of chloral hydrate, and their hearts were harvested for transplantation or explant studies.

Those experiments in which transplantation was carried out employed a protocol previously described (*1, 6*). Briefly, the aorta and pulmonary artery of the donated heart are joined end-to-side to the recipient abdominal aorta and inferior vena cava, resulting in a perfused, beating heart. Recipient animals were then immunosuppressed with cortisone acetate (Merck, Sharpe and Dohme Div., Merck and Co., West Point, PA), 125 mg/kg/day, and 0.2 ml of rabbit antimouse thymocyte serum (ATS) (kindly supplied by Henry Winn, Ph.D., Transplantation Unit, Massachusetts General Hospital, Boston, MA), twice weekly (*1, 5*). They were then observed for morbidity and mortality.

Explants of cardiac tissue were prepared by aseptically removing hearts from latently infected or NSG-inoculated mice and placing them in cold lactated Ringer's solution. Hearts were cut into 1×2-mm pieces and overlain onto secondary mouse embryo cultures as previously described (*2*). Cardiac tissue prepared the same way, was also seeded in wells without mouse embryo cultures. Aliquots of culture fluid were obtained throughout the 5–6-week culture period, stored at −70°C, and tested for the presence of virus by plaque assay (*2*).

Pretreatment of MCMV latently infected donor mice with cyclophosphamide or irradiation resulted in a significant fall in the peripheral white blood cell count. Whereas the untreated, latently infected donor mice had white blood cell counts comparable to uninfected animals of approximately 6200/mm^3, those irradiated 5 days previously had white blood cell counts of approximately 500/mm^3 and those who had received cyclophosphamide, approximately 1500/mm^3. These blood counts were determined at the time the donor's heart was removed for the transplantation and explant culture experiments. When hearts from both the pretreated and the untreated animals were transplanted into CMV seronegative recipients that were then immunosuppressed, lethal disseminated primary CMV infection resulted. There was no significant difference in the duration of survival in these animals among the three groups—that is, all animals, whether their donors were pretreated or not, succumbed from their disseminated primary CMV infection 17–20 days after cardiac transplant (Table 1).

Similarly, there was no significant difference in the recovery of active virus from cardiac explant cultures of latently infected cardiac tissue whether or not the animals had been pretreated.

TABLE 1. Effect of cyclophosphamide and irradiation treatment of donor mice latently infected with MCMV on the donor white blood cell count and the survival of recipients of hearts transplanted from these donors

Treatment	White blood cell count of donor (per mm^3)	n	Days of death of recipients of heart transplants[a]
Cyclophosphamide	1500±1050	8	19.25±2.9
Irradiation	510±150	8	20.50±5.5
Untreated	6200±620	7	17.40±2.3

[a] All recipients were MCMV-seronegative prior to transplant, and received immunosuppression with cortisone acetate, 125 mg/kg/day, and 0.2 ml of rabbit antimouse thymocyte serum twice weekly following transplantation.

TABLE 2. Reactivation of latent MCMV from cardiac explant cultures of hearts from BALB/C mice infected 4–6 months previously with sublethal doses of MCMV

Treatment	Explant + MEC[a] (No. wells pos./No.)		Explant only (No. wells pos./No.)	
	No tested	Hearts pos.	No. tested	Hearts pos.
Untreated	14/59 (24%)	5/10 (50%)	7/25 (28%)	6/10 (60%)
Cyclophosphamide	15/48 (31%)	5/8 (63%)	5/15 (31%)	4/8 (50%)
Irradiation	5/26 (19%)	3/5 (60%)	2/12 (18%)	2/5 (40%)
Uninfected	0/12	0/2	0/5	0/2
Uninfected + irradiation	0/11	0/2	0/3	0/2

[a] The explant is overlain onto secondary mouse embryo culture.

As delineated in Table 2, both the percentage of hearts from which virus was recovered and the percentage of wells that were positive were essentially identical, whether or not the animals had been pretreated.

We and others have previously demonstrated that mice seropositive for CMV—and, hence, latently infected with the virus—harbor latent virus within their hearts (*1, 3*). Transplanting of these hearts into seronegative recipients or placing these hearts into explant culture results in reactivation of the latent virus and—in the case of the transplant recipient—disseminated primary CMV infection. Epidemiologic information from human cardiac transplantation suggests that the human cytomegalovirus behaves in a similar fashion. Control and prevention of primary CMV infection could be accomplished by pretreatment of the donor to eliminate the latently infected cells, or it could require more intensive therapy of the transplant recipient. Pretreatment of the donor is most likely to be successful if the site of viral latency is not intrinsic cardiac tissue such as myocardial cells, fibroblasts, or vascular endothelium, but rather involves the passenger leukocytes, which may be present within any organ of the body and which are more amenable to elimination by donor pretreatment.

In these studies, we have attempted to determine if donor pretreatment aimed at the passenger leukocytes with two treatment programs that might be feasible for allograft donors—namely, high-dose cyclophosphamide or high-dose irradiation—might influence the rate of viral transmission. Unfortunately, neither donor pertreatment regimen significantly influenced the recovery of virus in the explant system or the outcome of transplantation when these hearts from pretreated animals were transplanted into seronegative recipients that were then immunosuppressed. Although this evidence is indirect, we suggest that the major site of viral latency within the heart is intrinsic cardiac tissue, and that efforts to control CMV infection in cardiac transplant recipients will have to be directed entirely at treatment or prophylaxis of the recipient, rather than pretreatment of the donor.

EILEEN J. WILSON
DONALD N. MEDEARIS
LESLIE V. BARRETT
ATUL BHAN
ROBERT H. RUBIN[2]
The Medical, Children's, and Pathology Services
Massachusetts General Hospital
The Departments of Medicine, Pediatrics, Pathology
The Harvard Medical School
Boston, Massachusetts 02114

[2] Reprint request should be addressed to: Dr. Robert H. Rubin, Infectious Disease Unit, Massachusetts General Hospital, Boston, MA 02114.

REFERENCES

1. Rubin RH, Wilson EJ, Barrett LV, Medearis DN. Primary cytomegalovirus infection following cardiac transplantation in a murine model. Transplantation 1984; 37: 306.
2. Wilson EJ, Medearis DN Jr, Barrett LV, Rubin RH. Activation of latent murine cytomegalovirus in cardiac explant and cell cultures. J Infect Dis (in press).
3. Shanley JD, Billingsley AM, Shelby J, Corry RJ. Transfer of murine cytomegalovirus by heart transplantation. Transplantation 1983; 36: 584.
4. Preiksaitis JK, Rosno S, Grumet C, Merigan TC. Infections due to herpes viruses in cardiac transplant recipients: role of the donor heart and immunosuppressive therapy. J Infect Dis 1983; 147: 974.
5. Jordan MC. Adverse effects of cytomegalovirus vaccination in mice. J Clin Invest 1980; 65: 798.
6. Corry RJ, Winn HJ, Russell PS. Primarily vascularized allografts of hearts in mice: the role of H-2D, H-2K, and non-H-2 antigens in rejection. Transplantation 1973; 16: 343.

Received 10 September 1985.
Accepted 9 October 1985.

EFFECT OF CYCLOSPORINE UPON THE FUNCTION OF ISCHEMICALLY DAMAGED KIDNEYS IN THE RAT

The efficacy of cyclosporine as a maintenance immunosuppressive agent in cadaver renal transplantation is now well established. The nephrotoxicity of this drug has been documented in several studies (1, 2) and, fortunately, this problem can usually be monitored with serum drug levels and reversed by appropriate dose reduction (*3*). One issue that remains controversial concerns the possible harmful effect of cyclosporine on initial cadaver graft function caused by its nephrotoxicity superimposed on renal ischemia incurred prior to transplantation. This concept implies that the combined effect of these two factors is more detrimental to renal function than either factor alone.

This problem ws first suggested in an early clinical study by Calne et al.—who, after observing posttransplant oliguria in 11 of 32 cadaver recipients treated with cyclosporine, recommended withholding the drug unless a prompt initial diuresis was present (*4*). This concept was then tested in a laboratory study by Homan et al., who found no harmful effect of cyclosporine on the function of ischemically damaged canine renal autografts (*5*). More recent clinical studies have yielded conflicting data. In the Canadian multicentered trial, a higher incidence of primary cadaver graft nonfunction was observed in recipients managed with cyclosporine (*6*). However, a report from Houston showed no difference in the incidence or outcome of posttransplant acute tubular necrosis in cyclosporine-versus-azothiaprine–treated recipients (*7*).

The purpose of the present study was to evaluate the individual and combined effects of cyclosporine and ischemia on renal function in an experimental rat model. Male Sprague-Dawley rats weighing 275–375 g were used. The animals were fed Purina Rodent Chow 5001 and were given free access to water prior to surgery. The rats were anesthetized with sodium pentobarbitol, 5 mg/100 g i.p. In all experiments, a midline abdominal incision was made and the right kidney removed. The left kidney was completely mobilized by dividing all perirenal attachments, and the renal artery and vein were dissected free. In animals subjected to renal ischemia, the renal artery was occluded for 60 min with a noncrushing microvascular clamp; the clamp was then removed and the abdomen was closed. In animals not subjected to renal ischemia, the kidney and renal vessels were mobilized but the artery was not occluded and the abdomen was then closed. All animals received 7 cc warm 5% dextrose and water i.p. at the end of the experiment. In animals that received cyclosporine (Sandimmune, oral solution) postoperatively, this was given orally each day at a dose of 50 mg/kg in 0.5 ml of 5% dextrose and water.

A total of 148 rats were employed in this study, and these animals were divided into four experimental groups. Group 1 (n=22) was a sham group in which no renal ischemia was sustained and no cyclosporine was given. Animals from group 2 (n=50) were subjected to 60 min of renal ischemia but did not receive cyclosporine. In group 3 (n=15), no renal ischemia was sustained, but cyclosporine, 50 mg/kg per day was given postoperatively. Animals from group 4 (n=61) were subjected to 60 min renal ischemia and also received cyclosporine, 50 mg/kg day postoperatively.

Within each study group, animals were sacrificed on days 0, 1, 2, 3, 4, or 11 following surgery. On the day of sacrifice, the rats were anesthetized with sodium pentobarbitol, 5 mg/100 g i.p. and blood samples were obtained through an aortic puncture. Serum blood urea nitrogen (BUN)* and creatinine (CR) were measured by reflectance spectrophotometry. Serum sodium and potassium were measured by an ion selective electrode. In animals receiving cyclosporine, cyclosporine whole-blood levels were measured by high pressure liquid chromatography (*8*); since cyclosporine was not administered on the day

* Abbreviations used: BUN, blood urea nitrogen; CR, creatinine.

TABLE 1. Mean biochemical and survival data for rats in four experimental groups

Group	Days following operation					
	0	1	2	3	4	11
1. Sham:						
No. animals	5	5			5	7
No. survived	5	5			5	7
Cr (mg/dl)	0.36±.1	.52±.1			.36±.1	.46±.1
BUN (mg/dl)	16±1	27±1			23±2	27±1.0
Na^+ (mEq/L)	137±1.0	132±1.5			143±1.1	142±.6
K^+ (mEq/L)	4.3±.1	3.4±.1			4.0±.1	3.8±.1
2. 60 min ischemia:						
No. animals		10	10	10	10	10
No. survived		10	10	10	10	9
Cr (mg/dl)		3.62±.3	2.28±.8	3.20±.6	.86±.2	.4±.1
BUN (mg/dl)		95±7	84±18	121±15	64±12	36±1
Na^+ (mEq/L)		136±1	137±.7	136±.6	137±.7	138±1.3
K^+ (mEq/L)		4.5±.5	3.5±.3	4.0±2	3.3±.2	4.4±.1
3. No ischemia and cyclosporine:						
No. animals		5			5	5
No. survived		5			5	5
Cr (mg/dl)		52±.06			.56±.1	.36±.1
BUN (mg/dl)		34±4			32±4	48±2
Na^+ (mEq/L)		134±2.6			144±1.4	138±.8
K^+ (mEq/L)		3.4±.2			4.0±.1	4.6±.3
Cyclosporine level (ng/ml)					3504	2844
4. 60 min ischemia and cyclosporine						
No. animals		11	10	10	10	20
No. survived		11	10	10	10	12
Cr (mg/dl)		3.7±.4	1.7±.7	2.8±.7	1.2±.2	1.04±.1
BUN (mg/dl)		120±8	99±16	118±13	94±12	86±6
Na^+ (mEq/L)		134±1.3	132±1.0	131±1.0	136±.7	140±3
K^+ (mEq/L)		4.6±.4	4.1±.6	3.8±.2	3.4±.2	5.0±.2
Cyclosporine level (ng/ml)		997			3003	3867

of sacrifice, these represent 24-hr blood trough levels of cyclosporine. The data were subjected to analysis of variance or Student's t test. The 0.05 level of probability was used as the criterion of statistical significance.

The mean renal function, electrolyte, and survival data for animals in the four experimental groups are presented in Table 1. The renal function and electrolyte data are presented only for surviving animals. In animals that underwent a sham operation and did not receive cyclosporine (group 1), there were no deaths, renal function did not change significantly, and electrolytes remained normal postoperatively. The results in animals that underwent a sham operation and then received cyclosporine postoperatively (group 3) were not significantly different from those in the latter group. In animals subjected to 60 min warm renal ischemia but not receiving cyclosporine (group 2), the mean postoperative CR and BUN levels were significantly elevated compared with group 1 on days 1 and 4 ($P<.05$), but had returned to the mean baseline level by day 11; mean electrolyte values in this group remained normal.

In animals subjected to 60 min of warm renal ischemia who then also received cyclosporine (group 4), the mean postoperative CR and BUN levels were significantly elevated compared with group 1 on days 1, 4, and 11 ($P<.05$) while the mean electrolyte values remained normal. There was no significant difference in the mean CR and BUN levels between groups 2 and 4 on days 1, 2, or 3. On day 4, the mean BUN level was significantly lower in group 2 (64±12 vs). 94±12, $P<.05$) but the mean CR levels were not significantly different in groups 2 and 4, although CR levels in group 4 were elevated. A significant difference in both values ($P<.05$) was present on day 11, at which time the mean CR and BUN had returned to the baseline level in group 2 (0.4±.1 and 36±1) but remained elevated in group 4 (1.04±.1 and 86±8).

The only deaths occurred in rats from group 2 (1 of 10) and group 4 (8 of 20) who were to have been sacrificed on day 11 after the operation. These animals all expired on the postoperative days 7–10, and the presumed cause of death was acute renal failure. The incidence of mortality beyond postoperative day 4 was significantly greater in group 4 compared with group 2 ($P<.05$).

The results of this experimental study demonstrate that the combination of renal ischemia and cyclosporine therapy is more damaging to renal function than either of these factors alone. Renal function was not affected by cyclosporine therapy alone but was significantly impaired by 60 min of ischemia. The combination of cyclosporine therapy and 60 min of ischemia was more detrimental to renal function than 60 min of ischemia alone. As evidence of this, there were more animal deaths from acute renal failure in the former group as well as more protracted elevations in the serum CR and BUN levels postoperatively. This additional renal damage was caused by the same dose of cyclosporine that, when given to animals with no renal ischemia and with comparable cyclosporine blood levels, did not impair renal function.

These experimental data support the concept that cyclosporine's nephrotoxic effect may be more pronounced in the presence of a recent renal ischemic insult, and that these two factors may act synergistically to produce more severe renal functional impairment than is caused by either alone. This concept requires further study in the clinical setting—and, if validated, argues against administering cyclosporine following cadaver transplantation until initial graft function is assured.

Ghassan Kanazi
Nicholas Stowe
Donald Steinmuller
Hwieh Ho-Hsieh
Andrew C. Novick[1]
The Section of Renal Transplantation
Cleveland Clinic Foundation
Cleveland, Ohio

[1] Address requests for reprints to: Andrew C. Novick, M.D., Head, Section of Renal Transplantation, Cleveland Clinic Foundation, 9500 Euclid Avenue, Cleveland, Ohio 44106.

REFERENCES

1. Klintman BG, Iwatsuki S, Starzl TE. Nephrotoxicity of cyclosporin A in liver and kidney transplantation. Lancet 1981; 1: 470.
2. Sweny P, Hopper J, Gross M, et al. Nephrotoxicity of cyclosporin. Lancet 1981; 1: 663.
3. Kahan BD, Van Buren CT, Lin SN, et al. Immunopharmacologic monitoring of cyclosporin A treated recipients of cadaver kidney allografts. Transplantation, 1982, 34: 36.
4. Calne RY, Rolles K, White DJG, et al. Cyclosporin initially as the only immunosuppressant in 34 recipients of cadaver organs. Lancet 1979; 2: 1033.
5. Homan WP, French ME, Morris PJ. Effect of cyclosporine A upon the function of ischemically damaged renal autografts in the dog. Transplantation 1980; 30: 228.
6. Stiller C. The Canadian trial of cyclosporine; cyclosporine therapy compared to standard immunosuppression in renal transplants; an exploration of nephrotoxicity. Transplant Proc 1983; 15: 2479.
7. Flechner SM, Payne WD, Van Buren C, Kerman R, Kahan BD. The effect of cyclosporine on early graft function in human renal transplantation. Transplantation 1983; 36: 268.
8. Sawchuk RJ, Cartier LO. Liquid-chromatographic determination of cyclosporine A in blood and plasma. Clin Chem 1981; 27: 1368.

Received 17 September 1985.
Accepted 1 October 1985.

ACCELERATED DEVELOPMENT OF SPONTANEOUS THYMIC LYMPHOMAS IN MALE AKR MICE RECEIVING CYCLOSPORINE[1]

Cyclosporine CsA* has rapidly become one of the most widely used immunosuppressive agents for clinical organ transplantation, but information concerning its long-term toxicological effects is relatively scarce (*1–3*). Dietary administration of CsA to rats and mice at doses comparable to clinical usage results in the marked reduction, or even loss, of the medullary components of the thymus (*4, 5*). The functional significance of the changes remains unknown.

The thymus plays an essential role in T cell lymphoma development in strains of mice with either a low or a high spontaneous incidence of this tumor, regardless of whether lymphoma develops spontaneously or is induced by chemicals,

* Abbreviations used: CsA, cyclosporine; PMA, phorbol-12-myristate-13-acetate.

[1]This work was supported by grants from the National Institutes of Health (CA 36175 and CA 18659).

radiation, and leukemogenic viruses (*6–8*). The development of spontaneous and induced lymphomas is effectively prevented by thymectomy (*9, 10*), and the implantation of thymuses into thymectomized mice restores their susceptibility to lymphoma development (*11–13*). We have recently demonstrated that CsA treatment markedly enhances the induction of thymic lymphomas in mice that have a low spontaneous incidence pretreated with a small dose of the carcinogen N-methyl-N-nitrosourea (*14*). We postulated that the disturbance of the thymic microenvironment induced by CsA exerted the pivotal role in promoting the induction of thymic lymphomas (*14*). In the present study, we investigated whether CsA treatment modifies the development of spontaneous thymic lymphoma in AKR mice that are known to have a high incidence of such tumors (*15*).

Male mice of the AKR/J strain, 6 weeks old and weighing 20–22 g were obtained from the Jackson Laboratory (Bar Harbor, ME). Five to six mice were housed in wire cages in a room maintained with 12-h light and dark cycles, a constant temperature of 20 ± 2°C and 50 ± 10% humidity. They were fed Purina Chow (Ralston, Purina, St. Louis, MO) and water ad libitum and acclimatized to the facility 10 days before the start of experimental diets. The mice were divided into two groups. Group 1 was given a basal diet (Dyet Inc., Bethlehem, PA) (*4*), and group 2 was given the same diet containing 0.015% cyclosporine (CsA, Sandoz, Ltd., Basel, Switzerland). CsA was mixed into the diet without the addition of any solvents, and both basal and CsA diets were pelleted.

Mice developing thymic lymphomas typically exhibited the clinical signs of respiratory distress due to compression of the thoracic organs, and mice with such symptoms were killed. Age-matched mice receiving a basal diet were also periodically killed at the same time. Complete autopsies were done, and the major organs were fixed in Stieves solution. The tissues were sectioned and stained with hematoxylin-eosin.

In AKR mice, the spontaneous thymic lymphomas develop with an incidence of 50–70% in males and 70–85% in females at the age of 8–9 months (*15*). In the present experiments, the first tumor in mice receiving a basal diet was noted in the 23rd week, and 33% of mice killed between 30 and 34 weeks of the experiment showed thymic lymphomas (Table 1). In the group of mice that received the CsA diet, the first thymic tumor was noted in the 17th week, and 72% of mice killed between 20 and 29 weeks showed thymic lymphomas. The incidence of the tumor in mice killed between 30 and 34 weeks was 100% (Table 1). The only other tumor found in either group of mice was one hepatocellular carcinoma in a mouse receiving a CsA diet.

The histological appearance of the thymic lymphomas in mice receiving the basal diet or the CsA diet was the same. It showed sheets of uniformly sized large lymphocytes or lymphoblasts with a high rate of mitosis (Fig. 1). They were also indistinguishable from those of the tumors induced in Swiss mice with a single injection of MNU followed by a CsA diet (*14*). The thymuses of mice that received a basal diet and did not develop thymic tumors were variable in size (12–16 mg net weight). Histologically they showed readily identifiable cortical and medullary components, although the relative proportions of these structures varied considerably from one animal to another (Fig. 2). Involution of the cortex, enlargement of the medulla, and frequent germinal center formation, which have been described as the prelymphomatous changes in the AKR thymus (*16*), were not observed.

The results of the these experiments, together with those reported earlier (*14*) demonstrate that CsA accelerates spontaneous development of thymic lymphomas, as well as development of lymphomas induced by an exogenously administered carcinogen. Although many factors have been suggested as being involved in radiation or chemically induced lymphomas and in spontaneous lymphomas developing in AKR mice, there is as yet no unified concept for the induction mechanism. We suggested that the enhancing effect of CsA on thymic lymphoma induction in carcinogen-initiated mice is mediated through its promoting action. In the classic concept of two-

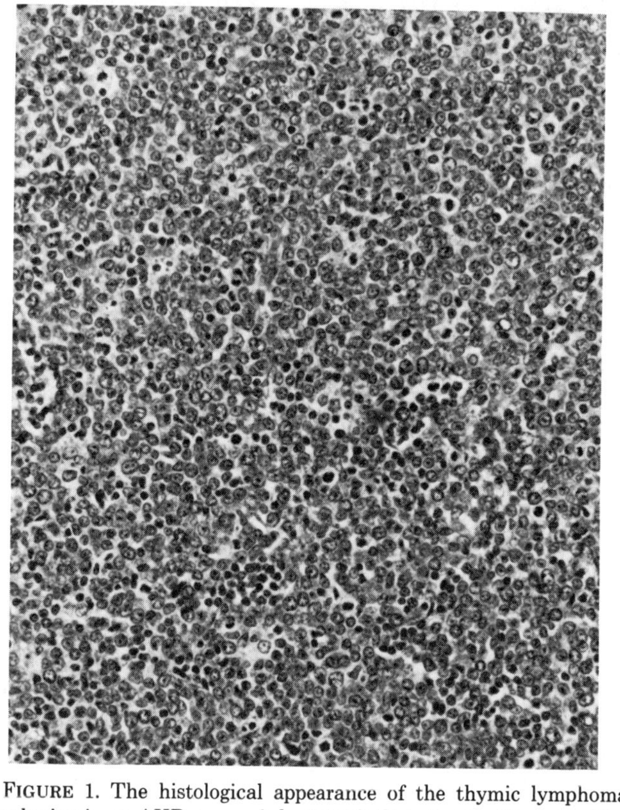

FIGURE 1. The histological appearance of the thymic lymphoma developing in an AKR mouse fed a 0.015% CsA diet for 28 weeks. The tumor is composed of uniformly sized lymphocytes and lymphoblasts with many mitotic figures (×350).

TABLE 1. Thymic lymphomas in AKR mice with or without cyclosporine treatment

Group	Treatment	Tumor Incidence[a]			Total	Average latent period (weeks)
		<19 weeks	20–29 weeks	30–34 weeks		
1	Basal diet	0/1	2/12 (17%)	3/9 (33%)	5/22 (23%)	30
2	CsA-diet	1/3[b]	13/18 (72%)[c]	9/9 (100%)[c]	23/30 (77%)[c]	27

[a] Number of lymphoma-bearing mice/number of mice examined.
[b] One mouse had hepatocellular carcinoma.
[c] The differences are significant ($P<0.005$) when compared with group 1 by the chi-square test.

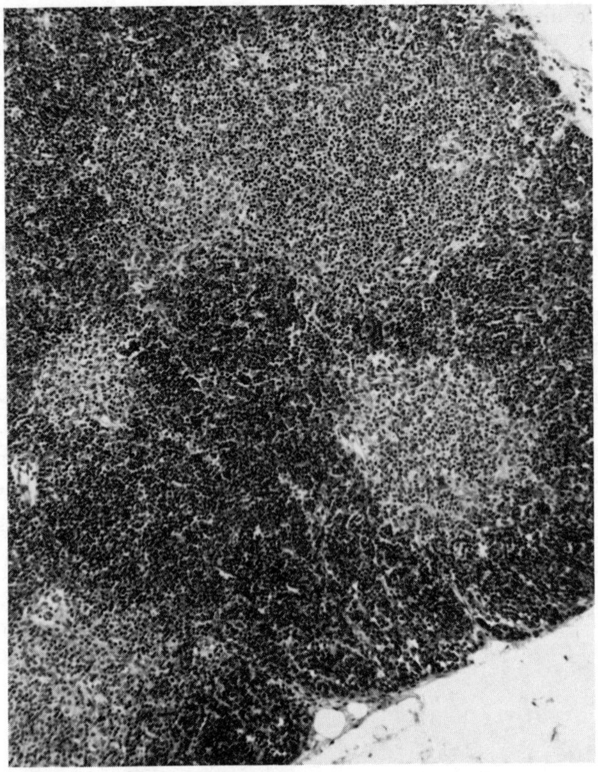

FIGURE 2. The histological appearance of the thymus of an AKR mouse fed a basal diet for 26 weeks. The cortical and medullary components of the thymus are readily apparent (×140).

stage chemical carcinogenesis, initiation involves possible mutationlike events induced by a carcinogen in a selected number of target cells, and promotion involves selective growth of initiated cells to overt neoplasms (*17, 18*). The high incidence of spontaneous thymic lymphomas in AKR mice suggests that this strain of mice harbor clones of initiated cells in the thymus. It is thus conceivable that the acceleration of lymphoma development in AKR mice receiving CsA may be due to its promotional effect. The biological phenomenon is analogous to the effect of phenobarbital, which is a well-known promoter of liver tumor induction in chemically initiated rats, and which enhances the development of spontaneous hepatomas in C3H mice that have a high incidence of such tumors (*19*).

Although the mechanism of tumor promotion is not known, one of the mechanisms is altered differentiation of target cells (*20, 21*). Phorbol-12-myristate-13-acetate (PMA) and related phorbol diesters, which are promoters in a two-stage skin carcinogenesis system, were found to alter cell differentiation in normal and transformed cells (*21*). Our suggestion that CsA may interfere with differentiation of T lymphocyte maturation in the thymus, and thereby exert a promotional effect, is based on two observations: the preferential effects of CsA on T cell functions (*2, 22*), and the morphological alterations of the thymus in CsA-treated animals (*4, 23*). The crucial question of what role promoter-induced alteration of differentiation plays in tumor promotion is still unresolved.

Endogenous murine retroviruses have been implicated as a possible etiological agent for the development of AKR spontaneous lymphomas, although the mechanism by which they might induce lymphomas is unknown (*15*). There are, however, suggestions that retroviruses associated with murine thymic lymphomas may not be directly transforming—rather they may contribute to lymphoma induction by an indirect mechanism (*24–26*). Recent studies (*27, 28*) indicate that in chemically induced or radiation-induced thymic lymphoma the transforming genes of these tumors are activated oncogenes of the ras family, which are not related murine leukemia viruses. Murine leukemia viruses associated with murine lymphomas may be involved in activation of these cellular oncogenes or in the expression of the activated oncogenes. At present there is no information regarding the effects of CsA on the expression of various forms of murine leukemia viruses, and such studies are necessary to clarify the roles of murine leukemia viruses and cyclosporine in the etiology of murine thymic lymphomas. Better understanding of the mechanism of CsA action in vivo is vital to its successful use in transplant patients.

In summary, dietary administration of CsA at a concentration of 0.015% to male AKR mice markedly enhanced the development of spontaneous thymic lymphomas. The tumors developed earlier, and a 100% incidence was obtained by 30 weeks of the dietary feeding. Comparison of the present results with those reported earlier suggests that CsA accelerates induction of the thymic lymphomas by promoter-like effects.

Acknowledgments. We thank Ms. Deborah L. Newman for preparation of the manuscript.

ATSUO HATTORI
MOHAN I. R. PERERA
LYNN A. WITKOWSKI
HEINZ W. KUNZ
THOMAS J. GILL III
HISASHI SHINOZUKA[2]
Department of Pathology
University of Pittsburgh School of Medicine
Pittsburgh, PA 15261

[2] To whom correspondence should be sent.

REFERENCES

1. Morris PJ. Cyclosporin A. Transplantation 1981; 38: 349.
2. Britton S. Palacios R. Cyclosporin A: usefulness, risks and mechanisms of action. Immunol Rev 1982; 65: 5.
3. Kahan BD. A powerful addition to the immunosuppressive armamentarium. Am J Kidney Dis 1984; 3: 444.
4. Demetris AJ, Nalesnik MA, Kunz HW, Gill TJ, Shinozuka H. Sequential analyses of the development of lymphoproliferative disorders in rats receiving cyclosporine. Transplantation 1984; 38: 239.
5. Shinozuka H, Demetris AJ, Witkowski LA, Perera MIR, Nalesnik MA, Gill TJ. Experimental model of cyclosporine-induced lymphoproliferative disorders. Fed Proc 1984; 43: 662.
6. Nagaya H. Thymus function in spontaneous lymphoid leukemia. I. Premature leukemogenesis in "young" thymectomized mice bearing "old" thymus grafts. J Immunol 1973; 111: 1048.
7. Zielinski CC, Waksal SD, Datta SK. Thymic epithelium is programmed to induce preleukemic changes in retrovirus expression and thymocyte differentiation in leukemia susceptible mice: studies on bone marrow and thymic chimeras. J Immunol 1982; 129: 882.
8. Schwartz RS, Datta SK, Hiai H, Morrissey PJ, Waksal SD. The role of abnormal T-lymphocyte differentiation in murine leukemia virus expression and leukemogenesis. In: Essex M, Tadaro G, Zur-Hansen H, eds. Viruses in naturally occurring cancers. Cold Spring Harbor, N.Y.: Cold Spring Harbor Press, 1980: 1199.
9. McEndy DP, Boon MD, Furth J. On the role of the thymus, spleen and gonads in the development of leukemia in a high-leukemia stock of mice. Cancer Res 1944; 4: 377.

10. Kaplan HS. Influence of thymectomy, splenectomy and gonadectomy on the incidence of radiation-induced lymphoid tumors in strain C57B1 mice. J Nat Cancer Inst 1950; 11: 83.
11. Hays EF. The role of thymus epithelial reticular cells in viral leukemogenesis. Cancer Res 1968; 28: 21.
12. Kaplan HS, Brown MB, Paull J. Influence of post-radiation thymectomy and of thymic implants on lymphoid tumor incidence on C57B1 mice. Cancer Res 1953; 13: 677.
13. Law LW. Increase in incidence of leukemia in hybrid mice bearing thymic transplants from a high leukemic strain. J Nat Cancer Inst 1952; 12: 789.
14. Shinozuka H, Gill TJ, Kunz HW, Witkowski LA, Demetris JA, Perera MIR. Enhancement of the induction of murine thymic lymphomas by cyclosporine, Transplantation 1986; 41: 377.
15. Gross L. Mouse leukemia in oncogenic viruses, vol 1, 3rd ed, New York: Pergamon Press, 1983: 305.
16. Metcalf D. Histologic and transplantation studies on preleukemic thymus of the AKR mouse. J Nat Cancer Inst 1966; 37: 425.
17. Boutwell RK. Some biological aspects of skin carcinogenesis. Prog Exp Tumor Res 1964; 4: 207.
18. Farber E. The multistep nature of cancer development. Cancer Res 1984; 44: 4217.
19. Peraino C, Fry RJM, Staffeldt E. Enhancement of spontaneous hepatic tumorigenesis in C3H mice by dietary phenobarbital. J Nat Cancer Inst 1973; 51: 1349.
20. Berenblum I. A speculative review: the probable nature of promoting action and its significance in the understanding of carcinogenesis. Cancer Res 1954; 14: 471.
21. Diamond L, O'Brien TG, Baird WM. Mechanisms of tumor promotion. Adv Cancer Res 1980; 32: 1.
22. White DJG, Plumb AM, Pawelec G, Brons G. Cyclosporin A: an immunosuppressive agent preferentially active against proliferating T cells. Transplantation 1979; 27: 55.
23. Cheney RT, Sprent J. Capacity of cyclosporine to induce autograft-versus-host disease and impair intrathymic T cell differentiation. Transplant Proc 1985; 17: 528.
24. Mayer A, Dorsch-Hasler K. Endogenous MuLV infection does not contribute to onset of radiation or carcinogen-induced murine thymoma. Nature 1982; 295: 253.
25. Ihle JN, Lee JC, Enjuanes L, Cicurel L, Horak I, Pepersack L. Chronic immunostimulation as a possible mechanism in type-C viral leukemogenesis in viruses. In: Essex M, Tadaro G, Zur-Hansen H, eds. Naturally occurring cancers. Cold Spring Harbor, N.Y.: Cold Spring Harbor Press, 1980: 1049.
26. Yanagihara K, Seyama T, Kamiya K, Inoh A, Yokoro K. Generation of lymphomageneic mouse type-C viruses from radiation- or chemically-induced non-producer T-cell lymphoma cell lines infected with non-oncogenic ecopropic virus. Japan J Cancer Res (Gann) 1985; 76: 331.
27. Guerrero I, Calzada P, Mayer A, Pellicer A. A molecular approach to leukemogenesis: mouse lymphomas contain an activated C-ras oncogene. Proc Nat Acad Sci USA 1984; 81: 202.
28. Guerrero I, Villastante A, D'Eustachio P, Pellicer A. Isolation, characterization, and chromosome assignment of mouse N-ras gene from carcinogen-induced thymic lymphoma. Science 1984; 225: 1041.

Received 10 September 1985.
Accepted 11 October 1985.

DONOR-TYPE MHC-POSITIVE CELLS IN THE HOST SPLEEN AFTER RAT ORGAN TRANSPLANTATION

Differences Between Pancreas and Heart Allograft Recipients[1]

Migratory bone-marrow–derived cells may contribute substantially to the immunogenicity of an organ allograft. Prolonged allograft survival has been demonstrated in several experimental models after depletion or inactivation of potential passenger cells (*1–3*). The cell type exerting passenger cell functions has not been unequivocally established so far. Much attention has been focused on antigen presentation by Ia-positive interstitial dendritic cells contained in an organ allograft. Theoretically, presentation of foreign histocompatibility antigens might take place in the allograft itself or in the recipient's lymphatic system, or both. In this study we demonstrate that intact donor-type major histocompatibility complex (MHC)*-positive cells may enter the recipient's immune system and can be found in the host spleen. Following pancreas transplantation the majority of these cells are lymphocytes and not Ia-positive dendritic cells. Large numbers of donor lymphocytes reached the recipient spleen only after pancreas transplantation and not after heart grafting.

A sequential immunohistological investigation of the distribution of donor class I and class II MHC antigens was performed in the spleens of rat pancreas and heart allograft recipients. In the strain combinations DA (RT1.$A^aB^aC^{av1}$)-to-LEW (RT1.$A^LB^LC^L$) and LEW-to-LEW.1U (RT1.$A^uB^uC^u$), rejection of heterotopic duct-ligated pancreas whole-organ allografts and accessory abdominal heart transplants regularly occurred within 10 days. Recipient spleens were removed at daily intervals from days 1–10 after transplantation, stored in liquid nitrogen, cut in a cryostat, and stained using an indirect immunoperoxidase procedure, as described previously (*4*). Donor class I MHC antigens in DA to LEW recipient spleens were demonstrated by the NDS 54 (previously MN 4–91–6) mouse antirat antibody applied in ascitic form (*5*). Donor type class II antigens were visualized by the F 17-23-2 antibody in LEW-to-LEW.1U recipient spleens (*6*). In addition, 0x6 antibody, which recognizes a monomorphic class II antigen determinant, was included (*7*). A1D2 mouse antirat monoclonal antibody as ascites does not react with antigens present in the rat lymphatic system and served as a control (*8*).

Following pancreas transplantation in the DA-to-LEW combination, there was a progressive influx of donor class I MHC-positive lymphocytes into the recipient's periarteriolar lymphatic sheath (PALS). On day 2 donor cells were evenly distributed throughout the PALS, and a smaller number of cells appeared in the corona of splenic follicles. By day 3 they were most numerous, with the majority of cells situated in the follicle corona and fewer cells in the PALS (Fig. 1a). Cells expressing donor class II MHC antigens were examined in LEW-to-LEW.1U pancreas recipients. In contrast to donor class I positive lymphocytes, cells expressing donor class II MHC antigens were not seen in the inner PALS, but appeared only in the outer part of the lymphatic sheath close to the marginal zone, and mostly in the follicle corona. The majority of donor class II MHC-positive cells were observed on days 4 and 5 after transplantation. They were almost exclusively situated in the follicle corona (Fig. 1b). There were about twice as many donor-type class I MHC-positive cells as class II MHC-positive ones. A direct comparison of cell numbers, however, was impossible

[1] This work was supported by Grants Ste 360/1-1 of the Deutsche Forschungsgemeinschaft and I/38510 of the Stiftung Volkswagenwerk.

* Abbreviations used: FDS, follicular dendritic cell: MHC, major histocompatibility complex; PALS, periarteriolar lymphatic sheath.

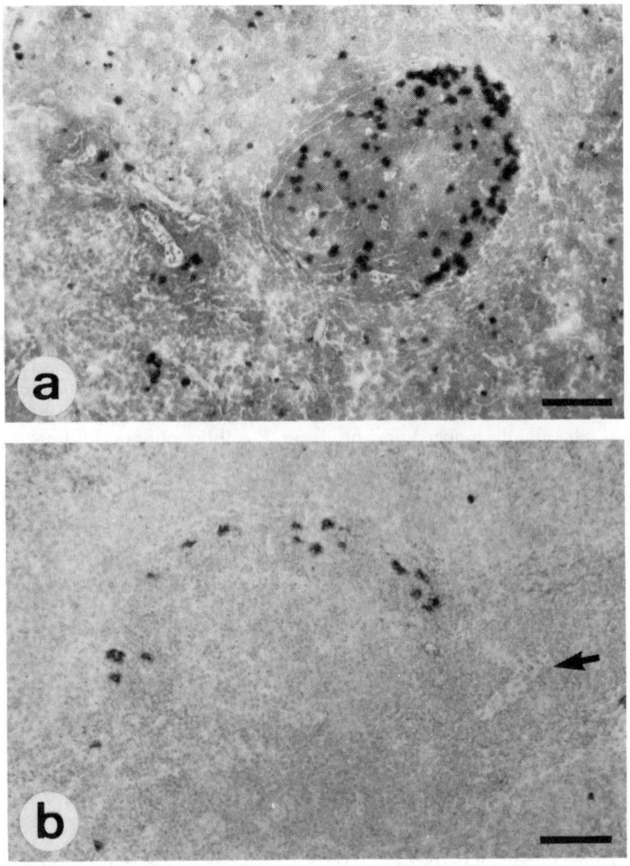

FIGURE 1. Indirect immunoperoxidase staining of (a) donor-derived class I MHC antigen-positive and (b) donor-derived class II MHC antigen-positive cells in the spleen of day 3 pancreas allograft recipients. Dark cells in the marginal zone and red pulp have endogenous peroxidase (Hemalum counterstain). Bar = 100 μm. (a): DA-to-LEW graft recipient: class I MHC-positive donor cells are found throughout the PALS and accumulate in the follicle corona (NDS 54 antibody). (b): LEW-to-LEW.1U graft recipient: donor class II MHC-positive cells are only situated in the follicle corona (F17-23-2 antibody). Arrow indicates central artery.

because of the different strain specificities of the antibodies employed. From days 4 and 5 on, no intact donor class I or class II MHC-positive cells were detected. However, at the outer border of the PALS, and in the follicle corona, several macrophagelike cells were visible containing granular donor type class I or class II MHC-reactive material. Surprisingly, a crescent-shaped reticular staining pattern with antidonor class I and class II MHC antibodies was observed in the outer part of the follicle center in certain follicles. This staining was first visible on days 3 and 4 after pancreas grafting, and became more intensive on days 5–10. In most cases it was clearly much more pronounced than the reticular background staining in follicle centers seen after omission of the first antibody. In addition, neither irrelevant A1D2 antibody ascites used in identical dilution nor RT1.A^a-specific NDS 54 ascites applied to LEW-to-LEW.1U spleen sections produced such a staining pattern. In the red pulp of the recipient's spleen no major accumulations of donor-type cells were detected, although during days 2–4 single cells appeared in this compartment. The red pulp was not investigated in detail in this study.

Following heart transplantation in the strain combinations DA-to-LEW and LEW-to-LEW.1U, there was no immigration of major numbers of donor cells into the recipient white pulp. There seemed to be very low numbers of dendritic shaped donor class I and class II MHC-positive cells present in the PALS on days 1 and 2. Not more than 5–10 of these cells were detected per spleen cross section. The reticular staining observed in the follicle centers of pancreas allograft recipients was also seen with class I and class II MHC reagents in heart allograft recipients from day 6 on.

Visualization of a monomorphic class II determinant with 0x6 antibody showed a substantial broadening of the Ia-positive marginal zone, and an increase in class II MHC-positive cells in the red pulp from days 1–10 in pancreas and heart graft recipients.

Our study demonstrates that, during the first 4–5 days after transplantation of fully allogeneic or MHC-incompatible whole-pancreas allografts in the rat, substantial numbers of donor-derived lymphocytes enter the traffic areas of the recipient's splenic white pulp. This phenomenon is not observed after heart grafting in the same strain combinations. It is obviously due to the great number of lymph nodes inevitably transplanted along with the pancreatic tissue. These lymph nodes can be well distinguished in paraffin sections of the graft and they undergo enlargement during acute rejection (unpublished observation). In contrast, no major lymph nodes are attached to the graft in heart transplantation. The donor cells reaching the heart recipient's white pulp during days 1–2 may well be emigrated interstitial dendritic cells, although their exact morphology was difficult to assess.

The distribution of donor type class I and class II MHC-positive cells observed in pancreas recipients corresponds to the differential migration patterns described by Nieuwenhuis and Ford (*9*) for rat T and B lymphocytes 24 hr after a single i.v. injection of radioactively labeled syngeneic lymphocytes. Thus we confirmed that there is no MHC restriction of the emigration of recirculating lymphocytes through vessel walls and in B-cell–T-cell segregation in the spleen (*10*). Unfortunately, the migration patterns of allogeneic B and T cells could not be investigated in more detail because the specificities of the antibodies used prevented double staining for donor class I and class II MHC antigens. Indirect comparison of recipient spleens in two different strain combinations indicates that, in the follicle corona, donor class I MHC-positive cells are much more abundant than cells carrying donor class II MHC antigens. This suggests that a substantial number of donor lymphocytes in this compartment are in fact T cells.

Using several nonhistological techniques and autoradiography, two groups have shown that, in rats, allogeneic lymphocytes are destroyed by an NK-like process during the first 12 hr after i.v. injection. This rapid killing of allogeneic lymphoid cells was assumed to be T-cell-independent, nonspecific, and critically dependent on the presence of the spleen (*10, 11*). In fact, it was demonstrated that there were no intact allogeneic cells present in the recipient spleen 24 hr after i.v. injection, and the radioactive label was taken up by phagocytic cells in the PALS (*10*). Our investigation, however, shows that allogeneic lymphocytes derived from pancreas grafts are virtually absent from the recipient spleen at 24 hr, but intact cells appear in great numbers two or three days later. The most likely cause of this late immigration is the destruction of the lymphatics draining the graft, which leads to discharge of lymph into the recipient's peritoneal cavity. It has been shown that lymphocytes injected into this site readily enter the recirculating pool

(*12*). Thus, the delayed arrival of donor cells in the recipient spleen would be due to an additional lymph node passage in this situation. Alternatively, lymphocytes may leave the grafted nodes by the venous route, a mechanism that has not been observed in normal rats (Pabst R, personal communication). The fact that detectable numbers of intact allogeneic lymphocytes are observed in the recipient spleen may be due to the continuous supply of cells from the transplanted lymph nodes, which may suffice to temporarily overcome the loss by nonspecific killing. Of course, we cannot exclude any phenomena occurring earlier than 24 hr after grafting. The modal transit time of syngeneic rat thoracic duct cells through the spleen is assumed to be in the range of 4–5 hr (*13*). Thus, we should have been able to detect the remnants of allogeneic cells on day 1, if they had been destroyed earlier. On days 4 and 5 macrophages in the PALS and follicle corona clearly contained large clumps of donor-type material. The location of these cells differed from that of typical interdigitating Ia-positive cells in the PALS—however, their exact nature remains to be defined.

The crescent-shaped reticular staining pattern observed in some follicle centers of pancreas and heart graft recipients after day 4 clearly requires a more detailed investigation. Obviously it is due to staining of follicular dendritic cells (FDCs) by donor-specific reagents. However, not all FDCs present in the follicle center are visualized, and not all splenic follicles are stained. The controls described seem to exclude that the phenomenon is due to Fc receptors on FDCs, nevertheless, some cases with high background staining were difficult to interpret, and a more rigorous demonstration of specificity is necessary. A fascinating hypothesis is that the staining is really due to complexes of allogeneic MHC antigenic material and antibody bound to FDCs in a way similar to that known for soluble antigens (*14*). If this is the case, a prolonged persistence of the pattern can be anticipated.

Irrespective of the role FDCs, our results offer a potential explanation for the differences in survival observed in pancreas and heart allografts in rat strain combinations with limited genetic incompatibility. Heart grafts incompatible at classic class I MHC antigens (RT1.A) or non-MHC antigens survived for more than 100 days, while pancreas grafts were acutely rejected using identical donor-recipient combinations (*15–17*). The transfer of major numbers of immunocompetent lymphocytes along with a pancreas graft may induce a competition of both host-versus-graft and graft-versus-host reactions, especially if the recipient is only partially histoincompatible with the donor.

Acknowledgments. We wish to thank R. Pabst, M.D., for helpful discussions, J. Fabre, Ph.D., for kindly providing the NDS 54 and F 17-23-2 antibodies, and G. S. Eisenbarth, M.D., for supplying the A1D2 ascites. P. Peschel and M. Giesecke provided technical assistance.

BIRTE STEINIGER[2]

JÜRGEN KLEMPNAUER

Zentrum Anatomie

Abteilung V and Klinik für Abdominal und Transplantationschirurgie

Hannover Medical School

Federal Republic of Germany

[2] Address reprint requests to: Birte Steiniger, M.D., Zentrum Anatomie, Abteilung V, 4150, Medizinische Hochschule, Postfach 610180, D-3000 Hannover 61, FRG.

REFERENCES

1. Lechler RI, Batchelor JR. Restoration of immunogenicity to passenger cell-depleted kidney allografts by the addition of donor strain dendritic cells. J Exp Med 1982; 155: 31.
2. Faustman D, Hauptfeld V, Lacy P, et al. Prolongation of murine islet allograft survival by pretreatment of islets with antibody directed to Ia determinants. Proc Natl Acad Sci USA 1981; 78: 5156.
3. Hart DNJ, Winearls CG, Fabre JW. Graft adaptation: studies on possible mechanisms in long-term surviving rat renal allografts. Transplantation 1980; 30: 73.
4. Steiniger B, Klempnauer J, Wonigeit K. Phenotype and histological distribution of interstitial dendritic cells in the rat pancreas, liver, heart and kidney. Transplantation 1984; 38: 169.
5. Milton AD, Fabre JW. Massive induction of donor type class I and class II MHC antigens in rejecting cardiac allografts in the rat. J Exp Med 1985; 161: 98.
6. Hart DNJ, Fabre JW. Major histocompatibility complex antigens in rat kidney, ureter and bladder. Transplantation 1981; 31: 318.
7. McMaster WR, Williams AF. Identification of Ia glycoproteins in rat thymus and purification from rat spleen. Eur J Immunol 1979; 9: 426.
8. Crump MA, Scearce R, Dobersen M, et al. Production and characterization of a cytotoxic monoclonal antibody reacting with rat islet cells. J Clin Invest 1982; 70: 659.
9. Nieuwenhuis P, Ford WL. Comparative migration of B- and T-lymphocytes in the rat spleen and lymph nodes. Cell Immunol 1976; 23: 254.
10. Rolstad B, Ford WL. The rapid elimination of allogeneic lymphocytes: relationship to established mechanisms of immunity and to lymphocyte traffic. Immunol Rev 1983; 73: 87.
11. Heslop B, McNeilage LJ. Natural cytotoxicity: early killing of allogeneic lymphocytes in rats. Immunol Rev 1983; 73: 35.
12. Binns RM, Pabst R, Licence ST. The behaviour of pig lymphocytes in vivo. In: Tumbleson ME, ed. Swine in biomedical research. (in press).
13. Smith ME, Ford WL. The recirculating lymphocyte pool of the rat: a systematic description of the migratory behaviour of recirculating lymphocytes. Immunology 1983; 49: 83.
14. Tew JG, Phipps RP, Mandel TE. The maintenance and regulation of the humoral immune response: persisting antigen and the role of follicular antigen-binding dendritic cells as accessory cells. Immunol Rev 1980; 53: 175.
15. Klempnauer J, Hoins L, Steiniger B, et al. Evidence for a differential importance of MHC and non-MHC alloantigens in pancreas and heart transplantation in the rat. Transplant Proc 1984; 16: 778.
16. Klempnauer J, Steiniger B, Wonigeit K, et al. Genetics of heart allograft rejection in the rat. Transplant Proc 1985; 17: 1897.
17. Klempnauer J, Wonigeit K, Steiniger B, et al. Pancreas whole organ transplantation in the rat: differential effect of individual MHC regions. Transplant Proc 1983; 15: 1308.

Received 24 September 1985.
Accepted 8 October 1985.

THE RATIONALE FOR ANTIMITOTIC TREATMENT PRIOR TO BONE MARROW TRANSPLANTATION

Empiricism has always played a major role in medicine. Very often in clinical practice procedures that work are adopted well before their rationale is clear and supported by observations derived in experimental systems. One example of this is the antimitotic regimen often used prior to bone marrow transplantation (*1, 2*). Although such treatment is quite logical when malignant or myeloproliferative disease is involved, there is no theoretical need for it in diseases like aplastic anemia (*3*). As a matter of fact, if aplastic anemia is due to reduced (or absent) activity in the hematopoietic stem cell compartment, infusion of marrow from a healthy identical twin should result in prompt hematologic recovery even without conditioning the recipient with antimitotic agents. Different authors, however, have reported several marrow grafts from identical twins in patients with acquired severe aplastic anemia (ASAA)* who did not recover following a simple infusion of syngeneic bone marrow (*4–6*). Surprisingly, when conditioned with cyclophosphamide, most of these patients did recover following a second infusion of syngeneic marrow. Camitta and his colleagues proposed that cyclophosphamide could inhibit a regulatory or immune mechanism suppressing normal stem cell growth and differentiation, or eradicate dysfunctional stem cells occupying critical marrow niches (*7*). Thomas and Storb (*8*) preferred the alternative that cyclophosphamide could overcome an autoimmune disorder underlying ASAA. In the course of studies of lymphocyte turnover, we came upon observations that could well provide the appropriate explanation and the experimental basis for this clinical practice. Thus we have found altered patterns of homing of autologous and grafted blood cells in mice submitted to an antimitotic regimen (*9*). We have used a new protocol of prolonged in vivo hydroxyurea (HU) administration that eliminates all cycling cells. Mice were injected twice a day for four consecutive days with HU at 1 mg/g body weight, a dose

* Abbreviations used: ASAA, acquired severe aplastic anemia; HU, hydroxyurea; RBC, red blood cells.

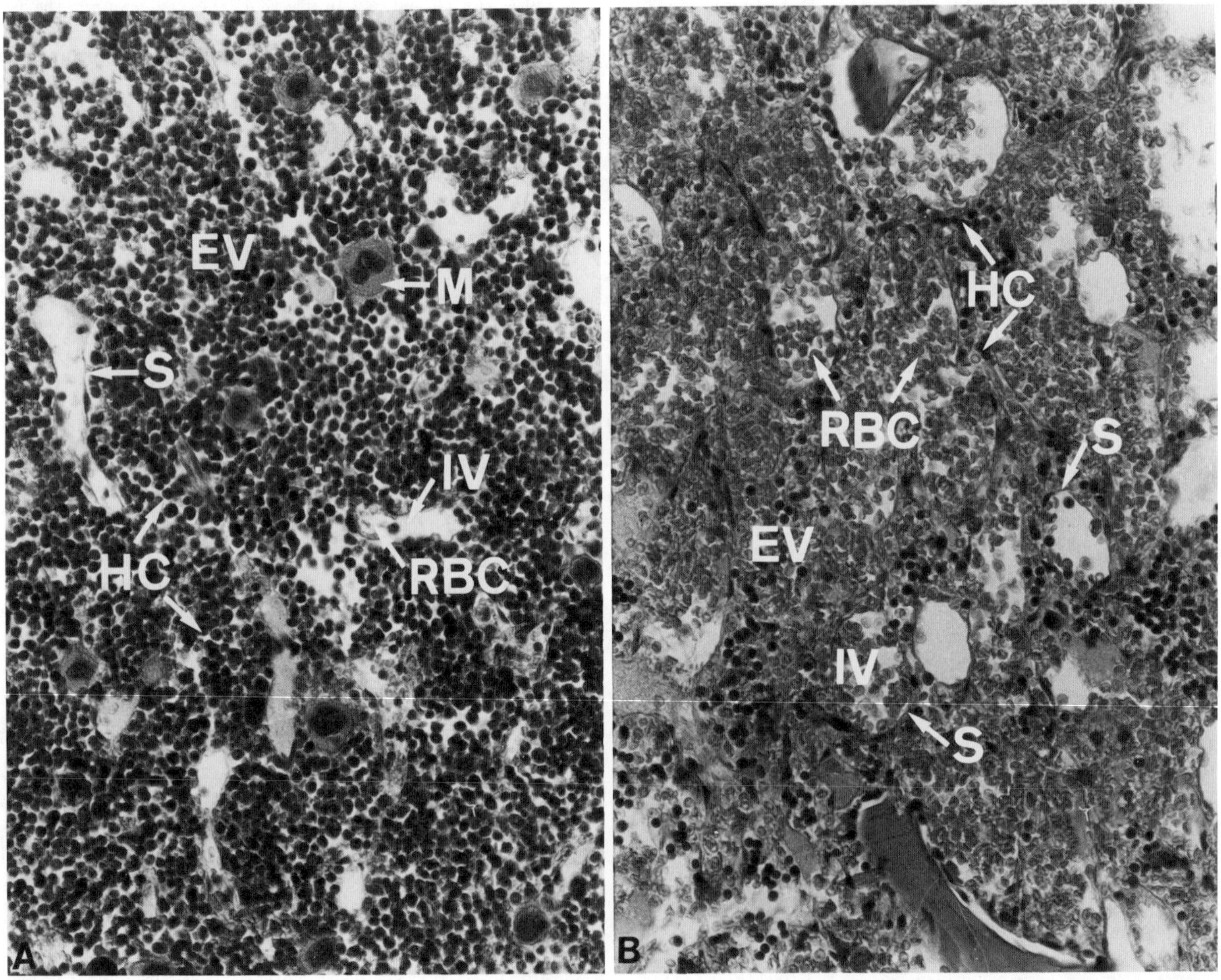

FIGURE 1. Overall view of bone marrow from 12-week-old C57BL/6 mice. (A) normal bone marrow; (B) bone marrow from HU-treated mice. EV: extravascular space; HC: hemopoietic cells; IV: intravascular space; M: megakaryocyte; RBC: red blood cells; S: sinus wall. After fixation, femurs were embedded in paraffin and all the different sections were mounted and stained (hematein and phloxin; ×200 [slightly reduced]).

previously established to kill all cycling cells when administered twice with a 7-hr interval (*10*). This treatment kills 99% of nonlymphoid nucleated bone marrow cells, and it eliminates peripheral short-lived lymphocytes (around 70% of B cells and 40% of T lymphocytes) (*11*). An increased concentration of mature red blood cells (RBC), as well as an abnormal distribution of T and B lymphocytes in bone marrow of HU-treated animals lead us to suspect that cell migration/homing patterns were altered by the antimitotic regimen. This was confirmed by injecting spleen and bone marrow cells i.v. into normal and HU-treated recipients. The recovery of grafted normal spleen cells in the spleen of HU-treated recipients was roughly 10 times lower than that obtained in normal recipients. In contrast, bone marrow of HU-treated animals was considerably more "permeable" to the homing of transfused cells, as 3 to 4 times more cells were recovered in the marrow of such recipients, no matter what the injected cells were (spleen or bone marrow cells from syngeneic or allogeneic donors) (*9*). It appeared, therefore, that the antimitotic treatment altered local conditions in bone marrow and allowed for a higher migration of circulating cells into this organ. The decrease in migration of cells into the spleen of HU-treated animals might be merely a secondary effect. Two possibilities, or a combination of them, could account for the altered migration and distribution of lymphocytes and RBC after this long-term HU-treatment: an alteration of the bone marrow-blood barrier achieved by the massive antimitotic administration leading to an enhanced permeability of the barrier and an expansion of the vascular sinuses in order to compensate for the relative emptiness of the extravascular space, with a consequent greater blood volume per shaft. This second hypothesis implies, however, that free bone marrow space left by HU treatment is the primary phenomenon leading to the enhanced cell migration into the marrow. In order to find an answer to these questions, morphological studies were performed. Figure 1 shows bone marrow tissues from normal (A) and HU-treated (B) C57BL/6 mice. The different types of blood cell precursors in the normal bone marrow are intermingled with one another as well as with fat cells and with fibroblasts. The whole tissue is richly supplied with thin-walled blood vessels that constitute part of the bone marrow blood barrier. As expected, mature RBC are absent from the extravascular space. Bone marrow from HU-treated animals (Fig. 1B) shows a marked difference in its overall pattern, as compared with normal marrow. Very few blood cell precursors are left, and a striking amount of RBC "fills up" the whole marrow tissue. Figure 2 shows another feature of bone marrow from HU-treated mice. Numerous adipose cells covering a great proportion of the marrow tissue are observed. Adipocytes are known to develop in the empty space of the marrow in chronic aplastic anemia (*12*). Although this study was performed after only four days of antimitotic regimen, a consistent part of the marrow tissue was already occupied by adipose cells. This observation rules out the possibility that RBC preferentially migrate to the marrow of HU-treated mice only to "fill up" the free bone marrow space.

A higher magnification of bone marrow from normal (A) and HU-treated (B) mice is shown in Figure 3. These pictures are centered on the marrow sinuses. A simple flattened endothelium lines the sinusoids of normal bone marrow separating intravascular and extravascular spaces. As shown in Figure 3B, marrow sinusoids were expanded and the sinus wall integrity seems affected by HU treatment. Moreover, an extravasation

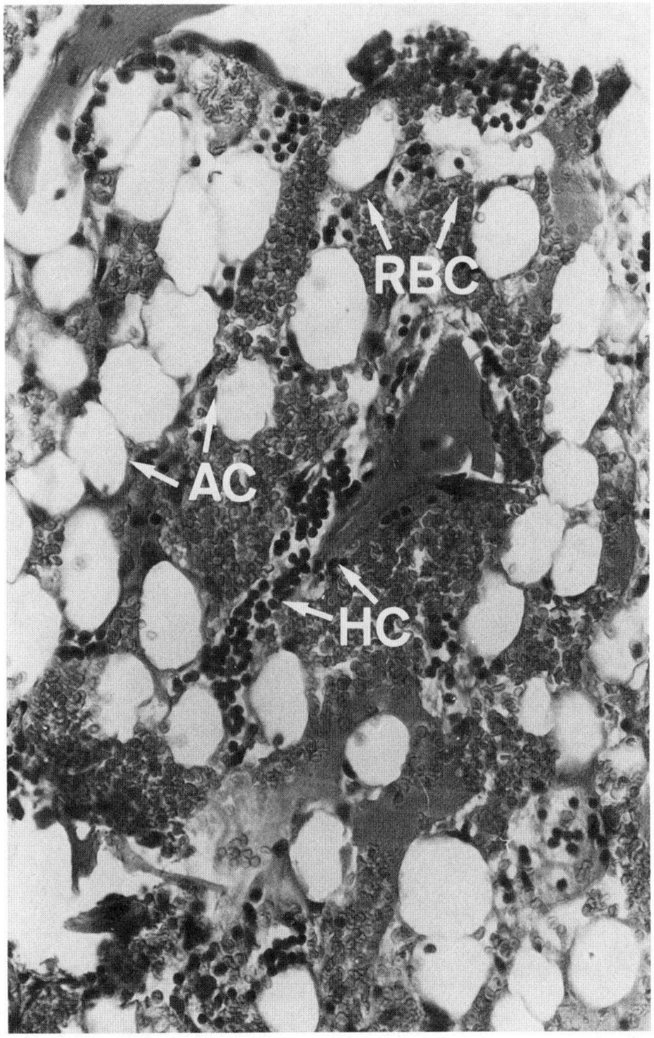

FIGURE 2. Bone marrow from HU-treated mice. AC: adipose cells; HC: hemopoietic cells; RBC: red blood cells (×200 [slightly reduced]).

of RBC was clearly observed leading to the presence of mature RBC in the extravascular space of bone marrow. It is impossible, however, to deduce from these observations the primary phenomenon leading to this modified marrow architecture. The most likely explanation would be an expansion of the marrow sinusoids followed by an extravasation of blood cells out of the vascular compartment.

The increased blood-to-marrow permeability resulting from the antimitotic treatment could explain the fact that transfused cells localize far more efficiently to the recipient marrow after HU administration. In other words, these observations support the hypothesis that one of the major benefits of antimitotic pretreatment of bone marrow recipients is an enhanced migration of donor blood cells to the marrow due to the marked histological and hemodynamical alterations of the marrow sinusoids. Although these results only stress the enhanced migration of transfused cells into the marrow and do not study stem cell development, they could be of importance when considering the possibility of antimitotic regimens prior to grafting individuals with hemopoietic precursors.

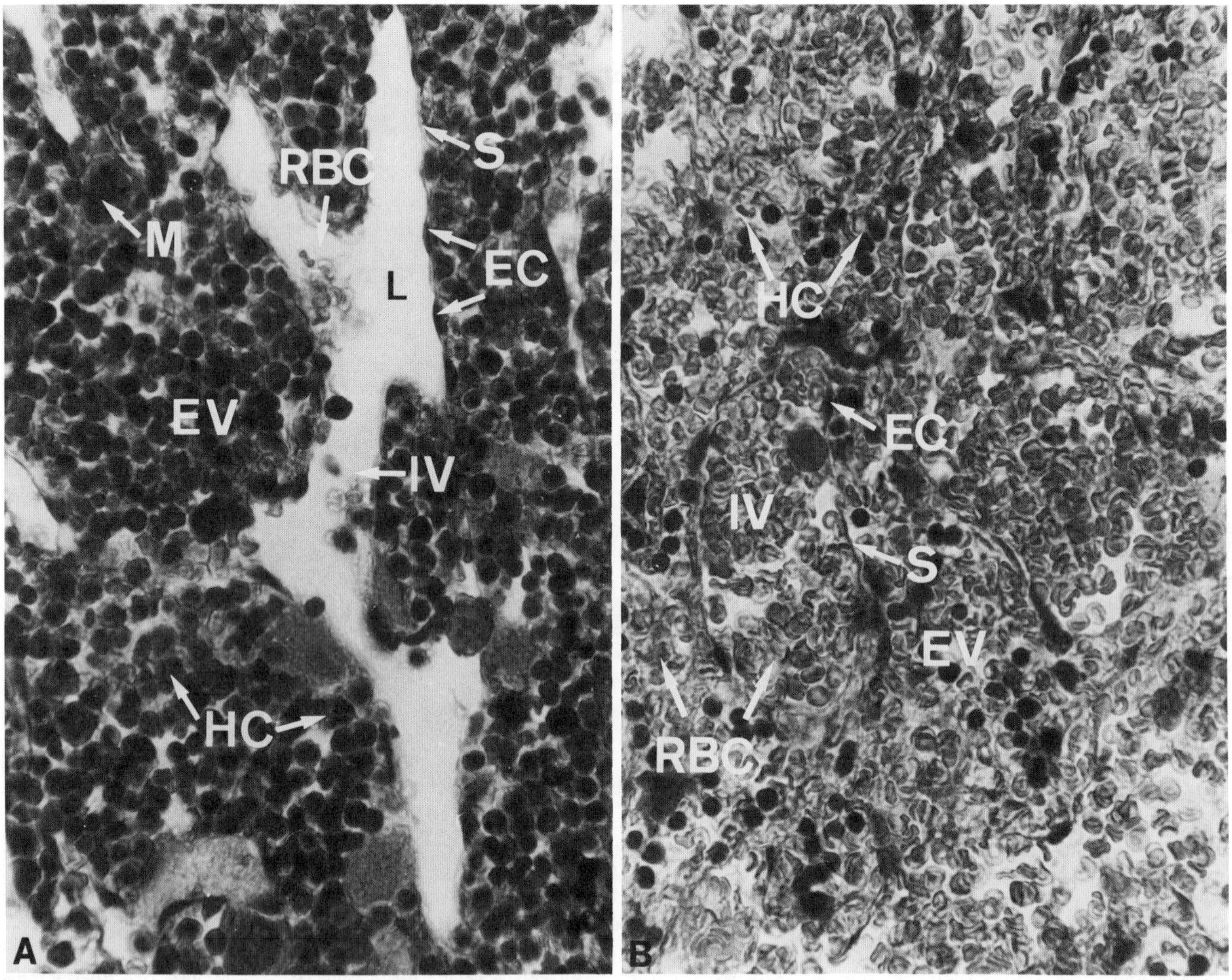

FIGURE 3. Bone marrow sinuses from normal (A) and HU-treated mice (B). EC: endothelial cells; EV: extravascular space; HC: hemopoietic cells; IV: intravascular space; L: lumen; M: megakaryocyte; RBC: red blood cells; S: sinus wall (×400 [slightly reduced]).

Acknowledgments. I thank Patrick Avé and Pierre Ravisse for their expertise in histological preparations, Miguel Coquis Rondon for his photographic skills, António Coutinho for critical reading of the manuscript, and Jacqueline Badella for excellent secretarial work.

MARTINE LÉVY[1]
Unité d'Immunobiologie
Département d'Immunologie
Institut Pasteur
F-75724 Paris Cédex 15
France

[1] Address correspondence to: Dr. Martine Lévy, Unité d'Immunobiologie, Institut Pasteur, 25 rue du Docteur Roux, 75724 Paris Cédex 15, France.

REFERENCES

1. Parkman R, Rappeport J, Camitta B, et al. Successful use of multiagent immunosuppression in the bone marrow transplantation of sensitized patients. Blood 1978; 52: 1163.
2. Devergie A, Gluckman E. Bone marrow transplantation in severe aplastic anemia following cytoxan and thoraco-abdominal irradiation. Exp Hematol 1982; 10 (suppl 10): 17.
3. Storb R, Thomas ED, Buckner CD, et al. Marrow transplantation for aplastic anemia. Semin Hematol 1984; 21: 27.
4. Applebaum FR, Fefer A, Cheever MA, et al. Treatment of aplastic anemia by bone marrow transplantation in identical twins. Blood 1980; 55: 1033.
5. Lu DP. Syngeneic bone marrow transplantation for treatment of aplastic anemia: report of a case and review of the literature. Exp Hematol 1981; 9: 257.
6. Appelbaum FR, Cheever MA, Fefer A, Storb R, Thomas ED. Recurrence of aplastic anemia following cyclophosphamide and syngeneic bone marrow transplantation: evidence for two mechanisms of graft failure. Blood 1985; 65: 553.
7. Camitta BM, Storb R, Thomas ED. Aplastic anemia. Pathogenesis, diagnosis, treatment and prognosis. N Engl J Med 1982; 306: 645.
8. Thomas ED, Storb R. Acquired severe aplastic anemia: progress and perplexity. Blood 1984; 64: 325.
9. Lévy M. Altered patterns of organ distribution of autologous and grafted blood cells in mice treated with hydroxyurea. Transplantation 1986; 41: 204.
10. Hodgson GS, Bradley TR, Martin RF, et al. Recovery of proliferating haemopoietic progenitor cells after killing by hydroxyurea. Cell Tissue Kinet 1975; 8: 51.
11. Lévy M. Long-lived lymphocytes include lipopolysaccharide reactive B cells. Cell Immunol 1985; 96: 290.
12. Thomas ED. Aplastic anaemia. Clin Haematol 1978; 7: 429.

Received 16 July 1985.
Accepted 19 September 1985.

CYCLOSPORINE AND FAMILIAL MEDITERRANEAN FEVER AMYLOIDOSIS

The discovery of cyclosporine has brought about a true revolution in the field of transplantation in general and kidney transplantation in particular. The most cautions report claims a 20% increase in survival (*1*), while in many centers, including our own, survival has practically doubled.

The drug, however, has its side effects (*1*); fortunately few cause major concern. Their appearance demands reduction or cessation of the cyclosporine treatment with or without cahnge to the azathioprine and steroid protocol.

This report deals with a special group of amyloidotic patients, sufferers of familial Mediterranean fever (FMF),* who displayed poor tolerance to the drug.

FMF is an autosomal recessive disorder common in Sephardic Jews, Armenians, Turks, and Arabs of the Levant. The disease manifests itself during the first or second decade of life and is characterized by two independent phenotypic characters: episodically recurrent, short-lived, febrile attacks accompanied by peritonitis, pleurisy, or synovitis; and systemic amyloidosis of the AA type, causing death from renal failure at an early age (*2*).

FMF-amyloidotic patients represent 6% of the candidates for renal transplantation in Israel—most of them being young patients in their third and fourth decade. Chronic colchicine treatment prevents febrile attacks and renal amyloidosis, and it has been recommended for all FMF patients over the last 12 years, with good results and no significant side effects (*2*).

Case 1. A 33-year-old FMF-amyloidotic North African patient was transplanted in May 1984. The patient was considered at very high risk because of malignant hypertension, severe left heart hypertrophy, and uremic pericarditis. After an anuric phase of 20 days, despite excellent renal perfusion shown by technetium scans, a profuse diuresis started, resulting in rapid decrease of serum creatinine levels below 1 mg%. He was treated initially with cyclosporine 10 mg/kg, prednisolone 30 mg per day, and colchicine. The massive antihypertensive treatment was gradually discontinued. In the second week he began complaining of severe disabling abdominal pains, vomiting, and anorexia. He responded only partially to antidiarrheal medications. He then developed right hip arthralgia and sudden sharp pains in both feet that required prolonged hospitalization. All symptoms receded when the daily dose of cyclosporine was sharply reduced. Today, ten months after transplantation, he receives cyclosporine 1 mg/kg/day, prednisolone 7.5 mg, and colchicine 1.5 mg/day. The serum creatinine is 0.8 mg%.

Case 2. A twenty-eight year old North African Jew with FMF-renal amyloidosis was given a renal transplant in November 1984 (from his younger brother) after completion of a donor-specific blood transfusion protocol. He was treated with cyclosporine 10 mg/kg body weight and low-dose steroids. The postoperative course was satisfactory, with good urinary output; a serum creatinine level of 0.9 mg% was reached within 9 days. During the third week the patient began complaining of sharp sudden leg pains, very severe abdominal pains, weakness, vomiting, diarrhea, and hypertension. Symptomatic treatment, increased colchicine and a reduced cyclosporine daily dose did not, however, alleviate the patient's pains.

Finally, in the fourth week, the medication was altered to azathioprine 150 mg and prednisolone 15 mg daily; only then did the abdominal pains and the diarrhea stop. The patient became normotensive and his appetite returned to normal. His serum creatinine level today is 0.8 mg%.

Case 3. A 36-year-old North African man underwent his first cadaveric renal transplantation in 1982. He was treated at that time with the standard Imuran + steroid regimen when he experienced a violent steroid unresponsive rejection accompanied by high fever and convulsions, that dictated urgent transplant nephrectomy.

In April 1984 he underwent his second renal transplantation. At that time cyclosporine was still unavailable to us, so he was treated with the old immunosuppressive regimen, azathioprine and steroids. For the first three weeks after transplantation the patient was anuric; he had daily spikes of fever up to 39.5°C that did not responded to i.v. boluses of steroids. During the third week cyclosporine became available to us and he was treated with 10 mg/kg body weight. The fever disappeared, there was profuse diuresis, and his serum creatinine levels dropped below 1 mg%. At the end of two weeks he began complaining of sharp leg pains, severe bouts of diarrhea, and cramping abdominal pains that responded poorly to analgesics. These pains were severe enough to prevent his discharge. The oral cyclosporine dose was reduced gradually to 5 mg/kg/day, but the abdominal pains and diarrhea persisted. He lost his appetite and 10 kg weight; he also developed mild jaundice (bilirubin 4.2 mg, mostly indirect). The jaundice and abdominal pains completely disappeared when the cyclosporine was discontinued. Today, one year after transplantation, the serum creatinine is 0.5 mg%, and his weight is normal. He takes 7.5 mg prednisolone and colchicine 1 mg per day.

Early results in renal transplantation in FMF-amylidotic patients with conventional immunosuppressive regimens have been presented elsewhere (*3*). Five of ten transplanted patients died, all of them during episodes of rejection. The deaths were related to massive steroid therapy. The other five who did not reject are well with functioning grafts.

Later experience with twenty-one transplantations in this particular high risk group of patients led us to the hypothesis that they may belong to a privileged group of "low responders" requiring relatively low-dose immunosuppression (steroids in particular). This approach has markedly reduced postoperative morbidity and mortality (*4*). In addition, routine colchicine treatment has abolished the FMF crises in almost all patients, thereby improving their quality of life (*3*).

The introduction of cyclosporine as the main immunosuppressive drug in renal transplantation has resulted in a remarkably low incidence of episodes of rejection, thus removing the need for i.v. administration of high doses of prednisolone. At the same time the require maintenance dose of prednisone has also been reduced at most centers, and some do without it altogether (*5, 6*).

Despite its remarkably attributes, cyclosporine has side effects that, in amyloidotic patients, are severe enough to dictate rapid diminution of the administered dose, its cessation, or change to azathioprine. The following complications appeared in all three cases by the end of the second week or the begining of the third: severe abdominal pains, anorexia, vomiting, diarrhea, sharp sudden leg pains, weakness and weight loss (Table 1). The abdominal pains, however, were not accompanied by the peritoneal signs typical of FMF crisis (*2*).

* Abbreviation used: FMF, familial Mediterranean fever.

TABLE 1. Cyclosporine and FMF amyloidosis

Case number	Side effects	Present status	Present treatment
1.	Severe abdominal pains Vomiting Diarrhea Severe weakness Anorexia Weight loss Sharp sudden leg pains	Serum creatinine 0.9 Works full time	Cyclosporine 1 m/kg Prednisone 7.5 mg Colchicine 1.5 mg
2.	Severe abdominal pains Diarrhea Severe weakness Vomiting Hypertension Sharp sudden leg pains	Serum creatinine 0.8 Normotensive Works full time	Azathioprine 150 mg Prednisone 10 mg Colchicine 1 mg
3.	Severe abdominal pains Diarrhea Vomiting Severe anorexia Weight loss (10 kg) Sharp sudden leg pains Mild jaundice	Serum creatinin 0.5 Chronic active hepatitis	Prednisone 7.5 mg Colchicine 1 mg

A fourth amyloidotic patient had his transplanted kidney removed on the 9th postoperative day because of severe jaundice, leukopenia, and thrombocytopenia. Besides cyclosporine, the patient was treated with inadvertantly high doses of ceftizoxime. He was found retrospectively to have an active cytomegalic viral infection. Whether the jaundice was a result of cyclosporine treatment, rejection, cytomegalovirus infection, or ceftizoxime intoxication is uncertain. The duration of cyclosporine treatment in this case was too short for signs of cyclosporine intolerance to occur.

One could be tempted to discourage the use of the drug in amyloidotic patients; however, some of these patients have lost their kidneys to rejection using conventional treatment (azathioprine and steroids), but they did not experience any episode of rejection when treated with cyclosporine (case 3).

Our counsel is to treat the amyloidotic patients initially with cyclosporine (10–12 mg/kg) and to expect the complications to occur in the third week; when they do occur, there is a choice to reduce the dose rapidly to very low levels (2 mg/kg or less), to switch to azathioprine, or simply to stop the cyclosporine. This should permit simple and safe management of the first two critical weeks, retaining the benefits of the steroid-sparing effect of cyclosporine, and thus avoiding the steroid toxicity that has, in the past, led to a very high morbidity and mortality in this particular group of patients (*3*, *4*).

An interesting question is whether or not cyclosporine affects amyloidosis or amyloidotic deposits. A partial answer may be found in experiments carried out in our laboratory. In murine experimental amyloidosis cyclosporine did not seem to affect the development of amyloidosis (see the accompanying Letter to the Editor, page 799).

Bruno Siegal[1]
Debora Zemer[2]
Mordechai Pras[2]
Transplantation Unit
Sheba Medical Center
Heller Institute of Medical Research
Sheba Medical Center
Tel-Hashomer, Israel

[1] Transplantation Unit.
[2] Heller Institute of Medical Research.

REFERENCES

1. Starzl TE. Clinical aspects of cyclosporin therapy. In: Kahan BD, ed. Cyclosporin. New York: Grune & Stratton, 1984.
2. Gafni J, Sohar E, Zemr D. Amyloid nephropathy. In: Hamburger, ed. Nephrology. New York: Wiley, 1979.
3. Jacob ET, Bar-Nathan N, Shapira Z, Gafni J. Renal transplantation in the amyloidosis of FMF. Arch Intern Med 1979; 139: 1135.
4. Jacob ET, Siegal B, Bar-Nathan N, Gafni J. Improving outlook for renal transplantation in amyloid nephropathy. Transplant Proc 1982; 14(1): 41.
5. Calne RY, White DIG, Evans DB. Cyclosporin A in cadaveric organ transplantation. Br Med J 1981; 282: 934.
6. Starzl TE, Hakala TR, Rosenthal JT. The Colorado-Pittsburgh cadaveric renal transplantation study with cyclosporin. Transplant Proc 1983; 25(4): 2459.

Received 23 August 1985.
Accepted 13 October 1985.

SUPEROXIDE DISMUTASE DECREASE IN CARDIAC TRANSPLANTS[1]

Genetic dissimilarity between donor and host determines the fate of a foreign organ transplanted into a human or animal host. When the two are very dissimilar, normal tissue architecture in the allograft is destroyed and the graft is rejected (1, 2). The molecular mechanism of graft rejection is unknown, but large inflammatory changes accompany, for example, cardiac tissue rejection—lympocytic myocarditis appears and the

[1] This work was supported by the New Brunswick (Canada) Heart Foundation, and by the Medical Research Council of Canada.

graft is infiltrated by monocytes and polymorphonuclear leukocytes (PMNLs)* (1, 3). The coupling mechanism between this inflammatory leukocyte infiltration and graft destruction is very poorly understood. There is, however, much evidence that activated PMNLs and monocytes can generate superoxide (respiratory burst), and that superoxide and the hydroxyl radical (formed from $O_2^{\cdot-}$ + H_2O_2) are toxic to biomolecules (4). Damage to membranes is a particular problem since a cascade of damage can propagate through the unsaturated portions of the lipids following initial radical attack (5).

Much attention has been focussed on the details of the inflammatory response of the host, but the transplanted organ itself is provided with an efficient antioxidative defense system. We reasoned that inflammatory damage to transplanted tissue and the eventual destruction of this tissue may involve inactivation of one or more of the antioxidative defense enzymes in the transplanted tissue. We were encouraged in this belief by a recent study showing that neutrophil depletion or pretreatment with superoxide dismutase (SOD) inhibited severe cardiovascular dysfunction in dogs treated with phorbol myristate acetate (a potent neutrophil activator) (6). SOD is one of the primary tissue defense enzymes, catalyzing dismutation of the superoxide radical in a reaction that can be summarized thus:

$$2O_2^{\cdot-} + 2H^+ \rightarrow H_2O_2 + O_2$$

Intraabdominal cardiac allografts exchanged between appropriate strains of inbred rats are an ideal in vivo system for controlled investigation of the pathogenesis of graft rejection because of the relative morphological and structural homogeneity of the myocardium, and the reproducibility, in time, of gross histological events of acute rejection. Male rats (250–300 g) from two inbred strains, Lewis (RT-1^l) and BN (RT-1^n) were used to perform syngeneic (Lewis→Lewis) and allogeneic (BN→Lewis) heart transplantations (isografts and allografts, respectively). Heterotopic cardiac allografts and isografts were transplanted to the great abdominal vessels of recipient animals using a modification of the method of Ono and Lindsey (7). Cardiac isografts survive indefinitely, but the allografts are totally rejected within 7 days.

Organs were removed and processed separately from transplanted and control animals on the 5th day posttransplantation since lymphoid cell infiltration of the allograft peaks at 5±2 days. The excised organs were: cardiac allograft and isograft, the graft recipient's own heart, the hearts of nontransplanted BN and Lewis control rats, and the spleens and livers of all graft recipients and Lewis control rats. These organs were chosen because the transplant recipient's own heart and liver are not intimately involved in the rejection process (and will serve as controls) while the spleen is. Molecular events seen in the cardiac allograft that are integral to rejection may be mirrored in the animal's spleen.

Enzyme activities were assayed in the supernatants of the Polytron treated tissues (12,000 ×g supernatant used for GSH.Px and SOD; 800 ×g supernatant for catalase [CAT]). SOD was assayed by the xanthine/xanthine oxidase/cytochrome c method of McCord and Fridovich (8). GSH.Px was assayed by the coupled glutathione reductase/NADPH method of Paglia and Valentine (9) using t-butyl hydroperoxide as substrate. CAT was assayed by the $KMnO_4$ method of Cohen et al. (10). Protein was measured by the method of Lowry et al. (11).

To measure protein synthesis, isograft and allograft recipients—as well as control Lewis and BN rats—were injected, i.v., 5 days posttransplantation with L-[^{35}S]-methionine (New England Nuclear) in saline (800 μCi/rat). After 2 hr the rats were sacrificed and tissues were homogenized in 5 ml of TRIS-EDTA, pH 7.4, on ice, and were centrifuged at 800 ×g for 10 min at 4°C. Sample aliquots from the resulting supernatants were incubated with pancreatic ribonuclease A (Sigma) at a final concentration 0.1 mg/ml and run in a 7–17% SDS gradient polyacrylamide slab gel (12). Equivalent radioactivity was loaded into each sample well of a gel. The gel was then processed for autoradiography by soaking in Enlightning (New England Nuclear), drying, and exposing to Kodak XAR-5 film for 6 weeks at −80°C.

Peroxidative damage to cardiac membranes was measured by the amount of thiobarbituric acid-reactive material in the 12,000 ×g supernatant of allograft homogenates (13).

SOD activities in the various cardiac tissues and in the livers and spleens of transplanted and nonoperated control animals are given in Table 1. Both specific and total SOD activities are greatly decreased in allografts (33–40% lower than control hearts), and specific SOD activity is decreased also in the spleens of allograft recipients (~53% lower). In the cardiac isograft there is a much smaller decrease in SOD levels. There appears to be an increase in total SOD activity in the transplant recipients' own hearts, as if in compensation for the general inflammatory response to the transplant operation. The dramatic decreases in SOD activities in cardiac allografts are not a general result of the trauma of surgery; they are seen only in the transplanted hearts of the genetically dissimilar transplantations and not in the transplant recipients' own hearts or in their livers.

The spleen is an organ important to the rejection process. Total SOD activity in the allograft recipients' spleen is statistically comparable to control spleen levels, but the specific SOD activity is decreased. This seems to indicate that SOD remains normal in the spleen but that the increased splenic activity associated with inflammatory response to the allograft is ac-

TABLE 1. SOD activity in rats' organs at 5 days posttransplantation

Organ	Specific activity U/mg protein	Total activity
Lewis control heart	13.1±1.7[a] (6)[b]	237±12
BN control heart	14.0±5.5 (4)	278±11[c]
Isograft recipient's own heart	13.5±1.9 (5)	264±43[d] ↑[f]
Cardiac isograft	10.7±2.4[c] (5) ↓[e]	207±18[c] ↓
Allograft recipient's own heart	12.4±1.5 (6)	264±20[c] ↑
Cardiac allograft	8.0±2.6[c] (6) ↓	185±38[c] ↓
Lewis control liver	11.4±2.5 (5)	2439±312
Isograft recipient's liver	10.3±1.6 (5)	2648±277
Allograft recipient's liver	11.1±3.0 (6)	2514±223
Lewis control spleen	11.8±4.0 (5)	189±29
Isograft recipient's spleen	8.8±2.6[d] (5) ↓	173 ± 40
Allograft recipient's spleen	5.6±2.1[c] (6) ↓	157 ± 44

[a] Mean ± SD.
[b] Number of rats tested.
[c] Values significantly different at $P = 0.05$ using Student's t test.
[d] Values significantly different at $P = 0.1$ using Student's t test.
[e] (↓) Decrease in activity relative to Lewis control.
[f] (↑) Increase in activity relative to Lewis control.

* Abbreviations used: CAT, catalase; GSH.Px, glutathione peroxidase; MDA, malonaldehyde; PMNLs, polymorphonuclear lymphocytes; SOD, superoxide dismutase; TBA, thiobarbituric acid.

TABLE 2. GSH.Px and CAT activity in rats' organs at 5 days posttransplantation

Organ	GSH.Px activity (U/mg protein)	Catalase activity (U/mg protein)
Lewis control heart	231±57[a] (5)[b]	1.8±0.4 (5)
BN control heart	178 (1)	2.7 (1)
Isograft recipient's own heart	239±60 (5)	1.8±0.5 (4)
Cardiac isograft	167±15 (5)	1.9±0.6 (4)
Allograft recipient's own heart	229±28 (3)	2.1±0.5 (3)
Cardiac allograft	237±54 (3)	1.6±0.1 (3)
Lewis control liver	351±98 (5)	21±7 (5)
Isograft recipient's liver	319±98 (5)	25±17 (4)
Allograft recipient's liver	553±262 (3)	33±10 (3)
Lewis control spleen	176±38 (5)	3.9±1.2 (5)
Isograft recipient's spleen	167±36 (5)	5.0±2.9 (5)
Allograft recipient's spleen	200±28 (3)	5.3±1.0 (3)

[a] Mean ± SD.
[b] Number of rats tested.

companied by increases in soluble proteins other than SOD.

Glutathione peroxidase (GSH.Px) and CAT, two other antioxidative enzymes, were unchanged or very little affected in the transplanted hearts (Table 2).

Decreases in SOD activity may be due to destruction of SOD in situ, to a decrease in SOD synthesis, or to a combination of the two. Autoradiography of tissue homogenates (taken on the 5th day posttransplantation) indicate comparable levels of protein synthesis in cardiac allografts, cardiac isografts, and nonoperated control hearts. We measured protein synthesis for only 2 hr on the 5th day posttransplantation, and this does not tell us about protein synthesis during the whole rejection period. But 5±2 days can be considered the peak time of host response to the allograft. As a first approximation the identical patterns of protein synthesis in the controls and allograft (which we found) indicate that decrease in the synthesis of SOD is not the primary cause of lower enzyme activities in the allografts.

Host response to the allograft involves mobilization of inflammatory cells at the graft site and a subsequent respiratory burst. The O_2^- thus generated can ultimately cause a cascade of oxidized products from a membrane, and these products include lipid hydroperoxides. We postulate that SOD in the allograft may be inactivated by continuous toxic-oxygen bombardment, and that radical and peroxide damage can then proceed unchecked by the enzyme defense system. That SOD can be inactivated in vivo by exposure to toxic oxygen products is supported by previous studies demonstrating inactivation of the enzyme by high levels of H_2O_2 in vitro (14).

We looked for biochemical evidence of increased membrane damage in cardiac allografts using the thiobarbituric (TBA) assay for malonaldehyde. In preliminary experiments we measured MDA levels in the allografts at 5 and 7 days posttransplantation. Two animals were sacrificed at 5 days—one with a nearly normal heart rate of the allograft and with nearly normal SOD levels, and the second representative of peak host response (slow heart rate and reduced SOD activity). A third animal was sacrificed at 7 days posttransplantation when the allograft had ceased to beat. MDA levels were dramatically increased (100% and 210%, respectively) over control levels in the latter two allografts. In these same animals, their own hearts had control animals' (not treated surgically) levels of MDA. While three animals do not constitute a statistically significant sample, these results do complement our findings of decreased levels of SOD.

We have demonstrated decreased activity of the primary antioxidative defense enzyme SOD in rat cardiac allografts, and also approximately normal levels of GSH.Px and CAT. There is no indication at 5 days posttransplantation that abnormally high or low protein synthesis is associated with the decreased enzyme activity in the allograft; rather it seems that the enzyme is inactivated in situ. Such inactivation may be caused by prolonged exposure to H_2O_2 or to other products of a prolonged inflammatory response. These results demonstrate a direct link between the inflammatory response of the host animal and destruction of the transplanted organ; they indicate that deregulation of an antioxidative defense enzyme, superoxide dismutase, is an early molecular event in cardiac allograft destruction.

M. KLOC
K. MAILER
S. STEPKOWSKI
Department of Chemistry
St. Mary's University
Department of Surgery
Dalhousie University
Halifax, Nova Scotia,
Canada B3H 3J5

REFERENCES

1. Forbes RDC, Guttmann RD. Pathogenetic studies of cardiac allograft rejection using inbred rat models. Immunol Rev 1984; 77: 5.
2. Häyry P. Intragraft events in allograft destruction. Transplantation 1984; 38: 1.
3. Häyry P, von Willebrand E, Parthenais E, Nemlander A, Soots A, Lautenschlager I, Alfoldy P, Renkonen R. The inflammatory mechanisms of alograft rejection. Immunol Rev 1984; 77: 85.
4. Halliwell B. Production of superoxide, hydrogen peroxide, and hydroxyl radicals by phagocytic cells: a cause of chronic inflammatory disease? Cell Biol Int Rep 1982; 6: 529.
5. Bielski BHJ, Arudi RL, Sutherland MW. A study of the reactivity of HO_2/O_2^- with unsaturated fatty acids. J Biol Chem 1983; 258: 4759.
6. Rowe GT, Eaton LR, Hess ML. Neutrophil-derived, oxygen free radical-mediated cardiovascular dysfunction. J Mol Cell Cardiol 1984; 16: 1075.
7. Ono K, Lindsey ES. Improved technique of heart transplantation in rats. J Thorac Cardiovasc Surg 1969; 57: 225.
8. McCord J, Fridovich I. Superoxide dismutases. An enzymic function for erythrocuprein. J Biol Chem 1969; 244: 6049.
9. Paglia DE, Valentine WN. Studies on the quantitative and qualitative characterization of erythrocyte glutathione peroxidase. J Lab Clin Med 1967; 70: 158.
10. Cohen C, Dembieci D, Marcus J. Measurement of catalase activity in tissue extracts. Anal Biochem 1970; 34: 30.
11. Lowry OH, Rosebrough NJ, Farr AL, Randall RJ. Protein measurement with the Folin phenol reagent. J Biol Chem 1951; 193: 265.
12. Laemmli UK. Cleavage of structural proteins during the assembly of the head of bacteriophage T4. Nature 1970; 227: 680.
13. Ohkawa H, Ohishi N, Yagi K. Assay for lipid peroxides in animal tissues by thiobarbituric acid reaction. Anal Biochem 1979; 95: 351.
14. Hodgson EK, Fridovich, I. The interaction of bovine erythrocyte superoxide dismutase with hydrogen peoxide: inactivation of the enzyme. Biochemistry 1975; 14: 5294.

Received 6 September 1985.
Accepted 1 October 1985.

ERYTHROMYCIN AND CYCLOSPORINE[1]

Cyclosporine is an important new drug that has gained widespread use in clinical transplantation (*1–3*). With its use, many important drug interactions have been recognized. Cyclosporine is metabolized primarily in the liver, at least in part by the hepatic P450 mixed oxidase system (*3*). Therefore, drugs that increase activity of this system, such as diphenylhydantoin and rifampin, have been demonstrated to cause abrupt decreases in cyclosporine blood levels that may lead to rejection (*4, 5*). Drugs that inhibit the P450 system, such as ketaconazole, cimetidine, and high-dose methylprednisolone, may lead to abrupt rises in blood cyclosporine that may precipitate toxicity of the drug (*6–9*). We report here another drug interaction, erythromycin with cyclosporine, that led to increased blood levels of cyclosporine in four patients and was associated with cyclosporine toxicity.

Patient one (R.Z.) received a cadaveric renal transplant and was maintained on cyclosporine and prednisone. Cyclosporine dosage was adjusted in the first 3 weeks posttransplant to achieve a whole-blood level, as measured by high-performance liquid chromatography, of 150–250 ng/ml. The patient was doing well until 3 weeks posttransplant when he became febrile and developed an interstitial pneumonia. Bronchoscopy was performed and bronchoalveolar lavage yielded a diagnosis of *Legionella pneumophila.* The patient was started on erythromycin 1 g i.v. every 6 hr. He recovered in 3 weeks from his pneumonia. Cyclosporine and erythromycin dosage, cyclosporine drug levels, and serum creatine are shown in Table 1. Cyclosporine drug levels increased 2 days after institution of erythromycin therapy. As indicated, cyclosporine was tapered until therapeutic levels were obtained. Note that the patient needed only 1/6 the dose of cyclosporine to obtain similar blood levels on day +15 compared with day +4. With the tapering of both cyclosporine and erythromycin, cyclosporine drug levels fell and the patient's renal function improved without further treatment. He is doing well 3 months posttransplant. His only neurological symptoms consisted of lethargy on days +8 to +12.

Patient two (D.N.) received a cadaveric transplant and was started on cyclosporine and prednisone. She did well initially but developed signs of rejection approximately 2 weeks posttransplant. A renal biopsy revealed no cellular rejection, but signs of acute humoral mediated rejection as demonstrated by antibody and complement deposition with vasculitis. Because of this, she was treated with plasmapheresis and cyclophosphamide according to an ongoing protocol in our center. She tolerated this well with minimal improvement in renal function and was discharged 5 weeks posttransplant on cyclosporine and prednisone. Four days later she was readmitted with fever and diffuse interstitial pulmonary infiltrates. She was started empirically on erythromycin and trimethoprim-sulfamethoxazole. Bronchoscopy was performed but no diagnosis could be made. Following the negative bronchoscopy, trimethoprim-sulfamethoxazole was discontinued (after only 2 doses) and erythromycin continued. Table 2 lists the cyclosporine and erythromycin dosages along with cyclosporine blood levels and serum creatinine levels. Two days after erythromycin was started, a tremor and an elevated cyclosporine blood level were noted. The level of 943 ng/ml reflects the dose of 400 mg given orally 12 hr previously. Because of this, her evening dose the next day (+1) was held. Despite this, the next drug level obtained (24 hr after an oral dose of 350 mg) was still elevated at 288 ng/ml (day +2). She was given an even smaller dose (70 mg i.v.) and a blood level 24 hr later was still elevated at 488 ng/ml (day +3). The patient was dialyzed on day +2 for three hr because of decreased renal function and fluid overload. The patient was asymptomatic during dialyses with no cramping, nausea, vomiting, or other symptoms suggesting dysequilibrium syndrome. During the entire day, the patient was drowsy and at 2 hr after dialysis 4 episodes of total unresponsiveness were noted. These lasted 5–15 min. Serum electrolytes and glucose were normal, blood pressure was 160/90 mm Hg, pulse was 70/min, and findings of a neurological exam were normal except for unresponsiveness even to deep pain. Lumbar puncture, electroencephalogram and head computerized tomography scan findings were all normal. The patient had cyclosporine stopped and azathioprine instituted. By the next day, the patient was alert and had no more episodes of unresponsiveness. On the day when she had her neurological symptoms, she received an i.v. dose of cyclosporine and started with a cyclosporine blood level of 288 ng/ml. Since her trough level 24 hr later was still 488 ng/ml, she must have had quite high peak blood levels during her neurological episodes. The next day she started with a cyclosporine blood level of 488 ng/ml, but experienced no symptoms as she was given no further cyclosporine. On day +4, the cyclosporine blood level was still 127 ng/ml despite the patient not receiving any drug for 48 hr. This suggests markedly prolonged metabolism of the drug in the presence of erythromycin. The patient recovered from her pneumonia and continues on azathioprine and prednisone with a creatinine level of 3.0 mg/dl.

TABLE 1. Patient one

Days[a]	Cyclosporine dose (mg)[b]	Erythromycin dose	Cyclosporine blood level (ng/ml)[c]	Serum creatinine (mg/dl)
−2	200 b.i.d./i.v.		275	2.4
−1	200 b.i.d./i.v.		270	2.2
0	200 b.i.d./i.v.	1 g i.v. q.i.d.[d]		2.1
+2	200 b.i.d./i.v.	1 g i.v. q.i.d.	421	2.7
+4	600 b.i.d./p.o.	1 g i.v. q.i.d.	437	3.0
+6	500 b.i.d./p.o.	1 g p.o. q.i.d.	948	2.7
+8	500/450/p.o.	1 g p.o. q.i.d.	1134	3.6
+9	450/400/p.o.	1 g p.o. q.i.d.	1426	3.8
+10	450/350/p.o.	1 g p.o. q.i.d.		4.4
+11	0	750 mg p.o. q.i.d.		5.5
+12	0	750 mg p.o. q.i.d.	255	6.9
+13	0	500 mg p.o. q.i.d.	307	5.0
+15	200 p.o.	500 mg p.o. q.i.d.	380	6.1
+17	200 p.o.	500 mg p.o. q.i.d.		6.3
+21	200 p.o.	500 mg p.o. q.i.d.	119	4.0
+28	200 p.o.	0	50	2.2
+88	400 p.o.	0	140	1.7

[a] Days are listed in relationship to the institution of erythromycin therapy.

[b] Cyclosporine dosages are shown in milligrams given every 12 hr (b.i.d.) or once a day as indicated. i.v. = intravenously given dose. p.o. = dose given orally. Pt. weight was 75 kg.

[c] Cyclosporine blood levels are whole-blood levels as measured by high-performance liquid chromatography. They were measured immediately prior to a dose and therefore represent the previous day's dose.

[d] q.i.d. = every 6 hr.

[1] This work was supported in part by the Veterans Administration.

TABLE 2. Patient two

Days[a]	Cyclosporine dose (mg)[b]	Erythromycin dose	Cyclosporine blood level (ng/ml)[c]	Serum creatinine symptoms (mg/dl)
−2	400 b.i.d./p.o.		150	3.8
−1	400 b.i.d./p.o.			4.0
0	400 b.i.d./p.o.	500 mg i.v. q.i.d.[d]	119	4.5
+1	350 p.o.	500 mg i.v. q.i.d.	943	5.0 Drowsiness and tremor
+2	70 i.v.	500 mg i.v. q.i.d.	288	3.8[e] Drowsiness, tremor, and unresponsiveness
+3	0	500 mg i.v. q.i.d.	488	4.2
+4	0	500 mg i.v. q.i.d.	127	4.3
+5	0	500 mg p.o. q.i.d.	69	3.2[e]
+7	0	500 mg p.o. q.i.d.	—	3.1

[a] See footnote [a] to Table 1.
[b] See footnote [b] to Table 1. Pt. weight was 80 kg.
[c] See footnote [c] to Table 1.
[d] See footnote [d] to Table 1.
[e] Represents a postdialysis creatinine level.

TABLE 3. Patient three

Days[a]	Cyclosporine dose (mg)[b]	Erythromycin dose	Cyclosporine blood level (ng/ml)[c]	Serum creatinine (mg/dl)
−18	300 p.o.	0	221	1.8
0	300 p.o.	500 mg p.o. b.i.d.[e]	—	1.6
+2	300 p.o.	500 mg p.o. b.i.d.	389	2.6
+3	350 p.o.	500 mg p.o. b.i.d.	346	2.4
+4	300 p.o.[d]	500 mg p.o. b.i.d.	360	3.7
+5	275 p.o.[d]	500 mg p.o. b.i.d.	379	3.4
+6	275 p.o.[d]	500 mg p.o. b.i.d.	404	3.5
+7	275 p.o.	500 mg p.o. b.i.d.	310	2.7
+8	275 p.o.	500 mg p.o. b.i.d.	653	2.7
+9	275 p.o.	0	421	2.2
+10	275 p.o.	0	334	1.5
+20	275 p.o.	0	164	1.7

[a] See footnote [a], Table 1.
[b] See footnote [b], Table 1. Pt. weight was 65 kg.
[c] See footnote [c], Table 1.
[d] Received 750 mg. methylprednisolone i.v.
[e] See footnote [d], Table 1.

TABLE 4. Patient four

Days[a]	Cyclosporine dose (mg)[b]	Erythromycin dose	Cyclosporine blood level (ng/ml)[c]	Serum creatinine (mg/dl)
−3	650 p.o.	0	297	3.4
−2	600 p.o.	0	337	3.8
−1	500 p.o.	500 i.v. once	205	3.9
0	0	500 i.v. q.i.d.[d]	171	4.5
+1	0	500 i.v. q.i.d.	—	4.9
+2	0	500 i.v. q.i.d.	193	5.2
+3	0	500 i.v. q.i.d.	—	4.8
+4	0	500 i.v. q.i.d.	159	4.3
+5	0	500 i.v. q.i.d.	174	3.6
+6	0	500 i.v. q.i.d.	149	3.1
+7	0	500 i.v. q.i.d.	122	2.9
+8	0	500 i.v. q.i.d.	107	2.4
+9	0	500 i.v. q.i.d.	72	2.2
+10	0	500 i.v. q.i.d.	71	2.1

[a] See footnote [a], Table 1.
[b] See footnote [b], Table 1. Pt. weight was 90 kg.
[c] See footnote [c], Table 1.
[d] See footnote [d], Table 1.

Patient three (D.B.) received a cadaveric renal transplant and was started on prednisone and cyclosporine. She did well with excellent graft function. At four months posttransplant, she was stable with a serum creatinine of 1.8 on 300 mg of cyclosporine (6 mg/kg). Her cyclosporine level was 221 ng/ml (Table 3). Her local physician started her on erythromycin for acne. Two days later she was noted to have an elevated creatinine and an elevated cyclosporine level. She was admitted to the hospital and treated for presumptive rejection. Her cyclosporine levels continued to be elevated until the erythromycin was discontinued. She is currently doing well on 275 mg of cyclosporine with a serum creatinine of 1.7.

The fourth patient demonstrates the potential for erythromycin to markedly prolong the clearance of cyclosporine. R.S. was doing well on cyclosporine and prednisone 5 months posttransplant. Because of a creatinine of 3.5 mg/dl, he was switched to azathioprine and prednisone. He continued with a creatinine of 3.0–3.5 mg/dl and was therefore started back on low-dose cyclosporine (3 mg/kg) and continued on azathioprine (2 mg/kg). He had a renal biopsy that demonstrated fibrosis. During this period his cyclosporine blood levels were 150–180 ng/ml. He became leukopenic, had his azathioprine discontinued, and developed severe *Legionella* pneumonia. He was started on erythromycin and, because of the severity of the pneumonia, all immunosuppression was withheld. Despite receiving no drug, his cyclosporine drug level six days later was 149 ng/ml (Table 4). This suggests markedly prolonged drug metabolism.

These four cases suggest that cyclosporine metabolism is inhibited by concomitant erythromycin administration. Three patients were started on the antibiotic because of proved or suspected *Legionella* infection. The fourth started erythromycin because of acne. They all had marked increases in cyclosporine blood levels with toxicity. Nephrotoxicity and neurotoxicity are recognized side effects of cyclosporine and may be related to blood levels of the drug (*1–3, 10, 11*). The interaction of erythromycin and cyclosporine could be predicted from what is known of the effect of erythromycin on the cytochrome P450 system. Erythromycin decreases cytochrome P-450 activity

(*12*), which has led to increased levels of another drug metabolized by this system, theophylline (*13*). This well known interaction has led to many cases of theophylline toxicity (*13*). Other possibilities may explain these observations. First, the infection itself in three of the patients may have altered the metabolism of the drug. Second, erythromycin may increase absorption or bioavailability by displacing cyclosporine from red blood cells. Patient three did receive methylprednisolone, a drug known to increase cyclosporine levels. However, this effect is usually transient, and our patient had elevated levels before the boluses. These levels persisted until erythromycin was discontinued. All of these possibilities—i.e., decreased metabolism, increased absorption, or increased bioavailability—need to be investigated with formal kinetic studies. Since our laboratory measures whole-blood cyclosporine utilizing a high-performance liquid chromatography the drug levels represent true cyclosporine and not metabolites. Thus, elevated cyclosporine levels must be due to increased absorption or decreased metabolism. Increased absorption could explain the findings in patients 1–3 but not patient 4. This patient had very prolonged metabolism of the drug. Our four cases suggest (along with the known effect of erythromycin on cytochrome P-450) that decreased metabolism of cyclosporine may occur with administration of erythromycin. Whatever the cause, clinicians should be aware that concomitant administration of cyclosporine and erythromycin may lead to increased levels of cyclosporine and toxicity.

Thomas A. Gonwa[2,3]
Dai D. Nghiem
James A. Schulak
Robert J. Corry
The Veterans Administration Medical Center
The Departments of Medicine and Surgery
University of Iowa
Iowa City, Iowa 52242

[2] T.A.G. is a research associate of the Veterans Administration.

[3] Reprint requests to T.A. Gonwa, 8E-26, Veteran's Administration Medical Center, Iowa City, Iowa 52240.

REFERENCES

1. Cohen DJ, Loertscher R, Rubin MF, Tilney NL, Carpenter CB, Strom TB. Cyclosporine: a new immunosuppressive agent for organ transplantation. Ann Intern Med 1984; 101: 667.
2. Tilney NL, Milford EL, Araujo J-L, Strom TB, Carpenter CB, Kirkman RL. Experience with cyclosporine and steroids in clinical renal transplantation. Ann Surg 1984; 200: 605.
3. Kahan BD, Van Buren CT, Flechner SM, Jarowenko M, Yasumara T, Rogers AJ, Yoshimura N, LeGrue S, Drath D, Kerman RH. Clinical and experimental studies with cyclosporine in renal transplantation. Surgery 1985; 97: 125.
4. Keown PA, Laupacis A, Carruthers G, Stawecki M, Koegler J, McKenzie FN, Wall W, Stitler CR. Interaction between Phenytoin and Cyclosporine following organ transplantation. Transplantation 1984; 38: 304.
5. Van Buren D, Wideman CA, Reid M, Gibbons S, Van Buren CT, Jarowenko M, Flechner SM, Frazier OH, Coolev DA, Kahan BD. The antagonistic effect of Refampin upon Cyclosporine bioavailability. Transplant Proc 1984; 16: 1642.
6. Wood AJ, Maurer G, Niederberger W, Beveridge T. Cyclosporine: pharmacokinetics metabolism, and drug interactions. Transplant Proc 1982; 14: 659.
7. White DJG, Blatchford NR, Cauwenbergh G. Cyclosporine and Ketoconazole. Transplantation 1984; 37: 214.
8. Ferguson RM, Sutherland DE, Simmons RL, Najarian JS, Ketoconazole. Cyclosporin metabolism and renal transplantation. Lancet 1982; 2: 882.
9. Boogaerts MA, Zacher P, Verwilghen RL. Cyclosporin methylprednisolone and convulsions. Lancet 1982; 2: 1216.
10. Atkinson K, Biggs J, Darveniza P, Boland J, Concannon A, Dodds A. Cyclosporine-associated central nervous system toxicity after allogeneic bone marrow transplantation. Transplantation 1984; 38: 34.
11. Wilczek H, Ringden O, Tyden G. Cyclosporine-associated central nervous system toxicity after renal transplantation. Transplantation 1984; 39: 110.
12. Donan G, Descatoire V, Pessayre D. Self-induction by erythromycin of its own transformation into a metabolite forming an inactive complex with reduced cytochrome P-450. J Pharmacol Exp Ther 1981; 218: 509.
13. Bukowskyj M, Nakatsu K, Munt PW. Theophylline reassessed. Ann Intern Med 1984; 101: 63.

Received 6 August 1985.
Accepted 1 October 1985.

0041-1337/86/4106-0800$02.00/0
TRANSPLANTATION

Vol. 41, No. 6
Printed in U.S.A.

Transplantation

LETTERS TO EDITOR

Repeated casein injections induce experimental amyloidosis in mice (*1*); the chemical type of this amyloidosis has proved to be AA, the same as in human amyloidosis associated with chronic infections, chronic inflammation, and the genetic form of familial Mediterranean fever (*2*).

Cyclosporine is a potent antirejection agent that was introduced in recent years for organ transplantation (*3, 4*). Since about 6–10% of renal transplanted patients in Israel suffer from amyloid nephropathy, we were concerned about the outcome of these transplanted patients receiving cyclosporine as the main antirejection agent, and we decided to examine its influence on the induction of experimental amyloidosis in mice.

In the first experiment, 22 male white Swiss mice received daily s.c. injections of 0.5 ml 12% casein 6 times per week, plus cyclosporine 2.5 mg in dextrose 5% (about 100 mg/kg) injected i.p. After one week the cyclosporine dose was reduced to 1.25 mg because the mice suffered from diarrhea and 4 died. The control group received casein injections s.c. and dextrose 5% i.p.

After 12 days the mice were killed. All mice in the experimental group, as well as the control group, developed splenic amyloidosis. There was no significant difference in the amount of amyloid deposited within the two groups. In a second experiment 9 white Swiss mice were injected with casein once a week and cyclosporine 2.5 mg three times per week. After 5 weeks the experimental group contained the same amount of splenic amyloidosis as the control group that did not receive cyclosporine.

We concluded that cyclosporine had no positive or negative influence on the development of experimental amyloidosis in mice.[1]

SHMUEL SHTRASBURG[2]
BRUNO SIEGAL[3]
DEBORAH ZEMER[2]
Heller Institute of Medical Research
Transplant Unit
Sheba Medical Center Tel-Hashomer, Israel

[1] This work was supported by Shauder Grant No. 06012601010000, Tel Aviv University.
[2] Heller Institute of Medical Research.
[3] Sheba Medical Center.

REFERENCES

1. Eriksen N, Ericsson LH, Pearsall D, Lagunoff D, Benditt EP. Mouse amyloid protein AA: homology with non-immunoglobulin protein of human and monkey amyloid substance. Proc Natl Acad Sci USA 1976; 73: 964.
2. Levin M, Franklin EC, Frangione B, Pras M. The amino acid sequence of a major non-immunoglobulin in component of some amyloid fibrils. J Clin Invest 1972; 51: 2773.
3. Calne RY, White DIG, Evans DB. Cyclosporin A in cadaveric organ transplantation. Br Med J 1981; 282: 934.
4. Strazl TE, Hakala TR, Rosenthal JT. The Colorado-Pittsburgh cadaveric renal transplantation study with cyclosporin. Transplant Proc 1983; 25(4): 2459.

The recent article by the Helsinki group, *Blood eosinophilia, steroids, and rejection* (*1*), suggests a very interesting association between blood eosinophilia and early rejection. The authors make a case with sequential eosinophile counts, fine-needle aspiration biopsies, and serum creatinine levels, for the correlation of eosinophilia with inflammatory renal changes—which, in turn, could be a reflection of increased specific immune reactivity. The significance of these observations in the overall immune response awaits further understanding.

I would like to stress the point, though, that eosinophilia may be related to other conditions—and, in tropical and subtropical countries, it could be the only early marker of some parasitic infections. We have previously highlighted the association of eosinophilia with parasitic infections, particularly *Strongyloides stercolaris*, in transplant recipients (*2*). In patients who develop eosinophilia, especially when associated with nonspecific abdominal distress, diarrhea, fever, or partial intestinal obstruction, strongyloidiasis should immediately enter the suspect list in the differential diagnosis. Failure to diagnose and treat such a condition (which normally does not require any attention) may, in the transplanted immunosuppressed patient, have catastrophic consequences. These considerations should be kept in mind when using eosinophilia as a marker of rejection.

E.A. SANTIAGO-DELPIN
Puerto Rico Transplant Program
San Juan, Puerto Rico

REFERENCES

1. Lautenshlager I, Von Willebrand E, Häyry P. Blood eosinophilia, steroids, and rejection. Transplantation 1985; 40: 354.
2. Santiago-Delpín EA, Rodríguez-Campos B, Ramírez-González RE, Miranda JL, Strongyloidiasis in the immunosuppressed host. Bol Asoc Med P Rico 1982; 74: 134.

ERRATA

There was an omission of one of the authors' names in the article entitled "Investigation of T and natural killer cell function with monoclonal antibodies" published in the January 1986 issue of *Transplantation*. The authors should have been listed as P.J. Thurlow, G. McArthur, I.F.C. McKenzie, and A.J.F. d'Apice. We apologize for any inconvenience that this may have caused.

In the article entitled "Cotton-wool exudates not observed in recipients of renal transplants treated with cyclosporine" by Oechslin et al., which appeared in the January 1986 issue of *Transplantation*, there is a typographical error on page 61, line 11. The sentence should read "Moreover, as far as we are aware, cotton-wool spots have *not* been observed in patients showing a rejection reaction to bone marrow transplants . . . ". We apologize for any inconvenience this may have caused.

AUTHOR INDEX

Achauer, B. M., 39
Ahonen, J., 410
Aigner, F., 412
Alejandro, R., 364
Alongi, S. V., 709
Altman, D. G., 713
Amadeo, J. H., 606
Andreoli, S. P., 63
Arens, L., 235
Arnall, J. C., 766
Arnold, R., 170
Ascher, N. L., 177, 214
Autenried, P., 413

Babayan, R. K., 536
Bach, J. F., 730
Bacher, J., 122
Bagchus, W. M., 739
Bagot, M., 316
Bakker, W. W., 739
Balfour, B., 96
Ballardie, F. W., 537
Baloh, R., 657
Balshi, J. D., 118
Bander, N. H., 593
Bansal, V. K., 404
Bar, S., 680
Barkley, S. C., 173
Barocci, S., 135, 199
Barrett, L. V., 781
Barry, J. M., 125
Baumal, R., 152
Beatty, P., 583
Beaudoin, R., 640
Bell, P. R. F., 652
Belzer, F. O., 544
Benear, J. B., 274
Bensinger, W. I., 602
Berden, J. H. M., 264
Bergstein, J., 63
Berndt, M. C., 565
Bewick, M., 276
Bhan, A., 781
Bielmann, D., 343
Bijma, A. M., 111
Bismuth, H., 398
Bitter-Suermann, H., 626
Black, K. S., 39
Blanchard, J. M., 527
Blank, M., 759
Blume, K. G., 268
Borland, A., 192
Bowen, A., 539
Bozdech, M. J., 544
Bradstock, K. F., 565
Brendel, W., 426
Bron, K. M., 539
Broomhead, A. F., 565
Brown, C. B., 464
Bruggeman, C. A., 695
Bruning, J. H., 695
Buckley, B. M., 335
Buckner, C. D., 602
Bucy, R. P., 661
Buice, R. G., 411
Bull, R. W., 111
Bunjes, D., 170
Burastero, S., 135
Buszta, C., 598

Buttifant, L., 96
Buurman, W. A., 33, 111, 156, 751

Cadoni, A., 135
Cain, G. R., 21
Campos, H., 730
Canafax, D. M., 177
Cardinet, G. H., III 21
Carlson, G. A., 688
Carozzi, S., 135
Carrozzi, S., 199
Carter, N. P., 468
Casellas, P., 356
Cavallini, M., 654
Celada, F., 135, 199
Champlin, R., 21
Chapman, J. R., 468
Chatenoud, L., 730
Chen, X., 495
Chkoff, N., 730
Chouvet, B., 340
Chow, S. S., 152
Christensen, E., 713
Chudzik, J., 659
Civin, C. I., 220
Clift, R. A., 602
Cobbold, S., 634
Cohen, A., 173
Cohen, A. D., 534
Cohen, J., 260
Cohen, Z., 266
Coles, M. I., 776
Collins, T., 141
Colvin, R. B., 572
Cook, D. J., 447
Cooper, B. A., 356
Cooper, D. K. C., 29
Cooper, E. L., 514
Cordon-Cardo, C., 593
Cordonnier, C., 316
Cornélissen, G., 654
Corry, R. J., 797
Cosimi, A. B., 572, 593
Crougneau, S., 398
Cuddon, P. A., 21

Daffin, L. E., 663
Dagher, F. J., 709
D'Amaro, J., 719
Dandavino, R., 55
Daniel, V., 454
Davie, J. M., 661
Dawson, P. J., 286
Deeg, H. J., 47, 111, 583
DeFazio, S. R., 26
Deierhoi, M. H., 546
Delmonico, F. L., 593
Demetris, A. J., 377
Dendle, T., 669
Dessi, V., 135, 199
DeWolf, A., 296, 388
Dibelius, A., 426
Dicke, K. A., 4, 129
Diven, W., 388
Donga, J., 739
Donnenberg, A. D., 220
Doveren, R. F. C., 33
Dowdy, S. F., 39

Doxiadis, I., 111
Drayson, M. T., 745
Dreikorn, K., 454
Droz, D., 730
Dubertret, L., 316
Dummer, J. S., 725
Duncan, W. R., 626
Duquesnoy, R. J., 620
Duran, L. W., 279

Eastwood, S. L., 534
Eklund, B., 410
Emond, J., 398
Epstein, R. B., 274
Ettenger, R. B., 133
Evans, D. J., 537

Fabre, J. W., 499
Farge, D., 55, 182
Fauser, A. A., 356
Fawzy, F. I., 478, 484
Feld, L. G., 664
Ferguson, R. M., 69, 75, 84, 349, 400
Fernando, O. N., 131
Fidelus, R. K., 187
Field, M. J., 529
Fiere, D., 340
Fildes, R. D., 664
Fine, R. N., 133, 173
Finstad, C. L., 593
First, M. R., 406
Fischer, S., 125
Fisher, M., 468
Flechner, S. M., 459
Flener, R., 716
Fontana, I., 199
Forbes, R. D. C., 55
Forman, S. J., 268
Foulks, G. N., 229
Frederick, D., 274
Fresco, R., 404
Fryd, D. S., 177
Fuller, B. J., 161
Fuller, T. C., 572
Fung, J., 620
Furnas, D. W., 39

Gale, R. P., 21
Gallagher, M. T., 268
Gassmann, W., 380
Gast, C. C., 719
Gibbons, C. P., 464
Gigou, M., 398
Gill, T. J., III, 377, 392, 784
Gimbrone, M. A., Jr., 141
Girard, B., 556
Glichlick, D., 579
Gloor, B., 60
Goehle, S., 328
Gokal, R., 262
Goldin, H., 755
Goldstein, G., 431, 730
Gonwa, T. A., 797
Gonzalez, G. A., 39
González, Z., 606
Goormastic, M., 598
Gordon, G., 644
Gore, S. M., 319

Gores, P. F., 271, 529, 648
Gottschalk, R., 489
Gozzo, J. G., 26
Gratama, J. W., 719
Gray, D. W. R., 699
Gray, T. A., 335
Green, C. J., 161
Greenleaf, G. E., 556
Gridelli, B., 388, 657
Griffin, R. J., 776
Griffith, B. P., 620, 725
Griño, J. M., 410
Groenewegen, G., 751
Gronau, C., 759
Grose, J. H., 640
Grosse-Wilde, H., 111
Gugenheim, J., 398
Guillen, F. J., 734
Guttmann, R. D., 55, 182
Guyotat, D., 340

Hackl, M., 412
Hahn, H. J., 44
Halberg, F., 654
Hall-Craggs, M., 709
Halloran, P. F., 413
Hancock, W. W., 734
Hanley, J. A., 182
Hano, J. E., 404
Hansen, W. P., 593
Hardesty, R. L., 620, 725
Harrison, C., 147
Hartner, W. C., 26
Hattori, A., 784
Häyry, P., 290, 410
Healing, G., 161
Heil, J. E., 177
Heils, J., 654
Heimpel, H., 170
Heit, W., 170
Henny, F. C., 442
Heslan, M., 316
Hess, A. D., 644
Hesse, U. J., 271, 395, 648
Hewitt, C. W., 39
Hilgard, H. R., 384
Himeno, K., 209
Ho, H-N, 392
Ho, M., 725
Hodgen, G. D., 122
Hoedemaeker, P., 739
Hoffman, R. A., 214
Ho-Hsieh, H., 782
Holt, D. W., 276
Horsburgh, T., 652
Horton, J. D., 766
Houssin, D., 398
Howard, E. B., 39
Howden, B., 147
Huber, C., 716
Hughes, W. G., 565
Hurst, R. D., 286
Hutchinson, I. V., 166, 547
Hyland, B. J., 214

Idelson, B. A., 536
Ildstad, S. T., 372
Ind, P. W., 260
Israel, L., 67

Jablonski, P., 147
Jaffers, G. J., 572
Janossy, G., 131
Jarowenko, M., 436
Jeng, L. B., 395
Jeong, G., 126
Jeunhomme, G. M. A. A., 751
Johnson, R. W. G., 262
Jonker, M., 431
Jordan, S. C., 133, 173
Joseph, S., 100
June, C. H., 47

Kabral, A., 565
Kahan, B. D., 436, 459
Kam, I., 296
Kamada, N., 396
Kamata, K., 495
Kanazi, G., 782
Kanitakis, J., 340
Kanz, L., 356
Karow, A. M., Jr., 669
Karwa, G., 579
Kaufman, C., 620
Kay, R., 464
Keisari, Y., 755
Kennedy, M. S., 47
Kerman, R., 436
Khauli, R. B., 598
Kiesche, A., 688
Kinnaert, P., 52
Klempnauer, J., 787
Kloc, M., 794
Kloting, I., 44
Klotz, L. H., 593
Knight, S. C., 96
Kodera, Y., 311
Koene, R. A. P., 264
Kohnert, K. D., 44
Kolb, H. J., 111
Koller, J., 412
Königsberger, H., 426
Konoeda, Y., 253
Koo, G. C., 126
Kootstra, G., 33, 156
Korinek, J. K., 129
Kornberger, R., 412
Kovarik, J., 716
Kozeny, G. A., 404
Kramer, W. G., 459
Kreeft, H. A. J. G., 719
Kreis, H., 730
Kretschmer, M., 328
Krumbacher, K., 111
Kunkl, A., 199
Kunz, H. W., 377, 392, 784
Kupiec-Weglinski, J. W., 734

Lachance, J., 640
Lackie, A. M., 360
Lacombe, M., 730
Lacy, P. E., 661
Ladiges, W., 111
Landmann, J., 60
Landsverk, J., 478, 484
Langer, B., 266
LaPointe, R., 388
Lapp, W. S., 238, 242
Laube, F., 44
Laughter, A. H., 187
Laurent, G., 356
Lawler, W., 262
Lee, H. M., 474
Lee, J. R., 122
Lee, K. K. W., 286
LeFever, A. V., 301
Lehnert, S., 675
Leichter, H. E., 133
Leiter, E., 716
Lemire, J. M., 173
Leunissen, K. M. L., 666
Levy, G. J., 583
Levy, J. P., 316
Lévy, M., 204
Lévy, M., 790
Libby, P., 141
Liesnard, C., 52
Lindsay, G. D., 67
Löhr, G. W., 356
Lorber, M. I., 459
Losslein, K. L., 111
Loughran, T. P., Jr., 47
Lucke, S., 44
Ludwin, D., 100, 120
Luft, B. J., 611
Lum, L. G., 583, 587
Lunec, J., 161
Lynch, S., 296

Macpherson, T. A., 392
MacSween, J. M., 534
Maes, N., 52
Magnusson, M., 598
Mailer, K., 794
Majoor, G. D., 92
Malik, S. T. A., 131
Mallick, N. P., 262
Manca, F., 199
Margreiter, R., 412, 716
Marsden, J. T., 276
Marshall, S. T., 688
Marshall, V. C., 147
Martin, D. C., 39
Martin, S., 262
Martin-Comin, J., 410
Masaki, Y., 495
Matas, A. J., 579
Matory, Y., 122
Mauduit, G., 340
Mauer, S. M., 664
Mayer, T. K., 67
Mayoral, J., 529
Mayumi, H., 209
McArthur, G., 104
McCabe, R. E., 611
McCann, R. L., 541
McDonald, M., 669
McGeorge, M. B., 474
McKenzie, I. F. C., 104
McMaster, P., 335
McNally, P. G., 464
McShane, P., 699
Medearis, D. N., 781
Mendez-Picon, G., 474
Mickey, M. R., 253
Mihatsch, M., 343
Milton, A. D., 499
Mintz, D. H., 364
Mistry, N., 652
Mitani, M., 209
Mitterschiffthaler, G., 412
Mizuno, S-I, 311
Mohanakumar, T., 474
Monaco, A. P., 26, 489
Montero, C. G., 725
Moorhead, J. F., 131
Morecki, S., 680
Morishima, Y., 311
Morris, P. J., 166, 468, 699
Mowat, A. M., 192
Mozes, M. R., 527
Müller-Ruchholtz, W., 380
Muller-Ruchholtz, W., 759
Murphy, G. F., 734

Naimark, A., 536
Najarian, J. S., 177, 271, 395, 648, 654
Nakamoto, S., 598
Neefe, J., 122
Neuberger, J., 713
Neuhaus, P., 431
Nghiem, D. D., 797
Nocera, A., 135
Noel, R., 640
Noga, S. J., 220
Nomoto, K., 209
Nooij, F. J. M., 431
Norman, D. J., 125
Novick, A. C., 598, 782
Novitzky, D., 29
Noyes, W. D., 128
Nusbacher, J., 67

O'Brien, J., 96
Oechslin, M., 60
Ohno, R., 311
Okubo, M., 495
Old, L. J., 593
Oldham, J. A., 319
Oliveira, D. B. G., 260
Oljans, P. J., 442
O'Neal, W. K., 536
Opelz, G., 454
Orloff, M. J., 556
Orosz, C. G., 69, 75, 84, 349, 400

Paganini, E., 598
Paradis, I. L., 725
Parfrey, N. A., 182
Parfrey, P. S., 55, 182
Park, M. S., 253
Parrott, D. M. V., 192
Paul, L. C., 442
Payne, W. D., 177
Pease, L. R., 279
Pegg, D. E., 396
Pellicci, R., 388
Pembrey, R. G., 421
Penkrot, R. J., 539
Perera, M. I. R., 377, 784
Perloff, L. J., 118
Permanetter, W., 426
Persson, A., 616
Pesce, A. J., 406
Pierce, J. A., 663
Pifer, L., 436
Pilarski, L. M., 521
Piper, D. J., 593
Pober, J. S., 141
Pohanka, E., 716
Pollak, R., 527
Pomerance, A., 776
Porter, K. A., 296
Posner, J. N., 709
Posner, M. P., 474
Pras, M., 793
Prendergast, M. M., 565
Prince, H. E., 235
Provisor, A. J., 63

Quinn, T., 579

Rabin, B. S., 620
Rae, D., 147
Raff, R. F., 111
Raftery, A. T., 464
Raftery, M. J., 131
Rajaraman, K., 534
Ramirez-González, R., 606
Ramsey, G., 67
Rao, K. M., 657
Rao, R., 669
Rees, A. J., 537
Reid, K. E., 276
Reidy, J. R., 126
Reiss, C. S., 141
Remington, J. S., 611
Renkonen, R., 290, 704
Rickles, F. R., 734
Rivé-Mora, E., 606
Roca, M., 410
Roch, P., 514
Rogerson, M. E., 276
Rose, M. L., 776
Rost, F., 52
Roy, R., 640
Rozing, J., 739
Rubin, R. H., 593, 781
Ruers, T. J. M., 156
Russell, P. S., 572, 593
Rybka, W. B., 675

Sachs, D. H., 372
Sadler, J. H., 709
Sakai, R. S., 173
Salusky, I. B., 133
Sanders, J., 583
Sandoz, P. F., 343
Sanfilippo, F., 229, 248, 508, 541
Sanghvi, A., 388, 657
Santiago-Delpín, E. A., 606, 800
Santos, G. W., 220, 644
Sao, H., 311
Sauer, M., 759
Scanlon, L., 388, 657
Schäfer, A. J., 454
Schang, T., 650
Schmeiser, T., 170
Schoch, G., 111
Schoutens-Serruys, E., 52
Schraut, W. H., 286
Schreiber, M. J., 598
Schroeder, T. J., 406
Schulak, J. A., 797
Schwartz, C. L., 220
Schwarz, M., 716
Scornik, J. C., 447
Sealey, M. M., 335
Seddik, M., 238, 242
Seemayer, T. A., 238, 242, 675
Segal, M. C., 539
Seltman, H., 388
Shaw, B., 388, 657
Shen, S. Y., 709
Shienvold, F. L., 364
Shih, C. C-Y., 301
Shinozuka, H., 377, 784
Shiobara, S., 587
Short, C. D., 262
Shtrashurg, S., 800
Siegal, B., 793, 800
Simmons, R. L., 177, 214
Simpkin, S., 161
Singal, D. P., 100, 111

Sirinek, L., 75, 84
Sirinek, L. P., 349, 400
Sitges-Serra
A., 648
Sitges-Serra, A., 271
Skolnick, M. L., 539
Slasky, B. S., 539
Slavin, S., 680
Slichter, S. J., 602
Smith, S. C. H., 335
Smits, J. F. M., 156
Snow, C., 384
Soberman, R., 579
Solders, G., 616
Sollinger, H. W., 544
Solomon, L. R., 262
Spencer, S. C., 499
Spielberger, M., 412
Spitzer, G., 4
Springate, J. E., 664
Spronken, E. E. M., 33
Srigley, J. R., 129
Stanacev, N. Z., 659
Starzl, T., 657
Starzl, T. E., 296, 388, 539
Steiniger, B., 787
Steinmuller, D., 782
Steinmuller, D. R., 598
Stephany, D., 372
Stepkowski, S. M., 626, 794
Stolear, J. C., 52
Storb, R., 111, 328, 583, 587
Stowe, N., 782
Strand, M. H., 177
Strauss, L. C., 220
Strijbosch, L., 33
Stroehlein, J. R., 129
Struyker-Boudier, H. A. J., 156
Stuhne-Sekalec, L., 659
Sullivan, K. M., 583
Summerton, C. B., 464
Sutherland, D. E. R., 177, 271, 395, 529, 648, 654
Sweny, P., 131

Tai, J., 531
Tamaki, T., 396
Tange, J. D., 147
Tanke, H. J., 442
Tavanlis, G., 147
Taylor, E., 384
Tellis, V. A., 579
Terasaka, R., 661
Terasaki, P. I., 253
Thiede, A., 650
Thiel, G., 60, 343
Thivolet, J., 340
Thomas, E. D., 583, 602
Thompson, C. B., 47
Thompson, R. E., 593
Thorner, P., 152
Thurlow, P. J., 104
Thys, J. P., 52
Tidman, N., 131
Tiggeler, R. G. W. L., 264
Tilkin, A-F, 316
Tilney, N. L., 734
Timmermann, W., 650
Ting, A., 468
Tiver, K., 565
Todo, S., 296
Tokuda, N., 209
Tolkoff-Rubin, N. E., 593
Tomlin, P., 335
Torres, A., 177
Toussaint, C., 52
Townsend, L., 274
Towpik, E., 734
Treseler, P. A., 229, 248, 508
Troppmair, J., 716
Truitt, R. L., 301
Tygstrup, N., 713
Tze, W. J., 531

Uchiyama, T., 495
Urban, P., 556
Valente, U., 135, 199
Van, H. V., 340
Van Boven, C. P. A., 695
Van Breda Vriesman, P. J. C., 92, 695
Van Buren, C. T., 459
Van der Linden, C. J., 33, 156
Van Der Linden, J. A., 719
Van der Sluis, R. F., 264
Van Dongen, J. J., 156
Van Es, L. A., 442
Van Heugten, J. G., 719
Van Hooff, J. P., 666
Van Leendert, R. J. M., 666
Van Suylichem, P., 431
Veitch, P. S., 652
Veith, F. J., 579
Vellekoop, L., 129
Venkataramanan, R., 296
Verdonck, L. F., 719
Vereerstraeten, P., 52
Verm, R. A., 129
Vernant, J. P., 316
Vertuno, L. L., 404
Vidt, D. G., 598
Vigeral, P., 730
Vismans, F-J. F. E., 666
Vogelsang, G. B., 644
Von Kolzynski, M., 380
Von Specht, B. U., 426
Von Willebrand, E., 410

Wadgymar, A., 413
Wadhwa, N. K., 406
Wakisaka, A., 253
Waldmann, H., 634
Walter, P., 426
Wangel, A., 290
Warren, H. S., 421
Warzock, R., 44
Wassef, R., 266
Watanabe, Y., 209
Weigensberg, M., 680
Weir, M. R., 709
Weiss, L., 680
Weiss, R., 579
Wellisch, D. K., 478, 484
Westbroek, D. L., 111
Whitsett, C. F., 663
Wicomb, W. N., 29
Wideman, C., 459
Wilczek, H., 616
Williams, G., 260, 537
Williams, R., 713
Wilson, D. R., 152
Wilson, E. J., 781
Winearls, C. G., 260, 537
Winn, H. J., 572
Witherspoon, R. P., 328, 587
Witkowski, L. A., 377, 784
Wobbes, T., 264
Wolcott, D. L., 478, 484
Wolfe, J. A., 541
Woloszczuk, W., 716
Wood, M. L., 489
Wottge, H. U., 759
Wottge, H-U, 380
Wren, S. M., 372
Wright, C., 268

Yacoub, M. H., 776
Yau, J. C., 129
Yee, G. C., 411
Yokomaku, S., 311
Yoshikawa, S., 311
Yum, M., 63

Zaia, J. A., 268
Zajko, A. B., 539
Zander, A. R., 129
Zeevi, A., 620
Zemer, D., 793, 800
Zerbe, T. R., 620
Zicca, A., 135
Zinn, N. E., 75, 84, 349, 400
Zwaan, F. E., 719

SUBJECT INDEX

Adenosine deaminase, binding protein (human), 593
Alloantibody, response, effect of blood transfusions on (rat) (Communication), 652
Alloantigen
  cellular immunity to (mouse), 384
  I-A, induction of intestinal phase of graft-versus-host reaction by Lyt 2^- cells activated by (mouse), 192
  interferon-gamma and neopterin levels during stimulation with (human), 716
  presentation by endothelial cells (dog), 751
  -specific cells, site of selection of (rat), 745
Allograft. *See also* Graft
  bowel, graft-versus-host disease induced by (rat), 286
  cornea, histocompatibility complex antigens to the immunogenicity of (rat), 508
  heart
    class I and class II histocompatibility complex antigens in rejecting (rat), 499
    effect of splenectomy on influence of pretransplant blood transfusions on survival (rat) (Communication), 527
    splenectomy and blood transfusions in (rat) (Communication), 118
  influence of OK709F treatment on survival (monkey), 431
  islet, immunogenicity of purified and unpurified (mouse) (Communication), 529
  kidney
    class I and class II histocompatibility complex antigens in rejecting (rat), 499
    cyclosporine-pretreated (dog) (Communication), 395
    cytolytic T cell line established from lymphocytes homing in a rejected (human) (Communication), 135
    decapsulation of (human) (Communication, 264
    effects of delayed function on recipients of (human), 177
    failure of platelet transfusion to improve survival (human), 468
    improved function and survival after blood transfusions (human), 640
    intrarenal hydrostatic pressure measurements in the diagnosis of rejection (human), 464
    prognostic value of eosinophil in rejection (human), 709
    role of histocompatibility antigens in survival (rat), 166
    treatment (rat), 156
    use of cyclosporine to prevent rejection (dog) (Communication), 654
  pancreas, endocrine function of (rat) (Communication), 650
  prolonged survival resulting from donor pretreatment with phytohemagglutinin-P (rat) (Communication), 120
  rejected, antitubular basement membrane antibody production by lymphocytes isolated from (human), 173
  rejection
    effect of third-party blood transfusions on (human) (Communication), 125
    in thymectomized mice, 209
  responses, second-set (earthworm), 514
  skin
    inhibition of rejection by cyclosporine (rat), 734
    rejection by L3/T4$^+$ and Lyt-2$^+$ T cell subsets (mouse), 634
  spleen, induction of tolerance by (rat), 626
  sponge matrix
    donor-specific antibody in (mouse), 349
    frequency of cytotoxic T lymphocytes in (mouse), 75
  thyroid, rejection (mouse), 421
  tissue, limb (rat), 39
Alloimmunization, platelet, plasma exchange for (human), 602
Alloreactivity
  mechanisms (mouse), 75, 84, 349
  prethymic T cells committed to (mouse), 759
Allospecificity
  of cytotoxic T lymphocytes in sponge matrix allografts, analysis by dilution (mouse), 84
  of T cells (human), 620
Allotransplantation, intrathecal, of pancreatic endocrine cells (rat) (Communication), 531
8-Aminoguanosine, prolongation of skin graft survival with (dog) (Communication), 274
Amyloidosis, familial Mediterranean fever, cyclosporine and (human) (Communication), 793
Anemia, aplastic, associated with mucocutaneous candidasis (human), 583
Antibody
  antigen-specific, responses of lymphocytes to tetanus toxoid after bone marrow transplantation (human), 587
  anti-HLA, kidney transplantation despite FACS crossmatch following plasma exchange (human) (Communication), 131
  antitubular basement membrane, production by lymphocytes isolated from a rejected allograft (human), 173
  donor-specific, in sponge matrix allografts (mouse), 349
  HTLV-III, immunosuppression in a kidney transplant recipient with (Communication), 260
  humoral, effect of mizoribine on production (mouse), 495
  mixed lymphocyte culture-inhibiting, after blood transfusions (mouse), 100
  monoclonal
    analysis of hemopoietic cells (dog, mouse), 565
    inhibition of H-Y-specific lymph node response by (mouse) (Communication), 127
    T and natural killer cell function with (human), 104
    therapy (human), 572
    used for monitoring of kidney transplant patients, 442
  monoclonal antithymocyte, binding to kidney (rat), 739
  nephritogenic, specificity of (rat), 739
  OK709F, influence on allograft survival (monkey), 431
  OKT3 monoclonal, in kidney recipients (human), 730
  pregnancy, determinants of HLA indicated by (human), 253
  serum, reactivity (human), 447
Antigen
  allogeneic, immune responses against (mouse), 209
  class I and class II histocompatibility complex, in rejecting heart and kidney allografts (rat), 499
  class II major histocompatibility complex, expression (human), 141
  class I major histocompatibility complex platelet transfusion of (human) (Communication), 648
  H, T cell response to (mouse), 521
  histocompatibility
    -disparate skin grafts (frog), 766
    expression of class I and class II (human), 776
    role in enhancement of kidney allograft survival by blood transfusion (rat), 166
  histocompatibility complex
    contribution to immunogenicity of corneal allografts (rat), 508
    expression by cells in the cornea (rat), 248
    role (rat), 229
  HLA DR, as prognostic indicator of kidney transplant survival (human) (Communication), 534
  Ia-like and Thy-1, role in bone marrow engraftment (dog, mouse), 565
  leukocyte, expression by cells in the cornea (rat), 248
  major histocompatibility complex and nonmajor histocompatibility complex, requirement on same erythrocyte for erythrocyte-mediated prolongation of kidney allograft survival (rat), 92
  Pa, localization on the placenta (rat), 392
  -specific antibody responses of lymphocytes to tetanus toxoid after bone marrow transplantation (human), 587
  thymus donor, tolerance to (frog), 766
  transplantation, relating structure to immune function (human) (Overview), 279
  tubular, diagnosis of tubular injury in kidney transplant patients by a urinary assay, 593
Antiglobulin test, associated with gamma globulin use in bone marrow transplant recipients (human) (Communication), 663

Antilymphocyte globulin
effect on kidney allograft (human), 177
treatment of steroid-resistant rejection in patients receiving cyclosporine, 579
Antilymphocyte serum, bone marrow and, skin graft prolongation with (mouse), 26
Antithymocyte globulin, for treatment of kidney transplant rejection (human) (Communication), 133
Artery, thrombosis after transplantation, Doppler ultrasound as screen for (human) (Communication), 539
Autograft, islet, comparison of spleen and kidney (dog) (Communication), 271
Autonomic system, dysfunction, in nondiabetic uremia (human), 616
Autotransplantation, free radical-induced damage in kidneys after (rabbit), 161
Azathioprine
effect on kidney allograft (human), 177
reduction, in kidney transplant patients with hepatitis, 55

Basement membrane, antibody production by lymphocytes isolated from a rejected allograft (human), 173
B cell, functional defect (mouse), 242
Bile, cyclosporine concentration in (human) (Communication), 657
Biopsy, endomyocardial, allospecificity of T cells grown from (human), 620
Bladder, extravasation of material in (human) (Communication), 536
Blood, whole units, effect of storage on lymphocyte surface markers in (human), 235
Blood cell, patterns of organ distribution of (mouse), 204
Blood concentrations, cyclosporine, in management of kidney transplant recipients (Communication), 276
Bone marrow
and antilymphocyte serum, skin graft prolongation with (mouse), 26
engraftment, role of Ia-like and Thy-1 antigens in (dog, mouse), 565
evaluation of the use of high-dose cytoreduction with (human) (Overview), 4
functional pre-T cells in (mouse), 238
grafting, regulation of immunoglobulin production after (human), 328
graft recipients, predictive test for graft-versus-host disease in (human), 316
of graft-versus-host-reactive mice, splenic colony-forming units in, 242
procedure for depletion of lymphocytes from (human), 220
purging with ricin A chain immunotoxin, reconstitution of hematopoiesis after (human), 356
transplant, plasma fibronectin after (human) (Communication), 128
transplantation
antigen-specific antibody responses of lymphocytes to tetanus toxoid after (human), 587
antimitotic treatment prior to (human) (Communication), 790
cellular immunity to vaccinations and herpes virus infections after (human), 719
histological and immunological changes in skin after (human), 340
manipulation of graft-versus-host disease for a graft-versus-leukemia effect after (mouse), 301
natural resistance to (mouse), 688
radiation nephritis following total-body irradiation and cyclophosphamide in preparation for (human), 63
reconstitution after (human), 583
transplantation (rat), 290, 704
transplant donors, psychological adjustment of, 484
transplant patients, correlation of hypomagnesemia with onset of cyclosporine-associated hypertension in, 47
transplant recipients
adaptation of (human), 478
antiglobulin tests associated with gamma globulin use in (human) (Communication), 663
Bone marrow cell, radiolabeled (mouse), 688
Bowel, allograft, graft-versus-host disease induced by (rat), 286
Brain death, impairment of kidney slice function following (pig), 29

Calcium, plasma-ionized, monitoring during liver transplantation (human), 335
Candidasis, mucocutaneous, aplastic anemia associated with (human), 583
Cell, -mediated lympholysis generation by alloactivated lymphocytes suppression (mouse), 69
Centrifugation elutriation procedure, for depletion of lymphocytes from bone marrow (human), 220
Chimera
lymphoid, development (rat), 39
suppressor cell-induced tolerance in (mouse), 680
Cholesterol, -phosphatidylinositol liposomes, encapsulation of cyclosporine by (Communication), 659
Cirrhosis
biliary, evaluation of liver transplantation for (human), 713
micronodular, graft-versus-host disease complicated by (human) (Communication), 129
Clone, alloreactive lines and, sensitivity to cyclosporine (human), 199
Coagulation, infrared contact, treatment of kidney allograft with (human) (Communication), 264
Commercialization in transplantation (Editorial), 1
Cornea
allograft, contribution of histocompatibility complex antigens to immunogenicity of (rat), 508
expression of histocompatibility complex and leukocyte antigens by cells in (rat), 248
Cotton, -wool exudates (human), 60
Crossmatch, FACS, kidney transplantation despite (human) (Communication), 131
Cyclophosphamide
in treatment of graft-versus-host disease (human), 170
radiation nephritis following total-body irradiation and (human), 63
Cyclosporine
alternative to cyclophosphamide in treatment of graft-versus-host disease (human), 170
and familial Mediterranean fever amyloidosis (human) (Communication), 793
and intralipid, interaction (dog) (Communication), 266
and kidney ischemic injury (rat), 152
and the ischemic kidney (rat), 147
antilymphocyte globulin treatment of steroid-resistant rejection in patients receiving, 579
-associated hypertension in marrow transplant patients, correlation of hypomagnesemia with onset of, 47
-associated microangiopathy in kidney transplantation (human) (Communication), 541
blood concentrations in management of kidney transplant recipients (Communication), 276
concentration in bile (human) (Communication), 657
effect on kidney allograft (human), 177
effect on prevention of rejection of islet xenografts (rat, mouse) (Communication), 661
effect on the function of damaged kidneys (rat) (Communication), 782
effect on thymic lymphomas (mouse) (Communication), 784
effects on endocrine pancreas (rat), 44
effects on induction of thymic lymphomas (mouse), 377
effects on *Toxoplasma gondii* (mouse), 611
encapsulation by phosphatidylinositol-cholesterol liposomes (Communication), 659
for steroid-resistant rejection of kidney grafts (human) (Communication), 537
immunosuppressant (mouse), 187
inhibition of skin allograft rejection by (rat), 734
kidney transplants treated with (human), 60
metabolism and pharmacokinetics (dog), 388
Nva^2-cyclosporine versus, liver transplantation under (dog), 296
pharmacokinetics of, demographic factors affecting (human), 459
-pretreated kidney allografts (dog) (Communication), 395
sensitivity of alloreactive lines and clones to (human), 199
sensitivity of dendritic cells to (rabbit), 96
use in reversal of diabetes (rat), 426
use in transplantation (human) (Communication), 797
use to prevent kidney allograft rejection (dog) (Communication), 654
Cytomegalovirus
effects of donor pretreatment on transmission of (mouse) (Communication), 781
infection, Leu-7-positive T lymphocytes during (human) (Communication), 268
transfer by heart and kidney transplants (rat), 695
Cytoreduction, high-dose, evaluation of the use (human) (Overview), 4

Decapsulation, spontaneous, of a kidney allograft (human) (Communication), 264
Dendritic cell, sensitivity to cyclosporine (rabbit), 96

Diabetes
advanced, reversal of metabolic abnormalities by whole pancreas transplantation (rat), 556
reversal by transplantation of islets and cyclosporine treatment (rat), 426
Diabetics, with end stage kidney disease survival of, 598
Dialysis, therapy (human), 598
Diary of Forthcoming Events, 139, 547
Dimethyl sulfoxide, transplantation of kidneys after treatment with (dog), 669
Diphosphonate, treatment of hyperparathyroidism with (human) (Communication), 666
Doppler ultrasound, as screen for liver artery thrombosis after transplantation (human) (Communication), 539
Drug, immunosuppressive, administration (rat), 156

Endocrine, function of pancreas allografts (rat) (Communication), 650
Endocrine cell, pancreatic, allotransplantation of (rat) (Communication), 531
Endothelial cell, alloantigen presentation by (dog), 751
Endothelium
immunogenicity (rat), 229
vascular, immunogenicity of (human), 141
Eosinophil, in kidney allograft rejection, prognostic value of (human), 709
Epidermal cell, -lymphocyte reaction (human), 316
Epithelium, corneal, immunogenicity (rat), 229
Errata, 667, 801
Erythrocyte, -mediated prolongation of kidney allograft survival (rat), 92
Erythromycin
prophylaxis for Legionnaire's disease in immunosuppressed patients, 52
use in transplantation (human) (Communication), 797
Esophagus, varices, graft-versus-host disease complicated by (human) (Communication), 129

FACS crossmatch, kidney transplantation despite (human) (Communication), 131
Familial Mediterranean fever, amyloidosis, cyclosporine and (human) (Communication), 793
Fibronectin, plasma, after bone marrow transplant (human) (Communication), 128
Fluid leakage, treatment with infrared contact coagulation (human) (Communication), 264

Gamma, level during stimulation with alloantigens (human), 716
Gamma globulin, use in bone marrow transplant recipients antiglobulin tests associated with (human) (Communication), 663
Globulin
antilymphocyte
effect on kidney allograft (human), 177
treatment of steroid-resistant rejection in patients receiving cyclosporine, 579
antithymocyte, for treatment of kidney transplant rejection (human) (Communication), 133
gamma, use in bone marrow transplant recipients (human) (Communication), 663
Graft. *See also* Allograft
injury, reversible (human) (Communication), 541
kidney
anti-Rh_o (D) in Rh-positive patients receiving, 67
cyclosporine for steroid-resistant rejection of (human) (Communication), 537
skin
histocompatibility antigen-disparate (frog), 796
prolongation of survival with 8-aminoguanosine (dog) (Communication), 274
prolongation with donor-strain bone marrow and antilymphocyte serum (mouse), 26
prolonged survival on nonimmunosuppressed hosts (monkey) (Communication), 122
Grafting, bone marrow, regulation of immunoglobulin production after (human), 328
Graft-versus-host disease
complicated by micronodular cirrhosis and esophageal varices (human) (Communication), 129
cyclosporine as alternative to cyclophosphamide in treatment of (human), 170
in bone marrow graft recipients, predictive test for (human), 316
induced by small bowel allografts (rat), 286
in recipient of a pancreas-spleen transplant (human) (Communication), 544
lymphoid cell subclasses in target organs during (rat), 704
manipulation (mouse), 301
role of helper and suppressor T cells in (human), 328
Graft-versus-host disease, treatment with thalidomide (rat), 644
Graft-versus-host reaction
amplification by irradiation (mouse), 675
and immune function (mouse), 238, 242
induction of intestinal phase (mouse), 192
oxidative burst potential exhibited by macrophages during (mouse), 755
Graft-versus-leukemia, effect, manipulation of graft-versus-host disease for (mouse), 301

Heart
allograft
class I and class II histocompatibility complex antigens in rejecting (rat), 499
effect of splenectomy on influence of pretransplant blood transfusions on survival (rat) (Communication), 527
splenectomy and blood transfusions in (rat) (Communication), 118
class I and class II histocompatibility antigens (human), 776
-lung transplant recipients, infections in (human), 725
transplant patients, allospecificity of T cells grown from (human), 620
transplants
and explants, effects of donor pretreatment on transmission of cytomegalovirus with (mouse) (Communication), 781
superoxide dismutase decrease in (rat) (Communication), 794
transfer of cytomegalovirus by (rat), 695
Hematopoiesis, after bone marrow purging with ricin A chain immunotoxin, reconstitution of (human), 356
Hematopoietic cell, transplantation, myasthenia gravis and polymyositis following (dog), 21
Hematuria, following kidney transplantation (human) (Communication), 664
Hemolymph transfer, assay for immunorecognition (cockroach, locust), 360
Hemopoietic cell, monoclonal antibody analysis (dog, mouse), 565
Hepatitis, reduction of azathioprine in kidney transplant patients with, 55
Herpes virus, infections, cellular immunity to (human), 719
Histocompatibility
antigen, role in enhancement of kidney allograft survival by blood transfusion (rat), 166
antigen-disparate skin grafts rejection of (frog), 766
antigens, expression of class I and class II (human), 776
Histocompatibility complex
antigens
contribution to immunogenicity of corneal allografts (rat), 508
expression by cells in the cornea (rat), 248
expression of class II (human), 141
in rejecting heart and kidney allografts (rat), 499
platelet transfusion of (human) (Communication), 648
requirement for major and nonmajor (rat), 92
role (rat), 229
-positive cells in spleen (rat) (Communication), 787
products, regulation of expression (human) (Overview), 413
HLA DR antigen, as prognostic indicator of kidney transplant survival (human) (Communication), 534
HLA loci, determinants of (human), 253
Hormone, therapy, reversibility of injury by (pig), 29
HTLV-III antibody, immunosuppression in a kidney transplant recipient with (Communication), 260
Hydrostatic pressure, measurements in the diagnosis of kidney allograft rejection (human), 464
Hydroxyurea, effect on blood cells (mouse), 204
Hypercalciuria, following kidney transplantation (human) (Communication), 664
Hyperglycemia, effect on islets transplanted to the kidney capsule site (rat), 699
Hyperparathyroidism, treatment with diphosphonate (human) (Communication), 666
Hypersensitivity, reactions in the small intestine (mouse), 192
Hypertension, cyclosporine-associated, in marrow transplant patients, 47

Hypomagnesemia, correlation with onset of cyclosporine-associated hypertension in marrow transplant patients, 47
Hyporeactivity, to transplantation across a species barrier, effect of T cell depletions in reconstitution on (mouse, rat), 372

Ia-bearing cell, in islets of Langerhans, identification (rat, dog, pig, human), 364
Immune function
  graft-versus-host reaction and (mouse), 238, 242
  relating structure of transplantation antigens to (human) (Overview), 279
Immune reactivity
  after allogeneic or isogeneic transfusion (mouse), 489
  after irradiation (rat), 380
Immune response, against allogeneic antigens (mouse), 209
Immunity
  cellular
    to alloantigens (mouse), 384
    to vaccinations and herpes virus infections after bone marrow transplantation (human), 719
Immunodeficiency, T cell (mouse), 238
Immunogenetics, report of the Third International Workshop (dog), 111
Immunogenicity
  of corneal allografts, contribution of histocompatibility complex antigens to (rat), 508
  of corneal epithelium, stroma, and endothelium (rat), 229
  of purified and unpurified islet allografts (mouse) (Communication), 529
  of vascular endothelium (human), 141
Immunoglobulin, production, regulation after bone marrow grafting (human), 328
Immunosuppressant, cyclosporine (mouse), 187
Immunosuppression
  in a kidney transplant recipient with HTLV-III antibodies (Communication), 260
  of anti-idiotypic and non-anti-idiotypic antibodies to OKT3 (human), 572
Immunosuppressive agent, use of OKT3 as (human), 730
Immunosuppressive drugs, administration (rat), 156
Immunotoxin, ricin A chain, reconstitution of hematopoiesis after bone marrow purging with (human), 356
Infection
  cytomegalovirus, Leu-7-positive T lymphocytes during (human) (Communication), 268
  herpes virus, cellular immunity to (human), 719
  in heart-lung transplant recipients (human), 725
  Pneumocystis carinii, methods for diagnosis in kidney allograft recipients, 436
  transplantation for hematologic malignancies (human) (Communication), 268
Infrared contact coagulation, treatment of kidney allograft with (human) (Communication), 264
Inhibition, of H-Y-specific lymph node response by monoclonal antibody (mouse) (Communication), 127
Interferon
  level during stimulation with alloantigens (human), 716
  production capacity, after bone transplantation (human), 311
Intestine, small, hypersensitivity reactions in (mouse), 192
Intralipid, cyclosporine and, interaction (dog) (Communication), 266
Irradiation
  amplification of graft-versus-host reaction by (mouse), 675
  immune reactivity after (rat), 380
  lymphoid, suppressor cell-induced tolerance in chimeras prepared with (mouse), 680
  total-body, radiation nephritis following (human), 63
Islet
  allogeneic, reversal of diabetes by transplantation of (rat), 426
  allograft, immunogenicity of purified and unpurified (mouse) (Communication), 529
  autograft, comparison of spleen and kidney (dog) (Communication), 271
  xenograft, effect of cyclosporine on prevention of rejection of (rat, mouse) (Communication), 661
Islets of Langerhans, identification of Ia-bearing cells in (rat, dog, pig, human), 364

Kidney
  allograft
    class I and class II histocompatibility complex antigens in rejecting (rat), 499
    cyclosporine-pretreated (dog) (Communication), 395
    cytolytic T cell line established from lymphocytes homing in a rejected (human) (Communication), 135
    decapsulation of (human) (Communication), 264
    effects of delayed function on recipients of (human), 177
    erythrocyte-mediated prolongation of survival (rat), 92
    failure of platelet transfusion to improve survival (human), 468
    improved function and survival after blood transfusions (human), 640
    intrarenal hydrostatic pressure measurements in the diagnosis of rejection (human), 464
    prognostic value of eosinophil in rejection (human), 709
    role of histocompatibility antigens in survival (rat), 166
    treatment (rat), 156
    use of cyclosporine to prevent rejection (dog) (Communication), 654
  allografted, analysis of T lymphocyte response in rejecting (dog), 33
  allograft recipients, methods for diagnosis of *Pneumocystis carinii* infection in, 436
  binding of monoclonal antithymocyte antibodies to (rat), 739
  capsule site, effect of hyperglycemia on islets transplanted to (rat), 699
  damaged, effect of cyclosporine on function of (rat) (Communication), 782
  disease, survival of diabetes with end stage, 598
  free radical-induced damage in, after hypothermic preservation and autotransplantation (rabbit), 161
  graft
    anti-Rh_o (D) in Rh-positive patients receiving, 67
    cyclosporine for steroid-resistant rejection of (human) (Communication), 537
  ischemic, cyclosporine and (rat), 147, 152
  islet autograft, comparison with spleen (dog) (Communication), 271
  recipients, use of OKT3 monoclonal antibody in (human), 730
  slice function, impairment following brain death (pig), 29
  transplant
    antithymocyte globulin for treatment of rejection (human) (Communication), 133
    effect of third-party blood transfusions on (human) (Communication), 125
    lymphokine responsiveness and HLA DR antigens as prognostic indicators of survival (human) (Communication), 534
    transfer of cytomegalovirus by (rat), 695
    treated with cyclosporine (human), 60
  transplantation
    assessment of plasma neopterin (human), 454
    cyclosporine-associated microangiopathy in (human) (Communication), 541
    despite positive FACS crossmatch following plasma exchange of anti-HLA antibodies (human) (Communication), 131
    hematuria and hypercalciuria following (human) (Communication), 664
    high- versus low-dose steroids in (human), 319
    importance of Lewis system in (human), 474
    living-related (human), 602
    platelet transfusion of class I major histocompatibility complex antigen before (human) (Communication), 648
    study (human), 616
  transplant patients
    monoclonal antibodies used for monitoring of, 442
    tubular injury in, 593
  transplant recipients
    cellular rejection in (Communication), 262
    cyclosporine blood components in the management of (Communication), 276
    decreased incidence of aseptic necrosis in (human), 182
    immunosuppression in (Communication), 260
  transplants, value of urinary sediment in the diagnosis of rejection in (human), 343

Legionnaire's disease, erythromycin prophylaxis for, in immunosuppressed patients, 52
Letters to the Editor, 800
Leukemia, lymphoma, spontaneous (mouse), 301

Leukocyte, antigen, expression by cells in the cornea (rat), 248
Lewis system, importance in kidney transplantation (human), 474
Liposomes, phosphatidylinositol-cholesterol, encapsulation of cyclosporine by (Communication), 659
Liver
  artery thrombosis after transplantation, Doppler ultrasound as screen for (human) (Communication), 539
  hypothermic preservation of the (rat) (Communication), 396
  transplantation
    for biliary cirrhosis, evaluation (human), 713
    plasma-ionized calcium monitoring during (human), 335
    under Nva^2-cyclosporine versus cyclosporine (dog), 296
Lumbricus terrestris, second-set allograft responses in, 514
Lung, -heart transplant recipients, infections in (human), 725
Lymphokine, responsiveness of prognostic indicator of kidney transplant survival (human) (Communication), 534
Lymph node
  H-Y-specific, inhibition of response by monoclonal antibody (mouse) (Communication), 127
  stimulated, entry of lymphocytes into (rat), 745
Lymphocyte
  alloactivated, suppression of cell-mediated lympholysis generation by (mouse), 69
  antigen-specific antibody responses of (human), 587
  B, activation in graft-versus-host disease (rat), 290
  culture-inhibiting antibodies after blood transfusions (mouse), 100
  cytolytic T cell line established from (human) (Communication), 135
  entry into stimulated lymph nodes (rat), 745
  -epidermal cell reaction (human), 316
  from bone marrow, procedure for depletion of (human), 220
  homing in a rejected kidney allograft, cytolytic T cell line established from (mouse) (Communication), 135
  isolated from a rejected allograft, antitubular basement membrane antibody production by (human), 173
  surface markers in whole blood units, effect of storage on (human), 235
  T
    allospecificity in sponge matrix allografts (mouse), 84
    analysis of response in rejecting allografted kidneys (dog), 33
    Leu-7-positive (human) (Communication), 268
    migration (mouse), 214
    serum antibody reactivity of patients with HLA-matched, 447
    subpopulation after bone marrow transplantation (human), 311
Lymphoid cell, subclasses in target organs during graft-versus-host disease (rat), 704
Lympholysis, cell-mediated, suppression by alloactivated lymphocytes (mouse), 69

Lymphoma
  leukemia, spontaneous (mouse), 301
  thymic
    effect of cyclosporine on (mouse) (Communication), 784
    effects of cyclosporine on induction of (mouse), 377
Lyt 2^- cell, induction of intestinal phase of graft-versus-host reaction by (mouse), 192
Lyt 2^+ cell, rejection of thyroid allografts by transfer of (mouse), 421

Macrophage, oxidative burst potential exhibited by (mouse), 755
Malignancy
  evaluation of the use of high-dose cytoreduction with marrow in (human) (Overview), 4
  hematologic, bone marrow transplantation for (human) (Communication), 268
Metabolism
  abnormalities of advanced diabetes reversal of (rat), 556
  effects of cyclosporine on (dog), 388
Microangiopathy, in kidney transplantation, cyclosporine-associated (human) (Communication), 541
Migration, activated T lymphocytes (mouse), 214
Mitosis, paralysis and recovery of locomotor function during (mouse), 214
Mizoribine, effect on humoral antibody production (mouse), 495
Myasthenia gravis, and polymyositis, following hematopoietic cell transplantation (dog), 21

Natual killer cell, T and, function with monoclonal antibodies (human), 104
Necrosis, aseptic, decreased incidence in kidney transplant recipients (human), 182
Neopterin
  level during stimulation with alloantigens (human), 716
  plasma, in kidney transplantation (human), 454
Nva^2-cyclosporine, versus cyclosporine, liver transplantation under (dog), 296

Pancreas
  allograft, endocrine function of (rat) (Communication), 650
  endocrine, effects of cyclosporine on (rat), 44
  -spleen transplant, graft-versus-host disease in recipient of (human) (Communication), 544
  transplantation, reversal of metabolic abnormalities of advanced diabetes by (rat), 556
Pharmacokinetics
  effects of cyclosporine on (dog), 388
  of cyclosporine, demographic factors affecting (human), 459
Phosphatidylinositol, -cholesterol liposomes, encapsulation of cyclosporine by (Communication), 659
Phytohemagglutinin-P, prolonged allograft survival resulting from donor pretreatment with (rat) (Communication), 120
Placenta, localization of the Pa antigen on (rat), 392

Plasma
  exchange of anti-HLA antibodies, kidney transplantation despite FACS crossmatch following (human) (Communication), 131
  -ionized calcium monitoring during liver transplantation (human), 335
  neopterin, in kidney transplantation assessment (human), 454
Plasma exchange, for platelet alloimmunization (human), 602
Plasma fibronectin, after bone marrow transplant (human) (Communication), 128
Platelet, alloimmunization, plasma exchange for (human), 602
Pneumocystis carinii, infection in kidney allograft recipients, methods for diagnosis of, 346
Polymyositis, myasthenia gravis and, following hematopoietic cell transplantation (dog), 21
Polyneuropathy, in nondiabetic uremia (human), 616
Prednisolone, ways of administering (rat), 156
Pregnancy, antibodies, determinants of HLA indicated by (human), 253
Preservation
  hypothermic
    free radical-induced damage in kidneys after (rabbit), 161
    of the liver (rat) (Communication), 396
  of the kidney (dog), 669
Pressure, hydrostatic, measurements in the diagnosis of kidney allograft rejection (human), 464
Protein, adenosine deaminase binding (human), 593
Protein kinase, activation (mouse), 187

Radiation nephritis, following total-body irradiation and cyclophosphamide (human), 63
Radioimmunoassay, pharmacokinetics of cyclosporine estimated by demographic factors affecting (human), 459
Reaction
  epidermal cell-lymphocyte (human), 316
  graft-versus-host
    amplification by irradiation (mouse), 675
    and immune function (mouse), 238, 242
    induction of intestinal phase (mouse), 192
  graft-versus-host reaction, oxidative burst potential exhibited by macrophages during (mouse), 755
  hypersensitivity, in the small intestine (mouse), 192
Reactivity
  immune
    after allogeneic or isogeneic transfusion (mouse), 489
    after irradiation (rat), 380
  serum antibody (human), 447
Reconstitution
  effect of T cell depletions in (mouse, rat), 372
  of hematopoiesis after bone marrow purging with ricin A chain immunotoxin (human), 372
Rejection
  allograft
    effect of third-party blood transfusions

Rejection—(*Continued*)
on (human) (Communication), 125
in thymectomized mice, 209
cellular, in kidney transplant recipients (Communication), 262
in kidney transplants, value of urinary sediment in the diagnosis of (human), 343
in patients receiving cyclosporine steroid-resistant, 579
kidney allograft
intrarenal hydrostatic pressure measurements in the diagnosis of (human), 464
prognostic value of eosinophil in (human), 709
use of cyclosporine to prevent (dog) (Communication), 654
kidney graft, cyclosporine for steroid-resistant (human) (Communication), 537
kidney transplant, antithymocyte globulin for treatment (human) (Communication), 133
of histocompatibility antigen-disparate skin grafts (frog), 766
of islet xenografts, effect of cyclosporine on prevention of (rat, mouse) (Communication), 661
of thyroid allografts by transfer of Lyt 2^+ cells (mouse), 421
skin allograft
by L3/$T4^+$ and Lyt-2^+ T cell subsets (mouse), 634
inhibition by cyclosporine (rat), 734
Response
alloantibody, effect of blood transfusions on (rat) (Communication), 652
allograft, second-set (earthworm), 514
immune, against allogeneic antigens (mouse), 209
lymph node, inhibition by monoclonal antibody (mouse) (Communication), 127
mitogenic (human), 640
T lymphocyte, analysis in rejecting allografted kidneys (dog), 33
Rh
-immunized donor, anti-Rh_o (D) in Rh-positive patients receiving kidney grafts from, 67
-positive patients receiving kidney grafts, anti-Rh_o (D) in, 67
Ricin A chain, immunotoxin, reconstitution of hematopoiesis after bone marrow purging with (human), 356

Serum
antibody reactivity (human), 447
antilymphocyte, skin graft prolongation with (mouse), 26
Skin
allograft
inhibition of rejection by cyclosporine (rat), 734
rejection by L3/$T4^+$ and Lyt-2^+ T cell subsets (mouse), 634
graft
histocompatibility antigen-disparate (frog), 766
prolongation of survival with 8-aminoguanosine (dog) (Communication), 274
prolongation with donor-strain bone marrow and antilymphocyte serum (mouse), 26
prolonged survival on non-immunosuppressed hosts (monkey) (Communication), 122
histological and immunological changes in (human), 340
Spleen
allograft, induction of tolerance by (rat), 626
colony-forming units in bone marrow of graft-versus-host-reactive mice, 242
donor-type major histocompatibility complex-positive cells in (rat) (Communication), 787
islet autograft, comparison with kidney (dog) (Communication), 271
-pancreas transplant, graft-versus-host disease in recipient of (human) (Communication), 544
Splenectomy
and blood transfusion in heart allografts (rat) (Communication), 118
effect on influence of pretransplant blood transfusions on heart allograft survival (rat) (Communication), 527
Sponge
matrix allograft, donor-specific antibody in (mouse), 349
matrix allografts
allospecificity of T lymphocytes in (mouse), 84
frequency of cytotoxic T lymphocytes in (mouse), 75
Steroid
in kidney transplantation, high- versus low-dose (human), 319
-resistant rejection in patients receiving cyclosporine antilymphocyte globulin treatment of, 579
-resistant rejection of kidney grafts, cyclosporine for (human) (Communication), 537
Storage, effect on lymphocyte surface markers in whole blood units (human), 235
Stroma, immunogenicity (rat), 229
Subset, T cell, skin allograft rejection by L3/$T4^+$ and Lyt-2^+ (mouse), 634
Superoxide dismutase, decrease in heart transplants (rat) (Communication), 794
Suppression, of cell-mediated lympholysis generation by alloactivated lymphocytes (mouse), 69
Suppressor cell, -induced tolerance in chimeras (mouse), 680

T cell
allospecificity of (human), 620
and natural killer cell function with monoclonal antibodies (human), 104
cytolytic, line established from lymphocytes homing in a rejected kidney allograft (human) (Communication), 135
depletions in reconstitution, effect on specific hyporeactivity to transplantation across a species barrier (mouse, rat), 372
helper and suppressor, role in graft-versus-host disease (human), 328
prethymic (mouse), 759
response to minor H antigens (mouse), 521
subsets, skin allograft rejection by L3/$T4^+$ and Lyt-2^+ (mouse), 634
suppressor
in allogeneic models (rat) (Overview), 547
populations (rat), 626
Tetanus, toxoid, antigen-specific antibody responses of lymphocytes to (human), 587
Thalidomide, treatment of graft-versus-host disease with (rat), 644
Thrombosis, artery, Doppler ultrasound as screen for (human) (Communication), 539
Thymectomy, allograft rejection and immune responses against allogeneic antigens after (mouse), 209
Thymus
donor antigens, tolerance to (frog), 766
lymphoma, effects of cyclosporine on (mouse), 377
lymphomas, effect of cyclosporine on (mouse) (Communication), 784
Thyroid, allograft, rejection (mouse), 421
Tissue, allograft, limb (rat), 39
Tolerance
induction by spleen allografts (rat), 626
suppressor cell-induced, in chimeras (mouse), 680
Toxoid, tetanus, antigen-specific antibody responses of lymphocytes to (human), 587
Toxoplasma gondii, effects of cyclosporine on (mouse), 611
Transfusion, blood
allogeneic or isogeneic, immune reactivity in (mouse), 489
effect on alloantibody response (rat) (Communication), 652
improved kidney allograft function and survival after (human), 640
influence on heart allograft survival (rat) (Communication), 527
lymphocyte culture-inhibiting antibodies after (mouse), 100
role of histocompatibility antigens in enhancement of kidney allograft survival by (rat), 166
splenectomy and, in heart allografts (rat) (Communication), 118
third-party, effect on allograft rejection in HLA-identical sibling kidney transplants (human) (Communication), 125
Transfusion, platelet
failure to improve kidney allograft survival (human), 468
of class I major histocompatibility complex antigen (human) (Communication), 648
Typing cell, analysis (dog), 111

Ultrasound, Doppler, as screen for liver artery thrombosis after transplantation (human) (Communication), 539
Uremia, nondiabetic, autonomic system dysfunction and polyneuropathy in (human), 616
Urinary sediment, in the diagnosis of rejection in kidney transplants, value (human), 343

Vaccination, cellular immunity to (human), 719
Varice, esophageal, graft-versus-host disease complicated by (human) (Communication), 129

Wool, -cotton exudates (human), 60

Xenograft, islet, effect of cyclosporine on prevention of rejection of (rat, mouse) (Communication), 661

Transplantation

Volume 42

BALTIMORE, MD.
1986

July 1986
Volume 42
Number 1

Transplantation

Official Journal of the Transplantation Society

Contents

EXPERIMENTAL TRANSPLANTATION

Prolonged survival of cardiac allografts in rats following the administration of heat-treated donor lymphocytes: A possible immunosuppressive role for class I major histocompatability complex antigens.
M.A. Baird, M.P. Bradley, and B.F. Heslop. 1

Serology of liver transplantation in the rat: I. Alloantibody responses and evidence for tolerance in a nonrejector combination.
N. Kamada and T. Shinomiya. 7

Correction of equine severe combined immunodeficiency by bone marrow transplantation.
C.M. Bue, W.C. Davis, N.S. Magnuson, V.D. Mottironi, H.D. Ochs, C.R. Wyatt, and L.E. Perryman. 14

Cure of malignant lymphoma in dogs with peripheral blood stem cell transplantation.
F.R. Appelbaum, H.J. Deeg, R. Storb, T.C. Graham, K. Charrier, and W. Bensinger. 19

CLINICAL TRANSPLANTATION

A prospective analysis of the accuracy and cost effectiveness of digital subtraction angiography for living-related renal donor evaluation.
J. McElroy, A.C. Novick, S.B. Streem, D. Steinmuller, B. Risius, C. Buszta, and D. Steinhilber. 23

Multivariate analysis of risk factors in cadaver donor kidney transplantation.
F. Sanfilippo, W.K. Vaughn, W.M. LeFor, and E.K. Spees. 28

Renal transplants from HLA-haploidentical living-related donors: The influence of donor-specific transfusions and different immunosuppressive regimens.
T. Leivestad, D. Albrechtsen, A. Flatmark, and E. Thorsby. 35

Immunogenetic and clinical factors affecting renal transplantation. A rigorous analysis of data recorded by the UK Transplant Service.
W.R. Gilks, B.A. Bradley, S.M. Gore, and N.H. Selwood for the users of the UK Transplant Service. 39

Analyzing transplant survival data.
W.R. Gilks, S.M. Gore, and B.A. Bradley. 46

Epstein-Barr virus infection and immunity in bone marrow transplant recipients.
D.H. Crawford, N. Mulholland, V. Iliescu, R. Hawkins, and R. Powles. 50

Potential utilization of a national HLA-typed donor pool for bone marrow transplantation.
R.P. Gale. 54

Marrow function reconstitution by fraction 3 of Percoll-density-gradient–separated cells.
H. Ekert, W.M. Ellis, G.M. Georgiou, D.M. Robertson, K. Tiedemann, and K.D. Waters. 58

IMMUNOBIOLOGY

Mutagenicity of cyclosporine: Induction of sister chromatid exchange in human cells.
K. Yuzawa, I. Kondo, K. Fukao, Y. Iwasaki, and H. Hamaguchi. 61

Immune transfer studies in canine allogeneic marrow graft donor-recipient pairs.
H. Grosse-Wilde, K. Krumbacher, F. Schüning, I. Doxiadis, H.K. Mahmoud, C. Emde, A. Schmidt-Weinmar, and U.W. Schaefer. 64

Rejection of murine cardiac allografts. I. Relative roles of major and minor antigens.
J.F. Burdick and L.W. Clow. 67

Depletion of T cells from human bone marrow using monoclonal antibodies and rabbit complement: A quantitative and functional analysis.
A. Rohatiner, R. Gelber, S.F. Schlossman, and J. Ritz. 73

The effect of Collins' solution on the function and structure of isolated proximal convoluted tubules from rabbit kidneys.
J.F. Figueiredo, D. Falkenstein, S.A. Draibe, D. Sigulem, and O.L. Ramos. 80

BRIEF COMMUNICATIONS

Liver transplantation in Crigler-Najjar syndrome: A case report.
H. Wolff, G. Otto, H. Giest. 84

Bile duct varices: An alternative to portoportal anastomosis in liver transplantation.
J.R. Hiatt, W.J. Quinones-Baldrich, K.P. Ramming, J.F. Lois, and R.W. Busuttil. 85

Prolongation of cardiac allograft survival with BN 52021, a specific antagonist of platelet-activating factor.
M. L. Foegh, B.S. Khirabadi, J.R. Rowles, P. Braquet, and P.W. Ramwell. 86

The specific distribution of glycolipid-based blood group A antigens in human kidney related to A_1/A_2, Lewis, and secretor status of single individuals.
M.E. Breimer and B.E. Samuelsson. 88

Hyperacute rejection of a renal allograft in the presence of anti-HLA-Cw5 antibody.
J.R. Chapman, C. Taylor, A. Ting, and P.J. Morris. 91

Urine cytology in relation to urinary tract malignancies in renal transplant patients.
A.M.M. Kootte, J. Zwartendijk, J.A.M. Beekhuis-Brussee, J.H. van Bockel, and L.C. Paul. . . . 93

The synergistic effect of cyclosporine and iloprost on survival of rat cardiac allografts.
J.R. Rowles, M.L. Foegh, B.S. Khirabadi, and P.W. Ramwell. 94

Induced tolerance to allogeneic pancreatic islet transplants.
B.S. Leibel, J.M. Martin, and W. Zingg. 96

Prolongation of canine cardiac allograft survival using donor-specific buffy coat pretransfusions.
P.A. Kurlansky, A.R. Dresdale, R. Pierson, R.P. McManus, R.E. Michler, H. Sachs, W.G. Thomas, H. Lau, M.A. Hardy, C. Marboe, K. Reemtsma, and E.A. Rose. 98

LETTERS TO THE EDITOR

The continuation of the debate on gene conversion.
J. Klein and L.R. Pease. 102

Cytotoxic T lymphocyte activity in sponge matrix allografts.
J.D. Tyler and C.G. Orosz. 105

Blood eosinophilia in transplant patients.
L.E. Ianhez, J. Sabbaga, J.F. de Araújo, F.J. de Paula, and E. Sabbaga. 107

DIARY OF FORTHCOMING EVENTS 107

Transplantation

Official Journal of the Transplantation Society

Transplantation (ISSN 0041—1337) is published monthly by Williams & Wilkins, 428 E. Preston Street, Baltimore, MD 21202. Second class postage paid at Baltimore, MD, and at additional mailing offices. Postmaster, send address changes (form 3579) to Williams & Wilkins, 428 E. Preston Street, Baltimore, MD 21202. Subscription rates $105.00 ($120.00 foreign); institutions $130.00 ($145.00 foreign); single copy $12.00 ($15.00 foreign). (Prices subject to change) Indexed by *Current Contents* and *Index Medicus*.

Transplantation

INSTRUCTIONS FOR AUTHORS

Articles dealing with completed research, and brief or preliminary reports designated as *Brief Communication* will be considered for publication. The latter should present new ideas or techniques or findings of special timeliness and significance. *Brief Communications* should not be divided into sections; it is recommended that the last paragraph be a summary and the entire double-spaced typewritten manuscript *including* tables and figures should not exceed 10 pages. *Letters to the Editor*, whether in commentary on articles appearing in TRANSPLANTATION or about other pertinent matters will also be considered. *Overview* articles should cover a topic of special interest in the field of transplantation. The *overview* should not exceed 4000 words and should not be divided in sections. The references should be done according to the instructions below for *References*. If and when manuscripts are accepted for publication, it will be necessary for The Williams & Wilkins Company to receive in writing the assignment of copyright from all authors of all manuscripts. Forms for this purpose will be supplied. *Submit an original, 2 copies, and 3 sets of illustrations.* Avoid extensive handwritten alterations. Failure to observe the format requested may delay processing of the manuscript.

Typescript must be *double-spaced throughout.* Use bond paper for the original copy. Maintain a minimum left margin of approximately 4 cm and a right margin of 2.5 cm. Number the pages in sequence.

Title page should carry the title, author's name under the title, and institution and address under the author's name. Include postal zone or "zip code" in the address. To avoid confusion in bibliographic indexing, it is preferable for authors to state given names in full.

Title should be concise (preferably not more than 15 words).

Summary of not more than 250 words is to be typed on a separate sheet.

Footnotes for the text should be typed double-spaced on a separate page, but all footnotes may be typed on the same page. Footnotes should be designated by superscript Arabic numbers and numbered in sequence. Footnotes should include source of support (cited as footnote to the title), current address, correspondence address, and abbreviations.

Abbreviations used in the text and their meanings should be listed alphabetically and typed double-spaced on a separate sheet of paper or on the page with other footnotes.

References should be typed double-spaced on a separate sheet. References should be numbered in the order in which they are cited in the text. Six or fewer authors should be listed. If there are seven or more, only the first three and "et al." should be listed. The titles of articles are to be included, and the journal names are to be abbreviated according to the *Index Medicus* style. Text citations of the references are placed in parentheses. Only papers that have been accepted for publication should be listed in the references. Manuscripts in preparation, unpublished observations, and personal communications should be referred to as such in the text. Completed manuscripts that have been submitted for publication may be cited as footnotes to the text. If the manuscript is subsequently in press, appropriate changes can be made in the galleys. The following are examples of the reference style:

1. Winearls CJ, Fabre JW, Millard PR, Morris PJ. Use of cyclophosphamide and enhancing serum to suppress renal allograft rejection in the rat. Transplantation 1979; 28: 271.
2. Osler AG. Complement: mechanisms and functions. Englewood Cliffs: Prentice Hall, 1976.
3. National Center for Health Sciences. Acute conditions: incidence and associated disability, United States July 1968–June 1969. Rockville, Md.: National Center for Health Statistics, 1972. (DHEW publication no. (HSN) 72-1036).

Tables should be typed *double-spaced throughout* (including column heads, footnotes, and data), each table on a separate sheet. Number the tables in sequence with Arabic numerals. For each table supply a concise descriptive heading. Designate explanatory footnotes by superscript lowercase Latin letters. Type footnotes immediately below the table to which they refer. All columns must carry concise headings descriptive of the data in the column. Photographs of tables are not acceptable. All tables are cited in the text in numerical order.

Figures (i.e., photomicrographs, charts, and graphs) are to be supplied as unmounted glossy photographic prints. Lettering on graphs should be large enough so that when the figure is reduced to the width of a single column (8.8 cm), the lettering is still legible (1.5 mm high for an 8.8-cm-wide figure). Photomicrographs and other photographs should be no larger than 8.8 cm in width, if possible. Number the figures in sequence in Arabic numbers. Figures should be labeled on the back with the author's name, figure number, and the word "top." All figures are cited in the text in numerical order. Figure legends, numbered to correspond with the figures, typed double-spaced, and assembled on a separate sheet are to be supplied for all figures. These legends should explain all symbols used on the figures and should indicate staining and magnification for photomicrographs.

Page charges. Authors will be charged $40.00 for each printed page per article. Under exceptional circumstances, page charges will be waived by the editors.

Submit manuscripts to either editorial office:

A. P. Monaco, M.D.
TRANSPLANTATION
North American Editorial Office
New England Deaconess Hospital
185 Pilgrim Road
Boston, Massachusetts 02215

J. R. Batchelor, M.D.
TRANSPLANTATION
European Editorial Office
Department of Immunology
Royal Postgraduate Medical School
Hammersmith Hospital
Ducane Road
London W12, England

Information for Subscribers

Published monthly, two volumes a year, beginning January and July.

Annual Subscription Rates—U. S. A. AND POSSESSIONS: personal, $105.00; institutional, $130.00; single copies, $12.00. FOREIGN: personal, $120.00; institutional, $145.00; single copies, $15.00. Institutional (multiple reader) rate applies to libraries, schools, hospitals, clinics, group practices, and federal commercial, and private institutions and organizations. A special in-training rate of $60.00 ($85.00 foreign) is available to residents, fellows, interns and students. (Prices subject to change) In requesting this rate, which is limited to three years, please give training status and name of institution. Subscribers may request that their copies be sent by air mail; the extra charge entailed for air service will be billed to the subscriber.

New and renewal subscriptions are entered to begin with the January or July issue. Correspondence regarding subscriptions should be addressed to the publishers.

Change of address. Publisher must be notified 60 days in advance. Undeliverable journals will be destroyed. Duplicates (if available) can be ordered from the publishers at the regular price of single issues.

Reprints of individual articles are available *only* from authors.

Microfilm. For availability, inquire of Williams & Wilkins.

Japanese Yen price is available from our sole agent: USACO Corporation, 13-12 Shimbashi 1-Chome, Minato-Ku, Tokyo 105, Japan, telephone 03-502-6471.

WILLIAMS & WILKINS

Publishers of Books and Periodicals in Medicine and the Allied Sciences
428 East Preston Street, Baltimore, Md. 21202, U.S.A.

AUTHOR INDEX

Albrechtsen, D., 35
Appelbaum, F. R., 19

Baird, M. A., 1
Beekhuis-Brusse, J. A. M., 93
Bensinger, W., 19
Bradley, B. A., 39, 46
Bradley, M. P., 1
Braquet, P., 86
Breimer, M. E., 88
Bue, C. M., 14
Burdick, J. F., 67
Busuttil, R. W., 85
Buszta, C., 23

Chapman, J. R., 91
Charrier, K., 19
Clow, L. W., 67
Crawford, D. H., 50

Davis, W. C., 14
De Araujo, J. F., 107
Deeg, H. J., 19
De Paula, F. J., 107
Doxiadis, I., 64
Draibe, S. A., 80
Dresdale, A. R., 98

Ekert, H., 58
Ellis, W. M., 58
Emde, C., 64

Falkenstein, D., 80
Figueiredo, J. F., 80
Flatmark, A., 35
Foegh, M. L., 86, 94
Fukao, K., 61

Gale, R. P., 54
Gelber, R., 73
Georgiou, G. M., 58
Giest, H., 84
Gilks, W. R., 39, 46
Gore, S. M., 39, 46
Graham, T. C., 19
Grosse-Wilde, H., 64

Hamaguchi, H., 61
Hardy, M. A., 98
Hawkins, R., 50
Heslop, B. F., 1
Hiatt, J. R., 85

Ianhez, L. E., 107
Iliescu, V., 50
Iwasaki, Y., 61

Kamada, N., 7
Khirabadi, B. S., 86, 94
Klein, J., 102
Kondo, I., 61
Kootte, A. M. M., 93
Krumbacher, K., 64
Kurlansky, P. A., 98

Lau, H., 98
LeFor, W. M., 28
Leibel, B. S., 96
Leivestad, T., 35
Lois, J. F., 85

Magnuson, N. S., 14
Mahmoud, H. K., 64
Marboe, C., 98
Martin, J. M., 96
McElroy, J., 23
McManus, R. P., 98
Michler, R. E., 98
Morris, P. J., 91
Mottironi, V. D., 14
Mulholland, N., 50

Novick, A. C., 23

Ochs, H. D., 14
Orosz, C. G., 105
Otto, G., 84

Paul, L. C., 93
Pease, L. R., 102
Perryman, L. E., 14
Pierson, R., 98
Powles, R., 50

Quinones-Baldrich, W. J., 85

Ramming, K. P., 85
Ramos, O. L., 80
Ramwell, P. W., 86, 94
Reemtsma, K., 98
Risius, B., 23
Ritz, J., 73
Robertson, D. M., 58
Rohatiner, A., 73
Rose, E. A., 98
Rowles, J. R., 86, 94

Sabbaga, E., 107
Sabbaga, J., 107
Sachs, H., 98
Samuelsson, B. E., 88
Sanfilippo, F., 28
Schaefer, U. W., 64
Schlossman, S. F., 73
Schmidt-Weinmar, A., 64
Schüning, F., 64
Selwood, N. H., 39
Shinomiya, T., 7
Sigulem, D., 80
Spees, E. K., 28
Steinhilber, D., 23
Steinmuller, D., 23
Storb, R., 19
Streem, S. B., 23

Taylor, C., 91
Thomas, W. G., 98
Thorsby, E., 35
Tiedemann, K., 58
Ting, A., 91
Tyler, J. D., 105

Van Bockel, J. H., 93
Vaughn, W. K., 28

Waters, K. D., 58
Wolff, H., 84
Wyatt, C. R., 14

Yuzawa, K., 61

Zingg, W., 96
Zwartendijk, J., 93

August 1986
Volume 42
Number 2

Transplantation

Official Journal of the Transplantation Society

Contents

OVERVIEW

Expression of class I transplantation antigens.
H.W. Harris and T.J. Gill III 109

EXPERIMENTAL TRANSPLANTATION

Bone marrow transplantation with T-cell-depleted grafts: I. Reconstitution of immunohemopoietic functions in lethally irradiated mice transplanted with unseparated or T-cell-depleted syngeneic bone marrow grafts.
M. Shalit, M. Ayalon, L. Weiss, B. Leshem, E. Kedar, and S. Slavin. 118

Preservation damage in liver transplantation: Influence of rapid cooling.
G. Otto, H. Wolff, I. Uerlings, and K. Gellert. 122

Glomerular damage after kidney preservation.
R. Lambert, M. Henry, B. Howden, P. Jablonski, D. Rae, G. Tavanlis, V. Marshall, and J. Tange. 125

Hepatocyte transplantation for enzyme deficiency disease in congenic rats.
J.P.A.M. Vroemen, W.A. Buurman, K.P.M. Heirwegh, C.J. van der Linden, and G. Kootstra. . 130

The chyloesophageal fistula: A new approach to thoracic duct drainage.
E.P.M. Williamson and R.A. Sells. 136

Evidence that Ia^{+} bone-marrow-derived cells are the stimulus for the intestinal phase of the murine graft-versus-host reaction.
A. McI. Mowat. 141

CLINICAL TRANSPLANTATION

Sequential analysis of HLA–class II antigen expression in human renal allografts: Induction of tubular class II antigens and correlation with clinical parameters.
S.V. Fuggle, D.L. McWhinnie, J. R. Chapman, H.M. Taylor, and P.J. Morris 144

Increased factor VIII as an index of vascular injury in cyclosporine nephrotoxicity.
Z. Brown, G.H. Neild, J.J. Willoughby, N.V. Somia, and S.J. Cameron. 150

Detrimental effect of cyclosporine on initial function of cadaver renal allografts following extended preservation: Results of a randomized prospective study.
A.C. Novick, H. Ho-Hsieh, D. Steinmuller, S.B. Streem, R.J. Cunningham, D. Steinhilber, M. Goormastic, and C. Buszta. 154

Characteristics and clinical relevance of autolymphocytotoxins in patients with aplastic anemia.
N. Carpentier, J. Fontannaz, M. Jeannet, C. Nissen, and B. Speck. 159

IMMUNOBIOLOGY

Functional activity of soluble antigen-specific helper T cell molecules: Requirement for separable entities for the induction of cytotoxic T cell and B cell responses.
J.F. Krowka, C. Shiozawa, E. Diener, and L. Pilarski. 162

Mediation of cellular recruitment in vivo by functionally distinct T cell clones.
D.W. Hanto, M.B. Widmer, and R.L. Simmons. 168

In vitro and in vivo cytotoxicity of T cells cloned from rejecting allografts.
M.E. Snider, L. Armstrong, J.L. Hudson, and D. Steinmuller. 171

Expression of donor class I major histocompatibility antigens on the vascular endothelium of mouse skin allografts.
R.M.W. de Waal, M.J.J.T. Bogman, I.M.H.A. Cornelissen, A.N. Vermeulen, and R.A.P. Koene. 178

Mechanisms of transplantation tolerance in B-cell-chimeric chickens: Impairment of Tolerance by T cell growth factor.
L. Lehtonen, O. Vainio, and P. Toivanen. 184

Development of suppressor lymphocytes during acute rejection of rat cardiac allografts and preservation of suppression by anti-IL-2 receptor monoclonal antibody.
T.M. Schneider, J.W. Kupiec-Weglinski, E. Towpik, W. Padberg, D. Araneda, T. Diamantstein, T.B. Strom, and N.L. Tilney. 191

Inability to transfer immune unresponsiveness of chickens bursectomized at 60 hours of incubation.
T. Veromaa, S. Jalkanen, K. Granfors, and P. Toivanen. 197

Prolonged skin allograft survival through enhancement effects on donor tissue.
H.L. Deutsch, H.D.J. Edington, C.M. McCullough, and P.H. Sugarbaker. 200

The effectiveness of anti-Ia-immunotoxins in the suppression of MLR.
K. Nakahara, D. Kaplan, M. Bjorn, and C. G. Fathman. 205

IMMUNOGENETICS, HISTOCOMPATIBILITY AND TISSUE ANTIGENS

Differences in immunoglobulin subclasses between dye exclusion and ^{51}Cr release complement-dependent lymphocytotoxicity assays.
P.R. McConnachie, J.F. Denegri, F.E. Lower, D.S. Torry, and J.A. McIntyre. 212

The genetic control of the antibody response to the Pa antigen in the rat.
H.W. Kunz and T.J. Gill, III. 217

BRIEF COMMUNICATIONS

Severe nephrotoxicity due to the combined use of Gentamicin and cyclosporine in renal allograft recipients.
A. Termeer, A.J. Hoitsma, and R.A.P. Koene. 220

Allogeneic bone marrow transplantation for X-linked lymphoproliferative syndrome.
A.H. Filipovich, B.R. Blazer, N.K.C. Ramsay, J.H. Kersey, L. Zelkowitz, S. Harada, and D.T. Purtilo. 222

Pretransplant antibody screening using lymphocytes frozen in microtest trays.
A. Schafer and G. Opelz. 224

Assessment of primarily vascularized cardiac allografts in mice.
R.A. Superina, W.N. Peugh, K.J. Wood, and P.J. Morris. 227

LETTERS TO EDITOR

Transmission of malaria by bone marrow transplantation.
F. Dharmasena and E.C. Gordon-Smith 228

September 1986
Volume 42
Number 3

Transplantation

Official Journal of the Transplantation Society

Contents

OVERVIEW

Increasing utilization of bone marrow transplantation.
M.M. Bortin and A.A. Rimm. 229

EXPERIMENTAL TRANSPLANTATION

Transplantation of the small bowel across MHC and non-MHC disparities in the rat.
M.D. Lee, H.W. Kunz, T.J. Gill III, D.A. Lloyd, and M.R. Rowe. 235

Monoclonal antibodies for the prevention of graft-versus-host disease and marrow graft rejection: The depletion of T cell subsets in vitro and in vivo.
S. Cobbold, G. Martin, and H. Waldmann. 239

Cure of murine thalassemia by bone marrow transplantation without eradication of endogenous stem cells.
G. Wagemaker, T.P. Visser, and D.W. van Bekkum. 248

CLINICAL TRANSPLANTATION

Characterization of antileukemia cells' cytotoxic effector function: Implications for monitoring natural killer responses following allogeneic bone marrow transplantation.
L. Delmon, A. Ythier, P. Moingeon, A. Nowill, C. Bayle, J.L. Pico, M. Hayat, J. Ritz, and Th. Hercend. 252

The contribution of large granular lymphocytes to B cell activation and differentiation after T-cell-depleted allogeneic bone marrow transplantation.
M.K. Brenner, J.E. Reittie, J. Ph. Grob, J.Z. Wimperis, S. Stephens, J. Patterson, A.V. Hoffbrand, and H.G. Prentice. 257

Immunosuppressive metabolites of cyclosporine in the blood of renal allograft recipients.
T.G. Rosano, B.M. Freed, J. Cerilli, and N. Lempert. 262

Prediction of crossmatch outcome in highly sensitized dialysis patients based on the identification of serum HLA antibodies.
J.W. Oldfather, C.B. Anderson, D.L. Phelan, D.E. Cross, A.M. Luger, and G.E. Rodey. 267

Transplantation of fetal fibroblasts and correction of enzymatic deficiencies in patients with Hunter's or Hurler's disorders.
M. Adinolfi, I. McColl, D. Chase, A.H. Fensom, K. Welsh, S. Brown, J. Marsh, M. Thick, and M. Dean. 271

Long-term survival and immunological tolerance of human epidermal allografts produced in culture.
J. Thivolet, M. Faure, A. Demidem, and G. Mauduit. 274

IMMUNOBIOLOGY

Drug-induced in vitro tolerance to allogeneic antigens: I. Establishment of a tolerance induction system in a fully allogeneic murine combination.
N. Tokuda, H. Gondo, H. Mayumi, K. Taniguchi, K. Himeno, and K. Nomoto. 281

Suppression of the immune response to allogeneic histocompatibility antigens by a single exposure to ultraviolet radiation.
S.E. Ullrich. 287

Induction of B cell tolerance in rats by large doses of allogeneic erythrocytes.
G.D. Majoor and P.J.C. van Breda-Vriesman 292

Enhancement of induction of intestinal adenocarcinomas by cyclosporine in rats given a single dose of N-methyl N-nitrosourea.
M.I.R. Perera, H.W. Kunz, T.J. Gill III, and H. Shinozuka. 297

Abrogation of immunosuppressive effect of donor spleen cells on renal allografts in the rat by irradiation or heat treatment.
D. Cranston, K.J. Wood, and P.J. Morris. 302

BRIEF COMMUNICATIONS

Intravascular coagulation and kidney donation.
K.M.L. Leunissen, Th.J.M. Ruers, F. Bosman, G. Kootstra, and J.P. Van Hooff. 307

Pilot study of Campath-1, a rat monoclonal antibody that fixes human complement, as an immunosuppressant in organ transplantation.
G. Hale, H. Waldmann, P. Friend, and R. Calne. 308

Ranitidine, cimetidine, and the cyclosporine-treated patient.
M.V. Jarowenko, C.T. van Buren, W.G. Kramer, M.I. Lorber, S.M. Flechner, and B.D. Kahan. 311

A shorter procedure for preparation of E-rosette-depleted bone marrow for transplantation.
Y. Reisner, W. Friedrich, and I. Fabian. 312

The use of phytohemagglutinin stimulated mononuclear cell subpopulations for HLA typing studies involving chronic myelogenous leukemia patients.
C. Callaway, D.H. Maurer, D. Brown, W. Fang, K.M. Fehir, and M.S. Pollack. 315

Inhibition of anti-CD3 (T3) antibody-induced activation of T cells by cyclosporine.
J. Bentin, D.A. Carson, J.H. Vaughan, and C.D. Tsoukas. 317

Development of bullous pemphigoid after allogeneic bone marrow transplantation: Report of a case.
M. Ueda, T. Mori, S. Shiobara, M. Harada, T. Yoshida, T. Matsuda, K. Hattori, H. Mizoguchi, K.M. Sullivan, and R.P. Witherspoon. 320

Histocompatibility loci associated with lymphocyte alloantigenic loci.
M.H. Henning and I.F.C. McKenzie. 322

Prolonged survival of cyclosporine-treated allogeneic hepatocellular implants.
H. Darby, C. Selden, and H.J. Hodgson. 325

Pancreaticoduodenal transplantation in the rat: A technique update.
S. Lee, M. Scott, and A.R. deMacedo. 327

A technique for heart-lung transplantation in mice.
S. Lee and D. Yancey. 329

Cuff technique for orthotopic liver transplantation in the rat: A simplified method for the suprahepatic vena cava anastomosis.
A. Settaf, J. Gugenhiem, D. Houssin, and H. Bismuth. 330

Erratum 332

Diary of Forth Coming Events 332

November 1986
Volume 42
Number 5

Transplantation®

Official Journal of the Transplantation Society

Contents

OVERVIEW

Cyclosporine in allogeneic bone marrow transplantation.
O. Ringdén 445

EXPERIMENTAL TRANSPLANTATION

Recovery of glomerular and tubular function in autotransplanted dog kidneys preserved by hypothermic storage or machine perfusion: Relation of initial function to long-term function.
C.M. Gregg, L.R. Cos, P. Saraf, C.W. Fridd, and C.A. Linke. 453

Early indices of warm ischemic damage in autotransplanted canine kidneys preserved by simple hypothermic storage.
C.M. Gregg, M.K. Lai, W.A. Mandour, and C.A. Linke. 458

Modulation of host defenses to pyogenic microorganisms by cyclosporine.
T.E. Miller and G. Findon. 463

Concanavalin A-dependent cell-mediated cytotoxicity in bronchoalveolar lavage fluid: Correlation with lung allograft rejection in mongrel dogs during cyclosporine dose tapering.
A.J. Norin, S.L. Kamholz, K.L. Pinsker, E.E. Emeson, and F.J. Veith. 466

CLINICAL TRANSPLANTATION

Adverse effect of splenectomy on the survival of patients with more than one kidney transplant.
F.S. Shofer, W.T. London, P. Lyons, S.J. Simonian, J.F. Burke, B.E. Jarrell, R.A. Grossman, and C.F. Barker. 473

Expression of HLA-DR antigens on peripheral blood T lymphocytes and renal graft tubular epithelial cells in association with rejection.
F.C. Henny, J.J. Weening, W.M. Baldwin, P.J. Oljans, H.J. Tanke, L.A. van Es, and L.C. Paul. 479

Pulmonary complications of orthotopic liver transplantation.
W.A. Jensen, R.M. Rose, S.M. Hammer, R.L. Jenkins, A. Bothe, Jr., P.N. Benotti, W.H. Dzik, P. Costello, U. Khettry, C. Trey, G.M. Eliopoulos, and A.W. Karchmer 484

Multivariate prediction model of kidney transplant success rates.
M. Hennige, C.O. Köhler, and G. Opelz. 491

TC-99M DTPA scans in renal allograft rejection and cyclosporine nephrotoxicity.
W. Gedroyc, D. Taube, I. Fogleman, G. Neild, S. Cameron, and M. Maisey. 494

Marrow graft rejection and veno-occlusive disease of the liver in patients with aplastic anemia conditioned with cyclophosphamide and cyclosporine.
H.J. Deeg, H.M. Shulman, E. Schmidt, G.C. Yee, E.D. Thomas, and R. Storb. 497

Modulation of the response to interleukin-2 in recipients of donor-specific transfusions under azathioprine immunosuppression.
J.D. Tyler, C.B. Anderson, and G.A. Sicard. 502

OKT3 monoclonal antibody plasma levels during therapy and the subsequent development of host antibodies to OKT3.
G. Goldstein, A.J. Fuccello, D.J. Norman, C.F. Shield, III, R.B. Colvin, and A.B. Cosimi. 507

The clinical course of IgA-nephropathy and Henoch-Schönlein purpura following renal transplantation.
U. Bachman, C. Biava, W. Amend, N. Feduska, J. Melzer, O. Salvatierra, and F. Vincenti. . . 511

Interstitial pneumonitis following autologous bone marrow transplantation.
R. Pecego, R. Hill, F.R. Appelbaum, D. Amos, C.D. Buckner, A. Fefer, and E.D. Thomas. . . . 515

Opportunistic strongyloidiasis in renal transplant recipients.
J.S. Morgan, W. Schaffner, and W.J. Stone. . . . 518

IMMUNOBIOLOGY

Suppression of B cell immunity to DNP by serotherapy with monoclonal anti-DNP antibodies: Effect of treatment schedule on the magnitude of specific suppression and its duration.
P.R. Beining, B. Merchant, E.F. Lizzio, and T. Hoffman. . . . 524

The splenic microenvironment and self recognition as factors in allograft rejection in rats: A study using Indium-111-labeled cells.
R. Pollak, J.M. Blanchard, and V.A. Lazda. . . . 528

The mechanism of prolonged graft survival following removal of the regional lymph node.
J.S. Wotherspoon and S.E. Dorsch. . . . 532

Allogeneic hepatocyte transplantation in the rat spleen under cyclosporine immunosuppression.
L. Makowka, G. Lee, C.S. Cobourn, E. Farber, J.A. Falk, and R.E. Falk. . . . 537

Further observations on transfusion collapse curves in inbred rats.
M.A. Baird and B.F. Heslop. . . . 542

The activity of suppressor cells in the spleen of murine bone marrow chimeras.
M. Imamura, T. Miyazaki, H. Fujimoto, T. Fukuhara, M. Kasai, T. Itaya, and K. Sakurada. . . . 548

BRIEF COMMUNICATIONS

Renal transplantation in patients with a history of heroin abuse.
M.J.V. Gordon, R. White, A.J. Matas, V.A. Tellis, D. Glicklich, T. Quinn, R. Soberman, and F.J. Veith. . . . 556

HLA-DP matching and graft-versus-host disease in allogeneic bone marrow transplantation.
G. Pawelec, G. Ehninger, H. Schmidt, and P. Wernet. . . . 558

Orthotopic liver transplantation for hepatobiliary malignancy: Report of three cases of special interest.
J.O. Colonna II, R.A. Ray, L.I. Goldstein, J.R. Hiatt, W. Quinones-Baldrich, K.P. Ramming, and R.W. Busuttil. . . . 561

Use of two donor-specific transfusions for living-related donor kidney transplantation.
R.T. Schweizer, S.A. Bartus, M.A. Rovelli, and L.M. Bow. . . . 562

Preliminary report of the effect in an animal model CSC. Microsurgically revascularized bone allografts with immunosuppression with cyclosporine.
M. Aebi, P. Regazzoni, S.M. Perren, and F. Harder. . . . 567

Effect of cyclosporine on islet xenograft survival in the BB/W rat.
H. Selawry, K. Whittington, and R. Fajaco. . . . 568

December 1986
Volume 42
Number 6

Transplantation®

Official Journal of the Transplantation Society

Contents

OVERVIEW

Failure of allogeneic canine marrow grafts after total-body irradiation: Allogeneic "resistance" versus transfusion-induced sensitization.
R. Storb and H.J. Deeg. 571

EXPERIMENTAL TRANSPLANTATION

Immunosuppressive activity of serum from liver-grafted rats.
N. Kamada, T. Shinomiya, T. Tamaki, and K. Ishiguro. 581

Cryopreservation of mouse pancreatic islets: Effects of fast cooling on islet B cell function and on the outcome of islet transplantation.
S. Sandler, Y. Kojima, and A. Andersson. 588

Prolongation of renal allograft survival in antilymphocyte-serum-treated dogs by postoperative injection of density-gradient-fractionated donor bone marrow.
W.C. Hartner, S.R. DeFazio, T. Maki, T.G. Markees, A.P. Monaco, and J.J. Gozzo. 593

CLINICAL TRANSPLANTATION

Renal transplantation in 45 patients with amyloidosis.
A. Pasternack, J. Ahonen, and B. Kuhlbäck. 598

A prospective study of unexplained nausea and vomiting after marrow transplantation.
G.D. Spencer, R.C. Hackman, G.B. McDonald, D.E. Amos, B.A. Cunningham, J.D. Meyers, and E.D. Thomas. 602

Immunoglobulin class and specificity of antibodies causing positive T cell crossmatches: Relationship to renal transplant outcome.
J.R. Chapman, C.J. Taylor, A. Ting, and P.J. Morris. 608

Small intestinal transplantation using cyclosporine: Report of a case.
Z. Cohen, R.E. Silverman, R. Wassef, G.A. Levy, M. Burnstein, J. Cullen, L. Makowka, B. Langer, and G.R. Greenberg. 613

IMMUNOBIOLOGY

Evidence that secondary mixed leukocyte culture supernatant mediates changes in cellular recruitment, blood flow and vascular permeability.
D. Hanto, J.T. Harty, R.A. Hoffman, and R.L. Simmons. 621

Evidence of a cyclosporine-binding protein in human erythrocytes.
R.P. Agarwal, R.A. McPherson, and G.A. Threatte. 627

Induction of antiidiotypic antibodies by blood transfusions: Characterization of T cell alloantigen-specific receptors by sera from transfused mice.
D.P. Singal, D. Ludwin, S. Joseph, M.A. Blajchman, F.A. Ofosu, and S-K. Liao. 632

Rejection of skin grafts and generation of cytotoxic T cells by mice depleted of $L3T4^+$ cells.
J. Woodcock, D. Wofsy, E. Eriksson, J.H. Scott, and W.E. Seaman. 636

The requirement for the renal transplant to induce allograft unresponsiveness by the combination of extracted histocompatibility antigen and cyclosporine.
N. Yoshimura and B.D. Kahan. 642

Human class II antigens: Implication of carbohydrate in the determinants recognized by several antihuman class II monoclonal antibodies.
R.L. Sparrow, H.A. Vaughan, and I.F.C. McKenzie. 647

Ultraviolet irradiation of canine dendritic cells prevents mitogen-induced cluster formation and lymphocyte proliferation.
J. Aprile and H.J. Deeg. 653

Inhibition of rat mixed lymphocyte pancreatic islet cultures with anti-la immunotoxin.
J. Shizuru, S. Ramakrishnan, T. Hunt, R.C. Merrell, and C.G. Fathman. 660

The role of resident accessory cells in corneal allograft rejection in the rabbit.
K.A. Williams, T.S. Mann, M. Lewis, and D.J. Coster. 667

Expression of HLA antigens on renal tubular cells in culture: I. Evidence that mixed lymphocyte culture supernatants and gamma interferon increase both class I and class II HLA antigens.
G.A. Bishop, B.M. Hall, M.G. Suranyi, D.J. Tiller, J.S. Horvath, and G.G. Duggin. 671

Comparison of the immunosuppressive effects of cyclosporine, lipid-soluble anesthetics, and calmodulin antagonists: Response to exogenous interleukin 2.
S.J. LeGrue and C.G. Munn. 679

BRIEF COMMUNICATIONS

The effect of irradiation of the donor spleen on rejection of porcine pancreaticoduodeno-splenic allografts.
D.C. Dafoe, D.A. Campbell, Jr., W.H. Marks, A. Borgstrom, A.S. Lichter, and J.G. Turcotte. . . 686

Suppression of host-versus-graft response in experimental biliary obstruction.
P.T. Roughneen, A.D. Kulkarni, D.J. Gouma, W.C. Fanslow, and B.J. Rowlands. 687

Isolation of rat pancreatic islets by ductal injection of collagenase.
R. Sutton, M. Peters, P. McShane, D.W.R. Gray, and P.J. Morris. 689

Enumeration of transferrin-receptor-expressing lymphocytes as a potential marker for rejection in human cardiac transplant recipients.
T. Mohanakumar, K. Hoshinaga, N.L. Wood, S. Szentpetery, and R.R. Lower. 691

The effect of repeated pregnancies on renal allograft function.
J.R. Scott, D.W. Branch, N.K. Kochenour, and R.M. Larkin 694

Assessment of factors associated with donor-specific sensitization in patients given donor-specific blood transfusions.
S. Vaidya, B.G. Sommer, E. Pagel, M. Koegel, and R.M. Ferguson. 695

Cell-mediated lympholysis in Kaposi's sarcoma after renal allograft: Report of two cases.
S.G. Rodríguez, R.S. Martín, H.A. Araujo, C.L. Alvarez, and M.D.C. Samaniego. 697

Immunofluorescence caused by cyclosporine in urinary exfoliative cytology from renal transplant recipients.
A.E. Larsen. 699

Stored-blood donor-specific transfusions with cyclosporine in distantly related and unrelated donor-recipient pairs.
T.R. Hefty and J.M. Barry 702

AUTHOR INDEX 704

SUBJECT INDEX 707

0041-1337/86/4201-0001$02.00/0
TRANSPLANTATION
Vol. 42, No. 1
Printed in U.S.A.

Transplantation

ARTICLES

PROLONGED SURVIVAL OF CARDIAC ALLOGRAFTS IN RATS FOLLOWING THE ADMINISTRATION OF HEAT-TREATED DONOR LYMPHOCYTES[1]

A POSSIBLE IMMUNOSUPPRESSIVE ROLE FOR CLASS I MAJOR HISTOCOMPATIBILITY COMPLEX ANTIGENS[1]

MARGARET A. BAIRD,[2] MARK P. BRADLEY, AND BARBARA F. HESLOP

Department of Surgery, University of Otago Medical School, Dunedin, New Zealand

Pretransplant transfusions of spleen and lymph node cells heated to 45°C or 50°C for 1 hr prolong the survival of subsequent donor-specific heart grafts in the fully allogeneic donor-host combination DA (RT1^a) → AS (RT1^l). The results are comparable to survival times recorded following pretransplant transfusions of purified donor specific red blood cells (RBC) in the same strain combination. Both class I and class II major histocompatibility complex (MHC) antigens are serologically detectable on heat-treated cells; by contrast only class I antigens are expressed on red blood cells. Although heat-treated cells stimulate alloantibody formation, they fail to provoke a proliferative response in an in vivo host-versus-graft assay. Both red blood cells and heat-treated inocula persist in the host for long periods, possibly an important consideration in relation to their capacity to prolong the survival of subsequent donor strain allografts.

The experimental data support the contention that class I MHC antigens can be immunosuppressive in the context of allografting. The present results recall the experiments carried out early in the century, which used heat-treated tumor cells to prolong the survival of subsequent viable tumor allografts, and which are sometimes cited as the first example of active enhancement.

The host response evoked by allogeneic class I antigens (equivalent to mouse H-2K and D) of the major histocompatibility complex (MHC)* has been studied using two different experimental approaches, each of which has provided a different view of the immunogenicity of these molecules. Thus, when mutant recombinant or congenic mouse strains are arranged so that donor and host (or stimulator and responder) differ with respect only to H-2K or H-2D antigens, these class I antigens are able to stimulate graft rejection, to provoke the production of alloantibodies, and to evoke and effect cell-mediated cytotoxicity (*1–3*). Implicit in the design of these immunogenetically elegant experiments has been the "silence" of MHC gene products not being tested, and with respect to which donor and host (or stimulator and responder) have been identical. The class I antigens under investigation in these experiments have been presented in cell populations such as skin grafts and lymphoid cell suspensions, which seem likely to have included macrophages and cells of the Langerhans and dendritic cell lineages.

An alternative approach to the function of allogeneic class I antigens has involved studying the immunogenicity of populations of cells such as purified red cells and platelets that express class I but not class II MHC antigens. These cells have not only been poorly immunogenic (*4–7*), but have led to prolonged survival of subsequent donor strain kidney, heart, and bone marrow allografts (*8–14*). While the substance mediating the immunosuppression in these experiments has not yet been identified with certainty, the specificity of the immunosuppression in some of these experiments has suggested a possible role for the class I antigens themselves (*7, 11*). Support for this idea comes from the observations of Kamada et al. (*15*) who reported that the specific immunosuppression that followed liver allografting in rats was apparently mediated by a molecule that was inactivated by a monoclonal antibody reactive with rat class I MHC antigen. The potential clinical usefulness of pretreatment schedules that fail to immunize and are specifically immunosuppressive prompted an examination of the effects of administering donor strain heat-treated lymphocytes in the context of organ grafting in rats.

Lymphocytes heated to 45°C for 1 hr continue to express MHC class I antigens and class II antigens, but the cells are functionally dead: they are unable to stimulate alloreactivity in vitro (*16, 17*), but are specifically able to inhibit in vitro alloreactivity (*18–21*). We report here that heat-killed lymph node cells and spleen cells specifically prolong the survival of donor strain heart allografts in rats, and have an immunosuppressive effect comparable to that of allogeneic red cells. Possible clinical implications of these findings are discussed.

MATERIALS AND METHODS

Animals. Rats were 2–8 months old and came from the departmental colony. The following inbred strains were used

* ALC, allogeneic lymphocyte cytotoxicity; ELISA, enzyme-linked immunosorbent assay; MHC, major histocompatibility complex; MLR, mixed lymphocyte reaction; NK, natural killer; PVP, polyvinylpyrrolidone; RBC, red blood cell.

[1] This work was supported by the Medical Research Council of New Zealand and the Royal Australasian College of Surgeons Foundation.

[2] Address correspondence to: M. A. Baird, Ph.D. Department of Surgery, Otago Medical School, P.O. Box 913, Dunedin, New Zealand.

(MHC haplotypes in parentheses): DA ($RT1^a$), AS ($RT1^l$), PVG ($RT1^c$), and AUG ($RT1^c$) together with $(DA\times AS)F_1$ hybrids. The origins and characteristics of these strains are detailed in standard listings (*22*).

Preparation and injection of red blood cells. Blood was collected into heparinized syringes by aortic puncture, diluted 1:1 in saline, and centrifuged three times through a double discontinuous Ficoll Hypaque density gradient as previously described (*23, 24*). This procedure regularly achieves 99.85% depletion of leukocytes (*24*). The cells were washed twice and diluted 1:1 in saline, following which 0.3 ml (approximately 1.8×10^9 red cells) was injected into the exposed lateral tail vein.

Preparation and injection of viable and heat-treated lymph node and spleen cells. Cervical, axillary, mesenteric, aortic, and iliac lymph nodes and spleens were harvested from donor rats. Cell suspensions were prepared by gently pressing these tissues through a stainless steel sieve into PBS + 10% fetal calf serum. The cells were washed twice, counted and adjusted to a concentration of 6×10^8/ml. Suspensions were divided in two. One part was injected i.v. (3×10^8 nucleated cells in 0.5 ml per rat), while the other was heated at 45°C or 50°C for 1 hr, washed twice, readjusted to 6×10^8/ml and injected as above. Cell viability was assessed by dye exclusion using Trypan blue in 0.8% saline.

Accessory heart grafts. Rats were anaesthetized with halothane and nitrous oxide. Hearts were grafted into the abdomen using a modification of the method of Silber (*25*). The left kidney was removed and the renal artery and ureter tied off. The donor pulmonary artery was joined end-to-end to the left renal vein, while the donor aorta was joined end-to-side to the host aorta. Graft survival was monitored by electrocardiography, the survival endpoint being the last day on which a tracing was obtainable. Tracings were obtained daily for the first 8 days after grafting, and at twice-weekly intervals thereafter.

Serological assay for the detection of Class I and Class II antigens. The urease enzyme-linked immunosorbent assay (ELISA) for detecting class I and class II MHC antigens was similar to the procedure for H-Y antigen (*26*). Briefly, heat-treated or fresh lymphocytes (5×10^4 per well) were dried onto 96-well plates (Nunc Immunoplate) overnight. Monoclonal antibodies directed against rat class I or class II MHC molecules (Y1/100 directed against $RT1.A^a$ and YRB/24 directed against $RT1.B^c$, crossreacting with $RT1.B^a$ and negative with $RT1.B^l$, Serotec, UK) were used as primary antibodies, and sheep anti-rat IgG conjugated with urease (Commonwealth Serum Laboratories, Melbourne) as the second antibody. The assay was developed with urease substrate (Commonwealth Serum Laboratories, Melbourne), which provides a yellow (negative) to purple (positive) color change. Each test was carried out using known positive and negative controls.

Quantitation of host-versus-graft reactivity by popliteal node assay. Lymph node cell suspensions were prepared as described above, centrifuged through Ficoll-paque (Pharmacia, Uppsala), and washed twice. Half a given suspension was injected into the left foot-pad of parental strain hosts, and the remaining half was heated at 45°C for 1 hr, prior to injection into the right foot-pad. Two cell doses were investigated, 2×10^7 and 12×10^7 in 0.1 ml saline. Controls received 0.1 ml saline. Four days after injection the popliteal nodes were harvested and weighed. The cellular kinetics of this test has been described in detail elsewhere (*27–30*).

Titration of hemagglutinating antibodies. Red blood cells (RBC) were prepared as a 2% suspension in 20% bovine serum albumin, and sera were serially diluted in polyvinylpyrrolidone (PVP) MW 160,000 as described elsewhere (*7*). Equal volumes of serum and RBC were drawn into microhematocrit tubes that were gently rocked at 30-min intervals and read macroscopically at 2 hr. Negative controls (cells from the serum donor strain) were included with each test.

Migration pattern of heat-treated lymph node cells. Cell suspensions were prepared from the lymph nodes of DA donors as described above, adjusted to a concentration of 10^8/ml and labeled with 40 μCi/ml of ^{51}Cr (sodium chromate (^{51}Cr) in sterile isotonic saline, Radiochemical Centre, Amersham, UK) for 30 min at 37°C. The cells were washed three times, and suspended at approximately 2×10^8/ml. Part of each suspension was used for i.v. injection (2×10^7 cells in 0.1 ml/rat) into groups of DA and AS hosts. The remainder of each suspension was heated to 45°C for 1 hr prior to injection at the same dosage into groups of AS hosts. Samples of the cell suspension were retained for calculation of the total radioactivity injected. Rats were killed either 24 or 48 hr or 7 days later, and lymph nodes (superficial and deep cervical, axillary, mesenteric, aortic, and iliac), spleen, liver, kidney, lung, blood (500 μl), and thymus removed. The radioactivity in these organs was measured in a gamma counter. Urine was collected from the groups of AS recipients killed 24 and 48 hr after injection. Results were expressed as a percentage of the total radioactivity injected.

RESULTS

Prolongation of survival of donor-strain heart grafts by pretransplant transfusion with heat-treated allogeneic lymphocytes or purified allogeneic red blood cells. Groups of AS strain rats were treated with three i.v. injections at weekly intervals (total dose approximately 9×10^8 cells) of fresh DA lymphocytes (lymph node and spleen cells), heat-treated DA lymphocytes (45°C or 50°C for 1 hr), fresh AS lymphocytes, heat-treated AS lymphocytes, or heat-treated PVG (third-party) lymphocytes. In a comparable experiment, groups of AS rats received 4 i.v. injections at weekly intervals of DA, AS, or PVG red cells (total dose approximately 7.2×10^9 cells). One week after the last injection all rats were grafted with auxiliary DA heart grafts, the survival of which was monitored electrocardiographically.

The results are summarized in Table 1. It is apparent that both heat-treated allogeneic lymphocytes and allogeneic red blood cells were able specifically to suppress the immune response to fully allogeneic heart grafts. Heat-treated cells had a less predictable immunosuppressive effect than did red cells, in that not all recipients of heat-treated cells showed prolonged survival of donor-strain heart allografts, whereas all recipients of allogeneic red cells showed prolonged graft survival.

The capacity of heat-treated and fresh allogeneic lymph node and spleen cells to provoke the production of hemagglutinating alloantibodies. Serum was collected from the AS rats in the above experiments after the final injection of cells, and again four days after they had received heart grafts. The results are shown in Figure 1. Hemagglutinin titers in pregraft sera were slightly higher in animals treated with live cells than in the recipients of heated cells. No antibodies were recorded after treatment with allogeneic red blood cells. Of the postgraft sera, no antibodies could be detected in AS rats pretreated with DA red cells. On the other hand, recipients of heat-treated cells showed no impairment of their capacity to produce hemaglutinins in response to DA heart grafts. Since only 50% of the cells in the suspension heated at 45°C for 1 hr excluded Trypan blue,

TABLE 1. The effects of various pretreatments on the survival of DA heterotopic heart grafts in AS hosts

Donor→host	Pretreatment[a]	Graft survival time (days)		Significance[d]
		Female hosts	Male hosts	
AS→AS	Nil	4×>100	4×>100	
DA→AS	Nil	6, 6, 6, 6, 7	6, 7, 7, 10, 16	
DA→AS	DA RBC	32, 46, 50, 52	21, 22, 27, 43	
DA→AS	AS RBC	6, 7, 7, 7, 8, 8	6, 6, 6, 6, 7, 7	
DA→AS	PVG RBC		6, 6, 7, 7, 7, 8	
DA→AS	DA heated lymphocytes	9, 11, 13, 32[b]	3[c]×>100 6, 10, 10, 14, >25, 2×>26, 2×>30[c]	
DA→AS	AS heated lymphocytes	4, 6, 6, 13[b]		
DA→AS	PVG heated lymphocytes	6, 6, 7, 7, 8, 8[b]		
DA→AS	DA fresh lymphocytes	1, 1, 1, 1, 4, 4, 5, 6		
DA→AS	AS fresh lymphocytes	4, 5, 9, 13		

[a] RBC = 4 iv injections at weekly intervals of purified red cells (total cells approximately 7.2×10^9)

Heated lymphocytes = 3 iv injections at weekly intervals of heated lymph node cells and spleen cells (total cells approximately 9×10^8): ([b] 45°C for 1 hr. [c] 50°C for 1 hr)

Fresh lymphocytes = 3 iv injections at weekly intervals of fresh lymph node cells and spleen cells (total cells approximately 9×10^8).

[d] The difference between the bracketed pairs was significant at the 1% level using Wilcoxon's test for unpaired samples.

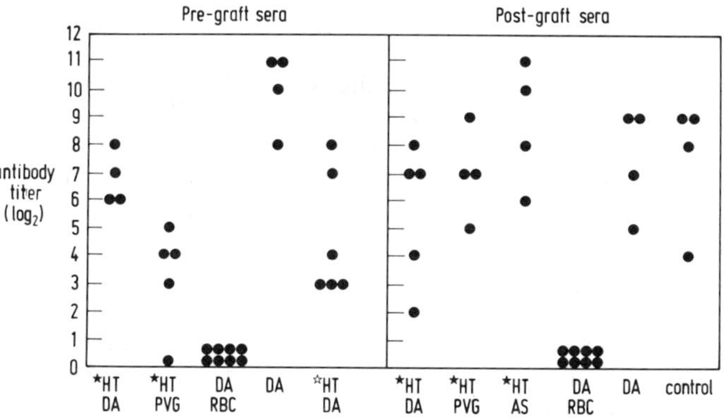

FIGURE 1. Hemaglutinin response to pretransplant transfusions of RBC or heat-treated lymphocytes and to subsequent heart allografts. Pregraft sera were taken from AS rats one week after the last of 3 i.v. injections of 3×10^8 donor strain (DA, PVG, and AS) spleen and lymph node cells prepared freshly or heat-treated at 45°C (★HT) or 50°C (☆HT) or 4 i.v. injections of 1.8×10^9 DA RBC. All recipients were grafted with DA hearts immediately after serum sampling. Postgraft sera were collected four days after allografting. "Control" sera were taken from untreated AS rats grafted with DA hearts.

another suspension heated at 50°C for 1 hr was examined for its capacity to provoke the production of alloantibodies. Both, however, evoked antibody responses (Fig. 1).

The finding that class II antigens on heat-treated cells are serologically detectable but functionally inactive in popliteal node assays. A urease ELISA using DA lymphocyte targets and doubling dilutions of a monoclonal antibody reactive against an MHC class II RT1.B[a] antigen (YRB/24: Serotec, UK), showed similar titration endpoints (1:6400) with both fresh and heat-treated targets. A monoclonal antibody reactive with a class I RT1.A[a] antigen (Y1/100: Serotec, UK) also reacted similarly with fresh and heated cells (titer 1:400) in a urease ELISA. Although these assays had relatively high levels of "background noise", there was a clear difference between DA and AS cells using both antibodies. Thus, both class I and class II antigens remained serologically identifiable despite heat treatment.

Popliteal node assays of host-versus-graft alloreactivity in vivo. Popliteal node enlargement was measured 4 days after the injection of fresh or heat-treated $(DA\times AS)F_1$ lymphocytes, or of saline alone, into the foot-pads of AS rats. Two doses of cells were examined, 2×10^7 and 12×10^7. The results are illustrated in Figure 2. It is apparent that the popliteal nodes draining the foot-pads injected with heat-treated cells showed no enlargement when compared with the popliteal nodes draining foot-pads injected with saline alone. On the other hand, popliteal nodes draining the foot-pads injected with fresh cells showed significant enlargement. These results were clearly demonstrable at the lower of the two doses and were not greatly altered by a six-fold increase in the dose of cells injected into the foot-pad. Thus, although class II antigens are identifiable on heated cells, they are unable to stimulate alloreactivity as measured by the popliteal node assay.

In relation to the practice of injecting fresh F_1 lymphocytes into the left foot-pad and heated F_1 lymphocytes into the right foot-pad in these experiments, it is noted that cells injected into one foot-pad have no effect on the weight of the contralateral popliteal node 4 days later (personal communication, the late W.L.Ford, and unpublished observations).

The capacity of heat-treated lymphocytes to migrate to the lymphoid organs. When suspensions of viable ^{51}Cr-labeled rat lymph node cells are injected i.v. into syngeneic or allogeneic hosts, they migrate in a pattern that is characteristic for the strain combination: the lymph nodes and spleen account for most of the label recovered from syngeneic or allogeneic recipients 24 hr after injection (*31*). Almost all the lymph node radioactivity represents viable cells (*32–35*). When the labeled cells are killed by heating to 56°C for half an hour, or by exposure to alloantibody prior to injection, or when debris or supernatant from freeze-thawed labeled cells is injected, the distribution of label changes in a characteristic fashion. Virtually no radioactivity is found in the lymph nodes, the spleen label is greatly reduced, liver radioactivity is increased, and large quantities of label are excreted in the urine (*33, 35*).

It is apparent from Table 2 that the distribution of label following the i.v. injection of 2×10^7 heat-treated (45°C for 1 hr) ^{51}Cr labeled DA lymphocytes into AS hosts was similar to that previously reported following the injection of dead cells and cell debris (*33, 35*). Compared with recipients of viable cell suspensions, animals that had received cells heated at 45°C for 1 hr showed significantly reduced lymph node and spleen radioactivity, and significantly increased liver and kidney label. It was thus concluded that lymphocytes heated to 45°C for 1 hr were functionally dead with respect to their capacity to migrate to the lymphoid organs. Table 2 also shows that a considerable proportion of the label remained in the body 7 days after injection, a point that is considered in the *Discussion* section in relation to the persistence of allogeneic red cells in the circulation.

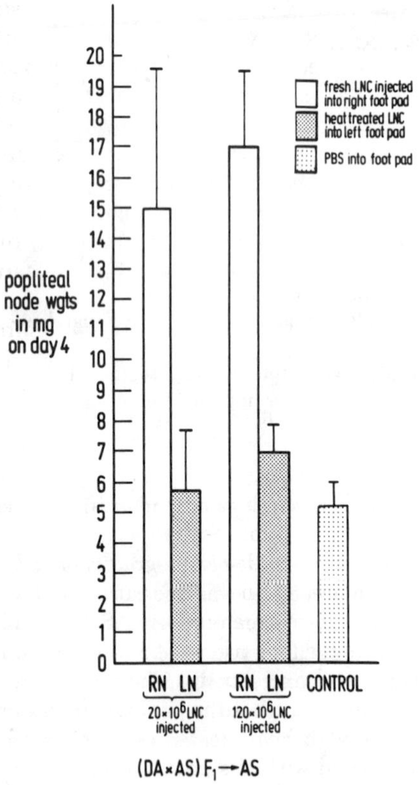

FIGURE 2. Popliteal node assay for in vivo host-versus-graft proliferative response to heat-treated (45°C for 1 hr) and fresh semiallogeneic lymphocytes.

The strain combination DA→AS was used throughout this series of experiments. It is noted, however, in connection with lymphocyte traffic studies, that unsensitized AS hosts regularly destroy a substantial proportion of i.v. injected viable DA lymph node cells as a result of allogeneic lymphocyte cytotoxicity (ALC), and a natural killer (NK)-like phenomenon (reviewed in *32, 36*). Thus, as a result of ALC substantially less radioactivity was present in the lymph nodes of AS hosts 24 hr after injection than was found in the lymph nodes of syngeneic (DA) recipients of the same cell suspension, and large quantities of label were excreted in the urine (Table 2). This is a typical result for the DA→AS strain combination (*31*). Nevertheless, the distribution of label characterizing ALC was clearly distinguishable from that associated with the injection of dead cells (*32*; Table 2).

DISCUSSION

These results confirm previous observations that heat-modified lymph node and spleen cells express class I and class II MHC antigens (*16*), but the cells are functionally dead (*21*). The inability of heat-treated cells, even at a very high dose (Fig. 2) to stimulate in popliteal node assays in vivo, parallels their inability to stimulate in mixed lymphocyte reaction (MLR) in vitro (*16, 17*). Likewise, their immunosuppressive effect in prolonging the survival of donor strain heart grafts (Table 1) probably represents an in vivo correlate of the inhibitory effect of heat-treated cells on the stimulatory capacity of fresh autologous cells in MLR (*18–21, 37*). The specificity of

TABLE 2. Distribution of radioactivity at various times after the injection of viable and heat-killed suspensions of ^{51}Cr-labeled DA lymph node cells

Donor→host[a]	Cell suspension	Time after injection	Mean radioactivity recovered (± SE) as a percentage of the total radioactivity from various sources					
			Lymph Nodes	Spleen	Liver	Kidneys	Total[b]	Urine[c]
DA→DA	Viable	24 hr	29.4 (1.2)	18.7 (0.6)	15.9 (0.3)	0.7 (0.03)	67.9 (0.6)	
DA→AS	Viable	24 hr	10.2 (0.2)	24.8 (0.4)	13.9 (0.12)	1.7 (0.04)	51.8 (0.5)	27.3 (1.8)
DA→AS	Heated (45°C for 1 hr)	24 hr	0.21[d] (0.05)	2.96[d] (0.05)	34.4[d] (2.4)	6.3[d] (0.1)	44.7 (2.5)	33 (1.6)
DA→AS	Viable	48 hr	7.4 (0.6)	22.3 (0.3)	14.1 (0.8)	2 (0.7)	46.4 (0.5)	35.4 (2.2)
DA→AS	Heated (45°C for 1 hr)	48 hr	0.24[d] (0.06)	3.16[d] (0.1)	32.8[d] (1.9)	6.3[d] (0.1)	43.2 (1.9)	38.1 (1.7)
DA→AS	Heated (45°C for 1 hr)	7 days	0.23 (0.17)	3.89 (0.17)	23.4 (0.7)	6.1 (0.09)	33.9 (0.9)	

[a] Groups contained 5–8 rats.

[b] Total for all organs counted (see the *Materials and Methods* section). Organs containing only small amounts of radioactivity have been excluded from this table.

[c] Total urine over the stated period.

[d] The difference between the figure indicated and the figure immediately above, which relates to the corresponding viable cell suspension, was highly significant $P<0.001$).

the immunosuppression afforded to heart allografts in rats (Table 1) implies a role for the MHC antigens. The specific immunosuppression following the administration of heat-treated cells may be analogous to the immunosuppression following the administration of purified red cells (*8–11*; Table 1) and platelets (*12–14*), both of which express class I but not class II MHC antigens. On the basis of in vitro experiments using heat-modified cells, Goeken (*21*) has suggested that T suppressor cells may be activated autonomously by class I antigens without the necessity for T cell help, and that suppressor T cells differ functionally from cytotoxic effector T cells in their requirement for help. On the basis of the same experiments, Goeken has also suggested that grafts which present mostly class I antigens may preferentially activate suppressor cells (*20*). While the use of heat-modified cells for specific immunosuppression has attracted relatively little attention in relation to organ allografts, it was nevertheless used by Flexner and Jobling as early as 1907 (*38*) to prolong the survival of tumor allografts. This work has previously been cited as the first example of active immunological enhancement (*39, 40*). It might be profitable to reexamine the other nonviable cellular inocula previously used to induce active enhancement (*39, 40*) with a view to their possible use as sources of class I MHC antigen.

The idea that MHC antigens can, in appropriate circumstances, be nonimmunogenic and immunosuppressive in adult hosts is not new, although a specific focus on the class I antigens (as opposed to other MHC antigens) is relatively recent. While in many instances it is difficult to comment on the relative extent to which a given graft or pretreatment inoculum (for example whole blood) expresses class I and class II antigens, there is, nevertheless, a series of experiments in which grafts known to express primarily class I MHC antigens have been not only poorly immunogenic but also specifically immunosuppressive. For instance, cultured endocrine allografts are accepted for long periods when transplanted under the renal capsule of allogeneic hosts (*41, 42*), and can in time impair the host's ability to reject subsequent allografts from the donor strain (*43*). Experimental liver grafts in pigs and rats are poorly immunogenic and often survive for long periods without immunosuppression (*44*). Both mouse and rat livers contain large quantities of class I antigen with only small quantities of class II antigen (*45, 46*). Liver allografts that have been accepted for long periods are able to condition pigs and rats to accept subsequent grafts of heart, kidney or skin from the same donor strain (*44, 47*). Additionally, allogeneic liver grafts transplanted into rats previously sensitized by a donor strain skin graft are not only frequently accepted, but may also allow a second skin graft to be retained in an apparently tolerated state (*47*). The immunosuppressive molecule in one series of rat liver grafts was apparently a class I antigen (*15*). Mouse liver cells have been shown to secrete a class I molecule rather than to express it on the cell membrane, and it has been suggested that this molecule might account for the immunosuppression effected by some liver grafts (*48*). The secreted molecule had some of the features of Qa molecules as well as H-2K and H-2D. Allogeneic kidneys that have been tolerated for a long period following passive enhancement, and that have lost their dendritic cells, are poorly immunogenic when retransplanted within the same species (*49, 50*)—they may also impair the immunological reactivity of their new hosts. It is noteworthy that long-tolerated kidney allografts express three times the quantity of class I antigen normally found in kidney (*51*). Soluble or semisoluble antigenic preparations from cell membranes may also be both poorly immunogenic and in some circumstances immunosuppressive. The class I antigenic content of at least some of these preparations in mice is suggested by their hemagglutinin-absorbing capacity (*52*).

Despite their inability to stimulate accelerated graft rejection or to cause popliteal node enlargement, the heat-killed cells used in the present experiments were able to stimulate the production of alloantibodies (Fig. 1). It seems unlikely that these results reflected the presence of a few viable class II bearing cells in the immunizing inoculum, since antibody production followed the injection of cells heated to 50°C for 1 hr (Fig. 1). Alloantibody production has likewise been reported in rats following the injection of a cell preparation which had been heated at 56°C for 1 hr and then homogenized (*53*). This suggests that a graft rejection reaction may call for a different presentation of antigen than is required for alloantibody production.

The possibility that class I antigens may be nonimmunogenic and immunosuppressive if presented in appropriate circumstances has implications for clinical transplantation: (1) as noted previously (*7, 11*) it provides a possible explanation for the protective effect of prior blood transfusion on subsequent kidney allografts in man, and (2) the observation that heat-treated cells express class I antigen in a poorly immunogenic form could possibly be exploited clinically, and might bypass some of the risks associated wtih blood transfusion. Obviously, a great deal more needs to be learned about the circumstances in which preparations expressing only (or primarily) class I antigens will evoke an immunosuppressive response. In connection with the two pretreatment inocula used in the present series, recipients were exposed to antigen (or putative antigen in the case of heat-treated cells) over a long period. When DA red cells are injected into unsensitized AS hosts, 48% of the red cells injected are present in the circulation one week later (*23*). Thus, 4 injections of red cells at weekly intervals would ensure that donor red cells remained in the circulation continuously for at least 5 weeks, and by inference (from red cell survival curves in rats) for substantially longer (*23*). In the case of heat modified ^{51}Cr-labeled lymph node cells, a substantial proportion of the injected label remained in the body 7 days after a single injection (Table 2), although it is uncertain whether this represented class I antigen recognizable as such by the immune system. Approximately 0.2% of the injected label was detectable in the blood 24 hr after injection, and 0.1% was present at 48 hr, but by 7 days the blood label did not exceed background levels of radioactivity (data not shown). Cultured thyroid allografts need to reside in their hosts for a long period before they evoke specific immunosuppression (*43*). The immunosuppressive effect of the present inocula might likewise have been related to the extent to which they persisted in the body.

Class I antigens in all the experiments cited above have been administered in the form of whole cells or of crude antigenic extracts. Considerable interest attaches to the results of administering purified preparations of class I antigens corresponding to mouse H-2K and D.

Acknowledgments. We thank Anne Williams, Anne-Marie Pulham, and Karen Skinner for their able technical assistance, and Noeleen Richardson for typing the manuscript.

REFERENCES

1. McKenzie IFC, Henning M. The immunogenecity of alloantigens of the various regions of the H-2 complex. Folia Biol (Praha) 1976; 22: 417.
2. Klein J. H-2 mutations: their genetics and effects on immune functions. Adv Immunol 1978; 26: 56.
3. Alter BJ, Katz SA, Bach FH. Cellular basis of response to K region Class I MHC disparities. Transplant Proc 1983; 15: 171.
4. Medawar PB. Isoantigens. In: Albert F, Lejeune-Ledant G, eds. Biological problems of grafting. Oxford: Blackwell, 1959: 8.
5. Owen RD. In: Albert F, Lejeune-Ledant G, eds. Biological problems of grafting. Oxford: Blackwell, 1959: 80.
6. Welsh KI, Burgos H, Batchelor JR. The immune response to allogeneic rat platelets; Ag-B antigens in matrix form lacking Ia. Eur J Immunol 1977; 7: 267.
7. Heslop B, Heslop H. Allogeneic red cells fail to induce haemagglutinating antibodies or cellular alloimmunity in rats and are immunosuppressive. Transplantation 1979; 28: 144.
8. Jeekel J, van Dongen G, Majoor G, Harder F. Enhancement of rat renal allograft with antibodies directed against erythrocyte-associated antigens (EAA). Transplant Proc 1977; 9: 969.
9. Martin DC, Hewitt CW, Osborne JG, Dowdy SE, Fristoe TL, Russell LA, Cote J. Enhanced kidney graft survival in rats by single or multiple blood transfusions and various blood products. Transplant Proc 1982; 14: 707.
10. Malik El, Fadil Malik ST, Sweny P, Moorhead JF. The enhancing and sensitizing effects of donor blood components, including dendritic cells, in a rat renal allograft model. Transplantation 1984; 38: 213.
11. Wood KJ, Evins J, Morris PJ. Suppression of rat renal allograft rejection in rats by Class I antigens on purified erythrocytes. Transplantation 1985; 39: 56.
12. Claas FHJ, Blankert JJ, Ruigrok R, Moerel L. Platelet transfusions can induce transplantation tolerance. Immunol Lett 1982; 5: 35.
13. Hibberd AD, Scott LJ. Allogeneic platelets increase the survival of rat renal allografts. Transplantation 1983; 35: 622.
14. Hibberd AD, Wood RA, Morris PJ. Pregraft allogeneic platelets are comparable with pregraft blood in prolonging the survival of rat renal allografts. Transplant Proc 1985; 17: 1655.
15. Kamada N, Brons G, Davies H. Fully allogeneic liver grafting in rats induces a state of systemic non-reactivity to donor transplantation antigens. Transplantation 1980; 29: 429.
16. Brewer JA, Hank JA, Wendel T, Schmeling GJ, Blank JL, Morrissey LW, Robins HI, Sondel PM. Heated lymphocytes express HLA-DR antigens despite their ability to stimulate in MLC. Tissue Antigens 1983; 22: 246.
17. Schellekens PTLX, Eijsvoogel VP. Lymphocyte transformation in vitro. III. Mechanism of stimulation in the mixed lymphocyte culture. Clin Exp Immunol 1970; 7: 229.
18. Sondel PM, Jacobson NW, Bach FH. Selective activation of human suppressor cells by a non-proliferative stimulus. Eur J Immunol 1977; 7: 38.
19. Burton RC, Fortin JL, Russell PS. T cell responses to alloantigens. I. Studies of in vivo and in vitro immunologic memory and suppression by limit dilution analysis. J Immunol 1980; 124: 2936.
20. Goeken NE. Preferential activation of human suppressor cells in vitro by heat-modified stimulators. Transplant Proc 1983; 15: 780.
21. Goeken NE, Eckerlie MK, Lioubin PJ, Staggs TS. Human T cell activation: role of Class I and Class II major histocompatibility complex antigens. Transplant Proc 1985; 27: 963.
22. Festing MFW. Inbred strains in biomedical research. London: Macmillan, 1979.
23. Baird MA, Heslop BF. Major histocompatibility complex-linked spleen-dependent transfusion "collapse curves" in inbred rats. Transplantation 1982; 34: 129.
24. Heslop HE. A method for preparing leucocyte depleted erythrocytes from rat blood. J Immunol Methods 1978; 22: 389.
25. Silber SJ. Microsurgery. Baltimore: Williams & Wilkins, 1979.
26. Bradley M, Heslop BF. An improved urease ELISA protocol for the screening of monoclonal H-Y antibodies. Proc U Otago Med Sch 1984; 62: 14.
27. Levine S. Local and regional forms of graft-versus-host disease in lymph nodes. Transplantation 1968; 6: 799.
28. Ford WL, Burr W, Simonsen M. A lymph node weight assay for the graft-versus-host activity of rat lymphoid cells. Transplantation 1970; 10: 258.
29. Dorsch SE, Roser B. A quantitative lymph node weight assay for allogeneic interactions in the rat. Aust J Exp Biol Med Sci 1974; 52: 253.
30. Markwick JR, Barnes RMR, Pegrum GD. Allogeneic cell interactions in the rat. I. Changes in the rate of cell proliferation during local graft-versus-host and host-versus-graft reactions. Cell Immunol 1977; 32: 52.
31. McNeilage LJ, Heslop BF, Heyworth MR, Gutman GA. Natural cytotoxicity in rats: strain distribution and genetics. Cell Immunol 1982; 72: 34.
32. Heslop BF, McNeilage LJ. Natural cytotoxicity: early killing of allogeneic lymphocytes in rats. Immunol Rev 1983; 73: 35.
33. Bainbridge DR, Brent L, Gowland G. Distribution of allogeneic ^{51}Cr labelled lymph node cells in mice. Transplantation 1966; 4: 138.
34. Heslop BF, Hardy BE. The distribution of ^{51}Cr-labelled syngeneic and allogeneic lymph node cells in the rat. Transplantation 1971; 11: 128.
35. Heslop BF, Hardy BE. In vivo damage to circulating lymphoid cells by alloimmune serum in rats. Transplantation 1972; 13: 364.
36. Rolstad B, Ford WL. The rapid elimination of allogeneic lymphocytes: relationship to established mechanisms of immunity and to lymphocyte traffic. Immunol Rev 1983; 73: 87.
37. Chui KM, Faanes RB, Choi YS. Activation of specific suppressor cells with heat-treated allogeneic tumor cells. Cell Immunol 1980; 49: 283.
38. Flexner S, Jobling JW. On the promoting influence of heated tumour emulsions on tumour growth. Proc Soc Exp Biol Med 1907; 4: 156.
39. Voisin GA. Immunological facilitation: a broadening of the concept of the enhancement phenomenon. Prog Allergy 1971; 15: 328.
40. Kaliss N. Immunological enhancement of tumour homografts in mice: a review. Cancer Res 1958; 18: 992.
41. Lafferty KJ, Bootes A, Dart G, Talmage DW. Effect of organ culture on the survival of thyroid allografts in mice. Transplantation 1976; 22: 138.
42. Lafferty KJ, Woolnough J. The origin and mechanism of the allograft reaction. Immunol Rev 1977; 55: 231.
43. Donohue JA, Andrus L, Bowen K, Simeonvic C, Prowse SJ, Lafferty KJ. Cultured thyroid allografts induce a state of partial tolerance in adult recipient mice. Transplantation 1983; 35: 62.
44. Calne RY, Sells RA, Pena JR, Davis DR. Induction of immunological tolerance by porcine liver allografts. Nature 1969; 223: 472.
45. Hart DNJ, Fabre JW. Quantitative studies on the tissue distribution of Ia and SD antigens in the DA and Lewis rat strains. Transplantation 1979; 27: 110.
46. Brent L, Bain AG, Butler R, Horsburgh R, Opara SC, Wood PJ. The antigenicity of purified liver parenchymal cells. Transplant Proc 1981; 13: 860.
47. Kamada N, Davies HS, Roser B. Reversal of transplantation immunity by liver grafting. Nature 1981; 292: 840.
48. Lee Maloy W, Coligan JE, Barra Y, Jay G. Detection of a secreted form of the murine H-2 Class I antigen with an antibody against its predicted carboxyl terminus. Proc Natl Acad Sci 1984; 81: 1216.
49. Lechler RI, Bachelor JR. Immunogenicity of retransplanted rat kidney allografts. J Exp Med 1982; 156: 1835.
50. Bachelor JR, Phillips BE, Grennan D. Suppressor cells and their

role in the survival of immunologically enhanced rat kidney allografts. Transplantation 1984; 37: 43.
51. Hart DNJ, Winearls CG, Fabre JW. Graft adaptation: studies on possible mechanisms in long-term surviving rat renal allografts. Transplantation 1980; 30: 73.
52. Hilgert I, Kristofova H. Immunogenic properties of cell-free tissue extracts in mice. Transplantation 1967; 5: 1256.
53. Butcher GW, Corvalan JR, Licence DR, Howard JC. Immune response genes controlling responsiveness to major transplantation antigens. Specific major histocompatibility complex-linked defect for antibody responses to Class I alloantigens. J Exp Med 1982; 155: 303.
Received 12 August 1985.
Accepted 24 October 1985.

0041-1337/86/4201-0007$02.00/0
TRANSPLANTATION
Vol. 42, No. 1

SEROLOGY OF LIVER TRANSPLANTATION IN THE RAT

I. ALLOANTIBODY RESPONSES AND EVIDENCE FOR TOLERANCE IN A NONREJECTOR COMBINATION[1]

NAOSHI KAMADA[2] AND TAKAHISA SHINOMIYA[3]

Department of Surgery, University of Cambridge and Addenbrooke's Hospital, Cambridge; and Mitsusbishi-Kasei Institute of Life Science, Machida-shi, Tokyo, Japan

The antibody response against class I and class II RT1 antigens has been studied in PVG rats grafted with DA liver. In this nonrejector combination, liver grafts survive permanently in all normal recipients and in about 50% of recipients presensitized by a DA skin graft, with concurrent induction of transplant tolerance for other DA organs and skin. Using a two-stage radioimmunoassay, the anti–class I (RT1A^a) levels in sera of normal PVG recipients of DA liver grafts were found to be low (maximal titer 1:50 serum dilution or less); after peaking at 2 weeks posttransplantation, they diminished to background levels by 6 weeks. The anti-RT1A^a response showed a close parallel to cell-mediated rejection events in the liver graft recipients. In contrast, anti–class II (RT1B^a/D^a) responses reached much higher titers (over 1:1000), which were maintained for several weeks before declining after 4 months. Similar observations were made in presensitized recipients. The induction of tolerance in the alloantibody response was indicated by the inability of DA skin grafts to restimulate anti-RT1 antibody in liver recipients. The observations support the picture of "split tolerance" indicated by previous cellular studies in this combination.

Previous publications have documented the remarkable ability of liver grafts between certain inbred strains of rats to survive and induce transplantation tolerance (*1–8*). Thus, in the combination of DA into PVG, liver grafts are never rejected, but instead induce a state of donor-specific unresponsiveness, such that grafts of other DA organs (heart, kidney) or skin are also be accepted (*3, 4, 6*). Moreover, even PVG rats presensitized against DA by skin grafting accept a DA liver graft permanently in 50% of cases, and of those long-term surviving animals half also become systemically tolerant of DA, as demonstrated by subsequent heart or skin grafting (*9*). Thus a liver graft can reverse an existing state of immunity, converting it into one of unresponsiveness. The mechanisms underlying liver-induced unresponsiveness are notable for their apparent complexity. Thus we have shown that liver grafting leads to specific deletion of T cell clones with the potential to reject DA tissue grafts, but that this deletion is selective, and leaves intact functions such as mixed lymphocyte and graft versus host reactivity (*10–12*). There is also evidence for soluble "blocking" factors in serum (*4, 11*) and an antigen-specific immunosuppressive activity in lymph of DA-liver grafted PVG rats (*13*).

In this article, we describe the alloantibody response to class I and class II antigens of the rat RT1 complex following liver grafting in the DA into PVG combination. A simplified genetic map of RT1, the rat major histocompatibility complex, is shown in Figure 1. All strong class I alloantigenic activity derives from the RT1A region, while class II (Ia) antigens are coded in the RT1B and RT1D regions (*14*). Class I (A region) antigens are widely expressed on body tissues, including red cells; the distribution of RT1B/D antigens, as with the Ia antigens of other species, is more restricted, being found principally on B cells, dendritic cells, some macrophages, Langerhans cells in the skin, and kidney proximal tubule cells—but not on red cells. RT1A antigens provoke cytotoxic T cell responses, but only weak proliferative responses (mixed lymphocyte response [MLR] and graft-versus-host reaction [GVHR]*), while RT1B/D antigens are potent stimulators of the latter. Strong antibody responses

[1] This work was supported by a grant from the Alex Foundation (Japan).

[2] Address correspondence to: Dr. Naoshi Kamada, Department of Transplantation and Research, Tokyo Medical School, Hachioji Medical Center, Tate-Machi, Hachioji City, Tokyo, Japan 193.

[3] Mitsubishi-Kasei Institute of Life Science.

* Abbreviations used: DAB-FCS, Dulbecco's phosphate-buffered saline (A and B) containing fetal calf serum; GVHR, graft-versus-host reaction; MHC, major histocompatibility complex; MLR, mixed lymphocyte response.

may occur to both classes of alloantigen in the rat after tissue grafting; anti–class I antibody is conveniently assayed by the results of red cell binding, while anti–class II can be assayed on lymph node cells.

There is one other report dealing in detail with the alloantibody response of liver grafted rats in this nonrejector combination (*15*). Using a complement-mediated cytotoxicity assay, the authors were virtually unable to detect antibody against class I RT1 antigens in PVG recipients of DA liver, but found that the response to class II antigens was high-titered and persistent. Here, we have extended these studies using a sensitive two-stage radioimmunoassay, and have been able to follow antibody responses in serum against class I and II alloantigens in normal and presensitized recipients for several weeks after liver grafting. The induction of tolerance in the alloantibody response after liver grafting has also been investigated and revealed interesting parallels with cellular mechanisms of unresponsiveness.

MATERIALS AND METHODS

Animals. DA (RT1^{a}), PVG (RT1^{c}), PVG.RT1^{a}, and PVG.R1 rats were obtained from OLAC (1976) Ltd., Bicester, Oxfordshire.

Transplantation. Orthotopic liver transplantation (DA donors, PVG recipients) was performed by our published technique (*16*). Rejection does not occur in this combination unless the recipient is presensitized (*9*).

Full-thickness orthotopic skin grafting was carried out according to the method of Roser and Ford (*17*). Grafts were inspected daily after the seventh day and scored as rejected on the first day of complete epithelial necrosis.

Cells. Rats were bled from a tail vein and the blood heparinized. After centrifugation through Ficoll, the leukocyte-containing interface was discarded, and the red cells resuspended and washed three times in Dulbecco's phosphate-buffered (A and B) saline containing 2% fetal calf serum (DAB/FCS).

Cervical lymph nodes were removed and a cell suspension prepared by passing through a fine mesh filter; the cells were washed three times in cold DAB/FCS and kept on ice until used.

Radioimmunoassays for alloantibodies. Antibodies against class I and class II donor (RT1^{a}) antigens in sera of DA-grafted PVG rats were detected by a two-stage binding assay using red cells or lymph node cells of the congenic strain PVG.RT1^{a} and radiolabelled sheep antirat immunoglobulin, as follows.

Anti–class I antibodies were assayed by red cell binding. Flexible 96-well microtiter plates (Dynatech Labs, VA; Cat. no. 1-220-24) were treated with 10% FCS for 10 min (a precaution against nonspecific binding of rat Ig), washed with distilled water and dried. Serial dilutions of rat sera under test were prepared in DAB/FCS and dispensed into the microtiter wells (50 μl per well); 50 μl of 2% red cells was added to each well and incubated for 1 hr at room temperature. The red cells were then washed 4 times in the wells by repeated centrifugation and resuspension in DAB/FCS. Then 100 μl of radioiodinated, affinity-purified sheep antibodies against rat immunoglobulin (Amersham International, Amersham, England, cat. no. IM. 132) was dispensed into each well (40,000 cpm per well) and incubated for 1 hr. The red cells were then again washed four times in the wells and finally transferred to clean wells and spun down. Individual wells containing red cells were cut out and radioactivity bound to each red cell pellet was counted in a gamma counter.

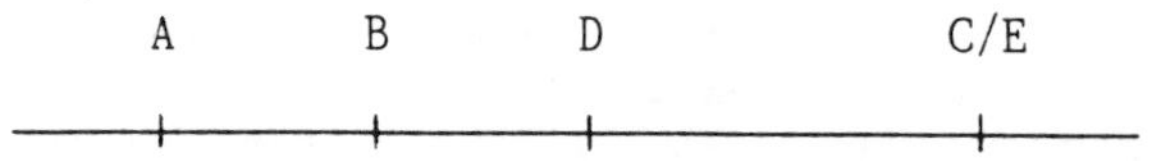

FIGURE 1. Map of the major histocompatibility complex of the rat, RT1. All the strong class I alloantigenic activity derives from the RT1A region, while RT1B and RT1D code for class II molecules. RT1C and RT1E are class I loci, not yet unequivocally separated, that are antigenically very weak and may be the equivalent of the mouse Qa/Tla region (*14*).

Anti–class II antibodies were assayed by lymph node cell binding. Rat sera were first exhaustively absorbed with red cells of the graft donor RT1 type to remove anti–class I activity. In practice, this generally involved at least four successive absorptions of 500 μl of serum with 50 μl packed DA red cells for 1 hr each time; absorption was confirmed by retitration of the serum against PVG.RT1^{a} red cells. The assay for anti–class II antibody followed the same protocol as the red cell binding assay above, but replaced red cells by 50 μl per well of lymph node cell suspension containing 10^7 cells per ml. All incubations were carried out in the cold.

Monoclonal alloantibody. The rat monoclonal anti-RT1A^{a} antibody R3/13 (*18*) was used as a positive control and reference standard for both the above assays; R3/13 supernatant was the generous gift of Dr. C. Milstein (Laboratory of Molecular Biology, Cambridge, England). The two binding radioimmunoassays, using red cells or lymph node cells, were of similar sensitivity in detecting R3/13.

RESULTS

Antibody response to class I RT1^{a} antigens after DA liver transplantation in normal PVG rats. The antibody response against class I (RT1A^{a}) alloantigens in normal PVG recipients (RT1^{c}) of DA liver was followed for several weeks posttransplantation. As noted above, liver grafts in this combination are never rejected, unless the recipient is sensitized against donor antigens by an earlier DA skin graft (*3, 9*). The progress of the response in one particular rat (No. 976) is shown in Figure 2 and is typical of several studied at the same time. The anti-RT1A^{a} response, as assayed by binding to PVG.RT1^{a} red cells, reached a peak during the first two weeks after liver grafting, but the titer was at all times low, with an endpoint of less than 1:50 serum dilution. Thereafter, the serum antibody level declined and by 6 weeks had returned to background (pretransplantation) levels. The specificity of this response for RT1A^{a} was confirmed by absorption of sera with PVG.R1 red cells—R1 being a recombinant haplotype with the A locus antigens of RT1^{a} and B/D antigens of RT1^{c} (*19*)—which completely removed all binding activity for PVG.RT1^{a} or DA red cells.

Antibody response to class I RT1^{a} antigens after DA liver transplantation in presensitized PVG rats. In PVG rats sensitized against DA antigens by skin grafting, the outcome of DA liver grafting is less predictable. In about half the animals, the liver is rejected, with death of recipients within 34 days of liver transplantation; in the remaining animals, the liver is accepted with long-term survival of the recipients, and in about half of these systemic tolerance of DA antigens can be demonstrated by permanent take of a skin or heart graft (*9, 12*). In a sensitized recipient that survived for more than 100 days after liver grafting and was again representative of several others studied (Figure 3, rat 987), serum anti-RT1A^{a} showed an initial fall in the first week after liver grafting, which can be attributed to

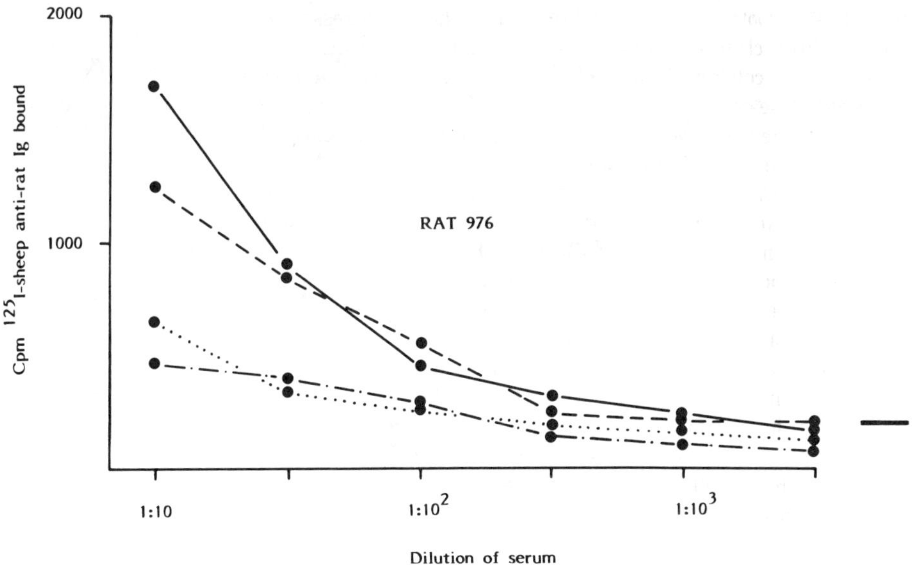

FIGURE 2. Antibody response to class I RT1[a] antigens in a normal PVG recipient of a DA liver graft (rat 976). Sera were taken 1 week (———), 2 weeks (------), 4 weeks (· · · · · ·), and 6 weeks (●-·-·-●) after liver transplantation and assayed by titration against PVG.RT1[a] red cells, with detection by ^{125}I-labeled sheep antirat Ig. Bar indicates background of assay.

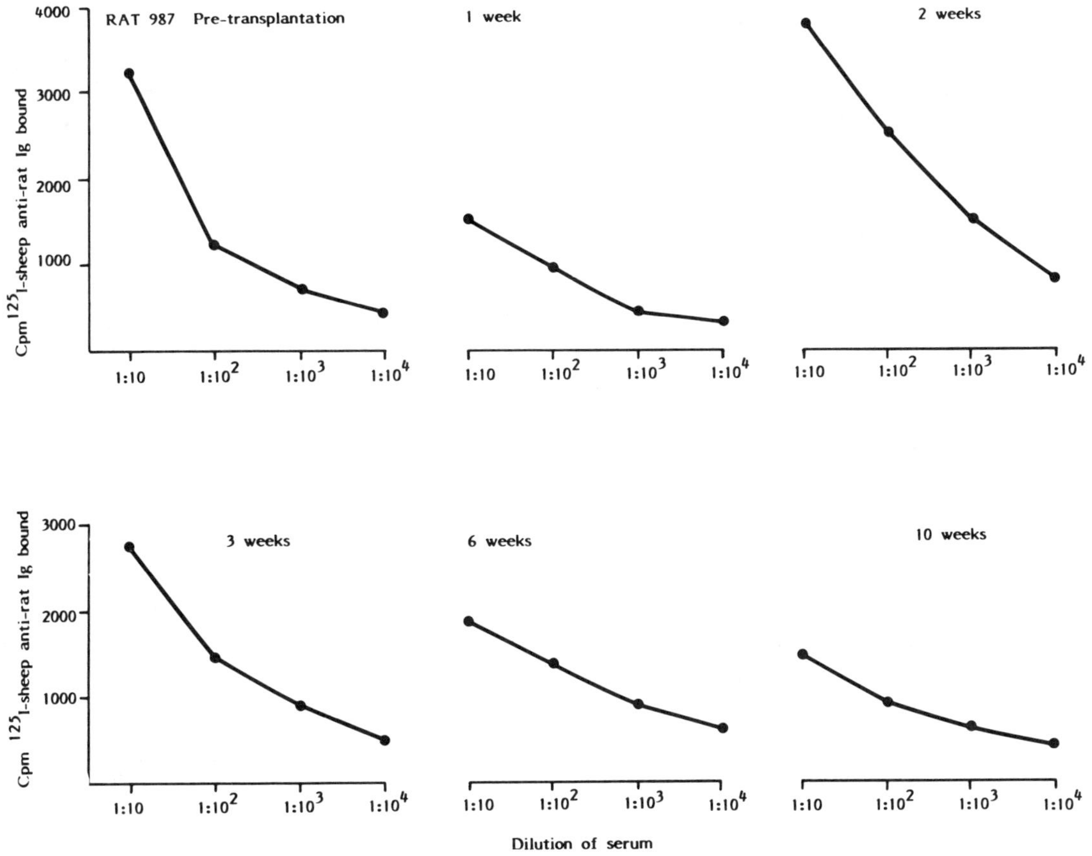

FIGURE 3. Antibody response to class I RT1[a] antigens in a PVG rat (987) sensitized by DA skin grafting and transplanted with a DA liver graft 4 weeks later. The skin graft was rejected in 9 days, but the liver graft survived permanently. Sera were taken immediately before and for several weeks after liver grafting, as shown, and assayed by titration against PVG.RT1[a] red cells, with detection by ^{125}I-labeled sheep antirat Ig.

the absorptive capacity of the liver; thereafter, the secondary response increased to peak at two weeks, but then fell away and by 10 weeks was below the pretransplantation level. It is interesting to compare this response with that in DA-sensitized, but non-liver-grafted controls (Figure 4). Instead of declining after 2–3 weeks, anti–class I antibody levels continued to increase for a surprisingly long time after DA skin grafting—e.g., at least two months in the animal shown and strongly maintained for over a year in others, even though the skin graft itself was rejected within 9 days. It is clear that the effect of a liver graft is first to restimulate and then to depress very significantly the anti–class I response in surviving animals.

Antibody response to class II RT1^a antigens after DA liver transplantation in normal or presensitized PVG rats. In contrast to the response to class I DA antigens, that against class II (RT1B^a/D^a) antigens in normal PVG recipients of a DA liver graft was somewhat slower to start, but then rose over a period of several weeks to attain titers of over 1:1000 serum dilution, as shown in Figure 5A (rat 976). Thereafter the anti–class II level remained high for some time, and only started to decline in the 4th month after liver transplantation. In DA-sensitized PVG recipients with long-term survival after DA liver grafting, a typical secondary response was seen, with a more rapid appearance and higher peak levels of anti–class II antibodies (Figure 5B, rat 987); here too, the serum titers were maintained at a high level very much longer than the anti-RT1A^a (class I) antibodies. Moreover, in both normal and sensitized recipients, the anti–class II response after liver grafting exceeded that in DA-skin-grafted, non-liver-grafted controls, the opposite result to that seen in the anti–class I response.

Anti-RT1^a response of liver graft recipients following DA skin grafting: evidence of tolerance. Following the acceptance of a DA liver graft by a normal PVG rat, a state of systemic unresponsiveness against DA antigens can be demonstrated by the unhindered specific acceptance of subsequent DA skin grafts (*3, 4, 8*). To investigate whether tolerance extended to the alloantibody response, sera from such liver-grafted, skin-grafted animals were assayed for anti–class I and anti–class II anti-RT1^a antibodies. DA skin grafts were placed on PVG recipients that had received a DA liver graft four months earlier; at this time, anti–class I antibody was undetectable in recipient sera by the red cell binding assay, while anti–class II titers were about a tenth of their peak level (endpoint about 1:100). At no point in the following three weeks was there any indication of a rise in serum antibody against RT1A^a antigen, suggesting that the liver graft had indeed successfully tolerized the antibody response to class I antigen. In the same animals, skin grafting also failed to stimulate secondary anti-RT1B^a/D^a responses, the existing anti–class II levels remaining approximately constant throughout the period of observation.

In the rats sensitized against DA before liver grafting, there was similar serological evidence for unresponsiveness toward class I antigen in 2 out of 3 animals, both of which accepted the second DA skin graft—but not in a third, which rejected the skin graft in 15 days. Thus the variability in induction of antibody unresponsiveness in this group evidently correlates with the similar variability in transplantation tolerance (*9, 12*). The anti–class II response in these rats was not boosted by the second-set skin graft, but as before remained at a significant level.

DISCUSSION

In this article we have traced the alloantibody responses against class I and class II RT1 antigens in individual PVG rats that have permanently accepted DA liver grafts. It is clear from the results in normal and presensitized recipients that class I and class II antigens in DA liver are both immunogenic in PVG and can stimulate primary and secondary responses; however, there are major differences in strength and duration of response against the two classes of molecule. The anti–class I response is the weaker of the two and shows a close correlation

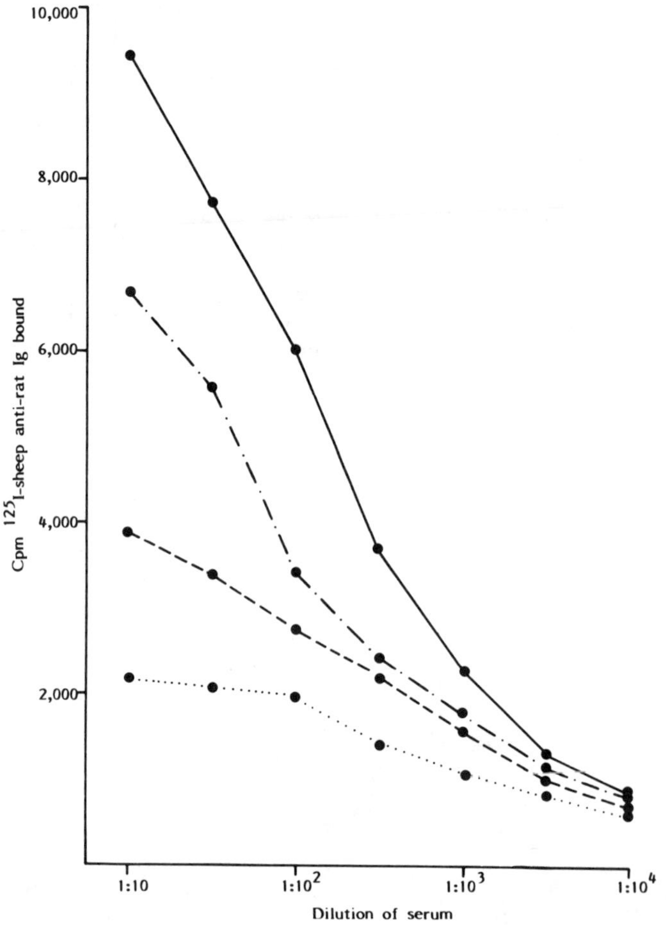

FIGURE 4. Antibody response to class I RT1^a antigens in a PVG rat after DA skin grafting. Sera were taken 1 week (· · · · · ·), 4 weeks (– – – – – –), 6 weeks (● – · – · – ●), and 10 weeks (———) after grafting and assayed by titration against PVG.RT1^a red cells, with detection by ^{125}I-labeled sheep antirat Ig.

with the establishment of transplantation tolerance in the liver recipient, while the anti–class II response is considerably greater both in titer and duration. In a normal (unsensitized) PVG recipient, the primary response against RT1A^a antigens is modest, as measured by serum antibody titers, and after peaking 1–2 weeks after liver grafting, gradually declines until it reaches pretransplantation levels. The disappearance of the response might indicate loss of RT1A antigens from the graft or their blocking by antibody; however, the failure to detect any trace of a secondary anti–class I response after skin grafting liver-transplanted rats indicates the induction of tolerance or specific immunosuppression. In contrast, primary antibody responses to RT1B^a/D^a antigens after liver grafting reach considerably stronger serum titers and are much longer lasting than those against RT1A^a; they only begin to decline in the fourth month after transplantation and they remained well above pretransplantation levels throughout this study. However, here too a subsequent skin graft failed to boost the antibody response, favoring the existence of an immunosuppressive mechanism. An identical pattern is seen in rats presensitized against DA and surviving for over 100 days after a DA liver graft. The anti–class I response is boosted, but decays after two weeks and

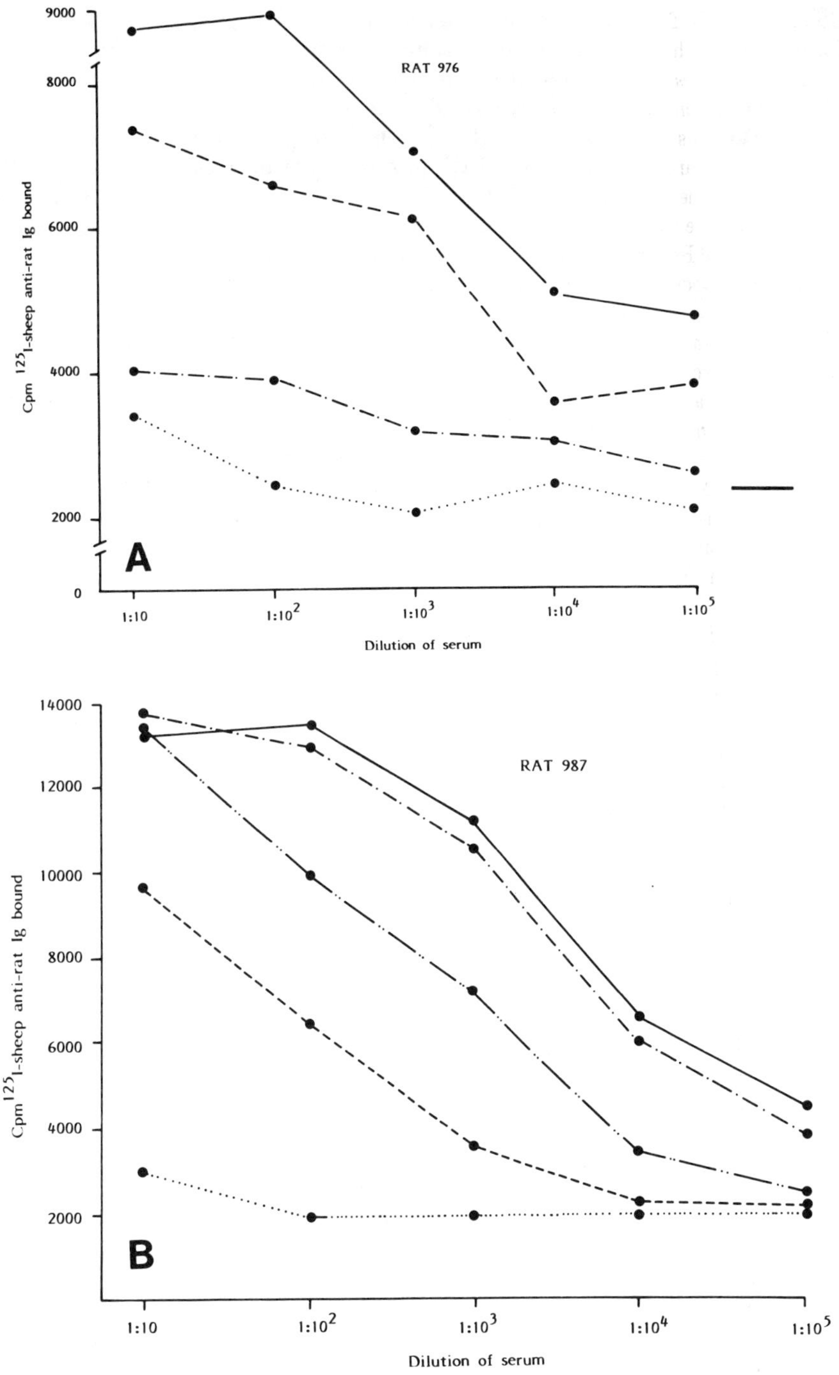

FIGURE 5. (A) Antibody response to class II RT1[a] antigens in a normal PVG recipient of a DA liver graft (rat 976). Sera were taken 1 week (· · · · · · ·), 2 weeks (●– · – · –●), 4 weeks (– – – – – –), and 6 weeks (———) after liver transplantation and assayed by titration against PVG.RT1[a] lymph node cells, with detection by ^{125}I-labeled sheep antirat Ig. (The background in this assay, indicated by the bar, is due to binding of the labeled anti-Ig reagent to rat B cells). (B) Antibody response to class II RT1[a] antigens in a PVG rat (987) sensitized by DA skin grafting and transplanted with a DA liver 4 weeks later (cf. Fig. 4). Sera shown were taken immediately before (· · · · ·) and 1 week (– – – – –), 2 weeks (●– · – · –●), 6 weeks (———), and 10 weeks (– · – · – · –) after liver grafting. Assay as above.

returns to pretransplantation levels (though not completely to background); it cannot be restimulated by further skin grafting, again indicating the establishment of tolerance and the effective reversal of the sensitized state (*9, 12*). The anti–class II response continues strongly for several weeks, but is also not restimulated by skin grafting.

Similar, though less extensive, results in the DA-into-PVG combination were reported by Zimmermann et al. using a complement-mediated cytotoxicity (Cr-release) assay to determine serum antibody levels (*15*). One drawback of using serum titers as an indicator of response after liver grafting is that an organ as large as the liver will undoubtedly act as an antigen adsorbent and remove an amount of antibody from the circulation that may be hard to quantify. Indeed, in all but one animal, Zimmermann et al. were unable to detect circulating anti–class I antibody by cytotoxicity, but could elute anti-RT1A from the graft with acid buffer (*15*). It is likely that the requirement for complement fixation in the Cr-release assay means that some serum antibody escapes detection. Our own findings suggest that, while absorption undoubtedly does occur and is evident, for example, in the transient reduction in serum anti-RT1A titer when presensitized PVG rats receive a DA liver graft (Fig. 3), the effect is probably not great enough to produce a complete or permanent masking of a response. Thus, using the two stage radioimmunoassay, which should detect all serum antibody classes, we have found anti–class I antibodies in all PVG sera within a week of DA-liver grafting, while a liver graft produced only a partial fall in serum titer in sensitized rats.

Compared with a DA skin graft, a DA liver graft is considerably less effective in stimulating an anti–class I response in PVG, even where the recipient has been presensitized, but is more effective than skin in induction of anti-class II antibodies. One factor influencing the nature of the alloantibody response is likely to be the amount and distribution of RT1 antigens on liver cells. In a quantitative study using absorption of alloantisera by liver homogenates (*20*), it was found that liver is considerably richer in class I than class II antigens, with about as much class I antigen as an equivalent weight of lymph node, but only 3% of the class II antigen of lymph node. The greater amount of class I antigen might contribute to the induction of tolerance. Binding of anti–class I antisera to liver cell suspensions suggested that the main repository of the antigen was on bile duct epithelial cells, while hepatocytes and vascular endothelium were negative (*21*). Using monoclonal anti-RT1 antibodies, the distribution of class II (Ia) antigens has been found to be restricted to dendritic cells around the portal tracts (*22*), though it has also been reported that Kupffer cells carry substantial amounts of class II antigen (*23*) and are the most immunogenic component when rat liver is fractionated (*23, 24*). Studies of dendritic cells in spleen and lymph nodes have shown that they act as important antigen-presenting cells (*25*) and this may explain the evident strong immunogenicity of class II antigens in liver. It is also possible that the level of RT1 antigens increases after transplantation as a result of the early transient rejection reaction (see below); thus, class II antigen has been found to be increased on bile duct epithelium and Kupffer cells in rat liver during GVHR (*26*), thought to be as a result of release of interferon by alloreactive T cells (*27*). Interestingly, the majority cells in the liver, the hepatocytes, appear to lack detectable RT1 antigens altogether.

The apparent ease with which the antibody response against class I DA antigens is suppressed or tolerized in PVG by liver grafting is also probably related to the inherited low responsiveness of the PVG strain. Butcher and colleagues have demonstrated a major histocompatibility complex (MHC)-linked immune response gene, Ir-RT1A^a, controlling alloantibody production against RT1A^a (*28*), rejection of skin allografts, in which RT1A^a is the only antigenic difference between graft donor and recipient, and generation of cytotoxic T cells (*29, 30*). PVG rats are genetic low responders against RT1A^a, while AO (RT1^u) and BN (RT1^n) are high responders. It is particularly interesting that DA liver grafts are acutely rejected by these latter two strains as well as by (PVG×AO)F_1 hybrids; although (BN×PVG)F_1 hybrids do not reject DA liver grafts, they mount a more vigorous response than PVG (*6, 30*). Thus, there is evident a close correlation between the potential to respond to RT1A^a and rejection of DA liver in these strains, even though whole-haplotype difference (i.e., RT1B/D as well as RT1A antigens) between donor and recipient is then involved. The nature of the alloantibody response in these other strains and F_1s following DA liver grafting has yet to be examined.

In our results, the anti-RT1A^a response in PVG recipients also shows a close parallel with the cell-mediated response within the graft itself (*6*). Although mild, there is clear evidence of a rejection reaction which reaches a peak 2 weeks after grafting, with mononuclear cell infiltration of portal tracts and sinusoids. By 4 weeks, however, the mononuclear invasion has virtually disappeared and the appearance of the liver after three months is normal (*6*). Similarly, the anti-RT1A^a antibody response peaks at about the same time, before diminishing to background levels over the subsequent weeks (Fig. 2). In contrast, the anti-R1B^a/D^a (class II antigen) response shows no correlation with the cellular rejection reaction, but instead increases over several weeks and remains at a high level thereafter (Fig. 5A).

We have noted that a state of systemic unresponsiveness develops in PVG recipients of DA liver grafts, such that simultaneous grafts of DA heart or kidney and subsequent grafts of DA skin are also accepted by the liver recipient (*3, 8, 32, 33*). The cellular basis for this state of transplantation tolerance induced by liver grafting has been studied in detail (*8*). In vivo, there is clear evidence from adoptive transfer assays for the deletion of alloreactive T cell clones responsible for graft rejection from the recirculating lymphocyte pool of liver graft recipients (*10, 11*); at the same time, GVH reactivity apparently remains unaffected, a situation that has been described as "split tolerance" (*10–12*). In vitro tests of T cell function support this picture: lymph node cells from DA-liver grafted PVG rats proliferate normally in mixed lymphocyte cultures when stimulated by irradiated DA spleen cells, but develop only very weak cytotoxic activity against DA targets (*4, 10, 11*). One interpretation of split tolerance is that class-I-reactive (cytotoxic) T cells are selectively eliminated by liver grafting, while class-II-reactive (proliferative) populations are unaffected (*8*). The serological findings reported here mirror this state of split or partial tolerance. Thus, to judge from the falling off in antibody levels at that time, tolerance in the anti–class I response seems to occur about 3 weeks after liver grafting; in contrast, the anti–class II response continues to increase. One can speculate that T cells responsible for delivering help to B cells in the antibody response to class I alloantigens may be among those deleted by the liver graft.

Finally, the possibility should also be considered that the high levels of anti–class II antibody that follow liver grafting in this combination contribute to the survival of the liver graft itself, or to that of subsequent tissue grafts, by enhancement mechanisms. Antibodies against rat class II antigens are potent mediators of enhancement (*33, 34*), and the rat is one of the species most susceptible to prolongation of graft survival by this means (*34*). Elsewhere, we have reported that passive transfer of serum from PVG rats with well-established, liver-induced tolerance of DA is able to prolong survival of (DA×PVG)F_1 heterotopic heart grafts in normal PVG recipients (*8, 11*), and that lymph from liver-grafted rats also has marked immunosuppressive properties (*13*). More recently, we have successfully prolonged the survival of fully allogeneic (DA) heart grafts in PVG recipients by means of relatively small amounts of serum from liver grafted rats (Kamada et al., *Transplantation*, in press). There are also similarities between split tolerance induced by liver grafting and the situation after enhancement, where proliferative T cell responses have been found to be normal in rats made unresponsive by enhancement (*34*). One interesting aspect of the anti–class II response that may reflect an immunoregulatory role is the observation that, although anti–class II antibody levels remain quite high for many weeks after liver grafting, they resist boosting by a subsequent skin graft. The possible part played by anti–class II antibody in liver-graft unresponsiveness and immunosuppression is worth further investigation.

Acknowledgments. We are grateful to Professor Roy Calne for his encouragement of our work on experimental liver grafting, to Dr. Cesar Milstein for a gift of monoclonal anti-RT1A[a] antibody (R3/13), and to Mrs. M. Thornburn and Miss N. Townley for preparation of figures.

REFERENCES

1. Houssin D, Gigou M, Szekely AM, Bismuth H. Spontaneous long-term survival of liver allograft in inbred rats. Transplant Proc 1979; 11: 567.
2. Houssin D, Gigou M, Franco D, Bismuth H, Charpentier B, Lang P, Martin E. Specific transplantation tolerance induced by spontaneously tolerated liver allograft in inbred strains of rat. Transplantation 1980; 29: 418.
3. Kamada N, Brons G, Davies HffS. Fully allogeneic liver grafting in rats induces a state of systemic nonreactivity to donor transplantation antigens. Transplantation 1980; 29: 429.
4. Kamada N, Davies HffS, Roser BJ. Fully allogeneic liver grafting and the induction of donor-specific unreactivity. Transplant Proc 1981; 13: 837.
5. Engemann R, Ulrichs K, Thiede A, Muller-Ruchholtz W, Hamelmann H. Value of a physiological liver transplant model in rats. Induction of specific graft tolerance in a fully allogeneic strain combination. Transplantation 1982; 33: 566.
6. Kamada N, Davies HffS, Wight D, Culank L, Roser B. Liver transplantation in the rat: biochemical and histological evidence of complete tolerance induction in nonrejector strains. Transplantation 1983; 35: 304.
7. Zimmermann FA, Knoll PP, Davies HffS, Gokel JM, Schmid T. The fate of orthotopic liver allografts in different rat strain combinations. Transplant Proc 1983; 25: 1272.
8. Kamada N. The immunology of experimental liver transplantation in the rat. Immunology 1985; 55: 369.
9. Kamada N, Davies HffS, Roser BJ. Reversal of transplantation immunity by liver grafting. Nature 1981; 282: 840.
10. Davies HffS, Kamada N, Roser BJ. Mechanisms of donor-specific unresponsiveness induced by liver grafting. Transplant Proc 1983; 15: 831.
11. Roser BJ, Kamada N, Zimmermann F, Davies HffS. Immunosuppressive effects of experimental liver allografts. In: Calne RY, ed. Liver transplantation: the Cambridge-King's College Hospital Experience. New York: Grune & Stratton, 1983: 35.
12. Kamada N, Shinomiya T. Clonal deletion as the mechanism of abrogation of immunological memory following liver grafting in rats. Immunology 1985; 55: 85.
13. Kamada N. Transfer of specific immunosuppression of graft rejection using lymph from tolerant, liver-grafted rats. Immunology 1985; 55: 241.
14. Howard JC. The major histocompatibility complex of the rat: a partial review. Metabolism 1983; 32: 41.
15. Zimmermann FA, Butcher GW, Davies HffS, Brons G, Kamada N, Turel O. Techniques for orthotopic liver transplantation in the rat and some studies of the immunologic responses to fully allogeneic liver grafts. Transplant Proc 1979; 11: 571.
16. Kamada N, Calne RY. A surgical experience with 530 liver transplants in the rat. Surgery 1983; 93: 64.
17. Roser BJ, Ford WL. Prolonged lymphocytopenia in the rat. Aust J Exp Biol Med Sci 1972; 50: 185.
18. Howard JC, Butcher GW, Licence DR, Galfre G, Wright B, Milstein C. Isolation of six monoclonal antibodies against rat histocompatibility antigens: clonal competition. Immunology 1980; 41: 131.
19. Butcher GW, Howard JC. A recombinant in the major histocompatibility complex of the rat. Nature 1977; 226: 362.
20. Hart DNJ, Fabre JW. Quantitative studies on the tissue distribution of Ia and SD antigens in the DA and Lewis rat strains. Transplantation 1979; 27: 110.
21. Lautenschlager I, Hayry P. Expression of the major histocompatibility complex antigens on different liver cellular components in rat and man. Scand J Immunol 1981; 14: 421.
22. Hart DNJ, Fabre JW. Demonstration and characteristics of Ia-positive cells in the interstitial connective tissues of rat heart and other tissues but not brain. J Exp Med 1981; 154: 347.
23. Lautenschlager I, Nyman N, Vaananen H, Lehto VP, Virtanen I, Hayry P. Antigenic and immunogenic components in rat liver. Scand J Immunol 1983; 17: 61.
24. Hayry P, Von Willebrand E, Parthenais E, et al. The inflammatory mechanisms of allograft rejection. Immunol Rev 1984; 77: 85.
25. Steinman RM, Nussenzweig MC. Dendritic cells: features and functions. Immunol Rev 1980; 53: 127.
26. Suitters AJ, Lampert IA. Class II antigen induction in the liver of rats with graft-versus-host disease. Transplantation 1984; 38: 194.
27. Steeg PS, Johnson HM, Oppenheim JJ. Regulation of murine macrophage Ia antigen expression by an immune interferon-like lymphokine: inhibitory effect of endotoxin. J Immunol 1982; 129; 2402.
28. Butcher GW, Corvalan JR, Licence DR, Howard JC. Immune response genes controlling responsiveness to major transplantation antigens. Specific major histocompatibility complex-linked defect for antibody responses to class I alloantigens. J Exp Med 1982; 155: 303.
29. Howard JC, Butcher GW. The mechanism of graft rejection and the concept of antigenic strength. Scand J Immunol 1981; 14: 687.
30. Butcher GW, Howard JC. Genetic control of transplant rejection. Transplantation 1982; 34: 161.
31. Kamada N, Wight DGD. Antigen-specific immunosuppression induced by liver transplantation in the rat. Transplantation 1984; 38: 217.
32. Kamada N. A description of cuff techniques for renal transplantation in the rat. Use in studies of tolerance induction during combined liver grafting. Transplantation 1985; 39: 93.
33. Davies DAL, Staines NA. A cardinal role for I-antigens (Ia) in immunological enhancement and the clinical implications. Transplant Rev 1976; 30: 18.
34. Stuart FP, Weiss A, Fitch FW. Induction and maintenance of immunological enhancement. In: Stuart FP, Fitch FW, eds. Immunological tolerance and enhancement. MTP Press, 1979: 29.

Received 25 June 1985.
Accepted 3 October 1985.

0041-1337/86/4201-0014$02.00/0
TRANSPLANTATION

Vol. 42, No. 1
Printed in U.S.A.

CORRECTION OF EQUINE SEVERE COMBINED IMMUNODEFICIENCY BY BONE MARROW TRANSPLANTATION[1]

CHARLES M. BUE,[2] WILLIAM C. DAVIS,[2] NANCY S. MAGNUSON,[2] VILMA D. MOTTIRONI,[3] HANS D. OCHS,[4] CAROL R. WYATT,[2] AND LANCE E. PERRYMAN[2,5]

Department of Veterinary Microbiology and Pathology, Washington State Universty, Pullman, Washington 99164-7040; Wadsworth Center for Laboratories and Research, New York State Department of Health, Albany, New York 12201; and Department of Pediatrics, University of Washington School of Medicine, Seattle, Washington 98195

A 32-day-old horse with severe combined immunodeficiency was transplanted with equine bone marrow cells in an attempt to establish immunologic responsiveness. A histocompatible, mixed-leukocyte-culture–nonreactive, sex-matched, full sibling was used as the donor. Recipient total lymphocyte count, T and B lymphocyte numbers, and response of peripheral blood mononuclear cells to phytolectin stimulation increased by 14 days following transplantation. Circulating lymphocytes exceeded 1000 cells/μl blood by 40 days posttransplantation, and by 170 days following transplantation, T and B lymphocyte numbers had reached normal values. The foal demonstrated significant primary and secondary antibody responses when immunized with bacteriophage ΦX 174 at 100 and 142 days posttransplantation. Concentrations of IgG and IgM remained within the normal range following cessation of i.v. plasma therapy 156 days after transplantation. More than 300 days following transplantation, the foal remains healthy and is growing normally. At no time during the posttransplant period was there detectable evidence of graft-versus-host disease.

Severe combined immunodeficiency (SCID)* is a disorder in which affected individuals are immunologically incompetent and succumb to overwhelming infection if untreated. SCID occurs in children (*1*), horses (2), and mice (*3*). SCID in the horse is the only outbred species animal model for the human disorder (*4*). Research on this model has been directed at elucidating the hereditary defect (*5–13*) and evaluating treatment protocols (*14, 15*) that might be applicable to infants with this disease. In addition, the equine model provides an opportunity to analyze the histocompatibility requirements essential for engraftment and to study the development of a fully competent immune system.

Severe combined immunodeficiency in the Arabian horse is characterized by lymphopenia, hypogammaglobulinemia, and lack of response by peripheral blood mononuclear cells to phytolectin stimulation (*5*). Foals with SCID fail to develop skin reactions to intradermal injections of phytohemagglutinin, keyhole limpet hemocyanin, or dinitrochlorobenzene (*16*), and their peripheral blood mononuclear cells fail to respond in mixed leukocyte culture (MLC) to lymphocytes from unrelated horses (*17*). Affected foals invariably succumb to overwhelming infection, usually within the first 5 months of life. The majority of these horses die of complications due to respiratory tract infections (*18*). SCID in the Arabian horse is inherited as an autosomal trait (*19–22*).

Attempts have been made to establish immunologic responsiveness in foals with SCID by transplantation of tissue containing hematopoietic stem cells. Other attempts using transplantation of fetal tissues have resulted in temporary engraftment, with some evidence of lymphocyte function (*15*). Transplantation of two SCID foals with bone marrow was unsuccessful (*23, 24*). None of these previous attempts has resulted in sustained engraftment with establishment of full immunologic function.

Here we report a foal with SCID who was given a bone marrow transplant from a histocompatible, MLC-nonreactive, sex-matched, full sibling donor in an attempt to establish immunologic responsiveness. The purpose of this study was to answer two fundamental questions regarding SCID in the horse: (1) Is the microenvironment in foals with SCID capable of supporting stem cells as they differentiate to functional lymphocytes? (2) Can SCID in the horse be corrected by transplantation of equine stem cells from an immunologically normal, histocompatible donor?

MATERIALS AND METHODS

Animals. SCID foals and normal foals were obtained from a herd of Arabian horses maintained at Washington State University. All adult horses in the herd are heterozygous for the SCID trait. The diagnosis of SCID was established by the following criteria: repeated peripheral blood lymphocyte counts of less than 1000 cells/μl, lack of serum IgM in samples taken before the foal was nursed, and lack of phytolectin responsiveness of peripheral blood mononuclear cells.

The bone marrow recipient SCID foal (A-1863) was placed with its dam in an isolation unit until 3 weeks of age when it was separated from the dam and moved to an individual isolation pen. Treatment consisted of weekly i.v. infusions of equine plasma containing antibodies to equine adenovirus, daily oral administration of sulfamethoxazole and trimethoprim, and injectable antibiotics when indicated.

Bone marrow donor horse A-1826 was a full sibling born the previous year.

[1] This work was supported by National Institutes of Health Grant HD 08886 from the Institute for Child Health and Human Development.

[2] Washington State University.
[3] New York State Department of Health.
[4] University of Washington School of Medicine.
[5] To whom correspondence should be sent.

* Abbreviations used: BSA, bovine serum albumin; ELA, equine lymphocyte antigen; FACS, fluorescence-activated cell sorter; MLC, mixed leukocyte culture; PBS, phosphate-buffered saline; PHA, phytohemagglutinin; PWM, pokeweed mitogen; SCID, severe combined immunodeficiency; SDH, sorbitol dehydrogenase.

Histocompatibility typing. MLC experiments were performed using methods previously described (*17*).

ELA typing was performed on peripheral blood mononuclear cells from the SCID foal, potential donor foals, their dams, and their sire. Blood samples were collected in bottles containing heparin and shipped to Albany, NY. ELA determinations were performed on 16 horses. They included 2 SCID foals, their dams, and one stallion who was the sire of all the foals tested. One SCID foal (A-1863) was a full sibling to a normal foal (A-1826). All samples were tested within 24 hr of bleeding.

Lymphocytes were isolated on a Ficoll-Isopaque gradient (*25*) and were ELA-typed against a panel of local antisera (*26*) and antisera from The Second International Workshop on Lymphocyte alloantigens of the Horse (*27*), defining specificities W1 to W10, by a standard microlymphocytotoxicity assay (*28*).

Preparation and administration of donor bone marrow. Bone marrow was collected from the donor in the following manner. The donor was given 100 units of heparin/kg body weight (Sigma, St. Louis, MO) i.v. At 5 min after injection, the animal was euthanized and exsanguinated. Bone marrow was collected by curettage from both humeruses and femurs (*29*) and placed in a beaker containing sterile Hanks' balanced salt solution with 20% Alsever's solution and penicillin/streptomycin (100 U and 100 μg/ml, respectively). Marrow tissue was minced with scissors and put through a stainless steel mesh screen to obtain a single-cell suspension. Cell suspensions obtained in this way were placed in 50 ml glass centrifuge tubes, underlaid with Ficoll-Hypaque, (Ficoll—Sigma, St. Louis, MO; Hypaque—Winthrop Labs, Menlo Park, CA) at a density of 1.079 g/ml, and centrifuged at 400 ×g for 40 min. After washing, the cells were resuspended in 270 ml of RPMI 1640, cell count and viability were assessed, and the cells were infused into the jugular vein through an indwelling catheter.

Analysis of lymphocyte subpopulations. The presence of T and B lymphocytes in the peripheral blood of recipient A-1863 was measured using three monoclonal antibodies specific for these equine lymphocyte subpopulations. HT23A and EqT3 react with epitopes expressed on the surface of mature equine T lymphocytes (Davis and Wyatt, unpublished observations). The monoclonal antibody 1.9/3.2 is specific for equine IgM, including that present on the surface of equine B lymphocytes (*30*). Evaluation of cells with monoclonal antibodies was carried out by placing 5×10^5 cells suspended in 25 μl of phosphate-buffered saline (PBS) containing 0.5% bovine serum albumin (BSA) and 10^{-3} M NaN_3 (PBS/BSA/NaN_3) into each of several wells of a 96-well round-bottomed microtiter plate (Flow Labs, McLean, VA), and 25 μl of ascitic fluid containing the monoclonal antibody of interest to each well. After incubation for 30 min at 4°C, the plate was centrifuged at 1500 RPM in a Beckman 3000 tabletop centrifuge for 5 min. The pellets were washed three times with 150 μl of PBS/BSA/NaN_3. Washed cells were resuspended in 100 μl of a 1:50 dilution of goat antimouse immunoglobulin antibody conjugated with fluorescein isothiocyanate (Cappel, Cochranville, PA) in PBS/BSA/NaN_3. The cells were incubated for 30 min at 4°C, after which they were washed twice using the same method as above. The percentage of cells binding a given antibody was determined by flow cytometric analysis using a Becton Dickinson fluorescence-activated cell sorter (FACS) 420 Research Analyzer.

Assessment of lymphocyte response to phytolectin stimulation. Lymphocytes were isolated from peripheral blood by density gradient centrifugation, and cultured in the presence of phytohemagglutinin ([PHA], Difco, Detroit, MI), concanavalin A ([Con A], Sigma, St. Louis, MO), and pokeweed mitogen ([PWM], Gibco, Grand Island, NY) as previously described (*16*). Incorporation of tritiated thymidine was measured in cells cultured a total of 72 hr.

Assessment of specific antibody production. To assess humoral immunity, recipient A-1863 was immunized with the T-cell-dependent antigen bacteriophage ΦX 174 at 100 and 142 days posttransplantation. Phage clearance and specific phage-neutralizing antibody activity was determined as previously described (*31, 32*). Antibody titers, expressed as rate of phage inactivation (K_v), were compared with those obtained following immunization of 4 SCID foals which had not been transplanted, and to those from 3 age-matched normal foals.

Posttransplant evaluation. During the posttransplant period, recipient A-1863 was monitored daily. The foal's body temperature was recorded, skin and mucocutaneous junctions of the mouth were examined for lesions indicative of GVHD (*33*), and the general condition of the foal assessed. Complete and differential leukocyte counts were performed twice weekly. As an indicator of hepatocyte necrosis, serum sorbitol dehydrogenase (SDH) activity was assayed twice weekly. Serum IgG and IgM quantitation (*2*), phytolectin stimulation assays, and flow cytometric analysis of peripheral blood mononuclear cells with HT23A, EqT3, and 1.9/3.2 were performed weekly.

RESULTS

ELA typing data from recipient A-1863, the bone marrow donor A-1826, and their parents are presented in Table 1. Mixed lymphocyte reactivity of bone marrow donor A-1826 to peripheral blood mononuclear cells from A-1863 and to those from a pool of unrelated horses is shown in Table 2. The data indicated these full siblings were histocompatible.

TABLE 1. ELA typing data

Horse	ELA phenotype
Sire	W5, W_[a]
Dam	W1, W9
Donor A-1826	W5[b] / W1
Recipient A-1863	W5[b] / W1

[a] Numbers indicate antigens detected using internationally recognized reagents obtained from multiparous mares of various breeds. "_" indicates a nondetectable antigen, or homozygosity for W5.

[b] Paternal haplotype appears above line, maternal haplotype appears below line.

TABLE 2. Reactivity of donor lymphocytes in mixed lymphocyte cultures

Stimulator cells[a]	Responder cells	cpm	Stimulation index
Recipient A-1863	Recipient A-1863	2557	1.0
Donor A-1826	Donor A-1826	2480	1.0
Recipient A-1863	Donor A-1826	3667	1.5
Pooled cells[b]	Donor A-1826	28,080	11.3
Donor A-1826	Recipient A-1863	4793	1.9
Pooled cells[b]	Recipient A-1863	4040	1.6

[a] Stimulator mononuclear cells were irradiated with 2000 rads from a ^{60}Co source.

[b] Equal numbers of mononuclear cells from 3 unrelated ponies were pooled and irradiated with 2000 rads.

Signs of lymphoid reconstitution were noted 12 days following transplantation with a significant rise in phytolectin responsiveness of peripheral blood mononuclear cells (Fig. 1). The lymphocyte count (Fig. 2) increased by day 14 as did B and T lymphocyte numbers (Fig. 3). There was a decrease in these parameters approximately 30 days following transplantation, followed by an increase by day 40. The lymphocyte count exceeded 1000 cells/μl by day 44 posttransplant. By day 170, total lymphocyte and T and B lymphocyte numbers had approached normal values. Plasma therapy was discontinued 156 days following transplantation. Figure 4 shows that, following an initial rise, IgG concentrations declined to less than 800 mg/dl following cessation of i.v. plasma treatment. Subsequently, IgG concentrations fluctuated, but never declined below the minimum normal value of 400 mg/dl. At 287 days following transplantation, T and B lymphocyte numbers, phytolectin responsiveness, and levels of IgG and IgM remained within the normal range (data not shown).

In Figure 5 and Table 3, the antibody responses by recipient A-1863 to primary and secondary immunizations with ΦX 174 are compared with the antibody responses exhibited by 3 normal foals and 4 untransplanted foals with SCID. In addition to a significant level of virus neutralizing antibody after both the primary and secondary immunization, recipient A-1863 exhibited an accelerated rate of virus clearance from serum following secondary virus injection. Circulating virus was undetectable 48 hr after injection, whereas in the 4 SCID foals which had not been transplanted, circulating virus persisted for more than 7 days. The maximum neutralizing antibody levels achieved by recipient A-1863, normal foals, and untransplanted foals with SCID following primary and secondary immunization with virus are given in Table 3. Table 3 also gives the percentage of IgG contributing to the total amount of neutralizing antibody present. The response to immunization with ΦX 174 was significant, albeit subnormal.

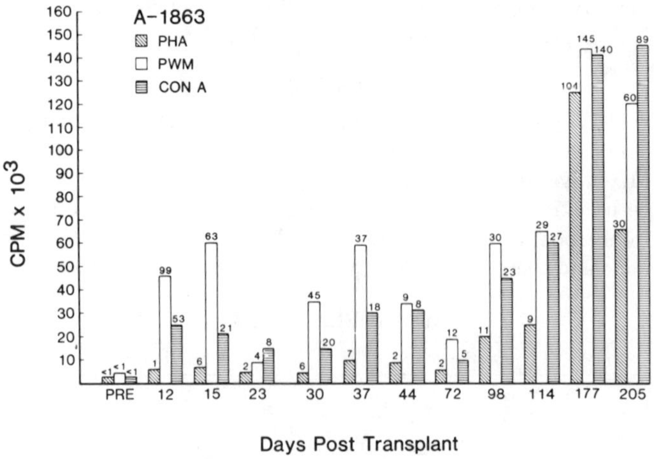

FIGURE 1. Response of peripheral blood mononuclear cells to phytolectin stimulation before and after transplantation.

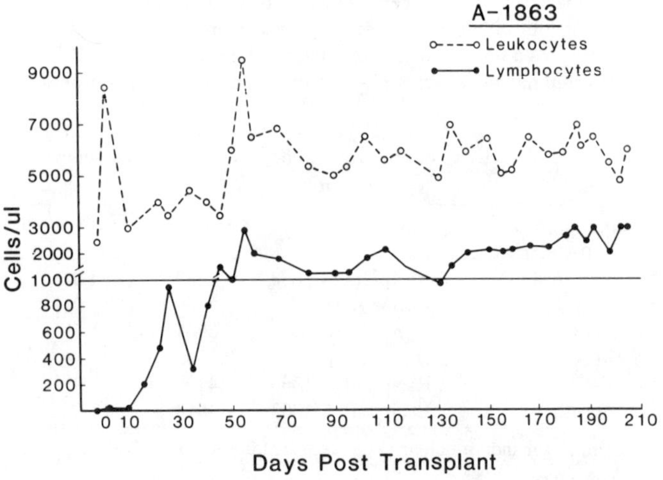

FIGURE 2. Lymphocyte and leukocyte counts before and after transplantation.

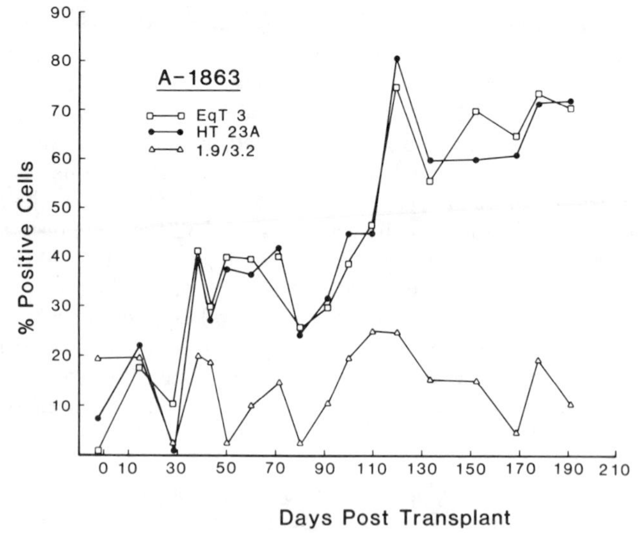

FIGURE 3. T and B lymphocyte numbers before and after transplantation.

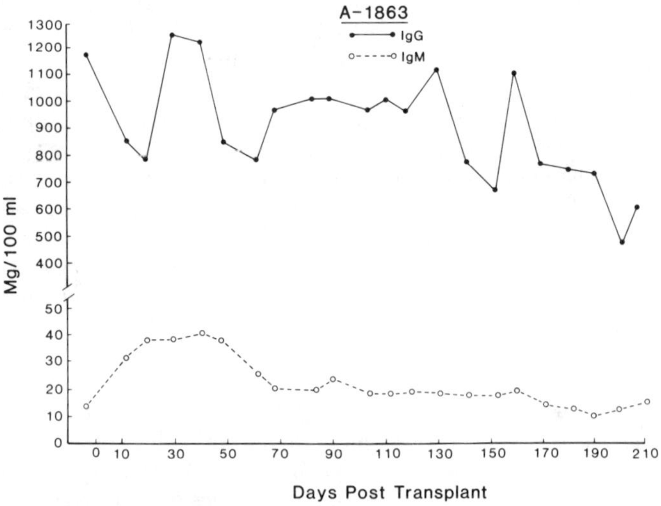

FIGURE 4. IgM and IgG concentrations before and after transplantation.

At no time during the posttransplant period has the foal exhibited signs of GVHD or shown signs of infection. The foal has survived more than 300 days following transplantation, is vigorous, and is gaining weight at a normal rate.

DISCUSSION

This experiment represents the first successful transplantation of hematopoietic stem cells resulting in sustained engraft-

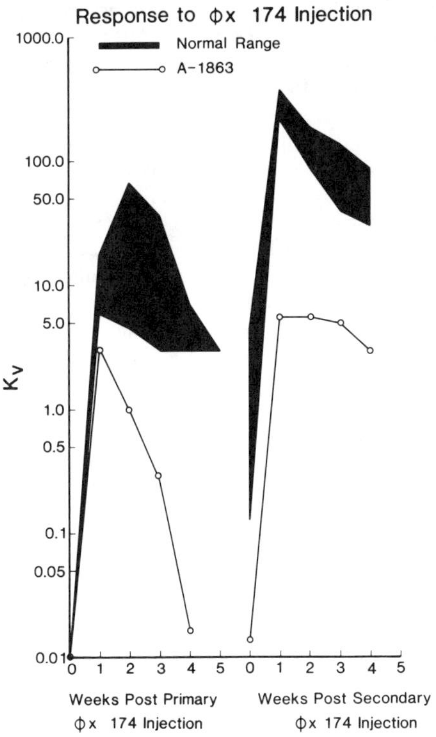

FIGURE 5. Primary and secondary responses following immunization with bacteriophage ΦX 174. The shaded area represents the range of responses of 3 normal foals; (○---○) response of SCID foal A-1863.

$$k_v = 2.3 \times \frac{\text{reciprocal of serum dilution}}{\text{time (minutes)}} \times \log \frac{\Phi\text{X 174 titer at start}}{\Phi\text{X titer at time T}}$$

TABLE 3. Summary of antibody responses to ΦX 174 injection

	Max Kv 1°[a]	Max Kv 2°[b]	% IgG 2°[c]
Normal foals:			
A-1561	17.9	364	73
A-1562	11.2	260	45
A-1564	63.0	229	81
Transplanted SCID foal:			
A-1863	2.88	5.40	1.4
Untransplanted SCID foals:			
A-1601	0.004	0.002	—
A-1609	0.004	0.002	—
A-1616	0.002	0.003	—
A-1624	0.002	0.003	—

[a] Maximum neutralizing antibody titer (Kv) following primary immunization where $Kv = 2.3 \times \frac{\text{reciprocal of serum dilution}}{\text{time (min)}} \times \log \frac{\Phi\text{X174 titer at start}}{\Phi\text{X174 titer at time T}}$.

[b] Maximum Kv following secondary immunization.

[c] The percentage of neutralizing antibody (Kv) of the IgG class following secondary immunization.

ment and establishment of immunologic responsiveness in the horse. There are at least two factors contributing to this success: (1) ELA matching of donor A-1826 and recipient A-1863 was performed. Previous attempts to select bone marrow donors for SCID foals involved mixed lymphocyte culture reactivity and matching of major blood group antigens between recipients and potential donors—however, ELA typing was not performed. Therefore, ELA typing might give better evidence of a suitable match than erythrocyte typing and mixed lymphocyte culture experiments. (2) Recipient A-1863 received 1.8×10^8 viable bone marrow cells/kg of body weight, whereas the foal reported by Ardans et al. received a total of 4×10^7, and the foal reported by Campbell et al. received 2×10^7 cells/kg on one occasion and 4×10^7 cells/kg on another. It is possible that a threshold number of donor cells must be given to a recipient before engraftment is successful. Any number below this threshold may be inadequate. The method of bone marrow cell collection may influence the actual number of stem cells administered. In the other unsuccessful attempts, bone marrow cells were collected by multiple aspirations that may have caused hemorrhage resulting in contamination of bone marrow tissue by peripheral blood cells. Furthermore, following collection, we performed density gradient centrifugation on donor bone marrow cells, removing neutrophils and further enriching for stem cells. Thus, the difference in number of administered stem cells might be even greater than the reported cell numbers suggest.

The results of this experiment provide answers to at least two important questions regarding SCID in horses: (1) Untreated bone marrow cells from an ELA-matched, MLC-nonreactive sibling donor can establish immunologic responsiveness in a foal with SCID. This is an important observation in that it demonstrates that SCID in horses can be corrected by the transplantation of normal stem cells; (2) SCID in the horse does not appear to be due to an inhospitable or inadequate microenvironment of the bone marrow and/or thymus. McGuire et al. reported that the basic thymic architecture was normal in SCID foals except for a paucity of identifiable lymphocytes (*8*). Furthermore, Splitter et al. reported that the hormonal activity of cell free extracts from thymic tissue of SCID foals was high enough to suggest that at least partial thymic function exists in these foals (*10*). The fact that transplantation of normal stem cells can correct SCID indicates that thymic tissue in SCID foals is functional and capable of processing cells destined to become T lymphocytes.

The posttransplant kinetics revealed a dramatic and sustained rise in lymphocyte count, which by day 50 following transplantation had reached normal levels. This correlates with the results of Gatti and coworkers who described a patient with SCID given a bone marrow transplant from his histocompatible full sister (*34*). In the SCID foal a significant rise in lymphocyte count was noted during the fourth week following transplantation. In the patient reported by Gatti, a normal percentage of lymphocytes was detected by 60 days following transplantation. Normal T lymphocyte numbers were detected in the peripheral circulation of A-1863 by 120 days following transplantation. These results are similar to the findings of Buckley and coworkers who reported normal T lymphocyte numbers by day 50 following transplantation of bone marrow from a histocompatible full sibling in a child with SCID (*35*). Recipient A-1863 demonstrated significant, but subnormal, antibody response to ΦX 174 100 days following transplantation. Similarly, patients with combined immunodeficiency receiving bone marrow transplants have exhibited abnormal antibody responses to ΦX 174 for more than a year following transplantation (*36–37*). The posttransplant appearance of immunoglobulins in recipient A-1863 can not be interpreted because the foal received plasma therapy until 156 days following transplantation. Collectively, the results indicate that the kinetics of immunological reconstitution in recipient A-1863 following transplantation are similar to those of humans given bone marrow transplants as a treatment for SCID.

We have established for the first time that SCID in horses can be corrected by transplantation of bone marrow from a histocompatible, full-sibling donor. This successful transplant has provided the first opportunity to study the posttransplant kinetics of immunologic reconstitution in a horse receiving a bone marrow transplant. A method of collecting and processing equine bone marrow tissue that allows for stem cell enrichment while reducing contamination by peripheral blood cells, and methods for monitoring equine immunologic reconstitution during the posttransplant period have been detailed.

We have performed transplants on foals with SCID using bone marrow from half-sibling donors, the cells of which were ELA-haploidentical and MLC-reactive to those of the recipients. Donor bone marrow cells were treated with HT23A, EqT3, and complement in an attempt to eliminate potentially alloreactive T lymphocytes prior to transplantation. These experiments have resulted in temporary engraftment without signs of graft-versus-host disease in 2 of 3 foals. Using these methods, it is now possible to further investigate the histocompatibility requirements between donors and recipients that may be necessary for immunologic reconstitution of foals with SCID when transplanted with bone marrow from partially matched donors.

Horses are the only known outbred species other than the human in which SCID occurs. By performing bone marrow transplants on foals with SCID, it will be possible to obtain information essential for elucidation of histocompatibility requirements between donors and recipients, for prevention of graft-versus-host disease, and for enhancement of graft survival that can be applied to this form of treatment for hematologic and oncologic disease in humans.

Note Added in proof. At 600 days posttransplantation, the subject of this report is growing normally, resisting infections, and has normal values for the immunologic parameters evaluated in the study. A tertiary injection of ΦX 174 was administered 383 days posttransplantation. The maximum antibody response was Kv = 121, and 81% of the detected antibody was IgG. These values approach those of normal horses following secondary immunization with ΦX 174 (Fig. 5 and Table 3).

Acknowledgments. We wish to thank A. Gallina, D.V.M., and M. Riggs, D.V.M., as well as P. Mason, K. Berg, and J. Ward for their assistance in collection and preparation of bone marrow.

REFERENCES

1. Cottier H. Copenhagen, Basle: Congress of the European Society for Hematology, 1957.
2. McGuire TC, Poppie MJ. Hypogammaglobulinemia and thymic hypoplasia in horses: a primary combined immunodeficiency disorder. Infect Immun 1973; 8: 272.
3. Bosma GC, Custer PR, Bosma MJ. A severe combined immunodeficiency mutation in the mouse. Nature 1983; 301: 527.
4. McGuire TC, Banks KL, Poppie MJ. Animal model: combined immunodeficiency in horses. Am J Pathol 1975; 80: 551.
5. McGuire TC, Banks KL, Poppie MJ. Combined immunodeficiency in horses: characterization of the lymphocyte defect. Clin Immunol Immunopathol 1975; 3: 555.
6. Banks KL, McGuire TC. Surface receptors on neutrophils and monocytes from immunodeficient and normal horses. Immunology 1975; 28: 581.
7. McGuire TC, Pollara B, Moore JJ, Poppie MJ. Evaluation of adenosine deaminase and other purine salvage enzymes in horses with combined immunodeficiency. Infect Immun 1976; 13: 995.
8. McGuire TC, Banks KL, Davis WC. Alterations of the thymus and other lymphoid tissue in young horses with combined immunodeficiency. Am J Pathol 1976; 84: 39.
9. Buening GM, Perryman LE, McGuire TC. Immunoglobulins and secretory component in the external secretions of foals with combined immunodeficiency. Infect Immun 1978; 19: 695.
10. Splitter GA, Incefy G, Iwata T, McGuire TC. Evaluation of functional thymic hormones in Arabian horses with severe combined immunodeficiency. Clin Exp Immunol 1979; 38: 37.
11. Yilma T, Perryman LE, McGuire TC. Deficiency of Interferon-gamma but not interferon-beta in Arabian foals with severe combined immunodeficiency. J Immunol 1982; 129: 931.
12. Magnuson NS, Perryman LE. Metabolic investigations of horses with severe combined immunodeficiency. N Y Acad Sci 1985; 451: 87.
13. Magnuson NS, Perryman LE, Suttle DP, Robinson JL, Mason PH, Marta KM. Metabolic investigations of fibroblasts from horses, Equus caballus, with herditary severe combined immunodeficiency. Comp Biochem Physiol 1985; 81B: 781.
14. Perryman LE, Buening GM, McGuire TC, Torbeck RL, Poppie MJ, Sale GE. Fetal tissue transplantation for immunotherapy of combined immunodeficiency in horses. Clin Immunol Immunopathol 1979; 12: 238.
15. Perryman LE, McGuire TC, Torbeck RL, Magnuson NS. Evaluation of fetal liver cell transplantation for immunoreconstitution of horses with severe combined immunodeficiency. Clin Immunol Immunopathol 1982; 23: 9.
16. Hodgin EC, McGuire TC, Perryman LE, Grant BD. Evaluation of delayed hypersensitivity responses in normal horses and immunodeficient foals. Am J Vet Res 1978; 39: 1161.
17. Perryman LE, McGuire TC. Mixed lymphocyte culture responses in combined immunodeficiency of horses. Transplantation 1978; 25: 50.
18. Perryman LE, McGuire TC, Crawford TB. Maintenance of foals with combined immunodeficiency: causes and control of secondary infections. Am J Vet Res 1978; 39: 1043.
19. Studdert MJ. Primary severe, combined immunodeficiency of Arabian foals. Aust Vet J 1978; 51: 109.
20. Poppie MJ, McGuire TC. Combined immunodeficiency in foals of Arabian breeding: evaluation of mode of inheritance and estimation of prevalence of affected foals and carrier mares and stallions. J Am Vet Med Assoc 1977; 170: 31.
21. Perryman LE, Torbeck RL. Combined immunodeficiency of Arabian horses: confirmation of autosomal recessive mode of inheritance. J Am Vet Med Assoc 1980; 176: 1250.
22. McGuire TC, Perryman LE. Combined immunodeficiency of Arabian foals. Immunologic defects in laboratory animals, vol 2. New York: Plenum Press, 1981: 185.
23. Ardans AA, Trommershausen-Smith A. Osburn BI, et al. Immunotherapy in two foals with combined immunodeficiency, resulting in graft versus host reaction. J Am Vet Med Assoc 1977; 170: 167.
24. Campbell TM, Studdert MJ, Ellis WM, Paton CM. Attempted reconstitution of a foal with primary severe combined immunodeficiency. Equine Vet J 1983; 15: 233.
25. Boyum A. Separation of leukocytes from blood and bone marrow. Scan J Clin Lab Invest 1968; 21: 109.
26. Mottironi VD, Perryman LE, Pollara B, et al. Major histocompatibility locus in the Arabian horse. Transplantation 1981; 31: 290.
27. Bailey E, Antczak DF, Bernoco D, et al. Joint report of the second international workshop on lymphocyte alloantigens of the horse, held 3–8 October 1982. Anim Blood Groups Biochem Genet 1984; 123.
28. Mittal KK, Mickey MR, Singal DP, Terasaki PI. Serotyping for homotransplantation. XVIII. Refinement of microdroplet lymphocyte cytotoxicity test. Transplantation 1968; 6: 913.
29. Sharp TG, Sachs DH, Matthews JG, Maples J, Woody JN, Rosen-

berg SA. Harvest of human bone marrow directly from bone. J Immunol Methods 1984; 69: 187.
30. McGuire TC, Perryman LE, Davis WC. Analysis of serum and lymphocyte surface IgM of healthy and immunodeficient horses with monoclonal antibodies. Am J Vet Res 1983; 44: 1284.
31. Uhr JW, Dancis J, Franklin EC, Finkelstein MS, Lewis EW. The antibody response to bacteriophage ΦX 174 in newborn premature infants. J Clin Invest 1962; 41: 1509.
32. Ochs HD, Davis SD, Wedgewood RJ. Immunologic responses to bacteriophage ΦX 174 in immunodeficiency diseases. J Clin Invest 1971; 50: 2559.
33. Perryman LE, Liu IKM. Graft versus host reactions in foals with combined immunodeficiency. Am J Vet Res 1980; 41: 187.
34. Gatti RA, Allen HD, Meuwissen HJ, Hong R, Good RA. Immunological reconstitution of sex-linked lymphopenic immunological deficiency. Lancet 1968; ii: 1366.
35. Buckley RH, Gard S, Haynes BF, et al. Severe combined immunodeficiency with natural killer (NK) cell predominance. Birth defects (original article series) 1983; 19: 101.
36. Ochs HD, Chen SH, Hoehn HW, Thomas ED. Bone marrow transplantation in adenosine deaminase deficiency: effect on immune fucntion and purine metabolism. Inborn errors of specific immunity. San Francisco: Academic Press, 1979.
37. Ochs HD, Lum LG, Johnson FL, Schiffman G, Wedgewood RJ, Storb R. Bone marrow transplantation in the Wiscott-Aldrich Syndrome: complete hematologic and immunologic reconstitution. Transplantation 1982; 34: 284.

Received 31 July 1985.
Accepted 30 October 1985.

0041-1337/86/4201-0019$02.00/0
TRANSPLANTATION

Vol. 42, No. 1
Printed in U.S.A.

CURE OF MALIGNANT LYMPHOMA IN DOGS WITH PERIPHERAL BLOOD STEM CELL TRANSPLANTATION[1]

FREDERICK R. APPELBAUM,[2] H. JOACHIM DEEG, RAINER STORB, THEODORE C. GRAHAM, KEITH CHARRIER, AND WILLIAM BENSINGER

The Fred Hutchinson Cancer Research Center and the University of Washington School of Medicine, Seattle, Washington 98104

Twelve dogs with spontaneous malignant lymphoma in chemotherapy-induced remission were treated with total-body irradiation (TBI) and transplantation of autologous peripheral blood mononuclear cells collected following chemotherapy-induced expansion of the stem cell pool. Four animals (33%) died of transplant-related complications, five (41%) relapsed, and three (25%) are long-term disease-free survivors. Recovery to 1000 white cells/mm^3 occurred by day 16 and dogs no longer required platelet transfusions by day 37. With the exception of delayed platelet recovery these results are virtually identical to those previously reported using autologous bone marrow transplantation for canine lymphoma. This study therefore suggests that autologous peripheral blood mononuclear cells collected following chemotherapy-induced expansion of the stem cell pool may offer a realistic alternative to autologous marrow transplantation in patients with malignant lymphoma for whom autologous marrow is not available.

Treatment with high-dose chemotherapy or chemoradiotherapy and autologous bone marrow transplantation can cure some patients of otherwise resistant malignant lymphoma and may have utility in the treatment of other malignancies as well (*1–3*). Marrow used for autologous transplantation is largely obtained from the anterior and posterior iliac crests while a small amount can be taken from the sternum. Some patients who would otherwise be candidates for autologous marrow transplantation may not have an available source of marrow if, for example, they have received prior radiotherapy to their iliac crests or if the crests are a site of obvious metastatic disease.

Hematopoietic stem cells in the peripheral blood are a potential alternative source of stem cells for use after marrow ablative therapy. Studies performed in normal mice, dogs, and monkeys have demonstrated that the transplantation of peripheral blood mononuclear cells after otherwise marrow ablative total-body irradiation (TBI) can result in recovery of normal hematopoiesis (*4–6*). Quantitative studies performed in the dog show that approximately 10 times more peripheral blood mononuclear cells than marrow cells are needed to protect an animal from the consequences of TBI; 0.5×10^8 nucleated bone marrow cells/kg are required to protect 100% of animals from 10 Gy TBI, while 6.0×10^8 peripheral blood mononuclear cells/kg are required to achieve similar survival (*7, 8*). The large number of peripheral blood mononuclear cells required for engraftment is a problem and initial attempts to use peripheral blood stem cells for transplantation in humans were unsuccessful in achieving full hematologic reconstitution, probably because too few cells were infused (*9, 10*).

The number of granulocyte-macrophage precursors (CFUc) in the peripheral blood can be increased by treatment with endotoxin or dextran sulfate, or following chemotherapy (*11–*

[1] This work was supported by PHS Grants CA 18105, CA 31787, and CA 15704 awarded by the National Cancer Institute, DHHS.

[2] Address correspondence to: Frederick R. Appelbaum, M.D., Fred Hutchinson Cancer Research Center, 1124 Columbia Street, Seattle, WA 98104.

13). Abrams et al. demonstrated that by collecting peripheral blood mononuclear cells 7–14 days after cyclophosphamide treatment, as few as 0.5×10^8 peripheral blood mononuclear cells/kg could protect dogs from otherwise lethal TBI (*14*). The use of this or other techniques to expand the pool of hematopoietic stem cells in the peripheral blood should, therefore, make autologous peripheral blood stem cell transplantation a practical alternative to the use of autologous marrow transplantation for the treatment of patients with malignant lymphoma.

In order to test this hypothesis, we have studied peripheral blood stem cell transplantation in dogs with malignant lymphoma. We have previously shown that with combination chemotherapy, complete remissions can be achieved in the majority of dogs with malignant lymphoma (*15*). If no further therapy is given after remission is achieved, the remission duration is short and all dogs relapse, usually within 100 days of treatment. If, however, after remission induction, autologous marrow is removed and the animal treated with 8.4 Gy TBI and reinfusion of autologous marrow, 24% of animals could be cured of their disease (*15–17*). In this study, we have taken a similar approach but have used hematopoietic stem cells collected from the peripheral blood instead of the marrow. The results demonstrate that peripheral blood stem cells can serve as an alternative to bone marrow for autologous transplantation following intensive therapy of malignant lymphoma.

MATERIALS AND METHODS

Dogs studied. Dogs suspected of having lymphoma were referred by veterinarians with the consent of the dogs' owners. All dogs had lymph node biopsies performed under general anesthesia to establish the diagnosis. Marrow aspirates and clot sections and peripheral blood smears were examined for evidence of lymphoma. Following the diagnosis of lymphoma, dogs were treated with combination chemotherapy to induce a clinical remission.

Chemotherapy. Chemotherapy consisted of nitrogen mustard, 0.2 mg/kg, on days 1 and 8; vincristine, 0.025 mg/kg, on days 1 and 8; prednisone, 2 mg/kg, on days 1–14; L-asparaginase, 250 u/kg, on days 1–14; and 6-mercaptopurine, 1 mg/kg on days 1–14 (*15*). Dogs that did not have a complete response after one cycle of therapy were treated with a second 14-day cycle. Parenteral fluids, antibiotics (ampicillin and amikacin or gentamicin), and transfusions of whole blood were administered as clinically indicated. Complete remission was defined as the absence of palpably enlarged peripheral lymph nodes or abdominal organomegaly and disappearance of malignant cells from the peripheral blood (or marrow if previously involved).

Collection of peripheral blood mononuclear cells. Approximately 7 days following the completion of chemotherapy, jugulocarotid arteriovenous shunts were placed for vascular access. Peripheral blood mononuclear cells were collected using a continuous flow blood cell separator (American Instrument Co., Inc. Silver Springs, MD). Blood flow rate through the separator was maintained at 40–60 ml/min, the bowl speed of the separator was kept at 1200 RPM, and the buffy coat was collected at 3 ml/min. The collection port was adjusted to obtain a buffy coat collection containing approximately 3 g/100 ml hemoglobin. Animals were leukapheresed for 3 hr or until 500 cc of buffy coat was obtained. During collection, animals were anticoagulated with heparin. The collected cells were respun in 15-cc siliconized conical tubes to remove excess red blood cells and plasma. An aliquot of the cells was analyzed for CFUc growth and the remaining cells were cryopreserved in 10% dimethyl sulfoxide as described elsewhere (*7, 8*). Following completion of the last leukapheresis, the arteriovenous shunt was tied off and then removed 7–10 days later.

CFUc assay. CFUc were assayed as previously described, except that post-endotoxin dog serum was used as the source of colony stimulating activity (*14*).

Total-body irradiation and transplantation. Within 14 days of stem cell collection, dogs were exposed to 8.4 Gy TBI given at 4 cGy/min by two opposing ^{60}Co sources. Within 4 hr following completion of irradiation, approximately 50% of the stem cell collection was thawed and rapidly infused, the remaining cells being given the following morning. Postirradiation supportive care consisted of parenterally administered Ringer's solution (50–100 ml/kg/day for 5–7 days); antibiotics, including ampicillin, gentamicin, and carbenicillin; and platelet transfusions as clinically indicated. The day of irradiation and first stem cell infusion is designated day 0.

Follow-up evaluation and statistical analysis. Following recovery of blood counts, dogs were returned to their owners with requests for monthly follow-up examinations by referring veterinarians—and, frequently, telephone follow-ups to owners of surviving dogs. Relapses were unambiguous and presented as obvious progressive lymphadenopathy. Remission duration and survival data were calculated using the method of Kaplan and Meier and compared using the log-rank procedure for failure data with censored observations (*18, 19*).

RESULTS

Twelve consecutive dogs that achieved complete remission following chemotherapy were entered into this study. Following remission induction, animals were leukapheresed on three consecutive days each. An average of 10.43 ± 9.75 (mean ± SD)$\times 10^8$ mononuclear cells/kg were collected per dog. The collections contained an average of 176 ± 115 CFUc per 10^6 mononuclear cells.

Within 14 days of leukapheresis, the 12 animals were treated with 8.4 Gy TBI at 4 cGy/min and reinfusion of their autologous peripheral blood cells. One animal (8%) died prior to engraftment. Three animals (25%) died following engraftment of transplant-related complications (hemorrhagic enteritis in one and pneumonia in 2). Five animals (42%) relapsed on days 42, 102, 105, 169, and 240 following transplant. Three dogs (25%) remain alive in continuous unmaintained remission at days 334, 631, and 727 from transplant. These results are shown in Table 1 and Figures 1 and 2 along with results obtained in a historical group of 38 dogs treated identically but with bone marrow rather than peripheral blood as the source of hematopoietic stem cells (*16*).

TABLE 1. Treatment of canine lymphoma using peripheral mononuclear cell or marrow transplantation

Stem cell source	Marrow	Peripheral blood
No. dogs	38	12
TBI dose (Gy)	8.4	8.4
TBI rate (cGy/min)	4	4
Death prior to engraftment (%)	2 (5%)	1 (8%)
Death from later transplant complications (%)	8 (21%)	3 (25%)
Relapse (%)	19 (50%)	5 (42%)
Long-term disease-free survival	9 (24%)	3 (25%)

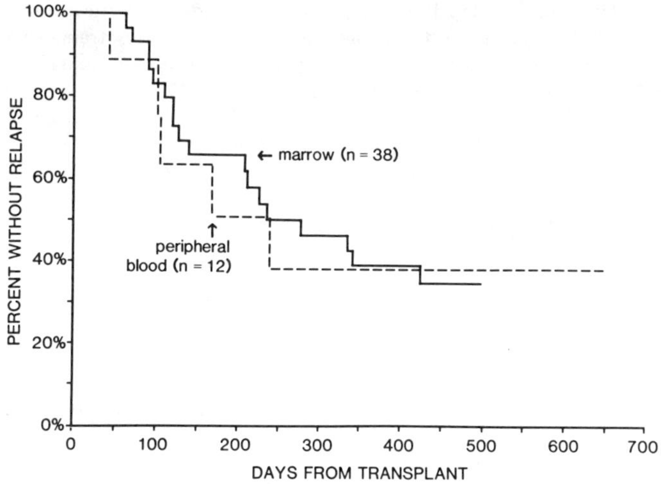

FIGURE 1. Kaplan-Meier product limit estimates for the probability of being in remission for dogs transplanted with peripheral blood (----) or marrow (———).

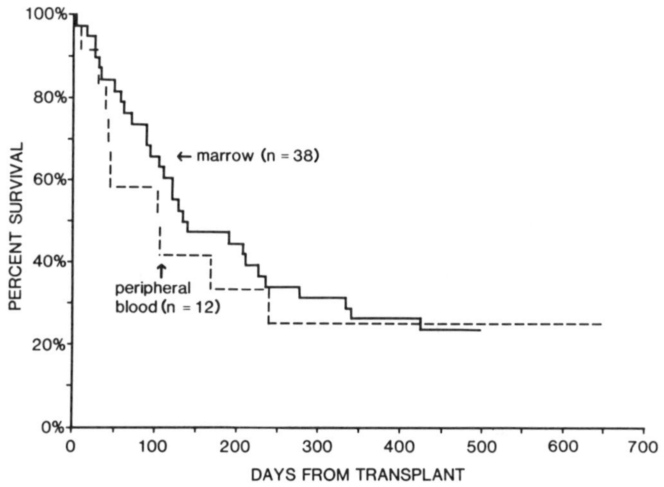

FIGURE 2. Kaplan-Meier product limit estimate for the probability of disease-free survival for dogs transplanted with peripheral blood (----) or marrow (———).

All animals were without evidence of disease in the marrow and peripheral blood at the time of transplantation. However, at the time of diagnosis 6 of the 12 animals had lymphoma in their marrow or peripheral blood. Prior hematogenous spread of disease did not appear to influence the chance of long-term survival in that 2 of the 3 long-term survivors initially presented with both marrow and peripheral blood involvement.

Granulocyte and white cell engraftment occurred rapidly and not particularly differently from observed following bone marrow transplantation. White counts reached $1000/mm^3$ at an average of 16.7±8.5 days posttransplant and granulocytes recovered to $500/mm^3$ by day 16.3±7.9. This rate of engraftment is not statistically different from that observed in 38 lymphoma dogs transplanted with autologous remission marrow who recovered to 1000 WBC/mm^3 by day 12.7±6.2. However, platelet engraftment was substantially slower in dogs receiving peripheral blood grafts. Dogs receiving peripheral blood grafts did not become independent of platelet transfusions until 37.1±13.1 days after grafting. This rate of recovery was slower than seen following bone marrow grafting, in which case dogs recovered in 20.4±13.6 days from transplant. However, despite this slower platelet recovery, the incidence of fatal bleeds (8%) was not different from what we had previously observed following marrow transplantation for canine lymphoma. Given the small number of dogs in this study, we were unable to detect a correlation between the rate of engraftment and either the number of cells or the number of CFUcs transplanted.

DISCUSSION

The ability to rescue normal animals from otherwise lethal total-body irradiation using autologous peripheral blood stem cells has been demonstrated in a number of animal models (*4–6*). However, the large number of cells necessary to ensure engraftment limits the practicality of this approach except in chronic myelogenous leukemia, in which the number of peripheral blood stem cells are dramatically increased as a consequence of the disease. The demonstration that methods exist to expand the pool of circulating stem cells using, for example, pretreatment of the donor with chemotherapy makes the use of peripheral blood stem cells a more realistic alternative. In this study we have demonstrated a similar outcome in the treatment of dogs with malignant lymphoma using TBI followed by autologous marrow or autologous peripheral blood stem cell transplantation. The proportion of animals dying early of transplant-related complications, the proportion relapsing—and, most important, the proportion cured—are similar using either marrow or peripheral blood. Three of 12 animals treated with TBI and peripheral blood stem cell transplantation are alive in complete remission at 334, 621, and 727 days from transplant. Since the latest relapse we have ever seen following marrow transplantation for canine lymphoma was at day 425, at least 2 and perhaps all 3 of these animals are, indeed, cured of their disease. The only definite difference between marrow and peripheral blood stem cell transplantation was slower platelet engraftment in recipients of peripheral blood stem cells. The reasons for slower platelet engraftment in the face of equal rates of white cell and granulocyte engraftment are unknown to us.

The use of autologous marrow to overcome otherwise lethal chemoradiotherapy is a well established approach. The surgical procedure used to obtain the marrow is, in general, safe and well tolerated (*20, 21*). The only compelling reason to consider the use of peripheral blood stem cells at present would be if marrow could not be obtained from the iliac crests, possibly because of prior radiotherapy, tumor involvement, or inability of the patient to undergo anesthesia. It is possible, however, that autologous peripheral blood stem cell transplantation could have advantages over autologous marrow transplantation in other settings. Contamination of marrow or peripheral blood with tumor stem cells undetectable by conventional means represents a potential source of relapse following transplantation. In certain diseases, such as malignant lymphoma and acute leukemia, malignant cells are seen earlier and more frequently in the marrow than in the peripheral blood, raising the possibility that autologous peripheral blood stem cell collections could be less often contaminated with tumor cells than marrow. This hypothesis has not been tested.

The observation that some dogs with malignant lymphoma can be cured with TBI and autologous peripheral blood stem cell transplantation suggests that a similar approach should work in man. Although previous studies attempting peripheral blood stem cell transplantation in man were disappointing, more recent reports using peripheral blood stem cells collected following chemotherapy to expand the pool of peripheral stem cells have been more encouraging. Reiffers et al. have reported one patient with acute nonlymphocytic leukemia who achieved full engraftment and a 6-month second remission following peripheral blood stem cell transplantation (*21*). Likewise, Korbling et al. have reported a patient with non-Hodgkin's lymphoma who engrafted following peripheral blood stem cell transplantation (*23*). Thus, this approach may offer a realistic alternative to autologous bone marrow transplantation, especially in patients for whom marrow is not available.

Acknowledgments. We thank Ray Colby, Dale Kalamasz, and Greg Davis for their help in caring for the animals, Lori Ausburn for her administrative help, and the veterinarians throughout the Pacific Northwest for referring animals for study. Schering Corporation (Bloomfield, NJ), Roerig-Pfizer Pharmaceuticals (New York, NY), Beecham Laboratories (Bristol, TN), Bristol Laboratories (Syracuse, NY), Burroughs-Wellcome Company (Research Triangle Park, NC) and Eli Lilly and Company (Indianapolis, IN) generously supplied Garamycin, Geopen, Ticar, Amikin, 6-mercaptopurine, and vincristine for these studies.

REFERENCES

1. Appelbaum FR, Herzig GP, Ziegler JL, Graw RG, Levine AS, Deisseroth AB. Successful engraftment of cryopreserved autologous bone marrow in patients with malignant lymphoma. Blood 1978; 52: 85.
2. Phillips GL, Herzig RH, Lazarus HM, et al. Treatment of resistant malignant lymphoma with cyclophosphamide, total body irradiation, and transplantation of cryopreserved autologous marrow. N Engl J Med 1984; 310: 1557.
3. Appelbaum FR, Buckner CD. Overview of the clinical relevance of autologous bone marrow transplantation. In: Dunton NJ, ed. Clinics in haematology. London: Saunders, (in press).
4. Goodman JW, Hodgson GS. Evidence for stem cells in the peripheral blood of mice. Blood 1962; 19: 702.
5. Cavins JA, Scheer SC, Thomas ED, Ferrebee JW. The recovery of lethally irradiated dogs given infusions of autologous leukocytes preserved at −80 C. Blood 1964; 23: 38.
6. Storb R, Graham TC, Epstein RB, Sale GE, Thomas ED. Demonstration of hemopoietic stem cells in the peripheral blood of baboons by cross circulation. Blood 1977; 50: 537.
7. Appelbaum FR, Herzig GP, Graw RG, et al. Study of cell dose and storage time on engraftment of cryopreserved autologous bone marrow in a canine model. Transplantation 1978; 26: 245.
8. Appelbaum FR. Hemopoietic reconstitution following autologous bone marrow and peripheral blood mononuclear cell infusions. Exp Hematol 1979; 7(suppl 5): 7.
9. Hershko C, Gale RP, Ho WG, Cline MJ. Cure of aplastic anaemia in paroxysmal nocturnal haemoglobinuria by marrow transfusion from identical twin: failure of peripheral-leucocyte transfusion to correct marrow aplasia. Lancet 1979; 1: 945.
10. Abrams RA, Glaubiger D, Appelbaum FR, Deisseroth AB. Result of attempted hematopoietic reconstitution using isologous, peripheral blood mononuclear cells: a case report. Blood 1980; 56: 516.
11. Cline MJ, Golde DW. Mobilization of hematopoietic stem cells (CFU-C) into the peripheral blood of man by endotoxin. Exp Hematol 1977; 5: 186.
12. Fliedner TM, Calvo W, Korbling M, Nothdurft W, Pflieger H, Ross W. Collection, storage and transfusion of blood stem cells for the treatment of hemopoietic failure. Blood Cells 1979; 5: 313.
13. Richman CM, Weiner RS, Yankee RA. Increase in circulating stem cells following chemotherapy in man. Blood 1976; 47: 1031.
14. Abrams RA, McCormack K, Bowles C, Deisseroth AB. Cyclophosphamide treatment expands the circulating hematopoietic stem cell pool in dogs. J Clin Invest 1981; 67: 1392.
15. Weiden PL, Storb R, Deeg HJ, Graham TC, Thomas ED. Prolonged disease-free survival in dogs with lymphoma after total-body irradiation and autologous marrow transplantation consolidation of combination-chemotherapy-induced remissions. Blood 1979; 54: 1039.
16. Appelbaum FR, Deeg HJ, Storb R, et al. Marrow transplant studies in dogs with malignant lymphoma. Transplantation 1985; 39: 499.
17. Deeg HJ, Appelbaum FR, Weiden PL, Hackman RC, Graham TC, Storb R. Autologous marrow transplantation as consolidation therapy for canine lymphoma: efficacy and toxicity of various regimens of total body irradiation. Am J Vet Res 1985; 46: 2016.
18. Kaplan EL, Meier P. Nonparametric estimation from incomplete observations. J Am Stat Assoc 1958; 53: 457.
19. Peto R, Peto J. Asymptotically efficient rank invariant test procedures (with discussions). J R Stat Soc A 1972; 135: 185.
20. Buckner CD, Clift RA, Sanders JE, et al. Marow harvesting from normal donors. Blood 1984; 64: 630.
21. Jin NR, Hill RS, Petersen FB, et al. Marrow harvesting for autologous marrow transplantation. Exp Hematol 1985; 13: 879.
22. Reiffers J, Bernard Ph, Vezon G, et al. Autografting with blood-derived stem cells in a patient with acute myeloid leukemia (A.M.L.) in relapse. 11th Annual Meeting of the EBMT (European Cooperative Group for Bone Marrow Transplantation) [Abstract]. 1985: 13.
23. Korbling M, Dorken B, Ho A, Maier WD, Hunstein W, Fliedner TM. Autologous transplantation of blood-derived hemopoietic stem cells after myeloablative treatment in a patient with Burkitt's lymphoma. Int J Cell Cloning 1985; 3: 224.

Received 11 September 1985.
Accepted 22 October 1985.

0041-1337/86/4201-0023$02.00/0
TRANSPLANTATION

Vol. 42, No. 1
Printed in U.S.A.

A PROSPECTIVE ANALYSIS OF THE ACCURACY AND COST-EFFECTIVENESS OF DIGITAL SUBTRACTION ANGIOGRAPHY FOR LIVING-RELATED RENAL DONOR EVALUATION

JOHN MCELROY, ANDREW C. NOVICK,[1] STEVAN B. STREEM, DONALD STEINMULLER, BARBARA RISIUS, CAROLINE BUSZTA, AND DIANE STEINHILBER

The Section of Renal Transplantation, Cleveland Clinic Foundation, Cleveland, Ohio 44106

From 1982 to 1984, we conducted a prospective study to evaluate the usefulness of i.v. renal digital subtraction angiography (DSA) for living-related donor (LRD) evaluation. Twenty-eight LRDs were evaluated with the traditional approach of intravenous pyelography (IVP) and standard catheter arteriography (SCA) (group 1). During the same period, 33 LRDs underwent renal DSA and IVP from a single i.v. contrast injection (group 2). If renal arterial imaging with DSA was considered satisfactory, no further radiographic studies were done (group 2-A, n = 23). If renal arterial imaging with DSA was not satisfactory, SCA was then obtained (group 2-B, n = 10).

DSA alone accurately defined the number and location of renal arteries in 21 of 23 patients from group 2-A, and in 5 of 10 patients from group 2-B. The major limitation of DSA was in patients with multiple renal arteries; accurate imaging was obtained in only 7 of these 13 patients (54%).

In group 2 overall, preoperative renal imaging was not accurate in 2 of 33 patients (6%); in both cases, an unsuspected polar artery was found at nephrectomy. The mean cost per patient of all radiographic renal imaging studies was $953.00 for group 2 and $1721.00 for group 1. These data suggest that the approach of preferentially evaluating LRDs with DSA-IVP, and obtaining SCA only if DSA yields poor visualization, is more cost-effective but not as accurate as the traditional policy of obtaining SCA and IVP in all cases.

The existing shortage of cadaveric organs for end-stage renal disease patients awaiting renal transplantation mandates the continued use of living-related donors who fulfill requisite medical and immunologic donor cirteria. This approach is further justified by the improved rate of graft success associated with transplantation from living-related versus cadaver donors, even during the present era of immunosuppression with cyclosporine (*1*).

Radiographic renal imaging is an accepted part of living-related renal donor evaluation. Intravenous pyelography (IVP)* is done to assess differential renal size and function as well as the status of the parenchyma and urinary collecting system. Renal angiography is necessary to assess the number, location, and patency of the arteries to both kidneys. The latter assessment has traditionally been done with standard catheter renal arteriography (SCA). More recently, intravenous digital subtraction angiography (DSA) has been proposed as an alternate, noninvasive, reliable technique. Yet there have been conflicting data on the efficacy of DSA in this group (*2–6*). We report herein the outcome of a prospective comparison of the relative accuracy and cost-effectiveness of DSA versus SCA in living-related renal donor evaluation.

MATERIALS AND METHODS

From 1982 to September 1984, 61 patients underwent living-related donor nephrectomy in our program. All of these patients underwent a thorough preliminary medical evaluation that included a careful history, physical examination, complete blood count and differential, PT, PTT, SMA-18, 3-hr glucose tolerance test, hepatitis screening, RPR test and STS, pap test for female patients, urinalysis, urine culture, 24-hr urine collection for creatinine clearance and protein, electrocardiogram and chest roentgenogram.

During this period, radiographic renal imaging was performed in 28 donors with the traditional approach of IVP and SCA (group 1); patients were hospitalized overnight to undergo the latter study. In performing SCA, an anteroposterior (A-P) flush aortogram and an A-P selective injection of each renal artery were done using a 6 French catheter; if renal arterial anatomy was not well delineated on A-P angiographic views, additional oblique projections were obtained. The average volume of contrast for performing SCA was 75 cc.

In the remaining 33 donors (group 2), radiographic renal imaging was preferentially done on an outpatient basis with DSA and IVP following an i.v. injection of 50 ml contrast material (meglumine diatrizoate). The basic technique for performing DSA is described in detail elsewhere (*7*). Briefly, following a plain abdominal roentgenogram, a 16-gauge cannula is introduced into the antecubital vein and advanced 6–8 inches. Glucagon 1 mg is administered i.v. for reduction of intestinal peristalsis. A preinjection fluoroscopic image is obtained and stored in computer memory as a "mask" image. The contrast material is injected rapidly at a rate of approximately 20 ml/sec for 2 sec yielding a total of 40 ml contrast per injection; this is followed by a 25 ml 5% dextrose flush. A second fluoroscopic image is obtained and stored in a second computer memory.The fluoroscopic images are converted by computer to digital data and then subtracted from each other. The digital sum is then reprocessed to print a real-time image that eliminates the mask image from the image with contrast, thus giving an image of the vasculature alone. These renal DSA studies were done with standard A-P views using a 9-inch diameter circular field size; if these views yielded suboptimal visualization of the renal arteries, then a second i.v. injection of contrast

[1] Address requests for reprints to Andrew C. Novick, M.D., Cleveland Clinic Foundation, 9500 Euclid Avenue, Cleveland, Ohio 44106.

* Abbreviations used: anteroposterior; DSA, digital subtraction angiography; IVP, intravenous pyelography; LRD, living-related donor; SCA, standard catheter arteriography.

material was given and oblique views were obtained. Most donors received two injections of contrast for an average contrast volume of 80 cc per DSA study. In all patients, when the DSA study was completed, serial abdominal roentgenograms were obtained to complete the pyelographic phase of the study.

In patients from group 2 undergoing evaluation with IVP and DSA, if renal arterial imaging with DSA was considered satisfactory, no further radiographic studies were performed (Fig. 1); there were 23 patients in this category (group 2-A). If renal arterial imaging with DSA was not considered satisfactory, the patient was hosptialized for performance of SCA; there were 10 patients in this category (group 2-B).

All SCA and DSA studies were carefully evaluated for the number, location, and patency of the renal arteries. The radiographic interpretations were correlated with intraoperative findings at the time of living-donor nephrectomy. The mean cost per patient of all radiographic renal imaging studies were calculated for donors in groups 1, 2-A, 2-B. For patients undergoing SCA, this figure includes the cost of hospitalization to perform the study.

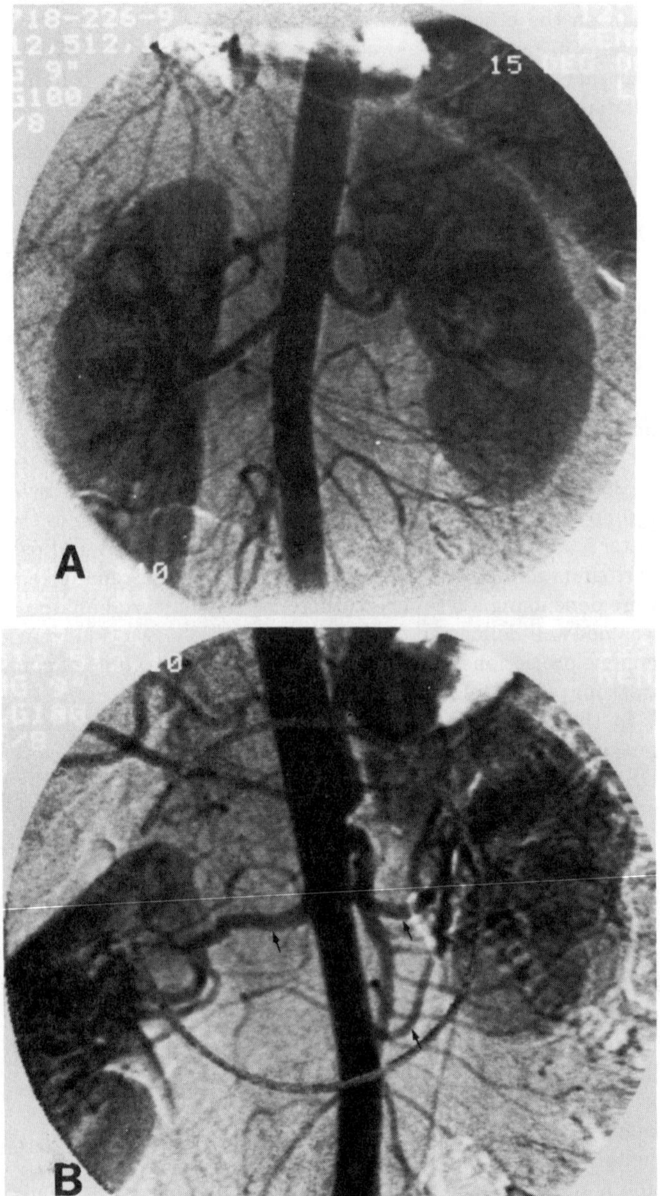

FIGURE 1. (A) DSA shows single artery to each kidney. (B) DSA shows single right renal artery and two left renal arteries (arrows).

RESULTS

The renal arteries of all patients in this study were normal with no evidence of stenosis or aneurysm formation. There were no complications of SCA or DSA. In particular, there were no cases of contrast-induced nephrotoxicity as determined by serum creatinine levels obtained before and after the study. All SCA studies accurately delineated renal arterial anatomy, and this was confirmed by findings at the time of nephrectomy. The results with SCA in this study are consistent with our earlier experience in 52 consecutive living-related renal donors who underwent SCA followed by nephrectomy from January 1979 to December 1981; intraoperative findings in these patients confirmed that SCA had accurately demonstrated the renal arterial anatomy in all cases.

The accuracy of DSA in group 2 patients is outlined in Table 1. Of 23 patients in whom DSA imaging of the renal arteries was considered satisfactory (group 2-A), two were found to have an unsuspected additional polar artery at the time of nephrectomy (Fig. 2). In both cases, extracorporeal renal vascular reconstruction was done (*8*) followed by successful transplantation into the recipient. There were 10 patients (group 2-B), in whom DSA imaging was considered suboptimal due to overlying mesenteric vessels or bowel gas. These patients were studied with SCA, which confirmed the impression upon DSA in 5 patients (Fig. 3) and yielded diagnostic information not observed upon DSA in 5 patients (Fig. 4); among the latter 5 patients, single and multiple renal arteries were present in 3 and 2 patients, respectively.

Table 2 illustrates the accuracy of DSA in imaging single or multiple renal arteries. DSA provided satisfactory visualization in 19 of 20 patients (95%) with single arteries bilaterally. The major limitation of DSA was in patients with multiple renal arteries unilaterally or bilaterally: accurate imaging was obtained in only 7 of these 13 patients (54%).

Overall, DSA provided accurate imaging of the renal arteries in 26 of 33 patients (79%). It is perhaps more relevant to examine the efficacy of our overall approach of preferentially using DSA to evalute renal arterial anatomy and obtaining SCA only if visualization upon DSA was suboptimal. With this approach, renal arterial anatomy was accurately delineated preoperatively in 31 of 33 patients (94%).

Table 3 outlines the mean cost per patient of all radiographic renal imaging studies performed in groups 1, 2-A and 2-B. The mean cost of this evaluation was $1721.00 for patients in group 1 evaluated with IVP and SCA alone. Not surprisingly, the mean cost was less ($418.00) for patients in group 2-A studied

TABLE 1. Accuracy of DSA for renal arterial imaging in living-related renal donors

	No. donors	DSA accurate	DSA inaccurate
Group 2-A	23	21	2
Group 2-B	10	5	5
Group 2-A & B	33	26 (79%)	7 (21%)

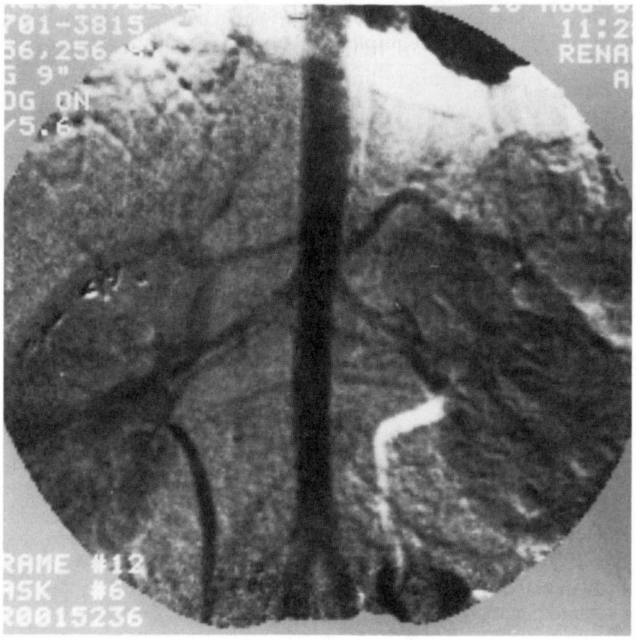

FIGURE 2. This DAS was considered satisfactory and demonstrates two right renal arteries and a single left renal artery. At the time of left donor nephrectomy, an additional unsuspected upper polar artery was found that had not been demonstrated upon DSA.

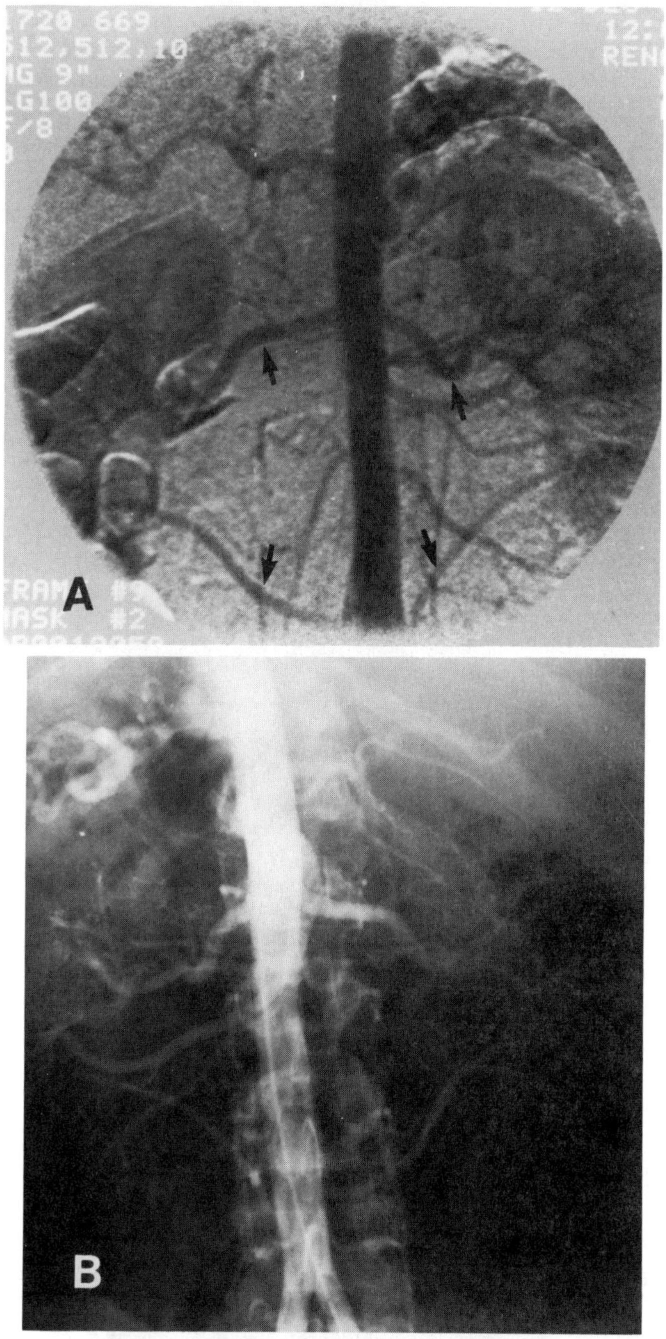

FIGURE 3. (A) Digital subtraction angiogram interpreted as showing two arteries to each kidney (arrows). (B) SCA was obtained to rule out the presence of additional renal arteries. The SCA confirms two arteries to each kidney.

with only a combined DSA-IVP, and was greater ($2182.00) for patients in group 2-B who underwent SCA in addition to DSA-IVP. Interestingly, the mean cost per patient of all donors from group 2 was still much less than that of donors from group 1 ($953.00 vs. $1721.00).

DISCUSSION

Digital subtraction angiography (DSA) is a relatively new technique for radiographic imaging of arterial anatomy following the injection of contrast material into a peripheral vein. This concept was originally proposed in 1939 by Robb and Steinberg (*9*), however, its usefulness was limited by the need for large doses of contrast and the relative insensitivity of standard radiographic film to small attenuation differences between tissues and contrast material. DSA ultimately developed from advances in digital image processing which, combined with radiographic techniques used in computed tomography, yielded contrast resolution ability previously not possible.

There are several advantages of DSA compared with standard catheter arteriography (SCA). DSA avoids the need for direct arterial cannulation, is more rapid to perform, can be done as an outpatient and is less expensive; in addition, an IVP can be simultaneously obtained from the same dose of contrast material. These attractive features spawned a number of studies on the efficacy of DSA for imaging of renal arteries in patients with suspected renovascular disease (*5, 10–13*); in these reports, the diagnostic accuracy of DSA ranged from 80–92%. In a study from our hospital, both renal DSA and SCA were obtained in 57 hypertensive patients (*7*); in 8 patients, DSA yielded a false radiographic interpretation, while in 49 patients DSA findings were identical to those obtained with SCA for an overall accuracy of 86%.

The use of DSA for living-related renal donor evaluation was a natural sequel to studies of its efficacy in delineating renal arterial anatomy. There are now several such reports, and, while DSA has provided accurate information in the majority of cases, there have been a small number of living-related donors in whom DSA alone proved unreliable in evaluating the number and location of renal arteries (*2–6*). The major deficiency of DSA in this setting has been a failure to uniformly visualize accessory renal arteries that occur in at least 20% of the population (*14*). Lack of awareness of this variation in vascular anatomy complicates performance of the transplant

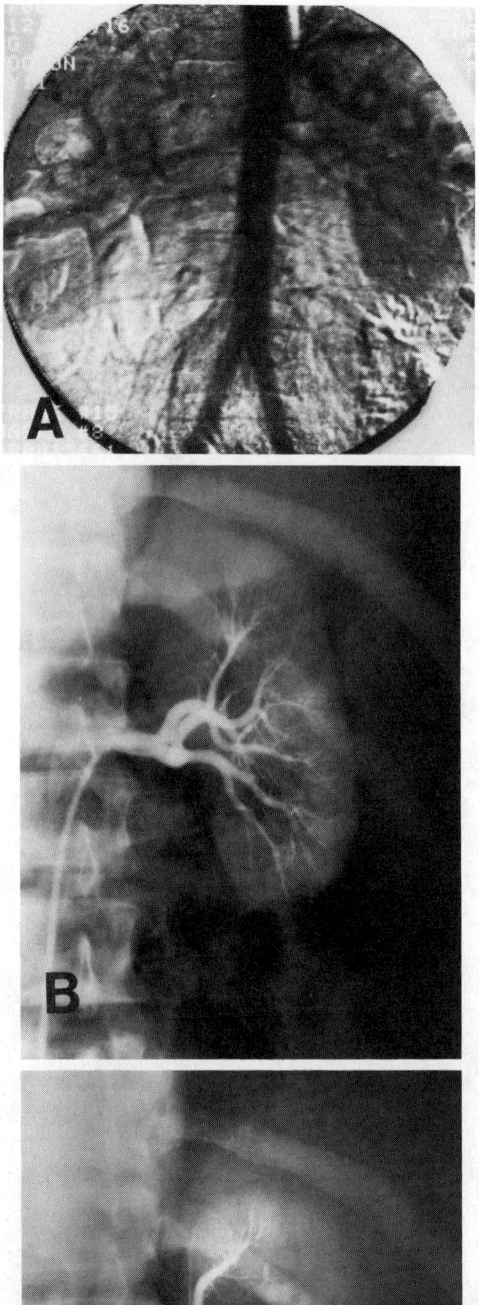

FIGURE 4. (A) This DSA was interpreted as showing two right renal arteries and a single left renal artery. The quality of renal arterial imaging was considered suboptimal and SCA was then also done. (B) Selective SCA of left main renal artery demonstrates an avascular area of the upper pole. (C) This area of the left upper pole is supplied by an additional polar artery, demonstrated upon selective SCA, that was not observed upon DSA.

TABLE 2. Accuracy of DSA in living-related donors with single or multiple renal arteries

No. renal arteries	No. donors	DSA accurate	DSA inaccurate
Single bilaterally	20	19	1
Multiple unilaterally	10	6	4
Multiple bilaterally	3	1	2

TABLE 3. Mean cost per patient of radiographic renal imaging for live-donor evaluation

	Group 1	Group 2-A	Group 2-B
Renal imaging studies:	IVP, SCA[a]	DSA/IVP	DSA/IVP
No. donors:	28	23	10
Mean cost per patient:	$1721	$418	$2182
		$953 for Groups 2-A & B combined	

[a] IVP = intravenous pyelography; DSA/IVP = combined digital subtraction angiogram and intravenous pyelography; SCA = Standard catheter angiography.

operation and may, in fact, compromise the outcome. In the present study, DSA was accurate in 26 of 33 donors (79%) overall, but was accurate in only 7 of 13 donors (54%) with multiple renal arteries. We conclude from these data that the diagnostic reliability of DSA alone is not sufficiently accurate for preoperative evaluation of living-related renal donors.

There are several reasons why DSA may provide poor visualization of the renal arteries. Overlying mesenteric vessels are a major cause of inadequate imaging that can occasionally be overcome by obtaining oblique views. Overlying bowel gas presents another problem even with routine preliminary administration of glucagon to inhibit peristalsis. Another cause of poor visualization is failure of the patient to suspend respiration during the study. A final potential problem with DSA is inadequate delivery of the contrast bolus to the renal vessels due to contrast extravasation at the injection site or performance of the Valsalva Maneuver, which can slow cardiac filling and cause trapping of contrast in the arm or neck veins.

If DSA alone is inadequate for living-related renal donor evaluation, then perhaps one should consider a policy of preferentially utilizing DSA but also obtaining SCA if DSA-imaging is deemed suboptimal. This would preserve the advantages of DSA for patients in whom high-quality imaging is obtained, while accepting that both DSA and SCA will be necessary in some patients. We undertook to evaluate this approach prospectively in the present study, comparing it with traditional living-donor renal arterial imaging with SCA alone. It is interesting that the mean per-patient cost of radiographic renal imaging with this approach was substantially reduced, even though 10 of 33 donors underwent both DSA and SCA. However, there were also 2 donors in the subgroup studied with DSA alone in whom a radiographically undetected polar renal artery was identified at the time of nephrectomy. In both cases, successful transplantation was ultimately accomplished after extracorporeal microvascular end-to-side anastomosis of the branch to the main renal artery.

In the present study, SCA accurately delineated the renal arterial anatomy in all 28 cases from group 1. Although SCA may occasionally prove inaccurate in these patients (*15*), our experience with SCA in 52 prior living-related donors also indicated reliable demonstration of renal arterial anatomy in all cases. When the accuracy of imaging with a technically satisfactory DSA study alone in the present study (21 of 23 patients) is compared with the accuracy of SCA alone in our program from 1979–1984 (80 of 80 patients), a statistically significant differences is observed ($P = .05$). Therefore, this prospective study suggests that the approach of preferentially evaluating living-related renal donors with DSA, and obtaining SCA only if DSA yields poor visualization, is more cost-effective than, but not as accurate as, the traditional policy of obtaining SCA in all cases. Based on these data, we have reverted to SCA exclusively in the evaluation of living renal donors in our program, and such studies are now also being performed on an out-patient basis, which has further reduced their cost (*16*).

REFERENCES

1. Monaco AP. Clinical kidney transplantation in 1984. Transplant Proc 1985; 17: 1.
2. Flechner SM, Sandler CM, Ben-Menachem Y, Van Buren CT, Kahan BD. Evaluation of living-related kidney donors using digital subtraction angiography. Cleve Clin Q, 1984; 51: 339.
3. Rabe FE, Smith EJ, Yune HY, Klatte EC, Leapman SB, Filo RS. Limitations of digital subtraction angiography in evaluating potential renal donors. Am J Rad 1983; 141: 91.
4. Hillman BJ, Zukoski CF, Ovitt TW, Ogden DA, Capp MP. Evaluation of potential renal donors and allograft recipients: digital video subtraction angiography. Am J Rad 1982; 138: 921.
5. Clark RA, Alexander ES. Digital subtraction angiography in the renal arteries: prospective comparison with conventional arteriography. Invest Radiol 1983; 18: 6.
6. Schmeller NT, Land W, Roth M. Letter to the editor. Transplantation 1984; 37: 221.
7. Zabbo A, Novick AC. Digital subtraction angiography for noninvasive imaging of the renal artery. Urol Clin North Am 1984; 11: 409.
8. Novick AC, Magnusson M. Multiple-artery renal transplantation: emphasis on extracorporeal methods of donor arterial repair. J Urol 1979; 122: 731.
9. Robb GP, Steinberg I. Visualization of the chambers of the heart, the pulmonary circulation and the great blood vessels in man: practical method. Am J Roentgenol 1939; 41: 1.
10. Gomes AS, Pais SO, Barbaric L. Digital subtraction angiography in the evaluation of hypertension. Am J Rad 1983; 140: 779.
11. Hillman BJ, Ovitt TW, Nudelman S, et al. Digital subtraction angiography of renal vascular abnormalities. Radiology 1981; 1939: 227.
12. Osborne RW, Goldstone T, Hillman BJ, et al. Digital video subtraction screening technique for renovascular hypertension. Surgery 1981; 90: 932.
13. Smith CW, Winfield AC, Price RP, et al: Evaluation of digital venous angiography for the diagnosis of renovascular hypertension. Radiology 1982; 144: 51.
14. Merklin RJ, Michaels NA. The variant renal blood supply with data on the inferior phrenic, ureteral, and gonadal arteries. J Int Coll Surg 1958; 29: 41.
15. Sherwood DT, Ruutu M, Chilsolm GD. Renal angiography problems in live kidney donors. Br J Radiol 1978; 51: 99.
16. Wolfel DA, Lovett BP, Ortenburger AI, Johnson LS, Sommerville DL. Outpatient arteriography: its safety and cost-effectiveness. Radiology 1984; 153: 363.

Received 15 May 1985.
Accepted 30 October 1985.

0041-1337/86/4201-0028$02.00/0
TRANSPLANTATION
Vol. 42, No. 1

Printed in U.S.A.

MULTIVARIATE ANALYSIS OF RISK FACTORS IN CADAVER DONOR KIDNEY TRANSPLANTATION

FRED SANFILIPPO,[1] WILLIAM K. VAUGHN,[2] WILLIAM M. LEFOR,[3] AND EVERETT K. SPEES[4]

South-Eastern Organ Procurement Foundation, Richmond, Virginia 23220[5]

Data collected prospectively on 3811 kidney transplants performed between June 1977 and July 1982 with follow-up to July 1984 by the 42 member institutions of the South-Eastern Organ Procurement foundation were analyzed to identify factors associated with graft and patient outcome in patients not receiving cyclosporine. Multivariate Cox regression analysis was used to examine the association and relative risk of 24 variables with three actuarial outcomes: overall graft failure, irreversible rejection, and patient death. Factors having no suggested association with any outcome included: recipient sex, history of pregnancy, blood group, and time on dialysis; organ preservation method, time and source; donor race; crossmatch test sensitivity; and annual center transplant rate. In decreasing order of relative risk, the factors most significantly associated with irreversible rejection were: loss of two or more prior grafts, low HLA-A,B match, lack of pretransplant blood transfusion, high (>60%) pretransplant sensitization to leukocyte (HLA) antigens, and delayed graft function. Splenectomy, insulin-dependent diabetes, and antilymphocyte serum therapy provided the greatest risk of patient death. Factors such as recipient age, race, and native nephrectomy had suggested associations with outcome. By adding each center as a separate covariate in the analysis, other center-dependent factors were quantitated and found in some cases to have a highly significant association with graft and patient outcome.

These results provide a basis for evaluating the potential risk of graft loss or patient death for those prospective cadaver kidney transplant recipients not being considered for cyclosporine therapy.

Despite more than 20 years of clinical experience with cadaver donor kidney transplantation, the relative importance of various factors that may affect patient and graft survival remains controversial. A number of practical and statistical problems have become apparent in attempting to properly analyze variables associated with transplant outcome. Since most studies have involved single-center observations, the limited number of patients generally available at one institution constrains the number of variables that can be examined. In addition, the potential for bias in patient selection, treatment, or other factors that cannot be controlled in single center analysis can significantly mask or amplify certain factors.

The common use of univariate analysis, or the exclusion of potentially confounding variables may also lead to inappropriate conclusions regarding transplant outcome. For example, HLA-A,B match level, prior graft loss, pretransplant blood transfusions, and the presence of preformed antileukocyte (HLA) antibodies are all highly interdependent variables and each is associated with graft survival (*1, 2*), so that proper analysis of any one of them must be stratified by the others. Retrospective accumulation of transplant data has also been shown to provide significant bias, especially in terms of the effect of HLA-A,B matching (*3*). Over the past 10–15 years there have been dramatic changes in the use of pretransplant transfusions and antirejection therapy. The frequency of retransplantation, and the average level of recipient presensitization, as well as other factors that could effect results if not considered in analysis of outcome. For example, the use of cyclosporine (CsA)* for maintenance immunosuppression of cadaver donor renal transplant recipients has only gained widespread use in the past 2–3 years, so that follow-up times on patients treated with CsA are limited. In addition, the criteria for use of CsA vary greatly among centers, providing substantial selection bias in evaluating patients receiving (or not receiving) CsA during this period. Finally, while most factors appear to influence short-term graft survival, others—such as HLA match (*2*) and perhaps CsA toxicity—have an increasing impact over time, so that length of available follow-up may effect the significance of certain factors.

The most useful type of analysis would therefore require a large, concordant patient population with long follow-up involving at least several centers; prospective, accurate, and complete acquisition of data concerning numerous factors on all transplants performed; and multivariate-type analysis to include patient, donor, and center variables. A recent study examined prognostic variables for overall graft failure in two distinct multicenter transplant populations not receiving CsA using multivariate analysis (*4*), but only a limited number of factors and patients were considered, and causes of irreversible graft rejection and patient death were not examined.

As a requirement for membership, the South-Eastern Organ Procurement Foundation (SEOPF) has required since June 1977 detailed prospective submission of data on all cadaver donor renal transplants performed by member institutions. Between June 1977 and July 1982 data on 3811 of 3874 patients transplanted by the 42 member institutions were entered into the central SEOPF computer, and follow-up information on these patients has been continuously recorded to the present. A recent study examined some of the variables in this data base using univariate analysis (*5*). In order to more comprehensively evaluate these data, we have used the Cox regression model for

[1] Departments of Pathology and Surgery, Duke University and Durham VA Medical Centers, Durham, NC 27710.

[2] Division of Biostatistics, Vanderbilt University, Nashville, TN 37232.

[3] Transplantation and Immunology Laboratory, University of South Florida, Tampa, FL 33612.

[4] Department of Surgery, The Johns Hopkins and Francis Scott Key Medical Centers, Baltimore, MD 21224.

[5] Address reprint requests to: South-Eastern Organ Procurement Foundation, P.O. Box 28060, Richmond, VA 23228.

* Abbreviations used: ALS, anti-lymphocyte serum; CsA, cyclosporine; PRA, panel-reactive antibody; SEOPF, South-Eastern Organ Procurement Foundation.

multivariate analysis of 24 distinct patient, donor, and center variables to identify associations with each of three different outcomes: overall graft failure, irreversible rejection, and patient death.

MATERIALS AND METHODS

Data base. Detailed information regarding SEOPF and the methods used by its members for matching donors and recipients, providing quality assurance of histocompatibility testing, and reporting donor, recipient, and follow-up information on each cadaver donor transplant performed has been previously reported (*2, 5–8*). Since June 1977, each member institution has been required to submit detailed information on all cadaver-donor transplants performed (regardless of donor organ source) to the central SEOPF office, where it is entered into a computer. Posttransplant follow-up information is also required at regular intervals (*2*). The completeness and accuracy of data obtained has been verified by cross-checking with financial records, and by random sampling comparisons between computerized data and hard-copy form, as well as between forms and patient charts (*2, 5*). Error rates of 0.07% and 0.36% were identified by random sample for discrepancies between information in the computer vs. on forms, and between the forms and patient chart, respectively (*2*). The patient population base used in this study is the same as that used for other recent studies (*2, 5, 9*), but includes a longer follow-up period (through July 1984). Thus, of 3874 cadaver renal transplants known to be performed during the patient entry period of June 1977–July 1982, data were not submitted on only 63 (1.6%). Although only a small number of patients received CsA before July 1982, to remove potential selection bias based on CsA therapy, all patients (183) transplanted at institutions that used CsA during the study period were excluded.

Statistical methods. Allograft failure and patient death rates were calculated by the actuarial life table method. Graft failure was calculated in two ways for each analysis: (1) overall graft failure, which includes all causes of graft loss with no exclusions as determined by return to maintenance dialysis, transplant nephrectomy, or patient death regardless of graft function; and (2) irreversible rejection, which includes as graft failures only cases in which failure was identified as any type of immune allograft rejection (hyperacute, accelerated acute, acute, or chronic). For analysis of graft survival by the latter method, (irreversible rejection only), patients with graft loss from causes other than irreversible rejection were censored (removed from the population at risk, but not considered a graft failure) at the time of graft loss.

The Cox regression model (*10*) was used to determine the significance of association between each covariate and outcome according to the formula: $\lambda(t; x_i) = \exp(x_i\beta_i)\lambda_o(t)$ where $\lambda(t; x_i)$ is the risk of occurrence—i.e., overall graft failure irreversible rejection, or patient death; $\lambda_o(t)$ is a baseline risk function; x_i are the covariates being considered; and β_i are the relative weights of association between each covariate and the risk of occurrence. The standardized regression coefficient Z_i for each covariate was calculated as $\beta_i \div$ standard error of β_i, and the likelihood ratio test was used to assess the significance of association between each covariate and risk of occurrence (i.e., β_i). The sign of each Z value indicates whether the association between outcome and the higher level of covariate assignment is positive or negative; the absolute value of Z indicates the weight of association. The relative risk for each covariate was calculated using the formula $\exp(\beta_i [x_{i2} - x_{i1}])$ where x_{i2} and x_{i1} are distinct levels of each covariate x_i. The 24 variables examined and levels assigned included: HLA-A, -B match (0, 1, 2, 3, 4); delayed graft function (0 = no; 1 = yes); pretransplant transfusion (0 = no; 1 = yes); recipient race (0 = white; 1 = nonwhite); sex (0 = female, 1 = male); prior grafts failed (0 = 0, 1 = 1, 2 = 2 or more); antilymphocyte serum (ALS) treatment posttransplant (0 = no; 1 = yes); peak (highest) percentage of panel-reactive antibody (PRA) pretransplant (0 = 0, 1 = 1–59%, 2 = ≥60%); pretransplant native bilateral nephrectomy (0 = no; 1 = yes); insulin-dependent diabetes (0 = no; 1 = yes); donor organ source (0 = local; 1 = shared); most recent (current) percentage of PRA pretransplant (0 = 0, 1 = 1–59%, 2 = ≥60%); age (1 = 2–14, 2 = 15–24, 3 = 25–44, 4 = 45–54, 5 = 55–89 years); recipient splenectomy pretransplant (0 = no, 1 = yes); history of pregnancy (0 = no, 1 = yes), blood group (0 = O, 1 = A, B or AB); time on dialysis pretransplant (months), donor race (0 = white, 1 = nonwhite); method of organ preservation (1 = ice only, 2 = ice and pump, or pump only); length of preservation (hours), year of transplant (1977, 1978, 1979, 1980, 1981, 1982); transplant rate (average transplant number per center per year); crossmatch sensitivity for each lab—calculated from interlaboratory proficiency tests = (false positive ÷ [true positive + false negative]) − false negative ÷ [true negative + false positive]); and center identification number. For several of the variables with multiple levels, a reference level was identified and each other level of that variable was entered as a separate covariate in the model, so that the risk associated with each level of the variable could be determined. Reference levels used were as follows: prior graft failure-0; HLA-A, B match-2; peak PRA-0; year of transplant-1981; age-25 to 44. In each case the reference level was that closest to the mean of the entire population, and by exclusion from the model represented a relative risk of 1.00. For center effects, code numbers were assigned to each center and were included as additional separate covariates, with one center (which had outcomes close to the mean) excluded as the reference level (i.e., relative risk of that center = 1.00). The goodness of fit of the Cox model to the data was determined by plotting the cumulative hazard of the residuals agains the residuals, which showed that the Cox model including all covariates fit the data extremely well. Computer programs used in these analyses were BMDP1L and BMDP2L (*11*).

RESULTS

Analysis of variables. As listed in Table 1, 24 separate factors were analyzed for associations with each of the outcomes considered. A covariate was considered as not having an association with outcome if the absolute Z value was <1.96 (P>0.05) or the relative risk was between 0.85 and 1.20. Of the patient (recipient) variables considered, five showed no suggested association with any outcome (i.e., overall graft failure, irreversible rejection, and patient death): sex, history of pregnancy, blood group, most recent (current) level of pretransplant presensitization (PRA), or length of time on dialysis. Four donor factors examined also were not associated with any outcome: donor race, method of organ preservation, the length of time of organ preservation, or the source (local vs. shared) of donor organ. Of the center-related variables, neither the relative sensitivity of crossmatch test used nor the number of transplants performed per year by the center had a suggested association with any outcome. As described in the *Materials and Methods* section the relative crossmatch sensitivity was calculated based on results of standardized cell and sera exchanges between laboratories for the study period, with a calculated range of −29.73 to 16.55. The range of transplant rates per year between centers was also substantial (5.7–80.7) with a mean of 30.7±4.9.

Overall graft failure. As shown in Table 2, several of the 24 variables examined showed a significant association with overall graft failure. Transplants performed in 1977, 1978, 1979 and 1980 also were associated with a significant ($Z>1.96$, $P<0.05$) relative risk (RR) compared to 1981, which was used as the reference level (RR = 1.00). Of the patient variables showing a significant association with outcome, failure of 2 or more prior grafts had the highest relative risk (RR = 1.506, $P<0.009$), followed by peak PRA≥60 (RR = 1.346, $P<0.003$). Using a reference level for HLA-A,B match of 2 (RR ≥ 1.00), patients with a 1 or a zero antigen match had a significantly higher risk of overall graft failure (RR = 1.161, 1.336 respectively). There was no suggested benefit of a 3 antigen match (compared to a 2 antigen match), although a 4 antigen match had a suggested benefit (RR = 0.85, P = NS). The other highest risk factors were delayed graft function (RR = 1.427, $P<0.0001$), no pretransplant blood transfusions (RR = 1.321, $P<0.0002$), and diabetes (RR = 1.318, $P<0.005$). Patients who lost 1 prior graft, were nonwhite, or between 45–54 years old had a modest but statistically significant ($P<0.05$) increased risk of overall graft failure. Only one center was associated with a statistically significant risk (RR = 1.457, p = 0.05) while 1 other with a significant benefit (RR = 0.704, $P<0.05$). The highest benefit associated with a center (RR = 0.624) was not statistically significant ($P = 0.058$). Native nephrectomy and ALS use were associated with modest suggested benefits (RR = 0.885, 0.937) but not at a statistically significant level, while splenectomy had a slight suggested risk (RR = 1.057, P = NS).

Irreversible graft rejection. Several different associations were found when graft outcome considering irreversible rejection rather than all causes of failure was examined. As shown in Table 3, the risks of prior graft failure, PRA≥60, and poor (0 or 1) HLA-A, B matching associated with irreversible rejection were substantially increased in comparison to their influence on overall graft failure. The association of pretransplant transfusion, delayed graft function, diabetes, native nephrectomy, year of transplant, age, and race were essentially unchanged, while ALS use and splenectomy were found to provide a significant benefit (RR = 0.763, 0.720, respectively). The risk of irreversible rejection was essentially equivalent for all age groups. Five centers were found to be associated with a statistically significant risk and one with a significant benefit.

Patient death. Only a few variables showed a significant association with patient death (Table 4). The highest risk (other than patient age) was associated with splenectomy (RR = 1.857, $P<0.004$) followed by diabetes (RR = 1.791, $P<0.003$) and use of ALS (RR = 1.665, $P<0.001$). Factors such as delayed graft function (RR = 1.267) and loss of 2 or more prior grafts (RR = 1.712) had risks that were suggestive statistically ($0.05<P<0.09$). Factors such as pretransplant transfusion, race, peak PRA, and nephrectomy had no suggested association with patient death. Considering HLA-A,B match, the lowest risk was seen at the reference level (HLA-A, B = 2; RR = 1.00) with the highest risk associated with a 4 antigen match (RR = 1.539, P = NS). A match level of 1 provided a moderate risk (RR = 1.371) that was statistically significant ($P<0.045$).

As would be expected, the oldest group of patients (55–89) had the highest risk of death (RR = 2.559, $P<10^{-4}$). In contrast, the lowest risk of death was found in the group between 15–24

TABLE 1. Association of variables examined by Cox regression analysis with graft or patient outcome

Associated with outcome	Not associated with outcome
HLA-A,B match	Recipient sex
Pretransplant transfusion	History of pregnancy
Prior graft failure	Recipient blood group
Diabetes	Current PRA[a]
Antilymphocyte serum therapy	Time on dialysis pretransplant
Peak PRA[a]	Donor race
Recipient age	Method of organ preservation
Recipient race	Time of organ preservation
Splenectomy	Organ procurement source (local/shared)
Native nephrectomy	
Delayed graft function	Center annual transplant rate
Year of transplantation	Center crossmatch test sensitivity
Transplant center	

[a] PRA denotes percentage of panel cells reactive with antibody.

TABLE 2. Relative influence of major factors associated with overall graft failure as determined by the Cox regression model

Variable (x_i)	Level	β Value	SE of β	Z value	P value	Relative risk[a]
Prior failed grafts	1	0.196	0.077	2.555	0.011	1.217
	≥2	0.410	0.156	2.634	0.009	1.506
HLA-A,B match	0	0.289	0.088	3.289	0.001	1.336
	1	0.150	0.071	2.097	0.036	1.161
	3	−0.033	0.089	−0.368	NS[b]	0.968
	4	−0.159	0.157	−1.012	NS	0.853
Peak PRA[b]	1–59	−0.030	0.067	−0.449	NS	0.970
	≥60	0.297	0.099	3.015	0.003	1.346
Pretransplant transfusion	None	0.326	0.085	3.831	0.0002	1.321
Diabetes	Yes	0.276	0.097	2.855	0.005	1.318
Race	Nonwhite	0.191	0.059	3.218	0.002	1.211
Delayed graft function	Yes	0.355	0.059	6.034	<0.0001	1.427
Age	45–54	0.158	0.0731	2.165	0.030	1.172
Center	Highest	0.376	0.192	1.958	0.050	1.457
	Lowest	−0.471	0.249	−1.895	0.058	0.624

[a] Relative risk values were obtained by comparing level identified for each variable against reference level for that variable (see the *Materials and Methods* and *Results* sections).

[b] PRA = percentage of panel cells reactive with antibody, NS = not significant.

TABLE 3. Relative influence of major factors associated with irreversible graft rejection as determined by the Cox regression model

Variable (x_i)	Level	β Value	SE of β	Z value	*P* value	Relative risk[a]
Prior failed grafts	1	0.343	0.092	3.731	0.0002	1.409
	≥2	0.634	0.185	3.427	0.0006	1.884
HLA-A,B match	0	0.430	0.106	4.046	<0.0001	1.538
	1	0.257	0.089	2.900	0.004	1.293
	3	−0.002	0.115	−0.015	NS[b]	0.998
	4	−0.194	0.200	−0.970	NS	0.824
Peak PRA[b]	1–59	−0.005	0.083	−0.062	NS	0.995
	≥60	0.392	0.119	3.294	0.001	1.479
Pretransplant transfusion	None	0.385	0.104	3.694	0.0003	1.377
Diabetes	Yes	0.252	0.120	2.108	0.034	1.287
Race	Nonwhite	0.156	0.074	1.978	0.048	1.157
Delayed graft function	Yes	0.320	0.073	4.362	<0.0001	1.377
Splenectomy	Yes	−0.329	0.176	−1.865	0.06	0.720
Antilymphocyte serum therapy	Yes	−0.270	0.095	−2.838	0.005	0.763
Center	Highest	0.895	0.230	3.886	<0.0001	2.447
	Lowest	−0.802	0.391	−2.052	0.041	0.449

[a] Relative risk values were obtained by comparing level identified for each variable against reference level for that variable (see the *Materials and Methods* section.

[b] PRA = percentage of panel cells reactive with antibody, NS = not significant.

TABLE 4. Relative influence of major factors associated with patient death as determined by the Cox regression model

Variable (x_i)	Level	β Value	SE of β	Z value	*P* value	Relative risk[a]
Splenectomy	Yes	0.619	0.211	2.929	0.0034	1.857
Diabetes	Yes	0.583	0.190	3.064	0.0023	1.791
Antilymphocyte serum therapy	Yes	0.510	0.148	3.459	0.0006	1.665
Prior failed grafts	1	−0.002	0.182	−0.013	NS[b]	0.998
	≥2	0.537	0.308	1.744	0.08	1.712
HLA-A,B match	0	0.182	0.209	0.870	NS	1.199
	1	0.316	0.157	2.016	0.045	1.371
	3	0.204	0.179	1.139	NS	1.227
	4	0.431	0.280	1.539	NS	1.539
Peak PRA[b]	1–59	−0.095	0.146	−0.648	NS	0.910
	≥60	0.272	0.215	1.262	NS	1.312
Delayed graft function	Yes	0.237	0.127	1.867	0.062	1.267
Age	2–14	−0.339	0.394	−0.861	NS	0.713
	15–24	−0.440	0.212	−2.074	0.040	0.644
	45–54	0.643	0.145	4.438	<0.0001	1.902
	55–89	0.940	0.190	4.936	<0.0001	2.559
Year of Transplant	1977	0.841	0.258	3.263	0.0011	2.319
	1978	0.754	0.231	3.257	0.0012	2.125
	1979	0.943	0.220	4.284	<0.0001	2.568
	1980	0.409	0.228	1.795	NS	1.505
	1982	0.164	0.385	0.426	NS	1.178
Center	Highest	0.443	0.401	1.105	NS	1.558
	Lowest	−0.864	0.302	−2.859	0.0043	0.422

[a] Relative risk values were obtained by comparing level identified for each variable against reference level for that variable (see the *Materials and Methods* section.

[b] PRA = percentage of panel cells reactive with antibody, NS = not significant.

years old (RR = 0.644, *P*<0.04) followed by the youngest age group (2–14), which had a RR = 0.713 (*P* = NS). The risk of death was lowest in patients transplanted most recently in 1981 or 1982 (RR = 1.00, 1.180), but highest in those transplanted in 1979 (RR = 2.568, *P*<0.0001). In terms of center-dependent factors, no center was associated with a statistically significant risk of patient death, whereas 3 centers were associated with a significant benefit.

High-risk patient subgroup analysis. To determine the relative risk of factors associated with irreversible rejection in certain high-risk patients, multivariate analysis was performed on defined patient subgroups. Patients were stratified into first-graft recipients and regrafted recipients, and analysis was performed considering 11 major variables as shown in Table 5. As indicated, in first-graft recipients poor (0,1 antigen) HLA-A,B matching provided a highly significant risk (RR = 1.70, 1.42 respectively) relative to a 2 antigen match, while good matching (3,4 antigens) provided no significant benefit. Alternatively, in regrafted patients, a 0 antigen match was associated with a suggested risk (RR = 1.50, *P* = NS) while a 4 antigen match provided a significant benefit (RR = 0.48, *P*<0.05).

Several other variables also showed differences in their relative risk or benefit between these two groups. The risk of high sensitization (PRA≥60) was greater in regrafted patients than first graft recipients (RR = 2.01 vs. 1.37), as was the risk of no pretransplant transfusions (RR = 1.73 vs. 1.32), and the benefit of ALS use (RR = 0.65 vs. 0.76). Conversely, race and native nephrectomy showed no significant risk or benefit in regrafted patients, whereas in first graft recipients nonwhites had a significant risk (RR = 1.23, $P<0.01$) and native nephrectomy provided a significant benefit (RR = 0.77, $P<0.02$). No significant differences in risk were seen between groups for delayed graft function, diabetes, patient age, or year of transplant.

In a similar manner, analysis was performed on patient subgroups considering all graft recipients who were highly sensitized (PRA≥60) or not highly sensitized (PRA = 0–59). Several differences between these groups were noted (Table 6). As with the other low-risk subset (first transplant recipients), poor (0,1 antigen) HLA-A,B matching in patients not highly sensitized provided a significant risk of irreversible rejection relative to a 2 antigen match, while no added benefit was seen with a higher (3 or 4 antigen) match. In the highly sensitized (PRA≥60) patient group, however, a 3 or 4 antigen match had a greater suggested benefit (RR = 0.77, 0.64, respectively, P = NS), while poor (0, 1 antigen) matching appeared to have a lesser risk (RR = 1.52, 1.19, respectively, P = NS). The most striking differences between groups were seen with native nephrectomy and splenectomy, both of which were associated with a significant benefit (RR = 0.79, $P<0.02$; RR = 0.65, $P<0.03$, respectively) in low-sensitized patients, but not in highly sensitized patients (RR = 1.07, 0.99, respectively). The benefit of ALS use appeared greater in high vs. less sensitized patients (RR = 0.55 vs. 0.77), while race (nonwhite) provided a significant risk ony in the less-sensitized group (RR = 1.20, $P<0.015$).

DISCUSSION

The relative importance of various factors potentially effecting graft and patient survival in cadaver renal transplants remains highly controversial. The influence of many factors has been examined by numerous single-center studies using univariate analysis, but because of the significant association among several of these variables, and the potentially confounding effects of other variables not included in these analyses, conclusions have been limited. One recent study (*4*) used multivariate analyses to examine several factors simultaneously, but was performed on a limited population with relatively short follow-up, and did not include many donor and center-dependent variables. In our own recent study on the influence of HLA-A, B matching (*2*) we reported the results of multivar-

TABLE 5. Influence of factors associated with irreversible graft rejection in first graft vs. regrafted recipients

Variable (x_i)[a]	Level	First transplant patients			Regrafted patients		
		Z value	*P* value	Relative risk	Z value	*P* value	Relative risk
HLA=A,B match	0	4.56	<0.0001	1.70	1.91	0.056	1.50
	1	3.66	0.0003	1.42	0.20	NS	1.04
	3	−0.04	NS[b]	1.00	−0.69	NS	0.87
	4	0.16	NS	1.04	−2.03	0.042	0.48
Peak PRA	1–59	−0.47	NS	0.96	1.41	NS	1.32
	≥60	2.01	0.045	1.37	3.25	0.0012	2.01
Native nephrectomy	Yes	−2.36	0.02	0.77	−0.24	NS	0.96
Splenectomy	Yes	−1.32	NS	0.76	−1.77	NS	0.62
Pretransplant transfusion	None	3.22	0.002	1.32	2.64	0.008	1.73
ALS use	Yes	−3.14	0.002	0.76	−2.72	0.007	0.65
Delayed graft function	Yes	4.26	0.0001	1.41	2.53	0.011	1.43
Race	Nonwhite	2.59	0.01	1.23	0.11	NS	1.02

[a] Other variables included in this analysis: diabetes, patient age, year of transplant (data not shown). PRA = percentage of panel cells reactive with antibody.

[b] NS = not significant.

TABLE 6. Influence of factors associated with irreversible graft rejection in high vs. low sensitized recipients

Variable (x_i)[a]	Level	PRA = 0–59[b]			PRA ≥ 60[b]		
		Z value	*P* value	Relative risk	Z value	*P* value	Relative risk
HLA=A,B match	0	4.43	<0.0001	1.62	1.49	NS	1.52
	1	3.36	0.0008	1.35	0.69	NS	1.19
	3	−0.03	NS[b]	1.00	−0.96	NS	0.77
	4	−0.19	NS	0.96	−1.05	NS	0.64
Prior failed grafts	1	3.41	0.0007	1.42	2.63	0.009	1.74
	≥2	2.89	0.004	1.94	1.83	NS	1.76
Native nephrectomy	Yes	−2.34	0.020	0.79	0.32	NS	1.07
Splenectomy	Yes	−2.26	0.024	0.65	−0.01	NS	0.99
Pretransplant transfusion	None	4.14	<0.0001	1.40	0.65	NS	1.23
ALS use	Yes	−3.25	0.0012	0.77	−2.74	0.006	0.55
Delayed graft function	Yes	4.47	<0.0001	1.39	1.52	NS	1.34
Race	Nonwhite	2.43	0.015	1.20	0.10	NS	1.02

[a] Other variables included in this analysis: diabetes, patient age, year of transplant (data not shown).

[b] PRA = percentage of panel cells reactive with antibody; NS = not significant.

iate Cox regression analysis including HLA-A, B match and 10 other variables, as well as center-dependent factors. However, several other variables were not included in that study, nor were results relating to overall graft survival and patient death. Furthermore, the incremental degree of risk or benefit associated with variables having discrete levels was not considered at that time, nor were effects in specific subgroups examined.

In terms of HLA matching, our results continue to show the importance of avoiding poor (0 or 1) HLA-A, B matches, and by including separate covariates for each match level, the significant relative risk of a 1 antigen as well as a 0 antigen match has now been identified. Our previous univariate analysis clearly identified the risk of irreversible rejection with a 0 antigen match (*2*) but suggested that 1,2, and 3 matches were essentially equivalent. The greater impact we found for HLA matching on irreversible rejection compared with all causes of graft failure supports the assumption that the risk of poor matching is largely from increased graft loss due to rejection. Multivariate analysis of certain high risk patient subgroups (e.g., high PRA, prior graft loss) also indicates that poor (0, 1 antigen) matching is most detrimental in the low-risk groups (PRA<60, first transplants) while good (3, 4 antigen) matching is most beneficial in high-risk patients (PRA≥60, retransplants).

Other factors relating to presensitization such as prior graft loss, blood transfusion, pregnancy, and PRA have been previously examined by us (*1*) and others (*3, 12, 13*) using univariate analysis—and, to a limited extent, by Krakauer et. al. (*4*) and us (*2*) using multivariate analysis. The risks we found to be associated with prior graft loss, presensitization, and no pretransplant transfusions are consistent with these previous results, while the absence of any independent risk associated with a prior history of pregnancy represents a new finding. The greater association of presensitization and prior graft failure (but not transfusion) with irreversible rejection vs. overall graft failure is provocative, and suggests that the first two factors predominantly provide an immunologic risk in terms of graft rejection, while the third is beneficial with regard to medical, surgical, and immunological factors. Subset analysis also confirms our previous findings using univariate analysis that high levels of presensitization (PRA) are most detrimental when associated with prior graft loss (*1*). Furthermore, the finding that loss of 2 or more prior grafts is associated with the highest relative risk for irreversible rejection (and a substantially increased risk compared with patients with one failed prior graft) indicates that such patients should be carefully considered as transplant candidates. Interestingly, the level of sensitization at the time of transplant (current PRA) showed no significant risk or benefit in the analysis. Although recent studies have indicated that sera representing historical (peak) PRA levels can be ignored for crossmatching against donor cells without an increased risk of hyperacute rejection (*14, 15*), our findings suggest that the peak, rather than most recent pretransplant PRA level, provides the better indicator of eventual graft rejection.

These results also confirm the significant risk of delayed graft function on eventual graft survival that has recently been reported (*9*). However, the finding that factors such as donor organ preservation method, time, and source, which have been associated with the rate of delayed graft function (*9*), are not themselves independent risk factors indicates that the risk of delayed graft function may be related more to reactions in the host rather than conditions affecting the donor organ prior to transplant. The significant association found between delayed graft function and irreversible graft rejection supports this conclusion.

The modest but significant risk of graft failure and irreversible rejection associated with recipient (but not donor) race is of interest since potential confounding variables such as HLA match, diabetes, and center effects are considered in the analysis. Possible explanations for this finding include differences related to native diseases, such as a higher incidence of hypertensive nephropathy in blacks, as well as socioeconomic factors that might effect compliance with therapy or consistent follow-up care.

Of related interest are the findings that native bilateral nephrectomy and splenectomy are associated with reduced irreversible graft rejection, especially in low-risk (first-transplant, PRA<60) patients. The apparent benefit of nephrectomy confirms our earlier report (*16*), which also indicated that the benefit was limited to first-graft recipients. Although the explanation for this association is still unclear, recent studies using a rat renal allograft model suggest that native kidneys may potentiate ischemic damage caused during organ harvest and preservation (*17*). The benefit of splenectomy has been controversial but reported previously in terms of reducing graft rejection (*18*). However, the substantial risks of sepsis and increased mortality associated with splenectomy have recently been recognized (*19, 20*) and support our findings that splenectomy, while beneficial in terms of reducing rejection, provides a major risk of patient death. Similarly, our findings support previous reports regarding the benefits of antilymphocyte serum in reducing rejection (*21, 22*), but also indicate the substantial risk of patient mortality associated with its use.

The inclusion of several center-related factors in this analysis helps reduce potential bias related to patient selection and treatment. The finding that transplant center activity (as measured by annual transplant rate per center) had no influence on outcome is of practical interest and supports the previous suggestion that the size of a transplant program per se is not a significant determinant of quality (*23*). Although smaller centers in this study may have had different, and possibly more stringent, criteria for patient and donor organ selection than larger centers, the inclusion of additional independent variable for each center in the analysis (as well as the many other variables that largely account for patient and donor criteria) strongly discount this qualification. Conversely, the significant risk or benefit associated with specific centers confirms that factors not otherwise identified by the other 23 variables in this analysis can presumably affect graft outcome. However, the risk or benefit associated with each center by this analysis should not necessarily be interpreted as a measure of its quality of care but rather as an indicator that different criteria are applied in patient and donor organ acceptance at different institutions. Major recipient factors such as overall health, motivation, secondary diseases, and socioeconomic status are not included in this analysis, and certainly would influence outcome in a center-dependent manner. Thus, the very strong impact of center effect we have found supports the inclusion of center-dependent variables for the proper analysis of outcome in renal transplantation.

Acknowledgments. We are indebted to the many persons at each SEOPF institution whose efforts have made it possible to assemble and analyze the SEOPF data base; to the staff of SEOPF—in particular, to Gene Pierce and Martha Diggs for managing the data base; and to N. Hall and M. Thomas for preparation of the manuscript.

REFERENCES

1. Sanfilippo F, Vaughn WK, Bollinger RR, Spees EK. The comparative effects of pregnancy, transfusion and prior graft rejection on sensitization and renal transplant results. Transplantation 1982; 34: 360.
2. Sanfilippo F, Vaughn WK, Spees EK, Light JA, LeFor WM. Benefits of HLA-A and HLA-B matching on graft and patient outcome after cadaveric donor renal transplantation. N Engl J Med 1984; 311: 358.
3. Opelz G, Terasaki PI. International histocompatibility workshop study on renal transplantation. In: Terasaki PI, ed. Histocompatibility testing 1980. Los Angeles: UCLA Tissue Typing Laboratory, 1980; 592.
4. Krakauer H, Spees EK, Vaughn WK, Grauman JS, Summe JP, Bailey RC. Assessment of prognostic factors and projection of outcomes in renal transplantation. Transplantation 1983; 36: 372.
5. McDonald JC, Vaughn WK, Filo RS, et al. Cadaver donor renal transplantation by centers of the South-Eastern Organ Procurement Foundation. Ann Surg 1984; 200: 535.
6. Heise ER, Biegel AA, MacQueen JM. HLA standardization and proficiency testing in the Southeastern Organ Procurement Foundation. Transplantation 1982; 33: 233.
7. Spees EK, Sanfilippo F, Goldman MR, Peters TG, Reitz BL, Vaughn WK. A comparison of kidney, heart and other organ procurement and sharing: the SEOPF experience. Heart Transplant 1983; 2: 212.
8. Spees EK, Mendez-Picon G, Vaughn WK, Reitz BA. Cadaver organ procurement and sharing by members of the South-Eastern Organ Procurement Foundation. Transplant Proc 1984; 16: 199.
9. Sanfilippo F, Vaughn WK, Spees EK, Lucas BA. The detrimental effects of delayed graft function in cadaver donor renal transplantation. Transplantation 1984; 38: 709.
10. Cox DR. Regression and life tables. J R Stat Soc 1972; 34: 187.
11. Dixon WJ, ed. BMDP Statistical Software. Berkeley: University of California, 1983.
12. Cicciarelli J, Terasaki PI. Sensitization patterns in transfused kidney transplant patients and their possible role in kidney graft survival. Transplant Proc 1983; 15: 1208.
13. Horimi T, Terasaki PI, Chia D, Sasaki N. Factors influencing the paradoxical effect of transfusions on kidney transplants. Transplantation 1983; 35: 320.
14. Cardella CJ, Falk JA. Graft outcome in patients with antibodies reactive with donor T and B cells. Transplant Proc 1983; 15: 1142.
15. Sanfilippo F, Vaughn WK, Spees EK, Bollinger RR. Cadaver renal transplantation ignoring peak reactive sera in patients with markedly decreasing pretransplant sensitization. Transplantation 1984; 38: 119.
16. Sanfilippo F, Vaughn WK, Spees EK. The association of native nephrectomy with decreased renal allograft rejection. Transplantation 1984; 37: 256.
17. Coffman TM, Sanfilippo FP, Brazy PC, Yarger WE, Klotman PE. Bilateral native nephrectomy improves renal isograft function in rats Kidney Int (in press).
18. Fryd DS, Sutherland DR, Simmons RL, Ferguson RM, Kjellstrand CM, Najarian JS. Results of a prospective randomized study on the effect of splenectomy versus no splenectomy in renal transplant patients. Transplant Proc 1981; 13: 48.
19. Peters TJ, Williams JW, Harmon HC, Rick LJ. Splenectomy and death in renal transplant patients. Arch Surg 1983; 118: 795.
20. Sutherland DER, Fryd DS, So SKS, Bentley FR, Asher NL, Simmons RL, Najarian JS. Long term effect of splenectomy versus no splenectomy in renal transplant patients. Transplantation 1984; 38: 619.
21. Mendez-Picon G, Spees EK, Vaughn WK, Niblack G, Williams GM, Filo RS, Heise G, Johnson K. Use of anti-lymphocyte serum for cadaveric transplantation: a prospective study of the Southeastern Organ Procurement Foundation (1977–1980). Transplant Proc 1982; 14: 120.
22. Griffin PJA, Williams GT, Salaman JR. Antilymphocytic globulin for the treatment of steroid non-responsive acute renal allograft rejection. Clin Nephrol 1984; 21: 115.
23. Sellers AL, Llach F, Franklin S, Gordon A, Fichman M. Renal transplantation in a community hospital. J Amer Med Assoc 1976; 236: 2866.
24. Gilks WR, Selwood N, Bradley BA. The variation among transplant center results in the United Kingdom and Ireland from 1977 to 1981. Transplantation 1984; 38: 235.

Received 29 July 1985.
Accepted 25 October 1985.

0041-1337/86/4201-0035$02.00/0
TRANSPLANTATION
Vol. 42, No. 1

Printed in U.S.A.

RENAL TRANSPLANTS FROM HLA-HAPLOIDENTICAL LIVING-RELATED DONORS

THE INFLUENCE OF DONOR-SPECIFIC TRANSFUSIONS AND DIFFERENT IMMUNOSUPPRESSIVE REGIMENS[1]

TORBJØRN LEIVESTAD,[2] DAGFINN ALBRECHTSEN, AUDUN FLATMARK, AND ERIK THORSBY

Institute of Transplantation Immunology and Surgical Department, The National Hospital, Oslo 1, Norway

A total of 151 potential recipients of kidney grafts from one-HLA-haplotype–mismatched MLC*-positive (RR>20%) donors treated during 1980–1984 was investigated. The recipients were divided retrospectively into four groups: (A) 42 patients who received pretransplant donor-specific transfusions (DST) and posttransplant azathioprine/prednisolone (DST-only); (B) 10 patients who received DST with azathioprine before and azathioprine/prednisolone after grafting (DST-aza); (C) 42 patients who received no pretreatment and azathiprione/prednisolone posttransplant (aza group) and (D) 57 patients who also received no pretreatment but cyclosporine/prednisolone posttransplant (CsA group).

DST-only led to persistently positive crossmatch in nine (21%) and transient positive crossmatch in two patients, while no sensitization occurred in the DST-aza group.

Posttransplant, early acute rejection episodes were frequent in the DST-only group, but no graft was lost to acute rejection during first year; one-year graft survival (GS) = 94%. Similar GS (93%) was obtained in the CsA group, while in the aza group poorer results were obtained; GS = 69%. In the DST-aza group clinical problems including serious infections were observed.

As CsA treatment without DST gave as high graft survival as in the DST groups, but avoided the sensitization risk by DST alone and the bone marrow complications of DST-aza, such treatment has become our preferred therapy for haploidentical renal transplants.

Since the start of our kidney transplantation program, we have preferred the use of one-HLA-haplotype–mismatched (haploidentical) living-related donors to cadaveric donor kidneys in all uremic patients not having a suitable HLA-identical sibling donor (*1*). We have previously reported that pretransplant blood transfusions from random donors improved graft survival in recipients of haploidentical kidneys, but did not result in graft survival comparable to that seen in recipients of HLA-identical sibling grafts (*2*). The introduction by the San Francisco group of donor-specific blood transfusions (DST) among recipients of haploidentical kidneys led to an excellent graft survival, but at the expense of a 30% antidonor sensitization precluding grafting (*3, 4*). Supplementing DST with concomitant azathioprine immunosuppression was, however, reported by Anderson et al. (*5*) to prevent sensitization without curtailing the graft survival.

During 1981–1983 we applied a DST protocol, without (1981–1982) or with (1983) azathioprine, in 52 patients. Studies of changes in cellular immune responsiveness induced by DST in some of these patients have been reported earlier (*6*). Here we report data on antibody sensitization and the clinical results of our DST program. The results are compared with those obtained in two groups not receiving DST: 42 patients receiving conventional immunosuppression (i.e., azathioprine and prednisolone) and 57 patients receiving CsA and prednisolone.

MATERIALS AND METHODS

Patients. This study includes 151 potential first graft recipients of a haploidentical living-related donor kidney treated from 1980 to 1984 and receiving four treatment protocols. Only cases in which there was mismatch for one detectable DR-antigen and/or in which standard one-way MLC test between recipient and donor was positive (RR>20%) are included. The four patient groups were comparable with respect to age (median 29 years, range 6–68), sex (male:female = 2:1) and pretransplant dialysis. In the DST-groups a higher proportion were previously untransfused (60% versus 31% in the aza group and 40% in the CsA group. $P<0.05$). Diabetic nephropathy was less frequent in the CsA group (11%) than in the DST groups (27%) and the aza group (26%), $P<0.05$.

DST groups. From 1981 to 1983, 52 patients were pretreated with DST. The donors were 34 parents, three offspring, and 15 siblings, all ABO-compatible and (with one exception) Rh-compatible with the recipients. All donors were negative in T and B lymphocyte crossmatch tests with recipient serum prior to the start of DST. At the start of DST 33 patients were on dialysis, while 10 additional entered hemodialysis before the day planned for grafting. Only 21 had received previous blood transfusions; four of the women had had previous pregnancies. The first 42 patients received DST alone (DST-only), while the last ten were given concomitant azathioprine (DST-aza).

Aza group. During 1980–1982, 42 patients received a haploidentical graft with conventional azathioprine/prednisolone immunosuppression. DST was not given due to Rh incompatibility (8 cases) or for logistic reasons; 18 were grafted during the last year prior to the introduction of DST.

CsA group. From January 1983 recipients of haploidentical grafts were randomized to DST-aza treatment or to CsA treatment without DST. When the DST-aza protocol was abandoned in August 1983, the CsA protocol was applied in all such recipients, thus the CsA group consisted of 57 patients grafted from 1983 to 1984.

DST protocol. Three transfusions, each of approximately 200 ml fresh whole blood (volume reduced according to recipient

[1] This work was supported by grants from the Norwegian Research Council of Sciences and the Humanities.

[2] Address correspondence to: T. Leivestad, Institute of Transplantation Immunology, Rikshospitalet, 0027 Oslo 1, Norway.

* Abbreviations used: aza, azathioprine; CsA, cyclosporine; DST, donor-specific transfusions; GS, graft survival; MLC, mixed-lymphocyte culture; PBM, peripheral blood mononuclear cells; PRA, panel-reactive antibodies.

body weight in the two children) from the potential kidney donor were given at two-week intervals. The patient with a Rh-incompatible donor was instead given buffy coats made by dextran sedimentation, supplemented with intramuscular anti-D (Rhesonativ; Kabi, Sweden). Additional random transfusions were avoided as far as possible, but two patients received buffy-coat-poor blood during the DST program. In the DST-aza patients, azathioprine, 2 mg/kg/day, with necessary adjustment as indicated by biweekly leukocyte counts, was instituted 2 days prior to the first DST and given until time of grafting.

Monitoring. Each DST was preceded by appropriate tests for red cell compatibility. Sera taken before each transfusion and two weeks following the last transfusion were tested in parallel for cytotoxic antibodies against fresh donor peripheral blood mononuclear cells (PBM) with the KN technique at 37°C (*7*) and against enriched donor T and B cells using the NIH technique (*8*) at 22°C and 37°C. All sera were also screened for red cell antibodies, and for cytotoxic antibodies against a panel of lymphocytes, using the KN technique with PBM and the NIH technique at 22°C with B cells. Grafting was performed only when the crossmatch against donor PBM, T, and B cells with serum taken just prior to transplantation was negative. Patients who, because of the development of antibodies or for other reasons, could not be transplanted with their potential donor were transferred to the cadaveric kidney transplant program unless another suitable living donor was at hand.

Grafting. Grafting was performed 3–21 (median 5) weeks after the third DST. The immunosuppression used was identical for the DST recipients and the aza group and consisted of azathioprine (5 mg/kg/day for two days pretransplant, 3 mg/kg i.v. during operation, and thereafter 200 mg/day with individual adjustment) and prednisolone (100 mg i.v. during operation, 40 mg/day for 8 weeks and then gradually reduced). Acute rejection episodes diagnosed by clinical criteria were treated with i.v. methylprednisolone (2 g first day, 1 g/day for two days, then 0.5–1 g/day as indicated). Clinically suspected recurrence of original kidney disease was confirmed by histological examination of graft biopsies.

The CsA group received CsA 15 mg/kg/day orally starting two days pretransplant, reduced to 13 mg/kg/day at 2 weeks, 11 mg/kg/day at 1 month, 9 mg/kg/day at 2 months, and further reduced according to toxicity or plasma CsA levels. Prednisolone was started on the day of transplantation, 100 mg/day tapered to 20 mg/day on day 9 and further to 10 mg/day at 3 months. Toxicity and rejection episodes were diagnosed by fine-needle aspiration biopsy, rejection episodes were treated with i.v. methylprednisolone (0.5 g on the first day, 0.25 g for the next three days).

TABLE 1. Pretransplant clinical course of DST recipients

	DST only	DST-aza	Total
Patients entered	42	10	52
Donor not used	1[a]	1[b]	2
Protocol stopped:			
Incomplete protocol		1[c]	1
Aza complication		3[c]	3
Positive crossmatch:			
Persistent	9 (21%)	0	9
Transient	2	0	2
Grafted as planned	32	5	37

[a] Psychiatric reasons.
[b] Car accident.
[c] Grafted with DST—donor with CsA immunosuppression.

RESULTS

Pretransplant clinical course in DST groups. This is illustrated in Table 1. No sensitization to erythrocyte antigens was seen, and except for moderate fever and chills in one patient who developed HLA antibodies to his donor, no complications were seen in the DST-only group. In the DST-aza group, one patient receiving buffy coats (due to Rh-incompatibility) did not take his azathioprine, but was not immunized and was grafted with his DST donor with CsA immunosuppression. Three patients developed severe leukopenia and thrombocytopenia with fever due to azathioprine toxicity during DST. One of them had a zoster outbreak and another a *Pneumocystis carinii* pneumonia. After 2–3 transfusions their pretreatment was stopped, and as the crossmatch still was negative, grafting was performed with the DST donor, using CsA. Thus, only five of the ten DST-aza recipients completed the protocol.

Sensitization. Nine (21%) of the 42 DST-only recipients, developed persistent cytotoxic antibodies to donor T and B cells, while two additional patients had a transiently positive crossmatch (Table 1). The time of antibody appearance and its maximal titer versus donor cells are given in Table 2.

Fifteen of the 42 DST-only recipients had a history of pre-

TABLE 2. Appearance of donor-specific and panel-reactive antibodies in eleven DST recipients

	Patient No.										
	1	2	3	4	5	6	7	8	9	10[a]	11[a]
Positive crossmatch following DST (DST No.)	1	1	3	3	3	1	1	1	2	1	1
Strength[b]											
KN	1	1	3	0	4	1	0	0	0	0	0
NIH-T	4	2	4	0	ND[d]	4	3	1	1	3	3
NIH-B	4	3	4	2	ND	3	3	1	1	3	2
PRA[c]											
KN	50%	40%	80%	0	20%	60%	0	0	0	0	0
NIH-B	50%	40%	ND	20%	40%	ND	ND	0	0	0	0

[a] Crossmatch again negative following third DST.
[b] Strength given as: 0 = <10%, 1 = 10–20%, 2 = 20–40%, 3 = 40–70%, and 4>70% cytotoxicity above negative control; most reactive serum.
[c] Panel reactive antibodies; percentage of positive reactions (strength 1–4) to panel of approximately 20 donors.
[d] ND: Not tested.

vious transfusions or pregnancies, and six of these (40%) developed a positive crossmatch (Table 3) compared with only three (11%) of the nontransfused and never-pregnant group of 27 ($P = 0.04$, Fisher's exact test).

Panel reactive antibodies (PRA) were detected after DST in six patients. In three they reacted with more than 50% of panel cells (PRA>50%). All of these had also been presensitized by pregnancies or random transfusions.

In the DST-aza recipients no sensitization to donor or panel cells could be demonstrated.

Postoperative course. All grafted recipients had primary diuresis and there were no hyperacute rejections. Further details are given in Table 4.

In the DST-only group, nine (28%) had no acute rejection episode during the first year. Acute rejection episodes started unusually early (range days 1–7, median day 2), compared with the aza group ($P<0.01$, two-tailed Wilcoxon two-sample rank sum test). The majority of episodes were rather easily reversed, although six patients (19%) needed 1–27 (median 12) dialysis treatments. No grafts were lost due to acute rejection. Since only five patients were grafted according to the protocol in the DST-aza group, this group is hard to evaluate, but all rejection episodes were easily reversed (Table 4).

In the aza group, acute rejection episodes started on median day 5 (range 1–50), in 17 cases (40%) necessitating dialysis, and in ten, rejection led to graft loss within the first three months. Only six recipients (14%) had no rejection episodes during first year. In the CsA group, acute rejection episodes were fewer; in 28 cases (49%) no rejection episode occurred during the first year. They also occurred later than in the aza group (range day 1–60, median day 10, ($P<0.01$), necessitating dialysis in five and leading to graft loss in three cases.

Graft survival. The overall results are given in Table 5. In the DST-only group, one graft was lost at 10 months due to chronic rejection and one at 28 months due to recurrent glomerulonephritis, while one patient died at 4 months with a functioning graft. The remaining patients and grafts are doing well with an observation time ranging from 54 to 30 months.

In the DST-aza group, three of five grafts were lost within the first year, one to recurrent kidney disease at 2 months and two due to patient death with functioning graft.

In the aza-group, one year GS was significantly lower than in the DST-only group, 69% ($P<0.01$). The subgroup of 29 having received previous transfusions fared somewhat better than the 13 nontransfused: GS 72% versus 62% ($P = 0.36$). The CsA group had a one year GS comparable to that of the DST-alone group.

Patients who developed donor-reactive antibodies. Nine patients were immunized to their DST donors, one of these was immunized to his mother during DST but was successfully grafted from the father, using CsA. Eight patients received cadaveric kidneys after a waiting period of 2–42 months. Of these, five have a functioning graft.

Patients with a transiently positive crossmatch. Two patients developed a positive T cell crossmatch following the first DST (patients 10 and 11 in Table 2), but became negative following the third DST. They were then grafted as planned. One had a mild, easily reversed rejection episode starting on day 2, the other has never experienced rejection.

Another patient was initially also immunized to his DST donor (patient 2 in Table 2), and was instead transplanted twice with cadaveric grafts which he rejected. His HLA profile is A19,28;B12,40;DR1,4 and that of his living-related donor A9,19;B27,40;DR4,—. The two cadaveric donors were: (1) A2,28;B17,40,DR4,7 and (2) A19,28;B15;DR4,6. His serum was then retested against the original DST-donor and was now found negative according to the KN and NIH tests against donor T and B cells, but his serum contained PRA reacting with 60% of the panel. He was grafted with the DST donor using CsA and has never experienced an acute rejection episode, although a slow rise of serum creatinine starting at 12 months may represent a slow chronic rejection.

DISCUSSION

The DST-only program clearly improved the results of one-HLA-haplotype–mismatched living-related grafts, the one year graft survival of 94% being significantly higher than for the aza group (also after exclusion of nontransfused patients). On the other hand the DST-only program led to donor-specific antibody formation in nine cases, precluding grafting.

TABLE 3. Influence of presensitization on DST-induced sensitization

	DST only			DST-aza
	Total	Presensitized[a]	Not presensitized	
No. patients	42	15	27	10
Positive crossmatch	9 (21%)	6 (40%)	3 (11%)	0
Panel antibodies	7 (17%)	4 (27%)	2 (7%)	0

[a] Patients with previous pregnancies and/or random transfusions.

TABLE 4. Start of first acute rejection episode in DST-treated patients and controls who were not pretreated

	DST only	DST-aza	Aza-group	CsA group
Transplanted	32	5	42	57
No acute rejection episode	9 (28%)	2	6 (14%)	28 (49%)
Rejection start				
Days 1–2	17 (53%)	1	6 (14%)	2 (4%)
Days 3–4	4 (13%)	0	4 (10%)	3 (5%)
Days 5–6	1 (3%)	0	17 (40%)	2 (4%)
Days 7–8	1 (3%)	0	6 (14%)	5 (9%)
Days 9–90	0	2	3 (7%)	17 (30%)
Posttransplant dialysis	6 (19%)	0	17 (40%)	5 (9%)
Graft loss from rejection within 3 months	0	0	12 (29%)	3 (5%)

TABLE 5. Graft survival and causes of graft loss within first year

	DST only (32)	DST-aza (5)	Aza group (42)	CsA group (57)
Graft survival:				
3 months	100%	60%	79%	93%
6 months	97%	60%	74%	93%
12 months	94%	40%	69%	93%
Graft loss first year:				
Acute rejection	0	0	12	3
Chronic rejection	1	0	0	0
Recurrent disease	0	1	0	0
Death (functioning graft)	1	2	1	1

Immunological consequences of DST could be detected in antibody development (Table 2) and altered T cell reactivity to donor (*6*) as well as in accelerated rejection episodes (Table 4).

Antibodies developed infrequently and were weak and of narrow specificity in the DST patients not presensitized by previous transfusions or pregnancies, they were strong and broadly reacting only in those also receiving random transfusions, in accordance with other reports (*4, 9, 10*). This calls for a restrictive transfusion policy in candidates for DST—and, when needed, filtered leukocyte-free blood should be used (*11, 12*).

The changes in donor-specific cellular immune responsiveness following DST-only have previously been reported (*6*). MLC reactivity toward the donor was specifically reduced in 87% of those tested, and in-vivo-generated MLC-suppressing cells were found in 73% of them. A comparable MLC reduction, but without evidence of MLC-suppressing cells, was found in three DST-aza recipients (unpublished observations). However, the MLC changes were the same in those who developed cytotoxic antibodies to the donor as in those who did not.

The posttransplant course demonstrated either an unusually early start of acute rejection or a total absence of rejection (Table 4). Thus, transfusions may serve as antigenic priming, resulting in secondary responses upon grafting; these, however, appear more easily reversible by immunosuppressive agents (*13*). The reasons for this are still unknown. We could not detect differences in the changes in donor-specific MLC responses between those who had early rejection episodes and those with a smooth posttransplant course. The higher frequency of acute episodes among our DST recipients compared with the San Francisco experience (*4*) may be due to the lower prednisolone dose used in our center.

Transient sensitization was seen in two cases—both were successfully grafted after the crossmatch had turned negative. Cochrum et al. (3) and Schweizer and Bow (*14*) have reported three cases of positive crossmatch induced by random transfusions that became negative following DST, while Salvatierra et al. (*4*) reported 14 similar patients where further DST failed to result in such desensitization. Thus, grafting may successfully be performed in the presence of a noncurrent positive, current negative crossmatch in accordance with the results reported by Cardella et al. for cadaveric grafts (*15*). Furthermore, a DST protocol may be tried in spite of preexisting antibodies, particularly when they are not strong, and a DST protocol may be completed even if antibodies develop intercurrently. In accordance with this, crossmatch-positive patients should be repeatedly retested.

No graft was lost due to acute rejection, and since there is also little other evidence that weak antibodies not disclosed in a routine crossmatch test play a role in acute rejection (*16*), the use of more sensitive techniques seems superfluous.

The addition of azathioprine during DST seemed to prevent antibody formation, which is in agreement with other reports (*5, 10*). The bone marrow depression caused by the azathioprine dose used varied, but severe leukopenia with serious infections in three patients led to our termination of this protocol. The minimum azathioprine dose necessary to prevent sensitization needs to be defined to avoid unnecessary bone marrow toxicity.

The use of CsA immunosuppression without DST in this patient group abolished the waiting time and meant less effort for donors and dialysis units. As the patients initially randomized to CsA treatment performed well (*17*), all our recipients of HLA-haploidentical living-related donor grafts since August 1983 have received CsA and no prior DST treatment, at present with a one-year GS of 93%. Only a careful evaluation of relative risks, complications, long-term results and costs among the different treatment protocols will tell which procedure should eventually be preferred.

Acknowledgments. The secretarial assistance of Kristi Goyer and Anne Mourier is gratefully acknowledged.

REFERENCES

1. Flatmark A, Thorsby E. The use of living related donors in kidney transplantation. Transplant Proc 1982; 14: 61.
2. Solheim BG, Flatmark A, Halvorsen S, Jervell J, Pape J, Thorsby E. Effect of blood transfusion on renal transplantation: study of 191 consecutive first transplants from living related donors. Transplantation 1980; 30: 281.
3. Cochrum KC, Hanes D, Potter D, et al. Donor-specific blood transfusions in HLA-D-disparate one-haplotype-related allografts. Transplant Proc 1979; 11: 1903.
4. Salvatierra O Jr, Vincenti F, Amend W, et al. Four-year experience with donor-specific blood transfusions. Transplant Proc 1983; 15: 924.
5. Anderson CB, Sicard GA, Etheredge EE. Pretreatment of renal allograft recipients with azathioprine and donor-specific blood products. Surgery 1982; 92: 315.
6. Leivestad T, Thorsby E. Effects of HLA-haploidentical blood transfusions on donor-specific immune responsiveness. Transplantation 1984; 37: 175.
7. Kissmeyer-Nielsen F, Kjerbye KE. Lymphocytotoxic microtechnique: purification of lymphocytes by flotation. In: Curtoni ES, Mattiuz PL, Tosi RM, et al, eds. Histocompatibility testing. Copenhagen: Munksgaard, 1967: 381.
8. NIAID manual of tissue typing techniques 1976–77. Bethesda, MD: DHEW publication No 76-545, 1976.
9. Mendez R, Iwaki Y, Mendez R, Bogaard T, Self B, Terasaki PI. Donor-specific blood transfusions: their immunologic effect and allograft outcome. Transplant Proc 1983; 15: 946.
10. Glass NR, Miller DT, Sollinger HW, Belzer FO. Comparative analysis of the DST and imuran-plus-DST protocols for live donor renal transplantation. Transplantation 1983; 36: 636.
11. Sirchia G, Parravicini A, Rebulla P, Greppi N, Scalamogna M, Morelati F. Effectiveness of red blood cells filtered through cotton wool to prevent antileukocyte antibody production in multitransfused patients. Vox Sang 1982; 42: 190.
12. Leivestad T. Production of leukocyte-poor blood. Experience with disposable filters (transl). Tidsskr Nor Laegeforen 1984; 104: 2175.
13. Terasaki PI. The beneficial transfusion effect on kidney graft survival attributed to clonal deletion. Transplantation 1984; 37: 119.
14. Schweizer RT, Bow LM. Successful kidney transplantation after loss of specific anti-donor antibodies. Transplantation 1983; 36: 71.
15. Cardella CJ, Falk JA, Nicholson MJ, et al. Successful renal transplantation in patients with T-cell reactivity to donor. Lancet 1982; 2: 1240.
16. Thorsby E. On the antibody crossmatch controversies. Transplant Proc 1985; 17: 1533.
17. Albrechtsen D, Soedal G, Berg KJ, et al. Cyclosporine in living related and cadaveric renal transplantation. Transplant Proc 1984; 16: 1191.

Received 2 September 1985.
Accepted 22 October 1985.

0041-1337/86/4201-0039$02.00/0
TRANSPLANTATION
Vol. 42, No. 1

Printed in U.S.A.

IMMUNOGENETIC AND CLINICAL FACTORS AFFECTING RENAL TRANSPLANTATION

A RIGOROUS ANALYSIS OF DATA RECORDED BY THE UK TRANSPLANT SERVICE[1]

WALTER R. GILKS,[2] BENJAMIN A. BRADLEY,[3] SHEILA M. GORE,[2] AND NEVILLE H. SELWOOD[4] FOR THE USERS OF THE UK TRANSPLANT SERVICE

United Kingdom Transplant Service, Bristol; and MRC Biostatistics Unit, Cambridge, United Kingdom

A total of 3653 first cadaver kidney transplants in nondiabetic recipients over 15 years of age, performed in 30 transplant centers throughout the United Kingdom between 1978 and 1983, were analyzed to discover which of many recorded recipient, donor, surgical, and tissue-matching variables were important for graft survival, and in which postoperative period they exerted their maximum influence. A considerable effort was invested in checking the validity of the data and the appropriateness of the statistical methods.

The duration of dialysis prior to transplantation was associated with a substantially reduced risk of graft failure, particularly at later postoperative times. Good HLA-B locus matching was also found to enhance graft survival—but, by contrast, HLA-A locus matching showed no significant effect on survival. Recipient age over 45 years, high serum reactivity, and grafts with anoxia time (the interval between circulatory arrest and perfusion with ice) exceeding 10 min were found to be associated with poor graft survival. Trends in survival were identified across calendar years of transplant, such that early graft failure (0–15 days) had increased in recent years, whereas later graft failure (>15 days) had declined.

Between January 1978 and July 1983, 3961 first cadaver kidney transplants performed in 30 transplant centers throughout the United Kingdom and Ireland were notified and were followed-up by the U.K. Transplant Service (UKTS).* This extensive database, containing recipient and donor details, tissue matching, and details of surgical procedure, provided a valuable opportunity to study the effects of these factors on graft survival.

The analysis was exploratory and attempted to discover not only which of the factors examined were important for graft survival, but also in which postoperative period these factors exerted their maximum influence. In order to avoid biases in estimation and consequent misinterpretations, the analysis made provision for transplant center individuality, used a multifactorial statistical technique; and validated the data and methods.

[1] This work was supported by a grant from the National Kidney Research Fund.

[2] MRC Biostatistics Unit.

[3] Address correspondence to: B. A. Bradley, M.B., Ch.B., Ph.D., U.K. Transplant Service, South Western Regional Transfusion Service, Southmead Road, Bristol BS10 5ND, U.K.

[4] U.K. Transplant Service.

*Abbreviations used: EDTA, European Dialysis and Transplant Association; UKTS, U.K. Transplant Service.

MATERIALS AND METHODS

The method of analysis (stratified piece-wise proportional hazards regression) enables the effects of pretransplant factors on graft survival to be estimated multifactorially, and allows multi-center data to be used without obscuring center individuality. These features reduce the possibility of bias in the estimated factor effects on graft survival, as described in the companion article (*1*), to which the reader is advised to refer. The assumptions embedded in the method and procedures for validating them on the data are also described there (*1*), together with definitions of the terms *hazard, baseline, factor effect*, and *z score*.

Graft failure was defined to include rejection or technical failure, deaths with functioning grafts being treated as lost to followup at the time of death. This choice seemed appropriate, since the distinction between technical failures and those due to rejection was not always clear-cut, and deaths with functioning grafts could have occurred for reasons unconnected with transplantation.

The European Dialysis and Transplant Association (EDTA) database, made available to us by kind permission of Dr. A. J. Wing, was used to check and enhance the quality of the UKTS data. Table 1 lists each factor analyzed, together with the percentage of recipients for whom the factor was unrecorded, unavailable, or unusable. Regrettably, information on pretransplant transfusions, nephrectomy, and splenectomy could not be utilized owing to a number of problems associated with these data.

Several factors in Table 1 were not recorded or not usable for substantial numbers of patients. For each of these factors a special "not available" category was created, and an effect for this category was estimated just as for the usual categories.

HLA-A and B locus mismatches were defined on the basis of the parent specificities, not their sub-specificities. Parent specificities were HLA-A1, 2, 3, 9, 10, 11, 19, 28, 29, 36; HLA-B5, 7, 8, 12, 13, 14, 15, 16, 17, 18, 21, 22, 27, 35, 37, 40, 41, 42, 46, 47, 53.

Both 118 recipients under the age of 15 and 168 recipients with multisystem disease were omitted from the analysis, because it was considered that these recipients could exhibit substantially atypical patterns of graft failure. A further 22 recipients with failure/death dates that were identifiably invalid were also omitted.

RESULTS

A total of 3653 first cadaver transplants remained after exclusions—and, of these, 1480 failed or died. A detailed breakdown of the causes and postoperative periods of failure is given in Table 2.

Of the factors listed in Table 1, only those in Table 3 were found to have a statistically significant effect on graft survival. Three recipient factors, no donor factors, one matching factor, and three surgical procedure factors from Table 3 jointly appear to be of importance; the z scores show that the evidence is strongest for the duration of dialysis and HLA-B-locus mismatching. Table 3 also includes two factors that do not have significant effects: HLA-A locus mismatches and year of transplant; the reasons for including these will become apparent.

The estimated effects of the "not available" categories of the factors in Table 3 were generally fairly small and not significant, and have been omitted from Table 3, but are shown for completeness in Table 4.

The effects in Table 3 were estimated under the assumption that their influence on graft survival was constant across postoperative time. Table 5 tests this assumption by reestimating these factor effects within each of four postoperative intervals, and it appears that several effects change in magnitude across postoperative time reflecting the changing postoperative environment to which these recipients are exposed. Overall, these changes with time in factor effects are highly significant (chi-square on 45 degrees of freedom for changes across postoperative time = 79.0, $P - 0.001$) so that the assumption of constant relative hazards is doubtful.

TABLE 1. Factors analyzed for their effects on graft survival, with percentage of recipients for whom each factor was unrecorded or unusable

Recipient:	Donor:
Age (4%)	Age (3%)
Sex (1%)	Sex (1%)
Blood group (−)	Blood group (−)
Rhesus (−)	Rhesus (4%)
Reaction frequency (80%)[a]	Cause of death (−)
Duration of pre-TX dialysis (20%)	Systolic BP (14%)
Primary renal disease (20%)	Length of hypotension (24%)
	Urea (16%)
	Creatinine (63%)
	Urine output (19%)
	Infection (12%)
	Length of ventilation (9%)
Matching:	Surgical:
Age matching (4%)	Local kidney/retyped (−)
Sex matching (1%)	Year of transplant (−)
Blood group matching (−)	Time of day (64%)
Rhesus matching (4%)	Left/right kidney (−)
HLA-A locus (1%)	Number of veins on graft (17%)
HLA-B locus (1%)	Whether veins were tied (26%)
HLA-DR locus (73%)[b]	Arterial anastomosis (13%)
HLA-B4/B6 (1%)	Perfusion result (13%)
Crossmatch result (2%)	Anoxia time[c] (68%)[d]
	Warm time[e] (28%)[d]
	Cold time[f] (64%)[d]
	Operative time[g] (64%)[d]

[a] Zeros and "not knowns" are indistinguishable.
[b] Available only for the more recent transplants.
[c] Between stopping donor ventilation and donor circulatory arrest.
[d] Other information on this factor was available, but not used in the analysis to avoid biases.
[e] Between donor circulatory arrest and perfusion of donor kidney with ice.
[f] Length of time donor kidney was in ice.
[g] Between removing donor kidney from ice and perfusing it with blood.

TABLE 2. Failures by cause group and deaths by graft function for each of four postoperative intervals

Cause	Postoperative interval (days)				
	0–15	16–40	41–100	100+	Total
Rejection	143	161	168	232	704
Technical failure	117	79	57	101	354
Unknown cause of failure[a]	92	46	41	—	179
Death with failed graft (earlier graft failure not recorded)	5	6	5	19	35
Death with functioning graft	12	22	50	101	185
Death with unknown graft function[a]	2	3	18	—	23
Total	371	317	339	453	1480

[a] Patients with no available EDTA follow-up.

TABLE 3. Estimated effects of the most important factors of graft survival among those in Table 1.

Factor	Estimated effect	Approximate SE	z score
Recipient age (baseline: 15–29 years)[a]:			
30–44	1.00	.07	−0.1
45+	1.15	.08	1.9
Duration of pretransplant dialysis (baseline: no dialysis) per year of dialysis	0.93	.02	−4.5
Reaction frequency (baseline: 1%–39%):			
40%–69%	1.09	.22	0.4
70%–100%	1.69	.32	2.7
A locus mismatches (baseline: no mismatches) per mismatch	0.99	.04	−0.3
B locus mismatches (baseline: no mismatches) per mismatch	1.20	.05	4.2
Anoxia time (baseline: 1–10 min) more than 10 min	1.22	.10	2.3
Warm time (baseline: 1–10 min) more than 10 min	0.80	.07	−2.7
Arterial anastomosis (baseline: one artery, one patch):			
One artery, no patch	1.03	.09	0.4
>1 Artery, all on 1 patch	1.02	.08	0.3
>1 Anastomosis	1.40	.19	2.4
Year of transplant (baseline: 1978) per year since 1978	1.00	.02	0.0

[a] The baseline for each factor has an effect of 1.00.

Recipient Factors

Recipient age. Recipients over 45 years of age have a slightly increased risk of graft failure: the estimated effect of 1.15 in Table 3 suggesting that, overall, the hazard for this age group is 15% higher than for recipients aged 15–29 years. Table 5 shows that the age effect is largest in the interval 41–100 days posttransplant.

Tables 3 and 5 understate the seriousness of the effect of age, since the risk of death without prior graft failure for older recipients is over three times that for recipients under 45 years of age. If *failure* is defined to include death with functioning graft then the estimated age effects are as in Table 6, from which it may be seen that, overall, the hazard for recipients over 45 is nearly 40% higher than for those aged between 15 and 29 years old.

TABLE 4. Estimated effects for the "not available" levels of factors.

Factor	Estimated effect	Approximate SE	z score
Recipient age (baseline: 15–29 years):			
Unknown	0.84	.16	−0.9
Duration of pretransplant dialysis (baseline: no dialysis):			
Unknown	1.02	.12	0.1
Reaction frequency (baseline: 1% to 39%):			
0% or unknown	1.13	.11	1.3
Anoxia time (baseline: 1–10 min):			
Unknown	0.99	.08	−0.1
Warm time (baseline: 1–10 min):			
Unknown	0.98	.08	−0.2
Arterial anastomosis (baseline: one artery, one patch):			
Unknown	1.09	.10	0.9

Duration of pretransplant dialysis. The effect on graft survival of the duration of pretransplant dialysis is highly statistically significant. The estimated effect of 0.93 in Table 3 indicates that recipients with one year of pretransplant dialysis have a hazard of failure that is 93% of that for recipients with no pretransplant dialysis, and recipients with 5 years of dialysis have a hazard that is $.93 \times .93 \times .93 \times .93 \times .93 = 0.7 = 70\%$ of that for recipients with no pretransplant dialysis. The implicit assumption here is that each additional year of pretransplant dialysis produces a further proportionate reduction in risk.

This assumption has been checked by creating several categories of duration of pretransplant dialysis (Table 7) and estimating an effect on graft survival within each. The results demonstrate a more or less steady decline in risk with duration of pretransplant dialysis, thus supporting the assumption (Table 7).

Table 5 shows that the dialysis effect is strongest in the period beyond 100 days posttransplant, and indicates that, in this period, recipients with 5 years of pretransplant dialysis have a hazard only 45% of that corresponding to no pretransplant dialysis.

Table 8 shows the results of including in the analysis a separate "duration of pretransplant dialysis" factor for each calendar year of transplantation. Although the dialysis effect for 1982 appears to be substantially weaker than for the preceding three years, there is, overall, no strong evidence for a calendar-time trend in the effects of pretransplant dialysis. Moreover, many of the 1982 transplantees had not been followed-up long enough for the predominantly late-acting dialysis effect to be observed in this cohort. Dialysis information was not available for transplants performed in 1983.

Table 8 also shows that the effect on graft survival of the

TABLE 5. Estimated effect on graft survival (with approximate SE), within each of four postoperative intervals, for the factors in Table 3

Factor	Estimated effect (with approximate SE)			
	0–15 Days	16–40 Days	41–100 Days	100+ Days
Recipient age (baseline: 15–29 years):				
30–44	1.00 (.14)	0.86 (.14)	1.33 (.22)	0.90 (.12)
45+	1.12 (.15)	1.16 (.17)	1.45 (.24)	1.00 (.14)
Duration of pretransplant dialysis (baseline: no dialysis) per year of dialysis[a]	1.00 (.03)	0.91 (.03)	0.95 (.03)	0.85 (.03)
Reaction frequency (baseline: 1% to 39%)				
40%–69%	1.19 (.36)	0.93 (.51)	0.71 (.34)	1.36 (.53)
70%–100%	1.24 (.39)	3.80 (1.5)	1.93 (.73)	0.73 (.45)
A locus mismatches (baseline: no mismatches) per mismatch	1.03 (.08)	1.00 (.09)	0.95 (.09)	0.96 (.08)
B locus mismatches (baseline: no mismatches) per mismatch	1.15 (.09)	1.31 (.12)	1.15 (.11)	1.22 (.10)
Anoxia time (baseline: 1–10 min) more than 10 min	1.08 (.18)	1.19 (.21)	1.29 (.23)	1.34 (.22)
Warm time (baseline: 1–10 min) more than 10 min	0.64 (.10)	0.81 (.15)	0.84 (.14)	0.90 (.14)
Arterial anastomosis (baseline: one artery, one patch):				
1 Artery, no patch	1.10 (.17)	1.02 (.18)	1.17 (.20)	0.86 (.14)
>1 Artery, all on one patch	1.14 (.15)	0.82 (.14)	1.16 (.19)	0.97 (.15)
>1 Anastomosis	1.32 (.36)	0.78 (.29)	1.61 (.43)	1.99 (.50)
Year of transplant (baseline: 1978) per year since 1978[a]	1.10 (.04)	0.97 (.04)	0.93 (.04)	1.00 (.05)

[a] Linear trend in estimated effects across postoperative intervals significant at 1% level.

TABLE 6. Estimated effects (with approximate SE) of recipient age—overall and within each of four postoperative intervals—where *failures* comprise all graft failures and all deaths

Factor	Estimated effect (with approximate SE)				
	Over all	0–15 Days	16–40 Days	41–100 Days	100+ Days
Recipient age (baseline: 15–29)					
30–44	1.02 (.07)	1.04 (.14)	0.89 (.14)	1.32 (.21)	0.93 (.12)
45+	1.36 (.09)	1.17 (.16)	1.26 (.18)	1.87 (.29)	1.34 (.16)

TABLE 7. Estimated effects on graft survival for each of several categories of duration of pretransplant dialysis (*no dialysis* is the baseline for comparison)

Duration of pretransplant dialysis	Number of recipients	Estimated effect	Approximate SE	z score
No dialysis	140	Baseline	—	—
1 Day–6 months	590	.83	.12	−1.3
6 Months–1 year	602	.79	.12	−1.6
1 Year–2 years	519	.68	.11	−2.6
2 Years–4 years	560	.72	.11	−2.2
Over 4 years	500	.54	.09	−3.9
Not available	742	1.02	.12	0.1

TABLE 8. Effects per year of dialysis on graft survival estimated for each calendar year of transplant and each HLA mismatch group.

Recipient group	Estimated "duration of dialysis" effect	Approximate SE	z score
Year of transplant:			
1978	.96	.03	−1.4
1979	.89	.04	−3.3
1980	.91	.03	−2.8
1981	.91	.03	−2.2
1982	.98	.03	−0.6
1983	No dialysis information		
HLA-B locus mismatches:			
0	.94	.03	−2.3
1	.93	.02	−3.2
2	.94	.03	−2.1

duration of pretransplant dialysis does not depend on the number of HLA-B locus mismatches between donor and recipient.

Reaction frequency. The risk of graft failure is substantially higher for recipients with a high antibody reaction frequency (i.e., recipients whose sera react positively with more than 70% of panel cells) than for recipients with a lower reaction frequency. Table 3 indicates that intermediate reaction frequency (40%–69% reactivity) does not produce significantly higher risks than low reaction frequency. The effect of reaction fruqency is strongest during the postoperative interval 16–40 days (Table 5), within which the risk of failure is nearly quadrupled for the recipients with high reactivity.

Matching factors: HLA-locus mismatches

The evidence supporting an HLA-B locus matching effect on graft survival is clear and strong in these data; by contrast, HLA-A locus matching appears not to add significantly to the explanation of graft survival. The benefits of HLA-DR locus matching could be as large as those for the B locus, but there is insufficient DR matching information in these data to establish this.

Implicit in the "per B locus mismatch" effect in Table 3 is the assumption that each additional B locus mismatch produces a further proportionate increase in the risk of graft failure. Table 9, in which a separate effect has been estimated for 1 and 2 B locus mismatches, shows this assumption to be fully justified. Thus it is estimated that the risk of failure for two B locus mismatches is 44% higher than for no B locus mismatches. This figure becomes 63% when only immunological failures are considered as failures (other failures and deaths being treated as lost-to-follow-up at the time of failure or death).

B locus mismatching effects appear to be constant over postoperative time (Table 5), and Table 10 shows that they are constant over calendar years of transplant as well as over several other subgroups: blood group "O" recipients appear to have a smaller B-mismatching effect than other patients, but the difference is not statistically significant; recipients with high or medium antibody reaction frequency have the same B-mismatching effect as those with low reaction frequency. (There were too few recipients with high reaction frequency to estimate a separate B-mismatching effect for these patients. There is also no trend in B-mismatching effects across centers grouped by their overall success rates or by their attainments in B locus matching (as measured for each center by the average number of B matches achieved).

Operation Factors

Anoxia time. Anoxia time (i.e., the time between stopping donor ventilation and donor circulatory arrest) exceeded 10 min in about one-third of all recipients for whom it was recorded. An anoxia time in excess of 10 min appears to have a detrimental effect on graft survival, and there is some suggestion in Table 5 that this effect is more pronounced in the later postoperative periods.

Warm ischemia time. Warm ischemia time (i.e., the time between donor circulatory arrest and perfusing the donor kidney with cooled solution) exceeds 10 min in the 72% of recipients for whom the information was recorded. A warm time in excess of 10 min apparently enhances graft survival, and the effect is mostly in the early postoperative period, reducing the hazard by about one-third in the first 15 days after transplantation.

The effect of warm time was estimated both for recipients with and for recipients without a recorded anoxia time, in order to investigate the possibility of a recording bias. The estimated warm time effects for these two groups (0.76 and 0.85) are not significantly different.

Arterial anastomosis. The estimated effects of this factor show that donor kidneys with an arterial patch are no more or less likely to succeed than those without a patch, provided that there is only one artery on the graft. Multiple arteries on the graft do not produce a disadvantage provided that they are all on a single patch. However, the 4% of donor kidneys that require more than one arterial anastomosis have significantly worse survival. (In an unknown number of grafts patches were removed before anastomosis: this suggests that our estimated effects for this factor are underestimated.)

Year of transplant. These data show no overall upward trend in graft survival between 1978 and 1983 (Table 3), although there has been a reduction in the proportion of transplants resulting in death with a functioning graft. However, in successive calendar years, graft survival rates have become significantly worse in the first two postoperative weeks, and significantly better in the interval 40–100 days posttransplant (Table 5). Table 11 shows these trends in more detail.

TABLE 11. Estimated effects on graft survival for each year of transplant (with 1978 as baseline for comparison) within each of several postoperative intervals

Year of transplant	Estimated effect (with approximate SE) in each postoperative interval				
	Overall	0–15 days	16–40 days	41–100 days	Over 100 days
1978	Baseline	Baseline	Baseline	Baseline	Baseline
1979	1.02 (.09)	1.20 (.23)	1.01 (.20)	0.94 (.18)	0.98 (.15)
1980	0.98 (.09)	1.05 (.19)	1.00 (.19)	0.84 (.16)	1.08 (.18)
1981	0.96 (.10)	1.13 (.22)	1.28 (.25)	0.66 (.15)	0.87 (.18)
1982	1.01 (.10)	1.46 (.27)	0.79 (.16)	0.79 (.16)	1.09 (.30)
1983	0.90 (.11)	1.67 (.36)	0.66 (.18)	0.64 (.18)	no data

DISCUSSION

Duration of pretransplant dialysis. The relationship between duration of pretransplant dialysis and reduced risk of graft failure extends similar observations made by others (*2–7*), although some have failed to find this relationship (*8–10*). It suggests that a minimum period of chronic hemodialysis might be beneficial prior to transplantation, but before such a radical deduction can be made alternative explanations of the phenomenon must be scrutinized. These include:

1. A surrogate effect for the quantity of blood transfusions received before transplantation. The longer the duration of pretransplant dialysis, the more units transfused (*2*). This explanation cannot be excluded, but the dialysis effect was apparent before blood transfusion gained wide acceptance as a conditioning regimen (*3*, *4*). Also, it has been argued that blood transfusions exert their maximum benefit during the early postoperative period (*11*); however, the dialysis duration effect exerts its maximum effect after the first 3 months.
2. Selection through sensitization and the crossmatch test. It is generally held that patients who are highly sensitized to HLA antigens wait longer before receiving a crossmatch-negative transplant. Thus patients with long dialysis duration may tend to be those receiving more compatible grafts. Since HLA matching and high sensitization were both taken into account by the multifactorial method when estimating the dialysis effect, this explanation can be discounted. Furthermore, patients with high serum reactivity had an increased risk of graft failure (Table 3).
3. An ill-defined selection mechanism. Knapp has suggested that long-surviving dialysis patients are robust individuals who were better able to withstand the rigors of transplantation (*12*). This explanation might be expected to be more relevant to patient survival, which was not tested here, than graft survival. In support of this, the data of Sanfilippo et al. indicate a positive association between death from infection and duration of dialysis (*13*).
4. Acquired immunological deficiency associated with chronic renal failure and hemodialysis that produces a long standing graft-protecting effect. Since 1956 patients suffering from chronic renal failure were seen to be immunodepressed, and subsequent experiments demonstrated that skin allografts to these patients were prolonged (*14*). These observations were confirmed in rats (*15*) and extended in patients by demonstrating reduced hypersensitivity skin test results (*16–21*). The phenomenon is reflected in vitro by depressed T cell responses to alloantigens (*22–26*)—and, although this is probably attributable to an intrinsic defect in the responsiveness of the blood T cell population, the plasma also carries suppressive factors (*24–28*). Some of these are dialyzable whereas others are retained by the membrane (*27–29*), and it has been suggested that because the plasma-depressive factors are not present in patients treated by peritoneal dialysis (*30*) plasticizers derived from the membrane

TABLE 9. Estimated effects on graft survival of B locus mismatches

Number of B locus mismatches	Estimated effect	Approximate SE	z score
1 Compared with 0	1.22	.09	3.0
2 Compared with 1	1.16	.09	2.2

TABLE 10. Effects per HLA-B locus mismatch on graft survival estimated for each calendar year of transplant, each recipient blood group, two recipient reaction frequency groups, groups of centers according to their success rate at 100 days, and groups of centers according to their rate of HLA-B locus matching

Recipient group	Estimated "per B locus mismatch" effect	Approximate SE	z score
Year of transplant:			
1978	1.22	.11	2.2
1979	1.17	.11	1.7
1980	1.22	.11	2.2
1981	1.17	.12	1.6
1982	1.27	.12	2.3
1983	1.00	.16	0.0
Recipient blood group:			
0	1.12	.06	1.9
A	1.17	.06	2.7
B	1.19	.13	1.7
AB	1.28	.18	1.8
Reaction frequency:			
0%–39%	1.21	.06	4.1
40%–100%	1.12	.19	0.7
Center success rate at 100 days:			
Highest 7 centers	1.34	.16	2.4
Next 8 centers	1.04	.09	0.5
Next 8 centers	1.21	.09	2.8
Lowest 7 centers	1.27	.12	2.5
Center rate of B matching:			
Highest 9 centers	1.15	.11	1.5
Next 14 centers	1.31	.08	4.2
Lowest 7 centers	1.06	.07	0.7

itself are responsible (*29*). The graft protective effect of chronic hemodialysis could therefore be attributable to a gradually decreasing immunocompetence that, although reversed after transplantation, allows specific graft protection to develop.

HLA mismatches. The HLA-B matching effect is exerted in all postoperative periods studied (Table 5), and it has been consistent throughout the years (Table 10). Moreover, it is evident in centers that have achieved a high proportion of HLA-B matches, as well as those with only a low rate of B matching (Table 10).

The observation that the number of HLA-A mismatches fails to correlate with graft failure, whereas HLA-B mismatches show a strong association is paradoxical. All class I structures share a common molecular make-up, thus there is no a priori reason to suppose that mismatches for one would be more or less potent than mismatches for the other. Nevertheless, several authors support the relative immunodominance of HLA-B over HLA-A (*31–33*). There are several alternative explanations of the HLA-A/B paradox:

1. That neither HLA-A nor B is immunodominant in rejection but that structures coded centromeric to HLA-B, and in strong linkage disequilibrium with it, are. These would include HLA-DR, DQ and DP products. Because of the recent introduction of HLA-DR matching and short duration of follow-up no data can be presented now.
2. A differential regulation of the expression of HLA locus products on renal vascular endothelium, such as to render HLA-B immunodominant over HLA-A. Although a number of studies confirm the expression of the "backbone" structure of HLA class I products on renal vascular endothelium (*34, 35*) there are no studies that compare the expression of HLA-A with HLA-B.

Reaction frequency. A total of 2.5% of recipients were known to carry "broad-spectrum" antibodies prior to transplantation that reacted against more than 70% of the population, and the possible contribution of pregnancy and blood transfusion demand further investigation. The risk of graft failure during the early postoperative period (0–15 days) in these highly sensitized recipients was little different from that in recipients with lower frequency antibodies. However, their risk of graft failure during the subsequent period (16–40 days) was quadrupled (ratio of hazards 3.80). Several possible explanations exist:

1. Technical difficulties with the crossmatch test might have led to false negative results. This would have been evidenced by an elevated risk of graft failure during the immediate postoperative period (0–15 days) rather than later.
2. Enhanced cellular immunity, the specificity of which is not accurately reflected in the lymphocytotoxic test, might coexist with humoral immunity. This concept is supported by a previous study in which a combined antigen (HLA-A2; male), which was recognized exclusively by cytotoxic T cells, was associated with poorer graft survival in sensitized but not in nonsensitized recipients (*36*).
3. Antibodies to kidney endothelium might coexist with lymphocytoxic antibodies, and their specificity would not necessarily be reflected in the cross match test. Although a dichotomy exists between lymphocytotoxic antibodies and those reacting with kidney endothelium (*35, 37, 38*), the incidence in the population of exclusive antirenal antibodies has not been investigated. One antibody that might be considered to exemplify this is the "monocyte-endothelial" antibody (*38*). Thus broad-spectrum patients might carry antibodies to donor endothelium that go undetected in the crossmatch test.

Ischemia and anoxia times. The definition of warm ischemia time by the UKTS has always attempted to distinguish between "anoxia time" and "warm ischemia" time. Furthermore, warm ischemia has never included the "warm up" time, recorded as "operative time." In this respect this study differs from others—for example, that by van Es et al. (*39*). The detrimental effect of anoxia and the protective effect of warm ischemia were therefore novel observations (*40*). In view of the incompleteness of recording of warm ischemic time—and especially anoxia time—these results must be viewed with some scepticism. If valid, the protective effect of warm ischemia might have been analogous to the phenomenon that the kidneys of hibernating squirrels can sustain longer periods of cold ischemia than the kidneys of nonhibernating squirrels (*41*), or the observation that seals' kidneys can withstand prolonged ischemia during dives (*42*).

Arterial anastomosis. Numerous techniques have been devised to resolve the problem of multiple renal arteries (*43, 44*). The present results indicate that multiple renal arteries on a single patch do not represent a disadvantage, but that multiple anastomoses do.

Year of transplant. During the period of study there was an overall trend toward improved graft survival, and a fall in patient mortality, but graft survival rates in the immediate postoperative period appear to have deteriorated. This might reflect a growing tendency for early abandonment of troublesome grafts, thereby avoiding the side effects of increased immunosuppressives, but it could also reflect a trend toward less aggressive and lower-dosage immunosuppressive regimens.

Conclusions. This analysis exemplifies how appropriate statistical methodology can be employed to extract more information from a renal transplant database than can be achieved by classic methods.

In particular, the analysis demonstrated the beneficial effects of dialysis duration and possibly warm ischemia, and showed clearly the benefits of HLA-B as opposed to HLA-A locus matching. Detrimental effects of recipient age, multiple arterial anastomoses, and a long duration of donor anoxia were also observed.

Acknowledgments. We gratefully acknowledge Professor Adrian F. M. Smith, Department of Mathematics, University of Nottingham, England for his contribution in setting up the project. Dr. Wing and his colleagues at EDTA are gratefully acknowledged in the text.

REFERENCES

1. Gilks WR, Gore SM, Bradley BA. Analyzing transplant survival data. Transplantation 1986; 42: 46.
2. Mebel M, Steger W, Richter K, et al. Long-term haemodialysis: an enhancing factor for cadaveric graft survival. Proc EDTA 1976; 14: 285.
3. Jacobs C, Brunner FP, Chantler C, et al. Combined report on regular dialysis and transplantation in Europe, VII, 1976. Proc EDTA 1977; 14: 3.
4. Wing AJ, Brunner FP, Brynger H, et al. Combined report on regular dialysis and transplantation in Europe, VIII, 1977. Proc EDTA 1978; 15: 3.
5. Brunner FP, Brynger H, Chantler C, et al. Combined report on regular dialysis and transplantation in Europe, IX, 1978. Proc EDTA 1979; 16: 2.

6. Brynger H, Brunner FP, Chantler C, et al. Combined report on regular dialysis and transplantation of children in Europe, 1979. Proc EDTA 1980; 17: 2.
7. Broyer M, Brunner FP, Brynger H, et al. Combined report on regular dialysis and transplantation in Europe, XII, 1981. Proc EDTA 1982; 19: 2.
8. Taylor R, Ting A, Briggs J. Renal transplantation in the United Kingdom and Ireland: the centre effect. Lancet 1985; 1: 798.
9. Fehrman I. Pretransplant blood transfusions and related kidney allograft survival. Transplantation 1982; 34: 46.
10. Rao KV, Anderson RC, O'Brien TJ. Factors contributing for improved graft survival in recipients of kidney transplants. Kidney Int 1983; 24: 210.
11. Terasaki PI, Perdue S, Ayoub G, Iwaki Y, Park MS, Mickey MR. Reduction of accelerated failures by transfusion. Transplant Proc 1982; 14: 251.
12. Knapp MS. Evaluating the treatment of renal failure by dialysis and transplantation. Lancet 1977; 2: 1068.
13. Sanfilippo F, Vaughn WK, Spees EK, et al. Influence of changes in pre-transplant sensitisation on patient and graft survival in cadaver renal transplantation. Transplantation 1984; 38: 124.
14. Dammin GJ, Couch NP, Murray JG. Prolonged skin homografts in uraemic patients. Ann NY Acad Sci 1956; 64: 967.
15. Morrison AB, Naness K, James R. Skin homograft survival in chronic renal insufficiency. Arch Pathol 1963; 75: 139.
16. Rolley RJ, Stenoff S, Williams GM, et al. Assessment of immunocompetency by DNCB sensitization prior to human renal allotransplantation. Surg Forum 1974; 25: 268.
17. Rolley RT, Sterioff S, Parks LC, et al. Delayed cutaneous hypersensitivity and human renal transplantation. Transplant Proc 1977; 9: 81.
18. Diamondopoulas AA, Briggs JD, Hamilton DNH. Cell-mediated immunity and sex. Lancet 1978; 1: 101.
19. Harris KR, O'Durny A, Walmsley B, et al. Dinitrochlorobenzene (DNCB) skin testing. No correlation with outcome of renal transplantation. Transplantation 1983, 15: 1154.
20. Rouxniantyeff M, Anderson CJ, Jacquet P, Kniker WJ. New in vitro methods to assay delayed cutaneous hypersensitivity. Transplant Clin Immunol 1979; 10: 297.
21. Kirkpatrick CA, Wilson WEC, Talmage DW. Immunologic studies in human organ transplantation. I. Observation and characterization of suppressed cutaneous reactivity in uremia. J Exp Med 1964; 119: 727.
22. Tourraine JL, Tourraine F, Revilland JP, et al. T-lymphocytes and serum inhibitors of cell-mediated immunity in renal insufficiency. Nephron 1975; 14: 195.
23. Elves MW, Israels MCG, Collinge M. An assessment of the MLR in renal failure. Lancet 1966; 1: 682.
24. Kasakura S, Lowenstein L. The effect of uremic blood on MLR and on cultures of leukocytes with PHA. Transplantation 1967; 5: 283.
25. Nelson DS, Penrose JM. Effect of hemodialysis and transplantation on inhibition of lymphocyte transformation by sera from uremic patients. Clin Immunol 1975; 4: 143.
26. Holdsworth SR, Fitzgerald MG, Hasking CS, Atkins RC. The effect of maintenance dialysis on lymphocyte function. I. Haemodialysis. Clin Exp Immunol 1978; 33: 95.
27. Abinko J, Omodera J, Sekino H. A peptide isolated from the haemodialysite of a uremic patient with immunodeficiency inhibits lymphocyte stimulation. J Appl Biochem 1981; 3: 562.
28. Kamata K, Okubo M, Sada M. Immunosuppressive factors in uraemic sera and composed of both dialysable and nondialysable components. Clin Exp Immunol 1983; 54: 277.
29. Gibson JP, Briggs WA, Boone BJ. Delivery of di-z-ethyexylphthulate to patients during haemodialysis. EJ Lab Clin Med 1976; 87: 519.
30. Atkins RC, Holdsworth R, Fitzgerald MG, Hoking CS. The effect of maintenance dialysis on lymphocyte function II. Peritoneal dialysis. Clin Exp Immunol 1978; 33: 102.
31. Oliver RT, Sachs JA, Festenstein H, Pegrum GD, Moorhead JF. Influence of HL-A matching, antigen strength, and immune responsiveness on outcome of 349 cadaver renal grafts. Lancet 1972; 2: 1381.
32. Dewar PJ, Wilkinson R, Elliott RW, et al. Superiority of B locus matching over other HLA matching in renal graft survival. Br Med J 1982; 284: 779.
33. Bashir HV, D'Apice A. Cadaver renal transplantation and HLA matching in Australia from 1971 to 1980. Transplantation 1982; 34: 183.
34. Baldwin WM III, Claas FHJ, van Es LA, van Rood JJ. Distribution of Endothelial-Monocyte and HLA antigens on renal vascular endothelium. Transplant Proc 1981; 13: 103.
35. Evans PR, Tricket LP, Smith JL, et al. The role of renal endothelial antigens and donor-specific antibodies in allograft rejection. Transplant Proc 1984; 16: 1181.
36. Galumy E, Bradley BA, Lansbergen Q, et al. The importance of H-Y incompatibility in human organ transplantation. Transplantation 1978; 25: 315.
37. Trickett LP, Evans PR, Spencer C, et al. Detection of donor-specific antibodies binding to endothelium in renal allografts using an indirect immunoperoxidase technique. Transplant Proc 1982; 14: 191.
38. Paul LC, van Es LA, Fleuren G. Demonstration of transplantation antigens on the endothelium of peritubular capillaries in renal allografts by the immunoperoxidase method. Transplantation 1979; 28: 72.
39. van Es A, Hermans J, van Bockel JH, et al. Effect of warm ischaemic time and HLA (A and B) matching on renal cadaveric graft survival and rejection episodes. Transplantation 1983; 36: 255.
40. Marshall VC. Renal preservation. In: Morris PJ, ed. Kidney transplantation: principles and practice. 2nd ed. New York: Grune and Stratton, 1984: 129.
41. Green CJ, Fuller BJ, Ross B, et al. Hibernatory animals as a model for hypothermic organ preservation. Proc Soc Cryobiol 1983; 20: 739.
42. Halasz NA, Elsner R, Garvie RS, Gratke GJ. Renal recovery from ischaemia: a comparative study of harbor seal and dog kidneys. Am J Physiol 1974; 227: 1331.
43. Merkel FK, Straus AK, Anderson O, et al. Microvascular techniques for polar artery reconstitution in kidney transplants. Surgery 1976; 79: 253.
44. Lee HM. Surgical techniques of renal transplantation. In: Morris PJ, ed. Kidney transplantation: principles and practice. 2nd ed. New York: Grune and Stratton, 1984: 129.

Received 25 January 1985.
Accepted 3 October 1985.

0041-1337/86/4201-0046$02.00/0
TRANSPLANTATION
Vol. 42, No. 1

ANALYZING TRANSPLANT SURVIVAL DATA[1]

WALTER R. GILKS,[2] SHEILA M. GORE,[2] AND BENJAMIN A. BRADLEY[3] For the Users of The United Kingdom Transplant Service

United Kingdom Transplant Service, Bristol; and MRC Biostatistics Unit, Cambridge, United Kingdom

Stratified proportional hazards regression is described as a method of estimating multifactorially preoperative factor effects on graft survival—and, at the same time, making due allowances for unknown transplant-center-specific influences. The multifactorial aspect of the method overcomes the biases inherent in analyzing transplant survival data one factor at a time, and stratification allows the data from many centers to be used simultaneously without the dangers associated with simple pooling of data from many sources. The proportionality and regression assumptions implicit in the method enable the data to be used efficiently, but must be validated on the data. Methods by which these assumptions may be relaxed are described—in particular, the stratified piece-wise proportional hazards regression method.

Many factors undoubtedly influence transplant survival rates; some of them are well documented and well recorded, such as HLA-B locus matching (*1*); some are suspected but difficult to measure, such as "clinical management" within a transplant center (*2*); others are unsuspected and unmeasured, and cannot be controlled except by randomization in prospective studies. Many analyses of effects on transplant survival have been published, yet most of these are single-center studies with few transplants, analyzing one factor at a time (i.e., unifactorially). This paper emphasizes the need for a multicenter, multifactorial (several factors simultaneously) approach and outlines an appropriate statistical methodology, known as "stratified (piece-wise) proportional hazards regression" (*3–5*). This method is a well-tried, widely applicable, and powerful development of two related methods of survival analysis: actuarial survival and the log-rank test (*6*). The method is applied to kidney graft survival in the U.K. and Ireland in the companion article (*1*).

Single-center studies have the advantage of not being complicated by substantial differences in clinical and other practices among centers. However, such studies rarely accumulate sufficient transplants to estimate reliably effects on graft survival. For example, even in a center with 400 transplants, there would be only a 50% chance of detecting an HLA-B locus matching effect of the size reported in the companion article (*1*) statistically significant at the 5% level. Multi-center studies overcome this lack of reliability. However, centers differ substantially in clinical practices and organization (*2*) and in their graft survival rates (*7*); analyses that fail to make provision for center individuality can promote serious misinterpretations. For example, if centers that attain a high average level of HLA-B locus matching also happen to be those with good survival due to a variety of undocumented clinical practices, then the apparent benefits of HLA-B locus matching will be exaggerated unless center individuality is properly accounted for in the analytical method.

The large number of transplants in a multi-center study enhances the usefulness of multifactorial analysis, which takes account of correlations between factors when estimating effects on graft survival (*8*). Unifactorial analyses cannot allow for these correlations and as a result may fail to identify some factors that affect graft survival while falsely identifying others. For example, in a univariate analysis, a long duration of pretransplant dialysis may have an apparent beneficial effect on kidney graft survival. However, this may be due entirely to the correlation between the duration of pretransplant dialysis and the number of pretransplant transfusions. A multifactorial analysis including both factors simultaneously would help to distinguish the benefits of each factor. It should be noted that a multifactorial approach is not advocated here purely to derive an elaborate predictor of graft survival for every configuration of patient/graft characteristics (although this can be produced as a by-product).

The stratified proportional hazards regression method enables factor effects on transplant survival to be estimated multifactorially, and at the same time makes provision for unrecorded aspects of center individuality. The strength of the method is that it embodies assumptions about factor effects in order to make efficient use of the data. However, unless these assumptions are validated they may represent weaknesses rather than strengths. Therefore, in the section on the statistical method, both the assumptions and methods of relaxing them are described.

The method described below applies only to preoperative and perioperative factors (such as tissue matching and number of pretransplant transfusions), although extensions of the method can accommodate postoperative factors, such as the number and timing of rejection episodes.

The Statistical Method

The stratified proportional hazards regression method, like many statistical methods, comprises two parts. First, a set of assumptions that specify a statistical model in terms of unknown coefficients (or parameters), and second, a method of estimating those coefficients using the data. In this section the model assumptions are described.[4] The method of estimation is too technical to present here, but may be found elsewhere (*3–5*). The method is included in the BMDP computer package (*9*).

Before describing the assumptions, three terms: *hazard*, *base-*

[1] This work was supported by a grant from the National Kidney Research Fund.

[2] MRC Biostatistics Unit.

[3] Address correspondence to: B. A. Bradley M.B., Ph.D., U.K. Transplant Service, South Western Regional Transfusion Service, Southmead Road, Bristol BS10 5ND, U.K.

[4] If s_t represents the actuarial survival rate at the beginning of day t (*6*) and f_t is the number of patients whose grafts failed on day *t*, then the estimated hazard of graft failure on day t is $h_t = f_t/s_t$. In principle the hazard rate can be computed for each of a number of patient

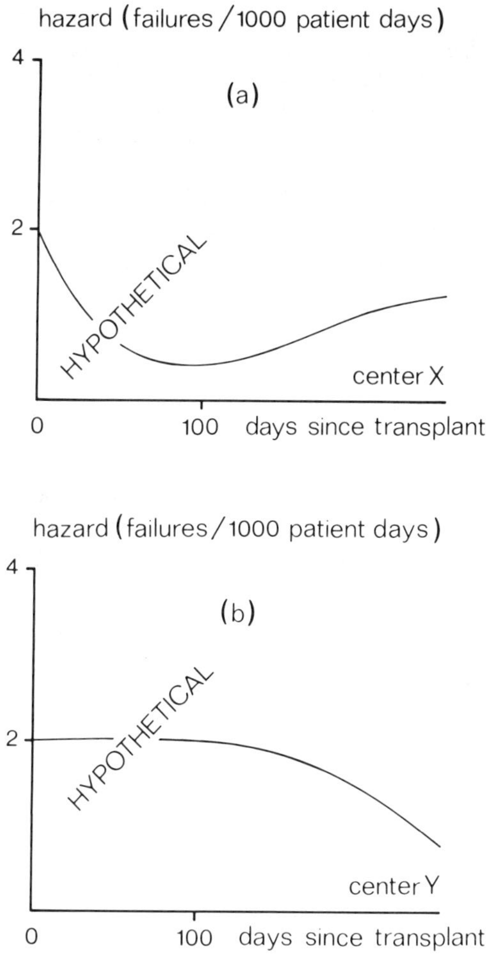

FIGURE 1. Hypothetical hazard curves (a) for center X, (b) for center Y.

line, and *effect* are introduced. Some hypothetical hazard patterns, illustrated in Figures 1–4, are used to explain the method clearly.

Hazard. The stratified proportional hazards regression model is most easily described in terms of the "hazard curve" rather than the more familiar life-table or actuarial survival curve. The hazard on day *t* is simply the failure rate during day *t* for recipients whose grafts were still functioning and who were not lost to follow-up at the end of the previous day. These daily hazards can be used to calculate actuarial survival (*8*);[4] In Figure 1a the (hypothetical) hazard for center X is initially high, indicating a high risk of immediate failure; then follows a relatively safe period, but after 100 days the hazard in center X slowly increases, indicating that, for patients surviving to 100 days, there are some hazardous times soon to be encountered.

The method allows each transplant center its own basic hazard curve. This is the "stratification" aspect of the method. For example, the hypothetical hazard curves for centers X and Y in Figure 1 differ in shape: in center Y, the hazard remains high up to 100 days, and then slowly decreases. The reason for allowing distinct hazard curves for each center is to accommodate the effects on transplant survival of the many unrecorded conditions and clinical practices that differ among transplant centers. Therefore the method does not attempt to explain these center differences directly.

Baseline. One category of each factor (it does not matter which) is chosen as a "*baseline*" for purposes of comparison. For example, if three categories of recipient age are defined (15–29, 30–44, and 45+ years), any one of these, for example the 15–29 years category, could be chosen as the baseline.

Effect. For a given factor (e.g., recipient age) on a given day posttransplant (e.g., 100 days) the "*effect*" of one category (eg., 45^+ years) relative to the baseline category (15–29 years) is the ratio of the corresponding hazards. This is illustrated in Figure 2a in which the (hypothetical) hazards for recipient age groups 45^+ years and 15–29 years at 100 days are 0.8 and 0.4 failures per 1000 patient days, respectively. Thus the effect of recipient age 45+ years (relative to the baseline) is 0.8/0.4 = 2.0—i.e., a doubling of the baseline hazard. Similarly, from Figure 2a, the

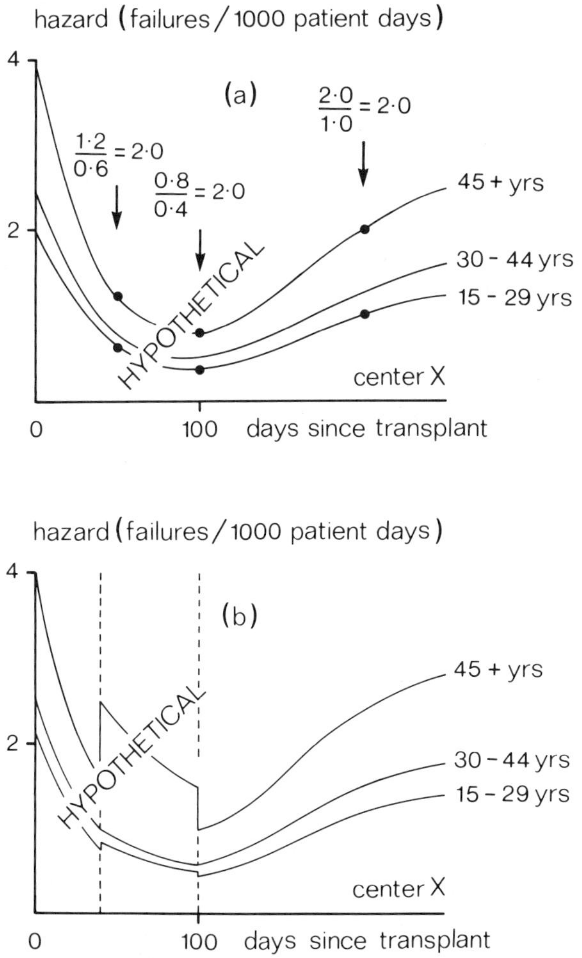

FIGURE 2. (a) Hypothetical estimated hazard curves for three categories of recipient age, (b) separately estimated within each of three discrete postoperative intervals.

subgroups, but in practice hazard rates based on small subgroups suffer too much from random variability to be of any use. Consequently the stratified proportional hazards regression model may be used to compare the hazards in different groups:

$$\log h_{t,c} = \log h_{o,t,c} + b_1x_1 + b_2x_2 + \ldots + b_nx_n$$

where $h_{t,c}$ is the hazard on day t in center c for a patient with factor values $x_1, x_2, \ldots, x_n$; where $h_{o,t,c}$ is the hazard on day t in center c for patients with the baseline values of each factor, and where $b_1, b_2, \ldots, b_n$ are the logarithms of the factor effects described in the text. Estimation of $b_1, b_2, \ldots, b_n$ and $h_{o,t,c}$ may be carried out as detailed elswhere (*3–5*). In the stratified piece-wise proportional hazards regression model the *b*s will differ in each interval.

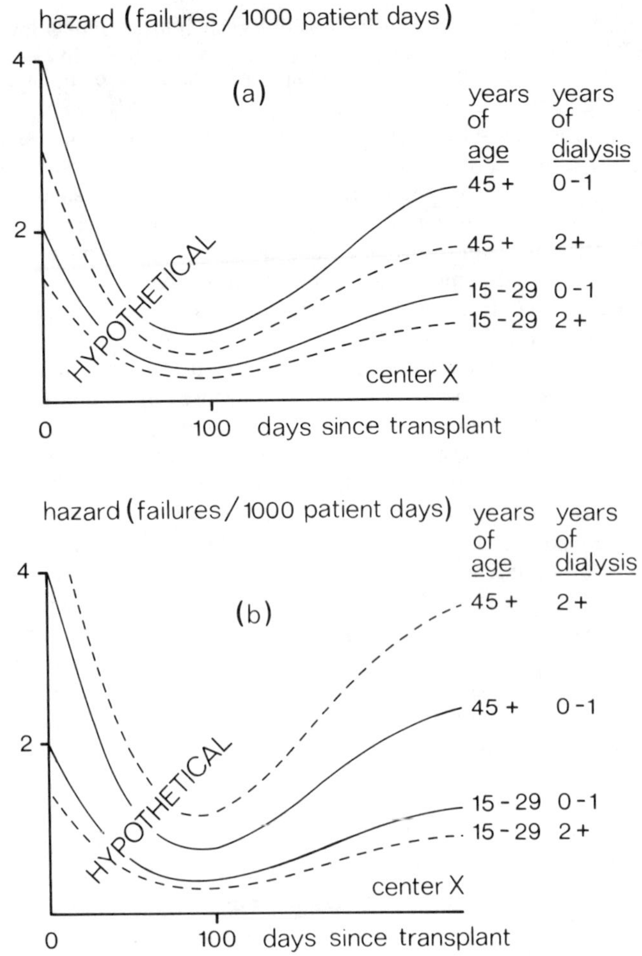

FIGURE 3. (a) Hypothetical estimated hazard curves for two categories of recipient age and two categories of duration of pretransplant dialysis, (b) with separate recipient age effects estimated for each category of duration of dialysis.

effect of age group 30–44 years at 100 days is 1.3. If these hypothetical effects were genuine they would indicate that, among patients surviving to 100 days, the risks of graft failure on that day increase with recipient age, other factors being equal. Note that an effect of 0.5 for a given category of a factor would mean that its hazard is half that of the baseline, and an effect of 1.0 would mean that its hazard is the same as that of the baseline, on that day. (Note that, in some texts and in BMDP (*9*), a factor effect is defined as the *logarithm* of the ratio of hazards).

Assumptions. The unknown coefficients to be estimated by the method are the factor effects. In practice, effects may vary across postoperative time and might also depend on other factors or on the transplant center. For example, the effect of recipient age 45+ years might increase at later postoperative times, or it might be larger among recipients with a long duration of pretransplant dialysis, or smaller in some centers than in others. Furthermore, substantial groups of homogenous patients with which to estimate these effects may not exist. Thus in order to estimate effects efficiently, three assumptions are made about them:

Assumption 1. Effects do not change across postoperative time. This is illustrated in Figure 2a, in which it can be seen that, as a result of this assumption, the (hypothetical) estimated effect of recipient age 45^+ years is the same (2.0) at all postoperative times (and similarly for age group 30–44 years where the effect is 1.3, 15–29 years being chosen as the baseline.) Thus the three curves are proportional. As a result of this proportional hazards assumption, all estimated hazard curves for any one center will be proportional to each other.

Now the proportional hazards assumption may not be valid. For example, age may exert a stronger detrimental influence in one postoperative interval than in others. The assumption can be relaxed by reestimating effects separately within discrete postoperative intervals (*8, 10*). (Within each interval, the estimation is performed only on patients whose grafts were still functioning at the start of the interval; all patients whose grafts were still functioning at the end of the interval are analyzed as if they were lost to follow-up at that time.) This is illustrated in Figure 2b, in which the estimated hazard curves for recipient age, estimated separately within each of three intervals, are by assumption proportional within each interval, yet are not proportional over the full time-span. (This is the stratified *piece-wise* proportional hazards regression model). For example, the (hypothetical) effect of age 45^+ years is greatest in the middle interval. If this hypothetical effect were genuine it would indicate that older recipients are, for some reason, particularly at risk in this middle time-interval, other factors being equal.

Assumption 2. The effects of one factor do not depend on

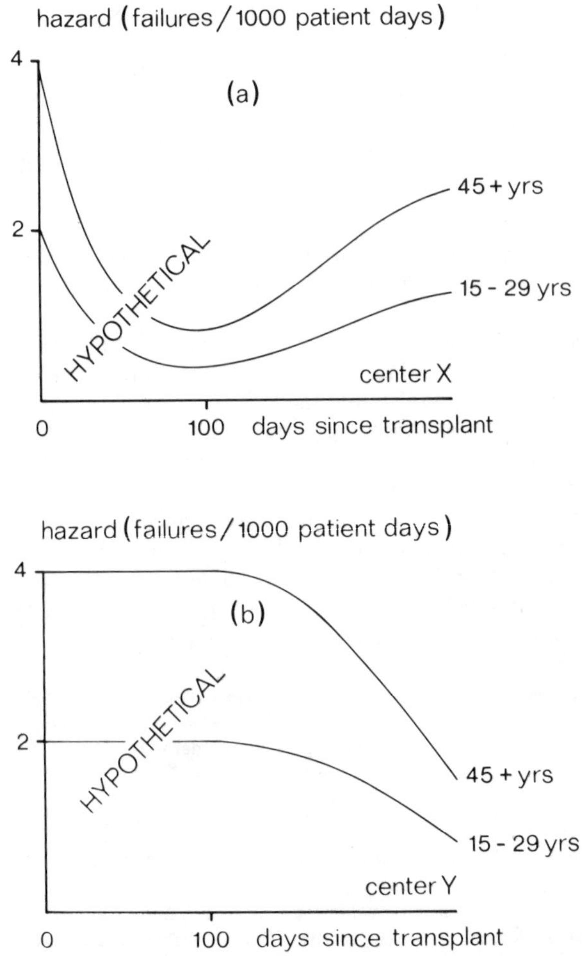

FIGURE 4. Hypothetical estimated hazards for two categories of recipient age (a) in center X, (b) in center Y.

other factors. (This is a regression assumption). This is illustrated in Figure 3a, which shows that, as a result of this assumption, the (hypothetical) estimated effect of recipient age 45^+ years is the same in each of two dialysis-duration groups. (Taking each dialysis group in turn it can be seen that the effect of age 45^+ years is 2.0 in each.) This assumption can be relaxed, for example, by estimating simultaneously a separate recipient age effect for each category of dialysis duration. This is illustrated in Figure 3b, in which the (hypothetical) estimated effect of recipient age 45^+ years is 2.0 for the 0–1 years of dialysis group, and is 3.0 for the 2+ years of dialysis group (taking the 15–29 years age group as the baseline age category, as before). If this hypothetical interaction between recipient age and dialysis duration were genuine it would indicate that older recipients are particularly at risk of graft failure if they have a long duration of pretransplant dialysis, other factors being equal.

Assumption 3. Effects do not differ among transplant centers, although the hazard curves themselves may differ. (This is also a regression assumption.) This is illustrated in Figure 4, in which the (hypothetical) estimated effect of recipient age 45^+ years is the same (2.0) in centers X and Y. This assumption can be relaxed by estimating simultaneously a separate recipient age effect for each of several groups of transplant centers.

RESULTS

Precision and evidence. In addition to the estimate of each factor effect, the method provides a measure of the precision of that estimate (its standard error) and a measure of the amount of evidence that the factor is relevant to graft survival (a *z score*). An extreme z score—outside the range (−2.0, +2.0)—indicates an estimated factor effect that is statistically significant ($P \leq 0.05$)—i.e., unlikely if the factor was irrelevant to graft survival.

DISCUSSION

Single-center studies often lack sufficient transplants to estimate reliably the effects of factors on transplant survival; pooled multi-center studies or unifactorial analyses can produce serious biases in estimating those effects, with consequential misinterpretations. The statistical method described here estimates factor effects multifactorially with appropriate allowances for unknown center factors. The proportionality and regression assumptions embedded in the method allow the data to be used efficiently, and can be relaxed when required. Note, however, that just as single-center studies may lack power and precision to identify factor effects, so multi-center studies may lack power and precision to identify interactions between factors. The method has been used to analyze kidney graft survival in the U.K. and Ireland in the companion article (*1*).

Acknowledgments. We gratefully acknowledge Professor Adrian F. M. Smith, Department of Mathematics, University of Nottingham, England, for his contribution in setting up the project.

REFERENCES

1. Gilks WR, Bradley BA, Gore SM, Selwood NH. Immunogenetic and clinical factors affecting renal transplantation: a rigorous analysis of data recorded by the UK Transplant Service. Transplantation 1986; 42: 39.
2. Taylor RM, Ting A, Briggs JD. Renal transplantation in the United Kingdom and Ireland—the center effect. Lancet 1985; 1, 8432: 798.
3. Cox DR. Regression models and life-tables. J R Stat Society 1972; 34: (series B) 187.
4. Kalbfleisch JD. Some extensions and applications of Cox's regression and life model. Paper presented at the Joint Statistical Meeting in Tallahassee, Florida, March 1974.
5. Kay R. Proportional hazard regression models and the analysis of censored survival data. Appl Stat 1977; 26: 227.
6. Peto R, Pike MC, Armitage P, et al. Design and analysis of randomised clinical trials requiring prolonged observation of each patient. II. Analysis and examples. Br J Cancer 1977; 35: 1.
7. Gilks WR, Selwood N, Bradley BA. The variation between transplant center results in the United Kingdom and Ireland from 1977 to 1981. Transplantation 1984; 38: 235.
8. Gore SM. Graft survival after renal transplantation: agenda for analysis. Kidney Int 1983; 24: 516.
9. BMDP Statistical Software. In: Dixon WJ, et al, eds. Berkeley: U California Press, 1983.
10. Gore SM, Pocock SJ, Kerr GR. Regression models and nonproportional hazards in the analysis of breast cancer survival. Appl Stat 1984; 33: 176.

Received 25 January 1985.
Accepted 3 October 1985.

0041-1337/86/4201-0050$02.00/0
TRANSPLANTATION
Vol. 42, No. 1

EPSTEIN-BARR VIRUS INFECTION AND IMMUNITY IN BONE MARROW TRANSPLANT RECIPIENTS

D.H. CRAWFORD,[1,2] N. MULHOLLAND,[1] V. ILIESCU,[1] R. HAWKINS,[1] AND R. POWLES[3]

Departments of Haematology and Oncology, and ICRF Human Tumour Immunology Group, Faculty of Clinical Sciences, University College, London; and Department of Haematology, Royal Marsden Hospital, Sutton, Surrey, England

Studies on patients for up to one year following allogeneic, HLA-matched bone marrow transplants have shown no increased incidence of salivary Epstein-Barr (EB) virus secretion and no significant rise in EB-virus-specific antibody titers. EB-virus-specific cytotoxic T cells could be detected in the peripheral blood of all patients by six months posttransplant. For up to one year posttransplantation in vitro EB virus infection of peripheral blood B lymphocytes from the majority of patients leads to an abortive infection followed by cell death, and without the establishment of continuously growing cell lines. This abnormality appeared to be due to patients' monocytes, which formed a defective feeder cell layer in culture, and it could be circumvented by culturing the EB-virus-infected B cells from patients on a feeder layer of x-irradiated adherent cells from normal peripheral blood. These findings may explain the relative lack of EB-virus-associated lymphoma seen in bone marrow transplant recipients when compared with other groups of transplant patients.

Epstein-Barr (EB)* virus is a ubiquitous human herpes virus that infects and immortalizes human B lymphocytes in vitro (*1*). Most individuals become infected with EB virus subclinically during childhood (*2*), but if primary infection is delayed until adolescence or early adult life it may be clinically manifest as infectious mononucleosis (*3*). Following primary infection the virus remains in the body as a lifelong, silent infection that can be detected as infectious virus particles in the saliva (*4*) and in a few circulating B lymphocytes that give rise to "spontaneous" B lymphoblastoid cell lines in culture (*5*). This latent infection is probably mainly controlled by memory T cells found in the peripheral blood of all seropositive individuals that can be stimulated to become specifically cytotoxic for EB-virus-infected B cells in vitro (*6*). This cytotoxicity is major histocompatibility complex (MHC)-restricted (*7*) and mediated by CD8-positive T cells (*8*). In immunosuppressed individuals "reactivation" of the latent EB virus infection may occur; this is manifest by increased secretion of salivary virus (*9*), raised EB-virus-specific serum antibody titers, an increased incidence of "spontaneously" derived lines in culture, and low or undetectable levels of circulating EB-virus-specific cytotoxic T cells (*10*). These patients have an increased incidence of B cell lymphoma, in which the malignant cells carry the EB virus genome (*11*). The lymphomas, which are often polyclonal in origin (*12*), have been reported in renal and cardiac transplant recipients (*11*), congenital immunodeficiencies (*13*), and the acquired immunodeficiency syndrome (*14*). In transplant recipients receiving cyclosporine, the drug has been shown to directly inactivate EB-virus-specific cytotoxic T cells, and it is suggested that this allows the accumulation of replicating EB-virus-infected cells in the body, leading directly to the evolution of polyclonal lymphoma (*10*).

Allogeneic bone marrow transplantation is a current form of therapy for acute myeloid leukemia, and it is usually given in association with total-body irradiation and immunosuppressive therapy (*15*). Reactivation of herpes viruses is known to occur under these conditions—and, in particular, cytomegalovirus causes high morbidity and mortality (*16*). However, despite an intensive immunosuppressive regimen, lymphomas developing posttransplantation are rare in these patients. In order to further investigate this observation, we have studied the latent EB virus infection and EB-virus-specific immunity in allogeneic bone marrow transplant recipients for up to two years posttransplantation.

MATERIALS AND METHODS

Patients. All patients were adults with acute myeloid leukemia (age range 14–41 years) who received HLA-matched, allogeneic bone marrow transplants at the Royal Marsden Hospital, Sutton, Surrey, between 1981 and 1984. Total-body irradiation of 9–10 GY was given prior to the transplant, and cyclosporine (4–12.5 mg/kg/day) was given for six months after transplantation. All donors and recipients were seropositive for antibodies to EB viral antigens.

Antibody titers. Serum antibodies to EB viral early antigen (*17*) and EB viral capsid antigen (*18*) were assayed by routine indirect immunofluorescence.

B cell lines (BCL). Peripheral blood mononuclear cells (PBM) separated from whole blood were T-cell-depleted (*19*) and infected with EB virus by resuspending cell pellets of up to 10^7 cells in 1 ml of culture supernatant from a B95-8 cell line[20] that had been filtered through a 0.45-μ filter and stored at −70°C. After a 1-hr incubation at 37°C, the cells were washed twice and cultured at 2×10^6/ml in RPM 1640 containing 10% fetal calf serum (FCS), 100 IU penicillin and streptomycin, and 2 mM glutamine in 0.2 ml volumes in flat microtiter wells with or without feeder cells.

Cell cultures. Cultures were incubated at 37°C in a humidified atmosphere containing 5% CO_2 in air, and were fed weekly by replacement of half the supernatant medium without disturbing the cell layer. The cultures were visualized weekly using an inverted microscope, and when proliferating foci of cells were seen they were subcultured and grown into BCL.

Feeder cells. PBM from normal individuals were x-irradiated at 2000 rads and plated in 0.1-ml volumes in flat-bottomed

* Abbreviations used: EB, Epstein-Barr, EBNA, EB viral nuclear antigen; FCS, fetal calf serum; MHC, major histocompatibility complex; PBM, peripheral blood mononuclear cells.

[1] University College.

[2] Royal Marsden Hospital.

[3] Address correspondence to: Dr. D.H. Crawford, Department of Virology, Royal Postgraduate Medical School, Du Cane Road, London W12 OHS.

wells at a concentration of 5×10^4/well. Supernatant medium and nonadherent cells were removed before test cells were added to the cultures. The cell-free supernatant from one-week cultures were added to some test cell cultures.

Natural killer (NK) cell assay. Fresh PBM were incubated with ^{51}Cr-labeled Raji cells at E:T ratios of 50:1, 25:1, 12.1, and 6.1 in an overnight assay. The supernatant medium was harvested and counted in a β counter. The percentage of specific ^{51}Cr release was calculated using the formula:

$$\% \frac{\%\text{ specific experimental }^{51}\text{Cr release (cpm)} - \text{spontaneous }^{51}\text{Cr release (cpm)}}{\%\text{ maximum }^{51}\text{Cr release (cpm)} - \text{spontaneous }^{51}\text{Cr release (cpm)}} \times 100$$

Human interferon α (HuINF α) assay. Culture supernatant medium was assayed for interferon using a radioimmunoassay (*21*).

EB viral nuclear antigen (EBNA). This was detected in fixed cells using anticomplimentary immunofluorescence (*22*).

Cytoplasmic immunoglobulin. This was detected in methanol-fixed cells using fluorescein-conjugated rabbit antibodies against IgM, IgG, and IgA (Dakepatts, Mercia Brocades Ltd., Byfleet, Surrey, UK).

Primary and secondary stimulation cultures. PBM were cultured with x-irradiated autologous BCL in a ratio of 40:1. After 10 days E-rosette-positive cells were separated and cultured with x-irradiated autologous BCL in a radio of 10:1 for a further 10 days (*7*).

EB-virus-specific cytotoxic assay. E-rosette-positive cells from stimulated cultures were incubated with ^{51}Cr-labeled target cells in ratios of 10:1, 5:1, 2.5:1, and 1:1. The target cells used were autologous BCL, allogeneic BCL, and K562. After four hours' incubation at 37°C the supernatant medium was harvested and counted in a β counter. The percentage of specific ^{51}Cr release was calculated using the formula stated for the NK cell assay (above).

Staining of PBM with monoclonal antibodies. This was carried out by indirect immunofluorescence using culture supernatant medium containing the following antibodies: BA-1 (*23*)—pan B cell, and OKM 1 (*24*)—monocyte-specific.

A goat antimouse fluorescein-conjugated second layer antibody (Nordic Immunological Laboratories Ltd., Maidenhead, Berkshire, UK) was used at a dilution of 1:40. The stained cells were analyzed on a fluorescence-activated cell sorter.

Assay for salivary EB virus. Saliva samples were diluted 1:1 with tissue culture medium and centrifuged 2000 rpm for 10 min. The supernatant medium was filtered through a 0.45-μ filter and stored at −70°C in 1-ml aliquots. These samples were used to infect cord blood PBM that were then plated in 0.2-ml volumes at 2×10^6 ml and scored for transformed foci after 6–8 weeks of culture.

RESULTS

Antibody titers to EB viral antigens. Serum antibody titers to viral capsid antigen (VCA) were measured in nine seropositive patients prior to transplantation and at 3, 6, 9, and 12 months posttransplantation. All the values were within the normal range, although a fall in antibody titer was noted at 3 and 6 months after transplant, and a return to a level one or two doubling dilutions above previous levels was general by one year.

Detection of salivary EB virus. Saliva samples from 25 patients were assayed for infectious EB virus prior to transplant and at three and six months posttransplantation. Three of the patients had detectable salivary virus prior to transplantation, whereas one had detectable virus at three months and two at six months. Normal seropositive control individuals showed 10% positivity.

PBM taken at monthly intervals for one year after BMT from nine recipients were infected with EB virus. During the first six months, PBM from only two patients showed evidence of transformation to EBNA-positive BCL. During the 6–9-month period, PBM from five out of nine patients yielded BCL after infection with EB virus. PBM taken from patients prior to or more than one year after transplantation and control cells all transformed into BCL following infection with EB virus.

PBM from six further BMT patients were T cell depleted by E rosetting prior to EB virus infection. No transformation was seen following EB virus infection of these cells taken monthly for a one-year period following BMT. In an attempt to explain these findings, a number of assays were carried out.

Numerical counting of BAI-positive cells in PBM samples showed B cell numbers of 1–10% in samples taken 1–2 months posttransplant; thereafter B cell numbers were within the normal limits of 5–25%. OKM_1-positive cells formed 10–30% of the total PBM at all times studied posttransplant.

NK cell activity in PBM from BMT recipients was measured prior to and at monthly intervals up to six months after transplantation, and was found to be low for 1–2 months posttransplant, after which it returned to within normal limits.

HuIFN α levels were measured in culture supernatant medium one week after EB virus infection of PBM or T-depleted PBM because this has been found to cause early die-back of proliferating foci (*25*). No detectable interferon was found in cultures from normal donors or BMT recipients.

The expression of EBNA and cytoplasmic immunoglobulin (IgM, IgG, IgA) was detected in EB-virus-infected, T-cell-depleted PBM from normal donors and BMT recipients during the first year posttransplant. In cultures from normal donors the percentage of EBNA-positive cells increased from 2% at day 2 to around 50% at day 7 and around 85% at day 12. In cultures containing PBM from BMT recipients around 2% of EBNA-positive cells were detected at day 2 after EB virus infection, but these cells died rapidly and no EBNA-positive cells were detected at days 5, 7, 9, and 12 (Fig. 1a).

Cytoplasmic IgM, IgG, and IgA containing cells from normal donors rose continuously in EB-virus-infected, T-cell-depleted cultures with a majority of IgM-containing cells, whereas no Ig-containing cells were seen in the cultures from BMT recipients (Fig. 1b).

When T-depleted PBM from BMT recipients were EB-virus-infected and added to a feeder layer of adherent cells from x-irradiated PBM (2000 rads) from a normal individual, EBNA expression, EB virus polyclonal activation, and continued cell growth occurred in a manner identical to that in PBM from normal individuals, with the emergence of BCL after a one-month period (Figure 1). The cell-free supernatant medium from x-irradiated normal PBM taken after one week of culture added to EB-virus-infected BMT PBM had no such effect.

All 10 patients studied recovered EB virus-specific cytotoxic T cell activity against the autologous BCL (derived prior to transplantation) by six months posttransplant (Fig. 2a). In three patients this activity could be detected by three months after BMT. In some cases the specific cytotoxicity was masked by NK cell activity after primary stimulation, but after second-

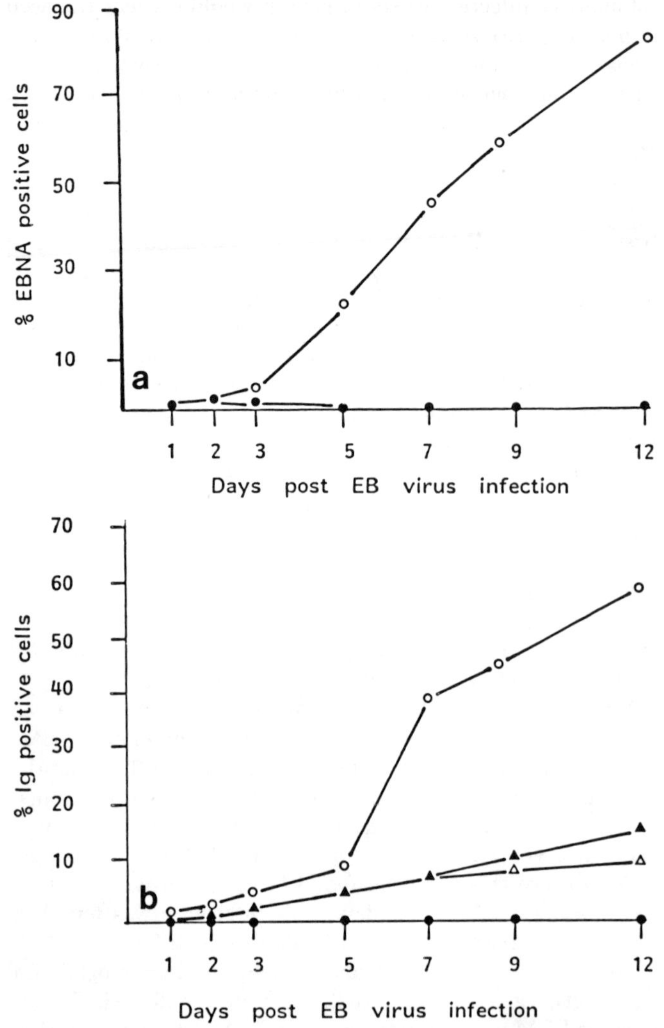

FIGURE 1. (a) % EBNA expression in EB-virus-infected E-rosette-negative PBM from a bone marrow transplant recipient (●——●) and a normal donor (○——○) over a 12-day period. (b) Percentage of cells staining for cytoplasmic immunoglobulin over a 12-day period following EB virus infection of E-rosette-negative PBM from a bone marrow transplant recipient (●——●) and a normal donor (IgM ○, IgG ▲, IgA △).

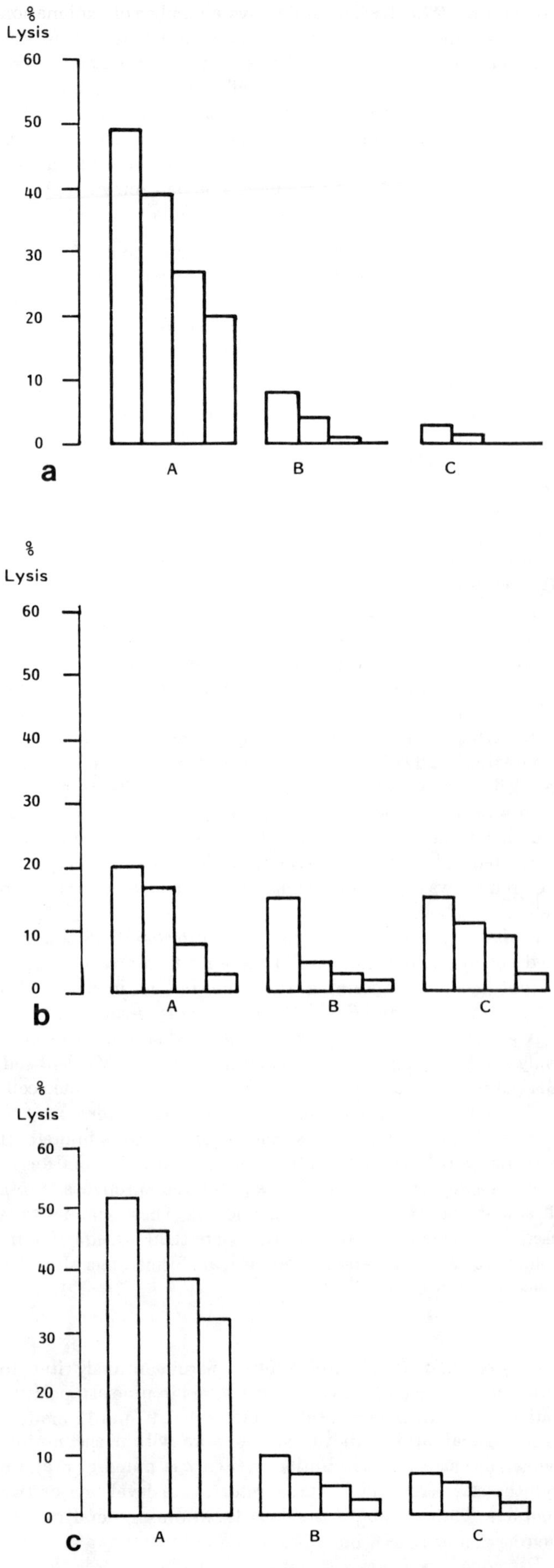

ary stimulation in vitro with the autologous x-irradiated BCL specific cytotoxicity could be clearly distinguished (Fig. 2b,c).

DISCUSSION

In vitro EB virus infection of peripheral blood B lymphocytes from normal individuals regularly gives rise to the outgrowth of BCL. Our results show that this is not the case following BMT, since no growth resulted from EB virus infection of PBM from 7 of 9 patients during the first six months after transplantation and 4 of 9 patients 6–12 months after trans-

FIGURE 2. Percentage of specific lysis of target cell lines by EB-virus-specific cytotoxic T cell lines grown in vitro from a BMT patient (a). Attacker:target ratios 10:1, 5:1, 2.5:1 and 1.25:1. Cell lines: A = autologous BCL, B = K562, C = allogeneic BCL. Percentage of specific lysis of target cell lines by EB-virus-specific cytotoxic T cell lines from a BMT patient after primary (b) and secondary (c) stimulation in vitro. Attacker:target ratios 10:1, 5:1, 2.5:1, and 1.25:1. Cell lines: A = autologous BCL, B = K562, C = allogeneic BCL.

plantation. This finding could have a number of explanations. The outgrowth of BCL from EB-virus-infected PBM from normal seropositive individuals may be inhibited by the presence of T cells stimulated in the culture to become specifically cytotoxic for EB-virus-infected autologous B cells. However, this is not the cause of the lack of outgrowth of BCL from PBM from BMT patients because the effect is not eliminated by removal of the T cells from the culture. Similarly, we have shown that this finding can not be explained by low B cell or monocyte numbers, excess NK cell activity early in the culture period, or α interferon production. The latter have been described as mechanisms of inhibition to the early outgrowth of BCL (*25*).

The finding of low levels of EBNA-positive cells early in the culture period (2% at two days) indicates that EB virus infection is taking place but that the cells do not become immortalized. A similar abortive infection has been reported after EB virus infection of chronic lymphatic leukemia cells (*26*). The cells are resistant to polyclonal activation by EB virus, and similar results have been found following pokeweed mitogen stimulation of PBM from BMT patients posttransplantation (*27*). Our results show that the addition of adherent cells from normal x-irradiated PBM allows the expression of EBNA, as well as cytoplasmic immunoglobulin and transformation into BCL of the EB-virus-infected B cells from BMT patients. The finding suggests that the defect following BMT is a monocyte defect—and, since normal numbers of OKM^+ cells are present, a qualitative rather than quantitative defect is likely. The finding that supernatant medium from one-week-old cultures of normal x-irradiated PBM does not support the growth of EB-virus-infected BMT B cells, suggests that the defect is not a soluble factor but in cellular contact. It has been known for many years that the outgrowth of BCL from normal cells is dependent on a feeder layer of monocytes or fibroblasts, and our data suggest that these cells are defective for up to one year after BMT. This may be due to the effects of total-body irradiation (about 1000 rads) or to cyclosporine treatment. However, irradiation a higher total dose of x-irradiation (2000 rads) is given to our normal PBM feeder layers supporting the outgrowth of BCL. Similarly, cyclosporine can be added to the culture medium without inhibition of cell growth (*28*). An alternative explanation is that the transplanted allogeneic monocytes are immature or nonfunctioning for a prolonged period.

Our data clearly show that, following HLA-matched, allogeneic bone marrow transplantation, T cells specifically cytotoxic for autologous EB-virus-infected B cells are absent from the peripheral blood for a 3–6-month period. Despite this lack of control cells, none of the patients in this study showed a rise in EB-virus-specific antibody titer of more than two doubling dilutions in the year following transplantation, and the percentage of patients with detectable salivary EB virus remained low during the first six months posttransplantation. Thus, in contrast to renal transplant patients, these patients did not show a "reactivation" of EB virus infection, even while being treated with cyclosporine, and no EB-virus-associated lymphomas have been observed in the patients transplanted at the Royal Marsden Hospital. These observations may be partly explained by our findings that, for up to one year posttransplantation, the in vitro EB virus infection of PBM or E-rosette-negative PBM leads to an abortive infection with transient expression of EBNA but without immortalization. If this type of abortive infection exists in vivo, it would prevent the accumulation of EB-virus-infected cells with the capacity for indefinite proliferation. The regeneration of EB-virus-specific cytotoxic T cells within six months would precede the recovery of this B cell abnormality in the vast majority of patients.

REFERENCES

1. Pope JH, Horne MK, Scott W. Transformation of foetal human leucocytes in vitro by filtrates of a human leukaemia cell line containing herpes like virus. Int J Cancer 1968; 3: 857.
2. Evans AS, Niederman JC, Cenabre LC, West B, Richards VA. A prospective evaluation of heterophile and EBV specific IgM antibody tests in clinical and subclinical infectious mononucleosis specificity and sensitivity of the tests and persistence of the antibodies. J Infect Dis 1975; 132: 546.
3. Henle G, Henle W, Diehl V. Relation of Burkitts tumour associated herpes-type virus to infectious mononucleosis. Proc Natl Acad Sci 1968; 59: 94.
4. Golden HD, Chang RS, Prescott W, Simpson E, Cooper TY. Leucocyte-transforming agent: prolonged excretion by patients with mononucleosis and excretion by normal individuals. J Infect Dis 1973; 127: 471.
5. Nilsson K, Klein G, Henle W, Henle G. The establishment of lymphoblastoid lines from adult and foetal human lymphoid cells and its dependence on EBV. Int J Cancer 1971; 8: 443.
6. Moss DJ, Rickinson AB, Pope JH. Long term T cell mediated immunity to Epstein-Barr virus in man. I. Complete regression of virus induced transformation in cultures of seropositive donor leucocytes. Int J Cancer 1978; 22: 662.
7. Moss DJ, Wallace LE, Rickinson AB, Epstein MA. Cytotoxic T cell recognition of Epstein Barr virus infected B cells. I. Specificity and HLA restriction of effector cells reactivated in vitro. Eur J Immunol 1981; 11: 686.
8. Crawford DH, Iliescu V, Edwards AJ, Beverley PCL. Characterisation of Epstein-Barr virus specific memory T cells from the peripheral blood of seropositive individuals. Br J Cancer 1983; 47: 681.
9. Strauch B, Siegel N, Andrews LL, Miller G. Oropharyngeal excretion of Epstein-Barr virus by renal transplant recipients, and other patients treated with immunosuppressive drugs. Lancet 1974; 1: 234.
10. Crawford DH, Edwards JBM, Sweny P, Janossy G, Hoffbrand AV. Long-term T-cell-mediated immunity to Epstein-Barr virus in renal-allograft recipients receiving cyclosporin A. Lancet 1981; 1: 10.
11. Crawford DH, Thomas JA, Janossy G, et al. Epstein Barr virus nuclear antigen positive lymphoma after cyclosporin A treatment in patients with renal allograft. Lancet 1980; 1: 1355.
12. Hanto DW, Frizzera G, Gajl-Peczalska KJ, et al. The Epstein Barr virus (EBV) in the pathogenesis of post transplant lymphoma. Transplant Proc 1981; 13: 756.
13. Henle W, Henle G. Consequences of persistent Epstein Barr virus infections. Cold Spring Harbor Symposium. Viruses in naturally occurring cancers, vol 7, 1980: 3–8.
14. Zeigler JL, Drew WL, Miner RC, et al. Outbreak of Burkitt's-like lymphoma in homosexual men. Lancet 1982; 2: 631.
15. Thomas ED, Clift RA, Buckner CD (for the Seattle Marrow Transplant Team). Marrow transplantation for patients with acute non-lymphoid leukaemia who achieve a first remission. Cancer Treat Rep 1982; 66: 143.
16. Nermair PE, Reeves W, Ray G, et al. A prospective analysis of interstitial pneumonia and opportunistic viral infection among recipients of allogeneic bone marrow grafts. J Infect Dis 1977; 136: 754.
17. Henle W, Henle G, Zajac BA, Pearson G, Waubke R, Scriba M. Differential reactivity of human serums with early antigen induced by Epstein-Barr virus. Science 1970; 169: 188.

18. Henle G, Henle W. Immunofluorescence in cells derived from Burkitt's lymphoma. J Bacteriol 1966; 91: 1248.
19. Kaplan ME, Clark C. An improved rosetting assay for detection of human T lymphocytes. J Immunol Methods 1974; 5: 131.
20. Miller G, Shope T, Lisco H, Stitt D, Lipman M. Epstein Barr virus: transformation cytopathic changes and viral antigens in squirrel monkey and marmoset leucocytes. Proc Natl Acad Sci USA 1972; 69: 383.
21. Secher DS. Immunoradiometric assay of human leukocyte interferon using monoclonal antibody. Nature 1981; 290: 501.
22. Reedman BM, Klein G. Cellular localisation of an Epstein Barr virus (EBV) associated complement fixing antigen in producer and non producer lymphoblastoid cell lines. Int J Cancer 1973; 11: 499.
23. Abrahamson CS, Kersey JH, Le Bieu TW. A monoclonal antibody (BA 1) reactive with cells of human B lymphocyte lineage. J Immunol 1981; 126: 83.
24. Breard J, Reinkerz EL, King PC, Goldstein G, Schossman SF. A monoclonal antibody reactive with human peripheral blood monocytes. J Immunol 1980; 124: 1943.
25. Thorley-Lawson DA. The transformation of adult but not newborn human lymphocytes by Epstein-Barr virus and phytohaemagglutinin is inhibited by interferon. The early suppression of Epstein Barr virus infection is mediated by interferon. J Immunol 1981; 126: 829.
26. Rickinson AB, Finerty S, Epstein MA. Interaction of Epstein-Barr virus with leukaemic B cells in vitro. I. Abortive infection and rare cell line established from chronic lymphatic leukaemic cells. Clin Exp Immunol 1982; 50: 347.
27. Witherspoon RP, Lum LG, Storb R, Thomas ED. In vitro regulation of immunoglobulin synthesis after human marrow transplantation. II. Deficient T and non-T lymphocyte function within 3–4 months of allogeneic, syngeneic, or autologous marrow grafting for haematologic malignancy. Blood 1982; 59: 844.
28. Crawford DH. Lymphomas after cyclosporin A treatment. In: Touraine JL, Traeger J, Betuel H, Brochier J, Dubernard JM, Revilloud JP, Triau R, eds. Transplantation and clinical immunology, XIII. Lyon: Excerpta Medica, 1981: 48.

Received 13 August 1985.
Accepted 22 October 1985.

0041-1337/86/4201-0054$02.00/0
TRANSPLANTATION
Vol. 42, No. 1
Printed in U.S.A.

POTENTIAL UTILIZATION OF A NATIONAL HLA-TYPED DONOR POOL FOR BONE MARROW TRANSPLANTATION[1,2]

ROBERT PETER GALE[3]

Department of Medicine, Division of Hematology and Oncology UCLA School of Medicine, Los Angeles, California 90024

Most individuals with diseases potentially treatable by bone marrow transplantation lack an HLA-identical sibling donor. The annual incidence of 11 diseases probably or possibly benefitted by bone marrow transplantation was corrected for patient and disease characteristics to determine annual adjusted incidences. These data were used to project the number of individuals who might receive transplants using an HLA-typed national bone marrow donor pool. Estimates of transplant outcome were then utilized to predict potential annual benefit. Approximately 12,000 individuals annually are predicted to be candidates for transplantation from a national donor pool. Using indicated projected benefits, this could result in benefit to approximately 5000 individuals. Such a pool may also be useful for individuals accidently exposed to radiation.

Bone marrow transplantation is increasingly used to treat immune disorders, aplastic anemia, and leukemia. Approximately 9000 transplants have been performed worldwide since 1970. Most successful transplants have utilized HLA-identical sibling donors. In some diseases, and under specified circumstances, bone marrow transplantation from an HLA-identical sibling has produced survival results comparable or superior to alternative therapies. In other diseases the use of bone marrow transplantation remains investigational (*1–4*).

Most patients who might benefit from a bone marrow transplantation lack an HLA-identical sibling donor. In the United States, the calculated likelihood of an individual having such a donor is approximately 30%. Alternative donors have been suggested in individuals without a sibling donor, including transplants for partially or fully HLA-matched related or unrelated donors and fetal liver cells.

In this study I analyzed the number of individuals in the United States who might benefit from bone marrow transplantation if suitable alternative donors were identified. Diseases were divided into those in which bone marrow transplantation is likely to be of benefit and those in which there is a possible but unproved benefit. Based on these estimates and predicted

* Abbreviations used: ALL, acute lymphoblastic leukemia; AML, acute myelogenous leukemia; CML, chronic myelogenous leukemia; DHHS, Department of Health and Human Services; NCI, National Cancer Institute; NHBLI, National Heart, Lung, and Blood Institute; NIAID, National Institutes of Allergy, Immunology, and Infectious Diseases; SCID, severe combined immune deficiency; SEER, Surveillance Epidemiology End Results.

[1] This work was supported in part by grant CA 23175 from the National Cancer Institute, NIH, USPHS, DHHS.

[2] These data were presented in part at the NIH Technology Assessment Conference in Bethesda, MD, May 13–15, 1985.

[3] Address correspondence to: Robert Peter Gale, M.D., Ph.D., Division of Hematology and Oncology, Department of Medicine, UCLA Center for the Health Sciences, Los Angeles, California 90024.

outcomes, it was possible to project potential survival benefit. These data should be useful in planning strategies to identify potential alternative donors for individuals with appropriate diseases who lack an HLA-identical sibling.

MATERIALS AND METHODS

Five diseases in which bone marrow transplantation is thought to produce results equivalent or superior to alternate therapies include aplastic anemia, acute lymphoblastic leukemia (ALL), * acute myelogenous leukemia (AML), chronic myelogenous leukemia (CML) and immune deficiency disorders such as severe combined immune deficiency (SCID), Wiskott-Aldrich syndrome, ataxia-telangectasia, and several less common disorders. Six diseases in which bone marrow transplantation has been suggested as a possible therapeutic modality are genetic disorders, Hodgkin and non-Hodgkin lymphoma, thalassemia, hemoglobinopathies, and multiple myeloma. Genetic disorders include a large number of genetically transmissible diseases, usually single enzyme deficiencies, in which involvement of bone-marrow-derived cells is a primary feature and in which transplantation of bone marrow cells has been reported to be beneficial in some instances.

Several data sources were used to analyze the annual incidence of these diseases in the United States. Cancer incidences were identified using data from the Surveillance Epidemiology End Results (SEER) of the National Cancer Institute (NCI) program (*5*) and American Cancer Society (*6*) and were updated to 1985 projected census figures. In the leukemias, these incidences were checked against estimates of the Leukemia Society of America and selected epidemologic studies. Incidence data for aplastic anemia were obtained from mortality records from the National Center for Health Statistics, estimates from the National Heart, Lung, and Blood Institute (NHLBI) and the Aplastic Anemia Foundation, and from selected epidemiologic studies (*7*). Data for immune disorders were based on recent reviews, estimates from the National Institutes of Allergy, Immunology, and Infectious Diseases (NIAID), and from personal communication. Incidence data for thalassemia and sickle cell anemia were based on estimated gene frequencies and were corrected for live births, sex, and race. Confirmation data were provided by the NHLBI, the Division of Material and Child Health, Department of Health and Human Services (DHHS) and the Cooley Anemia Foundation.

In each of the diseases indicated, data from the transplant literature were used to identify a subset of patients who might be potential recipients of bone marrow transplants based on results in recipients of HLA-identical grafts. For example, most data suggest that bone marrow transplantation in aplastic anemia is likely to be effective in individuals <40 years of age with the severe form of the disease. Of the 1400 annual cases of aplastic anemia, only 400 cases are severe and occur in individuals <40 years.

Data were also adjusted for the proportion of potential recipients projected to have an HLA-identical sibling. As indicated, this figure is approximately 30% in the United States. As a consequence, the pool of potential recipients was reduced to 70% of corrected incidence; most estimates were rounded to the nearest 25 or 50 as appropriate based on sample size. In some instances—such as SCID, thalassemia, and sickle cell anemia—the likelihood of a suitable donor may be less than 30% because of the probability of affected, related siblings. This is offset, to some extent, by the larger average kindred of families with thalassemia and sickle cell anemia.

The final calculation attempted to project potential benefit if these individuals received a bone marrow transplant from a donor from a theoretical HLA-typed donor pool. Outcome estimates were selected by discounting by 20% the 3–5-year disease-free survival results in comparable recipients of HLA-identical sibling transplants. Data were not corrected for performance status or other factors that might ultimately influence a critical assessment of the role of transplantation versus alternative therapies. In some disorders, such as hemoglobinopathies and multiple myeloma, there were insufficient data in HLA-identical siblings to project outcome. In the hemoglobinopathies, a figure similar to the outcome of thalassemia and aplastic anemia was selected.

RESULTS

Table 1 summarizes calculations in the five diseases in which bone marrow transplantation is reported to be of benefit in defined patient groups. The total annual incidence of these diseases is 16,400 cases. Correction of this figure for disease severity and age or remission status results in an adjusted annual incidence of 5200 cases. Of these, 2400 individuals are projected to have an HLA-identical sibling resulting in 2800 individuals who could potentially utilize an appropriate HLA-typed donor pool. If these transplants were undertaken with the indicated projected outcome, this would result in a potential benefit to 1200 individuals. Details regarding calculations to potential recipients with aplastic anemia, ALL, AML, and CML are indicated in Figures 1–4.

Table 2 summarizes similar calculations in seven diseases in which bone marrow transplantation is investigational but of possible benefit. The annual projected incidence of these disorders is 50,300 (the figure for thalassemia represents prevalence since annual incidence data are not available). Of these

TABLE 1. Potential recipients of HLA-matched unrelated transplants having diseases with proved benefit from transplantation

Disease[a]	Annual incidence	Transplant criteria[b]	Adjusted incidence	Potential recipients	Projected outcome	Projected benefit
Aplastic anemia	1400	Severe <40y	400	300	50%	150
ALL	2700	1st R >20y	2400	900	50%	350
		>1st R <40y			35%	
AML	8500	1st R <20y	1200	750	50%	275
		>1st R <40y			35%	
CML	3500	CP <50y	1000	700	50%	350
Immune	300	Severe <40y	200	150	50%	75
	16,400		5200	2800		1200

[a] ALL, acute lymphocytic leukemia; AML, acute myelogenous leukemia; CML, chronic myelogenous leukemia; immune, immune deficiency diseases.

[b] Transplant criteria: criteria of severe aplastic anemia (*9*); R, remission; y, years; CP, chronic phase.

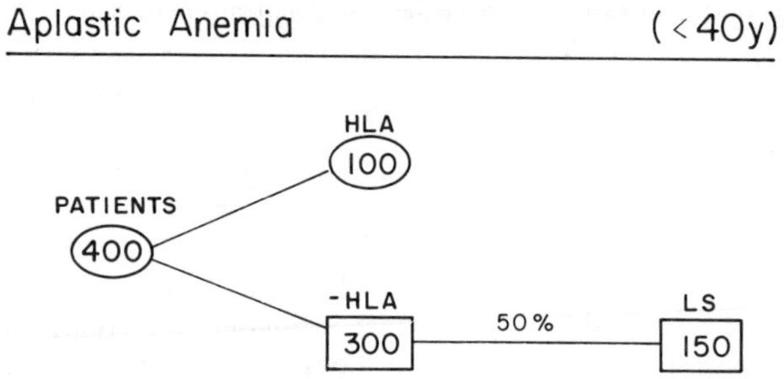

FIGURE 1. Potential recipients of bone marrow transplants for aplastic anemia in individuals <40 years. Of 400 patients, 100 are projected to have an HLA-identical sibling (HLA); 300 to lack suitable donors (−HLA). A projected benefit of 50% would result in 150 lives saved (LS).

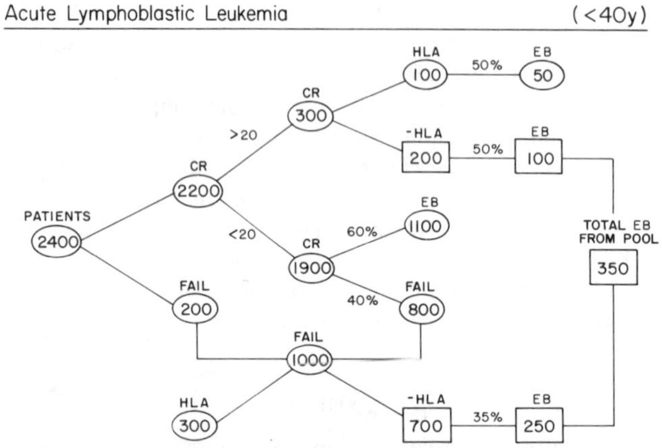

FIGURE 2. Potential recipients of bone marrow transplants for acute lymphocytic leukemia. Of 2400 patients, 2200 are projected to achieve complete remission (CR) with chemotherapy; 200 to fail to achieve complete remission (Fail). 300 of the CR patients are >20 years old and all are potential transplant candidates. A total of 100 have HLA-identical sibling donors (HLA) and 200 lack donors (−HLA). A projected benefit of 50% would result in 50 and 100 beneficiaries (EB) patients achieving CR (1900) <20 years and 60% are predicted to be cured by chemotherapy, resulting in 1100 beneficiaries (EB); 800 patients are projected to fail chemotherapy (Fail). Total initial and late failures are 1000 (Fail). A total of 300 individuals have HLA-identical sibling donors (HLA); 700 do not (−HLA). A projected 35% benefit would result in 250 beneficiaries (EB). Total estimated benefit from use of the donor pool for −HLA individuals is 350 (EB).

individuals, 14,900 have disease or age characteristics suggesting that they might be potential recipients of bone marrow transplants (8750 are potential recipients of transplants from a donor pool). If these individuals were transplanted, with the indicated projected outcomes, this would result in a benefit to 3600 individuals. Details of the specific calculation in Hodgkin disease and non-Hodgkin lymphoma are indicated in Figures 5 and 6. Of interest is a projected increase in the incidence of thalassemia and hemoglobinopathies in the United States as a consequence of the recent immigration of individuals from Southeast Asia (*8*).

DISCUSSION

In this study I review the number of individuals in the United States with selected diseases who are potential recipients of transplants from HLA-matched unrelated donors. These individuals are divided into two categories—those with diseases in which transplantation is generally regarded to be comparable or superior to alternative therapies and those with diseases in which transplantation may be useful, but for which sufficient data are not yet available for critical analyses. This division reflects a synthesis of currently available data from uncontrolled and controlled trials and may be considered overly optimistic or pessimistic by different investigators. It is important to emphasize that the designation of a disease as potentially treatable by bone marrow transplantation reflects results of transplants between HLA-identical siblings. Data using HLA-identical or partially matched unrelated donors are limited and can not be critically analyzed at present. It is unlikely, however, that survival results will exceed those achieved with HLA-identical siblings, and they may be inferior. If so, the criteria for transplantation from an HLA-matched unrelated donor may require revision. This caution applies to a greater extent in the disorders designated potentially treatable by transplantation since, in this setting, treatment from an HLA-identical sibling is of unproven efficacy. Despite these reservations, it is possible to predict the approximate number of individuals who might utilize the HLA-typed donor pool were

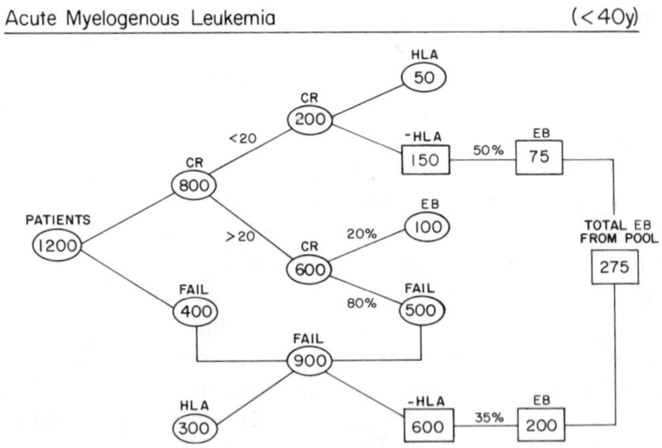

FIGURE 3. Potential recipients of bone marrow transplants for acute myelogenous leukemia. Of 1200, 800 are projected to achieve complete remission (CR) and 400 to fail to achieve complete remission (Fail). 200 of the CR patients are <20 years, of whom 50 have HLA-identical siblings (HLA) and 150 do not (−HLA). A projected 50% benefit would result in 75 beneficiaries (EB). Of the 600 complete remission patients >20 y, 20% or 100 will be cured by chemotherapy and 500 will relapse (Fail). The total patients who fail is projected to be 900. Of these 300 have HLA-identical siblings (HLA) and 600 do not (−HLA). A projected benefit of 35% results in 200 beneficiaries (EB). The total number of total beneficiaries from the pool is 275 (EB).

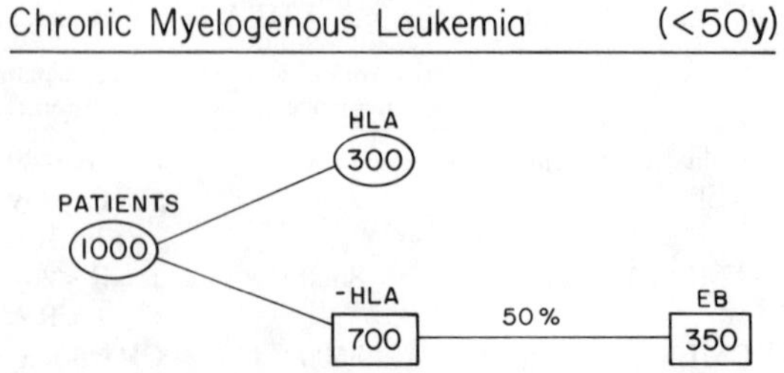

FIGURE 4. Potential recipients of bone marrow transplants for chronic myelogenous leukemia <50 years. Of 1000 patients, 300 will have an HLA-identical sibling (HLA) and 700 will not (−HLA). A projected 50% benefit would result in 350 beneficiaries (EB).

TABLE 2. Potential recipients of HLA-matched unrelated transplants having diseases of possible benefit from transplantation

Disease[a]	Annual incidence	Transplant criteria[b]	Adjusted incidence	Potential recipients	Projected outcome	Projected benefit
Genetic	1000	Severe <40y	1000	700	30%	200
Hodgkin	7750	Resistant <45y	1600	1100	30%	350
non-Hodgkin	22500	Resistant <45y	3800	2100	30%	700
Thalassemia	1000	Severe <40y	200	150	50%	75
Hemoglobinopathy	9050	Severe <40y	8000	4500	50%	2250
Myeloma	9000	<40y	300	200	20%	50
	50,300		14,900	8750		3600

[a] Genetic diseases; Hodgkin's and non-Hodgkin's lymphoma; β-thalassemia; hemoglobinopathy, hemoglobin SS, EE, and S-thal; multiple myeloma.

[b] Resistant; uncurable with conventional chemotherapy.

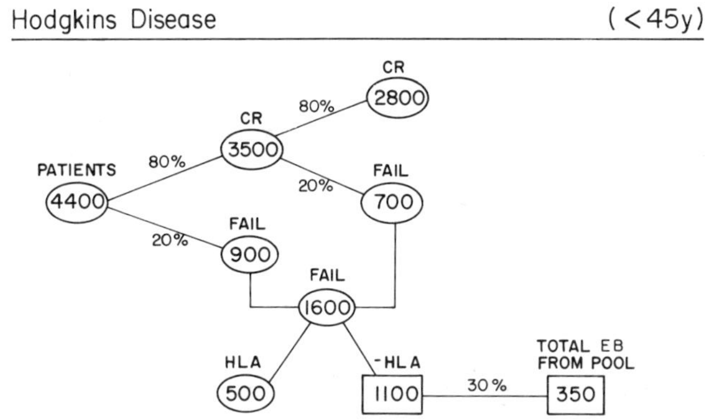

FIGURE 5. Potential recipients of bone marrow transplants for Hodgkin disease <45 years. Of 4400 patients 80% or 3500 will achieve complete remission (CR) and 900 will fail (Fail). An additional 20% of CR patients or 700 will relapse (Fail) for a total failure rate of 1600 (Fail). Of these 500 will have an HLA-identical sibling (HLA) and 1100 will not (−HLA). A projected 30% benefit would result in 350 beneficiaries (EB).

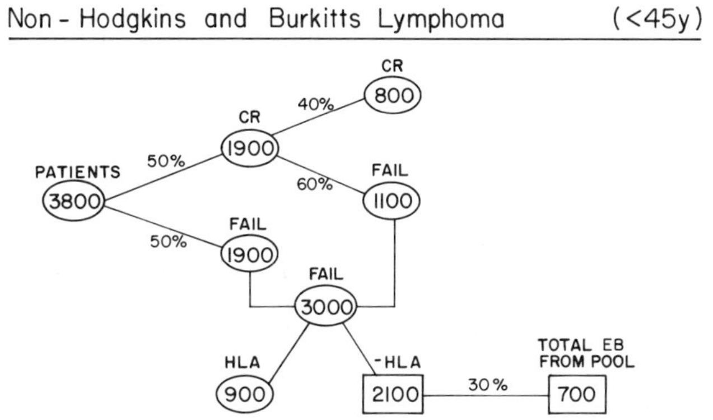

FIGURE 6. Potential recipients of bone marrow transplants for non-Hodgkin disease and Burkitt's lymphoma <45 years. Of 3800 patients, 1900 will achieve complete remission (CR) and 1900 will fail (Fail). Of the 1900 CR patients, 800 will subsequently relapse (Fail). Total failures are 3000 (Fail). Of these, 900 will have an HLA-identical sibling (HLA) and 2100 will not (−HLA). A projected benefit of 30% will result in 700 beneficiaries (EB).

it available. If all transplants are considered, this figure is approximately 12,000.

I also attempted to predict the number of individuals who might benefit if transplants from unrelated HLA-matched donors were performed. In diseases in which transplantation is regarded as likely to be beneficial, the proportion of long-term survivors was calculated by discounting by approximately 20% results obtained in HLA-identical sibling transplants. This resulted in an estimate of about 1275 individuals benefited. Calculations are less precise in diseases in which transplantation is not yet of proven benefit. I have estimated likely outcomes based on currently available, albeit incomplete, data. Again, it is likely that these figures will be regarded as either overly optimistic or pessimistic by different investigators. With these reservations, the estimated beneficial outcome in individuals with disease that may possibly be benefited by transplantation is 3600 and the total number of potential beneficiaries in both disease categories is about 5000.

Several assumptions, reviewed in the *Materials and Methods* section, were required for the calculations presented in this study. Nevertheless, these data provide a reasonable estimate of the number of individuals in the United States who might potentially utilize the HLA-typed unrelated donor pool were it available. These calculations assume that a potential donor can be identified for each recipient. It is unlikely that, regardless of pool size, such a projection will be achieved. It is relatively simple, however, to correct these data for the proportional numbers of HLA-matches achieved.

These data should be of use to individuals involved in bone marrow transplantation, histocompatibility testing, blood banking, and health care planning. Several regional HLA-typed donor pools currently exist and are increasingly used to provide donors for transplantation. Efforts are underway to centralize these data and increase the rate at which transplants from unrelated donors are performed—These data should prove useful in these planning efforts. Recent experience in the nuclear reactor accident at Chernobyl likewise suggests a potentially important use for an HLA-typed bone marrow donor pool.

Acknowledgments. The following persons assisted me greatly in the compilation of data related to this study: Dr. John Young, SEER, NCI, NIH, USPHS, DHHS; Drs. Harry Rosenberg and Francis Edmonds, NCHS, USPHS, DHHS; Ms. Marianne Jordan, Leukemia Society of America; Drs. Alan Levine and Anne Ball, NHLBI, NIH, USPHS DHHS; Dr. Jane Schutz, NIAID, NIH, USPHS, DHHS; Dr. Robertson Parkman, Los Angeles Children's Hospital; Dr. Carol Hyman, Cedar-Sinai Medical Center, Los Angeles; Dr. Moyses Szklo, Johns Hopkins University; Mr. Michael DiFilippo, Cooley Anemia Foundation.

REFERENCES

1. Gale RP, ed. Recent advances in bone marrow transplantation. New York: Liss, 1983.
2. van Rood JJ, Zwaan F, eds. Bone marrow transplantation. Semin Hematol 21: 1.
3. O'Reilly RJ. Allogeneic bone marrow transplantation: current status and future directions. Blood 1983; 62: 841.
4. Champlin RE, Gale RP. Role of bone marrow transplantation in the treatment of hematologic malignancies and solid tumors: critical review of syngeneic, autologous, and allogenic transplants. Cancer Treat Rep 1983; 68: 145.

5. Young JL Jr, Percy CL, Ajire AJ, eds. Surveillance epidemiology end results: incidence and mortality data 1973–77. NCI Monograph S7, USDHHA, PHS, NIH, NCI, Bethesda, MD, 1981.
6. Seidman H, Mashinski MH, Gelb SK, Silverberg E. Probabilities of eventually developing or dying of cancer, United States, 1985. Ca-A Cancer J Clinicians 1985; 35: 36.
7. Szklo M, Sensenbrenner L, Markowitz J, Weida S, Warm S, Linet M. Incidence of aplastic anemia in metropolitan Baltimore: a population based study. Blood in press.
8. Crocker AC, ed. Thalassemia in Southeast Asian refugees: public health planning aspects. Developmental Evaluation Clinic, Children's Hospital, Boston, MA.
9. Camitta B, O'Reilly R, Sensenbrenner L, et al. Antithoracic duct lymphocyte globulin therapy of severe aplastic anemia. Blood 1983; 62: 883.

Received 1 August 1985.
Accepted 7 November 1985.

0041-1337/86/4201-0058$02.00/0
TRANSPLANTATION

Vol. 42, No. 1
Printed in U.S.A.

MARROW FUNCTION RECONSTITUTION BY FRACTION 3 OF PERCOLL-DENSITY-GRADIENT–SEPARATED CELLS

HENRY EKERT,[1,2] W. MARY ELLIS,[1] GEORGE M. GEORGIOU,[3] DON M. ROBERTON,[3] KARIN TIEDEMANN,[1] AND KEITH D. WATERS[1]

Department of Clinical Haematology and Oncology, and Department of Immunology,† Royal Children's Hospital, Parkville, Victoria 3052, Australia*

Eight children with advanced tumors or acute myeloid leukemia were treated either with very-high-dose multi-agent chemotherapy (*4*) or marrow ablative high-dose melphalan (*4*) followed by autologous marrow rescue, using only fraction 3 from a Percoll-discontinuous density gradient separation of bone marrow buffy coats. Each patient received less than 20% of the number of cells usually reinfused from the buffy coat. The yield of CFU-c in Percoll gradient 3 was similar to the yield obtained from whole buffy coats of bone marrow. Reconstitution of marrow function with a neutrophil count >0.5×10⁹/L and platelet count >50×10⁹/L occurred in 7 patients in a medium time of 15 and 16 days, respectively—a time comparable to that following infusion of whole buffy coat in 20 other patients. In one patient, hemopoietic recovery was considerably delayed, suggesting that fraction 3 from the Percoll gradient had been relatively ineffective in marrow reconstitution. We conclude that fraction 3 from marrow separated on Percoll gradients has the advantages of small volume and good recovery of marrow stem cells and can promptly reconstitute marrow function in the majority of children treated with very-high-dose chemotherapy or marrow ablative doses of melphalan.

Very-high-dose chemotherapy for the treatment of solid tumors or leukemia may be followed by either allogeneic or autologous bone marrow transplantation. In autologous transplantation, it is usual to infuse the buffy coat of cryopreserved marrow (*1, 2*). The buffy coat contains blood and bone marrow cells, of which only a small minority are the progenitor cells required for marrow reconstitution. The cryopreservation medium usually contains 5% dimethylsulphoxide (DMSO),* and serum and reinfusion of considerable volumes is inconvenient and can be associated with the risk of anaphylactic reactions and considerable cell clumping, which increases with the duration of infusion. The expense of cryopreservation of buffy coats of harvested bone marrow is considerable, due to the large volumes that require freezing and storage. These problems could be reduced if only cells required for marrow reconstitution could be cryopreserved and reinfused.

Recent refinements of density gradient centrifugation techniques have shown that it is possible to concentrate in a single fraction cells that have proliferative potential for the granulocytic (CFU-c) and erythroid (BFU-E) series in bone marrow culture systems (*3, 4*). In the study reported here, we show that infusion of fraction 3 of Percoll discontinuous density gradient-separated cells from eight children treated with very-high-dose chemotherapy, resulted in reconstitution of marrow function in a time comparable to that following infusion of buffy coat in 21 other patients (*5*).

MATERIALS AND METHODS

Eight patients were entered in the study; three had abdominal non-Hodgkin's lymphoma, one rhabdomyosarcoma (RMS), two with neuroblastoma (NBL) and two with acute myeloid leukaemia (AML) (Table 1). On morphologic examination, the marrow was uninvolved with tumor cells. Marrow was harvested from the first four patients (*1–4*) before any chemotherapy was given. In the other four (*5–8*), marrow harvest was undertaken after remission induction and consolidation chemotherapy had been given. The high-dose chemotherapy programs used in

[1]Department of Clinical Haematology and Oncology.
[2]Address correspondence to: Dr. Henry Ekert, Director, Department of Clinical Haematology & Oncology, Royal Children's Hospital, Flemington Road, Parkville, Victoria 3052, Australia.
[3]Department of Immunology.

* Abbreviations used: AML, acute myeloid leukemia, BSA, bovine serum albumin; DMSO, dimethylsulfoxide; HBSS, Hanks' buffered saline solution; NBL, neuroblastoma; RMS, rhabdomyosarcoma.

these patients immediately prior to marrow transplantation are detailed in Table 1.

The procedures for bone marrow harvest, cryopreservation, storage, thawing, and reinfusion have been described previously (*2*). Briefly, 3×10^8 cells/kg of body weight were harvested by multiple small aspirates of bone marrow from anterior and posterior iliac crests. After aspiration, the marrow was filtered and the nucleated white cells or buffy coat were separated from red blood cells and plasma by centrifugation. The buffy coat was suspended in 10% DMSO and 20% fetal calf serum in Hanks' balanced salt solution (HBSS) in 5-ml ampoules and frozen at −1°C/min to −80°C. The buffy coat was then stored in liquid nitrogen until used. When required for reinfusion, the ampoules were thawed rapidly and the contents transferred to a bag, diluted 1:1 with HBSS, and mixed gently. The bag was then taken to the patient and reinfused rapidly.

The additional method of separation on discontinuous Percoll gradients has also been described in detail (*4, 6*). Bone marrow buffy coats were collected and evenly aliquoted over 16 discontinuous Percoll gradients for each patient. The Percoll gradients were made up of 2 ml each of 70, 60, 50, and 40% Percoll layered carefully over one another. Fraction 3, at the interface between 50 and 60%, which is enriched for progenitor cells, was collected, washed, cryopreserved, thawed, and reinfused. In patient number 5, fraction 3 was not cryopreserved, but was stored overnight at 4°C before reinfusion. CFU-c assays were carried out using a microassay (*5*) on leukocyte-conditioned medium underlayers as a source of colony-stimulating factor.

TABLE 1. Chemical data and chemotherapy

Patient no.	Age	Sex	Diagnosis	Chemotherapy	
				Drug	Dose
1	13	M	NHL[a]	VCR	1.5 mg/m^2×2
				CTX	1200 mg/m^2×4
				Ara-C	40 mg/m^2×12
				MTX	7.5 mg/m^2×3
2	3	F	NHL	As in 1	As in 1
3	11	F	NHL	As in 1	As in 1
4	9	M	Rhabdo.	CTX	1200 mg/m^2×4
				Adria	30 mg/m^2×3
				VCR	1.5 mg/m^2×2
5	9	F	Neuro.	Melphalan	150 mg/m^2
6	7½	F	Neuro.	Melphalan	150 mg/m^2
7	11½	M	AML	Melphalan	150 mg/m^2
8	3½	M	AML	Melphalan	150 mg/m^2

[a] VCR, vincristine; CTX, cytoxan; MTX, methotrexate; NHL, non-Hodgkin's lymphoma; Rhabdo., rhabdomyosarcoma; Neuro., neuroblastoma; AML, acute myeloid leukemia.

RESULTS

The total number of nucleated buffy coat cells applied to the Percoll gradients for each patient is shown in Table 2, together with the percentage recovery of the total cell number in fraction 3. The number of cells and CFU-c in the reinfusion inoculum per kilogram of body weight are also shown. Reconstitution of marrow function was monitored by daily full blood counts. The nadir of 0.1×10^9/L total white cells and less than 20×10^9/L platelets occurred on days 7 or 8 in all patients. Recovery of neutrophils to greater than 0.5×10^9/L occurred between days 12–18, and recovery of platelets to greater than 50×10^9/L by days 8–18 in all but one patient. In patient 5, recovery of neutrophils was delayed until day 25, and platelets until day 47.

In a historical control group of 20 patients, buffy coat was reinfused following high-dose multi-agent chemotherapy similar to that used in patients 1–4 and always incorporating cytoxan 1200 mg/m^2 given daily in 4 doses. Patients 9–18 had received no prior chemotherapy before marrow harvest and were therefore similar to patients 1–4. Hematologic reconstitution occurred in a similar time. Patients 19–29 had received prior chemotherapy before bone marrow harvest and are similar to patients 5–8. Hematologic reconstitution in these patients occurred in a similar time, but was delayed compared with that in patients who had not received chemotherapy before bone marrow harvest. Only the difference in platelet recovery time was statistically significant ($P<0.05$).

Clinically, the non-Hodgkin's lymphomas all responded with complete remission of tumor, but there was one early central nervous system relapse. The patient with rhabdomyosarcoma did not respond at all, and the patients with neuroblastoma and acute myeloid leukemia remain in remission. The duration of follow-up in these patients ranges from 1–18 months.

DISCUSSION

Although the median number of cells cryopreserved was less than 20% of the total number of nucleated cells, the CFU-c recovery was within the range seen for untreated buffy coats

TABLE 2. Results of cell separation on percoll gradients and hematologic recovery compared with buffy coat reinfusions

Patient no.	No. cells ×10^6/gradient	% Buffy coat	NO. cells ×10^8/kg reinfused	No. CFU-c ×10^4/kg	Hematologic recovery (days)	
					Neutrophils >0.5×10^9/L	Platelets >50×10^9/L
1	886	8	0.26	2.34	14	16
2	521	9	0.46	7.31	14	8
3	519	14	0.35	4.24	17	16
4	717	8	0.13	1.42	14	12
5	1075	4	0.21	2.46	25	47
6	922	17	0.26	1.52	12	12
7	722	20	0.47	4.25	17	17
8	700	11	0.52	7.03	18	18
Buffy coat reinfusions:						
9–18 (no prior chemotherapy)		100	Median 2.58, range 1.56–4.03	Median 7.28, range 0.53–32.71	Median 12, range 6–21	Median 13, range 6–23
19–29 (prior chemotherapy)		100	Median 2.17, range 1.08–2.93	Median 3.37, range 1.02–20.67	Median 17, range 9–28	Median 21, range 11–32

(Table 2). The time for recovery of hemopoietic function, as represented by a rise in neutrophil and platelet numbers in seven of the eight patients reported here, was also within the range of patients whose whole marrow buffy coat was cryopreserved and reinfused for both patients not previously treated with chemotherapy (N1–4 cf. 9–18; Table 2) and for those previously treated with chemotherapy (N5–8 cf. 19–29; Table 2).

The intensity of multi-agent chemotherapy in patients 1–4 and the dose of melphalan (140 mg/m^2) in patients 5–8 were such that if total bone marrow ablation was not achieved, the cellularity would have been reduced to such an extent that spontaneous recovery of hemopoiesis would have required at least 4, and more often 6, weeks. With the exception of patient 5, hemopoietic recovery occurred far more rapidly, providing evidence that fraction 3 from bone marrow separated on Percoll gradient of discontinuous density and osmolality did reconstitute marrow function in 7 out of 8 patients. In patient 5, one could argue that reinfusion of Percoll gradient 3 failed to accelerate hemopoietic recovery.

Density gradient separation of bone marrow prior to its use in transplantation has been reported previously using both bovine serum albumin (BSA) and Ficoll (*7, 8, 9*). In tube centrifugation methods using these materials, the gradients are readily overloaded resulting in the loss of large numbers of cells, and extensive washing of harvested cells is required because of the viscous nature of both BSA and Ficoll, again with considerable loss. These disadvantages led us to investigate the usefulness of Percoll for gradient separation. In two previous studies, we reported the use of a Percoll gradient of discontinuous density and osmolality for rapid separation of nucleated bone marrow cells (4, 6). The median cell recovery from fraction 3 from the Percoll gradient was 12.6% of the nucleated cell number applied for nine marrows studied, while that for cells from the same marrows applied to Ficoll-paque was 20.6% (*6*). The median CFU-c recoveries within these mononuclear cell fractions were $10.8\times10^4/10^9$ nucleated marrow cells applied to Percoll gradients and $11.3\times10^4/10^9$ nucleated marrow cells applied to Ficoll-paque gradients. The resulting enrichment for CFU-c on Percoll was 1.6 times that of Ficoll-paque. In a second study of seven marrows separated on Percoll, the median nucleated cell recovery on Percoll was 9.2% with a CFU-c recovery of $8.6\times10^4/10^9$ nucleated marrow cells applied (*4*). This again represents an enrichment for CFU-c recovery of 1.7 times that of the recovery for Ficoll-paque as described above. These median CFU-c recoveries are considerably higher than those from unfractionated marrow used for successful autologous transplantation in leukemic patients or patients with solid tumors as reported by Spitzer et al. (*10*), but are not as high as the median recovery of 25.3×10^4 CFU-c/10^9 nucleated cells following Ficoll-metrizoate separation on an IBM blood cell processor as reported by Gilmore et al. (*9*). However, this latter facility is not readily available in many laboratories.

In addition, the Percoll gradients described tolerate greater cell loads, with up to 1×10^9 nucleated cells being able to be applied to each 8-ml gradient. The lower cell recovery also results in a greater absolute depletion of T cells (*4*), a factor that may be of importance in allogeneic transplantation with respect to the avoidance of graft-versus-host disease. The lower total cell numbers recovered may allow more ready subsequent treatment of marrow with monoclonal antibodies in experimental approaches to marrow purging of immunocompetent or tumor cells (*11–14*). Other advantages of the small cell numbers are in cryopreservation with smaller volume storage requirements and the possibility of more rapid reinfusion.

By morphologic examination of Percoll gradients, we have observed that T cells, lymphoblasts, and neuroblastoma cells are concentrated in band 2 of the gradient, and depleted—but not eliminated—from band 3 (Macfarlane et al., unpublished observation).

REFERENCES

1. Appelbaum FR, Herzig GP, Ziegler JL, Graw RG, Levine AS, Deisseroth AB. Successful engraftment of cryopreserved autologous bone marrow in patients with malignant lymphoma. Blood 1978; 52: 85.
2. Ekert H, Ellis WM, Waters KD, Tauro GP. Autologous bone marrow rescue in the treatment of advanced tumours of childhood. Cancer 1982; 49: 603.
3. Ekert H, Tiedemann K, Waters KD, Ellis WM. Experience with high dose multiagent chemotherapy and autologous bone marrow rescue in the treatment of twenty-two children with advanced tumours. Aust Paediatr J 1984; 20: 195.
4. Ellis WM, Georgiou GM, Roberton DM, Johnson GR. The use of discontinuous Percoll gradients to separate populations of cells from human bone marrow and peripheral blood. J Immunol Methods 1984; 66: 9.
5. Ellis WM, Georgiou GM, Robertson DM, Turner JJ, Rendall KE. The development of a microassay for human committed progenitor cells. Int J Cell Cloning 1984; 2: 89.
6. Georgiou GM, Robertson DM, Ellis WM, Shen BJ, Ekert H, Hosking CS. CFU-c enrichment from human bone marrow using a discontinuous Percoll gradient and soy-bean agglutinin in comparison with Ficoll-paque. Clin Exp Immunol 1983; 53: 491.
7. Dicke KA, McCredie KB, Spitzer G, Zander A, Peters L, Verma JS, Stewart J, Keatirg M, Stevens EE. Autologous bone marrow transplantation in patients with adult acute leukemia in relapse. Transplantation 1978; 26: 169.
8. Wells JR, Sullivan A, Clive MJ. A technique for the separation and cryopreservation of myeloid stem cells from human bone marrow. Cryobiology 1979; 16: 201.
9. Gilmore MJML, Prentice HG, Blacklock HA, Ma JJF, Janossy G, Hoffbrand AV. A technique for rapid isolation of bone marrow mononuclear cells using Ficoll-metrizoate and the IBM 2991 blood cell processor. Br J Haematol 1982; 50: 619.
10. Spitzer G, Verma JS, Fisher R, Zander A, Vellekoop L, Litan J, McCredie KB, Dicke KA. The myeloid progenitor cell: its value in predicting hematopoietic recovery after autologous bone marrow transplantation. Blood 1980; 55: 317.
11. Prenctice HG, Blacklock HA, Janossy G, Bradstock KF, Skeggs J, Goldstein G, Hoffbrand AV. Use of anti-T-cell monoclonal antibody OKT3 to prevent acute graft versus host disease in allogeneic bone marrow transplantation for acute leukaemia. Lancet 1982; 2: 700.
12. Waldmann H, Polliak A, Hale G, et al. Elimination of graft versus host disease by in-vitro depletion of alloreactive lymphocytes with a monoclonal rat anti-human lymphocyte antibody (Campath-1). Lancet 1984; 2: 485.
13. Filipovich AH, Vallera DA, Youle RJ, Quinones RR, Neville JM, Kersey JM. Ex-vivo treatment of donor bone marrow with anti-T-cell immunotoxins for prevention of graft versus host disease. Lancet 1984; 1: 469.
14. Treleaven JG, Gibson FM, Ugelstad J, Rembaum A, Philips T, Caine GD, Kemshead JT. Removal of neuroblastoma cells from bone marrow with monoclonal antibody conjugated to magnetic microspheres. Lancet 1984; 1: 70.

Received 6 September 1985.
Accepted 15 October 1985.

0041-1337/86/4201-0061$02.00/0
TRANSPLANTATION
Vol. 42, No. 1

Printed in U.S.A.

MUTAGENICITY OF CYCLOSPORINE

INDUCTION OF SISTER CHROMATID EXCHANGE IN HUMAN CELLS[1]

KENJI YUZAWA, IKUKO KONDO,[2] KATASHI FUKAO, YOJI IWASAKI, AND HIDEO HAMAGUCHI[2, 3]

Department of Surgery, Institute of Clinical Medicine, and Department of Human Genetics, Institute of Basic Medical Sciences, University of Tsukuba, Niihari-gun, Ibaraki 305, Japan

To examine whether cyclosporine (CsA) has mutagenic potential against human cells, we analyzed sister chromatid exchange (SCE) induction by CsA using human lymphocytes in vitro. SCE frequencies increased significantly in the lymphocytes treated with 1 μg/ml and 5 μg/ml CsA, though the frequencies seemed to be less than one hundredth of those induced by mitomycin C (MMC). The value of induced SCE depended on CsA concentration. This result indicates that CsA has SCE inducibility. The data also suggest that CsA has a mutagenic effect on human lymphocytes.

Cyclosporine (CsA),* a cyclic undecapeptide of fungal origin, is a novel immunosuppressive drug with potent immunopharmacological properties (*1*). Compared with the conventional immunosuppressants in clinical use, such as azathioprine and cyclophosphamide, CsA represents an entirely new class of immunosuppressive drugs with its own physicochemical properties (*2*). The bulk of information on its mechanism of action points toward an effect on an early phase of the immune response, specifically, a preferential inhibition of the activation of T lymphocytes (*3–6*).

Development of malignant neoplasms is an important complication of immunosuppressive therapy in recipients of organ transplants (*7–9*). At a conservative estimate, the incidence of lymphoma in transplant patients treated with CsA was 0.7% (*10*). Although the exact mechanisms leading to the high risk of malignant neoplasms in organ transplant recipients have not been elucidated yet, multiple factors are probably involved in the etiology of the various tumors. They include disturbances of immunity, the oncogenic effects of immunosuppressive agents as mutagens, and possible cooncogenic properties of these compounds (*11*).

Conventional immunosuppressants, such as azathioprine and cyclophosphamide, have been reported to have cytostatic effects and mutagenicity (*12, 13*). The mutagenicity of immunosuppressants has been assessed in vitro using the Ames test, in which Salmonella is used (*14*), and in vivo by chromosomal analysis in experimental animals (*15*). In these analytical systems, CsA per se had no mutagenic effects (*16, 17*). However, the mutagenic potential of CsA for human cells has not been examined yet.

To examine whether CsA has a mutagenic potential for human cells, we analyzed the sister chromatid exchange (SCE) (*18, 19*) induction by CsA using human lymphocytes in vitro.

MATERIALS AND METHODS

CsA was kindly provided by Dr. E. Wiskott, Sandoz, Inc., Basel, Switzerland. It was dissolved in dimethylsulfoxide (DMSO, Wako Pure Chemical Industries, Ltd., Osaka, Japan) and diluted to an appropriate concentration (final concentration: 5, 1, 0.2, and 0.04 μg/ml) with culture medium, TC199 (Gibco) supplemented with 10% fetal calf serum. Heparinized peripheral blood lymphocytes were obtained from three healthy adults, a 28-year-old man (individual A), a 23-year-old woman (individual B) and a 29-year-old man (individual C) and cultured in medium with CsA for 2 hr at 37°C in a humidified atmosphere with 5% CO_2. Phytohemagglutinin P (PHA-P, Difco) and 5-bromodeoxyuridine (BrdU, Wako Pure Chemical Industries, Ltd., Osaka, Japan) were added to the culture medium and the cells were further cultured in the dark for 4 days at 37°C in a humidified atmosphere with 5% CO_2. After treatment with Colcemid (0.1 μg/ml) for 1 hr, the cells were collected, treated with 0.075 M KCl at 37°C for 20 min, and then fixed with methanol–acetic acid (3:1, v/v) according to standard methods (*20*). The cell suspensions were dropped onto dry slides, stained for 10 min with 0.5 μg/ml Hoechst 33258 (Hoechst) in 0.01 M phosphate-buffer solution, pH 7.0, containing 0.15 M NaCl and 0.3 M KCl, rinsed in distilled water, mounted with buffer under coverslips, and exposed to a UV light source (Panaball Ballastless Mercury Lamp, BH100-110V 100W, Matsushita Electric Industrial Company, Ltd., Osaka, Japan) for 30 min. The slides were then stained with 2% Giemsa (Merck Japan, Tokyo, Japan) in Sorensen's buffer, pH 7.0, for 10 min. Mitotic indexes were scored as numbers of metaphases versus total cell numbers for each concentration of CsA. SCEs in more than 30 metaphases were scored for each concentration of CsA. SCE values were subjected to statistical analysis using Student's t test (one-tailed). SCE values observed in the presence of 0.5% DMSO were used as controls, and those observed in the presence of 0.03 μg/ml mitomycin C (MMC) were used as a positive control.

RESULTS

Fig. 1 shows a typical SCE pattern in lymphocytes induced by 5 μg/ml CsA in which 15 SCEs are observed. As shown in Fig. 2, the mitotic index decreases remarkably in lymphocytes treated with a high concentration of CsA. This phenomenon has been reported previously (*4*). SCEs were scored in cells

[1] This work was supported by a Grant-in-Aid for Scientific Research from the Minstry of Education, Science and Culture, Japan.

[2] Department of Human Genetics.

[3] To whom correspondence and requests for reprints should be addressed, at Department of Human Genetics, Institute of Basic Medical Sciences, University of Tsukuba, Niihari-gun, Ibaraki 305, Japan.

* Abbreviations used: BrdU, 5-bromodeoxyuridine; CsA, cyclosporine (previously names cyclosporin A); DMSO, dimethylsulfoxide; MMC, mitomycin C; PHA-P, phytohemagglutinin P; SCE, sister chromatid exchange.

with metaphases under these proliferation-suppressed conditions. Table 1 presents the results of SCE induction by CsA. SCEs increased significantly in the presence of 5 μg/ml CsA in the cells from individuals A and B ($P<0.01$). In the cells from individual C, a sufficient number of metaphases were not analyzable at this concentration of CsA. SCE frequencies also increased significantly in the presence of 1 μg/ml CsA in cells from all three individuals ($P<0.01$). Furthermore, in the case of individual C, SCEs increased slightly but significantly even in 0.2 μg/ml CsA ($P<0.05$). The degree of SCE induction depended on the CsA concentration when more than 0.2 μg/ml CsA was used. To examine the reproducibility of the results, SCE induction by CsA was analyzed three months later, using lymphocytes from individual A. The result was very similar to that of the first experiment (Table 1). The number of SCEs induced by CsA seemed to be less than one hundredth of that induced by MMC: The SCE values induced by 5 μg/ml CsA were 12.5–15.3, compared to the SCE values induced by 0.03 μg/ml MMC of 16.4–22.5.

DISCUSSION

In the present study, it has been shown that SCE frequencies increased in lymphocytes treated with 1 μg/ml CsA in all three individuals examined. In addition, the frequencies became higher in lymphocytes from two individuals treated with 5 μg/ml CsA in which a sufficient number of metaphases were available for the SCE analysis. The elevated values were statistically significant ($P<0.01$) and depended on the CsA concentration. This result indicates that CsA has SCE inducibility in 1 μg/ml CsA, at least in vitro. Since mutagenic chemical agents induce chromosomal abnormalities and SCEs and since SCE occurs as a result of DNA damage, either directly or indirectly, by mutagenic agents (*21, 22*), the result also suggests that CsA may have a mutagenic effect on human lymphocytes.

Wide clinical usage of CsA has revealed some adverse effects.

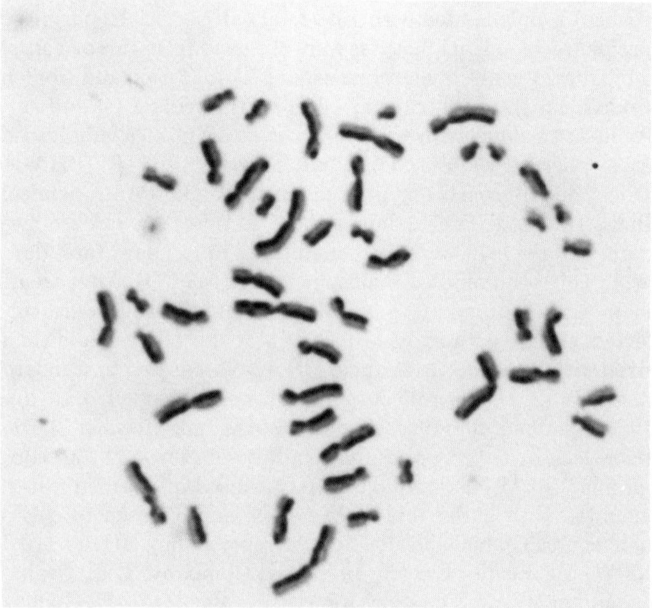

FIGURE 1. SCE pattern in a cell from individual A treated with 5 μg/ml cyclosporine (CsA) (Original magnification, ×1000).

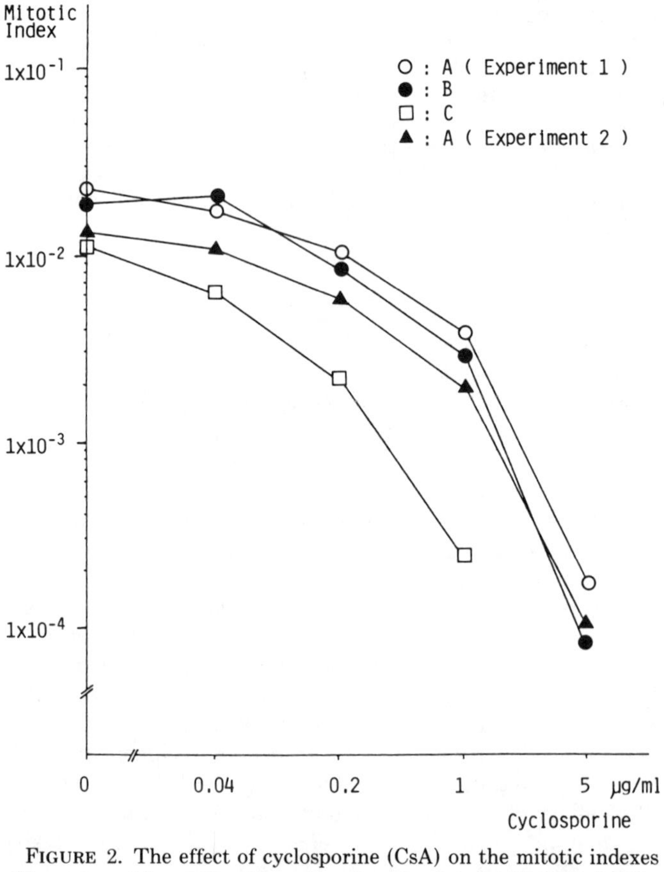

FIGURE 2. The effect of cyclosporine (CsA) on the mitotic indexes of human peripheral blood lymphocytes stimulated with PHA-P. The mitotic indexes were scored as the ration of numbers of metaphases to total cell numbers for each concentration of CsA. Lymphocytes were obtained from three healthy adults: individual A (○, ▲), individual B (●), and individual C (□).

TABLE 1. SCE induction by cyclosporine (CsA) in human peripheral blood lymphocytes from three individuals in vitro

Experimental conditions		SCEs/cell (mean ± SD)			
CsA (μg/ml)	DMSO (%)	A:28 y.o. man Experiment 1	A:28 y.o. man Experiment 2	B:23 y.o. woman	C:29 y.o. man
0	0	8.43±2.86	7.70±2.34	7.40±2.44	7.47±2.16
0	0.5	7.83±2.38	7.82±2.41	8.32±2.68	8.16±2.26
0.04	0.5	8.46±2.27 NS[a]	8.20±3.01 NS	8.60±2.24 NS	8.40±2.51 NS
0.2	0.5	8.12±2.46 NS	8.22±2.54 NS	9.30±2.17 NS	9.58±2.60[c]
1	0.5	10.29±3.05[b]	9.80±3.20[b]	11.90±2.44[b]	11.57±2.74[b]
5	0.5	13.97±2.51[b]	12.50±2.82[b]	15.32±4.37[b]	Not analyzable
MMC: 0.03 μg/ml	0	19.37±7.63	22.50±6.57	16.43±5.62	22.10±7.59

[a] NS: no significant difference.
[b] Statistically significant difference ($P<0.01$).
[c] Statistically significant difference ($P<0.05$).

The major adverse effects are nephrotoxicity, hyperkalemia, hepatotoxicity, lymphoma, gingival hyperplasia, hirsutism, and tremor (*23*). In reviewing the entire experience with lymphoma in CsA-treated organ recipients, 40 patients with lymphoma were reported in 5500 patients treated with CYA, and the incidence of lymphoma in patients was 0.7% (*10*). Generally, there is an increased incidence of malignancies following organ transplantation (*7–9*). The precise mechanism for this remains to be clarified. Conventional immunosuppressive agents, such as azathioprine and 6-mercaptopurine, have effects on DNA synthesis, and consequently have cytotoxic and mutagenic effects on human cells (*24*). On the other hand, it has been reported that CsA per se had no mutagenic effects in various experimental systems in which *Salmonella*, mice, and Chinese hamsters were used (*16*, *17*). Results of one study indicated that over-immunosuppression induced by CsA was a possible cause of lymphoma (*25*). However, the results of the present study suggest that CsA may have a mutagenic effect on human lymphocytes directly or indirectly. It is important to verify that CsA has a mutagenic effect on human lymphocytes as this may be a factor in the genesis of lymphoma.

Acknowledgments. We are grateful to Dr. E. Wiskott, Sandoz, Inc., Basel, Switzerland, for providing CsA as a powder; to Dr. Victor M. Darley-Usmar and Miss Y. Yamanouchi, Institute of Basic Medical Sciences, University of Tsukuba, for valuable suggestions and help; to Mr. M. Teranishi, Mr. M. Yamaguchi, and Mr. S. Abe for photographic assistance; and to Miss M. Sugawara, Miss H. Sukegawa, and Miss N. Morohashi for their help in typing the manuscript.

REFERENCES

1. Borel JF. Cyclosporin A: present experimental studies. Transplant Proc 1981; 13: 344.
2. Petcher TJ, Weber HP, Ruegger A. Crystal and molecular structure of an iododerivative of the cyclic undecapeptide cyclosporin A. Helv Chim Acta 1976; 59: 1480.
3. Palacios R. Mechanism of T cell activation: role and functional relationship of HLA-DR antigens and interleukins. Immunol Rev 1982; 63: 73.
4. Hess AD, Tutschka PJ, Santos GW. The effect of cyclosporin A on T lymphocyte subpopulations. In: White DJG, ed. Cyclosporin A. Amsterdam: Elsevier, 1982: 209.
5. Cammisuli S. The effect of cyclosporin A on cell interactions within the immune system. In: White DJG, ed. Cyclosporin A. Amsterdam: Elsevier, 1982: 243.
6. Bunjes D, Hardt C, Solbach W, Deusch K, Rollinghoff M, Wagner H. Studies on the mechanism of action of cyclosporin A in the murine and human T-cell response in vitro. In: White DJG, ed. Cyclosporin A. Amsterdam: Elsevier, 1982: 261.
7. Filipovich AH, Spector BH, Kersey J, Fraumeni J, Schottenfeld D, Stolley PD. Immunodeficiency in humans as a risk factor in the development of malignancy. Prev Med 1980; 9: 252.
8. Penn I. Malignancies associated with immunosuppressive or cytotoxic therapy. Surgery 1978; 83: 492.
9. Cleary ML. Depressed immunity and the development of cancer. Clin Exp Immunol 1981; 46: 459.
10. Beveridge T, Krupp P, McKibbin C. Letters to the Editor: lymphomas and limphoproliferative lesions developing under cyclosporin therapy. Lancet 1984; 1: 788.
11. Penn I. Lymphomas complicating organ transplantation. Transplant Proc 1983; 15: 2790.
12. Speck WT, Rosenkranz HS. Mutagenicity of azathioprine. Cancer Res 1976; 36: 108.
13. Seino Y, Nagao M, Yahagi T, et al. Mutagenicity of several classes of antitumor agents to Salmonella typhimurium TA 98, TA 100, and TA 92. Cancer Res 1978; 38: 2148.
14. Ames BN. The detection of chemical mutagens with enteric bacteria. In: Hollaender A, ed. Chemical mutagens, vol 1. New York: Plenum Press, 1971: 267.
15. Ad Hoc Committee on chromosome methodologists in mutation testing. Chromosome methodoligies in mutation testing. Toxicol Appl Pharmacol 1976; 36: 108.
16. Matter BE, Donatsch PP, Racube RR, Schmid B, Schmid W. Genotoxicity evaluation of cyclosporin A, a new immunosuppressive agent. Mutat Res 1982; 105: 257.
17. Ryffel B, Donatsch P, Madorin M, et al. Toxicological evaluation of cyclosporin A. Arch Toxicol 1983; 53: 107.
18. Gebhart E. Sister chromatid exchange (SCE) and structural chromosome aberration in mutagenicity testing. Human Genet 1981; 58: 235.
19. Latt SA. Microfluorometric detection of deoxyribonucleic acid replication in human metaphase chromosomes. Proc Natl Acad Sci USA 1973; 70: 3395.
20. Moorhead PS, Nowell PC, Mellman WJ, Battips DM, Hungerford DA. Chromosome preparations of leukocytes cultured from human peripheral blood. Exp Cell Res 1960; 20: 613.
21. Marin G, Prescott DM. The frequency of sister chromatid exchanges following exposure to varying doses of ^{3}H-thymidine or X-rays. J Cell Biol 1964; 21: 159.
22. Kato T. Induction of sister chromatid exchanges by UV light and its inhibition by caffeine. Exp Cell Res 1973; 82: 383.
23. Nelson PW. Cyclosporine. Surg Gynecol Obstet 1984; 159: 297.
24. Jensen MK. Chromosome studies in patients treated with azathioprine and amethopterin. Acta Med Scand 1967; 182: 447.
25. Cleary ML, Warnke R, Sklar J. Monoclonality of lymphoproliferative lesions in cardiac-transplant recipients. N Engl J Med 1984; 310: 477.

Received 17 July 1985.
Accepted 22 October 1985.

0041-1337/86/4201-0064$02.00/0
TRANSPLANTATION
Vol. 42, No. 1

Printed in U.S.A.

IMMUNE TRANSFER STUDIES IN CANINE ALLOGENEIC MARROW GRAFT DONOR-RECIPIENT PAIRS[1]

H. GROSSE-WILDE,[2] K. KRUMBACHER,[2] F. SCHÜNING,[3] I. DOXIADIS,[2] H.K. MAHMOUD,[3] C. EMDE,[3] A. SCHMIDT-WEINMAR,[3] AND U.W. SCHAEFER[3]

Department of Immunogenetics and Department of Internal Medicine (Tumor Research), University Hospital of Essen, D-4300 Essen 1, Federal Republic of Germany

Transfer of immunity occurring with bone marrow grafting was studied using the dog as a preclinical model. Allogeneic bone marrow transplantation (BMT) was performed between DLA-identical beagle littermates. The donors were immunized with tetanus toxoid (TT) or sheep red blood cells (SRBC), and their humoral response was monitored by hemagglutination. The recipients of bone marrow from TT-immunized donors showed a marked increase of antibody titer one week posttransplantation, while in the recipients of marrow from SRBC immunized donors the antibody titers were considerably lower. Within the following 60 days the antibody titers in both groups diminished gradually to pregrafting levels. Control experiments in which cell-free plasma from donors immunized with TT and SRBC respectively was transfused indicated that the initial rise of specific antibody titers after marrow grafting is likely to be due to a passive transfer of humoral immunity. A single challenge of these marrow graft recipients with the respective antigen 15–18 weeks posttransplantation led to a secondary type of humoral immune response. In addition, it could be demonstrated that transfer of memory against TT or SRBC was independent from the actual antibody titer and the time of vaccination of the donor. One dog was immunized with TT after serving as marrow donor. When the donor had shown an antibody response, a peripheral blood leukocytes (PBL) transfusion was given to his chimera. Subsequent challenge of the latter resulted in a secondary type of specific antibody response. This indicates that specific cellular-bound immunological memory can be transferred after BMT from the donor to his allogeneic bone marrow chimera by transfusion of peripheral blood leukocytes.

The data presented may be of importance in clinical BMT to protect patients during the phase of reduced immune reactivity by transfer of memory cells from histocompatible immunized donors.

In addition to the risk of development of graft-versus-host disease (GVHD)* human bone marrow graft recipients are especially threatened by viral, fungal, and bacterial infections because of a severe cellular and humoral immune deficiency. Therefore the problem of immunologic reconstitution after grafting remains a subject of intensive in vivo and in vitro studies.

Humoral and cell-mediated reactivity have been widely investigated in human and canine bone marrow chimeras (*1–4*). Depressed in vivo immune functions in the early postgrafting period, such as poor antibody responses and poor delayed-type hypersensitivity reactions correlate with abnormal in vitro reactions, such as disturbed immunoglobulin production and T cell function. The protection of transplanted patients during the period of greatest susceptibility to infections is possible with the administration of hyperimmunoglobulin (*5*).

We wished to study the transfer of cellular-bound immunocompetence inherent in bone marrow grafting. Earlier studies, concerning transfer of immunity with transplantation of bone marrow cells, were mainly carried out in inbred mice (*6–8*). These data, however, cannot be extrapolated to the human situation directly because of the different genetic background and the homing of immunocompetent cells.

The dog as an outbred animal model was therefore chosen to investigate whether specific immune memory can be transferred from a donor to radiation bone marrow chimeras.

MATERIALS AND METHODS

Animals and experimental groups. Litters of beagles were purchased from the breeding colonies of the University of Heidelberg and the University of Düsseldorf. The dogs were immunized against distemper, canine hepatitis, leptospirosis, and rabies, but their humoral response was not studied. Three bone marrow donors were immunized with tetanus toxoid (TT) and sheep red blood cells (SRBC), respectively. One of the TT-immunized donors was used twice to study transfer of immunity at different times after vaccination. A further dog was immunized with TT after bone marrow donation. In all, 8 bone marrow recipients and 7 donors were investigated.

Matching for histocompatibility antigens. Dog familes were typed for the canine major histocompatibility complex (DLA) by serology and by unidirectional MLC (*9*). All donor-recipient pairs were DLA-identical littermates.

Conditioning and bone marrow grafting. To achieve decontamination, dogs received oral, non absorbable antibiotics and antimycotics starting 14 days before transplantation. The transplantation conditioning regimen included 7 Gy total-body irradiation from a 60 Co source at a dose rate of 0.17 Gy/min. Bone marrow was infused on day 0 with a mononuclear cell count of $4–6\times10^8$/kg body weight. For the prevention of GVHD, methotrexate was given i.v. on days 1, 3, 6 and 11, and once weekly thereafter until day 100. Besides hematological reconstitution, sex chromosomes were used as a genetic marker to confirm engraftment.

[1] This work was supported by Deutsche Forschungsgemeinschaft SFB 102 TP E1 & E2.

[2] Department of Immunogenetics.

[3] Department of Internal Medicine (Tumor Research).

* Abbreviations used: BMT, bone marrow transplantation; DLA, dog leukocyte antigens; GVHD, graft-versus-host disease; MLC, mixed lymphocyte culture; Lf, lethal factor; PBL, peripheral blood leukocytes; PBS, phosphate-buffered saline; SRBC, sheep red blood cells; TT, tetanus toxoid.

Immunization procedures. Immunization of donors with TT was performed with tetanus vaccine for animals (Behringwerke Marburg, F.R.G.). The dogs received two i.m. injections of 1 ml TT (=30 lethal factor [Lf]) four weeks apart. Blood samples were taken once before immunization and weekly thereafter. Sera were stored at −80°C. For immunization of donors with SRBC, 2 ml of a 10% SRBC suspension in 0.9% saline was injected i.v. (*10*). Two booster injections with 0.5 ml of packed SRBC were given i.d. at three-week intervals. Recipients were challenged with 1 ml TT given i.m. or with 2 ml of 10% SRBC suspensions given i.v.

Hemagglutination assays. Humoral immune reactivity to TT was measured by passive hemagglutination of sensitized SRBC. The antigen used was a TT concentrate (1000 Lf/ml), kindly provided by Dr. Reber, Behringwerke Marburg (F.R.G.), which was conjugated to SRBC with glutaraldehyde (*11*). In pilot studies it was shown that the binding of 500 Lf to 10 ml of a 0.5% SRBC suspension yielded the best standardization of the assay. Two ml of a 2.5% suspension of SRBC was mixed with 4 ml of TT solution (125 Lf/ml) and 2 ml of 1% glutaraldehyde in phosphate-buffered saline (PBS), and incubated for 2 hr at 37°C. The sensitized SRBC were washed three times with PBS and adjusted to 0.5%. Before testing, sera were inactivated for 30 min. at 56°C and absorbed with washed untreated SRBC to remove natural hemagglutinins. Serum antibodies against SRBC were determined in microtiter plates by indirect hemagglutination using rabbit anti-dog-Ig (Medac, F.R.G.). After 15 hr incubation at room temperature, hemagglutination titers were registered.

RESULTS

Humoral immune response to TT. The first immunization of three donors with TT led to the development of slowly rising antibody levels over a period of four weeks. The second immunization yielded a rapid antibody increase one week later of up to 2^{14} (Fig. 1). After a slight decline during the following five weeks, the antibody titers remained stable for more than seven months. The sera of the respective marrow recipients showed a rise in antibody titers to 2^{6} within two weeks of transplantation. However, five weeks later the antibody titers dropped to values equivalent to those before grafting. The challenge of the recipients 16 weeks after grafting resulted in an antibody rise to titers of 2^{9} within one week. The titers remained at the same level throughout the time of observation, corresponding to those found in the donors.

Humoral immune response to SRBC. As shown in Figure 2, antibody formation against SRBC differed from the response to TT. A clear increase in antibody levels was already seen one week after primary immunization with SRBC. All sera of dogs tested contained variable (2^{2}-2^{5}) natural hemagglutinins against SRBC. The i.m. booster injections led to a peak of antibody production. Thereafter the antibodies decreased continuously. In marrow recipients of SRBC-immunized donors a slight and temporary rise of specific antibody titers was observed for three weeks. A challenge with SRBC given i.v. 14 weeks later induced antibody responses corresponding to those found in the donors after three immunizations.

Plasma transfer. From each donor immunized with TT or SRBC respectively, a plasma transfer was carried out to an unrelated dog without previous contact with the respective antigen. The cell free plasma was transfused on days 0, 9, and 10, corresponding to the bone marrow and blood transfusion regimen of transplantation. In the recipient of plasma from the TT-hyperimmunized donor an immediate rise in antibody titers to 2^{9} appeared. The transfusion of plasma containing SRBC antibodies resulted in only a small rise of antibody level in the recipient (Fig. 3).

Transfusion of PBL. One recipient was grafted with marrow

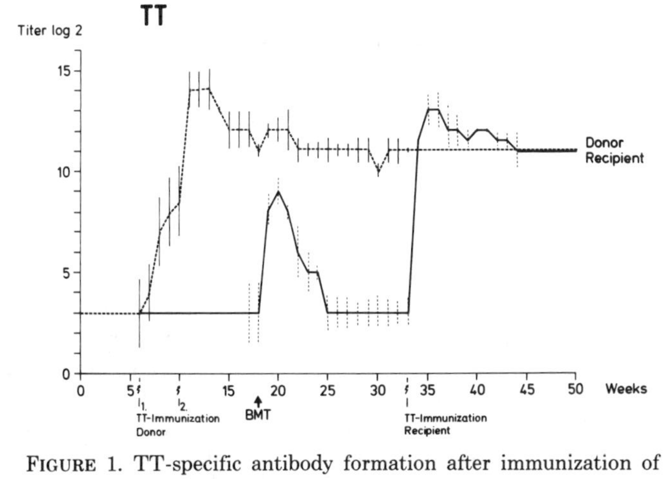

FIGURE 1. TT-specific antibody formation after immunization of three donors (-----), BMT, and one challenge of the respective recipients (———). Values are given as means ±SEM.

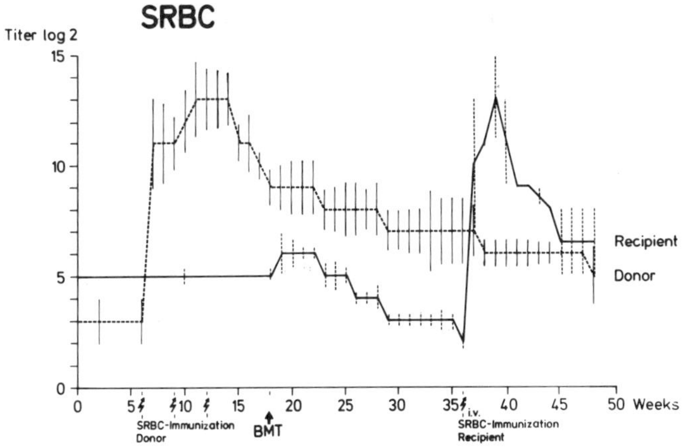

FIGURE 2. SRBC-specific antibody formation after immunization of three donors (-----), BMT, and one challenge of the respective recipients (———). Values are given as means ±SEM.

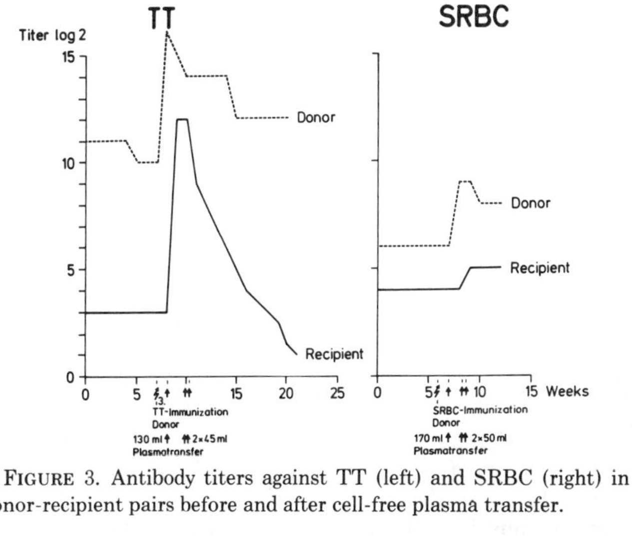

FIGURE 3. Antibody titers against TT (left) and SRBC (right) in donor-recipient pairs before and after cell-free plasma transfer.

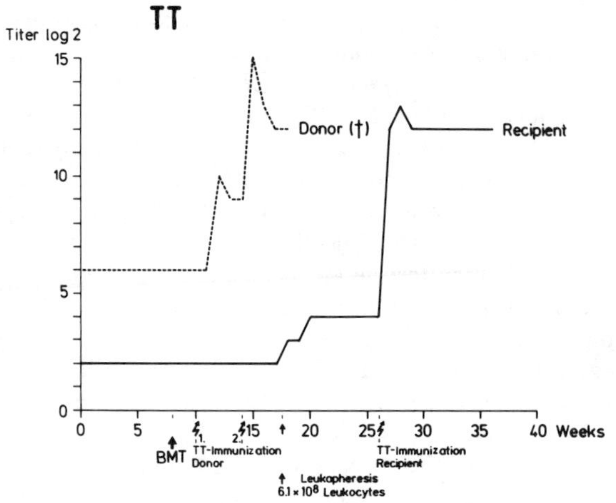

FIGURE 4. TT-specific antibody titers in a donor-recipient pair before and after BMT. The donor was immunized after marrow donation and served as leukocyte donor 10 weeks later. The recipient was challenged 8 weeks afterwards.

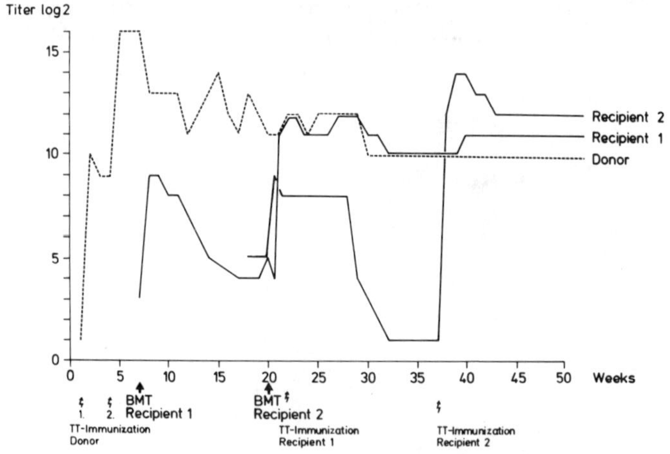

FIGURE 5. Antibody titers of one TT immunized marrow donor (-----) and his two marrow recipients (———) with antigen challenge at different intervals.

from a nonimmunized donor. The donor was then twice immunized with TT. Ten weeks after BMT, 6.1×10^8 PBL were transfused from the donor to the marrow recipient. Antigen challenge of the recipient 8 weeks later resulted in a secondary type of humoral immune response (Fig. 4).

Marrow transplantation at different times after vaccination of the donor. One TT-immunized dog was used as marrow donor for two recipients. The first marrow grafting was performed three weeks after the donor's second immunization, at which time it showed an antibody titer of 1:64,000. The same dog served again as marrow donor three months later, showing at this time an antibody titer of 1:2,000 (Fig. 5). After challenge, both recipients responded with an immediate rise in antibody titer, which is typical for a secondary type of humoral immune response. It may be of interest that the second recipient responded with a greater rise in antibody levels after challenge than the first recipient.

DISCUSSION

The transfer of immunity with bone marrow has been documented in the murine model (*5–7*). Our present study was designed to investigate the immune transfer with allogeneic marrow transplantation in a random bred animal model such as the dog. Our results clearly demonstrate that cellular bound memory against specific antigens is transferred with bone marrow stem cells in BMT. It has been suggested that a sufficient number of memory T cells may only be present in the donor marrow at specific times (*2*). In contrast, we found the secondary immune response of the recipients to be independent of the interval after immunization and the antibody titer of the donor at the time of transplantation.

We could demonstrate that the rise of specific antibodies in the recipient immediately after grafting is most likely due to passive transfer of antibodies with the bone marrow graft and the subsequent supportive blood transfusions. Approximately five weeks after grafting these antibodies disappear, which is in agreement with the known half-life of immunoglobulins. Thereafter the immune system of the recipient remains in a dormant state until antigen exposure. The fact that the antigen challenge results in a definite secondary type of humoral immune response can be taken as evidence that, with bone marrow, fully competent memory T and B cells are transferred. In absence of GVHD in all recipients, we have no plausible explanation why the donor immune system ceases its specific antibody production after being inoculated into the recipient, although its fully established immunological capacity is demonstrated by the secondary type of immune response after challenge. However, one must take into account that methotrexate was given until day 100 for preventing GVHD, and its immunosuppressive action may have affected the antibody production against TT and SRBC.

The comparison of specific antibody titers against TT and SRBC in these donors and recipients shows differences. The SRBC specific antibodies peak quickly and then decline continuously during 10 weeks. In contrast, the TT-specific antibody level remains stable over the period recorded. One explanation could be the physical difference between the two antigens studied. The SRBC, being a corpuscular antigen, is likely eliminated completely by the immune system, whereas TT molecules persist in a reduced but sufficient amount to continue stimulating specific antibody production. We can extend this assumption to the BMT model described above. The phenomenon of the quiescent specific immune capacity toward TT in the recipient of bone marrow from TT-immunized donors may be due to the absence of TT molecules in the recipient that would be needed for continuing antibody formation. This implies that the physiological site of the persisting TT molecules is not the bone marrow.

In a recent communication, Wahren et al. (*13*) found in human bone marrow chimeras that the transferred viral antibody production persisted usually only for a moderate length of time and seemed to have a finite life span. In only a few cases was an immune transfer of long duration seen. A similar course of humoral immunity was observed in our study with SRBC, whereas the TT response remained stable. However, our follow-up after challenge lasted only for 17 weeks.

Similar to the data available from syngeneic mice (*11*), in our experiments we found PBL of an immunized donor to be capable of transferring specific immunity to the bone marrow chimera. In extrapolation to human marrow transplantation, one would expect the immune transfer to occur after active immunization of the donor prior to BMT. For example, cytomegalovirus and herpes simplex virus natural immunity of the donor is caused by the donor's subclinical infection with the active virus, while in this case the active immunization is done with life-attenuated or killed vaccines, and thus will not cause any potential risk of severe infections to the recipient. As active immunization of human bone marrow recipients has proved to be ineffective until one year postgrafting, the concept of cellular-bound immune transfer from immunized donors deserves further extensive study in a preclinical model such as the dog.

Acknowledgments. We thank Ms. Marion Happel and Mr. Reiner Moog for their excellent technical assistance.

REFERENCES

1. Witherspoon RP, Storb R, Ochs HD, et al. Recovery of antibody production in human allogeneic marrow graft recipients: influence of time posttransplantation, the presence or absence of graft versus host disease and antithymocyte globulin treatment. Blood 1981; 58: 36.
2. Witherspoon RP, Lum LG, Storb R. Immunologic reconstitution after human bone marrow grafting. Semin Hematol 1984; 21:2.
3. Ochs HD, Storb R, Thomas ED, et al. Immunologic reactivity in canine marrow graft recipients. J Immunol 1974; 113:1039.
4. Abb J, Kolb HJ, Rodt HV, Grosse-Wilde H, Rieder J, Thierfelder S. In vitro and in vivo immune response to specific antigens in canine marrow graft recipients. Z. Immunitätsforschg 1977; 150: 152.
5. Kubanek B, Ernst P, Ostendorf P, Schäfer U, Wolf H. Preliminary data of a controlled trial of intravenous hyperimmune globulin in the prevention of cytomegalovirus infection in bone marrow transplant recipients. Transplant Proc 1985; 17:468.
6. Stoloff IL. The production of antibody to transferred bone marrow. J Immunol 1960; 85: 304.
7. Gengozian N, Makinodan T, Stekarchi JC. Transplantation of antibody forming cells in lethally irradiated mice. J Immunol 1961; 86: 113.
8. Stoner RD, Bond VP. Antibody formation by transplanted bone marrow, spleen, lymph nodes and thymus cells in irradiated recipients. J Immunol 1963; 91: 185.
9. Vriesendorp HM, Grosse-Wilde H, Dorf ME. The major histocompatibility system of the dog. In: Goetze D. The major histocompatibility system in man and animals. Berlin, Heidelberg, New York: Springer Verlag, 1977: 129.
10. Abb J, Netzel B, Rodt H, Grosse-Wilde H, Weger N, Thierfelder S. Hematologic and immunologic studies in dogs given nitrogen mustard. Blut 1977; 35: 51.
11. Baljer G, Thein P, Hechler H, et al. Untersuchungen zur intranasalen Schutzimpfung gegen Tetanus beim Pferd. Berl Münch Tierärztl Wochenschr 1982; 95: 208.
12. Rabin BS, Rose NR. Antibody formation by adoptively transferred mouse peripheral blood leucocytes. Immunology 1970; 18: 259.
13. Wahren B, Gahrton G, Linde A, et al. Transfer and persistence of viral antibody-producing cells in bone marrow transplantation. J Infect Dis 1984; 150: 358.

Received 1 August 1985.
Accepted 22 October 1985.

---

mic

0041-1337/86/4201-0067$02.00/0
TRANSPLANTATION
Vol. 42, No. 1

REJECTION OF MURINE CARDIAC ALLOGRAFTS

I. RELATIVE ROLES OF MAJOR AND MINOR ANTIGENS[1]

JAMES F. BURDICK AND LAWRENCE W. CLOW

Division of Transplantation and Vascular Surgery, Johns Hopkins University, Baltimore, Maryland

The relative contributions of incompatibilities for class I, class II, or minor antigens to primarily vascularized graft rejection have not been previously compared in large numbers of strains. In our experiments, murine primarily vascularized heterotopic cardiac graft rejection was studied in 16 donor-recipient strain combinations, representing different precisely defined major and/or minor histoincompatibilities. Complete major incompatibilities generally produced strong graft rejection, although it was confirmed that prolonged survival occurs in certain combinations that are incompatibile for class I, or class I plus class II, antigens. In addition, however, strong rejection of these grafts was produced in some recipient strains when the donor was incompatible only for minor antigens. This strong effect of minor antigens may reflect their strong stimulation of delayed-type hypersensitivity, whereas the influence of class II antigens seems more related to stimulation of mixed lymphocyte culture generation of lymphocyte-mediated cytotoxicity.

[1] This work was supported by funds from USPHS Grant AI-15081.

The genetic incompatibilities leading to experimental graft rejection are of interest because of what they imply about the mechanisms of sensitization and graft destruction, as well as their direct relevance to clinical transplantation. Minor antigen incompatibilities in the rat have been shown to produce rejection of skin and primarily vascularized cardiac allografts, although not as powerfully as a mismatch for the entire major histocompatibility complex (MHC),* RT-1, in the strains reported thus far (*1*). Extensive comparisons of results of primarily vascularized organ grafts using congenic pairs of mouse strains, in which the genetics of the minor antigens and the MHC are the best characterized, have not been reported. Most studies of graft rejection in the mouse have been with skin grafts, or nonvascularized organ implants (*2–4*). Some reports indicate that primarily vascularized organ grafts may be rejected less vigorously than skin (*2, 5, 6*). When primarily

* Abbreviations used: DTH, delayed-type hypersensitivity; 2-ME, 2-mercaptoethanol; MHC, major histocompatibility complex; MLC-LMC, mixed lymphocyte culture-lymphocyte mediated cytotoxicity; PBS, phosphate-buffered saline.

vascularized murine cardiac allografts were investigated by Corry and Russell (*6, 7*) they found that grafts incompatible for the entire H-2 in one combination, or for the K-plus-I region in another case, were rejected. The $B6AF_1$ recipients used in those studies also differ at H-9 with the C57BL/10 background of the congenic strains employed as donors. In one combination involving only minor antigens in the mouse, moderately strong rejection against primarily vascularized cardiac allografts was observed (*6*). Therefore, these previous data suggested that both major and minor antigens may stimulate strong rejection of primarily vascularized grafts.

In another approach to the assessment of in vivo reactivity against allogeneic tissue, we have confirmed previous data (*8*) suggesting that the effect of multiple minor antigens in the elicitation of murine delayed-type hypersensitivity (DTH) is particularly strong relative to the effect of the MHC in a large number of strains (*9–11*). This was unexpected in view of the predominate role played by the MHC in many allogeneic reactions, as exemplified by stimulation of MLC-lymphocyte mediated cytotoxicity (LMC). The strong DTH was not due to Mls incompatibility, and appeared to represent an additive effect of crossreactive responses against multiple minor antigens. Recently it has been questioned whether the process of graft rejection is more like DTH or more like MLC-LMC (*12–23*). It is thus of particular interest to establish more generally whether multiple minor antigens can cause strong primarily vascularized graft rejection, since if this is the case it seems possible that this aspect of graft rejection is due to a mechanism analogous to DTH.

The experiments described here were performed to systematically determine the influence of different antigen types in vascularized murine cardiac allograft rejection. The results in 16 strain combinations, including many congenic pairs, indicate an important role both for class II plus class I antigens, and for multiple minor antigens, in stimulating rejection. In addition, experiments revealing high or low responses with MLC-LMC and with DTH in some of these strain combinations confirmed that MLC-LMC is an analog of the effects of MHC incompatibility on graft rejection, whereas the data suggest that stimulation of graft rejection by multiple minor antigens is analogous to DTH.

MATERIALS AND METHODS

Male mice of the following strains were obtained from Jackson Laboratories, Bar Harbor, ME, and used between 2 and 6 months of age: B10.A., B10.BR, B10.D2/o, BALB/c, AKR, C3H/He, C3H.SW, and DBA/2. Breeding pairs of strains B10.T(6R), B10.MBR, B10.AQR, and B10.AKM were provided courtesy of David Sachs, M.D., and these mice were raised here.

Lymphocytes and target cells. Lymphocytes for the MLC and for sensitization in the DTH assay were prepared by teasing spleens apart in Dulbecco's phosphate-buffered saline (PBS) or tissue culture medium. The resultant suspension, after the clumps had settled, was counted and employed without erythrocyte lysis. Splenocytes used for challenge in DTH underwent brief erythrocyte lysis with NH_4C1 (*24*) and then were washed and filtered through a loose plug of nylon wool. The tumor lines RDM-4 (H-2^k carried in AKR animals) and P815 (H-2^d, carried in DBA/2 animals) were obtained from peritoneal lavages, washed, and resuspended for ^{51}CR-labeling as targets for LMC.

MLC-LMC assays. For MLC, twenty replicates of 10^6 irradiated stimulator splenocytes were mixed with 10^6 responder cells, in 2-ml aliquots, in RPMI 1640 (GIBCO, Grand Island, NY) with added glutamine, pen-strep, 25 mM hepes and 10% fetal calf serum (M.A. Bioproducts, Walkersville, MD). Stimulator cells were irradiated with 3000 rads from a cesium source. In one experiment 5×10^{-5} M 2-mercaptoenthanol (2-ME) was used in the MLC as indicated. The cells were harvested after 6 days in culture, washed, and employed as effector cells for LMC, by adding them to tumor target cells labeled with ^{51}Cr (Amersham Corp., Arlington Heights, IL) in the indicated effector:target (E:T) ratios in a total volume of 0.2 ml of Leibovitz's Medium L-15 (GIBCO) plus 10% fetal calf serum. Triplicates of 10^4 target cells per well in tissue culture plates (LinbrO U-bottomed, Flow Laboratories, McLean, VA) were employed. After three hours at 37°C in 5% CO_2, the plates were centrifuged for 10 min at 1000 g and then 0.1 ml of the supernatant was aspirated for gamma counting. The percentage of cytotoxicity was calculated by dividing twice the average number of cpm in the supernatant aliquot by the average of the total cpm initially present in aliquots containing 10^4 target cells.

DTH assays. The isotopic ear assay, as developed by Miller et al., was employed (*25*). Recipients were given cyclophosphamide 2 mg. i.p. on day −2; test groups were sensitized with injection s.c. of 5×10^7 viable allogeneic donor strain lymphocytes on day 0, and controls were left uninjected. On day 6, all test and control mice were anesthetized with chloral hydrate, and challenged with splenocytes from the sensitizing donor strain or another strain, using 4×10^6 cells in 0.01 ml PBS injected i.d. into the left ear pinna. Three hours later 0.1 uM of flourodeoxyuridine and then 2 μCi of ^{125}I-iododeoxyuridine (Amersham Corp., Arlington Heights, IL), was injected i.p. At 16–24 hr later the mice were sacrificed and the left and right ear pinnas removed by transection at the hairline. These were counted individually in a gamma counter and the results expressed for each group as the average of the ratio of the counts in the left (challenged) ear to the right ear (L/R). Statistical significance of differences between groups was assessed by the two-tailed *t* test.

Primarily vascularized cardiac allografts. Hearts were transplanted to the abdomens of the recipients as primarily vascularized grafts by the microvascular technique previously described (*6, 26*). The state of the grafts was determined by abdominal palpation of the graft pulse, graded as 0 to 4, which produces a reproducible evaluation. Short-term survival is over 95% in animals of the B10 background, but significantly poorer in other strains: about 20% survival in BALB/c recipients and 50% in DBA/2. Only animals that survived longer than five days were included in the studies. In certain combinations there was a decrement in pulse at 7–21 days, which then was at least partially restored, with subsequent long-term graft survival for two months or more; in these cases the listed survival time of the heart represents the eventual outcome, regardless of intermediate changes. Syngeneic hearts regularly survived indefinitely with strong impulses.

Histology. At the times indicated the hearts were removed, and histologic sections were prepared and stained with Hematoxylin and Eosin (courtesy of K. Solez, M.D.). One or two sagittal sections were reviewed for each specimen, and the percentage of residual nonrejected cardiac tissue estimated.

RESULTS

Heart graft survival in different strains. A listing of the primarily vascularized allogeneic cardiac grafts performed in these strains and carefully evaluated for survival by assessment of cardiac impulse, is shown in Table 1. There was some variability in the results, particularly if the rejection was not strong, which has also been noted for hepatic transplants in rats (*27*). However at least two major patterns were evident. In the mice in the group designated *rapid rejection*, the heartbeat began to decline by 1–2 weeks, and went on to permanent cessation in most recipients rather quickly, with a median survival time to rejection of two weeks or less. On the other hand, most hearts in recipients in the group designated *long-term survival*, after a transient decrement in impulse, exhibited at least partial restoration of the impulse, which was then palpable indefinitely. This finding in the B10.A recipients of B10.BR grafts is like the results previously reported with B10.BR hearts in $B6AF_1$ recipients (*6, 7, 26*), in which the H-2 incompatibility is the same. In addition, a few strain combinations (*intermediate rejection*) produced neither decisive rejection nor convincing long-term survival. The degree of rejection did not correlate completely with either MHC or minor antigen incompatibilities.

The histologic features of early rejection were characterized by typical interfasicular infiltrates and myocytolosis. More extensive rejection produced large masses of dense leukocyte infiltrate—and, later, a total destruction of the myocardial tissue.

The assessment of primarily vascularized graft survival was somewhat more difficult than with skin grafts, since the primarily vascularized grafts that were not rejected quickly and completely were capable of maintaining or reconstituting a pulse after severe partial rejection. This led to prolonged scoring of an intermittent or very weak pulse in certain strain combinations, unlike the complete cessation of impulse, or good long-term heart beat that occurred in other strain combinations. To determine the degree of rejection produced by different incompatibilities independent of palpation, the percentage of remaining nonrejected cardiac tissue in a series of grafts 2–3-months old was assessed histologically, and the results of this are shown in Table 2, with the strain listing organized as in Table 1. In general, it may be seen that these results paralleled the pattern found by palpation of the cardiac impulse—confirming, in particular, that the grafts that were thought on the basis of palpation to be beating strongly also had a moderate or large residual amount of normal cardiac tissue histologically. The only major discrepancy was in the B10·BR recipients of (H-2 incompatible) B10.D2 hearts, in which one graft appeared to have less residual viable tissue than would have been thought from palpation.

DTH results in different strains. In Figure 1 are shown examples of the DTH reactions found against some of the H-2 or multiple minor antigen differences employed in these studies. The striking finding was that incompatibility for multiple minor antigens produced a strong response, as compared with incompatibility at H-2 (*8, 9*). This was in marked contrast to the results with MLC-LMC involving major or minor incompatibilities, as shown below.

MLC-LMC results in different strains. In Figure 2 are shown the results of MLC-LMC assays against several strains chosen for incompatibility at major or minor loci, for comparison with the DTH and heart graft results. These results conformed to the usual finding that only strains with incompatibility for I region class II stimulatory antigens can produce strong responses in this assay. It is unclear whether MLC stimulation with added 2-ME is more or less artefactual than without this addition. Although specific stimulation by a partial H-2 incompatibility (syngeneic for Ia) became demonstrable when 2-ME was added to the MLC (Fig. 3, A and B), even with this the stimulation by multiple minor incompatibilities alone was very weak (Fig. 3, C).

TABLE 1. Survival of primarily vascularized cardiac grafts (palpation)

Recipient	Donor	Incompatability	Rejection day	Median
Rapid rejection (median <15 days):				
B10.D2	B10.BR	Entire H-2	7, 7, 10	7
B10.D2	DBA/2	Mult minor	6, 7, 8, 56+, 56+	8
B10.A	B10.T(6R)	H-2 K+I	6, 8, 8, 9, 15, 40	9
B10.A	AKR	H-2D + mult minor	6, 10, 10, 10, 17	10
B10.A	DBA/2	H-2 K+I + mult minor	7, 8, 8, 11, 12, 33, 56+, 56+, 56+	12
Balb/c	DBA/2	Mult minor	8, 11, 12, 16, 20, 56+	14
Intermediate rejection (median = 15–28 days):				
B10.A	B10.AQR	H-2 K	12, 12, 16, 19, 48	16
C3H/He	C3H.SW	Entire H-2	10, 10, 10, 31, 52, 54	21
B10.BR	B10.MBR	H-2 K+D	14, 21, 22, 24, 56+, 56+	23
DBA/2	Balb/c	Mult minor	5, 26, 56+	26
Long-term survival (median >28 days):				
B10.A	B10.D2	H-2 K+I	9, 27, 39, 56+, 56+	39
B10.BR	B10.AKM	H-2 D	23, 56, 56+	56
B10.A	B10.BR	H-2 D	10, 20, 56+, 56+, 56+, 56+, 56+	56+
B10.BR	B10.A	H-2 D	26, 56+, 56+, 56+, 56+	56+
B10.BR	AKR	Mult minor	28, 35, 42, 56+, 56+, 56+, 56+	56+
B10.BR	B10.D2	Entire H-2	13, 56+, 56+	56+
Syngeneic:				
C3H/He	C3H/He	—	56+, 56+, 56+	56+

TABLE 2. Survival of primarily vascularized grafts (histologic viability)

Recipient	Donor	Incompatability	Percentage viable	Median
Rapid rejection (median <15 days):				
B10.D2	B10.BR	Entire H-2	n.t.[a]	—
B10.D2	DBA/2	Mult minor	0, 0, 0, 5, 5	0
B10.A	B10.T(6R)	H-2 K+I	0, 5, 10, 10, 15, 65	10
B10.A	AKR	H-2D + mult minor	0, 0, 0, 0, 10, 50	0[b]
B10.A	DBA/2	H-2 K+I + mult minor	0, 0, 0, 0, 0, 10, 20	0
Balb/c	DBA/2	Mult minor	n.t.	—
Intermediate rejection (15–28 days):				
B10.A	B10.AQR	H-2 K	5, 5, 25, 25, 80	25
C3H/He	C3H.SW	Entire H-2	0, 5, 10, 20, 35	10
B10.BR	B10.MBR	H-2 K+D	20, 40, 55, 60, 85, 90	58
DBA/2	Balb/c	Mult minor	n.t.	—
Long-term survival (>28 days):				
B10.A	B10.D2	H-2 K+I	10, 10, 20, 25, 40, 55, 55, 60, 85	40
B10.BR	B10.AKM	H-2 D	10, 80, 95	80
B10.A	B10.BR	H-2 D	60, 100, 100, 100	100
B10.BR	B10.A	H-2 D	0, 0, 70, 80, 85, 95	75
B10.BR	AKR	Mult minor	90, 90	(90)
B10.BR	B10.D2	Entire H-2	0, 10, 95	10
Syngeneic:				
C3H.SW	C3H.SW	—	80, 90, 100	90

[a] n.t. = not tested.
[b] Scored at 8–11 days.

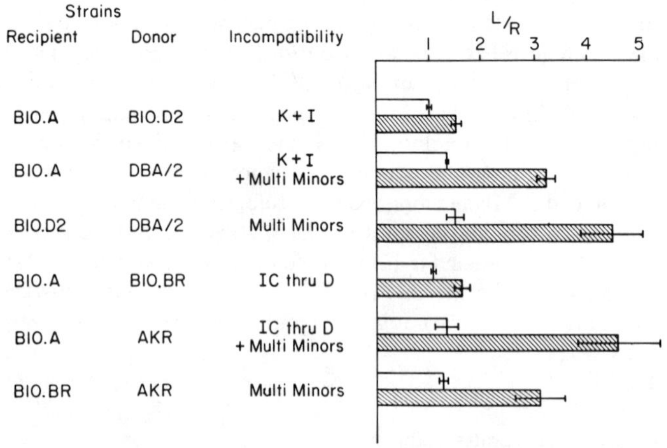

FIGURE 1. Effect of major and minor histocompatibilities on DTH. Sensitization and challenge were with the same, indicated, lymphocytes. Results expressed as L/R averages of four or five animals per group ± SEM. Clear bars: unsensitized controls; hatched bars: sensitized test groups. All differences between control and experimental groups significant to at least the $P<0.01$ level, calculated using the two tailed t test.

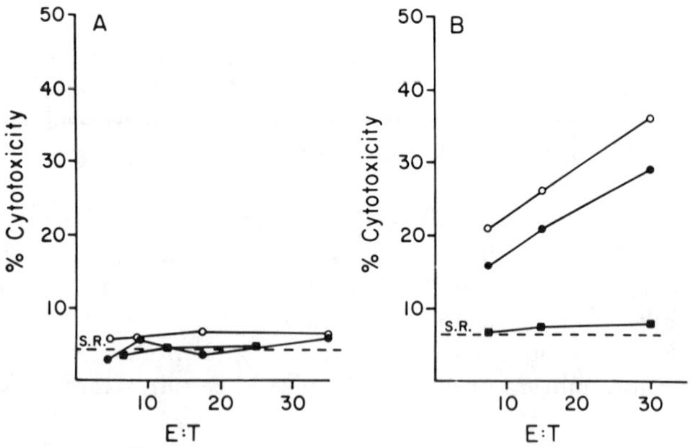

FIGURE 2. Results of major and minor antigen incompatibilities in MLC-LMC. The MLC portion was as indicated, and the effector cells were tested against RDM-4 target in panel A and P815 target cells in panel B. No 2-ME was employed in the tissue culture medium. Panel A: ● = B10.AαB10.BR, ○ = B10.AαAKR, ■ = B10.BRαAKR; Panel B: ● = B10.AαB10.D2, ○ = B10.AαDBA/2, ■ = B10.D2αDBA/2. The results are given ± SEM; SR = spontaneous release.

DISCUSSION

The use of multiple congenic strain pairs in our experiments allowed extension of previous data (*1, 6, 7, 26, 28*) on the role of histocompatibility antigens in cardiac graft rejection. As shown in Tables 1 and 2, there was not a strong concordance between graft survival and the degree of histoincompatibility as assessed in other ways. Strains that were incompatible at least at the K + I regions exhibited rapid or intermediate rejection in 4 of 6 pairs, but this major incompatibility allowed long-term survival in 2 combinations. In general, incompatibility only for other portions of H-2 produced weaker rejection. It was interesting that incompatibility for the I region was not strongly associated with severe rejection: certain strains matched at the I region with their donors still developed strong rejection. Furthermore, one of the strain combinations that resulted only in an intermediate degree of rejection, and two of the combinations that commonly produced long-term survival, involved H-2 I region incompatibility. However there was some tendency toward an additive effect of separate H-2 regions in producing rejection, as previously reported for the rat RT-1 subregions (*28*). Two of the 4 instances of isolated multiple minor incompatibilities, in strains compatible for H-2, resulted in severe rejection. It has been reported with certain rat strains that primarily vascularized cardiac grafts are unlike kidney grafts in that the hearts induce more uniformly strong rejection (*29*). However it is apparent from our results with this large number of strains that primarily vascularized hearts in some mouse strain pairs can exhibit prolonged survival in the face of histoincompatibilities that seem strong by other criteria.

The B10.BR hearts placed in B10.A recipients, and the AKR

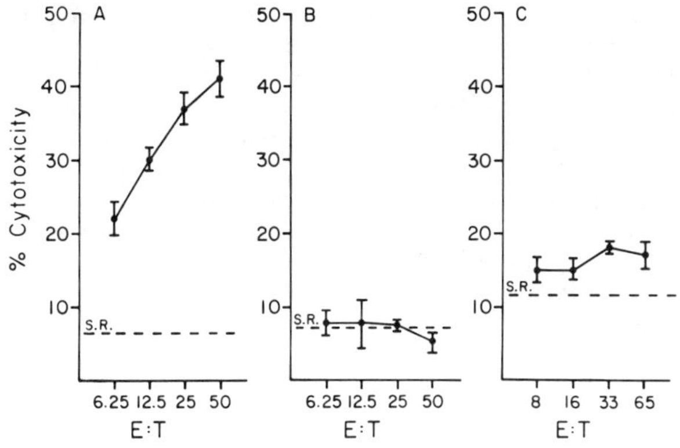

FIGURE 3. Result of employing 2-ME in the tissue culture medium during MLC generation of cytotoxicity. Subsequent LMC results given against target cells as indicated. Panel A: B10.AαB10.BR, RDM-4 target cells; Panel B: B10.AαB10.BR, P815 target cells; Panel C: B10.BRαAKR, RDM-4 target cells. The effector cells in panels A and B were the same, showing specificity for reaction only against RDM-4 target cells. The results are given ± SEM; SR = spontaneous release.

hearts placed in B10.BR recipients, which differ only for H-2D, or multiple minor antigens, respectively, were found to survive long-term in most instances; however, when AKR donors in B10·A recipients were employed, in which the multiple minor antigen incompatibilities were coupled with H-2D incompatibility, the hearts were promptly and permanently rejected. It therefore appears that the addition of the H-2D region incompatibility to the multiple minor antigen differences, neither of which was capable of producing severe permanent rejection independently, resulted in strong complete rejection due to the additive effects of these two types of incompatibility. This is not certain, however, since this experiment does not rule out an immune response gene for the minor antigens of AKR that is different in B10.A than in B10.BR, which could conceivably produce the result obtained.

The influence of minor antigens on graft rejection has been documented in the past. Skin graft rejection due to single minor antigens is typically detectable but rather weak, but multiple minor antigens may produce rather strong skin graft rejection (*1, 30, 31*). Similarly, strong graft-versus-host disease may be generated by multiple minor antigens (*22, 33*), and a synergism similar to that observed in our experiments for H-2D plus multiple minor antigens was reported for the combination of H-Y and H-2K (*34*) in the elicitation of graft-versus-host disease. Rejection of primarily vascularized cardiac allografts in rats may be caused by multiple minor antigens, although not as powerfully as a mismatch for the entire MHC (*1, 35*). Moderately strong rejection of primarily vascularized cardiac allografts was previously reported for one murine strain pair that was incompatible for minor antigens only (*6*). Multiple minor antigens reportedly can cause organ graft rejection to a varying degree in the few strains available for testing in other species as well (*36, 37*). Therefore the strong rejection produced by minor incompatibilities in several strain combinations in our experiments is not unprecedented. However our data in the mouse indicate that this is a stronger and more general effect than had previously been thought from experiments with a more limited number of strains in mice and other species in the past.

Two experimental analogs of graft rejection that are commonly discussed are DTH and MLC-LMC (*12–23*). These two responses to allogeneic tissue were not stimulated equally by the same incompatibilities in our experiments. Incompatibility for the I region was a strong stimulus for the in vitro generation of cytotoxicity, whereas DTH was strongly stimulated by multiple minor antigens. In all combinations tested that evinced rapid rejection, there was incompatibility either for the entire H-2 region, or for multiple minor antigens, or for a segment of H-2 plus multiple minor antigens. Therefore, in each of these cases, unlike other strains with only partial H-2 incompatibility, strong stimulation would be produced either in DTH (due to multiple minor antigens), or in MLC-LMC (due to H-2 I region incompatibility), or in both tests. Although the mechanism of rejection was not directly investigated in our experiments, these findings are consistent with the proposal that each of these experimental models represents an accurate analogue of one aspect of rejection. We have previously shown that Mls incompatibility is not an important factor in the strong stimulation produced in DTH by multiple minor antigens, since compatibility for the strong Mls allele does not diminish the DTH response, and responses are strong against strains that carry the weaker Mls alleles (*11*).

Situations that produce strong stimulation in DTH or in MLC-LMC, but in which strong graft rejection does not occur, may be the result of genetically determined differences in the ability of different strains to reject organ grafts. The strength of skin graft (*18, 38*) and tissue graft (*29, 39*) rejection in mice is reportedly controlled by immune response genes in some cases. The possibility that there is a difference between the recipients with the H-2^d haplotype and the H-2^k haplotype in immunologic responsiveness for rejection of primarily vascularized cardiac grafts was suggested by our data: all H-2^d recipients were in the rapid rejection or intermediate rejection groups, whereas all those of the H-2^k haplotype were in the intermediate rejection or long-term survival groups. In evaluating primarily vascularized grafts between rat strains congenic for different RT-1 haplotypes on the PVG background, the "strong response gene" (μ) seemed to partially control the strength of rejection (*28*). In somewhat different experiments we found a strain-dependent difference in immune responsiveness against primarily vascularized xenografts in immunosuppressed recipient mice (*40*), and there is apparently a non-SLA-linked immune response gene for rejection of grafts incompatible for minor antigens in miniature swine (*36*).

The immunologic status of the recipients of long-surviving grafts, as compared with other strain combinations in which the graft is quickly rejected, will be the subject of future reports.

REFERENCES

1. Katz SM, Liebert M, Gill TJ, Kunz HW, Cramer DV, Guttmann RD. The relative roles of MHC and non-MHC genes in heart and skin allograft survival. Transplantation 1983; 36: 96.
2. Warren RP, Lofgreen JS, Steinmuller D. Factors responsible for the differential survival of heart and skin allografts in inbred rats. Transplantation 1973; 16: 458.
3. Davis WC, McKenzie IFC, Melvold RW. A comparison of skin and heart graft rejection patterns in H-2 mutant mice. Transplantation 1980; 29: 189.
4. Klein J, Chiang C, Lofgreen J, Steinmuller D. Participation of H-2 regions in heart transplant rejection. Transplantation 1976; 22: 384.
5. Barker CF, Billingham RE. Comparison of the fates of Ag-B locus compatible homografts of skin and hearts in inbred rats. Nature 1970; 225: 851.

6. Corry RJ, Winn HJ, Russell PS. Primary vascularized allografts of hearts in mice. Transplantation 1973; 16: 343.
7. Corry RJ, Russell PS. New possibilities for organ allografting in the mouse. In: Calne RY, ed. *Immunological aspects of transplantation surgery*. New York: Wiley, 1973: 279.
8. Smith FI, Miller JFAP. Delayed-type hypersensitivity to allogeneic cells in mice. III. Sensitivity to cell-surface antigens coded by the major histocompatibility complex and by other genes. J Exp Med 1979; 150: 965.
9. Ohori P, Nadel S, Burdick JF. Two aspects of delayed type hypersensitivity are stimulated strongly by minor antigens. Transplantation 1983; 36: 581.
10. Burdick JF, Williams GM. Anergy for delayed type hypersensitivity in preleukemic AKR mice. J Natl Cancer Instit 1985; 84: 1089.
11. Burdick JF. Strong cellular immune responses induced in vivo against minor antigens in the mouse. Immunology (in press).
12. Gurley KE, Lowry RP. Role of delayed-type hypersensitivity (DTH) in renal allograft rejection. Transplant Proc 1983; 15: 339.
13. Christmas SE, MacPherson GG. The role of mononuclear phagocytes in cardiac allograft rejection in the rat. II. Characterization of mononuclear phagocytes extracted from rat cardiac allografts. Cell Immunol 1982; 69: 271.
14. Christmas SE, MacPherson GG. The role of mononuclear phagocytes in cardiac allograft rejection in the rat. III. The effect of cells extracted from rat cardiac allografts upon beating heart cell cultures. Cell Immunol 1982; 69: 281.
15. Dallman MJ, Mason DW, Webb M. The role of host and donor cells in the rejection of skin allografts by T cell-deprived rats injected with syngeneic T cells. Eur J Immunol 1982; 12: 511.
16. Gregory CD, Atkinson ME. Large agranular lymphocytes: early nonspecific effector cells in allograft rejection in the mouse. Immunology 1984; 53: 257.
17. Hurme M, Chandler PR, Hetherington CM, Simpson E. Cytotoxic T-cell responses to H-Y: correlation with the rejection of syngeneic male skin grafts. J Exp Med 1978; 147: 768.
18. Tyler JD, Galli SJ, Snider ME, Dvorak AM, Steinmuller D. Cloned Lyt-2^+ cytolytic T lymphocytes destroy allogeneic tissue in vivo. J Exp Med 1984; 159: 234.
19. LeFrancois L, Bevan MJ. A reexamination of the role of Lyt-2-positive T cells in murine skin graft rejection. J Exp Med 1984; 159: 57.
20. Bradley JA, Mason DW, Morris PJ. Evidence that rat renal allografts are rejected by cytotoxic T cells and not by non-specific effectors. Transplantation 1985; 39: 169.
21. Kim B, Rosenstein M, Weiland D, Eberlein TJ, Rosenberg SA. Clonal analysis of the lymphoid cells mediating skin allograft rejection: mediation of graft rejection in vivo by cloned Lyt-1^+2^-proliferative, noncytotoxic long-term cell lines. Transplantation 1983; 36: 525.
22. Lowry RP, Gurley KE. Immune mechanisms in organ allograft rejection. III. Cellular and humoral immunity in rejection of organ allografts transplanted across MHC subregion disparity RT1.B(RT1.D). Transplantation 1983; 36: 405.
23. Boyle W. An extension of the ^{51}Cr-release assay for the estimation of mouse cytotoxins. Transplantation 1968; 6: 761.
24. Smith F, Miller JF. Delayed-type hypersensitivity to allogeneic cells in mice. I. Requirements for optimal sensitivation and definition of the response. Int Arch Allergy Appl Immunol 1979; 58: 285.
25. Burdick JF, Russell PS. Antigenic requirements for induced rejection of long-surviving murine heart transplants. J Immunol 1982; 128: 1551.
26. Limmer J, Herbertson BM, Calne RY. Orthotopic rat liver transplantation using different combinations of four inbred strains. Eur Surg Res 1980; 12: 343.
27. Lowry RP, Blackburn JK. Studies on rejection of heart grafts bearing isolated RT1A-encoded class I disparities. Transplant Proc 1984; 16: 1118.
28. Paris AMI, Bishop C, Festenstein H, Gunther E. Non-major histocompatibility system immunogenetic influences on rat renal allograft survival. Transplantation 1978; 25: 252.
29. Graff RJ, Silvers WK, Billingham RE, Hildemann WH, Snell GD. The cumulative effect of histocompatibility antigens. Transplantation 1966; 4: 605.
30. Johnson LL, Bailey DW, Mobraaten LE. Genetics of histocompatibility in mice. II. Survey for interactions between minor (Non-H-2) antigens by skin grafting. Immunogenetics 1980; 11: 363.
31. Storb R, Weiden PL, Graham C, Lerner KG, Thomas ED. Marrow grafts between DLA-identical and homozygous unrelated dogs. Evidence for an additional locus involved in graft-versus-host disease. Transplantation 1977; 24: 165.
32. Korngold R, Sprent J. Lethal GVHD across minor histocompatibility barriers: nature of the effector cells and role of the H-2 complex. Immunol Rev 1983; 71: 5.
33. Elkins WL, Silvers WK. Synergistic interaction of H-Y and H-2K in elicitation of graft-versus-host responses. Transplantation 1982; 34: 71.
34. Hildemann WH, Mullen Y. The weaker the histoincompatibility, the greater the effectiveness of specific immunoblocking antibodies: a new immunogenic rule of transplantation. Transplant Proc 1973; 5: 617.
35. Pennington LR, Flye MW, Kirkman RL, Thistlethwaite JR, Williams GM, Sachs DH. Transplantation in miniature swine. X. Evidence for non-SLA-linked immune response gene(s) controlling rejection of SLA matched kidney allografts. Transplantation 1981; 32: 315.
36. Dausset J, Rapaport FT, Cannon FD, Ferrebee JW. Histocompatibility studies in a closely bred colony of dogs. III. Genetic definition of the DL-A system of canine histocompatibility, with particular reference to the comparative immunogenicity of the major transplantable organs. J Exp Med 1971; 134: 1222.
37. Wettstein PJ, Haughton G. The genetic control of the immune response to murine histocompatibility antigens. I. The response to H-4 alloantigens. Immunogenetics 1977; 4: 65.
38. Schultz JS, DeMott-Fribert R, Beals TF. Immunogenetic control of the response of female mice to male tissue grafts. Immunogenetics 1981; 12: 199.
39. Burdick JF, Jooste SV, Winn HJ. Variations in the responses of mouse strains to rat xenografts. J Immunol 1979; 123: 954.

Received 10 July 1985.
Accepted 29 October 1985.

0041-1337/86/4201-0073$02.00/0
TRANSPLANTATION
Copyright © 1986 by The Williams & Wilkins Co.

Vol. 42, No. 1
Printed in U.S.A.

DEPLETION OF T CELLS FROM HUMAN BONE MARROW USING MONOCLONAL ANTIBODIES AND RABBIT COMPLEMENT

A QUANTITATIVE AND FUNCTIONAL ANALYSIS[1]

AMA ROHATINER,[2,3] RICHARD GELBER, STUART F. SCHLOSSMAN, AND JEROME RITZ[4,5]

Divisions of Tumor Immunology and Biostatistics, Dana Farber Cancer Institute; Department of Medicine, Harvard Medical School; and Department of Biostatistics, Harvard School of Public Health, Boston, MA 02115

Graft-versus-host-disease (GVHD) remains the principal complication of allogeneic bone marrow transplantation. In animal models mature T lymphocytes have been shown to be responsible for GVHD and, therefore, in vitro treatment of donor bone marrow using monoclonal T cell specific antibodies and complement is currently being investigated as a strategy for the prevention of GVHD. In the present studies anti-T12 and anti-T11 monoclonal antibodies and rabbit complement were used to remove T lymphocytes from normal bone marrow. The efficacy of depletion was investigated by immunofluorescence assays and by in vitro culture of the residual cells using nonspecific mitogens or allogeneic B cells as the proliferative stimulus in the presence of lymphocyte-conditioned medium containing interleukin 2 (IL-2). Immunofluorescence analysis showed complete depletion of T12$^+$ and T11$^+$ cells after treatment with the respective antibodies and with the combination. Nevertheless, culture of treated bone marrow with phytohemagglutinin (PHA) or concanavalin A (Con A) and conditioned media containing IL-2 resulted in the proliferation of mature T cells (T3$^+$, T4$^+$ or T8$^+$, T11$^+$). Stimulation of treated marrow with allogeneic cells (Laz 388) resulted in the growth of a population with natural killer (NK) cell phenotype (T3$^-$, T11$^+$, NKH1$^+$). The latter population was found to be strongly cytotoxic against K562 cells, a standard NK target. As expected, NK cells that are T11$^+$ and T12$^-$ appeared to be more effected by in vitro treatment with anti-T11 than with anti-T12. A clonogenic assay was then used to quantitate the efficacy of target cell depletion in vitro. Three sequential incubations of bone marrow with either anti-T12 or anti-T11 plus complement resulted in depletion of 1–2 logs of clonogenic cells. Treatment with both antibodies concurrently resulted in elimination of 2–3 logs of clonogenic target cells. Although multiple treatments with both anti-T12 and anti-T11 were more effective than similar treatment with only one antibody, it remains to be established whether such combinations will be necessary in the clinical setting or whether more selective depletion of T cells without removal of NK cells might be optimal.

Allogeneic bone marrow transplantation is increasingly being utilized as a treatment modality for patients with hematologic malignancies. However, the morbidity and mortality of the transplant procedure remain appreciable, with graft-versus-host disease (GVHD)* being the principal complication. Despite current immunosuppressive therapies including corticosteroids, methotrexate, cyclosporine, and antithymocyte globulin, 50% of graft recipients who receive histocompatible marrow develop GVHD to a significant degree (*1, 2*). Furthermore, the severity of GVHD in patients receiving HLA-mismatched marrow effectively limits bone marrow transplantation to the 40% of patients with histocompatible donors.

It has been demonstrated in several experimental systems that the cells responsible for initiating GVHD are mature T lymphocytes (*3, 4*). In vitro treatment with conventional heteroantisera or with monoclonal antibodies and complement has been shown to be capable of selectively removing T lymphocytes from normal bone marrow (BM) without compromising hematopoietic reconstitution (*5, 6*). Moreover, in several animal models, T cell depletion has been followed by successful engraftment across major and minor histocompatibility barriers without the development of GVHD (*5–9*). Against this background, several clinical studies have commenced using various monoclonal antibodies and complement or monoclonal antibody-ricin conjugates to deplete allogeneic marrow of T lymphocytes prior to infusion (*10–16*). Initial results suggest that such in vitro treatment is not deleterious to marrow engraftment and that engraftment can occur without the development of GVHD in both histocompatible and haplotype-mismatched recipients.

The present work was undertaken to determine the efficacy of in vitro treatment with monoclonal antibodies and complement to deplete T cells from normal donor marrow. These studies have attempted to quantitate the extent of T cell depletion using in vitro culture techniques that are capable of expanding small residual populations not detectable by immunofluorescence assays and flow cytometer analysis. In so doing, both T cell and natural killer (NK) cell populations were analyzed separately by phenotypic markers and functional assays. The ability to deplete these different functional elements was evaluated for two monoclonal antibodies with different

[1] This work was supported in part by NIH Grants CA 34183 and CA 06516.

[2] AR is supported by the Imperial Cancer Research Fund, London.

[3] Present address: ICRF Dept. of Medical Oncology, St. Bartholomew's Hospital, London E.C.1.

[4] JR is a scholar of the Leukemia Society of America.

[5] Address correspondence to: Jerome Ritz, M.D., Division of Tumor Immunology, Dana-Farber Cancer Institute, 44 Binney Street, Boston, MA 02115.

* Abbreviations used: BM, bone marrow; CFU-GM, colony-forming unit—Granulocyte-macrophage; Con A, concanavalin A; GM-FITC, fluorescein-conjugated goat antimouse Fab IgC; GVHD, graft-versus-host disease; IL-2, interleukin 2; LCM, lymphocyte-conditioned medium; MNC, mononuclear cells; MR, maximal release; PB, peripheral blood; PHA, phytohemagglutinin; PMA, phorbol-myristate acetate; SR, spontaneous release.

specificities: anti-T12, a pan-T-cell antibody specific for a 120 Kd surface glycoprotein and anti-T11, an antibody specific for the sheep erythrocyte receptor antigen present on all cells within the T cell lineage. Both antibodies, or reagents with identical specificities, are currently being used in clinical trials (*10*, *12*, *15*).

MATERIALS AND METHODS

Cells. Normal BM and peripheral blood (PB) were obtained from volunteer donors and the mononuclear cell (MNC) fraction was isolated by Ficoll-Hypaque density gradient centrifugation.

Cell lines. LAZ 388 is an Epstein-Barr-virus–transformed B lymphoblastoid cell line. K562 was derived from a patient with blastic transformation of chronic myeloid leukemia.

Monoclonal antibodies. Anti-T12 is a IgM monoclonal antibody that activates rabbit complement and is specific for a cell-surface glycoprotein with a molecular weight of 120,000 daltons (*10*). Anti-T12 reacts with normal peripheral blood T cells and mature medullary thymocytes but is not reactive with less differentiated thymic T cells. Anti-T11 defines an antigen associated with the sheep erythrocyte receptor (*17*) that is expressed on all thymocytes and peripheral blood T lymphocytes. The vast majority of normal NK cells in peripheral blood also express T11 antigen. The antibody that was used in the lysis experiments is an IgG2b antibody that also activates complement-mediated lysis. Anti-T1 is reactive with the majority of peripheral blood T cells and a fraction of thymocytes (*18*); anti-T3 defines all functionally mature peripheral blood T lymphocytes (*19*); anti-T4 and anti-T8 characterize helper and cytotoxic/suppressor T cells, respectively (*18*); anti-T9 recognizes the transferrin receptor, which is present on erythroid precursors and activated lymphocytes (*20*, *21*). Anti-Ia is directed against a monomorphic HLA-DR antigen (*22*), anti-B1 is B-lymphocyte-specific (*23*); and anti-MO1, MY4, and MY8 recognize myelomonocytic differentiation antigens (*24*, *25*). Anti-NKH1(N901) reacts with a small population of cells in peripheral blood that morphologically appear as large granular lymphocytes (*26*, *27*). All peripheral blood cells with natural killer (NK) activity express this antigen. Ascites from a negative hybridoma clone, 8A7, was used as a control throughout.

Complement. Baby rabbit complement (Pel Freez, Rogers, AR) was used at a 1:10 dilution after screening for toxicity against human bone marrow using a standard chromium release assay and bone marrow culture for CFU-GM.

Treatment of bone marrow with antibody and complement. Antibodies were diluted in RPMI 1640 containing 2.5% human AB serum (2.5% AB RPMI) to a final antibody concentration of 20 μg/ml. Filter-sterilized rabbit complement was diluted (1:10) in RPMI 1640. After separation by Ficoll-Hypaque density sedimentation, BM MNC were washed twice and resuspended in the antibody solution to a concentration of 2×10^7cells/ml. Marrow was incubated for 30 min at room temperature with the negative antibody 8A7, with anti-T12 or anti-T11 alone, or with both anti-T12 and anti-T11. The cells were then spun down and resuspended in the equivalent volume of diluted complement. Incubation with complement was continued for 45 min at 37°C and the whole procedure repeated twice. After the final complement incubation, cells were washed twice and samples taken for further analysis.

Preparation of lymphocyte-conditioned medium (LCM) containing interleukin-2 (IL-2). MNC obtained from a peripheral blood buffy coat were incubated at 37°C for 4 hr at a concentration of 2.5×10^6 cells/ml with irradiated LAZ 388 cells (5×10^7 cell/ml) in 2.5% AB-RPMI with the addition 4 μg/ml phytohemaglutinnin (PHA) (Burroughs Wellcome and Co, Greensville, NC) and 5 ng/ml phorbol-myristate acetate (PMA) (Sigma Chemical Co., St. Louis, MO). After 4 hr, the cells were spun down, washed 4 times, resuspended in 2.5% AB RPMI, and incubated for 48 hr at 37°C. After centrifugation, the lymphocyte conditioned medium was harvested, filtered (0.45-μ), and stored at −70°C.

Culture of residual lymphocytes. After treatment with antibody and complement, cells were resuspended in RPMI 1640 containing 10% human AB serum, 1 mM pyruvate, and 2 mM 1-glutamine at a concentration of 1×10^6/ml, and 100 μl aliquots cultured in round-bottomed microtiter plates with medium alone, PHA 0.5 μg/ml, concanavalin A (Con A) 62.5 μg/ml, or irradiated LAZ 388 cells (1×10^5 cells/well). LCM (20 μl) were added to each well, so that the final LCM concentration was 10%. The cultures were fed every 3 days by removing 0.1 ml of medium and adding 0.1 ml of fresh medium containing 10% AB RPMI and 20% LCM. After 10–12 days, depending on the rate of growth, phenotypic analysis and NK assay were performed as described below.

Indirect immunofluorescence assay. Phenotypic analysis was performed by indirect immunofluorescence using specific monoclonal antibodies followed by fluorescein-conjugated goat antimouse Fab IgC(GM-FITC, Tago Inc. Burlington, CA) using standard techniques (*27*). Background fluorescence was determined by incubating cells with the negative antibody 8A7 followed by GM-FITC. Samples were analyzed on a fluorescence-activated cell sorter (FACS 1, Becton Dickinson, Mountain View, CA) or on an Epics V (Coulter Electronics, Hialeah, FL). A total of 10,000 cells were analyzed in each sample.

Assessment of NK activity. Effector cells were incubated with 5000 ^{51}Cr-labeled target cells at various effector:target cell ratios in V-bottomed microtiter plates. After 4 hr at 37°C, the plates were spun 3 min, 0.1 ml of supernatant was removed, and cytotoxicity determined by measurement of release of ^{51}Cr into the supernatant. Spontaneous release (SR) was determined by incubation of target cells with medium alone (5% AB RPMI 1640) and maximal release (MR) was determined by addition of detergent (1% NP-40) instead of antibody. All assays were done in triplicate. Specific cytotoxicity was calculated according to the following formula (equation 1):

$$\%\ \text{specific cytotoxicity} = \frac{(\text{experimental counts} - \text{SR})}{(\text{MR} - \text{SR})} \times 100$$

Limiting dilution assay. After treatment with antibody and complement, cells were resuspended in 10% AB RPMI in a volume equal to that which, after treatment with the control antibody, contained MNC at a concentration of 1×10^6 cells/ml. Six serial ten-fold dilutions were made using the same medium and 10 100 μl aliquots of each dilution plated in 96-well round-bottomed microtiter plates. The cells were then cultured with a feeder layer consisting of autologous PB MNC 10^5 cell/well + PHA or autologous PB MNC (5×10^4 cells/well) + LAZ 388 (5×10^4 cells/well). All feeder layer cells were irradiated (5000 rads) prior to plating. Feeder cells alone were plated as controls. 20 μl of 20% LCM was added to each well and the plates were incubated for 10 days at 37°C in 5% CO_2. The cultures were fed every 3–4 days as described above. On day 9, the cells were pulsed with ^{3}H-thymidine and harvested 18 hr later. Growth was assessed on the basis of ^{3}H-thymidine uptake. Any well with growth greater than the mean control well count +2SD was counted as positive. Plates were scored on the basis of the number of positive wells at each dilution, and the estimated number of T cell "clonogenic units" per 10^6 cells (θ) was calculated using the following formula (*28–29*):

$$\theta = \exp(-\gamma - m) \qquad \text{(equation 2)}$$

where γ = Euler's constant = 0.57722

$m = X_0 + d/2 - (d/n)\sum$

$X_0 = \log_e Z_0$

Z_0 = initial volume of marrow/well = 0.1 ml

$d = \log_e a$

a = dilution factor = 10

n = number of wells plated at each dilution = 10

$\sum$ = total number of positive wells

The probability of clonogenic unit growth in a well containing $\log_e$ dose (×) of cells was assumed to be given by the Poisson model as $1 - \exp(-\theta\exp[\times])$. Paired comparison t tests were based on the asymptotic normality of the Spearman estimators (m) for the mean $\log_e$ dose of cells required to achieve clonogenic unit growth. The assays were designed using a dilution factor of 10 and 10 wells per dilution to detect a difference in depletion of clonogenic units of .8 logs with statistical power 90% and a 0.05 level of significance. Plated concentrations ranged from 10^5 to 10^0 cells/well to ensure complete growth and no growth at the assay extremes, as required by the estimation procedure.

RESULTS

Phenotypic analysis following treatment with monoclonal antibody and complement. Initial evaluation of the effectiveness and specificity of antibody and complement-mediated depletion of T cells was carried out using indirect immunofluorescence assays with subsequent analysis by flow cytometry. As shown in Table 1, following treatment with anti-T12 and complement, the percentage of T12-positive cells fell to zero and there was a corresponding fall in the number of T cells detectable by other T cell markers (T3, T4, T8, and T11). Lysis with anti-T11 and complement resulted in apparent complete depletion of T11-positive cells though small numbers (2–4%) of residual T cells were again measurable by other T-cell-specific monoclonal antibodies (T3, T4, T8, and T12). Following lysis with the combination of antibodies, neither T11-positive nor T12-positive cells were detectable by phenotypic analysis. Nevertheless, residual T cells as measured by reactivity with anti-T3, anti-T4, and anti-T8 could still be detected—although in all instances the percentage of positive cells was relatively small. In most instances this low level of reactivity could not be reliably distinguished from nonspecific background fluorescence, especially since the multiple cycles of incubation with antibody and complement always resulted in increased levels of nonspecific fluorescence. In all T cell depletion experiments there was a concomitant increase in percentages of cells expressing myelomonocytic antigens, such as MO1, and there was no depletion of B lymphocytes as measured by reactivity with anti-B1.

TABLE 1. Phenotypic analysis of bone marrow mononuclear cells following treatment with anti-T-cell monoclonal antibodies and rabbit complement

Treatment	% Cells reactive with monoclonal antibody						
	T3	T4	T8	T11	T12	B1	Mo-1
Pretreatment[a]	17[c]	10	7	13	10	3	28
Anti-T12 + C′[b]	10	5	3	6	0	4	36
Anti-T11 + C′[b]	4	3	2	0	4	2	38
Anti-T11 + anti-T12 + C′[b]	6	3	2	0	0	3	34

[a] Values represent average of 15 different bone marrow samples.
[b] Values represent average of 5 different bone marrow samples.
[c] Percentage of cells reactive with monoclonal antibody by indirect immunofluorescence assay and flow cytometric analysis.

Characterization of residual T cells and NK cells following in vitro culture. Although flow cytometric analysis showed complete depletion of T12-positive and T11-positive cells following complement-mediated lysis with the respective antibodies, it was likely that small numbers of residual T cells might still be present. Antibody and complement-treated marrow cells were therefore cultured under conditions that would activate such residual cells and their proliferation was then induced and maintained using LCM containing interleukin 2 (IL-2). In order to maximize the identification and functional characterization of any residual cells, various activation conditions were used including PHA, Con A, and allogeneic cells. After 9–12 days in culture, sufficient cells were available in each instance for phenotypic and functional analysis.

As shown in Tables 2 and 3, regardless of which antibody was used for in vitro depletion, stimulation by either PHA or Con A led to the proliferation of cells with a mature T cell phenotype—i.e., cells that coexpressed T1, T3, and T11, with subsets expressing T4 or T8. Most of the cells were T9 and Ia-positive reflecting T cell activation. In contrast, culture in the presence of LAZ 388 resulted in the proliferation of a different phenotypic population of cells that were T11-positive and strongly NKH1-positive but T3-negative. This phenotype is characteristic of a population of cells in normal peripheral blood that have the morphology of large granular lymphocytes and have natural killer activity (*26–27*). These cultured cells, therefore, appear to represent a proliferating population of NK cells with a phenotype similar to that of various NK clones that have previously been characterized (*27*). Again the majority were Ia and T9-positive reflecting cell activation and proliferation. Testing with other T-cell-specific antibodies, anti-T1, -T4, -T8, and -T12, demonstrated low levels of reactivity, again consistent with the finding that these populations did not have a mature T cell phenotype. Culture with medium alone, that is, with no specific stimulus except for the addition of LCM, also resulted in the proliferation of a population with an NK cell phenotype ($T11^+$, $NKH1^+$, $T3^-$) in the three instances in which sufficient cells were obtained for further analysis. As expected, B lymphocytes, erythroid, and myeloid cells did not proliferate under these culture conditions, so that after 9–14 days in culture essentially all cells had either T cell or NK cell phenotype.

Regardless of which antibody was used for the initial lysis, two distinct populations of cells could be identified depending on the subsequent culture conditions. More detailed comparison of the phenotype of cells cultured after lysis with anti-T12 and anti-T11 did, however, reveal differences that reflected the different reactivities of the two antibodies used for T cell depletion. Cells stimulated with PHA or Con A expressed a mature T cell phenotype, but following treatment with anti-

TABLE 2. Phenotype of cultured cells following treatment with anti-T12 antibody and complement

Antigen	In vitro culture stimulation			
	Medium	LAZ 388	PHA	CON A
T1	4[a]±2.6	5±1.2	69±4.4	69±7.5
T3	12±4.5	9±6.2	71±5.3	64±2.1
T4	18±5.3	6±2.9	22±0.5	53±8.5
T8	0±0.6	9±6.5	16±0.8	18±8.2
T9	14±4.9	56±7.0	29±0.8	40±9.2
T11	92±1.3	82±2.6	94±0.8	97±0.8
T12	9±5.3	2±0.8	25±0.8	43±16.8
Ia	47±10.6	83±9.4	60±10.2	68±13.6
B1	0±0	1±0.8	0±0	0±0.4
NKH1	84±2.9	73±5.3	26±2.4	19±4.6
MY4	1±0.5	0±2.2	0±0	0±0.4

[a] The percentage of cells expressing each antigen was calculated using indirect immunofluorescence assay followed by flow cytometric analysis. Background reactivity (always less than 5%) was subtracted from each result. Each value represents the mean of 5 BM samples ±1 SD.

TABLE 3. Phenotype of cultured cells following treatment with anti-T11 antibody and complement

Antigen	In vitro culture stimulation		
	LAZ 388	PHA	CON A
T1	14[a]±6.2	74±7.8	90±3.6
T3	22±6.5	81±6.1	92±2.5
T4	25±2.4	63±6.9	73±4.6
T8	7±5.3	25±6.9	35±4.5
T9	65±3.7	64±4.1	72±3.7
T11	66±6.5	85±7.0	60±7.5
T12	4±3.3	68±18.2	69±7.8
Ia	91±1.1	59±6.5	33±3.3
B1	8±5.7	3±0.4	1±1.3
NKH1	69±2.8	5±1.2	4±0.8
MO1	22±1.2	3±1.6	5±0.5
MY4	2±0.4	3±1.3	5±0.6

[a] Proliferation following culture with conditioned medium alone was insufficient for phenotypic analysis. Each value represents the mean of 5 bone marrow samples ±1 SD.

T12, the percentage of residual T12-positive cells was lower than that observed following treatment with anti-T11 (mean values 25% vs. 68% with PHA and 43% vs. 69% with Con A). This appears to reflect weaker expression of the T12 antigen on the residual population that survived lysis with anti-T12 and complement. With regard to the NK cell population, following lysis with anti-T12 it was possible to induce proliferation of NK cells with T-cell-conditioned medium alone. However, despite identical culture conditions, no growth was observed following T11 lysis. This finding is consistent with the known expression of T11 antigen on the majority of normal NK cells, and indicates that T11 lysis affected NK cells more than treatment with anti-T12. The effect of anti-T11 treatment on NK cells was also noted following stimulation by PHA or Con-A. Here the percentage of cultured NKH1-positive cells was lower than that seen after treatment with anti-T12 (3–7% vs. 18–29%).

Cytotoxicity of cultured cells following monoclonal antibody and complement lysis. As noted previously, the residual cells expressed different phenotypes depending on the proliferative stimulus. These phenotypic differences suggested that cells cultured with LAZ 388 would have NK cell activity, whereas those with a mature T cell phenotype would not. Figure 1 shows the results of a cytotoxicity assay measuring natural killer activity for each of the cultured cell populations following lysis with anti-T12 plus complement. Similar results were obtained with cells cultured after treatment with anti-T11 plus complement (data not shown). In these experiments phenotype correlated well with functional activity, so that the NKH1-positive cells resulting from culture with LAZ 388 or with LCM alone exhibited marked cytotoxicity against K562 target cells, while the NKH1 negative cells cultured with PHA or Con A showed very little NK activity.

Quantitative analysis of T cell depletion with monoclonal antibody and complement. In vitro culture of antibody-treated marrow suggested that small numbers of $T12^+$ and $T11^+$ cells were still present despite complement-mediated lysis and apparent complete depletion by immunofluorescence analysis. In order to quantitate both the extent of depletion and the number of residual cells remaining following treatment, a clonogenic assay was developed using in vitro culture of cells at multiple cell concentrations. Similar assays have previously been used to quantitate depletion of tumor cell targets from normal bone marrow by treatment with monoclonal antibodies and complement (*29, 30*). In our studies this "limiting dilution assay" was performed under two different culture conditions using PHA and LAZ 388 to determine both the numbers of residual T cells and NK cells. Cells were cultured for 10 days in the presence of LCM and proliferation assessed by incorporation of ^3H thymidine.

A mathematical formula (equation 2) was used to estimate the number of residual T cell "clonogenic units" remaining after treatment with anti-T11 or anti-T12 alone, or the combination of antibodies. The number of cells lysed in each case was then calculated using the negative antibody 8A7 as a control (Table 4 and Figure 2). Following treatment with 8A7 and complement, a greater number of clonogenic units was detected on culture with LAZ 388 cells than with PHA (mean 1.9×10^5 vs. 3.3×10^4; $P = 0.001$). This reflects the strong allogeneic stimulation of mature T cells as well as NK cells by Laz 388 and represents a cloning efficiency of approximately 90%,

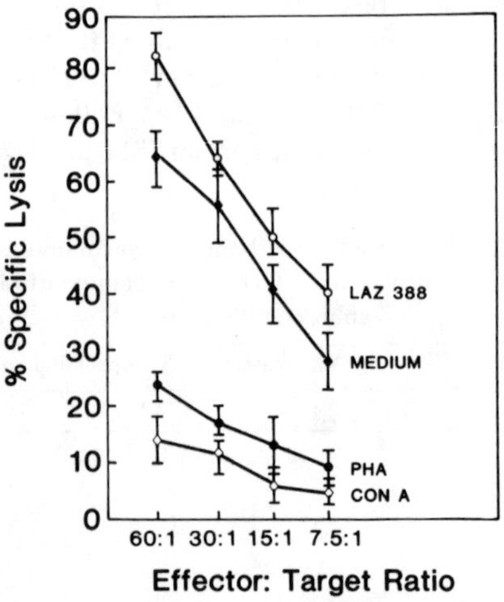

FIGURE 1. Cytotoxicity of bone marrow mononuclear cells cultured with irradiated LAZ 388 cells, medium alone, PHA, or Con A following treatment with anti-T12 and complement. Natural killer cell activity against K562 cells was assessed at 4 effector:target cell ratios.

TABLE 4. Depletion of T cell "clonogenic units" from bone marrow with monoclonal anti-T12 and anti-T11 plus complement

	8A7	Anti-T12	% Lysis	8A7	Anti-T11	% Lysis	8A7	Anti-T11 + anti-T12	% Lysis
PHA	2.8×10^3	7.1×10	97.49	4.9×10^3	8.6×10	98.24	3.2×10^4	3.3×10	99.89
	8.9×10^4	2.8×10^3	96.84	2.1×10^3	3.1×10^2	85.37	2.2×10^4	8.2×10	99.63
	3.5×10^4	8.9×10^2	97.49	7.7×10^4	2.0×10^3	97.41	4.4×10^4	2.2×10	99.95
	1.8×10^4	6.3×10	99.64	—	—	—	3.6×10^4	6.1×10	99.83
			mean[a] = 98.36			mean = 95.94			mean = 99.87
Laz 388	1.4×10^4	0.8×10	99.94	$\times10^4$	1.7×10^3	98.26	6.0×10^5	6.7×10	99.99
	3.5×10^5	1.1×10^4	96.84	4.8×10^3	1.0×10^2	97.86	4.8×10^4	7.5×10	99.84
	5.6×10^4	5.6×10^3	90	9.3×10^4	2.9×10^3	96.91	9.7×10^4	2.2×10	99.97
	4.4×10^5	3.3×10	99.99	—	—	—	3.3×10^5	3.0×10^2	99.92
			mean = 99.65			mean = 97.74			mean = 99.95

[a] Mean = 100% − geometric mean of the percentage of clonogenic units not lysed.

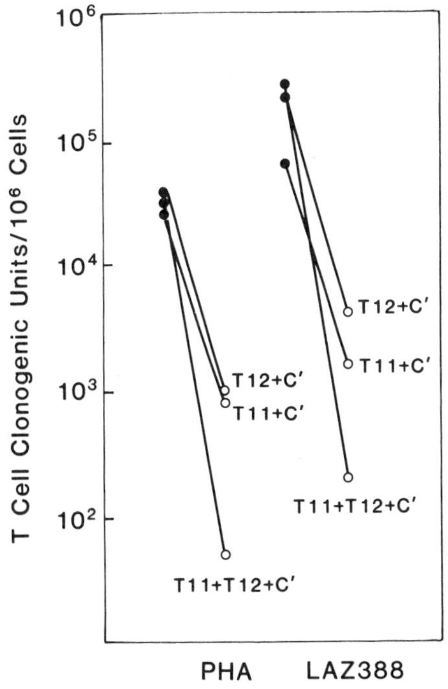

FIGURE 2. Depletion of T cell clonogenic units following treatment with monoclonal antibody and complement; (●) treatment with negative control antibody 8A7, plus complement. (○) Treatment with anti-T11 or anti-T12 plus complement. Marrow cells treated with negative control antibody or anti-T cell antibody were cultured with PHA or Laz 388 cells to stimulate cell proliferation, and the estimated number of clonogenic cells remaining was calculated as described in the *Materials and Methods* section. Results represent the mean of 11 different experiments shown in Table 4.

assuming that for each 10^6 BM MNC in the starting population, approximately 15–20% are T cells or NK cells. Using PHA stimulated cultures to measure the depletion of T cells, anti-T12 alone was capable of lysing between 1 and 2 logs of cells (geometric mean lytic efficiency: 98.36%). Treatment with anti-T11 alone was somewhat less efficient than anti-T12 alone and did not result in depletion of more than 2 logs of cells in any experiment (geometric mean lytic efficiency 94.94%). When anti-T11 and anti-T12 were used in combination, T cell depletion measured with PHA stimulation was enhanced compared with anti-T12 alone ($P = 0.01$) and with anti-T11 alone ($P = 0.002$). In each of 4 experiments, at least a 2-log depletion occurred, and in one instance greater than 3-log lysis was achieved (mean lytic efficiency 99.87%).

As shown by the in vitro culture experiments following T cell depletion Laz 388 stimulated assays measured NK cell depletion as well as T cell lysis. Treatment with anti-T12 alone gave variable degrees of lysis (range 90.00% to 99.99%), which may reflect variability in the numbers of NK cells in the starting populations. Treatment with anti-T11 gave more consistent results but was always less than 99% lysis. In contrast, use of both anti-T12 and anti-T11 resulted in a 3–4-log depletion (mean lytic efficiency 99.95%), significantly more than with anti-T11 ($P = 0.005$) and more consistently than with anti-T12 alone.

DISCUSSION

In contrast to current methods of posttransplant immunosuppression, in vitro treatment of allogeneic marrow to remove immunocompetent T lymphocytes offers an alternative strategy for prevention of GVHD. Although preincubation of donor marrow with single or multiple monoclonal anti-T-cell antibodies without complement has failed to prevent GVHD (*31, 32*), in vitro lysis of T cells using monoclonal antibodies and complement has been successful, as have other methods of T cell depletion (*33*). The preliminary results of such clinical trials in which patients have received T-cell-depleted allogeneic marrow are encouraging, with the majority of recipients not having developed severe GVHD despite infusion of histoincompatible marrow in some instances (*11–15, 33*).

Within the context of a clinical study to investigate the use of T cell depleted bone marrow for allogeneic transplantation, one objective of the present experiments was to determine whether any T12-positive cells remained following in vitro treatment with anti-T12 and complement. Phenotypic analysis of bone marrow before and after 3 cycles of treatment identical to that used in the clinical study suggested that complete removal of T12-positive cells was possible with the use of anti-T12 alone, though small numbers of residual T cells could be detected with other T-cell-specific monoclonal antibodies. The use of another lytic monoclonal antibody, anti-T11, and complement similarly resulted in the absence of detectable T11-positive cells, though some T12-positive cells remained. T cell depletion could be further enhanced by concurrent use of the two antibodies. However, the limitations of sensitivity using flow cytometric analysis, together with the inevitable increase in nonspecific background fluorescence associated with 3 cycles of in vitro treatment, made it probable that residual cells would persist. Similar results have been found using other methods for in vitro treatment (*34–36*), and in our studies this was confirmed by culture of the residual mononuclear cells under various conditions conducive to the proliferation of T lymphocytes. These experiments revealed the presence of cells that expressed a mature T cell phenotype in every instance despite apparent complete depletion by immunofluorescence analysis. Although it is likely that these cells simply reflect the presence of residual T cells, it is also possible that the mature T cells seen after in vitro culture of T-cell-depleted marrow are derived from immature T cells that have undergone differentiation as well as proliferation in vitro. This may be a more significant factor following anti-T12 depletion, since this reagent is only reactive with fully differentiated T cells. In this regard, the finding that T cells recovered following culture of anti-T12-treated marrow expressed less T12 antigen than those recovered following anti-T11 treatment, suggests that these cells are at least in part derived from a residual population that expresses less T12 antigen. Nonetheless, given the necessity for prolonged in vitro culture, it is impossible to accurately determine whether cultured T cells were derived from precursor cells or whether some cells simply remained viable despite in vitro treatment.

The implication for clinical studies of allogeneic bone marrow transplantation is that, despite in vitro depletion with antibody and complement, donor marrow will very likely contain small numbers of T cells capable of proliferating in vivo, and might be sufficient to cause clinical GVHD. In a murine model of GVHD in the context of minor histocompatibility antigen differences, the presence of 0.3–1% T cells in the donor spleen cell population was capable of causing GVHD (*6*). The number of residual T cells that would be capable of causing GVHD in humans is not known, however T cell depletion in the experiments that have been described indicated that the use of one monoclonal antibody alone often results in greater than 1% residual T cells. Only experiments that utilized both anti-T12 and anti-T11 in combination were consistently effective in removing greater than 99% of T cells. Fortunately, the results of the clinical studies to date suggest that, at least for patients receiving HLA-identical marrow grafts, the presence of a minimal number of T cells in the marrow inoculum may not be deleterious—and, indeed, it may be necessary for reconstitution of normal T cell function.

Whereas stimulation with PHA or Con A led to the proliferation of mature T lymphocytes, stimulation with allogeneic EB-virus-transformed B cells in the presence of LCM or LCM alone resulted in the growth of a population of cells with the characteristics of natural killer cells. These cultured cells expressed T11 and NKH1 but were generally T3-negative—a cell-surface phenotype known to be characteristic of human NK cells (*26*, *27*). It is of interest that some of the earliest cells to appear in the peripheral blood of patients who have received either autologous bone marrow that has been treated in vitro with the monoclonal antibody anti-B1 and complement (*37*) or allogeneic bone marrow that has been treated with anti-T12 and complement (*38*) are $T11^+$, $NKH1^+$ NK cells. Whether such cells could contribute, in some patients, to the clinical manifestations of GVHD remains to be established. Experimental studies in rodents have shown that augmentation of NK cell activity occurs during the acute graft-versus-host reaction (*39*) with recruitment of NK cells in both peripheral and intestinal lymphoid tissue (*40*). Moreover, others have reported (*41*, *42*) a correlation between high NK cell activity and the occurrence of acute GVHD in patients receiving allogeneic marrow, implying that the cells involved in GVHD are able to exert NK cell activity at some stage of their maturation. If this were the case, the use of an antibody such as anti-T11 might be helpful, as this reagent would result in depletion of NK cells as well as T cells. On the other hand, NK-active cells have not been directly implicated in the development of GVHD, and maintenance of NK cell activity may facilitate adequate immunological reconstitution.

Having defined the conditions for in vitro growth of mature T lymphocytes and NK cells, PHA and LAZ 388 were then used as the proliferative stimulus in a limiting dilution assay in order to quantitate the degree of lysis achieved. The assay here described is a procedure originally applied to the problem of estimating bacterial growth (*28*). In the present studies it was used to estimate the number of T cell clonogenic units per 10^6 cells that remain following in vitro treatment; the results of these experiments are summarized in Figure 2. Although there was some variation in the degree of lysis achieved with each antibody alone it appeared that the overall results with anti-T12 and anti-T11 were similar and resulted in a 1–2 log cell depletion. When the two antibodies were used concurrently, an additive effect was observed, so that in some cases greater than 99.9% lysis was achieved, representing over 3 logs of cell depletion.

Although treatment with both anti-T11 and anti-T12 plus complement in this in vitro model increased the extent of T cell depletion over that achieved with a single antibody, it is not known whether such combinations will be required in the clinical setting. Our studies suggest that the addition of anti-T11 to anti-T12 results in elimination of NK cells as well as T cells. The hypothesis that maximal lysis is optimal is an attractive one, but the presence of a certain minimal number of T cells or NK cells may be required for adequate immunologic reconstitution to take place. More complete elimination of both T and NK cells may not be more effective in preventing GVHD, but may result in slower and more defective immunologic reconstitution and an increased incidence of infectious complications posttransplant. In addition, donor NK cells have been implicated as potential mediators of antileukemia activity following allogeneic marrow transplantation (*38*).

Elimination of immunocompetent T lymphocytes from donor marrow appears to be a promising method for the prevention of acute GVHD in patients with histocompatible donors, and it is possible that this technique can also be successfully applied to patients receiving HLA-mismatched marrow. The availability of sensitive assays to quantitate the degree of lysis achieved will help in the development of effective methods of in vitro T cell depletion and the choice of specific monoclonal antibody reagents. The ability to measure residual viable NK cells as well as T cells will also facilitate the evaluation of clinical outcome and provide correlations with the incidence and severity of acute GVHD, rapidity of marrow engraftment, and the incidence of leukemia relapse following bone marrow transplantation.

Acknowledgments. We are very grateful to Mary Kornacki, David Leslie, and Herbert Levine for their assistance in performing the flow cytometric analyses.

REFERENCES

1. Thomas ED, Storb R, Clift RA, Fefer A, Johnson L, Neiman PE, et al. Bone marrow transplantation. N Engl J Med 1975; 292: 902.
2. Storb R, Prentice RL, Buckner CD, Clift RA, Appelbaum F, Deeg J, et al. Graft versus host disease and survival in patients with

aplastic anemia treated by marrow grafts from HLA-identical siblings. N Engl J Med 1983; 308: 302.
3. Tyan ML. Modification of severe graft-versus-host-disease with antisera to the theta antigen or to whole serum. Transplantation 1973; 15: 601.
4. Yunis EJ, Good RA, Smith J, Stutman O. Protection of lethally irradiated mice by spleen cells from neonatally thymectomized mice. Proc Natl Acad Sci UDA 1974; 71: 2544.
5. Rodt HV, Thierfelder S, Eulitz M. Anti-lymphocytic antibodies and marrow transplantion. III. Effect of heterologous anti-brain antibodies on acute secondary disease in mice. Eur J Immunol 1974; 4: 25.
6. Korngold R, Sprent J. Lethal graft-versus-host disease after bone marrow transplantation across minor histocompatibility barriers in mice. Prevention by removing mature T cells from marrow. J Exp Med 1978; 148: 1687.
7. Vallera DA, Youle RJ, Neville DM, Kersey JM. Bone marrow transplantation across major histocompatibility barriers. V. Protection of mice from lethal graft versus host disease by pretreatment of donor cells with monoclonal anti-Thy-1.2 coupled to the toxin Ricin. J Exp Med 1982; 155: 949.
8. Wagemaker G, Vriesendorp HM, Van Bekkum DW. Successful bone marrow transplantation across major histocompatibility barriers in rhesus monkeys. Transplant Proc 1981; 13: 875.
9. Vallera DA, Soderling CCB, Carlson GJ, Kersey JM. Bone marrow transplantation across major histocompatibility barriers in mice. Effect of elimination of T cells from donor grafts by treatment with monoclonal Thy1.2 plus complement or antibody alone. Transplantation 1981; 31: 218.
10. Reinherz EL, Geha R, Rappeport JM, Wilson M, Penta AC, Hussey RE, et al. Reconstitution after transplantation with T lymphocyte depleted HLA haplotype mismatched bone marrow for severe combined immunodeficiency. Proc Natl Acad Sci USA 1982; 79: 6047.
11. Filipovich AH, Vallera DA, Youle RJ, Quinones RR, Neville DM, Kersey JM, et al. Ex-vivo treatment of donor bone marrow with anti-T-cell immunotoxins for prevention of graft-versus-host disease. Lancet 1984; 1: 469.
12. Trigg ME, Billing R, Sondel PM, Dickerman JD, Erickson C, Finlay JL, et al. Depletion of T cells from human bone marrow with monoclonal CT-2 and complement. J Biol Res Modif 1984; 3: 406.
13. Prentice HG, Blacklock HA, Janossy G, Gilmore MJML, Price-Jones L, Tidmann, et al. Depletion of T lymphocytes in donor marrow prevents significant graft versus host disease in matched allogeneic leukaemic marrow transplant recipients. Lancet 1984; 1: 472.
14. Waldmann H, Polliak A, Hale G, Or R, Cividalli G, Weiss L, et al. Elimination of graft-versus-host disease by in vitro depletion of alloreactive lymphocytes with a monoclonal rat anti-human lymphocyte antibody (CAMPATH-1). Lancet 1984; 2: 483.
15. Herve P, Flesch M, Cahn JY, Racadot E, Plouvier E, Lamy B, et al. Removal of marrow T cells with OKT3-OKT11 monoclonal antibodies and complement to prevent Graft-versus-host disease: a pilot study in ten patients. Transplantation 1985; 39: 138.
16. Ritz J. Use of monoclonal antibodies in autologous and allogeneic bone marrow transplantation. Clin Haematol 1983; 12: 813.
17. Meuer SC, Hussey RE, Fabbi M, Fox D, Acuto O, Fitzgerald KA, et al. An alternative pathway of T cell activation: a functional role for the 50 kd T11 sheep erythrocyte receptor protein. Cell 1984; 36: 897.
18. Reinherz EL, Schlossman SF. The differentiation and function of human T lymphocytes: a review. Cell 1980; 19: 822.
19. Reinherz EL, Kung PC, Goldstein G, Schlossman SF. A monoclonal antibody with selective reactivity with functionally mature human thymocytes and all peripheral human T cells. J Immunol 1981; 123: 1312.
20. Reinherz EL, Kung PC, Goldstein G, Levey RM, Schlossman SF. Discrete stages of human intrathymic differentiation. Analysis of normal thymocytes and leukemic lymphoblasts of T cell lineage. Proc Natl Acad Sci USA 1980; 77: 1588.
21. Sutherland R, Delia D, Schneider C, Newman R, Kemshead J, Greaves M. Umbiquitous cell-surface glycoprotein on tumor cells is proliferation-associated receptor for transferrin. Proc Natl Acad Sci USA 1981; 78: 4515.
22. Nadler LM, Stashenko P, Hardy R, Pesando JM, Yunis EJ, Schlossman SF. Monoclonal antibodies defining serologically distinct HLA-D/DR-related Ia like antigens in man. Hum Immunol 1981; 1: 77.
23. Nadler LM, Stashenko P, Ritz J, Hardy R, Pesando JM, Schlossman SF. A unique cell surface antigen identifying lymphoid malignancies of B cell origin. J Clin Invest 1981; 67: 134.
24. Todd RF III, Nadler LM, Schlossman SF. Antigens on human monocytes identified by monoclonal antibodies. J Immunol 1981; 126: 1435.
25. Griffin JD, Ritz J, Nadler LM, Schlossman SF. Expression of myeloid differentiation antigens on normal and malignant cells. J Clin Invest 1981; 68: 932.
26. Griffin JD, Hercend T, Beveridge R, Schlossman SF. Characterization of an antigen expressed by human natural killer cells. J Immunol 1983; 130: 2947.
27. Hercend T, Griffin JD, Benussan A, Schmidt RE, Edson MA, Brennan A, et al. Generation of monoclonal antibodies to a human NK clone: characterization of two NK associated antigens; $NKH1_A$ and NKH2, expressed on subsets of large granular lymphocytes. J Clin Invest 1985; 75: 932.
28. Johnson EA, Brown BW. The Spearman estimator for serial dilution assays. Biometrics 1961; 17: 79.
29. Bast RC Jr, DeFabritiis P, Lipton J, Gelber R, Maver C, Nadler L, et al. Elimination of malignant clonogenic cells from human bone marrow using multiple monoclonal antibodies and complement. Cancer Res 1985; 45: 499.
30. DeFabritiis P, Bregni M, Lipton J, Greenberger J, Nadler L, Rothstein L, et al. Elimination of clonogenic Burkitt's lymphoma cells from human bone marrow using 4-hydroperoxycyclophosphamide in combination with monoclonal antibodies and complement. Blood 1985; 65: 1064.
31. Prentice HG, Janossy G, Skeggs D, Blacklock YA, Bradstock KF, Goldstein G, et al. Use of anti-T-cell monoclonal antibody OKT3 to prevent acute graft-versus-host disease in allogeneic bone-marrow transplantation for acute leukaemia. Lancet 1982; 1: 700.
32. Martin PJ, Hansen JA, Thomas ED. Preincubation of donor bone marrow cells with a combination of murine monoclonal anti-T-cell antibodies without complement does not prevent graft-versus-host disease after allogeneic marrow transplantation. J Clin Immunol 1984; 1: 18.
33. Reisner Y, Kapoor N, Kirkpatrick D, Pollack MS, Dupont B, Good RA, O'Reilly RJ. Transplantation for acute leukemia with HLA-A and B nonidentical parental marrow cell fractionated with soybean agglutinin and sheep red blood cells. Lancet 1981; 2: 327.
34. Levitt L, Kipps TJ, Engleman EG, Greenberg PL. Human bone marrow and peripheral blood T lymphocyte depletion: efficacy and effects of both T cells and monocytes on growth of hematopoietic progenitors. Blood 1985; 65: 663.
35. Moreau J, Miller RG. Growth at limiting dilution of human T cell colonies from T cell-depleted peripheral blood leukocytes. J Immunol 1983; 130: 1139.
36. Kernan NA, Flomenberg N, Collins NH, O'Reilly RJ, Dupont B. Quantitation of T lymphocytes in bone marrow by limiting dilution assay. Transplantation 1985; 40: 317.
37. Nadler LM, Takvorian T, Botnick L, Bast RC, Finberg R, Hellman S, et al. Anti-B1 monoclonal antibody and complement treated autologous bone marrow transplantation for relapsed B cell non-Hodgkin's lymphoma. Lancet 1984; 2: 427.
38. Hercend T, Takvorian T, Nowill A, Tantravahi R, Moingeon P,

Anderson KC, et al. Characterization of natural killer cells with anti-leukemia activity following allogeneic bone marrow transplantation. Blood 1986; 67: 722
39. Clancy J, Mauser L, Chapman AL. Level and temporal pattern of naturally cytolytic cells during acute graft-versus-host-disease (GVHD) in the rat. Cell Immunol 1983; 79: 1.
40. Borland A, Mowat A Mc I, Parrott DMV. Augmentation of intestinal and peripheral natural killer cell activity during the GVH reaction in mice. Transplantation 1983; 36: 513.
41. Dokhelar M-C, Wiels J, Lipinski M, Tetavd E, Deverigie A, Gluckman E, et al. Natural killer cell activity in human bone marrow recipients. Transplantation 1981; 31: 61.
42. Gratama JW, Lipovich-Oosterveer MA, Ronteltap C, Sinnige LGF, Janen J, Van Der Griend RJ, Bolhuis RLH. Natural immunity and graft-versus-host-disease. Transplantation 1985; 40: 256.

Received 2 January 1985.
Accepted 29 October 1985.

0041-1337/86/4201-0080$02.00/0
TRANSPLANTATION
Vol. 42, No. 1

Printed in U.S.A.

THE EFFECT OF COLLINS' SOLUTION ON THE FUNCTION AND STRUCTURE OF ISOLATED PROXIMAL CONVOLUTED TUBULES FROM RABBIT KIDNEYS[1]

J.F. FIGUEIREDO,[2] D. FALKENSTEIN, S.A. DRAIBE, D. SIGULEM, AND O.L. RAMOS

Renal Division, Department of Internal Medicine, Escola Paulista de Medicina, São Paulo, Brasil

Proximal convoluted tubules (PCTs) from rabbit cortical slices were perfused after preservation in Collins' solution with the in vitro microperfusion technique.

Under these conditions, after maneuvers of in vitro preservation, the following findings were observed: (1) Tubules were best preserved, functionally and morphologically, when bathed with Collins' solution peritubularly. (2) Tubular preservation was inadequate when the Collins' solution contacted only the luminal or luminal and peritubular sides.

These observations indicate a difference in the reactions of various cellular sides to the preservation process, suggesting that during preservation of the whole kidney, there are differences in the preservation of the various tissues of the organ.

Renal preservation, utilizing several techniques, has been widely used in clinical organ transplantation. Several solutions that preserve the function of isolated kidney have been designed for this purpose (*1, 2, 3*). Nevertheless, studies of the efficacy of preservation are usually assayed using whole-kidney function, and they have provided contradictory data. On the other hand, there are only a few studies of the effects of preservation on cell metabolism and function. It would be of interest to know the pathophysiological characteristics of preserved renal tissue in order to improve preservation techniques.

In previous reports, using the microperfusion technique of the in vitro isolated tubule, it has been shown that long-term storage of a rabbit's renal cortical slice in a Collins' and sodium phosphate buffer solution can keep the proximal tubules functionally and morphologically viable for several hours (*4, 5*).

Based on these data, several maneuvers for in vitro preservation were simulated, so that the preservation solution was in contact with various cellular sides of the tubule of the kidney (luminal, peritubular, and interstitial sides). Therefore, functional and morphological changes in the various cellular sides could be evaluated.

These maneuvers could indicate the delivering of a preservation solution in the several compartments of the kidney parenchyma.

The following theoretical methods for delivering the preservation solution into the renal tubule were considered (Fig. 1):

Group 1. Using the first method the preservation solution contacts the tubule only by the basolateral route (peritubular). This is similar to flushing the solution through the kidney by hydrostatic pressure during kidney preservation.

Group 2. Using the second method the preservation solution contacts the tubule through the luminal and peritubular routes. This is similar to perfusing the kidney by glomerular filtration, which could occur using high hydrostatic pressure or a pump.

Group 3. Using the third method, the preservation solution contacts the tubules only on the luminal side of the tubular cellular layer, which rarely could occur if all the preservation solution contacted the tubule by glomerular filtration.

The aim of the present study was to verify the direct effect of the Collins solution (*6*) on the convoluted proximal tubules and to see if there is a preferential way to preserve the cellular layer, considering that the precise distribution of preservation solutions in the various kidney tissues is still unknown.

[1]This work was supported by grants from Conselho Nacional de Desenvolvimento Científico e Tecnológico—CNPq, Fundação de Amparo à Pesquisa do Estado de São Paulo—FAPESP, and Instituto Paulista de Estudos e Pesquisas em Nefrologia e Hipertensão—Ipepenhi.

[2]Address correspondence to: José Francisco Figueiredo, M.D., Ph.D., Disciplina de Nefrologia, Escola Paulista de Medicina, Rua Botucatu, 740, 04023 São Paulo, SP, Brasil.

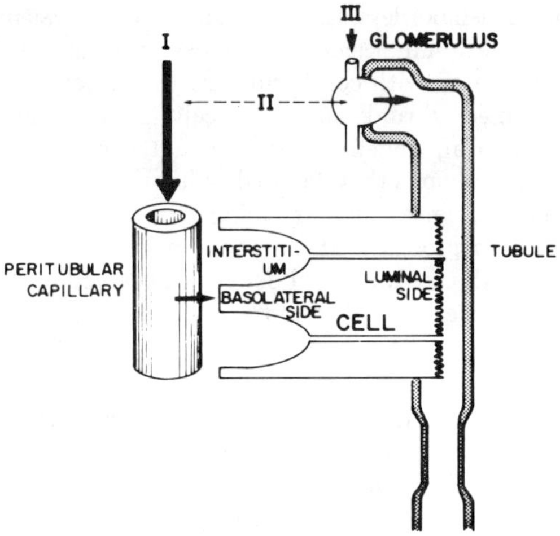

FIGURE 1. Possible methods for delivering the preservation solutions into the kidney parenchyma.

MATERIALS AND METHODS

Proximal convoluted tubules (PCTs)* were dissected from the cortical regions of the kidney and perfused by the method developed originally by Burg et al. (*7–9*).

Kidneys were removed from male white rabbits weighing 1.5–2.5 kg and cut into thin slices for tubule dissection; these were placed in a Petri dish with a modified Krebs-Henseleit solution containing 6.5 g/dl of fraction V bovine serum albumin (Miles Co.) at 4°C gassed with 95% O_2 plus 5% CO_2.

After dissection, the tubule was transferred into a special perfusion chamber and attached to a micropipette system—which on the perfusion side was composed of a holding pipette, a perfusion pipette, and a fluid exchange pipette connected to a fluid reservoir—that drove the perfusion flux by hydrostatic pressure. The collection side was composed of a holding pipette filled with oil and a constant-volume-bore collection pipette (Fig. 2). In the control and recovery perfusion period the tubule was bathed with a modified Krebs-Henseleit solution (KHA) with 6.5 g/dl of bovine serum albumin (Table 1) at 37°C, gassed with 95% O_2 plus 5% CO_2. The tubule was perfused by hydrostatic pressure with an ultrafiltrate of the bathing solution that had been passed through a Millipore-Pellicon membrane, PTGC 047-10, having a 10^4-dalton nominal molecular weight limit.

In each perfusion period, equilibration for at least 20 min was allowed before measurements were taken. The bath solution was changed continuously by an infusion pump system (Harvard, model 975). The perfusion solution was changed during the experiment by a special exchange pipette system (*9*).

Volume absorption (Jv, $nl \cdot min^{-1} \cdot mm^{-1}$) was determined using ^{14}C-Carboxy-inulin (New England Nuclear, Boston) according to the equation:

$$Jv = \frac{V_L}{L}\left(\frac{^{14}\text{C-inulin L}}{^{14}\text{C-inulin O}} - 1\right)$$

where: V_L ($nl \cdot min^{-1}$) is the collection rate; L (mm) is the length of the perfused tubule, measured at the end of the experiment, and ^{14}C-inulin$_L$/^{14}C-inulin$_O$ is the ratio of the concentration of the volume marker in the collected and perfused solutions, respectively.

The radioactivity of ^{14}C-inulin in the bath was monitored in each collection period, to detect possible leaks in the perfusion system or in the tubular epithelia. Under normal conditions, experiments with a leakage of more than 5% of the perfusion rate of ^{14}C-inulin are not acceptable.

The following experiments were designed to study the direct effect of Collins' solution (Table 1) on the peritubular or intraluminal side of proximal convoluted tubule:

Group 1. Proximal convoluted tubules (n = 7) were perfused in the control period with KHA solution at 37°C gassed with 95% O_2 plus 5% CO_2 at the peritubular and luminal side. In this period 3 samples were collected, at 10-min intervals, for Jv measurements. In the experimental (E) period, Collins' solution at 10°C, without gassing, was added to the peritubular side and the luminal side remaining filled with an ultrafiltrate of KHA solution, without perfusion pressure. This period lasted for 20 min without sample collection. The KHA solution was then added again to the peritubular side, at 37°C with gassing, and the recovery period performed.

Group 2. In this group, after a control period, the PCTs (n = 6) were perfused with Collins' solution at 10°C without gassing at the peritubular and luminal side, without perfusion pressure. Following this experimental period of 25 min, another period with a gassing KHA at 37°C at both sides was performed as the recovery period.

Group 3. In this group, in the experimental period, PCTs (n = 5) were perfused with KHA at 10°C without gassing at the peritubular side and with Collins' at 10°C at the luminal side without perfusion pressure. After 25 min under these

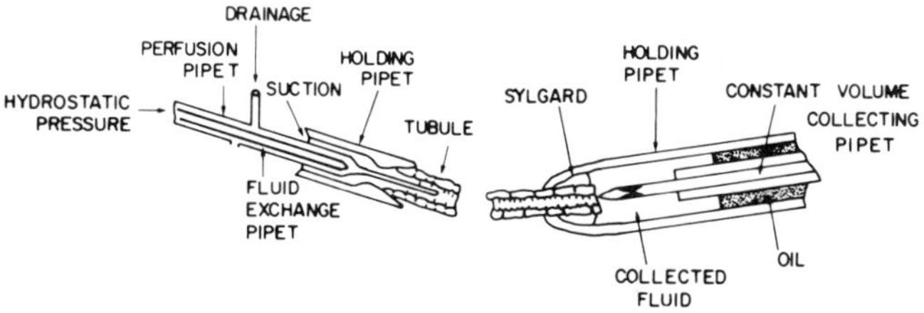

FIGURE 2. Microperfusion system.

TABLE 1. Composition of solutions (mM)

Solutions	Krebs-Henseleit with bovine albumin (KHA)	Collins' (C_2)
NaCl	105	—
$NaHCO_3$	25	10
$NaH_2C_2O_3$	10	—
NaH_2PO_4	1	—
KH_2PO_4	0.6	15
K_2HPO_4	—	40
KCl	5	15
$MgSO_4$	0.8	28
$CaCl_2$	2	—
Alanine	5	—
Glucose	8	139
Bovine albumin	6.5 g/dl	—
Osmolality (mOsm/kg H_2O)	290	330
pH at 25°C	7.4	7.0

* Without additives.

* Abbreviations used: KHA, Krebs-Henseleit albumin solution; PCT, proximal convoluted tubule.

experimental conditions, the recovery period with a gassing KHA at 37°C at both sides was performed in the tubule.

Results are expressed as an average of at least 3 collections in each period and were calculated from the average values for individual tubules and expressed as the mean ± SEM.

The statistical analyses were evaluated by the Student's *t* test and $P<0.05$ was taken as the level of statistical significance.

RESULTS

Functional aspects. The direct effects of Collins' (C_2) solution on the peritubular or luminal sides or on both sides of PCTs without perfusion pressure, are shown in Table 2.

Table 2 summarizes the mean of individual function values obtained in group 1. In this group (n = 7), during the control period, PCTs were perfused with KHA solution at 37°C at both sides at a perfusion rate of 12.1±0.7 $nl \cdot min^{-1}$ and the Jv was 1.15±0.24 $nl \cdot min^{-1} \cdot mm^{-1}$. During the experimental period, the maneuvers performed with the addition of C_2 solution at 10°C on the peritubular side seem to preserve the tubular function as shown in the recovery period. During this period, the Jv obtained was of 1.05±0.17 $nl \cdot min^{-1} \cdot mm^{-1}$ at a perfusion rate of 13.0±0.8 $nl \cdot min^{-1}$, values not different from the control.

In group 2 (n = 6) during the control period the Jv obtained was 1.21±0.31 $nl \cdot min^{-1} \cdot mm^{-1}$. Nevertheless, the experimental maneuver of addition of C_2 solution at 10°C at the luminal and peritubular sides decreased tubular function during the recovery period. During this period, the Jv decreased to 0.38±0.22 $nl \cdot min^{-1} \cdot mm^{-1}$ about 69% below the control period without significant change in the perfusion rate.

In group 3 (n = 5) the experimental condition of addition of C_2 at 10°C only at the luminal side markedly decreased tubular function. The Jv decreased from 0.83±0.18 in the control to 0.14±0.09 $nl \cdot min^{-1} \cdot mm^{-1}$ in the recovery period. Under this condition, a significant decrease in perfusion rate, from 13.6± 0.5 to 11.4±0.6 $nl \cdot min^{-1}$ ($P<0.05$) could be detected between the control and recovery periods.

Morphological aspects. Proximal convoluted tubules, when perfused with KHA on both sides, in the control period, showed a visible lumen by optical microscopy (100×), delimited by a pyramidal epithelial cellular layer that showed a defined brush border in the luminal side. Under experimental conditions in which the C_2 solution was added only at the peritubular, or at both tubular sides, as in groups 1 and 2, a marked decrease in the luminal diameter was observed, probably by cell swelling. This morphological aspect reverted in the recovery period, but the epithelial cells still showed morphological changes and undefined brush borders. In group 3, in which C_2 was in contact only with the luminal side, an increase was detected in the luminal diameter, with cell shrinkage. In the recovery period, cells remained shrunk and the cellular morphology was changed, with an undefined or interrupted brush border appearance and regions that denoted cellular exfoliation.

The morphological tubular changes in the recovery period were larger in groups 2 and 3 than in group 1. These data correlated with the functional behavior observed in the PCTs, under these experimental conditions.

TABLE 2. The effect of the Collins' solution at 10°C without gassing on rabbit proximal convoluted tubules fluid absorption (Jv) at the peritubular (group 1), both (group 2), or luminal (group 3) sides of the tubule without perfusion

Group	Perfusion time (min)			Perfusion rate (nl/min^{-1})		Jv ($nl/min^{-1}/mm^{-1}$)		Δ Jv %
	Control	Experimental	Recovery	Control	Recovery	Control	Recovery	
1 (n = 7)	60[a]	20	55	12.1	13.0	1.15	1.05	9
	±4	±1	±3	±0.7	±0.8	±0.24	±0.17	
2 (n = 6)	48	27	50	17.0	14.4	1.21	0.38[b]	69
	±4	±1	±1	±1.5	±0.1	±0.31	±0.22	
3 (n = 5)	48	28	51	13.6	11.4[b]	0.83	0.14[b]	83
	±2	±3	±4	±0.5	±0.6	±0.18	±0.09	

[a] Mean ± SEM.
[b] Paired *t* test ($P<0.05$).

DISCUSSION

These results indicate that different epithelial cells sides of the tubule react differently after perfusion, depending on the surface of the PCTs that had contact with the Collins' solution. It was observed that contact of the C_2 solution with the peritubular surface (group 1) resulted in the best preservation of tubular function and morphology. A possible reason for this could be that the basolateral membrane structure, which is poorly permeable to ions and molecules, could prevent the influx of ions of this solution into the cell (*2*). At the same time, the temperature of 10°C and the ionic composition of C_2 solution should inhibit the cellular "pumps," and ion exchange would only depend on passive flux due to ionic gradients. On the other hand, contact of the C_2 solution with the luminal side could lead to absorption of C_2 solution ions by the cell, which could change the internal cellular milieu and metabolism (*10*). This phenomenon probably causes cellular injury that could be reversible or not after reperfusion of the tubule.

The experimental condition in which C_2 solution contacted the peritubular side of the PCT could be similar to the conditions in the clinical situation when the kidney is flushed by hydrostatic pressure during its preparation for transplantation. Under these conditions the preservation solution probably reaches the nephron via the peritubular capillaries. Glomerular filtration is possibly abolished during kidney flushing, as shown by the fact that the preservation solution comes out by the renal vein and not through the ureter, during clinical preservation.

Our data indicated that if glomerular filtration could occur during kidney preservation, it would lead to cellular injury similar to that observed in groups 2 and 3. These injuries were noted by morphological aspects resembling acute tubular necrosis, and were demonstrated by a fall in fluid absorption and in perfusion rate. This fall in perfusion rate could denote cellular swelling or tubular obstruction by casts originating from cellular desquamation like that observed by Nórlen et al. in studies with micropuncture in preserved rat kidneys (*11*).

These data, although in the isolated tubule theoretically could be used for explanation of some very-well-established clinical technical maneuvers, aim to obtain the best kidney preservation.

For example, for flushing solution it was established that the height of the perfusion is about one meter and this maneuver probably could prevent glomerular filtration. Another theoretical conclusion that could be drawn from these data could be the explanation of why, during kidney preservation by pump, it is impossible to use any kind of flushing solution, but under this condition it is necessary to use plasmalike solutions.

Our functional and morphological results obtained with this technique show the necessity of more detailed investigations on the effect of preservation on the cellular layers of the nephron segments. Finally, these studies show general characteristics of the various kidney compartments that should be taken into consideration in order to have better kidney preservation.

We thank Mrs. Marina André da Silva and Aurea B. Michelotto for secretarial assistance.

REFERENCES

1. Belzer FO. Renal preservation. N Engl J Med 1974; 291: 402.
2. Belzer FO, Southard JH. The future of kidney preservation. Transplantation 1980; 30: 161.
3. Marshall, VC. Renal preservation prior to transplantation. Transplantation 1980; 30: 165.
4. Falkenstein D, Conti GT, Ajzen H, Draibe SA, Figueiredo JF. Properties of the isolated rabbit proximal convoluted tubule and pars recta after long-term storage in a modified Collins solution. Braz J Med Biol Res 1982; 15: 361.
5. Pirie SC, Potts DJ. Application of cold flush preservation to in vitro microperfusion studies of kidney tubules. Kidney Int 1985; 28: 982.
6. Collins GM, Bravo-Shugarman M, Terasaki PI. Kidney preservation for transplantation. Initial perfusion and 30 hours ice storage. Lancet 1969; 2: 1219.
7. Burg MB, Grantham J, Abramow M, Orloff J. Preparation and study of fragments of single rabbit nephrons. Am J Physiol 1966; 210(6): 1293.
8. Kokko JP, Burg MB, Orloff J. Characteristics of NaCl and water transport in the renal proximal tubule. J Clin Invest 1971; 50: 69.
9. Burg MB. Perfusion of isolated renal tubules. Yale J Biol Med 1972; 45: 321.
10. Southard JH, Belzer FO. Principles of renal preservation for transplantation. In: Marberger M, Dreikorn K, eds. Renal preservation, vol 8. Baltimore: Williams & Wilkins, 1983: 188.
11. Nórlen BJ, Engberg A, Källskog Ö, Wollgast M. Nephron function of the transplanted rat kidney. Kidney Int 1978; 14: 10.

Received 11 July 1985.
Accepted 16 October 1985.

0041-1337/86/4201-0084$02.00/0
TRANSPLANTATION
Vol. 42, No. 1

Printed in U.S.A.

LIVER TRANSPLANTATION IN CRIGLER-NAJJAR SYNDROME
A CASE REPORT

Starzl and coworkers have reported encouraging results after liver replacement in inborn metabolic disorders (*4, 5*). In 23 children with metabolic disorders, the survival rate was superior to the overall survival in pediatric recipients. Consequently inborn metabolic disorders were accepted as indications for liver transplantation by the Consensus Development Conference held in 1983 (*3*).

Usually transplantation is necessary because of metabolic insufficiency of the diseased organ. Correction of a metabolic disorder obtained by grafting a normal liver is an additional aim. We have performed a liver transplantation, in a child suffering from Crigler-Najjar syndrome.

Case report. The boy, who was born in 1974, suffered from an inborn metabolic disorder that became apparent from the fifth day of his life. After diagnosing the enzyme deficiency, treatment was started using phenobarbital. The bilirubin level never exceeded 15 mg%.

Initially, physical and mental development was only slightly inferior to normal. Later on psychomotoric reactions were retarded. Despite the additional administration of prednisone and ultraviolet light application, the bilirubin level increased up to 40 mg % until November 1981, and signs of kernicterus developed. The child became unconscious. Early in January 1982 generalized tonic-clonic convulsions were observed repeatedly. Not able to have another child, the parents of the boy wished to have a liver transplantation performed under any circumstances.

On January 22nd, 1982 a suitable liver was harvested from a 10 year old child who had died in a traffic accident. The liver transplantation was performed without any complication. Vessels were anastomosed in the following order: suprahepatic caval vein, portal vein (thereafter declamping), infrahepatic caval vein, and hepatic artery. Bile duct reconstruction was performed using mucosa suture technique (*6*) with a T tube placed as a stent.

The histological examination of the explanted diseased organ showed signs of cholostasis and reactive hepatitis. At biochemical examination glucuronyl transferase was not demonstrable. At the time of transplantation the boy's body weight amounted to 23 kg, his height to 122 cm. The graft function was normal immediately after transplantation. Increase in serum activity of liver enzymes was mild. Bilirubin level returned to normal within 4 days.

Despite the excellent clinical and paraclinical graft function, the brain stem damage persisted, with coma and convulsions. Anticonvulsive treatment proved to be difficult. For almost 5 months a permanent administration of phenytoin and distraneurine was necessary. Nutrition was performed parenterally as well as with a gastric tube.

Four weeks after transplantation a severe agranulocytosis became apparent. At that time immunosuppression performed with 20 mg azathioprine and 25 mg methylprednisone per day was reduced to methylprednisone only. As late as 4 months after transplantation, when a rejection crisis occurred, the patient was given Imuran again. Thereafter clinical and paraclinical signs of rejection were promptly reversed.

Three months after grafting, convulsive activities seen on the electroencephalogram decreased. In early May movements became coordinated successively and the patient started speaking again. At dismissal, immunosuppression consisted of 5 mg methylprednisone and 12.5 mg azathioprine per day. It has not been changed up to now. The T tube was removed after 6 months. Later on the the boy started attending a special school. In the meantime his height is 133 cm and his body weight 33 kg, which is within the 10th percentile. Brain stem disturbances have decreased considerably. However, ataxia remains, being noticeable in fine motoric movement.

In our patient hyperbilirubinemia was affected by phenobarbital. Therefore this Crigler-Najjar syndrome has to be classified as Type II (*1, 2*). On the other hand, the decreasing effect of treatment and the neurological damage are very seldom found in Type II. This emphasizes our limited pathophysiological understanding in this disorder.

By transplantation, the condition of a severely damaged patient with inborn metabolic error can be ameliorated considerably. But there is another aspect which is worth mentioning: in pediatric patients the regenerative capacity of the brain justifies every effort imaginable in treatment. In our patient an apparently lost life could be saved.

H. WOLFF[1]
G. OTTO[1]
H. GIEST
The Surgical Clinic of The Charité Hospital
Berlin, German Democratic Republic

[1]Address correspondence to: H. Wolff and G. Otto, Surgical Clinic of the Charité Hospital, Schumannstr. 20/21, GDR 1040 Berlin.

REFERENCES

1) Billing BH. Bilirubin metabolism. In: Schiff L, ed. Diseases of the liver. Philadelphia, Toronto: Lippincott 1975: 287.
2) Bloomer JR, Sharp HL. The liver in Crigler-Najjar syndrome, protoporphyria and other metabolic disorders. Hepatology 1984; 4: 18S.
3) Consensus Conference: Liver transplantation. JAMA 1983; 250: 2961.
4) Iwatsuki S, Shaw BW, Starzl TE. Liver transplantation for biliary atresia. World J Surg 1984; 8: 51.
5) Starzl TE, Iwatsuki S, Shaw BW, Gordon RD. Orthotopic liver transplantation in 1984. Transplantation Proc 1985; 17: 250.
6) Wolff H, Otto G, David H. Biliary tract reconstruction in liver transplantation. Transplantation Proc 1985; 17: 274.

Received 7 August 1985.
Accepted 15 October 1985.

BILE DUCT VARICES

An Alternative to Portoportal Anastomosis in Liver Transplantation

Thrombosis of the portal vein presents a substantial obstacle to orthotopic liver transplantation, and preoperative ultrasonography is performed routinely in an effort to identify this condition. Shaw et al. (*1*) have described vein grafting to the confluence of the superior mesenteric and splenic veins as a surgical option when a patent portal vein is absent. Spira and coworkers (*2*) have emphasized that portal vein occlusion may be manifested by variceal dilatation of veins in the wall of the common hepatic and common bile ducts. Recently, we managed an unsuspected portal vein occlusion encountered during liver transplantation by anastomosis of the donor portal vein to a large varix of this sort in the recipient porta hepatis.

The patient, a 37 year-old man with end-stage liver disease from idiopathic familial cirrhosis, was referred to UCLA as a candidate for hepatic transplantation. Ultrasonography of the porta hepatis was believed to confirm patency of the portal vein. At exploration, however, the portal vein remnant was represented by a fibrotic cord. A two centimeter thin-walled varix, probably the structure seen on ultrasonography, was identified inferolateral to the common bile duct. The varix was controlled just above the pancreas with a vascular clamp and an end-to-end anastomosis was constructed between the donor portal vein and the varix using 6–0 polypropylene suture. Patency and blood flow were confirmed intraoperatively with a doppler probe.

The patient's liver function has been good in the year following operation, and digital subtraction arteriography (Fig. 1) shows patency of the portal system and of the anastomosis from the confluence of two large varices to the donor portal vein.

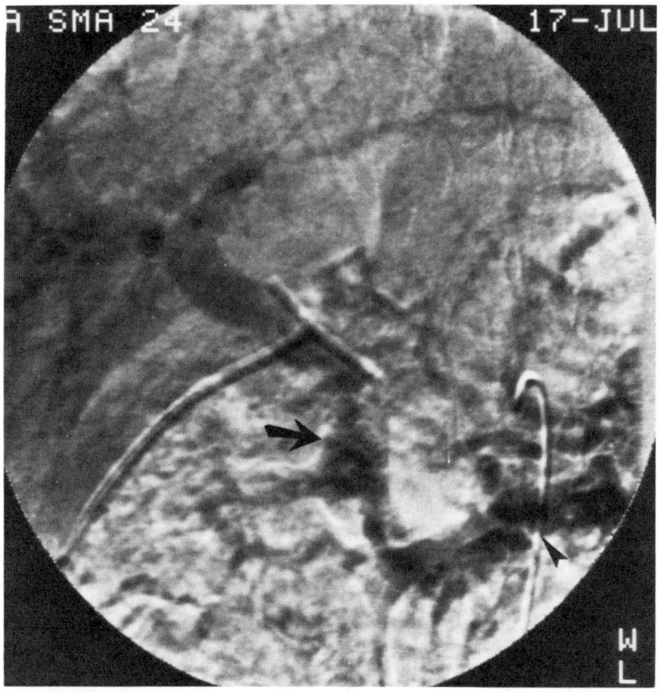

FIGURE 1. Venous phase of digital subtraction arteriogram with catheter positioned in superior mesenteric artery identifies flow from the superior mesenteric vein (arrowhead) to the liver via an anastomosis between the confluence of two large varices (arrow) and the donor portal vein. A t tube stents the common bile duct anastomosis.

Variceal distention of veins bridging portal and systemic circulations and occlusion of the portal vein itself represent two late sequelae of hepatic cirrhosis. When the portal vein is occluded in cirrhosis, varices in the porta hepatis may act to preserve hepatopetal flow. Such varices are demonstrable by arteriography and cholangiopancreatography (*2, 3*). Their clinical significance in nontransplant biliary surgery, including potential for injury and mistaken identity as the common duct, has been emphasized (*2*).

Candidacy for orthotopic liver transplantation should not be considered until a patent portal vein has been identified. Real-time ultrasonography is an acceptable method of documenting portal vein patency that avoids the risk of arteriography, particularly in small children in whom an arteriographic complication may be devastating. The patient reported by us illustrates a limitation of ultrasonography—the first false negative in 40 of our patients.

Shaw and the Pittsburgh liver transplant group have described a group of patients from their experience with thrombosed or small (less than 4 mm in diameter) portal veins. Successful transplantation has been accomplished using venous interposition between the donor portal vein and the confluence of the recipient superior mesenteric and splenic veins (*1*).

The surgeon performing orthotopic liver transplantation should anticipate the possibility of portal vein occlusion in cirrhotic patients, strive to identify this preoperatively, and understand the surgical options when the problem is encountered unexpectedly. One physiologic manifestation of the occlusion may be variceal dilatation of veins related to the wall of the common bile duct, and we present their use as an alternative to portoportal anastomosis when a suitable portal vein is absent.

Jonathan R. Hiatt
William J. Quinones-Baldrich
Kenneth P. Ramming
Juan F. Lois
Ronald W. Busuttil[1]
The Departments of Surgery and Radiology
UCLA Medical Center
Los Angeles, California

[1] Address correspondence to: Ronald W. Busuttil, M.D., Ph.D., Room 77-132 CHS, UCLA Medical Center, Los Angeles CA 90024.

REFERENCES

1. Shaw BW, Iwatsuki S, Bron K, Starzl TE. Portal vein grafts in hepatic transplantation. SGO 1985; 161: 66.
2. Spira R, Widrich WC, Keusch KD, Jackson BT, Katzman HE, Coello AA. Bile duct varices. Arch Surg 1985; 120: 1194.
3. Williams SM, Burnett DA, Mazer MJ. Radiographic demonstration of common bile duct varices. Gastrointest Radiol 1982; 7: 69.

Received 29 October 1985.
Accepted 8 November 1985.

PROLONGATION OF CARDIAC ALLOGRAFT SURVIVAL WITH BN 52021, A SPECIFIC ANTAGONIST OF PLATELET-ACTIVATING FACTOR

Platelet-activating factor ([PAF]* 1-O-alkyl-2[R]-acetyl-glycero-3-phosphorylcholine) is implicated as a mediator of inflammatory and acute allergic responses (*1*) and as contributing to the pathogenesis of antibody and complement-mediated hyperacute allograft rejection (*2*). PAF is released from platelets, polymorphonuclear leukocytes (PMN), basophils, macrophages, lymphocytes and endothelial cells (*3–6*). PAF causes peripheral vasodilation and increases vascular permeability (*7*); furthermore, PAF decreases coronary blood flow (*8*), which is related to a negative ionotropic effect (*10*). A possible role for PAF in acute graft rejection has not been explored but several possible mechanisms exists. Through increased vascular permeability, PAF may be implicated in the early events of cell recruitment to the allograft. PAF may also play a role in the cell-to-cell interaction within the graft.

It is with these considerations in mind that we have evaluated the effect of allograft survival of the recently identified PAF antagonist BN 52021 (9H-1,7a-[epoxymethano]-1H,6aH-cyclopenta[c]furo[2,3-b]furo-[3′,2′:3,4]cyclopental[1,2-d]furan-5,9-12-(4H)-trione,3-tert-butylhexahydro-4,-7b,-11hydroxy-8 methyl (Fig. 1) in a rat heterotopic cardiac transplant model. This compound is a natural product and is the most potent and specific PAF antagonist reported (*9*). BN 52021 has been studied extensively in a number of experimental pathophysiological models and found effective in inhibiting PAF-induced dye leakage (*7*), platelet aggregation, and immune challenge in response to IgG aggregates (*10*), as well as ovalbumin in passively sensitized rats (*10*). We report that this new PAF antagonist BN 52021 significantly prolongs survival of rat cardiac allografts.

Rats of the Lewis strain were recipients and Lewis × Brown Norway F_1 hybrids (L×B-NF_1) were donors. Heterotopic cardiac transplantation was performed as previously described (*12, 13*). Graft function was monitored daily by palpation through the abdominal wall and rejection was considered to be complete when no heartbeat was detected.

Azathioprine (Burroughs Wellcome, Triangle, NC) was prepared in 0.9% saline and administered i.p. Cyclosporin (CsA, Sandoz, East Hanover, NJ) was dissolved in olive oil and given once daily i.m. The PAF antagonist, BN 52021 (Henri Beaufour Institute, Paris, France), was dissolved in dimethylsulfoxide (DMSO) and administered twice daily with azathioprine and once daily with CsA. Prednisolone sodium phosphate (Merck, Sharp & Dohme, West Point, PA) was administered once daily.

The report consisted of two studies. In the first, the recipients following transplantation were randomly divided into five groups: group 1 (untreated controls, n=6) received saline (0.5 ml, i.p., daily); group 2 (n=4) received saline and the vehicle of the PAF antagonist—namely, DMSO (0.1 ml/daily i.m.); group 3 (n=4) were given azathioprine (5 mg/kg/daily in 0.5 ml saline i.p.) and DMSO; group 4 (n=11) were treated with azathioprine (5 mg/kg/daily, i.p.) and the PAF antagonist, BN 52021 (10 mg/kg/daily i.m. in DMSO); group 5, (n=5) received azathioprine and prednisolone (2 mg/kg/daily, i.p.) In the second study, the possibility of a synergistic effect of CsA and BN 5202 was explored. The animals were randomly divided into a further three groups: 6, 7, and 8. Group 6 (n=6) received CsA (0.5 mg/kg/daily i.m.); group 7 (n=7) received CsA (0.5 mg/kg/daily i.m.) + BN 52021 (10 mg/kg/daily i.m.) as above; and group 8 (n=6) received CsA (0.5 mg/kg/daily i.m.) + prednisolone (2 mg/kg/daily i.m.). The Newman-Keuls multiple range test was used for comparison between the groups. Statistical analysis was performed with the use of the Prophet Computer System (NIH, Division of Research Resources).

The allograft survival data of the first study are shown in Table 1. The saline-treated recipients (group 1) rejected their allografts 8.5±0.4 days posttransplantation. In the other control group (group 2, DMSO), allograft rejection was completed in 9.8±0.9 days and there was no significant difference in graft survival between these two control groups. In group 3 (azathioprine and DMSO), allograft rejection was significantly delayed (11.6±0.3 days) only when compared with saline treated animals. The combination of the PAF antagonist (BN 52021) and azathioprine (group 4) further delayed graft rejection to 14.8±0.6 days. Group 5 (azathioprine and prednisolone) exhibited an allograft survival of 12.8±0.4 days. The allograft survival in group 4 was significantly prolonged when compared with saline-treated (group 1, $P<0.01$), DMSO-treated (group 2, $P<0.01$), azathioprine-plus-DMSO–treated (group 3, $P<0.05$), and azathioprine-plus-prednisolone-treated rats (group 5, $P<0.05$).

In the second study (Table 2) CsA treatment (group 6) yielded an allograft survival time of 10.3±0.4 days. The allograft survival was significantly prolonged in the CsA–BN 52021 combination (group 7) and the CsA-prednisolone combination (group 8) to 14.0±0.5 and 18±2.9 days, respectively (P 0.05 for both groups) when compared with CsA treatment (group 6).

These data show for the first time that treatment of rat cardiac allograft recipients with a specific PAF antagonist (BN 52021) in combination with azathioprine or CsA significantly delays graft rejection. The doses of CsA and azathioprine did not by themselves prolong graft survival. This combination of azathioprine and PAF antagonist was more effective in prolonging graft survival in the cardiac allograft model used here than the traditional immunosuppressive combination of azathioprine and prednisolone. The combination of PAF antagonist and CsA improved allograft survival to the same degree as prednisolone and CsA.

Our data imply that PAF might be involved in cell-mediated graft rejection, and not only in hyperacute rejection as described by Ito et al. (*2*). The cellular response in allograft rejection involves activation of a variety of cells that have been found to release PAF. The protection against allograft rejection of both prednisolone and BN 52021 is interesting in relation to the finding that hydrocortisone inhibits the release of the PAF-precursor, lyso-PAF, from macrophages (*14*). One mechanism for involvement of PAF in organ rejection may be through an effect on calcium flux. PAF increases free intracellular Ca^{++} in a number of cells, including human platelets and human PMNs (*15*). If PAF has the same effect in lymphocytes, this may facilitate the initial activation of lymphocytes that is Ca^{++}-dependent (*16*). Calcium also activates phospholipase A_2 (*17*), which is one of the rate limiting steps for the release of arachidonic acid and thereby the formation of eicosanoids, PAF, in fact, releases eicosanoids from cells and tissues (*18*). The various eicosanoids have all been implicated in immune modulation (*19*). We have indirect evidence for the involve-

* Abbreviations used: AZA, azathioprine; CsA, cyclosporine; DMSO, dimethylsulfoxide; LxB-NF_1, Lewis × Brown Norway F_1 hybrids; PAF, platelet-activating factor; PMN, polymorphonuclearcytes; Predn, prednisolone.

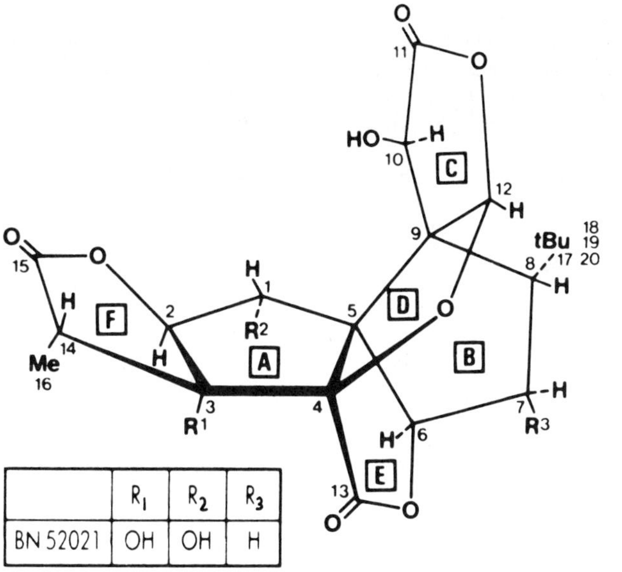

FIGURE 1. Chemical structure of the PAF-antagonist BN 52021.

TABLE 1. The effect of PAF antagonist (BN 52021) + azathioprine (AZA) treatment on cardiac allograft survival compared with controls and AZA + prednisolone

Group	n	Treatment	Daily dose	Survival—days (mean ± SEM)[a]
1	6	Saline	0.5 ml	8.5±0.4
2	4	Saline + DMSO	0.5 and 0.1 ml	9.8±0.9
3	4	AZA + DMSO	5 mg and 0.1 ml	11.6±0.3
4	6	AZA + BN 52021	5 and 10 mg	14.8±0.6
5	5	AZA + Predniso-lone	5 and 2 mg	12.8±0.4

[a] For *P* value see the *Results* section.

TABLE 2. The effect of cyclosporine (CsA) and PAF antagonist (BN 52021) treatment on cardiac allograft survival compared with CsA and prednisolone

Group	n	Treatment	Daily dose	Survival—days (mean ± SEM)[a]
6	11	CsA	0.5 mg	10.3±0.4
7	7	CsA + BN 52021	0.5 and 10 mg	14.0±0.5
8	6	CsA + Predniso-lone	0.5 and 2 mg	18.0±2.9

[a] For *P* value see the *Results* section.

ment of Ca^{++} in cell-mediated graft rejection in that both verapamil and nifedipine were found to prolong rat cardiac allograft survival when administered in combination with the same dose of azathioprine used in the present study (*20*). It is of interest that nifedipine caused a dose-dependent inhibition of the calcium-ionophore-induced release of PAF in human neutrophils (*21*). Thus our data are consistent with the idea that PAF elicits rejection, and that the response may be mediated via Ca^{++} influx. PAF also reduces coronary artery flow in the pig (*8*); thus a PAF antagonist is likely to maintain coronary flow. Rat platelets are atypical; unlike other species, PAF is not released from this blood element, and it does not aggregate the rat platelet (*22*); consequently in this transplant model the PAF antagonist exerts its effect through cells other than platelets.

The improved prolongation of cardiac graft survival in recipients treated with the novel and specific PAF antagonist BN 52021 combined with azathioprine or CsA, when compared with azathioprine or CsA administered by themselves, suggests a causal role for PAF in promoting cardiac allograft rejection. There are still no reports of PAF release during acute allograft rejection in the rat or in patients. Nevertheless the data described here suggests the possibility of new treatment modalities in which a PAF antagonist or PAF synthesis inhibitor could be used to lower the dosage of CsA or prednisolone.

MARIE L. FOEGH[1,2]
BIJAN S. KHIRABADI[3]
JOHN R. ROWLES[3]
PIERRE BRAQUET[4]
PETER W. RAMWELL[3]
Department of Surgery
Division of Transplantation
Department of Physiology and Biophysics
Georgetown University Medical Center
Washington, D.C., 20007

[1] Department of Surgery.
[2] Address correspondence to: Dr. Marie Foegh, Department of Surgery, Division of Transplantation, Georgetown University Medical Center, Kober Cogan Bldg. Room 206, Washington, D.C. 20007.
[3] Department of Physiology and Biophysics.
[4] I.H.B. Research Laboratories, Les Plessis-Robinson, France.

REFERENCES

1. Benveniste J. PAF-acether (platelet activating factor). Adv Prostaglandin Thromboxane Leukotriene Res 1985; 13: 11.
2. Ito S, Camussi G, Tetta C, Milgrom F, Andres G. Hyperacute allograft rejection in the rabbit. Lab Invest 1984; 51: 148.
3. Chignard M, LeConedic JP, Tence M, Vargaftig BB, Benveniste J. The role of platelet activating factor in platelet aggregation. Nature 1979; 179: 799.
4. Camussi G, Aglietta M, Coda R, Bussolino F, Piacibello W, Tetta C. Release of platelet-activating factor (PAF) and histamine. II. The cellular origin of human PAF: monocytes, polymorphonuclear neutrophils and basophils. Immunology 1981; 42: 191.
5. Camussi G, Aglietta M, Malavasi F, Tetta C, Piacibello W, Sanavio F, Bussolino F. The release of platelet activating factor from human endothelial cells in culture. J Immunol 1983; 131: 2397.
6. Bussolino F, Foa R, Malauasi F, Ferrando ML, Camussi G. Release of platelet activating factor (PAF)-like material from human lymphoid cell lines. Exp Hematol 1984; 12: 688
7. Inarrea P, Gomez-Cambronero J, Pascual J, Ponte MC, Hermando L, Sanchez-Crespo M. Synthesis of PAF-acether and blood volumes changes in Gram-negative sepsis. Immunopharmacology 1985; 9: 45.
8. Feuerstein G, Ramwell PW, Hayes E, Goldstein RE. Effect of platelet activating factor on coronary hemodynamics and coronary venous plasma levels of TXB2 6-keto-PGF_1 and leukotriene C4 immuno-reactivity in the intact domestic pig heart. Adv Prostaglandins Thromboxane Leukotriene Res 1985; 13: 19.
9. Braquet P. Treatment and prevention of PAF-acether-induced sickness by a new series of highly specific inhibitors. GB patent 8,418,424(1984); US patent 1984.
10. Sanchez-Crespo M, Fernandez-Gallardo S, Nieto ML, Baranis J, Braquet P. Inhibition of the vascular actions of immunoglobulin G aggregates by BN 52021, a highly specific antagonist of PAF-acether. Immunopharmacol 1985; 10: 69.
11. Nunez D, Chignard M, Korth R, et al. Specific inhibition of PAF-acether-induced Platelet activation by BN 52021 and comparison with the PAF-acether inhibitors Kadsurenone and CV3988. Eur J Pharmacol 1986; 123: 197.
12. Khirabadi BS, Foegh ML, Ramwell PW. Urine immunoreactive

thromboxane B2 in rat cardiac allograft rejection. Transplantation 1985; 39: 6.

13. Ono K, Lindsey ES. Improved technique of heart transplantation in rats. J Thorac Cardiovasc Surg 1969; 57: 225.
14. Parente L, Flower RJ. Hydrocortisone and "macrocortin" inhibit the zymosan-induced release of lyso-PAF from rat peritoneal leucocytes. Life Sci 1985; 36: 1225.
15. Flaherty JT, Swendsen CL, Lees CJ, McCall CE. Role of extracellular calcium and neutrophil degranulation responses to 1-0-alkyl- 2-0-acetyl-5n-glycero-3-phosphocholine. Am J Pathol 1981; 105: 107.
16. Tsien RY, Pozzan T, Rink TJ. Calcium homeostasis in intact lymphocytes: cytoplasmic free calcium monitored with a new intracellularly trapped fluorescent indicator. J Cell Biol 1982; 97: 325.
17. Graven PA, DeRubertis FR. Ca^{2+} Calmodulin-dependent release of arachidonic acid from renal medullary prostaglandin synthesis. J Biol Chem 1983; 258: 4814.
18. Voelkel NF, Worthen S, Reeves JT, Henson PN, Murphy RC. Nonimmunological production of leukotrienes induced by platelet-activating factor. Science 1982; 218: 286.
19. Foegh M, Alijani MR, Helfrich GB, Ramwell PW. Icosanoids and organ transplantation. Ann Clin Res 1984; 16: 318.
20. Foegh ML, Khirabadi BS, Ramwell PW. Prolongation of rat cardiac allograft survival by Ca^{++} blockers. Transplantation 1985; 40: 211.
21. Jouvin-Marche E, Cerrina J, Coeffier E, Duroux P, Beneveniste J. Effect of the Ca^{2+} antagonist nifedipine on the release of platelet-activating (PAF-acether), slow-reacting substance and -glucoronidase from human neutrophils. Eur J Pharmacol 1983; 89: 19.
22. Inarrea P, Gomez-Cambronero J, Nieto M, Crespo MS. Characteristics of the binding of platelet-activating factor to platelets of different animal species. Eur J Pharmacol 1985; 105: 309.

Received 10 September 1985.
Accepted 8 November 1985.

THE SPECIFIC DISTRIBUTION OF GLYCOLIPID-BASED BLOOD GROUP A ANTIGENS IN HUMAN KIDNEY RELATED TO A_1/A_2, LEWIS, AND SECRETOR STATUS OF SINGLE INDIVIDUALS

A Possible Molecular Explanation for the Successful Transplantation of A_2 Kidneys into O Recipients[1]

Blood group ABO compatibility has, during the whole era of kidney transplantation, been considered essential in selecting donors for renal homografts even if a few cases of incompatible grafts have functioned well (*1, 2*). This consensus was mainly based on an analogy with blood transfusions and the generally accepted idea of only two ABO antigens—A and B—with a wide tissue distribution throughout the body (*3–5*). Experiences with experimental skin transplantations (*6*) and incompatible kidney grafts (*1, 2*) have supported this view. However, skin grafts from blood group A_2 donors have not been rejected from blood group O or B donors (*6*). This was the stimulus for a clinical trial of transplanting A_2 kidneys into O recipients (*7*) that started in 1974. Until now, 17 such transplantations have been performed with conventional immunosuppression, and the outcome is comparable to that of ABO-compatible controls. A few successful blood group A_1-O transplantations with recipient plasmapheresis have also been reported (*8, 9*).

Blood group ABH antigens in human tissues have been classified as type 1 (Galβ1→3GlcNAc) or type 2 (Galβ1→4GlcNAc) according to the type of core saccharide (*10, 11*). Recently new types of blood group H and A glycolipids have been identified. A third type (Galβ1→3GalNAcα1→), found in human erythrocytes (*12*), has essentially a repetitive H/A epitope structure (Fig. 1). The fourth type (Galβ1→3GalNAcβ1→)—identified in human meconium (*13*), erythrocytes (*14, 15*), and kidney (*16*)—has the H disaccharide or the A trisaccharide, linked β1→3 to the galactosamine of globotetraosylceramide (blood group P antigen). These "globo-H" and "globo-A" compounds represent interesting examples of a previously unknown interaction between the blood group P and ABO systems. The chemical structures of the basic types of A glycolipids present in human tissues are shown in Figure 1. Blood group ABH glycolipids have a tissue-specific distribution. So in humans, for example, type 1 chain glycolipids dominate in intestinal epithelium (*17*) and type 2 chain compounds are the major ones present in erythrocytes (*11*), while the pancreas contains both types (*11, 17*). The fourth type ("globo-H/A") is present in very small amounts in erythrocytes (*14, 15*), but it makes up about half the glycolipid-based A antigens in the kidney (*16*).

The chemical basis for the difference between the A_1 and A_2 subgroups of blood group A is not entirely known, but it has been claimed (*10, 11*) that the difference is qualitative (type of core-saccharide-based A antigens) or quantitative (number of A determinants), or both. However, the type 3 chain antigen and the type "4" chain, or globo-A antigen, have recently (*12, 15*) been shown to be present in A_1 erythrocytes but almost absent in A_2 erythrocytes.

The biosynthesis of the ABH antigens is considered to be controlled by the *ABO*, *H*, and *Se* genes (*10, 11, 18–20*). The fucosyltransferase produced by the *H*-gene is restricted to acting upon type 2 chain substrates, while the enzyme produced or regulated by the *Se*-gene can act upon both type 1 and 2 substrates, although it prefers type 1 chain substrates (*18–20*). The A_1 and the A_2 genes produce 2 different galactosaminyltransferases (*21*), of which the A_2-gene-coded transferase has a lower efficiency in transferring galactosamine onto type 1 and 2 substrates (*21*; and Samuelsson B, unpublished data); we have recently shown that its efficiency in acting upon the globo-H substrate is low (Breimer ME, Larson G, Samuelsson B, manuscript in preparation).

The distribution of blood group A glycolipids in individual kidneys by immunochemical methods and its correlation with the blood group status of the donors are described here.

The human kidneys analyzed were obtained for transplantation but discarded for technical reasons or because of a lack of suitable recipients. The vascular tree of each kidney was rinsed with salt solution, and the kidneys were kept sterile at 4°C for up to 48 hr. Blood group typing of the donors was performed on erythrocytes by standard serological procedures. Total nonacid glycolipid fractions were prepared from the lyophilized tissue by chloroform-methanol extraction, mild alkaline hydrolysis, and column chromatography as described elsewhere (*22, 23*). The glycolipid fractions were analyzed with

[1] This work was supported by grants from the Swedish Medical Research Council (Nos. 6521 and 7131).

```
Type 1 chain

A-6-1   GalNAcα1→3Galβ1→3GlcNAcβ1→3Galβ1→4Glcβ1→1Ceramide
                  2
                  ↑
                Fucα1

Type 2 chain

A-6-2   GalNAcα1→3Galβ1→4GlcNAcβ1→3Galβ1→4Glcβ1→1Ceramide
                  2
                  ↑
                Fucα1

Type 3 chain

A-9-3   GalNAcα1→3Galβ1→3GalNAcα1→3Galβ1→4GlcNAcβ1→3Galβ1→4Glcβ1→1Ceramide
                  2                 2
                  ↑                 ↑
                Fucα1             Fucα1

Type 4 chain (Globo-A)

A-7-4   GalNAcα1→3Galβ1→3GalNAcβ1→3Galα1→4Galβ1→4Glcβ1→1Ceramide
                  2
                  ↑
                Fucα1
```

FIGURE 1. Structural formulas of the four basic blood group A glycolipids present in human tissues. The designation "type 1–4" refers to the core saccharide carrying the classic blood group A trisaccharide determinant. The shorthand designation stands for: blood group—number of sugar residues—type of carbohydrate chain. Thus A-6-1 means a type 1 chain blood group A hexaglycosylceramide.

high-performance thin-layer chromatography (HPTLC)* and stained with a chemical reagent (*23*). The antigenic reactivity of the glycolipids separated by HPTLC was tested using a modification of the method of Magnani et al. (*24, 25*). HPTLC plates (Merck, Darmstadt) were treated with primary antibody (mouse monoclonal anti-A, Dakopatts, Denmark) followed by ^{125}I-labeled secondary antibody (rabbit antimouse IgM). Plates were dried and autoradiographed. The mouse monoclonal anti-A antibody has been shown to react with all blood group A glycolipids tested (4–12 sugar components, types 1, 2, and "4" or the globo-series of carbohydrate chains, mono- and difucosyl structures); it has no crossreactivity against Forssman pentaglycosylceramide and a number of other glycolipids tested (Hansson G, Stromberg N, unpublished results).

The total amount of nonacid glycolipid isolated from each kidney was in the range of 61–195 mg, corresponding to 4.8–6.1 mg/g of dry tissue weight. Figure 2 shows the thin-layer chromatogram of the total nonacid glycolipid fractions from single kidneys (cases 1–9), two pure reference glycolipids (A-6-2 and globo-A), and a polar nonacid glycolipid fraction isolated from pooled human kidneys obtained at autopsy of blood group A individuals (lane A). The chemical detection (Figure 2 [left portion]) shows that globotriaosyl- and globotetraosylceramides (the P^k and P antigens, respectively) are the major glycolipids present in the kidneys, together with mono- and diglycosylceramides (*26*). The band migrating as a pentaglycosylceramide, present in all kidney fractions, consists to 75% of globotetraosylceramide having an additional terminal Galβ1-3 residue and to 25% of the X-5 glycolipid (type 2 chain isomer of the Le^a-pentaglycosylceramide) ([*26*] and Breimer, ME, manuscript in preparation). Lane A also shows a heptaglycosylceramide band that has been purified and structurally characterized as the globo-A glycolipid (Fig. 1) (*16*). This band was also seen in the total glycolipid fractions of cases 1, 2, 6, and 7 when large amounts of substance were applied on the plate. When the major glycolipids with 1–4 sugar residues were separated from the others by column chromatography, several other minor components migrating below the five-sugar region were seen, (*16, 26*). Minor glycolipids can, however, be detected in the total fraction by immunostaining directly on the thin-layer plate with various biological reagents (*24, 25*), as shown in Figure 2 (right portion), when monoclonal anti-A antibodies are used. The total polar glycolipid fraction isolated from kidneys obtained at autopsy (lane A) contain A active compounds with from 6 to about 16 sugar residues. This pattern reflects the total glycolipid content of several donors and contaminating glycolipids from blood cells and plasma trapped in the organ after death. For the single kidney fractions (cases 1–9), a nonspecific binding to globotriaosyl- and globotetraosylceramides is seen in all lanes. This phenomenon is occasionally seen with some antibodies when large amounts of substance are present in one spot on the plate. (Compare this with chemical detection.)

Both qualitative and quantitative differences in blood group A glycolipids are seen between individuals. As expected, blood group O individuals (cases 8 and 9) have no A antigens. Blood group A hexaglycosylceramides (type 1 and/or type 2 chains) are present—though the amounts vary—in all cases of blood group A. The globo-A antigen is present in cases 1, 2, 6, and 7, strongly reduced in case 3, and seems to be qualitatively lacking in cases 4 and 5. In the 8–9-sugar-chain region 2 bands are seen. Both are present in cases 1, 2, 6, and 7, while the slower moving is lacking in cases 3–5 and the faster moving is reduced in case 5 and lacking in case 4. The faster moving of the two bands discussed may be identical to the blood group A octaglycosyl ceramide earlier isolated from human erythrocytes (*11*). In addition, a weak staining of the anti-A antibody is seen in the 10–12 sugar region of cases 1–3. When a similar thin-layer plate was stained with a monoclonal anti-B antibody (not shown) a double band migrating as blood group B hexaglycosylceramides (type 1 and/or type 2 chain) was seen in cases 6 and 7. No band with the Rf value that would have been expected for a "globo-B" heptaglycosylceramide was seen. Immunostaining of the kidney glycosphingolipids (Fig. 2) was also performed using other monoclonal, as well as polyclonal, anti-A antisera. The results (not shown) were essentially identical with the ones shown (Fig. 2).

From the Lewis typing of the red blood cells, it may be concluded that cases 1, 2, 6, and 7 are secretor individuals, and that case 3 and 5 are nonsecretors (*27*). The Lewis status of case 4 and the blood group A subgroup of case 6 are lacking because the blood group serology was determined in local hospitals. When comparing the blood group status of the donors with their kidney blood group A glycolipid pattern, the following conclusions may tentatively be drawn: globo-A glycolipids, and possibly some related more slow-moving compounds (about 9 sugars), are produced in "large" amounts in A_1 secretors, in much smaller amounts in nonsecretors, and not at all in A_2 individuals—nonsecretor individuals, therefore, have smaller amounts of blood group A glycolipids, and this is even more pronounced for the A_2 individuals.

The exact effect of the secretor gene and the A_2 character on the A glycolipids, however, cannot be settled, because case 4 (A_2) was not typed for secretor or Lewis and case 5 is a nonsecretor. The number of glycolipid-based A-plus-B antigenic determinants in the A_1B secretor individuals is of the

* Abbreviation used: HPTLC, high-performance thin-layer chromatography.

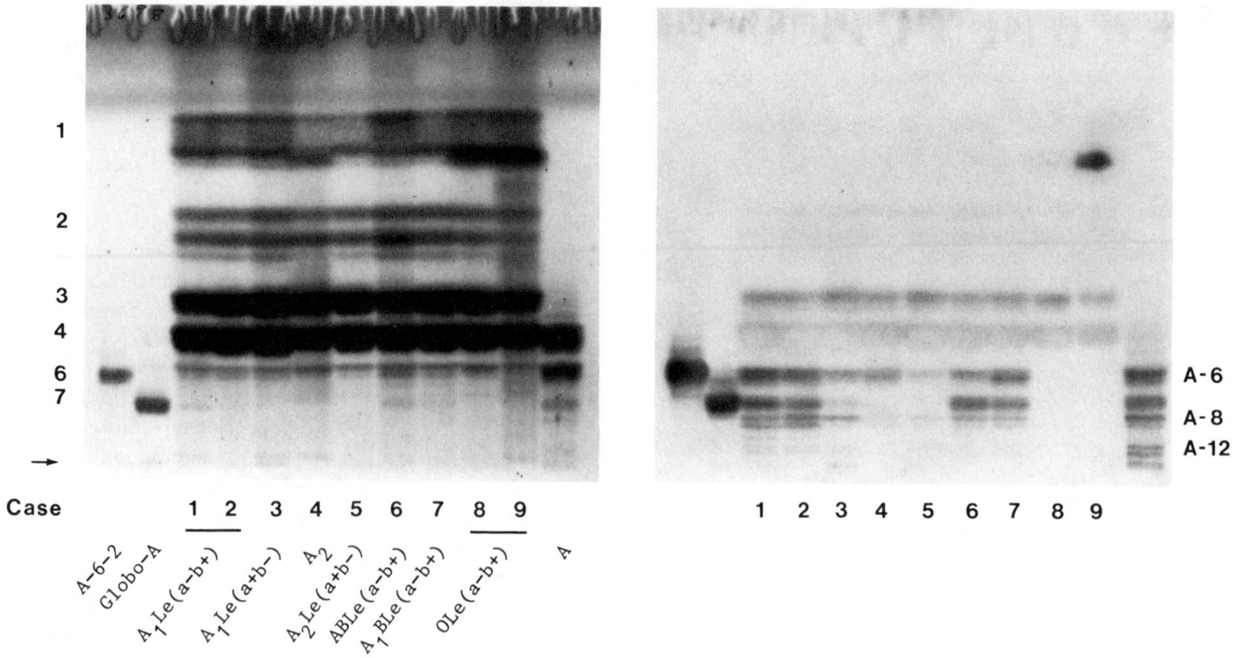

FIGURE 2. Thin-layer chromatogram of total nonacid glycolipid fractions isolated from kidneys of human individuals (cases 1–9). The blood groups of the donors' red blood cells are shown below each lane. For case 7, the red cells were typed as A_1B Le(a-b-). The kidney glycolipid portion contained, however, Le^b glycolipids in the same amounts as cases 1, 2, and 6. Lewis typing of red blood cells is known to be troublesome, and the expression of Lewis antigen is affected by other conditions such as alcohol abuse (*32*)—which was the case for this individual. Therefore, the blood group type of this individual is regarded as A_1B Le(a-b+). Lane A is a partly purified nonacid glycolipid fraction isolated from kidneys obtained at autopsy from several human individuals. Reference glycolipids are A-6-2 and globo-A (for structure see Fig. 1) isolated from the human pancreas (*17*) and kidneys (*16*), respectively. HPTLC plates were developed in chloroform: methanol:water, 60:35:8 (by volume). For detection, a chemical reagent (anisaldehyde [left chromatogram]) and autoradiography after binding with monoclonal anti-A antibody (right chromatogram) were used. The amount applied was 40 μg for cases 1–9, 10 μg for lane A, and 2 μg for the A-6-2 and globo-A compounds. The designation to the left indicates the number of sugar residues in each glycolipid band, and that to the right indicates the mobility of the different blood group A glycolipids shown.

same order of magnitude as A determinants in the A_1 secretors. This is probably due to a precursor competition between the *A* and *B* gene coded glycosyltransferases (*28*) and has the effect of a reduction in blood group A antigen expression. This competition may not occur for the globo series antigens, as epithelial cells from the urinary tract of a B secretor individual lack the expected "globo B" compound (as judged from immunostaining with anti-B antibodies and P-fimbriated *Escherichia coli*, Leffler H, personal communication).

Oriol et al. have shown, using the immunofluorescence technique, that the blood group A antigens of the kidney are located in vascular endothelium and in the convoluted distal tubules and collecting tubules (*29*). The A antigen in vascular endothelium was not found to be dependent on the secretor status of the individuals, while the distal and collecting tubules contained only A antigens in secretor individuals. It was also noted that the vascular endothelium of A_2 individuals contained fewer A antigens than that of A_1 individuals, but no data regarding the distal and collecting tubules in A_2 individuals was given (*29*). The biosynthesis of type 2 chain ABH antigens is largely independent of the secretor status of the individual (*10, 11, 18–20*). One may therefore predict that the type 2 chain blood group A hexaglycosyl- and octaglycosylceramides present in the kidneys (Fig. 2 [right portion]) are probably located in the vascular endothelium, while the globo-A structures (possibly secretor-dependent) are present in the distal and collecting tubules.

Some years ago it was shown that mismatching for the Lewis antigens also contributes to the rejection of kidney transplants (*30, 31*). The influence of secretor status on the number and type of A antigens present in the kidney, as demonstrated here, indicates that it may also be important to establish this serological parameter of kidney donors.

The successful transplantation of A_2 kidneys into O recipients (*7*) may be explained by the qualitative (lack of globo series A antigens) and quantitative difference in A determinants in the kidney. A better knowledge of the chemical structure, biosynthesis, and expression of blood group ABH, Lewis, and related carbohydrate antigens in the kidney may form the basis for an extension of the selection of donors for blood-group-incompatible transplantation in the future—thus solving problems such as the relative lack of grafts for O recipients (*7*).

Acknowledgment. H. Brynger is gratefully acknowledged for help with kidney material and for valuable discussions.

MICHAEL E. BREIMER
BO E. SAMUELSSON
Department of Surgery I
University of Göteborg
Sahlgrens Hospital
413 45 Göteborg
Department of Medical Biochemistry
University of Göteborg
S-400 33 Göteborg, Sweden

REFERENCES

1. Starzl TE, Marchiro TL, Holmes JH, et al. Renal homografts in patients with major donor-recipient blood group incompatibilities. Surgery 1964; 55: 195.
2. Wilhardt R, Tung KSK, Deodhar SD, Nakamoto S, Koleff WJ. ABO blood group incompatibility in human renal homotransplantation. Am J Clin Pathol 1969; 51: 15.
3. Glyn LE, Holborow EJ. Distribution of blood group substances in human tissues. Br Med Bull 1959; 15: 150.
4. Szulman AE. The histological distribution of blood group substances A and B in man. J Exp Med 1960; 111: 785.
5. Szulman AE. The histological distribution of blood group substances in man as disclosed by immunofluorescence. II. H antigen and its relation to A and B antigens. J Exp Med 1962; 115: 977.
6. Ceppellini R, Bigliani S, Curtoni ES, Leigheb G. Experimental allotransplantation in man. II. The role of A_1, A_2 and B antigens. III. Enhancement by circulating antibody. Transplant Proc 1969; 1: 390.
7. Brynger H, Rydberg L, Samuelsson B, Blohme I, Lindholm A, Sandberg L. Renal transplantation across a blood group barrier—A_2 kidneys to O recipients. Proc EDTA 1982; 19: 427.
8. Slapak M, Evans P, Trickett L, Harris KR, Gordon P, Matini A, Mocetin AJ. Can ABO-incompatible donors be used in renal transplantation? Transplant Proc 1984; 16: 75.
9. Alexandre GPJ, DeBruyer M, Morian M. 9th Meeting of American Society of Transplant Surgeons 1983 [Abstract].
10. Watkins WM. Genetics and biochemistry of some human blood groups. Proc R Soc Lond [Biol] 1978; 202: 31.
11. Hakomori S-i, Kobata A. Blood group antigens. In: Sela M, ed. Tissue antigens, vol 2. New York: Academic, 1974: 74.
12. Clausen H, Levery SB, Nudelman E, Tsuchiya S, Hakomori S-i. Repetitive A epitope (type 3 chain A) defined by blood group A_1-specific monoclonal antibody TH-I: chemical basis of qualitative A_1 and A_2 distinction. Proc Natl Acad Sci USA 1985; 82: 1199.
13. Karlsson K-A, Larson G. Molecular characterization of cell surface antigens of fetal tissue. J Biol Chem 1981; 256: 3512.
14. Kannagi R, Levery SB, Hakomori S-i. Blood group H antigen with globoseries structure: isolation and characterization from human blood group O erythrocytes. FEBS Lett 1984; 175: 397.
15. Clausen H, Watanabe K, Kannagi R. Blood group A glycolipid (A^x) with globoseries structure which is specific for blood group A_1 erythrocytes: one of the chemical bases for A_1 and A_2 distinction. Biochem Biophys Res Commun 1984; 124: 523.
16. Breimer ME, Jovall P-Å. Structural characterization of a blood group A heptaglycosylceramide with globo-series structure. FEBS Lett 1985; 179: 165.
17. Breimer ME. Tissue specificity of glycosphingolipids as expressed in pancreas and small intestine of blood group A and B human individuals. Arch Biochem Biophys 1984; 228: 71.
18. LePendue J. α-2-*L* Fucosyltransferase activities of human serum: properties of two distinct enzymes and their relationships with the genetics of H tissue antigens. In: Red cell membrane glycoconjugates and related genetic markers. Paris: Libraire Arnette, 1983: 183.
19. Betteridge A, Watkins WM. Variant forms of α-2-*L* fucosyltransferase in human submaxillary glands from blood group ABH "secretor" and "non-secretor" individuals. Glycoconj J 1984; 2: 61.
20. Kumazaki T, Yoshida A. Biochemical evidence that secretor gene, Se is a structural gene encoding a specific fucosyltransferase. Proc Natl Acad Sci USA 1984; 81: 4193.
21. Schachter H, Michaels MA, Tilley CA, Crookston MC, Crookston JH. Qualitative differences in the *N*-Acetyl-*D*-galactosaminyltransferases produced by human A^1 and A^2 genes. Proc Natl Acad Sci USA 1973; 70: 220.
22. Breimer ME, Hansson GC, Karlsson K-A, Leffler H. Glycosphingolipids and the differentiation of intestinal epithelium. Exp Cell Res 1981; 135: 1.
23. Breimer ME, Hansson GC, Karlsson K-A, Leffler H. Isolation and partial characterization of blood group A and H active glycosphingolipids of rat small intestine. J Biol Chem 1982; 257: 906.
24. Magnani JL, Smith DF, Ginsburg V. Detection of gangliosides that bind cholera toxin: direct binding of ^{125}I labeled toxin to thin layered chromatograms. Anal Biochem 1981; 109: 399.
25. Hansson GC, Karlsson K-A, Larson G, et al. Mouse monoclonal antibodies against human cancer cell lines with specificities for blood group and related antigens. J Biol Chem 1983; 258: 4091.
26. Breimer ME, Karlsson K-A. Chemical and immunological identification of glycolipid based blood group ABH and Lewis antigen in human kidney. Biochim Biophys Acta 1983; 755: 170.
27. Race RR, Sanger R. Blood groups in man. Boston: Blackwell, 1975: 323.
28. Watkins WM, Greenwell P. Dominance relationships of the genes at the *ABO* blood group locus. 18th Congress of the Int Soc Blood Transfusion, Munich, July 22–27, 1984, S. 36 [Abstract].
29. Bariety J, Oriol R, Hinglais N. Distribution of blood group antigen A in normal and pathologic human kidneys. Kidney Int 1981; 17: 820.
30. Oriol R, Cartron J, Yvart J. The Lewis system: new histocompatibility antigens in renal transplantation. Lancet 1978; 1: 574.
31. Oriol R, Oplez G, Chun C, Terasaki PI. The Lewis system and kidney transplantation. Transplantation 1981; 29: 397.
32. Stigendal L, Olsson R, Rydberg L, et al. Blood group Lewis phenotype on erythrocytes and in salivia in alcoholic pancreatitis and chronic liver disease. J Clin Pathol 1984; 37: 778.

Received 14 June 1985.
Accepted 25 October 1985.

HYPERACUTE REJECTION OF A RENAL ALLOGRAFT IN THE PRESENCE OF ANTI-HLA-Cw5 ANTIBODY[1]

Transplantation in the presence of a positive lymphocytotoxic crossmatch between recipient serum and donor lymphocytes has been contraindicated since reports in the late 1960s correlating donor specific reactivity with hyperacute rejection of the renal allograft (*1–3*). Studies clarifying the existence of autoreactive antibodies directed at T and B cells subsequently demonstrated that not all positive crossmatches were deleterious to the graft (*4, 5*). For some years we have thus had a policy of transplanting selected patients with autoantibodies in the presence of a positive T cell crossmatch, when we have considered that the crossmatch was due to autoantibody. In patients with both anti-HLA and autoantibodies we ensure full matching at the HLA A and B loci to reduce the chance that the crossmatch is due to the anti-HLA antibody (*6*).

In this paper we report the case of a man receiving his fourth renal transplant, which was matched at the A,B and DR loci. The patient was known to have both autoantibodies and HLA antibodies previously but the positive crossmatch with the serum taken on the day of the transplant was thought to be due to autoantibody alone because of the degree of HLA matching. Subsequent analysis revealed however that the patient had lost autoreactivity by the time of the fourth transplant but had retained 10–15% panel reactivity. The graft was hyperacutely rejected, and we therefore initiated this study to determine the specificity of antibody causing the positive crossmatch.

The HLA types of the patient, and his four grafts are detailed

[1] This work was supported by a grant from the Medical Research Council of the United Kingdom.

in Table 1, together with the number of days to graft failure. The fourth renal allograft, with a 20-hr, 39-min cold ischemia time, was anastamosed end-to-side to the right internal iliac artery with an end-to-side venous anastamosis to the right external iliac vein. Following removal of the clamps the kidney perfused well initially, but after 5–10 min became blue, and by 30 min was black and flabby despite good pulses at the hilum. By 1-hr later the kidney appeared to have improved, in that it was firm and perfusing patchily, and histology of a biopsy taken 30 min after opening the vascular clamps showed only interstitial edema. It was therefore left in-situ but never functioned, and the patient has refused graft nephrectomy. However, a subsequent biopsy taken before stopping immunosuppression revealed arterial edema and intimal proliferation with fibrinoid necrosis and lymphocytic infiltration of the walls. Glomeruli were hemorrhagic and there was extensive interstitial hemorrhage with a minor degree of lymphocytic infiltration.

The only detectable HLA mismatch in the fourth graft was Cw5, and we believe that the specificity of the antibody causing the positive crossmatch was HLA-Cw5. The serum collected just before transplantation that gave a positive crossmatch was shown to have HLA-Cw5 reactivity when tested against panels of both peripheral blood lymphocytes and cells from patients with chronic lymphatic leukemia (Table 2). Further evidence for the presence of an HLA-Cw5 antibody was obtained by testing the serum against selected cells that had HLA-A, B, and C antigens similar to those of the recipient, but either did or did not express Cw5 (Table 3). It can be seen that reactivity occurred only with targets expressing Cw5.

The antigenic stimulus for production of anti-Cw5 antibodies may have been the two previous grafts, which were mismatched for Cw5 (Table 1). Apart from the three previous grafts the only other known source of sensitization was two units of blood given at the time of the first transplant.

Since it is unusual to implicate a C locus antibody as a cause of hyperacute rejection further serological studies were undertaken to provide additional evidence. Cytotoxicity of anti-HLA class I antibodies can be inhibited specifcally by monoclonal antibodies directed at a monomorphic determinant of HLA class I antigens (*7*). The positive crossmatch against donor cells and against cells having the same HLA type as the donor were blocked specifically by the monoclonal antibody PA2.6, which reacts with a monomorphic determinant of HLA-ABC (*8*). This suggests that the positive crossmatch was indeed caused by an antibody directed at an HLA-ABC antigen expressed by the donor.

It is known that HLA-C locus antigens are lost from the surface of stored cells (*9*), and this characteristic was therefore used to demonstrate that the antibody was directed at a C locus antigen. Cytotoxicity was lost when cells from RM (Table 3), who is HLA-ABC and DR-identical with the donor, were stored at 22°C for 7 days. The stored cells also lost their reactivity with specific HLA-Cw5 sera used for typing, but retained both A and B locus specificities.

The C locus has been thought to be unimportant in tissue typing for renal transplantation, and one study has shown that C locus matching does not have an influence on renal allograft outcome (*10*). Attempts to deliberately immunize volunteers against C locus antigens have shown that they are only weakly immunogenic (*11*), and this is confirmed by the paucity of antibodies to the C locus in the sera of multiparous women.

Our data suggest, however, that there may be specific circumstances in which the C locus should be considered. The data presented here not only illustrate the relationship between antibody to class I Major histocompatibility complex antigens and hyperacute rejection, but also demonstrate that the C locus antigen can be relevant in renal transplantation if anti-HLA-C antibody is present in serum at the time of the operation.

TABLE 1. HLA-A, B, Bw, C, and DR antigens of recipient and donors

	HLA					Days to failure
	A	B	Bw	C	DR	
Patient	2, 3	7, 44	4, 6	–, 7	2, 7	
Donor 1	2, 3	7, 44	4, 6	5	1, 4	14
Donor 2	2, 3	15, 44	4, 6	5, 3	6, –	179
Donor 3	2, 3	7, –	–, 6	–, 7	2, 7	0
Donor 4	2, 3	7, 44	4, 6	5, 7	2, 7	Hyperacute

TABLE 2. Panel reactivity of serum collected on the day of transplantation

Cells	Cw 5-positive		Cw 5-negative	
	Positive cytotoxicity	Negative cytotoxicity	Positive cytotoxicity	Negative cytotoxicity
Peripheral blood lymphocytes	4	1	2	33
Chronic lymphatic leukemia cells	6	1	4	20
Totals	10	2	6	53

$Chi^2 = 30.58$ ($P<0.001$).

TABLE 3. (A) Positive T and B cell reactivity with serum from the day of transplantation

	HLA			
	A	B	Bw	C
Donor 4	2, 3	7, 44	4, 6	*5*, 7
RM	2, 3	7, 44	4, 6	*5*, 7
CeB	2, 3	7, 44	4, 6	*5*, 7
RD	*32*, 3	7, 44	4, 6	*5*, 7
DB	2, 3	7, 44	4, 6	*5*, –
ChB	2, 3	*17*, 44	4, –	*5*, –

TABLE 3. (B) Negative reactivity with serum from the day of transplantation

	HLA			
	A	B	Bw	C
Donor 3	2, 3	7, –	–, 6	–, 7
GW	2, 3	7, 44	4, 6	*2*, 7
IH	2, 3	7, *15*	–, 6	*3*, 7
RP	2, 3	7, –	–, 6	–, 7
JC	2, 3	7, *14*	4, 6	–, 7
MB	2, *11*	*62*, *39*	–, 6	*3*, 7

J. R. CHAPMAN[2]
C. TAYLOR
A. TING
P. J. MORRIS
Nuffield Department of Surgery
University of Oxford
John Radcliffe Hospital
Oxford, England, OX3 9DU

[2] Medical Research Council Training Fellow.

REFERENCES

1. Kissmeyer-Nielsen F, Olsen S, Petersen VP, Fjeldborg O. Hyperacute rejection of kidney allografts, associated with pre-existing antibodies against donor cells. Lancet 1966; 2: 662.
2. Williams GM, Hume DM, Page Hudson R, et al. "Hyperacute" renal-homograft rejection in man. N Engl J Med 1968; 279: 611.
3. Patel R, Terasaki P. Significance of the positive crossmatch test in kidney transplantion. N Engl J Med 1969; 280: 735.
4. Cross DE, Greiner R, Whittier FC. Importance of the autocontrol crossmatch in human renal transplantation. Transplantation 1976; 21: 307.
5. Morris PJ, Ting A. The crossmatch in renal transplantation. Tissue Antigens 1981; 17: 75.
6. Ting A, Morris PJ. Successful transplantation with a positive T and B cell crossmatch due to autoreactive antibodies. Tissue Antigens 1983; 21: 219.
7. Ellis SA, Taylor C, Hildreth JEK, McMichael AJ. An HLA Class I specific monoclonal antibody that fails to bind to part of the HLA-A series. Hum Immunol 1985; 13: 13.
8. Brodsky FM, Parham P, Branstable CJ, Crumpton MJ, Bodmer WF. Monoclonal antibodies for analysis of the HLA system. Immunol Rev 1979; 47: 3.
9. Loon J, Terasaki PI, Bernoco D. Loss of HLA-C locus specificities from stored lymphocytes and de novo synthesis following incubation at 37°C. Tissue Antigens 1981; 18: 349.
10. Solheim BG, Flatmark A, Enger E, Jervell J, Thorsby E. Influence of HLA-A, -B, -C and -D matching on the outcome of clinical kidney transplantation. Transplant Proc 1977; 9: 475.
11. Ferrara GB, Tosi R, Longo A, Castellani A, Viviani C, Carminati G. "Silent" allelles at the HLA C locus. J Immunol 1978; 121: 731.

Received 24 October 1985.
Accepted 29 October 1985.

URINE CYTOLOGY IN RELATION TO URINARY TRACT MALIGNANCIES IN RENAL TRANSPLANT PATIENTS

The following case report prompted us to study the diagnostic value of the cytological examination of the urine sediment from renal transplant patients. In 1982 a 45-year-old woman was referred for cadaveric renal transplantation; she had been on chronic hemodialysis since 1980 because of end-stage renal failure caused by analgesic nephropathy. Unilateral nephrectomy was performed in 1981 because of repeated urinary tract infections. Histological examination showed an end-stage kidney with no specific characteristics. Posttransplant immunosuppressive medication consisted of azathioprine and low-dose corticosteroids, as described elsewhere (*1*); an antirejection course of high-dose corticosteroids was initiated on day 5. Two months after transplantation, she was hospitalized because of repeated urinary tract infections and microscopic hematuria. Cytological examination of successive urine samples showed malignant cells. At cystoscopy, several small papillary lesions were noted and removed; histological examination revealed papillary transitional cell carcinoma (grade II). Subsequent cytological examinations performed at regular intervals indicated that the urine still contained malignant cells. At cystoscopy several months later papillary lesions were again found and removed; histologically, one of these lesions exhibited again papillary transitional cell carcinoma (grade I). One year after transplantation, cytological examination of the urine still revealed malignant urothelial cells, while multiple biopsies of bladder mucosa suggested the possibility of an in situ carcinoma; two months later, radical cystectomy was performed because repeated histological studies now indicated invasive bladder cancer. The transplanted ureter emptied via a ureteroenterostomy. Histologically the bladder did not contain any tumor tissue. One year after the cystectomy, the patient died of a hepatic carcinoma that resembled histologically the biopsy material obtained from the bladder 14 months before. A revised evaluation of the initial material indicated a transitional cell carcinoma (grade III). The transplanted kidney showed no abnormalities at autopsy; the renal pelvis and ureter contained no tumor tissue.

Although cytological examination of the urine sediment is useful for the diagnosis of neoplasms of the renal pelvis, ureter, and bladder in nontransplant patients, no data on its value for renal transplant recipients are, to our knowledge, available. We therefore undertook a cross-sectional, and partly longitudinal, study of the cytology of urine sediments from renal transplant patients on long-term immunosuppressive therapy. All patients who received a transplant before 1978 and routinely visited our outpatient clinic in 1983 and 1984 with a functioning graft were enrolled in the study. Between 1966 and 1978, 328 patients underwent transplantation; by 1983, 158 had a functioning graft, 78 had returned to dialysis, and 92 had died. Of the deceased, 6 had died of a malignant tumor (3 lymphoproliferative tumors, 1 melanoma, 1 breast cancer, 1 Ewing's sarcoma). Thirty-two patients visited another hospital for their posttransplant follow-up and were therefore not included in the study. Consequently, urine sediments from 126 patients without an acute rejection episode were examined.

A total of 275 urine specimens were examined cytologically over a 24-month period; the number of specimens per patient ranged from 2 to 4. A freshly voided, early morning urine sample (volume 5–30 ml) was collected, refrigerated, and processed by the cytopathology laboratory using cytocentrifugation and the Papanicolaou staining method. Slides were screened for morphologically abnormal cells; the results were classified according to Papanicolaou into 5 classes: class I, normal cells; class II, abnormal but benign cells; class III abnormal cells, possibly malignant; class IV, serious suspicion of malignancy; class V definitely malignant cells. A class IV or V classification was considered an indication for extensive urological studies.

The frequency distribution of the cytological classes of the 275 urine samples from 126 renal transplant patients is shown in Figure 1. In five cases, cells that were classified as Papanicolaou class IV/V were found in urine samples obtained 2–3 weeks apart. These findings were not associated with urinary tract infections, the use of cyclophosphamide or other medications, or chronic rejection. Extensive urologic examination, including intravenous pyelography and cystoscopy of all five patients as well as retrograde ureterography and selective lavage of the ureters in two cases, did not reveal a neoplasm. Urine specimens obtained 2–3 months later contained cells that were classified as class I–III only. At present, 18 months (range 17–23 months) after the urological studies, no signs of an urothelial tumor have emerged. One patient died in the follow-up period of a myocardial infarction; at autopsy no urinary tract carcinoma was found. Therefore no correlation between

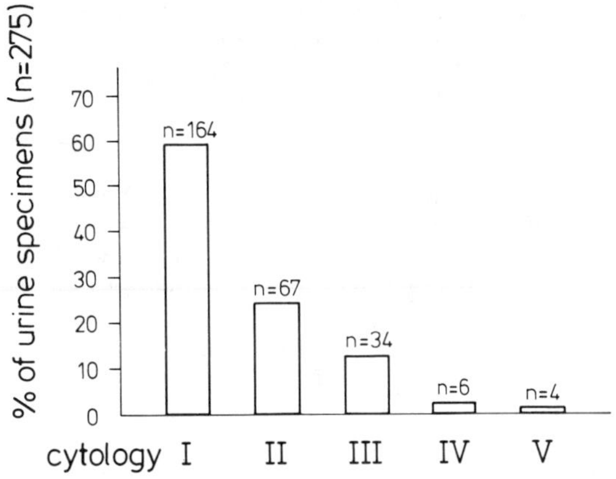

FIGURE 1. Frequency distribution of cytological classes of 275 urine samples from 126 renal transplant patients.

incidental positive cytological findings and urinary tract carcinoma in renal transplant patients could be demonstrated.

An increased incidence of epithelial and lymphoproliferative tumors has been recognized in renal transplant recipients (*2–4*). Since squamous cell carcinoma of the skin, lip, and cervix are the most prevalent (*2–5*), regular follow-up studies of the skin and cervical smears have been recommended (*5*). The risk of urinary tract carcinoma seems to increase following renal transplantation (*6*). This may, however, be attributable to the original disease rather than the transplantation, as was probably the case in our patient (*7*). Furthermore, pretransplant uraemia (*8–11*)—as well as posttransplant chronic immunostimulation, immunosuppressive treatment (*2–4*), and oncogenic viruses (*2–5*)—may cause or contribute to the increased incidence of posttransplant neoplasms.

In the present study, routine urine cytology suggested the possibility of an urinary tract carcinoma in 5 renal transplant recipients; however, extensive urological studies as well as clinical and postmortem follow-up data did not reveal a tumor. Moreover, in all cases the abnormal cells disappeared spontaneously within 2–3 months. On the other hand, the cytological findings remained definitely abnormal for our patient who ultimately died of disseminated urinary tract carcinoma. None of the 121 patients with repeatedly normal urine cytology exhibited signs of a carcinoma of the urinary tract in the 18-month follow-up period. It therefore appears that the urine of transplanted patients who have received long-term immunosuppressive medication may transiently show malignant cells in the absence of any demonstrable carcinoma. So far we have not been able to find an explanation, although one possibility would be that transient viral infections or virus reactivation in urinary tract epithelial cells caused the transiently positive urine cytological findings. We would suggest extensive urologic examination of renal transplant patients only whenever routine urine samples obtained over a 2–3-month period repeatedly show malignant cells.

ANTOINETTE M. M. KOOTTE[1,2]
JACOB ZWARTENDIJK[3]
JANNIE A. M. BEEKHUIS-BRUSSEE[3]
JOHAN H. VAN BOCKEL[4]
LEENDERT C. PAUL[1]
Departments of Nephrology, Urology and Surgery
University Hospital
Leiden, The Netherlands

[1] Department of Nephrology.
[2] Address correspondence to: A. M. M. Kootte, Department of Nephrology, University Hospital Leiden, 2333 AA Leiden, The Netherlands.
[3] Department of Urology.
[4] Department of Surgery.

REFERENCES

1. Van Hooff JP, Van Es A, Koolen MI, Kalff MW, Van den Broek PH, De Graeff J. Less aggressive rejection therapy and low-dose corticosteroids leading to satisfactory cadaveric kidney graft survival and low morbidity rate. Proc Eur Dial Transplant Assoc 1980; 17: 435.
2. Penn I, Starzl TE. Malignant tumors arising de novo in immunosuppressed organ transplant recipients. Transplantation 1972; 14: 407.
3. Hoover R, Fraumeni JF. Risk of cancer in renal transplant recipients. Lancet 1973; 2: 55.
4. Penn I. Depressed immunity and the development of cancer. Clin Exp Immunol 1981; 46: 459.
5. Blohmé I, Larkö O. Premalignant and malignant skin lesions in renal transplant patients. Transplantation 1984; 37: 165.
6. Sheil AGR, Flavel S, Disney APS, Mathew TH. Cancer in dialysis and transplant patients. Transplant Proc 1985; 13: 195.
7. Gonwa TA, Corbett WT, Schey HM, Buckalew VM. Analgesic-associated nephropathy and transitional cell carcinoma of the urinary tract. Ann Intern Med 1980; 93: 249.
8. Matas AJ, Kjellstrand CM, Simmons RL, Buselmeier TJ, Najarian JS. Increased incidence of malignancy during chronic renal failure. Lancet 1975; 1: 883.
9. Herr HW, Engen DE, Hostetler J. Malignancy in uremia: dialysis versus transplantation. J Urol 1979; 121: 584.
10. Miach PJ, Dawborn JK, Xipell J. Neoplasia in patients with chronic renal failure on long term dialysis. Clin Nephrol 1976; 5: 101.
11. Sutherland GA, Glass J, Gabriel R. Increased incidence of malignancy in chronic renal failure. Nephron 1977; 181: 182.

Received 16 July 1985.
Accepted 14 October 1985.

THE SYNERGISTIC EFFECT OF CYCLOSPORINE AND ILOPROST ON SURVIVAL OF RAT CARDIAC ALLOGRAFTS[1]

The two immunosuppressive drugs widely used in cardiac transplantation—namely, cyclosporine (CsA)* and prednisolone—possess extremely serious side effects. CsA induces nephrotoxicity and prednisolone causes aseptic bone necrosis. Therefore treatment modalities for reducing the dose of these drugs are of considerable clinical interest.

Some of the cyclooxygenase products of the 6 polyunsaturated fatty acids appear to be cytoprotective in a general sense. These products include prostacyclin (PGI_2) and the prostaglandins of the E series-i.e., PGE_1 and PGE_2—which possess prop-

Received 10 September 1985.
Accepted 7 November 1985.

* Abbreviations used: CsA, cyclosporine; PGI_2 prostacyclin; PGE_1, prostaglandin E_1; PGE_2, prostaglandin E_2.

[1] This work was supported by American Heart Association Grant 84-1147 and by National Institutes of Health Grant HL 32319.

erties indicating a beneficial role in transplantation of nonvascular (*1*) and vascularized grafts (*2–5*). These properties include stabilization of platelets and leukocytes sufficient to inhibit aggregation. Both PGI_2 and the PGE series are vasodilatory, and therefore lower peripheral resistance—but PGI_2 has a more prominent dilatory effect on the coronary artery tree in a wide range of species (*6*). Iloprost (Zk 36374, 5-[E]-1S, 5S,6R, 7R)-7-hydroxy-6-[E]-[3S,4RS]-3-hydroxy-4-methyl-oct-1-en-6-yn-yl-bicyclo 3.30-octan-3-ylidenpentanoic acid) is a chemically stable prostacyclin analogue that is reported to exert significant biochemical protective effects after myocardial ischemia consequent to experimental artery occlusion (*7*). Iloprost has also been shown to improve functional recovery of the isolated rat heart after hypothermic arrest (*8*). This carbacyclin analogue is reported to be more selective in inhibiting platelet aggregation than PGI_2 and with fewer systemic hemodynamic effects (*9*). Some of the CsA toxicity might be mediated by inhibition of PGI_2 synthesis in the vascular endothelium (*10*).

In addition to these potential beneficial vascular and hematological effects, a case can be made for the use of prostacyclin analogues in immunosuppression. PGI_2 inhibits lymphocyte proliferation in response to both antigens and mitogens (*11*), as well as decreasing Ia expression by murine macrophages (*12*). For these reasons we decided to evaluate to what degree iloprost can prolong graft survival in the presence of a minimal dose of CsA, which by itself does not increase survival. To this end we used the rat cardiac allograft model and showed that iloprost can indeed significantly increase graft survival in combination with low-dose CsA to the same extent as the combination of CsA and prednisolone.

Heterotopic cardiac transplantation was performed in rats (*13, 14*). This model has been characterized earlier in terms of different immunosuppressive regimens and the role of the different icosanoids (*15, 16*). Allograft survival was determined by daily palpation of heartbeat through the abdominal wall by an independent investigator. Rejection was defined as cessation of heartbeats. Lewis rats were recipients and Lewis Brown-Norway F_1 were donors. In the study described here, 28 rats were divided into five groups. Group 1 (n = 4) received the vehicle for CsA (olive oil, 0.1 ml/daily i.m.). Group 2 (n = 5) received iloprost (Schering, W. Berlin, Germany, 0.72 mg/kg, daily by osmotic pump). Group 3 (n = 9) were treated with CsA (Sandoz, East Hannover, NY, 0.5 mg/kg, daily i.m.). Group 4 (n = 5) received CsA (0.5 mg/kg, daily i.m.) and iloprost as above. Group 5 (n = 5) were given CsA (0.5 mg/kg, daily i.m.) and prednisolone (Merck, Sharp and Dohme, West Point, PA, 2 mg/kg, daily i.m.). Results are expressed as mean ±SEM. The Newman-Keuls multiple range test was used for comparison between the groups. Each experimental group was tested against each of the other groups.

The dose of CsA (0.5 mg/kg daily) was low enough not to significantly prolong allograft survival by itself. There was no significant difference in the graft survival of vehicle-treated (group 1), iloprost-treated (group 2) or CsA-treated rats (group 3). The combination of CsA and iloprost (group 4) improved graft survival significantly ($P<0.05$) to 14.2±1.4 days, as compared with groups 1, 2, or 3. The combination of CsA and prednisolone (group 5) significantly improved ($P<0.01$) allograft survival (18.0±2.9 days) when compared with groups 1, 2, or 3. The data are shown in Figure 1.

Prostacyclin has been employed successfully in patients with chronic kidney transplant rejection, in that the transplant

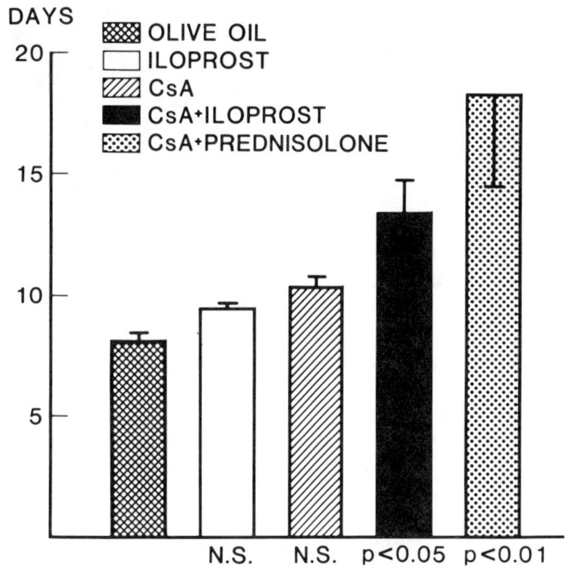

FIGURE 1. Cardiac allograft survival in days ±SEM in the five experimental groups. The combination of CsA and iloprost or CsA and prednisolone prolonged allograft survival significantly.

function was improved (*17*). In a rat heterotopic cardiac allograft model, prostacyclin significantly improved graft survival but only by 1.2–1.5 days (*5*). The allograft survival obtained in the present study by combining a low dose of CsA with iloprost was longer than that obtained when PGI_2 was used by itself (*5*). This survival had the same magnitude as seen in a similar model where azathioprine was combined with a PGE_1 analogue (*3*). Successful preservation of kidney graft function was obtained in the same histoincompatible strains as used in our study with daily administration of a PGE_1 analogue (*4*). These investigators also found that the PGE_1 analogue abrogated the capacity of the host animals to activate donor specific cytotoxic lymphocytes in vivo. The prostaglandin E compounds and PGI_2 are thought to exert their inhibitory effect on lymphocyte proliferation in vitro by increasing the intracellular level of cyclic AMP. More recently the inhibitory effect of the E prostaglandins has been suggested to be exerted by inhibition of interleukin-2 production (*18, 19*). Inhibition of interleukin-2 production has not yet been demonstrated for PGI_2 or its analogues, which are likely to be more potent than PGE_2 in inhibiting both mitogen and antigen-induced lymphocyte proliferation (*12*). Recently interleukin-1, but not interleukin 2, has been shown to induce synthesis of PGI_2 in human endothelial cells. The immunosuppressive effect of CsA is reported to be mediated through inhibition of interleukin 2 messenger RNA (*20*). Thus the synergistic effect of the low-dose CsA and the PGI_2 analogue, iloprost might be through these two mechanisms. This would strengthen the case for a CsA sparing effect of iloprost. The combination of CsA with either prednisone or iloprost showed a synergistic effect. This suggests the possibility of reducing or replacing prednisone with a stable long-acting prostacyclin analogue.

JOHN R. ROWLES
MARIE L. FOEGH[2]

[2] Address correspondence to: Marie Foegh, M.D., Department of Surgery, Division of Transplantation, Georgetown University Medical Center, Cober-Kogan Bldg. Room 206, Washington, D.C. 20007.

BIJAN S. KHIRABADI
PETER W. RAMWELL
Department of Surgery, Division of Transplantation
Department of Physiology and Biophysics
Georgetown University Medical Center
Washington, D.C. 20007

REFERENCES

1. Quagliata F, Lawrence VJW, Philips-Quagliata JM. Prostaglandin E_1 as a regulator of lymphocyte function. Cell Immunol 1973; 6: 457.
2. Strom TB, Carpenter CB, Crago EJ, Norris S, Devlin R, Peper RJ. Suppression of in vivo and in vitro alloimmunity by prostaglandins. Transplant Proc 1977; 9: 1075.
3. Kort WJ, Bonta IL, Adolfs MJP, Westbrook DL. Synergism of (15S-)-15-methyl-prostaglandin E with either azathioprine or prednisolone on the survival of hearts allografts in rats. Prostaglandins Leukotrienes Med 1982; 8: 661.
4. Strom TB, Carpenter CB. Prostaglandin as an effective antirejection therapy in rat renal allograft recipients. Transplantation 1983; 35: 279.
5. Shaw FL. Prolongation of rat allograft survival by treatment with prostacyclin or aspirin during acute rejection. Transplantation 1983; 35: 526.
6. Bunting S, Gryglewski R, Moncada S, Vane J. Arterial walls generate from prostaglandin endoperoxide a substance (prostaglandin X) which relaxes strips of mesenteric and coeliac arteries and inhibit platelet aggregation. Prostaglandins 1976; 12: 897.
7. Smith EF, Gallenkamper W, Beckmann R, Thomsen T, Mannesmann G, Schror K. Early and late administration of a PGI_2-analogue, ZK 36374 (iloprost): effects on myocardial preservation, collateral blood flow and infarct size. Cardiovasc Res 1984; 18: 163.
8. Gilst WHV, Boonstra PW, Terpstra JA, Wildevuur CRM, de-Langen CDJ. Improved functional recovery of the isolated rat heart after 24 hours of hypothermic arrest with a stable prostacyclin analogue (ZK 36374). J Mol Cell Cardiol 1983; 15: 789.
9. Stenzel JC, Buse M, Losert W. Comparison of the vasodepressor action of ZK 36 374, a stable prostacyclin derivative, PGI_2 and PGE_1 with their effect on platelet aggregation and bleeding time in rats. Prostaglandins Leukotrienes Med 1983; 10: 197.
10. Rossi V, Breviario F, Ghezzi P, Dejana E, Mantovani A. Prostacyclin synthesis induced in vascular cells by interleukin-1. Science 1985; 229: 174.
11. Leung KH, Michich E. Prostaglandin modulation of development of cell mediated immunity in culture. Nature 1981; 288: 597.
12. Snyder DS, Beller DI, Unanue ER. Prostaglandins modulate macrophage Ia expression. Nature 1982; 299: 163.
13. Ono K, Lindsey ES. Improved technique of heart transplantation in rats. J Thorac Cardiovasc Surg 1969; 57: 255.
14. Khirabadi BS, Foegh ML, Ramwell PW. Urine immunoreactive thromboxane B_2 in rat cardiac allograft rejection. Transplantation 1985; 39: 6.
15. Foegh ML, Alijani MR, Helfrich GB, Ramwell PW. Eicosanoids and organ transplantation. Ann Clin Res 1984; 16: 318.
16. Foegh ML, Khirabadi B, Ramwell PW. Prolongation of experimental cardiac allograft survival with thromboxane-related drugs. Transplantation 1985; 40: 124.
17. Leithner C, Sinzinger H, Schwarz M. Treatment of chronic kidney transplant rejection with prostacyclin: reduction of platelet deposition in the transplant; prolongation of platelet survival and improvement of transplant function. Prostaglandins 1981; 22: 783.
18. Rappaport RS, Dodge GR. Prostaglandin E inhibits the production of human interleukin 2. J Exp Med 1982; 155: 943.
19. Walker C, Kristensen F, Bettens F, DeWeck AL. Lymphokine regulation of activated (G_1) lymphocytes. I. Prostaglandin E_2-induced inhibition of interleukin 2 production. J Immunol 1983; 130: 1770.
20. Elliott JR, Lin Y, Mizel SB, Bleackley RC, Harnish DG, Paetkau V. Induction of interleukin 2 messenger RNA inhibited by cyclosporin A. Science 1984; 226: 1439.
21. Rossi V, Breviario F, Ghezzi P, Dejana E, Mantovani A. Prostacyclin synthesis induced in vascular cells by interleukin-1. Science 1985; 229: 174.

INDUCED TOLERANCE TO ALLOGENEIC PANCREATIC ISLET TRANSPLANTS[1]

Allograft transplantation depends on permanent immune suppression the side effects of which constitute a serious burden. In order to solve this problem we tried a new approach—namely, that of enhancing immunotolerance to transplanted islets of Langerhans by a process of adaptation. No immunosuppressive agents were used. In a preliminary project, outbred streptozotocin-diabetic Wistar rats followed a desensitization protocol for one year using whole pancreas from normal allogenic donor Wistar rats, at which time they were homografted through the portal vein with donor Wistar rat islets. Of the five treated animals, two became clinically and biochemically normal following transplantation and remained so for six months, at which time they were sacrificed and examined histologically. This revealed the presence of numerous well-granulated islets in the lumina of the portal vessels of the liver. None were seen in the failures or the "non-adapted" controls. Encouraged by these results we undertook the study reported here in which a larger number of animals with better-defined genetic incompatibility were used—namely, Lewis ($RT1^l$) and Wistar-Furth ($RT1^u$) strains.

Received 6 September 1985.
Accepted 7 November 1985.
[1] This work was supported by an S.L. Lunenfeld research grant.

A total of 40 inbred Wistar-Furth male rats of approximately 250 g body weight were made diabetic by injecting 70 mg/kg of streptozotocin i.p. Six noninjected animals of the same age were kept as normal controls. Of the streptozotocin-injected animals, 29 developed insulin-dependent diabetes. Five of them were used as diabetic controls and the remaining 24 rats were admitted to the tissue injection program. Once the diabetes and the respective insulin requirements of each animal were established after 4–6 weeks, pancreatic tissue inoculation was commenced.

Animals were housed in individual cages, in an air-conditioned room with a 12×12-hr light cycle, and fed with regular laboratory chow and water ad libitum. Body weight was measured each week. The urine was tested for glucose and ketones daily and the insulin dose adjusted accordingly in a combination of 0.5:1.5 units of regular and protamine-zinc insulins. At monthly intervals, blood samples for glucose and insulin determinations were drawn from a tail vein.

The material for the daily inoculations was prepared three times a week. From a normal inbred Lewis rat pancreas, 100 mg of the splenic portion were dissected out, placed in 5 ml saline plus 250 mg Ampicillin, and minced to a fine suspension suitable for injection through a 21-gauge needle and kept at 4°C. Before inoculation, the tissue suspension was diluted with saline to achieve the desired concentration in a volume of 0.5 ml per rat. Starting with a concentration of one-millionth of the estimated weight of the whole gland, the dose was doubled every two weeks. In 22 weeks it reached a concentration of 1/1000, which was maintained for a further 30 weeks. The inoculations were given every morning s.c. in the scruff of the neck.

Thirteen of the 24 initially diabetic animals recovered spontaneously from their diabetes while on the inoculation program. This was evident by the progressive reduction of insulin requirements associated with aglycosuria, normal glycemia, and insulinemia. The morphological regeneration of the pancreas and its normal insulin content were confirmed postmortem. Since this event was not related to our protocol but was a failure of streptozotocin dosage, and since it was not practical to reinject streptozotocin into these disparate animals and they no longer fitted our protocol, they were excluded from the study.

At the end of the one year's treatment, the 11 inoculated animals and the 5 diabetic noninoculated controls were transplanted with isolated islets. For each transplantation 500–800 islets were harvested from two donor normal Lewis rats (*1*) and injected into the portal vein via the splenic branch, under Penthrane anaesthesia (Two inoculated animals died of hemorrhage after surgery). Body weight, glycosuria, and glycemia were monitored after transplantation following the same schedule as before.

Autopsies were performed in all animals 5–6 months after transplantation. Histological observation of the islets was done on all pancreas and liver specimens, as well as on the area of tissue inoculation. Sections were stained with hematoxylin-eosin, aldehyde-thionine, and peroxidase immunohistochemical staining to differentiate the main three types of islet-secreting cells.

Blood glucose was measured using an automated Beckman glucose analyzer. Insulin was determined by immunoassay (*2*). Pancreatic insulin and insulin at the site of inoculation in the neck was extracted with acid alcohol and assessed by radioimmunoassay.

The results are summarized in Table 1. The daily pancreatic inoculations had no effect on the diabetic state, as judged by the insulin requirement. This was tested after the 22nd week of inoculation by reducing the required daily insulin dose to one-half. There was increased glycosuria and glycemia almost immediately, which necessitated restoration of the previous insulin therapy. The nonfasting blood glucose levels in the group, tested at different periods during the year, ranged from 243 to 365 mg/dl. The corresponding mean value in nondiabetic controls was 144 mg/dl.

Nine animals who had received a complete course of inoculations for a period of one year survived the allotransplantation. Of these, seven were cured of their diabetes within one month of transplantation and remained so until they were sacrificed approximately six months later for histological assessment. By this time they were indistinguishable from the normal matched controls.

The five diabetic controls that did not receive the pancreas injections but that had diabetic severity and insulin requirements similar to those of the inoculated group were also allotransplanted. All five controls rejected the transplanted islets. In the successfully transplanted animals the blood glucose levels returned to concentrations of <250 mg/dl. Plasma insulin measured at six months posttransplantation were within the normal range. In inoculated rats, the histological search for islets at the inoculation site in the neck, both by standard stainings and by immunohistochemistry, failed to identify islet cells. The insulin content in the acid-alcohol extraction of the area tissue was 6.5 μU/mg, which was not different from values in tissue distant from the injection site (5.6 μU/mg).

The histology of the host's pancreas in the successfully transplanted rats demonstrated a massive destruction of the

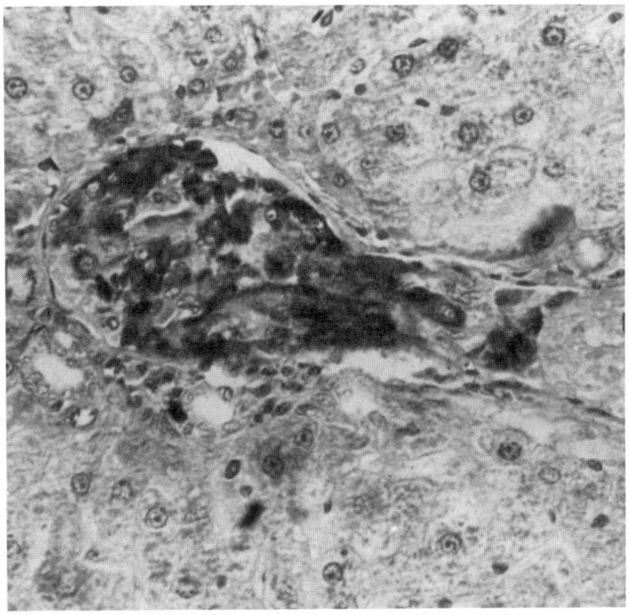

FIGURE 1. An islet of Langerhans lodged in the lumen of a portal vessel six months after transplantation. Well-granulated β cells (dark stain) are clearly seen (aldehyde-thionine stain, magnification approximately 240×).

TABLE 1. Allotransplantation of islets (Lewis) to Wistar-Furth rats (mean values ± SEM)

Group (No. animals)	Body weight (g): At transplant time	Body weight (g): At killing time	Glycosuria	Glycemia (mg/dl): At transplant time	Glycemia (mg/dl): At killing time	Plasma insulin at killing (μU/ml)	Pancreas insulin (mU/mg)
Normal control (6)		408±15.8	0		126±8.2	42±6.6	7.3±0.9
Transplanted diabetic control (5)	361±16.6	341±7.5	+ to +++ (continuously)	391±14.2	304±47.7	Exogenous insulin daily	0.5±0.3
Transplanted tissue-inoculated							
Unsuccessful (2)	372±16.5	342±14.1	+ to +++	359±15.2	364±6.5	Exogenous insulin daily	0.4±0.2
Successful (7)	344±13.1	375±13.2	0 (following transplant)	325±17.8	174±6.2	39±4.1	0.4±0.1

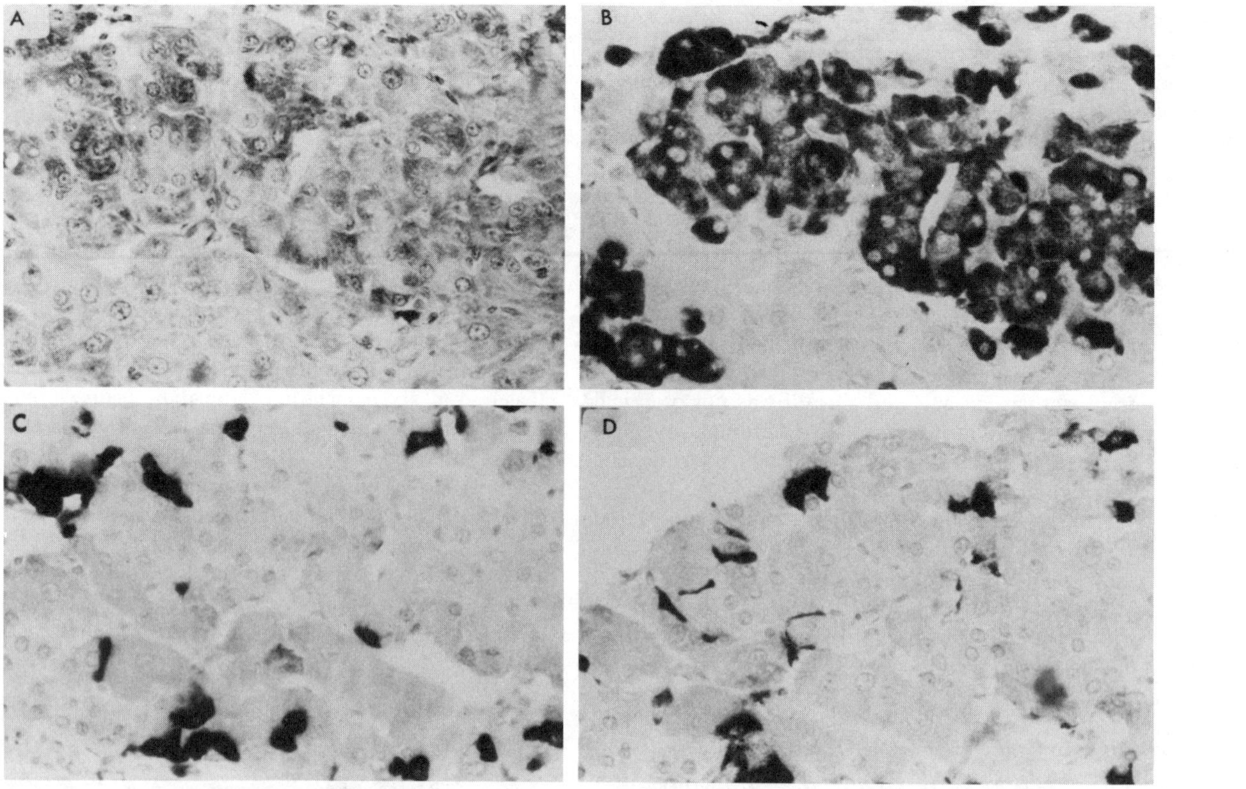

FIGURE 2. Serial sections of an intraportal transplanted islet: (A) Aldehyde-thionine stain; (B) β cells of the same islet detected by antiinsulin serum reacted with peroxidase-antiperoxidase reaction; (C) α cells identified by antiglucagon serum; and (D) somatostatin-secreting cells (D cells) reacted with the specific antiserum (magnification approximately 160×).

beta cells, induced by the streptozotocin administration. The insulin content in the acid-alcohol extracts of these same pancreases ranged from 0.03 to 0.8 μU/mg compared to 7.3 μU/mg in the nondiabetic control pancreases.

Histological examination of the liver of these same animals revealed the presence of many well-granulated islets within the lumen of the portal vessels (Fig. 1). By specific immunohistochemical staining for insulin, glucagon, and somatostatin of serial sections of the grafted islet, the presence of the three types of secretory cells can be identified (Fig. 2). No cellular infiltrates were present in or around the transplanted islet tissue.

In the preliminary experiment involving the outbred Wistar strain, two of five animals in which induced immune tolerance had been attempted by the technique described herein experienced successful islet cell allografts. Again, using a similar protocol across a well defined strong histocompatibility barrier—namely, inbred Lewis donors to inbred Wistar-Furth recipients, seven of nine animals had successful islet cell grafts.

In both series all of the noninoculated diabetic controls rejected their transplants. Also, no immunosuppression of recipient or special treatment of donor tissue was applied.

In conclusion, an alternative method of pancreatic islet transplantation has been introduced. It prevents rejection in a significant number of cases and avoids the use of immune suppression.

Further investigation will be necessary to determine how this procedure affects the immune system, whether or not it is useful for other organs, and whether it is applicable to man and other species.

Acknowledgments. We are grateful to Mrs. I. Burlon and I. Sun for their technical assistance.

Bernard S. Leibel
Julio M. Martin
Walter Zingg
Research Institute
The Hospital for Sick Children
Toronto, Ontario, Canada, M5G 1X8

REFERENCES

1. Lacy PE, Kostianovsky M. Method for the isolation of intact islets of Langerhans from rat pancreas. Diabetes 1967; 16: 35.
2. Herbert V, Lau KS, Gottlieb CW, Bleicher SJ. Coated charcoal immunoassay of insulin. J Clin Endocrinol Metab 1965; 25: 1375.

PROLONGATION OF CANINE CARDIAC ALLOGRAFT SURVIVAL USING DONOR-SPECIFIC BUFFY COAT PRETRANSFUSIONS

Blood transfusion has been demonstrated to prolong allograft survival in human kidney transplantation (*1*). This beneficial "transfusion effect" has been reported using random (*2*) and donor-specific transfusion (*3*), and has received extensive experimental support from animal models using skin (*4*), kidney (*5*), heart (*6*), and liver (*7*) allografts. Modifications of the pretransfusion approach have included blood component ther-

Received 1 August 1985.
Accepted 22 October 1985.

TABLE 1. Pretransfusion procedures in canine heterotopic heart transplants

Group	Pretransfusion[a]	Immunosuppression
Control	None	None
UVDBT	UV-irradiated donor buffy coat (1×10^9 cells) at −3, −2, −1 weeks	None
UVDBT (1/10)	UVDBT diluted 1/10 (1×10^8 cells)	None
UVDBT (1/100)	UVDBT diluted 1/100 (1×10^7 cells)	None
IS	None	Peritransplant: Azathioprine: 4 mg/kg/day Prednisone: 20 mg/day Posttransplant: Azathioprine 2 mg/kg/day Prednisone 20 mg/day
UVDBT-IS	UVDBT	Same as IS
DBT-IS	DBT-no UV irradiation	Same as IS
PIS	None	Pretransplant (−3, −2, −1 weeks): Azathioprine: 4 mg/kg/day Prednisone: 20 mg/day Peritransplant and Posttransplant: Same as IS
UVDBT-PIS	UVDBT	Same as PIS
DBT-PIS	DBT	Same as PIS

[a] Transfusion given at −3, −2, −1 weeks pretransplant.

apy, immunosuppression at the time of pretransfusion—and, most recently, ultraviolet irradiation of donor-specific blood elements (*8*). However, experience with heart transplant patients has been limited (*9*), and the effect of pretransfusion on cardiac allograft survival in a large animal model has not been documented.

We investigated the effect of donor-specific buffy coat pretransfusions in a canine heterotopic cardiac allograft model. In addition, the effect of ultraviolet irradiation of the donor buffy coat, and the role of immunosuppression at the time of pretransfusion were studied.

Heterotopic cardiac transplantation in outbred mongrel dogs was performed using our modification (*10*) of Jamieson's technique. (*11*) Allograft survival was monitored by the presence of an extra deflection on the daily electrocardiogram and the endpoint of rejection was defined as complete loss of the allograft signal. Prompt postrejection autopsy was performed on all recipients to evaluate the allograft and to exclude technical failure. Histologic examination was performed in a blind fashion to confirm rejection.

Buffy coat preparations of CPDA-anticoagulated blood were obtained by centrifugation and circulated through a monolayer grid either with or without ultraviolet radiation. Radiation was supplied by two Sylvania FS 20 lamps for 4 hr, to a total dosage of 9000 joules/m^2 per 1–3×10^9 cells. Cellular viability after ultraviolet (UV)* irradiation was confirmed by trypan blue exclusion. The inhibitory effect of UV irradiation on the stimulatory activity of dog peripheral blood lymphocytes was confirmed by mixed lymphocyte reaction (MLR) in a dose-response fashion.

Donor buffy coat preparations, either UV-irradiated (UVDBT) or nonirradiated (DBT), were transfused into recipient dogs at 3 weeks, 2 weeks, and 1 week prior to heart transplantation. Immunosuppression (IS), when given, consisted of perioperative azathioprine given orally at a dose of 4 mg/kg/day and prednisone 20 mg/day the day before, the day of, and the day after transplantation. Postoperatively, azathioprine at 2 mg/kg/day orally was combined with prednisone 20 mg/day.

Because of evidence indicating augmentation of the transfusion effect when combined with peritransfusion immunosuppression (*4*), a further experiment employed the above-described perioperative immunosuppressive regimen at the time of each of the three pretransplant transfusions, and then proceeded with the same perioperative and postoperative protocol described above (PIS).

To evaluate the possible contribution of antigen dosage, experiments were conducted with UV-irradiated buffy coat preparations at 1/10 and 1/100 of the cellular concentration. All treatment protocols are outlined in Table 1.

Statistical analysis of graft survival data (Table 2) was performed using the generalized Wilcoxon-Breslow test for comparison of censured data. Correction for multiple comparisons with the use of the Bonferone inequality test required a P value of 0.003 to achieve statistical significance.

UVDBT without IS did not, in any concentration tested, prolong allograft survival. There may have been a mild sensitizing effect to the UV treatment, as these grafts had shorter than control survival times (Fig. 1), however this difference was not significantly significant for the number of animals tested.

DBT-IS significantly prolonged allograft survival (P=0.0001 vs. control). UV irradiation of the donor infusion (UVDBT-IS) resulted in marked allograft prolongation in some animals but in early rejection in other animals (P=0.167 vs. controls).

DBT-PIS was the most successful regimen tested in prolonging heart allograft survival. However, comparison of this prolongation with DBT-IS (i.e., without peritransfusion immuno-

* Abbreviations used: DBT, donor buffy coat transfusion; IS, immunosuppression; MLR, mixed lymphocyte reaction; PIS, pretransplant, peritransfusion immunosuppression; UV, ultraviolet.

TABLE 2. Allograft survival with donor buffy-coat transfusion (DBT) in canine heterotopic heart transplants

Group	Number	Survival time (days)	P[b]
Control	7	7, 7, 8, 9, 10, 11, 11	
UVDBT	7	4, 4, 4, 5, 5, 8, 50	0.046
UVDBT (1/10)	5	6, 7, 11, 12, 14	0.564
UVDBT (1/100)	5	7, 8, 10, 11, 12	0.374
UVDBT-IS	7	1, 5, 14, 17, 25, 178[c], 251[d]	0.167
DBT-IS	7	11, 19, 23, 36, 37, 103,[d] 188[c]	0.001[b]
IS	6	15, 16, 16, 16, 23, 24	0.001[b]
UVDBT-PIS	7	9, 13, 14, 14, 273, 274,[d] 281[c]	0.004
DBT-PIS	6	14,[d] 19, 51, 209, 240, 259[c]	0.001[b]
PIS	6	6, 7, 8, 12, 15, 17	0.254

[a] See Table 1.
[b] P value compared with control; value of 0.003 significant.
[c] Still living at time of writing.
[d] Died from other causes without evidence of rejection.

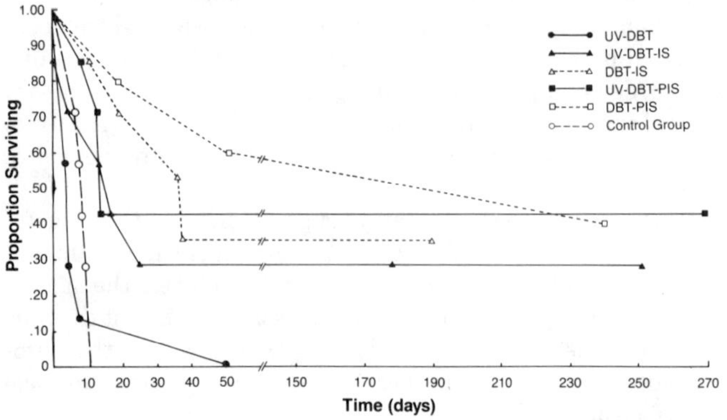

FIGURE 1. The sensitizing effect of UV irradiation on donor buffy pretransfusions is demonstrated. Heterotopic canine heart allograft survival was compared in animals given donor-specific buffy coat pretransfusions (DBT) and standard immunosuppression with azathioprine and prednisone both with (PIS) and without (IS) pretransplant, peritransfusion immunosuppression. UV irradiation of the buffy coat (UV-DBT) resulted in diminished allograft survival in both groups. Control animals received neither pretransfusion nor immunosuppression.

suppression) was not statistically significant with the number of animals tested.

The finding that pretransplant buffy coat transfusions significantly prolong heterotopic cardiac allograft survival in the outbred mongrel dog model corroborates clinical kidney transplant studies (*12*). The confirmation is important since extreme caution must be exercised in applying data from one organ or species to another—direct evidence must ultimately be obtained (*13*).

Although the beneficial effect of pretransfusion has been recognized for some time, considerable controversy persists regarding the mechanism of allograft prolongation. While most investigators propose clonal deletion (*14*), or induction of cellular (*6, 7*) or humoral (*15*) suppressive mechanisms, others maintain that pretransfusion merely preselects "low-response" recipients who might otherwise enjoy a more prolonged allograft survival (*16*). Clinical data suggest that selection does not adequately account for the observed transfusion benefit (*2*). In our model, all allograft recipients were pretransfused and subsequently transplanted, regardless of response status. Because graft survival was significantly prolonged, (Fig. 2) our findings do not support the selection theory as the sole explanation for the transfusion effect.

Though disappointing, the failure of UV-irradiated buffy coat transfusions to induce a state of donor-specific allograft acceptance was not surprising. Further study of UV-treatment of antigen-presenting cells has demonstrated the need for additional immunosuppression as the histoincompatibility of donor-recipient pairs increases (*17*). There is a suggestion from our data of increased sensitization in the UV-treated groups (Fig. 1), even in the presence of immunosuppression, although the number of experiments is too small to draw definitive conclusions. One possible explanation for this tendency could be that UV inactivation of the antigen presenting cell has interfered with the induction of a suppressor clone in a manner analogous to immunosuppression (*18*) or splenectomy (*6*) in other experimental models.

Given the considerable refinement of success with cyclosporine therapy, as well as the relatively unpredictable timing of the transplant procedure itself, the role of pretransfusion in clinical heart transplantation remains questionable. The additional benefit of transfusion in cyclosporine-treated kidney transplant recipients remains controversial. However, cyclosporine does not seem to serve as adequate immunosuppression when given alone, and has several documented side effects, occasionally requiring conversion to azathioprine in a few heart transplant patients. Therefore, any modality that would yield comparable or improved results at lower doses would clearly be welcome. The transfusion effect is generally believed to be maximal in the 1–6-month posttransfusion period (*19*), thus

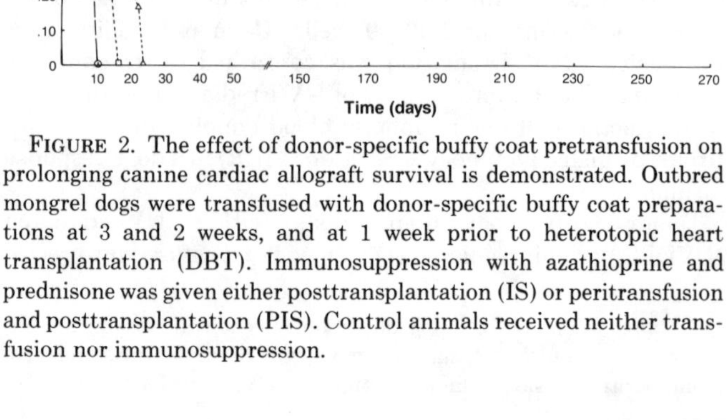

FIGURE 2. The effect of donor-specific buffy coat pretransfusion on prolonging canine cardiac allograft survival is demonstrated. Outbred mongrel dogs were transfused with donor-specific buffy coat preparations at 3 and 2 weeks, and at 1 week prior to heterotopic heart transplantation (DBT). Immunosuppression with azathioprine and prednisone was given either posttransplantation (IS) or peritransfusion and posttransplantation (PIS). Control animals received neither transfusion nor immunosuppression.

allowing for considerable flexibility in a pretransfusion regimen. Lastly, early success of pretransfusion in a xenograft model (*20*) magnifies the potential future value of any successful form of pretransplantation therapy.

In summary, we have demonstrated the beneficial effect of combining pretransplant donor-specific buffy coat transfusion, with azathioprine-prednisone immunosuppression on prolonging heterotopic cardiac allograft survival in the difficult outbred mongrel dog model. The effectiveness of this therapy and the failure of ultraviolet irradiation of pretransfused cells to improve our results have important implications for understanding the mechanism of the transfusion effect, and for improving our current approach to clinical transplantation.

PAUL A. KURLANSKY
ARTHUR R. DRESDALE
ROBIN PIERSON
ROBERT P. MCMANUS
ROBERT E. MICHLER
HENRY SACHS
WILLIAM G. THOMAS
HENRY LAU
MARK A. HARDY
CHARLES MARBOE
KEITH REEMTSMA
ERIC A. ROSE
Cardiac Transplantation Research Laboratory
Department of Surgery
Columbia University
College of Physicians & Surgeons
New York, New York 10032

REFERENCES

1. Opelz G, Terasaki PL. Dominant effect of transfusions on kidney graft survival. Transplantation 1980; 29: 153.
2. Pfaff WW, Fennell RS, Howard RJ, Ireland JF, Scornik JC. Planned random donor blood transfusion in preparation for transplantation. Transplantation 1984; 38: 701.
3. Anderson CB, Tyler JD, Sicare GA, Anderman CK, Rodey GE, Etheredge EE. Pretreatment of renal allograft recipients with immunosuppression and donor specific blood. Transplantation 1984; 38: 664.
4. Maki T, Okazaki H, Wood ML, Monaco AP. Mouse skin allograft model for study of pregraft blood transfusion. Transplant Proc 1982; 14: 394.
5. VanEs AA, Marquet RL, VanRood JJ, Balner H. Influence of a single blood transfusion on kidney allograft survival in unrelated rhesus monkeys. Transplantation 1978; 26: 325.
6. Shelby J, Wakely E, Corry RJ. Suppressor cell induction in donor-specific transfused mouse heart recipients. Surgery 1984; 96: 296.
7. Neuhaus P, Brolsch C, Neuhaus R, Lauchart W, Vonnahme F, Wonigeit K, Borlefts J, Balner H, Pichlmayr R. Pretransplant blood transfusions have a positive influence on liver graft survival in rhesus monkeys. Transplant Proc 1985; 17: 1129.
8. Lau H, Reemtsma K, Hardy MA. Pancreatic islet allograft prolongation by donor-specific blood transfusions treated with ultraviolet irradiation. Science 1983; 221: 754.
9. Katz MR, Goldman M, Barnhart G, Hastillo A, Szentpetery S, Wolfgang T, Hess M, Lower RR. Pretransplant transfusions in cardiac allograft recipients [Abstract]. Circulation 1984; 70(II):173.
10. Dresdale AR, Sachs H, Thomas W, Kurlansky P, Marboe C, Reemtsma KR, Rose EA. Heart allograft survival in outbred dogs treated with procarbazine hydrochloride and antithymocyte globulin. Transplantation 1985; 39: 15.
11. Jamieson SW, Burtan AN, Reitz BA, Shumway NE. A new method for heterotopic cardiac transplantation in the dog. J Surg Res 1982; 32: 150.
12. Okazaki H, Takahashi H, Miura K, Ishizaki M, Taguchi Y. Significant reduction of sensitization and improved allograft outcome with donor-specific buffy coat transfusion. Transplantation 1984; 37: 523.
13. Perloff LJ, Barker CF. Variable response to donor-specific blood transfusion in the rat. Transplantation 1984; 38: 178.
14. Terasaki P. The beneficial transfusion effect on kidney graft survival attributed to conal deletion. Transplantation 1984; 37: 119.
15. Singal DP, Joseph S, Ludwin D. Blood transfusion, suppressor cells and anti-idiotypic antibodies. Transplant Proc 1985; 17: 1104.
16. Iwaki Y, Kinukawa T, Terasaki PL, Mickey, MR, Ono Y. Donor-specific transfusion from unrelated dogs and evidence against the selection mechanism. Transplant Proc 1983; 15: 979.
17. Lau H, Reemtsma K, Hardy MA. The use of direct ultraviolet irradiation and cyclosporine in facilitating indefinite pancreatic islet allograft acceptance. Transplantation 1984; 38: 566.
18. Niessen GJCM, Marquet RL, Cobussen-Mathijssen A, Heijstek GA, Jeekel J. The blood transfusion effect in rats can be abolished by administration of cyclosporine A during transfusion. Transplant Proc 1983; 15: 1026.
19. Betuel H, Touraine JL, Malik MC, Bonnet MC, Carrie J, Dubernard JM, Traeger J. Kidney transplantation in patients submitted to deliberate transfusions to random transfusions and to thoracic duct drainage. Transplant Proc 1982; 14: 276.
20. Marquet RL, Vanes AA. Prolongation of baboon to rhesus kidney xenograft survival by pretransplant rhesus blood transfusions. Transplantation 1978; 25: 165.

0041-1337/86/4201-0102$02.00/0
TRANSPLANTATION

Vol. 42, No. 1
Printed in U.S.A.

Transplantation

Letters to Editor

THE CONTINUATION OF THE DEBATE ON GENE CONVERSION

In his defense of the gene conversion hypothesis, proposed as an explanation for the generation of major histocompatibility complex (MHC)* polymorphism, Larry R. Pease cites as evidence a short sequence coding for amino acid residues 130 through 150 in the class I α polypeptide chains (*1*). Since this stretch has become a *Paradestück* in the hands of the proponents of the gene conversion hypothesis, I must point out that the DNA sequence is most likely incorrect.

The stretch is purported to show that the *H-2D*^{b} gene is quite dissimilar in this segment to its allele L^d and quite similar to a nonallelic gene K^b. The presumption is therefore that the sharing of a stretch of nucleotide sequence between nonallelic genes (D^b and K^b) is the result of segmental exchange or "gene conversion." The crucial sequence in this comparison is that belonging to the L^d gene. This gene has been sequenced in two laboratories, by Evans et al. (*2*) and by Moore et al. (*3*). Pease quotes as a source of the sequence in his Figure 1 the Evans et al. paper, but in fact the sequence is from the Moore et al. paper. Had he used the Evans et al. sequence, the case for gene conversion would have all but disappeared.

I show the critical segment of the two L^d sequences in Table 1, together with additional mouse, human, rabbit, and pig class I sequences. The two sequences differ in six nucleotide pairs, and obviously one of them must be wrong. But which one? I would bet that the Moore et al. sequence—the same sequence that Pease used, attributing it to Evans et al.—is incorrect. The reasons for this conviction are apparent from Table 1. In this sequence, the codon specifying amino acid residue 136 is TTC, while in all other sequences the codon is GCG or a synonymous variant thereof. Where did the TTC codon come from? There is no gene to "donate" it and there are no intermediates to suggest its mutational derivation from the ancestral GCG codon. The TTC codon is absolutely foreign in the sequence and hence most likely represents a sequencing error.

Another difference between the two L^d sequences is in the codon specifying amino acid residue 139. Here, the Moore et al. sequence has a T and the Evans et al. sequence a C in the second position. Since virtually all the other H-2 sequences have a T in this position, it might be the Moore sequence that is correct here. But whether it is T or C at this position does not make much difference to our considerations.

The two remaining differences are in the codons specifying amino acid residues 140 and 141. In the Evans et al. sequence, these codons begin with a G, like all other codons in this position, whereas in the Moore et al. sequence they begin with a T. I find it extremely unlikely that mutations in adjacent codons would change the G to T in a single sequence, and again I am willing to bet that the Moore et al. sequence is incorrect.

If one compares the Evans et al. L^d sequence with the rest of the available sequences, one realizes that L^d is, as we would expect from alleles, almost identical with D^b, and K^b is different from D^b, again as we would expect from nonallelic genes. There is therefore not only no need, but also no basis for explaining the observed differences by gene conversion: they are all fully explained by point mutations and thus the *Paradestück* for gene conversion collapses in disgrace.

The real question is, however, which of the two sequences is correct. This question can be answered only by resequencing the controversial DNA stretch. But until this is done, I do not find it very scientific to choose only the one sequence that supports one's preconceived ideas and to pretend that there is no other sequence. As far as our knowledge stands at the moment, the DNA stretch depicted in Table 1 certainly does not support the hypothesis of segmental exchange between MHC genes.

In Table 2, I illustrate the second example quoted by Pease in support of the segmental exchange hypothesis. I have amended it, however, to include some other sequences of class I loci that are now known. This amendment is quite informative because it puts the sequences into a proper evolutionary perspective. Even for the few sequences that Pease selected for display, he had to admit that "the supporting evidence is far from clear" and that "this mixture of shared and divergent amino acid sequences might then be cited as evidence that selection maintains homologies among the proteins and that point mutations generate diversity in *H-2* genes." Table 2 shows that the changes can be explained very easily and quite naturally even without involving selection because, with two exceptions, they have occurred at the third (synonymous) position of the codons in the H-2 sequences. The most important point is, however, that similar changes occur in different species and so, unless one wants to postulate gene conversion between mouse and human genes, it is quite logical to postulate that the observed substitutions are the result of point mutations.

I dealt with the *H-2K*^{b} mutations as evidence for segmental exchange in my previous communication (*23*), so I will not repeat myself here, except to point out a fact that the proponents of the gene conversion hypothesis seem to forget. It is that most of the mutations were detected in F_1 hybrids and that, to establish congenic lines, the hybrids were then backcrossed repeatedly to one of the parental strains. In each backcross generation, the progeny was tested and the mutants were selected by skin grafting. Therefore for at least 12 generations selection pressure was applied that would have unwittingly picked out subsequent mutations. Such additional mutations probably caused more rapid rejection of the skin grafts—the individuals carrying them were, therefore, preferred for further mating. In this regard, it may be significant that the so-called *bg* series of mutants, in which only small changes occur and which even some of the proponents of the gene conversion hypothesis believe might be the result of point mutations, arose in C57BL/6 rather than an F_1 hybrid, and the mutants were, therefore, not backcrossed and selected for any number of generations. At any rate, as long as alternative explanations for the origin of *H-2* mutations have not been excluded, the mutations cannot be considered as proving segmental exchange in the K^b gene.

* Abbreviation used: MHC, major histocompatibility complex.

TABLE 1. The stretch of DNA sequence coding for amino acid residues 136 through 146. Identity with a nucleotide pair in the top line is indicated by a dash.[a]

	136				140					145	
H-2K^d	GCG	GCG	GAC	ACG	GCG	GCG	CTG	ATC	ACC	AGA	CGC
K^b	---	---	---	-T-	---	---	---	---	---	-A-	-A-
K^k	---	--C	---	-T-	---	---	---	---	---	-A-	-A-
K^{w29}	---	---	---	-T-	---	---	---	---	---	-A-	-A-
D^b	---	---	---	-T-	---	---	-A-	---	---	C--	---
D^d	---	---	---	-T-	---	---	-A-	---	---	C--	---
L^d (Moore)	TTC	---	---	-T-	T--	T--	-A-	---	---	C--	---
L^d (Evans)	---	---	---	---	---	---	-A-	---	---	C--	---
Q7^d	---	-T-	---	-T-	---	--A	-A-	---	---	C--	---
Q10^b	--A	---	---	GT-	---	---	A-T	---	---	C--	---
Q10^q	--A	---	---	GT-	---	---	A-T	---	---	C--	---
Tla^b	--A	--A	---	---	--A	--A	--A	---	---	---	A--
Tla^c	--A	--A	---	-T-	--A	--A	GA-	---	---	---	A--
HLA-A2	---	---	---	-T-	--A	--T	-A-	C-	---	-AG	-A-
A3	---	---	---	-T-	---	--T	-A-	---	---	-AG	---
Aw24	---	---	---	-T-	---	--T	-A-	---	---	-AG	---
B7	--C	---	---	---	--T	---	-A-	---	---	CAG	---
Bw58	---	---	---	---	---	--T	-A-	---	---	CAG	---
328	--C	---	---	--C	---	--T	-A-	---	---	CAG	---
RLA-1	---	---	---	---	---	--T	-A-	-A-	---	CAG	---
RLA-2	---	---	---	---	A-A	---	-A-	---	T--	-AG	---
SLA-1	---	---	---	-T-	---	--T	-A-	---	---	-AG	---
SLA-2	---	---	---	---	---	--T	-A-	---	---	-AG	---

[a] References: *H-2K^d* (*4*), *H-2K^b* (*5*), *H-2K^k* (*6*), *H-2K^{w29}* (*7*), *H-2D^b* (*8*), *H-2D^d* (*9*), *H-2L^d* (Moore) (*3*), *H-2L^d* (Evans) (*2*), *H-2Q7^d* (called by Steinmetz et al. 27.1 or *Q6* (*10*), *H-2Q10^b* (*11*), *H-2Q10^q* (*12*), *H-2T1a^b* (*13*), *H-2T1a^c* (*14*), *HLA-A2* (*15*), *HLA-A3* (*16*), *HLA-Aw24* [*17*), *HLA-B7* (*18*), *HLA-Bw58* (*19*), *HLA-323* (*20*), *RLA-1* (*21*), *RLA-2* (*21*), *SLA-1* (*22*), *SLA-2* (*23*).

TABLE 2. The stretch of DNA sequence coding for amino acid residues 94 through 110. Identity with a nucleotide pair in the top line is indicated by a dash. For references, see Table 1.

		95															110
H-2K^d	ACG	TTC	CAG	CGG	ATG	TTC	GGC	TGT	GAC	GTG	GGG	TCG	GAC	TGG	CGC	CTC	CTC
K^b	--T	A-T	---	GT-	--C	-CT	---	---	--A	C--	---	--C	---	G--	--A	---	---
K^k	---	---	--A	---	---	-A-	---	---	--G	---	---	---	---	---	---	---	---
K^{w29}	---	A--	---	---	---	-A-	---	---	---	---	---	---	---	G--	---	---	---
D^b	--A	C--	---	-AG	---	-CT	---	---	---	T--	---	---	---	---	---	---	---
D^d	--A	C--	---	T--	---	GCT	---	---	---	---	-A-	---	---	G--	---	---	---
L^d (Moore)	--A	C--	---	T--	---	-A-	---	---	---	---	---	---	---	G--	---	---	---
L^d (Evans)	--A	C--	---	T--	---	TA-	---	---	---	---	---	---	---	G--	---	---	---
Q7	--A	C--	--A	T--	---	-AT	---	---	---	A--	---	--C	---	G--	---	---	---
Q10^q	---	A--	---	T--	---	-AT	---	---	A-A	---	---	--C	---	G--	---	T--	---
Q10^b	---	A--	---	T--	---	-AT	---	---	A-A	---	---	--C	---	G--	---	T--	---
Tla^c	--C	A--	---	GT-	---	-AT	---	---	--G	---	-A-	-TC	TT-	G--	A--	---	T--
Tla^b	--C	A--	---	GT-	---	-AT	---	---	--G	---	-A-	-TC	TT-	G--	A--	---	T--
HLA-A2	--C	G--	---	A--	---	-AT	---	--C	---	---	---	---	---	---	---	T--	---
A3	--C	A--	---	ATA	---	-AT	---	--C	---	---	---	---	---	G--	---	T--	---
Aw24	--C	C--	---	AT-	---	--T	---	--C	---	---	---	---	---	G--	---	T--	---
B7	--C	C-T	---	A-C	---	-A-	--T	--C	---	---	---	C--	---	G--	---	---	---
Bw58	-TC	A--	---	A--	---	-AT	---	--C	---	---	---	C-C?	---	G--	---	---	---
JY328	--C	C--	---	A--	---	-CT	-C-	--C	---	---	---	C-C	---	G--	---	---	---
RLA-1	--T	---	G--	A G	---	--T	---	--C	--G	--C	T--	G--	--T	G--	---	T--	T--
RLA-2	--C	C--	G--	T--	---	-A-	---	--C	--G	--C	---	G--	---	G--	---	---	---
SLA-1	--C	C--	---	A-C	---	-AC	---	--C	T--	T--	--A	C-A	---	G--	-T-	---	---
SLA-2	--C	A--	---	ATC	---	-AC	---	--C	---	---	--A	C-A	---	G--	-TC	---	---

So once more: where is the evidence that gene conversion occurs in the MHC loci?

JAN KLEIN
Max-Planck-Institut für Biologie
Abteilung Immungenetik
Corrensstraße 42
7400 Tübingen 1
Federal Republic of Germany

REFERENCES

1. Pease LR. Diversity in H-2 genes encoding antigen-presenting molecules is generated by interactions between members of the major histocompatibility complex gene family. Transplantation 1985; 39: 227.
2. Evans GA, Margulis DH, Camerini-Otero RD, et al. Structure and expression of a mouse major histocompatibility antigen gene, *H-2L^d*. Proc Natl Acad Sci USA 1982; 79: 1984.

3. Moore KW, Sher BT, Sun YH, et al. DNA sequence of a gene encoding a BALB/c mouse L^d transplantation antigen. Science 1982; 215: 679.
4. Kvist S, Roberts L, Dobberstein B. Mouse histocompatibility genes: structure and organization of a K^d gene. EMBO J 1983; 2: 245.
5. Weiss E, Golden L, Zakut R, et al. The DNA sequence of the H-$2K^b$ gene: evidence for gene conversion as a mechanism for the generation of polymorphism in histocompatibility antigens. EMBO J 1983; 2: 453.
6. Arnold B, Burgert H-G, Archibald AL, et al. Complete nucleotide sequence of the murine H-$2K^k$ gene: comparison of three *H-2K* locus alleles. Nucleic Acid Res 1984; 12: 9473.
7. Morita T, Delarbre C, Kress M, et al. An *H-2K* gene of the t^{w32} mutant at the *T/t* complex is a close parent of an H-$2K^q$ gene. Immunogenetics 1985; 21: 367.
8. Reyes AA, Schöld M, Wallace RB. The complete amino acid sequence of the murine transplantation antigen H-$2D^b$ as deduced by molecular cloning. Immunogenetics 1982; 16: 1.
9. Sher BT, Nairn R, Coligan JE, et al. DNA sequence of the mouse H-$2D^d$ transplantation antigen gene. Proc Natl Acad Sci USA 1985; 82: 1175.
10. Steinmetz M, Moore KW, Frelinger JG, et al. A pseudogene homologous to mouse transplantation antigens: transplantation antigens are encoded by eight exons that correlate with protein domains. Cell 1981; 25: 683.
11. Mellor AL, Weiss EH, Kress M, et al. A nonpolymorphic class I gene in the murine major histocompatibility complex. Cell 1984; 36: 139.
12. Kress M, Cosman D, Khoury G, et al. Secretion of a transplantation-related antigen. Cell 1983; 34: 189.
13. Obata Y, Chen Y-T, Stockert E, et al. Structural analysis of *TL* genes of the mouse. Proc Natl Acad Sci USA 1985; 82: 5475.
14. Fisher DA, Hunt III SW, Hood L. Structure of a gene encoding a murine thymus leukemia antigen, and organization of *Tla* genes in the Balb/c mouse. J Exp Med 1985; 162: 528.
15. Koller BH, Orr HT. Cloning and complete sequence of an *HLA-A2* gene: analysis of two HLA-A alleles at the nucleotide level. J Immunol 1985; 134: 2727.
16. Strachan T, Sodoyer R, Damotte M, et al. Complete nucleotide sequence of a functional class I HLA gene, *HLA-A3:* implications for the evolution of *HLA* genes. EMBO J 1984; 3: 887.
17. N'Guyen C, Sodoyer R, Trucy J, et al. The *HLA-AW24* gene: sequence, surroundings, and comparison with the *HLA-A2* and *HLA-A3* genes. Immunogenetics 1985; 21: 479.
18. Orr HT, López de Castro JA, Parham P, et al. Comparison of amino acid sequences of two human histocompatibility antigens, HLA-A2 and HLA-B7: location of putative alloantigenic sites. Proc Natl Acad Sci USA 1979; 76: 4395.
19. Ways JP, Coppin HL, Parham P. The complete primary structure of HLA-Bw58. J Bioch Chem 1985; 260: 11924.
20. Srivastava R, Duceman BW, Biro PA, et al. Molecular organization of the class I genes of the human major histocompatibility complex. Immunol Rev 1985; 84: 93.
21. Tykocinski ML, Marche PN, Max EE, et al. Rabbit class I MHC genes: cDNA clones define full-length transcripts of an expressed gene and a putative pseudogene. J Immunol 1984; 133: 2261.
22. Satz ML, Wang L-C, Singer DS, et al. Structure and expression of two porcine genomic clones encoding class I MHC antigens. J Immunol 1985; 135: 2167.
23. Klein J. Gene conversion in Mhc genes? Transplantation 1984; 38: 327.

The structural analysis of the H-$2K^b$ class I variants has given rise to the hypothesis that genetic interactions among class I major histocompatibility complex (MHC)* genes contribute to the generation of diversity at the H-2 loci (*1, 2*). This argument is based on the nature of the nucleotide and amino acid substitutions that occur in the variant H-$2K^b$ molecules as well as the identification of exact duplicates of the variant sequences in potential donor genes within the Qa region of the murine MHC. The characteristics of the variants that suggest that a copy event rather than de novo random substitution underlies the generation of the variants are the following: (1) The mutations are complex; up to seven nucleotide changes have been observed in a single variant. (2) The multiple mutation sites that are seen within any given variant are clustered rather than randomly distributed throughout the domains of the transplantation antigen where antigenicity is determined. (3) The arrays of substitutions (including silent base substitutions) that occur in the variants are characteristic of other known class I sequences and have been identified elsewhere within the haplotype giving rise to the variants. (4) Some of the variants have recurred in independent matings. These findings were recently summarized in an overview in Transplantation (*2*). I would like to stress that I view these findings as suggesting that gene interactions contribute to the generation of diversity among the H-2 genes. The relative contribution of such events compared with random substitution, deletions, and insertions is not clear, but can be addressed experimentally.

Jan Klein has disagreed before (*3*) and continues to disagree now. In his current attack on the "gene conversion" hypothesis, Dr. Klein questions the validity of the sequence comparisons presented within my article (*2*) that are based on the H-$2L^d$ DNA sequence published by Moore and colleagues (*4*). I suggest that Dr. Klein's comments, while potentially meritorious in detail, do not deal with the important issues, and that his alternative explanation for the origin of the H-$2K^b$ variants cannot account for the data.

The major portion of Dr. Klein's criticism is focused on Figures 1 and 2 of my article (*2*). This is unfortunate because neither of these figures deals with the substance of the argument but instead represent an attempt to explain the issue under discussion to readers who do not normally follow the area. In Figure 1, I used an example from the literature (admittedly with misreference of the H-$2L^d$ sequence) to illustrate the nature of the argument advanced by others over the past several years to promulgate the "gene conversion" hypothesis. In defending his point of view, Dr. Klein failed to note my argument that comparisons among distantly related alleles of the *H-2* loci do not provide acceptable evidence for gene interactions within the MHC. Curiously this one area of agreement between Dr. Klein's point of view and my own draws the bulk of his criticism. The basis for this criticism is that Dr. Klein suspects that the sequence data published by Moore and colleagues (*4*) is incorrect. This may be true, although no one to my knowledge has proved his contention. Regardless, Dr. Klein's argument is irrelevant for two reasons. First, the sequences shown in Figure 1 of my article are an illustrative example, not the only piece of data advanced in support of the "gene conversion" hypothesis. Second (and most important), comparisons of the sort shown in Figure 1 are not very useful in evaluating the question of whether gene interactions contribute to diversity among H-2 loci. The main factors clouding such comparisons are that the genetic distance separating compared alleles is undefined and that the repertoire of potential donor sequences is uncharacterized. Therefore one is left with no way to evaluate how may changes have occurred at a given site and whether substitutions are the result of copy events or point mutations. In Figure 2 from my article I presented se-

* Abbreviation used: MHC, major histocompatibility complex.

quences from a different region of the same set of genes to illustrate what I perceive to be the typical relationship among the distantly related MHC genes and alleles. Dr. Klein's insinuation in his current letter that these comparisons (Figures 1 and 2) were advanced by me in support of the "gene conversion" hypothesis is totally false. To the contrary, I strongly suggest that such comparisons do not provide compelling evidence for or against the gene interaction hypothesis.

The meat of my argument was presented in Figure 3 (*2*). The basis of this argument is the observation that spontaneous MHC variants have occurred that contain nucleotide sequences that cannot be explained by random chance mutations, even if one supposes strong accompanying selection. In his letter, Dr. Klein suggests that because some of the variants—such as the one respresented in Figure 3—occurred in F_1 hybrid mice that were subsequently backcrossed at least 12 times, the complex nature of the mutations (seven nucleotide substitutions in the case of bml) could be accounted for by the accumulation of random mutations by unwitting selection during the backcross generations. Let us suppose that these random mutations occurred at a frequency of 10^{-3} per generation (a very generous estimate). For the moment, let us argue that each new mutant can be absolutely distinguished for the purpose of unwitting selection from the earlier mutants in the line. With luck 6000 mice would have to be screened to accumulate the additional six mutations. Even supposing that six additional mutations could have occurred during the backcross generations, how then does one account for the clustered array of the substitutions? The structural characterization of the *H-2K*^{b} variants has shown clearly that amino acid substitutions at many different positions within the first 180 amino acid residues influence histcompatibility. Why then should random mutations, which occur generation after generation as supposed by Dr. Klein, be directed to particular clusters (as in the cases of *bm1*, *bm4*, *bm8*, and *bm10*)? Furthermore, how does one account for the precise array of silent substitutions seen in the *bm1* variant? The statistical argument against random mutation as the etiological mechanism generating the variants is compelling. The mutation rate is much lower than 10^{-3}, the unwitting selection rate was surely far less than 100%, and many fewer than 500 mice were screened in each backcross generation during the breeding of the mutant congenic lines. For these reasons and those presented earlier (*1, 2*), the idea that the *H-2K*^{b} mutants as a group arose by random mutation simply is untenable.

As evidence supporting the hypothesis that the *H-2K*^{b} variants occurred by gene interactions I have cited the characterization of potential donor nucleotide sequences that are identical to the variant sequences within the mouse strain that gave rise to the mutants. Together with the profile of the variants themselves these findings strongly suggest that sequences encoded within the Qa region of the MHC were "templates" for the transfer of nucleotide sequence to the *H-2K*^{b} gene variants. This hypothesis does not pretend to explain MHC polymorphism. What the hypothesis says is that genetic interactions among class I MHC genes generates diversity. How diversity of this sort contributes to the evolution of *H-2* class I sequences remains to be seen.

LARRY R. PEASE
Department of Immunology
Mayo Medical School
Rochester, MN 55904

REFERENCES

1. Pease LR, Schulze DH, Pfaffenbach GM, Nathenson SG. Spontaneous H-2 mutants provide evidence that a copy mechanism analogous to gene conversion generates polymorphism in the major histocompatibility complex. Proc Natl Acad Sci USA 1983; 80: 242.
2. Pease LR. Diversity in H-2 genes encoding antigen-presenting molecules is generated by interactions between members of the major histocompatibility complex gene family. Transplantation 1985; 39: 227.
3. Klein J. Gene conversion in MHC genes. Transplantation 1984; 38: 327.
4. Moore KW, Sher BT, Sun YH, Eakle KA, Hood L. DNA sequence of a gene encoding a BALB/c mouse L^d transplantation antigen. Science 1982; 215: 679.

CYTOTOXIC T LYMPHOCYTE ACTIVITY IN TRANSPLANT PATIENTS

I would like to respond to two recent articles in *Transplantation* by Orosz et al. (*1, 2*) concerning cytotoxic T lymphocyte (CTL)* activity in sponge-matrix allografts. I believe that the authors have presented conclusions in those articles that are in direct contradiction to their data. The conclusions are: 1) that limiting dilution analysis (LDA) is a more sensitive technique than direct ^{51}Cr release assay (CRA) for assessing the extent of CTL activity in allografts and 2) that since their LDA show relatively few CTL (<1% frequency) within allografts, CTL are not a prominent component of the rejection process.

In the first article (*1*), the authors demonstrate, using a cloned C57B1/6 anti-DBA/2 CTL line, that the lytic activity of an effector population in the CRA is linearly proportional to the frequency of CTL within the effector population. A plot of the results of this experiment is presented in their Figure 5 (*1*), and from this plot the authors deduce that the CRA cannot detect CTL at a frequency of less than approximately 1/126. The authors conclude that the LDA must be more sensitive than the CRA since LDA experiments detected CTL frequencies of up to 1/100000.

Now consider the following: the authors did 9 experiments in which both LDA and CRA were performed on cells isolated from DBA/2 sponge allografts implanted in C57B1/6 hosts 13 days previously. I have extracted their results from two tables (Table 1 [*1*] and Table 2 [*2*]) and present them in Exhibit 1. The ID column identifies the respective table number and the corresponding animal number used by the authors. The first column of Exhibit 1 is the lytic activity (LU/10^6) of the cells as determined by CRA on the day of excision. The second column is the reciprocal of the CTL frequency as determined by LDA of the same cells. If one examines the CTL frequencies determined by LDA, it is readily apparent that, for most allografts, the CTL frequency (mean 1/187) is below the limit that should give detectable activity in CRA (i.e., <1/126). Nevertheless, in all 9 experiments significant CRA activity was detected (mean 18.7 LU/10^6 cells). If one assumes that the CTL present in the graft are no more potent than the CTL clone used to generate their Figure 5 (*1*)—which appears to be a conservative assumption since this clone was purposely chosen for its high lytic activity—one can use Figure 5 to estimate the minimal CTL frequency based on the CRA data. Simple inspection shows that Figure 5 can be reduced to the following

* Abbreviations used: CRA, ^{51}CR release assay; CTL, cytotoxic T lymphocyte; LDA, limiting dilution analysis.

EXHIBIT 1. CTL activity in sponge-matrix allografts

ID	LU/10E6 cells (CRA)	1/frequency (LDA)	1/frequency (CRA)	LU/10E6 CTL (LDA)
1–4	35.7	109	3	4000
1–5	6.2	233	17	1678
1–6	16.1	114	7	1949
1–7	18.1	222	6	4240
1–8	15.1	249	7	4009
1–9	31.2	49	4	1578
2–7	18.1	242	6	4622
2–8	18.1	295	6	5634
2–9	9.5	166	11	1743
Mean	18.7	187	6	3671
SD	9.4	81	4	845

linear equation:

Equation 1:

$$LU/10^6 \text{ effector cells} = LU/10^6 \text{ CTL} \times \text{CTL frequency} + \text{y-intercept}$$

For Figure 5 the $LU/10^6$ CTL can be shown to be approximately 120, and the y-intercept to be approximately minus 1. (Ideally the y-intercept should be zero but it is not because of the lower limit of detection of the CRA.) Thus rearrangement of Equation 1 to solve for CTL frequency yields:

Equation 2:

$$\text{CTL frequency} = (LU/10^6 \text{ cells} + 1) / 120$$

Application of Equation 2 to the data in column 1 of Exhibit 1 yields the results shown in column 3. Thus, the CRA data indicate that the mean CTL frequency for the graft cells is 1/6, or about 30-fold higher than detected by LDA (mean 1/187). Since both estimates cannot be correct, is it possible to determine which is more likely to be correct? Assuming that all of the CTL in the graft are detected by LDA and the CRA results reflect the activity of CTL present in the graft at the time of excision, one can estimate the lytic potency of the CTL present in the graft by further rearrangement of Equation 1:

Equation 3:

$$LU/10^6 \text{ CTL} = (LU/10^6 \text{ effector cells}/ \text{ CTL frequency}) - \text{y-intercept}$$

Application of Equation 3 to the data from column 1 ($LU/10^6$ effector cells) and column 2 (CTL frequency by LDA), assuming again a y-intercept value of minus 1, yields the results shown in column 4. These values indicate that if the LDA estimates of CTL frequency and the CRA estimates of their activity are correct, the graft CTL had on average over 3000 $LU/10^6$ CTL.

Hence, using the authors' own data, we are left with two very different conclusions:

1. The CRA results indicate that the CTL frequency is approximately 1/6 (17%) if one assumes the CTL in the graft have a lytic potency equivalent to the authors' cloned CTL (120 $LU/10^6$ CTL). Since the CTL clone was purposely chosen for its high lytic activity, it may well be that graft CTL are not this active, and thus the CTL frequency may be higher than 17% (all other things being equal the CTL frequency is inversely proportional to the lytic potency of the CTL [Equation 2]).
2. The LDA results indicate that the CTL frequency is approximately 1/187 (0.5%) and that the CTL have, on average, a lytic activity of over 3000 $LU/10^6$—approximately 25-fold greater potency than the authors' CTL clone. Since the authors contend that the LDA detects not only fully activated CTL but also CTL precursors and presumably memory CTL, the estimates of CTL potency may be too low, since they were based on the assumption that the LDA frequencies represented only activated CTL present at the time of the CRA.

Given this choice of alternatives, I find the first much easier to accept than the second. Thus, I believe that: (1) The authors have grossly underestimated the CTL frequency by LDA; consequently, at least in their hands, LDA is substantially less sensitive in detecting CTL activity than CRA; and (2) consequently, CTL are a prominent component of the allograft response. Moreover, since the authors' data (their Table 1 [*2*]) demonstrate that T cells represent about 21% of the infiltrating cells, the CTL component appears to be the principle T cell subset present (nearly 80% of T cells).

JOHN D. TYLER
Transplantation Laboratory
Department of Surgery
Washington University School of Medicine
St. Louis, Missouri 63110

REFERENCES

1. Orosz CG, Zinn NE, Sirinek L, Ferguson RM. In vivo mechanisms of alloreactivity: I. Frequency of donor-reactive cytotoxic T lymphocytes in sponge matrix allografts. Transplantation 1986; 41: 75.
2. Orosz CG, Zinn NE, Sirinek L, Ferguson RM. In vivo mechanisms of alloreactivity: II. Allospecificity of cytotoxic T lymphocytes in sponge matrix allografts by limiting dilution analysis. Transplantation 1986; 41: 84.

We have read with interest Dr. Tyler's analysis of our recently published data regarding the frequency of donor-reactive cytotoxic T lymphocytes (CTL)* in sponge matrix allografts. We were aware that more ^{51}Cr release assay (CRA)-detectable, donor-reactive cytolytic activity is mediated by cells recovered from sponge matrix allografts than would be expected on the basis of their limiting dilution analysis (LDA)-detectable, donor-reactive CTL frequency. This eventually caused us to question the premise that the CRA detects only cytolytic T lymphocytes. As first reported by Häyry and Roberts (*1*), this is not true for cells that infiltrate sponge matrix allografts, where non-T cells contribute significantly to CRA-detectable cytolytic activity. This fact, which is often overlooked, precludes extrapolation of CTL frequency from data obtained by CRA in the sponge matrix allograft system.

This fact was also a consideration when we designed our study of the relationship between CRA-detectable cytolytic activity and LDA-detectable CTL frequency. For that study we used a cloned cytolytic T cell line, since we could then be certain that observed cytolytic activity was mediated exclusively by CTL. Similar considerations have also caused us to examine the development of humoral immunity in sponge matrix allografts (*2*), since the accumulation of cells "armed" with donor-reactive antibodies could account for some of the reported non-CTL-mediated cytolytic activity in sponge matrix allografts.

* Abbreviations used: CRA, ^{51}Cr release assay; CTL, cytotoxic T lymphocyte; LDA, limiting dilution analysis.

Since Dr. Tyler's analysis rests entirely on the assumption that all CRA-detectable cytolytic activity reported in our experiments is mediated by CTL, we must disagree with his conclusions. Nonetheless, his analysis does illustrate the disparity between CTL frequency determined by LDA and CTL frequency predicted on the basis of CRA. Dr. Tyler's analysis reinforces our doubts concerning the prominence of donor-reactive CTL in allograft rejection, and further demonstrates that LDA is more valuable than CRA by illustrating a serious problem inherent in analyses of in vivo CTL behavior that are solely reliant on data obtained with the CRA.

Charles G. Orosz
Nancy E. Zinn
Lawrence P. Sirinek
Ronald M. Ferguson
Department of Surgery, Division of Transplantation and Therapeutic Immunology Program
Ohio State University
Columbus, Ohio 43210

REFERENCES

1. Roberts PJ, Hayry P. Effector mechanisms in allograft rejection. II. Density, electrophoresis, and size fractionation of allograft-infiltrating cells demonstrating several classes of killer cells. Cell Immunol 1977; 30: 236.
2. Sirinek LP, Zinn NE, Ferguson RM, Orosz CG. In vivo mechanisms of alloreactivity. III. Development of donor-specific antibody in sponge matrix allografts. Transplantation 1986; 41: 349.

Blood Eosinophilia in Transplant Patients

The article "Blood eosinophilia, steroids, and rejection" by Lautenschslager et al. (*1*) deserves some comment. Several patients had eosinophilia before the rejection episode, and in some cases, it was present more than 10 days before rejection. I suggest that this is because 40% of patients in dialysis have eosinophilia (*2*). In a group of 50 transplant patients treated with azathioprine and prednisone we found that 41 (82%) of the patients had a rejection crisis associated with blood eosinophilia. Another 12 patients (33%) had eosinophilia without rejection, and 8 of these 12 had eosinophilia in the pretransplant period. We also observed that, in some patients, the eosinophilia persisted, after the reversal of rejection (*3*).

We think that progressive eosinophilia in the posttransplant period, mainly in patients without pretransplant eosinophilia, suggests a rejection crisis; our data has also been confirmed in patients under cyclosporine treatment.

REFERENCES

1. Lautenschlager I, Von Willebrand E, Hayry P. Blood eosinophilia, steroids, and rejection. Transplantation 1985; 40: 354.
2. Hoy EW, Cestero RVM. Eosinophilia in maintenance hemodialysis. J Dialysis 1979; 3: 73.
3. Ianhez JE, Sabbaga J, Araujo JF, Paula FJ, Sabbaga E. Correlação entre eosinofilia sanguinea e crise de rejeição no transplante renal. J Bras Nefrol 1985; 7: 103.

Luiz Estevam Ianhez
Jorge Sabbaga
Jacinto Ferreira de Araújo
Flávio Jota de Paula
Emil Sabbaga
Unidade de Transplante Renal
Hospital das Clínicas F.M.U.S.P.
São Paulo
SP-CEP:05403, Brasil

DIARY OF FORTHCOMING EVENTS

Anyone organizing a meeting likely to be of interest to the readers of Transplantation may submit essential information about the meeting to any editorial office, which will consider its inclusion in the Diary of Events. This information should be received by the North American Editorial Office at least six months before the event. The Diary appears four times annually.

DATE	PLACE	SUBJECT	SECRETARIAT
July 30–Aug. 1	Amsterdam, The Netherlands	6th International Workshop on Alloantigenic systems in the rat	Dr. L.C. Paul Academisch Ziekenhuis Leiden Rijnsburgerweg 10 2333 AA Leiden, The Netherlands
August 3–8	Helsinki, Finland	XIth International Congress of the Transplantation Society	Dr. Pekka Hayry Transplantation Lab Univ. of Helsinki Haartmaninkatu 3 Helsinki, Finland
September 14–18	New Orleans, LA	12th Annual Meeting American Society for Histocompatibility and Immunogenetics	ASHI Central Office 211 East 43rd St. Suite 301 New York, N.Y. 10017
September 27	Leiden, The Netherlands	Eurotransplant Meeting	Marianne Franzen Eurotransplant Foundation c/o Blood bank University Hospital Rijnsburgerweg 10 2333 AA Leiden, The Netherlands

0041-1337/86/4202-0109$02.00/0
TRANSPLANTATION
Copyright © 1986 by The Williams & Wilkins Co.

Vol. 42, No. 2
Printed in U.S.A.

Transplantation

OVERVIEW

EXPRESSION OF CLASS I TRANSPLANTATION ANTIGENS[1]

HERBERT W. HARRIS[2] AND THOMAS J. GILL III

Department of Pathology, University of Pittsburgh School of Medicine, Pittsburgh, Pennsylvania 15261

Introduction

Recent advances in molecular immunology have led to an increased appreciation that the cellular interactions involved in the immune response are receptor-mediated phenomena involving complex regulatory mechanisms. Evidence has begun to emerge suggesting that an important component in this regulation involves the modulation of cell surface expression of the products encoded by the genes in the major histocompatibility complex (MHC).* These molecules have long been known to be the primary targets of the immune response to xenogeneic or allogeneic grafts and to serve as restriction elements in the recognition of exogenous antigens. Several recent overviews have discussed various aspects of the expression of transplantation antigens, including alloantigen expression on vascular endothelial cells (*1*) and modulation of this expression by interferon (*2*). A general review of the modulation of class I and class II antigens has also appeared recently (*3*). This review will focus on the class I transplantation antigens and will concentrate on the genetics and molecular biology of the regulation of their expression. It will also relate the expression of class I antigens to relevant issues in transplantation, oncology, reproductive immunology, and infectious diseases.

Biosynthesis of Class I Antigens

The biosynthesis of class I antigens is a complex process with many steps that, beginning at the level of transcription, may be subject to numerous regulatory influences. The activation of RNA synthesis by class I genes in the mouse is believed to occur at approximately day 10 of gestation (*4*). Very low levels of *H-2D* transcripts have been detected at earlier stages, and they were found to rise dramatically at or about day 10 (*5*). The F9 teratocarcinoma has been studied as a model for the developmental regulation of *H-2K* gene transcription. These cells fail to transcribe mRNA that is detectable using cDNA probes specific for the *H-2K* product, but when differentiation is induced with retinoic acid, *H-2K* transcripts may be found (*6*). This change is accompanied by a decrease in the DNase I sensitivity (*6*) and an increase in the methylation of the *H-2K* gene (*7*). Paradoxically, increases in DNase I sensitivity (*8*) and decreases in methylation (*9*) have been found to correlate with the developmental activation of several other genes. The transcriptional activation of class I heavy chain genes appears to be independent of β_2-microglobulin transcription, which has a different developmental time-course (*5*).

Recently, a detailed analysis of mouse class I promoter regions has been done (*10*). Sequence analysis revealed eight regions that are homologous to regulatory sites known to influence expression of eukaryotic genes. These include inverted repeats with homology to the GC-rich regions of SV40 and of HSV tk promoters, a sequence homologous to the SV40 enhancer, a sequence homologous to an adenovirus Ela enhancer, and a site similar to a consensus sequence found in heat shock protein promoters in *Drosophila.* Deletion analysis employing a series of constructs derived from the *H-2K*^{b} promoter indicated that at least two of these regions display enhancer-like activity in the experimental system. They were the region homologous to the GC-rich promoter and the region homologous to the SV40 enhancer, which are both conserved among mouse class I transplantation antigen genes. Interestingly, these sequences are not conserved among Qa region class I genes nor are they conserved in the β_2-microglobulin gene (*10*). The enhancer elements function well when introduced into cells that normally express *H-2* genes, but they function poorly in undifferentiated embryonal carcinoma cells that do not express *H-2* genes. This indicates that the enhancer activity is subject to external (*trans*-acting) regulation. When chloramphenicol acetyl transferase and thymidine kinase constructs controlled by *H-2K*^{b} promoters are introduced into undifferentiated embryonal carcinoma cells, these genes are transcribed at low levels, whereas complete class I genes are not transcribed at all (*11*). This finding adds further support to the idea that transcription is regulated by elements external to the promoter. However, the importance of transcriptional regulation has not been clearly established with regard to cell surface expression. Inhibition of transcription with actinomycin-D treatment for brief periods does not interfere with reexpression of HLA antigens on the surface of papain-treated lymphocytes (*12*). This suggests that subsequent steps in the processing of mRNA may be more important in the control of class I antigen expression.

RNA splicing affects the manner in which eukaryotic genes are expressed. For example, membrane-bound and secreted forms of immunoglobulin molecules arise from the use of alternate splicing signals in the processing of precursor mRNA transcripts (*13*). Evidence has accumulated that alternate splicing sites exist in MHC transcripts and that they may be important determinants in the expression of MHC antigens. A comparison of sequence data from mouse cDNA clones pH-2I

[1] Work in the authors' laboratory was supported by grants from the National Institutes of Health (CA 18659, HD 08662, HD 09880), the Tim Caracio Memorial Cancer Fund, and the Beaver County Cancer Society.

[2] H.W.H. is a fellow of the Culpepper Foundation.

* Abbreviations used: MHC, major histocompatibility complex; Pa, pregnancy-associated.

and pH-2II revealed a high degree of homology, except for the presence of an additional 139 base pair insert in pH-2II; this difference suggests that an intron present in pH-2II was removed from pH-2I (*14*). A similar analysis of cDNA clones mapped to the *H-2K* locus revealed two clones identical in sequence except for a short internal deletion (*15*). A more recent study of cDNA clones obtained from mouse liver demonstrated alternate splicing occurring at rates such that approximately 5–10% of the transcripts present in the liver lacked the third exon (*16*). Transfection of mouse fibroblast cell lines with the $H\text{-}2^d$ gene resulted in the appearance of at least two species of mRNA, as detected by S_1 mapping, which arose from alternate splicing of the transcript of this gene (*17*). Complete sequence data derived from genomic clones of the *H-2* genes have shown that several alternate splicing sites occur throughout these genes (*18*). The extent to which these alternate splicing sites are used has yet to be demonstrated, but their use could result in molecules that lack certain antigenic determinants or that are secreted rather than being inserted into the cell membrane. Secreted class I gene products have been detected (*19, 20*), and it is possible that the excision of hydrophobic domains through alternate splicing may have an important regulatory function in controlling cell surface expression. Alternate splicing of N-terminal domains could also vary the expression of individual antigenic determinants by producing truncated molecules lacking one or more determinants. Molecules that may have arisen from alternate splicing in this manner have been detected in the rat, where sequential immunodepletion with monoclonal antibodies has demonstrated the existence of a series of antigens distinguished by the number of determinants they carry (*21*). Using three monoclonal antibodies, distinct molecules were precipitated that differed by the presence of all three, two, or only one of the epitopes recognized by the monoclonal antibodies. The observation that they are expressed in fairly specific proportions (*22*) suggests that they are not merely cleavage products or senescent molecules that have lost one or more of their antigenic determinants.

Additional factors that may alter RNA processing and expression have been demonstrated. Sequence analysis of *H-2D* and *H-2L* genes revealed that they differ from the *H-2K* gene by the insertion of *Alu*-like repetitive elements in their 3′-noncoding sequence (*23*). Although the functional significance of the presence of these sequences is not clear, the ubiquity of these elements and their highly conserved sequences suggests that they are generated by reverse transcription of RNA molecules containing *Alu* sequences (*24, 25*). This indicates that these sequences could function as transposable elements inserting new genetic information at sites of integration. In the *H-2D* and *H-2L* genes, the *Alu* sequences are associated with the introduction of an additional polyadenylation signal that is used 20 times more frequently than other signals common to the *H-2K* gene (*23*). Because the H-2D and H-2L antigens are expressed at lower levels than the H-2K antigen, the use of this polyadenylation signal may result in mRNA molecules having less stability or translational efficiency.

Posttranslational Modification and Turnover

Subsequent steps in the biosynthesis of class I antigens involve their association with β_2-microglobulin, glycosylation and membrane insertion. Much evidence has accumulated to suggest that these processes are closely linked. Studies of the transport and maturation of HLA-A and -B antigens in lymphoblastoid cells lines indicate that nascent peptides are first inserted into the membrane of the endoplasmic reticulum and that association with β_2-microglobulin occurs within 5 min (*26*). The molecules are core-glycosylated, and during the next 20–25 minutes, terminal glycosylation occurs. Surface expression of the antigen follows 10–15 min later. A similar sequence of events is known to occur in murine cells (*27*). Pulse-chase experiments showed that the intracellular pool of class I molecules is relatively small and that the majority of newly synthesized molecules is transported rapidly to the surface (*28*). Once the mature molecules reach the cell surface, they are inserted into the membrane, where flow cytometric measurements showed that they exist as freely rotating monomers whose lateral mobility is probably restricted by cytoskeletal anchorage (*29*).

Several studies have shown that β_2-microglobulin plays a critical role in the process of posttranslational modification and intracellular transport. Comparison of the Raji cell line, which produces β_2-microglobulin and expresses class I heavy chains, with the Daudi cell line, which does neither, suggests that the event which is dependent upon β_2-microglobulin is terminal glycosylation (*30*). This is because Daudi cells have been found to contain heavy chains which are core-glycosylated but not terminally glycosylated (*30*). This finding is difficult to reconcile with the observation that inhibition of glycosylation by tunicamycin does not block cell surface expression (*31*). Another possibility is that the physical transport of heavy chains to the Golgi apparatus is the step where β_2-microglobulin plays its role. A study employing *Xenopus laevis* oocytes microinjected with translatable mRNA has shown that class I heavy chains accumulate in the endoplasmic reticulum in the absence of β_2-microglobulin (*32*). However, the exact relationship between β_2-microglobulin and intracellular transport is unclear. Recent experiments employing transfection of mouse L cells with $H\text{-}2L^d$ genes altered by site-directed mutagenesis showed that intracellular transport and surface expression can be disrupted by removal of the highly conserved disulfide bridge between cysteine-203 and cysteine-259 (*33*). Antigen encoded by the $H\text{-}2L^d$ gene was present in the cytoplasm in a glycosylated form partially associated with β_2-microglobulin. This finding suggests that additional factors beyond association with β_2-microglobulin are necessary for appropriate intracellular transport.

Although these phenomena indicate that β_2-microglobulin has a significant effect on class I antigen expression, a number of instances in which class I antigen expression takes place in the absence of β_2-microglobulin have been described. Several studies have presented evidence that class I heavy chains may exist in the cell membrane without being associated with β_2-microglobulin. Immunoprecipitation of the $H\text{-}2D^b$ heavy chain with either monoclonal antibodies or with alloantisera failed to coprecipitate any β_2-microglobulin, indicating that this molecule may exist largely in an unassociated form (*34*). A murine cell line has been found that fails to express β_2-microglobulin and most class I heavy chains with the one exception of the $H\text{-}2D^b$ molecule (*35*). In the Daudi cell line, molecules have been immunoprecipitated by monoclonal antibodies that recognize framework determinants shared by all class antigens (*36*); they appear to be a subset of human class I antigens which do not require β_2-microglobulin for their expression, but their identity is not well established.

Membrane-bound MHC molecules are shed from the cell

surface in the form of large particles containing membrane lipids (*37*). This shedding is dependent upon metabolic energy, and it is inhibited by colchicine, suggesting that it is an active process subject to cytoskeletal control (*38*). When cells are placed in culture, a significant fraction of the shed antigens is passively adsorbed by lymphocytes and macrophages (*39*). Adsorption of class I antigens is known to occur in vivo onto platelets, which acquire a considerable amount of antigen passively (*40*). Comparison of shedding rates in a series of inbred mice indicates that regulatory genes controlling shedding rates map within the MHC (*41*). In particular, a locus mapping to the left of the *I-A* region controls the rate of $H\text{-}2D^d$ shedding. These differential shedding rates might account for the preferential MHC restriction patterns seen with haptens, such as TNP, or with viral antigens that require, for immune recognition, a stable association with MHC antigens on the cell surface.

The dependence of MHC antigen expression on the cell cycle has been the source of controversy. Over the years, a number of studies dealing with the influence of cell cycle kinetics on the susceptibility of tumor cells to lysis by MHC-directed antibodies and cytotoxic T cells have been undertaken. This literature is difficult to interpret because of the many different methods used to determine cell cycle position and to measure antigen expression. Early studies using limiting dilution cytotoxicity indicated that expression was minimal during the S and G_1 phases (*42, 43*), but susceptibility of tumor cells to lysis by MHC-directed cytotoxic T cells did not seem to correlate with these changes in expression (*44*). A more recent study employing flow cytometric analysis of sorted populations of cells in each phase of the cell cycle indicated that only very small differences existed in the expression of K, D, and L products during the cycle (*45*). These small differences were attributed to changes in cell size, since the magnitude of the changes in expression was found to be similar to changes in surface area during the cell cycle as determined by light scattering measurements. These results have been extended by recent measurements that indicate that G_2/M cells express about 1.6 times as much class I antigen as G_0/G_1 cells, and that the surface area of G_2/M cells is approximately 1.5 times that of G_0/G_1 cells (*46*). This finding indicates that the average surface density of class I antigens is maintained throughout the cell cycle. Cytotoxic T cell clones directed at the products of each class I locus produces lysis that is independent of the stage of the target cell in its cycle. It appears, therefore, that the cell surface density of class I antigens remains relatively stable despite the multiplicity of structural and metobolic changes that occur during the cell cycle.

Genetic Regulation of Expression

Class I antigen expression has a complex genetic regulation, and the existence of specific regulatory genes has clearly been established. The nature of regulatory genes controlling class I antigen expression on the cell surface has been studied in somatic cell hybrids using a series of hybrid cell lines obtained from mouse/human fusions containing a portion of chromosome 6. Human class I gene transcripts were found, but no class II transcripts could be detected (*47*). Because the parental mouse line did not express class I antigens, the continued expression of human class I transcripts in the hybrid is evidence for the existence of *cis*-regulation of class I antigen expression by elements present on chromosome 6. Evidence for *trans*-regulation came from studies involving fusion of nonexpressing murine teratocarcinoma lines with normal mouse spleen cells. The *H-2K* and/or *H-2D* products from both parental haplotypes were expressed on hybrids after differentiation in vitro indicating *trans*-acting complementation of the expression-defective allele by genes derived from the normal spleen cells (*48*). Moreover, the existence of hybrids expressing either an *H-2K* or *H-2D* product, or both, indicates that the two loci are under independent control. Evidence for negative *trans*-regulation was obtained in a study of hybrids derived from the fusion of murine embryonal carcinoma cells with human melanoma cells. Although HLA antigens were expressed in the hybrids, the expression of murine H-2 antigens were suppressed suggesting the existence of *trans*-acting products from the melanoma line which inhibited the expression of the murine MHC genes (*49*).

The presence of multiple regulatory genes has recently been demonstrated in a series of hybrids constructed from human B-lymphoblastoid cell lines. Fusion of two expression-deficient lines resulted in an increased expression of HLA antigens from both parental lines, and the loss of chromosome 6 belonging to one parental line resulted in the reduced expression of HLA antigen derived from the other line (*50*). These results were explained by postulating the existence of at least two *trans*-acting factors, one of which is a product of chromosome 6.

Measurement of H-2K and H-2D expression in different haplotypes using assays for the binding of alloantisera to spleen cells indicated that the relative expression of antigens encoded by the *K* and *D* loci depended on the particular allele such that $D^b > K^d = K^k = K^b = D^q > D^d > K^q > D^k$ (*51*). The difference in binding varied from 10–70% and was thought to be consistent with (if not explanatory of) preferential restriction patterns observed for anti-viral and anti-hapten cytotoxic T cells. A recent study employing flow cytometric methods demonstrated that the *L* locus product was expressed at levels that were two-fold to three-fold lower than those of either the *K* and *D* loci (*52*). Differential expression that is locus-specific has also been demonstrated in the rat in which the expression order is $A^n >> E^w > F^a$ (*53*). A complete picture of expression differences among various haplotypes in the rat is hampered by the fact that only one allele of the *E* and *F* loci is currently known. In the *HLA* system, the *C* locus products appear to be expressed at significantly lower levels than those of the *A* or *B* loci (*54*).

The situation in F_1 hybrid mice is complicated by the fact that some alleles tend to dominate others, resulting in a level of expression that is very different from the predicted value of 50% of the parental level based on gene dosage effects (*55*). These quantitative differences in expression were also reflected in the degree to which target cells are recognized by cytotoxic T cells (*56*). A recent study in which monoclonal antibodies were used has called into question many of the results previously obtained with alloantisera. This study indicated that the resting level of class I antigens varied only slightly among inbred strains (*57*). However, it was noted that K^k expression increased with age and was higher in females than in males. Thus, turnover kinetics and differential shedding rates may be more important in determining cytotoxic T cell restriction phenomena insofar as viruses and haptens may require stable complex formation with class I molecules at the cell surface.

Tissue Distribution

Variation in class I antigen expression among different tissues has led to the suggestion that it may influence the manner in which grafts are rejected (*58*). Tissues bearing large quantities of class I antigens may be more suitable targets for cytotoxic T cells, whereas those bearing relatively small quantities are thought to be destroyed primarily by antibody-dependent effector mechanisms (*58*). Graft rejection consists of two processes occurring more or less simultaneously. First, there is the response directed at antigens expressed by parenchymal cells—which, in most cases, are class I MHC antigens. Second, there is a response directed at blood vessels, which is probably elicited by the class II antigens expressed on vascular endothelium. Therefore, class I expression, or the balance between class I and class II expression, has a significant impact on the graft rejection process.

Many reports have been published regarding tissue distribution, and the early work employing alloantisera has been, with several noteworthy exceptions, consistent with the more recent studies using monoclonal antibodies. In the human, estimation of the relative expression of HLA antigens has been undertaken using a quantitative absorption assay with radiolabeled monoclonal antibodies. It was found that the spleen carries the largest amount of class I antigens and that, relative to the spleen, bone marrow expresses 15%; kidney, 14%; liver, 9%; heart, 5%; and brain, 1% (*59*). Recent studies have indicated that the distribution of HLA class I antigens is somewhat more restricted than earlier work suggested. In particular, it has been reported that class I antigens are not expressed on cerebral cortex, cerebellum, sympathetic ganglia, hypophysis, parathyroid gland, thyroid, exocrine pancreas, hepatocytes, sperm, seminiferous tubules, skeletal muscle, and smooth muscle (*60*). In addition, gastric mucosa and pancreatic islet cells are only weakly positive, and no class I antigens are expressed on the corneal endothelium or on the duodenal glands of Brunner (*61*). These results stand in marked contrast to the idea that class I antigen expression is constitutive. The fact that many tissues do not express class I antigens raises a number of interesting questions in the area of clinical transplantation. For example, it is known that the outcome of corneal transplantation is influenced by matching at class I loci (*62*). However, the absence of class I antigen from corneal endothelium suggests that other factors, such as closely linked genes, may be involved in controlling the rejection process.

In the mouse and rat, a number of studies of the tissue distribution of class I antigens have been shown patterns of expression similar to those of the human. However, several cases of species-specificity of expression have been observed. In the mouse, consistently negative tissues included hepatocytes, adrenal glands, skeletal muscle, cardiac muscle, pancreatic islet cells, and nerves (*63*). The rat, like the mouse and human, has the largest amount of class I antigens on lymphoid tissues; liver has somewhat less, and the kidney expresses about 33% as much as the liver (*64*). Cardiac muscle has very low levels of both class I and class II antigens, and the vigor with which cardiac grafts are rejected in the rat may be due to the expression of heart-specific histocompatibility antigens. However, significant differences exist between the rat and mouse. The rat expresses a substantial amount of class I antigens on red blood cells amounting to approximately 15% of that found on lymphocytes, whereas in the mouse and the human, these cells express little or no class I antigen (*21*). Moreover, class I antigens are found on pancreatic islet cells and adrenal tissues, which are consistently negative in the mouse (*63*). Rat endothelium expresses no class I antigens, and many of the class II-positive cells found in these tissues are on passenger leukocytes (*65*). In addition to antigens that are expressed on the cell surface, a number of studies have demonstrated that soluble class I antigens are secreted by certain tissues, for example, the liver of the mouse (*66–68*). The function of these molecules is uncertain, but they may play a substantial role in shaping the immune responses to the transplanted organs that secrete them.

Class I Antigen Expression and Tumor Immunology

In recent years the expression of MHC antigens on tumor cells has received a great deal of attention, and much evidence has been developed suggesting that alterations in expression may play a crucial role in oncogenesis and metastasis. Perturbations in the expression of MHC antigens have been documented in many tumor lines—and, in most cases there is a partial or complete loss of antigens on the cell surface. Moreover, lack of antigen expression seems to be associated with the metastatic potential of the tumor. A series of mouse leukemia cell lines derived from the AKR strain was studied for expression of *H-2K* and *H-2D* products. Both increases and decreases in expression were reported among the various cell lines, as determined by immunofluorescent methods, but propagation of tumor cells in vivo was correlated with the decrease expression of the H-$2K^k$ product (*69*).

Neonatal rat kidney cells transformed by oncogenic adenovirus 12 and by nononcogenic adenovirus 5 were compared immunologically by producing antibodies to each line in BALB/c mice and by studying the immunoprecipitates obtained with these antibodies. The oncogenicity of the transformed cells was found to correlate with the absence of two proteins, one of which was identified as the RT1.A antigen (*70*). In a subsequent study, the blocking of RT1.A expression was mapped to a product of the early 1a region of the type 12 adenovirus genome, and this resulted in a substantial reduction in susceptibility to lysis by cytotoxic T cells (*71*). By contrast, mouse embryo cells transformed by type 12 adenovirus showed an increase in the rate of *H-2K* gene transcription (*72*). The basis for these divergent effects is not clear, but similar perturbations in MHC antigen expression have been demonstrated in other oncogenic virus models. Using SV40-transformed fibroblast lines transplanted into mice, a highly oncogenic cell line which resisted lysis by SV40-specific cytotoxic T cells was found to be deficient in H-$2K^k$ antigen expression (*73*).

Formation of metastases has been found to correlate strongly with altered MHC gene product expression in a number of tumor cell lines. Comparisons of class I antigen expression were made between the tumor cells found at the site of injection of methylcholanthrene-induced tumors and those found at the sites of lung metastases. The parent tumor lines expressed both the H-2^k and H-2^b haplotype antigens, whereas the cells derived from the metastases tended to express only H-2^k antigens (*74*). On the other hand, serial transplantation of H-2^k-negative clones resulted in the spontaneous expression of antigens from the *k* haplotypes, and this was associated with metastases (*75*). Taken together, these results suggest that the balance in the expression of certain MHC antigens may be important in conferring metastatic potential on tumor cells.

In a study involving the metastatic properties of the Lewis lung carcinoma, metastatic cells were found to express H-$2D^b$ antigens at high density but lacked H-$2K^b$ antigens (*76*). This difference in expression resulted in a relative resistance on the part of the tumor cells to lysis by anti-H-$2K^b$ cytotoxic cells. Subclones of the Lewis lung carcinoma carrying a low K^b/low D^b or a high K^b/high D^b phenotype were not metastatic; cells carrying a low K^b/high D^b phenotype were highly metastatic, and cells carrying a medium K^b/high D^b phenotype were intermediate in metastatic potential (*77*). Although the exact meaning of these results remains somewhat obscure, it seems that locus-specific imbalances in tumor expression of class I antigens plays an important role in the evasion of immune surveillance and in the development of metastases.

The mechanism by which MHC antigen expression is altered on tumor cells is not known, but a few insights have emerged recently. Although expression of individual loci may be altered independently, analysis of a series of AKR leukemia cell lines showed a consistent correlation among H-2K, H-2D and β_2-microglobulin mRNA levels, suggesting that perturbations of expression can affect coordinate expression of these molecules (*78*). Cell lines transformed by SV-40 and analyzed by Southern blotting using H-2-specific probes showed that mutations resulting in altered restriction endonuclease cleavage sites had occurred in the lines negative for H-$2K^k$ expression (*79*). The actual sites of integration of the SV-40 genome were not linked to the MHC, so that the mutations could not be directly attributed to the integration of the virus. Analysis of human cells infected with type 2 adenovirus indicated that a protein encoded by the adenovirus genome formed a complex with HLA class I proteins and prevented their terminal glycosylation and subsequent expression (*80*). A similar mechanism may be operative in adenovirus-transformed rodent cell lines.

The fact that diminished or altered MHC antigen expression has been associated with the more aggressive behavior of tumor cells has led to studies in which antigen expression was increased by the introduction of additional class I genes into tumor cells by transfection. A transplantable mouse leukemia line lacking H-$2K^k$ antigen but transfected with the *H-2K*^{k} gene was rejected (*81*). Transfection of adenovirus-transformed mouse cells with murine class I genes eliminated their oncogenic potential (*82*). A similar study involving transfection of H-2K-deficient murine fibrosarcoma lines dramatically reduced tumorigenicity and metastasis formation (*83*). Evidence that enhancement of class I antigen expression plays a role in the natural resistance to tumor growth comes from the observation that the cytotoxic monokine tumor necrosis factor is also a potent inducer of class I antigen synthesis (*84*). These observations indicate that the genes that regulate MHC antigen expression represent vulnerable sites within the genome of the cell. Mutagenic agents that impair MHC antigen expression could create conditions favoring the development of malignancy by altering the cell surface antigen phenotype, such that the cell evaded immune surveillance. Conversely, pharmacologic agents that induce expression of MHC genes in tumor cells—such as retinoic acid (*48*), immune interferon, and calcitriol (*85*)—may eventually play a role in inducing the rejection of tumors. A review of agents known to alter MHC antigen expression has recently been presented (*3*).

Class I Antigen Expression and Reproductive Immunology

The control of the expression of MHC antigens on the placenta is one of the central issues of reproductive immunology. The mouse placenta expresses class I antigens (*86*) but not class II antigens (*87*). No class II antigens are expressed on the human placenta (*88*), and villous trophoblast has been reported to express no class I antigens (*89*). However, class I antigens have been detected on the extravillous trophoblast (*90*), but they do not represent the full complement of these antigens since the private specificities of the HLA-A and B have not been detected (*91*). When placental tissue was separated into cytotrophoblast and syncytiotrophoblast fractions, HLA-A, B, and C antigens were found in the cytotrophoblast during early gestation (*92*). Placental tissues have low levels (ca. 15%) of class I antigen mRNA transcript in humans (*93*) and in mice (*94*). In the rat, a class I molecule carrying a broadly shared antigenic determinant has been demonstrated (*95*); it is probably the only class I antigen expressed on the surface of the placenta, and it is located on the basal trophoblast (*96*). It has been designated the Pa (pregnancy-associated) antigen, and it is encoded by a locus mapping near *RT1.A* and to the left of *RT1.B* (*97*), The maternal immune response to the Pa antigen or the injection of anti-Pa antibody during pregnancy does not cause fetal loss (*98*). The Pa antigen may stimulate a nondestructive immune response or even a suppressor response.

Class I Antigen Expression and Antiviral Immunity

The restriction of the immune response to viral antigens by class I antigens was initially demonstrated by mapping the immune response genes to viruses to the MHC (*99*). This concept was reinforced by the subsequent finding that unresponsiveness at the level of cytotoxic T cells could be mapped to the *K* and *D* loci in the mouse (*100*). Because of this association between antiviral immunity and class I loci, it might be expected that the regulation of expression of class I antigens would be influenced by the development of antiviral immunity. Among the most important mediators of the response to viral infections are the interferons, and they are powerful enhancers of the expression of both class I antigens and β_2-microglobulin (*101, 102*). The HLA class I transcripts are greatly increased by interferon in parallel with the changes in antigen expression on the cell surface (*103*). Analysis of the tissue specificity of gamma-interferon induction of class I antigen expression in the mouse revealed pronounced differences in responses. Heart, kidney and adrenal tissues showed a 4-fold to 8-fold increase in expression while the pancreas and small intestine responded with a 13-fold to 17-fold increase (*104*). The tissues that showed the least change were the spleen, liver and lung, and these tissues had the highest resting levels of class I antigens (*104*). Quantitative comparisons of mRNA expression indicated that induction of class I transcripts occurred at interferon concentrations over 100 times lower than those required to induce the viral inhibitor (2′-5′) oligo(A)-synthase, and this observation indicates the fundamental importance of class I antigen expression in antiviral immunity (*105*).

The mechanism by which interferons enhance expression of the class I antigens has been investigated extensively. Cell lines have been identified that are relatively resistant to interferon induction—and, among sensitive lines, cells in the G_0/G_1 phase appear to be more responsive (*106*). Using flow microfluorimetry, cell lines could be selected from human thymus leukemia cells that differed in the inducibility of class I antigen expression by interferon (*107*). These lines apparently arise from stable mutations in the regulatory genes that mediate the response to interferon. Induction of antigen expression occurs when mouse L cells are transfected with human MHC genes (*108*), even in the absence of upstream sequences and of variable lengths of coding sequences (*109*). This phenomenon has been attributed to posttranscriptional recombinations between the transcripts arising from the transfected genes and those of the host. Such recombinational events appear to be a property of mouse transfection systems (*110*). Because these truncated genes are regulated by interferon in the same manner as host MHC genes, interferon may exert its effects at a posttranscriptional level, such as mRNA stability. Alternatively, evidence that the regulatory site resides in the upstream promoter sequences comes from comparison of the HLA genes with another interferon-induced molecule, metallothionein II. A homologous sequence of approximately 30 base pairs found in the two genes may be a target site for interferon induction (*111*).

There is evidence that a number of viruses have the capacity to circumvent the protective enhancement of class I antigen expression elicited by interferon. The type 2 adenovirus produces a protein that forms a complex with newly synthesized MHC antigens and prevents their terminal glycosylation (*80*). Cells infected by this strain of adenovirus accumulate class I antigens in the perinuclear space, and this reflects an inhibition of intracellular transport that may be related to the blockade of terminal glycosylation (*112*). There is also evidence that different viruses can interact to alter class I antigen expression. Murine fibroblasts infected with Molony leukemia virus showed a 10-fold increase in class I antigen expression, while fibroblasts infected with Molony sarcoma virus alone or coinfected with both viruses showed no change in class I antigen expression (*113*). Although it is not clear whether perturbations in cell surface antigen expression play a significant role in the pathogenicity of viruses, assays of in vitro cytotoxicity suggest that target cell killing is a function that requires expression of both viral and MHC antigens (*114*). It is likely that the induction of class I antigens by interferon and the inhibition of their expression by some viruses are important determinants in the host-parasite relationship for viral pathogens.

Conclusion

The expression of class I antigens is a closely regulated process that is of central importance for many immunological phenomena. The detailed investigation of the molecular biology of their expression may serve as a useful model for the regulation of mammalian genes at the levels of transcription, mRNA processing, translation, and posttranslational processing. The complex phenomena of locus-specific and haplotype-specific variations in class I antigen expression and the demonstration of *cis-* and *trans*-regulatory elements indicate that class I regulation is likely to involve multiple interactive processes at all of these levels.

There is considerable evidence that quantitative and qualitative variation in class I antigen expression plays a major role in the immunological responses to transplanted organs, tumor surveillance, and antiviral immunity. Study of the regulation of class I expression at the molecular level can provide insights into many of the immunological processes involved in the acceptance or rejection of a transplant—be it an organ, a fetus, or a tumor. Because of the multifaceted role of the class I antigens, measurements of class I expression may also provide a useful diagnostic and prognostic index, and modulation of class I expression may become a useful therapeutic tool.

REFERENCES

1. Paul LC, Baldwin WM, van Es LA. Vascular endothelial antigens in renal transplantation. Transplantation 1985; 40: 117.
2. Pober JS, Collins T, Gimbrone MA, Libby P, Reiss CS. Inducible expression of class II major histocompatibility complex antigens and the immunogenicity of vascular endothelium. Transplantation, in press.
3. Halloran PF, Wadgymar A, Autenreid P. The regulation of expression of major histocompatibility complex products. Transplantation 1986; 41: 413.
4. Ozato K, Wan Y, Orrison BN. Mouse major histocompatibility class I gene expression begins at midsomite stage and is inducible in earlier-stage embryos by interferon. Proc Natl Acad Sci USA 1985; 82: 2427.
5. Morello D, Duprey P, Israel A, Babinet C. Asynchronous regulation of mouse H-2D and β_2-microglobulin RNA transcripts. Immunogenetics 1985; 22: 441.
6. Croce CM, Linnenbach A, Huebner K, Parnes JR, Margulies DH, Appella E, Seidman JG. Control of expression of histocompatibility antigens (H-2) and β_2-microglobulin in F9 teratocorcinoma stem cells. Proc Natl Acad Sci USA 1981; 78: 5754.
7. Tanaka K, Appella E, Jay G. Developmental activation of the H-2K gene is correlated with an increase in DNA methylation. Cell 1983; 35: 457.
8. Kunnath L, Locker J. DNase sensitivity of the rat α-fetoprotein genes. Nucleic Acids Res 1985; 13: 115.
9. Kunnath L, Locker J. Developmental changes in the methylation of rat albumin and α-fetoprotein genes. EMBO J 1983; 2: 317.
10. Kimura A, Israel A, LeBal O, Kourilsky P. Detailed analysis of the mouse H-2K^b promoter: enhancer-like sequences and their role in the regulation of class I gene expression. Cell 1986; 44: 261.
11. Daniel-Vedele F, Israel A, Benicourt C, Kourilsky P. Functional analysis of the mouse H-2K^b gene promoter in embryonal carcinoma cells. Immunogenetics 1985; 21: 601.
12. Turner MJ, Strominger JL, Sanderson AR. Enzymatic removal and re-expression of a histocompatibility antigen, HL-A2 at the surface of human peripheral lymphocytes. Proc Natl Acad Sci USA 1972; 69: 200.
13. Early P, Rogers J, Davis M, Calame K, Bond M, Wall R, Hood L. Two mRNAs can be produced from a single immunoglobulin mu gene by alternate RNA processing pathways. Cell 1980; 20: 313.
14. Steinmetz M, Moore KW, Frelinger JG, Sher BT, Shen F, Boyse EA, Hood L. A pseudogene homologous to mouse transplantation antigens: transplantation antigens are encoded by eight exons that correlate with protein domains. Cell 1981; 25: 683.
15. Kress M, Glaros D, Seidman JG, Khoury G, Jay G. Alternative RNA splicing in expression of the H-2K gene. Nature 1983; 306: 602.
16. Lalanne JL, Transy C, Guerin S, Darche S, Meulin P, Kourilsky P. Expression of class I genes in the major histocompatibility complex: identification of eight distinct mRNAs in DBA/2 mouse liver. Cell 1985; 41: 469.
17. Transy C, Lalanne J, Kourilsky P. Alternative splicing in the 5′ moiety of the H-2K^d gene transcript. EMBO J 1984; 3: 2383.
18. Sher BT, Nairn R, Coligan JE, Hood LE. DNA sequence of the mouse H-2D^d transplantation antigen gene. Proc Natl Acad Sci USA 1985; 82: 1175.
19. Kress M, Cosman D, Khoury G, Jay G. Secretion of a transplantation-related antigen. Cell 1983; 34: 189.
20. Maloy WL, Colligan JE, Barra Y, Jay G. Detection of a secreted form of the murine H-2 class I antigen with an antibody against its predicted carboxyl terminus. Proc Natl Acad Sci USA 1984; 81: 1216.
21. Misra DN, Kunz HW, Gill TJ III. Immunochemical evidence for multiple class I antigens coded by the MHC of the rat (RT1) and their differential expression on red blood cells and lymphocytes. J Immunogenet 1983; 10: 379.
22. Misra DN, Noeman SA, Kunz HW, Gill TJ III. Detection by monoclonal antibodies of antigens coded by the MHC and quantitative differences in their expression on erythrocytes

from different strains. Transplant Proc 1983; 15: 1549.
23. Kress M, Barra Y, Seidman JG, Khoury G, Jay G. Functional insertion of an Alu type 2 (B2 SINE) repetitive sequence in murine class I genes. Science 1984; 226: 974.
24. Schmid CW, Jelinik WR. The Alu family of dispersed repetitive sequences. Science 1982; 216: 1065.
25. Singer MF. SINEs and LINEs: highly repeated short and long interspersed sequences in mammalian genomes. Cell 1982; 28: 433.
26. Owen MJ, Kissonerghis A, Lodish HF. Biosynthesis of HLA-A and HLA-B antigens in vivo. J Biol Chem 1980; 255: 9678.
27. Dobberstein B, Garoff H, Warren G, Robinson PJ. Cell-free synthesis and membrane insertion of mouse H-2D^d histocompatibility antigen and β_2-microglobulin. Cell 1979; 17: 759.
28. Vitetta ES, Uhr JW. Synthesis of surface H-2 alloantigens in murine splenocytes. J Immunol 1975; 115: 374.
29. Damjanovich S, Tron L, Szollosi J, Zidovetzki R, Vaz LC, Regateiro F, Arndt-Jovin DJ, Jovin TM. Distribution and mobility of murine histocompatibility H-2K^k antigen in the cytoplasmic membrane. Proc Natl Acad Sci USA 1983; 80: 5985.
30. Sege K, Rask L, Peterson PA. Role of β_2-microglobulin in the intracellular processing of HLA antigens. Biochemistry 1981; 20: 4523.
31. Lindolfi NF, Rich RR, Cook R. Differential glycosylation requirements for the cell surface expression of class I molecules. J Immunol 1985; 134: 423.
32. Severinsson L, Peterson PA. β_2-microglobulin induces intracellular transport of human class I heavy chains in Xenopus laevis oocytes. J Cell Biol 1984; 99: 226.
33. Miyazaki J, Appella E, Ozato K. Intracellular transport blockage caused by disruption of the disulfide bridge in the third external of the major histocompatibility complex class I antigen. Proc Natl Acad Sci USA 1986; 83: 757.
34. Maloy WL, Hammerling G, Nathenson SG, Coligan JE. Comparison of alloantisera and hybridoma antibody for the purification of the H-2D^b murine histocompatibility antigen and preliminary molecular characterization of this antigen. J Immunol Methods 1980; 37: 287.
35. Potter TA, Boyer C, Schmitt-verhulst A, Golstein P, Rajan TV. Expression of H-2D^b on the cell surface in the absence of detectable β_2-microglobulin. J Exp Med 1984; 160: 317.
36. Quarata V, Walker LE, Ruberto MA, Pellegrino MA, Ferrone S. The free and the β_2-microglobulin-associated heavy chains of HLA-A, B alloantigens share the antigenic determinants recognized by the monoclonal antibody Q1/28. Immunogenetics 1981; 13: 285.
37. Emerson SG, Cone RE. I-A^k and H-2K^k antigens are shed as supramolecular articles in association with membrane lipids. J Immunol 1981; 127: 482.
38. Emerson SG, Cone RE. Regulation of murine B lymphocyte plasma membrane protein turnover and shedding. J Cell Physiol 1981; 109: 25.
39. Emerson SG, Cone RE. Absorption of shed I-K^k and H-2K^k antigens by lymphoid cells. Transplantation 1982; 33: 36.
40. Lalezari R, Driscoll AM. Ability of thrombocytes to acquire HLA specificity from plasma. Blood 1982; 59: 167.
41. Emerson SG, Murphy DB, Cone RE. Selective turnover and shedding of H-2K and H-2D antigens is controlled by the major histocompatibility complex. Implications for H-2-restricted recognition. J Exp Med 1980; 152: 783.
42. Pasternak CA, Warmsley AMH, Thomas DB. Structural alterations in the surface membrane during the cell cycle. J Cell Biol 1971; 50: 562.
43. Everson LK, Plocinik BA, Rogentine GN. HLA expression on the G1 and G2 cell-cycle stages of human lymphoid cells. J Natl Cancer Inst 1974; 53: 913.
44. Sanderson CJ, Thomas JA. The mechanism of T cell mediated cytotoxicity. III. Changes in target cell susceptibility during the cell cycle. Proc R Soc Lond [Biol] 1976; 194: 417.
45. Harris DT, Sekaly RP. Target cell susceptibility to immune lysis and expression of MHC antigens are independent of position in the cell cycle. J Immunol 1984; 133: 40.
46. Muller CP, Stephany DA, Wunderlich JR. Changes in mouse MHC expression during the cell cycle of Con A-treated spleen cells. J Immunol 1986; 136: 17.
47. Benham FJ, Quintero MA, Goodfellow PN. Human-mouse hybrids with an embryonal carcinoma phenotype continue to transcribe HLA-A,B,C. EMBO J 1983; 2: 1963.
48. Gmur R, Solter D, Knowles BB. Independent regulation of H-2K and H-2D gene expression in murine teratocarcinoma somatic cell hybrids. J Exp Med 1980; 151: 1349.
49. Den Boer WC, Van Der Kamp WM, Mulder MP. Expression of embryonic and MHC antigens in heterokaryons of murine embryonal carcinoma and human melanoma cells. Exp Cell Res 1984; 154: 25.
50. Salter RD, Howell DN, Cressewll P. Genes regulating HLA class I antigen expression in T-B lymphoblast hybrids. Immunogenetics 1985; 21: 235.
51. O'Neill HC, McKenzie FC. Quantitative variation in H-2-antigen expression. I. Estimation of H-2K and H-2D expression in different strains of mice. Immunogenetics 1980; 11: 225.
52. Potter TA, Hansen TH, Habberset R, Ozato K, Ahmed A. Flow microfluorometric analysis of H-2L expression. J Immunol 1981; 127: 580.
53. Misra DN, Kunz HW, Gill TJ III. Analysis of class I antigens in the rat by monoclonal antibodies. J Immunol 1985; 134: 2520.
54. Rask J, Lindblom JB, Peterson PA. Structural and immunological similarities between HLA antigens from three loci. Eur J Immunol 1976; 6: 93.
55. O'Neill HC, McKenzie FC. Quantitative variation in H-2-antigen expression. II. Evidence for a dominance pattern in H-2K and H-2D expression in F_1 hybrid mice. Immunogenetics 1980; 11: 241.
56. O'Neill HC, Blanden RV. Quantitative variation in the expression of paternally-derived H-2 antigens in F_1 hybrid mice affect T-cell responses. J Exp Med 1979; 148: 724.
57. Dower SK, Segal DM. Interaction of monoclonal antibodies with MHC class I antigens on mouse spleen cells. II. Levels of expression of H-2K, H-2D and H-2L in different mouse strains. J Immunol 1985; 134: 431.
58. Hayry P. Intragraft events in allograft destruction. Transplantation 1984; 38: 1.
59. Williams KA, Hart DJ, Fabre JW, Morris PJ. Distribution and quantitation of HLA-ABC and DR(Ia) antigens on human kidney and other tissues. Transplantation 1980; 29: 274.
60. Natali G, Bigotti A, Nicotra MR, Viora M, Manfredi D, Ferrone F. Distribution of human class I (HLA-A,B,C) histocompatibility antigens on normal and malignant tissues of nonlymphoid origin. Cancer Res 1984; 44: 4679.
61. Daar AS, Fuggle SV, Fabre JW, Ting A, Morris PJ. The detailed distribution of HLA-A,B,C antigens in normal human organs. Transplantation 1984; 38: 287.
62. Batchelor JR, Casey TA, Werb A, et al. Matching and corneal grafting. Lancet 1976; 1: 551.
63. Ponder BAJ, Wilkinson MM, Wood M, Westwood JH. Immunohistochemical demonstration of H-2 antigens in mouse tissue sections. J Histochem Cytochem 1983; 31: 911.
64. Hart DJ, Fabre JW. Quantitative studies on the tissue distribution of Ia and SD antigens in the DA and Lewis rat strains. Transplantation 1979; 27: 110.
65. Hart DJ, Newton MR, Reece-Smith H, Fabre JW, Morris PJ. Major histocompatibility complex antigens in the rat pancreas, isolated pancreatic islets, thyroid and adrenal. Transplantation 1983; 36: 431.
66. Lew AM, Maloy WL, Coligan JE. Characteristics of the expression of the murine soluble class I molecule (Q10). J Immunol 1986; 136: 254.
67. Mellor AL, Weiss EH, Kress M, Jay G, Flavell RA. A nonpoly-

morphic class I gene in the murine major histocompatibility complex. Cell 1984; 36: 139.

68. Cosman D, Khoury G, Jay G. Three classes of mouse H-2 messenger RNA distinguished by analysis of cDNA clones. Nature 1982; 295: 73.

69. Schmidt W, Alonso A, Leben L, Festenstein H. Differential regulation of H-2 antigen expression in tumors and its biologic consequences. Transplant Proc 1981; 13: 1814.

70. Schrier WP, Bernards R, Vaessen RTMJ, Houweling A, van der Eb AJ. Expression of class I major histocompatibility antigens switched off by highly oncogenic adenovirus 12 in transformed rat cells. Nature 1983; 305: 771.

71. Bernards R, Schrier PI, Houweling A, Bos JL, van der Eb AJ, Zijlstra M, Melief CJM. Tumorigenicity of cells transformed by adenovirus type 12 by evation of T-cell immunity. Nature 1983; 305: 776.

72. Rosenthal A, Wright S, Quade K, Gallimore P, Cedar H, Grosveld F. Increased MHC H-2K gene transcription in cultured mouse embryo cells after adenovirus infection. Nature 1985; 315: 579.

73. Gooding LR. Characterization of a progressive tumor from C3H fibroblasts transformed in vitro with SV40 virus. Immunoresistance in vivo correlates with phenotypic loss of H-$2K^k$. J Immunol 1982; 129: 1306.

74. Katzav S, deBaetselier P, Gorelik E, Feldman M, Segel S. Immunogenetic control of metastasis formation by a methylchloranthrene induced tumor (T10) in mice: differential expression of H-2 gene products. Transplant Proc 1981; 13: 742.

75. Katzav S, deBaetselier P, Tartakovsky B, Feldman M, Segel S. Alterations in major histocompatibility complex phenotypes of mouse cloned T10 sarcoma cells: association with shifts from nonmetastatic to metastatic cells. J Natl Cancer Inst 1983; 71: 317.

76. Isakov N, Katzav S, Feldman M, Segel S. Loss of expression of transplantation antigens encoded by the H-2K locus on Lewis lung carcinoma cells and its relevance to the tumor's metastatic properties. J Natl Cancer Inst 1983; 71: 139.

77. Eisenbach L, Feldman M, Segel S. MHC imbalance and metastatic spread in Lewis lung carcinoma clones. Int J Cancer 1983; 32: 113.

78. Schmidt W, Hensleing U, Bevec D, Alonso ADR, Festenstein H. Control of synthesis and expression of H-2 heavy chain and β_2-microglobulin in AKR leukemias. Immunogenetics 1985; 22: 483.

79. Rogers MJ, Gooding LR, Margulies DH, Evans GA. Analysis of a defect in the H-2 genes of SV40 transformed C3H fibroblasts that do not express H-$2K^k$. J Immunol 1983; 130: 2418.

80. Burgert H, Kvist S. An adenovirus type 2 glycoprotein blocks cell surface expression of human histocompatibility class I antigens. Cell 1985; 41: 987.

81. Hui K, Grosveld F, Festenstein H. Rejection of transplantable AKR leukemia cells following MHC DNA-mediated cell transformation. Nature 1984; 311: 750.

82. Tanaka K, Isselbacher KJ, Khoury G, Jay G. Reversal of oncogenesis by the expression of a major histocompatibility complex class I gene. Science 1985; 228: 26.

83. Wallich R, Bulbuc N, Hammerling GJ, Katzav S, Feldman M, Segel S. Abrogation of metastatic properties of tumor cells by de novo expression of H-2K antigens following H-2 gene transfection. Nature 1985; 315: 301.

84. Collins T, Lapierre LA, Fiers W, Strominger JL, Pober J. Recombinant human tumor necrosis factor increases mRNA levels and surface expression of HLA-A, B antigens in vascular endothelial cells and dermal fibroblasts in vitro. Proc Natl Acad Sci USA 1986; 83: 446.

85. Ball ED, Guyre PM, Glynn JM, Rigby WFC, Fanger MW. Modulation of class I HLA antigens on HL-60 promyelocytic leukemia cells by serum-free medium: re-induction by gamma IFN and 1,25-dihydroxyvitamin D3 (calcitriol). J Immunol 1984; 132: 2424.

86. Wegmann TG, Singh B, Carlson GA. Allogeneic placenta is a paternal strain antigen immunoabsorbant. J Immunol 1979; 123: 1020.

87. Chatterjee-Hasrouni S, Lala PK. MHC antigens on mouse trophoblast cells: paucity of Ia antigens despite the presence of H-2K and D. J Immunol 1980; 127: 2070.

88. Brami CJ, Sanyal MK, Dwyer JM, Johnson CC, Kohorn EI, Naftolin F. HLA-DR antigen on human trophoblast. Am J Reprod Immunol 1983; 3: 165.

89. Galbraith RM, Ferrara GB, Ades EW, Galbraith GMP. Differential expression of transplantation antigens within the normal human placental chorionic villus. Am J Reprod Immunol 1981; 1: 331.

90. Sunderland CA, Redman CWG, Stirrat GM. HLA-A,B,C antigens are expressed on nonvillous trophoblast of the early human placenta. J Immunol 1981; 127: 2614.

91. Redman CWG, McMichael AJ, Stirrat GM, Sunderland CA, Ting A. Class I major histocompatibility complex antigens on human extra-villous trophoblast. Immunology 1984; 52: 457.

92. Montgomery B, Peeyush LK. Ontogeny of the MHC antigens on human trophoblast cells during the first trimester of pregnancy. J Immunol 1983; 131: 2348.

93. Kawata M, Parnes JR, Herzenberg LA. Transcriptional control of HLA-A,B,C antigen in human placental cytotrophoblast using trophoblast-and HLA-specific monoclonal antibodies and the fluorescence-activated cell sorter. J Exp Med 1984; 160: 633.

94. Tanaka K, Ozato K, Parnes JR, Ramanthan L, Seidman JG. Control of H-2 antigen and β_2-microglobulin gene expression in mouse trophoblast. Proc Natl Acad Sci USA 1983; 80: 5597.

95. Ghani AM, Gill TJ III, Kunz HW, Misra DN. Elicitation of the maternal antibody response to the fetus by a broadly shared MHC class I antigenic determinant. Transplantation 1984; 37: 187.

96. Ghani AM, Gill TJ III, Kunz HW. Pregnancy-induced monoclonal antibody to a unique fetal antigen. Transplantation 1984; 37: 503.

97. Macpherson TA, Ho NH, Kunz HW, Gill TJ III. Localization of the Pa antigen on the placenta of the rat. Transplantation 1986; 41: 392.

98. Ghani AM, Gill TJ III, Misra DN, Kunz HW. The antibody response to the fetus and its genetic control: monoclonal antibodies to a unique fetal antigen. Transplant Proc 1985; 17: 1842.

99. Zinkernagel RM, Doherty PC. Restriction of in vitro T cell-mediated cytotoxicity in lymphocytic choriomeningitis within a syngeneic or semiallogeneic systems. Nature 1975; 248: 701.

100. Zinkernagel RM, Doherty PC. H-2 compatibility requirement for T-cell-mediated lysis of target cells infected with lymphocytic choriomeningitis virus. Different cytotoxic T-cell specificities are associated with structures coded for in H-2K or H-2D. J Exp Med 1975; 141: 1427.

101. Heron I, Hokland M, Berg K. Enhanced expression of β_2-microglobulin and HLA antigens on human lymphoid cells by interferon. Proc Natl Acad Sci USA 1978; 77: 6215.

102. Fellous M, Kamoun M, Gresser I, Bono RR. Enhanced expression of β_2-microglobulin and HLA antigens on interferon treated human lymphoid cells. Eur J Immunol 1979; 9: 446.

103. Fellous M, Nir U, Wallach D, Gilles M, Rubinstein M, Revel M. Interferon-dependent induction of mRNA for the major histocompatibility antigens in human fibroblasts and lymphoblastoid cells. Proc Natl Acad Sci USA 1982; 79: 3082.

104. Skoskiewick MJ, Colvin RB, Schneeberger EE, Russell PS. Widespread and selective induction of major histocompatibility complex-determined antigens in vivo by gamma interferon. J Exp Med 1985; 162: 1645.

105. Wallach D, Fellous M, Revel M. Preferential effect of gamma interferon on the synthesis of HLA antigens and their mRNAs in human cells. Nature 1982; 299: 833.

106. Basham TY, Bourgead MF, Creasy AA, Merigan TC. Interferon increases HLA synthesis in melanoma cells: interferon-resistant and sensitive cell lines. Proc Natl Acad Sci USA 1982; 79: 3265.
107. Burrone OR, Kefford RF, Gilmore D, Milstein C. Stimulation of HLA-A,B,C by interferon-α. The derivation of milt 4 variants and the differential expression of HLA-A,B,C subsets. EMBO J. 1985; 4: 2855.
108. Rosa F, LeBouteiller PP, Abadie A, Mishal Z, Lemonnier FA, Bourrel D, Lamotte M, Kalik J, Jourdan B, Fellous M. HLA class I genes inserted into murine cells are inducable by interferon. Eur J Immunol 1983; 13: 495.
109. Yoshie O, Schmidt H, Lengyl P, Reddy ESP, Morgan WR, Weissman SM. Transcripts of human HLA gene fragments lacking the 5′-terminal region in transfected mouse cells. Proc Natl Acad Sci USA 1984; 81: 649.
110. Goodenow RW, Stroynowsky I, McMillan M, Nicholson M, Eakle K, Sher BT, Davidson N, Hood L. Expression of complete transplantation antigens by mammalian cells transformed with truncated class I genes. Nature 1983; 301: 388.
111. Friedman RL, Stark GR. α-interferon-induced transcription of HLA and metallothionein genes containing homologous upstream sequences. Nature 1985; 314: 637.
112. Anderson M, Paabo S, Nilsson T, Peterson PA. Impaired intercellular transport of class I MHC antigens as a possible means for adenovirus to evade immune surveillance. Cell 1985; 43: 215.
113. Flyer DC, Burakoff SJ, Faller DV. Retrovirus-inducted changes in major histocompatibility complex antigen expression influence susceptibility to lysis by cytotoxic lymphocytes. J Immunol 1985; 135: 2287.
114. Zinkernagel RM, Doherty PC. MHC-restricted cytotoxic T cells: studies on the biological role of polymorphic major transplantation antigens determining T-cell restriction-specificity, function and responsiveness. Adv Immunol 1979; 27: 51.

0041-1337/86/4202-0118$02.00/0
TRANSPLANTATION
Vol. 42, No. 2
Printed in U.S.A.

Transplantation

ARTICLES

BONE MARROW TRANSPLANTATION WITH T-CELL-DEPLETED GRAFTS

I. RECONSTITUTION OF IMMUNOHEMOPOIETIC FUNCTIONS IN LETHALLY IRRADIATED MICE TRANSPLANTED WITH UNSEPARATED OR T-CELL-DEPLETED SYNGENEIC BONE MARROW GRAFTS[1]

M. SHALIT,[2] M. AYALON,[3] L. WEISS,[4] B. LESHEM,[3] E. KEDAR,[3] AND S. SLAVIN[4,5]

Departments of Medicine A and Bone Marrow Transplantation and Immunology Research, Hadassah University Hospital; and Lautenberg Center for General and Tumor Immunology, Hadassah-Hebrew University School of Medicine, Jerusalem, Israel

The potential role of donor's mature T lymphocytes on the recovery of various immunological functions and hematopoiesis was investigated in lethally irradiated BALB/c mice by studying reconstitution with normal, as compared with T-cell-depleted, syngeneic marrow grafts. Recovery of total, as well as mononuclear, peripheral white blood cell counts, platelets, hemoglobin levels, proportion of Thy 1.2$^+$ cells, responses to concanavalin A, phytohemagglutinin and lipopolysaccharide, mixed lymphocyte response, cell-mediated lympholysis response, anti-SRBC agglutinins and natural killer activity were basically similar in recipients of unmanipulated (as compared with T cell depleted) syngeneic marrow grafts. The data suggest that in a syngeneic murine bone marrow transplantation setting, mature donor T lymphocytes do not seem to play a major role in immunohemopoiesis. Normal T cell number and T-cell-dependent immune function can be readily regenerated out of the stem cell reservoir of adult donors following transplantation into lethally ablated recipients.

Bone marrow transplantation (BMT)* offers one of the major advances in the treatment of a large number of malignant and life-threatening, nonmalignant hematological disorders for which no specific alternative therapy exists. With BMT from allogeneic donors, one of the major problems confronting the therapist is graft versus host disease (GVHD), a disorder caused by mature committed T lymphocytes in the marrow graft reacting immunologically against host alloantigens (*1, 2*). Clinically significant GVHD occurs in about 70% of patients transplanted from histocompatible siblings, and results in death in 15–30% of them, despite the use of "optimal" prophylactic posttransplant immunosuppressive therapy (*3–5*).

Several experimental and clinical studies suggest that prevention of GVHD can be accomplished by in vitro removal of mature T lymphocytes from donor marrow prior to transplantation (*6–8*). Various methods have now been developed that are effective in depleting alloreactive T lymphocytes from murine and human marrow, achieving complete prevention of GVHD. These techniques include treatment of the marrow with different types of monoclonal anti-T-cell antibodies (*6–10*), depletion of lymphocytes forming rosettes with sheep red blood cells (SRBC) with or without agglutination with lectins (*11*), and treatment with immunotoxins (*12*). A critical question yet to be solved is whether T cell depletion in any way affects the immunologic or hematopoietic reconstitution of the recipients, since many immunohematopoietic functions were previously shown by in vitro studies to be T-cell-dependent.

The present study was undertaken to investigate the effects of removal of immunocompetent T cells from the bone marrow on syngeneic reconstitution of lethally irradiated mice during the first 8 weeks following BMT.

MATERIALS AND METHODS

Mice. BALB/c female mice aged 10–16 weeks were supplied by the Hebrew University-Hadassah Medical School Mouse Colony. They received acidified water without antibiotics and regular diet. All mice were maintained under standard conditions with no isolation.

Total-body irradiation. Irradiation was delivered by a Phillips x-ray unit (250 KV, 15 MA) at a rate of 50 rads/min, at a source-to-skin distance of 70 cm, through 0.25-mmCu and 1.0-mmAl filters. Animals were positioned in radiation chambers and exposed to a total dose of 650 rads, which was confirmed to be a lethal dose for BALB/c mice.

Bone marrow transplantation. Mice were sacrificed by cervical dislocation and long bones (femur, tibia, and humerus) were removed. Bone marrow was flushed from the marrow cavities

[1] This work was supported by a grant from the Joint Research Fund of the Hebrew University and Hadassah; the Roselle Herzog Fund for Cancer Research; the Chief Scientist's Office, Israel Ministry of Health; Basic Research Foundation, Israel Academy of Sciences; Israel Cancer Research Fund; Ruth Estrin Goldberg Memorial for Cancer Research; and the Lady Tata Memorial Trust.

[2] Department of Medicine A, Hadassah University Hospital.

[3] The Lautenberg Center for General and Tumor Immunology. Hadassah-Hebrew University School of Medicine.

[4] Department of Bone Marrow Transplantation and Immunology Research, Hadassah University Hospital.

[5] Address correspondence to: S. Salvin, M.D., Hadassah University Hospital, 91120 Jerusalem, Israel.

* Abbreviations used: BMT, bone marrow transplantation; Con A, concanavalin A; CML, cell-mediated lympholysis; FCS, fetal calf serum; GVHD, graft-versus-host disease; LPS, lipopolysaccharide; MLR, mixed lymphocyte reaction; NBS, newborn calf serum; NK, natural killer; PFC, plaque-forming cell; PHA, phytohemagglutinin; SRBC, sheep red blood cell; WBC, white blood cell.

with RPMI 1640 medium (Biolab, Jerusalem, Israel) using a 25-gauge needle. Cell suspensions were filtered through a fine nylon mesh and washed twice in RPMI 1640. Aliquots of 0.3 ml medium containing 10^7 nucleated cells were injected i.v. into recipient mice 24 hr after irradiation.

T lymphocyte depletion. Donor bone marrow cells were treated with monoclonal anti-Thy 1.2 antibody (Cedarlane Laboratories, Hornby, Ontario, Canada) and Low-Tox rabbit complement (Cedarlane Laboratories): Cells were adjusted to 10^7/ml in diluted (1:400) anti-Thy-1.2 antibody, and incubated for 30 min at 4°C with occasional agitation. Complement was added to pelleted cells at a final dilution of 1:8. Cells were incubated for 60 min at 37°C, pelleted, resuspended, and injected i.v. into recipients. Cell recovery was calculated and viability determined by trypan blue exclusion. The lytic efficacy of the antibody was monitored by testing the residual T cells with FITC-conjugated monoclonal anti-Thy-1.2 antibody (Bio-Yeda, Rehovot, Israel). More than 95% of T cells were consistently killed in the bone marrow inocula.

Mitogen assays. Washed spleen cells were resuspended in RPMI 1640 medium supplemented with glutamine (2 mM), penicillin (100 U/ml), streptomycin (100 μg/ml), 2-mercaptoethanol (5×10^{-5} M), and 5% fetal calf serum (FCS) to a final concentration of 2.5×10^5 cells/0.2 ml/well. Mitogens were added in final concentrations as follows: concanavalin A (Con A, 2× crystallized, Miles-Yeda) 5 μg/ml; phytohemagglutinin (PHA-P, Difco Lab, Detroit, MI) 10 μg/ml; and lipopolysaccharide (LPS, Difco) 50 μg/ml in 0.2-ml flat-bottomed microtiter plates (Nunc, Denmark). The culture plates were incubated at 37°C in a humidified 5% CO_2 in air incubator for 3 days. Samples were pulsed 16–18 hr before harvest with 1 μCi of ^{3}H-thymidine (1 mCi/ml, Nuclear Research Center, Negev, Israel) in 0.02 ml RPMI-1640. The cultures were harvested with an automatic harvester and ^{3}H-thymidine incorporation was measured using a Beckman scintillation counter. Samples were performed in triplicate, and the results were expressed as the percentage of normal responses to the same stimulus, according to the following formula:

$$\% = \frac{\text{cpm experimental} - \text{cpm background}}{\text{cpm normal} - \text{cpm background}} \times 100$$

Mixed lymphocyte reaction (MLR). Washed spleen cells were resuspended in complete medium containing 10% newborn calf serum (NBS) at a final concentration of 10^7/ml. Stimulating allogeneic C57BL/6 splenocytes irradiated with 2500 rads were suspended to the same concentration. Equal volumes (0.1 ml) of responding and stimulating cells (10^6 cells each) were mixed in 0.2 ml flat-bottomed microculture plates and incubated in a humidified 5% CO_2 in air incubator for 4 days. Samples were pulsed with 1 μCi of ^{3}H-thymidine for 16–18 hr before harvest. Results were expressed as percentage of normal response (see above).

Cell-mediated lympholysis (CML). Splenocytes (5×10^6) were cocultured with 1×10^6 irradiated (2500 rads) allogeneic C57BL/6 splenocytes for 5 days in 2 ml plates (Costar, Cambridge, MA) at 37°C. The cytotoxic activity of the sensitized splenocytes was assessed by a 4-hr ^{51}Cr release assay, using either 5×10^3 Con-A-induced lymphoblasts of C57BL/6 origin or H-2^b lymphoma target cells at effector/target cell ratios ranging from 1/2 to 100/1. The cytotoxic activity per culture, expressed in lytic units, was calculated as previously described (*13*).

Natural killer (NK) cell assay. Spleen cells were washed twice and resuspended in 10% FCS-RPMI medium at a final concentration of 2×10^6 cells/ml. The RL♂1 radiation induced lymphoma cell line was used as target. NK activity was determined by a direct ^{51}Cr release method (see CML).

In vivo immunization with sheep red blood cells (SRBC) and assay of serum hemagglutinins. Mice were injected intraperitoneally with 0.5 ml of 10% suspension of SRBC. Seven days later, mice were bled, the serum was separated, heat-inactivated and kept frozen until assayed.

Serial two-fold dilutions (starting at 1/5) of serum samples (50 μl) were incubated in U-shape 96-well microtiter plates (Nunc, Denmark) with 1% SRBC (20 μl) in the presence of 1% FCS. Hemagglutination titer (the last tube which showed 50% agglutination) was determined after a 30 min. incubation period at 37°C followed by a 2 hr. incubation at 4°C.

Percentage of T lymphocytes in the spleen. The percentage of T-cells in the spleens was determined by immunofluorescence using FITC-labeled monoclonal anti-Thy 1.2 antibody (Miles Yeda) (at 1:50) by microscopy.

Peripheral blood count. Mice were bled from the retro-orbital veins using heparin-coated glass capillaries. Blood samples were counted for hemoglobin, platelets and white blood cells in a Coulter counter. Blood smears were stained with giemza stain and absolute lymphocyte count in the peripheral blood was calculated.

Statistical analysis was carried out using the Student's t test.

RESULTS

Monitoring of various immunological and hematological parameters was carried out periodically for 8 weeks following BMT. Each analysis was performed with 3 or 4 individual test mice and age-matched normal control mice.

T cell content of untreated and T-cell-depleted marrow inocula. The proportions of T lymphocytes in the marrow samples of BALB/c mice in different experiments ranged between 5–12% (median 7%). The absolute number of T lymphocytes (median) infused into recipients of untreated marrow grafts was 5×10^5–1.2×10^6 (median 7×10^5). Recipients of T-lymphocyte-depleted marrow grafts received 10^7 bone marrow cells with less than 14×10^3 T lymphocytes per mouse, according to the sensitivity of the assay system.

Peripheral blood counts. Red blood cell counts were similar in recipients of T-cell-depleted marrow and those reconstituted with unmanipulated marrow grafts (Table 1). There was a decrease in platelet counts 10 days following irradiation with rapid recovery to low-normal levels as early as 17 days after BMT (Table 1). A sharp decrease in peripheral white blood cell and mononuclear cell counts followed whole-body irradiation and BMT. The slow recovery of the counts towards the normal range was essentially unaffected by T cell depletion. The white blood cell (WBC) counts of recipients of untreated, as compared with T-cell-depleted, marrow grafts were 1900 vs. 2100/mm^3; 3800 vs. 3200/mm^3; and 3800 vs. 4100/mm^3, respectively, 10, 17, and 24 days following BMT. Only the WBC counts on days 31 and 38 were significantly lower ($P<0.05$) in the T-cell-depleted group; 4200 vs. 7000/mm^3; and 4700 vs. 7500/mm^3, respectively. However, this would seem to be irrelevant since both levels are within the normal range, and normal levels were again detected on day +56 in both groups (6000 vs. 6400/mm^3). The rise in the absolute number of mononuclear cells in the

TABLE 1. Hematological and immunological profile of BALB/c mice reconstituted with untreated or T-cell-depleted marrow grafts following lethal whole-body irradiation

	Untreated marrow (day following transplantation)						T-cell-depleted marrow (day following transplantation)					
	10	17	24	31	38	56	10	17	24	31	38	56
White blood cells/mm³	1900	3800	3800	7000	7500	6000	2100	3200	4100	4200	4700	6400
Mononuclear cells/mm³	200	400	2500	4400	5000	4600	200	300	2400	3000	3600	4400
Hemoglobin (g/dl)	14	17	16	19	17	16	15	18	18	16	16	16
Platelets/mm³×10⁻⁵	5	13	11	10	11	10	6	12	10	12	10	10
Spleen T lymphocytes (%)	ND[a]	14±1	30±4	ND	27±1	31±0.5	ND	12±1	23±3	ND	29±0.5	28±1
Percentage of normal responsiveness												
Con A	ND	12±5	37±5	66±11	63±3	74±5	ND	9±3	27±7	64±14	77±6	69±3
PHA	ND	5±1	12±3	31±12	49±4	56±3	ND	3±2	14±5	44±10	41±5	56±4
LPS	ND	28±6	65±4	104±15	88±12	115±5	ND	37±10	68±9	134±18	112±10	103±6
MLR	ND	1	31±5	ND	34±6	41±4	ND	2	28±7	ND	30±5	36±4
CML	ND	ND	10±5	53±0.5	41±14	65±12	ND	ND	10±1	58±19	57±24	43±7
Percentage of normal anti-SRBC response	ND	4	4	25	50	50	ND	4	4	25	50	50
Percentage of normal NK activity	ND	66±13	160±17	107±12	112±9	ND	ND	198±23	176±8	138±8	177±30	ND

[a] ND: not done.

peripheral blood was similar in recipients of unseparated, as compared with T-cell-depleted marrow grafts (Table 1).

Analysis of percentage of T cells in the spleen revealed early recovery (day 24) to near-normal levels comparable in the two groups of untreated, as compared with T-cell-depleted marrow grafts: 30±4% vs. 23±3%; 27±1% vs. 29±0.5%; and 31±0.5% vs. 28±1% on days 24, 38, and 56 post-BMT, respectively.

Response to mitogens. Proliferative responses to T cell and B cell mitogens were similar in both groups (Table 1). Recovery of Con A responsiveness in the two groups preceded the recovery of PHA responsiveness. Con A response reached 60–80% of normal values within 5–6 weeks while PHA response reached only 56% at 8 weeks following BMT. Responsiveness to LPS recovered completely as early as day 31 after transplantation and even exceeded the control values, in recipients of untreated and T-cell-depleted marrow grafts.

MLR and CML assays. MLR showed a partial but identical recovery pattern in both experimental groups (Table 1). No MLR responses were obtained on day 17 post-BMT in both groups. MLR responsiveness reached 30% and 40% of control response in both experimental groups by days 24 and 56 post-BMT. Similar results were obtained in the CML assays: by day 24 post-BMT, only 10% of normal response was observed in both groups, and 50–65% of normal response was observed at 8 weeks after transplantation.

Anti-SRBC response. Anti-SRBC-agglutinin response was studied in recipients of untreated and T-cell-depleted marrow grafts (Table 1). Both experimental groups were capable of mounting an identical anti-SRBC response starting on day 31 post-BMT and reaching 50% of normal response by day 38 following transplantation.

NK activity assay. Recovery of NK activity against RL♂1 was complete at 17 days posttransplantation (Table 1). The NK activity of the T-cell-depleted group was somewhat higher than that of the untreated group at 17, 24, 31, and 38 days post-BMT, although this difference was significant only in the immediate posttransplant period, reaching 198 vs. 66% of normal response on day 17 post-BMT.

In other experiments (data not shown) we found normal phagocytic activity (bacteria, zymosan, latex particles) of peritoneal exudate cells in both groups as early as 10 days post-transplantation.

DISCUSSION

The kinetics of immunological reconstitution following transplantation of unmanipulated marrow grafts have previously been studied in experimental animals and humans. Marusic (*14*) studied the immune functions of mice for seven weeks after syngeneic marrow transplantation. Peripheral white blood cell counts returned to normal values within two weeks while mononuclear counts reached normal values at five weeks. Proliferative responses to T cell mitogens recovered completely six weeks following transplantation. In another report, Gregory and Lajtha (*15*) studied plaque-forming cells (PFC) in response to SRBC in lethally irradiated mice reconstituted with syngeneic marrow cells. Peak PFC response was demonstrated at ten weeks, reaching about 50% of normal value. Impaired proliferative responses to T cell mitogens were observed within the first three months following human marrow transplantation; these functions normalized by one year in most patients (*16, 17*). In contrast, cytotoxic/effector cells mediating antibody-dependent cellular cytotoxicity and natural killing activity returned to normal levels by 30 days after grafting (*18, 19*). Peripheral B and T lymphocyte counts and IgM and IgG levels reached normal values 3–4 months following transplantation (*16, 17, 20*). The immunohematopoietic reconstitution of mice (or humans) transplanted with T-cell-depleted bone marrow has been studied in far less detail. Onoe et al. (*21*) and Krown et al. (*22*) have demonstrated complete immunological reconstitution of chimeric mice transplanted with T-cell-depleted grafts from allogeneic donors 90–100 days post-transplantation. The only reduced function detected was primary PFC response against SRBC, however the secondary response was vigorous. No detailed analyses of immunohematopoietic functions at early times after BMT were performed in these studies.

The significance of the role of T lymphocytes mediated through hematopoietic factors, as well as T-dependent immunological functions, has recently been suggested in numerous studies. It therefore seems essential to determine whether transplantation of T-cell-depleted marrow grafts into lethally ablated recipients might result in impaired recovery of various hematopoietic or immune functions.

This study was designed to evaluate the rate and degree of recovery of various hematologic and immunological functions in lethally irradiated mice transplanted with syngeneic whole versus T-cell-depleted marrow grafts. The kinetics of reconstitution of proliferative responses to T cell and B cell mitogens, NK activity, MLR, CML, and antibody production—as well as peripheral blood count—were essentially identical in both experimental groups. The data suggest that BMT using T-cell-depleted grafts is effective and safe and that T-dependent functions are recovered from the T cell pool that develops out of the uncommitted stem cell reservoir.

Our conclusions justify autologous BMT with depletion of lymphocytes, T cells included. Such procedure is required for elimination of malignant lymphocytes from autologous marrow grafts in cases of acute lymphocytic leukemias and non-Hodgkin's lymphomas.

Our study also demonstrates that immunological functions in recipients of T-cell-depleted and unseparated marrow grafts recover at different rates. The first function to recover is NK activity, reaching higher than normal values as early as 17–24 days posttransplantation. Similar recovery patterns were observed by Doklehr (*23*) and Livnat et al. (*18*) in human bone marrow recipients. This may be attributed to relatively rapid maturation of NK cells—or, alternatively, to depletion of suppressor cells in the early posttransplantation period. Proliferative responses to the B cell mitogen (LPS) recovered relatively early—one month after transplantation—while the primary antibody response to SRBC reached only 50% of normal values. This may reflect complete restoration of fully functioning B cells bearing the LPS receptor with partial capability of antibody production to the T-dependent antigen (SRBC) employed here. T cell functions measured by proliferative responses to Con A and PHA and in MLR also showed different recovery patterns. Con A responsiveness reached 80% of normal values six weeks following transplantation, while PHA and MLR responsiveness reached 60% and 40%, respectively, during the same observation period. As has been previously reported (*24*) various T cell subpopulations respond differentially to mitogens. This phenomenon might be related to stages of differentiation (*25*). Thus, the kinetics of reconstitution of various immunological functions described here would be dependent on different stages of recovery of T cell subsets.

Allogeneic BMT is becoming a routine medical procedure for the treatment of an increasing number of malignant and nonmalignant disorders. It has recently been shown that T cell depletion from the marrow before transplantation is an essential condition for successful BMT, since only by this approach could GVHD, a major cause of morbidity and mortality, be prevented (*7–10*). In the early posttransplantation period, the host immune system is severely depressed due to the aggressive conditioning. During this time the recipient is vulnerable to opportunistic infections by bacteria, viruses, and fungi, which are occasionally fatal. Reconstitution of the immune functions depends on the appearance of fully functioning donor-derived immunocompetent cells in adequate numbers during the transition period from the host to the donor-type immune system. It has been suggested that low-grade immunity may be conferred by competent donor T cells infused with the marrow inoculum. These mature cells derived from donor marrow and peripheral blood may provide some protection until stem cells and lymphocyte precursors develop to maturity. Our study suggests that residual donor T lymphocytes may not be essential for recovery of immune functions in syngeneic, and hence autologous, marrow transplantation. The potential beneficial effects of donor-type T cells is currently under investigation. An essential question that has yet to be resolved is whether the T cell depletion procedure, which eliminates mature T cells from marrow inoculum, in any way affects the recovery of various immunological functions and recall of immunological responsiveness in the first weeks following allogeneic BMT. These questions are the subject of our present studies in experimental animals and in patients undergoing allogeneic BMT, as compared with autologous BMT.

REFERENCES

1. Korngold R, Sprent J. Lethal graft-versus-host disease after bone marrow transplantation across minor histocompatibility barriers in mice. J Exp Med 1978; 148: 1687.
2. Storb R, Thomas ED. Allogeneic bone marrow transplantation. Immunol Rev 1983; 71: 77.
3. Storb R, Prentice RI, Buckner CD, et al. Graft versus host disease and survival in patients with aplastic anemia treated by marrow grafts from HLA-identical siblings. Beneficial effect of a protective environment. N Engl J Med 1983; 308: 302.
4. Ramsey N, Kersey JH, Robinson LL, et al. A randomised study of the prevention of acute graft versus host disease. N Engl J Med 1982; 306: 392.
5. Storb R, Epstein RB, Graham TC, et al. Methotrexate regimens for control of graft versus host disease in dogs with allogeneic marrow grafts. Transplantation 1970; 9: 240.
6. Vallera DA, Soderling CCB, Carlson GJ, et al. Bone marrow transplantation across major histocompatibility barriers in mice. Effects of elimination of T cells from donor grafts by pretreatment with monoclonal Thy 1.2 plus complement or antibody alone. Transplantation 1981; 31: 218.
7. Waldmann H, Polliack A, Hale G, et al. Elimination of graft-versus-host disease by in-vitro depletion of alloreactive lymphocytes with a monoclonal rat anti-human lymphocyte antibody. Lancet 1984; 2: 483.
8. Prentice HG, Blacklock HA, Janossy G, et al. Depletion of T lymphocytes in donor marrow prevents significant graft-versus-host disease in matched allogeneic leukemic marrow transplant recipients. Lancet 1984; 1: 472.
9. Sharp TG, Sachs DH, Fauci AS, et al. T cell depletion of human bone marrow using monoclonal antibody and complement-mediated lysis. Transplantation 1983; 35: 112.
10. Spruce WE, McMillan R, Miller W, et al. Transplantation of T-lymphocyte-depleted bone marrow between HLA-mismatched individuals. Transplantation 1983; 36: 369.
11. Reisner Y, Kapoor N, Kirkpatrick D, et al. Transplantation for severe combined immunodeficiency with HLA-A,B,D,DR incompatible parental marrow cells fractionated by soybean agglutinin and sheep red blood cells. Blood 1983; 61: 341.
12. Fillipovich AH, Vallera DA, Youle RJ, et al. Ex-vivo treatment of donor bone-marrow with anti-T-cell immunotoxins for prevention of graft versus host disease. Lancet 1984; 1: 469.
13. Kedar E, Chriqui-Zeira E, Mitelman S. Methods for amplifying the induction and expression of cytotoxic response in vitro to syngeneic and autologous freshly-isolated solid tumors of mice. Cancer Immunol Immunother 1984; 18: 126.
14. Marusic M. Immunological recovery of thymectomized and sham-thymectomized lethally irradiated mice reconstituted with syngeneic bone marrow cells. Experientia 1979; 35: 683.
15. Gregory CJ, Lajtha LG. Recovery of immune responsiveness in lethally-irradiated mice protected with syngeneic marrow cells. Int J Radiat Biol 1970; 17: 117.
16. Storb R, Ochs HD, Weiden PL, et al. Immunologic reactivity in marrow grafts recipients. Transplant Proc 1976; 8: 637.

17. Gale RP, Opelz G, Mickey MR, et al. Immunodeficiency following allogeneic bone marrow transplantation. Transplant Proc 1978; 10: 223.
18. Livnat S, Seigneuzet M, Strob R, et al. Analysis of cytotoxic effector cell function in patients with leukemia or aplastic anemia before and after marrow transplantation. J Immunol 1980; 124: 481.
19. Lopez C, Kirkpatrick D, Livnat S, et al: Natural killer cells in bone marrow transplantation. Lancet 1980; 2: 1025.
20. Witherspoon RP, Lum LG, Storb R. Immunologic reconstitution after human marrow grafting. Semin Hematol 1984; 21: 2.
21. Onoe K, Fernandes G, Good RA. Humoral and cell-mediated immune responses in fully allogeneic bone marrow chimera in mice. J Exp Med 1980; 151: 115.
22. Krown SE, Coico R, Scheid MP, et al. Immune function in fully allogeneic mouse bone marrow chimeras. Clin Immunol Immunopathol 1981; 19: 268.
23. Dokhelar MC. Recovery of NK cell activity after bone-marrow transplantation. In: Herberman RB, ed. NK cells and other natural effector cells. New York: Academic Press, 1982: 1253.
24. Shortman K, von Boehmer H, Lipp J, et al. Subpopulations of T-lymphocytes. Transplant Rev 1975; 25: 193.
25. Stobo JD. Phytohemagglutin and concanavalin A: probes for murine T cell activation and differentiation. Transplant Rev 1972; 11: 60.

Received 12 July 1985.
Accepted 13 November 1985.

0041-1337/86/4202-0122$02.00/0
TRANSPLANTATION
Vol. 42, No. 2

PRESERVATION DAMAGE IN LIVER TRANSPLANTATION

INFLUENCE OF RAPID COOLING

G. OTTO,[1] H. WOLFF, I. UERLINGS, AND K. GELLERT

The Surgical Clinic and Pathological Institute of the Charité Hospital, Berlin, German Democratic Republic

Liver preservation and transplantation was performed in pigs. For flush perfusion cold (2°C) and warm (15°C) lactated Ringer's solution were compared. Administration of cold Ringer's resulted in a severe endothelial damage of sinusoids that was aggravated after recirculation, as shown by electron microscopic examination. Using warm Ringer's solution this alteration was limited. Liver parenchymal cells are impaired mainly during reflow as a consequence of microcirculatory disturbance. After cold flushing animals died within a few hours, whereas after flushing with warm Ringer's solution pigs survived definitively.

In our experience with 32 clinical liver transplantations at the Charité Hospital, Berlin, ischemic damage has been an important reason for graft failure. In 5 recipients preservation damage was the main cause of death and in 2 more patients it may have contributed to lethal complications (*15*). Also other transplantation teams have reported unsuccessful liver transplantation caused in part by graft ischemia (*4, 11, 13*).

In former experiments we reported the significance of hypoxia during liver preservation in pigs (*10*). Using a mixture of blood and lactated Ringer's solution we were able to mitigate the severe damage to sinusoidal endothelium that is observed as soon as after flush perfusion with Ringer's solution and that is responsible for poor graft function after recirculation. In this study, the influence of the temperature of the perfusate was investigated. Visualized by electron microscopic examination, the timing and type of preservation damage were of special interest.

[1]Address correspondence to: Doz.Dr.Sc.Med. G. Otto, Surgical Clinic of the Charité Hospital, GDR 1040 Berlin, Schumannstr. 20/21.

MATERIALS AND METHODS

Liver transplantation was performed in unselected minipigs weighing 20–25 kg. After preparation of the donor organ, flush perfusion was performed through the portal vein with intact arterial blood supply using 1000 ml of lactated Ringer's solution (2°C) containing 2000 IU heparin/L (R_c; *n=19) in group 1 and lactated Ringer's solution (15°C) containing 2000 IU heparin/L (R_w; n=8) in group 2.

After hepatectomy, the liver was placed in cold Ringer's solution and flushing was finished with 500 ml of R_c in groups 1 and 2. Thereafter grafts in group 1 were perfused with 500 ml of (A) Collins 2 (*6*) (n=8) or (B) plasma protein fraction (PPF; (*14*) (n=11). In group 2 no additional perfusion was performed.

The time of storage at 4°C amounted to 5–6 hr. Before and after flushing, after perfusion with Collins or PPF, after preservation, and at 1 and 24 hr after transplantation, biopsies were taken for electron microscopic examination.

RESULTS

Survival of animals was not influenced by the kind of storage (Collins or PPF) in group 1. It depended only on the kind of flushing. Survival time averaged 8.3 hr in 1A and 9.7 hr in IB compared with 41.6 days in group 2. The difference between

* Abbreviations used: PPF, plasma protein fraction; R_c, cold lactated Ringer's solution; R_w, warm lactated Ringer's solution.

groups 1 and 2 is highly significant ($P < 0.001$). In group 1, all animals recovered promptly after surgery. After several hours, urine production ceased and the animals became unconscious and died with respiratory distress, convulsions, or cardiac arrest.

After donor operation mild liver damage could be observed by electron microscopy. There were products of hepatocellular destruction within the sinusoidal space (shedding), a slight swelling of endothelium in some cases, and a slight vacuolization of the endoplasmic reticulum.

Further alterations occurred mainly within the sinusoids. As early as after flushing the endothelium was desquamated or it had a high electron density in group 1. The morphologic structures of the Dissé spaces and of the hepatocellular microvilli were destroyed (Fig. 1). Perfusion with Collins 2 or PPF caused no further visible alterations. The extent of this damage after storage was limited and did not depend on the preservation solution according to visual examination. At 1 hr and especially 24 hr after reflow the endothelial damage was pronounced (Fig. 2). Parenchymal necroses were apparent.

Using R_w for flushing, there was only minor sinusoidal alteration. Uncovered parenchymal cells and destroyed microvilli were rare. After storage, the endothelial destruction was similar to the condition after flushing. The extent of damage was slight even 24 hr after reflow (Fig. 3).

In spite of the partially severe alteration of the sinusoidal structures, liver parenchymal cells were comparatively well preserved. After storage a swelling of mitochondria and vacuolization of endoplasmic reticulum was visible but seemed to be reversible. Morphologically there was no apparent difference between Collins 2 or PPF storage.

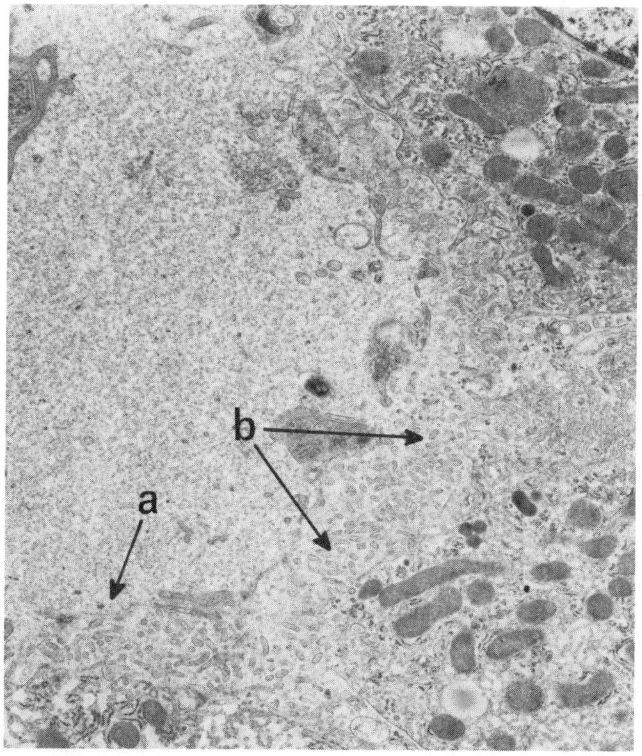

FIGURE 1. Porcine liver after flushing with R_c. Desquamation of endothelium (a), widened Dissé spaces with destroyed microvilli (b). Magnification 8000×.

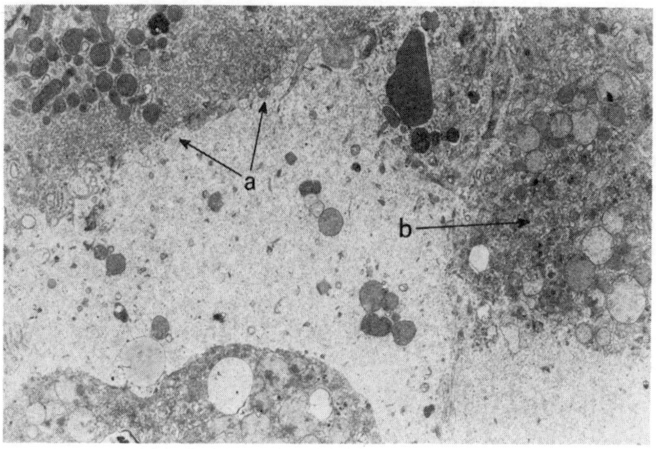

FIGURE 2. Porcine liver preserved with R_c and PPF solution 24 hr after reflow. Complete desquamation of endothelium (a), and beginning parenchymal cell necroses (b). Magnification 6000×.

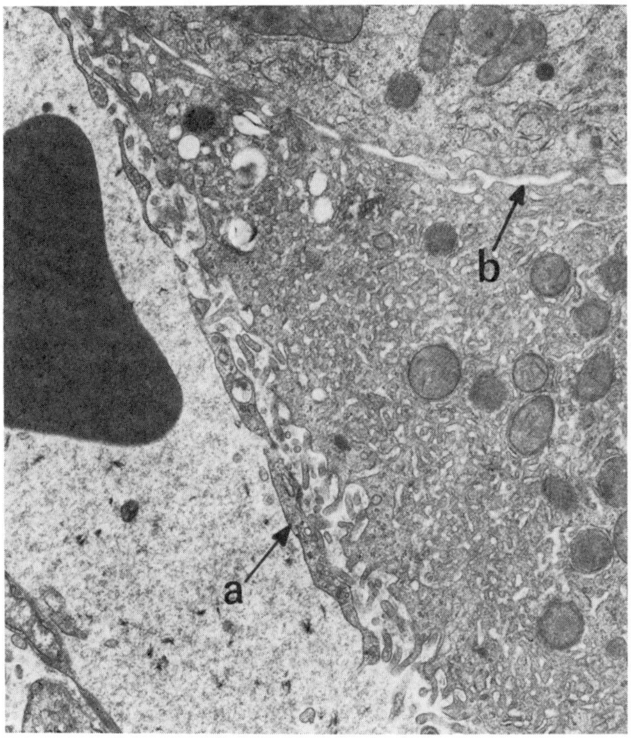

FIGURE 3. Porcine liver after R_w flushing and R_c storage 24 hr after reflow. Normal endothelium and Dissé spaces (a). Slight widening of interhepatocellular spaces (b). Magnification 10,000×.

DISCUSSION

Our preservation procedure in group 1 was based on the principles used in clinical liver transplantation: precooling of the organ by Ringer's flushing while the hepatic artery remains intact and storage after perfusion with Collins 2 or PPF solution (*4, 11, 12, 15*). The only difference in our technique was in the velocity of cooling. A liver temperature below 10°C was reached within 8 to 10 min.

The failure of this method in our experiments is in contrast to the results of other authors, and the discrepancy cannot be explained completely. Calne preserved porcine livers for more than 6 hr (*5*) and Benichou managed to preserve canine livers for up to 18 hr (*2*). On the other hand the survival rate in Bockhorn's experiments performed in pigs is extremely low (*3*) and Abouna has reported disappointing results in liver preservation (*1*). Based on extensive experience in pigs, Koristek pointed out that pigs survived only after preservation with blood/Ringer's (*7*). Possibly porcine liver is particularly susceptible to the preservation procedure. Thereby sinusoidal structures are damaged to a higher degree than liver parenchymal cells (*8*). This occurs mainly during flush perfusion and it increases significantly after reflow. During storage the extent of additional morphologic damage was slight and did not depend on Collins 2, PPF, or Ringer's solution. Therefore it is unlikely that the disappointing results in group 1 are due to Collins 2 or PPF storage, particularly as many livers in clinical preservation have been stored for this period in these solutions with good results.

The initial alteration could be prevented by administration of oxygen carriers in the preservation solution (*10*). As demonstrated here, the benefit from relatively warm oxygen free solution is very similar to that from red blood cells.

The mechanisms of this damage remain hypothetical. The sensitivity of vascular sphincters to cold may play an important role during the initial phase of preservation and inhibit the inflow of arterial blood into the sinusoidal system. Consequently the damage caused by cold flushing may be explained by the lack of oxygen in Ringer's solution and the consequences of sphincteric spasm. Both these mechanisms influence the condition of sinusoids. After reflow the endothelial destruction increases and limits hepatic function. Damage of hepatocytes occurs during storage too (*9*) but primarily this can be explained as a consequence of microcirculatory disturbance. This could be demonstrated 1 and 24 hr after transplantation.

From our results we conclude that: (1) rapid cooling is an important pathophysiological mechanism in porcine liver preservation; (2) endothelial cells are more susceptible to this damage than hepatocytes; (3) flushing and reflow are critical phases of preservation; (4) the pathomorphological appearance after gradual cooling is very similar to that after administration of red blood cells, so ischemia seems to be a basic pathophysiological mechanism; and (5) the demonstrated pathophysiological principles and processes may be of importance in clinical liver preservation too.

REFERENCES

1. Abouna GM, Hurwitz R, Serrou B. Organ preservation by Collins solution. Lancet 1971; 1: 1076.
2. Benichou J, Halgrimson CG, Weil R III, Koep LJ, Starzl TE. Canine and human liver preservation for 6–8 hours by cold perfusion. Transplantation 1977; 24: 407.
3. Bockhorn H. Die allogene Lebertransplantation. I. Morphologische und funktionelle Veränderungen in experimentellen Untersuchungen beim Schwein. Res Exp Med 1981; 178: 79.
4. Calne RY. Recent advances in clinical transplantation of the liver and pancreas. Transplant Proc 1983; 15: 1263.
5. Calne RY, Dunn DC, Herbertson BM, Bitter-Suermann H, Davis DR, Smith DP, Reitter FH. Preservation of the porcine liver. Transplant Proc 1974; 6: 289.
6. Collins GM, Bravo-Shugarman M, Terasaki PI. Kidney preservation for transportation. Initial perfusion and 30 hours ice storage. Lancet 1969; 2: 1219.
7. Koristek V. Experimental liver transplantation. Acta Fac Med Univ Brunen 1975.
8. Myagkaya G, van Veen H, James J. Ultrastructural changes in rat liver sinusoids during prolonged normothermic and hypothermic ischemia in vitro. Virchows Arch [Cell Pathol] 1984; 47: 361.
9. Otto G, David H, Wolff H, Wassilew G, Marx I. Elektronenmikroskopische Befunde während hypothermer Lagerungskonservierung der Leber. II. Morphometrie der Hepatozyten. Langenbecks Arch Chir 1981; 354: 125.
10. Otto G, Wolff H, David H. Preservation damage in liver transplantation: electronmicroscopic finding. Transplant Proc 1984; 16: 1247.
11. Pichlmayr R, Brölsch Ch, Neuhaus P, et al. Report on 68 human orthotopic liver transplantations with special reference to rejection phenomena. Transplant Proc 1983; 15: 1279.
12. Starzl TE, Hakala TR, Shaw BW Jr, Hardesty RL, Rosenthal TJ, Griffith BP, Iwatsuki Sh, Bahnson HT. A flexible procedure for multiple cadaveric organ procurement. Surg Gynecol Obstet 1984; 158: 223.
13. Starzl TE, Iwatsuki S, van Thiel D, et al. Evolution of liver transplantation. Hepatology 1982; 2: 614.
14. Wall WJ, Calne RY, Herbertson BM, Baker PG, Smith DP, Underwood J, Kostakis A, Williams R. Simple hypothermic preservation for transporting human livers long distances for transplantation. Transplantation 1977; 23: 210.
15. Wolff H, Otto G, David H, Friis E, Kranz D, Kunz B, Lohse W, Pahlig H, Schädlich M, Simon H, Winkler H, Witter H, Wolff K. Klinische Lebertransplantation in der DDR. Zentralbl Chir, 1985; 110:794.

Received 7 August 1985.
Accepted 15 November 1985.

0041-1337/86/4202-0125$02.00/0
TRANSPLANTATION
Vol. 42, No. 2

Printed in U.S.A.

GLOMERULAR DAMAGE AFTER KIDNEY PRESERVATION[1]

ROBERT LAMBERT,[2] MARK HENRY,[2] BRIAN HOWDEN, PAULA JABLONSKI,[3] DEREK RAE, GLORIA TAVANLIS, VERNON MARSHALL, AND JOHN TANGE[2]

Department of Surgery, Monash University and Prince Henry's Hospital; and Department of Pathology, University of Melbourne, Parkville, 3052, Australia

Severe proteinuria occurs during isolated organ perfusion of kidneys removed from SD and DA rats and subjected to 24-hr cold preservation. In both strains increased glomerular permeability was associated with changes in glomerular visceral epithelial cells, particularly cytoplasmic edema and detachment of cells from capillary basement membranes. Foot processes were intact and staining for sialoglycoprotein was retained. The changes were compatible with survival of the isograft kidney after transplantation, but moderate proteinuria was found in some rats after one month.

Protein loss in the urine during isolated organ perfusion is very much less in kidneys subjected to 4-hr cold preservation, and the glomerular epithelial cells are normal or show only minimal cytoplasmic edema on electron microscopy.

The experiment shows that significant damage to glomeruli may occur during preservation prior to transplantation, and the model itself can be usefully exploited to determine the relation between increased glomerular permeability to albumin and the associated changes in the glomerular capillary wall.

Kidney damage during preservation for renal transplantation is most obviously expressed as damage to proximal convoluted tubules (*1*) and this may give rise to interstitial nephritis after transplantation. These two lesions develop after renal ischemia, and since their severity is proportional to the duration of the ischemia (*2*) renal parenchymal scarring has been used to assess the efficacy of transplant preservation procedures (*3*). Much less attention has been paid to glomerular lesions—and, in our experience, although moderate proteinuria developed in some rats given renal isografts, glomerular damage did not affect survival or renal function (*4*).

However, a favorable outcome following renal transplantation might not preclude the existence of transient glomerular damage, and such damage might be revealed by ultrastructural studies and by functional changes during isolated kidney perfusion.

MATERIALS AND METHODS

Male outbred (Sprague Dawley) or inbred DA rats, 270–330 g body wt., were housed 5 to a cage and given a pellet diet and tap water to drink.

Rats were anesthetized with ether and given mannitol (0.1 g) i.v. A cannula (Portex pp10) was then inserted into the right ureter and the kidney, superior mesenteric artery, and aorta and origin of the renal artery dissected. Heparin (100 IU) was given i.v. just before cannulation of the renal artery via the mesenteric artery. The kidney was immediately flushed with 4–8 ml. of cold preservation solution at a maximum pressure of 100 mmHg and excised. The excised kidneys were either placed in a beaker of this solution at 0°C or perfused continuously (recycling volume = 7 ml) with the flushing solution at 4°C and at a flow rate of 18 ml/hr. The solution contained 5% bovine serum albumin, fraction V (Miles, Pentax), Na 84, K 78, Mg 40, citrate 54, sulphate 40, mannitol 50, and glucose 10 mmol/L; pH was 7.1 and osmolality 300 mOsm/kg.

At the end of the storage period (4 or 24 hr) renal function was tested by perfusion of the kidney at 37°C for 60 min with 100 ml 6.5% dialyzed bovine serum albumin in Krebs-Henseleit buffer. This perfusate was continuously gassed with 95% oxygen/5% carbon dioxide and contained glucose (10 mM); glycine (2.2 mM); glutamine (2.0 mM); alanine (1.9 mM); lysine and serine (1.0 mM each); arginine and cysteine (0.5 mM each); leucine (0.4 mM); phenylalanine, methionine, isoleucine, and valine (0.3 mM each); histidine, aspartate and asparagine (0.2 mM each); tryptophane (0.07 mM); and tyrosine (0.02 mM). Perfusion pressure was maintained at 80–90 mmHg. Control kidneys were perfused under the same conditions, without any preliminary storage period. Two kidney perfusions were always run concurrently. Function of the kidney was assessed by addition of ^{3}H-inulin (5 μc in 2 mg) to the perfusate and serial (10-min) collection of urine and plasma for the estimation of sodium, potassium, and ^{3}H radioactivity. Both plasma and urine protein were determined with the Biuret method.

For all kidneys the first 10-min specimen of urine was not included in the data because this includes urine in the cannula during the period of cold ischemic storage. The proteinuria data is based on the average of the five subsequent urine specimens. Functional parameters (inulin clearance, U/P inulin ratio, and percentage of sodium reabsorption) are the average of the best two values attained during the normothermic perfusion. These are obtained during the last 20 min of the normothermic perfusion of preserved kidneys. Means ± SEM are given throughout. The groups of data are compared using Wilcoxon's rank sum test.

After perfusion both preserved and control kidneys were immersion fixed by 1.25% gluteraldehyde in 0.1 M phosphate buffer and prepared for light and electron microscopy. Some preserved kidneys were prepared for morphological study, directly after preservation, without isolated kidney perfusion.

RESULTS

After 24 hr cold preservation, renal function was reduced during isolated organ perfusion in comparison with control kidneys (Tables 1 and 2). Glomerular filtration rate (inulin clearance) and percentage of Na reabsorption were reduced in

[1] This work was supported by grants from the National Health and Medical Research Council and the Monash University Special Fund.

[2] From the Department of Pathology, University of Melbourne.

[3] To whom correspondence and requests for reprints should be addressed, at the Department of Surgery, Prince Henry's Hospital, St. Kilda Road, Melbourne, Victoria, 3004, Australia.

TABLE 1. Renal function after isolated kidney perfusion following 24-hr cold preservation

Rat strain	SD	DA	SD	DA
Storage method	Ice	Ice	4°C perfusion	4°C perfusion
GFR (ml/min)	0.34±0.04	0.19±0.05	0.51±0.04	0.12±0.03
% Na reabsorption	53.5±2.1	63.4±3.9	58.9±2.3	63.5±3.0
Protein output (mg/hr)	465±73	224±51	711±78	168±29
Filtered fraction of protein	0.57±0.05	0.49±0.04	0.49±0.03	0.61±0.05
Number of experiments	15	7	21	8

TABLE 2. Proteinuria and renal function in isolated control kidneys perfused at 37°C

Rat strain	DA	SD
GFR (ml/min)	0.65±0.11	0.65±0.14
% Na reabsorption	97.6±1.1	98.1±0.4
Protein output (mg/hr)	17.0±12.0	14.0±5.0
Filtered fraction of protein	0.009±0.004	0.009±0.005
Number of experiments	5	4

TABLE 3. Proteinuria and renal function in 4-hr-preserved ice-stored kidneys perfused at 37°C

Rat strain	DA	SD
GFR (ml/min)	0.49±0.09	0.49±0.06
% Na reabsorption	96.3±0.9	97.3±0.7
Protein output (mg/hr)	25.0±5.0[a]	56.0±15.0
Filtered protein	0.017±0.004[a]	0.042±0.006
Number of experiments	4	6

[a] $P<0.01$, comparing DA and SD-preserved kidneys.

kidneys obtained from both SD and DA rats, and inulin clearance was significantly ($P<0.01$) lower in DA than in SD kidneys. The method of preservation, static or perfusion, did not affect function except in kidneys from SD rats, in which perfusion preservation significantly improved glomerular filtration rate.

Proteinuria was greater in SD than DA kidneys but this may have been influenced by their higher glomerular filtration rates. The filtered fraction of protein was not significantly affected by the strain of rat or method of preservation.

Renal function during isolated kidney perfusion after 4 hr cold preservation (Table 3) was much less impaired than after 24 hr; values for GFR and percentage of Na reabsorption were not significantly different from control values—but, while proteinuria was much less severe, it was increased over control values, although the increase was not statistically significant for DA kidneys.

On light microscopy there were striking changes in 24-hr-cold–preserved rat kidneys following isolated organ perfusion. Bowman's spaces and adjoining proximal convoluted tubule lumens were filled with protein (bovine serum albumin) (Fig. 1). Protein was also found in the distal nephron. The accumulation of protein in tubular lumens was more severe in SD than DA rats, but even in this strain was focal rather than diffuse, affecting some groups of glomeruli and tubules and not others.

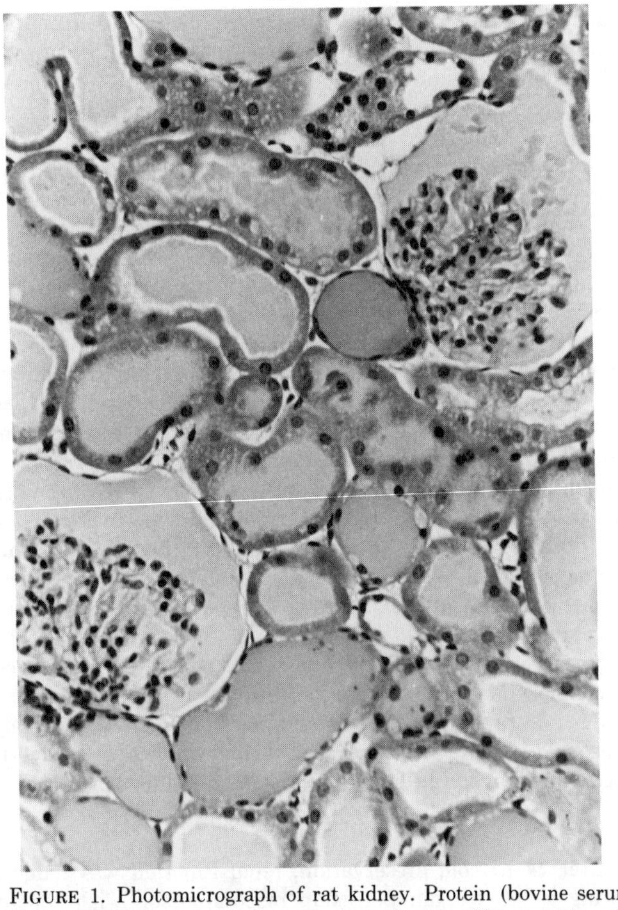

FIGURE 1. Photomicrograph of rat kidney. Protein (bovine serum albumin) fills Bowman's spaces and tubular lumens; SD rat, 24 hr cold perfusion preservation, isolated kidney perfusion (H&E × 250).

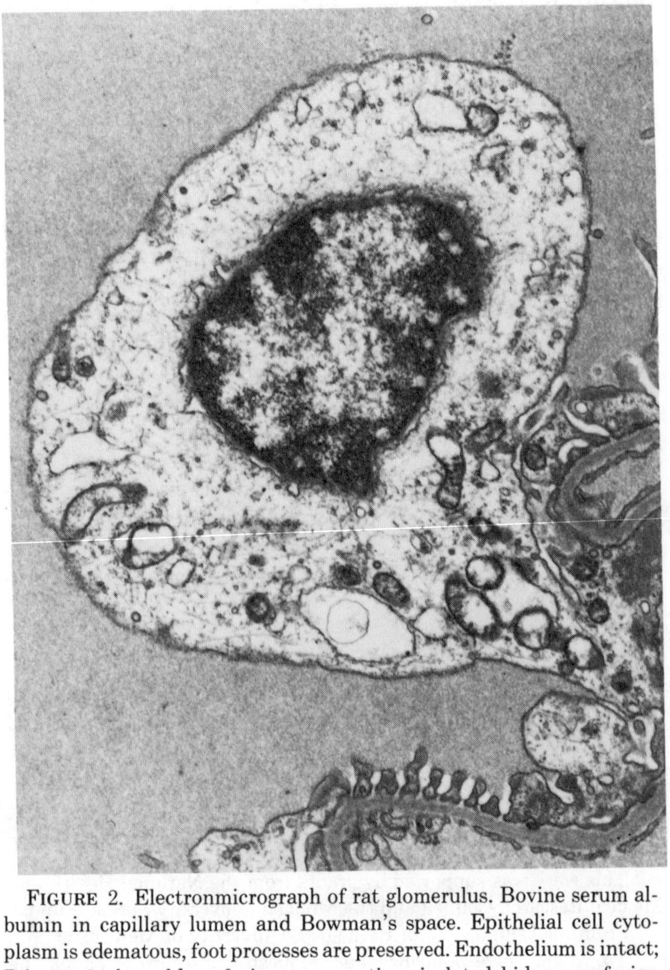

FIGURE 2. Electronmicrograph of rat glomerulus. Bovine serum albumin in capillary lumen and Bowman's space. Epithelial cell cytoplasm is edematous, foot processes are preserved. Endothelium is intact; DA rat, 24 hr cold perfusion preservation, isolated kidney perfusion (×11,000).

Some glomerular epithelial cells had swollen vacuolated cytoplasm, but tubular morphology was generally well preserved with the epithelium of the thick ascending limb free of lysosomal droplets. Neither the strain nor the method of preservation affected the histological appearances of preserved kidneys after isolated kidney perfusion. Protein was not present in tubule lumens of preserved kidneys not subjected to isolated organ perfusion; protein was present in Bowman's space after perfusion preservation but not after cold storage.

After 4 hr cold preservation followed by isolated kidney perfusion protein was again found in tubule lumens in both cortex and medulla, but in smaller amounts than at 24 hr. Only an occasional glomerulus had protein in Bowman's space. On electron microscopy particular attention was paid to glomeruli with protein in Bowman's space.

After 24 hr cold preservation and isolated kidney perfusion visceral glomerular epithelial cell cytoplasm was swollen and cell organelles and fibrils widely separated (Fig. 2). In some cells endoplasmic reticulum was widely dilated (Fig. 3), and in others large membrane lined spaces were present within cell outlines (Fig. 4). Other cells showed extensive microvillus formation (Fig. 5). Foot processes were largely intact but when the whole of a sectioned glomerulus was examined occasional cells or processes had become separated from capillary basement membrane (Fig. 3). Sometimes this change was found in

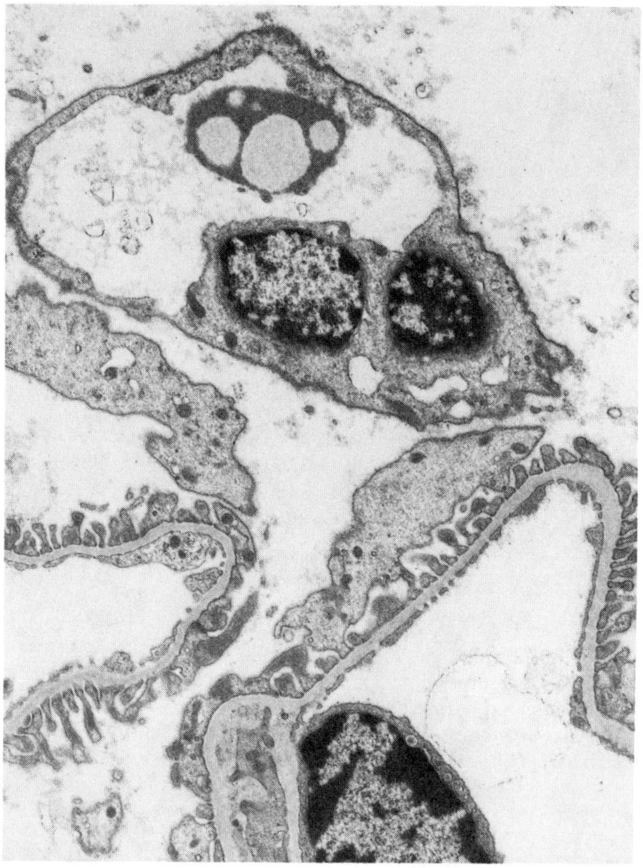

FIGURE 4. Electronmicrograph of rat glomerulus. There is a large membrane-bound space within the outlines of the glomerular epithelial cell. This contains an inclusion body. Foot processes and endothelium are preserved; SD rat, 24 hr cold perfusion preservation, isolated kidney perfusion (×6000).

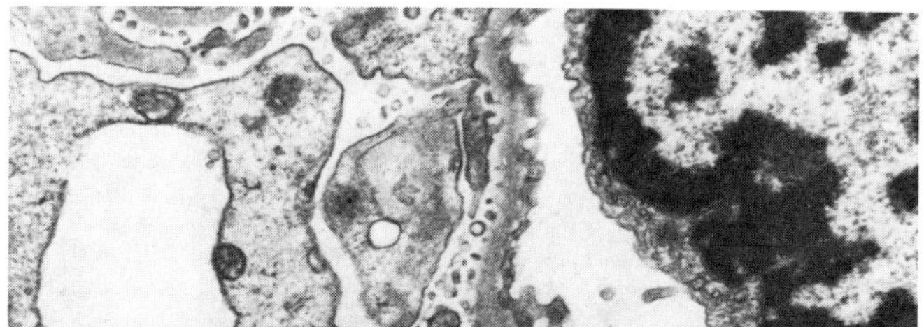

FIGURE 3. Electronmicrograph of rat glomerulus. The endoplasmic reticulum of the visceral epithelial cells is dilated. In the area where foot processes have become detached from capillary basement membrane there is extensive microvillus formation; SD rat, 24 hr cold perfusion preservation, isolated kidney perfusion (×12,500).

a number of capillaries (Fig. 6). The cell membranes retained their affinity for colloidal iron (Fig. 7), even when the cell processes were separated from capillary basement membranes (Fig. 8). However, bound bovine serum albumin may have contributed to the staining reactions of the damaged cell.

Endothelial cells were usually normal in appearance, but in some glomeruli endothelial cells showed compacted electron-dense cytoplasm (Fig. 6). There was microvillus formation and the endothelial fenestrae were irregular in size and pattern distribution over the capillary basement membrane. Axial cells and glomerular basement membranes were normal.

Similar appearances were shown by glomerular epithelial and endothelial cells in 24-hr-preserved kidneys not subjected to isolated kidney perfusion.

In glomeruli from kidneys preserved for 4 hr and then perfused, the epithelial cells showed only minimal cytoplasmic swelling. Foot processes were preserved. Even in glomeruli with albumin in Bowman's space, electron microscopy of the whole section failed to show epithelial cell detachment.

The ultrastructure of glomeruli from isolated perfused control kidneys was normal.

DISCUSSION

These experiments indicate that glomeruli from rat kidneys preserved for experimental renal transplantation show increased permeability to bovine serum albumin during isolated

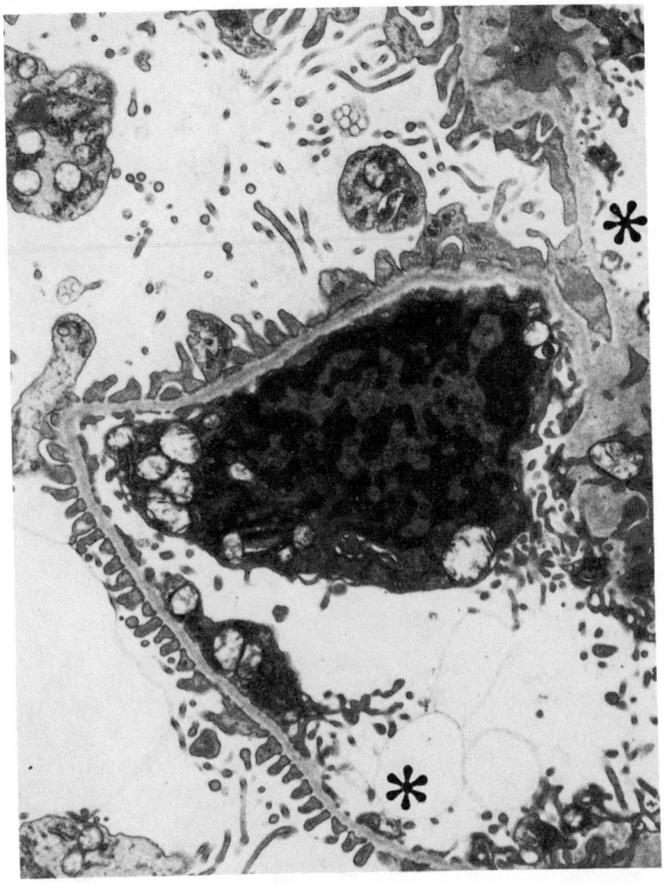

FIGURE 5. Electronmicrograph of rat glomerulus. Both endothelial and epithelial cells show extensive microvillus formation. Endothelial fenestrae are irregularly distributed over the capillary basement membrane (*); DA rat, 24 hr cold perfusion preservation, isolated kidney perfusion (×7000).

organ perfusion. At 24 hr protein loss in the urine was greater in SD than in DA kidneys but this probably reflects the lower GFR recorded in the DA kidney rather than any difference in glomerular permeability to protein. The severity of the proteinuria appeared to be related to the duration rather than the method of preservation (ice storage or cold perfusion), and it was very much greater after 24 hr than after 4 hr.

Protein loss after 24 hr was associated with changes in glomerular visceral epithelial cells. These consisted of cell swelling, microvillus formation and detachment of epithelium from capillary basement membranes. Foot processes were preserved and surface sialoglycoprotein staining retained even in the presence of epithelial cell detachment. Endothelial cell abnormalities were present in some glomeruli but increased glomerular permeability to bovine serum albumin occurred in the absence of glomerular endothelial cell lesions. The glomerular epithelial and endothelial cell changes can be seen after cold preservation alone and like the proteinuria, appear to be related to the duration of the preservation rather than to the method used. Moreover, proteinuria is present during isolated organ perfusion of kidneys stored in solutions free of colloid (Jablonski P, unpublished data). The appearances in preserved glomeruli are different from those recorded after warm renal ischemia with reflow (*5*) and similar appearances have been described after preservation by Andrews and Coffey (*1*); glomerular epithelial cell swelling, but not the endothelial cell changes, were prevented by the use of hypertonic preservation solutions (*1*). This is probably only a cosmetic effect, and tends to mask the underlying biochemical changes that attract water into the cell. The ultimate viability of glomerular cells, and of kidney cells generally, is shown by isograft survival figures after 24 hr preservation of 70% for SD rats and 100% for DA rats. Some rats with renal isografts, however, have appreciable proteinuria at one month (*4*). It is perhaps pertinent that rats with experimental myxedema also show extreme swelling of glomerular epithelial cytoplasm with preservation of foot processes (*6*).

One other factor probably contributes to the morphological changes in the glomerular epithelial cell. Spontaneous glomerular epithelial cell lesions, consisting of cystic malformations and droplet accumulation have been reported in rats from different laboratories (*7, 8*). The lesions are more prominent in older rats and are eventually associated with albuminuria and focal glomerulosclerosis (*9, 10*). These spontaneous lesions are found in a variety of strains but are more prevalent in some strains than others. The lesions are more obvious in perfusion fixed kidneys and under these circumstances may be demonstrated in rats 3 months old (*4*). The appearances of the lesion are identical with some of the epithelial cell lesions described in experimental models of glomerular disease, such as remnant

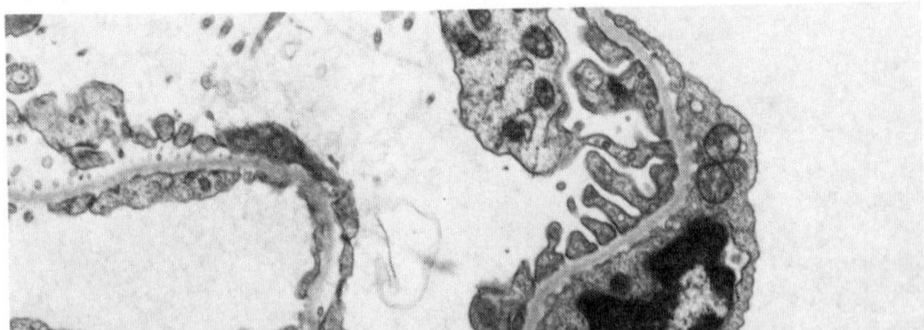

FIGURE 6. Electronmicrograph of rat glomerulus. There is extensive detachment of visceral epithelial cells and foot processes from some capillary walls but not from others. Endothelium shows minor damage; DA rat, 24 hr cold perfusion preservation (×7000).

nephropathy (*11*), overload proteinuria (*12*), and aminonucleoside nephrosis (*12*).

It is possible that enhanced filterability of bovine serum albumin (*13*) and increased perfusate flow to the glomerulus during isolated kidney perfusion might both make a significant extra contribution to protein loss in the presence of increased glomerular permeability. However, in this experiment, the major factor is likely to be the altered glomerular permeability—and, after 24 hr, this is associated with changes in the visceral glomerular epithelial cell. Protein appears in Bowman's space external to epithelial cells with intact foot processes and demonstrable sialoglycoprotein. However, elsewhere in the same glomerulus, epithelial cells have separated from glomerular basement membrane. Ryan and Karnovsky (*14*) have demonstrated focal loss of protein across the glomerular capillaries at these sites, and Alcorn and Ryan (*15*) have stressed the importance of such focal lesions as the principal determinant of glomerular proteinuria.

There appears to be considerable merit in this position, but it does embrace the corollary proposition that impaired function in the epithelial cell does not affect glomerular permeability until the cell is actually detached from the basement membrane. Stolte et al. (*16*) have shown that glomerular permeability is increased eightfold in the isolated perfused kidney in the absence of ultrastructural changes, and there is a further increase in glomerular permeability after 4 hr cold preservation and isolated kidney perfusion. This further increase also occurs

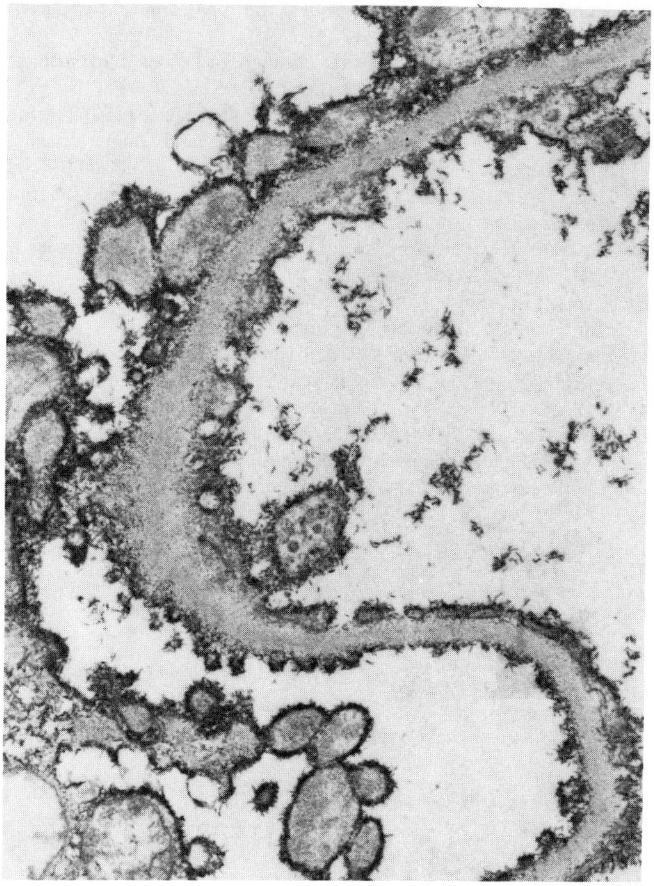

FIGURE 8. Electronmicrograph of rat glomerulus. Epithelial cells are detached from capillary basement membrane. Both detached epithelial cells and the endothelium show positive staining for sialoglycoprotein. DA rat, 24 hr cold perfusion preservation, isolated kidney perfusion (×18,000).

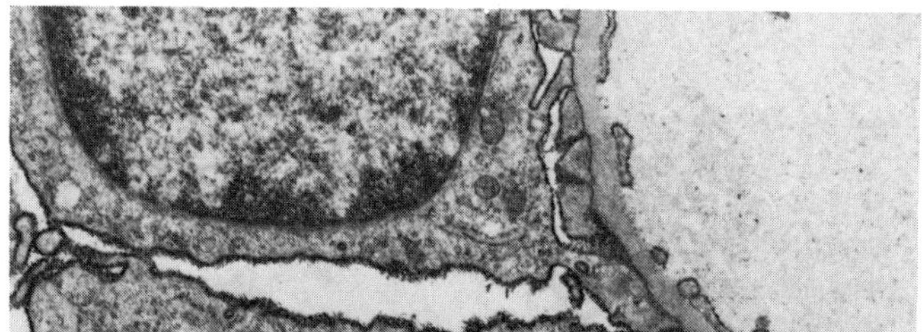

FIGURE 7. Electronmicrograph of rat glomerulus. Intact epithelial cells show positive staining for sialoglycoprotein; SD rat, 24 hr cold perfusion preservation, isolated kidney perfusion (×10,000).

in the absence of obvious ultrastructural glomerular changes. This suggests that both general and local factors may contribute to increased glomerular permeability. It should be possible, using graduated periods of glomerular preservation and isolated kidney perfusion, to sharply localize the onset of severe proteinuria and to define the nature of these associated glomerular lesions. This possibility is being actively investigated.

This research has demonstrated that damage to glomeruli can develop during preservation for renal transplantation. The lesions are partly reversible and do not affect isograft survival, but represent a further identifiable and potential complication of renal transplantation.

REFERENCES

1. Andrews PM, Coffey AK. Factors that improve the preservation of nephron morphology during cold storage. Lab Invest 1982; 46: 100.
2. Jablonski P, Howden BD, Rae DA, Birrell SC, Marshall VC, Tange J. An experimental model for assessment of renal recovery from warm ischaemia. Transplantation 1983; 35: 198.
3. Howden B, Rae D, Jablonski P, Marshall VC, Tange JD. Studies of renal preservation using a rat kidney transplant model. Evaluation of citrate flushing. Transplantation 1983; 35: 311.
4. Lambert R, Carroll N, Henry M, et al. Glomerular epithelial cell lesions in renal isografts. Pathol, in press.
5. Barnes JL, Osgood RW, Reineck J, Stein JH. Glomerular altera-

tions in an ischaemic model of acute renal failure. Lab Invest 1981; 45: 378.
6. Green CR, Ham KN, Tange JD. Glomerular lesions in experimental hypothyroidism. Arch Pathol 1974; 98: 156.
7. Kraus B, Cain H. Über eine spontane Nephropathie bei Wistarratten. Die licht-und elektronenmikroskopischen Glomerulumveränderungen. Virchows Arch [Pathol Anat] 1974; 363: 343.
8. Haley DP, Bulger RE. The ageing male rat: structure and function of the kidney. Am J Anat 1983; 167: 1.
9. Hirokawa H. Characterisation of age-associated kidney disease in Wistar rats. Mech Ageing Dev 1975; 4: 301.
10. Elema TD, Arends A. Focal and segmental glomerular hyalinosis and sclerosis in the rat. Lab Invest 1975; 33: 554.
11. Shimamura T, Morrison AB. A progressive glomerulosclerosis occurring in partial five-sixths nephrectomized rats. Am J Pathol 1975; 79: 95.
12. Lawrence GM, Brewer DB. A morphometric, biochemical and histochemical comparison of puromycin aminonucleoside and hyperalbuminaemic induced proteinuria in the female Wistar rat. J Pathol 1983; 139: 115.
13. Lawrence GM, Brewer DB. Glomerular ultrafiltration and tubular reabsorption of bovine serum albumin and derivatives with increased negative charge in the normal female Wistar rat. Clin Sci 1984; 66: 47.
14. Ryan GB, Karnovsky MJ. An ultrastructural study of the mechanisms of proteinuria in aminonucleoside nephrosis. Kidney Int 1975; 8: 219.
15. Alcorn D, Ryan CB. Distribution of anionic groups in the glomerular capillary wall in rat nephrotoxic nephritis and aminonucleoside nephrosis. Pathology 1981; 13: 37.
16. Stolte H, Schurek HJ, Alt JM. Glomerular albumin filtration: a comparison of micropuncture studies in the isolated perfusion rat kidney with in vivo experimental conditions. Kidney Int 1979; 16: 377.

Received 10 September 1985.
Accepted 11 November 1985.

0041-1337/86/4202-0130$02.00/0
TRANSPLANTATION Vol. 42, No. 2

Printed in U.S.A.

HEPATOCYTE TRANSPLANTATION FOR ENZYME DEFICIENCY DISEASE IN CONGENIC RATS

J. P. A. M. VROEMEN,[1,2] W. A. BUURMAN,[1] K. P. M. HEIRWEGH,[3] C. J. VAN DER LINDEN,[1] AND G. KOOTSTRA[1]

Department of Surgery, Biomedical Center, Annadal Hospital, University of Limburg, 6201 BX Maastricht, The Netherlands; and Department of Medical Reseach, University of Leuven, B-3000 Leuven, Belgium

Long-term effects of hepatocyte transplantation (HTX) in the treatment of enzyme deficiency disease were studied. Congenic enzyme-deficient (R/APfd-j/j) and non-enzyme-deficient (R/APfd) rats were used as recipients and donors, respectively. The R/APfd-j/j rat strain is congenitally deficient of bilirubin uridyldiphosphate (UDP)-glucuronyl transferase.

R/APfd-j/j rats underwent HTX by intrasplenic injection of 10^7 isolated R/APfd hepatocytes (group 1A). Another group of R/APfd-j/j rats was treated similarly, but underwent splenectomy after 11 weeks (group 1B). Controls consisted of R/APfd-j/j rats grafted with 10^7 R/APfd-j/j hepatocytes (group 2), and R/APfd-j/j rats that underwent a sham operation (group 3).

Total plasma bilirubin (TB) levels were significantly reduced in groups 1A and 1B during the experiment (both $P<0.01$). In the control groups TB reduction was not observed. Bile analyses at 30 weeks after HTX showed that in group 1A 13.7±2.7% of total biliary bilirubin was conjugated. In group 1B a significantly lower fraction was conjugated: 6.6±1.1% ($P<0.05$). Conjugated bilirubin was not found in bile of groups 2 and 3. Histology showed survival of hepatocytes in all spleens of rats of groups 1A, 1B and 2.

It is concluded that congenic hepatocytes from R/APfd donors are not rejected after transplantation into the R/APfd-j/j rat, and maintain long-term function. Splenectomy does not abolish, but does reduce, the therapeutic effect significantly, indicating that part of the transplanted hepatocytes maintains function in the enzyme-deficient host liver. The congenic R/APfd-j/j and R/APfd rat strains represent a new animal model for research in metabolic deficiency disease.

Experimental hepatocyte transplantation (HTX)* is receiving increasing attention as a possible treatment for acute hepatic failure or enzyme deficiency disease. This therapeutic approach is based on the assumption that grafted hepatocytes provide metabolic support for deficient hepatic function(s) (*1–8*).

Received 6 August 1985.
Accepted 14 November 1985.
[1] University of Limburg, The Netherlands.
[2] Address correspondence to: J.P.A.M. Vroemen, Department of Surgery, Annadal Hospital, P.O. Box 1918, 6201 BX Maastricht, The Netherlands.
[3] University of Leuven, Belgium.

* Abbreviations used; BDG, bilirubindiglucuronide; BMG, bilirubinmonoglucuronide; HTX, hepatocyte transplantation; MHC, major histocompatibility complex; PAS, periodic-acid–Schiff; TB, total plasma bilirubin; UDP, uridyldiphosphate.

Previously we showed that the Gunn rat, a rat strain with unconjugated hyperbilirubinemia due to a hereditary absolute deficiency of bilirubin uridyldiphosphate(UDP)-glucuronyl transferase activity, can be treated by intrasplenic hepatocyte transplantation. However, hepatocytes from nondeficient allogeneic donors are rejected by the Gunn rat, which renders the therapeutic effect only transient (*9*). This rejection of allogeneic hepatocytes transplanted into the rat spleen has recently been described in more detail (*10*). The outcome of previous studies raised the question of whether enzyme deficiency disease could be treated with permanent success if nondeficient donor hepatocytes were not rejected. In the experimental situation, transplantation of hepatocytes from congenic nondeficient donors would not only give an answer to this question, but would also provide a unique model for the study of DNA-transfer.

In order to obtain a new animal model to study HTX in the treatment of enzyme deficiency without interference of rejection, the recessive "jaundiced" gene of the GUNNXRPfd-j/j rat was transferred to the non-enzyme-deficient R/APfd rat by eight backcross-intercross cycles. This resulted in the congenic enzyme-deficient R/APfd-j/j strain (j/j stands for homozygously jaundiced).[4]

In the present work we investigated the long-term results of HTX in the enzyme-deficient R/APfd-j/j rat, with special interest in the effects of combined intransplenic and intraportal HTX.

MATERIALS AND METHODS

Animals. Adult R/APfd rats (250–350 g), obtained from the Proefdierencentrum Leuven, University of Leuven, Leuven, Belgium, served as hepatocyte donors. Adult R/APfd-j/j rats (300–350 g), from the same supplier, were used as hepatocyte recipients in all experiments. The latter strain was obtained after 8 backcross-intercross cycles of the R/APfd strain with the GUNNXRPfd-j/j strain. As a result, the genetic material of the R/APfd and R/APfd-j/j strains is identical, with the exception of the homozygous "jaundiced" gene in the R/APfd-j/j rat, and possibly a few genes belonging to the same linkage group 2. The major histocompatibility complex (MHC) determining genes are situated on linkage group 9. Consequently, the R/APfd and R/APfd-j/j strains (hereafter referred to as R/A and R/A-j/j strain, respectively) are congenic and histocompatible.[4]

Hepatocyte transplantation. Isolation of hepatocytes was performed by a modification of the two-step perfusion technique of Seglen (*11*). After cannulation of the portal vein, the liver was perfused with approximately 250 ml Ca^{++}-free Krebs-Henseleit solution at a flow rate of 20–25 ml/min. The perfusion was gassed with a mixture of O_2 and CO_2 (95:5), and kept constantly at 38°C at a pH of 7.4–7.5. During this perfusion the liver was excised without damaging the liver capsule. Subsequently, perfusion was started with a 0.05% collagenase (type IV, Sigma Chemicals, St. Louis, MO) and 5 mM Ca^{++}-ion containing Krebs-Henseleit solution. After 10 min of collagenase digestion, the swollen liver was disconnected from the perfusion apparatus, and the capsule was removed, thus freeing the isolated liver cells. This initial cell suspension was filtered through a 100-μm nylon sieve to eliminate cell clusters and connective tissue debris, and washed three times at 0–4°C. The cells were then counted and resuspended in Krebs-Henseleit solution containing 10 mg/ml fatty-acid-free bovine serum albumine (Sigma Chemicals, St. Louis, MO) to a concentration of 10^7 viable cells/ml. Cell viability was assessed by the trypan blue exclusion test, and ranged from 85% to 95%. Within 1 hr to 3 hr after hepatocyte isolation, 1 ml of the cell suspension (kept on ice) was injected into the spleen of the recipient rat in 30 sec. Hilar vessels of the spleen were not clamped. During the intrasplenic injection, suspension was observed flowing off via the splenic veins into the portal vein. In this way, combined intrasplenic and intraportal HTX was performed. Leakage of cell suspension and blood loss was minimized by tamponade of the injection site with a cotton-tip. Ether anesthesia was given to all animals undergoing the operation.

Experimental protocol. The experimental groups were divided as follows:

Group 1A: 14 R/A-j/j rats receiving 10^7 R/A hepatocytes
Group 1B: 8 R/A-j/j rats receiving 10^7 R/A hepatocytes, and undergoing splenectomy at 11 weeks post-HTX
Control groups were as follows
Group 2: 11 R/A-j/j rats receiving 10^7 R/A-j/j hepatocytes
Group 3: 12 R/A-j/j rats undergoing a sham operation (i.e., intrasplenic injection 1 ml Krebs-Henseleit solution)

Blood sampling and measurement of total body weight took place 3 days before HTX, on day 3 post-HTX, weekly till week 4, and at larger intervals till the end of the experiment at 30 weeks. Total plasma bilirubin (TB) level and hematocrit were determined in each blood sample. Blood samples, obtained at 30 weeks post-HTX, were also examined for the presence of bilirubin glucuronides. During the last weeks of the experiment 24-hr urine collections from the animals were obtained for assay on conjugated bilirubin. At the end of the experiment all animals were provided with a bile fistula. In all bile samples concentrations of bilirubin monoglucuronide (BMG), bilirubin di-glucuronide (BDG), and total bilirubin, were determined. After bile collection the animals were sacrificed. From each animal tissue specimens were obtained from spleen, liver, and right lung for histological examination.

Sampling procedures. Blood sampling was performed by paraorbital venipuncture under ether anesthesia, and 24-hr urine samples were obtained by housing the animals in metabolic cages. For bile collection the common bile duct was cannulated with silicone tubing. A bile fistula was created by exteriorizing this silicone cannula at the neck of the animal. This procedure succeeded in 13 (of 14) rats in group 1A, 6 (of 8) rats in group (1B), 9 (of 11) in group 2, and in 11 (of 12) in group 3. Failures in bile sampling were due to technical problems. Rats were allowed to recover from anesthesia before commencement of bile collection. During this collection (3 hr) rats were able to eat and drink, and to move freely in their cages. Bile was collected in tubes on ice in the semidark.

Analytical methods. Determination of TB levels was performed by spectrophotometry (Americal Optical Bilirubinometer, type 10211, Buffalo, NY). Serum, urine, and bile samples were examined for the presence of BMG and BDG, using the highly sensitive alkaline methanolysis method combined with high-pressure liquid chromatography, as described by Muraca and Blanckaert (*12*). This method allows specific detection of

[4] Leyten R, Vroemen JPAM, Blanckaert N, Heirwegh KPM. The congenic normal R/APfd and jaundiced R/APfd-j/j rat strains: a new animal model of hereditary nonhaemolytic unconjugated hyperbilirubinaemia due to defective bilirubin conjugation. (manuscript submitted for publication). R. Leyten is Director of Proefdierencentrum (Laboratory Animal Center), University of Leuven, de Croylaan 34, B-3030 Heverlee, Belgium.

small concentrations of BMG and BDG in the presence of unconjugated bilirubin (limits of detection 10 nM and 20 nM, respectively).

Histology. Spleen, liver, and lung tissue were fixed in 10% buffered formaldehyde, and embedded in paraffin. Histological examination of spleen, liver, and lung tissue was performed on routine 6-μm tissue sections, stained with hematoxylin and eosin (H&E) and by the periodic acid Schiff (PAS) procedure.

Statistical analysis. Comparison of TB levels and total body weight between the experimental groups was performed by repeated measures analysis of variance (two-factor mixed design), completed by post-hoc F-tests (*13*). For comparison between groups of bile analyses results and liver and spleen weights, the Mann-Whitney *U* test was used. Data within the same group were compared by means of the Wilcoxon rank test.

RESULTS

Assessment of graft function. TB levels (mean ± SEM) of the groups are shown in Figure 1. In groups 1A and 1B, the jaundiced enzyme-deficient rats transplanted with hepatocytes from congenic nondeficient donors, the course of TB levels had a biphasic appearance. During the first week a significant TB decrease was observed in these groups compared with the pre-HTX TB levels ($P<0.05$). Thereafter, TB returned to pretransplant levels. From week 6 onward a gradual decrease in TB was observed in both groups. Splenectomy in the animals of group 1B at 11 weeks post-HTX did not result in a rise of TB levels. This suggested that donor hepatocytes were functioning not only in the spleen but also in the liver. At the end of the experiment, both groups 1A and 1B demonstrated a statistically significant reduction of TB in comparison to pre-HTX values (both $P<0.01$). Mean TB was reduced from 154±4.5 μM to 123±4.3 μM in group 1A, and from 147±4.1 μM to 122±5.1 μM in group 1B. Jaundiced rats receiving enzyme-deficient hepatocytes or undergoing sham-treatment (groups 2 and 3, respectively), did not exhibit a decrease in TB levels. Both control groups showed a transient TB increase in the immediate post-transplant period. This phenomenon, observed before in jaundiced rats treated with liver cells from jaundiced donors (*9*), is most likely caused by increased bilirubin formation and/or additonal impairment of bilirubin excretory pathways after surgical trauma or infection.

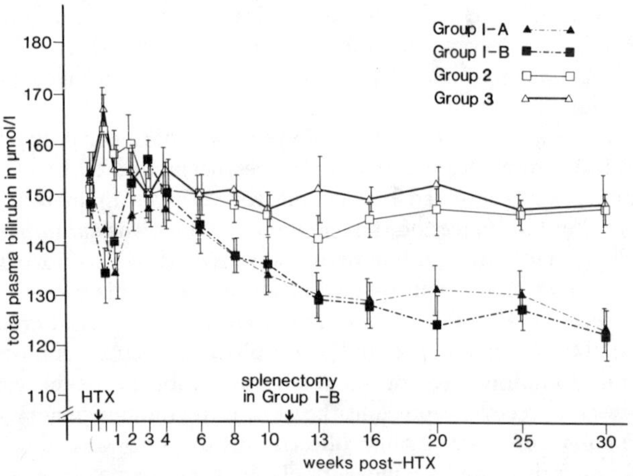

FIGURE 1. TB levels (mean ± SEM) during the experiment. Repeated measures analysis of variance demonstrated a significantly different course of TB change between the groups during the experiment ($F[1.61]=2.06$; $P<0.005$). Groups 1A vs. 1B and groups 2 vs. 3 did not differ significantly during the experiment (post-hoc F test; both $P>0.2$). The differences between groups 1A and 2, 1A and 3, 1B and 2, and 1B and 3 were statistically significant ($P<0.01$, $P<0.005$, $P<0.005$, and $P<0.001$, respectively).

Anemia due to frequent blood sampling was ruled out as a cause of reduced bilirubin formation and subsequent TB reduction. Hematocrits did not differ significantly between groups during the experiment and remained constant (range 0.45–0.52).

TB reduction caused by the presence of bilirubin UDP-glucuronlytransferase activity after transplantation with hepatocytes from nondeficient donors should imply the formation of bilirubin glucuronides. Biliary excretion of bilirubin glucuronides was demonstrated in all bile specimens from enzyme-deficient rats treated with nondeficient donor hepatocytes (groups 1A and 1B) at week 30. In group 1A 13.7 ± 2.7% (mean ± SEM) of biliary bilirubin was conjugated (range 5.3%–42.4%), with a mean biliary concentration of bilirbuin glucuronides of 1.95 μM. The mean biliary excretion of conjugated bilirubin in this group amounted to 6.9×10^{-4} μmol/100 g b.wt./hr. In group 1B (treatment identical to that of group 1A, plus splenectomy at week 11) the mean conjugated fraction of total biliary bilirubin was significantly smaller ($P<0.05$): 6.6±1.1% (range 4.6%–11.8%), the mean biliary concentration of bilirubin glucuronides being 1.07 μM. The mean biliary excretion of conjugated bilirubin was 3.6×10^{-4} μmol/100 g b.wt./hr. BMG exceeded BDG excretion in both groups 1A and 1B (both $P<0.05$). In group 1A BMG and BDG constituted 8.8±1.4% and 4.9±1.4%, respectively, of total biliary bilirubin. For group 1B these values were 5.6±1.0% and 1.0±0.1%. In bile from groups 2 and 3 bilirubin glucuronides were not found. These findings provided unequivocal evidence that transplantation of congenic nondeficient hepatocytes results in the persisting activity of the congenitally deficient enzyme in the host. The results of the bile analyses are summarized in Figure 2.

In serum of treated animals, conjugated bilirubin was virtually absent; at 30 weeks, when TB reduction was most significant, traces of conjugated bilirubin were found in only one animal of group 1A (200 nM BMG and 100 nM BDG) and in one animal of group 1B (400 nM BMG and 540 nM BDG). As expected, conjugated bilirubin was not found in serum samples of groups 2 and 3. Very low concentrations of unconjugated bilirubin were found in urine of jaundiced rats (range 0–540 nM). Only in one rat of group 1A was conjugated bilirubin detected (60 nM BMG and 30 nM BDG).

Total body weight. Statistically significant differences among the groups in weight gain were not observed. Considering normal weight gain as an important parameter for the overall state of health in rats, this finding is of importance.

Observations at autopsy. At autopsy attention was primarily focused on spleen and liver. Because of the theoretical possibility of migration of donor hepatocytes via the hepatic veins into the pulmonary vascular bed, lung tissue was also histologically studied. In all animals the peritoneal cavity was examined for the presence of ectopic liver tissue, but signs of inoculation of hepatocytes on the peritoneum were not found.

Spleen: The spleens of all rats that received donor hepatocytes—groups 1A, 1B, and 2—looked remarkably different from the spleens of the sham-operated animals of group 3, which had a normal macroscopic appearance. Spleens in groups 1A, and 2 (having received hepatocytes from normal and deficient

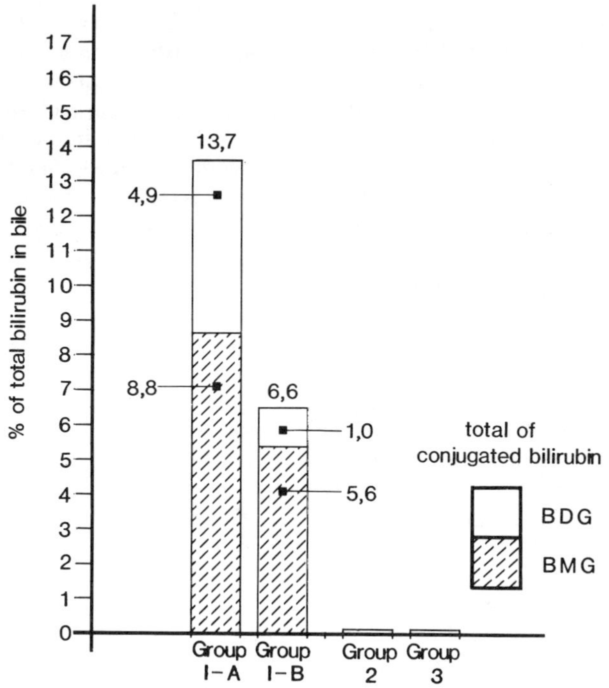

FIGURE 2. Results of the bile analyses. Conjugated bilirubin was only observed in group 1A and group 1B. The quantity of conjugated bilirubin is expressed as the percentage of total bilirubin in bile. Mean percentages are given. Formation of bilirubin glucuronides was more pronounced in group 1A than in group 1B ($P<0.05$). In both groups the formation of BMG exceeded that of BDG (both $P<0.05$).

TABLE 1. Liver and spleen weights at autopsy

	Liver weight[a]	Spleen weight[b]
Group 1A	12.117±667	252±15
Group 1B	12.193±417	470±14[c]
Group 2	13.251±584	295±14
Group 3	12.796±423	416±18

[a] Liver weights did not differ significantly between groups. All weights are in milligrams; mean values ±SEM are given.

[b] Spleen weights in groups 1A and 2 were significantly lower than in groups 1B and 3 (all $P<0.01$).

[c] Data at splenectomy 11 weeks post-HTX.

donors, respectively) contained white-brown consolidated areas, and were significantly smaller than spleens in group 1B (data at splenectomy 11 weeks post-HTX) or in group 3 (all $P<0.01$) (Table 1). Group 1B spleens were undergoing changes similar to, though less pronounced than, those in group 1A spleens, but were not yet reduced in weight, compared with the sham-operated control rats. Histological examination revealed morphologically intact hepatocytes in all spleens of groups 1A, 1B, and 2. Most cells retained their typical binuclear appearance (Fig. 3). PAS stain demonstrated the presence of glycogen granules in the hepatocyte cytoplasm, indicating the metabolic activity of these cells. Clusters of hepatocytes were dispersed in the red pulp of the spleen. Germinal centers remained intact. Definite histological proof of proliferative activity of transplanted hepatocytes was not observed, although sporadic mitotic figures were found in some animals. In some "hepatized" areas, signs of steatosis were observed (Fig. 4). These degenerative changes of the donor hepatocytes occurred in groups 1A, 1B, and 2.

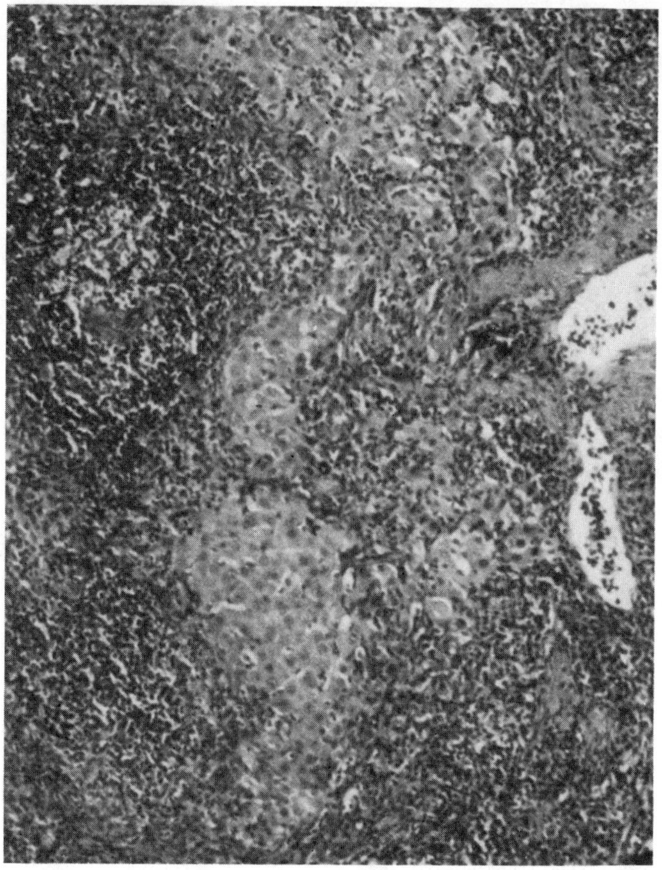

FIGURE 3. Congenic hepatocytes in the host spleen 30 weeks after transplantation (group 1A). Morphologically intact hepatocytes are found in the red pulp. Reconfiguration of the typical hepatic structure was not observed. PAS-positive granules into the cytoplasm of the grafted cells indicate intact glycogen metabolism (PAS, ×50).

Liver: Histological examination of livers did not reveal morphological differences between groups, and showed normal histological features. Grafted hepatocytes could not be distinguished in the recipient livers with the applied histological techniques.

Lung: Hepatocytes were not observed in lung tissue of transplanted rats.

DISCUSSION

Intraportal infusion of nondeficient isolated hepatocytes has been shown to reduce TB levels in the immunosuppressed Gunn rat (*6–8*). The authors of these previous reports suggested that donor hepatocytes provided bilirubin UDP-glucuronyl transferase activity, resulting in the fall of TB. The excretion of bilirubin conjugates, however, was not demonstrated in these studies. As a consequence, the abovementioned theory was not accepted by others, who believed that functional impairment of the reticuloendothelial system by hepatocyte debris caused prolonged red cell survival, reduced bilirubin formation and a subsequent fall in TB (*14*). This possibility seems unlikely, since our previous work provided unequivocal evidence for the formation of bilirubin glucuronides by surviving nondeficient donor hepatocytes in the HTX-treated Gunn rat (*9*). Moreover, here we demonstrate the long-term survival and conjugating capacity of the donor hepatocytes in both spleen and liver of the enzyme-deficient recipient.

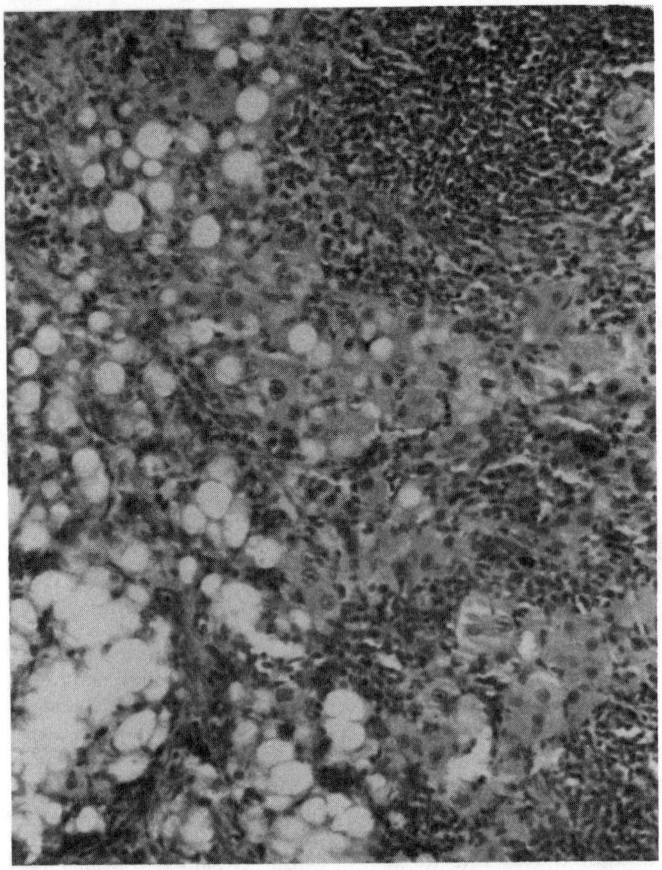

FIGURE 4. Congenic hepatocytes in the host spleen 30 weeks after transplantation (group 1A). In some of the areas of the red pulp populated with transplanted hepatocytes, signs of fatty infiltration of the grafted cells occurred. This degenerative change in hepatocytes is also encountered in liver steatosis (H&E, ×100).

From a physiological point of view, intraportal infusion of hepatocyte suspension would seem the most appropriate way of transplantation, offering the isolated hepatocytes the most physiological environment for nidation: i.e., the liver itself. However, intraportal HTX confronts the investigator with an important drawback: histological monitoring of graft behavior is technically difficult, because the donor hepatocytes cannot be easily distinguished from the host liver cells (*15, 16*). In order to avoid this problem in the study of HTX, another suitable recipient organ for isolated hepatocytes was required. It has been documented in syngeneic normal rats that the spleen may function as such an organ (*15–17*). After injection into the spleen, hepatocytes inoculate and survive in this organ, and even show proliferative activity. In spite of reports about the necessity of "hepatotrophic factors" from portal blood for unimpaired liver cell function (*18*), hepatocytes seem to thrive well in the splenic pulp, and remain biochemically active. Intrasplenic HTX allows routine histological monitoring of graft survival, and facilitates anatomical and cytochemical studies of the grafted cells.

These considerations led us to the conclusion that the optimal technique for HTX consisted of a combined intrasplenic and intraportal route of administration of the hepatocyte suspension. This technique was performed by intrasplenic injection of hepatocytes without clamping of the splenic hilar vessels. During infusion one can actually see the suspension flowing through the splenic veins into the portal circulation. Thus, only a part of the hepatocytes remain in the spleen. In this study the long-lasting metabolic activity of intraportally transplanted hepatocytes was assessed by performing a splenectomy in HTX-treated rats several weeks after the transplantation procedure. After splenectomy, bile of transplanted animals of group 1B still contained bilirubin glucuronides. The quantity of these bilirubin conjugates, however, was only about half of the quantity observed in group 1B. This provides evidence that a portion of the hepatocytes exerts its function in the spleen, and another part does so in the liver.

The fact that bilirubin glucuronides were not detectable in blood samples of rats of groups 1A and 1B (with the exception of 2 animals), but were present in bile of all these animals, seems contradictory at first sight. However, it is known that conjugated bilirubin, after i.v. administration to the congenitally jaundiced rat, is rapidly excreted via the biliary route, with a maximal biliary excretion of 5.75 μmol/100 g b.wt./hr (*19*). The mean biliary excretions of conjugated bilirubin in groups 1A and 1B, respectively, were calculated to be 8.300 and 16.500 times less. Therefore, it is conceivable that all conjugated bilirubin, produced by the nondeficient donor hepatocytes, is immediately excreted into bile of the host, and does not reach detectable concentrations in peripheral blood.

The explanation for the biphasic course of bilirubin levels in groups 1A and 1B is based on the histological data on syngeneic HTX of Kusano and Mito (*15, 16*). At the time of transplantation, virtually all hepatocytes are viable with intact metabolic functions. Approximately one week after transplantation many of the donor hepatocytes undergo necrosis, whereas others suffer cellular damage, rendering them temporarily nonfunctional. This sequence of events would explain the initial, but transient TB decrease in our study. After several weeks donor cells would gradually recover, regain their function, and might even start proliferating. This would account for the gradual fall in TB observed in this study 6 weeks post-HTX.

Our findings at autopsy were largely in accordance with those of other studies, with the exception of steatotic changes in some of the hepatized areas of the spleen after 30 weeks. This observation has not been reported thus far after intrasplenic HTX and is possibly indicative of degenerative changes in the ectopic liver cells, suggesting that the intrasplenic location of donor hepatocytes is not ideal after all. Lung biopsies did not reveal any signs of inoculation of hepatocytes. It is noteworthy in this respect that a recent report described the successful implantation of isolated rat liver cells in the lung parenchyma by infusing the cell suspension into the jugular vein (*20*).

In summary, we may conclude from the present data that the R/APfd-j/j and R/APfd rat strains provide an excellent model for transplantation research in the treatment of enzyme deficiency disease. Congenic hepatocytes from nondeficient R/APfd donors are not rejected after combined intrasplenic and intraportal HTX into the enzyme-deficient R/APfd-j/j rat, and maintain long-term function. This results in the appearance of the missing enzyme activity in the recipient. Splenectomy reduces, but does not abrogate, the therapeutic effect, indicating that part of the transplanted hepatocytes exert their metabolic function in the enzyme-deficient host liver.

In view of these results, HTX from the R/APfd strain to the R/APfd-j/j strain appears to be an excellent model for the study of gene transfer in mammalian cells (*21*). If gene transfer is performed in isolated R/APfd hepatocytes, and these transfected cells are subsequently transplanted to the R/APfd-j/j rat, the appearance of bilirubin glucuronides in the transplanted animal will indicate the functional presence of these grafted cells. Determination of the gene product will demonstrate whether or not the gene transfer has been successful. Another approach to the study of gene transfer is the autotransplantation of hepatocytes from the deficient rat, after transfection has provided the correct genetic information for the production of the missing enzyme. In the latter example, HTX with cells from congenic nondeficient donors may serve as a perfect control for the function of the autologous hepatocytes treated by gene transfer.

Sofar, the application of HTX for enzyme deficiency disease has only been studied in the congenitally juandiced rat. A complete normalization of TB levels has not been obtained by HTX. The required amount of nondeficient hepatocytes is probably too large to ever achieve conjugation of all bilirubin in the recipient. It would, therefore, be interesting to study HTX in a model of enzyme deficiency disease in which only a very small quantity of the missing enzyme activity is required to abolish all manifestations of disease. An example of such disease in the human is phenylketonuria. The presence of 5% of the normally available quantity of phenylalanine hydroxylase (a liver enzyme) would be sufficient for total cure in the phenylketonuric child (*22*). Unfortunately, an animal model of such disease is not available.

We expect that HTX, possibly in combination with gene transfer, will offer perspectives for future clinical use in—as yet—uncurable enzyme deficiency diseases.

Acknowledgments. We thank Mr. G. Michiels (Leuven) and Mr. P. Willems (Maastricht) for technical assistance, Mr. C. Voskamp (Maastricht) for preparing the figures, and Mrs. K. Spronck (Maastricht) for typing the manuscript. Ir. R. Leyten (Leuven) kindly provided the laboratory animals.

REFERENCES

1. Sutherland DER, Numata M, Matas AJ, Simmons RL, Najarian JS. Hepatocellular transplantation in acute liver failure. Surgery 1977; 82: 124.
2. Makowka L, Rotstein LE, Falk RE, et al. Allogeneic and xenogeneic hepatocyte transplantation in experimental hepatic failure. Transplantation 1980; 30: 429.
3. Makowka L, Rotstein LE, Falk RE, et al. Studies into the mechanism of reversal of experimental acute hepatic failure by hepatocyte transplantation. Can J Surg 1981; 24: 39.
4. Minato M, Houssin D, Demma I, et al. Transplantation of hepatocytes for treatment of surgically induced hepatic failure in the rat. Eur Surg Res 1984; 16: 162.
5. Cuervas-Mons V, Cienfuegos JA, Maganto P, et al. Time-related efficacy of liver cell isografts in fulminant hepatic failure. Transplantation 1984; 38: 23.
6. Matas AJ, Sutherland DER, Steffes MW, et al. Hepatocellular transplantation for metabolic deficiencies: decrease of plasma bilirubin in Gunn rats. Science 1976; 192; 892.
7. Sutherland DER, Matas AJ, Steffes MW, Simmons RL, Najarian JS. Transplantation of liver cells in an animal model of congenital enzyme deficiency disease: the Gunn rat. Transplant Proc 1977; 9: 317.
8. Groth CG, Arborgh B, Björken C, Sundberg B, Lundgren G. Correction of hyperbilirubinaemia in the glucuronyl-transferase-deficient rat by intraportal hepatocyte transplantation. Transplant Proc 1977; 9: 313.
9. Vroemen JPAM, Blanckaert N, Buurman WA, Heirwegh KPM, Kootstra G. Treatment of enzyme deficiency by hepatocyte transplantation in rats. J Surg Res 1985; 39: 267.
10. Ebata H, Iwao O, Mito M. Rejection of allogeneic hepatocytes and fetal hepatic tissue transplanted into the rat spleen. Transplantation 1985; 39: 221.
11. Seglen PO. Preparation of isolated rat liver cells. Methods Cell Biol 1976; 13: 29.
12. Muraca M, Blanckaert N. Liquid-chromatographic assay and identification of mono- and diester conjugates of bilirubin in normal serum. Clin Chem 1983; 29: 1767.
13. Bruning JL, Kintz BL. Computational handbook of statistics. 2nd ed. Glenview, Illinois: Scott, Foresman and Company, 1977.
14. Woods RJ, Parbhoo SP. An explanation for the reduction in bilirubin levels in congenitally jaundiced Gunn rats after transplantation of isolated hepatocytes. Eur Surg Res 1981; 13: 278.
15. Kusano M, Mito M. Observations on the fine structure of long-survived isolated hepatocytes inoculated into rat spleen. Gastroenterology 1982; 82: 616.
16. Mito M, Ebata M, Kusano M, Onishi T, Saito T, Sakamoto S. Morphology and function of isolated hepatocytes transplanted into rat spleen. Transplantation 1979; 28: 499.
17. Woods RJ, Fuller BJ, Attenburrow VD, Nutt LH, Hobbs KEF. Functional assessment of hepatocytes after transplantation into rat spleen. Transplantation 1982; 33: 123.
18. Starzl TE, Francavilla A, Halgrimson CG, et al. The origin, hormonal structure and action of hepatotrophic substances in portal venous blood. Surg Gynecol Obstet 1973; 137: 179.
19. Arias LM, Johnson L, Wolfson S. Biliary excretion of injected conjugated and unconjugated bilirubin by normal and Gunn rats. Am J Physiol 1961; 200: 1091.
20. Selden C, Gupta S, Johnstone R, Hodgson HJF. The pulmonary vascular bed as a site for implantation of isolated liver cells in inbred rats. Transplantation 1984; 38: 81.
21. Kucherlapati R, Skoultchi AI. Introduction of purified genes into mammalian cells. CRC Crit Rev Biochem 1984; 16: 349.
22. Bartholomé K. Genetics and biochemistry of the phenylketonuria-present state. Hum Genet 1979; 51: 241.

0041-1337/86/4202-0136$02.00/0
TRANSPLANTATION
Vol. 42, No. 2
Printed in U.S.A.

THE CHYLOESOPHAGEAL FISTULA

A New Approach to Thoracic Duct Drainage[1]

ERIC PAUL MICHAEL WILLIAMSON AND ROBERT A. SELLS

Renal Transplant Unit, Royal Liverpool Hospital, Liverpool L7 8XP, England

The main reason for the virtual abandonment of external thoracic duct drainage as an immunosuppressive measure is not its lack of efficacy, but the time-consuming technical problems of maintaining cannula patency and replacing the large obligatory losses of fluid and protein. In an effort to overcome these problems we have devised a method of diverting thoracic duct lymph internally into the esophagus of the sheep, our hypothesis being that fluid and protein should be resorbed, but lymphocytes and antibodies destroyed. By isolating that part of the venous system into which the thoracic duct drains and anastomosing this conduit to the cervical esophagus a chyloesophageal fistula was created. A mean patency of 19 days was demonstrated radiologically and there was a reproducible peripheral blood lymphopenia of over 50% of preoperative values at 4 weeks. Although plasma albumin levels fell from 37 g/L to 29 g/L at 1 week, they remained stable thereafter. No parenteral fluid or protein was administered, yet the animals remained well with no significant weight loss or overt signs of dehydration or hypoproteinemia. Skin allograft mean survival time was prolonged from 9 to 11.8 days (*P*<0.01).

Since Gowans first demonstrated the immunosuppressive potential of thoracic duct drainage, the technique has been used in man—but, because of technical problems, discomfort for the patient, and high hospital costs, it has not been widely adopted. We describe an experimental technique of internal lymph diversion in the sheep which, if applied in man, might overcome many of the disadvantages while retaining the considerable immunosuppressive potential of lymph diversion.

The physiology of lymphocyte recirculation was elucidated in the late 1950s by Gowans (*1*) and has recently been reviewed by Ford (*2*). Gowans' elegant experiments in rats demonstrated a population of long-lived small lymphocytes recirculating continuously between blood and lymph. He postulated that such cells might be immunologically competent (*3*) and showed not only that skin allograft survival was prolonged in rats depleted of thoracic duct lymph by external drainage (*4*), but also that there was a marked depression of antibody-mediated responses (*5*). These findings have been confirmed in a number of different allograft models in various species (*6–9*).

External thoracic duct drainage was introduced to clinical transplantation by Franksson in 1964 (*10*). Subsequently, a number of workers reported considerably improved graft survival times, fewer rejection episodes and reduced requirements for immunosuppression when using the technique (*11–15*). Some of these authors used no adjunctive immunosuppressive methods for up to 102 days (*11, 12*).

Furthermore, thoracic duct drainage is an effective immunosuppressive procedure for the highly sensitized patient. Starzl and others have successfully transplanted patients whose sera killed 100% of cells in their panel and who also had positive crossmatches with their donor's lymphocytes at the time of the operation (*17–19*). These are important observations, for they afford new opportunities for an increasing number of patients who might otherwise remain untransplantable.

Thoracic duct drainage has also been shown—by Machleder and Paulus, for example—to be of benefit in various autoimmune diseases such as rheumatoid arthritis and systemic lupus erythematosus. These authors also showed a remarkable prolongation of skin allograft survival in man to a mean of 124 days (*20*).

We have conceived a technique that could provide adequate thoracic duct drainage without the disadvantages of an external fistula; in this experiment, we divert the thoracic duct lymph of sheep into the gut and we monitor the immunological events thereafter. We hypothesize that lymphocytes and immunoglobulins should be destroyed by a combination of changes is osmolality and pH and the effects of digestive secretions, and that degradation products and water should be resorbed.

MATERIALS AND METHODS

One-year-old commercially available Welsh mountain and Clun Forest sheep of 25–35 kg were used. Preoperatively they were starved of food for 48 hr and water for 24 hr.

Operative details. All of the operation was carried out under general anesthesia, using full aseptic techniques. The object was to create a chyloesophageal fistula (COF*, group 1) to drain all thoracic duct lymph into the cervical esophagus via an isolated jugular venous conduit (n=14) or a silastic cannula and 3-way tap (n=3). Controls (group 2) were sham operations (n=6) and thoracic duct ligations (n=2).

Originally, a right lateral decubitus position was used, (n=6) but because of difficulties in the mobilization of the great veins a midline approach was adopted (n=8; Fig. 1). This was found to give much improved access to the confluence of the great veins in the root of the neck. The animal was positioned supine and a midline cervical incision made. The sternomandibularis muscles were retracted from the midline and an upper sternal split performed. The jugular vein was mobilized as it joined the brachial vein to form the innominate vein, and these vessels were all carefully cleaned to display the superior vena cava. There was considerable variation in the position of the thoracic duct termination. Although the duct passed behind the jugular vein at a constant point it frequently continued posteriorly for a few centimeters enclosed in the adventitial sheath before its termination so that the feasibility of applying the final tie (Fig.

Received 14 June 1985.
Accepted 15 November 1985.
[1] The Merseyside Association for Kidney Research.

* Abbreviations used: COF, chyloesophageal fistula;

2) to the innominate vein was largely governed by the precise anatomical arrangement. If this crucial tie obstructed the duct, an alternative procedure was employed, the vein being divided and the ends oversewn (Fig. 2). All tributaries of the left jugular and innominate veins were meticulously ligated (Fig. 1). This area was found to be richly supplied with lymph trunks, the most notable being the tracheal lymph trunks draining the head and neck. These arise in a lateral retropharyngel position and run caudally dorsolateral to the trachea. All these lymphatics were either carefully avoided or ligated, as failure to do so resulted in large collections of lymph in the wound. After ligation and division of the jugular vein 10 cm distal to its termination a consistently placed valve was disrupted using a fine nerve hook. When it had been confirmed that lymph was flowing from the vein it was anastomosed to the esophageal mucosa using a continuous fine (5–0) prolene suture. The muscular layers were approximated with one or two sutures, and a silicone cannula (outside diameter 1.3 mm) introduced into the conduit via the stump of a tributary and tied into position, (Figs. 1 and 2), the other end being tunneled to the exterior and secured in place with sutures. The wound was then closed in layers.

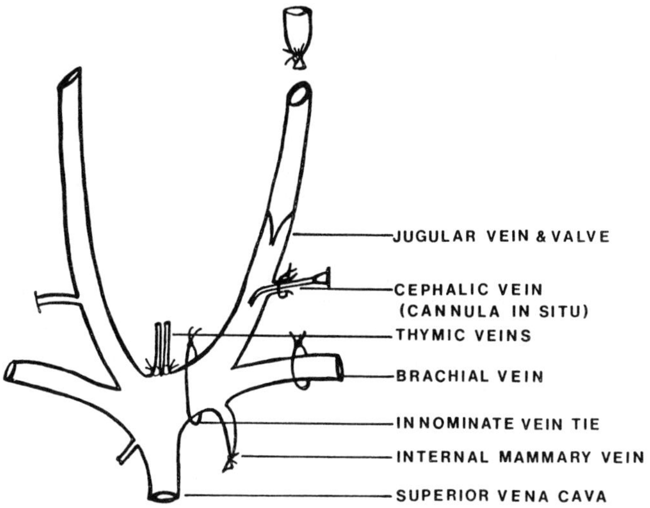

FIGURE 1. Midline approach to the great veins showing the main tributaries requiring ligation.

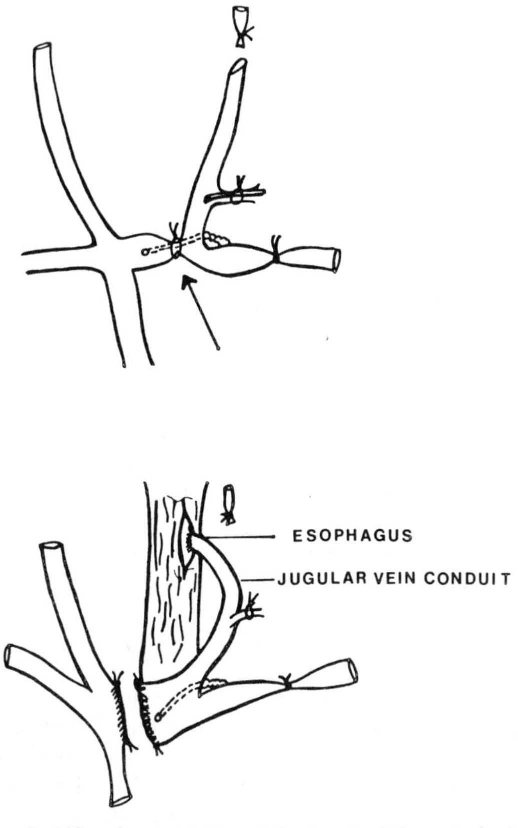

FIGURE 2. (Above) constriction of the terminal thoracic duct by the innominate vein ligature (arrow); (Below) division of the innominate vein at its termination and suture, to avoid obstruction of the thoracic duct.

A third technique was evaluated in which the thoracic duct was cannulated using silicone tubing (outside diameter 1.2 mm) that was brought externally and connected to a 3-way tap. A further length of tubing was connected to this, inserted through a stab wound into the esophagus, and secured with a purse-string suture.

In sham operations (group 2) the esophagus and veins were mobilized as in group 1 but no further procedure carried out (n=6). In two further cases of thoracic duct was ligated.

Postoperatively the sheep were allowed water, ewe and lamb nuts, and salt lick ad libitum. No hay or straw was allowed in order to reduce rumination. At no stage were parenteral infusions administered. The indwelling cannula was flushed at least twice daily with heparinized saline (1000 units in 100 ml).

Orthotopic skin grafts were performed in 15 animals—6 in group 2 and 9 in group 1. Autografts were always applied in conjunction with allografts and acted as controls. Grafts of almost full thickness were cut using a dermatome and applied to similarly prepared sites, either on the forelegs or the flank. Sutures and pressure bandages were used, in the initial stages, to hold them securely in placed.

Rejection was assessed macroscopically and microscopically, and was considered to have occurred when the graft lost its pliancy and became edematous and discolored. None of the allografts survived long enough for a convincing growth of wool to occur, but this did happen with the autografts. At 6 to 7 days both autografts and allografts sometimes became transiently edematous, but they regained pliancy when rolled between finger and thumb after 2–3 days.

In addition, paraffin sections of the biopsy specimens were stained with hematoxylin and eosin and evaluated blind by two independent observers, according to a five-point linear analogue scale, 0 representing no evidence of rejection and 5 complete necrosis.

Autopsies were performed on all animals at the time of sacrifice (either at least six weeks postoperatively after closure of the fistula or earlier because of wound infection).

RESULTS

Clinical condition. All animals appeared to be in normal health, with no overt signs of dehydration or wasting, and fed normally. None died postoperatively. Six animals, all in group 1, were sacrificed due to purulent wound infections at an average postoperative interval of 4 weeks. These appeared to be well and fed normally despite their infections.

Weight. Animals with a fistula (group 1) lost an average of 1.8 kg. over the first fortnight, but thereafter maintained a stable weight, until the fifth week. Sham-operated animals lost 0.7 kg. over the first 3 weeks—but, after 6 weeks, their weight had returned to preoperative levels (Table 1).

TABLE 1. Weights in kilograms

Group	Pre-COF	1 Week	2 Weeks	3 Weeks	4 Weeks	5 Weeks	6 Weeks
Group 1 (n=15)	29.0	28.0	27.1	27.1	27.0	26.8	26.3
Group 2a (n=6)	29.8	29.5	28.9	28.3	28.8	29.3	30.0

Fistula patency. In the group 1 animals with a venous conduit there was a mean patency of 19 days postoperatively, demonstrated radiographically (range 7–50 days). In group 1 animals with a 3-way tap there was a mean patency of 10 days (range 7–11 days).

Autopsies. The only abnormal findings were chylous pleural effusions in three animals, following obstruction of the fistula. The thoracic duct never appeared to be greatly dilated, even in animals in which it had been deliberately ligated. The esophageal mucosa at the site of the fistula showed a blind pit or a small ostium through which a probe could be passed, often after dislodging a small plug of vegetable matter. The lumen of the conduit was often difficult to find, being encased in thick fibrous tissue.

Histologically, this was seen to be an inflammatory reaction with an infiltrate of polymorphonuclear and monocytic cells and accompanying fibrous reaction.

Plasma proteins. Plasma albumin levels were unchanged in sham-operated animals, but fell during the first week after the formation of an internal fistula (Fig. 3). However, the level thereafter remained constant and the animals exibited no clinical ill-effects. Plasma globulin (Fig. 4) changed insignificantly in the control group, but there was a marked and consistent rise in experimental animals with a fistula.

White cell counts. There was no significant change in postoperative peripheral blood lymphocyte counts in sham-operated animals, and the fall in animals with a ligated thoracic duct was of doubtful significance. However, there was a sustained and uniform fall in animals with a COF (group 1), when compared with preoperative values. Also, when the absolute peripheral blood lymphocyte counts of group 1 and group 2 (sham) were compared at weekly intervals, there was a statistically significant fall in group 1 that was maintained over the six-week period (Mann-Whitney *U* test $P<0.001$). These results are shown in Table 2.

Skin grafts. The mean survival time in sham-operated animals was 9 days (SD: 0.63). The mean graft survival time in group 1 animals was 11.0 days (SD: 2.07). In this group, 1 animal was sacrificed because of a wound infection at 13 days, but had a nonrejected graft. These results are depicted in Table 3.

Microscopically also, the severity of the rejection process in group 1 animals was less, with a mean score of 2.0 compared with 3.0 in control animals.

DISCUSSION

Patency. We have succeeded in diverting the thoracic duct lymph into esophagus of the sheep for up to 50 days (mean 19 days) and have observed a sustained fall in peripheral blood lymphocyte levels and a prolongation of allograft survival in animals with demonstrably patent fistulae. Although much longer periods of thoracic duct cannulation have been achieved in man, they have not in animals, presumably because of the problems of restraint, hygiene, and lack of active cooperation. The sheep is not an ideal animal in this respect, because rumination ensures that the anastomosis is constantly bathed

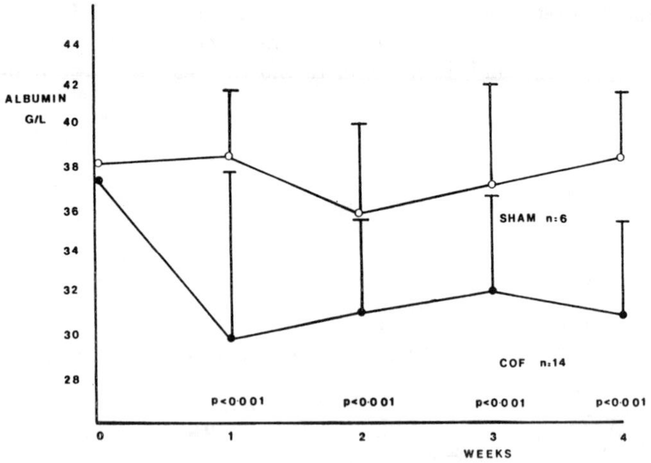

FIGURE 3. Plasma albumin concentration. (Open circles: sham, filled circles: chyloesophageal fistula—Mann-Whitney *U* test).

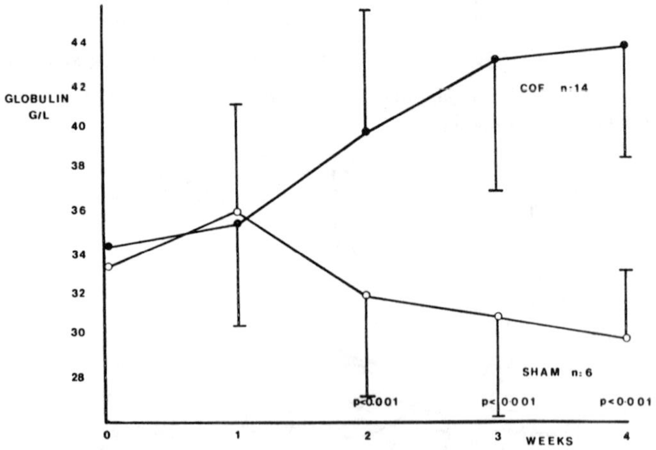

FIGURE 4. Plasma globulin concentration. (Open circles: sham, filled circles-chyloesophageal fistula—Mann-Whitney *U* test).

in infected partly digested material that may physically block the ostium of the fistula as well as lead to an ineradicable infection of the lymph and eventual clotting and fibrosis. Longer periods of patency would be anticipated in nonruminant species.

Peripheral blood lymphocyte count. The effect of external thoracic duct drainage on blood lymphocyte counts has been described by previous authors. In the rat there is a marked fall within three days to levels of up to 83% of preoperative values (*21*). In larger animals, however, the fall is less marked and less constant (*22–25*). The fall of 60% found in our model is in close accord with these values, although it is interesting to note that the deficit is maintained for some weeks after blockage of the fistula. In this context Machleder and Paulus (*20*) found that peripheral blood lymphocyte levels in man did not return to normal until 15 weeks after the cessation of external drainage. There are two possible explanations for this delay: first, the lymphocytes removed are long-lived cells and replenish-

TABLE 2. Peripheral blood white cell and lymphocyte counts[a]

	Pre	1 Week	2 Weeks	3 Weeks (n=16)	4 Weeks (n=13)	5 Weeks (n=9)	6 Weeks (n=9)
Group 1 (n=17):							
White cell count	10.0	8.6	8.7	8.1	8.4	10.2	8.5
Lymphocyte count	8.0 (2.8)	3.5 (1.6)[b]	3.9 (1.5)[b]	4.2 (1.8)[b]	3.9 (2.0)[b]	5.1 (2.5)[b]	4.3 (1.4)[b]
Group 2a (n=6):							
White cell count	7.8	6.8	6.7	5.9	6.0	5.8	5.3
Lymphocyte count	5.8 (0.8)	5.0 (0.6)[c]	5.4 (1.4)[c]	5.2 (0.9)[c]	5.2 (1.1)[c]	6.0 (1.0)[c]	4.3 (1.2)[d]
Group 2b (n=2):							
White cell count	9.6	7.3	8.2	8.2	6.7	7.6	6.4
Lymphocyte count	8.5 (2.0)	5.2 (3.4)[d]	7.0 (1.9)[c]	7.0 (4.1)[c]	6.5 (2.6)[c]	6.3 (3.1)[c]	5.0 (3.0)[d]

[a] The figures in parentheses indicate 1 SD. The *P* values denoted by the superscript letters refer to a comparison with the preoperative values within each group (Mann-Whitney *U* Test); group 1: COF, group 2a: sham, group 2b: ligation.

[b] $P<0.001$.

[c] *P* not significant.

[d] $P<0.01$.

TABLE 3. Skin graft survival times in days

	Sham	COF
Survival time	8, 9 (×4), 10	10, (×4), 11, 12 (×2), 13, 17
Mean survival time	9 (SD 0.63)	11.8 (SD 2.07) $P<0.01$

ment takes time and depends upon a number of factors, such as the degree of continuing or new antigenic stimulation; second, there is evidence from those animals in which thoracic duct ligation was performed that mere obstruction of the duct results in a more prolonged lymphopenia than that seen in control animals. Lee and Blalock both showed, in the cat, that thoracic duct ligation resulted in a fall in peripheral blood lymphocyte levels (up to 56% of normal values), the latter not being regained for 3 weeks. In control animals counts fell to similar levels, but returned to normal within four days (*26, 27*). Heath (*28*) in studies of lymphatic obstruction in sheep, has clearly shown that obstruction or disruption is bypassed by collaterals that grow from the duct concerned. Because the process is one of new vessel formation, rather than dilatation of existing channels, it takes 2–3 weeks for a functional collateral circulation to develop. During this time the number of small lymphocytes returned to the circulation is diminished. There is also clinical evidence (*29*) that early obstruction of an external thoracic duct fistula produces greater immunosuppression than prolonged but poor drainage.

Immunosuppression. There are a number of theoretical reasons for expecting immunosuppression following thoracic duct drainage. Not only is the absolute number of small recirculating lymphocytes depleted, but, as Bell and coworkers have shown (*30*), there is both an absolute reduction of T helper cells and a relative reduction when compared with T cytotoxic/suppressor cells. There is also an increase in the number of early thymocytes as revealed by the Okt10 monoclonal antibody. They speculate that this might represent a state of immunological immaturity "with optimal conditions for allograft tolerance." High Okt4/8 ratios have been shown to correlate well with graft survival (*31*) and the changes produced by thoracic duct drainage may simply represent a difference in the extent to which cytotoxic/suppressor and helper subsets recirculate. There is evidence, for example, that suppressor cells recirculate less than helper cells (*32–34*). Thoracic duct drainage also selectively depletes T cells, as compared with B cells, probably because the number of recirculating B cells is lower than the number of recirculating T cells (*30, 35, 36*).

There is some theoretical support for the hypothesis that thoracic duct drainage might be effective in the sensitized recipient, in that virgin or unsensitized B cells are not recoverable from the thoracic duct lymph of an intermediate recipient after injection, whereas B cells from a primed, sensitized donor are fully capable of recirculating (*37*). Memory B lymphocytes have been shown to be long-lived (*38*), and T cells need antigenic stimulation to enter the recirculating pool (*39*).

In this study, we have shown a prolongation of skin allograft survival following internal drainage of the thoracic duct. Prolongation of skin allograft survival following external thoracic duct drainage in animals has generally been found to be modest (*4, 9*) and the sheep allograft response seems to be a particularly strong one and resistant to other forms of immunosuppression (*40*).

These results were obtained despite the fact that no parenteral fluid or protein supplementation was needed or given at any stage. It was gratifying that the sheep remained clinically well with no signs of dehydration, apathy, or weakness. The fall in plasma albumin might be accounted for by hemodilution caused by a reduced tissue fluid oncotic pressure, consequent upon the continuous removal of protein-rich fluid from the tissue spaces while overall hydration is maintained. Wound infections were a problem in 6 animals (36%). This infection rate, not seen in control animals, could arise as a specific complication of the procedure, or it might be due to the immunosuppressed state of the animals.

Conclusion. We are encouraged by the feasibility of performing the chyloesophageal fistula in the sheep, although there are problems in maintaining long-term patency in this species that might not be expected in a nonruminant. Nonetheless, internal thoracic duct lymph diversion is associated with sustained lymphopenia and modest but significant prolongation of skin allograft survival while the animals remain healthy. The preparation successfully avoids the need for parenteral fluid replacement inherent in external thoracic duct drainage, inducing at the same time a state of immunosuppression.

We believe further evaluation is justified in a nonruminant species, with particular regard to the effect of internal thoracic duct drainage on hyperacute rejection in sensitized recipients.

Acknowledgments. We thank R.M. Binns, Ph.D., for his helpful advice, and the departments of Haematology, Chemical Pathology, and Immunology in the Royal Liverpool Hospital.

REFERENCES

1. Gowans JL. The recirculation of lymphocytes from blood to lymph in the rat. J Physiol (Lond) 1959; 146: 54.
2. Ford WL. Lymphocyte migration and immune responses. Prog Allergy 1975; 19: 1.
3. Gowans JL, McGregory DD, Cowen DM, Ford CE. Initiation of immune responses by small lymphocytes. Nature 1962; 196: 651.
4. McGregor DD, Gowans JL. Survival of homografts of skin in rats depleted of lymphocytes by chronic drainage from the thoracic duct. Lancet 1964; 1: 629.
5. McGregor DD, Gowans JL. The antibody response of rats depleted of lymphocytes by chronic drainage from the thoracic duct. J Exp Med 1963; 117: 303.
6. Woodruff MFA, Anderson NA. Effect of lymphocyte depletion by thoracic duct fistula and administration of anti-lymphocyte serum on the survival of skin homografts in rats. Nature 1963; 200: 702.
7. Singh L, Vega RE, Makin GS, Howard JM. External thoracic duct fistula and canine renal homograft. JAMA 1965; 191: 1009.
8. Fish JC, Tyson KR, Beathard GA, Sarles HE, Remmers AR, Ritzmann SE. Circualting lymphocyte depletion: effect on renal allograft survival in calves. Surgery 1970; 67: 969.
9. Samuelson JS, Fisher B, Fisher ER. Prolonged survival of skin homografts in dogs with thoracic duct fistula. Surg Forum 1963; 14: 192.
10. Franksson C. Letter to the editor. Lancet 1964; 1: 1331.
11. Franksson C, Lundgren G, Magnusson G, Ringden O. Drainage of thoracic duct lymph in renal transplant patients. Transplantation 1976; 21: 133.
12. Sarles HE, Remmers AR, Fish JC, et al. Depletion of lymphocytes for the protection of renal allografts. Arch Intern Med 1970; 125: 443.
13. Fish JC. Renal transplantation after thoracic duct drainage. Ann Surg 1981; 193: 752.
14. Murray JE, Wilson RE, Tilney NL, et al. Five years' experience in renal transplantation with immunosuppressive drugs: survival, function, complications, and the role of lymphocyte depletion by thoracic duct fistula. Ann Surg 1968; 168: 416.
15. Tilney NL, Atkinson JC, Murray JE. The immunosuppressive effect of thoracic duct drainage in human kidney transplantation. Ann Intern Med 1979; 72: 59.
16. Irvin GL, Carbone PP. Immunosuppression with lymph depletion in man. Surg Gynecol Obstet 1967; 124: 1283.
17. Johnson HK, Niblack GD, Tallent MB, Richie RE. Immunologic preparation for cadaver renal transplant by thoracic duct drainage. Transplant Proc 1977; 9: 1499.
18. Richie RE. Thoracic duct drainage in transplantation. Transplant Proc 1980; 12: 483.
19. Starzl TE, Koep LJ, Weil R, Halgrimson CG, Franks JJ. Thoracic duct drainage in organ transplantation: will it permit better immunosuppression? Transplant Proc 1979; 11: 276.
20. Machleder HI, Paulus H. Clinical and immunological alterations observed in patients undergoing long-term thoracic duct drainage. Surgery 1978; 84: 157.
21. Gowans JL. The effect of the continuous reinfusion of lymph and lymphocytes on the output of lymphocytes from the thoracic duct of unanesthetized rats. Br J Exp Pathol 1957; 338: 67.
22. Ellis F. Renal homograft response following thymectomy and thoracic duct drainage in goats. Transplantation 1967; 5: 21.
23. Fish JC, Mattingley AT, Ritzmann SE, Sarles HE, Remmers AR. Circulating lymphocyte depletion in the calf. Arch Surg 1969; 99: 664.
24. Fitts CT, Majeski JA, Sharbaugh RJ, Hargest TS, Graber CD, Henniger GR. Immunosuppression by thoracic duct filtration. Transplantation 1972; 14: 236.
25. Townsend CM, Fish JC, Vyvial T, Kiamar M, Ritzmann SE. Lymphocyte kinetics during depletion by thoracic duct drainage in calves. Transplantation 1970; 10: 284.
26. Lee FC. Changes in the number of small lymphocytes of the blood following ligation of the thoracic duct. J Exp Med 1922; 36: 247.
27. Blalock A, Robinson CS, Cunningham RS, Gray ME. Experimental studies on thoracic duct blockage. Arch Surg Chicago 1937; 34: 1049.
28. Heath T. Pathways of intestinal lymph drainage in normal sheep and in sheep following thoracic duct occlusion. Am J Anat 1964; 115: 569.
29. Franksson C, Blomstrand R. Drainage of the thoracic lymph duct during homologous kidney transplantation in man. Scand J Urol Nephrol 1967; 1: 123.
30. Bell JD, Marshall GD, Shaw BA, et al. Alterations in human thoracic duct lymphocytes during thoracic duct drainage. Transplant Proc 1983; 15: 677.
31. Cosimi AB, Colvin RB, Burton RC, et al. Monoclonal antibodies for immunologic monitoring and treatment in recipients of renal allografts. N Engl J Med 1981; 305: 308.
32. de Sousa M, Freitas A, Huber B, Cantor H, Boyse EA. Migratory patterns by Ly subsets of T lymphocytes in the mouse. Adv Exp Biol Med 1979; 51. New York: Plenum.
33. Beverley PCL. Lymphocyte heterogeneity: in Lever, Roelants, B and T cells in immune recognition 1977; 35. Wiley and Sons, London.
34. Hall JG, Morris B. The output of cells in lymph from the popliteal node of the sheep. Q J Exp Physiol 1962; 47: 360.
35. Frost H. The effect of antigen on the output of recirculating T and B lymphocytes from single nodes. Cell Immunol 1978; 37: 390.
36. Cahill RNP, Heron I, Poskitt DC, Trnka Z. Lymphocyte recirculation in the sheep foetus: functional interactions. Ciba Foundation Symposium 1980; 71: 1435.
37. Strober S. Initiation of antibody responses by different classes of lymphocytes, V, Fundamental changes in the physiological characteristics of virgin thymus-independent B lymphocytes and B memory cells. J Exp Med 1972; 136: 85.
38. Strober S, Dilley J. Biological characteristics of T and B lymphocytes in the rat. J Exp Med 1973; 137: 1275.
39. Miller JFAP, Mitchell GF. The thymus and antigen-reactive cells. Transplant Rev 1969; 1: 3.
40. Mitchell RM. Studies on renal transplantation in sheep. Aust NZ J Surg 1959; 28: 263.

0041-1337/86/4202-0141$02.00/0
TRANSPLANTATION

Vol. 42, No. 2
Printed in U.S.A.

EVIDENCE THAT Ia^+ BONE-MARROW-DERIVED CELLS ARE THE STIMULUS FOR THE INTESTINAL PHASE OF THE MURINE GRAFT-VERSUS-HOST REACTION[1]

ALLAN McI. MOWAT

Department of Bacteriology and Immunology, Western Infirmary, Glasgow, Scotland G11 6NT

We have investigated whether bone marrow (BM) or tissue-derived cells provide the stimulus for the intestinal phase of graft-versus-host reaction (GVHR) in F_1 mice injected with parental spleen cells. After injection of CBA cells, the characteristic increases in crypt length, crypt cell production rate (CCPR), and intraepithelial lymphocyte (IEL) count occurred in the jejunum of (CBA×BALB/c)F_1→CBA BM chimeras, but not in CBA→(CBA×BALB/c)F_1 BM chimeras. Thus, BM-derived cells alone can induce intestinal GVHR and, as similar intestinal alterations were found in (A.TH×A.TL)→A.TL BM chimeric mice after injection of A.TL spleen cells, we deduce that the BM-derived stimulator cells are Ia^+. We conclude that the intestinal pathology in this model of GVHR is an indirect effect of soluble mediators that are released during a local delayed-type hypersensitivity (DTH) reaction induced by recognition of Ia^+ passenger leukocytes within the mucosa.

The concept that allograft rejection and graft-versus-host reaction are caused by direct destruction of tissue cells by allospecific cytotoxic T lymphocytes (CTL)* has been challenged by recent evidence suggesting that delayed-type hypersensitivity is the prinicpal mechanism (*1, 2*). We have shown previously that $Lyt2^-$ cells activated by I-A alloantigens are responsible for the crypt hyperplasia and increased numbers of intraepithelial lymphocytes that characterise the intestinal phase of GVHR in unirradiated F_1 mice (*3*). These changes occur in the absence of specific CTL (*4*) and we, and others, have demonstrated that the mucosal alterations can occur as a "bystander phenomenon" in grafts of intestine that are syngeneic to the cells used to induce the GVHR (*5–7*). Thus, we have postulated that the intestinal pathology is due to a local DTH response induced by Ia^+ leukocytes within the mucosa (*7*). However, small intestinal epithelial cells may also be Ia^+ (*8, 9*) and it has not been proved that the stimulating cells are of bone marrow origin. Nor has it been determined whether allogeneic BM-derived cells are a prerequisite for the induction of intestinal GVHR or whether the stromal cells of the intestine can themselves stimulate alloreactive T cells. Therefore, the aims of this study were to examine directly the relative roles of BM and tissue-derived cells in inducing the intestinal phase of GVHR and to investigate whether the stimulator cells carry class II MHC alloantigens.

MATERIALS AND METHODS

Mice. CBA (H-2^k) and (CBA×BALB/c)F_1 (H-$2^{k\times d}$) mice were obtained from departmental stocks. A.TH(H-2^{t2}) and A.TL(H-2^{tl}) mice were obtained originally from Olac 1976 Ltd (Bicester, England) and then maintained in the department. Donors of spleen cells and BM aged 8–12 weeks were used, while BM recipients were first used when aged 12–16 weeks.

Preparation of cell suspensions. Spleens were trimmed free of surrounding tissues and placed in cold RPMl 1640 (Gibco Biocult) before mincing through a fine wire-mesh filter. After washing three times in medium, the cells were counted by phase contrast microscopy and adjusted to 3×10^8 viable cells/ml. Bone marrow cells were obtained from the femurs of mice by flushing through with RPMl 1640 and were washed three times before use.

Elimination of T lymphocytes from bone marrow. 10^7 cells/ml were incubated in 1:1000 monoclonal anti-Thy 1.2 (F7D5—Olac 1976) for 40 min at 4°C followed by 30 min in 1:10 rabbit complement (Low Tox M-Cedarlane) at 37°C. Treated cells were washed three times before use.

Preparation of bone marrow chimeras. Mice received 950 rads irradiation from a 300 keV X-ray source (Dynaray) at a distance of 100 cm and a dose rate of 250 rad/min. Immediately thereafter, mice were reconstituted with $1–1.6\times10^7$ anti Thy 1.2-treated bone marrow cells i.v. and maintained on drinking water containing 100 mg/L neomycin sulphate (Calbiochem) for the next four weeks. Mice were used for GVHR experiments after at least 3–4 months, when alloantibody testing showed that >99% of lymphoid cells were of donor origin. Normally, >98% chimeric mice survived until this time.

Induction of graft-versus-host reaction. Mice were injected with 6×10^7 parental spleen cells i.p. and the intestinal and systemic GVHR assessed near the peak of the intestinal GVHR, 12 days later (*7*). Control mice received only 0.2 ml RPMl 1640 i.p. Systemic GVHR was assessed using the spleen weight assay of Simonsen (*10*) as follows:

$$\text{Spleen index} = \frac{\text{relative spleen weight in experimental mouse (mg/10 g body wt.)}}{\text{mean relative spleen weight in controls}}$$

Measurement of intestinal GVHR. The presence of intestinal GVHR was assessed by the intraepithelial lymphocyte count and by measurements of mucosal architecture and epithelial cell proliferation kinetics, as described previously (*7*). Briefly, mice were killed at intervals after receiving 7.5 mg/kg colchicine ip (BDH Ltd) and 1-cm^2 pieces of jejunum removed 10 cm from the pylorus. IEL counts were performed on H and E–stained sections and expressed as IEL/100 epithelial cells, while mucosal architecture was assessed on tissues stained in bulk by the modified Feulgen reaction. Villus and crypt lengths were expressed in micrometers, and on the same sections, the number of metaphases per crypt was measured. The CCPR was

[1] This work was supported by MRC grant G8224559 CA.

* Abbreviations used: BM, bone marrow, CTL, cytotoxic T lymphocyte; DTH, delayed-type hypersensitivity; GVHR, graft-versus-host reaction; IEL, intraepithelial lymphocyte; MHC, major histocompatibility complex; MLR, mixed lymphocyte reaction.

then calculated by linear regression analysis of the relationship between the number of metaphases/crypt and the time after colchicine.

Statistics. Results expressed as means ±1 SD were compared by Student's *t* test except for crypt cell production rates, which were compared by covariance analysis.

RESULTS

Role of allogeneic bone cells in induction of GVHR. The ability of bone-marrow-derived cells to induce a GVHR was examined in (CBA×BALB/c)F_1→CBA BM chimeras by injecting 6×10^7 CBA spleen cells i.p. Nine days later, these mice had significant splenomegaly compared with controls (Table 1) and had significant increases both in crypt length (139.6±1.7 μm vs. 118.1±2.7 μm) and in crypt cell production rate (12.4±3.0 vs. 4.4±1.4) compared with controls (Fig. 1A). Furthermore, mice injected with parental spleen cells had increased numbers of IEL in the jejunum (Fig. 1B 19.5±3.3 vs. 13.0±2.2 IEL/100 epithelial cells). Villus atrophy was not seen in mice with GVHR. Thus, the presence of allogeneic F_1 BM-derived cells is sufficient to induce both systemic and intestinal GVHR in mice the tissues of which are syngeneic to the alloreactive donor cells.

Ability of allogeneic intestinal tissues to induce a local GVHR. In view of the GVHR induced by allogeneic BM cells in syngeneic intestine, it was important to assess whether allogeneic tissue-derived cells could stimulate a GVHR in the absence of allogeneic BM cells. Thus, we prepared CBA→(CBA×BALB/c)F_1 BM chimeric mice and induced a GVHR with 6×10^7 CBA spleen cells i.p. As reported previously (*11*) these mice had mild splenomegaly, which was considerably less than that found in F_1→CBA chimeras with GVHR (Table 1). When the intestinal phase of GVHR was assessed, mice injected with CBA spleen cells had crypt lengths and CCPR that were identical to control CBA→F_1 mice (Fig. 2A) and did not have an increased IEL count (Fig. 2B). Once again, mice with GVHR had no evidence of villus atrophy. Thus, the presence of allogeneic epithelial cells is not sufficient to stimulate the intestinal phase of GVHR in the absence of allogeneic bone-marrow-derived cells.

Evidence that bone-marrow-derived cells that induce intestinal GVHR are Ia$^+$. As we had shown previously that class II major histocompatibility complex (MHC) alloantigens were alone sufficient and necessary to induce intestinal GVHR (*3*) we examined whether the BM-derived cells required to stimulate GVHR carried class II MHC antigens. To do this we used A.TH and A.TL mice, which differ only at class II MHC loci, and prepared (A.TH×A.TL)F_1→A.TL BM chimeras. These mice were injected with A.TL spleen cells i.p. so that the only stimulus for a GVHR in these mice are the class II alloantigens expressed on BM-derived cells of F_1 origin. As shown in Figures 3A and B, these mice had significant increases in CCPR (22.8±0.9 vs. 12.4±0.3) and in IEL count (22.5±3.3 vs. 12.4±3.8) compared with controls. These mice also had longer crypts than controls but, as before, no villus atrophy was found in GVHR.

TABLE 1. Induction of systemic GVHR in (CBA×BALB/c)F_1→CBA and CBA→(CBA×BALB/c)F_1 bone marrow chimeras by injection of 6×10^7 CBA spleen cells

Chimeric Host	Group	Rel. spleen wt. (mg/10g wt.)[a]	Spleen index
F_1→CBA	Control	27.30±2.05	—
	GVHR	47.72±6.79	1.75±0.25
CBA→F_1	Control	23.1±3.04	—
	GVHR	31.5±4.3	1.37±0.18

[a] Relative spleen weights and spleen indices on day 12 of GVHR. Results shown are means ±1 SD for 6 mice/group.

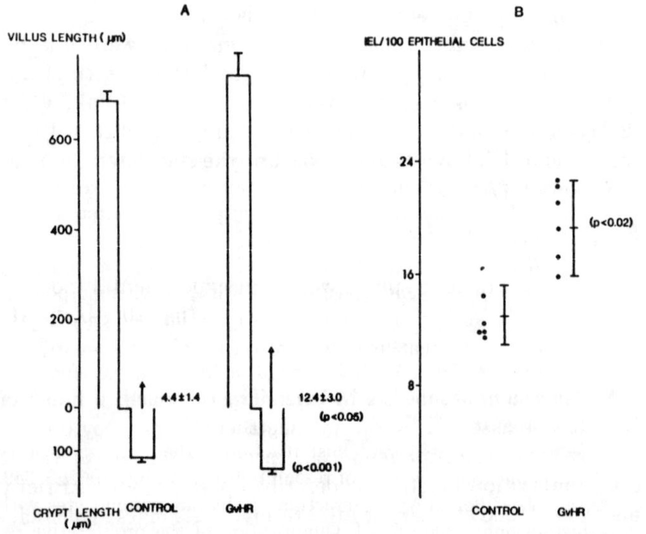

FIGURE 1. Intestinal phase of GVHR in (CBA×BALB/c)F_1→CBA chimeras 12 days after injection of 6×10^7 CBA spleen cells i.p. (A) mucosal architecture: bars represent mean villus and crypt lengths +1 SD and arrows represent CCPR ±1 SD; (B) intraepithelial lymphocyte counts: results are mean number of IEL/100 epithelial cells ±1 SD; 6 mice per group.

DISCUSSION

The results presented here show that the cells responsible for inducing the intestinal phase of GVHR in F_1 hybrid mice are of bone marrow origin and these carry alloantigens coded by the class II loci of the MHC. In contrast, the tissue cells of the intestine play no role in inducing the local GVHR and the intestinal pathology occurs as a "bystander phenomenon."

Tissue damage as a bystander phenomenon in GVHR has

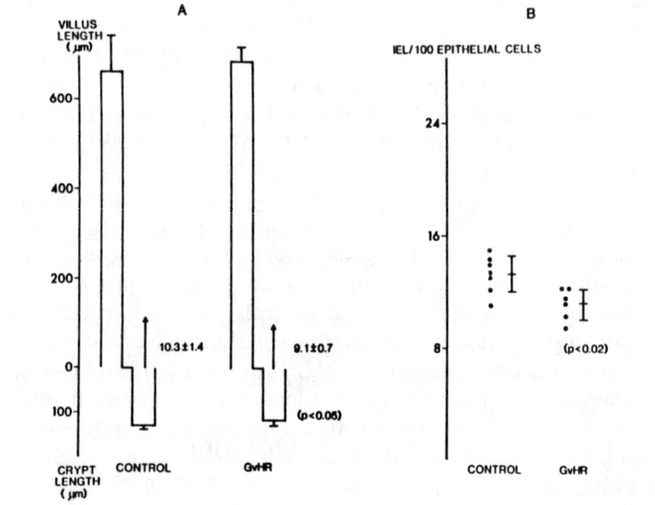

FIGURE 2. Intestinal phase of GVHR in CBA→(CBA×BALB/c)F_1 chimeras 12 days after injection of 6×10^7 CBA spleen cells. (A) mucosal architecture: bars represent mean villus and crypt lengths +1 SD and arrows represent CCPR ±1 SD; (B) intraepithelial lymphocyte counts: mean number of IEL/100 epithelial ±1 SD; 6 mice per group.

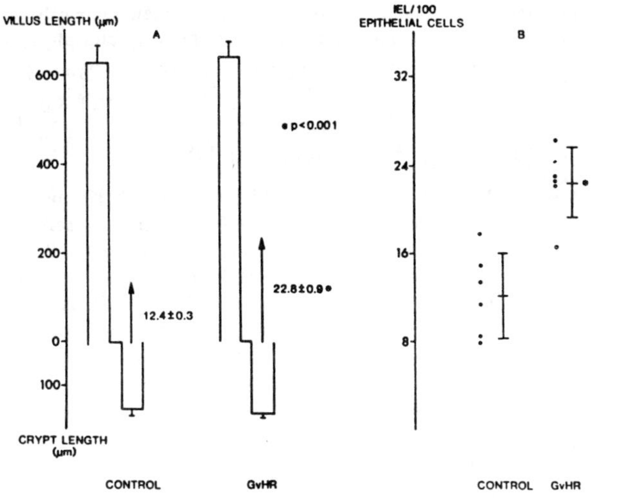

FIGURE 3. Intestinal phase of GVHR in (A.TH×A.TL)F_1→A.TL chimeras 12 days after injection of 6×10^7 A.TL spleen cells i.p. (A) mucosal architecture: bars represent mean villus and crypt lengths +1 SD and arrows represent CCPR ±1 SD; (B) intraepithelial lymphocyte counts: results shown are mean number of IEL/100 epithelial cells ±1 SD; 5 or 6 mice per group.

been shown to occur in kidney (*12*), skin (*13*), and intestine (*5–7*) that are syngeneic to the donor cells used to induce the GVHR. In addition, it has been shown that kidney and skin damage (*13, 14*) as well as splenomegaly (11), destruction of lymphoid tissues (*14*), and systemic lethal GVHR (*15–16*) can occur in F_1→P BM chimeras after injection of parental lymphoid cells. The present report is the first to identify the importance of allogeneic BM cells in the intestinal phase of GVHR and has also demonstrated that these stimulator cells carry class II MHC alloantigens. In contrast to these results, however, the single previous report that attempted to identify intestinal changes during a GVHR in F_1→P BM chimeric animals could find no damage in the gut (*14*). Nevertheless, these authors did not report the intestinal changes in detail—and, as they only examined the terminal stages of GVHR in dying animals, any gut damage specific to GVHR may have been overlooked. In contrast, our sensitive assays of intestinal pathology in otherwise healthy animals are able to follow the development of intestinal GVHR in these animals.

While our findings are entirely consistent with the concept that Ia^+ "passenger leukocytes" are critical for stimulating rejection of allogeneic tissues (*17*), we have not identified the BM-derived stimulator cell. However, it is reasonable to propose that Ia^+ dendritic cells will be responsible. Lymphoid dendritic cells are potent stimulators of alloreactive T cells (*18*) and BM-derived cells of this type are present within the intestinal mucosa and its draining lymph (*19, 20*). Furthermore, dendritic cells in intestinal lymph have been shown to stimulate a mixed lymphocyte reaction (MLR) in vitro (*19*) and can act as passenger leukocytes in the induction of kidney graft rejection (*21*). We are currently investigating whether lymphoid dendritic cells are indeed responsible for inducing intestinal GVHR.

The outstanding feature of our study was that intestinal tissues themselves could not induce a local GVHR, despite the facts that intestinal epithelium expresses both class I and II MHC antigens and class II expression on enterocytes is enhanced during a GVHR (*8, 9*). Although Ia^+ endothelial cells (*22*) and thyroid epithelial cells (*23*) have been shown to activate T cells, this has not been described for enterocytes. Thus, our findings are indirect evidence that expression of Ia antigens by gut epithelium does not necessarily confer the ability to activate T cells, and this requires direct investigation using isolated enterocytes. One further conclusion from our findings is that alloantigens shed from epithelial cells play no role in induction of the local GVHR. Processing and re-presentation of shed alloantigens by antigen-presenting cells that are syngeneic to the alloreactive T cells has been shown to be important in the MLR in vitro (*24*) and in allospecific DTH in vivo (*25*). However, in our hands, intestine of F_1 origin was unable to induce a GVHR in mice whose hemopoietic system was of parental origin, indicating that parental T cells did not respond to shed F_1 antigens presented on parental APC.

The intestinal alterations we have detailed are identical to those found in normal, allogeneic gut that are induced by $Lyt2^-$T cells (*3*) and occur in the absence of antihost CTL (*4*). Together, these features support the concept that the crypt hyperplasia and hypertrophy that characterize this model of GVHR are not secondary to direct destruction of enterocytes by allospecific CTL, but are due to "enteropathic lymphokines" released during a local DTH response (*7*). From the findings reported here we now conclude that this mucosal DTH response is induced by lymphoid cells of BM origin that activate class II MHC-restricted donor T lymphocytes.

REFERENCES

1. Mason DW. Subsets of T cells in the rat mediating lethal graft-versus-host disease. Transplantation 1981; 32: 222.
2. Loveland BE, McKenzie IFC. Which T cells cause graft rejection? Transplantation 1982; 33: 217.
3. Mowat AMcI, Borland A, Parrott DMV. Hypersensitivity reactions in the small intestine. VII. The intestinal phase of murine graft-versus-host reaction is induced by Lyt 2^- T cells activated by I-A alloantigens. Transplantation (in press).
4. Borland A, Mowat AMcI, Parrott DMV. Augmentation of intestinal and peripheral natural killer cell activity during the graft-versus-host reaction in mice. Transplantation 1983; 36: 513.
5. Elson CO, Reilly RW, Rosenberg IH. Small intestinal injury in the GVHR: an innocent bystander phenomenon. Gastroenterology 1977; 72: 886.
6. van Bekkum DW, Knaan S. Role of bacterial microflora in development of intestinal lesions from GVHR. J Natl Cancer Inst 1977; 58: 787.
7. Mowat AMcI, Ferguson A. Hypersensitivity reactions in the small intestine. VI. Pathogenesis of the graft-versus-host reaction in the small intestinal mucosa of the mouse. Transplantation 1981; 32: 238.
8. Mayrhofer G, Pugh CW, Barclay AN. The distribution, ontogeny and origin in the rat of Ia positive cells with dendritic morphology and of Ia antigen in epithelia, with special reference to the intestine. Eur J Immunol 1983; 13: 112.
9. Barclay AN, Mason DW. Induction of Ia antigen in rat epidermal cells and gut epithelium by immunological stimuli. J Exp Med 1982; 156: 1665.
10. Simonsen M. Graft versus host reactions. Their natural history and applicability as tools of research. Progr Allergy 1962; 6: 349.
11. Sprent J, Miller JFAP. Interaction of thymus lymphocytes with histoincompatible cells. I. Quantitation of the proliferative response of thymus cells. Cell Immunol 1972; 3: 361.
12. Streilein JW. Pathologic lesions of GvH disease in hamsters: antigenic target versus "innocent bystanders." Prog Exp Tumor Res 1972; 16: 396.
13. Elkins WL, Guttman RD. Pathogenesis of a local graft-versus-host reaction: immunogenicity of circulating host leucocytes. Science

1968; 159: 1250.

14. Cornelius EA, Martinez C, Yunis EJ, Good RA. Haematological and pathological changes induced in tolerant mice by the injection of syngeneic lymphoid cells. Transplantation 1968; 6: 33.
15. Hilgard HR, Martinez C, Good RA. Production of runt disease in tolerant mice by the injection of syngeneic lymphoid cells. J Exp Med 1965; 122: 1017.
16. Steinmuller D, Shelby J. Lymphoid target cell replacement and refractoriness to graft-versus-host disease. Transplantation 1980; 30: 313.
17. Lafferty KJ. Immunogenicity of foreign tissues. Transplantation 1980; 29: 179.
18. Steinman RM, Witmer MD. Lymphoid dendritic cells are potent stimulators of the primary mixed leucocyte reaction in mice. Proc Natl Acad Sci USA 1978; 75: 5132.
19. Mason DW, Pugh CW, Webb M. The rat mixed lymphocyte reaction: roles of a dendritic cell in intestinal lymph and T-cell subsets defined by monoclonal antibodies. Immunology 1981; 44: 75.
20. Wilders MM, Sminia T, Janse EM. Ontogeny of non-lymphoid and lymphoid cells in the rat gut with special reference to large mononuclear Ia-positive dendritic cells. Immunology 1983; 50: 303.
21. Lechler RI, Batchelor JR. Restoration of immunogenicity to passenger cell-depleted kidney allografts by the addition of donor strain dendritic cells. J Exp Med 1982; 155: 31.
22. Pober JS, Gimborne MA, Cotran RS, Reiss CS, Burakoff SJ, Fiers W, Ault KA. Ia expression by vascular endothelium is inducible by activated T cells and by human γ interferon. J Exp Med 1983; 157: 1339.
23. Londei M, Lamb JR, Bottazzo GF, Feldman M. Epithelial cells expressing aberrant MHC Class II determinants can present antigen to cloned human T cells. Nature 1984; 312: 639.
24. Rock KL, Barnes MC, Germain RN, Benacerraf B. The role of Ia molecules in the activation of T lymphocytes. II. Ia-restricted recognition of allo K/D antigens is required for class I MHC-stimulated mixed lymphocyte responses. J Immunol 1983; 130: 457.
25. Smith FI, Miller JFAP. Delayed-type hypersensitivity to allogeneic cells in mice. III. Sensitivity to cell-surface antigens coded by the major histocompatibility complex and by other genes. J Exp Med 1979; 150. 965.

Received 8 August 1985.
Accepted 25 October 1985.

0041-1337/86/4202-0144$02.00/0
TRANSPLANTATION Vol. 42, No. 2

Printed in U.S.A.

SEQUENTIAL ANALYSIS OF HLA–CLASS II ANTIGEN EXPRESSION IN HUMAN RENAL ALLOGRAFTS

INDUCTION OF TUBULAR CLASS II ANTIGENS AND CORRELATION WITH CLINICAL PARAMETERS[1]

SUSAN V. FUGGLE,[2] DOUGLAS L. MCWHINNIE, JEREMY R. CHAPMAN, HELEN M. TAYLOR, AND PETER J. MORRIS

Nuffield Department of Surgery, University of Oxford, John Radcliffe Hospital, Oxford OX3 9DU, England

The expression of HLA-class II antigens was assessed in 142 biopsies from 29 recipients of cadaveric renal allografts who received either short-term cyclosporine (n=12) or azathioprine and low-dose prednisolone (n=17). Biopsies were obtained before transplantation, routinely at days 7, 21, 90, and 365 after transplantation, and at other times as clinically indicated. Cryostat sections were labeled with monoclonal antibodies using an indirect immunoperoxidase technique.

In all biopsies HLA-class II antigens were expressed on glomeruli and intertubular structures. In pretransplant biopsies proximal tubules expressed class II antigens, whereas distal tubules were always negative. After transplantation three patterns of class II expression were recognized based on renal tubular class II staining: normal, focal increased, and generalized increased expression.

Sequential biopsy analysis showed fluctuating levels of expression in individual patients, which correlated with cellular infiltration and was associated with allograft rejection. 71% of biopsies obtained at day 90 from patients on conventional therapy showed increased class II expression compared with only 9% of biopsies from patients on cyclosporine immunosuppression. All patients with normal class II antigen expression in day 90 biopsies had well-functioning grafts two years after transplantation, whereas 3 of 9 with increased class II antigen expression had failed. Furthermore, all grafts failing from irreversible rejection before 90 days showed marked increase of class II antigen expression.

The increased class II antigen expression in renal allografts may be merely a marker of rejection or may have a role in the augmentation of the response, either in its induction or as a target for the effector arm of the reaction.

HLA class II (D region) antigens are a highly polymorphic family of membrane-bound glycoproteins (*1*). They play an intimate role in antigen recognition and subsequent cellular

[1] This work was supported by a grant from The Medical Research Council of the UK and the National Kidney Research Fund.

[2] Address correspondence to: Susan V. Fuggle, D. Phil., Nuffield Department of Surgery, John Radcliffe Hospital, Oxford, OX3 9DU, England.

reactions in an immune response (*2*). Incompatibilities between donor and recipient class II antigens provide a powerful stimulus of the rejection response. They are thus an important barrier to transplantation—and indeed matching of HLA-DR antigens that are part of the class II (D region) complex improves renal allograft survival (*3*).

Class II antigens have a restricted tissue distribution, being expressed primarily on B lymphocytes, monocytes, macrophages (*4*), Langerhans cells (*5*), dendritic cells (*6*)—and, in the human, on endothelium (*7*). Nevertheless, the expression of class II antigens is less restricted than previously thought, as shown in our own laboratories in the human, where class II is expressed on certain epithelial cells (*8, 9*). Furthermore, class II antigens are readily induced on cells on which they are not normally expressed (*10–14*). In vitro studies have demonstrated that the T-lymphocyte-derived interferon-γ plays a role in the induction of class II antigens (*15–18*).

Induction of class II antigens is of particular relevance to transplantation, since cells in which class II antigens have been induced may be able, in turn, to provide a further stimulus to the allograft response, as well as to become potential targets for the rejection process.

In human kidney HLA class II antigens are detected on glomerular endothelium and mesangium, intertubular capillaries, interstitial dendritic cells (*8, 19, 20*), and in some kidneys within the cytoplasm of the proximal tubules (*8*). Increased expression of class II antigens has been demonstrated in both murine (*21*) and human renal allografts in association with acute rejection (*22*).

We have compared the expression of HLA class II antigens in serial renal biopsies taken before, and at predetermined times after transplantation, in patients receiving either cyclosporine or azathioprine and prednisolone. The aim of the study was to see whether increased levels of class II antigens could be detected following transplantation—and, if so, to determine their relationship with rejection episodes and other clinical parameters.

MATERIALS AND METHODS

Biopsies. A total of 142 biopsies were obtained from 29 recipients of cadaver renal allografts. The patients were included in a controled trial comparing the immunosuppressive regimens of short-term cyclosporine (CsA)* and azathioprine and low-dose prednisolone (AP). Patients receiving CsA were converted to conventional therapy at three months. Acute rejection episodes were treated by the administration of 3–5 0.5 g-bolus doses of i.v. methylprednisolone.

Preanastomosis wedge biopsies were obtained from kidneys after donor nephrectomy and preservation but before graft insertion. Harvested kidneys were perfused with hypertonic citrate solution (13 kidneys) or with Collins' solution (14 kidneys). The perfusate in two of the kidneys was unknown. Cold ischemia times ranged from 11 to 28 hr. Post transplantation percutaneous needle core biopsies were routinely obtained at approximately 7, 21, 90, and 365 days after transplantation, and at other times as clinically indicated. A pretransplant biopsy and a minimum of three posttransplant biopsies were studied from each patient.

Biopsies were snap-frozen in liquid nitrogen and stored at −80°C. Serial 6-μ cryostat sections were transferred onto gelatinized multispot microscope slides (C.A. Hendley Ltd, Loughton, Essex, UK), air dried, fixed in acetone for 10 min at room temperature, and stored at −80°C.

Monoclonal antibodies. The following monoclonal antibodies were used:

NFKI: a monomorphic anti HLA-class II antibody (*8*)

F10-89-4: an antibody directed against the leukocyte-common (LC) antigen, present on monocytes, lymphocytes, and granulocytes (*23*)

Leu 4: a pan-T lymphocyte marker (*24*)

F3-20-7: a negative control antibody that recognizes the dog Thy-1 molecule and does not crossreact with human tissue (*25*)

Indirect immunoperoxidase staining. Tissue sections were incubated for 30 min with saturating concentrations of monoclonal antibodies in a humidified atmosphere at room temperature. Sections were washed in phosphate-buffered saline (PBS) and incubated for a further 30 min with the second antibody. This consisted of a rabbit antimouse immunoglobulin (1:100, Dako Immunoglobulins, Copenhagen, Denmark) in which antihuman immunoglobulin activity was blocked by the addition of 20% human AB serum. After further washing, the reaction was developed by incubation with a solution of diaminobenzidine tetrahydrochloride (Sigma Ltd., Poole, Dorset, UK) 6 mg/ml in PBS containing 3 μl/ml 10 vol. hydrogen peroxide for 8 min. The reaction was stopped by immersion in a large volume of PBS. The sections were counterstained with hematoxylin, dehydrated, and mounted in DPX (Raymond A. Lamb, London, UK) for microscopy.

Assessment of Immunoperoxidase Staining

All biopsies were assessed without knowledge of patient data.

HLA–class II antigens. Expression of class II antigens was studied on all structures within the kidney. The nature and intensity of class II antigen staining was assessed on glomeruli, intertubular structures, large vessel endothelium, renal tubules—and, where applicable, cellular infiltrate. Proximal tubules were distinguished from distal tubules by cellular morphology and nuclear distribution. In particular, proximal tubules were characterized by their small uneven lumen, surrounded by large cells with widely spaced nuclei (*26*).

Leukocytes and T lymphocytes. Morphometric analysis of the leukocyte-common and pan-T-cell staining was performed by a point counting method (*27*). The percentage area of a biopsy occupied by cells of each antigenic specificity was calculated (McWhinnie et al., unpublished observations). The results are expressed as the percentage area of the biopsy occupied by infiltrating leukocytes or T lymphocytes ±SEM (%).

Evaluation of Clinical Status

Since there are no absolute criteria for the diagnosis of acute rejection, particularly in patients treated with cyclosporine, an independent observer (H.M.T.) examined all patient records for the following five predetermined clinical criteria:

1. Graft tenderness or swelling
2. Pyrexia (in absence of infection)
3. Oliguria (in absence of ureteric obstruction) or decreasing urine output of approximately 10%/day on the two preceeding days
4. Rising creatinine of approximately 10%/day on two preceeding days, or dialysis
5. Response to course of i.v. methylprednisolone

A minimum of three positive criteria were required for the

* Abbreviations used: AP, azathioprine and low-dose prednisone; CsA, cyclosporine; LC, leukocyte-common; MHC, major histocompatibility complex; PBS, phosphate buffered saline.

diagnosis of rejection. Biopsies obtained within 2 days of a rejection episode were also defined as rejection biopsies. Histopathological criteria were not used to evaluate clinical status since cellular infiltrate of the biopsies was assessed as part of this study.

Statistical Analysis

Statistical analyses were performed using the Mann-Whitney *U* test.

RESULTS

Immunohistological Staining

HLA class II antigen expression. This is summarized in Table 1.

Pretransplant biopsies. (Fig. 1A) In all 29 pretransplant biopsies, HLA class II antigens were detected on the glomerular endothelium, mesangium, and intertubular structures (capillaries and interstitial dendritic cells [*8*]). In contrast, in large vessel endothelium and in renal tubules, there was variation, both within a biopsy and between biopsies in class II antigen expression. Many biopsies did not contain large vessels—but, when present, the staining was either weakly positive or negative. The cytoplasm of the proximal tubules was positive for class II antigens in 27 of 29 kidneys, while the distal tubules, collecting ducts, and loops of Henlé were negative in all biopsies studied.

Transplant biopsies. The glomeruli and intertubular structures were intensely stained for class II antigens in all 113 posttransplant biopsies. Three patterns of class II expression were determined in the posttransplant biopsies.

1. Generalized increase in class II antigen expression: (Fig. 1B) In 53 biopsies all of the renal tubules were intensely positive for HLA class II antigens. The endothelium of large vessels was also strongly stained. Marked infiltration by mononuclear cells, a large proportion of which were class-II-positive, was seen in most biopsies. When this infiltrate was present throughout the biopsy, intertubular capillaries and interstitial dendritic cells were often difficult to identify.

2. Focal increase in class II antigen expression: (Fig. 1C) In fourteen biopsies there were focal increases in class II antigen expression that were frequently perivascular or associated with a mononuclear cell infiltrate. In areas of increased expression, intensely positive proximal tubules, and sometimes distal tubules and large vessel endothelia could be

TABLE 1. Summary of class II antigen expression in normal kidneys before transplantation and in transplanted human kidneys

	Glomerulus and intertubular structures	Large vessel endothelium	Tubules	
			Proximal	Distal
Pretransplant biopsies	+[a]	w+[b] or −[c]	+ or −	−
Transplant biopsies:				
Generalized increase in class II antigen expression	+	+	+	+
Focal increase in class II antigen expression	+	±[d]	±	±
No increase in class II antigen expression	+	w+ or −	+ or −	−

[a] +: class II antigens expressed.
[b] w+: class II antigens weakly expressed.
[c] −: class II antigens undetected.
[d] ±: focal increase in class II antigen expression.

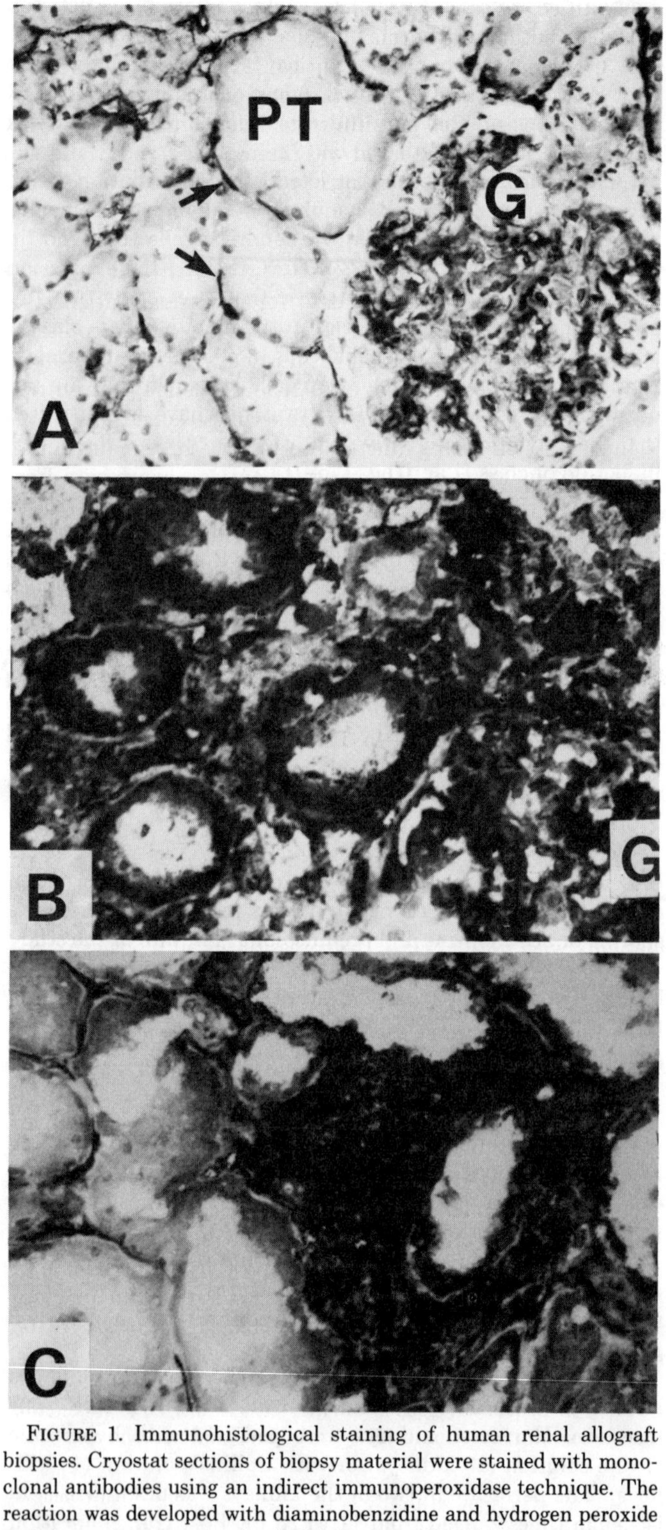

FIGURE 1. Immunohistological staining of human renal allograft biopsies. Cryostat sections of biopsy material were stained with monoclonal antibodies using an indirect immunoperoxidase technique. The reaction was developed with diaminobenzidine and hydrogen peroxide and the nuclei counterstained with hematoxylin. (A) Typical distribution of HLA-class II antigens in a preserved normal human kidney before transplantation. The glomerus (G) and intertubular structures (indicated by arrows) are intensely positive for class II antigens; the cytoplasm of proximal tubules (PT) is weakly positive (× 350). (B) Generalized increase in HLA-class II antigen expression in a renal transplant during a rejection episode. All of the renal tubules, the glomerulus (G), and interstitial infiltrate are intensely class-II-positive (× 350). (C) Focal increase in class II antigen expression in a posttransplant renal biopsy. The intensely class-II-positive cellular infiltrate is surrounded by renal tubules strongly stained for class II antigen (× 350)).

identified, while in other areas of the tissue section the class II distribution was normal.

3. No increase in class II antigen expression: No increase in class II staining was seen on any of the renal structures in 46 biopsies. Cellular infiltrate that contained an HLA class II positive component was often present, but there was no increased class II staining of renal tubules.

Sequential Analysis of HLA-Class II Antigen Expression in Renal Allografts

Analysis of the sequential data for individual patients revealed that increased levels of HLA-class II antigen expression can be induced in the allograft within 7 days of transplantation. Furthermore, once induced, class II antigens may return to a normal level of expression at variable times thereafter.

In 23 patients with a functioning graft at three months, four sequential patterns of HLA-class II antigen expression were identified (Table 2). In a further 5 patients acute rejection led to graft failure and nephrectomy within three months of transplantation. While early biopsies showed variable class II expression, at graft nephrectomy there was generalized increased class II expression in all patients. One patient died with a functioning graft at day 66 from *Pseudomonas* septicemia and fulminating cytomegalovirus infection, but no renal material was obtained at postmortem examination. All three previous biopsies had shown increased class II expression.

Association of Increased HLA-Class II Antigen Expression with Clinical Parameters

Immunosuppression. Seventeen patients were treated with AP and 12 patients received CsA therapy. Analysis of sequential patterns of HLA-class II expression revealed that six of seven patients with normal class II expression in all biopsies (Table 2, group 1) received CsA therapy, while six patients with increased antigen levels in all biopsies (Table 2, group 4) received AP immunosuppression. Groups 2 and 3 (Table 2) were composed of four of seven and one of three CsA-treated patients, respectively. Of patients who lost their graft within three months of transplantation, five of six received conventional AP therapy.

Analysis of the routine biopsies obtained at days 7, 21, and 90 is shown in Table 3. In biopsies obtained at day 7, 73% from patients treated with AP had increased class II expression, compared with 40% of those treated with CsA. At day 21 similar numbers of biopsies in this group demonstrated this phenomenon. By day 90 the percentage of biopsies in CsA-treated patients with increased class II expression had decreased to only 9%, while those treated with AP remained elevated as before. Both CsA and AP patients had similar numbers of rejection episodes (mean ± SEM: CsA 1.7±0.4; AP 2.0±0.2, NS).

TABLE 2. Sequential analysis of HLA class II antigen expression in renal allografts functioning at 3 months, and graft survival at 2 years[a]

	Early biopsies (within 30 days)	Day 90 biopsies	No. patients	No. grafts functioning at 2 years
Group 1	Normal	Normal	7	7
Group 2	Increased on at least one biopsy	Normal	7	7
Group 3	Normal on at least one biopsy	Increased	3	2
Group 4	Increased on all biopsies	Increased	6	4

[a] Five grafts removed before 90 days for irreversible rejection all showed generalized class II antigen expression.

TABLE 3. Influence of immunosuppressive therapy on HLA class II expression in renal allografts

Biopsy (days post transplant)	Cyclosporine		Azathioprine/Prednisolone	
	No. biopsies	% Biopsies with increased class II	No. biopsies	% Biopsies with increased class II
7	10	40%	15	73%
21	12	42%	16	88%
90	11	9%	14	71%

Graft status. Of 42 biopsies taken during clinical rejection, increased HLA class II expression was seen on 31 (74%), while the other 11 (26%) showed normal expression. Thirteen percent of the biopsies with increased class II and 64% of the biopsies with normal class II expression were from patients treated with CsA. In 71 biopsies from grafts with stable function, 22 (31%) showed a generalized increase in class II antigen expression, 14 (20%) a focal increase, and 35 (49%) normal class II antigen expression.

Patients with increased levels of HLA class II expression at day 90 had experienced a mean ± SEM of 2.5±0.3 rejection episodes, while patients with normal expression had only experienced 1.4±0.3 episodes of rejection (P=<0.02). Similarly a greater number of methylprednisolone pulses had been administered during this period to patients with increased expression at day 90 (mean ± SEM: normal expression 1.6±0.3 pulses, increased expression 3.1±0.3 pulses; P=<0.01).

Cellular infiltration. (Figure 2) In routine biopsies obtained at days 7, 21, and 90 the total infiltrating leukocytes and the T lymphocyte component of the cellular infiltrate were compared between grafts with increased (generalized) and normal class II expression. There were insufficient grafts with focally increased class II expression to allow a meaningful analysis. In biopsies with increased class II expression the magnitude of leukocyte infiltration did not significantly vary between day 7 (22.5±3.2%), day 21 (20.2±2.9%), and day 90 (18.0±3.1%) (Fig. 2a). However, in biopsies with normal levels of class II expression, the leukocyte infiltrate significantly decreased from 17.0±3.4% at day 7 to 5.0±1.3% by day 90 (P<0.003). Moreover, leukocyte infiltration in biopsies with normal class II distribution was significantly less than the infiltration in biopsies with increased class II expression at day 21 (8.3±1.4% vs. 20.1±2.9%, P<0.003) and day 90 (5.0±1.3% vs. 18.0±3.1 P<0.0006).

The T lymphocyte component of the cellular infiltration represented less than 40% of the infiltrating cells. However, the relationship between increased class II expression and T lymphocytes was similar to that described for the total infiltrating leukocytes. In biopsies with increased class II expression the infiltration did not differ with time, but in biopsies with normal expression there was a decrease in infiltration from day 7 through to day 90 (Fig. 2b).

Other clinical parameters. There was no correlation between the HLA class II antigen status of the transplanted kidney and the solution used to perfuse the donor kidney, the warm and cold ischemia times, the number of pregraft blood transfusions, or the number of HLA-DR antigens mismatched between donor and recipient.

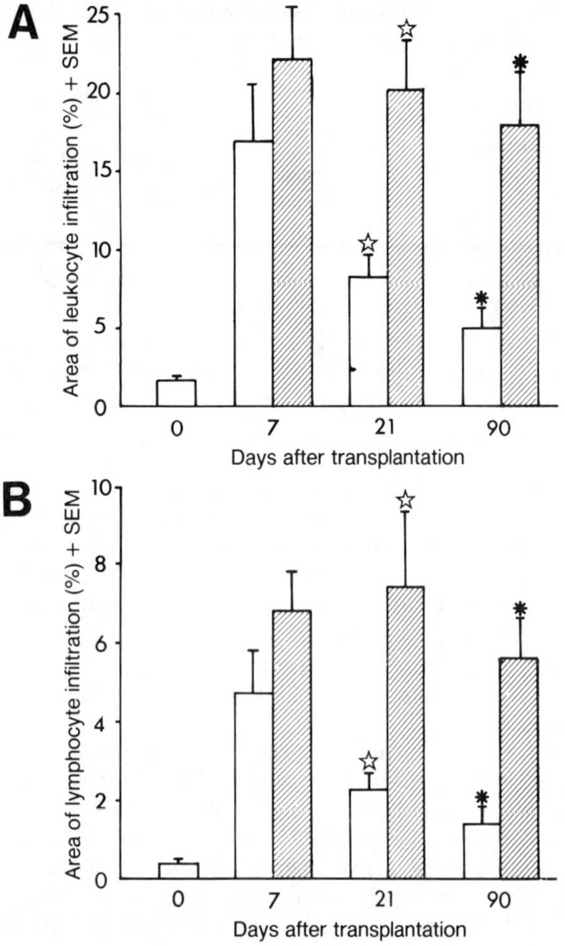

FIGURE 2. The degree of cellular infiltrate in renal allograft biopsies with normal HLA-class II expression (□) and increased HLA class II antigens (▨) ±SEM, expressed as the percentage of the area examined occupied by the infiltrating cells: (A) total infiltrating leukocytes; (B) T lymphocyte infiltration; (☆) $P<0.003$; (∗) $P<0.0006$).

Association of HLA-Class II Antigen Expression with Graft Survival at 2 Years

Allograft survival at two years was examined in 23 patients with a functioning graft at day 90 (Table 2, groups 1–4). There was 100% graft survival in kidneys with normal levels of class II antigens at day 90 (groups 1 and 2) irrespective of whether there had been increased levels during the first month. In groups 3 and 4, in which kidneys had increased class II antigen expression at day 90, 3 of 9 (33%) of the grafts had failed by two years.

DISCUSSION

Despite the presence of class II antigens in proximal tubules before transplantation, the current study clearly demonstrates that increased levels of class II antigens may be detected after transplantation. All the renal tubules may become intensely class-II-positive, as does weakly staining or nonstaining endothelium of large vessels. In addition focal increases in antigen expression were identified that were often perivascular or associated with a cellular infiltrate. Furthermore, once induced, class II antigen expression may return to a normal level: 7 of 16 grafts with increased antigen levels during the first month were normal at day 90.

The distribution of HLA class II antigens in the 29 pretransplant biopsies was consistent with our previous findings (*8*). HLA class II antigens were strongly expressed on the glomerular mesangium and endothelium, intertubular capillaries, and dendritic cells. The distal tubules were always negative, but the staining of proximal tubules varied among kidneys; positive in 27 kidneys and negative in two. The presence of HLA class II antigens on proximal tubules of normal kidney has been confirmed by other groups (*28, 29*) while Hall et al. (*22*) mention weak staining around the base of the tubular cells. However, these findings are at variance with other investigations (*19, 20, 30, 31*) in which class II antigens were not detected on proximal tubules. It is possible that the small numbers of kidneys studied by these groups did not express class II antigen on proximal tubules, although the results may reflect differences in the sensitivity of the staining techniques. One important variable is the anti-class-II antibody. A comparison of monoclonal anti-HLA-class-II antibodies as part of an international workshop revealed that although 79 antibodies detected class II antigens in the glomerulus and intertubular structures, 33% were unreactive with the proximal tubules (*32*). There are many possible explanations of these findings—e.g., antibody titer, antibody affinity, or epitope density.

Induction of class II antigens has been reported in pathological conditions such as thyroiditis (*13*) and primary biliary cirrhosis (*14*). In the field of transplantation, induced class II antigens have been detected in GVHD within skin and colonic epithelium (*10*), in kidney (*33*), and in liver (*34*). In rejecting skin grafts, aberrant expression of class II antigens has been described on epithelium (*35*) and on vascular endothelium (*12*). Takas et al. (*36*) have shown the presence of induced class II antigens on the bile duct epithelia during rejection of liver allografts. Studies of murine renal allografts have demonstrated class II induction in proximal tubules (*21*)—and, in the human, on all renal tubules (*22*) during allograft rejection.

Analysis of our data suggests an indirect rather than direct correlation between class II induction and rejection. In contrast to the reports of others (*22, 37*), there was not an absolute correlation between increased levels of class II antigens on renal tubules and clinical rejection. Of the rejection episodes, 26% were not accompanied by an increase in tubular class II antigen. However, patients with increased class II expression at 90 days had experienced more rejection episodes and courses of antirejection therapy than patients with normal class II expression. Once induced, class II antigens seem to persist for some weeks (*21*)—and it is, therefore, not surprising that during periods of stable graft function, both normal and increased class II expression was detected.

In this study the most significant association was between the degree of cellular infiltration and increased class II expression. Although biopsies with normal class II expression at days 21 and 90 contained marked leukocyte infiltration, the infiltrate in biopsies with increased class II expression was significantly greater. A similar association was seen with T lymphocyte infiltration, which is in accordance with T lymphocyte involvement in class II antigen induction in vivo. In GVHD, if the cell innoculum is depleted of T cells, class II induction is abrogated (*35*). In addition the T-lymphocyte-derived lymphokine interferon-γ has been shown in vitro to induce class II antigens on a variety of different cell types including macrophages (*15*), melanoma cells (*16*), endothelium, (*17*) and dermal fibroblasts (*18*). It is, therefore, possible that interferon-γ secreted by activated infiltrating cells may be responsible for the induction of tubular class II antigens in the renal allografts.

Induction of class II antigens was influenced quite markedly by the immunosuppressive therapy. It is of relevance that CsA has been shown to lead to failure of expression of class II major histocompatibility complex (MHC) antigens on canine arterial and venous endothelium in vitro (*38*) and in vivo in normal canine kidneys (*39*), suggesting that class II antigens are not constitutively expressed on endothelium. In this study patients receiving CsA had a lower incidence of increased class II expression than those treated with conventional AP therapy. One possible explanation for this observation is that CsA can inhibit interferon-γ release (*40*), perhaps by a dose-dependent mechanism—and may thereby diminish class II induction. Indeed class II was induced in 6 of our 12 CsA patients, and as patients in both groups had similar numbers of rejection episodes, this phenomenon was independent of rejection.

In vitro studies have demonstrated that cells on which class II antigens have been induced are able to function as antigen-presenting cells (*41, 42*). Indeed, transfection of mouse L cells with a human class II gene was sufficient to confer accessory cell function (*43*). Renal tubular cells expressing class II antigens may, therefore, act as antigen presenting cells and be an important stimulus of the rejection process. While endothelial cells, which have been shown to present antigens in certain circumstances (*42, 44*), express class II at the time of transplantation, the presence of induced tubular class II antigen may be of secondary importance in the stimulation of rejection. However, increased tubular class II would provide additional targets and may render the graft more vulnerable to destruction by effector mechanisms specific for class II antigens, leading to further damage of the renal parenchyma with tubular necrosis. However, if class II antigens did serve as additional targets for effector mechanisms, one would expect to see more histological evidence of glomerular damage in acute rejection—but this generally is not a striking feature of rejection episodes in renal transplantation. Nevertheless the association between CsA immunosuppressive therapy, the lower incidence of class II expression, and the better graft survival rate is quite impressive.

REFERENCES

1. Bodmer JG, Bodmer WF. Histocompatibility 1984. Immunol Today 1984; 5: 251.
2. Benacerraf B. Cellular interactions. In: Dorf ME, ed. The role of the major histocompatibility complex in immunobiology. Chichester: Wiley, 1981: 255.
3. Ting A, Morris PJ. A powerful effect of HLA-DR matching on survival of cadaver renal allografts. Lancet 1980; 2: 282.
4. Hammerling GJ. Tissue distribution of Ia antigens and their expression on lymphocyte subpopulations. Transplant Rev 1976; 30: 64.
5. Klareskog L, Tjernlund U, Forsum U, Peterson PA. Epidermal Langerhans cells express Ia antigens. Nature 1977; 268: 248.
6. Steinman RM, Kaplan G, Witmer MD, Cohn ZA. Identification of a novel cell type in peripheral lymphoid organs of mice. V. Purification of splenic dendritic cells, new surface markers and maintenance in vitro. J Exp Med 1979; 149: 1.
7. Hirschberg H, Moen T, Thorsby E. Specific destruction of human endothelial cell monolayers by anti-DRw antisera. Transplantation 1979; 28: 116.
8. Fuggle SV, Errasti P, Daar AS, Fabre JW, Ting A, Morris PJ. Localization of major histocompatibility complex (HLA-ABC and DR) antigens in 46 kidneys: differences in HLA-DR staining of tubules among kidneys. Transplantation 1983; 35: 385.
9. Daar AS, Fuggle SV, Fabre JW, Ting A, Morris PJ. The detailed distribution of MHC Class II antigens in normal human organs. Transplantation 1984; 38: 293.
10. Mason DW, Dallman M, Barclay AN. Graft-versus host disease induces expression of Ia antigen in rat epidermal cells and gut endothelium. Nature 1981; 293: 149.
11. Lampbert IA, Suitters AJ, Chisholm PM. Expression of Ia antigen on epidermal keratinocytes in GVHD. Nature 1981; 293: 149.
12. de Waal RMW, Bogmon MJJ, Maass CN, Cornelssen LMG, Tax WJM, Koene RAP. Variable expression of Ia antigens on the vascular endothelium of mouse skin allografts. Nature 1983; 303: 426.
13. Hanafusa T, Chiovato L, Doniach D, Pujol-Borrell R, Russell RCG, Bottazzo GF. Aberrant expression of HLA-DR antigen on thyrocytes in Graves disease: relevance for autoimmunity. Lancet 1983; 2: 1111.
14. Ballardini G, Bianchi FB, Doniach D, Mirakian R, Pisi E, Bottazzo GF. Aberrant expression of HLA-DR antigens on bile duct epithelium in primary biliary cirrhosis: relevance to pathogenesis. Lancet 1984; 2: 1009.
15. Steeg PS, Johnson HM, Oppenheim JJ. Regulation of murine macrophage Ia antigen expression by an immune interferon-like lymphokine: inhibitory effect of endotoxin. J Immunol 1982; 129: 2402.
16. Basham TY, Merigan TC. Recombinant interferon increases HLA-DR synthesis and expression. J Immunol 1983; 130: 1492.
17. Pober JS, Gimbrone MA, Cotran RS, Reiss CS, Burakoff SJ, Fiers W, Ault KA. Ia expression by vascular endothelium is inducible by activated T cells and by human interferon γ. J Exp Med 1983; 157: 1339.
18. Pober JS, Collins T, Gimbrone MA, et al. Lymphocytes recognize human vascular endothelial and dermal fibroblast Ia antigens induced by recombinant immune interferon. Nature 1983; 305: 726.
19. Scott H, Brandtzaeg P, Hirschberg M, Solheim BG, Thorsby E. Vascular and renal distribution of HLA-DR-like antigens. Tissue Antigens 1981; 18: 195.
20. Natali PG, DeMartino C, Quaranta V, et al. Expression of Ia-like antigens in normal human non-lymphoid tissues. Transplantation 1981; 31: 75.
21. Benson EM, Colvin RB, Russell PS. Induction of Ia antigens in murine renal transplants. J Immunol 1985; 134: 7.
22. Hall BM, Duggin GG, Phillips J, Bishop GA, Horvath JS, Tiller DJ. Increased expression of HLA-DR antigens on renal tubular cells in renal transplants: relevance to the rejection response. Lancet 1984; 2: 247.
23. Dalchau R, Kirkley J, Fabre JW. Monoclonal antibody to a human leukocyte-specific membrane glycoprotein probably homologous to the leukocyte-common (L-C) antigen of the rat. Eur J Immunol 1980; 10: 737.
24. Ledbetter JA, Evans RL, Lipinski M, Cunningham-Rundles C, Good RA, Herzenberg LA. Evolutionary conservation of surface molecules that distinguish T lymphocyte helper/inducer and T cytotoxic/suppressor subpopulations in mouse and man. J Exp Med 1981; 153: 310.
25. McKenzie JL, Fabre JW. Studies with a monoclonal antibody on the distribution of Thy-1 in the lymphoid and connective tissues of the dog. Transplantation 1981; 31: 275.
26. Bloom W, Fawcett DW. A textbook of histology. 10th ed. Philadelphia: Saunders, 1972.
27. Aherne WA, Dunnill MS. Morphometry. London: Arnold, 1982: 33.
28. Hancock WW, Kraft N, Atkins RC. The immunohistochemical demonstration of major histocompatibility antigens in the human kidney using monoclonal antibodies. Pathology 1982; 14: 409.
29. Evans PR, Trickett LP, Smith JL, MacIver AG, Tate D, Slapak M. Varying expression of major histocompatibility complex antigens on human renal endothelium and epithelium. Br J Pathol 1985; 66: 77.
30. Koyama K, Fukunishi T, Barcos M, Tanigaki N, Pressman D. Human Ia antigens in non-lymphoid organs. Immunology 1979; 38: 333.

31. Häyry P, von Willebrand E, Andersson LC. Expression of HLA-ABC and DR locus antigens on human kidney, endothelial, tubular and glomerular cells. Scand J Immunol 1980; 11: 303.
32. Fuggle SV, Carter NP, Ting A, Morris PJ. Studies on the tissue distribution of class II antigens. Dis Markers 1984; 2: 235.
33. Wadgymar A, Urmson J, Baumal R, Halloran PF. Changes in Ia expression in mouse kidney during acute graft-versus-host disease. J Immunol 1984; 132: 1826.
34. Suitters AJ, Lampbert IA. Class II induction in the liver of rats with graft-versus-host disease. Transplantation 1984; 38: 194.
35. Dallman MJ, Mason DW. Induction of Ia antigens on murine epidermal cells during the rejection of skin allografts. Transplantation 1983; 36: 222.
36. Takas L, Szende B, Monostori E, et al. Expression of HLA-DR antigens on bile duct cells of rejected liver transplants. Lancet 1983; 2: 1500.
37. Bishop GA, Hall BM, Phillips J, et al. Expression of HLA-DR antigens on renal tubular cells during rejection. Transplant Proc 1985; 17: 64.
38. Groenewegen G, Buurman WA, Jeunhomme GMAA, van der Linden CJ. Effect of cyclosporine on MHC–Class II antigen expression on arterial and venous endothelium in vitro. Transplantation 1985; 40: 21.
39. Groenewegen G. Vascular endothelial cells in immune reactions [Thesis]. University of Maastricht, 1985.
40. Reem GH, Cook LA, Vilcek J. Gamma interferon synthesis by human thymocytes and T lymphocytes inhibited by cyclosporin A. Science 1983; 221: 63.
41. Londei M, Lamb JR, Bottazzo GF, Feldmann M. Epithelial cells expressing aberrant MHC Class II determinants can present antigen to cloned human T cells. Nature 1984; 312: 639.
42. Groenewegen G, Buurman WA, Jeunhomme GMAA, van der Linden CJ, Vegt PA, Kootstra G. In vitro stimulation of lymphocytes by vascular endothelial cells. A study with canine arterial and venous endothelial cells. Transplantation 1984; 37: 206.
43. Austin P, Trowsdale J, Rudd C, Bodmer W, Feldmann M, Lamb J. Functional expression of HLA-DP genes transfected into mouse fibroblasts. Nature 1985; 313: 61.
44. Hirschberg H, Bergh OJ, Thorsby E. Antigen-presenting properties of human vascular endothelial cells. J Exp Med 1980; 152: 249s.

Received 26 September 1985.
Accepted 14 November 1985.

0041-1337/86/4202-0150$02.00/0
TRANSPLANTATION Vol. 42, No. 2

INCREASED FACTOR VIII AS AN INDEX OF VASCULAR INJURY IN CYCLOSPORINE NEPHROTOXICITY[1]

ZARIN BROWN, GUY H. NEILD,[2,3] JOHN J. WILLOUGHBY, NIKUNJI V. SOMIA, AND STEWART J. CAMERON

Renal Unit, Department of Medicine, Guy's Hospital, London SE1; and Institute of Urology, London WC2, England

Very high plasma concentrations of factor-VIII-related antigen (RAG) (VIII-RAG) were found in renal allograft recipients during periods of nephrotoxicity induced by cyclosporine. In eight recipients, who were investigated at weekly intervals, levels of factor-VIII-RAG fell toward normal as the dose of cyclosporine was reduced. Plasma levels of C-reactive protein, an acute phase reactant protein, were never raised in these recipients. These findings are further evidence that toxic doses of cyclosporine are associated with vascular injury.

The major complication of cyclosporine in renal transplantation is nephrotoxicity (*1*). The mechanism of acute nephrotoxicity is unknown but it is reversible and dose-dependent (*2, 3*). Cyclosporine is also associated with vascular injury and this effect may relate to its nephrotoxicity. A hemolytic uraemic syndrome (HUS)* may occur after both bone marrow (*4*) and liver transplantation (*5*). Renal allograft recipients receiving high doses of cyclosporine may develop glomerular capillary thrombosis (*6*) or a renal arteriolar vasculopathy, which is similar to the arteriolar lesion associated with severe hypertension or HUS (*7*). Following mismatched bone marrow transplantation there may be massive loss of endothelial integrity with pulmonary edema and fluid retention (*8*). Cyclosporine greatly enhances vascular injury that occurs in experimental acute serum sickness in rabbits (*9*), and accelerates renal arteriosclerosis in the spontaneously hypertensive rat (*10*). Factor-VIII-related antigen (VIII-RAG) is one of several proteins synthesized by the vascular endothelium (*11*). Increased blood levels of factor VIII-RAG have been found in diseases associated with vascular injury (*12–14*). To examine whether cyclosporine is implicated in renal vascular injury, we measured

[1] This work was supported by the Leukaemia Research Fund and by the special trustees of Guy's Hospital.
[2] Institute of Urology.
[3] Address correspondence to: GH Neild, M.D., M.R.C.P., St. Philip's Hospital, Sheffield St., London WC2 A2EX, England.

* Abbreviations used: AT III, antithrombin III; AZA, azathioprine; CRP, C-reactive protein; CsA, cyclosporine; ELISA, enzyme-linked immunosorbent assay; HUS, hemolytic uremic syndrome; Pred, prednisolone; RIA, radioimmunoassay; FVIII-C, factor VIII coagulant activity; FVIII-RAG, factor-VIII-related antigen.

plasma concentrations of factor-VIII-RAG in renal allograft recipients during periods of nephrotoxicity.

MATERIALS AND METHODS

Patients. Eight patients with nephrotoxicity were selected from a group of sixty consecutive renal allograft recipients who were immunosuppressed with cyclosporine and prednisolone. Their clinical details and the immunological status of donor and recipient have been reported (*15*). Our assessment of nephrotoxicity was based on clinical and morphological findings and the response to a reduction in the cyclosporine dose (*15*).

Immunosuppression. Cyclosporine (Sandimmun, Sandoz Ltd.) was given orally as a single daily dose in the following regimen: 14 mg/kg/day for 14 days, then 12 mg/kg/day until day 30, 10 mg/kg/day until day 60, 8 mg/kg/day until day 90, then 6 mg/kg/day. Prednisolone was given orally at a starting dose of 15 mg/m^2 tapering to a dose of 10 mg/m^2 at 6 months. Whole-blood cyclosporine levels (μg/L) were measured by radioimmunoassay (RIA), using the Sandoz RIA kit. Cyclosporine was given at 6.00 P.M., and blood levels were measured the following morning.

Methods. For this study patients were bled initially at weekly intervals and subsequently every two to four weeks at clinic attendances. Aliquots of serum and citrated plasma were stored at −70°C.

Factor-VIII-RAG was measured in citrated plasma by two methods:

1. "Rocket" immunoelectrophoresis (*16*) using rabbit antibody to human FVIII-RAG (Atlantic Antibodies) and standardized against the 9th British standard for factor VIII (National Institute for Biological Standards and Control, Hampstead).

2. Enzyme-linked immunoabsorbent assay (ELISA) (*17*). This method was modified by the use of 3,3′5,5′-tetramethylbenzidine dihydrochloride (Miles Ltd.) as a substrate solution.

C-reactive protein was determined by single radial immunodiffusion using goat antihuman C-reactive protein antibody and standardized using Calibrator 7 (Atlantic Antibodies). The lower limit of detection was 6 μg/ml.

Factor VIII coagulant activity (FVIII-C) was assayed by a one-stage technique (*18*) using factor-VIII-deficient plasma (Immuno Ltd.). Antithrombin III was measured in citrated plasma by a two-step colorimetric assay using the Diacrom AT III kit (Wellcome Diagnostics).

Renal function. Plasma urea and creatinine, plasma biochemistry, and hematological indices were monitored (*7*). Renal biopsies were performed routinely after one week, one month and one year, and for episodes of renal dysfunction. Renal dysfunction was defined as an episode of deteriorating renal function with a rise in plasma creatinine of more than 20% above the preceeding baseline value or an inappropriately high plasma creatinine that fell by 20% or more with the correct treatment. Episodes of dysfunction considered to be due to rejection were treated with pulses of 1 g methylprednisolone on three consecutive days. Episodes of dysfunction thought to be due to nephrotoxicity were treated by a reduction in the dose of cyclosporine of 2 mg/kg/day every seven days.

Controls. Control groups were (1) 21 healthy volunteers; (2) 10 patients on hemodialysis; (3) 19 transplant recipients who were maintained on prednisolone and azathioprine, including seven with creatinine levels of over 200 μmol/L and deteriorating function; and (4) 8 patients receiving prednisolone and cyclosporine who had neither rejection nor toxicity. These patients were followed for the same period as the 8 patients with nephrotoxicity. In addition we examined 6 plasma samples from 5 patients, within 2 days of a biopsy-proved diagnosis of rejection, which occurred 7 days or more after transplantation.

Statistics. Comparison of different groups was made by a Wilcoxon rank sum test.

RESULTS

During this study the cyclosporine levels were not used in our clinical management, and we used higher doses than at present. Several patients were nephrotoxic for a longer period than we would now permit.

Factor VIII-RAG (rocket) levels were measured retrospectively on serial samples from eight patients who had episodes of nephrotoxicity lasting at least 22 weeks and who never had evidence of rejection. Figure 1 shows their factor-VIII-RAG levels at the beginning of their nephrotoxic period, which occurred 5.8±2.4 weeks (mean ± SEM) after transplantation, and 44±11 weeks later, when they were either less toxic or considered no longer to be toxic. They were compared with the following groups (1) normal controls; (2) uremic controls; (3) transplant recipients receiving prednisolone and azathioprine with creatinine concentrations ranging from 80 to 550 μmol/L (205±73); (4) transplant recipients with stable function on prednisolone and cyclosporine studied during weeks 5 to 6 and after week 37. These data and the renal function at the time of study are summarized in Table 1. Serial data on a nephrotoxic individual is shown in Figure 2.

We found a very close correlation between factor-VIII-RAG levels as measured by "rockets" and ELISA up to levels of 4

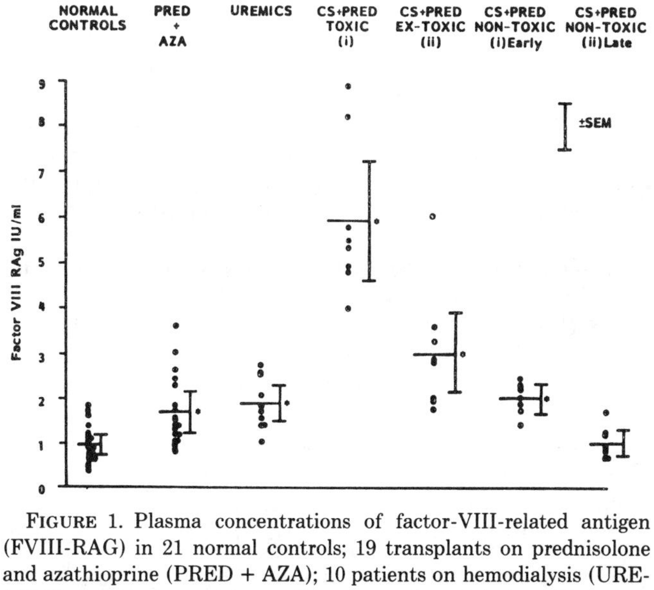

FIGURE 1. Plasma concentrations of factor-VIII-related antigen (FVIII-RAG) in 21 normal controls; 19 transplants on prednisolone and azathioprine (PRED + AZA); 10 patients on hemodialysis (UREMICS); 8 patients receiving cyclosporine and prednisolone (i) at start of toxicity: mean time after transplantation week 5.8 (CS + PRED TOXIC), and (ii) later when less toxic (CS + PRED EX-TOXIC): mean time week 44; 8 patients receiving cyclosporine and prednisolone who had neither rejection nor toxicity (CS + PRED NON-TOXIC) were studied (i) early: weeks 5–6, and (ii) later: mean week 37 (P <0.001 compared with normal controls).

TABLE 1. Clinical and hematological data

	n	FVIII RAg (IU/ml)	AT III (%)	FVIII C (IU/ml)	Creatinine (μmol/L)	CsA levels (μg/L)	CsA dose (mg/kg/day)
I. CsA + Pred.: toxic	8	5.9±1.36	155±15.0	1.5±0.6	215±54	1280±196	9.8±1.9
II. CsA + Pred.: ex-toxic	8	3.1±1.10	142±16.0	1.5±0.6	152±52	599±254	4.1±0.9
I. CsA + Pred.: nontoxic	8	2.0±0.26	116±13.6	1.4±1.1	182±54	559±208	9.5±0.6
II. CsA + Pred.: nontoxic	8	1.0±0.25	114±13.8	—	137±25	405±98	5.2±0.6
Pred + Aza	19	1.7±0.37	149±14.0	1.2±0.5	205±73	—	—
Uremics	10	1.9±0.38	121±13.0	—	1069±164	—	—
Normal controls	21	1.0±0.17	108±4.0	0.97±0.3	97±14	—	—

[a] Groups are the same as those in Figure 1. All results are shown as mean ± SEM. Cyclosporine levels are whole blood values measured by RIA.

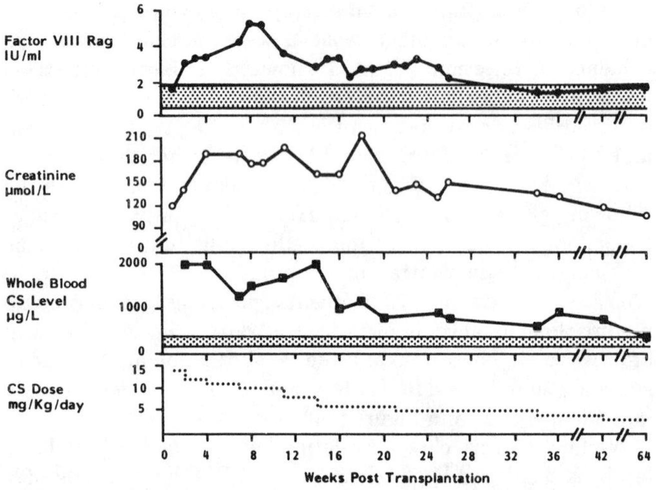

FIGURE 2. Serial data on one patient with cyclosporine nephrotoxicity. Hatched areas show normal range.

IU. Above this level the rocket method progressively overestimated the ELISA results.

Factor-VIII-C was not significantly raised in any group (Table 1). Antithrombin III was significantly raised in the nephrotoxic group compared with the nontoxic group at a comparable time, normal controls, and uremic controls (P=<0.001; Table 1).

In our normal population CRP levels were 9.6±2.3 μg/ml (mean ± SEM). We considered levels above 18 μg/ml to be raised. C-reactive protein was raised in the first week following transplant operation, as previously described (*19*). It was not subsequently raised in any of our patients who were nephrotoxic. We have examined 6 samples taken within 2 days of a diagnosis of rejection. Rejection occurred at day 16±4 (mean ± SEM), range day 9–21: CRP was raised in all cases 43.5±19 μg/ml (mean ± SEM), range 30–83. In these samples the mean factor-VIII-RAG was 2.8±0.8 IU/ml (mean ± SEM), range 1.5–4.

DISCUSSION

We found very high levels of factor-VIII-related antigen in renal allograft recipients during periods of cyclosporine nephrotoxicity. Factor-VIII-RAG is produced by the vascular endothelium and also by megakaryocytes (*11*). Raised levels are indicative of vascular injury (*12–14*).

Factor VIII coagulant activity (VIII-C) was not significantly raised. Like factor VIII-RAG, it is also an acute phase protein, but its site of synthesis is unknown (*20*). However, we do not believe that we have measured an acute phase protein response, since levels of the acute phase protein CRP were not raised. In uremia, all forms of factor VIII are raised (*21*), but this may be only a marker of an acute-phase protein response, rather than of vascular injury (*22*). Our nephrotoxic patients were not uremic; both their factor-VIII-RAG and antithrombin III levels were significantly higher than the uremic controls. Antithrombin III is also synthesized by the vascular endothelium (*23*); raised levels in our nephrotoxic patients are also indicative of vascular involvement.

There is evidence from both animal studies and allograft recipients that cyclosporine initiates or enhances vascular injury (*4–10*). It may enhance platelet-endothelial interaction (*7, 9*), and this might lead to endothelial injury. It has been reported that cyclosporine therapy is associated both with an increased tendency to thrombosis and with increased platelet aggregability (*24*). Hypercoagulability could be mediated by increased monocyte procoagulant activity (*25*). However, we can not exclude that cyclosporine may have a direct effect on the endothelium—either causing abnormal stimulation or a toxic injury.

Could the raised factor VIII levels be due to chronic vascular rejection? Our patients diagnosed as nephrotoxic had no morphological evidence of rejection in their renal biopsy material (*15*) and their renal function improved progressively as the dose of cyclosporine was reduced. None of our 60 transplant recipients who have received cyclosporine and who have been studied prospectively have had clinical and morphological evidence of chronic rejection within the first year, so we can not comment on what might occur in such a process. We have, however, studied seven patients who were receiving prednisolone and azathioprine and who had slowly and progressively deteriorating renal function. Their levels of factor-VIII-RAG were no higher than those on similar therapy with normal function.

We did not routinely examine patients during acute rejection. Acute-phase proteins may rise for 4–5 days during rejection (*19*). However, we found raised levels of CRP, in samples taken at least 7 days posttransplantation, in all patients who were rejecting. It is likely that one single measurement of a high level of factor-VIII-RAG reflects only endothelial injury, but the simultaneous measurement of CRP may permit one to distinguish rejection (with raised CRP) from nephrotoxicity (with normal CRP).

In samples in which the factor-VIII-RAG was highest we found the levels as measured by the rocket method were disproportionately raised compared with the ELISA method. In acute respiratory failure, a condition characterized by thrombosis and loss of endothelial integrity in the pulmonary microcirculation, this discrepancy has also been reported (*14*), and it has been suggested that the vascular endothelium may release an early, incomplete, or defective factor VIII molecule, or that normally synthesized factor VIII is altered in the circulation by proteolytic enzymes (*20, 14*).

In conclusion, we believe that the high levels of factor-VIII-RAG associated with cyclosporine-toxicity are due to enhanced production of factor-VIII-RAG by the vascular endothelium. Serial measurements of factor-VIII-RAG may be a useful guide in the management of nephrotoxicity.

Acknowledgments. Our thanks to Jane Needham and Cecilia Gillespie for technical assistance, and to Dr. Sam Machin for valuable discussions.

REFERENCES

1. Cyclosporin A as sole immunosuppressive agent in recipients of kidney allografts from cadaver donors: preliminary results of a European Multicentre Trial. Lancet 1982; 2: 57.
2. Klintmalm GBG, Iwatsuki S, Starzl TE. Nephrotoxicity of Cyclosporin A in liver and kidney transplant patients. Lancet 1981; 1: 470.
3. Hows JM, Chipping PM, Fairhead S, Smith J, Baughan A, Gordon-Smith EC. Nephrotoxicity in bone marrow transplant recipients treated with cyclosporin A. Br J Haematol 1983; 54: 69.
4. Shulman H, Striker G, Deeg HJ, Kennedy M, Storb R, Thomas ED. Nephrotoxicity of Cyclosporin A after allogeneic marrow transplantation: glomerular thromboses and tubular injury. N Engl J Med 1981; 305: 1392.
5. Bonser RS, Adu D, Franklin I, McMaster P. Cyclosporin-induced haemolytic uraemic syndrome in liver allograft recipient. Lancet 1984; 2: 1337.
6. Neild GH, Reuben R, Hartley RB, Cameron JS. Glomerular thrombi in renal allografts associated with Cyclosporin therapy. J Clin Pathol 1985; 38: 253.
7. Mihatsch MJ, Thiel G, Spichtin HP, et al. Morphological findings in kidney transplants after treatment with Cyclosporine. Transplant Proc 1983; 15: 2821.
8. Powles R, Pedrazzini A, Crofts M, Clink H, et al. Mismatched family bone marrow transplantation. Semin Haematol 1984; 21: 182.
9. Neild GH, Ivory K, Williams DG. Glomerular thrombosis and cortical infarction in Cyclosporin-treated rabbits with acute serum sickness. Br J Exp Pathol 1983; 65: 133.
10. Ryffel B, Siegel H, Mueller AM, Hauser R, Mihatsch MJ. Nephrotoxicity of cyclosporine in spontaneously hypertensive rats. Transplant Proc 1985; 17: 1430.
11. Jaffe EA. Endothelial cells and the biology of factor VIII. N Engl J Med 1977; 296: 377.
12. Jones RL, Peterson CM. The fluid phase of coagulation and the accelerated atherosclerosis of diabetes mellitus. Diabetes 1981; 30 (suppl 2): 33.
13. Kahaleh MB, Osborn I, LeRoy EC. Increased factor VIII/von Willebrand factor antigen and von Willebrand factor activity in scleroderma and in Raynaud's phenomenon. Ann Intern Med 1981; 94: 482.
14. Carvalho ACA, Bellman SM, Saullo VJ, Quinn D, Zapol WM. Altered factor VIII in acute respiratory failure. N Engl J Med 1982; 307: 1113.
15. Taube DH, Neild GH, Williams DG, Cameron JS, et al. Differentiation between allograft rejection and cyclosporin nephrotoxicity in renal allograft recipients. Lancet 1985; 2: 171.
16. Laurell CB. Quantitative estimation of proteins by electrophoresis in agarose gel containing antibody. Anal Biochem 1966; 15: 45.
17. Short PE, Williams CE, Picken AM, Hill FGH. Factor VIII related antigen: an improved enzyme immunoassay. Med Lab Sci 1982; 39: 351.
18. Austen DEG, Rhymes IL. In: A laboratory manual of blood coagulation. Oxford: Blackwell, 1980: 53.
19. Maury CPJ, Teppo A-M. Comparative study of serum amyloid-related protein SAA, C-reactive protein, and B2-microglobulin as markers of renal allograft rejection. Clin Nephrol 1984; 22: 284.
20. Lombardi R, Mannucci PM, Seghatchian MJ, Vicente V, Coppola R. Alterations of factor VIII/v Willebrand factor in clinical conditions associated with an increase in its plasma concentration. Br J Haematol 1981; 49: 61.
21. Deykin D. Uraemic bleeding (Nephrology forum). Kidney Int 1983; 24: 698.
22. Howard MA, Whitworth JA, Hendrix LE, Thomas KB, Firkin BG. Abnormal factor VIII in chronic renal failure. Med J Aust 1979; 1: 148.
23. Chan TK, Chan V. Antithrombin III, the major modulator of intravascular coagulation, is synthesized by human endothelial cells. Thromb Haemost 1981; 46(2): 504.
24. Vanrenterghem Y, Roels L, Lerut T, et al. Thrombo-embolic complications and haemostatic changes in cyclosporin-treated cadaveric kidney allograft recipients. Lancet 1985; 1: 99.
25. Carlsen E, Mallet AC, Prydz H. Effect of Cyclosporine A on procoagulant activity in mononuclear blood cells and monocytes in vitro. Clin Exp Immunol 1985; 60: 407.

Received 15 October 1985.
Accepted 14 November 1985.

0041-1337/86/4202-0154$02.00/0
TRANSPLANTATION
Vol. 42, No. 2

Printed in U.S.A.

DETRIMENTAL EFFECT OF CYCLOSPORINE ON INITIAL FUNCTION OF CADAVER RENAL ALLOGRAFTS FOLLOWING EXTENDED PRESERVATION

RESULTS OF A RANDOMIZED PROSPECTIVE STUDY

ANDREW C. NOVICK,[1] HWEI HO-HSIEH, DONALD STEINMULLER, STEVAN B. STREEM, ROBERT J. CUNNINGHAM, DIANE STEINHILBER, MARLENE GOORMASTIC, AND CAROLINE BUSZTA

The Section of Renal Transplantation, Cleveland Clinic Foundation, Cleveland, Ohio

We report herein the results of a randomized prospective trial comparing maintenance cyclosporine (CsA)-prednisone immunosuppression to a regimen of azathioprine-prednisone-antilymphocyte globulin (ALG) in cadaver renal transplant recipients. Fifty-six patients were entered into this study with 31 assigned to the ALG group and 25 to the CsA group. These two groups were well matched for most major determinants of graft outcome and the mean renal preservation time was 37 hr in each group. The incidence of acute tubular necrosis (ATN) was high in both groups (58% ALG, 72% CsA, NS). There were five cases of primary nonfunction in the CsA group and only one in the ALG group (P=.05). Of the kidneys that functioned, the mean serum creatinine nadir (1.5 vs. 2.2 mg/dl, P=.06) and the mean number of days to reach the serum creatinine nadir (24.2 vs. 43.3 days, P=.03) were both less in the ALG group. The actuarial one-year graft survival rate in the ALG and CsA groups is 78% and 48%, respectively (P<.05). This difference is mainly due to the large number of primary nonfunctioning grafts in the latter group, which we attribute to the effect of CsA's nephrotoxicity superimposed on renal ischemia incurred prior to transplantation. These data emphasize that, in order to realize the full benefit of CsA in cadaver transplantation, renewed emphasis must be placed on minimizing ischemic renal damage.

Cyclosporine, a fungal peptide metabolite, is the newest addition to the maintenance immunosuppressive armamentarium for preventing rejection folowing cadaver renal transplantation. There is little doubt that the use of this agent in combination with prednisone has yielded improved graft survival compared with conventional regimens involving azathioprine and prednisone (*1–3*). Nevertheless, a number of issues remain unresolved concerning the most useful application of cyclosporine in cadaver transplantation (*4*).

Several studies have shown no significant difference in graft or patient survival when comparing immunosuppression with cyclosporine-prednisone with conventional regimens incorporating antilymphocyte globulin (ALG)* (*5–7*). In this context, the advantage of cyclosporine has been in achieving a reduced incidence of rejection episodes and infections along with a shorter hospitalization time (*7*). These benefits have been weighed against its known nephrotoxicity, as manifested by elevated serum creatinine levels, and a greater incidence of hypertension in cyclosporine-treated patients (*7–9*).

Another controversial issue concerns a possible severe detrimental effect of cyclosporine on initial cadaver graft function caused by its nephrotoxicity superimposed on renal ischemia incurred during organ procurement or preservation. Some studies have observed such an effect while others have not (*6, 7, 10–15*).

When cyclosporine became available for general use in late 1983, we initiated a randomized prospective trial comparing maintenance cyclosporine-prednisone immunosuppression to our existing regimen of azathioprine-prednisone-ALG. The results in 56 consecutive cadaver transplant recipients entered into this trial are presented herein, with emphasis on measures of initial graft function and their effect on eventual graft outcome in these two groups.

MATERIALS AND METHODS

From December 1983 to September 1984, 56 cadaver renal transplants were performed at the Cleveland Clinic. All cadaver kidneys were procured from suitable heart-beating donors who were managed with a standard protocol including liberal hydration and administration of diuretic agents. All cadaver kidneys were removed with a warm ischemia time of <5 min, flushed with Collins-2 solution, and then preserved by hypothermic pulsatile perfusion using plasmanate as the perfusate. In all cases, viability criteria on perfusion were acceptable (*16*) and transplantation was performed with a revascularization time <45 min.

The selection and preparation of recipients for renal transplantation in our program have previously been described (*17–19*). HLA AB and DR antigens were determined for all donors and recipients. In all cases, the donor and recipient were red-cell compatible, with a negative current lymphocytotoxic cross-match. All recipients had received blood transfusions prior to transplantation. At the time of transplantation, patients were randomly assigned to an immunosuppressive regimen involving either cyclosporine (CsA) or Minnesota ALG. Permission for inclusion in the present study was obtained from each patient. In this study, 9 pairs of cadaver kidneys (i.e., both kidneys from the same donor) were transplanted; the recipient of one kidney from each pair was managed with CsA while the recipient of the second kidney from each pair was managed with ALG.

All patients received 1 g i.v. methylprednisolone (IVMP) in four divided doses on the day of transplantation. Maintenance

[1] Address requests for reprints to: Andrew C. Novick, M.D., Chairman, Organ Transplant Center, Cleveland Clinic Foundation, 9500 Euclid Avenue, Cleveland, Ohio 44106.

* Abbreviations used: ALG, antilymphocyte globulin; ATN, acute tubular necrosis; CsA, cyclosporine; IVMP, intravenous methylprednisolone.

immunosuppression in the ALG group (n=31) was with prednisone 30 mg/day with further tapering after two months, azathioprine 1–2 mg/kg/day, and ALG 20 mg/kg/day for the first 14 days; episodes of rejection were treated with a second course of ALG or IVMP—or, in some cases, cyclosporine.

Maintenance immunosuppression in the CsA groups (n=25) was with prednisone 30 mg/day with further tapering after two months, and oral cyclosporine 14 mg/kg/day commencing a few hours pretransplant. The oral cyclosporine dose was reduced to 12 mg/kg/day after two weeks, to 10 mg/kg/day after four weeks, and was then adjusted individually according to the level of renal function and 24-hr whole-blood trough CsA levels as determined by high-pressure liquid chromatography (*20*). Blood trough levels were obtained daily while in the hospital and dose adjustments were made to keep this level between 100 and 200 ng/ml. For patients unable to take oral medication initially postoperatively, i.v. cyclosporine was administered at a daily dose of 4–6 mg/kg/day. Figure 1 illustrates the mean daily oral dose of cyclosporine following transplantation for patients in this group. Episodes of rejection in this group were treated with either IVMP or ALG.

Acute tubular necrosis (ATN) was defined as the need for dialysis within the first week posttransplant. Several assessments were used in establishing a diagnosis of rejection including clinical signs, the serum creatinine level, isotope renography with hippuran, ultrasonography, computerized tomography, the serum CsA level, and allograft biopsy. For some patients in the CsA group with a mild elevation in the serum creatinine level, a trial of lowering the daily cyclosporine dose was attempted—and, if renal function improved, the episode was ascribed to cyclosporine nephrotoxicity. All instances of rejection in the CsA group were verified by a renal biopsy demonstrating characteristic histological criteria (*21*). Complete follow-up has been obtained in all patients and the posttransplant interval ranges from 8–17 months.

Univariate comparisons of demographic and clinical variables were done using the chi-square test or Students *t* test as appropriate. Graft survival estimates were calculated using the Kaplan-Meier Method (*22*). The generalized Wilcoxon statistic was used to test for curve differences (*23*). Multivariate graft survival comparisons after adjusting for differences in individual variables were done using the Cox proportional hazards regression model (*24*). Graft loss was considered to occur at the time of transplant nephrectomy, return to dialysis or death from any cause.

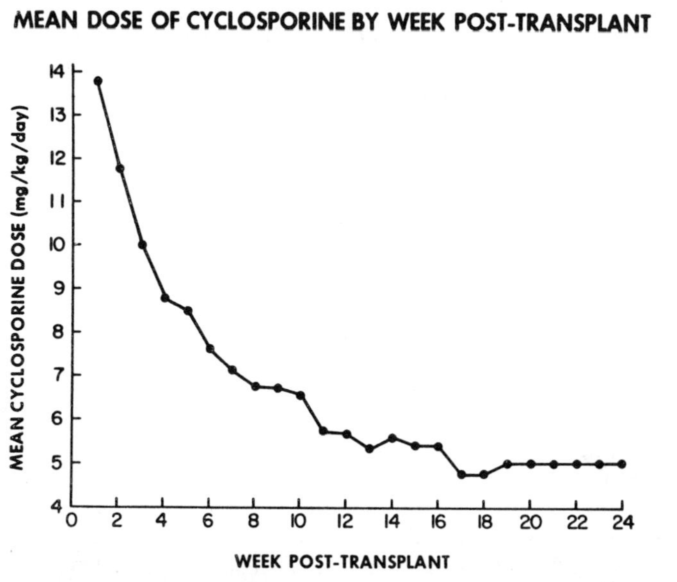

FIGURE 1. Mean daily oral dose of cyclosporine following cadaver renal transplantation for patients in the CsA group.

RESULTS

Of 56 patients in this study, 31 were assigned to the ALG group and 25 were assigned to the CsA group. The characteristics of patients in the two groups are detailed in Table 1, along with significance results for univariate comparisons between the two groups. There were more retransplants in the CsA group (P=.06) and more better DR-matched grafts in the ALG group (P=.02).

Early graft function. Renal preservation times and data relative to initial graft function in the two groups are described in Table 2. All but two kidneys in the study were preserved for >24 hr, and 38 kidneys (68%) were preserved for >36 hr. The mean preservation time for the ALG and CsA groups is identical (37.2 hr vs. 37.5 hr). The incidence of ATN was high in both groups (58% ALG, 72% CsA) with no significant difference. There were 5 cases of primary nonfunction in the CsA group and only 1 in the ALG group (P=.05). The six primary nonfunctioning kidneys were obtained from donors with ages of 12, 19, 25, 36, 47, and 58 years. These primary nonfunctioning kidneys were all removed 3–7 weeks posttransplant; in all cases, histopathologic study showed patchy cortical necrosis with no evidence of rejection or a primary vascular problem.

The mean blood trough CsA level during the first three days posttransplant was calculated for each patient in the CsA group. For the entire CsA group, this level ranged from 92 to 286 ng/ml (mean 169 ng/ml). The mean blood trough CsA level during

TABLE 1. Characteristics of patients in the ALG and cyclosporine groups

	ALG group (n = 31)	CsA group (n = 25)	P
Sex:			
Male	19	15	0.99
Female	12	10	
Mean recipient age (range), in years	36 (12–62)	40 (13–63)	0.20
Diabetes mellitus	3	3	0.78
Retransplants	2	6	0.06
Blood transfusions:			
0	0	0	
1–5	24	16	0.27
>5	7	9	
HLA AB match:			
<2	21	16	0.77
≥2	10	9	
HLA DR match:			
0 Ag	3	8	
1 Ag	17	15	0.02
2 Ag	11	2	
Source of cadaver kidney:			
Local	23	19	0.88
Imported	8	6	
Age (years) of cadaver donor:			
Range	4–56	7–58	0.91
Mean	27	27	

TABLE 2. Preservation time and initial graft function in ALG and cyclosporine groups

	ALG group (n = 31)	CsA group (n = 25)	P
Preservation time (hr):			
<24	1	1	0.99
24–36	9	7	
>36	21	17	
Range	19.3–46.1	23.4–49.3	
Mean	37.2	37.5	
ATN:	18 (58%)	18 (72%)	0.28
Primary Nonfunction	1	5	0.05
Mean No. dialyses[a]	5.06	5.83	0.34
Mean Scr nadir (mg/dl)[a,b]	1.5	2.2	0.06
Mean days to Scr nadir[a]	24.2	43.3	0.03

[a] Excluding primary nonfunctioning grafts.
[b] Scr = serum creatinine.

the first three days for the 5 patients with primary graft nonfunction was 102, 127, 146, 174, and 243 ng/ml.

Of the kidneys in both groups that functioned, there was no significant difference in the number of dialysis treatments that were necessary pending resolution of ATN. However, the mean serum creatinine nadir (1.5 vs. 2.2 mg/dl, P=.06) and the mean number of days to reach the serum creatinine nadir (24.2 vs. 43.3 days, P=.03) were both less in the ALG group.

Early graft function in paired kidney recipients. There were nine pairs of kidneys from the same cadaver donor in which one kidney from each pair was transplanted into a recipient managed with ALG and the other into a recipient managed with CsA. In these ALG and CsA subgroups, all factors relative to donor status, donor preparation, and procurement were identical. Within each pair of kidneys, the difference in preservation time ranged from 0–5 hr. In five pairs of kidneys, the graft allocated to an ALG patient was preserved longer; in three pairs of kidneys, the preservation time of each graft was identical (within 1 hr); in one pair of kidneys, the graft allocated to a CsA patient was preserved longer (3 hr).

The mean preservation time in these ALG and CsA subgroups is 38.4 hr and 36.3 hr, respectively (Table 3). There was one case of primary nonfunction in a CsA-treated patient. The serum creatinine nadir (1.45 vs. 2.65 mg/dl) and the mean number of days to reach the serum creatinine nadir (18.3 vs. 28.3 days) were both less in the ALG subgroup, but these differences were not statistically significant due to the small number of grafts. Figure 2 depicts the mean serum creatinine level following transplantation in these two subgroups; the changes in renal function reflect not only the rate and extent of recovery from renal ischemia but also the occurrence of rejection episodes within each subgroup.

Rejection episodes and graft outcome. The occurrence and timing of rejection episodes in the ALG and CsA groups is provided in Table 4. Rejection episodes occurred in 20 of 31 ALG patients (65%), including 9 patients who experienced rejection within the first 30 days posttransplant. Only 6 of 25 CsA patients (24%) developed an episode of rejection (P<.005).

Currently, 25 of 31 grafts in the ALG group and 14 of 25 grafts in the CsA group are functioning, with a mean follow-up interval of 12.3 and 11.6 months, respectively. The causes of graft loss are listed in Table 5. The actuarial one-year graft survival rate in the ALG and CsA groups is 78% and 48%, respectively (Fig. 3, P<.05). A multivariate analysis of graft survival after adjusting for differences in DR matches and retransplants still shows significantly improved graft survival in the ALG group compared with the CsA group (P=.02).

Among CsA-treated patients, equivalent one-year graft survival was observed with a preservation time <36 hr or >36 hr

TABLE 3. Preservation time and initial graft function in paired kidney recipients

	ALG group (n = 9)	CsA group (n = 9)	P
Preservation time (hr):			
Range	30.1–45.1	24.3–44.7	
Mean	38.4	36.3	
ATN	6	7	
Primary Non-Function	0	1	
Mean No. dialyses[a]	5.0	6.5	
Mean Scr nadir (mg/dl)[a,b]	1.45	2.65	NS[c]
Mean days to Scr nadir[a]	18.3	28.3	NS

[a] Excluding primary nonfunctioning grafts.
[b] Scr = serum creatinine.
[c] NS = not significant.

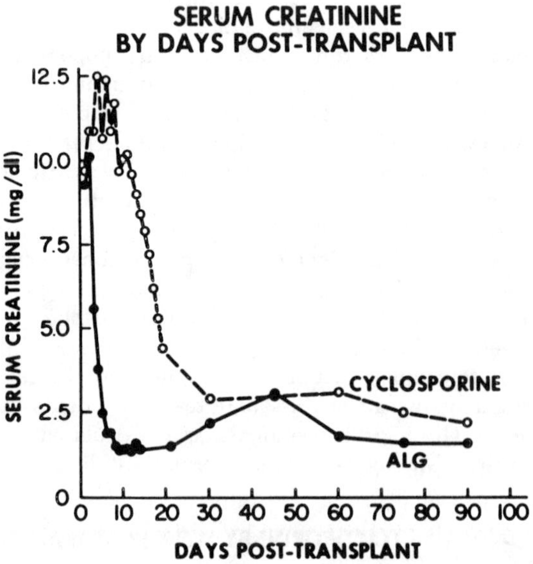

FIGURE 2. Mean serum creatinine level following transplantation in paired kidney recipients managed with cyclosporine or ALG.

TABLE 4. Rejection episodes and graft survival in ALG and cyclosporine groups

	ALG group (n = 31)	CsA group (n = 25)
No. rejections:		
0	11	19
1	12	6
2	7	0
>2	1	0
Days to onset of rejection:		
<30	9	4
30–60	7	0
>60	4	2
Mean	52.3	49.6
Functioning grafts:		
First transplants	23/29	10/19
Retransplants	2/2	4/6
Overall	25/31	14/25

TABLE 5. Causes of graft loss in ALG and cyclosporine groups

ALG group	CsA group
Rejection (2)	Rejection (3)
Primary Nonfunction (1)	Primary Nonfunction (5)
Heart failure (1)[a]	Myocardial infarction (1)[a]
Bowel perforation (1)[a]	Bowel perforation (1)
Urologic complication (1)	Tuberculosis (1)[a]

[a] Died with a functioning graft.

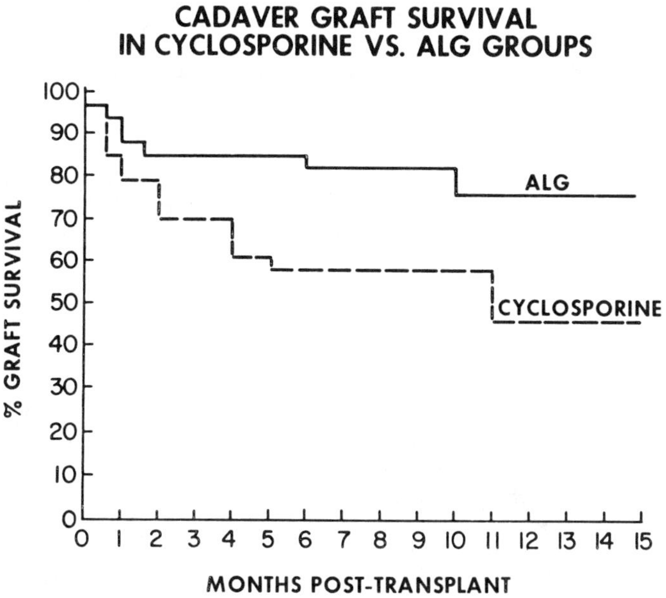

FIGURE 3. Actuarial cadaver graft survival following transplantation in ALG (n=31) and cyclosporine (n=25) groups. The difference is statistically significant ($P<.05$).

(50% vs. 47%). There was no correlation between DR antigen matching and graft outcome in this study. The actual six-month graft survival rate with 0, 1, and 2 DR-matched grafts is 73%, 75%, and 69% for the entire series; 67%, 88%, and 82% for the ALG group; and 75%, 60%, and 0% for the CsA group.

Currently, 52 of 56 patients are alive. Two patients have died in each group; all of the patients who died had a functioning graft at the time of death.

DISCUSSION

Following the initiation of clinical trials with cyclosporine as an immunosuppressive agent in cadaver renal transplantation, it soon became apparent that nephrotoxicity was a commonly observed side-effect. In one of the earliest studies by Calne et al. (*14*), posttransplant oliguria occurred in 11 of 32 patients treated with cyclosporine; the authors attributed this to nephrotoxicity and recommended withholding the drug unless a prompt initial diuresis was observed. Subsequent work in this country confirmed the renal toxicity of daily maintenance cyclosporine, while suggesting that this problem could be monitored with serum drug levels and reversed by appropriate dose reduction (*8, 9, 25*). In general, this policy has proven both judicious and effective, and significant permanent renal damage from long-term cyclosporine administration has not thus far been observed, although many patients have elevated serum creatinine levels.

Several recent studies have focused attention again on the problem alluded to in Calne's initial report, namely the harmful effect of cyclosporine's nephrotoxicity in the setting of a freshly transplanted cadaver kidney that has been subjected to prolonged ischemia. Although such ischemia might otherwise be tolerated with complete renal recovery, the combined effect of these two factors appears to cause permanent graft damage in some cases. In the Canadian multicenter trial (*13*), graft survival was impaired when cyclosporine was administered to recipients of cadaver kidneys preserved for >24 hr or with a revascularization time of >45 min; this effect was not present in patients managed with azathioprine. In this study, the incidence of primary graft nonfunction was also higher with cyclosporine therapy compared with azathioprine. In the Minnesota trial (*7*), cadaver graft survival was significantly lower in cyclosporine-treated patients whose grafts underwent ATN compared with those who did not undergo ATN; a significant difference was not observed when the same analysis was done for azathioprine-treated patients. Finally, a recent report from the International Collaborative Transplant Study indicated significantly better allograft survival with cyclosporine compared with conventional immunosuppression when the renal preservation time was <36 hr; however with >36 hr of renal preservation, graft survival with cyclosporine was markedly reduced—and, in fact, equal to that obtained with conventional therapy (*15*).

Reports from other groups have offered conflicting data relative to the above observations. In a combined study from three transplant centers in Boston, the incidence of ATN was significantly higher with cyclosporine compared with conventional immunosuppression, but this did not adversely effect graft outcome (*6*). A report from Houston indicated no difference in the incidence or outcome of ATN in cyclosporine versus azathioprine-treated recipients; in this study it is appropriate to note that the mean renal preservation time in both groups was approximately 20 hr (*10*).

Prior to the availability of cyclosporine, the most effective maintenance immunosuppressive protocol in our cadaver transplant program was with azathioprine-prednisone and adjunctive ALG (*26, 27*). In 1984, we reported a one-year graft success rate of 78% in 100 consecutive cadaver recipients managed with this regimen (*19*). During this era, there was no adverse effect of ATN, prolonged renal preservation up to 48 hr, or the use of imported kidneys on ultimate graft outcome (*18, 28*). The incidence of ATN following cadaver transplantation in our program has been stable for several years and is approximately 50%.

In the present study, we compared immunosuppression with cyclosporine-prednisone to our prior regimen of azathioprine-prednisone-ALG. These two groups were well matched for age, sex, diabetes, transfusions, use of local or imported kidneys, donor age, and HLA AB match with the donor. There were more retransplants and fewer 2 DR-matched grafts in the CsA group. All cadaver kidneys were preserved with pulsatile perfusion, and the mean preservation time was 37 hr in each group.

The most striking finding in this study is the difference in graft success between the ALG and CsA groups (78% vs. 48% at one year), which was mainly due to a large number of primary nonfunctioning grafts in the latter group. This difference in graft success was statistically significant ($P<.05$) even after adjusting for differences in DR matches and retransplants. Graft outcome was better in the ALG group despite the fact that these patients experienced more rejection episodes. If primary nonfunctioning grafts are eliminated from the analysis of graft success, a significant difference between the ALG and CsA groups is no longer present.

Even among cadaver kidneys that ultimately functioned following transplantation, the time to attainment of the serum creatinine nadir was significantly longer (P=.03) in the CsA group. The actual serum creatinine nadir achieved was also higher in the CsA group but this finding was only marginally significant. These latter observations are further reinforced by similar findings in a subgroup of paired grafts from the same cadaver donor in which the recipients of each pair of kidneys were allocated into opposite treatment groups. In this subgroup, all donor and preservation-related variables were identical for patients receiving CsA or ALG, and observed differences in initial function are only due to differences in posttransplant immunosuppression.

Since pulsatile perfusion was used exclusively as the method of preservation in this study, we are unable to comment on the relative merits of this method versus cold storage in conjunction with cyclosporine immunosuppression. Some reports have indicated that pulsatile perfusion is advantageous (*29, 30*) while others suggest that cold storage may be preferable (*10, 12*), and further studies are necessary to resolve this issue.

The results of this prospective trial support the concept that cyclosporine offers no advantage over conventional immunosuppressive regimens incorporating ALG—and that it may, in fact, be detrimental in recipients of cadaver kidneys with extended (>24 hr) renal preservation times. These data also argue in favor of withholding cyclosporine therapy posttransplant until initial graft function is assured, particularly in programs such as ours with a significant incidence of ATN. Recipients of grafts that undergo ATN can be more effectively managed initially with ALG; following resolution of ATN, conversion to cyclosporine therapy can be considered. This information also emphasizes that, in order to realize the full benefit of cyclosporine in cadaver renal transplantation, renewed emphasis must be placed on minimizing ischemic renal damage.

REFERENCES

1. Starzl TE, Hakala T, Rosenthal T, et al. The Colorado-Pittsburgh cadaveric renal transplantation study with cyclosporine. Transplant Proc 1983; 15: 2459.
2. Kahan BD, Van Buren C, Flechner SM, et al. Cyclosporine immunosuppression mitigates against immunologic risk factors in renal transplantation. Transplant Proc 1983; 15: 2469.
3. European Multicenter Trial Group. Cyclosporine in cadaveric renal transplantation: one-year follow-up of a multicenter trial. Lancet 1983; 2: 986.
4. Rapaport FT. Cyclosporine: panacea or mirage? Am J Kid Dis 1984; 3: 440.
5. Halloran PF, Ludwin D, Aprile M, et al. Randomized comparison between cyclosporine and conventional therapy plus Minnesota antilymphocyte globulin in cadaveric renal transplantation. Transplant Proc 1983; 15: 2513.
6. Cho SI, Bradley JW, Monaco AP, Tilney NL. Comparison of kidney transplant survival between patients treated with cyclosporine and those treated with azathioprine and antithymocyte globulin. Am J Surg 1984; 147: 518.
7. Najarian JS, Fryd DS, Strand M, et al. A single institution, randomized, prospective trial of cyclosporine versus azathioprine-antilymphocyte globulin for immunosuppression in renal allograft recipients. Ann Surg 1985; 201: 142.
8. Klintman GB, Iwatsuki S, Starzl TE. Nephrotoxicity of cyclosporin A in liver and kidney transplantation. Lancet 1981; 1: 470.
9. Sweny P, Hopper J, Gross M, et al. Nephrotoxicity of cyclosporin. Lancet 1981; 1: 663.
10. Flechner SM, Payne WD, Van Buren C, Kerman R, Kahan BD. The effect of cyclosporine on early graft function in human renal transplantation. Transplantation 1983; 36: 268.
11. Tilney NL, Milford EL, Araujo JL, Strom TB, Carpenter CB, Kirkman RL. Experience with cyclosporine and steroids in clinical renal transplantation. Ann Surg 1984; 200: 605.
12. Belitsky P for the Canadian Transplant Study Group. Initial nonfunction of cyclosporine-treated cadaver renal allografts preserved by single cold storage. Transplant Proc 1985; 17: 1485.
13. Stiller C. The Canadian trial of cyclosporine: cyclosporine therapy compared to standard immunosuppression in renal transplants: an exploration of nephrotoxicity. Transplant Proc 1983; 15: 2479.
14. Calne RY, Rolles K, White DJG, et al. Cyclosporin A initially as the only immunosuppressant in 34 recipients of cadaver organs. Lancet 1979; 2: 1033.
15. Opelz G for the Collaborative Transplant Study. The influence of ischemia times and HLA-DR matching and cyclosporine-treated cadaver kidney grafts. Transplant Proc 1985; 17: 1478.
16. Magnusson MO, Stowe NT. Controversy in organ preservation. Urol Clin North Am 1976; 3: 491.
17. Novick AC, Braun WE, Magnusson M, Stowe N. Current status of renal transplantation at the Cleveland Clinic. J Urol 1979; 122: 433.
18. Flechner SM, Novick AC, Steinmuller DG, et al. Determinants of allograft survival in 100 cadaver kidney transplants. J Urol 1982; 127: 1084.
19. Novick AC, Khauli RB, Braun WE, et al. Improved results of cadaver renal transplantation with azathioprine, prednisone and antilymphocyte globulin. J Urol 1984; 131: 636.
20. Sawchuk RJ, Cartier LO. Liquid-chromatographic determination of cyclosporine A in blood and plasma. Clin Chem 1981; 27: 1368.
21. Sibley RJ, Rynasiewicz JJ, Ferguson JM, et al. Morphology of cyclosporine nephrotoxicity and acute rejection in patients immunosuppressed with cyclosporine and prednisone. Surgery 1983; 94: 225.
22. Kaplan EL, Meier P. Nonparametric estimation from incomplete observations. J Am Stat Assoc 1958; 53: 457.
23. Breslow N. A generalized Kruskal-Walis test for comparing k samples subject to unequal patterns of censorship. Biometrika 1970; 57: 579.
24. Cox DR. Regression models and life tables. J Roy Stat Soc [Series B] 1970; 34: 187.
25. Kahan BD, Van Buren CT, Lin SN, et al. Immunopharmacologic monitoring of cyclosporin A treated recipients of cadaver kidney allografts. Transplantation 1982; 34: 36.
26. Novick AC, Braun WE, Steinmuller D, Buszta C, Greenstreet R, Kiser WS. A randomized prospective controlled double-blind evaluation of antilymphocyte globulin in cadaver renal transplantation. Transplantation 1983; 35: 175.
27. Novick AC, Streem SB, Braun WE, Steinmuller D, Goormastic M, Cunningham R. Prophylactic anti-lymphoblast globulin, low-dose prednisone, and anti-lymphoblast globulin for first-rejection: a steroid-sparing approach to immunosuppressive therapy. Transplant Proc 1983; 15: 599.
28. Smith C, Novick AC, Steinmuller D, et al. Recent trends in organ procurement for renal transplantation at the Cleveland Clinic. Cleve Clin Q 1984; 51: 345.
29. Manis T, Hong JH, Bronsther OL, Friedman EA, Butt KMH. Superior results with machine-perfused kidneys in cyclosporine-treated recipients. Transplant Proc 1985; 17: 1483.
30. Mittal VK, Kaplan MP, Rosenberg JC, Allaben RA, Toledo-Pereyra LH. Pulsatile perfusion: better than hypothermic storage with cyclosporine as an immunosuppressant. Dial Transplant 1985; 14: 136.

Received 13 June 1985.
Accepted 15 November 1985.

0041-1337/86/4202-0159$02.00/0
TRANSPLANTATION
Copyright © 1986 by The Williams & Wilkins Co.

Vol. 42, No. 2
Printed in U.S.A.

CHARACTERISTICS AND CLINICAL RELEVANCE OF AUTOLYMPHOCYTOTOXINS IN PATIENTS WITH APLASTIC ANEMIA[1,2]

NICOLE CARPENTIER,[3] JEAN FONTANNAZ, MICHEL JEANNET, CATHERINE NISSEN, AND BRUNO SPECK

Transplantation Immunology Unit, Division of Immunology and Allergology, Hôpital Cantonal Universitaire, Geneva; and Division of Hematology, Kantonsspital, Basle, Switzerland

Serum of 68 patients with aplastic anemia was tested for the presence of autolymphocytotoxins (auto-LTs). Prior to specific disease treatment, 16 patients (24%) displayed antibodies cytotoxic to their own lymphocytes. These antibodies had the characteristics of cold-reactive lymphocytotoxins. Their detection in patients' sera was found unrelated to a viral or toxic cause of the disease or the patients' HLA genotype. Broadly reactive anti-HLA antibodies were less frequent in pretreatment sera containing auto-LTs, suggesting that these autoantibodies could modulate alloantibody production. However, after specific disease treatment, the alloantibody frequency was comparable in patients with or without auto-LTs. We found no significant difference in response to antilymphocyte serum or bone marrow graft outcome in the patients in relation to the presence or absence of pretreatment auto-LTs. This observation suggests that the detection of these autoantibodies in aplastic anemia has no clinical relevance.

Several studies have documented the presence of antibodies to autologous lymphocytes in serum of normal subjects and patients with a wide variety of diseases (*1, 2, 3, 4*). These autoantibodies react more frequently with B than T lymphocytes, and at cold temperature; they generally belong to the IgM class of immunoglobulins. Some experiments have suggested that they are directed to surface IgM of B cells and may modulate lymphocyte function—such as, in particular, the production of alloantibodies in patients (*4, 5, 6,*).

So far, there has been only one report on non-HLA allo-LTs and auto-lymphocytotoxins (LTs)* in patients with aplastic anemia who were treated by bone marrow transplantation (BMT) (*7*). That study gave no evidence of pronostic significance of auto-LTs for the graft outcome.

The present study was also undertaken to determine whether auto-LTs could influence the response of aplastic patients to treatment with antilymphocyte serum or BMT.

MATERIALS AND METHODS

Patients. A group of 68 patients with severe aplastic anemia were studied. The mean age of the patients was 18.4±1.1 years (range: 5–49). The group comprised 48 male and 28 female patients. Based on the history, the disease could be related to a toxic cause in 3 cases and to a viral infection in 11 patients. In the other subjects, the origin of the anemia could not be recognized. Forty nine patients were treated with antilymphocyte globulin (ALG), while 19 patients were grafted with bone marrow from an HLA-identical sibling.

Detection of autolymphocytotoxins and allolymphocytotoxins. The standard microlymphocytotoxicity assay (*8*) was used to detect cytotoxic antibodies. A serum was judged to be cytotoxic if it killed more than 30% of target lymphocytes above a baseline cell death less than 15%. Pretreatment serum from all the patients was assayed for cytotoxicity to T and B autologous lymphocytes at 5°C and 37°C, and at serial dilutions to determine the titers of auto-LTs. In the patients undergoing transplantation, it was further assayed on B and T lymphocytes from the graft donors. Pretreatment sera from 13 patients with auto-LTs and 45 patients without such antibodies were also tested for cytotoxicity to a panel of allogeneic lymphocytes that was representative of all serologically recognized HLA specificities. This test, which mostly screened antibodies to T cell–HLA antigens, was repeated on posttreatment sera from the 13 patients with autoantibodies and in 29 of the negative patients. The percentage of positive serum reactions with the lymphocyte panel was used to express the degree of patients' alloimmunization.

HLA typing. HLA-A, B, and DR lymphocyte antigens were typed in the patients and in their family members by the same lymphocytotoxicity test using a large battery of antisera with well-defined HLA specificities.

RESULTS

Circulating antibodies cytotoxic to autologous lymphocytes were found in 16 of the 68 patients studied (24%). The detection of these autoantibodies was found unrelated to a toxic or viral cause of the anemia. The characteristics of serum reactivity in the 16 positive patients are depicted in Table 1. The auto-LTs were directed to B cells in all cases, and to T lymphocytes in 3 patients. Cold-reactive auto-LTs were more frequent and at higher titers than warm-reactive antibodies.

Serum reactivity against lymphocytes of the HLA-identical donors was studied before BMT in 19 patients. Serum from 4 of the 6 future recipients with auto-LTs showed a pattern of cytotoxicity to donor's lymphocytes similar to that to autologous B or T cells (Table 1), while the 13 patients without auto-LTs had a negative serum crossmatch with donor's lymphocytes.

Previous studies have suggested that auto-LTs can inhibit

[1] This paper was presented at The Annual Meeting of the Swiss Society of Hematology, Interlaken, May 9 and 10, 1985.

[2] This work was supported by Grants 3.834.083 and 3.904.083 from the Swiss National Scientific Research Foundation.

[3] Reprint requests should be sent to: N. Carpentier, M.D., Transplantation Immunology Unit, Hôpital Cantonal Universitaire, 1211 Geneva 4, Switzerland.

* Abbreviations used: ALG, antilymphocyte globulin; BMT, bone marrow transplantation; LTs, lymphocytotoxins.

alloantibody production (*4, 5, 6*). To investigate this possibility in aplastic anemia, pretreatment and posttreatment serum cytotoxicity to a panel of allogeneic lymphocytes were compared in patients with or without auto-LTs. Before the specific disease treatment, we recorded an incidence and intensity of positive serum reactions on the panel that was lower among the 13 patients with auto-LTs who were tested for alloantibodies than in the 45 patients without auto-LTs (Table 2). In contrast, after the treatment the degree of allosensitization in this auto-LTs-positive group was almost identical to the 29 negative patients who were re-tested.

Patients' genotypes were deduced from the data of the HLA-typing of their family members. Their possible relationship with the formation of auto-LTs was investigated. When compared, the frequencies of some HLA alleles differed among the patients with or without auto-LTs. There was an overrepresentation of HLA-A10, A11, B21, BW35, B40, DR5, and DRW6 in the patients with autoantibodies, while B15, B18, DR4, and DR7 were more frequent in those without such antibodies. However, when corrected for the number of antigens tested, the deviation of incidence of these alleles between the patients' groups or the patients and a normal population was no longer significant.

Our material was also analyzed to determine whether there were any correlations between the presence of auto-LTs or cytotoxic alloantibodies, and the patients' response to treatment. In the patients treated with BMT, the outcome of the graft and the patients' fate were comparable regardless of the presence of lymphocytotoxins (Table 3). Graft rejection only occurred in the patient who had both auto-LTs and allo-LTs, and a negative serum crossmatch on donor's lymphocytes. A positive crossmatch against the donor's cells observed in three other patients with autoantibodies did not prevent permanent engraftment. The rate of response to ALG-treatment was also almost similar in the patients with or without lymphocytotoxins before treatment. A complete recovery of self-hematopoiesis was even more frequently observed in the patients with lymphocytotoxins than in those without.

TABLE 1. Reactivity of serum autolymphocytotoxins in 16 patients with aplastic anemia

Patients	Titers of cytotoxins: To autologous lymphocytes B 5°	B 37°	T 5°	T 37°	To graft donor's lymphocytes B 5°C	B 37°C	T 5°C	T 37°C
BRA	1:4	1:4	0	0	0	0	0	0
WAC	0	1:8	0	0	0	1:8	0	0
DOR	0	1:8	0	0	0	1:8	0	0
BOE	1:2	0	0	0	1:2	0	0	0
MIR	1:32	1:16	0	0	1:16	1:16	0	0
DAL	1:2	0	0	0	0	0	0	0
RAM	1:2	1:1	0	0	ALG-treated			
EST	0	1:2	0	0	ALG-treated			
MEI	1:16	1:2	1:1	0	ALG-treated			
BEU	1:1	0	0	0	ALG-treated			
STA	1:2	0	0	0	ALG-treated			
COS	1:2	0	1:4	0	ALG-treated			
WIT	1:2	0	0	0	ALG-treated			
RUB	1:4	0	0	0	ALG-treated			
SOF	1:64	0	0	0	ALG-treated			
PUG	1:16	1:2	1:2	1:1	ALG-treated			
Total No.	13/16	8/16	3/16	1/16	2/6	3/6	0/6	0/6
positive %	81	50	19	6	33	50	0	0

TABLE 2. Pretreatment and posttreatment serum cytotoxic alloantibodies in aplastic patients with or without autolymphocytotoxins (autoLTs)

% Positive serum reactions on lymphocyte panel[a]	Before treatment: AutoLTs present	Before treatment: AutoLTs absent	After treatment: AutoLTs present	After treatment: AutoLTs absent
>90	0	7	4	9
50–89	2	6	3	11
<50	2	8	4	4
0	9	24	2	5
Total No. (%)	4 (31)	21 (47)	11 (85)	24 (83)

(Column headings spanned by "Numbers of patients with alloantibodies".)

[a] The percentage of positive reactions was considered as evaluating alloantibody levels; sera were tested on total allogeneic lymphocyte populations—therefore the test measures mostly anti-T-cell cytotoxicity.

DISCUSSION

The data indicate that 24% of the patients with aplastic anemia had circulating auto-LTs before specific treatment of the disease. This incidence of cytotoxic autoantibodies is above the 13% frequency previously reported in another aplastic patients' group (*7*). Taking into account the young age of most patients, it is much higher than the incidence (almost 0% in children and usually less that 15% in adults) of cold non-HLA lymphocytotoxins recorded in healthy individuals (*1, 3*).

The auto-LTs that were found, are temperature-sensitive with maximal activity at 5°C, and mostly react with B cells. Therefore they possess characteristics similar to cold-reactive, non-HLA, lymphocytotoxins previously detected in various disease states (*2, 3*), in kidney transplant recipients (*9*), in renal hemodialysis patients (*4*), and in some healthy subjects (*1, 3*).

TABLE 3. Evolution of patients with aplastic anemia in relation to pretreatment lymphocytotoxins

	BM-grafted: n	Graft take	GVHD	Death	ALG-treated: n	Self hematopoiesis: Complete	Self hematopoiesis: Partial	Death
AutoLTs	6	5 (83)[a]	3 (50)	3 (50)	10	7 (70)	2 (20)	1 (10)
AlloLTs	9	8 (89)	6 (67)	6 (67)	16	12 (75)	1 (6)	3 (19)
Total LTs	14	13 (93)[b]	9 (64)	8 (57)	23	16 (70)[c]	3 (13)	4 (17)
No LTs	5	5 (100)	3 (60)	3 (60)	26	13 (50)	6 (23)	7 (27)
Total	19	18 (95)	12 (63)	11 (58)	49	29 (59)	9 (18)	11 (23)

[a] Percentage of patients indicated in parentheses.

[b] Auto and allolymphocytotoxins (LTs) were associated in one case.

[c] Auto and alloLTs were associated in 3 cases.

Target antigens of auto-LTs could be—as suggested for some non-HLA allolymphocytotoxins (*5, 6*)—surface IgM of lymphocytes. However, there is at present no rigorous experimental data in favor of such a specificity, and some findings suggest that most auto-LTs recognize cell surface determinants other than IgM. For instance, auto-LTs present in hemodialyzed patients were found to bind to lymphocytes even after the removal of the membrane Ig and Fc receptors (*4*). In addition, absorption studies performed in aplastic anemia by Gluckman et al. (*7*) have further shown that non-HLA lymphocytotoxins could be removed from serum with B or T cells, which indicates that the target antigens involved were also shared by T cells.

The stimuli responsible for the frequent occurrence of auto-LTs in patients with certain diseases are unknown. In aplastic anemia the presence of these antibodies could reflect the autoimmune mechanisms that are suspected to cause the disease (*10–14*). Their significant development in normal individuals under immunizing circumstances (*15*) may also suggest that they are formed following B cell activation by various stimuli—in particular, viral infections or sensitization to alloantigens. However, our study and others' (*4, 7*) indicate that the detection of auto-LTs in patients is unrelated to a toxic or viral cause of the disease, or to alloimmunization induced by repeated transfusions.

The clinical relevance of the occurrence of cold, non-HLA lymphocytotoxins in diseases is still difficult to assess. Some observations have suggested that they may be of importance, particularly in transplantation. In kidney transplant recipients, a correlation of such lymphocytotoxins with a longer graft survival has indeed been observed (*9, 16–18*). This finding may be related to the lower levels of anti-HLA alloantibodies found in hemodialyzed patients with auto-LTs (*4*), which suggests that these autoantibodies can exert a suppressive effect on B cell function. The trend of a lesser degree of allosensitization that we recorded before specific treatment in aplastic patients with auto-LTs may support this concept. However, our data and others' (*4, 7*) indicate that cytotoxic autoantibodies do not prevent the production of alloantibodies during treatment. In addition, in the previous and present studies in aplastic anemia, there is no evidence of an association of auto-LTs with any peculiar clinical course, whether patients are treated with BMT or ALG. These findings suggest that the occurrence of such autoantibodies in this disease has no prognostic significance.

Acknowledgments. We are grateful to Dr. R. C. Atkins for reviewing this manuscript and to Mrs M. Carnal for her excellent secretarial assistance.

REFERENCES

1. Park MS, Terasaki PI, Bernoco D. Autoantibody against B lymphocytes. Lancet 1977; 2: 465.
2. Ozturk G, Terasaki PI. Non-HLA lymphocyte cytotoxins in various diseases. Tissue Antigens 1979; 14: 52.
3. Prou PO. Les lymphocytotoxines froides. Rev Française Transplant et Immunohématol 1979; 22: 167.
4. Lobo PI. Nature of autolymphocytotoxins present in renal hemodialysis patients. Their possible role in controlling alloantibody formation. Transplantation 1981; 32: 233.
5. Ozturk G, Terasaki PI. Cytotoxic antibodies against surface immunoglobulin. Transplantation 1980; 29: 140.
6. Takahashi H, Terasaki PI, Iwaki Y, Nakata S. Identification of surface IgM as the target antigen of cold lymphocytotoxins. Tissue Antigens 1980; 16: 176.
7. Gluckman E, Gluckman JC, Andersen E, Guillet J, Devergie A, Dausset J. Lymphocytotoxic antibodies after bone marrow transplantation in aplastic anemia. II. Non-HLA antibodies. Transplantation 1980; 29: 471.
8. Mittal KK, Mickey MR, Singal DP, Terasaki PI. Serotyping for homotransplantation. XVIII. Refinement of microdroplet cytotoxicity test. Transplantaion 1968; 6: 913.
9. Klouda PT, Jeannet M. Cold and warm antibodies and graft survival in kidney allograft recipients. Lancet 1976; 1: 876.
10. Nissen C, Cornu P, Gratwohl A, Speck B. Peripheral blood cells from patients with aplastic anemia in partial remission suppress growth of their own bone marrow precursor in culture. Br J Haematol 1980; 45: 233.
11. Nissen C, Gratwohl A, Speck B. Autoimmunity against bone marrow precursor cells. In: Engelfriet CP, van den Borne AEG, van Loghem JJ, eds. Immunohaematology. 1983.
12. Abdou NI. Plasma exchange in the treatment of aplastic anemia. Prog Clin Biol Res 1982; 106: 337.
13. Garcia A, Gudim IV, Noyola MC, Callejas RJ. Inhibidor circulante de la eritropoyesis en pacientes con anemia aplastic adquirida. Sangre 1984; 29: 15.
14. Gordon-Smith EC. Treatment of aplastic anemia. Prog Clin Biol Res 1984; 148: 335.
15. Naito S, Mickey MR, Hirato A, Terasaki PI. Autolymphocytotoxins following immunization by pregnancy, transplantation, and disease. Tissue Antigens 1971; 1: 219.
16. Lobo PI, Werstervelt FB, Rudolf LE. Kidney transplantation across positive B and T cell crossmatches. Transplantation 1978; 26: 84.
17. Iwaki Y, Terasaki PI, Park MS, Billing R. Enhancement of human kidney allografts by cold B lymphocyte cytotoxins. Lancet 1978; 1: 1228.
18. Ting A. Morris PJ. Renal transplantation on B-cell crossmatch with autoantibodies and alloantibodies. Lancet 1977; 2: 1095.

Received 23 June 1985.
Accepted 25 October 1985.

0041-1337/86/4202-0162$02.00/0
TRANSPLANTATION

Vol. 42, No. 2
Printed in U.S.A.

FUNCTIONAL ACTIVITY OF SOLUBLE ANTIGEN-SPECIFIC HELPER T CELL MOLECULES

REQUIREMENT FOR SEPARABLE ENTITIES FOR THE INDUCTION OF CYTOTOXIC T CELL AND B CELL RESPONSES[1]

JOHN F. KROWKA,[2,3] CHIAKI SHIOZAWA,[2,4] ERWIN DIENER,[2,4] AND LINDA M. PILARSKI[2,5]

The Department of Immunology and the MRC Group on Immunoregulation, University of Alberta, Edmonton, Alberta, Canada T6G 2H7

These studies constitute the first report of a comparison of the ability of a population of antigen-specific helper factors (ASHF) to induce cell-mediated and humoral immune responses. Supernatants of helper T lymphocyte (T_H) cell lines, were purified by antigen-affinity chromatography and tested for their ability to induce cytotoxic T lymphocyte (CTL) responses and IgM responses in vitro. The supernatant of a noncloned T_H line was found to contain two functionally distinct types of ASHF that are separable by anion-exchange chromatography: one factor triggers CTL resonses ($ASHF_{CTL}$), the other triggers IgM B cell responses ($ASHF_B$). Clone 4C6, derived from the parent line CHI, produces $ASHF_{CTL}$ but not $ASHF_B$. These observations could result from two entirely distinct ASHF or from the association of common antigen-specific subunits with different antigen-nonspecific subunits to make $ASHF_{CTL}$ or $ASHF_B$.

It has been demonstrated in a number of experimental systems that both cytotoxic T lymphocyte precursors (CTL_p)* and the precursors of antibody secreting B lymphocytes require inductive signals from helper T lymphocytes (T_H) to mediate their antigen-specific effector functions (*1, 2*). Both antigen-specific and antigen-nonspecific T-derived factors have been reported to participate in the induction of CTL and B cell responses (*3–11*). It is a plausible but unproved assumption that antigen-specific helper factors (ASHF) are soluble forms of T_H antigen receptors (T_HAR).

In previous reports we have demonstrated ASHF-mediated induction of both cytotoxic T lymphocytes (CTL) and primary IgM responses in vitro (*5, 9, 11*). The ASHF from the T cell line CHI, described in this report and characterized previously (*5, 11*) recognizes determinants expressed on chicken red blood cells (CRBC) of the B2 major histocompatibility complex (MHC) haplotype. In order to compare the B2-CRBC-specific induction of CTLp with the B2-CRBC-specific induction of IgM responses, we have modified the helper-dependent CTLp assay developed by Pilarski (*12*). The unique and adaptable system developed here (*5*) enables comparisons of the ability of a T_H population or its secreted products to trigger CTLp, with its ability to specifically help other classes of immune response to either soluble or cell-surface antigens.

The basic experimental system involves the use of low numbers of thymocytes as a source of responder cells where help is limiting (*12*). In order to generate CTL from the CTLp resident in a thymocyte population an exogeneous source of help is required that may be IL-2-containing material, antigen-specific helper cells, or ASHF (*5, 12–14*). In the experiments to be described, ASHF specific for CRBC are able to participate in the induction of CTLp specific for Class I H-2 alloantigens. Allogeneic stimulator cells pulsed with fragments of B2-CRBC present carrier determinants recognized by ASHF. Recognition of H-2-encoded alloantigens that are intrinsic to the stimulator cells, and of B2-CRBC antigens by CTLp and ASHF respectively, results in the delivery of an inductive signal to the alloreactive CTLp. Our system is basically analogous to induction systems in which the recognition of class II MHC-encoded antigens by T_H results in the differentiation of CTLp that recognize class I MHC-encoded antigens (*15, 16*).

Although CHI-derived ASHF triggers both CTLp and IgM responses in an antigen-specific manner, it was not known if our ASHF preparation contains two types of class-specific ASHF or if the same ASHF moiety is responsible for triggering both CTL and IgM responses. This type of comparative analysis has never been previously reported. By anion-exchange chromatography of CHI-derived, antigen-affinity purified supernatant, we have been able to separate the ASHF that trigger CTLp ($ASHF_{CTL}$) from the ASHF that triggers B cell responses ($ASHF_B$). In addition, we were able to show that ASHF purified from clone 4C6 efficiently triggers CTLp but does not specifically induce B cell responses, thus providing further evidence that $ASHF_{CTL}$ and $ASHF_B$ are distinct and separable entities.

MATERIALS AND METHODS

Animals and antigens. BALB/cCr, CBA/J, and (BALB/c×CBA/J)F_1 mice, bred at the Small Animal Centre, University of Alberta were 4–16 weeks old and were sex-matched in individual experiments. Erythrocytes were obtained from chickens homozygous for the B2 or B13 MHC haplotypes. Freeze-thaw antigen (FTA) was prepared as described previously (*5, 17*). Briefly, CRBC were lysed by 4 cycles of freezing in liquid N_2 and thawing at 37°C. Cellular debris was removed by centrifugation at 500×G for 5 min. Lipopolysaccharide (LPS) from Escherichia coli serotype 0.55.B5 (Sigma Chemical

[1] This work was supported grants from the Medical Research Council of Canada to L.M.P. and E.D.

[2] Department of Immunology.
[3] Recipient of Alberta Heritage Foundation for Medical Research Studentship.
[4] MRC group on Immunoregulation.
[5] Address correspondence to: L. M. Pilarski, Department of Immunology, University of Alberta, Edmonton, Alberta, Canada T6G 2H7.

* Abbreviations used: AFC, antibody-forming cell; ASHF, antigen-specific helper factors (subscripts CTL or B refer to the ability to help CTL or IgM responses, respectively); CRBC, chicken red blood cells; CTLp, cytotoxic T lymphocyte precursors; FCS, fetal calf serum; FTA, freeze-thaw antigen; IL-2, interleukin 2; LPS, lipopolysaccharide; MHC, major histocompatibility complex; NR, nonrosetted cells; RFC, rosette-forming cell; T_H, Helper T lymphocyte; pre-T_H, helper T cell precursor; T_HAR, T_H antigen receptor.

Co., St. Louis, MO) was used at a concentration of 10 μg/ml of culture medium.

Helper T cell lines. The phenotype of the clonally heterogenous cell line CHI, which recognizes B2 chicken MHC antigens, includes cells that are Thy 1^+, $Lyt1^+$, $Lyt2^+$, and Ia^+ (*1*). This cell line is maintained without antigen or accessory cells in RPMI-1640 medium (GIBCO, NY) containing $5{\times}10^{-5}$ M β-mercaptoethanol, 10% fetal calf serum ([FCS] GIBCO, NY) antibiotics, and an optimal concentration of partially-purified interleukin 2 (IL-2), prepared as described previously (*13, 18*). Clone 4C6 was derived from the parent line CHI by limiting dilution at a ratio of 0.2 cells per microculture well. CHI was originally derived from CBA/J (H-2^k) educated T cells (*5, 11*).

Preparation of antigen-specific helper factors. Supernatants from the Th line CHI were collected after 24–48 hr of culture and dialyzed against phosphate buffered saline (PBS). These supernatants were passed through antigen-affinity columns that consisted of B2 CRBC coupled to Sepharose 4B, as described previously (*11*). The bound material was eluted from the CRBC with 2M NaCl, dialyzed against PBS, and concentrated. This material is referred to as *Ca^{++}-sufficient* ASHF. *Ca^{++}-deficient* (i.e., "incomplete" ASHF) was prepared by dialyzing the Ca^{++}-sufficient ASHF against 0.01 M Hepes buffer (pH 7.4) containing 10^{-3} M Ethyleneglycol-bis-(β-aminoethyl ether) N,N′-tetraacetic acid (EGTA). This material was rechromatographed on a B2-CRBC-affinity column in the presence of 10^{-3} M EGTA. The bound material was eluted from the antigen-affinity column with 2M NaCl, exhaustively dialyzed against PBS, and concentrated. These ASHF preparations do not contain detectable amounts of IL-2, as measured by their inability to promote growth of an IL-2 dependent T cell line and the specificity of their inductive properties (*5*). The amount of ASHF required to trigger a CTL response represents the amount of material produced by 10^3 cells in a period of 24–48 hr. Although the ASHF preparations used here are enriched for helper activity (*11*) they cannot be considered to be pure; multiple bands are observed after SDS gel chromatography (Krowka JF, Pilarski LM, unpublished data). The ASHF do not contain CRBC antigen as they are derived from cell lines maintained in the absence of antigen; in addition, to prevent antigen carry over during the affinity purification, the sepharose-coupled CRBC are fixed with 0.2% glutaraldehyde (*11*). The specificity controls reported here indicate that B2 antigen is not provided by the ASHF preparation.

Ion exchange chromatography. Antigen-affinity-purified material was eluted from a DEAE-Sephacel column (1×9-cm; Pharmacia, Uppsala) by a linear concentration gradient of NaCl (0–0.5 M) in 0.05 M HEPES buffer (pH 7.5) (*11*). All fractions were dialyzed exhaustively against PBS before being assayed for helper activity in the induction of CTL or IgM responses. The DEAE elution profile of CHI-ASHF is illustrated in Figure 1. Protein concentrations were determined by absorbancy at 280 nm using bovine serum albumin as a standard. BSA and ASHF preparations were tested using both A_{280} absorbance and the Coomassie Blue colorimetric assay for protein (*19*) to establish the validity of BSA as a standard for monitoring absorbance of ASHF fractions. After pooling and concentration, each fraction was assayed for total protein by the Coomassie Blue method.

Assay for antigen-specific help for CTLp. As described previously (*5, 14*), $3{\times}10^5$ mouse splenic stimulator cells were incubated with the freeze-thaw antigen (FTA) from 10^6 CRBC in MEM (GIBCO, NY) with $5{\times}10^{-5}$ M β-mercaptoethanol but without FCS at 37°C for 2 hr in conical-bottomed Linbro microculture plates (Flow Laboratories, Rockville, MD). Unbound antigen and nonadherent cells were then removed by gently washing the cultures twice. Graded dilutions of ASHF in culture medium (MEM with $5{\times}10^{-5}$ M β-mercaptoethanol, 5% FCS, and antibiotics), culture medium, or an optimal concentration of partially purified IL-2 in culture medium were added to the adherent cells. Cultures were irradiated with 1500 rads prior to the addition of 1 or $2{\times}10^5$ responder thymocytes from 4–6-week-old mice, followed by incubation at 37°C in 10% CO_2-air atmosphere for 5 days. The total volume in each microculture well was 0.2 ml.

Cytotoxicity assay. Cytotoxicity generated against the murine MHC alloantigens on the stimulator cells was assayed using $5{\times}10^4$ concanavalin A (Con-A)-induced blast target cells per culture well in a standard ^{51}chromium release assay (*14*). Target cells in all cytotoxicity assays were not pulsed with any CRBC antigens. Values in tables represent the mean ±SE of six replicate wells per group.

Assay for antigen-specific help for B cells. Enrichment of CBA/J splenic B cells that recognize CRBC antigens by rosetting and culture techniques have been described previously (*9–11*). Briefly, mononuclear spleen cells were purified on an Isopaque-Ficoll (Pharmacia Fine Chemicals, Uppsala, Sweden) gradient prior to washing and incubation with B2 or B13 CRBC. After incubation, rosette-forming cells (RFC) and CRBC were separated from nonrosetted cells (NR) on an Isopaque-Ficoll gradient. After washing, $2{\times}10^3$ RFC, $1{\times}10^6$ irradiated (1500 rads) NR, and ASHF, LPS, or medium were cultured in Linbro microculture plates in Click's medium with 5% FCS. As described previously, NR provide antigen-nonspecific differentiation factors for RFC (*10*). The total volume in each microculture well was 0.2 ml. Cultures were tested after four days for the presence of antibody forming cells (AFC) by the direct hemolytic plaque assay of Cunningham and Szenberg (*20*) as described previously (*11*). IgM responses are expressed as AFC ± SE.

RESULTS

Triggering of both CTL and IgM responses by ASHF. Table 1 demonstrates that antigen-affinity purified supernatants from the cell line CHI are able to induce helper-dependent primary CTL responses and primary IgM responses in vitro in an antigen-specific manner.

Our ASHF assay system involves the generation of alloantigen-specific CTL. Previous experiments have demonstrated that ASHF is not a polyclonal activator and will trigger only those CTLp that are also recognizing antigen (*1, 5*). Fragments of B2-CRBC perform the function of "carrier" determinants recognized on the surface of the stimulator cells by ASHF. Table 1 demonstrates that significant CBA/J H-2^k CTL responses against BALB/c (H-2^d) alloantigens are induced by ASHF only when the (BALB/c×CBA) F_1 stimulator cells are pulsed with B2-CRBC FTA, but not when stimulator cells are pulsed with B13-CRBC FTA. Previous reports demonstrate that antigen-affinity purified ASHF contains no detectable IL-2 activity (*5, 11*).

The same preparation of ASHF is also able to preferentially induce primary IgM responses to B2-CRBC (Table 1), as previously described (*11*). Copurification of antigen-nonspecific B-cell-inductive lymphokines with ASHF may explain the weak triggering of AFC reactive with B13-CRBC. This nonspecific triggering never exceeded 33% of LPS-induced responses to

TABLE 1. Antigen-affinity-purified ASHF from the cell line CHI triggering both CTL and IgM responses in an antigen-specific manner[a]

Final dilution (μg protein): CHI-ASHF added to culture	CTL activity (% specific lysis of Balb targets/culture ±SE)		B cell activity (AFC/culture ±SE)	
	B2-FTA stimulators	B13-FTA stimulators	B2-CRBC	B13-CRBC
Without ASHF	<1	<1	4±4	4±2
1/20 (42)	34.6±6.0	5.3±1.7	92±8	44±11
1/60	NT	NT	316±24	156±41
1/200 (4.2)	32.8±4.7	<1	108±23	12±4
1/600	NT	NT	100±11	36±30
1/2,000 (0.42)	18.7±4.4	<1	NT	NT
1/20,000	<1	<1	NT	NT
LPS	NT	NT	276±30	472±39
IL-2	64.9±4.8	39.5±4.0	NT	NT

[a] Antigen-affinity-purified ASHF from the cell line CHI was tested for its ability to trigger CTL or AFC responses, as described in the *Materials and Methods* section and previously (*5, 11*). In the assay for help for CTLp, 10^5 CBA thymocytes were cultured with irradiated B2-FTA- or B13-FTA-pulsed (BALB/c×CBA/J)F_1 stimulators and ASHF, IL2, or medium. Note that at a dilution of 1/60, ASHF was capable of inducing a B2-specific AFC response equal in magnitude to the LPS control response. The B13-specific response amounts to only 33% of the LPS control. More details on the specificity of this factor are given elsewhere (*11*). NT = not tested.

B13-CRBC. The antigen specific AFC-inductive and CTL-inductive activity of CHI-ASHF has been confirmed in many experiments, as reported elsewhere (*1, 5, 11*).

Separation of antigen-specific helper factor activities for the induction of CTL and IgM responses by ion-exchange chromatography. To determine if the CTL and IgM responses were induced by two distinct ASHF moieties in the antigen-affinity purified supernatants, an aliquot of the ASHF preparation tested in the experiment shown in Table 1 was subjected to ion-exchange chromatography and each fraction tested for antigen-specific helper activity in the generation of CTL and AFC. The elution profile of CHI-ASHF from a DEAE-Sephacel anion-exchange column is illustrated in Figure 1. Although the specific ASHF activity is considerably increased by antigen-affinity chromatography (20–40-fold) (*11*) extraneous proteins are still present (Fig. 1).

Since we have observed that ASHF preparations help a CTL response most efficiently if the stimulator cells are of the same H-2 haplotype as the CHI T_H line (H-2^k) (*1, 5*), all ASHF fractions were assayed for activity on CTLp in cultures containing BALB/c (H-2^d) responder thymocytes and B2-CRBC-pulsed CBA/J (H-2^k) adherent stimulator cells. In parallel, triggering activity on CBA/J B cells was tested. Table 2 demonstrates that ASHF-activity in the induction of CTL responses ($ASHF_{CTL}$) occurs exclusively in DEAE-fraction E. In contrast, the ASHF activity that acts on B cells ($ASHF_B$) is contained in fraction C.

The data demonstrate the existence in CHI-ASHF of at lest two functionally distinct ASHF that are both specific for B2-CRBC antigens. Residual antigen-nonspecific AFC-inductive activity is concentrated in fraction B. A more detailed analysis of the ability of DEAE-fractionated CHI-ASHF to stimulate B cell proliferation and differentiation has been reported previously (*11*).

Preferential triggering of CTL but not IgM responses by ASHF derived from clone 4C6. Although CHI has been maintained in vitro for approximately two years, the cells of this line are phenotypically heterogeneous (*1*). To minimize heterogeneity, CHI was cloned by limiting dilution. We isolated a clone, 4C6, able to help the induction of thymocyte CTLp in a "carrier-specific" manner in response to B2-CRBC FTA-pulsed stimulator cells.

Table 3 demonstrates that unfractionated ASHF preparations from clone 4C6, or the DEAE-fraction "E" of 4C6-ASHF, can trigger CTLp but not B cells in an antigen-specific manner. Fraction E of 4C6-ASHF contains crossreactive or nonspecific factor(s) able to induce a small (10.5%) CTL response to B13-FTA-pulsed stimulators. However the CTL response to B2-FTA-pulsed stimulators was significantly greater (39.4%) ($P<0.0005$). The location of ASHF activity in DEAE-fraction "E" of both 4C6-ASHF and CHI-ASHF suggests that the same molecular species in both ASHF preparations is responsible for the carrier-specific induction of CTLp. In contrast to the highly efficient triggering of CTLp by 4C6-ASHF (106% of control IL2-stimulated CTLp), even the highest concentrations tested of the DEAE fractions obtained from this sample (Table 3) were only weakly active in the triggering of AFC responses (maximum 21% of control LPS-induced IgM AFC), and this activity was not antigen-specific. Clone 4C6 appears to secrete some antigen-nonspecific B cell-directed lymphokines that participate in the induction of AFC precursors. At 3-fold lower concentrations of the 4C6 ASHF fraction, efficient and specific triggering of CTLp was maintained but no induction of B cells was observed (data not shown).

Evidence that Ca^{++}-sufficient ASHF from clone 4C6 is stringently restricted to syngeneic adherent cells. Previous reports (*11*) demonstrate that ASHF consists of a minimum of two subunits held together by Ca^{++} that can be dissociated if Ca^{++} is removed by EGTA. In the CTL inductive system, complete (Ca^{++}-sufficient) ASHF is H-2 unrestricted; incomplete (Ca^{++}-deficient) ASHF is restricted by products encoded in the I region of the H-2 gene complex (*5*). This appears to be due to a requirement for syngeneic H-2-encoded products to reconstitute the CTL-inductive activity of antigen-binding moieties

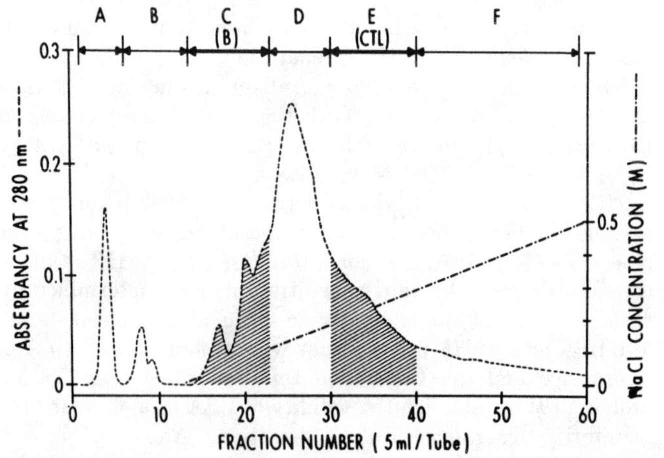

FIGURE 1. Protein elution profile of antigen-affinity-purified supernatant of the cell line CHI, subjected to DEAE-Sephacel chromatography. Among the pools of fractions (A to F), $ASHF_B$ and $ASHF_{CTL}$ activities were recovered from fractions C and E, respectively (see Table 2).

TABLE 2. Evidence that ASHF activities for CTL_p induction ($ASHF_{CTL}$) and for the induction of B cell IgM responses ($ASHF_B$) are separable by ion-exchange chromatography[a]

CHI-ASHF: DEAE fraction	Protein (μg/ml)	CTL activity (% specific lysis/culture ±SE)		B cell activity (AFC/culture ±SE)	
		B2-FTA stimulators	B13-FTA stimulators	B2-CRBC	B13-CRBC
Without ASHF		<1	<1	12±2	20±8
A	29	<1	<1	132±18	104±24
B	16	<1	<1	72±8	56±10
C	60	<1	<1	276±18	64±10
D	376	<1	<1	96±14	56±8
E	113	27.6±3.0	<1	32±8	24±4
F	83	9.6±1.3	8.5±2.1	78±12	56±8
LPS		NT	NT	244±20	312±40
IL-2		27.3±4.5	21.4±1.4	NT	NT

[a] The biological activities of $ASHF_{CTL}$ and $ASHF_B$ were recovered from distinct fractions after DEAE-Sephacel chromatography of antigen-affinity purified supernatant from the cell line CHI (Fig. 1). The total amount of protein recovered in the antigen-affinity-bound material was 8.6 mg. Recovery of protein from DEAE-Sephacel chromatography was 75%. A 1/60 final dilution of ASHF (1.0 μg protein-fraction C) for B cell culture and a 1/180 final dilution (0.63 μg protein-fraction E) for CTL culture are shown in this table. At no dilution tested were the antigen-specific B cell- or CTL-inductive activities found in fractions other than C or E, respectively (not shown). The unfractionated CHI-ASHF from which the DEAE-fractions were derived, was highly active and antigen-specific in its ability to trigger both CTL and AFC responses (Table 1). In the assay for CTL activity, BALB/c thymocyte responders were cultured with B2- or B13-CRBC FTA pulsed CBA stimulator cells. Cytotoxicity is expressed as % specific lysis of CBA targets.

TABLE 3. The inductive activities of DEAE-fractionated and unfractionated ASHF, derived from clone 4C6, indicating that $ASHF_{CTL}$ and $ASHF_B$ are distinct molecular species[a]

4C6-ASHF: DEAE fraction	Protein (μg/ml)	CTL activity % Specific lysis/culture ± SE		B cell activity	
		B2-FTA	B13-FTA	AFC/culture ± SE: B2-CRBC	Fraction of LPS-stimulated control
Without ASHF		3.9±4.7	<1	4±1	0.005
A	170	9.1±1.4	2.4±2.0	108±24	0.15
B	14	2.8±4.1	<1	24±6	0.03
C	92	<1	<1	152±44	0.21
D	391	5.8±3.4	9.9±4.0	60±10	0.08
E	176	39.4±2.5	10.5±1.0	76±4	0.10
F	60	1.1±2.5	<1	52±18	0.07
Unfractionated	800	57.3±4.0	9.4±3.8	148±2	0.20
LPS		NT	NT	732±30	1.0
IL-2		54.2±4.9	50.9±3.8	NT	NT

[a] Affinity-purified ASHF was prepared from supernatants of clone 4C6, followed by ion-exchange (DEAE) chromatography, performed as described in the *Materials and Methods* section. The elution profile of 4C6-ASHF was nearly identical to that of CHI-ASHF (Fig. 1). Experimental conditions are as described for Table 2. No fraction of 4C6-ASHF specifically triggered AFC responses at any dilution tested (not shown).

that have been affinity-purified in Ca^{++}-deficient conditions (incomplete ASHF). The number and type of H-2-encoded subunits present as part of complete or incomplete forms of ASHF are not known but these appear to include Ia (*21*). Purification of functional activity on antigen-affinity columns (*5, 11*) indicates that both contain antigen-binding moieties, presumably T_HAR. The phenotypic analysis of clone 4C6 (*1*), demonstrating very few Ia^+ cells, suggested that ASHF derived from 4C6 might be similar to the "incomplete" form of ASHF. Table 4 demonstrates that 4C6 ASHF, prepared under Ca^{++}-sufficient conditions, is even more stringently restricted in its requirements for syngeneic adherent cells than the "incomplete" (Ca^{++}-deficient) CHI-derived ASHF.

The most permissive assay system—i.e., the system that detects both complete and incomplete forms of ASHF—employs adherent stimulator cells expressing MHC-encoded antigens that are syngeneic to the CBA/J (H-2^k)-derived T_H line CHI (*5*). When using B2-FTA-pulsed CBA/J stimulators, antigen-specific triggering of BALB/c thymocytes by complete or incomplete CHI-ASHF or by 4C6 ASHF could be observed (Table 4, line 1). When responder and stimulator cells are allogeneic to the CHI-ASHF-producing cells, only the complete—not the incomplete—form of CHI-ASHF or 4C6-ASHF was able to trigger thymocyte CTLp (line 2).

The use of B10.BR stimulator cells demonstrates that 4C6-ASHF is not functionally identical to incomplete ASHF derived from CHI cells (line 3). Significant CTL responses were generated by incomplete CHI-ASHF but not by 4C6 ASHF in response to B2-FTA-pulsed B10.BR stimulators. The response of CBA/J thymocytes to B2-FTA-pulsed stimulator cells that were allogeneic to the ASHF-producing T_H provided further evidence that incomplete CHI-ASHF and 4C6-ASHF are different (lines 4 and 5). In these experiments, CBA/J CTLp were induced specifically in response to B2-FTA-pulsed BALB/c or B10 stimulators by either complete or incomplete CHI-ASHF but not by 4C6-ASHF. This suggests that syngeneic adherent cells from the responder thymocyte population were able to provide the "completor" subunits necessary to reconstitute the incomplete (Ca^{++}-deficient) CHI-ASHF, but not 4C6 ASHF.

The differences between 4C6-ASHF and the "incomplete"

TABLE 4. Stringent restriction of the function of ASHF from clone 4C6 to syngeneic adherent cells[a]

Type of thymocyte CTLp	Type of B2-FTA-pulsed stimulator cells	Ratio (% Specific Lysis ASHF:IL-2)		
		Complete ASHF (Ca^{++}-sufficient)	Incomplete ASHF (Ca^{++}-deficient)	4C6 ASHF
Allogeneic to ASHF:				
BALB/c	CBA	1.95 (28.3:14.5)	1.07 (27.3:25.4)	1.25 (45.1:36.2)
BALB/c	B10	1.09 (28.0:25.7)	<0.05 (<1.0:18.6)	<0.03 (<1.0:28.5)
BALB/c	B10.BR	—	0.35 (22.0:64.0)[b]	<0.02 (<1.0:56.4)
Syngeneic to ASHF:				
CBA	BALB/c	0.73 (36.2:49.4)	1.10 (23.3:21.4)	<0.05 (<1.0:21.2)
CBA	B10	0.90 (43.7:48.7)	1.40 (36.6:24.7)	<0.03 (<1.0:29.4)

[a] Three types of CBA-derived ASHF were compared with regard to their requirement for syngeneic stimulator cells. ASHF was purified from clone 4C6 (derived from the T_H line CHI) in the presence of Ca^{++}. The results for 4C6 ASHF were all derived from the same experiment. The ASHF-inducible CTL responses against target cells syngeneic to the stimulators are presented in comparison with the IL-2-inducible control responses in each experiment. ASHF preparations were assayed at several dilutions (not shown) with consistent results. All experiments included a specificity control to confirm the lack of induction with B13-FTA-pulsed stimulator cells. The results of several experiments are summarized. In all experiments, the response of thymocytes cultured with pulsed stimulator cells but without help was <1.0% specific lysis. All of these experiments have been repeated at least twice.

[b] Rows 1, 2, and 3, column 4 (incomplete ASHF) were parts of the same experiment (*5*).

ASHF prepared by treatment with EGTA followed by antigen-affinity chromatography of supernatants from the clonally heterogenous T_H line CHI are not clear. The DEAE elution profile of functionally active ASHF-CTL from CHI-ASHF and 4C6-ASHF indicates that both have similar electronegative charges (Tables 2 and 3 and Fig. 1). Both incomplete (Ca^{++}-deficient) CHI-ASHF and 4C6-ASHF require syngeneic H-2-encoded products for functional activity. However, the stringent requirements of 4C6-ASHF (Table 4) demonstrate that it may be even less complete than Ca^{++}-deficient CHI-ASHF.

DISCUSSION

In addition to the data presented in this report, a large body of evidence demonstrates that ASHF participate in the induction of cell-mediated and antibody-mediated immune responses (*1, 3, 5, 7, 9–11*). Antigen-specific binding and functional activity suggest that ASHF may be a soluble form of clonally expressed T_HAR. The observed homologies between T_HAR and immunoglobulins (*22, 23*) and the precedent of distinct membrane and secreted forms of μ, δ, and γ immunoglobulin heavy chains (*24–26*) suggest that similar splicing mechanisms may also be used to generate distinct forms of T_HAR α and/or β chains. A secreted form of T_HAR would extend the ability of T_H to deliver antigen-specific help beyond the limits of its cell membrane. Large gaps exist in our understanding of how T_H functions may selectively induce a particular class of immune response. Antigen-nonspecific lymphokines such as BCGF (*8*) or IL-2 (*27*) appear to exhibit target specificity in the activation of B or T lymphocytes. Our results suggest that $ASHF_{CTL}$ and $ASHF_B$ constitute antigen-specific primary inductive signals that selectively regulate the class of immunity activated by antigen.

Systems have not been developed previously to test in parallel the inductive effects of ASHF on cell-mediated and antibody-mediated immune responses. In this report the ASHF activities for CTL and B cell responses are demonstrated to be distinct and separable. Ion-exchange chromatography is able to resolve $ASHF_{CTL}$ and $ASHF_B$ into two separate entities. Further support for our distinction between $ASHF_{CTL}$ and $ASHF_B$ is provided by the evidence that the bulk of ASHF secreted by clone 4C6 is selective for the induction of CTLp but not for B cells. At present, our definition of $ASHF_{CTL}$ is operational. Our working assumption is that $ASHF_{CTL}$ interacts with the CTLp via mechanisms involving its constant region which by antigen-bridging is brought into close contact with the CTLp. Alternatively, it is possible that ASHF is triggering thymocyte T_H precursors (pre-T_H), which then trigger the CTLp. Regardless of whether ASHF acts directly on both the CTLp and the pre-T_H—or if it acts only indirectly via the induction of pre-T_H—our conclusions remain valid. The selectivity of fraction E and of 4C6 ASHF indicate that the chain of events leading to the generation of CTL involves antigen-specific collaborative events quite distinct from those leading to B cell induction. Experiments are in progress to define the mechanism(s) through which $ASHF_{CTL}$ is able to act.

It is clear that ASHF-CTL and ASHF-B are functionally distinct. The molecular basis for these differences, however, is not clear. The studies of Shiozawa et al. (*11*) demonstrate that ASHF-B consist of antigen-binding subunits and antigen-nonspecific subunits that are associated in the presence of Ca^{++}. Both types of subunits are required for functional activity. Analysis of effluents and eluates of ASHF purified on CRBC-affinity columns in the presence of EGTA demonstrated that both the effluent and the eluate fractions were required to functionally reconstitute the induction of B-cell proliferative responses or AFC activity (*11*). This is in contrast to CTLp induction, where the eluate alone is able to function provided that adherent cells syngeneic to the ASHF are provided (Table 4). This appears to be a reflection of the ability of the ASHF assay system to provide the second antigen-nonspecific subunit. The B cell system is nonpermissive for the detection of incomplete forms of ASHF (*11*).

The inability of fraction E to suppress an AFC response induced by fraction C indicates that an inhibitory mechanism is not responsible for the inactivity of fraction E in triggering AFC responses (Shiozawa C, Diener E, unpublished observations). However, the stringent requirements of 4C6-ASHF for syngenic H-2 products suggests that this form of ASHF is more incomplete than Ca^{++}-deficient CHI-ASHF. The 4C6-ASHF and the DEAE fraction E of CHI-ASHF may consist of "naked" T_HAR. We suggest that antigen-nonspecific subunits that may include Ia molecules are required to make this Fraction E 4C6 ASHF identical to the incomplete (Ca^{++}-deficient) CHI-ASHF. In the permissive CTL induction system (using syngeneic splenic adherent cells) all necessary antigen-nonspecific subunits are provided by adherent cells to form a "complete"

ASHF. Our observation that the AFC assay is nonpermissive and the CTLp assay is permissive for the detection of incomplete ASHF may explain the preferential CTLp inductive activity of Fraction E and 4C6 ASHF. It does not however, provide any obvious explanation for the inability of fraction C to trigger CTLp. Since unfractionated CHI-ASHF efficiently triggers CTL responses, it is unlikely that suppressive moieties present in fraction C are obscuring the effect(s) of ASHF-CTL present in this fraction. It is not clear why DEAE fraction C of CHI-ASHF is able to trigger AFC but not CTL responses.

A number of experiments suggest that ASHF consists of T_HAR and Ia antigens, (*1, 7*). In addition to the demonstration of antigen specificity in the binding of nominal antigen and in tests of functional activity, depletion of ASHF activity by anti-Ia antibodies supports this model (*20, 28*). A widely-held and probably correct view is that T_HAR are antigenically monovalent (*29*). It is our working hypothesis that functionally active ASHF consists of multimolecular complexes of T_HAR-related molecules (e.g., a secreted form of the T_HAR) and Ia antigens. It is possible that Ia antigens function as a polymorphic glue to aggregate antigenically monovalent T_HAR thereby allowing a high avidity interaction with antigen on an antigen-presenting cell through multipoint binding.

Previous experiments have demonstrated that both $ASHF_B$ and $ASHF_{CTL}$ consist of an antigen-binding subunit and a subunit (or subunits) that does not bind antigen (*5, 11*). Our experiments indicate that the interaction of both antigen-specific and antigen-nonspecific subunits is required for functional activity of the ASHF (*5, 11*). Thus, there are two possible explanations for our observation of distinct $ASHF_{CTL}$ and $ASHF_B$: there exist completely different ASHF isotypes, produced by two different subsets of class-specific T_H, or a single type of T_H-derived antigen-specific receptor associates with different numbers and/or types of antigen-nonspecific subunits, derived from adherent cells, to form either $ASHF_{CTL}$ or $ASHF_B$. The experiments to isolate and identify the subunits of $ASHF_{CTL}$ and $ASHF_B$ are currently in progress.

REFERENCES

1. Pilarski LM, Krowka JF. Regulation of the induction of cytotoxic T cells by antigen-specific T cells and by antigen-specific T cell factors. In: Watson JD, Marbrook J, eds. Recognition and regulation in cell-mediated immunity. New York: Marcel Dekker, 1985: 367.
2. Singer A, Hodes RJ. Mechanisms of T cell-B cell Interaction. Ann Rev Immunol 1983; 1: 211.
3. Kilburn DG, Talbot FO, Levy JG. Characteristics of an antigen-specific helper factor that enhances the in vitro generation of cytotoxic cells directed against a syngeneic tumor. J Immunol 1981; 127: 2465.
4. Plate JMD, McDaniel CA, Flaherty L, Stimpfling JH, Melvold RW, Martin NO. Antigen-specific soluble helper activity for murine major histocompatibility complex-encoded molecules. I. Kinetics of factor production after skin transplantation and genetic mapping of the H-2 region specificity. J Exp Med 1981; 156: 681.
5. Krowka JF, Shiozawa C, Diener E, Paetkau V, Pilarski LM. Induction of cytotoxic lymphocyte responses by antigen-specific helper factors. J Immunol 1984; 133: 2018.
6. Paetkau V, Shaw J, Mills G, Caplan B. Cellular origins and targets of costimulator (IL2). Immunol Rev 1980; 51: 157.
7. Germain R, Benacerraf B. Helper and suppressor T cell factors. Spring Sem Immunopath 1980; 3: 93.
8. Howard M, Paul WE. Regulation of B-cell growth and differentiation by soluble factors. Ann Rev Immunol 1983; 1: 307.
9. Shiozawa C, Longenecker BM, Diener E. In vitro cooperation of antigen-specific T cell-derived helper factor, B cells, and adherent cells or their secretory products in a primary IgM response to chicken MHC antigens. J Immunol 1980; 125: 68.
10. Jaworski MC, Shiozawa C, Diener E. Triggering of affinity-enriched B cells. Analysis of B cell stimulation by antigen-specific helper factor or lipopolysaccharide. Dissection into proliferative and differentiative signals. J Exp Med 1982; 155: 248.
11. Shiozawa C, Sawada S, Inazawa M, Diener E. Triggering of affinity-enriched B cells. II. Composition and B cell triggering properties of affinity-purified, antigen-specific, T cell derived helper factor. J Immunol 1984; 132: 1892.
12. Pilarski LM. A requirement for antigen-specific helper T cells in the generation of cytotoxic T cells from thymocyte precursors. J Exp Med 1977; 145: 709.
13. Shaw J, Caplan B, Paetkau V, Pilarski LM, Delovitch TL, McKenzie IFC. Cellular origins of co-stimulator (IL2) and its activity in cytotoxic T lymphocyte responses. J Immunol 1980; 124: 2231.
14. Baum LL, Pilarski LM. In vitro generation of antigen-specific helper T cells that collaborate with cytotoxic T-cell precursors. J Exp Med 1978; 1148: 1579.
15. Bach FH, Bach ML, Sondel PM. Differential function of major histocompatibility complex antigens in T-lymphocyte activation. Nature 1976; 259: 273.
16. Klein J, Juretic A, Baxevanis CN, Nagy ZA. The traditional and a new version of the mouse H-2 complex. Nature 1981; 291: 455.
17. Pilarski LM, Vergidis D. Cytotoxic T cell response to minor histocompatibility antigens: apparent lack of H-2 restriction in killers stimulated by membrane fragments. J Exp Med 1982; 156: 217.
18. Farrar JJ, Fuller-Farrar J, Simon PL, Hilfiker ML, Stadler BM, Farrar WL. Thymoma production of T cell growth factor (Interleukin 2). J Immunol 1980; 125: 2555.
19. Bradford MM. A rapid and sensitive method for the quantitation of microgram quantities of protein utilizing the principle of protein-dye binding. Anal Biochem 1976; 72: 248.
20. Cunningham A, Szenberg A. Further improvements in the plaque technique for detecting antibody forming cells. Immunology 1968; 14: 599.
21. Shiozawa C, Sonik S, Singh B, Diener E. Antigen specific T-cell derived helper factor. In: De Weck A, Oppenhein J. Biochemical characterization of lymphokines. New York: Academic, 1980: 557.
22. Hedrick SM, Nielsen EA, Kavaler J, Cohen DI, Davis MM. Sequence relationships between putative T-cell receptor polypeptides and immunoglobulins. Nature 1984; 308: 153.
23. Siu G, Clark SP, Yoshikai Y, et al. The human T cell antigen receptor is encoded by variable, diversity, and joining gene segments that rearrange to generate a complete V gene. Cell 1984; 37: 393.
24. Alt FW, Bothwell ALM, Knapp M, et al. Synthesis of secreted and membrane-bound immunoglobulin mu heavy chains is directed by mRNAs that differ at their 3′ ends. Cell 1980; 20: 293.
25. Fitzmaurice L, Owens J, Blattner FR, Cheng HL, Tucker PW, Mushinski JF. Mouse spleen and IgD-secreting plasmacytomas contain multiple IgD chain RNAs. Nature 1982; 296: 459.
26. Tyler BM, Cowman AF, Adams JM, Harris AW. Generation of long mRNA for membrane immunoglobulin γ2a chains by differential splicing. Nature 1981; 279: 406.
27. Pure E, Isakson PC, Paetkau V, Caplan B, Vitetta ES, Krammer PH. Interleukin 2 does not induce murine B cells to secrete Ig. J Immunol 1982; 129: 2420.
28. Lonai P, Puri J, Bitton S, Ben-Neriah Y, Givol D, Hammerling G. H-2 restricted helper factor secreted by cloned hybridoma cells. J Exp Med 1981; 154: 942.
29. Jensenius JC, Williams AF. The T lymphocyte antigen receptor: paradigm lost. Nature 1982; 300: 583.

Received 7 June 1985.
Accepted 8 Nov 1985.

0041-1337/4202-0168$02.00/0
TRANSPLANTATION
Vol. 42, No. 2

Printed in U.S.A.

MEDIATION OF CELLULAR RECRUITMENT IN VIVO BY FUNCTIONALLY DISTINCT T CELL CLONES[1]

DOUGLAS W. HANTO,[2] MICHAEL B. WIDMER,[3] AND RICHARD L. SIMMONS

The Department of Surgery and the Immunobiology Research Center, Department of Laboratory Medicine and Pathology, University of Minnesota Health Sciences Center, Minneapolis, Minnesota 55455

The ability of functionally distinct alloreactive T cell clones to mediate cellular recruitment in vivo was examined in a modified sponge matrix allograft model. Changes in cellular recruitment to paired healed s.c. urethane sponge grafts injected with cytolytic T lymphocyte (CTL), helper, or helper-independent CTL clones, or bulk resting mixed leukocyte culture (MLC) cells, and allogeneic or syngeneic blasts were studied. Injection of indium-111-labeled unsensitized cells i.v. was used to assess cellular recruitment to the graft site. All three alloreactive T cell clones and bulk MLC cells mediated preferential recruitment of circulating labeled cells when injected with allogeneic cells. The helper clone mediated significantly greater recruitment than the CTL clone. These results confirm at the clonal level our previous observations that populations of allosensitized cells enriched for either cytolytic or noncytolytic T lymphocytes can mediate cellular recruitment in vivo and extends them to include helper-cell-independent cytolytic T lymphocytes.

Recent studies from our laboratory have focused on the possible role of specifically allosensitized lymphocytes (SSL)* in mediating and amplifying graft rejection (*1–4*). Using bulk populations of SSL, we have shown that the in vivo interaction between sensitized T cells and target cells bearing the sensitizing alloantigens results in an increase in lymphocyte recruitment, blood flow, and vascular permeability at the graft site. We have postulated that these phenomena are the result of the secretion of one or more lymphokines by the responding SSL (*5*), resulting in the attraction of additional circulating lymphocytes, and thereby expanding the pool of both specifically sensitized and nonspecific inflammatory cells at the graft site. In studies performed to determine the role of lymphocyte subpopulations in this system, we found that whole populations, as well as populations treated with antibodies against Lyt-1 and Lyt-2 surface antigens and enriched for cytolytic and noncytolytic cells, were effective in the recruitment assay. To gain further insight into the functional characteristics of the cell type(s) responsible for recruitment, we examined, in the present study, the ability of functionally distinct alloreactive T cell clones to mediate cellular recruitment in vivo.

[1] This work was supported Grants AI16869 and AI19200 from the National Institutes of Health.

[2] To whom requests for reprints should be addressed, at Washington University School of Medicine, Department of Surgery, 4989 Barnes Hospital Plaza, St. Louis, MO 63110.

[3] Scholar of the Leukemia Society of America.

*Abbreviations used: B6, C57BL/6; Con A, concanavalin A; CTL, cytolytic T lymphocyte; DBA, DBA/2J; DTH, delayed-type hypersensitivity; IL-2, interleukin-2; LPS, lipopolysaccharide; MEM, minimal essential medium; MLC, mixed leukocyte culture; RI, recruitment index; SN, supernatant; SSL, specifically sensitized lymphocytes; TCGF, T cell growth factor.

MATERIALS AND METHODS

Mice and experimental design. Female C57BL/6 (B6,H-2^b) mice (Charles River Breeding Laboratories, Wilmington, MA) and DBA/2J (DBA,H-2^d) mice (The Jackson Laboratory, Bar Harbor, ME) were used at 8–12 weeks of age. Two cell-free urethane sponges were implanted s.c. on opposite sides of the lateral thorax in B6 mice. Thirteen days later, after neovascularization of the sponges had occurred, bulk B6 anti-DBA MLC cells or clones were injected (5×10^6) into both sponges. Specific-alloantigen-bearing LPS (lipopolysaccharide) blasts (DBA, 5×10^6) were injected into one sponge, and syngeneic blasts (B6, 5×10^6) into the opposite sponge. At 4 hr after sponge injection, indium-111-oxine-labeled unsensitized B6 spleen cells (*2*), were injected i.v. Sponges were removed and counted in a gamma counter one hour after i.v. injection to determine the relative accumulation of the labeled cells in the two sponges. The percentage of injected activity recovered in the sponge was calculated after correcting for the background count. The cellular recruitment index (RI), was calculated by dividing the percentage of injected activity recovered in each sponge matrix graft that was inoculated with B6 anti-DBA SSL and the specific DBA blasts by the percentage of injected activity in the sponge containing B6 anti-DBA SSL and the syngeneic B6 blasts.

$$\mathrm{RI} = \frac{\%\ \text{injected activity (anti-DBA SSL and DBA blasts)}}{\%\ \text{injected activity (anti-DBA SSL and B6 blasts)}}$$

The RI will equal 1.00 if the injected labeled cells enter the sponges at random. Values greater than 1.00 indicate preferential localization of labeled cells in the sponge matrix graft injected with the SSL and specific target.

T cell clones. T cell clones were derived by limiting dilution from 5-day B6 anti-DBA bulk mixed leukocyte culture (MLC) populations as previously described (*6*). Briefly, limiting dilution microcultures for cloning were seeded on day 5 of MLC with 0.25 B6 anti-DBA cells per well, 1×10^6 irradiated (2000 rads) DBA spleen cells and 30% (v/v) secondary MLC supernatant (2°MLC SN) as a source of growth factors. Cells from growth-positive microcultures were expanded and maintained by weekly subcultures in 16-mm Costar wells containing 6×10^6 irradiated (2000 rads) DBA spleen cells and 20% (v/v) 2°C MLC SN. The culture medium consisted of Dulbecco's modified Eagle's medium (DMEM) supplemented with 2% fetal bovine serum and additional amino acids. The functional characteristics of these clones in vitro were determined as previously described (*6, 7*) and are shown in Table 1. T cell clones for in vivo experiments were used on day 6 after previous subculture with antigen and 2° MLC SN. Control bulk MLC populations were used on day 14 after culture initiation. MLC populations and clones were harvested, washed, and suspended in supplemented DMEM at the desired concentration for sponge injection. Cells from bulk MLC and clones were tested in vitro at various effector cell/target cell ratios against ^{51}Cr-labeled DBA LPS blasts in a 4-hr assay (*2*).

LPS blasts. LPS blasts were obtained by culturing B6 or DBA spleen cells for 48 hr in supplemented minimal essential medium (MEM) with 40 μg/ml LPS. These cells were harvested, washed twice and resuspended in supplemented DMEM at the desired concentration for use as targets in cytotoxicity assays or for sponge injection.

Statistical analyses. The tabulated results are derived from multiple experiments. Values are expressed as the mean plus or minus standard error of the mean ($\bar{X} \pm SE$). Statistical significance was determined by the Wilcoxon two-tailed Student's *t* test. The P value of RI compared with 1.00 was calculated using the formula:

$$t = \frac{(RI - 1.00)}{SE} \text{ with } n - 1 \text{ degrees of freedom.}$$

RESULTS

Table 1 shows the functional characteristics in vitro of the clones used in these experiments. Cytolytic T lymphocyte (CTL) clone N1-5 is cytolytic for DBA cells but does not proliferate in tissue culture in response to antigenic stimulation without the overt addition of exogenous T cell growth factors (TCGF) or helper T cells that do proliferate and produce TCGF in response to antigenic stimulation. The helper-independent CTL clone N1-1 proliferates in a short-term assay and retains cytolytic activity when allostimulated without the addition of exogenous lymphokines (*6*). In addition clones N1-1 and N1-6 (helper T cell) release interleukin-2 (IL-2) when stimulated with specific alloantigen-bearing cells or Con-A, but clone N1-5 does not. These T cell clones, as well as unsensitized B6 spleen cells (negative control) and bulk MLC populations, were used in the experiments reported here. On the day of testing in vivo, the cells were also tested for cytolytic activity against DBA target cells. Figure 1 shows the cytolytic activity of the fresh spleen cell preparation, resting day-14 MLC cells, and the respective clones after in vitro expansion. These data confirm that the cytolytic activity of clones N1-1 and N1-5 was preserved during expansion. The unsensitized spleen cell preparation, bulk resting MLC cells, and helper cell clone (N1-6) had no significant cytolytic activity.

The results in Table 2 demonstrate the activity of these various populations in the recruitment assay. Labeled indicator cells accumulated equally in sponges injected with unsensitized spleen cells plus allogeneic or syngeneic LPS blasts. There was, however, a preferential increase in cell localization to the sponge grafts injected with blasts bearing the sensitizing alloantigen and each of the four groups of specifically sensitized lymphocytes, including bulk resting MLC cells, and all three functionally distinct T-cell clones. There was no significant difference in the ability of the bulk resting MLC cells, CTL, or helper-independent CTL clones to mediate cellular recruitment. There was significantly greater cellular recruitment mediated by the helper T cell clone compared with the CTL clone (P=0.049). These results confirm at the clonal level our previous observations that populations of sensitized cells enriched for either cytolytic or noncytolytic T lymphocytes can mediate cellular recruitment in vivo, and extend them to include the helper-cell-independent cytolytic T lymphocyte.

DISCUSSION

These findings have several implications for understanding the pathogenesis of allograft rejection. The relative importance of various functional subclasses of T lymphocytes in allograft and tumor rejection remains unclear (*8*). Some in vivo studies have employed adoptively transferred lymphocytes enriched for helper or cytolytic T cells on the basis of cell surface differentiation antigens. Some investigators have concluded that noncytolytic $Lyt\text{-}1^{+}2^{-}$ cells in the mouse (*9–11*) or $OX8^{-}$, $W3/25^{+}$ cells in the rat (*12*) are primarily responsible for allograft rejection. Allograft destruction in those experiments might be

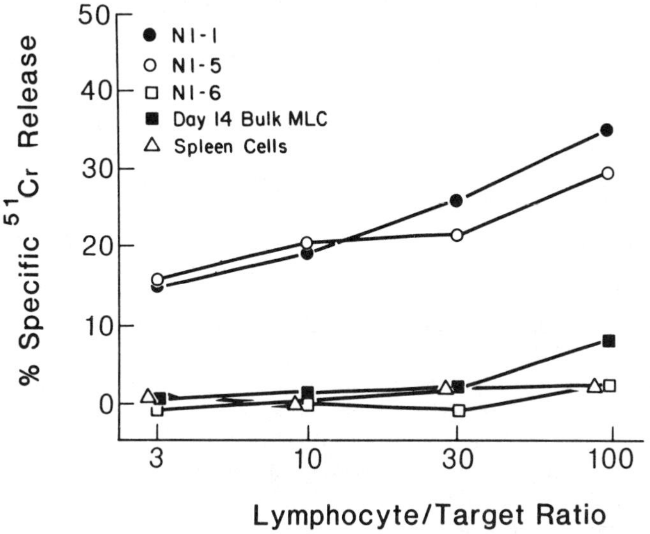

FIGURE 1. Cytolytic activity of T cell populations and clones. Cells were tested at various effector cell/target cell ratios for cytolytic activity against ^{51}Cr-labeled DBA LPS blast targets in a 4-hr assay.

TABLE 1. Functional characteristics in vitro of T cell clones

Clone	Specific cytolytic activity	Proliferative response to antigen	Requirement for exogenous TCGF[a] for proliferative response to antigen	Production of TCGF in response to antigen or Con A
N1-1 (helper-independent CTL)[b]	+	+	−	+
N1-5 (CTL)	+	+	+	−
N1-6 (helper T cell)	−	+	−	+

[a] T cell growth factors.
[b] Cytolytic T lymphocytes.

TABLE 2. Cellular recruitment properties[a] of lymphocyte populations and clones

Cells	Clone function	% ($\bar{X}$±SE) of i.v.-injected activity recovered in sponge		Recruitment index ($\bar{X}$±SE) (n)	P^b
		DBA targets	B6 targets		
Unsensitized spleen cells	—	0.48±.03	0.44±.02	1.10±.05[c] (16)	NS
Resting, day 14 bulk MLC	—	0.51±.03	0.36±.02	1.45±.06[d] (13)	<.001
Clone N1–1	Helper-independent CTL	0.57±.03	0.37±.02	1.52±.07[e] (11)	<.001
Clone N1–5	CTL	0.60±.03	0.42±.03	1.45±.07[f] (9)	<.001
Clone N1–6	Helper T Cell	0.66±.03	0.39±.01	1.70±.09[g] (9)	<.001

[a] Clones were derived by limiting dilution from 5-day B6 anti-DBA bulk MLC populations (*6*). DBA and B6 spleen cells were cultured for 2 days in LPS (40 μg/ml) and used as targets. Cloned cells were harvested on day 6 of expansion and 5×10^6 were injected with 5×10^6 DBA or B6 targets into plain sponge matrix grafts that had been implanted s.c. on opposite sides of the lateral thorax in B6 recipients 13 days earlier. At 4 hr after sponge injection, 20×10^6 ^{111}In-labeled fresh B6 spleen cells were injected i.v. Sponges were removed and counted 1 hr later.

[b] *P* value of RI compared with 1.00; NS = not significant.

[c,d,e,f,g] *P* values: [c] vs. [d,e,f,g] <0.05; [d] vs. [e,f] NS; [d] vs., [g] .02; [e] vs. [f,g] NS; [f] vs. [g] .049.

mediated either directly by these populations or the lymphokines they secrete, thus resembling a delayed-type hypersensitivity (DTH) reaction, or indirectly by recruitment of the actual effector cells to the site of the graft. A major criticism concerning the effector populations in those studies is that selection of the transferred cell population on the basis of cell surface antigen phenotype does not always predict their function. Other studies involving adoptive transfer of cloned T lymphocytes have demonstrated that cytolytic Lyt-2$^+$ cells are capable of mediating the rejection of syngeneic and allogeneic tumors, leading to the conclusion that graft destruction is the result of direct cell-mediated killing (*13, 14*). It is possible—and, in fact, likely—that several mechanisms are important in allograft rejection.

In previous studies using bulk populations, we demonstrated that the interaction between populations enriched for either cytolytic Lyt-2$^+$ or noncytolyic Lyt-2$^-$ cells and alloantigen results in an increase in cellular recruitment, blood flow, and vascular permeability locally at the graft site (*2–4*). Subsequent studies have shown that soluble factors present in 2° MLC supernatant are also capable of mediating these changes (*5*). Conventional inflammatory mediators such as serotonin, bradykinin, and histamine, which may be involved in DTH reactions do not however, alter lymphocyte recruitment in this model (*15*). Therefore, even though there are some similarities between these lymphokine mediated events in allograft rejection and DTH reactions, there are also clear differences.

The current data obtained with cloned T cells are consistent with the idea that any specifically sensitized lymphocyte, whether functionally a helper T cell or a CTL of the helper-dependent or independent type has the capacity, after interaction with the sensitizing alloantigen, to attract unsensitized cells out of the circulation. This cellular recruitment might be mediated by lymphokines elaborated by the T cell clones. Characterization of the lymphokine activities secreted by the three clones used in these experiments involved testing only for the presence of IL-2. The failure to detect IL-2 release by this particular CTL clone (N1-5) suggests that IL-2 is not the major mediator of lymphocyte recruitment in this case. Further in vitro characterization of the lymphokines produced by cloned T lymphocytes is required, wtih direct comparison of the effects of the clones and their lymphokines in vivo. These studies are presently in progress. An additional consideration in these studies concerns the nature of the cell population that accumulates at the site of interaction between the alloreactive cells and their targets. The identity of the subpopulation recruited this system has yet to be investigated; it is possible that different subpopulations may be recruited by the different types of T cells used as effectors.

We do not know precisely what role recruitment of circulating unsensitized cells plays in effecting a lethal insult to the allograft. We have previously postulated that a chance encounter between a few circulating specifically sensitized lymphocytes and alloantigen at the graft site may release lymphokines that mediate the accumulation of both sensitized and nonsensitized cells at the graft site. This is analogous to DTH reactions in which lymphokines are elaborated that have the capacity to inhibit cell migration, increase cellular infiltration, cause tissue damage, and increase local blood flow and vascular permeability (*16*). Such lymphokine-mediated phenomena may explain in part the nonspecificity and heterogeneity of the cellular infiltrate at the site of DTH reactions and in rejecting allografts. Furthermore expansion of the pool of SSL and other inflammatory cells at the graft site may be an important amplification mechanism in allograft rejection.

In conclusion, we have demonstrated that helper, cytolytic, and helper-independent cytolytic T cell clones are capable of mediating lymphocyte recruitment when exposed to the sensitizing alloantigen in vivo. It is likely that allograft rejection involves a combination of cell mediated killing by cytoxic cells and lymphokine secretion by cytotoxic and/or noncytotoxic cells that may cause direct tissue damage, changes in blood flow, and permeability, and an increase in cellular recruitment, thereby attracting additional circulating SSL and nonspecific inflammatory cells that amplify the host response.

Acknowledgments. We thank Birgitta Clinchy and John Harty for expert technical assistance.

REFERENCES

1. Hopt UT, Sullivan W, Hoffman R, Simmons RL. Migration and cell recruiting activity of specifically sensitized lymphocytes in sponge matrix allografts. Transplantation 1980; 30: 411.
2. Hanto DW, Hopt UT, Hoffman R, Simmons RL. Lymphocyte recruitment, regional blood flow, and vascular permeability at sites of allogeneic cellular interactions. J Immunol 1982; 129: 2437.
3. Hanto DW, Hopt UT, Hoffman R, Simmons RL. Recruitment of unsensitized circulating lymphocytes to sites of allogeneic cellular interactions. Transplantation 1982; 33: 541.
4. Hanto DW, Harty JT, Simmons RL. Lymphocyte recruitment properties of regional lymph node or spleen cells during skin allograft rejection. Transplantation 1983; 36: 578.

5. Hanto DW, Harty JT, Simmons RL. Soluble mediators generated by allogeneic stimulation increase lymphocyte recruitment, regional blood flow, and vascular permeability in vivo. Transplant Proc 1985; 17: 578.
6. Widmer MB, Bach FH. Antigen-driven helper cell-independent cloned cytolytic T lymphocytes. Nature 1981; 294: 750.
7. Widmer MB, Roopenian DC, Biel LW, Bach FH. Characterization of alloreactive T cell clones in vitro. In: von Boehmer H, Haas W, eds. T cell clones. New York: Elsevier, 1985.
8. Loveland BE, McKenzie IFC. Which T cells cause graft rejection? Transplantation 1982; 33: 217.
9. Loveland BE, Hogarth PM, Ceredig RH, McKenzie IFC. Cells mediating graft rejection in the mouse I. Lyt-1 cells mediate skin graft rejection. J Exp Med 1981; 153: 1044.
10. Loveland BE, McKenzie IFC. Cells mediating graft rejection in the mouse. II. The Ly phenotypes of cells producing tumor allograft rejection. Transplantation 1982; 33: 174.
11. Loveland BE, McKenzie IFC. Cells mediating graft rejection in the mouse. III. Ly-1$^+$ precursor T cells generate skin graft rejection. Transplantation 1982; 33: 407.
12. Dallman MJ, Mason DW, Webb M. The roles of host and donor cells in the rejection of skin allografts by T cell deprived rats injected with syngeneic T cells. Eur J Immunol 1982; 12: 511.
13. Engers HD, Glasebrook AL, Sorenson GD. Allogeneic tumor rejection induced by the intravenous injection of Lyt-2$^+$ cytolytic T lymphocyte clones. J Exp Med 1982; 156: 1280.
14. Engers HD, Lahaye T, Sorenson GD, et al. Functional activity in vivo of effector T cell populations. II. Anti-tumor activity inhibited by syngeneic anti-MoMULV-specific cytolytic T cell clones. J Immunol 1984; 133: 1664.
15. Hanto DW, Harty JT, Hoffman RA, Simmons RL. Secondary mixed leukocyte culture supernatant mediate changes in cellular recruitment, blood flow, and vascular permeability. Transplantation (in press).
16. Cohen S, Pick E, Oppenheim JJ, eds. Biology of the lymphokines. New York: Academic Press, 1979.

Received 17 October 1985.
Accepted 25 November 1985.

0041-1337/86/4202-0171$02.00/0
TRANSPLANTATION Vol. 42, No. 2

IN VITRO AND IN VIVO CYTOTOXICITY OF T CELLS CLONED FROM REJECTING ALLOGRAFTS[1]

MARY ELLEN SNIDER,[2,3] LORI ARMSTRONG,[4] JERRY L. HUDSON,[4] AND DAVID STEINMULLER[2,3,5]

The Histocompatibility Laboratory, Transplantation Society of Michigan, and the Flow Cytometry Laboratory, Department of Pathology, University of Michigan, Ann Arbor, Michigan

Epa-1 is a tissue-restricted, non–major histocompatibility (MHC) antigen that may be responsible for the extreme sensitivity of skin to allograft rejection and graft-versus-host disease (GVHD), especially with MHC-compatible donors and recipients. To confirm that Epa-1 serves as a target in allograft rejection and GVHD, we isolated Epa-1-specific cytotoxic T lymphocyte (CTL) clones completely in vivo from sponge-matrix allografts and from lymph nodes draining rejecting skin allografts. These clones induced GVHD-like skin lesions in antigen-specific, MHC-restricted fashion following intradermal inoculation into appropriate hosts. The in vivo–derived clones are conventional CTL since they are IL-2-dependent and express the Thy-1.2$^+$, Lyt-1$^-$, Lyt-2$^+$, L3T4$^-$ phenotype. The results of this study also are pertinent to the controversy over which T-cell subset actually mediates allograft immunity, since the intragraft isolation and subsequent cloning of conventional CTL that induce necrotizing skin lesions are direct evidence that CTL are the proximal mediators of allograft rejection.

Although it is well accepted that T cells mediate acute allograft rejection (*1*), there is controversy over which T-cell subset is responsible for the tissue destruction (*2*). One useful approach to elucidate the effector cell in question is to determine which T cell subset fulfills a form of Koch's postulates—namely, to find antigen specific effector cells at the site of rejection, to isolate and grow those cells in vitro, and to show that inoculation of the cells into appropriate hosts induces tissue destruction. We employed this approach within the context of a model allograft system.

The antigenic determinant inducing allograft rejection in our model is the tissue-restricted minor histocompatibility antigen Epa-1. Epa-1 is defined by cytotoxic T lymphocytes (CTL)*

[1] This work was supported by U.S.P.H.S. Research Grant AI21208 and funds from the EPICS Division, Coulter Corporation, Hialeah, FL.

[2] Transplantation Society of Michigan.
[3] Present address: Department of Surgery, University of Michigan School of Medicine, Ann Arbor, MI 48109.
[4] University of Michigan.
[5] Address correspondence to: Dr. David Steinmuller, 1520 MSRB I, University of Michigan Medical School, 1150 West Medical Center Drive, Ann Arbor, MI 48109.

* Abbreviations used: BSS, balanced salt solution; CSC, cultured spleen cells; CTL, cytotoxic T lymphocyte; EC, epidermal cells; FACS, fluorescence-activated cell sorter; FCS, fetal calf serum; GAR-FITC, fluorescein-conjugated goat antirat antibody; GVHD, graft-versus-host disease; ^{3}HTdR, tritiated thymidine; IL-2, interleukin 2; LNC, lymph node cells; 2-ME, 2-mercaptoethanol; MHC, major histocompatibility complex; PBS, phosphate-buffered saline.

that specifically lyse epidermal cells (EC), fibroblasts, and activated macrophages while not significantly affecting lymphocyte targets (3). Previously we isolated an Epa-1-specific CTL clone, 21-4, from a bulk culture population of primed spleen cells (4). This Lyt-2^+ CTL clone is antigen specific, H-2 restricted and IL-2 dependent (4, 5). However, since 21-4 was derived following an in vitro culturing period, we wanted to isolate effector cells at the site of a rejecting allograft to fulfill Koch's first postulate. To accomplish this we utilized the sponge matrix allograft model of Roberts and Häyry (6), which simplified the extraction of cells infiltrating the allograft. We also isolated cells from the lymph nodes draining rejecting skin allografts.

Allograft-infiltrating cells and cells from draining lymph nodes were assayed for CTL activity and subsequently cloned for further characterization. The propagation of antigen-specific cloned cell lines derived from the allografts fulfilled Koch's second postulate. The clones were found to be conventional CTL since they were L3T4a^-, Lyt-2^+, H-2-restricted, and IL-2-dependent. Moreover, these cloned CTL induced antigen-specific ulcerative lesions in vivo, thereby fulfilling all of Koch's postulates as mediators of allograft rejection. Some of our findings have been reported in preliminary form (7).

MATERIALS AND METHODS

Mice. C3H/HeJ (C3H; Epa-1^-, *H-2^k*) and CBA/J (CBA; Epa-1^+, *H-2^k*) mice of both sexes were purchased from the Jackson Laboratory, Bar Harbor, ME. B10.A(4R) (Epa-1^+, *H-2^{h4}*) and B10.0L (Epa-1^+, *H-2^{ol}*) male mice were generously provided by Chella David, Ph.D., of The Mayo Clinic, Rochester, MN.

Preparation of EC. EC were obtained from trypsinized mouse tail skin as previously described (8). Briefly, the skin was removed from the tail and incubated for 60 min at 37°C in a 0.5% solution of trypsin (No. 610-5095, GIBCO, Grand Island, NY) in Mishell-Dutton phosphate-buffered balanced salt solution (BSS) without calcium and magnesium. The dermis was peeled away from the epidermis with fine forceps and the EC were scraped off with glass probes into a BSS solution containing 10% fetal calf serum (FCS) and 0.025% crude DNase (No. D-0876, Sigma, St. Louis, MO). The cells were gently mixed to disrupt clumps and then pipetted through nylon mesh with 110-μ openings (Nitex No. HC-3-110, Tetko, Elmsford, NY) to remove any remaining clumps and debris. The cell suspension was centrifuged at 300×g for 10 min, and the pellet was resuspended in a small volume of BSS containing 10% FCS. Viable cells were enumerated by trypan blue dye exclusion.

Sponge matrix allografts. Urethane sponges (kindly provided by R. Simmons, M.D., and N. Ascher, M.D., of the University of Minnesota, Minneapolis, MN) were prepared as described by Ascher et al. (9). Briefly, 10×10×5-mm pieces were washed extensively with two 30-min boilings in distilled water, a 30-min soaking in acetone, a 30-min soaking in absolute ethanol, and two 30-min boilings in distilled water. The prepared sponges were placed in a glass petri dish and autoclaved for 20 min.

The original protocol described by Roberts and Häyry (6) was to allow an i.p.-implanted sponge to be naturally coated and impregnated with host cells and then to transplant the coated sponge s.c. to a desired allogeneic secondary host. However, a sponge also may be impregnated with donor cells by transplanting it s.c. into a host and injecting the desired allogeneic donor cells directly into the sponge matrix, as shown by Hanto et al. (10). Our preliminary experiments confirmed that injection of EC into sponges resulted in CTL influx that was comparable to the IP coating technique (data not shown). Hence, we adopted the following protocol. Sponges were soaked in serum-free BSS and then transplanted s.c. into the nucha of Epa-1^- C3H hosts that were untreated or previously immunized—the latter, by a single i.p. injection of 10^7 Epa-1^+ CBA EC. After 24 hr, 10^7 sterile CBA EC were injected into the sponge matrix in a volume of 0.2 ml serum-free BSS. At various intervals thereafter the sponge allografts were removed and placed in sterile BSS containing 10% FCS. Infiltrated cells were squeezed out of the sponges with sterile forceps into 35-mm Petri dishes. The sponges were placed in fresh media and squeezed to free cells two more times, and the cells were pipetted through the 110-μ nylon mesh to remove clumps and debris. The filtered suspensions were centrifuged at 300×g for 10 min, and the cell pellets were resuspended into small volumes of BSS plus 10% FCS for enumeration and dilution to the desired concentrations. Sponge cells from 2–3 hosts per group were pooled for each time point studied.

The brachial and axial nodes draining the site of sponge implantation or skin grafting were removed at various times from C3H hosts that received sponges impregnated with CBA EC or that were grafted bilaterally with CBA skin, as described elsewhere (11). Lymph nodes were teased in BSS containing 10% FCS, gently mixed, and pipetted through nylon mesh. The cell suspension was centrifuged at 300×g for 10 min, and the pellet was resuspended for enumeration. We used the method of Starzinski-Powitz et al. (12) to promote the differentiation of CTL precursors. These investigators demonstrated that T cells from lymph nodes draining the site of inoculation of hapten-conjugated syngenic cells resulted in hapten-specific CTL after culturing for three days without antigen. Moreover, we demonstrated the same phenomenon with T cells from lymph nodes draining the sites of skin allografts (13). Consequently, we tested cells from lymph nodes draining sponge or skin allografts for CTL activity directly as well as after three days in culture without antigen. The lymph node cells (LNC) were cultured under the same conditions as the cultured spleen cells (CSC) described below.

Cytotoxicity assays. CTL activity was measured in 3-hr ^{51}Cr release assays with either EC or CSC target cells, as described elsewhere (8). Previously we have shown that culturing spleen cells in medium with FCS and 2-mercaptoethanol (2-ME) for 2–3 days renders them as susceptible to lysis by Epa-1-specific CTL as mitogen-stimulated spleen cells (14). Therefore, C3H or CBA spleen cells were cultured for 2–3 days at a density of 2.5×10^6/ml in upright 25-cm^2 flasks in 20 ml of RPMI-1640 medium supplemented with 2 mM L-glutamine, 1 mM sodium pyruvate, 0.12 mM nonessential amino acids (GIBCO No. 320-1140), 25 mM HEPES buffer, 0.05 mM 2-ME, 100 U/ml penicillin, 100 μg/ml streptomycin, and 10% FCS. EC target cell suspensions were filtered through carefully washed glass wool packed in a 3-cc syringe barrel prior to labeling, as described elsewhere (8). Target cells were labeled by a 30-min incubation in a shaking water bath with $Na_2{}^{51}CrO_4$ (No. NE2-0305, New England Nuclear, Boston, MA) at 0.1 mCi/30×10^6 cells/ml in BSS containing 10% FCS. The labeled cells were washed four times, counted, and adjusted to 5×10^5 ml in the assay medium, Eagle's minimal essential medium with 10% FCS. The previously characterized Epa-1-specific CTL clone 21–4 (4) was utilized in several experiments as a positive effector-cell control. The effector cells were adjusted to 1.25×10^6 ml of assay medium and 0.2 ml/well was delivered to conical-bottomed 96-well plates (No. 3897, Costar, Cambridge, MA). The target cells were added with a 1.0 ml Hamilton syringe at 20 μl/well, resulting in an effector-to-target cell ratio of 25:1; then the trays were centrifuged at 50×g for 5 min. Following a 3-hr incubation at 37°C in a 5% CO_2-humidified incubator, 0.1 ml of the supernatant fluid was removed from the wells for gamma counting.

The maximum release of ^{51}Cr from labeled target cells was determined by incubating them in water for 3 hr to achieve hypotonic lysis. The percentage of specific lysis was defined as $I - N/X - B$, where I = mean ^{51}Cr release in the presence of immune effector cells, N = mean ^{51}Cr release in the presence of fresh normal syngeneic spleen cells, X = mean maximum ^{51}Cr release in water and B = machine background. Means were calculated from quadruplicate wells and the standard deviations never exceeded 10%.

Derivation of CTL clones. Sponge and LNC were cloned by micromanipulation of individual cells (*15*). Briefly, 1×10^4 cells were placed in a 60-mm dish containing 4 ml of BSS with 10% FCS, and several 4-fold dilutions were delivered into replicate plates. Each plate was chilled on an ice bath and examined under an inverted phase contrast microscope. A single cell in an isolated field was removed with a heat-drawn 10-μl capillary pipet and placed into a plate containing medium alone to confirm the presence of a single cell. Each single cell then was transferred to a microtiter well containing culture medium supplemented with 20% concanavalin-A-stimulated rat spleen cell supernatant (IL-2 medium) prepared as previously described (*4*) and "feeder cells," 5×10^5 irradiated (2500 rads) C3H spleen cells and 10^4 irradiated (4000 rads) CBA EC. After 7–10 days, half the contents of actively growing wells was transferred to a 16-mm diameter well of a 24-well tray (Costar No. 3424) containing 2 ml of IL-2 medium and fresh irradiated feeder cells. The microtiter wells were refed with IL-2 medium, and after allowing for regrowth the wells were assayed for CTL activity.

Proliferation assay. Proliferation of the cloned CTL was evaluated by the incorporation of tritiated thymidine (^{3}HTdR). Briefly, 1×10^4 CTL were cultured for 72 hr in 96-well flatbottomed plates (Costar No. 3596) with 2×10^3 irradiated (4000 rads) syngeneic C3H EC or allogeneic CBA EC stimulators. The mixed cultures were suspended in a total volume of 0.2 ml culture medium/well in the presence or absence of 20% IL-2 medium. Six hr prior to harvesting, the cells were pulsed with 1 μCi ^{3}HTdR of 6.7 Ci/mM, specific activity (TMM-199E, RPI, Mt. Prospect, IL). The cells were harvested on glass fiber filter paper and ^{3}H incorporation was measured by liquid scintillation spectrometry. All cultures were run in quadruplicate.

Fluorescence-activated cell sorter (FACS) analysis. FACS analysis of clone 58 and ND6 was conducted on the EPICS C flow cytometer (Coulter Corporation, Hialeah, FL). Feeder cells and debris were removed from cell preparations by Ficoll-Hypaque gradient centrifugation. Both cloned T cells were subjected to direct immunofluorescence and three T cell differentiation antigens were evaluated: Thy 1.2, Lyt-1, and Lyt-2. Clone 58 was also subjected to indirect immunofluorescence whereby a fourth antigen, L3T4a, was measured. Results are provided from the indirect labeling procedure, since a more complete cell surface phenotype was obtained with this technique. In the first step of the indirect procedure, 3×10^5 clones were stained with monoclonal rat antimouse Thy 1.2, Lyt-1, Lyt-2, and L3T4a (Nos. 1331, 1343, and 1353, respectively, Becton Dickenson, Mountain View, CA) and GK1.5 hybridoma culture supernatant, a generous gift from Dr. W. Wei, Michigan Cancer Foundation, Detroit, MI. Fluorescein-conjugated goat antirat (GAR-FITC; No. 1213-1721, Cappel Laboratory, Malvern, PA) monoclonal antibody was employed as the secondary fluorescent probe. MAS 051 monoclonal antibody (Accurate Chemical, Westbury, NY) was used as a negative control since it does not bind to mature peripheral T cells. After the clones were stained, they were fixed with paraformaldehyde and stored at 4°C until the flow cytometry was performed. Fluorescence was measured on a logrithmic amplification scale and the results are expressed in histogram form.

Evaluation of cloned CTL function in vivo. CTL cloned from sponge matrix allografts and draining lymph nodes were harvested from culture and the feeder cells removed by Ficoll-Hypaque sedimentation. The interface cells were washed four times with BSS containing 10% FCS and the desired number of cells ($5–10\times10^6$) was injected intradermally into (C3H×CBA) F_1 hybrid or syngeneic C3H control hosts in 30 μl of BSS. The injection sites were observed daily for the development of lesions, which were defined as grossly visible ulcerations of the skin (*5*).

RESULTS

Sponge allograft infiltrating cells. We examined the cellular response to Epa-1-disparate sponge allografts by enumerating the infiltrating cells and then evaluating their CTL activity. Sponges implanted into C3H hosts were impregnated with CBA EC, and the resulting infiltrating cells were squeezed out for evaluation. The average number of infiltrating cells removed from the sponge matrix allograft are shown in Table 1. Cell migration into the allografts peaked at two weeks in normal hosts and at one week for hosts previously immunized with CBA EC. Significant numbers of infiltrating cells were found for both groups up to three weeks after transplantation. By the fourth week, the cell yield decreased to that found in control syngeneically transplanted sponges at two weeks.

We then compared the CTL activity of sponge-derived cells taken from normal and immune hosts. Sponge matrix allografts were transplanted at weekly intervals into normal and immunized C3H mice and the infiltrated cells were removed and assayed for cytotoxic activity against allogeneic and syngeneic EC and CSC targets. The CTL activity of sponge cells from both groups was allo and EC-specific (Fig. 1). It peaked two

TABLE 1. The average cell yield from sponge matrix allografts[a]

Duration of sponge (weeks)	Number of viable cells $\times10^6$/sponge[b]	
	Normal hosts	Immune hosts[c]
1	12.2±1.9	21.3±0.6
2	27.9±2.0	17.1±1.9
3	16.2±4.2	8.6±0.5
4	5.8±0.1	6.1±1.5

[a] Sponge allografts implanted at weekly intervals were all removed, and the extracted cells counted on the day of the assay.

[b] Mean ±SD of 3–5 experiments per time point.

[c] C3H/He hosts were primed by an i.p. immunization of 1×10^7 CBA EC one week prior to sponge allograft implantation. The average number of cells recovered from three control syngeneically coated sponges was $5.3\pm1.0\times10^6$ at two weeks after transplantation.

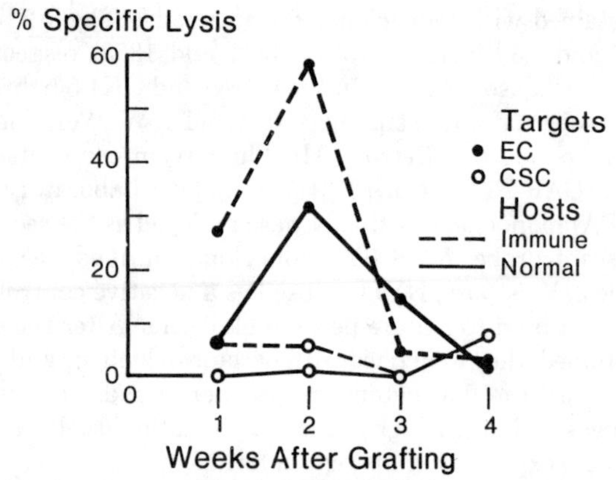

FIGURE 1. Cytotoxicity against CBA EC and CSC targets of sponge-derived cells evoked by transplanting sponge allografts containing CBA EC into C3H hosts. Normal and immune hosts were used, the latter were immunized by a single i.p. injection of 1×10^7 CBA EC. The effector-to-target cell ratio was 25:1 and the spontaneous ^{51}Cr release ranged from 11% to 16%. The results shown are typical of three replicate experiments.

weeks after transplantation, when cells from the normal and immunized hosts lysed 32% and 58% of the CBA EC targets, respectively. However, only the sponge-derived CTL from the immune hosts had significant activity at one week (27% lysis), and the intensity of their overall response was greater than the CTL activity from normal hosts throughout the time course.

Epa-1-specific CTL lyse CBA EC while not significantly affecting CBA lymphocytes or syngeneic C3H EC (*4*). This pattern of target cell susceptibility previously was shown to be directed against the Epa-1 determinant by extensive studies with large panels of mice (*14*) and by cloned CTL (*4*). In the present study, sponge cells from both normal and immune hosts readily lysed Epa-1$^+$ CBA EC but had neglible activity with CBA CSC and C3H EC and CSC (Fig. 1): the percentage of specific lysis of syngeneic EC and the CSC targets from both strains never exceeded 4%. Thus, the C3H hosts responded to the Epa-1$^+$ allografts with an influx of Epa-1-specific CTL.

Regional lymph node response to sponge allografts. Ascher et al. (*16*) have shown that precytotoxic cell recruitment into H-2-incompatible sponges occurs by day 5 after grafting, and that sponge effector cells become sensitized in the regional lymph nodes and then migrate to the allografts, even though no detectable CTL activity is found in the nodes until after allograft rejection. Therefore, we examined cells from lymph nodes draining the sites of sponge-allograft implantation for Epa-1-specific cytotoxic activity. Axillary and brachial lymph nodes were removed two weeks after implantation of Epa-1-disparate sponge allografts into normal C3H hosts, and the LNC were assayed for CTL activity. The cells had no measurable activity when assayed directly, but had CTL activity comparable to sponge-derived cells when assayed after three days in culture without antigen to promote CTL differentiation (Fig. 2). At an effector-to-target cell ratio of 25:1, the sponge cells and cultured LNC lysed 37% and 35% of the CBA EC targets, respectively, while the CBA CSC targets were not significantly affected by CTL of either type. This primary LNC response was Epa-1-specific since the lysis of syngeneic C3H EC and CSC targets did not exceed 3%. In contrast, culturing sponge cells without antigen did not result in an enhanced CTL response; in fact, the overall activity decreased from 37% to 14% at the effector-to-target cell ratio of 25:1 (data not shown), a phenomenon previously observed with T cells cultured from the spleens of skin-allografted hosts (*13*).

These data suggest that sponge-derived cells are fully differentiated CTL, and that the draining lymph node may be the source of precytotoxic effector cells. Therefore, a time course study was designed to compare the development of CTL activity in sponge allografts and the regional lymph nodes. Untreated C3H mice received Epa-1-disparate sponge allografts at various intervals and the sponges and draining lymph nodes were removed and the expressed cells assayed for CTL activity to determine the site of sensitization. Figure 3 shows that lymph-node-derived cells exhibited Epa-1-specific CTL activity prior to the sponge-derived cells: the CTL activity of cultured LNC peaked at ten days after transplantation (45% lysis) while 14 days were necessary to see the peak sponge cell activity (31% lysis). Moreover, the first detectable CTL activity was observed by day seven in the regional LNC preparation (15%). LNC assayed without any culturing period had no detectable activity throughout the 18-day time course (data not shown). Both cell preparations had negligible activity against syngeneic EC or CSC targets: the lysis of these targets did not exceed 8%. These data support the hypothesis that sensitization to Epa-1 occurs within the draining lymph nodes prior to CTL maturation within the allograft.

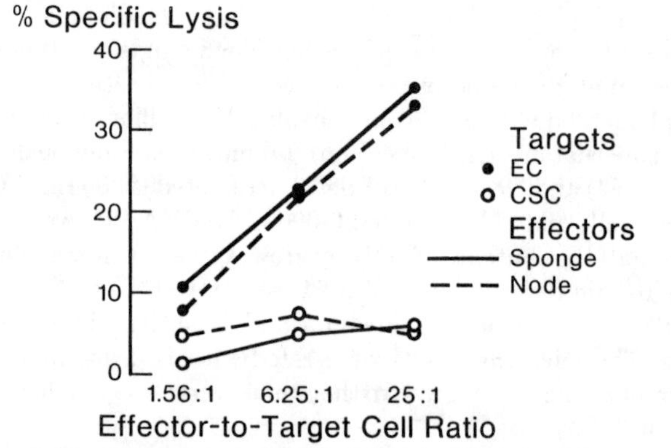

FIGURE 2. Cytotoxicity of C3H effector cells derived from sponge allografts and draining lymph nodes and assayed against CBA EC and CSC targets. The sponge was loaded with CBA EC two weeks prior to assay and normal hosts were used. The spontaneous ^{51}Cr release ranged from 10% to 17%. The results shown are typical of three replicate experiments.

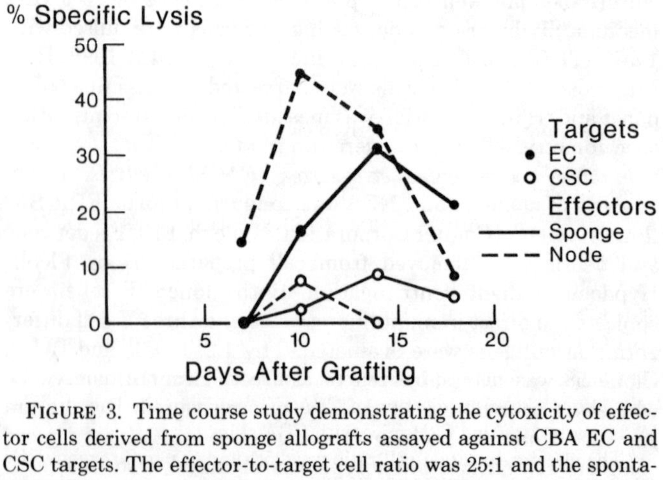

FIGURE 3. Time course study demonstrating the cytoxicity of effector cells derived from sponge allografts assayed against CBA EC and CSC targets. The effector-to-target cell ratio was 25:1 and the spontaneous ^{51}Cr release ranged from 9% to 16%. The results shown are typical of three replicate experiments.

Cloning of Epa-1-specific CTL. Clone 21–4 originally was derived from a bulk-culture primed spleen cell preparation by soft agar cloning (*4*) and subsequently was subcloned by micromanipulation (*5*). Because 21–4 was derived from an in vitro culture, we wanted to determine whether Epa-1-specific CTL clones could be generated completely in vivo. Hence, cells derived from lymph nodes draining Epa-1^+ skin allografts were assayed for Epa-1-specific cytotoxicity. Axillary lymph nodes were removed 13 days after CBA skin was transplanted bilaterally onto C3H mice. The cells were assayed immediately and after 3 and 5 days in culture without any antigenic stimulation. Epa-1-specific CTL were clearly present in the 3-day cultured LNC since the CSC targets were not significantly lysed, but nonspecific CTL were more prominent in the 5-day culture (Table 2). This prompted us to clone single cells by micromanipulation from the 3-day cultured LNC preparation, thus reducing the probability of cloning CTL that recognize antigens shared by lymphocytes and EC (*17*). In addition, single cells also were cloned from Epa-1-disparate sponge allografts two weeks after transplanting the sponges into normal C3H mice. Three clones, each originating from sponge allografts and lymph nodes, respectively, were selected by the ability to preferentially lyse CBA EC, while not affecting C3H EC or C3H and CBA CSC targets (Table 3); all of the CTL clones were Epa-1-specific.

In a previous study (*14*), a large panel of recombinant mouse strains on the Epa-1^+ C57BL/10 background were used to map the gene product restricting Epa-1-specific CTL to the K end of the *H-2* complex. We utilized two of the most informative strains, B10.A(4R) and B10.OL, to determine the H-2 restriction of the in-vivo-derived clones. Like the Epa-1-specific CTL clones studied previously (*4, 5*), all the present clones were restricted by the $H\text{-}2K^k$ gene product (Table 4).

To further characterize the Epa-1-specific CTL clones we

TABLE 2. CTL activity of LNC removed 13 days after skin grafting[a] (% specific lysis)[b]

CBA target cells	Culture time (days) 0	3	5
EC	0	31	45
CSC	0	10	38

[a] Axillary lymph nodes were removed and pooled from 3 C3H mice 13 days after the hosts were bilaterally grafted with CBA skin.

[b] The effector-to-target cell ratio was 25:1 and the spontaneous ^{51}Cr release ranged from 9% to 20%. This experiment was repeated three times with similar results.

TABLE 3. Alloantigen specificity of sponge allograft–derived and draining lymph node–derived clones[a] (% specific lysis[b])

Target cell	Sponge-derived clones			Lymph-node-derived clones		
	ID17	ND6	NR46	26	58	68
CBA EC	29	45	34	42	37	41
CBA CSC	0	0	3	6	2	−1
C3H EC	1	−1	0	1	0	2
C3H CSC	0	−2	−3	0	0	6

[a] Clones were derived by micromanipulation from the sponge allograft two weeks after injection of CBA EC and from the lymph nodes 13 days after grafting C3H mice with CBA skin.

[b] The effector-to-target cell ratio was 25:1 and the spontaneous ^{51}Cr release ranged from 12% to 22%. This experiment was repeated twice with similar results.

TABLE 4. H-2 restriction of cloned CTL (% specific lysis)[a]

Target EC	Epa-1	H-2			Sponge-derived clones		Lymph node derived clones		
		K	I	D	ND6	NR46	26	58	68
CBA	+	k	k	k	28	32	43	37	28
C3H	−	k	k	k	−5	−5	−6	−7	−7
B10.A(4R)	+	k	k/b	k	15	25	33	19	23
B10.0L	+	d	d	k	−1	−6	−8	−2	−8

[a] The effector-to-target cell ratio was 25:1 and the spontaneous ^{51}Cr release ranged from 17% to 21%. This experiment was repeated twice with similar results.

TABLE 5. Proliferation response of cloned CTL(^{3}HTdR incorporation[a])

Clone	IL-2	None	CBA EC	C3H EC
ND6	−	109±21	140±73	472±131
	+	52,682±6448	105,054±3560	77,229±8695
58	−	79±14	1128±387	359±87
	+	78,088±974	58,031±6409	71,482±9254
21-4	−	78±16	269±97	360±57
	+	6652±1205	27,787±2396	8638±686
None	−	297±184	232±52	NT[b]

[a] Mean cpm ± SD of quadruplicated cultures.

[b] NT = not tested.

examined their proliferative response with and without exogeneous IL-2. Conventional CTL require antigen and IL-2 to proliferate, but helper-cell independent CTL are driven by antigen to proliferate without the need for exogeneous IL-2 (*18*). All of our clones proliferated with IL-2-enriched medium present even in the absence of specific antigen (Table 5). Two of the three clones exhibited maximum proliferation in the presence of both IL-2 and Epa-1^+ EC. None of the clones showed any helper-cell independent characteristics since antigen stimulation alone did not elicit cell proliferation. Therefore, these minor antigen-specific clones appear to be conventional, IL-2-dependent CTL.

Flow cytometry. Flow cytometric analysis was done to determine the cell surface phenotype of cytotoxic clones isolated from sponge allografts and lymph nodes draining skin allografts. Lymph-node-derived clone 58 and sponge-derived clone ND6 were initially subjected to direct immunofluorescence to evaluate three differentiation antigens. Both clones were Thy 1.2^+, Lyt-1,$^-$ and Lyt-2^+ (data not shown). Subsequent experiments were done using indirect immunofluorescence to examine a fourth antigen, L3T4a, and data are presented from a represenative experiment. As seen in Figure 4, clone 58 as Thy 1.2^+, Lyt-1^-, Lyt-2^+, and L3T4a^-. The negative controls, MAS 051 antibody, GAR-FITC and PBS, were all negative. Thus, the clones stimulated by Epa-1-specific allografts express the classic CTL phenotype—i.e., they are Thy 1.2^+, Lyt-1^-, Lyt-2^+, and L3T4a^-.

In vivo tissue destruction. Clone 21–4 CTL induce ulcerating skin lesions when injected intradermally into appropriate hosts and must recognize both Epa-1 and the H-$2K^k$ restricting molecule in order to do so (*5*). Since all the in-vivo-derived clones displayed an identical pattern of target cell lysis to that of 21–4 in vitro, we tested their ability to mediate tissue destruction in vivo. Table 6 shows that every Epa-1^+ F_1 hybrid host tested developed a progressive skin lesion, but no lesions developed in the Epa-1^- syngeneic hosts.

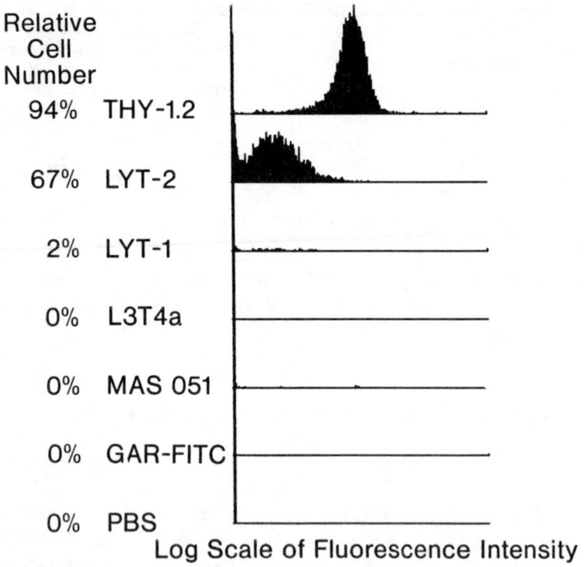

FIGURE 4. FACS analysis of Thy1.2, Lyt-1, Lyt-2, and L3T4a expression on clone 58. Three negative controls were used. The first control was cells incubated in only PBS. For the second negative control, cells were incubated with PBS for the first step and GAR-FITC was added to the second incubation period. For the last control, clone 58 was incubated with the negative control antibody, MAS051.

TABLE 6. Skin lesions evoked by cloned CTL[a]

Clone	Source	No. positive/No. tested[b]	
		(C3H×CBA)F_1 hosts	C3H hosts
26	Sponge	2/2	0/2
58	Sponge	11/11	0/3
ND6	Node	6/6	0/3
NR46	Node	6/6	0/3

[a] Hosts received 5×10^6 cloned CTL intradermally.
[b] Positive skin lesions progressed to ulceration within 5 days.

DISCUSSION

The results of this study provide further evidence of the role of Epa-1 in allograft rejection and GVHD. It is well known that EC are very susceptible to damage under these conditions (*14*), even when donors and hosts are matched for MHC antigens. Epa-1 antigens may be responsible for this extreme sensitivity of skin to allograft rejection and GVHD. They function in vivo as histocompatibility antigens since Epa disparity influences the fate of skin allografts (*19*) and Epa antigens serve as targets for necrotizing, GVHD-like skin lesions (*5*; Table 6). However, the ultimate test of the role of Epa-1 in allograft immunity was to isolate Epa-1-specific CTL completely in vivo, thereby fulfilling a form of Koch's postulates.

Primary responses to non-MHC alloantigens have been very difficult to demonstrate both in vitro (*20*) and in vivo (*21*). Indeed, both in vivo priming and in vitro boosting previously were required to generate CTL responses to Epa-1 (*14*). However, in the present study we were able to demonstrate that a primary response to Epa-1—and thus presumably to other non-MHC alloantigens—can occur entirely in vivo. The demonstration of EC-specific CTL derived from both sponge allografts and draining lymph nodes in normal hosts is prima facie evidence of a primary CTL response to Epa-1 in vivo. In characterizing this response, we also obtained evidence that CTL precursors arise in the draining lymph nodes and migrate to the allograft, where they mature into functional CTL. Moreover, we obtained further important evidence that Epa-1 serves as a target for allograft rejection and GVHD by showing that Epa-1-specific CTL clones derived from sponge allografts and from lymph nodes draining Epa-1 disparate skin grafts induce ulcerative skin lesions when injected into semiallogeneic hosts.

Our results also are pertinent to the controversy about which T cell subset mediates allograft immunity (*2*). Loveland et al. (*22*) reported that the adoptive transfer of helper T cells into thymectomized, irradiated, bone-marrow-reconstituted mice enabled these hosts to rejected skin allografts. This finding threatened the previously accepted assumption that CTL are the effector cells of allograft rejection. However, Loveland et al. inadvertently depleted cytotoxic T cells by their negative selection procedure in their attempts to adoptively transfer cells of the cytotoxic phenotype. Thus, their conclusion that CTL do not mediate allograft rejection was premature. Nevertheless, this prompted many other investigators to study the roles of helper and cytotoxic T cell subsets in allograft immunity, as recently reviewed by one of us (*2*). For example, Dallman et al. (*23*) showed that the helper but not the cytotoxic T cell subset could adoptively transfer skin allograft immunity in rats. However, they found significant numbers of cells with the cytotoxic phenotype infiltrating skin allografts in hosts reconstituted with the helper subset. This suggested either that the helper cell preparation was contaminated with CTL or that the helper cells stimulated the differentiation of CTL precursor in the hosts. LeFrancois and Bevan (*24*) subsequently addressed these very possibilities by transferring allograft immunity between mouse strains with different Thy-1 alleles that enabled CTL of host and donor origin to be distinguished. They found that CTL were mostly of host origin when the recipients were reconstituted with the helper cell subset, thereby proving that CTL precursors were activated in hosts given helper T cells. In addition, LeFrancois and Bevan also found that the negative selection procedures were not totally effective because anti-Lyt-2 monoclonal antibody and complement treatment did not eliminate all CTL from the transferred helper T cell population. In another study, Heidecke et al. (*25*) demonstrated synergy between helper and cytotoxic T cell subsets to produce allograft rejection in T-cell-deprived rats. Reestablishment of acute rejection capacity approaching that seen in intact hosts required the adoptive transfer either of unfractionated T cells or both T cell subsets and a course of IL-2 treatment. These findings and others reviewed elsewhere (*2*) indicate that both T cell subsets are necessary to promote rejection, the helper T cell probably stimulating the CTL that actually kill allogeneic cells. If this is the case, then the CTL still remains as the proximal mediator of allograft rejection.

We examined the role of the CTL in this regard—first by isolating them at the site of rejecting allografts and then by studying the capacity of cloned, allograft-derived CTL to mediate tissue destruction in vivo. We isolated and cloned Epa-1-specific CTL from sponge matrix allografts loaded with Epa-1-disparate EC and from the lymph nodes draining the site of Epa-1^+ skin allografts. These effector cells are conventional CTL because they lyse Epa-1^+ EC in vitro in an H-2-restricted fashion, they are dependent on an exogenous source of IL-2 for growth, and they have the Thy-1^+, L3T4a^-, Lyt-1^-, Lyt-2^+ phenotype. The intradermal injection of these in-vivo-derived CTL into semiallogeneic hosts induced ulcerative skin lesions.

Thus, we have directly proved that CTL infiltrating allografts or those present in lymph nodes draining rejecting allografts can mediate allogeneic tissue destruction in vivo. In conclusion, our results support the view that cytotoxic T cells mediate allograft rejection, though they do not exclude the possibility that other effector mechanisms contribute to graft destruction.

Acknowledgments. We thank Lois A. Gannon for expert assistance in preparing the manuscript.

REFERENCES

1. Steinmuller D. The immune response to a tissue allograft. In: Morris PJ, ed. Tissue transplantation, clinical surgery international. Edinburgh: Churchill Livingstone, 1982: 14.
2. Steinmuller D: Which T cells mediate allograft rejection? Transplantation 1985; 40: 229.
3. Burlingham WJ, Snider ME, Tyler JD, Steinmuller D. Lysis of mouse macrophages, fibroblasts and epidermal cells by epidermal alloantigen-specific cytotoxic T lymphocytes: effect of culture and inflammatory agents on Epa-1 expression. Cell Immunol 1984; 87: 553.
4. Tyler JD, Steinmuller D. Establishment of cytolytic T lymphocyte clones to epidermal alloantigen Epa-1. Transplantation 1982; 34: 140.
5. Tyler JD, Galli SJ, Snider ME, Dvorak AM, Steinmuller D. Clones Lyt-2^+ cytolytic T lymphocytes destroy allogeneic tissue in vivo. J Exp Med 1984; 159: 234.
6. Roberts PJ, Häyry P. Sponge matrix allografts: a model for analysis of killer cells infiltrating mouse allografts. Transplantation 1976; 21: 437.
7. Snider ME, Steinmuller D. In vivo isolation of minor alloantigen-specific cytotoxic lymphocytes. Transplant Proc 1985; 17: 596.
8. Steinmuller D, Tyler JD. Evidence of skin-specific alloantigens in cell-mediated cytotoxicity reactions. Transplant Proc 1980; 12: 107.
9. Ascher NL, Ferguson RM, Hoffman R, Simmons RL. Partial characterization of cytotoxic cells infiltrating sponge matrix allografts. Transplantation 1979; 27: 254.
10. Hanto DW, Hopt UT, Hoffman R, Simmons RL. Recruitment of unsensitized circulating lymphocytes to sites of allogeneic cellular interactions. Transplantation 1982; 33: 541.
11. Steinmuller D. Skin grafting. In: Di Sabato G, Langone JJ, van Vanakis H, eds. Methods in enzymology, vol 108. Immunochemical techniques, chap 3, part G, separation and characterization of lymphoid cells. New York: Academic Press, 1984: 20.
12. Starzinski-Powitz A, Pfizenmaier K, Rollinghoff M, Wagner H. In vitro sensitization of T cells to hapter-conjugated syngeneic structures of major histocompatibility complex. I. Effect of in vitro culture upon generation of cytotoxic T lymphocytes. Eur J Immunol 1976; 6: 799.
13. Steinmuller D, Santee LJ, Krco CJ. Augmentation of cell-mediated cytotoxicity by short-term in vitro precultivation of effector cells. Transplant Proc 1979; 11: 834.
14. Steinmuller D, Tyler JD, David CS. Cell-mediated cytotoxicity to non-MHC alloantigens on mouse epidermal cells. I. H-2 restricted reactions among strains sharing the H-2^k haplotype. J Immunol 1981; 126: 1747.
15. Zagury D, Bernard J, Thierness N, Feldman M, Berke G. Isolation and characterization of individual functionally reactive cytotoxic T lymphocytes: conjugation killing and recycling at the single cell level. Eur J Immunol 1975; 5: 818.
16. Ascher N, Chen S, Hoffman RA, Simmons RL. Maturation of cytotoxic T cells within sponge matrix allografts. J Immunol 1983; 131: 617.
17. Tyler JD, Steinmuller D, Burlingham WJ. Cell mediated cytotoxicity to non-MHC alloantigens on mouse epidermal cells. IV. An alloantigen shared with B cells but not T cells. Cell Immunol 1982; 68: 93.
18. Widmer MB, Bach FH. Antigen-driven helper cell-independent cloned cytolytic T lymphocytes. Nature 1981; 294: 705.
19. Steinmuller D, Tyler JD, Waddick KG, Burlingham WJ. Epidermal alloantigen and the survival of mouse skin allografts. Transplantation 1982; 33: 308.
20. McPhail S, Yron I, Stutman O. Primary in vitro cytotoxic T cell response to non-major histocompatibility complex antigens in normal mice. J Exp Med 1982; 156: 610.
21. Korngold R, Doherty PC. The localized primary cytotoxic T-cell response to cells expressing minor histocompatibility differences. Scand J Immunol 1984; 19: 175.
22. Loveland BE, Hogarth PM, Ceredig R, McKenzie IFC. Cells mediating graft rejection in the mouse. I. Lyt-1 cells mediate skin graft rejection. J Exp Med 1981; 153: 1044.
23. Dallman MJ, Mason DW, Webb M. The roles of host and donor cells in the rejection of skin allografts by T cell-depleted rats injected with syngeneic T cells. Eur J Immunol 1982; 12: 511.
24. LeFrancois L, Bevan MJ. A reexamination of the role of Lyt-2-positive T cells in murine skin graft rejection. J Exp Med 1984; 159: 57.
25. Heidecke CD, Kupiec-Weglinski JW, Lear PA, Abbud-Filho M, Araujo JL, Araneda D, Strom TB, Tilney NL. Interactions between T lymphocyte subsets supported by interleukin 2-rich lyphokines produce acute rejection of vascularized cardiac allografts in T cell deprived rats. J Immunol 1984; 133: 582.

Received 4 October 1985.
Accepted 20 November 1985.

0041-1337/86/4202-0178$02.00/0
TRANSPLANTATION
Vol. 42, No. 2

Printed in U.S.A.

EXPRESSION OF DONOR CLASS I MAJOR HISTOCOMPATIBILITY ANTIGENS ON THE VASCULAR ENDOTHELIUM OF MOUSE SKIN ALLOGRAFTS

ROB M. W. DE WAAL,[1] M. JOSÉ J. T. BOGMAN, INE M. H. A. CORNELISSEN, ARNO N. VERMEULEN,[2] AND ROBERT A. P. KOENE[3]

The Department of Pathology and The Department of Medicine, Division of Nephrology, and The Department of Parasitology, Sint Radboud Hospital, University of Nijmegen, The Netherlands

The expression of a class I MHC antigen on the vascular endothelium of mouse skin allografts was assessed by in vivo uptake of radiolabeled monoclonal anti-class-I antibody in the grafts after i.v. injection into the recipients. Endothelial localization of the bound antibodies was demonstrated via double-labeling immunofluorescence microscopy using factor-VIII-related antigen as a marker for endothelial cells. Treatment of recipients with cyclosporine was accompanied by low levels of class I antigen expression in the grafts, and similarly low levels were measured in grafts carried by nude recipients in the complete absence of rejection. Withdrawal of immunosuppressive therapy was followed by an increased class I antigen expression in the donor skin. An increase was also observed in skin grafts undergoing first-set rejection. We conclude that the expression of class I antigens on the capillary endothelium of mouse skin allografts in vivo is variable and is under influence of the immune status of the recipient.

Murine class I major histocompatibility complex (MHC)* antigens are membrane-bound glycoproteins that are coded for by the K, D, and L region, and also by the Qa-Tla-region of the murine H-2 complex. They consist of a 45,000 dalton polypeptide heavy chain that is anchored in the cell membrane, and is nonconvalently associated with a smaller polypeptide chain of 12,000-dalton β2-microglobulin. In the physiological situation, class I molecules are thought to be involved in the immune response against virally infected cells, functioning as restriction elements in T-cell-mediated cell lysis. They are expressed on the surface of the majority of nucleated cells and have their analogues in the human HLA-A, -B, and -C antigens (*1*).

In the transplantation situation both allogeneic class I and class II antigens can evoke an immune response in the host leading to rejection of the allografted tissue, which is illustrated in mice by the rejection of skin allografts transplanted between strains that differ only at the K or D region or at the I region of the H-2 complex (*2*). The primary targets for rejection are the vessels of the graft (*3–6*). Vascular endothelial cells carry both class I and class II MHC antigens, and we showed in an earlier study that the levels of class II antigen expression on these cells are variable (*7*). Class I antigens are expressed on cultured unstimulated human endothelial cells (*8*). The expression levels are enhanced after in vitro exposure to immune interferon (*9*). These findings suggest that, analogously to the situation for class II antigens, there may be variations in the expression of endothelial class I MHC antigens in vivo as well, especially in the transplantation situation, in which T cell activation is accompanied by the production of immune interferon. Therefore we have studied the expression of a class I MHC antigen in vivo in a model similar to that used for the study of class II MHC antigen expression (*7*). The results show that the levels of expression vary under influence of the immune status of the recipient.

MATERIALS AND METHODS

Animals. Inbred strains of congenic C57BL/10 (H-2^b), B10.BR (H-2^k), B10.D2(H-2^d), and B10.A (H-2^a) mice were originally obtained from the Jackson Laboratory (Bar Harbor, ME), A.TL (H-2^{tl}), and C3H.OH (H-202) mice from the Dutch Cancer Institute (Antoni van Leeuwenhoekhuis, Amsterdam), A.AL (H-2^{al}) mice from the Weizmann Institute (Rehovot, Israel), and BALB/c (H-2^d) mice from The National Institutes of Health (Bethesda, MD). The strains were kept in our animal house by continuous brother-sister matings. BALB/c nu/nu (H-2^d), B10.LP (H-2^b), and B10.LP nu/nu mice were purchased from the Radiobiological Institute of TNO (Rijswijk, The Netherlands), and AKR (H-2^k), B10.M (H-2^f), BALB/K (H-2^k), and B10.AQR (H-2^{yl}) mice from Olac Ltd. (Blackthorn, Bicester, UK).

Antibodies. Anti-class-I and class II monoclonal IgG2 antibodies were raised in our laboratory in the BALB/c anti BALB/K (H-2^d anti H-2^k) combination, and the corresponding cell clones were immortalized by fusion with the Sp2/O Ag14 myeloma according to standard procedures described elsewhere (*10*). Rabbit antiserum directed against human factor-VIII-related antigen was purchased from the Central Laboratory of the Red Cross Blood Transfusion Service (Amsterdam) and goat antiserum directed against rabbit Ig, TRITC-conjugated, from Cappel Laboratories (West Chester, PA). The N-hydroxysuccinimide ester of biotin, and FITC-conjugated avidin were obtained from Sigma Chemical Company (St. Louis, MO).

Cytotoxic assay. The in vitro cytotoxic activity of the monoclonal anti-class-I antibody on lymphoid cells of different mouse strains was determined in a two-stage dye exclusion

* Abbreviations used: BSA, bovine serum albumin; CsA, cyclosporine; FITC, fluorescein isothiocyanate; GAR-TRITC, goat antirabbit immunoglobulin serum conjugated with TRITC; IF, immunofluorescence; SDS-PAGE, sodium dodecyl sulphate polyacrylamide gel electrophoresis; MHC, major histocompatibility complex; PBS, phosphate-buffered saline; PBS/BSA/azide, PBS containing 1% BSA and 0.1% sodium azide; TRITC, tetraethylrhodamine isothiocyanate.

[1] Address correspondence to: Rob M. W. de Waal, Ph.D., Department of Pathology, Sint Radboud Hospital, P.O. Box 9101, 6500 HB Nijmegen, The Netherlands.

[2] Department of Parasitology.

[3] Division of Nephrology.

microcytotoxicity assay, as published previously (*11*). The titer of the antibody in this test was 5×10^5.

Immunoprecipitation. For the immunoprecipitation of class I molecules, thymus cells were surface-labeled according to the lactoperoxidase technique (*12, 13*).

Antibody labeling. Monoclonal anti-class-I IgG2b was radioiodinated and biotinylated as described previously (*7, 14, 15*).

Binding assays. Binding of the monoclonal anti-class-I antibody to murine lymphoid cells was tested in vitro in the indirect IF test or in the radioactive binding assay, using standard techniques.

Skin grafting. Standardized (8×8-mm) squares of donor tail skin were grafted onto the right dorsal flank of recipient mice by a modified "fitted graft" technique (*11*).

Immunosuppression. In part of the protocols the graft recipients were immunosuppressed by treatment with cyclosporine (Sandoz Ltd, Basel, Switzerland). The drug was dissolved in olive oil, at a concentration of 20 mg/ml, and was administered orally in a daily dose of 75 mg/kg body weight.

Indirect immunofluorescence. Recipient BALB/c mice, carrying both A.TL and B10.D2 skin grafts, were injected with 0.1 ml of phosphate buffered saline (PBS) containing 100 μg biotinylated monoclonal anti-class-I IgG and 0.1% bovine serum albumin (BSA). After 4 hr the mice were sacrificed and the grafts were removed and immediately frozen in liquid nitrogen. For indirect immunofluorescence (IF) staining, cryosections, 4–5 μm thick, were incubated in 500-fold diluted avidin conjugated with fluorescein isothiocyanate (FITC) (Sigma Chemical Company) in PBS/0.1% BSA for 30 min, and washed. Subsequently the tissue sections were incubated with rabbit antiserum against human factor-VIII-related antigen, which cross-reacts with murine factor VIII antigen, in a 100-fold dilution, washed, and developed with goat antirabbit Ig conjugated with tetraethylrhodamine (GAR-TRITC), 50-fold diluted. After washing, these sections were mounted in Aquamount (Gurr, BDH Chemicals, Poole, England), and examined under a Leitz Dialux fluorescence microscope equipped with epiillumination and filter combinations for FITC and TRITC fluorescence.

In vivo binding studies. Uptake of radiolabeled anti-class-I IgG in allografts in vivo was determined by i.v. injection of the radiolabeled antibody in the recipient mice. Then .1 ml of PBS/0.1% BSA, containing $1–5 \times 10^5$ cpm of label, corresponding to approximately 100 ng of IgG, was injected via the tail vein in BALB/c recipients of A.TL and B10.D2 grafts. To determine the amount of radioactivity in the graft, the animals were killed, the grafts removed, and the emission of gamma radiation was quantitated using a LKB compugamma counter (LKB, Turku, Finland).

RESULTS

Specificity of the monoclonal antibody. Cellulose-acetate electrophoresis of the monoclonal antibody showed a single discrete band in the gamma region. Immunoelectrophoretic analysis revealed the presence of an IgG monoclonal protein—which, using specific antisubclass antisera, proved to be of the IgG 2b subclass, type kappa. The specificity of the antibody was investigated with the complement-dependent cytotoxicity assay or the indirect IF test. A positive reaction was observed with cells of the b, k, p, s, m, a, yl, tl, al, and o2 haplotypes and a negative reaction with cells of the d and f haplotypes. These results indicate that the antibody recognizes the H-2.5 public antigen, a determinant shared by K and D region class I molecules (*16*). In our experiments, the reaction with the K region product was shown by binding of the antibody to B10.AQR ($H-2^{yl}$) cells and the reaction with the D region product by binding to C3H.OH($H-2^{o2}$) cells.

Immunoprecipitation studies confirmed the anti-class-I specificity. Sodium dodecyl sulphate–polyacrylamide gel electrophoresis (SDS-PAGE) analysis of the molecules precipitated from B10.A thymocyte lysate by the monoclonal antibody demonstrated that both the 45,000 and the 12,000 dalton subunit representing the heavy chain of the class I molecule and β2-microglobulin, respectively, were detectable. These molecules were not precipitated by a previously described (*7*) anti-class-II monoclonal antibody in a parallel control precipitation experiment. No specific precipitation was observed with thymocyte lysate of B10.D2 control cells.

Binding of the anti-class-I antibody to murine skin allografts in vivo. For the in vivo studies of class I antigen expression, A.TL or B10.A mice were used as donors of the test grafts and B10.D2 mice for control grafts. The A.TL and B10.A strains express the class I antigenic determinant recognized by the monoclonal antibody, while B10.D2 does not. BALB/c mice, which are also negative for the class I antigenic determinant, were used as recipients. To test the in vivo binding in the grafts, monoclonal anti-class-I IgG, purified by protein A affinity chromatography, was labeled with ^{125}I and aliquots containing 1.2×10^5 c.p.m. of radiolabel were injected i.v. into otherwise untreated BALB/c recipients of both an A.TL and a B10.D2 skin graft, on several days after transplantation. Figure 1 shows that there is, on day 5 after transplantation, specific binding to the A.TL graft, whereas the control B10.D2 graft only shows background levels. A high binding level in the A.TL graft is measurable at 4 hr after injection, and maximal at 8 hr. After 8 hr, the binding gradually declines, indicating a loss of radiolabel from the graft. The binding of an unrelated radiolabeled

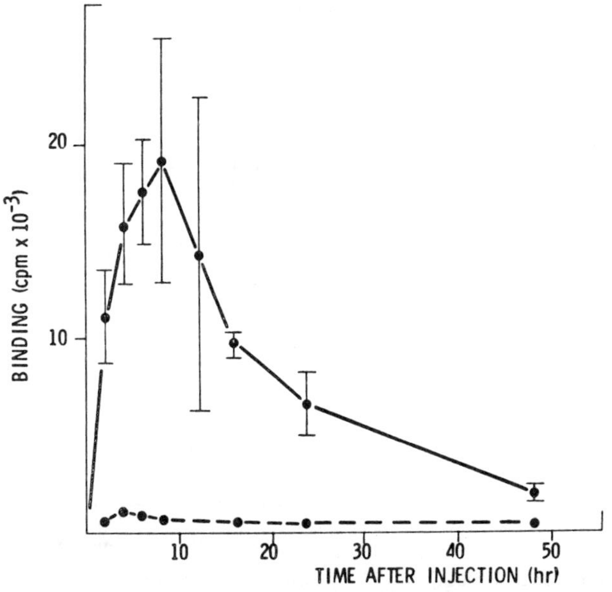

FIGURE 1. Binding of ^{125}I-labeled anti-class-I IgG to A.TL (●——●) and B10.D2 (●– – –●) skin allografts in vivo on day 5 after transplantation. Each point represents the mean of the values measured in 3 grafts; the bars represent the standard deviations. Injected radioactivity: 10^5 c.p.m. per mouse.

monoclonal antibody (WT3, directed against human T lymphocytes) was always negative (not shown). Although maximal binding values were obtained after 8 hr, we found considerable standard deviations at this time in these and other experiments. Therefore, in all subsequent experiments the uptake of radiolabel was assessed in grafts removed after 4 hr.

Immunohistological localization of the bound anti-class-I antibody. BALB/c recipients of A.TL and B10.D2 skin allografts were injected i.v. on day 5 after transplantation with biotin-conjugated anti-class-I IgG. The grafts were removed after 4 hr and prepared for immunohistological analysis. Binding of the anti-class-I antibody exclusively occurred on the endothelial cells in the A.TL grafts, and overlapped with the localization of factor-VIII-related antigen, used as a marker for endothelial cells (*17, 18*). In the B10.D2 grafts and in the recipient tissues, no specific binding was observed. We concluded from this finding that the specific uptake of radiolabel in an A.TL skin allograft after i.v. injection of radioiodinated monoclonal anti class I antibody can be regarded as a measure for the expression of donor class I antigens on the cells of the vascular endothelium.

Binding of the anti-class-I antibody on different days after transplantation. The in vivo uptake of radiolabeled anti-class-I antibody in A.TL skin grafts was determined in otherwise untreated BALB/c recipients. Fig. 2 shows that maximal binding is observed at days 5 and 6 after transplantation. After day 6 the amount of bound radioactivity rapidly diminished to a background level at day 9. This decrease is accompanied by gradual rejection of the graft (median survival time: 9.2±1.1 day, n = 10).

Binding of anti-class-I antibody in vivo in skin allografts carried by immunosuppressed and nu/nu recipients. In B10.D2 recipients of A.TL skin allografts, cellular rejection was postponed by daily administration of cyclosporine (CsA) (*19*). The binding capacity of the allografts for anti-class-I IgG was monitored by performing the in vivo binding assay on different days after transplantation. Maximal binding was measured at days 5 and 8 after transplantation (Fig. 3). At day 9 there is a

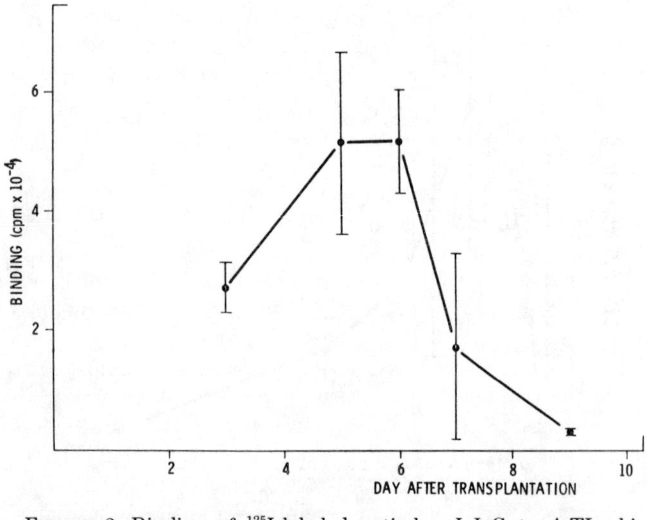

FIGURE 2. Binding of ^{125}I-labeled anti-class-I IgG to A.TL skin allografts in vivo on different days after transplantation. Recipient BALB/c mice were injected i.v. with 5×10^5 c.p.m. of radiolabel. Grafts were removed after 4 hr. Each point represents the mean value of measurements in four different grafts. The bars indicate the standard deviations.

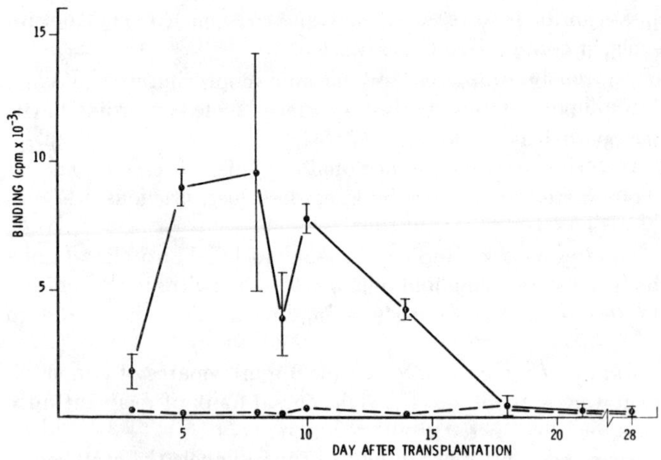

FIGURE 3. Binding of ^{125}I-labeled anti-class-I IgG to A.TL (●–●) and BALB/c (●– – –●) skin allografts on immunosuppressed B10.D2 recipients in vivo on different days after transplantation. Recipient mice were treated daily with cyclosporine. Injected radioactivity: 6×10^4 c.p.m. per mouse. Grafts were removed after 4 hr. Each point is the mean of measurements in two grafts; the range is indicated by the vertical bar.

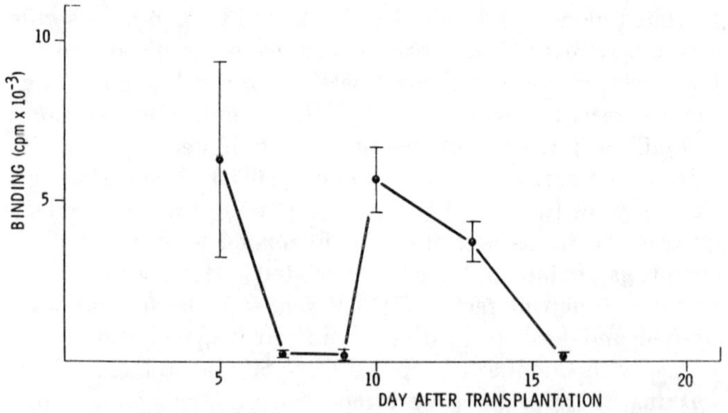

FIGURE 4. Binding of ^{125}I-labeled anti-class-I IgG to A.TL skin allografts on BALB/c nu/nu recipients in vivo on different days after transplantation. Injected radioactivity: 6×10^4 c.p.m. per mouse. Grafts were removed after 4 hr. Each point represents the mean value of the measurements in two grafts as given by the vertical bars.

suggestion of transient decrease, which in this experiment clearly cannot be considered significant, but which was confirmed in subsequent experiments. At day 10 the binding was high again, but after this time it gradually decreased to background levels at day 18. All grafts in these CsA-treated recipients had a macroscopically healthy appearance without signs of rejection at any time during the experiment.

In A.TL grafts carried by BALB/c nu/nu recipients, we found comparable results, as is shown in Figure 4. After an initial high binding value at day 5 and a temporary decline at day 7 to 9, we saw high levels at day 10 that gradually decreased to control levels at day 16 in skin grafts that were in healthy condition. This experiment was repeated twice in BALB/c nu/nu recipients carrying B10.BR skin allografts and the same pattern of class I antigen expression was observed, including the transient decrease of binding at days 7–9. We also assessed the expression of the donor endothelial class I antigen in B10.BR skin allografts after a more prolonged residence on BALB/c nu/nu recipients. Table 1 shows that on day 471 after transplantation very low levels of uptake of radiolabeled anti-class-I antibody were observed, comparable to the background levels in control B10.D2 skin allografts of the same age. Simultaneously the binding of the antibody to 5-day-old B10.BR skin allografts after injection of the recipients with an equal dose of the labeled antibody was tested as a positive control. In these grafts high levels of binding were measured.

The low binding of anti-class-I antibody to long-standing skin allografts was confirmed by immunofluorescence (IF). After a residence of 48 days on BALB/c nu/nu recipients, A.TL skin grafts (n = 4) did not show detectable binding of the anti-class-I IgG, conjugated with biotin.

To confirm the influence of the immune status of the recipient on the expression of donor endothelial class I MHC antigens, tail skin from B10.LP (H-2^b) donor mice was transplanted onto both normal and nude BALB/c recipients. The B10.LP strain gives a positive reaction with the monoclonal anti-class-I antibody used, while the BALB/c strain is negative. The results are given in Table 2, showing that on day 5 after transplantation the binding levels are significantly higher in skin grafts placed on normal BALB/c recipients than in skin grafts carried by BALB/c nu/nu recipients.

Reexpression of endothelial class I antigens after withdrawal of cyclosporine therapy. Donor tail skin from B10.A mice was transplanted onto B10.D2 recipients. The B10.A strain reacts with the monoclonal anti-class-I antibody, whereas the B10.D2 strain does not. All recipients were treated with CsA daily, for 3 weeks. At this time CsA administration was stopped in half the group while in the other half it was continued. From here on the binding of ^{125}I-labeled anti-class-I antibody in the grafts was determined on different days. Figure 5 shows that in recipients receiving CsA throughout, the uptake of radiolabel remained at a low level, whereas in the group in which CsA administration was discontinued, an enhanced class I antibody binding was found.

TABLE 1. Binding of radiolabeled anti-class-I monoclonal antibody in long-standing mouse skin allografts carried by nu/nu recipients[a]

Donor	Day after transplantation	n[b]	Binding (cpm)
B10.BR	471	2	147, 149
B10.D2	471	2	169, 108
B10.BR	5	5	5551, 7967, 6792, 7975, 4918
B10.D2	5	5	272, 230, 286, 170, 215

[a] BALB/c nu/nu recipients of both a B10.BR and a B10.D2 skin allograft were injected on the above mentioned days after transplantation with 10^5 cpm of radiolabeled monoclonal anti class I IgG.

[b] Number of skin grafts measured.

TABLE 2. Influence of the recipient's immune status on class I MHC antigen expression on the vascular endothelium of mouse skin allografts

Donor	Recipient[a]	n[b]	Binding ± SD (cpm)	Level of significance[c]
B10.LP	BALB/c	10	4208±1415	P=0.001
B10.LP	BALB/c nu/nu	8	2140±391	
B10.D2	BALB/c	5	825±162	

[a] 3.10^5 cpm of radiolabeled anti-class-I IgG was injected on day 5 after transplantation into otherwise untreated recipients. Grafts were removed after 4 hr.

[b] Number of recipient animals (each carrying one skin allograft).

[c] Statistical significance of differences between mean binding values were calculated according to Student's t test.

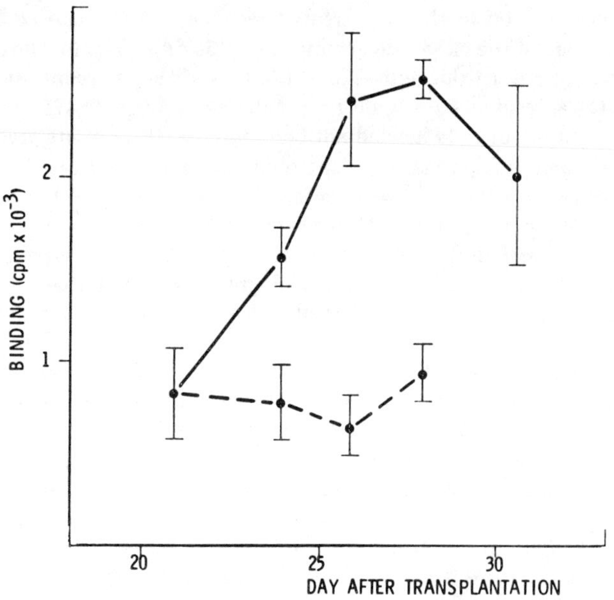

FIGURE 5. Binding of ^{125}I-labeled anti-class-I IgG to B10.A allografts on B10.D2 recipients in vivo on different days after transplantation. The recipients were treated daily with 75 mg/kg CsA, orally, for three weeks. On day 21 after transplantation, CsA administration was stopped in 8 recipient mice (●——●). Control mice received CsA throughout (●- - -●). Injected radioactivity: 1.5×10^4 c.p.m. per mouse. Grafts were removed after 4 hr. Each point represents the mean value of the measurements in two skin grafts, as given by the bars.

DISCUSSION

In this study we investigated influences on the expression of a class I MHC antigen on the vascular endothelium of mouse skin allografts. The kinetics of binding of radiolabeled anti-class-I IgG to donor vascular endothelium showed that a maximal binding was reached at 8 hr after injection (Fig. 1). After reaching this maximum, the levels of binding diminished, indicating a loss of bound radiolabel from the grafts. This loss might be caused by release of the labeled antibodies, or by shedding of antigen-antibody complexes from the endothelial cell surface. The release of such complexes from kidney allografts after infusion of polyclonal alloantibodies was reported earlier (*20*). In the present study the mechanism underlying the loss of radiolabel was not further investigated.

When we followed the in vivo uptake of radiolabeled anti-class-I antibodies in the grafts carried by normal immunocompetent recipients in the course of time after transplantation, maximal binding was seen at days 5 and 6 after transplantation (Fig. 2). Lower levels before this time can be explained by the fact that the connection between the blood vessels of donor and recipient is still incomplete during the first four days after transplantation (*21, 22*). At day 9 only control levels were observed, probably as a consequence of vascular damage and obstruction caused by the rejection process. When rejection was prevented by treatment of recipients with CsA, the highest binding levels were seen at day 7 after transplantation (Fig. 3), which correlates well with our previous finding that, in immunosuppressed animals, the vulnerability for antibody-mediated rejection is maximal on this day (*22*). Although in these mice no rejection occurred the binding levels gradually diminished after 10 days. In A.TL skin grafts transplanted onto nude mice, a similar pattern was observed (Fig. 4), with decrease of binding levels to control values after two weeks. This indicates that the decrease seen in the CsA-treated recipients is not caused by masking of the class I determinant by this drug. The low levels seem to persist during the total lifespan of the recipient mice. After a residence on nude recipients for as long as 471 days, the uptake of radiolabeled antibody in B10.BR skin allografts was comparable to that in control grafts (Table 1). In both the B10.D2 and the nude recipients we saw a temporary decrease in uptake around day 9 after transplantation. In previous studies we found that antibody responses can be observed in nude recipients of mouse skin allografts (*23*), but that these are weak, transient, and completely extinguished after three weeks (*24*). This temporary formation of antidonor antibodies may have blocked the binding of the labeled antibody. Whether such an antibody formation can also explain the transient decrease in the CsA-treated B10.D2 recipients deserves further study.

Variability in expression of class I antigens in vitro both in cultured cells and cell lines has repeatedly been described (*25–31*). Gamma-interferon, a product of activated T lymphocytes was found to be responsible for in vitro enhancement of class I antigen expression (*30, 31*). Variable expression of class I antigens was also reported for cultured human endothelial cells (*8, 9*). Our findings indicate that the expression of class I antigens on endothelial cells in healthy skin allografts is also variable in vivo. It is not clear whether the decrease in expression observed in immunoincompetent hosts implies a complete disappearance of these class I MHC antigens from the donor endothelial cells. Low levels of expression may escape from detection because of lack of sensitivity of the technique used. It has been suggested that cells in vitro may loose class I antigens completely if cultured in serum-free medium (*32*). Reexpression occurred after exposure to interferon-γ. Induction of HLA class I antigens in vitro on cells that normally lack these antigens was reported recently (*33*), and a similar induction was found in vivo in allografted heart (*34*) and liver (*35*) tissue. Therefore, the low levels of expression that we found in long-standing allografts probably represent basic, low levels on skin endothelium in an unstimulated environment, although modulation of class I antigen cannot be excluded.

In two experiments we found that activation of the immune system was accompanied by an increase in class I antigen expression. It is shown in Table 2 that in skin allografts from B10.LP donors that were transplanted onto BALB/c recipients an enhanced expression of class I antigens in the donor tissue could be observed, in comparison with grafts transplanted onto BALB/c nu/nu recipients. More important, withdrawal of CsA therapy, which leads to graft rejection within 10–13 days (*36*), induced a rise in the class I antigen expression levels in the graft (Fig. 5).

The diminished expression of donor class I antigens on graft endothelium in immunosuppressed animals offers a new explanation for the so-called adaptation phenomenon. This phenomenon is characterized by a decreased vulnerability of long-surviving allografts and xenografts for both humoral (*37–41*) and cellular (*42–46*) effector mechanisms. It has been proposed that in long-standing skin grafts this is caused by replacement of donor endothelium in the graft vessels by that of the host (*41*). Decreased expression of donor MHC antigens could be another mechanism in adaptation. This possibility has been formerly rejected, because in homogenates of established kidney allografts normal or increased amounts of MHC antigens could be measured (*46*). Since it has been shown, however, that the microvasculature is the primary target of rejection (*3–6*), it can be assumed that especially the endothelial MHC antigen expression, and not the MHC expression in the whole tissue, determines the susceptibility of the graft for rejection.

It seems most likely that the low expression of class I antigens in long-standing grafts represents a normal, quiescent state that is regained after a period of heightened expression induced by the transplantation procedure and the accompanying rejection process. This variability can also explain why long-standing skin grafts after retransplantation are sensitive to antibody-mediated rejection in an almost unimpaired fashion (*39*), a phenomenon that is not in keeping with the hypothesis of replacement of donor by host endothelium. Our findings do not allow conclusions at this point, since with our technique the assessment of the expression in vivo in the vessels of nontransplanted skin is not possible.

Although it is clear that the immune status of the recipient affects donor class I antigen expression, the inductive stimulus itself was not identified in our study. However, from the fact that nude mice lack T-cell-dependent immunity, and that CsA primarily inhibits stimulated T lymphocytes it can be deduced that activation of T lymphocytes in the recipients is an important factor governing the expression of donor endothelial class I antigens.

In general, the expression of class I and also class II antigens on the vascular endothelium of allografts seems to be a factor of major importance in the determination of the survival of the grafts. The results of our studies imply that the host and the graft are mutually influencing each other, which provides a new and more dynamic picture of the processes taking place during graft rejection and graft adaptation.

Acknowledgments. We thank W. Roeffen for generous help in the immunoprecipitation analysis, W. Tax, Ph.D., for his kind gift of the monoclonal antibodies, Mrs. C. Maass for skillful technical assistance and Mrs. J. van Rennes and Y. Stammes for preparation of the manuscript. Cyclosporine was generously provided by Sandoz Ltd (Basle, Switzerland). We appreciate the help of the staff of the animal laboratory (Mr. J. Koedam and colleagues).

REFERENCES

1. Ploegh HL, Orr HT, Strominger JL. Major histocompatibility antigens: the human (HLA-A,-B,-C) and murine (H-2K, H-2D) class I molecules. Cell 1981; 24: 287.
2. McKenzie IFC, Henning MM. The H-2 complex: immunogenicity and enhancement studies of H-2K region alloantigens. J Immunogenet 1977; 4: 249.
3. Anderson ND, Wyllie RG, Shaker IJ. Pathogenesis of vascular injury in rejecting rat renal allografts. Johns Hopkins Med J 1977; 144: 135.
4. Dvorak HF, Mihm Jr MC, Dvorak RG, Barnes BA, Manseau EJ, SJ Galli. Rejection of first-set skin allografts in man. The microvasculature is the critical target of the immune response. J Exp Med 1979; 150: 322.
5. Dvorak HF, Mihm Jr MC, Dvorak AM, Barnes BA, Galli SJ. The microvasculature is the critical target of the immune response in vascularized skin allograft rejection. J Invest Dermatol 1980; 74: 280.
6. Forbes RDC, Guttmann RD, Gomersall M, Hibberd J. A controlled serial ultrastructural tracer study of first-set cardiac allograft rejection in the rat. Evidence that the microvascular endothelium is the primary target of graft destruction. Am J Pathol 1983; 111: 184.
7. de Waal RMW, Bogman MJJ, Maass CN, Cornelissen LMHA, Tax WJM, Koene RAP. Variable expression of Ia antigens on

the vascular endothelium of mouse skin allografts. Nature 1983; 303: 426.

8. Pober JS, Gimbrone MA Jr, Cotran RS, Reiss CS, Burakoff SJ, Fiers W, Ault KA. Ia expression by vascular endothelium is inducible by activated T-cells and by human γ-interferon. J Exp Med 1983; 157: 1339.
9. Pober JS, Collins T, Gimbrone MA Jr, Cotran RS, Gitlin JD, Fiers W, Clayberger C, Krensky AM, Burakoff BJ, Reiss CS. Lymphocytes recognize human vascular endothelial and dermal fibroblast Ia antigens induced by recombinant immune interferon. Nature 1983; 305: 726.
10. Tax WJM, Willems HW, Kibbelaar MDA, de Groot J, Capel PJA, de Waal RMW, Reekers P, Koene RAP. Monoclonal antibodies against human thymocytes and T lymphocytes. In: Peeters H, ed. Protides of the biological fluids, 29th coloquium. Oxford and New York: Pergamon Press, 1981: 701.
11. Berden JHM, Gerlag PGG, Hagemann JFHM, Koene RAP. Role of antiserum and complement in the acute antibody-mediated rejection of mouse skin allografts in strain combinations with increasing histoincompatibility. Transplantation 1977; 24: 175.
12. Pink JRL, Ziegler A. Radiolabeling and immunoprecipitation of cell-surface macromolecules. In: Lefkovits I, Pernis B, eds. Immunological methods. London: Academic Press, 1979: 169.
13. Vitetta ES, Poulik MD, Klein J, Uhr JW. Beta 2-microglobulin is selectively associated with H-2 and TL alloantigens on murine lymphoid cells. J Exp Med 1976; 144: 179.
14. Hunter WM, Greenwood FC. Preparation of 131-I labelled human growth hormone of high specific activity. Nature 1962; 194: 495.
15. Pohlit HM, Haas W, von Boehmer H. Haptenation of viable biological carriers. In: Lefkovits I, Pernis B, eds. Immunological methods. London: Academic Press, 1979: 181.
16. Klein J, Figueroa F, David CS. H-2 haplotypes, genes and antigens: second listing. II. The H-2 complex. Immunogenetics 1983; 17: 553.
17. Hoyer LW, de los Santos RP, Hoyer JR. Antihemophilic factor antigen. Localization in endothelial cells by immunofluorescent microscopy. J Clin Invest 1973; 52: 2737.
18. Bloom AL, Giddings JC, Wilks CJ. Factor VIII on the vascular intima: possible importance in hemostasis and thrombosis. Nature New Biol 1973; 241: 217.
19. Lems SPM, Koene RAP. Prolongation of mouse skin allograft survival by cyclosporin A: graft rejection after withdrawal of therapy. IRCS Med Sci 1979; 7: 184.
20. Fine RN, Batchelor JR, French ME, Shumak KH. The uptake of 125-I labeled rat alloantibody and its loss after combination with antigen. Transplantation 1973; 16: 641.
21. Zarem HA. The microcirculatory events within full-thickness skin allografts (homografts) in mice. Surgery 1969; 66: 392.
22. Gerlag PGG, Koene RAP, Hagemann JFHM, Wijdeveld PGAB. Hyperacute rejection of skin allografts in the mouse. The sensitivity of ingrowing skin grafts to the action of alloantibody and complement. Transplantation 1975; 20: 308.
23. Koene RAP, Gerlag PGG, Jansen JJ, Hagemann JFH, Wijdeveld PGAB. Rejection of skin grafts in the nude mouse. Nature 1974; 251: 69.
24. Capel PJA, Lems SPM, Koene RAP. Antibody response to allogeneic and xenogeneic skin grafts in nude mice. In: Reed ND, ed. Proceedings third int workshop on nude mice. New York: Gustav Fisher, 1982: 275.
25. Vignaux F, Gresser I. Differential effects of interferon on the expression of H-2K, H-2D, and Ia antigens of mouse lymphocytes. J Immunol 1977; 118: 721.
26. Heron I, Hokland M, Berg K. Enhanced expression of B-2-microglobulin and HLA antigens on human lymphoid cells by interferon. Proc Natl Acad Sci USA 1979; 75: 6215.
27. Fellous M, Kamoun M, Gresser I, Bono R. Enhanced expression of HLA antigens and B_2-microglobulin on interferon-treated human lymphoid cells. Eur J Immunol 1979; 9: 446.
28. Inai K, Ng A, Glassy MC, Ferrone S. Differential effect of interferon on the expression of tumor-associated antigens and histocompatibility antigens on human melanoma cells: relationship to susceptibility to immune lysis mediated by monoclonal antibodies. J Immunol 1981; 127: 505.
29. Liao S, Kwong PC, Khosravi M, Bent PB. Enhanced expression of melanoma-associated antigens and B2-microglobulin on cultured human melanoma cells by interferon. JNCI 1982; 68: 19.
30. Wong GHW, Clark-Lewis I, McKimm-Breschkin JL, Harris AW, Schrader JW. Interferon-induces enhanced expression of Ia and H-2 antigens on B lymphoid, macrophage, and myeloid cell lines. J Immunol 1983; 131: 788.
31. Wallach D, Fellous M, Revel M. Preferential effect of γ interferon on the synthesis of HLA antigens and their mRNA's in human cells. Nature 1982; 299: 833.
32. Ball ED, Guyre PM, Glynn JM, Rigby WFC, Fanger MW. Modulation of class I HLA antigens on HL-60 promyelocytic leukemia cells by serum-free medium: re-induction by gamma-IFN and 1,25-dihydroxyvitamin D3 (calcitriol). J Immunol 1984; 132: 2424.
33. Sutherland J, Mannoni P, Rosa F, Huyat D, Turner AR, Fellous M. Induction of the expression of HLA class I antigens on K562 by interferons and sodium butyrate. Hum Immunol 1985; 12: 65.
34. Milton AD, Fabre JW. Massive induction of donor-type class I and class II major histocompatibility complex antigens in rejecting cardiac allografts in the rat. J Exp Med 1985; 161: 98.
35. Nagafuchi Y, Hobbs KEF, Thomas HC, Scheuer PJ. Expression of beta-2-microglobulin on hepatocytes after liver transplantation. Lancet 1985; 8428: 551.
36. Lems SPM, Capel PJA, Koene RAP. Rejection of long-surviving mouse skin allografts after withdrawal of cyclosporin A therapy. Transplant Proc 1980; 12: 283.
37. Jooste SV, Winn HJ, Russel PS. Destruction of rat skin grafts by humoral antibody. Transplant Proc 1973; 5: 713.
38. Jooste SV, Winn HJ. Acute destruction of rat skin grafts by alloantisera. J Immunol 1975; 114: 933.
39. Gerlag PGG, Capel PJA, Hagemann JFHM, Koene RAP. Adaptation of skin grafts in the mouse to antibody-mediated rejection. J Immunol 1980; 125: 583.
40. Burdick JF, Russell PS, Winn HJ. Sensitivity of long-standing xenografts of rat hearts to humoral antibodies. J Immunol 1979; 123: 1732.
41. Jooste SV, Colvin RB, Winn HJ. The vascular bed as the primary target of the destruction of skin grafts by antiserum. II. Loss of sensitivity to antiserum in long-term xenografts of skin. J Exp Med 1981; 154: 1332.
42. Nirmul G, Severin C, Taub RN. Adaptation of skin allografts in mice treated with anti-lymphocyte serum. Transplantation 1972; 13: 27.
43. McKenzie IFC, Koene RAP, Winn HJ. Evidence of adaptation in skin grafts in enhanced irradiated mice. Transplantation 1972; 14: 661.
44. Stuart FP, Fitch FW, Rowley DA. Specific suppression of renal allograft rejection by treatment with antibody and antigen. Transplant Proc 1970; 2: 483.
45. Batchelor JR, Welsh KI, Maynard A, Burgos H. Failure of long-surviving passively enhanced kidney allografts to provoke T-dependent alloimmunity. I. Retransplantation of (AS×AUG)F1 kidneys into secondary AS recipients. J Exp Med 1979; 150: 455.
46. Hart DNJ, Winearls CG, Fabre JW. Graft adaptation: studies on possible mechanisms in long-term surviving rat renal allograft. Transplantation 1980; 30: 73.

Received 23 April 1985.
Accepted 11 November 1985.

0041-1337/86/4202-0184$02.00/0
TRANSPLANTATION Vol. 42, No. 2
 Printed in U.S.A.

MECHANISMS OF TRANSPLANTATION TOLERANCE IN B-CELL-CHIMERIC CHICKENS

IMPAIRMENT OF TOLERANCE BY T CELL GROWTH FACTOR[1]

LASSE LEHTONEN,[2] OLLI VAINIO, AND PAAVO TOIVANEN

Department of Medical Microbiology, Turku University, SF-20520 Turku, Finland

Transplantation tolerance was induced in cyclophosphamide-treated, B-cell-depleted chickens by transfer of allogeneic bursal cells. To study the presence of specific suppressor cells in tolerant birds, mitomycin-C-treated peripheral blood lymphocytes (PBL) from tolerant recipients were cocultured in mixed lymphocyte cultures of normal syngeneic responder and allogeneic stimulator cells. No evidence of suppression was detected, since responses in cultures with tolerant cocultured cells were on the same level as the mixed lymphocyte reaction (MLR) of normal responders without cocultured cells. However, responses in cultures with normal cocultured cells were significantly higher. If cocultured cells were not treated with mitomycin C, responses to tolerizing alloantigen were equally high in cultures with tolerant cocultured cells as in cultures with normal cocultured cells. Likewise, when lymphocytes from tolerant chickens were mixed with normal syngeneic cells in graft-versus-host (GVH) splenomegaly assay, no suppression was detected, but the GVH reaction was even stronger than the reaction induced by the mixture of cells from two normal chickens. Furthermore, administration of chicken T cell growth factor (TCGF) into the cultures enhanced considerably the MLR of tolerant cells against the tolerizing alloantigen, but not against syngeneic or third-party stimulator cells. These results indicate that the transplantation tolerance in B-cell-chimeric chickens is due to lack of alloantigen-specific helper cells. When exogenous help is offered to tolerant cells either by normal syngeneic cells or by exogenous TCGF, the reactivity of tolerant cells against the tolerogen is reestablished.

We have started a series of experiments to study the acquired immunological tolerance in chickens. In a previous report we showed that transplantation of allogeneic bursal cells into B-cell-depleted recipients induces specific unresponsiveness for donor line alloantigens though only immature bursal cells from 4-day-old donors can induce a stable state of B cell chimerism detectable in peripheral blood of the recipients (*1*). We have now studied further the regulatory mechanisms of tolerance in this experimental model, which is analogous to mammalian models of neonatal tolerance.

The presence of regulatory T cell subpopulations in chicken has been shown in various functional assays (*2*). The characterization of suppressor and helper cells has, however, been difficult because no specific antisera have been available to these chicken T cell subsets (*3*). In the present study we have used MLR and GVH splenomegaly assay as model systems for the detection of regulatory T cells subsets (*4–6*) in tolerant chickens. Regulatory cell effects on MLR were studied in coculture experiments, where cells from tolerant and normal chickens were added into mixed lymphocyte cultures of syngeneic normal responder and allogeneic stimulator cells. The effect of tolerant cells on GVH reactivity of normal cells was determined in mixing experiments (*6*). In addition, the effect of exogenous chicken TCGF on MLR of tolerant chickens was determined (*7, 8*).

The mechanisms maintaining neonatal tolerance in mammals have been of interest to many research groups during the recent years. In this report we present evidence on deletion of alloantigen-specific helper functions as the mechanism of transplantation tolerance in B-cell-chimeric chickens.

MATERIALS AND METHODS

Chickens. H.B2 and H.B15 major histocompatibility complex (B-complex) homozygous chickens from the colonies of the Department of Medical Microbiology, Turku University, were used in this study (*9*). H.B14 line chickens were used as third-party antigen controls in MLR.

Induction of tolerance and its testing. H.B15 chickens treated with cyclophosphamide (4 mg i.p. on four consecutive days after hatching) were transplanted at the age of 4 days with allogeneic bursal cells from 4-day-old H.B2 donors (bursal stem cells) as described elsewhere (*1*). The degree of B-lymphoid chimerism in peripheral blood was determined and the reactivity of the recipients to antigenic stimulation by donor type histocompatibility antigens in MLR and skin graft test, as well as their graft-versus-host (GVH)* competence in splenomegaly assay were tested (*1*). Six H.B15 chickens, which were highly tolerant for H.B2 line alloantigens in the mixed-lymphocyte reaction (MLR) and GVH assay were used in further experiments. All these chickens were also chimeric having their B cells of H.B2 orgin. The number of donor line B cells was 10–16% of peripheral blood lymphocytes (PBL) 31 weeks after transplantation of bursal cells, when measured with a specific anti-B-F2 alloantiserum in a triple-layer immunofluorescence method as described previously (*1*).

Mixed lymphocyte reaction. The MLR assay was performed as described previously (*1*). Stimulator cells from peripheral blood of normal chickens were prepared by low-speed centrifugation (10, 11). The leukocyte-containing plasma was col-

[1] This work was supported by grants from The Research and Science Foundation of Farmos Oy and from the Sigrid Jusélius Foundation.

[2] To whom correspondence and reprint requests should be addressed.

* Abbreviations used: Con A, concavalin A; FITC, fluorescein isothiocyanate; GVH, graft-versus-host; IL-2, interleukin 2; MLR, mixed lymphocyte reaction; norm., normal; NCS, normal chicken serum; PBL, peripheral blood lymphocytes; PBS, phosphate-buffered saline; pT_c, precursors of cytotoxic T cells; TCGF, T cell growth factor; tol., tolerant.

lected and centrifuged for 10 min at 1200 rpm. The supernatant was removed and the leukocyte pellet was washed once more with phosphate-buffered saline (PBS) supplemented with 1% normal chicken serum (NCS). Cells were resuspended in RPMI-1640 medium supplemented with L-glutamine (2 mM, Gibco Europe, Glasgow, UK), sodium pyruvate (1 mM, Gibco), essential amino acids (0.8 × final, Gibco), nonessential amino acids (0.4 × final, Gibco), penicillin (100 U/ml), streptomycin (100 μg/ml), 2-mercaptoethanol (5×10^{-5} M), $NaHCO_3$ (0.75 g/L of medium) and 2.5% fresh NCS, and treated for 30 min at 40°C with 50 μg/ml mitomycin C (Sigma M-0503, St. Louis, MO). Thereafter cells were washed three times with PBS and resuspended in the complete culture medium (as described above) at a density of 1.0×10^{7} cells/ml. Responder cells were isolated at the same way and resuspended in the complete culture medium at a density of 2.5×10^{6} cells/ml. To study the effect of tolerant cells on MLR of normal H.B15 responders against H.B2 and H.B14 stimulators, cocultured cells from normal H.B15 control chickens and from H.B15 chickens tolerant for H.B2 alloantigens were added into MLR assay. Cocultured cells were isolated as described above. Mitomycin-C-treated and untreated cocultured cells were used in each experiment, and they were resuspended in complete medium at a density of 2.5×10^{6} cells/ml. MLR was set up in triplicate by adding 100 μl of each cell suspension to wells of U-bottomed microtiter plate (Nunc, Roskilde, Denmark). Cocultured cells and responder cells were used in 1:1 ratio in all experiments. Responder cells from four H.B15 individuals were used in each experiment. The reactivity of responder cells without cocultured cells was tested in the same experiment. Mitomycin-C-treated cocultured cells had no reactivity when incubated with stimulator cells. The MLR of untreated cocultured cells with stimulator cells was also checked (Table 1). After 5 days of incubation at 40°C in a 5% CO_2-air humidified atmosphere each culture was pulsed with 20 μl (0.25 μCi) of ^{125}I-labeled 5-iodo-2′-deoxyuridine (The Radiochemical Centre Amersham, UK, specific activity 90–110 mCi/mg), and 5-fluoro-2′-deoxyuridine (Fluka, Buchs, Switzerland) was added to the culture in a final concentration of 10^{-6} M to increase the uptake of the isotope, as described elsewhere (*12*). After 6 hr of incubation the cells were harvested onto filter paper with a multiple-channel cell harvester (Brandel, Gaithersburg, MD). Dried paper discs were placed into vials and counted for 1 min with a gamma counter (LKB Wallac, Turku, Finland).

GVH reaction in mixing experiments. The GVH splenomegaly assay was performed as described elsewhere (*1, 3, 13*). Cells from tolerant and normal chickens were mixed in various combinations to study the effect of tolerant cells on GVH competence of normal cells and vice versa (*6*). In brief, PBL from normal H.B2, H.B15, and H.B2-tolerant H.B15 chickens were separated by slow speed centrifugation and resuspended in RPMI-1640 (Gibco Europe, Glasgow, UK). Cells of two chickens were then mixed in 1:1 ratio and 100 μl of the cell mixture containing 3.0×10^{6} cells was injected i.v. into 13-day-old H.B2 embryos. Three or 4 embryos were injected with each cell combination tested. The GVH competence of each chicken used was also tested separately by injecting 1.5×10^{6} cells per embryo. In some experiments only 2 or 3 embryos could be used to test the GVH competence of individual control chickens. The splenomegaly induced by allogeneic cells was, however, always great, and no GVH reaction could be induced by syngeneic cells. Five days after injection the embryos were killed and the body and the spleen were weighed. The results are given as the mean of the relative weights of the spleen (spleen weight in milligrams per 100 grams of body weight). Spleens from uninjected embryos served as controls.

TABLE 1. MLR of normal and tolerant chickens used as cell donors in coculture experiments[a]

Responder cells	Number of chickens	Stimulator cells		Background[b]
		H.B2	H.B14	
Normal H.B15	6	19,975±8647[c]	6722±1775	142±36
$H.B15_{H.B2\text{-tol.}}$	6	425±195	15,899±5734	309±72

[a] All mixed lymphocyte cultures were performed simultaneously on the same plate with the corresponding coculture experiment.

[b] Background = cpm of responder cells cultured with medium.

[c] Expressed as mean of net cpm ±SEM. Net cpm = (cpm of responder cells cultured with mitomycin-C-treated stimulator cells) − (cpm of responder cells cultured with medium).

Production of TCGF. TCGF containing culture supernatant was prepared by stimulating chicken spleen cells (3.0×10^{6} ml) with 2 μg/ml concavalin A (Con A) (Pharmacia Fine Chemicals, Uppsala, Sweden) as described elsewhere (*14*). Cells were cultured in serum-free McCoy's 5A medium (Gibco Europe, Glasgow, UK) supplemented as described previously (*14*) in 75-cm^2 tissue culture flasks (Nunc, Roskilde, Denmark). After 48 hr of incubation cells were spun down and 40 mg/ml methyl-alfa-D-mannoside (Sigma Chemical Co, St. Louis, MO) was added to supernatants. TCGF containing supernatants were assayed for their ability to support the proliferation of TCGF-dependent long-term cultured T cell line and Con A blasts as described previously (*14*).

Administration of TCGF into mixed lymphocyte cultures. One-way MLR was set up as described above. Responder cells were cultured with mitomycin-C-treated stimulator cells either with or without the presence of 0.5% T cell growth factor (TCGF) containing supernatant. This concentration could still induce a significant proliferation of the cells of the T cell line and of Con A blasts (*14*), but not of unstimulated PBL.

Statistics. Student's t test was used for the comparison of means in GVH assay and in TCGF experiments. The paired t test was used to evaluate the results of MLR coculture experiments.

RESULTS

Suppressor activity of cells from tolerant chickens. Regulating activity of the mitomycin-C-treated cocultured cells from normal H.B15 and H.B2-tolerant H.B15 chickens (Table 1) was assayed in one-way MLR tests. When stimulated with the tolerizing alloantigen the responses detected were significantly lower ($P<0.001$ by paired t test) in cultures with tolerant cells as regulators than in cultures with normal cocultured cells and the mean percentage of suppression (% suppression = 100 × [1 - cpm in cultures with tolerant cells as regulators per cpm in cultures with normal cells as regulators]) was 35.5% (Table 2A). Only in four cultures of 24 was the response higher with tolerant cells than with normal cells. However, the reactivity observed in the presence of tolerant cells was not reduced when compared with the reactivity of the H.B15 responders without cocultured cells. When third-party stimulator cells (H.B14) were used, no difference could be detected between normal and tolerant cocultured cells (Table 2B). We interpret these findings to indicate that tolerant cells show no suppressor activity, whereas addition of normal cells increases MLR responses.

TABLE 2. (A) Suppressor cell activity of mitomycin-C-treated[a] cocultured cells from H.B15 chickens tolerant for H.B2 alloantigens: effect of tolerant cells on MLR of normal syngeneic H.B15 responders against the tolerizing alloantigen

Cocultured cells		H.B15 responders stimulated with H.B2 cells				
		I[b]	II	III	IV	Mean % of suppression[c]
None		29,164[e]	40,126	10,422	4,738	
Norm.	(H.B15$_1$)	33,551	48,872	19,764	31,435	47.2
Tol.	(704)[d]	22,233	29,979	3658	20,411	
None		30,203	46,755	56,443	30,943	
Norm.	(H.B15$_2$)	33,947	47,603	70,789	34,966	5.3
Tol.	(705)	34,260	36,989	88,014	27,045	
None		20,302	38,129	12,247	16,439	
Norm.	(H.B15$_3$)	38,032	54,917	19,635	32,673	39.5
Tol.	(708)	19,299	37,388	15,193	14,947	
None		1889	874	5550	5615	
Norm.	(H.B15$_4$)	2540	7330	18,132	25,493	63.0
Tol.	(709)	1081	1088	3554	18,132	
None		26,698	2582	1786	6803	
Norm.	(H.B15$_5$)	13,548	9135	4645	21,500	−0.1
Tol.	(711)	14,645	8322	5738	16,699	
None		29,212	4805	971	2685	
Norm.	(H.B15$_6$)	13,416	9697	16,609	12,852	58.1
Tol.	(712)	9628	2674	5513	4498	
					Mean	35.5
					SEM	±6.4
					Total number =	24

[a] Cocultured cells were treated with mitomycin C (50 μg/ml) for 30 min at 40 °C.

[b] Peripheral blood lymphocytes from 4 individual H.B15 chickens (I–IV) were used as responders to test the effect of cocultured cells on allogeneic MLR.

[c] % suppression = 100 × (1 − [cpm in cultures with tolerant cells as regulators per cpm in cultures with normal cells as regulators]). Negative values of suppression represent enhancement.

[d] 704–712 are H.B15 chickens transplanted with H.B2 bursa cells four days posthatching. Their B cells are of donor orgin and they are highly tolerant for H.B2 line alloantigens.

[e] Each individual value represents the mean cpm of triplicate cultures. The statistics associated with the difference between these values were determined with paired t test and are presented in the text.

Effect of untreated tolerant cells on MLR of normal syngeneic responders. When cocultured cells were not treated with mitomycin C, the responses to tolerizing alloantigen were as high in the cultures with tolerant cells as in the cultures with normal cocultured cells (Table 3A). The mean suppression was −2.4%, indicating that the responses were even slightly higher in cultures with tolerant cells than in cultures with normal cocultured cells. This result was somewhat surprising, because tolerant cells had only a low response to bursa cell donor line alloantigens when stimulated alone, and a weaker response would have been expected in cultures with tolerant cells. The lack of difference between the cultures could not be explained by crowding of cells since the addition of cocultured cells in most instances caused a clear increase in uptake of the isotope. The responses in cultures with tolerant cocultured cells were significantly higher ($P<0.01$ by paired t test) than in cultures without cocultured cells (Table 2A). Also when responses in cultures with untreated tolerant cocultured cells were compared with responses with mitomycin-C-treated cocultured cells (Table 2A), a significant increase ($P<0.001$) was detected. The recovery of the response of tolerant cells in MLR can be explained by the fact that normal syngeneic responders in the cultures can offer "help" for alloantigen-specific T lymphocyte precursors of tolerant chickens.

When third-party stimulator cells (H.B14) were used, the H.B15 MLR responses in cocultures with tolerant cells were significantly higher ($P<0.001$) than with normal cells. In 21 cultures with tolerant cells the response was higher and in 3 cultures lower than in the corresponding culture with normal cocultured cells. The mean enhancement was 85.3% (Table 3B). Although the response of tolerant cells to H.B14 stimulation in normal one-way MLR is somewhat higher than that of normal H.B15 cells used as cocultured cells (Tables 1 and 4), the difference in coculture MLR experiments was unexpectedly great. This result is probably explained by the multiple stimulation of normal H.B15 responder cells with H.B2-chimeric H.B15 cocultured cells and H.B14 stimulator cells. The tolerant cocultured cells contained at least 2.5×10^4 H.B2 line B cells per culture, which can induce some additional proliferation in the cultures. In addition, it is possible that tolerant cells contain relatively more helper cells or T lymphocyte precursors, which are specific for H.B14 line alloantigens, while helper cells specific for H.B2 line alloantigens are deleted in these chickens.

Effect of tolerant cells on GVH competence of normal cells.

TABLE 2. (B) Suppressor cell activity of mitomycin-C-treated cocultured cells from H.B15 chickens tolerant for H.B2 alloantigens: effect of tolerant cells on MLR of normal syngeneic H.B15 responders against third-party alloantigen[a]

Cocultured cells		H.B15 responders stimulated with H.B14 cells: I	II	III	IV	Mean % of suppression
None		2688	10,776	11,000	13,640	
Norm.	($H.B15_1$)	12,925	5757	2857	7194	0.6
Tol.	(704)	2120	7394	4752	6209	
None		2848	18,261	15,210	2171	
Norm.	($H.B15_2$)	7298	16,126	24,498	1270	9.6
Tol.	(705)	7454	11,259	9334	1928	
None		41,888	25,190	23,226	8969	
Norm.	($H.B15_3$)	37,741	27,954	19,695	9103	−16.0
Tol.	(708)	38,742	33,423	23,148	11,288	
None		11,000	1289	8982	13,640	
Norm.	($H.B15_4$)	11,933	1288	3334	11,693	23.6
Tol.	(709)	9682	1067	2138	9247	
None		27,443	15,541	11,000	27,417	
Norm.	($H.B15_5$)	35,026	19,429	11,223	10,053	−31.7
Tol.	(711)	29,359	16,660	8355	28,452	
None		13,342	4588	4446	1317	
Norm.	($H.B15_6$)	30,888	8609	2529	1640	−33.3
Tol.	(712)	29,089	7350	7538	909	
					Mean	−7.9
					SEM	±13.3
					Total number =	24

[a] See footnotes to Table 2A.

The GVH competence of H.B2-tolerant H.B15 cells and normal cells was studied in mixing experiments, where tolerant and normal H.B15 cells were injected in a ratio of 1:1 with normal H.B2 or H.B15 cells into 13-day-old H.B2 embryos (Table 5). The splenomegaly of H.B2 recipients induced by H.B2-tolerant H.B15 cells alone (mean of relative spleen weights was 122.2 mg/100 g body weight) was significantly higher ($P<0.001$ by Student's t test) than the splenomegaly induced by H.B2 cells (79.0), but significantly lower ($P<0.005$) than the splenomegaly induced by normal H.B15 cells (394.5). When whole blood was injected in our previous studies, the difference in GVH competence against H.B2 embryos was insignificant between normal H.B2 chickens and H.B15 chickens tolerant for H.B2 line alloantigens (*1*). If H.B2 cells were mixed with cells from another H.B2 donor or with H.B2-tolerant H.B15 cells, the splenomegaly induced was somewhat greater (101.0 and 145.4, respectively) than with H.B2 cells alone, but the difference between these two groups was insignificant. Instead, the splenomegaly induced by mixed H.B2 and H.B15 cells was great (300.4) and it differed significantly ($P<0.001$) from the splenomegaly induced by the mixture of H.B2 and H.B2-tolerant H.B15 cells (145.4). When tolerant cells were combined with syngeneic H.B15 cells from normal donors, the GVH reaction detected was very strong (492.8), even—although not significantly—stronger than the GVH reaction induced by a mixture of cells from two normal H.B15 chickens (433.1). The splenomegaly induced by tolerant and normal H.B15 cells (492.8) also differed significantly ($P<0.02$) from the splenomegaly induced by the mixture of normal H.B15 and H.B2 cells (300.4).

These results indicate that the response of normal H.B15 cells was not inhibited in the presence of tolerant cells. Rather the response of tolerant cells was potentiated in the presence of normal syngeneic cells, which again indicates the role of alloantigen-specific helper cells in the tolerance of these chickens. If adequate helper function is offered to tolerant cells by normal syngeneic cells, the GVH reactivity of tolerant cells is reestablished.

MLR of tolerant cells in the presence of exogenous TCGF. It is known that T cell growth factor can substitute for T cell help in some circumstances (*7, 15*). We have studied the effect of exogenous TCGF on MLR of tolerant cells (Table 4). In the absence of TCGF tolerant chickens were unable to generate MLR against the tolerogen. The difference in reactivity against H.B2 line stimulators was insignificant between tolerant and H.B2 line responders, and highly significant ($P<0.005$ by Student's t test) between tolerant and normal H.B15 cells. When exogenous TCGF was added, the difference between the response of normal and tolerant cells was still significant ($P<0.005$), although the MLR response of tolerant cells was now much higher. However, the MLR response of tolerant cells to H.B2 line stimulation in the presence of TCGF rose significantly higher ($P<0.001$) than the response of H.B2 line responder cells. The addition of TCGF did not have much effect on the response of tolerant cells to third-party (H.B14) stimulation. Instead, the responses of normal H.B2 and H.B15 cells were clearly affected. This might be explained by the relatively higher number of H.B14-specific helper cells in tolerant chickens, which would lead to saturation of H.B14 reactive lympho-

TABLE 3. (A) Effect of untreated cells from tolerant chickens on MLR of normal syngeneic H.B15 responders against the tolerizing alloantigen[a]

Cocultured cells		H.B15 responders stimulated with H.B2 cells				
		I	II	III	IV	Mean % of suppression
Norm.	(H.B15$_1$)	39,403	39,031	69,290	42,142	42.4
Tol.	(704)	23,256	39,522	11,000	22,762	
Norm.	(H.B15$_2$)	45,322	78,026	47,634	44,239	7.0
Tol.	(705)	32,257	46,545	76,943	35,305	
Norm.	(H.B15$_3$)	61,639	64,265	51,353	46,569	46.3
Tol.	(708)	37,718	46,386	18,660	31,413	
Norm.	(H.B15$_4$)	17,143	15,575	28,543	34,631	22.0
Tol.	(709)	12,199	15,267	14,077	32,459	
Norm.	(H.B15$_5$)	6613	4611	8140	16,882	−116.8
Tol.	(711)	19,494	9545	14,800	31,008	
Norm.	(H.B15$_6$)	24,353	13,626	7901	15,695	−15.4
Tol.	(712)	17,650	21,344	8951	18,736	
					Mean	−2.4
					SEM	±13.3
					Total number =	24

[a] See footnotes to Table 2A.

cytes with endogenous help. The increase in reactivity in the presence of TCGF may also partly be due to activation of T lymphocyte precursors with low avidity to stimulating antigen (*7*). Exogenous TCGF increased also the background proliferation of responder cells. The proliferation was highest in cultures with tolerant cells, which results probably from the activation of H.B15 line T lymphocyte precursors against the H.B2-line B lymphocytes. Stimulation with syngeneic cells induced only low MLR responses even in the presence of TCGF.

DISCUSSION

We have previously shown that transplantation of pure B cells from neonatal bursa of Fabricius to B-cell-depleted, cyclophosphamide-treated, newly hatched chickens induces a stable lymphoid chimerism and transplantation tolerance to donor line alloantigens (*1*). Our present study looks further into the mechanisms of tolerance in this experimental model. The results obtained indicate that an active suppressor mechanism is not involved in the maintenance of tolerance, but the tolerance is rather due to the lack of alloantigen-specific helper functions.

We performed cell mixing experiments to test the possible presence of suppressor cells in tolerant chickens. If the tolerance in our experimental system resulted from suppressor cell activity or from suppressive factors, as has been described in several other models of tolerance (*16–26*), the MLR of normal responder cells should be reduced when cocultured with tolerant cells. However, no impairment in MLR of responder cells against the tolerizing alloantigen in the presence of tolerant cocultured cells could be detected. No suppressive action of tolerant cells could be detected in the GVH assay either. The GVH reaction observed in the splenomegaly assay was even stronger when tolerant cells were mixed with normal syngeneic cells than when cells from two normal chickens were combined. These results are in agreement with previously reported data that the unresponsive state can not be transferred in vitro in cell mixing experiments (*4*, *27*, *28*).

There is now evidence that in mice neonatally tolerized to whole H-2 or class II differences the suppressor mechanism is superimposed on clonal deletion of alloantigen-specific helper cells (*7*, *29*). Clonal deletion of helper cells is also suggested by our present experiments with chickens. We found out that mitomycin-C-treated cocultured cells from normal chickens potentiated the MLR of normal syngeneic responders against the tolerizing alloantigen, whereas tolerant cocultured cells did not have any effect on the response of normal cells. Since MLR to allogeneic stimulation is dependent on production of interleukin-2 (IL-2) in the cultures (*30*), the lack of IL-2 producers in tolerant cocultured cells is a possible explanation for this observation. On the other hand, when cocultured cells were not treated with mitomycin C, the MLR response to the tolerizing alloantigen was enhanced by both normal and tolerant cocultured cells to the same extent. This indicates that even tolerant chickens have precursors of MLR-reactive cells that can be stimulated in the presence of normal cells. The evident recovery of responses can not be explained, if total lack of such precursors resulting from clonal deletion is assumed, but it supports the conclusion that the lack of alloantigen-specific helper cells plays a role in maintenance of tolerance. Even the finding that a remarkable GVH reaction was induced, when tolerant cells were injected together with normal syngeneic cells into allogeneic embryos of tolerizing line, can be explained by the help offered by the normal cells to GVH-unresponsive tolerant cells. The reactivity of tolerant cells in MLR and in the GVH assay in the presence of normal syngeneic cells is thus most probably due to the activity of normal helper cells or to factors (including TCGF) produced by them.

There are reports showing that the tolerant state can be overcome by the addition of TCGF in vitro or even in vivo (*7*,

TABLE 3. (B) Effect of untreated cells from tolerant chickens on MLR of normal syngeneic H.B15 responders against third-party alloantigen[a]

Cocultured cells		H.B15 responders stimulated with H.B14 cells: I	II	III	IV	Mean % of suppression
Norm.	($H.B15_1$)	16,404	9105	4701	6420	−131.1
Tol.	(704)	14,000	6752	14,757	21,899	
Norm.	($H.B15_2$)	6866	8132	15,813	4780	−19.6
Tol.	(705)	11,631	8610	11,255	6456	
Norm.	($H.B15_3$)	34,978	50,887	25,005	8390	−44.4
Tol.	(708)	36,916	99,415	28,799	19,250	
Norm.	($H.B15_4$)	10,005	12,951	4665	15,068	−74.9
Tol.	(709)	24,414	34,354	7452	22,374	
Norm.	($H.B15_5$)	44,760	42,427	8634	9558	−94.8
Tol.	(711)	49,930	73,300	16,658	31,191	
Norm.	($H.B15_6$)	34,302	26,507	7146	876	−146.7
Tol.	(712)	52,001	38,199	12,841	4252	
						Mean −85.3
						SEM ±19.7
						Total number = 24

[a] See footnotes to Table 2A.

TABLE 4. Effect of exogenous T cell growth factor (TCGF) on MLR of tolerant chickens

Responder cells	Number of chickens	TCGF[a]	Stimulator cells: H.B15	H.B2	H.B14	Background[b]
Normal H.B15	11	−	22±59[c]	22,447±4270	9480±1475	80±20
		+	867±521	34,443±3695	18,237±2657	668±109
$H.B15_{H.B2\text{-}tol.}$	6	−	195±161	361±227	14,642±1032	84±20
		+	1341±819	14,505±3229	14,823±4448	2162±724
Normal H.B2	8	−	8480±2867	54±24	4801±1295	72±19
		+	19,800±3530	1073±402	12,503±2324	810±142

[a] MLR was carried out in the presence (+) or absence (−) of a final concentration of 0.5% of pretested TCGF containing Con A culture supernatant.

[b] Background = cpm of responder cells cultured with medium.

[c] Expressed as mean of net cpm ± SEM. Net cpm = (cpm of responder cells cultured with mitomycin-C-treated stimulator cells) − (cpm of responder cells cultured with medium).

28, 31, 32). However, contradictory results have also been obtained (*27*). In the present work we wanted to test the hypothesis that the effect of normal cells on the reactivity of tolerant cells described above is attributed to the effect of TCGF produced by normal cells. Our results show clearly that exogenous TCGF increases considerably the MLR response of tolerant cells to tolerizing alloantigen, though the level of reactivity of normal cells is not quite obtained. This probably indicates a reduction of precursors of MLR-reactive cells specific for tolerogen in tolerant chickens. The effect of TCGF on MLR of tolerant cells against syngeneic or third-party stimulator is much weaker.

Chicken TCGF used in our experiments closely resembles mammalian IL-2. It has a molecular weight of approximately 13,000 as determined by gel filtration on Sephadex G-100 (*14*). Chicken TCGF activity from the Con A culture supernatant can be absorbed both by the long-term-cultured T cell line and by Con A blasts indicating the presence of TCGF receptors on both cell populations. In addition, chicken TCGF is definitely a product of T cells, since agammaglobulinemic birds also produced TCGF upon Con A stimulation (*14*). In mammalian species IL-2, produced mainly by helper T cells following stimulation with class II MHC antigen-bearing cells, activates precursors of cytotoxic T cells (pT_c) and allows their proliferation and differentation into mature cytotoxic lymphocytes (*33*). Deletion of helper cell activity leads to immunological unresponsiveness (*33*), although all tolerogen-specific pT_c were not eliminated (*7, 34, 35*). Our present results are in agreement with results obtained from mammalian models showing that deletion of IL-2-producing helper cells is responsible for the maintenance of tolerance (*7, 27–29*). However, further studies are needed to verify more precisely the role of regulatory T cells and frequencies of pT_c during transplantation tolerance in chickens.

TABLE 5. GVH competence of leukocytes from tolerant chickens in mixing experiments[a]

Cell donors[b]	Number of donors[c]	Total cell number per embryo	Relative spleen weight of H.B2 line host embryos 5 days postinjection[d]
Normal H.B2	11	1.5×10^6	79.0±4.9[e]
Normal H.B15	13	1.5×10^6	394.5±56.1
$H.B15_{H.B2\text{-}tol.}$	6	1.5×10^6	122.2±3.8
Normal H.B2 with normal H.B2	4	3.0×10^6	101.0±11.4
Normal H.B2 with normal H.B15	6	3.0×10^6	300.4±23.8
Normal H.B2 with $H.B15_{H.B2\text{-}tol.}$	6	3.0×10^6	145.4±19.5
Normal H.B15 with normal H.B15	8	3.0×10^6	433.1±64.8
Normal H.B15 with $H.B15_{H.B2\text{-}tol.}$	12	3.0×10^6	492.8±46.6
—	—	—	44.0±4.0[f]

[a] Cells from tolerant and normal chickens were mixed in equal numbers.

[b] Control chickens used in combinations were also tested alone. Various control chickens were used in combinations with tolerant and other control chickens.

[c] Number of chickens or combinations tested.

[d] 2–4 13-day-old embryos were injected with indicated number of isolated PBL from each chicken tested and the mean of the relative weight of spleens (spleen weight in milligrams per 100 g body weight) five days after injection was considered the splenomegaly value for the chicken.

[e] Mean ±SEM.

[f] Mean ±SEM of ten uninjected control embryos.

A disturbed TCGF production has recently been reported to play a role in autoimmunity in the chicken (*36*). Obese strain chickens, which are affected with spontaneously occurring autoimmune thyroiditis similar to human Hashimoto's thyroiditis (*37*), have enhanced response to Con A stimulation due to hyperproduction of TCGF (*36*). The defect underlying this hyperproduction may be possibly in nonspecific suppressor factors that regulate TCGF production in normal chickens (*38*). When obese strain chickens are tolerized with thyroglobulin at hatching, the severity of thyroiditis is reduced significantly (*39*). If tolerance to thyroglobulin results from deletion of TCGF-producing helper cells as our results on allotolerance with B-cell-chimeric chickens indicate, the inhibition of thyroiditis is explained by the reduction of TCGF during the lymphocyte recognition of self-antigens. The results with obese strain chickens indicate the important role of IL-2 in self-tolerance and support the conception, presented by Malkowsky et al., that presence of IL-2 during antigen recognition plays a critical role in the induction of tolerance (*31, 32*).

In summary, the stable lymphoid chimerism mediates a prolonged exposure to the tolerizing alloantigen in our experimental system (*1*). The presence of T cells is not a prerequisite for tolerance induction since the unresponsiveness is induced with pure B cells. The mechanisms underlying the tolerant state included at least functional inactivation of the T cell population (helper T cells) producing TCGF and possibly also a reduction in the number of pT_c. We could not find any evidence of a suppressor mechanism in cell mixing experiments. Instead, the unresponsiveness of tolerant cells was abrogated in vitro by addition of normal cells or exogenous TCGF. These results in an avian model emphasize further the role of TCGF in the induction and maintenance of transplantation tolerance.

Acknowledgments. We thank Ms. Päivi Jalonen and Ms. Raija Ojala for excellent technical assistance.

REFERENCES

1. Lehtonen L, Vainio O, Eerola E, Toivanen P. Lymphoid cell chimerism and transplantation tolerance induced by bursal and postbursal cells. Transplantation 1985; 40: 398.
2. Chi DS, Thorbecke GJ. Supressor cells and other T-lymphocytes. In: Toivanen A, Toivanen P, eds. Avian immunology, basis and praxis. Boca Raton, FL: CRC Press, (in press).
3. Traill KN, Böck G, Boyd RL, Ratheiser K, Wick G. Ontogeny of surface markers on functionally distinct T cell subsets in the chicken. Eur J Immunol 1984; 14: 61.
4. Gruchalla RS, Streilein JW. Analysis of neonatally induced tolerance of H-2 alloantigens. II. Failure to detect alloantigen-specific T-lymphocyte precursors and suppressors. Immunogenetics 1982; 15: 111.
5. Damle NK, Mohagheghpour N, Kansas GS, Fishwild DM, Engleman EG. Immunoregulatory T cell circuits in man. Identification of a distinct T cell subpopulation of the helper/inducer lineage that amplifies the development of alloantigen-specific suppressor T cells. J Immunol 1985; 134: 235.
6. Rouse BT, Warner NL. The role of suppressor cells in avian allogeneic tolerance: implications for the pathogenesis of Marek's disease. J Immunol 1974; 113: 904.
7. Wood PJ, Strome PG, Streilein JW. Clonal analysis of helper and effector T-cell function in neonatal transplantation tolerance: clonal deletion of helper cells determines lack of in vitro responsiveness. Immunogenetics 1984; 20: 185.
8. Schwartz DH, Doherty PC. Induction of early alloantigen tolerance in thymus and spleen. Thymus 1984; 6: 105.
9. Briles WE, Bumstead N, Ewert DL, et al. Nomenclature for chicken major histocompatibility (B) complex. Immunogenetics 1982; 15: 441.
10. Hudson L, Roitt JM. Immunofluorescent detection of surface antigens specific to T and B lymphocytes in the chicken. Eur J Immunol 1973; 3: 63.
11. Vainio O, Ratcliffe MJH. Proliferation of chicken peripheral blood leukocytes in response to pokeweed mitogen is macrophage dependent. Cell Immunol 1984; 85: 235.
12. Lassila O, Eskola J, Toivanen P. A micromethod for stimulation of chicken lymphocytes in vitro using whole blood. Clin Exp Immunol 1976; 26: 641.
13. Simonsen M. Alloagression in chickens. Acta Pathol Microbiol Scand [C] 1975; 83: 1.
14. Vainio O, Ratcliffe MJH, Leanderson T. Chicken T cell growth factor: use in the generation of long-term cultured T cell line and biochemical characterization. Scand J Immunol 1986; 23: 135.
15. Good ME, Nossal GJV. Functional clonal deletion and suppression as complementary mechanisms operative in adult hapten-induced cytotoxic T cell tolerance. J Immunol 1983; 131: 2662.
16. Dorsch S, Roser B. Recirculating suppressor T cells in transplantation tolerance in the rat. Immunol Rev 1979; 46: 55.
17. Dorsch S, Roser B. Suppressor cells in transplantation tolerance. I. Analysis of the suppressor status of neonatally and adoptively tolerized rats. Transplantation 1982; 33: 518.
18. Dorsch S, Roser B. Suppressor cells in transplantation tolerance. II. Identification and possible mode of action of chimeric suppressor T cells. Transplantation 1982; 33: 525.
19. Holán V, Chutna J, Hašek M. Specific suppressor of antigen-reactive cells in neonatal transplantation tolerance. Nature 1978; 274; 895.
20. Hilgert J. The involvement of activated specific suppressor T cells in maintenance of transplantation tolerance. Immunol Rev 1979; 46: 27.
21. Gorczynski RM, MacRae S. Suppression of cytotoxic response to

histoincompatible cells. I. Evidence for two types of T lymphocyte-derived suppressors acting at different stages in the induction of a cytotoxic response. J Immunol 1979; 122: 737.
22. Gorczynski RM, MacRae S. Suppression of cytotoxic response to histoincompatible cells. II. Analysis of the role of two independent T suppressor pools in maintenance of neonatally induced allograft tolerance in mice. J Immunol 1979; 122: 747.
23. Streilein JW, Gruchalla RS. Analysis of neonatally induced tolerance of H-2 alloantigens. I. Adoptive transfer indicates that tolerance of class I and class II antigens is maintained by distinct mechanisms. Immunogenetics 1981; 12: 161.
24. Stephenson SP, Roser B. The molecular basis of transplantation tolerance. Transplant Proc 1985; 17: 1145.
25. Lancaster F, Chui YL, Batchelor JR. Anti-idiotypic T cells suppress rejection of renal allografts in rats. Nature 1985; 315: 336.
26. Hall BM. Mechanisms maintaining enhancement of allografts. I. Demonstration of a specific suppressor cell. J Exp Med 1985; 161: 123.
27. Feng HM, Glasebrook AL, Engers HD, Louis JA. Clonal analysis of T cell unresponsiveness to alloantigens induced by neonatal injection of F_1 spleen cells into parental mice. J Immunol 1983; 131: 2165.
28. Carnaud C, Ishizaka ST, Stutman O. Early loss of precursors of CTL and IL-2-producing cells in the development of neonatal tolerance to alloantigens. J Immunol 1984; 133: 45.
29. Wood PJ, Strome P, Streilein JW. Clonal frequencies of alloreactive cells in mice tolerant of H-2. Transplant Proc 1985; 17: 1137.
30. Ilonen J, Karttunen R. The production of interleukin 2 as a measure of reactivity in mixed lymphocyte cultures. Immunobiology 1984; 167: 399.
31. Malkowský M, Medawar PB. Is immunological tolerance (nonresponsiveness) a consequence of interleukin 2 deficit during the recognition of antigen? Immunol Today 1984; 5: 340.
32. Malkowský M, Medawar PB, Thatcher DR, et al. Acquired immunological tolerance of foreign cells in impaired by recombinant interleukin 2 or vitamin A acetate. Proc Natl Acad Sci USA 1985; 82: 536.
33. Wood PJ, Streilein JW. Immunogenetic basis of acquired transplantation tolerance. Transplantation 1984; 37: 223.
34. Stockinger B. Cytotoxic T-cell precursors revealed in neonatally tolerant mice. Proc Natl Acad Sci USA 1984; 81: 220.
35. Heeg K, Wagner H. Analysis of immunological tolerance to major histocompatibility antigens. I. High frequencies of tolerogen-specific cytotoxic T lymphocyte precursors in mice neonatally tolerized to class I major histocompatibility complex antigens. Eur J Immunol 1985; 15: 25.
36. Schauenstein K, Krömer G, Sundick RS, Wick G. Enhanced response to Con A and production of TCGF by lymphocytes of obese strain (OS) chickens with spontaneous autoimmune thyroiditis. J Immunol 1985; 134: 872.
37. Wick G, Boyd R, Hála K, Thunold S, Kofler H. Pathogenesis of spontaneous autoimmune thyreoiditis in Obese strain (OS) chickens. Review. Clin Exp Immunol 1982; 47: 1
38. Krömer G, Schauenstein K, Neu N, Stricker K, Wick G. In vitro T cell hyperreactivity in Obese strain chickens is due to a defect in nonspecific suppressor mechanism(s). J Immunol 1985; 135: 2458.
39. Sanker AJ, Clark CR, Sundick RS. The induction of tolerance to thyroglobulin significantly reduces the severity of thyreoiditis in obese strain chickens. J Immunol 1985; 135: 281.

Received 12 September 1985.
Accepted 12 November 1985.

0041-1337/86/4202-0191$02.00/0
TRANSPLANTATION
Vol. 42, No. 2
Printed in U.S.A.

DEVELOPMENT OF SUPPRESSOR LYMPHOCYTES DURING ACUTE REJECTION OF RAT CARDIAC ALLOGRAFTS AND PRESERVATION OF SUPPRESSION BY ANTI-IL-2-RECEPTOR MONOCLONAL ANTIBODY[1]

TOBIN M. SCHNEIDER,[2,3] JERZY W. KUPIEC-WEGLINSKI,[2] EDWARD TOWPIK,[2] WINFRIED PADBERG,[2,4] DORIAN ARANEDA,[2] TIBOR DIAMANTSTEIN,[5] TERRY B. STROM,[6] AND NICHOLAS L. TILNEY[2,7]

The Surgical Research Laboratory, Harvard Medical School, and The Department of Surgery, Brigham and Women's Hospital, Boston, Massachusetts; The Department of Medicine, Beth Israel Hospital, Boston, Massachusetts; and The Immunological Research Unit, Klinikum Steglitz, Freie Universitat Berlin, West Germany

Suppressor activity was investigated in rats undergoing acute rejection of heterotopic cardiac allografts. Spleen cells were harvested at 7 days from LEW rats rejecting (LEW×BN)F_1 heart grafts and fractionated into their T, T suppressor/cytotoxic, and T helper subpopulations. Transfer of alloimmune unseparated spleen

[1] This work was supported by NIH Grant 5 RO1 AI 19071-11.
[2] Harvard Medical School and Brigham and Women's Hospital.
[3] Current address: Department of Surgery, Stanford University Hospital, Stanford, CA 94305.
[4] Supported by Deutsche Forschungsgemeinschaft grant Pa 313/1-1.
[5] Freie Universitat.
[6] Beth Israel Hospital.
[7] Address correspondence to: Nicholas L. Tilney, M.D., Department of Surgery, Brigham and Women's Hospital, 75 Francis St., Boston, MA 02115.

cells to syngeneic recipients of (Lew×BN)F_1 test grafts accelerated rejection from 8 to 6.5 days ($P<0.01$). Graft survival was prolonged to about 15 days ($P<0.005$) after transfer of the splenic T suppressor/cytotoxic fraction. Treatment of test graft recipients with ART-18, a mouse antirat monoclonal antibody directed against the rat interleukin 2 receptor on the surface of activated lymphocytes, increased graft survival to about 3 weeks ($P<0.005$), and to about 23 days ($P<0.005$) when test graft recipients were treated with ART 18 following transfer of alloimmune unseparated spleen cells. In contrast, ART-18 treatment of test graft recipients already injected with T suppressor/cytotoxic cells had no additive effect. Increased production of endogenous interleukin 2 occurred concomitantly with the onset of rejection in these animals; interleukin 2 release declined during the late stages of rejection when suppressor activity had increased. Similarly, in T-cell-depleted (B) rats, allograft rejection could be produced by immune reconstitution with sensitized lymphocytes, but could be significantly delayed by prior transfer of suppressor cells. These data document the presence of potent suppressor activity in the acutely rejecting host and suggest that the suppressor mechanisms are inhibited less than effector mechanisms by interleukin-2-receptor–targeted therapy.

The host responses to a vascularized organ allograft include complex cellular interactions among lymphocytes that recognize and become activated by foreign antigens, then proliferate and differentiate into various subpopulations with effector or suppressor functions. Suppressor T cells (Ts)* play an important role in the induction and maintenance of antigen specific allograft "tolerance" (*1, 2*) and in various models of immunological unresponsiveness (*3, 4*). Treatment with cyclosporine also produces donor-specific host unresponsiveness (*5–7*) by blunting the development of effector lymphocytes, as well as allowing the gradual emergence of antigen-specific Ts (*8–11*); Ts have also been found in rejecting allografts in untreated hosts as early as 7 days after transplantation (*12*). Despite these observations, however, the significance of Ts found in immunologically unresponsiveness hosts and their relationship to those generated during rejection are unclear.

Although the presumed role of Ts in acute rejection is to stop the inflammatory process and return the host to immunological homeostasis, effector mechanisms transcend those of suppression, at least until graft destruction has been completed. Activated T helper cells produce interleukin 2 (IL-2), a lymphokine that binds to IL-2 receptors (IL-2R) on T cells, and that is required for the growth, maintenance, and proliferation of resting T cells, and the development of cytotoxic T cells (Tc) and their response to alloantigen (*13*). Thus any modulating effect of Ts on host alloreactivity is overcome by IL-2-stimulated effector activity mediating graft rejection. In contrast, IL-2R-targeted therapy with monoclonal antibody inhibits T cell proliferation and maturation of alloantigen-induced Tc in vitro (*14*), resulting in prolonged allograft survival in vivo (*15, 16*).

The present studies were undertaken to clarify both the development of Ts in acute rejection and their potential role in prolonging graft survival. In addition, the T-cell-deficient B rat was used to observe and manipulate Ts activity in an animal that is immunologically inert and lacking effector activity. As Ts are also spared following IL-2R targeted therapy, a mechanism for generation of Ts independent of IL-2 is proposed. Inferences drawn from these and related studies suggest that the development of Ts may be a critical facet of the overall host responses against allografted tissues.

* Abbreviations used: Con A, concanavalin A; FITC, fluorescein-conjugated isothiocyanate; IL-2, interleukin 2; IL-2R, interleukin 2 receptors; sT, sensitized T cells; sSL, sensitized spleen cells; sLNC, sensitized lymph node cells; sTh, sensitized T helper cells; sTs/c, sensitized T suppressor cytotoxic cells; Ts, T suppressor; Th, T helper-inducer; Ts/c, T suppressor-cytotoxic.

MATERIALS AND METHODS

Animals. Inbred male rats (Microbiological Associates, Walkersville, MD) were used in all experiments, Lewis rats (LEW, $RT1^l$) as recipients of organ allografts, Lewis × Brown Norway hybrids (LEW×BN)F_1 as heart donors. Brown Norway (BN, $RT1^n$) rats served as donors for skin grafts, and Wistar Furth (WF, $RT1^u$) as third-party heart donors.

Heart grafting. Heterotopic cardiac allografts were anastomosed to the infrarenal abdominal great vessels by standard microvascular techniques (*17*). Graft size and ventricular contractions were assessed daily by palpation through the recipient flank. Rejection was defined as the time of complete cessation of myocardial contractions. If questionable, the graft was visualized directly at laparotomy.

The T-cell-deprived B rat. B rats were produced as described previously (*18*). LEW rats underwent thymectomy at 6–7 weeks, then were lethally irradiated with 750 rads total-body x-radiation 4 weeks later. Immediately following x-radiation, the animals were reconstituted with bone marrow cells from syngeneic, thymectomized, profoundly thoracic-duct-drained donors. After 4 weeks of recovery, (LEW×BN)F_1 heart grafts were transplanted. Only healthy rats with well-functioning grafts (>3 weeks) were used for transfer experiments. Cachectic animals or those that failed to gain weight were excluded from further studies.

Preparation of lymphocyte populations. Spleen or lymph nodes were teased apart and the cells expressed through 60-gauge wire mesh into RPMI 1640 medium supplemented with 5 mM N-2-hydroxyethylpiperazine-N-2-ethanesulfonic acid (HEPES), 10% heat-inactivated fetal calf serum, and 2 mM L-glutamine. Specifically sensitized spleen cells (sSL) were harvested from LEW rats acutely rejecting (LEW×BN)F_1 heart grafts transplanted 7 days previously; sensitized lymph node lymphocytes (sLNL) were prepared from draining axillary and cervical nodes of LEW rats rejecting BN skin grafts placed 10 days before. Cells were filtered through cotton wool, erythrocytes were lysed with hypotonic (0.83%) ammonium chloride (pH 7.21), and lymphocytes were washed thrice to remove debris. Cell viability, checked with trypan blue, was always >90%.

Monoclonal antibodies (MoAb). W3/25 (Sera-lab, Accurate Chemicals, Westbury, NY) is a mouse IgG directed against the rat T helper/inducer subset (Th); OX-8 (Sera-lab) mouse IgG labels the suppressor/cytotoxic (Ts/c) subset (*19*). ART-18 is a mouse antirat IgG monoclonal antibody (protein concentration 10 mg/ml containing 5 mg/ml of pure antibody) directed against the rat IL-2R (*20*). It was administered i.v., 300 μg/kg/day for 14 days.

Preparation of T cell subpopulations. Purified T cells were prepared by passage of sSL over nylon-wool columns as described elsewhere (*21*). After washing, the sensitized T cells (sT) were incubated with saturating concentrations of W3/25, washed again, and then passed through 10-ml Degalan V26 bead columns (Degussa, NJ) coated with goat antimouse IgG (Cappell Laboratories, Cochranville, PA). T lymphocytes, negatively selected Ts/c (W3/25−), and Th (W3/25+) were used in adoptive transfer experiments.

Cell markers. Aliquots of the separated subpopulations were incubated with W3/25 or OX-8 on ice for 1 hr, washed, and resuspended in fluorescein isothiocyanate (FITC)-conjugated rabbit antimouse IgG (Tago Inc., Burlingame, CA). Preparations were then inspected by indirect immunofluorescence microscopy; purity was usually >90% for the desired subset, and contamination less than 1% for the alternative subset.

IL-2 activity. Monodispersed splenic lymphocytes in RPMI 1640 medium plus 10 μg/ml of concanavalin A (Con A, Sigma Chemical Co., St. Louis, MO) were incubated for 48 hr at 37°C in 5% CO_2. The supernatants were harvested and stored at −20° until analysis. IL-2 activity was measured using the method of Gillis et al. (*22*). Briefly, the supernatants were diluted repetitively two-fold in microtiter plates and 4×10^3 IL-dependent CTLL-2 cells added to make a final volume of 0.2 ml. Cells and supernatants were incubated at 37°C for 20 hr, pulsed with 1 μCi ^{3}H-TdR, and then harvested 4 hr later. After counting in a liquid scintillation spectrophotometer, IL-2 activity was calculated by probit analysis and compared with a reference standard. IL-2 units were calculated according to the formula:

$$\text{Il-2 units} = \frac{\text{reciprocal titer of sample at 50\% max cpm of control}}{\text{reciprocal titer of 50\% max cpm of control}}$$

Statistical analysis. Graft survival data were compared using Student's *t* test. IL-2 assays were compared using the Mann-Whitney rank order test for nonparametric data. $P<0.05$ was considered significant.

RESULTS

Three experimental adoptive transfer protocols were tested to assess suppressor activity developing during the course of acute rejection. sSL from unmodified heart grafted hosts were fractionated into sT, sTs/c, and sTh cells. In the first series of studies, effector potency of the cells was ascertained by transferring the individual populations (70×10^6) to groups of untreated syngeneic LEW rats transplanted with (LEW×BN)F_1 test cardiac allografts the same day. Survival of the test grafts was monitored and compared with similar animals receiving lymphocyte subsets from unsensitized rats. The second series of studies was designed to determine the effects of IL-2R-targeted therapy on the development of suppressor activity; groups of test graft recipients received sSL, sT, or sTs/c plus a course of ART-18. The recipients were sacrificed at 7 or 14 days, and spleen supernatants were tested for IL-2 production. In the third series of experiments, sTs/c were administered to B rats bearing long-standing (LEW×BN)F_1 cardiac allografts. These were then reconstituted 1 or 2 weeks later with 10^8 sLNL. As immunocompetency can be restored by transfer of sLNL, prolongation of graft survival was taken as evidence of suppressor activity in the inoculum. There were 4–6 animals in each group.

Effect of transferred cells on allograft survival. (LEW×BN)F_1 cardiac allografts were rejected acutely by untreated LEW hosts in a mean survival time (MST)±SD=8±1 days. sSL harvested at the time of acute allograft rejection from unmodified recipients and transferred into syngeneic animals, accelerated test graft rejection in a second-set manner (6.5±.6 days, $P<0.01$). Although the test grafts were rejected in 9±1 days following transfer of sT, their survival in animals treated with the sTs/c subpopulation (W3/25−) was prolonged to 15±3 days ($P<0.005$). In contrast, transfer of unsensitized Ts/c failed to modify graft survival (10.7±1 days). Specificity studies were performed by transfer of sSL or sTs/c from LEW rats that had rejected WF heart grafts; when these third-party cell populations were transferred to LEW hosts of (LEW×BN)F_1 grafts, rejection time was not affected (9±1 days). Thus, although whole sSL accelerated rejection of test grafts, transfer of the sTs/c fraction prolonged their survival significantly in an immunologically specific manner.

The effect of ART-18 plus transferred cells. The effect of administration of anti IL-2R MoAb was then assessed in a similar test system. A course of ART-18 alone for 14 days prolonged allograft survival to 21±1 days (*16*). Test graft recipients receiving sSL or sT on the day of grafting were also treated with ART-18; graft survival was significantly lengthened when compared with that of animals not receiving the antibody (23±5 days vs. 6.5±0.6, and 23±4 vs. 9±1 days, respectively, $P<0.005$, Fig. 1). Histologically, dramatic preservation of myocardial structure in animals receiving cell transfers plus ART 18 was noted 14 days after transplantation (Fig. 2); although there was moderate lymphocytic infiltration, the extensive myonecrosis occurring in acutely rejected hearts was absent. In contrast, combining ART-18 therapy with transfer of sTs/c produced rejection in 14±1 days, similar to that following transfer of sTs/c alone (Fig. 3). Thus, ART-18 increases graft survival only when whole T lymphocytes are transferred; it does not complement the effect of transferred Ts/c.

Ts activity in B rats. Cardiac allografts survive indefinitely in T-cell-depleted B rats (*23*); however, reconstitution with 10^8 sLNL caused rejection in 13±1 days. In contrast, when sTs/c (70×10^6) were transferred 7 days prior to immune restoration with sLNL, allograft survival was prolonged significantly (17± 3 days, $P<0.025$). When sTs/c were resident in B recipients for 14 days prior to immune restoration a further potentiation of the suppressive effect was noted, with graft survival prolonged to 21±2 days ($P<0.005$, Fig. 4). B recipients given sTs/c without immune reconstitution with sLNL never rejected their grafts. Administration of Th (W3/25$^+$, 70×10^6) to B rats bearing long-standing (LEW×BN)F_1 cardiac allografts invariably produced

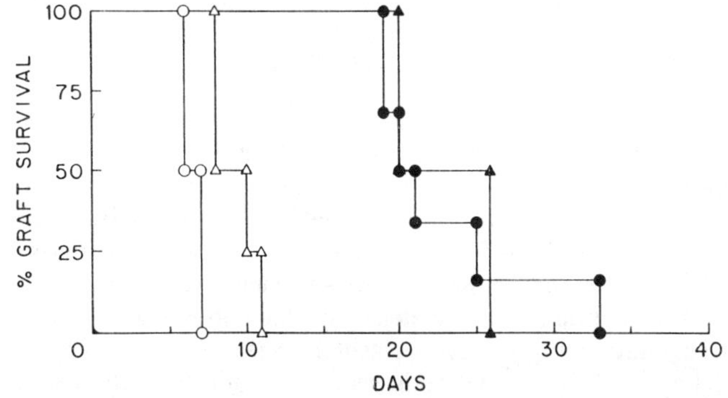

FIGURE 1. Survival curves for test LBN cardiac allografts in LEW recipients after adoptive transfer of sensitized splenic lymphocyte populations ± ART-18, 300 μg/kg/day × 14 days. (○) sSS; (△) sT; (●) sSL+ART-18; (▲) sT+ART-18.

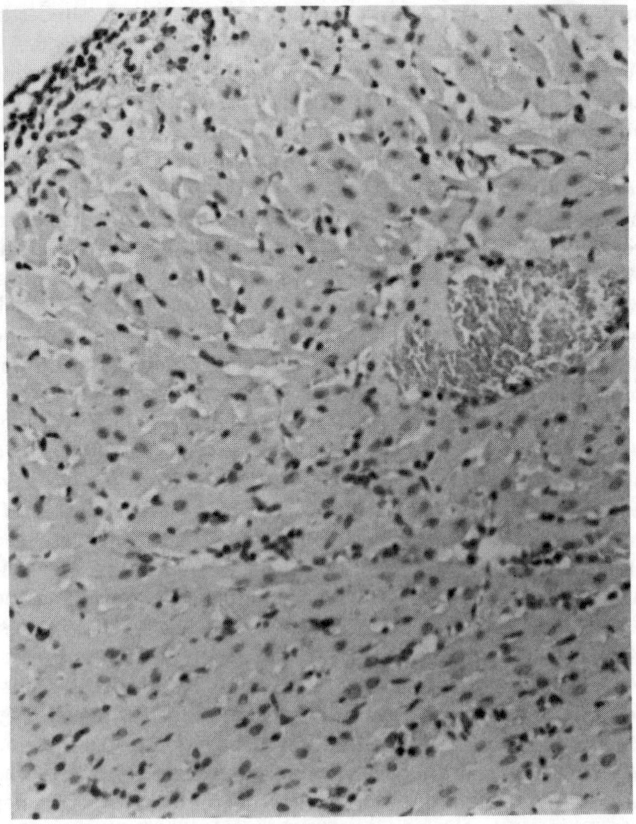

FIGURE 2. 40× photomicrograph of LBN test cardiac allograft in LEW recipient 14 days after transplantation and adoptive transfer of 70×10^6 sSL and treatment with ART-18, 300 μg/kg/day × 14 days. There is preservation of myocardial structure and absence of necrosis.

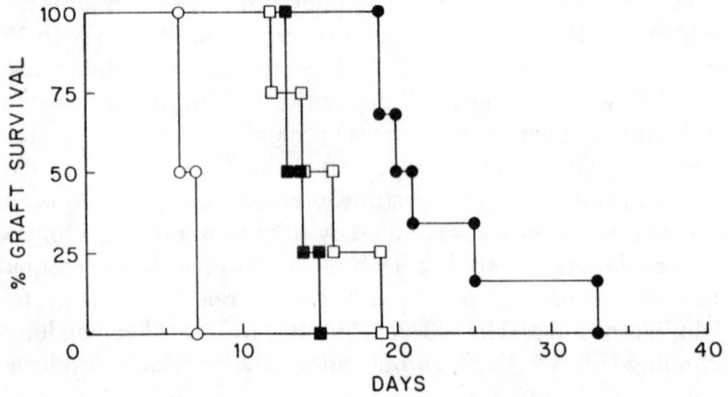

FIGURE 3. Survival curves for test LBN cardiac allografts in LEW recipients after adoptive transfer of sensitized splenic lymphocyte populations ± ART-18, 300 μg/kg/day × 14 days. (○) sSL; (□) sTs/c; (●) sSL+ART-18; (■) sTs/c+ART-18.

rejection within 13 days. Addition of a course of ART-18 beginning on the day of Th transfer delayed rejection until 36± 5 days ($P<0.001$), confirming mediation of rejection by IL-2R-producing Th. Thus, in the B rat sTs/c extended graft survival, whereas sTh and/or their products produced rejection.

IL-2 bioactivity. Having demonstrated potent suppressor activity developing in vivo in acutely rejecting hosts, we next determined IL-2 activity released by spleen cells of the various recipient groups following lymphocyte transfer (Table 1). IL-2 activity was low (0.16 U) in test graft recipients during the period of graft prolongation produced by transfer of antigen-specific Ts/c from acutely rejecting hosts; however, by the time of test graft rejection at 14 days, the IL-2 activity had markedly increased (0.64 U). Production of endogenous IL-2 was high at 7 days (accelerated rejection) and 14 days (after peak rejection) following transfer of sSL (0.44, $P<0.003$ and 0.68, $p<0.05$, respectively) into test graft recipients. In contrast, IL-2 levels were low (0.14 U) in test animals given sSL+ART-18 at 7 days and were not detected at 14 days. Similarly, IL-2 levels markedly depressed in the untreated B rat, return toward normal only after immune reconstitution (*24*). Thus, in all treatment groups, IL-2 bioactivity correlated closely with the rejection status of the recipient, being low during periods of good graft function and rising during active rejection.

DISCUSSION

The emergence of antigen-specific suppressor cells (Ts) within the W3/25− OX8+ Ts/c fraction in host lymphoid tissues may be responsible both for increased allograft survival in various rat models (*4, 6–9, 12, 25, 26*) and in the reversal of the acute rejection process (*12*). Spleens of animals acutely rejecting their grafts at 7 days contain both activated Th and Ts/c (*12, 19*). Three observations were made by transferring sensitized spleen cell populations to test graft recipients: transfer of sensitized whole spleen cells produced accelerated, second-set rejection; transfer of unfractionated sT did not affect the tempo of acute rejection, implicating a role either for the deleted B cells or macrophages in accelerated rejection, as well as the offsetting effects of effector cells and suppressor cells in the remaining T lymphocyte population; sTs/c significantly

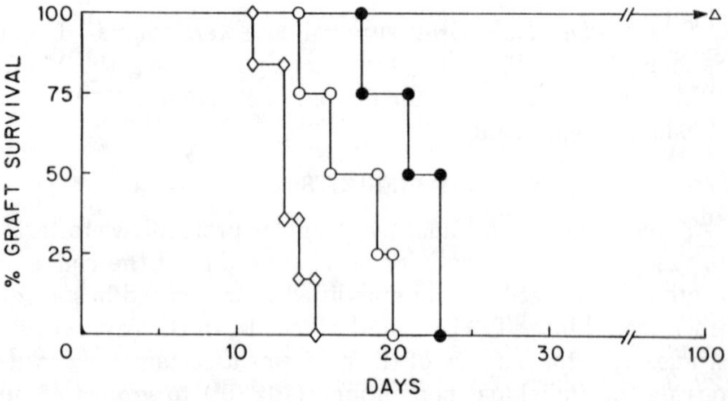

FIGURE 4. Survival curves in B recipients of LBN cardiac allografts after immune reconstitution and adoptive transfer of sensitized suppressor lymphocytes. (△) Indefinite survival in untreated B rats; (◇) Immune reconstitution with 10^8 sLNC; (○) Adoptive transfer of 70×10^6 sTs/c 1 week before immune reconstitution with sLNC; (●) Adoptive transfer of 70×10^6 sTs/c 2 weeks before immune reconstitution with sLNC.

TABLE 1. Interleukin 2 bioactivity[a] in LEW recipients of $(LEW\times BN)F_1$ test cardiac allografts 7 or 14 days after adoptive transfer of sensitized splenic lymphocyte populations ± ART-18 MoAb[a]

	sSL		sTs/c: − ART 18
	− ART 18	+ ART 18	
7 Days	0.44	0.14	0.16
14 Days	0.68	0.00	0.64

[a] Each value represents the mean of 4–7 experiments. Lymphokine levels are expressed in units of IL-2 elaborated by spleen cells and are calculated by probit analysis; control IL-2 reference standard = 1.00 unit; control IL-2 production in untreated graft recipients = 0.09 unit.

prolonged survival of test grafts. In addition, when tested in a mixed lymphocyte reaction coculture assay, lymphocytes from host peripheral blood and spleen potently suppressed proliferation of naive syngeneic responder cells (*27*). Thus, during the rejection process, the graft recipient develops alloantigen specific immunomodulating mechanisms that cannot overcome the effector pathway to graft destruction, but that may limit the extent of the ongoing response and restore host homeostasis once the process is completed.

We investigated the unopposed functional activity of Ts/c in graft recipients by using B rats with their depressed or absent effector activity. B rats reject their grafts in an acute tempo only following reconstitution with sensitized Th+Ts/c+IL-2-conditioned medium (*28*). In the present studies, transfer of syngeneic sTs/c prior to this reconstitution prolonged graft survival, presumably by allowing engraftment of antigen-specific Ts clones in the immunodeficient animals before administration of the effector components. Indeed, increasing the period of residence of sTs/c before transfer of sensitized effector cells caused a parallel increase in allograft survival. Attempts to show even more dramatic prolongation by transfer of sTs/c more than 2 weeks before immune reconstitution were unsuccessful; however, B rats are severely T-cell-depleted, and permanent engraftment of Ts clone may require T cell–T cell interactions and lymphokine production that can occur only in fully immunocompetent hosts.

Allograft survival can also be prolonged in these animals by administration of anti-IL-2R ART-18 MoAb (*16*). Indeed, IL-2-targeted therapy plus transfer of sSl prolonged allograft survival even more dramatically; in contrast, anti-IL-2R treatment plus transfer of sTs/c did not increase graft survival beyond the effect attributable to Ts alone. Presumably, ART-18 either blocks the IL-2R of Th and Tc or destroys the IL-2R+ cells directly, while not affecting the stimulus to the Ts clone. Thus, we suggest that Ts do not express IL-2R during this early period of rejection. However, since the Ts clone may not yet be fully activated, permanent tolerance is not achieved and the graft is eventually rejected.

The correlation of decreased endogenous IL-2 activity and graft survival supports the concept that regulation of this lymphokine is critical to the development of allograft tolerance (*29, 30*). Similarly, temporary depression of IL-2 levels occurs in grafted rats during cyclosporine treatment (*24, 31*). As IL-2 is required for activation, growth and proliferation of Th and Tc (*32–34*), any agent that blocks IL-2R or destroys IL-2R+ cells, either at the release stage (cyclosporine) or at the receptor stage (ART-18) should be effective in reducing helper-induced cell-mediated rejection or in stimulating Ts clones; these activities result in prolonged graft survival. In the mouse, monoclonal IL-2R MoAb inhibits the proliferation of T cells in response to alloantigen and mitogen, as well as the development of cytotoxic T cell effector responses (*35*); in the rat, ART-18 functions in a similar manner (*20*). Alternatively, as every proliferating T cell bears IL-2R, attenuation or removal of Th and Tc would yield the same result. The selective sparing of Ts may relate to dysynchronous IL-2R expression.

Development of antigen specific Ts in host unresponsiveness to allografts also occurs in various immunomodulated animal models. Batchelor et al. found suppression mounted by spleen cells from both cyclosporine-treated and immunologically enhanced rats in vitro and in vivo (*25, 36*). Other studies in an enhancement model confirmed Ts activity both in naive and in irradiated test graft recipients (*3*). Hendry et al. were able to prolong test graft survival in normal rats following transfer of lymphocytes from enhanced rat recipients of cardiac allografts (*37*). Slavin et al. described a suppressor effect in animals bearing indefinitely surviving allografts following total-lymphoid irradiation (*26*). In the mouse, treatment with monoclonal anti-Ia antibody results in increased graft survival and transferrable suppression of delayed hypersensitivity responses (*38*). Decline of suppression correlated with onset of rejection. Most recently, Hall et al. investigated suppressor activity in cyclosporine-treated animals and found Ts to inhibit the ability of LNL to restore rejection in irradiated rats akin to the B rat model (*6*), while Dorsch and Roser reported similar results using neonatally tolerized rats as donors of Ts (*39, 40*).

The complex adoptive transfer model used in the present studies has allowed detection of Ts in untreated, allografted animals. Detection of such Ts has heretofore been difficult due to the overriding primacy of the effector cascade. The effect of Ts is antigen-specific. This subpopulation may be less dependent on IL-2 than the helper-cytotoxic pathway, may respond to stimuli independent of IL-2 since blockade of IL-2R does not inhibit development of the antigen specific Ts clone, and may have dysynchronous expression of IL-2R densities. Cotner et al. have emphasized that virtually all proliferating, S-phase human T lymphocytes express IL-2R (*41*). In contrast, failure of the anti IL-2R, anti-Tac antibody, to block selective human T cell proliferation to mitogens has suggested an IL-2-independent activation pathway for T cells analagous to that proposed here (*42*). IL-3 is a likely candidate; it affects immature T cells and generates IL-2-responding populations and is not a growth requirement for Tc (*31, 43*).

REFERENCES

1. Streilein JW. Suppressor cells are necessary for tolerance. Transplant Proc 1985; 17: 1558.
2. Brent L, Horsburgh T, Wood PJ. Induction of suppressor cells and allograft tolerance. Transplant Proc 1980; 12: 464.
3. Hall BM. Mechanisms maintaining enhancement of allografts. I. Demonstration of a specific suppressor cell. J Exp Med 1985; 161: 123.
4. Tutschka PJ, Hess AD, Beschorner WE, Santos GW. Suppressor cells in transplantation tolerance. I. Suppressor cells in the mechanism of tolerance in radiation chimeras. Transplantation 1981; 32: 203.
5. Kupiec-Weglinski JW, Filho MA, Strom TB, Tilney NL. Sparing of suppressor cells: a critical action of cyclosporine. Transplantation 1984; 38: 97.
6. Hall BM, Helbart MF, Dorsch SE. Suppressor T cells in rats with prolonged cardiac allograft survival after treatment with cyclosporine. Transplantation 1984; 37: 595.
7. Bordes-Aznar J, Kupiec-Weglinski JW, Duarte AJS, Milford EL, Strom TB, Tilney NL. Function and migration of suppressor lymphocytes from cyclosporine-treated heart graft recipients. Transplantation 1983; 35: 185.
8. Hutchinson IF, Shadur CA, Duarte AJS, Strom TB, Tilney NL. Cyclosporin A spares selectively lymphocytes with donor-specific suppressor characteristics. Transplantation 1981; 32: 210.
9. Kupiec-Weglinski JW, Lear PA, Strom TB, Tilney NL. Population of cyclophosphamide-sensitive T suppressor cells maintain cyclosporine-induced allograft survival. Transplant Proc 1983; 15: 2357.
10. Nagao T, White DJG, Calne RY. Kinetics of unresponsiveness induced by a short course of cyclosporin A. Transplantation 1982; 33: 31.
11. Bordes-Aznar J, Lear PA, Strom TB, Tilney NL, Kupiec-Weglinski

JW. Kinetics of cyclosporin-A-induced unresponsiveness to cardiac allografts in rats. Transplant Proc 1983; 15: 500.
12. Araujo JL, Kupic-Weglinski JW, Araneda D, Towpik E, Heidecke CD, Williams JM, Tilney NL. Phenotype, activation status and suppressor activity of host lymphocytes during acute rejection and after cyclosporine induced unresponsiveness of rat cardiac allografts. Transplantation 1985; 40: 278.
13. Farrar JJ, Benjamin WR, Hilfiker ML, Howard M, Farrar WL, Fuller-Farrar J. The biochemistry, biology, and role of interleukin 2 in the induction of cytotoxic T cell and antibody forming responses. Immunol Rev 1982; 63: 129.
14. Depper JM, Leonard WJ, Robb RJ, Waldmann TA, Greene WC. Blockade of the interleukin 2 receptor by anti-Tac antibody: inhibition of human lymphocyte activation. J Immunol 1983; 131: 690.
15. Kirkman RL, Barrett LV, Gaulton GN, Kelley VE, Ythier A, Strom TB. Administration of an anti-interleukin 2 receptor antibody prolongs cardiac allograft survival in mice. J Exp Med 1985; 162: 358.
16. Kupiec-Weglinski JW, Diamantstein T, Tilney NL, Strom TB. Anti-interleukin 2 receptor monoclonal antibody therapy spares T suppressor cells and prevents/reverses acute allograft rejection. Proc Nat Acad Sci USA 1986; 83: 2624.
17. Ono K, Lindsey ES. Improved technique of heart transplantation in rats. J Thorac Cardiovasc Surg 1969; 7: 225.
18. Schneider TM, Kupiec-Weglinski JW, Towpik E, Strom TB, Tilney NL. Studies on mechanisms of acute rejection of vascularized organ allografts. Hum Immunol 1986; 15: 320.
19. Mason DW, Arthur RP, Dallman MJ, Green JR, Spickett GR, Thomas ML. Functions of rat T lymphocyte subsets isolated by means of monoclonal antibodies. Immunol Rev 1983; 74: 57.
20. Osawa H, Diamantstein T. The characteristics of a monoclonal antibody that binds specifically to rat T lymphoblasts and inhibits IL 2 receptor functions. J Immunol 1983; 130: 51.
21. Duarte AJS, Carpenter CB, Strom TB. Expression of T cell differentiation antigens and Ia on rat cytotoxic T lymphocytes. J Immunol 1982; 128: 580.
22. Gillis S, Ferm MM, Ou W, Smith KA. T cell growth factor: parameters of production and a quantitative microassay for activity. J Immunol 1978; 120: 2027.
23. Lear PA, Heidecke CD, Kupiec-Weglinski JW, Araneda D, Strom TB, Tilney NL. Restoration of allograft responsiveness in B rats. II. Requirements for lymphoid populations and lymphokine. Transplantation 1983; 36: 412.
24. Kupiec-Weglinski JW, Heidecke CD, Araujo JL, Abbud-Filho M, Towpik E, Araneda D, Strom TB, Tilney NL. Behavior of helper T lymphocytes in cyclosporine-mediated long-term graft acceptance in the rat. Cell Immunol 1985; 93: 168.
25. Lancaster F, Chui YL, Batchelor JR. Anti-idiotypic T cells suppress rejection of renal allografts in rats. Nature 1985; 315: 336.
26. Slavin S, Reitz C, Bieber H, et al. Transplantation tolerance in adult rats using total lymphoid irradiation (TLI): permanent survival of skin, heart and marrow allografts. J Exp Med 1978; 147: 700.
27. Uhteg LC, Salomon DR, Rocher LL, Kupiec-Weglinski JW, Araujo JL, Rubin MF, Tilney NL, Carpenter CB. Cyclosporine-induced transplantation unresponsiveness in rat cardiac allograft recipients: in vitro determination of helper and suppressor activity. J Immunol 1985; 135: 1800.
28. Heideicke CD, Kupiec-Weglinski JW, Lear PA, Abbud-Filho M, Araujo JL, Araneda D, Strom TB, Tilney NL. Interactions between T lymphocyte subsets supported by interleukin 2 rich lymphokines produce acute rejection of vascularized cardiac allografts in T cell deprived rats. J Immunol 1984; 133: 582.
29. Bunjes D, Hardt C, Rollinghoff M, Wagner H. Cyclosporine mediates immunosuppression of primary T cell responses by impairing the release of interleukin 1 and interleukin 2. Eur J Immunol 1981; 11: 657.
30. Andrus L, Lafferty KJ. Inhibition of T-cell activation by cyclosporin A. Scand J Immunol 1982; 15: 449.
31. Abbud-Filho M, Kupiec-Weglinski JW, Araujo JL, Heidecke CD, Tilney NL, Strom TB. Cyclosporine therapy of rat heart allograft recipients and release of interleukins (IL 1, IL 2, IL 3): a role for IL 3 in graft tolerance? J Immunol 1984; 133: 2582.
32. Wagner H, Rollinghoff M. T-T cell interactions during in vitro cytotoxic allograft responses. I. Soluble products from activated Ly^{1+} T cells trigger autonomously antigen primed Ly^{23+} T cells to proliferation and cytolytic activity. J Exp Med 1978; 148: 1523.
33. Farrar JJ, Simon PL, Koopman WJ, Fuller-Bonar J. Biochemical relationship of thymocyte mitogenic function and factors enhancing humoral and cell mediated immune responses. J Immunol 1978; 121: 1353.
34. Mannel DN, Mizel SB, Diamantstein T, Falk W. Induction of interleukin 2 responsiveness in thymocytes by synergistic action of interleukin 1 and interleukin 2. J Immunol 1985; 134: 3108.
35. Malek TR, Ortega GR, Jakway JP, Chan C, Shevach EM. The murine IL-2 receptor. II. Monoclonal anti IL-2 receptor antibodies as specific inhibitors of T cell function in vitro. J Immunol 1984; 133: 1976.
36. Batchelor JR, Phillips BE, Grennan D. Suppressor cells and their role in the survival of immunologically enhanced rat kidney allografts. Transplantation 1984; 37: 43.
37. Hendry WS, Tilney NL, Baldwin WM III, et al. Transfer of specific unresponsiveness to organ allografts by thymocytes. J Exp Med 1979; 149: 1042.
38. Williams IR, Perry LL. Regulation of transplantation immunity in vivo by monoclonal antibodies recognizing host class II restriction elements. II. Effects of anti-Ia immunotherapy on host T cell responses to graft alloantigens. J Immunol 1985; 134: 2942.
39. Dorsch S, Roser B. Suppressor cells in transplantation tolerance. I. Analysis of the suppressor status of neonatally and adoptively tolerized rats. Transplantation 1982; 33: 518.
40. Dorsch S, Roser B. Suppressor cells in transplantation tolerance. II. Identification and probable mode of action of chimeric suppressor T cells. Transplantation 1982; 33: 525.
41. Cotner T, Williams JM, Christenson L, et al. Simultaneous flow cytometric analysis of human T cell activation as expression and DNA content. J Exp Med 1983; 157: 461.
42. Koretzky GA, Daniele RP, Greene WC, Nowell P. Evidence for an interleukin-independent pathway for human lymphocyte activation. Proc Natl Acad Sci USA 1983; 80: 3444.
43. Ihle JN, Reber L, Keller J, Lee JC, Hapel AJ. Interleukin 3: possible roles in the regulation of lymphocyte differentiation and growth. Immunol Rev 1982; 63: 5.

Received 4 October 1985.
Accepted 14 November 1985.

0041-1337/86/4202-0197$02.00/0
TRANSPLANTATION
Vol. 42, No. 2

INABILITY TO TRANSFER IMMUNE UNRESPONSIVENESS OF CHICKENS BURSECTOMIZED AT 60 HOURS OF INCUBATION[1]

TIMO VEROMAA,[2] SIRPA JALKANEN,[3] KAISA GRANFORS, AND PAAVO TOIVANEN

Department of Medical Microbiology, University of Turku, SF-20520 Turku, Finland

Chickens surgically bursectomized (Bx)* at 60 hours of incubation have been found unable to produce specific antibodies, in spite of close-to-normal serum immunoglobulin levels. Suppressor cell overactivity as a reason for the impaired antibody production in the Bx chickens has not been ruled out. In the present work, we have studied whether the state of immune unresponsiveness of the Bx chickens can be transferred to normal chickens by transfer of bone marrow cells. Bone marrow cells from 10-week-old Bx or control (Co) chickens were grafted into x-ray-irradiated histocompatible 5–12-day-old normal recipients. After the transplantation the recipients were immunized with a pool of five antigens, and the antibody responses were quantitated by ELISA. The inability of the Bx chickens to produce specific antibodies could not be transferred to normal chickens by transfer of bone marrow cells, as no differences in the antibody responses between the two recipient groups were observed. The results indicate that suppressor cells do not play a role in preventing specific antibody formation in the Bx chickens.

It has recently been demonstrated that chickens surgically bursectomized (Bx) at 60 hr of incubation have plasma cells and are able to produce serum immunoglobulins. However, Bx chickens have been found unable to produce specific antibodies to a variety of different antigens even after heavy immunization (*1–3*).

Suppressor cell overactivity as a reason for the impaired antibody production in the Bx chickens has not been ruled out. Suppressor cells have been reported to maintain agammaglobulinemia in x-ray-irradiated and neonatally bursectomized chickens transplanted with bone marrow or spleen cells from agammaglobulinemic donors (*4, 5*). In the present work, we have studied whether the state of immune unresponsiveness of the Bx chickens can be transferred to normal chickens by transfer of bone marrow cells.

MATERIALS AND METHODS

Experimental design. Bone marrow cells from 10-week-old Bx or Co chickens were grafted to normal, 5–12-day-old histocompatible recipients that were given 5 Gy whole-body x-ray irradiation prior to grafting. After the grafting, the recipients were immunized three times with one week intervals, starting at the age of six weeks and using five different antigens. Control groups included normal chickens and chickens only receiving irradiation. The antibody responses of the four groups of chickens were quantitated by ELISA.

Chickens. Fertilized eggs from the line H.B15 kept at the Department of Medical Microbiology, Turku University, were used. The incubation of the eggs and the care of the birds were as described previously (*6*).

Bursectomy. Bursectomy at 60 hr of incubation was carried out according to the previously described technique (*2*). Briefly, the operation was performed under aseptic conditions using microsurgery scissors just before the amniotic membrane begins to cover the caudal part. The tail bud was cut off caudally to the leg buds. Hatchability of the operated embryos was 10–20% with 2% surviving beyond the first week of life.

Completeness of the bursectomy. To verify that the Bx chickens did not produce antibodies, they were immunized at the age of six weeks with 1 ml of 5% concentrate of chicken red blood cells. MHC (major histocompatibility complex) phenotypes of the cells used were B 13/15, 19/21, 15/y (y representing an unnamed allotype), and they were administered i.p. four times with one-week intervals. Serum samples were collected prior to first immunization and thereafter with one-week intervals. The occurrence of anti-MHC-antibodies was tested by microtitration using 25-μl volumes of the serum to be titrated and 0.25% red blood cells of other chicken strains. The diluent was 10% normal chicken serum tested to be free from any anti-MHC-antibodies. The plates were incubated for 1 hr at 37°C and then for 24 hr at 4°C before reading.

Autopsies were carried out at the age of 10 weeks. To determine the completeness of the bursectomy, the whole cloacal region was dissected out, fixed with 10% neutral buffered formalin, and embedded in paraffin. Serial sections cut throughout the region were stained with hematoxylin and eosin.

Preparation and transplantation of cells. The donors were sacrificed by exsanguination at the age of 10 weeks. Single-cell suspensions from the bone marrow were prepared as described earlier (*6*). Viability of the cells to be transplanted was determined by exclusion of 0.25% trypan blue. The number of the cells injected was based on the counts of viable cells (always >90%); immature and mature erythrocytes were excluded. Cells of 10-week-old Bx or Co donors (10^8) were injected i.v. in a 1.0-ml volume into the jugular vein of histocompatible normal irradiated recipients.

Antigens and immunizations. The bone marrow recipients and x-ray-irradiated and normal controls were immunized at the age of 6 weeks with *Escherichia coli* lipopolysaccharide (LPS), levan, tetanus toxoid, and dinitrophenyl-bovine serum albumin (DNP_7-BSA). The origin and amount of the antigens given at a time were as follows: *E coli* LPS (lipopolysaccharide W, *E coli* 055:B5, Difco Laboratories, Detroit, MI) 10 μg; native levan prepared from *Corynebacterium levaniformis* as described

[1] This work was supported by a grant from the Sigrid Jusélius Foundation.

[2] To whom correspondence and reprint requests should be sent.

[3] Present address: Department of Pathology, Stanford University, Stanford, CA, 94305.

* Abbreviations used: Bx: bursectomized at 60 hours of incubation; Co: control; MHC: major histocompatibility complex; LPS: lipopolysaccharide; DNP_7-BSA: dinitrophenyl-bovine serum albumin; GVH: graft-versus-host; ELISA: enzyme-linked immunosorbent assay.

previously (*7, 8*) 100 ng; tetanus vaccine (The National Health Institute, Helsinki, Finland, 10 Lf/ml tetanus toxoid) 1 ml of 1:20 dilution; and DNP_7-BSA prepared according to the method of Eisen (*9*) 1 mg. Each antigen was administered i.p. three times with one-week intervals. Serum samples were collected before the first immunization and after the second and third immunization.

Determination of specific antibodies. Serum IgM, IgG, and IgA class antibodies were quantitated by an enzyme-linked immunosorbent assay (ELISA) as described previously (*1*). The concentration of antibodies in the sample is expressed as relative ELISA units, where 1 unit is 1/100 of the corresponding antibody concentration in the positive reference serum.

RESULTS

Completeness of the bursectomy. All Bx birds appeared typically tailless. At the autopsy no macroscopic or microscopic remnants of bursal tissue were detected. The Bx chickens did not respond to the immunization with a pool of chicken red blood cells, as tested by the microtitration method, whereas the normal animals produced a vigorous response (not shown).

Antibody responses of the recipients of the bone marrow cells and their controls. All birds responded equally well to the immunization. No statistically significant differences in the antibody responses to DNP_7-BSA, LPS, levan, or tetanus toxoid between the recipients of Bx bone marrow cells and the recipients of normal bone marrow cells were observed. Responses in all animal groups were excellent against LPS, tetanus toxoid, DNP, and BSA, whereas antibody titers against levan were lower but still clearly detectable. Figure 1 shows the responses against LPS and tetanus toxoid; responses against DNP, BSA, and levan were similar (not shown). No differences between the two recipient groups of 5-day-old and 12-day-old chickens were observed; therefore, combined results are presented.

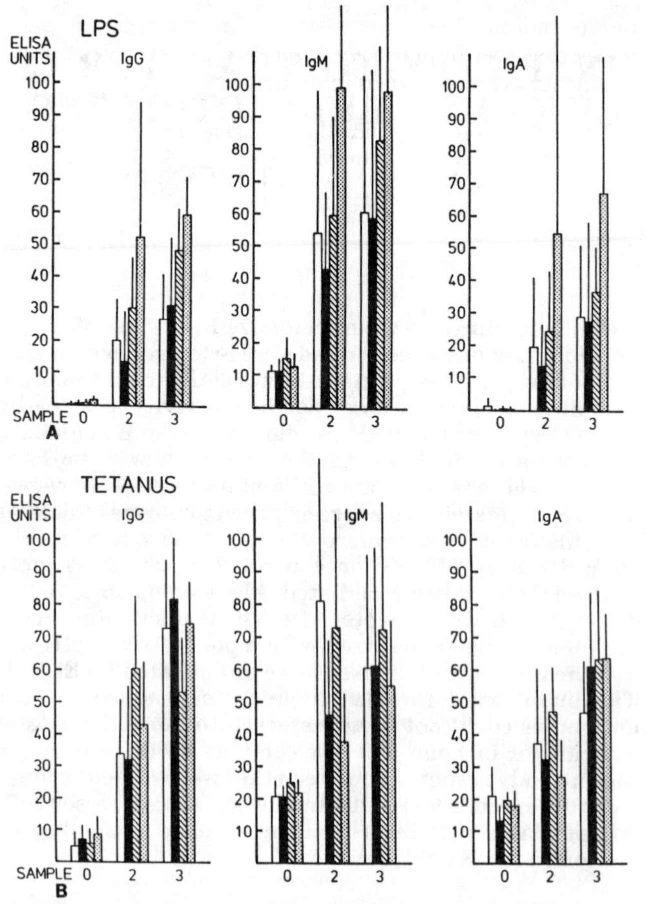

FIGURE 1. Antibody responses against (A) LPS and (B) tetanus toxoid. Sample 0 was collected prior to immunization, and samples 2 and 3 were collected one week after the second and third immunization, respectively. Arithmetic means + SD (n=5–11) of ELISA units are given. (White columns) x-ray-irradiated recipients of Bx bone marrow; (black columns) x-ray-irradiated recipients of Co bone marrow; (striped columns) x-ray-irradiated controls; (dotted columns) normal controls—no transplantation, no irradiation.

DISCUSSION

The inability of the Bx chickens to produce specific antibodies could not be transferred to normal, irradiated chickens by transfer of bone marrow cells. Such a transferable suppression has been described by Blaese et al. (*4*) who used surgical bursectomy one day posthatching combined with x-ray irradiation to produce agammaglobulinemic chickens. Bone marrow cells from these animals were grafted into irradiated recipients, and persistent agammaglobulinemia, characterized by inability to produce antibodies and by progressive loss of serum IgG and IgM, was developed. These observations of transferable suppression were confirmed by Palladino et al. (*5*) who used spleen cells obtained from agammaglobulinemic chickens, which had been embryonically bursectomized by testosterone followed by cyclophosphamide given posthatching. Similarly, Kermani-Arab and Leslie (*10*) used treatment with antichicken IgM antibody embryonically and surgical bursectomy at hatching to produce agammaglobulinemic chickens. Transplantation of lymphoid cells from these animals rendered the recipients severely hypogammaglobulinemic or agammaglobulinemic.

Lawrence et al. (*11*) also demonstrated serial transfer of IgA deficiency caused by IgA specific suppressor T cells. Chanh et al. (*12*) could show that IgG specific suppressor cells are responsible for an inherited IgG deficiency in UCD 140 line chickens and that B complex (major histocompatibility complex) homology was not required for suppression. On the contrary, it has been shown (*13*) that thymus cells from 7–11-week-old neonatally bursectomized donors have significantly less suppressive activity than thymus cells from normal or sham-bursectomized donors of the same age; skin graft rejection and graft-versus-host (GVH) reactivity were applied for testing. However, all methods of bursectomy described above result in a total B cell depletion and hypogammaglobulinemia or agammaglobulinemia. In contrast, in the chickens surgically bursectomized at 60 hr of incubation the B cell morphology and function are quite normal, the most remarkable deficiency being inability to produce specific antibodies. In patients suppressor cells able to prevent specific antibody formation have been described (*14, 15*). However, the suppression was not complete but selective, allowing a few specificities to develop. In Bx chickens no specific antibodies to any antigen have so far been found.

Bx chickens have a markedly decreased serum IgG level (*16*) but it seems unlikely that this could be due to IgG-specific suppressor cells—at least the possible suppressor effect cannot be transferred to normal chickens by transfer of bone marrow cells. The T cell system in the Bx chickens seems to be undisturbed (*1, 3, 17*), and apparently the defect is not due to impaired antigen presentation (*18*). Altogether, the present results indicate that suppressor cells do not play a role in preventing specific antibody formation in the chickens surgically bursectomized at 60 hr of incubation.

Acknowledgments. We thank Marjo Vesanto, Tarja Puurunen, and Soile Niittoaho for expert technical assistance.

REFERENCES

1. Granfors K, Martin C, Lassila O, Suvitaival R, Toivanen A, Toivanen P. Immune capacity of the chicken bursectomized at 60 h of incubation. Production of the immunoglobulins and specific antibodies. Clin Immunol Immunopathol 1982; 23: 459.
2. Jalkanen S, Granfors K, Jalkanen M, Toivanen P. Immune capacity of the chicken bursectomized at 60 hr of incubation: surface immunoglobulin and B-L (Ia-like) antigen bearing cells. J Immunol 1983; 130: 2038.
3. Jalkanen S, Korpela R, Granfors K, Toivanen P. Immune capacity of the chicken bursectomized at 60 hr of incubation. Cytoplasmic immunoglobulins and histological findings. Clin Immunol Immunopathol 1984; 30: 41.
4. Blaese RM, Weiden PL, Koski I, Dooley N. Infectious agammaglobulinemia: transmission of immunodeficiency with grafts of agammaglobulinemic cells. J Exp Med 1974; 140: 1097.
5. Palladino MA, Lerman SP, Thorbecke GJ. Transfer of hypogammaglobulinemia in two inbred chicken strains by spleen cells from bursectomized donors. J Immunol 1976; 116: 1673.
6. Toivanen P, Toivanen A. Bursal and postbursal stem cells in chicken. Functional characteristics. Eur J Immunol 1973; 3: 585.
7. Miranda JJ. Studies of immunological paralysis. IX. The immunogenicity and tolerogenicity of levan (polyfructose) in mice. Immunology 1972; 23: 829.
8. Moreno C, Courtenay BM, Howard JG. Molecular size and structure in relation to tolerogenicity of small fructosans (levans). Immunochemistry 1976; 13: 429.
9. Eisen HN, Belman S, Carsten ME. Reaction of 2.4-dinitrobenzenesulfonic acid with free amino groups of proteins. J Am Chem Soc 1953; 75: 4583.
10. Kermani-Arab V, Leslie GA. Suppression of immunoglobulin synthesis by transplantation of T cells from anti-μ bursectomized chickens into normal recipients. J Immunol 1977; 119: 530.
11. Lawrence EC, Arnaud-Battandier F, Koski IR, Dooley NJ, Muchmore AV, Blaese RM. Tissue distribution of immunoglobulin secreting cells in normal and IgA-deficient chickens. J Immunol 1979; 123: 1767.
12. Chanh TC, Benedict AA, Tam LQ, Abplanalp H, Gershwin ME. Inherited 7S immunoglobulin deficiency in chickens. Presence of suppressor T cells that suppress synthesis of 7S immunoglobulin but not IgM. J Immunol 1980; 125: 108.
13. Droege W. The antigen-inexperienced thymic suppressor cell: a class of lymphocytes in the young chicken thymus that inhibits antibody production and cell-mediated immune responses. Eur J Immunol 1976; 6: 279.
14. Rothbach C, Nagel J, Rabin B, Fireman P. Antibody deficiency with normal immunoglobulins. J Pediatr 1979; 94: 250.
15. Saxon A, Kobayashi RH, Stevens RH, Singer AD, Stiehm ER, Siegel SC. In vitro analysis of humoral immunity in antibody deficiency with normal immunoglobulins. Clin Immunol Immunopathol 1980; 17: 235.
16. Jalkanen S, Granfors K, Jalkanen M, Toivanen P. Immune capacity of the chicken bursectomized at 60 hr of incubation. Failure to produce immune, natural and autoantibodies in spite of immunoglobulin production. Cell Immunol 1983; 80: 363.
17. Eerola E, Jalkanen S, Granfors K, Toivanen A. Immune capacity of the chicken bursectomized at 60 hr of incubation. Mitogen induced cell proliferation and immunoglobulin secretion. J Immunol 1983; 131: 120.
18. Eerola E, Granfors K, Jalkanen S, Toivanen A. Immune capacity of the chicken bursectomized at 60 hr of incubation. Effect of adherent cells on the production of immunoglobulins and specific antibodies in vitro. Clin Immunol Immunopathol 1984; 31: 202.

Received 8 October 1985.
Accepted 8 November 1985.

0041-1337/86/4202-0200$02.00/0
TRANSPLANTATION
Vol. 42, No. 2

Printed in U.S.A.

PROLONGED SKIN ALLOGRAFT SURVIVAL THROUGH ENHANCEMENT EFFECTS ON DONOR TISSUE

HARVEY L. DEUTSCH, HOWARD D. J. EDINGTON, CHRISTOPHER M. MCCULLOUGH, AND PAUL H. SUGARBAKER[1]

The Colorectal Cancer Section, Surgery Branch, Division of Cancer Treatment, National Cancer Institute, National Institutes of Health, Bethesda, Maryland, 20205

A skin allograft retransplantation model was utilized to study the mechanism of immunological enhancement in a murine system. Enhancement was accomplished by treating allografted recipients with host antidonor serum (B6AF$_1$ anti-B10.D2 alloantiserum). Grafts from enhanced or untreated hosts were retransplanted after seven days onto a second recipient. Enhanced retransplanted grafts had significantly prolonged survival as compared with unenhanced grafts. The survival of enhanced retransplanted grafts was as prolonged as that of primary skin grafts on antiserum-treated hosts. Splenocytes harvested from recipients of enhanced retransplanted allografts showed delayed and diminished development of T cell responses to graft alloantigens. Sensitization of the second recipient abrogated prolonged survival of enhanced retransplanted grafts. Also, enhancement prevented sensitization of allografted recipients. One interpretation of these studies suggests that a sensitization block is a sufficient mechanism of skin allograft enhancement. The site of action of antisera is within the graft itself. Decreased T cell responses in the host are indirect effects of diminished antigenicity of enhanced grafts. Further studies of immunological enhancement should be directed to the graft, not toward the graft recipient.

The concept of immunological enhancement was introduced by Kaliss and coworkers in 1956 (*1*, *2*). Snell and colleagues attempted to define the mechanism of immunological enhancement; they suggested afferent (sensitization block), efferent (effector cell block), or central (immunologic tolerance) mechanisms that were responsible for this phenomenon (*3*). In 1972 Jeekel, McKenzie, and Winn described a convenient system for further exploring the mechanism of immunologic enhancement. They used the prolonged survival of skin allografts as an in vivo endpoint by which to measure the effects of enhancing alloantisera (*4*). Sugarbaker and Chang, using this skin allograft model, showed that alloantiserum delayed and depressed cellular immune responses from a skin allograft in treated mice (*5*). McCullough and coworkers attempted to define the effects of alloantiserum on a normal mouse. They could find no suppressive effects on the alloserum-treated host. Rather, in a retransplantation model, the prolonged survival of skin allografts were found to be expressed within the graft itself (*6*). Recently, some investigators have suggested that alloantiserum prolongs graft survival by eliminating passenger cells bearing Ia determinates from the skin allograft (*7*, *8*). As noted by Billingham, selective immunosuppression rather than total modification of the immune system and its resultant undesirable sequelae, would greatly improve the outlook for clinical transplantation. In this study we show, using a skin allograft retransplantation model, that the effects of enhancing serum are directly on the grafted tissue and result in a sensitization block of the host. Alloserum is shown to prevent the sensitization of a skin allograft recipient. These data, when taken together, should focus the attention of further research away from immunosuppressive effects of enhancement on the host and toward the effects of alloserum on the graft itself.

MATERIALS AND METHODS

Animals. Male mice of the strain B10.D2/oSn (B10.D2), B10.BR/SgSn (B10.BR), and B6AF$_1$ were obtained from the Jackson Laboratory, Bar Harbor, ME and maintained on chow ad libitum. Animals were housed individually. As shown in Table 1, the H-2 differences between B10.D2 donor and B6AF$_1$ recipient are at the H-2K specificity 31, plus subregions I-A, I-J, and I-E. The H-2 differences of B10.D2 donor with B10.BR recipient include the entire major histocompatibility complex (MHC).*

Alloantiserum. Production of alloantiserum is fully described elsewhere (*6*). Briefly, B6AF$_1$ anti-B10.D2 alloantiserum was raised by weekly i.p. injections of a cell suspension of B10.D2 thymocytes, splenocytes, and mesenteric lymph nodes into B6AF$_1$ mice. After seven weekly injections, B6AF$_1$ mice were bled by tail vein and sera was collected. Serum showing 50% cytotoxicity at a dilution of 1:512 was pooled and used as enhancing serum.

Skin grafting. Skin grafts were performed as previously described, utilizing an uncovered skin graft technique (*10*). B10.D2 allografts were prepared from the ventral mouse ear and grafted onto the prepared lateral thoracic cage of B6AF$_1$ recipients. Grafts were sutured in place with 6–0 silk. All recipients were anesthesized by i.p. sodium pentobarbital. Enhancement was accomplished by i.p. injection of recipients with 0.3 ml of alloantisera on days 1 and 4 after skin grafting. On day 7 after grafting, the primary recipients had their grafts excised with the inclusion of a 2-mm rim of recipient tissue, retransplanted onto the prepared lateral thoracic cage of second recipients, and sutured in place with 6–0 silk. Retransplanted grafts were covered with petroleum gauze and a plaster cast (Johnson and Johnson, New Brunswick, NJ) (*8*). At seven days after transplantation, gauze and plaster casts were removed and the graft left uncovered. Scoring was accomplished using a system based on the percentage of graft remaining intact and shrinkage. The day of retransplantation was defined as day 0

[1]Address correspondence to: Paul H. Sugarbaker, M.D., Head, Colorectal Cancer Section, Surgery Branch, National Cancer Institute, Bldg. 10, Rm. 2B07, Bethesda, MD, 20205.

* Abbreviations used: MHC, major histocompatibility complex; MST, mean survival time.

TABLE 1. H-2 differences of B10.D2 donor mice with B10.BR and $B6AF_1$ recipients

	H-2 region							
	K	I-A	I-J	I-E	I-C	S	G	D
Donor B10.D2	d	d	d	d	d	d	d	d
Recipient	k	k	k	k	d	d	d	d
$B6AF_1$	b	b	b	b	b	b	b	b
Donor B10.BR	k	k	k	k	k	k	k	k

of graft survival. Grafts were scored daily on a 0–4 scale. A score of 1+ was assigned to animals that had 1–25% of their graft rejected; 2+ indicated 26–50% rejection, etc. Grafts that had shrunk to 50% or less of their original size or over 50% rejected were recorded as having rejected the allograft. Primary grafts are referred to here as *parked* grafts.

Cell-mediated lympholysis. Cell-mediated lympholysis was carried out as described by Brunner et al. (*11*). Spleens were harvested and made into a single-cell suspension with passage through 40-gauge wire mesh. Spleen cells were washed and diluted to an appropriate concentration in complete media: RPMI 1640 (Grand Island Biological Co., NY), plus 7.5% heat-inactivated fetal calf serum (Grand Island Biological Co.), 100 units/ml of penicillin G, and 100 μg/ml streptomycin (Media Unit, NIH, Bethesda, MD). Red blood cells were lysed with ACK Lysing Buffer (Media Unit, NIH) for 2 min and centrifuged at 150 g for 10 min, and then washed three times with complete media. Cells were counted by Trypan blue exclusion and diluted to 5×10^6 cells/ml. Target cells consisted of i.p.-passaged P815 mastocytoma tumor ($H\text{-}2^d$). Targets were incubated with 200 $\mu Ci^{51}Cr$ for 45 min at 37°C and then washed three times. Targets were counted and readjusted to 1×10^5 cells/ml. Effector cells were serially diluted eight times from 5×10^6 cells/ml. Effectors and targets were mixed in a 96-well microtiter plate to a total volume of 0.2 ml per well (Linbro Scientific, McLean, VA). Each effector-to-target ratio was subjected to triplicate analysis. Microtiter plates were centrifuged at 150 g for 5 min and incubated for 4 hr at 37°C in 5% CO_2. Harvesting was preceeded by centrifugation at 10 min, and supernatant was collected with the Titertek supernatant collecting system (Flow Laboratory, Skatron Inc., Sterling, VA). Samples were counted in a gamma counter.

Percentage of release of ^{51}Cr was calculated by the following equation:

$$\frac{\text{counts supernatant} - \text{counts spontaneous release}}{\text{total counts}} \times 100$$

Data. All groups consisted of at least four animals, with each experiment carried out at least twice. The Wilcoxon test was utilized with a two-tailed level of significance. Survival data is given as mean survival time (MST) ±1 SD.

RESULTS

Persistence of effect of alloantiserum after retransplantation of enhanced allograft onto naive second recipient. The effectiveness of enhancing alloantiserum is well established in prolonging skin allograft survival. B10.D2 allografts on untreated $B6AF_1$ recipients had a mean survival time of 11±0.4 days, as compared with enhanced recipients with a mean survival time of 16.4±0.9 days (data not shown). The difference in survival of these two groups was statistically significant at a P value of 0.01. Figure 1 shows the survival of enhanced and untreated B10.D2 grafts that were retransplanted at seven days onto naive $B6AF_1$ recipients. Allografts taken from enhanced mice and transferred to second recipients showed a mean survival time of 17±1.7 days, whereas the survival of unenhanced retransplanted grafts was 9.6±1.1 days. This was statistically significant at a P value of 0.008. These data suggest that the essential features of enhancement are contained within the enhanced allograft itself, in that the effect of alloantiserum can be transferred with the enhanced allograft. Host effects of alloantiserum, although they may exist, are not necessary for prolonged skin graft survival.

A similar experiment with grafts retransplanted to $B6AF_1$ recipients after four days on the primary host was performed. MST of enhanced retransplanted skin grafts is 16.0±0.5 and unenhanced 12.0±1.1. This was statistically significant at a P value of .0093. Effective enhancement after retransplantation was seen even after limited parking of the skin graft on the primary host.

Immunogenicity of retransplanted allograft altered by alloantiserum. Splenocytes were harvested from recipients of enhanced retransplanted allografts at days 12, 14, 16, and 18 after retransplantation and from unenhanced retransplanted recipients at days 8, 10, 12, and 14. These days were selected for assay of cell-mediated cytotoxicity because grafts are rejected during this time. Splenocytes were harvested from 2 mice, pooled and assayed for cytotoxicity at an effector-to-target ratio of 50:1. Figure 2 shows that the cytotoxicity of spleen cells harvested from animals bearing enhanced retransplanted skin grafts was markedly reduced and delayed in the generation of high levels of specific cytotoxicity in vitro. Thus it appears that recognition of B10.D2 alloantigens by the second host was reduced when grafts were exposed to specific alloantiserum in the primary host.

If B10.BR skin grafts were placed on $B6AF_1$ recipients, treatment of the primary host with $B6AF_1$ anti-B10.D2 anti-

	PRIMARY RECIPIENT	DONOR SKIN	SECOND RECIPIENT	MST ON SECOND RECIPIENT	p VALUE
—	ENHANCED $B6AF_1$	B10.D2	$B6AF_1$	17 ± 1.7	.008
- -	$B6AF_1$			9.6 ± 1.1	

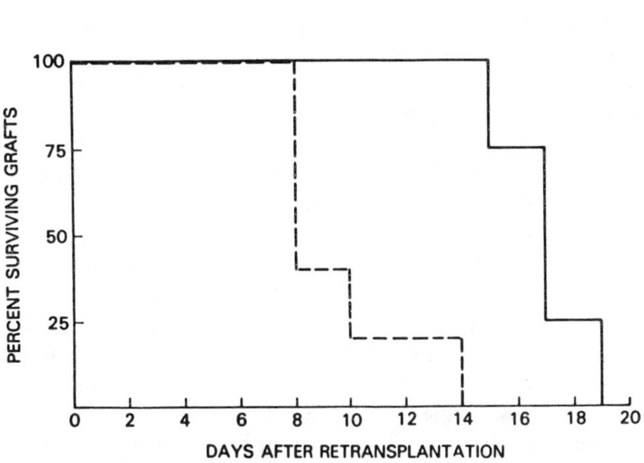

FIGURE 1. Persistence of effect of antisera after retransplantation of an enhanced allograft to a second naive recipient. Primary $B6AF_1$ recipients were skin-grafted with B10.D2 allografts; half the mice were treated with 0.3 ml of antisera i.p. on days 1 and 4 after grafting. On day seven, parked allografts were retransplanted to untreated $B6AF_1$ recipients. MST of retransplanted allografts on second recipients was determined.

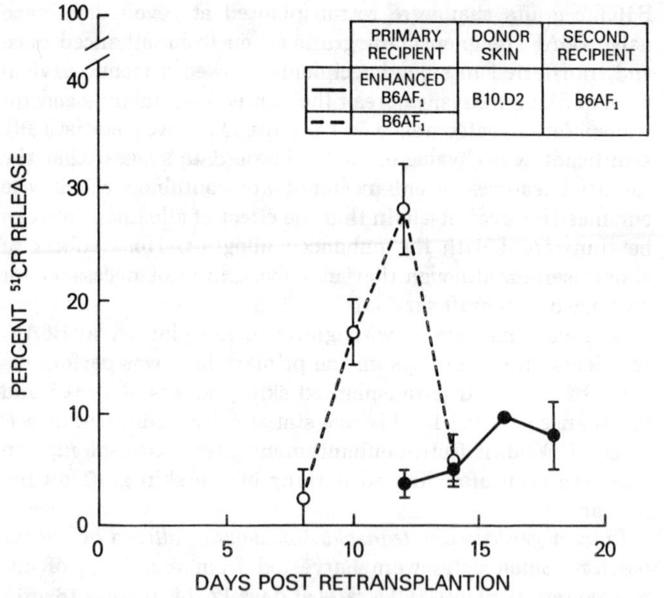

FIGURE 2. Splenocytes from recipients of enhanced retransplanted allografts showed delayed and diminished T cell cytotoxicity toward a ^{51}Cr-labeled donor syngeneic target cell. A ^{51}Cr release assay was performed on days 12, 14, 16, and 18 after retransplantation in the enhanced group and on days 8, 10, 12, and 14 after retransplantation in the unenhanced group.

serum did not result in a diminished cytoxicity to B10.BR alloantigens. Also survival of B10.BR primary or retransplanted skin grafts was not prolonged by $B6AF_1$ anti-B10.D2 antisera (data not shown).

Failure of enhancement with B10.BR mice used as the second recipient. B10.D2 skin allografts were excised at day seven from enhanced or unenhanced primary $B6AF_1$ recipients and retransplanted onto naive B10.BR recipients. As shown in Figure 3, the MST of the enhanced allografts on the B10.BR recipient was 9.3±0.71 days, as compared with 8.0±0 days for unenhanced grafts. There was no statistically significant difference in survival between the enhanced and unenhanced groups. These data suggest that all the MHC differences between the B10.D2 donor and B10.BR recipient must be reactive with enhancing alloantiserum for enhancement to be effective. Enhancing sera directed only at one part of the H-2 region was ineffective in prolonging graft survival.

Prior sensitization of second recipient abrogating prolonged survival of enhanced retransplanted grafts. B10.D2 allografts parked on enhanced or unenhanced $B6AF_1$ primary recipients were retransplanted at day 7 onto sensitized $B6AF_1$ recipients. The sensitized recipients had received B10.D2 skin allografts 13 days previously, and the skin grafts were completely rejected. The retransplanted grafts were placed on the opposite flank of the recipients. As shown in Figure 4, no difference in survival was observed for enhanced or unenhanced retransplanted skin grafts on these sensitized second recipients and second-set rejection was evident. Thus, once an animal was primed to a particular alloantigen, the enhancing effect of alloantisera in the retransplantation model was not observed.

Prevention of host sensitization by skin allograft by enhancing alloantisera. $B6AF_1$ recipients were skin-grafted with B10.D2 allografts, and half the animals were enhanced at days 1 and 4 after grafting. After seven days, these allografts were excised and the graft bed closed. Fourteen days after removal of the first graft a second B10.D2 allograft was placed on these mice. Survival of the second grafts on enhanced mice was 12.8±1.0 days. Unenhanced recipients showed second set rejection of the second skin allograft, with MST of 8.8±1.1 days. These differences are statistically significant at the P=.034 level (Fig. 5). Alloantiserum-treated recipients were not sensitized; their

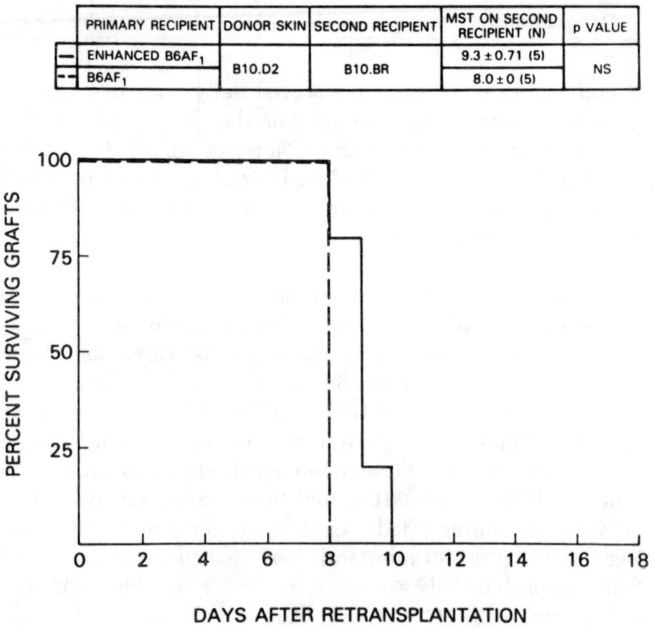

FIGURE 3. All histoincompatible antigens between donor and recipient must be reactive with alloantisera for enhancement to occur. Enhanced or unenhanced primary $B6AF_1$ recipients were skin-grafted with B10.D2 grafts, and seven days later retransplanted to naive B10.BR second recipients. No difference in graft survival was noted.

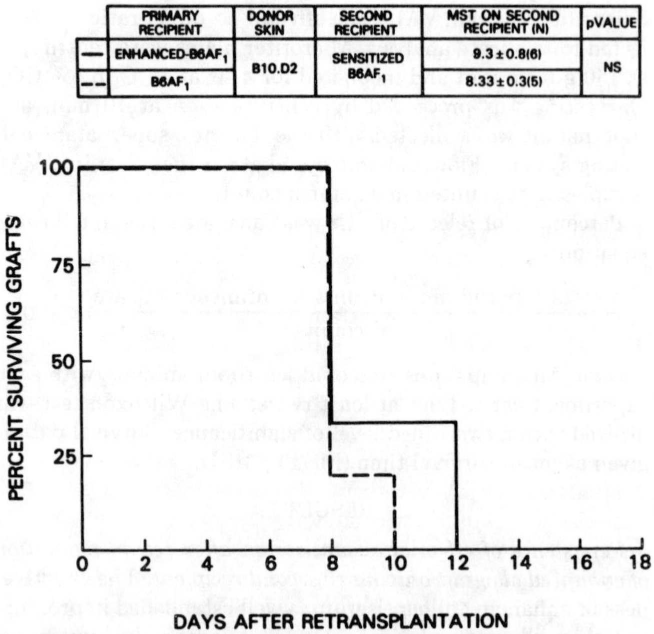

FIGURE 4. Sensitization of second recipients abrogated prolongation of survival of enhanced retransplanted allografts. $B6AF_1$ primary recipients were grafted with B10.D2 allografts, and half the group was treated with antisera on days 1 and 4. Seven days later, these allografts were retransplanted to sensitized $B6AF_1$ recipients that had completely rejected B10.D2 allografts. Second-set rejection was observed.

RECIPIENT	DONOR SKIN	TREATMENT AT DAY 7	TREATMENT AT DAY 21	MST OF SECOND GRAFT (N)	p VALUE
ENHANCED B6AF$_1$	B10.D2	GRAFT EXCISED AND GRAFT BED CLOSED	REGRAFTED WITH B10.D2 SKIN	12.8 ± 1.0 (5)	.037
B6AF$_1$				8.83 ± 1.1 (6)	

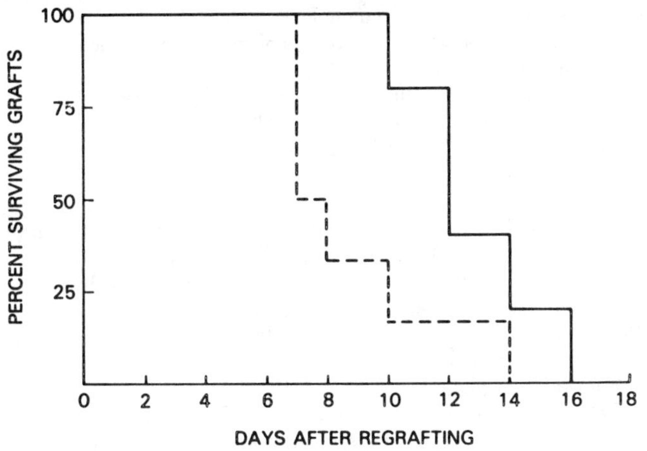

FIGURE 5. Enhancement prevents host sensitization by a skin allograft. Enhanced or unenhanced primary B6AF$_1$ recipients were skin grafted with B10.D2 grafts. Seven days later grafts were excised and the graft bed sutured closed. Fourteen days after graft excision, the same recipients were regrafted with new B10.D2 allografts. MST of the second B10.D2 allografts on previously enhanced and grafted recipients showed the survival expected of primary allografts. Untreated recipients showed second-set rejection.

grafts showed the survival time expected of a primary untreated skin allograft. Thus, alloantiserum was able to prevent sensitization of the host for the seven days while these mice were bearing B10.D2 skin allografts.

DISCUSSION

A number of investigators have shown that immunological enhancement, as first described in a tumor system by Kalis et al., is applicable to murine skin and to primarily vascularized organ allograft models (*1, 2, 12*). Jeekel, McKenzie, and Winn were able to prolong skin allograft survival from approximately 10 to 15 days (*4*). Corry et al. achieved enhancement in the heart allograft model with similar prolongation of graft survival (*13*). However, studies undertaken to elicit the mechanism of passive enhancement have focused on modification or alteration of the host immune system by the host antidonor alloantisera. The technique of skin allograft retransplantation as described in this report and elsewhere permitted us to study the effect of enhancement on the grafted tissue in the absence of effect on the host (*14*). As is evident from our retransplantation data, passive enhancement was transferable with the grafted tissue. Prolongation of enhanced allograft survival after retransplantation to a second host was equally as prolonged as primary skin grafts on antisera-treated hosts. Moreover, to our surprise, the effect of antiserum on a parked allograft was noted as early as four days after grafting onto the primary host.

One may conclude that delayed and diminished T cell cytotoxicity in the second recipient is evidence for the alteration of graft immunogenicity. This finding was only evident in the host of the treated retransplanted allograft. Peak splenic cytotoxicity was noted at day 12 for the second host of the untreated graft and was delayed until day 16 for the recipient of the enhanced retransplanted graft. Sugarbaker and Chang and others have shown similar modification of host T cell cytotoxicity in the primary allograft model (*5, 15*). Also, they demonstrated that enhancing alloantibody interferes with the specific accumulation of cytotoxic T cells in the skin allograft (*16*). One explanation, espoused by Hutchinson and Zola, suggested depletion of antigen reactive cells by the interaction with antibody complexes resulting in opsonization of these cells by the liver (*17*). However, our data derived from in vivo and in vitro experiments suggests that it is not the host's responses that are altered by enhancing alloantiserum—rather the host's reaction to the grafted tissue was modified by alloantiserum (*6*). Batchelor and coworkers made similar observations in the rat model (*18–19*). They attributed the decreased immunogenicity of the passively enhanced retransplanted renal allograft to the elimination of the immunogenic donor passenger cells. Studies are in progress to determine the effect, if any, of alloantiserum in altering the number of Ia-positive Langerhans cells in the epidermis of treated donor allografts.

B6AF$_1$ mice differ from B10.D2 donor mice at the H-2K specificity 31, as well as IA, I-J, and I-E regions. However, the difference between B10.D2 donor and B10.BR recipients are across the entire MHC. The retransplantation of an allograft that was enhanced on a B6AF$_1$ primary recipient to a naive B10.BR recipient showed no prolongation of graft survival when compared with untreated controls. Even though the B10.D2 allograft on the primary recipient had antibody directed at its K and I-A, regions of the MHC, there was no enhancing effect seen with retransplantation to a B10.BR recipient. Hence, to cause prolonged survival of a retransplanted graft it appeared that all histoincompatible antigens between donor and recipient had to be reactive with enhancing serum. Staines et al. demonstrated that antibodies directed against Ia antigens appear to be the major specificity involved in enhancement (*20*). In addition, McKenzie and Hennings reported that I-A and I-B differences are more important for enhancing effect that other differences (*21, 22*). However, our retransplantation data suggest that antiserum directed only at H-2K or only at Ia region antigens is inadequate for enhancement in this strain combination.

A potential problem with this experiment concerns B10.BR host responses to the B6AF$_1$ rim of skin retransplanted with the B10.D2 skin graft. B6AF$_1$ alloantigens from the primary host may sufficiently contaminate the skin graft so that enhanced B10.D2 grafts fail to show prolonged survival—i.e., anti-B6 responses. This seems unlikely for C57BL/6 grafts or C57BL/10 mice are never rejected (*4*). It seems more likely that H-2^d antigens at the K end of the MHC complex in the enhanced grafts bring about the primary allograft rejection. Also, it is possible that B10.D2 grafts can never be enhanced on B10.BR mice because of the strength of the histoincompatible MHC antigens.

In the primary skin graft model, McKenzie et al. showed that second set rejection of skin grafts occurred in previously grafted animals and was not prevented by intermittent or continuous alloantiserum administration (*15*). Our retransplantation model showed similar effects. We were unable to demonstrate inhibition of second-set rejection by retransplantation of a previously enhanced graft to a second recipient that had been sensitized by rejecting a relevant skin graft. In this study, prior sensitization to the relevent antigen was sufficient to nullify the modifying enhancing properties of previously enhanced grafts. It appears that once a host's immune system has been primed to a specific alloantigen, its immunologic memory to that antigen cannot be overcome by the transfer of enhancing properties of the antisera-treated allograft. In addition, this data would suggest that an efferent mechanism of enhancement is unlikely.

Despite our inability to overcome prior host sensitization with an enhanced retransplantated allograft, we were able to prevent sensitization of the primary recipient. Enhanced hosts with grafts were excised at day seven and regrafted two weeks later with a fresh graft did not exhibit second-set rejection. In fact these second grafts showed a survival time expected in a primary untreated skin allograft recipient. As expected, a control group of untreated recipients showed second-set graft rejection. These results, along with those previously shown, argue against an efferent mechanism of enhancement and strongly suggest that a sensitization block (afferent mechanism of enhancement) operates in this model.

REFERENCES

1. Kaliss N, Kandutsch AA. Acceptance of tumor homografts by mice injected with antiserum. Proc Soc Exp Biol Med 1956; 91: 118.
2. Kalis N. Immunological enhancement of tumor homografts in mice: a review. Cancer Res 1958; 18: 992.
3. Snell GD, Winn HJ, Stimpfling JH, Parker SJ. Depression by antibody of the immune response to homografts and its role in immunological enhancement. J Exp Med 1960; 112: 293.
4. Jeekel J, McKenzie IFC, Winn HJ. Immunological enhancement of skin grafts in the mouse. J Immunol 1972; 108: 1017.
5. Sugarbaker PH, Chang AE. Enhancing alloantibody effective during sensitization but not effector phase of skin graft rejection. Transplantation 1979; 28: 63.
6. McCullough CS, Sugarbaker PH, Matthews WS. Effects of passive enhancement on graft and host: graft adaptation by alloantibody at the mechanism of prolonged skin allograft survival. Transplantation 1984; 37: 91.
7. Hart DNJ, Fabre JW. Mechanism of induction of passive enhancement. Transplantation 1982; 33: 319.
8. Sugarbaker PH, McCullough CS, Deutsch HL. Retransplantation of murine skin allografts: assessment of treatment effects on the allograft in the absence of effects on the host. J Immunol Methods 1984; 72: 361.
9. Billingham RE. The feasibility of altering the immunogenicity of grafts. J Invest Dermatol 1976; 67: 149.
10. Sugarbaker PH, Change AE. Uncovered skin grafts in mice. J Immunol Methods 1979; 31: 167.
11. Brunner KT, Mauel J, Rudolf H, Chaupis B. Studies of allograft immunity in mice. I. Induction, development and in vitro assay of cellular immunity. Immunology 1970; 18: 501.
12. French ME, Batchelor JR. Immunological enhancement of rat kidney grafts. Lancet 1969; 2: 1103.
13. Corry RJ, Winn HJ, Russell PS. Heart transplantation in cogenic strains of mice. Transplant Proc 1973; 5: 733.
14. Silvers WK, Billingham RE, Sanford BH. The H-Y transplantation antigen: a Y-linked or sex influenced factor. Nature 1968; 220: 40B.
15. McKenzie IFC, Koene R, Winn HJ. Mechanism of skin graft enhancement in the mouse. Transplant Proc 1971; 3: 712.
16. Chang AE, Sugarbaker PH. Abrogation of T-cell homing by alloantibody. Transplantation 1980; 29: 127.
17. Hutchinson IV, Zol AH, Batchelor JR. Immunological enhancement of rat renal allografts using rabbit antisera with specificity for rat transplantation antigens. Transplantation 1976; 22: 273.
18. Batchelor JR, Welsh KI, et al. Failure of long surviving passively enhanced kidney allografts to provoke T-dependent alloimmunity. I. Retransplantation of $(AS\times AUG)F_1$ kidneys into secondary AS recipients. J Exp Med 1979; 150: 455.
19. Welsh KI, Batchelor JR, et al. Failure of long surviving passively enhanced kidney allografts to provoke T-dependent alloimmunity. II. Retransplantation of $(AS\times AUG)F_1$ kidneys from AS recipients into $(AS\times WF)F_1$ secondary hosts. J Exp Med 1979; 150: 465.
20. Staines DA, Guy K, Davies DAL. The dominant role of Ia antibodies in the passive enhancement of H-2 incompatible skin grafts. Eur J Immunol 1975; 5: 782.
21. McKenzie IFC, Henning MM. The H-2 complex: immunogenicity and enhancement studies of H-2K regional alloantigens. J Immunogenet 1977; 4: 249.
22. McKenzie IFC, Henning MM. The differential destructive and enhancing effects of anti-H-2K, H-2D, and anti-Ia antisera on murine skin allografts. J Exp Med 1978; 147: 611.

Received 21 November 1984.
Accepted 13 November 1985.

0041-1337/86/4202-0205$02.00/0
TRANSPLANTATION
Copyright © 1986 by The Williams & Wilkins Co.

Vol. 42, No. 2
Printed in U.S.A.

THE EFFECTIVENESS OF ANTI-Ia-IMMUNOTOXINS IN THE SUPPRESSION OF MLR[1,2]

KAZUHIKO NAKAHARA,[3] DONALD KAPLAN,[4] MIKE BJORN,[4] AND C. GARRISON FATHMAN[5,6]

Division of Immunology, Department of Medicine, Stanford University Medical Center, Stanford, California 94305; and Cetus Corporation, Emeryville, California 94608

The potential use of a mouse anti-Ia monoclonal antibody conjugated with a plant toxin as an immunosuppressive agent for organ transplantation was examined by studying the mixed lymphocyte reaction (MLR). In initial observations in a murine system utilizing strains A/J and C57B1/6 (B6), it was shown that a rich-toxin-conjugated anti-I-E^k monoclonal antibody (13.4-immunotoxin) would kill Ia-bearing cells of strain A/J (I-E^k)—but not of strain B6, the cells of which lack I-E determinants. Studies reported here demonstrated that 13.4-immunotoxin effectively removed stimulatory cells from the I-E-bearing spleen cells but had no effect on spleen cells lacking I-E determinants or responder lymph node cells (I-E$^+$ or I-E$^-$) similarly treated (i.e., 1 μg/10^6 cells). Taking advantage of the finding that such anti-I-E antibodies react with rat spleen cells bearing class II major histocompatibility complex molecules, we utilized these toxin-conjugated antibodies to inhibit MLR in rats. Assuming that the MLR is an in vitro representative of graft rejection, we suggest that such immunotoxins might be useful for pretreatment of organ allografts for transplantation across major histocompatibility barriers.

In 1957, Snell suggested that passenger leukocytes contained in organ allografts might play a particularly significant role in the induction of transplantation immunity (*1*). This concept was supported by the observation that the survival of allografts could be prolonged by culture in vitro that removed passenger leukocytes prior to transplantation (*2–6*). Additional support for this hypothesis came from the following observations: (1) injection of donor lymphoid cells would allow prompt rejection of successfully transplanted allografts (*7–9*); (2) allografts taken from donors pretreated with radiation, immunosuppressive drugs, or steroids showed a reduced ability to immunize the hosts (*10–16*); and (3) allograft survival could be shown to be prolonged by pretreatment of donor grafts with leukocidal reagents, including antilymphocyte serum (*17, 18*). These observations support the possibility that passenger leukocytes are involved in the initiation of immune rejection. The hypothesis examined in this paper is that class II major histocompatibility complex (MHC)[6] products (Ia antigens) are solely responsible for the initiation of alloaggression, and that removal of such Ia bearing cells will effectively eliminate stimulation in mixed lymphocyte cultures between Ia-disparate lymphoid cell populations.

The central role of Ia products in T cell recognition has been thoroughly demonstrated. Thus, T cell proliferative responses to antigen (*19, 20*) and T-cell-dependent antibody responses in vitro (*21*) have been shown to be inhibited by antibodies directed against such Ia determinants of the antigen-presenting cell. In our laboratory, utilizing alloreactive and antigen-specific T cell clones, it has been demonstrated that I-region-encoded mixed lymphocyte reaction (MLR)-stimulating determinants, Ia antigens, and immune response genes are all associated with the same cell surface products and are indistinguishable (*22–26*). Elsewhere, it has been shown that antisera directed to Ia determinants enhance skin and kidney allografts (*27–28*). Recently, it has been demonstrated that allograft survival can be prolonged by pretreatment with heterologous anti-Ia antisera and complement in allo-organ transplants in murine heart and islet cell transplants (*9, 29*).

Central to the use of toxin-conjugated antibodies was the experimental demonstration that a number of proteins, including ricin, abrin, and diphtheria toxin act as cytotoxins. As a result of their lack of specificity, however, none of these toxic substances could be used as cytotoxic agents for therapy. The demonstrated specificity of interactions of hormones and antibodies with their specific receptors or ligands, respectively, raised the possibility of construction of targeted cytotoxins. The availability of highly specific monoclonal antibodies that demonstrate selective specificity for certain cell-surface antigens has greatly increased interest in the use of such cytotoxins. Toxic conjugates have allowed a variety of innovative approaches to immunotherapy as is evidenced by the large number of laboratories involved in constructing and characterizing such immunotoxin conjugates (*30–50*). In the present study, the potential effectiveness of a mouse anti-Ia monoclonal antibody conjugated with ricin for use in organ transplantation was examined by studying mixed lymphocyte reactions.

MATERIALS AND METHODS

Mice. A/J (H-2^k) and C57B1/6 (B6, H-2^b) mice were obtained from Jackson Laboratories, Bar Harbor, ME. Adult male mice, aged 12–18 weeks, were used.

[1] This work was supported in part by the National Institutes of Health Grants AI 18705 and 18716, and by the Kroc Foundation and Cetus Corporation.

[2] This article was previously published in *Transplantation* 1985; 40: 62; it is reprinted here with revised figures.

[3] Current address: First Department of Internal Medicine, Faculty of Medicine, University of Tokyo, Tokyo, Japan.

[4] Cetus Corporation.

[5] Stanford University Medical Center.

[6] Address correspondence to: C. Garrison Fathman, M.D., Division of Immunology, Department of Medicine, Stanford University Medical Center, Stanford, CA 94305.

[6] Abbreviations used: LBN: (Lewis×Brown Norway) F_1 rats; MLR: mixed lymphocyte reaction; MHC: major histocompatibility complex; PBS: phosphate-buffered saline; RTA: ricin toxin A chain; 13.4-RTA: immunotoxin conjugate of RTA to monoclonal antibody 13.4 with SPDP; SPDP: N-succinimidyl-3-(2-pyridyldithio) propionate; SDS-PAGE: Sodium dodecyl sulfate polyacrylomide gel electrophoresis.

Rats. Male ACI rats, 11–18 weeks of age, weighing 200–280 g were obtained from Simonsen Laboratories, Gilroy, CA. Male Lewis×Brown Norway (LBN) F_1 rats, 12–18 weeks of age and 300–400 g were obtained from Harlan Sprague-Dawley Company, Walkersville, MD.

Monoclonal antibody. The monoclonal antibody 13.4 used in this study was generously provided by Gunter Hammerling, Ph.D., Heidelberg, FRG, and purified by Brian Fendly, Cetus Immune Corporation, Palo Alto, CA; it has been described previously (*51*). This antibody reacts with the I-E^k molecule and has been associated with specificity Ia.7.

The 13.4-ricin conjugate (13.4-immunotoxin). Monoclonal antibody 13.4 (2 mg/ml in phosphate-buffered saline [PBS]) was derivatized with the heterobifunctional cross-linking reagent N-succinimidyl-3-(2-pyridyldithio) propionate (SPDP; Pharmacia, Piscatway, NJ) (*45, 52*). SPDP (0.075 ml, 20 mM) in absolute ethanol was added to each milliliter of antibody solution, followed by incubation at room temperature for 30 min. The derivatized antibody was extensively dialyzed against PBS at 4°C to remove residual unreactive SPDP, then analyzed for pyridine-2-disulfide content, as described by Carlsson et al (*52*). An average of 4 such residues was found per molecule of antibody.

Ricin A chain (RTA) was purchased from EY Labs, San Mateo, CA. This RTA was essentially nontoxic to a variety of 3cultured cell lines, requiring a dose of 0.1 μM to inhibit protein synthesis by 50%. RTA (0.8 mg/ml) was freshly reduced by adding dithiothreitol (1 M; pH 7.0) to a final concentration of 50 mM. Following incubation for 30 min at room temperature, the reduced RTA was desalted on a G-25 column equilibrated in PBS. Fractions containing the highest protein concentrations were pooled. The reduced, desalted RTA was then mixed with derivatized antibody. Final concentrations of derivatized antibody and RTA were 4.4 μM and 10 μM, respectively. The conjugate mixture was incubated at room temperature for 1 hr, then stored at 4°C. Successful conjugation was demonstrated by sodium dodecyl sulfate polyacrylamide gel electrophoresis (SDS-PAGE) and by the spectrophotometric determination of the quantity of pyridine-2-thione released upon mixing the derivatized antibody with RTA (*52*). An average of 1.5 molecules of RTA were covalently coupled to each molecule of antibody. Subsequent analysis suggested that whole ricin or B chain was present in this commercial preparation of ricin A chain at a concentration of 1:1000 by lactose inhibition experiments, so we refer to the product as 13.4-immunotoxin.

Cell preparation. Spleen and lymph node cells were teased in RPMI 1640 (Gibco, Grand Island, NY) supplemented with 10% fetal calf serum (M.A. Bioproducts, Walkersville, MD). 40 μM

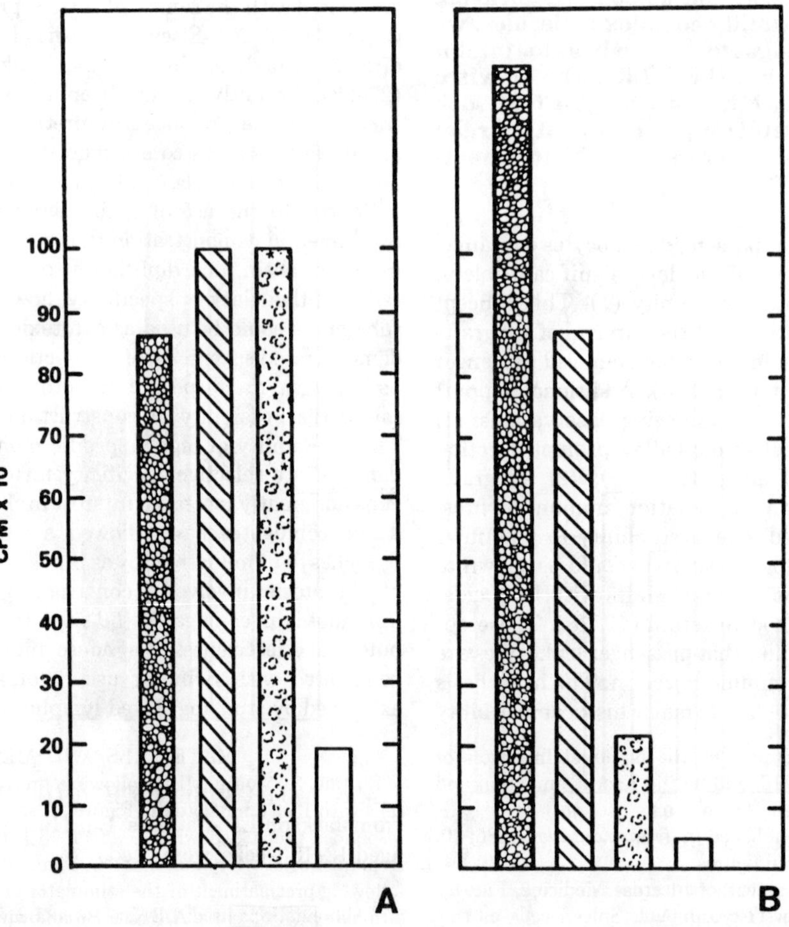

FIGURE 1. Mouse MLR following pretreatment of stimulator cells with 13.4-immunotoxin. Spleen cells, as the stimulator, were treated with 1 μg of 13.4-immunotoxin or the same dose of toxin-unconjugated 13.4 per 1 × 10^6 spleen cells for 10 min at 37°C. (A) the A/J anti-B6 MLR; (B) the B6 anti-A/J MLR. ( ) = treated with the 13.4-immunotoxin; ( ) = treated with toxin unconjugated 13.4; ( ) = allogeneic MLR treated with phosphate-buffered saline for a positive control; ( ) = syngeneic MLR treated with PBS for a negative control.

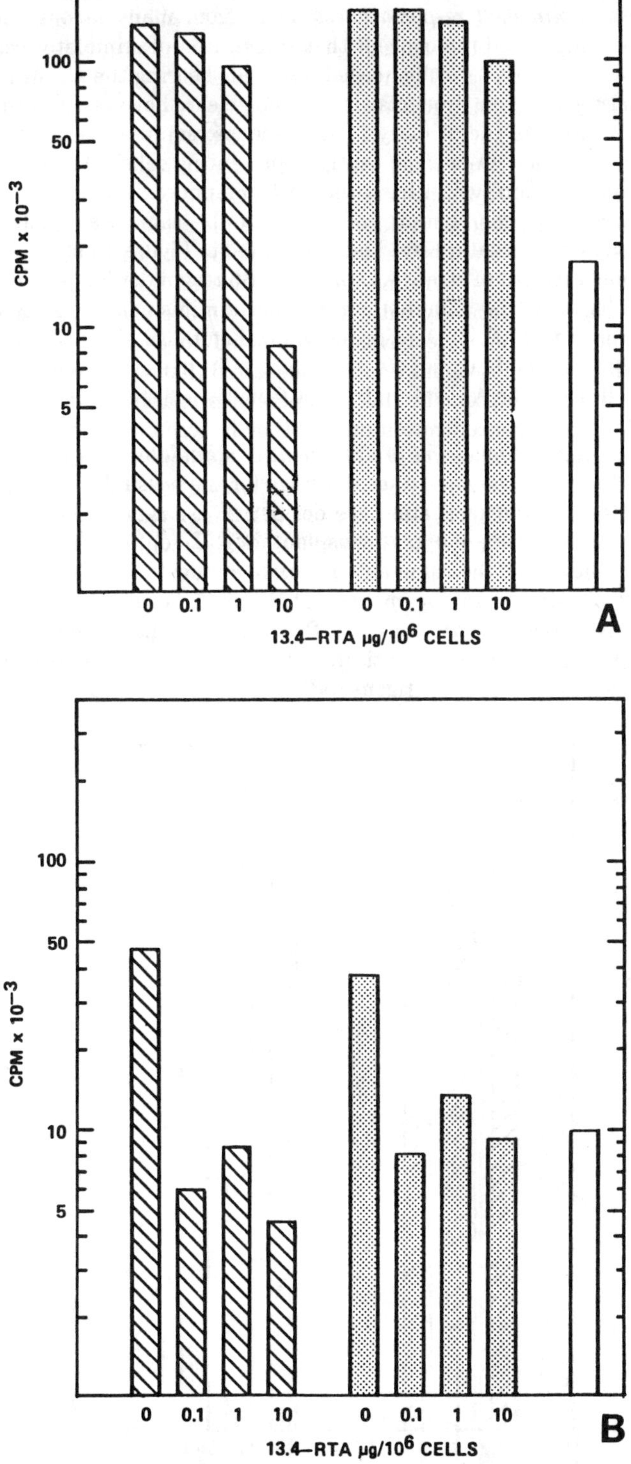

FIGURE 2. Mouse MLR with or without lactose. Figure 2A shows A/J anti-B6 and Figure 2B shows B6 anti-A/J. Spleen cells as the stimulator were treated with 0, 0.1, 1, and 10 μg of the 13.4-immunotoxin per 1 × 10^6 spleen cells for 10 min at 37°C in the presence ( ) or in the absence ( ) of 100 mM lactose; ( ) syngeneic MLR, A/J anti-A/J (A), B6 anti-B6 (B).

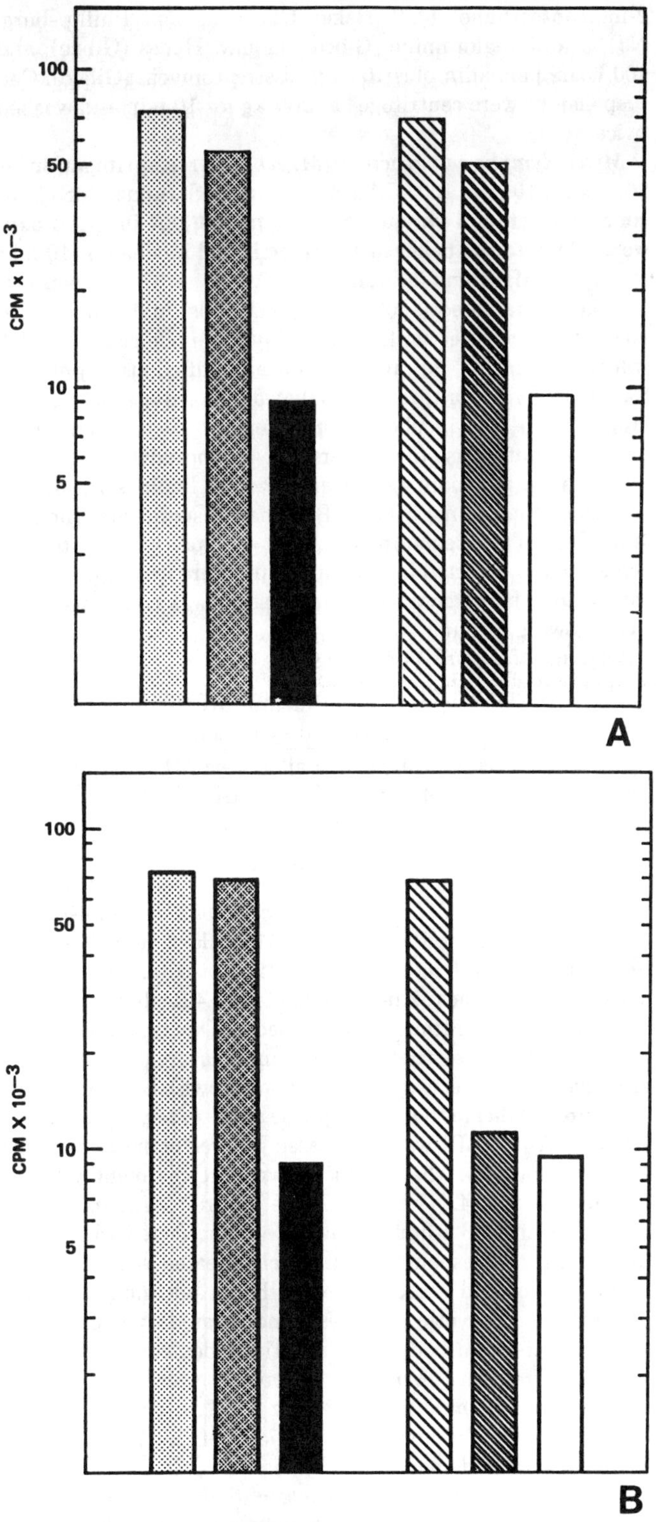

FIGURE 3. Mouse MLR following pretreatment of the responder cells with 13.4-immunotoxin. Figure 3A shows lymph node cells as the responder pretreated with 1 μg of 13.4-immunotoxin per 1 × 10^6 responder cells for 10 min at 37°C. Figure 3B shows data of the MLR following pretreatment of the stimulator cells under these same conditions. ( ) = A/J anti-B6 following pretreatment with 13.4-immunotoxin; ( ) = B6 and anti-A/J following pretreatment with 13.4-immunotoxin; ( ) = untreated A/J anti-B6; ( ) untreated B6 anti-A/J; ( ) A/J anti-A/J; ( ) B6 anti-B6.

2-mercaptoethanol (J.T. Baker Chemical Co., Phillipsburg, NJ), 2 mM L-glutamine (Gibco), 12 mM Hepes (Gibco), and 100 U/ml penicillin plus 100 μg/ml streptomycin (Gibco). Cell suspensions were centrifuged at 200 ×g for 10 min and washed twice.

Mixed lymphocyte reaction (MLR). After centrifugation at 200 ×g for 10 min, 100 mM lactose (Sigma, St. Louis, MS) final concentration and various amounts of the 13.4-immunotoxin were added to the pellet of spleen cells and incubated (10 min for mouse MLR and 60 min for rat MLR) at 37°C. Then 1×10^6 viable irradiated (3300 rads) spleen cells[7] in 0.1 ml culture media were cultured with 0.5×10^6 lymph node cells (1×10^6 spleen cells in Fig. 3a) at 37°C in a humidified atmosphere of 5% CO_2/95% air for three days, labeled with tritiated thymidine (1 μCi/well) and incubated for a further 18 hr. Cells were harvested onto glass fiber filters (M.A. Bioproducts) and thymidine incorporation was determined by liquid scintillation counting (Beckman LS 6800, Beckman Instruments, Inc., Irvine, CA). These experiments were set up in triplicate and deviations of reported incorporated cpm were less than 10% of the mean. The percentage of suppression was calculated with the following formula:

percentage of suppression

$$= \left[1 - \frac{\text{cpm of experimental MLR-cpm of untreated syngeneic MLR}}{\text{cpm of untreated allogeneic MLR-cpm of untreated syngeneic MLR}}\right] \times 100$$

RESULTS

Pretreatment of MLR stimulator cells with the 13.4-immunotoxin. In initial studies, the 10×10^7 cells were pelleted and pretreated with 100 μg of the 13.4-immunotoxin in 50 μl or the same amount of the toxin-unconjugated 13.4 for 10 min at 37°C and were washed 3 times in MLR media. This time was chosen from initial studies that showed 4 min pretreatment was as effective as 4 hr pretreatment (data not shown). Data presented in Figure 1 indicate that the response of the experimental group (B6 anti-A/J MLR) was suppressed by pretreatment with the 13.4-immunotoxin when compared with pretreatment with the unconjugated 13.4. The cpm of the control MLR using A/J responder and B6 stimulator cells was unaffected when compared with the response between cells treated with the 13.4-immunotoxin and those treated with the unconjugated 13.4. From these observations, it was demonstrated that toxin-conjugated anti-Ia antibody could effectively deplete MLR stimulator cells from an I-E-positive spleen.

Immunotoxin inhibition of mouse MLR in the presence of lactose. Despite the apparent specificity of the 13.4-immunotoxin conjugates demonstrated by the data presented in Figure 1, the possibility existed that contaminant ricin toxin (either whole ricin or free ricin B chains) might persist in such antibody ricin A chain toxin conjugates (*29*). Data presented in Figure 2 supports this premise. These data show the results of A/J-anti B6 and B6 anti-A/J MLRs in the presence and absence of 100 mM lactose. Stimulator cells were incubated with varying amounts of 13.4-immunotoxin from 0.1 to 10 μg per 10^6 cells, as above. In the control A/J anti-B6 MLR, the response was suppressed at a concentration of 10 μg of the 13.4-immunotoxin per 1×10^6 stimulator cells in the absence of lactose. In the presence of lactose, this suppression of stimulation was relieved, supporting our hypothesis that there were contaminant ricin molecules (or free B chains) in the 13.4-immunotoxin preparation. Because of the possibility of whole toxin and/or free B chain contaminants in the 13.4-immunotoxin preparations, we added 100 mM lactose to all subsequent assays in vitro.

Pretreatment of responder cells with 13.4-immunotoxin without diminished responsiveness. Data from many laboratories had supported the concept that recognition of stimulator cells by alloreactive T cells needed only cells bearing the allostimulating I region products. It was not clear, however, whether initiation of the primary MLR response required the presence of syngeneic Ia-bearing "antigen-presenting cells". To address this question, we utilized the 13.4-immunotoxin conjugate to treat responder lymph node cells in the same way that we treated stimulator cells. Data presented in Figure 3A show that pretreatment of strain A/J or strain B6 responder lymph nodes cells with 13.4-immunotoxin did not diminish their ability to respond in MLR. Data presented in Figure 3B show that this same antibody conjugate was effective in depleting stimulator cells from the A/J spleen but not from the B6 spleen (as in Fig. 1).

Rat MLR following pretreatment of stimulator cells with the 13.4-immunotoxin. To set the stage for the possibility of organ allograft transplantation, we decided to use rats as the model system for ease of organ transplantation. To do this, we needed to show that the same anti-Ia toxin conjugate system we had demonstrated in the mouse MLR would be effective in rat mixed lymphocyte cultures. Previous data had shown that certain mouse anti-Ia antisera crossreact with rat class II major histocompatibility antigens (*53*). So spleen cells from rats were

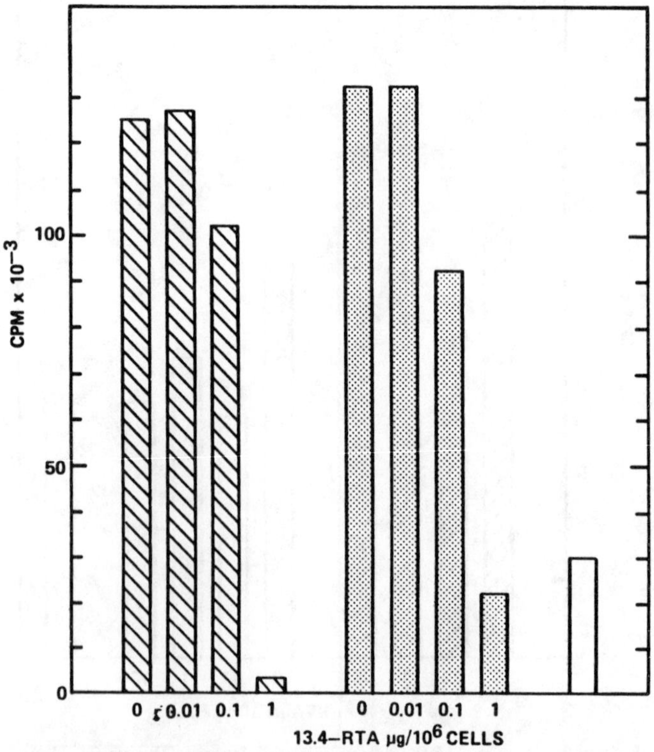

FIGURE 4. Rat MLR by pretreatment of stimulator cells with 13.4-immunotoxin in the presence or in the absence of lactose. Spleen cells from LBN rats were treated with 0, 0.01, 0.1, and 1 μg of 13.4-immunotoxin per 1×10^6 spleen cells for 60 min at 37°C in the presence (dotted) or absence (hatched) of 100 mM lactose. (open) = syngeneic MLR for a negative control. Lymph node cells (1×10^5) from ACI rats were used for responder cells.

pretreated with varying amounts of 13.4-immunotoxin for 60 min at 37°C prior to culture (Fig. 4). Such pretreatment with 13.4-immunotoxin was done in the presence of 100 mM lactose. Data obtained from the rat MLR was very similar to that presented for the murine system. 1 μg of 13.4-immunotoxin suppressed the ability of 1×10^6 rat spleen cells to stimulate a mixed lymphocyte culture as effectively as in the murine mixed lymphocyte culture. These data are presented as percentages of suppression of MLR using rat spleen cells pretreated with 13.4-immunotoxin. The percentage of suppression was calculated using the formula described in the *Materials and Methods* section. Complete suppression was obtained by pretreatment of rat spleen cells with 13.4-immunotoxin, whereas no suppression was observed using as pretreatment control antibody that had not been conjugated (Fig. 5).

DISCUSSION

Data presented in this article have demonstrated that pretreatment of spleen cells with murine anti-Ia monoclonal antibody 13.4 (anti I-E^k) conjugated with commercially prepared ricin A chain (but not unconjugated antibody) specifically removed the stimulator cell population from mixed lymphocyte cultures. Data presented in Figure 1 show that 13.4-immunotoxin effectively depleted stimulator cells from the spleen cell preparation and demonstrated specificity for the I-E^k molecule. Crossreactivity of anti-I-E antibodies with rat splenocytes had been previously demonstrated (*53*). We reconfirmed these data in our present study and have shown that the 13.4-imunotoxin is effective in removing stimulator cells from rat spleen cells following pretreatment with immunotoxin conjugates in the presence of lactose. These data suggest the possibility of using such murine anti-Ia antibodies for organ pretreatment in rodent organ allograft transplant systems.

Of particular interest was the finding that pretreatment of responder cells with 13.4-immunotoxin under conditions identical to those utilized to totally remove the stimulator cell population, showed no effect on the ability of lymph node cells to respond to MLR (Fig. 3). Thus, these data suggest that responder T cells can proliferate to allogeneic class II MHC products in the absence of syngeneic Ia-bearing cells.

Like many toxic proteins produced by bacteria and plants, ricin consists of two chains, the A chain and the B chain. The A chain is the active chain and the B chain is the binding chain (*29, 54–56*). The A chain inhibits protein synthesis on ribosomes and the B chain binds to galactose residues of the cell membrane and thereby helps the A chain to penetrate into the

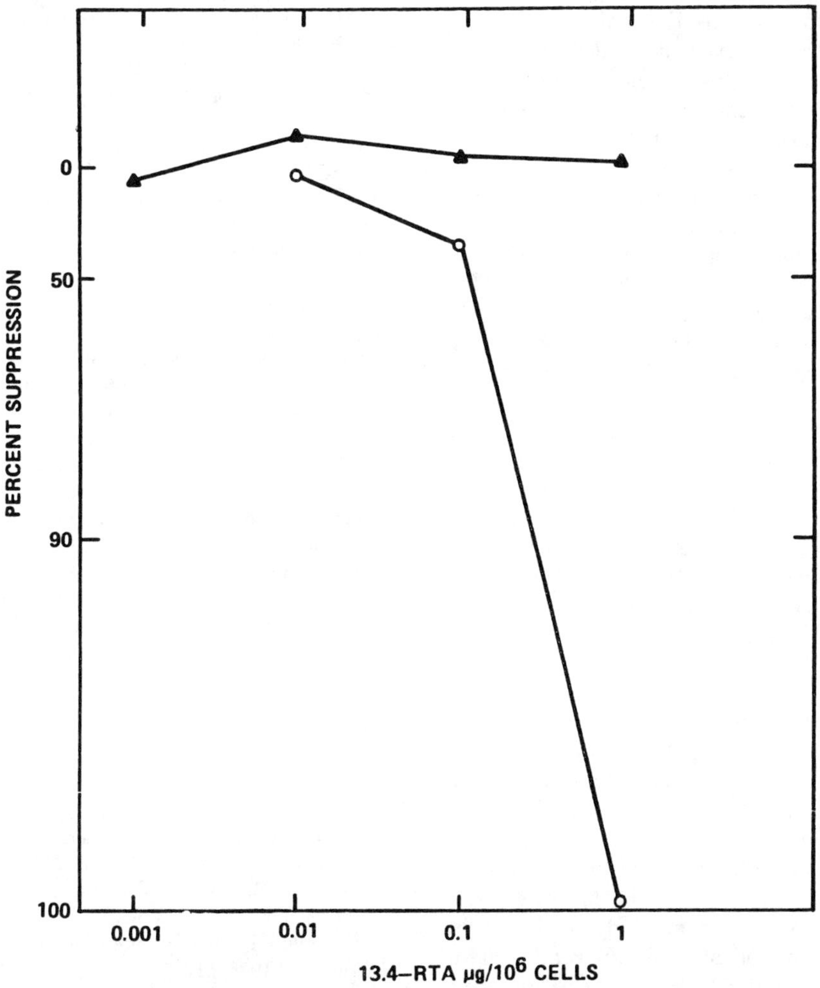

FIGURE 5. Percentage of suppression of rat MLR. Spleen cells from LBN rats used as stimulator cells were treated with serial concentrations of 13.4-immunotoxin or toxin unconjugated 13.4 only. (○——○) = percentage of suppression by 13.4-immunotoxin; (▲——▲) = percentage of suppression by 13.4 only. Results of triplicate cultures of one of three similar experiments are presented above. The cpm of syngeneic control was 1256; allogeneic control of 0% suppression was 26,711.

cytoplasm to reach the ribosomes. The B chain binds to almost all mammalian cells, so whole ricin toxin shows little selective specificity. In recent years, the possibility of replacing the B chain of toxins with other binding moieties (hormones or antibodies) having a different specificity has been explored. Although such toxin conjugates are usually not as toxic as intact toxin, they are highly toxic compared with the original hormones, antibodies, or A chain alone (*56–59*). Toxin A chains conjugated with monoclonal antibodies have been shown to exhibit highly specific reactions in elimination of target cells as previously reported (*44–47*). However, it has also been reported that some conjugates of antibody and the toxin A chain do not have the ability to kill target cells (*42, 50, 60*). The monoclonal anti-Ia antibody 13.4 conjugated with the ricin A chain used in these experiments, however, is highly cytotoxic. The selective cytotoxicity of this conjugate suggests that it is specific for the I-E region product recognized by antibody 13.4 but that the commerical preparation of ricin A chain was probably contaminated with ricin B chain or with whole toxin.

The nonspecific toxicity of immunotoxin conjugates containing whole ricin toxin that contains both the A chain and the B chain is usually blocked by carrying out the incubation in the presence of lactose, which has been shown to compete for the binding of the toxin to galactose residues on the cell surface (*39, 40, 42, 50, 59, 61*). If antibodies are conjugated with the toxin A chain and utilized to treat cells, the addition of lactose is theoretically not necessary. However, in our data, as shown in Figure 2, the MLR response in the absence of lactose was suppressed nonspecifically, even though our toxin conjugate did not show obvious evidence of contaminating B chains or whole ricin when analyzed by electrophoresis on SDS gel (data not shown). Vitetta et al. have also indicated that, when tested for toxicity in mice, trace contamination with B chains or ricin can occasionally be detected following purification of A chains, with no evidence of contaminating B chains on SDS gel (*29*). We therefore concluded that whole ricin or B chain contaminated our ricin toxin A chain preparation however the use of lactose in the cultures blocked the binding of the "contaminant" B chain.

Progress in organ transplantation—including kidney, heart, and bone marrow allografts—has been made over the past 20 years because of the development of new approaches including irradiation, immunosuppressants, antithymocyte globulin, and monoclonal antibodies. Recently reports of the clinical application of monoclonal antibodies directed against human T cells in renal allografts have appeared (*62, 63*). Though preliminary, the authors conclude that these observations warrant further study. Additionally, a marked prolongation of murine pancreatic islet cell and heart allograft survival across major histocompatibility complex barriers by pretreatment with a heterologous anti-Ia anti-serum and complement prior to transplantation has been reported recently (*9, 30*). By pretreatment of donor bone marrow cells with monoclonal anti-Thy-1.2 coupled with whole ricin, a successful murine bone marrow transplantation across major histocompatibility barriers has been reported (*50*). We have demonstrated, in this article, the first trial of a mouse anti-Ia monoclonal antibody immunotoxin to deplete stimulator cells from rodent MLR. From these data, we conclude that such α Ia-immunotoxins might be useful to pretreat selected organ allografts for transplantation across major histocompatibility barriers.

Acknowledgments. We thank P. Diane Infante, Koulin Chou, and Leigh Scalapino (Cetus Corporation) for their expert technical assistance and John Frelinger, Ph.D., and Susan Conner for the SDS-PAGE. We acknowledge the kind supply of rats from Dennis Modry, M.D., and Grant Hoyt, and we offer special thanks to Robyn Kizer and Diane O'Neill for their careful and patient secretarial assistance in the preparation of the manuscript.

REFERENCES

1. Snell GD. The homograft reaction. Annu Rev Microbiol 1957; 2: 439.
2. Sollinger HW, Burkholder PM, Ramus WR, Bach FH. Prolonged survival of xenografts after organ culture. Surgery 1977; 81: 74.
3. Lacy PE, Davie JM, Finke EH. Prolongation of islet allograft survival following *in vitro* culture (24°C) and a single injection of ALS. Science 1979; 204; 312.
4. Lacy PE, David JM, Finke EH. Prolongation of islet xenograft survival without continuous immunosuppression. Science 1980; 209: 283.
5. Lafferty KJ, Cooley MA, Woolnough J, Walker KZ. Thyroid allograft immunogenicity is reduced after a period in organ culture. Science 1975; 188: 259.
6. Steinmuller D. Passenger leukocytes and the immunogenicity of skin allografts: a critical reevaluation. Transplant Proc 1982; 8: 1094.
7. Lacy PE, Davie JM, Finke ED. Induction of rejection of successful allografts of rat islets by donor peritoneal exudate cells. Transplantation 1979; 28: 415.
8. Talmage DW, Dart G, Radovich J, Lafferty KJ. Activation of transplant immunity: effect of donor leukocytes on thyroid allograft rejection. Science 1976; 191: 385.
9. Faustman D, Hauptfeld V, Lacy P, Davie J. Prolongation of murine islet allograft survival by pretreatment of islets with antibody directed to Ia determinants. Proc Natl Acad Sci USA 1982; 78: 5156.
10. Stuart FP, Garrick T, Holter A, Lynch A, Bastien E. Delayed rejection of renal allografts in the rat and dog by reduction of passenger leukocytes. Surgery 1971; 70: 128.
11. Guttmann RD, Lindquist RR. Renal transplantation in inbred rat: XI. Reduction of allograft immunogenicity by cytotoxic drug pretreatment of donors. Transplantation 1969; 8: 490.
12. Varkarakis MJ, Sampson D, Brede HD, Murphy GP. The immunosuppressive effect of procarbazine hydrochloride in canine renal allografts. Transplantation 1972; 13: 42.
13. Zincke H, Woods JE. Attempted immunological alteration of canine renal allograft donors. Transplantation 1974; 18: 480.
14. Beyer MM, Friedman EA. Prolonged survival of rabbit skin and kidney allografts following donor treatment with cytosine arabinoside. Transplantation 1975; 19: 60.
15. Soots A, Hayry P. Prolongation of rat cardiac allograft survival by donor pretreatment. Transplantation 1978, 25: 259.
16. Swistel AJ, McCabe RE, Lorico DR, Wildstein A, Fitzpatrick HF. The effect of donor pretreatment and low-dose immunosuppression on the 24-hour preserved canine renal allograft. Transplant Proc 1979; 11: 1673.
17. Freeman JS, Chamberlain EC, Reemtsma K, Steinmuller D. Prolongation of rat heart allografts by donor pretreatment with immunosuppressive agents. Transplant Proc 1971; 3: 580.
18. Oluwole S, Hardy MA, Wang T, et al. Donor pretreatment: rat heart allograft survival and measurement of passenger leukocyte depletion with indium-111. Transplantation 1980; 30: 31.
19. Schwartz RH, David CS, Sachs DH, Paul WE. T lymphocyte-enriched murine peritoneal exudate cells: III. Inhibition of antigen-induced T lymphocyte proliferation with anti-Ia antisera. J Immunol 1976; 117: 531.
20. Longo DL, Schwartz RH. Inhibition of antigen-induced proliferation of T cells from radiation-induced bone marrow chimeras by a monoclonal antibody directed against an Ia determinant on the antigen-presenting cell. Proc Natl Acad Sci USA 1981; 78: 514.
21. Frelinger JA, Niederhuber JE, Shreffler DC. Inhibition of immune

response *in vitro* by specific antiserums to Ia antigens. Science 1975; 188: 268.
22. Fathman CG, Hengartner H. Crossreactive mixed lymphocyte reaction determinants recognized by cloned alloreactive T cells. Proc Natl Acad Sci USA 1979; 76: 5863.
23. Fathman CG, Kimoto M, Melvold R, David CS. Reconstitution of Ir genes, Ia antigens, and mixed lymphocyte reaction determinants by gene complementation. Proc Natl Acad Sci USA 1981; 78: 1853.
24. Fathman CG. Hybrid I region antigens. Transplantation 1980; 30: 1.
25. Fathman CG, Kimoto M. Studies utilizing murine T cell clones: Ir genes, Ia antigens and MLR stimulating determinants. Immunol Rev 1981; 54: 57.
26. Fathman CG, Frelinger JG. T-lymphocyte clones. Annu Rev Immunol 1983; 1: 633.
27. Davies DAL, Staines NA. A cardinal role for I-region antigens (Ia) in immunological enhancement, and the clinical implications. Transplant Rev 1976; 30: 18.
28. McKenzie IFC, Henning MM. The I region transplantation antigens: immunogenicity and enhancement. J Immunogenetics 1977; 4: 259.
29. Faustman D, Kraus P, Lacy PE, Finke EH, Davie JM. Survival of heart allografts in non-immunosuppressed murine recipients by pretreatment of the donor tissue with anti-Ia antibodies. Transplantation 1982; 34; 302.
30. Vitetta ES, Krolich KA, Miyama-Inaba M, Cushley W, Uhr JW. Immunotoxins: a new approach to cancer therapy. Science 1983; 219: 644.
31. Jansen FK, Blythman HE, Carriere D, et al. High specific cytotoxicity of antibody-toxin hybrid molecules (immunotoxins) for target cells. Immunol Lett 1980; 2: 97.
32. Masuho Y, Hara T. Target-cell cytotoxicity of a hybrid of Fab′ of immunoglobulin and A-chain of ricin. Gan 1980; 71: 759.
33. Raso V, Griffin T. Specific cytotoxicity of a human immunoglobulin-directed Fab′-ricin A chain conjugate. J Immunol 1980; 125: 2610.
34. Raso V. Antibody mediated delivery of toxic molecules to antigen bearing target cells. Immunol Rev 1982; 62: 93.
35. Thorpe PE, Ross WCJ, Cumber AJ, Hinson CA, Edwards DC, Davies AJS. Toxicity of diphtheria toxin for lymphoblastoid cells in increased by conjugation to antilymphocytic globulin. Nature 1978; 271: 752.
36. Ross WCJ, Thorpe PE, Cumber AJ, Edwards DC, Hinson CA, Davies AJS. Increased toxicity of diphtheria toxin for human lymphoblastoid cells following covalent linkage to anti-(human lymphocyte) globulin or its $F(ab')_2$ fragment. Eur J Biochem 1980; 104: 381.
37. Gilliland DG, Collier RJ. A model system involving anti-concanavalin A for antibody targeting of diphtheria toxin fragment A. Cancer Res 1980; 40: 3564.
38. Masuho Y, Hara T, Noguchi T. Preparation of a hybrid of fragment Fab′ of antibody and fragment A of diphtheria toxin and its cytotoxicity. Biochem Biophys Commun 1979; 90: 320.
39. Thorpe PE, Cumber AJ, Williams N, Edwards DC, Ross WCJ, Davies AJS. Abrogation of the non-specific toxicity of abrin conjugated to anti-lymphocyte globulin. Clin Exp Immunol 1981; 43: 195.
40. Youle RJ, Neville Jr. DM. Anti-Thy 1.2 monoclonal antibody linked to ricin is a potent cell-type-specific toxin. Proc Natl Acad Sci USA 1980; 77: 5483.
41. Blythman HE, Casellas P, Gros O, et al. Immunotoxins: Hybrid molecules of monoclonal antibodies and a toxin subunit specifically kill tumor cells. Nature 1981; 290 :145.
42. Thorpe PE, Mason DW, Brown ANF, et al. Selective killing of malignant cells in a leukemic rat bone marrow using an antibody-ricin conjugate. Nature 1981; 297: 594.
43. Houston LL, Nowinski RC. Cell-specificity cytotoxicity expressed by a conjugate of ricin and murine monoclonal antibody directed against Thy 1.1 antigen: Cancer Res 1981; 41: 3913.
44. Krolick KA, Villemez C, Isakson P, Uhr JW, Vitetta ES. Selective killing of normal or neoplastic B cells by antibodies coupled to the A chain of ricin. Proc Natl Acad Sci USA 1980; 77: 5419.
45. Gilliland DG, Steplewski Z, Collier RJ, Mitchell KF, Chang TH, Koprowski H. Antibody-directed cytotonic agents: use of monoclonal antibody to direct the action of toxin A chains to colorectal carcinoma cells. Proc Natl Acad Sci USA 1980; 77: 4539.
46. Roso V, Ritz J, Basala M, Schlossman SF. Monoclonal antibody-ricin A chain conjugate selectively cytotoxic for cells bearing the common acute lymphoblastic leukemia antigen. Cancer Res 1982; 42: 457.
47. Oeltmann TN, Forbes JT. Inhibition of mouse spleen cell function of diphthelia toxin fragment A coupled to anti-mouse Thy 1.2 and by ricin A chain coupled to anti-mouse IgM. Arch Biochem Biophys 1981; 209: 362.
48. Thorpe PE, Brown ANF, Ross WCJ, et al. Cytotoxicity acquired by conjugation of an anti-Thy 1.1 monoclonal antibody and the ribosome-inactivating protein, gelonin. Eur J Biochem 1981; 116: 447.
49. Krolick KA, Uhr JW, Vitetta ES. Selective killing of leukemia cells by antibody-toxin conjugates: implications for autologous bone marrow transplantation. Nature 1982; 295: 604.
50. Vallera DA, Youle RJ, Neville DM, Jr., Kersey JH. Bone marrow transplantation across major histocompatibility barriers: I. Protection of mice from lethal graft-vs.-host disease by pretreatment of donor cells with monoclonal anti-Thy-1.2 coupled to the toxin ricin. J Exp Med 1982; 155: 949.
51. Hammerling GJ, Hammerling U, Lemke H. Isolation of twelve monoclonal antibodies against Ia and H-2 antigens: serological characterization and reactivity with B and T lymphocytes. Immunogenetics 1979; 8: 433.
52. Carlsson J, Drevin N, Axen R. Protein thiolation and reversible protein-protein conjugation. N-succinimidyl 3-(2-pyridyldithio) propionate, a new heterobifunctional reagent. Biochem J 1978; 173; 723.
53. Wettstein PJ, Frelinger JG, Hood L. Serological and biochemical characterization of rat (RT 1) class II molecules with restricted mouse anti-Ia sera. Immunogenetics 1981; 13: 93.
54. Olsnes S, Pihl A. Different biological properties of the two constituent peptide chains of ricin, a toxic protein inhibiting protein synthesis. Biochem. 1973; 12: 3121.
55. Olsnes S, Pihl A. Chimeric toxins. Pharmacol Ther 1981; 15: 355.
56. Jansen FK, Blythman HE, Carriere D, Casellas P, et al. Immunotoxins: hybrid molecules combining high specificity and potent cytotoxicity. Immunol Rev 1982; 62: 185.
57. Neville DM Jr., Youle RJ. Monoclonal antibody-ricin or ricin A chain hybrids: kinetics analysis of cell killing for tumor therapy. Immunol Rev 1982; 62: 75.
58. Thorpe PE, Ross WCJ. The preparation and cytotoxic properties of antibody-toxin conjugates. Immunol Rev 1982; 62: 119.
59. Houston LL. Transport of ricin A chain after prior treatment of mouse leukemia cells with ricin B chain. J Biol Chem 1982; 257: 1532.
60. Mason DW, Thorpe PE, Ross WCJ. Elimination of leukemic cells from rodent bone marrow *in vitro* with antibody-ricin conjugates: implications for autologous marrow transplantation in man. Cancer Surv 1982; 1: 389.
61. Olsnes S, Saltvedt E, Pihl A. Isolation and comparison of galactose-binding lectins from Abrus precatorius and Ricius communis. J Biol Chem 1974; 249: 802.
62. Cosimi AB, Colvin RB, Burton RC, et al. Use of monoclonal antibodies to T-cell subsets for immunologic monitoring and treatment in recipients of renal allografts. N Engl J Med 1981; 305: 308.
63. Russell PS. New approach to the use of antibodies for immunosuppression. Transplant Proc 1982; 14: 506.

Received 21 February 1984.
Accepted 10 December 1984.

0041-1337/86/4202-0212$02.00/0
TRANSPLANTATION
Vol. 42, No. 2
Printed in U.S.A.

DIFFERENCES IN IMMUNOGLOBULIN SUBCLASSES BETWEEN DYE EXCLUSION AND ^{51}Cr RELEASE COMPLEMENT-DEPENDENT LYMPHOCYTOTOXICITY ASSAYS

P. R. McCONNACHIE,[1,2] J. F. DENEGRI,[1] F. E. LOWER,[3] D. S. TORRY,[4] AND J. A. McINTYRE[5]

Immunotransplant Laboratory, Division of Hematopathology, Vancouver General Hospital, Vancouver, British Columbia, Canada V5Z 1M9; Immunotransplant Laboratory, Memorial Medical Center, Springfield, Illinois 62781; and Departments of Microbiology and Obstetrics and Gynecology, Southern Illinois University School of Medicine, Springfield, Illinois 62708

Paradoxical differences previously noted between lymphocytotoxicity detected by dye exclusion at room temperature (CDCE) or by ^{51}Cr release (CDC^{51}Cr) at 37°C in maternal antipaternal complement-dependent lymphocytoxicity have suggested that CDCE and CDC^{51}Cr at 37°C, but not at 20°C, may detect different immunological antibody-antigen interactions. Reactions in the two test systems against the same target cells were compared in sera from known immune dialysis patients, secondary aborting women, and refractory platelet recipients before and after heat treatment of sera, absorption with solid-phase heparin, anti-light-chain augmentation, and the addition of murine monoclonal anti-IgG subclass antibodies. The results demonstrate significant differences between the two tests using the same target and sera. Further, the results imply the presence of an inhibitor and an inhibitor of inhibitor in sera. The involvement of different immunoglobulin subclasses was shown in the two tests. These data demonstrate the necessity for further study of the nature of the differences in the mechanisms of these clinically important antibody-detecting systems.

Microlymphocytotoxicity or complement-dependent lymphocytotoxicity measured by dye exclusion (*1*) (CDCE)* is the standard tissue typing and transplant crossmatch test. Over recent years the test has been modified in various ways for increased sensitivity (*2–4*) but the endpoint is still loss of membrane integrity assessed by microscopic evaluation of the proportion of swollen target cells containing dye. The same endpoint of loss of membrane integrity can also be detected more quantitatively through the release of ^{51}Cr as chromate ion in the ^{51}Cr release assay described by Rogentine (*5*), which has been shown to correlate extremely closely with CDCE. The ^{51}Cr release complement-dependent lymphocytotoxicity assay (CDC^{51}Cr) when positive at 37°C in the presence of a negative pretransplant CDCE crossmatch is associated with decreased renal graft survival (*6–8*), and for that reason has been thought to be more sensitive than, or different from, CDCE. In our studies of maternal antipaternal immunity in women described as secondary aborters, we have detected paradoxical differences between the reaction patterns of CDCE and CDC^{51}Cr (*9, 10*). These differences suggest that CDC^{51}Cr at 37°C and CDCE at 20°C do not detect the same immunological interactions. Our studies of this phenomenon are detailed in this investigation.

MATERIALS AND METHODS

Three sources of sera were used for comparisons of CDCE and CDC^{51}Cr reactions. These were chronic hemodialysis patients (*35*), women with repeated spontaneous abortions who had been classified as secondary aborters (*15*), and patients who had received multiple platelet transfusions for thrombocytopenia (*3*). All sera were known to be reactive to various members of a 51-member HLA select lymphocyte panel by CDCE. The lymphocyte panel members and the husbands of the secondary aborters provided target lymphocytes for the comparative tests.

CDCE was performed by the modified two-step method (*4*) with a wash prior to the addition of complement. In some tests CDCE was done with and without the wash step. The CDC^{51}Cr assay was modified from the Rogentine method (*5*) by incubation at 37°C (*6*) and by using diluted complement titrated to reduce spontaneous lysis. The original Rogentine method for CDC^{51}Cr involved a 10 min room temperature incubation of 0.020 ml serum and 5×10^4 ^{51}Cr-labeled lymphocytes in 0.025 ml of cell culture medium in duplicate 12×75 mm glass tubes. Undiluted complement, 0.025 ml was then added, and incubation proceeded for a further 2 hr at room temperature. In our modified method, the target cell preparation was the same, but we increased the test serum volume to 0.050 ml and used the complement at a pretested dilution (1/10 or 1/20) in medium 199–10% fetal calf serum (FCS) in a volume of 0.2 ml. The three test constituents were added together and test incubation was for 3.5 hr at 37°C in 5% CO_2 in air. The test reaction was stopped with the addition of 2 ml 4°C Hanks' balanced salt solution (HBSS) and centrifugation for 7 min at 1500×G at 4°C. Supernatants were decanted into empty tubes. For each test, both supernatant tubes and tubes containing cell pellets (residual) were counted in a gamma counter with a ^{51}Cr window. Test ^{51}Cr release was (cpm supernatant ÷ [cpm supernatant + cpm residual]) × 100. Mean test release of duplicate tubes was expressed as percentage of maximum release by the formula:

$$\frac{(\text{test release} - \text{spontaneous release})}{(\text{maximum release} - \text{spontaneous release})} \times 100.$$

[1] Vancouver General Hospital.

[2] To whom correspondence should be addressed, at Immunotransplant Laboratory, Memorial Medical Center, 800 North Rutledge, Springfield, Illinois 62781.

[3] Memorial Medical Center.

[4] Department of Microbiology, Southern Illinois University School of Medicine, Springfield IL 62708.

[5] Department of Obstetrics and Gynecology, Southern Illinois University School of Medicine. Current address; Methodist Center for Reproduction and Transplantation Immunology, Methodist Hospital, Indianapolis Indiana 46202.

* Abbreviations used: ADCC, antibody-dependent cell-mediated cytotoxicity; CDC, complement-dependent lymphocytotoxicity; CDCE, complement-dependent lymphocytotoxicity by dye exclusion; FCS, fetal calf serum; HBSS, Hanks' balanced salt solution.

Maximum release was obtained in 2% triton X. We considered 10% of maximum ^{51}Cr release to be positive. Background or spontaneous release was generally 4–10% and was that obtained when FCS was substituted for test serum.

A number of sera from each group were tested against the same ^{51}Cr-labeled targets in a complement-independent, antibody-dependent cell-mediated cytotoxicity assay (ADCC) (*6*). The only difference between ADCC and our modified CDC^{51}Cr was the substitution of a known normal effector cell preparation (1×10^6 lymphocytes in 0.2 ml 199–10% FCS) for the complement dilution. For ADCC, spontaneous release was that obtained with normal effector cells and known nonreactive AB serum in place of the test serum. All other assay conditions were the same as for CDC^{51}Cr. All effector cells used were previously known to react with the particular antiserum–target cell combinations tested.

We examined the effects of the following treatments on CDCE, CDC^{51}Cr and some ADCC reactions of known positive sera against the same target cells. Sera were heat treated at 56° for 30 min to test for inhibitory activity (*11*) or were absorbed with equal volumes of solid-phase heparin conjugated to sepharose CL 6B (Pharmacia). The rationale for the use of solid-phase heparin as an absorbent is that s.c. heparin injections twice a day have been shown to prevent recurrent secondary spontaneous abortions (*13*) and recent evidence has demonstrated that control of in vitro CDCE/CDC^{51}Cr is under the influence of serum inhibitors and regulatory molecules including heparin (*16*). Absorptions were at room temperature for 1 hr on a rocking platform. Sera were removed from the absorbent following 5-min centrifugations at 6000 ×G. The control absorbent was a human normal serum—Sepharose CL-6B preparation. Sequential known nonreactive serum samples from one hemodialysis patient were tested in CDCE and CDC^{51}Cr against the same target cell to which subsequent samples were demonstrably positive. The negative samples were tested with the antiglobulin augmentation method in CDCE (*12*), which was adapted to CDC^{51}Cr as follows: Target cells and test sera were incubated together for 30 min and then washed ("flick" method for CDCE, added medium plus centrifugation and decanting for CDC^{51}Cr). Equal amounts of pretitrated subcytotoxic antikappa (Atlantic antibody) were added, followed by complement and normal incubation. This was to see if weak or negative CDC^{51}Cr reactions could be augmented by antikappa, as has been demonstrated in CDCE. In other experiments 1:10 dilutions of monoclonal anti-IgG$_1$, anti-IgG$_2$, anti-IgG$_3$, or anti-IgG$_4$ monoclonal antibodies (Gibco, Grand Island, NY) were added to 0.002 ml or 0.025 ml quantity to CDCE and CDC^{51}Cr assays prior to the addition of target cells and complement to test for differences in IgG subclass involvement in the two test systems. The monoclonal antibodies were all of the IgG$_1$ subclass.

RESULTS

Because of previous studies that had demonstrated that pretransplant crossmatches in hemodialysis patients' sera can be negative by CDCE and positive to the same donor cell by CDC^{51}Cr (*7, 8*), we chose 110 sera from 35 multitransfused dialysis patients and tested the sera by both tests in parallel against 4–5 target lymphocytes. The results were compared by chi square analysis, (Table 1). which indicated that the distribution of concordant and discordant pairs of reactions deviated significantly from what would be predicted by chance. Both tests were positive in the same serum in 26% of the 291 positive tests, CDCE alone was positive in 32%, and CDC^{51}Cr alone was positive in 42%. Since we had determined in the previous studies with serum titrations that prozone was not a factor when one test was positive and the other negative, we proceeded with further studies to examine the differences between the two tests.

The effect of heat treatment of 6 sera tested in all three systems is shown in Table 2. Sera VB, HO, and WH were from patients who had developed lymphocytotoxic antibodies following multiple platelet transfusions for thrombocytopenia. The others were from secondary aborters. Platelet recipients' sera were tested against panel lymphocytes and aborters against paternal lymphocytes. Heat-treated sera were tested with and without the wash step in all three test systems.

There are three points to be made in this set of results. First, it is clear that in the untreated sera all three tests are independent of each other. A strong CDCE does not predict strong CDC^{51}Cr or ADCC (serum HO$_1$) and ADCC does not predict CDCE (WK). Second, heat treatment of sera produced different results in the complement-dependent test systems. Only 1 of 8 positive CDCE reactions was heat sensitive but all positive CDC^{51}Cr reactions (8/8) were severely affected. The decrease in ^{51}Cr release ranged from 55–100%; the mean decrease was 79±18%. Only 2 of 7 ADCC reactions were heat-sensitive. Third, the singular CDCE reaction that was heat-sensitive was

TABLE 1. Comparison of CDCE versus CDC^{51}Cr in 110 sera from dialysis patients against 5 target cells

CDCE reactions	CDC^{51}Cr reactions	
	Positive[a]	Negative
Positive[a]	77	92
Negative	122	238

Chi square = 6.66
$.005<P<001$

[a] A positive reaction in CDC^{51}Cr was 10% of maximum ^{51}Cr release or greater. A positive CDCE reaction was a cytotoxicity score of 4 or more.

TABLE 2. Effect of heating sera at 56°C for 30 min on CDCE, CDC^{51}Cr, and ADCC reactions

Serum	Cytotoxicity[b] in CDCE		% Max ^{51}Cr Release			
			CDC^{51}Cr		ADCC	
	Untreated	56°C	Untreated	56°C	Untreated	56°C
VB$_1$[a]	8,8	8,8	35.6	0[d]	14.2	0[e]
VB$_2$	8,8	8,8	50.1	13.2[d]	20.0	7.5[e]
HO$_1$	8,8	2,2[c]	3.3	0.5	2.2	2.8
HO$_2$	8,8	8,8	26.3	2.9[d]	27.4	23.2
WH	8,8	8,8	22.9	5.4[c]	5.3	4.0
NM	8,8	8,8	50.3	5.5[c]	17.1	12.9
BW$_1$	8,8	8,8	42.5	8.7[c]	60.2	53.1
BW$_2$	8,8	8,8	32.5	0[c]	16.2	12.6
WK	1,1	1,1	10.3	4.6[c]	24.8	25.3

[a] Subscript numbers refer to the same serum tested against different targets.
[b] Cytotoxicity expressed in standard 1–8 range, duplicate reactions: 1, 0–10% cytotoxicity; 2, 11–20%; 4, 21–50%; 6, 51–80%; 8, 81–100%.
[c] A wash step restored activity to original level.
[d] A wash step failed to restore activity to original level.
[e] A wash step restored activity to greater than 50% of original level.

restored to original levels when a wash step was added (HO_1). This was not the case with the heat-sensitive $CDC^{51}Cr$ reactions of sera VB and HO_2. A wash step restored activity only to 4.2%, 4.0%, and 5.6%, respectively. In the remaining sera—WH, NM, BW, BW_2, and WK—a wash step returned ^{51}Cr release to within 3–5% of untreated levels. These differential effects of heat treatment and wash steps in different sera in different tests suggest biological rather than physical differences between the test systems, as all sera were tested undiluted in this experiment.

Heparin has been successfully used as a treatment to prevent secondary recurrent abortion (*13*). For that reason we had previously used heparin absorption in the strong $CDC^{51}Cr$ that was so prevalent in secondary aborters. This is shown in 8 secondary aborters' antipaternal $CDC^{51}Cr$ (Table 3). Heparin absorption reduced $CDC^{51}Cr$ significantly in all 8 sera (mean reduction 95%±8.5). The addition of a wash step restored serum reactivity to original levels or above in all sera. There was no significant effect of heparin absorption on ADCC (data not shown, mean reduction 18.1%±7.8). A different effect was seen when the same sera were tested against a 51-member HLA select frozen lymphocyte panel in CDCE (Table 4). Three patterns were apparent in the heparin-absorbed sera; reactions of a given serum against certain individual panel cells remained unchanged to some extent in all sera (except serum WK, in which all reactions became negative), some positive reactions became negative, and some previously negative reactions became positive. The mean change of panel reactivity was a loss of 40.8% ± 25% of the positive reactions. Another interesting point was that the reactions of two sera, FM and WK, were only positive against panel cells sharing HLA antigens with the respective husbands of the women. Exposure of the sera to solid-phase heparin reduced positive reactions to negative on 6 of the previously positive 13 panel cells for serum FM, and reduced positive reactions to negative on all 13 previously positive cells for serum WK. Different panel cells were involved in the positive reaction with the two sera.

TABLE 3. Effect of absorptions with solid-phase heparin on maternal antipaternal $CDC^{51}Cr$

	% ^{51}Cr release	
	Before heparin absorption	After heparin absorption[a]
KC	66	0
PM	61	3.7
FM	21.9	0
BW	60	1.4
AM	70.8	16.6
WK	27.7	0
BM	67.1	0

[a] A wash step restored activity to original level or greater.

TABLE 4. Effect of exposure of serum to solid-phase heparin on dye exclusion cytotoxicity in a 51-member lymphocyte panel

Sera	Serum reactivity to panel			
	Before heparin absorption	After heparin absorption	% Reactivity	
			Lost	Gained
KC	40/51[b]	24/51	40	
PM	26/51	29/51	19.2	4.5
FM[a]	13/51	7/51	46.5	
BW	24/50	14/50	42	14.3
AM	35/51	32/51	8.6	3.1
WK[a]	13/51	0/51	100	
BM	25/51	20/51	24	3.2

[a] Panel reactivity explicable in terms of paternal HLA antigens.
[b] Positive reactions/total reactions; 4,6,8 reactions were considered positive.

Another comparison of CDCE and $CDC^{51}Cr$ was carried out with sequential serum samples from a dialysis patient. The sera were chosen to cover 6 monthly samples prior to a positive reaction developing in CDCE (Table 5). $CDC^{51}Cr$ never was positive against the target cell used. We attempted to augment weak or negative CDCE and $CDC^{51}Cr$ in the sera preceding the known positive specimens using a 1/400 dilution of anti–kappa-light-chain antibody. Antikappa augmented CDCE reactions in 4 specimens in the 4 months preceding the known positive specimens but in no sample was $CDC^{51}Cr$ converted to positive.

We then examined the effect of adding equal volumes of murine IgG_1, monoclonal anti-IgG subclass antibodies to titrated sera in antipaternal CDCE and $CDC^{51}Cr$. The dilutions chosen were peak CDCE (1/16) and the next dilution (1/32), and peak $CDC^{51}Cr$ (1/4). Then 1 μl of monoclonal antibody was added to the maternal serum dilution in CDCE and 50 μl in $CDC^{51}Cr$. Adding anti-IgG subclass antibodies produced different results in CDCE and $CDC^{51}Cr$ (Table 6). Anti-IgG_1 blocked both CDCE and $CDC^{51}Cr$ completely. Anti-IgG_3 had a detectable blocking effect only in $CDC^{51}Cr$. The blocking of CDCE by anti-IgG_1 was most evident at the 1/32 serum dilution but was quite apparent at 1/16. Although it is difficult to quantitate visual cytotoxicity, the mean reduction in CDCE with added anti-IgG_1 was 66% at 1/16 and 81% at 1/32. This was quite comparable to the 88 and 94% blocking of $CDC^{51}Cr$ by anti-IgG_1. By the same form of calculation ([mean cytotoxicity score with anti-IgG ÷ mean cytotoxicity score untreated] −1) anti-IgG_3 only produced a 6% decrease in CDCE at 1/32 as compared with 45% in $CDC^{51}Cr$. Although there seemed to be an inhibition of CDCE at 1/32 by anti-IgG_2 (31%) we did not consider this significant as 4 of the 6 replicates were still more than 50% cytotoxic and there was no detectable effect at the 1/16 dilution. Repeated tests of serum samples from two other secondary aborters confirmed the 80–90% and 40–45% inhibition of antipaternal $CDC^{51}Cr$ by anti-IgG_1 and anti-IgG_3, respectively.[6]

DISCUSSION

These studies were stimulated by the observation that neither a positive CDCE nor positive $CDC^{51}Cr$ at 37°C in the same

TABLE 5. Antiglobulin enhancement of weak or negative CDCE and $CDC^{51}Cr$

Serum date	Normal test CDCE[a]	$CDC^{51}Cr^b$	Anti-kappa added (1/100)	
			CDCE[a]	$CDC^{51}Cr^b$
Jan	11	4.3	22	2.1
Feb	11	6.5	22	4.0
Mar	11	7.0	64	2.6
Apr	11	1.5	44	1.0
May	11	1.7	44	2.0
Jun	11	ND	88	ND
Jul	66	ND	88	ND
Aug	68	ND	88	ND

[a] Results expressed as duplicate standard lymphocytotoxicity scores.
[b] Results expressed as mean % max. ^{51}Cr release from duplicate tubes.

TABLE 6. Effect of added anti-IgG subclass monoclonal antibodies on maternal antipaternal CDCE and $CDC^{51}Cr$

Added anti-IgG	Cytotoxicity scores in CDCE[a]	% ^{51}Cr release in $CDC^{51}Cr$		
	Serum 1 (1/16)[c]	Serum (1/32)	Serum (1/4)	Serum[b] (1/4)
None	8 8 8 8 8 8	6 4 6 6 6 4	19.0	30
Anti-IgG_1 (1/10)[c]	2 4 2 4 2 2 (66.0%)[d]	1 1 1 1 1 1 (81.0%)[d]	2.3 (88%)[d]	1.7 (94%)[d]
Anti-IgG_2 (1/10)	6 6 8 8 8 8	6 2 4 2 4 4	20.5	26.3
Anti-IgG_3 (1/10)	8 8 6 6 6 6	6 6 4 4 6 4	10.5 (45%)[d]	18.0 (40%)[d]
Anti-IgG_4 (1/10)	6 8 8 8 6 6	6 6 6 6 6 4	18.6	24.9

[a] 1; 0–10% cytotoxicity, 2; 11–20%, 4; 21–50%, 6; 51–80%, 8; 81–100%. Six replicate reactions were recorded.

[b] Two subsequent monthly serum samples from the same secondary aborter were tested.

[c] Maternal serum or anti subclass antibody dilution in fetal calf serum.

[d] % inhibition of $CDC^{51}Cr$ or CDCE.

serum predicted that the other would be positive against the same target cell, in spite of the high correlation between the two test systems demonstrated by chi-square. This indicates that the two tests may be detecting either common or associated but different factors. However, the differences in reactions were sufficient to support exploration of potential biological differences between the two tests. Neither prozone (*11*) nor relative sensitivity differences (*5*) would explain the high frequency of either test being positive and the other negative with the same serum and complement against the same target cell. Heat treatment of sera demonstrated significant differences between the two tests; CDCE was inhibited by heat treatment in only 1 of 8 tests but $CDC^{51}Cr$ was markedly inhibited or blocked in 8 of 9 tests.

That the effect of heat treatment was reversible with the addition of a wash step (i.e., a two-stage test) was not surprising as this has been previously described as caused by anticomplementary factors produced by heating (*11*) or by long-term storage of serum (*14*). However, we observed that a wash step did not uniformly restore $CDC^{51}Cr$ activity in heat-treated sera from the platelet-transfused patients but it did restore $CDC^{51}Cr$ activity to the original level in spontaneous aborters' sera, and CDCE reactivity was also restored to original levels with a wash step in both groups of sera. Similar losses of $CDC^{51}Cr$ activity were obtained following serum absorption with solid-phase heparin-sepharose. This was used because of preliminary successes using s.c. heparin to prevent recurrent abortion in women described immunologically as secondary aborters (*13*). Again, a wash step in heparin-absorbed sera prior to the addition of complement restored $CDC^{51}Cr$ activity to or beyond original levels. It is not likely that this effect produced both by heat treatment and exposure to solid-phase heparin is due to induced anticomplementary factors because exogenous complement is added in both systems. Rather, a more tenable hypothesis would require serum factors capable of inhibiting antibody-complement interactions and other factors capable of inhibiting the inhibitor (*15*). Thus, both heat treatment and solid-phase heparin absorption could alter or inactivate the "inhibitor of the inhibitor," permitting the previously inactive inhibitor to block the antibody complement interaction. The wash step removes that inhibitor, thus restoring antibody activity to original levels.

At this point we must emphasize that a wash step in $CDC^{51}Cr$ does not significantly increase ^{51}Cr release in a number of the sera–target cell combinations shown in the upper right quadrant of Table 1—i.e., where CDCE was strongly positive (60–100% cytotoxicity) and $CDC^{51}Cr$ was weak (less than 10% ^{51}Cr release). Four such sera were retested with a wash step added in $CDC^{51}Cr$, and in only 1 was the ^{51}Cr release greater than 10% after the wash (data not shown). This, plus the previously noted failure of a wash step to restore positive ^{51}Cr release lost after heat treatment in the platelet recipient sera amplifies the noted differences between the two test systems. A potential explanation of this difference between the two systems relates to the much greater uptake of ^{51}Cr by monocytes and non-T cells compared with T cells (*17*). This could explain a negative CDCE with a positive $CDC^{51}Cr$ by B cells and not T cells releasing isotope, but it would not explain the reverse situation, which was the case in 32% of the sera screened (Table 1). We have also noted in the other studies two instances of positive CDCE to B cells (40–60% cytotoxicity) that was negative by CDCE against the whole cell population (12–20% cytotoxicity) and was also negative in $CDC^{51}Cr$ against the whole cell population (^{51}Cr release less than 4%). We cannot, therefore, explain all instances of $CDC^{51}Cr$-positive CDCE-negative reactions on the basis of differential uptake and release of ^{51}Cr by non-T and T lymphocytes, although we recognize that this may be the case in some of the 42% of screened sera (lower left quadrant of Table 1).

Where heparin absorption reduced $CDC^{51}Cr$ activity to secondary aborters paternal target cells by approximately 80%, the effect on CDCE against panel lymphocytes was strikingly different. Although there was a net decrease in CDCE reactivity of approximately 40% it is notable that new reactions appeared after heparin absorption in 4 of the 7 sera tested. This again points out that perhaps $CDC^{51}Cr$ and CDCE detect different antibodies. It is possible that $CDC^{51}Cr$ primarily detects a non-HLA antipaternal antibody possibly directed at TLX specificities (*13*) and that CDCE detects both anti-TLX and anti-HLA. Heparin absorption may result in selective inhibition of one or the other form of antibody. This concept of selective inhibition becomes important with respect to the two sera noted in Table 4, in which the panel reactivity before heparin absorption could be accounted for by reactive panel cells sharing paternal HLA antigens (Bw35 and Cw4 for serum FM and A3 B17 for serum WK). That heparin absorption could remove 50–100% of the activity of what could be operationally defined as HLA bi-specific sera is not fully understood, and is under further investigation.

Another difference between the two test systems was illustrated by the failure of anti-light-chain antibody to enhance weak or negative $CDC^{51}Cr$ reactions in parallel with CDCE reactions in a sequential series of sera from one dialysis patient. This could be explained if the developing weak antibody were anti-HLA rather than anti-TLX and $CDC^{51}Cr$ preferentially detected anti-TLX.

The use of anti-subclass antibodies demonstrated a clear difference between CDCE and CDC^{51}Cr with respect to one secondary aborter reacting to her husband's lymphocytes. The only clear reduction of CDCE was with added anti-IgG_1, but in CDC^{51}Cr anti-IgG_1—and, to a lesser extent, anti-IgG_3—reproducibly decreased CDC^{51}Cr reactivity. It should be noted that the serum tested was an extremely powerful antipaternal serum. The dilutions used were selected from titration studies for maximum cytotoxicity in CDC^{51}Cr and at maximum cytotoxicity and the next dilution for CDCE. These data suggest that in this particular serum both CDCE and CDC^{51}Cr detect an antipaternal IgG_1 but CDC^{51}Cr at 37°C also detects an antipaternal IgG_3.

At this stage of investigation the data support the contention that the differences observed between the two test systems reflect biological differences in terms of the action of different immunoglobulin molecules and their interactions with apparent inhibitory regulatory mechanisms within serum.

These data indicate the necessity for further in-depth study of the nature of the mechanisms of these clinically important antibody detecting test systems.

REFERENCES

1. Mittal KK, Mickey MR, Singal DP, Terasaki PI. Serotyping for homotransplant. Refinement of microdroplet lymphocyte cytotoxicity tests. Transplantation 1968; 6: 913.
2. Ting A, Hasegawa T, Ferrone S, et al. Presensitization detected by sensitve crossmatch tests. Transplant Proc 1973; 5: 813.
3. Johnson AH. Antiglobulin microcytoxicity test. NIAID manual of tissue typing techniques. Ray JG, ed. NIH publication #80-545, 1979.
4. Amos DB. NIH modified technique. NIAID manual of tissue typing techniques. Ray JG, ed. NIH publication #80-545, 1979.
5. Rogentine GN, Plocinik BA. Application of the ^{51}Cr cytotoxicity technique to the analysis of human lymphocyte isoantigens. Transplantation 1967; 5: 1323.
6. McConnachie PR, Finch WT, Birtch AG. Monitoring and prediction rejection. Transplant Proc 1978; 10: 543.
7. Kerman R, Van Buren CT, Flechner S, Kahan BD. Visual, ^{51}Cr release and flow cytometry crossmatch results and graft survival. Transplant Proc 1984; 16: 1430.
8. McConnachie PR, Finch WT, Birtch AG. CDC^{51}Cr: a predictor of kidney graft rejection. Transplant Proc 1984; 16: 1448.
9. McConnachie PR, McIntyre JA. Maternal antipaternal immunity in couples predisposed to repeated pregnancy losses. Am J Reprod Immunol 1984; 5: 145.
10. McIntyre JA, McConnachie RP, Taylor CG, Faulk WP. Clinical immunologic and genetic definitions of primary and secondary recurrent spontaneous abortions. Fertil Steril 1984; 42: 849.
11. Ferrone S, Tosi RM, Centis D. Anticomplementary factors affecting the lymphocytotoxicity test. In: Histocompatibility testing. Copenhagen: Munksgaard, 1967: 357.
12. Fuller TC, Cosimi AB, Russell PS. Use of antiglobulin ATG reagent for detection of low levels of alloantibody. Transplant Proc 1978; 10: 463.
13. McIntyre, JA, Faulk WP, Nicholls-Johnson VR, Taylor CG. Immunological testing and immunotherapy in recurrent spontaneous abortions. Obstet Gynecol 1986; 67: 169.
14. Van der Weerdt CM, Veenhoven-von Riesz LE, Englefriet CP. Difficulties encountered in the production and testing of monospecific cytoxic lymphocyte antisera. In: Histocompatibility testing. Copenhagen: Munksgaard, 1970: 339.
15. McIntyre JA, Faulk WP. Antibody responses in secondary aborting women: effect of inhibitors in blood. Am J Repro Imm Micro 1985; 9: 113.
16. Torry DS, McIntyre JA, Faulk WP, McConnachie PR. Inhibitors of complement-mediated cytotoxicity in normal and secondary aborter sera. Am J Repro Immun Micro 1986; 10: 53.
17. Kovithavongs T, Dossetor JB. Difference in ^{51}Cr uptake and release by T and non-T lymphocytes and its significance in interpreting some discrepant results of ^{51}Cr release cytotoxic assays. Transplantation 1977; 23: 505.

Received 5 June 1985.
Accepted 8 Nov. 1985.

0041-1337/86/4202-0217$02.00/0
TRANSPLANTATION
Vol. 42, No. 2
Printed in U.S.A.

THE GENETIC CONTROL OF THE ANTIBODY RESPONSE TO THE Pa ANTIGEN IN THE RAT[1]

HEINZ W. KUNZ AND THOMAS J. GILL III

Department of Pathology, University of Pittsburgh School of Medicine, Pittsburgh, Pennsylvania 15261

The antibody response to the pregnancy-associated (Pa) antigen in the pregnant female segregated with the major histocompatibility complex (MHC) when the female progeny in the (PVG×WF)F_1×PVG testcross, in which the PVG strain is a low responder to Pa and the WF strain is a high responder, were mated to DA male rats. These results show that non-MHC immune response genes do not play a role, or at least any significant role, in the immune response to the paternal component of the placental antigens: the response approximates a unigenic trait with simple Mendelian segregation. Serological analysis showed that the antibodies formed by both the high responder (GMT 15, titer 1:32,768) and low responder (GMT 3, titer 1:8) female rats were directed against the Pa antigen. These findings show that the genetic control mechanism and the specificity of the antibody elicited by the placental antigen Pa are different from those in the responses to organ grafts and to soluble antigens.

The antibody response to the paternal component of the placental antigens is directed against the Pa antigen, which is a unique class I antigen encoded by the major histocompatibility complex (MHC)* and which has a pattern of antigenic specificity different from that of the classic class I transplantation antigens (*1, 2*). It is present on the basal trophoblast of placentae from the *a, d, f, b,* and *m* haplotypes and absent from placentae from the *c, g, h, l, k, n,* and *u* haplotypes (*3*). No antibody response has been detected in the reciprocal strain combinations that have been examined—i.e., Pa(+) anti-Pa(−), and this observation suggests that the allele to the gene encoding the Pa antigen is a null allele.

Genetic control of the antibody response to the Pa antigen has been studied in the *u*×*a* (2,4,5) and *n*×*a* (1) strain combinations (maternal strain written first) by using the appropriate congenic animal as the maternal strain. These experiments showed that a major component of the genetic control was linked to the MHC, but they did not rule out a significant role for non-MHC genes in regulating the magnitude of the immune response, since congenic strains with only two different backgrounds were studied (*1, 4*). Such a regulatory role for non-MHC immune responses (Ir) genes has been demonstrated in the antibody response to a variety of antigens—e.g., synthetic polypeptides (*6–8*). The issue is further complicated by the observation that a semiallogeneic placenta carrying the Pa antigen does not necessarily elicit an antibody response in a Pa(−) maternal strain (e.g., PVG×DA [*1, 9*]). Hence, the absence of the Pa antigen in a given strain does not necessarily imply that the strain has the Ir genes necessary to recognize the Pa antigen.

As with all antibody responses studied by sensitive enough techniques, there are high and low responders to placental antigens rather than an absolute presence or absence of an antibody response. Previous studies (*1*) showed that the WF×DA (*u*×*a*) strain combination was a high responder: the average anti-Pa antibody response was greater than 1:2048 (GMT 11), and 100% of pregnant female rats responded. By contrast, the PVG×DA (*c*×*a*) strain combination was a low responder combination with an average anti-Pa antibody response less than 1:4 (GMT 2), and less than 60% of the pregnant female rats responded.

The present study was undertaken for two reasons. First, the genetic control of the antibody response to the Pa antigen was examined in a testcross between the F_1 hybrid of a high and low responder to the Pa antigen and the low responder strain in order to determine whether both MHC-linked and non-MHC Ir genes were involved. Second, the specificity of the antigen eliciting the antibody response in the low responders—i.e., whether it was also against the Pa antigen, was examined.

MATERIALS AND METHODS

All the rats used in this study were obtained from our colony at the University of Pittsburgh School of Medicine. The testcross used to study the segregation of the antibody responses was generated by mating (PVG×WF)F_1 hybrid female rats with PVG male rats and then mating the female progeny with DA male rats. The WF strain is a high responder to the Pa antigen, whereas the PVG strain is a low responder. The mating scheme and the antibody responses predicted for different genetic control mechanisms are shown in Figure 1.

The antibody responses to the matings with the DA male rats were tested at 5–7 days postpartum, which is the time when the maximal titers are obtained, by hemagglutination in Ficoll and by cytotoxicity (*1*). Their magnitude was expressed as the geometric mean titer (GMT) of the logarithm to the base 2, so that titers could be averaged and compared. The specificity of the antibody response was tested using red blood cells from rats of various haplotypes, and the strains used are listed in Table 1.

The litter sizes in each mating were recorded at birth to examine whether there was any difference between the high-responder and low-responder progeny of the testcross.

RESULTS

The antibody response to the Pa antigen segregated with the *u* haplotype, and there was no evidence for a significant effect on the magnitude of the immune response by non-MHC genes (Table 2). All the antibodies in both the high and low responders were hemagglutinating, and approximately 20% of the high-responder female rats also made cytotoxic antibodies in all three pregnancies. None of the low responders made cytotoxic antibodies in any of the pregnancies. The high responders had a GMT of approximately 15 (titer 1:32,768) and 100% of

[1] This work was supported by Grants HD 08662 and HD 09880 from the National Institutes of Health.

* Abbreviations used: GMT, geometric mean titer; Ir, immune response; MHC, major histocompatibility complex; Pa, pregnancy-associated.

the female rats responded, whereas the low responders had a maximal GMT of approximately 3 (titer 1:8) and 60% or less of the female rats responded.

Analysis of the antibody response in both the high and low responders showed that the antibody in each case was elicited by the Pa antigen (Table 3). The antibody in the high-responder *c/u*×*a/a* mating reacted with the *a*, *o* (*RT1.A*^{d}), *f*, *b*, and *m* haplotypes and was directed against an MHC antigen because it reacted with BN.1A but not with DA.1N. There was also a very small amount of crossreactivity with the *k* haplotype in some sera of the second and third pregnancies (1:64 compared with 1:262,144 for the reactivity with *a*). The antibody response in the low responders was also against the Pa antigen: it reacted with the *a*, *o* (*RT1.A*^{d}) and *f* haplotypes. The lack of reactivity with the *b* and *m* haplotypes is expected with such a low level of responsiveness, since the anti-Pa antibodies react much more strongly with the *a*, *d*, *f* group than with the *b*, *m* group (*1*).

The litter sizes at birth were not significantly different for the *c/u*×*a/a* and *c/c*×*a/a* matings of the testcross, and they were generally somewhat larger than those of the F_1 hybrids and those of the inbred DA strain (Table 4).

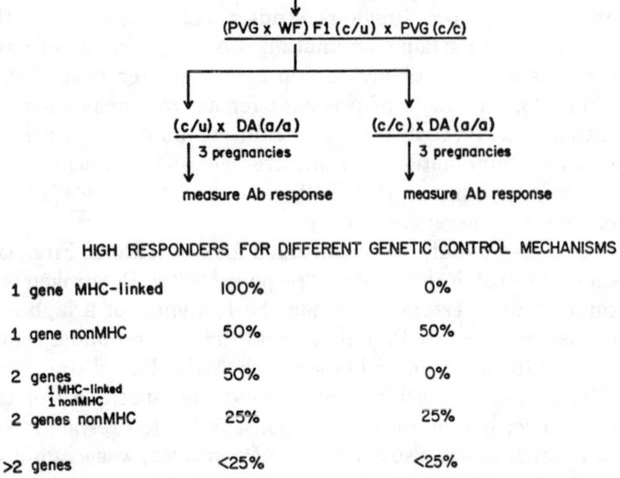

FIGURE 1. The mating scheme of the testcross used to study the genetic control of the antibody response to the Pa antigen and the interpretation of the possible results. The latter gives the percentage of high responders predicted to occur in each of the two matings for a given genetic control mechanism.

TABLE 1. Haplotypes of strains used for serological testing and for mating

Haplotype	Strain	Haplotype	Strain
a	DA	*h*	BN.1H(HW)
	BN.1A(DA)	*k*	BN.1K(WKA)
b	BN.1B(BUF)	*l*	BN.1L(LEW)
c	PVG	*m*	BN.1M(MNR)
	BN.1C(AUG)	*n*	DA.1N(BN)
o[a]	BN.1O(MR)	*u*	WF
f	BN.1F(AS2)		BN.1U(WF)
g	BN.1G(KGH)		

[a] RT1.A^{d}B^{d}D^{a}E^{-}.

DISCUSSION

The antibody response of the pregnant female rat to the paternally derived Pa antigen is controlled exclusively, or almost so, by an MHC-linked immune response gene (Fig. 1): it is the closest to a unigenic antibody response trait with simple Mendelian segregation seen in the rat. The antibody response of the heterozygous *c/u* female rats to the fetuses sired by DA male rats was as high as that of WF (*u/u*) female rats mated with DA male rats (*1*). This finding is different from the response to soluble antigens—e.g., synthetic polypeptides—in which the antibody response of the heterozygotes is approximately half or less that of the corresponding high responder strain (*6, 10*). This difference may also be a manifestation of the unique unigenic genetic control mechanism regulating the response to the fetus.

The anti-Pa antibody response was lower in the first pregnancy compared with the second and third pregnancies, as noted previously (*2*), so there is some evidence for an anamnestic response after the first pregnancy, but not after the second pregnancy. The antibody specificity in both the high and low responders was the same—i.e., to the Pa antigen. The presence of a high or low anti-Pa antibody response, however, did not effect the litter sizes of the animals.

There are some striking differences between the immune response to the Pa antigen in pregnancy and the immune response to soluble antigens (*6–8*) and to tissue antigens (*11*). First, the Pa antigen carries only a broadly shared public specificity, whereas the classic class I transplantation antigens have a series of histogenetically active private specificities. Second, the gene encoding the Pa antigen does not appear to have an allelic specificity, since there is no antibody response in the reciprocal Pa(+) × Pa(−) mating (*1, 2, 9*). By contrast, the class I transplantation antigens have a whole series of reciprocal specificities. Third, if a strain does not carry the Pa antigen, it does not necessarily have the Ir genes to recognize the Pa antigen. For example, the PVG strain is Pa(−), but it does not mount a significant antibody response against the

TABLE 2. Antibody responses in various matings[a]

Mating[b]	Pregnancy 1			Pregnancy 2			Pregnancy 3		
	Responders/ total animals	GMT	±SD	Responders/ total animals	GMT	±SD	Responders/ total animals	GMT	±SD
WF×DA[c]	7/7	11.29	4.19	6/6	11.12	3.31	6/6	12.00	4.43
PVG×DA	2/9	1.00	2.35	3/9	0.78	1.39	4/7	1.43	1.40
(PVG×WF)×DA									
c/u×*a/a*[d]	18/20	6.20	3.16	20/20	14.74	2.51	20/20	14.40	2.91
c/c×*a/a*[e]	9/21	1.76[f]	2.43	13/21	3.10[f]	3.16	7/21	1.00[f]	1.82

[a] Data are the geometric mean titers (GMT) of the hemagglutination assays.

[b] Female strain written first.

[c] (*1*).

[d] 20% of the antibody in all three pregnancies was also cytotoxic.

[e] None of the antibody in any of the three pregnancies was cytotoxic.

[f] Significantly lower ($P < 0.001$) than *c/u*×*a/a*.

TABLE 3. Serological analysis of antibodies in the sera of high and low responders[a]

Haplotype of mated females	Pregnancy	Haplotype of cells used for absorption	Haplotype of cells in test panel											
			a	*b*	*c*	*o*[b]	*f*	*g*	*h*	*k*	*l*	*m*	*n*	*u*
c/u[c]	1	None	12	0	0	14	14	0	0	0	0	14	0	0
		o[b]	0	0	0	0	0	0	0	0	0	0	0	0
	2	None	18	13	0	17	18	0	0	6	0	16	0	0
		o	0	0	0	0	0	0	0	0	0	0	0	0
	3	None	17	13	0	19	15	0	0	6	0	15	0	0
		o	0	0	0	0	0	0	0	0	0	0	0	0
c/c[d]	1	None	2	0	0	3	0	0	0	0	0	0	0	0
		o	0	0	0	0	0	0	0	0	0	0	0	0
	2	None	4	0	0	5	4	0	0	0	0	0	0	0
		o	0	0	0	0	0	0	0	0	0	0	0	0
	3	None	4	0	0	5	3	0	0	4	0	0	0	0
		o	0	0	0	0	0	0	0	0	0	0	0	0

[a] Geometric mean titers (GMT) of the hemagglutination assays.
[b] RT1.A^{d}.
[c] 6–7 sera in each pregnancy pooled.
[d] 4–6 antibody-containing sera in each pregnancy pooled.

TABLE 4. Litter sizes at birth in the different matings

Mating[a]	Pregnancy 1			Pregnancy 2			Pregnancy 3		
	No.	Mean	±SD	No.	Mean	±SD	No.	Mean	±SD
DA×DA[b]	14	7.50	1.16	14	7.07	2.16	14	6.86	2.50
WF×DA[b]	9	8.33	1.66	5	7.80	1.48	5	3.00	3.00
PVG×DA	10	7.00	3.50	10	9.40	1.71	9	8.00	2.74
(PVG×WF)×DA									
c/u×*a/a*	19	9.21	2.46	20	9.65	3.15	20	9.30	2.38
c/c×*a/a*	21	10.52	2.50	21	10.00	2.02	21	10.19	2.32

[a] Female strain written first.
[b] *(1)*.

Pa(+) DA strain. In organ transplant situations, this is not generally true. Fourth, the antibody response to the Pa antigen is under essentially unigenic Mendelian control rather than under the polygenic control that regulates the response to soluble antigens *(6–8)* and to tissue antigens *(11)*. Finally, the antibody response to the Pa antigen in the serum of the pregnant animal appears to be monoclonal, since its serological reactivity parallels that of the monoclonal antibodies derived from the splenic lymphocytes of pregnant rats *(1, 2)*. By contrast, the antibody response to organ transplants is quite heterogeneous.

The antigenic structure of the placenta is different from that of the parenchymal organs, and this difference may be the key to its acceptance by the mother. Studies in other species also show that their placentae have a broadly shared class I antigen similar to the Pa antigen on their surfaces and interfacing with the maternal blood *(3)*, so this structure appears to reflect a general mechanism for escaping immune destruction. The role of the immune response in the process of implantation is still controversial, but if it does play a role, the unique nature of the major placental antigen will be critical to it. Further comparative examination of the genetic control mechanisms involved in the immune response to the Pa antigen and of those involved in the immune response to organ grafts will provide greater insight into both processes, and may provide novel ways of controlling both.

Acknowledgments. We thank Professor D. B. Amos for his helpful discussions.

REFERENCES

1. Ghani AM, Gill TJ III, Kunz HW, Misra DN. Elicitation of the maternal antibody response to the fetus by a broadly shared MHC class I antigenic determinant. Transplantation 1984; 37: 187.
2. Ghani AM, Kunz HW, Gill TJ III. Pregnancy-induced monoclonal antibody to a unique fetal antigen. Transplantation 1984; 37: 503.
3. Macpherson TA, Ho HN, Kunz HW, Gill TJ III. Localization of the Pa antigen on the placenta of the rat. Transplantation 1986; 41: 392.
4. Smith RN, Sternlicht M, Butcher GW. The alloantibody response in the allogeneically pregnant rat. I. The primary and secondary responses and detection of Ir gene control. J Immunol 1982; 129: 771.
5. Smith RN, Margolies RT, Sternlicht M. The alloantibody response in the allogeneically pregnant rat. II. Primary pregnancy-induced anti-RT1.A^{a} alloantibodies. J Immunol 1982; 129: 777.
6. Gill TJ III, Kunz HW, Stechschulte DJ, Austin KF. Genetic and cellular factors in the immune response. I. Genetic control of the antibody response to poly $Glu^{52}Lys^{33}Tyr^{15}$ in the inbred rat strains ACI and F344. J Immunol 1970; 105: 14.
7. Davis BK, Kunz HW, Shonnard JW, Gill TJ III. MHC-linked and nonMHC-linked immune response genes in the rat. Transplant Proc 1981; 13: 1046.
8. Sieber WK Jr, Wagener DK, Gill TJ III, Kunz HW, Eddy GE. The effect of maternal responder status on the genetic control of the antibody response. J Immunogenet 1980; 7: 173.
9. Gill TJ III. Immunity and pregnancy. CRC Crit Rev Immunol 1985; 5: 201.
10. Davis BK, Kunz HW, Shonnard JW, Gill TJ III. Immune response to poly ($Glu^{52}Lys^{33}Tyr^{15}$) in congenic rats. Transplant Proc 1981; 13: 1378.
11. Butcher GW, Howard JC. Genetic control of transplant rejection. Transplantation 1982; 34: 161.

Received 19 September 1985.
Accepted 14 November 1985.

0041-1337/86/4202-0220$02.00/0
TRANSPLANTATION
Vol. 42, No. 2

Printed in U.S.A.

SEVERE NEPHROTOXICITY CAUSED BY THE COMBINED USE OF GENTAMICIN AND CYCLOSPORINE IN RENAL ALLOGRAFT RECIPIENTS

After renal transplantation patients are at increased risk of infection due to the use of immunosuppressive drugs to prevent rejection. Several studies have shown the beneficial effect of intraoperative antibiotic prophylaxis on wound infections and other infections (*1, 2*). However, some chemotherapeutics or antibiotics are potentially nephrotoxic, especially when used in combination with cyclosporine. The incidence of nephrotoxicity by cyclosporine has been shown to increase if the drug is combined with cotrimoxazole, trimethoprim, or amphotericin B (*3–6*). We have recently observed that the combination of cyclosporine with gentamicin, used either prophylactically or therapeutically, also results in severe nephrotoxicity.

Since 1979 we had treated our transplant recipients with a single prophylactic gift of gentamicin (1.5 mg/kg i.m.) and lincomycin (600 mg i.m.) immediately before transplantation. When cyclosporine became available, the combined use of this nephrotoxic drug with the prophylactic administration of gentamicin/lincomycin resulted in a dramatic increase of the incidence of acute tubular necrosis (ATN)* in our center (Table 1). The incidence of ATN before the use of the combination of gentamicin/lincomycin and cyclosporine had become as low as 5%, after the introduction of a new hydration protocol as previously reported (*7*). When antibiotic prophylaxis was changed to a combination of 2000 mg ceftazidime, plus 1000 mg ampicillin, plus 600 mg lincomycin, given as a single dose immediately before transplantation, the incidence of ATN decreased again to 10%. Cyclosporine was administered i.v. during the first two days in a dose of 5 mg/kg body weight. Thereafter it was given orally in a dose of 17.5 mg/kg body weight, and this dose was decreased every fortnight with 2 mg/kg.

Severe nephrotoxicity due to the combination of cyclosporine and gentamicin was also observed in three patients who received the antibiotic later after transplantation.

Case 1. A seven-year-old boy received immunosuppression with cyclosporine and low-dose prednisone after transplantation (Fig. 1). He suffered twice from an acute rejection—the first treated with rabbit antithymocyte globulin and the second with high oral doses of prednisone—but two months after transplantation stable renal function was reached with a serum creatinine value of 80 μmol/L. At that time he received 7.5 mg/kg cyclosporine daily, and blood levels were rather low (65 ng/ml of whole blood). Treatment with i.v. gentamicin was then started because of a urinary tract infection with *Pseudomonas aeruginosa.* The infection was present for 2 days before the start of the treatment. Serum creatinine had remained stable during this period. After having received two doses of 30 mg (1.5 mg/kg body weight) of gentamicin the patient became completely anuric on the first treatment day. Gentamicin injections were discontinued, and diuresis returned gradually during the day thereafter. The serum creatinine level increased over two days to 242 μmol/L, and decreased gradually to normal levels thereafter without any further treatment. Subsequently, the urinary tract infection was successfully treated with ceftazidime without further problems.

Case 2. Seven days after renal transplantation a 10-year-old girl received prophylactic gentamicin before cystoscopy. She had stable renal function with a serum creatinine level of 100 μmol/L. The cyclosporine dose was at that time 17.5 mg/kg daily, and the cyclosporine trough levels were 500 ng/ml of whole blood. After a single dose of 35 mg gentamicin (1.5 mg/kg body weight) the urinary output decreased by more than 50% for four days. Serum creatinine increased to a maximum level of 450 μmol/L and decreased thereafter to 150 μmol/L within 5 days.

Case 3. One month after transplantation, when he used 13.5 mg/kg cyclosporine daily, a 40-year-old male patient had a serum creatinine level of 300 μmol/L. His cyclosporine trough levels ranged between 150 ng/ml and 1000 ng/ml of whole blood. He received a seven-day course of gentamicin because of flucloxacillin-resistant high fever. Gentamicin was started six days after an operation during which an anastomosis of the host's ureter with the pyelum of the graft was made because of urinary leakage (the serum creatinine level being 600 μmol/L at that time). Urinary output decreased significantly (more than 60%) from the third day of antibiotic treatment, and the serum creatinine level increased from that day (200 μmol/L) to 480 μmol/L eight days later, despite normal gentamicin levels and reduction of the cyclosporine dose). After discontinuation of gentamicin, diuresis gradually increased and the serum creatinine level decreased in one week to 225 μmol/L.

From May 1983 until March 1985 gentamicin has been administered concomitantly with cyclosporine to 11 patients, seven times as a single prophylactic dose before a surgical procedure, four times as a therapeutic course because of infection. Apart from the three patients presented here, there were two additional cases in which a substantial loss of renal function occurred after a single dose of gentamicin, but in which other etiologic factors could not be excluded with complete certainty. Four cases were not evaluable because they underwent intermittent hemodialysis at the time of administration. In the two remaining patients, one of whom received a single dose and the other a therapeutic course of 5 days, no significant changes in serum creatinine levels were found.

From these results it is obvious that the combination of cyclosporine with gentamicin can be very hazardous, not only perioperatively, but also later in the course after renal transplantation. This is conceivable because both drugs are notoriously nephrotoxic. However, the deleterious effects of this combination on renal function in human renal transplant recipients has not been reported before. In rats, the toxic effects of combined administration of cyclosporine and gentamicin are well established (*8, 9*). In these animals the renal damage caused by gentamicin, as well as cyclosporine, is dose-related and involves the proximal tubule. Gentamicin induces necrosis

* Abbreviation used: ATN, acute tubular necrosis.

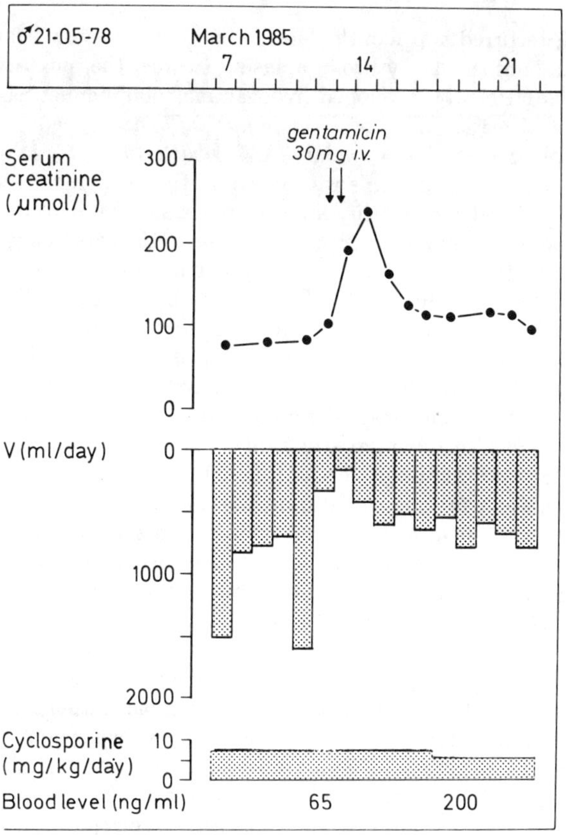

FIGURE 1. Case 1. Severe nephrotoxicity caused by the combined use of gentamicin and cyclosporine.

TABLE 1. Incidence of ATN after renal transplantation

Antibiotics	Cyclosporine	Patients with ATN[a]	Duration of ATN (days [mean ± SD])
Gentamicin and Lincomycin	No	1/21 (5)	1
Gentamicin and Lincomycin	Yes	6/9 (67)	14.0±2.6
Ceftazidime and Ampicillin and Lincomycin	Yes	5/48 (10)	12.6±1.9

[a] Patients with ATN/total number of patients. Percentages are given in parentheses.

of the convoluted segment, and cyclosporine causes vacuolization of the straight segment (*8*). When the two drugs are administered together, both the biochemical and the morphological parameters of renal damage are altered more than would be expected from simple summation of their individual effects. High-dose therapy causes ATN with acute renal failure, and there is significant reduction of renal function even with the lowest-dosage combinations (*9*). Although serum levels of neither drug were measured in these experiments, it was postulated that the effects they cause when given together are a reflection of higher-than-usual serum concentrations of one or both drugs. The onset of renal failure would result in further increases in circulating drug levels (*8, 9*). This can only be true for gentamicin, because cyclosporine is metabolized in the liver and excreted in feces. In human bone marrow recipients, high serum trough levels of cyclosporine combined with therapeutic serum levels of aminoglycoside are reported to be a risk factor for renal failure (*10*). In our patients toxic levels of cyclosporine were not seen. It seems that high or toxic serum levels of either drug are not required, and that the mere combination of two nephrotoxic drugs is sufficient to induce renal damage. The immediate onset of renal failure with anuria after two doses of gentamicin as seen in our first patient is highly unusual for this drug. In fact, suggests a renovascular pathogenesis. However, the precise mechanism of nephrotoxicity caused by the combined use of gentamicin and cyclosporine remains unclear at this moment. Our results also demonstrate that cyclosporine can be safely combined with ceftazidime. This is in accordance with experimental data in rats, showing that concomitant administration of cyclosporine and cephalosporines did not result in acute renal failure.

ARIËN TERMEER
ANDRIES J. HOITSMA
ROBERT A. P. KOENE
Division of Nephrology
Department of Internal Medicine
St. Radboud Hospital
Nijmegen, Holland

REFERENCES

1. Tilney NL, Strom TB, Vineyard GC, Merril JP. Factors contributing to the declining mortality rate in renal transplantation. N Engl J Med 1978; 299: 1321.
2. Novick AC. The value of intraoperative antibiotics in preventing renal transplant wound infections. J Urol 1981; 125: 151.
3. Thompson JF, Chalmers DHK, Hunnisett AGW, Wood RFM, Morris PJ. Nephrotoxicity of trimethoprim and cotrimoxazole in renal allograft recipients treated with cyclosporine. Transplantation 1983; 36: 204.
4. Nyberg G, Gäbel H, Althoff P, Björk S, Herlitz H, Brynger H. Adverse effect of trimethoprim on kidney function in renal transplant patients. Lancet 1984; 1: 394.
5. Ringdén O, Myrenfors P, Klintmalm G, Tydén G, Öst L. Nephrotoxicity by cotrimoxazole and cyclosporin in transplanted patients. Lancet 1984; 1: 1016.
6. Kennedy MS, Deeg HJ, Siegel M, Crowley JJ, Storb R, Thomas ED. Acute renal toxicity with combined use of amphotericin B and cyclosporine after marrow transplantation. Transplantation 1983; 35: 211.
7. Tiggeler RGWL, Berden JHM, Hoitsma AJ, Koene RAP. Prevention of acute tubular necrosis in cadaveric kidney transplantation by the combined use of mannitol and moderate hydration. Ann Surg 1985; 201: 246.
8. Whiting PH, Simpson JG, Davidson RJL, Thomson AW. The toxic effects of combined administration of cyclosporin A and gentamicin. Br J Exp Pathol 1982; 63: 554.
9. Whiting PH, Simpson JG. The enhancement of cyclosporin A-induced nephrotoxicity by gentamicin. Biochem Pharmacol 1983; 32: 2025.
10. Hows JM, Palmer S, Want S, Dearden C, Gordon-Smith EC. Serum levels of cyclosporin A and nephrotoxicity in bone-marrow transplant patients. Lancet 1981; 2: 145.
11. Whiting PH, Thomson W, Simpson JG. Renal and hepatic function in rats treated with cyclosporin A in combination with gentamicin or cephalosporin antibiotics. Br J Exp Pathol 1983; 64: 693.

Received 20 September 1985.
Accepted 15 November 1985.

ALLOGENEIC BONE MARROW TRANSPLANTATION FOR X-LINKED LYMPHOPROLIFERATIVE SYNDROME[1]

X-linked lymphoproliferative syndrome (XLP),* a lethal genetic immunodeficiency, was described in 1975 as Duncan's disease, after the family name of the original kindred (*1*). Male patients with XLP are susceptible to fatal complications from Epstein-Barr virus (EBV) infection. Previous studies have revealed (*2, 3*) that: (1) male patients experience a variety of pathologic sequelae (proliferative and aproliferative) after exposure to EBV if they survive their primary exposure; (2) surviving male patients suffer from progressive defects in cell-mediated immunity that can lead to a variety of infectious diseases; and (3) female heterozygotes for the XLP trait generally exhibit abnormal antibody responses to EBV following primary EBV infection. The average life expectancy for male patients in the "Duncan" kindred has been 9.7 years. Deaths have resulted from acute infectious mononucleosis, malignancies of B lymphocytes that harbor the EBV genome, agammaglobulinemia, or aplastic anemia (*2*).

Bone marrow transplantation (BMT) has been successful in treating patients with severe or partial congenital X-linked immunodeficiencies, such as severe combined immunodeficiency and Wiskott-Aldrich syndrome, when sibling donors (both unaffected individuals and carriers of the x-linked trait) have been used (*4–6*). We reasoned that marrow transplantation could also immunoreconstitute patients suffering from XLP. This report describes the results of the first bone marrow transplantation undertaken for treatment of XLP.

UPN 274, a man, was first evaluated for immunodeficiency disease in 1974 when he was found to have an elevated IgM and a low IgA level following silent infection by EBV. No antibodies against EBV or T cell cytotoxic response to EBV-infected cells, as measured by the regression of EBV-infected B cells in the presence of autologous T cells, were detected. However, peripheral mononuclear cells formed spontaneous Epstein-Barr nuclear antigen (EBNA)–positive lymphoblastoid cell lines in vitro, and the virus was excreted in saliva and throat secretions. He was maternally related to six male cousins who had died from complications of EBV infection (*1*).

Before the first documented episode of EBV infection, UPN 274 had a history of infectious problems including neonatal moniliasis, recurrent otitis media, and meningococcal meningitis at 8 years of age. At 11 years, he silently became infected with EBV from a sister who had acute infectious mononucleosis (IM). At age 14, UPN 274 developed encephalitis of undetermined cause. He suffered from chronic upper respiratory symptoms, intermittent fevers, and headaches without specific diagnoses. Anemia (Hb 4.4 gm/dl) in association with anti-i autoantibody occurred in December 1981 when the patient was 18 years old. Nine weeks later generalized lymphadenopathy and fevers signaled the onset of IM. His peripheral blood lymphocytes underwent a reversal of the T cell subset proportions as he recovered from the IM and the inverted OKT4/OKT8 ratio (0.2–1.1) persisted throughout the remainder of his life. The anemia, which temporarily reversed during this course of IM, recurred two months later, when bone marrow examination confirmed erythroid aplasia. During the next nine months UPN 274 developed hypogammaglobulinemia, pansinusitis, three episodes of *Hemophilus influenzae* pneumonia, and a pleural effusion secondary to *Mycobacterium* tuberculosis. He was maintained with antituberculous therapy, transfusions of packed red blood cells, and i.v. immunoglobulin until he underwent bone marrow transplantation at 19 years of age.

During the years prior to transplant spontaneous B lymphoblastoid cell lines (BLCL) were readily and repeatedly obtained from this patient's peripheral blood mononuclear cell populations (*7*). UPN 274 also developed progressive loss of natural killer (NK) function (*8*). His delayed onset of infectious mononucleosis and progressive loss of NK function and the acquisition of other immune defects were unusual events in the expected natural history for XLP (*2, 3*).

Permission for transplantation was obtained under a bone marrow transplantation protocol for patients with lethal immunodeficiencies who have genotypically histocompatible donors (approved by the Committee on the Use of Human Subjects at the University of Minnesota). UPN 274 was treated in a private high-efficiency particulate air filtration room on the bone marrow transplant unit at the University of Minnesota. He was started on oral trimethoprim/sulfamethoxazole prophylaxis before cytoreduction. A bone marrow biopsy obtained before cytoreduction demonstrated moderate hypocellularity with a paucity of erythroid elements. Pretransplant conditioning consisted of i.v. cyclophosphamide (60 mg/kg/day $\times$ 2), followed two days later by 7.5 Gy total-body irradiation. UPN 274 received 3×10^8 nucleated marrow cells/kg from his EBV-seropositive histocompatible (HLA, mixed lymphocyte culture (MLC)-identical) sister, who had previously recovered uneventfully from infectious mononucleosis. Posttransplant prophylaxis for acute graft-versus-host disease (GVHD) consisted of antithymocyte globulin, prednisone, and methotrexate (*9*). The posttransplant course was complicated by *Streptococcus mitis* sepsis, herpes simplex stomatitis, and gastric inflammation of unknown cause during the first three weeks. White blood count engraftment (three consecutive days with absolute WBC$\geq$1000/mm^3) was recorded on day 25 posttransplant and cytogenetic examination of the bone marrow on day 28 posttransplant demonstrated all female (donor) cells. The patient was discharged on day 40 posttransplant. Rash, low-grade fevers, nausea, and vomiting signalled the onset of acute GVHD. Liver biopsy performed 46 days posttransplant was consistent with grade II GVHD. Oral prednisone (60 mg/M^2 day) was started on day 51 posttransplant, with subsequent rapid resolution of symptoms. Two weeks after return to his home, he began to experience headaches and high fevers. Hepatic dysfunction, encephalopathy, and disseminated intravascular coagulopathy progressed rapidly despite broad spectrum antibiotic therapy and the patient died 84 days posttransplant.

Autopsy demonstrated submassive hepatic necrosis caused by adenovirus (which was cultured from many organs) (*10*). The majority of hepatocytes contained intranuclear viral inclusions consistent with adenovirus infection. Careful examination of lymph nodes and other lymphoid organs did not reveal foci of lymphoma or other malignancy. Bone marrow sections showed mild hypocellularity but full maturation of the erythroid series. Retrospective analyses of serum samples obtained pretransplant and sequentially posttransplant revealed no detectable antibody titres to adenovirus.

[1] This work was supported by NIAMDDK-AM 00959, NIH P01-CA 21737 (AHF), PHS CA30196, Nebraska Department of Health LB506, and the Lymphoproliferative Research Fund (DTP).

* Abbreviations used: BCBL, B lymphoblastoid cell line; BMT, bone marrow transplantation; EBV, Epstein-Barr virus; GVHD, graft-versus-host disease; IM, infectious mononucleosis; NK, natural killer; SCID, severe combined immunodeficiency; XLP, x-linked lymphoproliferative syndrome.

Data comparing immune function pretransplant and posttransplant are listed in Table 1. Prior to BMT serum immunoglobulin levels were all below normal limits despite immunoglobulin infusions. UPN 274 had not demonstrated detectable anti-EBV antibodies (anti-VCA IgG, IgM, or IgA; anti EA: DR, D, or anti-EBNA) despite a history of episodes of exposure to EBV at age 11 and clinical infectious mononucleosis at age 18 (*2*). During the second posttransplant month and after transfusions had ceased, concentrations of IgG, IgM, and IgA achieved normal levels (immunoglobulin transfusions had ceased at the time of BMT) and low levels of anti-EBNA and anti-VCA IgG antibody were detected for the only time during his course. After the institution of prednisone therapy for treatment of GVHD, EBV titers again reverted to the negative range. Quantitation of lymphocyte subsets pretransplant demonstrated a paucity of circulating B cells by determination of lymphocytes expressing polyvalent surface IgG for monoclonal antibody B^1 (*11*), but normal absolute numbers of T lymphocytes and a mild inversion of the T_4/T_8 ratio. By seven weeks posttransplant, lymphocyte counts achieved normal values of both T and B cells. A persistent T_4/T_8 inversion was documented. Several attempts at establishing spontaneous BLCL posttransplant were unsuccessful. (There was no outgrowth of EBV-transformed cells from posttransplant specimens.) Evidence for pulmonary or reactivated cytomegalovirus infection was never demonstrated. The acquired abnormality in NK activity was corrected after marrow transplantation as measured on two occasions (Table 1). Extensive studies of B cell function in the pretransplant period had suggested the possibility of secondary (acquired) T cell suppression of terminal differentiation of B lymphocytes as a probable cause of the progressive hypogammaglobulinemia that UPN 274 experienced (*12, 13*). A partial defect intrinsic to the B lymphocyte population could not be excluded. After engraftment of donor cells immunoglobulin synthesis normalized despite the persistent preponderance of T lymphocytes with the "suppressor" ($OKT8^+$) phenotype.

The underlying genetic defect in the x-linked lymphoproliferative syndrome, as with most hereditary immunodeficiencies, has not yet been defined on a molecular level. Precedents have been set for correction of lethal genetic disorders (both x-linked and non-x-linked) by providing permanent engraftment of metabolically normal marrow precursor cells from related individuals (*4, 5, 6*). Similarly, successful BMT can correct acquired diseases such as idiopathic aplastic anemia. UPN 274, a young man with XLP, had a documented history of genetically determined immunodeficiency, as well as the secondary abnormalities of red cell aplasia and hypogammaglobulinemia prior to transplantation (*1–3*). In the brief period posttransplant, the immunologic and hematologic defects were successfully reversed with engraftment of normal donor cells.

TABLE 1. Immunologic function in X-LP before and after bone marrow transplantation

	Pre-BMT[a]	Post-BMT[b]
Serum immunoglobulins:		
IgG (mg/dl)	448[c]	840
IgM (mg/dl)	7	57
IgA (mg/dl)	17	248
EBV antibody titers:		
Anti-EBNA	<1:5	1:10
Anti-VCA IgG	<1:10 or 1:10	1:40
Anti-VCA IgM	<1:2	1:2
Lymphocyte quantitation:		
Absolute T cell count	2358/mm^3	1114/mm^3
Absolute B cell count	31/mm^3	120/mm^3
T_4/T_8 ratio	37.5/44.5	13.3/50.2
NK function	≤20% Normal controls	Normal ×2

[a] Within 1 month of BMT.
[b] 5–8 weeks post-BMT.
[c] Patient was receiving i.v. immunoglobulin.

A number of issues faced us in preparing for marrow transplantation of this patient with XLP. As with other patients who have long histories of prior immunodeficiency and multiple infections, the risk of an intercurrent life-threatening infection in UPN 274 was considered to be significant. Thus, prophylactic triomethoprim/sulfamethoxazole and antitubercular therapy continued until the time of his death. The risks of reactivation of EBV infection in the form of life-threatening infectious mononucleosis or posttransplant lymphoma were also considered. EBV infection as a primary or reactivated process has rarely been reported in the BMT setting and has not been fatal (*14, 15*). Posttransplant lymphoproliferative disorders of donor (or unknown) origin have developed in several patients with leukemia when there was donor recipient mismatching and GVHD (*16, 17*). Fatal EBV-associated lymphoproliferative disorders involving recipient cells have also been demonstrated in children with severe combined immunodeficiency (SCID) who received thymic epithelial grafts (*18, 19*) or failed engraftment of mismatched bone marrow (*20*). As a rule, these recipients remained relatively immunodeficient posttransplant. On the other hand, a review of 45 children with SCID or Wiskott-Aldrich syndrome who were successfully immunoreconstituted by BMT revealed that none of the patients had yet developed malignant lymphoma after grafting (*21*). This finding encouraged us to attempt BMT on UPN 274 because two of his maternal cousins had died of malignant lymphoma (*1*).

Selection of a safe but effective pretransplant conditioning protocol was another concern in the treatment of UPN 274. We elected to use cyclophosphamide and total-body irradiation, a regimen that had shown little toxicity in young patients with acute nonlymphocytic leukemia (ANLL) (*22*) and achieved reliable engraftment in patients who had received prior blood transfusions. Bone marrow examination 28 days posttransplant confirmed complete engraftment with donor-type cells. Moderate GVHD (an anticipated complication in approximately half of matched recipients in their late teens) ensued, but was effectively controlled with prednisone therapy.

It is possible that the posttransplant immunosuppression used for GVHD prophylaxis—and, later, for therapy—may have increased this patient's risk of disseminated adenovirus infection. GVHD, and the variety of attendant opportunistic infections with this complication and/or its therapy, continues to pose a major obstacle to the successful long-term outcome of adults undergoing allogeneic bone marrow transplantation.

Nonetheless, the observations of immunologic improvement afforded in the early posttransplant course of this patient provide reason for optimism that marrow transplantation can be used for treatment of the primary and secondary complications of genetic immunodeficiency–XLP.

Acknowledgments. We owe a great debt to the many friends and individuals involved in the care of this patient, including associates of the XLP registry, family members, and nursing and house staff at the University of Minnesota Hospitals. Special thanks to Dr. T.A. Waldmann, Metabolism Branch, NIH for studies of in vitro immunoglobulin synthesis; Dr. W.T. Ulburg, Kalamazoo, MI, for performing the autopsy; and C.L. Krawczak and J. Gfrerer for providing editorial assistance in preparing the manuscript.

A.H. Filipovich[2,3]
B.R. Blazar[3,4]
N.K.C. Ramsay[3]
J.H. Kersey[4]
L. Zelkowitz
S. Harada[5]
D.T. Purtilo[5]
Bone Marrow Transplant Team
University of Minnesota
Minneapolis, Minnesota 55455
Department of Pathology
University of Nebraska College of Medicine
Omaha, Nebraska 68105

[2] Address correspondence to: A.H. Filipovich, M.D., Box 261 Mayo, University Hospitals & Clinics, 420 Delaware St. SE, Minneapolis, MN 55455.

[3] Bone Marrow Transplant Team, University of Minnesota. Recipient of Grant IN-13W-16 from the American Cancer Society.

[4] Bruce Blazar is a fellow of the Leukemia Society of America, Inc. and is a recipient of Clinical Investigator Award 1 K08 AM01509 from the National Institutes of Health.

[5] The XLP Registry, Department of Pathology, University of Nebraska College of Medicine.

REFERENCES

1. Purtilo DT, Cassel CK, Yang JPS, Harper R, Stephenson SR, Landing BH, Vawter GF. X-linked recessive progressive combined variable immunodeficiency (Duncan's disease). Lancet 1975; 1: 935.
2. Harada S, Tatsumi E, Lipscomb HL, Purtilo DT. Responses to Epstein-Barr virus in immune deficient patients. In: Purtilo DT, ed. Immune deficiency and cancer: Epstein-Barr virus and lymphoproliferative malignancies. New York: Plenum Press, 1984: 123.
3. Purtilo DT, Zelkowitz L, Harada S, Brooks CD, Bechtold T, Saemundsen AK, Lipscomb HL, Yetz J, Rogers G. Delayed onset of infectious mononucleosis associated with acquired agammaglobulinemia and red cell aplasia. Ann Intern Med 1984; 101: 180.
4. Bortin MM, Rimm AA. Severe combined immunodeficiency disease: characterization of the disease and results of transplantation. JAMA 1977; 238: 591.
5. Parkman R, Rappeport J, Geha R, Belli J, Cassady R, Levey R, Nathan DG, Rosen FS. Complete correction of Wiskott-Aldrich syndrome by allogeneic bone-marrow transplantation. N Engl J Med 1978; 298: 921.
6. Kapoor N, Kirkpatrick D, Blaese RM, Oleske J, Hilgartner MH, Chaganti, Good RA, O'Reilly RJ. Reconstitution of normal megakaryocytopoiesis and immunologic functions in Wiskott-Aldrich syndrome by marrow transplantation following myeloablation and immunosuppression with busulfan and cyclophosphamide. Blood 1981; 57: 692.
7. Harada S, Bechtold T, Purtilo DT. Cell-mediated immunity to Epstein-Barr virus (EBV) and natural killer (NK)-cell activity in X-linked lymphoproliferative syndrome. Int J Cancer 1982; 216: 739.
8. Lipinski M, Virelizier J-L, Tursz T, Griscelli C. Natural killer and killer cell activities in patients with primary immunodeficiencies or defects in immune interferon production. Eur J Immunol 1980; 10: 246.
9. Ramsay NKC, Kersey JH, Robison LL, McGlave P, Woods WG, Krivit W, Kim T, Goldman A, Nesbit M. A randomized study of the prevention of acute graft-versus-host disease. N Engl J Med 1982; 306: 392.
10. Purtilo DT, White R, Filipovich AH, Kersey J, Zelkowitz L. Fulminant liver failure induced by adenovirus post bone marrow transplantation. Letter to editor. N Engl J Med 1985; 312: 1707.
11. Nadler LM, Ritz J, Hardy R, Pesando JM, Schlossman SF, Stashenko P. A unique cell surface antigen identifying lymphoid malignancies of B cell origin. J Clin Invest 1981; 67: 134.
12. Lindsten T, Seeley JK, Kasamoto K, Yetz J, Harada S, Bechtold T, Rogers G, Purtilo DT. Immunodeficiency in the X-linked lymphoproliferative syndrome. II. Immuno-regulatory T cell defects. J Immunol 1982; 129: 2536.
13. Waldmann TA, Broder S. Polyclonal B cell activators in the study of the regulation of immunoglobulin synthesis in the human system. Adv Immunol 1982; 32: 1.
14. Meyers JD, Atkinson K. Infections in bone marrow transplantation. Clin Haematol 1983; 12: 791.
15. Lange B, Henle W, Meyers JD, et al. Epstein-Barr virus-related serology in marrow transplant recipients. Int J Cancer 1980; 26: 151.
16. Gossett TC, Gale RP, Fleischman H, Austin GE, Sparkes RS, Taylor CR. Immunoblastic sarcoma in donor cells after bone-marrow transplantation. N Engl J Med 1979; 300: 904.
17. Schubach WH, Hackman R, Neiman PE, Miller G, Thomas ED. A monoclonal immunoblastic sarcoma in donor cells bearing Epstein-Barr virus genomes following allogeneic marrow grafting for acute lymphoblastic leukemia. Blood 1982; 60: 180.
18. Borzy MS, Hong R, Horowitz SD, Gilbert E, Kaufman D, DeMendonca W, Oxelius V-A, Dictor M, Pachman L. Fatal lymphoma after transplantation of cultured thymus in children with combined immunodeficiency disease. N Engl J Med 1979; 301: 565.
19. Reece ER, Gartner JG, Seemayer TA, Joncas JH, Pagano JS. Epstein-Barr virus in a malignant lymhoproliferative disorder of B-cells occurring after thymic epithelial transplantation for combined immunodeficiency. Cancer Res 1981; 41: 4243.
20. Shearer WT, Ritz J, Finegold MJ, et al. Epstein-Barr virus-associated B-cell proliferations of diverse clonal origins after bone marrow transplantation in a 12-year-old patient with severe combined immunodeficiency. N Eng J Med 1985; 312: 1151.
21. Neudorf SML, Filipovich AH, Kersey JH. Immunoreconstitution by bone marrow transplantation decreases lymphoproliferative malignancies in Wiskott-Aldrich and severe combined deficiency syndrome. In: Purtilo DT, ed. Immune deficiency and cancer: Epstein-Barr virus and lymphoproliferative malignancies. New York: Plenum Press, 1984: 471.
22. Kersey JH, Ramsay NKC, Kim TH, McGlave PB, Krivit W, Levitt S, Filipovich AH, Woods WG, O'Leary M, Coccia P, Nesbit ME. Allogeneic bone marrow transplantation in acute nonlymphocytic leukemia: a pilot study. Blood 1982; 60: 400.

Received 12 August 1985.
Accepted 25 November 1985.

PRETRANSPLANT ANTIBODY SCREENING USING LYMPHOCYTES FROZEN IN MICROTEST TRAYS

Potential transplant recipients may be presensitized to transplantation antigens because of their exposure to blood transfusions, pregnancies, or previous transplants. Routine screening of the patients' serum for the presence of lymphocytotoxic antibodies, therefore, is a standard procedure. If antibodies against a cell panel are detected, care must be taken to eliminate kidney donors who possess antigens against which the potential recipient's antibodies react. The direct lymphocytotoxic crossmatch test serves as a last decisive check before going ahead with the transplant operation. Patients with broadly reactive antibodies are extremely difficult to transplant because they are crossmatch-positive against most potential donors. Even if the crossmatch is negative, reports indicate that a presensitized recipient is at an increased risk of graft failure (*1, 2*).

We recently reported on the advantage of using lymphocytes prefrozen in microtest trays for antibody screening (*3*). Using this technique, screening against a large cell panel can be performed rapidly. A single microtest tray allows testing for antibodies against a panel of 50 cell donors within approximately 4 hr. We report here the serum screening of 141 patients on our local waiting list using, in parallel, frozen lymphocyte trays and conventional techniques. The overall correlation of test results was good, but we noticed a somewhat greater sensitivity of tray-frozen cells for B cell antibodies.

The method of preparing and using frozen lymphocyte trays has been published in detail (*3*). Sera obtained from 141 patients on our transplant waiting list were tested on a set of trays that contained cells of 50 randomly selected blood donors. The same sera were tested conventionally against 50 fresh lymphocyte samples obtained from another group of random blood donors, either without further separation, or after separation into B and T lymphocytes. B cell testing was carried out at 5°C and 37°C to distinguish "warm-reactive" from "cold-reactive" antibodies. An increase of at least 10% panel reactivity at 5°C as compared with 37°C was taken to indicate the presence of "B-cold" antibodies. Reactions giving >10% kill above background were counted as positive.

The results obtained with frozen lymphocyte trays showed very good agreement with those obtained with conventional testing of unseparated lymphocytes, although there were some interesting differences. Of the 141 sera, 111 were entirely negative with both techniques. The reactivity of 30 sera that were positive in one or both tests is illustrated in Figure 1. Interestingly, of 3 sera that showed greatly increased reactivity on frozen trays as compared with the conventional technique, 2 contained B-warm antibodies and 1 contained B-cold antibodies. Figure 1 shows that the overall sensitivity of frozen tray testing was somewhat greater, resulting in a shift to the right of the best fit line of regression ($y=2.03+0.79\times$). Excluding the 3 outlyers (strong B cell reactivity) a correlation of $R=0.928$ was obtained.

Testing against panels of B and T cells revealed that 22 of the 30 sera identified as antibody-positive by their reactions against unseparated cells contained T cell antibodies, whereas 8 sera contained primarily B cell antibodies, 4 of which were B-cold and 4 were B-warm. In addition, another 46 sera that had been classified initially as antibody-negative showed evidence for B cell reactivity (21 B-warm, 25 B-cold). However, the B reaction scores of these sera were much weaker than those of the 8 sera that were found positive against unseparated cells also.

Our results demonstrate that, in an everyday situation in which the sera of 141 potential transplant recipients were tested, frozen lymphocyte trays gave results comparable to those obtained with conventional screening techniques. The sensitivity of frozen tray screening was somewhat greater, confirming our initial observation (*3*). This is probably due to a somewhat increased sensitivity for detection of B cell antibodies, probably because of a relative enrichment of B cell targets during the washing of frozen-thawed trays due to their better adherence to plastic. However, as shown here, only strong B cell antibodies give positive reactions and such sera are rare. With respect to a subsequent transplant, the detection of strongly reactive B cell antibodies may even be advantageous, as deleterious effects of strong B-warm antibodies have been reported (*4*). In our opinion, the frozen tray technique represents an important improvement over conventional techniques for the rapid detection of lymphocytotoxic antibodies in potential transplant recipients.

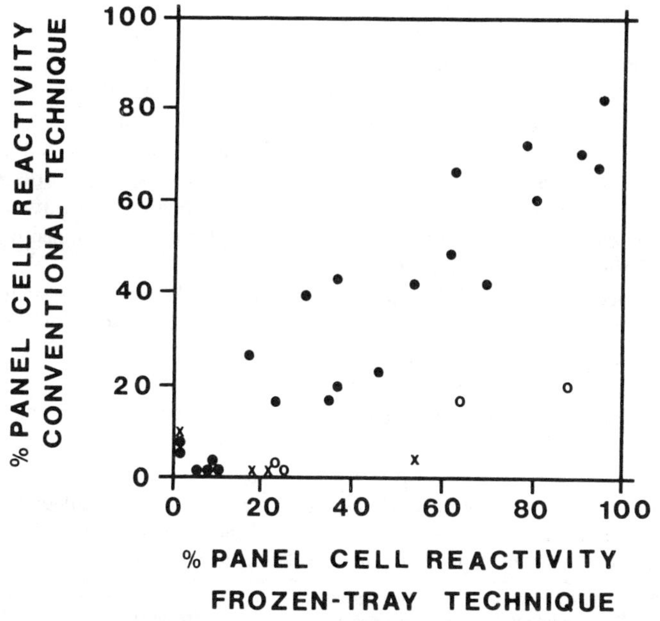

FIGURE 1. Percentages of lymphocytotoxic antibody reactivity against unselected panels of lymphocytes. Each dot represents one serum's reactivity in the conventional screening test and in the frozen tray technique. Sera with >5% reactivity against panel are plotted. Overall, serum reactivity was somewhat greater with frozen trays: (●) = serum with T cell antibodies, (○) = serum containing primarily B-warm antibodies, (×) = serum containing primarily B-cold antibodies (determined in conventional screening).

Acknowledgments. The excellent technical assistance of Karin Kotelmann and Gisela Günther is gratefully acknowledged.

AXEL SCHÄFER
GERHARD OPELZ
Department of Transplantation Immunology
Institute of Immunology
University of Heidelberg
Heidelberg, West Germany

REFERENCES

1. Terasaki PI, Mickey MR, Kreisler M. Presensitization and kidney transplant failures. Postgrad Med J 1971; 47: 89.
2. Opelz G, Mickey MR, Terasaki PI. HLA matching and cadaver kidney transplant survival in North America. Transplantation 1977; 23: 490.
3. Ruder H, Opelz G, Lenhard V, et al. A rapid screening technique for lymphocytotoxic antibodies using tray-frozen lymphocytes. Cryobiology 1984; 21: 480.
4. Ayoub G, Park MS, Terasaki PI, et al. B-cell antibodies and crossmatching. Transplantation 1980; 29: 227.

Received 11 October 1985.
Accepted 11 November 1985.

ASSESSMENT OF PRIMARILY VASCULARIZED CARDIAC ALLOGRAFTS IN MICE[1]

The large number of genetically well-defined inbred and congenic strains of mice (*1*), and the recent availability of cloned H-2 gene products (2) makes the mouse an ideal animal with which to study graft rejection and the ways in which the rejection response can be modified.

The first description of a primarily vascularized transplant model in the mouse was in 1973 when Corry et al. (*3*) studied the behavior of heterotopically transplanted hearts across different histocompatibility barriers. We have recently successfully developed a primarily vascularized heart model in the mouse to supplement our studies with the rat model. However having mastered the technical problems, we found difficulties in determining the exact point of rejection.

Direct abdominal palpation of heterotopically transplanted hearts has been the most popular method of assessing allograft viability in the rat and mouse models (*4–6*). When the mouse model was developed, rejection was defined as the first noticeable decline in the intensity of allograft pulsations as determined by abdominal palpation (*3*). Later, the criteria for determining rejection were redefined and the endpoint of graft function was the day when all palpable contractions ceased (*7*).

We think that, in the mouse, reliance upon palpation alone for the assessment of cardiac allograft function has serious drawbacks (since palpation is a subjective measure) and that this method of monitoring should be used in conjunction with a more objective test of cardiac allograft function as this animal model becomes more widely used to study graft rejection. We have chosen electrocardiographic monitoring as an alternate method of assessment. In this report we discuss our findings using this method, which clearly demonstrate that electrocardiograph (ECG)* monitoring and palpation combine to provide an objective and reliable method for the assessment of cardiac allograft function. Using the data obtained we propose a new index of cardiac allograft function based on ECG criteria.

Unrelated and congenic strains of mice (C3H/He, C57BL/10, B10.BR, DBA/2, B10.D2, BALB/c, B10.A(4R) were supplied by Olac 1976 Limited (Shaw's Farm, Bicester, Oxon, England) or our own animal house facilities.

The operative technique was similar to that used by Corry et al. (*3*). After the induction of satisfactory anesthesia by the i.p. injection of 0.1 ml/10 g body weight of a 3.6% chloral hydrate solution, the infrarenal aorta and inferior vena cava (IVC) were prepared for anastomosis. The donor heart was then harvested from the heparinized donor. Donor-to-recipient aorta and donor pulmonary artery–to–recipient IVC were anastomosed end-to-side with a 10–0 continuous nylon suture. Onset of allograft pulsations was usually almost immediate following the resumption of coronary perfusion.

Allograft assessment was carried out in all cases in two ways: by palpation and by electrocardiography. Daily abdominal palpation, performed by two independent observers, in the awake animal was used to grade the cardiac impulses from 4+ (strong, easily palpable contractions) to 0 (no palpable contractions).

ECGs were taken twice weekly, or more often when allografts were judged to be on the point of rejecting. Anesthesia was induced as described above. Then 27-gauge needles attached to ECG leads I, II, and III were placed s.c. in the left and right axillae and in the right groin. The ECG of the recipient's own heart was thus taken. The axillary leads were then repositioned on the anterior abdominal wall on either side of the allograft and its ECG recorded.

An index of graft function was obtained by dividing the number of beats per minute of the transplanted heart by the number of beats per minute of the animal's native heart as determined by the ECG. The ratio thus obtained compensated for variability in the frequency of contraction of the allograft caused by differing depths of sedation that affected the native heart in an identical way. This ratio was then compared with the traditional method of graft assessment performed by abdominal palpation. Particularly interesting were the instances when different conclusions on the state of allograft viability were reached depending on which method of assessment was used.

A total of 230 ECGs were performed on mice transplanted over a period of four months, and 54 grafts were judged as having 4+ pulsations, 33 as 3+, 55 as 2+, and 88 as 1+ at the time of the ECG. Mean ratio values obtained using the ECG were calculated for the four groups of allografts categorized according to palpational assessment (Table 1). The differences between the mean ratio values for the four groups were significant ($P<0.02$), except for that between the 2+ and 1+ group ($P<0.06$). Mean ratio values for each category correlated well with declining scores as assessed by palpation (r=0.97), although a wide range of ratio values existed within each category (Fig. 1).

The only consistent ECG change occurring during rejection was a slowing in the frequency of contraction of the rejecting graft (Fig. 2). The frequency of contractions of newly grafted hearts always approached or surpassed the frequency of contraction of the native heart. Rejecting hearts often had ratios below 0.7. Voltage changes were found to be unreliable indicators of rejection because the height of the QRS wave changed dramatically depending on the position of the allograft or the location of the abdominal leads.

Discrepancies between the two methods of assessment were not uncommon. Eighteen grafts judged to be 1+ by palpation by two independent observers, had no electrical activity present on ECG. Laparotomies performed in these instances always revealed rejected grafts with no visible muscular contractions, thus confirming the ECG findings. In these cases, the impression of viability conveyed by palpation had been the result of the rapid passive expansion of the grafts by the transmission of the aortic systolic pressure.

Occasionally, QRS complexes were obtained from grafts with no palpable pulsations; laparotomies in these cases showed small patches of contracting muscle, usually near the aortic root, that were not large enough to be detected by palpation. These allografts were nevertheless considered rejected since not enough functioning muscle was present to generate a pal-

TABLE 1. The relationship between the strength of cardiac allograft pulsation, as determined by palpation, and the ratio of the frequency of the cardiac allograft to that of the native heart

Number of allografts	Strength of pulsation	Allograft/native heart frequency
54	4+	0.91±0.1[a]
33	3+	0.84±0.1[a]
55	2+	0.69±0.2[a]
88	1+	0.66±0.2[a]

[a] Results are expressed as the mean ±SD. Differences between the means are significant ($P<0.02$), except for that between the 2+ and the 1+ group.

[1] This work was supported by a grant from the Medical Research Council of the UK.

* Abbreviations used: ECG, electrocardiography; IVC, inferior vena cava.

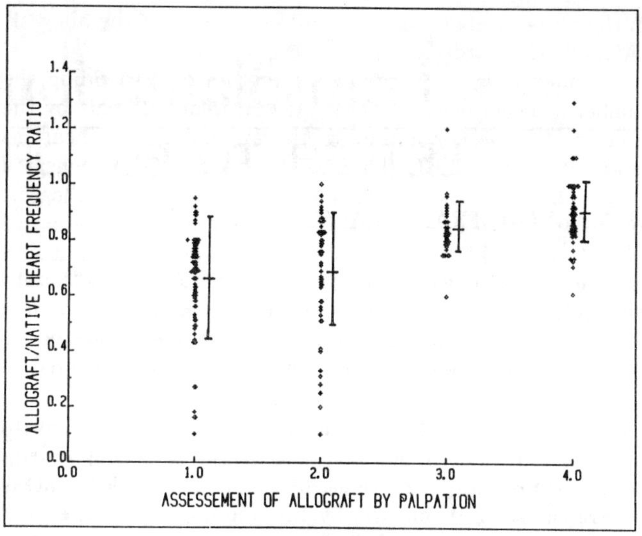

FIGURE 1. Ratio values for 230 ECGs plotted against the scores for pulsations obtained by palpation. Horizontal lines next to each column represent mean ratio values for each assessment by palpation score ± SD.

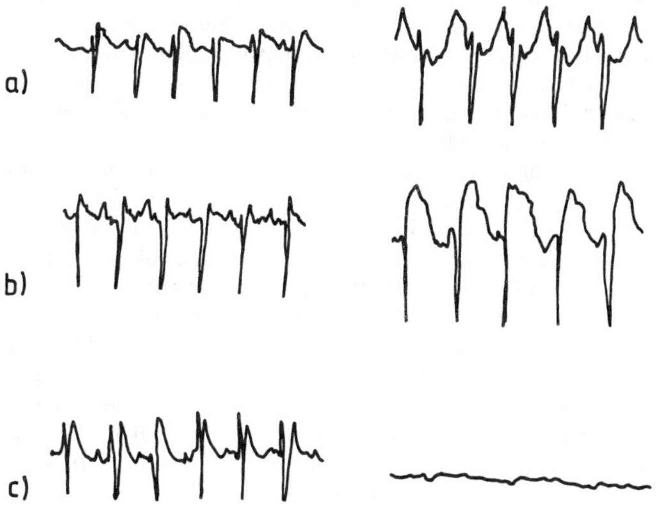

FIGURE 2. Serial ECGs taken over a period of two weeks, with the native heart traces on the left and the allograft traces on the right. The transplanted heart first slows down (b) and then stops (c), whereas the native heart remains unchanged. The small deflections seen in the ECG of the allograft in (c) are the electrical impulses of the native heart picked up by the abdominal leads. The origin of these deflections sometimes seen on the tracing obtained by the leads placed in the abdominal positions is obvious because the frequency of these deflections is identical to that of the QRS complex in the native heart ECG.

pable pulse. Histological examination of 1+ allografts with no ECG activity always revealed the typical changes of irreversible rejection, including dense mononuclear cell infiltration, interstitial edema, and hemorrhage.

Hearts have commonly been used as heterotopic vascularized allografts in rats, but have rarely been used in mice because the operation is more difficult. Having developed the mouse heterotopic heart allograft model in Oxford, we decided to use final cessation of allograft activity as our endpoint for determining rejection. But, as our familiarity with the model increased, it became apparent that mistakes were being made in the assessment of graft function when we relied solely on the method of abdominal palpation.

In 17% of allografts judged to be 1+ by palpation, no ECG could be obtained. These hearts were rejected both macroscopically and microscopically. Rapid passive expansion of these hearts by the aortic systolic pressure had led to the mistaken impression that they were still contracting. This passive motion could be stopped by direct occlusion of the proximal aorta. Attempts to occlude the aorta in the awake animal by abdominal compression generally resulted in a struggling animal the graft of which could not be assessed at all.

Whenever the rejection of a cardiac allograft does not lead to the formation of an intracardiac thrombus, the ventricles may continue to be passively distended by the transmission of aortic pulsations. These pulsations can then be easily felt through the very thin abdominal wall of mice, and the observer can be convinced that the allograft is still viable. By using the ECG, however, objective evidence concerning the state of the allograft is obtained. Moreover, the ECG ratio can be used to characterize allograft function at any one time in an objective manner, and allograft behavior can be compared between different groups of recipients.

We think that if the use of the heterotopic heart allograft model in the mouse becomes more common, it will be essential that the criteria by which function is assessed are standardized in order to minimize errors always inherent in subjective methods of assessment of graft function. In our opinion, this type of allograft must have both palpable pulse and electrical activity to be considered still functional. This dual method of assessment, as well as providing an objective index of cardiac function, has eliminated the most commonly made error in our hands, which was to mistake a rejected passively expanded graft for a weakly functioning one.

RICCARDO A. SUPERINA[2]
WILIAM N. PEUGH
KATHRYN J. WOOD[3]
PETER J. MORRIS
Nuffield Department of Surgery
University of Oxford
John Radcliffe Hospital
Oxford OX3 9DU, England

[2] RAS is supported by the R. Samuel McLaughlin Foundation, Toronto, Canada.

[3] Address correspondence to: Dr. K. J. Wood, Nuffield Dept. of Surgery, John Radcliffe Hospital, Oxford, OX3 9DU.

REFERENCES

1. Klein J, Figueroa F, Nazz ZA. Genetics of the MHC: the final act. Annu Rev Immunol 1983; 1: 119.
2. Hood L, Steinmetz M, Malinser B. Genes and the MHC of the mouse. Annu Rev Immunol 1983; 1: 529.
3. Corry RJ, Winn HJ, Russel PS. Primarily vascularized allografts of hearts in mice. Transplantation 1973; 16: 343.
4. Miller CM, Martinelli GP, Racelis D, Schanzer H. Prolongation of rat cardiac allografts by pre-transplant administration of blood transfusions and cyclosporin A. Transplantation 1982; 33: 335.
5. Marquet RL, Heysteck GA, Tinbergen WJ. Specific inhibition of organ allograft rejection by donor blood. Transplant Proc 1971; 3: 708.
6. Von Bekkum DW, Heysteck GA, Marquet RC. Effects of immunosuppression treatment on rejection of heart allografts in rats. Transplantation 1969; 8: 678.
7. Shelby J, Wakely E, Corry RJ. Suppressor cell induction in donor-specific transfused mouse heart recipients. Surgery 1984; 96: 296.

Received 24 January 1985.
Accepted 12 November 1985.

0041-1337/86/4202-0228$02.00/0
TRANSPLANTATION

Vol. 42, No. 2
Printed in U.S.A.

TRANSMISSION OF MALARIA BY BONE MARROW TRANSPLANTATION

Infection frequently occurs as a consequence of bone marrow transplantation (BMT). * It is related in part to the process of marrow ablation which results in neutropenia and immune deficiency. The speed of marrow engraftment and return of immune competence are the principal factors determining the infectious complications that occur after BMT. Bacterial and fungal infections are usual during the immediate post-BMT period of neutropenia, and after this period viral infections such as cytomegalovirus or herpes zoster are more frequent, although bacterial infections due to encapsulated organisms can also occur "late" after transplantation (*1*). These infections can be exogenous—i.e., acquired from outside the BMT recipient; transferred from the donor bone marrow; or acquired from the environment or caused by endogenous latent bacterial, protozoal, or fungal infections, such as tuberculosis, toxoplasmosis or coccidioidomycosis, which can become active during BMT.

Transmission of malaria by BMT has not been previously recognized although theoretically the risks are identical to the transmission of infected blood products. We have experience of a case of malaria transmitted by this route and wish to outline the subsequent successful measures used to prevent transmission of malaria by BMT.

A 27-year-old Nigerian woman with aplastic anaemia of five years duration was admitted for bone marrow transplantation. She had been resident in Great Britain since 1981 and had returned from holiday in Nigeria in June 1984. She had received daily proguanil prophylaxis during her stay in Nigeria and was administered ten tablets of chloroquine sulphate 200 mg base as a therapeutic course on her return. Blood films at this stage did not show any malarial parasites. The donor was her HLA-identical brother, a Nigerian resident of the same blood group as the recipient. He had not received any antimalarial therapy. Thin and thick blood films from the donor failed to demonstrate any malarial parasites. Films made from the bone marrow likewise revealed no parasites. Bone marrow was admixed with dimethylsulfoxide and cryopreserved at −196°C in liquid nitrogen for three weeks prior to administration. Transplantation was carried out at the beginning of November. After infusion of the transplant, the recipient developed loin pain and hemoglobinuria. This was thought to have been caused by the process of freezing and thawing of the marrow, which had led to red cell destruction with liberation of hemoglobin into the intravascular compartment. Engraftment occurred at day 11 post-transplant but graft failure was apparent 26 days after transplantation.

The donor was reharvested and the marrow infused 29 days after the first transplant without prior manipulation of the marrow. Again thin and thick blood films from the peripheral blood and marrow of the donor did not reveal any malaria parasites. Six days after the second transplant the recipient became febrile. These high fevers did not respond to therapy with ceftazidime, amikacin, vancomycin, or amphotericin B administered in sequence. Blood films revealed Plasmodium falciparum. Effective therapy could not be administered as death occurred. Autopsy was not permitted.

Accidental transmission of malaria is documented following blood transfusion (*2*). With the increase in frequency of bone marrow transplants and the use of donors from endemic areas, the transmission of malaria by this route deserves attention. Acquired immunity to malarial parasites in endemic areas leads to absence of detectable parasitemia but an inability completely to sterilize the infection, a phenomenon that has been termed *premunition* (*3*). Blood products including bone marrow from these individuals has the potential for transmission of malaria as demonstrated in our patient. Recrudescence of a latent malarial infection was unlikely as adequate chloroquine therapy was given to the recipient prior to transplantation and chloroquine resistance has not been reported in Nigeria (*4*). Malarial infection did not follow the first transplant as the process of cryopreservation of the marrow had apparently led to rupture of the red cells and thus to nonviability of the parasites.

As there is a potential risk of transmission of malaria by this route we have subsequently established a policy of treating the bone marrow donors from malarious areas prior to bone marrow harvest. Therapeutic courses of chloroquine or quinine have been used depending on the drug sensitivity of the malarial parasites in the area of residence of the donor. In addition recipients who originated from malarious areas have been given therapeutic courses of appropriate antimalarial treatment. These measures appear to have been successful in the prevention of malaria transmission by BMT.

Acknowledgments. We thank the London School of Hygiene and Tropical Medicine for technical help.

FINELLA DHARMASENA
E.C. GORDON-SMITH
Royal Postgraduate Medical School
University of London
Hammersmith Hospital
London W12 OHS, England

REFERENCES

1. Winston DJ, Schiffman G, Wang DC, et al. Pneumococcal infections after human bone marrow transplantation. Ann Intern Med 1979; 91: 835.
2. World Health Organization, Geneva. Malaria control–a reoriented strategy. WHO Chronicles 1978; 32: 226.
3. Sergent E. Latent infection and premunition: some definitions of microbiology and immunology. In: Garnham PCC, Pirce AE, Roitt IM, eds. Immunity to protozoa. Oxford: Blackwell, 1963: 38.
4. World Health Organization, Geneva. Malaria risk in international travel. WHO Weekly Epidemiological Record 1984; 29: 221.

* Abbreviations used: BMT, bone marrow transplantation.

0041-1337/86/4203-0229$02.00/0
TRANSPLANTATION

Vol. 42, No. 3
Printed in U.S.A.

Transplantation
OVERVIEW

INCREASING UTILIZATION OF BONE MARROW TRANSPLANTATION[1]

MORTIMER M. BORTIN[2] AND ALFRED A. RIMM

International Bone Marrow Transplant Registry, The Department of Medicine and the Division of Biostatistics/Clinical Epidemiology, Medical College of Wisconsin, Milwaukee, Wisconsin 53226

Prior to 1969 there were approximately 200 patients reported in the scientific literature who received bone marrow or fetal tissue transplants (*1*). All had advanced disease, and only a few showed clear evidence of engraftment with improvement or cure. In 1970 the future of bone marrow transplantation was in doubt. Many investigators directed their efforts to other fields because results had been so disappointing. Others persisted because of promising results in animal experiments (*2–5*), and because of the finding in 1968 that several immunodeficiency diseases could be treated successfully with allogeneic bone marrow transplantation when donor and recipient were identical or closely matched for HLA (*6–8*).

Since the early 1970s, increased activity in the field has been largely the result of progressively improving results. Most stem from advances in the following areas: understanding of the immunobiology and immunogenetics of bone marrow transplantation; methods for histocompatibility testing; pretransplant immunosuppressive preparative regimens; and posttransplant patient care. In addition to the clinical epidemiologic research programs of the International Bone Marrow Transplantation Registry (IBMTR),* periodic surveys are conducted to determine activity in the field worldwide. We present data documenting the growth in the use of bone marrow transplantation during the past 30 years, particularly in the leukemias.

The IBMTR maintains a roster of active bone marrow transplant teams. Several mechanisms are used to ensure identification of all teams. First, most teams presently report detailed information regarding their consecutive bone marrow transplant experience to the IBMTR. Second, using the U.S. National Library of Medicine as a resource, the biomedical literature is screened monthly for articles on clinical bone marow transplantation to identify new teams. Third, the IBMTR maintains a booth at annual meetings of the International Society for Experimental Hematology and encourages new teams to identify themselves. Fourth, the 24 members of the Advisory Committee of the IBMTR help to identify small or beginning teams that have not yet published reports of their work. The IBMTR roster of 162 active bone marrow transplant teams is presented in Table 1. This list is believed to represent essentially all institutions worldwide that had a bone marrow transplant program in 1984. There undoubtedly were existing transplant teams, particularly in remote areas or areas of restricted international contact, that unintentionally are not listed.

Data regarding the number of patients receiving bone marrow transplants were derived from several sources. For the period prior to 1968, the data are based on patients reported in the medical literature (*1*). Between 1969 and 1982 our estimates were obtained from cases reported to the IMBTR, data provided by several large teams that do not participate in the IBMTR research program, and reviews of the medical literature. Data for 1983 and 1984 were obtained by surveying the 162 known active bone marrow transplant teams (Table 1). The response rate was 100%. Teams were requested to provide information regarding the number of patients transplanted and the disease for which each transplant was performed. Data were collected for transplants of bone marrow from allogeneic or identical twin donors and for transplants of other hematopoietic or lymphopoietic tissues, such as fetal liver cells, fetal thymus, or cultured thymic epithelium. Less than 5% of the patients received transplants of tissues other than bone marrow, and use of the term "bone marrow" in this report includes these patients. Patients receiving autologous bone marrow were not included in the surveys.

Although the data are based on information compiled from a variety of sources, rather than from a review of hospital records, we believe the estimates are close approximations of the actual number of patients worldwide who have received bone marrow transplants. Data provided in response to our surveys were cross-checked against data in the IBMTR and/or the literature.

Growth in the field of bone marrow transplantation is reflected by the annual increase in the number of patients transplanted—and, to a lesser extent, by the number of new teams. This increase can be divided into four distinct periods (Table 2).

* Abbreviation used: IBMTR, International Bone Marrow Transplant Registry.

[1] This work was supported by Grant 1PO1 CA/AM 40053 from the National Cancer Institute, DHHS: Contract N01-AI-62530 from the National Institute of Allergy and Infectious Diseases, DHHS; Grant AM 33752 from the National Institute of Arthritis, Diabetes, Digestive and Kidney Diseases, DHHS; Contract BI6-084-US from the Commission of the European Communities; and grants from the Jacob and Hilda Blaustein Foundation, Charles E. Culpeper Foundation, William Randolph Hearst Foundation, RGK Foundation, Ambrose Monell Foundation, Samuel Roberts Noble Foundation, Elsa U. Pardee Foundation, Sandoz, Inc., and the Swiss Cancer League.

[2] Address reprint requests to: Mortimer M. Bortin, M.D., International Bone Marrow Transplant Registry, Medical College of Wisconsin, P.O. Box 26509, Milwaukee, WI 53226.

TABLE 1. Roster of known bone marrow transplant teams, 1984

Institution	City	State
A. United States:		
Children's Hospital	Little Rock	Arkansas
Alta Bates Hospital	Berkeley	California
City of Hope National Medical Center	Duarte	California
Scripps Clinic & Research Foundation	La Jolla	California
Children's Hospital	Los Angeles	California
UCLA Department of Medicine	Los Angeles	California
UCLA Department of Pediatrics	Los Angeles	California
Children's Hospital	Oakland	California
Children's Hospital	San Diego	California
Pacific Medical Center	San Francisco	California
University of California	San Francisco	California
University of Colorado	Denver	Colorado
University of Florida	Gainesville	Florida
All Children's Hospital	St. Petersburg	Florida
Emory University	Atlanta	Georgia
St. Francis Hospital	Honolulu	Hawaii
University of Iowa	Iowa City	Iowa
Rush Presbyterian–St. Luke's	Chicago	Illinois
Loyola University Medical Center	Maywood	Illinois
University of Kansas	Kansas City	Kansas
University of Kentucky	Lexington	Kentucky
Tulane Medical Center	New Orleans	Louisiana
Louisiana State Medical Center	New Orleans	Louisiana
Harvard Medical School	Boston	Massachusetts
Johns Hopkins Oncology Center	Baltimore	Maryland
NIH, NIAID	Bethesda	Maryland
Wayne State University	Detroit	Michigan
University of Minnesota	Minneapolis	Minnesota
Mayo Clinic	Rochester	Minnesota
Washington University	St. Louis	Missouri
Duke University Medical Center	Durham	North Carolina
University of Nebraska	Omaha	Nebraska
Bishop Clarkson Memorial Hospital	Omaha	Nebraska
Roswell Park Memorial Institute	Buffalo	New York
Sloan-Kettering Cancer Center	New York	New York
University of Cincinnati	Cincinnati	Ohio
Children's Hospital	Cincinnati	Ohio
Cleveland Clinic Foundation	Cleveland	Ohio
Case–Western Reserve University	Cleveland	Ohio
Ohio State University	Columbus	Ohio
Oklahoma Teaching Hospitals	Oklahoma City	Oklahoma
University of Oklahoma	Oklahoma City	Oklahoma
Oregon University	Portland	Oregon
Children's Hospital	Philadelphia	Pennsylvania
Hahnemann University	Philadelphia	Pennsylvania
St. Jude Children's Research Hospital	Memphis	Tennessee
White Hall Medical Center	Chattanooga	Tennessee
M.D. Anderson Hospital	Houston	Texas
Baylor College of Medicine	Houston	Texas
Children's Hospital	Houston	Texas
Wilford Hall Medical Center	Lackland	Texas
Leland R. Cowan Cancer Clinic	Murray	Utah
Fred Hutchinson Cancer Center	Seattle	Washington
U. Wisconsin Department of Medicine	Madison	Wisconsin
U. Wisconsin Department of Pediatrics	Madison	Wisconsin
Children's Hospital	Milwaukee	Wisconsin
Medical College of Wisconsin	Milwaukee	Wisconsin

TABLE 1—*continued*

Institution	City	Country
B. Europe:		
Med. Univ.-Klinik	Vienna	Austria
Cliniques Universitaires Saint-Luc	Brussels	Belgium
Academisch Ziekenhuis St. Rafael	Leuven	Belgium
Rigshospitalet	Copenhagen	Denmark
University of Helsinki	Helsinki	Finland
Turku University	Turku	Finland
Universitaire d'Angers	Angers	France
Centre Reg. de Transfus. Sanguine	Besancon	France
University of Bordeaux	Bordeaux	France
Henri Mondor Hospital	Creteil	France
Hôpital Debrousse	Lyon	France
Hôpital Eduoard Herriot	Lyon	France
Centre Leon Berard	Lyon	France
Institut J. Paoli Calmettes	Marseille	France
Hôpital Saint Jacques	Besancon	France
Centre Hospitalier Regional de Nancy	Nancy	France
Hôpital Saint-Louis	Paris	France
Hôpital Saint-Antoine	Paris	France
Hôpital des Enfants Malades	Paris	France
Hôpital Jean Bernard	Poiters	France
Hôpital Bellevue	Saint Etienne	France
Hôpital Purpan	Toulouse	France
Groupe Hôpital Paul-Brousse	Villejuif	France
Karl Marx Universitat	Leipzig	East Germany
University of Essen	Essen	West Germany
Kinderklinik Medizinischen Hochschule	Hannover	West Germany
Medizinishe und Poliklinik	Kiel	West Germany
Medizinische Universitats Klinik I	Cologne	West Germany
U. Munich, Medizinische Klinik III	Munich	West Germany
Universitats-Kinderklinik	Munich	West Germany
Medizinische Universitatsklinik	Tubingen	West Germany
Universitat Ulm	Ulm/Donau	West Germany
Institute of Haematology	Budapest	Hungary
Semmelweis University	Budapest	Hungary
St. James Hospital	Dublin	Ireland
St. Orsola University Hospital	Bologna	Italy
Ospedale San Martino	Genoa	Italy
University of Milan	Milan	Italy
Università-Ospedale di Parma	Parma	Italy
Ospedale Riuniti di Pesaro	Pesaro	Italy
Hospital of Pescara	Pescara	Italy
Universita delgi Studi la Sapineza	Rome	Italy
Universita delgi Studi di Roma	Rome	Italy
U. Leiden Department of Medicine	Leiden	Netherlands
U. Leiden Department of Pediatrics	Leiden	Netherlands
Katholieke Universiteit	Nijmegen	Netherlands
Dr. Daniel Den Hoed Cancer Center	Rotterdam	Netherlands
University of Oslo	Oslo	Norway
University of Barcelona	Barcelona	Spain
Reina Sofia Hospital	Cordoba	Spain
Clinica Puerta de Hierro	Madrid	Spain
Hospital de la Princesa	Madrid	Spain
Medico Marques de Valdecilla	Santander	Spain
Seguridad Social la Fe	Valencia	Spain
Huddinge Hospital	Huddinge	Sweden
Kantonsspital	Basel	Switzerland

TABLE 1—*continued*

Institution	City	Country
Kantonsspital	Zurich	Switzerland
Kinderspital	Zurich	Switzerland
Queen Elizabeth Medical Center	Birmingham	United Kingdom
Royal Infirmary of Edinburgh	Edinburgh	United Kingdom
Glasgow Royal Infirmary	Glasgow	United Kingdom
St. James University Hospital	Leeds	United Kingdom
Charing Cross Hospital	London	United Kingdom
Hammersmith Hospital	London	United Kingdom
Hospitals for Sick Children	London	United Kingdom
The London Clinic	London	United Kingdom
Royal Free Hospital	London	United Kingdom
Royal Marsden Hospital	London	United Kingdom
University College Hospital	London	United Kingdom
University of London	London	United Kingdom
Westminster Hospital	London	United Kingdom
Royal Victoria Infirmary	Newcastle	United Kingdom
University Hospital	Belgrade	Yugoslavia
Klinka za Unutrasnje bolesti KBC-Rebro	Zagreb	Yugoslavia
C. Other locations:		
Institute of Medical Science	Adelaide	Australia
St. Vincent's Hospital	Darlinghurst	Australia
Royal Perth Hospital	Perth	Australia
Prince of Wales Children's Hospital	Randwick	Australia
Institute of Clinical Pathology	Westmead	Australia
Queen Elizabeth Hospital	Woodville	Australia
Hospital de Clinicas	Parana	Brazil
Tom Baker Cancer Center	Calgary	Canada
McMaster University	Ontario	Canada
Children's Hospital	Montreal	Canada
Hôpital Maisonneuve-Rosemont	Montreal	Canada
Montreal General Hospital	Montreal	Canada
Royal Victoria Hospital	Montreal	Canada
Hospital for Sick Children	Toronto	Canada
Ontario Cancer Institute	Toronto	Canada
Beijing Medical College	Beijing	China
Lanzhou General Hospital	Lanzhou	China
Tata Memorial Hospital	Bombay	India
Hadassah University Hospital	Jerusalem	Israel
Shari Zedek Hospital	Jerusalem	Israel
Tel Hashomer Hospital	Tel Aviv	Israel
Tokai University	Kanagawa	Japan
Kanazawa University	Kanazawa-shi	Japan
Daini Red Cross Hospital	Nagoya	Japan
Niigata University	Niigata	Japan
Center for Adult Diseases	Osaka	Japan
Jichi Medical School	Tochigi	Japan
University of Tokyo	Tokyo	Japan
Catholic Medical School	Seoul	Korea
Christchurch Hospital	Christchurch	New Zealand
King Faisal Hospital	Riyadh	Saudi Arabia
University of Cape Town	Cape Town	S. Africa

Lorenz et al. (*2*) reported in 1951 that mice and guinea pigs could survive supralethal doses of total-body irradiation if given i.v. infusions of bone marrow cells from donors of the same species postirradiation. From this discovery until 1968 there were reports of 203 human bone marrow transplants in the scientific literature (*1*) E. Donnall Thomas, M.D. Seattle, estimates that at least an equal number of bone marrow transplants were attempted in this same interval, but not reported (personal communication).

TABLE 2. Activity in the field of bone marrow transplantation

Period	Patients Transplanted[a]	New Teams[a]
1. 1955–1968	2–64	<2
2. 1969–1978	80–199	5–12
3. 1979–1981	400–874	6–17
4. 1982–1984	1450–2398	25–28

[a] Annual number.

In the following decade, 1969–1978, approximately 1350 patients worldwide received bone marrow transplants. During this interval, 80–200 patients were transplanted annually. The estimated number of patients transplanted in the three years from 1979 to 1981 was 1825, with annual activity ranging from 400 to 875 patients treated. For the three years 1982–1984 there were approximately 6067 patients who received bone marrow transplants: 1450 in 1982, 2219 in 1983, and 2398 in 1984.

The annual cumulative number of patients receiving bone marrow transplants, as well as the annual number of active bone marrow transplant teams are shown in Figure 1. Note that in the seven-year period 1978–1984 there was a twelvefold increase in patients transplanted, from 199 in 1978 to 2398 in 1984.

From the available data we estimate that 9445 patients received bone marrow transplants in the 30-year period 1955–1984, and 4617 (49%) were transplanted in 1983 and 1984. The distribution of patients by disease category and geographic location of teams performing the transplants for 1983 and 1984 are presented in Table 3.

Further evidence of rapid growth in the field of bone marrow transplantation is the recent increase in the number of new teams being formed (Fig. 1). In the 26 years from 1955 through 1980, approximately 104 teams entered the field, an average of four per year. Between 1981 and 1984, 95 new teams entered the field. Of the 199 institutions that have had a bone marrow transplantation program, 162 continue to have active teams, and 59% of these were initiated in the past four years. Since 1955, 37 teams disbanded.

To evaluate team size, we analyzed the total number of patients transplanted per team in 1983 and 1984 (Table 4). Of the 162 active bone marrow transplant teams, 66 (41%) transplanted 10 or fewer patients, while eight teams (5%) transplanted more than 100 patients in this two-year interval.

Data reported to the IBMTR since 1969 have shown a marked increase in the use of transplantation for malignant disease, in comparison with nonmalignant disease (Table 5). Prior to July 1980, 72% of the transplants were performed for nonmalignant diseases; since then 77% of the transplants were for patients with malignancies, primarily leukemia.

The data presented demonstrate progressive growth in the field of bone marrow transplantation in the past 30 years, as measured by a steady annual increase in the number of patients being transplanted and in the number of new teams entering the field. Several factors seem to be primarily responsible for this trend.

Prior to 1980, bone marrow transplantation was widely viewed as an experimental procedure. Transplants were largely restricted to patients with advanced disease who had failed to respond to other modes of therapy. With reports from several centers (*9, 10*) that 5–20% of patients with end-stage leukemia could achieve long-term disease-free survival via bone marrow transplantation, an increasing number of leukemia patients, especially those known to have a poor prognosis on chemotherapy, were transplanted in earlier stages of their disease (*11–16*). Reports that bone marrow transplantation had a high probability for improvement or cure in selected cases of severe aplastic anemia (*17*) and severe combined immunodeficiency disease (*18*) also spurred growth in the field. Progressively improving results have resulted in bone marrow transplantation being accepted by many physicians as a therapeutic option, with referral of increasing numbers of patients to transplant teams.

Among patients who might benefit from bone marrow transplantation, only about 35–40% have an HLA-identical sibling who can serve as a donor. Prior to 1980, almost all transplants were restricted to donors and recipients who were HLA-identical siblings. Since then, an increasing number of teams have been investigating the use of other family members or unrelated donors who are fully or partially HLA-matched with the recipient when no HLA-identical silbing is available. Early results (*19–23*) have been encouraging, and this also has contributed to increasing activity in the field.

Another consideration that has led to increased utilization of bone marrow transplantation has been improved understanding of risk factors for transplant-related causes of treatment failure, such as early infectious complications (*24, 25*), graft-versus-host disease (*26, 27*), and interstitial pneumonitis (*28, 29*). It is now possible to avoid certain risks. When this is not possible, patients who are at high risk for a specific complication can often be identified pretransplant, and special precautions may then be taken to reduce the risk.

General supportive measures, such as experienced and skilled nursing personnel, hyperalimentation, laminar airflow isolation, improved antimicrobials, infectious disease surveillance, and psychological support, as well as other improvements in patient care also have played an important role in the increased

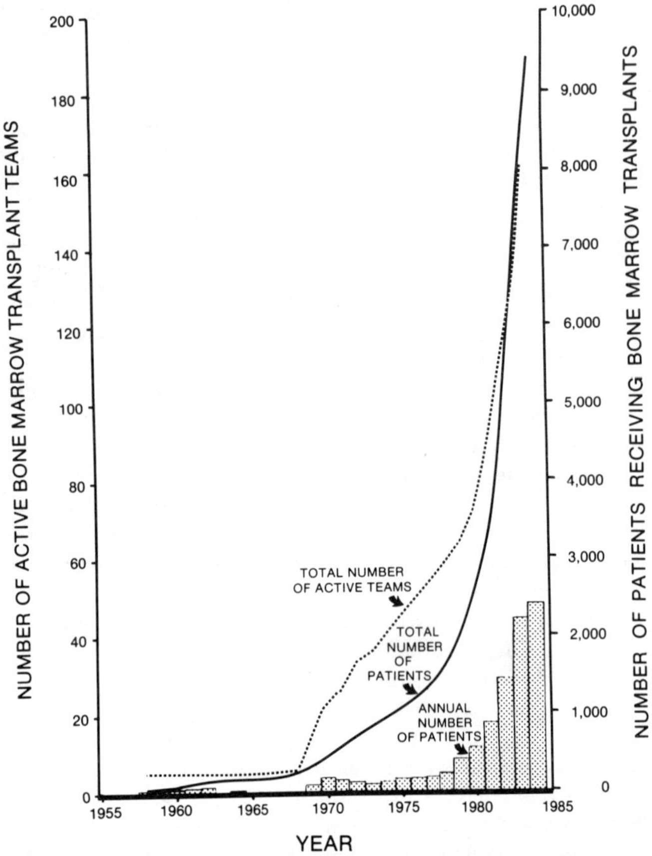

FIGURE 1. Vertical bars represent number of patients who received bone marrow transplants annually. Solid line indicates cumulative number of patients who received bone marrow transplants from 1958 through 1984. Dashed line represents cumulative number of active bone marrow transplant teams from 1958 through 1984.

TABLE 4. Team size as reflected by total number of patients receiving bone marrow transplants in 1983 and 1984

Location	No. Patients transplanted in 1983 and 1984					Total teams
	≤10	11–20	21–50	51–100	>100	
USA	27[a]	7	11	8	4	57
Europe	22	18	21	9	3	73
Other[b]	17	7	5	2	1	32
Total:	66	32	37	19	8	162

[a] Indicates that 27 teams located in the United States performed bone marrow transplants for 10 or fewer patients in 1983 and 1984.

[b] Includes teams in Australia, Brazil, Canada, China, India, Israel, Japan, Korea, New Zealand, Saudi Arabia, and South Africa.

TABLE 5. Proportion of patients treated with bone marrow transplantation by disease category[a] as reported to the International Bone Marrow Transplant Registry

Interval	N	Malignancies	Hematopoietic disorders	Rare diseases
7/69–6/80	699	28%	47%	25%
7/80–6/85	3187	77%	18%	5%

[a] The disease category of *malignancies* refers to leukemia, lymphoma, and other malignant diseases; *hematopoietic disorders* refers to severe aplastic anemia, thalassemia major, and other nonmalignant disorders of hematopoiesis; *rare diseases* refers to immunodeficiency, lysosomal storage, and other rare genetic disorders.

TABLE 3. Results of IBMTR survey showing number of patients (%) receiving allogeneic or syngeneic bone marrow transplants in 1983 and 1984 by location of team and disease category treated.[a]

Location	Disease category—1983			Total	Disease category—1984			Total
	Malignancies	Hematopoietic disorders	Rare diseases		Malignancies	Hematopoietic disorders	Rare diseases	
USA	812 (84)	96 (10)	62 (6)	970	856 (85)	82 (8)	62 (6)	1000
Europe	730 (75)	128 (13)	110 (11)	968	885 (81)	145 (13)	64 (6)	1094
Other	230 (82)	41 (14)	10 (4)	281	257 (85)	37 (12)	10 (3)	304
Total:	1772 (80)	265 (12)	182 (8)	2219	1998 (83)	264 (11)	136 (6)	2398

[a] The disease category of *malignancies* refers to leukemia, lymphoma, and other malignant diseases; *hematopoietic disorders* refers to severe aplastic anemia, thalassemia major, and other nonmalignant disorders of hematopoiesis; *rare diseases* refers to immunodeficiency, lysosomal storage, and other rare genetic disorders.

safety—and, hence, the increased use of bone marrow transplantation.

In the past 30 years, there have been striking changes in the proportion of patients treated with bone marrow transplantation for malignant versus nonmalignant diseases. In the years prior to 1980, 72% of patients reported to the IBMTR were transplanted for nonmalignant diseases. Since 1980 77% of transplants were for malignant diseases. Thus, while the absolute numbers of patients transplanted for rare diseases and hematopoietic disorders have doubled and tripled in the past five years, the number being transplanted for malignancies has increased 24-fold.

Several factors were cited in this review that account in part for the recent rapid rise in the use of bone marrow transplantation. These, and several additional considerations lead us to believe that, at least in the immediate future, the field will continue to expand at a rapid rate. In comparison with other forms of therapy, bone marrow transplantation now appears to offer an impressive disease-free survival advantage for selected patients with several hematologic malignancies. Among these are those under 40 years of age who have an HLA-identical sibling donor and are transplanted for chronic myelogenous leukemia while in the chronic phase of their disease (*30*), and those transplanted for acute lymphoblastic leukemia in second remission—or in first remission, if adults (*31*). A proportion of patients with genetic disorders, such as thalassemia major and lysosomal storage diseases also have been shown to respond favorably to bone marrow transplantation (*32–34*). Perhaps the single most important factor that is likely to result in a further increase in the application of bone marrow transplantation is expansion of the pool of appropriate donors to include related and unrelated individuals who are partially or fully matched with the patient at HLA (*19–23*).

Acknowledgments. This 30th report from the International Bone Marrow Transplant Registry was prepared for the Advisory Committee: Robert Peter Gale, M.D., Ph.D., Los Angeles (Chairman); Fritz H. Bach, M.D., Minneapolis; A. John Barrett, M.D., London: Dirk W. van Bekkum, M.D., Ph.D., Rijswijk; James C. Biggs, M.D., Sydney; Karl G. Blume, M.D., Los Angeles; Mortimer M. Bortin, M.D., Milwaukee; Karel A. Dicke, M.D., Ph.D., Houston; Eliane Gluckman, M.D., Paris; John M. Goldman, M.D., London; Robert A. Good, M.D., Ph.D., St. Petersburg; Roger H. Herzig, M.D., Cleveland; Richard Hong, M.D., Madison; John H. Kersey, M.D., Minneapolis; Hans-Jochem Kolb, M.D., Munich; Alberto M. Marmont, M.D., Genoa; Tohru Masaoka, M.D., Osaka; Hans A. Messner, M.D., Ph.D., Toronto; Richard J. O'Reilly, M.D., New York; Ray L. Powles, M.D., London; Alfred A. Rimm, Ph.D., Milwaukee; Olle Ringden, M.D., Ph.D., Stockholm; Jon J. van Rood, M.D., Ph.D., Leiden; Ciril T. Rozman, M.D., Barcelona; Bruno Speck, M.D., Basel; Roy S. Weiner, M.D., Gainesville; and Ferdinand E. Zwaan, M.D., Ph.D., Leiden.

We thank Ms. D'Etta Koser and Ms. Sharon Gurgul for help with data analysis and Ms. Karen Witkowski for help in preparation of the manuscript.

REFERENCES

1. Bortin MM. A compendium of reported human bone marrow transplants. Transplantation 1970; 9: 571.
2. Lorenz E, Uphoff D, Reid TR, Shelton E. Modification of irradiation injury in mice and guinea pigs by bone marrow injections. J Natl Cancer Inst 1951; 12: 197.
3. Yunis EJ, Hilgaard HR, Martinez C, Good RA. Studies on immunologic reconstitution of thymectomized mice. J Exp Med 1965; 121: 607.
4. Epstein RB, Bryant J, Thomas ED. Cytogenetic demonstration of permanent tolerance in adult outbred dogs. Transplantation 1967; 5: 267.
5. van Bekkum DW, deVries JJ. Radiation chimaeras. London: Logos Press, 1967.
6. Bach FH, Albertini RJ, Joe P, Anderson JJ, Bortin MM. Bone marrow transplantation in a patient with Wiskott-Aldrich syndrome. Lancet 1968; 2: 1364.
7. Gatti RA, Allen HD, Meuwissen HJ, et al. Immunological reconstitution of sex-linked lymphopenic immunological deficiency. Lancet 1968; 2: 1366.
8. deKoning J, Dooren LJ, van Bekkum Dw, et al. Transplantation of bone-marrow cells and fetal thymus in an infant with lymphopenic immunological deficiency. Lancet 1969; 1: 1223.
9. Thomas ED, Buckner CD, Banaji M, et al. One hundred patients with acute leukemia treated by chemotherapy, total body irradiation, and allogeneic marrow transplantation. Blood 1977; 49: 511.
10. Bortin MM, Rimm AA. Bone marrow transplantation for acute myeloblastic leukemia. JAMA 1978; 240: 1246.
11. Thomas ED, Buckner CD, Clift RA, et al. Marrow transplantation for acute nonlymphoblastic leukemia in first remission. N Engl J Med 1979; 301: 597.
12. Blume KG, Beutler E, Bross KJ, et al. Bone marrow ablation and allogeneic marrow transplantation in acute leukemia. N Engl J Med 1980; 302: 1041.
13. Gale RP. Clinical trials of bone marrow transplantation in leukemia. In: Gale RP, Fox DF, eds. Biology of bone marrow transplantation. New York: Academic, 1980: 11.
14. Forman SJ, Spruce WE, Farbstein MJ, et al. Bone marrow ablation followed by allogeneic marrow grafting during first complete remission of acute nonlymphoblastic leukemia. Blood 1983; 439.
15. Kersey JH, Ramsay NKC, Kim T, et al. Allogeneic bone marrow transplantation in acute nonlymphoblastic leukemia: a pilot study. Blood 1981; 60: 400.
16. Powles RL, Clink HM, Bandini G, et al. The place of bone marrow transplantation in acute myelogenous leukemia. Lancet 1980; 1: 1047.
17. Storb R, Thomas ED, Buckner CD, et al. Marrow transplantation in 30 untransfused patients with severe aplastic anemia. Ann Intern Med 1980; 92: 30.
18. Bortin MM, Rimm AA. Severe combined immunodeficiency disease. Characterization of the disease and results of transplantation. JAMA 1977; 238: 591.
19. Storch S, Gale RP, Champlin R, Ho W, et al. Partially mismatched marrow transplantation for acute leukemia and aplastic anemia. In: Gale RP, ed. Recent advances in bone marrow transplantation. New York: Alan R. Liss, 1983: 785.
20. Powles RL, Kay HEM, Morgenstern GR, et al. Mismatched family donors for bone-marrow transplantation as treatment for acute leukemia. Lancet 1983; 1: 612.
21. Gingrich RD, Howe CWS, Goeken NE, et al. The use of partially matched, unrelated donors in clinical bone marrow transplantation. Transplantation 1985; 39: 526.
22. Filipovich AH, Ramsay NKC, Arthur DC, McGlave P, Kim T, Kersey JH. Allogeneic bone marrow transplantation with related donors other than HLA MLC-matched siblings, and the use of antithymocyte globulin, prednisone, and methotrexate for prophylaxis of graft-versus-host disease. Transplantation 1985; 39: 282.
23. Beatty PG, Clift RA, Mickelson EM, et al. Marrow transplantation from related donors other than HLA-identical siblings. N Engl J Med 1985; 313: 765.
24. Winston DJ, Gale RP, Meyer DV, Young LS and the UCLA Bone Marrow Transplantation Group. Infectious complications of human bone marrow transplantation. Medicine 1979; 58: 1
25. Zaia JA. Infections. In: Blume KG, Petz LD, eds. Clinical bone marrow transplantation. New York: Churchill Livingstone, 1983: 131.
26. Ringden O, Nilson B, Bolme P, et al. Factors associated with severe acute graft-versus-host disease (GVHD). Exp Hematol 1984;

12(suppl 15): 49.

27. Atkinson K, Farrell C, Chapman G, Downs K, Penny R, Biggs J. Female marrow donors increase the risk of acute graft-versus-host disease: effect of donor age and parity and analysis of cell subpopulation in the donor marrow inoculum. Br J Hematol (in press).
28. Meyers JD, Flournoy N, Thomas ED. Nonbacterial pneumonia after allogeneic marrow transplantation: a review of ten years' experience. Rev Infect Dis 1982; 4: 1119.
29. Bortin MM, Kay HEM, Gale RP, Rimm AA. Factors associated with interstitial pneumonitis after bone marrow transplantation for acute leukemia. Lancet 1982; 1: 437.
30. Speck B, Bortin MM, Champlin R, et al. Allogeneic bone marrow transplantation for chronic myelogenous leukemia. Lancet 1984; 1: 665.
31. Gale RP, Kersey JH, Bortin MM, et al. Bone marrow transplantation for acute lymphoblastic leukemia. Lancet 1983; 2: 663.
32. Lucarelli G, Polchi P, Izzi T, et al. Marrow transplantation for thalassemia after treatment with busulphan and cyclosphosphamide. Exp Hematol 1984; 12(suppl 15): 95.
33. Joshi R, Barrett AJ, Ingram L, et al. Bone marrow transplantation for beta thalassemia major. Exp Hematol 1984; 12(suppl 15): 97.
34. Hobbs JR: Correction of 34 genetic diseases by displacement bone marrow transplantation. Plasma Ther Transfus Technol 1985; 6: 221.

0041-1337/86/4203-0235$02.00/0
TRANSPLANTATION
Copyright © 1986 by The Williams & Wilkins Co.

Vol. 42, No. 3
Printed in U.S.A.

Transplantation

ARTICLES

TRANSPLANTATION OF THE SMALL BOWEL ACROSS MHC AND NON-MHC DISPARITIES IN THE RAT[1]

MYUNG DUK LEE, HEINZ W. KUNZ, THOMAS J. GILL III, DAVID A. LLOYD, AND MARC R. ROWE

Department of Surgery, Children's Hospital of Pittsburgh; and Department of Pathology, University of Pittsburgh School of Medicine, Pittsburgh, Pennsylvania 15261

Using congenic strains of rats, the effect on the rejection of small bowel transplants across isolated major histocompatibility complex (MHC) and nonMHC antigenic disparities was examined. The medial survival time of small bowel grafts across MHC differences in the LEW anti-LEW.1N and LEW.1N anti-LEW strain combinations was 14 and 12 days, respectively. The median survival time across the nonMHC antigenic difference in the BN anti-DA.1N strain combination was 20 days, which was significantly longer than the rejection time across the MHC differences (P<0.005). Both hemagglutinating and cytotoxic antibodies were produced in all three strain combinations, but the magnitude of the response varied considerably and did not correlate with the time of rejection. In the case of MHC differences, the antibody was directed against both class I and class II antigens, and with the nonMHC difference, the greatest response was directed against the major blood group antigen RT2.

Transplantation of the small bowel is potentially an important therapeutic approach for the treatment of inflammatory bowel disease, vascular accidents, trauma, and cancer—and it is an important adjunct to other procedures, such as pancreas transplantation. However, small bowel transplantation presents a variety of surgical and immunological difficulties (*1*). The surgical problems lie in the fragility of the bowel tissue and the complexity of its microvasculature. The immunological problems are both the host-versus-graft reaction and the graft-versus-host reaction caused by the lymphocytes in the Peyer's patches.

Studies on the transplantation of the small bowel in the rat have used the surgical technique of Monchik and Russell (*2*), or a slight modification thereof, and combinations either of inbred strains or of F_1 hybrids and inbred strains (*2–5*). In all but one report (*4*), the genetic disparities included both major histocompatibility complex (MHC)* and nonMHC differences. Rejection was assessed by criteria ranging from stomal necrosis of the transplant to death of the animal; despite these differences, there was reasonable agreement about the rejection times. Recently, more sophisticated electrophysiological and morphological techniques have been used to assess the progressive changes in the bowel transplant that lead to overt rejection (*6*).

It is critical to define the immunological parameters of rejection as a prelude to further analysis of the mechanisms involved in rejection, and as a means to identify the causes of graft failure as being due either to surgical or to immunological factors. In addition, cyclosporine prolongs the rejection time of small bowel transplants (*6–8*), and this effect may be under genetic control as it is in skin graft rejection (*9*). Hence, the major genetic barriers to bowel transplantation must be clearly identified, so that appropriate immunosuppressive regimens can be designed. This research exploits the availability of a variety of congenic strains of rats to assess the relative roles of MHC and nonMHC antigens in rejection. It also analyzes the antibody responses accompanying rejection.

MATERIALS AND METHODS

Animals. All of the animals used in this study came from our colony at the University of Pittsburgh School of Medicine. The various strains and their haplotypes are listed in Table 1. Male rats weighing 150–250 g were used in all studies, and four experimental groups with specific genetic disparities were established with 5–7 animals each: LEW anti-LEW (control), BN-anti-DA.1N (nonMHC), LEW anti-LEW.1N (MHC), and LEW.1N anti-LEW (MHC).

Transplantation. The animals were fasted for at least 12 h prior to operation, but had free access to water. Open-drop ether anesthesia was used, and the surgical technique was that of the heterotopic auxillary small bowel transplant (*2, 10*). A 20-cm segment of distal jejunum was isolated, preserving the mesenteric pedicle, and perfused with chilled Ringer-lactate solution containing 10,000 units/L of heparin by a cannula placed in the distal aorta. The isolated loop of bowel was removed with a vascular pedicle comprising the portal vein, superior mesenteric artery, and a segment of aorta; irrigated with phosphate-buffered saline, and stored at 4°C in the perfusion fluid.

The anesthetized recipient animal was given fluid through the right common jugular vein. A vertical abdominal incision was used to expose the infrarenal aorta and inferior vena cava, and then heparin (100 units/kg) was given by i.v. injection. The aorta and vena cava were occluded 1 cm distal to the left renal vein using a vascular clamp, and an end-to-side anastomosis was made between the donor portal vein and the recipient inferior vena cava and between the donor superior mesenteric

* Abbreviations used: MHC, major histocompatibility complex; RBC, red blood cell.

[1]This work was supported by grants CA 18659 and HD 08662 from the National Institutes of Health, and by grants from the Tim Caracio Memorial Cancer Fund and the Beaver County Cancer Society.

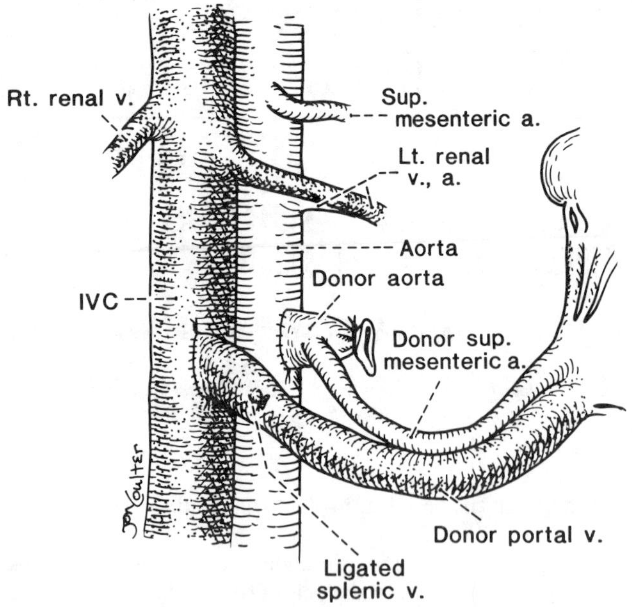

FIGURE 1. Diagram showing the surgical attachment of the small bowel as a heterotopic axillary graft. The donor superior mesenteric artery was positioned so that it lies toward the animal's right and across the inferior vena cava. This position avoids torsion of the donor portal vein.

TABLE 1. Strains used for transplantation and for serological analysis

Strain	Haplotype at different loci						
	RT1	RT2	RT3	RT6	RT7	RT8	RT9
DA	*a*	*b*	*a*	*b*	*a*	*b*	*a*
BUF	*b*	*a*	*b*	*a*	*b*	*b*	*a*
ALB	*b*	*b*	*b*	*b*	*b*	*b*	*a*
PVG.2A (AUG)	*c*	*a*	*a*	*a*	*a*	*b*	*a*
AUG.2B (PVG)	*c*	*b*	*a*	*b*	*a*	*b*	*a*
LEW	*l*	*a*	*a*	*a*	*a*	*b*	*a*
BN	*n*	*a*	*b*	*b*	*a*	*b*	*a*
DA.1N (BN)	*n*	*b*	*a*	*b*	*a*	*b*	*a*
LEW.1N (BN)	*n*	*a*	*a*	*a*	*a*	*b*	*a*

artery and the recipient aorta, using 9–0 ethylon sutures for the venous anastomosis and 8–0 proline sutures for the arterial anastomosis (Fig. 1). After completing the vascular anastomoses, but before releasing the vascular clamp, 1.5 ml of warm 0.15 M NaCl was injected i.v. The two ends of the grafted intestine were brought out through the anterior abdominal wall as jejunostomies to create a Thiry-Vella loop. The cold ischemia time was 40–55 min, and the major vessels of the recipient were occluded for 20–30 minutes.

After operation, the animals were housed individually, and for the first 18 hr they were infused with 2.5% glucose and 0.5% NaCl through the jugular catheter at 120 ml/kg/24 hr. They were returned to regular feeding and drinking thereafter, and ampicillin, 50 mg/kg/24 hr, was given by i.v. injection for three days after operation. The animals were evaluated daily for stoma viability, consumption of food and water, and body weight. In the strain combinations used here, graft survival beyond 72 hr was attained in 90% of the animals.

Evaluation of immune response. The major criterion for rejection of the graft was closing of the jejunal stoma; coincidentally, a palpable abdominal mass developed behind the stoma. Thereafter, the animal's food intake decreased and it lost weight. Histological examination of the stoma at this time showed both acute and chronic inflammation. The significance of the differences in rejection times was assessed by the Mann-Whitney *U* test.

The antibody responses were measured at one, two, and three months after transplantation by hemagglutination in Ficoll and by cytotoxicity using splenic lymphocytes (*11*); the data at two months are given in Table 2. The sera were analyzed for the presence of antibodies to class I and class II antigens by absorption with red blood cells (RBC) of the appropriate strain using three to five volumes of red cells to one volume of serum: all of the class I reactivity was removed. Separation of T and B cells was done on nylon-wool columns (*12*). The data were recorded as the titer and the strength (0 to +++) of hemagglutination, and as the titer and percentage of killing for cytotoxicity.

RESULTS

Small bowel transplants are rejected across both isolated MHC and nonMHC differences (Table 2). Rejection is slower ($P<0.005$) across a purely nonMHC difference than across an MHC difference alone. Reciprocal grafting across the LEW/LEW.1N difference gave rejection times which did not differ significantly. An antibody response occurred in all strain combinations tested, and it remained at a fairly stable level from one to three months after grafting. The antibody response did not, however, correlate with rejection, and there was no correlation between the production of hemagglutinating and cytotoxic antibody. The strongest cytotoxic antibody response occurred in the LEW.1N anti-LEW combination—whereas there was only a low cytotoxic response in two of the six grafted animals in the reciprocal strain combination.

The cytotoxic antibody response in the LEW.1N anti-LEW combination was made against both class I and class II antigens. The unabsorbed antiserum killed 90% of LEW splenic lymphocytes— and, when it was absorbed with LEW red blood cells, lymphocyte killing was reduced to 50–60%. In addition, the unabsorbed antiserum reacted with both T and B cells. The antibody response to nonMHC antigens in the BN anti-DA.1N strain combination was directed mainly against RT2, which is the major blood group antigen in the rat, and to a lesser extent against nonRT2 antigens (Table 3). When the antiserum was absorbed with $RT2^a$ red blood cells, all of the antibody was removed, within the limits of detection—whereas when it was absorbed with $RT2^b$ red blood cells, the titer was decreased but not eliminated. These findings are consistent with the removal of the nonRT2 antibodies leaving only the antibodies to $RT2^a$ in the absorbed antiserum.

DISCUSSION

Small bowel transplantation elicits a strong antibody response against both MHC and nonMHC antigens, but the type and magnitude of the response do not correlate with graft rejection. The definition of rejection that we used produces consistent and reproducible results, and the median survival times in this study are consistent with those from other studies in the literature (Table 4). This consistency indicates that once a clear indication of rejection occurs, the inevitable sequence of events leading to the loss of the graft is initiated. The similarity of the rejection times across MHC plus nonMHC

TABLE 2. Rejection of small bowel transplants across disparities at MHC and nonMHC loci

Strain combination (genetic disparity)	Graft survival (days)	Hemagglutination		Cytotoxicity[a]	
		Titer	Strength	Titer	Percentage of lymphocytes killed
LEW anti-LEW (none)	>218	0		0	
	>219	0		0	
	>232	0		0	
	>234	0		0	
	>256	0		0	
	MST >232				
BN anti-DA.1N (nonMHC)	20	64	+	0	
	20	32	+	0	
	20	64	+	0	
	21	64	++	64	70
	24	128	++	0	
	MST 20				
LEW anti-LEW.1N (MHC)	9	1024	++	0	
	12	0		0	
	13	2048	++	128	90
	14	ND[b]			
	14	256	++	0	
	16	128	+	0	
	16	2048	++	16	90
	MST 14				
LEW.1N anti-LEW (MHC)	10	1024	++	32	90
	10	2048	++	256	90
	12	1024	++	128	90
	12	2048	++	64	90
	13	512	++	32	90
	14	64	+	4	90
	14	>4096	++	>512	90
	MST 12				

[a] Splenic lymphocytes.
[b] (ND) not done.

TABLE 3. Serological analysis of antibodies in a transplantation combination differing only at nonMHC loci

Panel of test cells		BN anti-DA.1N antisera[a]	
Strain	RT2	Unabsorbed	Absorbed with PVG.2A RBC
BUF	*a*	16 (±)	0
PVG.2A	*a*	128 (++)	0
LEW	*a*	32 (±)	0
ALB	*b*	128 (++)	32 (++)
AUG.2B	*b*	64 (++)	16 (++)
DA.1N	*b*	64 (++)	8 (++)

[a] Titer (strength of agglutination).

differences and those across MHC differences alone show that the MHC differences are the dominate genetic barrier. The slower rejection time across purely nonMHC differences supports this conclusion.

The rejection times of small bowel transplants are generally longer than those for heart and skin rejection across the same genetic differences (Table 5). They are comparable to the median survival time of bone marrow transplants across MHC differences but are shorter for such transplants across nonMHC differences. The major blood group antigen RT2 is not a histocompatibility barrier to transplantation of the heart, skin, and bone marrow. Preliminary studies of small bowel transplants using the PVG.2A anti-PVG strain combination (RT2 disparate only) indicates that the same is true for small bowel transplantation. Thus, matching for blood groups is not critical for the survival of organ transplants in rats. The deleterious effect of mismatching ABO blood groups in the transplantation of some human organs, e.g., kidney, but not in others, e.g., liver, appears to be caused by antibody-mediated mechanisms involving natural hemagglutinins, which are not present in rats, and not to tissue histoincompatibility. In the rat, the nature of the antibody response to the small bowel is the same as in the heart, skin, and bone marrow.

The results presented here and those in the literature suggest that three principles are useful in approaching small bowel transplantation in any species, including the human. First, matching for MHC antigens should be done, especially in view of the potential for both host-versus-graft and graft-versus-host reactions. Further attempts to identify the nonMHC antigens involved in rejection should be made, because the effects of immunosuppressive agents may be different depending upon the genetic barrier crossed (*9*). Second, the diagnosis of rejection is probably best made by mucosal biopsy—as in the endomyocardial biopsy technique for the heart—and some of the morphological criteria of rejection have already been identified (*7*). Third, the most convenient and safe test for rejection would be a test of bowel function—such as the transport of small molecules across the mucosa—and the physiological complexity of the small bowel should provide ample opportunity to develop such a test.

Note added in proof. After this article was submitted, another report on the transplantation of small bowel in the LEW-to-(LEW×BN)F_1 hybrid strain combination appeared (*19*). The findings are consistent with those reported here.

TABLE 4. Graft survival of small bowel transplants across various antigenic differences[a,b]

Strain combination		Monchik and Russel (2)	Telford and Corry (3)	Thiede and Deltz (4)	Kirkman et al. (5)	Pomposelli et al. (13)	Antigenic disparity
Recipient	Donor						
(LEW×BN)F_1	LEW	17 (12–20)			14 (9–17)	16	MHC
LEW	(LEW×BN)F_1	9 (6–12)	12 (9–14)		8 (7–10)		MHC + nonMHC
LEW	BN	8 (7–9)		10±2[c]			MHC + nonMHC
BN	LEW	11 (9–13)					MHC + nonMHC
LEW	F344			20±3[c]			nonMHC + Tla
Criterion of rejection:		Death	Stomal necrosis	Death	Palpable mass of indurated bowel	Death	

[a] All transplants were performed by the technique of Monchik and Russell (2), as were the transplants reported in this article: heterotopic transplant of the small bowel, or a portion thereof, as an auxillary organ.
[b] Data are given as the median survival times and the range of rejection times, except as noted.
[c] Average survival time ± 95% confidence limits.

TABLE 5. Graft survival of different organs across MHC and nonMHC disparities in different strain combinations

Genetic disparity		Median survival times (range) in days[a]			
MHC	NonMHC	Small bowel	Heart[b]	Skin[b]	Bone marrow
A, B, D	None	12 (10–14)	6 (6)	17 (15–20)	14 (14–28)
		14 (9–16)	7 (6–8)	9 (8–10)	14 (14–35)
		17 (12–20)	7 (7–8)	10 (9–10)	
None	All	20 (20–24)	11 (10–13)	18 (16–20)	Highly variable[c]
			13 (12–14)	14 (13–16)	
			14 (13–17)	23 (20–26)	
			16 (15–17)	16 (14–19)	
None	RT2 only	(>90)[d]	>125	>200	>250
			>125	>200	>250

[a] References (2, *14–18*) and this article.
[b] Heart and skin grafts were in the same strain combinations.
[c] From <180 to >250 days in a variety of strain combinations.
[d] Preliminary data from the PVG.2A anti-PVG strain combination.

Acknowledgment. We thank Trish Boyle for her technical assistance.

REFERENCES

1. Kirkman RL. Small bowel transplantation. Transplantation 1984; 37: 429.
2. Monchik GJ, Russell PS. Transplantation of small bowel in the rat: technical and immunological considerations. Surgery 1971; 70: 693.
3. Telford GL, Corry RJ. Immunological enhancement of rat small intestinal allografts. Arch Surg 1978; 113: 615.
4. Thiede A, Deltz E. Morphological reaction in transplanted small intestines using immunogenetically defined rat strain combinations. Langenbecks Arch Chir 1978; 340: 119.
5. Kirkman RL, Lear PA, Madara JL, Tilney NL. Small intestine transplantation in the rat—immunology and function. Surgery 1984; 96: 280.
6. Madara JL, Kirkman RL. Structural and functional evolution of jejunal allograft rejection in rats and the ameliorating effects of cyclosporine therapy. J Clin Invest 1985; 75: 502.
7. Schwartz MZ, Flye MW, Rostyk B, Storozuk MS. Effect of cyclosporin A on growth and function of transplanted fetal rat intestine. Surg Forum, 1982; 33: 341.
8. Craddock GN, Nordgreen SR, Reznick RK, et al. Small bowel transplantation in the dog using cyclosporine. Transplantation 1983; 35: 284.
9. Pinto M, Gill TJ III, Kunz HW. Prolongation of skin graft survival across different genetic barriers in rats with cyclosporine—and its potentiation by Bordetella pertussis vaccine. Transplantation 1983; 36: 171.
10. Harmel RP Jr. A simplified technique of small intestinal transplantation in the rat. J Pediatr Surg 1984; 19: 400.
11. Ghani A, Gill TJ III, Kunz HW, Misra DN. Elicitation of the maternal antibody response to the fetus by a broadly shared MHC class I antigenic determinant. Transplantation 1984; 37: 187.
12. Ohhashi T, Iwabuchi K, Natori T, Nakagawa Y, Kikuchi Y, Aizawa M. The B region-associated antigens and MLR phenotypes in the Japanese inbred strains of rats. Transplantation 1981; 8: 191.
13. Pomposelli F, Maki T, Kiyoizumi T, Gaber L, Balogh K, Monaco AP. Induction of graft-versus-host disease by small intestinal allotransplantation in rats. Transplantation 1985; 40: 343.
14. Katz SM, Liebert M, Gill TJ III, Kunz HW, Cramer DV, Guttmann RD. The relative roles of MHC and non-MHC genes in heart and skin allograft survival. Transplantation 1983; 36: 96.
15. Katz SM, Cramer DV, Kunz HW, Gill TJ III. Effect of major histocompatibility complex genetic disparities on cardiac and skin graft rejection in the rat. Transplantation 1983; 36: 463.
16. Pinto M, Gill TJ III, Kunz HW III, Dixon-McCarthy B. The relative roles of MHC and nonMHC antigens in bone marrow transplantation in rats. Transplantation 1983; 35: 607.
17. Oaks MK, Cramer DV. The genetics of bone marrow transplantation in the rat. Transplantation 1985; 39: 69.
18. Oaks MK, Cramer DV. Chronic graft-versus-host disease in rats after syngeneic bone marrow transplantation. Transplantation 1985; 39: 504.
19. Schraut WH, Lee KKW, Dawson PJ, Hup RD. Graft-versus-host disease induced by small bowel allografts: clinical course and pathology. Transplantation 1986; 41: 286.

Received 24 September 1985.
Accepted 2 December 1985.

0041-1337/86/4203-0239$02.00/0
TRANSPLANTATION
Vol. 42, No. 3
Printed in U.S.A.

MONOCLONAL ANTIBODIES FOR THE PREVENTION OF GRAFT-VERSUS-HOST DISEASE AND MARROW GRAFT REJECTION

THE DEPLETION OF T CELL SUBSETS IN VITRO AND IN VIVO[1]

STEVE COBBOLD[2], GILLY MARTIN, AND HERMAN WALDMANN

Division of Immunology, Department of Pathology, University of Cambridge, Cambridge CB2 1QP, United Kingdom

One of the major complications of allogeneic bone marrow transplantation is graft-versus-host disease. This can be avoided by removing the mature T cells from the marrow, most conveniently by the use of monoclonal antibodies. However, T cell purging results in an increased tendency for the recipient to reject the donor marrow. We have developed monoclonal antibodies to L3/T4 and Lyt-2 that specifically deplete functional T cell subsets in mice. We demonstrate that such reagents can be used to control both graft-versus-host disease and marrow rejection in mouse models of bone marrow transplantation across one-haplotype or two-haplotype major histocompatibility differences. Such strategies to abrogate host resistance, by administration of anti-T-cell monoclonal antibodies to the recipient, may complement marrow T cell purging for human allogeneic bone marrow transplantation.

The transplantation of allogeneic bone marrow poses problems unique in the field of organ grafting because of the presence of two mutually aggressive sets of immune cells. The recipients immune system attempts to reject the "invading" bone marrow (host-versus-graft reaction; [HVGR])* while the immunocompetent cells in the graft react against the recipient causing graft-versus-host disease (GVHD). Most bone marrow transplant patients, particularly those with neoplastic disease, are given cytoreductive treatment, including irradiation, which plays an important part in reducing the hosts' ability to reject (*1*). Graft-versus-host disease can also be reduced by eliminating mature T cells from the donor marrow, with, for example, monoclonal antibodies in vitro (*2–4*). However, it seems that there is a reciprocal interference between graft-versus-host and host-versus-graft reactions (*1*), the extent of which is related to the genetic disparity between donor and host. This means that for mismatched marrow transplantation, or in sensitized recipients, unacceptably high levels of irradiation may be needed to ensure engraftment in the absence of GVHD (*5–9*). In the past this reciprocal nature of the interactions between donor and host has made it difficult to investigate the mechanisms causing GVHD and marrow rejection, and the role played by different subsets of T cells. The recent development of monoclonal antibodies that can specifically deplete functional T cell subsets in mice (*10*) allowed us to independently manipulate T cells in the donor marrow or in the recipient animals. We could then investigate, using the well-developed mouse models of bone marrow transplantation, how therapeutic monoclonal antibodies might be used to manipulate T cell subsets, with the aim of avoiding both GVHD and marrow rejection.

Firstly, let us consider the problem of graft-versus-host disease. In mice, removal of mature T cells from donor marrow, either with antilymphocyte sera (*11–13*) or with monoclonal anti-Thy-1 (*14–16*) and heterologous complement in vitro, leads to a substantial reduction in lethal graft-versus-host disease. However, it is unclear whether GVHD is due to any single functional population of T cells. It has been suggested that Lyt-2^+ cytotoxic T lymphocytes (CTL) are the primary cause of graft-versus-host reactions across minor antigen differences (*17*), while both Lyt-1^+ and Lyt-2^+ cells must be removed from the marrow for transplantation across major histocompatibility complex (MHC) mismatches. However, the interpretation of these results must be questioned because of the uncertain effects of monoclonal anti-Lyt-1, an antigen expressed at different levels on all T cells (*18*). The recent availability of monoclonal antibodies that are effective in vivo to both L3/T4 and Lyt-2 (*10*), the functional equivalents of OKT4 and OKT8 in man (*19, 20*), allows an analysis of the role of T cell subsets in GVHD that should be directly applicable to clinical transplantation.

It is clear that GVHD can be avoided by removal of the T cells from the donor marrow, but we then have to consider the increased tendency for the host to reject the incoming marrow. The resistance to bone marrow grafting would seem to be broadly divisible into two types—first, the phenomenon of *syngeneic resistance*, usually ascribed to NK cells (*21*), a problem that we do not approach in the experiments described here; and second, the rejection of allogeneic cells, which may be due to conventional, but radioresistant mechanisms of rejection. It has been shown that both L3/$T4^+$ and Lyt-2^+ T cells play a part in rejecting allogeneic skin grafts, the former in naive mice and the latter in primed hosts (*22*). This was accomplished by manipulating the T cell subsets in vivo with selected monoclonal antibodies to the appropriate antigens (*10, 23*), an approach that we extend to the recipients of bone marrow.

We exploit a number of defined donor-host relationships in

[1]This work was supported by the Medical Research Council, U.K.

[2]Address correspondence to: S.P. Cobbold MA., Ph.D., Division of Immunology, Level-3, Laboratories Block, New Addenbrooke's Hospital, Hills Road, Cambridge. CB2 2QQ, U.K.

* Abbreviations used: ADCC, antibody-dependent cell-mediated cytotoxicity; ATX, adult thymectomized; BMT, bone marrow transplant; BSA, bovine serum albumin; CTL, cytotoxic T lymphocyte; FITC, fluorescein isothiocyanate; GVH(D), graft-versus-host (disease); HA, hemagglutination; HEPES, N-2-hydroxyethylpiperazine- N′-2-hydroxypropanesulfonic acid; HVG(R), host-versus-graft (reaction); MAb, monoclonal antibody; MeSH, 2-mercaptoethanol; MHC, major histocompatibility complex; NK, natural killer; PBS, phosphate-buffered saline; SRBC, sheep red blood cell.

the mouse model in order to separate the different contributions to survival of GVHD, rejection, and possible failure of an H-2 incompatible chimeric immune system. With respect to GVHD, we first show that fully allogeneic (MHC and minor-antigen-mismatched) parent→F_1 lethal graft-versus-host reactions (where the recipient is tolerant of donor cells) are due mainly to Lyt-2^+ cells, although L3/T4^+ cells may influence the severity of this effect. We also demonstrate that GVHD can be avoided either by T cell depletion of the donor mice, or by simply coating the marrow at the time of infusion. We then investigate the situation where there is a potential for both GVHD and rejection. In one haplotype mismatches—the situation most comparable with parent-to-child grafts in man—or in the two-haplotype ("A into B") system often studied in mice, we show that survival is improved by eliminating T cells in the recipient, as well as from the donor marrow. In both types of mismatch, after eliminating GVHD, removing the host's ability to reject leads to long-term survival, complete chimerism, and immunocompetence. Under conditions where the ability to reject is reduced, we also show that it is necessary to remove both L3/T4^+ and Lyt-2^+ cells from the marrow to avoid death from graft-versus-host disease.

MATERIALS AND METHODS

Mice. CBA/CaH, BALB/c, (CBA×BALB/c)F_1, C57B1/10, (CBA×B10)F_1, and SJL×BALB/c)F_1 mice, and (DA×LOU)F_1 rats, were bred and maintained under conventional conditions at the animal facility of the Department of Pathology at the University of Cambridge.

In vivo T cell subset depletion with monoclonal antibodies. Mice were adult-thymectomized (ATX) by the method of Monaco et al. [*24*] at 5–6 weeks of age, and allowed to recover at least 10 days. Randomly selected mice were given two i.v. injections, 5–7 days apart, of monoclonal rat IgG2b antibodies to T cell antigens. These were in the form of partially purified antibody (50% $(NH_4)_2SO_4$ precipitation) from ascitic fluids produced by growing the Y3/Ag1.2.3-derived (*25*) hybridomas YTS 154.7 (anti-Thy-1), YTS 121.5 (anti-Lyt-1), YTS 191.1 (anti-L3/T4), and YTS 169.4 (anti-Lyt-2) (*10*) in pristane-primed (DA×LOU)F_1 rats. Each mouse received 0.2 ml at 10 mg protein/ml in phosphate-buffered saline (PBS), equivalent to 200–500 μg of active monoclonal antibody (MAb) per injection. These mice were used as bone marrow and spleen cell donors after a further three weeks (minimum) to ensure antibody clearance.

Bone marrow transplantation. Groups of recipient mice were taken at 8–20 weeks old. When experiments were too large to age-match and sex-match all mice, they were divided equally between each experimental group. Before transplantation each group received a 10 day course of oral metronidazole followed by 5–7 days of tetracycline (Terramycin, Pfizer, UK; 50 mg/L in the drinking water). In some experimental groups these animals were given monoclonal antibodies (YTS 191.1 and YTS 169.4, 1 mg protein/ml PBS, equivalent to 20–50 μg active MAb i.v.) at the time of starting terramycin (5–7 days before irradiation). Recipient mice were given 850 rads at 38 rads/min from an x-ray source (220KV, Dept. of Pathology, Cambridge, UK), on day 0 of transplantation, and rested for four hours before being given bone marrow (1×10^7) and spleen 1×10^7 cells i.v. (in a volume of 0.2 ml HEPES buffered Eagle's medium). The marrow was prepared from donor femurs, and mixed with an equal number of spleen cells from the same donors (ATX-depleted, or normal mice as appropriate). In some cases monoclonal antibodies (YTS 154.7 at 2 mg protein/ml, or YTS 191.1 or YTS 169.4 at 0.1 mg protein/ml) were added to the bone marrow and spleen cells 5–15 min before injection.

Transplanted mice were divided into cages of 2–3 animals and given acidified (pH2) drinking water–unless, when stated, terramycin drinking water—or biweekly i.m. injections of gentamicin (80 μg) were given. Mice were individually weighed twice each week following transplantation, and the progress of each group was compared with that of mice given syngeneic bone marrow and spleen cells as follows:

$$\%\text{ syngeneic group weight}^{dn} = \frac{\Sigma(\text{ex. weights}^{dn}) \times \Sigma(\text{syn. weights}^{d0})}{\Sigma(\text{syn. weights}^{dn}) \times \Sigma(\text{ex. weights}^{d0})} \times 100$$

where Σ = the sum of; Ex. weights = individual experimental weights, syn. weights = individual syngeneic weights, dn = day n after transplant, d0 = day 0 of transplant. Mice that died were counted as having zero weight. Statistical significance between groups was estimated by the value of *P* obtained from chi-squared at one degree of freedom as calculated by the log-rank (nonparametric) method (*26*) applied to individual survival times.

Skin grafts. Bone marrow transplanted mice were grafted after day 100 with skin from donor, recipient, and third-party strains, side by side in the same graft bed. Small pieces (approx. 10×5-mm) of tail skin were placed in a prepared bed on the lateral thoracic wall of recipient mice. These were held in place by Vaseline-impregnated gauze and plaster bandage, which were removed after 10 days, and the grafts were examined daily for rejection. In all cases the central recipient-type graft was fully accepted. Rejection was considered complete when no viable part of an individual graft remained. Mice were maintained on terramycin drinking water for three weeks from skin grafting if not already receiving antibiotics.

Antibody responses. The primary antibody response to sheep red blood cells (SRBC) was determined by challenging mice i.p. with 0.2 ml 10% washed SRBC in PBS. After 10 days the mice were bled from the tail vein, and the serum hemagglutination (HA) titers determined—either directly (total IgM and IgG antibody) or in the presence of 0.1M 2-mercaptoethanol (IgG antibody). Secondary responses were similarly measured after reimmunizing with SRBC one month later.

H-2 typing. Transplanted mice were tested for the level of donor and recipient-type leukocytes by a modification of the method of Chandler et al. (*27*). Briefly, peripheral blood cells were obtained from 2–3 drops of venous blood (tail vein) by water lysis. These were tested with monoclonal antibody supernatants to H-$2K^kD^k$ (clone 12-2-2S [*28*]), H-$2K^b$ (clone 28-13-3S [*29*]), and H-$2D^d$ (clone 34-4-21S [*30*]), and used for cytolysis in the presence of unabsorbed, selected guinea-pig or rabbit serum as a source of complement (1/50 dilutions). The proportion of cells killed was estimated in the presence of fluorescein diacetate (live cells fluoresce green) and propidium iodide (dead cells fluoresce red).

In the case of BALB/c-into-CBA chimeras (and the CBA syngeneic controls), the following immunofluorescence method was used to detect any residual recipient (H-2^k) cells in the peripheral blood. Fresh whole blood (from the tail vein) was used to make thin smears on microscope slides. After 30 min air drying, these were sequentially fixed in acetone (5 min) and ethanol (1 min) with air drying (10 min) after each step. Nonspecific binding was blocked by incubation in PBS 1% bovine serum albumin (BSA) for 1 hr. These slides were incubated with 200 μl of a rat IgG2b monoclonal antibody that reacts with H-2^k but not H-2^d (R1-21.1 [*31*]) for 30 min in a humid box, with rocking. The slides were washed with PBS 0.1% BSA, three times over 5 min, and then incubated as above with a monoclonal antirat IgG2b(*32*) coupled to FITC (NORIG 7.16.2-FITC, 5 μg/ml; Sera-Lab, UK) in PBS 0.1% BSA containing 0.5 μg/ml propidium iodide. After washing as above—and then in PBS—the slides were mounted in 90% glycerol 10% PBS containing 1 mg/ml p-phenylenediamine (to stop quenching) and observed on a Leitz fluorescence microscope (50 × water immersion objective) with filter block H2 (long-pass 515 nm). Cell nuclei were seen to fluoresce orange/red, so that neutrophils (often autofluorescent) and mononuclear cells could be distinguished. Positively stained cells showed a bright green ring (weaker fluorescence could be distinguished from autofluorescence by further observation with a high-performance filter block such as a Leitz L2 (band-pass 525/20 nm).

RESULTS

Graft-versus-host disease in MHC-disparate parent into F_1 marrow transplants. Graft-versus-host disease in inbred animals can be studied in the absence of rejection by grafting parental bone marrow to F_1 recipients—which are, of course, tolerant of the donor histocompatibility antigens. There are three ways in which mature T cells could be removed with monoclonal antibodies from the marrow in order to avoid GVHD: first, the antibodies could be used to deplete T cells in vitro with, for example, complement prior to administration; second, the contaminating T cells could be coated with antibody in vitro and eliminated in vivo by opsonization; and third, the T cells could be eliminated from the donor animals in advance of transplantation. Each of these methods has different practical or experimental advantages: donor depletion allows the transplant to be performed without any antibody present; in vitro depletion is easily monitored; and coating for in vivo opsonization is the simplest, involving the least manipulation of the marrow. We show that, with appropriate monoclonal antibodies, in vivo depletion of donor animals and simple coating for opsonization in the recipient, are equally effective at eliminating the T cells causing GVHD.

Adult thymectomized T-cell-subset–depleted CBA mice (*10*) were used as the source of bone marrow and spleen cells in the experiment shown in Figure 1A, while cells from normal mice were simply coated with the appropriate rat IgG2b monoclonal antibodies in vitro (Figure 1B). In both cases the cells were transplanted into lethally irradiated (850 rads) (CBA×BALB/c)F_1. It can be seen in both experiments that either pan-T or Lyt-2 depletion of donor cells protected the recipients from lethal GVHD (median survival of the GVH group = 14 days; pan-T or Lyt-2-depleted group 95% survival >100 days; $P \leq 0.0001$),—while removal of the L3/T4$^+$ population gave only partial protection (58% survival >100 days, compared with the GVH group; $P < 0.0001$, compared with Lyt-2 or the pan-T group ($P < 0.001$). Adding Lyt-2-depleted cells back to the L3/T4-depleted inoculum decreased the overall survival again (25% >day 100; Fig. 1A), although GVHD was still delayed compared with controls—probably due to a different ratio of cell types in the mixture (median survival = 29 days; compared with the GVH group median survival = 14 days, $P \leq 0.17$—not a signifi-

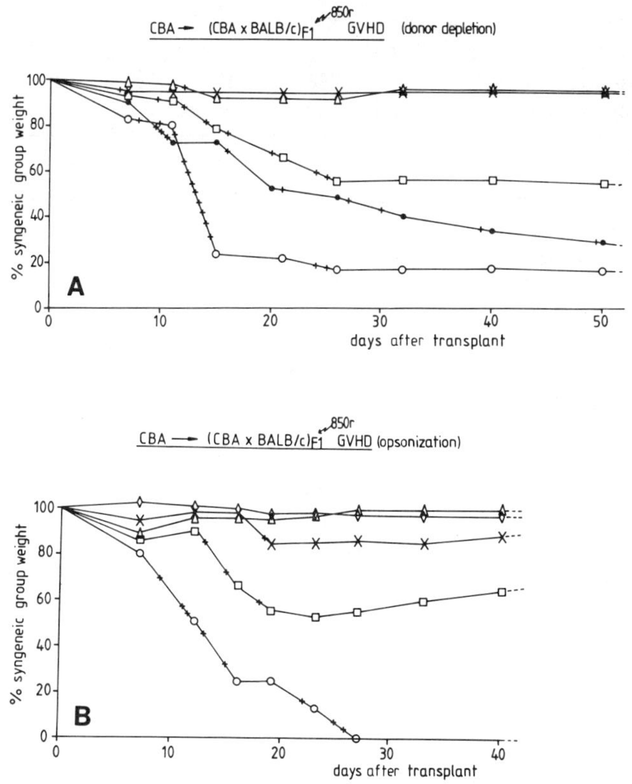

FIGURE 1. Graft-versus-host disease in mismatched parent-into-F_1 marrow transplants. (A) Spleen and bone marrow cells (10^7 of each) were obtained from adult-thymectomized, T-cell-subset–depleted mice, as described in the *Materials and Methods* section. These were injected i.v. into lethally irradiated (850 rads) (CBA×BALB/c)F_1 recipients (12–16 animals per group). (B) Spleen and bone marrow cells (10^7 of each) were obtained from normal CBA mice and monoclonal antibodies to different T cell antigens added just before transfer to recipient mice (for opsonization) as above (8 animals per group). The following groups were tested: (○) GVHD controls with no monoclonal antibody; (◇) anti-Thy-1 (YTS 154.7); (□) anti-L3/T4 (YTS 191.1); (△) anti-Lyt-2 (YTS 169.4); (X) anti-L3/T4 and anti-Lyt-2 (pan-T-cell depletion); and (●) an equal mix of cells from anti-L3/T4-depleted and anti-Lyt-2-depleted mice. (+) indicates the death of individual animals.

cant difference). These results suggest that Lyt-2$^+$ cells are a major cause of lethal GVHD in this model, but that the severity of the disease may be influenced by a contribution from L3/T4$^+$ cells. It should be noted, however, that the recipients of Lyt-2-depleted marrow and spleen all had temporary alopecia at 2–4 weeks posttransplant (but no signs of wasting or weight loss in either experiment), which was not observed in animals receiving pan-T-depleted donor cells (anti-Lyt-2 + anti-L3/T4).

It is clear from these experiments that the rat IgG2b monoclonal antibodies are equally effective at eliminating the T cells in vivo, either by simple coating and opsonization in the recipient, or by injection and depletion of the donor mice. The latter observation allowed us to independently deplete the T cells from donor or recipient mice. This allowed us, for the first time, to truly separate the normally reciprocal interactions of GVHD and marrow rejection, and to investigate the roles of different T cells in each.

Depletion of donor and recipient T cells in one-haplotype-mismatched marrow grafts. The most common mismatched bone marrow allograft used in a clinical setting is that from parent to child, a situation that can be modeled using the one-haplotype difference between two F_1 strains of mice—for example, $(CBA \times B10)F_1$ and $(CBA \times BALB/c)F_1$. This combination leads to the potential for both GVH and rejection (HVG) reactions, while the shared haplotype should allow normal cooperation resulting from common H-2 restriction elements between donor and recipient cells. (Previously it had been suggested that two-haplotype-mismatched, chimeric T cells fail to cooperate with presenting cells, leading to poor long-term survival [33, 34]). Adult thymectomized and T-cell-depleted (anti-L3/T4 plus anti-Lyt-2) $(CBA \times B10)F_1$ mice were used as donors for the marrow and spleen, which was transplanted into lethally irradiated $(CBA \times BALB/c)F_1$ euthymic recipients. One group of these recipients had been given 20–40 μg of monoclonal antibodies to both L3/T4 and Lyt-2 antigens, sufficient to deplete the T cells by >90% [10]. This was performed seven days before the transplant in order to allow clearance of the antibody in vivo (antibody could not be detected in the serum or on cells at this time [results not shown]). The results in Figure 2 show that depletion of the donor cells only delayed mortality (GVH median survival = 11.5 days, depleted donor-group median survival = 17.5 days; $P \leq 0.002$) compared with the GVHD controls (which received undepleted cells). However, when both the donor and the recipient had been depleted of all T cells, a number of animals became long-term survivors (47% survival >130 days, compared with the depleted donor group: $P \leq 0.002$). If these mice received undepleted donor cells, rapid mortality was observed that was identical to that of the GVHD controls. This suggests that the monoclonal antibodies given to the recipient reduced the tendency for marrow rejection in the absence of GVHD by further immunosuppressing the host T cells. Therefore, to improve the conditions for allogenic bone marrow transplantation, monoclonal antibodies can be used to deplete the T cells from both the donor marrow and the recipient.

Having eliminated GVHD and marrow rejection in the construction of allogeneic bone marrow chimeras, it was of interest

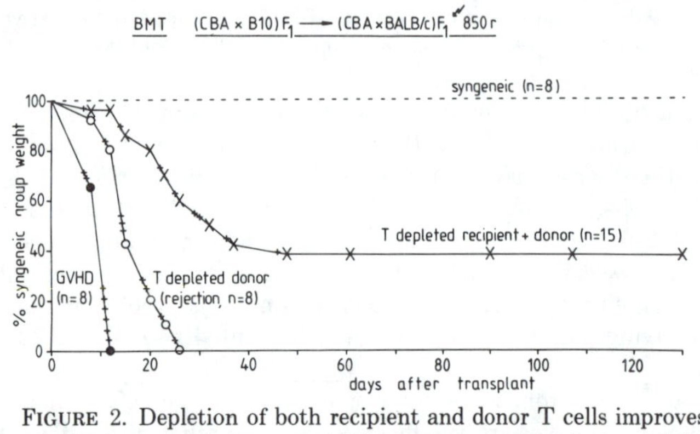

FIGURE 2. Depletion of both recipient and donor T cells improves survival of one-haplotype-mismatched marrow transplants. Adult-thymectomized $(CBA \times B10)F_1$ mice were used as donors for bone marrow and spleen cells (10^7 of each). These were not depleted in the GVHD control group (●), but in other groups were given antibody to eliminate L3/T4+ and Lyt-2+ cells (YTS 191.1 plus YTS 169.4, as described in the *Materials and Methods* section). Donor cells were given i.v. to lethally irradiated $(CBA \times BALB/c)F_1$ euthymic recipients (4 hr after 850 rads), either undepleted (○) or pre-depleted (X) with anti-L3/T4 (YTS 191.1) plus anti-Lyt-2 (YTS 169.4) seven days before transplantation. The syngeneic group (normal CBA×BALB/c recipients) received the same number of spleen and marrow cells from $(CBA \times BALB/c)F_1$ mice. (+) indicates the death of individual animals.

to establish the immunological status of such animals. In the past there has been considerable debate over the poor ability of allogeneic chimeras to mount normal immune responses (33–35). In particular it has not been clear whether this relates to chronic or subclinical GVH and HVG reactions, or whether new T cells have had to mature in an environment where the presenting cells express H-2 restriction elements different from the nonhemopoietic cells, leading to inappropriate immune responses. The latter point should apply only to two-haplotype-mismatched chimeras where the H-2 antigens on donor and recipient are entirely incompatible. To investigate this question of immunocompetence further, we followed the long-term survival in the two-haplotype mismatch after elimination of GVHD and marrow rejection, using in vivo T cell depletion as described above.

Improvement of survival of two-haplotype-mismatched chimeras after depletion of donor and recipient T cells. Two experiments were performed using separate depletion of the donor BALB/c and recipient CBA mice (different at both haplotypes) with monoclonal anti-L3/T4 plus anti-Lyt-2. The results shown in Figure 3A were very similar to those obtained in the

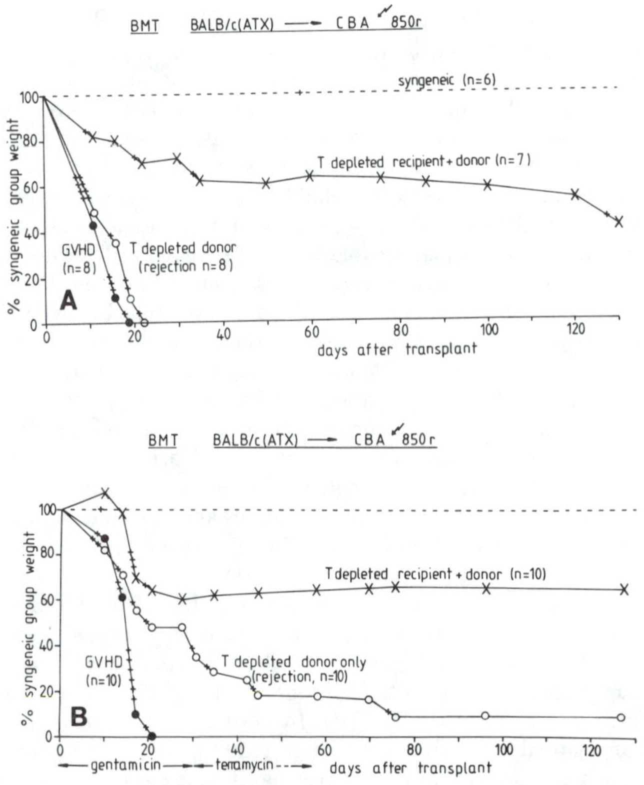

FIGURE 3. Depletion of both recipient and donor T cells improves survival of two-haplotype-mismatched marrow transplants. Adult thymectomized BALB/c mice were used as donors for bone marrow and spleen cells (10^7 of each). These were not depleted in the GVHD control group (●), but in other groups they were given antibody to eliminate L3/T4+ and Lyt-2+ cells (YTS 191.1 plus YTS 169.4, as described in the *Materials and Methods* section). Donor cells were given i.v. to lethally irradiated CBA euthymic recipients (4 hr after 850 rads), either undepleted (○) or predepleted (X) with anti-L3/T4 (YTS 191.1) plus anti-Lyt-2 (YTS 169.4) five days before transplantation. (A) All mice maintained on pH2 drinking water in conventional conditions; (B) all mice given gentamicin (i.m.) days 0–30 and oxytetracycline in drinking water from day 31. (+) indicates the death of individual animals.

one-haplotype model described above, with long-term survival depending on depletion of both donor and recipient T cells, to avoid GVHD (GVHD group compared with donor and recipient depletion: $P \leq 0.007$) and rejection (donor and recipient depletion compared with just donor depletion; $P \leq 0.01$), respectively. The second experiment, shown in Figure 3B, differed slightly in that antibiotics were given continuously to the recipient animals. In this case depletion of just the donor T cells was a little more effective at prolonging survival (not significant: GVHD group compared with T-depleted group: $P \leq 0.14$), but the majority of animals still died eventually, presumably because of late graft failure by rejection. Depletion of both donor and recipient T cells again gave a high proportion of long-term survivors (donor and recipient depletion compared with donor depletion only; $P \leq 0.04$) which was not significantly different from the syngeneic group survival ($P \leq 0.19$). It should be noted that in the experiment without antibiotics some weight loss (and one death) was observed after day +100, which was not seen in the experiment in Figure 3B. It is well known that the level of infections is a major factor determining survival after marrow transplants, and that mismatched chimeras can be produced in "germ-free" conditions without any T cell depletion (*36, 37*). It is, however, not clear how infections may influence the interactions between GVHD and marrow rejection.

Immunocompetence and chimerism after allogeneic bone marrow transplantation. Transplanted mice that survived beyond day +100 were investigated for the level of chimerism, specific tolerance to donor skin grafts, and immunocompetence, as assessed by rejection of third-party skin grafts and antibody responses to sheep red blood cells (SRBC). The data are shown in Table 1. With respect to chimerism, all allogeneic recipients tested showed no evidence of autologous hemopoiesis, demonstrating that the donor marrow was fully accepted. Also, when tested, the chimeras were specifically tolerant of donor-type skin while third-party (e.g., H-2^s) allogeneic skin was vigorously rejected. All the chimeras were able to make significant levels of agglutinating antibody (IgM and IgG) to SRBC in both primary and secondary responses. The latter is in contrast with reports in the literature, in which primary anti-SRBC responses were said to be absent in such allo-(strain A into strain B) chimeras (*35, 38, 39*). This demonstrates that—at least at the T, B, and presenting cell level—the chimeric cells are able to successfully cooperate in an immune response, presumably in an H-2 restricted manner. It is, however, still possible that responses to viral infections in recipient tissues (bearing an H-2 type different from that of hemopoietic cells) would be impaired by inappropriate presentation—leading to late death, as suggested by Rayfield et al. (*34*). Perhaps the most important point, however, is that the one-haplotype mismatches, which are more relevant to human bone marrow transplantation, showed perfectly normal immune reconstitution.

The above results demonstrate that depletion of all donor and recipient T cells allows the acceptance of allogeneic marrow in the absence of GVHD, with the creation of immunocompetent chimeras. The question remained as to whether it was necessary to eliminate all T cells—or, as suggested by the earlier parent→F_1 experiments, whether it would be sufficient to eliminate only one T cell subset. With regard to rejection of allogeneic cells, we have previously shown that both T cell subsets are intimately involved in rejecting skin grafts, particularly if the recipient has been primed (*22*). Most bone marrow transplant patients will have been primed by multiple blood transfusions, so it seemed unlikely that removing only one subset would reliably reduce marrow rejection in a clinical setting. We therefore concentrated on using totally depleted recipients to test whether removing just the Lyt-2$^+$ or L3/T4$^+$ cells from donor marrow would be sufficient to eliminate GVHD in the absence of rejection, as this might be beneficial to the recipient by transferring some donor acquired immunity or providing a potential for the so-called graft-versus-leukemia effect (*36*).

Graft-versus-host disease in T-depleted recipients caused by both T cell subsets. In the past, attempts to investigate which subsets cause GVHD in fully mismatched models have been frustrated by the contribution of graft rejection to mortality. Depleting the marrow of all T cells or just one subset often delayed death, but long-term survival was generally still poor ([*33, 34*)] and our own unpublished results). However, by using T-depleted recipients, and adult thymectomized, T-cell-subset-depleted donors, it can be seen that the best survival was obtained by eliminating all T cells (Fig. 4: median survival GVHD group = 13.5 days; group depleted of all T cells, 57% survival >130 days: $P \leq 0.003$). Removal of just the L3/T4$^+$ or

TABLE 1. Chimerism and immunocompetence after bone marrow transplantation with both donor and recipient T cell depletion

	Chimerism (mean cytotoxic index)[a]				Primary anti-SRBC responses (Log_2 HA titer)[b]		Secondary anti-SRBC responses (Log_2 HA titer)[b]		Skin graft survival (days)		
	k	d	b	Type	Total	MeSH res.	Total	MeSH res.	CBA	B10	SJL×BALB/c
CBA → CBA	*95*	7	11	—	10.0±1[d]	6.9±0.5	10.0±1	10.0±0	← ND[e] →		
BALB/c → CBA	0	*74*	0	donor[c] (n = 7)	6.4±2	3.5±2	8.7±1	7.7±2	← ND →		
(CBA×BALB/c)F_1 → (CBA×BALB/c)F_1	*89*	*75*	11	—	10.0±1	7.6±1	10.0±1	10.0±0	>99	12±0	<11
(CBA×B10)F_1 → (CBA×BALB/c)F_1	*94*	4	*64*	donor (n = 6)	9.8±1	7.3±1	9.7±1	9.7±1	>99	>99	15±1

[a] $$\text{Cytotoxic index} = \frac{\%\ \text{experimental kill} - \%\ \text{background kill}}{\%\ \text{control kill} - \%\ \text{background kill}} \times 100$$

where controls % kill/% background kill were; CBA+anti-H2k = 87/8, BALB/c+anti-H2d = 36/10, B10+anti-H2b = 72/6.

[b] Background hemagglutination titers before immunization ≤2 (total) and <1 (MeSH resistance).

[c] Confirmed <1% recipient H-2k immunofluorescence with rat MAb R1-21.1.

[d] Figures quoted give mean ± SD with 5–8 mice/group.

[e] Not determined.

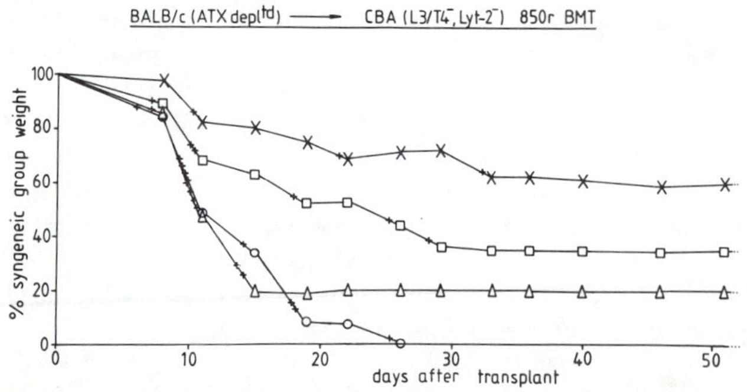

FIGURE 4. Graft-versus-host disease in two-haplotype-mismatched bone marrow transplants with T-depleted recipients. Recipient euthymic CBA mice were depleted of T cells five days before transplantation by i.v. administration of anti-L3/T4 and anti-Lyt-2 as described in the *Materials and Methods* section. At 4 hr after lethal irradiation (850 rads) these were given i.v. bone marrow and spleen cells (10^7 of each) from adult-thymectomized T-cell-subset-depleted mice in the following groups (8–9 mice per group): (O) undepleted donor mice (GVHD controls); (Δ) Lyt-2$^+$ cell depletion; (□) L3/T4$^+$ cell depletion, (X) both L3/T4$^+$ and Lyt-2$^+$ cell depletion. (+) indicates the death of individual animals.

Lyt-2$^+$ cells was not as effective (compared with the GVHD group: median survival L3/T4-depleted group = 22.5 days: $P \leq 0.07$; median survival Lyt-2-depleted group = 13.0 days; $P \leq 0.9$), while failure to deplete T cells in either the donor or the recipient again lead to rapid death, as observed previously (Fig. 3).

To summarize all the above results, it seems that mismatched bone marrow transplantation can be achieved to produce immunocompetent allogeneic chimeras, using monoclonal antibodies to deplete all the mature T cells in both the donor and the recipient.

DISCUSSION

The successful transplantation of allogeneic marrow depends on a number of factors. First, the donor marrow must be obtained in sufficient quantity to supply enough stem cells to repopulate the recipient's hemopoietic system—any manipulations designed to eliminate graft-versus-host disease by removing mature T cells must, therefore, not reduce the stem cell compartment and risk inadequate repopulation. Second, the recipient must be appropriately conditioned to receive the donor marrow. This will normally involve a combination of cytotoxic drugs and radiotherapy, with the threefold aim of "creating space" for the new marrow, immunosuppressing the recipient to avoid marrow rejection, and agressively eliminating residual disease—the latter being the therapeutic basis for performing the transplant in the case of patients with neoplastic disease. If all the above aims are achieved without serious complications through infections or nonspecific toxicity of the cytoreduction, the transplanted stem cells should regenerate all the different hemopoietic cells, including a new immune system. This is the critical point for the generation of healthy, immunocompetent chimerism—the new T cells must be processed, presumably by the thymus, to recognize as self both the recipient antigens and those of the new hemopoietic system. A failure to recognize both sets of self antigens would lead to a reduced ability to recognize foreign antigens (which are seen in the context of self by MHC-restricted T cells) and the possibility of autoreactivity. In the same way, any mature T cells "left over" from the donor or recipient will have a tendency to cause GVH or HVG reactions that may well compromise the generation of tolerant T cells and lead to an ineffective immune system. It is, therefore, important to remove as many T cells as possible from both the donor marrow and the recipient. Monoclonal antibodies have been in use for some time to remove T cells from the donor marrow, but it has often been assumed that lethal irradiation would be sufficient to immunosuppress the recipient. It is now clear that this is not the case, even in matched siblings, where T-depletion of donor marrow has lead to rejection (*1, 4, 6, 8, 9*). We have demonstrated here that monoclonal antibodies can also be used in the recipient to deplete T cells as an adjunct to the normal cytoreductive therapy, avoiding rejection and allowing a new, effective immune system to develop.

In the experiments described above we used separate depletion of the donor and recipient T cells to distinguish GVHD and rejection. However, for practical purposes, the simplest method of depleting both sets of T cells would be to add a vast excess of monoclonal antibody that would then be injected with the marrow into the recipient. This can be achieved in mice with, for example, the rat IgG2b monoclonal anti-Thy-1 (YTS 154.7) to create either fully allogeneic two-haplotype C57/B16→CBA (*40, 41*) or one-haplotype (CBA×B10)F_1→(CBA×BALB/c)F_1 chimeras (% syngeneic group weight at day +200: Thy-1-treated group (n = 10), [87%] GVHD controls (n = 10), [9%]: $P \leq 0.0001$, results not shown). The minimum amount of antibody required to ensure a high proportion of long-term survivors (approx. 100 μg/mouse of YTS 154.7) was similar to the minimum dose required to deplete a mouse by >90%, and was in vast excess (>100-fold) over that needed to lyse the marrow T cells (in vitro with added complement). This suggests that the antibody is again increasing survival by reducing T cells in both the donor inoculum and the recipient by opsonization in vivo. It is possible that a similar mechanism may apply to previous reports of successful allogeneic transplants in mice with reagents such as antilymphocyte globulin (*13*). In such cases recipients could be depleted by antibody directly or by "arming" antibody-dependent cellular cytotoxicity mechanisms in the coated donor marrow.

In the past a number of questions have been raised concerning the immunocompetence of allogeneic chimeras. In particular these have involved the problems of H-2 restriction in two-haplotype-mismatched combinations. There has been much argument over the role of different cells in the thymus in determining whether new T cells are restricted to recipient thymic H-2 antigens (*42, 33*), or donor H-2, on repopulating presenting cells, or a combination of both (*43, 44*). If maturing T cells are restricted only to recipient thymic antigens, they may be unable to cooperate with donor-type antigen-presenting and B cells, leading to poor antibody responses, as observed by Onoe et al. (*35*). However, if the T cells are restricted only by donor antigen-presenting cells they may be unable to react against viruses in recipient tissues, leading to poor long-term survival (*34*). The pattern of H-2 restriction actually observed may be critically influenced by any residual mature T cells in the donor marrow or in the recipient, and by the balance of GVH and HVG reactions. The two-haplotype-mismatched chimeras generated by depleting T cells in the donor and the recipient were shown to be generally immunocompetent—and, if maintained on simple antibiotics (oxytetracycline in the drinking water), they remained as healthy as syngeneic controls for extended periods (>200 days). It remains to be seen whether a more detailed investigation of such immunocompetent chimeras will resolve some of the arguments concerning the maturation and restriction of T cells in the thymus. The possible problems of T cells being selected for recognition of inappropriate MHC alleles should not apply to the one-haplotype mismatch because one set of parental MHC genes is shared between the donor and recipient, but the need to eliminate GVH and HVG reactions remains the same.

We have argued above that, for an effective new immune system to develop, it is necessary to remove all the T cells in both the donor and recipient. If it were possible to remove just those T cells responsible for GVHD and marrow rejection there might be the added advantages of transferring donor acquired immunity and a graft-versus-leukemia reaction. T cells can be divided into two major subsets—restricted either to class I or to class II MHC antigens—which, in the mouse, express the Lyt-2 or L3/T4 molecules, respectively. There has been considerable debate over which of these subsets is responsible for allogeneic reactions in vivo—and, in particular, which rejects allografts or causes GVHD. We show here that both T cell subsets are capable of causing GVHD, with the Lyt-2^+ cells of major importance in the CBA→(CBA×BALB/c)F_1 model, while in the two-haplotype difference, using T-depleted recipients, the best survival was obtained by removing both L3/T4$^+$ and Lyt-2^+ cells from the marrow. There have been conflicting reports concerning the T cell subsets causing GVHD across minor, compared with major, histocompatibility differences (*17, 45–47*). For example, Korngold and Sprent (*17*) suggest that Lyt-2^+ cells are responsible for anti-non-MHC (minor antigen) GVHD, while Lyt-1 (or, more recently, L3/T4 [*48*]) positive cells were said to cause GVHD against complete P→F_1 mismatches, comparable to the combination where we show Lyt-2^+ cell dependence. Our results are reminiscent of the P→F_1 model of Gleichmann et al. (*49*), where Lyt-2^+ cells seem to cause acute, lethal GVHD, and Lyt-1^+ (L3/T4$^+$) cells lead to a form of chronic GVHD with autoimmune reactions suggested by the temporary alopecia in our Lyt-2-depleted marrow group. Gleichmann suggests that although the F_1 recipients are tolerant—and, therefore, unable to reject the incoming marrow—the shared parental haplotype could lead to anomolous interactions, either helping or suppressing certain aspects of GVH. It remains to be determined whether T-cell-depleted F_1 recipients produce similar results, or allow both subsets to cause GVHD as in the depleted two-haplotype-mismatched hosts. One interpretation of all these findings is that both T cell subsets can independently cause GVHD—the Lyt-2^+ cells directed against pure class I MHC differences and the L3/T4$^+$ cells against MHC class II (*48*). When there are multiple antigen differences, the particular strain combination and conditioning regimen would then determine the relative stimulation of class I or class II MHC-restricted responses in the context of different minor histocompatibility antigens. When applying these results to bone marrow transplant in man, when the genetic differences and other factors are generally ill-defined, the only sure way to eliminate GVHD would be to eliminate both T cell subsets from the marrow.

Having considered the T cells causing GVHD, let us now turn to the T cells in the recipient that can reject the marrow graft. We have recently shown that both T cell subsets are intimately involved in the classic rejection of allogeneic skin-grafts across either major or minor histocompatibility differences (*22*). There is considerable evidence to show that T cells remaining after lethal irradiation could reject by these classic mechanisms. Sado et al. (*50*) have shown that different mouse strains exhibit a remarkable variation in the amount of radiation needed to eliminate T cell responses (CBA mice, for example, are relatively resistant). Suman et al. (*51*) demonstrated that, even in radiation chimeras primarily of donor origin, a high proportion of dividing cells in the lymph node were from the recipient. It therefore seems logical that the use of monoclonal antibodies that suppress the rejection of allogeneic skin grafts in vivo should also reduce any tendency of the recipients to reject bone marrow transplants. Indeed, it has been previously demonstrated that the use of anti-Thy-1 in vivo reduced early rejection of allogeneic marrow in the recipient spleen (*52*). However, the authors were not certain whether the antibody was acting mainly on T cells or on other resistance mechanisms, such as NK cells.

It has been suggested that failure of marrow engraftment does not necessarily involve the classic T cell mechanisms of rejection, but instead rather ill-defined mechanisms sometimes referred to as *syngeneic resistance*, which are often linked with NK cells (*21, 53*). Warner and Dennert (*54*) have recently reported that NK cells may operate through antibody-dependent cell-mediated cytotoxicity (ADCC) to reject allogeneic bone marrow. However, all these data are based on assays that measure the short-term proliferation of cells in the spleen, which may not be a reliable indicator of full hemopoietic recovery and long-term survival (*1*). The interpretation of syngeneic resistance is complicated and may involve many factors, such as the need to make "space" for incoming marrow, the efficiency of stem cells to home to appropriate sites for hemopoiesis, and possible idiotypic reactions between donor and recipient immune systems. However, such factors may also play a role in reducing the efficiency of allogeneic marrow transplantation—and, in particular, natural cytotoxicity (*55*) and inappropriate homing via asialoglycoprotein receptors (*56*) have been implicated. The manipulation of these forms of resistance, combined with the suppression of allogeneic rejection, may further increase the reliability of marrow transplantation in circumstances in which the number of available stem cells is limited.

So far we have considered the resistance and rejection of allogeneic marrow as a function of the recipient. The donor marrow itself will, of course, influence these reactions in a number of ways. Apart from the effects of T cells, which we will assume have been removed to eliminate GVHD, there will be other cells that may influence whether the developing chimera becomes tolerant of the donor antigens. In particular, there may be two types of important cell: antigen-presenting cells, which may have both tolerizing and stimulating roles, and the so-called *veto* cells (which may be T or non-T cells) with the ability to abort responses to themselves (*57–59*). It should be noted that in all our experiments a mixture of marrow and spleen cells was used (to simulate the blood-contaminated marrow used in man), and this may provide presenting and veto cells different from pure marrow—where, it should be noted, T cell depletion of the recipient gave a less clear-cut improvement in survival (our own unpublished results). In practical terms it is possible that appropriate manipulations of the marrow could change the balance of veto and antigen presentation to further increase the chance of grafting smaller numbers of marrow stem cells.

In summary, our results show that appropriate monoclonal antibodies can be used to deplete T cells, not only in the donor marrow but also in the recipient. This avoids GVHD and reduces the tendency for rejection of the transplant, leading to the improved long-term survival of stable, immunocompetent chimeras.

REFERENCES

1. Vriesendorp HM. Engraftment of haemopoietic cells. Bone marrow transplantation. Biological mechanisms and clinical practice. In: van Bekkum DW, Lowenberg B, eds. New York: Marcel Dekker, 1985; 73.
2. Reisner Y, Kapoor N, Kirkpatrick D, et al. Transplantation for acute leukemia with HLA-A and B nonidentical parental marrow cells fractionated with soybean agglutinin and sheep red blood cells. Lancet 1981; 2: 327.
3. Prentice HG, Blacklock HA, Janossy G, et al. Depletion of T lymphocytes in donor marrow prevents significant graft versus host disease in matched allogeneic leukemic marrow transplant recipients. Lancet 1984; 1: 472.
4. Waldmann H, Or R, Hale G, et al. Elimination of graft versus host disease by in vitro depletion of alloreactive lymphocytes using a monoclonal rat anti-human lymphocyte antibody (CAMPATH-1). Lancet 1984; 2: 483.
5. Sondel PM, Bozdech MJ, Trigg ME, et al. Additional immunosuppression allows engraftment following HLA-mismatched T cell-depleted bone marrow transplantation for leukemia. Transplant Proc 1985; 17: 460.
6. O'Reilly RJ, Collins NH, Kernan N, et al. Transplantation of marrow-depleted T cells by soybean lectin agglutination and E-rosette depletion: major histocompatibility complex-related graft resistance in leukemic transplant recipients. Transplant Proc 1985; 17: 455.
7. Storb R, Prentice RL, Thomas ED, et al. Factors associated with graft rejection after HLA-identical transplantation for aplastic anaemia. Br J Haematol 1983; 55: 573.
8. Slavin S, Waldmann H, Or R, et al. Prevention of graft-versus-host disease in allogeneic bone marrow transplantation for leukemia by T cell depletion in vitro prior to transplantation. Transplant Proc 1985; 17: 465.
9. Martin PJ, Hansen JA, Buckner CD, et al. Effects of in vitro depletion of T cells in HLA-identical allogeneic marrow grafts. Blood 1985; 66: 664.
10. Cobbold SP, Jayasuriya A, Nash A, Prospero TD, Waldmann H. Therapy with monoclonal antibodies by elimination of T-cell subsets in vivo. Nature 1984; 312: 548.
11. Trentin JJ, Judd KP. Prevention of acute graft versus host mortality with spleen absorbed antithymocyte globulin. Transplant Proc 1973; 5: 865.
12. Rodt H, Thierfelder S, Eulitz M. Anti-lymphocyte antibodies and marrow transplantation. III. Effect of heterologous anti-brain antibodies on acute secondary disease in mice. Eur J Immunol 1974; 4: 25.
13. Muller-Ruchholtz W, Wottge HU, Muller-Hermelink HK. Bone marrow transplantation in rats across strong histocompatibility barriers by selective elimination of lymphoid cells in donor marrow. Transplant Proc. 1976; 8: 537.
14. Vallera DA, Soderling CCR, Carlson GJ, Kersey JH. Bone marrow transplantation across major histocompatibility barriers in mice. Effect of elimination of T cells from donor grafts by pre treatment with monoclonal anti-Thy-1 plus complement or antibody alone. Transplantation 1981; 31: 218.
15. Onoe K, Yasumizu R, Oh-Ishi T, et al. Specific elimination of the T lineage cells: effect of in vitro treatment with anti-Thy 1 serum without complement on the adoptive cell transfer system. J Immunol Methods 1982; 49: 315.
16. OKunewick JP, Meredith RP, Braunschweiger PG, et al. Definition and prevention of graft-versus-host disease with the use of monoclonal antibodies. Exp Hematol 1982; 10: 12.
17. Korngold R, Sprent J Lethal GVHD across minor histocompatibility barriers: nature of the effector cells and role of the H2 complex. Immunol Rev 1983; 71: 5.
18. Ledbetter JA, Rouse RV, Spedding, Micklem H, Herzenberg LA. T cell subsets defined by expression of Lyt-1, 2, 3 and Thy-1 antigens: two parameter immunofluorescence and cytotoxicity analysis with monoclonal antibodies modifies current views. J Exp Med 1980; 152: 280.
19. Dialynas DP, Quan ZS, Wall KA, et al. Characterization of the murine T cell surface molecule designated L3T4, identified by monoclonal antibody GK1.5: similarity of L3T4 to the human Leu3/T4 molecule. J Immunol 1983; 131: 2445.
20. Ledbetter JA, Evans RL, Lipinski M, et al. Evolutionary conservation of surface molecules that distinguish T lymphocyte helper/inducer and cytotoxic/suppressor subpopulations in mouse and man. J Exp Med 1981; 153: 310.
21. Cudkowicz G, Bennett M. Peculiar immunobiology of bone marrow allografts. II. Rejection of parental grafts by resistant F1 hybrid mice. J Exp Med 1971; 134: 1513.
22. Cobbold SP, Waldmann H. Skin allograft rejection by both L3/T4+ and Lyt-2+ T cell subsets. Transplantation 1986; 41: 634.
23. Cobbold SP, Waldmann H. Immunosuppression with monoclonal antibodies: rules for effective serotherapy. Adv Exp Med 1985; 186: 789.
24. Monaco AP, Wood ML, Russel PS. Studies on heterologous anti-lymphocyte serum in mice. III. Immunologic tolerance and chimerism produced across the H-2 locus with adult thymectomy and anti-lymphocyte serum. Ann NY Acad Sci 1966; 129: 190.
25. Galfre G, Milstein C, Wright B. Rat x rat hybrid myelomas and a monoclonal anti-Fd portion of mouse IgG. Nature 1979; 277: 131.
26. Peto R, Pike MC, Armitage P, et al. Design and analysis of randomized clinical trials requiring prolonged observation of each patient. 2. Analysis and examples. Br J Cancer 1977; 35: 1.
27. Chandler P, Matsunaga T, Benjamin D, Simpson E. Use and functional properties of peripheral blood lymphocytes in mice. J Immunol Methods 1979; 31: 341.
28. Ozato K, Mayer N, Sachs DH. Hybridoma cell lines secreting monoclonal antibodies to mouse H-2 and Ia antigens. J Immunol 1980; 124: 533.
29. Ozato K, Sachs DH. Monoclonal antibodies to mouse MHC antigens. III. Hybridoma antibodies reacting to antigens of the H-2b haplotype reveal genetic control of isotype expression. J Immunol 1981; 126: 317.
30. Ozato K, Mayer NM, Sachs DH. Monoclonal antibodies to mouse major histocompatibility complex antigens. IV. A series of hybridoma clones producing anti-H-2d antibodies and an examination of expression of H-2d antigens on the surface of these cells. Transplantation 1982; 34: 113.
31. Koch S, Koch N, Robinson P, Hammerling G. Comparison of allogeneic and xenogeneic determinants on the H-2Kk molecule. Transplantation 1983; 36: 177.
32. Aqel, NM, Clark M, Cobbold SP, Waldmann H. Immunological screening in the selection of monoclonal antibodies: the use of the isotype-specific antiglobulins. J Immunol Methods 1984; 69: 207.
33. Zinkernagel RM, Althage A, Callahan G, Welsh RM. On the immunocompetence of H-2 incompatible bone marrow chimeras. J Immunol 1980; 124: 2356.
34. Rayfield LS, Brent L. Tolerance, immunocompetence, and secondary disease in fully allogeneic radiation chimeras. Transplantation 1983; 36: 183.
35. Onoe K, Fernandes G, Good RA. Humoral and cell-mediated immune responses in fully allogeneic bone marrow chimera in

mice. J Exp Med 1980; 151: 115.
36. Truitt RT, Pollard M. Allogeneic bone marrow chimerism in germ-free mice. IV. Therapy of "Hodgkin's-like" reticulum cell sarcoma in SJL mice. Transplantation 1976; 21: 12.
37. Muto M, Sdo T, Aizawa S, Kamisaku H, Kubo E. Bone marrow transplantation across the major histocompatibility barrier in specific-pathogen-free mice: effects of intact versus T cell-depleted bone marrow on the expression of anti-host reaction in the recipient spleens. J Immunol 1981; 127: 2421.
38. Onoe K, Yasumizu R, Oh-ishi T, Kakinuma M, Good RA, Morikawa K. Restricted antibody formation to sheep erythrocytes of allogeneic bone marrow chimeras histoincompatible at the K end of the H-2 complex. J Exp Med 1981; 153: 1009.
39. Ildstad ST, Wren SM, Bluestone JA, Barbieri SA, Sachs DH. Characterization of mixed allogeneic chimeras. Immunocompetence, in vitro reactivity, and genetic specificity of tolerance. J Exp Med 1985; 162: 231.
40. Cobbold SP, Thierfelder S, Waldmann H. Immunosuppression with monoclonal antibodies: a model to determine the rules for effective serotherapy. Mol Biol Med 1983; 1: 285.
41. Thierfelder S, Cobbold S, Kummer U, Waldmann H, Schuh R. Antilymphocyte antibodies and marrow transplantation. VII. Two out of nine complement fixing monoclonal anti-Thy-1 antibodies require no admixture of complement for suppression of graft-versus-host reactions. Exp Hematol 1985, 13: 948.
42. Zinkernagel RM, Doherty PC. Immunological surveillance against altered self components by sensitised T lymphocytes in lymphocytic choriomeningitis. Nature 1974; 251: 547.
43. Waldmann H, Munro A, Maurer PH. The role of MHC gene products in the development of the T-cell repertoire. Immunology of bone marrow transplantation. In: Thierfelder S, Rodt H, Kolb HJ, eds. Springer-Verlag, Berlin, Heidelberg: 1980; Haematology and blood transfusion. 25, 93.
44. Longo DL, Schwartz RH. T-cell specificity for H-2 and Ir gene phenotype correlates with the phenotype of thymic antigen-presenting cells. Nature 1980; 287: 44.
45. OKunewick JP, Buffo MJ, Kociban DL. Possible independent complementary roles for Lyt-1+ and Lyt-2+ T-cells in mouse minor histocompatibility (MiHL) GvH reaction. Exp Hematol 1985; 13: 429.
46. Rolink AG, Pals ST, Gleichmann E. Allosuppressor and allohelper T cells in acute and chronic graft-vs.-host disease. J Exp Med 1983; 157: 755.
47. Mason DW. Subsets of T cells in the rat mediating lethal graft-versus-host disease. Transplantation 1981; 32: 222.
48. Korngold R, Sprent J. Surface markers of T cells causing lethal graft-versus-host disease to class I versus class II H-2 differences. J Immunol 1985; 135: 3004.
49. Gleichmann E, Pals ST, Rolink AG, Radaszkiewicz T, Gleichmann H. Graft-versus-host reactions: clues to the etiopathology of a spectrum of immunological diseases. Immunol Today 1984; 5: 324.
50. Sado T, Kamisaku H, Kubo E. Strain difference in the radiosensitivity of immunocompetent cells and its influence on the residual host-vs-graft reaction in lethally irradiated mice grafted with semiallogeneic bone marrow. J Immunol 1985; 134: 704.
51. Suman L, Silobrcic V, Kastelan A. Chimerism in lymph nodes of F1 into irradiated parental recipient chimaeras rejecting skin allografts from the other parent. Transplantation 1978; 25: 302.
52. von Melchner H, Bartlett PF. Mechanisms of early allogeneic marrow graft rejection. Immunol Rev 1983; 71: 31.
53. Waterfall M, Rayfield LS, Brent L. Abrogation of resistance to bone marrow transplantation by induction of specific tolerance in natural killer cells? Nature 1984; 311: 663.
54. Warner JF, Dennert G. Bone marrow graft rejection as a function of antibody-directed natural killer cells. J Exp Med 1985; 161: 563.
55. Ford WL, Rolstad B, Fossum S. The elimination of allogeneic lymphocytes: a useful model of natural killer cell activity in vivo? Immunol Today 1984; 5: 227.
56. Samlowski E, Daynes RA. Bone marrow engraftment is enhanced by competitive inhibition of the hepatic asialoglycoprotein receptor. Proc Natl Acad Sci USA 1985; 82: 2508.
57. Fink PJ, Rammensee HG, Benedetto JD, Staerz UD, LeFrancois L, Bevan MJ. Studies on the mechanism of suppression of primary cytotoxic responses by cloned cytotoxic T lymphocytes. J Immunol 1984; 133: 1769.
58. Fink PJ, Rammensee HG, Bevan MJ. Cloned cytolytic T cells can suppress primary cytotoxic responses directed against them. J Immunol 1984; 133: 1775.
59. Muraoka S, Miller RG. Cells in bone marrow and in T cell colonies grown from bone marrow can suppress generation of cytotoxic T lymphocytes directed against their self antigens. J Exp Med 1980; 152: 54.

Received 16 September 1985.
Accepted 1 December 1985.

0041-1337/86/4203-0248$02.00/0
TRANSPLANTATION
Copyright © 1986 by The Williams & Wilkins Co.

Vol. 42, No. 3
Printed in U.S.A.

CURE OF MURINE THALASSEMIA BY BONE MARROW TRANSPLANTATION WITHOUT ERADICATION OF ENDOGENOUS STEM CELLS[1]

GERARD WAGEMAKER,[2,3,4] TRUDI P. VISSER,[2] AND DIRK W. VAN BEKKUM[2,4]

Radiobiological Institute TNO, Rijswijk; and Department of Radiobiology, Erasmus University, Rotterdam, The Netherlands

α-Thalassemic heterozygous (Hbath/+) mice were used to investigate the possible selective advantage of transplanted normal (+/+) hemopoietic cells. Without conditioning by total-body irradiation (TBI), infusion of large numbers of normal bone marrow cells failed to correct the thalassemic peripheral blood phenotype. Since the recipients' stem cells are normal with respect to number and differentiation capacity, it was thought that the transplanted stem cells were not able to lodge, or that they were not stimulated to proliferate. Therefore, a nonlethal dose of TBI was given to temporarily reduce endogenous stem cell numbers and hemopoiesis. TBI doses of 2 or 3 Gy followed by infusion of normal bone marrow cells proved to be effective in replacing the thalassemic red cells by normal red cells, whereas a dose of 1 Gy was ineffective. It is concluded that cure of thalassemia by bone marrow transplantation does not necessarily require eradication of thalassemic stem cells. Consequently, the objectives of conditioning regimens for bone marrow transplantation of thalassemic patients (and possibly other nonmalignant hemopoietic disorders) should be reconsidered.

As a result of relative protection of heterozygous phenotypes against malaria, the thalassemias belong to the most common genetic diseases of humans. Current therapy fails to be curative. Bone marrow transplantation is a demonstrated effective therapy in young people (*1*, *3*), but has not found widespread application in view of the risks of the immunological complications. Gene therapy, using autologous bone marrow cells, has been proposed as a valid alternative future approach (*2*, *3*).

The present study, using α-thalassemic heterozygous (Hbath/+) mice (*4*), was done to define the conditions required for acceptance of and cure by normal syngeneic bone marrow cells (comparable to autologous cells in humans), as a prelude to the gene therapy approach. The mutation of these mice is a deletion of both nonallelic α-genes (*5*) and is lethal in the homozygous state (*4*). In heterozygotes, the mutation causes a microcytic, hypochromic anemia with reticulocytosis and erythrocytosis; the red cells have a shortened life-span (*6*). The study is based on the hypothesis that the shortened life-span of the thalassemic erythrocytes results in a preponderance of the +/+ phenotype in mixed hemopoietic chimeras, which are defined by coexistence of donor-and-recipient–derived hemopoietic stem cells and their progeny.

It has been proposed that two separate objectives need to be achieved by the conditioning regimen preparing thalassemia patients for acceptance of an allogeneic bone marrow graft; first, the thalassemic stem cell population must be damaged sufficiently to be incapable of regeneration; and second, there must be adequate immunosuppression to achieve allogeneic engraftment (*1*). This approach seems logical, especially by the clear analogy to the objectives of the conditioning regimens used for leukemia patients. Other clinical investigators have adopted the same reasoning for the treatment of a variety of nonmalignant, congenital disorders by bone marrow transplantation (*7*). However, the necessity of complete ablation of the thalassemic (but not malignant) stem cells has not been proved. Experimental separation of the two objectives can only be achieved using semiallogeneic or syngeneic normal donor cells, thereby avoiding the need for immunosuppression of the recipient. There is no way to perform such studies in an outbred species like man. Therefore, the inbred thalassemic mice used in this study also provided the first opportunity to study the necessity of marrow ablation in the preparation of a thalassemia patient for bone marrow transplantation.

MATERIALS AND METHODS

α-Thalassemic male heterozygous (Hbath/$^{+}$) mice from stock 352HB (*4*) were kindly provided by Dr. R. A. Popp (The Oak Ridge National Laboratory) in 1981, and since inbred into BALB/c mice by backcrossing. For the present study, female mice, aged approximately 12 weeks, of the 6th to 10th generation of backcrossing were used. Normal female BALB/c mice of the same age groups served as +/+ donors. In this way, the genetic disparity between donor and recipient is close to that of a syngeneic combination—and, at most, equivalent to a P → F_1 combination; in neither case is rejection of grafted cells expected to occur.

Total body irradiation (TBI)* was given using a two-source 800 Ci ^{137}Cs gamma irradiation facility at a dose rate of 0.82 Gy/min, one day prior to transplantation, as previously described (*8*).

Bone marrow cell suspensions were prepared as reported earlier (*8*) and administered i.v. in numbers given in the *Results* section.

Blood samples were obtained by tail bleeding at two-week intervals for the first three months after transplantation, and thereafter at three-month intervals. Blood cell values were determined by standard methods. Analysis of the red cell size profiles was done as described elsewhere (*9*) by using an Elzone

[1] This work was supported in part by a program grant of The Netherlands Foundation for Medical Research, FUNGO, which is subsidized by The Netherlands Organization for the Advancement of Pure Research ZWO.

[2] Radiobiological Institute TNO.

[3] Address correspondence to: Dr. G. Wagemaker, ℅ Radiobiological Institute TNO, P.O. Box 5815, 2280 HV Rijswijk, The Netherlands.

[4] Erasmus University.

* Abbreviation used: TBI, total-body irradiation.

Particle Channelyzer attached to a 256-channel pulse height analyzer; the calibrated volume increment per channel was 0.871 fl. Cure of thalassemia was defined as a rise of the hematocrit to normal values, disappearance of erythrocytosis and reticulocytosis, and disappearance of microcytosis. The peripheral blood cell values were determined by standard methods.

RESULTS

Bone marrow transplantation resulted in rapid cure of supralethally (9 Gy) irradiated thalassemic recipients (Table 1), leading to a correction of the thalassemic peripheral blood phenotype as shown in Figure 1. However, without prior irradiation of the recipients, no cures were observed, although very large numbers of bone marrow cells were infused (Table 1).

The latter observation contrasts with results using another genetically anemic mutant, W/W^v, which can be cured by bone marrow transplantation without prior irradiation (*10*). In this mutant, the anemia is caused by defective self-replication and differentiation of the hemopoietic stem cells, which results in a greatly reduced number of stem cells (*9*). The thalassemic mice, in contrast, have normal numbers of stem cells with a normal repopulation capacity (*11*). Therefore it was decided to temporarily reduce the number of endogenous stem cells of thalassemic recipient mice by a nonlethal dose of TBI. Table 1 demonstrates that this approach proved to be successful in recipients conditioned with 2 and 3 Gy TBI, whereas recipients that received 1 Gy TBI maintained their thalassemic peripheral blood phenotype. An example of the conversion of erythrocyte size in a mouse conditioned with 2 Gy TBI and transplanted with 10^7 bone marrow cells is shown in Figure 2. The near-normal peripheral blood red cell values of cured mice are given in Table 2.

Since the latter experiments were done with relatively large numbers of transplanted bone marrow cells, the minimum number of bone marrow cells required for cure at the irradiation dose of 3 Gy was determined. Conversion to a normal red blood cell phenotype required 10^6 bone marrow cells per mouse, whereas infusion of 3×10^5 cells resulted in 1 cure in 4 mice transplanted (Table 3).

TABLE 1. Transplantation of $Hba^{th}/+$ mice by infusion of +/+ bone marrow cells using various conditioning regimens[a]

	Cures per total tested						
	0.5	1	1.5	2	2.5	6	12 months
Conditioning with 9 Gy TBI (cell dose):							
10^5	0/3	3/3	3/3	10/10	10/10	10/10	10/10
10^6	0/3	3/3	3/3	10/10	10/10	10/10	10/10
No TBI given (cell dose):							
3×10^7	0/3	0/3	0/3	0/10	0/10	0/10	0/7
10^7	0/3	0/3	0/3	0/10	0/10	0/10	0/7
10^6	0/3	0/3	0/3	0/10	0/10	0/10	0/7
10^5	0/3	0/3	0/3	0/10	0/10	0/10	0/7
Nonlethal TBI, 10^7 cells per mouse (irradiation dose [Gy]):							
1	0/4	0/4	0/4	0/4	0/4	0/4	0/4
2	0/4	0/4	0/4	4/4	9/13	13/13	4/4
3	0/4	0/4	4/4	4/4	4/4	4/4	4/4

[a] Experiments 1 and 2 were simultaneously done and involved 10 mice per exprimental group. If the whole group was not tested for cure, mice were randomly selected. In experiment 2 three mice were sacrificed per group for a retransplantation experiment, which failed to demonstrate the presence of the infused donor cells. Experiment 3 involved 4 mice per experimental group; the 2 Gy group was supplemented with data from another, ongoing experiment, which involved 9 mice.

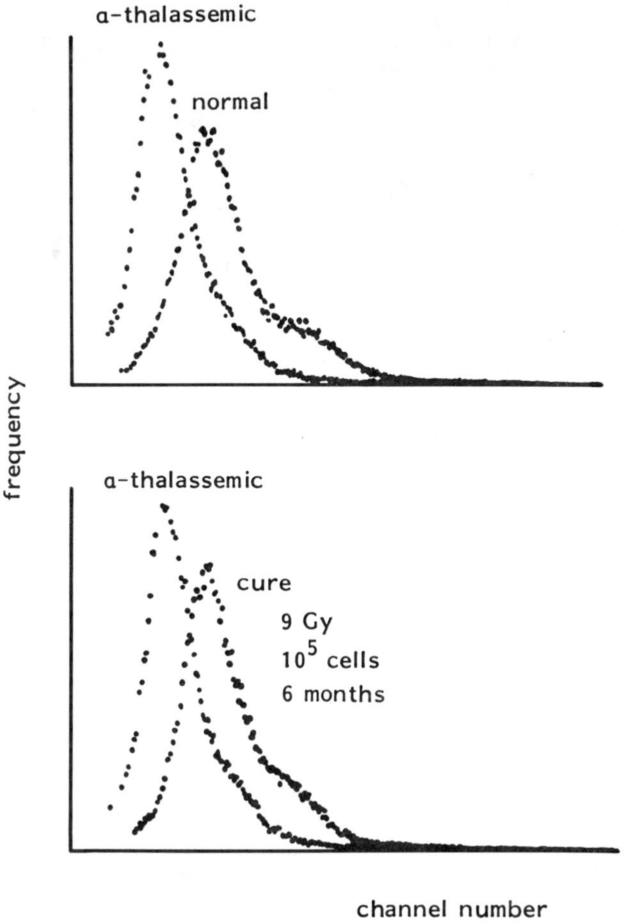

FIGURE 1. Upper panel: erythrocyte size distributions of normal BALB/c and $Hba^{th}/+$ mice. The mean corpuscular volume of normal erythrocytes was 51±2 fl and that of $HbA^{th}/+$ mice 37±1 fl. Lower panel: conversion to a normal red cell phenotype by bone marrow transplantation following a lethal dose of TBI.

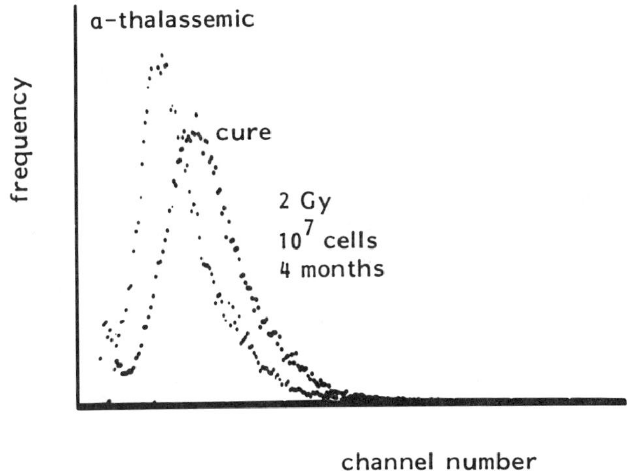

FIGURE 2. Conversion to a normal red cell phenotype by bone marrow transplantation following a nonlethal dose of TBI.

TABLE 2. Peripheral blood red cell characteristics of Hbath/+ mice transplanted with 10^7 +/+ bone marrow cells after 3 Gy TBI determined 6 months after transplantation[a]

	Hbath/+	+/+	Transplanted
Erythrocytes (10^{12}/L)	9.5±0.2	8.9±0.2	9.1±0.2
Hematocrit (%)	35±1	47±3	44±2
Corpuscular volume (fl)	37±1	51±2	48±3
Reticulocytes	7.2±2.9	2.4±0.6	2.9±0.8

[a] Mean values ± SD.

TABLE 3. Number of +/+ bone marrow cells required for cure of Hbath/+ mice following 3 Gy TBI[a]

Cell dose	Cures per total tested	
	3 Months	5 Months
10^7	4/4	4/4
3×10^6	4/4	4/4
10^6	4/4	4/4
3×10^5	1/4	1/4
10^5	0/4	0/4

[a] The experiment involved 4 mice per experimental group.

DISCUSSION

These experiments demonstrate that thalassemia can be cured by infusion of relatively low numbers of bone marrow cells following a nonlethal dose of TBI. This is most readily explained by assuming that, with the near-syngeneic donors used in this mouse model, the procedure results in mixed hemopoietic chimerism with a selective advantage of the infused normal cells along the erythroid maturation pathway. Since no other marker for hemopoietic chimerism was incorporated in the present experiments, the degree of chimerism in other hemopoietic differentiation pathways is as yet unknown. The results provide direct evidence that complete eradication of thalassemic stem cells is not required for cure of thalassemia by bone marrow transplantation. Hence, engraftment failures reported in the few human thalassemia patients who have been treated with bone marrow transplantation (*3*, *12*) should be attributed to insufficient immunosuppressive therapy rather than incomplete marrow ablation, which is strongly corroborated by the fact that the majority of the failures occurred in older individuals with, necessarily, a considerable (hyper) transfusion history.

Thus, the findings demonstrate that the conditioning regimen for thalassemic recipients of allogeneic bone marrow cells should not necessarily involve the potentially lethal stage of marrow ablation. However, as yet no conditioning regimen has been developed that allows for acceptance of a bone marrow graft in patients without eradication of normal hemopoietic stem cells.

Earlier it was stated, based on research in this laboratory, that conditioning of transplant patients has three objectives; first, to create sufficient space in the bone marrow; second, to provide sufficient immunosuppression for prevention of rejection; and third, in case of malignancy, to achieve tumor eradication (*13*). In fact, the objective of marrow ablation is thought to be imperative only in case of hemopoietic malignancy. In the donor-recipient combination chosen for the experiments described here, only space is relevant. Table 4 gives a comparison between the calculated number of Hbath/+ bone marrow cells that survive the nonlethal doses of irradiation used, and

TABLE 4. The calculated residual number of Hbath/+ bone marrow cells in comparison to, respectively, the smallest effective and the largest ineffective number of +/+ bone marrow cells observed at various doses of nonlethal gamma irradiation

Irradiation dose (Gy)	Residual number of bone marrow cells[a]	Smallest effective number of cells infused	Largest ineffective number of cells infused
0	2×10^8[b]	—	3×10^7 (7)[c]
1	1.5×10^8	—	10^7 (15)
3	2×10^7	10^6 (20)	3×10^5 (60)

[a] Calculation based on a D_0 value of 1 Gy and an extrapolation number of 2 for CFU-S and repopulating stem cells exposed to gamma rays (*22*, *23*); these values are in agreement with most data in the literature (*24*).

[b] Calculated on the assumption that 1 femoral shaft contains 8.5% of total mouse hemopoietic bone marrow cells.

[c] In parentheses: the calculated ratio of recipient to donor cells.

the infused number of +/+ bone marrow cells. At an irradiation dose of 3 Gy, the smallest effective number of +/+ cells is 20–60-fold lower than the calculated number of residual Hbath/+ bone marrow cells. This agrees well with the ratio of 30 observed by Barker and MacFarlane in direct competition experiments using lethally irradiated recipient mice (*14*), especially if it is taken into account that not all grafted cells will reach an appropriate hemopoietic site. Since a similar or more favorable ratio of donor-to-recipient cells in, respectively, the 1-Gy-irradiated and the nonirradiated recipients was not effective (Table 4), these experiments provide the first direct evidence that the creation of space in the recipient's bone marrow is a realistic requirement for acceptance of a bone marrow graft. The results indicate that a conditioning regimen equivalent to an irradiation dose of 2 Gy is sufficient to meet this requirement.

Unirradiated recipients failed to show chimerism by the thalassemia marker used here. This is in agreement with earlier studies (*15*, *16*, *17*), which demonstrated that large numbers of syngeneic cells infused in unirradiated mice result in only <1% to maximally 3% bone marrow chimerism. Recently, values around 10% bone marrow chimerism have been reported following infusion of 10^8 bone marrow cells (*18*). It should be strongly emphasized that this number of cells is equivalent to approximately half the recipient's bone marrow and cannot be considered practical for therapeutic purposes. In combination with the data presented in Table 4, this recent observation also suggests that 10^8 cells per mouse would be the minimum effective cell number required for cure of unirradiated thalassemic recipients. This implies that the unirradiated and 3-Gy-irradiated groups differ at least 100-fold in absolute cell numbers required for cure, and at least 10-fold in the ratio of residual-to-infused effective cell numbers. Obviously, such differences far exceed some uncertainty in the estimates of residual cell numbers after nonlethal irradiation shown in Table 4, while any uncertainty in the estimated number of bone marrow cells in unirradiated mice would only affect the absolute values of the calculated ratios and not their relative differences. Therefore uncertainty in the estimates of bone marrow cell numbers in unirradiated or nonlethally irradiated mice does not detract from our conclusion that the creation of space is a realistic requirement for acceptance of a bone marrow graft. Whether "space" must be considered a direct spatial requirement for infused hemopoietic stem cells to lodge in hemopoietic organs, or whether it merely reflects lack of proliferation of grafted stem cells in unconditioned recipients because of lack of stem cell demand remains to be investigated.

Insertion of normal globin genes in the hemopoietic stem cells of thalassemia patients is a valid option for future therapy. In that case, autologous cells are being grafted. The near syngeneic donor-recipient combination used in the present murine model is directly comparable to autologous transplantation in humans. Therefore, the results reveal a strategy for the conditioning regimen and an estimate of the cell numbers required for the successful application of such a therapy. The observed ratio between normal and thalassemic cells that results in effective replacement of the thalassemic phenotype appeared to be more extreme than could be expected from the difference in life-span between normal and thalassemic erythrocytes alone. In fact, approximately 5% of normal cells suffice to cure the mice. This finding suggests that thalassemic erythrocyte precursors have a growth disadvantage compared with normal cells, indicating that inserted normal globin genes, if expressed during erythropoietic maturation, may—in contrast to what might have been expected (*3*)—confer a growth advantage on thalassemic cells along the erythroid maturation pathway. As a consequence, a selectable marker gene might not be required. However, the results also show that the method to be chosen for globin gene transfer should be highly efficient to provide the relatively large numbers (approximately 4×10^7/kg body weight) of "repaired" cells required for cure.

Mixed (or split) chimerism is normally observed after transplantation for severe combined immunodeficiency—only the affected lymphocyte pathway(s) being replaced by donor cells (*19*). Establishment of this type of chimerism does not seem to be dependent on the underlying lesion causing SCID. Also, in CBA/N mice only the defective B lymphocyte lineage appeared to be replaced by donor cells following infusion of histocompatible spleen cells without prior conditioning (*20*). Similar cases have been observed after transplantation of normal cells for murine osteopetrosis, in which the affected osteoclasts had been replaced by donor cells and hemopoiesis remained of recipient type (*21*). Therefore it is thought that the above considerations are not unique for thalassemia but may as well apply to various other congenital, nonmalignant hemopoietic diseases.

Acknowledgments. We are indebted to Dr. R. A. Popp for his kind sharing of $Hba^{th}/+$ mice and to Mr. J. Westhof for expert breeding of these mice; to Mr. W. Slingerland for measuring erythrocyte size distributions; and to Dr. L. C. J. Dorssers for critically reading the manuscript.

REFERENCES

1. Thomas ED, Buckner CD, Sanders JE, et al. Marrow transplantation for thalassemia. Lancet 1982; 2: 227.
2. Mercola KE, Cline MJ. The potentials of inserting new genetic information. N Engl J Med 1980; 303: 1297.
3. Nienhuis AW, Anagnou NP, Ley TJ. Advances in thalassemia research. Blood 1984; 63: 738.
4. Russell LB, Russell WL, Popp RA, Vaughan C, Jacobson KB. Radiation induced mutations at mouse hemoglobin loci. Proc Natl Acad Sci USA 1976; 73: 2843.
5. Whitney JB, Martinell J, Popp RA, Russell LB, Anderson WF. Deletions in the α-globin gene complex in α-thalassemic mice. Proc Natl Acad Sci 1981; 78: 7644
6. Popp RA, Francis MC, Bradshaw BS. Erythrocyte life-span in alpha thalassemic mice. Birth defects: original article series 1978; 14: 181.
7. Parkman R, Rappeport JM, Hellman S, et al. Busulfan and total body irradiation as antihematopoietic stem cell agents in the preparation of patients with congenital bone marrow disorders for allogeneic bone marrow transplantation. Blood 1984; 64: 852.
8. Van Bekkum DW, De Vries MJ. Radiation chimaeras. New York, London: Academic and Logos Prss, 1967.
9. Merchav S, Wagemaker G, Van Bekkum DW. Reconstitution of the defective stem cell differentiation of W/W^v mice by infection with Rauscher leukemia virus. J Natl Cancer Inst 1985; 75: 361.
10. Bernstein SE, Russell ES. Implantation of normal blood-forming tissue in genetically anemic mice, without X-irradiation of the host. Proc Soc Exp Biol Med 1959; 101: 769.
11. Wagemaker G, Visser TP. Enumeration of stem cells and progenitor cells in alpha-thalassemic mice reveals lack of specific regulation of stem cell differentiation. Exp Hematol 1986; 14: 303.
12. Lucarelli G, Polchi P, Izzi T, et al. Allogeneic marrow transplantation for thalassemia. Exp Hematol 1984; 12: 676.
13. Vriesendorp HM, Van Bekkum DW. Role of total body irradiation in conditioning for bone marrow transplantation. In: Thierfelder S, Rodt H, Kolb HJ, eds. Immunobiology of bone marrow transplantation. Berlin: Springer Verlag, 1980: 359.
14. Barker JE, McFarland EC. The stem cells of alpha thalassemic mice. Exp Hematol 1984; 12: 285.
15. Micklem HS, Clarke CM, Evans EP, Ford CE. Fate of chromosome marked mouse bone marrow cells transfused into normally syngeneic recipients. Transplantation 1968; 6: 299.
16. Takada A, Takada Y, Ambrus JL. Proliferation of donor spleen and bone marrow cells in the spleens and bone marrows of unirradiated and irradiated adult mice. Proc Soc Exp Biol Med 1970; 136: 222.
17. Takada Y, Takada A. Proliferation of donor hematopoietic cells in irradiated and unirradiated host mice. Transplantation 1971; 12: 334.
18. Saxe DF, Boggs SS, Boggs DR. Transplantation of chromosomally marked syngeneic marrow cells into mice not subjected to hematopoietic stem cell depletion. Exp Hematol 1984; 12: 277.
19. Dooren LJ, Vossen JM. Severe combined immunodeficiency: reconstitution of the immune system following bone marrow transplantation. In: Van Bekkum DW, Lowenberg B, eds. Bone marrow transplantation. New York, Basel: Marcel Dekker, 1985: 351.
20. Volf D, Sensenbrenner LL, Sharkis SJ, et al. Induction of partial chimerisme in nonirradiated B-lymphocyte deficient CBA/N mice. J Exp Med 1978; 147: 940.
21. Loutit JF, Nisbett NW. The origin of osteoclasts. Immunobiology 1982; 161: 193.
22. Till JE, McCulloch EA. A direct measurement of the radiation sensitivity of normal mouse bone marrow cells. Radiat Res 1961; 14: 213.
23. McCulloch EA, Till JE. The radiation sensitivity of normal mouse bone marrow cells, determined by quantitative marrow transplantation into irradiated mice. Radiat Res 1960; 13: 115.
24. Hendry JH, Lord BI. The analysis of the early and late response to cytotoxic insults in the hemopoietic cell hierarchy. In: Potten CS, Hendry JH. Cytotoxic insult to tissue. Edinburgh: Churchill Livingstone, 1983: 1.

Received 19 September 1985.
Accepted 21 November 1985.

0041-1337/86/4303-0252$02.00/0
TRANSPLANTATION

Vol. 42, No. 3
Printed in U.S.A.

CHARACTERIZATION OF ANTILEUKEMIA CELLS' CYTOTOXIC EFFECTOR FUNCTION

IMPLICATIONS FOR MONITORING NATURAL KILLER RESPONSES FOLLOWING ALLOGENEIC BONE MARROW TRANSPLANTATION[1]

L. DELMON, A. YTHIER, P. MOINGEON, A. NOWILL, C. BAYLE, J.L. PICO, M. HAYAT, J. RITZ,[2] AND TH. HERCEND[3,4]

Unité de Biologie Cellulaire et Service d'Hématologie, Institut Gustave-Roussy, Villejuif, France

We have studied here cytotoxic function of three cloned cell lines—TC12, 48, and 50—derived from circulating lymphocytes that were potentially able to eliminate residual tumor cells in a patient transplanted for treatment of acute lymphocytic leukemia. These cloned cells, which have both phenotypic and functional characteristics of natural killer lymphocytes, were tested in chromium release assays against a panel of 16 uncultured populations of leukemia cells. In addition, their activity was compared with that of cloned and uncloned NK cells from normal individuals.

It was found that TC clones induced a much weaker degree of killing against fresh tumor cells compared with conventional NK target cell lines such as K562 or MOLT4. In addition, there was great heterogeneity in their individual lytic capacity against the various leukemia blasts (TC12, 48, and 50 cells killed in a significant fashion, respectively 7, 1, and 4 of the 16 leukemias), reflecting the functional diversity of normal NK cell populations. Thus, for a fraction of leukemias, there was no correlation between lytic ability of TC cells and that of uncloned lymphokine-activated large granular lymphocytes from normal peripheral blood.

Together, these results support the view that direct identification of patients' cytotoxic lymphocytes screened against in vivo relevant tumor cells is necessary to evaluate potentially beneficial immunologic responses in the context of bone marrow transplantation.

Intensive chemotherapy and total body irradiation followed by allogeneic bone marrow transplantation (ABMT)* is an effective therapeutic modality for various forms of leukemias (*1–5*). While ablative treatment programs certainly provide the major therapeutic contribution for eradication of leukemia, it has been postulated that immunological reconstitution with allogeneic lymphocytes may exert an adjuvant antitumor effect. This hypothesis was strenghtened by data showing that patients who develop graft-versus-host disease (GVHD) have a decreased risk of leukemia relapse when compared with patients who do not develop GVHD (*6–7*).However cellular mechanisms potentially responsible for graft-versus-leukemia effects have not been identified.

Recently, we have studied immune reconstitution in one patient transplanted for treatment of a T cell acute lymphocytic leukemia, in whose case large numbers of pure tumor had been cryopreserved during the acute phase of the disease (*8*). Following ABMT, we demonstrated the existence of peripheral blood lymphocytes able to destroy thawed uncultured recipient's blasts. Meanwhile the patient did not develop any significant graft-versus-host disease, and it was suggested that cells with antitumor activity were not necessarily identical to those mediating GVHD. Lymphocytes responsible for antileukemic activity were characterized using cloning techniques. Antileukemic clones were found to be phenotypically heterogeneous but all expressed a pan-natural-killer (NK)–associated antigen, NKH1A (*9*). Moreover they were shown to display a strong cytotoxic activity against NK-susceptible hematopoietic cell lines, such as K562 and MOL T4 (*8*).

Here we have further characterized antileukemic activity displayed by three of these cloned cell lines termed *TC12*, *TC48*, and *TC50*. A panel of 16 uncultured pure tumor cell populations was obtained from patients with either lymphoid or myeloid leukemia. Cytotoxicity assays were performed against the blasts, using as effector cells TC clones, or cloned NK lymphocytes derived from normal donors, or uncloned circulating lymphocytes of healthy individuals. It was found that individual TC clones, as well as normal NK cells, were very heterogeneous with respect to their capacity of lysing additional populations of allogeneic leukemia cells.

MATERIALS AND METHODS

Uncloned effector cells. Peripheral blood mononuclear cells (PBMC) were obtained from normal human volunteers by Ficoll-Hypaque density gradient centrifugation. Adherent cells were removed by applying PBMC suspension to sterilized nylon-wool columns. Nylon-wool-nonadherent PBMC were then separated by centrifugation on a Percoll discontinuous density gradient (Pharmacia; Uppsala, Sweden) according to the method described by Timonen et al. (*10*). Briefly six concentrations of sterilized Percoll diluted in medium were prepared, ranging from 31% to 47% (respectively 31, 34, 37, 41, 45, and 47%). After layering 2 ml of each solution into 15-ml conical test tubes, 10^8 cells in 1.5 ml of RPMI 1640 medium were applied on top of the gradient, and the tubes were spun at 550 g for 30 min at room temperature. Fractions were numbered 0–5 corresponding to cells harvested at each interface from the top to the bottom of the tube. Fraction 2 (F2 cells) and fraction 4 (F4 cells) were studied in the present experiments. F2 cells

[1] This work was supported in part by Contrat de Recherche Clinique N85D28, Institut Gustave-Roussy.

[2] Division of Tumor Immunology, Dana Farber Cancer Institute, Boston, MA, a scholar of the Leukemia Society of America.

[3] Thierry Hercend is a special fellow of the Leukemia Society of America.

[4] Address correspondence to: Th. Hercend, M.D., Ph.D., Unité de Biologie Cellulaire, Institut Gustave-Roussy, rue Camille Desmoulins, 94805 Villejuif, France.

* Abbreviations used: ABMT, allogeneic bone marrow transplantation; EBV, Epstein-Barr virus; GVHD, graft-versus-host disease; γIF, gamma interferon; LCM, lymphocyte-conditioned medium; LGL, large granular lymphocytes; PBMC, peripheral blood mononuclear cells; r-IL2, recombinant interleukin 2.

were chosen because they contained high percentages of large granular lymphocytes (LGL) (65–80%) when analyzed with Giemsa-stained cytocentrifuged cell smears. In addition NK cytotoxicity against K562 target cells was found to be maximal in this particular fraction. F4 cells containing more than 95% small lymphocytes and exerting no NK activity against K562 cells served as a control group. More than 90% F4 cells were found to react with anti-T3 monoclonal antibody. Approximately 5–10% of the input was recovered in F2 fractions, whereas 20–30% of the cells were present in F4—yielding an usual F2/F4 cell ratio of approximately 0.3. Following purification, PBMC, F2, and F4 were cryopreserved with a final concentration of 20% human AB serum and 10% DMSO. Recombinant IL2 (Biogen Inc., Courtesy of T. Strom) and purified recombinant gamma-interferon (Courtesy of Dr. Strom) were used for pretreatment of effector cells.

Cytotoxic clones. Methods for generation of cloned cell lines without preselected specificity have been described in detail (*11–13*). Briefly, for initial cloning, cells are usually seeded at 1 or 0.5. cells/well on a feeder layer of autologous or allogeneic irradiated (5000 rads) PBMC plus PHA (2 μg/ml) and/or allogeneic irradiated (5000 rads) EBV-transformed B cells. Colonies are expanded by addition of culture medium containing LCM (10–15% final dilution) every 3 days. LCM is produced followig stimulation of whole PBMC at a concentration of 2.5 10^6 c/ml by a combination of PHA, PMA, and irradiated EBV-transformed B cells as previously described (*11*). Cells are washed 4 times after 3 h to remove the mitogens, and supernatants are harvested after 40 h of incubation at 37°C.

Clones described in these studies have been subcloned at least 3 times at 100 cells/well. They all have a homogenous phenotype when tested with a series of monoclonal antibodies. Phenotypes are stable and have been controlled after each subcloning procedure. Of the clones used here, JT3, JT9, and JTB18 have been previously described (*9, 11–13*). TC12, TC48, and TC50 were derived from peripheral blood lymphocytes of a leukemic patient during early reconstitution following allogeneic bone marrow transplantation. Cell surface phenotypes have been determined using indirect immunofluorescent assays and subsequent cytofluorometric analysis. Anti-T3 defines all mature T lymphocytes in human peripheral blood. T4 and T8 antigens are expressed on reciprocal subpopulations of circulating T lymphocytes. Anti-T11 defines an antigen associated with the sheep erythrocyte receptor (*14*). NKH1A (*9*) is a pan-NK-associated marker, whereas NKH2 (*9*) is expressed on a subpopulation of circulating LGL and a fraction of human NK clones. The reactivity of the clones with these 6 monoclonal antibodies (Mab) is shown in Table 1. All Mab reacted with less than 5% or more than 90% of cloned cells in each case. As shown in Table 1, TC48 represents an uncommon lymphocyte reacting only with anti-NKH1A. TC12, TC50, and JTB18 clones have a more usual NK-associated phenotype. Indeed they coexpress both T11 and NKH1A antigens. JT3 has an additional common NK phenotype reacting with anti-T11, anti-NKH1A, and anti-NKH2. JT9 represents a minor subset of cells that coexpress T3, T8, and T11 antigens—as well as the NK-associated structure NKH1A.

TABLE 1. Surface phenotype of cloned cytotoxic cell lines

Clone	T3[a]	T4	T8	T11	NKH1A	NKH2
TC12	−	−	−	+	+	−
TC48	−	−	−	−	+	−
TC50	−	−	−	+	+	−
JT3	−[b]	−	−	+	+	+
JT9	+	−	+	+	+	−
JTB18	−	−	−	+	+	−

[a] Expression of antigens determined by indirect immunofluorescence reactivity with specific monoclonal antibodies.

[b] (−) <5% of cells reactive; (+) >90% of cells reactive.

Target cells. Two continuously growing cell lines have been used in this study. K562 was established from a patient with chronic myelogenous leukemia. MOLT 4 is a T cell leukemia line. Fresh leukemia cells were cryopreserved using a final concentration of 20% human AB serum and 10% DMSO.

Cytotoxicity assays. Cytotoxic activity was measured in a standard 4-hr chromium release assay. Effector–to–target cell ratios inducing maximal cytotoxicity were determined in preliminary experiments and subsequently used throughout the study. E/T ratios of 40:1 and 10:1 were used with uncloned and cloned effector cells, respectively. The percentage of specific cytotoxicity was calculated as previously described (*11*). Results are expressed as the mean of triplicate cultures.

RESULTS

For the present studies, initial selection of the patients depended upon white blood cell counts and/or percentages of circulating blasts. Indeed substantial numbers of leukemic cells were necessary to standardize and reproduce the experiments. A critical point here was to ensure that target cells were actually leukemia cells and not contaminating normal cells. Peripheral blood was treated by Ficoll density gradient centrifugation prior to cryopreservation in multiple identical aliquots. For each tumor cell population, one aliquot was thawed and immediately incubated for 2 hr at 37° C in the presence of ^{51}chromium. Cells were subsequently washed and cytocentrifuge smears were prepared. Final selection was based upon morphological analysis of the labeled samples, and only those containing at least 90% blasts with perfect viability were considered for further studies. According to these criteria, 16 tumor cell populations have been tested here, including 11 acute myeloid leukemias with a majority of undifferentiated M1 cases and 6 acute lymphoblastic leukemias (Table 2).

Susceptibility of leukemia cells to human NK clones. Clones TC12, 48, and 50 were assayed for cytotoxicity against the selected leukemia cell populations. JT3, JT9, and JTB18 cloned cells lines (which have been isolated from circulating NK cells of healthy individuals—see the *Material and Methods* section and Table 1) were tested in parallel.

As shown in Table 3, leukemic blasts were generally much less susceptible to TC clones than conventional in-vitro-established NK target cell lines, such as MOLT4 or K562. Furthermore TC lymphocytes were not more efficient in killing fresh tumor cells than cloned NK cells from normal donors. Specifically, there was no cytotoxicity greater than 50% against any leukemia using short term ^{51}chromium release at an optimal effector–to–target cell ratio.

An additional finding was the heterogeneity of the clones with respect to their capacity of destroying the various populations of leukemia cells. For example, JT3 lymphocytes—which are highly cytotoxic against multiple tumor cells lines (*13*), including MOLT4 and K562—had virtually no activity against most fresh leukemia blasts. In contrast, TC12, TC50, and JTB18 demonstrated a significant degree of killing (++ ⩾15%) against, respectively, 7, 4, and 7 leukemias of the 16 selected cases. TC48 cells, which were cytotoxic against relevant residual blasts potentially present in the transplanted

TABLE 2. Leukemias tested as target cells in cytotoxicity assays

Leukemia	Patients	Type[a]	Age	Sex	WBC/mm	% Tumor cells[b]
AML	RAV	M1	17	M	397000	95
	MA5	M1	20	F	93000	95
	JAN	M1	36	F	165000	90
	COC	M1	37	F	77000	90
	DEC	M1	44	F	184000	95
	ALG	M1	45	M	7300	90
	MAND[c]	M2	18	F	1000	100
	FED	M2	68	F	182000	100
	GIU	M5	13	M	186000	95
	BEN	M5	25	F	46000	100
	TAN	M5	27	F	25000	90
ALL	MAR	L1	8	F	48000	100
	COR	L1	10	F	59000	90
	RIC	L2	9	M	83000	90
	TUR	L2	11	M	19000	100
	LAR	L2	13	M	165000	100

[a] According to the FAB morphological classification.

[b] Percentage of tumor cells on cytocentrifuge smears following Ficoll-Hypaque density gradient centrifugation, cryopreservation, thawing and chromium labeling.

[c] For this patient sufficient number of bone marrow leukemia cells were available for studies.

patient, had little if any effect on all additional leukemias, excluding MAR. This later population of tumor cells was clearly the most susceptible, and at least a minor degree of lysis was measured with each clone including JT3 and JT9. Finally, note that cases relatively susceptible to TC12 and TC50 clones included M1 (ALG), M2 (FED), and M5 (TAN) acute myeloid leukemias, as well as lymphoblastic leukemias (MAR).

Susceptibility of leukemia blasts to resting and lymphokine-activated natural killing. The panel of leukemia blasts was tested for susceptibility to natural cytotoxicity mediated by three cell fractions isolated from normal donors' peripheral blood (see the *Materials and Methods* section): peripheral blood mononuclear cells, Percoll fraction 2 enriched in large granular lymphocytes, and Percoll fraction 4 containing exclusively small lymphocytes. To standardize experiments, these fractions were cryopreserved immediately after separation. Thus, it was possible to test simultaneously selected effector cells from several donors against the panel of leukemias, and to compare results obtained under identical experimental conditions. Prior to cytotoxicity assays, each cell fraction was thawed and incubated for 18 hr in medium or optimal doses, determined in previous experiments (*15*), of recombinant IL-2 (36 ng/ml) or recombinant gamma interferon (500 units/ml).

Results obtained with small lymphocytes are not presented in Table 4 because there was no cytotoxicity at all in these fractions (either resting or lymphokine activated) against any of the tested leukemias. As expected LGL cytotoxicity was greater than that of peripheral blood mononuclear cells. Moreover, the degree of killing induced by the different fractions was clearly enhanced following r-IL2 and γ IF treatment, although this later lymphokine was slightly less efficient. Susceptibility of individual leukemia was virtually identical for the 3 normal donors presented here, who had been preselected because their thawed IL-2-stimulated LGL fraction induced a lysis greater than 50% in standard NK assays against K562 cells. It was found (Table 4) that only one population of leukemic blasts (MAR) was almost as susceptible to peripheral blood natural killing as K562. In 9 of 16 cases, (MAS, JAN, DEC, GIU, BEN, TAN, COR, RIC, and TUR) there was no significant cytotoxicity in any fraction studied, including IL-2-activated LGL. Blasts from 6 patients (RAV, COC, ALG, FED, MAN, and LAR) presented a degree of susceptibility that was best demonstrated using IL-2-stimulated LGL as effector cells. In this latter group, were included undifferentiated myeloid blasts (RAV, COC, and ALG) and more heterogeneous myeloid tumor populations (FED and MAN), as well as lymphoblasts (LAR).

Note that correlation was loose comparing results obtained with uncloned and cloned effector cells. For example, there was little if any killing against blasts such as COR, TAN, or DEC by peripheral blood—whereas these leukemias were relatively susceptible to TC12 and JTB18. This suggested that functional effects of individual, possibly minor, NK subsets may not be detected using heterogeneous populations of uncloned effector cells. Conversely in the limited panel tested, there were no clones representative of those circulating effector cells that were able to lyse LAR cells rather efficiently.

DISCUSSION

We have studied here three clones, TC12, TC48, and TC50, derived from circulating lymphocytes that were potentially able to eliminate residual tumor cells in a transplanted patient. These cytotoxic lymphocytes were tested against a panel of fresh leukemia cell populations. Susceptibility of uncultured tumor cells to TC clones was generally lower than that of conventional in-vitro-established cell lines, such as K562 or MOLT-4. In addition, TC lymphocytes did not display stronger cytotoxicity against leukemias compared with additional populations of normal NK cells. Individually, it was found that

TABLE 3. Susceptibility of leukemia cells to cytotoxic clones

Target cells	Effector cells[a]					
	JT3	JT9	JTB18	TC12	TC48	TC50
K562	++++[b]	++++	++++	++++	++++	++++
MOLT4	++++	++++	++++	++++	++++	++++
RAV	−	−	++	+	+	+
MAS	−	−	NT[d]	+	−	+
JAN	−	−	+	+	−	+
COC	−	+	++	++	−	+
DEC	−	+	+	++	−	+
ALG	−	+	++	++	+	++
MAN	−	++	+	+	−	+
FED	−	−	+++	++	+	++
GIU	−	+	−	−	−	+
BEN	−	+	−	+	−	+
TAN	−	+	++	++	+	++
MAR	+	++	+++	+++	+++	++
COR	−	+	++	++	−	+
RIC	−	−	+	+	−	−
TUR	−	−	−	+	−	−
LAR	−	−	+	+	−	+
JAP[c]	−	+	NT	+++	+++	+++

[a] E/T ratio 10:1, 4-hr assays. Results presented are representative of at least two separate experiments for each clone and each target cells.

[b] Percentage of specificity is expressed as follows: (−) <5, (+) ≥ 5, (++) ≥ 15, (+++) ≥ 30, (++++) ≥ 50.

[c] TC clones have been identified (*8*) in patient JAP, using his own leukemia blasts as target cells. Results presented here are retrospective because JAP tumor cells are no longer available for studies.

[d] (NT) not tested.

TABLE 4. Susceptibility of leukemia cells to resting and lymphokine-activated peripheral blood natural killing

Effector cells[a]		Target cells																
		K562	RAV	MAS	JAN	COC	DEC	ALG	MAN	FED	GIU	BEN	TAN	MAR	COR	RIC	TUR	LAR
DONOR 1:																		
PBMC	M	+[b]	−	−	−	−	−	−	−	−	−	−	−	−	−	−	−	−
	IL2	+	−	−	−	−	−	−	−	−	−	−	+	+	−	−	−	−
	IF	+	−	NT	−	−	−	−	−	+	−	−	−	+	−	−	−	−
LGL	M	++	+	−	−	−	−	−	+	+	−	−	−	+	−	−	−	+
	IL2	++++	++	−	−	++	−	−	++	+	−	−	+	+++	−	−	+	++
	IF	++	−	NT	−	+	−	−	+	+	−	−	−	++	−	−	−	+
DONOR 2:																		
PBMC	M	+	+	−	−	−	−	−	−	+	−	−	−	−	−	−	−	−
	IL2	+++	++	−	−	+	−	+	+	+	−	−	−	+++	−	−	−	++
	IF	+	+	NT	−	−	−	−	−	+	−	−	−	++	−	−	−	+
LGL	M	++	+	−	−	+	−	−	+	+	−	−	−	++	−	−	−	++
	IL2	++++	+++	+	+	+++	−	++	++	++	−	+	+	++++	+	−	+	+++
	IF	++	++	NT	+	+	−	−	+	++	−	−	−	+++	−	−	−	++
DONOR 3:																		
PBMC	M	+	−	−	−	−	−	−	−	−	−	−	−	−	−	−	−	+
	IL2	+++	+	−	−	+	−	−	+	+	+	−	−	++	+	−	−	++
	IF	++	+	NT	−	−	−	−	+	+	+	−	−	+	−	−	−	+
LGL	M	++	+	−	−	+	−	−	+	+	−	−	−	+	−	−	−	+
	IL2	++++	++	−	+	++	−	+	++	++	+	+	+	+++	+	−	+	++
	IF	+++	+	NT	−	+	−	−	+	+	−	−	−	++	−	−	−	++

[a] E/T ratio 40:1, 4-hr assay. Results presented are representative of three separate experiments for each group of effector cells (for example LGL-IF) and each target cells. Effector cells were treated with medium (M), r-IL2 (36 ng/ml), or purified interferon (500 units/ml) for 18 hr prior to addition of chromium-labeled target cells.

[b] Percentage of specific cytotoxicity is expressed as follows: (−) <5, (+) ≥5, (++) ≥15, (+++) ≥30, (++++) ≥50.

TC12 and TC50 mediated a moderate but significant killing against, respectively, 7 and 4 of 16 leukemias. A relatively broad cytotoxicity was also obtained with normal uncloned large granular lymphocytes stimulated by interleukin 2 and with one clone, JTB18, derived from a normal donor. In contrast, TC48 cells that were strongly lytic toward tumor cells of the transplanted patient had a substantial activity against only one additional leukemia. This functional heterogeneity was further shown with two clones, JT3 and JT9, derived from healthy individuals.

In the context of allogeneic bone marrow transplantation, NK active lymphocytes have been implicated in a number of immunologic responses. For example, it has been reported that NK cells in the host can mediate resistance to an allogeneic marrow graft (*16–18*). It has also been suggested that natural killer lymphocytes from the donor may contribute to graft-versus-host disease (*19–20*) (GVHD), whereas other studies found no correlation between circulating activity against K562 cells and GVHD (*21*). Finally, a large number of transplanted patients have been studied in an attempt to correlate peripheral blood cytotoxicity against K562 cells and the frequency of leukemia relapse. Statistical analysis concluded that there was no relationship between NK cell activity and recurrent leukemia (*21*). In fact, these conflicting or negative results may well be secondary to methodological problems in connection with the heterogeneity of NK cytotoxic reactions. Indeed, it is now well-established that natural killing is mediated by several—if not many—subsets of effector cells (*22*). Specifically, the role of NK active lymphocytes as potential antileukemic effectors in transplanted patients should be reevaluated in light of the present studies. They strongly suggest that the cytotoxicity of uncloned effector cells toward highly susceptible cell lines, such as K562, is irrelevant in evaluating antitumor activity. For example, following BMT the preponderance of cells such as JT3 with a very common NK-associated phenotype would generate positive results using conventional NK target cell lines without any expected antileukemic effect. In this regard, note that TC clones were obtained by isolation from peripheral blood of the transplanted patient cloned colonies without preselected specificity. Screening procedures indicated that less than 40% of colonies cytotoxic against K562 displayed antileukemic activity (*8*).

Our experiments in accordance with previous reports (*23–25*) showed that a fraction of fresh leukemia blasts is moderately but consistently killed by uncloned lymphokine-activated NK effector cells from normal peripheral blood. In addition, there was no evidence that relevant antileukemic TC lymphocytes induced a stronger degree of killing than normal NK cells. Leukemias susceptible to peripheral blood cytotoxicity could, therefore, represent more appropriate target cells for prospective clinical studies than conventional cultured cell lines. However, clonal analysis demonstrated here a major heterogeneity in lysis of individual leukemias by monoclonal populations of effector cells. In addition, the distribution of unique NK subsets dividing and expanding in the process of immune reconstitution following BMT may well differ from that of healthy individuals. It is, therefore, likely that using one given leukemia as a representative target cell for monitoring antitumor activity in a group of patients would generate misleading results. For example, the relevant TC lymphocytes would not have been selected with target cells such as RAV or LAR, which are well killed by normal peripheral blood LGL.

The recent identification of human NK cells with direct antitumor activity again raises the question of whether immunological mechanisms contribute to leukemia eradication in some transplanted patients. To substantiate this hypothesis, appropriate in vitro parameters have to be correlated with a decreased risk of leukemia relapse. The present results strongly suggest that direct experimental systems assaying the patient's effector cells against the patient's tumor cells must be used exclusively. Of course, this represents a major restriction because it excludes from studies cases in which sufficient numbers of pure cryopreserved tumor cells are not available. Furthermore, specific activity measured against fresh leukemic blasts in short-term chromium release assays is low (which, incidentally, may lead to underestimation [26] of the actual antitumor effects of cytotoxic cells). Thus the presence of minor subsets of antileukemic lymphocytes with potential in vivo relevance may not be detected using uncloned populations of effector cells. It is, therefore, possible that laborious cloning procedures will have to be employed for positive identification of antileukemic cells in order to accurately delineate groups of patients with clinically beneficial immunological responses.

Acknowledgments. We thank Mrs. M. Guillard and E. Leclercq for excellent technical assistance, and Mrs. D. Rivierre for skillful assistance in the preparation of the manuscript.

REFERENCES

1. Thomas ED, Storb R, Clift RA, et al. Bone marrow transplantation. N Engl J Med 1975; 292: 832.
2. Blume KG, Beutler E, Bross KJ, et al. Bone marrow ablation and allogeneic marrow transplantation in acute leukemia. N Engl J Med 1980; 302: 1041.
3. Johnson FL, Thomas ED, Clark BS, et al. A comparison of marrow transplantation with chemotherapy for children with acute lymphoblastic leukemia in second or subsequent remission. N Engl J Med 1981; 305: 846.
4. Dinsmore R, Kirkpatrick D, Flomenberg N, et al. Allogeneic bone marrow transplantation for patients with acute non lymphocytic leukemia. Blood 1984; 63: 649.
5. Appelbaum FR, Dahlberg S, Thomas ED, et al. Bone marrow transplantation or chemotherapy after remission induction for adults with acute non lymphoblastic leukemia. Ann Intern Med 1984; 101: 581.
6. Weiden PL, Flournoy N, Thomas, ED, et al. Antileukemic effect of graft-versus-host disease in human recipients of allogeneic marrow grafts. N Engl J Med 1979; 300: 1068.
7. Weiden PL, Sullivan KM, Flournoy N, et al. Antileukemic effect of chronic graft-versus-host disease. N Engl J Med 1981; 304: 1529.
8. Hercend TH, Takvorian T, Nowill A. Tantravahi R, Moingeon P, Anderson KC, Murray C, Bohuon C, Ythier A, Ritz J. Characterization of natural killer cells with anti-leukemia activity following allogeneic bone marrow transplantation. Blood 1986; 67: 22.
9. Hercend TH, Griffin JD, Bensussan A, et al. Generation of monoclonal antibodies to a human NK clone: characterization of two NK associated antigens, NKH1A (200KD) and NKH2 (60KD), expressed on subsets of large granular lymphocytes. J Clin Invest 1985; 75: 932.
10. Timonen T, Saskela E. Isolatoin of human natural killer lymphocytes by discontinuous gradient centrifugation. J Immunol Methods 1980; 36: 285.
11. Hercend TH, Meuer SC, Reinherz SF, Schlossman SF, Ritz J. Generation of a cloned NK cell line derived from the "null cell" fraction of human peripheral blood. J Immunol 1982; 129: 1299.
12. Hercend TH, Reinherz EL, Meuer SC, Schlossman SF, Ritz J. Phenotypic and functional heterogeneity of human cloned natural killer cell lines. Nature 1983; 301: 158.
13. Hercend TH, Meuer SC, Brennan A, et al. Identification of a clonally restricted 90KD heterodimer on the two human cloned natural killer cell lines: its role in cytotoxicity effector function. JEM 1983; 158: 1547.
14. Reinherz EL, Meuer SC, Fitzgerald KA, et al. Antigen recognition by human T lymphocytes is linked to surface expression of the T3 molecular complex. Cell 1982; 30: 735.
15. Ythier A, Delmon L, Reinherz EL, et al. Proliferative responses of circulating human NK cells: delineation of an unique pathway involving both direct and helper signals. Eur J Immunol (in press).
16. Warner JF, Dennert G. Effects of a cloned cell line with NK activity on bone marrow transplants, tumor development and metastasis in vivo. Nature 1982; 300: 31.
17. Harrison DE, Carlson GA. Effects of the beige mutation and irradiation on natural resistance to marrow grafts. J Immunol 1983; 130: 484.
18. Rolstad B, Benestad HB. The "natural resistance" to bone marrow allografts in normal and athymic nude rats. Rapid cytotoxic reactions both in vivo and in vitro. Eur J Immunol 1984; 14: 793.
19. Dokhelar MC, Wiels J, Lipinski M, et al. Natural killer cell activity in human bone marrow recipients. Transplantation 1981; 31: 61.
20. Borland A, Mowat A, Parrott DMV. Augmentation of intestinal and peripheral natural killer cell activity during the graft-versus-host reaction in mice. Transplantation 1983; 36: 513.
21. Livnat S, Seigneuret M, Storb R, Prentice RL. Analysis of cytotoxic effector cell function in patients with leukemia or aplastic anemia before and after marrow transplantation. J Immunol 1980; 124: 481.
22. Ortaldo JR, Herberman R. Heterogeneity of natural killer cells. Annu Rev Immunol 1984; 2: 359.
23. Pattengale PK, Gidlund M, Nilssow K, et al. Lysis of fresh human B lymphocyte derived leukemia by interferon activated natural killer (NK) cells. Int J Cancer 1982; 1: 7.
24. Moore M, Taylor GM, White WJ. Susceptibility of human leukemias to cell mediated cytotoxicity by interferon treated allogeneic lymphocytes. Cancer Immunol Immunother 1982; 13: 56.
25. Pattengale PK, Sundstrom C, Yu A, Levine A. Lysis of fresh leukemic blasts by interferon activated human natural killer cells. Natl Immun Cell Growth Regul 1984/84; 3: 165.
26. Beran M, Hansson M, Kiessling R. Human Natural Killer cells can inhibit clonogenic growth of fresh leukemic cells. Blood 1983; 61: 596.

Received 15 October 1985.
Accepted 12 December 1985.

0041-1337/86/4203-0257$02.00/0
TRANSPLANTATION
Vol. 42, No. 3
Printed in U.S.A.

THE CONTRIBUTION OF LARGE GRANULAR LYMPHOCYTES TO B CELL ACTIVATION AND DIFFERENTIATION AFTER T-CELL-DEPLETED ALLOGENEIC BONE MARROW TRANSPLANTATION

M. K. BRENNER,[1,2] J. E. REITTIE,[2] J-P. GROB,[4] J. Z. WIMPERIS, S. STEPHENS,[5] J. PATTERSON,[1] A. V. HOFFBRAND, AND H. G. PRENTICE

Department of Haematology, Royal Free Hospital, Hampstead, London, NW3 20G, England

Immunoglobulin and specific antibody levels are well maintained in the recipients of T-cell-depleted allogeneic bone marrow transplants (BMT), even though up to 99% of mature T cells are removed from the donor graft. For 3–8 weeks after the procedure, natural killer (NK) cells with an activated pattern of target cell killing have been shown to circulate in the recipient. This study investigates whether these recipient NK cells spontaneously secrete lymphokines that modulate B cell function in a way analogous to that of in-vitro-activated NK cells from normal individuals. Large granular lymphocytes (LGLs) (which contain a high proportion of NK cells) have been prepared from the peripheral blood of 11 recipients of T-cell-depleted major-histocompatibility-complex–matched allografts. In the first 4–6 weeks after BMT these LGLs were found spontaneously to secrete interleukin 2, interferon gamma and B cell differentiation factor. While secretion of these factors declines by 20–24 weeks after BMT, the quantitities are still greater than those seen from control donors. Patient LGLs are also able to activate autologous (donor) B cells, rendering them potentially responsive to the secreted factors. It appears likely that activated NK cells (or LGL) play a significant role in maintaining B cell function in vivo after T-cell-depleted BMT.

While depletion of mature T cells from allogeneic donor marrow has proved to be successful in preventing both acute and chronic graft versus host disease (GVHD) (*1*), the monoclonal antibodies used to achieve this removal not only are specific for the alloreactive T lymphocytes responsible for GVHD, but also eliminate helper T cells (*2*). It has been unclear, therefore, how the procedure might affect subsequent recipient B cell function. After conventional bone marrow transplantation (BMT), B cell function remains severely depressed for 6–18 months (*3, 4*). We have shown that, paradoxically, T depletion may actually enhance the recovery of total immunoglobulin and of specific antibody responses (*5–7*). Although recipients of T-depleted marrow synthesize high titers of antibody as rapidly as 3 weeks after BMT, the source of help for these B cell responses has been unclear (*5, 6*). While it is possible that radiation and cytotoxic-drug-resistant recipient T helper cells or residual donor T lymphocytes may both contribute, the numbers of such cells detected early after BMT are low (*2*).

Investigation of natural killer (NK) cell activity following T-depleted BMT (*8*) led us to consider a third source of help. NK function is rapidly restored in the recipients of T-depleted allografts; moreover, these NK cells are functionally activated and possess the capacity to kill targets, such as lymphoblastoid cell lines that are not normally destroyed by "resting" NK cells (*8*). It has recently become apparent that NK cells activated in vitro have the capacity to secrete a range of lymphokines, including interleukins 1 and 2 (IL-1 and 2) (*9, 10*), gamma interferon (gamma IFN) (*11*) and B cell growth and differentiation factors (BCGF + BCDF) (*12, 13*): these NK cells may also activate B lymphocytes (*12*).

We have now investigated whether NK cells, with their activated pattern of target cell killing, also spontaneously secrete factors that are capable of modulating B cell development after BMT.

In man, the bulk of NK activity is contained within cells defined morphologically as large granular lymphocytes (LGL). The results of the present study show that cultures of LGLs obtained within the first 6 weeks after BMT secrete biologically significant quantities of IL2, BCDF, and gamma IFN, and that these cells also possess the capacity to activate autologous (donor) B cells and so render them responsive to the factors that the LGLs secrete.

MATERIALS AND METHODS

Patient details. Eleven patients were studied 4–6 weeks after BMT, and 6 of these were restudied at 20–24 weeks: 1 had chronic granulocytic leukemia (CGL) in chronic phase, 2 had CGL in accelerated phase: 2 had common acute lymphoblastic leukemia (cALL), one in first remission, one in second. Two patients had thymic (T)ALL in first or second remission, and two patients were in first remission of acute myeloblastic

[1] Supported by the Leukemia Research Fund.

[2] Address correspondence to: Dr. M. K. Brenner, Department of Haematology, Royal Free Hospital, Pond Street, Hampstead, London, NW3 2QG, England.

[3] Supported by the Wellcome Trust.

[4] Supported by The Royal Society, The Swiss and Vaudoise League Against Cancer, The Swiss National Fund For Scientific Research, and the EORTC.

[5] Division of Communicable Diseases, Clinical Research Centre, Harrow, Middx.

* Abbreviations used: ALG, antilymphocyte globulin; AML, acute myoblastic leukemia; BCDF, B cell differentiation factor; BCGF, B cell growth factor; BMT, bone marrow transplantation; cALL, common acute lymphoblastic leukemia; CGL, chronic granulocytic leukemia; FCS, fetal calf serum; GVHD, graft-versus-host disease; IFN, interferon; IL-1,2; interleukin 1,2; LGL, large granular lymphocyte; McAb, monoclonal antibody; MHC, major histocompatibility complex; MLR, mixed lymphocyte reaction; MNC, mononuclear cells; NK, natural killer; PWM, pokeweed mitogen; SAA, severe aplastic anemia; SRBC, sheep red blood cells; T, thymic; TBI, total-body irradiation.

leukemia (AML). Finally, one patient had beta-thalassemia major, and one severe aplastic anemia (SAA). All donors and recipients were major histocompatibility complex (MHC)-matched and mixed lymphocyte reaction (MLR)-nonreactive. Patients with leukemia in first remission or the chronic phase of CGL were conditioned with cyclophosphamide 60 mg/kg/×2 (+ Mesna) (*14*); those in 2nd remission or accelerated phase CGL received 45 mg cyclophosphamide ×2 and cytosine arabinoside 3 g/m^2 b.d. for 3 days. All leukemia patients also received total-body irradiation (TBI) given in a single dose at 15 cGy/min (the midplane received dose rate) to a planned maximum dose of 750 cGy to the lung (midplane) (*14*). The patients with thalassemia major and SAA were conditioned with busulphan 4 mg/kg for 2 days, cyclophosphamide 50 mg/kg for 4 days and antilymphocyte globulin (ALG) for 5 days. The median age of recipients was 20 years (mean = 21.9). The median age of the nine donors investigated was 28 years (mean = 24). T lymphocyte depletion was carried out as previously described (*14*), using two monoclonal antibodies, RFT8 (anti-CD_8) and MBG6 (anti-CD_6), and rabbit complement. Median T depletion was 98.3% (mean = 98.5%) and median T cell numbers infused were 0.036×10^8/kg (mean = 0.034×10^8/kg). Eight patients had no GVHD, 2 had grade I, and 1 had grade II GVHD (Seattle criteria). All grafts were self-sustaining.

Media. The serum-free culture medium used was modified from that of Iscove and Melcher (*15, 16*).

Cell preparation. Venous blood (60 ml) was removed from donors or from the BMT recipients 4–6 and 20–24 weeks after the procedure. After defibrination, the blood was mixed with equal volumes of RPMI and layered onto Ficoll hypaque. Following centrifugation the interface mononuclear cells (MNC) were washed ×2 and adjusted to 5×10^6/ml in RPMI + 10% fetal calf serum (FCS). 5-ml aliquots were incubated for 90 min at 37°C in 5-cm petri dishes (Nunc). Nonadherent cells were removed and depleted of T cells by rosetting with neuraminidase-treated sheep red blood cells (SRBC) and further Ficoll hypaque centrifugation. The T cells were freed of SRBC using ammonium chloride solution. The interface cells were rerosetted—and, after repeat Ficoll-hypaque centrifugation, contained <2% CD_3-positive lymphocytes and 5–15% monocytoid cells. They showed no response to pokeweed mitogen (PWM) (*17, 18*) and were used as the nominal B cell population. The LGL-enriched fractions were obtained from adherent-cell-depleted MNC using a discontinuous Percoll density gradient (*19*). Briefly, Percoll solutions at 45%, 42.5%, 40%, and 37.5% were layered into 10-ml tubes, and 1.5 ± 10^7 adherent-cell-depleted MNC in 2 ml RPMI + FCS were layered on top. The tubes were centrifuged at 650 ×g for 30 min. To obtain sufficient cells in the early post-BMT period, the top two cell layers were taken: to enable a comparison to be made between patient and donor LGLs this protocol was followed for all preparations. Although this produced 5–20% monocyte contamination, these cells do not contribute to the functional effects of LGLs either normally (*10*) or after BMT (data not shown).

Immunofluorescence staining (Table 1). The proportion of NK cells in the MNC and LGL fractions was assessed by counting the number of cells expressing NK-associated surface antigens in an indirect immunofluorescence assay and microscope analysis. The monoclonal antibody (McAb) used was Leu 11b (Becton Dickenson), which reacts with an antigen present on most LGLs and virtually all lymphocytes with NK function (*20*). In addition, the number of T helper-inducer cells in the LGL fraction was assessed by counting the number of cells expressing the T4 (CD4) antigen using the Leu 3a McAb (BD). A microplate method was used with fluorescein isothiocyanate (FITC)-conjugated goat F $(ab)_2$ antimouse immunoglobulin as second reagent.

Cell culture techniques. Preparation of LGL supernatants: LGLs prepared as above were cultured at 2×10^6/ml in serum-free medium for 72 hr. The cultures were spun—and, after filtration through a 0.22-μ membrane, the supernatants were stored at −70°C before testing them at 10% and 40% of final culture volume.

Measurement of lymphokine content of LGL supernatants: To determine BCDF activity, the lymphoblastoid cell line CESS (*21*) was used at 10^3 cells/flat-bottomed well in Nunc 96-well plates in 200 μl of serum-free medium. To these wells were added varying concentrations of either a laboratory standard of known BCDF activity or the test supernatant. After 72 hr incubation the quantity of IgG present in the supernatant was measured by solid-phase ELISA. The activity of the unknown supernatant was assessed by comparing the curve of Ig produced with the Ig produced by a laboratory standard. One unit of BCDF activity was defined as the quantity needed to induce 33% maximal IgG production by CESS.

IL-2 was measured using an IL-2-dependent T cell line as previously described (*22*). Results were standardized against recombinant IL-2 (Biogen).

IFN-gamma was measured using a monoclonal antibody based immunoradiometric assay (*23*), (SUCROSEP IRMA, Boots-Celltech Diagnostics Ltd, Slough, UK). Assays were set up according to the protocol provided by the manufacturer. Briefly, IFN-gamma standards, or cell culture supernatants, were diluted in tissue culture medium and dispensed in 200 μl volumes into assay tubes. To these were added 50 μl ^{125}I-monoclonal mouse antihuman IFN-gamma. After 2 hr at room temperature, 50 μl solid-phase antibody (polyclonal sheep antihuman IFN-gamma-coupled sephacryl particles) was added. Tubes were shaken for 2 hr and unbound ^{125}1-anti-IFN-gamma was removed using the sucrose-layering separation method (*24*). The remaining bound ^{125}1 was counted on a gamma-counter (NE 1600, Nuclear Enterprises, Paisley, Scotland). The assay standard had been calibrated against the NIH human IFN-gamma reference preparation (Cg23 901 530, obtained from NIH, Bethesda, MD). The minimum sensitivity of the assay was 1 U/ml IFN-gamma.

Coculture of NK cells and B cells for immunoglobulin production. LGLs from the recipient and autologous B cells (from the bone marrow donor) were cocultured at a 1:1 ratio in 200 μl flat-bottomed wells (Nunc) containing 150 μl of Iscove's medium at a final cell concentration of 10^6/ml. To some wells a lectin-free supernatant with known B cell differentiation activity, prepared as described previously (*25*), was added at 10% final volume. As a positive control, donor B cells were also cocultured with donor irradiated T cells at a 1:4 ratio (*26*). IgG and IgM produced were measured using an enzyme-linked immunosorbent assay in which plastic plates (M129A Dynatech) were coated with class-specific antiglobulin, and the quantity of Ig bound measured using alkaline-phosphatase-conjugated class-specific antibody (Sigma). The specificity controls and standard described previously were used (*26*).

RESULTS

Phenotype of LGLs. Cells were obtained from three groups: donors, recipients at 4–6 weeks post-BMT, and recipients at 18–24 weeks post-BMT (Table 1). The proportion of lymphocytes in the MNC and LGL populations that appeared as LGLs was similar to the proportion positive for the NK cell marker detected by Leu 11b. The proportion of cells that is morphologically LGL or positive for Leu 11b is not significantly different among groups.

Lymphokine secretion by LGL. LGLs prepared from normal donors do not secrete detectable quantities of IL-2, gamma interferon, or BCDF when they are cultured in serum-free medium for 72 h (Fig. 1). In contrast, LGLs obtained 4–6 weeks post-BMT almost invariably secrete significant quantities of these factors in the absence of any further stimulation (Fig. 1). While the quantities of lymphokines produced showed considerable variation among individuals, secretion of a high level of any one factor was not predictive of high-level secretion of any other factor. By 20–24 weeks post-BMT spontaneous secretion was reduced, although recipient cells still produced greater quantities than donor LGLs (Fig. 1).

LGL activation of B cells. A previous clonal analysis of activated LGLs from normal individuals indicated that some clones secreted B cell differentiation factors and were also able to activate target B cells, rendering them responsive to these differentiation factors (*12*). Thus coculture of these LGL clones with B cells led to the production of substantial quantities of immunoglobulin (*12*). In contrast, coculture of uncloned LGLs from marrow recipients with autologous (donor) B cells does not induce significant immunoglobulin synthesis, even when the LGLs have been shown to secrete BCDF spontaneously (Table 2). However, if exogenous BCDF is added to the cocultures then high levels of IgM and IgG are produced; B cells cultured alone do not respond to added BCDF (Table 2). Thus, patient LGLs are capable of rendering autologous B cells factor-responsive—but, in the culture conditions chosen, they do not induce differentiation of these activated, BCDF-responsive, B cells.

DISCUSSION

Recipients of T-cell-depleted marrow show rapid reconstitution of B cell function. Total Ig levels (*5*) and antigen-induced specific antibody responses (*6, 7*) are soon restored, despite intensive pretransplant conditioning and the removal of up to 99% of donor T cells (*1*). Reconstitution occurs at a time when few T cells with mature helper phenotype are present in peripheral blood or marrow (*2*), and we have investigated the possibility that "help" for these B cells is provided by activated large granular lymphocytes (LGLs) with NK function.

TABLE 1. Phenotype of large granular lymphocytes

Source of cells	Preparation	% Cells of LGL morphology (mean ± SD)	% Cells LEU 11b-positive (mean ± SD)
Normal donor	PBM[a]	15.0±5.2	16.5±3.8
Recipient (4–6 weeks)	PBM	10.8±3.0	13.0±6.3
Recipient (18–24 weeks [n = 5])	PBM	15.0±10	20.0±4.7
Normal donor	LGL	69.0±10.4	64.2±10.2
Recipient (4–6 weeks)	LGL	62.3±8.2	56.4±9.2
Recipient (18–24 weeks)	LGL	46.7±23.1 n = 6	60.3±5.0

[a] Adherent-cell-depleted. Recipient LGL contained no detectable CD_4-positive cells. Donor LGL contained <1% CD_4 positive lymphocytes.

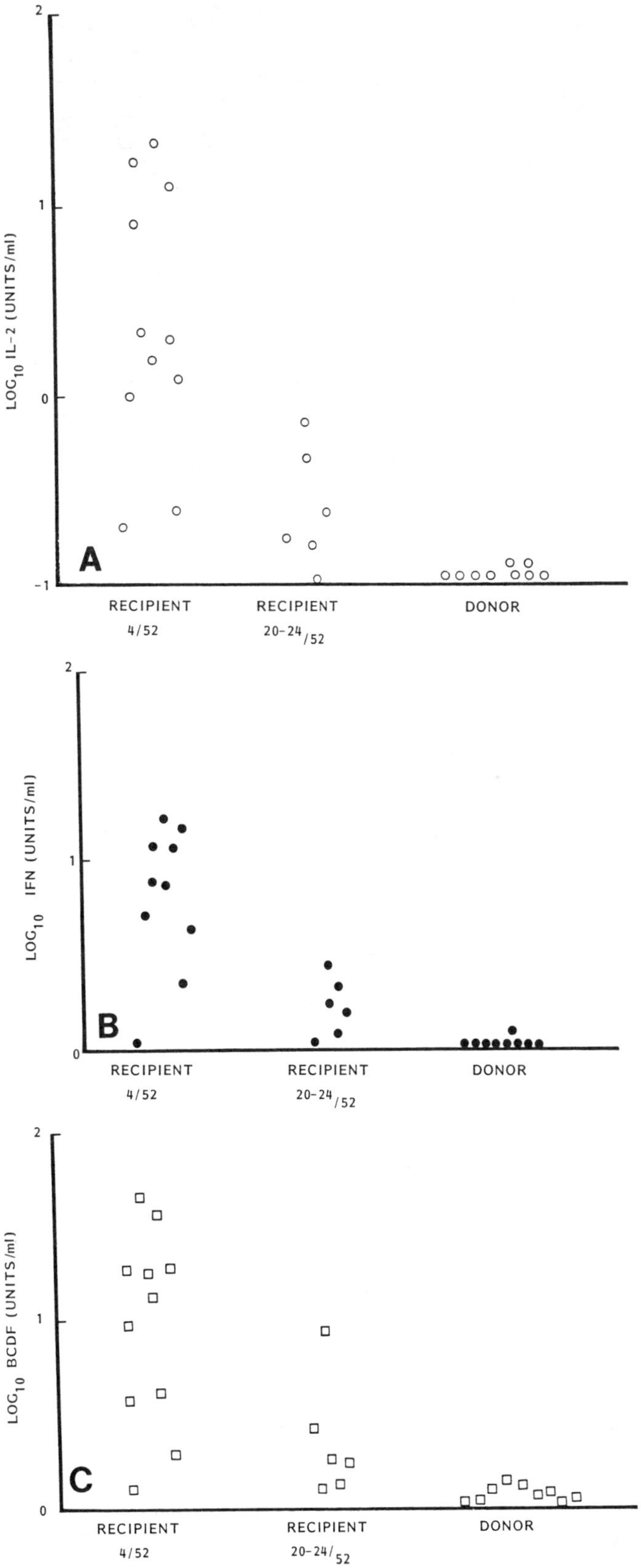

FIGURE 1. LGL supernatants from transplant recipients at 4–6 weeks after BMT (group 1), from recipients at 20–24 weeks after BMT (group 2), or normal donors (group 3) were assayed for their IL-2, IFN-gamma, and BCDF content, as described in the *Materials and Methods* section. Analysis of variance indicated the following significant differences among the groups: (A) IL-2; 1×2 (P<0.05), 1×3 (P<0.001), 2×3 (P<0.01); (B) IFN-gamma: 1×2 (P<0.01), 1×3 (P<0.001), 2×3 (P<0.01); (C) BCDF: 1×2 (P<0.05), 1×3 (P<0.001), 2×3 (P<0.05).

TABLE 2. Effects of adding differentiation factor to cocultures of B cells and LGL

Cells cultured[a]	Factor added[b]	Donor/recipient 1[c]		Donor/recipient 2[c]	
		IgM	IgG	IgM	IgG
B	−	0.15	<0.1	0.22	0.11
B	+	1.32	0.64	0.87	0.52
LGL	−	<0.1	<0.1	<0.1	<0.1
LGL	+	<0.1	<0.1	<0.1	<0.1
B+LGL	−	0.2	<0.1	0.38	0.14
B+LGL	+	7.63	3.43	9.80	4.12
B+T	−	0.48	0.26	0.30	0.29
B+T	+	11.22	6.36	14.78	5.10

[a] Cell cultures were carried out as described in the *Materials and Methods* section using donor B cells and recipient LGL or (as a positive control) donor B cells and donor-irradiated (2000 rads) T cells. T cells alone produced no detectable Ig.

[b] Differentiation factor (see the *Materials and Methods* section) was added at 10% of final culture volume.

[c] Results (μg/ml) shown are the means of triplicate cultures in two representative donor/recipient pairs taken at 4 weeks after BMT. Paired t testing shows a highly significant effect for adding LGL to B cells cultured in the presence of factor ($P<0.001$).

Most previous accounts of the interaction of fresh LGL/NK cells and LGL clones with B lymphocytes have focused on their capacity to inhibit B cell growth and differentiation (*12, 27, 28*). However, when LGLs are activated, although they retain their NK function, they also secrete at least four lymphokines—IL-1, IL-2, BCGF, and BCDF—that can augment B cell growth and differentiation (*9, 10, 12, 13*). Moreover, clonal analysis of normal LGLs with NK activity demonstrates not only that some of these cells secrete stimulatory factors, but that they can also induce B lymphocytes to become factor-responsive (*12*). We have previously shown that in the first month after BMT, NK cells with an "activated" pattern of target cell killing circulate in the peripheral blood (*8*). Our present data demonstrate that these activated cells also spontaneously secrete in vitro readily detectable quantities of IL2, gamma IFN, and BCDF. While the titers produced are substantially lower than those observed when LGLs are activated by mitogens in vitro (*9, 10*), the quantities are biologically significant (*29*). Coculture of these lymphokine-secreting LGL with autologous (donor) B cells induces immunoglobulin secretion, but only when the cultures are supplemented with additional BCDF (Table 2). Thus, despite lymphokine secretion and their capacity to render B cells responsive to differentiation factors, these LGLs by themselves are incapable of inducing in vitro all the differentiation steps required for immunoglobulin to be secreted. It is likely that this failure is a reflection of the underlying heterogeneity of the LGL population, which contains cells and produces factors that are inhibitory as well as stimulatory (*11, 27, 28*). Certainly, while activated LGL from normal donors also render B cells factor responsive, unambiguous helper activity is most readily seen in vitro only when the function of individual LGL clones is analyzed (*12*).

It seems likely that the activated LGLs studied here are of donor rather than recipient origin, as all sex-mismatched patients had dividing lymphocyte and Leu-7-positive cells of donor phenotype by 6 weeks post-BMT (*30*). However, NK activity is particularly resistant to cytotoxic drugs and to radiation, such that some nondividing LGLs may be of recipient origin; a study of DNA polymorphisms in a purified LGL population should resolve this issue.

The capacity of LGLs to activate B cells seems to be a direct property of the LGLs themselves, rather than to be dependent on contaminating T helper cells. In the post-transplant period the LGL population contains no detectable CD4-positive cells, while the B-enriched population contains a maximum of 2% CD3-positive cells (*17, 18*). There is no reason why any residual T cells should be stimulated under the coculture conditions chosen: dividing cells in both the LGL-enriched and non-T population are of donor origin, and even if cells of recipient origin are present, all donors and recipients studied were MHC-identical and MLR-unreactive. Under such circumstances it seems unlikely that residual T cells would provide significant helper effects. Residual monocytes, however, form up to 20% of both the LGL and B-enriched population, and may be indirectly involved in the events leading to B cell activation.

The in vivo signal for LGL activation is unclear. Activation does not correlate with clinically detectable GVHD or with virus infection (*8*), and the most likely possibilities are that it represents stimulation of donor LGL by recipient tissue specific alloantigens (or vice versa), or that it is a consequence of depleting the T cell population responsible for down-regulating self-activation by lymphokine-secreting LGL.

By 6 months after transplantation, NK cells with an activated killing pattern have disappeared from the peripheral blood (*8*). Similarly LGLs at this time secrete lower quantities of lymphokines with B cell activity. By now, however, T4 numbers are near-normal (*2*) and help for antibody synthesis is presumably of a more conventional nature.

We believe that LGL (or NK) activation of B lymphocytes is unlikely to be of significance only in bone marrow transplant recipients. It seems more probable that such activation represents another route by which mature B cells can be readily recruited and induced to differentiate when the immune system is exposed to antigen challenge.

Acknowledgment. We thank Mrs. Megan Evans for secretarial help in typing this manuscript.

REFERENCES

1. Prentice HG, Blacklock HA, Janossy G, et al. Depletion of T lymphocytes in donor marrow prevents significant graft-versus-host disease in matched allogeneic leukaemic marrow transplant recipients. Lancet 1984, 1: 472.
2. Janossy G, Grob J-P, Favrot M, et al. T cell regeneration after transplantation of T-cell depleted allogeneic bone marrow. Clin Exp Immunol 1986; 63: 385.
3. Elfenbein GJ, Anderson PN, Humphrey RL, Mullins GM, Sensenbrenner LL, Wards JR, Santos GW. Immune system reconstituion following allogeneic bone marrow transplantation in man: a multiparameter analysis. Transplant Proc 1976; 8: 641.
4. Noel DR, Witherspoon RP, Storb R, et al. Does graft versus host disease influence the tempo of immunologic recovery after allogeneic human marrow transplantation? An observation on 56 long term survivors. Blood 1978; 51: 1087.
5. Brenner MK, Wimperis JZ, Reittie JE, et al. Recovery of immunoglobulin isotypes after T cell depleted bone marrow transplantation. Br J Haematol (in press).
6. Wimperis JZ, Brenner MK, Patterson J, Reittie JE, Hoffbrand AV, Prentice HG. Transfer of a functional B cell immune system following T cell depleted allogeneic bone marrow transplantation. Lancet 1986 i 339.
7. Wimperis JZ, Berry NJ, Brenner MK, Grundy J, Hoffbrand AV,

Griffiths PD, Prentice HG. Production of anti-cytomegalovirus antibody following T-cell depleted bone marrow transplant. Br J Haematol (in press).
8. Rooney CM, Wimperis JZ, Brenner MK, Patterson J, Hoffbrand AV, Prentice HG. Natural killer activity following T cell depleted allogeneic bone marrow transplantation. Br J Haematol 1986; 62: 413.
9. Kasahara T, Djeu JY, Dougherty SF, Oppenheim JJ. Interleukin 2 mediated immune interferon (IFN-gamma) production by human T cells and T cell subsets. J Immunol 1983; 130: 1784.
10. Scala G, Allavena P, Djeu JY, Kasahara T, Ortaldo JR. Human large granular lymphocytes are potent producers of Interleukin I. Nature 1984; 309: 56.
11. Djeu JY, Stocks N, Zoon K, Stanton GJ, Timonen T, Herberman RB. Positive self-regulation of cytotoxicity in human natural killer cells by production of interferon upon exposure to influenza and herpes viruses. J Exp Med 1982; 156: 1222.
12. Vyakarnam A, Brenner MK, Reittie JE, Lachmann PJ. Human cell clones with NK function activate B cells and secrete B cell differentiation factor. Eur J Immunol 1985; 15: 606.
13. Pistoia V, Cozzolino F, Tarcia M, Castigli E, Ferrarini M. Production of B cell growth factor by a Leu^{7+} $OKM1^{+}$ Non-T cell with the features of large granular lymphocytes. J Immunol 1985; 134: 3179.
14. Prentice HG. A review of the current status and techniques of allogeneic bone marrow transplantation for treatment of leukaemia. J Clin Pathol 1983; 36: 1207.
15. Iscove NN, Melchers F. Complete replacement of serum by albumin, transferrin and soybean lipid in cultures of lipopolysaccaride-reactive B lymphocytes. J Exp Med 1978; 147: 923.
16. Farrant J, Newton CA, North ME, Weyman C, Brenner MK. Production of antibody by human B cells under serum free conditions. J Immunol Methods 1984; 68: 25.
17. Insel RA, Merler E. The necessity for T cell help for human tonsil B cell responses to PWM: induction of DNA synthesis, immunoglobulin and specific antibody production with a T cell helper factor produced with PWM. J Immunol 1977; 118: 2009.
18. Keightley RG, Cooper MD, Lawton AR. The T cell dependence of B cell differentiation induced by PWM. J Immunol 1976; 117: 1539.
19. Timonen T, Saksela E. Isolation of human NK cells by density gradient centrifugation. J Immunol Methods 1980; 36: 285.
20. Lanier LL, Le AM, Phillips JH, Warner NL, Babcock GF. Subpopulations of human natural killer cells defined by expression of the Leu-7 (HNK-1) and Leu-11 (NK-15) antigens. J Immunol 1983; 131: 1789.
21. Muraguchi A, Kishimoto T, Yoshitsugu M, Kuritani T, Kaieda T, Yashizaki K, Yamamura Y. T cell replacing factor—(TRF) induced IgG secretion in a human B blastoid cell line and demonstration of a receptor for TRF. J Immunol 1981; 127: 412.
22. Gillis S, Ferm M, Ou W, Smith K. T cell growth factor: parameters of production and a quantitative microassay. J Immunol 1978; 120: 2027.
23. Page CD, Abbott SR. Experience with highly sensitive immunoradiometric assays for interferon in human serum [Abstract]. Antiviral Res 1984; 1: 76.
24. Wright JF, Hunter WM. The sucrose layering separation: a non-centrifugation system. In: Hunter WM, Corrie JET, eds. Immunoassays for clinical chemistry. Edinburgh: Churchill Livingstone, 1983: 170.
25. Brenner MK, North ME, Weyman C, Farrant J. The interaction of specific T cell help and non-specific B cell growth factors in the induction of antigen specific responses in human lymphocytes, studied in serum free micro-cultures. Immunology 1983; 50: 377.
26. Brenner MK, Munro AJ. T cell help in human in vitro antibody producing systems: role of inhibitory T cells in masking allogeneic help. Cell Immunol 1981; 57: 280.
27. Arai S, Yamamoto H, Itah K, Kumagai K. Suppressive effect of human natural killer cells on pokeweed mitogen-induced B cell differentiation. J Immunol 1983; 131: 651.
28. Abbruzzo LF, Rowley DA. Homeostasis of the antibody response: immunoregulation of NK cells. Science 1983; 222: 581.
29. Itoh K, Shiba K, Shimiza Y, Suzuki R, Kumagai K. Generation of activated killer-cells by recombinant interleukin 2 in combination with interferon gamma. J Immunol 1985; 134: 3124.
30. Walker H, Singer CRJ, Patterson J, Goldstone AH, Prentice HG. The significance of host haemopoietic cells detected by cytogenetic analysis of bone marrow from recipients of bone marrow transplants. Br J Haematol (in press).

Received 2 September 1985.
Accepted 21 November 1985.

0041-1337/86/4203-0262$02.00/0
TRANSPLANTATION
Vol. 42, No. 3

Printed in U.S.A.

IMMUNOSUPPRESSIVE METABOLITES OF CYCLOSPORINE IN THE BLOOD OF RENAL ALLOGRAFT RECIPIENTS[1]

THOMAS G. ROSANO,[2] BRIAN M. FREED,[3] JAMES CERILLI,[4] AND NEIL LEMPERT[4]

Departments of Clinical Chemistry, Biochemistry, and Surgery, Albany Medical College and Albany Medical Center Hospital, Albany, New York 12208

Cyclosporine levels by radioimmunoassay (RIA) and high-performance liquid chromatography (HPLC) were monitored in serial blood samples (n=177) from 11 renal allograft recipients. HPLC analysis revealed three primary metabolites of CsA (M17, M1, and M21) in peak and trough blood samples; M17 was the preponderant metabolite. In 4 patients on whom serial metabolite assays were performed, M17 was found in the blood at 86–2004 ng/ml; M1 and M21 were found at up to 100 ng/ml. The immunosuppressive properties of purified metabolites M1, M17, M21, and M8 (which was not detected in the blood) were compared with CsA. M17—and, to a lesser extent, M1 and M21—were found to inhibit the in vitro response of human mononuclear cells in the mixed leukocyte culture and in mitogen (phytohemagglutinin [PHA], concanavalin A [Con A], and pokeweed mitogen [PWM]) assays at 1000 ng/ml. M8 exhibited no in vitro inhibitory activity. M17 was further tested at 10–1000 ng/ml in PHA and mixed lymphocyte culture (MLC) assays. M17 had considerably less inhibitory activity (12–43%) than CsA (18–70%) in the PHA assay. However, in MLC experiments M17 blocked the proliferative response by 39–72% at 100–800 ng/ml, which approached the degree of inhibition exhibited by CsA (63–87%). In 34 of 37 (92%) patient blood samples, the level of metabolite M17 was found to exceed the parent drug level and could not be measured accurately by RIA. The observed in vitro immunosuppressive activity of metabolites (particularly M17) and their presence in the blood of renal allograft recipients suggest a possible role for these metabolites in the immunopharmacology of CsA.

Cyclosporine (CsA)* is a potent immunosuppressive agent that selectively inhibits T cell responses. CsA reduces the incidence of rejection episodes in renal allograft recipients (*1–3*), decreases the requirement for adjunctive steroid therapy (*2, 4, 5*), and has resulted in a significant improvement in graft survival (*2, 6–8*). The major drawback to the use of CsA is the relatively high incidence of nephrotoxicity, which has necessitated the careful monitoring of CsA levels in the blood. Unfortunately, it has not been possible to establish a well-defined therapeutic window for CsA because nephrotoxicity may occur over a wide range of CsA levels (*9*).

Very little is known about the molecular mechanisms by which CsA induces immunosuppression or nephrotoxicity. However, it has recently been shown that induction of cytochrome P-450 with Aroclor 1254, which presumably causes an increase in metabolism of CsA, results in a decrease in nephrotoxicity without affecting the level of immunosuppression (*10–12*)—the authors suggest that renal tubular damage is due to the parent CsA molecule rather than the metabolites. It is therefore possible that the inability to establish a therapeutic window for CsA may be due to the fact that the relative contributions of CsA metabolites in immunosuppression and nephrotoxicity are not known.

It is often assumed that the radioimmunoassay (RIA) method measures the amount of CsA and metabolites in the blood (*13–15*). Several investigators have attempted to use the difference between the CsA level determined by high-performance liquid chromatography (HPLC), which is specific for CsA, and RIA as an indication of the level of metabolites in the blood (*16, 17*). However, of the nine CsA metabolites isolated from human urine (*18*), only one (M17) has been shown to exhibit significant crossreactivity with the antibody used in the RIA (*19*). Furthermore, the immunosuppressive properties of these metabolites and their presence in the blood of renal allograft recipients have not been demonstrated. We report here on the HPLC detection of three primary metabolites of CsA in the blood of renal allograft recipients, and the degree to which these metabolites suppress human T cell responses in vitro.

MATERIALS AND METHODS

Patients. From January 1984 to January 1985, 42 end-stage renal disease patients received cadaveric renal allografts with CsA as the primary immunosuppressive agent. From January to September 1984, CsA (5 mg/kg/day in two doses given at 12-hr intervals) was initiated when the patient had achieved good renal function. Prednisone was given initially as a 300-mg bolus and then adjusted to give the patient 30 mg/day during the first month posttransplant and 20 mg/day during the second month. Patients with good renal function were then maintained on 10 mg prednisone/day. Whole-blood RIA for CsA was performed daily while the patient was in the hospital, then thrice-weekly on an outpatient basis during the next month. The frequency of CsA monitoring was decreased to

[1] This work was supported by the James Hilton Manning and Emma Austin Manning Foundation, and by the National Kidney Foundation of Northeastern New York.

[2] Address correspondence to: Thomas G. Rosano, Ph.D., Department of Clinical Chemistry, Albany Medical Center Hospital, Albany, NY 12208.

[3] From the Transplantation Immunology Laboratory, Department of Surgery, Albany Medical College, Albany, New York 12208.

[4] From the Division of Renal Transplantation, Department of Surgery, Albany Medical College, Albany, New York 12208.

* Abbreviations used: Con A, concanavalin A; CsA, cyclosporine A; CsC, cyclosporine C; CsD, cyclosporine D; HBSS, Hanks' balanced salt solution; HPLC, high-performance liquid chromatography; ^{3}H-thymidine, tritiated thymidine; M1, (4-hydroxy-N-methyl-L-leucine[9]) cyclosporine; M8, ([N-methyl-]2-amino-3,8-dihydroxy-6,7-dehydro-4-methyl-octenoic acid[1])(4-hydroxy-N-methyl-L-leucine[9])cyclosporine; M17, ([N-methyl-]2-amino-3,8-dihydroxy-6,7-dehydro-4-methyl-octenoic acid[1]) cyclosporine; M21, (N-demethylated leucine[4]) cyclosporine; MLC, mixed leukocyte culture; PBMC, peripheral blood mononuclear cells; PHA, phytohemagglutinin; PWM, pokeweed mitogen; RIA, radioimmunoassay.

weekly, biweekly, and then to monthly in the absence of complications. Patients transplanted between September 1984 and January 1985 also received a 4 mg/kg of azathioprine preoperatively, which was immediately tapered to 1 mg/kg and adjusted when needed to maintain a WBC count of >5,000 cells/cc.

RIA analysis of CsA. RIA analysis (*19*) of whole-blood hemolysates was performed with reagents and methods from Sandoz Ltd., Basel, Switzerland. All analyses were performed in duplicate. The coefficient of variation for CsA analysis by this method ranged from 4 to 11%.

HPLC analysis of CsA. Quantitative analysis of CsA levels by HPLC was performed as previously described (*15*). Briefly, isocratic separation of CsA and the internal standard (CsD) was performed on a Zorbax CN column (DuPont Instruments, Wilmington, DE) with a mobile phase containing acetonitrile/methanol/water (34/18/48 by volume). A column flow rate of 0.75 ml/min at 60°C was maintained. Sample extraction was performed by the method of Carruthers et al. (*14*). The coefficient of variation for CsA analysis by this method ranged from 4% to 6%.

HPLC analysis of CsA metabolites. The HPLC analysis of CsA described above did not allow adequate separation of CsA metabolites. To identify and quantitate metabolites, the following HPLC method was developed. Sample preparation was performed by a modification of the ether extraction procedure reported by Carruthers et al. (*14*). Modifications included the substitution of CsC as the internal standard and ether extraction under alkaline conditions prior to acid conditions. HPLC-grade diethyl ether was necessary to eliminate components in the ether that coelute with CsA metabolites. Recovery of the metabolites was >90% under these conditions. Chromatographic separation of these metabolites was performed with a reverse-phase CN column (DuPont Instruments, Wilmington, DE) maintained at 70°C. The mobile phase consisted of 35% (v/v) acetonitrile/water and its flow rate was 1.5 ml/min. UV-detection was set at 210 nm with 0.02 attenuation units full scale. The peak height ratio method was used for quantitation. Purified M1, M17, and M21 (*18*) used in identification and quantitation of CsA metabolites were a generous gift of G. Maurer, Ph.D., and W. Neiderberger, Ph.D., (Biopharmaceutical Dept, Sandoz Ltd, Basel, Switzerland). The metabolites were reconstituted in absolute methanol and the concentrations determined gravimetrically with an automatic electrobalance (Cahn Model 4700, Cerritos, CA). For standard material, blood from nonmedicated volunteers was spiked with purified M1, M17, and M21.

Crossreactivity of M17 in the RIA. Crossreactivity of M17 in the RIA was determined by dilution studies with hemolyzed blood samples containing pure CsA or M17. Blood used in the study was obtained from healthy nonmedicated volunteers. The initial concentrations of CsA and M17 used in the dilution studies were 1900 ng/ml and 2390 ng/ml, respectively.

Renal transplant patient samples. Serial CsA levels were analyzed in whole-blood hemolysates from 11 patients who had received cadaveric renal allografts. CsA levels were monitored by RIA and HPLC for each patient over a period ranging from 12 to 83 days. Except for the peak blood sample (drawn 4 hr after the oral dose) all bloods were drawn just prior to the subsequent dose and are referred to as trough samples. Serial samples from patients 2, 3, 10, and 11 were also analyzed for the level of CsA metabolites. All samples were stored frozen until analyzed.

Assays for in vitro immunosuppressive activity. Whole blood (20 ml) was collected in heparinized syringes from normal volunteers and diluted with an equal volume of Hanks' balanced salt solution (HBSS). The blood was then layered over 10 ml of Ficoll-Paque (Pharmacia, Piscataway, NJ) and centrifuged at 400 ×g for 40 min. The peripheral blood mononuclear cells (PBMC) were removed from the Ficoll interface and washed three times in HBSS. The cells were resuspended to 10^6 cells/ml in RPMI-1640 (MA Bioproducts, Walkersville, MD) containing 100 units/ml of penicillin and 100 μg/ml of streptomycin. In mitogen assays, 2×10^5 cells (0.2 ml) in media supplemented with 10% agamma human serum (KC Biologicals, Lenexa, KS) were plated in 96-well flat-bottomed plates (Costar). The cells were stimulated with phytohemagglutinin (PHA, Burroughs-Wellcome HA-15, 250 μg/ml), concanavalin A (Con A, Sigma, 10 μg/ml), or pokeweed mitogen (PWM, Gibco, 100 μg/ml) and incubated at 37°C in humidified 6% CO_2/94% air. Then 48 hr later (6 days later in the PWM assay) the wells were pulsed with 0.6 μCi of ^{3}H-thymidine (NEN Research Products, Boston, MA; specific activity 1.9 Ci/mmol) for 18 hr and harvested onto glass fiber filters using a Mash II cell harvester (MA Bioproducts). The disks were placed into scintillation vials with 3 ml of scintillation fluid (Econofluor, NEN) and counted in a liquid scintillation counter (Beckman).

The mixed leukocyte culture (MLC) was performed by culturing 10^5 responder PBMC with 10^5 irradiated (3000 rads, cesium source) stimulator cells in media supplemented with 20% autologous plasma in flat-bottomed tissue culture plates. The plates were incubated for 5 days at 37°C, then pulsed and harvested as described for the mitogen assays.

The effects of CsA and its metabolites on proliferation in the in vitro assays were determined by adding the agents to the cultures prior to the addition of the mitogens or stimulator cells. CsA, M1, M8, M17, and M21 were reconstituted in methanol and diluted in RPMI-1640 to the concentrations shown in the Figures 1–6. Methanol diluted in the same manner (300–500 fold) exhibited no inhibitory activity in any of the assays.

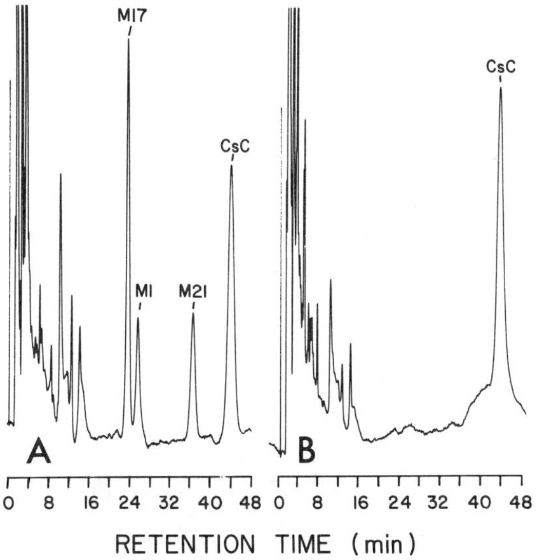

FIGURE 1. Separation of CsA metabolites by HPLC. Chromatogram (A) is from blood spiked with purified M17 (870 ng/ml), M1 (290 ng/ml), and M21 (790 ng/ml). Chromatogram (B) is a control blood obtained from a nonmedicated volunteer. CsC was included in both samples as the internal standard.

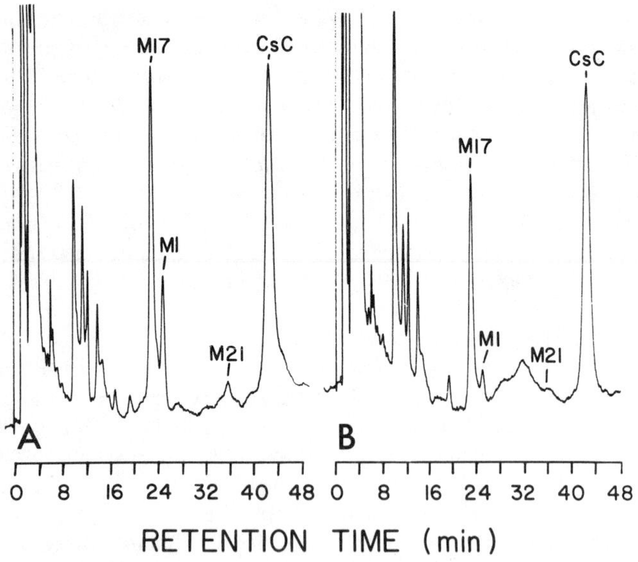

FIGURE 2. HPLC analysis of CsA metabolites in peak and trough samples from a renal allograft recipient. Samples were drawn 4 hr (A, peak) and 24 h (B, trough) after an oral dose of CsA. The peak sample contained M17 (620 ng/ml), M1 (260 ng/ml), and M21 (80 ng/ml). The trough sample contained M17 (464 ng/ml) and M1 (53 ng/ml), but no detectable amount of M21. The CsA peak elutes at approximately 60 min and is not shown in these chromatograms.

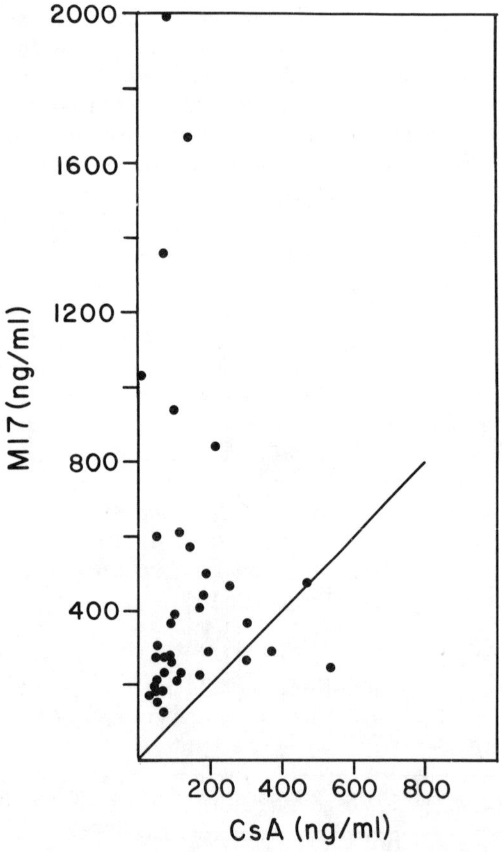

FIGURE 3. Comparison of CsA and M17 levels in renal allograft recipients. Serial trough blood samples (n=37) were obtained from 4 patients and analyzed for both CsA and metabolites by HPLC. The diagonal line represents equivalence between CsA and M17.

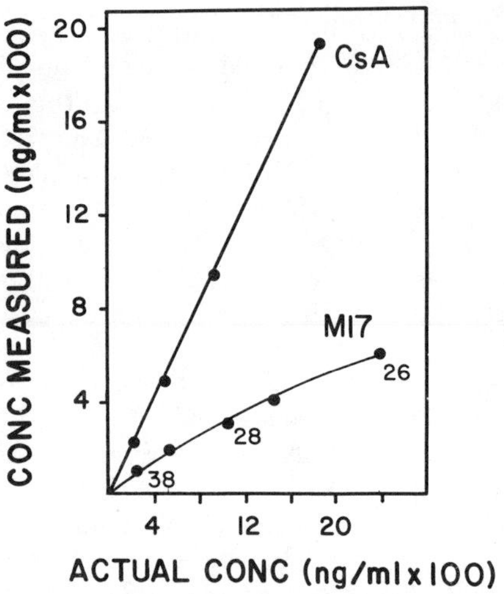

FIGURE 4. Crossreactivity of M17 in the CsA radioimmunoassay. CsA and M17 were added to whole blood in the concentrations shown. The blood samples were analyzed by RIA for apparent CsA concentration. The numbers adjacent to the points represent the percentage of the actual M17 concentration detected by RIA.

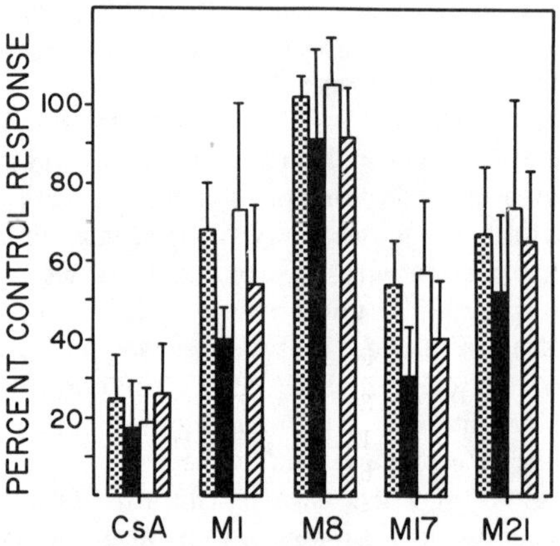

FIGURE 5. Immunosuppressive activity of CsA and metabolites in vitro. Data are expressed as the mean ±SD. The compounds were reconstituted in absolute methanol and diluted to a final concentration of 1000 ng/ml in the culture wells. Methanol diluted appropriately exhibited no inhibitory activity (control response). Data are presented as the percentage of control response in PHA (checkered boxes, n=6), Con A (black boxes, n=6), PWM (open boxes, n=4), and MLC (slashed boxes, n=12) assays. Individual assays were performed in triplicate.

Statistics. The MLC data were analyzed by Student's *t* test for unpaired data.

RESULTS

Comparison of CsA levels by RIA and HPLC. A comparison of CsA levels measured by HPLC, and RIA in 177 blood samples from 11 renal allograft recipients was performed. In all the samples, the level of CsA measured by RIA was greater than the level measured by HPLC (data not shown). A similar comparison with CsA-spiked blood from nonmedicated volunteers resulted in equivalent levels by RIA and HPLC, indicating a high degree of correlation between the two assays in the absence of metabolites. The percentage of the RIA levels that was actually due to CsA is shown in Table 1. From these studies, we determined that the actual amount of CsA in the blood varied from 6% to 81% of the level measured by RIA.

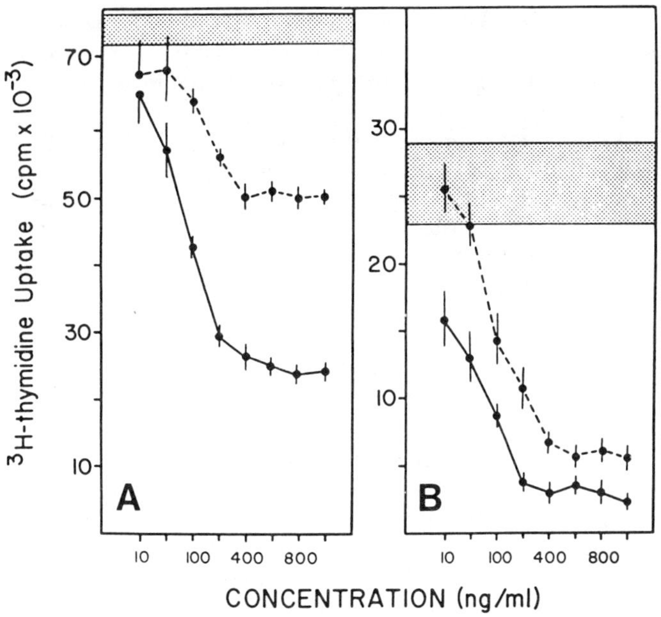

FIGURE 6. Effect of CsA and M17 on PHA and MLC responses. CsA and M17 were added to the cultures at 10–1000 ng/ml. The cells were then stimulated with PHA (A) or allogeneic cells (B). The mean ±SD of ^{3}H-thymidine uptake for cells treated with CsA (●——●) and M17 (●- - -●) are shown in reference to 1 SD of the control response (shaded area).

TABLE 1. Percentage of RIA level resulting from CsA

Patient	n	[CsA (HPLC)/CsA (RIA)] × 100		Days posttransplant
		Mean	Range	
1	21	38	(23–51)	2–30
2	10	14	(6–24)	10–20
3	6	62	(34–78)	3–12
4	22	44	(31–70)	3–24
5	24	36	(23–60)	1–24
6	13	48	(34–64)	107–186
7	32	59	(36–81)	3–83
8	13	36	(22–44)	244–272
9	16	37	(28–54)	5–124
10	14	33	(12–59)	239–256
11	6	39	(28–60)	158–179
Control[a]	20	98	(91–105)	—

[a] Control data were obtained from 20 analyses of a CsA-supplemented blood pool from nonmedicated volunteers.

Variations in this percentage were observed among the patients and even in blood samples from the same patient drawn on different days.

Identification and quantitation of CsA metabolites in blood. Analysis of blood samples using the HPLC method for CsA revealed additional unresolved peaks with retention times similar to those of the primary metabolites of CsA (M1, M17, M21). A chromatographic method was therefore developed for the measurement of primary metabolites. This procedure allowed the separation of M1, M17, and M21 in blood spiked with purified metabolites (Fig. 1A). A typical analysis of blood for nonmedicated volunteers demonstrated the specificity of the assay (Fig. 1B). The primary metabolites of CsA were identified in blood from renal allograft recipients treated with CsA. Typical metabolite patterns in peak and trough blood samples are shown in Figure 2. M17 was the preponderant metabolite in peak and trough blood samples, followed by lesser amounts of M1. M21 was found only in blood samples containing high levels of M17. The concentration of metabolites was determined in serial trough samples (n=37) in 4 renal allograft recipients. The level of M17 ranged from 80 ng/ml to 2004 ng/ml. Levels of M17 above 800 ng/ml were observed in blood samples from only one of the four patients. M1 and M21 were found at concentrations below 100 ng/ml. No significant correlation was observed between the level of M17 and CsA as measured by HPLC (Fig. 3). In 34 of 37 samples, the level of M17 exceeded the level of CsA.

Immunocrossreactivity of CsA metabolite 17. To determine the extent of RIA crossreactivity by M17, we performed a series of RIA analyses on medication-free blood spiked with pure CsA or M17. In a comparative dilution experiment, the measurement of CsA was linear over the entire dilution range while dilutions of M17 showed a nonlinear response (Fig. 4). The absolute concentration of M17 was greatly underestimated by the RIA method. RIA crossreactivity ranged from 26% to 38%, and it decreased as the concentration of M17 increased. The extent of error in the RIA estimation of M17 levels therefore increased with increasing concentrations of the metabolite.

In vitro immunosuppressive activity of CsA and metabolites. CsA and four metabolites (M1, M8, M17, and M21) were assayed initially at 1000 ng/ml for in vitro inhibition of the response of PBMC to PHA, Con A, PWM, and allogeneic cells (MLC). As can be seen in Figure 5, CsA inhibited all responses to 17–26% of the control. M17 inhibited PHA and PWM responses to only 54–57% of control, but inhibition in the Con A (30.7±12.7%) and MLC (39.7±15.8%) assays approached the level of inhibition exhibited by CsA. M1 and M21 exhibited significant immunosuppressive activity in the PHA, Con A, and MLC assays, but were considerably less inhibitory than either CsA or M17. M8 exhibited virtually no suppressive activity.

The MLC is of particular interest in these studies in that it is an in vitro model of the immune response to allografts. CsA exhibited significantly more suppressive activity (25.9±12.6% of the control) than M17 (39.7±15.8%; P=0.02). However, M17 was significantly more suppressive than either M1 (54.2±17.5%; P=0.04) or M21 (65.1±17.7%; P=0.001). Neither CsA nor any of the metabolites were toxic to the cells at the concentrations tested (data not shown).

CsA and M17 were then assayed in PHA and MLC experiments to determine their inhibitory effects over a range of therapeutic concentrations. As can be seen in Figure 6, CsA was considerably more suppressive than M17 in the PHA assay. However, in the MLC, M17 was only slightly less inhibitory than CsA in the 100–1000 ng/ml range.

DISCUSSION

The importance of CsA metabolites in the immunopharmacology of CsA therapy is largely unknown. Based on findings of MLC-inhibitory activity in the serum of CsA-treated renal allograft recipients when only low levels of the parent drug were detected, it has been suggested that metabolites of CsA may contribute significant immunosuppressive activity (*20, 21*). Freeman et al. (*22*) have recently identified metabolites M17 and M18 in the blood of normal individuals treated with CsA and phenytoin, but the metabolism of CsA in the absence of phenytoin was not studied. Maurer identified metabolites

M1, M8, M10, M17, M18, and M21 in the blood of normal volunteers given oral doses of CsA (*23*). We now report the identification of three CsA metabolites (M1, M17, and M21) in the blood of renal allograft recipients treated with CsA; all three are primary metabolites according to the pathways proposed by Maurer et al. (*18*). M17, formed by hydroxylation of the side chain of amino acid 1, appeared to be the preponderant metabolite. This finding is consistent with data reported by Maurer on the metabolism of ^{3}H-cyclosporine by human subjects following an oral administration of the drug (*23*). M1, formed by hydroxylation of the methyl leucine in position 8, was present in lower concentrations than M17—and M21, a demethylated derivative of CsA, was detectable only when high levels of M17 were found. Our chromatographic analysis demonstrated that the level of metabolites usually exceeded the level of the parent compound in patients on CsA therapy. A significant amount of metabolites appeared within 4 hr of oral administration of CsA, suggesting the drug was metabolized rapidly.

Other investigators (*13, 14*) have demonstrated crossreactive interference in the RIA, presumed to be due to CsA metabolites. Our data are consistent with these reports—and, in addition, demonstrate significant interindividual and intraindividual variation in the amount of crossreactants. Donatsch et al. (*19*) have shown that, of the major metabolites, M17 has by far the greatest degree of crossreactivity with the antibody used in the RIA. However, the RIA greatly underestimated the actual concentration of M17, and the extent of the error was directly proportional to the concentration of the metabolite. When the metabolites in the blood of renal allograft recipients were below the limit of detection by HPLC, the correlation between CsA levels measured by RIA and HPLC was good. When the level of metabolites was high, a significant discrepancy was observed between CsA levels measured by the two assays. For example, a blood sample from a renal allograft recipient had 294 ng/ml CsA when measured by RIA. When analyzed by HPLC methods, the blood contained 84 ng/ml CsA and 2004 ng/ml of M17. It is clear from these studies that the RIA is not an accurate method by which to estimate the level of metabolites in the blood.

We have also demonstrated that M17 exhibits a considerable amount of immunosuppressive activity in vitro. Although M17 was not as inhibitory as CsA, we have also shown that the concentration of M17 in the blood may exceed that of CsA by greater than 20-fold. M17 may therefore be contributing a significant amount of immunosuppressive activity in the CsA-treated patient. It is interesting to note that the hydroxylation of amino acid 1 (M17) or amino acid 9 (M1) in the CsA molecule did not completely abolish its immunosuppressive activity, but hydroxylation of both amino acids results in a secondary metabolite (M8) that exhibits no inhibitory activity in vitro.

It has recently been demonstrated that enhancing the activity of the cytochrome P-450 system with Aroclor 1254 resulted in decreased nephrotoxicity without altering the level of immunosuppression (*10–12*). These studies did not identify specific metabolites of CsA, so it is not possible to determine which were immunosuppressive or nephrotoxic. However, it is clear that it will be important to determine the extent to which CsA metabolites are nephrotoxic, since the answer to this question may have far-reaching implications for the future of CsA therapy. Indeed, recent reports have suggested that nephrotoxicity is an irreversible chronic condition that threatens the use of CsA as an immunosuppressive agent (*24*). Protocols that reduce CsA nephrotoxicity without drastically altering the level of immunosuppression will therefore greatly improve the therapeutic efficacy of this drug.

We have not been able to study the in vivo immunosuppressive activity of M17 or any of the other metabolites because only small quantities have been available to us. Nevertheless, the high concentration of M17 in the blood of renal allograft recipients indicates the potential importance of this metabolite in patient therapy.

The practical implications for patient monitoring and for further studies into the biological importance of CsA metabolites are evident from our findings. The apparent immunosuppressive activity of M17 suggests that monitoring the level of M17 in the blood of renal allograft recipients may be important. Recent studies by Rogers et al. (*21*) have demonstrated the presence of an immunosuppressive factor, or factors, in the serum of patients treated with CsA. Patients who generated this factor, the characteristics of which appear to be similar to those of CsA, exhibited significantly fewer rejection episodes than patients without the factor. It is possible that the factor discovered by these investigators is metabolite M17. However, Freeman et al. (*22*) reported that only a small portion of the total M17 could be detected in plasma. Furthermore, using purified M17 spiked into whole blood, we observed that >90% of the M17 was distributed into the cell compartment (data not shown). These findings suggest that the factor reported by Rogers et al. may be yet another immunosuppressive metabolite of the parent compound. Further studies are needed to define the in vivo immunosuppressive properties of M17 and other metabolites, as well as the roles of these metabolites in CsA therapy.

Acknowledgments. We gratefully acknowledge the technical assistance of Mrs. Priscilla Yadegari and Ms. Diane Hayes.

REFERENCES

1. Baldwin WM, Hutchinson LF, Meijer CJLM, Tilney NL. Immune responses to organ allografts. III. Marked decrease in medullary thymocytes and splenic T lymphocytes after cyclosporin A treatment. Transplantation 1981; 31: 117.
2. Najarian JS, Strand M, Fryd DS, et al. Comparison of cyclosporine versus azathioprine-antilymphocyte globulin in renal transplantation. Transplant Proc 1983; 15: 2463.
3. Bunzendahl H, Wonigeit K, Klempnauer J, Brolsh C, Pichlmayr R. Cyclosporine and steroids: effects on clinical course after renal allotransplantation. Transplant Proc 1983; 15: 2531.
4. Starzl TE, Hakala TR, Rosenthal JT, Iwatsuki S, Shaw BW. The Colorado-Pittsburgh cadaveric renal transplantation study with cyclosporine. Transplant Proc 1983; 15: 2459.
5. Squifflet JP, Pirson Y, Jamart J, Wallemacq P, Westelinck K, Alexandre GPJ. Cyclosporine in cadaver renal transplantation at a center with good results using conventional treatment. Transplant Proc 1985; 17: 1212.
6. Stiller C. The Canadian trial of cyclosporine. Cyclosporine therapy compared to standard immunosuppression in renal transplants: an exploration of nephrotoxicity. Transplant Proc 1983; 15: 2479.
7. Sells RA. A prospective randomized substitutive trial of cyclosporine as a prophylactic agent in human renal transplant rejection. Transplant Proc 1983; 15: 2495.
8. Johnson RWG, Wise WH, Bakram A, et al. A four-year prospective study of cyclosporine in cadaver renal transplantation. Transplant Proc 1985; 17: 1197.
9. Loertscher R, Abbud-Filho M, Strom TB. Cyclosporine: a promising immunosuppressive agent. Drug Ther 1984; (July): 16.

10. Cunningham C, Whiting PH, Burke MD, Wheatley DN, Simpson JG. Increasing the hepatic metabolism of cyclosporine abolishes nephrotoxicity. Transplant Proc 1983; 15: 2712.
11. Cunningham C, Gavin MP, Whiting PH, et al. Serum cyclosporine levels, hepatic drug metabolism, and renal tubulotoxicity. Biochem Pharmacol 1984; 33: 2857.
12. Thompson AW, Whiting PH, Simpson JG. Cyclosporine: immunology, toxicity, and pharmacology in experimental animals. Agents Actions 1984; 15: 306.
13. Abisch E, Beveridge T, Gratwohl A, et al. Cyclosporin A: correlation between HPLC and RIA serum levels. Pharm Weekbl (Sci) 1982; 4: 84.
14. Carruthers SG, Freeman DJ, Koegler JC, et al. Simplified liquid chromatographic analysis for cyclosporine A and comparison with radioimmunoassay. Clin Chem 1983; 29: 180.
15. Rosano TG. Effect of hematocrit on cyclosporine (cyclosporin A) in whole blood and plasma cyclosporine levels in renal transplant patients. Clin Chem 1985; 31: 410.
16. Robinson WT, Schran HF, Barry EP. Methods to measure cyclosporine levels: high pressure liquid chromatography, radioimmunoassay, and correlation. Transplant Proc 1983; 15: 2403.
17. Yee GC, Kennedy MS, Storb R, Thomas ED. Pharmacokinetics of intravenous cyclosporine in bone marrow transplant patients. Comparison of two methods. Transplantation 1984; 38: 511.
18. Maurer G, Loosli HR, Schreier E, Keller B. Disposition of cyclosporine in several animal species and man. I. Structural elucidation of its metabolites. Drug Metab Dispos 1984; 12: 120.
19. Donatsch P, Abisch E, Homberger M, Traber R, Trapp M, Voges R. A radioimmunoassay to measure cyclosporin A in plasma and serum samples. J Immunoassay 1981; 2: 19.
20. Fidelus RK, Ferguson RM. The immunosuppressive action of cyclosporine (CyA) as evaluated in 24-hour kinetic profiles. Transplant Proc 1983; 15: 1921.
21. Rogers AJ, Yoshimura N, Kerman RH, Kahan BD. Immunopharmacodynamic evaluation of cyclosporine-treated renal allograft recipients. Transplantation 1984; 38: 657.
22. Freeman DJ, Laupacis A, Keown PA, Stiller CR, Carruthers SG. Evaluation of cyclosporin-phenytoin interaction with observations on cyclosporin metabolites. Br J Clin Pharmacol 1984; 18: 887.
23. Maurer G. Metabolism of cyclosporine. Transplant Proc 1985; 17: 19.
24. Strom TB, Loertscher R. Cyclosporine-induced nephrotoxicity. Inevitable and intractable? N Engl J Med 1985; 311: 728.

Received 20 May 1985.
Accepted 9 December 1985.

0041-1337/86/4203-0267$02.00/0
TRANSPLANTATION

Vol. 42, No. 3
Printed in U.S.A.

PREDICTION OF CROSSMATCH OUTCOME IN HIGHLY SENSITIZED DIALYSIS PATIENTS BASED ON THE IDENTIFICATION OF SERUM HLA ANTIBODIES[1]

JOHN W. OLDFATHER,[2] CHARLES B. ANDERSON, DONNA L. PHELAN, DONALD E. CROSS, ALAN M. LUGER, AND GLENN E. RODEY

Missouri Illinois Regional Blood Services, American Red Cross, St. Louis 63108; Departments of Pathology, Medicine, and Surgery, Washington University School of Medicine, St. Louis 63110; Midwest Organ Bank, Kansas City, Missouri 64111; and Department of Pathology, University of Missouri, Columbia, Missouri 65201

High levels of allosensitization (>50%), which often occur in dialysis patients awaiting renal transplant, make donor selection difficult. Such patients may be included in elaborate protocols in which they are crossmatched with all available ABO compatible donors, or crossmatching may be deferred until a very-well-matched donor becomes available. The former approach of random crossmatching is costly and inefficient, while the latter approach may overlook crossmatch-compatible donors. We believe that the identification of antibodies present in highly reactive sera and the use of this information in donor selection would increase the frequency of crossmatch-negative donors for these patients. In this study eleven sera, reactive with 70% to 100% of a random cell panel, were obtained from multiply transfused dialysis patients. Sera were analyzed by standard (CDC) and antiglobulin augmented (AHG-CDC) lymphocytotoxicity, and by differential absorption with HLA-typed platelets. All sera contained only one or two antibodies directed against the high frequency public HLA epitopes, accounting for 85% to 100% of each serum's total reactivity. These characterized sera were crossmatched with 114 random normal donors. The frequency of negative crossmatches was 20.5%. However, if the serum antibody data had been used to preselect donors for crossmatch—that is, to exclude donors that were likely to be positive—the negative crossmatch frequency would have increased to 86.4%. The use of the serum analysis data in donor selection would have reduced the total number of required crossmatches by 78%. Serum analysis correctly predicted the outcome of 95.6% of crossmatches performed with an average of 3% false positives and 1.3% false negatives. This approach to donor selection reduces

[1] This work was supported by a grant from the Missouri Kidney Program, and by NIH Grant Ro1-AM-27895.

[2] Address correspondence to: John W. Oldfather, Ph.D., Department of Pathology, Jewish Hospital, 217 E. Chestnut Street, Louisville, KY 40202.

unnecessary crossmatching and increases the likelihood of finding crossmatch-compatible donors for highly reactive patients.

Dialysis patients who are awaiting renal transplants often become allosensitized to HLA class I antigens. Many of these patients develop reactivity against a large percentage of the random population (>50%), as demonstrated by monthly serum screens. HLA allosensitization by pregnancy, previous transplants, or multiple transfusions often leads to the production of broadly reactive antibodies (*1*). In patients immunized by multiple transfusion, the high reactivity is due to the production of antibodies directed against the shared public determinants (epitopes) present on the HLA class I heavy chain, distinct from the private determinants (*2*). Since the public epitopes are shared by several HLA gene products, they are present in the population in higher frequency than the unique private epitopes—and, therefore, antibodies directed against the public epitopes can result in sera that are highly reactive (Table 1). Highly sensitized dialysis patients whom we have studied tend to make only 1 to 3 antibodies against these high-frequency public epitopes rather than multiple, low-frequency antibodies against the private determinants (*2*). The likelihood of procuring crossmatch-compatible, unrelated kidneys for such patients is low. One approach to this problem is to crossmatch these highly reactive patients against all ABO-compatible kidney donors. This results in performing many unnecessary crossmatches with no increase in the efficiency of finding crossmatch-negative donors. Another approach is to crossmatch only kidneys that are well matched with the recipient. The polymorphism of the HLA-A and -B locus gene products makes such matches infrequent. Furthermore, this latter approach misses the occasional crossmatch-compatible donors who are not well matched for HLA-A and -B locus antigens.

In this study, we characterized the public antibodies present in highly reactive sera by the antiglobulin-augmented lymphocytotoxic technique and by differential absorption with HLA-typed platelets. We determined the value of such analyses to predict crossmatch outcome, to reduce unnecessary crossmatching, and to increase the likelihood of finding a crossmatch-compatible donor for the highly sensitized patient.

MATERIALS AND METHODS

Serum analysis. Eleven sera were selected for study from our population of dialysis patients awaiting kidneys from cadaveric donors. All sera reacted with more than 50% of a 36–42-cell normal lymphocytic panel. Screening was performed by both standard complement dependent lymphocytotoxicity (CDC)* (*3*) and by the antihuman-globulin-augmented modification (AHG-CDC) of the standard method (*4*). The AHG-CDC technique is more sensitive and overrides the cytotoxicity-negative absorption-positive (CYNAP) phenomenon, resulting in a more accurate analysis of the serum's reactivity. The standard assay is included in this study for parallel comparisons. Since antibodies to the high-frequency class I public epitopes are prevalent in the sensitized, multiply transfused patient, our preliminary analysis of a serum's reactivity begins with the assumption that it will be restricted to one or two of the known public determinants. Listed in Table 1 are the major public determinants that are shared by the designated HLA-A and -B locus gene products. In the event that specificity could not be assigned by the direct analysis of the reactivity pattern, sera were absorbed with relevant HLA-typed platelets (*2, 4*). The appropriate platelet was selected for absorption by mismatching only one public epitope between the platelet and serum donor phenotypes. A single mismatch would be more likely to remove only one antibody if several antibodies were present. Absorptions with irrelevant platelets were included as a control for nonspecific absorption. The absorbed serum and the acid-eluted antibody from the platelets were screened on a panel of 36–42 cells. The absorption process was continued sequentially until all reactivity was accounted for, or until no reactivity remained in the absorbed serum.

Crossmatch protocol. Characterized sera were crossmatched blindly against 114 donor T lymphocytes by CDC and AHG-CDC techniques at room temperature. Crossmatches were performed in triplicate at serum dilutions of $^1/_1$, $^1/_2$, and $^1/_4$. The crossmatch was considered positive with any reproducible reactivity above the reactivity of the negative control.

TABLE 1. Major public determinants present on HLA-A and -B locus gene products

Public epitopes	Associated private epitopes	Frequency (%)[a]	Reference
1C	A1,3,10,11,w19	79	Unpublished data
2C	A2,9,28	66	(6)
28C	A28,w33,w34,26	20	(6)
5C	B5,15,35,18	48	(7)
7C	B7,w22,27,w42,13,40	45	(8)
8C	B8,14,18,39	37	Unpublished data
12C	B12,21,13,40	43	Unpublished data
17C	B15,17	20	(9)
Bw4		79	(10)
Bw6		87	(10)

[a] North American white population.

RESULTS

The eleven sera included in this study were reactive with 58–94% of cells on our standard screening panel by AHG-CDC, as compared with 8–62% by the CDC technique (Table 2). Specificity assignments were made by inspection or computer analysis of screen results. Some sera ($^6/_{11}$) were further characterized by absorption with relevant HLA-typed platelets if specificities could not be determined because of complexity or degree of reactivity. All sera were found to contain more reactivity when tested by AHG-CDC and all possessed antibodies to one or two of the high frequency public epitopes. In only two sera, AB and LN, was additional activity against private epitopes detected. Specificity assignments based only on CDC screens were always incomplete and did not reflect the serum's total range of reactivity. The score value is the percentage of total reactivity that is accounted for by given specificity assignments. Sera in this study had scores ranging from 70% to 100%, with an average of 91.3%. Low score values indicate the presence of additional undefined antibody reactivity.

The results of retrospective crossmatching between the eleven highly reactive sera and random, normal donors are shown in Tables 3 and 4. Crossmatch predictions from either CDC serum analysis (Table 3) or AHG-CDC serum analysis (Table 4) are compared with observed crossmatch outcomes.

* Abbreviations used in this article: AHG-CDC, antihuman-globulin-augmented complement-dependent lymphocytotoxicity; CDC, standard complement-dependent lymphocytotoxicity; CM, crossmatch; CYNAP, cytotoxicity-negative absorption-positive phenomenon.

TABLE 2. Serum analysis summary

Serum	CDC (% spec.)[b]	AHG-CDC (% spec.)	Score (%)[c]
TA[a]	62 A1,A10	93 A1,10,11 A2,28	93
AB[a]	40 B7,Bw42	80 7C A2,28 A1[d]	98
LM[a]	60 2C	83 2C Bw4	92
LN[a]	36 A2,B7	93 7C A2,28 B12[d]	84
MF	19 B12	72 12C	70
DS	38 B12	63 12C	100
DD	34 B7	58 7C	89
PD	22 B27	60 7C	95
ME	13 B7	69 7C 12C	100
DR[a]	8 A2	94 2C 12C	83
AF[a]	64 2C	75 2C 7C	100

[a] Specificities determined by differential absorption with HLA-typed platelets.
[b] Percentage of reactivity determined on a panel of cells from 36 normal donors.
[c] Percentage of total reactivity accounted for by the assigned specificities.
[d] Antibodies to private epitopes.

TABLE 3. Comparison of observed CDC crossmatch (CM) outcome[a] with the predicted outcome based on CDC serum analysis

		Predicted CM Result[b] +	Predicted CM Result[b] −	
Observed CM outcome	+	132	31	163
	−	3	94	97
		135	125	260

[a] Four characterized sera were tested against 65 normal donors.
[b] Predicted results were determined by comparing serum analysis data with the HLA phenotype of the donor.

TABLE 4. Comparison of observed AHG-CDC crossmatch (CM) outcome[a] with the predicted outcome based on AHG-CDC serum analysis

		Predicted CM Result[b] +	Predicted CM Result[b] −	
Observed CM outcome	+	456	18	474
	−	8	114	122
		464	132	596

[a] Eleven characterized sera were tested against 114 normal donors.
[b] Predicted results were determined by comparing serum analysis data with the HLA phenotype of the donor.

Predicted crossmatch results were determined by comparing the antibody specificities identified by serum analysis with the phenotype of the donor. When the antiglobulin-augmented assay was used to characterize a serum's reactivity (Table 4), the correlation between the predicted and observed AHG-CDC crossmatch outcome was 95.6% (Table 5). Of 596 total crossmatches performed, there was concordance with 456 positive crossmatches and 114 negative crossmatches. The correlation between predicted and observed crossmatch results decreased when sera were characterized by CDC and compared with CDC crossmatches. The CDC serum analysis correctly predicted 132 positive crossmatches and 94 negative crossmatches (Table 3). However, 31 positive crossmatches were incorrectly predicted to be negative by CDC antibody analysis resulting in a predictive value of 85.9% (Table 5). The number of false-positive (i.e., predicted negative but observed positive) crossmatches was 4-fold higher when CDC serum analysis was used for prediction, as compared with the AHG-CDC analysis. When the comparison of CDC serum analysis and AHG-CDC crossmatches was made, the number of unpredicted positive crossmatches increased to 80 of 260 crossmatches (10-fold higher than the AHG-CDC analysis). This underscores our observation that the CDC assay alone is not sufficient for serum analysis. In this study crossreacting specificities, as well as entire crossreacting groups, would not have been detected if the sera had not also been screened by AHG-CDC (Table 2).

TABLE 5. Predictive value of CDC as AHG-CDC serum analysis

Serum analysis	Crossmatch	% Correlation
CDC	CDC	85.9
CDC	AHG-CDC	68.8
AHG-CDC	AHG-CDC	96.6

[a] Percentage of correctly predicted crossmatches (both positive and negative).

One of the most important results of serum analysis preselection of donors is its effect on negative crossmatch frequency. Of 596 crossmatches, 20.5% were negative when donors were selected randomly. The negative crossmatch frequency was markedly increased to 86.4% when the AHG-CDC serum analysis was used to preselect donors who were likely to be crossmatch-negative. Furthermore, this preselection process reduces the number of crossmatches performed from 596 to 132 (78% reduction). Only 8 negative crossmatches of 596 total (1.3%) were missed by preselection.

DISCUSSION

This study confirms our previous observation that the highly allosensitized state in dialysis patients is due to the development of antibodies to the high-frequency public HLA determinants (*2*). Accurate analysis of these highly reactive sera cannot be done using only CDC primarily because of the CYNAP phenomenon that frequently occurs with public antibodies. Antiglobulin augmentation of the CDC assay both increases its sensitivity and overrides CYNAP (*4*). Furthermore, it has been shown that this increased sensitivity is HLA-specific and not due to random reactivity (*4*). Our serum analyses consistently showed that the AHG-CDC assay resulted in a higher percentage of reactivities than did the CDC technique—but, more importantly, complete patterns of antibody reactivity were developed by AHG-CDC, and only in this way could the actual specificity be determined. Indeed, in seven of eleven sera one or more antibodies would have been overlooked entirely if we had only used the standard cytotoxic assay for serum analysis (Table 2).

One of the objectives of this study was to determine whether the results of serum analysis (CDC or AHG-CDC) could be used to predict the outcome of a crossmatch (CDC or AHG-

CDC) event with a given donor. This is, if reactivity to an HLA determinant were specifically identified in the serum, would the crossmatch result correlate with the expression of that determinant on donor cells. Conversely, we wished to determine which of these techniques was accurate to a level that would result in acceptably low numbers of unexpected positive crossmatches that were not predicted by the serum analysis. CDC serum analysis proved to be less predictive than the AHG-CDC analysis of their respective crossmatch outcomes. In fact, the former technique resulted in a 4-fold higher rate of unexpected positive crossmatches (12% vs. 3%). These false-positive results were probably due to undefined antibody reactivity. However, the difference in frequency of false positives between assay systems is very likely a function of the unpredictable influence of the CYNAP phenomenon on the CDC technique. The effects of CYNAP are avoided when the assay is antiglobulin-modified.

Analysis of HLA antibodies in the sera of highly alloimmunized dialysis patients can be a valuable tool for prospectively selecting donor/recipient combinations. In this study the overall rate of occurrence of a negative crossmatch among random donors was 20.5%. If this donor population had been preselected to exclude phenotypes that were likely to be reactive with the analyzed sera, the negative crossmatch frequency would have risen to 86.4%. The total number of required crossmatches would have been reduced from 596 to 132 (78% reduction).

In our experience it is not necessary to perform a complete analysis on a highly reactive serum each month, but only when there has been a significant change in the percentage of reactivity or pattern of reactivity. After the initial complete analysis, most changes in specificity can be identified by inspection of monthly serum screens without further platelet absorption. In our program virtually all highly reactive patients (>50%) have required no more than one platelet absorption analysis—and, in approximately half these patients, only the computer analysis of the monthly screen data was necessary to make specificity assignments. Therefore, the identification of serum antibodies adds little or no additional cost when calculated on a per-patient-per-month basis. In fact, we estimate that this approach is less costly (both in labor and materials) than the preparation of monthly current crossmatch trays on all patients and the mass crossmatching process on all ABO-compatible recipients when a kidney becomes available. Both approaches (that is, recipient selection based on serum antibody identification and recipient selection based on random crossmatching in preloaded trays) require very similar amounts of a technologist's time at the time of organ harvest, since both involve a two-stage procedure of initial (preloaded monthly sera or selected sera) and final (current serum) crossmatching. Current sera for final crossmatching are usually diluted and plated after recipient selection. The serum analysis approach is also of value in the procurement of nonlocal kidneys. Generally, cells for crossmatching cannot be obtained without actually importing the kidney at considerable cost. Therefore, a method that can predict the final crossmatch outcome 97% of the time would be extremely useful and would result in greater confidence in the chances for transplanting the imported kidney. The potentially crossmatch-negative donors, who are overlooked in some centers because of less-than-perfect phenotype matches, could now be considered in view of a patient's serum analysis. (This premise was recently confirmed by Delmonico et al [5].) Such an approach to donor/recipient matching could result in the successful transplantation of kidneys in many more of the highly allosensitized dialysis patients and a reduction in unnecessary crossmatching.

REFERENCES

1. Scornik J, Ireland J, Howard R, Pfaff W. Assessment of the risk for broad sensitization by blood transfusion. Transplantation 1984; 37: 249.
2. Oldfather J, Mora A, Phelan D, et al. The occurrence of crossreactive "public" antibodies in the sera of highly sensitized dialysis patients. Transplant Proc 1983; 15: 1212.
3. Terasaki PI, McClelland JD. Microdroplet assay of human serum cytotoxins. Nature 1964; 204: 998.
4. Fuller T, Phelan D, Gebel H, Rodey G. The antigenic specificity of antibody reactive in the antiglobulin-augmented lymphocytotoxicity test. Transplantation 1982; 34: 24.
5. Delmonico FL, Fuller A, Cosimi AB, et al. New approaches to donor crossmatching and successful transplantation of highly sensitized patients. Transplantation 1983; 36: 629.
6. Oldfather JW, Gebel HM, Holmes DJ, Rodey GE. Detection of two distinct public specificities on HLA-A28 bearing lymphocytes. Tissue Antigens 1983; 22: 16.
7. Schwartz BD, Luehrman LK, Lee J, Rodey GE. A public antigen determinant in the HLA-B5 cross-reacting group. A basis for cross-reactivity and a possible link with Behcet's disease. Hum Immunol 1980; 1: 37.
8. Schwartz BD, Luehrman LK, Rodey GE. Public antigenic determinant on a family of HLA-B molecules. Basis for cross-reactivity and a possible link with disease predisposition. J Clin Invest 1979; 64: 938.
9. Schwartz BD, Luehrman LK, Lee J, Rodey GE. HLA serological cross-reactivity: HLA-B15 has two public antigens. Hum Immunol 1980; 4: 331.
10. Ayres J, Cresswell P. HLA-B specificities and w4, w6 specificities are on the same polypeptide. Eur J Immunol 1976; 6: 794.

Received 19 August 1985.
Accepted 5 December 1985.

0041-1337/86/4203-0271$02.00/0
TRANSPLANTATION
Vol. 42, No. 3
Printed in U.S.A.

TRANSPLANTATION OF FETAL FIBROBLASTS AND CORRECTION OF ENZYMATIC DEFICIENCIES IN PATIENTS WITH HUNTER'S OR HURLER'S DISORDERS[1]

MATTEO ADINOLFI,[2] IAN MCCOLL,[3] DIANE CHASE,[2] ANTHONY H. FENSOM,[2] KEN WELSH,[4] SUSAN BROWN, JANE MARSH,[2] MICHAEL THICK,[3,4] AND MICHAEL DEAN[5]

Paediatric Research Unit, The Prince Philip Research Laboratories; Department of Surgery, Tissue Typing Unit, United Medical Schools of Guy's and St Thomas's Hospitals; and Division of Biochemistry, Kennedy Institute of Rheumatology, London, United Kingdom

An attempt was made at correcting the specific lysosomal enzyme deficiencies in 7 children with Hunter's or Hurler's diseases by transplantation of fetal fibroblasts. In spite of pretreating the young patients with stored blood, following a procedure employed successfully to avoid rejection of kidneys from incompatible donors, the use of serum-free media for culturing the cells before being harvested and incubation of the cells with chorionic gonadotrophin, the transplantation of fetal fibroblasts was not associated with biochemical or clinical changes. None of the seven patients showed immune reactions against the transplanted cells, HLA antigens, or the missing enzymes.

The mucopolysaccharidoses are a group of inborn errors of metabolism in which a deficiency of a lysosomal enzyme results in the accumulation of glycosaminoglycans (GAGs)* in lysosomes, and their excessive excretion in urine (*1*).

During the past fifteen years, several attempts have been made to correct some of these deficiencies, with conflicting results. Treatment with plasma or leukocyte infusions have not been successful, and transplantation of patients with Hunter's or Hurler's diseases with cultured fibroblasts from normal individuals have produced contradictory results (*2–4*). While, for example, Dean and collaborators (*5, 6*) noticed an increase in the low-molecular-weight GAGs and oligosaccharide fragments in the transplanted patients, Gibbs et al (*7*) could not detect major biochemical changes or clinical improvements following the transplant of fibroblasts. They also noticed that the combined administration of prednisolone and azathioprine could induce per se an increased excretion of low molecular weight GAGs.

In both groups of investigations the transplanted fibroblasts from normal individuals were not HLA-compatible. In fact, since fibroblasts do not express HLA-DR antigens, Gibbs et al (*7*) deliberately injected HLA A, B and C-incompatible cells. The transplantation procedures involved fibroblasts that had been cultured in media containing calf serum; they were washed just before being injected.

Under these conditions fibroblasts absorb the calf plasma proteins present in the medium, which cannot be removed even by repeated washing, and may induce an immune response after transplantation (*8*).

Since failure to correct lysosomal enzyme deficiencies by transplantation of adult fibroblasts may also be attributable to the expression on these cells of minor histocompatibility antigens, we have transplanted patients with Hunter's or Hurler's diseases with human fetal fibroblasts that did not express HLA DR antigens and produced only small quantities of HLA A antigens. These cells were cultured in serum-free medium for 48 hr before being transplanted and incubated in a suspension of human chorionic gonadotropin (HCG) hormone. This hormone was used since previous experiments had shown that human skin grafts were not readily rejected when treated with HCG hormone and transplanted into the guinea pig (*9*). Finally, in order to avoid rejection mediated by minor histocompatibility antigens, the young patients were repeatedly transfused with small aliquots of stored red cells, following a procedure that has been proved to avoid rejection of histologically incompatible kidney transplants (*10–12*).

MATERIALS AND METHODS

Patients. The present trial was performed on a group of six young patients with Hunter's and one with Hurler's disease (Table 1). Of these patients, S.L. and M.H. had been transplanted with amniotic epithelial cells during a previous study (*13*). The diagnoses were established biochemically by demonstrating the specific deficiency of α-L iduronate sulphate sulphatase or α-iduronidase in white cells (*14*). Abnormal excretion of GAGs was also detectable in the urine (*6*).

TABLE 1. Details of seven patients transplanted with human fetal fibroblasts

Name	Date of birth (month/year)	Date of transplant (month/year)	Number of cells transplanted (millions)	Disease
G.P.	12.71	2.83	160	Hunter
		11.83	250	
G.R.	7.79	3.83	200	Hunter
S.H.	10.74	3.83	230	
		11.83	200	Hunter
C.A.	9.79	3.83	230	Hunter
M.H.	10.76	11.83	250	Hunter
L.B.	5.77	3.83	220	Hunter
J.B.	1.83	11.83	500	Hurler

[1] This work was supported by Action Research, The Medical Research Council, and The Mucopolysaccharidosis Society.

[2] Paediatric Research Unit, The Prince Philip Research Laboratories.

[3] Department of Surgery.

[4] Tissue Typing Unit United Medical Schools of Guy's and St. Thomas's Hospitals.

[5] Kennedy Institute of Rheumatology.

* Abbreviations used: GAG, glycosaminoglycan; HCG, human chorionic gonadotropin.

Samples of blood were repeatedly collected before starting the treatment, and no variations in the levels of the specific lysosomal enzyme were noticed. Soon after the transplants, blood was collected, at short intervals of 4–7 days and then for 8–10 months at monthly intervals. Leukocytes, separated from whole blood treated with heparin, were washed, separated into small aliquots, and stored at −50°C for no more than 3–4 weeks before being tested. The specific levels of α-L iduronate sulphate sulphatase and α-iduronidase were also measured in sera.

Enzyme assay. The activities of α-L-iduronate sulphate sulphatase and α-iduronidase were measured as previously described (*1, 6, 14*).

The assay for α-L-iduronate sulphate sulphatase was performed at Guy's Hospital and at the Kennedy Institute using similar procedures; only the time was protracted for 20 hr for the assays carried out at the Kennedy Institute. The urinary glycoconjugates were separated into polymeric glycosaminoglycans and oligosaccharide fractions, and their levels estimated as previously described (*8*).

Immunological tests. Pretransplantation blood transfusions: All children to be transplanted and their parents were serologically typed for the blood groups ABO and Rh and for the HLA A, B, C, and DR system using conventional techniques (*15, 16*).

Pretransplantation blood transfusions were performed as previously described (*10*). Briefly, one pint of blood from a compatible (ABO and Rh) donor was collected in ACD, divided into three aliquots, and stored at +4°C. After one week, one aliquot of "leukocyte-poor" blood was transfused. This was followed by another two transfusions at one week intervals.

Samples of sera were tested before the 2nd and 3rd transfusion, and one week after the 3rd transfusion to detect the presence of antibodies against red cell or HLA antigens.

Immune response to HLA antigens following transplantation of fetal fibroblasts: Samples of blood were collected from the patient after the transplant at intervals of one month for 7–8 months. Sera were then tested for the presence of cytotoxic antibodies again HLA antigens using a panel of 60 donors.

At least two sera from each patient were also tested by indirect immunofluorescence technique against the fetal fibroblasts that had been used for transplantation. Expression of HLA A, B, C, and DR antigens on the surface of the human fetal fibroblasts to be transplanted was investigated using two monomorphic antisera, W6/32 and DA2 as previously described (*17*). Further investigations were also performed by absorbing antisera, after appropriate dilutions, against various HLA antigens with the fetal fibroblasts, and then testing the absorbed and untreated sera against a selected panel of donor lymphocytes (*16*). Before being transplanted, random samples of fibroblasts were tested to establish whether macrophages or monocytes were still present in the cultures, using specific monoclonal antibodies and the immunoperoxidase method by one of us (K.W.), but such contaminating cells could not be detected.

Fetal fibroblasts. Fibroblasts from two human fetuses about 16 weeks old were initially tested to establish their suitability for transplantation. Simultaneously, the MRC5 fibroblast line (kindly donated by Dr. P. Jacobs, MRC Unit, Mill Hill, London) was cultured and tested. All three samples of fetal cells proved to be suitable for the purpose of culturing a large number of cells in a short period. The fibroblast cultures were performed in an incubator that had not been previously used and was kept in an isolated room. The cells were cultured in Eagle's minimal essential medium with 10% calf serum buffered with Hepes and sodium bicarbonate. The medium was changed every 3 days. Periodically, and just before being transplanted, samples of fibroblasts were collected and tested for possible bacteria and *Mycoplasma* contamination. The cells were also assayed to confirm that the synthesis of lysomal enzymes was still as efficient as at the beginning of the in vitro cultures.

Before being transplanted, confluent cells were kept for 48 hr in serum-free Iscove's (Flow Laboratories, UK) medium, which was changed twice over a period of 24 hr. The cells were collected mechanically and washed twice in Iscove's medium. They were suspended in a sterile saline solution and incubated for about 1 hr with HCG (10,000 units). After being washed once, the cells were injected s.c. in four sites (*5, 6*). Data concerning the number of fetal fibroblasts transplanted are shown in Table 1.

Follow-up of the patients after the transplant. Enzyme assays for α-L-iduronate sulphate sulphatase or α-iduronidase were performed on white cells collected at intervals of about one month over a period ranging from 8 to 12 months. Further samples were collected at intervals of 2–3 months, for a total period of observation that varied from 13 to 22 weeks. Samples of urine were also collected and GAG levels were estimated (*1, 6*).

Although the aim of the present investigation was exclusively to establish whether a specific enzyme deficiency could be corrected in patients with Hunter's or Hurler's diseases, complete physical examinations were performed before and after the transplants. All the children were repeatedly assessed by a pediatric otologist and an ophthalmologist. Before being transplanted, they were also seen by a clinical psychologist, and they were reexamined a few months (*6–8*) after the transplant.

RESULTS

Levels of lysosomal enzymes. The levels of α-iduronidase and α-L-iduronate sulphate sulphatase were estimated in white cells and serum before the transfusions of "stored" blood and one week after the transfusions of the 3rd aliquot. No increase in enzyme values was observed following the transfusion of ABO and Rh-compatible blood.

Samples of white cells and sera were tested for α-L-iduronate sulphate sulphatase activity in duplicate at Guy's Hospital and at the Kennedy Institute after the transplantation of fibroblasts. At least one sample from a normal adult individual was used as a control and at least one sample from a patient with the specific lysosomal enzyme deficiency was included in each set of tests.

While the results collected at Guy's suggested that after the transplant none of the 7 transplanted children showed, at any time, an increase of either α-iduronidase or α-L-iduronate sulphate sulphatase, the results of the estimations carried out at the Kennedy Institute pointed to increased values of α-L-iduronate sulphate sulphatase in 3 patients with Hunter's disease. However, the levels of the enzyme in white cells varied markedly from sample to sample in the same subject over several months.

Excretion of GAGs and oligosaccharides in urine. Samples of urine were collected and examined before transplantation, and at least every 2 months following the transplant of fetal fibroblasts. No consistent changes in the excretion of total GAGs or oligosaccharides was observed. The occasional variations were not correlated with apparent increases of α-L-iduronate sulphate sulphatase observed in the white cell samples tested at the Kennedy Institute.

Clinical observations. All 7 patients tolerated the injection of fibroblasts without side effects. Only one (G.P.) showed a moderate rash around the injected area, which lasted 48 hr. No clinical improvement was noticed during the period of observation lasting from 13 to 22 months. In one child (M.H.), reduced mobility of articulation was noticed. In the child with Hurler's disease (J.B.), corneal opacity was not affected by the transplant.

Immunological investigations. Sera were collected from each patient before transfusion of stored red cells, one week after the third transfusion of blood, and at intervals of about 4 weeks during the first 6 months following the transplant of fetal fibroblasts. Samples collected before and after the transplants were tested against lymphocytes from a panel of 60 selected donors. Cytotoxic HLA antibodies were not demonstrated after blood transfusion or the transplantation of fetal fibroblasts.

When selected sera obtained after the transplant were tested by indirect immunofluorescence against the fetal fibroblasts cultured in vitro, no positive staining was observed. Two children (G.P. and S.H.) received a second transplant of fetal fibroblasts without showing signs of immunological reaction at the sites of inoculation.

Selected sera collected before and after the transplants were also tested for the presence of antibodies that could precipitate and/or inhibit α-L-iduronate sulphate sulphatase. Briefly, extracts containing the enzyme were mixed with the sera, and after incubation the precipitates and supernatants were tested for residual enzyme activity. No reduction of the biological activity of α-L-iduronate sulphate sulphatase was detected using the sera of the transplanted patients.

DISCUSSION

The rationale for using fibroblast transplantation for the correction of lysosomal storage diseases is based on the demonstration that several lysosomal enzymes are released from normal cells and taken up by deficient host cells via a specific receptor (*18*). This had been repeatedly demonstrated in vitro using fibroblasts from patients with Hurler's or Hunter's diseases (*14*, *17*) and it is assumed that similar uptake will also occur in vivo once normal fibroblasts are transplanted in a child with α-iduronidase or α-L-iduronate sulphate sulphatase deficiency. The second assumption is that fibroblasts are not likely to induce immunization and to be rejected, since they do not express HLA DR antigens (*18*, *19*).

In previous studies either apparently HLA compatible or incompatible fibroblasts from normal adult individuals were used (*5–7*) with controversial results. Despite opinions expressed about the transient changes of the levels of white-cell-specific lysosomal enzyme observed in a few patients following the transplants, this therapy has not induced prolonged biochemical or clinical improvement.

Failure of this corrective therapy may be due to various reasons. Perhaps too few cells were transplanted to induce measurable biochemical changes. Alternatively, fibroblasts from normal adults, even if HLA compatible, may be rejected because they adsorb calf antigens from the media used during the in vitro culture (*8*).

The present trial was planned based on the assumptions that (A) pretreatment with stored blood could avoid immune rejection; (B) fetal fibroblasts, not expressing HLA DR antigens and poorly expressing HLA ABC antigen, had a better chance to survive an immunological reaction of the host; (C) cells maintained in serum-free medium for at least 24 hr before being transplanted should be contaminated with only a minimal amount of calf plasma proteins; (D) fibroblasts incubated with HCG, claimed to protect human skin from being rapidly rejected when transplanted into guinea pigs (*9*), should not be promptly rejected even if containing minor histocompatibility antigens.

In spite of these procedures, the transplantation of fetal fibroblast did not correct the specific enzyme deficiencies of young patients with Hunter's or Hurler's diseases.

Sporadic and modest increases of α-L-iduronate sulphate sulphatase were observed by one of us (M.D.) in three of the six patients with Hunter's disease who received transplants, but these variations were not associated with changes in the urinary excretions of GAGs.

Recently Manca et al. (*20*), have observed an immune reaction specific against the fibroblasts of a patient rejecting a transplanted kidney. The immune reaction was claimed to be directed against an antigen expressed exclusively on the fibroblasts of the donor. However, we were unable to detect evidence for immune response against the transplanted cells; in fact, when sera from the treated patients were tested against a panel of lymphocytes from 60 normal donors, cytotoxic antibodies could not be detected. Furthermore, sera from the transplanted patients did not contain antibodies against the transplanted fibroblasts. Antibodies against the missing enzyme were also absent in the posttransplantation sera, as judged by the precipitation method.

If failure to correct the enzyme deficiencies responsible for Hunter's or Hurler's diseases, observed in the present study or in trials based on the use of fibroblasts from normal adult individuals, cannot be attributed to an immune response, the possibility of a reaction to residual bovine plasma proteins adsorbed by the cells cannot be excluded. Other causes of failure may be the limited number of cells transplanted—as compared with the total cell body of the young patient—or with inhibitors affecting the half-life of the transplanted enzyme. However, preliminary studies have shown that inhibitors of α-L-iduronate sulphate sulphatase were present neither in the sera of 3 children transplanted with fetal fibroblasts, nor in other young untreated patients (Chase D, Adinolfi M, unpublished observations).

Unfortunately, the absence of suitable markers on the surface of the fetal fibroblasts did not allow us to follow their fate after being transplanted, and the lack of suitable animal models for Hunter's or Hurler's disease has made it difficult to establish with certainty the causes of the failure to correct these lysosomal storage diseases by means of transplantation (*8*).

Acknowledgment. We thank Christine Lavery and all members of the families who have collaborated in our study.

REFERENCES

1. Benson PF, Fensom AH. Prevention and treatment of biochemical genetic disorders. In: Adinolfi M, Benson PF, Giannelli F, Seller MY. Paediatric research: London: Heinemann, 1982.
2. Di Ferrante N, Nichols BL, Donnelly PU, Neri G, Hrgovcic R, Berglund RK. Induced degradation of glycosaminoglycans in Hurler's and Hunter's syndromes by plasma infusion. Proc Natl Acad Sci USA 1971; 68: 303.
3. Erickson RP, Sandman R, Robertson WVP, Epstein CJ. Inefficacy of fresh frozen plasma therapy of mucopolysaccharidosis II. III. Pediatrics 1972; 50: 693.
4. Dean MF, Benson PF, Muir H. Mobilisation of glycosaminoglycans by plasma infusion in mucopolysaccharidosis type III: two types of response. Nature (New Biol) 1973; 243: 143.

5. Dean MF, Muir H, Benson PF, Button LR, Roylston A, Mowbray J. Enzyme replacement therapy by fibroblast transplantation in a case of Hunter syndrome. Nature 1976; 261: 323.
6. Dean MF, Stevens RL, Muir H, Benson PF, Button LR, Anderson RL, Boylston A, Mowbray J. Enzyme replacement therapy by fibroblast transplantations. J Clin Invest 1979; 63: 138.
7. Gibbs DA, Spellacy E, Tompkins R, Watts RWE, Mowbray JF. A clinical trial of fibroblast transplantation for the treatment of mucopolysaccharidoses. J Inherited Metab Dis 1983; 6: 62.
8. Adinolfi M, Brown S. Strategies for the correction of enzymatic deficiencies in patients with mucopolysaccharidoses. Dev Med Child Neurol 1984; 26: 401.
9. Loke YW. Immunology and immunopathology of the human foetal-maternal interaction. Holland: Elsevier-North, 1978.
10. Persijn GG, Cohen B, Lansbergen Q, van Rood JJ. Retrospective studies on the effect of blood transfusion in renal transplantation in the Netherlands. Transplantation 1978; 28: 396.
11. Persijn GG, D'Aurato J, van Rood JJ. Pretransplant blood transfusion and long-term renal allograft survival. Lancet 1984; 2: 1043.
12. Terasaki PI. The beneficial transfusions effect of kidney graft survival attributed to clonal deletion. Transplantation 1984; 37: 119.
13. Akle C, McColl I, Dean M, Adinolfi M, Brown S, Fensom AH. Marsh J, Welsh K. Transplantation of amniotic epithelial membranes in patients with mucopolysaccharidoses. Expl Clin Immunogenet 1985; 2: 43.
14. Benson PF, Fensom AH. Genetic biochemical disorders. Oxford, New York, Toronto: Oxford University Press, 1985.
15. Mollison PL. Blood transfusion in clinical medicine. Oxford: Blackwell, 1967.
16. Welsh KI, Batchelor JR. Assays for antibodies against histocompatibility antigens. In: Weir, ed. Handbook of experimental immunology. Oxford: Blackwell, 1978.
17. Adinolfi M, Akle C, McColl I, Fensom AH, Tansley L, Connolly P, Hsi BL, Faulk, WP, Travers P, Bodmer WF. Expression of HLA antigens, β_2 microglobulin and enzymes by human amniotic epithelial cells. Nature 1982; 295: 325.
18. Neufield EF. The uptake of enzymes into lysosomes: an overview. Birth Defects 1980; 16(1): 77.
19. Espimark A, Möller E. Tissue typing of cells in culture. Histocompatibility typing of diploid fibroblast cultures by the mixed hemadsorption (MH) test. Tissue Antigens 1978; 11: 273.
20. Manca F, Barocci S, Kunki A, Gurreri G, Celada F. Recognition of donor fibroblasts antigens by lymphocytes homing in the human grafted kidney. Transplantation 1983; 36: 670.

Received 12 September 1985.
Accepted 21 November 1985.

0041-1337/86/4203-0274$02.00/0
TRANSPLANTATION

Vol. 42, No. 3
Printed in U.S.A.

LONG-TERM SURVIVAL AND IMMUNOLOGICAL TOLERANCE OF HUMAN EPIDERMAL ALLOGRAFTS PRODUCED IN CULTURE[1,2]

JEAN THIVOLET,[3] MICHEL FAURE, AÏCHA DEMIDEM, AND GILLES MAUDUIT

Inserm U.209, Clinique Dermatologique et Immunologie, Lyon, France

Human epidermal cells from a small skin specimen can be grown in culture into multilayered sheets suitable for the permanent coverage of large burn wounds when used as epidermal autografts. We report here on the long-term survival of such cultured epidermal sheets used as epidermal allografts (EAG) across a major histocompatibility barrier in three nonimmunosuppressed adult patients, suffering from large chronic grafted leg ulcers, where the EAG have been placed to cover the conventional split-thickness skin autograft donor site. The absence of rejection was based upon clinical, histological, and immunopathological observation of the allografted sites at various intervals after grafting of the EAG. The identity of the epidermal cells on the grafted area with cultured cells from allogeneic donor was then established after blood substance typing by indirect immunofluorescence.

Furthermore, epidermal cells from cultured sheets, but not control human cells from freshly excised normal epidermis, failed to stimulate the recipient peripheral blood cells in the mixed epidermal cell lymphocyte culture reaction, a finding that is related to the complete absence of class-II-antigen–bearing cells in cultured epidermis. This absence of T cell stimulation was noted not only on the day of grafting but throughout the follow-up. Altogether, these findings show that Langerhans cell and other class-II-antigen–bearing cell-depleted cultured epidermal allografts, are tolerated in unrelated recipients. EAG may serve as a skin substitute in patients with large wounds or burns. Since EAG may be grown continuously, the coverage of burns may not then be limited by the availability of the donor site, or by the time necessary to produce epidermal tissue in cultures.

[1] This work was supported in part by a grant from the Caisses d'Assurance des Professions Libérales, Section Province, Lyon, France.
[2] This work was carried out with the agreement of the Ethical Committee of Claude Bernard University, Lyon.
[3] Address correspondence to: Pr. J. Thivolet, Inserm U.209, Clinique Dermatologique et Immunologie, Pavillon R, Hôpital E. Herriot, 69374 Lyon Cx 08, France.

Epidermal cells (keratinocytes) can be grown in vitro and produce thin living epithelia suitable for grafting. A human skin biopsy specimen of 2 cm^2 can then be expanded in surface area by a factor of 10,000 in three to four weeks (*1*). Epidermis produced in vitro has been used successfully for permanent autografts in patients with large burns (*2, 3*). In fact, the use of cultured grafts from autologous epidermal cells may be limited not by the availability of suitable donor sites but by the time required for the growth of the cells in vitro.

The fact that this reconstituted epidermis are devoid of Langerhans cells and other class-II-antigen–expressing cells, strongly suggests that they may be used as allografts for burn wounds. In a preliminary report, we studied the in vivo survival of human epidermal allograft (EAG)* produced in vitro from a male donor skin sample and grafted onto a genetically dissimilar female recipient (*4*). No evidence of graft rejection could be noted. A similar finding has also been shown by Hefton et al. (*5*) using another epidermal cell culture system to obtain human epidermal sheets suitable for grafting. Since such long-term survival of conventional human skin allograft has never been clearly demonstrated in normal nonimmunosuppressed patients, we studied, in 3 patients grafted with non compatible EAG produced in vitro, both the survival of the EAG and the in vitro response of lymphocytes from the recipients to the keratinocytes from the donors.

MATERIALS AND METHODS

Experimental protocol. Epidermal cell (EC) cultures, grafting of epidermal sheets, and clinical and biological follow-up have been conducted as follows. Briefly, EAG were obtained by cultivating epidermal cells (keratinocytes) from epidermal cell suspensions from donors (D). Recipients of EAG were patients suffering from large chronic leg ulcers covered with conventional split-thickness skin autograft. Afterwards, EAG produced in vitro were placed on the recipient (R) donor site. At various intervals after grafting, skin biopsies were taken from EAG for histological and immunopathological examination. In parallel, mixed epidermal lymphocyte cultures (MELC) were conducted on the day of grafting, and every two weeks thereafter, with suspensions of EC from the donor and peripheral blood lymphocytes (PBL) from the recipient; aliquots of cultured EC were kept frozen until their use in MELC.

Patients. Epidermal cells used to produce EAG were obtained from normal adult human skin samples in three male patients undergoing plastic surgery (donors [D]). Recipients (R) of allografts were three women (R1, R2, R3), whose ages ranged from 52 to 79 years, suffering of large chronic leg ulcers. In each case 120-cm^2 split-thickness skin graft from their left forearm was excised, meshed to expand the surface area, and placed as an autograft on the leg ulcer, while EAG from the respective donor were placed on the autograft donor site as dressing. Tissue and blood typing of the donor and recipient in each pair are given in Table 1.

Preparation of cultured epithelia. Epidermal epithelia were cultured according to the method described by Howard Green (*3, 6*). Briefly, a full-thickness skin sample measuring 2 cm^2 was obtained from a plastic surgery operation, placed in culture medium, and transferred to the laboratory for cultivation. After removal of as much subcutaneous tissue and dermis as possible, the tissue was minced and trypsinized. Then 75-cm^2 culture flasks already containing 1.5×10^6 lethally irradiated 3T3 cells were inoculated with over 10^6 EC each. The cultures were fed with 3:1 mixture of Dulbecco-Vogt modification of Eagle's medium and Ham's F-12 medium. Supplements were as follows: fetal calf serum 10%, hydrocortisone 0.4 μg/ml, insulin 5 μg/ml, triiodothyronine, 2×10^{-9} M, choleragen 10^{-10} M, and adenine 8×10^{-4} M. The cultures were incubated at 37°C in an atmosphere containing 10% CO_2. After 3 days, epidermal growth factor (EGF) was added to the medium to 10 ng/ml. The medium was changed twice weekly until the cultures became confluent (between 10 and 14 days). To prepare graftable secondary cultures, subconfluent primary cultures were trypsinized and the cells were transferred to flasks of the same size containing irradiated 3T3 cells. These cultures were maintained in the same way as the primary cultures. One or two days before the cultures were scheduled for grafting, the spent medium was changed and the cultures were refed with medium from which choleragen was omitted.

TABLE 1. Tissue and blood typing (ABO/RH) of donors (D) and recipients (R)

	R1	D1	R2	D2	R3	D3
Blood typing (ABO/RH)	A_1/−	0/+	0/−	0/−	0/+	A_1/+
Tissue typing:						
HLA A	25/29	2/32	2/3	32/33	2/11	2/11
HLA B	51/44	13/35	14/44	14/39	7/38	18/44
HLA C	W3 −	W4 −	− −	− −	− −	W3 −
HLA DR	4 −	7/W_{11}	4/7	1 −	W_{13} −	ND[a]

[a] (ND) not done.

Grafting. Confluent secondary cultures destined for grafting were detached intact from the surface of the tissue culture dish, using the enzyme dispase II, 1.2 μ/ml of serum-free medium. The epithelium was then washed with serum-free medium and placed basal side up on a 4.5×6.0-cm rectangle of vaseline gauze in a 100-mm Petri dish. The edges of the epithelium were secured to the gauze with metallic surgical clips. Serum-free medium was added to cover the basal surface of the epithelium and the dishes containing the grafts were transported to the bedside.

Epithelial grafts with the vaseline gauze covering were placed on the prepared site with the basal layer directed against the recipient bed, then held in place by a single layer of vaseline gauze overlaid with several layers of nonimpregnated gauze. The gauzes were removed 5 days after grafting; the dressing was then changed daily for 10 days. Thereafter the grafts were left exposed.

Clinical and immunopathological follow-up. Clinical follow up started at the first dressing and was carried out daily during the first 4 weeks, then weekly for the next 2 months.

Skin biopsies were performed under local anesthesia on days 14, 28, and 42 using a 4-mm punch. The skin specimen was cut into two pieces. One was fixed in 10% buffered formalin, embedded in paraffin, stained with hematoxylin-eosin, and examined under conventional microscopy. The other was frozen in liquid nitrogen and stored at −80°C to be used for immunofluorescence (IF) analysis.

Indirect immunofluorescence (IIF) studies were performed

* Abbreviations used: CEC, cultured epidermal cells; D, donor(s); EAG, epidermal allografts; EC, epidermal cells; EGF, epidermal growth factor; IF, immunofluorescence; IIF, indirect immunofluorescence; MCA, monoclonal antibody(ies); MELC, mixed epidermal lymphocyte culture; PB, peripheral blood; PRL, peripheral blood lymphocytes; R, recipient(s).

using (1) monoclonal antibodies (MCA) to various cell membrane determinants: OKT_3 (Ortho Pharmaceutical Corp., Raritan, NJ); Leu 2a, Leu 3a (Becton-Dickinson, Mountain View, CA) to T cell subpopulations; OKT6 (Ortho, Raritan, NJ) specific for Langerhans cells among EC and BL_2 (J. Brochier INSERM U80, Lyon, FR) to HLA-DR antigen (7); and (2) rabbit antibodies and human antiserum to the dermoepidermal junction constituents (type IV collagen (I. Pasteur, Lyon, FR), laminin (BRL, MA) and basal membrane zone (BMZ) antigens in the first step, then the appropriate FITC-conjugated antibody. Slides were viewed under a Zeiss fluorescence microscope with epiillumination.

Demonstration of blood group antigens expressed by EC in EAG. Blood group substances are known to be expressed by human epidermal cells in the upper Malpighian layers (*8*). Taking advantage of the dissimilarities between donor and recipient (Table 1), indirect IF using MCA against blood group A (Centre National Transfusion Sanguine, Paris, FR, dilution 1/10) was performed on days 14 and 42 after grafting on sections of skin samples taken from the allografted site. As controls, normal human skin specimens from group A patients were studied.

Mixed epidermal lymphocyte cultures. Allogeneic MELC were carried out for every donor and recipient pair. Cells from confluent EAG were resuspended after trypsinization on the day of grafting. EC aliquots were also kept frozen to be used in subsequent MELC. MELC were performed as already described (*9, 10*). Briefly, in each well, 1×10^5 peripheral blood cells (PB cells) from the recipient were co-cultivated with 1×10^5 EC in 0.2 ml RPMI 1640 + 15% heat-inactivated AB human serum, 2 mM-L glutamine and antibodies at 37°C in a 5% CO_2, 5% H_2O atmosphere. As controls, PB cells alone were cultured under conditions otherwise identical to those of MELC. Cultures were established in triplicate. After 5 days of culture, ^3H-thymidine was added (1 μCl/well), and the cells harvested 18 hr later. Thymidine uptake was evaluated by means of liquid scintillation counting and expressed as mean c.p.m. of triplicates. MELC were initiated on the day of grafting, and at 14, 28, and 42 days after grafting. As controls, 3 kinds of allogeneic MELC were also conducted: (1) cultured EC against control allogeneic PB cells (5 healthy adult volunteers unrelated to donors or EAG recipients); (2) EC isolated from normal adult human skin against the recipient PB cells; (3) the same control EC suspensions against control allogeneic PB cells.

RESULTS

EAG. When ready for grafting, the cultured epithelial sheets ranged in thickness from four to seven cell layers (Fig. 1). These epithelial sheets were composed of a basal cell layer and a few suprabasal keratinocyte layers; neither melanocytes, nor Langerhans cells could be noted on histological, immunopathological, or electronmicroscopy examination of these epidermal sheets after their dispase detachment from the culture flasks.

Clinical examination. When the Vaseline gauze was removed 5 days after grafting, EAG were visible as a very thin translucent sheet. This contrasted with the pink-redness of the surrounding wound dermal areas that had not been grafted after surgical removal of split-thickness tissue for conventional autografting. Over the next two weeks, grafts thickened, spread outward, and merged with each other and with the surrounding normal skin. These clinical observations were similar to those otherwise noted using EAG as autografts (*2, 3*). Neither inflammatory symptoms, nor signs of graft rejection could be observed at any time during the 3 month follow-up in any of the three cases (5 months for patient 1). No retraction could be noted, and the intermediate term quality seemed excellent.

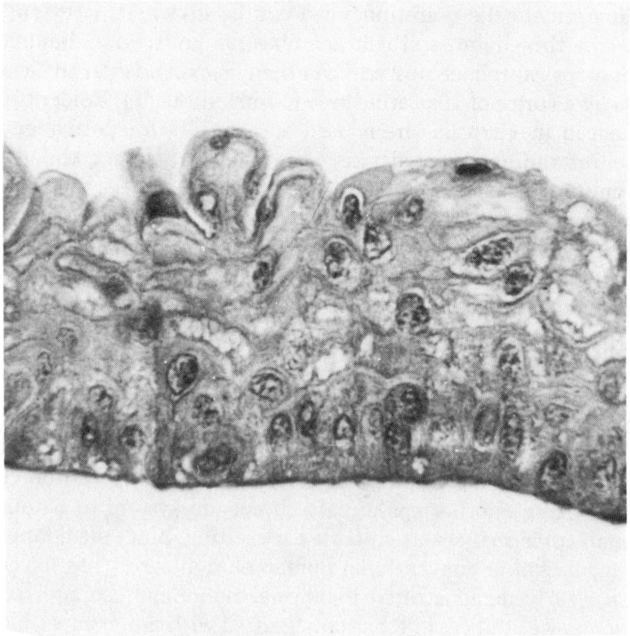

FIGURE 1. Cultured epidermal sheet (H&E; ×100). Note the basal cell layer and 6–7 suprabasal layers.

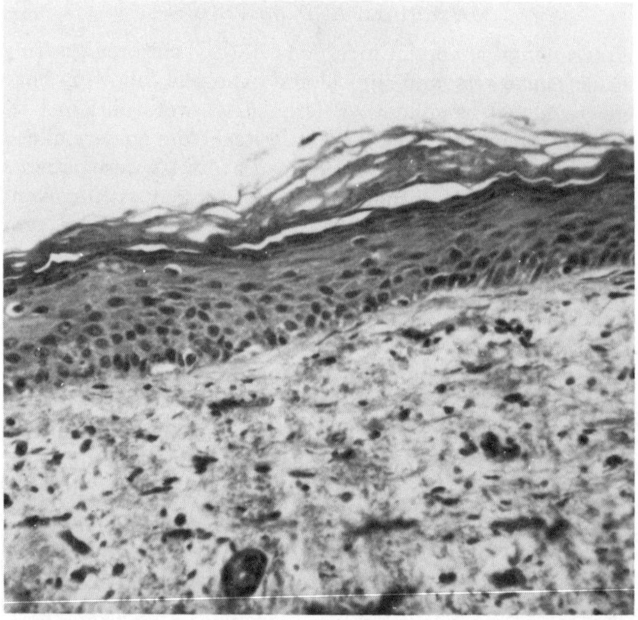

FIGURE 2. Biopsy of the graft at day 28 (H&E; ×25) showing a fully stratified epidermis with a mild orthokeratosis in surface. Note the absence of rete ridges and a moderate dermal infiltration of mononuclear cells.

Histology and immunopathological examinations. Skin samples taken 14 days after grafting showed that the grafted area was completely covered by a slightly hypertrophic epidermis that did not show rete ridges or adnexal structures (Fig. 2). The dermoepidermal junction was linear—and, by IF analysis, the three major components of the junction (i.e., basal membrane zone antigen, laminin, and type IV collagen) were present (Figs. 3–5). Above the basal cell layer, where no necrosis could be noted, a stratum spinosum of generally more than 10 cell layers, a well-represented stratum granulosum, and a mild orthokeratosis in the surface were noted. No inflammatory mononuclear cells invading the epidermis were present. Such a structure, similar to that noted in the case of grafting surgical or burn wounds with autologous epithelium (*2*), suggested that healing was not the result of ingrowth of residual epithelial elements. The underlying dermis corresponding to the graft bed was edematous, with a number of large capillaries somewhat turgescent, surrounded by mild lymphoplasmocytic infiltrates. The

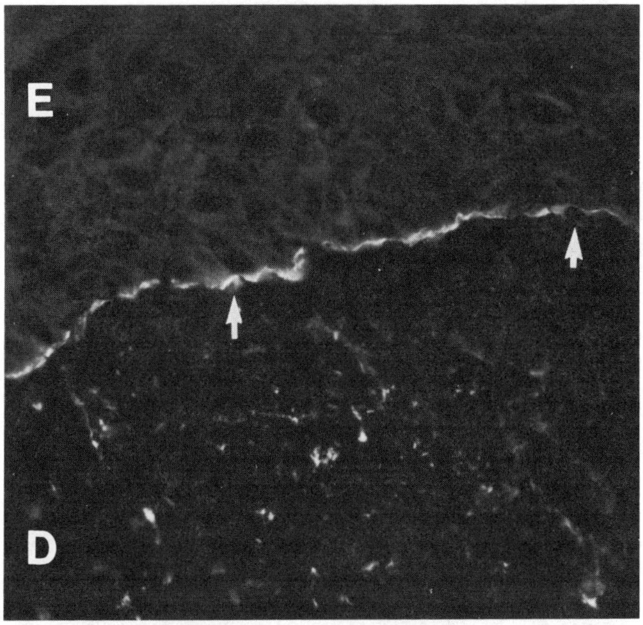

FIGURE 3. Indirect IF: basal membrane zone antigens (arrow). (E) epidermis; (D) dermis (×40).

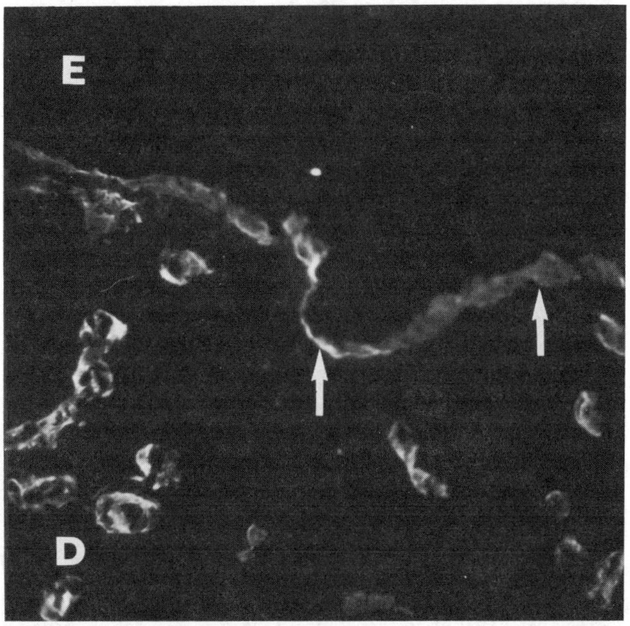

FIGURE 4. Indirect IF: laminin (arrows) at the dermoepidermal junction (×40). (E) epidermis; (D) dermis.

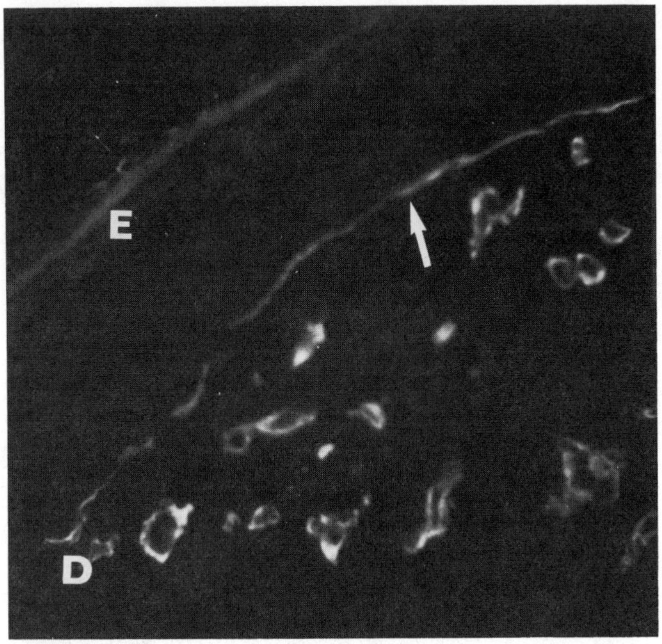

FIGURE 5. Indirect IF: collagen IV (arrow) at the dermoepidermal junction (×40). (E) epidermis; (D) dermis.

following skin samples at days 28 and 42 showed similar features and were identical for each patient grafted. Dermal inflammation remained mild-to-moderate. These dermal cellular infiltrates were noted by IF to contain T3, T4, and T8-positive cells. Numerous class-II-antigen–expressing cells were seen in the dermis. Most of them corresponded to mononuclear cells, which lacked the T6-specific marker of Langerhans cells, and were presumably "activated" mononuclear cells. A few of them were OKT6-positive, a finding noted only in one case (pair 2), 14 days after grafting, together with OKT6 and HLA-DR-positive dispersed dentritic cells scattered throughout the epidermal malpighian layers. Contrasting with the unusual presence of OKT6-positive dermal cells, Langerhans cells were noted in every patient, as early as the first skin biopsy and throughout the following skin examinations. Since cultured EAG do not contain Langerhans cells, this reappearance of Langerhans cells among the epidermal cells in the very first few weeks after grafting, which has previously been noted when grafting with autologous epithelium (*2*), is likely due to a colonization of the epidermis by Langerhans cells from a circulating pool of donor cells originating in the bone marrow (*11*).

Demonstration of blood group substance on EAG keratinocytes. In pairs 1 and 3 (Table 1) donor and recipient were dissimilar in term of blood group substance typing; investigation of the identity of the epidermis corresponding to the allografted area was performed on pair 1. Using MCA instead of polyclonal antibodies, blood group substances may be demonstrated by IF on frozen sections without trypsinization; they are strongly expressed in upper epidermal layers as well as in dermal vessels and glands, as shown in Fig. 6 by an A blood group control. Skin sections obtained from the grafted area 14 and 42 days after grafting R1 ($A1^+$) with EAG grown in vitro from D1 (0) keratinocytes were reacted with anti A MCA by IF. As illustrated in Fig. 7, no labeling of the epidermis could be noted, in contrast with the strong fluorescence of dermal structures, which demonstrated that, at least 42 days after grafting, the

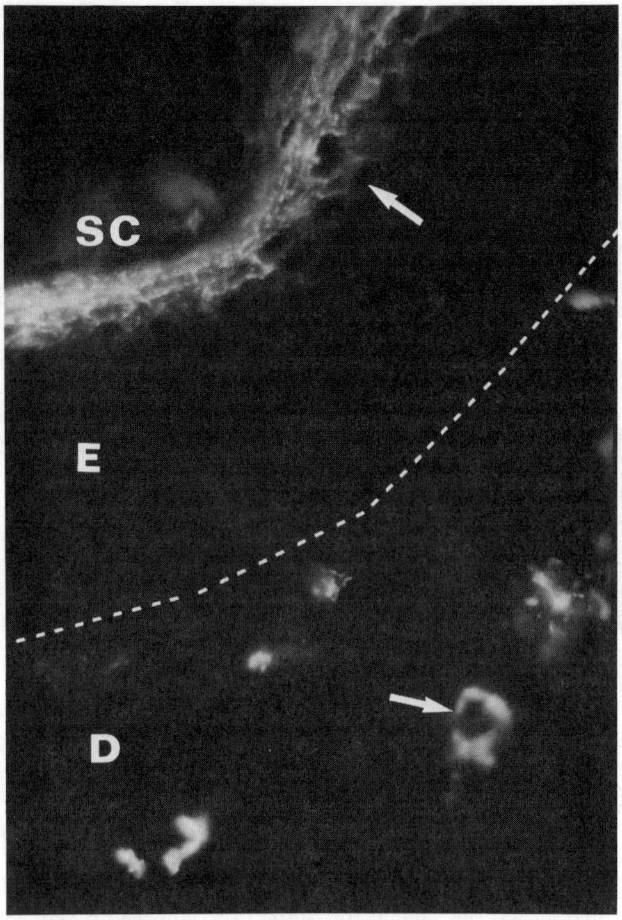

FIGURE 6. Blood group antigen A (arrows) in normal skin. Indirect immunofluorescence (×40). (SC) stratum corneum; (E) epidermis; (D) dermis. Note the presence of blood group substance in the granular layer and in dermal vessels.

epidermis present at the grafting area was really the cultured epithelium and had not been replaced by epidermal cells from the recipient.

MELC. Results of lymphocyte proliferation in MELC were expressed by the stimulation indexes (SI)—i.e., in each case, the ratios of the cpm counts in MELC to those obtained when PB cells were cultured in the absence of EC, since insignificant counts are obtained when EC are cultured alone (*9*). As shown in Fig. 8, when tested in MELC on the day of grafting, EC from cultured epithelia failed to stimulate not only PBL from the recipient but also unrelated allogeneic control PBL (SI = 1). In contrast, when tested against control allogeneic EC suspensions, the proliferative responses of the cells from the recipients were similar to those noted using cells from five unrelated donors. SI in recipients 1, 2, and 3 were respectively 6, 37, and 18; those obtained with control PB cells ranged from 7 to 25. During the following six weeks, a very low response was noted when PBL from the recipients were tested in MELC in the presence of cultured EC from the donors (pairs 1 and 2) (Fig. 8). This contrasted with the rate of proliferation noted when control EC were used as stimulating cells. This very low response did not increase from the second to the sixth week. In pair 3, no response (SI = 1) was even noted at 4 weeks and 9 weeks after grafting when PB cells from the recipients were tested against EC from the skin donor (Fig. 8). In each case, when present, these responses were very weak. Nevertheless they contrasted with the absence of proliferation when control PB cells were tested against EC from cultured epithelia.

DISCUSSION

This data shows that, in each of the three patients studied, long-term survival of in-vitro-produced human epidermal allografts has been achieved across a major histocompatibility barrier. This demonstration is based upon various criteria. No clinical or histological symptom of rejection could be noted during the few months following grafting. As early as day 6 after grafting, the EAG were visible as a very thin translucent sheet that contrasted with the uncovered area. EAG continued to thicken from week to week. The histological patterns were similar to those previously noted with epidermal sheets produced in vitro used as autografts (*2, 3*). They were those of a mature multilayered epidermis that contained all cell layers—but rete ridges were lacking, as were, for example, adnexal structures, sebaceous glands, and hair follicles. The similarity between these features and those noted when the same cultured epidermis is used for autografts (*2*) strongly suggests that EAG had not been replaced by epithelial cells from the recipients when histological examinations were performed. However, the identity of keratinocytes of long-term living grafts cannot be established without the help of biological markers. Such a control, based upon a dissimilarity between blood group sub-

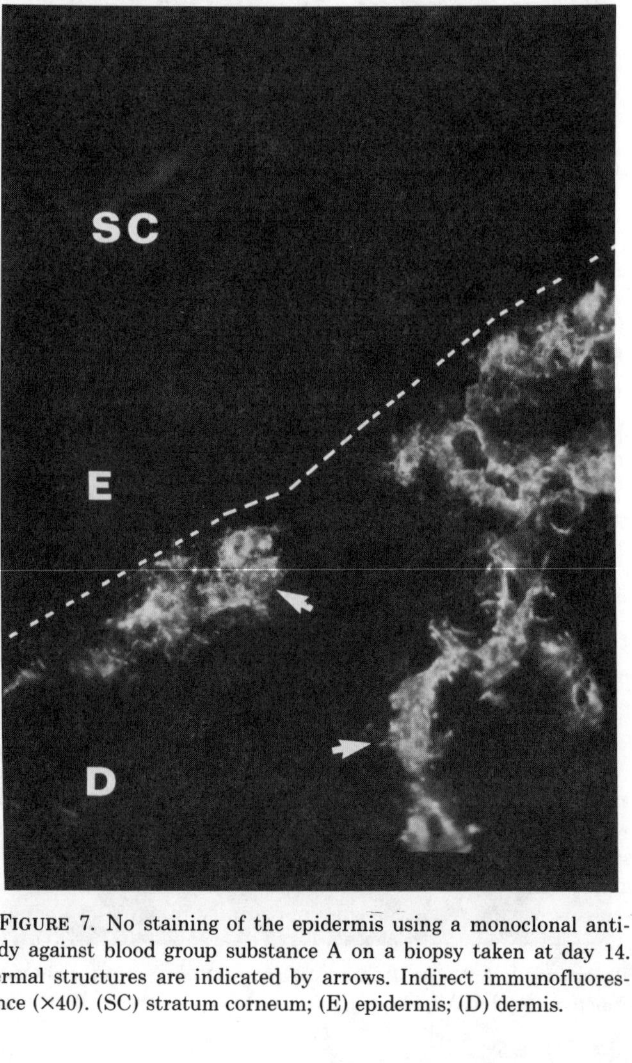

FIGURE 7. No staining of the epidermis using a monoclonal antibody against blood group substance A on a biopsy taken at day 14. Dermal structures are indicated by arrows. Indirect immunofluorescence (×40). (SC) stratum corneum; (E) epidermis; (D) dermis.

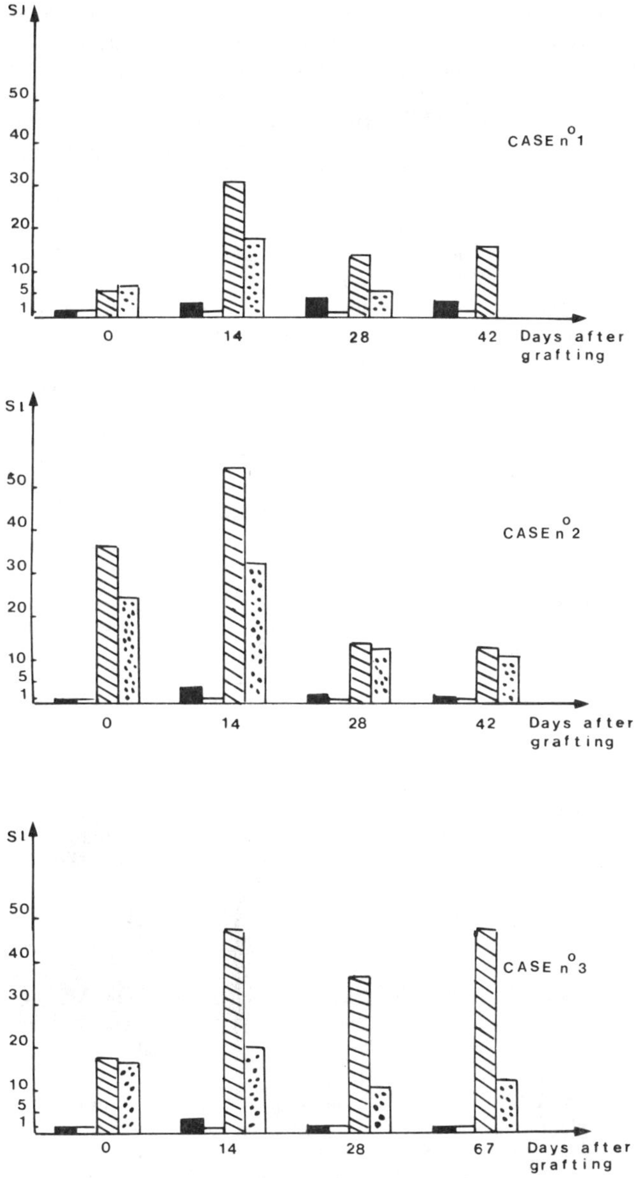

FIGURE 8. Results in allogeneic mixed epidermal cell–lymphocyte cultures. (■) PBL from the recipient and cultured epidermal cells (CEC) from the donor. (□) Control allogeneic PBL and cultured epidermal cells. (▨) PBL from the recipient and allogeneic unrelated epidermal cells (epidermal cells obtained from skin specimens, not from cultures, and containing HLA-DR(+)Langerhans cells. (⊠) Control PBL and allogeneic unrelated epidermal cells.

$$\text{SI} = \text{stimulation index, i.e.} = \frac{\text{cpm of PBL in MELC}}{\text{cpm of PBL alone}}$$

Note that CEC are unable to stimulate control allogeneic PBL (□) or PBL from the recipients (■) (day 0) and that no—or only a weak—proliferative response of the recipient PBL to CEC is observed in MELC conducted 14, 28, 42, or 67 days after grafting (■).

stances, has been achieved in pair 1, and shows that no A substance from the recipient was expressed by epidermal cells at the site where grafts had been performed. For technical reasons, we did not have the opportunity to conduct a similar IF study on the grafted area of patient 3 with anti-A MCA. This would have been the mirror-image experiment for the data obtained in patient 1, and would have covered all possible objections about the origin of the epithelial cells in the donor area (e.g., that epidermal cells do not express blood group substances for physiological reasons, such as extensive cell division or inflammation in the underlying dermis during the healing process). Studies are now in progress to study other similar pairs (A donors and O recipients), but also using karyotyping as a further control of this identity between cultured epidermal cells and keratinocytes present at the graft site months after the covering of the wound.

In vitro responses in the mixed epidermal lymphocyte cultures correlated well the prolonged survival. In MELC, PBL proliferate upon stimulation with allogeneic epidermal cells (*10*). The response depends upon the presence of class II antigen expressing Langerhans cells among the allogeneic cell suspensions used as stimulating cells (*10, 12, 13*). The MELC has been demonstrated to be identical to the classic one-way mixed lymphocyte culture reaction (*14*). In the present study, cultured epidermal cells from each donor failed to stimulate allogeneic PBL—either cells from the recipients or cells from unrelated individuals—a finding that can be related to the lack of Langerhans cells (*14, 15*), which are the only epidermal cells that express the class II antigen in normal noninflammatory epidermis (*16*), in the epithelial cultures used as allografts, and as a source of stimulating cells in MELC. Only a very weak stimulation—or even an absence of response (pair 3)—of the recipient cells was noted in MELC that was conducted 2, 4, and 6 weeks after grafting, but it did not increase with time, and was not within the allogeneic response ranges noted when the same cells were induced to proliferate in response to unrelated Langerhans-cell-undepleted epidermal cell suspensions. These findings show that immunocompetent cells from the recipients are not able to recognize and to be stimulated by Langerhans-cell-depleted epidermal cells from the epidermal cultures, even after these epidermal grafts have been used as allografts. However, the very weak stimulation that could be observed contrasted with the absence of allostimulation noted both at the time of grafting and when unrelated allogeneic PBL were tested against the cultured cells. This suggests that, even in the absence of class-II-antigen–positive cells in the EAG, the grafted keratinocytes were able to induce a kind of minor sensitization in the recipient. This was not sufficient to lead to a full allogeneic response—as evidenced by the minor proliferation in MELC two weeks after the introduction of the EAG into the recipients—or to the rejection of the grafts, as noted clinically. Moreover, only mild inflammatory infiltrates were noted on skin biopsies performed at various intervals. No sign of vasculitis, or epidermal damage due to a mononuclear attack of the epidermis could be observed. When Langerhans cells were present (OKT6 and HLA-DR-positive cells), they were located among the dermal infiltrates, or they were occasionally seen in the epidermis. We also noted similar histological findings when using identical cultured epidermal material as autografts—which suggests that such immunopathological observations do not follow the introduction of allogeneic keratinocytes into the recipient; more likely they are due to a nonspecific inflammatory reaction secondary to the surgical trauma and the healing process.

These results must be considered in the light of the immune response to the allograft (*17*). The initiation requires that class-II-antigen–bearing cells are present as stimulatory cells. In a skin allograft, Langerhans and other class-II-positive cells play a major role in immunorecognition and graft injection (*16*).

Contrasting with epidermal cell suspensions obtained from normal skin, cultured epidermis contains only keratinocytes, and no dendritic or other DR-positive cells are present (*14, 15*). This is a unique model of an allograft in the nonimmunodepressed patient (*17, 18*). In the present study, the possibility of an acquired induced immunotolerance cannot be excluded. The investigation of this hypothesis is in progress.

Former investigators (*19, 20*) have reported variable prolongation of nonsyngeneic graft survival of pancreatic, thyroid, ovarian tissue, or skin that had been maintained in vitro prior to transplantation. In man, Hefton et al. (*5*) used epidermal allografts, after in vitro EC cultures, with a rapid healing; however, they did not study the immune response of recipients or give any evidence of the identity of the epidermal coverage present at the site of grafting weeks after transplantation. The present work provides the first evidence that cultured human EAG are tolerated, are not immunologically rejected, and do not induce a significant immune response.

Some applications of these results may be considered. Contrasting with other epidermal cell cultures, including that used by Hefton et al. in their previous report (*5, 21, 22*), the culture system used in the present and some other studies (*1, 2*) provides, from a tiny skin biopsy sample, a sufficient number of epidermal sheets to cover the entire body surface (*2*). Cultured human EAG may be prepared in advance and kept frozen, and serve as permanent substitute skin in the coverage of large burn wounds. Thus, the use of cultured EAG should not be limited by the availability of suitable donor sites and the time required for the growth of the cells in vitro. Results may be extended to other varieties of epithelial cells—such as pancreatic, hepatic, and thymic epithelial cells. Last, but not least, this model could provide the opportunity for studying in depth the mechanisms of acquired tolerance.

Acknowledgments. We thank D. Bemelmans, M.D., D. M. Chabanon, M.D., M. Gaucherand, and C. Ohrt, for their technical assistance, and Pr. J. P. Revillard for his excellent advice in the preparation of this work.

REFERENCES

1. Green H, Kehinde O, Thomas J. Growth of cultured human epidermal cells into multiple epithelia suitable for grafting. Proc Natl Acad Sci USA 1979; 76: 5665.
2. Gallico GG, O'Connor NE, Compton CC, Kehinde O, Green H. Permanent coverage of large burn wounds with autologous cultured human epithelium. N Engl J Med 1984; 311: 448.
3. O'Connor NE, Gallico G, Compton C, Kehinde O, Green H. Grafting of burns with cultured epithelium prepared from autologous epidermal cells. II. Intermediate term results on three pediatric patients. In: Hunt TK, Heppenstall KB, Pines E, Rovee D, eds. Soft and Hard tissue repair: biological and clinical aspects, vol 2. New York: Praeger Scientific, 1984: 283.
4. Thivolet J, Faure M, Demidem A, Mauduit G. Cultured human epidermal allografts are not rejected for a long period. Arch Dermatol Res 1986; 278: 252.
5. Hefton JM, Madden MR, Finkelstein JL, Shires GT. Grafting of burn patients with allografts of cultured epidermal cells. Lancet 1983; 2: 428.
6. Rheinwald JG, Green H. Serial cultivation of strains of human epidermal keratinocytes: the formation of keratinizing colonies from single cells. Cell 1975; 6: 331.
7. Faure M, Frappaz A, Schmitt D, Dezutter-Dambuyant C, Thivolet J. Role of HLA-DR bearing Langerhans and epidermal indeterminate cells in the in vitro generation of alloreactive cytotoxic T cells in man. Cell Immunol 1984; 83: 271.
8. Dabelsteen E, Buschard K, Hakomori S, Young WW. Pattern of distribution of blood group antigens on human epidermal cells during maturation. J Invest Dermatol 1984; 82: 13.
9. Czernielewski J, Faure M, Schmitt D, Thivolet J. Cultures mixtes lymphocytes-cellules épidermiques (CMLE) autologues et allogéniques chez l'homme: approche in vitro des intéractions lymphoépidermiques. Pathol Biol 1982; 30: 688.
10. Faure M, Schmitt D, Dezutter-Dambuyant C, Frappaz A, Gaucherand M, Thivolet J. In vitro studies of human epidermal antigen presenting cells. The mixed skin lymphocyte reaction: an in vitro model for the generation of alloreactive cytotoxic T cells by human epidermal cells. Br J Dermatol 1984; 111(S27): 11.
11. Katz SI, Tamaki K, Sachs DH. Epidermal Langerhans cells are derived from cells originating in bone marrow. Nature 1979; 282: 324.
12. Stingl G, Katz SI, Shevach EM, Rosenthal AS, Green I. Analogous functions of macrophages and Langerhans cells in the initiation of the immune response. J Invest Dermatol 1978; 71: 59.
13. Hirschberg H, Braathen LR, Thorsby E. Antigen presentation by vascular endothelial and epidermal Langerhans cells: the role of HLA-DR. Immunol Rev 1982; 66: 57.
14. Tanaka S, Sakai A. Stimulation of allogeneic lymphocytes by skin epidermal cells in the rat. Transplantation 1979; 27: 194.
15. Czernielewski J, Demarchez M, Prunieras M. Human Langerhans cells in epidermal cell culture, in vitro skin explants and skin grafts onto "Nude" mice. Arch Dermatol Res 1984; 276: 288.
16. Demidem A, Faure M, Dezutter-Dambuyant C, Thivolet J. Loss of allogeneic T cell activating ability and Langerhans cells markers in human epidermal cell cultures. Clin Immunol Immunopathol 1986; 38: 319.
17. Dezutter-Dambuyant C, Cordier G, Schmitt D, Faure M, Laquoi C, Thivolet J. Quantitative evaluation of two distinct cell populations expressing HLA-DR antigens in normal human epidermis. Br J Dermatol 1984; 111: 1.
18. Wood PJ, Streilein JW. Immunogenetic basis of acquired transplantation tolerance. Transplantation 1984; 37: 223.
19. Lafferty KJ, Woolnough J. The origin and mechanism of the allograft rejection. Immunol Rev 1977; 35: 231.
20. Lafferty KJ, Bootes A, Dart G, Talmage DW. Effect of organ culture on the survival of thyroid allografts in mice. Transplantation 1976; 22: 138.
21. Hegre OD, Hickey GE, Marshall S, Serie JR. Modification of allograft immunogenecity in perinatal islets isolated and purified in vitro. Transplantation 1984; 37: 227.
22. Eisinger M, Lee JS, Hefton JM, Darzynkiewicz Z, Chiao JW, De Harven E. Human epidermal cell cultures: growth and differentiation in the absence of dermal components or medium supplements. Proc Natl Acad Sci USA 1979; 76: 5340.
23. Faure M, Eisinger M, Bystryn JC. Decreased expression of epidermal cytoplasmic antigens in cultured human keratinocytes. J Invest Dermatol 1981; 76: 347.

Received 8 October 1985.
Accepted 28 November 1985.

0041-1337/86/4203-0281$02.00/0
TRANSPLANTATION
Vol. 42, No. 3

Printed in U.S.A.

DRUG-INDUCED IN VITRO TOLERANCE TO ALLOGENEIC ANTIGENS

I. Establishment of a Tolerance Induction System in a Fully Allogeneic Murine Combination[1]

Noriaki Tokuda,[2] Hisashi Gondo, Hisanori Mayumi, Kazuto Taniguchi, Kunisuke Himeno, and Kikuo Nomoto

Department of Immunology, Medical Institute of Bioregulation, Kyushu University, Fukuoka, Japan

C3H/HeSlc (H-2^k) spleen cells were cultured with mitomycin C (MMC)-treated C57BL/6CrSlc (H-2^b) spleen cells for 2 days and incubated with 5-fluorouracil (5-FU) for a further 9 hr. Thereafter, those C3H/He spleen cells were recultured with the same allogeneic cells for 5 days. Cell-mediated cytotoxicity (CMC) and mixed lymphocyte reaction (MLR) were profoundly suppressed, antigen-specifically, in such C3H/He spleen cells. In contrast, interleukin 2(IL-2) production was not impaired in the restimulating mixed lymphocyte culture (MLC) with C57BL/6. Moreover, an adequate amount of exogenous IL-2 added to the restimulating MLC did not lead to a restoration of the depressed CMC. Suppressor cell activity in the CMC assay was not detected in the C3H/He spleen cells exposed to such a tolerance induction. These results suggest that the unresponsiveness to alloantigens in CMC and MLR was induced through a clonal deletion mechanism, and there may exist a 5-FU-resistant—thus less-proliferative—cell population that can produce IL-2 even after the tolerance induction.

Despite the extensive clinical use of cyclosporine (*1*), conventional antimitotic drugs, such as cyclophosphamide (CY)* (*2*), azathioprine (*3*), and methotrexate (*4*) are effective as immunosuppressive agents for patients receiving grafts of allogeneic organs or bone marrow cells. As their immunosuppressive activities are nonspecific, the patients are in an immunosuppressive state also against various microorganisms, when the drugs are prescribed for long periods postoperatively. We reported an experimental induction of specific tolerance to allografts in various murine combinations in vivo by giving i.v. viable allo-spleen cell antigens plus i.p. CY 2 days later (*5–11*). In this system, a profound tolerance to skin allografts was induced in H-2-matched combinations and was maintained without any immunosuppressive treatments after grafting (*10, 11*). In contrast, a profound tolerance could not be induced in H-2-mismatched combinations using the same method, although tumor allograft tolerance was induced and maintained for long periods (*5–9*).

As deduced from an analysis of the in vivo system, the mechanism of this form of tolerance seems to be a clonal elimination (*5–11*). The preimmunization with allogeneic antigens may elicit cell division of the reactive clones and the dividing cells would be destroyed by the antimitotic drug CY given 2 days after the antigen stimulation (*5–11*). Furthermore, the difficulty of tolerance induction to skin allografts in H-2-mismatched combinations may be ascribed to the existence of a less-proliferative—thus resistant to CY—population that appears to be responsible for some types of cell-mediated immunity (*5–10*).

In order to establish an in vitro model for further analysis of this in vivo system, we attempted to induce tolerance to alloantigens in vitro, using a method consisting of in vitro presensitization with fully allogeneic antigens plus treatment with 5-fluorouracil (5-FU). This drug was used since CY is not active in vitro (*12*) and 5-FU seems to have little or no influence on nonproliferating cells (*13, 14*). With this in vitro system, cell-mediated cytotoxicity (CMC) and the mixed lymphocyte reaction (MLR) against fully allogeneic antigens were profoundly reduced in the responder cells. The ability to produce interleukin 2 (IL-2) was preserved after the tolerance induction.

MATERIALS AND METHODS

Animals. Inbred male C3H/HeSlc (H-2^k, Mls^c), C57BL/6CrSlc (H-2^b, Mls^b) and DBA/2CrSlc (H-2^c, Mls^a) mice, were obtained from the Shizuoka Laboratory Animal Center (Shizuoka, Japan). Mice 8–12 weeks of age were used for all experiments. Only C3H/He mice were used as the responders.

Cell culture to induce tolerance. Spleen cells were used as responders or stimulators in mixed lymphocyte cultures (MLC). Responder cells (3×10^7) were cocultured with mitomycin C (MMC)-treated (40 μg/ml for 30 min) stimulator cells (1.5×10^7) in 5 ml of RPMI 1640 (GIBCO, Grand Island, NY) medium, supplemented with 10% NU-serum (Collaborative Research, Inc., Lexington, MA), 5×10^{-5} M 2-mercaptoethanol, and antibiotics (100 U/ml penicillin and 100 μg/ml streptomycin) (i.e., complete RPMI medium) in a culture flask (Falcon 3002). Cultures were incubated in a humidified atmosphere containing 5% CO_2 at 37°C.

Presensitization in vitro with allogeneic cells was carried out for 1–3 days before treatment with 5-FU. MMC-treated syngeneic spleen cells were used as control stimulators in presensitization.

Treatment with 5-FU. For this purpose, 1 ml of various concentrations of 5-fluorouracil (5-FU, Kyowa Hakko, Tokyo, Japan), diluted in the complete RPMI medium described above,

[1] This work was supported by a Grant-in Aid for Scientific Research from the Ministry of Education, Science and Culture, Japan.

[2] Address correspondence to: Noriaki Tokuda M.D., Department of Immunology, Medical Institute of Bioregulation, Kyushu University 69, 3-1-1 Maidashi, Higashi-ku, Fukuoka 812, Japan.

* Abbreviations used: CMC, cell-mediated cytotoxicity; Con A, concanavalin A; CY, cyclophosphamide; 5-FU, 5-fluorouracil; IL-2, interleukin 2; MLC, mixed lymphocyte culture(s); MLR, mixed lymphocyte reaction(s); MMC, mitomycin C.

was added to the cultures 1–3 days after the in vitro presensitization of the responders, and 1 ml of the complete RPMI medium was added to all the cultures that were not treated with 5-FU. The cultured cells were washed three times with Hanks' balanced salt solution and then used as responders in the in vitro restimulation with allogeneic cells.

Assay for CMC. After in vitro restimulation for 5 days, the cultures were harvested. The culture condition of the restimulating MLC was the same as that described for the tolerance induction culture. The assay for cytotoxic activity was carried out with a standard microcytotoxicity assay. Concanavalin A (Con A, type IV, Sigma Chemical Co., St. Louis, MO) stimulated spleen cells (5 μg/ml Con A, 5×10^6 cells/ml for 48 hr) were labeled with ^{51}Cr (100 μCi) for 1 hr at 37°C and were used as the target cells. Effector cells and target cells (2×10^4) were incubated in a round-bottomed microplate (Corning, 25850) for 4 hr at 37°C. The complete RPMI medium described above was used for this assay. The amount of ^{51}Cr released in 0.1 ml of supernatant was measured by a well type gamma counter. The percentage of ^{51}Cr-release was calculated by the following formula:

$$\% \text{ cytotoxicity} = \frac{\text{experimental release} - \text{control release}}{\text{maximum release} - \text{control release}} \times 100$$

The maximum release was determined by incubating the target cells with 10% triton X (Wako Pure Chemical Co., Osaka, Japan). The control release was determined by incubating targets with spleen cells from naive mice. The control release was in the range of 15–24% of the maximum release. The data were expressed as the mean value of 6 samples ±SD.

IL-2 source and addition of IL-2 into the restimulating MLC for CMC assay. Rat T cell growth factor (Collaborative Research Inc., Lexington, MA) was used as a source of exogenous IL-2, and was added to the restimulating MLC for CMC assay at a final concentration of 10% (28 half-maximal units/ml).

Assay for IL-2 activity. After tolerance induction, the responder cells were restimulated with antigens homologous to the tolerogen, the third-party antigens, or Con A. MLC supernatants were harvested on the third day of the restimulating MLC described above. Con A supernatants were obtained by stimulating responder cells with Con A (5 μg/ml Con A, 5×10^6 cells/ml) for 24 hr. HT-2 cells, an IL-2 dependent T cell line, were used as targets for the IL-2 assay. HT-2 cells (5×10^3 cells/well) and an aliquot volume of the MLC supernatant (0.1 ml) or the Con A supernatant (0.1 ml) were cocultured in a flat-bottomed microplate for 24 hr. At 6 hr before harvesting, 1 μCi of ^3H-thymidine was added to each well. In this assay also the complete RPMI medium was used. The ^3H-thymidine uptake was measured by a liquid scintillation counter. The IL-2 titer of the supernatants was represented by a half-maximal unit, using a probit analysis (*15*). HT-2 cells were kindly provided by Ross E. Longley, Oklahoma Medical Research Foundation, Ph.D.

Assay for mixed lymphocyte reaction (MLR). The in vitro cultured cells presensitized and treated with 5-FU were used as the responder cells. The responder cells (6×10^5 cells/0.1 ml) and stimulator cells (3×10^5 cells/0.1 ml) were cocultured in a flat-bottomed microplate (Corning 25860) in a humidified atmosphere containing 5% CO_2 at 37°C. The complete RPMI medium described above was used for this assay. Pulse labeling with ^3H-thymidine (1 μCi/well) was carried out 6 hr before harvesting. The results were represented by net cpm/min and stimulation index. The stimulation index was calculated as follows;

$$\text{stimulation index} = \frac{\text{cpm in the presence of MMC-treated allogeneic cells}}{\text{cpm in the presence of MMC-treated syngeneic cells}}$$

The data were expressed as the mean value of triplicate samples ±SD.

Statistics. Student's t test was used for statistical evaluation. A P value of less than 0.05 was considered significant.

RESULTS

Preliminary selections of timing for 5-FU treatment, concentration of 5-FU, and duration of 5-FU treatment. At the initiation of the experiments, we observed by trial and error the optimal conditions for three distinct factors required to induce an optimal tolerant state in vitro. The first factor was the timing of 5-FU treatment after presensitization with allogeneic cells. According to our in vivo results (*5*), the optimal timing of CY treatment was 1–3 days after antigen stimulation. Thus, we tentatively chose 24 hr after initiation of presensitizing MLC because we presumed that the antigen presentation and resulting cell division would occur more smoothly in in vitro MLC than in vivo. The second and third factors were the concentration of 5-FU and the duration of the 5-FU exposure in the presensitizing MLC. Using CMC as a parameter of tolerance, we examined various combinations of concentration and duration, to obtain optimal conditions of tolerance induction, in which the CMC in the tolerized responder cells would be minimized and the CMC in control responder cells (we used responder cells cultured with syngeneic cells for the same period as the presensitization and treated with 5-FU as controls) would be maximized. Consequently, we chose a relatively low concentration (5 μg/ml) and a long exposure period (9 hr) (data not shown). The quality and dose of allogeneic antigens for presensitizing MLC may be another factor related to induction in in vitro tolerance but we fixed this factor, as described in the *Materials and Methods* section, for the purpose of simplicity. Based on these preliminary data, we further examined the conditions described above, to achieve an optimal tolerant state.

Optimal duration for presensitization to induce tolerance. C3H/He spleen cells were cultured with C57BL/6 spleen cells for 1–3 days, then 5-FU was added at a final concentration of 5 μg/ml, and the preparations were cultured for another 9 hr. After washing with Hanks' balanced salt solution, the responders were restimulated with C57BL/6 spleen cells for 5 days and then assayed for cytotoxicity. The activity of CMC against the allogeneic cells was considerably suppressed when the responders were presensitized for two days (Table 1).

Optimal concentration of 5-FU to induce tolerance. Various concentrations of 5-FU were added to the cultures after presensitization of C3H/He spleen cells with C57BL/6 for two days. The responder cells were incubated in the presence of various concentrations of 5-FU for 9 hr. CMC in the groups of cells presensitized with C57BL/6 spleen cells and treated with 5-FU was reduced as the concentration of 5-FU increased (Table 2, lines 1–3). On the other hand, CMC in the groups presensitized with syngeneic cells and treated with 5-FU showed high levels of activities (Table 2, lines 5–7). From this experiment, the optimal concentration of 5-FU required to induce tolerance was confirmed to be 5 μg/ml, and we did not examine a higher

TABLE 1. Optimal duration for presensitization to induce tolerance in C3H/He spleen cells

Presensitization[a]		Treatment with 5-FU[b]		restimulation[c]	% Cytotoxicity to C57BL/6 Con A blasts	
Antigen	Duration	Conc.	duration[d]		50:1[e]	25:1
C57BL/6	24 hr	5 μg/ml	9 hr	C57BL/6	14.6±1.7[f,g]	8.8±1.4[g]
C57BL/6	48 hr	5 μg/ml	9 hr	C57BL/6	0.8±1.0[g]	−1.1±2.8[g]
C57BL/6	72 hr	5 μg/ml	9 hr	C57BL/6	7.6±2.0[g]	3.5±1.8[g]
—	—	—	—	C57BL/6[h]	67.7±2.1	63.2±8.4

[a] C3H/He spleen cells were presensitized with MMC-treated C57BL/6 spleen cells for 1–3 days.
[b] The responders presensitized with allogeneic cells were treated with 5-FU at a concentration of 5 μg/ml for 9 hr.
[c] Restimulation was carried out for 5 days, using MMC-treated C57BL/6 spleen cells as the stimulators.
[d] Concentration.
[e] Effector:target ratio.
[f] Mean ± SD.
[g] Significantly different from control ($P<0.01$).
[h] Untreated normal spleen cells were used as responders (positive control).

concentration, since the degree of tolerance induced in the presence of this concentration of 5-FU appeared to be sufficient for further analytical studies.

When we compared the data on four groups (italicized in Table 2 [lines 1, 4, 5, and 8]) as a presensitization-plus-5-FU group (line 1), a presensitized control group (line 4), a 5-FU control group (line 5), and an untreated culture control group (line 8), tolerance to C57BL/6 with respect to CMC in C3H/He spleen cells was obtained only when the responder cells were presensitized with C57BL/6 and treated with 5-FU. This nature of tolerance induction in vitro is compatible with our previous results obtained in vivo (*5–8*, *10*).

Optimal duration of 5-FU treatment to induce tolerance, and the effect of IL-2 added to the restimulating MLC on CMC. To determine the appropriate duration of 5-FU treatment required to induce unresponsiveness in CMC, C3H/He spleen cells were incubated with 5-FU for 6–12 hr at a concentration of 5 μg/ml, after the presensitization with MMC-treated C57BL/6 spleen cells for 2 days (Table 3). CMC of the presensitized responder cells was depressed, as the duration of treatment with 5-FU increased, and sufficient tolerance to C57BL/6 was achieved only when the responder cells were presensitized with the homologous antigens and treated with 5 μg/ml of 5-FU for more than 9 hr (lines 2 and 3). However, when the duration of 5-FU exposure was increased up to 12 hr, a nonspecific suppression of CMC became significant (line 6). Moreover, the number of surviving cells after the treatment with 5-FU for 12 hr was significantly smaller than that for 9 hr, in both the tolerized group (line 3) and the 5-FU control group (line 6). Therefore, the optimal duration of 5-FU treatment was estimated to be 9 hr. We concluded that the optimal conditions required to induce in vitro tolerance in C3H/He spleen cells to C57BL/6 were as follows: duration of presensitizing culture—48 hr, concentration of 5-FU—5 μg/ml, and duration of 5-FU exposure—9 hr. These conditions were used for tolerance induction in the following experiments. However, these optimal conditions did depend on the responder strains (data not shown).

In this experiment, we also examined the restoring effect of exogenous IL-2 added to the restimulating MLC on CMC in order to elucidate whether the abrogation of CMC could be ascribed to depressed IL-2 production. As shown in Table 3, the addition of exogenous IL-2 did not restore the depressed CMC in the tolerized groups (lines 2 and 3), whereas it did so in nonspecifically depressed groups (lines 4–6). Therefore the tolerant state could not ascribe to depressed IL-2 production.

TABLE 2. Optimal concentration of 5-FU to induce tolerance in C3H/He spleen cells

Presensitization (2 days)[a]	Conc. of 5-FU (μg/ml)[b]	Restimulation[c]	% Cytotoxicity to C57BL/6 Con A blasts	
			100:1	50:1
C57BL/6	5	*C57BL/6*	0.8±2.1[d]	−0.6±0.5[d]
C57BL/6	3	C57BL/6	4.3±0.5[d]	3.1±0.5[d]
C57BL/6	1	C57BL/6	14.8±1.8[d]	13.6±2.8[d]
C57BL/6	0	*C57BL/6*	56.8±4.4	57.2±2.9
C3H/He	5	*C57BL/6*	65.1±0.7	65.8±2.3
C3H/He	3	C57BL/6	63.4±1.3	54.2±1.4
C3H/He	1	C57BL/6	64.6±2.4	60.2±4.8
C3H/He	0	*C57BL/6*	31.4±1.4	30.7±1.1
—	—	C57BL/6[e]	69.7±2.1	66.0±2.1

[a] C3H/He spleen cells were presensitized with MMC-treated C57BL/6 or C3H/He spleen cells for 2 days.
[b] Final concentration of 5-FU in the cultures.
[c] See footnote *c* of Table 1.
[d] Significantly different from the data without treatment with 5-FU ($P<0.01$).
[e] Untreated normal spleen cells were used as responders (positive control).

IL-2 production in C3H/He spleen cells after tolerance induction. As indicated by the foregoing results, the elimination of reactive cytotoxic T cell precursor populations seems plausible. However, it was not definitely determined whether the reactive helper T cell population is also eliminated by the tolerance induction. We next examined the IL-2 producing ability of the responder presensitized and treated with 5-FU.

These results are shown in Table 4. In this experiment, we prepared only a 5-FU control group as the control, because the highest level of CMC was detected in this group, as described above (Table 2, line 5). IL-2 production in responder cells after tolerance induction to C57BL/6 was maintained normally in the MLC with C57BL/6 compared with the 5-FU control group (Table 4), thereby suggesting that the helper T cell population remained appreciably intact even after tolerance induction. IL-2 production in the responder cells tolerized to C57BL/6 was also maintained normally in the MLC, with the third-party antigen (DBA/2) and in the culture with Con A (Table 4).

Specificity of tolerance in CMC assay. In order to demonstrate that C3H/He responder cells from restimulating MLC with C57BL/6 do kill C57BL/6 in a specific manner, the responder cells were examined for their CMC activity against DBA/2 Con A blasts (Table 5). After restimulating MLC with C57BL/6,

TABLE 3. Optimal duration of treatment with 5-FU to induce tolerance in C3H/He spleen cells, and the effect of IL-2 added to the restimulating MLC on CMC

Presensitization (2 days)	Treatment with 5-FU[a]		Restimulation[b]	% Cytotoxicity to C57BL/6 Con A blast			
				Normal restimulating MLC		Addition of IL-2 in the restimulating MLC[c]	
	Conc.	Duration		50:1	25:1	50:1	25:1
C57BL/6	5 μg/ml	6 hr	C57BL/6	7.6±1.3	4.8±0.7	13.3±1.1	9.7±1.3
C57BL/6	5 μg/ml	9 hr	C57BL/6	2.6±1.0	2.1±0.9	2.7±1.4	2.8±1.3
C57BL/6	5 μg/ml	12 hr	C57BL/6	1.2±0.5	1.7±1.2	0.4±0.9	2.0±1.2
C3H/He	5 μg/ml	6 hr	C57BL/6	44.1±2.6	29.4±3.3	58.4±1.7	44.7±2.6
C3H/He	5 μg/ml	9 hr	C57BL/6	21.0±0.3	13.3±1.0	46.8±3.1	32.1±2.2
C3H/He	5 μg/ml	12 hr	C57BL/6	16.0±1.4	6.4±1.3	49.7±3.5	31.0±0.5
—	—	—	C57BL/6[d]	72.0±5.9	63.3±2.0	ND[e]	ND

[a] C3H/He spleen cells were presensitized with MMC-treated C57BL/6 or C3H/He spleen cells for 2 days and treated with 5-FU for 6, 9, or 12 hr.
[b] See footnote *c* of Table 1.
[c] IL-2 was added to the cultures at the concentration of 10% (28 U/ml).
[d] Untreated normal spleen cells were used as responders (positive control).
[e] Not done.

TABLE 4. IL-2 producing ability in C3H/He spleen cells presensitized with C57BL/6 and treated with 5-FU

Presentitization (2 days)	Treatment with 5-FU		Titer of IL-2[a] stimulator[b]		
	Conc.	Duration	C57BL/2	DBA/2	Con A
C57BL/6	5 μg/ml	9 hr	2.7 U/ml	4.3 U/ml	6.1 U/ml
C3H/He	5 μg/ml	9 hr	2.9 U/ml	3.3 U/ml	4.6 U/ml

[a] Titer of IL-2 was assessed by a probit analysis, using HT-2 cells.
[b] C57BL/6, DBA/2 spleen cells or Con A were used as stimulators to raise endogenous IL-2. MLC supernatants, after stimulation with MMC-treated DBA/2 or C57BL/6 spleen cells, were harvested on the third day of the restimulating MLC. Con A supernatants were obtained by stimulating cells with Con A (5 μg/ml, 5×10^6 cells/ml) for 24 hr.

high levels of CMC activity against C57BL/6 were detected in the presensitized control (line 1), untreated culture control (line 3), and 5-FU control (line 4) groups. However, CMC against DBA/2 was not detected in all three control groups. In the presensitized-plus-5-FU group (line 2), CMC against C57BL/6 or DBA/2 was not detected. In contrast, the responder cells from the naive positive control group showed a weak level of CMC activity against the third-party targets (line 5). The same result was obtained when we used EL-4 (H-2^b) and P815 (H-2^d) tumor cells as the target cells (data not shown).

Next, C3H/He spleen cells tolerized to C57BL/6 were examined for their ability to provoke CMC against the third-party antigens (DBA/2). After the MLC with DBA/2 for 5 days, an appreciable level of CMC against DBA/2 was detected in the tolerant group, as compared with 5-FU control group (Table 6).

Lack of suppressor cells in tolerized responder cells. In vivo tolerance induction by our method was ascribed to a clonal deletion and not to the contribution of suppressor cells (*5*). In this in vitro system, we could exclude the contribution of suppressor cells, as shown in the following experiment. Spleen cells from naive C3H/He mice were mixed with C3H/He spleen cells tolerized to C57BL/6 immediately before restimulating MLC with C57BL/6 (Table 7, line 3). CMC was not suppressed in this group compared with a group not mixed with the tolerized cells (line 2 versus line 3). In other words, the unresponsiveness of the tolerized responder cells was abrogated by adding naive syngeneic cells to the culture (line 1 versus line 3). These results suggest that the mechanism of this in vitro tolerance to fully allogeneic antigens is clonal elimination and not induction of suppressor cells.

Abrogated MLR after tolerance induction and its specificity. As described in the *Introduction*, the mechanism of this type of tolerance, determined using antimitotic drugs, is considered to be destruction of dividing cells in which the division is provoked by presensitization with allogeneic antigens. If so, the activity of lymphocyte proliferation of the responders, presensitized and treated with 5-FU, should be profoundly reduced. Such was the case, as shown in Figure 1. The cell proliferation in the tolerized responder cells was extremely weak compared with events in the control groups (naive cells not precultured and the 5-FU controls). This unresponsiveness of the tolerized responder cells in MLR was also tolerogen-specific (Table 8).

DISCUSSION

In contrast to the in vivo tolerance induction to alloantigens, there are only a few reports on in vitro systems, such as a hot-pulse technique (*16–18*), and a bromodeoxyuridine and light method (*19–22*). On the basis of our prevous results in vivo (*5–11*), we designed a system for the in vitro induction of specific unresponsiveness to allogeneic antigens in CMC and MLR. Here the responder cells were presensitized with allogeneic antigens and treated with 5-FU.

The mechanism of this in vitro specific tolerance in CMC is considered to be clonal elimination, as described above, because the tolerance was achieved only in the presensitization-plus-5-FU groups (Table 2). The possibilities that the tolerance was induced by presensitizing MLC alone (such as suppressor cell induction) or by 5-FU alone (nonspecific suppression) were excluded. Moreover, probable induction of suppressor cells in the tolerant group was excluded in other experiments (Table 6). Since the tolerance in CMC was associated with profound depression of MLR throughout the restimulating MLC period (Fig. 1), the proposal that the division is provoked by presensitization with allogeneic antigens and is destroyed by the antimitotic drug—and, as a result, that the reactive cell population is clonally eliminated (*6, 8, 10*)—seems plausible.

In contrast to the tolerance-inducible—i.e., highly proliferative and antimitotic drug-sensitive—cell population, we reported the existence of a cell population that is less proliferative in response to H-2-mismatched antigens in the in vivo system

TABLE 5. Specificity of CMC

Presensitization (2 days)	Treatment with 5-FU		Restimulation	% Cytotoxicity to Con A blasts			
				C57BL/6		DBA/2	
	Conc.	Duration		50:1	25:1	50:1	25:1
C57BL/6	0 μg/ml	9 hr	C57BL/6	27.5±3.0	25.8±4.5	−4.0±5.3	−2.5±1.0
C57BL/6	5 μg/ml	9 hr	C57BL/6	−1.9±4.2	0.7±5.2	−2.0±6.9	−5.3±10.0
C3H/He	0 μg/ml	9 hr	C57BL/6	61.8±5.7	57.0±5.4	−3.2±3.7	−2.1±8.8
C3H/He	5 μg/ml	9 hr	C57BL/6	31.3±3.9	31.5±4.4	−5.5±7.7	−0.8±6.5
—	—	—	C57BL/6[a]	49.9±4.8	46.0±4.8	8.3±5.0	6.6±3.0

[a] Untreated normal spleen cells were used as responders (positive control).

TABLE 6. Specificity of unresponsiveness in CMC assay

Presensitization (2 days)	Treatment with 5-FU		% Cytotoxicity to Con A blasts Stimulator cells in restimulation[a]			
			C57BL/6		DBA/2	
	Conc.	Duration	50:1	25:1	50:1	25:1
C57BL/6	5 μg/ml	9 hr	−5.2±8.3[b]	−7.2±7.4[b]	27.1±12.0	24.9±5.1
C3H/He	5 μg/ml	9 hr	28.0±10.4	21.2±8.7	46.6±7.5	36.6±10.6

[a] C57BL/6 or DBA/2 spleen cells were used as the stimulators in the restimulating MLC and as targets for CMC assay.
[b] Significantly different from control ($P<0.01$).

TABLE 7. Lack of suppressor cells in C3H/He spleen cells presensitized with C57BL/6 and treated with 5-FU

No. responder cells		Stimulator cells	% Cytotoxicity to C57BL/6 Con A blasts[c]	
Presensitized and 5-FU-treated cells[a]	Naive cells[b]		50:1	25:1
2×10^7	—	C57BL/6	1.9±1.7	1.7±2.4
—	2×10^7	C57BL/6	24.3±2.7	18.2±2.1
2×10^7	2×10^7	C57BL/6	39.2±2.0	21.3±2.2
4×10^7	—	C57BL/6	5.4±1.8	0.9±2.2
—	4×10^7	C57BL/6	51.4±3.5	33.7±2.9

[a] C3H/He spleen cells were presensitized with MMC-treated C57BL/6 spleen cells for 2 days and treated with 5-FU (5 μg/ml) for 9 hr.
[b] Naive cells were obtained from normal C3H/He mice.
[c] Responder cells were cocultured with stimulator cells (C57BL/6) for 5 days and then assayed for cytotoxicity.

TABLE 8. Specificity of unresponsiveness in the MLR assay

Presensitization (2 days)	Treatment with 5-FU		^{3}H-thymidine uptake[a] stimulator cells in restimulation[b]	
	Conc.	Duration	C57BL/6	DBA/2
C57BL/6	5 μg/ml	9 hr	3672±826[c] (0.8±0.2)	49800±3720 (10.8±0.8)
C3H/He	5 μg/ml	9 hr	17000±2050 (15.6±1.9)	47700±373 (43.8±3.4)
—	—	—[d]	10300±7280 (84.1±5.9)	89700±3260 (73.0±2.7)

[a] The assay of ^{3}H-thymidine uptake was done 4 days after restimulation.
[b] MMC-treated C57BL/6 or DBA/2 spleen cells were used as stimulators in the restimulating MLC.
[c] Net cpm (stimulation index).
[d] Untreated normal spleen cells were used as responders (positive control).

(*5–10*)—and, thus, is CY-resistant. This population is considered to be responsible for some types of cell-mediated immunity, such as delayed foot-pad reaction and a part of CMC (*5–8, 10*). Although there are differences between the in vivo and in vitro systems (see below), a 5-FU-resistant, less-proliferative, cell population that can still produce IL-2 after tolerance induction in vitro was identified in the present study. IL-2-producing cells may be helper T cells that bear the phenotype of Lyt-1$^+$ (*23, 24*), although this proposal has been questioned (*25*). We have not yet done the Lyt-marker analysis—however, the 5-FU-resistant cells are probably helper T cells. According to reports by other investigators (*26, 27*), lymphocyte cell lines obtained by the limiting dilution method were relatively proliferative, and many of such cell lines were helper T cells. There is some inconsistency between such findings and our result. However, we tentatively consider that most of helper T cells may be less proliferative. This explanation is compatible with the fact that helper T cells are usually radioresistant (*25*).

If we compare the in vitro tolerance induction system with the in vivo system in the same murine combination disparate in both H-2 and non H-2 antigens, the tolerance in CMC may be more profound in the in vitro than in the in vivo system, because a low level of CMC was detectable even after the tolerance induction in vivo but not in vitro. This remaining CMC activity after the in vivo tolerance induction could not be abrogated completely even when we increased the dose of CY up to 200 mg/kg (unpublished data). Further increments in the CY dose were not given because high doses have untoward effects in the recipient mice (another reason for establishing an in vitro system). Other possibilities are that the restimulating MLC was carried out immediately after tolerance induction culture in vitro, while the CMC assay in vivo was usually done 2–4 weeks after the tolerance induction according to another schedule (*5, 6, 8, 10*). Moreover, in the in vitro system, there is no influence of primary lymphoid organs, such as the bone marrow and thymus, on the tolerance induction (*8, 10*).

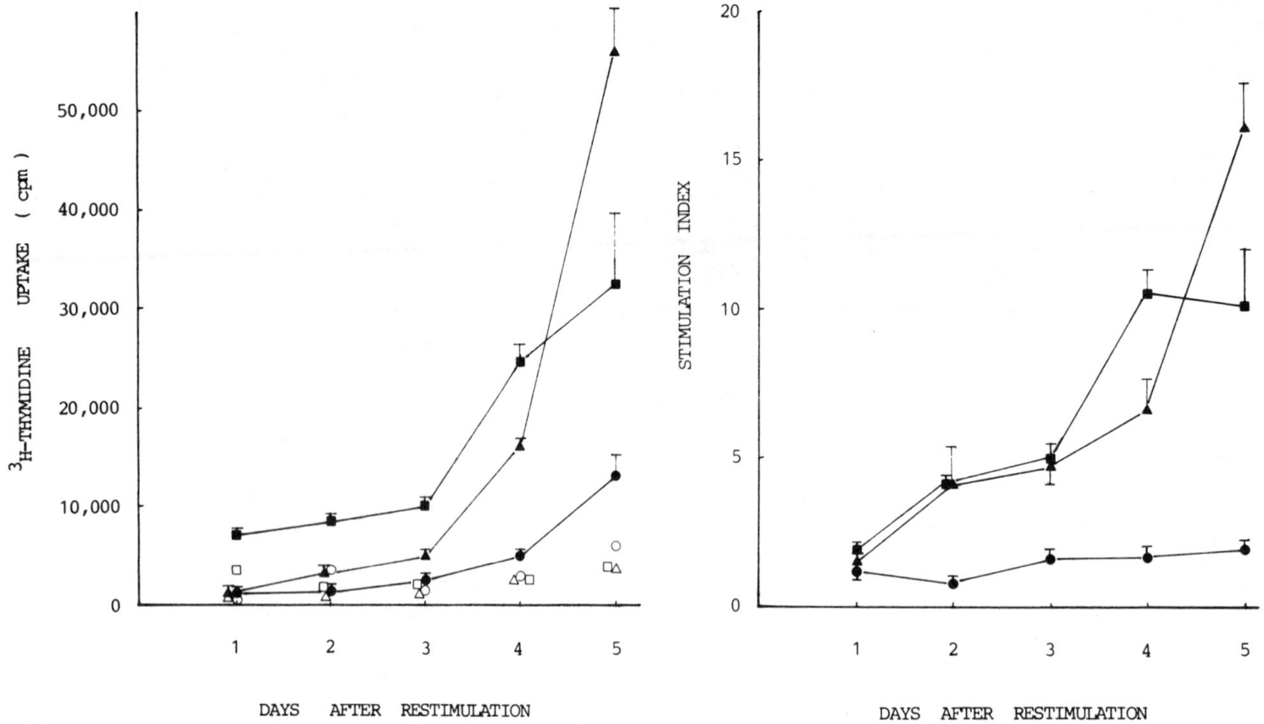

FIGURE 1. Abrogated MLR in C3H/He spleen cells presensitized with C57BL/6 and treated with 5-FU (9 hr). C3H/He spleen cells presensitized with C57BL/6 (2 days) and treated with 5-FU (9 hr) (○), C3H/He spleen cells presensitized with C3H/He (2 days) and treated with 5-FU (9 hr) (△), or naive C3H/He spleen cells without the preceding culture (□) were used as responders. These cells were stimulated with MMC-treated C57BL/6 (black symbols) and C3H/He (white symbols) spleen cells for one to five days. Proliferation was assessed by ^{3}H-thymidine uptake. Data were expressed by net cpm (left) and stimulation index (right). Vertical bars represent standard deviations.

Acknowledgment. We thank Ms. M. Ohara of Kyushu University for comments on the manuscript.

REFERENCES

1. Borel JF, Feurer C, Gubler HU, Stahelin H. Biological effects of cyclosporin A: a new lymphocytic agent. Agents Action 1976; 6: 468.
2. Storb R, Thomas ED, Weiden PL, et al. One hundred ten patients with aplastic anemia treated by marrow transplantation in Seattle. Transplant Proc 1978; 10: 135.
3. Starzl TE, Marchioro TL, Wadel WR. The reversal of rejection in human renal homografts with subsequent development of homograft tolerance. Surg Gynecol Obstet 1963; 117: 385.
4. Appelbaum FR, Clift RA, Buckner CD, et al. Allogeneic marrow transplantation for acute nonlymphoblastic leukemia after first relapse. Blood 1983; 61: 949.
5. Shin T, Mayumi H, Himeno K, Sanui H, Nomoto K. Drug-induced tolerance to allografts in mice. I. Difference between tumor and skin grafts. Transplantation 1984; 37: 580.
6. Mayumi H, Shin T, Himeno K, Nomoto K. Drug-induced tolerance to allografts in mice. II. Tolerance to tumor allografts of large doses associated with rejection of skin allografts and tumor allografts of small doses. Immunobiology 1985; 169: 147.
7. Shin T, Himeno K, Mayumi H, Nomoto K. Drug-induced tolerance to allografts in mice. III. Prolongation of skin graft survival by tolerance induction in congeneic mice disparate in the major H-2 antigens. Transplantation 1985; 39: 333.
8. Mayumi H, Himeno K, Shin T, Nomoto K. Drug-induced tolerance to allografts in mice. IV. Mechanisms and kinetics of cyclophosphamide-induced tolerance. Transplantation 1985; 39: 209.
9. Mayumi H, Kayashima K, Shin T, Nomoto K. Drug-induced tolerance to allografts in mice. V. Prolongation of skin graft survival in tolerant mice with combined immunosuppressive treatments. Transplantation 1985; 39: 335.
10. Mayumi H, Himeno K, Shin T, Nomoto K. Drug-induced tolerance to allografts in mice. VI. Tolerance induction in H-2 haplotype-identical strain combinations in mice. Transplantation 1985; 40: 188.
11. Mayumi H, Himeno K, Tokuda N, Nomoto K. Drug-induced tolerance to allografts in mice. VIII. Effect of thymectomy and/or splenectomy on tolerance induction in a H-2 haplotype-identical strain combination. Transplantation (in press)
12. Hill DL. Pharmacology. In: A review of cyclophosphamide. Springfield: Charles C Thomas, 1975: 60.
13. Lin H. Differential lethal effect of cytotoxic agents on proliferating and nonproliferating lymphoid cells. Cancer Res 1973; 33: 1716.
14. Lin H. Schedule-dependent effect of phase-specific cytotoxic agents on production of hemolytic plaque-forming cells. J Natl Cancer Institute 1976; 56: 95.
15. Gillis S, Ferm MM, Ou W, Smith KA. T cell growth factor: parameters of production and a quantitative microassay for activity. J Immunol 1978; 120: 2027.
16. Dutton RW, Mishell RI. Cell population and cell proliferation in the in vitro response of normal mouse spleen to heterologous erythrocytes. Analysis by the hot pulse technique. J Exp Med 1967; 126: 443.
17. Peavy DL, Pierce CW. Cell-mediated immune response in vitro. III. Elimination of specific cytotoxic lymphocyte responses by ^{3}H-thymidine suicide. J Immunol 1975; 115: 1521.
18. Cantor H, Jandinski J. The relationship of cell division to the generation of cytotoxic activity in mixed lymphocyte culture. J Exp Med 1974; 140: 1712.
19. Zoschke DC, Bach FH. Specificity of antigen recognition by human lymphocytes in vitro. Science 1970; 170: 1404.

20. Janewy CA, Murphy PD, Kemp J, Wigzell H. T cell specific for hapten-modified self are precommited for self major histocompatibility complex antigens before encounter with the hapten. J Exp Med 1978; 147: 1065.
21. Maryanski JL, Cerottini J, Brunner KT. Susceptibility of proliferating cytolytic T lymphocytes to 33258 Hoechst-modified BudR and light treatment: quantitation of the residual precursor cells by limiting dilution analysis. J Immunol 1980; 124: 839.
22. Rammensee H-G, Bevan MJ. Evidence from in vitro studies that tolerance to self antigens is MHC-restricted. Nature 1984; 308: 741.
23. Klein J. Mixed lymphocyte reaction. In: Immunology: the science of self-nonself discrimination. New York: Wiley-Interscience, 1982: 457.
24. Hogarth PM, McKenzie IFC. Lymphocyte antigens. In: Paul EW, ed. Immunogenetics. New York: Raven Press, 1984: 169.
25. Pilarski LM, McKenzie FC. Requirement for help in the generation of alloantigen-specific helper cells. Transplantation 1985; 40: 305.
26. Glasebrook AL, Fitch FW. Alloreactive cloned T cell lines. I. Interaction between cloned amplifier and cytolytic T cell lines. J Exp Med 1980; 151: 876.
27. Watson J. Continuous proliferation of murine antigen-specific helper T lymphocytes in culture. J Exp Med 1979; 150: 1510.

Received 29 July 1985.
Accepted 16 December 1985.

0041-1337/86/4203-0287$02.00/0
TRANSPLANTATION
Vol. 42, No. 3

Printed in U.S.A.

SUPPRESSION OF THE IMMUNE RESPONSE TO ALLOGENEIC HISTOCOMPATIBILITY ANTIGENS BY A SINGLE EXPOSURE TO ULTRAVIOLET RADIATION[1]

STEPHEN E. ULLRICH[2]

Department of Immunology, The University of Texas M. D. Anderson Hospital and Tumor Institute at Houston, Texas 77030

Sensitization of C3H mice with allogeneic BALB/c spleen cells after a single exposure to ultraviolet (UV) radiation renders the mice incapable of generating an effective delayed-type hypersensitivity (DTH) response against BALB/c cells. In addition to the depressed DTH response, spleen cells from the UV-irradiated mice are unable to proliferate to alloantigen in a one-way mixed lymphocyte reaction (MLR). This inability to respond to alloantigen appears to be mediated by suppressor T cells, in that nylon-wool-nonadherent cells from the spleens of the UV-irradiated mice could suppress the MLR response of normal spleen cells to allogeneic spleen cells. In addition, the amount of interleukin-2 (IL-2) in the supernatants of the suppressed MLR cultures was also decreased. In all cases, the observed suppression was specific for the antigen used to sensitize the UV-irradiated animals. These data suggest that UV radiation can be used as an agent to induce a selective suppression of immune reactivity against allogeneic cells.

Ultraviolet (UV)* radiation is a highly selective immunosuppressive agent (*1*). Chronic exposure of mice to UV radiation results in the induction of highly antigenic skin cancers (*2*). Long before the primary tumors arise, suppressor T lymphocytes can be found in the lymphoid organs of these mice (*3*, *4*).These suppressor cells have been implicated in the development of the primary UV-induced tumors (*5*) as well as the inability to reject the transplanted tumors (*3*, *4*). The suppressive activity of these cells is highly selective. Only the rejection of UV-induced tumors is suppressed. The rejection of other syngeneic tumors is unaffected (*4*). In all other respects the immune status of these mice (i.e., antibody formation, mitogen reactivity, generation of cytotoxic lymphocytes, and allograft rejection) appears to be normal (*6*, *7*, *8*).

The exact mechanism by which UV radiation suppresses the immune response is not entirely clear. In addition to the induction of suppressor cells, UV radiation has been shown to cause an impairment in antigen-presenting cell (APC) function. Greene et al. (*9*) demonstrated that immunization of UV-irradiated mice with hapten-modified APC isolated from UV-treated animals failed to induce a hapten-specific delayed-type hypersensitivity (DTH) response. Subsequent studies by Letvin et al. (*10*) demonstrated a correlation between impairment of APC function with a decrease in the numbers of I-A-positive cells in the spleens of UV-irradiated mice. In addition, Greene et al. (*9*) also reported that immunization of a UV-irradiated mouse with UV-treated haptenated APC not only failed to induce DTH but rather caused the induction of hapten-specific suppressor T cells. A similar finding was reported by Sauder et al. (*11*). Immunization with hapten-modified UV-irradiated epidermal cells resulted in a decreased DTH response with the appearance of suppressor T cells. Recently, Granstein (*12*) has reported that a novel I-J-bearing UV-resistant APC in the

[1] This work was supported by Grant RR5511-22 from the National Institutes of Health, funds from the Kleberg Foundation, and funds from U. T. M. D. Anderson Annual Campaign, a project of The University of Texas Cancer Fund Board of Visitors.

[2] Address correspondence to: Stephen E. Ullrich, Ph.D., Department of Immunology, HMB 178, The University of Texas M. D. Anderson Hospital and Tumor Institute, 6723 Bertner Avenue, Houston, TX 77030.

* Abbreviations used: APC, antigen-presenting cell; CHS, contact hypersensitivity; DTH, delayed-type hypersensitivity; IL-2 interleukin-2; MLR, mixed lymphocyte reaction; NR, nonirradiated controls; SRBC, sheep erythrocytes; UV, ultraviolet.

epidermis activates suppressor cells rather than the helper cell pathway. These findings point out the UV-induced alteration in APC function and suggest that the effect of UV radiation on APC function and the induction of suppressor T cells may be linked.

Our studies have been concerned with understanding the immunosuppression that results after a single exposure to UV radiation. After a single exposure to UV radiation, mice are incapable of responding to contact allergens applied to distant unirradiated skin. Associated with this suppression of contact hypersensitivity (CHS) is a defect in splenic APC function (*13*), as well as the induction of suppressor T cells (*14*). In order to activate the suppressive pathway at least two signals are required: exposure to UV radiation and epicutaneous sensitization with hapten (*15, 16*). Exposure to UV radiation alone, or epicutaneous sensitization with an immunogenic dose of hapten, will not induce suppression. Our recent studies have been concerned with the nature of the antigenic stimulus required to induce suppression after exposure to UV radiation. We have reported that the s.c. sensitization of a UV-irradiated mouse with complex antigens, such as proteins or sheep erythrocytes, can also activate the suppressive pathway (*17*). The epicutaneous application of hapten or the sensitization with hapten-modified cells is not an absolute requirement to induce suppression in this system. These findings suggest that suppression of the immune response to a variety of complex cellular antigens may be accomplished by the s.c. sensitization of a UV-irradiated mouse. Here we test this hypothesis by examining the effect UV radiation has on DTH to allogeneic spleen cells. We found that DTH to alloantigen could be depressed by a single exposure of mice to UV radiation five days prior to sensitization. This depression was reflected by the inability of spleen cells from these mice to proliferate in a one-way mixed lymphocyte response (MLR). In addition, spleen cells from the UV-irradiated mice could suppress the MLR of normal cells to alloantigen in an antigen-specific manner.

MATERIALS AND METHODS

Animals. Specific-pathogen-free female C3H/HeN Cr (MTV^-), BALB/c AnN, and C57BL/6N mice were supplied by the National Cancer Institute, Frederick Cancer Research Facility Animal Production Area. The mice were housed and cared for according to the guidelines set forth by the Guide for the Care and Use of Laboratory Animals (Department of Health and Human Services Publication No. (NIH) 78-23).

Treatment of mice with UV radiation. These methods have been published in detail elsewhere (*16*). Briefly, the dorsal hair of the mice was removed with electric clippers. The animals were then exposed for 3 hr to UVB (280–320 nm) radiation. The source of the radiation was a bank of six FS-40 sunlamps. The total incident dose of radiation received by the mice was 30–40 kJ/m^2.

Induction of DTH to alloantigen. A modification of the procedure of Liew (*18*) was used. BALB/c nucleated spleen cells (10^8) were injected s.c. into two sites on each flank of each recipient C3H mouse. Six days later, the footpad thickness of the sensitized mice was measured by the use of an engineer's micrometer (Swiss Precision Instruments, Los Angeles, CA). The mice were then challenged by the injection of 10^7 BALB/c spleen cells into each hind footpad, and 24 hr later, the footpad swelling in response to the challenge was determined. The background response was determined by measuring the footpad swelling observed in mice that were not sensitized with antigen but were challenged with 10^7 spleen cells. The specific footpad swelling was calculated by subtracting the footpad swelling found in the nonsensitized controls from that observed in the sensitized animals. All UV irradiation was done 5 days prior to antigenic sensitization.

Generation of an MLR in vitro. Whole spleen cells from C3H, UV-treated mice sensitized with BALB/c spleen cells or cells from nonirradiated (NR), C3H mice also sensitized with BALB/c cells were used as responder cells in a one-way MLR. The stimulator cells were either mitomycin-C-treated (50 $\mu g/ml/10^7$ cells, incubated for 30 min at 37°C) BALB/c or C57BL/6 spleen cells. The stimulator and responder cells were suspended in RPMI 1640 medium supplemented with 10% fetal calf serum, 5×10^{-5}M 2 mercaptoethanol, 100 units/ml penicillin, 100 $\mu g/ml$ streptomycin, 2 mM L-glutamine, vitamins, nonessential amino acids, and 10 mM Hepes buffer (GIBCO, Grand Island, NY). In general, 2×10^5 responder cells and 2×10^5 stimulator cells were cultured together in a U-bottomed 96-well microtiter dish for 5 days at 37°C. During the last 18 hr of culture, 1 μCi/well of tritiated thymidine was added (ICN Radiochemical, Irvine, CA). The radioactivity incorporated by the responder cells was determined by harvesting the cells into glass fiber filters followed by liquid scintillation counting.

Determination of suppressor cell activity. Spleen cells from UV-irradiated and NR control mice were passed through nylon-wool columns according to the procedure described by Julius et al. (*19*). The nonadherent fraction was then added to cultures containing responder cells from normal C3H mice and mitomycin-C-treated C57BL/6 or BALB/c stimulator cells. These cells were then cultured together for 5 days in 96-well microtiter dishes, as described above.

The effect of UV irradiation on the generation of IL-2. The proliferation of an IL-2-dependent cell line, HT-2 ([*20*] generously provided by Dr. Susan Rich, Baylor College of Medicine) was used to measure IL-2 activity. Mixed lymphocyte cultures consisting of 10^7 responder cells from UV-treated mice were cultured with 10^7 mitomycin-C-treated stimulator cells for 3 days in 24-well cluster dishes. Serial dilutions of the supernatant from the MLR cultures were then added to 5000 HT-2 cells in 96-well microtiter dishes. The cells were cultured for 24 hr; during the last 6 hr of culture, 1 μCi/well of tritiated thymidine was added. The radioactivity incorporated by the HT-2 cells was measured as described above. As a positive control for these experiments, various dilutions of partially purified rat IL-2 (Collaborative Research, Lexington, MA) were added to the HT-2 cells.

RESULTS

The effects of UV radiation on the DTH response to alloantigen are shown in Table 1. Sensitization of NR C3H mice with either BALB/c or C57BL/6 spleen cells generated a positive DTH response. Exposure of the mice to UV radiation 5 days prior to sensitization resulted in a significant ($P<.001$) depression of the DTH response. This experiment has been repeated 4 times, with the levels of depression ranging from 43% to 61% of the response found in the NR controls.

The ability of spleen cells from the UV-irradiated mice to proliferate in response to allogeneic spleen cells, as measured using a one-way MLR, are shown in Table 2. When the responder cells were isolated from the NR mice, significant proliferation developed in response to the BALB/c stimulator

TABLE 1. Effect of UV radiation on the DTH response to alloantigen

UV[a]	Sensitization[b]	Δ Footpad swelling[c]	Specific footpad swelling[d]	% Suppression[e]
–	–	11.5±6.6	–	–
–	BALB/c cells	35.6±4.9	24.1	0
+	BALB/c cells	23.8±7.4	12.3	49 (P<.001)[f]
–	–	2.2±1.6	–	–
–	C57BL/6 cells	62.8±11.1	60.6	0
+	C57BL/6 cells	36.6±9.5	34.4	44 (P<.001)

[a] 30–40 kJ/m^2 (280–320 nm).
[b] 10^8 NSC injected s.c.
[c] Difference in footpad thickness 24 hr after challenge with 10^7 NSC; mean value ± SE; N = 10; units = CM×10^{-3}.
[d] Δ Footpad swelling of sensitized mice minus Δ footpad swelling of unsensitized mice.
[e] $(1 - \frac{\text{[specific footpad swelling of UV-treated mice]}}{\text{specific footpad swelling of control mice}} \times 100.$
[f] Two-tailed Student's t test, UV-treated vs. NR mice.

TABLE 2. Effect of UV radiation on MLR to alloantigen

Treatment of C3H mice		Stimulator Cells in vitro[c]	CPM[d]	% Suppression[e]
UV[a]	Sensitization in vivo[b]			
–	+	–	4079±91	–
–	+	BALB/c	30751±3845	–
–	+	C57BL/6	28352±3738	–
+	+	–	4775±695	–
+	–	BALB/c	35334±278	0
+	+	BALB/c	4523±1005	85 (P<.001)[f]
+	+	C57BL/6	41650±5714	0

[a] 30–40 kJ/m^2.
[b] 10^8 BALB/c spleen cells injected s.c.
[c] 2×10^5 mitomycin-C-treated spleen cells.
[d] cpm ± SE from triplicate samples.
[e] See footnotes for Table 1.
[f] Two-tailed Student's t test, UV-treated mice vs. NR controls.

cells. However, exposure to UV radiation before sensitization resulted in an 85% depression of the proliferative response. The antigen specificity of the UV-induced depression was also examined. When spleen cells isolated from UV-irradiated C3H mice sensitized with BALB/c cells were cultured with C57BL/6 stimulator cells, rather than BALB/c stimulator cells, a proliferative response was generated. Also note that when the mice were exposed to UV radiation but were not sensitized with allogeneic spleen cells, no depression of the proliferative response was seen.

A second characteristic of UV-induced immunosuppression, in addition to antigen specificity, is the induction of suppressor T lymphocytes (*3–5*). The existence of suppressor cells in the spleens of mice with depressed DTH response was examined by adding nylon-wool-nonadherent spleen cells to MLR cultures. The data from this experiment are presented in Table 3. The addition of cells from UV-irradiated mice to one-way MLR cultures using normal C3H cells as responder cells and BALB/c cells as stimulator cells, caused a significant suppression (P<.001) of the proliferation of the C3H cells. The level of suppression was related to the number of suppressor cells used. The addition of the suppressor cells isolated from the spleens of UV-irradiated mice sensitized with BALB/c cells had no suppressive effect on the proliferative response of normal C3H lymphocytes to C57BL/6 cells. In fact, the addition of suppressor cells from UV-irradiated mice caused an enhancement of the proliferative response. This probably reflects an increased number of effector cells in the cultures capable of responding to the allogeneic C57BL/6 cells. These data indicate that an antigen-specific suppressor cell is generated in the spleens of UV-irradiated mice sensitized with allogeneic spleen cells.

The effect of UV radiation on the generation of IL-2 was also tested, and the data from this experiment (Fig. 1) demonstrate that sensitization of UV-irradiated animals depresses the ability of their spleen cells to generate IL-2. When spleen cells isolated from mice with depressed DTH and proliferative response to allogeneic BALB/c cells were cultured with BALB/c stimulator cells, the generation of IL-2 was also depressed. When these cells were cultured with C57BL/6 cells, instead of BALB/c cells, IL-2 was generated. The response of NR cells cultured with C57BL/6 cells or BALB/c cells was similar to the response seen when responder cells from the UV-irradiated mice were cultured with C57BL/6 cells (data not shown).

DISCUSSION

The immunosuppressive activity of UV radiation has been examined by a number of investigators (*21*). In general, exposure to UV radiation results in a systemic, specific, suppression of immune reactivity (*1*). The study presented here shows that sensitization of UV-irradiated mice with allogeneic spleen cells results in a specific unresponsiveness to the antigen used for sensitization. This was demonstrated using in vivo (DTH) and in vitro (MLR and generation of IL-2) parameters of immune reactivity. In all situations tested, the suppression was specific for the antigen originally used to sensitize the UV-irradiated animal. The majority of the experiments presented here have used allogeneic BALB/c spleen cells to sensitize C3H mice. The reciprocal experiments— sensitization of UV-irradiated C3H mice with C57BL/6 cells—have also been performed, with similar results (data not shown).

TABLE 3. Antigen-specific suppressor cells in the spleens of UV-irradiated mice

Stimulator Cells[a]	UV Cells[b]	NR Cells[c]	CPM[d]	% Suppression[e]	P<[f]
BALB/c	–	–	76615±6025	–	
BALB/c	–	4×10^5	81720±6888	0	
BALB/c	–	2×10^5	75443±6410	0	
BALB/c	–	1×10^5	60937±9226	20	.01
BALB/c	4×10^5	–	21538±4970	72	.001
BALB/c	2×10^5	–	33316±2194	57	.001
BALB/c	1×10^5	–	37043±9362	52	.001
C57BL/6	–	–	79131±5359	–	
C57BL/6	–	4×10^5	123733±15117	0	
C57BL/6	–	2×10^5	130866±10033	0	
C57BL/6	–	1×10^5	98246±6648	0	
C57BL/6	4×10^5	–	102640±7240	0	
C57BL/6	2×10^5	–	111894±5084	0	
C57BL/6	1×10^5	–	90342±6098	0	

[a] 2×10^5 spleen cells.
[b] Nylon-wool-purified cells from UV-irradiated mice sensitized with 10^8 BALB/c spleen cells.
[c] Nylon-wool-purified cells from NR mice sensitized with 10^8 BALB/c spleen cells.
[d] cpm ± SE from triplicate samples.
[e] See footnotes for Table 1.
[f] Two-tailed Student's t test, cultures with UV-treated or NR cells vs. cultures with stimulator and responder cells only.

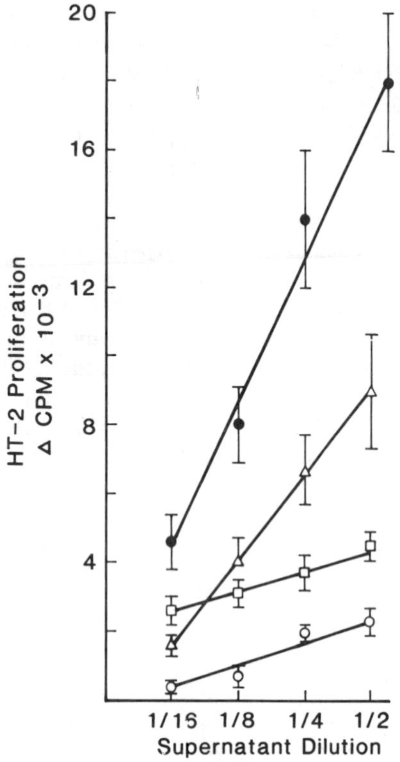

FIGURE 1. UV-induced suppression of the generation of IL-2 in response to allogeneic stimulation. Spleen cells from C3H UV-irradiated mice, sensitized with BALB/c spleen cells were cultured with C57BL/6 stimulator cells (△——△) or BALB/c stimulator cells (□——□), or they were cultured alone (○——○) for 3 days. Supernatants were collected, and their ability to support the proliferation of HT-2 was determined. The response of HT-2 cells to serial dilutions of an IL-2 preparation is also shown (●——●). The 1:2 supernatant dilution corresponds to 0.1 units/well of IL-2.

As pointed out previously, exposure to UV radiation results in the impairment of APC function by a decrease in the number of I-A-positive cells (*9, 10*) and the induction of suppressor T cells (*3, 4, 14*). From the data presented in Tables 1 and 2, it is impossible to distinguish the mechanism causing the hyporesponsiveness in the UV-irradiated animals. It is possible that the inability to generate DTH and MLR responses is due to a defect in APC function or the induction of suppressor cells. The data presented in Table 3 suggest that the activation of suppressor cells may play a role in the UV-induced unresponsiveness. In this experiment the response of normal spleen cells to alloantigen was suppressed in an antigen-specific manner by nylon-wool-purified cells isolated from the UV-irradiated animals. It is difficult to reconcile the antigen specificity of the UV-induced hyporesponsiveness shown in Tables 2 and 3 and Figure 1 solely with a defect in antigen presentation. In all probability a situation is occurring here that is similar to that described by others (*9, 11, 12*)—a UV-induced impairment in APC function is activating antigen specific suppressor cells. The identity of this suppressor cell is not entirely clear. Because they were isolated from whole spleen cell populations by procedures that are generally used to enrich for T lymphocytes, it is possible that the suppressor cells are T cells. Studies to examine the phenotype of the suppressor cells are currently in progress.

The effect of UV radiation on lymphokine production was also examined. A potential problem with measuring IL-2 activity in a supernatant fluid is that the activity is a measure of the net balance between IL-2 production and consumption. While it is possible that the decreased level of IL-2 in the supernatant of cells isolated from UV-irradiated mice might reflect an increased consumption of the lymphokine, we do not believe this is the case for the following reason. Parallel cultures were set up measuring IL-2 production or T cell proliferation in response to allogeneic stimulation. Both IL-2 activity (Fig. 1) and T cell proliferation (Table 1) were depressed—in fact, the MLR response was reduced to background levels. Therefore, it seems unlikely that IL-2 would be consumed by T cells in cultures where T cell proliferation is totally shut down. These data also suggest that the impairment of T helper cell function may be involved in the UV-induced immunosuppression.

Previous studies have demonstrated that the ability of UV-irradiated mice to respond to allogeneic cells in the MLR is normal (*6*). This appears to contradict the data reported here. However, there is a fundamental difference in the experimental protocol used in this study that explains this discrepancy. The irradiation and sensitization protocols used in this report were patterned after those used previously to demonstrate the systemic suppression of CHS after a single exposure to UV radiation (*14–16*). It is clear from these studies that two signals, UV radiation and antigenic stimulation, are required to activate the suppressive pathway. In this study when the UV-irradiated mice were sensitized with allogeneic spleen cells DTH and MLR were depressed. On the other hand, when the UV-irradiated mice were not sensitized with allogeneic cells, the MLR generated was comparable to the response observed when cells from NR mice were used (Table 2). These data suggest that the suppression of the MLR response was not observed in previous studies because the second signal, antigenic stimulation was not administered.

Not only are two signals required to activate suppression but they must be administered in a prescribed sequence. The mice must be irradiated first and then 3 to 15 days later the animals must be sensitized (*13*). Reversal of these treatments, antigenic sensitization followed by UV radiation, does not activate the suppressive pathway (*15*). A possible mechanism may involve the inhibition of normal APC function by UV radiation. When antigen is introduced it then comes into contact with a UV resistant cell similar, if not identical, to the one described by Granstein (*12*). This cell then presents the antigen to suppressor T cells. This mechanism would explain why the sensitization of mice with an immunogenic dose of antigen after UV radiation results in suppression rather than immunization. It would explain the antigen specificity of the suppression and also explain why sensitization must follow UV irradiation and not vice versa.

It is possible that the suppression of immune reactivity after a single exposure to UV radiation may have potential clinical applications. An advantage in using UV radiation to induce immunosuppression is that the antigenic specificity of the resulting suppression is determined by the choice of the antigen used to sensitize the mice (Tables 2 and 3, Fig. 1); the route of sensitization (*17, 22*); and the time course between UV irradiation and sensitization (*13*). Therefore, by manipulating these conditions, the investigator can choose the specificity of the resulting immunosuppression.

A second potential advantage in using UV radiation to induce suppression is that the suppressor cells induced may also suppress allograft rejection. This is suggested by recent studies on the range of activity of the suppressor T cells induced by hapten sensitization of UV-irradiated mice. Once induced, these cells suppress the CHS response, the generation of cytotoxic T lymphocytes, and antibody formation (*22*). In addition, the proliferation of T cells to hapten-modified splenic adherent cells is also suppressed (*16*). It is possible that the suppressor cells induced by the allogeneic sensitization of UV-irradiated mice may also exhibit a wide range of activity. If so, these cells may also suppress allograft rejection. Experiments to test this hypothesis are currently in progress. However, preliminary results have demonstrated that the survival of allogeneic fetal cardiac grafts is prolonged after UV irradiation and allogeneic sensitization of the recipient mice (Ullrich SE, unpublished observation).

There have been a number of reports recently that point out the potential therapeutic value of the UV-induced modulation of immune function. Lau et al. (*23*) have demonstrated that in vitro exposure of islet of Langerhans to UV radiation altered their immunogenicity, without adversely affecting their endocrine function, and resulted in the prolonged survival of the grafts in allogeneic diabetic animals. A concomitant reduction in blood glucose levels was noted. Hauser et al. (*24*) demonstrated that the induction of experimental allergic encephalomyelitis in mice could be prevented by prior exposure to UV radiation. Morison and Pike (*25*) found that a single exposure to UV radiation could suppress a graft-versus-host reaction. Also, Spellman et al. (*26*) found that specific tolerance to protein antigens could be induced by the topical application of the antigen to UV-irradiated skin. The specific suppression of the response to alloantigens, as reported here, may be yet another example of the potential therapeutic application of UV radiation.

Acknowledgments. I thank M. L. Kripke for her critical review of this manuscript, and acknowledge the technical assistance of Jacqueline Walker and the secretarial help of Helen Farr.

REFERENCES

1. Kripke ML. Immunologic unresponsiveness induced by ultraviolet radiation. Immunol Rev 1984; 80: 87.
2. Kripke ML. Antigenicity of murine skin tumors included by ultraviolet light. JNCI 1974; 53: 1333.
3. Spellman CW, Daynes RA. Modification of immunologic potential by ultraviolet radiation. II. Generation of suppressor cells in short term UV-irradiated mice. Transplantation 1977; 24: 120.
4. Fisher MS, Kripke ML. Further studies on the tumor-specific suppressor cells induced by ultraviolet radiation. J Immunol 1978; 121: 1139.
5. Fisher MS, Kripke ML. Suppressor T lymphocytes control the development of primary skin cancers in ultraviolet-irradiated mice. Science 1982; 216: 1133.
6. Spellman CW, Woodward JG, Daynes RA. Modification of immunological potential by ultraviolet radiation. I. Immune status of short term UV-irradiated mice. Tranpslantation 1977; 24: 112.
7. Kripke ML, Lofgreen JS, Beard J, Jessup JM, Fisher MS. In vivo immune response of mice during carcinogenesis by ultraviolet irradiation. JNCI 1977; 59: 1227.
8. Norbury KC, Kripke ML, Budman MB. In vitro reactivity of macrophages and lymphocytes from ultraviolet-irradiated mice. JNCI 1977; 59: 1231.
9. Greene MI, Sy MS, Kripke ML, Benacerraf B. Impairment of antigen-presenting cell function by ultraviolet radiation. Proc Natl Acad Sci USA 1979; 76: 6591.
10. Letvin NL, Nepon JT, Greene MI, Benacerraf B, Germain RN. Loss of Ia-bearing splenic adherent cells after whole body ultraviolet irradiation. J Immunol 1980; 125: 2550.
11. Sauder DN, Tamaki K, Moshell AN, Fujiwara H, Katz SI. Induction of tolerance to topically applied TNCB using TNP-conjugate ultraviolet light-irradiated epidermal cells. J Immunol 1981; 127: 261.
12. Granstein RD. Epidermal cells are responsible for transferable suppressor cell generation after immunization of mice with ultraviolet radiation-treated epidermal cells. J Invest Dermatol 1985; 84: 206.
13. Noonan FP, Kripke ML, Pedersen GM, Greene MI. Suppression of contact hypersensitivity in mice by ultraviolet irradiation is associated with defective antigen presentation. Immunology 1981; 43: 527.
14. Noonan FP, DeFabo EC, Kripke ML. Suppression of contact hypersensitivity by UV radiation and its relationship to UV-induced suppression of tumor immunity. Photochem Photobiol 1981; 34: 683.
15. Kripke ML, Morison WL, Parrish JA. Systemic suppression of contact hypersensitivity in mice by psoralen plus UVA radiation. J Invest Dermatol 1983; 81: 87.
16. Ullrich SE. Suppression of lymphoproliferation by hapten-specific suppressor T lymphocytes from mice exposed to ultraviolet radiation. Immunology 1985; 54: 343.
17. Ullrich, SE, Azizi E, Kripke ML. Suppression of the induction of delayed-type hypersensitivity reactions in mice by a single exposure to ultraviolet radiation. Photochem Photobiol 1986; 43: 633.
18. Liew FY. Regulation of delayed-type hypersensitivity. VI. Antigen-specific suppresor T cells and suppressor factor for delayed-type hypersensitivity to histocompatibility antigens. Transplantation 1982; 33: 69.
19. Julius MH, Simpson E, Herzenberg LA. A rapid method for the isolation of functional thymus-derived lymphocytes. Eur J Immunol 1973; 3: 645.
20. Watson J. Continuous proliferation of murine antigen-specific helper T lymphycytes in culture. J Exp Med 1979; 150: 1510.
21. Parrish JA. The effect of ultraviolet radiation on the immune system. Albuquerque, NM: Johnson and Johnson, Baby Products, 1983.
22. Ullrich SE, Gee GK, Kripke ML. Suppressor lymphocytes induced by epicutaneous sensitization of UV-irradiated mice control multiple immunologic pathyways. Immunology (in press).
23. Lau H, Reemtsma K, Hardy MA. Prolongation of rat islet allograft survival by direct ultraviolet irradiation of the graft. Science 1984; 223: 607.
24. Hauser SL, Weiner HL, Che M, Shapiro ME, Gilles F, Letvin NL. Prevention of experimental allergic encephalomyelitis (EAE) in the SJL/J mouse by whole body ultraviolet irradiation. J Immunol 1984; 132: 1276.
25. Morison WL, Pike RA. Suppression of graft-versus-host reactivity in the mouse popliteal node by UVB radiation. J Invest Dermatol 1985; 84: 483.
26. Spellman CW, Anderson WL, Bernhard EJ, Tomasi TB. Suppression of antibody responses to topically applied antigens by ultraviolet light irradiation. J Exp Med 1984; 160: 1891.

Received 1 November 1985.
Accepted 17 December 1985.

0041-1337/86/4203-0292$02.00/0
TRANSPLANTATION
Vol. 42, No. 3
Printed in U.S.A.

INDUCTION OF B CELL TOLERANCE IN RATS BY LARGE DOSES OF ALLOGENEIC ERYTHROCYTES

GERARD D. MAJOOR[1] AND PETER J.C. VAN BREDA VRIESMAN

Department of Immunology, University of Limburg, Maastricht, The Netherlands

Several studies have now confirmed our original observation that transfusions of large doses of donor-specific allogeneic erythrocytes (E) induce humoral unresponsiveness to E-associated antigens (including major histocompatibility complex (MHC) class I antigens) in rats, which is associated with prolonged survival of subsequently inserted renal grafts. To examine whether this tolerance was due to induction of suppressor (T) cells or to anergy or deletion of antigen-specific B cells, an in vitro system was developed that allowed generation of primary immune responses of rat splenocytes to allogeneic erythrocytes. Cocultivation of B and non-B cells from tolerant and normal rats in this system showed that E transfusions had induced B cell tolerance in the recipients; no evidence was obtained that suppressor T cells were involved in the maintenance of unresponsiveness. On the contrary, non-B cells from tolerant rats could "help" normal B cells for antibody formation to allogeneic E.

In vivo, tolerance to allogeneic E could be broken in one rat strain combination by skin allografts. Therefore, the state of B cell tolerance induced by E transfusions may be referred to as "reversible clonal anergy."

In spite of several years of intensive research, the mechanisms involved in prolongation of human kidney graft survival by blood transfusions given prior to transplantation have not been elucidated (*1, 2*). In an experimental approach we have studied the effects of pretransplant transfusions of highly purified erythrocytes (E)* on renal allograft survival in rats. Our studies in the LEW-to-BN rat strain combination have demonstrated that infusions of 10^{10} LEW E per 100 g body weight induced humoral tolerance to LEW E-associated antigens (BN tol. LEW rats) and were associated with markedly prolonged survival of subsequently inserted LEW kidney grafts (*3*). Similar observations were recently reported by others using different rat strain combinations (*4, 5*). In these studies beneficial effects of E transfusions on kidney graft survival were only demonstrable if E administered and kidney grafts derived from the same donor strain. This finding excluded nonspecific effects of E or E breakdown products in these models (*6*).

Neither the mechanism by which transfusions of donor E prolonged rat renal allograft survival, nor the way in which allogeneic E induced humoral tolerance is known. LEW kidneys transplanted into BN tol. LEW rats did not break tolerance; since the development of vasculonecrotic lesions in rejecting LEW renal allografts was associated with the presence of antidonor IgG hemagglutinins we have proposed that prolonged graft survival could be due to the absence of such antibodies (*3, 7*). However, transfusions of E from LEW.1N and BN.1L MHC congenic rats to BN recipients did not prolong LEW renal allograft survival to the extent seen in BN tol. LEW rats, in spite of the absence of antidonor IgG hemagglutinins in both types of recipients (*8*). Therefore, E transfusions must interfere with other immune reactions involved in graft rejection—e.g., cytotoxic T lymphocytes (CTL) or delayed-type hypersensitivity (DTH)—as well. It has been shown for example that the number of CTL in renal allografts residing in donor E-transfused rats was decreased (*9*). On the other hand, we did not obtain evidence for modified CTL responses in BN tol. LEW hosts of LEW kidney grafts (*3*).

As a working hypothesis, we have suggested that transfusions of allogeneic E induced suppressor T cells in rats specifically controlling immune reactions involved in kidney graft rejection, including antidonor hemagglutinin responses (*3*). In this study, we have examined the hypothesis that humoral tolerance induced by large doses of allogeneic E is due to the induction of suppressor (T) cells or to clonal anergy or deletion of antigen-specific B cells. For this purpose, we have adapted the in vitro model of Rosenberg et al. (*10*) for rat primary antibody responses to sheep E for responses to allogeneic E. Due to the relatively low density of major histocompatibility complex (MHC) class I antigens on LEW E (*11, 12*), and the often weak responses of BN lymphocytes in vitro (*13*), this study had to be performed using LEW responder lymphocytes and DA E as antigen. In this combination, as in the LEW-to-BN combination, transfusions of DA E have been shown to prolong survival of DA kidney grafts in LEW hosts (*4*).

MATERIALS AND METHODS

Rats. LEW ($RT1^l$) and BN ($RT1^n$) rats were obtained from specific-pathogen-free (SPF) lines kept at the Department of Animal Services of the University of Limburg. SPF LEW.1N ($RT1^n$ on the LEW genetic background), LEW.1A ($RT1^a$), and DA ($RT1^a$) rats were purchased from the Zentralinstitut für Versuchstiere, Hannover, F.R.G. BN.1L ($RT1^l$) rats were kindly donated by Dr. T.J. Gill III, Pittsburgh PA. Only male rats were used.

Purification of E and induction of tolerance. The procedure for the purification of E has previously been described in detail (*14*). Tolerance to allogeneic E was induced by two or three infusions of 10^{10} E spaced two weeks apart. The first infusion was administered when the recipients were about one month of age (weight 80–100 g).

Culture medium (CM). Sodium-bicarbonate-buffered RPMI-1640 (GIBCO; Breda, the Netherlands) was supplemented with 0.1 M D-glucose, 0.25 mM Na-pyruvate, 2% (v/v) MEM amino

[1] Address correspondence to: G.D. Majoor, Department of Immunology, University of Limburg, Biomedical Center, P.O. Box 616, 6200 MD Maastricht, The Netherlands.

* Abbreviations used: AFC, antibody-forming cell; AFCF, AFC focus; CM, culture medium, Con A sup., concanavalin A supernatant; CTL, cytotoxic T lymphocyte; DTH, delayed-type hypersensitivity; E, erythrocyte; IL-2, interleukin 2; MAb, monoclonal antibody; MHC, major histocompatibility complex; PBS, phosphate-buffered saline; SPF, specific-pathogen-free.

acids (50×), 4% (v/v) nonessential amino acids (100×), 1.7 mM glutamine, 10 mM N′-2-hydroxyethylpiperazine-N′-ethanosulfonic acid (HEPES), 50 μM 2-mercaptoethanol, 50 μg/ml gentamycin, and 10% heat-inactivated fetal calf serum. If the medium was supplemented with supernatant from concanavalin-A-stimulated rat spleen cells (Con A sup) (10%, v/v) 25 mM α-methyl-D-mannoside was also added. The pH of the medium was finally readjusted to 7.3.

Sources of interleukin-2 (IL-2). Supernatant from LEW spleen cells cultured for 24 hr at 5×10⁶/ml in the presence of 5 μg Con A was used as a source of IL-2. Potency of the supernatant was determined by titration on mouse CTLL cells and measuring proliferation of these IL-2-dependent cells by ^{3}H-thymidine incorporation as described by Nagelkerken et al. (*15*). Recombinant human IL-2 was kindly donated by Drs. Fierz and De Vos, University of Gent, Belgium. It was established in our laboratory to contain 400,000 units/ml.

Culture system. Spleen cells were prepared as previously described (*16*). Cells were cultured in CM overnight in plastic culture flasks to allow adherence of macrophages (*17*). Nonadherent cells were collected and separated into B and non-B cells, as indicated below, or cultured unseparated at 5×10^6/ml in CM in cluster wells (Costar No. 3524) together with 5×10^6 washed DA E. CM was supplemented either with 10% Con-A sup. or 25 μl recombinant human IL-2 diluted 1:50. Except when specified otherwise, cultures were kept for 3 days at an angle of 30°; at that time 1.0 ml CM was added. The cells were resuspended, and culturing was continued for two more days in the horizontal position.

Cell separation. Nonadherent spleen cells were separated into B and non-B cells according to a modification of the "panning" technique of Wysocki and Sato (*18*). For this purpose, plastic petri dishes were coated with purified goat antimouse IgG. Cell suspensions to be separated were treated with OX-12 (mouse monoclonal antibody [MAb] to rat κ light chain; Serotec, Bicester, UK), and His 14 (mouse MAb to a rat B cell differentiation marker) (*19*). His 14 was kindly donated by Dr. F. Kroese. At the end of the cell separation procedure, cells were washed and samples were taken for analysis in a fluorescence-activated cell sorter (FACS IV, Becton-Dickinson). Usually about 80% of the positively selected cells were OX-12$^+$, His 14$^+$ (B cells); 90% of the nonadherent cells were W3/13$^+$ (a marker for rat peripheral T cells) (*20*).

Antibody-forming cell (AFC) assay. LEW anti-DA E AFC were enumerated in an antibody-forming cell focus (AFCF) assay, as recently described (*16*). Since only about 2×10^6 viable cells were recovered after 5 days in culture, the assay was scaled down to 35-mm plastic petri dishes. In brief, viable cells were recovered from individual cultures by centrifugation on Ficoll-Isopaque (d = 1.090) (viable cell yield 89±7.6%). Cells were washed twice and resuspended in 1.0 ml balanced salt solution for withdrawal of a 50-μl sample for automated cell counting (Coulter Counter model ZF). Cells were pelleted again and resuspended in 1.0 ml 0.6% agarose at 37°C. Each suspension was next transferred to a 35-mm petri dish (Falcon No. 3001F) coated with affinity-purified rabbit anti-rat IgM antibody. This antibody preparation (SLM-2) was prepared and generously provided by Dr. H. Bazin. After sedimentation of the cells at 37°C, the agarose was solidified at room temperature and incubation was continued at 37°C for 2.5 hr. The agarose layer was removed, and 5×10^7 DA E in 2.0 ml phosphate-buffered saline (PBS) were introduced per dish, followed by 1.5 hr of incubation at room temperature. Unbound E were carefully washed away, and bound E were fixed with 0.25% (v/v) glutaraldehyde in PBS. Washed and dried dishes were examined with an inverted microscope with dark field illumination, and foci of E were counted.

Hemagglutination assay. Hemagglutinins were determined in a dextran-facilitated assay (*21*).

Skin transplantation. Full-thickness skin grafts of about 1×1-cm were taken from the abdomen of 2 months old donor rats and inserted on the back of the recipients. The graft was protected for 7 days by a bandage, and inspected on that day and each of the following days for signs of rejection.

Statistics. *P* values were determined using Student's *t* test.

RESULTS

Culture conditions. Generation of LEW anti-DA E antibody-forming cells (AFC) was dependent on the addition of the cultures of external growth or differentiation factors contained in Con A sup. (Table 1). Although batches of Con A sup. were routinely tested for potency to support T cell proliferation and only satisfactory batches were used, marked variation in the efficacy of individual batches of Con A sup. to support generation of AFC was noticed. Therefore an attempt was made to replace Con A sup. by recombinant (human) IL-2. This preparation was shown to support formation of LEW anti-DA E AFC at final dilutions of 1:400 and 1:2000 (Fig. 1); a dilution

TABLE 1. Evidence that LEW anti-DA E responses in vitro are IL-2-dependent and antigen-specific

Exp.	Group	Antigen	Source of IL-2	AFCF/well visualized		
				With DA E	With sheep E	With LEW E
1.	1[a]	—	—	2,4	1	0
	2	5×10^6 DA E	—	2,4	2	0
	3	5×10^6 DA E	Con A sup. (rat)	96,145	0	0
	4	5×10^6 purified DA E	Con A sup. (rat)	78,162	0	0
	5	1.5×10^3 DA leucocytes[b]	Con A sup. (rat)	1,2	0	0
2.	1	5×10^6 DA E	—	0,2,2,3	ND[c]	ND
	2	—	Recombinant IL-2 (human)	4	ND	ND
	3	5×10^6 DA E	Recombinant IL-2 (human)	86,113,134,137	ND	ND
	3a	5×10^6 DA E	Recombinant IL-2 (human)	274,286,347,514	ND	ND

[a] At variance with the culture system described in the *Materials and Methods* section, cultures in Exps. 1, and 2, groups 1–3 were cultured for five days in the horizontal position.

[b] The number of leukocytes is equivalent to that contained in 5×10^6 nonpurified DA E.

[c] (ND) not done.

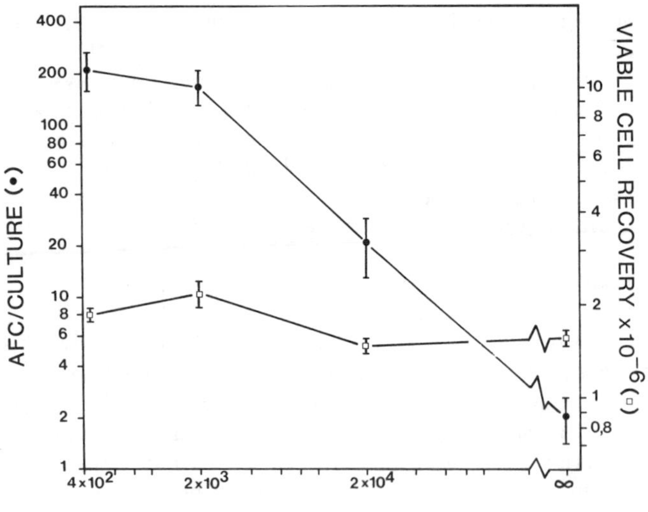

FIGURE 1. Dose-response relationship for addition of recombinant human IL-2 to cultures of LEW nonadherent spleen cells and DA E. (●) mean number of anti DA AFC/culture; (□) mean number of viable cells/culture. Determinations were performed after 5 days in culture. Vertical bars represent ±SEM.

of 1:2000 was chosen for subsequent experimentation. In the absence of antigen few or no AFCF were detected, indicating that the recombinant IL-2 preparations did not aspecifically promote the development of AFC (Table 1).

Specificity and kinetics. LEW anti-DA E responses did not result from stimulation by DA leukocytes present among the E used for antigen-priming of the cultures (Table 1). Purified DA E were as effective in stimulating AFC formation as DA E containing white blood cells; moreover, addition of DA leukocytes (purified from 5×10^6 E by brief treatment of the cells with a .15 mM NH_4Cl solution) to LEW spleen cells did not yield DA E-specific AFC. Sheep E or LEW E used instead of DA E for visualization of AFCF developed very few, if any, foci thus reconfirming specificity of the in vitro anti-DAE response. In a separate experiment pooled anti-DA E AFC were analyzed for specificity for RT1.A[a] antigens. Similar numbers of AFCF were developed using LEW.1A instead of DA as indicator E (248 and 276 AFCF/culture, respectively), indicating that in vitro anti-DA E responses were also directed to RT1.A[a] antigens. The kinetics of the primary anti-DA E response is shown in Fig. 2. Although the mean number of AFCF was somewhat higher on day 6 than on day 5, the optimum response per 10^6 viable cells was detected after 5 days in culture. Hence, day 5 was selected for measuring anti-DA AFCF.

Splenic B cells from LEW tol. DA rats do not respond to DA E. Neither unseparated spleen cells from LEW tol. DA rats, nor B cells purified therefrom, responded to DA-E in vitro. (Table 2, groups 2 and 4). Addition of non-B spleen cells from normal LEW rats to B cells tol. DA did not restore anti-DA E responses (Table 2, group 8). On the contrary, in exps. 1 and 2 addition of DA tol. B cells to normal non-B spleen cells appeared to suppress residual responses of the latter. However, this suppression was not statistically significant. In exp. 3, residual responses of non-B cells from normal LEW spleens were almost eliminated by combining the MAbs His 14 and OX-12 for B cell purification. The magnitudes of all other responses in this experiment were comparable to those obtained in exps. 1 and 2.

Failure to demonstrate suppressor cell activity in spleens of LEW tol. DA rats. Two experiments were designed to explore whether suppressor cells were involved in the maintenance of humoral tolerance to DA E in LEW rats given injections of 10^{10} purified DA E. In the first approach, attempts were made to demonstrate putative suppressor cells by coculturing spleen cells from DA tol. and unmodified LEW rats. Cocultivation of LEW spleen cells with 20% or 50% spleen cells from LEW tol. DA rats did not significantly reduce anti-DA E AFC responses, as compared with the response of corresponding numbers of LEW spleen cells cultured alone (Table 3).

For the second approach, B cells were purified from normal LEW spleen and added to B-cell-depleted splenocytes from LEW tol. DA rats. Numbers of B and non-B cells cultured

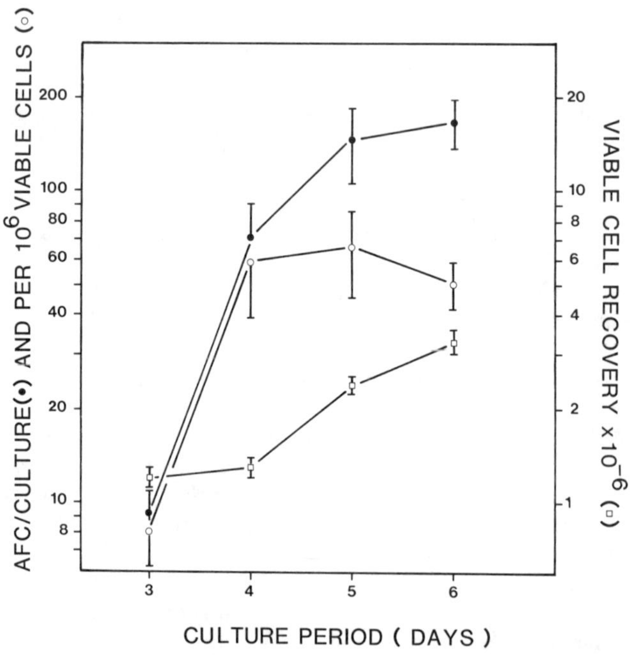

FIGURE 2. Kinetics of the AFC response of LEW nonadherent spleen cells to DA E in vitro. (●) mean number of anti-DA AFC/culture; (○) mean number of anti-DA AFC/10^6 viable cells; (□) mean number of viable cells/culture. Vertical bars represent ±SEM.

TABLE 2. Inability of splenic B cells from LEW tol. DA rats to respond to DA E, although non-B cells support anti-DA E responses of normal LEW B cells

Group	LEW spleen cells cultured[a]	No. of wells/ experiment	No. of anti-DA AFCF (mean ± SEM)		
			Exp. 1	Exp. 2	Exp. 3
1	5×10^6	4–6	269±68	135±55	185±46
2	5×10^6 DA tol.	3	3±1	1±1	1±1
3	2.2×10^6 B[b]	6	77±29	34±8	87±29
4	2.2×10^6 DA tol. B[b]	3–6	2±1	1±0	3±1
5	2.8×10^6 B-depleted	6	37±16	54±26	6±4
6	2.8×10^6 DA tol. B-depleted	3	5±2	1±0	2±1
7	2.2×10^6 B+2.8×10^6 DA tol. B-depleted	6	225±53	256±50	320±26
8	2.2×10^6 DA tol. B+2.8×10^6 B-depleted	6	13±2	7±4	12±7

[a] All cultures additionally contained 5×10^6 DA E.

[b] B cells were positively selected with MAb OX-12 in Exps. 1 and 2, and with MAbs OX-12 and His 14 in Exp. 3.

derived from their relative proportions among splenic lymphocytes. In 3 individual experiments anti-DA E responses in such cultures were comparable with, or even stronger than, those of unseparated LEW spleen cells (Table 2, groups 7 and 1, respectively). Addition of non-B cells from LEW tol. DA rats to purified normal B cells increased anti-DA E responses significantly (Table 2, groups 3 vs. 7, P; Exp. 1: <0.05, Exp. 2: <0.002, Exp. 3: <0.001). Thus, instead of exerting suppression, splenic non-B cells from LEW tol. DA rats were capable of providing "help" for normal B cells to develop into DA-E specific AFC.

Effects of skin allografts on the maintenance of tolerance to donor strain E in vivo. LEW kidneys grafted into BN tol. LEW rats have previously been demonstrated not to break established humoral unresponsiveness to LEW E-associated antigens (*3*). However, Heslop and Heslop had noticed earlier anti-DA hemagglutinin responses in BS recipients given 3 nonimmunogenic doses of 5×10^9 purified DA E prior to a DA skin graft (*22*). Therefore, LEW and DA skin grafts were grafted to BN tol. LEW and LEW tol. DA rats, respectively, to establish whether these grafts could break tolerance to donor E-associated antigens. As shown in Table 4, survival of skin grafts was little or not at all prolonged after transfusions of donor strain E in both rat strain combinations. However, as opposed to DA skin grafts on LEW tol. DA hosts, LEW skin grafts broke tolerance for LEW E-associated antigens (including $RT1.A^l$) in BN tol. LEW rats.

DISCUSSION

This study was designed to determine the mechanisms involved in the maintenance of humoral tolerance induced by infusions of large doses of allogeneic E in rats. Data obtained from in vitro studies indicated that i.v. administration of doses of 10^{10} DA E to young LEW rats induced B cell tolerance, and that suppressor T cells were not involved in the maintenance of tolerance.

As stated in a preliminary report (*23*) the in vitro response of LEW spleen cells to DA MHC class I antigens showed strong resemblance to the primary in vitro response of LEW spleen cells to sheep E described by Rosenberg et al. (*10*). This similarity corroborates the conclusion of others, reached in different experimental systems, that humoral responses to allogeneic MHC antigens are not essentially different from responses to other T-cell-dependent antigens (*24, 25*). In the culture system described here and by Rosenberg et al. (*10*) development of primary alloantibody responses depended on the addition of an external source of IL-2. Use of recombinant (human) IL-2 strongly suggested that IL-2 is the effective factor in this preparation. Aspecific stimulatory effects of bacterial factors (i.e., lipopolysaccharides) possibly present in recombinant preparations were ruled out by demonstrating that, in the absence of antigen, few—if any—AFC to DA E were generated.

Apart from being an effective T cell growth factor IL-2 has recently been shown also to be effective as a B cell growth and differentiation factor (*26, 27*). This may explain why AFC could be generated in cultures of purified B cells and DA E, although addition of splenic non-B cells from LEW tol. DA rats significantly increased such responses. Since FACS analysis of purified B cells indicated that about 20% non-B cells were present, it could also be argued that T cells possibly contaminating the B cells delivered help for anti-DA E responses. If this were true, IL-2 may have acted rather as a B cell and T helper cell mitogen than as a B cell differentiation factor in the cultures.

The data presented in this paper are compatible with the explanation that infusion of large amounts of DA E into young LEW rats induced B cell tolerance, and that at the time of assay (about two weeks after the last infusion of DA E) no suppressor T cells were present. The absence of suppressor T cells from LEW tol. DA rats was a somewhat surprising finding as our model resembled the xenogeneic model (i.v. injection of large doses of sheep E in mice) used by Gershon and Kondo, in which activity of suppressor T cells was demonstrated for the first time (*28*). However, more recently Kuroiwa et al. showed that priming of AKR mice with sheep E and weekly boosting with hamster E induced B cell tolerance (*29*). On the other hand, substitution of hamster E given for the first booster by formalin-fixed hamster E elicited antigen-specific suppressor T cells in C57B1/6 mice. Thus, depending on the combination of antigen and recipient used, either B cell tolerance or suppressor T cells may cause unresponsiveness. Furthermore, sensitivity of B cells for tolerization has been shown to vary depending on the type of carrier and the density of haptens per carrier molecule employed (*30, 31*). Different mechanisms of humoral unresponsiveness induced by xenogeneic or allogeneic E may reflect similar effects of cell-associated antigens on the induction of tolerance in rodent recipients.

Our data do not reveal the mechanism by which allogeneic E induced B cell tolerance in rats. According to current concepts of induction of B cell tolerance (*32*) it is conceivable that introduction of large amounts of allogeneic E tolerized both peripheral mature antigen-specific B cells and, due to "spillover" to the bone marrow, immature B cells. In young recipients, as used in this study, the balance between immature and mature B cells may quantitatively be in favor of the former. Pre-B cells and immature B cells are generally thought to be more sensitive to tolerization than mature B cells (*33, 34*). This may explain why tolerization is attained easily using one-month-old recipients.

Grafting of LEW skin onto BN tol. LEW recipients elicited antibody responses to LEW E-associated antigens. Absorption

TABLE 3. Evidence that cocultivation of normal LEW spleen cells with spleen cells from rats tol. DA does not suppress anti-DA E responses

Group	LEW spleen cells cultured[a]	No. anti-DA AFCF (mean ± SEM)
1	5×10^6	225±60
2	4×10^6	366±27
3	2.5×10^6	302±67
4	5×10^6 DA tol.	1±1
5	$4\times10^6+1\times10^6$ DA tol.	441±92
6	$2.5\times10^6+2.5\times10^6$ DA tol.	274±88

[a] All cultures (5 per group) additionally contained 5×10^6 DA E.

TABLE 4. Rejection of skin grafts by recipients tolerized with donor-strain E

Recipient strain	Donor strain	Donor-E tolerant	n	Graft rejection time (range in days)	Antidonor hemagglutinins 7 and 14 days posttransplantation (range $\log_2$ titers)
BN	LEW	No	4	8	12
		Yes	4	9–10	5–8[a]
LEW	DA	No	4	12–13	9–11
		Yes	4	12–13	0

[a] Anti-LEW hemagglutinins were eliminated after absorption with BN.1L E.

with BN.1L E completely removed the hemagglutinating capacity of these antisera, indicating that the antibodies were directed to RT1.A[l] antigens. These data indicated that B cell tolerance to LEW E in BN rats was reversible. Therefore, the state of tolerance induced by transfusions of allogeneic E may be best characterized as a reversible state of "clonal anergy" (*35*).

We conclude, from the data presented in this study and in a previous report (*8*), that B cell tolerance to donor E-associated alloantigens cannot by itself explain the prolonged survival of subsequently inserted kidney grafts. Presumably, infusions of large doses of allogeneic E not only induced specific B cell tolerance but interfered with some other component(s) of the host antigraft immune response.

Acknowledgments. We thank Marie-José W. H. van de Gaar for technical assistance, Mrs. Francine Teng-Vangrootloon for typing the manuscript, and Mr. Eep van Dam for skin transplantations.

REFERENCES

1. Opelz G. Current relevance of the transfusion effect in renal transplantation. Transplant Proc 1985; 17: 1015.
2. Teresaki PI. The beneficial transfusion effect on kidney graft survival attributed to clonal deletion. Transplantation 1984; 37: 119.
3. Majoor GD, van de Gaar M-JWH, Vlek LFM, van Breda Vriesman PJC. The role of antibody in rat renal allograft rejection. I. Absence of antibody to erythrocyte-associated antigens is associated with enhanced renal allograft survival. Transplantation 1981; 31: 369.
4. Wood KJ, Evins J, Morris PJ. Suppression of renal allograft rejection in the rat by class I antigens on purified erythrocytes. Transplantation 1985; 39: 56.
5. El-Malik F, Malik STA, Varghese Z, Sweny P, Moorhead JF. The enhancing and sensitizing effects of donor blood components, including dendritic cells, in a rat renal allograft model. Transplantation 1984; 38: 213.
6. Keown PA, Descamps B. Improved renal allograft survival after blood transfusion: a nonspecific, erythrocyte-mediated immunoregulatory process? Lancet 1979; 1: 20.
7. Majoor GD, van Breda Vriesman PJC. Role of antibody in rat renal allograft rejection. II. Failure to enhance renal allografts by sensitization to donor class I antigens presented by donor strain erythrocytes. Transplantation 1983; 35: 121.
8. Majoor GD, van Breda Vriesman PJC. Both MHC and non-MHC antigens residing on the same erythrocyte are required for donor-erythrocyte-mediated prolongation of the rat renal allograft survival. Transplantation 1986; 41: 92.
9. Wood KJ, Morris PJ. Purified erythrocytes suppress rejection of renal allografts in the rat and inhibit the accumulation of specific cytotoxic T cells in the graft. Transplant Proc 1985; 17: 1925.
10. Rosenberg JS, Gilman SC, Feldman JD. Regulation of rat B cell responses by T cell subsets and Interleukin-2. J Immunol 1982; 129: 996.
11. Hart DNJ, Fabre JW. Problems in the use of erythrocytes for RT1.A typing studies, probably due to quantitative differences in RT1.A antigen expression in different strains. Transplant Proc 1981; 13: 1329.
12. Begovitch AB, Blankenhorn EP, Winters BA, Gasser DL. Genetic control of the expression of class I molecules on rat erythrocytes. Immunogenetics 1983; 18: 45.
13. Shonnard JW, Davis BK, Netherey L, Cramer DV. In vitro responses of BN strain inbred rats. Transplant Proc 1981; 13: 1390.
14. Majoor GD, van de Gaar M-JWH, van Breda Vriesman PJC, Günther E. Rat erythrocytes elicit antibody formation against RT1.A region-determined antigens in allogeneic recipients. Immunology 1981; 43: 467.
15. Nagelkerken L, Henfling M, van Breda Vriesman P. Accessory cell function of thoracic duct non-lymphoid cells, dendritic cells and splenic adherent cells in the Brown Norway rat. Cell Immunol 1985; 93: 520.
16. Majoor GD. Enumeration of rat allospecific antibody-producing cells by a solid-phase antibody forming cell focus (AFCF) assay. J Immunol Methods 1984; 71: 37.
17. Weiss A, Fitch FW. Suppression of the plaque-forming cell response by macrophages present in the normal rat spleen. J Immunol 1978; 120: 357.
18. Wysocki LJ, Sato VL. "Panning" for lymphocytes: a method for cell selection. Proc Natl Acad Sci USA 1978; 75: 2844.
19. Kroese FGM, Opstelten D, Wubbena AS, et al. Monoclonal antibodies to rat B lymphocyte (sub-) populations. In: Klaus GGB, ed. Microenvironments in lymphoid systems. New York: Plenum, 1985: 81.
20. Williams AF, Galfre G, Milstein C. Analysis of cell surfaces by xenogeneic myeloma-hybrid antibodies: differentiation antigens of rat lymphocytes. Cell 1977; 12: 663.
21. Günther E, Stark O. The major histocompatibility system of the rat Ag-B or H-1 system. In: Götze D, ed. The major histocompatibility system in man and animals. Berlin: Springer-Verlag, 1977: 207.
22. Heslop BF, Heslop HE. Allogeneic red blood cells fail to induce haemagglutinating antibodies or cellular alloimmunity in rats and are immunosuppressive. Transplantation 1979; 28: 144.
23. Majoor GD, van de Gaar M-JWH. Primary in vitro response to major histocompatibility complex class I alloantigens. Transplant Proc 1985; 17: 1847.
24. Butcher GW, Corvalan JR, Licence DR, Howard JC. Immune response genes controlling responsiveness to major transplantation antigens. J Exp Med 1982; 155: 303.
25. Antoine JC, Howard JC. Study of the in vitro secondary alloantibody immune response of rats to RT1.A[a] class I alloantigens. Transplant Proc 1983; 15: 1591.
26. Zubler RH, Lowenthal JW, Erard F, Hashimoto N, Devos R, MacDonald HR. Activated B cells express receptors for, and proliferate in response to, pure Interleukin 2. J Exp Med 1984; 160: 1170.
27. Nakanishi K, Malek TR, Smith KA, Hamaoka T, Shevach EM, Paul WE. Both Interleukin 2 and a second T cell-derived factor in EL-4 supernatant have activity as differentiation factors in IgM synthesis. J Exp Med 1984; 160: 1605.
28. Gershon RK, Kondo K. Infectious immunological tolerance. Immunology 1971; 21: 903.
29. Kuroiwa A, Nomoto K, Takeya K. Mechanisms of antigen-specific unresponsiveness to heterologous erythrocytes in mice: deletion of B cell clone and generation of suppressor T cells. Cell Immunol 1979: 47: 79.
30. Pike BL, Battye FL, Nossal GJV. Effect of hapten valency and carrier composition on the tolerogenic potential of hapten-protein conjugates. J Immunol 1981; 126: 89.
31. Waters CA, Diener E. Tolerance induction during ontogeny. II. Distinct unresponsive states in immature mice question the generality of clonal abortion. Eur J Immunol 1983; 13: 928.
32. Nossal GJV. Cellular mechanisms of immunologic tolerance. In: Paul WE, ed. Annual Rev Immunol 1983; 1: 33.
33. McIntosh KR, Segre D. B- and T-cell tolerance induction in young-adult and old-mice. Cell Immunol 1976; 20: 230.
34. Klinman NR, Schrater AF, Katz DH. Immature B cells as the target for in vivo tolerance induction. J Immunol 1980; 126: 1970.
35. Nossal GJV, Pike BJ. Clonal anergy: persistence in tolerant mice of antigen-binding B lymphocytes incapable of responding to antigen or mitogen. Proc Natl Acad Sci USA 1980; 77: 1602.

Received 8 October 1985.
Accepted 12 December 1985.

0041-1337/86/4203-0297$02.00/0
TRANSPLANTATION

Vol. 42, No. 3
Printed in U.S.A.

ENHANCEMENT OF INDUCTION OF INTESTINAL ADENOCARCINOMAS BY CYCLOSPORINE IN RATS GIVEN A SINGLE DOSE OF N-METHYL N-NITROSOUREA[1]

MOHAN I. R. PERERA, HEINZ W. KUNZ, THOMAS J. GILL III, AND HISASHI SHINOZUKA[2]

Department of Pathology, University of Pittsburgh School of Medicine, Pittsburgh, Pennsylvania 15261

Dietary administration of cyclosporine (CsA) to rats induces lymphoproliferative disorders involving the gut lymphoid plaques with frequent mucosal ulceration. In this study, we investigated whether administration of a known chemical carcinogen prior to CsA treatment modifies the development of the lesions induced by CsA. Male Sprague-Dawley rats were given either a single i.p. injection of N-methyl N-nitrosourea (MNU) (25 mg/kg) or the solvent—and one week thereafter they were fed a diet containing 0.011% CsA. Control rats were fed a basal diet with or without prior MNU treatment. Of the rats that received MNU and CsA, 60% developed adenocarcinomas of the small and large intestine arising in the regions of the intestinal lymphoid plaques. Only 1 of 12 rats given MNU followed by a basal diet developed adenocarcinoma. No tumors developed in rats treated with CsA alone, but there was atypical proliferation of the intestinal mucosa in conjunction with lymphoid hyperplasia of the gut. The mucosal damage secondary to CsA-induced lymphoid lesions probably acted as a promoting stimulus for the development of intestinal carcinomas.

Cyclosporine (CsA)* a fungal metabolite of *Trichoderma polysporum*, is an effective immunosuppressant with low myelotoxicity (*1*). It has been used successfully as the primary drug to suppress the rejection of organ transplants (*2, 3*). The mechanism of action of CsA is not known, and it is thought to act by inhibiting the expression of antigen-induced signals necessary for the generation of T-cell-dependent immune responses (*4, 5*).

In experimental studies, chronic administration of CsA to rats and mice has led to morphological alterations of several lymphoid organs—the thymus, spleen, lymph nodes, and gut-associated lymphoid tissues (*6, 7*). In rats receiving CsA, striking changes were observed in the gut-associated lymphoid tissues; these consisted of marked enlargement caused by proliferation of atypical lymphoid cells and ulceration of the overlying epithelial cells (*6*). More recently, we demonstrated that CsA treatment markedly enhanced the induction of thymic lymphomas in mice pretreated with a small dose of carcinogen (*8*). In the present study similar experiments were conducted in rats to test whether CsA modifies the lymphoproliferative lesions in the gut. Contrary to our expectation, the target organ of tumor development by CsA was shifted to the intestinal mucosa.

MATERIALS AND METHODS

Male Sprague-Dawley rats (Hilltop Laboratories, Pittsburgh, PA) weighing 100–120 g were individually caged in a room with temperature and humidity control and a 12-hr light/dark cycle. They were fed Purina Chow (Ralston Purina, St. Louis, MO) and water ad libitum, and were acclimatized to the facility 7 days before the start of experiments.

The rats were divided into four groups. Two groups of 10–12 rats each were given a single i.p. injection of N-methyl N-nitrosourea (MNU; K&K Laboratories, Plainview, NY) dissolved in 10% ethanol and citrate buffer, pH 5.0, at a dose of 25 mg/kg body weight. The other two groups of 11 or 12 rats each received the solvent alone. One week later, one group of rats that received MNU and one group that received only the vehicle were placed on a basal diet (Dyets Inc., Bethlehem, PA) (*6*) containing 0.011% cyclosporine (CsA, Sandoz, Ltd., Basel, Switzerland). Two similar groups were given a basal diet. The CsA was mixed into the diet without the addition of any solvents, and both the CsA and basal diets were pelleted.

Food intakes were measured 3 days every week for the first 6 weeks. The animals were weighed every week during the first 10 weeks, and every 2–3 weeks thereafter up to the 30th week. The rats exhibiting rapid weight loss or clinical signs of general weakness were killed during the course of the experiments, and the experiments were terminated 34 weeks after the beginning of CsA feeding. When the animals were killed complete autopsies were done, and tissues from the thymus, mesenteric lymph nodes, intestinal lymphoid plaques, spleen, lung, kidney, and liver were fixed in stieve's solution solution. The tissues were sectioned and stained with hematoxylin and eosin.

RESULTS

No differences in the amount of food consumption were noted among the four groups of rats. In the first 6 weeks of the experiments, each group of rats consumed an average of 19–24 g of the diet per rat per day. In rats given a CsA diet, the daily intake of CsA by a rat during the initial 6-week period was 6.2–8.5 mg/kg body weight. The groups of rats that received a CsA diet continuously showed less gain in body weight compared with the group of rats that received a basal diet without MNU (Fig. 1). The differences were apparent after 10 weeks of the dietary treatment ($P<0.01$ by the Student's t test). Rats that received an MNU injection and were maintained on a basal diet showed a significant reduction in weight gain between 10 and 17 weeks ($P<0.01$) but regained their weight to approximately that of the basal diet group without MNU after 18

[1] This work was supported by grants from the National Institute of Health (CA 36175 and CA 18659).

[2] To whom correspondence should be sent at Department of Pathology, University of Pittsburgh, School of Medicine, Pittsburgh PA 15261.

* Abbreviations used: CsA, cyclosporine; MNU, N-methyl-N-nitrosourea.

weeks. The rats that developed intestinal carcinomas consistently showed a rapid weight loss.

Tumor incidence. Table 1 summarizes the incidence of intestinal adenocarcinomas in the four groups of rats. No intestinal tumors were observed in rats that received a CsA diet or a basal diet without MNU pretreatment (groups 3 and 4). Six of 10 rats that received a single injection of MNU and were maintained on a CsA diet (group 2) developed intestinal tumors (Fig. 2). The earliest tumor was noted in the 22nd week of the dietary treatment. All the tumors were sessile, ranging in greatest dimension between 7 mm. and 12 mm. Of six tumor-bearing rats, two had a tumor in the lower portion of the ileum. Four rats developed tumors in the ascending and transverse colon, and two of these four rats developed two tumors each in the colon. The tumors frequently caused intestinal obstruction and marked dilatation of the intestine proximal to the tumors. Of the 12 rats given a single injection of MNU and maintained on a basal diet (group 1), one rat developed an intestinal carcinoma in the 33rd week of the experiment. One rat from each group that received an MNU-injection developed a subcutaneous tumor on the side of chest wall. These tumors were adenocarcinomas, most probably of breast origin.

Histology. The major histological changes associated with the development of intestinal tumors in rats maintained on a CsA diet were in the gut-associated lymphoid plaques. These changes will be described in detail, and the pertinent changes in other organs will be mentioned briefly.

In the groups of rats maintained on a basal diet, the gut-associated lymphoid plaques were well preserved; they consisted of lymphoid aggregates in the submucosa and well-defined, serosally based germinal centers surrounded by small lymphocytes forming a subluminal caps (Fig. 3). The overlying epithelium showed intact intestinal villi. In rats maintained on a CsA diet without prior MNU treatment over 24 weeks, many of the gut-associated lymphoid plaques were hypertrophic and showed varying degrees of elevation from the mucosal surface. The regular patterns of the germinal centers and the lymphoid caps

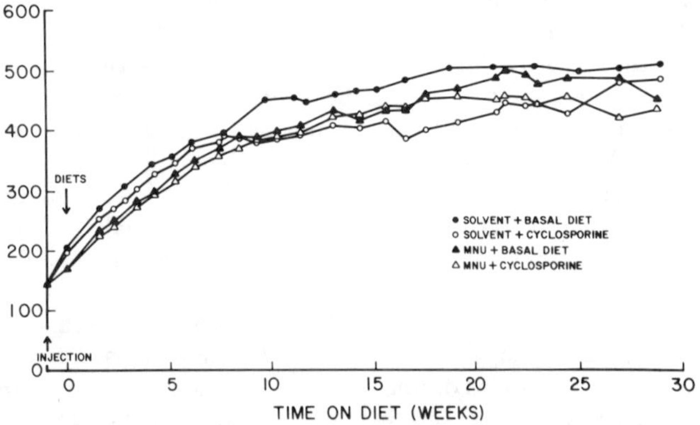

FIGURE 1. Changes in body weight of rats given four regimens of treatment. Each point represents the mean of 10–12 rats in the first 20 weeks. Between 20 and 30 weeks, 5 rats were killed in the group given MNU and maintained on the basal diet, and 3 or 4 rats were each from the other groups. The standard error of the mean for each point was less than 14% of the mean. The differences between the group given the solvent + basal diet and the groups given the solvent + cyclosporine and MNU + cyclosporine are significant ($P<0.01$) and 10 weeks. The differences between the group given the solvent + basal diet and the group given MNU + basal diet are significant ($P<0.01$) between 10 and 17 weeks.

TABLE 1. Incidence of intestinal adenocarcinomas

Group	Treatment		No. rats	No. rats with intestinal carcinomas	Mean latent period (weeks)
	MNU[a]	CsA[b]			
1	+	−	12	1 (8.6%)[c]	33
2	+	+	10	6 (60.0%)	26
3	−	−	10	0	—
4	−	+	12	0	—

[a] MNU: a single i.p. injection (2.5 mg/100g body weight).
[b] CsA: 0.011% in the diet.
[c] $P<0.05$ between group 1 and 2 by the chi-square test.

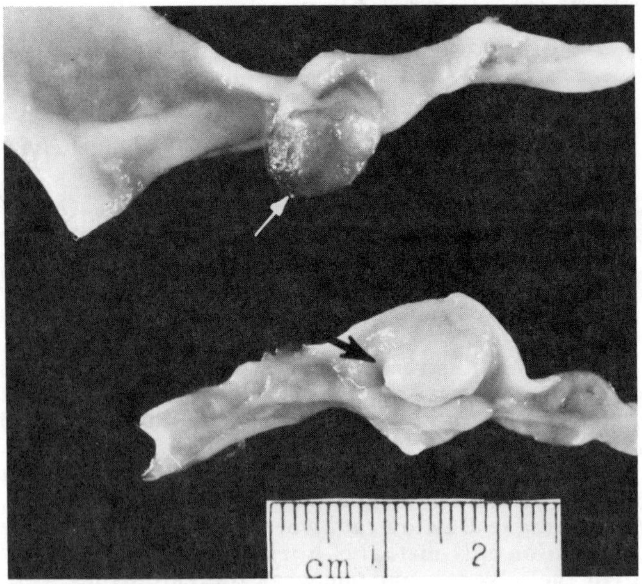

FIGURE 2. Gross appearance of colonic adenocarcinomas (arrows) in a rat given a single injection of MNU and maintained on a CsA diet for 26 weeks. Both tumors are sessile and protruding into the colonic lumena.

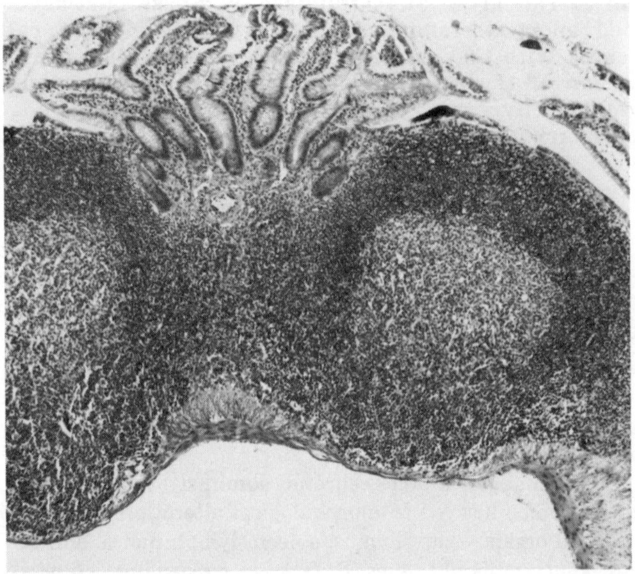

FIGURE 3. Microscopic appearance of the gut-associated lymphoid plaque of a rat maintained on a basal diet for 31 weeks. Well-defined germinal centers are surrounded by small lymphocytes and form subliminal caps (×63).

were obscured by proliferating large lymphocytes and immunoblasts (Fig. 4). The intestinal villi covering the lymphoid tissue were frequently flattened, and there was downward growth of mucosal glands into the lymphoid tissue (Fig. 4). Clusters of mucosal glands were frequently seen in the lymphoid tissue close to the serosal surfaces (Fig. 5), and these glands showed a high rate of mitosis in the epithelial cells (Fig. 6).

The changes in the gut-associated lymphoid tissues of the MNU-treated rats maintained on a CsA diet were more pronounced, exhibiting extensive downward growth of atypical mucosal glands (Fig. 7). Many glands embedded in the lymphoid tissues were cystically dilated and filled with mucinous material (Fig. 7). In addition, the epithelium associated with the lymphoid plaques frequently showed marked atypia of the mucosal glands suggestive of premalignant changes (Fig. 8). All the intestinal tumors were typical adenocarcinomas with varying degrees of mucin production and dense fibrous stroma (Fig. 9). Although lymphoid cells were seen at the periphery of the tumors, the tumors themselves showed rather scant lymphocytic infiltration. In one tumor, the stroma showed metaplastic bone formation (Fig. 10). Metastatic adenocarcinomas were found in the mesenteric lymph nodes of one rat.

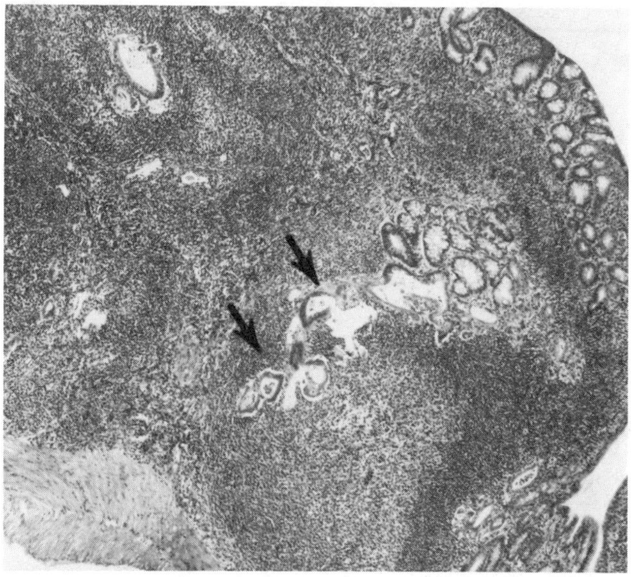

FIGURE 4. Microscopic appearance of the hypertropic colonic gut-associated lymphoid plaque of a rat maintained on the CsA diet for 28 weeks. The normal patterns of the germinal centers are obscured by proliferating lymphoid cells. The mucosa is flattened, and there are clusters of mucosal glands growing downward into the lymphoid tissues (×63).

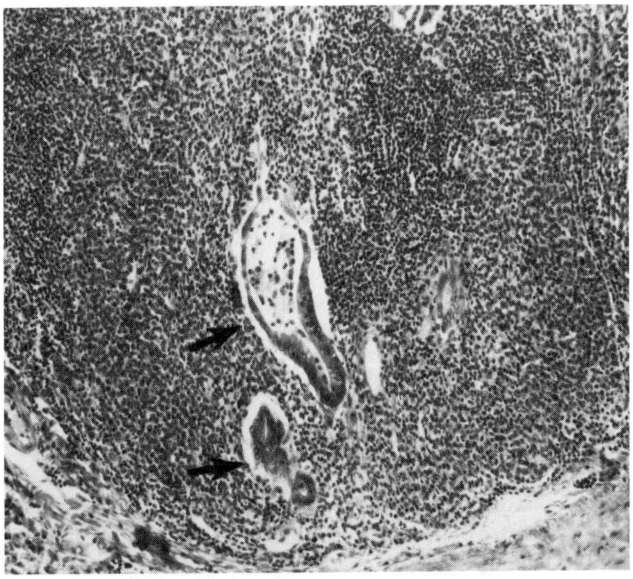

FIGURE 5. Microscopic appearance of the colonic gut-associated lymphoid plaque of a rat maintained on the CsA diet for 28 weeks. A few mucosal glands (arrows) are seen very close to the serosa (×140).

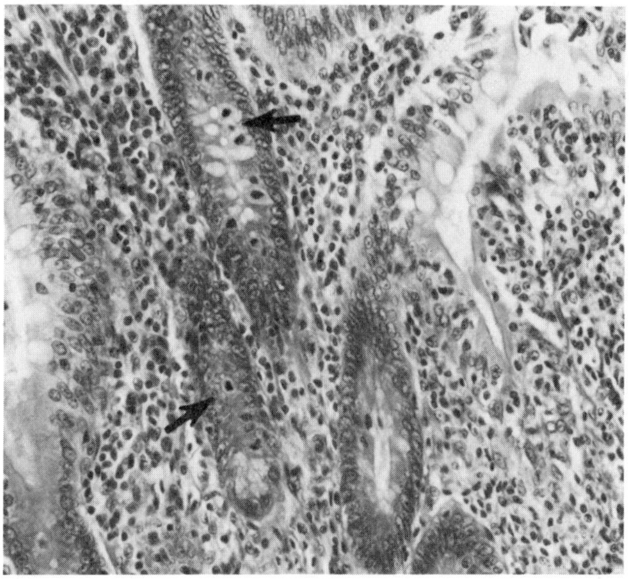

FIGURE 6. Microscopic appearance of the colonic mucosa adjacent to the gut-associated lymphoid plaque in a rat maintained on the CsA diet for 30 weeks. The glandular epithelium shows a high rate of mitosis (arrows) (×312).

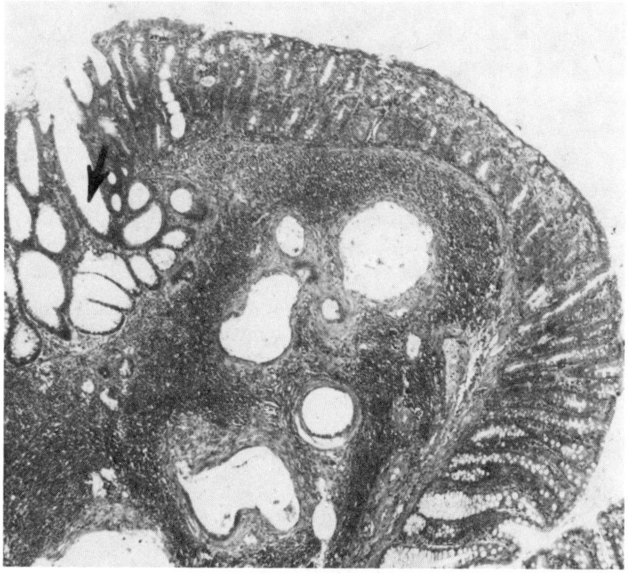

FIGURE 7. Microscopic appearance of a colonic gut-associated lymphoid plaque in a rat given a single injection of MNU and maintained on the CsA diet for 26 weeks. The plaque is hypertrophic and protruding into the lumen. Many mucosal glands are embedded in the lymphoid tissue and are cystically dilated. Hyperplastic mucosal glands (arrows) are also seen (×63).

The thymuses and the kidneys were the organs that consistently showed morphological alterations in the rats given a CsA diet, with or without prior MNU treatment. The thymuses showed varying degrees of medullary atrophy (*6*), and the kidneys showed signs of chronic interstitial nephritis characterized by the presence of scattered, cystically dilated tubules containing colloid casts and focal lymphocytic infiltration (Fig. 11).

DISCUSSION

This study was initiated to test whether CsA enhances the induction of lymphoid tumors, particularly in the gut, when animals are pretreated with a known chemical carcinogen: the results were completely unexpected and are described for the first time. MNU has been used for the induction of colonic tumors in experimental animals, but many studies employed repeated doses and direct intrarectal administration (*9–12*). We are not aware of any reports that a single i.p. injection of MNU resulted in the selective induction of intestinal tumors. In the present experiment, the high incidence of adenocarcinomas of the small and large intestine was obtained after a single i.p. injection of a relatively small dose of MNU (25 mg/kg body weight) when animals were kept on the diet containing CsA. The most likely explanation for the enhancement of the

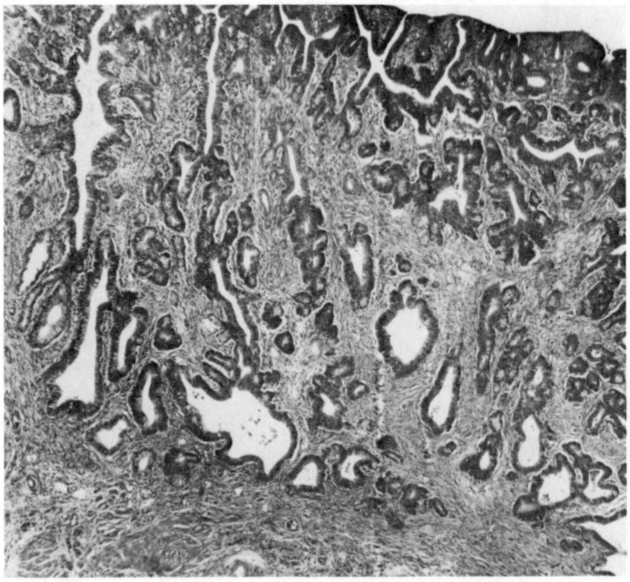

FIGURE 8. Microscopic appearance of atypical hyperplastic colonic mucosa adjacent to the gut-associated lymphoid plaque of a rat given a single injection of MNU and maintained on the CsA diet for 28 weeks (×58).

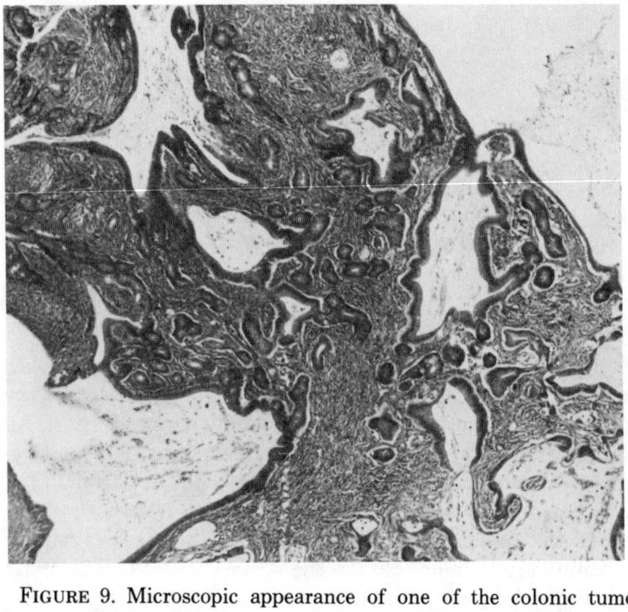

FIGURE 9. Microscopic appearance of one of the colonic tumor shown in Figure 2. It is a mucin-producing adenocarcinoma (×50).

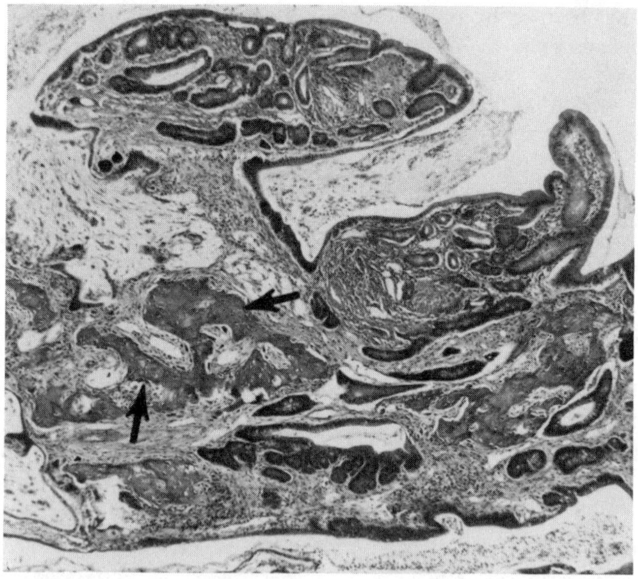

FIGURE 10. Microscopic appearance of the colonic tumor in a rat given a single injection of MNU and maintained on the CsA diet for 28 weeks. A typical adenocarcinoma and bony metaplasia (arrows) in the stroma are present (×63).

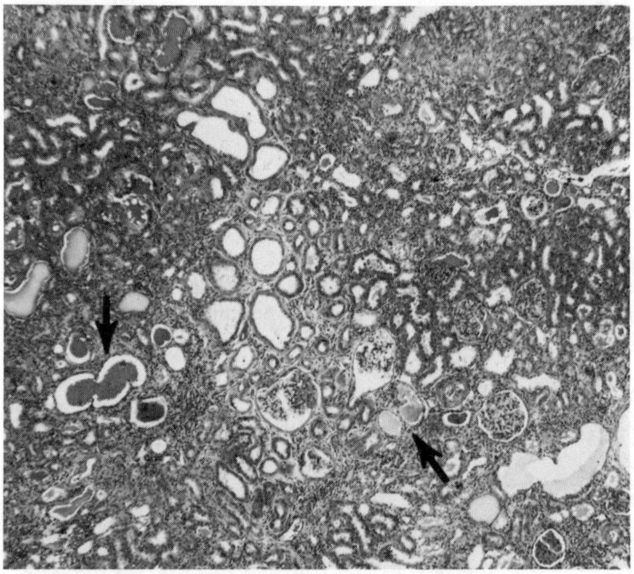

FIGURE 11. Microscopic appearance of the kidney of a rat maintained on the CsA diet for 33 weeks. The tubules show varying degrees of dilatation, and some contain colloid casts (arrows). There is slight interstitial fibrosis, as well as scattered lymphocytic infiltration. The glomeruli appear to be intact (×56).

intestinal tumor induction would be that it is secondary to the selective effect of CsA on the gut-associated lymphoid plaques.

Earlier we demonstrated that short-term feeding of CsA mixed in the diet caused marked alterations of the gut-associated lymphoid plaques, which consisted of blurring of the germinal centers, proliferation of lymphoid cells, and mucosal ulceration (*6*). The long-term effects could not be assessed in these studies because of the toxicity of CsA. By lowering of the CsA concentration in the diet, we were able to maintain rats for more than 30 weeks with only minor retardation of gain in body weight (Fig. 1). Although histological evidence of chronic pyelonephritis was noted in many animals on the CsA diet, it did not appear to cause death from renal failure, despite the well-documented renal toxicity of CsA (*13, 14*). The changes in the gut-associated lymphoid plaques involved both the lymphoid tissues and the covering epithelium. The changes in the latter were manifested by the distortion of the villi, flattening of the mucosa, downward growth of mucosal glands into the lymphoid tissue, and a high rate of mitosis in the epithelial cells of these glands. These changes strongly suggest that repeated injury and repair might have taken place in the epithelial cells associated with lymphoid tissue. In organ transplant patients receiving CsA and subsequently developing intestinal lymphomas, the mucosa adjacent to the lymphomatous nodules of the intestine showed changes similar to those described here (Nalesnik AM, personal communication).

As expected, the changes in the gut-associated lymphoid plaques induced by CsA in the MNU-treated rats were more severe than those in rats that did not receive MNU—particularly with respect to cellular and glandular atypia. Atypical mucosa suggestive of precancerous lesions was frequently associated with the lymphoid plaques. Based on these observations, we suggest that the adenocarcinomas developing in the gut under the present experimental conditions may originate from the areas of atypical mucosa associated with lymphoid plaques. The question of whether intestinal tumors arise in the regions of the gut-associated lymphoid plaques has been debated even in the conventional experimental model of the induction of colonic tumors by chemical carcinogens. Analysis of the spatial association of colon tumors induced by chemicals in relation to organized lymphoid aggregates led several investigators to suggest that experimentally induced colonic carcinomas arise at sites containing preexisting gut-associated lymphoid plaques (*15–17*).

Based on the current concept that cancer development is a multistep process broadly divisible into initiation and promotion (*18, 19*), it is reasonable to postulate that in the present experiment MNU served as the initiating agent and that the changes associated with CsA treatment exerted a promoting stimulus. Whether the CsA effects are mediated through simple mucosal damage and repair, which provides regenerative stimuli to the epithelial cells, or through more complex interactions of epithelial cells and lymphoid cells remains to be clarified. The epithelium overlying the gut-associated lymphoid plaques contains specialized cells termed "*M*" cells (*20, 21*). It is not known whether carcinogens or CsA selectively interact with these cells and cause the preferential development of adenocarcinomas in these sites. Sulfated polysaccharides, such as degraded carrageenan and dextran sulfate sodium, have been shown to induce colonic tumors in experimental animals (*22, 23*). There has been a suggestion that these compounds may act as tumor promoters rather than carcinogens that interact directly with DNA (*24*). Considering the known immunomodulatory effects of sulfated polysaccharides (*25–27*), their effects on the gut-associated lymphoid plaques and the overlying epithelium should be examined in light of the studies reported here. The experimental model of intestinal adenocarcinoma induction employing CsA, as described here, may be useful in analyzing many of the unanswered questions regarding the pathogenesis of intestinal carcinogenesis.

Finally, the results of the present experiments stand in sharp contrast to those of identical experiments conducted in mice. Feeding a CsA diet to mice initiated with a small dose of MNU markedly enhanced the development of thymic lymphomas (*8*). No such tumors were induced in rats, even though the experimental protocols were identical. Further studies are needed to clarify the significance of species difference in target organ specificity for the induction of cancer by CsA.

Acknowledgments. We thank Ms. Lynn A. Witkowski for her technical assistance, and Ms. Deborah L. Newman for preparation of the manuscript.

REFERENCES

1. Borel JF, Feurer C, Magnee C, Stahelin H. Effects of the new antilymphocytic peptide cyclosporin A in animals. Immunology 1977; 32: 1017.
2. Morris PJ. Cyclosporin A. Transplantation 1981; 38: 349.
3. Calne RY. Immunosuppression for organ grafting—observation with cyclosporine A. Immunol Rev 1979; 46: 113.
4. White DJG, Plumb AM, Pawelec G, Brons G. Cyclosporin A: an immunosuppressive agent preferentially active against proliferating T cells. Transplantation 1979; 27: 55.
5. Britton S, Palacios R. Cyclosporin A: usefulness, risks and mechanisms of action. Immunol Rev 1982; 65: 5.
6. Demetris AJ, Nalesnik MA, Kunz HW, Gill TJ, Shinozuka H. Sequential analyses of the development of lymphoproliferative disorders in rats receiving cyclosporine. Transplantation 1984; 38: 239.
7. Shinozuka H, Demetris AJ, Witkowski LA, Perera MIR, Nalesnik MA, Gill TJ. Experimental model of cyclosporine-induced lymphoproliferative disorders. Fed Proc 1984; 43: 662.
8. Shinozuka H, Gill TJ, Kunz HW, Witkowski LA, Demetris JA, Perera MIR. Enhancement of the induction of murine thymic lymphomas by cyclosporine. Transplantation 1986; 41: 377.
9. Reddy BS, Watanabe K, Wesiburger JH. Effect of high fat diet on colon carcinogenesis in F344 rats treated with 1,2-dimethylhydrazine, methylazoxymethanol acetate or methylnitrosourea. Cancer Res 1977; 37: 4156.
10. Lev R, Herp A. Pathogenesis of rat colon carcinomas induced by N-methyl-N-nitrosourea. J Natl Cancer Inst 1978; 61: 779.
11. Ward JM, Sporn MB, Wenk ML, Smith JM, Feeser D, Dean RJ. Dose response to intrarectal administration of N-methyl-N-nitrosourea and histopathologic evaluation of the effect of two retinoids on colon lesions induced in rats. J Natl Cancer Inst 1978; 60: 1489.
12. Weese JL, Starling JR, Turner JH. Development of a carcinogen induced rat colon cancer with lymph node metastases. Dis Colon Rectum 1983; 26: 573.
13. Ryffel B. Experimental toxicological studies with cyclosporin A. In: White DJG, ed. Proceedings of an international conference on Cyclosporin A. Cambridge, MA: Elsevier, 1982: 45.
14. Thomson AW, Whiting PH, Simpson JG. Pathobiology of cyclosporin A in experimental animals. In: White DJG, ed. Proceedings of an international conference on Cyclosporin A. Cambridge, MA: Elsevier, 1982: 177.
15. Bland PW, Britton DC. Colonic lymphoid tissue and its influence on tumor induction in dimethylhydrazine-treated rats. Br J Cancer 1981; 44: 275.

16. Nauss KM, Locniskar M, Pavlina T, Newberne PM. Morphology and distribution of 1,2-dimethylhydrazine dihydrochloride-induced colon tumors and their relationship to gut-associated lymphoid tissue in the rat. J Natl Cancer Inst 1984; 73: 915.
17. Deasy JM, Steele G, Ross DS, Lahey SJ, Wilson RE, Madara J. Gut-associated lymphoid tissue and dimethylhydrazine-induced colorectal carcinoma in the Wistar/Furth rat. J Surg Oncol 1983; 24: 36.
18. Pitot HC, Serica AE. The stages of initiation and promotion in hepatocarcinogenesis. Biochim Biophys Acta 1980; 605: 191.
19. Farber E. The multistep nature of cancer development. Cancer Res 1984; 44: 4217.
20. Owen RL, Jones AL. Epithelial cell specialization within human Peyer's patches: an ultrastructural study of intestinal lymphoid follicles. Gastroenterology 1974; 66: 189.
21. Smith MW, Peacock MA. "M" cell distribution in follicle-associated epithelium of mouse Peyer's patch. Am J Anat 1980; 159: 167.
22. Iatropoulos MJ, Goldberg L, Coulston F. Intestinal carcinogenesis in rats using 1,2 dimethylhydrazine with or without degraded carrageenan. Exp Mol Pathol 1975; 23: 386.
23. Hirono I, Kuhara K, Hosaka S, Tomizawa S, Goldberg L. Induction of intestinal tumors in rats by dextran sulfate sodium. J Natl Cancer Inst 1981; 66: 579.
24. Hirono I, Ueno I, Aiso S, Yamaji T, Goldberg L. Enhancing effect of dextran sulfate sodium on colorectal carcinogenesis by 1,2-dimethylhydrazine in rats. Gan 1983; 74: 493.
25. Thomson AW, Brent L, Fowler EF. Carrageenan and the immune response. Lancet 1981; 1: 671.
26. Larsen B. The biological effects of carrageenan and other sulphated polysaccharides with particular attention to immunological and cancerological properties. Ugeskr Laeger 1982; 144: 860.
27. Bergstedt-Lindqvist S, Fernandez C, Severinson E. A synergistic polyclonal response to dextran sulphate and lipopoly-saccharide immunoglobulin secretion and cell requirements. Scand J Immunol 1982; 15: 439.

Received 4 October 1985.
Accepted 2 December 1985.

0041-1337/86/4203-0302$02.00/0
TRANSPLANTATION Vol. 42, No. 3

ABROGATION OF THE IMMUNOSUPPRESSIVE EFFECT OF DONOR SPLEEN CELLS ON RENAL ALLOGRAFTS IN THE RAT BY IRRADIATION OR HEAT TREATMENT[1]

DAVID CRANSTON,[2] KATHRYN J. WOOD,[3] AND PETER J. MORRIS

Nuffield Department of Surgery, University of Oxford, John Radcliffe Hospital, Oxford, United Kingdom

In the donor-recipient strain combination Lewis ($RT1^l$) to Dark Agouti ($RT1^a$), indefinite renal allograft survival (MST> 100 days) was induced by pretreating recipient animals i.v. with 10^6 to 10^8 viable spleen lymphocytes, seven days before transplantation. Pretreatment with 10^4 or 10^5 cells was ineffective (MST 10 days). However when 10^7 live, but heat-treated (55°C for 10 min) or irradiated (1000 rads) cells were used, all the animals rejected the allograft in a normal fashion (MST 10 and 11 days, respectively). Median survival time of third-party controls was 10 days.

The relative amount of cell surface major histocompatibility antigens (class I and class II) expressed by the three spleen cell preparations was investigated using monoclonal antibodies and fluorescence activated cell sorter analysis and found to be similar. After 24 hr in culture, only 1% of heat-treated and 10% of irradiated cells were viable, in contrast to 75% of untreated splenocytes. Trafficking of these lymphocytes in recipient animals was investigated by ^{51}chromium labeling of the cells: 30% of lymphocytes had localized in the liver within 3 hr with little difference in localization among the different cell preparations. But, although 20% of normal and irradiated cells localized in the spleen within 3 hr, at no stage were more than 5% of the heat-treated cells found in the spleen. It is suggested that the length of time viable donor lymphocytes remain in the recipient circulation is important in the induction of specific immunosuppression by spleen lymphocytes.

The beneficial effect of preoperative blood transfusion in renal transplantation is well established (*1*, *2*), although the underlying mechanism remains obscure. In the rat, renal allografts have been enhanced by pretreatment with cells of donor origin from lymph node, bone marrow and spleen (*3–6*); whole blood (*7–8*); and cellular components of blood (*9–13*). In contrast to the clinical phenomenon, this enhancement in the rat can be shown to be immunologically specific.

A number of hypotheses have been advanced to explain these effects in both the induction and maintenance phase of the suppression. They include the formation of antiidiotype antibodies (*14*), Fc-receptor-blocking antibodies (*15*), anti-Ia-blocking antibodies (*16*), and the induction of suppressor cells (*17*). A suppressor cell mechanism now seems to be the most likely mechanism to explain the specific immunosuppression induced by whole blood in the rat (*17*). Although there is no

[1] This work was supported by a grant from the Medical Research Council.
[2] The Hanson Surgical Research Fellow.
[3] Address correspondence to: Dr. Kathryn J. Wood, Nuffield Dept. of Surgery, John Radcliffe Hospital, Oxford, OX3 9DU U.K.

doubt that the (MHC)* is important, the different cell types that have been shown to cause the induction of suppression differ in their expression of MHC antigens. The precise role of class I and class II antigens in enhancement is not yet clear, although it has been shown beyond doubt that highly purified erythrocytes that express class I antigen alone can be used to induce suppression of allograft rejection, as well as cells expressing both class I and class II molecules (*13*).

In this study we have confirmed the immunosuppressive effect of whole spleen cells in the LEW-to-DA strain combination and sought to modify the cells by heat treatment or irradiation of the lymphocytes prior to pretreatment of the allograft recipient. We have then compared two aspects of the treated cells with normal cells—namely, viability after treatment and the localization of both treated and normal chromium-labeled cells in vivo.

MATERIALS AND METHODS

Animals. Inbred male Lewis ($RT1^l$–LEW), Dark Agouti ($RT1^a$–DA), and Brown Norway ($RT1^n$–BN) rats between 10 and 30 weeks of age were used in all experiments. All animals were maintained at the John Radcliffe Hospital, Oxford, where the DA and LEW rats were bred. BN rats were purchased from Olac, U.K.

Transplantation. Allogeneic kidneys were transplanted into the left orthotopic site with end-to-end anastomosis of the blood vessels and ureter, essentially as described previously (*18*). A seven-day contralateral nephrectomy was performed. Transplant function was assessed by serum urea estimations on days 0 (the time of transplantation), 7, 10, and 14—and subsequently at weekly intervals.

Preparation of spleen cells. The spleen was teased through a 500-μ gauge sieve into 10 ml of phosphate-buffered saline (PBS). The suspension was transferred to a 50-ml falcon tube, and the large particles allowed to settle. The supernatant was centrifuged at 1000 rpm for 10 min, and the cells washed twice in PBS. Contaminating red blood cells were lysed by resuspending the cells in 2 ml of tris ammonium chloride and incubating them at room temperature for 5 min. The suspension was then diluted to 50 ml with PBS, and centrifuged at 1000 rpm for 10 min. The cells were washed twice in PBS and resuspended at 10^8 cells/ml in 0.5% (w/v) bovine serum albumin in PBS. Immediately before pretreatment of the recipient animals, the cells were washed and resuspended in normal saline.

Pretreatment. The LEW recipients were injected i.v. with different doses of cells in 1 ml of normal saline into the femoral vein or dorsal vein of the penis seven days or one day before transplantation. Some animals were given two or three i.v. doses during the seven days before transplantation.

Heat treatment and irradiation. Heat treatment was carried out by placing the cells in a 20-ml plastic container in a water bath at 55°C for 10 min. Cells to be irradiated were given 1000 rads, at a dose of 500 rads/min, in a gamma irradiator (Gamma cell 1000, Isomedix Inc., Parsippany, NJ). The cells were treated immediately before injection into the recipients.

Cell viability. The cells were checked for viability immediately before injection into the recipient by staining with florescein diacetate (FDA) and ethidium bromide (EB). Those cells that were cultured in RPMI 1640 for 24 hr were also assessed in a similar fashion, before and after the culture period.

Fluorescence analysis of cell surface MHC antigens. Donor spleen lymphocytes (10^6 in 50 μl 0.5% BSA/PBS) were incubated with a saturating concentration (10 μg/ml) of three monoclonal antibodies: F16.44.11 (anti-class-I), F17.44.11 (anti-class-II) and MRC OX1 (anti-leukocyte-common antigen). A negative control was included in each assay. Using affinity-purified goat antimouse antibody, conjugated to fluorescein isothiocyanate (FITC) (Sigma, U.K.) blocked with 10% (v/v) normal rat serum, the cells were examined by flow cytometry on a cytofluograf (System 50 L, Ortho Diagnostic Inc., Boston, MA).

Traffic of ^{51}Cr-labeled allogeneic cells. A method similar to that first described by Bainbridge et al. (*19*) for mice, and Heslop and Hardy (*20*) for rats was used. The donor spleen lymphocytes were taken and labeled in vitro with ^{51}chromium at a concentration of 10 μCi/10^8 cells/ml. After incubation for 90 min at 37°C the cells were layered over 5 ml fetal calf serum and centrifuged at 1000 rpm at 4°C for 10 min. The supernatant was discarded and the cells washed three times in normal saline before being resuspended at 10^7 cells/ml. The cells were counted in a gamma counter before being injected i.v. into groups of syngeneic and allogeneic recipients. The animals were killed at 3, 24, and 72 hr, and one week after injection, and the different organs removed and counted in a gamma counter. Three animals were used at each time point. The localization in each tissue was expressed as a percentage of the counts in the injected cells.

Statistics. The significance of all comparisons was assessed by the Mann-Whitney *U* test.

RESULTS

Pretreatment with normal donor spleen cells. DA rats pretreated 7 days before transplantation with a single i.v. dose of 10^6, 10^7, or 10^8 donor LEW spleen cells accepted a LEW kidney indefinitely (Table 1); 10^5 or 10^4 cells were ineffective. The effect was donor-specific as 10^7 BN cells did not influence the rejection of LEW kidneys.

In contrast, pretreatment the day before transplantation failed to produce any significant enhancement (Table 2). Of the seven animals given 10^8 donor spleen cells the day before transplantation, two survived for 42 and 43 days, respectively. However both animals had persistantly elevated ureas (>200 mg%) following the delayed nephrectomy on day 7 (results not shown).

Pretreatment with heat-treated and irradiated cells. Heat-treated (55°C for 10 min) LEW splenocytes (10^7) failed to prolong allograft survival (Table 3). These cells were not immediately killed by the heat treatment, 50% being viable at the time of injection (Table 4). But following a 24 hr period of culture in vitro there were virtually no viable cells.

Similarly, splenocytes irradiated with 1000 rads failed to enhance—although viability at the time of injection was similar to that of untreated cells (Tables 3 and 4). These cells die more slowly in vitro than do the heat-killed cells. After 24 hr of culture, 10% were still viable, in contrast to 1% of the heat-treated cells. But in marked contrast, 70% of the untreated cells were viable.

Although a single dose of irradiated cells seven days before transplantation fails to induce prolongation of graft survival, multiple doses of irradiated cells will enhance it (Table 5). A

* Abbreviations used: BN, Brown Norway; DA, Dark Agouti; EB, ethidium bromide; FDA, fluorescein diacetate; FITC, fluorescein isothiocyanate; LEW, Lewis; MHC, major histocompatibility complex; MST, median survival time; PBS, phosphate-buffered saline.

TABLE 1. Pretreatment of recipient animals i.v. with various numbers of donor spleen cells 7 days before transplantation

Donor to recipient	Strain of donor cells	Dose of donor cells	Number of animals	Survival	MST (days)	P value[a]
LEW-to-DA	LEW	10^8	5	>100 (×5)	>100	<0.004
	LEW	10^7	8	70,[b] >100 (×7)	>100	<0.004
	LEW	10^6	5	>100 (×5)	>100	<0.004
	LEW	10^5	5	10,11,11,10,10	10	
	LEW	10^4	2	10,10	10	
	—	—	5	10,10,10,10,11	10	
	BN	10^7	5	10,10,10,10,10	10	

[a] P values were obtained using the Mann-Whitney U test by comparing the group of animals pretreated with donor spleen cells with those treated with third-party cells.
[b] Not rejected MST – median survival time.

TABLE 2. Pretreatment of DA rats with LEW spleen cells i.v. 1 day before transplantation of a LEW kidney

Dose of donor cells	Number of animals	Survival (days)	MST[a] (days)
10^8	7	10,10,10,11,11,42,[b] 43[b]	10
10^7	2	10,10	10

[a] (MST) median survival time.
[b] With high ureas.

TABLE 3. Pretreatment of DA rats with 10^7 heat-treated (55°C for 10 min) or irradiated (1000 rads) LEW spleen cells i.v. 7 days before transplantation of a LEW kidney

Treatment	Number of animals	Survival (days)	MST[a]
Heat-treated	6	10,10,10,10,10,11	10
Irradiated	5	11,11,11,11,12	11

[a] (MST) median survival time.

TABLE 4. Viability of normal, heat-treated, and irradiated cells on injection and after being cultured in vitro for 24 hr.[a]

	On injection	24 hr in culture
Normal	85% ±5	70% ±10
Irradiated	85% ±5	10% ±4
Heat-treated	50% ±10	1% ±1

[a] The results are reported as the mean value for 10 high power fields ± 1 SD. The cells were stained with fluorescein diacetate and ethidium bromide.

TABLE 5. Pretreatment of DA rats with multiple doses of irradiated (1000 rads) LEW cells i.v. at different times before transplantation of a LEW kidney

Day before transplant −7	−5	−3	Total cell dose	No. animals	Survival	MST[a]
10^7	10^7	10^7	3×10^7	5	>100 (×5)	>100
10^7	—	10^7	2×10^7	8	9,12,13[b],13,13,19 >100, >100	13[c]
10^6	10^6	10^6	3×10^6	4	>100 (×4)	>100
10^6	—	10^6	2×10^6	2	10,11	10
—	—	—	—	5	10,10,10,10,11	10

[a] (MST) median survival time.
[b] Technical failure.
[c] $P = 0.034$ compared with controls.

total dose of 3×10^7 cells or 3×10^6 cells given in 3 doses during the seven days prior to transplantation results in indefinite graft survival (MST>100 days). The blood ureas are more elevated at 10 days and take longer to return to normal levels than those in the animals pretreated with normal cells (results not shown). The effect is less marked with two doses of a total of 2×10^7 cells (MST 13 days) or 2×10^6 cells (MST 10 days) (Table 4).

The influence of treatment on the expression of MHC antigens. There was no difference in the cell surface expression of class I or class II MHC antigens by the spleen leukocytes immediately after irradiation, although after heat treatment a slight reduction was observed in the amount of class I antigen expressed (Table 6).

Trafficking experiments. Figure 1 shows the results of the trafficking experiments of ^{51}chromium-labeled LEW splenocytes after i.v. injection of the cells in syngeneic and allogeneic recipients. Most of the cells pass through the lungs quickly, although the heat-treated allogeneic cells seemed to be delayed for longer than the other preparations of cells, which may be due to clumping of these cells following heat treatment (results not shown). Within 3 hr, 30% of lymphocytes localized in the liver, and over the next few days the counts decreased to 20% of that injected. There was little difference among the three cell types in their localization in the liver (Fig. 1, A and B). This is in direct contrast to the spleen: 20% of the normal and irradiated lymphocytes were found in the spleen within 3 hr, but at no stage did more than 5% of the heat-treated cells, either allogeneic or syngeneic, localize in the spleen (Fig. 1, C and D).

DISCUSSION

In these experiments, DA rats pretreated with a single i.v. injection of LEW spleen leukocytes showed suppression of rejection and enhanced survival of LEW kidneys. The results are comparable to previous studies in different strain combinations. Guttman et al. (*3*) showed that a single i.v. injection of 10^7 cells from thymus, spleen, lymph nodes, or whole blood 5–7 days before transplantation in the (LEW×BN)F_1-to-LEW strain combination resulted in suppression of rejection. Ockner et al. demonstrated a similar effect with bone marrow cells (*4*). Lauchart et al. (*11*) and El-Malik et al. (*12*) have examined the enhancing role of B and T lymphocyte subpopulations—in a cardiac and renal allograft model, respectively—and shown that the enhancement is produced by the B cell, and not the T cell, subpopulation. However it should be noted that our own current experiments in a different strain combination do not confirm these findings.

The timing of the pretreatment is important in this model, for although pretreatment at or immediately before transplantation would be the ideal protocol for clinical use, pretreatment

TABLE 6. The surface major histocompatibility antigens present on untreated, heat-treated, and irradiated cells immediately after treatment (expressed as percentages of cells labeled)

	Normal	Heat	Irradiated
Negative control (0.5% BSA/PBS)	6.9	3.2	3.1
F16	96.5	82.7	96.3
F17	25.6	28.5	25.5
OX1	96.4	93.1	98.3

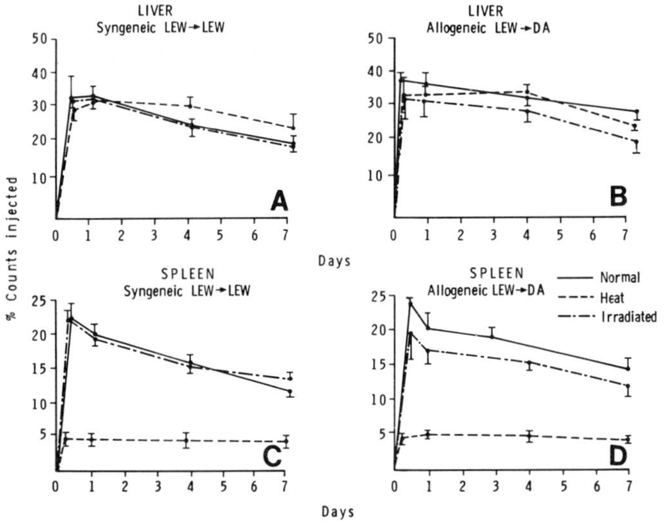

FIGURE 1. Trafficking of ^{51}Cr-labeled spleen lymphocytes into the liver (A, B) and spleen (C, D) of syngeneic and allogeneic recipients. Expressed as a percentage of the counts injected ±SEM.

one day before transplantation was much less effective in this model (Table 2). Stuart et al. (*5*) found that 10^8 viable spleen cells 24 hr before transplant in the $(LEW \times BN)F_1$-to-LEW combination (with immediate nephrectomy) caused increased graft survival, but the animals had persistently high blood ureas. Silber et al. (*6*) demonstrated indefinite survival with 1.5×10^8 donor spleen cells in the $(LEW \times DA)F_1$-to-DA combination, but this is a weak histocompatibility barrier. Our results showed prolonged survival in two of eight animals treated with 10^8 spleen cells one day before transplantation, but both these animals had persistently high blood ureas (Table 2). Thus it is apparent that the i.v. injection of splenocytes needs to be at least some days before the transplantation of the renal allograft.

Both heat treatment and irradiation of the spleen cells were found to abrogate the enhancement effect of a single injection of cells, with recipient animals rejecting their grafts in the same time as the controls (Table 3). Exposure of cells to heat has been shown to damage DNA, RNA, proteins, nucleoproteins, lipids, chromosomes, nucleoli, membranes, lysosomes, and microtubules—as well as a large variety of biosynthetic pathways and metabolic functions within the cell (*21*), and differing degrees of heat will produce these effects to differing degrees. However in our experiments, heating to 55°C resulted in the immediate death of 50% of cells, and no cells were viable after 24 hr in culture. It could be assumed that few viable cells persisted after i.v. injection.

Lymphocytes are among the most radiosensitive of all mammalian cells. They are also unusual with regard to the time of cell death following irradiation. Whereas most cells exposed to low or moderate doses of irradiation do not die until the time of first or second cell division (mitotic death), some subpopulations of lymphocytes die soon after exposure (interphase death) (*22*). The mechanisms involved in interphase death are poorly understood, as is the physical and chemical basis for the remakable sensitivity of the lymphocyte. Furthermore, specific subpopulations of lymphocytes differ in their sensitivity to irradiation. In particular, B cells irradiated and maintained in tissue culture survive less well than do T cells treated in an identical fashion (*23*), and B cells exhibit radiation-induced morphological abnormalities at lower doses than do T cells (*24*). B cells are more radiosensitive than T cells, as judged by their ability to home to secondary lymphoid tissues and recirculate in a normal manner (*23*). This is of particular interest in view of previous reports that B cells will cause enhancement of both cardiac and renal allografts in the rat, but T cells fail to do so (*11, 12*). So it is possible that the irradiation of the spleen cells led to a selective depletion of B cells, thus abrogating the enhancing effect.

Although most of the irradiated, and 50% of the heat-treated, cells appear viable on injection they probably die faster than normal cells. Studies on the kinetics of cell death in tumor lines indicate a contrast between direct heat death, which is rapid and essentially complete within 24–48 hr and irradiation-induced death which is observed after a delay period of several days (*25*). Although a substantial number of heat treated and irradiated cells were alive at the time of injection, they may be dying more quickly than normal cells. The death of all heat-treated and most of the irradiated cells during 24 hr of culture supports that suggestion. As the time when viable cells are present in the recipient circulation may have a role to play in the induction and maintenance of enhancement, experiments using normal and treated cells labeled with ^{51}Cr were undertaken to attempt to resolve this question.

There was a marked difference in the trafficking of heat-treated cells, in contrast to normal or irradiated cells, that essentially followed a similar pattern in both syngeneic and allogeneic recipients. Heslop and Hardy (*20*) have found a difference when lymphocyte distribution in allogeneic recipients is compared with that in syngeneic animals, with more label being recovered from the spleen than the lymph nodes in allogeneic recipients and the reverse being true in syngeneic animals. Interestingly, they found that no label was recovered from the lymph nodes when heat-treated cells were injected. This was found also to be the case in the mesenteric group of nodes that we studied (results not shown). There is evidence to suggest that allogeneic cells are not killed in the lymph nodes, and that the radioactivity in the lymph nodes accurately reflects live cells (*26*). Allogeneic cells that fail to reach the lymph nodes may be eliminated within 48 hr (*27*). The elimination is due to natural cytotoxicity and depends on the presence of an intact spleen (*27*).

Whether the extent of radioactivity in an organ continues to reflect the number of living donor cells remains a debatable point. Although it seems quite possible that, after the death of ^{51}Cr-labeled cells in tissues, their radioactivity may be incorporated into macrophages (*28*), cells that are destroyed in the circulation probably do not have their ^{51}chromium reutilized, and it is excreted in the urine (*28*).

This trafficking data supports the hypothesis that heat-treated cells are eliminated more quickly from the recipient—hence the abrogation of the enhancing effect. But it does not explain the difference in the enhancing effect between normal and irradiated cells. Initially it was thought that the chromium labeling itself could have the same effect as irradiation, and that the so called normal cells labeled with chromium were behaving as irradiated cells. However, with smaller doses of chromium, as used in this study, similar results were obtained, and it seems unlikely that this is the explanation. In view of other workers' experience with irradiation and lymphocyte subsets, it may be that apparently normal localization of irradiated cells reflects the localization of T cells rather than B cells, the latter being more radiation-sensitive. This might also explain why lower doses of irradiation do not abrogate the enhancing effect, if one postulates that B cells are surviving, at least for a sufficient length of time to cause the required enhancement. Furthermore we have shown that multiple doses of irradiated cells do induce prolonged graft survival, and the mechanism of this may be that it effectively lengthens the time that viable cells, especially B cells, are presented to the recipient.

From these studies it appears that pretreatment with spleen leukocytes i.v. must take place some days before renal allografting if enhancement is to occur. Little attention has been focused on the fate of donor cells once they are in the recipient circulation in relation to the mechanism of tolerance induction—and, although it has been assumed in the past that the majority of these cells are rapidly destroyed, some may be surviving. The abrogation of enhancement by heat treatment or irradiation of the spleen cells is probably due to death of the cells soon after injection—consequently, viability of the injected cells for some undetermined period within the lymphoid circulation is necessary for enhancement to occur.

REFERENCES

1. Opelz G, Terasaki PI. Poor kidney transplant survival in recipients with frozen blood transfusions or no transfusions. Lancet 1974; 2: 696.
2. Opelz G. Blood transfusions and renal transplantation. In: Morris PJ, ed. Kidney transplantation: principles and practice. 2nd ed. London, New York: Grune & Stratton, 1984: 323.
3. Guttmann RD, Lindquist RR, Kawabe K, Ockner SA. Renal transplantation in the inbred rat. Further observations on the induction of enhancement by active immunization. Transplantation 1972; 13: 15.
4. Ockner SA, Guttmann RD, Lindquist RR. Renal transplantation in the inbred rat. Modification of rejection by active immunization with bone marrow cells. Transplantation 1970; 9: 30.
5. Stuart FP, Saitoh T, Fitch FW. Rejection of renal allografts: specific immunologic suppression. Science 1968; 160: 1463.
6. Silber SJ, Miller JFAP, Morris PJ. Graft-versus-host reactivity and renal allograft survival in rats given allogeneic spleen cells or spleen allografts. Transplantation 1976; 22: 160.
7. Fabre JW, Morris PJ. The effect of donor strain blood pretreatment on renal allograft rejection in rats. Transplantation 1972; 14: 608.
8. Marquet RL, Heystek GA, Tinbergen WJ. Specific inhibition of organ allograft rejection by donor blood. Transplant Proc 1971; 3: 708.
9. Welsh KI, Burgos H, Batchelor JR. The immune response to allogeneic rat platelets (Ag-B antigens) in matrix form lacking Ia. Eur J Immunol 1977; 7: 267.
10. Jenkins AM, Woodruff MFA. The effect of prior administration of donor strain blood or blood constituents on the survival of cardiac allografts in rats. Transplantation 1971; 12: 57.
11. Lauchart W, Alkins BJ, Davies DAL. Only B lymphocytes induce active enhancement of rat cardiac allografts. Transplantation 1980; 29: 259.
12. El-Malik F, Malik STA, Varghese Z, Sweny P, Moorhead JF. The enhancing and sensitizing effects of donor blood components, including dendritic cells, in a rat renal allograft model. Transplantation 1984; 38: 213.
13. Wood KJ, Evins J, Morris PJ. Suppression of renal allograft rejection in the rat by class I antigens on purified erythrocytes. Transplantation 1985; 39: 56.
14. Fagnilli L, Singal DP. Blood transfusions may induce anti-T cell receptor antibodies in renal patients. Transplant Proc 1982; 14: 319.
15. McLeod AM, Power DA, Mason RJ, Stewart KN, Shewan WG, Edward N, Catto GR. Possible mechanism of action of transfusion effect in renal transplantation. Lancet 1982; 2: 468.
16. Davies DAL, Staines NA. A cardinal role for I region antigens (Ia) in immunological enhancement and the clinical implications. Transplant Rev 1976; 30: 18.
17. Hutchinson IV, Wood KJ, Morris PJ. Suppressor cells present in rat kidney allografts in untreated or blood transfused recipients. (Submitted.).
18. Fabre J, Lim SH, Morris PJ. Renal transplantation in the rat: details of a technique. Aust NZ J Surg 1971; 41: 69.
19. Bainbridge DR, Brent L, Gowland G. Distribution of allogeneic 51Cr-labelled lymph node cells in mice. Transplantation 1966; 4: 2.
20. Heslop BF, Hardy BE. The distribution of 51Cr-labeled syngeneic and allogeneic lymph node cells in the rat. Transplantation 1971; 11: 128.
21. Thrall DE, Gerweck LE, Gillette EL, Dewey WC. Response of cells in vitro and tissues in vivo to hyperthermia and x-irradiation. In: Lett JT, Adler H, eds. Advances in radiation biology, vol 6. New York: Academic, 1976: 1.
22. Anderson RE, Standefer JC. Radiation injury in the immune system. In: Potten CS, Hendry JH, eds. Cytotoxic insult to tissues: effect on cell lineages. London: Churchill Livingstone, 1983: 67.
23. Anderson RE, Sprent J, Miller JFAP. Radiosensitivity of T and B lymphocytes. I. Effect of irradiation on cell migration. Eur J Immunol 1974; 4: 199.
24. Anderson RE, Standefer JC, Scaletti JV. Radiosensitivity of defined populations of lymphocytes. VI. Functional, structural and biochemical consequences of in vitro radiation. Cell Immunol 1977; 33: 45.
25. Mivechi NF, Hofer KG. Evidence for separate modes of action in thermal radiosensitization and direct thermal cell death. Cancer 1983; 51: 38.
26. Heslop BF, McNeilage J. Natural cytotoxicity: early killing of allogeneic lymphocytes in rats. Immunol Rev 1983; 73: 35.
27. McNeilage LJ, Heslop BF. Lymphocyte homing in syngeneic and unsensitized MHC compatible allogeneic hosts. I. Evidence for both syngeneic self-recognition and early killing of allogeneic cells. Cell Immunol 1980; 50: 58.
28. Rolstad B, Ford WL. The rapid elimination of allogeneic lymphocytes: relationship to established mechanisms of immunity and to lymphocyte traffic. Immunol Rev 1983; 73: 87.

Received 12 November 1985.
Accepted 28 November 1985.

0041-1337/86/4203-0307$02.00/0
TRANSPLANTATION
Vol. 42, No. 3

Printed in U.S.A.

Transplantation

BRIEF COMMUNICATIONS

INTRAVASCULAR COAGULATION AND KIDNEY DONATION[1]

Cadaveric kidneys from a donor with intravascular coagulation are generally not accepted for grafting. We report here the outcome after grafting the kidneys of a donor with intravascular coagulation. The donor was 19 years old with a femoral shaft fracture and severe brain damage after a trauma. Laboratory investigations before donor nephrectomy showed a decreased number of thrombocytes: 70×10^9/L ($150<n<350\times10^9$), a decreased fibrinogen content: 0.7 g/L ($1.7<n<4.0$), and increased fibrin degradation products: 70 mg/L ($n<10$ mg/L), and even so fragmentocytes were seen. Renal function was normal at the time of donor nephrectomy (creatinine 0.9 mg%). Routine histopathological study of the kidney biopsy showed no abnormalities, however trichrome stains showed glomerular capillary fibrin deposits.

In spite of the likelihood of intravascular coagulation in the donor, we decided to transplant both kidneys. The first kidney was transplanted in a 56-year-old man. Immunosuppression consisted of cyclosporine 10 mg/kg/day and prednisolone 10 mg/day, both orally. A kidney biopsy 1 hr after transplantation showed massive fibrin deposition in the glomeruli (Fig. 1). After 7 days, diuresis was 150 ml/24 hr, and another biopsy was taken. Histological examination now showed an interstitial rejection—however, there were no fibrin thrombi in the glomerular capillaries (Fig. 2). Antirejection treatment with Solumedrol did improve kidney function to a creatinine clearance of 25 ml/min at 21 days. After conversion to azathioprine (2 mg/kg/day) and prednisolone (10 mg/day orally) the creatinine clearance improved to ±40 ml/min.

The second kidney was transplanted in a 51-year-old woman.

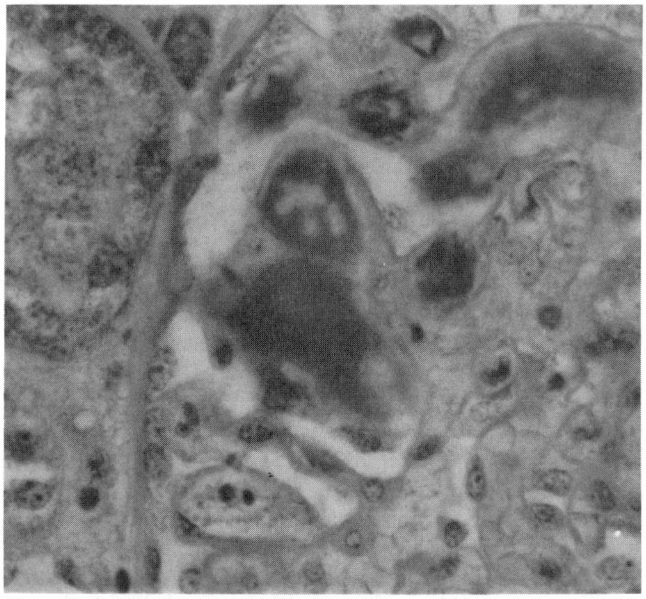

FIGURE 1. Kidney biopsy taken 1 hr after transplantation. Note the fibrin thrombi in the glomerular capillaries.

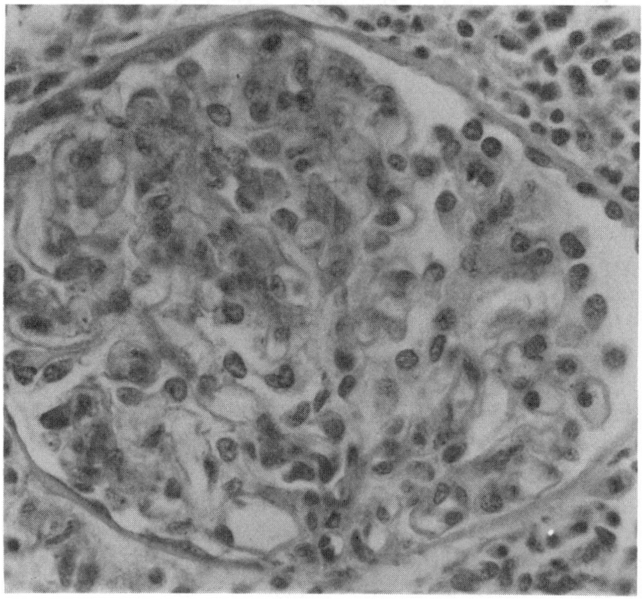

FIGURE 2. Kidney biopsy taken 7 days after transplantation. There are no fibrin thrombi in the glomerular capillaries anymore.

Immunosuppression consisted of azathioprine 2 mg/kg/day and prednisolone in an initial dose of 1.5 mg/kg/day tapered in 3 weeks to 20 mg/day. In a biopsy taken 1 hr after transplantation, massive depositions of fibrin in glomerular capillaries were seen. In the first days after transplantation, a rejection crisis was treated with steroids in high doses—thereafter kidney function improved to a creatinine clearance of ±50 ml/min. At six months after transplantation a kidney biopsy was performed. The histopathological study of the biopsy showed normal glomerular capillaries.

In conclusion, both kidneys transplanted from a donor with diffuse intravascular coagulation and with histopathological evidence of fibrin thrombi in glomerular capillaries (*1, 2*) function adequately now 10 months after transplantation. One kidney was biopsied 7 days posttransplantation and did not show fibrin thrombi or glomerular damage. These observations show that fibrin thrombi in glomerular capillaries of a donor kidney can be resolved by the fibrinolytic system of the recipient. However good kidney function and a kidney biopsy are necessary prior to transplantation to exclude renal cortical necrosis as a consequence of severe intravascular coagulation (*3*). Renal cortical necrosis, however, is an unusual occurrence in patients with an established disseminated intravascular coagulation (*4, 5*).

K.M.L. LEUNISSEN[2]

[1] This work was supported by the Dutch Kidney Foundation.

TH.J.M. RUERS[3]
F. BOSMAN[4]
G. KOOTSTRA[3]
J.P. VAN HOOFF[2]
Departments of Nephrology, Surgery, and Pathology
University Hospital
Maastricht, The Netherlands

[2] Department of Nephrology.
[3] Department of Surgery.
[4] Department of Pathology.

REFERENCES

1. Haanen C, Holdrinet A, Wijdeveld P. Intravascular clotting and acute renal failure. Pathogenesis and clinical findings with renal failure. Stuttgart: Thieme, 1971: 132.
2. Haanen C. Gedissimineerde intravasale stolling. Ned Tijdschrift Geneeskunde 1976; 120: 381.
3. Mathin RA, Gary NE. Acute cortical necrosis. Case report and review of literature. Am J Med 1974; 56: 110.
4. Colman RW, Robboy SJ, Minna JD. Disseminated intravascular coagulation. (DIC): an approach. Am J Med 1972; 52: 679.
5. Robboy SJ, Colman RW, Minna JD. Pathology of disseminated intravascular coagulation (DIC): analysis of 26 cases. Hum Pathol 1972; 3: 327.

Received 10 October 1985.
Accepted 11 November 1985.

PILOT STUDY OF CAMPATH-1, A RAT MONOCLONAL ANTIBODY THAT FIXES HUMAN COMPLEMENT, AS AN IMMUNOSUPPRESSANT IN ORGAN TRANSPLANTATION[1]

Graft rejection is still a significant problem in clinical transplantation, and there is a need for immunosuppressants that do not have the potential toxic side-effects associated with steroids or cyclosporine (CsA*). The ultimate objective is to achieve donor-specific tolerance rather than the present global immunosuppression, so that increased susceptibility to infection can be avoided. At present, however, this is a distant goal, and recently attention has focused on the use of monoclonal antibodies as alternative immunosuppressants.

Here we study the use of a rat monoclonal antibody, CAMPATH-1, in the treatment and prophylaxis of rejection in patients receiving kidney, pancreas, or liver transplants. CAMPATH-1 (IgM) recognizes >95% of human peripheral mononuclear cells (T cells, B cells, and monocytes) and is particularly effective at lysis of lymphocytes with human complement (*1*). This makes it a novel candidate for clinical trials, despite its broad specificity, because there is no information concerning the use or effectiveness in vivo of human-complement-fixing monoclonal antibodies. CAMPATH-1 has already been used successfully for the removal of T cells from bone marrow in vitro to prevent graft-versus-host disease (*2*). Preliminary trials in monkeys and patients with leukemia have shown that it can deplete circulating lymphocytes, probably by complement-mediated lysis, but without harmful side-effects (*3*).

To evaluate the effectiveness of any proposed new immunosuppressant, a randomized controlled trial is essential—however, the relative success of current kidney transplantation means that a large number of patients would be needed. We therefore first carried out this pilot study in selected patients to examine the practicality of antibody administration and to discover any untoward side-effects that might be caused by CAMPATH-1 by virtue of its specificity or complement-fixing ability. In addition we wished to know whether there was sufficient indication of its effectiveness to justify a more extensive controlled trial.

Transplantation of kidney, pancreas and liver was carried out as previously described (4–6). Routine immunosuppression for kidney and combined kidney/pancreas grafts consisted of CsA 4 mg/kg/day i.v. from the first postoperative day, changing to 17 mg/kg/day orally when bowel function returned. For liver grafts, prednisolone, 1 mg/kg/day and azathioprine, 1.5 mg/kg/day were given i.v. initially and then orally. CAMPATH-1 was purified from rat ascitic fluid by precipitation with ammonium sulphate (*3*) and administered i.v. at 0.5 mg/ml in 0.9% saline over a period of 1–3 hr (25 mg for adults, 12.5 mg for children, and 7.5 mg for infants). At the first injection, a test dose of 1 mg was given, followed by an observation period of 30 min in case of acute reactions. Initially a cautious policy of discontinuing antibody treatment after any kind of acute reaction was adopted, but later, if reactions were observed, subsequent doses of antibody were given with no side-effects if preceded by 100 mg of hydrocortisone or 4 mg of oral chlorpheniramine.

Treatment of acute rejection. An initial test of the safety and efficacy of therapy with CAMPATH-1 was carried out in a 29-year-old male patient with presumed steroid-resistant rejection of a kidney graft (Fig. 1). The graft was tender and had not functioned satisfactorily since transplantation; the serum creatinine level was > 1000 μmol/L, urine output was <100 ml/day, and regular dialysis was necessary. A biopsy on day 9 showed acute tubular necrosis with possible evidence of rejection; biopsies on days 19 and 25 showed moderate cellular rejection. There was only a slight response to two 3-day courses of methylprednisolone (1 g/day) and conversion of maintenance immunosuppression had little effect. On day 29, serotherapy with CAMPATH-1 was commenced, and 25 mg of antibody was given each day for nine days. During this period good diuresis was established and the serum creatinine level fell to near normal levels, despite the fact that prednisolone levels were simultaneously being reduced. Peripheral blood counts of red cells, platelets, and neutrophils did not change significantly during antibody therapy. The lymphocyte count was low at the beginning of treatment but there was an observable drop immediately after each injection of antibody. Nevertheless, the level was restored after 24 hr, and at the end of nine days treatment it was about the same as at the beginning (Fig. 2). The level of hemolytic complement showed slight fluctuations that seemed to correlate with the injections of CAMPATH-1, but were probably insignificant. (This is in contrast with the very large fluctuations seen during serotherapy of patients with high numbers of circulating lymphocytes [*3*].) Anti-rat-Ig antibodies were detectable on day 10 and increased sharply during the next seven days. No adverse reactions to the injections were observed. The kidney continues to function well two years later.

[1] This work was supported by the Medical Research Council.
* Abbreviation used: CsA, cyclosporine.

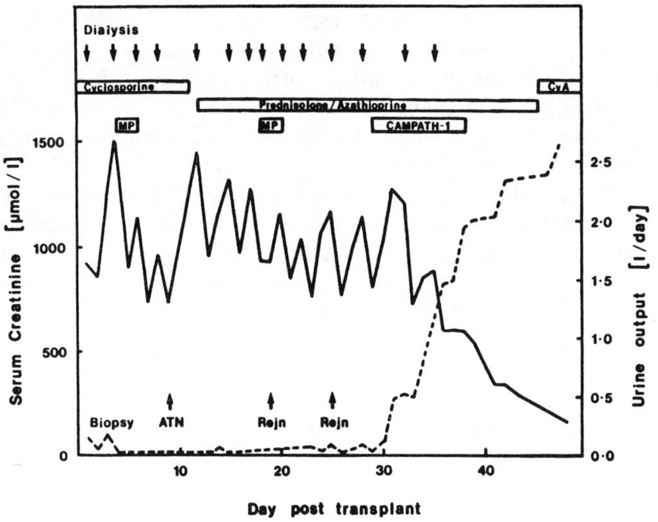

FIGURE 1. Treatment of kidney graft rejection with CAMPATH-1. Following kidney transplantation urine output (-----) remained very low, serum creatinine (——) was high and regular dialysis was necessary (↓). Two courses of treatment with methylprednisolone (MP) and conversion from CsA to prednisolone/azathioprine had little effect. CAMPATH-1 was given i.v. at 25 mg/day for nine days, and after a satisfactory response, maintainance immunosuppression reverted to CsA.

Five other patients received CAMPATH-1 for presumed rejection episodes but the results were not evaluable because three experienced some reactions resulting in discontinuation of treatment, and in the others subsequent investigations suggested that CsA toxicity and not rejection was the cause of poor function.

Prophylactic treatment: kidney plus pancreas. Eleven patients receiving combined kidney and pancreas grafts were treated with CAMPATH-1, 25 mg twice a day, starting on day 0 or day 1 posttransplant, in addition to routine immunosuppression with CsA. Two patients were treated for 5 days and 8 for 10 days. All the pancreas grafts were carried out using the paratopic technique (*5*). Pancreas grafts in three patients became infarcted within a few days of operation and were removed; one of these patients subsequently died from sepsis. The remaining 8 pancreatic grafts functioned satisfactorily (*7*) and the kidney grafts in all 10 surviving patients were functioning at six months, although one was subsequently lost due to chronic rejection. This was a poor-prognosis group of patients; not only were they diabetic with microvascular complications but also no attempt was made to match for HLA. During the ten days of antibody treatment there was one probable rejection episode and one possible rejection episode (not confirmed by biopsy); a total frequency of 0.18 episodes/patient. This compares favorably with a frequency of 0.48 episodes/patient in a group of 50 first-time kidney cadaver graft recipients treated with CsA alone, and it was correlated with a lower use of steroids in the first 10 days for the antibody-treated patients. However, in the period from 10 days to 6 months after cessation of antibody treatment, rejection episodes were somewhat more numerous in the pancreas + kidney group (1.2 episodes/patient) than in the conventionally treated kidney group (0.7 episodes/patient).

Prophylactic treatment: liver. Thirty-six liver graft recipients were treated with a single dose of CAMPATH-1 daily for ten days, starting on day 2 or day 3 posttransplant. The incidence of acute rejection was hard to determine because biopsies were rarely performed, but the survival at 3 months of the CAMPATH-1-treated patients (69%) appeared to be improved when compared with a historical group of 49 patients (49%). This group consisted of all other liver grafts since January 1980, excluding retransplants and patients who died in the first three days. Comparison of the two life tables by the log-rank test (*8*) gave a chi-squared value of 4.2, which implies a significance level for the difference of $P = 0.04$. Survival at one year was still better in the CAMPATH-1 treated patients (50%) than in the historical group (37%), but the difference then was less marked ($P = 0.12$). The two groups are neither matched nor randomized, and the control group contained only 3 patients aged < 16 years, whereas the antibody-treated group included 13 children. However when only adult patients in each group were considered, the life tables were indistinguishable, although the significance of the difference was then diminished because the number of patients was smaller.

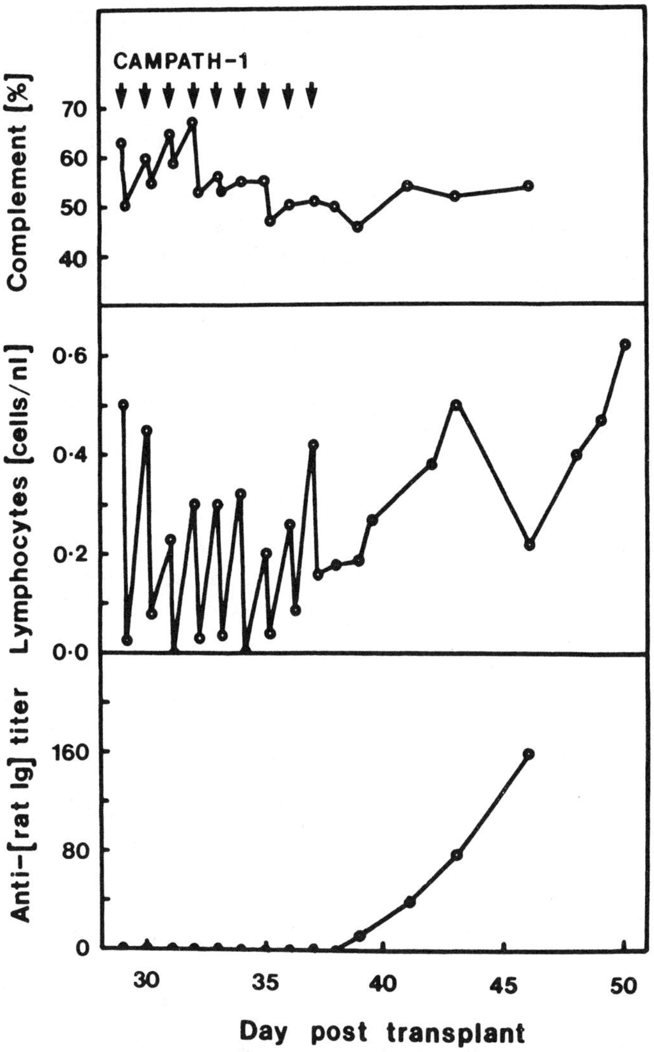

FIGURE 2. Effects of CAMPATH-1 injections during treatment of graft rejection. CAMPATH-1 was given at 25 mg/day (↓), as shown in Figure 1. Total hemolytic complement was assayed by lysis of red cells and expressed as a percentage of the activity of a standard batch of normal human serum. Absolute lymphocyte counts were calculated from total white cell counts and differential cell counts. Anti-rat-Ig titer was measured by agglutination of red cells coupled with CAMPATH-1 antibody.

Effects of CAMPATH-1 injections. Four patients experienced relatively mild reactions associated with the main dose (but not the test dose), consisting of nausea, flush, wheezes, urticaria, or rigor. In three cases treatment was discontinued, but in the other it was continued with no problem when 100 mg of hydrocortisone was given prior to each injection. One patient showed a more severe reaction to the 1-mg test dose, consisting of chill, wheeze, and tachycardia which was treated with a combination of hydrocortisone, chlorpheniramine, and adrenalin. The antibody had inadvertently been diluted in dextrose-saline, the low ionic strength of which had caused the IgM to precipitate. It is likely that large aggregates of the antibody were responsible for the acute reaction. Two other patients also required treatment for reactions possibly associated with the first dose of antibody, and in all these three cases antibody therapy was discontinued. Thus antibody treatment was discontinued in a total of six patients (not included in the analysis) all within the first seven months of study. Since then patients have received CAMPATH-1 without any serious problems. Steroids prevent anaphylactic-type reactions to antibody injections, so it was not surprising that virtually all of the reactions noted were in patients who received CsA as the main immunosuppressant, and very uncommon in the liver transplant patients who received prednisolone during the time when antibody was given.

In all patients blood counts were monitored daily but the antibody treatment did not appear to have any effect on the levels of red cells, platelets, or neutrophils. Daily serum samples were tested for anti-rat-Ig in five patients, and in each case an antiglobulin response was detectable, beginning between days 7 and 11 (Fig. 2). These patients had all received CsA as a standard immunosuppressant. The titers (40–320) were small compared with a hyperimmune rabbit serum (approx 100,000) but would be adequate to neutralize any further antibody injections (*3*).

Several monoclonal antibodies of different specificities have been tested clinically for their potential immunosuppressive effects in transplantation (*9–11*). The mouse IgG2a antibody OKT3 appears to be very effective for treatment of rejection episodes (*12–14*), and prophylactic treatment with OKT3 may also be effective (*15*). A potentially superior strategy that might produce long-term tolerance could be the specific clonal deletion of alloreactive cells during an aggressive response, using a monoclonal antibody specific for activated T cells (*9*). Early results with such a reagent were very encouraging (*16*), though further studies were less successful (*17*).

These antibodies are thought to operate by opsonization or by interference with cell function, and the possible role of complement for cell lysis with monoclonal antibodies has not been investigated. Here we have shown that a human-complement-fixing antibody can safely be used in transplant patients, and there is some evidence to suggest that it does cause cell lysis in vivo. The side effects observed in a few patients were no more severe than those seen with other monoclonal antibodies that do not fix human complement (*12, 18*). These reactions, which are also seen with antilymphocyte globulin, are often thought to be mainly a consequence of cell lysis (*12, 19*). As expected, the majority of patients tested showed an anti-rat-Ig response, which would probably prohibit extended or repeat courses of treatment by neutralization—though did not promote acute sensitivity or serum sickness. The antiglobulin response to monoclonal antibodies has already been documented, and CAMPATH-1 is not unusual in this respect.

Three pieces of evidence suggest that CAMPATH-1 might have some therapeutic value in control of rejection: (1) reversal of acute rejection in one patient correlated with antibody treatment (Fig. 1); (2) there was a low incidence of early rejection episodes and relatively good graft survival in combined kidney and pancreas recipients treated prophylactically with CAMPATH-1 and CsA (These patients are a high-risk group because not only are they diabetic, but also no attempt was made to match for HLA type.); and (3) Liver transplant patients who received prophylactic CAMPATH-1 plus azathioprine/prednisolone showed slightly improved survival compared with the historical group. However, at present we cannot rule out alternative explanations for these findings and the only way to demonstrate clearly a clinical effect will be by means of a randomized, controlled trial that is now in progress.

Acknowledgments. We gratefully acknowledge the expertise of many clinical and nursing colleagues at Addenbrooke's Hospital, Cambridge and King's College Hospital London, and thank Penny Lovat for expert technical assistance.

GEOFFREY HALE[2,3]
HERMAN WALDMANN[2]
PETER FRIEND[4]
ROY CALNE[4]
Department of Pathology
University of Cambridge
Cambridge CB2 1QP
Department of Surgery
University of Cambridge
Addenbrooke's Hospital
Cambridge CB2 2QQ, United Kingdom

[2] Department of Pathology.
[3] Address correspondence to: Dr. G. Hale, Division of Immunology, Level 3, Laboratories Block, Addenbrooke's Hospital, Hills Road, Cambridge CB2 1QP, United Kingdom.
[4] Department of Surgery.

REFERENCES

1. Hale G, Bright S, Chumbley G, et al. Removal of T cells from bone marrow for transplantation: a monoclonal antilymphocyte antibody that fixes human complement. Blood 1983; 62: 873.
2. Waldmann H, Or R, Hale G, et al. Elimination of graft versus host disease by in vitro depletion of alloreactive lymphocytes using a monoclonal rat anti-human lymphocyte antibody (CAMPATH-1). Lancet 1984; 2: 483.
3. Hale G, Swirsky DM, Hayhoe FGJ, Waldmann H. Effects of monoclonal anti-lymphocyte antibodies in vivo in monkeys and humans. Mol Biol Med 1983; 1: 321.
4. Calne RY. A colour atlas of renal transplantation. London: Wolfe Medical, 1984.
5. Calne RY. Paratopic segmental pancreas grafting: a technique with portal venous drainage. Lancet 1984; 1: 595.
6. Calne RY. Recipient operation. In: Calne RY, ed. Liver transplantation. New York: Grune & Stratton, 1983: 155.
7. Calne RY, Brons IGM. Observations on paratopic segmental pancreas grafting with splenic venous drainage. Transplant Proc 1985; 17: 340.
8. Peto R, Pike MC, Armitage P, et al. Design and analysis of randomized clinical trials requiring prolonged observation of each patient. II. Analysis and examples. Br J Cancer 1977; 35: 1.
9. Kirkman RL, Araujo JL, Busch GJ, et al. Treatment of acute renal allograft rejection with monoclonal anti-T12 antibody. Transplantation 1983; 36: 620.
10. Cosimi AB. Treatment of rejection: antithymocyte globulin versus monoclonal antibodies. Transplant Proc 1985; 17: 1526.

11. Terasaki P, Cats S, Cicciarelli J, et al. Use of monoclonal antibodies for kidney transplant patients. Transplant Proc 1985; 17: 1521.
12. Cosimi AB, Burton RC, Colvin RB, et al. Treatment of acute renal allograft rejection with OKT3 monoclonal antibody. Transplantation 1981; 32: 535.
13. Norman DJ, Barry JM, Henell K, Funnell MB, Goldstein G, Bohannon L. Reversal of acute allograft rejection with monoclonal antibody. Transplant Proc 1985; 17: 39.
14. Ortho Multicenter Transplant Study Group. A randomized trial of OKT3 monoclonal antibody for acute rejection of cadaveric renal allografts N Engl J Med 1985; 313: 337.
15. Kreis H, Chkoff H, Vigeral P, et al. Prophylactic treatment of allograft recipients with monoclonal anti-T3 cell antibody. Transplant Proc 1985; 17: 1315.
16. Takahashi H, Okazaki H, Terasaki PI, et al. Reversal of transplant rejection by monoclonal antiblast antibody. Lancet 1983; 2: 1155.
17. Takahashi H, Okazaki H, Terasaki PI, et al. Follow-up on initial trials of kidney transplant rejection reversal by a monoclonal antiblast antibody. Transplant Proc 1985; 17: 69.
18. Levy R, Miller RA. Biological and clinical implications of lymphocyte hybridomas: tumor therapy with monoclonal antibodies. Annu Rev Med 1983; 34: 107.
19. Nelson PW, Cosimi AB, Delmonico FL, et al. Antithymocyte globulin as the primary treatment for renal allograft rejection. Transplantation 1983; 36: 587.

Received 4 September 1985.
Accepted 1 December 1985.

RANITIDINE, CIMETIDINE, AND THE CYCLOSPORINE-TREATED RECIPIENT

While the advent of cyclosporine (CsA)* has had significant impact on renal transplantation, the improved success rate is partially offset by the nephrotoxicity of CsA, particularly in the presence of high drug levels (e.g., >200 ng/ml serum by radioimmunoassay [RIA]) (*1*). Not only does CsA cause impaired graft function, but this nephrotoxicity also complicates the diagnosis of rejection. Furthermore, the situation may be compounded by the concomitant use of other nephrotoxic agents. Among the gastrointestinal causes contributing significantly to morbidity in renal transplantation, peptic ulcer disease is the preponderant single entity frequently requiring H-2 antagonist therapy (*2, 3*). Routine cimetidine prophylaxis of renal allograft recipients has been advocated in patients immunosuppressed with azathioprine-prednisone (*4*). This communication assesses whether the use of cimetidine (CM) or ranitidine (RAN) in CsA-prednisone immunosuppressed patients alters CsA metabolism or causes synergistic nephrotoxicity.

This review of 325 renal and 52 cardiac allograft recipients immunosuppressed with CsA-prednisone excludes patients who were either clearly nephrotoxic from CsA per se or undergoing allograft rejection at the time of initiation of CM or RAN therapy. Additionally, individuals receiving other nephrotoxic agents or drugs known to affect CsA metabolism were excluded from the review. These criteria were met by 13 allograft recipients (7 renal and 6 cardiac), who were undergoing treatment with either CM or RAN under CsA-prednisone immunosuppression.

In the renal group the mean blood urea nitrogen (BUN) and serum creatinine (Cr) prior to the initiation of CM or RAN therapy was 42±20 mg/dl and 2.28±0.79 mg/dl, and during H-2 antagonist therapy, 42±20 mg/dl and 3.22±1.19 mg/dl. While there was no change in BUN, the increase in serum creatinine was significant ($P<0.01$). In contradistinction to all renal allograft patients, who displayed an increased serum creatinine, only two of the six cardiac allograft recipients exhibited increased serum creatinine levels upon initiation of H-2 antagonist therapy. One of these two patients developed renal failure requiring dialysis. The renal function returned to pretreatment levels (BUN/creatinine 15/1.2 mg/dl) within two weeks of cessation of RAN therapy (Table 1). The reproducibility of the H-2 blocker effect on the renal function of CsA-treated recipients was demonstrated in two renal allograft recipients. One patient had CM instituted and then discontinued on two separate occasions with the same degree of renal dysfunction each time. A second renal allograft recipient had a similar course with the substitution of CM for RAN on different occasions in the same course of H-2 blocker therapy.

TABLE 1. Serum BUN and creatinine prior to and during CM or RAN therapy in renal and cardiac allograft recipients

	Serum BUN/creatinine (mg/dl)			
	Off H-2 blocker		On H-2 blocker	
	BUN	Creatinine	BUN	Creatinine
A. Renal allograft patients:				
1.	39	2.2	26	3.3
2.	37	2.0	42	2.8
3.	95	3.6	48	5.1
4.	23	1.8	26	2.0
5.	34	1.5	37	2.2
6.	20	1.4	21	1.8
7.[a]	27	1.7	34	2.7
8.	51	2.7	64	3.9
9.[b]	55	3.6	85	5.2
Mean serum BUN/creatinine	42±20	2.28±0.79	42±20[d]	3.22±1.19[e]
B. Cardiac allograft recipients:				
1.[c]	28	1.5	62	9.1
2.	30	1.8	19	1.2
3.	20	1.7	40	3.5
4.[d]	17	1.2	15	1.0
5.[d]	22	1.8	24	1.8
6.[d]	35	2.3	26	1.4
Mean serum BUN/creatinine	25.2±5.9	1.72±0.33	31±16[d]	2.36±2.13[d]

[a] Same patient as 6 treated with H-2 antagonist on a separate occasion.
[b] No change in serum creatinine elevation in this patient when RAN was substituded for cimetidine.
[c] This recipient required dialysis until RAN was discontinued.
[d] Comparison of pretherapy versus posttherapy, not a significant difference.
[e] Comparison of pretherapy versus posttherapy significant at the level $P<0.01$.

The mean (cardiac and renal combined) CsA serum trough levels (by RIA) (*5*) prior to and during H-2 antagonist therapy were 153±94 ng/ml and 93±29 ng/ml at CsA doses of 7.1±2.8 mg/kg and 6.1±2.8 mg/kg, respectively. There was no significant difference between CsA pharmacokinetic parameters ob-

* Abbreviations used: BUN, blood urea nitrogen; CM, cimetidine; Cr, creatinine; CsA, cyclosporine; RAN, ranitidine.

served prior to and during H-2 antagonist therapy in two immunosuppressed allograft recipients (Table 2).

CM and RAN are potent agents for the inhibition of gastric secretion (*4*). However, there is an estimated 1/100,000 incidence of renal failure from interstitial nephritis occurring in nontransplant patients receiving CM. An increased serum creatinine has been observed to a lesser extent, but the findings are not uniform (*6, 7*). Contrariwise studying a group of ten nontransplant patients, Yeung et al. (*8*) found a significant increase in endogenous creatinine clearance upon RAN treatment. The ten patients in their CM group exhibited no change in serum creatinine or in endogenous creatinine clearance (*8*). In contrast to our findings with CM or RAN in CsA-treated patients, Garvin et al. found no change in the mean serum creatinine of renal allograft recipients immunosuppressed with azathioprine-prednisone; 2.82 mg/dl pretherapy with CM and 2.85 mg/dl following six weeks of CM treatment (*3*). The data presented herein suggest an impact of CM and RAN on renal function, as reflected by BUN and serum creatinine in a segment of allograft recipients immunosuppressed with CsA. Although this decrement was not uniform in cardiac recipients, there was a consistent deterioration of allograft renal function, as measured by serum creatinine, in kidney recipients that was not associated with altered CsA disposition parameters.

TABLE 2. Pharmacokinetic parameters observed in two renal allograft recipients with and without H-2 antagonist therapy

Parameter	PO values ± SD		t^a
	On CM/RAN	Off CM/RAN	
	(n = 3)	(n = 4)	
Patient No. 1:			
AUC/dose	765±230	558±153	1.44
$t_{1/2}$ (hours)	10.7±2.59	9.03±4.17	0.60
Cmax (ng/ml)	1334±1089	634±219	1.29
tp (hours)	2.2±1.04	3.0±1.41	0.82
	(n = 1)	(n = 6)	
Patient No. 2:			
AUC/dose	561	1707±1000	
$t_{1/2}$ (hours)	5.44	5.91±2.45	
Cmax (ng/ml)	1342	1504±884	
tp (hours)	1	2.3±1.03	

[a] No significant difference found.

MARK V. JAROWENKO[1]
CHARLES T. VAN BUREN[1]
WILLIAM G. KRAMER[2]
MARC I. LORBER[1]
STUART M. FLECHNER[1]
AND BARRY D. KAHAN[1,3]
The Division of Immunology and Organ Transplantation
Department of Surgery
The University of Texas Medical School at Houston
University of Houston College of Pharmacy
Houston, Texas 77030

[1] The University of Texas Medical School at Houston.
[2] University of Houston College of Pharmacy.
[3] To whom correspondence should be directed, at Suite 6240 MSMB, 6431 Fannin Street, Houston, TX 77030.

REFERENCES

1. Kahan BD, Van Buren CT, Flechner SM, et al. Clinical and experimental studies with cyclosporine in renal transplantation. Surgery 1985; 97: 125.
2. Ahonen J, Paimeda H, Kauste A, Hayry P, Eklund B, Petterson E. Ranitidine and cimetidine in renal transplantation: a clinical trial. Int J Tissue React 1983; 5: 373.
3. Garvin PJ, Carney K, Castaneda M, Codd JE. Peptic ulcer disease following transplantation: the role of cimetidine. Am J Surg 1982; 114: 545.
4. van Roemund HPC, Tiggeler RGWL, Berden JHM, van Lier HJJ, Koene RAP. Cimetidine prophylaxis after renal transplantation. Clin Nephrol 1981; 18: 39.
5. Donatsch P, Abisch E, Homberger M, Traber R, Trapp M, Voges R. Cyclosporin A in plasma and serum samples. Immunoassay 1981; 2: 19.
6. Rowley-Jones D. Cimetidine-induced renal failure (letter). Br J Med 1982; 285: 1422.
7. Santoro JJ, Pitone JM, Biondi RJ, Chiesa JC, Pecora AA. Cimetidine-induced acute renal failure (letter). Br Med J 1982; 285: 975.
8. Yeung CK, Wong KL, Ng MT, Lgi CL. Effects of cimetidine, ranitidine and antacid on renal function. Clin Ther 1984; 6: 620.

Received 6 September 1985.
Accepted 13 December 1985.

A SHORTER PROCEDURE FOR PREPARATION OF E-ROSETTE-DEPLETED BONE MARROW FOR TRANSPLANTATION[1]

Studies in murine models of marrow transplantation have demonstrated that graft-versus-host disease (GVHD)* is initiated by thymus-derived T lymphocytes of donor origin (*1, 2*). During the past decade, significant progress has been made in developing techniques to allow transplants of histoincompatible marrow without risk of GVHD (*3–7*). In previous studies we demonstrated that depletion of T cells from murine marrow with lectins permitted transplantation across major histocompatability barriers without GVHD (*7*). Using this approach we were able to achieve an effective depletion of alloreactive T lymphocytes from both primate (*8*) and human (*9*) marrow. To date, O'Reilly et al. (*10*) have applied this fractionation technique for transplants in twelve patients with severe combined immune deficiency (SCID) and 20 patients with late-stage leukemia resistant to chemotherapy, who lacked HLA identical sibling donors. During the past two years, this technique has also been applied successfully in various centers throughout the world (*11–16*).

The method consists of four main steps: (1) selective removal of red blood cells by gravity sedimentation in Hetastarch; (2) agglutination of bone marrow cells with soybean agglutinin (SBA) and subsequent differential sedimentation of agglutinated cells (SBA^+); (3) removal of E-rosette-forming T cells

[1] This work was supported by a grant from the Leukemia Foundation, Chicago, and by the Israel Cancer Research Fund, New York.

* Abbreviations used: GVHD, graft-versus-host disease; CFU-GM, myeloid progenitor cells; SBA, soybean agglutinin; SCID, severe combined immune deficiency; SRBC, sheep red blood cells.

from the SBA⁻ fraction by centrifugation over Ficoll-Hypaque; and (4) removal of the trace of residual T cells (<0.5%) in the SBA⁻E⁻ fraction by separation of cells forming E rosettes with neuraminidase-treated sheep red blood cells (SRBC).

Recently it has been shown that when T cells are removed by a one-step E-rosetting procedure involving SRBC treated either with neuraminidase (*12*) or with 2-aminoethylisothiouronium bromide hydrobromide (AET) (*10*), GVHD can be avoided. Although this shortens the bone marrow purification procedure by about 3 hr, the length of time that is still required to process the large volumes of bone marrow necessary for human grafts (over 10 hr) remains a serious problem calling for further improvement.

A limiting step of the current method is the E-rosetting with SRBC. This procedure is laborious and time-consuming for the following reasons: (1) the low leukocyte concentration used ($5–10\times10^6$ cells/ml), which is unsuitable for processing the large volume of bone marrow needed for transplantation (on the average about 24 tubes of 50 ml each are required when the cell mixture of SBA⁻ bone marrow cells and SRBC is layered onto Ficoll); (2) the incubation for 1 hr in ice of the bone marrow-SRBC mixture; and (3) the gentle procedure needed to resuspend the cells in each tube.

Gmelig-Meyling and Ballieux described a fast E-rosetting method (*17*) in which human peripheral blood mononuclear cells are mixed with SRBC, layered directly on a Ficoll-Metrizoate mixture of higher specific gravity (1.090) than Ficoll-Hypaque (1.077), and centrifuged at high speed (1200 ×g) for 30 min. E rosettes are presumably formed in this procedure by collisions of T cells with SRBC at the Ficoll-Metrizoate interface. In the present study we describe a modification of this technique that we find more suitable for the preparation of bone marrow for transplantation.

In preliminary studies with human peripheral blood leukocytes, various parameters of the methodology described by Gmelig-Meyling and Ballieux (*17*) were optimized (data not shown). Based on these preliminary results we began our investigations on large-scale bone marrow preparations using the following modifications: (1) neuraminidase-treated SRBC were used instead of untreated SRBC; (2) regular speed centrifugation (400 ×g) on Ficoll-Hypaque (specific gravity 1.077) for 30 min was used instead of high-speed centrifugation (1200 ×g) on Ficoll-Metrizoate with a high specific gravity of 1.090; (3) the range of leukocyte concentrations were between $10–40\times10^6$/ml with optimum T cell depletion at 15×10^6/ml.

The preparation of neuraminidase-treated SRBC and the leukocyte-rich fraction from human bone marrow, as well as the isolation of SBA⁻ marrow cells, are carried out as previously described (*9*). Following these two initial steps, SBA⁻ bone marrow cells are resuspended in 20 ml medium M-199 (Bio-Lab, Jerusalem) at $10–40\times10^6$ cells/ml with 5 ml of a 10–50% suspension of neuraminidase-treated SRBC. The cell suspension is then layered on top of 20 ml Ficoll-Hypaque (specific gravity = 1.077), and centrifuged for 30 min at 400 ×g. The nonrosetting mononuclear cells are collected from the Ficoll-Hypaque interface and washed twice with M-199.

Table 1 shows the effect of bone marrow concentration on total cell recovery, percentage of remaining E-rosette-forming cells, and CFU-GM recovery. As can be seen, high stem cell recoveries were obtained at 15×10^6 cells/ml and 40×10^6 cells/ml, whereas T cell depletion was slightly less efficient at 40×10^6 cells/ml.

TABLE 1. E-rosetting of bone marrow cells prior to lectin separation: effect of bone marrow cell concentration

	Bone marrow concentration ($\times10^6$/ml)	Fraction	Nucleated cells ($\times10^8$)	CFU-GM ($\times10^6$)[a]	E rosettes (%)[b]	E rosettes ($\times10^6$)
Exp. 1	40	Before	9.5	2.1	19	180
		After	4.2	2.0	0.1	0.42
		Recovery (%)	44	95		0.23
Exp. 2	40	Before	7.1	1.6	14	99
		After	2.9	1.9	0.2	0.58
		Recovery (%)	40	118		0.58
Exp. 3	40	Before	11.3	2.4	22	248
		After	5.9	1.8	0.3	1.77
		Recovery (%)	52	75		0.71
Mean recovery (%) Exp. 1–3			45	96		0.50
Exp. 4	15	Before	11.3	4.1	18	203
		After	5.2	4.0	<0.1	0.15
		Recovery (%)	40	95		0.07
Exp. 5	15	Before	10	2.3	22	220
		After	1.5	2.1	<0.1	0.045
		Recovery (%)	15	91		0.20
Exp. 6	15	Before	225	79	18	4050
		After	50	73	<0.1	1.5
		Recovery (%)	22	92		0.037
Exp. 7	15	Before	122	38	14	1708
		After	20	17	<0.1	0.6
		Recovery (%)	16	44		0.035
Exp. 8	15	Before	98	31	12	1176
		After	18	41	<0.1	0.56
		Recovery (%)	18	131		0.047
Mean recovery (%) Exp. 4–8			22	90		0.091

[a] A total of 1×10^5 cells/ml of the various fractions were cultured essentially as previously described (*18*) in Iscove's modified Dulbecco's medium, 30% fetal calf serum, 15% placental conditioned medium, and 5×10^{-5} M 2-mercaptoethanol in a final concentration of 0.9% methylcellulose. The cells were plated in 1-ml portions in a 35-mm tissue culture dish (Lux Scientific Corporation, Thousand Oaks, CA). Cultures were incubated at 37°C in a humidified atmosphere of air-5% CO_2 for 10 days. Colonies were scored using an inverted microscope.

[b] The assay for detection of E-rosette-forming cells was performed as previously described (*19*); <0.1% E rosettes means that an occasional rosette was seen on screening a slide with approximately 1×10^4 cells (maximally 3 per slide).

The effectiveness of the fast E rosette method in removing T cells from the SBA⁻ cell fraction obtained after differential agglutination with SBA, using a bone marrow concentration of 15×10^6/ml, is demonstrated in Table 2.

In nine large-scale experiments, the percentage of remaining T cells did not exceed 0.1%, a criterion that was set from our experience with the previous method to ascertain successful transplant without GVHD. Indeed, in 5 consecutive transplants of HLA-haploidentical bone marrow depleted of T cells by SBA agglutination and E-rosetting according to the fast method described here, in only one patient was a transient grade 1 GVHD observed (Table 3).

The number of SBA⁻ cells that have to be processed by

TABLE 2. E-rosetting of SBA^- bone marrow cells

	Bone marrow cells[a]	Nucleated cells ($\times 10^8$)	CFU-GM ($\times 10^6$)	E-Rosettes %[b]
Exp. 1	Unseparated	250	74	ND
	SBA^-	43	20	7
	SBA^-E^-	18	30	<0.1
	Recovery %	41	150	
Exp. 2	Unseparated	200	25	ND
	SBA^-	20	18	14
	SBA^-E^-	12.4	19	<0.1
	Recovery %	62	105	
Exp. 3	Unseparated	217	50	ND
	SBA^-	25	20	24
	SBA^-E^-	14	19	<0.1
	Recovery %	56	95	
Exp. 4	Unseparated	138	21	ND
	SBA^-	21	ND	33
	SBA^-E^-	10.5	10	<0.1
	Recovery %	50	—	
Exp. 5	Unseparated	156	53	ND
	SBA^-	22	32	4
	SBA^-E^-	10	24	<0.1
	Recovery %	45	75	
Exp. 6	Unseparated	131	26	ND
	SBA^-	25	ND	14
	SBA^-E^-	15	9.3	<0.1
	Recovery %	60	—	
Exp. 7	Unseparated	120	55	15
	SBA^-	9	10	12
	SBA^-E^-	3.6	19	<0.1
	Recovery %	40	190	
Exp. 8	Unseparated	237	30	
	SBA^-	40	30	
	SBA^-E^-	17	20	
	Recovery %	42	66	
Exp. 9	Unseparated	159	40	22
	SBA^-	43	26	10
	SBA^-E^-	18	48	0
	Recovery %	41	184	
Mean recovery (%)		48	123	

[a] Recovery is expressed as a percentage of SBA^-E^- cells out of the initial number of SBA^- cells. Unseparated cells tested are after the gravity sedimentation step.

[b] As in footnote [b] in Table 1.

TABLE 3. HLA-mismatched marrow transplants in severe combined immunodeficiency (SCID) using the new fractionation procedure

Patient	Donor	Cell engrafted	GVHD	Status
UPN 11	Father	T	—	Well >18 months
UPN 12[a]	Mother	T, B, hemopoietic	—	Well >15 months
UPN 13[a]	Mother	T, B, hemopoietic	—	Well >12 months
UPN 14	Father	T	Grade 1[b]	Well >11 months
UPN 15	Father	T	—	Well >12 months

[a] Cytoreduced with Busulfan (2 mg/kg/day ×4), anti-T cell gelulin (ATG, 40 mg/kg/day ×4), and cyclophosphamide (50 mg/kg/day ×4).

[b] Transient nonspecific skin rash that lacked characteristic histological signs of GVHD and disappeared with prednisone treatment at 2 mg/kg/day for 1 week.

E-rosetting with SRBC in a regular bone marrow transplant is 2–5×10^9 cells. According to the current, unmodified procedure these cells are divided into 20–50 tubes at a concentration of 5×10^6/ml and then incubated with SRBC for 1 hr on ice. In the new modified procedure, which we have now tested, the SBA^- cells are divided into only 6–20 tubes and are layered on Ficoll without prior incubation on ice—thus avoiding the tedious procedure of gently resuspending many cell pellets following this incubation. Using the new technique the whole bone marrow purification procedure, including red cell removal by dextran sedimentation, SBA agglutination, and E-rosetting with SRBC, can be finished within 6 hr.

Our experience with this method already suggests that it is highly reproducible. However, it is recommended that the T cell contamination in the purified cell fraction be tested by a 30-min E-rosette assay (*18*) prior to transplantation, and that the fast E-rosetting step be repeated whenever T cell contamination exceeds 0.1%.

Acknowledgments. We thank Ruth Dror, Renate Weitmann, and Esther Ruber for skillful technical assistance, and Dvorah Ochert for help in preparing the manuscript.

YAIR REISNER[2]
WILHELM FRIEDRICH[3]
INA FABIAN[4]
Department of Biophysics
The Weizmann Institute of Science
Rehovot, Israel
Department of Pediatrics
University of Ulm, Federal Republic of Germany
Department of Histology and Cell Biology
Sackler School of Medicine
Tel Aviv University, Israel

[2] Address correspondence to: Y. Reisner, Ph.D., Department of Biophysics, The Weizmann Institute of Science, Rehovot 76100, Israel.

[3] University of Ulm.

[4] Sackler School of Medicine.

REFERENCES

1. Uphoff DE. Preclusion of secondary phase of irradiation syndrome by inoculation of fetal hematopoietic tissue following lethal total-body X irradiation. J Natl Cancer Inst 1958; 20: 625.
2. Yunis EJ, Good RA, Smith J, Stutman O. Protection of lethally irradiated mice by spleen cells from neonatally thymectomized mice. Proc Natl Acad Sci USA 1974; 71: 2544.
3. Dicke KA, van Bekkum DW. Allogeneic bone marrow transplantation after elimination of immunocompetent cells by means of density gradient centrifugation. Transplant Proc 1971; 3: 666.
4. Von Boehmer H, Sprent J, Nahbolz M. Tolerance to histocompatibility determinants in tetraparental bone marrow chimeras. J Exp Med 1975; 141: 322.
5. Rich RR, Kirkpatrick CH, Smith TK. Simultaneous suppression of responses to allogeneic tissue in vitro and in vivo. Cell Immunol 1972; 5: 190.
6. Dexter TM, Spooner E. Loss of immunoreactivity in long term bone marrow culture. Nature 1978; 275: 135.
7. Reisner Y, Itzicovitch L, Meshorer A, Sharon N. Hemopoietic stem cell transplantation using mouse bone-marrow and spleen cells fractionated by lectins. Proc Natl Acad Sci USA 1978; 75: 2933.
8. Reisner Y, Kapoor N, O'Reilly RJ, Good RA. Allogeneic bone marrow transplantation using stem cells fractionated by lectins. VI. In vitro analysis of human and monkey bone soybean agglutinin. Lancet 1980; 2: 1320.
9. Reisner Y, Kapoor N, Kirkpatrick D, et al. Transplantation for acute leukaemia with HLA-A and B non-identical parental marrow cells fractionated with soybean agglutinin and sheep red blood cells. Lancet 1981; 2: 327.

10. O'Reilly RJ, Collins NH, Kernan N, et al. Transplantation of marrow-depleted of T-cells by soybean lectin agglutination and E-rosette depletion: major histocompatibility complex-related graft resistance in leukemic transplant recipients. Transplant Proc 1985; 17: 455.
11. Friedrich W, Goldmann SF, Vetter U, et al. Immunoreconstitution in severe immunodeficiency following transplantation of HLA-haploidentical, T-cell depleted bone marrow. Lancet 1984; 1: 761.
12. Friedrich W, Goldmann SF, Ebell W, et al. Severe combined immunodeficiency: treatment by bone marrow transplantation in 15 infants using HLA-haploidentical donors. Eur J Pediatr 1985; 144: 125.
13. Slavin S, Waldmann H, Or R, et al. Prevention of graft-versus-host disease in allogeneic bone marrow transplantation for leukemia by T-cell depletion in vitro prior to transplantation. Transplant Proc 1985; 17: 465.
14. Filipovich AH, Ramsay NKC, McGlave P, et al. Mismatched bone marrow transplantation: use of related donors other than HLA MLC identical siblings and T cell depletion. In: Gale RP, ed. Recent advances in bone marrow transplantation. New York: Alan R. Liss, 1983: 769.
15. Cowan M, Ammann A, Wara D, et al. Mismatched bone marrow transplantation using soybean agglutinin negative marrow cells. Pediatr Res 1984; 18(4, part 2): 254A.
16. Newland AC, Kearney JW, Hughes AF, Yeatman NWJ. Allogeneic transplantation in adults with acute leukaemia using soybean agglutinin fractionated bone marrow. Exp Hematol 1983; 11(S14): 191.
17. Gmelig-Meyling F, Ballieux RE. Simplified procedure for the separation of human T and non-T cells. Vox Sang 1977; 33: 5.
18. Brain P, Gordon J, Willetts WA. Rosette formation by peripheral blood lymphocytes. Clin Exp Immunol 1970; 6: 681.
19. Fauser AA, Messner HA. Granuloerythropoietic colonies in human bone marrow, peripheral blood and cord blood. Blood 1978; 52: 1243.

Received 21 August 1985.
Accepted 5 December 1985.

THE USE OF PHYTOHEMAGGLUTININ-STIMULATED MONONUCLEAR CELL SUBPOPULATIONS FOR HLA TYPING STUDIES INVOLVING CHRONIC MYELOGENOUS LEUKEMIA PATIENTS[1]

It has been our own experience, and that of several other laboratories performing histocompatibility testing for potential bone marrow transplantation recipients, that mononuclear cells from patients with chronic myelogenous leukemia (CML)* are often extraordinarily difficult to allotype for HLA DR antigens and/or to utilize in mixed leukocyte culture (MLC) tests. The vast majority of peripheral blood mononuclear cells (MNC) from these patients are abnormal cells, and very few normal B cells or monocytes expressing class II molecules can be isolated for determination of DR (and DQ) allotypes. When (irradiated) CML patient MNC are utilized as stimulator cells in MLC they often either fail to stimulate unrelated responder cells (Table 1) or they continue to incorporate such large amounts of thymidine spontaneously that the potential alloreactivity of cells from related potential bone marrow donors cannot be evaluated with conventional radiolabeled thymidine measurements of proliferative responses (not shown). We obtained a few successful MLC tests by enrichment for the nonblastic peripheral blood cells for use as stimulator cells by density gradient separations (unpublished data), but these less blastic cells also usually tended to stimulate allogeneic cells poorly.

To solve these problems, it was apparent from earlier studies of healthy individuals, that class-II-positive activated (normal) T cells from these patients might be able to be used as test cells. Methods for activating T cells from healthy donors that had been tried included incubation with pooled irradiated MNC (*1*), or pokeweed mitogen (PWM) (*2*). In preliminary comparative experiments with control cells, we found, however, that pooled MNC induced relatively little DR expression (not shown) and that residual pokeweed mitogen caused high nonspecific stimulation of fresh autologous responder cells (see below). We next tried to induce class II antigens on CML patients' T cells with gamma interferon (IF-gamma), which we and others have shown induces class II antigens on many different kinds of cells—including subpopulations of monocytes (*3*), dermal fibroblasts (*4*), endothelial cells (*5*), and melanoma cells (*6*)—that do not constitutively express these determinants. Approximately 8% of T cells isolated after 6 days of stimulation of patient MNC with gamma interferon (1000 U/ml) reacted with the monomorphic anti-DR antibody L243 (courtesy of R. Levy, M.D., (*7*) using flow cytometric techniques. However, although, these "T cells" could elicit weak proliferative responses of allogeneic cells (not shown), they did not proliferate, and for many patients there were too few cells to use for all the needed studies. Moreover, there was insufficient class II expression to obtain DR allotypes with conventional serological techniques and the DR-positive cells could have represented a low level of contaminating monocytes. (T cells isolated from CML patients after gamma interferon treatment of their MNC by positive selection of the cells forming

TABLE 1. Results from a representative CML patient mixed leukocyte culture test

Responder MNC	Stimulator cells (mean cpm ^{3}H thymidine[a])			
	VT-MNC CML patient[b]	AL-MNC Control	JF-MNC Control	Medium
VT-CML patient	*1463*	1947	1217	1370
AL-control	453	*357*	5745	330
JF-control	425	4790	*290*	543
Medium	530	390	343	45

[a] In this and subsequent tables, MLC tests were performed with standard conditions in which 50,000 irradiated stimulator MNC were incubated with 50,000 responder MNC, in triplicate, in RPMI 1640 (Gibco) supplemented with 15% pooled AB serum, glutamine, and antibiotics in 96-well round-bottomed microtiter plates (Costar) at 37°C for 5 days. Then 1 μCi ^{3}H thymidine (specific activity 2 Ci/mmol, Amersham, Arlington Heights, IL) was added for the final 18 hr of culture. Cultures were then harvested for scintillation counting by standard techniques. Autologous controls are in italics.

[b] Note that this representative CML patient's MNC fail to stimulate allogeneic responses or to proliferate (above background) in response to allogeneic cells.

* Abbreviations used: AET, 2-aminoethyl isothiouronium bromide hydrobromide; CM, conditioned medium; CML, chronic myelogenous luekemia; IF-gamma, gamma interferon; MLC, mixed leukocyte culture; MNC, mononuclear cells; PHA, phytohemagglutinin.

[1] This work was supported in part by National Institutes of Health Grants CA-37888, AM-33988, AM-33990, and AI-21289.

rosettes with AET-treated sheep red blood cells (E-rosette cells) by standard techniques (*8*) were only about 80% pure.)

Since phytohemagglutinin (PHA) treatment of normal MNC can also yield a population of class-II-positive, activated T cells (*9, 10*) we then tried to utilize unseparated CML patient MNC in similar experiments. Unseparated MNC from four CML patients were incubated for six days with PHA, and T cells were subsequently isolated as described above. The patient "T cell" preparations were sometimes only 60–80% positive after staining with the monoclonal pan-T-cell antibody Leu-5 (Bectin Dickenson Monoclonal Center, Inc., Mountain View, CA), probably because of the presence of "sticky" contaminating leukemic cells. The cells were, nevertheless, always over 40% DR-positive after staining with the L243 monoclonal anti DR antibody, and they could be isolated in sufficient numbers for both DR typing and MLC studies. However, these activated T cells had relatively poor viability (approximately 50–65%) and could not easily be used for serological DR typing.

We subsequently decided to isolate patients' T cells prior to incubation with PHA—and, since it is well known that PHA activation of healthy donor T cells requires the presence of monocytes or other antigen-presenting cells, we utilized a mixture of adherent cells and T cells to try to obtain activated T cells from CML patients (although there might have been sufficient numbers of contaminating monocytes to present antigen anyway). Adherent cells were obtained by incubating MNC in 35-mm flat-bottomed 6-well trays (Costar, Cambridge, MA) for one hour at 37°C (8×10⁶ cells/well). Nonadherent cells were then utilized for the sterile isolation of T cells with AET-treated sheep red blood cells. These T cells were added back to the wells containing the adherent cells at a final concentration of 1×10^6 T cells/ml, 4 ml/well. PHA (Wellcome Laboratories, Ltd, Buckingham, England) was added at a final concentration of 0.1 μg/ml or 1.0 μg/ml, and the cultures were incubated for six days at 37°C before harvesting. In order to obtain maximum induction of class II antigens, "conditioned medium" (CM) prepared from 5×10^6/ml fresh spleen cells—incubated for 40 h with 1 μg/ml PHA, 1 ng/ml PMA, and 1.3×10^6/ml irradiated Daudi cells—was added at a final concentration of 3% for the final 3 days of culture.

Typical cell yields for CML patients and controls utilizing the procedures described above are shown in Table 2. These cells were always at least 40% positive for the L243 DR marker. Although some patients had very poor recovery of T cells, and although proliferative responses with 0.1 μg/ml PHA yielded fewer cells than with 1.0 μg/ml PHA, there were sufficient numbers of viable cells obtained in all cases to perform all tests required. These cells could also be easily typed for DR alloantigens in all but one of seven cases, and the control donor's typing results were exactly the same as those found previously in tests using B cells. In one case, a repeat test with longer incubation times was necessary, and it can be anticipated that all patients (including HA, Table 2) might be successfully DR-allotyped with modified test conditions. Although the activated T cells could be less easily typed for HLA A,B,C antigens than cells obtained prior to PHA incubation, that problem was easily resolved by utilizing some of the positively selected T cells that were not incubated with PHA for the HLA A,B,C typing. The lower concentrations of PHA, 0.1 μg/ml, worked better for activation of T cells utilized in MLC tests because residual

TABLE 2. Representative cell yields obtained from CML patients and controls

Sample ID and DR type[a]	Clinical status	MNC number	Viable E rosette T cell yield (%)[b]	Viable PHA stimulated T cell yield–%
AR-DR5,7	CML	106×10^6	3×10^6 (3%)	1.0 μg/ml PHA—60%
CH-DR1,3	CML	662×10^6	25×10^6 (4%)	1.0 μg/ml PHA—138%
				0.1 μg/ml PHA—68%
RM-DR2,7	CML	383×10^6	70×10^6 (18%)	0.1 μg/ml PHA—69%
DC-DR7	CML	78×10^6	33×10^6 (42%)	0.1 μg/ml PHA—55%
HA-DR?[d]	CML	780×10^6	147×10^6 (19%)	0.1 μg/ml PHA—3%
RC-DR2,4	Control	70×10^6	10×10^6 (14%)	1.0 μg/ml PHA—196%
				0.1 μg/ml PHA—138%
DB-DR3,w6	Control	63×10^6	41×10^6 (65%)	0.1 μg/ml PHA—176%

[a] DR allotypes obtained from serological tests utilizing PHA-activated T cells.

[b] As noted in the text, the rosette-forming T cells from patients were from 60–80% (while those from the controls were over 95% pure).

[c] Mixtures of positively selected T cells and adherent monocytes were incubated for 6 days at 37°C with 0.1 or 1.0 μg/ml PHA as noted. The percentage yield is based on the number of T cells at the start of the PHA incubation present period.

[d] This patient's PHA incubated T cells failed to show sufficient reactivity with DR typing sera for antigen assignments to be made.

TABLE 3. Representative results for a mixed leukocyte culture test for PHA-activated T cells[a]

Responder MNC	Stimulator cells (mean cpm ^{3}H thymidine)[b]						
	T cells A (0.1 μg/ml PHA)[c]			T cells A (1.0 μg/ml PHA)			T cells (PWM)
	without CM	+3% CM day 0	+3% CM day 3	without CM	+3% CM day 0	+3% CM day 3	
A	*820*	*1060*	*383*	*9800*	*18063*	*16673*	*47660*
B	5880	3330	7056	17840	35976	25736	52736
C	16850	7480	13880	26033	37226	36023	67120
Medium	573	360	405	1026	866	1430	900

[a] Autologous controls are in italics. Test conditions are as described in Table 1.

[b] T cells were isolated and incubated for 6 days with autologous monocytes and 0.1 μg/ml PHA or 1.0 μg/ml PHA, with or without conditioned medium, or PWM.

[c] Since autologous MNC did not respond to 0.1 μg/ml PHA-treated autologous cells, residual PHA was not the cause for the allogeneic responses in this case. (At 1.0 μg/ml, there is residual PHA detected. Residual PWM also caused a highly elevated "autologous" response.)

PHA from cells incubated at the higher concentration apparently caused nonspecific proliferation of the responder cells (Table 3), but 1.0 μg/ml PHA worked better for DR allotyping.

Typical (MLC) results obtained with 0.1 μg/ml and 1.0 μg/ml PHA-treated T cells are shown in Table 3, in comparison with results obtained for PWM-treated T cells, and with and without the addition of CM at day 0 or day 3. The results indicate that the 0.1 μg/ml concentration of PHA, with or without added CM, can induce sufficient DR expression on the normal T cells of CML patients to allow them to be successfully used for critical MLC tests in bone marrow transplantation.

Acknowledgement. We thank Lucy Stewart for her expert typing and editorial assistance.

CYNTHIA CALLAWAY[2]
DAVID H. MAURER
DENOLA BROWN
WENDY FANG
KIM M. FEHIR
MARILYN S. POLLACK
Histocompatibility Laboratory and Departments of Microbiology and Immunology and Medicine
The Methodist Hospital and Baylor College of Medicine
Houston, Texas 77030

[2] Address correspondence to: Cynthia Callaway, Histocompatibility Laboratory F501, The Methodist Hospital, Houston, TX 77030.

REFERENCES

1. Suciu-Foca E, Susinno E, McKiernan P, Rohowsky C, Weiner J, Rubinstein P. DRw determinants on human T cells primed against allogeneic lymphocytes. Transplant Proc 1978; 4: 845.
2. Rich RR, Abramson SL, Seldin MF, Puck JM, Levy R. Role of Ia-positive cells in induction of secondary human immune responses to haptens in vitro. J Exp Med 1980, 152: 218s.
3. Basham T, Smith W, Lanier L, Morhenn V, Merigan T. Regulation of expression of class II major histocompatibility antigens on human peripheral blood monocytes and Langerhans cells by interferon. Hum Immunol 1984; 10: 83.
4. Maurer DH, Collins WE, Hanke JH, Van M, Rich RR, Pollack MS. Class II positive human dermal fibroblasts restimulate cloned allospecific T cells but fail to stimulate primary allogeneic lymphoproliferation. Hum Immunol 1985; 14: 245.
5. Pober JS, Gimbrone MA Jr, Cotran RS, Reiss CS, Burakoff SJ, Fiers W, Ault KA. Ia expression by vascular endothelium is inducible by activated T cells and by human interferon. J Exp Med 1983; 157: 1339.
6. Pollack MS, Chin-Louie J, Moshief RD. Functional characteristics and differential expression of class II DR, DS and SB antigens on human melanoma cell lines. Hum Immunol 1984; 9: 75.
7. Lampson LA, Levy R. Two populations of Ia-like molecules on a human B cell line. J Immunol 1980; 125: 293.
8. Suciu-Foca N, Khan R, Zachary AA, Braun WE. Preparation of T lymphocytes for MLC culture. In: Zachary AA, Braun WE, eds. The AACHT laboratory manual. Am Assoc Clin Hist Test 1981: I-11-1.
9. Ko HS, Fu SM, Winchester RJ, Yu DTY, Kunkel HG. Ia determinants on stimulated human T lymphocytes: occurrence on mitogen- and antigen-activated T cells. J Exp Med 1979; 150: 246.
10. Reinherz EL, Kung PG, Pesando JM, Goldstein G, Schlossman SF. Ia determinants on human T cell subsets defined by monoclonal antibodies: activation stimuli required for expression. J Exp Med 1979; 150: 1472.

Received 6 September 1985.
Accepted 2 December 1985.

INHIBITION OF ANTI-CD3 (T3) ANTIBODY-INDUCED ACTIVATION OF T CELLS BY CYCLOSPORINE[1]

Accumulated evidence indicates that optimal activation of T lymphocytes requires the participation of two signals. Our recent report, as well as data from others, have demonstrated that for human resting T cell activation one signal can be provided by antibodies to the CD3* complex, and the other by interleukin 2 (IL-2) (*1–3*). The CD3 complex is associated with the antigen receptor on the cell surface, and is intimately involved with the T cell activation process (*4–6*). Antibodies reactive with this complex are believed to trigger IL2-receptor expression.

In the present investigation, we have used the drug cyclosporine (CsA), a fungal metabolite with clinically proved immunosuppressive activity (*7–9*), in an attempt to dissect the activation of T cells by anti-CD3 antibodies and IL-2. We found that CsA interferes with the signal delivered by anti-CD3 antibodies, thus inhibiting both cellular proliferation and expression of IL-2 receptors.

Cell cultures were performed in RPMI 1640 medium supplemented with 2% heat-inactivated fetal calf serum (FCS), 100 units/ml penicillin, 100 μg/ml streptomycin, and 2 mM L-glutamine (all from M.A., Bioproducts, Los Angeles, CA). The anti-CD3 monoclonal antibody (MoAb) used was 64.1 (New England Nuclear Corp., Boston, MA) (*10*). Recombinant IL-2 (RIL2) produced in *Escherichia coli* (*11*) was generously provided by Cetus Corp. (Emeryville, CA). IL-2 (lot Lp 227) was shown by the supplier to be 98% pure by sodium dodecyl sulfate polyacrylamide gel electrophoresis and contained less than 0.02 ng endotoxin/mg IL-2. One unit of IL-2 activity is the amount producing half-maximal growth of an IL-2-dependent cell line. Monoclonal antibodies reactive with the T4 (helper/inducer) and T8 (cytotoxic/suppressor) T cell subsets used as supernatant fluids—harvested from hybridoma cell cultures CRL 8002 and CRL 8014, respectively—were obtained from the American Type Culture Collection. Fluorescein-conjugated antihuman IL-2 receptor monoclonal antibody (clone 2A3) was purchased from Becton Dickinson (Mountain View, CA). Cyclosporine was provided by Sandoz Ltd., (Basel, Switzerland) and was dissolved in absolute ethanol. Dilutions of the drug were made in culture medium. Control cultures contained ethanol alone at the same concentrations.

Purification of peripheral blood T lymphocytes was performed as previously described (*2*). Briefly, mononuclear cells from normal healthy donors were isolated by Hypaque-Ficoll density gradient, and T cells obtained by rosetting with neuraminidase-treated sheep erythrocytes. Contaminating monocytes were removed by two cycles of carbonyl iron treatment (*12, 13*). Proliferation of T cells was determined by culturing 2×10^5 cells per triplicate microtiter tray well (Costar No. 3596,

[1] This work was supported in part by National Institutes of Health Grants AM 21175, AM 36010 and RR 00833; by the University of California Task Force on AIDS, and by a grant from the Lilly Research Laboratories. This is publication number 4172BCR from the Research Institute of Scripps Clinic.

* Abbreviations: CD3: cluster of differentiation 3; FCS, fetal calf serum; IL-2: interleukin 2; CsA: cyclosporine; MoAb: monoclonal antibody.

TABLE 1. Effect of cyclosporine on proliferation and IL2-receptor expression

Addition	[^{3}H]-thymidine uptake (cpm×10^{-3})[a]	Percentage of receptor positive cells[b]
Medium	0.15±0.03	2.1
64.1	1.31±0.21	8.8
IL-2	1.33±0.44	4.4
64.1 + IL-2	45.64±10.32	37.5
64.1 + IL-2 + CsA 10 ng/ml	40.82±7.83	32.5
64.1 + IL-2 + CsA 100 ng/ml	28.90±6.27	24.3
64.1 + IL-2 + CsA 1000 ng/ml	3.92±0.98	9.2
64.1 + IL-2 + CsA 25,000 ng/ml	0.66±0.40	7.7

[a] Purified T cells, 2×10^5, were incubated in microtiter plate wells with monoclonal antibody 64.1 (50 ng/ml) and/or recombinant IL-2 (7.5 U/ml) in the presence or absence of various concentrations of CSA for 3 days. Proliferation was assessed by addition of [^{3}H]-thymidine (1 μCi/well) during the last 5 hr of the incubation period. Results are expressed as averages of triplicate determination (± SD).

[b] The IL2 receptor was assessed with a fluorescein-conjugated anti-IL2 receptor monoclonal antibody and cytofluorographic analysis in the FACS IV. The results are representative of four replicate experiments.

Cambridge, MA), in the presence or absence of various concentrations of CsA, and by adding [^{3}H]-thymidine (1 μCi/well) during the last 5 hr of incubation. Detection of IL-2 receptors was assessed by immunofluorescence staining and flow cytometry (*14*).

Resting peripheral blood lymphocytes can be induced to proliferate only in the presence of both anti-CD3 antibody 64.1 and IL-2. Either signal alone is not an efficient activator (*1, 2*). The results in Table 1 confirm these data and further demonstrate that CsA can inhibit the proliferation in a dose-dependent manner. In addition, CsA inhibits the expression of IL-2 receptors, as determined by immunofluorescence analysis with monoclonal anti-IL2 receptor antibody (Table 1). Inhibition of proliferation and IL-2 receptor expression was not due to competition for binding of CsA and anti-CD3 or anti-IL2 receptor antibodies (data not shown).

In order to determine whether CsA interferes with the signals delivered by antibody 64.1 or IL-2, or both, we performed the experiments described below. Cultures of purified T cells were incubated with antibody 64.1 and IL-2 for various periods before addition of CsA. Alternatively, cultures were incubated with antibody alone for various times before addition of both CsA and IL-2. We observed that the delay of CsA addition caused a time-related abrogation of its antiproliferative effect (Fig. 1A). Furthermore, delaying both CsA and IL-2 additions produced an identical time-related inhibition of the antiproliferative effect (Fig. 1B). It is of interest that delaying CsA addition even for 1 hr caused noticeable abrogation of the drug's inhibitory effect (Fig. 1, A and B). Delaying addition for 24 hr rendered activated T cells insensitive to inhibition by the drug (Fig. 1, A and B). In other experiments where CsA was added at culture initiation, the inhibitory effect of the drug was unhindered regardless of when antibody or IL-2 was added (Fig. 1, C and D). The amount of CsA used in these studies (100 ng/ml) was similar to that found in serum during chronic administration (*15*). The above data suggest that, at least for the time points tested, CsA interferes with the signal(s) initiated by anti-CD3 antibody but not with the events mediated by IL-2. If the latter were the case, delaying addition of both CsA and IL-2 should not have resulted in abrogation of inhibition (Fig. 1B).

We wished to determine whether the antiproliferative effect of CsA had any T cell subset specificity. To this end, we enriched for T4 (helper/inducer) or T8 (cytotoxic/suppressor) positive subpopulations by indirect immunofluorescence staining with the respective monoclonal antibody, followed by sorting in the cytofluorograph (FACS IV). Two types of experiments were performed: staining with antibody OKT4 or staining with antibody OKT8 followed by sorting. It can be seen in Fig. 2 that either type of manipulation produced enriched and depleted subpopulations with sensitivities similar to the antiproliferative effects of CsA (50–60% inhibition).

The in vitro activation of resting peripheral T cells by antibodies to the CD3 molecular complex and IL-2 is independent of monocyte participation and does not have an absolute requirement for crosslinking of CD3 molecules (*2*). In the present investigation, we demonstrated that this two-step activation process is inhibited by the immunosuppressive drug CsA. It is

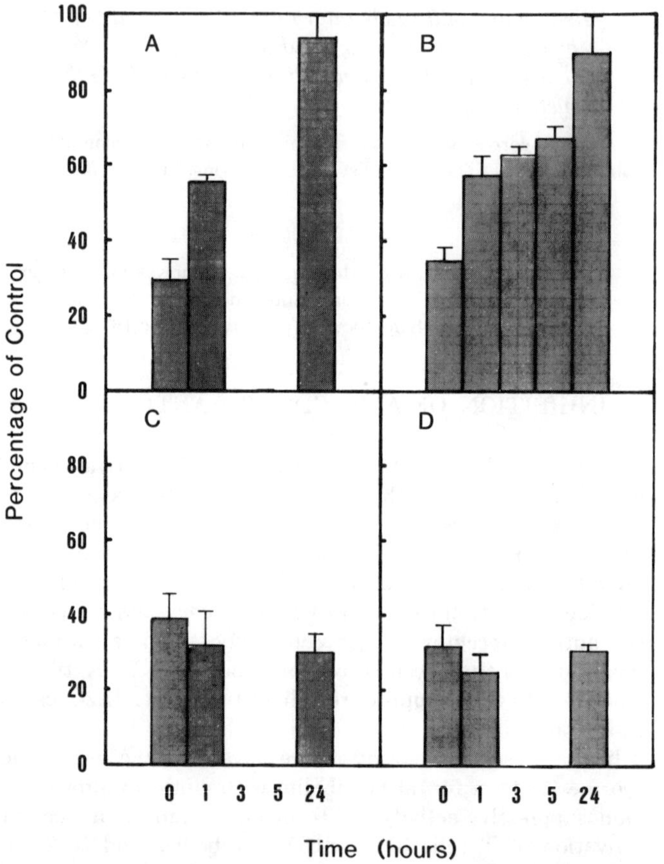

FIGURE 1. Time kinetics of CsA addition. Purified T cells, 2×10^5 per microtiter tray well, were incubated under the following protocols: (A) antibody 64.1 (50 ng/ml) and IL-2 (7.5 U/ml) for various times before addition of CsA (100 ng/ml); (B) antibody 64.1 (50 ng/ml) alone for various times before addition of CsA (100 ng/ml) and IL-2 (7.5 U/ml); (C) antibody 64.1 (50 ng/ml) and CsA (100 ng/ml) before addition of IL-2 (7.5 U/ml); (D), IL-2 (7.5 U/ml) and CsA (100 ng/ml) before addition of antibody 64.1 (50 ng/ml). After the second addition, incubation was continued for 3 days. Control cultures were incubated in a similar fashion without CsA. Proliferation was assessed by [^{3}H]-thymidine incorporation during the last 5 hr of incubation. The data represent the mean (± SD) of triplicate determinations. The results of (B) are those of three replicate experiments. The rest of the data are from one experiment.

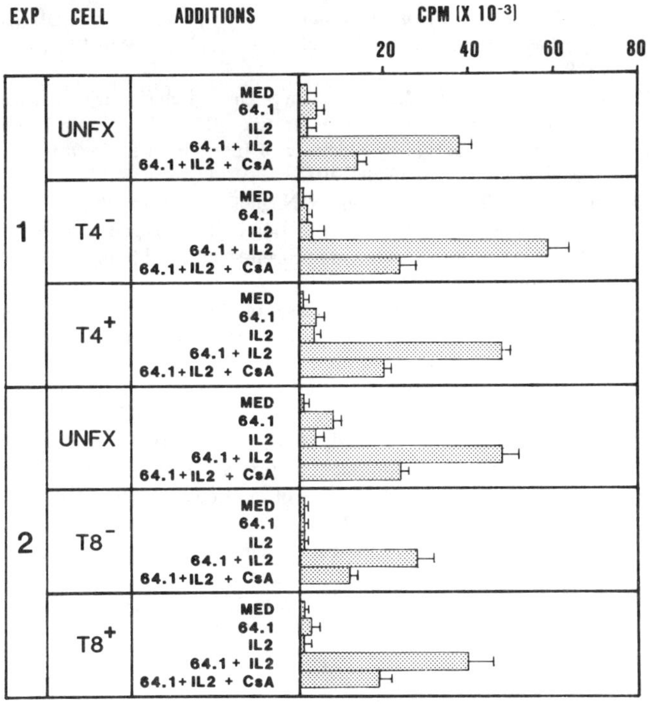

FIGURE 2. The antiproliferative effect of CsA on T cell subsets. Populations enriched in T4-positive or T8-positive T cells were obtained by incubating purified T lymphocytes either with antibody OKT4 (experiment 1) or OKT8 (experiment 2) followed by fluorescein-conjugated goat antimouse immunoglobulin and sorting in the cytofluorograph (FACS IV) into positive and negative populations. The fractionated populations were >90% pure. The sorted cells were cultured under the conditions noted for 3 days. Proliferation was assessed by adding [^{3}H]-thymidine during the last 5 hr of incubation.

of interest that CsA inhibits not only cellular proliferation, but also expression of IL-2 receptors. There is some controversy concerning whether CsA can inhibit expression of IL-2 receptors. Studies using already activated cells (tumor lines or mitogen activated lymphocytes) have indicated that CsA specifically inhibits IL-2 production (*16–19*) without any significant effects on IL-2 receptor expression (*17, 20–22*). In view of the present findings with resting cells, it is possible that the state of cellular activation is a critical determinant of the outcome of CsA-mediated inhibition of IL-2 receptor expression.

The association of the CD3 molecular complex with the antigen receptor heterodimer on the surfaces of T cells and the activating properties of anti-CD3 antibodies have prompted the hypothesis that this complex serves as a transducer of the antigenic signal (*4–6*). The ability of anti-CD3 antibodies to render T cells sensitive to the growth-promoting effects of IL-2 suggests that the CD3 complex initiates IL-2 receptor expression. In previous studies, however, incubation of T cells with anti-CD3 antibody alone did not result in any reproducible detection of IL-2 receptors (*1, 2*). Since receptors were assayed by indirect immunofluorescence using monoclonal anti-IL-2 receptor antibody, lack of detection may reflect limitations in the sensitivity of this particular assay system. Our data suggest that CsA primarily affects the step(s) activated by anti-CD3 antibody.

In a randomized clinical trail the results of which were recently published (*23*), the monoclonal anti-CD3 antibody OKT3 was used to treat acute rejection of cadaveric renal transplants. Patients undergoing acute rejection received OKT3 daily with concomitant lowering of the dosage of other immunosuppressive drugs or with conventional steroids. It was found that the OKT3-treated group had a significantly higher rate of reversal of rejections than the steroid-treated group. Other monoclonal anti-T-cell antibodies have been also used in renal allograft rejection (*24–26*). Although they have resulted in removal of T cells, they have not produced the striking results obtained with OKT3 (*24–26*). This could very well be due to the unique relationship of the CD3 complex to T cell activation. Anti-CD3 antibody treatment is always performed in conjunction with other immunosuppressive drugs. In view of our present data with CsA, one should exercise caution in the selection of the concomitant drug regimen. Thus study of the effects of immunosuppressive drugs on T cell activation in an in vitro system, such as the one used in this study, may provide valuable information in deciding the best immunosuppressive strategy in clinical transplantation.

In summary, the activation of peripheral T lymphocytes by antibodies to the CD3 complex and IL-2 is inhibited by the immunosuppressive drug CsA. The inhibition seems to be exerted at the step that is activated by anti-CD3 antibodies. Furthermore, CsA has no preferential effects on any particular T cell subset.

Acknowledgments. We thank Don McQuitty and Susan Stone for the FACS analysis. We are also grateful to our GCRC staff for providing the blood specimens and our BCR Word Processing Center for preparing the manuscript.

JACQUES BENTIN[2]
DENNIS A. CARSON
JOHN H. VAUGHAN
CONSTANTINE D. TSOUKAS
Department of Basic and Clinical Research
Scripps Clinic and Research Foundation
La Jolla, California 92037

[2] Jacques Bentin is supported in part by a grant from Fond de la Recherche Scientifique Medicale (FRSM), Brussels, Belgium.

REFERENCES

1. Palacios R. Mechanisms by which accessory cells contribute in growth of resting T lymphocytes initiated by OKT3 antibody. Eur J Immunol 1985; 15: 645.
2. Tsoukas CD, Landgraf B, Bentin J, et al. Activation of resting T lymphocytes by anti-CD3 (T3) antibodies in the absence of monocytes. J Immunol 1985; 135: 1719.
3. Schwab R, Crow MK, Russo C, Weksler ME. Requirements for T cell activation by OKT3 monoclonal antibody: role of modulation of T3 molecules and interleukin 1. J Immunol 1985; 135: 1714.
4. Meuer SC, Fitzgerald KA, Hussey RE, Hodgdon JC, Schlossman SF, Reinherz EL. Clonotypic structures involved in antigen-specific human T cell function. Relationship to the T3 molecular complex. J Exp Med 1983; 157: 705.
5. Weiss A, Imboden J, Wiskocil R, Stobo J. The role of T3 in the activation of human T cells. J Clin Immunol 1984; 4: 165.
6. Tsoukas CD, Valentine M, Lotz M, Vaughan JH, Carson DA. The role of the T3 molecular complex in antigen recognition and subsequent activation events. Immunol Today 1984; 5: 311.
7. Borel JF. The history of cyclosporin A and its significance. In: White DJG, ed. Cyclosporin A: proceedings of an international conference on Cyclosporin A. New York: Elsevier, 1983: 5.
8. Kahan BD. Cyclosporin: the agent and its actions. Transplant Proc 1985; 17(suppl 1): 5.

9. Shevach EM. The effects of cyclosporin A on the immune system. Ann Rev Immunol 1985; 3: 397.
10. Hansen JA, Martin PJ, Beatty PG, Clark EA, Ledbetter JA. Human T lymphocyte cell surface molecules defined by the workshop monoclonal antibodies (T cell protocol). In: Bernard A, Boumodl A, Danoset J, Milsteon C, Schlossman SF, eds. Leukocyte typing: human leukocyte differentiation antigens detected by monoclonal antibodies. New York: Springer Verlag, 1984: 195.
11. Wang A, Lu SD, Mark DF. Site-specific mutagenesis of the human interleukin 2 gene: structure-function analysis of the cysteine residues. Science 1984; 224: 1431.
12. Wahl SM, Rosenstreich DC, Oppenheim JJ. Separation of human lymphocytes by E rosette sedimentation. In: Bloom BR, David JR, eds. In vitro methods in cell mediated and tumor immunity. New York: Academic, 1976: 231.
13. Lee KC. Carbonyl iron powder. In: Mishell BB, Shiigi SM, eds. Selected methods in cellular immunology. San Francisco: WH Freeman, 1980: 179.
14. Julius MD, Sweet RG, Fathman CG, Herzenberg LA. Fuorescence activated cell sorting and its applications. In: Richmond CR, Petersen DF, Mullamy PF, Anderson EC, eds. Mammalian cells: probes and problems. Proceedings of the first Los Alamos Life Science Symposium AEC Series, 1974: 107.
15. Keown PA, Stiller CR, Ulan RA, et al. Immunological and pharmacological monitoring in the clinical use of cyclosporin A. Lancet 1981; 1: 686.
16. Elliott JF, Lin Y, Mizel SB, Bleackley RC, Harnish DG, Paetkan V. Induction of interleukin 2 messenger RNA inhibited by cyclosporin A. Science 1984; 226: 1439.
17. Kronke M, Leonard WJ, Depper JM, et al. Cyclosporin A inhibits T-cell growth factor gene expression at the level of mRNA transcription. Proc Natl Acad Sci USA 1984; 81: 5214.
18. Granelli-Piperno A, Inaba K, Steinman RM. Stimulation of lymphokine release from lymphoblasts. Requirement for mRNA synthesis and inhibition by cyclosporin A. J Exp Med 1984; 160: 1792.
19. Kermani-Arab V, Salehmoghaddam S, Danovitch G, Hirji K, Rezai A. Mediation of the antiproliferative effect of cyclosporin on human lymphocytes by blockade of interleukin 2 biosynthesis. Transplantation 1985; 39: 439.
20. Miyawaki T, Yachie A, Ohzeki S, Nagaoki T, Taniguchi N. Cyclosporin A does not prevent expression of Tac antigen, a probable TCGF receptor molecule, on mitogen-stimulated human T cells. J Immunol 1983; 133: 244.
21. Dos Reis GA, Shevach EM. Effect of cyclosporin A on T cell function in vitro: the mechanism of suppression of T cell proliferation depends on the nature of the T cell stimulus as well as the differentiation state of the responding T cell. J Immunol 1982; 129: 2360.
22. Buntjes D, Hardt C, Rollinghoff M, Wagner H. Cyclosporin A mediates immunosuppression of primary cytotoxic T cell responses by impairing the release of interleukin 1 and interleukin 2. Eur J Immunol 1981; 8: 657.
23. Ortho Multicenter Transplant Study Group. A randomized clinical trial of OKT3 monoclonal antibody for acute rejection of cadaveric renal transplants. N Engl J Med 1985; 313: 337.
24. Thurlaw PJ, Lovering E, d'Apice AJF, McKenzie IFC. A monoclonal anti-pan-T-cell antibody in vitro and in vivo studies. Transplantation 1983; 36: 293.
25. Takahashi H, Okazaki H, Terasaki PI, et al. Reversal of transplant rejection by monoclonal antiblast antibody. Lancet 1983; 2: 1155.
26. Kirkman RL, Aranjo JL, Busch GJ, et al. Treatment of acute renal allograft rejection with monoclonal anti-T12 antibody. Transplantation 1983; 36: 620.

Received 13 November 1985.
Accepted 9 December 1985.

DEVELOPMENT OF BULLOUS PEMPHIGOID AFTER ALLOGENEIC BONE MARROW TRANSPLANTATION

REPORT OF A CASE[1]

Allogeneic bone marrow transplantation (BMT)* is used with increasing success in the treatment of leukemia and severe aplastic anemia. Generalized mottled erythematous rash, papulosquamous plaques, desquamation, hyperpigmentation, leukoderma, and partial alopecia are common cutaneous manifestations in the initial features of the generalized type of chronic graft-vs.-host disease (GVHD), which usually does not include bullous skin lesions (*1–3*). Bullous pemphigoid (BP) is considered to be one of the autoimmune cutaneous diseases. It is characterized by the presence of antibasement-membrane-zone (BMZ) antibodies in the serum, and it involves skin lesions (*4*). We report a case of BP that developed 3 months after allogeneic marrow transplantation in the absence of any clinical or histologic evidence for chronic graft-versus-host disease.

A-46-year-old man was referred to us on May 29, 1982 because of throat pain and generalized formation of bullae. He had been treated with high-dose cyclophosphamide and total-body irradiation, followed by allogeneic marrow transplantation from his HLA-identical brother, which was performed for the treatment of acute myelogenous leukemia during first remission at the Fred Hutchinson Cancer Research Center on January 28, 1982. He received methotrexate (MTX) weekly for the prevention of acute GVHD (*5*). In addition, on day 0 he received a subcutaneous implant of cultured thymic tissue that was matched with his HLA type. This was done as part of a study to control chronic GVHD (*6*). He was seropositive for cytomegalovirus (CMV) before transplantation, and CMV was isolated from his urine on multiple occasions after transplantation. The clinical course following BMT was uncomplicated by the development of acute or chronic GVHD or interstitial pneumonitis. He returned to Japan on May 2, 1982 (day 94 post-transplant). Early in May, he noticed a bullous lesion on his anterior chest and pain on swallowing. The bullae became generalized and throat pain increased. He lost 2 kg of his body weight in one month due to impaired oral intake. On May 26, he vomited a tissue fragment, which was identified histologically as esophageal mucosa showing mild inflammatory change. He was hospitalized on May 29.

Physical examination revealed widely-spread bullous lesions in various stages of the disease. Some of these lesions were also observed in the oral mucosa and palpebral conjunctiva. The

[1]This work was supported in part by grants-in-aid for Cancer Research from the Ministry of Health and Welfare (58-6) and the Ministry of Education, Science and Culture (59010028); by the Japanese Government; and by the Fifth Research Grant from Japanese Foundation for Multidisciplinary Treatment of Cancer.

* Abbreviations used: BMT, bone marrow transplantation; BMZ, basement membrane zone; BP, bullous pemphigoid; CMV, cytomegalovirus; GVHD, graft-versus-host disease; IL-2, interleukin 2; MTX, metthrotrenate; PHA, phytohemagglutinin; PWM, pokeweed nitogen.

liver edge was palpable 2 cm below the right costal margin; it was smooth, normal in consistency, and not tender.

Liver function tests showed slight elevation of alkaline phosphatase (467 IU/L; normal range; 88–271) and γ-glutamyl transpeptidase (314 IU/L; normal range, 4–43), while serum levels of total bilirubin and transaminases were within normal limits. Serum levels of IgG, IgM, and IgA moderately decreased; IgG was 895 mg/dL (normal range: 1325–1773), IgM 90 mg/dL (normal range: 99–229), and IgA 68 mg/dl (normal range: 140–316). Antinuclear, antimitochondrial, anti-smooth-muscle and anti–extractable-nuclear-antigen antibodies were not detected in the serum.

The presence of subbasilar bullae was histologically demonstrated in the biopsied specimens of the skin, and no associated degenerative necrotic changes were seen in the basal layer, epidermis, or skin appendages. By fluorescent staining, deposits of IgG and C′3 were identified in the dermoepidermal junction. IgM deposits were not found in the junction. Furthermore, the patient's serum contained an IgG antibody that bound with BMZ of guinea pig lip (titer 1:40), whereas the antibody was not detected in the serum from his marrow donor.

Endoscopic examination performed on June 1 revealed severely erosive esophagitis with hemorrhage. Web formation and sclerotic changes (*7*) were not observed endoscopically. Mild scattered lymphocytic infiltration was observed in the subepithelial layers of the biopsied esophageal tissues. The deposits of IgG and C′3 were also identified on the basal layer. IgM deposits were absent. Histological findings of the bullous lesions in the skin and esophagus—which lacked signs of epithelial cell necrosis and inflammation of other skin appendages such as sweat glands, hair follicles, or submucosal glandual structures—were highly compatible with those of bullous pemphigoid and not with those of chronic GVHD. Treatment with prednisolone (1 mg/kg/day) and azathioprine (50 mg/day) was started on June 2. Azathioprine was discontinued on June 14 because of the elevations in serum transaminase levels, which subsequently returned to normal. The outcome was excellent, and both skin and esophageal lesions completely disappeared early in July. The patient was discharged on July 12 and prednisolone treatment was tapered.

Before the prednisolone therapy was started, functions of T and non-T cells were evaluated by using the pokeweed mitogen (PWM)-induced immunoglobulin synthesis in vitro as described previously (*8*). The patient's non-T cells failed to produce Ig in vitro with the help of normal T cells. There was no significant suppressor T cell function. T cell subset analysis using monoclonal antibodies showed a marked decrease of OKT4-positive cells to 16.9% (normal range: 28.4–47.0) and slight increase of OKT8-positive cells to 30.9% (normal range: 16.6–28.2) among peripheral blood mononuclear cells. Proliferative responses to mitogens were significantly decreased. Responses to phytohemagglutinin (PHA) were 2026 cpm (normal range 117,000 ± 33,000 cpm), and those to concanavalin A were 2372 cpm (normal range 79,000 ± 17,000 cpm), respectively (*9*). Interleukin 2 (IL-2) producing capacity (*10*) was also depressed to 16% of normal control.

GVHD in allogeneic marrow graft recipients is a systemic illness characterized by acute and chronic forms. During the acute phase, the skin, liver and gastrointestinal tract are preferentially involved. The skin manifestations are erythema, edema, and desquamation (*2, 5*). These skin changes are accompanied by histologic findings of basement membrane desposits of IgM and C′3, and epithelial cell necrosis (*11*). The chronic form of GVHD is mainfested usually more than 2–3 months after transplantation. The skin lesions include papulosquamous plaques on skin and buccal mucosa, alopecia, hyperpigmentation, and s.c. scarring that leads to joint contractures (*1, 3, 5*). The skin and mucosal lesions in chronic GVHD are characterized by histologic evidence of epithelial cell necrosis, lymphocytic infiltration of skin appendages, and fibrosis (*3*). IgM and complement deposits in the dermoepidermal junction are common in patients with chronic GVHD, but IgG deposits in the dermoepidermal junction are nonspecific and are found in normal skin and in skin of patients with or without GVHD (*11*).

In this patient, both skin and esophageal bullae developed around day 100 posttransplant, which coincided with the usual time of the onset of chronic GVHD (*1*); varicella zoster infection may also occur around this time. Multiple cultures of the bullous fluid were negative for varicella zoster virus, and serological studies were not diagnostic. Histological and immunofluorescent studies of the biopsied specimens from the skin and esophagus were highly compatible with bullous pemphigoid (*4*) but not compatible with chronic GVHD (*3*). Although the development of anti-basement membrane IgG antibodies is a possible manifestation of underlying chronic GVHD, this possibility is unlikely becacuse IgM deposits on the BMZ, which have been reported in patients with cutaneous chronic GVHD (*11*), were not detected in this patient. There was no clinical evidence suggesting the presence of chronic GVHD. Furthermore, biopsied specimens from the skin, liver, and oral mucosa revealed no histological evidence compatible with chronic GVHD.

Bullous pemphigoid is a chronic autoimmune blistering skin disease characterized by the deposition of immunoglobulins and/or complement at the BMZ. The majority of patients with this disease have circulating IgG antibody against the BMZ of the skin (*4*). Recently, pemphigoid antigen was extracted directly from normal human skin and partially characterized (*12*). Thus, concerning the development of BP, it is hypothesized that anti-BMZ antibody initially binds to the antigen in the lamina lucida, followed by complement activation and release of anaphylatoxins, which activate tissue mast cells to release eosinophil chemotactic factor (*4*). Migrating eosinophils release lysozomal enzymes which degrade BMZ structures and result in the loss of dermoepidermal adherence. Some immunological abnormalities have been reported in patients with BP to explain the production of anti-BMZ autoantibodies. These include abnormalities such as decrease of suppressor T cells (*13*), low responsiveness to PHA (*14*), and deficiency in IL-2 production (*15*). In this case, similar abnormal findings were observed in mitogenic responses and IL-2 production. Although the circulating OKT8-positive cells with a suppressor/cytotoxic phenotype were slightly increased in this patient's peripheral blood, their suppressor function in in vitro Ig synthesis was not detected—moreover T-helper and non-T cell functions were also decreased. From these observations, it is suggested that such disorders of immune regulation may play a role in permitting the generation of autoantibodies against BMZ as in other autoimmune diseases. Still remaining to be explained is the mechanism of antigen presentation that triggered the events leading to bullous pemphigoid in this patient.

Acknowledgments. We thank Dr. T. Kaminaga, Dr. S. Tanabe, and

Dr. M. Takada for their comments and discussion about bullous pemphigoid and immunofluorescent diagnostic study.

MIKIO UEDA[2]
TAKAO MORI
SHINTARO SHIOBARA
MINE HARADA
TAKASHI YOSHIDA
TAMOTSU MATSUDA
KEN-ICHI HATTORI[3]
HIDEAKI MIZOGUCHI[4]
KEITH M. SULLIVAN[5]
ROBERT P. WITHERSPOON[5]
The Kanazawa University Bone Marrow Transplant Team
Department of Medicine and Blood Transfusion Service
Kanazawa University School of Medicine
Kanazawa 920, Japan

[2] Address correspondence to: Mikio Ueda, M.D., Third Department of Medicine, Kanazawa University School of Medicine, Kanazawa 920, Japan.

[3] Red Cross Blood Center of Ishikawa Prefecture.

[4] Division of Hematology, Department of Medicine, Tokyo Women's Medical College, Tokyo, Japan.

[5] The Departments of Pathology and Medicine, University of Washington School of Medicine, and the Fred Hutchinson Cancer Research Center, Seattle, Washington, 98101.

REFERENCES

1. Shulman HM, Sale GE, Lerner KG, et al. Chronic cutaneous graft-versus-host disease in man. Am J Pathol 1978; 91: 545.
2. Saurat JH. Cutaneous manifestations of graft-versus-host disease. Int J Dermatol 1981; 20: 249.
3. Shulman HM, Sullivan KM, Weiden PL, et al. Chronic graft-versus-host syndrome in man. A long-term clinicopathologic study of 20 Seattle patients. Am J Med 1980; 69: 204.
4. Sams Jr WM, Gammon WR. Mechanism of lesion production in pemphigus and pemphigoid. J Am Acad Dermatol 1982; 6: 431.
5. Thomas ED, Storb R, Clift RA, et al. Bone marrow transplantation. N Engl J Med 1975; 292: 832, 895.
6. Atkinson K, Storb R, Ochs HD, et al. Thymus transplantation after allogeneic bone marrow graft to prevent chronic graft-versus-host disease in humans. Transplantation 19; 33: 168.
7. McDonald GB, Sullivan KM, Schuffler MD, et al. Esophageal abnormalities in chronic graft-versus-host disease in humans. Gastroenterology 1981; 80: 914.
8. Witherspoon RP, Lum LG, Storb R, et al. In vitro regulation of immunoglobulin synthesis after human marrow transplantation. II. Deficient T and non-T lymphocyte function within 3–4 months of allogeneic, syngeneic, or autologous marrow grafting for hematologic malignancy. Blood 1982; 59: 844.
9. Ueda M, Harada M, Shiobara S, et al. T lymphocyte reconstitution in long-term survivors after allogeneic and autologous marrow transplantation. Transplantation 1984; 37: 552.
10. Ruscetti FW, Gallo RC. Human T lymphocyte growth factor: regulation of growth and function of T lymphocytes. Blood 1981; 57: 379.
11. Tsoi MS, Storb R, Jones E, et al. Deposition of IgM and complement at the dermo-epidermal junction in acute and chronic cutaneous graft-vs-host disease in man. J Immunol 1978; 120: 1485.
12. Stanley JR, Woodley DT, Katz SI. Identification and partial characterization of pemphigoid antigen extracted from normal human skin. J Invest Dermatol 1984; 82: 108.
13. Hovmark A, Asbrink E. An immunological study of patients with bullous pemphigoid. Acta Derm Venereol (Stockh) 1982; 62: 201.
14. Ahmed AR. Lymphocyte studies in bullous pemphigoid. J Dermatol 1981; 8: 385.
15. Ahmed AR, Hijri K, Kermani VA. Interleukin-2 production in bullous pemphigoid. Arch Dermatol Res 1984; 276: 330.

Received 22 October 1985.
Accepted 26 November 1985.

HISTOCOMPATIBILITY LOCI ASSOCIATED WITH LYMPHOCYTE ALLOANTIGENIC LOCI

Several *H* (histocompatibility) loci have previously been identified to be associated with the *Ly-1*, *Ly-2*, *Ly-3*, and *Thy-1* loci in mice, as skin grafts exchanged between congenic pairs are rejected and lead to antibody formation to the appropriate surface alloantigen. The *H* loci associated with the *Ly-1*, *Ly-2*, *Ly-3*, *Ly-4*, *Ly-6*, and *Thy-1* loci have now been examined in several newer C57BL/6 congenic strains in nonprimed, primed, and hyperimmune mice. The results show that—except for *Ly-4*, which is linked to the *H-3* locus and for Thy-1 antigens, which are present on epidermal cells—while none of the *Ly* loci have histocompatibility effects in one set of congenic strains, they were noted in another set of different origin. In addition, grafts exchanged between the two different *Ly-1* or *Ly-2* congenic strains were rejected, indicating the presence of *H* genes separate from, but linked to *Ly-1* and *Ly-2* loci in these strains. The *Ly-1*, *Ly-2*, *Ly-3*, and *Ly-6* loci are presumably linked to, but distinct from several of the ubiquitous non-H-2 histocompatibility loci.

Histocompatibility (*H*) loci in the mouse are traditionally defined by the rejection of skin grafts, although this necessarily restricts their definition to those alloantigenic determinants expressed on dermal tissue, including those of general (e.g., H-2), or restricted distribution (e.g., Ia antigens), or those specific to skin (*Skn* loci). It was therefore of interest to note that loci, coding for determinants that were apparently lymphocyte-specific also led to skin graft rejection—e.g., *Thy-1*, *Ly-1*, *Ly-2*, *Ly-3*, and *T1a* (*1–3*). These loci were called *H(Ly-1)*, *H(Ly-2)*, *H(Ly-2, Ly-3)*, and *H(T1a)* (*1*). One of these determinants, Thy-1, has subsequently been found to be present on epidermal tissue (*4*)—but for others, such as *Ly-1*, and *Ly-2* the specificities are clearly lymphocyte-restricted (*3, 5*). It was concluded, at least for the *Ly-1* and *Ly-2* loci, that the H genes were probably linked to, but separate from these loci and were included in the production of the congenic strain. With the development of additional strains, congenic for the *Ly-1*, *Ly-2*, *Ly-4*, *Ly-6*, and *Thy-1* loci, the association of *H* and *Ly* loci has been reexamined. We find that only the *Ly-4* and *Thy-1* loci are also *H* loci—the newer *Ly-1* and *Ly-2* congenic strains do not carry *H* loci different from those of the parent, and neither does the C3H.B6-*Ly-6*^{b} congenic strain.

The mice were obtained from M. Cherry, Ph.D., Jackson Laboratory, Bar Harbor, ME, were: B6-*Ly-1*^{a} (n12,F21); B6.PL(75NS)-*Ly-2*^{a} (n10,F21); C3H.B6-*Ly-6*^{b} (n8,F13); B6.PL(74NS)-*Thy-1*^{a} (n10,F18)—and, from Dr. E.A. Boyse, Sloan Kettering Institute, NY: B6.*Ly-1*^{a} (n17,F>10); B6-*Ly-2*^{a} (n16,F>10); and B6-*Ly-2*^{a}-*Ly-3*^{a} (n17,F>10). It should be noted that the Cherry B6-*Ly-1*^{a} strain was of mixed origin, whereas B6.PL(75NS) obtained the *Ly-2a* allele from PL. The C57BL/6 Boyse strains received the *Ly-1a* and *Ly-2a* loci from C3H, and *Ly-2*^{a}, *Ly-3*^{a} loci from RF. The A.AL-*Thy-1*^{a} (n11,F>9) and A.AL-*Thy-1*^{b} (n11,F>9) strains were obtained from Dr. D. Schreffler, Department of Genetics, University of St. Louis, St. Louis, MO (*6*). (n = No. of generations of backcrossing to produce the congenic ines; F = No. of brother × sister crosses; for some strains complete records were not available). Skin grafts were performed by grafting tail skin on to the dorsum and were considered to be rejected when all epithelium had disappeared. Immunizations were performed by injecting mice with approximately 10^7 spleen and lymph node cells i.p. weekly for 10–15 weeks. Female mice were used for all experiments.

Ly-1. It has previously been reported (*1*) that skin graft rejection occurred in congenic mice differing at the *Ly-1* locus because of the *H(Ly-1)* locus incompatibility, which was considered to have segregated with the *Ly-1* locus during the production of the congenic strain. These studies were performed using the Boyse congenic strain (B6-Lyt-1.1/Boy = B6-*Ly-1*^{a}), and the studies herein were performed using both this subline and that produced by Cherry (B6-*Ly-1*^{a}/Cy). It should be noted that the C57BL/6 strain used in both sets of experiments reported herein was C57BL/6By, rather than C57BL/6Boy or Cy, but this does not appear to have affected the results.

The *H(Ly-1)* locus could not be detected when skin grafts were exchanged between C57BL/6 and B6-*Ly-1*^{a}/Cy in either direction (Table 1), using naive or hyperimmune (expts. 1 and 5) mice and periods of observation of >100 days. The use of F_1 hybrid recipient mice, such as (C57BL/6×BALB/c)F_1 or (B6-*Ly-1*^{a}×C3H)F_1, to overcome any "*Ir* gene" effects in the response of the homozygotes also made no difference when the Cherry subline was used (expts. 2 and 6) (Table 1). When the Boyse subline was used, naive mice did not reject their grafts, whereas hyperimmune mice mostly rejected their grafts in 20–30 days (expts. 3 and 7). Graft rejection was also apparent using hyperimmune F_1 hybrid recipient mice, especially when (C57BL/6×BALB/c)F_1 mice received B6-Ly-1^a/Boy skin grafts (expt. 4). By contrast, when (B6-*Ly-1*^{a}/Boy×C3H)F_1 hyperimmune mice (expt. 8) received C57BL/6 grafts, no rejection occurred. This is difficult to explain, as the *Ly-1*^{a} allele in the congenic strain was also derived from C3H. Presumably nonresponder *Ir* gene alleles were introduced into this F_1 hybrid by the use of the C3H strain.

In toto then, the results demonstrate that there was no *H* difference (for skin grafts) associated with the *Ly-1* locus when the Cherry subline was used, but that it was present in studies involving the Boyse subline. It was clear that the Boyse strain carried an additional *H* locus—either linked to *Ly-1* or present as a "passenger" locus. This was confirmed by the final study in which B6-*Ly-1*^{a}/Cy grafts were not rejected by B6-Ly-1^a (expt. 9), whereas the *H* gene was revealed by grafting in the reciprocal direction (expt. 10)—but, again, only in hyperimmune mice. The results demonstrate that there is no histocompatibility conferred in skin grafts by an *Ly-1* incompatibility, and that the Boyse subline carries an H locus not present in the Cherry sub-line or in C57BL/6, although whether this locus was linked to *Ly-1* was not determined.

Ly-2. Grafts exchanged between C57BL/6 and the Ly-2/Cy congenic strains were not rejected when performed in either direction, using naive or hyperimmune mice or when F_1 recipient hybrids were used (expts. 11, 12, 15 and 16). Thus, there is no *H* locus difference between these strains, and the *H-Ly-2* locus could not be identified. When the Boyse *Ly-2* strains were used, there was no rejection in naive mice in grafts exchanged in either direction (expts. 13 and 17) but hyperimmune mice rejected their grafts, some quite rapidly (expts. 13

TABLE 1. Graft rejection in Ly-1 and Ly-2 congenic strains

Expt.	Donor → recipient	Median survival time of grafts in (days ± SE [No. Reject./total No.]) First set	Immunized
Ly-1.1:			
1	B6-*Ly-1*^{a}/Cy→B6	NR[a]	NR
2	B6-*Ly-1*^{a}/Cy→(B6×BALB/c)F_1	NR	NR
3	B6-*Ly-1*^{a}/Boy→B6	NR	21.6±3.8 (8/8)
4	B6-*Ly-1*^{a}/Boy→(B6×BALB/C)F_1	NR	24.7±5.2 (3/7)
Ly-1.2:			
5	B6→B6-*Ly-1*^{a}/Cy	NR	NR
6	B6→(B6-*Ly-1*^{a}/Cy×C3H)F_1	NR	NR
7	B6→B6-*Ly-1*^{a}/Boy	NR	28.7±5.2 (4/7)
8	B6→(B6-*Ly-1*^{a}/Boy×C3H)F_1		NRNR
9	B6-Ly-1a/Cy→B6-Ly-1^a/Cy	NR	NR
10	B6-Ly-1a/Boy→B6-Ly-1a/Cy	NR	39.6±7.8 (14/15)
Ly-2.1:			
11	B6.PL(75NS)/Cy→B6	NR	NR
12	B6.PL(75NS)/Cy→(B6×BALB/c)F_1	NR	NR
13	B6-*Ly-2*^{a}/Boy→B6	NR	21.7±4.2 (8/10)
14	B6-*Ly-2*^{a}/Boy→(B6×BALB/c)F_1	51.2±8.7 (3/7)	24.1±4.3 (9/12)
Ly-2.2:			
15	B6→B10.PL(75NS)Cy	NR	NR
16	B6→(B6.PL(75NS)Cy×C3H)F_1	NR	NR
17	B6→B6-*Ly-2*^{a}/Boy	NR	14.7±1.6 (11/11)
18	B6→(B6-*Ly-2*^{a}×C3H)F_1	NR	12.8±2.8 (7/8)
19	B6.PL(75NS)Cy→B6-Ly-2^a Boy	NR	13.8±2.1 (7/7)
20	B6-Ly-2^a/Boy→B6.PL(75NS)Cy	NR	21.7±3.7 (8/8)
21	B6.PL(75NS)/Cy→B6-Ly-2^a-3^a/Boy	NR	NR
22	B6-Ly-2^a-3^a→B6.PL(75NS)Cy	NR	22.7±2.9 (5/7)

[a] (NR) not rejected.

and 17). When F_1 hybrid recipients were used, graft rejection occurred in a proportion of naive or hyperimmune recipients (expts. 14 and 18) but nonimmune (B6-Ly-2^a/Boy×C3H)F_1 mice did not reject C57BL/6 grafts (expt. 18). The two *Ly-2* congenic strains therefore differed—one being associated with an *H* locus different from that of C57BL/6 and B6.PL(75NS). This was confirmed by the reciprocal rejection noted when hyperimmune *Ly-2* congenic mice of one *Ly-2* congenic strain rejected grafts from the other strain (expts. 19 and 20). When a different Boyse *Ly-2* congenic line was used (B6-Ly-2^a, 3_a) there was no rejection of B6.PL(75NS) grafts by naive or immune mice (expt. 21), but in the reciprocal direction hyperimmune mice rapidly rejected their grafts (expt. 22). As in the *Ly-1* locus, it can be concluded that there is an *H* locus associated with—but distinct from—*Ly-2* in the Boyse strains; this *H* locus cannot be identified in the Cherry subline.

Ly-4. The *Ly-4* locus is closely linked (and possibly identical with) the H-3 locus (*7*), and it was therefore not surprising that graft rejection occurred between *Ly-4* congenic strains (Table 2) in 20–40 days (expts. 23 and 24). The contribution of *Ly-4* to this is impossible to assess as the relationship of these two loci is not clear, and the presence of Ly-4.1 or Ly-4.2 specificities on epidermal cells has not been examined. However, as stated previously (*7*), Ly-4.2 antibody is not produced when graft rejection occurs between H-3/Ly-4-incompatible strains or when (BALB/c×SWR)F_1 mice reject B10.D2 grafts. (This is the combination used for producing Ly-4.2 antibody.) In addition, the use of anti-Ly-4.2 antibody, passively, administered in an attempt to enhance skin grafts in this combination, was without effect. The *Ly-4* locus is therefore one example of the close linkage of an *H* locus and *Ly* locus that leads to the rejection of skin grafts.

Ly-6. Grafts exchanged between *Ly-6* congenic mice were not rejected, whether donors were naive or hyperimmune, or when appropriate F_1 hybrid mice were used, and when both alleles of *Ly-6* were examined (Table 2, expts. 25–27). Thus, in the C3H mice congenic for *Ly-6*, there is no *H* locus associated with the *Ly-6* locus. By contrast, a recent report (*8*) has indicated the presence of an *H* locus difference between BALB/c and BALB.DAG—a strain congenic for *Ly-6.2* (DAG) on a BALB/c background. The discussion for the *Ly-1* and *Ly-2* loci could also apply here, and could indicate a locus closely linked to, but separated from, *Ly-6* that is present in the BALB/c congenic line but absent from the C3H.B6 line. Alternatively, this locus could be present as a nonlinked passenger locus in the BALB/c strain. In addition, C57BL/6 and C3H could well have the same allele at the "*H(Ly-6)*" locus, in which case rejection would not occur. Provided that the genetic background has no influence on the results, then it is clear that *Ly-6* is not present as an H antigen for skin grafts. However in some strains these can have an associated *H* locus.

Thy-1. Earlier studies demonstrated an *H* locus associated with or identical to the *Thy-1* locus, as grafts were rejected in *Thy-1* congenic strains, anti-Thy-1 antibodies were produced, and the Thy-1 antigen was demonstrated to be present on epithelial cells (*23*). Several new *Thy-1* congenic strains were examined: A.AL-*Thy-1^a*, A.AL-*Thy-1^b* grafts were not rejected by naive mice, whereas rejection occurred in hyperimmune mice (expts. 28 and 31). Also (A.AL-*Thy-1^b*×B10.A)F_1 hybrid mice rejected their grafts when nonprimed, but not when hyperimmune (expt. 29)—a phenomenon previously noted (*9*) within the *Thy-1* locus. However (A.AL-*Thy-1^a*×RF)F_1 mice did not reject A.AL-*Thy-1^b* grafts whether naive or immune (expt. 32). The other *Thy-1* congenic strain, B6.PL(74NS)-*Thy-1^a*, was also examined where grafts with the Thy-1.1 specificity were not rejected (expt. 30), whereas rapid rejection occurred in the opposite direction (expt. 33). The studies clearly demonstrate the existence of an H(*Thy*) locus, with rejection occurring in both of these congenic *Thy-1* strains. As one of the components of the skin-epidermal cell is Thy-1^+, it is not unreasonable to consider that Thy-1^+ on these cells is the target for graft rejection, thus describing the H(*Thy*) locus (*4*). By contrast, epidermal cells are Ly-1^-, Ly-2^-, Ly-3^- (*4*), and when skin grafts are performed there is no product on skin to cause rejection.

Thus several quite different skin graft rejection responses

TABLE 2. Graft rejection in Ly-4, Ly-6, and Thy-1 congenic strains

Expt.	Donor→recipient	Median survival time of grafts (days ± SE [No. reject.)/total No.])	
		First Set	Immunized
Ly-4.2:			
23	C57BL/10→B10.C(28NX)	23.6±4.9 (10/10)	NT[b]
	→B10.LPa	21.4±5.3 (8/8)	NT
	→B10.C-H-3^c	24.6±4.6 (9/10)	NT
Ly-4.1:			
24	B6.C(28NX)→C57BL/10	43.4±8.7 (5/7)	NT
Ly-6.1:			
25	C3H→C3H.B6-Ly-6^b	NR[a]	NR
26	C3H→(C3H.B6-Ly-6^b×B6)F_1	NR	NR
Ly-6.2:			
27	C3H.B6-*Ly-6^b*→(C3H×BALB/c)F_1	NR	NR
Thy-1.1:			
28	A.AL-*Thy-1^a*→A.AL-*Thy-1^b*	NR	NT
29	A.AL-*Thy-1^a*→(A.AL-*Thy-1^b*×B10.A)F_1	35.2±4.3 (10/12)	NR
30	B6.PL(74NS)→B6	NR	NT
Thy-1.2:			
31	A.AL-*Thy-1^b*→A.AL-*Thy-1^a*	NR	33.1±4.6 (14/17)
32	A.AL-Thy-1^b→(A.AL-Thy-1a×RF)F_1	NR	NR
33	B6→B6.PL(74NS)	20.7±7.7 (5/10)	15.8±2.1 (8/8)

[a] (NR) not rejected.
[b] (NT) not tested.

were noted, not for differences emanating from the *Ly-1, 2, 6* loci when the Cherry strains were used—but the H(*Ly-1*) and H(*Ly-2*) loci were again identified in the Boyse strains. It is clear that none of these three loci code for alloantigens present on skin, but they are associated with an *H* locus, which is not surprising because of the large number and ubiquitous distribution of these loci. By contrast, the *Ly-4* and *Thy-1* loci are either closely associated with H loci or are in fact H loci themselves. There is, therefore, not a prior reason for *H* loci—detected by skin grafting—to be necessarily associated with lymphocyte alloantigens. It should be noted that while *H* genes traditionally refer to the rejection of skin grafts, this definition is unnecessarily restrictive, and we would expect graft rejection to occur at differences arising from incompatibilities at the *Ly-1, 2,* and *6* loci if lymphoid tissues were used, rather than skin grafts.

Margaret M. Henning
Ian F. C. McKenzie
Research Centre for Cancer and Transplantation
Department of Pathology
The University of Melbourne
Parkville, Victoria 3052, Australia

REFERENCES

1. Flaherty L, Bennett D. Histocompatibilities found between congenic strains which differ at loci determining differentiation antigens. Transplantation 1973; 16: 505.
2. John M, Carswell E, Boyse EA, Alexander G. Production of ϕ antibody by mice that fail to reject θ: incompatible skin grafts. Nature 1972; 238: 57.
3. Staines NA, O'Neill GJ. Comparative immunogenicity of Thy-1.1 and Thy-1.2 antigens. J Immunogenet 1975; 2: 223.
4. Scheid M, Boyse EA, Carswell EA, Old LJ. Serologically demonstratable alloantigens of mouse epidermal cells. J Exp Med 1972; 135: 938.
5. McKenzie IFC, Potter TA. Murine lymphocyte surface antigens. Adv Immunol 1979; 27: 178.
6. Klein J. List of congenic strains of mice I Lines with differences at alloantigenic loci. Transplantation 1973; 15: 137.
7. Potter TA, McKenzie IFC, Cherry MC. Murine Lymphocyte Alloantigens: the Ly-4 locus. J Immunogenet 1981; 8: 15.
8. Berumen L, Sachs JA, Festenstein H. DAG (Ly-6.2) effect on skin grafts, antibody and MLC utilising congenic BALB. DAG. Immunogenetics 1981; 12: 415.
9. Flaherty L, Bennett D. The unusual fate of second skin grafts across an H(T1a) barrier. Transplantation 1973; 16: 682.

Received 16 July 1985.
Accepted 12 December 1985.

PROLONGED SURVIVAL OF CYCLOSPORINE-TREATED ALLOGENEIC HEPATOCELLULAR IMPLANTS[1]

Models for the survival and eventual proliferation of syngeneic rat hepatocytes implanted into rat spleens are well established (*1, 2*), but little is known about the survival of allogeneic cells. There has been one report of rapid rejection of F344 ($RT1^l$) rat hepatocytes when implanted into Lewis ($RT1^l$) and WKA ($RT1^k$) rat spleens—rejection occurring by day 4 and within 24 hr, respectively (*3*). In this communication we confirm rapid rejection of DA ($RT1^a$) hepatocytes from August ($RT1^c$) spleens, and present evidence that oral cyclosporine prevents this.

Male inbred August and DA rats were used throughout the experiments and kept under standard laboratory conditions. Hepatocytes were isolated by a two-step, noncirculating, collagenase perfusion procedure modified from Seglen (*4*), using 0.025% collagenase (s.a. 0.15 U/mg). Dispersed cells were purified by differential centrifugation, and the hepatocytes implanted directly into the splenic tissue of recipients. The spleen was exposed by a small left subcostal incision and 0.2 ml cell suspension, containing 2×10^6 viable hepatocytes, injected directly into the inferior end of the spleen, through a 25-gauge needle. Temporary hemostasis was achieved by clamping the vessels at the splenic hilus, and a catgut ligature prevented leakage from the injection site. Duplicate 5-μm-thick, transverse cryostat sections were cut at 800-μm intervals through the implanted spleen and stained for the presence of hepatocytes using haematoxylin and eosin and indirect immunofluorescence with a polyclonal rabbit antibody raised against a rat liver cell membrane preparation and fluorescein-isothiocyanate-labeled sheep antirabbit immunoglobulin.

In preliminary experiments, the survival pattern of DA ($RT1^a$) hepatocytes implanted into unprotected August ($RT1^c$) recipients was determined. Liver cells were found in the spleens of all 7 animals sacrificed 24 h after implantation. By 4 days, hepatocytes could only be positively identified in 1 of 8 spleens tested; and no surviving allogeneic cells could be found within longer-term spleens—a further 21 implants of up to 1 month's duration being tested. The effect of cyclosporine treatment on this survival pattern was then investigated.

From day −2, 6 August rats were given cyclosporine (Sandoz, Basel, Switzerland) at 25 mg/kg, daily, by gavage. The drug was diluted to 10 mg/ml in olive oil, and 6 control animals received the appropriate volume of olive oil alone. On day 0, each rat was implanted with 2×10^6 DA hepatocytes. Cyclosporine (or olive oil) continued to be administered daily until the animals were sacrificed—3 test and 3 control on days 4 and 14 after transplantation.

Unprotected animals. No surviving hepatocytes were found in any of the control grafts at 4 or 14 days. Splenic tissue surrounding the implant site was necrotic and associated with extensive polymorphonuclear leucocyte infiltration extending well into the splenic pulp (Fig. 1).

Cyclosporine-treated animals. Hepatocytes were positively identified in all cyclosporine spleens. There was minimal necrosis associated with the area of implantation at 4 days, largely resolved in the 14 day implants. The number of surviving cells seen in each spleen varied widely, with a general impression of fewer hepatocytes at 14 days than at 4. The liver cells were found scattered over a small region of splenic red pulp, rarely in groups of more than two or three, except where trapped in trabeculae, or in close proximity to some other morphological feature (Fig. 2).

A long-term rejection study is currently underway, and DA hepatocytes have now been positively identified in the spleens of chronically dosed, cyclosporine-treated August recipients 28 days after implantation.

The rapid rejection of hepatocytes from the splenic pulp—completed by 4 days in the DA($RT1^a$) to August ($RT1^c$) com-

[1] This work was supported by a grant from the Medical Research Council.

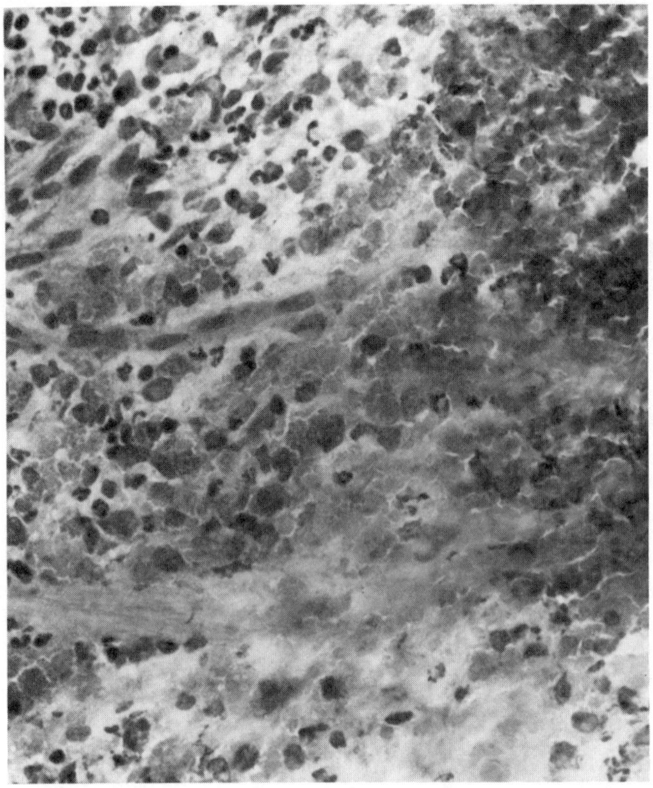

FIGURE 1. Unprotected August rat spleen, 4 days after implantation of 2×10^6 DA rat hepatocytes. The liver cells have been rejected and the implant area has become necrotic and infiltrated by cells (H&E; ×150).

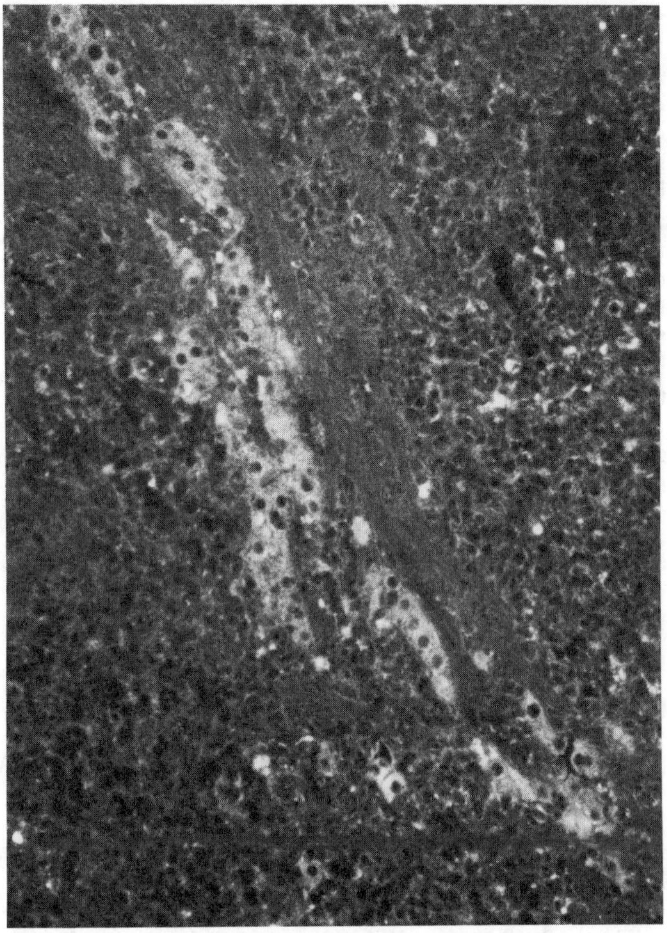

FIGURE 2. Cyclosporine-treated August rat spleen, 14 days after implantation of 2×10^6 DA rat hepatocytes. (cyclosporine at 25 mm/kg daily from day −2). Groups of hepatocytes lie up against trabeculae traversing the red pulp (immunofluorescent labelling; ×100).

bination used here, and occurring within 24 h in the markedly incompatible F344($RT1^l$) to WKA($RT1^k$) strain combination used by Ebata et al. (3)—presumably reflects an immunologically mediated process based on histocompatibility differences. Ebata et al. suggest a dominant role for humoral immunity in this rejection process, on the evidence of a lack of lymphoid cell infiltration within the graft. The rapidity of the rejection process however, argues against this, and in our experiments the grafted cells were surrounded by a pleomorphic cell infiltrate. There was a prominent polymorphonuclear leukocyte presence, but the contribution of lymphocytic cells to the process was difficult to assess, as such cells are present within the normal spleen. We are currently undertaking further experiments to define the contribution of different types of cell-mediated immunity to the rejection process. Natural killer cell cytotoxicity is a rapidly occurring process—but, at least by analogy with allogeneic lymphocyte cytotoxicity, is not affected in rats by cyclosporine at doses similar to those used here (*5*). T-cell-mediated rejection seems likely, although experiments on rat pancreatic islet cell transplantation—in which macrophage-mediated rejection was suggested in a system inhibitable by cyclosporine—indicate that this possibility should also be explored (*6*).

Acknowledgment. Dr. J. F. Borel of Sandoz Products Limited, Basel, Switzerland, kindly donated the cyclosporine used in this study.

HELEN DARBY
CLARE SELDEN
HUMPHREY J. HODGSON[2]

Department of Medicine
Royal Postgraduate Medical School
Hammersmith Hospital
London W12 OHS

[2] Address reprint requests and correspondence to: H. J. F. Hodgson, M.D., Department of Medicine, Royal Postgraduate Medical School, London W12 OHS.

REFERENCES

1. Woods RJ, Fuller BJ, Attenburrow VD, Nutt LH, Hobbs KEF. Functional assessment of hepatocytes after transplantation into rat spleen. Transplantation 1982; 33: 123.
2. Darby H, Johnstone R, Gupta S, Selden C, Hodgson HJ. Hepatocyte survival after implantation into the splenic pulp of syngeneic rats. Clin Sci 1985; 68(suppl II): 65p.
3. Ebata H, Oikawa I, Mito M. Rejection of allogeneic hepatocytes and fetal hepatic tissue transplanted into rat spleen. Transplantation 1985; 39: 221.
4. Seglen PO. Preparation of isolated rat liver cells. Methods Cell Biol 1976; 13: 29.
5. Heslop BF, McNeilage LJ, Sengupta S. Allogeneic lymphocyte cytotoxicity in rats: the effects of various pharmacological agents. Immunology 1984; 53: 43.
6. Bell PRF, Wood REM, Peters M, Nash JR. Comparison of various methods of chemical immunosuppression in islet cell transplantation. Transplant Proc 1980; 12: 291.

Received 29 October 1985.
Accepted 21 November 1985.

PANCREATICODUODENAL TRANSPLANTATION IN THE RAT

A Technique Update[1]

Pancreas transplantation is rapidly becoming accepted as a viable treatment in diabetic patients who have developed, or are at risk of developing, the potentially fatal complications of diabetes mellitus. Although pancreatic transplantations are being performed at many major centers throughout the world, the overall one-year graft survival rate is still only around 25%. The problem is essentially two-fold: graft failure due to rejection, and graft malfunction secondary to technical problems. In order to address these and other problems, it is necessary to return to the laboratory and assess the situation in a tried and tested animal model.

In our laboratory we have used microsurgical techniques to perform over one thousand pancreas transplants in the rat. In freshly alloxan-induced diabetic rats receiving a syngeneic transplant, our operative mortality is low, and our one-year graft survival rate is over 60%. In allografted animals, the one-year survival is lower, primarily due to the side effects of our present long-term immunosuppressive regimen. Although we have performed a large number of duct-ligated pancreas transplants, the majority of our work has been with pancreaticoduodenal grafts, as we think that this is the model that most closely resembles the present clinical situation—namely, whole organ grafts with enteric conduit drainage of the exocrine secretions of the gland. We present here our current technique with the refinements that have been developed through the experience of the senior author since the method was first described (*1*). This model is a well-tried and proved preparation for studies in pancreatic transplantation, a fact that is borne out by the number of investigators who have used this technique in their studies (*2–6*).

Anesthesia. There are a large number of short-acting anesthetic agents available, but in our laboratory we prefer ether inhalation, as it is easily controlled and quickly reversible.

Donor operation. The so-called no touch technique must be exercised throughout the entire transplant operation, but particularly harvesting the donor pancreas (Fig. 2a).

The abdomen is entered via a midline incision and the intestines are retracted to the left of the rat. The duodenum is gently picked up with non-toothed thumb forceps; the ligament of Trietz is cut, and the duodenum is freed from the ascending colon; this latter stage is achieved by holding the colon in a rubber-shod clamp while the duodenum is picked up with thumb forceps, and the fibrous band between the two structures is divided along the colon—thus freeing the ventral surface of the pancreas from the colon. The right and middle colic vessels are divided between ligatures at this time. The stomach is now reflected up onto the chest wall and held in place with a curved hemostat, and the intestines are transferred to the right side of the rat.

The aorta at the level of the celiac and superior mesenteric arteries is carefully dissected free from the surrounding structures, and the left adrenal vessels are ligated close to the aorta and cut. The lumbar branches of the aorta (usually one or two pairs) are ligated and divided, freeing the aorta from the underlying structures. The superior branch of the splenic artery and the left gastric artery are ligated together and cut distally. Splenectomy is then performed following placement of serial ligatures on the vessels at the splenic hilum.

At this time the border between the omental fat and pancreas should be identified, and the small vessels running between these two structures must be ligated and divided. This procedure continues along the greater curvature of the stomach until the region of the pylorus is reached, where a heavy tie is placed around the pyloric ring and the stomach is divided proximally. (After division of the esophagus, the stomach can be discarded.) The bile duct and hepatic artery should now be identified in the porta hepatis, where they are ligated and divided.

The intestines are once more retracted to the left of the rat and the right renal artery (which arises laterally from the aorta at the level of the superior mesenteric artery) is ligated and divided. The mesenteric vein (portal vein) is now ligated and divided at the distal margin of the pancreas.

A loose ligature is placed around the aorta just below the superior mesenteric artery and a clamp is applied to the aorta 1 cm above the celiac axis. A fine needle is introduced into the aorta distal to the ligature and the graft is perfused until bloodless with 3–4 ml of cold (7°C) saline. Following withdrawal of the needle, the ligature is pulled tight and an aortic segment is obtained by cutting below the clamp and ligature. The duodenum is divided at the obvious vascular demarcation line. The portal vein is cut at the liver hilum in an oblique fashion, leaving a small piece of liver on the right corner of the vein. (This helps later to find the portal vein and ensure correct orientation of the venous anastomosis.) The graft can now be lifted from the animal and placed in cold saline.

Recipient operation. After entering the abdomen via a midline incision, the intestine are retracted to the left of the rat and the aorta and inferior vena cava (IVC)* are dissected free from each other (Fig. 2b). If the gonadal vessels arise in a position that could ultimately jeopardize the graft anastomosis, they should be ligated and divided.

The infrarenal aorta and IVC are clamped together, and a venotomy is made at the 7–11 o'clock position. An elliptical excision is made in the anterior wall of the aorta and the openings are flushed with saline to remove fibrinous clots. The graft is taken from the cold saline and laid in the recipient rat's right flank with the head of the pancreas in the inferior position. The size of the aortic opening is adjusted according to the diameter of the donor aorta. (The aortotomy should be slightly larger than the diameter of the donor aorta.) An end-to-side aortoaortic anastomosis is fashioned, using a continuous suture technique with 9–0 or 10–0 sutures. After suturing the anterior edges of the two aorts, the graft is reflected to the left of the rat, thus enabling completion of the posterior wall. The size of the IVC venotomy is tailored to the diameter of the portal vein. Following correct orientation of the portal vein, the small piece of liver is removed; if the septum still exists between the two branches of the portal vein it is divided, thus making a larger portal vein opening (Fig. 1). Following placement of two stay sutures, the venous anastomosis is performed without moving the graft from the left side—the posterior wall being anastomosed from the inside of the vessels and the anterior wall being closed classically.

[1] This is publication No. 4181 IMM from the Research Institute of Scripps Clinic, La Jolla, California. The work was supported by NIH Grant AM 33125.

* Abbreviation used: IVC, inferior vena cava.

Following completion of the vascular anastomosis, the graft is replaced in the right flank, the anastomotic lines are checked (under high power) for gaps or tears, and the clamp is released. The clamp should be released slowly while two small gauze pads are placed over the anastomoses. The pads should be left in place for approximately 3 min. If, however, the gauze becomes soaked with blood within the first minute, the clamp should be reapplied and the bleeding points located. After successful anastomosis, the duodenum and pancreas should have returned to their normal pink color, and the mesenteric vessels should be pulsating (Fig. 2).

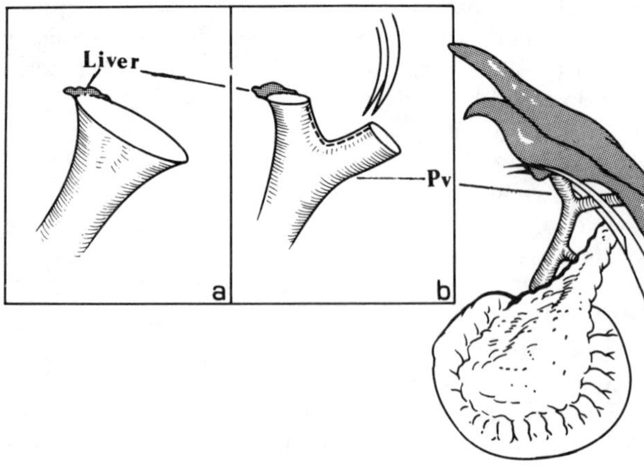

FIGURE 1. Preparation of the portal vein. (a) Final product with small piece of liver attached to aid orientation and identification. (b) Division of the septum between right and left branches. (c) Division of the vein high in the liver hilum.

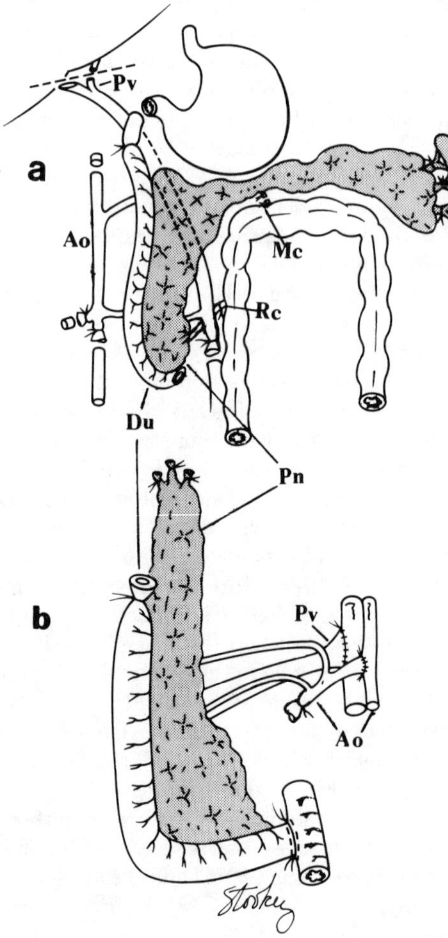

FIGURE 2. Schematic plan of donor harvest (a) and pancreaticoduodenal transplantation (b).

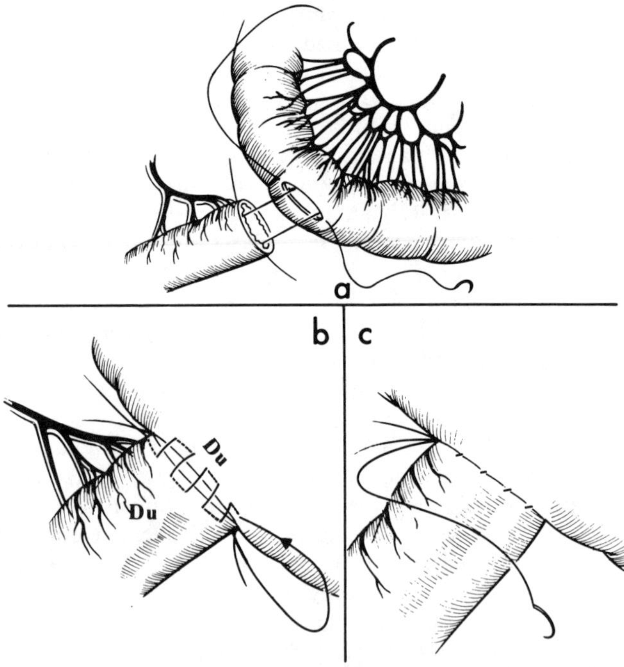

FIGURE 3. End-to-side duodenoduodenostomy, using a modified Connell suture.

An end-to-side duodenoduodenostomy is now performed using a Connell-type technique with 7–0 silk (Fig. 3). When there is perfect hemostasis, an i.v. injection of saline (3–5 ml) is made via the dorsal vein of the penis. This helps combat postoperative shock. The intestines are placed back into the abdomen and the wound is closed with a 3–0 silk continuous suture.

Graft failure due to technical problems is a frustrating and annoying occurrence—and, unfortunately, it is a common occurrence, even in the hands of people experienced in microsurgical techniques. Our experience has shown us that there are a number of points, if adhered to, that will decrease the incidence of this problem.

1. It is essential that the pancreas itself is not directly manipulated, as the ensuing trauma results in pancreatitis and subsequent graft failure. A "no-touch" technique must be used. This is achieved by using the duodenum to pick up the graft and by leaving ligatures long, thus enabling them to be used as "pancreatic retractors" when the gland needs repositioning.

2. When performing the splenectomy, or separating pancreas from stomach and omentum, pancreatic tissue must not be included in any ligatures.

3. All small vessels on and around the pancreas (particularly those between pancreas and omentum) must be ligated meticulously; pancreatic hematomas are common sequelae if this is not done, and graft failure will follow.

4. The portal vein outlet must be adequate to prevent graft congestion. As mentioned in the operative technique, this can be achieved by cutting the portal vein beyond its bifurcation, and then dividing the septum (Fig. 1). Graft congestion can also be prevented by ensuring correct orientation of the portal vein by means of leaving a piece of liver on one edge of the vein.

5. Postoperative care of the rat is very important. The rat should be kept warm until fully awake, and postoperative shock can be avoided by giving an i.v. injection of saline at the end of the procedure.

6. Above all, during the operation extreme care must be taken with all tissues; in particular, hemorrhage should be kept to a minimum, as there is a direct correlation between lack of blood loss and survival.

This model of pancreatic transplantation is well tried and tested, and if the pitfalls outlined are scrupulously avoided the success rate of the technique is very high, making it ideal for studies designed to assess the problems of clinical pancreatic transplantation.

SUN LEE
MICHAEL SCOTT
ARTHUR R. DEMACEDO
Department of Immunology
Scripps Clinic and Research Foundation
La Jolla, California 92037
Department of Surgery
University of California
San Diego, California 92103

REFERENCES

1. Lee S, Tung KSK, Koopmans H, Chandler JG, Orloff MJ. Pancreatico-duodenal transplantation in the rat. Transplantation 1972; 13: 421.
2. Bell RH, Fernandez-Cruz L, Brimm J, Sayers HA, Lee S, Orloff MJ. Prevention by whole pancreas transplantation of glomerular basement membrane thickening in alloxan diabetes. Surgery 1980; 88: 31.
3. Hirose K, Osterby R, Nozawa M, Gundersen HJG. Development of glomerular lesions in experimental long-term diabetes in the rat. Kidney Int 1982; 21: 689.
4. Brekke IB, Schmidt E, Schmidt FW. Effect of pancreas transplantation on liver carbohydrate metabolism. J Clin Chem Clin Biochem 1982; 20: 81.
5. Orloff MJ, Lee S, Carters AC, Grambort DE, Storck LG, Knox D. Long term studies of pancreas transplantation in experimental diabetes mellitus. Ann Surg 1975; 182: 198.
6. Weil R, Nozawa M, Koss M, et al. Effect of pancreas transplantation on diabetic nephropathy in rats. Surg Forum 1974; 25: 386.

Received 13 November 1985.
Accepted 20 December 1985.

A TECHNIQUE FOR HEART-LUNG TRANSPLANTATION IN MICE[1]

Fulmer and colleagues (*1*) first observed that neonatal or fetal mouse hearts implanted s.c. into the mouse ear survived and pulsated continuously. Jirsch et al. (*2*) and Judd et al. (*3, 4*) have extensively studied rejection and tolerance of mouse heart allografts using Fulmer's transplantation technique. This unique mouse heart implantation technique is so simple to perform that even those who are not microsurgeons can perform it without difficulty.

Revascularized heterotopic mouse heart transplantation was reported in 1973 by Corry and associates (*5*); this operation was modified from the technique of rat heart transplantation described by Abbott et al. (*6*), Ono et al. (*7*), and Tomita (*8*). It is so complicated and difficult to perform that this operative technique has never been as popular as Abbott's. Recently, Blanchard and Pollak (*9*) have shown some improvement in the survival of mouse heart grafts using a modified revascularization technique; the number of anastomoses of major blood vessels is the same as that used by Corry et al. (*5*). In order to master this transplantation skill, one needs extensive microvascular surgical training. The purpose of this communication is to introduce a simpler technique of transplanting the mouse heart so that someone who can perform rat heart transplants could also master the operating technique in the mouse. Using a modified Fox-Montorsi (*10*) technique, we were able to transplant rat heart-lung by aortoaortic anastomosis alone (*11*). This technique has been extended to mouse heart-lung transplantation to investigate the mode of rejection of these organs and the technique is described.

It is essential to have the proper microsurgical instruments to pursue this technique: a modified Castroviejo needle holder (narrow jaw), curved and straight jeweler's forceps, iris scissors, straight iris forceps, a modified posterior capsulotomy cystitome (Sharpoint, Reading, PA) a miniature Satinsky clamp, 10–0 microsutures, a 2-ml syringe with 27-gauge and 30-gauge needles. Ligatures (6–0) and routine instruments for thoracotomy and laparotomy are also needed, and all surgical maneuvers are made under a 10–16× magnification. A clean technique is used throughout the procedure.

Under ether anesthesia, the donor animal is placed on its back, a bilateral subcostal incision is made by cutting through the diaphragm, and a bilateral axillary line incision is made to lift up the thoracic cage. At this time the internal mammary vessels are not damaged, and no major bleeding is encountered. The thymus is gently dissected from the major blood vessels and the right superior vena cava (SVC)* is ligated close to the heart. The aorta is dissected free from underlying structures and cut at the innominate artery, and the SVC is cut above the ligature. The left SVC and azygos vein are ligated and cut distally. Perfusion of the heart-lung is made by injecting 1–1½ ml of cold saline (7°C) via the inferior vena cava (IVC) rather slowly so that the heart will pulsate and expel all bloody perfusate through the aorta. It is also essential to perfuse slowly so that no pulmonary edema occurs. A ligature is placed around the hilum of the left upper lung lobe and the lobe is resected. The trachea is cut at the aortic arch level and peeled downward from the esophagus, and the IVC is cut below the tie. The heart-lung is placed in saline.

Under ether anesthesia, the recipient is prepared surgically and placed on its back, and a midline incision is made, avoiding any epigastric vessels and tributary bleeding. The intestines are retracted to the left (they may be exteriorized) and the aorta above the iliac bifurcation is cleaned. There is no need for separation of the aorta and IVC, and no need for sacrificing any lumbar branches. With the straight iris forceps, the aorta is picked up and clamped with the Satinsky clamp longitudinally. During this maneuver, the IVC contents are milked away from the aorta so that the anastomosis is easier for the operator. Using the cystitome (modified), an aortotomy is done on the aorta and flushed with saline. At this time the graft trachea is cut at the bronchial bifurcation. The bronchi are also cut longitudinally to promote bronchoalveolar secretions into the abdominal cavity after the transplantation. The heart-lung is placed in the right lower quadrant of the abdomen. The graft's aorta is flushed with saline, and an end-to-side aortoaortic anastomosis is performed using a continuous suture technique with 10–0 suture. Four stitches are usually needed on each side,

[1] This is publication No. 4165 IMM from the Research Institute of Scripps Clinic, La Jolla, California.

* Abbreviations used: IVC, inferior vena cava; SVC, superior vena cava.

in addition to the stay sutures. The suture lines are gently pressed with a cotton swab and the clamp is released. The heart will begin to turn pink and to pulsate. A fluid supplement of 0.25 ml of 5% dextrose/saline is given through the tail vein or through the jugular vein. The amount may be increased if fluid loss is detected. At this time atrial dilatation may occur, in which case the dilated atrium is squeezed using two cotton swabs to promote the heartbeat. When there is evidence of regular heartbeat, all lung lobes except the right upper lobe may be resected after the ligation of each hilum. One lung lobe may function as a reservoir. The abdomen is closed with 4–0 suture, and the animal is kept warm for at least 2 hr.

It is anticipated that the blood entering through the aorta during the diastolic phase of the graft will pass through the coronary arteries, then the coronary sinus, right ventricle, pulmonary circulation, left atrium, and left ventricle in that order—then it will finally enter the graft's aorta to recipient's aorta at the systolic phase of the graft's heartbeat. The initial mortality is high because of the animal's size and total blood volume.

Sun Lee
Diane Yancey
Department of Immunology
Research Institute of Scripps Clinic
La Jolla, California 92037

REFERENCES

1. Fulmer RI, Carmer AT, Liebelt RA, Liebelt AG. Transplantation of cardiac tissue into mouse heart. Am J Anat 1963; 113: 273.
2. Jirsch DW, Kraft N. Cellular immunity in vitro and heterotopic transplantation of the mouse heart. Transplantation 1972; 14: 395.
3. Judd KP, Allen CT Jr, Guiberteau MJ, Trentin JJ: Prolongation of murine cardiac allografts with antilymphocytic serum. Transplant Proc 1969; 1: 470.
4. Judd KP, Trentin JJ. Cardiac transplantation in mice. V. Prolongation of allografts with cell-free extracts and antilymphocytic globulin. Transplantation 1973; 16: 351.
5. Corry RJ, Winn H, Russell PS. Primary vascularized allografts of heart in mice. Transplantation 1973; 16: 343.
6. Abbott CP, Lindsey ES, Creech O Jr, DeWitt CW. A technique for heart transplantation in the rat. Arch Surg 1964; 89: 645.
7. Ono K, Lindsey ES, Creech O. Transplanted rat heart. Local graft irradiation. Transplantation 1969; 7: 176.
8. Tomita F. Heart transplantation in the rat. Sapporo Med 1966; 30: 165.
9. Blanchard JM, Pollack R. Techniques for perfusion and storage of heterotopic heart transplantation in mice. Microsurg 1985; 6: 169.
10. Fox U, Montorsi M. A technical modification of heart-lung transplantation in rats. J Microsurg 1980; 1: 377.
11. Lee S, Lee D, Curtis GP, Orloff MJ. A simplified heterotopic rat heart transplantation. J Microsurg 1981; 2: 294.

Received 1 November 1985.
Accepted 17 December 1985.

CUFF TECHNIQUE FOR ORTHOTOPIC LIVER TRANSPLANTATION IN THE RAT

A Simplified Method For The Suprahepatic Vena Cava Anastomosis

The liver has a privileged status with regard to allograft rejection. In several species—including the pig (*1*), the monkey (*2*), and the rat (*3*)—it has been demonstrated that in contrast with other organ allografts (skin, kidney, or heart), liver allografts can survive indefinitely without immunosuppression. The main advantage in using rat for the study of liver allograft rejection is that several combinations of inbred rats are available in which genetic disparities are clearly defined and permit precise immunological studies. However, orthotopic liver transplantation in the rat involves a difficult and skillful surgical technique. The initial technique described by Lee et al. (*4, 5*) requires a long microsurgical training. The two anastomoses of the suprahepatic vena cava and the portal vein should be performed quickly in order to minimize warm ischemic damage to the liver and damage to the recipient. The application of the cuff technique for vascular anastomosis—as originally described by Payr (*6*) and more recently applied to orthotopic (*7, 8*), heterotopic (*9, 10*), liver, renal (*11*), and pancreas (*12*) transplantation in the rat—has simplified this problem. However, in the technique of Kamada et al. (*7*), only the portal anastomosis was performed using this technique. Miyata et al. (*8*) later described use of the cuff technique for the three vascular anastomoses. However the introduction of the cuff into the recipient's suprahepatic vena cava is difficult due to the short length of vena cava lying between the liver and the diaphragm. To overcome this problem, we have developed a technique in which the intrahepatic segment of the vena cava is approached by a partial hepatectomy, which renders the introduction of the suprahepatic vena cava cuff easier and safer.

Adult male Sprague Dawley rats were purchased from Charles River (France). The animals were anesthetized with ether, and the operation was performed under clean but nonsterile conditions. Harvesting, cooling, and introduction of the cuff in the three vessels (infrahepatic vena cava, suprahepatic vena cava, and portal vein) of the donor's liver was nearly identical to the technique described by Miyata et al. In the recipient, the abdomen was opened via a midline incision. After mobilization of the liver, the hepatic artery was doubly ligated and divided. The portal vein and the infrahepatic vena cava were crossclamped with a Satinski clamp. A partial hepatectomy removing the median lobe (*13*) was performed in order to approach the intra hepatic vena cava and to open it (Fig. 1). The donor's liver was then positioned orthotopically. The lumen of the vena cava was washed with Ringer's solution to prevent air embolism, and the cuff was placed into the recipient's intrahepatic vena cava (Fig. 2). The anastomosis was completed with a circular 7.0 silk ligature over the cuff. At this time, the recipient's liver was removed. Portal and infrahepatic vena cava anastomoses were performed according to the techniques described by Kamada (*7*) and Miyata (*8*). Biliary anastomosis was performed using a polyethylene tube introduced and secured in the two bile ducts and completed by an end-to-end continuous suture. During the operation, oxygen was administered via an intranasal catheter. An i.v. drip was established using the penile vein. Postoperatively, the animals were warmed under infrared lamps in their cages for 2–3 hr, and allowed normal food and water ad libitum. Up to the 3rd postoperative day, glucose was added to their water (100 g/L) and 2 mg of gentamicin was injected i.m. every day.

A total of 28 orthotopic liver grafts have been performed

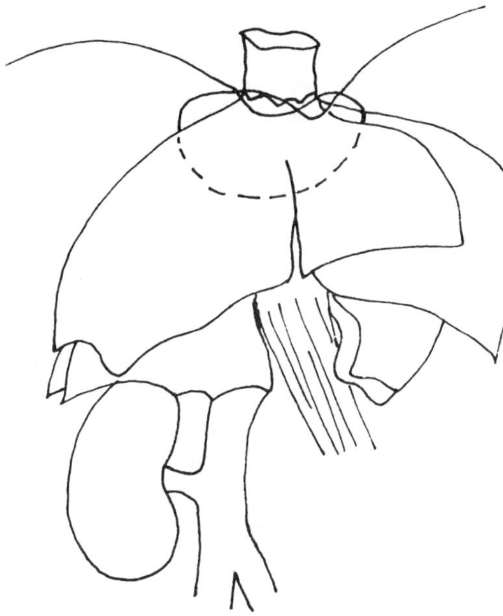

FIGURE 1. Resection of the median lobe of the recipient's liver.

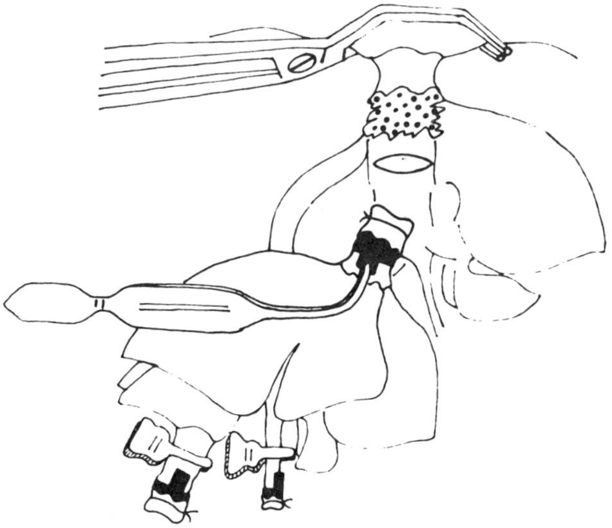

FIGURE 2. Introduction of the donor's suprahepatic vena cava cuff into the recipient's intrahepatic vena cava.

using the technique; 12 of them were performed to assess the technique. All the 16 grafts performed since the technique was established survived the operation. One animal died in the first postoperative day from disruption of the suprahepatic anastomosis. Four animals died at 6, 7, 22, and 25 days postoperatively from biliary leakage; this complication was later avoided by using a polyethylene tube introduced in the two biliary ducts. Eleven animals (70%) survived more than two months. The recipient operation usually lasted 60 min. The longest lasted 70 min and the shortest 45 min. Mean portal vein occlusion time was 11 min (8–15 min). Average time of cuff fixation on the vessels of the donor liver was 11 min (7–15 min). Mean vena cava occlusion time was 12 min, 30 sec. (10–16 minutes). The principal difficulty in liver transplantation in rats is to reduce the portal vein clamping time. Portal vein clamping time longer than 25 min is usually fatal. Using our technqiue, the portal vein clamping time is very short (11 min), comparing favorably with those reported by Kamada (16 min) and by Miyata (13.6 min).

The suprahepatic vena cava anastomosis is perhaps the most formidable technical challenge encountered in the course of a liver transplantation procedure in man (*14, 15*) and in large animals (*16*) because of the short length of the suprahepatic vena cava. In the rat, in which precise immunological studies can be performed, the cuff technique, by reducing clamping time, greatly improves survival figures. However the introduction of the cuff in the short suprahepatic vena cava of the recipient seemed somewhat difficult to us. The modification described has provided a reliable means for rapidly performing the suprahepatic vena cava anastomosis.

A. SETTAF
J. GUGENHEIM[1]
D. HOUSSIN
H. BISMUTH
Groupe de Recherche de Chirurgie Hépatique
Hôpital Paul Brousse
Villejuif, 94800 France

[1] Address requests for reprints to: J. Gugenheim, Groupe de Recherche de Chirurgie Hépatique, Hôpital Paul Brousse, 14 avenue Paul Vaillant Couturier, 94800 Villejuif, France.

REFERENCES

1. Cordier G, Garnier H, Clot JP, et al. Biologie expérimentale: greffe de foie chez le porc: approche chirurgicale. CR Acad Sci 1965; 260: 5621.
2. Calne RY, Davis DR, Pena JR, et al Hepatic allografts and xenografts in primates. Lancet 1970; 1: 103.
3. Houssin D, Charpentier B, Gugenheim J, et al. Spontaneous longterm acceptance of RT 1 incompatible liver allografts in inbred rats. Analysis of the immune status. Transplantation 1983; 36: 615.
4. Lee S, Charters AC, Chandler, JG. A technique for orthotopic liver transplantation in the rat. Transplantation 1973; 16: 664.
5. Lee S, Charters AC, Orloff RJ. Simplified technique for orthotopic liver transplantation in the rat. Am J Surg 1975; 30: 38.
6. Payr E. Beitrage zu technick der blutgefass und nervennhat nebst mittheilungen uber die Verwvendung eines resorbirbaren metalles in der chirurgie. Arch Klin Chir 1900; 62: 67.
7. Kamada N, Calne RY. Orthotopic liver transplantation in the rat: techique using cuff for portal vein anastomosis and biliary drainage. Transplantation 1979; 28: 47.
8. Miyata M, Fischer IM, Fuhs M, Irselhard W, Kassai Y. A simple method for orthotopic liver transplantation in the rat. Transplantation 1980; 30: 335.
9. Marni A, Ferrero ME. Heterotopic liver grafting in the rat. A simplified method using cuff techniques. Transplantation 1985; 39: 329.
10. Mulher GA. Simple method for heterotopic auxiliary liver transplantation in the rat. Transplantation 1983; 36: 221.
11. Kamada N. A description of cuff techniques for renal transplantation in the rat: use in studies of tolerance induction during combined liver grafting. Transplantation 1985; 39: 93.
12. Volan MS, Lindsey NS, Savas CP, Slater DN, Fox M. Pancreatic transplantation in the rat: a simplified method using aortic interposition and cuff technique. Transplantation 1982; 33: 327.
13. Lambert R. In: Surgery of digestive system in the rat. Springfield: 1965; 57.
14. Starzl TE, Koep LJ, Weil R III, Halgrimson CG. Development of a suprahepatic recipient vena cava cuff for liver transplantation. Surg Gynecol Obstet 1979; 149: 76.
15. Raju S, Didlake R. Suprahepatic vena cava cuff in liver transplantation. Transplantation 1984; 37: 110.
16. Woodle ES, Hunter GC, Ward RE. The diaphragmatic vena cava cuff in hepatic transplantation. Transplantation 1985; 39: 105.

Received 26 November 1985.
Accepted 17 December 1985.

DIARY OF FORTHCOMING EVENTS

Anyone organizing a meeting likely to be of interest to the readers of *Transplantation* may submit essential information about the meeting to any editorial office, which will consider its inclusion in the Diary of Events. This information should be received by the North American Editorial Office at least six months before the event. The Diary appears four times annually.

DATE	PLACE	SUBJECT	SECRETARIAT
1986			
November 2	Chicago, IL	AASLD Liver Transplantation Meeting	Louise Ince Charles Slack, Invc. 6900 Grove Rd. Thorofare, N.J. 08086
1987			
April 26–May 1	Keystone, CO	UCLA Symposium—The T Cell Receptor	UCLA Symposia Molecular Biology Inst. Univ. of California Los Angeles, CA 90024
June 11–13	Gothenburg, Sweden	3rd Congress of European Society of Organ Transplantation	Hans Brynger, M.D. Transplant Unit Sahlgrenska Sjukhuset S-413 45 Gothenburg, Sweden

ERRATUM

In an article entitled "Skin allograft rejection by L3/T4$^+$ and Lyt-2$^+$ T cell subsets" by S. Cobbold and H. Waldmann in the May 1986 issue of *Transplantation*, there is an omission in the references on page 639. The journal citation in reference 26 should be Adv Exp Med 1985; 186: 789. We apologize for any inconvenience that this may have caused.

0041-1337/86/4205-0445$02.00/0
TRANSPLANTATION
Vol. 42, No. 5

Printed in U.S.A.

Transplantation
OVERVIEW

CYCLOSPORINE IN ALLOGENEIC BONE MARROW TRANSPLANTATION[1]

OLLE RINGDÉN[2]

Departments of Clinical Immunology and Transplantation Surgery, Karolinska Institute, Huddinge Hospital, S-141 86 Huddinge, Sweden

Cyclosporine (CsA)* is a fungal metabolite with potent immunosuppressive properties (*1–4*). In renal transplantation, multicenter trials have shown that CsA considerably improves graft and patient survival compared with conventional therapy (*5, 6*). Furthermore, with the use of CsA, increasing numbers of successful liver (*7*) and heart transplants have been performed (*8*). However, in allogeneic bone marrow transplantation the role of CsA is less well defined. CsA was initially used in allogeneic bone marrow transplantation by Powles et al. (*9, 10*). The first reports suggested a favorable outcome in marrow transplant patients treated with CsA, having a decrease in the incidence of severe graft-versus-host disease (GVHD) and improved survival compared with historic controls treated with methotrexate (MTX) (*11–16*). More recently, randomized trials have been reported (*17–21*). However, these have failed to show an improvement in the survival rate and a decline in the incidence of GVHD using CsA compared with conventional prophylaxis using MTX. A review of CsA, its use in experimental transplantation, and its mechanism of action has been reported by Morris (*22*). In this survey I shall, therefore, discuss studies of CsA that are relevant to its use in clinical bone marrow transplantation.

Pharmacology. The pharmacology of CsA was recently extensively reviewed by Kahan (*23*). Therefore, in this article, the value of pharmacological monitoring in bone marrow transplantation (BMT) patients is emphasized. When CsA is taken orally it is administered in an olive-oil solution. Peak concentrations in serum are obtained after 3 to 4 hr. Bioavailability ranges from 20% to 50% (mean 34%) (*24*). In blood, CsA is distributed in the following way: 50% is bound to the erythrocytes, 4–9% is bound to lymphocytes, 10–20% is bound to leukocytes, and 30–40% is found in plasma. Of the total amount of plasma, 5% is free and 90% is protein-bound. At room temperature the CsA plasma level falls, and it stabilizes after 1 hr at approximately half the plasma level found at 37°C (*25, 26*). The highest tissue concentration of CsA occurs in fat. High concentrations of CsA are also noted in the liver, kidneys, pancreas, adrenals, and lymph nodes (*26, 27*). About 99% of CsA is metabolized in the liver and excreted in the bile (*24*). An enterohepatic circulation was found in one-third of the patients examined (*28*). In addition to CsA, 10–12 smaller metabolites are identified in plasma and 17 metabolites in urine (*24*). CsA concentrations can be determined by radioimmunoassay (RIA) or by high-performance liquid chromatography (HPLC) (*23, 28–32*). Using RIA before marrow transplantation, it was found that the CsA clearance was 10 ± 5 L/hr (mean ± SE), the half-life was 26 ± 15 hr, and the bioavailability was 16 ± 10% (*32*).

In allogeneic marrow transplantation CsA is used mainly for the prevention of GVHD. CsA is generally given as a continuous i.v. infusion or divided into 2 or 3 doses one day before transplantation in doses ranging from 2.5 to 7.5 mg/kg/day. CsA is given i.v. until the patients can take oral medication. Oral CsA is given initially in an amount of 12.5 mg/kg/day divided into two doses. In most centers CsA is given for the first 6 months after transplantation, but in a few the drug is given for 12 months (*10–21, 33–37*). When MTX was used as prophylaxis against GVHD, acute GVHD was not seen more than 2 months after transplantation (*38*). However, in patients treated with CsA, acute GVHD may appear as late as 1 year after transplantation (*36, 37*). When this occurred it was easily reversed, in most cases by reintroduction of the drug. In patients with aplastic anemia treated with CsA, late graft failures were reported by Hows et al. 4–7.5 months after BMT after discontinuation of CsA (*39*). When CsA prophylaxis was prolonged to 12 months, no late failures were reported. Accordingly we have treated 9 consecutive patients with aplastic anemia undergoing BMT with CsA prophylaxis for 12 months. All are alive now and none have had a graft failure. It may therefore be advisable to continue CsA prophylaxis for 1 year in patients undergoing BMT for aplastic anemia in order to avoid late failures. We treated patients undergoing BMT for hematological malignancies with CsA for 12 months in the hope of preventing chronic GVHD (*21*). However, the incidence of chronic GVHD was 30% which is similar to that reported using MTX or CsA for 6 months as prophylaxis (*17, 18, 21, 40, 41*).

The value of following CsA serum concentrations has not

[1]This work was supported by grants from the Swedish Medical Research Council, the Baltzar von Platen Foundation Barncancerfonden, Jennyfonden, and The Karolinska Institute.

[2]Address correspondence to: Olle Ringdén, M.D., Department of Transplantation Surgery, Huddinge Hospital, S-141 86 Huddinge, Sweden.

* ALL, acute lymphoblastic leukemia; ANLL, acute nonlymphoblastic leukemia; BMT, bone marrow transplantation; CML, chronic myeloid leukemia; CsA, cyclosporine; EBMT, European Group for Bone Marrow Transplantation; GVHD, graft-versus-host disease; HPLC, high-performance liquid chromatography; IBMTR, International Bone Marrow Transplantation Registry; MTX, methotrexate; RIA, Radioimmunoassay.

been definitely established: several authors have noted the absence of a therapeutic window (*42–44*). Some investigators report a correlation between high CsA concentrations early after transplantation and nephrotoxicity (*36, 44–48*). Kennedy and coworkers in Seattle note that, during the first 4 weeks after BMT, patients with trough levels of CsA of <150, 150–250, and >250 ng/ml have an incidence of renal dysfunction of 73%, 95%, and 100%—and it develops at a median of 46, 29, and 20 days after transplantation (*47*). Gluckman et al., on the other hand, found no correlation between CsA concentrations in plasma and signs of nephrotoxicity and hepatotoxicity (*48*). Hows et al. have shown that high serum concentrations of CsA of >500 ng/ml are potentially nephrotoxic and suggest that early nephrotoxicity can be avoided by maintaining the CsA at levels between 100 and 400 ng/ml, using RIA (*44*).

Divergent results have been reported regarding a correlation between low CsA plasma concentrations and GVHD (*36, 42–48*). Gratwohl et al. showed that CsA plasma levels were the same in patients without GVHD and in those with various grades of acute GVHD (*36*). Gluckman et al., on the other hand, reported a correlation between plasma levels and GVHD: in patients with GVHD, the mean plasma level was 84 ± 62 ng/ml and in those without GVHD the level was 211 ± 63 ng/ml (P<0.001) (*48*).

The value of following the CsA levels to avoid toxicity or GVHD remains to be established. Since CsA is bound with high affinity to lymphocytes (*49*), the effector cells of GVHD, it can hardly be expected that the plasma levels should show a direct correlation with the therapeutic effect. In this respect whole-blood levels do not seem to be better than serum levels (*42, 43*). However, it is important to determine the CsA levels in BMT patients during malabsorption of CsA caused by enteritis—in order to ensure absorption—and during liver dysfunction—in order to avoid excessively high levels (*50–52*).

CsA has been reported to interact with a number of drugs. An increase in the CsA plasma concentration is induced by ketoconazole (*53–57*), diltiazem (*58*), danazol, norethisteron, and low-dose oral contraceptives (*59*), as well as after the administration of high doses of methylprednisolone (*60, 61*). Prednisolone affects the CsA metabolism and CsA affects prednisolone metabolism by reducing the prednisolone clearance (*60–62*). A reduced CsA concentration occurs after rifampicin (*63*) and antiepileptic medication with phenytoin (*64*). These interactions may be due to the fact that these drugs, like CsA, use the hepatic hydroxylating P-450 enzyme system for their metabolism.

The nephrotoxic agents that have been shown to potentiate the nephrotoxic effect by CsA include aminoglucosides (*44, 65*), diltiazem (*58*), amphotericin-B (*66*), melphalan (*57*), trimethoprim, and trimethoprim-sulphamethoxazole (*46, 67, 68*).

Side-effects. An anaphylactic reaction to i.v. CsA, probably caused by the i.v. preparation cremophor, was reported in a BMT patient (*69*). A similar reaction was reported in a renal transplant recipient (*70*).

The most disturbing side-effect of CsA is nephrotoxicity, which has been reported in 70–100% of the patients (*17, 21, 34, 36, 44, 71, 72*). Nephrotoxicity is reversible on dose reduction and is most easily monitored by following the serum creatinine levels. Dialysis has occasionally been necessary (*17, 34, 46, 73*). Schulman et al. described glomerular thrombosis and tubular injury in 3 BMT patients with renal insufficiency who were treated with CsA (*74*). In our experience BMT patients with 1½ years of CsA therapy have normal serum creatinine levels (*21*); so far there seems to be no reason to suspect any lasting renal damage in these BMT patients, such as interstitial fibrosis which was found in the kidneys of recipients of renal (*75, 76*) and heart (*77*) allografts who were on continuous long-term CsA medication.

Hepatotoxicity induced by CsA is difficult to diagnose in BMT patients. This is because there may be alternative explanations of liver dysfunction, such as GVHD, venoocclusive liver disease, hepatitis, chemotherapy and/or irradiation. Among the first 5 patients treated with CsA because of established GVHD 4 died, and they all had liver damage (*9*). Autopsies revealed centrilobular necrosis of the liver, which is typical of drug-induced toxicity. Tutschka et al. found that 14 of 22 patients treated with CsA had an increase in serum bilirubin values, and in 8 of them CsA may have contributed to this (*34*). Atkinson et al. reported that 86% of their patients had had one or more episodes of hyperbilirubinemia, and that CsA was responsible for 34% of the episodes (*51*). CsA patients have also been reported to have higher bilirubin values than those of historic controls who were treated with methotrexate (*71*). In our studies 6 of 30 patients had signs of hepatotoxicity in association with CsA-induced nephrotoxicity. The liver abnormalities normalized after the doses were reduced (*21*).

Reversible central nervous system toxicity has been noted (*78*), and this and other neurological disturbances may be aggravated by CsA-induced hypomagnesemia (*79, 80*). Tremor, a common side-effect of CsA treatment, is seen in 23–100% of the patients (*21, 33, 34, 44, 71*). Hypertension has been reported in 23–60% of CsA-treated BMT patients (*21, 33, 81, 82*). In a randomized study from Seattle, a 60% incidence of hypertension was found in patients treated with CsA, as compared with 20% in patients treated with MTX (P<0.0001) (*82*). Treatment with steroids was also associated with hypertension, but age was of no importance in this study. Animal experiments suggest that CsA induces stimulation of the renin-angiotensin-aldosterone system (*83, 84*). However, this is probably not the reason for hypertension in CsA-treated BMT patients, since Ferrant et al. found that the renin-angiotensin-aldosterone system was not stimulated in CsA-treated BMT patients with hypertension (*85*). Recently a correlation was reported between hypomagnesemia and hypertension in CsA-treated BMT patients (*86*). Ferrant et al. also found that fluid retention did not contribute to hypertension (*85*). Fluid retention, on the other hand, was estimated by Barrett et al. to occur in 40% of BMT patients treated with CsA, and in 20% of these the CsA dose was reduced (*33*).

That it is difficult to define hirsutism is evidenced by the variability in frequency that is reported: it ranges from 9% to 100% (*21, 33, 34, 44, 71*). In our experience the incidence of hirsutism in BMT patients seems higher than that in renal transplant recipients (*21, 87*). This may due to the fact that hirsutism is commoner in younger patients on CsA (*87*)—and that BMT patients, in general, are younger than the recipients of renal grafts.

CsA may induce nausea, vomiting, and anorexia. Since these side-effects are commonly seen after chemotherapy and total-body irradiation they are not well defined. However, an incidence of 80% to which CsA medication may have contributed was reported and a dose reduction was necessary in 10% of the patients (*33*). Gingival hyperplasia is not commonly studied but seems to occur in about 20% of BMT patients (*21, 33*), which is the same frequency as that noted in renal transplant recipients (*87*).

The most severe problem associated with CsA therapy is the development of lymphoma (*88*)—which, in general, is increased in allograft recipients (*89*). Patients who develop lymphoma during CsA therapy show increased antibody titers against Epstein-Barr virus, and this viral antigen is also found in the tumor cells (*90, 91*). In vitro human B cells can transform to Epstein-Barr-virus–positive cell lines in the presence of CsA (*92*). This may be due to the fact that CsA abrogates the natural T cell immunity that should prevent the growth of Epstein-Barr-virus–infected B cells. A similar process may lie behind the development of lymphoma in some CsA patients. A poorly differentiated lymphocytic lymphoma developed 6 months after BMT in a patient treated with CsA (*93*). However, the incidence of lymphoma in BMT patients treated with CsA was only 0.2%, which is lower than the figure for recipients of whole-organ allografts (*94*).

The "capillary leakage syndrome" is seen in recipients of bone marrow from HLA mismatched donors treated with CsA (*73, 95, 96*). This complication, which is fatal, is characterized by pulmonary edema, convulsions, intravascular hemolysis, and renal failure. In recipients of HLA-matched marrow and in patients treated with MTX it is not seen so often. However, it is reported that the antifungal drug mepartricin-sodiumlaurylsulfate has contributed to this syndrome in some CsA-treated recipients of HLA-matched marrow (*97*). The pulmonary capillary leakage syndrome has also been reported in liver transplant recipients treated with i.v. CsA (*98*).

Effect on survival and GVHD. Powles and coworkers initially used CsA to treat GVHD, but 4 of 5 patients died of liver failure (*9*). Thereafter they used CsA as a prophylaxis against GVHD (*10*). This first prophylactic trial included 23 patients. In three of them, CsA was discontinued after a brief treatment, and all 3 died of acute GVHD. Only one of the remaining patients died of GVHD. Following this series, several uncontrolled trials using CsA as prophylaxis against GVHD were reported(*11–16, 33–35, 37, 48, 57, 71, 72, 99–102*). In some of these trials the CsA-treated patients were compared with historic controls treated with MTX (*11–71*). Most of the investigators found a favorable effect on the survival rate and less serious GVHD in the CsA patients. For instance, Bacigalupo et al. reported severe acute GVHD in 3 of 24 CsA-treated patients compared with 8 of 21 historic controls treated with MTX (P=0.04) (*71*). The one-year survival rate was 72% in the CsA patients and 52% in the MTX patients (NS). In BMT patients with ANLL in first remission who were treated with CsA at the Royal Marsden Hospital, the long-term survival rate was the same as in ANLL patients who received MTX in Seattle (*100, 103*). The patients at the Royal Marsden Hospital tended to have a lower death rate from GVHD, but a higher incidence of relapses. It may therefore be speculated that CsA, which seemed to effectively prevent GVHD in this trial, also reduced the beneficial graft-versus-leukemia effect associated with GVHD (*104, 105*).

The improvement in the survival rate compared with historic controls was especially striking in patients with aplastic anemia: long-term survival in CsA-treated patients improved by about 30% compared with historic controls treated with MTX (*11, 13–15*). Hows et al. reported that 14% of the CsA patients died of GVHD, as against 36% of the previous MTX patients (*13*). Another advantage of CsA was the decrease in the incidence of rejections. Rejections have been a main problem in BMT for severe aplastic anemia. However, after the discontinuation of CsA, late failures have been reported in patients with aplastic anemia, as mentioned above (*39*).

The initially promising results of using CsA to prevent GVHD initiated the use of this drug in HLA-mismatched transplantations. The group from Royal Marsden Hospital has the largest experience using CsA in mismatched transplantation. Using one-haplotype-mismatched family donors, about one-third of the patients became long-term survivors (*95*). However, in patients above 20 years of age the outcome was very poor.

CsA was also used to treat acute GVHD (*9, 106, 107*). The group from Seattle studied 48 patients with hematological malignancies who developed grades II–IV acute GVHD during prophylaxis with MTX (*106*). Patients treated with a combination of CsA and antithymocyte globulin had a 6-month survival rate of 67% compared with 25% in patients treated with CsA in combination with antithymocyte globulin and methylprednisolone. In another study from Seattle, patients who had grades II–IV acute GVHD despite MTX prophylaxis were randomized to methylprednisolone or CsA treatment for at least 2 weeks (*107*). In the CsA group the response rate was 61% compared with 41% in the patients treated with methylprednisolone (P<0.05). These two trials from Seattle suggest that CsA is useful in the treatment of established acute GVHD and is at least as effective as methylprednisolone in this respect.

Several multicenter analyses were performed to compare the outcome in BMT patients treated with CsA with those receiving MTX (*108–114*). The International Bone Marrow Transplant Registry (IBMTR) reported that in patients with ANLL in first remission, grades II–IV acute GVHD accurred in 42% of the patients treated with MTX, compared with 30% of those treated with CsA (NS) (*108*). In one report from the European Group for Bone Marrow Transplantation (EBMT), including 134 leukemic patients treated with CsA and 124 comparable patients treated with MTX, the two groups had the same actuarial 3-year survival rate (*109*). The incidence of acute GVHD was slightly higher in the CsA patients (P=0.02), but there was no difference in the grading of GVHD. In a later analysis from EBMT in patients with ANLL, the incidence of acute GVHD was 70% for CsA patients compared with 60% for MTX patients (P=0.006) (110). Among 192 patients with ALL, the EBMT reported a 67% incidence of acute GVHD compared with 63% in patients treated with MTX (P=0.03) (111). In a more recent EBMT report on leukemia, patients on CsA prophylaxis did significantly better than patients on MTX prophylaxis (ANLL (P=0.006), ALL (P=0.02) (*112*). In patients with aplastic anemia the EBMT reported that the 1-year survival rate was 55% in patients treated with MTX, and 70% in patients treated with CsA (*113*). In 27 patients treated with MTX prophylaxis and thoracoabdominal irradiation the 1-year survival rate was 73% compared with 90% in 14 patients treated with CsA prophylaxis and receiving thoracoabdominal irradiation. In a recent EBMT report on aplastic anemia, the incidence of grades II–IV acute GVHD was 58% in CsA-treated patients and 55% in MTX-treated patients. The long-term survival rates were 71% and 55% in the two groups (*114*).

When CsA prophylaxis against GVHD was compared with MTX in randomized trials, there were no differences in the incidence of grades II–IV acute GVHD, chronic GVHD, or survival (Table 1) (*17–21*). The only exception was a study of patients over 30 years of age with a relapse of leukemia, in which those randomized to MTX had an actuarial incidence of GVHD of 71% compared with 45% among those receiving CsA (*20*). Thus, contrary to the preliminary uncontrolled reports and some of the international multicenter analyses, the randomized trials revealed no beneficial effect on the severity of GVHD or the survival rate using CsA, as compared with MTX.

Relative advantages and disadvantages of using cyclosporine vs. methotrexate. One advantage of using CsA, as compared with MTX, is a faster engraftment. The reason for this is that CsA, unlike MTX, is not myelotoxic (*115*). CsA patients have been reported to have an earlier engraftment with respect to neutrophils (*116, 117*), granulocytes (*17, 20, 21, 71, 117*), leukocytes (*21, 116, 117*), thrombocytes (*17, 20, 71, 116*), and reticulocytes (*21, 116*). Some centers have reported that for CsA patients this probably resulted in fewer days with fever (*117*), fewer infections (*71*), a reduced need for granulocyte transfusions (*117*), fewer days with systemic antibiotics (*71*), and a more rapid discharge from the hospital (*17*). However, in some of the randomized trials no differences between CsA-treated and MTX-treated patients regarding engraftment (*18*), requirements for transfusions (*18, 21*), or time in the hospital were reported (*18, 21*). In five randomized trials it was noted that CsA-treated patients had mucositis less often than MTX-treated patients (*17, 18, 20, 21, 117*).

Multicenter analysis performed by the IBMTR and EBMT showed that patients with leukemia receiving a high-dose rate of total-body irradiation (>6 cGy/min) had an increase incidence of interstitial pneumonitis if they were treated with MTX than if they were treated with CsA (*109, 118*). At lower dosc rates of total body irradiation there was no difference in the incidence of interstitial pneumonitis.

An increased risk of relapse after BMT for ANLL patients treated with CsA compared with those receiving MTX was reported by EBMT (*109, 110*). In these studies some centers that mainly use CsA were compared with other centers that use MTX. Since the conditioning before BMT, especially regarding total-body irradiation, may differ at different centers this observation has to be treated with caution. However, data from a randomized trial in patients with advanced leukemia showed that CsA-treated patients had a 70% incidence of relapse as compared with 37% for MTX-treated patients (Table 1) (*20*). This difference was statistically significant ($P<0.05$) and points in the same direction as the report from EBMT. However, in 4 randomized trials there was no difference in relapse frequency between patients treated with CsA and with MTX (Table 1) (*17–19, 21*).

Future use of cyclosporine in bone marrow transplantation. In solid organ transplantation the use of CsA has considerably improved graft and patient survival rates (*5–8*). In organ transplantation, CsA is often combined with prednisolone, as introduced by Starzl et al. (*119*). Recently a combination of CsA prednisolone, and azathioprine has been shown to produce good results in renal transplant recipients (*120–122*). However, in other studies the results of triple therapy have not been better than with CsA alone in renal allograft recipients (*123*).

In BMT, randomized trials showed no decrease in the incidence of GVHD or the survival rates of patients treated with CsA alone compared with MTX (*17–21*). Thus, CsA used alone may not be the best treatment for GVHD. Experiments in dogs have shown that a combination of CsA with ony 4 initial doses of MTX reduced the incidence of GVHD and improved the survival rate after BMT (*124*). This treatment was also evaluated in man in prospective randomized trials. Recently Storb et al. reported that patients with ANLL in first remission or CML in first chronic phase who were treated with this combination of CsA and MTX had a significantly decreased incidence of grades II–IV acute GVHD—33% compared with 54% in patients treated with CsA alone (*125*). The two-year actuarial survival was 80% in patients treated with the combination therapy compared with 55% in those treated with CsA alone ($P<0.05$). The group from Seattle has also treated patients suffering from severe aplastic anemia with the combination of CsA and four doses of MTX, and compared this with conventional MTX treatment in a randomized controlled trial (*126*). Patients treated with combination therapy had less acute GVHD and a better survival rate than those treated with MTX alone.

Survival figures similar to those reported by the Seattle group using a combination of CsA and MTX (*125*) were reported in preliminary trials using T cell depletion in patients with acute leukemia in first remission (*127*) and CML in first chronic phase (*128*). Although T cell depletion of the bone marrow seems to effectively prevent GVHD, the risk of graft rejection and relapse seems to be greater than when pharmacological immunosuppression in used (*129–131*).

In BMT patients CsA has also been combined with methylprednisolone (*132*). Patients treated with this combination were compared in a randomized trial with those treated with methylprednisolone and cyclophosphamide. There was no statistically significant difference between the two groups in the overall survival rate, but it was suggested that CsA and methylprednisolone more effectively prevented grade II acute

TABLE 1. Results of five randomized trials comparing cyclosporine (CsA) and methotrexate (MTX) as prophylaxis against graft-versus-host disease

Diagnosis	Study	Reference No.	No. patients with CSP/MTX	% Patients treated with CSP/MTX: Grade II-IV acute GVHD	Chronic GVHD	Interstitial pneumonitis	Relapse	Survival (actuarial at 3 years [*17, 18, 21*])
ANLL	(Seattle)	(*17*)	36/39	33/56	50/47	25/20	14/10	61/47
CML	(Seattle)	(*18*)	25/30	42/46	50/63	20/13	4/4	62/66
Acute leukemia	(Sidney)	(*19*)	20/16	45/19	73/57	15/13	17/0	50/81[b]
Leukemia in relapse	(Seattle)	(*20*)	26/30	45/71[a]	50/64	15/23	70/37[a]	15/17[b]
Hematological malignancies	(Stockholm)	(*21*)	30/29	40/22	30/39	10/21	13/7	58/69
Total			137/137	41/47	49/51	18/19	20/14	52/55[b]

[a] $P<0.05$.
[b] Absolute survival.

GVHD. The combination of CsA and prednisone was also compared with MTX and prednisone in a prospective randomized trial in 107 patients with leukemia (*133*). The combination of CsA and prednisone was superior in preventing GVHD.

Until now CsA has in many cases been used as the sole immunosuppressive treatment to prevent GVHD after BMT. The trials that use a combination of CsA and MTX or prednisolone look very promising and show CsA definitely has a future role in the prevention of GVHD. The optimal use of CsA has yet to be determined. The ultimate goal in the prophylaxis and prevention of GVHD is to produce a minimal GVHD and maximal graft-versus-leukemia effect. However, this may prove impossible. The question of whether the highest patient survival rate can be achieved by pharmacological immunosuppression, or marrow manipulation, or a combination of the two remains to be answered.

REFERENCES

1. Borel JF, Feurer C, Gubler HU, Stähelin H. Biological effects of Cyclosporin A: a new antilymphocytic agent. Agents Actions 1976; 96: 468.
2. Borel JF, Feurer C, Magnée C, Stähelin H. Effects of the new antilymphocytic peptide Cyclosporin A in animals. Immunology 1977; 32: 1017.
3. Borel JF, Meszros J. Skin transplantation in mice and dogs: effect of cyclosporin A dihydrocyclosporin C. Transplantation 1980; 29: 161.
4. Borel J. The history of Cyclosporin A and its significans. In: White DJG, ed. Cyclosporin A. New York: Elsevier, 1982: 4.
5. European Multicentre Trial Group. Cyclosporin in cadaveric renal transplantation: one-year follow-up of a multicentre trial. Lancet 1983; 2: 986.
6. Canadian Multicentre Transplant Study Group. A randomized clinical trial of cyclosporine in cadaveric renal transplantation. N Engl J Med 1983; 309: 809.
7. Starzl TE, Iwatsuki S, Klintmalm G, Schröter GPJ, Weil R III, Koep LJ, Porter KA. Liver transplantation, 1980, with particular reference to cyclosporin A. Transplant Proc 1981; 13: 281.
8. Shumway NE. Recent advances in cardiac transplantation. Transplant Proc 1983; 15: 1221.
9. Powles RL, Barrett AJ, Clink HEM, et al. Cyclosporin A for the treatment of graft-versus-host disease in man. Lancet 1978; 2: 1327.
10. Powles RL, Clink HM, Spence D, et al. Cyclosporin A to prevent graft-versus-host disease in man after allogeneic bone-marrow transplantation. Lancet 1980; 1: 327.
11. Kendra JR, Barrett AJ. Comparison of methotrexate and cyclosporin A in the prevention of graft versus host disease in leukaemia transplants. In: Touraine JL, Gluckman E, Griscelli C, eds. Bone marrow transplantation in Europe II. Amsterdam: Elsevier, 1981: 165.
12. Powles RL, Morgenstern GR. Cyclosporin A to prevent graft-versus-host disease in man following HLA/MLC matched allogeneic bone marrow transplantation. In: White DJG, ed. Cyclosporin A. Amsterdam: Elsevier, 1982: 485.
13. Hows JM, Palmer S, Gordon-Smith EC. Use of cyclosporin A in allogeneic bone marrow transplantation for severe aplastic anemia. Transplantation 1982; 33a: 383.
14. Kendra JR, Lucas CF, Chambers D, et al. Bone marrow transplantation for severe aplastic anaemia. A review of the Westminster experience of 24 cases. Clin Lab Haematol 1983; 5: 131.
15. Speck B, Gratwohl A, Nissen C, et al. Knochenmark transplantation bei Leukämie und aplastischer Anämie. Schweiz Med Wochenschr 1983; 113: 622.
16. Vitale V, Bacigalupo A, Frassoni F, et al. Fractionated total body irradiation (fTBI) in marrow transplantation for leukemia. Br J Haematol 1983; 55: 547.
17. Deeg HJ, Storb R, Thomas ED, et al. Cyclosporine as prophylaxis for graft-versus-host disease: a randomized study in patients undergoing marrow transplantation for acute nonlymphoblastic leukemia. Blood 1985; 65: 1325.
18. Storb R, Deeg HJ, Thomas ED, et al. Marrow transplantation for chronic myelocytic leukemia: a controlled trial of cyclosporine versus methotrexate for prophylaxis of graft-versus-host disease. Blood 1985; 66: 698.
19. Biggs J, Atkinson K, Gillett E, Downs K, Concannon A, Dodds A. A randomised prospective trial comparing cyclosporin and methotrexate given for prophylaxis of graft-versus-host disease after bone marrow transplantation. Transplant Proc 1986; 18: 253.
20. Irle C, Deeg HJ, Buckner CD, et al. Marrow transplantation for leukemia following fractionated total body irradiation: a comparative trial of methotrexate and cyclosporine. Leuk Res 1985; 9: 1255.
21. Ringdén O, Bäckman L, Lönnqvist B, et al. A randomized trial comparing the use of cyclosporin and methotrexate for graft-versus-host disease prophylaxis in bone marrow transplant recipients with hematologic malignancies. Bone Marrow Transplant 1986; 1: 41.
22. Morris PJ. Cyclosporin A. Transplantation 1981; 32: 349.
23. Kahan BD. Individualization of cyclosporine therapy using pharmacokinetic and pharmacodynamic parameters. Transplantation 1985; 40: 457.
24. Beveridge T. Pharmacokinetics and metabolism of cyclosporin A. In: White DJG, ed. Cyclosporin A. New York: Elsevier, 1982: 35.
25. Niederberger W, Lemaire M, Maurer G, et al. Distribution and binding of cyclosporine in blood and tissues. Transplant Proc 1983; 15: 2419.
26. Atkinson K, Boland J, Britton K, Biggs J. Blood and tissue distribution of cyclosporine in humans and mice. Transplant Proc 1983; 15: 2430.
27. Ried M, Gibbons S, Kwok D, et al. Cyclosporine levels in human tissues of patients treated for one week to one year. Transplant Proc 1983; 15: 434.
28. Kahan BD, Ried M, Newburger J. Pharmacokinetics of cyclosporine in human renal transplantation. Transplant Proc 1983; 15: 446.
29. Donatsch P, Abisch E, Homberger M, et al. A radioimmunoassay to measure cyclosporin A in plasma and serum samples. J Immunoassay 1981; 2: 19.
30. Niederberger W, Schaub P, Beveridge T. High-performance liquid chromatographic determination of cyclosporin A in human plasma and urine. J Chromatogr Biomed Appl 1980; 182: 454.
31. Yee GC, Kennedy MS, Storb R, Thomas ED. Pharmacokinetics of intravenous cyclosporine in bone marrow transplant patients. Transplantation 1984; 38: 511.
32. Bertault P, Maraninchi D, Carcassonne Y, et al. Clinical pharmacokinetics of ciclosporin A in bone marrow transplantation patients. Cancer Chemother Pharmacol 1985; 15: 76.
33. Barrett AJ, Kendra JR, Lucas CF, et al. Cyclosporine A as prophylaxis against graft-versus-host disease in 36 patients. Br Med J 1982; 285: 162.
34. Tutschka PJ, Beschorner WE, Hess AD, Santos GW. Cyclosporin-A to prevent graft-versus-host disease: a pilot study in 22 patients receiving allogeneic marrow transplants. Blood 1983; 61: 318.
35. Biggs J, Atkinson K, Concannon A, et al. Bone marrow transplantation in 33 patients with malignant blood diseases and severe aplastic anaemia. Med J Aust 1983; 70(2): 120.
36. Gratwohl A, Speck B, Wenk M, et al. Cyclosporine in human bone marrow transplantation. Transplantation 1983; 36: 40.
37. Speck B, Gratwohl A, Osterwalder B, et al. Experience with 100 allogeneic marrow grafts using cyclosporin-A (CYA) for prophylaxis against GvHD. Exp Hematol 1985; 13(suppl 17): 126.
38. Thomas ED, Storb R, Clift RA, et al. Bone marrow transplanta-

tion. N Engl J Med 1975; 292: 832.

39. Hows J, Palmer S, Gordon-Smith EC. Cyclcosporine and graft failure following bone marrow transplantation for severe aplastic anaemia. Br J Haematol 1985; 60: 611.
40. Sullivan KM, Schulman HM, Storb R, et al. Chronic graft-versus-host disease in 52 patients: adverse natural course and successful treatment with combination immunosuppression. Blood 1981; 57: 2.
41. Ringdén O, Paulin T, Lönnqvist B, Nilsson B. An analysis of factors predisposing to chronic graft-versus-host disease. Exp Hematol 1985; 13: 1962.
42. Biggs JC, Atkinson K, Britton K, Downs K. The use of cyclosporine in human marrow transplantation: absence of a therapeutic window. Transplant Proc 1985; 17: 1239.
43. Bacigalupo A, Di Giorgio F, Frassoni F, et al. Cyclosporin A serum and blood levels in marrow graft recipients: correlation with administered dose, serum creatinine and graft-versus-host disease. Acta Haematol (Basel) 1984; 72: 155.
44. Hows JM, Chipping PM, Fairhead S, et al. Nephrotoxicity in bone marrow transplant recipients treated with Cyclosporin A. Br J Haematol 1983; 54: 69.
45. Lindholm A, Ringdén O, Lönnqvist B. The role of cyclosporine doses and plasma levels for efficacy and toxicity in bone marrow transplant recipients. Transplantation (in press).
46. Kennedy MS, Deeg HJ, Storb R, Thomas ED. Cyclosporine in marrow transplantation: concentration-dependent toxicity and immunosuppression in vivo. Transplant Proc 1983; 15: 471.
47. Kennedy MS, Yee GC, McGuire TR, et al. Correlation of serum cyclosporine concentration with renal dysfunction in marrow transplant recipients. Transplantation 1985; 40: 249.
48. Gluckman E, Lokiec R, Devergie A. Pharmacokinetic monitoring of cyclosporine in allogeneic bone marrow transplant. Transplant Proc 1985; 17: 500.
49. Ryffel B, Donatsch P, Götz U, Tschopp A. Cyclosporin-A receptor on mouse lymphocytes. Immunology 1980; 41: 913.
50. Atkinson K, Biggs JC, Britton K, et al. Oral administration of cyclosporin A for recipients of allogeneic marrow transplants: implications of oral gut dysfunction. Br J Haematol 1984; 56: 223.
51. Atkinson K, Biggs JC, Dodds AJ, Concannon AJ. Cyclosporin-associated hepatotoxicity after allogeneic marrow transplantation in man: differentiation from other causes of posttransplant liver disease. Transplant Proc 1983; 15(suppl 1): 545.
52. Yee GC, Kennedy MS, Storb R, Thomas ED. Effect of hepatic dysfunction on oral cyclosporin pharmacokinetics in marrow transplant patients. Blood 1984; 64: 1277.
53. Cunningham C, Burke MD, Whiting PH, et al. Ketokonazole, cyclosporin, and the kidney. Lancet 1982; 2: 1464.
54. Daneshmend TK. Ketaconazole-cyclosporin interaction. Lancet 1982; 2: 1342.
55. Dieperink H, Møller J. Ketoconazole and cyclosporin. Lancet 1982; 2: 1217.
56. Gluckman E, Devergie A, Lokiec F, et al. Nephrotoxicity of cyclosporin A in bone-marrow transplantation. Lancet 1981; 2: 144.
57. Morgenstern GR, Powles R, Robinson B, McElwain TJ. Cyclosporin interaction with ketoconazole and melphalan. Lancet 1982; 2: 1342.
58. Pochet JM, Pirson Y. Cyclosporin-Diltiazem interaction. Lancet 1986; 1: 979.
59. Ross WB, Roberts D, Griffin PJA, Salaman JR. Cyclosporin interaction with danazol and norethisterone. Lancet 1986; 1: 330.
60. Klintmalm G, Säwe J. Administration of high doses of methylprednisolone increases the cyclosporine plasma levels in renal transplant recipients. Lancet 1984; 1: 731.
61. Öst L, Klintmalm G, Ringdén O. Mutual interaction between prednisolone and cyclosporin in renal transplant patients. Transplant Proc 1985; 17: 1252.
62. Öst L. Effects of cyclosporin on prednisolone metabolism. Lancet 1984; 1: 45.
63. Langhoff E, Madsen S. Rapid metabolism of cyclosporin and prednisone in kidney transplant patients on tuberculostatic treatment. Lancet 1983; 2: 1303.
64. Keown PA, Stiller CR, Laupacis AL, et al. The effects and side-effects of cyclosporine: relationship to drug pharmacokinetics. Transplant Proc 1982; 14: 659.
65. Hows J, Harris R, Palmer S, Gordon-Smith EC. Immunosuppression with Cyclosporin A in allogeneic bone marrow transplantation for severe aplastic anemia: preliminary studies. Br J Haematol 1981; 48: 227.
66. Kennedy MS, Deeg HJ, Siegel M, et al. Acute renal toxicity with combined use of amphotericin B and cyclosporine after marrow transplantation. Transplantation 1983; 35: 211.
67. Thompson JF, Chalmers DHK, Hinnitsett AGW, et al. Nephrotoxicity of trimethoprim and cotrimoxazole in renal allograft recipients treated with cyclosporin. Transplantation 1983; 36: 204.
68. Ringdén O, Myrenfors P, Klintmalm G, et al. Nephrotoxicity by Co-trimoxazole and cyclosporin in transplanted patients. Lancet 1984; 1: 1016.
69. Chapuis B, Helg C, Jeannet M, et al. Anaphylactic reaction to intravenous cyclosporine. N Engl J Med 1985; 312: 1259.
70. Kahan BD, Wideman CA, Flechner S, Van Buren CT. Anaphylactic reaction to intravenous cyclosporine. Lancet 1984; 1: 52.
71. Bacigalupo A, Frassoni F, van Lint MT, et al. Cyclosporin A in marrow transplantation for leukemia and aplastic anemia. Exp Haematol 1985; 13: 244.
72. Hows JM, Palmer S, Gordon-Smith EC. Use of cyclosporin A in allogeneic bone marrow transplantation for severe aplastic anemia. Transplantation 1982; 33: 383.
73. Atkinson K, Biggs JC, Hayes J, et al. Cyclosporin A associated nephrotoxicity in the first 100 days after allogeneic bone marrow transplantation: three distinct syndromes. Br J Haematol 1983; 54: 59.
74. Shulman H, Striker G, Deeg HJ, et al. Nephrotoxicity of cyclosporin A after allogeneic marrow transplantation. Glomerular thromboses and tubular injury. N Engl J Med 1981; 305: 1392.
75. Klintmalm G, Bohman SO, Sundelin B, et al. Interstitital fibrosis in renal allografts after 12 to 46 months of cyclosporin treatment; beneficial effects of lower doses early after transplantation. Lancet 1984; 2: 950.
76. Bohman SO, Klintmalm G, Ringdén O, et al. Interstitial fibrosis in human kidney grafts after 12 to 46 months of cyclosporine therapy. Transplant Proc 1985; 17: 1168.
77. Myers BD, Ross J, Newton L, et al. Cyclosporine-associated chronic nephropathy. N Engl J Med 1984; 311: 699.
78. Atkinson K, Biggs J, Darveniza P, et al. Cyclosporine-associated central nervous system toxicity after allogeneic bone marrow transplantation. Transplantation 1984; 38: 34.
79. June CH, Thompson CB, Kennedy MS, et al. Profound hypomagnesemia and renal magnesium wasting associated with the use of cyclosporine for marrow transplantation. Transplantation 1985; 39: 620.
80. Thompson CB, June CH, Sullivan KM, Thomas ED. Association between cyclosporin neurotoxicity and hypomagnesaemia. Lancet 1984; 2: 116.
81. Lokiec F, Devergie A, Gluckman E. Cyclosporine therapy: clinical and biological events. Exp Hematol 1984; 12(suppl 15): 68.
82. Loughran TP, Deeg HJ, Dahlberg S, et al. Incidence of hypertension after marrow transplantation among 112 patients randomized to either cyclosporine or methotrexate as graft-versus-host disease prophylaxis. Br J Haematol 1985; 59: 547.
83. Baxter CR, Duggin GG, Willis NS, et al. Cyclosporin A-induced increases in renin storage and release. Res Commun Chem Pathol Pharmacol 1982; 37: 305.

84. Siegl H, Ryffel B. Effect of Cyclosporin on renin-angiotensin-aldosterone system. Lancet 1982; 2: 1274.
85. Ferrant A, De Plaen JF, Uten M, Michaux JL. Cyclosporine induced hypertension in bone marrow transplantation: absence of stimulation of the renin-angiotensin-aldosterone system. Exp Hematol 1984; 12(suppl 15): 70.
86. June CH, Thompson CB, Kennedy MS, Loughran TP Jr, Deeg HJ. Correlation of hypomagnesemia with the onset of cyclosporine-associated hypertension in marrow transplant patients. Transplantation 1986; 41: 48.
87. Ringdén O, Öst L, Klintmalm G, et al. Improved outcome in renal transplant recipients above 55 years of age treated with cyclosporine A and low doses of steroids. Transplant Proc 1983; 15: 2815.
88. Calne RY, Rolles K, Thiru S, et al. Cyclosporin A initially as the only immunosuppressant in 34 recipients of cadaveric organs. Lancet 1979; 2: 1033.
89. Penn I. Lymphomas complicating organ transplantation. Transplant Proc 1983; 15: 2790.
90. Starzl TE, Nalesnik MA, Porter KA, et al. Reversability of lymphomas and lymphoproliferative lesions developing under cyclosporin-steroid therapy. Lancet 1984; 1: 583.
91. Crawford DH, Thomas JA, Janossy G, et al. Epstein Barr virus nuclear antigen positive lymphoma after cyclosporin A treatment in patient with renal allograft. Lancet 1980; 1: 1355.
92. Bird G, McLachlan S, Britton S. Cyclosporin A promotes spontaneous outgrowth in vitro of Epstein-Barr virus induced B cell lines. Nature 1981; 289: 300.
93. Bloom RE, Brennan JK, Sullivan JL, et al. Lymphoma of host origin in a marrow transplant recipient in remission of acute myeloid leukemia and receiving cyclosporin A. Am J Hematol 1985; 18: 73.
94. Beveridge T, Krupp P, McKibbin C. Lymphoma and lymphoproliferative lesions developing under cyclosporin therapy. Lancet 1984; 1: 788.
95. Powles RL, Morgenstern GR, Kay HEM, et al. Mismatched family donors for bone-marrow transplantation as treatment for acute leukaemia. Lancet 1983; 1: 612.
96. Tydén G, Ringdén O, Lundgren G. Treatment of mismatch bone-marrow transplantation syndrome. Lancet 1983; 2: 1278.
97. Marmont AAM, Van Lint MT, Frassoni F, Bacigalupo A. Adult respiratory distress syndrome (ARDS) after BMT in patients receiving cyclosporin A. Exp Hematol 1984; 12(suppl 15): 73.
98. Powell-Jackson PR, Carmichael FJL, Calne RY, Williams R. Adult respiratory distress syndrome and convulsions associated with administration of cyclosporine in liver transplant recipients. Transplantation 1984; 38: 241.
99. Morgenstern GR. Cyclosporin A for the prevention of graft versus host disease following allogeneic bone marrow transplantation in man. Blut 1980; 41: 177.
100. Powles RL, Morgenstern G, Clink HM, et al. The place of bone-marrow transplantation in acute myelogenous leukaemia. Lancet 1980; 1: 1047.
101. Speck B, Gratwohl A, Nissen C, et al. Cyclosporin A for prophylaxis of GVH in clinical bone marrow transplantation. In: Baum SJ, Ledney GD, Khan A, eds. Experimental hematology today 1981. Basel: Karger, 1981: 117.
102. Speck B, Gratwohl A, Nissen C, et al. Bone marrow grafting for leukaemia and aplastic anaemia. In: White DJG, ed. Cyclosporin A. Amsterdam: Elsevier, 1982: 491.
103. Thomas ED, Buckner ED, Clift RA, et al. Marrow transplantation for acute nonlymphoblastic leukemia in first remission. N Engl J Med 1979; 301: 597.
104. Weiden PL, Flournoy N, Thomas ED, et al. Anti-leukemic effect of graft-versus-host disease in human recipients of allogeneic-marrow grafts. N Engl J Med 1979; 300: 1068.
105. Weiden PL, Sullivan K, Flournoy N, et al. Antileukemic effect of chronic graft-versus-host disease. Contribution to improved survival after allogeneic marrow transplantation. N Engl J Med 1981; 304: 1529.
106. Deeg HJ, Loughran TP, Storb R, et al. Treatment of human acute graft-versus-host disease with antithymocyte globulin and cyclosporine with or without methylprednisolone. Transplantation 1985; 40: 162.
107. Kennedy MS, Deeg HJ, Storb R, et al. Treatment of acute graft-versus-host disease after allogeneic marrow transplantation. Randomized study comparing corticosteroids and cyclosporine. Am J Med 1985; 78: 978.
108. Gale RP, Kay HE, Rimm AA, Bortin MM. Bone-marrow transplantation for acute leukaemia in first remission. Lancet 1982; 2: 1006.
109. Zwaan FE, Hermans J. Report of the EBMT leukemia working party. Exp Hematol 1983; 11(suppl 13): 3.
110. Zwaan FE, Hermans J, Barrett AJ, Speck B. Bone marrow transplantation for acute nonlymphoblastic leukaemia: a survey of the European Group for Bone Marrow Transplantation (EGBMT) Br J Haematol 1984; 56: 645.
111. Zwaan FE, Hermans J, Barrett AJ, Speck B. Bone marrow transplantation for acute lymphoblastic leukaemia: a survey of the European Group for Bone Marrow Transplantation (EGBMT). Br J Haematol 1984; 58: 33.
112. Zwaan FE, Hermans J, Lyklema A. Bone marrow transplantation for leukemia in Europe: Factors influencing the possibility of long-term leukemia-free survival. Exp Hematol 1985; 13(suppl 17): 3.
113. Gluckman E. Report of the European bone marrow transplantation group: aplastic anemia working party. Exp Hematol 1983; 11(suppl 13): 45.
114. Bacigalupo A, Di Giorgio F, Congiu M, et al. Treatment of severe aplastic anemia in Europe 1970–1983: a report of the EBMT SAA Working Party. Exp Haematol 1985; 13(suppl 17): 56.
115. Hellman A, Goldman JM. Effects of cyclosporin A on human granulopoiesis in vitro. Transplantation 1980; 30: 386.
116. Hows JM, Kaffaf S, Palmer S, Harris R, et al. Regeneration of peripheral blood cells following allogeneic bone marrow transplantation for severe aplastic anaemia. Br J Haematol 1982; 52: 551.
117. Atkinson K, Biggs JC, Ting A, et al. Cyclosporin A is associated with faster engraftment and less mucositis than methotrexate after allogeneic bone marrow transplantation. Br J Haematol 1983; 53: 265.
118. Bortin MM, Kay HEM, Gale RP, Rimm AA. Factors associated with interstitial pneumonitis after bone-marrow transplantation for acute leukaemia. Lancet 1982; 1: 437.
119. Starzl TE, Klintmalm GBGF, Weil R III, et al. Cyclosporin-A and steroid therapy in 66 cadaver kidney recipients. Surg Gynecol Obstet 1981; 153: 486.
120. Fries D, Kechrid C, Charpentier B, Hammouche M, Moulin B. A prospective study of a triple association: cyclosporine, corticosteroids and azathioprine in immunologically high-risk transplantation. Transplant Proc 1985; 17: 1231.
121. Slapak M, Geoghegan T, Digard N, Ahmed K, Sharman VL, Crockett R. The use of low dose cyclosporine in combination with azathioprine and steroids in renal transplantation. Transplant Proc 1985; 17: 1222.
122. Simmons RL, Canafax DM, Strand M, et al. Management of cyclosporine nephrotoxicity after renal transplantation: use of low doses of cyclosporine, azathioprine and prednisone. Transplant Proc 1985; 17(suppl 1): 266.
123. Salaman JR, Griffin PJA. Immunosuppression with a combination of cyclosporin, azathioprine, and prednisolone may be unsafe. Lancet 1985; 2: 1066.
124. Deeg HJ, Storb R, Appelbaum FR, et al. Combined immunosuppression with cyclosporine and methotrexate in dogs given bone marrow grafts from DLA-haploidentical littermates. Transplantation 1984; 37: 62.

125. Storb R, Deeg J, Whitehead J, et al. Methotrexate and cyclosporine compared with cyclosporine alone for prophylaxis of acute graft-versus host disease after marrow transplantation for leukemia. N Engl J Med 1986; 314: 729.
126. Storb R, Deeg HJ, Farewell V, et al. Marrow transplantation for severe aplastic anemia: methotrexate alone compared with a combination of methotrexate and cyclosporine for prevention of acute graft-versus-host disease. Blood 1986; 68: 119.
127. Prentice HG, Blacklock MA, Janossy G, et al. Depletion of T lymphocytes in donor marrow prevents significant graft-versus-host disease in matched allogeneic leukemic marrow transplant recipients. Lancet 1984; 1: 472.
128. Hows J, Apperley J, Yin J, et al. T-cell depletion with campath 1 to prevent GVHD. Exp Hematol 1985; 13(suppl 17): 114.
129. Mitsuyasu RT, Champlin RE, Ho WG, et al. Prospective randomized controlled trial of ex vivo treatment of donor bone marrow with monoclonal anti-T cell antibody and complement for prevention of graft-versus-host disease: a preliminary report. Transplant Proc 1985; 17: 482.
130. Patterson J, Prentice HG, Gilmore M, et al. Analysis of rejection in HLA matched T-depleted bone marrow transplants. Exp Hematol 1985; 13(suppl 17): 117.
131. Trigg ME, Billing R, Sondel PM, et al. Clinical trial depleting T lymphocytes from donor marrow for matched and mismatched allogeneic bone marrow transplants. Cancer Treat Rep 1985; 69: 377.
132. Santos GW, Brookmeyer R, Saral R, Tutschka PJ. Cyclosporine (CsA) versus cyclophosphamide (CY)-prevention of graft-versus-host disease (GVHD) [Abstract 254]. Exp Hematol 1985; 13: 427.
133. Blume KG, Forman SJ, Krance RA, et al. A prospective randomized study on acute graft-versus-host disese in 107 patients with leukemia: methotrexate/prednisone versus cyclosporin A/prednisone. Transplant Proc (in press).

0041-1337/86/4205-0453$02.00/0
TRANSPLANTATION
Copyright © 1986 by The Williams & Wilkins Co.

Vol. 42, No. 5
Printed in U.S.A.

Transplantation
ARTICLES

RECOVERY OF GLOMERULAR AND TUBULAR FUNCTION IN AUTOTRANSPLANTED DOG KIDNEYS PRESERVED BY HYPOTHERMIC STORAGE OR MACHINE PERFUSION

RELATION OF INITIAL FUNCTION TO LONG-TERM FUNCTION[1]

CHRISTINE M. GREGG,[2] LOUIS R. COS,[3] PRADEEP SARAF,[3] CHARLOTTE W. FRIDD,[3] AND CHARLES A. LINKE[3,4]

Department of Biology, The Pennsylvania State University, University Park, Pennsylvania 16802; and Department of Urology, University of Rochester School of Medicine and Dentistry, Rochester, New York 14642

Sixteen male dogs had split renal function studies prior to unilateral nephrectomy and autotransplant. Kidneys were preserved for 24 hr by either simple hypothermic storage in Collins C2 solution (SHS) or machine-perfused (MP) on a Waters machine (MOX 100) with plasmanate perfusate. Renal function studies were repeated at 1 hr and at 7, 14, and 28 days, and the statistical relationship between initial and 1-month function was determined for a number of parameters. All MP kidneys functioned immediately, whereas ⅓ of SHS kidneys had delayed function. Recovery was more rapid in MP kidneys and was essentially complete by 14 days, at which time MP kidneys had higher rates of creatinine clearance and sodium reabsorption. However, by one month 3/7 MP kidneys ($P = 0.15$ compared with SHS) had lower creatinine clearance rates than at 2 weeks, and para-aminohippurate (PAH) clearance and fractional sodium reabsorption were significantly decreased. During the same period SHS kidneys either showed continued improvement or maintained stable function. Thus, by one month there were no differences between the groups in clearances of creatinine and PAH, plasma creatinine and blood urea nitrogen concentrations, or fractional reabsorption of sodium, potassium, and water. For SHS kidneys, the 1-hr creatinine clearance and the absolute rate of sodium reabsorption were strong predictors of the eventual function of the kidneys at one month (r = 0.93 and r = .83, $P<0.05$, respectively). No such correlations were found in MP kidneys (r = <.01, $P>0.9$ for both variables). The data show that MP results in significantly better function early after transplant, but this advantage does not persist, and that SHS kidneys early function is a good predictor of long-term recovery, but this is not true for MP kidneys.

Simple hypothermic storage is used by many hospitals to preserve kidneys prior to transplant. The composition of the preservation solution is critically important and evaluation of new or modified solutions is best done by assessing the long-term function of the transplanted organ. However, possible compositional modifications are numerous, and testing each in chronic studies is both expensive and impractical. It would be useful to know if there are any indices of renal function that could be measured shortly after transplant and that are well correlated with the long-term outcome. This would allow more efficient screening of new or modified preservation solutions.

Therefore, several parameters of glomerular and tubular function were measured before nephrectomy and again at 1 hr, 7 days, 14 days, and 28 days. Patterns of functional recovery were characterized at each time and the statistical relationship of initial function to 1-month function was determined for a number of variables. Two well-established preservation methods were used: simple hypothermic storage (SHS)* in Collins solution and machine perfusion (MP). Autotransplantation was used to preclude the problem of rejection, and animals were carefully followed clinically to verify that changes in function after transplant were not due to complications such as infection.

MATERIALS AND METHODS

Surgical procedures and infusions. Sixteen male dogs were premedicated with 1 mg atropine and anesthetized with pentobarbital. An i.v. hydrating solution of 2.5% dextrose in 0.45% saline was given 75 ml/hr throughout the procedure. A femoral artery cutdown was done in order to monitor blood pressure and for blood sampling. Priming doses of creatinine (125 mg/kg) and para-aminohippuric acid (PAH, 6.6 mg/kg) were given, followed by infusion of an isotonic maintenance solution containing 3.4 mg/ml creatinine, 0.6 mg/ml PAH, and 5% mannitol given at 0.3 ml/min/kg. Prior to opening the abdomen a bolus of 12.5 g of mannitol was given i.v. Both ureters were cannulated with No. 5 feeding tubes.

After 45 min of equilibration, renal function (see below) was measured separately in each kidney. The clearance infusion

[1] This work was supported by the Henry C. Buswell Fund for Urology Research.

[2] The Pennsylvania State University.

[3] University of Rochester School of Medicine and Dentistry.

[4] Address reprint requests to: Charles A. Linke, M.D., Department of Urology, Box 656, University of Rochester School of Medicine and Dentistry, 601 Elmood Avenue, Rochester, NY 14642.

* Abbreviations used: BUN, blood urea nitrogen; GFR, glomerular filtration rate; MP, machine-perfused; PAH, para-aminohippuric acid; SHS, simple hypothermic storage.

was discontinued and mannitol was infused at 12.5 g/hr until the renal artery was clamped. Left transperitoneal nephrectomy was done and the kidney was flushed with 250 ml Collins C2 solution from a height of 1 meter. Warm ischemia time for SHS and MP kidneys was 8±1 min and 6±2 min, respectively. Kidneys were preserved for 24 hr by SHS at 4°C in C2 solution or were perfused at 7°C with plasmanate perfusate and a Waters machine (MOX 100). Other details of the perfusion technique have been described previously (*1*).

After a contralateral transperitoneal nephrectomy, the preserved kidney was autotransplanted into the right iliac fossa using the iliac artery and vein. The Politano-Leadbetter technique (*2*) was used for the ureteroneocystostomy and a bladder hitch was also constructed. No ureteral stent or bladder drainage catheter was used. The kidney was kept chilled during the revascularization procedure.

Renal function studies. Renal function was measured separately for each kidney just prior to nephrectomy and in the transplanted kidney at 1 hr and at 7, 14, and 28 days. Posttransplant function was expressed as a percentage of the preharvest function for that same kidney. Parameters measured each time were: clearances of creatinine and PAH as well as the absolute and fractional reabsorption of sodium, glucose, potassium, and water. The mean of three successive clearance periods was used. Prior to nephrectomy clearance periods were 10 min, and after transplant, 20 min. The rate of infusion of the clearance solution was also decreased appropriately after transplant and increased as function recovered. Other routine laboratory tests were: complete blood count, blood urea nitrogen (BUN), plasma creatinine concentration, urinalysis, and urine osmolality.

Sodium reabsorption was quantified because approximately 90% of the energy production of the kidney is utilized to transport sodium from tubular fluid to blood and because the reabsorption of many other substances is linked to sodium reabsorption either directly or indirectly (*3, 4*). Since it is reabsorbed only in the proximal tubule (*4*), the presence of glycosuria in the absence of hyperglycemia is evidence of decreased proximal tubular transport capacity and/or increased tubular permeability (*5*).

Analytical techniques. Creatinine and PAH were measured on deproteinized samples of plasma and urine with a Technicon Autoanalyzer using the methods of Folin and Wu (*6*) and Bratton and Marshall (*7*), respectively. Glucose was determined with a Yellow Springs glucose analyzer, osmolality by freezing-point depression (Osmette osmometer), and sodium and potassium by flame photometry (Instrumentation Laboratories). Clearances and fractional reabsorption of water and electrolytes were calculated using standard formulas (*8*). Fractional reabsorption or excretion refers to the fraction (expressed as a percentage) of the filtered load of a substance (creatinine clearance rate × plasma concentration) that was reabsorbed or excreted.

Data analysis. Analysis of variance was used to test for differences between groups at any given point when the variances were similar. If variances were unequal (such as immediately after transplant when some kidneys did not function), the distribution-free Wilcoxon rank sum test was used as a substitute (*9*). When there were two variables of classification for the two groups (such as immediate versus delayed function). Fisher's exact test (*9*) was used. In order to relate early (1-hr) and late (1-month) function, values at each time were ranked and Spearman's rank order correlation coefficient was calculated (*9*). Standard parametric correlation coefficients between certain variables were also determined. Dogs were randomly assigned to the 2 groups and the function results were not known until the entire series was completed.

RESULTS

Absolute values for preharvest, initial (1-hr) and 1-month posttransplant function are summarized in Table 1. There were no differences prior to transplant. Two deaths occurred during the study due to intussusception and anesthesia. Since the deaths were not related to renal failure, all available data have been included. Bacteriuria was present at some point in about half the dogs in each group, but there were no major urinary tract infections or other surgical complications. All kidneys in both groups exhibited significant glycosuria (18–88 mg/dl) immediately after transplant, but never thereafter.

TABLE 1. Preharvest (control), initial (1–2 hr), and final (1 month) renal function in autotransplanted dog kidneys preserved by simple hypothermic storage (SHS) or machine perfusion (MP)

Time	Group	CR CL[a] (ml/min)	PAH CL (ml/min)	UFR (ml/min)	% Reabsorption		BW (kg)	KW (g)
					Na	H_2O		
Control	SHS	46.2	133	2.7	98.3	93.9	23.5	74.6
	(9)	±4.5	±10	±.3	±.3	±0.8	±2.1	±7.3
	MP	40.8	146	3.1	96.5	91.2	22.7	67.6
	(7)	±5.8	±18	±.1	±.8	±1.6	±1.4	±9.9
1–2 hr.	SHS	6.4	16	1.5	62.3	48.9	—	—
	(9)	±1.9	±4	±.5	±15.6	±15.7		
	MP	8.0	33[b]	1.8	93.8[c]	77.8[c]	—	—
	(7)	±.9	±7	±.3	±1.6	±5.2		
1 Month	SHS	37.0	129	2.8	96.6	90.6	22.9	92.9
	(7)	±6.6	±15	±.2	±1.4	±2.1	±2.2	±11.1
	MP	37.0	125	3.7	95.3	88.8	23.0	88.7
	(7)	±4.8	±15	±.3	±0.6	±1.7	±1.4	±6.3

Data are mean ± SEM. All rates are normalized to 100 g kidney weight (KW).

[a] Abbreviations not previously used: (CR CL) creatinine clearance rate; (UFR) urine flow rate; (BW) body weight.

[b] $P<0.05$ compared with SHS at the same time.

[c] $P<0.10$ compared with SHS at the same time.

Patterns of functional recovery. After transplant, all MP kidneys functioned immediately and urine flow averaged 1.8 ± 0.3 ml/min/100 g kidney weight. In contrast, 3/9 SHS kidneys ($P = 0.15$ compared with SHS) produced <1 ml of urine in the first 2 hr and had very low rates of creatinine clearance. Still, the group means for creatinine clearance were not different initially ($P = 0.45$, Table 1). Fractional sodium reabsorption tended to be higher in MP kidneys ($P = 0.06$, Table 1), and PAH clearance was almost 2-fold greater ($P<0.05$, Table 1). MP kidneys also had a much lower rate of fractional potassium excretion (73% ± 14% of the filtered load vs. 124% ± 8% for SHS, $P<0.05$).

Although renal function improved progressively in both groups (Figs. 1–3, MP kidneys recovered more rapidly. Serum creatinine levels were significantly lower after one week in MP kidneys (2.4 ± 0.3 for MP vs. 7.1 ± 2.2 for SHS kidneys, $P<0.05$), but not different thereafter. After two weeks of recovery, both creatinine clearance (Fig. 1) and the absolute rate of sodium reabsorption were higher in MP kidneys (Fig. 2). However, when the data were factored for the difference in filtered load, the fractional rates of sodium reabsorption (expressed as a percentage) were not different (98.6% ± 0.4% for MP and 95.5% ± 1.8% for SHS). PAH clearances for the two groups (Fig. 3) were also not different at any time other than at 1 hr (Table 1).

From 2 to 4 weeks posttransplant, some aspects of MP kidney function declined. Three of seven dogs had a decrease in creatinine clearance at 4 weeks compared with two weeks ($P = 0.15$ compared with SHS; Fisher's exact test). However, there was no difference in the mean values at two and four weeks in MP kidneys, primarily because one dog had a 48% increase in creatinine clearance during this same period. However, PAH clearance (Fig. 3) and fractional sodium reabsorption were lower at one month than at two weeks. Fractional sodium reabsorption was 98.6% ± 0.4% at two weeks and 95.3% ± 0.6% at one month ($P<0.05$).

In contrast, the function of SHS kidneys continued to improve from two to four weeks (Figs. 1–3). Thus, by one month

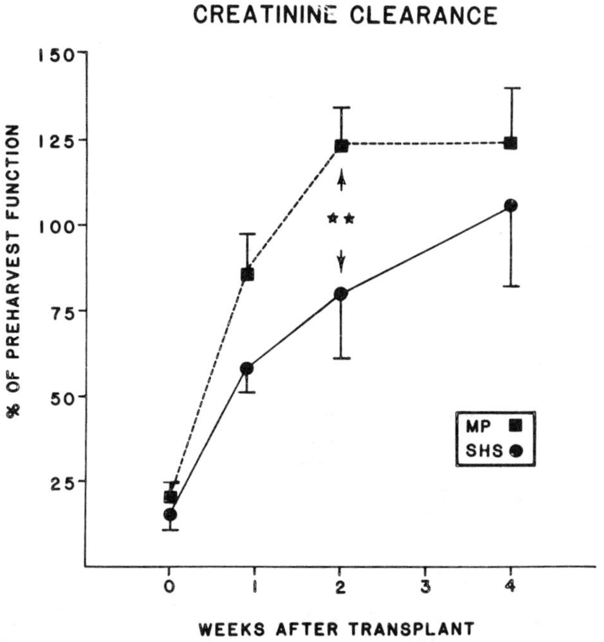

FIGURE 1. Posttransplant creatinine clearance rates expressed as a percentage of the preharvest value for the same kidney. (MP) machine perfused (n=7); (SHS) simple hypothermic storage (n=7); (**) $P<0.01$, SHS compared with MP at the same time.

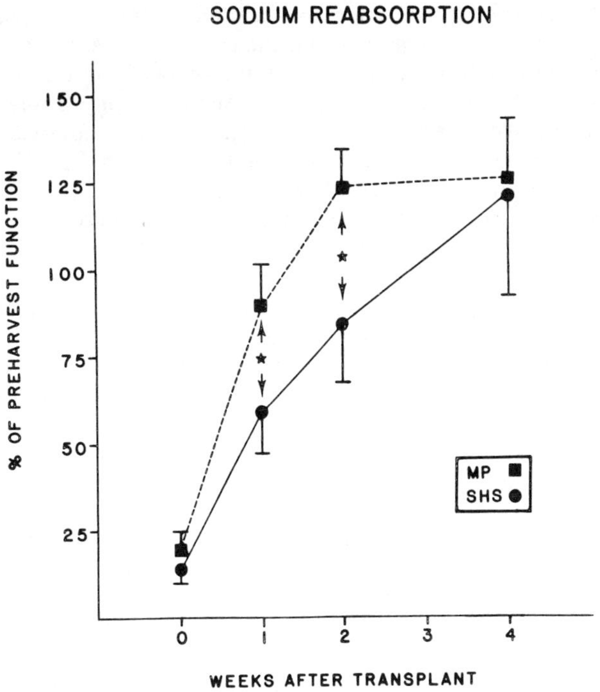

FIGURE 2. Rate of absolute sodium reabsorption after transplant expressed as a percentage of the preharvest value for the same kidney. (MP) machine perfused (n=7); (SHS) simple hypothermic storage (n=7); (*) $P<0.05$, SHS compared with MP at the same time.

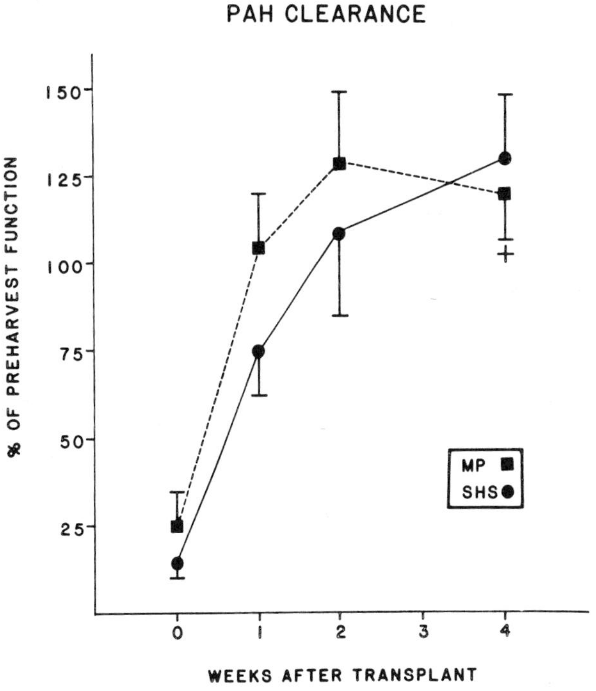

FIGURE 3. Posttransplant clearance rates for para-aminohippuric acid (PAH) expressed as a percentage of the preharvest value for the same kidney. (MP) machine perfused (n=7); (SHS) simple hypothermic storage (n=7); (+) value different from that of 2 weeks.

after transplant, there were no longer any differences between MP and SHS kidneys in the clearance rates of creatinine and PAH; urine flow rate; fractional reabsorption of sodium, potassium, and water; body weight; or kidney weight (Table 1). Plasma creatinine concentration and blood urea nitrogen levels were also very similar at that time (data not shown). Thus, although MP kidneys have better initial function, this advantage does not persist if SHS kidneys are given sufficient time to recover.

Relationship of initial function to final function. Results of the statistical correlation between 1-hr and 1-month function are shown in Table 2. MP kidneys had no significant relationships between initial and final ranks or absolute values for any of the several parameters measured. In contrast, SHS kidneys had a very high positive correlation (r = .93, $P<0.025$) between the rank values for initial and final creatinine clearances. This relationship was also present (r = .77, $P<0.05$) when actual creatinine clearance rates were used in the calculation. As expected, the initial absolute rate of sodium reabsorption was also highly predictive of the more long-term function (Table 2). Again, this was not true for MP kidneys, perhaps because of the decline in function from 2 to 4 weeks posttransplant that occurred in some of these kidneys.

Although there were also significant relationships for fractional reabsorption of sodium and water in SHS kidneys, this relationship did not appear to be quite as reliable, since the rank correlation was not strong (Table 2). The significance of the absolute correlation was largely due to two kidneys that had very low initial values. Although it may well be that a low rate of fractional sodium reabsorption 1–2 hr after transplant is a poor prognostic sign, our data are not strong enough to make that assertion with confidence. In a related study we did find that fractional sodium reabsorption 1–2 hr after transplant was markedly decreased in kidneys subjected to 30 min of warm ischemia prior to preservation (*10*). However, after a few days of recovery, fractional sodium reabsorption in this study was not a good index of eventual recovery since it was high and quite constant after one week—even in kidneys with the lowest rates of creatinine clearance and absolute sodium reabsorption. Thus, for kidneys preserved by SHS, the initial creatinine clearance and the absolute rate of sodium reabsorption were the best predictors (in the absence of other complications) of the ultimate function of the transplanted kidney. More data are required before concluding that initial fractional sodium reabsorption is also a useful predictor, but results with SHS-preserved kidneys in this study are consistent with that possibility.

Since creatinine clearance was a useful marker, we also determined what other variables were best correlated with the creatinine clearance rate (Table 3). For this analysis, all values from 1 hr to 1 month were used and each group was examined separately. As expected, there were many significant correlations, but two were much better than the others independent of the preservation method (Table 3). The absolute rate of sodium reabsorption was almost perfectly correlated with the creatinine clearance rate and the urine osmolality also had quite a strong positive relationship. Kidneys with very low initial function almost invariably had hypotonic urine (Fig. 4), but after one week of recovery both groups were able to form hypertonic urine.

TABLE 2. Correlation of initial function with 1-month function for various parameters of renal function in autotranplanted kidneys preserved for 24 hr by simple hypothermic storage (SHS) or machine perfusion (MP)

Variable	Rank correlation		Absolute correlation	
	SHS (7)	MP (7)	SHS (7)	MP (7)
CR CL	.93[b]	<.10	.77[c]	.12
PAH CL	.50	.64	.62	−.35
UFR	.32	<.10	.46	−.20
Na R	.83[c]	<.10	.68	.01
% Na R[a]	.61	−.78	.89[d]	−.45
% H_2O R	.50	.35	.79[c]	−.26
% K EX	.36	<.10	.68	.01

Values are the correlation coefficient (r). Number of pairs is (n).

[a] % = fractional reabsorption (R) or excretion (EX) of sodium (Na) and potassium (K); higher values for r are required for significance when the rank correlation coefficient is used.

[b] $P<0.025$.

[c] $P<0.05$.

[d] $P<0.001$; see the *Results* section for qualification.

DISCUSSION

Recovery of both glomerular and tubular function was more rapid in MP kidneys, and function in this group was clearly superior at two weeks posttransplant. Other workers have also reported that early function is superior in MP kidneys for 1–2 weeks after transplant (*1, 11*). However, after one month of recovery, there were no longer any systematic differences in function. This result was also seen by Kraemer et al. (*1*), but only glomerular filtration rate was measured in that study. In both our groups, recovery of tubular reabsorption of sodium closely paralleled recovery of glomerular filtration rate (GFR).

TABLE 3. Correlation of various parameters of renal function with the rate of creatinine clearance in autotransplanted kidneys preserved for 24 hr by simple hypothermic storage (SHS) or machine perfusion (MP)[a]

	Na R	% Na R	UFR	Uosm[c]	[Na]u[d]	[K]u
SHS (24)	.99[b]	.38	.70[b]	.79[b]	.41	−.28
MP (28)	.99[b]	.39	.48	.78[b]	.57	−.01

[a] Values are the correlation coefficient (r). The number of pairs is (n). All values in both groups except [K]u are significant at $P < 0.05$.

[b] Correlations significant at $P < 0.0001$.

[c] (Uosm) urine osmolality.

[d] ([ ]u) urinary concentration.

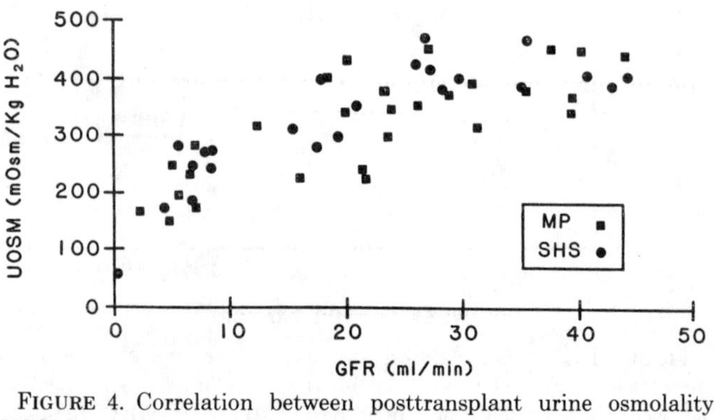

FIGURE 4. Correlation between posttransplant urine osmolality (UOSM) and the rate of creatinine clearance (GFR). R=.79 and r=.78 ($P<0.0001$) for SHS and MP, respectively.

The correlation between GFR and the absolute rate of sodium reabsorption was identical for kidneys preserved by either technique (r = 0.99, $P<0.001$). This was to be expected since both GFR and the absolute rate of reabsorption increased together, while the fractional reabsorption remained high and virtually constant after the first week. Functional recovery in this model is probably essentially complete at one month, since Kraemer et al. (*1*) observed no further improvement in clearances of creatinine or inulin from 30 to 60 days in autotransplanted dog kidneys preserved by either SHS or MP.

A major purpose of this work was to discover if there were any parameters of initial renal function that could be used to predict the eventual performance of the graft (assuming no unrelated complications supervened). Of the several parameters of glomerular and tubular function measured, only creatinine clearance and the absolute rate of sodium reabsorption were highly predictive of later performance. This is not surprising since both are primary activities of the kidney and most aspects of renal function are directly or indirectly coupled to the rate of sodium reabsorption (*3, 4*). What was unexpected was that there were not similar correlations between initial and final function in MP kidneys.

The failure to find any useful predictors for MP kidneys may be due to the fact that the function of MP kidneys was less variable. That is to say, there was not as wide a range of initial and final values as was present in SHS kidneys. Correlations were best exposed when there is a relatively wide range of values for both variables. Second, some aspects of MP function decreased from 2 to 4 weeks posttransplant, so that there was poor correlation between initial and final ranks. It should be said that despite the small decreases, final function was still excellent in all MP kidneys at one month. Therefore, the interpretation of the lack of correlation between initial and final function is not easily made. It may be that the small decline in function is a harbinger of some slowly developing pathological change related to the perfusion process (*12*), or it may simply mean that function has stabilized after a condition of relative hyperemia which was present at two weeks. Other studies will be required to clarify whether the apparent decline in function is biologically significant. The purpose of this work was not to demonstrate the superiority of one preservation method over another, but rather to observe whether improved early function with a new or modified SHS preservation solution is a reasonable basis for proceeding to chronic survival studies.

It may be argued by some that in humans kidneys with excellent initial function may ultimately fail. However, rejection and/or other complications may account in large part for the apparent lack of relationship between early and late function in some human studies. Other workers (*13, 14*) have reported that there is a significant correlation between initial and eventual renal function in humans transplanted with cadaver kidneys. Whenever animal models that minimize or control for the problem of rejection are used, there is a clear relationship between immediate and long-term function in kidneys preserved by SHS. That is, the early (1–2 hr after transplant) creatinine or inulin clearance rate is consistently lower in kidneys damaged by warm ischemia (*10, 15, 16*), and/or by preservation techniques known to produce poor long-term results. These include prolonged storage by SHS (*17, 18*), or the use of different preservation solutions and/or pharmacological additives (*18–21*). For example, in our laboratory when the sodium and potassium concentrations of Collins solution were reversed (i.e. high sodium-low potassium), initial creatinine clearance was decreased by an additional 60–70% (unpublished results).

We conclude that in SHS-preserved kidneys both the initial creatinine clearance and the absolute rate of sodium reabsorption are excellent indices of the degree of recovery of renal function to be anticipated (assuming no complications supervene). Thus, improved early function provides a strong rationale for proceeding to the essential and costly chronic survival studies that are required to demonstrate unequivocally the superiority of one method over another. Although improved early function in MP kidneys may also be indicative of better long-term recovery, our data do not permit that conclusion.

Acknowledgments. We thank the late Dominic Femiano, Rose Sanders, and Susan Schoen for their excellent technical assistance.

REFERENCES

1. Kraemer GK, Panner BJ, Linke CA. Bilateral cervical transplantation of canine kidneys for study of canine renal preservation. Urology 1976; 8: 352.
2. Politano VA, Leadbetter WF. An operative technique for the correction of vesicoureteral reflux. J Urol 1958; 79: 932.
3. Weinstein AM, Windhager EE. Sodium transport along the proximal tubule. In: Seldin DW, Giebisch G, eds. The kidney: physiology and pathophysiology. New York: Raven Press, 1985: 1033.
4. Hierholzer K. Sodium reabsorption in the distal tubular system. In: Seldin DW, Giebisch G, eds. The kidney: physiology and pathophysiology. New York: Raven Press, 1985: 1063.
5. Small A, Bell RT, Filo RS. Abnormal tubular permeability in hypothermic perfused kidneys. J Appl Physiol 1975; 38: 615.
6. Folin O, Wu H. A system of blood analysis. J Biol Chem 1919; 38: 81.
7. Bratton AC, Marshall EK Jr. A new coupling component for sulfanilamide determination. J Biol Chem 1938; 128: 537.
8. Sullivan LP, Grantham JJ. Physiology of the kidney. Philadelphia: Lea & Febiger, 1982: 41.
9. Steel RGD, Torrie JH. Principles and procedures of statistics. New York: McGraw-Hill, 1962: 358.
10. Lai MK, Mandour WA, Gregg CM, Linke CA. Inosine pretreatment in canine renal preservation. Transplantation 1979; 28: 261.
11. Small A, Feduska NJ, Leapman SB. Function of autotransplanted kidneys after 24-hour preservation by hypothermic pulsatile perfusion or simple cold storage. Transplantation 1978; 26: 228.
12. Opelz G, Terasaki PI. Advantage of cold storage over machine perfusion for preservation of cadaver kidneys. Transplantation 1982; 33: 64.
13. Davidson JM, Uldall PR, Ross Taylor RM. Relation of immediate posttransplant renal function to long-term function in cadaver kidney recipients. Transplantation 1977; 23: 310.
14. Opelz G, Sasaki N, Terasaki PI. Prediction of long-term kidney transplant survival by monitoring early graft function and clinical grades. Transplantation 1978; 25: 212.
15. Noble MJ, Magnusson MO, Stowe NT, Novick AC, Straffon RA. Preservation of ischemically damaged canine kidneys: cold storage versus perfusion. Invest Urol 1980; 17: 503.
16. Denham BS, Linke CA, Fridd CW. Twenty-four hour canine renal preservation by pulsatile perfusion, hypothermic storage, and combinations of the two methods. Transplant Proc 1977; 9: 1553.
17. Grundmann R, Strumper R, Eichmann J, Pichlmaier H. The immediate function of the kidney after 24- to 72-hour preservation. Transplantation 1977; 23: 437.
18. Fischer JH, Knupfer P, Beyer M. Flush solution 2, a new concept for one- to three-day hypothermic storage preservation. Transplantation 1985; 39: 122.

19. Khuri FJ, Panner B, Linke CA, Cockett ATK. Comparison of Sacks II solution and modified Collins solution (Ursol) in simple cold preservation of canine kidneys. J Surg Res 1975; 19: 361.
20. Rashid HA, Panner BJ, Linke CA. Effect of pharmacological doses of methylprednisolone on preservation of renal function. J Surg Res 1975; 18: 21.
21. Howden B, Rae D, Jablonski P, Marshall VC, Tange J. Studies of renal preservation using a rat kidney transplant model: evaluation of citrate flushing. Transplantation 1983; 35: 311.

Received 12 December 1985.
Accepted 27 January 1986.

0041-1337/86/4205-0458$02.00/0
TRANSPLANTATION

Vol. 42, No. 5
Printed in U.S.A.

EARLY INDICES OF WARM ISCHEMIC DAMAGE IN AUTOTRANSPLANTED CANINE KIDNEYS PRESERVED BY SIMPLE HYPOTHERMIC STORAGE[1]

CHRISTINE M. GREGG,[2] MING K. LAI,[3] W. ANTHONY MANDOUR,[3] AND CHARLES A. LINKE[3,4]

Department of Biology, The Pennsylvania State University, University Park, Pennsylvania 16802; Department of Urology, University of Rochester School of Medicine and Dentistry, Rochester, New York 14642

After measurement of normal renal function, dog kidneys (n = 52) were subjected to 3, 15, or 30 min of normothermic warm ischemia (WI). After 24 hr of preservation by simple hypothermic storage (SHS) in a modified Collins solution, autotransplant was done and renal function was again measured beginning at 1 hr. Compared with preharvest values, kidneys with minimal (3 min) WI had (1) significantly decreased clearances of creatinine (Cr) and para-aminohippuric acid (PAH), PAH extraction, absolute and fractional Na reabsorption, Na excretion, and urinary Na concentration; (2) no change in urine flow rate or K excretion; and (3) significantly increased fractional excretion of Na, K, and H_2O. Compared with minimal WI, 30-min WI produced further significant decreases in clearances of Cr, PAH, and PAH extraction; and further increases in fractional excretion of Na, K, and H_2O. Urine flow was also decreased by about half and urine Na concentration rose significantly. Several parameters were very significantly correlated with the length of WI, but the most reliable index was the fractional reabsorption of Na. When several functional parameters were used together, kidneys with significant (30 min) WI prior to preservation could be identified with a high degree of statistical reliability.

The use of cyclosporine in kidney transplant recipients has increased markedly in recent years. However, the nephrotoxic properties of this drug are well-known, and close monitoring is essential when renal function is compromised. The diagnosis of early graft failure is often difficult since there are several potential causes of anuria or oliguria. Ischemic acute tubular necrosis is always a potential problem since known or unknown episodes of normothermic ischemia may occur in cadaver donors. It would be useful to have statistically reliable criteria that would permit identification of kidneys with significant warm ischemic damage shortly after transplant. Such knowledge should permit more intelligent management of the immunosuppressive regimen.

In order to discover if there were functional criteria that would clearly identify kidneys with significant warm ischemic damage, we measured several parameters of glomerular and tubular function in normal and ischemically damaged kidneys starting 1 hr after transplant. Prior to transplant, all kidneys were preserved for 24 hr by simple hypothermic storage (SHS) in order to simulate a reasonable clinical situation. Autotransplant was used to circumvent problems of rejection. Changes in function were correlated with the length of warm ischemia (WI)* and the results were compared with published data obtained in patients experiencing known acute rejection (*1*).

The data show that many aspects of glomerular and tubular function are impaired by simple hypothermic storage (SHS), and that several of these functional changes were highly correlated with the length of WI prior to preservation. By combining several parameters, the damaged kidneys could be identified statistically with a probability of >99%.

MATERIALS AND METHODS

Mongrel dogs of either sex (n = 26) weighing 20.4±1.1 kg were premedicated with atropine 1 mg and Innovar Vet (fentanyl and droperidal) 0.1 ml/kg. Anesthesia was induced with i.v. sodium pentobarbital 10 mg/kg supplemented as necessary. Ringer's lactate was given i.v. at 75 ml/hr throughout, since pilot studies showed that there was substantial insensible water

[1] This work was supported by the Henry C. Buswell Fund for Urology Research.
[2] The Pennsylvania State University.
[3] University of Rochester School of Medicine and Dentistry.
[4] Address reprint requests to Charles A. Linke, M.D., Department of Urology, University of Rochester School of Medicine and Dentistry, 601 Elmwood Avenue, Rochester, NY 14642.

* Abbreviations used: GFR, glomerular filtration rate; PAH, paraaminohippuric acid; RPF, renal plasma flow; SHS, simple hypothermic storage; UFR, urine flow rate; WI, warm ischemia.

loss during this procedure. The femoral artery was cannulated to obtain blood samples and for measurement of mean arterial pressure (Sanborn 267 transducer and 269 recorder). Mannitol 12.5 g i.v. was given as a bolus prior to laparotomy and then infused continuously at 12.5 g/hr until nephrectomy was completed. Priming doses of creatinine and sodium para-aminohippuric acid (PAH) were followed by a maintenance infusion containing creatinine 3.4 mg/ml and PAH 0.6 mg/ml in 0.9% NaCl (0.3 ml/kg/min). Both ureters were cannulated so individual kidney function could be measured.

After 45 min of equilibration, clearances of creatinine and PAH were measured during two 10-min periods, and the values were averaged. Plasma samples were taken at the midpoint of each period. Sodium (Na) and potassium (K) handling were also quantified. Following the clearance measurements, the infusion of PAH and creatinine was discontinued.

Kidneys were subjected to minimal (2–3 min), 15 min, or 30 min of warm ischemia (WI). This was done by completely mobilizing the kidney and ureter, severing all blood vessels, and leaving the kidney in the abdominal cavity for the specified period. Both kidneys were subjected to the same period of warm ischemia. Dogs were randomly assigned to groups, and the order of kidney harvest (right or left kidney removed first) and the order of reimplantation were also randomized. Kidneys were promptly immersed in chilled (4°C) 0.9% saline, flushed from a height of 1 meter with 250 ml of cold (4°C) Ursol (*2*) without methylprednisolone, and stored cold for 24 hr. After nephrectomy animals were left with a positive fluid balance of about 300 ml to reduce dehydration from insensible water loss in case they did not drink spontaneously.

The next day, both kidneys were autotransplanted into the neck after the method of Kraemer et al. (*3*), excluding the formation of a skin pouch. Briefly, this technique involves end-to-end anastomosis of the renal artery to the common carotid artery, and the renal vein to the external jugular vein. During the entire anastomosis the kidneys were kept immersed in an ice slush of 0.9% saline. Revascularization required 30–40 min/kidney. All vascular clamps were removed at the same time so that recirculation began simultaneously. Because of initial bleeding from the anastomosic site, 5 animals required transfusion of whole blood and/or additional amounts of Ringer's lactate in order to maintain blood pressure. These animals were distributed among the three groups (2: minimal WI; 1: 15-min WI; and 2: 30-min WI).

At 1 hr after unclamping, split-kidney function was measured during three 20-min periods and the values were averaged. Preparation of the dog was identical to the preharvest procedure except that the maintenance infusion of PAH and creatinine was decreased to 0.075 ml/kg/min because pilot studies showed clearance of both substances to be decreased after kidney preservation and transplant. Blood samples were also taken from the femoral artery and both renal veins to permit measurement of PAH extraction and calculation of RPF. The blood was immediately cooled and centrifuged and the plasma was promptly removed.

Chemical analyses. Concentrations of PAH and creatinine were measured in deproteinized samples of urine and plasma using a Technicon Autoanalyzer and an automation of the methods of Folin and Wu (*4*), and Bratton and Marshall (*5*), respectively. Na and K were measured in plasma and urine by flame photometry (Instrumentation Laboratories, Model 343) using lithium as the internal standard.

Calculations. Clearances of creatinine and PAH and fractional handling of water and electrolytes were calculated using the usual formulas (*6*). Glomerular filtration rate (GFR) was considered to be equal to the clearance of creatinine. The percentage of extraction of PAH by each kidney was calculated as: $([RA_{PAH} - RV_{PAH}]/RA_{PAH}) \times 100\%$, where RA_{PAH} and RV_{PAH} are the renal arterial and renal venous plasma concentrations of PAH, respectively. Following transplantation, the renal plasma flow (RPF) was estimated by the formula: $(U_{PAH} \times UFR)/(RA_{PAH} - RV_{PAH})$, where U_{PAH} is the urinary concentration of PAH, UFR is the urine flow rate, and the other symbols are as previously given. Fractional reabsorption or excretion of a substance refers to the fraction of the filtered load (GFR × plasma concentration) reabsorbed or excreted. UFR/GFR was used to calculate fractional water handling.

Statistical analysis. The paired *t* test was used to compare preharvest and posttransplant function in the same kidney. One-way analysis of variance and the Scheffe test (*7*) were used to detect differences either before or after transplant among the three groups (minimal, 15-min, or 30-min WI). Calculation of correlation coefficients and linear regression analysis was done using standard techniques; n is the number of kidneys unless otherwise specified. The data were not factored for dog weight since this was similar in all groups (21 ± 2, 20.5 ± 1.8 and 19.6 ± 1.8 kg for minimal, 15-min, and 30-min WI, respectively).

RESULTS

Data are mean ± SEM and all differences mentioned hereafter are significant at $P<0.05$ unless stated otherwise. Absolute values for preharvest function are shown in Table 1 and the

TABLE 1. Effect of prepreservation warm ischemia (WI) on initial posttransplant function in kidneys preserved for 24 hr by simple hypothermic storage

Parameter	Minimal WI (n=16)		15-min WI (n=14)		30-min WI (n=22)	
	Before[a]	After	Before	After	Before	After
Cr Cl	34.5	8.8[e]	34.9	7.8[e]	28.4	4.2[e,f,g]
(ml/min)[b]	±2.9	±.7	±2.4	±.7	±2.2	±.5
PAH Cl	114	32.1[e]	123	29.1[e]	111	12.6[e,f,g]
(ml/min)	±5	±3.8	±8	±4.9	±7	±2.3
PAH Cl/Cr Cl	3.6	3.7	3.7	3.6	4.0	2.8[e]
	±.2	±.4	±.2	±.3	±.2	±.2
UFR (ml/min)	4.0	3.4	5.0	3.8	4.9	2.7[e]
	±.3	±.3	±.4	±.4	±.3	±.3
UFR/CrCl	86.9	61.4[e]	85.1	46.5[e,f]	81.1	35.0[e,f]
	±1.3	±1.2	±1.1	±3.6	±1.3	±2.9
Na Reab.	4481	938[e]	4885	871[e]	3914	222[e,f]
(μEq/min)	±437	±165	±671	±88	±762	±46
% Na Reab.[c]	91.8	85.6[e]	92.5	77.6[e]	92.7	34.1[e,f,g]
	±0.5	±1.0	±1.2	±4.9	±1.7	±6.0
K Excr.[d]	67.0	59.0	43.0	75.0[e]	29.0	42.0[e]
(μEq/min)	±3.0	±7.0	±7.0	±4.0	±6.0	±9.0
% K Excr.	57.1	134[e]	33.3	174[e,f]	37.7	182[e,f]
	±4.3	±3	±6.2	±12	±8.2	±12

[a] (Before) preharvest value; (after) initial postransplant value.
[b] (Cr Cl) creatinine clearance rate.
[c] (% Reabsorption) fraction of the filtered load that was reabsorbed ×100%.
[d] Groups significantly different prior to transplant.
[e] Different from preharvest, $P<0.05$.
[f] Different from minimal WI, $P<0.05$.
[g] Different from 15-min WI, $P<0.05$.

posttransplant functions, expressed as a percentage of preharvest are in Table 2. There were no differences prior to transplant except for absolute and fractional K excretion (Tables 1 and 2).

Effects of cold ischemia alone. At 1–2 hr after transplant, clearances of PAH and creatinine were both about 28% of preharvest values (Table 2, Fig. 1, A and C). The percentage of PAH extraction was markedly reduced from 85–90% before nephrectomy to 14.4%±2.2% after transplant. Urine flow rate (Fig. 1B) was unchanged, but a much smaller fraction of the total glomerular filtrate was reabsorbed. Fractional water reabsorption was only 71%±2% of preharvest levels, even at the greatly reduced GFR (Table 2, Fig. 1A).

Although fractional Na reabsorption appeared to be only slightly lower (93.3% ± 1.0% of preharvest), the absolute rate of Na reabsorption was markedly impaired (21.5%±2% of preharvest). Urine Na concentration fell significantly (from 78.5± 6.4 mEq/L to 52.6±3.1 mEq/L) after transplantation, and urinary Na excretion was less than half the preharvest value (41.4% ± 6.1%). In contrast, fractional excretion of potassium rose markedly (Fig. 2A) and there was net K secretion. However, the absolute rate of potassium excretion was slightly but not significantly lower then preharvest (89%±10%, Fig. 2B). Potassium excretion/ml of GFR thus increased from 2.0 ± 0.2 μEq/min to 7.1±0.2 μEq/min.

In summary, the effects of cold ischemia alone were: (1) decreases in clearances of creatinine and PAH, percentage of PAH extraction, absolute and fractional Na and H_2O reabsorption, and urine Na concentration; (2) no change in urine flow and absolute K excretion; and (3) significant increases in fractional K excretion and urinary K concentration.

Effects of warm and cold ischemia. Warm ischemia for 15 min produced a number of additional small changes, but most of these were not significant when compared with the minimal ischemia group (Fig. 1, Table 2). The exceptions were a substantial further fall in the percentage of PAH extraction (Fig. 1D) and a substantial rise in both fractional and absolute K excretion (Fig. 2). Absolute K excretion was approximately double the preharvest value (Table 2). Both absolute and fractional rates of Na reabsorption tended to be decreased by 15 min of ischemia but not significantly so (Table 2). Urine flow was unchanged (Fig. 1B).

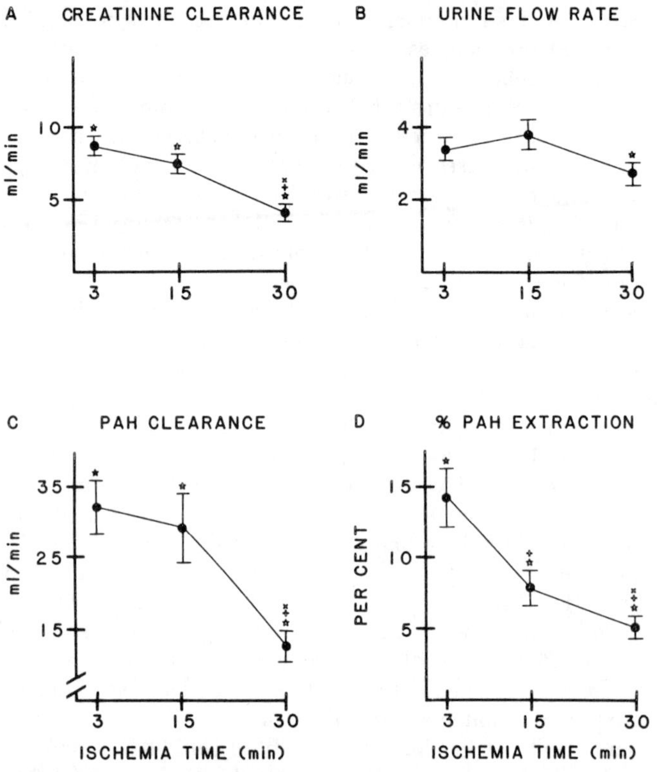

FIGURE 1. Initial (1-hr) posttransplant renal function in kidneys subjected to minimal (3 min), 15-min, or 30-min normothermic ischemia prior to 24 hr of cold storage in a modified Collins' solution. (*) significantly different from preharvest ($P<0.05$); (+) significantly different from minimal warm ischemia (WI) ($P<0.05$); (x) significantly different from 15-min WI.

TABLE 2. Posttransplant renal function expressed as a percentage of the preharvest value

Parameter	Warm ischemia time		
	Minimal (n=16)	15-min (n=14)	30-min (n=22)
Cr Cl	27.8[c] ±2.6	22.9[c] ±2.6	16.7[c,d] ±2.1
PAH Cl	28.4[c] ±3.0	24.8[c] ±4.4	12.5[c,d,e] ±2.1
UFR	90.3 ±9.1	80.7 ±9.9	55.9[c,d,e] ±5.9
UFR/CrCl	71.2[c] ±2.4	54.6[c,d] ±4.2	41.7[c,d,e] ±4.0
Na R	21.5[c] ±2.0	18.9[c] ±2.2	7.7[c,d,e] ±2.2
Fx Na R[a]	93.3[c] ±1.0	83.7[c] ±4.1	48.5[c,d] ±6.0
Na E	41.4[c] ±6.9	69.9 ±17.4	104.0 ±21.0
K E[b]	88.5 ±10.0	209.0[c,d] ±44.0	145.0[c,d] ±7.0
Fx K E[a]	267.0[c] ±18.0	611.0[c,d] ±98.0	835.0[c,d] ±257.0

[a] Fx = fraction of filtered load reabsorbed (R) or excreted (E).
[b] Groups significantly different prior to transplant.
[c] Different from preharvest, $p < 0.05$.
[d] Different from minimal warm ischemia, $p < 0.05$.
[e] Different from 15 min warm ischemia, $p < 0.05$.

Thirty minutes of WI produced additional marked changes in function, some of which were significant even when compared with 15 min of ischemia (Table 2). Specifically, clearances of creatinine (Fig. 1A), PAH (Fig. 1C), and percentage of PAH extraction (Fig. 1D) were all further reduced compared with 15 min WI. The absolute urine flow rate (Fig. 1B) also decreased from 15 min to 30 min WI so that urine flow was less than preharvest in this group alone. When expressed as a percentage of preharvest (Table 2) urine flow in the 30-min WI group was lower than in the minimal WI kidneys. Even so, urine flow was still quite good.

Figure 2A shows that fractional excretion of Na, water and K all rose as the period of warm ischemia increased. As expected, the effect for Na and water is clearly proportional to the length of warm ischemia. Absolute Na excretion (Fig. 2B) also increased progressively with ischemia. In the 30-min WI group, the rate of Na excretion was equal to preharvest levels (Fig. 2B) even though the filtered load was less than 20% of the normal value (Table 2). After 30 min WI the urine Na concentration was also significantly higher (63±9 mEq/L preharvest vs. 89±6 mEq/L after transplant).

The analysis of K excretion patterns was complicated by

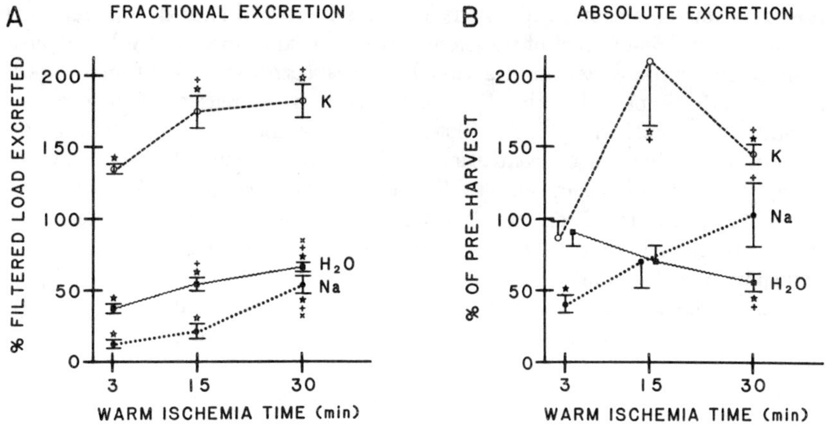

FIGURE 2. Excretion of Na, K, and H_2O as a function of WI time. Fractional excretion is the percentage of the filtered load excreted. Absolute excretion is the mass or volume excreted each minute expressed as the percentage of the preharvest value for that same kidney. (*) significantly different from preharvest ($P<0.05$); (+) significantly different from minimal warm ischemia (WI) ($P<0.05$); (x) significantly different from 15-min WI.

variation among the groups during the preharvest period. However, some differences were clear, such as the change from net reabsorption in control periods to net secretion after transplant. However, the increase in absolute (Table 2, Fig. 2B) and fractional K excretion (Fig. 2A) appeared to be maximal after 15-min WI. The rate of K excretion/ml GFR tended to increase as a function of warm ischemia time but there was no significant difference between the 15-min and 30-min WI groups (data not shown).

There were also differences between the groups in the time it took to flush the kidneys with 250 ml preservation solution. The flush time for kidneys with 30-min WI was higher than that seen with minimal WI (27±2 min vs. 17±2 min, $P<0.005$).

TABLE 3. Linear regression analysis of selected parameters as a function of warm ischemia time

Parameter	n[a]	r	Slope ± SE	Intercept ± SE	P
Cr Cl	52	−0.62	−2.3±0.4	32±3	<.0001
Na R	18	−0.75	−27.5±6.0	1125±116	<.0001
% Na R	18	−0.83	−1.5±0.2	92±5	<.000025
UFR/ Cr Cl	52	−0.69	−1.5±0.2	69±4	<.0001
Flush time[b]	40	+0.57	0.36±0.09	15.5±2.0	<.0002

[a] (n) = number of kidneys; (r) correlation coefficient; (P) significance of regression; see Table 1 for other abbreviations.

[b] (flush time) minutes to flush 250 ml preservation solution through kidney.

DISCUSSION

The data show that many aspects of glomerular and tubular function are significantly decreased by 24 hr of simple hypothermic preservation—most notably clearances of creatinine and PAH, percentage of PAH extraction, and sodium and water reabsorption. Subsequent studies (Gregg et al., manuscript in preparation) have revealed that after 24 hr of hypothermic storage, glucose reabsorption is also markedly impaired, the urine is isotonic to plasma (even in the presence of high levels of antidiuretic hormone), and protein excretion is increased 10-fold. Thus, these kidneys have most of the clinical symptoms of acute tubular necrosis, with the possible exception that renal blood flow may not be markedly reduced. Calculation of RPF (see the *Materials and Methods* section) gave values of 203±28 ml/min, 228±18 ml/min, and 216±19 ml/min for minimal, 15-min, and 30-min WI, respectively, all of which are significantly higher than preharvest. It should be realized that the error in calculating RPF may be substantial because of the low extraction rate for PAH (Fig. 1D), so that these values should be used advisedly. Even so, if the error were as great as 100% (which is unlikely), RPF would still calculate to be about 100 ml/min in each group. Another point that is evident from the data is that clearance of PAH is a very poor estimator of RPF in transplanted kidneys. Estimation of RPF by clearance of PAH assumes a high extraction for PAH, but our data clearly show that there is a dramatic reduction in this parameter after transplant.

With warm ischemia prior to SHS, many additional changes were observed. Linear regression analysis was used to determine which parameters were most closely related to the duration of WI time (Table 3). Although all the variables listed were significantly correlated with the length of WI, some had much less variability (reflected by a higher value for r), and were therefore more reliable indices of ischemic damage. Taken together, the data indicate that kidneys with significant WI damage prior to SHS could be statistically distinguished from kidneys with minimal ischemia with a high degree of confidence. Of kidneys with 30-min WI, 99% had the following characteristics:

1. Creatinine clearance <5.5 ml/min
2. Na reabsorption <341 μEq/min
3. Fractional Na reabsorption <61%
4. Fractional water reabsorption <43%
5. Flush time >22 min (for 250 ml at a height of 1 meter).

Clearance of exogenous creatinine was fairly well correlated with WI time, but it was not the most sensitive index of damage. Over 90% of dogs with minimal WI had GFR of 6.4 ml/min or above, whereas less than 10% of dogs with 30-min WI had clearances that high. The absolute rate of sodium reabsorption was also a fairly good index, but this variable is highly dependent on the GFR. The percentage of PAH extraction was a very sensitive indicator of WI damage, in that it decreased dramatically (compared with minimal WI) WI after only 15 min (Fig. 1D). However, there was little further change from 15 to 30 min, so that it was not well correlated with the WI time. UFR per se was also not a particularly sensitive index of ischemic damage since it was little affected (Table 2) until 30 min WI. UFR was most useful when combined with other factors. For example, a low UFR (<2 ml/min) coupled with a urine sodium of 70 mEq or above was highly characteristic of kidneys with significant WI damage.

The fractional rate of Na reabsorption was clearly the best index of ischemic damage (Table 3). This has also been demonstrated using an isolated perfused rat kidney (*8*) subjected to variable periods of warm ischemia (but not hypothermic perservation). The progressively larger fractional water excretion that was also prominent as the WI time increased is an inevitable accompaniment of the increased solute excretion.

As might be predicted, as fractional Na reabsorption was progressively impaired, urine Na concentration increased steadily ($r = -0.97$, $n = 18$, $P<.000001$). In the kidneys with 30 min WI, urine Na concentration was always at least 70 mEq/L. One would expect that at a low filtered load, urine Na should be low if tubular reabsorptive mechanisms are relatively intact and high if there is extensive tubular damage to both transport processes and membrane permeability. This prediction is supported by the report that after 2 hr of WI, rats had an extremely low GFR, and urine Na concentrations were approximately equal to plasma (*9*).

The signs of WI-induced acute tubular necrosis that we observed differ in several respects from those reported to accompany acute renal failure induced by rejection (*1*). The earliest retrospective signs of acute rejection involved changes in Na handling that were present even before a measurable rise in serum creatinine (*1*). Differences in renal function during acute rejection and ischemia-induced acute tubular necrosis are summarized in Table 4. The most characteristic differences are found in the handling of Na. Ischemia-induced acute tubular necrosis was associated with a high fractional (and absolute) rate of Na excretion, and urine Na concentration was relatively high, whereas the reverse was true during acute rejection.

In summary, the data indicate that there are characteristic changes in renal function that occur after various periods of WI. Cadaver kidneys displaying all the aforementioned functional criteria within 1 to 2 hr after transplantation are highly likely to have significant warm ischemic damage, particularly if functional changes due to accumulation of toxic substances in the donor can be ruled out. Advance knowledge of such warm ischemic damage should permit more intelligent clinical management.

TABLE 4. Summary of functional changes in transplanted kidneys after 30 min of warm ischemia (WI) prior to preservation and during acute rejection[a, b]

Parameter	30-min WI	Acute rejection[a]
Cr Cl[a]	↓	↓
RPF	↑ or no change	↓
F_xE Na	↑	↓
$[Na]_u$	>70 mEq/L	<20 mEq/L
UFR	↓	↓

[a] SOURCE: (*1*).
[b] See Tables 1 and 2 for abbreviations.

Acknowledgments. We thank the late Dominic Femiano, Charlotte Fridd, Fred Norway, and Rose Sanders for this expert technical assistance.

REFERENCES

1. Hong CD, Kapoor BS, First MR, Pollak VE, Alexander JW. Fractional excretion of Na after renal transplantation. Kidney Int 1979; 16: 167.
2. Wu MS, Linke CA, Panner B, Roberts A, Cockett ATK. Early evaluation of renal function after prolonged hypothermic preservation. Invest Urol 1973; 11: 154.
3. Kraemer GK, Panner BJ, Linke CA. Bilateral cervical transplantation of canine kidneys for study of canine renal preservation. Urology 1976; 8: 532.
4. Folin O, Wu H. A system of blood analysis. J Biol Chem 1919; 38: 81.
5. Bratton AC, Marshall EK Jr. A new coupling component for sulfanilamide determination. J Biol Chem 1938; 128: 537.
6. Sullivan LP, Grantham JJ. Physiology of the kidney. Philadelphia: Lea & Febiger 1982; 41.
7. Scheffe HA. A method of judging all contrasts in the analysis of variance. Biometrika 1953; 40: 87.
8. Marshall V, Ross B, Bishop M, Morris P. Evaluation of renal perfusion using the isolated perfused rat kidney: ischemic damage and the effects of inosine. Transplantation 1976; 26: 315.
9. Chiu PJS, Long JF. Urinary excretion and tissue accumulation of gentamicin and PAH in postischemic rat kidneys. Kidney Int 1979; 15: 618.

Received 12 December 1985.
Accepted 27 January 1986.

0041-1337/86/4205-0463$02.00/0
TRANSPLANTATION
Vol. 42, No. 5
Printed in U.S.A.

MODULATION OF HOST DEFENSES AGAINST PYOGENIC MICROORGANISMS BY CYCLOSPORINE[1]

THOMAS E. MILLER[2] AND GLENNE FINDON

Department of Medicine, University of Auckland, Auckland, New Zealand

Modulation of T cell activity by cyclosporine (CsA) predictably predisposes the host to infection with intracellular pathogens normally controlled by cell-mediated immune mechanisms. Little attention, however, has been paid to the effect of this agent on other cellular defense components associated with pathogens such as *Escherichia coli, Pseudomonas aeruginosa,* and *Staphylococcus aureus.* In the present experiments CsA administration exacerbated acute experimentally induced renal infection and led to a 100-fold increase in bacterial numbers. Furthermore, at a time when lesions in the control group were resolving, CsA-treated animals exhibited purulent abscesses involving up to 80% of the surface area of the kidney. Circulating leukocyte numbers were not reduced in CsA-treated hosts and the mechanism for provocation of infection remains to be explained.

The discovery of the fungal metabolite cyclosporine (CsA)* and its use as an immunosuppressive agent in organ transplantation represents a major advance in this field. CsA lacks the marrow-depressing activity of the more cytotoxic agents used to suppress the immune response, and is thought to act early in the process of T cell activation through its effect on suppressor T cells (*1*). Because infection is a major cause of mortality and morbidity in patients undergoing organ transplantation, the effect of immunosuppressive agents on host defense mechanisms is of considerable importance. CsA is believed to have a selective effect on T cells, and hence cell-mediated immunity (CMI). This component of the immune system is largely responsible for host defense to infection with intracellular pathogens *(Listeria monocytogenes,* Herpes simplex, *Toxoplasma gondii, Pneumocystis carinii, Mycobacterium sp.)*—and, to date, interest has focused on the association between infection with these agents and CsA administration. Surprisingly little attention has been paid to the effect of CsA on other cellular components of the host defense system, although recent surveys have shown a high incidence of infection with pyogenic extracellular microorganisms (*2–5*). Host defenses against these pathogens are not usually affected by agents that depress only CMI, suggesting that CsA additionally affects other defense mechanisms, although experimental evidence for this is lacking. We have attempted to provide this by studying the effect of CsA on renal infection in an animal model of pyelonephritis.

[1] This work was supported by The Medical Research Council of New Zealand.

[2] Address correspondence to: T.E. Miller, Ph.D. Department of Medicine Auckland Hospital, Park Road, Auckland, New Zealand.

* Abbreviations used: CMI, cell-mediated immunity; CsA, cyclosporine; DA, dark agouti.

MATERIALS AND METHODS

Experimental host. Female rats weighing 180–250 g were obtained from an inbred colony of a dark agouti (DA) strain.

Induction of pyelonephritis. Pyelonephritis was induced in both kidneys, as previously described (*6*), by the direct inoculation of *E coli 075* into the renal parenchyma of the surgically exposed kidney. A glass microcapillary pipette was used to inject two 5-μl aliquots of inoculum into the kidney, giving a mean challenge of 2200±700 viable bacteria per organ.

Cyclosporine administration. Cyclosporine, Sandoz Ltd., Basle, Switzerland, was provided in powder form, and dissolved, with constant stirring, in warm ethyl alcohol diluted 1:10 in olive oil. The appropriate dose was administered by i.m. injection of 0.1 ml into the thigh. In the first experiment, 5 groups of animals received a loading dose of 100 mg/kg, followed by 50 mg/kg every second day until sacrificed. All received a bacterial challenge on the 7th day, and the groups were sacrificed in turn on the 1st, 3rd, 7th, and 10th days after challenge. Corresponding groups that were challenged, but received carrier oil only, served as controls. In a second experiment, doses of 3, 6, 12.5, 25, and 50 mg/kg were given to different groups and the same doses repeated on alternate days for a total of 7 doses. Bacterial challenge was carried out on the 7th day, and the animals were sacrificed 7 days later. A control group was challenged, but received carrier material only. Preliminary experiments had shown that a 5–7-day exposure to CsA before challenge was necessary to affect host defenses.

Quantitative evaluation of gross pathological changes. Quantitation of the external gross pathology was made using a paper profile of the kidney, which was divided into 10 equal wedge-shaped areas. Renal lesions and scar formation were shaded in on the kidney profile following direct visual inspection of the kidney at autopsy. When lesions existed on both sides of the kidney, two profiles were used. Each division of the profile therefore equaled 5% of the total kidney surface. Gross pathological changes were expressed as a percentage of the total kidney surface.

Bacterial content of renal tissue. Serial 10-fold dilutions of whole homogenized kidneys were incorporated in nutrient agar pour plates to obtain the bacterial count per gram of wet renal tissue.

Peripheral blood leukocytes. Total and differential leukocyte counts were carried out on the venous blood of uninfected and infected animals, both CsA and carrier-treated.

Statistical analysis. Data was subjected to analysis by Wilcoxon's sum of ranks method for nonparametric data.

RESULTS

Acute pyelonephritis. CsA administration (50 mg/kg) did not affect bacterial numbers in the kidney 24 hr after challenge, but up to a 100-fold increase in bacterial numbers was demonstrable over a 10-day period (Fig. 1). The lesion size increased markedly in CsA-treated animals, and by 10 days involved over

65% of the surface of the kidney in half the kidneys examined, compared with 10% for the controls (Figs. 2 and 3).

Dose response. Seven days after challenge, low doses of CsA (3 and 6 mg/kg) had a minimal effect on bacterial numbers in the kidney, but animals treated with 12.5 mg/kg doses showed a 10-fold increase over controls. A 100-fold increase was found in the 50 mg/kg group (Fig. 4). Lesion size followed a similar trend and increased progressively, to involve up to 55% of the kidney surface at the highest dose of CsA (Fig. 5).

Peripheral blood leukocytes in CsA-treated animals. To examine the possibility that provocation of infection could be ascribed to CsA-induced leukopenia, peripheral blood leukocyte counts were carried out on pyelonephritic and control animals—both CsA and carrier-treated. CsA administration (50 mg/kg) led to a considerable increase in peripheral blood leukocytes of pyelonephritic animals compared with untreated pyelonephritic animals (32×10^9/L vs. 17×10^9/L). Circulating neutrophils accounted for most of the increase, but there was also an increase in lymphocyte numbers (Fig. 6).

DISCUSSION

Prevention of rejection by suppression of the immune response is the aim of the management of patients undergoing organ transplantation. Therapy with CsA, either alone or with

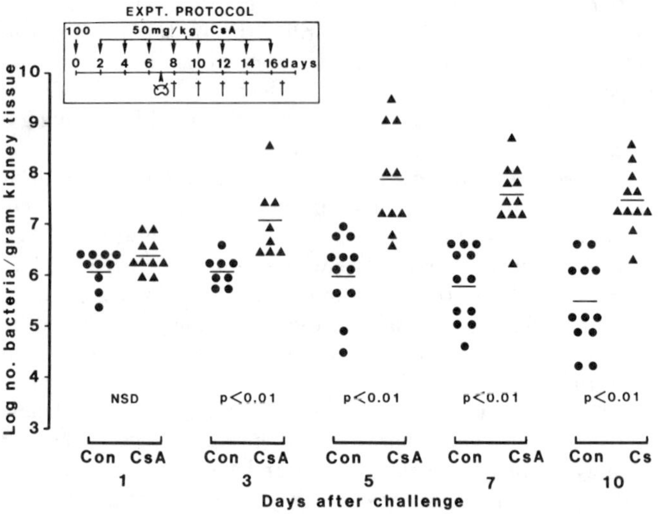

FIGURE 1. Effect of CsA (50 mg/kg every other day) on the bacterial count of kidney tissue at varying intervals after bacterial challenge.

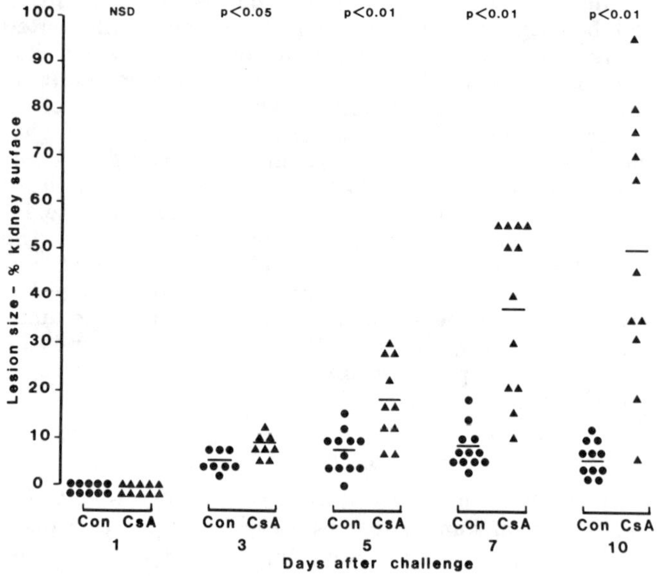

FIGURE 2. CsA administration (50 mg/kg every other day) enhances lesion size in acute experimental pyelonephritis.

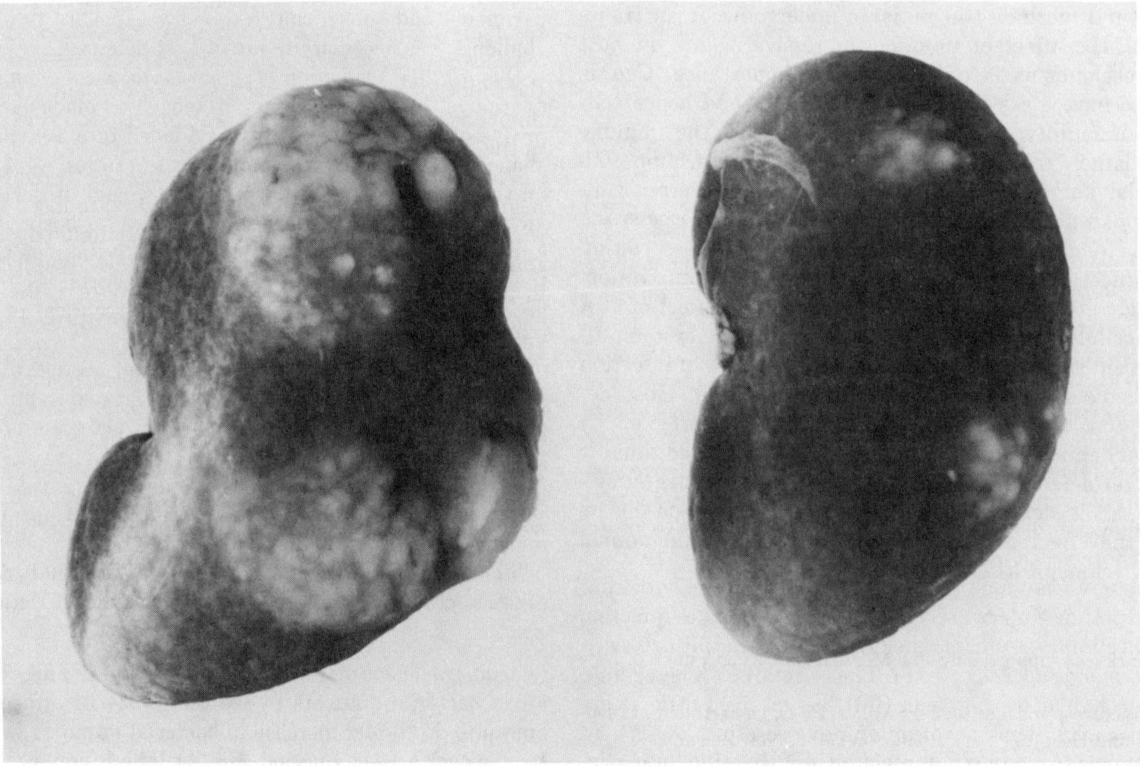

FIGURE 3. Provocation of lesion formation in acute pyelonephritis: untreated host (right) CsA-treated (left).

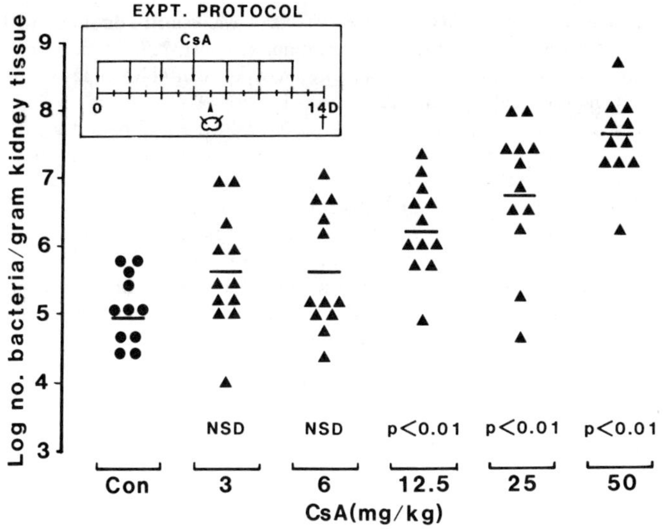

FIGURE 4. The effect of various doses of CsA on the bacterial count of kidney tissue 7 days after bacterial challenge. For statistical purposes, CsA-treated groups were compared with the carrier-treated controls.

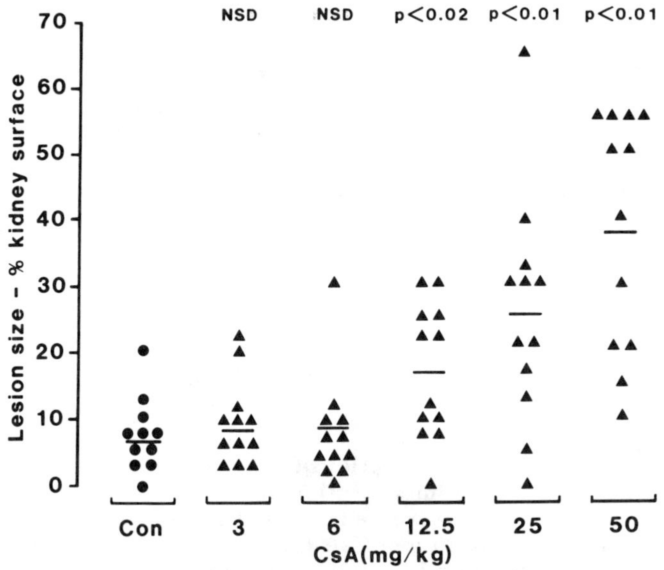

FIGURE 5. The effect of different doses of CsA on lesion size in acute pyelonephritis. For statistical purposes, CsA-treated groups were compared with the carrier-treated controls.

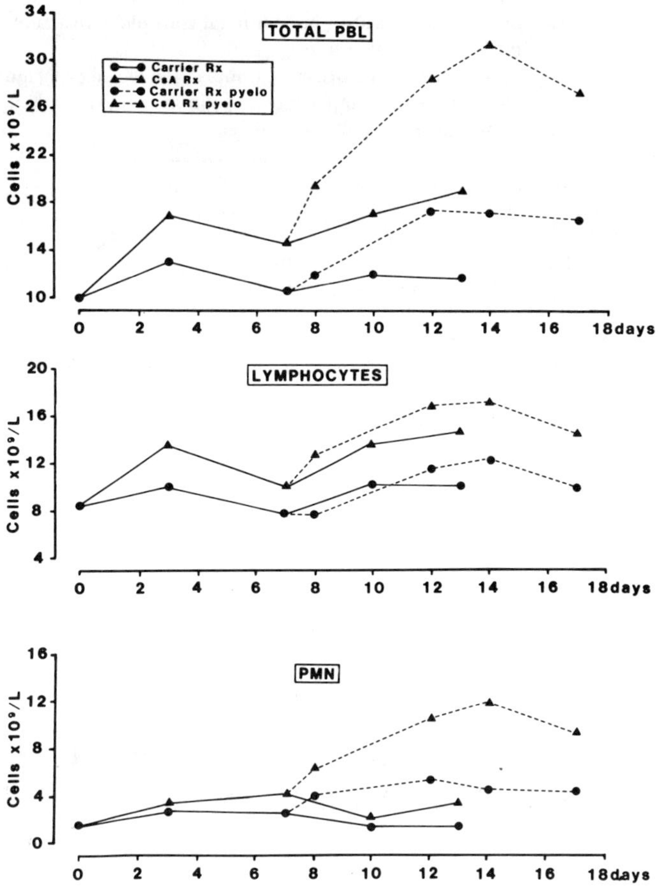

FIGURE 6. Effect of CsA (50 mg/kg) on peripheral blood leukocytes in normal and pyelonephritic animals.

other agents, appears to have advantages over earlier regimens because of its more specific action on lymphocyte subtypes and its comparative lack of marrow toxicity. While some of the early trials of CsA in renal transplantation showed an increase in infection-related problems, recent clinical experience suggests a similar incidence and pattern of infection in both patients managed on conventional immunosuppressive protocols and those receiving CsA (*2–5*). Studies showing that administration of CsA suppresses CMI are compatible with clinical and experimental observations that CsA provokes infection with intracellular organisms including *P carinii*, influenza virus, and *L monocytogenes* (*7–11*). The effect of CsA on cellular defense mechanisms other than CMI has received little attention. Our results, demonstrating an adverse effect of CsA on host resistance to acute renal infection, are therefore of particular significance. Bacterial numbers in renal tissue increased up to 100-fold in infected animals receiving CsA—and, at ten days after challenge when lesions in the control group were resolving, animals treated with 50 mg/kg CsA exhibited purulent abscesses, some involving up to 80% of the surface area of the kidney. Even at doses 4 times lower than this, bacterial numbers and lesion activation were increased over those found in the control groups.

The mechanism by which host resistance to pyogenic organisms is reduced by CsA is not clear. A drug-induced leukopenia would provide an explanation, but the maximum dose used was considered to be the equivalent of a "clinically effective dose" in man and was not known to cause any hematological, biochemical, or histopathological changes in treated animal hosts (*12*). In fact, circulating leukocyte numbers in animals treated with CsA increased, and the bacteriological results have been reproduced with dosages of CsA as low as 25% of the clinically effective dosage. Provocation of infection by CsA-induced, nonspecific cytoreductive activity therefore seems unlikely, and an alternative explanation—which takes account of an effect on noncellular defense mechanisms—needs to be considered.

Acknowledgments. Cyclosporine was kindly provided by Sandoz Ltd. Ms. Jacqueline Minett assisted with the preparation of the manuscript.

REFERENCES

1. Britton S, Palacios R. Cyclosporin A—usefulness, risks and mechanism of action. Immunol Rev 1982; 65: 5.
2. Sells RA. A prospective randomized substitutive trial of cyclospor-

ine as a prophylactic agent in human renal transplant rejection. Transplant Proc 1983; 15: 2495.
3. Najarian JS, Strand M, Fryd DS, et al. Comparison of cyclosporine versus azathioprine–antilymphocyte globulin in renal transplantation. Transplant Proc 1983; 15: 2463.
4. Sheil AGR, Hall BM, Tiller DJ, et al. Australian trial of cyclosporine (CsA) in cadaveric donor renal transplantation. Transplant Proc 1983; 15: 2485.
5. Sutherland DER, Payne WD, Fryd DS, et al. Comparison of cyclosporine and azathioprine for immunosuppression in diabetic and nondiabetic renal allograft recipients. Transplant Proc 1985; 17: 1204.
6. Miller TE, Robinson KB. Experimental pyelonephritis: a new method for inducing pyelonephritis in the rat. J Infect Dis 1973; 127: 307.
7. Hughes WT, Smith B. Provocation of infection due to *Pneumocystis carinii* by cyclosporin A. J Infect Dis 1982; 145: 767.
8. Schiltknecht E, Ada GL. *In vivo* effects of cyclosporine on influenza A virus–infected mice. Cell Immunol 1985; 91: 227.
9. Cook RM. Activity of cyclosporin A in experimental influenza virus infection in mice. Agents Actions 1983; 13: 98.
10. Schaffner A, Douglas H, Davis CE. Models of T cell deficiency in listeriosis: the effects of cortisone and cyclosporin A on normal and nude BALB/c mice. J Immunol 1983; 131: 450.
11. Hardy AM, Wajszczuk CP, Hakala TR, Rosenthal JT, Starzl TE, Ho M. Infection in renal transplant recipients on cyclosporine: *Pneumocystis* pneumonia. Transplant Proc 1983; 15: 2773.
12. Thomson AW, Whiting PH, Cameron ID, Lessels SE, Simpson JG. A toxicological study in rats receiving immunotherapeutic doses of cyclosporin A. Transplantation 1981; 31: 121.

Received 29 October 1985.
Accepted 11 February 1986.

0041-1337/86/4205-0466$02.00/0
TRANSPLANTATION
Vol. 42, No. 5
Printed in U.S.A.

CONCANAVALIN A–DEPENDENT CELL-MEDIATED CYTOTOXICITY IN BRONCHOALVEOLAR LAVAGE FLUID

CORRELATION WITH LUNG ALLOGRAFT REJECTION IN MONGREL DOGS DURING CYCLOSPORINE DOSE TAPERING[1]

ALLEN J. NORIN,[2] STEPHAN L. KAMHOLZ, KENNETH L. PINSKER, EUGENE E. EMESON,[3] AND FRANK J. VEITH

The Departments of Surgery, Microbiology and Immunology, and Medicine, Montefiore Medical Center–Albert Einstein College of Medicine, Bronx, New York 10467

Although cyclosporine (CsA) is widely used as the primary agent for inhibiting the rejection of organ allografts in man, the ideal immunosuppressive regimen for utilizing this drug is still uncertain. To investigate this question, a concanavalin A (con A)-dependent cell-mediated cytotoxicity (CDCMC) assay was used to examine the development of intragraft and peripheral blood cytolytic T lymphocyte activity during CsA dose tapering. These studies were conducted in a canine single-lung transplantation model that facilitates serial examination of intragraft effector cells by bronchoalveolar lavage (BAL). A remarkable correlation of increased intragraft CDCMC and clinical evidence of lung allograft rejection was observed during CsA dose tapering in some recipients. In other recipients CDCMC remained low and evidence of rejection was not observed during drug tapering. In contrast, peripheral blood CDCMC did not correlate well with evidence of rejection. Rejection phenomena observed after termination of CsA therapy were reversed by resumption of CsA treatment but were not reversed by administration of methylprednisolone. Furthermore, the increased level of CDCMC was diminished by reinstitution of CsA therapy at the initial dosage. Following termination of CsA therapy, a prolonged period of unresponsiveness was observed in nearly two-thirds of the recipients, and 60% of these latter dogs had unlimited survival of their lung allografts (median >496 days). Intragraft CDCMC remained low during the periods of unresponsiveness and increased upon onset of rejection. We conclude that measurement of intragraft CDCMC is a useful in vitro method of monitoring lung allograft rejection, and therefore provides a technique for adjusting CsA dosage schedules to achieve maximally effective immunosuppression. The use of this assay for monitoring rejection of other organ grafts requires further investigation.

Cyclosporine (CsA),* a potent and specific inhibitor of T-lymphocyte-mediated responses (*1*), has recently come into wide use as the major immunosuppressive agent in human

[1] This work was supported in part by grants from the U.S. Public Health Service (HL 17417) and The James Hilton Manning and Emma Austin Manning Foundation.

[2] Address correspondence to: Allen J. Norin, Ph.D., Montefiore Medical Center, 111 East 210th Street, Bronx, NY 10467.

[3] Present address: Department of Pathology, University of Illinois College of Medicine, Chicago, IL 60612.

* Abbreviations used: BAL, bronchoalveolar lavage; CDCMC, concanavalin-A-dependent cell-mediated cytotoxicity; con A, concanavalin A; CsA, cyclosporine; CTL, cytolytic T lymphocyte; lymph, lymphocytes, MØ, macrophages; PMN, polymorphonuclear leukocytes; NK, natural killer cells; RIA, radioimmunoassay.

organ transplantation (*2–5*). However, despite extensive experimental and clinical experience, the most effective treatment protocol utilizing this drug is still uncertain (*2*). In this regard, determination of appropriate immunosuppressive dosage and toxic drug dosage are primary issues (*6–8*). In this report we investigated a procedure for determining an effective immunosuppressive dosage schedule for administration of CsA. The strategy employed was to develop an in vitro assay for monitoring alloreactivity during CsA dose tapering that correlated with evidence of rejection. Such an assay might provide information for adjusting the dosage of CsA. A single lung transplantation model was utilized in unmatched mongrel dogs to assess this procedure. This experimental system provides an outbred experimental model similar in genetic heterogeneity to man. Furthermore, transplantation of a single lung affords the capability of serially sampling intragraft effector cells by the relatively benign procedure of bronchoalveolar lavage (BAL). Recipients survive severe rejection episodes sustained by the respiratory function of the normal contralateral lung, permitting analysis of intragraft effector cells during such periods. In vitro analyses of cells obtained from the graft itself were viewed as having the most likely possibility of detecting effectors of allograft destruction (*9*). For comparative purposes the function of peripheral blood cells was also determined.

An in vitro assay for detecting impending graft destruction in CsA-treated recipients should have three important features: it should measure an effector mechanism involved in the process of rejection, this activity should be exquisitely sensitive to the drug, and the methodology should be readily adaptable from an experimental setting to man. We therefore examined the association of cytolytic T lymphocyte (CTL) activity with clinical evidence of lung allograft rejection, since CTL have been shown to be important cell components involved in the destruction of organ allografts (*10, 11*). The generation of alloreactive CTL is also markedly inhibited by CsA (*12, 13*).

In the present study, CTL activity was measured by a concanavalin-A-dependent cell-mediated cytotoxicity (CDCMC) assay that was developed for use in the dog (*14*). This assay is believed to detect the total T cell cytolytic activity of a lymphocyte population since the lectin substitutes for alloantigens in the binding phase of the lytic reaction (*15, 16*). As such, the CDCMC assay may be useful for assessing rejection in outbred species since numerous antigenic differences may evoke a wide variety of specific cytolytic cell responses. Furthermore, CDCMC assays utilize standard cell lines as targets, which may eliminate the need for extensive storage of frozen donor cells.

This report demonstrates a close association between increased intragraft CDCMC activity and clinical evidence of lung allograft rejection after CsA dose tapering. Resumption of CsA therapy after drug tapering usually resulted in decreased CDCMC activity and diminution in rejection phenomena. As a consequence of the use of this approach, CsA treatment could be discontinued permanently in a substantial proportion of lung allograft recipients without evidence of graft destruction. Such recipients demonstrated persistently low levels of CDCMC.

MATERIALS AND METHODS

Lung transplantation and immunosuppressive therapy. Left lung transplantation was performed in 20–25-kg male mongrel dogs (Biomedical Associates, Inc., Friedenburg, PA) utilizing unrelated donors, as described in detail elsewhere (*17, 18*). Donor-recipient pairs were size-matched, but no other procedures (e.g., DLA, MLR typing) were used to select combinations, although pretransplant proliferative and cytotoxicity assays were performed on mixed lymphocyte cultures. CsA powder (Sandoz Ltd., Basel, Switzerland) was dissolved in corn oil for oral administration. In the more recent studies, CsA was received as a 100 mg/ml solution and diluted to the appropriate concentration with corn oil before oral administration. CsA was given initially at 17 mg/kg/day for 21 days, 13 mg/kg/day for 14 days, 9 mg/kg/day for 7 days, and 7 mg/kg/day thereafter unless stated otherwise. Cyclosporine serum levels were determined utilizing the standard radioimmunoassay (RIA) kit obtained from Sandoz (*19*). Lung allograft recipients treated with this CsA dose-tapering schedule were given corticosteroid therapy when evidence of rejection was detected (methylprednisolone, i.m. for 3 days at 1 g/day for acute rejection and oral prednisone, 40 mg/day tapered to 20 mg/day for maintenance therapy).

Clinical evaluation of rejection. Evidence of rejection was determined by previously described procedures (*17, 20–23*). In brief, plain chest roentgenograms were performed on a weekly basis, more frequently when abnormalities were detected, and before other diagnostic procedures. As a measure of blood flow through the transplanted lung, radionuclide perfusion scans were performed in lightly anesthetized recipients using ^{99}Tc (3 mCi) macroaggregated albumin, 10–90 μm, (New England Nuclear, Boston, MA). The perfusion scans were usually performed three times during the initial 100-day period after transplantation, and at least twice yearly thereafter. Open-lung biopsy specimens were obtained and processed using standard techniques.

Bronchoalveolar lavage. BAL was performed in pentobarbital-anesthetized lung allograft recipients as previously described (*22, 24*). Aliquots of heparinized isotonic NaCl (50 ml) were instilled into the right lower lobe of the normal lung through the channel of a fiberoptic bronchoscope (Machida, FBS6TL) until a 100-ml return was collected by suction. The lavage was then repeated in the left lower lobe of the transplanted lung. BAL cells were washed two times with Hanks' balanced salt solution without Ca^{+2} and Mg^{+2} (Grand Island Biological Co., Grand Island, NY) and analyzed immediately for total and differential cell counts by addition of 40 μl of 0.1% crystal violet stain (in 0.1 M citric acid) to 120 μl of the cell suspension. This rapid method for identifying and quantitating BAL cells yields 25–50% greater lymphocyte counts than standard Wright-Giemsa-stained cytocentrifuge preparations, and appears to more accurately reflect the cell composition of lung washings, as suggested by the studies of Saltini et al. (*25*).

Cell mediated cytotoxicity assays. CTL activity was measured as reported previously (*14, 26*). Washed BAL cells or Ficoll-Hypaque-isolated peripheral blood leukocytes were enriched for T lymphocytes by the nylon column technique and suspended in RPMI-1640 medium with 15% fetal bovine serum, penicillin (100 IU/ml), streptomycin (100 μg/ml), glutamine (2 mM), and 2-mercaptoethanol (5×10^{-5} M) (RPMI-complete). The human lymphoblastoid cell line, Raji, was used as the target in the CDCMC assay. 100 μl of effector cells was added to 100 μl of ^{51}Cr-labeled Raji cells and incubated with 10 μg/ml of concanavalin A (con A) (Miles, Elkhart, IN) in a 96-well microtiter plate (Nunc, Roskilde, Denmark). When the effector cell concentration utilized was 5 or 10×10^6 cells/ml, plates with round-bottomed wells were used, whereas V-bottomed plates were used at effector cell concentrations of 2.5×10^6 or less. Effector-target cell mixtures were not sedimented by centrifugation before or after incubation. Effector-to-target cell ratios were varied from 100:1 to 6.25:1, with the number of target cells kept constant. After 3 hr incubation at 37°C, 100 μl of culture supernatant was harvested from triplicate samples and the ^{51}Cr radioactivity determined in a gamma spectrophotometer (Searle Analytic 1185, Des Plaines, IL). The percentage of cytotoxicity was calculated by the formula: (cpm experimental − cpm spontaneous release) × 100 ÷ (cpm maximum release − cpm spontaneous release). The spontaneous release was determined in wells with target cells and 100 μl of RPMI-complete, while maximum release was determined in wells with target cells and 100 μl of 2% sodium dodecyl sulfate. The spontaneous release was usually 5–10% of the maximum release.

RESULTS

Effect of cyclosporine dose tapering on intragraft CDCMC activity and lung allograft rejection. Values of CDCMC were compiled for 20 canine lung allograft recipients following the initial CsA dose tapering protocol as described above. Based on this data three response groups were noted, as shown in Figure 1. Most canine lung allograft recipients receiving 17 mg/kg/day of CsA during the initial treatment period of 21 days had less than 15% CDCMC activity in BAL fluid. Following CsA dose tapering to ≤13 mg/kg/day the majority of lung recipients (22) had increased intragraft CDCMC activity that ranged from 24% to 60%, (response group 1). In contrast, 5 of the 20 lung allograft recipients retained low levels of intragraft CDCMC activity after the initial reduction in CsA dosage (response group 2). Evidence of graft rejection following CsA dose tapering is summarized in Table 1. All recipients exhibiting increased CDCMC activity after dose tapering (response group 1) had evidence of graft rejection as assessed by chest roentgenogram, perfusion scans of the lung, and open lung biopsies. Significantly, recipients without increased intragraft CDCMC activity (response group 2) also had no evidence of rejection as a result of CsA dose tapering (Table 1).

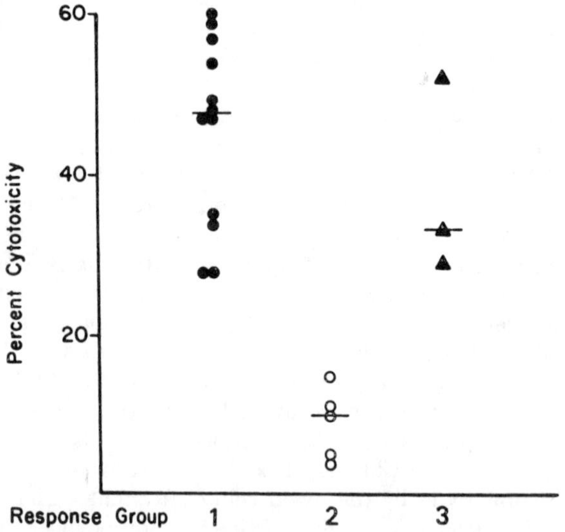

FIGURE 1. Intragraft concanavalin-A-dependent cell-mediated cytotoxicity: response to cyclosporine dose tapering. Lung allograft recipients in response groups 1 and 2 were treated for 21 days with CsA (17 mg/kg/day). The dose was then usually reduced to 13 mg/kg/day × 3 weeks and then to 9 mg/kg/day × 2 weeks. However, the CsA dose of some recipients in response group 1 was not reduced to 9 mg/kg/day due to the severity of rejection. CDCMC was analyzed at least one week after each dose tapering. The values reported were the highest levels of CDCMC observed. The initial dose of CsA was not reduced in recipients of response group 3 due to the severity of rejection. The CDCMC values reported for these recipients were obtained 14–20 days after transplantation. (Horizontal bar = median).

In three of the 20 canine lung allograft recipients, high levels of CDCMC activity were observed during the initial course of treatment with 17 mg/kg/day of CsA (response group 3, Fig. 1, and Table 1). Cytological examination of BAL fluid from the allografts revealed increased total cell counts and increased percentages of leukocytes (Table 2). These recipients had early evidence of graft destruction that could not be reversed by high-dose methylprednisolone therapy. CsA peak and trough levels in two of these recipients were found to be in the same range as those of graft recipients with healthy lung allografts receiving an identical dose of CsA (1600–2200 ng/ml peak and 150–300 ng/ml trough).

Termination of cyclosporine therapy: effect on intragraft CDCMC activity and lung allograft survival. The effect of discontinuing CsA therapy was studied in 11 canine lung transplant recipients with well-functioning allografts (i.e., blood flow >70% predicted) more than 60 days after transplantation. Six of these recipients were initially found to be in response group 1, and five of the recipients were in response group 2 (Table 3). All recipients in response group 2 (except No. 23) received a second course (30–60 days) of CsA treatment at 17 mg/kg/day. Recipient No. 23 had a minimal alveolar infiltrate on chest roentgenograms and relatively low CDCMC activity (28%) after CsA dose tapering to 7 mg/kg/day, and was therefore not treated with an additional course of 17 mg/kg/day CsA. Recipients in response group 2 were receiving 7 mg/kg/day of CsA at the time drug therapy was terminated.

Of the 11 lung transplant recipients, three (Nos. 44, 47, and 49) promptly rejected their allografts after cessation of CsA therapy. A representative study of one of these lung allograft

TABLE 1. Evidence of rejection and intragraft CDCMC activity associated with cyclosporine dose tapering in canine lung allograft recipients

Response group	n	Median CDCMC after CsA dose tapering	Recipients with increased rejection after CsA tapering[a]
1	12	47%	12
2	5	13%	0
3	3	32%[b]	NA

[a] Evidence of rejection was assessed by chest roentgenograms, radionuclide blood perfusion scans of the lung, and evaluation of open lung biopsy specimens.

[b] Recipients in this response group had evidence of graft destruction while receiving high-dose CsA therapy; (NA) not applicable.

TABLE 2. Cell content in BAL fluid of a lung allograft recipient exhibiting rejection while receiving high-dose cyclosporine treatment[a]

Lung	Differential cell count (percentage)			Cells/ml (BAL×10^{-5})
	Lymph	PMN	MØ	
Allograft	3	50	47	8
Normal	4	13	83	1

[a] This recipient was treated with a single daily oral dose of CsA at 17 mg/kg for 13 days. A total of 100 ml of BAL fluid was collected and cells were enumerated in a hemocytometer with a crystal violet stain, as described in detail in the *Materials and Methods* section.

TABLE 3. Lung allograft survival after termination of cyclosporine therapy[a]

Recipient	Response group	Allograft survival (days)		Allograft failure after CsA stopped
		Total	After CsA stopped	
44	1	115	13	Yes
47	2	134	16	Yes
49	1	74	13	Yes
23	1	190	95	Yes
37	1	302	145	Yes
46	2	196	99	Yes
1	2	>1053	>654	No
15	2	>415	>210	No
19	2	>1206	>1062	No
40	1	>586	>496	No
52	2	>264	>137	No

[a] Recipients Nos. 37, 40, 44, 46, and 47 were treated with an additional course of CsA at 17 mg/kg/day after the initial dose-tapering protocol (described in the *Materials and Methods* section), before cessation of drug treatment. The other recipients were treated with a maintenance dose of CsA, 7 mg/kg/day (after dose tapering) before termination of drug treatment. Total survival = days after transplantation when lung allografts were rejected or the experiment was terminated. Recipients Nos. 1 and 15 were killed for study at days 1053 and 415, respectively.

recipients (No. 44) demonstrating alterations in CDCMC activity during the posttransplantation period is shown in Figure 2, panel A. The rapid onset of a diffuse alveolar infiltrate in the allografted lung was observed during the initial CsA dose tapering procedure (day 49). CsA therapy, at 17 mg/kg/day was immediately reinstituted and the rejection episode resolved within 10 days. On day 80 BAL studies indicated an increase in CDCMC activity in both the transplanted lung (57%) and the normal lung (33%). Cytological examination of BAL fluid revealed increases in total cell count and PMN leukocytes in both lungs. Although antibiotics and additional immunosuppressive therapy were not administered during this period, this reaction diminished by 91 days after transplantation, as demonstrated by reduced inflammatory cells in BAL fluid (Table 4) and reduction in CDCMC activity to 24% in the transplant and 15% in the normal lung. The chest roentgenogram continued to be relatively normal. Subsequently, CsA therapy was terminated at 96 days after transplantation. At 109 days intragraft CDCMC had increased to 48% but peripheral blood CDCMC was unchanged (Fig. 2, panel A). Increased PMN leukocytes were observed in BAL fluid (Table 4) and evidence of rejection was seen on chest roentgenograms (alveolar infiltrate) and in an open lung biopsy as diffuse intraalveolar exudate of cells and fibrin.

Following cessation of CsA therapy, three other lung allograft recipients (Nos. 23, 37, and 46) had a prolonged period of unresponsiveness before evidence of rejection was observed. CDCMC activity during the post transplant period of one of these recipients (No. 46) is shown in Figure 2, panel B. Intragraft cytolytic activity remained at a low level following the initial tapering schedule but increased at 99 days after CsA treatment was discontinued. Peripheral blood CDCMC activity also increased at this time. The BAL fluid from the allograft had an increased percentage of lymphocytes and increased total cell numbers during the entire postoperative period (Table 5). Cell content data were therefore not associated with clinical evidence of rejection and were independent of the increase in CDCMC seen on day 159 (Fig. 2, panel B).

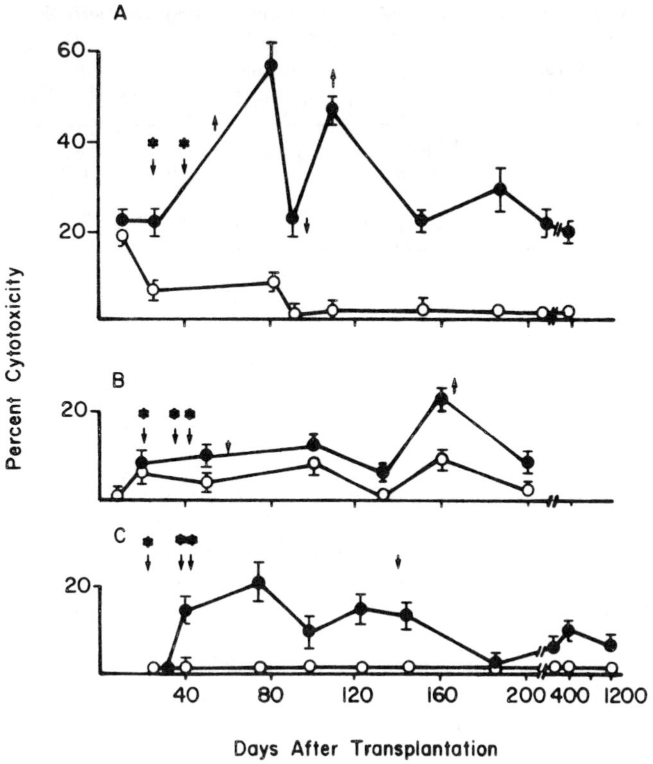

FIGURE 2. Serial intragraft and peripheral blood concanavalin-A-dependent cell-mediated cytotoxicity levels after lung transplantation. Activity in BAL fluid (●); activity in peripheral blood (○); (↨) reduction in CsA dose; (↓) termination of CsA therapy; (↑) resumption of CsA treatment at 17 mg/kg/day. (Panel A) profile of activity of recipient No. 44 showing an increase of CDCMC immediately after termination of CsA therapy and decreased CDCMC following resumption of 17 mg/kg/day CsA; (Panel B) recipient No. 46 showing a prolonged period of low CDCMC after termination of CsA treatment. Increased activity seen at 159 days was reduced following additional CsA treatment; (Panel C) profile of activity of recipient No. 19 showing a permanently low level of CDCMC after cessation of CsA treatment.

TABLE 4. Cell content of BAL fluid of lung allograft recipient No. 44

Days after transplantation	Lung	Differential cell count (percentage)			Cells/ml ($BAL\times10^{-5}$)
		Lymph	PMN	MØ	
91	Allograft	15	2	83	4
	Normal	22	3	75	3
109	Allograft	10	50	40	4
	Normal	13	15	72	3
151	Allograft	18	9	73	9
	Normal	14	2	84	5

Of the 11 recipients studied, 5 have had permanent survival of their lung allografts after CsA therapy was discontinued (Table 3). Among the unresponsive recipients, 4 were initially found to be in response group 2. The other permanently unresponsive recipient (No. 40) had significant evidence of lung allograft rejection and 35% CDCMC activity in BAL fluid after the initial CsA dose tapering. Following a second course of CsA therapy, as described above, CDCMC activity stabilized at 10%, and cessation of drug treatment was accomplished without subsequent evidence of graft destruction. Representative serial studies of CDCMC during the course of the posttransplantation

TABLE 5. Cell content of BAL fluid of lung allograft recipient No. 46

Days after transplantation	Lung	Differential cell count (percentage)			Cells/ml (BAL×10^−5)
		Lymph	PMN	MØ	
50	Allograft	47	1	52	14
	Normal	19	3	79	0.2
133	Allograft	32	6	62	14
	Normal	12	1	87	3
159	Allograft	43	10	47	8
229	Allograft	36	10	54	5
	Normal	20	4	76	1

period of one of the permanently unresponsive recipients (No. 19) is shown in Figure 2, panel C. CDCMC activity in BAL fluid reached a peak value of 19% at 77 days after transplantation and gradually declined to 7%. Less than 2% CDCMC was detected in peripheral blood lymphocyte preparations during the entire study period. Blood flow to the allografted lung at 1206 days after transplantation was about 80% of the normal flow to the left lung of autografted dogs. This level of fractional blood flow to the allografted lung was typical of the other long-term-tolerant recipients. Cytological examination of the BAL fluid revealed relatively normal differential and total cell content (Table 6).

Effect of additional high-dose cyclosporine treatment on intragraft CDCMC activity and lung allograft rejection after dose tapering. Studies were conducted to determine whether reinstitution of treatment with the initial dose of CsA, 17 mg/kg/day, would reverse increased intragraft CDCMC and graft rejection resulting from reduction in CsA dosage. A group of 5 recipients were selected for this investigation who exhibited increased CDCMC activity in BAL fluid and evidence of rejection following reduction or termination of CsA therapy (Table 7); 4 of the recipients (Nos. 37, 40, 44, and 47) were from response group 1, and one recipient was from response group 2 (No. 46). All of these recipients had improvement of chest roentgenograms and increased blood flow to the lung allograft 7–10 days and 2–4 weeks, respectively, after reinstitution of CsA treatment at 17 mg/kg/day. The intragraft CDCMC activity had decreased to levels observed prior to CsA dose tapering in each of the recipients following the additional treatment of 17 mg/kg/day CsA for 4 weeks. In three recipients (Nos. 37, 44, and 47), rejection, occuring after termination of CsA therapy was not reversed by treatment with methylprednisolone (1 g × 4 days). This unsuccessful steroid treatment was begun 5 days prior to reinstitution of CsA therapy. Methylprednisolone was shown to reverse lung allograft rejection in 3–4 days in lung allograft recipients receiving 7–13 mg/kg/day CsA (*20–22*). In these cases it is possible that the steroid treatment acted with CsA to reverse rejection. However, CsA at 17 mg/kg/day was effective in reversing rejection in recipients Nos. 40 and 46 without steroid treatment.

DISCUSSION

The data in this report demonstrate a striking positive correlation between clinical evidence of lung allograft rejection and increased intragraft CDCMC occurring after CsA dose tapering. Corticosteroid resistant rejection phenomena were reversed, and the level of CDCMC decreased by reinstitution of CsA therapy at 17 mg/kg/day. This latter observation is in agreement with the findings of Deeg et al. (*27*) who have shown that resumption of CsA therapy reversed the rejection process in a canine skin allograft model. Canine lung recipients that had no evidence of graft destruction following termination of CsA therapy maintained a low level of intragraft CDCMC. Taken together these results suggest that intragraft CDCMC may provide a functional assay of immune activity against lung allografts in an outbred species.

The CDCMC assay has been shown to detect alloreactive human CTL generated in vitro and human CTL generated in vivo (*28, 29*). The development of a reliable in vitro assay to monitor rejection would be important in assessing CsA-treated recipients, in view of recent data demonstrating that trough plasma levels of the drug do not correlate with the degree of immunosuppression (*8*). Results of the CDCMC assay, must, however, be evaluated in relationship to clinical parameters, since 2 of 40 lung allograft recipients had a transient increase in intragraft cytolytic activity without manifestations of graft destruction. In these cases (e.g., recipient No. 44) a clinical diagnosis of nonbacterial bilateral pneumonia is consistent with the presumption of viral-induced lung CTL detected by the CDCMC assay (*16, 28, 30*).

It is uncertain whether the CDCMC assay will be useful in monitoring rejection of other allografted organs since the lung is uniquely suited for serial sampling of intragraft effector cells (by BAL). Monitoring of the peripheral blood for alloreactivity might provide a suitable alternative; however, in most canine lung allograft recipients the CDCMC activity of BAL lymphocytes, but not peripheral blood lymphocytes, correlated with evidence of rejection. Low levels of peripheral blood CDCMC were observed between 2 and 4 weeks after transplantation and usually decreased thereafter regardless of rejection phenomena. Buurman, et al. (*31*) have shown the absence of mature CTL in the blood of untreated canine recipients undergoing renal allograft rejection. Migration of CTL to the graft was suggested

TABLE 6. Cell content in BAL fluid of untreated lung allograft recipient No. 19

Days after transplantation	Lung	Differential cell count (percentage)			Cells/ml (BAL×10^−5)
		Lymph	PMN	MØ	
144	Allograft	40	3	57	5.6
	Normal	27	3	70	1.3
1328	Allograft	30	19	51	6.4
	Normal	33	4	63	3.5

TABLE 7. Effect of additional high-dose cyclosporine treatment on CDCMC of T cells in BAL of lung allograft recipients[a]

Recipient	Percent cytotoxicity		
	After 1st treatment[a]	After termination of treatment	After 2nd treatment
37	7	38	8
40	21	35[b]	18
44	28	47	25
46	8	22	8
47	15	30	16

[a] CDCMC was evaluated at 21–35 days after transplantation.
[b] The CsA dose was 13 mg/kg/day.

as a cause for this observation. Keown, et al. (*32*) have observed reduced peripheral blood CTL activity in CsA-prednisone treated human renal allograft recipients relative to recipients receiving azathioprine-prednisone in the initial 4-week period after transplantation. CTL activity in peripheral blood was absent in the CsA group after 4 weeks and was not detectable in the azathioprine group after 12 weeks. In contrast, experiments analyzing the level of specific CTL precursors in peripheral blood have suggested an association with graft rejection (*26, 31*). Further analyses of intragraft and peripheral blood CTL activity and quantification of CTL precursors are currently under investigation in the canine lung allograft model and may clarify some of these issues.

Nearly two-thirds of the CsA-treated canine lung allograft recipients had a significant period of unresponsiveness following cessation of drug therapy. The period of tolerance was essentially unlimited in about half these recipients (median >496 days). In contrast, skin and renal allografts in mongrel dogs were rejected following termination of CsA therapy (*27, 33*). These findings may be explained by the short duration of treatment (≤21 days), an inadequate initial dose of CsA (<17 mg/kg/day) and/or organ-specific immune reactions. Our results in mongrel dogs are noteworthy in that a relationship was demonstrated between dose and duration of treatment, and induction of unresponsiveness (i.e., some dogs only became unresponsive after additional CsA treatment following the initial dose-tapering schedule). A number of reports have demonstrated the induction of an unresponsive state following CsA treatment of rats, rabbits, and pigs (*34–37*). More recently, Birkeland (*38*) presented a case report of a human recipient who experienced a period of unresponsiveness to a renal allograft. The adequacy of low levels of CsA to provide maintenance therapy to long-term surviving human renal allograft recipients (*8*) may be explained by induction of a state of tolerance in response to the initial high dose of CsA. The finding of unlimited lung allograft survival after termination of CsA treatment in a substantial proportion of recipients of an outbred species provides evidence justifying similar clinical trials in man.

A number of studies have demonstrated that lectin-dependent cell-mediated cytotoxicity assays identify functionally mature CTL. Lectin-dependent killing is inhibited by treatment of effector cells with antibodies against T cell surface antigens with or without complement treatment (*15, 39*). Cell separation procedures using nylon columns or erythrocyte rosetting also suggest that the CDCMC assay identifies CTL (*14, 15*). Natural killer (NK) and antibody-dependent cell-mediated cytotoxicity are not detected by the CDCMC assay in that these activities are usually relatively high in peripheral blood of normal individuals, whereas CDCMC activity is usually less than 5% (*14, 29, 40, 41*). Additionally, depletion of human NK activity by treatment with anti-leu-11b (*40*) and complement had no effect on CDCMC (*29*). Although Meuer et al. (*42*) have shown that cloned OKT_4^+ and OKT_8^+ CTL lines are detected by CDCMC, it is possible that other types of killer lymphocytes function in this cytolytic assay, such as those described by Grimm et al. (*43*) and Karre et al. (*44*).

A high degree of heterogeneity was revealed in the response of canine lung allograft recipients to CsA dose tapering with regard to clinical evidence of rejection and induction of unresponsiveness. This finding is not surprising in view of the genetic disparities among individuals of an outbred species such as the dog. Our observations further emphasize the need to individualize CsA treatment protocols (*2, 8*). In addition to monitoring CsA blood levels to minimize toxicity, the in vitro monitoring of cell-mediated immune function against the graft is an important element in assessing effective immunosuppression. Results of monitoring CDCMC in the canine lung allograft model suggest the feasibility of adjusting the CsA dosage according to data obtained by this functional immune assay.

Acknowledgments. We acknowledge the expert surgical technique of Michael Torres and Israel Colon and the invaluable laboratory work of Rimma Mushnitsky and Rattan Cherwoo. Cyclosporine blood levels were kindly determined in the tissue-typing laboratory at Montefiore Medical Center by Dr. Sandra Nehlsen-Cannarella. We also thank Steven Levine for preparing the manuscript.

REFERENCES

1. Shevach EM. The effects of cyclosporin A on the immune system. Ann Rev Immunol 1985; 3: 397.
2. Canadian Multicentre Transplant Study Group. A randomized clinical trial of cyclosporine in cadaveric renal transplantation. N Engl J Med 1983; 309: 809.
3. Starzl TE, Klintmaln GB, Porter KA, Iwatsuki S, Schroter GPJ. Liver transplantation with the use of cyclosporin A and prednisone. N Engl J Med 1982; 306: 557.
4. Oyer PE, Stinson EB, Jamieson SW, et al. Cyclosporin A in cardiac allografting: a preliminary experience. Transplant Proc 1983; 15: 1247.
5. Reitz BA, Wallwork JL, Hunt SA, et al. Heart-lung transplantation: successful therapy for patients with pulmonary vascular disease. N Engl J Med 1982; 306: 557.
6. Kahan BD, Van Buren CT, Liu SN. Immunopharmacological monitoring of cyclosporin A-treated recipients of cadaveric kidney allografts. Transplantation 1982; 34: 36.
7. Cohen DJ, Loertscher R, Rubin MF, Tilney ML, Carpenter CB, Strom TB. Cyclosporine: a new immunosuppressive agent for organ transplantation. Ann Intern Med 1984; 101: 667.
8. Klintmaln G, Sawe J, Ringden O, von Bahr C, Magnusson A. Cyclosporine plasma levels in renal transplant patients. Association with renal toxicity and allograft rejection. Transplantation 1985; 39: 132.
9. Hayry P. Intragraft events in allograft destruction. Transplantation 1984; 38: 1.
10. Bradley JA, Mason DW, Morris PJ. Evidence that rat renal allografts are rejected by cytotoxic T cells and not by nonspecific effectors. Transplantation 1985; 39: 169.
11. Tyler JD, Galli SJ, Snider ME, Dvorak AM, Steinmuller D. Cloned Lyt-2^+ cytolytic T lymphocytes destroy allogenic tissue in vivo. J Exp Med 1984; 159: 234.
12. Hess AD, Tutschka PJ. Effect of cyclosporin A on human lymphocyte responses in vitro. I. Cyclosporin A allows for expression of alloantigen activated suppressor cells while preferentially inhibiting the induction of cytolytic effector lymphocytes in MLR. J Immunol 1980; 124: 2601.
13. Heeg K, Deusch K, Solback W, Bunjes D, Wagner H. Frequency analysis of cyclosporine-sensitive cytotoxic T lymphocyte precursors. Transplantation 1984; 38: 532.
14. Emeson EE, Norin AJ, Veith FJ. Lectin-dependent cell-mediated cytotoxicity: a new and simple method to quantitate cytotoxic T cell activity in dogs. Transplantation 1982; 33: 365.
15. Bonavida B, Bradley T, Fan J, Hiserodt J, Effros R, Wexler H. Molecular interactions in T-cell mediated cytotoxicity. Immunol Rev 1983; 72: 119.
16. Henkart PA. Mechanisms of lymphocyte-mediated cytotoxicity. Ann Rev Immunol 1985; 3: 31.
17. Veith FJ, Sinha SBP, Dougherty JC, et al. Nature and evolution of lung allograft rejection with and without immunosuppression.

J Thorac Cardiovasc Surg 1972; 63: 509.
18. Veith FJ, Richards K. Improved technique for canine lung transplantation. Ann Surg 1973; 171: 553.
19. Nehlsen-Cannarella S, Veith FJ, Kamholz SL, et al. Variable tempo of cyclosporine peaks and troughs in lung transplant recipient: importance of frequent monitoring. Transplant Proc 1983; 15: 2450.
20. Norin A, Emeson EE, Montefusco CM, Pinsker KL, Kamholz SL, Veith FJ. Improved survival of transplanted lungs in mongrel dogs treated with cyclosporin A. Transplantation 1981; 32: 259.
21. Veith FJ, Norin AJ, Montefusco CM, et al. Cyclosporin A in experimental lung transplantation. Transplantation 1981; 32: 474.
22. Norin AJ, Emeson EE, Kamholz SL, et al. Cyclosporin A as the initial immunosuppressive agent for canine lung transplantation: short and long term assessment of rejection phenomena. Transplantation 1982; 34: 372.
23. Norin AJ, Emeson EE, Veith FJ. Unresponsiveness to lung allografts in mongrel dogs after cyclosporin A therapy. Transplant Proc 1983; 15: 508.
24. Pinsker KL, Norin A, Kamholz SL, Schreiber K, Montefusco CM, Veith FJ. Cell content in repetitive canine bronchoalveolar lavage. Acta Cytol 1980; 24: 558.
25. Saltini C, Hance AJ, Ferrans V, Basset F, Bitterman P, Crystal RG. Comparison of millipore filter and cytocentrifuge methods of quantifying bronchoalveolar lavage. NIH Workshop International Conference on Bronchoalveolar Lavage, Columbia, Md, May 1984.
26. Norin AJ, Emeson EE, Veith FJ. Studies on T cells from cyclosporine-induced unresponsive dog lung allograft recipients: reduced lymphocyte-mediated cytotoxicity but not reduced mixed lymphocyte reactivity. Transplant Proc 1983; 15: 2979.
27. Deeg HJ, Storb R, Gerhard-Miller L, Shulman HM, Weiden PL, Thomas ED. Cyclosporin A, a powerful immunosuppressant in vivo and in vitro in the dog, fails to induce tolerance. Transplantation 1980; 29: 230.
28. Bonavida B, Robins A, Saxon A. Lectin-dependent cellular cytotoxicity in man. Transplantation 1977; 23: 261.
29. Norin A, Karpel J, Fleitman J, Kamholz S, Pinsker K. Concanavalin A dependent cell mediated cytotoxicity in bronchoalveolar lavage fluid of patients with interstitial lung diseases: evidence of cytolytic T lymphocyte activity. Chest 1986; 89: 144S.
30. Doherty PC, Blanden RV, Zinkernagel R. Specificity of virus immune effector T cells for H-2K or H-2D compatibility interactions. Implications for H-antigen diversity. Transplant Rev 1976; 29: 89.
31. Buurman WA, Daeman AJJM, Groenewegen G, Doses RJMM, vander Linden CJ, Vegt PA. Limiting dilution analysis of canine alloantigen-reactive T lymphocytes. Transplantation 1983; 35: 363.
32. Keown PA, Essery-Rice G, Hellstron A, Sinclair NR, Stiller CR. Inhibition of human in vivo cytolytic T lymphocyte generation by cyclosporine following organ transplantation. Transplantation 1985; 40: 45.
33. Homan WP, French ME, Mallard PR, Morris PJ. A study of eleven drug regimens using cyclosporin A to suppress renal allografts in the dog. Transplant Proc 1981; 13: 397.
34. Nagao T, White DJG, Calne RY. Kinetics of unresponsiveness induced by a short course of cyclosporin A. Transplantation 1982; 33: 31.
35. Bordes-Aznar J, Lear PA, Strom TB, Tilney NL, Kupiec-Weglinski JW. Kinetics of cyclosporin A-induced unresponsiveness to cardiac allografts in rats. Transplant Proc 1983; 15: 500.
36. Green CJ, Allison AC, Precious S. Induction of specific tolerance in rabbits by kidney allografting and short period of cyclosporin A treatment. Lancet 1979; 2: 123.
37. Calne RY, White DJ, Rolles K, Smith DP, Herbertson B. Prolonged survival of pig orthotopic heart grafts treated with cyclosporin A. Lancet 1978; 1: 1183.
38. Birkeland SA. Withdrawal of cyclosporine treatment one year after renal transplantation. Transplantation 1985; 39: 677.
39. Bevan MJ, Cohn M. Cytotoxic effects of antigen and mitogen induced T cells on various targets. J Immunol 1975; 114: 559.
40. Lanier LL, Engleman EG, Gatenby P, Babcok CP, Warner NL, Hereberg LA. Correlation of functional properties of human lymphoid cell subsets and surface marker phenotypes using multiparameter analysis and flow cytometry. Immunol Rev 1983; 74: 143.
41. Ortaldo JR, Oldham RK, Cannon GC, Herberman RB. Specificity of natural cytotoxic reactivity of normal human lymphocytes against a myeloid leukemia cell line. J Natl Cancer Inst 1977; 59: 77.
42. Meuer SC, Hussey RE, Hodgdon JC, Hercend T, Schlossman SF, Reinherz EL. Surface structures involved in target recognition by human cytotoxic T lymphocytes. Science 1982; 218: 471.
43. Grimm EA, Mazumder A, Zhang HZ, Rosenberg SA. Lymphokine-activated killer cell phenomena. Lysis of natural killer-resistant fresh solid tumor cells by interleukin-2-activated autologous human peripheral blood lymphocytes. J Exp Med 1982; 155: 1823.
44. Karre K, Seeley JK, Eriksson E, Burton RC, Kiessling R. Anomalous Thy 1^+ killer cells in allogeneic and F_1-anti parental mixed leukocyte culture. Relation to natural killer cells and allospecific cytotoxic T lymphocytes. J Exp Med 1983; 156: 385.

Received 13 November 1985.
Accepted 7 February 1986.

0041-1337/861/4205-0473$02.00/0
TRANSPLANTATION
Vol. 42, No. 5
Printed in U.S.A.

ADVERSE EFFECT OF SPLENECTOMY ON THE SURVIVAL OF PATIENTS WITH MORE THAN ONE KIDNEY TRANSPLANT[1]

FRANCES S. SHOFER,[2] W. THOMAS LONDON,[2,3] PATRICIA LYONS,[4] SIMON J. SIMONIAN,[4] JAMES F. BURKE,[5] BRUCE E. JARRELL,[5] ROBERT A. GROSSMAN,[6] AND CLYDE F. BARKER[6]

Institute for Cancer Research, Fox Chase Cancer Center, Philadelphia 19111; Hahnemann University Hospital, Philadelphia 19102; Thomas Jefferson University Hospital, Philadelphia 19107; and Hospital of the University of Pennsylvania, Philadelphia, Pennsylvania 19104

Risk factors associated with death were identified in a cohort of patients who received 2 or more kidney transplants. Data on 19 variables were collected by chart review on 774 patients who received allografts between 1973 and 1980 at any one of 3 hospitals in Philadelphia. 124 of the patients received two or more transplants and were followed for a minimum of 1.5 years.

Modified life table analyses of single variables indicated that 7 factors—splenectomy, donor source, age, transplant hospital, number of HLA mismatches, donor sex, and survival time of the prior graft—were significantly related to patient survival. Using all 19 variables, the proportional hazards model was fit to the data. The characteristics most related to survival were splenectomy (*P*<.001), donor source (*P* = .0022), and age (*P* = .0015). The other 4 factors that were significant on univariate analysis were not significant in this multivariate analysis. The relative risk of death was 5.5 for patients who had had a splenectomy compared with those who had not had a splenectomy.

Patients who had received more than one transplant were compared with patients who had received only one transplant, and a subset of recipients of primary transplants who returned to dialysis after primary graft failure. Survival of patients who had received one transplant was approximately the same as that of the retransplanted population. When the proportional hazards model was fit to the populations that received one transplant and compared with the model for the retransplanted group, only age and donor source were common to all three models. The effect of splenectomy on survival was significant for the total population of primary transplant recipients but had no effect on the survival of the subset of recipients whose kidney grafts had failed and were returned to hemodialysis.

Infection accounted for 45% of the deaths among splenectomized, retransplanted patients. A higher percentage of septic deaths occurred in patients whose grafts were functioning at the time of death when compared with patients who had returned to dialysis after secondary graft failure.

Although retransplantation alone is not associated with an increased mortality, retransplantation in splenectomized patients carries a high risk of death.

Over the past 15 years, transplantation mortality has significantly decreased. In 1968, patient survival at one year was 58%—whereas in 1982, 86% of the patients receiving a cadaver graft survived to one year (*1, 2*). This dramatic decline is related to a progressive decrease in the number of septic deaths brought about by a better appreciation of the risks and limitations of immunosuppressive drugs and the use of broad spectrum antibiotics prophylactically (*3*).

Unfortunately, improvement in graft survival had not paralleled that of patient survival. In 1982, cadaver graft survival was 56% at one year, which was only a small increase over the survival rate in 1968, 48% (*1, 2*). As a result of the decline in patient mortality and continuing high rate of graft loss, many patients who have a failed first graft can be rehabilitated to receive another. Although the number of patients awaiting retransplantation has steadily increased, approximately one-third are actually transplanted again (between 10% and 20% of all transplants) thereby making retransplanted recipients a relatively small population. The number of reported series of such patients is, likewise, small.

Little is known about the risk factors affecting the survival of retransplanted recipients. Although, other investigators have not reported an increase in mortality in this group when compared with primary transplant recipients (*4–8*), subgroups of retransplanted patients may have an increased risk of death. The objective of this study was to identify specific risk factors associated with an increase in mortality rate in a cohort of patients who had received more than one kidney transplant. In addition, a comparison was made between the survival of retransplanted patients with the survival of patients who only received one transplant.

MATERIALS AND METHODS

All patients transplanted at any one of three hospitals in Philadelphia (Hahnemann University Hospital, Hospital of the University of Pennsylvania, and Thomas Jefferson University Hospital) between January 1, 1973 and December 31, 1980 were eligible for the study. Entry into the study was taken as date of transplant. Endpoint was date of death or March 15, 1982, whichever came first. Follow-up periods ranged from 1.5 to 9 years. Data on 20 variables thought to influence graft and/or patient survival was collected retrospectively from the charts of 774 patients (Table 1).

[1] This work was supported in part by USPHS Grants CA-06551, CA-22780, RR-05539, and CA-06927 from the National Institutes of Health, and by an appropriation from the Commonwealth of Pennsylvania.

[2] University of Pennsylvania School of Veterinary Medicine.

[3] To whom reprint requests should be addressed at Fox Chase Cancer Center.

[4] Hahnemann University Hospital.

[5] Thomas Jefferson University Hospital.

[6] Hospital of the University of Pennsylvania.

TABLE 1. Variables screened for association with patient survival

Variable	Categories
ABO blood type	O type/non O type
Age I (years)	Continuous
Age II (years)	0–30/31–45/>45
Dialysis time I (months)	<6, 6–12, 12–36, >36
Dialysis time II (years)	0–1/>1
Donor race	Black/other than black
Donor sex	Male/female
Donor source	Cadaver/parent or child/sibling
Graft status	Rejected/functioning
HBsAg status	HBsAg (−)/HBsAg (+)
Anti-HBs status prior to tx	Anti-HBs (+)/anti-HBs (−)
HLA-A,B mismatches I	0–1/2/3–4 antigens mismatched
HLA-A,B mismatches II	0–2/3–4 antigens mismatched
HLA-A,B mismatches III	0–2 cadaver/3–4 cadaver/1rd
Hospital of transplant	Hospitals, A, B, C
Hospital B	No/yes
Nephrectomy prior to transplant	No/yes
Number of transplants	2/more than 2
Preoperative blood transfusions	No/yes
Primary diagnosis I	By disease
Primary diagnosis II	Systemic/nonsystemic
Primary graft survival (months) I	Continuous
Primary graft survival (months) I	None/>0 months
Recipient race	Black/other than black
Recipient sex	Male/female
Splenectomy prior to transplant	No/yes
Year of last transplant I	Continuous from 1973 to 1980
Year of last transplant II	1973–74/1975–77/1978–80
Year of primary transplant I	Continuous from 1967 to 1980
Year of primary transplant II	<1973/1974–1977/1978–80

Of the 774 patients, 352 experienced a primary graft failure and were returned to dialysis. Of these, 150 were retransplanted, the rest remained on dialysis. A total of 26 patients were excluded from the retransplanted population because they were retransplanted elsewhere or the retransplant operation occurred after December 1980, the end of the entry period for the study. Therefore, the study group consisted of 124 patients, of whom 113 were second transplants, 9 were third, and 2 were fourth transplants.

In the second part of the study, the retransplanted population was compared with patients who received only one transplant (n = 623) and to a subset of that group including only recipients who returned to dialysis after a primary graft failure and were not known to have been retransplanted during the study period (n = 202).

Several statistical techniques were employed. Univariate analysis was accomplished by estimating the survival function by the life table method for each prognostic variable. Because of the large number of clinically relevant variables and the relationships between them, multivariate techniques were used to identify the factors that have the greatest effect on survival. For these reasons Cox's proportional hazards model as implemented by the Biomedical Data Program Statistical Software (BMDP, University of California at Los Angeles) was employed to identify and quantify the relationship between survival and a set of explanatory variables or prognostic factors. The model of best fit was determined by the maximum partial likelihood ratio test. To assess the relationship between cause of death and other factors, log linear analysis as implemented by BMDP was used.

RESULTS

For each of the 20 prognostic variables, retransplanted recipients were grouped according to subsets of the variables, and survival curves for the subgroups were estimated by the life table method. Using this technique, 7 factors—age, donor source, number of HLA mismatches, pretransplant splenectomy, transplant hospital, donor sex, and survival time of prior transplant—were of prognostic significance (Table 2).

The five-year survival for recipients over 45 years of age at the time of their last transplant was 26%, compared with 69% and 78% for the categories 31–45 years and 30 years or less, respectively. The differences between the 3 age groups are constant for the first 4 years, with a decrease in survival in the oldest age group, in the interval 4–4.5 years (data not shown, but roughly indicated in Table 2).

For donor source, as expected, mortality was higher among recipients of grafts from cadaver donors: 84% of the recipients who received a subsequent transplant from a relative survived to five years compared with 61% of the cadaver-donor recipients. This difference started from the onset of retransplantation and continued throughout the posttransplant period.

Recipients who had had a splenectomy had considerably poorer survival than those who had not (Fig. 1). Indications for removal of the spleen in these patients were splenic enlargement and leukopenia. In addition, in one of the hospitals, splenectomy was performed routinely until early 1974. Five years after transplantation only 37% of the splenectomized

TABLE 2. Summary survival data for 7 variables significantly related to survival in recipients who received more than one transplant

Prognostic variable	Number of patients (%)	Percentage surviving		
		1 Year	2 Years	5 Years
Age (years) II:				
<31	50 (40)	88	85	78
31–45	55 (44)	78	74	69
>45	19 (15)	68	62	26
Donor source:				
Cadaver	104 (84)	78	73	61
Living-related	21 (16)	95	95	84
HLA:				
0–2 mismatches	87 (70)	85	81	70
3–4 mismatches	37 (30)	77	66	52
Splenectomy:				
No	89 (72)	88	85	78
Yes	35 (28)	62	56	37
Transplant hospital:				
A	51 (41)	69	66	50
B	57 (46)	91	89	85
C	16 (13)	81	67	52
Donor sex (excludes living-related):				
Male	67 (64)	84	82	68
Female	37 (36)	67	58	47
Prior graft survival time:				
<One month	26 (21)	96	96	84
One month plus	97 (79)	76	71	58

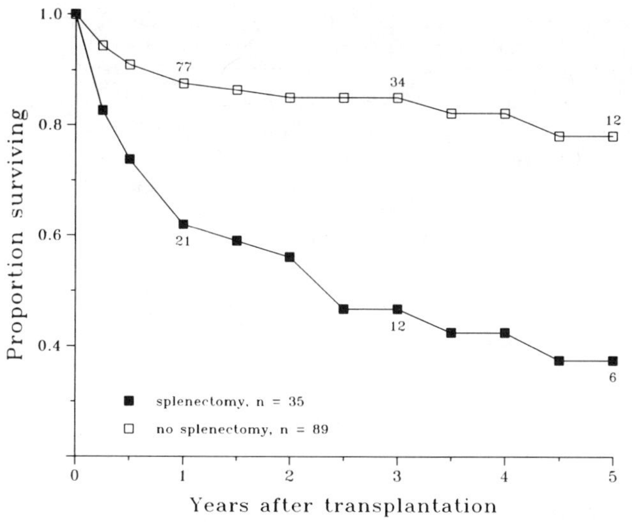

FIGURE 1. Patient survival after retransplantation: effect of splenectomy. The number of patients at risk at 1, 3, and 5 years is indicated below each curve ($P<0.001$ for the Breslow and Mantel-Cox tests, indicating that survival in nonsplenectomized patients is superior to that in patients receiving a splenectomy). For splenectomized patients the average age was 34.4 years; 77.1% received a cadaver kidney. For nonsplenectomized patients the average age was 33.8 years, 86.5% received a cadaver kidney.

recipients were still alive, compared with 78% of nonsplenectomized patients.

Using all 20 variables, the proportional hazards model was fit to the data. The characteristics most related to survival in order of entry into the equation were splenectomy ($P<0.0001$), age ($P = .0015$), and donor source ($P = .0022$) (Table 3). The other 4 factors that were significant on univariate analysis were not significant in this multivariate analysis, apparently because they were related to other factors that were significant. For example, on initial analysis of hospital where the transplant operation was performed, Hospital B had approximately 30% better survival at 5 years than Hospitals A or C. Because hospitals differ markedly in their treatment and patient populations, hospital of transplantation was evaluated for associations with the 3 variables (splenectomy, age, donor source) that were significant in the proportional hazards model. Of the three factors, there was an association between splenectomy and hospital; 10.5% of the recipients at Hospital B had a splenectomy compared with 53% and 12.5% in Hospitals A and C, respectively. This explains the difference in survival between Hospital B and A but not between B and C. The latter difference was accounted for by age; a significantly higher proportion of patients over 45 years of age (31.3%) were retransplanted at Hospital C compared with Hospital B (8.8%).

In the proportional hazards model favorable characteristics were no pretransplant splenectomy, a kidney graft from a living-related donor, and a young age (25 years) at time of retransplant. Unfavorable characteristics were: pretransplant splenectomy, a cadaver-donor kidney, and an older age (50 years) at time of retransplant. The relative risk for each variable was calculated by considering these favorable or unfavorable values of that variable, assuming the other variables were at their average value. For example, the risk of death for a recipient who had a splenectomy is 5.5 times greater than that for a recipient without a splenectomy. Likewise, a recipient of a cadaver-donor kidney has a 4.3-times greater risk of dying than the recipient of a kidney from a living-related donor, and a 50-year-old recipient has a 4.0 times greater risk of death compared with a 25-year-old recipient.

The retransplanted population was then compared with patients who received only one transplant, and a subset of this group that included only those recipients who returned to dialysis after primary graft failure and were not retransplanted during the entry period. Survival rates of these populations were approximately the same as that of the retransplanted population (Fig. 2). For the chronically dialyzed patient, survival rates were higher at 1 year, (87%) and lower at 5 years (52%), but neither of these differences was statistically significant.

Because no difference in survival was found in retransplanted patients when compared with patients who received one transplant, it was of interest to determine if the same prognostic variables were related to survival. When the data from the 202 recipients with failed primary renal grafts, who remained on maintenance hemodialysis were fitted to Cox's model, only age and donor source were common to both models). (Year of transplant and underlying disease were also included in the model of best fit for recipients returning to maintenance hemodialysis after graft failure.) Because splenectomy was not included in this model we looked at this risk factor alone in

TABLE 3. Variables related to survival from time of retransplantation[a]

Prognostic variable	Approximate chi-square	Significance level (P)
Splenectomy	22.41	<.0001
Age I	10.06	.0015
Donor source	9.03	.0022
Hospital	2.03	.1528
HLA mismatches	0.16	.6926
Donor sex	1.42	.2335
Prior graft survival time	1.43	.2325

[a] Proportional hazards model—Cox.

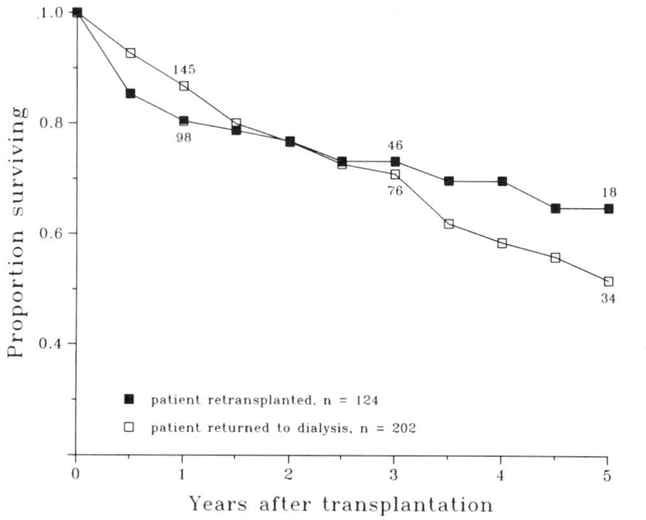

FIGURE 2. Relationship of treatment to patient survival in patients experiencing a primary graft failure. The number of patients at risk at 1, 3, and 5 years is indicated by the number above or below each curve (P values for the Breslow and Mantel-Cox test were .8892 and .3398, respectively).

these dialysis patients. On survival analysis there was no significant difference between splenectomized and nonsplenectomized patients who returned to dialysis after primary graft failure ($P = .7111$ and .8931 for the Breslow and Mantel-Cox tests, respectively).

When the data from the 623 recipients who received only a primary transplant were fitted to Cox's model and compared with the model of best fit for the retransplanted population, splenectomy in addition to donor source and age were common to both models. (The model of best fit for primary transplant recipients included two other factors—underlying disease and number of HLA mismatches.) Using the same set of favorable and unfavorable patient characteristics as were used in Cox's model for retransplantation, the relative risks for all three common factors were considerably less than those observed in patients receiving more than one transplant. For example, the relative risk of splenectomy in regrafted patients was 5.5 times greater than in nonsplenectomized recipients, whereas the relative risk for splenectomized primary transplanted recipients as compared with nonsplenectomized recipients was only 1.85 (Table 4). Univariate analysis of splenectomy confirms this observation. As illustrated in Figure 3, the magnitude of the difference at 5 years between splenectomized and nonsplenectomized retransplanted patients is considerably greater than the difference between splenectomized and nonsplenectomized primary transplant patients (40% vs. 10%).

The last variable examined was cause of death. Of the 124 patients, there were 35 deaths during the follow-up period. Infection accounted for the majority of deaths (37.1%). Other factors in transplantation have been known to influence cause of death. Two such factors were recipient's graft status at the time of death and pretransplant splenectomy. In Table 5 one can see a relationship between graft status and cause of death, as all patients whose death was due to infection died with a functioning graft. Furthermore, the majority of transplant deaths (59%)—that is patients who did not return to dialysis—was due to infection.

Although splenectomy and cause of death were not directly related, there appears to be an association within the subgroup of recipients who died a transplant death (i.e., were not on dialysis at the time of death). Of the 13 patients who died of infection in this group, 9 (69%) of them had been splenectomized. In addition the majority of the deaths (45%) among splenectomized recipients was due to infection.

TABLE 4. Comparison of relative risks in retransplanted patients and patients with only one transplant for selected variables[a]

Prognostic variable	Ratio of Risks	
	Retransplanted group (124)	Primary transplant only group (623)
Splenectomy	5.54	1.85
Age I	3.97	2.00
Donor source	3.60	1.97

[a] Favorable characteristics: no splenectomy, 25 years of age, living-related donor; unfavorable characteristics: splenectomy, 50 years of age, cadaver donor.

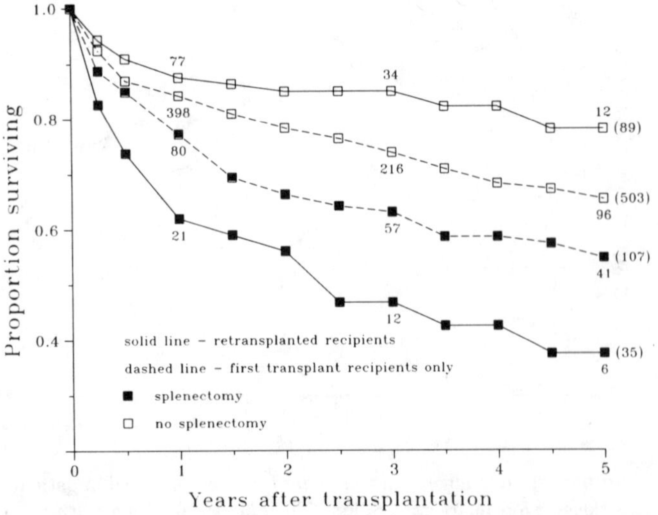

FIGURE 3. Comparison of patient survival by number of transplants: effect of splenectomy. The number of patients at risk at 1, 3, and 5 years is indicated above or below each curve. Numbers in parentheses represent the total number of patients at risk for that group.

TABLE 5. Log linear model for the factors graft status, splenectomy, and cause of death for retransplanted patients

Graft status[a]	Cause of death	Splenectomy		
		No	Yes	Total
Rejected	Infection	0	0	0
	Cardiovascular	3	0	3
	GI bleeding	1	0	1
	Other/unknown	5	4	9
	Total	9	4	13
Functioning	Infection	4	9	13
	Cardiovascular	1	2	3
	GI bleeding	1	3	4
	Other/unknown	0	2	2
	Total	6	16	22

[a] Refers to whether patient was on dialysis at time of death or died transplant death.

DISCUSSION

In agreement with other investigators, we did not find an increased mortality associated with retransplantation when compared with primary transplantation. The two-year mortality rate was approximately 20% for both groups. In other studies that examined retransplantation, the mortality ranged from 11% to 30% (*4–8*).

Although mortality experience is similar, the factors affecting survival in retransplanted recipients appear to be different. Underlying disease, number of HLA mismatches, and chronological year of transplantation influenced the survival of recipients of primary transplants (as indicated by Cox's models) but were not of significance in the retransplant population. Pretransplant splenectomy, donor source, and age were the only factors associated with the survival of retransplanted patients. Not only were the risk factors different, but the strengths of association with survival were also different. When compared, all three risk factors—age, donor source, and splenectomy—had a far greater influence on survival of the retransplanted group than in the primary transplant group.

Within the retransplanted group, a subgroup was identified that had a low mortality risk. Patients who were young, received a second kidney from a relative, and were not splenectomized had the lowest risk of death (estimated mortality at 4.5 years was 0.03%). On the other hand, asplenic older patients who received a cadaver kidney were at highest risk of death. The estimated mortality at one year was approximately 80%. Age of the patient and availability of a suitable donor kidney from a relative are not risk factors that can be altered. Whether to attempt transplantation on these potential recipients with an estimated survival of 62.8% at 4.5 years is a decision left to the recipient and transplant team.

However, splenectomy, which has by far the greatest influence on patient survival can be controlled. In the past, the rationale for splenic removal in transplantation was that it reduced lymphoid mass and increased the recipient's tolerance to azathioprine treatment. Several series (the Chicago group, Schulak and Stuart [*9, 10*] and Vertuno et al. [*11*]; Milwaukee group, Kauffman et al. [*12*]; and the Minnesota group Fryd et al. [*13*]) have shown that splenectomy does alter immunologic function and impairs the ability of patients to reject renal allografts. These investigators advocated pretransplant splenectomy because of a significant improvement in graft survival rates among their asplenic patients when compared with a comparable group of recipients who were not splenectomized. In a recent reanalysis of the Minnesota randomized prospective trial of splenectomy, Sutherland and colleagues demonstrated no effect of splenectomy on long-term (5-year) graft survival rates, with no detrimental effect on patients survival (*14*).

On the other hand, because removal of the spleen leads to depressed ability to clear bacteria and particulate antigens from the circulation, the splenectomized patient is at increased risk of death from overwhelming infection. A number of studies support this conclusion. O'Neal et al. (*15*) reported on 256 patients who underwent splenectomy (not necessarily transplant patients) and determined that death from sepsis in asplenic adults was 540 times as prevalent as death due to sepsis in the population at large. In the transplant literature, Rai et al. (*16*) demonstrated a significantly higher mortality in asplenic transplant recipients beginning at 1 year posttransplant. Two recent series (Alexander et al. (*17*) and Peters et al. (*18*)) that examined splenectomy and death in renal transplant patients also found an adverse effect of splenectomy on patient survival following primary renal transplantation. Both groups reported an excess number of deaths due to septicemia in their asplenic patients.

As demonstrated, the results of this study on retransplanted recipients are in agreement with the latter. At five years, only 37% of the splenectomized patients were still alive, compared with 78% of nonsplenectomized patients. In addition a higher proportion of the deaths due to infection were in the asplenic group (69%). Similarly, Spees et al. (*7*), in a report examining selective and therapeutic factors affecting multiple cadaveric kidney transplant success, found a reduced patient survival rate in both primary and secondary transplant recipients who had had pretransplant splenectomies. To date, the only other report that specifically addressed the issue of splenectomy in retransplanted recipients was that of Pierce and Hume (*19*). These authors recommended splenectomy before retransplantation because they demonstrated a beneficial effect on their retransplanted population but not on their primary transplant population. The number of asplenic patients was small (*5*) and the study was done in the early days of transplantation. A helpful association between splenectomy and graft survival could not be found in a later study by Hume and colleagues that included 25 patients (*20*).

Presence of splenectomy as a risk factor in either primary or subsequent transplantation and the absence of this effect on survival in patients returning to dialysis suggests that it is the combination of immunosuppressive therapy (all patients with a functioning renal allograft take immunosuppressive drugs to prevent rejection) and splenectomy that affects mortality. In support of this, Schwartz et al. (*21*), in a study examining postsplenectomy sepsis and mortality, reported the highest risk of infection in patients who, in addition to their splenectomy, had received chemotherapy, radiation, immunosuppressive therapy—or any combination of the three. Patients who were at lowest risk of infection were those who had a splenectomy as a result of trauma with no additional risk factors—e.g., chemotherapy.

Further support for the relationship between splenectomy combined with immunosuppressive therapy and infection can be seen on examination of cause of death. First, septicemia is more often associated with a transplant death (graft still functioning at time of death) than a dialysis death (graft lost, recipient died on dialysis). In this study, for the recipients who died with a functioning regraft, 59% of the deaths were due to septicemia when compared with all other causes. Of the thirteen retransplant recipients who died a dialysis death there were no known deaths due to infection. Several studies comparing causes of death in transplant and dialysis populations have also presented similar results (*22, 23*). Krumlovsky and colleagues reported that 16 of 22 deaths in their transplant population were due to infectious causes, compared with zero deaths of 10 in the dialysis population. Virtually all of their transplant deaths could be attributed to the transplant procedure and its complications, whereas most dialysis deaths were related to the underlying disease. Although Tilney et al. (*3*) have reported a decline in deaths caused by sepsis because of improved patient care and management of immunosuppressive therapy, infection is still a major cause of death in transplant patients.

Since 1977 a 14-valent, polysaccharide vaccine against pneumococcal infection (*Streptococcus pneumoniae*) has been available, and its use in splenectomized patients is recommended (*24*). More recently, the vaccine has been broadened to include 23 antigenic types (*25*). The use of these vaccines may reduce the risk of infections as a cause of death in splenectomized, retransplanted patients. Further investigation will be required to determine if this is the case.

In summary, three factors have been shown to be consistently related to patient survival in a retransplanted population. They are splenectomy, donor source, and age—of which splenectomy has the strongest association. There does not appear to be an increased mortality associated with retransplantation itself, although the factors affecting survival of these recipients are different. It is the combination of splenectomy and immunosuppressive therapy that negatively affects patient survival.

Acknowledgments. We gratefully acknowledge the statistical advice of Drs. E.D. Lustbader and S. Litwin.

REFERENCES

1. Advisory Committee to the Renal Transplant Registry. The 9th Report of the Human Transplant Registry. JAMA 1972; 220: 253.
2. Krakauer H, Grauman JS, McMullan MR, Creede CC. The recent U.S. experience in the treatment of end-stage renal disease by dialysis and transplantation. N Engl J Med 1983; 308: 1558.
3. Tilney NL, Strom TB, Vineyard GC, Merrill JP. Factors contributing to the declining mortality rate in renal transplantation. N Engl J Med 1978; 299: 1321.

4. Ascher NL, Ahrenholz DH, Simmons RL, Najarian JS. 100 second renal allografts from a single transplantation institution. Transplantation 1979; 27: 30.
5. Gifford RRM, Sutherland DER, Fryd DS, Simmons RL, Najarian JS. Duration of first renal allograft survival as indicator of second allograft outcome. Surgery 1980; 88: 611.
6. Potaux L, Aparicio M, leGuillou M. 30 cases of second renal transplants. Eur Urol 1981; 7: 201.
7. Spees EK, Vaughn WK, McDonald JC, et al. Why do secondary cadaver renal transplants succeed? Results of the South-Eastern Organ Procurement Foundation prospective study, 1977–1982. J Urol 1983; 129: 484.
8. Waltzer WC, Zincke H, Sterioff S, Offord KP. Renal transplantation after failure of a first graft. Surg Gyn Obstet 1981; 152: 476.
9. Stuart FP, Reckard CR, Ketel BL, Schulak JA. Effect of splenectomy on first cadaver kidney transplants. Ann Surg 1980; 191: 553.
10. Schulak JA, Hill JL, Reckard CR, Simonian SJ, Stuart FP. Infectious and functional consequences of splenectomy in adult renal transplant recipients. J Surg Res 1978; 25: 404.
11. Vertuno LL, Bansal VK, Hano JE, Giacchino JL, Geis WP. The role of splenectomy in cadaveric renal transplantation. Nephron 1981; 27: 273.
12. Kauffman HM, Swanson MK, McGregor WR, Rodgers RE, Fox PS. Splenectomy in renal transplantation. Surg Gyn Obstet 1974; 139: 33.
13. Fryd DS, Sutherland DER, Simmons RL, Ferguson CM, Kjellstrand CM, Najarian JS. Results of a prospective randomized study on the effect of splenectomy versus no splenectomy in renal transplant patients. Transplant Proc 1981; 13: 48.
14. Sutherland DER, Fryd DS, Bentley FR, Najarian JS. Longterm effect of splenectomy versus no splenectomy in renal transplant patients: re-analysis of a randomized prospective study. Transplant Proc 1985; 17: 136.
15. O'Neal BJ, McDonald JC. The risk of sepsis in the asplenic adult. Ann Surg 1981; 194: 775.
16. Rai GS, Wilkinson R, Taylor RMR, Uldall PR, Kerr DNS. Adverse effect of splenectomy in renal transplantation. Clin Nephrol 1978; 9: 194.
17. Peters TG, Williams JW, Harmon HC, Britt LG. Splenectomy and death in renal transplant patients. Arch Surg 1983; 118: 795.
18. Alexander JW, First, MR, Majeski JA, et al. The late adverse effect of splenectomy on patient survival following cadaveric renal transplantation. Transplantation 1984; 37: 467.
19. Pierce JC, Hume DH. The effect of splenectomy on the survival of first and second renal homotransplants in man. Surg Gyn Obstet 1968; 1300.
20. Hume DM. The immunological consequences of organ homotransplantation in man. Harvey Lect 1968–1969; 64: 261.
21. Schwartz PE, Sterioff S, Mucha P, Melton LP, Offord KP. Postsplenectomy sepsis and mortality in adults. JAMA 1982; 248: 2279.
22. Vincenti F, Amend W, Feduska NJ, Duca RM, Salvatierra O. Improved outcome following renal transplantation with reduction in the immunosuppression therapy for rejection episodes. Am J Med 1980; 69: 107.
23. Krumlovsky FA, del Greco F, Simon MM, Roguska J. Morbidity and mortality of chronic hemodialysis compared to renal transplantation. Trans Am Soc Artif Intern Organs 1975; 21: 102.
24. Austrian R, Douglas RM, Schiffman G. Prevention of pneumococcal pneumonia by vaccination. Trans Assoc Am Physicians 1976; 89: 184.
25. CDC Update: pneumococcal polysaccharide vaccine usage—United States. MMWR 1984; 33: 273.

Received 5 November 1985.
Accepted 10 February 1986.

0041-1337/86/4205-0479$02.00/0
TRANSPLANTATION
Vol. 42, No. 5

EXPRESSION OF HLA-DR ANTIGENS ON PERIPHERAL BLOOD T LYMPHOCYTES AND RENAL GRAFT TUBULAR EPITHELIAL CELLS IN ASSOCIATION WITH REJECTION[1]

FELIX C. HENNY,[2,3] JAN J. WEENING,[4] WILLIAM M. BALDWIN,[2] PAUL J. OLJANS,[5] HANS J. TANKE,[5] LEENDERT A. VAN ES,[2] AND LEENDERT C. PAUL[2]

Departments of Nephrology, Pathology, and Histochemistry and Cytochemistry, University Hospital Leiden, The Netherlands

Since the expression of HLA-DR antigens on peripheral blood T lymphocytes and renal graft tubular epithelial cells may be associated with immunological stimulation, we investigated the expression of these antigens on blood T lymphocytes and graft tubular epithelium in 84 renal transplant patients. Peripheral blood T lymphocytes were monitored by flow cytometry during the first 3 months after transplantation. Since the DR⁺ lymphocytes were selected by a double-labeling technique used for the Leu2a phenotype, the majority of the DR⁺ lymphocytes were also Leu2a⁺ with a small percentage of unidentified Leu2a⁻ lymphocytes. Forty-one patients were treated with cyclosporine (CsA) and 43 with azathioprine (Aza), while both groups received low-dose steroids. Frozen sections of 57 renal biopsies from 43 patients (21 on CsA and 22 on Aza) were stained for HLA-DR antigens. In the Aza group, clinical rejection episodes correlated with an increased percentage of DR⁺ peripheral lymphocytes (P=0.0005), and the expression of DR antigens on graft epithelial cells (P<0.001). In the CsA group, no relation between the expression of DR antigens on blood lymphocytes and clinical rejection episodes was evident, and the correlation between tubular DR staining and clinical rejection episodes was weaker than in the Aza group (P=0.03). In both the Aza and CsA group, an increase in DR⁺ peripheral lymphocytes correlated with positive staining of the renal tubular cells for HLA-DR antigens (P<0.001).

Monitoring of peripheral blood T lymphocyte subpopulations with monoclonal antibodies (mAbs)* may be useful for the management of rejection episodes in renal transplant recipients (*1, 2*). No consensus has been achieved, however, regarding the correlation between the T lymphocyte subpopulation ratios and the occurrence of rejection episodes (*2–4*). Since in-vivo-activated T cells express activation markers, such as class II antigens (*5*), some investigators have measured activated T cells in renal transplant recipients and found that the appearance of such markers correlates with rejection episodes or cytomegalovirus (CMV) infections in patients treated with Aza (*6–8*). In CsA-treated patients this correlation is weaker (*6*), which perhaps can be explained by the observation that CsA inhibits the appearance of activation markers after in vitro stimulation (*9, 10*). We recently reported that shortly after transplantation the percentage of "cytotoxic-suppressor" (Leu2a-positive) T cells that are HLA-DR-positive may exceed a 6% baseline value found for control subjects, while the percentage of HLA-DR-positive cells of the "helper-inducer" phenotype (Leu3a-positive) varies widely (*11*). Furthermore, others have found that the expression of class II antigens on renal tubular epithelial cells appears to correlate with rejection (*12*).

The aim of our study was to analyze whether the expression of HLA-DR antigens on peripheral blood T lymphocytes correlates with HLA-DR expression on renal graft tubular epithelial cells and to investigate the correlation of both with graft rejection.

MATERIALS AND METHODS

Patients. A group of 84 renal allograft recipients were studied during the first 3 months after transplantation; 41 were treated with CsA and 43 with Aza, while both groups received low-dose steroids, as described previously (*13*). Most patients (n=64) were randomly selected for either CsA (n=33) or Aza therapy (n=31) as part of a prospective trial. Patients who were 60 years of age or older and those who received a cadaveric graft with more than two HLA (A+B) mismatches routinely were given CsA (n=8), whereas patients who received a kidney from a living-related donor were given Aza (n=12). One or more transfusions of leukocyte-poor blood were administered to all patients before transplantation. CsA was given in a dose of 16 mg/kg/day tapered to 10 mg/kg/day over 3 months, according to a standard schedule and depending on CsA blood levels and renal function (*13*). The dosage of Aza was usually 2–2.5 mg/kg/day. In the CsA group rejection episodes were treated with 3 bolus injections of methylprednisolone; for the Aza group, rejection therapy consisted of rabbit antithymocyte globulin (RATG) or a higher dosage of prednisone. Diagnosis of rejection was based on clinical parameters, and other causes of renal dysfunction were excluded insofar as possible. The diagnosis of rejection was made independently of the experimental data presented in this paper.

Differentiation between CsA nephrotoxicity and rejection was achieved by observing the effect of a lower CsA dose on the serum creatinine concentration. When further deterioration of graft function occurred, rejection was suspected.

[1] This work was supported by a grant from The Dutch Kidney Foundation (No. C81.308).

[2] Department of Nephrology.

[3] Address correspondence to: F.C. Henny, Department of Nephrology, Building 32, University Hospital Leiden, 2333 AA Leiden, The Netherlands.

[4] Department of Pathology.

[5] Department of Histochemistry and Cytochemistry.

* Abbreviations used: Aza, azathioprine; CMV, cytomegalovirus; CsA, cyclosporine; FACS, fluorescence-activated cell sorter; FITC, fluorescein-isothiocyanate; IAHT, immune adherence hemagglutination technique; IFA, immunofluorescence assay; mAbs, monoclonal antibodies; PE, phycoerythrin; RATG, rabbit antithymocyte globulin.

Furthermore, in 57 instances a graft biopsy was taken before antirejection therapy was instituted. Diagnosis of CMV infection was based on a four-fold or more increase in the titer of antibodies against CMV (as determined by an immune adherence hemagglutination technique (IAHT)), the appearance of IgM antibodies against CMV (as determined by an immunofluorescence assay (IgM-IFA)) or positive CMV cultures. HLA-DR expression on circulating T lymphocytes was assessed 3 times a week during hospitalization and once a week during the outpatient follow-up period. During antirejection therapy, no monitoring was performed because of the lymphopenia that is usually observed during this treatment.

Pretransplantation blood samples from 59 patients were analyzed for HLA-DR expression on the T lymphocytes. For control purposes, DR expression was studied in 10 healthy controls and 20 renal allograft recipients with a stable graft function more than 6 months after transplantation. In a retrospective analysis, the expression of HLA-DR antigens on the circulating T lymphocytes was correlated with clinical rejection episodes that were defined by the institution of antirejection therapy.

Frozen sections of 57 renal biopsies obtained from 43 patients within 3 months of transplantation (21 CsA and 22 Aza) were analyzed retrospectively for HLA-DR expression on renal tubular cells.

Antisera. The following monoclonal antibodies were used: Leu2a, which reacts with the suppressor/cytotoxic subset (*14*), and the antibody designated anti-HLA-DR, which reacts with nonpolymorphic determinants of class II molecules on normal B cells and B cell lines, monocytes as well as activated T lymphocytes (*15*). The Leu2a mAB was conjugated directly with fluorescein isothiocyanate (FITC) and the anti-HLA-DR mAb with red fluorescent phycoerythrin (PE).

For staining of the biopsies by the indirect immunoperoxidase technique, the unconjugated anti-HLA-DR mAb was used together with a rabbit anti-mouse-IgG antiserum tagged with horseradish peroxidase (Dakopatts, Denmark). The Leu and anti-HLA-DR mAbs were purchased from Becton Dickinson Laboratory Systems, Mechelen, Belgium.

Analysis of peripheral blood T lymphocytes. Mononuclear cells were isolated, monocyte-depleted, and stained with both the FITC-conjugated Leu2a mAb (10 μg/ml) and the PE-conjugated anti-HLA-DR MAb (10 μg/ml) as described elsewhere (*11*). The cells were analyzed by 2 color flow cytometry using a fluorescence-activated cell sorter (FACS IV, Becton Dickinson, Sunnyvale, CA). A three-parameter analysis was performed to determine the percentage of Leu2a$^+$ cells that coexpress HLA-DR antigens. The Leu2a$^+$ cells were identified on the basis of their forward light scatter and their green FITC-fluorescence, and the cells coexpressing HLA-DR by the simultaneous red fluorescence of the PE-conjugated anti-HLA-DR (*11*). Control experiments with an HLA-DR-positive B cell line showed that there was no emission from the PE-labeled cells through the interference filter in the green channel. In the course of the study, however, we found that sometimes a small percentage of the very bright red fluorescent cells (0.1–1% of the total lymphocytes; see the *Results* section) emitted fluorescence in the green channel. Since, therefore, not all DR$^+$ cells are Leu2a$^+$ we choose to express all data as the percentage of DR$^+$ (originally also interpreted as Leu2a$^+$) cells of the total lymphocyte population.

Staining of tissue sections. For demonstration of HLA-DR antigens on renal tubular epithelial cells, an indirect immunoperoxidase technique was used, as described previously (*16*). The sections were incubated first with anti HLA-DR mAb (diluted in PBS; 1:80) and then with rabbit antimouse IgG tagged with horseradish peroxidase (diluted in 20% normal human serum; 1:80). The sections were not counterstained.

All specimens were examined by three independent investigators without prior knowledge of the clinical or the pathological diagnosis. Tubular DR staining was graded as + when most of the tubules (proximal and distal) throughout the entire

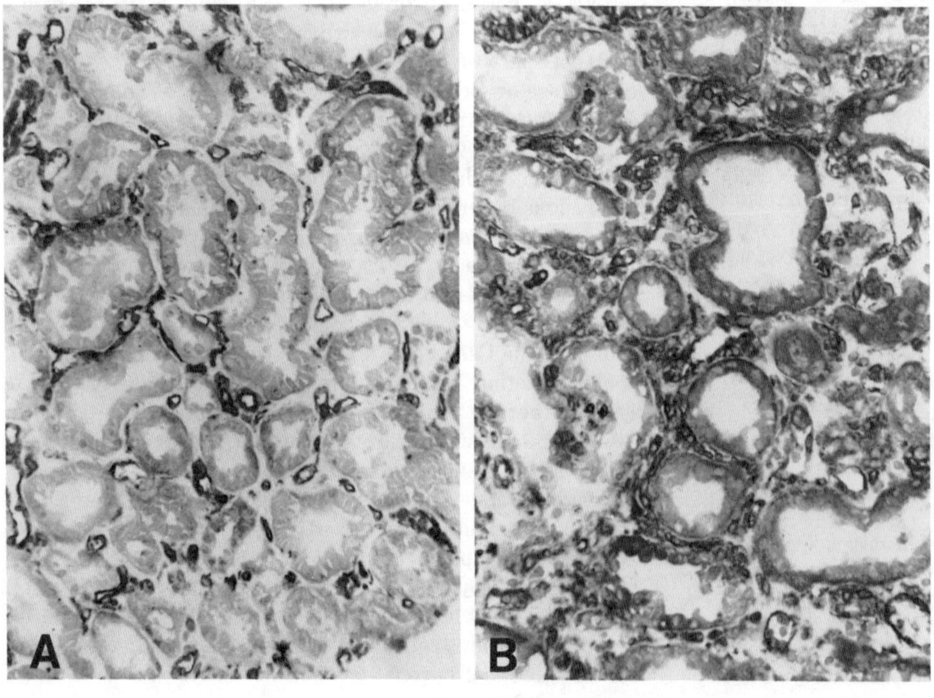

FIGURE 1. Photomicrographs of renal allograft biopsy specimens stained for HLA-DR antigen by an indirect immunoperoxidase technique: Stained cells appear black; (A) staining of structures in the interstitium only and (B) staining of both interstitium and tubular cells (400 ×).

section were positive, ± when only some of the tubules were weakly positive, and – when all tubules were negative compared with the positive staining of the interstitium (Fig. 1).

RESULTS

HLA-DR expression on peripheral blood T lymphocytes. Among the renal recipients studied during the first 3 months after transplantation, the percentage of DR^+ cells within the $Leu2a^+$ population varied from 1% to 56%, whereas the maximum percentage for controls was 6%, as described previously (*11*). When these data were analyzed in terms of the percentage of $Leu2a^+DR^+$ cells of the total lymphocyte population, the corresponding percentages were 0–11.5% and 0.8%, respectively. Among 20 additional controls with a stable graft function more than 6 months after transplantation, less than 1% (0.5± 0.2; mean ±SD) DR^+Leu2a^+ cells were found. We therefore considered 1% as the cut off point for analysis of the experimental data (Fig. 2). In 40 additional samples, in which the percentage of Dr^+Leu2a^+ cells varied from 0% to 3%, electronic compensation of the FACS for $Leu2a^-$, DR^+ cells showed that a maximum of 1% of the bright PE fluorescent cells were $Leu2a^-$ but had passed through the green channel. This implies that the percentages of DR^+ cells illustrated in Figure 2 are mainly $Leu2a^+DR^+$ cells with a small percentage of very strongly DR^+ but $Leu2a^-$ cells. Just prior to transplantation the percentage of DR^+ cells in dialysis patients varied considerably; the maximum percentage recorded was 6%. No correlation between the percentage of DR^+ cells before transplantation and either the development of an increased DR expression after transplantation or graft rejection was found. For the group of patients treated with Aza, retrospective analysis showed a correlation (P=0.0005) between an increased percentage of DR^+ cells after transplantation and the occurrence of a rejection episode, as defined by initiation of antirejection therapy (Fig. 2).

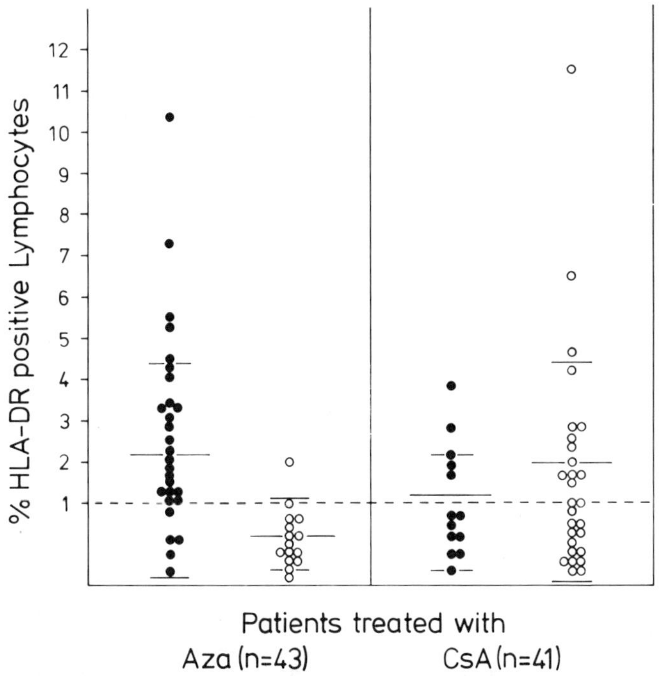

FIGURE 2. Percentages of DR^+ cells in patients treated with Aza (left) and CsA (right): (●) value before antirejection therapy; (○) highest value in patients without antirejection therapy. 23/28 patients treated with Aza had ≧1% DR^+ cells before antirejection therapy, and 13/15 patients without antirejection therapy never had ≧1% DR^+ cells (P=0.0005; Fisher's test). 5/13 patients treated with CsA had ≧1% DR^+ cells before antirejection therapy and 13/28 patients without antirejection therapy never had ≧1% DR^+ cells (P=0.31; Fisher's test).

A total of 23 of the 25 patients who developed ≧1% DR^+ cells in one or more consecutive samples received antirejection treatment. The interval between the first blood sample in which an increased DR^+ expression was observed and the start of rejection therapy varied from 1 to 14 days. Patients (n=6) with ≧1% DR^+ cells before transplantation who did not undergo a rejection episode exhibited normalization of the percentage of DR^+ cells within 10 days. In 17 of the 23 patients with increased DR expression, rejection was reversible, and after completion of antirejection therapy the percentage of DR^+ cells was less than 1%. Five patients received antirejection therapy without a prior increment in DR expression; in all cases therapy was started within 10 days of transplantation. Two patients exhibited a period (a minimum of 2 consecutive samples) of increased DR expression but did not require antirejection therapy; in both cases a symptomatic CMV infection was diagnosed on the basis of IgM antibody formation.

For patients treated with CsA, no correlation between DR expression and the initiation of antirejection therapy was found; only 5 of the 20 patients who exhibited increased DR expression required antirejection treatment, whereas 8 of the 21 patients who never showed increased DR expression received antirejection therapy. In the latter group, one patient experienced a secondary CMV infection without the formation of IgM antibodies against CMV. Of the 15 patients who exhibited increased DR expression without a clinical rejection episode, 2 had CMV infections with an IgM antibody response, 1 had a leakage of the transplant ureter, and 8 suffered a deterioration of graft function attributed to CsA nephrotoxicity. The 4 remaining patients had a stable graft function without signs of a CMV infection.

The incidence of periods of increased DR expression did not differ between the two treatment groups: 25 of 43 patients in the Aza group and 20 of 41 in the CsA group showed periods with increased DR expression. However, more patients received one or more antirejection treatments in the Aza group than in the CsA group—28 of the 43 patients in the Aza group (65.1%) versus 13 of the 41 patients in the patients in the CsA group (31.7%) (P=0.004; Fig. 2).

HLA-DR expression on graft tubular epithelial cells. The DR staining of 7 of the 57 renal biopsy sections could not be evaluated for technical reasons. The graft tubular epithelial cells in 24 biopsies were scored DR-positive unanimously (7 from the CsA and 17 from the Aza group), 18 were scored DR-negative unanimously (12 CsA and 6 Aza), and 8 (6 CsA and 2 Aza) were scored ± unanimously, or negative by one and positive or ± by the other examiners. When we analyzed only the biopsies with a unanimous score, a correlation was found (P<0.001) between DR expression in the tubular cells and rejection therapy for the Aza group (Table 1); only 1 DR-negative patient required antirejection treatment. For the CsA-treated patients this correlation was weaker (P=0.03; Table 1); 5 of the 12 patients who received antirejection therapy were DR-negative. Retrospective analysis of the light microscopy findings and the response to the antirejection treatment sug-

TABLE 1. Correlation between HLA-DR staining of renal tubular cells and rejection treatments for patients treated with azathioprine (Aza) or cyclosporine (CsA)

Treatment	Rejection	No rejection	P value (Fischer's test)
Patients treated with Aza:			
Tubular cells DR-positive	17	0	
Tubular cells DR-negative	1	5	<0.01
Patients treated with CsA:			
Tubular cells DR-positive	7	0	
Tubular cells DR-negative	5	7	0.03

TABLE 2. Correlation between HLA-DR staining of renal tubular cells and the percentage of DR$^+$ cells within the peripheral blood for 34 renal allograft recipients

	DR$^+$ cells within the peripheral blood		Total
	≧1%	<1%	
Tubular cells:			
DR-positive	17	2[a]	19
DR-negative	3	12[a]	14
Total	20	14	34

[a] P<0.001; Fischer's test.

gested, however, that the renal dysfunction was attributable to CsA nephrotoxicity rather than rejection. In 4/7 patients with a positive DR stain, rejection was irreversible. In 34 cases DR expression on peripheral lymphocytes was determined within 2 days of the biopsy. For both the Aza and the CsA-treated patients, a correlation was found between DR expression on peripheral blood cells and DR expression in the renal tubular cells of the graft (P<0.001; Table 2).

DISCUSSION

In the present study we have demonstrated that after transplantation the expression of HLA-DR antigens on peripheral lymphocytes correlates with clinical rejection episodes for renal transplant recipients treated with Aza (Fig. 2). Although we previously reported on DR$^+$ cells within the Leu2a$^+$ population (*11*), in this paper we have expressed all data as percentage of DR$^+$ cells of the total lymphocyte population because we recently found that a small percentage of the very strongly DR$^+$ cells are Leu2a$^-$ but emit fluorescence in the green FITC channel. Although the majority of DR$^+$ cells are indeed Leu2a$^+$, further experiments are in progress to determine whether the Leu2a$^-$Dr$^+$ cells belong to the "cytotoxic-suppressor" T cells with a modulated membrane structure in which the Leu2a epitope is not recognized, as shown previously (*11*). The low percentage of these cells and the fact that these very bright PE-fluorescent cells were not detected with the control B cell-line makes it unlikely that these DR$^+$Leu2a$^-$ cells are B cells.

All Aza-treated patients who received antirejection treatment while having <1% DR$^+$ cells were treated within 10 days of transplantation. Either heavier immunosuppression during this period or undetected pretransplant donor-specific presensitization may be responsible for this phenomenon, although we have no data to support either possibility. Both of the Aza-treated patients who showed increased DR expression but did not require antirejection therapy experienced a primary CMV infection; we have previously reported the expression of HLA-DR antigens on OKT 8$^+$ cells during such infections (*8*).

For CsA-treated patients no correlation between an increased DR expression on peripheral lymphocytes and clinical rejection episodes was found. However rejection is more difficult to diagnose in CsA-treated patients because of the nephrotoxic side effects of the drug (*13*). In some patients a deterioration of graft function resulting from CsA nephrotoxicity may have been treated as a rejection episode and vice-versa. It is of interest that the percentage of HLA-DR$^+$ T cells may increase in CsA-treated patients, which indicates that the drug does not prevent the appearance of the HLA-DR activation marker on T lymphocytes in vivo, as shown by others in vitro (*9, 10*). The episodes of increased DR expression in the CsA-treated patients who did not require antirejection therapy may reflect an immune activation of either suppressor cells or a mixture of both suppressor and cytotoxic cells that does not impair graft function to such an extent that additional therapy is necessary.

As mentioned, CMV infections may also lead to expression of class II antigens on T cells of the "cytotoxic-suppressor" phenotype (*8, 17, 18*). An increased percentage of DR$^+$ cells appears to occur with a primary or recurrent CMV infection only in association with an IgM antibody response to the virus. One patient with a serious secondary infection but without an IgM response did not exhibit increased DR expression. Although asymptomatic CMV infections may have caused a greater increase in DR expression in the CsA group than in the Aza group, we assume that this is unlikely since the sera of the recently transplanted patients are screened weekly for evidence of CMV infections.

The percentage of DR$^+$ lymphocytes prior to transplantation varied widely. Although a recent study of patients with aplastic anemia (*19*) showed that blood transfusions induce increased percentages of DR$^+$ Leu2a$^+$ cells that may be activated suppressor T lymphocytes, we found no correlation between the number of pretransplant blood transfusions and the percentage of DR$^+$ cells (data not shown). On the other hand, hemodialysis, continuous ambulatory peritoneal dialysis, or other as yet unknown factors could be responsible for the expression of HLA-DR antigens on circulating T lymphocytes before transplantation. The decrease in DR expression to normal values within 10 days of transplantation found for Aza-treated patients without a rejection episode could be due to immunosuppressive therapy. Pretransplant DR expression showed no correlation with graft outcome or the number of rejection episodes (data not shown).

The expression of HLA-DR antigens on graft tubular epithelium, especially distal epithelial cells, in association with rejection episodes is in agreement with the observations of Hall et al. (*12*). For nontransplanted kidneys, they and others found no DR antigens in or on tubular epithelial cells (*12, 20, 21*), whereas others reported only a faint staining within proximal tubular cells (*22, 23*). Whether these antigens are of donor or recipient origin is currently unknown but studies in animals have shown that tubular class II antigens in transplanted kidneys are of donor origin (*24–26*). Although a significantly higher percentage of biopsies was negative for HLA-DR in the CsA-treated group than in the Aza-treated group (12/19 vs. 6/23, respectively; Table 1), CsA obviously did not prevent the appearance of these antigens on tubular epithelial cells. The correlation between the expression of HLA-DR antigens on the recipient lymphocytes and the tubular epithelial cells of the graft (Table 2) suggests a relationship between these events. A likely possibility is that an alloactivation of recipient T lymphocytes by donor class-II-positive cells results in the production of lymphokines, including γ interferon. In addition to the recruitment of immune and inflammatory mediators to the site of their release within the graft, such soluble factors may also enhance the production and expression of several gene products, such as class II antigens, by the tubular cells, as has been shown for several cell types (*27, 28*).

In summary, in the present study a correlation was found between rejection episodes in Aza-treated renal transplant recipients and the expression of HLA-DR antigens on preponderantly Leu2a$^+$ peripheral lymphocytes as well as graft renal tubular cells. The lack of such a correlation for CsA-treated patients is probably not related to the capacity of CsA to prevent the appearance of HLA-DR antigens on these cells, but rather to the difficult differentiation between rejection episodes and CsA nephrotoxicity on the one hand and the appearance of activation markers without evident functional deterioration on the other. Further prospective studies are needed to determine whether the expression of HLA-DR on peripheral T lymphocytes and/or graft tubular epithelial cells can be used to differentiate CsA nephrotoxicity from rejection.

REFERENCES

1. Cosimi AB. Diagnostic and therapeutic applications of monoclonal antibodies to human T-cell subsets in renal transplant recipients. Urol Clin North Am 1983; 10: 289.
2. Van Es A, Tanke NJ, Baldwin WM III, Oljans PJ, Ploem JS, Van Es LA. Ratios of T lymphocyte subpopulations predict survival of cadaveric renal allografts in adult patients on low-dose corticosteroid therapy. Clin Exp Immunol 1983; 52: 13.
3. Cosimi AB, Colvin RB, Burton RC, et al. Monoclonal antibodies for immunologic monitoring and treatment in recipients of renal allografts. N Engl J Med 1981; 305: 308.
4. Ellis TM, Lee HM, Mohanakumar T. Alterations in human regulatory T-lymphocyte subpopulations after renal allografting. J Immunol 1981; 127: 2199.
5. Evans RL, Faldetta TJ, Humphreys RE, Pratt DM, Yunis EJ, Schlossman SF. Peripheral human T cells sensitized in mixed leucocyte culture synthesize and express Ia-like antigens. J Exp Med 1978; 148: 1440.
6. Carter NP, Cullen PR, Thompson JF, Bewick ALT, Wood RFM, Morris PJ. Monitoring lymphocyte subpopulation in renal allograft recipients. Transplant Proc 1983; 15: 1157.
7. Mazaheri R, Keown P, Laupacis A, Howson W, Sinclair N, Stiller CR. Lymphocyte subsets in the allograft recipient. II. Examination of Ia-reactivity and cell size in acute rejection. Transplant Proc 1983; 15: 1976.
8. Van Es A, Baldwin WM, Oljans PJ, Tanke HJ, Ploem JS, Van Es LA. Expression of HLA-DR on T lymphocytes following renal transplantation, and association with graft rejection episodes and cytomegalovirus infection. Transplantation 1984; 37: 65.
9. Palacios R, Möller G. Cyclosporin A blocks receptors for HLA-DR antigens on T cells. Nature 1981; 290: 792.
10. Leapman SB, Strong DM, Filo RS, Smith EJ, Brandt GL. Cyclosporin A prevents the appearance of cell surface "activation" antigens. Transplantation 1982; 34: 94.
11. Henny FC, Oljans PJ, Tanke HJ, Paul LC, Van Es LA. Comparison of monoclonal antibodies used for immunological monitoring of renal transplant recipients. Transplantation 1986; 41: 422.
12. Hall BM, Bishop GA, Duggin GG, Horvath JS, Philips J, Tiller DJ. Increased expression of HLA-DR antigens on renal tubular cells in renal transplants: relevance to the rejection response. Lancet 1984; 2: 247.
13. Henny FC, Kleinbloesem CH, Moolenaar AJ, Paul LC, Breimer DD, Van Es LA. Pharmacokinetics and nephrotoxicity of Cyclosporin A in renal transplant recipients. Transplantation 1985; 40: 117.
14. Engleman EG, Benike CJ, Glickman E, Evans RL. Antibodies to membrane structures that distinguish suppressor/cytotoxic and helper T lymphocyte subpopulations block the mixed leucocyte reaction in man. J Exp Med 1981; 154: 193.
15. Lampson LA, Levy R. Two populations of Ia-like molecules on a human B cell line. J Immunol 1980; 125: 293.
16. Van Es A, Meyer CJLM, Oljans PJ, Tanke HJ, Van Es La. Mononuclear cells in renal allografts. Correlation with peripheral blood T lymphocyte subpopulations and graft prognosis. Transplantation 1984; 37: 134.
17. O'Toole CM, Carvalho GS, Cranage MP, Large S. Immune responses in cardiac transplantation. I. Detection of activated T Ia$^+$ cells in the blood during herpes virus infections. Clin Exp Immunol 1984; 57: 671.
18. Carney WP, Iacoviello V, Hirsch MS. Functional properties of T lymphocytes and their subsets in cytomegalovirus mononucleosis. J Immunol 1983; 130: 390.
19. Zoumbos NC, Gascón P, Djeu JY, Trost SR, Young NS. Circulating activated suppressor T lymphocytes in aplastic anemia. N Engl J Med 1985; 312: 257.
20. Häyry P, von Willebrand E, Andersson LC. Expression of HLA-ABC and -DR locus antigens on human kidney endothelial, tubular and glomerular cells. Scand J Immunol 1980; 11: 303.
21. Scott H, Brandtzaeg P, Hirschberg H, Solheim BG, Thorsby E. Vascular and renal distribution of HLA-DR-like antigens. Tissue Antigens 1981; 18: 195.
22. Hancock WW, Kraft N, Atkins RC. The immuno-histochemical demonstration of major histocompatibility antigens in the human kidney using monoclonal antibodies. Pathology 1982; 14: 409.
23. Fuggle SV, Errasti P, Daar AS, Fabre JW, Ting A, Morris PJ. Localization of major histocompatibility complex (HLA-ABC and DR) antigens in 46 kidneys. Transplantation 1983; 35: 385.
24. Hart DNJ, Fabre JW. Endogenously produced Ia antigens within cells of convoluted tubules of rat kidney. J Immunol 1981; 126: 2109.
25. Benson EM, Colvin RB, Russell PS. Induction of Ia antigens in murine renal transplants. J Immunol 1985; 134: 7.
26. Mayrhofer G, Schon-Hegrad A. Ia antigens in rat kidney, with special reference to their expression in tubular epithelium. J Exp Med 1983; 157: 2097.
27. Pober JS, Gimbrone MA, Cotran RS, et al. Ia expression by vascular endothelium is inductible by activated T cells and by human γ interferon. J Exp Med 1983; 157: 1339.
28. Rosa F, Fellous M. The effect of gamma-interferon on MHC antigens. Immunol Today 1984; 5: 261.

Received 8 October 1985.
Accepted 30 January 1986.

0041-1337/86/4205-0484$02.00/0
TRANSPLANTATION
Vol. 42, No. 5
Printed in U.S.A.

PULMONARY COMPLICATIONS OF ORTHOTOPIC LIVER TRANSPLANTATION

WILLIAM A. JENSEN,[1,2] RICHARD M. ROSE, SCOTT M. HAMMER, ROGER L. JENKINS, ALBERT BOTHE JR., PETER N. BENOTTI, WALTER H. DZIK, PHILIP COSTELLO, URMILA KHETTRY, CHARLES TREY, GEORGE M. ELIOPOULOS, AND ADOLF W. KARCHMER

Departments of Medicine, Surgery, Radiology, and Pathology, New England Deaconess Hospital, and Harvard Medical School, Boston, Massachusetts 02215

Pulmonary complications following orthotopic liver transplantation (OLT) were prospectively evaluated in 18 individuals transplanted at the New England Deaconess Hospital. Of sixteen patients who survived the immediate postoperative period, 12 (75%) sustained a pulmonary complication. Of these complications, 64% were noninfectious—whereas 22% were infectious, and 14% probably infectious. Six of eight documented infections were caused by viruses of the herpes group. In four cases of viral pneumonitis other pulmonary pathogens were isolated (fungi-3, protozoan-1, bacteria-1). Unlike noninfectious complications, pulmonary infections were associated with a fatal outcome in five of six patients who died after OLT. Pulmonary complications are frequent and serious occurrences after OLT, and contribute to both the morbidity and mortality of this procedure. Compared with pulmonary complications seen after transplantation of other organs, OLT was associated with a higher proportion of noninfectious complications but a similar spectrum of pulmonary infections.

Orthotopic liver transplantation (OLT)* is now an accepted form of therapy for certain categories of end-stage liver disease (*1*). Although the first human OLT was performed in 1963 (*2*), it was not until 1967 that a transplant recipient had prolonged survival (*3*). Technical improvements in the surgical aspects of transplantation and the introduction of cyclosporine, a potent and specific inhibitor of graft rejection derived from the fungus *Trichoderma polysporum*, have contributed to improved survival following OLT described in recent reports (*4–6*). Despite these advances, technical complications of surgery, graft rejection, and infection remain major problems among transplant recipients (*7*).

Pulmonary disorders are a potential source of morbidity and mortality following OLT (*8*). Extensive upper abdominal operation and prolonged immunosuppressive therapy both predispose OLT recipients to respiratory complications. To investigate the frequency and nature of pulmonary complications during OLT, we prospectively evaluated 18 individuals undergoing OLT at the New England Deaconess Hospital.

[1] Address correspondence to: William Jensen, M.D., Division of Pulmonary Medicine, New England Deaconess Hospital, 185 Pilgrim Road, Boston, MA 02215.

[2] Fellow of the American Lung Association.

* Abbreviations used: ARDS, adult respiratory distress syndrome; CMV, cytomegalovirus; HSV, herpes simplex virus; ICU, intensive care unit; LT, liver transplant; solumedrol, methylprednisilone sodium succinate; OLT, orthotopic liver transplantation.

METHODS

Prospective Clinical Evaluation

Candidates for OLT were evaluated preoperatively by a study team consisting of transplant surgeons and medical specialists in the fields of pulmonary medicine, infectious disease, and gastroenterology. Prior to evaluation, all candidates gave written informed consent to a protocol for OLT approved by the hospital's institutional review board. Preoperative evaluation consisted of a history and physical exam by each team member. Particular attention was given to the nature and duration of liver disease and prior pulmonary or infectious disorders. All individuals had selected preoperative laboratory studies. In addition, preoperative pulmonary function studies were performed on a Med-Graphics 7200 system. These studies included spirometry, determination of lung volumes by the technique of nitrogen washout, single-breath diffusion capacity for carbon monoxide, and arterial blood gas analysis on room air. Values were compared with well-defined standards to derive the percentage of predicted based on the individual's sex, age, height, and weight (*9–12*).

Postoperatively, clinical evaluation was performed prospectively by members of the study team. All patients were assigned a number corresponding to their order of transplantation and are identified in this communication by the liver transplant (LT) number.

Pulmonary complications were categorized according to the following definitions.

Infectious complications. These were fever and pulmonary infiltrate with isolation or identification of a specific microorganism. Bacterial pneumonia was confirmed by a compatible sputum Gram stain, isolation of a bacterial pathogen in sputum and/or blood cultures, and response to specific antimicrobial therapy. Viral, fungal, or protozoan pneumonia was diagnosed on the basis of tissue obtained at open-lung biopsy or autopsy.

Noninfectious complication. This was a pulmonary disorder requiring therapeutic intervention, but for which there was no evidence of active infection by either clinical evaluation or microbiologic studies.

Data collection was facilitated by the use of standardized forms that were periodically updated by a member of the study team.

Diagnosis of Pulmonary Complications

A uniform approach to identifying the basis of pulmonary complications was employed throughout the study. For individuals with pleural effusion, this included a differential cell count and determination of the pleural fluid concentration of lactic dehydrogenase, total protein, glucose, and amylase. All pleural fluid specimens were cultured for bacteria (aerobic/anaerobic), fungi, and mycobacteria.

For individuals with pulmonary parenchymal disorders, extensive efforts were made to obtain lower respiratory tract secretions for microbiologic analysis. When possible, spontaneously expectorated sputum was examined. Patients who were unable to produce sputum underwent attempts to induce respiratory secretions by hydration, inhalation of fine-particle saline aerosol, and/or postural drainage. In individuals with nondiagnostic studies based on examination of expectorated or induced sputum, fiberoptic bronchoscopy was performed if bedside assessment of cardiac and fluid status failed to suggest the presence of cardiogenic pulmonary edema. Because of the frequent occurrence of coagulopathy in OLT recipients, bronchoalveolar lavage and endobronchial brushings were performed in place of transbronchial biopsy. In instances of persistent pulmonary infiltration in which fiberoptic bronchoscopy did not yield a specific diagnosis, open-lung biopsy was performed. Bronchoalveolar lavage material and lung biopsy specimens were examined for the presence of common and opportunistic pathogens by culture and special stains, in addition to cytologic and histologic evaluation for other processes such as neoplasia (*13*).

Immunosuppression and Graft Rejection

All OLT recipients received prednisone and cyclosporine to suppress graft rejection. The initial doses of cyclosporine were 6 mg/kg/day i.v. overlapping with 15 mg/kg/day p.o. as oral intake resumed. Attempts were made to maintain serum cyclosporine levels of 100–300 μg/ml (radioimmunoassay). After an initial 1 g i.v. bolus of methylprednisolone sodium succinate (solumedrol) at the time of graft implantation, steroids were tapered from a first-day dose of 200 mg solumedrol to 20 mg by the sixth postoperative day. The most intensive immunosuppressive therapy was maintained during the first three months following OLT. Thereafter, immunosuppression was modified on an individual basis according to the frequency and severity of graft rejection. Prednisone and cyclosporine were continued in all OLT recipients for the duration of the study. Suspected or proved episodes of rejection were treated by single or repetitive doses of i.v. solumedrol (range 500–1000 mg/day), or a six-day course of oral prednisone beginning with 200 mg/day and tapering to 20 mg/day. Refractory episodes of rejection were managed by the administration of OKT3 monoclonal antibodies (Ortho Pharmaceuticals) or the addition of azathioprine.

Graft rejection was suspected on clinical grounds when any of the following were present: diminished quality or quantity of bile output, rising serum bilirubin or transaminase values, unexplained fever, and leukocytosis. A presumptive diagnosis of rejection was made if a combination of these findings was present and there was no evidence of mechanical obstruction to the biliary anastomosis, systemic or hepatic infection, or hepatic drug toxicity. Clinically suspected episodes of graft rejection were confirmed in the majority of cases by the histologic appearance of a percutaneous biopsy of the graft (*14*). Beginning in July 1984, all patients underwent regularly scheduled protocol graft biopsies with additional biopsies obtained at weekly intervals during any period of abnormal liver function.

Statistical Analysis

Fisher's exact probability test was employed to determine whether individual risk factors correlated with the development of any pulmonary complication, infectious pulmonary complications, or noninfectious pulmonary complications. The following risk factors were analyzed: history of pulmonary disease, abnormal preoperative pulmonary function tests, and abnormal preoperative chest roentgenogram. Analysis of variance was employed to determine whether intraoperative units of transfused packed red blood cells and platelets or duration of operation correlated with the development of infectious pulmonary complications or noninfectious pulmonary complications.

RESULTS

Patient characteristics. A total of 6 men and 12 women with an average age of 46 years (range 26–60 years) underwent OLT. End-stage primary biliary cirrhosis (10 patients) was the most common reason for transplantation, followed by chronic active hepatitis (4 patients), sclerosing cholangitis (2 patients), and submassive hepatic necrosis (2 patients).

Six patients had no history of pulmonary disease. Eight had a history of cigarette smoking, and one of the cigarette smokers also had a history of asbestos exposure. In one patient each, the following were found: valvulotomy for pulmonic stenosis, multiple rib and vertebral compression fractures secondary to osteoporosis, right lung lobectomy for granulomatous disease, and nonspecific pneumonitis two years prior to transplantation.

Preoperative pulmonary function assessment. Pulmonary function tests were obtained in 13 individuals. In eight, all tests were normal. Five individuals had restriction of lung volumes that could be related clinically to the presence of ascites. The alveolar-arterial O_2 gradient was normal in 11 individuals and abnormal in four (abnormal: more than 10 mm Hg greater than predicted). The chest roentgenogram was normal in seven cases. Abnormalities noted on plain chest films included the presence of small pleural effusions (2 cases), subsegmental atelectasis (6 cases), elevated right hemidiaphragm (2 cases), and biapical emphysematous changes (1 case).

Transplant surgery and its complications. OLT necessitated a complex and lengthy operation. This was reflected by the mean duration of the operative procedure, which was 13 hr (range 6.5–18.5 hr). Patients required various amounts of blood product replacement during surgery: the mean number of units of packed red blood cells transfused was 50, with a median of 32 units, and a range of 9–199 units. Intraoperative red blood cell salvage was routinely performed in all cases with two cell-savers (Haemonetics, Inc., Braintree, MA) (*15*, *16*). Platelet requirements were also extensive: the mean units of platelets transfused was 42, with a median of 30 units, and a range of 0–120 units. Assisted venovenous bypass was used in all patients except one (LT No. 17), in whom technical problems precluded its use. In 12 operations, there were no serious intraoperative complications. The other nine procedures were complicated by: hypotension (6), hemorrhage and coagulopathy (5), hypercalcemia (1), hyperkalemia (1), and various technical complications (3). Two individuals died during the operation. In one, this was attributable to uncontrollable bleeding during the hepatectomy; in the other, death was related to primary graft nonfunction (preservation injury).

The postoperative course was complicated in the majority of cases. This was reflected in extensive utilization of intensive care unit (ICU) resources (mean days in ICU: 26.8, range 2–112). Nearly half of ICU days were spent on mechanical ventilation (mean days on ventilator: 12.6, range 1–56).

Graft rejection. Eleven episodes of graft rejection in 10 patients were documented pathologically by liver biopsy. A second OLT was necessary in two cases for uncontrollable rejection, and in one instance as a result of primary graft nonfunction (preservation injury). These 11 episodes of graft rejection did not occur within 2 weeks of any documented infectious episodes. However, episodes of liver dysfunction did occur in association with infection when no liver biopsy was obtained. In 4 individuals with documented respiratory infection, empiric steroids had been administered prior to the recognition of pneumonitis.

Pulmonary complications. Sixteen patients surviving the immediate postoperative period were followed for a mean of 8.2 months (range 2 weeks to 20 months). Of these patients, 75% (12/16) suffered a pulmonary complication. Of those with a pulmonary complication, 8% (1/12) had a single complication, while 92% (11/12) suffered multiple complications. Overall, there were 36 pulmonary complications in 12 patients: 22% (8/36) were infectious, 14% (5/36) probably infectious, and 64% (23/36) noninfectious. Individual complications are detailed in Table 1. No correlation could be found between risk of pulmonary complication following OLT and prior abnormality in the pulmonary history, preoperative pulmonary function studies, preoperative chest roentgenogram, duration of the operation, or units of blood and platelets transfused during the operation.

Infectious pulmonary complications. Viruses of the herpes group were the most frequently encountered pulmonary pathogens. Cytomegalovirus (CMV) pneumonitis developed in four cases, while herpes simplex virus pneumonitis and tracheobronchitis were documented in one case each. In two instances, CMV pneumonitis was diagnosed postmortem. Two cases of CMV pneumonia were diagnosed by open-lung biopsy—one of which was treated with an experimental antiviral drug 9-(1, 3-dihydroxy-2-propoxymethyl) guanine (BW B759U, Burroughs Wellcome Co., Research Triangle Park, NC). Herpes simplex virus (HSV) pneumonitis diagnosed by open-lung biopsy in one patient was treated with i.v. acyclovir for one week prior to the patient's death from disseminated aspergillosis. In another patient, the diagnosis of HSV tracheobronchitis was suggested by a bronchoscopic exam showing erythema and edema of central airways and a four-fold rise in serum antibodies to HSV during the course of a clinical illness characterized by fever and nonproductive cough. These viral respiratory tract infections occurred as early as two weeks and as late as 15 months posttransplantation (Fig. 1).

Fungal pathogens were the next most common cause of infectious pneumonitis. There were two cases of *Candida albicans* pneumonitis and two cases of *Aspergillus fumigatus* pneumonitis. These infections were diagnosed postmortem (3 cases) or by open-lung biopsy (1 case). Each case of fungal pneumonitis occurred six weeks or longer after initial transplantation (Fig. 1).

Bacterial pneumonitis occurred in two individuals within three weeks of the transplant operation. *Staphylococcus aureus* pneumonia was diagnosed by gram stain and sputum culture in a patient with a compatible illness who responded to pathogen-specific antibiotic therapy. *Klebsiella oxytoca* pneumonia was diagnosed antemortem based on a pulmonary infiltrate and positive blood and sputum cultures; this was confirmed by tissue examination postmortem.

Coexistent viral and fungal infection was present in three cases: HSV and *A fumigatus*; CMV and *A fumigatus*; CMV and *C albicans*. In the individual with *K oxytoca* pneumonia, CMV was also found in postmortem examination of the lungs.

Only one patient had pneumonia due to a protozoan, *Pneumocystis carinii*, which was a copathogen with CMV and *A fumigatus*.

"Probably infectious" pulmonary complications. There were five instances in which pulmonary complications were categorized as probably infectious. Three involved focal pulmonary infiltrates associated with fever that resolved on empiric antibiotic therapy. In two other cases, pulmonary infiltrate and fever were associated with positive buffy coat cultures for CMV. These patients improved as the intensity of immunosuppressive therapy was decreased.

Noninfectious pulmonary complications. Twenty-three complications were judged to be noninfectious. In general, localized complications such as hemothorax, atelectasis, or pleural effusion occurred in the immediate postoperative period and could be directly attributed to mechanical derangements of the chest wall or diaphragm resulting from the transplant operation.

Adult respiratory distress syndrome occurred in three individuals. It was of interest that these cases did not occur in the immediate postoperative period, in spite of the complicated nature of transplant surgery and the large transfusion requirement of the majority of transplant recipients. In two of these three patients, a predisposing condition for adult respiratory distress syndrome was identified: in one case it was temporally associated with the toxic shock syndrome, and in the other with bacteremia due to *Enterobacter aerogenes*.

Pulmonary calcification was a late postoperative finding in two individuals. In one, a chronic right lower lobe infiltrate of several months duration was found to contain diffuse calcification by open lung biopsy. In the other, a homogenous, rounded, left upper lobe infiltrate developed approximately five months after OLT. A technetium-99 methylene diphosphonate bone scan showed increased uptake in the infiltrate and needle aspiration revealed calcification. In neither case were pathogenic organisms or abnormal cytologic specimens obtained.

Fatalities. Six individuals died in the postoperative period. One postoperative fatality was due to graft rejection. In the remaining five fatal cases, death was attributed to overwhelming systemic infection that was associated in each instance with the presence of active pneumonitis (Table 2).

DISCUSSION

Pulmonary complications are frequent and serious occurrences during OLT. In our experience, 75% of transplant recipients have sustained a pulmonary complication. In 92% of these cases, multiple complications have been observed. Although these episodes undoubtedly contributed to the overall morbidity of OLT, it was difficult to assess the impact of pulmonary complications per se on morbidity, since transplant recipients also sustained a myriad of nonpulmonary complications such as graft rejection, extrapulmonary infection, and bleeding. Nevertheless, respiratory infection did play a prominent role in the fatal cases in this series. In five of the six patients who died in the postoperative period, respiratory infection was suspected clinically and documented postmortem, although in all five cases death was attributed to systemic infection (Table 2).

We tried to identify patient characteristics that would predict an increased likelihood of developing a pulmonary complica-

TABLE 1. Pulmonary complications

Liver transplant[a] (LT)	Infectious	Probably infectious	Noninfectious	Total
LT1	*Staphylococcus aureus* pneumonitis (19)[b] Herpes simplex virus (436) and *Aspergillus fumigatus* pneumonitis (443)	Left upper lobe aspiration pneumonitis (1)	Right hemothorax following liver biopsy (400) Tracheostomy secondary to prolonged mechanical ventilation (436) Pulmonary calcification right lower lobe (413)	6
LT2			Deep venous thrombosis (8) Right hemothorax complicating anticoagulant therapy (12) ARDS (27) Hemoptysis (27)	4
LT5	*Klebsiella oxytoca* (13) and cytomegalovirus pneumonitis (44)		Tracheostomy secondary to prolonged mechanical ventilation (32)	2
LT6	Cytomegalovirus tracheitis and pneumonitis (23)		ARDS associated with enterobacter bacteremia (6) Right lower lobe atelectasis (10)	3
LT7	Herpes simplex virus tracheitis (12)	Right retrocardiac infiltrate resolved with antibiotic therapy (17)	Large right pleural effusion (2) Tracheostomy secondary to stridor (12)	4
LT8				0
LT9				0
LT10			ARDS associated with toxic shock syndrome (20) Right lower and middle lobe atelectasis (25)	2
LT11	Cytomegalovirus and *Candida albicans* pneumonitis (93)		Hemothorax following open lung biopsy (99) Tracheostomy secondary to prolonged mechanical ventilation (105) Subglottic narrowing (213)	4
LT12			Bilateral large pleural effusions (14) Pulmonary calcification left upper lobe (118)	2
LT13	*Candida albicans* pneumonitis (54)	Bibasilar infiltrates resolved with antibiotic therapy (12)	Tracheostomy secondary to prolonged mechanical ventilation (28) Bilateral large effusions (43)	4
LT14		Left upper lobe infiltrate associated with positive buffy coat culture for cytomegalovirus (23) Bilateral interstitial infiltrate associated with positive buffy coat culture for cytomegalovirus (135)		2
LT15	Cytomegalovirus and *Pneumocystis carinii* pneumonitis and *Aspergillus fumigatus* pneumonitis (45)		Right lower lobe collapse (11)	2
LT16			Congestive heart failure (1)	1
LT17				0
LT18				0
Totals	8	5	23	36
% Total complications	22%	14%	64%	

[a] Only the sixteen patients surviving the immediate postoperative period included.
[b] Numbers in parentheses refer to postoperative day of complication listed.

tion. However, no statistically significant correlations were observed. The inability to correlate these parameters with the likelihood of developing pulmonary complications could reflect the small number of patients studied and/or the high incidence of pulmonary complications in this series. It was not possible to assess the relationship of postoperative pulmonary complications to episodes of graft rejection, since a uniform approach to episodes of liver dysfunction had only recently been implemented.

Unlike the experience with respiratory disorders occurring during the course of transplantation with other organs such as kidney (*17–19*), bone marrow (*20, 21*), and heart (*22, 23*), the

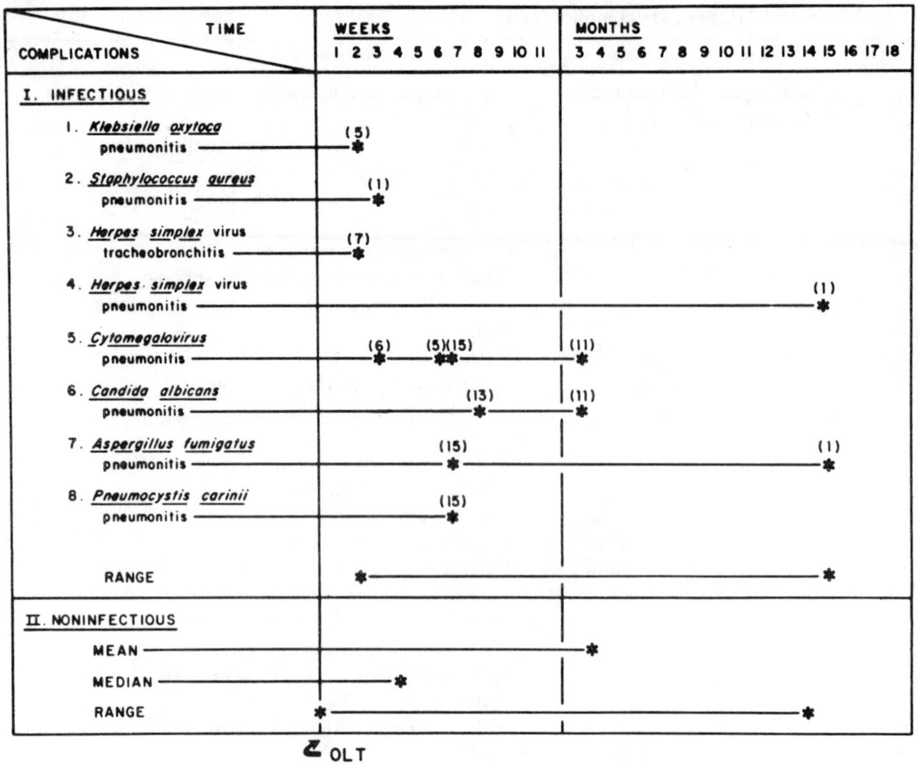

FIGURE 1. Time course of pulmonary complications in patients undergoing orthotopic liver transplantation. Numbers in parenthesis refer to the liver transplant (LT) number.

TABLE 2. Characteristics of fatalities associated with pneumonitis

Liver transplant (LT) number	Time of death	Cause of death	Lung findings Postmortem
LT6	23 Days	Refractory hypotension due to candidemia and disseminated cytomegalovirus	Cytomegalovirus pneumonitis, tracheitis
LT5	44 Days	Polymicrobial sepsis due to bowel infarction and perforation	Cytomegalovirus pneumonitis, *Klebsiella oxytoca* pneumonitis
LT15	45 Days	Disseminated cytomegalovirus and aspergillosis, intraabdominal hemorrhage	*Aspergillus fumigatus* pneumonitis, (cytomegalovirus and *Pneumocystis carinii* pneumonitis, 2 days antemortem by open-lung biopsy)
LT13	54 Days	Refractory hypotension due to candidemia and infarcted bowel	*Candida albicans* pneumonitis
LT1	443 Days	Disseminated aspergillosis	*Aspergillus fumigatus* pneumonitis (herpes simplex virus pneumonitis 1 week antemortem by open lung biopsy

majority of pulmonary complications we identified following OLT were noninfectious in origin. In many of these cases, the appearance of a focal pulmonary disorder such as atelectesis, hemothorax, or pleural effusion appeared to be causally related to mechanical derangements of the chest wall or diaphragm following the operation. Adult respiratory distress syndrome (ARDS) was an infrequent and late postoperative occurrence among these patients. The low incidence of postoperative ARDS was a surprising finding in these patients. Multiple factors related to OLT predispose graft recipients to postoperative ARDS: massive blood and crystalloid infusions, intraoperative hypotension, prolonged operation, liver failure, disseminated intravascular coagulation, infection, and the use of cyclosporine (*24*). Of these various risk factors, massive blood transfusion has had the longest and most controversial relationship to postoperative pulmonary insufficiency. Studies initially implicated microemboli of particulate material found in stored blood (*25*), and led to the use of microaggregate blood filters during massive transfusion (*26*). However, the absence of clear evidence of microemboli in the lungs of massively transfused patients (*27*) led to the suggestion that vasoactive substances released from transfused platelets and leukocytes produced ARDS by altering the permeability of the pulmonary capillaries (*28*). Although a microaggregate filter (20-μ) was used to filter red cell products in our patients, standard filters (170-μ) were used to administer the large quantities of leukocyte-rich platelet transfusions (mean: 42 units, median: 30 units, range: 0–120 units) given to OLT recipients. The low incidence of postoperative ARDS in our experience strongly argues against a role for transfused leukocyte or platelet-derived vasoactive substances in the pathogenesis of ARDS. However, it is also possible that the infrequent occurrence of ARDS in these individuals is related to intraoperative treatment with steroids, since animal studies suggest that prior exposure to corticosteroids may be effective in preventing ARDS in response to a well-defined injury (*29*).

One potential late pulmonary complication of massive transfusion may have been the development of pulmonary calcification. In one of two individuals (LT No. 1) with this finding, hypercalcemia (serum calcium 27.3 mg/dl) developed intraoperatively following multiple infusions of calcium chloride to counteract the chelating effect of the citrate anticoagulant in banked blood. As a result, this individual required treatment with mithramycin and calcitonin. Citrate, the anticoagulant in banked blood, is metabolized by the liver (*30*) and lowers the plasma ionized calcium by a direct chelating effect. Extensive transfusion during OLT may result in a large citrate load that is poorly metabolized secondary to hepatic dysfunction. As a result, severe depression of the serum ionized calcium occurs during the operation, which necessitates the use of repeated calcium infusions. As the capacity of the transplanted liver to metabolize citrate increases, rebound hypercalcemia may be observed, as in case LT No. 1. Other features of these two cases that may have contributed to the development of pulmonary calcification are postoperative renal dysfunction, which can impair calcium and phosphate excretion by the kidney; use of supplemental vitamin D for hepatic osteodystrophy secondary to primary biliary cirrhosis; and persistent postoperative metabolic alkalosis, possibly secondary to delayed metabolism of the blood anticoagulant citrate. Although these mechanisms might have contributed to a persistently elevated calcium phosphate product and a tendency to deposit calcium salts in tissues, ectopic calcification was restricted to the lung in the one patient (LT No. 1) who came to postmortem examination. This suggests that pulmonary calcification may result from metabolic abnormalities as well as local alterations in the lung, such as prior injury ("dystrophic" calcification) (*31*).

Infectious complications accounted for a smaller proportion of pulmonary complications than noninfectious ones in the series. However, respiratory infection appeared to have a greater impact on survival: five of six individuals dying in the postoperative period had respiratory infection associated with related or unrelated systemic infection (Table 2). The spectrum of respiratory pathogens found in OLT recipients was similar to that described in other transplant settings (*17–23*). Two of eight definite episodes of respiratory infection were solely attributable to CMV or HSV. In the remaining cases, pathogenic fungi, bacteria, and protozoa were isolated in four, two, and one instance each. In four of six cases in which fungi, bacteria, or protozoa were present, coexistent viral infection with HSV or CMV was documented. Therefore, herpes virus infections accounted for, or contributed to, the development of proved respiratory infection in six of eight episodes of infectious pneumonia in this series.

A variety of factors may have contributed to the development of serious viral infection in OLT recipients. Immunosuppression with corticosteroids and cyclosporine may have predisposed to reactivation of latent viral infection. Recent in vitro studies suggest that, despite its initial promise as a selective inhibitor of graft rejection, cyclosporine may depress T-helper cell production of lymphokines (*32, 33*), substances that play a critical role in host defense (*34*). Cyclosporine is further implicated by recent clinical studies showing no decrease in the incidence of viral infections in transplant recipients receiving cyclosporine compared with a group receiving azathioprine (*35*). Although we did not specifically evaluate the role of blood product transfusions or the graft in the transmission of primary CMV infection to OLT recipients, previous studies have shown an increased incidence of CMV infection in immunosuppressed individuals who received leukocyte transfusions (*36*), and in CMV seronegative renal transplant recipients who received a graft from a seropositive donor (*37*). Blood transfusions may also have transmitted human T cell lymphotropic virus (HTLV-III) to some OLT recipients (*38*). If so, the effects of this virus on the immune system could further contribute to the development of pneumonitis with opportunistic organisms. The possibility of HTLV-III infection complicating the course of OLT is currently under investigation.

There were four episodes of fungal pneumonitis in this series, and all were fatal except one case of *C albicans*. They occurred from six weeks to fifteen months postoperatively. A recent review of fungal infections in liver transplant recipients by Wajszczuk et al. outlines the importance of these infections and describes a number of predisposing factors, including use of antibiotics and corticosteroids, frequency and duration of operative procedures, and type of underlying liver disease (*39*). Only one of our patients with *C albicans* pneumonitis (LT No. 15) received preoperative antibiotics—however, two patients (LT No. 13 and LT No. 15) received preoperative steroids. Duration of the operation did not appear to be a risk factor for fungal pneumonitis in our series, since only one of our four cases had an operation that lasted longer than the mean. Boluses of solumedrol and broad spectrum antibiotics were given to three of four of our cases prior to the development of fungal pneumonitis, and this is in agreement with Wajszczuk's conclusions. Three of our cases had extensive posttransplantation operative procedures, including open lung biopsies and laparotomies. Unlike Wajszczuk's series in which primary biliary cirrhosis was associated with a lower incidence of fungal infection, three of our four cases had primary biliary cirrhosis.

The time of onset of pneumonitis in the posttransplant period was of limited value in differentiating infectious from noninfectious complications (Fig. 1). Of the noninfectious complications, 50% occurred within one month of the operation; in the majority, the mechanical effects of the operation on the chest wall and diaphragm resulted in focal radiologic abnormalities in the lower lung fields. Of the definite cases of infectious pneumonitis, 50% occurred within four weeks of transplantation. However, these cases were generally associated with diffuse or multiple focal radiologic abnormalities. It is of interest to note that two of four episodes of infection occurring within the first three weeks following transplantation were associated with herpes viruses (1 HSV, 1 CMV). Although, in renal transplant recipients, HSV infection commonly occurs in the first month posttransplantation, the peak occurrence of CMV infection is one to four months following transplantation (*18*). However, HSV and CMV infection in bone marrow transplant recipients have been shown to occur in the first postoperative month (*20, 21*).

In this series, pulmonary disorders contributed substantially to the morbidity and mortality of OLT. Compared with pulmonary complications in other transplant settings, recipients of OLT had more frequent noninfectious complications and a comparable proportion of serious infections. Identification of a large number of noninfectious complications occurring in close relationship to transplantation may lead to refinements in surgical technique and postoperative care that will diminish the number and severity of these noninfectious complications in the future. We have recently instituted an aggressive policy of graft biopsy to help better differentiate rejection from other types of liver graft dysfunction, in the hope of reducing the level of administered immunosuppression. Better understanding of the basis for serious viral infection during OLT could lead to new strategies for prevention and therapy that will no doubt have a substantial impact on patient survival.

Acknowledgments. We acknowledge Ms. Karen L. Celia for her excellent preparation of the manuscript, Mr. Hugh Wheeler for assisting with the statistical analysis, and the house staff and nursing staff of the New England Deaconess Hospital for their excellent care of these patients.

REFERENCES

1. Van Thiel DH, Schade RR, Starzl TE. After 20 years liver transplantation comes of age. Ann Int Med 1983; 99: 854.
2. Starzl TE, Marchioro TL, VonKaulla KN, et al. Homotransplantation of the liver in humans. Surg Gynecol Obstet 1963; 117: 659.
3. Starzl TE, Groth CT, Brettschneider L, et al. Orthotopic homotransplantation of the human liver. Ann Surg 1968; 169: 392.
4. Borel JF, Feurer C, Magnee C, Stahelin H. Effects of the new antilymphocytic peptide cyclosporin-A in animals. Immunology 1977; 32: 1017.
5. Starzl TE, Klintmalm GBG, Porter KA, et al. Liver transplantation with use of cyclosporin-A and prednisone. N Engl J Med 1981; 305: 266.
6. Starzl TE, Iwatsuki S, Van Thiel DH. Evolution of liver transplantation. Hepatology 1982; 2: 614.
7. Iwatsuki S, Shaw BW, Starzl TE. Current status of hepatic transplantation. Semin Liver Dis 1983; 3: 173.
8. Krowka MJ, Cortese DA. Pulmonary aspects of chronic liver disease and liver transplantation. Mayo Clin Proc 1985; 60: 407.
9. Knudson RJ, Lebowitz MD, Holberg CJ, Burrows B. Changes in the normal maximal expiratory flow-volume curve with growth and aging. Am Rev Resp Dis 1983; 127: 725.
10. Goldman HI, Becklake MR. Respiratory function tests: normal values at median altitudes and the prediction of normal results. Am Rev Tuberc Pulm Dis 1959; 79: 457.
11. Crapo RO, Morris AH. Standardized single breath normal values for carbon monoxide diffusing capacity. Am Rev Resp Dis 1981; 123: 185.
12. Mellemgaard K. The alveolar-arterial oxygen difference: its size and components in normal man. Acta Physiol Scand 1966; 67: 10.
13. Stover DE, Zaman MB, Hajou SI, Lange M, Gold J, Armstrong D. Bronchoalveolar lavage in the diagnosis of diffuse infiltrates in the immunosuppressed host. Ann Intern Med 1984; 101: 1.
14. Snover DC, Sibley RK, Freese DK, et al. Orthotopic liver transplantation: a pathological study of 63 serial liver biopsies from 17 patients with special reference to the diagnostic features and natural history of rejection. Hepatology 1984; 4: 1212.
15. Dzik WH, Jenkins RL. Use of intraoperative blood salvage in orthotopic liver transplantation. Arch Surg 1985; 120: 946.
16. Jenkins RL, Benotti PN, Bothe A, Rossi RL. Liver transplantation. Surg Clin North Am 1985; 65: 103.
17. Ramsey PG, Rubin RH, Tolkoff-Rubin NE, Cosimi AB, Russell PS, Greene R. The renal transplant patient with fever and pulmonary infiltrates: etiology, clinical manifestations and management. Medicine (Baltimore) 1980; 59: 206.
18. Rubin RH, Wolfson JS, Cosimi AB, Tolkoff-Rubin NE. Infection in the renal transplant recipient. Am J Med 1981; 70: 405.
19. Peterson PK, Feguson R, Fryd DS, et al. Infectious diseases in hospitalized renal transplant recipients: a prospective study of a complex and evolving problem. Medicine (Baltimore) 1982; 61: 360.
20. Winston DJ, Gale RP, Meyer DV, Young LS. Infectious complications of human bone marrow transplantation. Medicine (Baltimore) 1979; 58: 1.
21. Meyers JD, Flournoy N, Thomas ED. Nonbacterial pneumonia after allogeneic marrow transplantation: a review of ten years' experience. Rev Infect Dis 1982; 4: 1119.
22. Montgomery JR, Barrett FF, Williams TW. Infectious complications in cardiac transplant patients. Transplant Proc 1973; V: 1239.
23. Mason JW, Stinson EB, Hunt SA, Schroeder JS, Rider AK. Infections after cardiac transplantation: relation to rejection therapy. Ann Intern Med 1976; 85: 69.
24. Powell-Jackson PR, Carmichael FJL, Calne RY, Williams R: Adult respiratory distress syndrome and convulsions associated with administration of cyclosporine in liver transplant recipients. Transplantation 1984; 38: 341.
25. Jenevein EP, Weiss DL. Platelet microemboli associated with massive blood transfusion. Am J Pathol 1964; 45: 313.
26. Reul GJ, Beall AC, Greenberg SD. Protection of the pulmonary microvasculature by fine screen blood filtration. Chest 1974; 66: 4.
27. Martin AM, Simmons RL, Heisterkamp CA. Respiratory insufficiency in combat casualties: I. Pathologic changes in the lungs of patients dying of wounds. Ann Surg 1969; 170: 30.
28. Bredenberg CE. Does a relationship exist between massive blood transfusions and the adult respiratory distress syndrome? Vox Sang 1977; 32: 311.
29. Katsuyuki K, Wax SD, Watts WR. Effects of methylprednisolone on pulmonary microcirculation. Surg Gynecol Obstet 1974; 139: 1.
30. Collins JA. Massive blood transfusion. Clin Haematol 1976; 5: 201.
31. Felson B, Schwarz J, Lukin RR, Hawkins HH. Idiopathic pulmonary ossification. Radiology 1984; 153: 303.
32. Dupont E, Huygen K, Schandene L. Influence of in vivo immunosuppressive drugs on production of lymphokines. Transplantation 1985; 39: 143.
33. Kaufman Y, Chang AE, Robb RJ. Mechanism of action of cyclosporin A: inhibition of lymphokine secretion studied with antigen-stimulated T-cell hybridomas. J Immunol 1984; 133: 3107.
34. David JR, David RR. Cellular hypersensitivity and immunity, inhibition of macrophage migration and the lymphocyte mediators. Prog Allergy 1972; 16: 300.
35. Dummer SJ, Hardy A, Poorsatter A, Ho M. Early infections in kidney, heart and liver transplant recipients on cyclosporine. Transplantation 1983; 36: 259.
36. Winston DJ, Winston HG, Clifford HL, et al. Cytomegalovirus infections associated with leukocyte transfusions. Ann Intern Med 1980; 93: 671.
37. Betts RF, Freeman RB, Douglas GR, Talley TE, Rundell B. Transmission of cytomegalovirus infection with renal allograft. Kidney Int 1975; 8: 387.
38. Amman AJ, Wara DW, Dritz S, et al. Acquired immunodeficiency in an infant: possible transmission by means of blood products. Lancet 1983; 1: 767.
39. Wajszczuk CP, Dummer SJ, Ho M, et al. Fungal infections in liver transplants recipients. Transplantation 1985; 40: 347.

Received 12 December 1985.
Accepted 10 February 1986.

0041-1337/86/4205-0491$02.00/0
TRANSPLANTATION
Vol. 42, No. 5
Printed in U.S.A.

MULTIVARIATE PREDICTION MODEL OF KIDNEY TRANSPLANT SUCCESS RATES

M. HENNIGE,[1] C. O. KÖHLER,[2] AND G. OPELZ[1]

Department of Transplantation Immunology, Institute of Immunology, University of Heidelberg; and Computing Department, German Cancer Research Center, Heidelberg, West Germany

An excellent correlation of predicted and observed cadaver kidney graft survival rates was obtained using a nine-factor computer model. A total of 924 recipients for whom a >80% 1-year survival rate was predicted had an observed rate of 84.6%, whereas 179 recipients with a predicted 1-year success rate of <40% had an observed rate of 38.2%. Our model gives improved results as compared with previously published methods. We anticipate that the model's predictive power can be further refined, and that patient selection and organ sharing will benefit from the application of sophisticated computer models for the prediction of transplant success.

The outcome of renal transplantation is influenced by many factors. If several factors are considered simultaneously it is very difficult, if not impossible, for the physician evaluating a potential recipient to estimate the likelihood of success. Mickey et al. first reported on a successful computer model for the prediction of transplant success rates (*1*). However, the model was deficient in that only a small fraction of patients could be categorized as very good risks. Using the Cox regression method, we were able to develop a much improved model for the prediction of transplant success. We report here our model's technical details and its efficacy in predicting graft outcome in a series of 5619 cadaver kidney transplants performed in 1983 and 1984.

MATERIALS AND METHODS

Data of the Collaborative Transplant Study, a voluntary international study in which over 200 transplant centers in 31 countries are participating (*2*), served as basis for our computations. Only first and second cadaver donor transplants were included. We used the Cox regression model, characterized by its survivor function:

$$F(t_i X) = F_0(t)^{\exp(x\beta)}$$

which is equivalent to the hazard function model (*3*). The coefficient vector β was estimated by the method of partial likelihood using the program package SURVIVAL (*4*). Likelihood function was calculated as follows:

$$L(\beta) = \prod_{i=1,k} \left[\frac{\exp(X_{(i)}\beta)}{\sum_{l \in R(t_{(i)})} \exp(X_{(l)}\beta)} \right]$$

where $R(t_{(i)})$ is the number of individuals at risk at time $t_{(i)}$.

[1] University of Heidelberg.

[2] German Cancer Research Center.

The base line survivor function $F_0(t)$ was estimated using the formula:

$$F_0(t) = \prod_{i/t_{(i)}<T} \alpha_i$$

where, if only a single failure occurs at $t_{(i)}$:

$$\alpha_i = \left[1 - \left(\frac{\exp(x_{(i)}\beta)}{\sum_{l \in R(t_{(i)})} \exp(x_{(l)}\beta)} \right) \right]^{\exp(-x_{(i)}\beta)}$$

If more failures occur, α_i is determined by iteration (*5*).

Because of storage limitations in our computer during the computation of coefficient vector β, we had to find a practical balance between the number of factors that could be included and the number of transplants used for our computation of the individual factors' weight. To achieve good reliability, we aimed at using at least 1000 transplants for the weight computations. For our model, we selected the nine "strongest" factors that, based on single-variable analyses, had been found to influence graft survival, and we performed the weight computation of individual factors on 1200 transplants performed in 1982.

According to their influence in single variable analyses, the nine factors were coded as follows:

1. Transplant number: 0, 1, 2, 3
2. HLA-B+DR mismatches: 0, 1, 2, 3, 4
3. Pretransplant blood transfusions: 0 Tf: 0; 1 Tf: 1; >20 Tf: 2; 2–20 Tf: 3;
4. Immunosuppressive protocol: cyclosporine: 0; no cyclosporine: 1
5. Percentage of latest cytotoxic antibodies: <50%: 0; ≥50%: 1
6. Original disease: diabetes mellitus: 0; nephrosçlerosis: 1; other: 2
7. General pretransplant evaluation of patient: good: 0; moderate: 1; poor: 2
8. Days previous graft functioned: <1 year: 0; ≥1 year: 1
9. Center effect—3-month graft survival rates: 91–100%: 0; 81–90%: 1; 71–80%: 2; 61–70%: 3; 51–60%: 4; <51%: 5

The computed weights used in the model for stepwise increases in risk within patient subgroups were: transplant number: 0.0421; number of HLA-B and HLA-DR mismatches: 0.1288; number of pretransplant blood transfusions: −0.01231; immunosuppression with or without cyclosporine: 0.4475; percentage of lymphocytotoxic antibody reactivity in the latest pretransplant serum: 0.1930; presence of diabetes mellitus or nephrosclerosis: −0.1368; general pretransplant evaluation status: 0.3407; duration of the previous graft when retransplants were considered: 0.2405; and overall center performance: 0.2395.

Our predictive function is:

$$F(t;x)=F_0(t)\,(\exp[0.0421X_1 + 0.1288X_2 - 0.1231X_3 + 0.4475X_4 + 0.1930X_5 - 0.1368X_6 + 0.3407X_7 + 0.2405X_8 + 0.2395X_9)$$

where $F_{0(t)}$ is the estimated base-line survivor function and X_i are the assigned codes of individual factors.

Table 1 lists the degree of the 9 factors' dependence computed from the covariance matrix. Only variables X_1 (transplant number) and X_8 (duration of previous graft) showed a high degree of correlation as indicated by the correlation coefficient −0.766. Since duration of a previous graft can be utilized only when retransplants are considered, this is an expected finding. Table 1 shows that the other covariables used for computation exerted a largely independent influence. Expected but overall relatively weak correlations were found between the presence of high preformed lymphocytotoxic antibodies and transplant number (retransplants are more often done in presensitized patients), and between the general evaluation status and original disease (diabetic recipients are usually classified as higher risks) (Table 1).

RESULTS

The computation of each individual variable's weight had been based on 1200 cadaver transplants performed in 1982. To simulate prospective evaluation of our model, we applied it to 5619 transplants performed in 1983 and 1984. The transplants were categorized into six groups according to their predicted rate of one-year graft survival, ranging from <40% to >80% one-year success. We then proceeded to compute actuarial survival rates according to the method of Kaplan and Meier (*6*). An excellent fit of predicted and observed survival rates was obtained (Fig. 1). Most important, the discriminative power was improved compared with previous models. Mickey et al.'s model placed 10% of patients in the category with a >70% one-year predicted success rate, and the actually observed rate was only 67% (*1*). In contrast, 16.5% of transplants analyzed with our current model were placed in the >80% category, and the observed one-year survival rate of this group was 84.6% (Fig. 1).

When another set of transplants, rather than grafts performed in 1982, was used for the initial computation of each covariable's weight, only insignificant changes in the model's predictive power were observed. Thus, in this multicenter material of well over 5000 transplants, our model appeared quite stable. Reduction in the number of covariables used in the model resulted in a decrease of discriminative power.

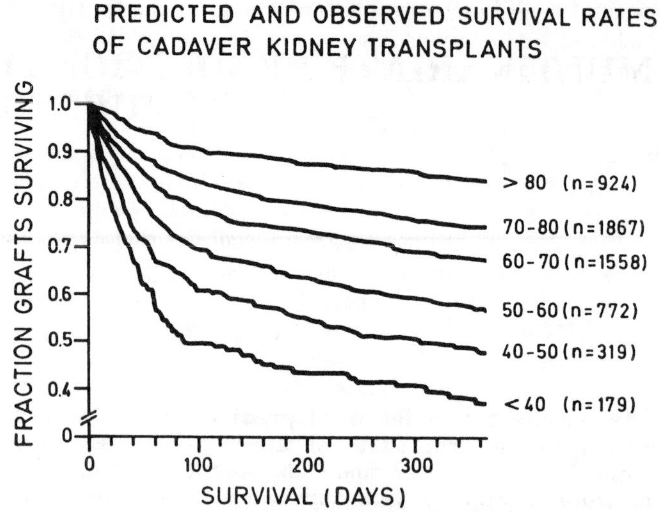

FIGURE 1. Actuarial cadaver transplant survival curves computed by the method of Kaplan and Meier (*5*) for subgroups of recipients for whom likelihood of graft outcome at one year had been predicted in the 9-factor model. Predicted ranges of one-year success rates and numbers of patients studied are indicated at the ends of curves. The prediction model was based on results of 1200 transplants performed in 1982, results shown are those of 5619 transplants done in 1983 and 1984.

DISCUSSION

The decision whether to go ahead with a kidney transplant depends on the likelihood of success. Only under rare circumstances will a patient or a physician accept an extremely high likelihood of failure. Because many factors influence the outcome of a renal transplant, it is very difficult to make an accurate risk assessment, especially under the stress condition of a sudden cadaver kidney offer. We demonstrate here that, using sophisticated statistical methods, a nine-variable prediction model allows the quite accurate pretransplant assessment of risk of failure. Only one of the nine factors included in our model is subjective to some extent: the patient's general pretransplant evaluation status as a candidate for transplantation. This evaluation has been requested routinely on the Collaborative Transplant Study questionnaire, and the three-stage categorization in "good," "mediocre," and "poor" transplant candidates correlates with observed graft survival rates. Our computations were based on the assumption that the requested "pretransplant" evaluation indeed was made prior to transplantation and not thereafter. The evaluation can be made well

TABLE 1. Correlation matrix of factors[a]

	x1	x2	x3	x4	x5	x6	x7	x8	x9
x1	1	.033	.052	−.001	−.285	−.053	.047	−.766	−.035
x2		1	−.049	−.063	.041	−.073	−.070	−.008	−.066
x3			1	−.129	.031	.081	.006	−.051	.014
x4				1	.008	.046	.074	.023	−.132
x5					1	−.051	−.069	.115	.067
x6						1	.242	−.017	−.037
x7							1	.007	−.002
x8								1	−.004
x9									1

[a] (x1) transplant number; (x2) mismatches HLA B+DR; (x3) pretransplant blood transfusions; (x4) immunosuppressive protocol; (x5) percentage lymphocytotoxic antibodies; (x6) original disease; (x7) general evaluation status; (x8) duration of previous graft; (x9) overall center performance.

ahead of the actual transplant operation; for the purpose of likelihood computation, this variable can be carried on the transplant candidate waiting list.

Accurate prediction of success rates has obvious advantages. If the predicted likelihood of success is low, it may be desirable to wait for a kidney with a better HLA match, or it might be desirable to transfuse the recipient, etc. Unfortunately, only some variables used in the prediction model can be influenced. Nevertheless, one obvious advantage would be that emphasis on HLA matching could be applied selectively in patients in whom a benefit could be expected. That certain patient categories benefit more from HLA matching than others has been reported (7).

Although the statistical model reported here provides a useful starting point for practical implementation, a few words of caution are indicated with respect to the model's applicability to individual centers' data. The model was developed and tested on the data base provided by over 200 transplant centers participating in the Collaborative Transplant Study. A very good fit of predicted and observed outcome was obtained in this collective material. This does not necessarily mean that each individual center's data agreed with the overall evaluation. If special selection or treatment procedures were used at some centers, deviations from the computations shown here would be expected. Therefore, before adopting this model for prospective use at a given center, it should be tested on the center's retrospective cases whether the model is suitable. Of course, this is particularly true for centers not represented in the Collaborative Transplant Study.

Our model of success rate prediction is still not ideal. Even though we obtained a very good fit of predicted and observed rates, improvement of the model's discriminative power is desirable. Ideally, most patients should be moved from the categories of intermediate success to the extremes of excellent or poor predicted success. To achieve that, the inclusion of additional variables and a finer definition of already included variables will be necessary. Simulation models should allow one or more factors' substitution for others (for example, when a kidney is offered for a patient, one might compute the expected improvement in graft survival if the patient waited for a kidney with one or two fewer HLA mismatches). In the future, complex computer programs that consider multiple variables in a large transplant population could aid in assigning specific treatment strategies and in achieving optimum kidney distribution, which should result in better overall transplant survival.

Acknowledgments. The cooperation of over 200 transplant centers in providing the data on which this work was based is gratefully acknowledged. We thank Prof. E. Weber of the German Cancer Research Center for providing statistical software.

REFERENCES

1. Mickey MR, Opelz G, Terasaki PI. Prospective estimates of probability of success of kidney transplants. Transplant Proc 1978; 11: 1914.
2. Opelz G. Influence of HLA matching, blood transfusions, and presensitization in cyclosporine-treated transplant recipients. Transplant Proc 1985; 17: 2179.
3. Cox DR. Regression models and life tables. J R Stat Soc [Ser B] 1972; 34: 187.
4. Edler L, Wahrendorf J. Berger J. Survival: a program package for the statistical analysis of censored survival times. Statist Software Newsletter 1981; 7: 110.
5. Kalbfleisch JD, Pretice RL. The statistical analysis of failure time data. New York: Wiley, 1980.
6. Kaplan EL, Meier P. Nonparametric estimation from incomplete observations. Am Stat Assoc. 1958; 53: 457.
7. Opelz G, Terasaki PI. Factors influencing effect of HLA matching on cadaver kidney transplants. Transplant Proc 1977; 9: 1795.

Received 28 October 1985.
Accepted 2 February 1986.

0041-1337/86/4205-0494$02.00/0
TRANSPLANTATION
Vol. 42, No. 5
Printed in U.S.A.

TC-99M DTPA SCANS IN RENAL ALLOGRAFT REJECTION AND CYCLOSPORINE NEPHROTOXICITY

WLADYSLAW GEDROYC,[1] DAVID TAUBE,[2] IGNAC FOGLEMAN, GUY NEILD,[3] STEWART CAMERON, AND MICHAEL MAISEY

Departments of Radiological Sciences and Nephrology, Guy's Hospital, London SE1, England

Renal allograft dysfunction arising from rejection or cyclosporine (CsA) nephrotoxicity can currently only be distinguished reliably by allograft biopsy. We have assessed Technetium (Tc)-99m diethylamine pentacetic acid (DTPA) scanning in 30 CsA-treated patients with allograft dysfunction. Scintigrams were performed during 20 biopsy-proved episodes of rejection and during 14 episodes of CsA nephrotoxicity. These results were compared with the scintigrams of 15 allografts showing stable function.

Quantitative indices expressing allograft perfusion (flow index) and function (uptake index) derived from the DTPA scintigrams showed no significant differences between the groups of patients with rejection, CsA nephrotoxicity, or stable or improving function. Similarly, the flow and uptake indices of individual allografts obtained during periods of stable or improving function and then during episodes of dysfunction due to rejection or CsA nephrotoxicity did not significantly change.

We conclude that Tc-99m DTPA scintigrams are of limited value in the management of allograft dysfunction in patients immunosuppressed with CsA.

Although cyclosporine (CsA)* is a potent immunosuppressive agent, its value is limited by nephrotoxicity, particularly in renal transplantation where allograft dysfunction may be due to rejection or CsA nephrotoxicity. At present, the most accurate method of differentiating rejection from CsA nephrotoxicity is allograft biopsy (*1–3*). This technique, however, may be complicated by hemorrhage, arteriovenous fistula formation, or even graft loss—and there is a need for a rapid, accurate, noninvasive method of differentiating rejection from CsA nephrotoxicity. Other less-invasive methods that have been studied are fine-needle aspiration (*2, 4*), intrarenal pressure monitoring (*5, 6*), and CsA whole-blood or plasma concentration determinations (*1, 7, 8*). None of these techniques however, is as yet of sufficient reliable diagnostic accuracy to allow confident differentiation of rejection from CsA nephrotoxicity.

Radionuclide assessment of allograft dysfunction may provide an accurate, noninvasive method of differentiating rejection from CsA nephrotoxicity. Tc-99m DTPA scintigrams have been used with success by our group (*9*) to evaluate allograft dysfunction in patients treated with azathioprine, and the purpose of this study was to assess this technique in CsA-treated renal transplant patients. We have therefore studied patients with well-defined rejection and CsA nephrotoxicity, and have compared these with scintigrams obtained at times of stable or improving allograft function.

MATERIALS AND METHODS

Patients. A group of 43 patients was studied. All patients were immunosuppressed with cyclosporine and prednisolone as previously described (*1*). Rejection was diagnosed histologically as previously described (*1, 2*) and treated with 1 g methylprednisolone given i.v. on three successive days. When severe, a course of antilymphocyte globulin (Hoechst) was administered. All patients in this study with rejection responded to this antirejection therapy.

CsA nephrotoxicity was diagnosed histologically as previously described (*1, 2*). The dose of CsA was reduced by 2 mg/kg/day on each occasion. All episodes of CsA nephrotoxicity in this study responded to CsA dose reduction. A total of 15 allografts were studied during periods of stable or improving function with sequential scintigrams bracketing the biopsy. These patients were studied at the time of routine allograft biopsy at one week, four weeks, and at one year posttransplantation. For inclusion in this study, the patients had stable or improving function, as judged by the plasma creatinine for three days prior to biopsy and ten days following biopsy.

Radionuclide scanning. We have used the method previously described by Hilson et al. (*9*). Briefly, the supine patient is imaged with a gamma camera positioned over the area of the renal transplant and bladder. A dose of 370 MBq of Tc-99m DTPA is injected into a peripheral vein as a bolus. The first image (perfusion) is recorded for 30 sec from the time of bolus injection; the next image, at 2 min, is recorded for 300,000 counts on a standard-field camera. The time taken for this image is noted, and subsequent images at 5 min, 10 min, and 20 min are recorded for the same length of time.

Quantitation. The flow (perfusion) and uptake indices were calculated as described below. The study is recorded by a dedicated computer at a frame rate of one per second for 30 sec, followed by one per minute for ten min. At the end of the study, regions of interest (ROI) are defined over the transplant, the iliac artery, and a background area. Time-activity curves are generated from these ROIs, and the areas under the arterial and renal curves up to the peak of the arterial curve are calculated. The index is then derived from the formula:

$$\text{perfusion index} = \frac{\text{area under arterial curve to peak}}{\text{area under renal curve}} \times 100$$

Normal values of this index should lie between 100 and 150, and the higher the index, the worse the perfusion.

[2] Present address: Renal Unit, Dulwich Hospital, East Dulwich Grove, London SE 22.

[3] Present address: Institute of Urology, St Phillip's Hospital, Sheffield Street, London WC2.

[1] Address requests for reprints to: Dr. W. Gedroyc, Department of Radiology, Guy's Hospital, London SE1.

* Abbreviations used: CsA, cyclosporine; DTPA, diethylamine pentacetic acid; ROI, region of interest; Tc, technetium-99 m.

TABLE 1. Interpretation by means of nuclear medicine compared with actual and biopsy diagnosis

Number of patient episodes	Actual diagnosis	Nuclear Medicine diagnosis
15	Stable/improving	5 Worsening (33%)
		10 Unchanged(66%)
14	CsA toxicity	4 Worsening (29%)
		6 Unchanged(43%)
		4 ATN (28%)
20	Rejection	8 Worsening (40%
		4 Unchanged(20%)
		8 ATN (40%)

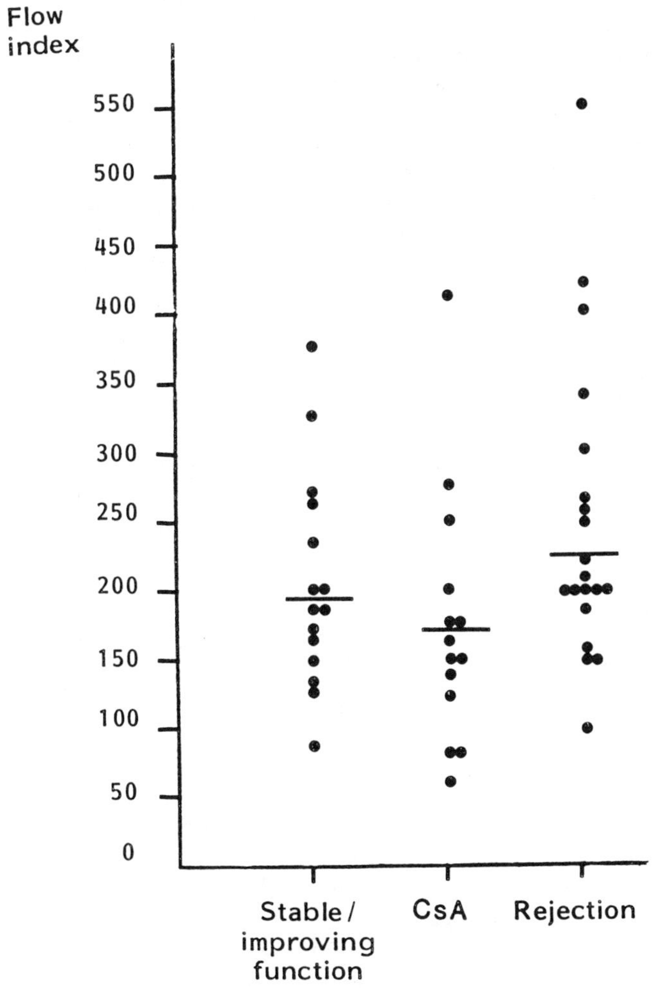

FIGURE 1. Flow index values of all patients studied.

The uptake index is calculated by obtaining the exact amount of counts acquired in the 30-sec frame—that is, between the first and second minute of the scintigram, subtracting the background and then dividing by the background. This results in an index of selective uptake that reflects renal function.

ROI for each patient for both flow and uptake index were stored on computer and were used again in subsequent examinations to optimize the reproducibility of studies.

Interpretation of Tc-99m DTPA scintigrams. All the Tc-99m DTPA scintigrams included in this study were assessed retrospectively. The nuclear medicine interpretations derived from the scintigram images and quantitative results were categorized into one of the following three groups:

1. Stable appearances (flow and perfusion indices showing no significant worsening)
2. Worsening appearances (change in flow and perfusion indices greater than the computer-derived standard deviation for each figure)
3. appearances suggesting acute tubular necrosis (good initial perfusion with little excretion and fading of the renal blood pool by 10 min)

These scintigram diagnoses are compared with the actual biopsy diagnoses in Table 1.

Statistical analysis. Wilcoxon's rank sum test was used to assess the differences in flow and uptake indices between the groups of patients with rejection, CsA nephrotoxicity, and stable or improving function. The signed rank sum test was used to assess changes in individual patients' flow and uptake indices during episodes of rejection, CsA nephrototoxicity, and stable or improving function.

RESULTS

A total of 49 patient episodes were studied with scintigrams performed either on the day of allograft biopsy or within two days before or three days after biopsy. Scans were performed during 20 rejection episodes, 14 during episodes of CsA nephrotoxicity and 15 during episodes of stable or improving function. Figures 1 and 2 show that there were no significant differences in flow or uptake indices between the individual

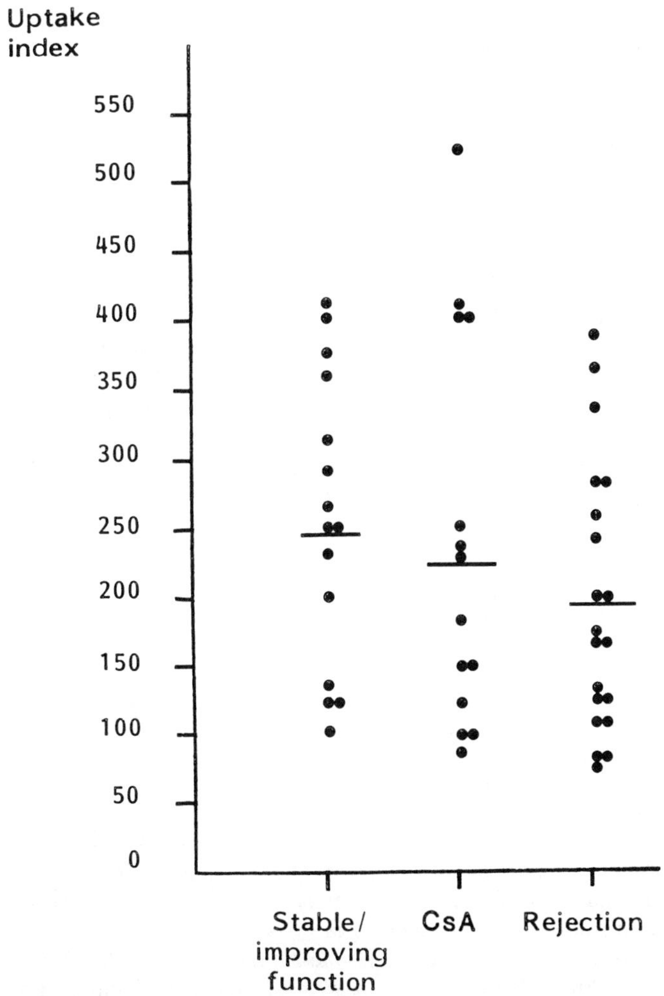

FIGURE 2. Uptake index values of all patients studied.

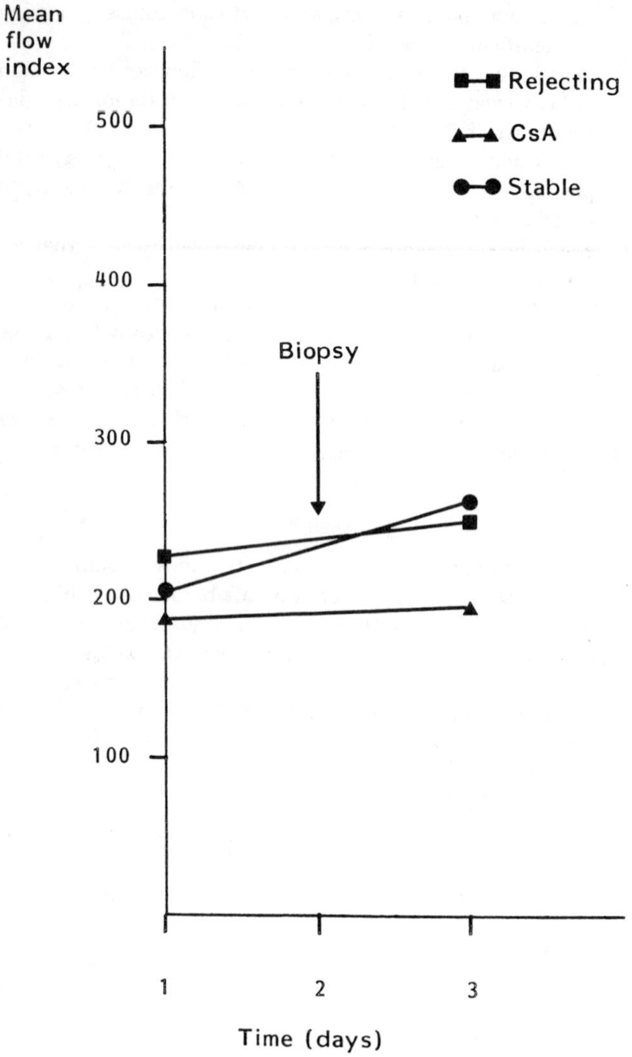

FIGURE 3. Mean flow index values bracketing dysfunction episodes.

groups. In this study, 18 episodes of rejection and 11 CsA nephrotoxicity episodes in 26 patients were assessed sequentially before and after the dysfunction episodes. Figures 3 and 4 show that the flow and uptake indices did not significantly alter during these periods. Table 1 shows the results of the blind and retrospective assessment of 49 scintigrams. There was agreement between the nuclear medicine findings and the biopsy findings in 66% of the scintigrams performed during episodes of stable or improving function; 29% of the CsA nephrotoxicity episodes, and 40% of the rejection episodes.

DISCUSSION

This study indicates that dynamic Tc-99m DTPA scintigrams were of no clinical value in discriminating rejection from CsA nephrotoxicity in a carefully defined group of patients with renal allograft dysfunction.

This contrasts with our previous study of azathioprine-treated, renal allograft recipients (*9*) in whom Tc-99m DTPA dynamic scanning was successfully used to differentiate rejection from acute tubular necrosis.

There are at least two possible explanations for this difference. First, CsA may interfere with the uptake and handling of Tc-99m DTPA by the kidney. In animal experiments, CsA causes reduced renal blood flow (*10*). This may explain why there was no difference in flow index in patients with CsA nephrotoxicity when compared with patients with rejection in whom the flow index was known to be impaired. Second, the group of patients in this study, although small, was very well defined, in that the cause of allograft dysfunction was based on histological examination of the kidney in every case. In the previous study (*9*) very few biopsies were performed, and the diagnosis of rejection was based on a minimum of two of the classic physical signs attributed to rejection. We are aware of only two other radionuclide studies of CsA-treated renal allografts (*11*, *12*). Although there have been scintigram studies on the nephrotoxic effects of CsA in liver transplant patients (*13*). In the first by Prescott et al. (*11*), two patients with CsA nephrotoxicity were investigated with iodinated hippurate radionuclide studies. The results were interpreted as rejection on the basis of previous experience in allografts treated with azathioprine. This further supports our disappointing findings that the radionuclide appearances of rejection are similar to those found during episodes of CsA nephrotoxicity. The second report by Wijeyesinghe et al. (*12*) used Tc-99m tin colloid and only included one transplant with probable CsA nephrotoxicity. It was thought that these results were not relevant to our study.

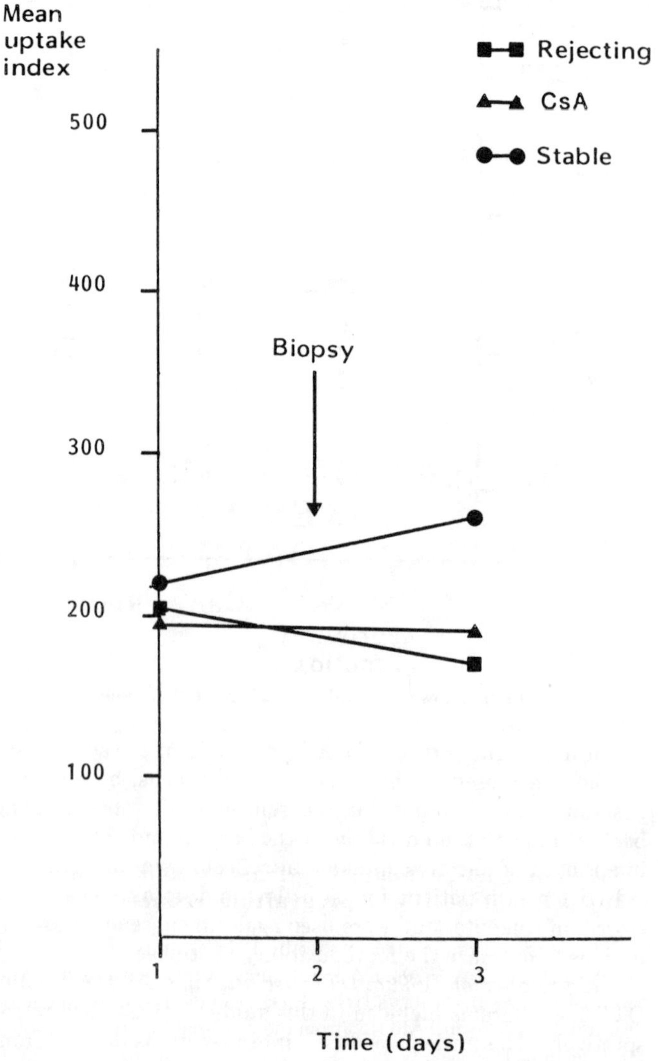

FIGURE 4. Mean uptake index values bracketing dysfunction episodes.

Thus, at present, we believe that when CsA is used the value of Tc-99m DTPA scintigrams is limited in the event of allograft dysfunction—other than ensuring that the graft is still perfused, and that there is evidence of renal tract obstruction or urinary leakage. Currently, there are no noninvasive methods of differentiating CsA nephrotoxicity from rejection available, and biopsy remains the only reliable means of making this distinction at present.

Acknowledgments. We gratefully acknowledge help received from the physicians and surgeons of Guy's Hospital renal unit in the compilation of the data in this study.

REFERENCES

1. Taube DH, Neild GH, Williams DG, et al. Differentiation between allograft rejection and cyclosporin A nephrotoxicity in renal transplant recipients. Lancet 1985; ii: 171.
2. Taube D, Neild G, Hobby P, Holt D, Welsh K, Cameron JS. A comparison of the clinical, histopathological, cytologic and biochemical features of renal transplant rejection, cyclosporin A nephrotoxicity and stable renal function. Transplant Proc 1985; 17: 179.
3. Sibley RF, Ryansiewicz J, Ferguson RM, et al. Morphology of cyclosporine nephrotoxicity and acute rejection in patients immunosuppressed with cyclosporine and prednisolone. Surgery 1983; 94: 225.
4. Von Willebrand E, Hayry P. Cyclosporin A deposits in renal allografts. Lancet 1983; ii: 189.
5. Salaman JR, Griffin PJA. Fine needle intra-renal manometry: a new test for rejection in cyclosporin-treated recipients of kidney transplants. Lancet 1983; ii: 709.
6. Wagner E, Pichlmayr R, Wonigeit K, Klempnallerd-Buzzendahl H, Lauchert W. Differentiation between rejection and cyclosporin-A nephrotoxicity by monitoring interstitial pressure in human renal allografts. Transplant Proc 1983; 15: 9.
7. Klintmalm G, Bergstrand A, Ringden O, et al. Graft biopsy for the differentiation between nephrotoxicity and rejection in cyclosporin A treated renal transplant recipients. Transplant Proc 1983; 15: 493.
8. Flechner SM, Van Buren C, Kerman RH, Kahan BD. The nephrotoxicity of cyclosporine in renal transplant recipients. Transplant Proc 1983; 13: 2689.
9. Hilson AJ, Maisey MN, Brown CB, et al. Dynamic renal transplant imaging with Tc-99m DTPA supplemented by a transplant perfusion index in the management of renal transplants. J Nuclear Med 1978; 19: 994.
10. Paller MS, Murray BM, Ferris TF. Decreased renal blood flow after cyclosporine infusion. Kidney Int 1985; 27: 346.
11. Prescott MC, Testa HJ, Lawson RS, Johnson R. The effect of cyclosporin A on the results of radionuclide investigations of kidney function in renal transplant recipients. In: Joekes AM, Constable AR, Brown NJG, Tauxe WN, eds. Radionuclides in nephrology. New York:Grune & Stratton, 1982: 275.
12. Wijeyesinghe ECR, Hawkins T, Keavey P, Wilkinson R. Technetium-99m tin colloid—its value in the diagnosis of renal transplant rejection and its potential for differentiating cyclosporin nephrotoxicity. Kidney Int 1985; 27: 351.
13. Klintmalm BG, Klingensmith WC, Iwatsuki I, Schröter GPJ, Starzl TE. Technetium-99M DTPA and ^{131}I-hippuran findings in liver transplant recipients treated with cyclosporin A. Radiology 1982; 142: 199.

Received 22 November 1985.
Accepted 4 February 1986.

0041-1337/86/4205-0497$02.00/0
TRANSPLANTATION
Vol. 42, No. 5
Printed in U.S.A.

MARROW GRAFT REJECTION AND VENO-OCCLUSIVE DISEASE OF THE LIVER IN PATIENTS WITH APLASTIC ANEMIA CONDITIONED WITH CYCLOPHOSPHAMIDE AND CYCLOSPORINE[1]

H. JOACHIM DEEG,[2] HOWARD M. SHULMAN, ELIZABETH SCHMIDT, GARY C. YEE, E. DONNALL THOMAS AND RAINER STORB

The Fred Hutchinson Cancer Research Center; The Swedish Hospital Medical Center; and the Departments of Medicine and Pathology, University of Washington School of Medicine, Seattle, Washington

Based on studies in multiply transfused dogs showing that cyclosporine (CsA) pregrafting reduced the incidence of rejection, we treated 11 multiply transfused patients with severe aplastic anemia with CsA, 12.5–20 mg/kg/day i.m. on days −6 to −1, and cyclophosphamide, 50 mg/kg/day i.v. on days −5 to −2, followed on day 0 by a marrow graft from an HLA-identical sibling donor. Patients were not given additional infusions of buffy coat cells from their marrow donors. As postgrafting prophylaxis for graft-versus-host disease 10 patients were given CsA, 12.5 mg/kg/day orally, and one patient was given a standard regimen of intermittent metho-

[1] This work was supported in part by PHS Grants CA 30924, CA 18029, CA 33252, CA 15704, CA 18221, and CA 09319 awarded by the National Cancer Institute, DHHS. E.D. Thomas is the recipient of Research Cancer Award AI02425 from the National Institute of Allergy and Infectious Diseases.

[2] Address correspondence to: H.J. Deeg, M.D., Lombardi Cancer Research Center, 3800 Reservoir Road NW, Washington, D.C., 20007.

trexate. Among 10 evaluable patients, 2 rejected their marrow grafts. Eight patients had sustained engraftment. Two of these developed severe veno-occlusive disease of the liver, a complication previously observed only in patients conditioned with total-body irradiation but not in more than 200 patients with aplastic anemia conditioned with cyclophosphamide without the addition of CsA. These data indicate that conditioning of patients with cyclophosphamide and concurrent CsA does not uniformly prevent graft rejection and can result in severe hepatic toxicity.

The success of allogeneic marrow transplantation in patients with aplastic anemia depends to a large extent on the efficacy of the conditioning regimen in suppressing the patient's immune response, thereby preventing graft rejection. In untransfused patients a regimen consisting of cyclophosphamide followed by marrow infusion from an HLA-identical donor resulted in engraftment in more than 90% of patients and more than 80% are surviving (*1*). In patients who had received transfusions of blood products before transplantation, the infusion of donor buffy-coat cells in addition to marrow reduced the incidence of marrow graft rejection from more than 30% to less than 15% and survival improved from 43 to 70% (*2*). However, despite the use of methotrexate (MTX)* after grafting, the addition of buffy coat cells led to a significant increase of chronic graft-versus-host disease (GVHD) (*3*).

Cyclosporine (CsA) has been shown in animal models and in clinical studies to be a potent immunosuppressant (*4–9*). In the present study of 11 patients with aplastic anemia, we investigated whether CsA given concurrently with cyclophosphamide might facilitate engraftment and prevent rejection, as shown in multiply transfused dogs (*10*) and as suggested by preliminary clinical results in multiply transfused patients (*7, 11*). Our results show that with this regimen the incidence of rejection was not reduced below that observed in recent patients conditioned with cyclophosphamide alone (*12*). In addition, this regimen was associated with severe hepatotoxicity.

MATERIALS AND METHODS

From December 1980 through July 1981, 11 consecutive patients with severe aplastic anemia, 13–42 (median 27) years of age, were entered into this study. Eight were male and three female. Nine were white and two Native American. The duration of their aplastic anemia was 0.25–3 (median 0.5) months. It was probably drug-related in three and of unknown etiology in eight patients. All had been previously transfused with 0–16 (median 6) units of red blood cells, 0–110 (median 18) units of platelets, or both. Five patients were refractory to transfusions with random-donor platelets. Three patients (unique patient numbers [UPNs] 1338, 1434, and 1464) had had pregnancies. None of the 11 patients had received treatment other than transfusion support before referral for marrow transplantation. At the time of transplantation the patients' granulocyte counts were 0.05–1.7 (median 0.3) $\times 10^9$/L, platelets 0.4–5.3 (median 8.1) $\times 10^9$/L, hematocrit 9–34.5% (median 23.6%), and corrected reticulocyte counts 0.1–2.3% (median 1.0%). Marrow cellularity for erythroid, myeloid, and megakaryocytic series was 0–5% (median 4%), 0–5% (median 3%), and 0–20% (median 0%), respectively.

* Abbreviations used: AAT, aspartate aminotransferase; AP, alkaline phosphatase; BUN, blood urea nitrogen; CsA, cyclosporine; GVHD, graft-versus-host disease; MTX, methotrexate; VOD, veno-occlusive disease.

All patients were given marrow grafts from HLA-identical siblings (*1, 2*). The donors were 12–43 (median 23) years old and were of the same sex in four instances and of opposite sex in seven. In one patient there was a minor and in one a major ABO incompatibility between donor and recipient.

The immunosuppressive regimens used are summarized in Table 1. One patient was given regimen 1 and 10 were given regimen 2. All patients were given i.v. cyclophosphamide, 50 mg/kg/day for four doses (days −5 to −2), followed within 36 hr by the infusion of 1.7–4.3 (median 2.9) $\times 10^8$ marrow cells/kg (*1, 2*). None of the patients received donor buffy coat cells following the marrow infusion (*13*). Postgrafting CsA was gradually tapered as described (*8, 9*). An i.v. preparation of CsA was not available at the time of this study. Methods of assessing allogeneic engraftment by erythrocyte antigen and isoenzyme determinations, and cytogenetic analyses of marrow and peripheral blood lymphocytes have been described (*1, 2*).

Acute GVHD was treated by an increase of the dose of CsA (one patient) or the administration of prednisone at 2 mg/kg/day (three patients) (*14*). In two patients chronic GVHD was treated with prednisone, initially 1 mg/kg per day, then every other day, either alone or in combination with azathioprine, 1.5 mg/kg per day (*15*).

Serum CsA levels were determined by radioimmunoassay as described (*16*).

The protocols and consent forms were approved by the Institutional Review Board of the Fred Hutchinson Cancer Research Center.

RESULTS

Engraftment and survival. Results are summarized in Table 2. One patient (UPN 1364) died too early to be evaluated for engraftment and two patients, one given MTX (UPN 1405) and one given CsA after grafting (UPN 1321) failed to achieve sustained engraftment. Both of these patients had successful second grafts after conditioning with cyclophosphamide and antithymocyte globulin, but both ultimately died. Eight patients had sustained engraftment documented at 7–38 (median 14) days by marrow aspiration. The data on acute and chronic GVHD are summarized in Table 2.

Four patients are alive and well 1395, 1543, 1555, and 1606 days after transplantation. All have normal hematologic parameters.

Toxicity

Hepatic toxicity. Elevations of serum alkaline phosphatase (AP) and aspartate aminotransferase (AAT) to more than twice normal were seen in seven and six patients, respectively. In six patients serum bilirubin rose to above 34 μmol/L (2 mg%). In all but two patients these abnormalities were short-lasting and resolved despite continued treatment with CsA. Patients UPN 1338 and 1464 developed the clinical picture of veno-occlusive disease (VOD) of the liver. Patient UPN 1338 had a rise in serum bilirubin to 11.5 mg% in week two and a peak of 46.6 mg% in week five. Concurrently AP and AAT rose to peaks of 195 and 3682 IU/L, respectively. Along with a deterioration in hepatic function, she developed anuric renal failure and required hemodialysis for 6 weeks. Her bilirubin subsequently declined and AP rose to values of approximately 1000 IU/L, clinically consistent with chronic GVHD. She died on day 241 from an intestinal hemorrhage.

Patient UPN 1464 had a rise of serum bilirubin to 16.4 mg% in week 2 and 74.1 mg% in week 5. AP and AAT rose to peak

TABLE 1. Immunosuppressive regimens[a]

Regimen	Pregrafting cyclosporine[b]	Postgrafting	
		Cyclosporine	Methotrexate
1	12.5 mg/kg/day i.m. (days −6 to −1)	No	15 mg/m² (day 1) 10 mg/m² (days 3, 6, 11, 18 . . . 102) i.v.
2	20 mg/kg/day i.m. (days −6 to −1)	12.5 mg/kg/day p.o. (days 0–50, then taper to day 180)	No

[a] All patients were given cyclophosphamide, 50 mg/kg/day i.v. on days −5 to −2.
[b] The dose of CsA was adjusted to serum creatinine levels. When the creatinine rose to >1.5 mg% (>133 μmol/L), CsA was reduced by 25–50%. When creatinine rose to ≥2.0 mg% (177 μmol/L), CsA was stopped and reinstituted only when renal function improved to a creatinine <2.0 mg% (177 μmol/L).

TABLE 2. Data on 11 patients with aplastic anemia given pregrafting cyclophosphamide and cyclosporine and HLA-identical marrow grafts

Immunosuppressive regimen	UPN	Age (years)/sex	In vitro tests of sensitization: RR/CR[a]	Sustained engraftment	GVHD: Acute, after first graft (grade/day of onset)	GVHD: Chronic (organs involved)[b]	Outcome (Karnofsky score)	Survival (days)[f]
1	1405	13/M	−/−	−	0	NA[c]	Died; severe GVHD after second graft; systemic adenovirus (type 5) infection	128
2	1312	42/M	−/+	+	III/62	NA	Died; renal failure; GVHD; cytomegalovirus enteritis, bowel perforation, septicemia	134
	1321	21/M	+/+	−	0	Yes (S,L,M)	Died; chronic GVHD after second graft	1010
	1329	14/M	+/+	+	I/30	No	Alive, restrictive pulmonary disease (80%)	>1606
	1338	27/F	−/+	+	0	Yes (S,L,M)	Died; renal failure, veno-occlusive disease of the liver, chronic GVHD, intestinal hemorrhage	241
	1367	27/M	+/+	+	0	No	Alive and well (100%)	>1555
	1365	29/M	−/+	+	II/11	Yes (S,M,G)	Died; chronic GVHD, multiple infections, septicemia, intracranial hemorrhage[e]	258
	1377	23/M	−/−	+	0	No	Alive and well (100%)	>1543
	1364	13/M	−/NT	TE[d]	NA	NA	Died; idiopathic interstitial pneumonitis	8
	1434	34/F	−/−	+	I/23	No	Alive and well (100%)	>1395
	1464	35/F	−/−	+	0	NA	Died; renal failure, veno-occlusive disease of the liver, septicemia	39

[a] (RR) relative response in mixed leukocyte culture; (CR) chromium release in cytotoxicity assay; (NT) not tested.
[b] (S) skin; (LC) liver; (G) gut; (M) mucosa; (E) eye.
[c] (NA) not applicable.
[d] (TE) too early to be evaluated.
[e] Clinical diagnosis; no autopsy was performed.
[f] Survival as of June 1, 1985.

values of 546 and 595 IU/L, respectively. Concurrently she developed anuric renal failure requiring hemodialysis until her death. She died on day 39 from septicemia.

Renal toxicity. Excluding patient UPN 1364 who died on day 8 and patient UPN 1405 who received CsA before grafting only, all 9 patients had a rise of serum creatinine and blood urea nitrogen (BUN). Eight doubled their baseline creatinine and three required hemodialysis. In one patient (UPN 1312), renal failure, apparently not related to CsA, followed the infusion of ABO-incompatible marrow and hemolysis. Reduction of the dose of CsA 5–45 days after transplantation was necessary in all but one patient (UPN 1367).

All patients also received vancomycin, five received amphotericin B, and two aminoglycosides that may have contributed to renal dysfunction. The four living patients have normal creatinine clearances.

CSA Serum Levels

Serum levels, as determined by radioimmunoassay (*16*), varied widely from patient to patient and occasionally from day to day. Of note was a comparison of CsA levels between the two patients developing VOD and the remaining 9 patients without VOD. The trough CsA levels in the 2 VOD patients during the first 2 weeks of CsA administration (32 observations) ranged from 0–1856, mean (±SD) 388±379 ng/ml compared with 0–888, mean (±SD) 171±189 ng/ml in the remaining patients

(66 observations) ($P<0.01$ by Mann Whitney U test). Elevated levels in VOD patients persisted even after discontinuation of CsA on days 5 and 8, respectively—presumably as a manifestation of impaired hepatic clearance (*17*).

Histologic Studies

Because of the known renal toxicity of CsA (*18*) and hepatic toxicities observed clinically in the present study our interest focused on those organs. Relevant histologic specimens were reviewed. Patient 1338 had two percutaneous liver biopsies on day 96 and day 171. Both biopsies had findings of VOD and GVHD. The VOD changes were those of long-standing lesions with fibrous obliteration of lumina of the small central venules (Fig. 1). The GVHD changes became progressively worse in the later biopsy, showing cholangiolar cholestasis, increasing bile duct injury with atypia, degeneration and dropout, and portal inflammation with bridging fibrosis. No tissue was available for examination from the second patient with the clinical syndrome of VOD of the liver (UPN 1464). Postmortem necropsy sections of liver from patients UPN 1405 and 1312 had changes of severe hepatic GVHD, while findings of VOD were absent. The kidneys from both autopsied patients had severe acute tubular interstitial injury with candida microabscess present in UPN 1312.

DISCUSSION

This report describes the results of a pilot study of the usefulness of CsA for the prevention of marrow graft rejection. The CsA regimens were based on two observations. First, we had shown in dogs that transfusion-related sensitization and subsequent marrow graft rejection could be overcome by the administration of CsA to the marrow recipient for 6 days before marrow infusion (*10*). Second, preliminary clinical trials suggested that patients given CsA instead of MTX had a reduced incidence of marrow graft rejection (*7, 11*).

Although the number of patients involved in the present study was small, two observations were of note. Of 10 evaluable patients given CsA pregrafting (and no donor buffy coat cells following marrow infusion), 2 failed to achieve sustained engraftment. This incidence was comparable to the 19.7% incidence of graft rejection in a recent analysis of patients conditioned with cyclophosphamide only, without the addition of donor buffy coat cells to the marrow inoculum (*2*). However,

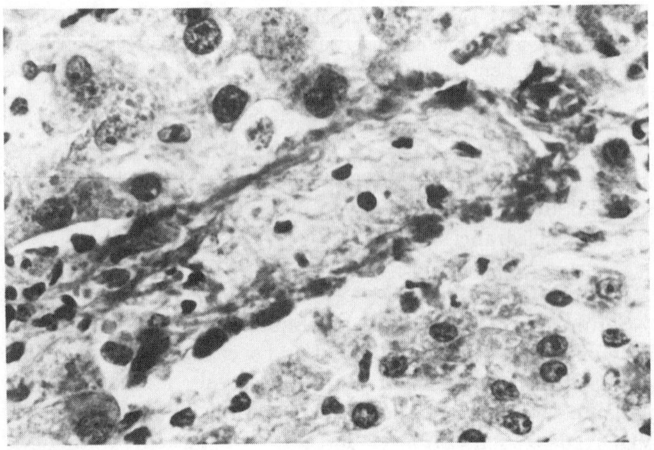

FIGURE 1. Liver biopsy on day 96 showing fibrous obliteration of central hepatic venule (CV). Trichrome stain; original magnification ×130.

the present CsA regimen was associated with severe toxicity, and overall results were not superior to those obtained with cyclophosphamide alone and inferior to those obtained with cyclophosphamide and the addition of donor buffy coat cells. Thus, we have to conclude that our regimen, as administered, cannot be recommended for transplant conditioning of patients with severe aplastic anemia.

Renal toxicity is a well-described side effect of CsA (*4, 19, 20*). Hepatic toxicity, however, including the occurrence of VOD of the liver in two patients appeared more severe than previously reported (*8, 21, 22*). In one patient VOD was proved by biopsy (*23*). In the second patient the clinical features were diagnostic, as shown by McDonald et al. who validated parameters of clinical diagnosis of VOD (*24*).

VOD has been observed in patients undergoing marrow transplantation after aggressive conditioning regimens almost exclusively involving the use of total-body irradiation, but VOD in patients treated with high doses of alkylating agents and not given irradiation is rare (*25, 26*). In particular, we have not, as yet, observed a single case of VOD in more than 200 patients with aplastic anemia conditioned for transplantation with a standard regimen of cyclophosphamide, 4×50 mg/kg as used in the present study, and not given CsA.

In previous studies from this (*18*) and other institutions (*22*), histologic changes in the liver of marrow transplant recipients consistent with CsA-induced hepatotoxicity have been described. The changes consisted of centrilobular hepatocyte atrophy and degeneration, both nonspecific findings. We propose that the administration of cyclophosphamide concurrently with CsA was responsible for additional toxicity leading to the unusual occurrence of VOD in two patients. Although both CsA and cyclophosphamide, when administered alone, are occasionally associated with hepatic dysfunction, when given in combination, each may mutually potentiate the hepatotoxicity of the other. Cyclophosphamide has been reported to depress hepatic microsomal enzymes (*27*), which are presumably responsible for CsA metabolism. Similarly CsA has been reported to reduce hepatic cytochrome P-450 levels in animals (*28*). As a result increased concentrations of cyclophosphamide, CsA (or their toxic metabolites), or both may be responsible for the apparent increased hepatotoxicity. High and sustained levels of CsA given prior to conditioning may render centrilobular hepatocytes more susceptible to the potentially toxic effects of active cyclophosphamide metabolites. The higher CsA levels in patients developing VOD would be in agreement with such a hypothesis, but we were unable to determine whether elevated levels resulted in increased hepatic toxicity—or, vice versa, whether hepatic damage (possibly of another etiology) resulted in further accumulation of CsA in the blood (*17*). One might speculate that the administration of CsA as an i.m. injection, a preparation no longer available, also might have contributed to sustained levels of CsA because of its slow release from the i.m. depot.

Alternatively CsA might amplify the cascade of basic events that may result in VOD. Recent studies in patients after marrow transplantation suggest that coagulation factors are involved in the pathogenesis of VOD (*29*). Using immunohistochemical techniques, we found deposits of factor VIII and fibrinogen in central hepatic venules, the subendothelial space, and at the interface of venules and hepatocytes. Vanrenterghem et al. (*30*), studying kidney graft recipients, observed an increased incidence of thromboembolic complications in patients treated with CsA as compared with those treated with steroids.

Among other findings, CsA-treated patients had elevated concentrations of factor VIII and fibrinogen, and increased adenosine-5′-diphosphate-induced platelet aggregation. In addition, one study found reduced prostacyclin production in the presence of CsA (*31*). These findings and previous reports on capillary thromboses after CsA (*18, 22*) suggest that CsA-related coagulation abnormalities, when superimposed on chemotherapy-induced injury in the liver, can result in the development of VOD.

Acknowledgments. We thank the physicians, nurses, ward clerks, secretaries, and technologists of the Adult Leukemia Center and the Swedish Hospital Medical Center, the patients' referring physicians—and, most importantly, the patients—for their cooperation in this study.

REFERENCES

1. Storb R, Thomas ED, Buckner CD, et al. Marrow transplantation in thirty "untransfused" patients with severe aplastic anemia. Ann Intern Med 1980; 92: 30.
2. Storb R, Doney KC, Thomas ED, et al. Marrow transplantation with or without donor buffy coat cells for 65 transfused aplastic anemia patients. Blood 1982; 59: 236.
3. Storb R, Prentice RL, Sullivan KM, et al. Predictive factors in chronic graft-versus-host disease in patients with aplastic anemia treated by marrow transplantation from HLA-identical siblings. Ann Intern Med 1983; 98: 461.
4. Cohen DJ, Loertscher R, Rubin MF, Tilney NL, Carpenter CB, Strom TB. Cyclosporine: a new immunosuppressive agent for organ transplantation. Ann Intern Med 1984; 101: 667.
5. Tutschka PJ, Beschorner WE, Allison AC, Burns WH, Santos GW. Use of cyclosporin A in allogeneic bone marrow transplantation in the rat. Nature 1979; 280: 148.
6. Deeg HJ, Storb R, Gerhard-Miller L, Shulman HM, Weiden PL, Thomas ED. Cyclosporin A, a powerful immunosuppressant in vivo and in vitro in the dog, fails to induce tolerance. Transplantation 1980; 29: 230.
7. Hows J, Harris R, Palmer S, Gordon-Smith EC. Immunosuppression with Cyclosporin A in allogeneic bone marrow transplantation for severe aplastic anaemia: preliminary studies. Br J Haematol 1981; 48: 227.
8. Deeg HJ, Storb R, Thomas ED, et al. Cyclosporine as prophylaxis for graft-versus-host disease: a randomized study in patients undergoing marrow transplantation for acute nonlymphoblastic leukemia. Blood 1985; 65: 1325.
9. Powles RL, Clink HM, Spence D, et al. Cyclosporin A to prevent graft-versus-host disease in man after allogeneic bone marrow transplantation. Lancet 1980; 1: 327.
10. Storb R, Deeg HJ, Atkinson K, et al. Cyclosporin-A abrogates transfusion-induced sensitization and prevents marrow graft rejection in DLA-identical canine littermates. Blood 1982; 60: 524.
11. Bacigalupo A, Frassoni F, van Lint MT, et al. Cyclosporin A in marrow transplantation for leukemia and aplastic anemia. Exp Hematol 1985; 13: 244.
12. Sanders JE, Whitehead J, Storb R, et al. Marrow transplant experience for children with aplastic anemia. Pediatrics, 1986; 77: 179.
13. Storb R, Thomas ED, Buckner CD, et al. Allogeneic marrow grafting for treatment of aplastic anemia. Blood 1974; 43: 157.
14. Doney KC, Weiden PL, Storb R, Thomas ED. Treatment of graft-versus-host disease in human allogeneic marrow graft recipients: a randomized trial comparing antithymocyte globulin and corticosteroids. Am J Hematol 1981; 11: 1.
15. Sullivan KM, Shulman HM, Storb R, et al. Chronic graft-versus-host disease in 52 patients: adverse natural course and successful treatment with combination immunosuppression. Blood 1981; 57: 267.
16. Donatsch P, Abisch E, Homberger M, Traber R, Trapp M, Voges R. A radio-immunoassay to measure cyclosporin A in plasma and serum samples. J Immunoassay 1981; 2: 19.
17. Yee GC, Kennedy MS, Storb RS, Thomas ED. Pharmacokinetics of intravenous cyclosporine in bone marrow transplant patients. Transplantation 1984; 38: 511.
18. Shulman H, Striker G, Deeg HJ, Kennedy M, Storb R, Thomas ED. Nephrotoxicity of cyclosporin A after allogeneic marrow transplantation. N Engl J Med 1981; 305: 1392.
19. Bennett WM, Pulliam JP. Cyclosporine nephrotoxicity. Ann Intern Med 1983; 99: 851.
20. Hows JM, Smith JM, Baughan A, Gordon-Smith EC. Nephrotoxicity in marrow graft recipients treated with cyclosporine. Transplant Proc 1983; 15: 2708.
21. Atkinson K, Biggs J, Dodds A, Concannon A. Cyclosporine-associated hepatotoxicity after allogeneic marrow transplantation in man: differentiation from other causes of posttransplant liver disease. Transplant Proc 1983; 15: 2761.
22. Tutschka PJ, Beschorner WE, Hess AD, Santos GW. Cyclosporin-A to prevent graft-versus-host disease: a pilot study in 22 patients receiving allogeneic marrow transplants. Blood 1983; 61: 318.
23. Shulman HM, McDonald GB, Matthews D, et al. An analysis of hepatic venocclusive disease and centrilobular hepatic degeneration following bone marrow transplantation. Gastroenterology 1980; 79: 1178.
24. McDonald GB, Sharma P, Matthews DE, Shulman HM, Thomas ED. Venocclusive disease of the liver after bone marrow transplantation: diagnosis, incidence, and predisposing factors. Hepatology 1984; 4: 116.
25. Shulman HM, McDonald GB. Liver disease after marrow transplantation. In: Sale GE, Shulman H, eds. The pathology of marrow transplantation. New York: Year Book, 1984: 104.
26. Ludwig J. Drug effects on the liver: a tabular compilation of drugs and drug-related hepatic diseases. Dig Dis Sci 1979; 24: 785.
27. Gurtoo HL, Marinello AJ, Struck RF, Paul B, Dahms RP. Studies on the mechanism of denaturation of cytochrome P-450 by cyclophosphamide and its metabolites. J Biol Chem 1981; 256: 11691.
28. Cunningham C, Whiting PH, Burke MD, Wheatley DN, Simpson JG. Increasing the hepatic metabolism of cyclosporine abolishes nephrotoxicity. Transplant Proc 1983; 15: 2712.
29. Shulman HM, Gown AM. An immunohistochemical study of liver disease after bone marrow transplant. Lab Invest 1985; 52: 61A.
30. Vanrenterghem Y, Roels L, Lerut T, Gruwez J, Michielsen P. Thromboembolic complications and haemostatic changes in cyclosporin-treated cadaveric kidney allograft recipients. Lancet 1985; 1: 999.
31. Neild GH, Rocchi G, Imberti L, et al. Effect of cyclosporine on prostacyclin synthesis by vascular tissue in rabbits. Transplant Proc 1983; 15: 2398.

Received 24 September 1985.
Accepted 7 February 1986.

0041-1337/86/4205-0502$02.00/0
TRANSPLANTATION
Vol. 42, No. 5

Printed in U.S.A.

MODULATION OF THE RESPONSE TO INTERLEUKIN 2 IN RECIPIENTS OF DONOR-SPECIFIC TRANSFUSIONS UNDER AZATHIOPRINE IMMUNOSUPPRESSION[1]

JOHN D. TYLER,[2] CHARLES B. ANDERSON, AND GREGORIO A. SICARD

Department of Surgery, Washington University School of Medicine St. Louis, Missouri 63110

The effect of plasma from recipients of donor-specific tranfusions given under azathioprine immunosuppression (DST+A) on the response to IL-2 was examined. Pre-DST+A plasma markedly enhanced the proliferative response to suboptimal doses of IL-2 by IL-2-dependent T cells, such that maximal responsiveness was achieved at lower IL-2 doses, as compared with normal plasma. Post-DST+A plasma also enhanced the response to suboptimal IL-2 doses. However at saturating IL-2 doses, the maximum response was markedly inhibited by post-DST+A plasma as compared with normal or pre-DST+A plasma. Neither toxicity nor inhibition of the IL-2 response was observed when the IL-2-dependent indicator cells were preincubated in post-DST+A plasma prior to an IL-2 dose-response assay. Of the recipients whose plasma was examined, nearly all exhibited some degree of inhibition (range: 8–50% inhibition) of the response to saturating levels of IL-2. Only one renal allograft has been lost in these recipients due to rejection, and this was an accelerated acute rejection in a recipient who had rejected 2 previous allografts and who developed a "transient" positive crossmatch to his donor during DST+A. The results suggest that inhibition of IL-2 responsiveness may be a frequent consequence of DST+A, and that the inhibition is dependent on an IL-2-mediated effect distinct from proliferation. Thus, such inhibition may contribute to the salutary effect of DST+A on renal transplantation.

Donor-specific transfusions under azathioprine immunosuppression (DST+A)* have led to significant prolongation of subsequent renal allograft survival (*1–3*). The mechanism(s) underlying the benefit of DST+A remains poorly understood, however recent results from this laboratory indicate that down-modulation of the allogeneic response is involved—the principle evidence being that of decreased reactivity to donor antigens following DST+A, as measured by the mixed lymphocyte reaction (MLR [*4*]) and more recently by limiting dilution analyses.[3] In the course of studies designed to elucidate the mechanism of decreased MLR, we quantitated the production of interleukin-2 (IL-2) by recipient PBL during the MLR; as a function of the recipient's status (before or after DST+A) and of the plasma source used to supplement the MLR cultures (recipient or control). In order to quantitate IL-2 production, it was necessary to generate standard dose-response curves with a known IL-2 source under media conditions similar to those of the MLR supernatant fluids being tested—i.e., in the presence of recipient or normal plasma. Unexpectedly, we observed that recipient plasma had a highly predictable effect on the absolute level of proliferation exhibited by the IL-2-responsive indicator cells.

MATERIALS AND METHODS

HLA-nonidentical recipients were given 3 transfusions consisting of 200 ml of donor blood at approximately 2-week intervals while receiving daily azathioprine immunosuppression that began 2–7 days prior to the first transfusion (*1–3*). Renal transplantation was performed 1–2 weeks (mean 9 days) following the last transfusion. All recipients had a negative crossmatch to their donor at the time of transplantation. IL-2 dose-response assays were conducted as follows: 2000 HT-2 cells (murine IL-2-dependent T cells [*5*] from exponentially growing cultures were washed once in balanced salt solution and added to triplicate 0.2-ml cultures containing various doses of IL-2. Culture media consisted of RPMI 1640 supplemented with antibiotics, Na pyruvate, nonessential amino acids, L-glutamine and 20% (v/v) normal or recipient plasma (*4*) or fetal calf serum (FCS, HyClone Laboratories, Logan, UT). Recipient plasma samples were collected from heparinized blood prior to the initiation of azathioprine immunosuppression (pre-DST+A), and after the completion of the transfusions but prior to renal transplantation (post-DST+A). Normal plasma consisted either of heparinized plasma collected simultaneously from the prospective donor or a pool collected from 12 healthy individuals. Plasma samples were passed through a 0.45-μ filter and stored at −70°C until used. The IL-2 source was a single batch of 48-hr culture supernatant fluid from phytohemagglutinin-stimulated human spleen cells that had been previously calibrated with the NCI-BRMP reference reagent ISDP-841 (*6*). The cultures were incubated for 24 hr at 37°C in 5% CO_2, and proliferation was assessed by ^{3}H-thymidine incorporation (1 μCi/well) during the final 6 hr of culture. Results are expressed as net dpm, as determined by liquid scintillation spectrometry, and subtraction of ^{3}H-thymidine incorporation by HT-2 cells incubated without IL-2. Linear regression analyses of log dose-response curves and statistical analyses of differences in means by *t* tests and of medians by Wilcoxon sign-rank tests were performed using RS/1 software (BBN Research Systems, Cambridge, MA) on a VAX 11/780 computer (Digital Equipment Corporation, Maynard, MA).

[1] This work was supported by USPHS Grant AM 27895, and by funds from the Missouri Kidney Program.

[2] To whom correspondence should be addressed, at: Department of Surgery University of Tennessee, 1924 Alcoa Highway Knoxville, TN 37920.

* Abbreviations used: DST+A, donor-specific transfusions under azathioprine immunosuppression; FCS, fetal calf serum; IL-2 interleukin 2; 2-ME, 2-mercaptoethanol; MLR, mixed lymphocyte reaction; NCI-BRMP, National Cancer Institute-Biological Response Modifiers Program, Frederick, MD; PBL, peripheral blood lymphocytes.

[3] Tyler, JD, Anderson CB and Sicard GA. Donor-specific transfusions under azathioprine immunosuppression: down-modulation of allogeneic responses (Manuscript submitted for publication).

RESULTS

Our initial purpose was to quantitate the production of IL-2 in anti-donor MLR cultures as a function of the recipient's status (before or after DST+A) and of the plasma (recipient or control) used to supplement the MLR cultures. The quantitation of IL-2 in the MLR culture supernatant fluids required the generation of a standard curve with a known IL-2 source. This was accomplished by measuring the proliferative response of the IL-2-dependent T cell line HT-2 (*5*) to varying suboptimal (titratable) doses of a precalibrated IL-2 source in parallel with proliferation of HT-2 cells in MLR supernatant fluids. In order to accurately compare the test response with the standard curve, we generated the standard curves in media identical to that used to supplement the MLR cultures.

Preliminary inspection of the IL-2 standard curves generated in the presence of recipient plasma (22 experiments) revealed a propensity for elevated proliferative responses as compared with identical assays conducted in control plasma. Since the enhancing effect, when observed, was present at all IL-2 doses initially employed (0.6–2.4 U/ml), we chose to demonstrate the individual results as the response theoretically occurring at an intermediate dose of 1U/ml IL-2. This response was calculated from linear regression analysis of individual log dose-response curves—all correlation coefficients (r-values) were >.91. As shown in Table 1, Pre-DST+A plasma from 7 of 11 recipients enhanced the IL-2 response, as compared with concurrent controls, resulting in significant elevation of both the mean ($P<.03$) and median ($P<.05$) proliferative response. Post-DST+A plasma from 9 of the 11 recipients enhanced the response, resulting in even more pronounced difference in the mean ($P<.002$) and median ($P<.01$) response as compared with controls. These results suggested that plasma from renal transplant candidates possessed IL-2-response–modulating properties, and also that such modulation might be more pronounced following DST+A. However, rigorous consideration of the latter possibility was hampered by several deficiencies in the initial experiments: First, the various recipient plasma samples were not tested concurrently and consequently experimental variation in terms of the absolute response of the controls was substantial. Second, the control plasma used in each experiment was obtained simultaneously from the donor, and therefore the post-DST+A results might have been skewed by effects of repetitive blood donation on donor plasma. Third, the dose range of IL-2 utilized was chosen to cover a titratable range (i.e., suboptimal range) and therefore did not provide information concerning effects of recipient plasma at optimal IL-2 doses. The latter was of particular concern since enhanced responsiveness to IL-2 would appear to be antithetical to induction of decreased alloreactivity via DST+A.

TABLE 1. Effect of recipient plasma on the response to IL-2

ID	Net dpm[a]			
	Pre-DST+A plasma		Post-DST+A plasma	
	Recipient	Control[b]	Recipient	Control
AH	66036	62239	20511	10552
CA	14628	14526	51565	34465
CO	18323	10036	8868	2378
EZ	17480	26224	55517	32503
KE	16549	11179	13359	12567
LA	21217	12640	41486	33295
ST	11442	10963	4686	1082
TY	18778	11210	13990	5276
WE	8118	4818	13963	6004
WO	35214	28145	24732	19051
WR	8993	8030	6290	8666
Mean	21525	18183	23179	15076
Median	17480	11210	13990	10552

[a] Net response of 2000 HT-2 cells at 1 U/ml IL-2 as calculated from linear regression analyses of log-dose response curves.

[b] Donor plasma.

Consequently, we examined the effect of recipient plasma over an extended range of IL-2 doses in parallel with a single pool of plasma collected from 12 healthy individuals and with fetal calf serum (FCS). All pre-DST+A samples were assayed concurrently, as were post-DST+A samples. As shown in Figure 1A, pre-DST+A plasma markedly enhanced the proliferative response at all suboptimal IL-2 doses as compared with normal plasma, and at all doses compared with FCS. Background responses in the absence of IL-2 were essentially identical for all groups and were subtracted from the IL-2-stimulated response, hence the enhancement is not due to IL-2-like activity in pre-DST+A plasma. The relatively poor response in FCS can be attributed to omission of 2 mercaptoethanol (2-ME), which we and others (*7*) have found to substantially augment IL-2 responses by HT-2 cells. However, since 2-ME was not added to the plasma samples, the enhanced IL-2 response in recipient plasma cannot be easily ascribed to a deficiency of the normal plasma because it was superior to FCS. The similarity of the shapes of the dose-response curves and the maximum responses in recipient and normal plasma indicate that the overall effect of pre-DST+A plasma is to increase the potency of IL-2 to trigger proliferation without altering its maximum efficacy.

The effect of post-DST+A recipient plasma on the IL-2 dose-response curve is depicted in Figure 1B. As with pre-DST+A plasma, post DST+A plasma significantly enhanced the response at IL-2 doses of 6 U/ml or less. However, in contrast to pre-DST+A plasma, the maximum response at optimal IL-2 doses was significantly lower in post-DST+A plasma than in normal plasma. Hence, post-DST+A plasma appears to contain both stimulatory and inhibitory properties, depending on the IL-2 dose employed.

Table 2 depicts the effect of each individual recipients post-DST+A plasma on the IL-2 response at 12 U/ml, which represents the dose at which the maximal response occurred in normal plasma (Figure 1, A and B)—i.e., the saturating IL-2 dose. Some degree of inhibition was observed in post-DST+A plasma of all recipients and inhibition was highly significant ($P<.05$) in all but one (KE).

In order to compare the effects of pre-DST+A and post-DST+A plasma of the recipients, the data depicted in Figure 1, A and B is reexpressed in Figure 1C as the percentage of the maximum proliferative response observed in normal plasma in the concurrent experiment. The validity of this normalization of the data is justified by the fact that the shapes of the resulting dose-response curves shown in Figure 1C are virtually indistinguishable from their counterparts in Figure 1, A and B—and identical normalization of the data from the concurrent normal controls resulted in 2 virtually identical curves (not shown). As is evident from Figure 1C, the striking difference between pre-DST+A and post-DST+A plasma lies in the marked inhibition of the maximal response by post-DST+A plasma. This inhibition would appear not to be due to direct antiproliferative or toxic effects of post-DST+A plasma, (e.g., via residual azathioprine), since proliferation was not inhibited at suboptimal doses

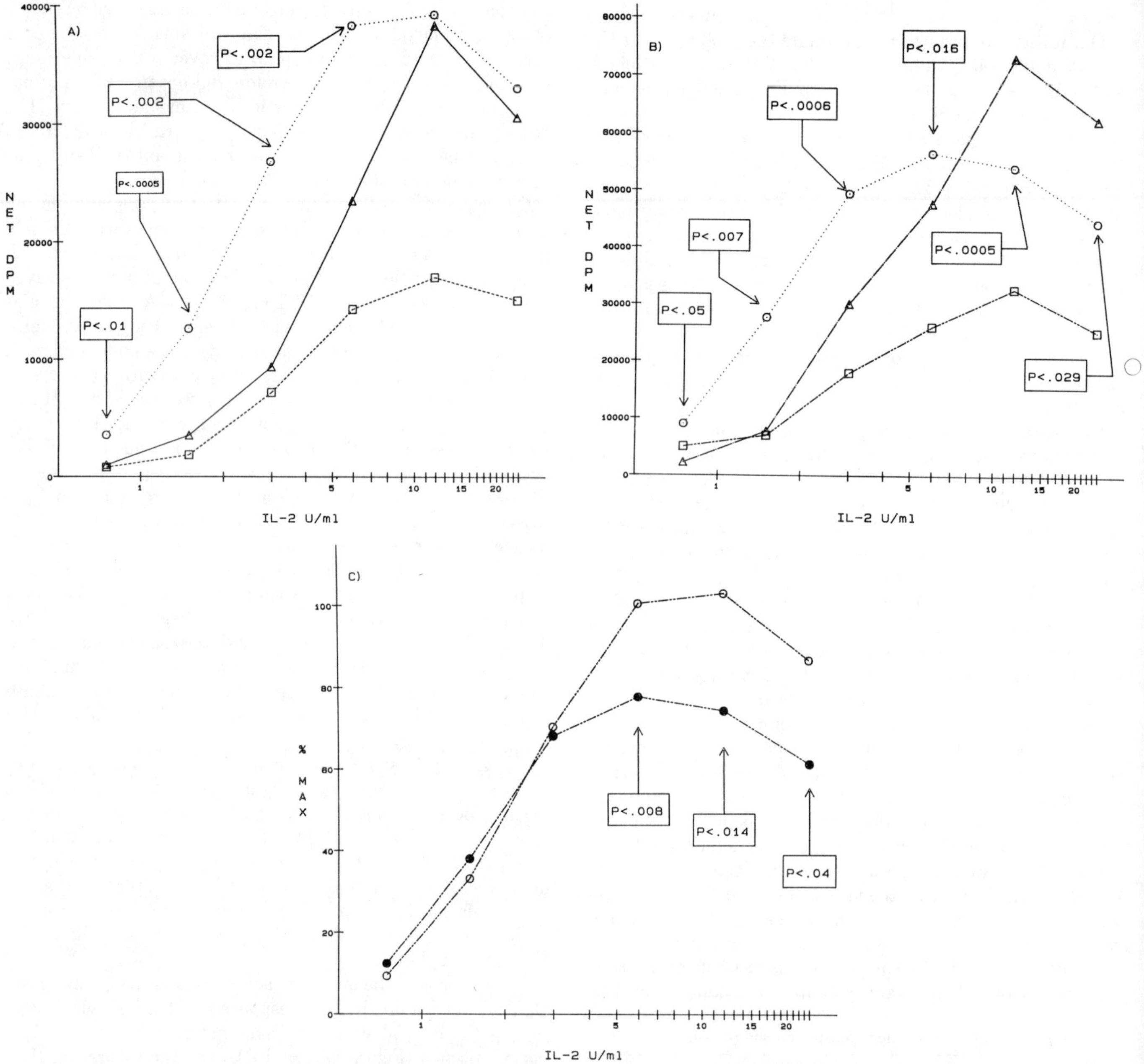

FIGURE 1. (A) The response to IL-2 in the presence of pre-DST+A plasma (mean of 9 recipients) (open circle); pooled normal plasma (open triangle); or FCS (open square). *P* values shown are from one-tailed unpaired *t* tests between recipient and normal plasma. (B) The response to IL-2 in the presence of recipient post-DST+A plasma (mean of same 9 recipients as Fig. 1A) (open circle); pooled normal plasma (open triangle); or FCS (open square). *P* values are from one-tailed unpaired *t* tests between recipient and normal plasma. (C) The response to IL-2 in pre-DST+A plasma (open circle); or post-DST+A plasma (closed circle). Values are expressed as the percentage of the maximum proliferative response observed in normal plasma in the concurrent experiment. *P* values are from paired one-tailed *t* tests.

of IL-2. In a limited number of similar experiments, the immunoaffinity purified NCI-BRMP reference reagent IL-2, ISDP-841 (*6*), was utilized as the standard IL-2 source and results qualitatively identical to those in Figure 1 were obtained (data not shown). Hence the inhibitory activity of post-DST+A plasma appears to be dependent on an IL-2-mediated effect, and not on one of the other lymphokines that may be present in the crude IL-2 source used for the present studies. Taken together, these observations suggested that post-DST+A plasma inhibits IL-2-mediated proliferation by modulation of an IL-2-dependent process that has pronounced effects on proliferation only at or near saturating levels of IL-2.

With this in mind, we examined whether inhibition of IL-2-induced proliferation would be mimicked by preincubation of the IL-2 indicator cells in post-DST+A plasma in the absence of IL-2. Accordingly, HT-2 cells (2×10^6/ml) were incubated at 37°C in 5% CO_2 for 6 hr in complete culture medium containing 20% post DST+A plasma, normal plasma, or FCS—but lacking IL-2. Following incubation the viability of all 3 cell preparations was greater than 95%, as assessed by trypan-blue dye exclusion. The cells were washed thrice and then added to an IL-2 dose-response assay supplemented with normal plasma. As shown in Figure 2, no significant difference in response occurred following preincubation with post-DST+A plasma as compared

TABLE 2. Inhibitory effects of post-DST+A plasma on the response to saturating doses of IL-2

Plasma source	Net dpm[a]		Percentage of inhibition[b]	P value[c]
	Mean	SD		
TY	36402	1001	50	.0005
CO	45407	3794	38	.00245
WR	47272	152	35	.0005
ST	48584	2182	33	.000838
WO	52051	3556	28	.003673
WE	60539	3187	17	.008076
CA	62142	3274	15	.011287
KE	64372	6473	12	.068551
LA	66807	3617	8	.041189
Normal	72745	467	Mean 26+/−14	.0005

[a] ^{3}H-thymidine incorporation by 2000 HT-2 cells cultured in 12 U/ml IL-2 and 20% plasma.

[b] As compared with normal control response.

[c] Paired one-tailed t test of the difference in mean dpm between the recipient and normal control.

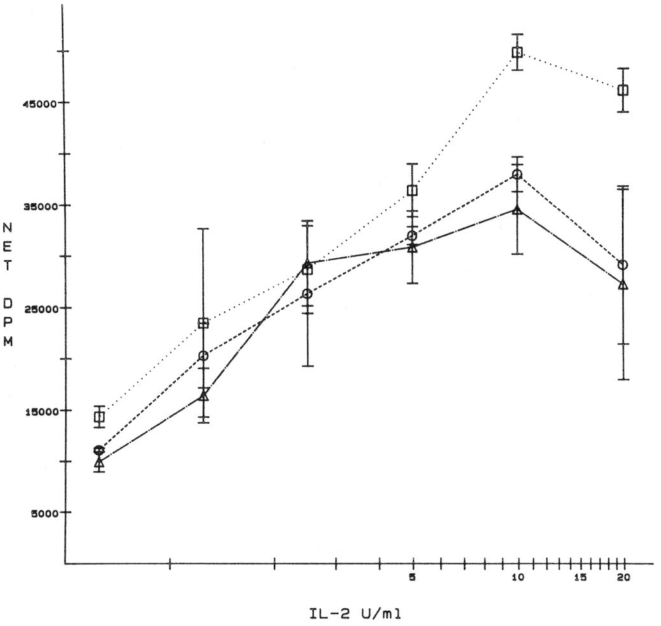

FIGURE 2. The effect of preincubation of HT-2 cells in post-DST+A plasma (open circle) normal plasma (open triangle), or FCS (open square) on the subsequent response to IL-2 in normal plasma. Each point represents the mean of two experiments each consisting of triplicate determinations.

with normal plasma, although both did induce inhibition at high IL-2 doses, as compared with FCS. The results are concordant with the notion that the inhibitory effect of post-DST+A plasma is dependent on IL-2-mediated effects. Additionally, the results demonstrate that post-DST+A plasma has no overt toxicity on the HT-2 indicator cells.

DISCUSSION

The results reported herein demonstrate that plasma obtained from renal transplant candidates has pronounced modulating effects on the proliferative response to IL-2. In view of the well-recognized impaired immune reactivity of patients with renal failure (*8–12*), it was surprising to observe that their plasma consistently enhanced proliferation at suboptimal doses of IL-2 (Fig. 1, A and B). However, such results may reflect an underlying disorder of immune regulation in these patients that manifests as immune deficiency in vivo. The IL-2 dose-response curves in pre-DST+A plasma and normal plasma (Fig. 1A) are analogous to dose-response curves exhibited by two agonists of equal maximal efficacy but of differing potency (*13*). Stimulation of the IL-2 response via C3b receptor interactions has been reported (*14*). This possible explanation for the enhancing effects of pre-DST+A plasma requires further investigation. Alternatively, the different dose-response curves may reflect the presence of a competitive antagonist in normal plasma that is absent from pre-DST+A plasma. Several investigators have reported soluble mediators in normal mouse serum/plasma that block the response to IL-2 (*15–18*); soluble IL-2 receptors have also been detected in normal human serum (*19*). Honda et al. (*20*) recently characterized a competitive IL-2 inhibitor released by concanavalin-A-stimulated murine T cells with an apparent M.W. of 11,000 to 12,000 daltons, which they consider to be an in vitro analogue of the IL-2 inhibitor present in normal serum or plasma. Preliminary tests suggest that such an IL-2 inhibitor may be present in normal, but not pre-DST+A, plasma—since simple dialysis markedly enhanced the subsequent IL-2 response in normal, but not pre-DST+A plasma. Because the dose-response curves in pre-DST+A and post-DST+A plasma at suboptimal doses are essentially identical (Fig. 1C), it seems probable that the mechanism underlying the stimulatory effects of pre-DST+A and post-DST+A plasma are similar.

From the standpoint of down-modulation of alloreactivity and improved renal allograft survival in recipients of DST+A, the inhibitory effect of post-DST+A plasma on the response to saturating levels of IL-2 is of particular interest. The inhibitory activity does not appear to be the result of direct toxic or antiproliferative effects of post-DST+A plasma, since inhibition is only observed at or near optimal doses of IL-2 (Fig. 1, B and C). Moreover, the inhibitory activity appears to require an IL-2-mediated effect (Fig. 2). Taken together these findings suggest that post-DST+A plasma interferes with an IL-2-dependent response at or near saturating levels of IL-2. An attractive candidate for such a process is the IL-2-induced upregulation of the IL-2 receptor on activated T cells (*21–24*)—i.e., IL-2 may regulate the proliferative response by influencing the expression of IL-2 receptors.

The mechanism underlying inhibition of the IL-2 response at saturating levels of IL-2 is currently under investigation in this laboratory. Since both DST and azathioprine are employed in our pre-renal-transplant conditioning regimen, it will be of interest to determine which may be more influential in inducing the inhibitory activity. Direct addition of azathioprine (1250 to 0.08 ng/ml) to IL-2 response assays has resulted in either no effect (low doses) or inhibition (moderate-to-high doses) of the proliferative response at both suboptimal and optimal IL-2 doses. Moreover, addition of plasma taken from a recipient prior to DST but after initiation of azathioprine immunosuppression exhibited no inhibition at any dose of IL-2. Hence, our preliminary results suggest that the selective inhibition observed in post-DST+A plasma is not a direct or acute effect of azathioprine—however, chronic and secondary effects of azathioprine immunosuppression cannot be discounted.

Extrapolation of our in vitro observations to the in vivo situation is hampered by a lack of information concerning physiologic levels of IL-2 produced in vivo. However, based on measurements of IL-2 production during in vitro MLR cultures of DST+A recipients (*4*, unpublished observations), the levels of IL-2 required to demonstrate inhibition by post-DST+A plasma would not appear to be physiologically excessive. Thus, one might predict that proliferation of IL-2 responsive alloreactive T cells would be inhibited in vivo during and/or following DST+A.

Of the 11 patients studied in this report, only 1 graft has been lost due to rejection—mean follow-up 12.2±2.7 months. This recipient (WR, Table 2) developed irreversible accelerated rejection at 12 days posttransplant, had rejected 2 previous transplants, and developed a "transient" positive crossmatch to his donor during DST+A. However, the effect of his post-DST+A plasma on IL-2 responsiveness showed no significant deviation from the mean profile exhibited by all recipients (Fig. 1, B and C), and it was among the most inhibitory at saturating doses of IL-2 (Table 2). Remarkably, a significant degree of inhibitory activity at high IL-2 doses was observed in the presence of post DST+A plasma in 10 of 11 recipients examined. Thus, it is possible that the development of IL-2 response inhibition is a frequent consequence of DST+A and may help to explain its salutary effect on renal transplantation. We are currently assessing the effect of posttransplantation plasma on IL-2 responses to determine if persistence of the activity correlates with superior allograft function.

REFERENCES

1. Newton WT, Anderson CB. Planned preimmunization of renal allograft recipients. Surgery 1973; 74: 430.
2. Anderson CB, Sicard GA, Etheredge EE. Pretreatment of renal allograft recipients with azathioprine and donor-specific blood products. Surgery 1982; 92: 315.
3. Anderson CB, Tyler JD, Sicard GA, Anderman CK, Rodey GE, Etheredge EE. Renal allograft recipient pretreatment with immunosuppression and donor-specific blood. Transplant Proc 1985; 17: 1047.
4. Tyler JD, Anderson CB, Sicard GA, Murphy MK, Anderman CK, Etheredge EE. Decreased mixed lymphocyte reactivity toward donor antigens following donor-specific transfusions combined with azathioprine immunosuppression. Transplant Proc 1985; 17: 1053.
5. Watson J. Continuous proliferation of murine antigen-specific helper T lymphocytes in culture. J Exp Med 1979; 150: 1510.
6. Robb RJ, Kutny RM, Chowdhry V. Purification and partial sequence analysis of human T-cell growth factor. Proc Natl Acad Sci USA 1983; 80: 5990.
7. Shipley GD, Abraham RT, Swanson BM, McHugh YE, Handwerger BS. Regulation of growth of an interleukin 2 (IL-2)-dependent murine T-cell clone (HT-2) in a defined serum-free medium. Cell Immunol 1985; 93: 459.
8. Kirkpatrick CH, Wilson WEC, Talmage DW. Immunologic studies in human organ transplantation. I. Observation and characterization of suppressed cutaneous reactivity in uremia. J Exp Med 1964; 119: 727.
9. Gordon A. Uremia. Curr Nephrol 1977; 1: 229.
10. d'Apice AJF, Coovadia HM, Mackay IR. Suppressor cells in stable dialysis and transplant patients. Nephron 1982; 31: 343.
11. Hsu CCS. Circulating lymphocyte inhibitors in liver diseases and uremia: concept of humoral immunoregulation and technical factors in inhibitor assays. In: Neubauer RH, ed. Naturally occurring biological immunosuppressive factors and their relationship to disease. Boca Raton, FL: CRC Press, 1979.
12. Gibbs JH, Robertson AJ, Brown RA, et al. Mitogen-stimulated lymphocyte growth and chronic uraemia. J Clin Lab Immunol 1982; 9: 19.
13. Gilman AG, Mayer SE, Melmon KL. Pharmacodynamics: mechanisms of drug action and the relationship between drug concentration and effect. In: Gilman AG, Goodman LS, Gilman A, eds. The pharmacological basis of therapeutics. 6th ed. New York: Macmillan, 1980.
14. Erdel A, Spaeth E, Alsenz J, et al. Role of C3b receptors in the enhancement of interleukin-2 dependent T-cell proliferation. Mol Immunol 1984; 21: 1215.
15. Hardt C, Rollinghoff M, Pfizenmaier K, Mosmann H, Wagner H. Lyt-23^+ cyclophosphamide-sensitive T cells regulate the activity of an interleukin 2 inhibitor in vivo. J Exp Med 1981; 154: 262.
16. Wagner H, Hardt C, Heeg K, Pfizenmaier K, Stotter H, Rollinghoff. The in vivo effects of interleukin 2 (TCGF). Immunobiology 1982; 161: 139.
17. Gautam SC, Hilfiker ML, Battisto JR. In vivo development of cytolytic t lymphocytes (CTL) to hapten-altered self: Mls-disparate cells facilitate the response by neutralizing IL 2 inhibitor. J Immunol 1983; 130: 533.
18. Maca RD. Inhibition of interleukin-2-induced proliferation of mouse T cells by normal mouse serum. J Biol Response Mod 1983; 2: 360.
19. Rubin LA, Kurman CC, Fritz ME, Nelson DL. Serum levels of soluble interleukin-2 receptor are elevated in patients with certain lymphoreticular malignancies. Clin Res 1985; 33: 457A.
20. Honda M, Chan C, Shevach EM. Characterization and partial purification of a specific interleukin 2 inhibitor. J Immunol 1985; 135: 1834.
21. Smith KA, Cantrell DA. Interleukin 2 regulates its own receptor. Proc Natl Acad Sci USA 1985; 82: 864.
22. Malek TR, Ashwell JD. Interleukin 2 upregulates expression of its receptor of a T cell clone. J Exp Med 1985; 161: 1575.
23. Wakasugi H, Bertoglio J, Tursz T, Fradelizi D. Il 2 receptor induction of human T lymphocytes: role for IL 2 and monocytes. J Immunol 1985; 135: 321.
24. Depper JM, Leonard WJ, Drogula C, Kronke M, Waldmann TA, Greene WC. Interleukin 2 (IL-2) augments transcription of the IL-2 receptor gene. Proc Natl Acad Sci USA 1985; 82: 4230.

Received 5 December 1985.
Accepted 6 February 1986.

0041-1337/86/4205-0507$02.00/0
TRANSPLANTATION
Copyright © 1986 by The Williams & Wilkins Co.

Vol. 42, No. 5
Printed in U.S.A.

OKT3 MONOCLONAL ANTIBODY PLASMA LEVELS DURING THERAPY AND THE SUBSEQUENT DEVELOPMENT OF HOST ANTIBODIES TO OKT3

GIDEON GOLDSTEIN,[1,2] ANTHONY J. FUCCELLO, DOUGLAS J. NORMAN,[3] CHARLES F. SHIELD III,[4] ROBERT B. COLVIN,[5] AND A. BENEDICT COSIMI

Immunobiology Division, Ortho Pharmaceutical Corporation, Raritan, New Jersey; 08869; Oregon Health Sciences University, Portland, Oregon 97201; St. Francis Regional Medical Center, Wichita Kansas 67214; and Massachusetts General Hospital, Boston, Massachusetts 02114

OKT3 levels and the presence of human antibodies to OKT3 were determined in the plasma of 66 patients receiving OKT3 monoclonal antibody (5 mg i.v. daily) for the treatment of acute renal allograft rejection. Plasma 24-hr trough levels of OKT3 rose over the first three days and then remained in a steady state over the remainder of the 14-day period of OKT3 therapy, with a mean level of 902±71 ng/ml (mean + SEM). On termination of OKT3 therapy plasma levels of OKT3 dropped to very low levels after 3 days. Host antibodies, usually of low titer, developed in a number of patients, usually 2–3 weeks after the start of OKT3 therapy. 37/43 patients (86%) who recieved OKT3 alone developed IgG anti-OKT3 antibodies; 9/23 patients (39%) who received Cytoxan in addition to OKT3 developed IgG anti-OKT3 antibodies, a significantly lower (*P* = 0.0002) incidence. The present regimens permitted maintenance of adequate levels of circulating OKT3 for 2 weeks, a sufficient time to reverse acute renal allograft rejection in most patients.

OKT3 is an IgG_{2A} murine monoclonal antibody that reacts with a 20,000 dalton protein associated with the human T cell antigen receptor (*1–4*). Interaction of OKT3 with its target protein blocks the function of T cells (*5*) and i.v. injections of OKT3 are effective in reversing acute rejection of renal allografts (*6*) and in preventing renal allograft rejection during the period of OKT3 administration (*7*).

However, like other murine monoclonal antibodies administered therapeutically in man (*8–13*), OKT3 does induce an antibody response in the recipient (*7, 14–18*), and these host antibodies have the potential to consume the administered OKT3 and prevent its therapeutic effect of blocking T cell killing and reversing rejection of the renal allograft. The incidence, rapidity of development, and titer of the host antibody response to OKT3 appears to be related to the use of concomitant immunosuppressive medications. In renal transplant patients treated with OKT3, 5 mg i.v. daily, with no other immunosuppressive medications (prophylactic regimen) 4/6 (67%) developed antibodies by the ninth day of treatment (*17*). In renal transplant patients similarly treated prophylactically with OKT3 with concomitant azathioprine and low-dose steroids 11/11 (100%) developed antibodies but did so later, 10 did so at 28–30 days, and one—presensitized as evidenced by a positive skin test before therapy—at 14 days (*17*). In patients with acute renal allograft rejection treated with OKT3, with lowering of steroids and azathioprine, 9/11 (82%) developed antibodies, usually after the fourteenth dose (*15*). A feature of the antibody response to OKT3 was the presence of both antimouse immunoglobulin isotype and anti-OKT3 idiotype antibodies (*15–17*).

It is considered that the therapeutic effectiveness of OKT3 in reversing acute renal rejection is related to the effect of this particular monoclonal antibody in blocking killing of the renal allograft cells by cytotoxic T cells of the recipient. The blocking effects of OKT3 on T cell killing in vitro are dependent on its concentration in the medium (*5*); by analogy the effective concentration of OKT3 in the body would be an important consideration in determining its effectiveness in blocking cellular rejection of the renal allograft. This article presents data on plasma levels of OKT3 during a first course of therapy with OKT3 and records the late development of antibodies to OKT3 that could affect plasma levels if prolonged or repeated therapy with OKT3 were contemplated.

MATERIALS AND METHODS

Patients. All patients were renal transplant patients being treated with OKT3 for acute renal allograft rejection. The treatment regimen has been described previously (*6*), and 43 patients (OKT3 alone) were from this reported study. Briefly, maintenance prednisone and azathioprine were lowered upon diagnosis of acute rejection, and daily i.v. injections of 5 mg OKT3 were given for 14 days, with subsequent reinstitution of azathioprine and prednisone after 14 days for maintenance immunosuppression. An additional 23 patients (OKT3 plus Cytoxan) were treated by a similar protocol with 5 mg OKT3 i.v. for 10 days; in addition Cytoxan, 400 mg i.v., was given on day 0 (3 patients only), and on days 7, 10, and 13 after starting OKT3.

Plasma samples. Plasma samples were obtained before the first injection of OKT3 and, throughout treatment, 24 hr after the previous injection of OKT3 (prior to the next injection of OKT3). In addition some samples were obtained 1 hr after the first dose, at daily intervals after the last dose, and at weekly intervals thereafter. Plasma was freshly separated then stored frozen at −20°C until assayed.

Plasma OKT3 levels. Plasma OKT3 levels were determined in a sandwich enzyme-linked immunosorbent assay (ELISA). The first layer was affinity-purified goat antimouse IgG (Jackson Immunoresearch Labs, Avondale, PA) coated on polyvinyl microtiter plates (Dynatech Labs, Alexandria, VA). The inter-

[1] Ortho Pharmaceutical Corporation.

[2] Requests for reprints should be sent to: Gideon Goldstein, M.D., Ph.D., Immunobiology Division, Ortho Pharmaceutical Corporation, Route 202, P.O. Box 300, Raritan, NJ 08869-0602.

[3] Oregon Health Sciences University.

[4] St. Francis Regional Medical Center.

[5] Massachusetts General Hospital.

mediate layer was plasma diluted 1/8 or OKT3 standards in a similar plasma dilution. Binding was detected with affinity-purified goat antimouse IgG coupled to alkaline phosphatase. The chromogen was p-nitrophenyl phosphate in 10% diethanolamine buffer, pH 9.8—the reaction being halted with 2.5 N NaOH; absorbance at 405 nm was measured using a MR600 automatic plate reader (Dynatech Labs, Alexandria, VA). OKT3 levels were determined by comparison with the standard OKT3 curves.

Antibodies to OKT3. Host antibodies to OKT3 were also determined in a sandwich ELISA technique. In this instance the layers were as follows: (1) OKT3 coated polyvinyl plates, (2) plasma dilutions, and (3) alkaline-phosphatase-linked goat antihuman IgG, IgM, or IgE. The goat antihuman immunoglobulin reagents were affinity-purified to eliminate reactivity with mouse immunoglobulins or other human immunoglobulin isotypes. Color development and absorbancy measurement were as above. Titer was determined by defining a positive test as one in which absorbance was equal to or greater than twice the absorbance of negative controls. For IgG anti-OKT3 antibodies titers of less than 100 gave high nonspecific background, so that 100 was the lowest titer that could be clearly detected as positive.

RESULTS

Plasma samples were obtained from 66 patients, 43 treated with OKT3 alone for a mean duration of 14 days and 23 treated with OKT3 plus Cytoxan for a mean duration of 10 days. Plasma levels of OKT3 did not differ significantly between the 2 groups, and the data for plasma OKT3 is therefore presented for the entire pool of 66 patients. In contrast, antibody responses to OKT3 differed markedly between the 2 groups, and these are presently separately.

Plasma OKT3 levels. The plasma OKT3 level at 1 hr after the first injection was 996±98 ng/ml (n = 60) and fell to 104±52 ng/ml at 24 hr (day 1, Fig. 1). Subsequently the 24-hr trough level of plasma OKT3 rose to 837±160 ng/ml by day 3 and remained in a steady state during the remaining period of treatment (3–14 days) with a mean value of 902±71 ng/ml, n = 66 (Fig. 1).

After cessation of therapy the mean trough level of plasma OKT3 was 996±99 ng/ml at 24 hr and then fell over the two subsequent 24-hr periods to 356 ng/ml and 12±9 ng/ml respectively (Fig. 2).

Host antibodies to OKT3. Table 1 summarizes the incidence of patients developing antibodies to OKT3. The highest incidence of antibodies were of the IgG isotype, and these were present in higher titers then IgM and IgE antibodies (see below). The incidence of IgG antibodies to OKT3 plus Cytoxan patients (39%) was significantly lower ($P = 0.0002$) than in patients treated with OKT3 alone (86%) (Table 1).

Figure 3 summarizes the highest titers of IgG antibodies to OKT3. These data show that fewer OKT3-plus-Cytoxan patients developed antibodies, in comparison with the group treated with OKT3 alone, and that the majority of patients in both groups who did develop antibodies had the lowest detectable titer of 100.

9/43 (21%) of patients treated with OKT3 alone developed IgM anti-OKT3 antibodies; these were 3 patients with maximum titers of 50 and 6 with highest titers of 100. 3/22 (14%) of OKT3-plus-Cytoxan–treated patients developed IgM anti-OKT3 antibodies, and these all had titers of 100. 10/35 (29%) of OKT3-alone-treated patients developed IgE anti-OKT3 antibodies; these were 3 patients with maximum titers of 10 and 7 with highest titers of 20.

Figure 4 displays the time of first appearance of IgG anti-

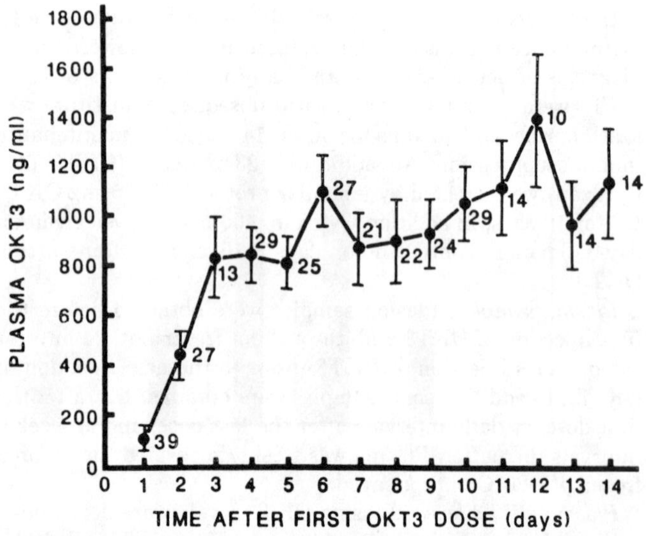

FIGURE 1. Plasma levels of OKT3 (mean ± SEM, n shown beside each point) 24 hr after each 5-mg i.v. dose. The first dose was given on day 0, so that day 1 represents levels 24 hr after the first dose.

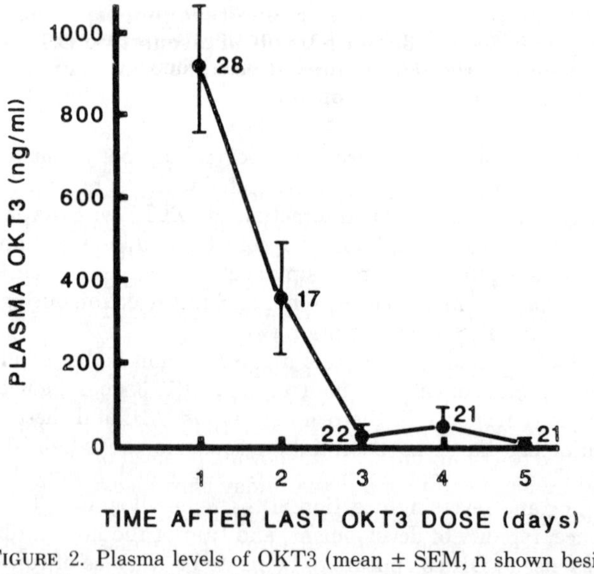

FIGURE 2. Plasma levels of OKT3 (mean ± SEM, n shown beside each point) at 24-hr intervals after the last 5-mg i.v. dose of a daily course of OKT3 treatment. Day 1 represents levels 24 hr after the last dose.

TABLE 1. Incidence of patients developing detectable IgG, IgM, or IgE antibodies to OKT3 after treatment with OKT3 or OKT3 plus Cytoxan

Treatment	Host antibodies to OKT3 and their isotopes (incidence [percentage])		
	IgG	IgM	IgE
OKT3 alone	37/43 (86)	9/43 (21)	10/35 (29)
OKT3 plus Cytoxan	9/23 (39)[a]	3/22 (14)	Not tested

[a] $P = 0.0002$, Fisher's exact test.

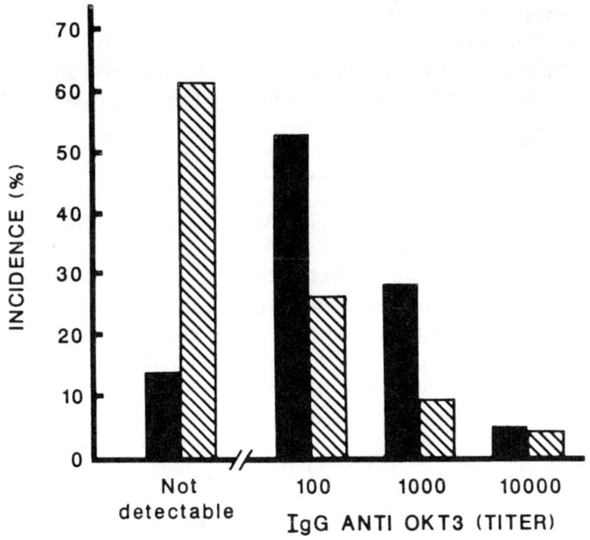

FIGURE 3. Highest titers of IgG anti-OKT3 antibodies in patients treated with OKT3 alone (solid bars) or OKT3 plus Cytoxan (hatched bars).

OKT3 antibodies. Only 2 patients (in the OKT3-only group) developed antibodies prior to 2 weeks. Both patients reversed their acute rejection; one maintained good long-term graft function, and the other developed early rerejection one week later that was uncontrollable, the graft being eventually lost.

The majority of patients in both groups who developed antibodies did so at 2–3 weeks. The time to peak titer was similar in both groups, being 20±2 days for the OKT3-only group and 23±3 days for the OKT3-plus-Cytoxan group.

DISCUSSION

OKT3 monoclonal antibody has been successfully used to treat acute renal allograft rejection in patients who have not received previous therapy with a murine monoclonal antibody (*6*). The recommended dosage schedule for OKT3 was 5 mg i.v. daily for 10 to 14 days, and the present study established that significant levels of OKT3 were maintained in the blood with this regimen. Peak levels of OKT3 would be expected to occur within 1 min of the injection by i.v. push; levels at this time were not measured in the present study. However, on the first day mean plasma OKT3 was 1002 ng/ml at 1 hr and dropped to 104 ng/ml at 24 hr, showing removal of OKT3 from the circulation quite unlike the 10-day half-life expected for an inert, unreactive antigen in the circulation (*19*). The major mechanism of removal of OKT3 from the circulation is almost certainly binding to T3 antigen on circulating T cells. This binding can be demonstrated within minutes of the injection of OKT3, and there is a rapid drop in circulating T cells as these opsonized cells are removed by the reticuloendothelial system (*20, 21*). Major consumption of OKT3 by this mechanism clearly occurred during the initial days of OKT3 therapy, a time when all the T3 antigen of circulating T cells was available for binding. This was evidenced by the lowest 24-hr trough level of plasma OKT3 of 104 ng/ml after the first injection, and subsequent rises of the 24-hr trough levels of OKT3 to 837 mg/ml after the third injection, with approximately steady state conditions thereafter. Following the last injection of OKT3, the levels of plasma OKT3 fell from 920 to 356 to 12 ng/ml over successive 24 hr periods and, concomitant with this, levels of OKT3^{+} T cells rose in the circulation. These findings suggest that T cell production is occurring throughout therapy with OKT3, and that this daily production of T3^{+} T cells is the major factor causing consumption of the daily injected OKT3.

Treatment with OKT3 was previously shown to be highly effective in blocking cell-mediated rejection in that 94% of acute renal allograft rejections were reversed (*6*). Other monoclonal antibodies that react with T cells and, like OKT3, cause their removal from the circulation, do not give similar high reversal rates (*22–24*). This suggests that depletion of circulating T cells cannot be the major mechanism whereby OKT3 blocks cellular rejection and highlights the pharmacological action of OKT3 in blocking T cell function. OKT3 reacts with, and thereby blocks the function of, the T3 antigen of human T cells (*5*), a structure associated with the T cell antigen receptor and necessary for signal transduction and T cell function (*2–4*). In vitro OKT3, at concentrations of 1000 ng/ml, blocks killing of specific targets by cytotoxic T cells (*5, 25, 26*). Since in vivo trough levels of OKT3 were 902 ng/ml, the levels during most of the time of treatment would have been considerably higher and certainly consistent with the concentrations of OKT3 required to block killing by cytotoxic T cells in vitro. The present study establishes that the regimen of OKT3 administration used—5 mg i.v. daily for 10 to 14 days—provides, in patients who have not previously received murine monoclonal antibodies, circulating levels of OKT3 that would block killing by cytotoxic T cells in vitro. These data are consistent with the clinical findings of high reversal rates of acute renal allograft rejection with this regimen of OKT3 administration, and they further focus on the pharmacological action of OKT3 in producing a highly selective block of T cell function.

Development of host antibodies to OKT3 would be another theoretical mechanism leading to lowering of circulating OKT3 levels, since it is well known that the development of host antibodies to an injected immunogen leads to an accelerated immune elimination and rapid removal of the immunogen from the circulation (*19*). Host antibodies to OKT3 did develop, despite the high efficacy of OKT3 in blocking T-cell-mediated cellular rejection of the renal allograft. The development of

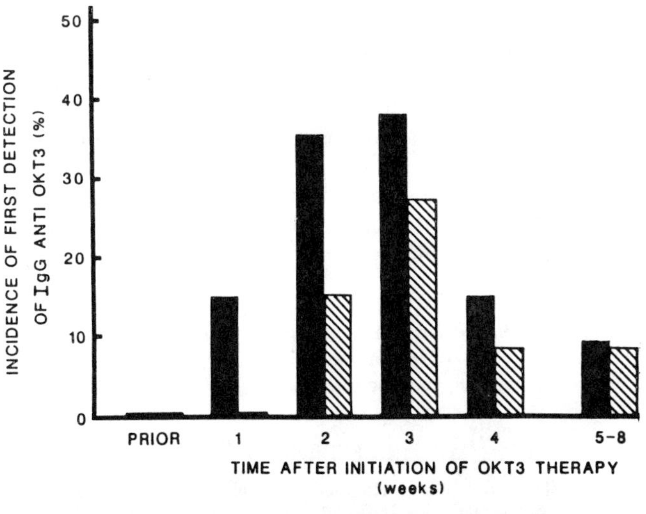

FIGURE 4. Times after initiation of OKT3 treatment when IgG anti-OKT3 antibodies were first detected. Solid bars denote patients treated with OKT3 alone, hatched bars denote those treated with OKT3 plus Cytoxan.

antibodies to immunoglobulin is generally considered to be T-cell-dependent, and the development of antibodies to OKT3 despite effective blockade of cell-mediated T cell function was a surprising finding. Perhaps a small residuum of T cell help is adequate to support B cell function and antibody formation or, alternatively, the presentation to B cells of OKT3 during monocyte phagocytosis of OKT3 opsonized T cells could have been adequate to stimulate antibody formation.

Antibodies to OKT3 have not produced significant symptoms of hypersensitivity, anaphylaxis, or serum sickness (*6*), so that their main significance is their potential for reducing levels of circulating OKT3. With the present protocols this effect was not significant during a 2-week course of treatment in patients previously unexposed to OKT3, but antibody development clearly must be considered in relation to the potential use of OKT3 for repeated or prolonged courses of treatment.

One approach would be to inhibit antibody formation to OKT3 with concomitant immunosuppressive treatments. It has already been shown that concomitant conventional immunosuppressive drugs affect the incidence and rapidity of development of antibodies to OKT3 (see above). The present study shows that Cytoxan, given for the most part toward the end of therapy with OKT3, reduced the incidence of IgG antibodies to OKT3 from 86% to 39%. Cytoxan is known to have selective and potent actions in inhibiting B cell function (*27*), and it is possible that this approach could be refined further.

Another approach is to increase the dose or frequency of administration of OKT3. Repeated courses of polyclonal antithymocyte globulin are administered despite the regular formation of host antibodies. The usual dose is large, on the order of 1 gm, so that this dose would still provide adequate levels of pertinent immunoglobulins despite complexing of host antibodies and injected immunoglobulin. The development of serum sickness in many patients retreated with polyclonal antithymocyte globulin raises a potential problem using the approach of higher and more frequent doses of OKT3 in patients with host antibodies.

The present study did not differentiate between antiisotype and antiidiotype antibodies to OKT3, but it is known that both types of antibody develop in most patients treated with OKT3 (*15, 16*). It has been shown that antiidiotype antibodies interfere with binding of OKT3 to T cells, whereas antiisotype antibodies do not (*16*). Furthermore, in an unusual patient who developed only antiisotype antibodies to OKT3 during therapy, plasma levels of OKT3 were not affected (*16*). This raises the possibility of yet another approach to the repeated or prolonged treatment with OKT3 of patients with antibodies to OKT3—the use of functionally equivalent antibodies of differing idiotypes to react with T3 and institute or maintain blockade of T cell function in the presence of antiidiotypic antibodies to OKT3.

Acknowledgments. We thank Ms. Linda Barnes, Dr. Huei Tsai, and Ms. Pien Nagy for control and analysis of the data, and Ms. Nancy Lawery for typing the manuscript.

REFERENCES

1. Kung PC, Goldstein G, Reinherz EL, Schlossman SF. Monoclonal antibodies defining distinctive human T-cell surface antigens. Science 1979; 206: 347.
2. Van den Elsen P, Shepley BA, Borst J, et al. Isolation of cDNA clones encoding the 20K T3 glycoprotein of human T cell receptor complex. Nature 1984; 312: 413.
3. Reinherz EL, Meuer S, Fitzgerald KA, Hussey RE, Levine H, Schlossman SF. Antigen recognition by human T lymphocytes is linked to surface expression of the T3 molecular complex. Cell 1982; 30: 735.
4. Imboden JB, Stobo JD. Transmembrane signalling by the T cell antigen receptor. J Exp Med 1985; 161: 446.
5. Chang TW, Kung PC, Gingras SP, Goldstein G. Does OKT3 monoclonal antibody react with an antigen-recognition structure on human T cells. Proc Natl Acad Sci USA 1981; 78: 1805.
6. Goldstein G, Schindler J, Tsai H, et al. A randomized clinical trial of OKT3 monoclonal antibody for acute rejection of cadaveric renal transplants. N Engl J Med 1985; 313: 337.
7. Kreis H, Chkoff N, Vigeral P, et al. Prophylactic treatment of allograft recipients with a monoclonal anti-T3+ cell antibody. Transplant Proc 1985; 17: 1315.
8. Sears HF, Herlyn D, Steplewski Z, Koprowski H. Effects of monoclonal antibody immunotherapy on patients with gastrointestinal adenocarcinoma. J Biol Resp Modif 1984; 3: 138.
9. Stratte PT, Miller RA, Amyx HL, Asher DM, Levy R. In vivo effects of murine monoclonal anti-human T cell antibodies in subhuman primates. J Biol Resp Modif 1982; 1: 137.
10. Sears HF, Mattis J, Herlyn D, et al. Phase-I clinical trial of monoclonal antibody in treatment of gastrointestinal tumours. Lancet 1982; 1: 762.
11. Shawler DL, Bartholomew RM, Smith LM, Dillman RO. Human immune response to multiple injections of murine monclonal IgG. J Immunol 1985; 135: 1530.
12. Dillman RO, Shawler DL, Dillman JB, Royston I. Therapy of chronic lymphocytic leukemia and cutaneous T-cell lymphoma with T101 monoclonal antibody. J Clin Oncol 1984; 2: 881.
13. Miller RA, Oseroff AR, Stratte PT, Levy R. Monoclonal antibody therapeutic trials in seven patients with T-cell lymphoma. Blood 1983; 62: 988.
14. Chatenoud L, Baudrihaye MF, Kreis H, Goldstein G, Schindler J, Bach JF. Human in vivo antigenic modulation induced by the anti-T cell OKT3 monoclonal antibody. Eur J Immunol 1982; 12: 979.
15. Jaffers GJ, Colvin RB, Cosimi AB, et al. The human immune response to murine OKT3 monoclonal antibody. Transplant Proc 1983; 15: 646.
16. Baudrihaye MF, Chatenoud L, Kreis H, Goldstein G, Bach JF. Unusually restricted anti-isotype human immune response to OKT3 antibody. Eur J Immunol 1984; 14: 686.
17. Chatenoud L, Baudrihaye MF, Kreis H, Goldstein G, Bach JF. The restricted human response to the murine monoclonal OKT3 antibody. Transplant Proc 1985; 17: 558.
18. Nelson PW, Jaffers GJ, Fuller TC, Cosimi AB, Colvin RB. Reduction of immune response to OKT3 monoclonal antibody. Transplant Proc 1985; 17: 644.
19. Dixon FJ. Experimental serum sickness. In: Samter M, ed. Immunological diseases. Boston: Little, Brown, 1965: 253.
20. Colvin RB, Cosimi AB, Burton RC, et al. Immunologic monitoring and therapy with monoclonal antibodies to T lymphocytes in renal allograft recipients. In: Proc of 8th Int Congr Nephrol, Athens 1981: 990.
21. Miller RA, Maloney DG, McKillop J, Levy R. In vivo effects of murine hybridoma monoclonal antibody in a patient with T-cell leukemia. Blood 1982; 58: 78.
22. Carpenter CB, Milford EL, Reinherz EL, et al. Monoclonal anti-T12 antibody as therapy for renal allograft rejection. Trans Assoc Am Physicians 1983; 16: 84.
23. Takahashi H, Okazaki H, Terasaki PI, et al. Reversal of transplant rejection by monoclonal antiblast antibody. Lancet 1983; 2: 1155.
24. Thurlow PJ, Lovering E, d'Apice AJF, McKenzie IFC. A monoclonal anti-pan-T-cell antibody: in vitro and in vivo studies. Transplantation 1983; 36: 293.
25. Biddison WE, Rao PE, Talle MA, Goldstein G, Shaw S. Possible

involvement of the T4 molecule in T cell recognition of class II HLA antigens: evidence from studies of CTL-target cell binding. J Exp Med 1984; 159: 783.
26. Biddison WE, Rao PE, Talle MA, Boselli CM, Goldstein G. Distinct epitopes on the T8 molecule are differentially involved in cytotoxic T cell function. Hum Immunol 1984; 9: 117.
27. Cupps TR, Edgar LC, Fauci AS. Suppression of human B lymphocyte function by cyclophosphamide. J Immunol 1982; 128: 2453.

Received 23 October 1985.
Accepted 6 February 1986.

0041-1337/86/4205-0511$02.00/0
TRANSPLANTATION
Vol. 42, No. 5
Printed in U.S.A.

THE CLINICAL COURSE OF IgA-NEPHROPATHY AND HENOCH-SCHÖNLEIN PURPURA FOLLOWING RENAL TRANSPLANTATION

ULLA BACHMAN, CLAUDE BIAVA, WILLIAM AMEND, NICHOLAS FEDUSKA, JULIET MELZER, OSCAR SALVATIERRA, AND FLAVIO VINCENTI[1]

Kidney Transplant Service and Department of Pathology, University of California Medical Center, San Francisco, California 94143

Recurrence of IgA-nephropathy and Henoch-Schönlein purpura is a common finding after renal transplantation. From 1970 to 1984, 1788 transplants were performed at our center. 13 patients had IgA-nephropathy and 3 patients had Henoch-Schönlein purpura. No patient with Henoch-Schönlein purpura had a proved recurrence. Six patients with IgA-nephropathy had a recurrence of IgA disease in the allograft within 3 to 8 months of transplantation. Three patients with a recurrence have retained their kidneys with stable renal function (follow-up of 1.7–2.7 years). Two of these patients lost their graft from severe rejection. One patient, who received an HLA-identical transplant, lost the graft from recurrent IgA disease associated with crescenteric glomerulonephritis. We found no difference in the prevalence of HLA-B 35 among the IgA patients compared with our total transplant population. IgA patients who received living related transplants had a higher recurrence rate of IgA in their allograft when compared with recipients of cadaveric kidneys (83% vs. 14%). Some caution is recommended in using related donors, especially HLA-identical siblings in patients with renal failure secondary to IgA-nephropathy.

Several types of glomerulonephritis, among them IgA-nephropathy and Henoch-Schönlein purpura are known to recur in the transplanted kidney (*1*). IgA-nephropathy has usually been regarded to be a relatively benign disease with few cases developing end stage renal disease (*2*). In recent years, however, this view has changed as the follow-up of these patients has been longer (*3*). Both children and adults with this nephropathy have developed uremia, the reported incidence varying between 10–50% of the patients (*4, 5*). In countries where the incidence of IgA-nephropathy is high—for instance, France, Japan, Australia, and Singapore—IgA-nephropathy is the original disease in a considerable number of uremic patients. While the clinical course of IgA-nephropathy in the native kidneys has been extensively documented, there are relatively few reports about the outcome of patients with IgA-nephropathy after renal transplantation, with only one study providing follow-up data of the outcome (*6*).

The recurrence rate of IgA in the renal allograft is considered to be high, approaching 50% of patients (*1, 6*). Usually the clinical picture of the recurrent disease has been benign, with graft loss due to rejection or recurrent disease being very low. Treatment of IgA-nephropathy with immunosuppressive agents has usually not been successful (*7*) and treatment of recurrent disease has not been tried. A recurrence of Henoch-Schönlein purpura has also been reported in some cases, the incidence rate being about 30% (*1*). Since Henoch-Schönlein purpura and IgA-nephropathy share the same renal pathological changes, and the clinical manifestations of the renal disease are very similar, the same disease process may underly the two conditions. The aim of this study is to further characterize the clinical course and outcome of transplanted patients with IgA-nephropathy and Henoch-Schönlein purpura, as the outcome of our cases seems to differ in some respects from those reported by other authors.

MATERIALS AND METHODS

Patient population. From 1968 through May of 1984, 2093 transplantations were performed at the University of California, San Francisco. The percentage of graft survival was calculated by actuarial methods, and it is expressed as percentage of survival plus or minus standard error.

Methods. All tissue specimens were routinely subject to light, immunofluorescent, and electron microscopy. Immunofluorescent studies were performed using a standard technique, and specimens were stained with fluoresceinated antisera to IgG, IgM, IgA, C_3, C_4, albumin, and fibrinogen. Processing for electron microscopy included primary fixation with glutaraldehyde,

[1] To whom requests for reprints should be addressed.

postfixation in osmium tetraoxide, and dehydration in ethanol with subsequent embedding in aryldite.

RESULTS

Overall transplant population. Figure 1 shows the underlying disorders responsible for end-stage renal disease in our patient population. IgA-nephropathy was present in 13 patients, and Henoch-Schönlein purpura in 3 patients. The diagnosis of IgA-nephropathy and Henoch-Schönlein purpura was established by the pathologic findings on kidney biopsy. In addition, the diagnosis in patients with Henoch-Schönlein purpura was supported by clinical findings. None of the patients had serological or clinical evidence of systemic lupus erythematosus.

Patients with IgA-nephropathy. There were 12 men and one woman with IgA-nephropathy, with a mean age of 28 years (range 11–38 years). The mean duration of the original disease from onset to uremia was 7 years (range 1–26 years). Only one of the 13 patients with IgA-nephropathy was black.

Six patients were transplanted with a living-related kidney. Two of these patients had HLA-identical sibling donors, while three of the patients received one-haplotype-matched kidneys following donor-specific blood transfusions according to our previously reported protocol (*8*). Seven patients received cadaveric kidneys. HLA-B 35 was present in three of the 13 patients (21%). The prevalence of HLA-B 35 in our transplant population is 17%. A summary of the data following transplantation is given in Table 1.

Graft and patient survival. All patients are alive. Four pa-

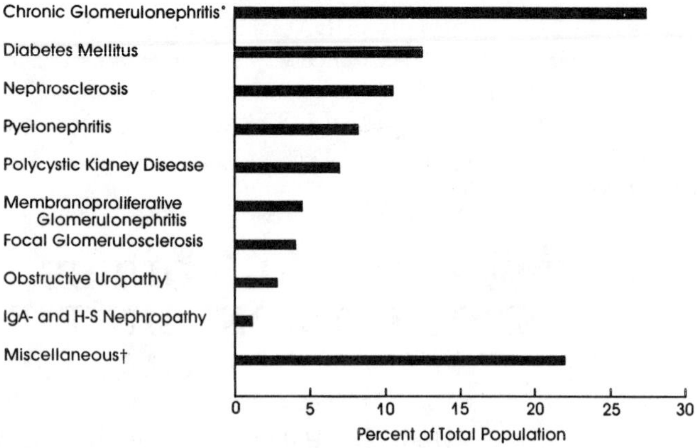

FIGURE 1. Underlying disorders responsible for renal failure in patients undergoing kidney transplantation.

TABLE 1. Clinical data of patients after renal transplantation

Case No.	Date	Donor	Interval to onset of clinical IgA	Interval to histological diagnosis	Follow-up as of July 1984		
					Proteinuria	Hematuria	S. Creat.[a]
1[a]	11/82	Living: 2 mismatches, DST	–	7 Months: recurrent IgA	Neg.	Neg.	1.7
2[a]	11/68	Living: 2 mismatches	4 Months	4 Months: no IgA at 243 months: recurrent IgA + rejection	Tx Nx 11/80	(chronic rejection)	
3[a]	10/79	Cadaver	3 Months	4 Months: recurrent IgA + rejection	Hemodialysis	3/80	
4[a]	11/81	Living: 2 mismatches, DST	1 Month	1 Month: recurrent IgA	Neg.	2–5	1.9
5[a]	6/80	Living: HLA-identical	1 Month	3 Months: recurrent IgA	Tx Nx 11/82	(recurrent IgA)	
6[a]	11/81	Living: 1 mismatch, DST	8 Months	32 Months: recurrent IgA	Pos.	25–50	1.8
7	4/83	Cadaver	13 Months	1 Month: acute rejection + minimal IgA	Pos.	Neg.	1.1
8	11/77	Cadaver	15 Months	16 Months: rejection + minimal IgA	Tx Nx 8/80	(chronic rejection)	
9	5/83	Living: HLA-identical	–	–	Neg.	Neg.	3.1 rejection
10	3/81	Cadaver	–	12 Months: rejection, no IgA	Pos.	25–50	1.9
11[b]	12/83	Cadaver	–	1 Month: no IgA	Neg.	Neg.	1.7
12[b]	3/84	Cadaver	–	1 Month: no IgA	Neg.	Neg.	1.4
13[b]	1/84	Cadaver	–	1 Month: no IgA	Neg.	Neg.	1.8
14[c]	1/68	Living	60 Months	–	Pos.	Neg.	1.7
15[c]	1/81	Cadaver	24 Months	–	Pos.	Neg.	1.0
16[b,c]	4/84	Cadaver	–	1 Month: no IgA	Neg.	Neg.	2.4

(S. Creat.) serum creatinine (mg/dl); (Tx Nx) nephrectomy of allograft; (DST) donor-specific blood transfusions.

[a] Recurrence of IgA disease.

[b] Cyclosporine.

[c] Henoch-Schönlein purpura.

tients have lost their grafts—3 because of rejection and 1 as a result of recurrent IgA-nephropathy in the graft. IgA deposits were also seen in 2 of the rejected grafts in sufficient amounts to be consistent with a recurrence of IgA. Nine patients who have retained their grafts have an average follow-up of 17 months (range 3–40 months).

Recurrence of IgA-nephropathy in the graft. Six patients (cases 1–6) had a recurrence of IgA-nephropathy in the graft. usually the diagnosis of recurrence was suspected when there was a reappearance of proteinuria, less often hematuria. The onsert of proteinuria was noticed 1–8 months after transplantation. A biopsy of the allograft was usually made shortly thereafter. No additional immunosuppressive therapy was given when the overall impression was that of recurrence. Of the 6 patients with a recurrence, 5 had a kidney from a living-related donor. Three patients now followed 1.7–2.7 years posttransplant have had stable renal function; 3 patients have lost their grafts, 2 from rejection and 1 from recurrent IgA-nephropathy.

Graft loss due to recurrent IgA-nephropathy. The patient who lost his kidney as a result of IgA-nephropathy is a 22-year-old man. He originally developed proteinuria and hematuria in early 1979, and a renal biopsy revealed IgA-nephropathy with segmental or global sclerosis of the glomeruli. He progressed rapidly to end-stage and was transplanted in June 1980 with a kidney from an HLA-identical sibling. One month after transplantation he had a rejection that responded to increased doses of steroids. Three months after transplantation he developed nephrotic-range proteinuria. A biopsy of the allograft revealed positive immunofluorescent staining for IgA. There were no electron-dense deposits in the mesangial areas. The light microscopy showed open glomerular capillary tufts, and the capillary lumina were open. There was a moderate degree of mesangial cellularity. The clincial course was stable until January of 1982, when the serum creatinine rose and a second biopsy was performed. The histopathological studies showed similar but more advanced disease compared with the previous biopsy. In addition, there were numerous electron-dense deposits in the mesangium. Several of the glomeruli were now partly or completely sclerosed. In less than a year he progressed to uremia, and a nephrectomy was performed in November of 1982. Histological examination of the allograft showed active IgA nephropathy with more severe mesangial proliferation associated with crescent formation in 50% of the glomeruli.

Patients without proved recurrence. Biopsies were done on two patients because rejection was suspected. In one patient the biopsy was performed only 10 days after transplantation, and trace amounts of mesangial IgA were found. In the other patient no IgA deposits were seen. Another three patients have had routine biopsies before discharge, usually one month after transplantation, because they were treated with cyclosporine. No IgA was found in these biopsies, and there has been no clinical evidence of recurrence. However the follow-up is rather short—3–6 months. Only one patient has not had a biopsy. This patient has recently had a severe rejection caused by discontinuing the immunosuppressive therapy.

Patients with Henoch-Schönlein purpura. Three patients with this diagnosis received transplants, two men and one woman, with a mean age of 21.8 years (range 13–30 years). The mean duration of the original disease from onset to uremia was 5.3 years (range 3–9 years). The first patient had a biopsy at one month after transplantation which showed no IgA (Table 1). The other two patients have proteinura which appeared after 24 and 60 months respectively; both have stable renal function after a follow-up of 3.5 and 16 years, respectively.

DISCUSSION

In most cases the recurrent IgA-nephropathy in the renal allograft appears to follow a different clinical course and differs in its prognosis from the original disease that destroyed the patient's native kidneys. In the only follow-up of patients with recurrent IgA-nephropathy reported, there have been no graft losses (*6*). The results from our center do not fully confirm this impression. Although the patient survival is 100%, 4 of 13 grafts were lost—two cadaver kidneys and two living-related kidneys. Three losses were from rejection and one was from recurrent IgA disease. Our graft loss is thus higher than that reported in the literature (*1*, *6*). Among all the reported cases in the literature only one graft was lost from current IgA disease (*9*). In this patient the progression of the disease was slow and she lost her graft 7 years after transplantation with a cadaveric kidney. Our patient who lost the kidney because of recurrent IgA disease had another clinical picture, being transplanted with a kidney from his HLA-identical sibling. He lost his kidney 2 years after transplantation, but evidence of a recurrence was suspected as early as 3 months after transplantation and was confirmed by biopsy after 4 months. The outcome of transplantation in this patient seems to be an exception to the usually benign course of recurrent IGA nephropathy (Table 2). In our two patients who had evidence of rejection and recurrent disease, the graft losses were considered to be due to rejection. The diagnosis of a recurrence is based on the histopathological findings of focal mesangial deposits of IgA—and also, often, of IgG. In the absence of a confirmed diagnosis in the native kidneys, IgA deposits in the graft can also be due to de novo nephropathy or IgA deposits already present in the donor kidney before transplantation (*10*, *11*). In the case described by Tolkoff-Rubin et al. (*10*), IgA deposits were found in the donor kidney, although the HLA-identical donor was completely asymptomatic. When using cadaveric kidneys there is also a risk of preexisting nephropathy, as 10% of clinically normal kidneys are described as having unsuspected glomerular disease (*11*). However, preexisting IgA disease may not always be deleterious. In some donor kidneys the IgA-nephropathy disappeared within 2–4 weeks posttransplantation (*12*).

The recurrence rate of IgA disease in our patients is 38%. This is in accordance with the findings of others who have reported that up to 50% of the patients have a recurrence (*1*,

TABLE 2. Summary of the literature 1975–1984

Reference	No. Patients with recurring IgA	Graft loss caused by IgA	Living-related transplants in patients with recurrent IgA	Cadaveric transplants in patients with recurrent IgA
Mathew et al., 1975 (*9*)	2/?	1	1	1
Seigler et al., 1977 (*22*)	3/?	0	3	0
Morzycka et al., 1982 (*23*)	1/5 (20%)	0	1	0
Berger et al., 1984 (*6*)	17/32 (53%)	0	9 (69%)	8 (42%)
Backman et al., this study	6/13 (46%)	1	5 (83%)	1 (14%)

6). Routine biopsies in all transplanted patients with IgA-nephropathy may reveal a higher incidence of recurrence, since some patients may be clinically asymptomatic. In our patients the first sign was usually proteinura that appeared within 4 months of transplantation. In several of the patients reported by Berger et al. (*2*) the recurrence was suspected and diagnosed within 6 months after transplantation.

The reason why one of our patients lost his HLA-identical graft from recurrent disease relatively early after transplantation is difficult to explain. One explanation for the rapid recurrence is that there might be some genetic predisposition to acquire the disease. This has also been suggested for the original disease. The association of some HLA antigens, especially HLA-B 35 and HLA-DR4, with IgA-nephropathy has been considered to be strong and also to be related to the outcome of the disease (*13, 14*). However, other studies have not demonstrated an association between IgA nephropathy and any HLA antigen (*15, 16*). We found only three patients with HLA-B 35, a prevalence that is not different from that of our total transplantation population. Only one of these patients had a recurrence. Even if there is no clear cut-proof of a specific HLA-antigen being linked to this disease, there might be some other genetic factor associated with IgA-nephropathy. IgA-nephropathy has been described in several HLA-identical siblings (*10, 17, 18*).

Of our 6 patients with a recurrence, 5 were transplanted with a kidney from a living-related donor. This 83% frequency of recurrence in living-related transplants is quite different when compared with the 14% recurrence rate in patients transplanted with a cadaveric kidney. Although we did not obtain a biopsy from the donor kidney at the time of transplantation, it is unlikely that the IgA disease in the recipients kidneys was already present in the donors. Renal function, including urine analysis was normal in all donors prior to transplantation—and, following donation, none of the donors have developed any renal abnormalities. Review of the literature shows that the majority of IgA recurrences have occurred in recipients of living-related kidneys (Table 2).

Histopathologically there is no difficulty in differentiating IgA-nephropathy from rejection, but sometimes both diseases are present in the allograft. That was the case in two of our patients. An important point to consider is whether the presence of IgA in the allograft can promote a rejection, as has been suggested by Sanfilippo et al. (*11*); 3 of their 4 cases transplanted with a kidney with known IgA-nephropathy had an early and irreversible rejection.

The clinical course of the recurrent disease seems, in most cases, to be more benign than that of the original disease. Also, the clinical symptoms are not always prominent or may even be missing. This is in contrast to the clinical course of IgA disease in the native kidneys, which progressed to end-stage renal disease. The possibility of an effect of the immunosuppressive therapy on the outcome of the recurrent disease must be considered. Even if conventional immunusuppressive therapy did not prevent a recurrence it might have modified its course. Whether the new immunosuppressive agent cyclosporine will have any influence on the course of the original disease or the recurrent glomerulopathy is unknown. Three of our patients treated with cyclosporine have so far exhibited no evidence of a recurrence after up to 6 months' follow-up.

Although recurrence of IgA-nephropathy in the renal allograft usually has a benign course, our results show that a recurrence of IgA in the renal allograft ended with graft loss in 50% of the patients. More observations are needed to further confirm this impression.

A recurrence of Henoch-Schönlein purpura has been reported in a few cases, the incidence being somewhat lower than that for IgA-nephropathy (*1, 19, 20*). As in IgA-nephropathy, most patients seem to have a benign course. At our center only three patients with Henoch-Schönlein purpura have been transplanted. Although recurrence has not been proved in our patients, two of them have proteinuria that appeared at a later stage than that in our patients with IgA-nephropathy. Renal function has been stable for several years, reflecting a benign course. However, a few patients reported in the literature have lost their grafts as a result of recurrent disease (*1*). The risk of losing a graft because of recurrent disease is thought to increase if transplantation is performed before, or too shortly after, the active purpura has subsided (*1*). A recurrence of only the renal symptoms can also be due to the development of IgA-nephropathy in the graft, which confirms the close pathogenetic interrelationship between the two diseases (*20, 21*). The overall prognosis of renal transplantation in patients with IgA nephropathy or Henoch-Schönlein disease is good but not entirely benign. Some caution is recommended in using related donors, especially HLA-identical siblings, because of the high recurrence rate in patients transplanted with a living-related kidney.

REFERENCES

1. Cameron JS. Glomerulonephritis in renal transplants. Transplantation 1982; 34: 237.
2. Berger J, Yaneva H, Nabarra B, Barbanel C. Recurrence of mesangial deposition of IgA after renal transplantation. Kidney Int 1975; 7: 232.
3. Berger J, Yaneva H, Crosnier J. La glomerulonephrite a depots mesangiaux d'IgA: une cause frequente d'insuffisance renale terminale. Nouv Presse Med 1980; 9: 219.
4. van der Peet J, Arisz L, Brentjens AR, et al. Clinical, pathological and therapeutic aspects of IgA-nephropathy in adults. Clin Nephrol 1977; 8: 335.
5. Southwest Pediatric Nephrology Study Group. A multicenter study of IgA-nephropathy in children. Kidney Int 1982; 22: 643.
6. Berger J, Noel LH, Nabarra B. Recurrence of mesangial IgA nephropathy after renal transplantation. Contr Nephrol 1984; 40: 195.
7. Clarkson AR, Seymour AE, Chan YL, et al. Clinical, pathological and therapeutic aspects of IgA nephropathy. In: Kincaid-Smith P, d'Apice AJ, eds. Progress in glomerulonephritis. New York: Wiley, 1979: 247.
8. Salvatierra O, Vincenti F, Amend W, et al. Deliberate donor specific blood transfusions prior to living related renal transplantation. Ann Surg 1980; 192: 543.
9. Mathew TH, Mathews DC, Hobbs JB, Kincaid-Smith P. Glomerular lesions after renal transplantation. Am J Med 1975; 59: 177.
10. Tolkoff-Rubin NE, Cosimi AB, Fuller T, Rubin RH, Colvin RB. IgA-nephropathy in HLA-identical siblings. Transplantation 1978; 26: 430.
11. Sanfilippo F, Croker BP, Bollinger RR. Fate of four cadaveric donor renal allografts with mesangial IgA deposits. Transplantation 1982; 33: 370.
12. Silva FG, Chanter P, Oirani CL, Hardy MA. Disappearance of glomerular mesangial IgA deposits after renal allograft transplantation. Transplantation 1982; 33: 214.
13. Hiki Y, Kobayashi Y, Tateno S, Sada M, Kashiwagi M. Strong association of HLA-DR4 with benign IgA nephropathy. Nephron 1982; 32: 222.
14. Berthoux FC, Gagne A, Sabatier JC, et al. HLA Bw35 and mes-

angial IgA glomerulonephritis. N Engl J Med 1978; 298: 1034.
15. Brettle RP, Peters DK, Batchelor JR. Mesangial IgA glomerulonephritis and HLA antigens. N Engl J Med 1978; 299: 200.
16. Richman AV, Mahoney JJ, Fuller TJ. Higher prevalence of HLA-B12 in patients with IgA-nephropathy. Ann Intern Med 1979; 29: 201.
17. Sabatier JC, Genin C, Cessenat H, et al. Mesangial IgA glomerulonephritis in HLA-identical brothers. Clin Nephrol 1979; 11: 90.
18. Katz A, Karan-Colas S, Falk JA. Family study in IgA nephritis: the possible role of IgA antigens. Transplantation 1980; 29: 505.
19. Baliah T, Kim KH, Anthone S, Anthone R, Montes M, Andres GA. Recurrence of Henoch-Schonlein's purpura glomerulonephritis in transplanted kidneys. Transplantation 1974; 18: 343.
20. Levy MR, Moussa AR, Habib R, Sagnadoux MF, Broyer M. Anaphylactoid purpura nephritis and transplantation. Kidney Int 1982; 22: 326.
21. Weiss JH, Blathena B, Curtis JJ, Lucas BA, Luke RG. A possible relationship between Henoch-Schonlein's syndrome and IgA-nephropathy (Berger's disease). Nephron 1979; 22: 582.
22. Seigler JF, Ward FE, McCoy RE, Weinert JC, Gunnells JC, Stickel DL. Long-term results with forty-five related renal allograft recipient genotypically identical for HLA. Surgery 1977; 81: 274.
23. Morzycka M, Croker BP, Seigler HF, Tisher CC. Revaluation of recurrent glomerulonephritis in kidney allografts. Am J Med 1982; 72: 588.

Received 6 September 1985.
Accepted 3 February 1986.

0041-1337/86/4205-0515$02.00/0
TRANSPLANTATION
Vol. 42, No. 5
Printed in U.S.A.

INTERSTITIAL PNEUMONITIS FOLLOWING AUTOLOGOUS BONE MARROW TRANSPLANTATION[1]

RICARDO PECEGO, ROGER HILL, FREDERICK R. APPELBAUM,[2] DEBORAH AMOS, C. DEAN BUCKNER, ALEXANDER FEFER, AND E. DONNALL THOMAS[3]

The Fred Hutchinson Cancer Research Center and the University of Washington School of Medicine, Seattle, Washington 98104

The incidence of interstitial pneumonitis (IP) was reviewed in 70 consecutive patients who received autologous marrow transplants for hematologic malignancies. All patients were treated with total-body irradiation (TBI), with or without other chemotherapeutic agents. Seven patients (10%) developed IP, 3 were due to cytomegalovirus, 1 due to *Pneumomcystis carinii*, and 3 of unknown cause (idiopathic). Risk factors for developing IP were increasing age and a prior history of irradiation to the chest. The use of methotrexate posttransplant did not increase the incidence of IP.

Interstital pneumonitis (IP)* is a major cause of morbidity and mortality following marrow transplantation (*1–3*). IP occurs in 20–40% of patients treated with cyclophosphamide (Cy), total-body irradiation (TBI) and allogeneic marrow transplantation for hematologic malignancies; it is fatal in approximately 50% of cases. Two-thirds of cases are associated with known pathogens, most often cytomegalovirus (CMV), much less frequently other viral pathogens or *Pneumocystis carinii* (*4*, *5*). The incidence of IP among patients treated for hematologic malignancies with similar preparative regimens who receive syngeneic rather than allogeneic transplantation is considerably reduced (17%), due primarily to the rarity of CMV (*6*). In allogeneic marrow recipients the incidence of IP due to CMV is highest in patients with acute graft-versus-host disease (*1–3*), while the incidence of idiopathic IP is identical in recipients of allogeneic or syngeneic marrow (*2*, *6*).

Autologous marrow transplantation has been used increasingly to treat patients with hematologic malignancies. The purpose of this analysis was to determine the incidence, mortality, and risk factors associated with the development of IP following autologous marrow transplantation in patients with hematologic malignancies.

MATERIALS AND METHODS

Between November 1978 and March 1985, 70 patients with acute leukemia or malignant lymphoma received autologous marrow transplants. The median age was 27 (range 4–61) years. Eighteen patients had acute lymphoblastic leukemia (ALL), 23 had acute nonlymphoblastic leukemia (ANL), and 29 patients had malignant lymphoma (ML). Cy, 60 mg/kg/day on two consecutive days, was given prior to TBI to 62 patients. One patient received high-dose cytosine arabinoside (Ara-C) 3 gm/m^2 q.12 hr ×6 days and TBI, one patient received nitrogen mustard (1 mg/kg) and TBI, one patient received, 1,3-bis(2-chloroethyl)1-nitrosourea (BCNU) (600 mg) plus Cy, and five

[1] This work was supported by PHS Grants CA 26828, CA 18029, CA 15704, CA 18221, and CA 30924, awarded by the National Cancer Institute, DHHS.

[2] Address correspondence to: Dr. Frederick R. Appelbaum, Division of Oncology, Fred Hutchinson Cancer Research Center, 1124 Columbia Street, Seattle, WA 98104.

[3] Dr. Thomas is a recipient of a Research Career Award AI 02425 from the National Institute of Allergy and Infectious Diseases.

* Abbreviations used: ALL, acute lymphoblastic leukemia; ANL, acute nonlymphoblastic leukemia; Ara-C, cytosine arabinoside; BCNU, 1,3,-bis(2-chloroethyl)1-nitrosourea; Cy, cyclophosphamide; IP, interstitial pneumonitis; ML, malignant lymphoma, MTX, methotrexate; TBI, total-body irradiation.

patients received TBI only. Twelve patients received a single dose of TBI of 10 Gy, and 58 patients received 12 Gy (six 2 Gy daily fractions) or 15.75 Gy (seven 2.25 Gy daily fractions). TBI was delivered at 7.5 cGy/min from dual opposing Co^{60} sources at a dose rate of 5–8 cGy/min. Twenty-six patients received posttransplant i.v. methotrexate (MTX) on a schedule developed for allogeneic marrow transplant recipients (*7*).

Eight patients had received radiation therapy to the chest a median of 11.5 months (range 18 days to 16 years) prior to transplant. Pretransplant sera from 46 patients were tested for antibody to CMV. Seroconversion was defined as a fourfold or greater increase in the titer. The criteria used for the classification of IP have been published elsewhere (*1*). Only first episodes of pneumonitis were considered. Patients who relapsed with their malignancy following transplant were, from then on, no longer considered to be at risk for IP. This was done in order to avoid confusing the effects of the transplant regimen with those of subsequent tumor progression and therapy. The day of marrow infusion was designated day 0.

The incidence of IP and its relationship with assorted variables (disease type, relapse status, age, prior radiation, and sex) were tested by chi-square, Fisher's exact test, and stepwise logistic regression analysis. The logistic regression model included the main effects and interactions between both age and sex and disease type and relapse status. All factors and interactions were allowed to enter and exit the model, depending on their significance.

RESULTS

Tables 1–4 present the results of this analysis. Table 1 compares the results of previously published data for the incidence of IP in syngeneic and allogeneic marrow transplant recipients. All cases of IP in autologous marrow transplant recipients were diagnosed histologically by open lung biopsy or at autopsy, and all were fatal. The incidence of CMV IP was significantly lower in patients receiving autologous marrow than in allogeneic marrow recipients ($P<0.05$). Cytomegaloviral pneumonitis in autologous marrow recipients was not significantly higher than in twins ($P>0.05$).

The median day of onset of IP was 27 days (range 10–117) after transplantation. Among patients with CMV idiopathic and pneumocystis pneumonitis, the median time of onset was 58 days (32–117), 16 days (10–21), and 30 days, respectively.

TABLE 1. Incidence of nonbacterial pneumonia after allogeneic, syngeneic, and autologous marrow transplantation[a]

Type of pneumonia	No. (%) patients with pneumonia after transplant		
	Autologous	Syngeneic[b]	Allogeneic[c]
Idiopathic	3 (4.3)	11 (11)	63 (12)
CMV	3 (4.3)	0	85 (16)
Pneumocystis carinii	1 (1.4)	1 (1)	34 (6)
Other viral pneumonias	0	1 (1)	16 (3)
Clinically diagnosed	0	4 (4)	32 (6)
TOTAL	7 (10)	17 (17)	215 (41)
Number of patients	70	100	525

[a] Entries represent number of patients (proportion) with each pneumonia type. Categories are not mutually exclusive and patients may be listed under more than one type (e.g., cytomegalovirus and *P carinii*.

[b] *See* (*1*).

[c] *See* (*7*).

TABLE 2. Occurrence of interstitial pneumonitis by patient age

Age (years)	No. patients studied	Etiology of IP (No. patients)		
		CMV	*Pneumocystis*	Idiopathic
<10	12	0	0	0
10–20	16	1	0	0
21–30	11	1	0	2
>30	31	1	1	1

TABLE 3. Prior irradiation[a] and interstitial pneumonitis

	Prior irradiation (No. patients)	
	Yes (n = 8)	No (n = 62)
Idiopathic	3	0
CMV	1	2
Pneumocystis carinii	1	0
Total	5	2
	$P = .0003$	

[a] Mantle or mediastinum irradiation.

Table 2 shows the age distribution and incidence of IP. The trend toward increased IP with age was significant ($P<0.05$).

Eight patients (all with malignant lymphoma) had received radiotherapy to the chest, usually as mantle or mediastinal therapy. Five of these patients developed interstitial pneumonitis, 3 idiopathic, 1 caused by CMV, and 1 resulting from *P carinii* (Table 3). The incidence of IP in patients receiving prior radiotherapy to the chest was higher than in patients without prior radiotherapy ($P<0.001$). Twenty-six patients received posttransplant MTX, and none developed IP. Seven of 44 patients who did not receive MTX developed IP. Table 4 reviews the seven cases of IP.

In the stepwise logistic regression analysis, only prior chest irradiation was significantly associated with the development of IP. However, only patients with malignant lymphoma had received prior irradiation and patients with malignant lymphoma tended to be older, making it impossible to evaluate the independent effects of irradiation, disease type, and age.

Pretransplant and posttransplant sera from 46 patients were available for determination of antibody to CMV. Twenty-seven patients did not have antibody to CMV on admission and 19 of those patients' sera were negative throughout the posttransplant period. One of these 19 seronegative patients developed IP caused by CMV. IP resulting from CMV developed in 1 of the 8 patients who seroconverted. Pretransplant and posttransplant sera for CMV antibody were not available in one patient who developed IP due to CMV.

DISCUSSION

The overall incidence of IP reported here (10%) for autologous marrow recipients was lower than that reported in allogeneic marrow recipients and similar to that seen in syngeneic marrow recipients (*1, 2, 3, 6*). Idiopathic IP is generally considered to be a consequence of chemoradiotherapy, since the incidence is similar in allogeneic and syngeneic marrow transplant recipients receiving the same Cy and TBI regimen (*1, 2, 8, 9*). The incidence of idiopathic IP in autologous marrow recipients in our study was 4.3%. The observation that all 3 cases of idiopathic IP following autologous transplantation occurred in patients who had received prior radiotherapy to the

TABLE 4. Characteristics of patients who developed interstitial pneumonitis, and clinical outcome[a]

UPN	Age	Diagnosis	Phase of disease	Prior radiation	Regimen	Survival (days)	Diagnosis
1189	27	ML	Relapse	No	BCNU + Cy + 10.0 Gy	56	CMV
1278	36	ML	Relapse	Mantle-40 Gy	15.75 Gy	16	Idiopathic
1324	52	ML	Relapse	Mantle-24 Gy	Cy + 12 Gy	47	*P carinii*
1362	35	ANL	Remission	No	Cy + 12 Gy	116	CMV
1446	26	ML	Relapse	Mantle- 40 Gy	Cy + 15.75 Gy	31	Idiopathic
1803	30	ML	Relapse	TNI + Mantle 40 Gy	Cy + 12 Gy	33	Idiopathic
2277	16	ML	Relapse	Mediastinum 20 Gy	Cy + 12 Gy	77	CMV

[a] (ML) malignant lymphoma; (ANL) acute nonlymphoblastic leukemia; (ALL) acute lymphoblastic leukemia; (Cy) cyclophosphamide 60 mg/kg ×2; (Gy) total dose of irradiation; (UPN) unique patient number; (BCNU) 1,3 BIS(2-chloroethyl)1-nitrosourea; (TNI) total nodal irradiation; (regimen) chemotherapy and total-body irradiation.

chest is consistent with the hypothesis that idiopathic IP is a consequence of the treatment regimen. This is also confirmed by recent observations that allogeneic marrow transplant recipients treated with fractionated TBI have a lower incidence of idiopathic IP than those receiving TBI in a single dose (*2*, *4*, *10*). In a more recent retrospective analysis of 350 patients receiving fractionated TBI and allogeneic marrow the incidence of idiopathic IP was 3.7% (unpublished observations).

Interstitial pneumonitis due to CMV is generally considered to occur in transplant recipients as a consequence of immunodeficiency, which is more pronounced in patients with graft-versus-host disease. Among 100 twin transplants previously reported, IP due to CMV was not observed (*6*). This has been reconfirmed in an analysis of an additional 26 patients with ALL, ANL, or ML who received syngeneic transplants following treatment regimens similar to that used for the autologous transplants reported here (unpublished observations). Of these 26 patients, 2 developed idiopathic IP and 2 had clinical IP (no biopsy or autopsy). There were no documented cases of CMV IP. In contrast, IP caused by CMV occurred in 17% of the most recent retrospective series of 350 patients receiving allogeneic transplants (unpublished observations). In studies reported here we have found that the incidence of IP due to CMV was less in recipients of autologous marrow transplantation (4%) than in recipients of allogeneic transplants (16–17%). Whether or not there is a significant difference in the incidence of IP resulting from CMV between recipients of autologous marrow (4%) and syngeneic marrow will probably not be known until larger patient numbers have accrued in both groups. It might be anticipated that IP caused by CMV would be higher in autologous marrow recipients due to immunosuppression caused by the underlying disease or because of exposure to chemotherapy. Recipients of syngeneic marrow on the other hand may be relatively protected by immunity transmitted with the twin's marrow.

The use of MTX posttransplant has been suggested to contribute to the incidence of IP (*1*, *11*). However, in this study 26 patients were treated with MTX and there was no IP. This observation suggests that the use of posttransplant MTX does not, of itself, cause IP and suggests that the increased incidence of CMV pneumonia observed in allogeneic recipients is due to GVHD and not its treatment (*1*, *2*).

Among recipients of autologous marrow prior chest irradiation and increasing age appeared to influence the incidence of IP. Of 8 autologous patients who received chest radiotherapy prior to TBI, 5 developed IP, and 3 of these were idiopathic. The finding of an increased incidence of IP in patients with prior chest irradiation is consistent with the observations of others (*8*, *9*, *12–14*). As in twin and allogeneic marrow recipients, IP appeared to be more common in older patients.

REFERENCES

1. Meyers JD, Flournoy N, Thomas ED. Nonbacterial pneumonia after allogeneic marrow transplantation: a review of ten years' experience. Rev Infect Dis 1982; 4: 1119.
2. Meyers JD, Flournoy N, Wade JC, et al. Biology of interstitial pneumonia after marrow transplantation. In: Gale RP, ed. Recent advances in bone marrow transplantation. New York: Liss, 1983: 405.
3. Neiman PE, Reeves W, Ray G, et al. A prospective analysis of interstitial pneumonia and opportunistic viral infection among recipients of allogeneic bone marrow grafts. J Infect Dis 1977; 136: 754.
4. Buckner CD, Meyers JD, Springmeyer SC, et al. Pulmonary complications of marrow transplantation. Review of the Seattle Experience. Exp Hematol 1984; 12(suppl 15): 1.
5. Cardozo BL, Hagenbeek A. Interstitial pneumonitis following bone marrow transplantation: pathogenesis and therapeutic considerations. Eur J Cancer Clin Oncol 1985; 21: 43.
6. Appelbaum FR, Meyers JD, Fefer A, et al. Nonbacterial nonfungal pneumonia following marrow transplantation in 100 identical twins. Transplantation 1982; 33: 265.
7. Thomas ED, Storb R, Clift RA, et al. Bone-marrow transplantation. N Engl J Med 1975; 292: 832.
8. Keane TJ, Van Dyk J, Rider WD. Idiopathic interstitial pneumonia following bone marrow transplantation: the relationship with total body irradiation. Int J Radiat Oncol Biol Phys 1981; 7: 1365.
9. Kim TH, Rybka WB, Lehnert S, Podgorsak EB, Freeman CR. Interstitial pneumonitis following total body irradiation for bone marrow transplantation using two different dose rates. Int J Radiat Oncol Biol Phys 1985; 11: 1285.
10. Thomas ED, Clift RA, Hersman J, et al. Marrow transplantation for acute nonlymphoblastic leukemia in first remission using fractionated or single-dose irradiation. Int J Radiat Oncol Biol Phys 1982; 8: 817.
11. Bortin MM, Kay HEM, Gale RP, Rimm AA. Factors associated with interstitial pneumonitis after bone-marrow transplantation for acute leukaemia. Lancet 1982; 1: 437.
12. Pino y Torres JL, Bross DS, Lam WC, Wharam MD, Santos GW, Order SE. Risk factors in interstitial pneumonitis following allogeneic bone marrow transplantation. Int J Radiat Oncol Biol Phys 1982; 8: 1301.
13. Salazar OM, Rubin P, Keller B, Scarantino C. Systemic (half body) radiation therapy: response and toxicity. Int J Radiat Oncol Biol Phys 1978; 4: 937.
14. Song CW, Kim TH, Khan FM, Kersey JH, Levitt SH. Radiobiological basis of total body irradiation with different dose rate and fractionation: repair capacity of hemopoietic cells. Int J Radiat Oncol Biol Phys 1981; 7: 1695.

0041-1337/86/4205-0518$02.00/0
TRANSPLANTATION
Copyright © 1986 by The Williams & Wilkins Co.
Vol. 42, No. 5
Printed in U.S.A.

OPPORTUNISTIC STRONGYLOIDIASIS IN RENAL TRANSPLANT RECIPIENTS[1]

JAMES S. MORGAN,[2] WILLIAM SCHAFFNER, AND WILLIAM J. STONE[3]

Department of Medicine, Vanderbilt University School of Medicine and Medical Service, Veterans Administration Medical Center, Nashville, Tennessee

Eight patients with severe strongyloidiasis complicating renal transplantation are reported. Twenty-one additional cases from the English-language literature are reviewed. In this setting, systemic strongyloidiasis is an often baffling illness involving multiple organ systems that is frequently complicated by serious bacterial infection. Bacteremia, meningitis, urinary tract infection, and pneumonia resulting from enteric organisms are common. In order to make the diagnosis, larvae must be sought by direct microscopy of stool, upper intestinal fluid, sputum, urine, or biopsy specimens.

Treatment with oral thiabendazole in prolonged or repeated courses is recommended. Effective parenteral therapy is not available. Following treatment, previously parasitized patients must be tested at regular intervals to detect therapeutic failure or reinfection. Screening of patients awaiting renal transplantation for chronic intestinal strongyloidiasis is suggested. Improvement of the observed 52% mortality will depend upon heightened awareness by physicians caring for renal transplant candidates, and upon improved therapeutic regimens.

Although strongyloidiasis is not commonly recognized as a complication of renal transplantation, many cases have been reported (*1–20*). *Strongyloides stercoralis* is an intestinal nematode of man with a worldwide distribution (*21*). Chronic subclinical infection may persist for decades in the normal host (*22–24*), only to become life-threatening in the immunocompromised state (*25, 26*).

Lacking a classic clinical syndrome, strongyloidiasis is one of the great imitators. The diagnosis is often serendipitously made while searching for other diseases. This review discusses the spectrum of clinical disease produced by *S stercoralis* in renal transplant recipients.

Background. Strongyloidiasis is endemic in the tropics but occurs with surprising frequency in many temperate regions (*26–29*). The parasite has been found in at least 36 states (*30*). *S stercoralis* has both exogenous and endogenous life cycles (Fig. 1). The exogenous cycle is the predominant mode of transmission. Rhabditiform larvae are passed in the stool where they molt in the soil within 24 hr and become infectious filariform larvae that are capable of penetrating skin. Penetration of intact skin usually occurs in the feet, sometimes along hair follicles on other parts of the body. Entry into the lymphatics and veins allows passage to the lungs, where larvae burrow into the alveoli, migrate actively up the bronchial tree, are swallowed, and are delivered to the duodenum and proximal jejunum. Once in the intestines, larvae molt into parthenogenic adult female *S stercoralis* that embed themselves into the subepithelial mucosa and begin laying up to 40 eggs per day. These eggs develop into rhabditiform larvae which pass out in the stool, perpetuating the exogenous cycle. Eggs are rarely found in the stool.

Filariform larvae can cause an endogenous cycle through autoinfection, usually in the perianal area, but also by invasion through the colon (Fig. 1). Autoinfection permits chronic host parasitism in climates where free-living larvae may not be found. This endogenous cycle increases the worm burden and may lead to disseminated disease.

Hyperinfection is an augmentation of the normal life cycle that is seen in heavily infected or compromised hosts. When host defenses are compromised, enhanced metamorphosis into invasive filariform larvae allows increased penetration within the proximal intestine, exacerbating the worm burden. *Dissemination* occurs when filariform larvae migrate outside the lungs and gastrointestinal tract, exceeding the boundaries of the normal life cycle. Bacteremia can accompany hyperinfection or dissemination. As tissues are disrupted by invading worms, it is postulated that enteric bacteria are transported into the circulation either on the surface of the larval integument or as excreta from the larval intestinal tract.

MATERIALS AND METHODS

Cases in renal transplant recipients were collected from the literature between 1971 and 1984 and from the records of the Vanderbilt University Hospital and the Nashville Veterans Administration Medical Center between 1972 and 1984. Eight cases were identified from the Vanderbilt-affiliated hospitals, four of which were previously published (*19, 20*). These 8 patients represented 0.7% of the 1068 renal transplants performed at our two institutions from 1972 to 1984. An additional 21 cases were found in the English literature (*1–18*).

All patients were recipients of living-related or cadaveric renal transplants. All patients received additional immunosuppressive treatment for episodes of rejection. These agents included prednisone, methylprednisolone, azathioprine, cyclophosphamide, local irradiation, actinomycin D, and antilymphocyte serum. Infection with *S stercoralis* was documented in one or more of the following specimens: stool, sputum, duodenal aspirate, urine, and bronchial brushings. In one case the diagnosis was made at autopsy (*3*).

Case Reports

Case 1. A 9-year-old girl, who lived in Tennessee and had not been abroad, developed renal failure in September 1979. Hemodialysis was initiated and bilateral nephrectomies were performed in January 1980, prior to living-related renal transplantation in March 1980. Postoperative immunosuppressive

[1] This work was supported by The Veterans Administration.

[2] Present Address: Liver Study Unit, Yale University School of Medicine, New Haven, CT 06510.

[3] Address reprint requests to: William J. Stone, M.D., VA Medical Center, Nashville, TN 37203.

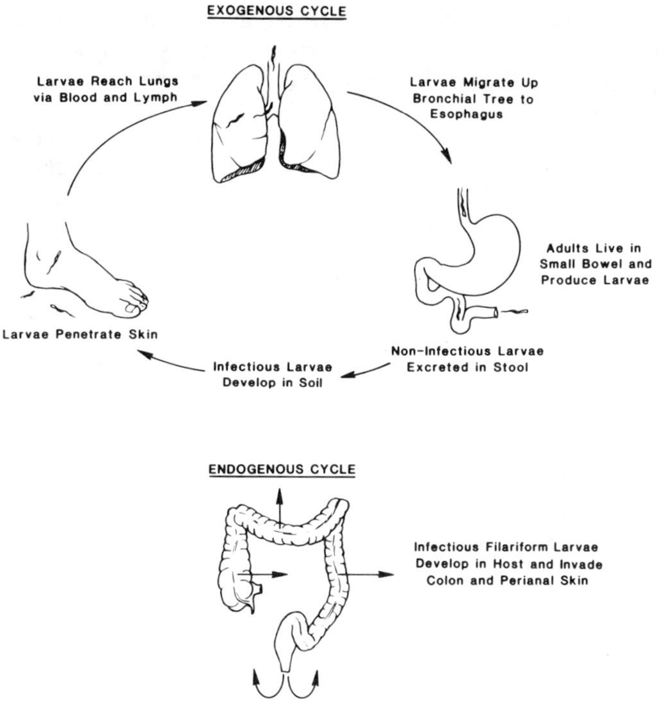

FIGURE 1. The life cycle of *Strongyloides stercoralis*. The exogenous cycle is characterized by rhabditiform larvae from human stool being transformed into invasive filariform larvae through an external phase. Man is then infected through cutaneous contact with soil. The endogenous cycle results from filariform larvae forming within or on the human host and invading the intestine or skin immediately (autoinfection).

therapy included azathioprine, glucocorticoids, irradiation, and antilymphocyte serum. Renal function remained satisfactory until transplant rejection with a serum creatinine of 12 mg/dl, was noted in January 1982.

The patient was below the 5th percentile for her age in height and weight. Peripheral differential leukocyte counts contained 6–13% eosinophils. Azathioprine, glucocorticoids, irradiation, and antilymphocyte serum were given. Peritoneal dialysis was instituted. The patient's course was uneventful until the 23rd hospital day when she developed high fever, severe abdominal pain, ileus, and rebound tenderness while on tapering doses of glucocorticoids and antilymphocyte serum. Cloudy peritoneal dialysate was noted, with an elevated white blood cell count of 4475/mm^3 (41% neutrophils and 59% mononuclear cells). Cultures of peritoneal fluid grew *Escherichia coli*. Blood cultures showed no growth.

After initial improvement with antibiotics, the patient experienced recurrent fever and abdominal pain with vomiting and hypertension. She became tachypneic and developed a productive cough with bloody sputum. A chest roentgenogram was clear. An upper gastrointestinal series demonstrated a filling defect in the duodenum suggesting an ulcer. A repeat chest roentgenogram showed bilateral pulmonary infiltrates. Previously declining peritoneal fluid leukocytes increased to 6600/cu mm. On the 29th hospital day *S stercoralis* larvae were detected in the peritoneal fluid (Fig. 2)—and, subsequently, in duodenal aspirate, a urine specimen, and stool examinations. Further past medical history indicated that the patient had previously been infected with ascaris. Review of the upper gastrointestinal series suggested probable ascaris worms. Therapy was instituted with thiabendazole 50 mg/kg/day, (500 mg/day), and later increased to 900 mg/day. On the second day of antihelminthic therapy the patient coughed up a large ascaris worm. Because of continued nausea, vomiting, and suspected poor thiabendazole absorption, mebendazole, pyrantil, and piperazine were added.

The patient's subsequent course was marked by unrelenting deterioration. She developed a headache, progressive obtundation, hypotension, lactic acidosis, and a maculopapular rash. Chest roentgenogram demonstrated progression of the bilateral infiltrates. Lumbar puncture showed 22 leukocytes with 80% mononuclear cells and 20% segmented cells. Cerebrospinal fluid grew *E coli*. The patient developed a tonic clonic seizure and became unresponsive.

Daily samples of urine, peritoneal fluid, and duodenal aspirate continued to contain motile strongyloides larvae despite antihelminthic therapy. Peritoneal fluid also grew *Streptococcus faecalis*. Lumbar puncture again showed white blood cells, but was culture-negative. Larvae were never detected in the cerebrospinal fluid. Peripheral blood eosinophilia increased to 40%. Nonmotile worms were noted in the peritoneal fluid on the 37th hospital day, the 9th day of antihelminthic therapy, and in duodenal aspirate on the 38th day. On the 40th hospital day blood cultures grew *Pseudomonas aeruginosa*. On the 42nd

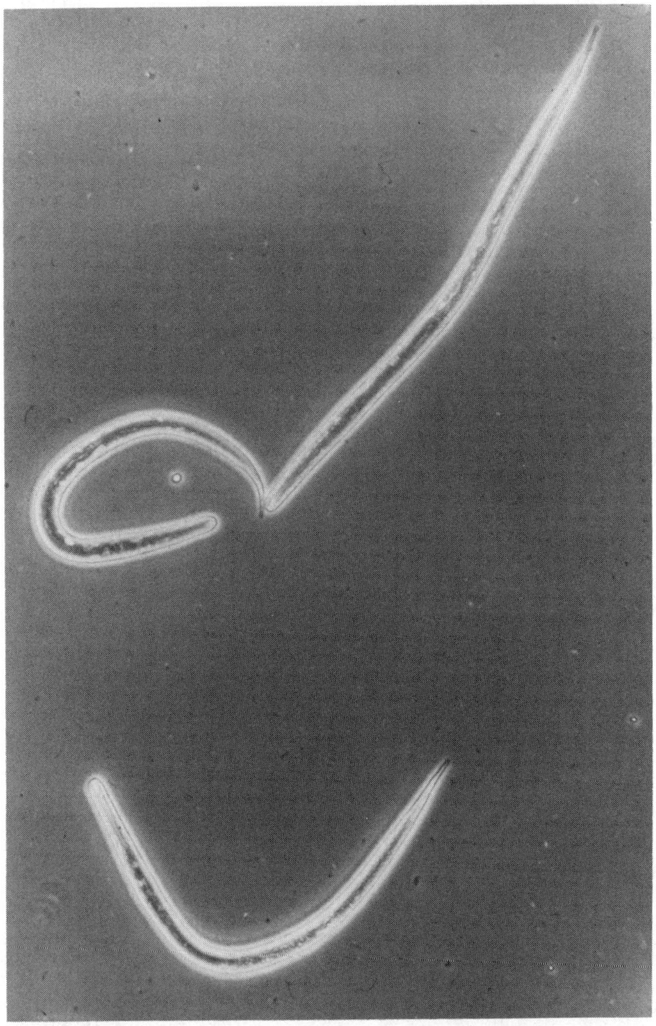

FIGURE 2. Rhabditiform larvae of *Strongyloides stercoralis* from peritoneal fluid of case 1 (magnification ×100 [slightly reduced]).

hospital day the patient developed a complex ventricular arrhythmia and died. No autopsy was performed.

This child developed a rapidly fatal illness in the second year after renal transplantation. Disseminated strongyloidiasis resulted from immunosuppressive therapy of transplant rejection and was extremely resistant to therapy with available antihelminthics. Bacterial peritonitis, pneumonia, bacteremia, and meningitis contributed to her death and were refractory to appropriate antibiotics. Inadequate drug absorption from the gastrointestinal tract and lack of parenteral therapy of strongyloidiasis were factors in the fatal outcome.

Cases 2–4. Three other unreported cases of strongyloidiasis have been seen in renal transplant recipients at our institutions from 1972 to 1984. A 38-year-old man died of disseminated aspergillosis only 3 months after a renal transplant. Larvae of *S stercoralis* were abundant in his duodenum at autopsy despite 3 prior courses of thiabendazole. A 24-year-old man with a peripheral blood eosinophilia of 14% was found to have *S stercoralis* larvae in his stool shortly before transplantation. A two-day course of thiabendazole eradicated the parasitism, which may have been caused by pica. Finally, a 54-year-old man nearly died of multiple infections during a stormy, 3-month hospitalization following renal transplantation. Cytomegalovirus, Herpesvirus hominis, hepatitis B virus and intestinal *S stercoralis* infection were documented. He recovered after thiabendazole and reduced immunosuppression. This patient was the only one of the three who had been outside the U.S.A., having served in the South Pacific during World War II.

RESULTS

A total of 41 episodes of documented infection with *S stercoralis* have been reported in 29 renal transplant recipients. They ranged in age from 9 to 54 years with an average age of 35; 24 were male. Eleven patients were born and raised in tropical or semitropical climates outside the continental United States (*1–3, 6, 10–12, 15–17, 19*). However, 9 of these patients were living in Britain or the continental U.S.A. when diagnosed.

Pretransplant evaluation. Evidence of parasitic disease was present in over half the cases prior to transplantation. Eosinophilia (5–53%) was noted in the peripheral blood of 11 patients (*2, 4, 7, 11, 13, 14, 19, 20*, case 3). Chronic gastrointestinal symptoms were mentioned in 2 cases and had been present in both for many years (2, 20). Three patients had documented strongyloidiasis prior to transplantation (*6, 14, 19*). In another patient a previous history of ascariasis was known (case 1). One patient regularly ate dirt (case 3).

In spite of evidence of parasitic disease, examination for ova and parasites was rarely pursued before transplantation. One of three patients with known previous strongyloidiasis was not screened prior to transplantation and was only reevaluated when hyperinfection supervened (*19*). Most of the patients born abroad or with eosinophilia had no specific preoperative evaluation (*3, 5, 8–10, 16–18*, and cases 2 and 3). Stool examination for ova and parasites was performed in only 5 of 29 cases prior to transplantation. Multiple stool examinations were mentioned in only one instance, and in this case no diagnosis was made (*14*). Only 3 of the 6 patients screened for parasites were diagnosed and treated (*6, 19*, and case 3).

Initial presentation. The onset of symptoms was usually associated with intensive immunosuppressive therapy, either in immediate posttransplantation regimens or during acute rejection episodes. The interval from transplantation to initial symptoms was less than one month in 5 cases, between one and three months in 18 cases, greater than 3 months in 3 cases, and unknown in 3 cases.

Clinical symptoms ultimately attributable to strongyloidiasis appeared in a variety of forms that were often misleading. Initial presentations included gastrointestinal complaints (11 cases), pulmonary symptoms (9 cases), bacteremia (3 cases), meningitis (2 cases), rash (2 cases), peritonitis (1 case), and fever of unknown origin (1 case). Fever was part of the initial symptom complex in at least 17 patients. Gastrointestinal symptoms included abdominal cramping, distention, anorexia, nausea, vomiting, pain, diarrhea, ulceration, and bleeding. Pulmonary symptoms most commonly included cough, sputum production, hemoptysis, wheezing, dyspnea, tachypnea, and pleuritic chest pain. Bacteremia usually was accompanied by fever, chills, intermittent confusion and obtundation, as well as hypotension. Meningitis was suggested by fever, headaches, altered mental status, and agitation. Two patients were first seen with fever and rash (*9*). In one instance a blotchy macular pruritic rash appeared on the trunk, buttocks, and thighs with progression to large confluent ecchymotic areas when scratched. In another case a nonpruritic rash appeared on the trunk as multiple round erythematous macules that blanched with pressure and gradually became more confluent. Abdominal pain and cloudy peritoneal dialysate were the initial findings in case 1.

Diagnosis. When these renal transplant recipients first became ill with strongyloidiasis, parasitic disease was usually not included in the differential diagnosis. Identification of *S stercoralis* within 5 days of initial symptoms was reported in only 5 of 29 cases (17%) (*2, 4, 12, 16*). Other diagnoses considered were cytomegalovirus infection, primary bacterial meningitis, primary bacterial pneumonia, sepsis resulting from varying causes, small bowel obstruction, acute pancreatitis, peptic ulcer disease, viral syndrome, primary bacterial peritonitis, and drug rash.

The diagnosis was serendipitous in half the cases. However, conventional diagnostic tests, when applied, were usually successful in finding strongyloidiasis (Table 1). In 11 cases, the diagnosis was confirmed by more than one test (*5–7, 9, 11, 12, 14–16, 19*, and cases 1, 2). Although peripheral blood eosinophilia was an important clue in several patients, only 10 of 29 cases (34%) had more than 10% eosinophils on peripheral smear. In a unique report, two cadaveric transplant recipients

TABLE 1. Identification of *Strongyloides stercoralis* in 29 Renal Transplant Recipients

Diagnostic test	Initial diagnosis	All specimens
Stool for ova and parasites	25	31
Sputum for cytology	6	9
Duodenal aspirate	3	7
Urine	2	3
Bronchoscopic aspirate	1	2
Peritoneal fluid	1	1
Wound	0	1
Blind loop fluid	0	1
Unknown	1	1
Autopsy	2	2
TOTAL	41 Episodes	58 Identifications

developed simultaneous strongyloidiasis that was diagnosed in the 10th posttransplant week (*9*). Both kidneys came from the same donor. Stool examination provided the diagnosis in one patient and urine microscopy in the other. The possibility of transmission of strongyloidiasis by the donated kidneys was suggested.

Identification of organisms. As shown in Table 1, strongyloides larvae were recovered from the lungs, gastrointestinal tract, genitourinary tract, peritoneum, and other sites. Larvae were not identified in the cerebrospinal fluid of the six cases of bacterial meningitis reported here. Both larvae and adult worms were identified in 6 of the 9 autopsies performed (*3, 4, 9, 11, 12*, and case 2). Histologic examination revealed *S stercoralis* in the pulmonary alveoli and vascular spaces, duodenum and duodenal ulcers, lymphatic vessels and mucosa of the small bowel, pancreas and peripancreatic lymph nodes, and portal spaces of the liver. In one case larval forms were distributed throughout the body (*11*). A more complete description of autopsy findings has been reported elsewhere (*19*).

Most bacterial organisms identified were of enteric origin. Positive cultures were seen in the blood of 11 patients (15 isolates), the sputum of 4 patients with pneumonia (6 isolates), the cerebrospinal fluid of 4 patients (4 isolates), the wounds of 2 patients (5 isolates), the urine of 3 patients (3 isolates), and the peritoneal fluid of one patient (3 isolates) (Table 2). Two additional cases of presumed bacterial meningitis were culture negative (*5, 13*). They may have represented strongyloides meningitis.

Twelve of the 29 cases (40%) had hyperinfection without systemic illness. Seven of these 12 patients had symptoms confined to the gastrointestinal tract, 4 were limited to the respiratory tract, and one had combined symptoms. In an additional seven cases of hyperinfection, sepsis was associated with gastrointestinal (2 cases), or combined (5 cases) symptoms. Dissemination was present in 10 patients. Seven had evidence of meningitis, 3 had documentation of strongyloides larvae in the urine, and one had larvae discovered in a transplant nephrectomy wound.

Therapy. Treatment in all cases was begun with thiabendazole. The usual initial course consisted of 25 mg/kg body weight twice daily for 3–5 days. Follow-up and retreatment were highly variable. Recurrence was generally associated with a single course of therapy and limited or no follow-up. In a few cases of unrelenting gradual deterioration and death, ongoing therapy failed to eradicate larvae from body fluids. In fact, on occasion, living worms were recovered from sputum and duodenal aspirates after a full course of therapy (case 1). Usually, when thiabendazole was unsuccessful in eradicating worm burdens, other antihelminthic agents were also ineffective. In patients who recovered from their initial illness, however, a lower incidence of recurrence seems to have corresponded with ongoing courses of therapy.

Mortality. Fifteen of the 29 patients died (52%). Recurrent or persistent strongyloidiasis, bacteremia, and dissemination were associated with a 70% mortality rate. Decreased mortality was observed in patients with no evidence of transplant rejection.

TABLE 2. Bacterial isolates in 29 renal transplant recipients with strongyloidiasis

Problem	Organism	Reference	No. isolates
Bacteremia	*Escherichia coli*	(*1, 19, 10*)	3
	Bacteroides fragilis	(*6, 8*)	2
	Streptococcus faecalis	(*11, 19*)	2
	Alkaligines faecalis	(*3*)	1
	Pseudomonas aeruginosa	Case 1	1
	Klebsiella pneumoniae	(*10, 15*)	2
	Enterobacter cloacae	(*6*)	1
	"Gram-negative bacilli"	(*11, 15, 17*)	*3*
Pneumonia	*Eikenella corrodens*	(*9*)	1
	P aeruginosa	(*9*)	1
	Hemophilus influenzae	(*15*)	1
	K pneumoniae	(*15*)	1
	E coli	(*19*)	1
	"Gram-negative bacilli"	(*14*)	*1*
Meningitis	*S faecalis*	(*4*)	1
	Proteus morganii	(*10*)	1
	E coli	Case 1	1
	"Gram-negative bacilli"	(*17*)	1
	Culture negative	(*5, 13*)	*2*
Urinary tract Infection	*K pneumoniae*	(*9*)	2
	S faecalis	(*19*)	*1*
Peritonitis	*E coli*	Case 1	1
	S faecalis	Case 1	*1*
Wound	*B fragilis*	(*7*)	1
	E coli	(*7, 5*)	2
	S faecalis	(*7, 5*)	*2*

DISCUSSION

Opportunistic infection with *S stercoralis* is a potentially preventable cause of disease and death in renal transplant recipients. Strongyloidiasis is usually present in its chronic gastrointestinal form when the patient is transplanted, but it is not diagnosed because of nonspecific or absent symptoms. During posttransplant immunosuppression, a devastating and deceptive illness may occur at varying intervals. A bewildering array of complaints and serious bacterial infections mimic many other diseases. Clinicians may be misled in a number of ways, chiefly by unfamiliarity with systemic strongyloidiasis.

The various manifestations of strongyloidiasis correlate well with the parasitic life cycle. Pruritus ani and larva currens correspond with autoinfection. Cough, wheezing, and hemoptysis indicate accelerating metamorphosis and increasing worm burden in the pulmonary phase. The amount of watery mucous diarrhea and gastrointestinal bleeding correspond with the intensity and duration of infection (*31*). Bacteremia suggests active worm migration within tissues. Meningitis, peritonitis, or genitourinary symptoms indicate heavy infection, aggressive invasion due to diminished host defenses, and a poor prognosis.

Delay in the diagnosis of strongyloidiasis has been associated with increased morbidity and mortality (*26*). The diagnosis of strongyloidiasis was delayed five or more days in 17 cases (66%). One diagnosis was made only at autopsy. Earlier detection and prompt therapy should reduce the complications and mortality in renal transplant patients. Other factors increasing the risk of mortality were increased steroid therapy (*32*), persisting parasitism, disseminated disease, bacteremia, and concurrent illness.

Several stumbling blocks delay the early diagnosis of strongyloidiasis. First, a history of recent travel to the tropics is usually not obtained, the significance of possible remote exposure abroad is not appreciated, and there is an unfamiliarity with strongyloidiasis in temperature zones. Chronic strongyloidiasis may be completely asymptomatic prior to immuno suppression and escape detection. Vietnam veterans may harbor this parasite and have undiagnosed disease (*33*). Immigrants, refugees, and travelers from tropical and subtropical regions may also have subclinical strongyloidiasis. Second, eosinophilia may be absent in the transplant candidate with subclinical infection. Immunosuppression may induce eosinopenia even when symptomatic disease is present. Thus, while an elevated eosinophil count should be investigated, the absence of eosinophilia should not be considered as evidence against strongyloidiasis. Third, stool examinations for ova and parasites are often negative in the presence of infection. Although the likelihood of false negatives declines as the worm burden increases, asymptomatic normal hosts with strongyloidiasis have larvae detected in only about 27% of stool specimens (*34*). Fourth, the variety of symptoms commonly suggests other diagnoses. Nausea, vomiting, anorexia, abdominal cramping, weight loss, and diarrhea may be attributed to acute gastroenteritis, peptic ulcer disease, or transplant medications. Fever, cough, and hemoptysis in the presence of roentgenographic infiltrates suggest other etiologies. Fifth, the emergence of bacterial infection may offer an explanation for signs and symptoms without identifying the cause of recurrent bacterial complications. Accordingly, persistent bacterial infection despite appropriate antibiotic therapy (especially bacteremia, meningitis, and peritonitis) should prompt further evaluation for underlying strongyloidiasis. Sixth, some diagnostic tests are underutilized or performed inappropriately. The value of sputum cytology in diagnosing the pulmonary phase of strongyloidiasis may have a broader application than is currently recognized. Since the life cycle of *S stercoralis* involves the lungs, the yield of this test increases proportionately with the degree of autoinfection and increasing worm burden. Intestinal aspirates that sample gastric rather than duodenal contents will yield false negatives. Nasogastric tubes may sample acidic gastric juices inhospitable to larvae. The string Enterotest (Hedeco, Palo Alto, California) more reliably samples the duodenum and proximal jejunum in the absence of dysmotility syndromes (*19*). However, a wet prep of the intestinal contents must be examined promptly. A Miller-Abbott tube affords documentation of duodenal position with fluoroscopy and provides samples with a higher diagnostic yield.

Once the diagnosis of strongyloidiasis is obtained, obstacles to eradication post further risks to the patient. Therapeutic failures suggest that an adequate antihelminthic regimen is not well established, particularly in immunocompromised hosts. Depressed cell-mediated immunity due to immunosuppression probably diminishes the effect of medical therapy (*35, 36*). Malnutrition, in some cases caused or compounded by a heavy worm burden in the small bowel with secondary protein-losing enteropathies, may further hamper cell-mediated immunity needed to eliminate infection (*37–38*). In addition, the increased worm burden found in disseminated cases may require an extended course of therapy for eradication. Poor absorption of the oral agent may contribute to subtherapeutic drug levels and ineffective therapy in some patients. Anatomic features such as the appendix, diverticula, or surgically created blind loops are recognized as havens inaccessible to oral antihelminthics (*19*). All antihelminthics with activity against *S stercoralis* are oral agents. Effective parenteral drug therapy is not currently available. There is preliminary evidence that cyclosporine has antiparasitic properties against *S stercoralis* (*39*). Reinfection could also occur following treatment. This would be most likely in endemic regions where family members are infected or in patients with pica (case 3). Perianal skin soilage, an avenue of autoinfection, may harbor filariform larvae not exposed to systemic antihelminthic therapy. Until more effective agents are available, repeated cycles of thiabendazole will be necessary to avoid life-threatening complications of repeated infection. Family members may also require treatment. Household dogs and cats may be a further reservoir of strongyloidiasis (*31*).

Beyond the period of intense immunosuppression, the risk of systemic strongyloidiasis diminishes. Most major morbidity and death occurred 1–3 months posttransplantation. Although transplant recipients may again develop chronic, subclinical infection following treatment, it appears that once they are no longer intensely immunosuppressed the risk of strongyloidiasis resembles that of any normal host. As in case 1, however, subsequent immunosuppression may be complicated by sudden reemergence of life-threatening illness.

The cost-effectiveness of screening and prophylaxis is worthy of mention. The 8 cases of strongyloidiasis in renal transplant recipients documented between 1972 and 1984 at the Nashville Veterans Administration Medical Center and the Vanderbilt University Hospital represented about 1% of the total transplant population. Although this figure may be an underestimate, the incidence could be less outside an endemic region. At this writing, four stool specimens examined for ova and parasites would cost a renal transplant candidate $68 at Vanderbilt. Additional evaluation with a sputum Papanicolaou-stained smear and string Enterotest duodenal aspirate would cost about $65. One 3-day course of thiabendazole, 25 mg/kg/day twice daily for 5 days, in a 70 kg man would cost $7. While reluctant to increase expenses, we consider that this evaluation is warranted, particularly when the patient has traveled to or resides in an endemic region. Screening prior to transplantation allows early detection, treatment of uncomplicated infection, and thorough follow-up. We prefer screening and therapy when indicated rather than blind prophylaxis. Life-threatening recurrences have been observed following detection and treatment of strongyloidiasis. Prophylaxis without screening may lead to omission of careful follow-up and allow systemic illness to develop.

Recommendations

Pretransplant evaluation.

1. All renal transplant candidates should submit at least 4 stools for ova and parasite examination prior to being activated. These patients should also submit 4 stools every six months while on the active list.
2. Residents, or former residents, of endemic areas should receive more thorough screening—e.g., Papanicolaou-stained smears of sputum and duodenal aspirate. Family members should be considered possible sources of transmission and submit specimens.

Posttransplant evaluation.

1. Include strongyloidiasis in the differential diagnosis of any rash, fever, pulmonary infiltrate, gastrointestinal illness, or bacterial infection. Investigate promptly.
2. Regard eosinophilia as a marker for helminthic infection, especially while immunosuppressed, until proved other-

wise. Do not eliminate strongyloidiasis from the differential diagnosis in the absence of eosinophilia.

3. Regard any bacterial infection due to enteric organisms as a possible complication of larval migration.
4. Be persistent in examining stool, sputum, and upper intestinal aspirates if the setting is at all suggestive of strongyloidiasis.

Therapy.

1. Treat transplant candidates for longer courses. We suggest an initial dose of thiabendazole 25 mg/kg/day twice daily for 3 days. Recheck stools following treatment and at regular bimonthly intervals for six months. Retreat if necessary. Monthly suppressive treatment may be required.
2. Treat transplant recipients for even longer courses. We suggest two cycles of thiabendazole 25 mg/kg/day twice daily for 5 days, with a 3 day interval between cycles. Recheck stools following treatment and at regular bimonthly intervals for one year. Monthly treatment, thiabendazole 25 mg/kg/day twice daily for 2 days, is recommended until larvae have been absent from screening specimens for six months.
3. Educate patients regarding pathogenesis.
4. In complicated cases both bacterial and parasitic infection must be treated.
5. When strongyloidiasis is diagnosed in a patient, educate health care workers regarding potential parasitic transmission by specimens, clothing, and contaminated bedding.

Acknowledgments. Expert secretarial assistance was provided by Mrs. Thelma Knickerbocker. Dr. G. Stephen Nace critically reviewed the manuscript. The patients were cared for by the many physicians of the Renal Transplant Service.

REFERENCES

1. White JV, Garvey G, Hardy MA. Fatal strongyloidiasis after renal transplantation: a complication of immunosuppression. Am Surg 1982; 48: 39.
2. Schumaker JD, Band JD, Lensmeyer GL, Craig WA. Thiabendazole treatment of severe strongyloidiasis in a hemodialyzed patient. Ann Intern Med 1978; 89: 644.
3. Fagundes LA, Busato O, Brentano L. Strongyloidiasis: fatal complication of renal transplantation. Lancet 1971; 2: 439.
4. Scoggin CH, Call NB. Acute respiratory failure due to disseminated strongyloidiasis in a renal transplant recipient. Ann Intern Med 1977; 87: 456.
5. Boram LH, Keller KF, Justus DE, Collins JP. Strongyloidiasis in immunosuppressed patients. Am J Clin Pathol 1981; 76: 778.
6. Venizelos PC, Lopata M, Bardawil WA, Sharp JT. Respiratory failure due to Strongyloides stercoralis in a patient with a renal transplant. Chest 1980; 78: 104.
7. Powell RW, Moss JP, Nagar D, et al. Strongyloidiasis in immunocompromised hosts. Presentation as massive lower gastrointestinal bleeding. Arch Intern Med 1980; 140: 1061.
8. Leapman SB, Rosenberg JB, Filo RS, Smith EJ. Strongyloides stercoralis in chronic renal failure: safe therapy with thiabendazole. South Med J 1980; 73: 1400.
9. Hoy WE, Roberts NJ, Bryson MF, et al. Transmission of strongyloidiasis by kidney transplant? Disseminated strongyloidiasis in both recipients of kidney allografts from a single cadaver donor. JAMA 1981; 246: 1937.
10. Meyers AM, Shapiro DJ, Milne FJ, Myburgh JA, Rabkin R. Strongyloides stercoralis hyperinfection in a renal allograft recipient. S Afr Med J 1976; 50: 1301.
11. Fowler CG, Lindsay I, Lewin J, Sweny P, Fernando ON, Moorhead JF. Recurrent hyperinfestation with Strongyloides stercoralis in a renal allograft recipient. Br Med J 1982; 285: 1394.
12. Weller IVD, Copland P, Gabriel R. Strongyloides stercoralis infection in renal transplant recipients. Br Med J 1981; 282: 524.
13. Vishwanath S, Baker RA, Mansheim BJ. Strongyloides infection and meningitis in an immunocompromised host. Am J Trop Med Hyg 1982; 31: 857.
14. DeVault GA, Brown ST, Montoya SF, King JW, Rohr MS, McDonald JC. Disseminated strongyloidiasis complicating acute renal allograft rejection. Prolonged thiabendazole administration and successful retransplantation. Transplantation 1982; 34: 220.
15. Hirschmann JR, Plorde JJ, Ochi RF. Fever and pulmonary infiltrates in a patient with a renal transplant. West J Med 1984; 140: 914.
16. Narasimhan N, Piering WF, Kauffman HM, Lemann J. Letter to the editor. Transplantation 1983; 36: 472.
17. Hooper DC, Pruitt AA, Rubin RH. Central nervous system infection in the chronically immunosuppressed. Medicine (Baltimore) 1982; 61: 166.
18. Bauer LA, Raisys VA, Watts MT, Ballinger J. The pharmockinetics of thiabendazole and its metabolites in an anephric patient undergoing hemodialysis and hemoperfusion. J Clin Pharmacol 1982; 22: 276.
19. Scowden EB, Schaffner W, Stone WJ. Overwhelming strongyloidiasis. An unappreciated opportunistic infection. Medicine 1978; 57: 527.
20. Stone WJ, Schaffner W. Strongyloidiasis in the compromised host. Internal Medicine for the Specialist 1982; 3: 48.
21. Gelman AC. Distribution of selected communicable diseases in the tropical and subtropical areas of the world. In: Hunter GW, Swartzwelder JC, Clyde DF, eds. Tropical medicine. Philadelphia: Saunders, 1976: 843.
22. Pelletier LL. Chronic strongyloidiasis in World War II Far East ex-prisoners of war. Am J Trop Med Hyg 1984; 33: 55.
23. Gill GV, Bell DR. Strongyloides stercoralis infection in former Far East prisoners of war. Br Med J 1979; 2: 572.
24. Grove DI. Strongyloidiasis in allied ex-prisoners of war in southeast Asia. Br Med J 1980; 1: 598.
25. Rivera E, Maldonado N, Velez-Garcia E, Grillo AJ, Malaret G. Hyperinfection syndrome with Strongyloides stercoralis. Ann Intern Med 1970; 72: 199.
26. Igra-Siegman Y, Kapila R, Sen P, Kaminski ZC, Louria DB. Syndrome of hyperinfection with Strongyloides stercoralis. Rev Infect Dis 1981; 3: 397.
27. Milder JE, Walzer PD, Kilgore G, Rutherford I, Klein M. Clinical features of Strongyloides stercoralis infection in an endemic are of the United States. Gastroenterology 1981; 80: 1481.
28. Schultz MG. The surveillance of parasitic diseases in the United States. Am J Trop Med Hyg 1974; 23: 744.
29. Amir-Ahmadi H, Braun P, Neva FA, Gottlieb LS, Zamcheck N. Strongyloidiasis at the Boston City Hospital. Emphasis on gastrointestinal pathophysiology and successful therapy with thiabendazole. Am J Dig Dis 1968; 13: 959.
30. Intestinal parasite surveillance. In: Jones WE, ed. Annual summary 1978. Center for Disease Control, Atlanta, GA. 1979: 9.
31. The Rhabditida: strongyloides and related forms. In: Beaver PC, Jung RL, Cupp EW, eds. Clinical parasitology. Philadelphia: Lea & Febiger, 1984: 253.
32. Davidson RA, Fletcher RH, Chapman LE. Risk factors for strongyloidiasis. A case-controlled study. Arch Intern Med 1984; 144: 321.
33. Pelletier LL, Gabre-Kidan T. Chronic strongyloidiasis in Vietnam veterans. Am J Med 1985; 78: 139.
34. Jones CA. Clinical studies in human strongyloidiasis. I. Semeiology. Gastroenterology 1950; 16: 743.
35. Dwork KG, Jaffe JR, Lieberman HD. Strongyloidiasis with massive hyperinfection. NY State J Med 1975; 75: 1230.

36. Purtilo DT, Meyers WM, Connor DH. Fatal strongyloidiasis in immunosuppressed patients. Am J Med 1974; 56: 488.
37. Milner PF, Irvine RA, Barton CJ, Bras G, Richards R. Intestinal malabsorption in Strongyloides stercoralis infestation. Gut 1965; 6: 574.
38. O'Brien W. Intestinal malabsorption in acute infection with Strongyloides stercoralis. Trans Roy Soc Trop Med Hyg 1975; 69: 69.
39. Schad GA. Cyclosporine may eliminate the threat of overwhelming strongyloidiasis in immunosuppressed patients. J Infect Dis 1986; 153: 178.

Received 15 October 1985.
Accepted 27 January 1986.

0041-1337/86/4205-0524$02.00/0
TRANSPLANTATION

Vol. 42, No. 5
Printed in U.S.A.

SUPPRESSION OF B CELL IMMUNITY TO DNP BY SEROTHERAPY WITH MONOCLONAL ANTI-DNP ANTIBODIES

EFFECT OF THE TREATMENT SCHEDULE ON THE MAGNITUDE OF SPECIFIC SUPPRESSION AND ITS DURATION

PAUL R. BEINING,[1] BRUCE MERCHANT, ELAINE F. LIZZIO, AND THOMAS HOFFMAN

Laboratory of Cell Biology, Center for Drugs and Biologics, Office of Biologics Research and Review, Food and Drug Administration, Bethesda, Maryland 20892; and Department of Biology, University of Scranton, Scranton, Pennsylvania 18510

The effect of prior administration of anti-DNP (N-[2,4-dinitrophenyl]-B-alanylglycylglycine) monoclonal antibodies on the humoral immune response of BALB/c mice was examined. One-time administration of a "cocktail" of two anti-DNP monoclonals resulted in suppression of the IgM anti-DNP response for one week after challenge but not longer. Maximal suppression of anti-DNP IgM plaque-forming cells was achieved by administration of antibody 1–2 weeks before challenge with DNP. Maximal suppression of serum IgM antibody was seen by administration of antibody 2–3 weeks before challenge with antigen. Following one-time administration of suppressive monoclonal antibody, the serum IgG antibody response to DNP was suppressed beginning 2 weeks after immunization and remained so for up to 241 days despite continual booster injections of antigen. Although most effective suppression of the humoral anti-DNP response was seen in animals receiving their single dose of suppressive antibody 2 weeks before first exposure to antigen, suppression of the IgG response was evident at all intervals examined up to 232 days in mice given monoclonal antibody between 0.1 day and 30 days before antigen, but not at earlier times. These findings suggest that regulatory networks, rather than the masking of antigenic determinants by passively administered antibody, play a role in antibody-mediated immunoregulation. They may be of use in designing strategies for optimizing immunosuppression protocols in clinical studies.

The capacity of passively administered antibody to selectively suppress immune responses is well established (*1, 2*). Although its mechanism is very poorly understood, this approach has been utilized for the past two decades for prevention of erythroblastosis fetalis in the Rh-positive progeny of Rh-negative mothers (*3*). A number of mechanisms have been proposed to account for this phenomenon; they include the masking or neutralization of antigenic determinants (*1*), the formation of antiidiotype antibody (*4, 5*), and the opsonization of antigen-reactive cells (*6*). Passively administered antibodies can also be utilized to selectively suppress the rejection of long-term renal allografts (*7*); to suppress the development of isohemagglutinins in sensitized transfusion recipients (*8*); and to suppress the development of anti-double stranded DNA antibody in a model of murine lupus erythematosus (*9*).

There seems to be good general agreement that antibody-mediated selective immune suppression (AMI)* is effective in suppressing primary antibody responses (*10*). Secondary immune responses are less susceptible to suppression (*11*). Most of the aforementioned information was gained through the use of polyclonal antisera. In this study, we sought to ascertain whether monoclonal antibodies might be effective in suppressing primary, or possibly secondary, immune responses to the hapten dinitrophenyl (DNP) in a murine model.

MATERIALS AND METHODS

Animals. Six-week-old female BALB/cAnN CRL BR mice were obtained rom Charles River Laboratories (Kingston, NY). They were housed in cages in groups of five and fed water and chow ad libitum.

Monoclonal Antibodies (MoAb). MoAb designated as "A4" and "C1" were derived from CBA/N or BALB/c mice, respectively, which had been immunized with a total dose of 500 μgm DNP (N-2, 4-dinitrophenyl)-B-ananylglycylglycine) coupled to keyhold limpet hemocyanin (KLH, Calbiochem-Behring, San Diego, CA) (*12*) on Bentonite (Sigma, St. Louis, MO). Spleen cells were fused with NS-1 myeloma cells and hybridomas prepared by the method of Kohler and Milstein (*13*). Screening

[1] University of Scranton.

* Abbreviation used: AMI, antibody-mediated selective immune suppression; BSA, bovine serum albumin; DNP, dinitrophenyl; DRBC, duck red blood cell; HA, hemagglutination; KLH, keyhole limpet hemocyanin; 2-ME, 2-mercaptoethanol; PFC, plaque-forming cell; SRBC, sheep red blood cell.

was performed by a spot assay of hemolysis (*13*). A4 was shown to be IgG_1k and Cl was determined to be $Ig_{2b}k$ by radial diffusion in agar using antiimmunoglobulin reagents (Cappel Laboratories, Kensington, MD). Ascites fluids from pristane-primed mice injected with hybridoma cells was used as a source of monoclonal antibody.

Immunization procedures. Groups of ten mice were injected i.v. with monoclonal antibody on days 58 (group 1), 44 (group 2), 30 (group 3), 23 (group 4), 16 (group 5), 10 (group 6), 6 (group 7) or 0.1 (group 8) before their first exposure to antigen. Antibody (0.1 ml each of undiluted A4 and Cl anti-DNP monoclonal antibody [2.9 μgm IgG, 0.2 ml total]), which had a hemagglutination titer of 1:16,000 was administered only once to each group. One group received no antibody (group 9) (positive control).

Following antibody administration to the 0.1-day group, all groups received 100×10[6] dinitrophenylated (*12*) duck red blood cells (DNP-DRBC) i.p. As a negative control, one group of mice received (for the first and only time) the A-4 and C-1 antibody but no antigen. Four days later, half the mice in each group were sacrificed, and their spleens were removed and assayed for plaque forming cells (PFC) according to the procedure described below. The other half of the mice from each group, except group 10, were boosted with DNP-DRBC antigen. This procedure was performed at intervals (initially weekly, then less frequently) up to 416 days after initial challenge with antigen.

Immune cell plaque-forming cell (PFC) assay. Numbers of antibody-producing PFC were analyzed by a modification of the technique of localized hemolysis in gel (*14*). Briefly, 0.9% Agar (1.8 g BactoAgar [Difco Laboratories, Detroit, MI], plus 100 ml distilled water) combined with 100 ml Eagle's medium ([2x], NIH Media Supply) was mixed with 20 ml 1% DEAE Dextran (Pharmacia Fine Chemicals, Piscataway, NJ) in Tris-buffered saline, pH 7.4, plus 10 ml 0.5% bovine serum albumin (BSA, Fraction V, Miles Laboratories, Kankokee, IL) in Tris-buffered saline, pH 7.4. Then 2 ml of this mixture was added to 15×100-mm glass test tubes and incubated at 56°C for 10 min, followed by 10 min at 45°C. Next, 0.2 ml of 10% DNP-conjugated (*13*) or unconjugated (background) sheep red blood cells (SRBC) plus 0.2 ml spleen cell suspension (50 × 10[6]/ml) was added, mixed, then poured into 100×15-mm Petri dishes that were subsequently incubated at 37°C for 1 hr. Finally, 3 ml of 10% guinea pig complement (Baltimore Biological Laboratories, Cockeysville, MD) reconstituted in Tris-buffered saline was overlayed on the agar and incubated for an additional 1 hr. Plaques were scored using a mechanical counter (Fisher Scientific, Silver Spring, MD).

Hemagglutination for IgG or IgM antibodies. Hemagglutination (HA) was performed using SRBC alone or coupled with DNP (*12*). Briefly, 25 μl 5% fetal bovine serum (with or without 0.1 M 2-mercaptoethanol [2-ME, Sigma, St. Louis, MO]) was mixed with 25 μl test serum and serially diluted in two-fold steps. Then 25 μl 0.5% SRBC was added and the plates incubated for 3 hr at room temperature or overnight at 4°C. Titer was scored as the end-point dilution for unequivocal (1+) agglutination. IgM IM anti-DNP monoclonals with known titers showed no hemagglutination when so treated with 2-ME.

Statistics. Statistical analysis was performed using Stat-Pak programs developed by BRIGHT Software (New Brunswick, NJ). Duncan's multiple range test (*15*) was used to determine significance between groups when Bartlett's test (*16*) determined no heterogeneity of variance.

RESULTS

Effect of passive administration of monoclonal anti-DNP antibodies on the IgM response to DNP-DRBC. Preliminary experiments were undertaken to establish the ability of monoclonal anti-DNP antibodies to suppress humoral immune responses of BALB/c mice to DNP-coupled duck erythrocytes (*13*). Ascites fluid (0.05 cc) from five different hybridomas, which reacted with DNP, was injected i.v. 2 h prior to immunization of mice with 100×10[6] DNP-DRBC. The two hybridoma ascites fluids (A4 and Cl) that caused the greatest reduction of PFC (data not shown), were used in subsequent experiments that addressed the magnitude and duration of suppression by antibody administered prior to immunization.

Individual BALB/c mice were given (on only one occasion) an i.v. dose ("cocktail") of 0.2 ml PBS containing 0.05 ml each of C-1 and A-4 monoclonal anti-DNP antibodies at various intervals, as described in the *Materials and Methods* section. Four days after immunization with DNP-DRBC, half the mice in all the groups were sacrificed; their spleens were removed and assayed for cells secreting anti-DNP IgM antibody vs. DNP (Fig. 1). Maximal suppression of IgM PFC was achieved by antibody administration 6 days prior to challenge with antigen. The result in this group was not statistically different from those achieved by administration of antibody on days −0.1, −10, −16, and −23. Suppression, significantly different from that of group 9 (the positive control that received no monoclonal antibody), was seen with animals given antibody up to 30 days before antigenic challenge. Group 10 (the negative control that received no DNP-DRBC) animals showed no PFC (data not shown).

The remaining mice were maintained over the course of 416 days and studied for their ability to produce serum antibody as assayed by hemagglutination. Serum IgM antibody (sensitive to 2-ME) against DNP at 7 days postimmunization was lowest in mice that had received antibody 23 or 16 days before challenge with antigen (Fig. 2). As with the PFC response, suppres-

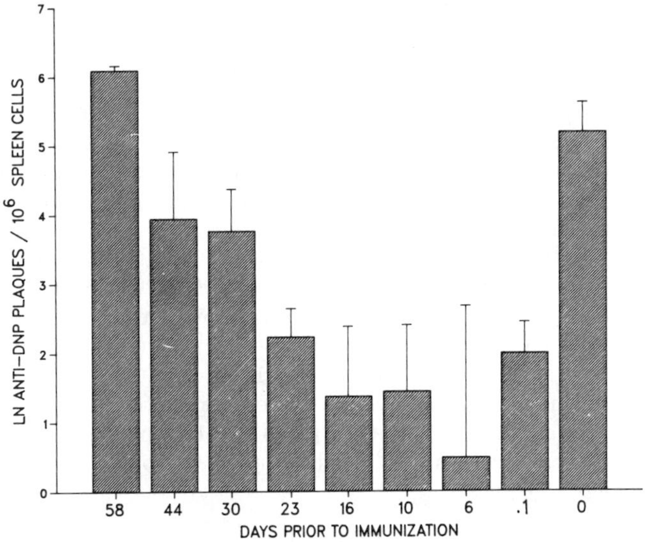

FIGURE 1. Suppression of IgM-PFC by monoclonal antibody cocktail. Eight groups of BALB/c mice (n=5) were administered 0.1 cc of ascites fluid containing MoAbs i.v. at the times indicated, prior to i.p. immunization with 100×10[6] DNP-conjugated duck red blood cells. Four days after receiving antigen, the animals were sacrificed and the spleens removed for assay of anti-DNP PFC as described in the *Materials and Methods* section. Error limits describe 1 SEM of the pooled sample.

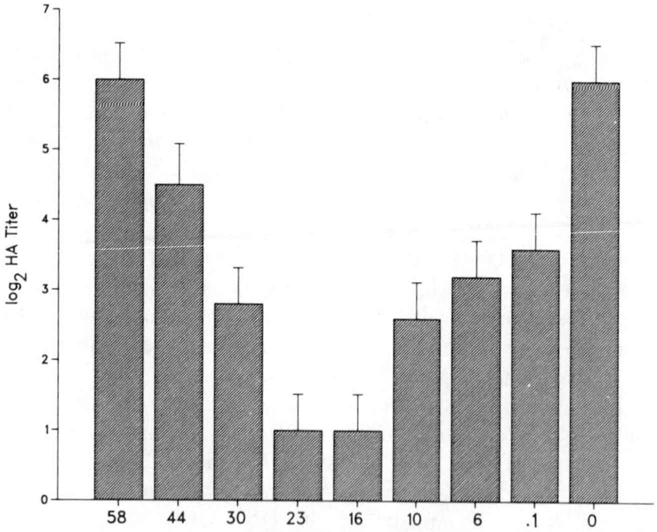

FIGURE 2. Suppression of serum IgM anti-DNP titer by monoclonal antibody. Mice were treated as shown in Fig. 1. Results are HA titers achieved on day 7 postimmunization. Error limits describe 1 SEM of the pooled sample.

sion that differed significantly from group 9 (positive control) was achieved by administration of antibody at all intervals between 0.1 day and 30 days prior to challenge with antigen. The IgM anti-DNP response measured at later times failed to show significant differences from (positive) control (data not shown). Group 10, which received only one injection of monoclonal antibody, showed no significant hemagglutination titer during the course of the study.

Effect of passive administration of MoAb cocktail on the IgG response to DNP-DRBC. Sera of mice were also tested for serum hemagglutination activity that was insensitive to 2-ME treatment (IgG) at intervals up to 416 days after initial immunization. Figure 3 depicts the IgG hemagglutination titers observed over the entire course of the study. Suppression of the IgG anti-DNP response was seen as early as two weeks in all groups receiving monoclonal antibody. Significant suppression was seen as late as 232 days after immunization despite the repeated administration of "booster" doses of DNP-DRBC. For ease of comparison, rank order of suppression among the groups over the entire course of the HA study is listed in Table 1, along with an indication (underlined) of the significance of differences between them. Greatest suppression (statistically significant) was seen in animals treated 16 or 10 days prior to initial challenge with antigen. Groups 1 and 2, which received antibody 58 or 44 days, respectively, before antigen challenge showed no difference in mean IgG titer compared with untreated animals subsequent to day 14 after initial immunization. One may appreciate that there exists noticeable cycling in the marginally suppressed group 2 (44d) and group 3 (30 days) compared with the firmly suppressed groups, especially group 6 (10 days).

DISCUSSION

This study describes the suppression of humoral responses to DNP-DRBC by passive administration of monoclonal antibody. IgM responses, measured by PFC or hemagglutination tests, were suppressed for one week by the administration of monoclonal antibody up to 30 days prior to immunization. IgG responses, measured by HA, were effectively suppressed by administration of antibody up to 30 days before challenge, but were suppressed maximally by monoclonal antibody given originally at 10 days or 16 days prior to challenge. IgG suppression was maintained for 232 days despite eight booster injections of antigen.

Preliminary experiments in our laboratory demonstrated that the administration of monoclonal anti-DNP antibodies could suppress primary immune responses when administered immediately before immunization. Secondary responses could not be inhibited (unpublished observations). Although unique monoclonals could suppress the response if given alone, optimal suppression of the polyclonal response was achieved by a mixture of two monoclonals. We therefore chose to use two monoclonals to achieve optimal conditions for suppression in the time-course study described here.

The superior results achieved with antibody administered 1–2 weeks prior to immunization might be considered surprising in light of other studies (*2*) and the clinical practice of giving anti-Rh antibody immediately before delivery (*3*). Nevertheless, suppression of the IgM anti-DNP response was more pronounced when antibodies were given at 10–16 days rather than 0.1 day before exposure to antigen. Similarly, IgG responses were consistently suppressed to a greater extent when MoAb were given 10–16 days before antigen. It was clear, however, that administration of monoclonals up to 0.1 day before antigen (but not 44 days or more before antigen), produced significant suppression. The effectiveness of MoAb given well before antigen makes unlikely explanations such as the masking of antigenic determinants as the mechanism for such suppression and favors the implication that regulatory networks (antiidiotype antibody or suppressor cells) may be involved.

The frequent reexposure to antigen during early development of the IgG response attempted here may well have elicited

TABLE 1. Duncan's multiple range test for serum IgG response

Bleeding (days after initial challenge with DNP-DRBC)	Ranking[a]								
7	6	9	5	7	8	4	3	2	1
14	5	6	4	7	8	1	2	3	9
21	6	5	8	4	7	2	3	1	9
28	6	5	7	4	8	3	2	1	9
48	5	3	7	4	6	8	2	1	9
62	5	7	6	4	8	3	2	9	1
90	6	5	7	4	8	3	2	9	1
118	7	5	6	4	3	8	2	1	9
232	6	5	3	4	7	8	2	9	1
416	8	5	6	3	1	4	7	2	9

[a] Group numbers assigned as in the *Materials and Methods* section. Those with common underlining were not statistically different from one another.

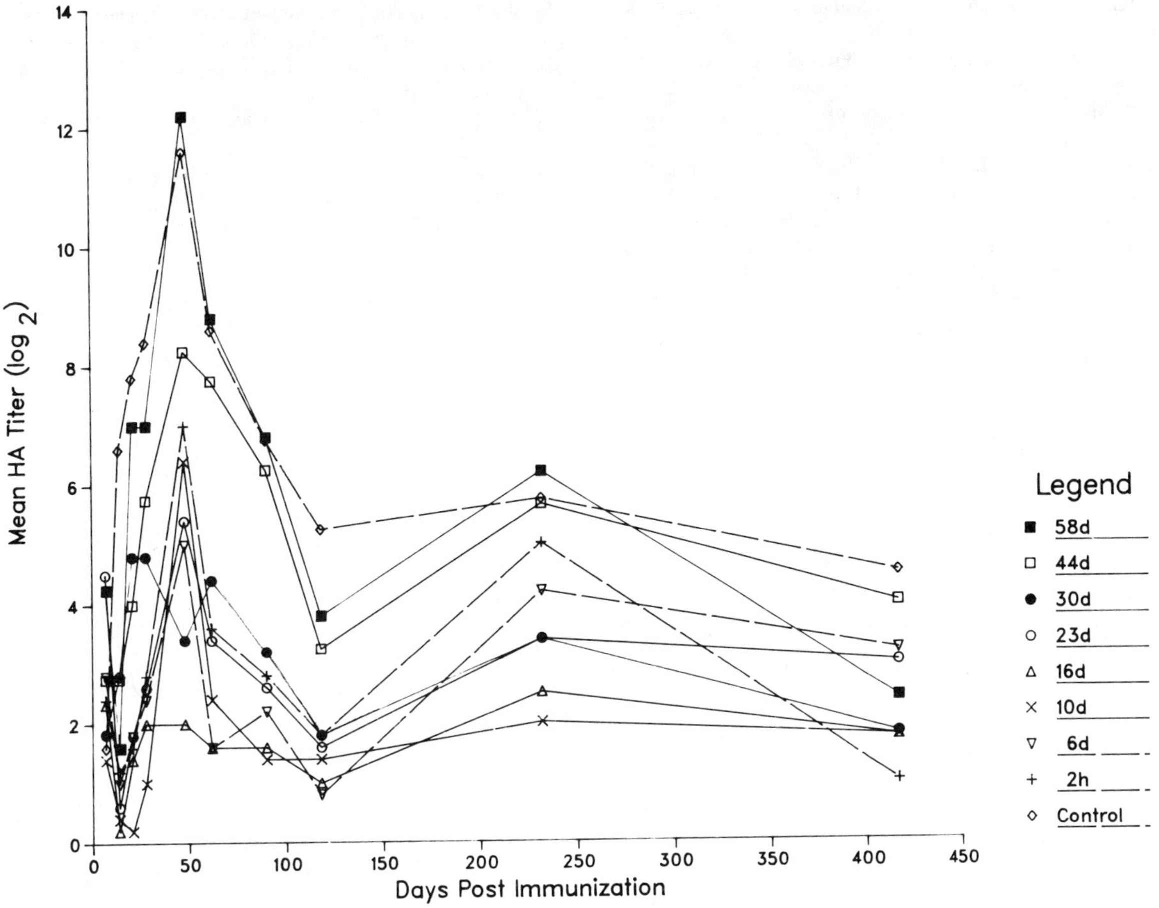

FIGURE 3. Time course of 2ME-resistant anti-DNP response over 415 days postimmunization. Mice identical to those described in Fig. 2 were bled serially at 7, 14, 21, 28, 48, 62, 90, 118, 232, and 416 days after immunization and then boosted immediately after each bleeding with 100×10^6 DNP-DRBC. One mouse in the −44-days group died unexplainably at 7 days; one other died after 118 days. One mouse in the positive control group died after 61 days; another two died after 23 days. One mouse from the −16-days group and one from the −10-days group died after 118 days.

control mechanisms not ordinarily observed in most previous studies. Nevertheless, precedent exists for the kind of broad suppression observed in this study. Monoclonal antibodies of a certain idiotype or polyclonal sera with reactivity against a limited portion of an antigen have been shown to suppress polyclonal antibody responses, as in the case of antibodies directed against fragments of BSA (*17*). Investigations are in progress to determine the idiotypic specificity of the monoclonals employed in this study.

Our study underscores the consideration that time intervals need to be well chosen when considering antibody-mediated immunosuppression for new clinical protocols, particularly those employing new monoclonals. For uses in transplantation, such as enhancing allograft survival, these issues need to be examined carefully.

Current efforts in our laboratory address the possible cellular nature of the immunosuppression observed, using cell-transfer techniques. The use of single, unique monoclonals is also under study. It is hoped that these results will contribute to a more sagacious clinical use of monoclonal antibodies.

Acknowledgments. Many thanks to Mike Hanson for technical assistance and Patricia Haggerty for secretarial assistance. Elizabeth Peters originated the hybridomes. B. Golding, S. Epstein, K. Stein, and P. Baker provided helpful discussion and critical comments.

REFERENCES

1. Henry C, Jerne NK. Competition of 19S and 7S antigen receptors in the regulation of the primary immune response. J Exp Med 1968; 128: 133.
2. Fitch FW. Selective suppression of immune responses. Regulation of antibody formation and cell-mediated immunity by antibody. Prog Allergy 1975; 19: 195.
3. Pollack W, Gorman JG, Freda WJ, Ascari WQ, Allen AE, Baker WJ. Results of clinical trials of RhoGAM in women. Transfusion 1968; 8: 151.
4. Bona C, Paul WE. Cellular basis of regulation of expression of idiotype. J Exp Med 1979; 149: 592.
5. Sy MS, Dietz MH, Germain RN, Benacerraf B, Greene MI. Antigen-and receptor-driven regulatory mechanisms. J Exp Med 1980; 151: 1183.
6. Hutchinson IV. Antigen-reactive cell opsonization (ARCO) and its role in antibody mediated immune suppression. Immunol Rev 1980; 49: 167.
7. Morris PJ. Suppression of rejection of organ allografts by alloantibody. Immunol Rev 1980; 49: 93.
8. Nilsson IM, Sundqvist SB. Suppression of secondary antibody response by intravenous immunoglobulin and development of tolerance in a patient with haemophilia B and antibodies. Scand J Haemotol 1984; 40 suppl: 33.
9. Hahn BH, Ebling FN. Suppression of NZB/NZW murine nephritis by administration of a syngeneic monoclonal antibody to DNA:

possible role of anti-idiotypic antibodies. J Clin Invest 1983; 71: 1728.

10. Rowley DA, Fitch FW, Stuart FP, Kohler H, Cosenza H. Specific suppression of immune responses. Science 1973; 181: 1138.
11. Uhr JW, Moller G. Regulatory effect of antibody on the immune response. Adv Immunol 1968; 8: 81.
12. Inman JK, Merchant B, Claflin L, Tacey SE. Coupling of large haptens to proteins and cell surfaces: preparation of stable, optimally sensitized erythrocytes for hapten-specific hemolytic plaque assays. Immunochemistry 1973; 10: 165.
13. Köhler G, Milstein C. Derivations of specific antibody producing tissue culture and tumor lines by cell fusion. Eur J Immunol 1976; 6: 511.
14. Jerne, NK. Towards a network theory of the immune system. Ann Immunol (Paris) 1974; 125c: 373.
15. Abramowitz M, Stegun IA. Handbood of mathematical functions. New York: Dover, 1964.
16. Duncan, DB. Multiple range and multiple F-tests. Biometrics 1955; 11: 1.
17. Krieger NJ, Pesce A, Michael JG. Immunoregulation of the anti-bovine serum albumin response by polyclonal and monoclonal antibodies. Cell Immunol 1983; 80: 279.

Received 18 November 1985.
Accepted 10 February 1986.

0041-1337/86/4205-0528$02.00/0
TRANSPLANTATION

Vol. 42, No. 5
Printed in U.S.A.

THE SPLENIC MICROENVIRONMENT AND SELF RECOGNITION AS FACTORS IN ALLOGRAFT REJECTION IN RATS

A STUDY USING INDIUM-111–LABELED CELLS

RAYMOND POLLAK, JACQUELINE M. BLANCHARD, AND VELTA A. LAZDA

University of Illinois College of Medicine at Chicago, Department of Surgery, Division of Transplantation, Chicago, IL 60680

Splenectomy facilitates organ allograft survival in some rat strains, and in weak donor-recipient histoincompatible pairs. We have found using a heart spleen "twin" graft model, using ACI rats as recipients and Lewis rats as donors, that the transplanted heart will survive in most recipients after delayed host splenectomy. The presence of a viable mass of splenic tissue will allow rejection to proceed only when the transplanted spleen is of host origin, and not when it comes from the donor (i.e., when it is allogeneic). The use of ^{111}In-labeled cells has allowed us to show that lymphocyte traffic and trapping is markedly altered in the transplanted allogeneic spleens, when compared with control transplanted syngeneic spleens. Thus, despite the presence of the splenic "microenvironment," cardiac allograft rejection does not occur in the absence of syngeneic splenic tissue. We conclude that the role of the spleen in the immune response is to facilitate the recognition of self and the acquisition of alloreactivity in weak responder rat strains and donor-recipient pairs.

Splenectomy has been shown to facilitate organ allograft survival in some, but not all, rat strain combinations (*1–3*). This enhanced survival, especially with delayed host splenectomy after transplantation, is most pronounced in weakly histoincompatible donor-recipient pairs, or when the recipient rat is a weak responder strain. To explain these observations it has been suggested that in some genetic nonresponder strains exposed to soluble antigens or alloantigens, and in weakly histoincompatible donor-recipient pairs, the spleen provides an essential microenvironment that favors the production of enhanced ratios of activated suppressor to effector cells, as well as the development of high-affinity cytotoxic cells that react with alloantigens on the target organ (*1, 4*). Strong responder strains, may fail to generate both suppressor and high-affinity cytotoxic cells, but can destroy allografts using low-affinity cytotoxic cells, possibly aided by greater alloantigen density on the donor organ in strongly histoincompatible pairs. Thus, the spleen might not be an essential requirement in the latter situation.

Our own previous data using a heart and spleen "twin" graft model have supported these findings, in that ACI recipients of Lewis heart and spleen twin grafts will permanently accept these allografts in 64% of instances after delayed (postoperative day 3) host splenectomy (*5, 6*). The reverse situation—i.e., Lewis recipients of ACI twin heart and spleen grafts and delayed posttransplant splenectomy in the host—almost always results in early rejection of the allograft (in 7–10 days) with no differences noted when compared with appropriate controls (*6*).

To explain the role of the splenic microenvironment further we studied the migration patterns of host lymphocytes labeled with Indium-111 in a rat heart and spleen twin allograft model combined with delayed host splenectomy. Our data suggest that in weak responder rat strains, the splenic microenvironment is important if rejection is to occur, as it provides a possible mechanism for self-recognition and alloantigen sensitization.

MATERIALS AND METHODS

Rats. Inbred 300–400 g retired breeder male Lewis (RT^l) rats, and ACI (RT1^a) rats were obtained from Harlan-Sprague Dawley, Inc. (Indianapolis, IN) and Laboratory Supply Inc. (Indianapolis, IN), respectively. Both strains were used as heart or spleen donors when appropriate.

Operative technique. Heterotopic cardiac allograft placement was performed under ether anesthesia after the method of Ono and Lindsey (*7*). In brief, the ascending aorta and pulmonary artery were anastomosed to the great vessels in the abdomen with ischemic times of less than 30 min. Graft function was assessed by daily palpation of the abdomen. Rejection was established by the absence of palpable ventricular activity.

Spleen allograft placement was performed after the method described by Blanchard and Tauber (*5*). In brief, the spleen is harvested on a pedicle of the splenic artery attached to an aortic cuff, and the splenic vein attached to the remnant of the portal vein. The aortic cuff and portal vein are anastomosed to the great abdominal vessels of the recipient using microvascular techniques above the placement of the heterotopic cardiac allograft.

Posttransplant host splenectomy was performed three days after initial heart and spleen implantation by opening the abdomen through an upper midline incision. The splenic vascular pedicle was ligated with fine suture material and the spleen removed.

Cell preparation. Spleens were harvested from 2–4 rats using sterile technique. They were suspended in cold (4°C) normal saline and were then pressed through a stainless steel wire mesh. The resulting preparation was passed through fine nylon gauze to remove retained clumps, and washed once in saline (200 ×g for 10 min). The Cell suspension was resuspended in saline, layered over Ficoll-Hypaque (LSM, Litton Bionetics, Kensington, MD) and centrifuged for 30 min at 400 ×g at 24°C. Cells at the interface were harvested, washed twice in saline, and resuspended in saline to a final concentration of $1–2\times10^7$ cells/ml. Viability was judged to be greater than 95% by trypan blue exclusion.

Cell labeling with Indium-111 oxine. Prepared splenocytes were suspended at $1–2\times10^7$ cell/ml in normal saline and incubated with 50 $\mu c/10^7$ cells of Indium-111 oxine (Medi-Physics, Arlington Heights, IL) for 20 min at room temperature. Cells were then washed twice in normal saline and resuspended to 2×10^7 cells/ml in normal saline. Cell viability was maintained at greater than 90% although labeling efficiency varied from 35–80%.

Assessment of labeled cell migration in vivo. Under ether anesthesia 2×10^7 labeled cells in 1 ml of normal saline were injected into the tail vein of the recipient rat at day 2 and again at day 6 after heart and spleen twin graft implantation. The rats were allowed to recover and were placed in metabolic cages with food and water ad libitum. Within 24 hr of injection, the rat was sacrificed and the recipient heart and spleen, as well as donor heart and spleen, were removed. The organs were weighed and placed in an auto-gamma spectrometer (Packard Model 5260) for quantitative estimation of the radioactivity present in each organ. Localization of the labeled cells in the various tissues was expressed as the percentage of injected Indium-111 per gram of tissue.

RESULTS

Group 1: ACI recipients of syngeneic heart and spleen twin grafts. From Table 1 it is evident that, in the nontransplanted situation, almost all the injected labeled lymphocytes are localized to the native host spleen. When the rats are injected at day 6 after twin graft transplantation, and after native host splenectomy, few lymphocytes are found in the viable beating syngeneic heart. Most of the labeled cells are recovered from the transplanted vascularized spleen graft.

Group 2: ACI recipients of single Lewis cardiac allografts: no host splenectomy. This group of ACI rats was injected at various times with labeled syngeneic cells after single cardiac allograft placement. It is apparent (Table 1) that the native spleen takes up a large percentage of the cells, but that significant numbers accumulate in the transplanted heart as rejection proceeds and is complete in all rats by 10 days.

Group 3: ACI recipients of single Lewis cardiac allografts and syngeneic spleen, together with host splenectomy on posttransplant day 3. This group of ACI rats was injected with labeled syngeneic cells at days 2, 7, and 10 after transplantation with a syngeneic spleen but alloheart. Posttransplant host splenectomy was performed in all recipients on day 3. From Table 1 it is apparent that most of the inoculum is localized to the donor and recipient spleen. Significant numbers also accumulate in the donor heart as compared with the recipient heart. This again allows rejection of the heart to be complete by 10 days in all recipients.

Group 4: ACI recipients of Lewis heart and spleen allografts, with host splenectomy on post transplant day 3. This group of ACI rats was injected with labeled syngeneic cells on postoperative days 2, 3, 6, 9, 14, 27, and 29 after twin allograft placement. All rats had posttransplant host splenectomy on day 3 posttransplantation. Cells localized to the donor spleen in larger numbers earlier in the posttransplant course than they did later on. Labeled cells also accumulated in the donor heart in numbers similar to those seen in earlier groups, but were not able to affect cardiac function or mount a rejection response to the allografted tissue. No heart in this group showed evidence of clinical rejection at 30 days, at which time all animals had been sacrificed.

Group 5: ACI recipients of Lewis heart allografts with or without host splenectomy 3 days posttransplantation. Five ACI recipients of Lewis heart allografts rejected the heart at 13.2± 1.095 days when splenectomy was performed 3 days posttransplantation. These data were compared with a control group of 9 ACI recipients of Lew cardiac allografts that did not undergo posttransplant splenectomy, and rejected the hearts at 10.0± 0.7 days ($P<0.01$).

Group 6: ACI recipients of heart and spleen twin grafts from Lewis donors with no host splenectomy. Mean survival time of the allografted hearts in this group was 19.7±10.9 days (n = 12) ($P = 0.01$, when compared with control rats in group 5).

DISCUSSION

Our previous work had demonstrated that Lewis cardiac allografts had been permanently accepted in 64% of ACI recipients that had had a host splenectomy three days after transplantation of an allogeneic heart and spleen twin graft. Control ACI rats reject these cardiac allografts in 10 days. ACI rats splenectomized at posttransplant day 3 reject the allograft significantly later (group 5). The addition of the allogeneic spleen as part of the twin graft prolongs cardiac allograft survival in nonsplenectomized ACI recipients (group 6), but does not result in permanent acceptance unlike the situation in the splenectomized ACI recipient of the twin graft. This latter finding is of interest as pretransplant or peritransplant conditioning of potential recipients by donor-specific splenocytes or peripheral blood transfusion has been shown to prolong allograft survival (*3, 8–10*). This phenomenon is true for both strong and weak responder strains and strong and weak donor-

TABLE 1. Isotope counts in ACI recipients of Lewis cardiac allografts infused with ^{111}In-labeled lymphocytes

Group	Transplant day	N	% administered dose/g of tissue						Outcome of cardiac transplant
			Native heart	Donor heart (syn/allo)[a]	Donor Heart To Native Heart	P[b]	Native spleen	Donor spleen (syn/allo)[a]	
1	0	2	0.0967±0.0091	—	—	—	39.0188±5.9130	—	Prolonged function
	8	2	0.1077±0.0280	0.1987±0.0418	1.8450	0.09	—	14.4110±2.3390	
2	3	2	0.1062±0.0154	0.8659±0.1040	8.1530	0.001	79.13±1.09	—	Uniform rejection—10days
	7	2	0.0604±0.0010	0.1562±0.0057	2.5860	0.001	29.22±12.16	—	
	10	2	0.0624±0.0091	0.2661±0.0404	4.2640	0.02	45.20±2.92	—	
3	3	2	0.0325±0.0014	0.2274±0.0419	6.9970	0.02	11.3754±1.57	15.9970±1.0140	Uniform rejection—10 days
	7	2	0.0492±0.0027	0.1762±0.0317	3.5813	0.03	—	27.9814±3.4230	
	10	2	0.0649±0.0011	0.2323±0.0121	3.5794	0.003	—	9.2462±0.6990	
4	3	2	0.0686±0.0121	0.1512±0.0218	2.2041	0.04	11.8265±2.317	8.5213±0.1470	
	4	2	0.1015±0.0068	0.2258±0.0076	2.2224	0.003	—	2.8240±0.3180	
	7	1	0.0500—	0.2064—	4.1280	—	—	2.8190—	
	10	1	0.0681—	0.5200—	7.6358	—	—	2.1198—	No rejection noted in any instances
	15	2	0.0701±0.0174	0.2512±0.0371	3.5834	0.02	—	1.5400±0.0990	
	28	1	0.0842—	0.1756—	2.0855	—	—	1.5770—	
	30	1	0.0521—	0.2080—	3.9923	—	—	1.5150—	

[a] (Syn/allo) syngeneic/allogeneic organ transplanted; refer to the *Results* section in the text for explanation of groups.
[b] (*P*) significance of transplanted heart count compared with native heart count.

recipient pairs. Among a number of proposed theories, the mechanism currently favored to explain this effect is that the conditioning regimen followed by the implantation of the allografted tissue results in the production of suppressor cells (*11*, *12*). These suppressor cells are then responsible for the prolongation of allograft survival seen in both man and experimental models. The most convincing evidence for the presence and efficacy of these suppressor cells is their ability to prolong allograft survival in well-controlled adoptive transfer experiments (*12*). Thus the prolongation of cardiac allograft survival seen in rats that retain the native spleen in the presence of the twin heart spleen allograft (group 6), might also be explained by the suppressor cell mechanism. Weaker responder strains, however, have an absolute requirement for the presence of the spleen for the conditioning regimen to be effective, and it is known that some genetic nonresponders produce large numbers of suppressor cells in response to soluble or alloantigens (*3*, *4*).

Similarly, it is known that weak responder strains or weakly incompatible donor-recipient pairs require the presence of the host spleen in order to mount an effective immune response to allografted tissues (*1*, *3*). The explanation for this phenomenon has been that the host spleen provided the correct microenvironment, or allowed cells of lower affinity sufficient time and surface area to become sensitized to allografted tissue bearing lower surface antigen density (*1*).

The use of Indium-111-labeled syngeneic lymphocytes has allowed us to dissect these phenomena in greater detail. Indium-111-labeled lymphocyte injected into recipients of transplanted hearts has been successfully used to study the cell kinetics, specificity, and mechanisms of cardiac allograft rejection in rats (*13*, *14*). We adopted this technique in an attempt to explain the permanent acceptance of cardiac allografts in splenectomized ACI rats that were the recipients of Lewis heart and spleen twin grafts. It appears that, in the nontransplanted ACI rats, labeled cells injected into the tail vein accumulate in large numbers in the host spleen, whence they migrate to the periphery (group 1). Similarly, when syngeneic heart and spleen twin grafts are transplanted with native host splenectomy, many of the labeled syngeneic lymphocytes are found in the transplanted spleen. The transplanted heart and native heart do not differ significantly in the number of labeled cells they harbor. When an allogeneic heart is transplanted, injected syngeneic lymphocytes again migrate to the host spleen and accumulate in the transplanted heart in significant numbers (group 2). By days 4–7 a peak is reached, with resulting uniform rejection of the heart in 10 days—the native heart remaining uninvolved in the infiltrative process. Although splenectomy prolongs cardiac allograft survival somewhat (group 5), provision of a syngeneic spleen with a transplanted allogeneic heart (group 3) again results in prompt rejection at 10 days with many cells accumulating in the transplanted spleen and effecting rejection of the transplanted heart. Of extreme interest, however, is the fact that in splenectomized ACI recipients of an allogeneic heart and spleen, the presence of the splenic microenvironment is not sufficient to mount an effective immune response (group 4). Moreover, it appears that labeled lymphocytes reaching the spleen do not stay there for an appreciable length of time as compared with syngeneic controls. This implies that they failed to recognize an antigenic surface characteristic that would trap them in the spleen (i.e., self-recognition) and so allow for the attainment of alloreactivity to the transplanted tissue. Thus, although the allografted heart accumulates more labeled cells than the native heart, their effect appears to be minimal and the hearts continue to function without being rejected—an observation also recently made by others (*15*).

From these experiments, the role of the spleen in mediating an effective immune response to allografted tissue in weak responder strains or weakly histoincompatible donor recipient pairs appears to be to serve as the primary site for the recognition of "self" by immunocompetent cells, and to provide a suitable microenvironment and surface area for immunocompetent cells to circulate and acquire alloreactivity. The presence of a viable but "foreign" spleen in ACI recipient rats, in the absence of the native syngeneic spleen, does not confer on the recipient rat the ability to reject allografted tissue, and so results in permanent allograft acceptance in the majority of animals studied.

Acknowledgment. We thank Ms. Suzanne M. Renfroe for her careful and attentive work in the preparation of the manuscript.

REFERENCES

1. Fabre JW, Batchelor JR. The role of the spleen in the rejection and enhancement of renal allografts in the rat. Transplantation 1975; 20: 219.
2. Souther SG, Morris RE, Vistnes LM. Prolongation of rat cardiac allograft survival by splenectomy following transplantation. Transplantation 1974; 17: 317.
3. Birinyi LK, Baldwin WM III, Tilney NL. Influence of selective splenectomy on survival of cardiac and skin allografts in enhanced rats. Transplantation 1980; 30: 59.
4. Benacerraf B, Kapp JA, Debre P, Pierce CW, de la Croix F. The stimulation of specific suppressor T cells in genetic non-responder mice by linear random copolymers of L-amino acids. Transplant Rev 1975; 26: 21.
5. Blanchard JM, Tauber JW. Heart and spleen twin grafts in rats. J Microsurg 1980; 1: 381.
6. Tauber JW, Blanchard JM. Heart and spleen twin grafts in rats. II. Delayed host splenectomy. J Microsurg 1981; 2: 261.
7. Ono K, Lindsey ES. Improved technique of heart transplantation in rats. J Thorac Cardiovasc Surg 1969; 57: 223.
8. Martin DC, Hewitt CW, Osborne JC, et al. Enhanced kidney graft survival in rats by single or multiple blood transfusions and various blood products. Transplant Proc 1982; 14: 407.
9. Stuart FP, Scollard DM, McKearn TJ, Fitch FW. Cellular and humoral immunity after allogeneic renal transplantation in the rat. V. Appearance of anti-idiotypic antibody and its relationship to cellular immunity after treatment with donor spleen cells and alloantibody. Transplantation 1976; 22: 455.
10. Soulillou JP, Blandin F, Gunther E, Lemoine E. Genetics of the blood transfusion effect on heart allografts in rats. Transplantation 1984; 38: 63.
11. Hall BM. Mechanisms maintaining enhancement of allografts. I. Demonstration of a specific suppressor cell. J Exp Med 1985; 161: 123.
12. Batchelor JR, Philipps BE, Grennah D. Suppressor cells and their role in the survival of immunologically enhanced rat kidney allografts. Transplantation 1984; 37: 43.
13. Oluwole S, Wang T, Fawwaz R, et al. Use of Indium-111-labeled cells in measurement of cellular dynamics of experimental cardiac allograft rejection. Transplantation 1981; 31: 51.
14. Cox JH, Chisholm PM, Yacoub MH. The specificity of the lymphocyte infiltrate in rat cardiac allografts. Transplant Proc 1985; 17: 235.
15. Kupiec-Weglinski JW, de Sousa M, Tilney NL. The importance of lymphocyte migration patterns in experimental organ transplantation. Transplantation 1985; 40: 1.

Received 1 November 1985.
Accepted 10 February 1986.

0041-1337/86/4205-0532$02.00/0
TRANSPLANTATION

Vol. 42, No. 5
Printed in U.S.A.

THE MECHANISM OF PROLONGED GRAFT SURVIVAL FOLLOWING REMOVAL OF THE REGIONAL LYMPH NODE[1]

J. S. WOTHERSPOON AND S. E. DORSCH

The Pathology Department, The University of Sydney, N. S. W. 2006, Australia

The immune responsiveness of rats in which the rejection of RT-1-incompatible neonatal heart grafts had been prevented by removal of the draining lymph node was examined. It was found that within three days of node removal animals developed a state of specific unresponsiveness characterized by the failure to reject secondary grafts made into the contralateral leg with intact draining nodes. Studies of recipients with long-surviving grafts revealed that their serum contained significant levels of cytotoxic alloantibody although their cells behaved like those from naive donors in mixed lymphocyte interactions, graft-versus-host responses, and adoptive allograft assays. There was no evidence for the presence of sensitized T cells or suppressor T cells in the tissues of recipients with long-surviving grafts. The findings support the suggestion that prolonged graft survival following node removal is due to enhancement actively induced by the passage of graft antigen into the circulation at a time when the induction of the cell-mediated response has been aborted by removal of the node regional to the graft.

The regional lymph node (LN)* draining the site of a secondarily vascularized allograft is critically involved in the development of the immune response to the graft (*1–3*). Removal of the LN draining an RT-1-incompatible neonatal heart (NNH) grafted in the plantar space of an adult rat causes a highly significant delay in graft rejection (*4*). The effect is maximal when the LN is removed 4 days after graft implantation, is specific, and extends to second grafts implanted at a site distant from the primary graft—and from which the lymphatic drainage has not been interrupted (*4*). The results of studies of the immune status of hosts in which prolonged allograft survival has been induced by removal of the regional LN draining the graft are given here.

MATERIALS AND METHODS

Rats. Inbred rats of the DA (RT-1[a]), PVG (RT-1[c]), WF (RT-1[u]) and BN (RT-1[n]) strains were obtained from the Blackburn Animal House, University of Sydney.

Cells. LN cells (LNC) were obtained by crushing excised nodes into Dulbecco's phosphate buffered saline (Oxoid Ltd., London, U. K.) containing 2.5% v/v fetal calf serum (Flow Laboratories, Sydney, Australia) (DAB/FCS). The resulting suspension was filtered through sterile gauze and washed twice. Spleen cells (SpC) were similarly prepared. All manipulations were performed at 22°C.

Neonatal heart grafts. The NNH grafting technique is a modification of that described by Fulmer et al. (*5*). Hearts were removed from neonatal rats within 48 hr of birth and implanted in the plantar space of the hind foot of adult recipients as previously described (*4*). Graft survival was monitored every second day by electrocardiographic (ECG) tracing. The time of graft rejection was taken as the first day that no ECG activity was recorded and expressed as the median survival time (MST) and range of rejection time for each experimental group.

Popliteal LN removal. The skin overlying the popliteal space was incised. The space was opened by blunt dissection and the node carefully removed. The skin was closed with a single suture and sprayed with antibiotic (Neotracin, Ethnor Ltd., Sydney, Australia).

Irradiation. Animals and cell suspensions were irradiated in a ^{60}Co source under conditions previously described (*4*).

Local GVH assay. The popliteal LN (PLN) weight assay of Ford, Burr, and Simonsen (*6*) was used. F_1 hybrids were injected with 5×10^6 cells in 0.1 ml in the foot-pad. The PLN was removed on day 7, stripped of adipose tissue and weighed to an accuracy of 0.1 mg. Weights are expressed as the arithmetic mean ± 1 SE.

Mixed lymphocyte interaction (MLI). Cellular proliferation was assayed using a microculture technique. Responder cell populations were assayed against both specific and third-party stimulator cells. The latter were mixed LNC and SpC, mitotically inactivated with 9.5 Gy irradiation. Triplicate cultures were prepared containing 4×10^5 responder cells and 2×10^5 stimulator cells in RPMI 1640 medium (GIBCO, Grand Island, NY) supplemented with 100 U/ml penicillin, 100 μg/ml streptomycin, 2 mM glutamine, 2.5 μg/ml amphotericin B, 2.5×10^{-3} 2-mercaptoethanol and 5% v/v DA serum. Cultures were incubated at 37°C in a 5% CO_2 atmosphere. Cellular proliferation was assessed by addition of 25 μl of 0.5 μCi/ml tritiated thymidine (Radiochemical Centre Ltd., Amersham, U. K.) per well 4 hr before harvest. Cells were harvested onto glass fiber discs, and label incorporation was measured by liquid scintillation.

Adoptive restoration of allograft reactivity. Alloimmune competence was tested in vivo by the adoptive allograft assay of Dorsch and Roser (*7*) using NNHs as indicator grafts. Assay animals were irradiated with 9.0 Gy, grafted in the foot-pad with an allogeneic NNH, then injected i.v. with the cell population to be tested. Graft survival was monitored as described.

Complement-mediated antibody cytotoxicity. Cytotoxic serum antibody was assayed using the method of Howard and Scott (*8*). Cell viability was determined by fluorescent microscopy after addition of 10 μl of staining solution containing 1 μg/ml acridine orange and 5 μg/ml ethidium bromide in DAB/FCS. Under 480 nm excitation live cells stained green and dead cells

[1] This work was supported by grants from the Consolidated Medical Research Fund, University of Sydney, and by a grant from the National Health and Medical Research Council of Australia.

* Abbreviations used: DAB/FCS, Dulbecco's buffered saline with 2.5% v/v fetal calf serum; ECG, electrocardiograph; GVH, graft-versus-host; MHC, major histocompatibility complex; MLI, mixed lymphocyte interaction; MST, medium survival time; NNH, neonatal heart; PLN, popliteal lymph node; SpC, spleen cell.

stained orange. Results are expressed as the antibody titer resulting in 50% cytotoxicity of the assay cells.

Statistics. As the tempo of graft rejection does not follow a normal distribution, graft survival times for two experimental groups were compared according to the Wilcoxon/Mann-Whitney rank sum test to determine the significance probability *p*. Other results were compared using the Student's *t* Test.

RESULTS

Effect of Removal of the PLN Draining An NNH Allograft

Removal of the regional LN draining an NNH allograft implanted in the hind foot-pad of adult recipients during the inductive stages of the immune response results in the prolongation of graft survival (*4*). Figure 1 shows the cumulative results of experiments comparing the survival times of PVG NNHs in DA recipients from which the draining LNs were removed, 4 days after graft implantation, with the survival times in control animals. In the former, the median survival time was 49 days with a range of 21–74 days (MST 49 [21–74]), which was significantly greater than the normal survival time of PVG NNH in DA rats (MST 17 [13–27]).

Effect of Node Removal on Graft Survival in Sensitized Recipients

To determine whether node removal had any effect in animals in which specific immune induction had previously occurred, the effect of node removal in graft recipients that had previously been sensitized to the graft antigens was examined.

A group of 8 DA rats that had previously rejected a PVG NNH and 4 that had rejected a WF NNH were challenged with a PVG NNH in the ungrafted foot-pad. Four days later the PLN draining the secondary PVG NNH was removed from 4 of the former and all of the latter recipients.

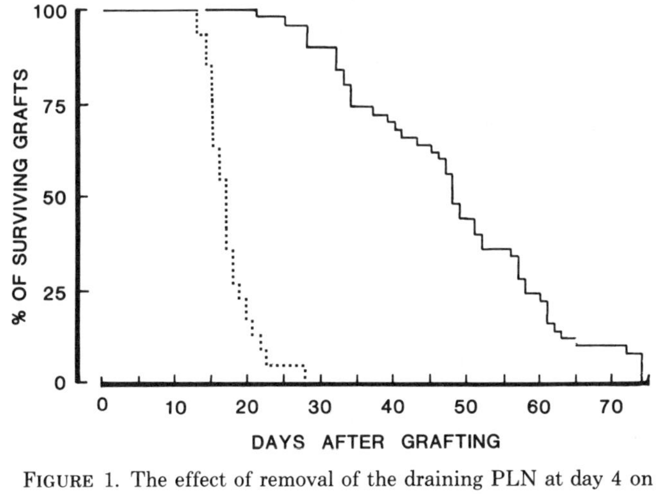

FIGURE 1. The effect of removal of the draining PLN at day 4 on the survival of PVG NNHs in DA rats. Graft survival time in DA recipients from which the node draining the PVG NNH has been removed (——) is significantly greater than that in control recipients (. . . . . .) (P<0.01).

The survival time of the secondary grafts in all groups is shown in Table 1. Specifically sensitized recipients from which the PLN draining the second graft had been removed showed second-set rejection tempo (MST 12 [10–12]) similar to that in specifically sensitized animals with intact nodes (MST 11.5 [10–13]). Recipients sensitized to WF antigens showed prolonged survival (MST 25 [19–31]) of the PVG graft from which the PLN had been removed. It was concluded that in previously sensitized hosts, LN removal does not prolong the survival of grafts bearing the sensitizing alloantigen. The rejection of grafts implanted after node removal was next examined.

The Effect of Node Removal on The Survival of Secondary Grafts

A group of 18 DA rats was grafted in one foot-pad with a PVG NNH. Four days later the PLN draining the grafts were removed from all recipients and 6 recipients were regrafted in the contralateral foot-pad with a second PVG NNH. Of the remaining recipients, 6 were similarly regrafted after a further 3 days and 6 were not regrafted. Survival times of all grafts were monitored and appear in Table 2. Control recipients, which were not regrafted, showed the expected prolonged survival of the primary graft following removal of its draining node (MST 43 [32–74] days). Recipients implanted with a second PVG NNH on the day the node draining the primary graft was removed rejected both primary and secondary grafts with a tempo that was within the range of normal rejection times (Fig. 1). In the group in which implantation of the second PVG NNH was delayed for 3 days after node removal rejection of both primary and secondary grafts was delayed (MST 33 [30–52] and 28 [18–40] days, respectively). The specificity of delayed rejection of secondary grafts implanted 3 days after the removal of the LN draining a primary graft was confirmed by examining the survival of secondary WF grafts in DA recipients from which the node draining a primary PVG graft had been removed. The results appear in Table 2. WF NNHs implanted 3 days after the node draining a PVG NNH had been removed were rejected in first-set tempo (MST 14 [10–14]). The primary PVG NNH showed the expected prolongation of survival (MST 46 [30–66]).

Skin grafts did not show extended survival in recipients in which prolonged survival of NNH grafts had been induced by removal of the PLN. Two groups of 5 DA recipients were grafted with PVG NNHs; in one group the draining PLN was removed 4 days later, and both groups were grafted with PVG skin 10 days later.

The skin grafts in both groups were rejected with an MST of 7 (7) days although the group from which the node had been

TABLE 1. The effect of removal of the PLN draining an NNH allograft on graft survival time in specifically sensitized DA recipients

Primary NNH graft	Secondary NNH graft				
	Donor	Day 4 PLN Removed	Day of graft rejection	MST (range)	P
PVG	PVG	–	10 (2), 13 (2)[a]	11.5 (10–13)	NSD
PVG	PVG	+	10, 12, (3)	12 (10–12)	0.01>P>0.005
WF	PVG	+	19, 22, 28, 31	25 (19–31)	

[a] Numbers in parentheses are number of individuals.

removed showed significantly prolonged NNH graft survival (MST 35 [35–39] days).

Alloimmune Responsiveness of Lymphocytes from Rats with Prolonged NNH Graft Survival

In order to elucidate the mechanism of prolonged graft survival following node removal, the cellular and humoral responses of recipients in which graft survival had been prolonged by node removal were compared with those of recipients that had rejected a graft.

Adoptive allograft assay. PVG NNHs were grafted into 8 DA recipients, and 4 days later 4 of these recipients had the PLN draining the graft removed. Nineteen days later, when grafts in the latter group were still showing normal ECG activity, and those in the control group had been ECG-negative for 7 days, LNC and SpC were obtained from each group and compared with cells from normal donors for their capacity to restore NNH graft rejection to irradiated DA assay rats.

Groups of 5 DA assay rats were irradiated with 9.0 Gy, grafted with PVG NNHs, and injected with aliquots of 5×10^7 LNC or SpC from each of the experimental groups or from normal DA donors. A further group of DA rats was irradiated and grafted, but not given cells. The grafts in all 7 groups were monitored.

The rejection times appear in Table 3. As expected, irradiated assay rats not restored with cells showed very prolonged survival of the indicator grafts. The MST of grafts in irradiated assay rats given LNC or SpC from donors in which graft survival had been prolonged by removal of the draining node was not significantly different from the MST of grafts in irradiated recipients given cells from normal donors. Recipients of LNC or SpC from donors that had rejected grafts showed significantly accelerated graft rejection compared with that of animals given normal cells.

GVH and MLI assays. LNC and SpC from DA rats in which PVG NNH graft survival had been prolonged to 25 days by removal of the PLN were compared with cells from DA recipients that had been grafted at the same time and had rejected the graft 10 days previously, and cells from normal DA donors in the local GVH assay (Table 4) and in MLI (Fig. 2). In each case, cells were tested for reactivity against specific (PVG) and third-party (BN) alloantigen.

The GVH response of LNC from recipients with prolonged NNH graft survival was similar to that of normal LNC. The response of SpC was specifically increased and resembled that of cells from donors that had rejected a PVG NNH graft (Table 4). LNC from donors with prolonged graft survival showed a normal proliferative response to PVG alloantigen in MLI assays, whereas cells from donors that had rejected a PVG NNH had a specifically reduced response. The results of MLI assays using SpC were difficult to interpret. SpC from animals that had rejected grafts showed increased proliferation in the response to specific and third party antigen. The response of SpC from animals with prolonged graft survival was slightly greater than that of naive cells but less than that of sensitized cells.

Alloantibody response. A total of 8 DA rats were grafted with PVG NNH grafts. Four days later the PLNs draining the grafts of 4 recipients were removed. The nodes were left in situ in 4 control recipients. All animals were bled twice weekly and the sera were assayed for the presence of cytotoxic antibody against PVG alloantigen. The results appear in Figure 3.

In the control group, specific antibody was detectable in the serum 10 days after grafting. Antibody titers remained high until the time of graft rejection (day 20) and fell to undetectable levels during the following 7 days. In recipients from which the PLN had been removed, there was a slight delay in the development of cytotoxic antibody, after which the response was biphasic. Titers fell at the time when antibody ceased to be detected in the serum of the control group but rose again prior

TABLE 2. Effect of removal of the PLN draining a primary NNH allograft on the survival of secondary NNH grafts

Primary graft (day 0)				Secondary graft			
NNH donor	PLN removed	MST (range)	P	NNH donor	Day implanted	MST (range)	P
PVG	+	43 (32–74)	0.01>P>0.005				
PVG	+	21 (21)		PVG	4	17 (13–17)	
PVG	+	33 (30–52)	NSD	PVG	7	28 (18–40)	0.01>P>0.005
PVG	+	46 (30–66)	0.01>P>0.005	WF	7	14 (10–14)	NSD
PVG	–	14 (12–26)		WF	0	12 (12)	

TABLE 3. The capacity of cells from NNH-grafted donors to adoptively restore NNH allograft rejection to irradiated syngeneic recipients

NNH grafted donor		Cell source	Day of graft rejection (number of recipients)	MST (range) of NNH grafts in irradiated recipients	P
Day 4 PLN removed	Graft rejected				
		—[a]	45, 47, 51, 63, 70	51 (45–70)	
		LN[b]	21, 30, 42, 45, 50	42 (21–50)	e
+	–	LN	35 (2), 37, 40, 45	36 (35–45)	c
–	+	LN	14, 17, 19, 23, 28	19 (14–28)	d
		SP[b]	28, 30, 35, 42, 46	35 (28–46)	
+	–	SP	29, 34 (2), 45	34 (29–45)	c
–	+	SP	19, 21, 26 (2)	23.5 (19–26)	d

[a] Unrestored control recipient.
[b] Normal DA donor.
[c] Survival time, NSD from control group, given cells from normal donor.
[d] Survival time significantly different (0.01>P>0.005) from control group given cells from normal donor.
[e] Survival time significantly different (0.05>P>0.01) from group not restored with cells.

TABLE 4. The local GVH responsiveness of cells from NNH-grafted donors

NNH grafted donor		Cell source	PLN weight (mg) [mean ± SD]			
Day 4 PLN removed	Graft rejected		DA×PVG F_1 hybrid	P^b	DA×BN F_1 hybrid	P^b
		LN[a]	33.0±2.2		69.7±4.4	
+	−	LN	31.7±3.7	NSD	51.6±9.0	NSD
−	+	LN	44.6±4.3	$0.02>P>0.01$	66.1±4.1	NSD
		SP[a]	12.9±0.8		60.0±2.3	
+	−	SP	19.6±1.7	$0.005>P>.001$	57.8±6.2	NSD
−	+	SP	20.0±1.6	$0.005>P>.001$		

[a] Cells from normal ungrafted DA rats.

[b] P values were calculated using the Student's t test, and in each case relate to the difference between the indicated PLN weight and the control values resulting from the injection of the same number of cells from ungrafted DA rats.

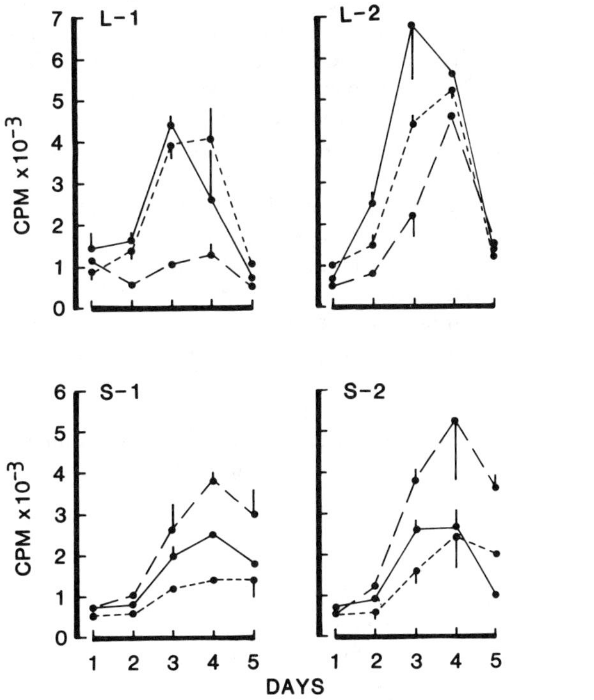

FIGURE 2. The MLI responsiveness of cells from NNH grafted donors. The MLI responsiveness of cells from DA recipients in which PVG NNH graft survival was prolonged to >24 days by removal of the PLN 4 days after grafting (——) was compared with the responsiveness of cells from recipients that had rejected their grafts (– – –) and cells from normal donors (- - - - -). The responsiveness of LNC (L) and SpC (S) against PVG (1) and BN (2) stimulator cells is shown. LNC from donors with prolonged graft survival show normal MLI responsiveness and SpC show a slight increase in the response to PVG alloantigen. LNC from donors that have rejected an NNH graft show a specifically decreased response to PVG; the response of SpC from these donors to specific (PVG) and third-party (BN) alloantigens is increased.

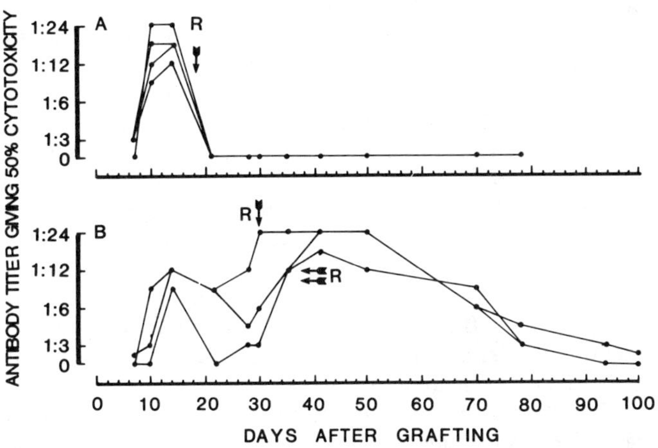

FIGURE 3. Specific alloantibody response in serum of DA recipients of PVG NNH allografts. (A) In control recipients alloantibody was detectable 7 days after grafting. The titer was maximal several days before the time of graft rejection (R ➼), after which it rapidly fell to undetectable levels. (B) Recipients from which the PLN had been removed 4 days after grafting showed a slight delay in the appearance of specific alloantibody in the serum. Titers were lower than those in the control group and fell slightly at the time grafts in the control group rejected, but rose again at the time their own grafts were rejected. Antibody was detectable in the serum for 50 days after graft rejection.

to graft rejection (29–37 days) and thereafter antibody remained detectable for more than 50 days.

DISCUSSION

Regional lymph nodes play a vital role in the immune response to peripheral antigen. Studies of the efferent lymph from the node draining a site of antigenic challenge have suggested that the normal development and systemic propagation of the immune response to protein antigens are critically dependent upon the temporal and anatomical relationships between peripheral antigen, the regional node, and the secondary nodes (*9*). There is abundant evidence that the normal development of the immune response to freely grafted tissue is dependent on lymphatic connections between the graft bed and lymphoid tissue. Skin grafts on sites with absent or poor lymphatic drainage enjoy prolonged survival (*10, 11*) and if lymphatic drainage between a skin graft and the draining LN is temporarily interrupted, graft rejection is delayed by the time required for alternative drainage to be established (*12*). The plantar space in the rat drains by a single lymphatic vessel to the PLN (*13*). As removal of the PLN only briefly interrupts the lymphatic connections from the foot-pad (*4*), it is obvious that prolonged graft survival following node removal must be the result of the actual loss of the node and/or lymphatic disruption at a critical point in the sequence of events leading to immune induction. The assumption that node removal specifically interferes with the inductive phase of the immune response is supported by the finding that node removal has no effect on graft survival in sensitized hosts.

The mechanism by which node removal interferes with induction may depend upon the loss of effective antigenic stimulation. In recent years it has been postulated that MHC class-II-antigen–bearing cells in grafted tissues are the major antigenic stimulus. Grafts depleted of passenger leukocytes (*14*) or dendritic cells (*15*) enjoy prolonged survival. Compared with skin or adult heart tissue, rat NNH tissue contains relatively few class-II-positive cells (unpublished observation), and this may account for the slow first set rejection tempo of NNH grafts relative to that of skin or adult heart grafts (*7, 16*). It may also be relevant to the effect of node removal on NNH graft survival. The MHC class-II-bearing dendritic cells, which are thought to be essential for normal immune induction, have a high rate of turnover in the tissues (*17*). Removal of the node draining an NNH graft 4 days after grafting would remove both graft antigen, which has reached the node by that time, and host cells, which have made initial contact with antigen either in the graft or in the node. This would effectively abort the inductive events essential for the ultimate production of effector and memory cells. If, by the time lymphatic connections are reestablished, the graft no longer contains sufficient antigen-presenting cells to reinitiate immune induction, it would not be rejected.

Such loss of immunogenicity could account for the survival of primary grafts following removal of the draining node but some other mechanism must be postulated to explain the specifically prolonged survival of secondary grafts with intact draining nodes. If the latter are implanted on the day the node draining the primary graft is removed, both grafts are rejected but if 3 days are allowed to elapse between node removal and implantation of the secondary graft, both the primary and the secondary grafts show prolonged survival in spite of the presence of the node draining the latter.

These findings suggest that a state of specific immunosuppression develops following node removal. The observation that, following node removal, animals mount a measurable alloantibody response—although graft rejection is significantly delayed—suggests that suppression might be antibody-mediated.

The humoral immune response in allograft recipients varies according to the nature of the grafted tissue, the method of grafting, and the antigens involved (*18*). It is well recognized that enhanced recipients do manifest cytotoxic antigraft antibody responses in the presence of surviving grafts, although antibodies are not always detectable throughout the life of the graft (*18*). In normal recipients of NNH grafts, serum antibody levels fall rapidly after graft rejection. In recipients from which the node draining the graft is removed there is a slight delay in the appearance of cytotoxic alloantibodies. After an initial peak, the antibody titers fall, but they rise again between 30 and 37 days when the grafts are rejected. Cytotoxic alloantibody levels subsequently remain elevated for a further 50 days. The initial delayed and reduced antibody response in these animals is similar to the response in actively enhanced animals (*18*). The prolonged time-course of the humoral response may be a consequence of prolonged exposure to the MHC class I antigens expressed on the long-surviving grafts.

The reactivity of cells from rats with long-surviving grafts is similar to that of animals bearing enhanced grafts (*19*). Proliferative responses in the local GVH assay and in MLI assays are normal or slightly increased, confirming that the cell populations are not clonally deleted (*4*), and the adoptive allograft assay reveals no evidence for the presence of sensitized T cells (*20*) or suppressor cells (*21*). Irradiated assay rats restored with LNC or SpC from animals with long-surviving grafts reject their indicator grafts with the same tempo as control recipients restored with the same number of cells from normal donors.

The observation that animals with long-surviving primary grafts reject secondary skin grafts, although they retain secondary NNH grafts, is not inconsistent with enhancement (*18*). Furthermore, as both skin and NNH grafts are free grafts, it supports the view that factors related to the mode of transplantation are not the only determinants of susceptibility to enhancement (*18*). We suggest that the mechanism by which specific immunosuppression is induced by node removal is similar to that operating in actively induced enhancement.

We have previously shown that anastomoses between the host circulation and vessels in NNH grafts are established within 2 to 4 days of grafting (*4*). Thus small amounts of graft antigen could directly enter the host circulation at the time when the induction of cell-mediated immunity in the regional node has been aborted by node removal. By the time lymphatic connections between the graft and the remaining lymphoid tissue are reestablished, small amounts of circulating alloantigen may have induced sufficient enhancing antibody to prevent immune induction by the original, now suboptimally, immunogenic graft. By day 7 actively induced antibody-mediated enhancement might be sufficiently established to prevent induction of cell-mediated immunity by secondary grafts of NNH tissue with intact draining nodes.

We thus propose that immunosuppression following node removal is induced and maintained by circulating antibody produced in response to small amounts of antigen released from the graft into the circulation at a time when normal cell-mediated immunity has been aborted by the removal of the draining node.

REFERENCES

1. Billingham RE, Brent L, Medawar PB. Quantitative studies on tissue transplantation immunity. II. The origin, strength and duration of actively and adoptively acquired immunity. Proc R Soc Lond (Biol) 1954; 143: 58.
2. Scothorne RJ, McGregor IA. Cellular changes in lymph nodes and spleen following skin homografting in the rabbit. J Anat 1955; 89: 283.
3. Pedersen NC, Adams EP, Morris B. The response of the lymphoid system to renal allografts in sheep. Transplantation 1975; 19: 400.
4. Dorsch S, Wotherspoon J, Keith I, Roser B. The role of the regional lymph node in the response to secondarily vascularised grafts. Transplantation 1983; 35: 231.
5. Fulmer RI, Cramer AT, Liebelt RA, Liebelt AG. Transplantation of cardiac tissue into the mouse ear. Am J Anat 1963; 113: 273.
6. Ford WL, Burr W, Simonsen M. A lymph node weight assay for the graft versus host activity of rat lymphoid cells. Transplantation 1970; 10: 258.
7. Dorsch S, Roser B. The adoptive transfer of first set allograft responses by recirculating small lymphocytes in the rat. Aust J Exp Biol Med Sci 1974; 52: 33.
8. Howard JC, Scott DW. The identification of sera distinguishing marrow derived and thymus derived lymphocytes in the rat thoracic duct. Immunology 1974; 27: 903.
9. Fahy VA, Gerber HA, Morris B, Trevella W, Zukoski CF. The function of lymph nodes in the formulation of lymph. Monogr Allergy 1980; 16: 82.
10. Barker CF, Billginham RE. Immunologically privileged sites. Adv Immunol 1977; 25: 1.
11. Tilney NL, Gowans JL. The sensitisation of rats by allografts

transplanted on alymphatic pedicles of skin. J Exp Med 1971; 133: 951.
12. Lambert PB, Frank HA, Bellman S. Farnsworth D. The role of the lymph trunks in the response to allogeneic skin transplants. Transplantation 1965; 3: 62.
13. Tilney NL. Patterns of lymphatic drainage in the adult laboratory rat. J Anat 1971; 109: 369.
14. Lafferty KJ, Prowse SJ, Simeonovic CJ, Warren HS. Immunology of tissue transplantation: a return to the passenger leukocyte concept. Annu Rev Immunol 1983; 1: 143.
15. Lechler RI, Batchelor JR. Restoration of immunogenicity to passenger cell depleted kidney allografts by the addition of donor strain dendritic cells. J Exp Med 1982; 155: 31.
16. Hall BM, Dorsch S, Roser B. The cellular basis of allograft rejection in vivo. I. The cellular requirements for the first set rejection of heart grafts. J Exp Med 1978; 148: 878.
17. Harte DNJ, Fabre JW. Demonstration and characterization of Ia positive dendritic cells in the interstitial connective tissues of rat heart and other tissues but not brain. J Exp Med 1981; 154: 347.
18. Carpenter CB, d'Apice AJF, Abbas AK. Antibodies in the rejection and enhancement of organ allografts. Adv Immunol 1976; 22: 1.
19. Hall BM. The cellular basis of the maintenance of passive enhancement. Transplant Proc 1981; 13: 640.
20. Hall BM, Dorsch S, Roser B. The cellular basis of allograft rejection in vivo. II. The nature of memory cells mediating second set heart graft rejection. J Exp Med 1978; 148: 890.
21. Dorsch S, Roser B. Recirculating suppressor T cells in transplantation tolerance. J Exp Med 1977; 145: 1144.

Received 29 October 1985.
Accepted 30 January 1986.

0041-1337/86/4205-0537$02.00/0
TRANSPLANTATION Vol. 42, No. 5

Printed in U.S.A.

ALLOGENEIC HEPATOCYTE TRANSPLANTATION IN THE RAT SPLEEN UNDER CYCLOSPORINE IMMUNOSUPPRESSION[1]

LEONARD MAKOWKA,[2,3] GEORGE LEE,[4] CHRISTOPHER S. COBOURN,[2] EMMANUEL FARBER,[4] JUDITH A. FALK,[2] AND RUDOLF E. FALK[2,5]

Departments of Surgery and Pathology, University of Toronto, Toronto, Ontario, Canada

An innovative approach for stimulating the rapid growth of allogeneic hepatocytes implanted into splenic tissue with maintenance of the structural integrity is described. Single cell suspensions of hepatocytes from normal male ACI-strain rats (RTI[a]) were injected (2×10^6 cells) into the spleen of allogeneic male Fischer (RTI[1]) recipient rats. A 70% partial hepatectomy (PH) was performed at the same time as hepatocyte transplantation. Animals were treated for 4 days prior to, and 1 day after, transplantation with a feeding regimen containing 0.05% 2-acetylaminofluorene (AAF) to inhibit regeneration of the residual host liver. Animals received cyclosporine (CsA) 3 mg/kg/day s.c. posttransplantation. Histological examination of a standard longitudinal section of the recipient spleen two days posttransplant revealed an approximately 0.54-mm^2 area replaced by hepatocytes. By 7 days this had increased to $0.97\pm.15$ mm^2. Without CsA administration, hepatocytes were undetected at 7 days. Both PH and AAF treatment were necessary for successful colonization and sustained proliferation. Withdrawal of CsA treatment at 10 days after transplantation resulted in rapid rejection of established hepatocytes. This study demonstrates that rapid colonization of the rat spleen with allogeneic hepatocytes can be achieved, and that the viability and structural integrity of these transplanted cells can be maintained for at least 14 days using cyclosporine immunosuppression.

[1] This work was supported by the Medical Research Council of Canada.
[2] Department of Surgery, University of Toronto, Toronto, Ontario, Canada.
[3] Recipient of a Centennial Fellowship from the Medical Research Council of Canada. Present Address: Department of Transplantation Surgery, University of Pittsburgh, Pittsburgh PA, 15213.
[4] Department of Pathology, University of Toronto, Toronto, Ontario, Canada.
[5] Address reprint requests to: R.E. Falk, M.D., Department of General Surgery, 1-046 Mullock-Larkin Wing, Toronto General Hospital, Toronto, Ontario, Canada M5G-2C4. Dr. Falk is a Career investigator with the Medical Research Council of Canada.

Numerous studies have established the spleen as a favorable site for the survival and growth of single-cell suspensions of hepatocytes (*1–3*). Dispersed hepatocytes transplanted into the spleen of syngeneic recipients engrafted and proliferated in the splenic parenchyma and maintained functional (*4*) and structural integrity (*5*). We have confirmed these studies and further demonstrated that hepatocytes proliferating in the spleen retain the activities of several enzymes—such as phosphatase, nonspecific esterase, and epoxide hydrolase—as well as those enzymes participating in the metabolic detoxification of the hepatotoxin carbon tetrachloride (Lee G., unpublished observation). These cells resembled normal hepatocytes by light and electron microscopic evaluation, with a normal array of organelles and the presence of intracytoplasmic glycogen (*6*). We have monitored the growth characteristics of intrasplenic transplanted hepatocytes over the entire life span of recipient rats (i.e., 2–3 years), and the extent of growth ranged from 20–40% of the splenic volume, which is in accordance with the observations made by Mito et al. (7). In no instances have there been any morphological or behavioral changes in the hepatocytes suggesting malignant transformation. One interesting phenomenon observed in our studies was that hepatocytes maintained in rat spleens responded to partial hepatectomy (PH)* performed upon the recipient by proliferating (6). This was confirmed by the demonstration of incorporation of tritiated thymidine in their nuclei and the presence of numerous mitoses. These findings suggested that the "signal" for proliferation in response to partial hepatectomy was not localized, but rather systemic. This proliferation was maintained for a more prolonged period only if the rats had been treated with a diet containing 0.05% 2-acetylaminofluorene (AAF), which acted by inhibiting the regenerative response of the host liver and thereby prolonging the proliferative stimulus to the transplanted cells (6).

The present studies were performed to determine if allogeneic hepatocytes could be similarly transplanted and maintained in the spleen of recipient rats immunosuppressed by cyclosporine (CsA). The implications of these studies for advancing the understanding of the pathophysiology and the treatment of liver diseases will be discussed.

MATERIALS AND METHODS

Animals. Male Fischer (F344:RTI[l]) strain rats, weighing 130–150 g were used as recipients in all studies. Male ACI (RTI[a]) strain rats weighing 180–200 g were used as histoincompatable donors of hepatocytes. All animals were acclimatized to a 12-hr light and dark cycle for at least 1 week prior to commencement of experimentation. Water and standard laboratory chow were administered ad libitum.

Drugs. Rat chow containing 0.05% AAF was purchased from Dyets Inc., Bethlehem, PA. CsA was obtained from Sandoz Co., Montreal, Quebec, diluted with saline immediately prior to administration, and given daily by s.c. injection at a dose of 3 mg/kg body weight.

Techniques of intrasplenic hepatocyte transplantation. We have previously described our technique for the intrasplenic transplantation of hepatocytes (6). Briefly this involves the initial disassociation of the donor liver by collagenase digestion into a single-cell suspension, as originally described by Berry and Friend (8). The cell suspension is subsequently subjected to repeated low-speed centrifugation to yield a final fraction enriched with viable hepatocytes. An inoculum of 0.2 ml. containing 2×10^6 viable hepatocytes is injected directly into the splenic parenchyma of recipient rats. A microvascular clamp is temporarily applied to the hilar vessels during the injection procedure and also at the injection site to minimize leakage of cells.

Assessment of hepatocyte growth. A standard longitudinal section (1–2-mm-thick) was cut along the midlongitudinal axis of the spleen and fixed in 10% buffered formalin for routine histological examination. Morphometric analysis was carried out on a Leitz ASM Image Analyzer on standard hematoxylin-and-eosin–stained sections. The total area of hepatocytes in relation to a standard section of spleen was determined in square millimeters and expressed as the mean ± standard error. When only 2 animals were analyzed, individual values as well as the mean are given without SE.

Experimental design. Experiment 1: Recipient rats (F344) with donor (ACI) liver cells transplanted into the spleen were divided into two groups. In group A, the recipients received daily CsA beginning at the time of hepatocyte transplantation. In group B, the recipient rats received saline and served as the control. All animals were sacrificed at 7 days posttransplantation and the spleens analyzed for the presence of hepatocytes.

Experiment 2: Recipient rats were subjected to 70% PH using the technique originally described by Higgins and Anderson (9), and then immediately underwent intrasplenic hepatocyte transplantation. They were then divided into two groups. In group A, the recipient rats received daily CsA, while recipients in group B received an equivalent amount of saline. Animals were sacrificed at 2, 4, and 7 days posttransplantation.

Experiment 3: All recipient rats were fed a dietary regimen containing AAF for 5 days. On the fourth day, all recipients underwent PH and immediately received an injection of donor liver cells directly into the spleen. The recipients were divided into two groups. In group A, the recipients received daily CsA treatment while recipients in group B received saline. Animals were sacrificed at 2 and 7 days posttransplantation.

Experiment 4: All recipients received treatment similar to that described in experiment 3, except that PH was not performed. Animals were sacrificed at 2 and 7 days posttransplantation.

Experiment 5: All recipients were treated according to the protocol described in experiment 3, except that all recipients received daily administration of CsA. At 7 days posttransplantation, the recipients were divided into two groups. In group A, the recipients continued to receive daily CsA injections. In group B, CsA was withdrawn. Animals were sacrificed at 2, 4, 7, 10, and 14 days posttransplantation.

RESULTS

Experiment 1 (Fig. 1). Hepatocytes were not detected at either 2 or 7 days after transplantation regardless of CsA administration.

Experiment 2 (Fig. 2). At 2 days posttransplantation colonies of hepatocytes were detected in both groups of recipients. However, at days 4 and 7, hepatocytes were present only in recipients receiving CsA. This observation suggests that PH is a requirement for the establishment of the hepatocytes in the spleen, and that rejection of the grafted hepatocytes occurred between days 2 and 4 posttransplantation in nonimmunosuppressed recipients. Furthermore, there was no appreciable in-

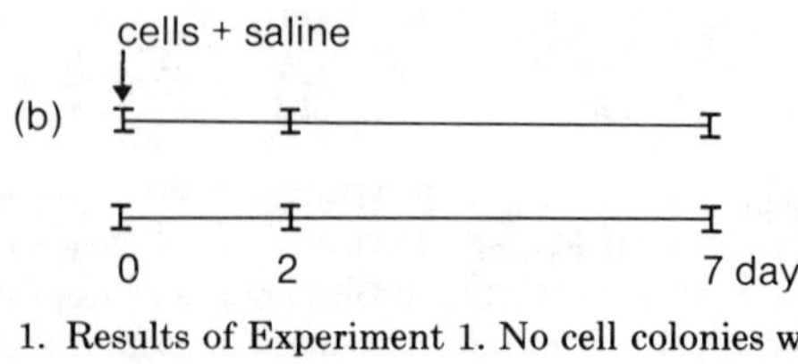

FIGURE 1. Results of Experiment 1. No cell colonies were detected at either 2 or 7 days; (CsA) cyclosporine.

* Abbreviations used: AAF, 2-acetylaminofluorene; CsA, cyclosporine; HPF, hepatocyte proliferation factor; PH, partial hepatectomy.

Experiment 2

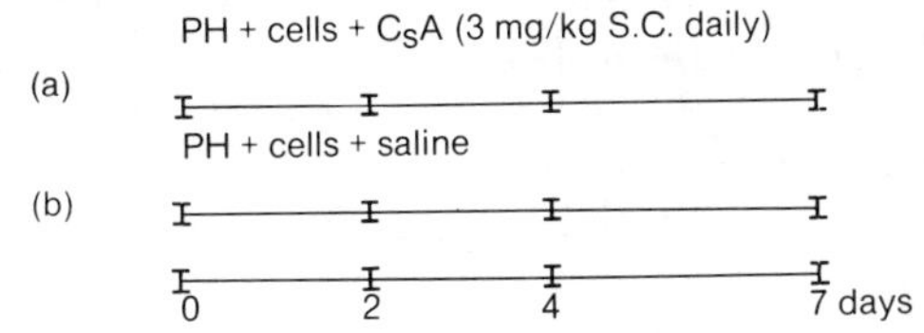

Results:

Time after Transplantation (days)	Total area of a standard spleen section colonised by hepatocytes. ($mm^2 \pm$ SE)	
	With C_SA	Without C_SA
2	0.35 0.16 x = 0.26	0.15 0.66 x = 0.41
4	0.23 ± .04(3)	NOT detectable (3)
7	0.21 ± .08(4)	NOT detectable (6)

FIGURE 2. Results of experiment 2; (CsA) cyclosporine; (PH) 70% partial hepatectomy, No. in brackets = No. of rats analyzed.

Experiment 3

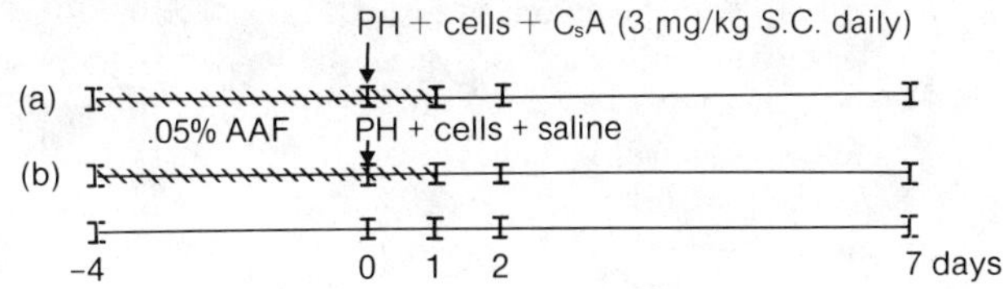

Results:

Time after Transplantation (days)	Total area of a standard spleen section colonised by hepatocytes. ($mm^2 \pm$ SE)	
	With C_SA	Without C_SA
2	0.42 0.66 x = 0.54	0.39 0.53 x = 0.46
7	0.97 ± .15(7)	NOT detectable (8)

FIGURE 3. Results of experiment 3; (CsA) cyclosporine; (PH) 70% partial hepatectomy; (AAF) 0.05% 2-acetylaminofluorene; No. in brackets = No. of rats analyzed.

crease in the extent of liver growth between days 2 and 7 in the immunosuppressed recipients (0.26 vs. 0.21 mm^2).

Experiment 3 (Fig. 3). At 2 days posttransplantation colonies of hepatocytes were detected in both groups of recipients, regardless of CsA administration (0.54 mm^2 and 0.46 mm^2). However at day 7, hepatocytes were present only in CsA-treated recipients. The extent of colonization in the immunosuppressed recipients at day 7 was about 5-fold greater than that observed in recipients in experiment 2, in which the recipient received PH without AAF treatment (0.97±0.15 mm^2 vs. 0.21 mm^2). In addition to the difference in the extent of growth, morphologic differences were also observed in the hepatocytes. In experiment 2, in which recipients received PH but no AAF treatment, the transplanted hepatocytes were arranged in the spleen as small islands containing 10–15 cells. The cells were atrophic and contained scanty cytoplasm. Mitoses were rarely seen (Fig. 4). In contrast, hepatocytes transplanted into the spleen under the PH and AAF protocol (experiment 3), were arranged in much larger aggregates (Fig. 5). Furthermore, the cells retained their normal morphology, with large nuclei and abundant cytoplasm. Mitoses were frequently encountered. This finding suggests that although PH is critical for the initial establishment of allogeneic hepatocytes in the spleen, appreciable growth of hepatocytes with normal morphology is achieved only when the proliferative stimulus provided by PH is prolonged by treatment with the AAF diet (Fig. 3B).

Experiment 4 (Fig. 6). Hepatocytes were not detected in either group of rats. This is consistent with the hypothesis proposed earlier that PH is essential for the initial establishment of allogeneic hepatocytes in the spleen.

Experiment 5 (Fig. 7). This experiment was designed to determine if maintenance of transplanted hepatocytes in the spleen required the continuous administration of CsA. Hepatocytes were present in the spleens of both groups of animals at 10 days posttransplantation (0.95±0.28 mm^2 and 0.64±0.20 mm^2) but were present on day 14 only in the group of rats that continued to receive daily CsA (0.97±0.49 mm^2 vs. not detectable). This suggests that CsA is necessary for the continued proliferation and viability of the transplanted hepatocytes and that its withdrawal leads to rejection of the hepatocytes. Note also that there was continued proliferation of hepatocytes up to 7 days in the presence of AAF treatment, which is consistent with the results of experiment 3.

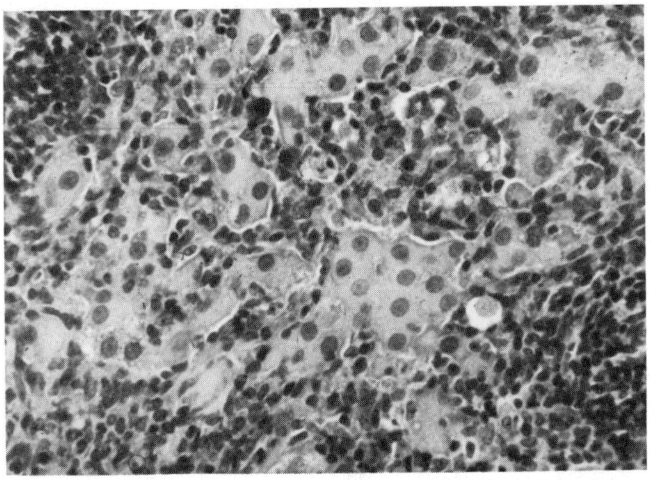

FIGURE 4. Hepatocytes transplanted into the splenic pulp of rats who received PH but not AAF. Notice the atrophic appearance and scanty cytoplasm. (H&E; ×375).

DISCUSSION

The experimental transplantation of hepatocytes, either as liver fragments or single-cell suspensions, into various ectopic sites in autologous and syngeneic recipients has been performed by several investigators in the past (*10–12*). This approach has been employed in our earlier studies as a means of analyzing various aspects of hepatic biology and physiology—in particular, mechanisms relating to liver regeneration and carcinogenesis (*13*). Recent studies have considered clinically oriented applications of hepatocyte transplantation—such as a method of replacement therapy for hepatic enzyme deficient diseases (*14*) and as a method of treatment of acute, fulminant hepatic failure (*15*). We recently described a new approach for stimulating the rapid growth of transplanted rat hepatocytes in the spleen of syngeneic recipients (*6*). This consisted of performing a 70% PH in the recipient rats immediately before intrasplenic hepatocyte transplantation. The proliferative stimulus created was sustained by inhibiting the host's residual liver fragment from regenerating by treating the recipients with a dietary regimen containing 0.05% AAF for one week before and one week after transplantation. Histological examination one week

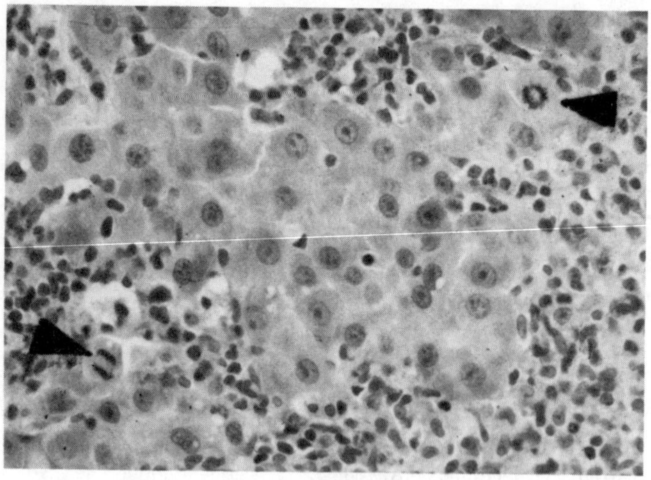

FIGURE 5. Hepatocytes transplanted into the splenic pulp of rats treated with PH and AAF. These cells are arranged in larger aggregates than those in Fig. 2 and have large nuclei. Mitoses are indicated by the arrows. (H&E; ×375).

Experiment 4

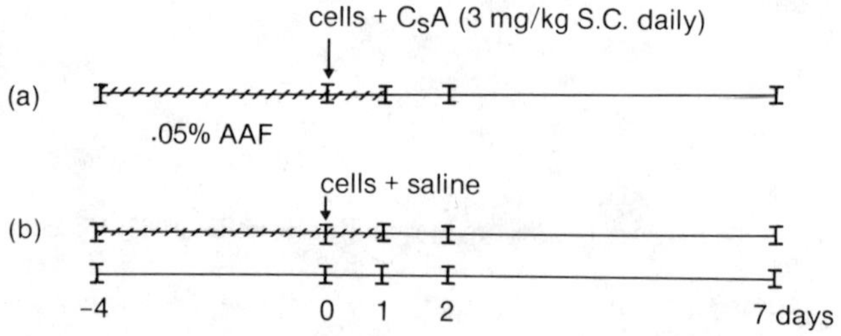

Results: No cell colonies were detected at either 2 or 7 days post-transplanatation.

FIGURE 6. Results of experiment 4; (CsA) cyclosporine; (AAF) 0.05% 2-acetylaminofluorene.

after transplantation revealed a 10-fold increase in liver mass in the spleens of such recipients when compared with recipients that were only partially hepatectomized but did not receive AAF. Therefore, it was demonstrated that—by maintaining a continuous proliferative stimulus—rapid hepatization of the spleen with viable syngeneic hepatocytes was produced.

This approach was continued in the present set of experiments and extended to study the feasibility of maintaining allogeneic hepatocytes in the spleen using CsA-induced immunosuppression. Results from our present experiments confirm that pretreatment with a dietary regimen of AAF is necessary to maintain the hepatic regenerative stimulus induced by a 70% partial hepatectomy in the donor. Treatment with AAF did not appear to inhibit the proliferation of the transplanted intrasplenic hepatocytes. Previous work has shown that in order for the AAF to inhibit proliferation, it must be given for 4–7 days prior to the onset of the proliferative stimulus. In addition, we have also shown that dividing hepatocytes are resistant to the inhibiting effect of AAF (*16*). The newly transplanted hepatocytes were not exposed to the AAF for a sufficient length of time, and were provided with the proliferative stimulus of partial hepatectomy immediately. Therefore

Experiment 5

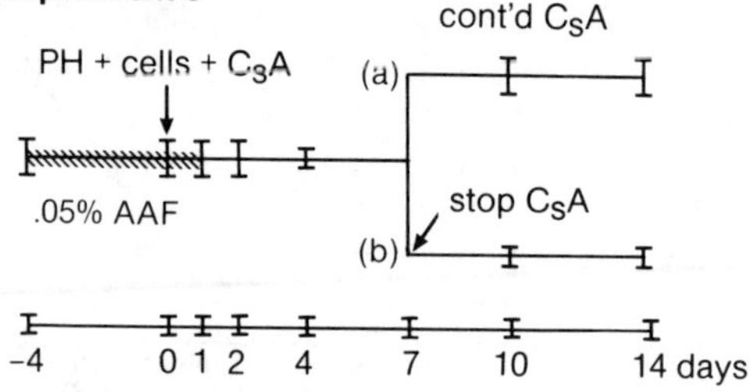

Results:

Effect of withdrawal of C_SA on established allogeneic hepatocytes in spleen. ($mm^2 \pm$ SE)

2 days	4 days	7 days	10 days	14 days
0.42, 0.60, $\bar{x}$ = 0.51	0.38, 0.59, $\bar{x}$ = 0.49	0.83 ± 0.08 (6)	cont'd C_SA: 0.95 ± 0.28 (3)	0.97 ± 0.49 (3)
			stop C_SA: 0.64 ± 0.23 (3)	NOT detectable (3)

FIGURE 7. Results of experiment 5; (CsA) cyclosporine; (PH) 70% partial hepatectomy; (AAF) 0.05% 2-acetylaminofluorene; No. in brackets = No. of rats analyzed.

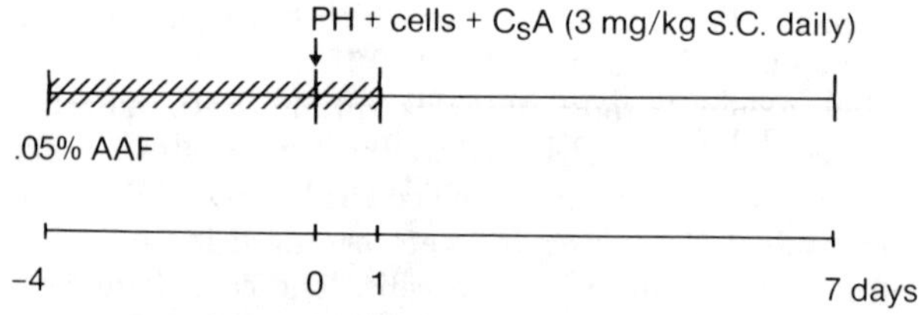

FIGURE 8. Treatment protocol for recipient rats for successful establishment and growth of allogeneic hepatocytes in spleens; (CsA) cyclosporine, (PH) 70% partial hepatectomy; (AAF) 0.05% 2-acetylaminofluorene.

they were able to show the desired growth within the spleen.

The hepatectomy was necessary to permit the initial, successful intrasplenic establishment of the hepatocytes. Continued daily CsA is essential to maintain established hepatocytes in this allogeneic model. Withdrawal of CsA leads to rapid disappearance and presumably rejection of the hepatocytes. This observation is in accordance with the recent report by Ebata et al. (*17*) that allogeneic intrasplenic hepatocytes were rejected after 2–4 days. A summary of the most successful protocol used in our present studies is depicted in Fig. 8.

This study provides a further advance toward the clinical application of hepatocyte transplantation. Maintenance of viability and continued proliferation using CsA immunosuppression in an allogeneic, rather than syngeneic, model correlates more closely with potential human hepatocyte transplantation. Congenital hepatic enzyme deficiencies such as Crigler-Najjar syndrome, Rotor syndrome, and alpha-1-antitrypsin deficiency provide suitable conditions for such application. The intraportal route of hepatocyte administration may be limited by the quantity of hepatocytes that can be transplanted by this route without interfering with the host liver blood supply (*18*), as well as by the development of coagulopathy and portal hypertension, as has already been described for pancreatic islet cell transplantation via this route (*19*). Long-term survival of intrasplenic syngeneic hepatocytes has been demonstrated in numerous reports (*5, 6, 20*). Experience with intrasplenic allogeneic hepatocyte transplantation combined with immunosuppression has not yet been described. Sutherland et al. have used heterozygous donors for hepatocyte transplantation into the homozygous Gunn rat, which lacks bilirubin uridine diphosphate glucuronyl transferase, using both the intraportal (*21*) and the intrasplenic routes (*18*). These authors achieved beneficial but temporary results consisting of transient decrease in the bilirubin levels (*18*). The potential for a more sustained decrease in bilirubin levels in Gunn rats using the methods of allogeneic hepatocyte transplantation described here is currently being evaluated in our laboratory.

Hepatocyte transplantation has been successfully applied as therapy for acute hepatic failure by Cuervas-Mons et al. (*22*). However their model is limited by the use of syngeneic cells. The model reported here may prove to be the next logical application for the treatment of this condition.

This technique should also allow further evaluation of hepatic-derived growth factors, which are currently being evaluated by many authors as well as ourselves (*23–25*). The availability of a factor capable of stimulating hepatocyte proliferation may replace the need for the PH and AAF. These interventions are cumbersome, potentially dangerous (i.e., AAF is a known carcinogen), and limit the clinical usefulness of this therapy. Hepatocyte proliferation factor(s) (HPF) have been shown to stimulate hepatic growth, as measured by in vivo and in vitro assays (*23*). They appear to be heat stable and have a molecular weight of approximately 26,000 (*24*). Regular i.p. injections of HPF after intrasplenic hepatocyte transplantation may result in hepatocyte proliferation as seen in this model, and is currently being evaluated.

In summary, this report has demonstrated the successful engraftment and maintenance of allogeneic hepatocytes in the spleen of rats with the ability to induce marked proliferation. These hepatocytes can remain viable for at least 14 days when CsA immunosuppression is maintained. Further characterization and study of this and similar models may give insight into the understanding of normal and abnormal liver pathophysiology. It may also allow the development of a clinically applicable form of treatment for situations requiring hepatic enzyme replacement or for acute hepatic failure. Characterization of the rejection reaction in the nonimmunosuppressed rats would provide a good model to study the cellular events in liver rejection.

REFERENCES

1. Mito M, Ebata H, Onishi T, Kusano M, Ono M. Survival of hepatocytes transplanted into the spleens of rats and dogs. Eur Surg Res 1977; 9: 166.
2. Mito M, Ebata M, Kusano T, Onishi T, Hiratsuka M, Saito T. Studies on ectopic liver utilizing hepatocyte transplantation into the rat spleen. Transplant Proc 1979; 1: 585.
3. Woods RJ, Fuller BJ, Attenburrow D, Nutt LH, Hobbs KEF. Functional assessment of hepatocytes after transplantation into rat spleen. Transplantation 1982; 33: 123.
4. Cuervas-Mons V, Cienfuegos J, Maganto P, et al. Long-term evaluation of isolated syngeneic hepatocytes transplanted into the normal rat spleen by Tc-99M-HIDA scintigraphy. Transplantation 1985; 39: 87.
5. Kusano M, Mito M. Observation of long-survived isolated hepatocytes inoculated into rat spleen. Gastroenterology 1982; 82: 616.
6. Finkelstein SD, Lee G, Medline A, et al. An experimental method for rapid growth of liver in spleen. Am J Pathol 1983; 110: 119.
7. Mito M, Ebata H, Kusano M, Onishi T, Saito T, Sakamato S. Morphology and function of isolated hepatocytes transplanted into the rat spleen. Transplantation 1979; 28: 499.
8. Berry MN, Friend SD. High-yield preparation of isolated rat liver parenchymal cells: a biochemical and fine structural study. J Cell Biol 1969; 43: 506.
9. Higgins GM, Anderson RM. Experimental pathology of the liver. Arch Pathol 1931; 12: 186.
10. Makowka L, Rotstein RE, Falk RE, et al. Allogeneic and xenogeneic hepatocyte transplantation. Transplant Proceed 1981; 13: 855.
11. Sutherland DER, Numata M, Matas AJ, Simmons RL, Najarian JS. Hepatocellular transplantation in acute liver failure. Surgery 1977; 82: 124.
12. Rugstad HE, Robinson SH, Yannoni C, Tashjian AH. Transfer of bilirubin uridine diphosphate-glucuronyltransferase to enzyme-deficient rats. Science 1970; 170: 553.
13. Lee G, Medline A, Finkelstein S, Makowka L, Farber E. Transplantation of hepatocytes from normal and preneoplastic livers into spleens of syngeneic host rats. Transplantation 1983; 36: 218.
14. Groth CG, Arborgh B, Bjorken C, Sundberg B, Lundgren G. Correction of hyperbilirubinemia in the glucuronyltransferase-deficient rat by intraportal hepatocyte transplantation. Transplant Proc 1977; 9: 313.
15. Baumgartner D, LaPlante-O'Neill PM, Sutherland DER, Najarian JS. Effects of intrasplenic injection of hepatocytes, hepatocyte fragments and hepatocyte culture supernatants on D-galactosamine induced liver failure in rats. Eur Surg Res 1983; 15: 129.
16. Roberts E, Ahluwalia MB, Lee G, Chan C, Sarma DSR, Farber E. Resistance to hepatotoxins acquired by hepatocytes during liver regeneration. Cancer Res 1983; 43: 28.
17. Ebata H, Oikawa I, Mito M. Rejection of allogeneic hepatocytes and fetal hepatic tissue transplanted into the rat spleen. Transplantation 1985; 39: 221.
18. Sutherland DER, Sommer BG, Hong C, Numata M, Najarian JS. Liver cell transplantation. Hepatic biliary and pancreatic surgery. Chicago: Year Book, 1980.
19. Traverso LW, Abou-Zamzam AM, Longmire WP Jr. Human pancreatic cell autotransplantation following total pancreatectomy. Ann Surg 1981; 193: 191.
20. Ebata H, Mito M. Intrasplenic fetal rat hepatic tissue isotransplantation. Transplantation 1985; 39: 77.
21. Matas AJ, Sutherland DER, Steffes MW, et al. Hepatocellular transplantation for metabolic deficiencies: decrease of plasma bilirubin in Gunn rats. Science 1976; 192: 892.
22. Cuervas-Mons V, Cienfuegos P, Maganto P, et al. Time-related efficacy of liver cell isografts in fulminant hepatic failure. Transplantation 1984; 38: 23.
23. Schwartz LC, Makowka L, Falk JA, Falk RE. The characterization and partial purification of hepatocyte proliferation factor, (in press).
24. Morley CGD, Kingdon HS. Identification and partial characterization of a DNA synthesis stimulating factor from the serum of partially hepatectomized rats. Biochem Biophys Acta 1973; 308: 260.
25. LaBreque DR. In vitro stimulation of cell growth by hepatic stimulator substance. Am J Physiol 1982; 242: G289.

Received 20 November 1985.
Accepted 7 February 1986.

0041-1337/86/4205-0542$02.00/0
TRANSPLANTATION
Vol. 42, No. 5

Printed in U.S.A.

FURTHER OBSERVATIONS ON TRANSFUSION COLLAPSE CURVES IN INBRED RATS[1]

MARGARET A. BAIRD[2] AND BARBARA F. HESLOP

Department of Surgery, University of Otago Medical School, Dunedin, New Zealad

Transfused allogeneic red blood cells (RBC) are very rapidly cleared from the host circulation in some strain combinations among inbred rats. The phenomenon, termed *collapse curve clearance*, an analogy with its human counterpart, is spleen-dependent. Allogeneic ^{51}Cr-labeled red cells taken up by the spleen are retained for at least 6 weeks, and appear to represent a pool of intact cells that are destroyed no more quickly than syngeneic red cells. Sequential transfusions delivered at weekly intervals gradually abrogate rapid clearance, but a longer interval between injections allows the collapse curve pattern to persist. Increasing the dosage of donor red cells above the standard dose used in these experiments decreases the clearance rate, while reducing the dosage further accelerates clearance. Several attempts to implicate anti-RBC antibody, and to correlate the presence of such antibody with accelerated clearance, have failed. The grafting of an additional syngeneic spleen neither increases the proportion of allogeneic RBC removed from the circulation, nor reverses a temporary paralysis of the phenomenon induced by red cell overloading. These experiments imply that rapid clearance of allogeneic red cells is not mediated by a purely cellular mechanism, but that it requires a humoral substance that is readily exhausted, but fairly quickly replenished. The possibility that the rat equivalent of the H-2.7 mouse antigen might be responsible was considered, but appropriate experiments on mice have failed to support this idea. The findings in these experiments strengthen the analogy to the clinical event.

In most allogeneic strain combinations among inbred rats, transfused donor red blood cells (RBC)* survive in the host for as long as syngeneic RBC (*1*). However, in 14 of the 78 strain combinations tested, allogeneic RBC are removed very rapidly from the blood (*1*). This accelerated clearance is linked to the major histocompatibility complex of the donor, but not to that of the host. The non–major histocompatibility complex (MHC) rat RBC alloantigens RT2, RT3, and RT8 are not implicated, since most donor/host strain combinations exhibiting rapid clearance share the same antigens at these loci (*2*). A role for the rat equivalent of the mouse H-2.7 antigen (a C4d fragment that becomes passively attached to red cells in some inbred strains [*3*]) has been suggested but not established (*1*): this possibility is further addressed in the present communication. The RBC clearance patterns observed in rats are similar to the collapse curves recorded in hematological literature, where apparently compatible transfused blood is removed very rapidly from the recipient circulation in the absence of detectable antibody (*4*). The human phenomenon is usually associated with the transfusion of small volumes of cells; one study recorded collapse curve clearance in 30% of patients receiving less than 10 ml (*5*), compared with only 5% transfused with therapeutic volumes (*6*). Despite putative host sensitization, successive transfusions from the same donor often survive normally (*5*). The cause of the subnormal red cell survival in man is unknown. Attempts to implicate humoral antibody as a mediator of rapid clearance have so far been unsuccessful in man (*7*), rat (*1*), and mouse, in which abruptly shortened RBC survival has also been observed (*8*).

In this communication we further clarify the mechanism of accelerated clearance of allogeneic RBC. We also examine the possibility that the H-2.7 antigen in mice is a determinant of rapid clearance.

MATERIALS AND METHODS

Animals. All rats were 2–8 months old and came from the departmental colony. The following inbred strains were used, the MHC haplotypes being indicated in parentheses: AS2 ($RT1^f$), AUG ($RT1^c$), BS ($RT1^l$), HS ($RT1^l$), PVG ($RT1^c$), $(AUG \times AS2)F_1$, plus progeny from an $(AUG \times AS2)F_1 \times AS2$ backcross population with the phenotype $RT1.A^{ff}$, concurrently in use in the genetic analysis of the collapse curve phenomenon. Mice from the congenic lines B10.A ($H\text{-}2^a$), B10.P ($H\text{-}2^p$), and B10.S ($H\text{-}2^s$) were bred from pairs generously provided by James Watson, Ph.D., (Auckland Medical School, N.Z.) and David Sachs, M.D., (National Institutes of Health, Bethesda, MD).

Preparation and injection of ^{51}Cr Labeled RBC. Rat blood was collected into heparinized syringes by aortic puncture, diluted 1:1 in saline, and centrifuged three times through a double discontinuous density gradient, a procedure that regularly achieves 99.85% depletion of leukocytes (*9*). The resultant cell pellet was diluted 1:1 in saline and labeled for 2 hr at 37°C with 200 μCi/ml ^{51}Cr (sodium chromate in aqueous solution containing 0.9% sodium chloride; the Radio Chemical Centre, Amersham, UK). The cells were washed 3 times and the pellet diluted 1:1 in saline, following which 0.15 ml (approximately 8.6×10^8 red cells) were injected into the exposed lateral tail vein. This dosage is referred to as the *normal dose*. Other doses studied were 8.6×10^9 cells injected in 1.25 ml and 8.6×10^7 cells injected in 0.15 ml. Unless otherwise specified, the normal dose of cells was injected. A given suspension was injected into groups of allogeneic recipients and syngeneic controls, each group consisting of 4–12 animals (sex stated in the data). Mouse erythrocytes were collected from the brachial artery in heparinized pipettes, purified and labeled at 600 μCi/ml for 30 min at 37°C. Cells were then spun down, washed twice, and diluted 1:20 in

[1]This work was supported by the Medical Research Council of New Zealand.

[2]Address correspondence to: M.A. Baird, Ph.D., Department of Surgery, Otago Medical School, P.O. Box 913, Dunedin, New Zealand.

* Abbreviations used: EDTA, ethylenediaminotetraacetate; MHC, major histocompatibility complex; PBS, phosphate-buffered saline; RBC, red blood cells.

saline. Then 0.15 ml was injected i.v. into each mouse, a dose approximately equivalent on the basis of RBC/weight to that administered to rats.

Measurement of radioactivity. Blood was collected from a lateral tail vein at various times after RBC injection into four 20 μl pipettes (Acupipettes, Dale Diagnostics, Miami, FL), and radioactivity was measured in a well-type scintillation counter. After subtraction of background radioactivity, individual counts were corrected for radionuclide decay and expressed as a percentage of the count recorded from the blood of the same animal on day 1 (i.e., one day after the injection of labeled cells). The rationale for this timing has been explained previously (*1*). In order to determine the radioactivity in spleen, animals were sacrificed at various intervals after injection of labeled cells, and spleens were harvested and counted. In spleen graft experiments liver and kidney were also harvested and counted. After subtracting the background radioactivity and correcting for radionuclide decay, organ radioactivity was expressed as a percentage of the total radioactivity injected, the latter figure being calculated from the radioactivity recorded in four 20-μl blood samples from the original suspension of labeled red cells. When multiple RBC transfusions were administered prior to harvesting spleens, organ radioactivity was expressed simply as counts per minute corrected for background only.

Spleen grafting. Spleens from AUG male donors were grafted into syngeneic male recipients using microsurgical techniques. The recipient's left kidney was removed and the renal vein and artery were rejoined end-to-end to the donor splenic vein and artery. Total ischemic times ranged from 30 to 40 min.

Separation of adherent and nonadherent populations from spleen cell suspensions. Spleens were removed from AUG hosts that had received ^{51}Cr-labeled AS2 red cells 14 days previously, and counted. A cell suspension prepared by passing sliced spleen through a stainless steel sieve into phosphate-buffered saline (PBS) + 10% fetal calf serum was counted and then treated with Tris-buffered isotonic ammonium chloride at 37°C for 5 min, spun down, and washed twice. The suspension was reconstituted to 25×10^6 cells/ml and distributed in 10 ml aliquots into 90-mm petri dishes that were covered and incubated at 37°C for 2 hr. Nonadherent cells were then gently resuspended and decanted. The plates were washed twice and adherent cells removed with warm (37°C) trypsin 1% in ethylenediaminotetraacetate (EDTA) (*10*).

Titration of hemagglutinins. Red cells were prepared as 2% suspension in 20% bovine serum albumin and sera were serially diluted in 1% polyvinylpyrrolidone (K60, GAF Corporation New York, NY). Equal volumes of serum and cells were drawn into microhemacrit tubes, rocked gently at 30-min intervals, and read at 2 hr. Negative controls (i.e., cells from the serum donor strain) were included in every batch of tests.

RESULTS

Splenic sequestration and retention of ^{51}Cr Label. To investigate how long donor RBC cleared from the host circulation are retained in the spleen, groups of allogeneic (BS) and syngeneic (AS2) hosts were splenectomized 3, 4, 5, and 6 weeks after receiving ^{51}Cr AS2 RBC. Spleens were counted and the radioactivity present expressed as a percentage of that injected on day 0. Figure 1 shows that while splenic radioactivity increased gradually from 15% to approximately 20% of the injected ^{51}Cr in syngeneic hosts over the period, the 40% sequestered in allogeneic hosts in the initial 3 weeks did not vary significantly over the remaining 21 days. It then became necessary to ascertain whether this radioactivity was within phagocytic cells or associated with intact erythrocytes. ^{51}Cr released from lysed RBC in vivo is quickly excreted and not reutilized (*1, 11*), but when RBC are phagocytosed in the spleen, the label may conceivably be retained by resident cells. This has been shown to occur when labeled lymphocytes are broken down in the spleen (*12*).

Allogeneic RBC are sequestered in the spleen for long periods. In order to determine the cellular location of ^{51}Cr within the spleen, cell suspensions prepared from the spleens of AUG or (AS2×AUG)F_1 hosts 14 days after the administration of labeled backcross (AS2×AUG)F_1×AS2 (RT1.A^{ff}) RBC were counted, following which the RBC were lysed. (The reason for using backcross donors is outlined in the *Materials and Methods* section; in the context of these experiments RT1.A^{ff} red cells are treated similarly, irrespective of whether they come from a backcross or a parental-strain (AS2) donor, and F_1 hosts are equivalent to syngeneic hosts (*13*). The radioactivity in the cell pellet before and after RBC depletion was expressed as a percentage of the injected cpm. Adherent and nonadherent populations making up the cell pellet were separated and counted. The results are summarized in Table 1. Approximately 56% of the injected radioactivity in AUG hosts was found to be associated with the spleen and 22% with the cell pellet—i.e., the cellular component of the spleen. When the cell pellet was depleted of RBC, approximately 8% of the injected radioactivity remained. The greater part of this remaining radioactivity was associated with the nonadherent cell pellet. Control suspensions from the spleens of (AUG×AS2)F_1 syngeneic hosts contained approximately half the radioactivity present in the spleens of AUG hosts. Just over one-quarter of the total organ radioactivity remained after RBC lysis—and, again, most of this was associated with the nonadherent population.

These results indicate a pool of intact RBC within the spleen of both syngeneic and allogeneic hosts. The pool is, however, substantially larger in the allogeneic spleens. Since the rate of excretion of the label is similar in both syngeneic and allogeneic hosts (*1*), it can be deduced that the destruction of red cells proceeds no more rapidly in allogeneic than in syngeneic hosts.

Effect of multiple injections on RBC survival on collapse curve donor/host combinations. To find out whether multiple injections of allogeneic RBC effect a change in their clearance pattern from the host circulation, four injections of purified

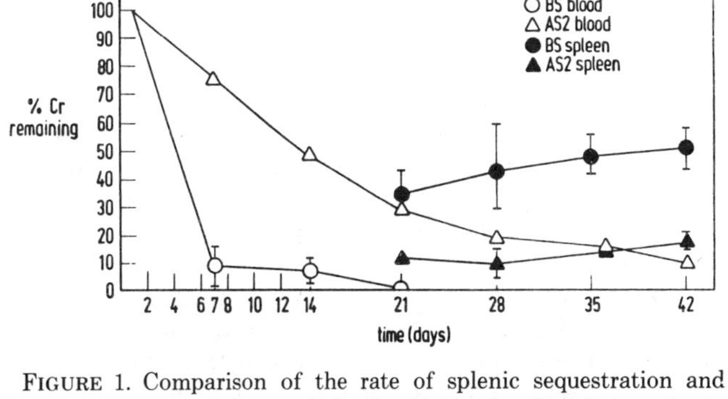

FIGURE 1. Comparison of the rate of splenic sequestration and retention of injected donor (AS2 ♀) red blood cell radioactivity in syngeneic (AS2 ♂♀) and allogeneic (BS ♀) hosts. Open symbols (△, ○) represent radioactivity in host circulation, closed symbols (▲, ●) radioactivity in spleen. Vertical bars represent standard deviation.

TABLE 1. Donor RBC radioactivity associated with intact RBC, and adherent and nonadherent spleen cell populations in syngeneic and allogeneic hosts 14 days after transfusion[a]

Donor strain	Host strain	Spleen	Spleen cell pellet	RBC-depleted spleen cells	Nonadherent spleen cells	Adherent spleen cells
(♀)	(♀)					
(AUG×AS2)F_1×AS2	AUG n2	56.3±1.9	21.8±3.9	8.1±1.2	7.5±1.4	0.7±0.1
	(AUG×AS2)F_1 n2	27.6±2.5	8.9±0.8	2.5±0.4	2.0±0.4	0.3±0.1

[a] cpm expressed as a percentage of injected cpm (corrected for background radioactivity and radionucleide decay). All data are mean ± SD. Mean percentage of day 1 radioactivity *in circulation* persisting on day 14 in AUG hosts: 6±6n2; and F_1 hosts: 45±1n2.

AS2 RBC were administered i.v. at weekly intervals to groups (n = 4) of AUG and AS2 hosts. The ^{51}Cr remaining in the host circulation (expressed as a percentage of that recorded on day 1) was monitored for seven weeks. Figure 2 shows that three injections were sufficient to convert the rapid clearance pattern characteristic of a collapse curve donor/host combination to a survival pattern indistinguishable from that seen in syngeneic hosts. Syngeneic and allogeneic hosts had similar levels of blood radioactivity four weeks after the fourth transfusion. When the immunization schedule was altered so that there was a three-week interval between the first and second injection, and a three-month interval between the second and third injections, collapse curve clearance was not impaired (Fig. 2). Several explanations could account for these observations: (1) rapid clearance required a small quantity of a humoral factor that was quickly exhausted, but which was replenished; (2) multiple transfusions brought about a state of active suppression of the production of a humoral factor; or (3) the limited capacity of the host spleen to sequestrate allogeneic RBC, coupled with a slow turnover rate, meant that a large proportion of the cells remained in circulation.

Hemagglutinating antibody response to RBC transfusions. To further investigate the possible relationship between donor RBC survival and antidonor RBC antibody, sera collected from AUG hosts before and after transfusion with AS2 RBC, were tested for anti-AS2 hemagglutinins. No antibodies were detectable in normal AUG hosts, and low titers were recorded three days after injection (Fig. 3). Titers in sera from animals receiving multiple transfusions dropped after the second injection—in 2/4 animals they were reduced to zero. This low response remained even after 5, 8, and 9 transfusions, and increasing the dose had no effect on the antibody titer. Sera from HS hosts transfused with PVG RBC were also tested for hemagglutinating antibody at intervals over the first fourteen days. This combination shows the typical "syngeneic" clearance pattern: 82% of day 1 donor RBC label remains in the host circulation on day 4 (*1*). However, hemagglutinin titers were comparable to those in the collapse curve combination AS2→AUG (Fig. 3). This finding implies that the dramatically shortened donor RBC survival in collapse curve combinations is not related to antidonor antibody in the host, and that the decreasing hemagglutinin titers observed following multiple transfusions are not causally related to the decreasing splenic sequestration that accompanies them (Figs. 2 and 3).

Effect of dose on clearance rates. When the dose of purified ^{51}Cr-labeled AS2 RBC was increased tenfold, the rate of clearance by AUG rats was significantly slower than that observed with the normal dose of RBC (Fig. 4). Conversely, reducing the normal dose tenfold accelerated the rate of clearance (Fig. 4). Collapse curve clearance is thus a function of the number of RBC transfused. This suggests that the host effector mechanism has a limited capacity to sequestrate allogeneic RBC in the spleen.

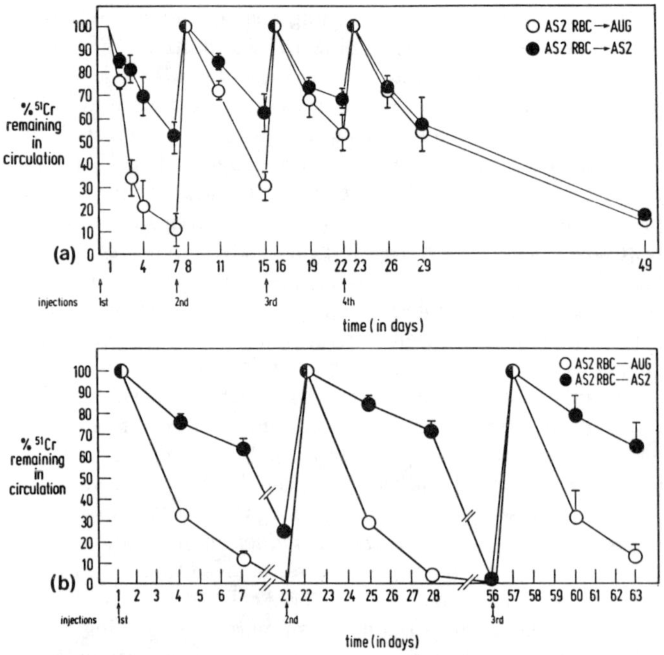

FIGURE 2. Effect of multiple transfusions on collapse curve clearance (AS2 ♀→AUG♂♀): (a) weekly transfusions convert rapid clearance to the syngeneic pattern; (b) intervals of 3 and 5 weeks between transfusions retain collapse curve clearance; Vertical bars represent standard deviation.

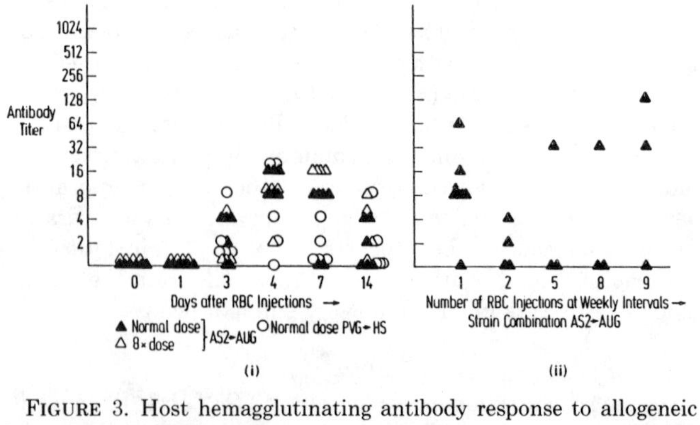

FIGURE 3. Host hemagglutinating antibody response to allogeneic donor RBC. The antibody titer was assayed following (i) a single RBC transfusion in allogeneic strain combinations representing rapid (AS2 ♀ → Aug ♂♀) and syngeneic-type (PVG ♂ → HS ♂) clearance patterns and (II) multiple RBC transfusions.

Lack of an effect of grafting an additional syngeneic spleen on the rate of clearance of allogeneic red cells. The spleen is necessary for the rapid clearance of allogeneic red cells (*1*). It is uncertain whether splenic sequestration represents a response to a membrane determinant on allogeneic red cells, or to a humoral factor (which presumably reacts with a red cell membrane determinant, as rapid clearance is immunogenetically specific). The following spleen grafting experiments were designed to distinguish between these alternatives. When AUG hosts were grafted with an additional syngeneic spleen labeled AUG red cells subsequently injected i.v. were shared approximately equally between the 2 spleens (Fig. 5c)—i.e., the grafted spleen functioned similarly to the natural spleen; and the proportion of allogeneic AS2-labeled red cells removed from the circulation was not significantly increased over the figure recorded in ungrafted controls—i.e., the doubling of the hypothetical effector cell population did not cause more red cells to be sequestrated (Fig. 5a). The two spleens sequestrated allogeneic cells approximately equally (Fig. 5c). No alteration in the distribution of syngeneic and allogeneic radioactivity to the liver and kidney resulted from the presence of an additional spleen (Fig. 5b). The unilateral nephrectomy that was a prerequisite to spleen grafting had no effect on the clearance of allogeneic red cells (data not shown).

In a further series of experiments AUG hosts were given 4 injections of unlabeled AS2 red cells at weekly intervals, the total dose being such as to effect a temporary "paralysis" of the rapid clearance effector mechanism (as in Fig. 2a). An additional AUG spleen was then grafted, followed by a dose of ^{51}Cr-labeled AS2 red cells. Control animals for this experiment were spleen-grafted, but did not receive prior injections of red cells. It was argued that, if rapid clearance were mediated by cells alone, the availability of an additional AUG spleen should allow the labeled AS2 red cells to be cleared in accelerated fashion. On the other hand, if rapid clearance required a circulating humoral factor (which had been temporarily depleted by the unlabeled cells administered earlier) the quantity of plasma in a spleen graft was unlikely to be sufficient to replenish it adequately. Figure 6a shows that the presence of an additional spleen did not abrogate the temporary "paralysis" of rapid clearance effected by repeated doses of red cells. Figure 6b elaborates upon the distribution of splenic radioactivity in the same animals. It is apparent that the relative proportion of radioactivity entering the normal and grafted spleens was approximately similar in the test (blocked by prior RBC injections) and control (nonblocked) hosts. The larger total splenic recovery in the control hosts probably reflects the absence of prior blocking injections of RBC in these animals. Figure 7 represents the results of an experiment designed to eliminate the possibility that the prior blocking injections of red cells paralyzed the capacity of both the natural and the subsequent grafted spleens to sequestrate the labeled RBC in the final injection. The experiment involved giving 3 doses of labeled AS2 RBC to hosts with natural and grafted (on day 21) spleens, and to normal hosts (Fig. 7a). It is apparent from Figure 7b that a single spleen (control) was capable of accommodating at least as many red cells as were accommodated in the 2 spleens

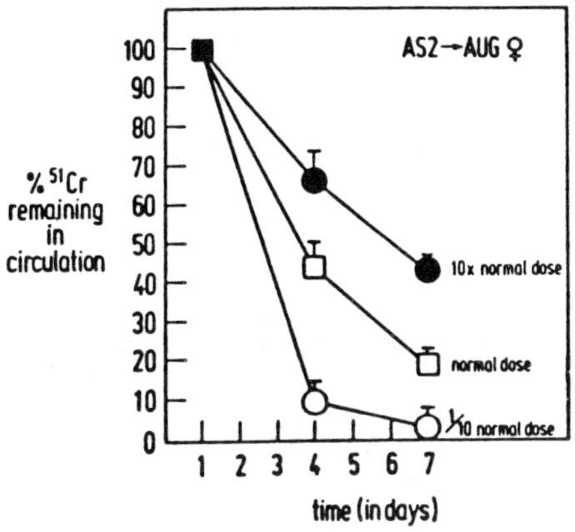

FIGURE 4. Rate of clearance of RBC in a collapse curve donor/host combination (AS2 ♀ → AUG ♀) is dose-dependent. Vertical bars represent standard deviation.

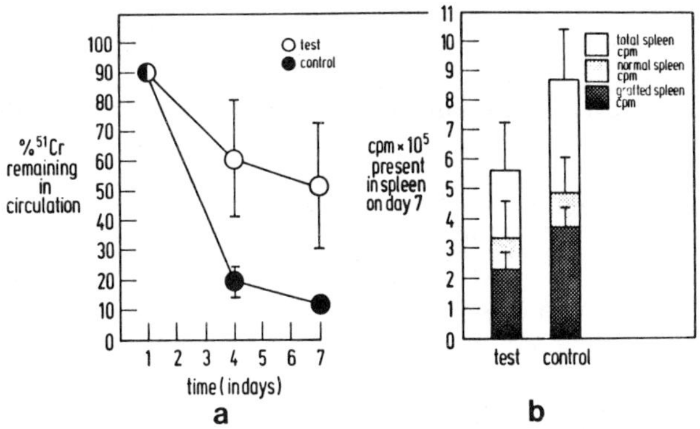

FIGURE 6. Syngeneic spleen grafting in the host after multiple transfusions of allogeneic RBC fails to effect a reversion to the collapse curve clearance pattern. Vertical bars represent standard deviation. (a) survival of ^{51}Cr-labeled AS2 RBC in AUG hosts that had received four transfusions of unlabelled AS2 RBC at weekly intervals followed by a syngeneic spleen graft (○—○, *test*) or a syngeneic spleen graft only (●—●, *control*). Each group comprised five male rats; (b) radioactivity present in grafted and normal AUG spleens harvested seven days after the injection of ^{51}Cr AS2 RBC.

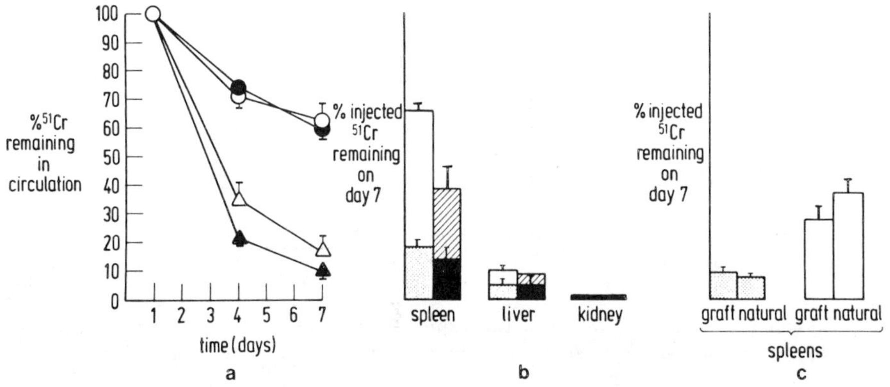

FIGURE 5 Effect of a syngeneic spleen graft in the host on the clearance (a) and sequestration (b, c) of a subsequent transfusion of ^{51}Cr-labeled allogeneic or syngeneic RBC. Vertical bars represent standard deviation. (a): (●) AUG RBC → AUG with AUG spleen graft (n = 3, ♂), (○) AUG RBC → AUG (n = 3, ♂), (▲) AS2 RBC → AUG with AUG spleen graft (n = 3, ♂), (△) AS2 RBC → AUG (n = 3, ♂); (b): (c): (□) AS2 RBC → AUG with AUG spleen graft (n = 3, ♂), (▨) AUG RBC → AUG with AUG spleen graft (n = 3 ♂), (▨) AS2 RBC → AUG (n = 3 ♂), (■) AUG RBC → AUG (n = 3 ♂).

of the test series. Thus, grafting accessory spleens to AUG hosts after they had received multiple transfusions of AS2 RBC did not reverse the depressed clearance rate, although the grafted and natural spleens were functionally equivalent to each other.

Taken together, these spleen grafting experiments suggest that splenic sequestration of allogeneic red cells is not purely a cellular phenomenon; it requires the presence of a humoral factor that can readily be exhausted.

Failure of donor-host incompatibility with respect to the H-2.7 antigen in congenic mouse strains to account for the accelerated clearance of allogeneic RBC. Because the H-2.7 antigen in mice is MHC-linked and is expressed on RBC—thereby having two of the attributes of the rat collapse curve determinant—it was previously postulated (*1*) that donor-host incompatibility with respect to the rat equivalent of this antigen might account for the rapid clearance of allogeneic red cells in rats. The H-2.7 antigen is a determinant on the C4d fragment of C4 and is adsorbed onto mouse red cells (*3*). A rat analogue has yet to be identified. To investigate a possible correlation between the presence of the MHC-linked H-2.7 antigen on mouse red blood cells and their survival on H-2-negative hosts, RBC from congenic mice positive for H-2.7 (B10.S, B10.P) were injected into H-2.7-negative hosts (B10.AS), and vice versa. The dose of RBC was calculated as corresponding on an RBC:weight basis to the standard dose used in rats. All three strains are derived from the same background strain, C57BL10. From Table 2 it can be seen that the H-2.7-positive RBC are cleared at approximately the same rate from H-2.7-negative hosts, H-2.7-positive hosts, and syngeneic hosts. Similarly, when donor and host are reversed and H-2-negative RBC are injected into H-2.7-positive hosts, no increase in clearance is

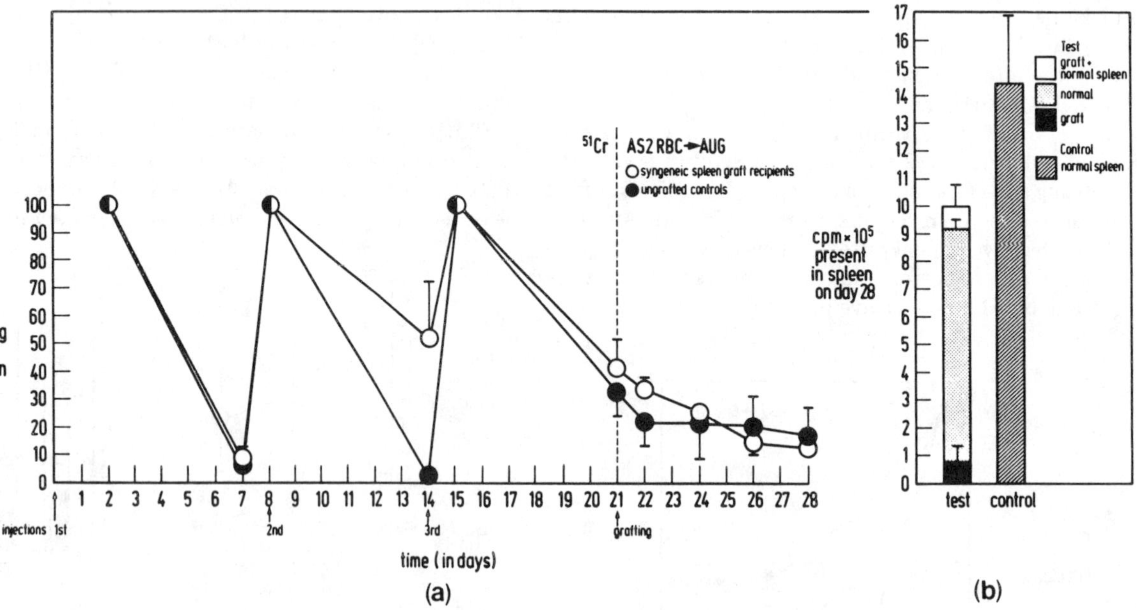

FIGURE 7. Multiple transfusions of allogeneic RBC, administered before the host is grafted with a syngeneic spleen, do not prevent sequestration of RBC transfused after grafting (Fig. 6). Vertical bars represent standard deviation. (a) survival of ^{51}Cr AS2 RBC in AUG hosts before and after syngeneic spleen grafting (○—○), and in ungrafted controls (●—●). Each group, comprising three male rats, received three transfusions of labeled RBC at weekly intervals; (b) radioactivity present in grafted and normal AUG spleens harvested 28 days after the first ^{51}Cr AS2 RBC transfusion (accessory spleens harvested 7 days after grafting).

TABLE 2. Survival of RBC in donor/host combinations differing in the H-2.7 phenotype

Donor strain (♀)	Recipient strain (♂ ♀)	Day 4			Day 7		
		Mean[a]	SD	Number in group	Mean[a]	SD	Number in group
B10.A	B10.A	80	12	6	60	13	6
(H-2.7-negative)	B10.P	72	8	6	55	10	6
	B10.S	75	16	6	58	12	6
B10.P	B10.P	79	7	8	66[b]	5	8
(H-2.7-positive)	B10.A	66	20	8	47[b]	17	8
	B10.S	87	3	4	68	5	4
B10.S	B10.S	71	10	8	59	11	8
(H-2.7-positive)	B10.A	70	8	5	58	9	5
	B10.P	69	13	6	61	8	6

[a] ^{51}Cr donor RBC label in host circulation expressed as a percentage of the day 1 radioactivity.

[b] The Student's t test was used to assess the significance of differences between the percentage of radioactivity remaining in congenic hosts and syngeneic controls. A significant difference was found only in the combination indicated ($0.02>P>0.01$).

observed. Hence, donor-host incompatibility with respect to H-2.7 is not accompanied by rapid clearance of allogeneic red cells in mice.

DISCUSSION

The experiments described here indicate that dramatically shortened survival of transfused allogeneic RBC in some donor-host combinations among inbred rats is brought about by sequestration of the red cells in the spleen, in which they persist for long periods in an apparently intact state. They are subsequently destroyed at approximately the same rate as syngeneic cells. While the rapid clearance of red cells does not occur in the absence of a spleen, nevertheless the spleen does not sequester large numbers of allogeneic red cells in the absence of a humoral factor that probably occurs naturally in the host. It can be depleted fairly readily by increasing the number of transfused cells or the frequency of transfusion (Figs. 2 and 4), but is replenished within a few weeks of depletion (Fig. 2). The main points relating to collapse curve clearance that remain to be resolved are the nature of the humoral factor, the nature of the MHC-linked red cell determinant with which the humoral factor is presumed to interact (since accelerated clearance is linked to the MHC of the donor (*1*), and the intrasplenic process by which sequestration is effected.

With respect to the humoral factor, antibody is the obvious candidate—either as naturally occurring antibody already present in the serum of unsensitized hosts, or as antibody produced in response to the transfused red cells. Günther et al. (*14*) have reported the existence of fluctuating levels of naturally occurring anti-RT1.A antibodies in some inbred strains. These may be antibodies to environmental antigens that simply crossreact with some RT1.A antigens, or they may reflect an intrinsic activity of the immune system. However, all attempts to demonstrate the presence of such antibodies in host strains exhibiting collapse curve clearance in our laboratory have failed, although assays were of comparable sensitivity. It seemed unlikely that host sensitization to transfused allogeneic erythrocytes resulted in accelerated clearance since accelerated clearance of allogeneic red cells was well under way three days after transfusion, when hemagglutinin titers were very low (Figs. 2 and 3) and comparable titers of antidonor antibody were also present in allogeneic strain combinations that did not exhibit collapse curve clearance. The latter result accords with Möller's finding in mice (*8*). Other workers have recorded relatively high antibody responses to allogeneic RBC one week after transfusion in a different strain combination, LEW→BN (*15*). However, in experiments in which RBC survival was also monitored, accelerated clearance did not become apparent until day 7 (*16*). In this situation it could more reasonably be argued that antibody produced in response to donor RBC eventually impaired their survival. It may be relevant that patterns similar to this have also been observed in our laboratory in three strain combinations in which LEW was the donor (unpublished observations).

While experiments reported here and in previous publications have failed to implicate antibody, the importance of a humoral factor has clearly been indicated. The possibility that this might be the rat analogue of mouse H-2.7 has not been excluded, although the experiments on mouse strains congenic for H-2.7 (Table 2) provides no circumstantial evidence to support this idea. The possibility that complement components are responsible for collapse curve clearance, however, remains attractive and will bear closer examination. Whatever the nature of the humoral factor, it does not exert its effect immediately—there is a lag period of at least 24 hr before allogeneic red cells are rapidly removed from the circulation ([1], Fig. 2).

A naturally occurring cellular mechanism possibly contributes to the ultimate sequestration of red cells by the spleen, but this mechanism is ineffective in the absence of the humoral factor (Figs. 6 and 7). The allogeneic red cells are not rapidly destroyed in the spleen—they are mainly intact at 3 weeks. The small quantity of label in the adherent cell population of the spleen suggests that very few allogeneic red cells have been phagocytosed (Table 1). On the evidence of the rate of excretion of radioactivity (*1*), the subsequent destruction of allogeneic red cells sequestered in the spleen proceeds at a rate indistinguishable from that of syngeneic red cells.

Retention of intact donor RBC within the spleen for relatively long periods poses some queries. How are these cells selectively retained? Mollison has suggested that clinical collapse curve clearance could be brought about by direct interaction between foreign donor cells and host mononuclear cells (*7*), but this does not appear to be the case in the rat. What part of the spleen is occupied by the pools of red cells? It has been noted that pooling may occur where the RBC are abnormal due to the removal of surface lipid components or blocking of surface sulph-hydryl groups (*17*, *18*), in which case the RBC accumulate in the pulp spaces of the spleen. Autoradiography using appropriately labeled donor RBC may provide some answers to our questions. What is the MHC-linked factor that distinguishes one haplotype from another with respect to accelerated clearance? A backcross analysis currently in progress using (AS2×AUG)F_1×AS2 backcross donors and AUG hosts has so far (175 donors) failed to separate the collapse curve determinant from RT1.A.

The dosage data presented here strengthen the analogy between the rat and the human phenomenon. Increasing the dose (ten times the normal dose used in these experiments is equivalent to a therapeutic transfusion to a 70-kg man) decreases the rate. At the normal dose second, third, and fourth transfusions from the same donor strain may be cleared at a reduced rate. When there is an extended interval between injections, the accelerated clearance pattern persists. It thus seems likely that transfusion collapse curves in the rat represent a valid model of the human condition (*4–6*).

Acknowledgments. We thank Anne Williams for doing the spleen grafts, and Karen Skinner and Anne Marie McCarthy for other technical assistance. The H-2.7 congenic mice were generous gifts from David Sachs, M.D., and James Watson, Ph.D.

REFERENCES

1. Baird MA, Heslop BF. Major histocompatibility complex-linked spleen-dependent transfusion "collapse curves" in inbred rats. Transplantation 1982; 34: 129.
2. Heslop BF, Baird MA, Elliot GS. Red cell alloantigens of the Dunedin inbred rat strains. Proc Univ Otago Med Sch 1981; 59: 16.
3. Klein J, Figueroa F, Klein D. H-2 haplotypes, genes and antigens: second listing. I. Non H-2 loci on chromosome 17. Immunogenetics 1982; 16: 285.
4. Mollison PL. Blood transfusion in clinical medicine. 3rd ed. Oxford: Blackwell, 1961: 484.
5. Adner PL, Foconi S, Sjölin S. Immunization after intravenous injection of small amounts of ^{51}Cr-labelled red cells. Br J Haematol 1963; 9: 288.

6. Szymanski IO, Valeri CR. Lifespan of preserved red cells. Vox Sang 1971; 21: 97.
7. Mollison PL. Blood transfusion in clinical medicine. 6th ed. Oxford: Blackwell, 1979.
8. Möller G. Survival of H-2 incompatible mouse erythrocytes in untreated and isoimmune recipients. Immunology 1965; 8: 360.
9. Heslop HE. A method for preparing leucocyte depleted erythrocytes from rat blood. J Immunol Methods 1978; 22: 389.
10. Heslop BF, Lyttle VA. Hyperplasia of donor cells in rejecting weakly antigenic skin grafts. Proc R Soc Lond Biol 1976; 193: 209.
11. Ebaugh FG, Emerson CP, Ross JF. The use of radioactive chromium 51 as an erythrocyte tagging agent for the determination of red cell survival in vivo. J Clin Invest 1953; 32: 1260.
12. Rolstad B, Ford W. The rapid elimination of allogeneic lymphocytes: relationship to established mechanisms of immunity to lymphocyte traffic. Immunol Rev 1983; 73: 87.
13. Baird MA, Heslop BF. The gene coding for the rat transfusion "collapse curve" is very close to RTI.A. Transplant Proc (in press).
14. Günther E, Elsasser-Beile U, Hedrich HJ. Occurrence of antibodies against RT1.A antigens in normal rat sera. Transplant Proc 1983; 15: 1560.
15. Majoor GD, van de Gaar M-JWH, Vlek LFM, van Breda Vriesman PJC. The role of antibody in rat renal allograft rejection. Transplantation 1981a; 31: 369.
16. Majoor GD. The role of antibody in renal allograft rejection. Belgium: Michiels Tongeren, 1981.
17. Harris IM, McAlister JM, Prankerd TAJ. The relationship of abnormal red cells to the normal spleen. Clin Sci 1957; 16: 223.
18. Jacobs HS, Jandl JH. Effects of sulphydryl inhibition on red blood cells. II. Studies in vivo. J Clin Invest 1962; 41: 1514.

Received 25 October 1985.
Accepted 3 February 1986.

0041-1337/86/4205-0548$02.00/0
TRANSPLANTATION
Vol. 42, No. 5
Printed in U.S.A.

THE ACTIVITY OF SUPPRESSOR CELLS IN THE SPLEEN OF MURINE BONE MARROW CHIMERAS[1]

MASAHIRO IMAMURA,[2,3] TAMOTSU MIYAZAKI,[2] HISAO FUJIMOTO,[2] TAKASHI FUKUHARA,[2] MASAHARU KASAI,[2] TOSHIYUKI ITAYA,[4] AND KEISUKE SAKURADA[2]

The Third Department of Internal Medicine and The Laboratory of Pathology, Cancer Institute, Hokkaido University School of Medicine, Sapporo 060, Japan

An intrasplenic injection (i.s.) of BALB/c bone marrow cells induces a higher survival rate than an intravenous injection (i.v.) in irradiated C3H/He recipients. Coculture experiments revealed the presence of alloantigen-specific and nonspecific suppressor cells in the spleens of mice injected i.s. and i.v. Suppressor activity decreased 50–60 days after bone marrow transplantation in i.v. chimeras, while there was no decrease in i.s. chimeras. In vitro suppressor activity was correlated with in vivo activity. Histopathological changes in the liver were examined. A total of 28% of the i.v. chimeras showed severe changes compared with 6% of the i.s. chimeras. The spleen indices of i.v. and i.s. chimeras were compared. Although there was no statistically significant difference between the spleen indices of i.v. chimeras and those of i.s. chimeras, spleen indices of i.v. chimeras tended to be higher than those of i.s. chimeras. These results show that suppressor cells in i.s. chimeras appear to inhibit graft-versus-host reactions more efficiently. Furthermore, an adoptive transfer assay showed that suppressor cells detected in i.s. chimeras were effective in vivo. We therefore suggest that suppressor cells detected in vitro correlate with in vivo activity and may play some role in the induction and maintenance of transplantation tolerance.

It has been reported that splenectomy prior to receiving an allograft abolishes immunological enhancement (*1–5*). Furthermore, a splenectomy performed prior to receiving an allograft induces increased graft-versus-host reactions (GVHRs)* (*6–8*), indicating that the spleen may exert an immunosuppressive influence on donor histocompatibility-antigen-reactive cells and that GVHRs may be depressed in its absence (*9*). In our previous work, intrasplenic (i.s.) bone marrow transplantation (BMT) of lethally irradiated mice induced longer survival than did intravenous (i.v.) BMT (*10*); similar results have also been obtained by Monaco et al. (*11*). We have not examined the mechanisms that cause such a beneficial effect.

[1] This work was supported in part by the Research Grant for Idiopathic Disorders of Hematopoietic Organs Research Committee from the Ministry of Health and Welfare of Japan, and by a Grant-in-Aid for Scientific Research (No. 5857109) from the Ministry of Education, Science and Culture of Japan.

[2] Third Department of Internal Medicine.
[3] Address correspondence to: Dr. Masahiro Imamura, The Third Department of Internal Medicine, Hokkaido University School of Medicine, Kita-15, Nishi-7, Kita-ku, Sapporo 060, Japan.
[4] Cancer Institute.

* Abbreviations used: BMT, bone marrow transplantation; Con A, concanavalin A; CML, cell-mediated lympholysis; GVHR (GVHD) graft versus host reaction (disease); Hepes, N-2-hydroxy-piperazine-N′-2-ethane-sulfonic acid; i.s. chimera, chimera created by intrasplenic bone marrow transplantation; i.v. chimera, chimera created by intravenous bone marrow transplantation; MLR, mixed lymphocyte reaction; SPF, specific-pathogen-free; ^{3}H-TdR, tritiated thymidine.

The important role played by suppressor cells in inducing and maintaining transplantation tolerance has been reported (*12–21*), although some investigators conclude that these are just bystander effects that do not induce any beneficial effect in maintaining transplantation tolerance (*22–27*). Clonal deletion (*28*) and serum blocking factors have also been thought to be candidates for the maintenance of transplantation tolerance (*29–31*), although the latter may not be important in the maintenance of the stable chimeric state (*32–34*). We therefore examined the presence of suppressor cells in mice receiving marrow using a mixed lymphocyte reaction (MLR) coculture assay, since this assay system has been used by several investigators (*12, 14, 17–21*). As we show here, bone marrow chimeras created by i.v. or i.s. injection possess alloantigen-specific and nonspecific suppressor cells in the spleen. Since the suppressor activity in these chimeras did not show any significant difference 30 to 40 days after BMT, we examined the time course of suppressor activity to determine whether there was any significant difference in the magnitude of suppression in i.v. and i.s. chimeras. In addition, we also examined the role of suppressor cells in vivo.

MATERIALS AND METHODS

Mice. Inbred BALB/c(H-2^d), C3H/He(H-2^k), and C57BL/6(H-2^b) mice were purchased from Shizuoka Agricultural Cooperative Association for Laboratory Animals (Hamamatsu, Shizuoka, Japan). Mice 2–4 months old were used in a laminar air flow room. All the mice used were specific-pathogen-free (SPF). Sado et al. (*35*) have reported that almost all lethally x-irradiated SPF mice are able to survive for a long period, even when they are injected i.v. with allogeneic bone marrow cells containing mature T cells. In our hands, however, some of the lethally x-irradiated SPF mice that received allogeneic bone marrow cells by i.v. injection survived for only a short period. This difference may be caused by different handling of the SPF mice. SPF mice in our laboratory were moved from the laminar air flow room into a conventional room for irradiation. Furthermore, they received food that was not sterilized. Since bacterial growth in the liver or the spleen was seen by microscopic examinations in mice receiving only x-irradiation, the situation of our SPF mice was similar to the conventional one.

Bone marrow transplantation. The method of bone marrow transplantation has been described previously (*10*). Briefly, 10–20 million BALB/c bone marrow cells obtained from the femoral and tibial cavities were injected i.s. or i.v. into x-irradiated (925–950 rads) C3H/He mice within 6 hr after x-irradiation without the elimination of mature T cells by anti-Thy1.2 antibody. The spleen was approached via a transverse left subcostal incision, and the exposed spleen was lifted out gently with forceps. Using a 1.0-ml syringe and a 27¾-gauge needle, 0.1 ml of cell suspension was injected directly into the splenic parenchyma. All the recipients were given drinking water with antibiotics for 3 weeks after x-irradiation.

Mixed lymphocyte reaction (MLR). Spleen cells were removed aseptically and teased into RPMI 1640 medium (Nissui Pharmaceutical Co., Ltd., Tokyo, Japan) supplemented with 10 mM Hepes, 2 mM glutamine, penicillin (100 units/ml), streptomycin (100 μg/ml), 5×10^{-5}M 2-mercaptoethanol and 10% heat-inactivated fetal bovine serum (Grand Island Biological Co., NY). The spleen suspensions were strained through gauze mesh. Stimulating cells were treated with 2000 rads x-irradiation. Cultures were performed in flat-bottomed, 96-well microtiter plates (Flow Laboratories, Inc., Hamden, CN). From 10^5 to 5×10^5 stimulating and from 10^5 to 5×10^5 responding cells were cultured in 200 μl of media. In the control cultures, responding cells were cultured with syngeneic stimulating cells. All the cultures were set up in triplicate. After 5 days' culture, 1 μCi of ^{3}H-thymidine (New England Nuclear, Boston, MA) was added to each well. The cells were harvested 6 hr later on paper filters with a multisample harvester. Filters were dried, dispensed into vials containing 2 ml of scintillation fluid, and counted in a liquid scintillation counter. The stimulation index of the responding cells was calculated as the ratio of the mean ^{3}H count incorporated in cultures containing x-irradiated allogeneic stimulating cells divided by the mean ^{3}H count incorporated in cultures containing x-irradiated syngeneic stimulating cells.

MLR coculture experiments. Utilizing the MLR system, spleen cells from chimeras were used in cocultures to assay for suppressor cells. The spleen cells came from chimeras that showed donor-type chimerism after H-2 typing using anti-H-2 antiserum. As controls, spleen cells from various strains of normal mice, including (BALB/c×C3H/He) F_1, were added to MLR cultures. Since (BALB/c×C3H/He) chimeras were shown to be closer to BALB/c mice than (BALB/c×C3H/He) F_1 mice in their alloantigen specificity (Table 1), spleen cells from BALB/c mice appeared to be the best control when determining the suppressor activity of chimeric spleen cells. Therefore, when calculating the percentage of suppression, MLR cocultured with spleen cells from the donor strain—i.e., BALB/c—of chimeras was used. A responder-to-coculture cell ratio of 1:0.25 was used, unless otherwise stated. The percentage of suppression was calculated as follows:

% suppression =

$$1 - \frac{^3\text{H thymidine incorporation of (responder cells + stimulator cells + chimeric spleen cells}}{^3\text{H thymidine incorporation of (responder cells + stimulator cells + donor spleen cells of chimeras}} \times 100$$

Generation of cytotoxic cells. The method for generating cytotoxic cells has been described elsewhere (*36*). Briefly, 25×10^6 spleen cells from BALB/c mice were cocultured with 2000-rad x-irradiated spleen cells from C3H/He or C57BL/6 mice mixed with 6.25×10^6 spleen cells from normal BALB/c mice or chimeras. Five days later, they were harvested and adjusted to give an effector-to-target ratio of 64:1. Concanvalin A (Con A) (Pharmacia Fine Chemicals, Uppsala, Sweden) activated lymphoblasts were used as target cells. They were labeled with sodium chromate 51 (New England Nuclear, Boston, MA), and 10^4 target cells were put into each well. After 4–5 hr of incubation with effector cells, the radioactivity in the supernatant was counted by a gamma counter. The percentage of specific immune lysis was calculated as follows:

% specific immune lysis

$$= \left[\frac{\text{cpm in experimental group} - \text{mineral release}}{\text{maximal release} - \text{minimal release}}\right] \times 100$$

Suppressor factors in supernatants from a 2-day culture of chimeric spleen cells. To determine whether suppressor activity is present in the culture supernatant taken from chimeric spleen cells, 50 μl of supernatant from a 2-day culture of chimeric spleen cells at a concentration of 2.5×10^6 cells/ml was added to 200 μl of BALB/c anti-C3H/He or BALB/c anti-C57BL/6 MLR on day 2. On day 5, 1 μCi of ^{3}H-TdR was added to each well of flat-bottomed 96-well microtiter plates; 6 hr later they were harvested with a semiautomated multiharvester.

Microscopic examination of the liver. For histopathologic examination, the livers from sacrificed chimeras were fixed in a 10% formalin solution and embedded in paraffin. Four μ-thick sections were prepared and routinely stained with hematoxylin and eosin. Histopathological changes in the liver due to GVHR were classified into three groups (severe, moderate, and no change). *Severe* change indicates massive necrosis and diffuse infiltration of lymphocytes and polymorphonuclear cells. *Moderate* change indicates focal necrosis and localized infiltration of lymphocytes and polymorphonuclear cells.

Spleen index. When the chimeras were killed for coculture experiments, their body and spleen weights were recorded. The spleen index was calculated as follows:

$$\text{spleen index} = \frac{\text{spleen weight}}{\text{body weight}} \times 10^{-3}$$

Adoptive transfer assay. C3H/He mice were lethally x-irradiated (925 rads) and injected with 10^7 spleen cells from BALB/c mice mixed with 5×10^6 spleen cells from (BALB/c×C3H/He) i.s. chimeras or BALB/c mice in exp. 1. In another experiment, lethally x-irradiated C3H/He mice were injected with 3×10^6 bone marrow cells and 5×10^5 spleen cells from BALB/c mice, mixed with 5×10^5 spleen cells from (BALB/c×C3H/He) i.s. chimeras.

RESULTS

MLRs using spleen cells from chimeras as stimulators. When spleen cells from BALB/c mice were stimulated with x-irradiated spleen cells from (BALB/c→C3H/He) chimeras created by i.v. or i.s. transplantation, the ^{3}H-TdR incorporation was similar to that in the control, thus indicating a low stimulation index (Table 1). In contrast, a strong MLR was observed when spleen cells from BALB/c mice were stimulated with x-irradiated spleen cells from C3H/He or C57BL/6 mice. Spleen cells from C3H/He or C57BL/6 mice responded to x-irradiated spleen cells from (BALB/c→C3H/He) chimeras, although the responses were weaker than those to x-irradiated spleen cells from BALB/c mice, particularly in Exp. 1 (Table 1) (2.9 or 2.4 vs. 6.0 stimulation indices for the C3H/He responder and 4.2 or 1.3 vs. 6.0 stimulation indices for the C57BL/6 responder).

Decreased MLRs of responder cells from chimeras. As shown in Table 2, spleen cells from (BALB/c→C3H/He) chimeras created by i.v. or i.s. transplantation showed poor MLRs against x-irradiated spleen cells from donor, recipient, and third-party mice shortly after bone marrow transplantation. Although MLRs against spleen cells from third-party mice tended to increase gradually until 72 days after bone marrow transplantation, the MLRs against spleen cells from donor and recipient mice were always low, indicating that the immunological tolerance to recipient antigens as well as donor antigens was established in the chimeric hosts.

The presence of suppressor cells in spleen cells from i.v. and i.s. chimeras. The presence of suppressor cells in the spleens of chimeras was examined by means of MLR coculture assays. Spleen cells from BALB/c mice were stimulated with x-irradiated spleen cells from C3H/He mice and cocultured with spleen cells from BALB/c, (BALB/c × C3H/He) F_1, C3H/He or C57BL/6 mice as controls, or with spleen cells from chimeras as the suppressor source. When compared with cocultures with normal spleen cells from BALB/c mice, 89% and 95% suppression against BALB/c anti C3H/He MLR was observed by coculturing with spleen cells from (BALB/c→C3H/He) i.v. and i.s. chimeras, respectively (Table 3). This suppressor activity was partially abrogated by 2000-rad x-irradiation, but not completely. Similarly, 65% and 78% suppression against BALB/c anti-C57BL/6 MLR was observed by coculturing with spleen cells from (BALB/c→C3H/He) i.v. and i.s. chimeras, respectively. In this case, more radiosensitive suppressor cells were detected, although in another experiment more radioresistant suppressor cells were detected (data not shown).

Although radioresistant suppressor cells were found, we usually used nonirradiated cells in coculture since radiosensitive suppressor activity would be lost and this could play some role in vivo.

Dose-response characteristics of suppressor cells. We examined whether the same population of suppressor cells could

TABLE 1. Mixed lymphocyte reactions caused by using spleen cells from chimeras as the stimulator

Responder	Stimulator (^{3}H-TdR incorporation [cpm] ± SD)				
	BALB/c	C3H/He	C57BL/6	i.v. Chimera	i.s. Chimera
Exp. 1:[a]					
BALB/c	6,594±553	100,782±18,689 (15.3)[c]	79,702±25,973 (12.1)	6,138±846 (0.9)	4,080±1,060 (0.6)
C3H/He	36,000±8,384 (6.0)	6,039±1,052	78,203±17,494 (12.9)	17,800±2,717 (2.9)	14,573±1,021 (2.4)
C57BL/6	20,852±6,366 (6.0)	12,314±2,626 (3.5)	3,484±1,028	14,531±2,113 (4.2)	4,378±463 (1.3)
Exp. 2:[b]					
BALB/c	16,385±1,318	86,453±2,765 (5.3)	78,022±6,788 (4.8)	26,845±4,836 (1.6)	18,709±6,123 (1.1)
C3H/He	95,925±6,508 (4.1)	23,535±3,631	102,407±3,865 (4.4)	83,307±7,677 (3.5)	58,079±4,867 (2.5)
C57BL/6	52,275±10,150 (3.3)	43,342±8,866 (2.7)	16,010±3,344	53,686±6,559 (3.4)	43,469±5,882 (2.7)

[a] Spleen cells from chimeras 43 days after BMT were used as the stimulator in Exp. 1.

[b] Spleen cells from chimeras 72 days after BMT were used as the stimulator in Exp. 2.

[c] Numbers in parentheses indicate stimulation indices.

TABLE 2. Decreased MLRs against spleen cells from third-party mice

Responder	Stimulator (^{3}H-TdR incorporation [cpm] ± SD)			
	(BALB/c→C3H/He) chimera	BALB/c	C3H/He	C57BL/6
Exp. 1 (day 37):				
i.v. Chimera	2,095±275	1,808±716 (0.9)[a]	1,770±16 (0.9)	1,441±57 (0.7)
i.s. Chimera	2,650±214	3,211±557 (1.2)	4,221±284 (1.6)	4,890±354 (1.8)
Exp. 2 (day 43):				
i.v. Chimera	5,707±542	6,337±481 (1.1)	8,217±1,867 (1.4)	7,443±309 (1.3)
i.s. Chimera	3,740±120	5,118±110 (1.4)	6,090±372 (1.6)	6,461±325 (1.7)
Exp. 3 (day 54):				
i.v. Chimera	1,992±602	2,047±218 (1.1)	2,073±591 (1.2)	5,929±1,317 (3.3)
i.s. Chimera	1,472±122	1,584±166 (1.1)	1,838±300 (1.2)	2,687±478 (1.8)
Exp. 4 (day 72):				
i.v. Chimera	50,315±1,516	23,577±259 (0.5)	30,365±2,332 (0.6)	71,003±2,867 (1.4)
i.s. Chimera	31,224±7,924	17,753±1,427 (0.6)	29,462±4,631 (0.9)	60,772±9,948 (1.9)

[a] Numbers in parentheses indicate stimulation indices.

TABLE 3. Radioresistant suppressor cells detected in the spleen of chimeras

Responder	Stimulator	Cocultured cells	^{3}H-TdR incorporation (cpm) ± SD	% Suppression
BALB/c	BALB/c	None	2,164±842	
BALB/c	C3H/He	None	13,571±1,899	
BALB/c	C3H/He	BALB/c	16,634±356	
BALB/c	C3H/He	C3H/He	12,666±748	
BALB/c	C3H/He	C57BL/6	14,328±1,007	
BALB/c	C3H/He	(BALB/c×C3H/He)F_1	13,049±1,268	
BALB/c	C3H/He	(BALB/c→C3H/He)i.v.[a]	1,851±933	89%
BALB/c	C3H/He	(BALB/c→C3H/He)i.s.[a]	819±65	95%
BALB/c	C3H/He	BALB/c_x[b]	6,658±736	
BALB/c	C3H/He	(BALB/c×C3H/He)F_{1x}	7,132±1,030	
BALB/c	C3H/He	(BALB/c→C3H/He)i.v.$_x$	3,817±684	43%
BALB/c	C3H/He	(BALB/c→C3H/He)i.s.$_x$	2,692±328	60%
BALB/c	C57BL/6	None	10,573±789	
BALB/c	C57BL/6	BALB/c	13,095±319	
BALB/c	C57BL/6	C3H/He	14,086±1,860	
BALB/c	C57BL/6	C57BL/6	10,513±289	
BALB/c	C57BL/6	(BALB/c×C3H/He)F_1	7,943±642	
BALB/c	C57BL/6	(BALB/c→C3H/He)i.v.	4,645±93	65%
BALB/c	C57BL/6	(BALB/c→C3H/He)i.s.	2,868±65	78%
BALB/c	C57BL/6	BALB/c_x	12,500±198	
BALB/c	C57BL/6	(BALB/c×C3H/He)F_{1x}	14,618±114	
BALB/c	C57BL/6	(BALB/c→C3H/He)i.v.$_x$	11,422±2,273	8%
BALB/c	C57BL/6	(BALB/c→C3H/He)i.s.$_x$	8,425±274	32%

[a] Spleen cells from chimeras 72 days after BMT were used.
[b] Spleen cells from chimeras that received 2000 rads x-irradiation.

suppress antidonor, antirecipient and anti-third-party MLR. To rule out any suppressive effect of cell crowding, we analyzed the dose response characteristics of suppression in various MLRs. When the responder-to-coculture cell ratio was adjusted to 1:0.75, antidonor and antirecipient MLR were suppressed to approximately 85–90% (Fig. 1). In contrast, the suppression against anti-third-party MLR was 40%–65%. When the ratio was reduced to 1:0.25, a strong suppressor activity (about 60%) was shown against antidonor and antirecipient MLR. However, only weak suppressor activity against anti-third-party MLR was shown. Furthermore, when the responder-to-coculture cell ratio was reduced to 1:0.125, the suppressor activity against antidonor MLR was almost nil, although appreciable suppressor activity against antirecipient MLR was still detected.

Inhibition of the generation of cytotoxic cells by spleen cells from chimeras. Spleen cells from (BALB/c→C3H/He) i.v. or i.s. chimeras were assayed for their ability to suppress the CML response of BALB/c to C3H/He. As shown in Table 4, no cytotoxic activity was observed against the BALB/c target, although the C3H/He targets were killed by BALB/c anti-C3H/He effector cells, showing 25.5% and 23.2% specific immune lysis. When spleen cells from i.v. and i.s. chimeras were added on day 0, the percentage of specific immune lysis was markedly reduced. BALB/c anti-C57BL/6 effector cells killed the C57BL/6 targets, showing 23.1% or 22.4% specific immune lysis, and the addition of spleen cells from i.v. and i.s. chimeras significantly reduced the cytotoxic activity.

Suppressor factor in 2-day culture supernatant of spleen cells from chimeras. Supernatant from 2 day cultures of spleen cells from normal or chimeric mice, 50 μl, was added to 200 μl of BALB/c anti-C3H/He or BALB/c anti-C57BL/6 MLR. As shown in Table 5, spleen cells from i.v. and i.s. chimeras induced 54% and 82% suppression of BALB/c anti-C3H/He MLR, while supernatants from these chimeras induced 61% and 37% suppression, respectively.

Similarly, supernatants from i.v. and i.s. chimeras induced 60% and 74% suppression of BALB/c anti-C57BL/6 MLR, respectively.

Time course studies of suppressor activities using MLR coculture assays. Suppressor activity against BALB/c anti-C3H/He MLR in (BALB/c→C3H/He) i.v. and i.s. chimeras is shown in Fig. 2. Suppressor activity in i.v. and i.s. chimeras was compar-

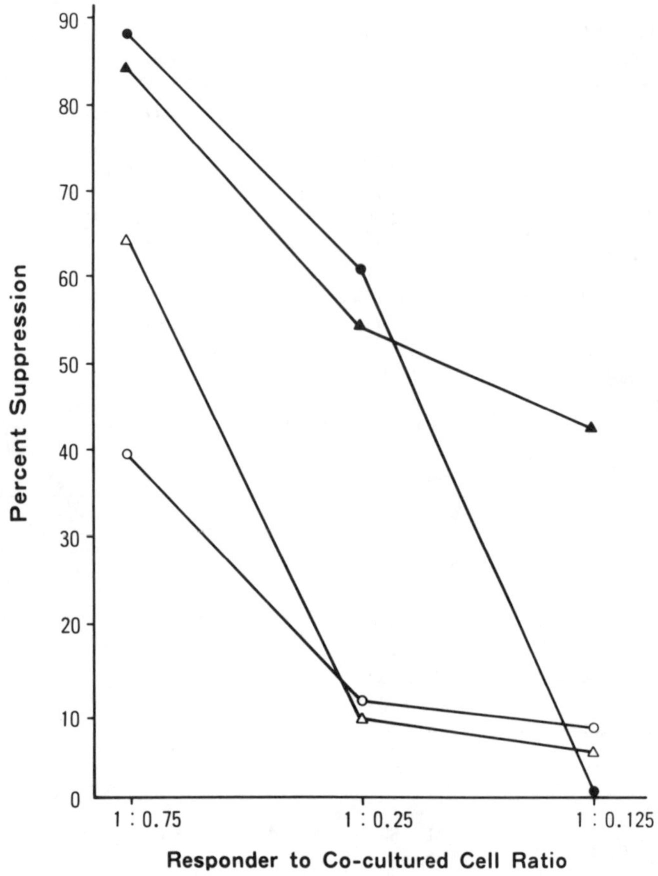

FIGURE 1. Dose response characteristics of suppressor activities against BALB/c anti-C3H/He MLR (▲—▲), BALB/c anti-C57BL/6 MLR (●—●), C3H/He anti-BALB/c MLR (△—△), and C3H/He-anti C57BL/6 MLR (○—○).

TABLE 4. Inhibition of the generation of cytotoxic cells

MLR	Cocultured cells	Target cells (% specific immune lysis)		
		BALB/c	C3H/He	C57BL/6
Exp. 1:[a]				
BALB/c anti C3H/He	BALB/c	0.0	22.5	4.5
BALB/c anti C3H/He	i.v. Chimera	0.0	0.0	2.5
BALB/c anti C3H/He	i.s. Chimera	0.0	3.2	2.0
BALB/c anti C57BL/6	BALB/c	3.3	4.1	23.1
BALB/c anti C57BL/6	i.v. Chimera	2.5	2.3	1.4
BALB/c anti C57BL/6	i.s. Chimera	0.0	1.1	1.3
Exp. 2:[b]				
BALB/c anti C3H/He	BALB/c	−1.3	23.2	6.4
BALB/c anti C3H/He	i.v. Chimera	−2.5	0.0	−1.2
BALB/c anti C3H/He	i.v. Chimera	−1.3	1.8	−0.7
BALB/c anti C3H/He	i.s. Chimera	3.8	0.0	1.5
BALB/c anti C3H/He	i.s. Chimera	−3.2	−3.2	0.7
BALB/c anti C57BL/6	BALB/c	0.0	0.0	22.4
BALB/c anti C57BL/6	i.v. Chimera	2.4	1.1	5.1
BALB/c anti C57BL/6	i.v. Chimera	2.2	2.8	3.6
BALB/c anti C57BL/6	i.s. Chimera	1.3	0.0	−1.4
BALB/c anti C57BL/6	i.s. Chimera	3.5	5.3	7.2

[a] Spleen cells from (BALB/c→C3H/He) chimeras that showed donor-type chimerism 61 days after BMT were used in Exp. 1.

[b] Spleen cells from (BALB/c→C3H/He) chimeras that showed donor-type chimerism 68 days after BMT were used in Exp. 2.

TABLE 5. Suppressor factor in culture supernatant of spleen cells from chimeras

Responder	Stimulator	Cocultured cells	^{3}H-TdR incorporation (cpm) ± SD	% Suppression
BALB/c	BALB/c	None	895±81	
BALB/c	C3H/He	BALB/c	7,498±882	
BALB/c	C3H/He	(BALB/c→C3H/He)i.v.[a]	3,470±711	54%
BALB/c	C3H/He	(BALB/c→C3H/He)i.s.	1,379±814	82%
BALB/c	C3H/He	BALB/c sup.[b]	2,405±445	
BALB/c	C3H/He	(BALB/c→C3H/He)i.v. sup.	945±100	61%
BALB/c	C3H/He	BALB/c→C3H/He)i.s. sup.	1,504±471	37%
BALB/c	C57BL/6	BALB/c	12,463±1,598	
BALB/c	C57BL/6	(BALB/c→C3H/He)i.v.	4,854±445	61%
BALB/c	C57BL/6	(BALB/c→C3H/He)i.s.	2,170±204	83%
BALB/c	C57BL/6	BALB/c sup.	3,042±698	
BALB/c	C57BL/6	(BALB/c→C3H/He)i.v. sup.	1,222±494	60%
BALB/c	C57BL/6	(BALB/c→C3H/He)i.s. sup.	791±45	74%

[a] Spleen cells from chimeras 40 days after BMT were used.

[b] Supernatant from 2-day culture of normal spleen cells from BALB/c mice or chimeric spleen cells.

ably high at 40 days after BMT, and decreased at days 50–60, followed by a marked increase of suppressor activity at day 70. Although there was no statistically significant difference between the suppressor activity in i.v. and i.s. chimeras at each time point, the suppressor activity at days 50–60 was significantly different ($P<0.01$ and $P<0.05$, respectively) from that at day 70 in the i.v. chimeras, though not in the i.s. chimeras.

Histopathological changes in the liver of i.v. and i.s. chimeras. Histopathological changes caused by GVHD were compared in i.v. and i.s. chimeras. Three groups were classified by the degree of GVHR. *Severe* change indicates massive necrosis and diffuse infiltration of lymphocytes and polymorphonuclear cells while *moderate* change indicates focal necrosis and localized infiltration of lymphocytes and polymorphonuclear cells. According to this classification, 28% of the i.v. chimeras showed severe change and 22% showed moderate change (Table 6). In contrast, only 6% of the i.s. chimeras showed severe change and 29% showed moderate change. No change was observed in 50% of the i.v. chimeras and 65% of the i.s. chimeras. These results suggest that there was a smaller effect on the livers of the i.s. chimeras than on the livers of the i.v. chimeras.

Spleen indices and kinetics. Spleen indices in the i.v. chimeras declined with time, but increased at day 70, running parallel to the kinetics of suppressor activity in the BALB/c anti-C3H/He MLR (Figs. 2 and 3). Spleen indices in the i.s. chimeras declined gradually with time and then reached a plateau. The kinetics were similar to the kinetics of suppressor activity in the BALB/c anti-C3H/He MLR. Chimeras with a typical runting syndrome showed a high spleen index (data not shown).

Adoptive transfer assay using chimeric spleen cells. In order to determine whether suppressor cells function in vivo, lethally x-irradiated C3H/He mice were injected with 10^7 spleen cells from BALB/c mice plus 5×10^6 spleen cells from (BALB/c→C3H/He) i.s. chimeras, or 5×10^6 spleen cells from BALB/c mice. As shown in Table 7, mean survival times of 13.3 days and 7.6 days were observed in the former and the

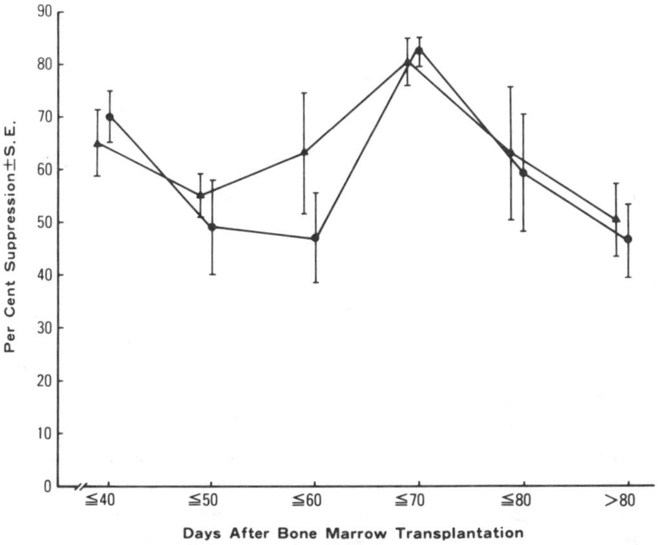

FIGURE 2. Time course of suppressor activities against BALB/c anti-C3H/He MLR. Suppressor activity in spleen cells from (BALB/c→C3H/He) i.v. chimeras (●—●). Suppressor activity in spleen cells from (BALB/c→C3H/He) i.s. chimeras (▲—▲). There were statistically significant differences in suppressor activities of i.v. chimeras between days 50 and 70 ($P<0.01$), and between days 60 and 70 ($P<0.05$), as determined by a *t* test.

TABLE 6. Histopathological changes in the liver of i.v. and i.s. chimeras

Chimera[a]	Magnitude of histopathological changes in the liver		
	Severe change	Moderate change	No change
i.v.	9/32 (28.1%)	7/32 (21.9%)	16/32 (50.0%)
i.s.	3/52 (5.8%)	15/52 (28.8%)	34/52 (65.4%)

[a] Chimeras 18 days to 269 days after bone marrow transplantation were used for the histopathological examination.

latter group, respectively. Similarly, when lethally x-irradiated C3H/He mice were injected with 3×10^6 bone marrow cells and 5×10^5 spleen cells from BALB/c mice, admixed with 5×10^5 spleen cells from (BALB/c→C3H/He) i.s. chimeras, the mean survival time was 9.8 days, and 2 of the 6 mice survived more than 30 days after BMT. In contrast, a mean survival time of 4.6 days was observed in the control group.

DISCUSSION

When spleen cells taken from i.v. or i.s. chimeras were used as responders in MLR shortly after bone marrow transplantation, low ^{3}H-TdR incorporation was always observed. Although the decreased response to donor and recipient antigens may be due to immunological tolerance, this would not be the case for the response to third-party antigens. We therefore suggest that suppressor cells may be generated in chimeras, although other possibilities also remain to be examined.

In terms of alloantigen specificity, both alloantigen-specific and nonspecific cells were observed in the spleens of i.v. and i.s. chimeras. According to dose response characteristics, alloantigen-specific suppressor cells may be different from alloantigen-nonspecific suppressor cells. Tutschka et al. (*19*) have reported that suppressor T cells responsible for the induction and maintenance of transplantation tolerance undergo a sequence of developmental steps from an alloantigen-nonspecific to an alloantigen-specific suppressor cell system that ultimately undergoes a clonal deletion. A similar change from nonspecific suppressor cells to specific suppressor cells has been reported by Slavin and Strober (*17*) who suggested that spleen cells from young chimeras 30–40 days after BMT inhibited the MLR nonspecifically, while spleen cells from old chimeras inhibited the MLR specifically. In our case, it is not at present clear whether nonspecific suppressor cells mature to specific suppressor cells. Regardless of the presence or absence of maturation of nonspecific suppressor cells into specific suppressor cells, there might be at least three suppressor cell populations—i.e., the first one for antidonor MLR, the second one for antirecipient MLR, and the third one for anti-third-party MLR. This possibility has been suggested by the finding of dose response characteristics that showed stronger suppressor activities against antidonor and antirecipient MLR than against anti-third-party MLR, although this was not always the case. There is, however, still some doubt as to whether nonspecific suppressor cells against anti-third-party MLR may also inhibit antidonor and antirecipient MLR. This uncertainty could be cleared up by using suppressor T cell clones.

According to time course studies of MLR coculture assays, there was a statistically significant decrease in suppressor activity in the i.v. chimeras 50–60 days after BMT. However, there was no decrease in suppressor activity in the i.s. chimeras in the same period. This is the only difference that could be detected in suppressor activity between i.v. and i.s. chimeras. Although this difference may be related to survival rates, there

TABLE 7. Adoptive transfer assay using spleen cells from i.s. chimeras

GVHR-inducing cells	Putative suppressor cells	Survival (days)	Mean ± SD
Exp. 1:			
BALB/c spleen cells[a]	None	7,8,8,9,9	8.2±0.8
BALB/c spleen cells[a]	BALB/c spleen cells[b]	6,7,7,8,8 8,8,8,8	7.6±0.7
BALB/c spleen cells[a]	(BALB/c→C3H/He)i.s. chimeric spleen cells[c]	8,8,8,8,9 13,25,27	13.3±7.5[f]
Exp. 2:			
BALB/c bone marrow cells +BALB/c spleen cells[a]	None	4,4,4,5,6	4.6±0.8
BALB/c bone marrow cells +BALB/c spleen cells[d]	(BALB/c→C3H/He)i.s. chimeric spleen cells[e]	5,6,7,21 >30,>30	>16.5±10.9[f]

[a] Spleen cells from BALB/c mice at a cell concentration of 10^7 cells/mouse were transferred into X-irradiated (925 rads) C3H/He mice.

[b] Spleen cells from BALB/c mice at a cell concentration of 5×10^6/mouse were mixed as control.

[c] Spleen cells from (BALB/c→C3H/He) i.s. chimeras 112 days after bone marrow transplantation were mixed as a suppressor source at a cell concentration of 5×10^6/mouse.

[d] BALB/c bone marrow cells (3×10^6/mouse) mixed with BALB/c spleen cells (5×10^5/mouse) were transferred into x-irradiated (925 rads) C3H/He mice.

[e] Spleen cells from (BALB/c→C3H/He) i.s. chimeras 204 days after bone marrow transplantation at a cell concentration of 5×10^5/mouse were mixed as suppressor source.

[f] There was a statistically significant difference ($P<0.05$) in mean survival days between the control and experimental group as determined by a *t* test.

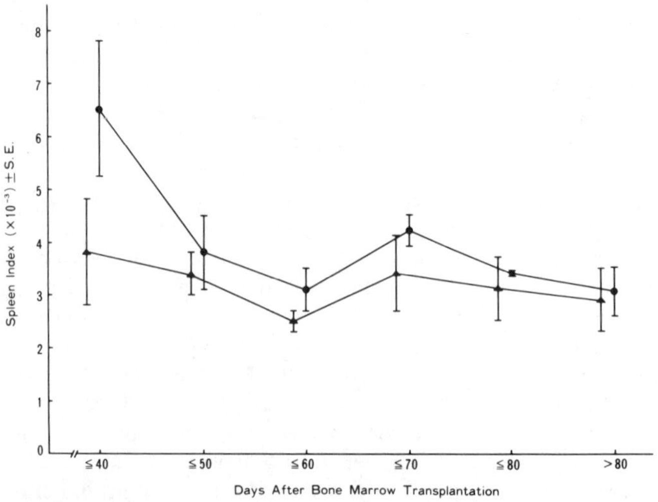

FIGURE 3. Time course of spleen indices. Spleen index of (BALB/c→C3H/He) i.v. chimeras (●—●) and spleen index of (BALB/c→C3H/He) i.s. chimeras (▲—▲).

is no direct evidence for that. At present, it is not yet clear why the i.s. chimeras had a weaker GVHR (e.g., a smaller change in the livers and a lower spleen index) than the i.v. chimeras, or why the suppressor activity in the i.s. chimeras remained in a comparably constant state for a long time, although it indicates that putting the marrow in the splenic environment induced these beneficial effects in the hosts.

It is unlikely that suppressor cells detected in MLR are mediated by antidonor or antihost cytotoxic T lymphocytes. Muto et al. (*37*) have reported that antidonor or antihost reactivity has been found even in chimeras that were tolerant to donor and recipient type antigens in MLR when their spleen cells were transferred into lethally x-irradiated donor or recipient mice. Spleen cells from chimeras seldom killed the BALB/c or C3H/He target cells at a E:T ratio of 50:1 (data not shown). In addition, there was no significant difference in cell yields between responder cells cocultured with spleen cells from normal mice and cells cocultured with spleen cells from chimeras 5 days after culturing (data not shown). This does not mean that spleen cells from chimeras kill responder cells, leading to decreased ^{3}H-TdR incorporation. Nevertheless, it does not completely rule out the possibility that decreased ^{3}H-TdR incorporation may be mediated by a reduction in the number of stimulator cells following the death of stimulator cells as a result of the cocultured cells. Therefore we tried to inactivate the possible cytotoxic activity in chimeric spleen cells by 2000-rad x-irradiation. Suppressor activity still remained after x-irradiation, although some suppressor activity was abrogated by this procedure. Since radiosensitive suppressor cells may play some role in vivo, we usually examined suppressor activities in coculture experiments without irradiating suppressor cells. In addition, since a factor derived from nonirradiated spleen cells showed a suppressor effect, it was suggested that irradiation should not be used.

An adoptive transfer assay suggested that suppressor cells detected in vitro MLR would function in vivo. Furthermore, GVHRs in the i.s. chimeras were weaker than those in the i.v. chimeras as determined by survival rates, histopathological changes in the liver, spleen index, and suppressor activity. Taken together, it might be reasonable to conclude that one of the factors suppressing GVHR might be the suppressor cells.

In conclusion, alloantigen-specific and nonspecific suppressor cells were generated in the spleens of i.v. and i.s. chimeras. They suppressed not only ^{3}H-TdR incorporation of responder cells but also the generation of cytotoxic cells. Furthermore, a 2-day culture supernatant from chimeric spleen cells exhibited suppressor activity, indicating that they secrete suppressor factors. Although there was no good correlation between the suppressor activity and histopathological changes in the liver, the results of an adoptive transfer assay suggested that suppressor cells function in vivo as well as in vitro. Furthermore, time course studies of the suppressor activity in i.v. and i.s. chimeras showed some differences in kinetics. These differences may be responsible for the beneficial effects of i.s. transplantation.

Acknowledgments. We thank Sachimi Nishikawa and Miho Sakai for typing the manuscript, and Haruyo Seki and Keiko Sano for secretarial assistance. We also deeply appreciate Dr. Norio Azumi, Laboratory of Surgical Pathology, Stanford University Medical Center, for his histopathological examinations.

REFERENCES

1. Enomoto K, Lucas Z. Immunological enhancement of renal allografts in the rat. III. Role of the spleen. Transplantation 1973; 15: 8.
2. Fabre JW, Batchelor JR. The role of the spleen in the rejection and enhancement of renal allografts in the rat. Transplantation 1975; 20: 219.
3. Kaplan HJ, Streilein JW. Do immunologically privileged sites require a functioning spleen? Nature 1974; 251: 353.
4. Levinson AI, Silvers WK. Effect of splenectomy on the induction of high degrees of tolerance to skin allografts in rats. Cell Immunol 1973; 6: 149.
5. Streilein JW, Grebe SC, Kaplan HJ, Streilein JS. An immunoregulatory role for the spleen in transplantation. Transplan Proc 1975; 7: 349.
6. Levine S. Graft-versus-host disease. Liver involvement in splenectomized rats. Transplantation 1968; 6: 294.
7. Bain GO, Suen WY, Remington DW, Pinno E. Liver infiltration in the graft-versus-host reaction. Transplantation 1969; 8: 83.
8. Gershon RK, Lance EM, Kondo K. Immuno-regulatory role of spleen localizing thymocytes. J Immunol 1974; 112: 546.
9. Grebe SC, Streilein JW. Graft-versus-host disease: a review. Adv Immunol 1976; 22: 120.
10. Imamura M, Miyazaki T, Okabe M, et al. Effect of intrasplenic injection of allogeneic bone marrow cells on the survival of lethally X-irradiated mice. Transplantation 1983; 35: 19.
11. Monaco AP, Gozzo JJ, Wood ML, Liegeois A. Use of low doses of homozygous allogeneic bone marrow cells to induce tolerance with antilymphocyte serum (ALS): tolerance by intraorgan injection. Transplant Proc 1971; 3: 680.
12. Tsoi MS, Storb R, Dobbs S, Santos E, Thomas ED. Specific suppressor cells and immune response to host antigens in long-term human allogeneic marrow recipients: implications for the mechanisms of graft-host tolerance and chronic graft-versus-host disease. Transplant Proc 1981; 13: 237.
13. Weiden PL, Storb R, Tsoi MS, Graham TC, Lerner KG, Thomas ED. Infusion of donor lymphocytes into stable canine radiation chimeras: implications for mechanism of transplantation tolerance. J Immunol 1976; 116: 1212.
14. Tsoi MS, Storb R, Dobbs S, Thomas ED. Specific suppressor cells in graft-host tolerance of HLA identical marrow transplantation. Nature 1981; 292: 355.
15. Hilgert J. The involvement of activated specific suppressor T cells in maintenance of transplantation tolerance. Immunol Rev 1979; 46: 27.
16. Tutschka PJ, Hutihns GW, Santos GW. Suppressor cells as possible mediators of immune function after marrow transplantation. In: Bamm SJ, Ledney GD, eds. Experimental Hematology New York: Springer, 1979: 113.
17. Slavin M, Strober S. Induction of allograft tolerance after total lymphoid irradiation (TLI): development of suppressor cells of the mixed leukocyte reaction (MLR). J Immunol 1979; 123: 942.
18. King DP, Strober S, Kaplan HS. Suppression of the mixed leukocyte response and of graft-vs-host disease by spleen cells following total lymphoid irradiation (TLI). J Immunol 1981; 126: 1140.
19. Tutschka PJ, Hess AD, Beschorner WE, Santos GW. Suppressor cells in transplantation tolerance. I. Suppressor cells in the mechanism of tolerance in radiation chimera. Transplantation 1981; 32: 203.
20. Tutschka PJ, Ki PF, Beschorner WE, Hess AD, Santos GW. Suppressor cells in transplantation tolerance. II. Maturation of suppressor cells in the bone marrow chimera. Transplantation 1981; 32: 321.
21. Tutschka PJ, Hess AD, Beshorner WE, Santos GW. Suppressor cells in transplantation tolerance. III. The role of antigen in the maintenance of transplantation tolerance. Transplantation 1982; 33: 510.
22. Basten A, Miller JFAP, Johnson P. T cell-dependent suppression of anti-hapten antibody response. Transplant Rev 1975; 26: 130.
23. Doyle MV, Parks DE, Weigle WO. Specific transient suppression of the immune response by HGG tolerant spleen cells. II. Effector cells and target cells. J Immunol 1976; 117: 1152.
24. Benjamin DC. Evidence for specific suppression in the maintenance of immunologic tolerance. J Exp Med 1975; 141: 635.
25. Parks DE, Doyle MV, Weigle WO. Induction and mode of action of suppression cells generated against human gamma globulin. I. An immunologic unresponsive state devoid of demonstrable suppressor cells. J Exp Med 1979; 148: 625.
26. Parks DE, Shaller DA, Weigle WO. Induction and mode of action of suppressor cells generated against human gamma globulin. II. Effect of colchicine. J Exp Med 1979; 149: 1168.
27. Loblay RH, Groth BF, Pritchard-Briscoe H, Basten A. Suppressor T cell memory. II. The role of memory suppressor T cells in the tolerance to human gamma globulin. J Exp Med 1983; 157: 957.
28. Nossal GJ, Pike BL. Functional clonal deletion in immunological tolerance to major histocompatibility complex antigens. Proc Natl Acad Sci USA 1981; 78: 3844.
29. Voisin GA, Kinsky R, Maillard J. Protection against homologous disease in hybrid mice by passive and active immunological enhancement facilitation. Transplantation 1968; 6: 187.
30. Hellström I, Hellström KE, Strob R, Thomas ED. Colony inhibition of fibroblasts from chimeric dogs mediated by the dogs' own lymphocytes and specifically abrogated by their serum. Proc Natl Acad Sci USA 1970; 66: 65.
31. Heron I. Is transplantation tolerance in the rat serum-mediated? Transplantation 1973; 15: 534.
32. Tsoi MS, Storb R, Weiden PL, Graham TC, Schroeder ML, Thomas ED. Canine marrow transplantation: are serum blocking factors necessary to maintain the stable chimeric state? J Immunol 1975; 114: 531.
33. Tsoi MS, Storb R, Weiden P, Santos E, Kopecky KJ, Thomas ED. Sequential studies of cell inhibition of host fibroblasts in 51 patients given HLA-identical marrow grafts. J Immunol 1982; 128: 239.
34. Tsoi MS, Storb R, Jones E, et al. Deposition of IgM and complement at the dermoepidermal junction in acute and chronic graft-versus-host disease in man. J Immunol 1978; 120: 1485.
35. Sado T, Kamisaku H. Allogeneic radiation chimeras induced in SPF mice: some immunobiological insights into immunologic dysfunctions and instabilities. Acta Haematol Japan 1977; 40: 900.
36. Imamura M, Gipson TG, Bensky N, Justice R, Martin WJ. Lung tumor-reactive cytotoxic lymphocytes generated in mixed lymphocyte reaction between C3HfeB/Hen ($H\text{-}2^{kb}$) and C3H/He ($H\text{-}2^{k}$) strain mice. J Immunol 1979; 122: 1863.
37. Muto M, Sado T, Aizawa S, Kamisaku H, Kubo E. Transplantation across the major histocompatibility barrier in specific-pathogen-free mice: effects of intact versus T cell-depleted bone marrow on the expression of anti-host reaction in the recipient spleens. J Immunol 1981; 127: 2421.

Received 10 July 1985.
Accepted 22 January 1986.

0041-1337/86/4205-0556$02.00/0
TRANSPLANTATION
Vol. 42, No. 5

Printed in U.S.A.

Transplantation

BRIEF COMMUNICATIONS

RENAL TRANSPLANTATION IN PATIENTS WITH A HISTORY OF HEROIN ABUSE

Recent improvement in cadaver graft survival has resulted in an upsurge in interest in transplantation. Patients who have been on dialysis for a number of years are increasingly requesting transplantation; yet the availability of cadaver kidneys has not significantly increased. As a result, cadaver kidneys are again becoming a scarce medical resource. As such, they should be utilized to provide the maximum benefit.

Former heroin addicts are potentially a high-risk group for transplantation. These patients have previously demonstrated irresponsible behavior. In addition, heroin, either by itself or because of associated impurities, has been implicated as a cause of renal failure. Both short and long-term patient and graft survival could be compromised by lack of compliance as well as by continued intravenous abuse of drugs. However, many addicts who discontinue use of the drug do not return to their addiction and such patients frequently demonstrate compliant behavior while on hemodialysis. A question remains, however, as to whether these individuals should be accepted for renal transplantation without regard to their history of heroin addiction. In this study, we compared the results of transplantation in a selected group of former heroin addicts with results in a matched control group.

Between June 1967, and April 1985, 665 patients underwent renal transplantation at Montefiore Medical Center. During this period patient selection criteria and immunosuppressive protocols have gradually evolved. For example, routine pretransplant blood transfusions were given to all patients starting in 1979, and cyclosporine was introduced in 1983. Since the inception of the program, patients with a history of drug abuse were accepted for transplantation if there was no longer any evidence of drug use and if the patients were compliant with their dialysis regimen.

The charts of all patients receiving renal transplants were reviewed. Twenty-one patients who were known heroin addicts (by chart documentation or by direct interview) were selected for detailed study and will henceforth be referred to as the *study group*. Patients whose drug abuse could not be confirmed by chart review or by interview were excluded from the study. The study group includes patients whose renal failure was thought to be secondary to the drug abuse and those whose renal disease was attributed to other causes. The 21 patients received 25 cadaver transplants (20 first, 5 second). Data for first and second transplants were considered separately.

For each first-transplant recipient in the study group, two matched control patients were selected (40 patients). The controls were all first-transplant recipients and were selected to match for age (±5 years), date of transplantation (±10 months), race, and donor source. There were no diabetic recipients in the study or control groups. When two controls could not be found for each patient, only one parameter was allowed to deviate in order to identify a second control patient. In nine controls, the age bracket was extended to up to nine years; five controls differed in race from their study counterparts and one differed in sex.

There was a uniform distribution of transplants to patients with a history of heroin abuse throughout the period from 1972 to 1985 (Table 1). The mean age (±SD) of the study group was 34.9 (±7.6) years (range 20–48), whereas the mean age of the control group was 35.1 (±8.2) years (range 18–50). There were 15 black and five white patients in the study group, and 26 black and 14 white patients in the control group. Three of the 20 study group patients and seven of the 40 controls were female.

One-year and four-year patient survivals were 95% and 77%, respectively, in the study group, and 95% and 88% in the control group (NS). The causes of death in the study group (5) and the control group (8) did not significantly differ, with the leading cause of death in both groups being infection. One-year and four-year graft survivals were 65% and 44%, respectively, in the study group and 64% and 51% in the control group. One-year first cadaver graft survival for all patients at our institution has steadily improved over the last five years and is currently >80%. In patients with functioning grafts mean serum creatinine at 12, 24, and 48 months was 2.2, 2.4, and 1.4, respectively, in the study group and 2.1, 2.7, and 1.2, respectively, in the control group (NS).

The pathogenesis of graft loss in the 10 study patients who ultimately lost their grafts was chronic rejection in seven, acute rejection in one, and stopping medications in two. In the control group, graft loss was secondary to chronic rejection in 14, sepsis in one, and recurrent disease in one (NS).

There was an average of 1.5 treated rejection episodes per patient in the study group as compared with 2.5 in the remainder of the patients. There was an average of 1.1 infectious complications per patient (4 local viral, 2 systemic viral, 14 bacterial including urinary tract infections, 1 TB) in the study group, similar to that seen in the controls. Two patients in the study group and three controls died of an infectious cause. In the study group, one patient died secondary to systemic viral infection 2.5 months posttransplant. The second death was due to pneumonia 41 months posttransplant and 8 months after returning to dialysis.

Five former drug abusers received second transplants. Four of these five are alive 2–12 years following their second transplant. One-year graft survival was 50% in this group of patients, similar to our overall graft survival for retransplants during the same time period. One of these patients received a third transplant that never functioned.

Of the 20 former addicts in the study group, 15 are still alive and eight have functioning kidneys (3 months to 12 years posttransplant) (Table 1). One patient has returned to using intravenous heroin since his transplant. His kidney continues to have good function 4.5 years after transplantation despite noncompliance with his medications. In the remaining patients, there is no evidence of return to heroin abuse at any time after transplantation; however, two patients did lose their kidneys secondary to noncompliance with immunosuppressive medications.

TABLE 1. Transplantation data

Patient number	Sex	Age at time of transplant	Date of transplant	Outcome
1	M	20	5/24/72	Died at 18.5 months with graft function from unknown causes, at home
2	F	25	10/10/72	Died at 44 months with graft function from trauma
3	M	45	4/1/73	Returned to dialysis at 1.5 months
4	M	24	4/7/73	Returned to dialysis at 20 months
5	M	27	2/11/76	Returned to dialysis at 53 months
6	M	32	5/11/76	Returned to dialysis at one month; died at 2.5 months from infection
7	M	33	8/21/79	Returned to dialysis at one month; died at 24.5 months from unknown cause
8	M	39	10/27/79	Alive with graft function
9	M	34	8/10/80	Alive with graft function
10	M	41	12/9/80	Returned to dialysis at 33 months; died at 41 months from infection
11	M	44	1/26/81	Returned to dialysis at three months
12	F	43	3/18/81	Alive with function
13	M	31	1/27/82	Returned to dialysis at three months
14	M	32	5/29/83	Returned to dialysis at four months
15	M	48	9/28/83	Returned to dialysis at 13.5 months
16	M	36	10/7/83	Alive with function
17	M	36	1/14/84	Alive with function
18	F	33	3/17/84	Alive with function
19	M	43	2/1/85	Alive with function
20	M	32	2/28/85	Returned to dialysis at two months

The moral and practical implication surrounding the decision as to who should receive renal transplants has plagued transplant surgeons since the first transplant was performed. The ability to identify patients at high risk for transplantation would result in a more efficient use of available kidneys. It has been suggested that former heroin addicts are one of these high-risk groups. Their potentially altered immunological state may increase their posttransplant complication rate. Their previous behavior raises doubts regarding the probability of their return to heroin use and the reliability of their future compliance with medical regimens.

Rao et al., in 1978, described 11 patients with heroin nephropathy who received four cadaver and seven living-related transplants. After a mean follow-up of 14 months, three had died, two others had lost their kidneys to rejection, and two patients had resumed heroin use (*1*). Ross et al., reported a series of eight addicted patients who received renal transplants, with a one-year patient survival rate of 100% and a graft survival rate of 75% (*2*). Stevens et al., reported on 20 transplants in 15 patients who were formerly addicted. There was an 87% one-year patient survival in this group and a 65% one-year graft survival (*3*).

Wc have also shown acceptable patient and graft survival in a carefully selected group of former heroin abusers. Of significance, however, is the large number of patients in our series, the longer follow-up, and the inclusion of a matched control group which, when compared with our study group, did not reveal any statistically significant differences in patient or graft survival. In addition, there was no difference in the rate of infectious complications or in cause of graft loss.

We believe that a past history of heroin addiction in patients showing evidence of being "drug-free" should not be considered a contraindication to renal transplantation.

MICHAEL J.V. GORDON
RONALD WHITE
ARTHUR J. MATAS[1]
VIVIAN A. TELLIS
DAN GLICKLICH
THERESA QUINN
ROBERT SOBERMAN
FRANK J. VEITH
Department of Surgery
Montefiore Medical Center
New York, New York 10467

[1] Address reprint requests to: Arthur J. Matas, M.D., Department of Surgery, Montefiore Medical Center, 111 East 210th Street, New York, NY 10467.

REFERENCES

1. Rao L, et al. Experience with 100 renal transplants. J Med Assoc Thai 1978; 1: 131.
2. Ross G, et al. Renal transplantation in the end stage renal disease of drug abuse. J Urol 1983; 129: 14.
3. Stevens J, et al. Renal transplantation in heroin addicts. Surg Gynecol Obstet 1983; 156: 651.

Received 20 November 1985.
Accepted 5 February 1986.

HLA-DP MATCHING AND GRAFT-VERSUS-HOST DISEASE IN ALLOGENEIC BONE MARROW TRANSPLANTATION[1]

Allogeneic bone marrow transplantation (BMT)* for the treatment of hematological malignancies and severe aplastic anemia has developed from an experimental procedure to a standard therapeutic approach over the past 10 years. The greatest experience so far has been acquired in transplanting HLA-identical sibling BM (*1*) in order to minimize graft-versus-host disease (GVHD). Nonetheless, in transplantation of BM from sources other than identical twins, acute (a) and chronic (c) GVHD cannot be consistently avoided, even under cyclosporine prophylaxis. This problem has gained further prominence with the introduction of HLA-haploidentical family BMT, and even HLA-phenoidentical unrelated-donor BMT. One approach to overcoming life-threating GVHD has been to deplete the BM of mature T cells prior to transplantation, which has resulted in significant reductions of the incidence and severity of aGVHD (*2*). However, delayed take or late rejection of the transplant may present a further problem when applying this technique (*3*). A long-standing theoretical possibility to avoid GVHD remains an improved method for tissue typing of donor and recipient in order to match for a greater range of—and/or the most important—transplantation antigens. However, one cause of GVHD is generally accepted to be mismatching for multiple "minor" transplantation antigens (*4*), which could provide insuperable problems of matching. Although several examples have now been reported in which cells from patients with GVHD have been shown to recognize minor antigens (*5–7*), such demonstrations require selective in vitro culture and/or cloning techniques to isolate the effector cells. Thus, their direct relevance for GVHD in vivo remains questionable. On the other hand, major histocompatibility complex (MHC) matching in most transplantation centers relies upon establishing identity at the class I HLA-A, B, and C loci, and at the class II locus HLA-DR, by serological techniques, and demonstrating mutual cellular nonreactivity in one-way and two-way mixed lymphocyte cultures (MLC). In addition, typing for the "supertypic" DRw52 and DRw53 specificities and the DQ locus products, has recently increased the potential discriminatory power of serological typing. Linkage disequilibrium is so high between DR, DRw, and DQ, however, that typing for the latter would not really be expected to improve matching. Some years ago, a new allelic member of the MHC class II gene family was described in man, and provisionally designated "SB" for "secondary B" cell antigen (*8*). It received this designation because its products could be detected only by secondary proliferative (primed lymphocyte typing, PLT) or cytotoxic responses of appropriately sensitized lymphocytes. This class II gene system, now recognized as HLA-DP (*9*), is encoded centromeric to DR/DQ (*10*), and its alleles are in very weak, or absent, linkage disequilibrium with the rest of the MHC (*11, 12*). The contribution of DP products to stimulation in primary MLC, even in the absence of strongly immunogenic DR/Dw differences, is weak or negligible (*8, 12*)—thus MLC typing of patients' families for BMT donor selection would not necessarily be informative for differences between recipient and donor at HLA-DP. Thus far, no reports have appeared to indicate that HLA-DP, as a major histocompatibility antigen, actually behaves as a transplantation antigen in contributing to organ rejection or GVHD (*13*). One possible anecdotal exception to this statement may be the reference to a case of severe aGVHD in the face of a DP-mismatched transplant cited by E. Möller et al. (*14*). These authors argued that, since a recombination between HLA-DR/DQ and DP is not infrequent, a sizeable proportion of BMT is carried out between DP-incompatible siblings. Thus, severe aGVHD could often be a result of DP-mismatch, rather than minor antigen incompatibility.

In order to approach the question of the potential relevance of HLA-DP matching to the incidence and severity of aGVHD or cGVHD in a clinical context, retrospective PLT typing for HLA-DPw1 through DPw5 was performed on 36 Tübingen BMT donor/recipent pairs. The results of DP typing of the donors and of the recipients before transplantation are shown in Table 1, together with an assessment of the worst grade of aGVHD that the patients suffered, their respective cGVHD status, and survival after transplantation. It is clear from these results that severe aGVHD and cGVHD can still develop in the face of a known match at the HLA-DP locus. In many instances, patient and donor shared the extremely common (in the white population, [*12*]) DPw4 specificity, which is suspected of being heterogeneous (*11, 15*). In these cases, it could be argued that there might well be differences between donor and recipient DPw4 subtypes, but that these were not detectable by the PLT reagents employed in this study. The application of finely discriminatory T cell clones (*15*) could help to resolve this question. Nonetheless, there are also clear cases where donor/recipient identity for the less common, remarkably homogeneous DPw specificities (DPw1, w2, w3, w5, [*13, 16*]) still resulted in severe aGVHD. Thus, for example, patients UPN 5 and UPN 18, carrying DPw2/5 and DPw2/2, suffered aGVHD grades III and II, respectively, despite being grafted with DP-matched BM.

In the material presented here there were only 3 cases of DP nonidentity between donor and recipient. In one case, in the family of patient UPN 4, the DPw2/4 donor was the mother of the DPw4/4 recipient. (Figure 1A shows the pedigree.) This situation of F_1-to-parent would not be predicted to result in recognition of the host by the grafted cells (unless DPw4 heterogeneity was present). In the family of patient UPN 47 (Fig. 1B), again the donor typed DPw2/4 and the recipient DPw4/4. In this case, the data, including GLO typing, are consistent with recombination on the maternal haplotype resulting in the inheritance of DPw2 instread of DPw4 by the patient's sister, the donor. In the third case, in the family of patient UPN 10 (Fig. 1C), an interesting situation has arisen that cannot be explained by crossing-over. Three repeated typing experiments failed to indicate the presence of either maternal haplotype-encoded DPw specificity (DPw2 or 3) in the patient, although her cells were perfectly capable of restimulating anti-DPw4 reagents responding to paternal haplotype-encoded products. This resulted, therefore, in a typing of DPw4/blank for the patient, but DPw3/4 for the donor. Despite this difference, the patient did not experience aGVHD or

* Abbreviations used: aGVHD, acute GVHD, BM, bone marrow; BMT, BM transplantation; cGVHD, chronic GVHD; GVHD, graft-versus-host disease; MHC, major histocompatibility complex; MLC, mixed lymphocyte cultures; PLT, primed lymphocyte typing.

[1] This work was supported by the Deutsche forschungsgemeinschaft, SFB 120, A1, B1.

TABLE 1. DP typing of HLA-A,B,C,DR,Dw identical recipient-donor pairs in allogeneic BMT, arranged in order of severity of aGVHD[a]

UPN	Age	Sex	Diagnosis	GVHD prophylaxis	DP type		GVHD		Survival (days)	Cause of death/K.I.
					Patient	Donor	Acute	Chronic		
94	14	m	ALL	Csa	4	4	IV	–	+36	50
5	25	m	SAA	MTX	2/5	2/5	III	–	34	P, aGVHD
26	21	m	ANLL	ATG/MTX	4	4	III	–	93	S
72	17	m	ALL	ATG/Csa	3	3	III	E	335	S, GVHD
73	15	m	CML	ATG/Csa	4/4	4/4	III	0	+362	100
38	43	f	ANLL	Csa	4	4	II	E	143	CMV-P
44	29	f	ANLL	ATG/Csa	3/bl	3/bl	II	–	57	CMV-P
91	24	m	ANLL	Csa	2	2	II	–	+96	100
60	20	m	ALL	ATG/Csa	4/4	4/4	II	L	301	R
75	25	m	CML	ATG/Csa	4	4	II	E	+327	60
18	5	m	ALL	ATG/MTX	2/2	2/2	II	0	+1689	100
29	24	f	ANLL	ATG/MTX	3	3	I	0	+1383	100
47	23	m	CML	ATG/MTX	4/4	2/4	I	E	254	VZV-P
9	12	m	SAA	MTX	2/3	2/3	I	E	303	VZV-P
57	5	m	CML	ATG/MTX	4/4	4/4	I	0	+726	100
63	19	m	SAA	Csa	4	4	I	L	+523	100
76	44	m	CML	ATG/CSA	2,3	2,3	I	L	+299	80
65	20	m	CML	Csa	4	4	I	0	+523	100
67	20	m	CML	Csa	1,3	1,3	I	0	+481	100
69	15	f	CML	ATG/Csa	1	1	I	0	+432	100
74	26	m	ANLL	ATG/Csa	4	4	I	0	+341	100
80	24	m	SAA	Csa	2,4	2,4	I	0	+243	100
81	38	f	ALL	Csa	2,5	2,5	I	–	106	R
85	18	m	ALL	Csa	4/4	4/4	I	0	+166	100
88	27	f	ANLL	Csa	4	4	I	0	+138	100
95	37	m	ANLL	Csa	4/4	4/4	I	–	+29	100
58	18	m	CML	ATG/Csa	4	4	I	L	+711	100
93	11	m	ALL	Csa	2/4	2/4	I	–	+54	100
77	14	m	ANLL	ATG/Csa	2,4	2,4	0	0	+285	100
10	21	f	AUL	ATG/MTX	4/bl	3/4	0	–	64	I-P
24	17	m	ANLL	ATG/MTX	5	5	0	0	827	R
37	30	f	ANLL	ATG/Csa	2	2	0	–	24	A-P
48	24	m	CML	ATG/Csa	4	4	0	0	+921	100
4	29	m	AUL	MTX	4/4	2/4	0	–	21	P
20	13	f	ALL	–	2/2	2/2	0	0[b]	421	R
89	21	m	ALL	–	2/4	2/4	0	0[b]	+124	100

[a] HLA-DP genotyping (a/b) or phenotyping (a,b) was performed on HLA-A,B,C,DR,Dw-genotyped mononuclear cells from donor-recipient siblings (except the family of patient UPN 4 where the donor was the mother), using the PLT reagents described elsewhere (*8*, *11*), after expansion in IL-2-containing medium (*15*). Two independent PLT reagents were employed for the definition of each specificity, and resulting data were analyzed by a centroid cluster program (*8*, *15*). When both PLT reagents for a particular DP specifically demonstrated significant positive clustering of arithmetic and log-transformed data, that specificity was assigned. Absence of a typable specificity (in genotyped material) is indicated as bl. Survival times are as of 18.12.1985. (K.I.) Karnovsky index for patients currently alive; (L) limited; (E) extensive; (MTX) methotrexate; (ATG) antithymocyte globulin; (Csa) cyclosporine; (ALL) acute lymphocytic leukemia; (ANLL) acute nonlymphocytic leukemia; (CML) chronic myelogenous leukemia; (SAA) severe aplastic anemia; (P) pneumonia; (S) sepsis; (CMV) cytomegalovirus; (VZV) varicella zoster virus; (A) *Aspergillus*; (I) interstitial; (R) relapse. Clinical assessment of GVHD was performed following the Seattle classification.

[b] Syngeneic BMT.

cGVHD. The reason for the lack of maternal-haplotype-encoded DPw product by the patient is unknown, and requires molecular genetic analysis.

Thus, in summary, from these results in families unselected for HLA recombinational events (excluding families of UPN 10, 20, and 89), the recombination frequency between HLA-DR/DQ and DP is 1/66 or 1.5%. This agrees very well with previous estimates (*13*), but is lower than the estimate of 3.3% made by studying HTC derived from selected consanguineous families (*17*), and is considerably less than seen in populations selected only for homozygosity at HLA-D (HTC), in which 24% typed for two different DP specificities (*18*). The figure for HLA-A,B,C,DR,Dw-matched, DP-mismatched unrelated donors would thus be expected to fall between these values. Although in the family material presented here, no DP differences between donor and recipient that would be expected to lead to recognition and to contribute to GVHD were found after excluding syngeneic BMT, numerous incidences of varying degrees of aGVHD (≥ grade II, 11/34 [32%]; including grade I, 28/34 [82%]) and cGVHD (9/24 [38%]) have been observed in the face of DPw compatibility. Although these data obviously could not exclude a role for DP differences were the recipients to have expressed DP antigens potentially recognizable by the graft, they do suggest that HLA-DP matching is of little prognostic benefit in avoiding GVHD in HLA-matched sibling combinations. If HLA-DP does not contribute critically to GVHD, this would be reassuring to know in the context of increasing application of unrelated HLA-matched (i.e., HLA-

Family pedigrees.

A) Fam. patient UPN 4.

Father	Mother (donor)
a) 2, -, 44, 5, 4, 1	c) 2, 5, 44, -, 4, 1
b) 2, 4, 35, -, 4, 2	d) 2, -, 44, 5, 2, 2

Sister	Brother	Patient
a) 2, -, 44, 5, 4, 1	b) 2, 4, 35, -, 4, 2	a) 2, -, 44, 5, 4, 1
d) 2, -, 44, 5, 2, 2	d) 2, -, 44, 5, 2, 2	c) 2, 5, 44, -, 4, 1

B) Fam. patient UPN 47.

Father	Mother
a) 31, 3, 60, 4, 4, 1	c) 2, 3, 62, (4), 2, 2
b) 3, 3, 7, 5, (4), 2	d) 3, 7, 7, (4), 4, (2)

Donor	Patient
a) 31, 3, 60, 4, 4, 1	a) 31, 3, 60, 4, 4, 1
c) 2, 3, 62, (4), 2, 2	c/d) 2, 3, 62, (4), 4, 2

C) Fam. patient UPN 10.1*

Father	Mother
a) 2, -, 17, 7, 4	c) 25, -, 18, 3, 2
b) 29, -, 44, 3, (4)	d) -, 2, 13, 1, 3

Donor	Patient
a) 2, -, 17, 7, 4	a) 2, -, 17, 7, 4
d) -, 2, 13, 1, 3	d) -, 2, 13, 1, blank.

FIGURE 1. Order of loci: HLA-A, C, B, DR, DP, GLO. (*) GLO typing not informative

A,B,C,DR and MLC-matched) donor transplantation for patients without related donors—in whom, as discussed above, the incidence of mismatch at DP is certainly greater than within a family.

Acknowledgments. The generous gift of PLT reagents from S. Shaw is gratefully acknowledged. Technical assistance was provided by A. Rehbein, I. Balko, and E. Schneider, and computer programming by M. Blaurock. We acknowledge the critical contribution to this study of our clinical colleagues responsible for the Tübingen BMT program.

GRAHAM PAWELEC
GERHARD EHNINGER
HELMUT SCHMIDT
PETER WERNET
Immunology Laboratory
Medizinische Klinik
D-7400 Tübingen, Federal Republic of Germany

REFERENCES

1. Beatty PG, Clift RA, Mickelson EM, et al. Marrow transplantation from related donors other than HLA-identical siblings. N Engl J Med 1985; 313: 765.
2. Rodt H, Kolb HJ, Netzel B, et al. Effect of anti-T cell globulin on GVHD in leukemic patients treated with BMT. Transplant Proc 1981; 13: 257.
3. Martin PJ, Hansen JA, Buckner CD, et al. Effects of in vitro depletion of T cells in HLA-identical allogeneic marrow grafts. Blood 1985; 66: 664.
4. Korngold R, Sprent J. Lethal GVHD across minor histocompatibility barriers: nature of the effector cells and role of the H-2 complex. Immunol Rev 1983; 71: 5.
5. Goulmy E, Gratama JW, Blokland E, Zwaan FE, van Rood JJ. A minor transplantation antigen detected by MHC-restricted cytotoxic T lymphocytes during graft versus host disease. Nature 1983; 302: 159.
6. Irle C, Beatty PG, Mickelson E, Thomas ED, Hansen JA. Alloreactive T cell responses between HLA-identical siblings. Detection of anti-minor histocompatibility T cell clones induced in vivo. Transplantation 1985; 40: 329.
7. Goulmy E, Blokland E, Gratama JW, Zwaan FE, van Rood JJ. Detection of minor histocompatibility antigens by MHC-restricted cytotoxic T lymphocytes generated during graft versus host disease. Exp Hematol 1984; 12(suppl 15): 77.
8. Shaw S, Johnson AH, Shearer GM. Evidence for a new segregant series of B cell antigens that are encoded in the HLA-D region and that stimulate secondary proliferative and cytotoxic responses. J Exp Med 1980; 152: 565.
9. Bodmer WF. The HLA system, 1984. In: Albert ED, Bauer MP, Mayr WR, eds. Histocompatibility testing 1984. Heidelberg: Springer Verlag, 1984: 11.
10. Kavathas P, DeMars R, Bach FH, Shaw S. SB: a new HLA-linked human histocompatibility gene defined using HLA mutant cell lines. Nature 1981; 293: 747.
11. Shaw S, Duquesnoy R, Smith PL. Population studies of the HLA-linked SB antigens. Immunogenetics 1981; 14: 153.
12. Pawelec G, Shaw S, Schneider M, et al. Population studies of the HLA-linked SB antigens and their relative importance in MLC typing: analysis of HLA-D homozygous typing cells and normal heterozygous populations. Hum Immunol 1982; 5: 215.
13. Sanchez-Perez M, Shaw S. HLA-DP: current status. In: Solheim BG, Möller E, Ferrone S, eds. HLA class II antigens. A comprehensive review of structure and function. Berlin: Springer, 1986: 83.
14. Möller E, Carlsson B, Wallin J. Distinct or overlapping functions of human class II genes? Scand J Immunol 1984; 22: 483.
15. Pawelec G, Shaw S, Wernet P. Analysis of the HLA-linked SB gene system with cloned and uncloned alloreactive T cell lines. Immunogenetics 1982; 15: 187.
16. Pawelec G, Shaw S, Schneider M, Rehbein A, Wernet P. Homogeneity of the HLA-linked SB2 and SB3 specificities demonstrated by cloned alloreactive T cells. Immunogenetics 1983; 17: 179.
17. Termijtelen A, Merakhan P, Shaw S, van Rood JJ. Mapping SB in relation to HLA and GLO using cells from first cousin marriage offspring. Immunogenetics 1983; 18: 503.
18. Wernet P, Shaw S, Brautbar C, Westphal E, Pawelec G. SB types of HLA-D homozygous typing cells. Immunogenetics 1983; 18: 547.

Received 14 January 1986.
Accepted 28 January 1986.

ORTHOTOPIC LIVER TRANSPLANTATION FOR HEPATOBILIARY MALIGNANCY

Report of Three Cases of Special Interest

The following experience with liver replacement in the presence of primary hepatobiliary malignancy has recently been reported by Iwatsuki et al. (*1*):

Malignancy principle indication for OLT: 41
Overall survival (4 months to 8⅔ years): 11 (27%)
Potentially cured by OLT: 27
Developed recurrence (median onset 8 months): 20 (74%)
Malignancy incidental to other liver disease: 13
Overall survival (median 16 months): 12 (92%)
Developed recurrence: 0

Based on their experience, a refinement in the role of liver replacement in cancer therapy can be anticipated. We report three cases of malignancy treated at UCLA with liver replacement the outcome of which is in contrast to that reported in the Denver/Pittsburgh series.

Since February 1984, we have performed orthotopic liver transplantation in 45 patients. Eight of our patients have had hepatobiliary neoplasms (Table 1). Our first recipient (OLT 1) was a 44-year-old man with a primary hepatic schwannoma. Although his initial postoperative course was quite encouraging, he subsequently developed widespread lymphatic and pulmonary metastases and died four months postoperatively. OLT 4 was a 41-year-old woman with a primary hepatoma. Her course was complicated by graft failure necessitating retransplantation. She died 32 days postoperatively with cerebral anoxia. There was no evidence of tumor recurrence at postmortem examination. OLT 6 is a girl who underwent transplantation at age 18½ months for an unresectable hepatoblastoma. Expert slide review confirmed the tumor to be in the favorable histology group, so she received no adjuvant chemotherapy. She is now 17 months posttransplant without evidence of recurrence. OLT 9 is a 17-month-old child with a giant hemangioendothelioma of the liver that was unresponsive to chemotherapy and right hepatic artery embolization. She is now 15 months posttransplant without evidence of recurrence. OLT 28 is a 50-year-old man with chronic active hepatitis B complicated by multifocal hepatocellular carcinoma. He is without recurrence now, 6 months postoperatively. The course of these five patients is in accordance with the Denver/Pittsburgh experience. The three patients in our series we find to be of particular interest include a 15-year-old girl with metastatic leiomyosarcoma, a 7½-year-old boy with tyrosinemia and hepatoma, and a 52-year-old woman with sclerosing cholangitis and cholangiocarcinoma.

Patient 1. OLT 2 is a 15-year-old girl who was diagnosed in May 1983 as having gastric leiomyosarcoma. She underwent partial gastrectomy at our center. Intraoperatively bilobar hepatic metastases were noted. A few paragastric nodes contained tumor, but there was no spread to celiac or paraaortic nodes. Postoperatively she was treated with chemotherapy. She received courses of Vincristine and Actinomycin plus Cytoxan alternating with courses of Vincristine and Adriamycin plus Cytoxan. Follow-up abdominal computerized tomography (CT)* scans showed minimal response initially and then mild progression within the liver. Multigated acquisition scan showed a modest diminution in her cardiac function (though still within normal limits) after a total Adriamycin dose of only 275 mg (200 mg/m^2).

Because there were no other options for treatment, liver replacement was decided upon. Preoperative CT scan revealed two large lesions involving both lobes and no evidence of extrahepatic disease in the abdomen or thorax. Hepatic transplantation was performed, and at exploration regional lymph nodes were examined by frozen section and found to be free of tumor. Histological examination of her liver confirmed the diagnosis of multifocal metastatic leiomyosarcoma. No adjuvant chemotherapy has been given and her immunosuppression is standard with cyclosporine and low-dose prednisone. Her postoperative course was uneventful and she is without known recurrence 21 months after transplant.

Patient 2. OLT 11 was a 7½-year-old boy diagnosed in infancy as having tyrosinemia. Dietary measures allowed reasonable neurologic development. He did, however, develop progressive cirrhosis, and several months prior to transplantation, hepatoma was discovered. CT scan revealed enlarged retroperitoneal lymph nodes. When a suitable liver became available he was explored, with a plan to abort should evidence of extrahepatic disease be found. All enlarged nodes and several normal-appearing nodes were examined by frozen section. There was no evidence of tumor spread, so total hepatectomy and orthotopic liver transplantation were carried out. Permanent section confirmed the presence of multifocal, moderately well-differentiated hepatocellular carcinoma in the liver. Examination of the lymph nodes revealed only sinus histiocytosis. However, tumor thrombus was found in one of the hepatic veins. Clonogenic assay was performed, but no agent was found to be particularly effective. Likewise, a monoclonal antibody that reacted with his tumor was not found. The postoperative course was uncomplicated and the child was discharged in 3½ weeks. A rejection episode responded to a steroid cycle seven weeks after transplantation. Four weeks later it was discovered that his alpha fetoprotein level had increased fourfold. CT scan revealed multiple abdominal, mediastinal, and pulmonary metastases. The child was begun on chemotherapy, but did not demonstrate any significant response and died 11 months postoperatively. He represents an example of aggressive tumor growth in a hepatocellular carcinoma found incidental to a nonmalignant cause of end-stage liver disease.

Patient 3. OLT 18 is a 52-year-old woman with end-stage liver disease secondary to sclerosing cholangitis. She underwent orthotopic liver transplantation in early February 1985. On gross examination there was no evidence of malignancy in her native liver. However, histologic examination revealed a mucinous adenocarcinoma arising in the extrahepatic bile duct with perineural and vascular invasion. Margins of resection were clear. We elected not to use adjuvant chemotherapy and did not alter our usual immunosuppressive regimen. Although her postoperative course was complicated by acute renal failure and reoperation for intrathoracic bleeding, she was discharged on the forty-first postoperative day. At ten months posttransplant there has been no evidence of tumor recurrence.

This case is of particular interest for two reasons. First, no cases of sclerosing cholangitis were included among the thirteen patients with malignancies incidental to nonneoplastic liver

* Abbreviation used: CT, computerized tomography.

TABLE 1. UCLA experience with OLT in the presence of hepatobiliary neoplasm

Patient	Neoplasm	Associated Liver Disease	Outcome
OLT 1 (44, male)	Hepatic schwannoma	None	Died, recurrent tumor 4 months postop.
OLT 2 (15, female)	Metastic gastric leiomyosarcoma	None	Alive, no recurrence 21 months postop.
OLT 4 (41, female)	Primary hepatoma	None	Died, no recurrence 32 days postop.
OLT 6 (18 months, female)	Hepatoblastoma	None	Alive, no recurrence 17 months postop.
OLT 9 (17 months, female)	Hemangioendothelioma	None	Alive, no recurrence 15 months postop.
OLT 11 (7½, male)	Hepatoma	Tyrosinemia	Died, recurrent tumor 11 months postop.
OLT 18 (52, female)	Bile duct cancer	Sclerosing cholangitis	Alive, no recurrence 10 months postop.
OLT 28 (50, male)	Multifocal hepatocellular carcinoma	Chronic active hepatitis B	Alive, no recurrence 6 months postop.

disease in Iwatsuki's report. Second, all the incidental malignancies in the reported series were intrahepatic, whereas our patient had a tumor arising in her common bile duct. All patients with bile duct cancer in the Denver/Pittsburgh series who survived beyond the early postoperative period subsequently died with recurrent tumor. A single patient with sclerosing cholangitis and bile duct cancer developed recurrence at 10 months and died 12 months after transplantation. In contrast to our patient, the presence of the tumor was the primary indication for transplantation. We also note that one patient transplanted for bile duct cancer did not develop a recurrence until 42 months postoperatively. Continued, close follow-up of our patient will be essential.

The results of a large series of liver transplantation in the presence of hepatobiliary malignancy have recently been reported. Several conclusions can be drawn from this study. However, even in our much smaller experience, three of eight cases differed from the trends established in this series. The role of liver transplantation in cancer therapy will undergo further refinement in the years to come. Decisions as to the suitability of patients for transplantation will continue to be made on an individual basis.

JOHN O. COLONNA II
RICHARD A. RAY
LEONARD I. GOLDSTEIN
JONATHAN R. HIATT
WILLIAM QUINONES-BALDRICH
KENNETH P. RAMMING
AND RONALD W. BUSUTTIL[1]
Departments of Surgery, Medicine, and Pathology
UCLA Center for The Health Sciences
Los Angeles, California

[1] Address correspondence to: Ronald W. Busuttil, M.D., Ph.D., Professor of Surgery, Director, Liver Transplant Program, UCLA Center for the Health Sciences, 10833 LeConte Ave., Los Angeles, CA 90024.

Acknowledgments. We acknowledge the assistance of Ms. Lisa Conti in the preparation of the manuscript.

REFERENCES

1. Iwatsuki S, Gordon RD, Shaw BW, Starzl TE. The role of liver transplantation in cancer therapy. Ann Surg 1985; 202(4): 401.

Received 16 December 1985.
Accepted 24 January 1986.

USE OF TWO DONOR-SPECIFIC TRANSFUSIONS FOR LIVING-RELATED DONOR KIDNEY TRANSPLANTATION

The technique of donor-specific transfusions (DST)* for poorly matched living-related donors has been a remarkable advance in kidney transplantation. The first clinical use of this concept was a pretransplant infusion of donor-histocompatible antigen by Newton and Anderson (*1*). The use of whole-blood transfusions for this purpose was developed by Salvetierra and his associates in San Francisco (*2*). Their protocol consisted of three 200-cc transfusions of whole blood from the potential kidney donor administered to the prospective recipient at two-week intervals. While sensitization to donor histocompatible antigen occurred in approximately 30% of the recipients, those not developing sensitization and ultimately receiving the kidney transplants did remarkably well. Graft survival at two years has been in the 90% range (*3*). In contrast, their historical control group with similarly matched kidney transplant recipients has a one-year graft survival of only 56%.

* Abbreviations used: DST, donor-specific transfusion; MLC, mixed-lymphocyte culture.

Attempts to reduce the sensitization rate have been described by several centers. One method that has had some success is the concurrent administration of azathioprine along with the donor-specific transfusions (*4*). In most cases, azathioprine was continued up to and beyond the time of the transplant. Another method to lessen sensitization has been the use of stored blood, which apparently modifies the antigen presentation (*5*).

In analysis of the sensitization pattern following DST, Salvetierra et al. noted that in 27% of patients who became sensitized against donor histocompatible antigens, the sensitization was detected only after the third DST (*3*).

In developing a method to prevent sensitization against the rhesus antigen in situations where the donor is Rh (+) and the recipient is Rh (−), we used only two DST along with the administration of anti-Rh immune globulin (*6*). None of the eight patients became sensitized to donor T or B cells. We therefore wondered if only two DST would minimize sensitization to donor histocompatible antigens in all patients. Another concern was whether or not the immunologic advantage of DST would be maintained with the abbreviated transfusion protocol.

Patients considered for living-related kidney transplantation in which there was a one-haplotype or greater antigenic difference between the donor and recipient were considered for DST. Mixed lymphocyte cultures (MLC) were performed in all cases. DST were used when the MLC stimulation index was greater than eight. The MLC method was a modified bidirectional macro system after Cochrum et al (*7*). Each DST consisted of approximately 200 cc of freshly drawn ABO-compatible whole blood at two-week intervals.

Beginning in October 1979, five of the 22 consecutive DST recipients received two DST; the other 17 received 3 DST. Since June 1982, all recipients have been given only two DST. Half these patients were also given azathioprine, 200 mg, on the day of DST and on the subsequent day. Prednisone, 25 mg/day, was also given with the azathioprine. Recipient serum was tested for antidonor cytotoxic antibody six weeks after the last DST and again immediately prior to transplantation. Cytotoxicity crossmatches against donor T and B cells were performed at room temperature and at 37°C. An antiglobulin-augmented method (*8*) was used for the anti-T-cell crossmatch.

Immunosuppression of the kidney transplant recipient was with azathioprine and prednisone in all cases. Cyclosporine in a low-dose range was also given to nine of the most recent recipients. Rejection episodes were reversed with i.v. methylprednisolone. Two patients received antithymocyte globulin for steroid-resistant rejection activity. Other characteristics of these two study groups, three DST vs. two DST, are shown in Table 1.

The results are summarized in Table 2. Sensitization to donor T lymphocytes has been essentially the same in the two groups, 2/17 (12%) for the three-DST group vs. 2/34 (6%) in the two-DST group. There was no difference in the degree of sensitization in the two subgroups of the two DST recipients, those receiving azathioprine and prednisone vs. no treatment at the time of DST.

Fifteen of three DST patients have received kidney transplants and 30 of the two DST group were transplanted. There was one early death in each group; both were due to pneumonia. One-year graft survival is 93% (3 DST) vs. 97% (2 DST). Overall, of the 45 transplants only one patient lost the graft from rejection when immunosuppression had been maintained. One patient discontinued immunosuppression and rejected the kidney transplant.

Of the four patients developing antidonor T cell cytotoxic antibody, two in each group, one was a multipara, another was a female patient showing sensitization prior to DST, and two were young patients not uremic at the time of DST—i.e., not yet on dialysis therapy.

We have been very pleased with the results of donor-specific transfusions despite the 8% sensitization rate. Of the four patients becoming sensitized, three have been successfully transplanted with cadaver kidneys with follow-up periods of between six months and three years. Our historical control group of 32 one-haplotype-matched living-related kidney transplant recipients had a one-year graft survival of 68%, compared with an overall graft survival of 89% (40/45) in the DST recipients.

TABLE 1. Characteristics of study groups

Characteristic	3 DST	2 DST
No. transfused	17	34
Males	14 (82%)	26 (76%)
Females	5	8
No. transplanted	15	30
No. transplanted with diabetes mellitus	2	10
	6/15 (40%)	14/30 (47%)
age > 45	4	4
No. transfused with third-party blood	17	33
	—	
Mean no transfusions/patient	10	8
Follow-up	All >2 years	29/30 >1 year; 21/30 >2 years
Mean MLC stimulation index: (modified macro method: SI 8 = high)	14.1	21.9

TABLE 2. Sensitization and graft survival of study groups

Transfusion groups	3 DST		2 DST	
Total no. sensitized	2/17 (12%)		2/34 (6%)	
Immunosuppression with DST	None		A. No treatment (n=17) No. sensitized: 1 (6%) B. Aza & Pred (n=17) No. sensitized: 1 (6%)	
Characteristics of sensitized patients	1. Multiparous female patient 2. Female patient sensitized to Pre-DST 3rd-party blood transfusions		1. 12 year old boy 2. 17 year old girl (Neither on dialysis during DST)	
No. transplanted	15		30	
Rejections	1st year: 0; 2nd year: 0		1st year: 0; 2nd year: 2[a]	
Deaths	1	0	1	0
Graft survival (includes death)	93%	93%	97%	86%
Patient survival	93%	93%	97%	95%
Current mean serum creatinine	1.3 mg/dl		1.6 mg/dl	
Fate of sensitized patients	1. Cadaver kidney transplant—rejected 2. Cadaver kidney transplant—functioning at 3 years		1. Cadaver kidney transplant—functioning at 3 years 2. Cadaver kidney transplant—functioning at 6 months	

[a] One patient discontinued immunosuppressive medication.

An analysis of rejection activity, as determined by the frequency of rejection episodes and their severity, showed no significant difference between the three-DST patients and those receiving two DST. However, four of the patients in the two-DST group who received azothioprine and prednisone with the DST, had considerable rejection activity. Two of these appeared to be losing their transplants from repeated rejection episodes until they were started on low-dose cyclosporine. Therefore we are not convinced that concommitant azothioprine is a useful measure, at least as we used it.

Since the sensitization rate in both the two-DST and three-DST groups was quite low, we could not demonstrate an immunologic advantage of using only two DST. The sensitized patients were the ones described as "responders" (*9*). Approximately 80% of the 51 transfused patients were male, and there was only one patient receiving a secondary transplant. It is, therefore, not surprising that the sensitization rate for the entire DST group of patients was quite low. The number of DST could not have had much effect upon the sensitization rate.

An additional factor may have been the liberal use of third-party blood transfusions in all of these patients. Only one of the DST recipients did not receive some third-party blood prior to beginning DST transfusions. The well known effect of third-party transfusions upon the success rate of kidney transplantation was undoubtedly present, and may also have contributed to the low sensitization rate to DST.

One might, therefore, conclude that only third-party transfusions should be administered, since even an 8% sensitization rate against DST donors might be lessened. Our concern with this idea is that when we studied our historical control group, we found that a large number of third-party blood transfusions had been administered to those patients. Yet the graft survival rate was not as good as that seen in the DST recipients, and the frequency and severity of rejection episodes were considerably greater.

Despite the 20% improved graft survival, the steroid-sparing affect of DST is, in our opinion, the greatest reason for continuing this method of immunoalteration. The infrequent and mild rejection episodes, which are almost all easily reversed with a modest boost in immunosuppression, is a phenomenon seen only in transplants from HLA-identical siblings and in the recipients of DST. It is the primary reason why so few serious infectious complications developed in the DST patients. This was true despite the fact that there was a large number of poor risk patients receiving DST. For example, 18% of our DST patients were over 45 years of age and 20/45 (45%) had type I diabetes mellitus. Whether or not cyclosporine will make DST obsolete remains to be seen. It is our impression that DST plus cyclosporine is presently the best approach for these living-related kidney transplant patients.

In conclusion, we have found that the administration of only two DST provides essentially the same results as three DST with respect to sensitization to T and B cells of the donor, and to graft and patient survival. Giving only two DST causes less inconvenience to the living-related kidney donor and shortens the work-up time.

R. T. Schweizer[1]
S. A. Bartus
M. A. Rovelli
L. M. Bow
Transplantation Service
Department of Surgery
Hartford Hospital and the University of Connecticut School of Medicine
Hartford, CT 06115

[1] Address correspondence to: Robert T. Schweizer, M.D., Surgical Research Laboratory, Hartford Hospital, Hartford, CT 06155.

REFERENCES

1. Newton WT, Anderson CB. Planned pre-immunization of renal allograft recipients. Surgery 1973; 74: 430.
2. Salvetierra O, Vincenti F, Amend W, et al. Deliberate donor-specific blood transfusion prior to living related renal transplantation: a new approach. Ann Surg 1980; 192: 543.
3. Salvetierra O, Iwaki Y, Vincenti F, et al. Incidence, characteristics, and outcome of recipients sensitized after donor-specific blood transfusions. Transplantation 1981; 32: 528.
4. Anderson CB, Tyler JD, Sicard GA, et al. Renal allograft recipient pre-treatment with immunosuppression and donor-specific blood. Transplant Proc 1985; 17: 1047.
5. Light JA, Metz S, Oddenino T, et al. Fresh versus stored blood in donor specific transfusion. Transplant Proc 1982; 14: 296.
6. Schweizer RT, Bartus SA, Silver H, et al. Kidney transplantation using donor specific blood despite Rh incompatibility. Transplantation 1981; 32: 345.
7. Cochrum KC, Salvetierra O, Belzer FO. Correlation between MLC stimulation and graft survival in living related and cadaver transplants. Ann Surg 1974; 180: 617.
8. Johnson AH. NIAID manual of tissue typing techniques. 1979–1980; 178.
9. Opelz G, Graver B, Mickey MR, et al. Lymphocytotoxic antibody responses to transfusions in potential kidney transplant recipients. Transplantation 1981; 32: 177.

Received 7 January 1986.
Accepted 27 January 1986.

MICROSURGICALLY REVASCULARIZED BONE ALLOGRAFTS WITH IMMUNOSUPPRESSION WITH CYCLOSPORINE

Preliminary Report of the Effect in an Animal Model CSC

Segmental defects in diaphysial bone resulting from congenital deformity, trauma, or tumor resection remain a challenging therapeutic problem. (*1–4*). To bridge such defects, cancellous grafts, vascularized and nonvascularized cortical autografts, and nonvascularized segmental allografts have been used. These vascularized autografts have several advantages as compared with avascular grafts (*5–8*). Autograft harvesting, however, creates an additional lesion in the patient and the procedure has its own morbidity. Bone allografting, therefore, seems a promising alternative in the treatment of large segmental bone defects and in the context of hemijoint and whole-joint replacement. Mankin and others (*2, 9*) have transplanted nonvascularized allografts without immunosuppression in man, but such transplants have an overall complication rate of about 15% (infections, nonunions, and fatigue fractures). From heterotopic transplants (*9–13*) information can be obtained concerning the behavior of the allograft alone, but graft incorporation in a bone defect cannot be studied. Primarily vascularized allografts have been studied in heterotopic whole-limb (*1*, *14*) or hemijoint transplant models (*4*, *15*), mostly in rodents. Without immunosuppression, and across major histocompatibility barriers, the failure rate has been unacceptably high. The fate of primarily vascularized diaphyseal allografts with and without immunosuppression and complete periosteal stripping is not yet well known.

Deep freezing—and, to a lesser degree, freeze drying—markedly reduce the ability of allografts to evoke an immune response in the graft recipient (*16*), but at the expense of graft viability. The presently available data suggest that the optimal conditions for successful segmental bone allografting include: mechanical stability between an orthotopic graft and recipient bone (*12*, *17*, *18*), immediate revascularization in order to maintain graft viability, and immunosuppression (*13*, *19*, *20*). The objectives of this study were to investigate the bone healing pattern of large, segmental, orthotopic, weight-bearing bone allografts in a technically standardized model and to analyze possible benefits of microvascular techniques and short-term steroid-free immunosuppression on the viability and remodeling of the graft.

A group of 38 mature, unmatched, unrelated mongrel dogs of both sexes, weighing between 25 and 35 kg were used. The dogs were divided into 6 recipient groups:

1. Autografts without microvascular anastomosis (A,− [n = 5] as controls for nonvascularized grafts)
2. Autografts with microvascular anastomosis (A,+ [n = 5] as controls for vascularized grafts)
3. Allografts without microvascular anastomosis (A1,− [n = 8])
4. Allografts with microvascular anastomosis (A1,+ [n = 7])
5. Allografts without microvascular anastomosis and immunosuppression (A1−, Cy [n = 7])
6. Allografts with microvascular anastomosis and immunosuppression (A1,+, Cy [n = 6])

The surgical procedure consists of transplanting an 8-cm long diaphyseal segment from the midshaft of the donor tibia (Fig. 1). The nutrient vessels were carefully preserved either alone or with a vessel segment of the cranial tibial vessels when a vascular anastomosis was planned. The periosteum of the graft was always completely stripped. The total ischemia time averaged 2½ hr. For internal fixation, the smallest possible number of screws to achieve the necessary stability for immediate weight bearing was implanted, in order to avoid interference with revascularizastion of the graft. A total of 3 screws was placed proximally and distally in the 12-hole, 3.5-Dynamic Compression Plates, a lag screw across each osteotomy, and a short central screw in the graft (Fig. 1).

The microvascular end-to-side anastomoses were made between the cranial tibial artery and vein of the recipient and the nutrient vessels of the grafts. The anastomoses were done by separate sutures with 10–0 nylon (Supramid DM 202, SSC, 8212 Neuhausen a/Rhf., Switzerland).

The immunosuppressive regimen consisted of cyclosporine during the first 4 weeks postoperatively, starting i.v. during the operation, followed by a daily dose of 20 mg/kg body weight for the first 2 weeks and 15/kg body weight during the second 2 weeks (*19*). From the first postoperative day on, the medication was hand-fed. Serum levels of cyclosporine were measured at 0, 14, and 28 days postoperatively (therapeutic range in dogs

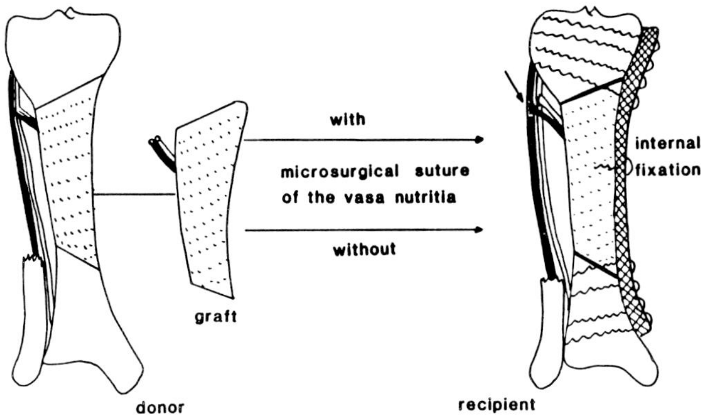

FIGURE 1. Scheme of the surgical procedure.

600–1200 ng/ml serum). The animals were allowed immediate full weight bearing.

Bone healing and viability were assessed by using 4 fluorochrome labels: xylenol orange injected at 3 and 16 weeks, calcein green at 6 weeks, Alzarin complexon at 9 weeks, and tetracycline at 12 weeks. These fluorochrome labels are only incorporated into the bone when living osteocytes are present (*21*). Prior to sacrifice at 20 weeks postoperative, all animals were injected with Disulfine blue i.v. Control angiography of the hind limbs was only performed in the group with microvascular anastomosis at 20 weeks. The tibias were removed and analyzed by radiographs and computerized tomography scans. Roentgenograms were taken at regular intervals during the postoperative course. Those at 20 weeks were analyzed and scored according to Powell and Goldberg (*22*). The score is based on the healing pattern of the 2 osteotomies (host-graft junctions) and the radiological aspect of the graft itself. The highest score is 7 (2 points each for the proximal and distal healed osteotomy and 3 points for an intact graft). Longitudinal and transverse sections of the removed tibias were prepared in order to document the graft-host interface healing, and the viability and degree of perfusion of the graft, by use of fluorescent micrographs, disulfine blue staining, and histomorphological analysis.

Figure 2 demonstrates the radiological score (at 20 weeks) according to Powell and Goldberg. The vascularized autografts had the highest (*9*, *11*), the nonimmunosuppressed allograft the lowest (*1*, *3*) score. All nonvascularized grafts had a lower score than the vascularized match, but the difference did not reach statistical significance. A significant difference existed ony between the vascularized allograft groups with (group 6) and without (group 4) immunosuppression. (One graft each in groups 5 and 6 showed a strong resorption—in fact, it is only in these 2 animals that cyclosporine had to be omitted for several days because of recurrent vomiting.) The most significant resorption and destruction of the graft itself is found in the revascularized allograft group without immunosuppression (*11*), causing the low score.

Figure 3 shows the results of the vital staining with disulfine. With a simple, semiquantitative scoring system we analyzed the presence of stained vessels in the periosteal, cortical, endosteal, and medullary canal areas of a cross section through the center of the graft. We could make out the following rank:

1. Autografts without vascular anastomoses
2., 3. Autografts with vascular anastomoses and allografts with vascular anastomoses and cyclosporine
4. Allografts without vascular anastomoses and cyclosporin.
5. Allografts without vascular anastomoses
6. Allografts with vascular anastomosis

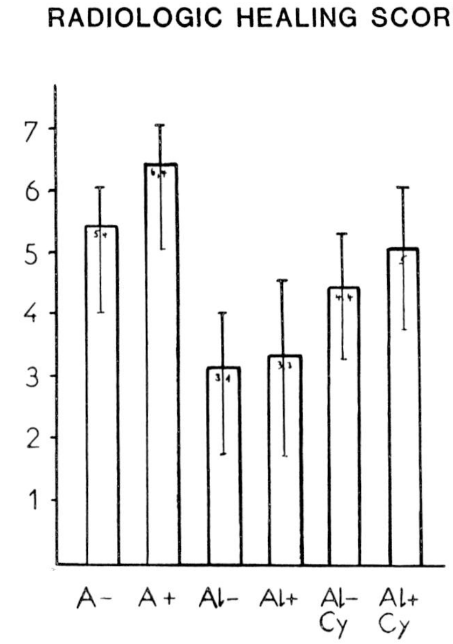

FIGURE 2. Radiologic healing score (maximal score 1—7 (p+d+g): (p) proximal graft-host interface; (d) distal graft-host interface; (g) graft; (p+d) interface healed [2], delayed union [1], no healing [0]; (g) normal architecture active reorganization, no resorption [3], [2], resorption defects [1], sequester formation [0].

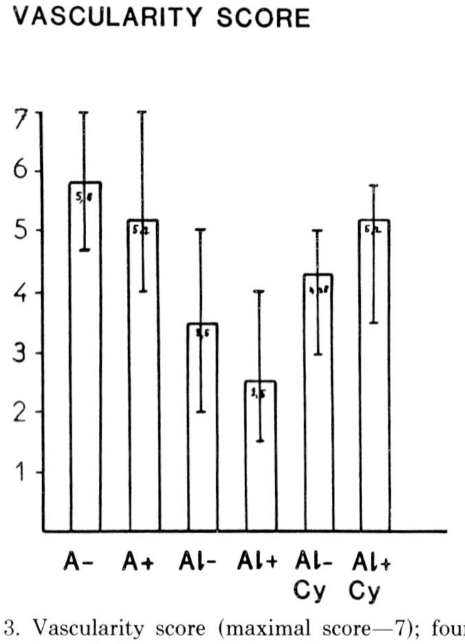

FIGURE 3. Vascularity score (maximal score—7); four areas of a cross-section through the center of the graft were measured: periosteal: max. 2 points, cortical: max. 2 points, endosteal: max. 2 points, medullary: max. 1 point; stained, dilated vessels with active remodelling:2; stained, normal vessels with reduced remodelling:1; no stained vessels:0. (A−) autograft without revascularization; (A+) autograft with revascularization; (A1−) allograft without revascularization; (A1+) allograft with revascularization; (A1−/Cy) allograft without revascularization + cyclosporine; (A1+/Cy) allograft with revascularization.

The scores of the immunosuppressed allografts differ significantly from these without immunosuppression and are in a range close to the nonvascularized autografts. In group 3 the grafts have only a periosteal blue-stained rim, whereas in group 4 some staining was regularly found also in the endosteal area.

Figure 4 shows chronologically the number of newly formed osteons in 4 segments of a cross-section through the center of the graft. Not only is the mean number of osteons per square millimeter higher in the autografted groups than in the allograft groups, but the formation of new osteons also starts earlier. Within the autograft groups a higher number of osteons was found in the grafts without anastomosis. In the allografts with microvascular anastomosis (groups 4 and 6) the ones with immunosuppression (group 6) show an earlier onset and a higher amount of new bone formation. In the allografts without anastomosis (groups 3 and 5) this difference is not significant.

The healing of osteotomies (the graft-recipient junction) was only disturbed in the nonimmunosuppressed allografts (groups 3 and 4)—particularly in the vascularized ones. The technique of internal fixation being the same in all groups, bone resorption and secondary instability (caused by the rejection reaction at this site) seems to be the cause of impaired bone healing in group 4. Without bone resorption (group 3) a stable internal fixation results in undisturbed healing at the level of the graft-recipient junction. This concurs with clinical experience (*2*). However, a healed osteotomy is not identical with viability of the whole graft.

In our nonvascularized, nonimmunosuppressed group (group 3), the osteotomies healed, although the graft itself was mostly a dead-spacer that was only very slowly replaced by 2 creeping substitutions, starting from the periphery toward the medullary canal.

The vital staining with disulfine blue has been proved to provide valid information about the actual vascularity of the bone (*21*). Disulfine disperses within the perfused vascular network and the corresponding pericapillary space. The living osteocyte is considered the connecting element between the pericapillary and the interstitial spaces. An even staining, therefore, means a good actual vascularity—primary (microvascular anastomosis) or secondary—resulting from an active remodeling and new bone formation.

By the remodeling process, nonperfused bone is replaced by new bone. It has been experimentally shown that the impairment of bone perfusion after a fracture (or osteotomy) is caused both by vascular severance produced by the osteotomy (or fracture) and by the application of the plate on the diaphysis for internal fixation (*21*). Subsequently, the areas of increased remodeling correspond to the primarily avascular areas with

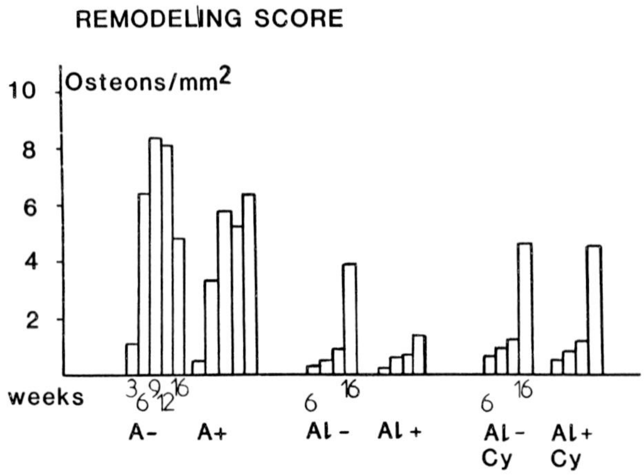

FIGURE 4. Remodeling score: average number of newly formed osteons per square millimeter in a cross-section through the center of the graft.

no disfulfine staining. The bone remodeling is characterized by the presence of osteoid, produced only by viable osteocytes. Accumulation of fluorochrome-labeled osteoid in the osteons therefore demonstrates viability of bone. The four labels given at different times postoperatively allow a chronological analysis of the remodeling pattern (*23*). The higher remodeling rate and the higher vascularity score of group 1 as compared with group 2 is understandable: in group 2 a better primary graft perfusion is allowed by immediate microsurgical revascularization, the total ischemic damage, though, being less important than in group 1. Therefore a smaller mass of bone needs to be remodelled. On the contrary, in the nonimmunosuppressed allografts (group 3 + 4)—with and without microsurgical anastomosis—the low staining score (below 4) indicates poor perfusion of the graft at 20 weeks. In group 3 the biggest part of the graft corresponds to a dead, nonperfused spacer. The remodeling is very slow and starts from the periosteal region (centripetally). Restoration of the medullary blood flow and a subsequent centrifugal remodeling cannot be observed in group 3. Allograft vasculitis, resulting from rejection, as found by Yaremchuk (*4, 15*) is probably the reason for it. The small amount of endosteal staining and remodeling in group 4 would then suggest that the microvascular anastomosis provided some medullary perfusion for the short period before its occlusion, which was most likely due to vasculitis. Without sequential angiography or isotopic evaluation we are, for the time being, not able to determine exactly how long the microvascular anastomoses remained patent during the postoperative period. In the autografts, 4 of 5 microvascular anastomosis remained open, producing the effects already described. Early occlusion of the microvasculature must be supposed in the allograft groups, due to rejection vasculitis, (groups 3 and 4) and due to the immunosuppressive regimen, which was limited to 4 weeks in these pilot experiments (groups 5 and 6). However, apparently even this short patency period of the microvasculature is sufficient to produce some effects—e.g., increased graft resorption and reduced new bone formation in group 4 compared with group 3.

Even after this short period of immunosuppression, as proposed by Burchardt (*19*), our allografts tend to match the autografts (higher healing score, higher vascularity score, less bone resorption). Experiments presently underway tend to indicate that long-term immunosuppression favorably influences this tendency of allografts to resemble autografts.

In conclusion these preliminary experiments indicate that histoincompatibility is the limiting factor for bone graft survival. Primary stable internal fixation allows rapid bone healing at the graft-recipient junction, if important bone resorption—due to graft rejection—does not cause a secondary instability. Short-term immunosuppression improves graft survival, but longer immunosuppression is necessary to obtain the full benefit of primary microcrovascular anastomoses and to induce the allograft to be incorporated in a way very much like that of analogous autografts.

M. Aebi
P. Regazzoni
S.M. Perren
F. Harder
Department of Orthopedic Surgery
University of Berne
Department of Surgery
University of Basle
Laboratory for Experimental Surgery
Swiss Research Institute
Davos, Switzerland

REFERENCES

1. Lipson RA, Kawano H, Halloran PF, McKee NH, Pritzker KPH, Langer F. Vascularized limb transplantation in the rat. I. Results with syngeneic grafts. Transplantation 1983; 35: 293.
2. Mankin HR. Complications of allograft surgery: In: Friedländer GE, Mankin HJ, Sell KW, eds. Osteochondrial allografts. Boston/Toronto: Little, Brown, 1983; 259.
3. Weiland AJ, Daniel RK. Microvascular anastomoses for bone grafts in the treatment of massive defects in bone. J Bone Joint Surg 1979; 61-A: 98.
4. Yaremchuk MJ, Sedacca T, May JW Jr. Vascularized knee allograft transplantation in a rabbit model. Trans Orthop Res Soc 1982; 7: 174.
5. Ostrup LT, Frederickson JM. Distant transfer of a free, living bone graft by microvascular anastomoses. Plast Reconstr Surg 1974; 54: 274.
6. Taylor GI, Miller GDH, Ham FJ. The free vascularized bone graft. Plast Reconstr Surg 1975; 55: 533.
7. Verdin PJ, Davy DT, Shaffer JW, Field GA. Relationships among mechanical and morphological properties in vascularized canine allografts. Trans Orthop Res Soc 1984; 9: 240.
8. Weiland AJ, Berggren A, Moore JR. Fate of revascularized bone grafts. In: Friedländer GE, Mankin HJ, Sell KW, eds. Osteochondral allografts. Boston/Toronto: Little, Brown, 1983: 113.
9. Goldberg VM, Porter BB, Lance EM. Transplantation of the canine knee joint on a vascular pedicle. J Bone Joint Surg 1980; 62-A:414.
10. Burwell RG. The fate of freeze-dried bone allografts. Transplant Proc 1976; 8(suppl 1): 95.
11. Elves MW. Humoral immune response to allografts of bone. Int Arch Allergy Appl Immunol 1974; 47: 708.
12. Moore JR, Phillips TW, Weiland AJ, McDonald DF. Influence of immunotherapy on allogenic transplants of bone revascularized by microvascular anastomoses. Trans Orthop Res Soc 1982; 7:175.
13. Moore JR, Phillips TW, Weiland AJ, Randolph MA. Allogenic transplant of bone revascularized by microvascular anastomoses: a preliminary study. J Orthopaedic Res 1984; 1: 352.
14. Lipson RA, Kawano H, Halloran PF, Pritzker KPH, Langer F. Vascularized limb transplantation in the rat. II. Results with allogeneic grafts. Transplantation 1983; 35: 300.
15. Yaremchuk MJ, Sedacca T, Schiller AL, May JW Jr. Vascular knee allograft transplantation in a rabbit model. Plast Reconstr Surg
16. Friedlander GE, Strong DM, Sell KW. Studies on the antigenicity of bone. J Bone Joint Surg 1976; 58-A: 854.
17. Burchhardt H. Biology of cortical bone graft incorporation. In: Friedlaneder GE, Mankin HJ, Sell KW, eds. Osteochondral allografts. Boston/Toronto: Little, Brown, 1983: 51.
18. Hutzschenreuter P. Beschleunigte Einheilung von allogenen Knochentransplantaten durch Praesensibilisierung des Empfängers und stabile Osteosynthese. Langenbecks Arch Chir 1972; 331: 321.
19. Burchardt H, Glowczewskie FP, Enneking WF. Short-term immunosuppression with fres segmental fibrular allografts in dogs. J Bone Joint Surg 1981; 63-A: 411.
20. Stewart JA, Langer F, Halloran P, Gross AE. Vascularized bone and joint transplantation in the rat: the effect of antilymphocyte serum and Cyclosoporin immunosuppression. Trans Orthop Res Soc 1984; 9: 266.
21. Gunst M. Die Blutversorgung der Kortikalis nach Verplattung der

intakten Kaninchentibia [Dissertation]. Basel, Switzerland: Universität Basel, 1977.
22. Powell AE, Bos GD, Goldberg VM, Zika JM, Heiple KG. Immune responses to bone allografts. In: Friedländer GE, Mankin HJ, Sell KW, eds. Osteochondral allografts. Boston/Toronto: Little, Brown, 1983.
23. Rahn BA. Die polychrome Sequenzmarkierung. Habilitationsschrift. Freiburg, West Germany: Universität Freiburg, 1976.

Received 7 January 1986.
Accepted 28 January 1986.

EFFECT OF CYCLOSPORINE ON ISLET XENOGRAFT SURVIVAL IN THE BB/W RAT[1]

Cyclosporine is a potent immunosuppressive agent used for the induction of long-term survival of grafted organs such as the heart, the kidney, liver, and bone marrow (*1*, *2*). Whereas the drug is quite effective in causing extended survival of whole organ transplants, it has been of limited usefullness in preventing immunological destruction of islet allografts (*3*, *4*). Isolated, dispersed islet preparations are unusually immunogenic and high doses of immunosuppressive agents and/or continuous immunotherapy have been required for the prevention of rejection of these cells. Indeed islet allografts, especially in the spontaneously diabetic BB/W rat, have been so difficult to accomplish that this approach has been given up more and more in favor of whole or segmental pancreas transplantation.

We have recently reported that the organ site used for the injection of isolated adult islets profoundly affects the outcome of these allografts in the minimally immunosuppressed rat (*5*). Our studies indicated that the cryptorchid testis—compared with other organs such as the liver, subrenal capsule, and the testis in its original, scrotal position—is the most suitable organ site for indefinite islet allograft survival in rats with streptozotocin-induced (*6*) and with spontaneously occurring diabetes mellitus (*5*). The cryptorchid testis appears to be an exceptionally immunologically privileged site and its use has proven particularly beneficial with regard to the need for immunosuppression. For example, it was shown that small amounts of antilymphocyte serum (ALS)* given over a short period following transplantation were sufficient to induce a state of permanent unresponsiveness in recipients with intratesticular islet allografts (*5*).

In view of this past experience the aim of the present study was to compare intrahepatic with intratesticular islet xenograft survival in the BB/W rat using two immunosuppressive agents, ALS and cyclosporine.

The recipients of islet xenografts were male BB/W rats with spontaneous diabetes mellitus of 30–90 days duration. The rats were obtained courtesy of A. Like, M.D., Worcester, MA. Only rats with plasma glucose concentrations of 375 mg/dl or more were grafted. Islets were isolated from male and female Golden Syrian hamsters using a collagenase digestion technique of Ballinger and Lacy (*7*). Following separation on at least two Ficoll gradients in tandem (*8*), the islets were transferred to biologic grade Petri dishes and incubated in CMRL-1066 medium at 35°C. After 3 to 4 days of culturing the islets were hand-picked under a stereomicroscope and each diabetic BB/W rat received an intraportal or an intratesticular injection of a total of 10 islets/g body weight, as previously described (*6*). A rat was considered cured of the diabetic process if it had a plasma glucose level equal to or less than 150 mg/dl. A total of 37 BB/W rats were divided into 6 groups and treated as follows:

Group 1. Five rats received intraportal injections of islets and an intraperitoneal injection of 1 ml ALS immediately posttransplantation and at 5-day intervals, for a total of 6 doses or until they reverted to a hyperglycemic state.

Group 2. Seven rats were given identical intraportal injections of islets and immediately postoperatively an i.v. injection of 25 mg/kg cyclosporine (Sandoz Ltd), followed by daily i.m. injections of 25 mg/kg of cyclosporine times 6, and then daily s.c. injections of 7 mg/kg of the drug for another 10 days. Immunosuppressive therapy was then discontinued.

Group 3. Four rats received intratesticular islet xenografts with the testes in their original scrotal position and an intraperitoneal injection of 1 ml ALS immediately after the operation and at 5-day intervals as outlined for group 1.

Group 4. Five rats were given abdominal intratesticular islet xenografts and no immunosuppressive therapy posttransplantation.

Group 5. Seven rats received abdominal intratesticular islet xenografts and ALS therapy as outlined above.

Group 6. Nine rats were given abdominal, intratesticular islet xenografts and cyclosporine therapy identical to the protocol outlined for group 2.

Orchiectomies were carried out on 2 normoglycemic rats in group 6 on days 30 and 32, respectively, after transplantation. The testes were fixed in formalin and prepared for histologic examination. Immunoperoxidase stains specific for insulin and C-peptide were also carried out, in addition to the standard hematoxylin and eosin stains.

The results are shown in Table 1: Xenograft survival of islets injected into the liver of ALS treated rats ranged between 3 and 5 days, with a mean of 3.8 days (group 1). Xenograft survival of intraportally injected and cyclosporine-treated rats ranged between 4 and 16, with a mean of 9.7 days. Five of the rats in this group died 4–12 days following transplantation. Prior to death they appeared ill and lost weight; 2 had breathing difficulties. Autopsies were done on these rats: 2 apparently died of lobar pneumonia. A microscopic examination of the livers of 2 of these rats showed massive congestion with a few foci of fatty changes. These findings, however, did not explain the cause of death in these animals. Only 2 rats in this group remained alive and normoglycemic for 13 and 16 days, respectively, before an abrupt reversal to a hyperglycemic state occurred (group 2). None of the 4 rats that were given intratesticular islet xenografts with the testes in their original scrotal position became normoglycemic. On the third day following transplantation these rats were reoperated and the grafted testes were anchored into the abdominal cavity. No other therapy was given. All 4 of these rats promptly became normoglycemic within the next 24 hr and remained so for a mean of an additional 6.5 days before an abrupt reversal to the diabetic process occurred in all of them (group 3). Graft survival of hamster islets injected into the abdominal testes without any immunosuppression ranged between 3 and 11 days with a mean of 8.0 days (group 4). Xenograft survival of islets injected into the cryptorchid testes in rats given minimal ALS therapy was not much longer and ranged from 8 to 15 days with a mean of 11.1 days. One of these animals died hypoglycemic on day 8

[1] This work was supported in part by Juvenile Diabetes Project Transplant, Miami, FL.

* Abbreviations used: ALS, antilymphocytre serum.

after transplantation (group 5). The recipients of cryptorchid islet xenografts and cyclosporine for 17 days following transplantation had a strikingly extended survival ranging between 3 and 40 days with a mean of 27.3 days. Of the 9 grafted rats, 7 were considered cured of the diabetic process (normoglycemia for periods equal to or more than 29 days). One of the rats in this group died hypoglycemic on day 3, and another was found dead in its metabolic cage on day 10 after transplantation; the cause of death was unknown (group 6).

The 2 rats that were orchiectomized on days 30 and 32 after transplantation immediately became hyperglycemic and died in acute diabetic ketoacidosis within 3 days. Figure 1 is a photomicrograph of the testis of the rat that had been xenografted for 30 days and illustrates the presence of well-preserved islet tissue under the testicular capsule in close association with the seminiferous tubules. The tubules appear necrotic with an absence of spermatogenesis. Intact, well-preserved islet cells are visible, and these cells also stained positive with an immunoperoxidase stain specific for insulin and C-peptide. There is no evidence of a cellular infiltrate either within the testis or in close proximity to the islet cells.

TABLE 1. Duration of normoglycemia in spontaneously diabetic BB/W rats transplanted with hamster islets

Group	Organ site	Treatment of recipients	Duration of normoglycemia (days)
1	Liver	ALS[a]	3, 3, 4, 4, 5
2	Liver	Cyclosporine[b]	4,[c] 6,[d] 8,[c] 9,[c] 12,[d] 13, 16
3	Scrotal testis	ALS	0, 0, 0, 0,
4	Cryptorchid testis	None	3, 7, 8, 11, 11
5	Cryptorchid testis	ALS	8,[e] 8, 9, 11, 13, 14, 15,
6	Cryptorchid testis	Cyclosporine[b]	3,[e] 10,[c] 30,[f] 32,[f] 29, 31, 33, 38, 40

[a] (ALS) 1 ml i.p. at 5-day intervals.

[b] (Cyclosporine) 25 mg/kg i.v. ×1 + 25 mg/kg i.m. ×6 + 7 mg/kg s.c. ×10.

[c] Died, cause unknown.

[d] Died, with pneumonia.

[e] Died hypoglycemic.

[f] Orchiectomy.

Our results show that prolonged islet xenograft survival can be achieved in the BB/W rat with cyclosporine therapy. These data also reemphasize the importance of the organ site used for the injection of the islets. As we have previously reported the abdominal testis is a superior organ site for the functional survival of islet allografts (*5*); this now also holds true for islet xenografts in the BB/W rat. In our experience the intraportal embolization of islets in the BB/W rat does not lead to prolonged survival of islet allografts or xenografts, regardless of whether ALS or cyclosporine is used as the immunosuppressive agent. In fact, 5 of the 7 rats that were given intraportal injections of islet xenografts and cyclosporine died rather acutely within 12 days following transplantation. Even though the cause of death of three of these rats remains unclear it was most likely related to cyclosporine toxicity since the rats that were given identical intrahepatic islet xenografts and ALS posttransplantation did not encounter the same fate. On the other hand the rats that were given cryptorchid islet xenografts tolerated the drug quite well, and 7 of these animals became normoglycemic and remained so for periods ranging from 29 to 40 days. These findings indicate an apparent differential effect of cyclosporine toxicity that depends upon the organ site used for the injection of the islet xenografts. Although we have no explanation for these observations, it is well known that cyclosporine is concentrated and metabolized by the liver (*1*). It is thus possible that the combined effects of the grafting of foreign cells into the liver in conjunction with very elevated tissue levels of cyclosporine caused by the i.v. and i.m. injections of the drug may have resulted in acute liver failure and death in these rats. We are unaware of similar reports on this aspect of cyclosporine toxicity. The only other data, to our knowledge, on islet xenograft survival in the rat were recently published

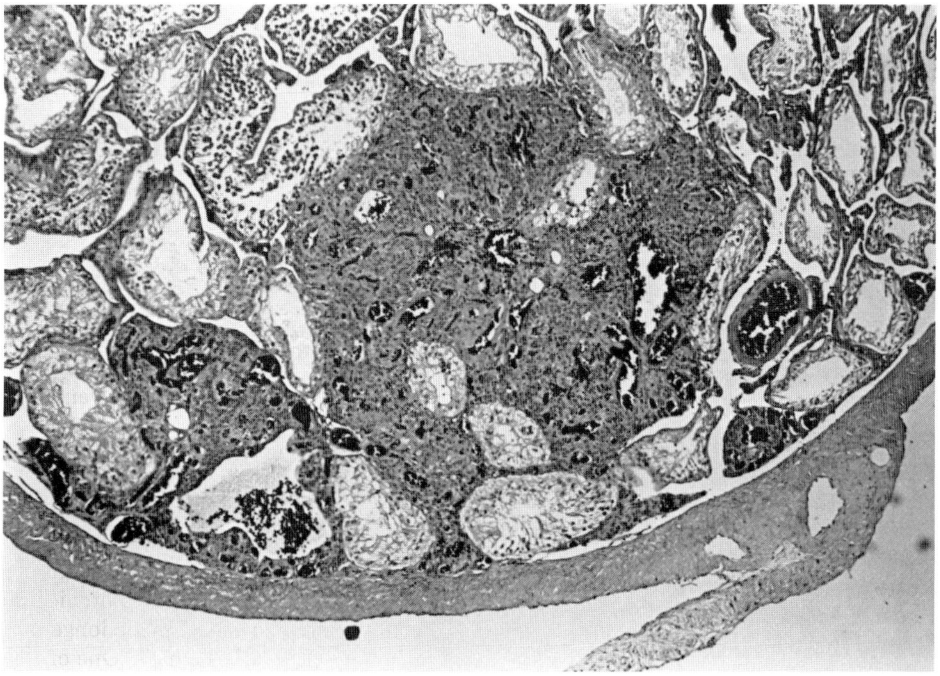

FIGURE 1. Photomicrograph of a cryptorchid islet xenograft in a BB/W rat 30 days after transplantation. Intact islet cells are visible under the testicular capsule and surrounding the seminiferous tubules. The tubules appear necrotic, with an absence of spermatogenesis. There is no cellular infiltrate either within the testis or in the vicinity of the islet cells. (hematoxylin and eosin; × 40).

by Nakajima and his coworkers (*9*). These investigators injected hamster islets intraportally into streptozotocin-induced diabetic rats and obtained a modest prolongation of islet xenograft survival, a mean of 14 days in 6 rats treated with 40 mg/kg/day of cyclosporine. It should be noted that none of their rats apparently died of cyclosporine toxicity even at this high dose, but they administered the drug by mouth rather than by intramuscular injection and this may have accounted for their results.

Previous research has shown that upon discontinuation of cyclosporine in rats with islet allografts, rejection of the islets take place very rapidly (*3, 4*). In our experience, however, normoglycemic rats with abdominal intratesticular islet xenografts and those with a short course of cyclosporine continued to have functional grafts for periods ranging between 12 and 22 days when they were completely off immunosuppression. These data suggest that cyrptorchid islet xenografts, in conjunction with short-term cyclosporine therapy, resulted in a state of unresponsiveness in the recipients, albeit of a short duration. It is thus conceivable that, by increasing the initial dose or by prolonging the period of cyclosporine administration, long-term islet xenograft survival may be induced in the BB/W rat.

In conclusion, we have shown that BB/W rats can be cured of type 1 diabetes with cryptorchid islet xenografts and concomitant cyclosporine therapy. Much doubt has been raised with regard to the feasibility of islet allografts because of the unusual immunogenicity of these tissues. But the cryptochid testis is an unusually immunologically privileged site and has proved to be the most effective organ site for the functional survival of both islet allografts and xenografts in the BB/W rat. We have recently completed histologic studies on rat testes that had been anchored in the abdominal cavity for 2 years, and we were unable to show any evidence of a malignant transformation of these cells (Selawry H, unpublished data). If these observations can be duplicated in a higher animal species such as the monkey, then this approach to islet transplantation may become clinically relevant.

HELENA SELAWRY[2]
KAREN WHITTINGTON
RITA FAJACO
Veterans Administration Medical Center
Miami, Florida 33125

[2] Address correspondence to: Helena Selawry, M.D., Veterans Administration Medical Center, Research 151, 1201 N.W. 16th Street, Miami, FL 33125.

REFERENCES

1. Cohen DJ, Loertscher R, Rubin MF, Tilney NL, Carpenter CB, Strom TB. Cyclosporine: a new immunosuppressive agent for organ transplantation. Ann Intern Med 1984; 101: 667.
2. Morris PJ. The impact of cyclosporin A on transplantation. Chicago: Year Book, 1984: 99.
3. Garvey JF, McShane P, Poole MD, Millard PR, Morris PJ. The effect of cyclosporin A on experimental pancreas allografts in the rat. Transplant Proc 1980; 12: 266.
4. Bell PR, Wood RF, Peters M, Nash JR. Comparison of various methods of chemical immunosuppression in islet cell transplantation. Transplant Proc 1980; 12: 291.
5. Selawry H, Fajaco R, Whittington K. Intratesticular islet allografts in the spontaneously diabetic BB/W rat. Diabetes 1985; 34: 1019.
6. Selawry HP, Whittington K. Extended allograft survival of islets grafted into the intra-abdominally placed testis. Diabetes 1984; 33: 405.
7. Ballinger WF, Lacy PE. Transplantation of intact pancreatic islets in the rat. Surgery 1972; 72: 175.
8. Selawry H, Mui MM, Paul RD, Diastasio JA. Improved allograft survival using highly enriched populations of rat islets. Transplantation 1984; 37: 202.
9. Nakajima Y, Kessler M, Nakano H, Lie TS. Restoration of T cell responsiveness to interleukin-2 in recipients of pancreatic islet xenografts treated with cyclosporine. Transplantation 1985; 40: 73.

Received 20 November 1985.
Accepted 29 January 1986.

0041-1337/86/4206-0571$02.00/0
TRANSPLANTATION
Vol. 42, No. 6

Printed in U.S.A.

Transplantation
OVERVIEW

FAILURE OF ALLOGENEIC CANINE MARROW GRAFTS AFTER TOTAL-BODY IRRADIATION

ALLOGENEIC "RESISTANCE" VERSUS TRANSFUSION-INDUCED SENSITIZATION[1]

RAINER STORB AND H. JOACHIM DEEG

Fred Hutchinson Cancer Research Center and Division of Oncology, University of Washington Department of Medicine, Seattle, Washington 98104

INTRODUCTION

Unlike transplantation of solid organs, successful bone marrow transplantation requires the crossing of a bidirectional barrier made up of both host-versus-graft and graft-versus-host reactions. Factors governing the success in crossing these barriers include the effectiveness of the immunosuppressive regimen used to condition a recipient for grafting, the degree of histocompatibility matching between donor and recipient, the composition of the cells used in the hematopoietic graft, and the nature of the postgrafting immunosuppression. This overview will address the first of the two barriers, host-versus-graft reactions, on the basis of data obtained mostly in a random bred canine model of marrow transplantation (*1–3*).

Host-versus-graft reactions may result in failure of sustained hemopoietic engraftment, a complication that usually will lead to death from marrow aplasia induced by the conditioning regimen. Graft failure can occur almost immediately with no evidence of graft function as illustrated by the hematologic changes depicted in Figure 1. In other cases, good initial graft function may precede late graft failure manifested by a decline of blood cell counts and development of marrow aplasia (Figure 2). For comparison, Figure 3 illustrates the blood cell counts in a dog with sustained hemopoietic engraftment and "permanent" repopulation of the hemopoietic and immune systems by cells of donor origin.

Two distinct mechanisms can lead to the same endpoint, graft failure. One, termed *graft resistance*, reflects the action of host cells that are insensitive to the usual doses of total-body irradiation (TBI)* and do not require prior sensitization to donor histocompatibility antigens in order to destroy the foreign marrow graft. We will show that these host cells may not be typical T cells and that they target on codominantly inherited donor antigens associated with the major histocompatibility complex (MHC). The other mechanism involves sensitization of recipients to minor and/or major histocompatibility antigens of the marrow donor before transplantation—usually via transfusions of blood products, but also through pregnancy. In contrast to transplantation of kidney (*4*), preceding transfusions may jeopardize rather than facilitate a subsequent marrow graft through the action of specifically sensitized T cells. Once sensitized, host T cells are less likely to be eradicated by high-dose TBI, enabling them to destroy the transplanted marrow.

This overview will outline the characteristic features of each of the two mechanisms involved in graft failure, graft resistance and transfusion-induced sensitization, as they present themselves in canine marrow transplantation. Dogs in these studies are defined by dog leukocyte antigen (DLA) typing as described (*5–7*). Recipients are conditioned with a minimum of 9.2 Gy of TBI delivered at a rate of 7 cGy/min from two opposing ^{60}CO sources, a dose that is more than twice the LD99 in this laboratory (4 Gy) (*8, 9*). Similarities to and differences from murine *hybrid resistance* will be discussed, as will be relevant data from clinical marrow transplantation, in particular transplants from HLA-nonidentical donors and those of T-cell-depleted marrow.

GRAFT "RESISTANCE"

"Resistance" to marrow grafts renders the infused marrow incapable of sustained engraftment in a recipient treated with an otherwise lethal dose of immunosuppression. Resistance is typically seen with DLA-nonidentical transplants but can occur under special circumstances even with grafts between DLA-identical littermates.

DLA-Nonidentical Marrow Grafts

The role of the major histocompatibility complex (MHC). Table 1 shows that marrow transplants between DLA-identical littermates following 9.2 Gy of TBI generally result in sustained engraftment (*10–14*). However, graft failure is the rule in recipients of marrow from DLA-nonidentical littermate or unrelated donors (*1, 10, 12–14*). These results suggest an involvement of MHC antigens in resistance to marrow grafts. However, the 50% incidence of graft failure in dogs given marrow grafts from DLA homozygous and phenotypically DLA-identical unrelated donors, higher than that seen in genotypically DLA-identical littermates, argues against such an interpretation (*1, 15*). Rather it suggests that one or more additional loci close to but not identical with DLA-A, -B, and -D play a role in graft resistance. Attempts to uncover the antigens through additional

[1] This work was supported by PHS grants CA 31787, CA 18221, HL 33859, HL 36444 (formerly CA 30924), and CA 15704, awarded by the National Cancer Institute, and the National Heart, Lung, and Blood Institute, DHHS.

* Abbreviations used: DLA, dog leukocyte antigen; HLA, human leukocyte antigen; MHC, major histocompatibility complex; NK, natural killer; SCID, severe combined immunodeficiency; TBI, total-body irradiation.

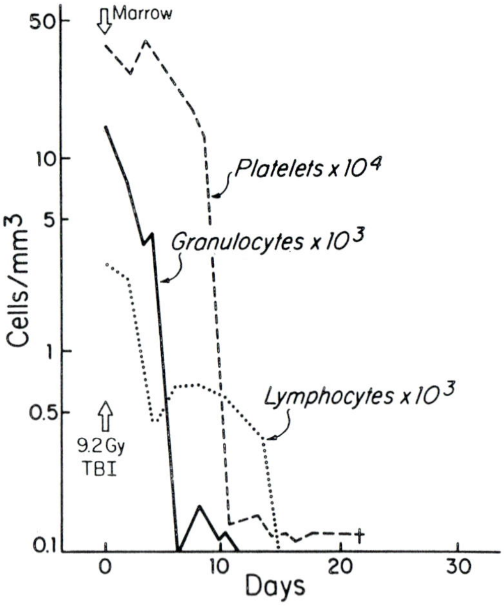

FIGURE 1. Hematological changes in a dog given 9.2 Gy of total-body irradiation (TBI) and an infusion of 3.8×10[8] marrow cells/kg from an unrelated DLA-nonidentical donor.

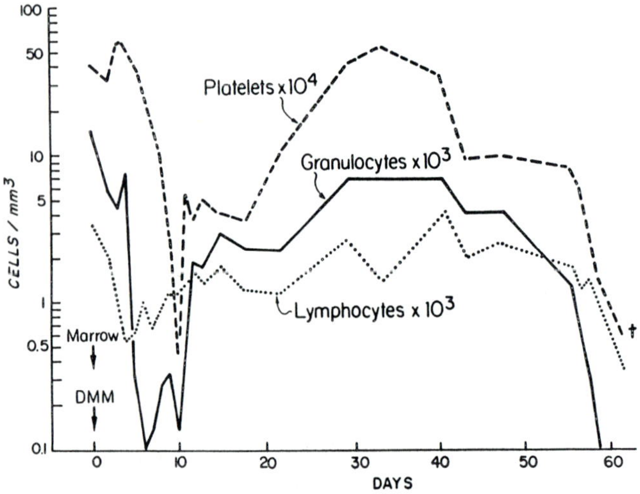

FIGURE 2. Hematological changes in a dog given 10 mg dimethylbusulfan (DMM)/kg i.v. followed by infusion of marrow and peripheral blood leukocytes from a DLA-identical littermate.

histocompatibility tests including primed lymphocyte typing, cell mediated lympholysis assays and typing of donor and recipient cells with a panel of cytotoxic cells, all failed (*16, 17*).

Evidence that T cells facilitate marrow engraftment. Consistent and sustained hemopoietic engraftment can be achieved in all donor-recipient combinations when viable peripheral blood leukocytes are infused in addition to the marrow inoculum (Table 2) (*18, 19*). The heterogeneous population of cells present in the peripheral blood includes mononuclear cells (both pluripotent hemopoietic stem cells and immunologically active cells) and granulocytes that may serve as a source of histocompatibility antigens. Possible mechanisms in the production of the prompt and permanent marrow grafts with blood leukocytes added to marrow include: 1. the administration of increased numbers of stem cells (*20*); 2. the potentiation of tolerance by a large amount of donor antigen provided by the

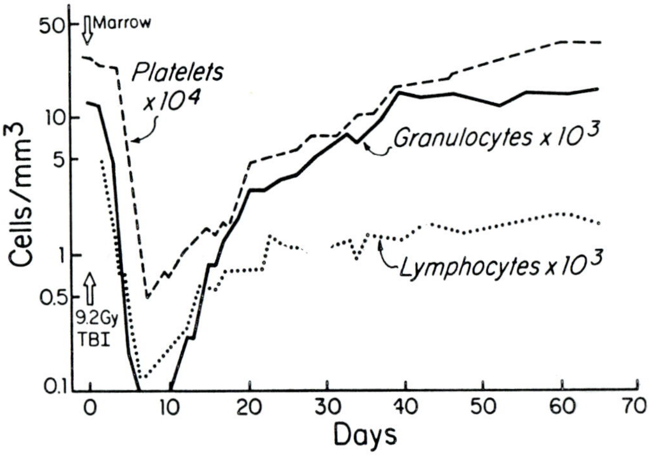

FIGURE 3. Hematological changes in a dog given 9.2 Gy of total-body irradiation (TBI) and 3.6×10[8] marrow cells/kg from a DLA-identical littermate.

TABLE 1. Dogs given 9.2 Gy total-body irradiation at 7 cGy/min followed within 4 hr by infusion of ≤4×10[8] marrow cells/kg

Marrow donor	Number of dogs studied	% With sustained graft
Littermate		
DLA-identical[a]	21	95
DLA-nonidentical[b]	12	8
Unrelated		
DLA-identical[c]	16	50
DLA-nonidentical[d]	36	8

[a] Genotypically identical.

[b] Includes both one and two DLA haplotype differences; five of the DLA-nonidentical littermates were conditioned with 11.5 Gy of total-body irradiation; all five rejected their grafts.

[c] Phenotypically identical.

[d] Different for two DLA haplotypes. Six of the 36 were conditioned with 10 Gy at 10cGy/min; five of the six rejected their grafts.

TABLE 2. Dogs given 9.2 Gy total-body irradiation at 7 cGy/min followed within 4 hr by infusion of ≤4×10[8] marrow cells/kg (In addition, recipients were given infusions of mononuclear cells from peripheral blood or thoracic duct lymph of the marrow donor.)

Marrow donor[a]	Number of dogs studied	Additional donor cells infused	% With sustained graft
Littermate			
DLA-identical	34	Viable PBL[b]	100
DLA-nonidentical	83	Viable PBL	95
Unrelated			
DLA-identical	13	Viable PBL	92
DLA-nonidentical	75	Viable PBL	91
	6	Irradiated PBL[c]	0
	8	Thoracic duct lymphocytes[d]	100

[a] For further detail see Table 1.

[b] PBL: peripheral blood leukocytes; a mean of 1.8×10[8] nucleated cells/kg were infused on days 1 and 2 after marrow grafting.

[c] Irradiated with 3000 rads from a Cesium source.

[d] Dogs were given a mean of 7.7×10[8] cells/kg on days 1 and 2 after marrow grafting.

infused cells; 3. the suppression of residual host immune reactivity by the immunocompetent cells infused via a graft-versus-host reaction; and 4. enhancement of donor stem cell growth via mononuclear cells.

The first possibility was ruled out by showing that resistance can also be abrogated when thoracic duct lymphocytes are substituted for peripheral blood leukocytes (*21*). Canine thoracic duct lymph, in contrast to peripheral blood, does not contain hemopoietic stem cells capable of protecting dogs against irradiation injury (*22*). Failure of in-vitro-irradiated leukocytes to overcome resistance excluded the second possibility (*1, 12*). It is as yet not possible to distinguish between the third and fourth possibilities. Current studies are directed toward elucidating whether the lymphocytes facilitating allogeneic marrow engraftment in vivo are identical with those found to enhance canine erythroid colony growth in vitro (*23–25*). Similar cells involved in enhancement of human burst-forming erythroid colony growth in vitro have been reported to be T lymphocytes (*26*). It is not known whether mononuclear cells useful in facilitating engraftment are distinct from those causing graft-versus-host disease.

The question of which host cells are involved in resistance to DLA-nonidentical grafts. When canine recipients were treated before TBI with a course of antithymocyte serum either alone or combined with procarbazine, only a slight increase in the engraftment incidence was seen (Table 3) (*1, 12*). This failure of anti-T-cell reagents to enhance engraftment was disappointing and argued against a primary involvement of T cells in graft resistance. In keeping with this interpretation was the finding that pretreatment of recipients by donor antigen followed by high-dose methotrexate before TBI was also ineffective in overcoming resistance (Table 3) (*1*). Methotrexate given in this way is very effective in suppressing other immune responses including those to sheep red blood cells and keyhole limpet hemocyanin in dogs.

Results in cyclosporine-treated dogs also supported the possibility that host cells mediating graft resistance were non-T cells (Table 4). Most dogs given marrow and peripheral blood leukocytes from DLA-nonidentical unrelated donors engrafted regardless of whether they received postgrafting immunosuppression with methotrexate, azathioprine, or 6-mercaptopurine (*27, 28*, and unpublished data). In contrast, dogs given cyclosporine postgrafting for the most part failed to engraft (*29, 30*). Apparently, cyclosporine inhibited the graft-facilitating effect of infused donor T lymphocytes, while not suppressing those host cells that mediate graft resistance. Adding methotrexate to cyclosporine postgrafting resulted in uniform engraftment, suggesting that methotrexate functions in a manner different from that of cyclosporine by inhibiting the proliferation of host cells causing graft failure, but not interfering to the same degree with the effect of donor T lymphocytes (*30, 31*). It is not clear why methotrexate is effective while another antimetabolite, azathioprine, is not.

What cells mediate graft resistance if not T cells? Are they cells of macrophage lineage or NK-like cells? We tested the possibility that these cells express Ia-like antigens on their surface, and attempted to abrogate resistance by treating recipients before or after TBI and marrow grafting with the monoclonal antibody 7.2 (directed against monomorphic Ia-framework structure; reactivity not blocked by antithymocyte serum) (*32*). Results were in keeping with our speculation (*33*). Half of the dogs so treated had sustained engraftment (Table 3). The mechanisms through which antibody to an Ia-like antigen overcame resistance are unknown, but could include destruction of cells by murine antibody and canine complement or antibody-dependent cell-mediated cytotoxicity, or blocking of relevant receptors on host cells. We favor the latter explanation since canine complement is not cytotoxic and canine mononuclear cells are incapable of antibody-dependent cell mediated cytotoxicity when combined with murine monoclonal antibody in vitro. Perhaps more specific and more effective antibodies can be developed.

Observations in dogs undergoing graft rejection revealed the presence of spontaneously proliferating large granular lymphocytes of host origin and early T cell lineage in marrow and peripheral blood (*34*). These cells were capable of suppressing in vitro hemopoietic colony growth of marrow donor origin. Stimulated by this finding, the possible role of macrophages in resistance, and the previous demonstration of an inhibiting effect of postgrafting methotrexate on pulmonary macrophage

TABLE 3. Dogs given 9.2 Gy total-body irradiation at 7 cGy/min followed by infusion of $\leq 4\times10^8$ marrow cells/kg from an unrelated DLA-nonidentical donor

Additional treatment: Before marrow graft	Additional treatment: After marrow graft	Number of dogs studied	% With sustained grafts
—	—	36	8
ATS + procarbazine[a]	—	15	26
Donor antigen followed by MTX[b]	—	3	0
Silica[c]	—	8	25
8.8 Gy TBI[d]	—	10	100
Anti-Ia mcAb[e]	—	8	50
—	Anti-Ia mcAb[e]	6	50
—	MTX[f]	10	60

[a] ATS: Rabbit antithymocyte serum was either given at 0.5 ml/kg daily on days −9 to −4 or at 0.6 ml/kg on days −7, −5, −3 combined with procarbazine, 12.5 mg/kg on days −8, −6, −4. In a number of cases, recipients were "primed" with donor blood transfusions one week before the first dose of procarbazine.

[b] Dogs were given 100 ml of marrow donor blood on day −3 followed by MTX (methotrexate), 0.6 mg/kg on days −2 and −1.

[c] 100 mg/kg i.v. 18 hr after irradiation and 6 hr before marrow infusion.

[d] Total dose delivered was 18 Gy in 3 fractions of 6 Gy each at intervals of 48 hr.

[e] mcABb 7.2 at 0.2 mg/kg/day, days −5 to 0 or days −1 to +3.

[f] 0.4 mg/kg on days 1, 3, 6, 11.

TABLE 4. Dogs given 9.2 Gy total-body irradiation at 7 cGy/min followed by infusion of $\leq 4\times10^8$ marrow cells/kg from an unrelated DLA-nonidentical donor on day 0 and 1.8×10^9 peripheral blood leukocytes/kg from the marrow donor on days 1 and 2

Postgrafting immunosuppression	Number of dogs studied	% Dogs with sustained graft
None	75	91
MTX[a]	55	91
CsA[b]	13	39
MTX + CsA[c]	31	97
Azath. or 6-MP[d]	10	90
Azath. + CsA[e]	10	50

[a] MTX: methotrexate, 0.4 mg/kg days 1, 3, 6, 11, and once weekly until day 102.

[b] CsA: cyclosporine, 15 mg/kg day 1 with gradual dose reduction through day 100.

[c] MTX, 0.4 mg/kg, days 1, 3, 6, 11 and CsA as above.

[d] Azath.: azathioprine, 6-MP=6-mercaptopurine, both at 1 mg/kg/day from day 1 to 100.

[e] Azathioprine, 1 mg/kg/day, days 1 to 11, CsA as above.

kinetics after TBI and marrow grafting (*35*), we reexplored the usefulness of this drug for overcoming resistance. Six of ten dogs given marrow grafts (no buffy coat cells) and postgrafting methotrexate showed sustained engraftment (*36*), confirming the notion that resistance is mediated by cells capable of proliferating even after high-dose TBI (Table 3). Further studies are required to determine whether macrophages, large granular lymphocytes, or both cell types play a role in graft resistance.

Resistance overcome by very high doses of TBI. Further studies showed that the term "resistance to marrow grafts" applies only to the conventionally used doses of TBI. When the dose of TBI was increased to 18 Gy, sustained engraftment was seen in all DLA-nonidentical dogs, indicating complete or near complete inactivation or destruction of host cells mediating graft resistance (Table 3) (*37*). It was of concern, however, that grafts of marrow depleted of T cells by treatment with monoclonal antibody and complement were not consistently successful even at this very high dose of TBI (unpublished data). Because of potential long-term sequelae, very high dose TBI may not be practical, and other less toxic approaches to overcome resistance are desirable.

Comparison with murine hybrid resistance. Hemopoietic histocompatibility antigens involved in hybrid resistance have been described in mice (*38–40*). Specific abrogation of hybrid resistance to parent marrow has been achieved in adult F_1 mice by injecting parental spleen cells. Similarly, the addition of thymocytes but not of lymph node lymphocytes to the marrow inoculum was effective (*41–43*). Comparable studies on thoracic duct lymphocytes have not been carried out in mice. Graft-versus-host disease appeared not to be a prerequisite for the abrogation of hybrid resistance since thymocytes from donor mice "tolerant" to the host were reported to be equally effective (*43*). The "amplifier" cell among the thymocytes that enhances hemopoiesis has not been identified (*44*). In contrast to the present findings in dogs, the infusion of additional parental murine spleen cells made incapable of division by exposure to 10,000 rads of in vitro irradiation also enhanced engraftment. The mechanisms underlying this effect are unknown.

While control through MHC-associated genes seems to be the case for both species, a noncodominant inheritance is postulated in mouse (*38–40*), while canine antigens appear to be inherited in a codominant fashion (*1, 15*).

Resistance to marrow grafts in mice can be nonspecifically abrogated by split-dose irradiation, injection of radioactive strontium, cyclophosphamide, *Corynebacterium parvum*, antimacrophage agents such as silica and purified carageenan, and xenogeneic antimouse sera—e.g., horse, rabbit, or goat antisera raised against lymphocytes, brain, bone marrow, or macrophages (*45–49*).

Many of the manipulations capable of overcoming hybrid resistance in mice were not effective in dogs. This is shown by our studies shown in Table 3 (*1, 12*) and those of Vriesendorp et al. (*50–52*). Pretreatment of recipients with *C parvum*, and cyclophosphamide and L-asparaginase, as well as a delay of the marrow infusion by three to five days after TBI, failed to enhance engraftment in dogs (*51, 52*). The use of the "antimacrophage" agent, silica particles, gave equivocal results in dogs, with benefit reported by Vriesendorp et al. (*50*) and marginal effectiveness seen by us (Table 3) (*1, 12*).

Observations in man and in nonhuman primates. Results in these species have shown a high incidence of sustained engraftment of unmodified marrow following high-dose chemoradiation therapy (*53–55*), presumably due to the fact that human and primate marrow, in contrast to canine and murine marrow, contains a sizable proportion of mature T cells. These T cells might have the same graft-enhancing effect as the added peripheral blood lymphocytes in mice and dogs. Nevertheless, 15% of human patients given haploidentical grafts from family members for leukemia show failure of sustained engraftment (Table 5) (*54, 56*). In vitro removal of T cells from the haploidentical marrow grafts in patients with leukemia resulted in graft failure rates of 35–40% (Table 5) (*57–61*). Better engraftment was seen when the conditioning regimen was intensified, although limiting nonhemopoietic toxicity has been noted (*57, 58*). Generally, the engraftment rate of T-cell-depleted haploidentical marrow was much better in children with congenital severe combined immunodeficiency (SCID), providing circumstantial evidence of a role of T cells in resistance (*62, 63*). However, in a number of SCID patients a conditioning regimen was needed for engraftment to occur, grafts were slow to take, and B cells were often not reconstituted. It remains to be seen to what extent data in SCID patients can be extrapolated to patients with other diagnoses.

Conclusions. Taken together, results in dogs to date suggest that resistance to DLA-nonidentical marrow grafts is targeted against codominantly inherited MHC-associated antigens distinct from DLA-A, -B and -D. The host effector cells appear to be of non-T cell lineage, express Ia-like surface antigens, are capable of proliferating after TBI, are to some degree susceptible to postgrafting methotrexate and treatment by anti-Ia antibody, and can be inactivated by very high doses of fractionated TBI (18 Gy). It is conceivable that more than one cell population participates in the eventual destruction of the marrow graft. Cells from the blood of dogs undergoing graft rejection and harvested on day 10 after TBI, showing characteristics of large granular lymphocytes of T cell lineage, are capable of suppressing donor marrow growth in vitro (*34*). Inhibition of marrow colony formation by human natural killer cells has also been reported (*64*). Resistance to marrow grafts, mediated by a "natural" immune system, may permit host T cells that have survived TBI to become sensitized and expand, thereby enabling them to become the dominant cell type seen at the time of rejection. Radioresistant clonable T cells have been described by Reisner et al. in monkeys (*65*). Others go as far as to equate marrow graft rejection to skin graft rejection (*3*). Regardless of the host mechanism involved, the addition of viable donor lymphoid cells to the marrow inoculum consistently results in sustained engraftment. It remains to be determined whether a

TABLE 5. Incidence of marrow graft failure among patients with leukemia given high dose chemotherapy combined with TBI

Transplant team	Marrow donor[a]	No. patients studied	T cell depletion of marrow	% With graft failure
Seattle	HLA-identical sib (*68*)	728	No	0.1
		20	Yes	35
	Haploidentical (*54*)	105	No	5
Los Angeles	HLA-identical sib (*69*)	20	No	0
		20	Yes	30
Wisconsin	Haploidentical (*58*)	22	Yes	36
New York	Haploidentical (*59*)	20	Yes	40

[a] Donors are family members in all cases (references in parentheses).

donor lymphoid cell can be identified that is capable of enhancing engraftment without causing graft-versus-host disease.

DLA-Identical Marrow Grafts

As shown in Table 1, failure of engraftment was generally not a problem in recipients of DLA-identical littermate marrow following 9.2 Gy of total body irradiation. However, when the dose of radiation was lowered to 5 Gy or dogs were given suboptimal immunosuppression with the chemotherapeutic agent dimethylbusulfan, failure of sustained engraftment was frequently seen (*3*, *66*). Table 6 shows results of experiments in dogs given a dose of 10 mg of dimethylbusulfan per kilogram (the "lethal" dose in dogs is 7.5 mg/kg) (*67*). Four of sixteen recipients of DLA-identical marrow failed to show evidence of hematopoietic engraftment, while four rejected their grafts after initial evidence of engraftment (see also Fig. 2). Only eight of the 16 showed sustained engraftment. Resistance to grafts from DLA-identical littermates was suppressed in 12 of 13 cases by additional treatment of recipients with antithymocyte serum alone or combined with procarbazine (Table 6) (*66*). Increasing numbers of host T lymphocytes could be documented in rejecting dogs.

Taken together, these results suggest that resistance to DLA-identical littermate grafts is caused by T cells susceptible both to TBI at 9.2 Gy and to antithymocyte serum in addition to dimethylbusulfan. In agreement with this interpretation was the finding that postgrafting cyclosporine did not interfere with engraftment of DLA-identical littermate marrow, in contrast to results with DLA-nonidentical marrow (*29*). Findings in DLA-identical littermates are at variance with those in DLA-nonidentical grafts, where non-T cells seem to play a primary role in graft resistance.

Grafts between human HLA-identical siblings have generally been successful, and resistance has not played a major role. For example, in a series of 728 patients with hematological malignancies given chemotherapy combined with TBI, the graft failure rate was 0.1% (Table 5) (*68*). However, recent studies have reported failure of engraftment in 30–35% of patients given T cell-depleted HLA-identical marrow grafts (Table 5) (*68*, *69*). Concurrent with the increased rate of graft failure, a reduction has been noted in the incidence of graft-versus-host disease. Some graft-versus-host disease may be needed for consistent engraftment with the currently used conditioning programs. Initial results suggest that more intensive conditioning of recipients may decrease the graft failure rate, although toxicity limits with this approach have been encountered.

Alternatively, as suggested by in vitro studies in human patients by Kernan et al. (*70*) and the in vivo studies in dimethylbusulfan-treated dogs (*66*), it may become possible to reduce graft failure by treating recipients with antibodies directed at T cells mediating resistance to HLA-identical grafts.

TABLE 6. Dogs given 10 mg dimethylbusulfan/kg and infusion of $\leq 4\times10^8$ marrow cells/kg from a DLA-identical littermate on day 1 and 1.8×10^9 peripheral blood leukocytes from the marrow donor on days 2 and 3. All were given standard methotrexate postgrafting

Additional treatment	Number of dogs studied	% Dogs with sustained graft
None	16	50
Antithymocyte serum (ATS)[a]	10	90
Procarbazine/ATS[b]	3	100

[a] ATS, 0.6 ml/kg, days −6 to −1.
[b] Procarbazine, 12.5 mg/kg, days −7, −5, −3, and ATS, 0.5 ml/kg, days −6, −4, −2.

TRANSFUSION-INDUCED SENSITIZATION

Prior transfusions are thought to enhance the survival of kidney grafts (*4*). In contrast, transfusions jeopardize the success of subsequent marrow grafts, even when donor and recipient are identical for the antigens of the MHC (*71*). Apparently, recipient T lymphocytes can become sensitized to minor and major histocompatibility antigens of the marrow donor via transfusions. The infused marrow would meet with a secondary immune response that is more radioresistant than a primary response. Consequently, memory T cells will survive in numbers sufficient to destroy the marrow graft.

Results in DLA-identical littermates. Table 7 illustrates experimental findings in DLA-identical littermates. Without preceding transfusions, 58 of 59 recipients showed sustained hemopoietic engraftment (*72*). When recipients were given one whole-blood transfusion from the marrow donor 10 days before transplantation, 73% of them rejected the marrow graft (*72*, *73*). Administration of three transfusions from the donor 24, 17, and 10 days before transplantation resulted in graft rejection in all cases (*72*). Contrary to the findings made with graft resistance, the infusion of viable buffy coat cells in addition to the marrow inoculum did not alter this 100% incidence of graft rejection in presensitized recipients (*72*). Apparently, three preceding transfusions provided a very strong immunological stimulus that was neither abrogated by radiation nor by additional buffy coat cell transfusions.

The 100% incidence of rejection after three transfusions of whole blood from the marrow donor (21 out of 21 instances)

TABLE 7. Results of marrow grafts between DLA-identical littermates after 9.2 Gy total-body irradiation with or without preceding transfusions (tx) from the marrow donor

Treatment	Donor PBL in addition to marrow	Number of dogs studied	% With rejection
No preceding tx	No	21	5
	Yes	38	0
One whole-blood tx, day −10[a]	Yes	18	73
Three whole-blood tx, days −24, −17, −10[a]	No	8	100
	Yes	13	100
Three leukocyte-poor platelet tx, days −24, −17, −10[b]	Yes	15	47
Three leukocyte-poor red cell tx, days −24, −17, −10[c]	Yes	14	36
4.2×10^3 mononuclear peripheral blood cells/kg tx, days −24, −17, −10[d]	Yes	7	57
Three injections of donor skin epithelial cells, days −24, −17, −10[e]	Yes	6	100

[a] 50 ml heparinized whole blood injected i.v.
[b] Median of 1.8×10^8 platelets/kg/transfusion, "contaminated" by a median of 6.7×10^3 mononuclear cells/kg (i.v.).
[c] Median of 3.1 ml packed red cells/kg/transfusion, "contaminated" by a median of 1.7×10^4 mononuclear cells/kg (i.v.).
[d] Ficoll-Hypaque separated mononuclear cells (i.v.); total number injected 12.5×10^3/kg.
[e] 1.1×10^6 viable epithelial cells/kg s.c.

suggests that at least two polymorphic histocompatibility systems outside of DLA are involved in sensitization (*72*). (The probability of encountering 21 of 21 rejections if only one polymorphic locus were involved is <.008; the likelihood for more than two loci is <.29, by the binomial significance test.) Therefore, attempts at unraveling the genetics of these antigen systems by in vitro tests of immunity would be difficult. Only 73% of dogs rejected after a single whole-blood transfusion from the DLA-identical littermate donor, while 25% had sustained engraftment. This is in keeping with the possibility of one important "minor" histocompatibility system requiring less intense immunization.

The conclusion that polymorphic "minor" antigens are involved is consistent with the finding that transfusions from unrelated DLA-nonidentical donors can immunize a recipient against a subsequent marrow graft from a DLA-identical littermate (Table 8) (*74*). In that situation, rejection of the marrow graft might be expected only when one or more of the blood transfusion donors and the marrow donor share "minor" antigens not present in the recipient. Whether additionally fortuitous matching of donor and recipient for Ia antigens is required is unknown. An even more pronounced effect of unrelated transfusions is seen in DLA-nonidentical littermates (Table 8) (*75*).

The observation that dogs given subcutaneous and intradermal injections of skin epithelial cells from the marrow donor rejected a subsequent DLA-identical marrow graft indicates that the expression of antigens mediating rejection is not restricted to hematopoietic cells, but extends to at least one other tissue (Table 7) (*72*). Skin epithelial cells cultured overnight in plastic dishes were chosen for the study because they would not be expected to contain nonepidermal cells in numbers sufficient to obscure the interpretation of results. Although contamination by leukocytes cannot be completely ruled out by morphological examination, canine skin epithelial cells so treated failed to stimulate lymphocytes from unrelated donors in vitro in mixed leukocyte culture.

More than half the recipients given transfusions of leukocyte-poor platelets or red blood cells from the marrow donor showed sustained hematopoietic engraftment (Table 7) (*72*). This result is somewhat surprising and suggests that platelets and red blood cells exhibit only some, not all, of the non-DLA antigens

TABLE 8. Results of hemopoietic grafts between littermates after 9.2 Gy TBI with or without preceding transfusions (tx) from unrelated dogs. (All DLA-nonidentical littermates were given peripheral blood leukocytes in addition to the marrow graft.)

Marrow donor-recipient combination	Preceding whole-blood transfusions	Number of dogs studied	% With rejection
DLA-identical littermates	No	59	2
	3 tx[a] from random unrelated donors, days −24, −17, −10	11	27
DLA-nonidentical littermates	No	12	0
	3 tx[a] from random unrelated donors, days −24, −17, −10	8	63

[a] 50 ml herparinized blood from each of 3 donors on each occasion i.v.

involved in sensitization and rejection—or, alternatively, that they express none of the antigens, and sensitization and rejection are due to mononuclear cell contamination that is on the order of 1.5×10^5 cells per dog. The latter explanation is supported by the finding that rejection can be seen after injections of only 12.5×10^3 mononuclear peripheral blood cells per kilogram (Table 7) (*76*).

Results in DLA-nonidentical dogs. Further studies in DLA-nonidentical unrelated donor-recipient pairs examined the effect of timing of preceding blood transfusions on sensitization to hemopoietic grafts (Table 9) (*75, 77, 78*). Rejection was most likely with the transfusion given 24 hr before TBI (86% rejection). A total of 75% of the dogs rejected when the transfusion was given on day −10, and 50% rejected when the transfusion was given 3 months before transplantation. Rejections seen in dogs transfused 24 hr before TBI, in all likelihood, represent primary immune responses. It is known that irradiation is most effective as an immunosuppressive agent when administered before antigen exposure. This has been most clearly shown in the primary humoral antibody response to several different antigens. In several systems exposure to antigen at critical times before irradiation resulted in a heightened immune response (*79*). The increased incidence of rejections in dogs transfused 3 months before grafting must be a reflection of a secondary immune response that also is not adequately suppressed by irradiation.

Prevention and suppression of transfusion-induced sensitization to the marrow graft. Other studies, done both in recipients of marrow from DLA-identical littermates and in DLA-nonidentical unrelated dogs were aimed at prevention or suppression of transfusion-induced sensitization, thereby permitting sustained engraftment (Table 10). Some of the manipulations found to be effective in overcoming resistance were not effective in suppressing transfusion-induced sensitization—e.g., postgrafting methotrexate (*75*). Conversely, manipulations ineffective in overcoming resistance were effective in abrogating transfusion-induced sensitization—e.g., cyclosporine and procarbazine/antithymocyte serum (*80–82*). These findings further support the speculation that two distinctly different mechanisms are operative in graft resistance and transfusion-induced sensitization.

Prevention of sensitization was also accomplished by exposure of the transfused whole blood to ultraviolet light (Table 10) (*83*). Dogs receiving blood irradiated with ultraviolet light all engrafted, while control dogs (Table 7) and those receiving sham irradiated blood products (Table 10) all failed to engraft. The exact mechanism by which this result is achieved is unknown, but in vitro and in vivo data are consistent with the possibility that cell surface Ia function of accessory cells is altered (*84*) or that other cell surface determinants, presumably non-DLA histocompatibility antigens, are modified by ultraviolet light exposure, thus escaping recognition by the recipient.

Comparison with results in other species. Similar to observations in dogs, studies in mice (*85–87*) and monkeys (*88*) have shown that blood transfusions prior to transplant frequently result in subsequent marrow graft rejection with conditioning regimens that otherwise lead to sustained engraftment.

Assessment of an impact of pretransplant transfusion on graft outcome in man appears to depend to some extent upon the underlying diagnosis for which the patient has been transplanted. In patients with hematologic malignancies conditioned with intensive treatment regimens including TBI, and given an

HLA-identical marrow graft, no adverse effect of pretransplant transfusions has been observed. However, in patients with severe aplastic anemia conditioned with cyclophosphamide only, strong correlations exist between pretransplant transfusions and subsequent rejection of HLA-identical marrow (*89–91*). More intensive conditioning regimens including TBI, total lymphoid irradiation, thoracoabdominal irradiation, procarbazine/antithymocyte globulin, and postgrafting cyclosporine have been employed to overcome transfusion-induced sensitization (*92–100*).

Conclusions. Pretransplant transfusions, especially from the prospective marrow donor, jeopardize the success of a subsequent marrow graft. Apparently transfusions result in recipient sensitization to histocompatibility antigens expressed on peripheral blood and marrow cells. At the time of transplantation, the patient's immune system recognizes the respective antigens expressed on donor marrow cells and mounts a memory response. This memory response appears to be mediated by T lymphocytes and is more difficult to suppress than a primary immune response.

TABLE 9. Results of bone marrow grafts between DLA-nonidentical unrelated dogs after 9.2 Gy of total-body irradiation with or without preceding transfusion from the marrow donor. (All recipients were given viable donor PBL infusions in addition to the marrow inoculum.)

Preceding transfusion	Number of dogs studied	% With rejection
No	75	9
One whole-blood transfusion:[a]		
Day −1	7	86
Day −10	12	75
Day −90	16	50

[a] 50 ml heparinized whole blood i.v.; days before marrow graft.

TABLE 10. Results of hemopoietic grafts in dogs given 9.2 Gy TBI with or without preceding transfusions from the marrow donors: attempts at preventing graft rejection by additional immunosuppressive therapy before or after grafting and by ultraviolet light (UV) exposure of blood products

Marrow donor-recipient combination	Preceding whole-blood transfusions[a] (tx) from marrow donor	Additional treatment	Number of dogs studied	% with rejection
DLA-identical littermates	3 tx, days −24, −17, −10	Cyclosporine[b]	9	22
	3 tx, days −24, −17, −10	UV irradiation[c] of tx blood	10	0
	3 tx, days −24, −17, −10	Sham irradiation of tx blood	4	100
DLA-nonidentical, unrelated	No	None	7	0
	1 tx, day −10	None	5	100
	No	MTX[d]	11	9
	1 tx, day −10	MTX[d]	5	100
	2 tx, days −20, −13	None	10	70
	2 tx, days −20, −13	ATS[e]	10	50
	2 tx, days −20, −13	Pro[f]	8	50
	2 tx, days −20, −13	Pro[f] + ATS[e]	10	10
	6 tx, days −50 to −15	None	15	73
	6 tx, days −50 to −15	Pro[f] + ATS[e]	15	20

[a] 50 ml heparinized whole blood i.v. on each occasion except in the last 2 groups, in which 75% of dogs were given platelet transfusions derived from 50 ml whole blood.

[b] Cyclosporine, 20 mg/kg/day i.m. on days −5 to 0.

[c] 1.35J/cm^2 of UV-B light from a germicidal lamp.

[d] MTX: methotrexate, 0.4 mg/kg i.v. on days 1, 3, 6, and 11 after marrow graft.

[e] ATS: rabbit antithymocyte serum, 0.6 ml/kg s.c. on days −7, −5, −3.

[f] Pro: procarbazine, 12.5 mg/kg i.v. on days −8, −6, and −4.

REFERENCES

1. Storb R, Weiden PL, Graham TC, Thomas ED. Failure of engraftment and graft-versus-host disease after canine marrow transplantation: two phenomena linked to but not exclusively determined by known antigens of the major histocompatibility complex. Transplant Proc 1978; 10: 113.
2. Deeg HJ, Storb R, Thomas ED. Marrow graft studies in dogs: factors influencing resistance to engraftment and graft-versus-host disease. Surv Immunol Res 1982; 1: 148.
3. Vriesendorp HM, Wagemaker G, van Bekkum DW. Engraftment of allogeneic bone marrow. Transplant Proc 1981; 13: 643.
4. Opelz G, for the Collaborative Transplant Study. Current relevance of the transfusion effect in renal transplantation. Transplant Proc 1985; 17: 1015.
5. Albert ED, Erickson VM, Graham TC, et al. Serology and genetics of the DL-A system. I. Establishment of specificities. Tissue Antigens 1973; 3; 417.
6. Bull RW, Vriesendorp HM, Cech R, et al. Joint report of the Third International Workshop on Canine Immunogenetics. II. Analysis of the serological typing of cells. Transplantation (in press).
7. Deeg HJ, Raff RF, Grosse-Wilde H, et al. Joint report of the Third International Workshop on Canine Immunogenetics. I. Analysis of homozygous typing cells (HTCs). Transplantation 1986; 41: 111.
8. Thomas ED, LeBlond R, Graham T, Storb R. Marrow infusions in dogs given midlethal or lethal irradiation. Radiat Res 1970; 41: 113.
9. Deeg HJ, Storb R, Weiden PL, et al. High dose total body irradiation and autologous marrow reconstitution in dogs: dose

rate related acute toxicity and fractionation dependent long-term survival. Radiat Res 1981; 88: 385.

10. Epstein RB, Storb R, Ragde H, Thomas ED. Cytotoxic typing antisera for marrow grafting in littermate dogs. Transplantation 1968; 6: 45.
11. Storb R, Rudolph RH, Thomas ED. Marrow grafts between canine siblings matched by serotyping and mixed leukocyte culture. J Clin Invest 1971; 50: 1272.
12. Weiden PL, Storb R, Graham TC, Sale GE, Thomas ED. Resistance to DLA-nonidentical marrow grafts in lethally irradiated dogs. Transplant Proc 1977; 9: 285.
13. Vriesendorp HM, Zurcher C, van Bekkum DW. Engraftment of allogeneic dog bone marrow. Transplant Proc 1975; 7: 465.
14. Vriesendorp HM, Klapwijk WM, van Kessel AMC, Zurcher C, van Bekkum DW. Lasting engraftment of histoincompatible bone marrow cells in dogs. Transplantation 1981; 31: 347.
15. Deeg HJ, Storb R, Raff RF, Weiden PL, DeRose S, Thomas ED. Marrow grafts between phenotypically DLA-identical and haploidentical unrelated dogs: additional antigens controlling engraftment are not detected by cell-mediated lympholysis. Transplantation 1982; 33: 17.
16. Ladiges WC, Raff RF, Brown S, Deeg HJ, Storb R. The canine major histocompatibility complex: supertypic specificities defined by the primed lymphocyte test (PLT). Immunogenetics 1984; 19: 359.
17. Raff RF, Storb R, Ladiges WC, Deeg HJ. Recognition of target cell determinants associated with DLA-D-locus-encoded antigens by canine cytotoxic lymphocytes. Transplantation 1985; 40: 323.
18. Storb R, Epstein RB, Bryant J, Ragde H, Thomas ED. Marrow grafts by combined marrow and leukocyte infusions in unrelated dogs selected by histocompatibility typing. Transplantation 1968; 6: 587.
19. Storb R, Deeg HJ. Contributions of the dog model in marrow transplantation. Plasma Ther Transfus Technol 1985; 6: 303.
20. Storb R, Epstein RB, Ragde H, Bryant J, Thomas ED. Marrow engraftment by allogeneic leukocytes in lethally irradiated dogs. Blood 1967; 30: 805.
21. Deeg HJ, Storb R, Weiden PL, et al. Abrogation of resistance to and enhancement of DLA-nonidentical unrelated marrow grafts in lethally irradiated dogs by thoracic duct lymphocytes. Blood 1979; 53: 552.
22. Storb R, Epstein RB, Thomas ED. Marrow repopulating ability of peripheral blood cells compared to thoracic duct cells. Blood 1968; 32: 662.
23. Torok-Storb BJ, Storb R, Graham TC, Prentice RL, Weiden PL, Adamson JW. Erythropoiesis in vitro: effect of normal versus "transfusion-sensitized" mononuclear cells. Blood 1978; 52: 706.
24. Torok-Storb BJ, Storb R, Deeg HJ, et al. Growth in vitro of donor marrow cultured with recipient lymphocytes predicts the fate of marrow grafts in transfused DLA-identical dogs. Blood 1979; 53: 104.
25. Torok-Storb BJ, Hansen JA. Modulation of in vitro BFU-E growth by normal Ia-positive T cells is restricted by HLA-DR (Letter). Nature 1982; 298: 473.
26. Nathan DG, Chess L, Hillman DG, et al. Human erythroid burst-forming unit: T-cell requirement for proliferation in vitro. J Exp Med 1978; 147: 324.
27. Storb R, Kolb HJ, Graham TC, et al. Marrow grafts between histoincompatible canine family members. Eur J Clin Biol Res 1972; 17: 680.
28. Storb R, Epstein RB, Graham TC, Thomas ED. Methotrexate regimens for control of graft-versus-host disease in dogs with allogeneic marrow grafts. Transplantation 1970; 9: 240.
29. Deeg HJ, Storb R, Weiden PL, Graham T, Atkinson K, Thomas ED. Cyclosporin A: effect on marrow engraftment and graft-versus-host disease in dogs. Transplant Proc 1981; 13: 402.
30. Deeg HJ, Storb R, Weiden PL, et al. Cyclosporin A and methotrexate in canine marrow transplantation: engraftment, graft-versus-host disease and induction of tolerance. Transplantation 1982; 34: 30.
31. Deeg HJ, Storb R, Appelbaum FR, Kennedy MS, Graham TC, Thomas ED. Combined immunosuppression with cyclosporine and methotrexate in dogs given bone marrow grafts from DLA-haploidentical littermates. Transplantation 1984; 37: 62.
32. Deeg HJ, Wulff JC, DeRose S, et al. Unusual distribution of Ia-like antigens on canine lymphocytes. Immunogenetics 1982; 16: 445.
33. Deeg HJ, Storb R, Szer J, Appelbaum FR, Hackman RC, Thomas ED. Facilitation of DLA nonidentical marrow by treatment of the recipient with monoclonal anti-Ia antibody. Transplant Proc 1985; 17: 493.
34. Raff RF, Deeg HJ, Loughran TP, et al. Characterization of host cells involved in resistance to marrow grafts in dogs transplanted from unrelated DLA-nonidentical donors. Blood (in press).
35. Springmeyer SC, Kopecky KJ, Deeg HJ, Whitehead J, Altman LC, Storb R. Pulmonary bronchoalveolar cell and protein kinetics in dogs given total body irradiation, autologous marrow grafts and methotrexate. Transplantation 1984; 37: 336.
36. Deeg HJ, Storb R, Raff R, Weiden PL, Graham TC, Thomas ED. Resistance to allogeneic marrow grafts in dogs: effect of DLA matching, buffy coat cells, methotrexate, cyclosporin A and fractionated total body irradiation [Abstract No. 163]. Exp Hematol 1981; 9(suppl 9): 97.
37. Deeg HJ, Storb R, Shulman HM, Weiden PL, Graham TC, Thomas ED. Engraftment of DLA-nonidentical unrelated canine marrow after high-dose fractionated total body irradiation. Transplantation 1982; 33: 443.
38. Cudkowicz G. Natural resistance to foreign hemopoietic and leukemia grafts (discussion). In: Cudkowicz G, Landy M, Shearer GM, eds. Natural resistance systems against foreign cells, tumors, and microbes. New York: Academic Press, 1978: 3.
39. Daley JP, Nakamura I. Natural resistance to lethally irradiated F_1 hybrid mice to parental marrow grafts is a function of H-2/Hh-restricted effectors. J Exp Med 1984; 159: 1132.
40. Lotzova E. Resistance to parental, allogeneic and xenogeneic hemopoietic grafts in irradiated mice. Exp Hematol 1977; 5: 215.
41. Goodman JW, Congdon CC. Blood-marrow mixtures in irradiated mice: effect of blood injections on bone marrow transplantation in lethally irradiated mice. Arch Pathol 1961; 72 (18): 32.
42. Goodman JW, Shinpock SG. Influence of thymus cells on erythropoiesis of parental marrow in irradiated hybrid mice. Proc Soc Exp Biol Med 1968; 129: 417.
43. Goodman JW, Shinpock SG. Interaction between T lymphocytes and hemopoietic stem cells: a critical mini-review. In: Gale RP, Fox CF, eds. Biology of bone marrow transplantation. ICN-UCLA Symp Mol Cell Biol, vol 17. New York: Academic Press, 1980: 461.
44. Goodman JW, Basford NL, Shinpock SG, Chambers ZE. An amplifier cell in hemopoiesis. Exp Hematol 1978; 6: 151.
45. Gallagher MT, Datta SK, Trentin JJ. Genetic resistance to bone marrow transplantation as a leukemia-lymphoma defense mechanism: correlation of in vivo lymphoma resistance and in vitro NK activity. Biomedicine 1980; 33: 73.
46. Bennett MJ. Prevention of marrow allograft rejection with radioactive strontium: evidence for marrow-dependent effector cells. J Immunol 1973; 110: 510.
47. Kiessling R, Hochman PS, Haller G, Shearer GM, Wigzell H, Cudkowicz G. Evidence for a similar or common mechanism for natural killer cell activity and resistance to hemopoietic grafts. Eur J Immunol 1977; 7: 655.
48. Rolstad B, Benestad HB. The "natural resistance" to bone marrow allografts in normal and athymic nude rats: rapid cytotoxic reactions both in vivo and in vitro. Eur J Immunol 1984; 14: 793.
49. Cudkowicz G, Yung YP. Abrogation of resistance to foreign body

marrow grafts by carrageenans. I. Studies with the anti-macrophage agent Seakem carrageenan. J Immunol 1977; 119: 483.

50. Vriesendorp HM, Lowenberg B, Visser TP, Knaan S, van Bekkum DW. Influence of genetic resistance and silica particles on survival after bone marrow transplantation. Transplant Proc 1976; 8: 483.
51. Vriesendorp HM, Klapwijk WM, Heidt PJ, Hogeweg B, Zurcher C, von Bekkum DW. Factors controlling the engraftment of transplanted dog bone marrow cells. Tissue Antigens 1982; 20: 63.
52. Vriesendrop HM, Zurcher C, Bull RW, et al. Take and graft-versus-host reactions of allogeneic bone marrow in tissue-typed dogs. Transplant Proc 1975; 7(suppl 1): 849.
53. Thomas ED, Storb R, Clift RA, et al. Bone-marrow transplantation. N Engl J Med 1975; 292: 832, 895.
54. Beatty PG, Clift RA, Mickelson EM, et al. Marrow transplantation from related donors other than HLA-identical siblings. N Engl J Med 1985; 313: 765.
55. van Bekkum DW, Lowenberg B, eds. Bone marrow transplantation: biological mechanisms and clinical practice. New York: Dekker, 1985.
56. Hansen JA, Beatty PG, Anasetti C, et al. Treatment of leukemia by marrow transplantation from donors other than HLA genotypically identical siblings. In: Gale RP, Champlin R, eds. Recent advances in bone marrow transplantation. UCLA Symp Mol Cell Biol, New Series, vol 53. New York: AR Liss (in press).
57. Sondel PM, Hank JA, Trigg ME, et al. Transplantation of HLA-haploidentical T-cell-depleted marrow for leukemia: autologous marrow recovery with specific immune sensitization to donor antigens. Exp Hematol 1986; 14: 278.
58. Bozdech MJ, Sondel PM, Trigg ME, et al. Transplantation of HLA-identical T-cell-depleted marrow for leukemia: addition of cytosine arabinoside to the pretransplant conditioning prevents rejection. Exp Hematol 1985; 13: 1201.
59. O'Reilly RJ, Collins NH, Kernan N, et al. Transplantation of marrow-depleted T cells by soybean lectin agglutination and E-rosette depletion: major histocompatibility complex-related graft resistance in leukemic transplant patients. Transplant Proc 1985; 17: 455.
60. Reisner Y, Kapoor N, Kirkpatrick D, et al. Transplantation for acute leukaemia with HLA-A and B nonidentical parental marrow cells fractionated with soybean agglutinin and sheep red blood cells. Lancet 1981; 2: 327.
61. Filipovich AH, Ramsay NKC, Arthur DC, McGlave P, Kim T, Kersey JH. Allogeneic bone marrow transplantation with related donors other than HLA MLC-matched siblings, and the use of antithymocyte globulin, prednisone, and methotrexate for prophylaxis of graft-versus-host disease. Transplantation 1985; 39: 282.
62. Reisner Y, Kapoor N, O'Reilly RJ, Good RA. Allogeneic bone marrow transplantation using stem cells fractionated by lectins. VI. In vitro analysis of human and monkey bone marrow cells fractionated by sheep red blood cells and soybean agglutin. Lancet 1980; 2: 1320.
63. Friedrich W, Goldmann SF, Vetter U, et al. Immunoreconstitution in severe combined immunodeficiency after transplantation of HLA-haploidentical, T-cell-depleted bone marrow. Lancet 1984; 1: 761.
64. Degliantoni G, Perussia B, Mangoni L, Trinchieri G. Inhibition of bone marrow colony formation by human natural killer cells and by natural killer cell-derived colony-inhibiting activity. J Exp Med 1985; 161: 1152.
65. Reisner Y, Ben-Bassat I, Douer D, Kaploon A, Schwartz E, Ramot B. A primate pre-clinical model for bone marrow transplantation. Definitive proof for host radio-resistant clonable T cells [Abstract No. 2]. Exp Hematol 1985; 13: 321.
66. Storb R, Weiden PL, Graham TC, Lerner KG, Nelson N, Thomas ED. Hemopoietic grafts between DLA-identical canine littermates following dimethyl myleran: evidence for resistance to grafts not associated with DLA and abrogated by antithymocyte serum. Transplantation 1977; 24: 349.
67. Kolb HJ, Storb R, Weiden PL, et al. Immunologic, toxicologic and marrow transplantation studies in dogs given dimethyl myleran. Biomedicine 1974; 20: 341.
68. Martin PJ, Hansen JA, Buckner CD, et al. Effects of in vitro depletion of T cells in HLA-identical allogeneic marrow grafts. Blood 1985; 66: 664.
69. Mitsuyasu RT, Champlin RE, Gale RP, et al. Depletion of T-lymphocytes from donor bone marrow for the prevention of graft-versus-host disease following bone marrow transplantation: a prospective randomized double blind trial. Ann Intern Med (in press).
70. Kernan NA, Flomenberg N, Dupont B, O'Reilly RJ. Identification of cytotoxic T lymphocytes in patients rejecting T cell depleted bone marrow transplants for leukemia. Blood 1984; 64: 216a.
71. Storb R, Weiden PL. Transfusion problems associated with transplantation. Semin Hematol 1981; 18: 163.
72. Storb R, Weiden PL, Deeg HJ, et al. Rejection of marrow from DLA-identical canine littermates given transfusions before grafting: antigens involved are expressed on leukocytes and skin epithelial cells but not on platelets and red blood cells. Blood 1979; 54: 477.
73. Storb R, Epstein RB, Rudolph RH, Thomas ED. The effect of prior transfusion on marrow grafts between histocompatible canine siblings. J Immunol 1970; 105: 627.
74. Storb R, Rudolph RH, Graham TC, Thomas ED. The influence of transfusions from unrelated donors upon marrow grafts between histocompatible canine siblings. J Immunol 1971; 107: 409.
75. Storb R, Kolb HJ, Graham TC, Kane PJ, Thomas ED. The effect of prior blood transfusions on hemopoietic grafts from histoincompatible canine littermates. Transplantation 1972; 14: 248.
76. Deeg HJ, Torok-Storb BJ, Storb R, et al. Rejection of DLA-identical canine littermate marrow after transfusion-induced sensitization: antigens involved are expressed on cotton-wool adherent but not on nonadherent mononuclear cells, granulocytes, or thoracic duct lymphocytes. In: Baum SJ, Ledney GD, Khan A, eds. Experimental hematology today. Basel: Karger, 1981: 31.
77. Weiden PL, Storb R, Kolb HJ, Graham TC, Kao G, Thomas ED. Effect of time on sensitization to hemopoietic grafts by preceding blood transfusions. Transplantation 1975; 19: 240.
78. Storb R, Kolb HJ, Graham TC, Erickson V, Thomas ED. The effect of buffy coat-poor blood transfusion on subsequent hemopoietic grafts. Transplantation 1973; 15: 129.
79. Taliaferro WH, Taliaferro LG, Jaroslow BN, eds. Radiation and immune mechanisms. New York: Academic Press, 1964.
80. Storb R, Floersheim GL, Weiden PL, et al. Effect of prior blood transfusions on marrow grafts: abrogation of sensitization by procarbazine and antithymocyte serum. J Immunol 1974; 112: 1508.
81. Weiden PL, Storb R, Slichter S, Warren RP, Sale GE. Effect of six weekly transfusions on canine marrow grafts: tests for sensitization and abrogation of sensitization by procarbazine and antithymocyte serum. J Immunol 1976; 117: 143.
82. Storb R, Deeg HJ, Atkinson K, et al. Cyclosporin-A abrogates transfusion-induced sensitization and prevents marrow graft rejection in DLA-identical canine littermates. Blood 1982; 60: 524.
83. Deeg HJ, Aprile J, Graham TC, Appelbaum FR, Storb R. Ultraviolet irradiation of blood prevents transfusion-induced sensitization and marrow graft rejection in dogs. Blood 1986; 67: 537.
84. Aprile JA, Deeg HJ. UV irradiation of canine dendritic cells prevents mitogen induced cluster formation and lymphocyte proliferation. Transplantation (in press).
85. da Costa H, Amiel JL, Mathe G. Immunisation contre des greffes de cellules hematopoietiques allogeniques par des transfusions de sang anterieures. Vox Sang 1964; 9: 420.

86. Barnes DWH, Loutit JF. What is the recovery factor in spleen? Nucleonics 1954; 12: 68.
87. Santos GW, Sensenbrenner LL. A sensitive and quantitative assay for non-H-2 histocompatibility antigens. Exp Hematol 1971; 21: 19.
88. van Putten LM, van Bekkum DW, de Vries MJ, Balner H. The effect of preceding blood transplants on the fate of homologous bone marrow grafts in lethally irradiated monkeys. Blood 1967; 30: 749.
89. Storb R, Prentice RL, Thomas ED. Marrow transplantation for treatment of aplastic anemia: an analysis of factors associated with graft rejection. N Engl J Med 1977; 296: 61.
90. Storb R, Prentice RL, Thomas ED, et al. Factors associated with graft rejection after HLA-identical marrow transplantation for aplastic anaemia. Br J Haematol 1983; 55: 573.
91. Storb R, Thomas ED, Buckner CD, et al. Marrow transplantation in thirty "untransfused" patients with severe aplastic anemia. Ann Intern Med 1980; 92: 30.
92. Storb R, Doney KC, Thomas ED, et al. Marrow transplantation with or without donor buffy coat cells for 65 transfused aplastic anemia patients. Blood 1982; 59: 236.
93. Ramsay NKC, Kim TH, McGlave P, et al. Total lymphoid irradiation and cyclophosphamide conditioning prior to bone marrow transplantation for patients with severe aplastic anemia. Blood 1983; 62: 622.
94. Parkman R, Rappeport J, Camitta B, Levey RH, Nathan DG. Successful use of multiagent immunosuppression in the bone marrow transplantation of sensitized patients. Blood 1978; 52: 1163.
95. Gluckman E, Barrett AJ, Arcese W, Devergie A, Degoulet P. Bone marrow transplantation in severe aplastic anaemia: a survey of the European Group for Bone Marrow Transplantation. Br J Haematol 1981; 49: 165.
96. UCLA Bone Marrow Transplant Team: Gale RP, Ho W, Feig S, et al. Prevention of graft rejection following bone marrow transplantation. Blood 1981; 57: 9.
97. Elfenbein GJ, Mellits ED, Santos GW, et al. Engraftment and survival after allogeneic bone marrow transplantation for severe aplastic anemia. Transplant Proc 1983; 15: 1412.
98. Hows JM, Palmer S, Gordon-Smith EC. Cyclosporine and graft failure following bone marrow transplantation for severe aplastic anemia. Br J Haematol 1985; 60: 611.
99. Devergie A, Gluckman E. Bone marrow transplantation in severe aplastic anemia following cytoxan and thoraco-abdominal irradiation. Exp Hematol 1982; 10(suppl 10): 17.
100. Bortin MM, Gale RP, Rimm AA, for the Advisory Committee of the International Bone Marrow Transplant Registry. Allogeneic bone marrow transplantation for 144 patients with severe aplastic anemia. JAMA 1981; 245; 1132.

0041-1337/86/4206-0581$02.00/0
TRANSPLANTATION

Vol. 42, No. 6
Printed in U.S.A.

Transplantation
ARTICLES

IMMUNOSUPPRESSIVE ACTIVITY OF SERUM FROM LIVER-GRAFTED RATS

PASSIVE ENHANCEMENT OF FULLY ALLOGENEIC HEART GRAFTS AND INDUCTION OF SYSTEMIC TOLERANCE[1]

NAOSHI KAMADA,[2] TAKAHISA SHINOMIYA,[3] TOHRU TAMAKI, AND KOICHI ISHIGURO[3]

Department of Surgery, University of Cambridge, Addenbrooke's Hospital, Cambridge, England; and Mitsubishi-Kasei Institute of Life Sciences, Minamiooya 11, Machida, Tokyo 194, Japan

Immunological enhancement of allogeneic heart graft survival by serum from rats tolerized by liver grafting has been studied. Serum taken from long-term-surviving PVG rats carrying orthotopic DA liver transplants (OLT serum) was able to increase the survival time of PVG.RT1^a heterotopic heart grafts in PVG recipients. Administration of 1 ml of OLT serum at the time of heart grafting led to permanent survival of the grafts in all animals. The recipients became systemically tolerant of RT1^a and several weeks later were able to accept permanently skin grafts from the same donor strain, while rejecting third-party grafts. Enhancement appeared to be mediated initially by IgG antibodies in the OLT serum against class II donor RT1^a antigens; significant enhancement was produced by as little as 100 μg of antibody. Recipient alloantibody responses following enhancement were studied and showed selective suppression of the anti-class-I (RT1A^a) antibody levels, while the anti-class-II antibody response was apparently unaffected. The implications of these results for mechanisms of unresponsiveness following enhancement and liver transplantation are discussed.

In previous papers, we have documented the survival of orthotopic DA (RT1^a) liver grafts in PVG (RT1^c) rats (*1–8*). Such grafts are not rejected (unless the recipient has been presensitized) but induce a state of systemic, DA-specific transplantation tolerance. The recipient serum (OLT serum)* contains a high level of antibodies to class II RT1^a alloantigens (*1, 9*) while, in contrast, the level of anti-class-I alloantibodies is very low and we have described evidence that the anti-class-I response is effectively tolerized after liver grafting (*1*). This serological picture mirrors the partial or "split" tolerant state seen in cellular reactivity (*1, 10–12*). Thus, while DA-liver-grafted PVG rats display donor specific unresponsiveness in graft rejection and fail to generate cytotoxic T cells in vitro, their potential to mount mixed lymphocyte and graft-versus-host reactions against DA (in the absence of OLT serum) is apparently normal (*10–12*). It is possible that the strong anti-class-II alloantibody response that follows liver grafting in this combination is central to the survival of the liver graft and the manifestations of transplantation tolerance in vivo. Antibodies against rat class II antigens are known to be potent mediators of enhancement and the rat is one of the species most susceptible to prolongation of graft survival by this means (*13–15*). Elsewhere, we have reported that passive transfer of serum from PVG rats with well-established, liver-induced tolerance of DA is able to prolong survival of (DA×PVG)F_1 heterotopic heart grafts in normal PVG recipients (*1*), and that lymph from liver-grafted rats also has marked immunosuppressive properties in vivo (*16*). Moreover, there are parallels between split tolerance induced by liver grafting and the situation after enhancement, where proliferative T cell responses have been found to be normal in rats made unresponsive by enhancement (*14*). In this paper, we have investigated further the enhancing effects of OLT serum and describe its ability to bring about permanent survival of fully allogeneic PVG.RT1^a heart grafts in PVG recipients and induction of systemic transplantation tolerance.

[1] This work was supported by a grant from the Alex Foundation (Japan).

[2] Address correspondence to: Dr. Naoshi Kamada, Department of Transplantation and Research, Tokyo Medical School, Hachioji Medical Centre, Tate-Machi, Hachioji City, Tokyo, Japan 193.

[3] Mitsubishi-Kasei Institute of Life Sciences.

* Abbreviations used: HPLC, high-performance liquid chromatography; OLT, orthotopic liver transplant.

MATERIALS AND METHODS

Animals. Rats, 8–16 weeks of age, of the following strains were obtained from OLAC (1976) Ltd., Bicester, Oxfordshire, UK: PVG (RT1^c), DA (RT1^a), WAG (RT1^u), the PVG congenic strains PVG.RT1^a and PVG.R1, and (DA×PVG)F_1 hybrids.

Surgical procedures. Orthotopic liver transplantation (OLT) was performed by our previously published techniques (*17*) generally using DA rats as donors and PVG rats as recipients; rejection does not occur in this combination. Heterotopic auxiliary heart grafting was performed in the neck using the method of Heron (*18*). Rejection was defined by cessation of heart beat on neck palpation and confirmed by histological examination of the grafts. Full-thickness skin grafting was carried out according to the method of Roser and Ford (*19*). Grafts were inspected daily after the seventh day and scored as rejected on the first day of complete epithelial necrosis.

OLT serum and IgG. The rat serum used in this study was a pool obtained from PVG recipients of DA liver grafts sacrificed 2–4 months after OLT. The IgG fraction was isolated by gel filtration on Sephadex G-200 (Pharmacia, Sweden) followed by ammonium sulphate precipitation and DEAE ion exchange high-performance liquid chromatography (HPLC). Pooled serum (9 ml) was applied to a G-200 column of dimensions 2.4 cm ID × 90 cm; peak IgG-containing fractions were pooled, precipitated with ammonium sulphate (40% satn.) and dialyzed against 50 mM Na-phosphate buffer, pH 7.6. IgG was further purified by HPLC (Tri Rotar-4 system, Japan spectroscopic Co. Ltd., Tokyo) using a prepacked column (7.5 mm ID × 75 mm) of a DEAE ion exchange resin (DEAE-5PW, Toyo Soda Manufacturing Co. Ltd., Tokyo) in 50 mM Na-phosphate, pH 7.6. The nonabsorbed protein peak (IgG) was collected and concentrated by ultrafiltration. IgG concentrations were estimated by enzyme linked immunosorbent assay (*20*).

Radioimmunoassays for rat alloantibodies. Antibodies against class I and class II donor ($RT1^a$) antigens in IgG purified from sera of $PVG.RT1^a$-grafted PVG rats were detected by a two-stage binding assay using respectively DA ($RT1^a$) red cells or lymph node cells and radiolabeled sheep anti-rat immunoglobulin, as follows.

Anti-class-I antibodies were assayed by red cell binding. Flexible 96-well microtiter plates (Dynatech Labs, Cat. No. 1–220–24) were treated with 10% fetal calf serum (FCS) for 10 min (a precaution against nonspecific binding of rat Ig), washed with distilled water, and dried. Serial dilutions of rat sera under test were prepared in PBS/2% FCS and dispensed into the microtiter wells (50 μl per well); 50 μl of 2% red cells was added to each well and incubated for 1 hr at room temperature. The red cells were then washed 4 times in the wells by repeated centrifugation and resuspension in PBS/FCS. Radioiodinated, affinity-purified sheep antibodies against rat Ig (100 μl) (Amersham International, Amersham, England, Cat. No. IM. 132) was then dispensed into each well (40,000 cpm per well) and incubated for a further 1 hr. The red cells were then again washed four times in the wells and finally transferred to clean wells and spun down. Individual wells containing red cells were cut out and radioactivity bound to each red cell pellet counted in a gamma counter.

Anti-class-II antibodies were assayed by lymph node cell binding. Rat sera were first exhaustively absorbed with red cells of the graft donor RT1 type to remove anti-class-I activity (four successive absorptions of 500 μl of serum with 50 μl packed DA red cells for 1 hr each time) and absorption was confirmed by retitration of the serum against DA red cells. The assay for anti-class-II antibody followed the same protocol as the red cell binding assay above, but replacing red cells by 50 μl per well of lymph node cell suspension 10^7 cells/ml. All incubations were carried out in the cold.

The rat monoclonal anti-$RT1A^a$ antibody R3/13 (*19*) was used as a positive control and reference standard for both the above assays; R3/13 supernatant was the generous gift of Dr. C. Milstein (Laboratory of Molecular Biology, Cambridge). The radioimmunoassays using red cells or lymph node cells were of similar sensitivity in detecting R3/13.

Absorption of OLT IgG by red cells. IgG purified from OLT serum was absorbed, as indicated in the *Results* section, with $PVG.RT1^a$ red cells to remove anti-class-I $RT1^a$ antibodies. IgG at 12 mg/ml was absorbed 4 times with packed, ficoll-separated $PVG.RT1^a$ red cells (100 μl/ml IgG) for 1 hr at room temperature, followed by removal of the red cells by centrifugation. Complete absorption of anti-class-I antibody was confirmed by radioimmunoassay.

RESULTS

Survival of $PVG.RT1^a$ allografts in normal PVG recipients. The behavior of $PVG.RT1^a$ liver, heart, and skin grafts in PVG recipients is identical to that of DA grafts, with which they share RT1 haplotype. As shown in Table 1, liver grafts in this combination are not rejected, whereas heterotopic heart grafts and skin grafts are rejected acutely.

Enhancement of semiallogeneic $(DA \times PVG)F_1$ heart grafts in PVG recipients by OLT serum. We have previously reported the increased survival of semiallogeneic heterotopic heart grafts in this combination when the recipients were inoculated with serum from DA-liver grafted PVG rats (*1, 11*); this observation was repeated using the new pool of OLT serum from the same combination prepared for the present experiments. The result, shown in Table 2, was that inoculation of 0.5 ml of OLT serum immediately after heart grafting led to permanent acceptance of the graft in 5/7 recipients; survival time in the remaining two recipients was not significantly different from that in the untreated controls.

Enhancement of fully allogeneic $PVG.RT1^a$ heart grafts in PVG recipients by OLT serum. Having established the effectiveness of the OLT serum pool in enhancement in a semiallogeneic combination, we turned to the fully allogeneic combination of $PVG.RT1^a$ hearts grafted into PVG. Different amounts of OLT serum were inoculated intravenously into the recipients, either as single injections immediately after grafting or as two injections, the first immediately after grafting and the second two days later. The effect on heart graft survival was dose-dependent, as shown in Figure 1. Permanent survival in a total of 11/11 animals was produced by inoculation of 1 ml of OLT serum, either as a single dose (group b) or divided into two doses (group c). A single inoculation of 0.5 ml caused permanent acceptance of the heart graft in 10/14 recipients (group d); the mean survival time in the remaining 4 was 21± 7.1 days. When the serum inoculation was reduced to 0.25 ml, no heart grafts were accepted permanently, but all showed significantly increased survival times (group e; MST 16.3±1.8 days compared with control of 8.4±0.5 days). The specific nature of the enhancement was shown by third-party (WAG) heart grafts, the survival of which on PVG recipients was not improved by inoculation of 1 ml OLT serum (group f). No

TABLE 1. Survival times of grafts of $PVG.RT1^a$ heart, skin, and liver in individual normal PVG recipients

Organ	Survival time (days [MST±SD])[a]
Heart	8, 8, 8, 8, 9, 9, 9 (8.4±0.5)
Skin	8, 8, 8, 9, 9, 9 (8.5±0.5)
Liver	>100 (6 grafts)

[a] Mean survival time ± SD.

TABLE 2. Enhancement of $(DA \times PVG)F_1$ heart grafts in PVG recipients by OLT serum

Treatment of recipient	Survival time in individual rats (days)
None	8, 9, 9, 10, 10, 12, 14, 15
0.5 ml OLT serum[a]	14, 16, >100 (5 grafts)

[a] Administered immediately after heterotopic heart graft.

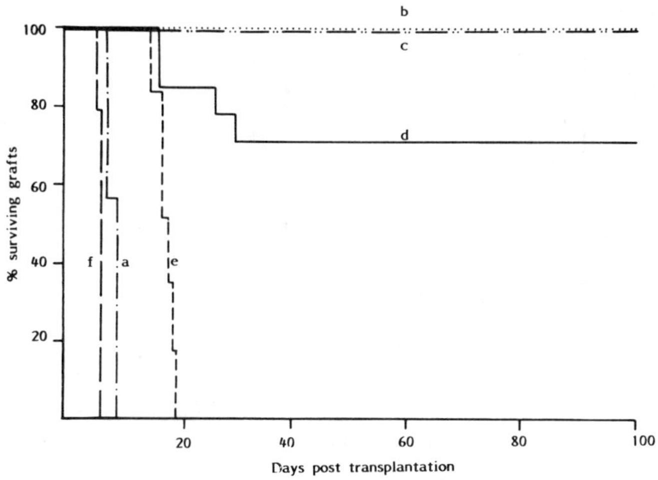

FIGURE 1. Enhancement of survival of PVG.RT1[a] heterotopic heart grafts on PVG recipients by OLT serum. Survival of PVG.RT1[a] heart grafts (a) on untreated PVG recipients; (b) on PVG rats given 1 ml OLT serum immediately after grafting; (c) on PVG rats given 0.5 ml OLT serum immediately after grafting and 0.5 ml two days later; (d) on PVG rats given 0.5 ml OLT serum immediately after grafting; and (e) on PVG rats given 0.25 ml OLT serum immediately after grafting. (f) Survival of WAG (3rd-party) heterotopic heart grafts on PVG rats given 1 ml OLT serum immediately after grafting. The same pool of OLT serum, from PVG rats carrying DA liver transplants was used throughout.

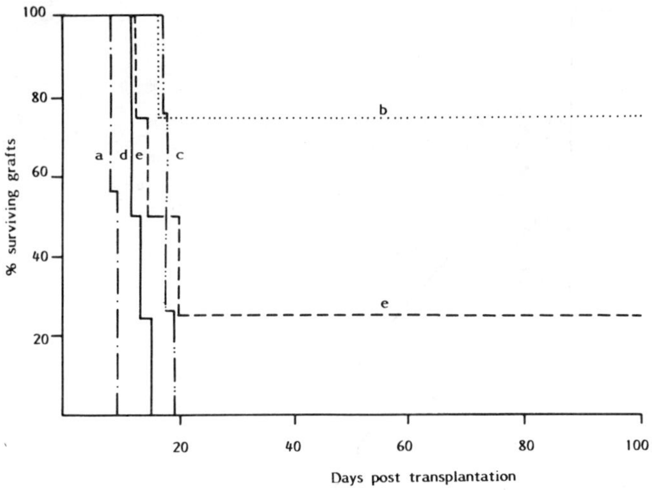

FIGURE 2. Enhancement of PVG.RT1[a] heterotopic heart grafts on PVG recipients by the IgG fraction of OLT serum (OLT IgG). Survival of PVG.RT1[a] heart grafts (a) on untreated PVG recipients; (b) on PVG rats given 12 mg OLT IgG immediately after grafting; (c) on PVG rats given 6 mg OLT IgG immediately after grafting; (d) on PVG rats given 6 mg OLT IgG absorbed with PVG.RT1[a] red cells; and (e) on PVG rats given 12 mg OLT IgG absorbed with PVG.RT1[a] red cells.

enhancing effect was shown by inoculation of 1 ml normal DA serum or 1 ml of serum taken from PVG rats 4 weeks after DA skin grafting (data not shown).

Enhancement of PVG.RT1[a] heart grafts in PVG recipients by purified IgG from OLT serum and anti-class-II alloantibody. The IgG fraction purified from the OLT serum pool by gel filtration and ion exchange chromatography showed the same enhancing properties as whole serum, with the same quantitative effectiveness (Fig. 2). Thus, inoculation of 12 mg IgG per recipient, the equivalent of 0.5 ml serum, led to permanent take of fully allogeneic heart grafts in 3/4 recipients (group b), while 6 mg/rat led to a more modest improvement in survival time (group c, MST 16±0.7 days). Enhancement was also achieved using IG from which antibodies to class I RT1[a] alloantigens had been removed by absorption with PVG.RT1[a] red cells, though there appeared to be some reduction in effectiveness compared with the unabsorbed IgG (groups d and e). In view of the small numbers of rats used (4 per group) the significance of this reduction is uncertain. The result supports the view that the class II antibodies present in OLT serum in high titer (*1, 9*) are the principal agents of enhancement (*15*).

Evidence for systemic tolerance following enhancement by OLT serum or IgG. The responsiveness of PVG rats with permanently surviving PVG.RT1[a] heterotopic heart grafts after enhancement by OLT serum or IgG was tested by grafts of PVG.RT1[a] and WAG skin. PVG.RT1[a] skin grafts were accepted indefinitely by all the enhanced rats (Fig. 3, groups b and c), compared with the normal rejection time of 8.5 days (Table 1), while third-party skin grafts on the same rats were rejected acutely (Fig. 3). This observation demonstrates that enhancement by OLT serum or its purified IgG fraction leads to an apparent state of specific, systemic transplantation tolerance.

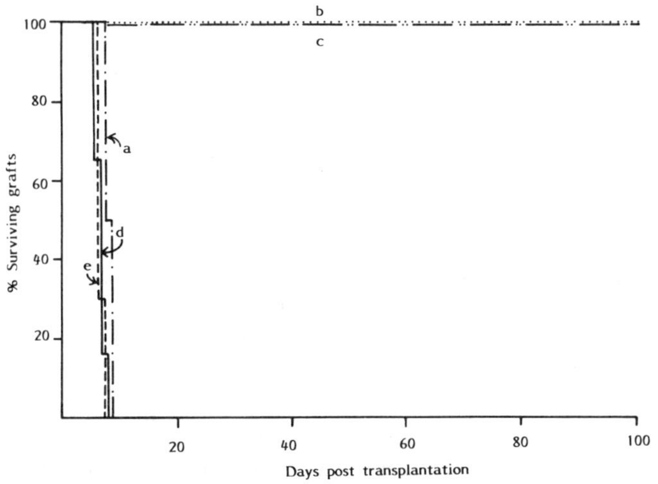

FIGURE 3. Survival of skin grafts on PVG rats carrying long-term-surviving PVG.RT1[a] heterotopic heart grafts. Survival of PVG.RT1[a] skin grafts (a) on untreated PVG recipients; (b) on PVG rats carrying PVG.RT1[a] heterotopic heart grafts for 80 days, the survival of the heart grafts having been enhanced by 1 ml OLT serum; (c) on PVG rats carrying PVG.RT1[a] heterotopic heart grafts for 80 days, the survival of the heart grafts having been enhanced by 12 mg OLT IgG. Survival of WAG skin grafts (d) on normal PVG rats and (e) on PVG rats carrying PVG.RT1[a] heterotopic heart grafts for 80 days, the survival of the heart grafts having been enhanced by 1 ml OLT serum.

Alloantibody responses in PVG rats following enhancement of PVG.RT1[a] heart grafts. Antibody levels against class I and class II RT1[a] antigens were assayed in normal and enhanced PVG recipients of PVG.RT1[a] heart grafts. All sera were taken 80 days after grafting. In the normal recipients, where the heart grafts were rejected within 9 days, good alloantibody responses to class I and class II antigens were still detectable at 80 days, the titers for both being in the range of 1:100–1:1000 serum dilution (Figs. 4a, 5a). In rats in which heart graft survival was enhanced by OLT serum or OLT IgG, the class I response was

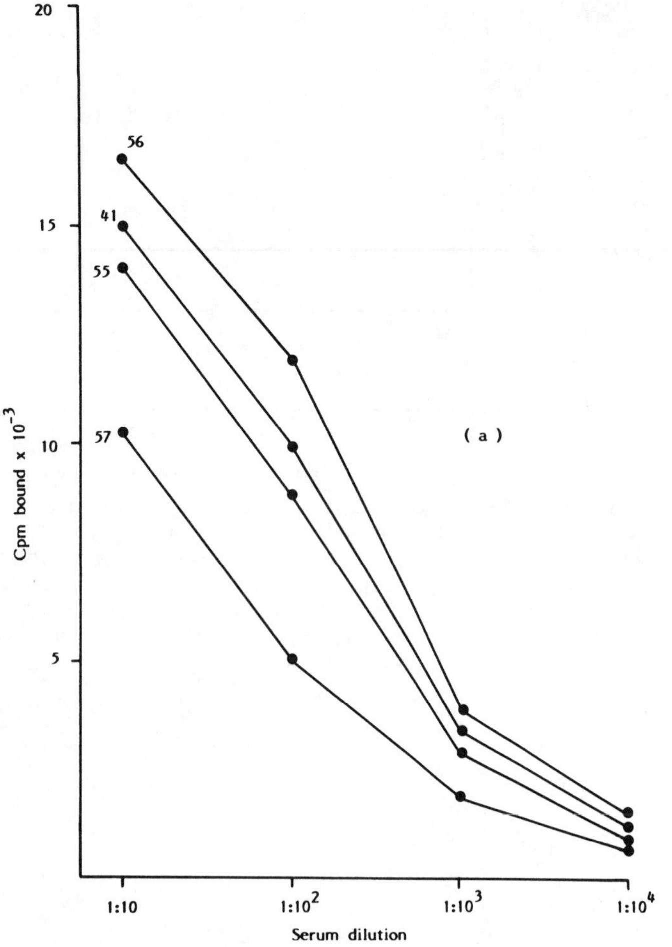

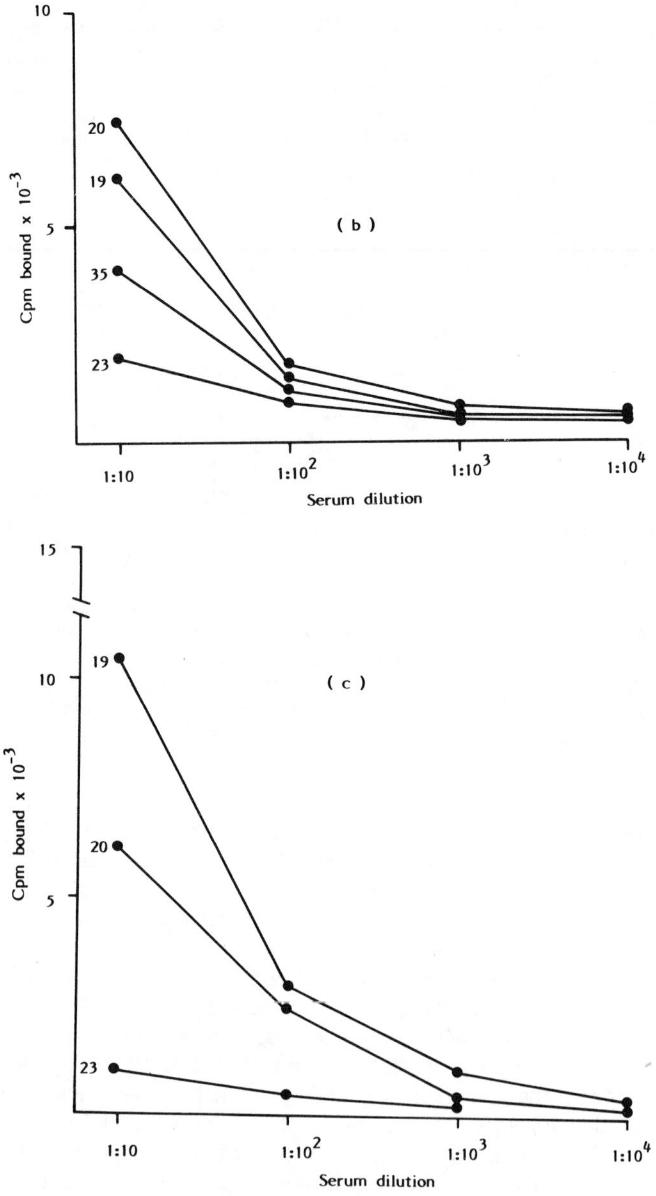

FIGURE 4. Antibody response against class I $RT1^a$ antigens in PVG recipients of PVG.$RT1^a$ heart grafts, as detected by radioimmunoassay. (a) Titration of sera from 4 untreated PVG recipients of PVG.$RT1^a$ heterotopic heart grafts. The grafts were all rejected within 9 days. Sera were taken 80 days postgrafting and assayed for antibodies binding to DA ($RT1^a$) red cells, with detection by ^{125}I-labeled sheep antirat Ig. The number beside each profile identifies an individual rat. (b) Titration of sera from 4 PVG recipients of PVG.$RT1^a$ heterotopic heart grafts, the survival of which was enhanced by 1 ml OLT serum. These grafts survived indefinitely; sera were taken 80 days postgrafting and assayed as above. (c) Titration of sera from 3 PVG recipients of PVG.$RT1^a$ heart grafts enhanced by 1 ml OLT serum, following a PVG.$RT1^a$ skin graft. Skin grafting was performed 80 days after heart grafting; neither the heart grafts nor the skin grafts were rejected. Sera were taken 30 days after skin grafting and titrated as above.

markedly reduced, being barely detectable in some cases, and with a maximum end-point of about 1:10 in others (Fig. 4b); in contrast, the anti-class-II response was seemingly unaffected and was maintained at a high level after enhancement (Fig. 5b). Antibody levels were also examined 30 days after skin grafting in the enhanced group. In 1/3 rats there was evidence for a slightly increased anti-class-I response after skin grafting, while in the other two, there was no discernible rise (Fig. 4c). On the other hand, the anti-class-II antibody levels in the same rats were significantly boosted by skin grafting (Fig. 5c). It thus appears that the tolerant state of these animals is also reflected in their anti-class-I alloantibody responses, but not in their anti-class-II responses.

DISCUSSION

Here we have demonstrated that passive transfer of serum from PVG recipients of DA liver grafts, or its purified IgG fraction, can enhance survival of fully allogeneic PVG.$RT1^a$ heart grafts in PVG recipients. At the highest doses of serum used (1 ml per recipient), heart grafts took permanently in all animals. The degree of enhancement was related to the dose of serum administered. The minimum required for permanent graft acceptance was 0.5 ml per rat; 0.25 ml caused significant prolongation of heart graft survival, but the grafts were all rejected within 19 days. The effectiveness of the purified IgG after absorption with PVG.$RT1^a$ red cells indicated that the enhancing agent is probably IgG antibody against class II $RT1^a$ antigens. The anti-class-II antibody content of the serum was estimated as about 400 μg/ml; thus, to secure permanent acceptance of a heart graft in this combination requires about 200 μg of antibody per rat (mean weight 250 g), while 100 μg produces a significant prolongation. This indicates that a circulating level of only 20–40 μg anti-class-II antibody/ml will

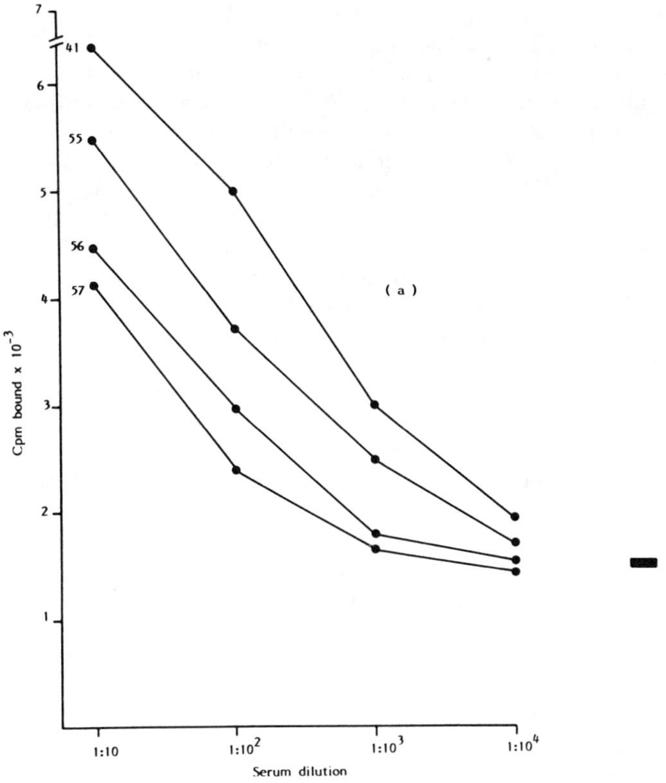

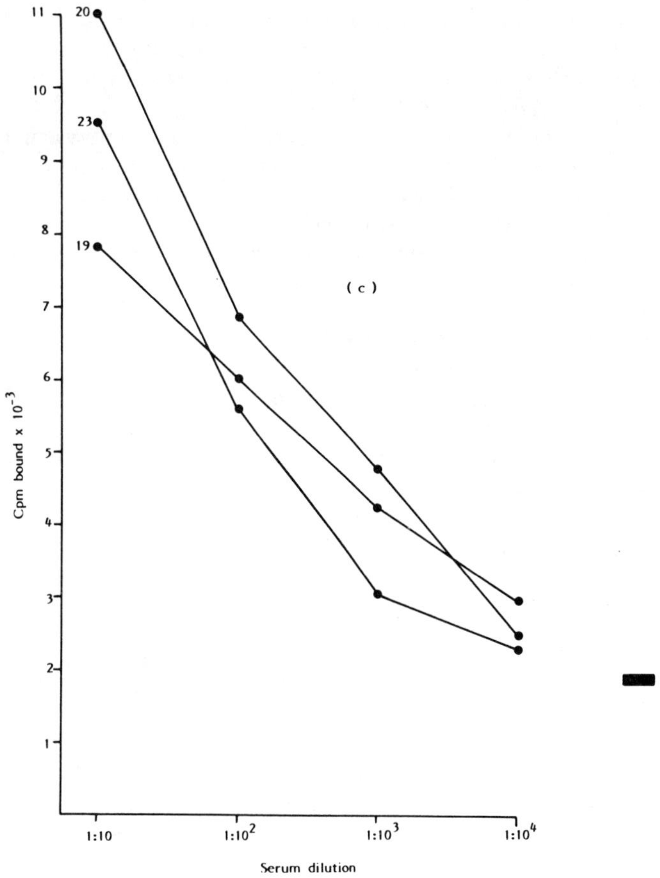

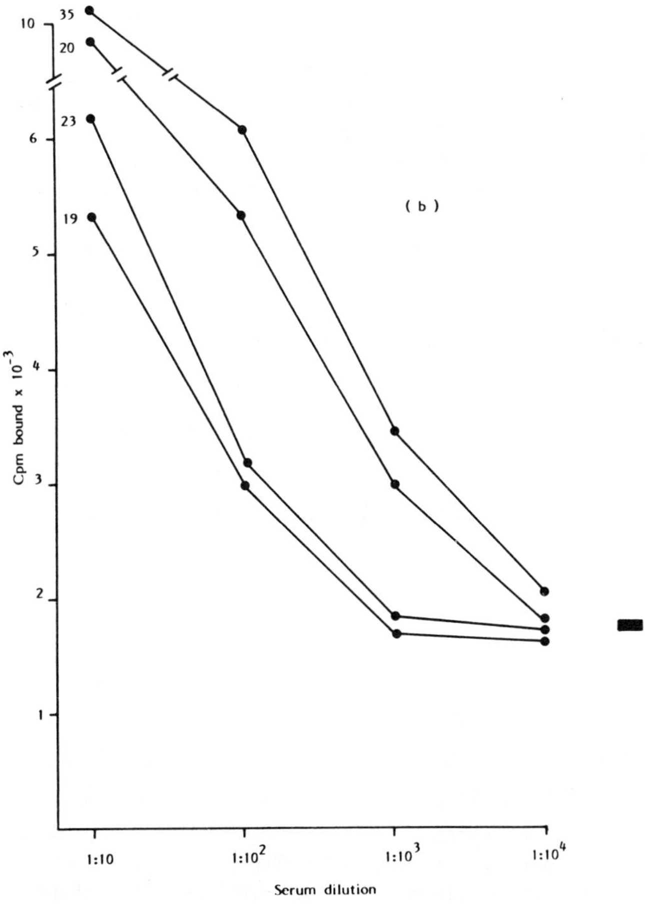

FIGURE 5. Antibody response against class II RT1^a antigens in PVG recipients of PVG.RT1^a heart grafts, as detected by radioimmunoassay. Sera in (a), (b), and (c) were the same as those in Fig. 4 (a), (b), and (c) respectively. Assays were performed against DA lymph node cells, the sera having first been absorbed with DA red cells to remove anti-class-I activity. Detection was by ^{125}I-labeled sheep anti-rat Ig. The bar represents the background of the assay, which is higher with lymph node cells than red cells due to binding of the radiolabeled anti-Ig reagent to rat B cells.

cause permanent acceptance of a PVG.RT1[a] heart graft in a PVG rat. The effectiveness of anti-class-II antibodies in enhancement of cardiac, as well as other, allografts in the rat is well recognized (*14, 15, 21*).

The unresponsiveness associated with enhancement was not confined to the grafted heart. Thus, PVG rats with long-term surviving PVG.RT1[a] heart grafts were systemically tolerant of RT1[a] antigens, as demonstrated by their permanent acceptance of RT1[a] skin grafts, while rejecting skin from third-party donors. Transplantation tolerance has been demonstrated in several rat combinations following enhancement (*15, 22*) and is regarded as part of the "maintenance" phase of enhancement (*15, 23*). It is, however, not invariably found; for example, in experiments similar in design to our own, Tilney and Bell observed that AS rats with enhanced, long-term heterotopic (AUG×AS)F_1 heart allografts failed to accept skin grafts of the heart donor type (*24*).

The serological picture following enhancement by OLT serum is of particular interest. After heterotopic PVG.RT1[a] heart grafting in normal PVG rats, there are good and roughly equal serum antibody responses against class I and class II RT1[a] antigens; although the grafts are rejected within 9 days, antibody levels are still high 80 days posttransplantation. Where a heart graft has taken permanently as a result of enhancement, the anti-class-I levels at 80 days are less than 10% those of nonenhanced controls, but anti-class-II levels are undiminished (Figs. 4 and 5). This latter point deserves special emphasis and is relevant to the possible mechanisms involved in enhancement induction (below). Moreover, there was very poor restimulation of anti-class-I antibody after PVG.RT1[a] skin grafting on PVG rats carrying enhanced heart grafts, while anti-class-II antibodies were clearly boosted. This apparent state of partial tolerance to RT1[a] antigens after enhancement by OLT serum resembles that following liver grafting itself in the same combination (*1*). It is well known that enhancement leads to suppression of the primary cytotoxic antibody response (*15, 22, 23*), though some of the assays used may limit detection to anti-class-I antibodies. Interestingly, in the paper already cited, Tilney and Bell succeeded in transferring enhancement with serum from rats carrying long-term heterotopic heart grafts, indicating a significant level of anti-class-II antibody (*24*). However, it is rather unusual to be able to transfer enhancement by serum from animals with long-surviving, enhanced grafts, suggesting that the recipient anti-class-II response is also often suppressed.

Our results accord with the view that recognition of class II (Ia) antigens is often required for induction of an anti-class-I response (*23, 25*). As a confirmation of this requirement in rejection of heart grafts, we have found that PVG.R1 heart allografts survive indefinitely in untreated PVG recipients (N.K., unpublished data), R1 having the recombinant r1 haplotype (RT1A[a]/B[c]D[c]), which presents only the class I RT1A[a] difference from PVG (RT1[c]). An obvious possible effect of passively transferred anti-class-II antibodies would be to mask class II antigens in the graft and prevent their recognition by helper T cells; alternatively, it has been proposed that the antibodies lead to removal of Ia-bearing interstitial dendritic cells (*26*), a major immunogenic source of class II antigen in organ grafts, or to opsonization of the Ia-reactive lymphocytes themselves after binding of Ia-antibody complexes (*27*). However, these last two hypotheses are difficult to accept here in view of the strength of the anti-class-II response in the enhanced recipients. The masking hypothesis, though often dismissed as unlikely due to the small amounts of antibody required for enhancement (*15, 26*), would seem to accord best with our observations, since eventual disappearance of the enhancing antibody by shedding or metabolism would allow the anti-class-II response to occur. During the period when class II antigens are not available on the heart graft, tolerance of RT1[a] antigens is evidently induced, and this may be related to the fact that PVG is a genetic low responder to RT1A[a] (*28*). The cellular basis of the state of partial (class-I-specific) tolerance remains to be investigated. While it is conceivable that it is entirely brought about by the high level of anti-class-II antibody—i.e., "autoenhancement," the long-term survival of fully allogeneic skin grafts on the enhanced recipients is more compatible with cellular unresponsiveness against class I antigens, since survival of skin grafts is generally difficult to prolong to this extent by antibody alone.

The close resemblance between the serological findings following enhancement and liver grafting raises the question of how far unresponsiveness associated with liver transplantation is antibody-dependent. When a DA liver is transplanted into a PVG rat, the anti-class-I response is minimal and short-lived and cannot be restimulated by skin grafting, while the anti-class-II response is strongly maintained over many weeks (*1, 9*). Two arguments could be brought against a crucial role for anti-class-II antibody in liver-induced tolerance. The first involves the time coruse of events: systemic transplantation tolerance is induced while the antibody response is still in its early stages (*1, 3*) and heart and kidney grafts are protected from rejection from the first day of liver transplantation (*7, 8*). Second, liver-induced tolerance of skin grafts correlates closely with clonal deletion of alloreactive recirculating T cells, as studied by adoptive transfer assay (*10–12*). However, the present finding that relatively small amounts of OLT serum can lead to enhancement must lend support to a role for anti-class-II antibody in the maintenance of unresponsiveness after liver grafting, and possibly in the processes involved in its induction as well. It will be of particular interest to know whether clonal deletion of alloreactive T cells can be demonstrated in recipients of OLT serum after allografting, as this would make the parallel between liver graft induced tolerance and enhancement in this combination virtually complete.

Acknowledgments. We are grateful to Professor Roy Calne (Cambridge) and Drs. K. Wakabayashi and T. Uchiyamada (Tokyo) for their encouragement of our work on experimental liver grafting and to Mrs. M. Thorburn and Miss N. Townley for preparation of figures.

REFERENCES

1. Kamada N. The immunology of experimental liver transplantation in the rat. Immunology 1985; 55: 369.
2. Kamada N, Brons G, Davies HffS. Fully allogeneic liver grafting in rats induces a state of systemic nonreactivity to donor transplantation antigens. Transplantation 1980; 29: 429.
3. Kamada N, Davies HffS, Wight D, Culank L, Roser B. Liver transplantation in the rat: biochemical and histological evidence of complete tolerance induction in nonrejector strains. Transplantation 1983; 35: 304.
4. Kamada N, Davies HffS, Roser BJ. Reversal of transplantation immunity by liver grafting. Nature 1981; 292: 840.
5. Zimmerman FA, Knoll PP, Davies HffS, Gokel JM, Schmid T.

The fate of orthotopic liver allografts in different rat strain combinations. Transplant Proc 1983; 25: 1272.
6. Kamada N, Davies HffS, Roser BJ. Fuly allogeneic liver grafting and the induction of donor-specific unreactivity. Transplant Proc 1981; 13: 837.
7. Kamada N, Wight DGD. Antigen-specific immunosuppression induced by liver transplantation in the rat. Transplantation 1984; 38: 217.
8. Kamada N. A description of cuff techniques for renal transplantation in the rat. Use in studies of tolerance induction during combined liver grafting. Transplantation 1985; 39: 93.
9. Zimmermann FA, Butcher GW, Davies HffS, Brons G, Kamada N, Turel O. Techniques for orthotopic liver transplantation in the rat and some studies of the immunologic responses to fully allogeneic liver grafts. Transplant Proc 1979; 11: 571.
10. Davies HffS, Kamada N, Roser BJ. Mechanisms of donor-specific unresponsiveness induced by liver grafting. Transplant Proc 1983; 15: 831.
11. Roser BJ, Kamada N, Zimmermann F, Davies HffS. Immunosuppressive effects of experimental liver allografts. In: Calne RY, ed. Liver transplantation: the Cambridge-King's College Hospital experience. New York: Grune & Stratton, 1983: 35.
12. Kamada N, Shinomiya T. Clonal deletion as the mechanism of abrogation of immunological memory following liver grafting in rats. Immunology 1985; 55: 85.
13. Stuart FP, Weiss A, Fitch FW. Induction and maintenance of immunological enhancement. In: Stuart FP, Fitch FW, eds. Immunological tolerance and enhancement. MPT Press, 1979: p 29.
14. Morris PJ. Suppression of rejection of organ allografts by alloantibody. Immunol Rev 1980; 49: 93.
15. Davies DAL. Enhancement. In: Calne RY, ed. Transplantation immunology, clinical and experimental. New York: Oxford University Press, 1984: 208.
16. Kamada N. Transfer of specific immunosuppression of graft rejection using lymph from tolerant, liver-grafted rats. Immunology 1985; 55: 241.
17. Kamada N, Calne RY. A surgical experience with 530 liver transplants in the rat. Surgery 1983; 93: 64.
18. Heron I. A technique for accesory cervical heart transplantation in rabbits and rats. Acta Pathol Microbiol Scand 1971; 79: 366.
19. Roser BJ, Ford WL. Prolonged lymphocytopenia in the rat. Aust J Exp Biol Med Sci 1972; 50: 185.
20. Engvall E, Perlmann P. Enzyme linked immunosorbent assay (ELISA) quantitative assay of immunoglobulin G. Immunochemistry 19 ; 8: 871.
21. Davies DAL, Alkins BJ. What abrogates heart transplant rejection in immunological enhancement? Nature 1974; 247: 294.
22. Batchelor JR, Welsh KI, Burgos H. Immunological enhancement. Transplant Proc 1977; 9: 931.
23. Batchelor JR. Immune mechanisms responsible for the prolonged kidney allograft survival in immunlogical enhancement. Transplant Proc 1981; 13: 562.
24. Tilney NL, Bell PRF. Studies on enhancement of cardiac and renal allografts in the rat. Transplantation 1974; 18: 31.
25. Bach FH, Roopenian DC, Wee SL, Biel LW, Isakov N, Widmer MB. T-cell responses to MHC and non-MHC antigens: reexamining the LD-SD concept. Prog Immunol 1983; 5: 1449.
26. Hart DNJ, Fabre JW. Mechanisms of induction of passive enhancement. Evidence for an interaction of enhancing antibody with donor interstitial dendritic cells. Transplantation 1982; 33: 319.
27. Hutchinson IV. Antigen-reactive cell opsonisation (ARCO) and its role in antibody-mediated immune suppression. Immunol Rev 1980; 49: 167.
28. Butcher GW, Corvalan JR, Licence DR, Howard JC. Immune response genes controlling responsiveness to major transplantation antigens. Specific major histocompatibility complex-linked defect for antibody responses to class I alloantigens. J Exp Med 1982; 155: 303.
29. Howard JC, Butcher GW. The mechanism of graft rejection and the concept of antigenic strength. Scand J Immunol 1981; 14: 687.

Received 4 September 1985.
Accepted 1 February 1986.

0041-1337/86/4206-0588$02.00/0
TRANSPLANTATION
Vol. 42, No. 6

Printed in U.S.A.

CRYOPRESERVATION OF MOUSE PANCREATIC ISLETS

EFFECTS OF FAST COOLING ON ISLET B CELL FUNCTION AND ON THE OUTCOME OF ISLET TRANSPLANTATION[1]

STELLAN SANDLER,[2] YASUHIKO KOJIMA,[3] AND ARNE ANDERSSON

Dept of Medical Cell Biology, Uppsala University, Biomedicum, S-751 23 Uppsala, Sweden

In most previous studies of cryopreserved isolated pancreatic islets, a slow cooling rate has been employed. We recently observed that faster cooling (5°C/min) resulted in better functional islet preservation than cooling at 0.5°C/min. We found that a culture period after the collagenase isolation of the islets, but prior to freezing, is crucial for the preservation of the islet B cell function. In the present investigation the function of isolated mouse pancreatic islets cooled in Hanks' solution supplemented with 2 M dimethylsulphoxide was compared with that of nonfrozen, cultured islets prepared from the same donors. The islets were cultured in RPMI 1640 + 10% calf serum for 3 days before freezing, and for 3 days after rapid thawing at 37°C. Islets were cooled at rates of 5, 15, or 25°C/min to 70°C and then plunged into liquid nitrogen. All three groups of cryopreserved islets responded with insulin secretion when challenged with high glucose concentrations in batch-type incubations. In further experiments it was found that glucose-stimulated (pro)insulin biosynthesis in islets frozen at 25°C/min was the same as that in the controls. Similar observations were made with respect to glucose-stimulated insulin release in perifusion experiments. However, a 30% reduction in insulin content was observed in the rapidly frozen islets. There was no difference in the replicatory capacity of the islets cells in vitro, as determined by an autoradiographic technique, between control islets and islets cooled at 5°C or 25°C/min. Intrasplenic implantation of 600–800 cryopreserved syngeneic islets into alloxan-diabetic mice led to complete or partial normalization of the hyperglycemia in seven of nine mice. When splenectomy was performed in five animals the serum glucose concentrations increased promptly. We conclude that relatively rapid cooling rates may be useful for cryopreservation of isolated pancreatic islets.

In most previous attempts to cryopreserve isolated pancreatic islets, a relatively slow cooling rate (<1°C/min) has been employed (*1–12*). It has been assumed that freezing such a microorgan as the pancreatic islets requires a slow cooling rate to avoid intracellular ice crystal formation and subsequent freeze damage of the B cells. However, some authors have demonstrated that the B cell function is preserved even when much faster cooling rates are used (*13, 14*). In line with this observation we found in a previous study that isolated mouse islets frozen at a rate of 5°C/min functioned better than those frozen at only 0.5°C/min (*15*). Moreover, successful cryopreservation of collagenase-isolated islets seems to benefit from a culture period before freezing both if the islets are cooled slowly (*6*) and if they are cooled at a more rapid rate (*16*).

In the present study the structure and function of mouse pancreatic islets cooled at even more rapid rates, which from a clinical and practical point of view might be preferable, have been investigated. The islet function in vitro was examined by assaying insulin release during either batch-type incubations or perifusion, (pro)insulin biosynthesis, and the insulin content. In addition, islet cell replicatory rates in vitro and in vivo following transplantation were determined by an autoradiographic technique. Finally, the ability of cryopreserved islets to normalize hyperglycemia was tested after islet transplantation into alloxan-diabetic syngeneic recipients.

MATERIALS AND METHODS

Animals. Pancreatic islets were isolated by a collagenase digestion technique (*17*) from adult male NMRI mice (Anticimex AB, Sollentuna, Sweden), starved overnight. For the transplantation experiments male inbred C57BL/6 mice originally obtained from the Jackson Laboratory, Bar Harbor, ME, aged 3–4 months, were used. The animals were allowed free access to tap water and laboratory chow (Ewos, Anticimex, Type R3, Södertälje, Sweden) throughout the experiments.

Islet culture and freeze-thawing procedure. After isolation and prior to freezing, islets were maintained for 3 days free-floating in culture medium RPMI 1640 (Flow Laboratories Ltd., Irvine, Scotland) supplemented with benzylpenicillin (100 U/ml) (Astra Läkemedel, Södertälje, Sweden), streptomycin (0.1 mg/ml) (Glaxo Laboratories Ltd., Greenford, Middlesex, England), and 10% calf serum (v/v) (Statens Bakteriologiska Laboratorium, Stockholm, Sweden). The cultures were kept at 37°C in humidified air + 5% CO_2. The culture medium was changed after 2 days.

After culture, freezing was performed, using a programmable temperature controller (Planer Minifreezer, Model R202/200R, Planer Products Ltd., Sunbury-on-Thames, England). Groups of about 150 islets were transferred at room temperature to sterilized glass ampoules containing 0.4 ml of Hanks' solution (Statens Bakteriologiska Laboratorium) supplemented with antibiotics as described above and 2 M dimethylsulphoxide

[1] This work was supported by grants from the Swedish Medical Research Council (12X-109; 17X-7501; K86-12P-7680-01), the Juvenile Diabetes Foundation International, the Swedish Diabetes Association, the Nordic Insulin Fund, the Swedish Society of Medicine, the Åke Wiberg Foundation, the Clas Groschinsky Memorial Foundation, and the O.E. and Edla Johansson Foundation.

[2] Address correspondence to: Dr. S. Sandler, Dept of Medical Cell Biology, Biomedicum, P.O. Box 571, S-751 23 Uppsala, Sweden.

[3] Present address: The First Department of Surgery, Fukui Medical School, 23-Shimoaizuki, Matsuoka-cho, Yoshida-gun, Fukui 910-11, Japan.

(Me_2SO)* (Sigma Chemicals, St Louis, MO) as a cryoprotective agent. Initially the islets were cooled at a rate of 8°C/min from room temperature to 0°C. The temperature was maintained for 20 min at 0°C to permit permeation of Me_2SO. Cooling was then continued at the selected rates down to −70°C, after which the ampoules were plunged into liquid nitrogen.

After storage at −196°C for 1 hr, the islets were thawed by stirring the glass ampoules in a water bath at 37°C. When the ice had just melted, the contents of the ampoules were poured into culture dishes containing 10 ml of culture medium, resulting in a dilution of Me_2SO down to less than 0.08 M. Finally 5 ml of culture medium was removed from the dishes and the frozen-thawed islets were cultured for another 3 days before further experiments. Groups of control islets were obtained from the same islet isolations as the frozen-thawed islets, but were maintained in culture for 6 days without any further treatment, except for exchange of medium every second day.

Islet insulin release. Duplicate groups of ten islets each were incubated for 3 consecutive hours at 37°C (O_2:CO_2; 95:5) during slow shaking in sealed glass vials (*18*) containing 0.25 ml of a bicarbonate-buffered medium (*19*) supplemented with bovine albumin (2 mg/ml; Miles Laboratories, Slough, England) and 10 mM HEPES (Sigma), hereafter referred to as KRBH. During the first and second hours the medium contained 1.67 mM glucose and during the third hour 16.7 mM glucose. The incubation medium was carefully removed after each 1-hr incubation and the insulin concentration of the medium was determined by radioimmunoassay (*20*), using mouse crystalline insulin as standard (Novo A/S, Copenhagen, Denmark) and ^{125}I-labeled insulin (Novo) as tracer. For measurements of the islet insulin content, groups of ten islets were sonicated in 0.50 ml of acid ethanol (15 ml of 12 M HCl in 70% ethanol); after extraction overnight at +4°C, the samples were stored at −20°C before insulin determination.

Islet perifusion. With minor alterations, the technique described by Lacy et al. (*21*) was used. Islets were perifused with KRBH supplemented with 0.5 mg/ml albumin and either 1.67 or 16.7 mM glucose. The flow rate of the perifusate was 1 ml/min and the insulin content of each effluent fraction was assayed as described above.

Islet (pro)insulin biosynthesis. Groups of ten islets in duplicate were placed in multiwell plates (well volume, 0.4 ml; Linbro Scientific, Hamden, CO) containing 0.1 ml of KRBH supplemented with 16.7 mM glucose and L-(4,5-^{3}H)leucine (sp.act. 50 μCi/ml; Amersham International, Amersham, England), and incubated for 120 min at 37°C (air + 5% CO_2). After incubation the islets were washed in Hanks' solution containing 10 mM nonlabeled leucine, and sonicated in 0.2 ml of redistilled water. The amounts of labeled islet (pro)insulin and other proteins in the homogenates were estimated by an immune-binding procedure (*22*).

Islet cell replication. During the last 18 hr of culture after thawing, and on the sixth day of culture in the case of the nonfrozen control islets, the culture medium was supplemented with 1 μCi/ml (^{3}H-methyl)thymidine (sp.act 5 Ci/mmol; Amersham International, Amersham, England). The islets were then rinsed and washed in Hanks' solution containing 10 mM nonradioactive thymidine and fixed in Bouin's solution, embedded in paraffin and cut into 7-μm sections. After removal of the paraffin, the sectioned islets were dipped in Kodak NTB-2 emulsion (Kodak AB, Sollentuna, Sweden) and exposed for 1 week at 4°C in tightly sealed boxes. The slides were then developed in Kodak D-19 at 20°C for 6 min, fixed in Kodak F-24 for 10 min, and finally stained with hematoxylin and mounted. To determine the islet cell labeling index, the number of radioactively labeled nuclei was counted at a magnification of ×1000 and expressed as a percentage of the total number of nuclei scored. A minimum of 1000 nuclei were counted in each islet preparation. The labeled islet nuclei were easily distinguishable by the large number of grains covering them. When the islet cell replication was estimated in transplanted islets, the recipient mice were injected with 30 μCi ^{3}H-thymidine 6 weeks after grafting. Then 60 min later the animals were killed and the areas beneath the renal capsule where the grafts were deposited were localized, removed, fixed, and processed for autoradiography essentially as described above, with the exception that the dipped sections were exposed for 5 weeks.

Islet transplantation. Male C57BL/6 mice rendered diabetic by alloxan (75 mg/kg body weight, i.v.) served as recipients. Donor islets were isolated from syngeneic female C57BL/6 mice, cryopreserved, and cultured for 3 days after thawing. About 600–800 islets were suspended in Hanks' solution and injected, using a microinfusion set, into the spleens of nine ether-anesthetized mice. Blood samples were taken by retroorbital sinus puncture before implantation, and on days 3, 7, 14, 21, and 28 after grafting. The glucose concentration in the blood samples was assayed by a glucose oxidase method, using an automated analyzer (Glucose Analyzer 2, Beckman Instruments, Fullerton, CA). In five animals splenectomy was performed on day 28 and the animals were killed on day 35, in order to investigate the effects of transplanted islets on the glucose homeostasis. The mice were killed by cervical dislocation after the last blood sample had been taken and the spleens were fixed in Bouin's solution and embedded in paraffin. Splenic sections (7-μm thick) were cut and stained with hematoxylin-eosin, and the morphology of the implanted islets was examined by light microscopy. To estimate the degree of islet cell replication in transplanted islets, groups of about 500 cryopreserved islets or nonfrozen cultured control islets were deposited under the renal capsule of ether-anesthetized alloxan-diabetic syngeneic mice, using a braking pipette. The animals were followed up for 6 weeks with serum glucose determinations and finally injected with ^{3}H-thymidine (see above).

Statistical analyses. Results are expressed as means ± SEM. Groups of data were compared with the paired and unpaired Student's *t* test.

RESULTS

Effects of different fast cooling rates on insulin release from cryopreserved islets. Islets were cultured for 3 days and then cooled at rates of 5, 15, or 25°C/min. After thawing and a further 3 days of culture it was found that all three groups of cryopreserved islets responded to a high glucose concentration with an increase in insulin secretion comparable to that of nonfrozen and cultured control islets (Table 1). The basal insulin release from islets cryopreserved at a cooling rate of

*Abbreviations used: HEPES, N-2-hydroxyethylpiperazine-N′-2-ethanesulphonic acid; KRBH, Krebs-Ringer bicarbonate buffer supplemented with 10 mM HEPES and 2 mg/ml albumin; Me_2SO, dimethylsulphoxide.

TABLE 1. Effects of various cooling rates on glucose-stimulated insulin release[a]

Cooling rate (°C/min)	5	15	25	Cultured controls
Insulin release (ng insulin/1 hr/10 islets):				
First hour (1.67 mM glucose)	6.8±2.2[b]	1.7±0.3	3.1±1.4	1.2±0.2
Second hour (1.67 mM glucose)	6.3±2.5[b]	3.7±1.0	2.7±0.7	0.8±0.2
Third hour (16.7 mM glucose)	29.6±5.2	42.3±7.0	46.2±8.5	33.4±5.1
Number of observations	10	10	10	8

[a] Islets were cultured in medium RPMI 1640 + 10% calf serum for 3 days before and after cryopreservation. Insulin released to the incubation medium was measured by radioimmunoassay. Values are given as means ± SEM.
[b] $P<0.05$ compared with cultured controls.

5°C/min was increased in comparison with that of nonfrozen cultured islets. Islets cooled at 25°C/min were employed in further in vitro experiments, since such islets had a glucose-induced insulin release at least as high as those cooled at 15°C/min.

Pro(insulin) biosynthesis and dynamics of insulin release by islets cooled at 25°C/min. Data on islet (pro)insulin biosynthesis and on perifusion of islets cooled at 5°C/min have been published recently (*15*). The rate of glucose-stimulated (pro)insulin biosynthesis in cryopreserved islets was similar to that in nonfrozen islets (Table 2). Furthermore, the percentage of contribution of newly synthesized (pro)insulin to the total pool of newly synthesized proteins in cryopreserved islets was comparable to that in cultured control islets.

The insulin content of cryopreserved islets was decreased, however, by about 30% (Table 2). Cryopreserved islets responded promptly with markedly increased insulin release when challenged with a high glucose concentration during perifusion (Fig. 1). The insulin response was of the same order of magnitude as that of nonfrozen islets and was sustained during the high-glucose stimulation. When the glucose concentration of the perifusate was lowered, the insulin release from both groups of islets returned to the basal level.

Effects of rapid cooling rates of islets on the rates of DNA replication of cryopreserved islets in vivo and in vitro. The labeling index of islets cooled at 5°C/min and subsequently transplanted was twice as high as that of nonfrozen, transplanted islets (Table 3). The labeling index of islets cooled at 25°C/min was also higher than that of the controls, but this difference did not attain statistical significance. It should be noted that the serum glucose concentrations of the animals that received about 500 transplanted cryopreserved islets were elevated (28.6±1.4 mM (5°C/min); 29.8±2.0 mM (25°C/min)) at the time of ^{3}H-thymidine administration 6 weeks after transplantation, whereas the animals submitted to grafting with nonfrozen islets were essentially normoglycemic (11.0±1.8 mM). However, when the different groups of islets were incubated in vitro in the presence of ^{3}H-thymidine for 18 hr at the same glucose concentration—i.e., 11.1 mM—the labeling index of the islet cells was about 1.2% in all groups (Table 3).

Transplantation of islets frozen at 25°C/min. Intrasplenic transplantation of about 600–800 syngeneic islets frozen at 25°C/min was attempted in nine alloxan-diabetic C57BL/6 mice. The mean serum glucose concentrations are shown in Fig. 2. When examining each recipient in more detail, it was found that all animals exhibited an initial improvement in the hyperglycemic state and three animals became normoglycemic within one week. In four mice an approximately 40% reduction of the serum glucose concentrations was noted during the first week, but gradually these animals became more hyperglycemic.

TABLE 2. (Pro)insulin biosynthesis and insulin content in cryopreserved mouse pancreatic islets cooled at 25°C/min and nonfrozen cultured control islets[a]

	Cryopreserved islets	Cultured control islets
(Pro)insulin biosynthesis (cpm × 10^{-3}/2 hr/20 islets)	12.6±1.8 (7)	15.3±1.2 (6)
Fraction (pro)insulin biosynthesis of total protein biosynthesis (%)	24.1±1.6 (7)	28.9±4.6 (6)
Islet insulin content (ng insulin/10 islets)	375±43 (8)[b]	523±61 (6)

[a] Islets were cultured for 3 days before and after cryopreservation. (Pro)insulin biosynthesis was estimated by measuring the incorporation of tritiated leucine at 16.7 mM glucose into (pro)insulin using an immune-binding technique and TCA-precipitable proteins (total protein biosynthesis). The insulin content was assessed by radioimmunoassay following extraction in acid ethanol. Numbers of experiments are given in parentheses. Values are given as means ± SEM.
[b] $P<0.05$ compared with cultured controls.

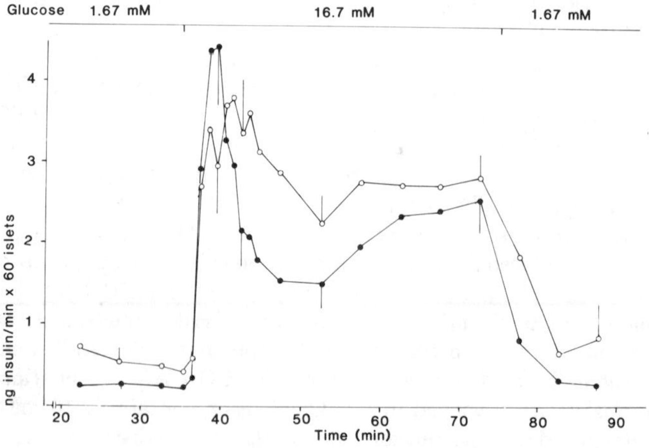

FIGURE 1. Insulin secretion by perifused islets cooled at a rate of 25°C/min (open circles) and by nonfrozen cultured islets (filled circles). Data are the means of seven and six experiments, respectively. SEM are given at some points on the curves.

Two mice showed a partial "cure," which was accompanied by moderately elevated serum glucose concentrations. When splenectomy was performed in five of the transplant recipients, the serum glucose concentrations increased markedly. Morphologically the fixed spleens displayed well-preserved pancreatic islets in the splenic parenchyma in all of the "cured" or partially "cured" animals (Fig. 3). In the "noncured" diabetic animals no or only few islets were found in the splenic sections. Some

TABLE 3. Effects of different cooling rates on the DNA replication of cryopreserved mouse islet cells in vivo and in vitro[a]

Cooling rate (°C/min)	5	25	Cultured controls
Labeling index (% of total number of nuclei scored):			
In vivo	1.00±0.15[b] (3)	0.82±0.30 (4)	0.42±0.07 (3)
In vitro	1.24±0.14 (7)	1.19±0.15 (8)	1.48±0.21 (8)

[a] Islets were cultured in medium RPMI 1640 + 10% calf serum for 3 days before and after cryopreservation. The islet cell replicatory rates in vitro were determined after addition of ^{3}H-thymidine, 1 μCi/ml, during the last 18 hr of culture. The replicatory activity in vivo was measured in islets transplanted beneath the renal capsule of alloxan-diabetic syngeneic mice. Six weeks after the islet transplantation the animals were injected with 30 μCi ^{3}H-thymidine i.p. and the animals were killed after 60 min. The graft-bearing section of the kidney was localized, fixed, and processed for autoradiography. Values are given as means ± SEM and numbers of observations are given within parentheses.

[b] $P<0.05$ as compared with cultured nonfrozen control islets.

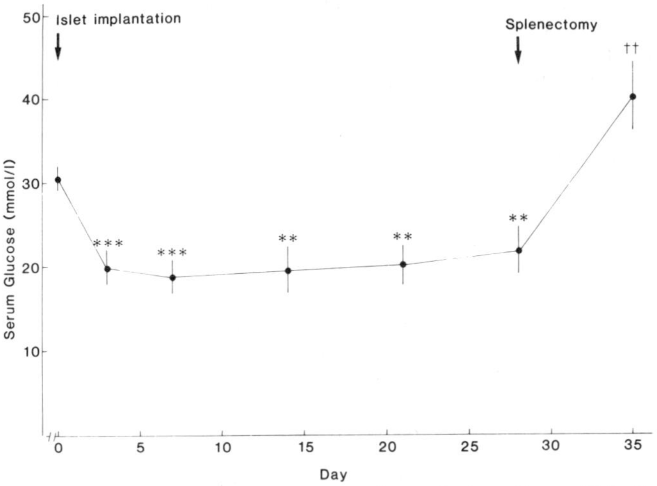

FIGURE 2. Serum glucose concentrations of nine alloxan-diabetic C57BL/6 mice implanted intrasplenically on day 0 with about 600 syngeneic islets cryopreserved at a cooling rate of 25°C/min. Splenectomy was performed in five animals on day 28. Values are given as means ± SEM. (**) and (***) indicate $P<0.01$ and $P<0.001$ compared with day 0 (unpaired Student's t test). (++) denotes $P<0.01$ (Student's paired t test) for comparison of serum glucose concentrations on days 28 and 35 in the five mice that were splenectomized.

of the latter animals showed signs of degeneration and cellular infiltration of the splenic islets.

DISCUSSION

Several freezing protocols for cryopreservation of pancreatic B cells have been presented during the last years, as recently reviewed by Bank (*23*). In particular there have been wide variations in the optimal cooling rate reported by different authors. This may be explained in many ways. First, different B cell preparations have been used—e.g., fetal rat pancreatic fragments (*24*), isolated islets prepared by collagenase digestion and Ficoll centrifugation (*1–4*), hand-picked collagenase-isolated islets (*6, 7, 15, 16*), and mechanically prepared islets without previous collagenase treatment (*12*). Second, there may be differences between the optimal cooling rates for B cells obtained from different experimental animals. Third, variations in the use of a cryoprotectant and the mode of its addition and its removal from the islets during or after thawing may lead to significantly different opinions on what is an optimal cooling rate. Finally, there may be variations in the selection, performance and interpretations of the viability tests applied to frozen-thawed islets. Some theoretical points may also be considered in this context—for example, whether the pancreatic islets should be regarded as a complex organ with different osmotic barriers for the cells located in the periphery and in the center of the islet, or whether the cells of the intact islet are permeable to water during the freeze-thawing processes to the same extent as when they are in a single-cell suspension. If the former is true, this would probably favor a slow cooling rate when freezing pancreatic islets.

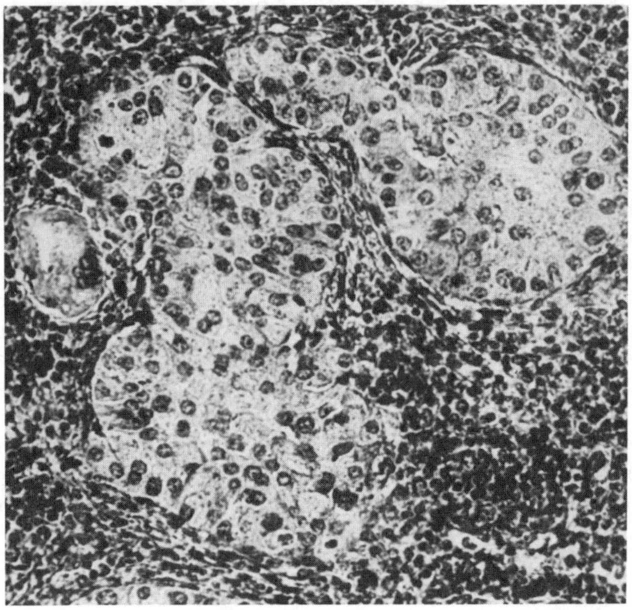

FIGURE 3. Light micrograph of cryopreserved islets implanted into the spleen of an alloxan-diabetic mouse (×350).

The data of the present study suggest that well-preserved islet B cell function can be maintained despite the use of a fairly rapid cooling rate (25°C/min). This is thus in good accordance with the recent findings of Taylor and Benton (*11*). Previously we found that the functional preservation was better in slowly cooled islets (0.5°C/min) than in more rapidly cooled ones (*6*). The somewhat contradictory results may in part be due to the fact that in the present and a recent study (*16*) we used a higher concentration of Me_2SO. Furthermore, the equipment used for rapid freezing in our first study provided less-well-controlled cooling rates than the currently used programmable freezer.

In the present investigation we found a reduction in the insulin content of the frozen-thawed islets compared with that of the nonfrozen cultured ones. This was also the case in our previous studies, both with slowly (0.5°C/min) and with more rapidly frozen (5°C/min) islets (*15, 16*). On the other hand, the functional capacities of the cryopreserved islets as reflected by the rates of (pro)insulin biosynthesis and rates of insulin release were equal to those of the nonfrozen islets when expressed on a per-islet basis. The reduction of the insulin content of the cryopreserved islets most probably reflects a decreased number of B cells in each cryopreserved islet. Indeed, in a recent investigation we observed a slight decrease in the DNA content of islets cooled at 25°C/min under conditions identical to those used in this study (*25*).

Besides a slight decrease in the number of cells in each islet there is also a small reduction in the number of freeze-thawed islets that survive the entire storage procedure. In a current study aimed at elucidating the efficacy of different biological supplements as additives to the islet cryopreservation medium we found that, with the present procedure, about 80% of the islets cooled at a rate of 25°C/min survived (Sandler and Andersson, manuscript in preparation). The corresponding figure for nonfrozen control islets cultured for the same period was 90%, a reduction which is, however, maintained more or less constantly. Thus, with very prolonged storage periods the present cryopreservation technique may prove to be superior to in vitro culture in terms of recovery.

The fact that the majority of the diabetic animals into which cryopreserved islets were transplanted failed to become normoglycemic suggests that the implanted number of functional B cells in these recipients was too low. Usually 500–600 healthy syngeneic islets are sufficient to cure mice of the C57BL/6 strain (*26*). It was nevertheless obvious that the transplanted cryopreserved islets contributed to reducing the diabetic state, in that the splenectomized animals showed a prompt elevation of their serum glucose concentrations. Since a reduction in the replicatory capacity of the islet cells in response to prolonged glucose stimulation following transplantation into a diabetic recipient animal may be a hindrance for normalization of the hyperglycemia (*27*), the replicatory activity of the cells of the cryopreserved islets was determined. It should be noted in this context that previously, and also in this study, we observed islet cell nuclei grouped into clusters after cryopreservation, suggesting specific freeze injuries (*15*). However, in the present study there was no difference in the autoradiographic labeling indices between the cryopreserved and nonfrozen cultured control islets in vitro. This is important, since a successful cure of human diabetics by transplantation using cryopreserved human islets will depend greatly on the growth abilities of the graft.

It is now quite obvious that pancreatic B cells may be cryopreserved using widely varying cooling rates. Depending on how the B cells are isolated and prepared, a period of tissue culture both before freezing and after thawing may be crucial (*16*). So far, reports on successful cryopreservation of human B cells are sparse (*5, 28*). Further investigation in this field must await the development of improved methods for isolation of islets from the human pancreas, or techniques for growing of human B cells in vitro. Promising results in this area have recently been published (*29, 30*).

Acknowledgments. We thank A-B. Andersson, C. Bittkowski, E. Forsbeck, and A. Nordin for excellent technical assistance and L. Bryngelsson and A. Snellman for careful preparation of the manuscript.

REFERENCES

1. Rajotte RV, Stewart HL, Voss WAG, Shnithka TK, Dossetor JB. Viability studies on frozen-thawed rat islets of Langerhans. Cryobiology 1977; 14: 116.
2. Rajotte RV, Scharp DW, Molnar GD, Preston R. Feasibility of low temperature banking for pancreatic islet cell transplantation. In: Federlin K, Bretzel RG, eds. Islet isolation, culture and cryopreservation. Stuttgart: Thieme, 1981: 124.
3. Rajotte RV, Warnock GL, Bruch LC, Procyshyn AW. Transplantation of cryopreserved and fresh rat islets and canine pancreatic fragments. Cryobiology 1983; 20: 169.
4. Rajotte RV, Eng P, Warnock GL, Kneteman NN. Cryopreservation of insulin-producing tissue in rats and dogs. World J Surg 1984; 8: 179.
5. Bretzel RG, Schneider J, Dobroschke J, Schwemmele K, Pfeiffer EF, Federlin K. Islet transplantation in experimental diabetes of the rat. VII. Cryopreservation of rat and human islets. Preliminary results. Horm Metab Res 1980; 12: 274.
6. Sandler S, Nilsson B, Borg LAH, et al. Structure and function of cryopreserved mouse pancreatic islets. In: Federlin K, Bretzel RG, eds. Islet isolation, culture and cryopreservation. Stuttgart: Thieme, 1981; 138.
7. Sandler S, Nilsson B, Petersson B, Hellerström C, Andersson A. Functional characteristics of cryopreserved mouse pancreatic islets. Horm Metab Res [Suppl] 1982; 12: 71.
8. Ferguson J, Allsopp RH, Taylor RMR, Johnston IDA. Isolation and long term preservation of pancreatic islets from mouse, rat and guinea pig. Diabetologia 1972; 12: 115.
9. Nakagawara G, Kojima Y, Mizukami T, Ono S, Miyazaki I. Transplantation of cryopreserved pancreatic islets into the portal vein. Transplant Proc 1981; 13: 1503.
10. McKay DB, Karow AM. A functional analysis on isolated rat islets of Langerhans: effects of dimethylsulfoxide and low-temperature preservation. Cryobiology 1983; 20: 41.
11. Taylor MJ, Duffy TJ, Davidsson PJ, Morgan SRA. Slow cooling of isolated rat islets of Langerhans in the presence of dimethyl sulfoxide or glycerol: effect upon the dynamic patterns of insulin release. Cryo-Lett 1982; 3: 148.
12. Wise MH, Yates A, Gordon C, Johnson RWG. Subzero preservation of mechanically prepared porcine islets of Langerhans. Response to a glucose challenge in vitro. Cryobiology 1983; 20: 211.
13. Bank HL, Davis RF, Emerson D. Cryogenic preservation of isolated rat islets of Langerhans: effect of cooling and warming rates. Diabetologia 1979; 16: 195.
14. Taylor MJ, Benton MJ. Interaction of cooling rate and warming rate during cryopreservation of isolated rat islets of Langerhans: some preliminary observations. Cryobiology 1983; 20: 713.
15. Andersson A, Sandler S. Viability tests of cryopreserved endocrine pancreatic cells. Cryobiology 1983; 20: 161.
16. Sandler S, Andersson A. The significance of culture for successful cryopreservation of isolated pancreatic islets of Langerhans. Cryobiology 1984; 21: 503.
17. Howell SL, Taylor KW. Potassium ions and the secretion of insulin by islets of Langerhans incubated in vitro. Biochem J 1968; 108: 17.
18. Keen H, Field JB, Pastan IH. A simple method for in vitro metabolic studies using small volumes of tissue and medium. Metabolism 1963; 12: 143.
19. Krebs HA, Henseleit K. Untersuchungen über die Harnstoffbildung im Tierkörper. Hoppe Seylers Z Physiol Chem 1932; 210: 33.
20. Heding LG. Determination of total serum insulin (IRI) in insulin-treated patients. Diabetologia 1972; 8: 260.
21. Lacy PE, Walker MM, Fink CJ. Perifusion of isolated rat islets in vitro. Participation of the microtubular system in the biphasic release of insulin. Diabetes 1972; 21: 987.
22. Berne C. Anti-insulin serum coupled to Sepharose 4B as a tool for the investigation of insulin biosynthesis in the B-cells of obese hyperglycemic mice. Endocrinology 1975; 97: 1241.
23. Bank HL. Cryobiology of isolated islets of Langerhans circa 1982. Cryobiology 1984; 20: 119.
24. Mazur P, Kemp JA, Miller RH. Survival of fetal pancreas frozen to −78° and −196°C. Proc Natl Acad Sci USA 1976; 73: 4105.
25. Kojima Y, Sandler S, Andersson A, Nakagawara G. Cryopreservation of cultured mouse pancreatic islets: effects of different

freezing media on islet viability. Low Temp Med 1985; 11: 47.
26. Andersson A, Eriksson U, Petersson B, Reibring L, Swenne I. Failure of successful intrasplenic transplantation of islets from lean mice to cure obese-hyperglycaemic mice, despite islet growth. Diabetologia 1981; 20: 237.
27. Swenne I, Andersson A. Effect of genetic background on the capacity for islet cell replication in mice. Diabetologia 1984; 27: 464.
28. Sandler S, Andersson A, Hellerström C, et al. Preservation of morphology, insulin biosynthesis and insulin release of cryopreserved human fetal pancreas. Diabetes 1982; 31: 238.
29. Gray DWR, McShane P, Grant A, Morris PJ. A method for isolation of islets of Langerhans from the human pancreas. Diabetes 1984; 33: 1055.
30. Sandler S, Andersson A, Schnell A, et al. Tissue culture of human fetal pancreas: development and function of B-cells in vitro and transplantation of explants to nude mice. Diabetes 1985; 34: 1137.

Received 12 December 1985.
Accepted 27 February 1986.

0041-1337/86/4206-0593$02.00/0
TRANSPLANTATION
Vol. 42, No. 6

PROLONGATION OF RENAL ALLOGRAFT SURVIVAL IN ANTILYMPHOCYTE-SERUM–TREATED DOGS BY POSTOPERATIVE INJECTION OF DENSITY-GRADIENT–FRACTIONATED DONOR BONE MARROW[1]

WILLIAM C. HARTNER,[2] SALLY R. DE FAZIO,[2] TAKASHI MAKI,[3] THOMAS G. MARKEES,[2] ANTHONY P. MONACO,[3] AND JAMES J. GOZZO[2,4]

College of Pharmacy and Allied Health, Northeastern University, Boston 02115, and Cancer Research Institute, New England Deaconess Hospital, Boston, Massachusetts 02215

Posttransplant injection of fractionated donor bone marrow cells results in the prolonged survival of mouse skin allografts. In this investigation, we extended the study to the use of donor bone marrow fractionated by density-gradient centrifugation in a larger animal model, canine renal transplantation. Renal allografts were placed in outbred, histoincompatible dogs treated daily with rabbit or horse antilymphocyte serum (ALS) from days −6 to +7 relative to kidney transplantation on day 0. Fresh, unfractionated donor bone marrow (BM) or a bone marrow fraction (BM Fr3) produced by centrifugation in a discontinuous Percoll density gradient was intravenously infused into recipients on days +13 or +14. Alternatively, frozen/thawed (F/Th) BM or BM Fr3 was infused after storage at −80°C for two weeks. BM Fr3 and unfractionated BM significantly (*P*<0.005) prolonged for median allograft function time (MFT) beyond the controls treated only with ALS (46 and 35 days vs. 18 days). The longer MFT with BM Fr3 was achieved with 20–40% of the unfractionated BM cell dose. In addition, BM Fr3-treated dogs exhibited a slower rate of loss of kidney function. F/Th BM was as effective as fresh BM in prolonging graft survival. A reduced mixed lymphocyte response to donor and third-party cells and markedly reduced responsiveness to Con A, PHA, and pokeweed mitogens at 30–45 days posttransplant suggested that animals were nonspecifically immunosuppressed during this period. By 60 days posttransplant, in two dogs treated with BM Fr3, the MLR to third-party cells, but not to donor cells, and the responsiveness to mitogens had returned to pre-ALS treatment values. Thus, treatment with ALS combined with fresh or F/Th BM that has been fractionated is an effective method for the prolongation of kidney allografts in dogs. The development of specific, long-term immunosuppression induced by fractionated bone marrow and success with F/Th BM in this canine renal allograft model suggests that application to human transplantation may be effective with fresh or F/Th BM fractions obtained from living-related or cadaveric donors.

Treatment with antilymphocyte serum (ALS)* plus donor bone marrow represents an effective means of prolonging allograft survival (*1*). This treatment involves the use of minimal

[1] This work was supported by Grants Am 33466 and AI 14551 from the National Institutes of Health.
[2] Northeastern University.
[3] New England Deaconess Hospital.
[4] Address correspondence to: Dr. J. J. Gozzo, College of Pharmacy and Allied Health, Room 110 Mugar Hall, Northeastern University, 360 Huntington Avenue, Boston, MA 02115.

* Abbreviations used: ALS, antilymphocyte serum; BM, bone marrow; BMC, bone marrow cells; BM Fr3, bone marrow fraction 3; Con A, concanavalin A; DMEM, Dulbecco's modified Eagle's medium; DMSO, dimethylsulfoxide; HBSS-H HEPES-buffered Hanks' balanced salt solution; F/Th, frozen/thawed; MFT, median allograft function time; MLC, mixed lymphocyte culture MLR, mixed lymphocyte reaction; PHA, phytohemagglutinin; PWM, pokeweed mitogen; RBC, red blood cells.

immunosuppression given only at the time of grafting, does not involve pretreatment of the recipient far in advance of the transplant, and can result in donor-specific immunosuppression. In the course of extensive studies using this protocol in a mouse skin allograft model, we have demonstrated that donor-specific suppressor cells can be recovered from animals bearing long-term surviving grafts (*2*), and that the reactivity of these animals toward third-party donors is not impaired (*3*). In addition to the application in a mouse skin allograft model, this protocol has been shown to be effective in renal transplantation in dogs (*4*), monkeys (*5*), and—in a preliminary clinical application—in humans (*6*).

Additional studies in our laboratory have focused on the preparation of fractions of the donor bone marrow to be used in this protocol. We have shown that fractions enriched for cells active in graft prolongation can be prepared by velocity sedimentation at unit gravity in stabilizing gradients of bovine serum albumin (*7*) or Ficoll (*8*). Although this method effectively separates cells on the basis of size, its capacity for handling large numbers of cells is severely limited, and thus restricted in its usefulness for large animals and in clinical situations. For this reason, we have recently investigated the use of discontinuous density gradient centrifugation in Percoll for the fractionation of mouse bone marrow (*9*).[5] Using a four-step gradient, we produced three nucleated cell fractions and a cell pellet that consisted primarily of erythrocytes. Cells with the ability to prolong skin allograft survival in ALS-treated mice were found largely in the nucleated cell fraction with the lowest density and represented approximately 10% of the recovered cells.

In the present investigation, we extended the study of the effect of donor bone marrow prepared by density gradient centrifugation to a larger animal model, canine renal transplantation. Fractions of donor bone marrow, both fresh and preserved by freezing, were compared with unfractionated bone marrow to assess their ability to prolong graft survival beyond that induced by treatment with ALS alone.

MATERIALS AND METHODS

Animals. Dogs of both sexes and of mixed breeds were obtained from Thorsen Breeding Lab, Westboro, MA, or Buckshire Corp., Perkasie, PA. The body weight of recipients was between 7 and 14 kg and that of donors between 10 and 15 kg. Dogs were screened for the presence of parasites during an isolation period. They were caged singly in the central animal quarters with a 12:12 light:dark cycle. Food consisted of commercial dog meal (Purina) supplemented with canned meat; water was available ad libitum.

Dog renal transplantation. Recipient dogs were treated with oral antibiotics (Velosef, Cephadrin [Squibb] 1000 mg) one day prior to the operation and 7 days postoperatively (500 mg/day). Anesthesia was induced with 20 mg/kg of i.v. Thymidal sodium (Bio-tal, Biocentics Co.) and was maintained with Halothane/N_2O gas. Lactated Ringer's solution was administered during operations. The donor kidney was flushed with 20 ml of heparinized lactated Ringer's (4°C) and placed in ice cold lactated Ringer's until transfer to the recipient. The ischemia time was approximately 30 min. The donor kidney was placed in the recipient's lower abdominal cavity. An end-to-end renal–to–common-iliac-artery and an end-to-side renal–to–common-iliac-vein anastomosis were performed. A ureteroneocystostomy reestablished the ureteral continuity. The dog's own kidneys were removed at the time of transplantation.

Recipient monitoring. Daily blood lymphocyte and leukocyte counts during ALS treatment were compared with pretransplant, pre-ALS treatment values. The data are presented only for dogs that had pretransplant blood lymphocyte counts averaging 10% or less of the pre-ALS treatment counts. The onset of rejection usually occurred during the posttransplant ALS treatment period in dogs with pretransplant lymphocyte counts ≧20% of the pre-ALS treatment counts. Pretransplant mixed lymphocyte reactions of the donor and recipient were used to confirm their histoincompatability. Posttransplant mixed lymphocyte reactions (MLR) were also used to confirm immunosuppression and to monitor immunological recovery.

Kidney function was assessed by daily serum creatinine determinations from a kit (Sigma Diagnostics) based on the method of Heinegard and Tiderstrom (*10*). Additionally, the graft was palpated for signs and degree of swelling. The urine volume and adequacy of hydration were noted daily, and dogs were given subcutaneous fluids in the posttransplant period if dehydrated.

Grafted kidneys were defined as rejected and dogs were evaluated for sacrifice when serum creatinine values exceeded 10 mg/dl (870 μM). The median allograft function time (MFT), defined as the median days posttransplant with a serum creatinine ≦10 mg/dl, was estimated by the method of Litchfield (*11*). The significance of the differences between two treatments was estimated with the Mann-Whitney *U* test (*12*). Animals were examined postmortem for the cause of kidney failure, and kidney sections were preserved in buffered 10% formaldehyde for histological examination.

Antilymphocyte serum (ALS). Rabbit antidog lymphocyte serum (rabbit ALS) was prepared in New Zealand White rabbits with dog mesenteric lymph node cells as described previously (*13*). Batches of rabbit ALS had lymphagglutination titers greater than 1:256. Serum was absorbed twice with 50–60 ml of washed canine red blood cells (RBC)/L of serum at 37°C for 30 min. After absorption, the hemagglutination titer was typically reduced from 1:1024 to 1:64. Horse antidog lymphocyte serum (horse ALS) was prepared as described elsewhere (*14*).

Bone marrow collection and infusion. Ribs were aseptically removed from the exsanguinated donor dog immediately following the second kidney donation. Marrow cells were expressed from the ribs with forceps and flushed into a Petri dish with HEPES-buffered Hanks' balanced salt solution (pH 7.4, MA Bioproducts, HBSS-H), centrifuged at 500 g for 5 min and washed twice. Nucleated cells were counted with crystal violet in 3% acetic acid and viability was estimated by eosin Y exclusion. RBC were not removed. Fresh, whole bone marrow cells and Percoll-fractionated bone marrow cells (see below) were infused i.v. at $30–50\times10^6$ nucleated cells/ml in HBSS-H over a 10–20-min period.

Bone marrow fractionation by Percoll density gradient centrifugation. A stock 90% Percoll solution (334 mosM) was prepared with HBSS-H as described by Shields et al. (*15*). Discontinuous gradients of Percoll (Pharmacia) were prepared in 15 ml polypropylene centrifuge tubes (Corning) by modification of a method described elsewhere.[5] The tubes were first

[5] Hartner WC, De Fazio SR, Monaco AP, Gozzo JJ. Prolongation of graft survival in ALS-treated mice by donor-specific bone marrow: unit gravity velocity sedimentation of the active bone marrow cells (manuscript submitted for publication).

filled with a 2.0 ml suspension of 100×10^6 nucleated bone marrow cells plus erythrocytes. Care was taken that this suspension was free of cell clumps, debris, and fat. Next, underlayers were added, first of 40% of the Percoll stock diluted in HBSS-H (density, 1.046 g/L; refractive index, 1.3425); and then of 52.5% stock Percoll diluted in HBSS-H (density 1.064 g/L; refractive index, 1.3450). Sufficient tubes were prepared to accommodate approximately 120% of the bone marrow cells that would be administered to the recipient animal were the marrow not fractionated. Extra cells were included to adjust for the 15–20% cell loss encountered during this procedure. After centrifuging the tubes at 400 g for 25 min, the cells found in the interface between the 40 and 52.5% Percoll layers were harvested by pipette and washed in HBSS-H. The resulting cell fraction is referred to here as "fraction 3" because it corresponds to the fraction in mouse bone marrow that is most active in prolonging graft survival—and, like BM fraction 3 of mouse, it was markedly heterogeneous but enriched with small-to-medium-sized cells of the lymphocytic type (*9*).

Bone marrow cell freezing, storage, and thawing for infusion. Bone marrow cells were resuspended in chilled Dulbecco's modified Eagle's medium (DMEM, MA Bioproducts) supplemented with 20% heat-inactivated dog serum at 60–100×10^6 nucleated cells/ml. Prior to freezing, the cell suspension was mixed with an equal volume of DMEM, 20% dog serum, and 20% dimethyl sulfoxide (DMSO, Sigma) at 4°C. Cells were frozen with a Linde Biological Freezer system in freezing vials (Nunc, Corning) at −2° to −3°C/min to approximately −20°C, and thereafter at −10°C/min to −70°C. Cells were stored at −80° until thawing. Cells for infusion into transplant recipients were thawed rapidly in a 37°C water bath to 0°C and diluted 1:1 with iced DMEM. Cell counts and viability were estimated as described above. The cell suspension was kept on ice until infused. Frozen/thawed unfractionated BMC and BM fraction 3 were infused i.v. at 10–25×10^6 viable, nucleated cells/ml over a 10–20-minute period.

Mixed lymphocyte reaction (MLR). Peripheral blood was collected in tubes containing preservative-free heparin. The buffy coat was separated with Histopaque-1077 (Sigma) by centrifugation and washed in HBSS-H.

Bone marrow cells to be used as stimulators in the MLR were stored frozen at −80°C as described above. Aliquots (1.5 ml) of frozen BMC were thawed rapidly at 37°C, and the DMSO was diluted slowly at room temperature by the addition of 1.5 ml HBSS-H containing 5% heat-inactivated dog serum every 10 min over 1 hr. The cells were centrifuged and resuspended in HBSS-H. Cell viability was estimated by eosin Y exclusion.

The MLR was performed by mixing 5.0×10^4 peripheral blood lymphocytes (responders) with 5.0×10^4 mitomycin-C-treated peripheral blood lymphocytes or BMC (stimulators) in 0.2 ml medium. The medium consisted of DMEM supplemented with 0.2 mM L-glutamine, 50 μg/ml gentamicin, and 10% heat-inactivated heterologous dog serum. All dog sera were pretested to confirm their ability to support MLR proliferation. All cultures were performed in triplicate in 96-well round-bottomed microtiter plates (Corning). After five days incubation at 37°C in a humid 7% CO_2 atmosphere, each culture was pulsed with 2 μCi of tritiated thymidine (2 Ci/mM, New England Nuclear), incubated for 20 hr longer, and harvested onto glass fiber filters with a Mini MASH unit (MA Bioproducts). Thymidine incorporation was measured in a beta scintillation counter (Packard Instruments). The results were expressed as mean counts/min (cpm) of triplicate cultures. Statistical outliers were excluded by the method of Leiblein (*16*).

The MLR stimulation index (SI) was calculated as:

$$SI = \frac{\text{mean cpm of MLR with allogeneic cells as stimulators}}{\text{mean cpm of MLR with autologous cells as stimulators}}$$

Mitogen stimulation of peripheral blood lymphocytes (5×10^4 in 0.2 ml medium) was done on the same schedule as the MLR with the following mitogens (Sigma): concanavalin A (Con A) at 1.0, 2.0 and 4.0 μg/ml; phytohemagglutinin (PHA) at 2.5, 5.0, and 10 μg/ml; and pokeweed mitogen (PWM) at 1.25, 2.5, and 5.0 μg/ml. Control values for unstimulated cultures were obtained from wells containing 5×10^4 cells in 0.2 ml medium without mitogens.

Dog treatment protocol. Mixed lymphocyte reactions were performed 1–2 weeks prior to dog preparation for transplantation. Dogs were immunosuppressed with 2 ml/kg, s.c., of rabbit ALS or horse ALS (2 or 3 ml/kg) from day −6 through day +7 relative to renal allografting on day 0. Rabbit ALS doses were increased by up to 50% when lymphocyte counts were not depressed to ≦10% of pretransplant lymphocyte counts. Bone marrow cells were routinely infused on days +13–+14 (6–7 days after ALS treatment).

RESULTS

Allograft prolongation. The effects of bone marrow treatments in prolonging renal allografts were assessed functionally (Fig. 1). ALS treatment alone prolonged the MFT approximately 1 week beyond that of untreated dogs (18 days vs. 10–12 days). Bone marrow fraction 3 prolonged the MFT considerably beyond that of the control dogs receiving ALS alone (46 days vs. 18 days, $P<0.005$).

The MFT of dogs treated with fractionated bone marrow was increased 11 days compared with unfractionated BMC-treated animals (46 compared to 35 days, although $P>0.05$).

The extended graft survival in dogs treated with fraction 3 was achieved with relatively lower cell doses. The fraction 3 doses administered were proportional to the number recovered from 10^8 unfractionated BMC/kg used as the fractionation starting material (i.e., 20–40% of the doses of unfractionated BMC, $\overline{X}\pm SD = 31\pm6\%$).

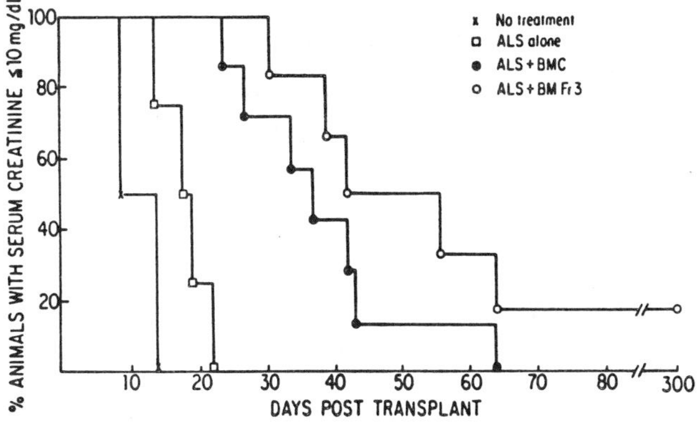

FIGURE 1. The duration of survival with a serum creatinine ≦10 mg/dl in kidney allografted dogs. Daily ALS treatment was from day −6 through day +7 relative to kidney allografting on day 0. Unfractionated bone marrow (BMC) at 3–10×10^7 viable cells/kg, or fraction 3 bone marrow (BM Fr3) at 2–4–10^7 viable cells/kg was administered at days +13 or +14. The number of dogs was: 2 with no treatment, 4 with ALS alone, 7 with ALS and BMC, and 6 with ALS and BM Fr3.

Dogs treated with unfractionated or fractionated BMC that had been frozen and stored at −80°C for two weeks also had prolonged allograft survival (Table 1, Fig. 1). These dogs had graft survival times that were comparable to dogs treated with nonfrozen bone marrow, although they received one-third to one-half the BMC of dogs receiving fresh unfractionated marrow.

Two of four dogs in the ALS-alone treatment group and three of seven dogs in the unfractionated BMC group treated with horse ALS had graft survival at least as long as that seen in the dogs treated with rabbit ALS alone (Table 1). More typically, however, treatment with horse ALS depressed lymphocyte counts inconsistently from dog to dog, and six additional horse-ALS-treated dogs (data not shown) showed the onset of marked rises of serum creatinine values during the ALS treatment period or within two days of the period's end. The six dogs had high (>20% of pre-ALS values) lymphocyte counts.

Apparent rejection-related 3–4-fold increases in kidney size always preceded rises of serum creatinine by 1–3 days for all treatment groups.

An overall picture of the time course of change in, and state of, allograft function is presented in Figure 2. Animals treated with ALS alone show a simple time course of serum creatinine changes. The pattern shown in animals treated with unfractionated BMC is complicated by the strong effect of the BMC on the course of four incipient rejection episodes. Bone marrow treatment led to the reversal of rising creatinine values, which were as high as 3.6 mg/dl at the time of cell infusion in these four BMC-treated animals and equalled 1.6 in the longest-surviving BM Fr3-treated case. Clearly, deterioration of kidney function remained reversible in early rejection episodes. Spontaneous reversals of rises in creatinine values were not seen in any control animals treated with ALS. Overall, the rate of loss of kidney function appeared to be lower with fraction 3 marrow than with the unfractionated marrow.

Mixed lymphocyte reactions. Dogs receiving bone marrow were unresponsive in MLR to both donor (SI=1.2±1.1) and third-party (SI=1.2±1.1) at 30–45 days posttransplant compared with pretransplant dogs tested (SI=6.0±2.5). In two animals, the MLR to the donor cells was specifically suppressed 60 days posttransplant, while that to third-party stimulators was not (SI of 1.4 and 1.2 vs. 8.7 and 4.1). Responsiveness to all three mitogens (Con A, PHA, and PWM) was reduced at least 3–20-fold 30–45 days posttransplant. Mitogen responsiveness approached pretransplant levels at 60 days posttransplant in animals with specific unresponsiveness. The MLR and the mitogen responsiveness were not correlated with graft status as estimated from serum creatinine values (Fig. 2) and by kidney size estimates (data not shown).

TABLE 1. Effect of bone marrow fractionation on the functional survival of kidney allografts

Bone marrow (BM) treatment group[a]	Survival of individual with serum creatinine ≦10 mg/dl (days)	MFT (days)[c]
No treatment	9, 14	—
ALS alone	14, 18, 19,[b] 22,[b]	18
Unfractionated BM + ALS	24, 34,[b] 37, 42,[b] 64	35[d]
Unfractionated BM + ALS (frozen/thawed)	29,[b] 43	
BM fraction 3 + ALS	31, 39, 42, 64, 300	46[d,e]
BM fraction 3 + ALS (frozen/thawed)	56	

[a] Dose of viable cells: unfractionated BM at 6.0±0.8×10^7/kg; BM Fr 3 at 3.1±0.6×10^7/kg.

[b] ALS used was horse ALS. All others received rabbit ALS.

[c] MFT: median kidney functional time, defined as the median day posttransplant with a serum creatinine ≦10 mg/dl. (*10*).

[d] *P*<0.005 compared with ALS alone. (Mann-Whitney *U* test).

[e] *P*>0.05 compared with unfractionated BM + ALS.

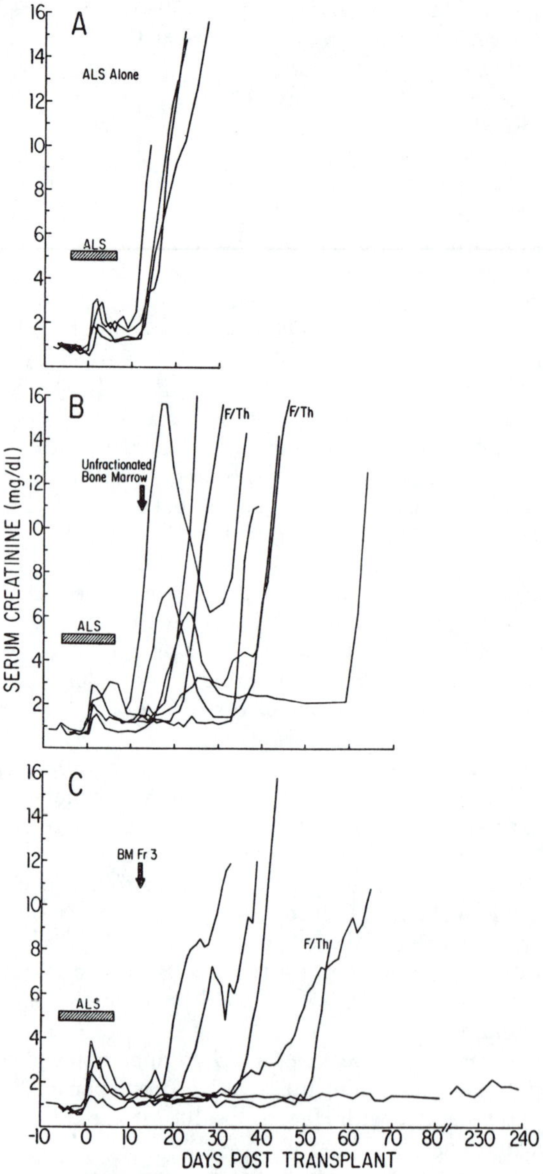

FIGURE 2. Summary of the time course of creatinine values for individual recipients following kidney transplantation. All animals received daily injections of ALS from days −6 to +7 relative to kidney allografting on day 0. (A) control animals receiving ALS alone; (B) animals treated with ALS and unfractionated bone marrow on days +13 or +14; (C) animals treated with ALS and bone marrow fraction 3 on days +13 or +14. F/Th indicates that the frozen bone marrow cells had been thawed and administered after 13–14 days' storage at −80°C.

DISCUSSION

Treatment of outbred histoincompatible dogs with ALS and a low-density fraction of donor bone marrow is effective in extending renal allograft functional survival. The suggestion that the MFT increased with the use of density-gradient-fractionated bone marrow when compared with unfractionated BMC is reinforced by the fact that significant prolongation was produced with relatively lower doses of cells than in the unfractionated BMC group. The prolonged survival observed with fraction 3 cells may be partially related to the removal of harmful, irrelevant, and dead cells found in whole bone marrow cell preparations.

Posttransplant MLR data revealed a condition of nonspecific immunosuppression followed, in two long-surviving dogs, by a state of donor-specific suppression. These observations of specific immunosuppression suggest that treatment with ALS plus BMC may be developed into an effective means for allograft prolongation that does not require chronic, nonspecific immunosuppression. Thus, one could avoid the growth-related problems observed in children receiving immunosuppressive treatment as well as complications associated with such treatment in both children and adults (*17*, *18*).

One major difference was noted between the separation by discontinuous density centrifugation of dog bone marrow cells and that of mouse cells (*9*). Mouse bone marrow fraction 3, which is enriched for cells active in allograft prolongation, consists of only 10% of the cells that can be recovered during the procedure. In contrast, dog bone marrow fraction 3 represents 20–40% of recoverable cells. Thus, this separation procedure in dogs may not be as efficient in reducing the load of irrelevant cells as in mice. In addition, we have noted during the separation of peripheral blood leukocytes from these outbred dogs that there is much more overlap between the densities of granulocytic and mononuclear cells than is found in humans or mice (unpublished observation). The relatively poor density-dependent separation of canine bone marrow probably results from a similar overlap; when fraction 3 cells have been refractionated on a continuous gradient, relatively little improvement in resolution was noted (unpublished observation). It appears that canine cells may be unique in this regard, however. Preliminary fractionation of monkey and human bone marrow in our laboratory indicates that cells from these species behave similarly to those from the mouse during density gradient centrifugation.

An increase of creatinine values before infusion of BMC did not seem to shorten the duration of allograft function. The mechanism of the immediate immunosuppressive effect of BMC during early rejection is not known at present, However, unfractionated bone marrow or fraction 3 plus ALS is clearly a powerful factor in the prolongation of allografts in dogs.

The optimal time for BMC infusion is apparently limited to a few days following the course of peritransplant ALS treatment. Caridis, et al. (*4*) obtained significant renal allograft prolongation in dogs with unfractionated BMC given three days after ALS treatment. We confirmed the effectiveness of bone marrow at three days with one dog (34 days survival) and have established that unfractionated BMC or fraction 3 may be given as late as 7 days after ALS treatment.

Percoll fractionation of BMC is perhaps not as effective in excluding nonprolonging cells or enriching for prolonging cells as gravity sedimentation.[5] However, the cells separated by this method are effective in prolonging allografts, and the method has a practical advantage in the preparation of large numbers of cells. The speed and simplicity of this separation procedure make it suitable for large animal and human transplantation.

Finally, these results in dogs suggest that clinical trials reported recently by Monaco et al. (*6*) with fresh donor whole bone marrow may possibly be extended with lower doses of fractionated bone marrow that has been obtained from living-related or cadaveric donors at the time of transplant and stored frozen until the time for infusion.

Acknowledgments. We gratefully acknowledge the support and technical assistance of D. Smith, R.G. Laurence, S.G. Sexton, and S.D. Chase of the Northeastern University Animal Care Facility.

REFERENCES

1. Monaco AP, Liegeois A, Wood ML, Clark AW. Active enhancement of tissue allografts with antilymphocyte serum and bone marrow. Adv Nephrology 1975; 5: 135.
2. Maki T, Gottschalk R, Wood ML, Monaco AP. Specific unresponsiveness to skin allografts in anti-lymphocyte serum-treated, marrow injected mice: participation of donor marrow-derived suppressor cells. J Immunol 1981; 127: 1433.
3. Wood ML, Monaco AP. Suppressor cells in specific unresponsiveness to skin allografts in ALS-treated, marrow-injected mice. Transplantation 1980; 29: 196.
4. Caridis T, Liegeois A, Barrett I, Monaco AP. Enhanced survival of canine renal allografts of ALS-treated dogs given bone marrow. Transplant Proc 1973; 5: 671.
5. Thomas JM, Carver FM, Foil MB, et al. Renal allograft tolerance induced with ATG and donor bone marrow in outbred rhesus monkeys. Transplantation 1983; 36: 104.
6. Monaco AP, Wood ML, Maki T, Madras PN, Sahyoun AI, Simpson MA. Attempt to induce unresponsiveness to human renal allografts with antilymphocyte globulin and donor specific bone marrow. Transplant Proc 1985; 17: 1312.
7. Gozzo JJ, Litvin DA, Bhatnagar YM, Monaco AP. Fractionated bone marrow: use of a lymphocyte-containing fraction for skin allograft prolongation in antilymphocyte serum-(ALS) treated mice. Transplant Proc 1981; 13: 592.
8. Gozzo JJ, Crowley M, Maki T, Monaco AP. Functional characteristics of Ficoll-separated mouse bone marrow cell population involved in skin allograft prolongation. J Immunol 1982; 129: 1584.
9. De Fazio SR, Hartner WC, Monaco AP, Gozzo JJ. Prolongation of graft survival in ALS-treated mice by donor-specific bone marrow: density-gradient fractionation of the active bone marrow cells. Transplantation (in press).
10. Heinegard D, Tiderstrom G. Determination of serum creatinine by a direct colorimetric method. Clin Chim Acta 1973; 43: 305.
11. Litchfield JT. A method for rapid graphic solution of time-percent effect curves. J Pharmacol Exp Ther 1949; 97: 339.
12. Goldstein A. Biostatistics. New York: MacMillan, 1964: 55.
13. Gozzo J, Wood M, Monaco AP. Studies on ALS in mice. VIII. Effect of immunizing cell type and dose on immunosuppressive potency and content of irrelevant antibody. Transplantation 1972; 14: 358.
14. Monaco AP, Abbott WM, Othersen HB, et al. Antiserum to lymphocytes: prolonged survival of canine renal allografts. Science 1966; 153: 1264.
15. Shields JM, Haston WS, Wilkinson PC. Separation of mouse lymphoblasts by discontinuous density centrifugation on Percoll gradients. J Immunol Methods 1983; 59: 159.
16. Lieblein J. The closest two out of three observations. Contributions to order statistics. New York: Wiley 1962: 129.
17. Blohme I, Brynger H. Malignant disease in renal transplant patients. Transplantation 1985; 39: 23.
18. Penn I, Makowski EL, Harris P. Parenthood following renal transplantation. Kidney Int 1980; 18: 221.

Received 31 October 1985.
Accepted 20 February 1986.

0041-1337/86/4206-0598$02.00/0
TRANSPLANTATION
Vol. 42, No. 6

RENAL TRANSPLANTATION IN 45 PATIENTS WITH AMYLOIDOSIS

A. PASTERNACK,[1] J. AHONEN, AND B. KUHLBÄCK

Fourth Department of Surgery and Fourth Department of Medicine, Helsinki University Central Hospital, Helsinki; and Department of Clinical Sciences, University of Tampere, Tampere, Finland

The results of renal transplantation in patients with amyloidosis were studied in 45 patients receiving primary cadaver grafts at a single center between March 1973 and October 1981. A control group of 45 patients with glomerulonephritis receiving primary cadaver grafts during the same period was also studied. These were matched according to the number of A and B locus incompatibilities and the date of transplantation.

The 3-year survival of the patients with amyloidosis was statistically significantly inferior (51%) to that of the controls (79%). Age over 40 years was the major factor determining low survival in these patients. Mortality was concentrated in the early posttransplantation period. The 3-year graft survival rate was the same in amyloidotics (38%) and controls (45%); with death of patients not included in graft loss, the corresponding figures were 53% and 49%.

Appearance of amyloid in the transplant was established by biopsy in four patients at 11–37 months of follow-up. Renal transplants functioning for more than one year were calculated to incur a minimum risk of 20% of acquiring amyloid.

When renal amyloidosis has progressed to end-stage renal failure, most patients have severe effects of systemic amyloidosis or of the underlying disease. Therefore renal transplantation may not be regarded as a suitable mode of treatment. The first successful renal transplantations in patients with renal amyloidosis were reported by Belzer et al. in 1968 (*1*) and Cohen et al. in 1971 (*2*). Since then about 60 patients with renal amyloidosis are known to have received renal transplants (*3–12*). Most reports are on few cases or a small series (*1–3, 9–11*) or summarize the experiences of many centers (*4–6*). The existing data on patient survival and on the fate of the grafts (*6, 8, 12*) do not provide sufficient information to justify large-scale renal transplantation in amyloidosis. A study from a single center with uniform transplantation procedures is clearly needed. In this communication we report a controlled one-center study on the outcome of 45 primary renal transplantations in patients with amyloidosis.

MATERIALS AND METHODS

Patients. Between March 1973 and October 1981, 45 patients with amyloidosis (28 men, 17 women) received primary cadaver kidney transplants.

Three patients had primary amyloidosis; in 33 amyloidosis was secondary to rheumatoid arthritis or some other chronic polyarthritis; and in 9 it was secondary to some other chronic inflammatory disease. Amyloidosis was diagnosed by renal biopsy in 29 and by biopsy of the spleen or rectal mucosa in 15 of the patients. In one patient the diagnosis was made on clinical grounds. The mean age at the time of transplantation was 45.4±12.4 (SD) years (range 22–67).

A control group was formed of 45 patients (32 men, 13 women) with end-stage renal failure due to chronic glomerulonephritis who received primary cadaver kidney transplants during the same period as the amyloidotics. The controls were selected from the transplantation cases, filed by date of operation, by taking for each patient with amyloidosis the closest patient with glomerulonephritis who had the same number of mismatched HLA-A and B locus antigens with the donor as did the amyloidotic patient. The mean age of the control group at the time of transplantation was 36.2±13.5 (SD) years (range 11–68).

The minimum follow-up for both groups of patients was 2 months (January 1982).

Dialysis and transfusion data. Twelve of the patients with amyloidosis and 7 of the patients with glomerulonephritis underwent kidney transplantation without any preceding dialysis treatment. Seven of the amyloidotics and two of the patients with glomerulonephritis were treated by peritoneal dialysis prior to transplantation (1–10 and 6 and 8 months, respectively). The remaining patients were treated by chronic intermittent hemodialysis prior to transplantation. The mean time on hemodialysis was 7.6±11.0 (SD) months in the patients with amyloidosis (n=26) and 9.3±7.7 (SD) months in the patients with glomerulonephritis (n=36).

Nineteen of the patients with amyloidosis and 17 of those with glomerulonephritis had never received any blood transfusions. More than 10 blood units had been transfused into 7 patients with amyloidosis and 5 patients with glomerulonephritis. In the remaining patients of both groups the number of blood units transfused was, in general, between one and four.

Tissue typing. Ten patients in each group received 0-mismatched kidneys (HLA-A,B); 16 patients had three, 18 patients two, and one patient in each group only one HLA antigen in common with the donor.

Transplantation data. The kidneys were transplanted extraperitoneally into the iliac vessels. The internal iliac artery was in most cases used for an end-to-end anastomosis. The ureter was implanted into the fundus of the bladder.

Mean ischemia time, from starting the cold perfusion of the graft to reestablishment of the circulation was 28.5±11.2 (SD) hr in the amyloidosis group and 28.2±14.4 (SD) hr in the glomerulonephritis group.

Immunosuppression. In almost all patients standard immunosuppression with methylprednisolone and azathioprine was used. Methylprednisolone was given in decreasing doses so that at about half a year after transplantation the maintenance dose was 8–16 mg every second day. Azathioprine was usually given in a dose of 150 mg daily, depending on the leukocyte and

[1]Address correspondence to: A. Pasternack, M.D., Department of Clinical Sciences, University of Tampere, SF-33520 Tampere, Finland.

thrombocyte counts. Acute rejection episodes were treated with bolus doses of methylprednisolone i.v. 0.5 g on the first, 0.25 on the second, and 0.25 on the third day. One patient with amyloidosis and 2 with glomerulonephritis were given cyclosporine alone instead of the above standard immunosuppressive regimen. One of the patients with amyloidosis and 3 of those with glomerulonephritis had cyclosporine combined with methylprednisolone.

Studies for amyloid in the grafts. Grafts removed by operation and at autopsy, as well as percutaneous biopsies of the grafts, were studied for the presence of amyloid by staining the tissue specimens with alkaline Congo red and examining them in polarized light. Fine-needle aspiration biopsy specimens of the grafts were studied by electron microscopy as described earlier (*13, 14*).

Statistical analysis. The life-table method was used to assess patient and graft survival. Graft survival was estimated in two ways: 1. graft losses included those due to death of patient, and 2. death with a functioning graft was taken as graft survival. Statistical significance was evaluated by the log-rank test. Mean values were compared with Student's t test.

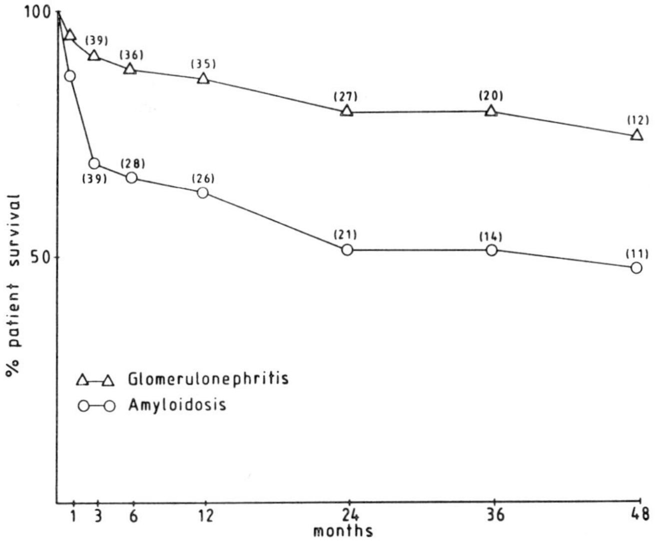

FIGURE 1. Actuarial patient survival after cadaver kidney transplantation in 45 patients with amyloidosis and 45 patient with glomerulonephritis.

RESULTS

Patient and graft survival rates. The actuarial patient and primary graft survival for the 45 amyloidotics and 45 glomerulonephritic controls are shown in Figures 1 and 2 and Table 1.

As regards survival, the patients with amyloidosis were statistically significantly inferior to the controls. The marked difference between the groups was established within the first 3 months, which reflects the high proportion of early deaths in the amyloidosis group. The 3-, 6-, and 12-month patient survival rates for patients with amyloidosis of two age groups, ≤40 years and ≥41 years, were 93, 93, and 57, 54, and 50%, respectively. In the glomerulonephritics the corresponding rates were 93, 93, and 89 and 86, 78, and 78%. Altogether 23 patients with amyloidosis and 10 with glomerulonephritis died during the follow-up. The mean age at death of the amyloidotics was 48.4±12.8 (SD) and 43.9±15.8 (SD) in the glomerulonephritics. This difference was not statistically significant.

Patient survival was not adversely influenced by the fact that some of the patients did not receive dialysis prior to transplantation. Mean patient survival in the 12 amyloidosis patients who underwent transplantation without preceding dialysis was 34.5±31.6 (SD) months, while it was 18.4±19.3 (SD) months in the 33 amyloidotics who received maintenance dialysis prior to transplantation ($P<0.05$).

The graft survival rates were similar in the patients with amyloidosis and those with glomerulonephritis. If death with a functioning graft was taken as graft survival, the rates were somewhat higher in the amyloidotics than in the glomerulonephritics. Graft survival rates were of about the same magnitude in patients grouped by age (≤40 years vs. ≥41 years), HLA incompatibility (0–1 incompatibility vs. 2–3 incompatibilities) or pretransplant blood transfusions (no transfusion vs. ≥1 transfusion).

Causes of death. The causes of death in the 23 patients with amyloidosis and the 10 controls with glomerulonephritis are presented in Table 2. In both groups the main causes of death were cardiovascular and infectious complications. Septic infection as a consequence of acute rejection or its treatment was the cause of death in six of the patients with amyloidosis and two with glomerulonephritis. Three patients with amyloidosis and one with glomerulonephritis died from coronary infarction. Four patients with amyloidosis died from late complications of generalized amyloidosis. In these patients the final stage was preceded by graft failure due to one of the following causes:

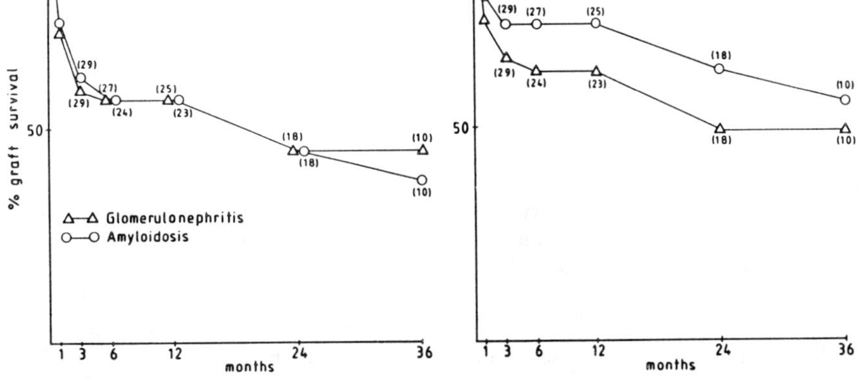

FIGURE 2. Actuarial graft survival for cadaver kidney transplants in 45 patients with amyloidosis and 45 patients with glomerulonephritis. (a) patient death included in graft loss; (b) patient death not included in graft loss.

TABLE 1. Actuarial patient and graft survival rates after renal transplantation in 45 patients with amyloidosis and 45 patients with glomerulonephritis

	Patient survival					Graft survival (patient death included in graft loss)				Graft survival (patient death not included in graft loss)			
	1-year	2-year	3-year	4-year	*P*	1-year	2-year	3-year	*P*	1-year	2-year	3-year	*P*
Amyloidotics	63	51	51	47	0.005	57	45	38	NS	74	63	53	NS
Glomerulonephritics	86	79	79	74		57	45	45		63	49	49	

TABLE 2. Causes of death

Cause of death	Amyloidotics	Glomerulonephritics
Cardiovascular disease	7	3
Infection	8	4
Generalized amyloidosis	4	
Other	4	3
Total	23	10

TABLE 3. Causes of graft failure

Graft failure	Amyloidotics	Glomerulonephritics
Patient died with functioning graft	9	3
Rejection	12	19
Operative and vascular complication	2	1
De novo glomerulonephritis or amyloidosis of graft	4	0
Total	27	23

appearance of amyloid in the graft, de novo membranous glomerulonephritis, chronic rejection, or irreversible acute rejection.

Causes of graft failure and recurrence of amyloid. The causes of graft failure in the 27 patients with amyloidosis and the 23 controls with glomerulonephritis are presented in Table 3. Death of a patient with a functioning graft was responsible for graft failure in 9 of the amyloidotics (33%) and 3 of the controls (13%). Five of the controls and 10 of the amyloidotics never experienced an acute rejection episode. Otherwise there were no clear differences between the groups in the frequency of single or repeated, reversible or irreversible acute rejection episodes. Chronic rejection was diagnosed in 6 amyloidotics and 10 glomerulonephritics. In the amyloidotics 44% of the graft losses were due to rejection. In the glomerulonephritic control group, as much as 83% of the losses were directly related to rejection.

At the end of the follow-up 13 of the 45 grafts were functioning without proteinuria and they were not studied for the presence of amyloid. The median follow-up of these grafts was 19 months (range 2–52). In one patient dying at 24 months with a nonfunctioning graft, autopsy was not performed. Because of proteinuria (≥1.0 g/24 hr) in three patients, or as part of a previous systematic study (*15*), 10 grafts were studied by fine-needle aspiration biopsy and one by conventional transcutaneous biopsy.

In 15 of the 23 patients who died, the grafts were studied for the presence of amyloid at autopsy. Five grafts were surgically removed and examined within 2 months of transplantation. One graft in which biopsy had revealed membranous glomerulonephritis at 21 months was removed at 32 months and found to have the same lesion and no amyloid. Histological evidence of the presence or absence of amyloid in the graft was available for 31 of the patients. The number of grafts studied and the findings in them at various times after transplantation are shown in Table 4.

Table 5 lists the data of the four patients with occurrence of amyloidosis in the graft. In two of them this complication resulted in loss of the graft. In two patients, also shown in the table, de novo membranous glomerulonephritis was considered to be the cause of graft failure.

TABLE 4. Findings of amyloid or membranous glomerulonephritis in the graft in relation to time after transplantation

Findings in the graft	Time after transplantation (months)	
	0–12	13–52
Histological study made:		
Amyloid		4
Membranous glomerulonephritis		2
No amyloid	19	6
Histological study not made, clinically no signs of amyloid	5	9

DISCUSSION

This study was based on a series of 45 patients with amyloidosis and the same number of controls with glomerulonephritis. It is, to our knowledge, the largest series hitherto reported from a single center. The controls were chosen to match the amyloidotics with regard to HLA-AB match grades—and, as far as possible, with regard to transplantation strategies. Unfortunately, matching for age and sex was not possible. On this basis it was possible to estimate survival rates by the life-table method and to examine several factors thought to be of prognostic importance.

Our study confirmed the impression of a low patient survival that has been expressed by previous authors (*5, 6, 8, 12*). In our series this was clearly due to the large number of deaths in the early posttransplantation period among patients over 40 years of age. Although amyloidotics over 40 years of age had remarkably shorter survival time than the glomerulonephritics of the same age group, the mean ages at death did not differ. Death of the patients with amyloidosis was often related to rejection, its treatment and subsequent infections—which are very poorly tolerated by these patients. In some of the patients complications of systemic amyloid were important prognostic factors. Probably many of the cardiovascular deaths were also related to widespread amyloidosis.

It was remarkable that so many of the patients with amyloidosis died with a functioning graft; graft survival per se was, if anything, even better than in the glomerulonephritic controls. Similar results have been obtained in some of the earlier studies. Kennedy and Castro (*6*) compared the results of 24

TABLE 5. Data of the patients with occurrence of amyloid in the graft and de novo membranous glomerulonephritis

Patient	Sex	Age (years)	Original disease	Graft complication	Time after transplantation (months)	Method of diagnosis
EV	M	26	Ankylosing spondylitis	Amyloid[a]	11	FNAB[b]
KV	F	55	Rheumatoid arthritis	Membranous glomerulonephritis[a]	14	FNAB
AS	F	62	Rheumatoid arthritis	Membranous glomerulonephritis[a]	21	FNAB
TT	M	27	Rheumatoid arthritis	Amyloid[a]	24	Renal biopsy
PP	M	38	Ankylosing spondylitis	Amyloid	28	FNAB
LS	F	45	Primary amyloidosis	Amyloid	37	FNAB

[a] Responsible for graft failure.
[b] FNAB: fine-needle aspiration biopsy of the graft.

renal transplants in patients with amyloidosis with the total of 19,631 transplantations reported to the American College of Surgeons/NIH Registry. Death with a functioning graft was about twice as frequent in the amyloidosis group as in the controls. Pras et al. (*12*) recently reported their experiences of renal transplantation in 20 patients with amyloidosis; 19 had familial Mediterranean fever. They compared actuarial survival rates with those of their patients without amyloidosis of the same era. Graft survival at 5 years was 60% in the amyloidotics and 47% in the nonamyloidotics. They also noted that at 12 months the number of acute rejection episodes per graft was 3.2 in the amyloidotics and 4.7 in the nonamyloidotic patients. We did not observe a clear difference between our groups in the frequency of rejection. The tendency, however, was toward fewer episodes in the amyloidotics, and rejection was a less important cause of graft failure in the amyloidotics than in the glomerulonephritic patients.

Recurrence of amyloid has been reported in 10 of about 60 renal transplants (*4–12*). It is impossible, however, to draw any exact conclusions about the true incidence, because most reports are on few or single cases, and larger series seem to have many patients in common. No systematic search for amyloid recurrence has usually been made. In our previous study we found three recurrences in 12 grafts in which fine-needle aspiration biopsy was done once or twice 10–68 months after transplantation (*15*). Eleven of these grafts are included in the present study. In this study 31 grafts were studied histologically for the presence of amyloid. Amyloid was found in 4 and membranous glomerulonephritis in 2 of the 12 grafts that were studied one year after transplantation or later. Six were found to be negative, and the 9 grafts that were not studied histologically had no clinical signs indicative of a recurrence. Thus it seems that, in patients with amyloidosis, renal transplants surviving for one year or more have a minimum chance of about 20% of acquiring amyloid. As most of the grafts surviving for less than one year were lost very soon after transplantation we cannot make any estimations of the risk of amyloid during the first posttransplantation year. A review of the literature and of our own patients does not reveal any special features common to the patients whose grafts acquired amyloid. Thus the determining factors remain obscure.

REFERENCES

1. Beltzer F, Ashby B, Gulyassy P, Powell M. Successful seventeen-hour preservation and transplantation of human cadaver kidney. N Engl J Med 1968; 278: 608.
2. Cohen A, Briccetti A, Harrington J, Mannick J. Renal transplantation in two cases of amyloidosis. Lancet 1971; 2: 513.
3. Pletka P, Cohen L, Hulme B, et al. Cadaveric renal transplantation. Lancet 1969; 1: 1.
4. ACS/NIH Renal Transplant Registry. JAMA 1975; 232: 148.
5. Jones NF. Renal amyloidosis: pathogenesis and therapy. Clin Nephrol 1976; 6: 459.
6. Kennedy CL, Castro JE. Transplantation for renal amyloidosis. Transplantation 1977; 24: 382.
7. Jacob ET, Bar-Nathan N, Shapira Z, Gafni J. Renal transplantation in the amyloidosis of familial Mediterranean fever. Arch Intern Med 1979; 139: 1135.
8. Kuhlbäck B, Falck H, Törnroth T, Wallenius M, Lindström BL, Pasternack A. Renal transplantation in amyloidosis. Acta Med Scand 1979; 205: 169.
9. Dorman TD, Gamelli RL, Benziger JR, Trainer TD, Foster RS. Systemic amyloidosis involving two renal transplants. Hum Pathol 1981; 12: 735.
10. Giraud P, Adone D, Durand D, Delsol G, That HT, Suc JM. Transplantation rénale dans la maladie périodique. Relation d'un cas et revue de la littérature. Ann Med Interne Paris 1981; 132: 507.
11. Touraine JL, Vital-Durand D, Malik MC, Blanc N, Traeger J. Récidive amyloide sur le transplant rénale malgré la colchicine au cours d'une maladie périodique. Ann Med Interne Paris 1981; 132: 511.
12. Pras M, Gafni J, Jacob ET, Cabili S, Zemer D, Sohar E. Recent advances in familial Mediterranean fever. Adv Nephrol 1984; 13: 261.
13. Pasternack A, Helin H, Törnroth T, Rantala J, Väisänen J, Rahka R. Aspiration biopsy of the kidney with a new fine needle: a way to obtain glomeruli for morphological study. Clin Nephrol 1978; 10: 79.
14. Helin H, Pasternack A, Rantala I. Rapid processing of renal glomeruli for electron microscopy. J Clin Pathol 1979; 32: 516.
15. Helin H, Pasternack A, Falck H, Kuhlbäck B. Recurrence of renal amyloid and de novo membranous glomerulonephritis after transplantation. Transplantation 1981; 32: 6.

Received 16 January 1986.
Accepted 28 February 1986.

0041-1337/86/4206-0602$02.00/0
TRANSPLANTATION
Vol. 42, No. 6
Printed in U.S.A.

A PROSPECTIVE STUDY OF UNEXPLAINED NAUSEA AND VOMITING AFTER MARROW TRANSPLANTATION[1,2]

GERALD D. SPENCER, ROBERT C. HACKMAN, GEORGE B. MCDONALD,[3] DEBORAH E. AMOS, BETH A. CUNNINGHAM, JOEL D. MEYERS, AND E. DONNALL THOMAS

The Departments of Medicine and Pathology, the Fred Hutchinson Cancer Research Center; the Veterans Administration Medical Center; and the University of Washington School of Medicine, Seattle, Washington

We prospectively studied patients with enigmatic nausea and vomiting after allogeneic marrow transplantation to define the causes of this syndrome. Fifty consecutive episodes of persistent vomiting were investigated using physical examination and laboratory tests, endoscopic biopsies and brushings, and clinical follow-up for four weeks. Potential causes of vomiting were identified in 39 of the 50 cases (78%). Fifteen cases had gastrointestinal infections (mainly herpesviruses), 13 had unsuspected acute intestinal graft-versus-host disease (GVHD), 8 had intestinal infection plus acute GVHD, and 3 had other causes (subdural hematomas, bacteremia, and encephalitis). In the remaining 11 cases, no cause of vomiting was found. Endoscopy was necessary for diagnosis in 36 cases and required a combination of methods: routine histology, cytology, viral culture, and immunohistology using monoclonal antibodies to cytomegalovirus (CMV) and herpes simplex virus type 1. Patients with unexplained vomiting or intestinal GVHD had significant improvement of nausea and vomiting over the four-week observation period, but those with CMV did not ($P = .01$).

We conclude that most allogeneic marrow transplant patients with enigmatic nausea and vomiting have gastrointestinal herpesvirus infections, acute GVHD, or both. Untreated CMV infections and persistent GVHD are associated with protracted vomiting in these patients.

Persistent nausea and vomiting are common after marrow transplantation and cause significant morbidity. Transient vomiting is usual after high-dose cyclophosphamide (*1*) and total-body irradiation before transplantation, but approximately one-third of our patients experience persistent nausea and vomiting during the third through the seventh weeks posttransplant. Our marrow transplant patients require parenteral nutrition for an average of two months, and persistent nausea is the most common reason for their inability to eat (*2*). Besides nutritional impairment and prolongation of hospitalization, repetitive vomiting can also lead to important medical and psychological problems (*3*).

Although chemoradiation therapy, severe acute graft-versus-host disease (GVHD),* and medications may lead to nausea, persistent vomiting cannot be explained in many cases and is often attributed to psychological causes. Some cases, however, may represent unrecognized GVHD or gastrointestinal infections. For example, we recently found nausea and vomiting as presenting symptoms in 11 of 17 patients with viral esophagitis after transplant (*4*). To better define the causes of enigmatic vomiting in this population, we performed a careful history and physical examination and gastrointestinal endoscopy with biopsies in patients with persistent, unexplained vomiting more than two weeks after allogeneic marrow transplantation. This interval was chosen to allow time for recovery from chemoradiation effects. We studied biopsies with immunohistology using monoclonal antibodies to cytomegalovirus (CMV) and herpes simplex virus (HSV) type 1, since esophageal infection with these viruses had previously proved difficult to diagnose (*4*). Immunohistology with these monoclonal antibodies has been shown to be a highly sensitive and specific method for the diagnosis of CMV pneumonia and mucocutaneous HSV infections (*5, 6*).

METHODS

Transplant Procedure

During the study period of June 1983 to September 1984, 261 patients with hematologic malignancies and 34 with aplastic anemia received allogeneic marrow transplants. Pretransplant conditioning consisted of total-body irradiation plus cyclophosphamide for malignancies, or cyclophosphamide alone for aplastic anemia, as previously described (*7–9*). Daily cyclosporine or intermittent methotrexate was given during the first 100 days for prophylaxis of GVHD (*10*).

Patient Selection

During the study period we entered 44 allogeneic transplant patients with unexplained nausea and vomiting into the study protocol described below. Forty-one patients had malignancies, two had preleukemia, and one had aplastic anemia. Six of these 44 patients were studied a second time because of severe vomiting three weeks or more after their initial examinations for a total of 50 studies in 44 patients.

Nausea and vomiting for seven consecutive days two weeks or more after allogeneic marrow transplant was required for entry into the study. Patients also had to be at least 12 years of age and medically stable, with platelet count ≥40,000/mm^3 after platelet transfusions. Patients entered did not have clinically obvious moderate or severe acute GVHD (clinical stage II or worse) (*7*), a temporal association of symptoms with

[1] Portions of this research have been published in abstract form (Gastroenterology 1984; 86: 1263, and Gastroenterology 1985; 88: 1596).

[2] This research was supported by grants CA 18029, CA 15704, and CA 30924 from the National Cancer Institute, DHHS, and by the Veterans Administration. Dr. Thomas is a recipient of Research Career Award A1 02425 from the National Institute of Allergy and Infectious Diseases.

[3] Address correspondence to: George B. McDonald, M.D., VAMC—Medical Service, 1660 South Columbian Way, Seattle, Washington 98108.

* Abbreviations used: CMV, cytomegalovirus; GVHD, graft-versus-host disease; HSV, herpes simplex virus.

medications (e.g., cyclosporine, amphotericin, interferon, methotrexate, oral antibiotics), or known acute medical illnesses that could explain nausea and vomiting (e.g., gastrointestinal or systemic infection, pancreatitis, ileus, central nervous system disorders, electrolyte derangements). Informed consent was obtained from all patients.

Study Protocol

Patients meeting entry criteria were interviewed and examined by one of us (G.D.S.). The severity of nausea and vomiting was recorded daily during the week before endoscopy and the three-week period after endoscopy. Severity of nausea and vomiting was scored in the following way:

(0) No nausea or vomiting.

(1) Infrequent nausea and vomiting, occasionally requiring antiemetic therapy; minor effect on performance status.

(2) Frequent nausea with at least 2 episodes of vomiting more than 8 hr apart, requiring frequent antiemetic therapy; moderate reduction in performance.

(3) Constant nausea and vomiting throughout the day, requiring frequent, often continuous antiemetic therapy; marked reduction in performance.

Mean weekly scores for severity of nausea and vomiting were obtained by dividing the sum of the daily severity scores (coded 0–3) by 7.

All patients underwent endoscopic examinations of the esophagus, stomach, and duodenum with a gas-sterilized Olympus GIF-XQ endoscope. Eighteen of these patients were also examined with a sterile rigid or Fujinon SIG-E2 flexible sigmoidoscope because they had diarrhea as well as vomiting. Duodenal biopsies were routinely performed in 48 of the 50 endoscopies. Rectal biopsies were done in all 18 sigmoidoscopies, regardless of mucosal appearance. Esophageal and gastric biopsies and brushings were performed only when the mucosa appeared abnormal. Esophageal specimens were obtained in 43 and gastric specimens in 12 of the 50. Endoscopic specimens were obtained from both the edge and base of ulcers. Separate biopsy specimens from each site sampled were fixed in Bouin's solution for histology, frozen in isopentane for immunohistology, and placed in transport medium for viral culture. Separate esophageal and gastric brushings were air-dried and fixed in ethanol for routine cytology and in acetone for immunofluorescence microscopy. All endoscopies were performed by one observer (G.D.S.).

Patients were followed on a daily basis for three weeks after endoscopy to detect other conditions causing nausea and vomiting, and to identify pneumonia caused by CMV.

Processing and Interpretation of Specimens

Routine histology. Sections of 5μ were cut from paraffin-embedded endoscopic biopsies and stained with hematoxylin and eosin, methenamine silver, and Brown and Hopps (tissue Gram) stains. Brushings were stained with Papanicolaou, Gram, and methenamine silver stains. Mean numbers of biopsies from each endoscopy for permanent sections were 2.5 (range 1–6) from the esophagus, 1.6 (range 1–4) from the stomach and duodenum, and 2.5 (range 1–5) from the rectum. Approximately 20 serial sections from each biopsy were stained with hematoxylin and eosin. CMV infection was diagnosed if large cells containing amphophilic intranuclear inclusions and multiple smaller intracytoplasmic inclusions were present. HSV infection was diagnosed when multinucleated giant cells, cells undergoing ballooning degeneration, or cells with ground-glass nuclei and eosinophilic intranuclear inclusions were seen. Fungal infection was demonstrated by budding yeast, pseudohyphae, and inflammatory cells in smears or biopsies. Necrosis of individual epithelial cells (apoptosis) in intestinal crypts, gastric glands, or the basal layer of esophageal squamous mucosa was necessary for the diagnosis of acute gastrointestinal GVHD (*11–14*). GVHD was not diagnosed if epithelial cell necrosis occurred within foci of acute inflammation or infection. Skin and liver GVHD were diagnosed histologically by published criteria (*12, 15–17*).

Immunohistology. Frozen mucosal biopsies were stored in Optimal Cutting Temperature Compound (Miles Laboratories, Inc., Elkhart, IN) at −70°C. Frozen sections of 6μ and smears of brushings were analyzed by indirect immunofluorescence using mouse ascites monoclonal antibodies 6-C5 to CMV (diluted 1:4000) and 3-G11 to HSV-1 (1:500) (Genetic Systems Corp., Seattle, WA) followed by fluorescein-conjugated goat antimouse antibody (Tago, Inc., Burlington, CA) (*5, 6*). Mean numbers of biopsies from each endoscopy analyzed by immunofluorescence were 1.6 (range 1–4) from the esophagus, 1.2 (range 1–2) from the stomach, 1.7 (range 1–4) from the duodenum, and 1.7 (range 1–3) from the rectum. Usually one section from each biopsy was analyzed for each virus.

Viral cultures. Biopsies were homogenized and inoculated into duplicate tubes of human diploid fibroblasts. Oropharyngeal viral cultures were obtained on or near the day of endoscopy in 47 of the 50 cases. Viral cultures were observed for 6 weeks before being considered negative. CMV and HSV were distinguished by their characteristic cytopathic effects and the range of cell lines infected. HSV isolates were confirmed and typed by indirect immunofluorescence using murine monoclonal antibodies (Genetic Systems Corp., Seattle, WA).

Statistical Methods

Mean weekly scores for severity of nausea and vomiting were compared in three groups of patients with different findings at endoscopy (GVHD, CMV, and unexplained). Assumptions of normality and equal variances were tested by analysis of skewness and kurtosis, and by Hartley's test (*18*). A repeated measures analysis of variance was computed on log-transformed weekly scores (*18*). Duncan's multiple range test was used to further analyze differences detected in the analysis of variance. A one-way analysis of variance was used to compare the mean day of endoscopy for the three groups, and the repeated measures analysis of variance was recomputed using day of endoscopy as a covariate (*18, 19*).

RESULTS

Causes of Nausea and Vomiting

Potential causes of nausea and vomiting were identified in 39 of the 50 cases (78%), 36 by endoscopy or sigmoidoidoscopy and 3 by clinical follow-up (Table 1). In the remaining 11 cases, vomiting was unexplained. Of the 6 patients who had endoscopy repeated for persistent or recurrent vomiting, 5 had different findings at the second endoscopy (Table 2).

Gastrointestinal infections. Gastrointestinal infections occurred alone in 15 cases and in combination with acute intes-

TABLE 1. Signs, symptoms, and endoscopic findings in 50 episodes of persistent vomiting

Causes of nausea and vomiting	n	Clinical and laboratory findings					Endoscopic findings		
		Dysphagia (n)	Fever >38.5°C (n)	Skin GVHD (n)	Stool volume (ml/d) median (range)	Bilirubin (mg/dl) median (range)	Day median (range)[a]	Esophagitis (n)	Cardia gastritis (n)
Gastrointestinal infection alone	15	5	4	4	50 (0–375)	1.2 (0.3–8.4)	53 (27–123)	13	4
Acute intestinal GVHD alone	13	4	3	10	312 (0–1848)	1.4 (0.3–11.7)	28 (19–76)	11	6
Acute GVHD plus infection	8	2	3	6	103 (0–613)	3.9 (0.5–19.4)	51 (34–77)	8	5
Conditions found in follow-up	3	0	1	1	175 (0–412)	1.0 (0.9–1.7)	62 (42–74)	1	1
Unexplained	11	0	1	4	113 (0–653)	1.1 (0.7–6.7)	51 (15–84)	10	8

[a] Day of endoscopy; day 0 is the day of marrow grafting.

TABLE 2. Findings in six patients who had endoscopy repeated for severe vomiting

UPN*	First endoscopy	Therapy	Second endoscopy	Interval in days
2121	*C difficile* colitis	Vancomycin	CMV	24
2088	Normal—unexplained	None	CMV + fungus + GVHD	21
1974	HSV + CMV + GVHD	Acyclovir, cyclosporine	HSV	35
2046	CMV + GVHD	Cyclosporine	Normal—unexplained	32
2077	GVHD	Cyclosporine, prednisolone	HSV + CMV + fungus	48
2115	CMV	None	CMV	22

* Unique patient number.

TABLE 3. Intestinal infection in 23 patients with persistent vomiting

Sites	Single organism		Multiple organisms		
	CMV	HSV	CMV + fungus	CMV + HSV	CMV + HSV + fungus
Esophagus only	6	2	1		1
Esophagus + intestine	9	1		1[a]	
Intestine only[b]	1				

[a] Esophageal HSV and enteric CMV.
[b] Plus 1 case of *C difficile* colitis.

TABLE 4. Sensitivity of diagnostic tests for esophageal and intestinal herpesvirus infections[a]

Test	Number of patients with positive test in esophagus		Number of patients with positive test in intestine	
	CMV (n=17)	HSV (n=5)	CMV (n=11)	HSV (n=1)
Immunofluorescence	6 (35%)[b]	3 (60%)[b]	1 (9%)	1 (100%)
Histology	13 (76%)	1 (20%)	2 (18%)	0 (0%)
Cytology	0 (0%)	3 (60%)	—	—
Culture	10 (59%)	3 (60%)	11 (100%)	0 (0%)

[a] Each patient had each test; number in parentheses is sensitivity of test.
[b] Includes one patient with brushing positive.

tinal GVHD in 8 others (Table 1). The site(s) of infection and causative agent(s) in these 23 cases are shown in Table 3. The presentation of gastrointestinal infections one to four months after transplant was quite nonspecific and variable. Fever was present in only 7 of 23 cases; however, in some of these, fever of unknown origin was a major clinical concern. Only 7 of 21 patients with infective esophagitis complained of dysphagia or chest discomfort, but some of these required continuous intravenous morphine for constant, burning chest pain. Five patients with HSV infection were treated with intravenous acyclovir, and 2 improved; 3 others did not, probably because each had concurrent GVHD or CMV infection. One patient with painful CMV esophagitis received acyclovir and intravenous immune globulin without improvement.

Only 1 of the 18 patients with CMV gastrointestinal infections developed biopsy-confirmed CMV pneumonia and 2 others recovered from suspected CMV pneumonias. Confirmed CMV pneumonia also occurred in 3 of 13 patients with intestinal GVHD alone and in none of 13 patients with neither GVHD or gastrointestinal CMV.

Routine histology or viral culture of biopsy material appeared to be most sensitive in detecting CMV infections (Table 4). However, more biopsies were obtained from each organ for routine histology than for immunohistology, and approximately 20 permanent sections from each biopsy versus 1 frozen section were analyzed for evidence of viral infection. Also, frozen sections of esophagus from seven patients consisted only of squamous epithelium without lamina propria or submucosa. Mucus occasionally produced a nonspecific fluorescent background which complicated analysis of intestinal specimens. Immunofluorescence, cytology and culture each detected three of the five cases of herpetic esophagitis. Immunofluorescence provided essential confirmatory evidence in one patient with suspicious but nondiagnostic cytology. Another patient with herpetic esophagitis had a duodenal biopsy positive for HSV by immunofluorescence but negative by histology and culture. HSV infections were type 1 in four cases with typing available.

Oropharyngeal cultures were obtained within 7 days of endoscopy in 45 cases and within 10 days of endoscopy in 2 others. Cultures were not done in 3 cases. Oropharyngeal cultures correctly predicted the presence or absence and type of viral gastrointestinal infection in 37 of the 47 cases (79%). In most cases of CMV infection, culture results were not available until weeks after endoscopy, however.

Acute intestinal GVHD. Acute GVHD occurred alone in 13 cases and was present in combination with infection in 8 others. Skin GVHD was seen in 16 of 21 cases (76%) with gastrointestinal GVHD and in 9 of 29 (31%) without gastrointestinal GVHD. Median stool volume was somewhat higher in cases with gastrointestinal GVHD, but overlap among groups was great; only 2 of the 21 cases with gastrointestinal GVHD had stool volumes over 500 ml/day, the minimum level recognized in the current clinical staging classification (*13*). Serum bilirubin also was not discriminatory because of overlap with other groups. However, patients with gastrointestinal GVHD and no infection had an earlier onset of vomiting than did patients with CMV alone (mean day of endoscopy was 33.5±5.8 vs. 54.3±5.5, $P = .05$). Patients with unexplained vomiting were endoscoped later than those with GVHD and earlier than those with CMV, but not significantly so.

Most patients did not receive additional immunosuppressive therapy for acute intestinal GVHD diagnosed by endoscopy because of the lack of diarrheal illness in most, as well as the frequent presence of simultaneous infections discovered at endoscopy. However, some received treatment during the postendoscopy observation for progressive intestinal GVHD or severe involvement of skin or liver. Six of 13 patients with GVHD alone had progression of intestinal GVHD, but seven remained at stage 0. Progression of intestinal GVHD was associated with diarrhea and worsening of nausea and vomiting.

The accuracy of upper gastrointestinal (gastric or duodenal) and rectal biopsies were compared in 11 patients with histologic evidence of intestinal GVHD who had simultaneous biopsies at both sites. Rectal and gastroduodenal biopsies were discordant in 8 of 11 cases and agreed in 3 cases.

Conditions discovered during follow-up. Three patients with neither GVHD nor infections at endoscopy had causes of nausea and vomiting discovered soon after endoscopy. One patient with bilateral subdural hematomas had resolution of nausea and vomiting after craniotomies. Another patient had *Staphylococcus epidermidis* bacteremia; vomiting ceased after antibiotic treatment and removal of an infected central venous catheter. A third patient developed a slowly progressive encephalitis of unknown cause with cognitive and cranial nerve deficits and very high cerebrospinal fluid protein; nausea and vomiting slowly resolved with improvement of the encephalitis.

Unexplained nausea and vomiting. Eleven patients with persistent nausea and vomiting had neither GVHD nor infections at endoscopy and had no other causes discovered during follow-up.

Follow-up of Patients with GVHD, CMV, and Unexplained Vomiting

Patients with gastrointestinal GVHD alone and those with unexplained vomiting improved significantly over the four-week observation period ($P = .01$), but those with CMV alone were unchanged (Table 5). Patients with GVHD alone had more severe presenting symptoms than those with CMV ($P = .05$). At the end of the four-week observation period, patients with GVHD alone and CMV alone had similarly severe nausea, but those with unexplained nausea and vomiting had significantly less severe symptoms ($P = .05$).

TABLE 5. Average severity of nausea and vomiting by week in three groups of patients[a]

Group	n	Week relative to endoscopy			
		−1	1	2	3
CMV alone	10[b]	1.50	1.57	1.26	1.16
GVHD alone	13	2.07[c]	1.46[d]	1.06[d]	1.12[d]
Unexplained	11	1.83	1.43	0.88[c]	0.66[c,d]

[a] 0: none; 1: mild; 2: moderate; 3: severe.
[b] Second study of UPN 2115 was dropped from this analysis.
[c] Significantly different from CMV group in same week ($P = .05$).
[d] Significantly different from week-1 in same group ($P = .01$).

TABLE 6. Causes of esophagitis in 43 endoscopies

Esophageal infections		21
CMV	15*	
HSV	4	
CMV + Fungus	1	
CMV + HSV + Fungus	1	
Acute esophageal GVHD alone		3
Idiopathic		19

* 1 patient had both CMV and acute esophageal GVHD.

Endoscopic Abnormalities

Esophageal ulcerations or erosions were present in 43 of the 50 cases, usually associated with infection or acute esophageal GVHD (Table 6). Nineteen cases of esophagitis had neither and presumably represented reflux esophagitis. Diffuse, shallow ulceration of the distal esophagus was the most common endoscopic finding in CMV esophagitis, but was not specific for this. Herpetic esophagitis could sometimes be recognized by shallow, oval ulcers with elevated margins in the midesophagus. The two cases of fungal esophagitis lacked characteristic pseudomembranous plaques. Dysphagia was usually absent in patients with esophagitis (Table 1). Major upper gastrointestinal bleeding occurred in 4 of the 50 cases and was always due to esophageal ulceration.

Inflammation of the gastric cardia was present in 24 of the 50 cases (Table 1). This appeared as erythema, edema, and submucosal hemorrhage, sometimes extending into the gastric fundus and body. Biopsies showed only nonspecific inflammation and hemorrhage, without evidence of infection or GVHD, suggesting that these changes were due to the trauma of repeated retching (*20*).

Duodenal and rectal mucosa were usually normal or only slightly reddened in appearance, even when acute GVHD or CMV was present.

Complications of Endoscopy

Two examinations resulted in complications. One patient bled from an ulcerated rectal biopsy site 16 days after grasp forceps biopsy and required transanal ligation of the bleeding artery. A second patient with 40,000 platelets/mm^3 developed a massive hematoma of the descending duodenum after biopsies and required duodenal resection below the ampulla of Vater. Although he recovered from this operation, he later died of CMV pneumonia.

DISCUSSION

Nausea and vomiting are common after allogeneic marrow transplantation, may persist for weeks or months, and result in significant morbidity and cost. This study shows that in a majority of patients with enigmatic vomiting, a specific diagnosis can be made by endoscopy and clinical follow-up. Specific causes of nausea and vomiting were identified in 37 (78%) of 50 consecutive cases. Recognition of these conditions provided useful clinical information leading to avoidance of potentially harmful immunosuppression in infected patients, specific antimicrobial therapy for non-CMV infections, evacuation of subdural hematomas in one patient, acid reduction therapy in patients with reflux esophagitis, and early recognition of intestinal GVHD in patients with progressive disease. Useful prognostic information was also derived regarding CMV infection: CMV gastrointestinal infection is associated with protracted nausea and vomiting but infrequently leads to CMV pneumonia.

Whether or not the conditions identified actually caused nausea and vomiting, or were merely present by coincidence because infections and GVHD are common after marrow transplantation, cannot be determined in a study of this nature. A specific answer to this question would have required endoscopic biopsies in asymptomatic marrow transplant patients. However, the observation that patients with gastrointestinal CMV infection have more protracted nausea and vomiting suggests a causal role for this organism. Nausea and vomiting were found in 11 of 17 marrow transplant patients with viral esophagitis endoscoped for indications other than vomiting in our recent retrospective review (*4*). Of 11 patients with vomiting in that study, 6 had CMV esophagitis, 3 had HSV esophagitis, and 2 had both CMV and HSV. Nausea and vomiting also occur in CMV enteritis (*21–23*). Mid-gut infection with CMV is common in marrow transplant patients, and can lead to ulceration, perforation, bleeding, and protein loss (*14, 21–25*). HSV infection was less common than CMV in the present series, possibly because of the frequent use of prophylactic acyclovir, or because HSV esophagitis is less likely to cause vomiting.

Accurate diagnosis of gastrointestinal infections required a combination of endoscopic biopsies, brushings, and cultures, a conclusion also reached in our recent study of esophageal infections (*4*). The significant contribution of immunohistology to the rapid diagnosis of CMV pneumonia prompted this application to endoscopically obtained biopsies (*5*). Although in the present study this technique demonstrated CMV infection less frequently than did routine histology or culture, it appeared quite sensitive in light of the relatively small amount of tissue analyzed. In seven patients, the esophageal frozen biopsy consisted only of squamous epithelium. These biopsies were inadequate, since esophageal CMV is usually identified in scattered endothelial cells and fibroblasts within the lamina propria, but only rarely in the epithelium (*24*). The effectiveness of immunohistology was further reduced by nonspecific fluorescence produced by intestinal mucus. Viral oropharyngeal culture accurately predicted the presence or absence and type of viral gastrointestinal infection in almost 80% of cases, but a major limitation of viral cultures is the several weeks often required for isolation and identification (*25, 26*). Precise identification of herpesvirus intestinal infections is important since acyclovir is effective therapy for HSV infections, and dihydroxy propoxymethyl guanine, a new antiviral agent, has shown promise against CMV (*27, 28*).

Mechanisms of nausea and vomiting in severe acute GVHD (clinical stages II to IV) remain undefined, but many of these cases have small intestinal mucosal denudation, transmural inflammation, and abnormal motility (*14, 29–31*). The observation that nausea and vomiting are common manifestations of clinically unsuspected GVHD apparent only on histologic examination suggests that nausea may result from relatively minimal intestinal involvement or may not be related to the extent of mucosal ulceration. Upper gastrointestinal (duodenal or gastric) biopsies often showed acute GVHD when rectal biopsies were normal and vice versa. This discrepancy probably results from the patchy distribution of early GVHD lesions and the tendency of GVHD to be less severe in the proximal and distal gut (*13, 14, 30, 31*).

In 11 (22%) of the 50 cases, nausea and vomiting remained unexplained even after endoscopy and clinical follow-up. These patients could have had unresolved chemoradiation conditioning effects, other conditions that could not be discovered by the methods used in this study, or psychological causes of nausea and vomiting. Effects of conditioning on the intestine are unlikely to cause nausea and vomiting more than 2 weeks after transplant. Postconditioning diarrhea usually resolves by this time, and intestinal absorptive function and protein loss return to normal unless early acute GVHD supervenes (*11, 14, 32, 33*). Furthermore, characteristic histologic features of intestinal chemoradiation toxicity—nuclear atypia, flattened crypt epithelium, and abnormal surface cells (*12*)—were not seen in any patient. However, the study methods would not have detected abnormal gastrointestinal motility as a potential cause of unexplained vomiting (*34*). For example, gastric emptying may be delayed by high-calorie parenteral nutrion; drugs (including antiemetics) with anticholinergic effects, narcotic analgesics, total-body irradiation, viral gastroenteritis, and reflux esophagitis (*35–39*).

The findings of this prospective study suggest that causes of enigmatic nausea and vomiting can be found in approximately three-fourths of allogeneic marrow recipients studied by endoscopy and clinical follow-up. Unsuspected gastrointestinal diseases, chiefly herpesvirus infections and acute GVHD, should be considered before attributing enigmatic vomiting to psychological causes. The advent of effective antiviral drugs makes diagnosis of specific infections important and offers hope of relief of protracted nausea and vomiting in some marrow transplant patients.

Acknowledgments. We are indebted to Mary D. Browne for her technical skills and to the physicians, nurses, and ward clerks who cared for these patients.

REFERENCES

1. Fetting JH, Grochow LB, Folstein MF, Ettinger DS, Colvin M. The course of nausea and vomiting after high-dose cyclophosphamide. Cancer Treat Rep 1983; 66: 1487.
2. Lenssen P, Moe GL, Cheney CL, Aker SN, Deeg HJ. Parenteral nutrition in marrow transplant recipients after discharge from the hospital. Exp Hematol 1983; 11: 974.
3. Laszlo J. Antiemetics and cancer chemotherapy. Baltimore: Williams & Wilkins, 1983.
4. McDonald GB, Sharma P, Hackman RC, Meyers JD, Thomas ED. Esophageal infections in immunosuppressed patients after marrow transplantation. Gastroenterology 1985; 88: 1111.
5. Hackman RC, Myerson D, Meyers JD, et al. Rapid diagnosis of cytomegalovirus pneumonia by tissue immunofluorescence with a murine monoclonal antibody. J Infect Dis 1985; 151: 325.
6. Goldstein LC, Corey L, McDougall JK, Tolentino E, Nowinski RC. Monoclonal antibodies to herpes simplex viruses: use in antigenic typing and rapid diagnosis. J Infect Dis 1983; 147: 829.

7. Thomas ED, Storb R, Clift RA, et al. Bone-marrow transplantation. N Engl J Med 1975; 292: 832.
8. Storb R, Doney KC, Thomas ED, et al. Marrow transplantation with or without donor buffy coat cells for 65 transfused aplastic anemia patients. Blood 1982; 59: 236.
9. Buckner CD, Clift RA, Thomas ED, et al. Allogeneic marrow transplantation for acute non-lymphoblastic leukemia in relapse using fractionated total body irradiation. Leuk Res 1982; 6: 389.
10. Deeg HJ, Storb R, Thomas ED, et al. Cyclosporine as prophylaxis for graft-versus-host disease: a randomized study in patients undergoing marrow transplantation for acute nonlymphoblastic leukemia. Blood 1985; 65: 1325.
11. Epstein RJ, McDonald GB, Sale GE, Shulman HM, Thomas ED. The diagnostic accuracy of the rectal biopsy in acute graft-versus-host disease: a prospective study of thirteen patients. Gastroenterology 1980; 78: 764.
12. Weiden PL. Graft-vs-host disease in allogeneic marrow transplantation. In: Gale RP, Fox CF, eds. Biology of bone marrow transplantation. New York: Academic, 1980: 37.
13. Snover DC, Weisdorf SA, Vercellotti GM, Rank B, Hutton S, McGlave P. A histopathologic study of gastric and small intestinal graft-versus-host disease following allogeneic bone marrow transplantation. Hum Pathol 1985; 16: 387.
14. McDonald GB, Sale GE. The human gastrointestinal tract after allogeneic marrow transplantation. In: Sale GE, Shulman HM, eds. The pathology of bone marrow transplantation. New York: Masson, 1984: 77.
15. Snover DC, Weisdorf SA, Ramsay NK, McGlave P, Kersey JH. Hepatic graft versus host disease: a study of the predictive value of liver biopsy in diagnosis. Hepatology 1984; 4: 123.
16. Shulman HM, McDonald GB. Liver disease after marrow transplantation. In: Sale GE, Shulman HM, eds. The pathology of bone marrow transplantation. New York: Masson, 1984: 104.
17. Shulman HM, Sale GE. Pathology of acute and chronic cutaneous GVHD. In: Sale GE, Shulman HE, eds. The pathology of bone marrow transplantation. New York: Masson, 1984; 40.
18. Ott L. An introduction to statistical methods and data analysis. Boston: Duxbury, 1977.
19. Winer BG. Statistical principles in experimental design. New York: McGraw-Hill, 1962.
20. Miller G. Gastric mucosal prolapse (Lett). Dig Dis Sci 1985; 30: 505.
21. Tytgat GN, Huibregtse K, Schellekens PTA, Feltkamp-Vroom TH. Clinical and immunologic observations in a patient with late onset immunodeficiency. Gastroenterology 1979; 76: 1458.
22. Tajima T. An autopsy case of primary cytomegalic inclusion enteritis with remarkable hypoproteinemia. Acta Pathol Jpn 1974; 24: 151.
23. Simmons RL, Matas AJ, Rattazzi LC, Balfour HH, Howard RJ, Najarian JS. Clinical characteristics of the lethal cytomegalovirus infection following renal transplantation. Surgery 1977; 82: 537.
24. Myerson D, Hackman RC, Nelson JA, Ward DC, McDougall JK. Widespread presence of histologically occult cytomegalovirus. Hum Pathol 1984; 15: 430.
25. Spencer GD, Shulman HM, Myerson D, Thomas ED, McDonald GB. Diffuse intestinal ulceration after marrow transplantation: a clinical-pathological study of 13 patients. Human Pathol 1986; 17: 621.
26. Stagno S, Pass RF, Reynolds DW, Alford CA. Diagnosis of cytomegalovirus infections. In: Nahmias AJ, Dowdle WR, Schinazi RF, eds. The human herpesviruses. New York: Elsevier; 1981: 363.
27. Shepp DH, Dandliker PS, deMiranda P, et al. Activity of 9-[2-hydroxy-1-(hydroxymethyl) ethoxymethyl] guanine in the treatment of cytomegalovirus pneumonia. Ann Intern Med 1985; 103: 368.
28. Masur H, Lane HC, Palestine A, et al. Effect of 9-(1,3-dihydroxy-2-propoxymethyl) guanine on serious cytomegalovirus disease in eight immunosuppressed homosexual men. Ann Intern Med 1986; 104: 41.
29. McDonald GB. Graft-versus-host-disease: effects on the intestine. In: Chadwick VS, Phillips SF, eds. The small intestine. London: Butterworth, 1982: 203.
30. Beschorner WE, Yardley JH, Tutschka P, Santos G. Deficiency of intestinal immunity with graft-versus-host disease in humans. J Infect Dis 1981; 144: 38.
31. Sale GE, McDonald GB, Shulman HM, Thomas ED. Gastrointestinal graft-versus-host disease in man: a clinicopathologic study of the rectal biopsy. Am J Surg Pathol 1979; 3: 291.
32. Weisdorf SA, Salati LM, Longsdorf JA, Ramsay NKC, Sharp HL. Graft-versus-host disease of the intestine: a protein losing enteropathy characterized by fecal alpha-1-antitrypsin. Gastroenterology 1983; 85: 1076.
33. Chatti N, Jobin G, Perreault C, Lebrun M. Protein losing enteropathy and malabsorption in patients undergoing allogeneic bone marrow transplantation [Abstract]. Gastroenterology 1984; 86: 1045.
34. Malagelada JR, Camilleri M. Unexplained vomiting: a diagnostic challenge. Ann Intern Med 1984; 101: 211.
35. MacGregor IL, Wiley ZD, Lavigne ME, Way LE. Slowed rate of gastric emptying of solid food in man by high caloric parenteral nutrition. Am J Surg 1979; 138: 652.
36. Minami H, McCallum RW. The physiology and pathophysiology of gastric emptying in humans. Gastroenterology 1984; 86: 1592.
37. Dubois A, Jacobus JP, Grissom MP, Eng RR, Conklin JJ. Altered gastric emptying and prevention of radiation-induced vomiting in dogs. Gastroenterology 1984; 86: 444.
38. Meeroff JC, Schreiber DS, Trier JS, Blacklow NR. Abnormal gastric motor function in viral gastroenteritis. Ann Intern Med 1980; 92: 370.
39. McCallum RW, Berkowitz DM, Lerner E. Gastric emptying in patients with gastroesophageal reflux. Gastroenterology 1981; 80: 285.

Received 29 October 1985.
Accepted 3 March 1986.

0041-1337/86/4206-0608$02.00/0
TRANSPLANTATION
Vol. 42, No. 6

IMMUNOGLOBULIN CLASS AND SPECIFICITY OF ANTIBODIES CAUSING POSITIVE T CELL CROSSMATCHES

RELATIONSHIP TO RENAL TRANSPLANT OUTCOME[1]

J.R. CHAPMAN, C.J. TAYLOR, A. TING, AND P.J. MORRIS

Nuffield Department of Surgery, University of Oxford, John Radcliffe Hospital, Headington, Oxford, OX3 9DU, England

A group of 42 renal transplants performed in the presence of a T-cell-positive crossmatch were analyzed to determine the class and specificity of the donor-reactive cytotoxic antibodies. Dithiothreitol (DTT) was used to reduce IgM antibodies and a monoclonal antibody directed at a monomorphic determinant present on all HLA class I antigens (PA2.6) was used to inhibit cytotoxicity of anti-HLA class I antibodies. Sera from 26 of the positive crossmatches were considered to be autoreactive, and the positive crossmatch proved to be due to IgM and not directed at HLA class I in each case. One year graft survival was 100% in the 5 living-related and 60% in the 21 cadaver donor transplants, of which 10 were regrafts. Of the 42 positive crossmatches, 16 were not due to autoantibody. One was positive in the current serum taken at the time of transplantation, and this graft was rejected hyperacutely, while 15 were positive with peak but not current serum samples. Of the positive crossmatches, 12 were inhibited by PA2.6 demonstrating that they were directed at HLA class I antigens. PA2.6 inhibition could not be shown in 3 and in 1 DTT reduction was technically unsatisfactory. While 4 of the 7 positive crossmatches due to IgM antibodies were successful, the 7 transplants performed with positive crossmatches due to IgG antibodies all failed. DTT reduction and inhibition of cytotoxicity by PA2.6 helps to define positive crossmatches with donor T cells that are not associated with graft failure. Transplantation in the presence of a peak positive T cell crossmatch due to an anti-HLA antibody might only be successful if the antibody in the peak serum is of the IgM class.

A positive T cell crossmatch assessed by a lymphocytotoxicity assay between the patient's serum and the renal donor's lymphocytes remains the best predictor of poor graft outcome, but does not (*1–3*)—and has never (*4–6*)—implied immediate graft failure in every case. Increasing numbers of sensitized patients are appearing on the waiting lists of most transplant centers (*7*), and for those who are highly sensitized the best hope of achieving a successful graft is to exploit some of the exceptions to the general rule. Two situations have been distinguished in which the chance of a successful outcome is higher than the chance of failure. The first is when the positive crossmatch is due to autoantibody—and this is perhaps most clearly demonstrable in the HLA identical living-related transplants that have been successfully performed despite a positive T cell crossmatch with serum taken on the day of the transplant (*8*). The second is when a positive crossmatch, not due to autoantibody, occurs with serum taken at the peak of a patient's sensitization some months or years before the transplant, but is negative with serum taken at the time of transplantation (*9*). In both these situations however, a number of grafts still fail rapidly because of rejection, especially in the case of regrafts, and it is possible that this is because of imperfect definition of relevant and irrelevant antibodies. A number of patients develop autoantibodies alone but many have both autoantibodies and anti-HLA antibodies, and in this situation it can be more difficult to ensure that a positive crossmatch is only due to the autoantibody. Graft survival in recipients of first grafts with a peak positive crossmatch is better than in recipients of regrafts (*9*), and this might imply that the peak positive crossmatch cannot always be ignored if a previous graft has been rejected.

Since 1976 we have had a policy in Oxford of transplanting patients in the presence of a positive T cell crossmatch with the donor, when we have believed that is has been due to autoantibody. In the past two years we have also performed a number of transplants in patients with a peak positive, current negative T cell crossmatch that was not due to autoantibody. We report here an analysis of this series of peak positive current negative crossmatch transplants. We have used dithiothreitol (DTT)* reduction to determine whether the antibody was of the IgG or IgM class. In addition we have determined whether the target of the antibody was HLA class I antigen or not by inhibition of the crossmatch with a noncytotoxic monoclonal antibody directed at a monomorphic determinant of HLA class I antigens. The aim of the study was to determine whether these tests helped to distinguish between peak positive current crossmatches associated with success and those associated with failure.

MATERIALS AND METHODS

Serological techniques. The standard lymphocytotoxicity assay employed donor spleen or lymph node T and B lymphocytes separated with neuraminidase treated sheep red blood cells. The complement dependent cytotoxicity assay (CDC) was performed in a standard microtiter plate with 1 μl of serum and 1 μl of donor cells at a concentration of 2×10^6/ml incubated for 30 min at 22°C. Rabbit complement was added for a further incubation of 2 hr at 22°C. Cell lysis was assessed under phase contrast microscopy using eosin dye exclusion. Lysis of more than 25% of the cells above background in duplicate or triplicate wells was considered positive for the purpose of defining the titer of diluted sera.

Serum samples were collected from patients at monthly intervals or more frequently after blood transfusion or after

[1] This work was supported by a grant from the Medical Research Council of the United Kingdom. JRC is an MRC Training Fellow.

* Abbreviations used: CDC, complement-dependent cytotoxicity; CLL, chronic lymphatic leukemia; DTT, dithiothreitol; 2-ME, 2-mercaptoethanol; PBL, peripheral blood lymphocytes; PBS, phosphate-buffered saline.

transplantation. These sera were screened routinely against panels of 40 different peripheral blood lymphocytes (PBL) and cells from 30 patients with chronic lymphatic leukemia (CLL), since autoreactive antibodies do not react or react sparingly with CLL cells (*10*). In addition many of the samples were screened against panels of T and B lymphocytes separated from the panel of PBL. Serum samples selected for crossmatching included those with the highest panel reactivities and the current samples. In all cases donor lymphocytes were preserved in liquid nitrogen and further analysis was performed with stored sera and donor cells.

Determination of immunoglobulin class. The reducing agent DTT was used to reduce IgM antibodies. DTT has been used in the study of antibodies to red cell antigens as a less obnoxious reagent than 2 mercaptoethanol (2-ME) (*11–14*). Sera in 1-μl volumes were dispensed onto a microtiter plate as neat serum and as doubling dilutions in Terasaki Park Medium (Gibco, Paisley, Scotland) to beyond the endpoint of cytotoxicity. Duplicate wells were left untreated, had 1 μl of 0.01M DTT added, or had 1 μl of phosphate-buffered saline (PBS) added. The trays were incubated for 30 min at 37°C before addition of the test cells for 30 min at 22°C. Rabbit complement with 0.002 M cystine was added and incubated for a further 2 hours at 22°C. Cell lysis was assessed using the same technique as above. A known IgM autoantibody was tested with each batch of DTT to confirm digestion.

Inhibition of antibodies to HLA class I antigens. Donor cells were suspended at a concentration of 2×10^6/ml and three equal aliquots were taken. The first remained untreated to act as control cells, while the second and third were centrifuged and resuspended in the same volume of a saturating concentration of the noncytotoxic mouse monoclonal antibody PA2.6 (*15*). This antibody is directed at a monomorphic determinant of all HLA class I antigens. Following incubation for 1 hr at 22°C the second aliquot was placed at 4°C, and the third washed and incubated for a further hour at 4°C with an affinity purified $F(ab')_2$ fragment of goat antimouse IgG heavy and light chains (Pel Freeze, Rogers, Arkansas). Finally the third aliquot was washed and resuspended in Terasaki Park medium at the original concentration. The three aliquots were tested in duplicate against the selected sera neat and in doubling dilutions using the standard cytotoxicity assay as above. On each occasion one or more known specific anti-HLA sera were used to confirm successful inhibition of cytotoxicity.

Renal transplantation. Patients receiving renal allografts with positive crossmatches that, at the time of transplantation were thought to be due to autoantibodies, were immunosuppressed in the same way as those with negative crossmatches. The majority received either azathioprine and low dose prednisolone or cyclosporine for 90 days with conversion to azathioprine and prednisolone (*16*). The group who were transplanted with a peak positive, current negative crossmatch that was not due to autoantibody all received cyclosporine and prednisolone, some having azathioprine in addition. Acute rejection was treated with bolus doses of 0.5 G methylprednisolone in all groups.

RESULTS

Control sera. A total of 25 sera, obtained mainly from multiparous women, that had previously been extensively characterized for use as reagents for tissue typing at the HLA-A, B, and C loci were reduced with DTT. The titer of lymphocytotoxicity of the untreated serum was compared with the titer of the serum after reduction with DTT for 30 min at 37°C (Table 1). In 13 combinations of serum and lymphocytes there was no change in the titer; in 14 combinations there was a decrease in titer by one dilution; in no serum was the reduction more than one titer and no serum lost cytotoxicity when tested neat.

A total of 21 autoreactive sera had been collected from patients awaiting renal transplantation following screening on panel cells and confirmation of autoreactivity with the patients' own lymphocytes. In contrast to the results with anti-HLA sera, when DTT was used to reduce the 21 sera with autoantibodies directed at both T and B cells, autologous cytotoxicity was completely abolished in 20. The one incompletely reduced autoreactive serum was reduced from a titer of 1/1024 to a kill of only 25% of the cells in neat serum. The highest titer of the other autoantibodies tested was 1/32, by comparison, emphasizing the most unusual nature of this one serum.

Inhibition of cytotoxicity by the monoclonal antibody PA2.6 was also tested with 25 sera directed at specific HLA-A, B, and C antigens (Table 1). There sera were used with a wide variety of cells including fresh peripheral blood lymphocytes, fresh lymph node or spleen lymphocytes, and frozen/thawed cells from those sources, in a total of 97 combinations. In each case cytotoxicity was inhibited by more than one doubling dilution, and in the majority of combinations using fresh cells, cytotoxicity was completely inhibited using PA2.6 with the addition of the goat antimouse antibody. In contrast the technique was not able to inhibit by more than one doubling dilution, the cytotoxicity of 17 sera containing autoantibodies using autologous cell targets, and in 12 cases the titer was actually unchanged.

On the basis of these experiments the criterion chosen for DTT reduction was that all cytotoxicity should be removed in neat serum. The criterion for inhibition by PA2.6 was that cytotoxicity should be completely removed or reduced by more than one doubling dilution. These definitions were then used for interpretation of the renal transplant crossmatches.

To test the ability of these techniques to discriminate between antibodies when present in a single serum sample, we studied the family of a patient awaiting renal transplantation. The sera of this highly sensitized patient was known to have both autoreactivity and antibodies to class I antigens as a result of previous testing with autologous cells and panels of normal cells and cells from patients with CLL. She had a positive crossmatch with all of her six siblings; one of these was HLA-identical, three were haploidentical, and two did not share either haplotype. DTT reduction and inhibition by PA2.6 were

TABLE 1. Control sera reactions using specific anti-HLA sera and target cells expressing the relevant antigens, and autoreactive sera and autologous target cells after DTT reduction or inhibition of cytotoxicity by the monoclonal antibody PA2.6 (antisera reacting with the following specificities: HLA A 1, 3, 9, 10, 11, 32; HLA B 7, 8, 12, 15, 35, 51; HLA Bw6, Cw3, Cw4)

A. DTT reduction	Number of sera	Number of test combinations	Negative with neat serum
Anti-HLA sera	25	27	0
Autoreactive sera	21	21	20

B. Inhibition with PA2.6	Number of sera	Number of test combinations	Number of tests reduced by more than one dilution
Anti-HLA sera	25	97	97
Autoreactive sera	17	17	0

used to distinguish between the anti-HLA antibody and the autoantibody when the serum was tested with autologous cells and those of her six siblings (Table 2). The autologous and HLA-identical lymphocyte reactions were DTT-reduced and not inhibited by PA2.6 implying an IgM non-HLA antibody—while reactivity to the five mismatched siblings was inhibited by PA2.6 and not DTT-reduced, implying an IgG anti-HLA antibody.

TABLE 2. Results from testing the serum from a highly sensitized patient known to have both autoantibody and anti-HLA antibody in a single serum against autologous cells and cells from the patient's six siblings

Lymphocytes	Cytotoxicity	Reduction by DTT	Inhibited by PA2.6
Patient	+	Yes	No
Siblings:			
HLA-identical	+	Yes	No
1-haplotype match	+	No	Yes
1-haplotype match	+	No	Yes
1-haplotype match	+	No	Yes
Complete mismatch	+	No	Yes
Complete mismatch	+	No	Yes

Transplant crossmatches. A total of 42 transplants performed in 41 patients across positive T cell crossmatches had both the relevant serum from the patient available and viable lymphocytes from the donor stored in liquid nitrogen. One transplant has been followed for only two months, but the remaining grafts have failed or been followed for more than 3 months, and all but five have been followed for more than one year after transplantation.

Positive crossmatches due to non-HLA antibodies. A total of 26 transplants had positive crossmatches that were reduced completely by DTT and were not inhibited by PA2.6 (Table 3). Of these transplants, 5 were from living-related donors and 21 were from cadaver donors; 9 of these crossmatches were positive with serum taken at the time of transplantation and 17 were only positive with the peak reactive serum and were negative when current serum samples were tested. All five recipients of living-related grafts had autoantibody in the relevant serum

TABLE 3. Positive T cell crossmatches caused by autoantibodies[a]

	Graft No. for patient	Autotest	Donor crossmatch		Reduced by DTT	Inhibited by PA2.6	Outcome	Graft histology
			Peak	Current				
1	1 LRD	TB	+	+	Y	N	Success	
2	1 LRD	TB	+	+	Y	ND	Success	
3	1 LRD	TB	+	+	Y	N	Success	
4	1 LRD	TB	+	−	Y	N	Success	
5	1 LRD	TB	+	+	Y	N	Success	
6	1	TB	+	−	Y	N	Died with functioning graft day 27	
7	3	TB	+	+	Y	N	Fail day 0	Acute rejection
8	1	TB	+	+	Y	N	Died with functioning graft day 71	
9	2	TB	+	−	Y	N	Success	
10	1	TB	+	−	Y	N	Success	
11	2	TB	+	−	Y	N	Success	
12	1	TB	+	+	Y	N	Success	
13	1	TB	+	+	Y	N	Success	
14	2	TB	+	−	Y	N	Faill day 8	Acute rejection
15	1	TB	+	−	Y	N	Success	
16	1	TB	+	−	Y	N	Fail day 356	Chronic rejection
17	1	TB	+	−	Y	N	Success	
18	1	TB	+	−	Y	N	Fail day 0	Ischemia
19	2	TB	+	−	Y	N	Fail day 97	Chronic rejection
20	2	TB	+	−	Y	N	Success	
21	1	TB	+	+	Y	N	Success	
22	3	TB	+	−	Y	N	Fail day 680	Chronic rejection
23	2	TB	+	−	(Y)	N	Success	
24	2	B	+	−	Y	N	Success	
25	1	TB	+	−	Y	N	Success	
26	2	TB	+	−	Y	N	Fail day 0	Acute rejection

[a] TB: positive T and B cell autoreactivity; Y: reduced by DTT; (Y): reduced from a titer of 1/1024 to 25% kill in neat serum by DTT; N: not inhibited by PA2.6; LRD: living-related donor; ND: not done.

and all the grafts are functioning. Of the 21 recipients of cadaver kidneys, 20 had autoantibodies that reacted with both T and B lymphocytes. One patient (No. 24, Table 3) had autoantibody reactive with her B, but not T, lymphocytes. The graft was HLA-compatible with the recipient and it had thus been thought that this crossmatch was not due to an anti-HLA antibody. However she would be included as a nonautoreactive peak positive current negative crossmatch in most series. Of the 21 grafts, 4 were lost within two weeks, 3 (all regrafts) were lost from rejection—and 1, which had a cold ischemia time of 45 hr, never functioned and did not have evidence of acute rejection on histology. There were 2 patients who died with functioning grafts, one from sepsis and the other from a myocardial infarct, within the first three months; 3 further grafts (1 first graft and 2 regrafts) were lost from chronic rejection at 97, 356, and 680 days. Graft survival was thus 72% at three months, and 60% at one year for the cadaver grafts, ten of which were regrafts, while the living-related grafts had a 100% one-year survival rate. It is worthy of note that only 3 grafts were lost from rejection in the first few weeks after transplantation.

Positive crossmatches due to anti-HLA antibodies. The monoclonal antibody PA2.6 inhibited cytotoxicity in 13 instances, confirming that these positive crossmatches were due to antibody directed at MHC class I products (Table 4). In one patient (number 42) the activity was present in serum taken on the day of the transplant. This patient, who has already been reported in detail (*17*), suffered hyperacute rejection of the graft with anti-HLA Cw-5 activity in the current serum sample. In the remaining 12 positive crossmatches, the activity was present in the peak but not current sera. It was thought that 11 were directed at HLA antigens because of the absence of autoreactivity and 1 had both anti-HLA and autoantibody. A further 3 patients have been transplanted with peak positive crossmatches when autoantibody has not been detected. Patient No. 31 had a crossmatch that was neither DTT-reduced nor inhibited by PA2.6—but, because of the high number of contaminating B cells in the preparation, this may have been due to IgG antibody directed at class II antigens. Patient No. 32 had a crossmatch that was not DTT-reduced, but inhibition with PA2.6 was technically unsatisfactory because of high levels of background cytotoxicity (although the reactivity was likely to be directed at HLA class I and was IgG). The crossmatch for patient No. 41 was clearly detectable using fresh T lymphocytes but was too weak to reproduce reliably with the higher levels of background cytotoxicity associated with the use of frozen/thawed cells.

The sera reactivity in a total of seven positive crossmatches was not reduced by DTT (Nos. 27–33, Table 4), implying that this reactivity was due to anti-HLA class I IgG antibodies. All 7 failed immediately or within weeks of transplantation. By contrast 4 of the 7 transplants in which the positive crossmatch appeared to be due to IgM anti-HLA (Nos. 34–40, Table 4) were successful; 2 rejected early and 1 failed on day 87.

DISCUSSION

The study has demonstrated that reduction with DTT and inhibition of cytotoxicity with a noncytotoxic monoclonal antibody are simple and reproducible techniques. They enable distinction to be made between both IgG and IgM anti-HLA class I antibodies and IgM non-HLA autoreactive antibodies in the sera of patients awaiting renal transplantation. DTT reduction adds 30 min to the duration of a standard lymphocytotoxicity test and can be interpreted on the basis of the result with undiluted serum in all but the most exceptional situations. Inhibition with PA2.6 adds betwen 2 and 3 hr and requires careful titration of all the reagents involved, but is a reliable technique that could be used in all tissue typing laboratories.

Our data using known sera and reactions that can be interpreted independently of these techniques have shown that all T cell autoantibodies tested were predominantly or exclusively IgM, and that 25 of our tissue typing anti-sera are IgG. PA2.6 inhibited all the allosera with known specificities for HLA-A,

TABLE 4. Relationship between class and specificity of antibodies causing a positive crossmatch and graft outcome[a]

	Graft No. for patient	Crossmatch		Reduced by DTT	Inhibited by PA2.6	Outcome	Graft histology
		Donor	Auto				
Peak positive current negative crossmatches (nonautoreactive):							
27	2	TB	—	N	Y	Fail day 0	Acute rejection
28	1	TB	—	N	Y	Fail day 7	Acute rejection
29	2	TB	—	N	Y	Fail day 29	Acute rejection
30	3	TB	TB	N	Y	Fail day 9	Acute rejection
31	1	TB	—	N	N	Fail day 44	Acute rejection
32	2	TB	—	N	?	Fail day 0	Acute rejection
33	3	TB	—	N	Y	Fail day 0	Acute rejection
34	2	TB	—	Y	Y	Success	
35	2	TB	—	Y	Y	Success	
36	2	TB	—	Y	Y	Success	
37	3	TB	—	Y	Y	Success	
38	2	TB	—	Y	Y	Fail day 83	Chronic rejection
39	2	TB	—	Y	Y	Fail day 4	Acute rejection
40	3	TB	—	Y	Y	Fail day 43	Acute rejection
41	2	TB	—	?	?	Success	
Current positive non-autoreactive crossmatch:[b]							
42	4	TB	—	N	Y	Fail day 0	Hyperacute rejection

[a] ?: technically unsatisfactory test; N: No; Y: Yes; TB: positive test with donor or auto T and B lymphocytes.

[b] Anti-HLA Cw-5 antibody (*17*).

B, and C locus antigens that were tested, but it has not inhibited any of the autoantibodies. In a patient known to have both autoantibody and anti-HLA antibody in the same serum sample the two techniques distinguish between the reactions with autologous or HLA identical cells and those with mismatched cells.

Retrospective analysis of positive crossmatches with donor T and B lymphocytes in transplants performed during the past eight years has confirmed that none of the crossmatches thought to be due to autoantibody could be inhibited by PA2.6 and all were due to IgM antibodies. Graft survival of transplants performed under these circumstances was acceptable, with all living-related grafts functioning and 72% of the cadaver grafts functioning at three months. Only three of the cadaver grafts were acutely rejected. Two of these were HLA-compatible regrafts in patients who had acutely rejected previous grafts and it is possible that these represented sensitization to minor histocompatibility antigens. It would seem, therefore, that the two techniques were able to select transplants performed in the presence of a positive crossmatch with either current or only peak serum, which were associated with reasonable success rates in highly sensitized and therefore high-risk patients. Prospective application of this approach on a wider basis might permit a considerable number of patients to be transplanted who would otherwise not receive kidneys.

The relevance of a peak positive current negative crossmatch not due to autoantibody has been questioned by the consistent experience from Toronto over the past six years (*9, 18*). Cardella and Falk have demonstrated that graft survival, in their experience, is the same for those with a peak positive crossmatch transplant (but current negative) as for those with a completely negative crossmatch. If the patients are divided into those receiving a first kidney and those receiving a regraft the success rate is much lower in regrafted patients. None of the crossmatches in their report were thought to be due to autoantibody. Thus the impetus for ignoring the crossmatch with previously positive sera and considering only recent sera gained considerable ground (*19*). In Oxford our overall experience has demonstrated that it is possible to transplant patients in the presence of a peak positive current negative crossmatch not due to autoantibody. However a number of grafts have been rejected rapidly and only five of 15 such grafts have been successful. It would seem that the peak positive crossmatch did have biological relevance in this subgroup of patients, all but two of whom received their second or third regraft.

We were able to confirm that the peak positive crossmatch was indeed directed at HLA class I antigens in all but three of our patients. These antibodies were further subdivided by DTT reduction into IgG and IgM. It was striking to note that there were no successful grafts when the peak positive crossmatch was due to an IgG antibody. There were successes and failures when the antibody was IgM. The number of patients involved is too small to draw firm conclusions, but clearly it does suggest that extreme caution is warranted in transplanting a kidney into a patient with a peak positive current negative crossmatch when the positive crossmatch is due to anti-HLA class I IgG antibody.

A degree of support, however, comes from the work with 2-ME by Ayoub and his colleagues who found a peak positive crossmatch in 18 patients with sera not tested at the time of the original transplant (*20*). These sera were treated with 2-ME, which—like DTT—preferentially reduces IgM antibodies; 6 of the crossmatches were negative after treatment of the sera with 2-ME and all grafts functioned for more than six months; 12 remained positive despite 2-ME, and 2 had prolonged graft survival. This technique may either have detected autoantibodies (since autologous crossmatches were not done), which are largely IgM (*21, 22*), or it may have differentiated IgG from IgM anti-HLA antibodies. Whichever is true, the data suggests that positive crossmatches due to IgM are associated with a better outcome than those due to IgG.

It is interesting to speculate on the possible biological significance of these observations. In the mouse the humoral response to the H-2 antigens appears to be thymus-dependent, in that both neonatal and adult thymectomy prevent an IgG response to H-2 antigens, but the IgM response remains unaltered (*23*). It is conceivable that the peak positive crossmatch, when it is due to an IgG anti-HLA antibody, acts as a serological marker for the presence of T cell memory. In contrast, when only an IgM HLA antibody exists in previous sera this may reflect the absence of memory T cells and hence a renal transplant would induce a first set reaction rather than the second set reaction that would be expected in a specifically sensitized patient. An IgM response may be relatively common after exposure to HLA antigens because of the immunodepression produced by uremia in these patients. Certainly the response to flagellin in transplant patients tends to be IgM only (*24*), and antibody produced as a result of a failed graft can be exclusively IgM (*25*). This interpretation would imply that while detection of antibody present at the time of transplantation is important to prevent direct antibody mediated damage to the graft, detection of antibody present only in serum remote from the day of transplantation could act as a marker of cellular reactivity.

In conclusion, we suggest that the use of DTT reduction and inhibition of cytotoxicity by a monoclonal antibody to HLA class I antigens may help to define positive crossmatches that are not associated with graft failure. While we agree that it is possible to transplant patients successfully despite a peak positive current negative crossmatch directed at donor HLA class I antigens, this may only be successful if the reactivity of the antibody is of the IgM class.

REFERENCES

1. Cross DE, Greiner R, Whittier FC. Importance of the autocontrol crossmatch in human renal transplantation. Transplantation 1976; 21:307.
2. Morris PJ, Ting A, Oliver DO, Williams K, Dunnill MS. Renal transplantation and a positive serological crossmatch. Lancet 1977; 1: 1288.
3. Ting A, Morris PJ. Successful transplantation with a positive T and B cell crossmatch. Tissue Antigens 1983; 21:219.
4. Patel R, Terasaki PI. Significance of the positive crossmatch test in kidney transplantation. N Engl J Med 1969; 280: 735.
5. Williams GM, Hume DM, Page Hudson R, Morris PJ, Kano K, Milgrom F. "Hyperacute" renal-homograft rejection in man. N Engl J Med 1968; 279: 611.
6. Heale WF, Morris PJ, Bennett RC, Mortensen PJ, Ting A. Leukocyte antigens in renal transplantation 8. Successful renal transplantation in the presence of a positive crossmatch. Med J Aust 1969; 2: 382.
7. Cheigh JS, Fotino M, Stubenbord WT, Suhanthiran M, Riggio RR, Saal SD. Declining transplantability of prospective kidney transplant recipients. JAMA 1981; 246: 135.
8. Chapman JR, Ting A, Morris PJ. Analysis of 126 positive crossmatch transplants. Transplant Proc 1985; 17: 2472.

9. Falk JA, Cardella CJ, Halloran P, Robinette M, Arbus G, Bear R. Transplantation can be performed with a positive (non-current) crossmatch. Transplant Proc 1985; 17: 1530.
10. Ting A, Morris PJ. Reactivity of autolymphocytotoxic antibodies from dialysis patients with lymphocytes from chronic lymphatic leukemia (CLL) patients. Transplantation 1978; 25: 31.
11. Pirofsky B, Rosner ER. DTT test: a new method to differentiate IgM and IgG erythrocyte antibodies. Vox Sang 1974; 27: 480.
12. Olsen PR, Weiben J, O'Leary JJ, Moscowitz AJ, McCullough J. A simple technique for the inactivation of IgM antibodies using dithiothreitol. Vox Sang 1976; 30: 149.
13. Knight RC. Measuring IgG anti-A/B titres using dithiothreitol (DTT). J Clin Pathol 1978; 31: 283.
14. Okuno T, Kondelis N. Evaluation of dithiothreitol (DTT) for inactivation of IgM antibodies. J Clin Pathol 1978; 31: 1152.
15. Brodsky FM, Parham P, Barnstable CJ, Crumpton MJ, Bodmer WF. Monoclonal antibodies for analysis of the HLA system. Immunol Rev 1979; 47: 3.
16. Chapman JR, Morris PJ. Cyclosporine nephrotoxicity and the consequences of conversion to azathioprine. Transplant Proc 1985; 17: 254.
17. Chapman JR, Taylor CJ, Ting A, Morris PJ. Hyperacute rejection of a renal allograft in the presence of anti-HLA-Cw5 antibody. Transplantation 1986; 42: 91.
18. Cardella CJ, Falk JA, Nicholson MJ, Harding M, Cook GT. Successful renal transplantation in patients with T-cell reactivity to donor. Lancet 1982; 2: 1240.
19. Goeken NE. Outcome of renal transplantation following a positive crossmatch with historical sera: the second analysis of the ASHI survey. Transplant Proc 1985; 17: 2443.
20. Ayoub GM, Terasaki PI, Tonai RJ. Improvements in detection of sensitization. Transplant Proc 1983; 15: 1202.
21. Lobo PI. Nature for autolymphocytotoxins present in renal haemodialysis patients. Their possible role in controlling alloantibody formation. Transplantation 1981; 32: 233.
22. Ting A, Morris PJ. Current status of crossmatching in clinical transplantation. In: Morris PJ, Tilney NL, eds. Progress in transplantation 2. Edinburgh: Churchill Livingstone, 1985: 44.
23. Klein J, Livnat S, Hauptfeld V, Jerabek L, Weissman I. Production of anti-H2 antibodies in thymectomized mice. Eur J Immunol 1974; 4: 41.
24. Rowley MJ, Mackay IR, Mckenzie IFC. Antibody production in immunosuppressed recipients of renal allografts. Lancet 1969; 2: 708.
25. Stocker JW, McKenzie IFC, Morris PJ. IgM activity in human lymphocytotoxic sera after renal transplantation. Nature 1969; 222: 483.

Received 24 January 1986.
Accepted 26 February 1986.

0041-1337/86/4206-0613$02.00/0
TRANSPLANTATION
Vol. 42, No. 6

SMALL INTESTINAL TRANSPLANTATION USING CYCLOSPORINE

REPORT OF A CASE[1]

ZANE COHEN,[2] RICHARD E. SILVERMAN, RAMSES WASSEF, GARY A. LEVY, MARCUS BURNSTEIN, JAMES CULLEN, LEONARD MAKOWKA, BERNARD LANGER, AND GORDON R. GREENBERG

The Divisions of General Surgery and Pathology, Toronto General Hospital; and the Department of Surgery, University of Toronto, Canada

A case of small intestinal allotransplantation is described. Cyclosporine and Solumedrol were used for immunosuppression. A hemolytic episode occurred, caused by anti-A antibodies derived from graft lymphocytes. Sudden severe encephalopathy developed on the ninth postoperative day, followed by intractable hypotension and death. Hepatic and splenic microinfarcts were identified on postmortem examination. Allograft rejection was identified by serial stomal biopsies and correlated with a rise in monocyte procoagulant activity, a potentially useful serologic marker of rejection. The absence of an anatomic circuit for recycling of cyclosporine did not alter serum radioimmunoassay/high-performance liquid chromatography ratios.

Attempts at clinical small intestinal transplantation using conventional immunosuppression have been unsuccessful. Seven such transplants have been reported in the literature, using combinations of prednisone, Imuran, and antilymphocyte globulin (*1–5*). Five of the patients died or underwent graft removal within 9 days because of technical failure, progression of preexisting disease, or sepsis. Rejection phenomena were documented in the other 2 cases. All 7 patients died, with the longest survivor living 76 days, but without adequate graft function.

[1] This work was supported by grants from the Medical Research Council of Canada and the Lawrence and Elsie Pifko Foundation, Toronto, Canada.

[2] Address reprint requests to: Z. Cohen, M.D., F.R.C.S.(C), F.A.C.S., Toronto General Hospital, 101 College Street, Eaton 9-242, Toronto, Canada.

The introduction of Cyclosporine (CsA)* has been associated with a marked improvement in the results of kidney, heart, and liver transplantation (*6*). As well, increased survival in CsA-treated canine, rat, and pig models receiving small intestinal allografts has been reported from several laboratories (*7–9*). Because of these recent results, we have been prepared to offer clinical small bowel transplantation as an experimental alternative to highly selected patients who have insufficient functional small intestine, and in whom a reasonable quality of life with long-term home parenteral nutrition cannot be achieved.

The following report describes the first human small intestinal transplant using cyclosporine and prednisone immunosuppression.

MATERIALS AND METHODS

Case history. The patient, a 26-year-old woman, was initially diagnosed as having Gardner's syndrome in 1978. There was no family history of adenomatosis coli. In 1979 a colectomy and ileorectal anastomosis were performed. However, because of continuing rectal bleeding a proctectomy with conventional ileostomy was required in 1980. There was no evidence of malignancy in either surgical specimen.

In 1981, the patient was investigated for abdominal pain and weight loss. The clinical impression of a midabdominal mass was confirmed by CT scan, which localized the lesion to the mesentery of the small bowel. A fine-needle biopsy of the lesion revealed the presence of fibrous tissue consistent with a diagnosis of desmoid tumor. Because of continuing abdominal pain exacerbated by eating, and progressive weight loss, the patient was treated in hospital with total parenteral nutrition. After regaining 35 pounds she was discharged on a home TPN program, but still required narcotic analgesics for pain control.

Over the next year, the patient was frequently hospitalized for recurrent episodes of dehydration secondary to high ileostomy output, as well as for TPN line sepsis, pain control, and depression. A trial of Clinoril did not produce objective evidence of tumor regression or symptomatic improvement in her obstructive symptoms. Radiotherapy was considered, but it was thought to present a significant risk of enteritis with little chance of benefit. Surgical resection of the desmoid tumor was planned in December, 1983. At laparotomy a 7×10×10-cm firm, pale tumor mass was found at the base of the small bowel mesentery encasing the superior mesenteric vessels and encroaching upon several loops of jejunum. Resection appeared to be possible, but only with sacrifice of these vessels and the entire small intestine. At that time it was thought that a further trial of home TPN was warranted.

However, postoperatively her pain progressed and her chronic small bowel obstruction persisted. Four months later another laparotomy was performed and the tumor was completely excised, along with the entire small bowel from the ligament of Treitz. The 4th part of the duodenum was anastomosed to the stomach, and a gastrostomy tube was placed. Truncal vagotomy and pyloroplasty and cholecystectomy were also performed. The patient had an uncomplicated recovery, and experienced marked amelioration of her abdominal pain. However two brief trials of home TPN were failures, with rehospitalization necessary for the treatment of dehydration and severe depression. Thereafter, she remained in hospital until the time of transplantation, completely dependent on hospital staff for her nutrition, and with no viable functional life outside the hospital setting.

Experimental small intestinal transplantation was suggested as a possible therapeutic alternative. A clinical program of small intestinal transplantation was approved by the Research Ethics Committee at the Toronto General Hospital in 1984. After much discussion with the patient and her family, it was decided to proceed with transplantation.

Small intestinal transplantation. In April 1985, a donor (blood group O) small intestine became available from a 10-year-old boy pronounced dead with massive head injuries sustained in an automobile accident. The prospective recipient was blood group A. Tissue typing indicated two matching class I antigens and no matching class II antigens. The technique of harvesting the small intestine had been developed and tested in brain-dead kidney donors. The entire small bowel from proximal jejunum to terminal ileum was harvested on a vascular pedicle of superior mesenteric artery (SMA) with aortic cuff and superior mesenteric vein (SMV). Both kidneys and the cardiac valves were also harvested for transplantation purposes. The excised specimen was then perfused ex vivo with heparinized Collins' solution at 4°C. Blanching of the vessels occurred immediately, followed by blanching of the entire small intestine within 3 min.

Simultaneous laparotomy was performed on the recipient after premedication with Netilmycin and Metronidazole, cyclosporine (2 mg/kg), and Solumedrol (30 mg). There was no evidence of recurrent desmoid tumor. The entire small bowel was transplanted. The SMA on its aortic cuff was anastomosed to the recipient aorta, and the SMV anastomosed to the recipient inferior vena cava. Excellent revascularization of the graft was seen. Both ends of the intestine were exteriorized as stomas; the proximal end in the left upper quadrant, and the distal end in the right lower quadrant. Total ischemic time from graft removal to revascularization was 85 min.

Postoperative course. The patient's early postoperative course was satisfactory. CsA was administered intravenously, initially in divided doses totalling 6–9 mg/kg/day—and, beginning on the 4th day, as a continuous infusion of 4 mg/kg/day to maintain a serum trough level between 200–300 μg/L (Fig. 1). Solumedrol dosage was gradually tapered to 10 mg b.i.d. by the 6th postoperative day. The intestinal allograft stomas were biopsied daily.

On the 4th day increasing jaundice was noted, associated with a rise in the serum bilirubin to 118 μg/L (normal = 2–20 μg/L), borderline elevation in serum alkaline phosphatase, and normal aspartate aminotransferase (AST) levels. A brisk red blood cell hemolytic reaction occurred on the 6th day with a fall in hemoglobin from 100 to 72 g/L. The patient's urine turned bright red and was found to contain free hemoglobin. High titers of anti-A antibody were identified in the serum, most likely produced by "primed" lymphocytes originating in the intestinal graft. The patient was transfused with 4 units of washed, irradiated type O packed red blood cells, following which her hemoglobin stabilized and her urine gradually cleared. She required 2 more units of similar type blood 2 days

* Abbreviations used: AST, aspartate aminotransferase; CMV, cytomegalovirus; CsA, cyclosporine; CsT, cyclosporine plus crossreactive metabolites; CT, computerized tomography; GVHD, graft-versus-host disease; HPLC, high-pressure liquid chromatography; IL-1, interleukin 1; IL-2, interleukin 2; LPS, lipopolysaccharide; PBM, peripheral blood mononuclear cells; PCA, procoagulant activity; RIA, radioimmunoassay; SMA, superior mesenteric artery; SMV, superior mesenteric vein; TPN, total parenteral nutrition.

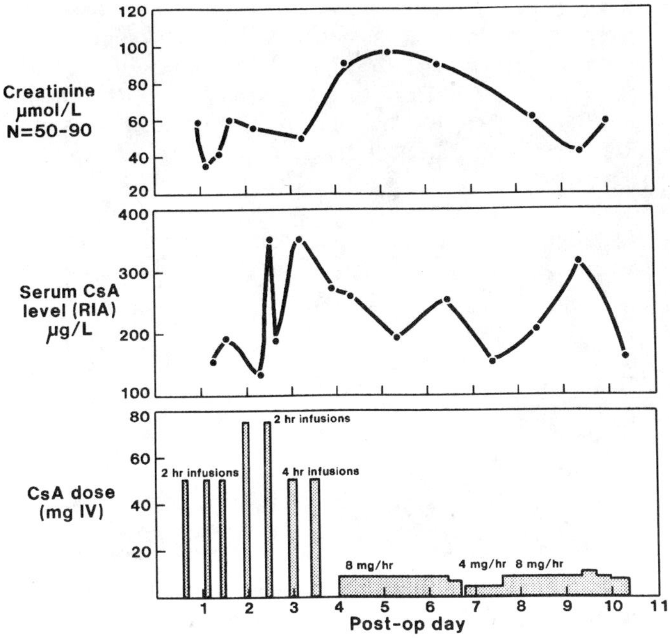

FIGURE 1. Lower panel shows cyclosporine dosage regimen. Initially bolus doses of 100 mg were given over 2 hr, then 150 mg over 2 hr, and later 200 mg over infusion periods of 4 hr. Beginning on day 4, a continuous infusion was used (patient weight—50 kg). Middle panel depicts cyclosporine trough levels measured by RIA. Upper panel shows postoperative serum creatinine; a slight elevation was seen on days 4–6.

later to maintain an adequate hemoglobin level. The serum bilirubin rose over the next few days and reached a plateau at 273 μg/L.

On the evening of the 9th postoperative day, several minutes after complaining of light-headedness, the patient suddenly collapsed and became deeply comatose. Her pupils initially were deviated to the left, then became central, fixed, and dilated. She became unresponsive with no spontaneous movements, and required endotracheal intubation and assisted ventilation. Blood pressure and heart rate at this time were 110/60 and 130, respectively. There had been no seizure activity associated with the event. A CT scan of the head was normal, as was cerebrospinal fluid examination. Serum electrolytes, including calcium and magnesium, were at normal levels.

The following morning the patient developed severe hypotension leading to a cardiac arrest from which she was resuscitated. Thereafter inotropic support was required for adequate blood pressure. Neurologically, only brainstem reflexes were present. At this point it was decided to remove the bowel transplant in the event that a severe graft-versus-host reaction was the cause of the encephalopathy. The graft was found to be viable, and the vascular anastomoses were intact. The patient's general condition continued to deteriorate, and she died the next day.

Allograft monitoring. Both the jejunal and ileal stomas were biopsied daily using a bronchoscopy forceps. Immediate frozen, as well as routine paraffin sections were evaluated.

Immunologic monitoring. Peripheral blood mononuclear cells were isolated from heparinized specimens. Assays were carried out measuring procoagulant activity (PCA), and interleukin-1 (IL-1) and interleukin-2 (IL-2) production. Mononuclear cell separation was accomplished by centrifugation over Ficoll-Hypaque and by selective adherence to fibronectin-coated plates as previously reported (*10*). Procoagulant activity was assayed by mononuclear cell capacity to shorten the spontaneous clotting time of human plasma in a one-stage clotting assay (*11*). Sera from the patient and normal controls were assayed daily for IL-1 activity. In addition, isolated monocytes were stimulated with *Escherichia coli* lipopolysaccharide (LPS, *E coli* 014) and assayed for inducible IL-1 activity in a costimulator assay (*12*). Spontaneous IL-2 activity in the serum, as well as inducible IL-2 activity in patient peripheral blood mononuclear cells exposed to Con A were measured by the method described by Gillis (*13*), utilizing an IL-2-dependent cell line (CTLL) provided by G. Mills (Hospital for Sick Children, Toronto).

Cyclosporine levels in serum and gastrostomy drainage. Daily serum trough CsA levels were measured using the radioimmunoassay (RIA) kit supplied by the manufacturer. On the 3rd postoperative day, serum and gastrostomy drainage CsA levels were determined hourly during, and at 0.5, 1, 2, 3, 4, 6, 8, and 10 hr after, a 4-hr infusion of CsA at a dose of 50 mg/hr. RIA and high performance liquid chromatography (HPLC) levels were measured. HPLC was performed using a Waters HPL chromatograph after acid and base extraction (University Hospital, London, Ontario, Canada). The flow rate was 1.5 ml/min., and the CsA peak was read at a 210 nm wavelength.

RESULTS

Daily graft biopsies. Both stomas had a normal appearance on gross inspection throughout the postoperative course. There was good correlation between frozen and paraffin sections taken daily. Histologic examination was considered normal on the first 3 days. On the 4th day slight changes were noted, consisting of minor blunting of the villi and an increased number of lymphocytes in the lamina propria. Biopsies from days 4–8 showed a mild-to-moderate lymphocytic infiltrate in the lamina propria. Minor blunting of villi was seen, and the epithelial layer remained entirely normal. On the 9th day, the infiltrate increased significantly, consistent with heightened rejection activity. The epithelial layer was unaffected (Fig. 2).

Immunologic responses. For the first 6 days following transplantation no procoagulant activity (PCA) was found in patient peripheral blood mononuclear cells (PBM) or control PBM. On the 9th day, correlating with an increasing lymphocytic infiltration of the allograft, a significant rise in patient PCA was present, with a further marked increase on the following day (Fig. 3). Control PBM continued to show no PCA. The activity was localized to the monocyte, as determined when cells were subfractionated and assayed. Spontaneous IL-1 and IL-2 activity could not be detected in the patient's serum nor was it inducible in patient PBM throughout the postoperative course. This was in contrast to inducible activity in a normal control. Due to a limited amount of blood, inducible activity levels were not determined on the last 2 days, at a time when PCA changes were noted.

Cyclosporine studies. Figure 1 depicts serum CsA trough levels measured by RIA, and the dosing regimen employed. Initially, i.v. doses of 100–200 mg were given over 2–4 hr twice daily. Beginning on the 4th day a continuous infusion of 8 mg/hr (4 mg/kg/day) was used. This was temporarily adjusted downward at the onset of a hemolytic episode on the 6th day. Trough levels of CsA were reasonably well maintained within the desired range of 200–300 μg/L. The serum creatinine was within

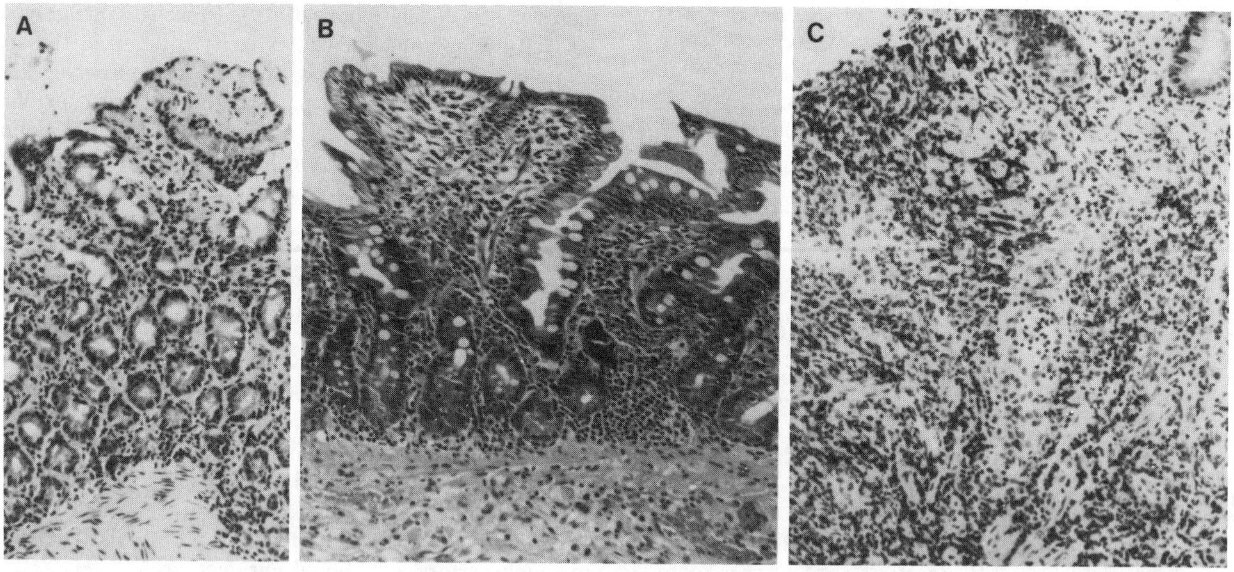

FIGURE 2. Stomal biopsies taken on 2nd (A), 5th (B), and 9th (C) postoperative days. The early biopsy is relatively normal. The biopsy done on day 5 displays mild blunting of the villi associated with increased cellularity in the lamina propria, primarily consisting of lymphocytes. The biopsy on day 9 shows heavy infiltration by lymphocytes. (Some degree of variability was present in the histologic appearances—the micrographs are representative of areas with the most severe changes.) (H&E; ×80).

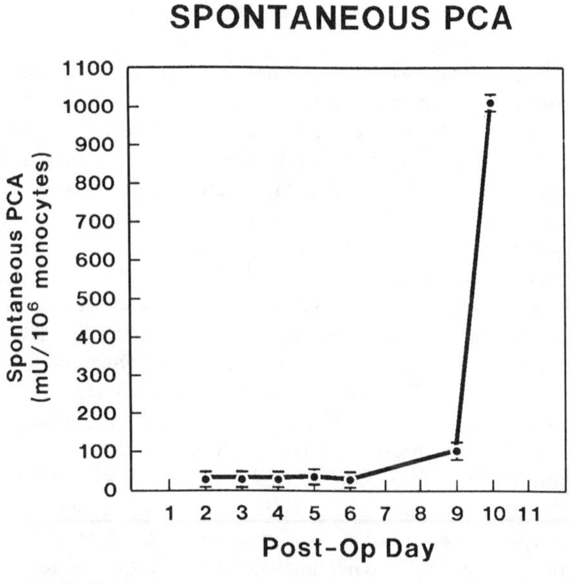

FIGURE 3. Spontaneous procoagulant activity in milliunits per 10^6 patient monocytes. Activity became elevated on the 9th postoperative day, and increased markedly on the 10th postoperative day.

TABLE 1. Cyclosporine levels (μg/L)[a]

Time (hr)		Serum RIA	Serum HPLC	Gastrostomy RIA	Gastrostomy HPLC
CsA (50 mg/hr)	0	329	78	4720	410
	1	390	157	6310	475
	2	324	256	5950	475
	3	437	198	6140	450
	4	888	823	6520	520
	4.5	957	766	6440	490
	5	647	421	5870	490
	6	501	182	4020	270
	7	445	136	7430	510
	8	595	113	6470	505
	10	328	89	8050	435
	12	150	66	7540	430
	14	368	90	11540	580

[a] CsA levels in serum and gastrostomy fluid. On the 3rd postoperative day, specimens were collected during a 4-hr infusion of 200 mg of CsA and at .5, 1, 2, 3, 4, 6, 8, and 10 hr afterward.

normal limits except for a slight rise on days 4–6, and preterminally on day 10 (Fig. 1).

Table 1 shows CsA levels in serum and gastrostomy drainage following infusion. Gastrostomy drainage levels were essentially representative of bile levels. Serum RIA levels varied from 150 to 957 μg/L 30 min after stopping the infusion. The ratio of total CsA (CsT = CsA + metabolites) to CsA in the serum as reflected in the RIA/HPLC ratio varied from 4.2:1 at trough to 1.1:1 at peak levels. CsT measurements in the gastrostomy drainage ranged between 4020 and 11,540 μg/L. The RIA/HPLC ratio varied from 11.5:1 to 19.9:1.

Intestinal graft pathology. Following removal of the intestinal allograft the mucosa was grossly intact throughout the length of the bowel. The proximal end had a thickened hemorrhagic appearance, the result of multiple biopsies.

Microscopically, a diffuse lymphoid infiltrate varying from mild to moderate was seen within the lamina propria and muscularis. Areas of blunting of villi and focal mucosal necrosis were present. The mesentery was involved with a similar mononuclear infiltrate, and small mesenteric vessels contained thrombi at various stages of evolution. The mesenteric lymph nodes showed evidence of reactive hyperplasia. The findings were compatible with a moderate rejection process (Fig. 4A,B).

Necropsy results. The most striking findings were related to the liver, spleen, and brain. The liver was enlarged, weighing 1950 g. Microscopically, diffuse cholestatic changes were seen, as well as a diffuse pattern of microinfarcts. These were predominantly zone 3 lesions, suggestive of hypoperfusion or ischemia. In some areas an advanced polymorphonuclear infiltrate was present, suggesting that the microinfarcts were more than 36 hr old, and preceded the patient's collapse. Electron microscopy failed to reveal evidence of arteritis or fibrin deposition (Fig. 5).

The spleen was also enlarged, weighing 550 g. The lower pole was grossly infarcted. A similar diffuse pattern of microinfarction was seen, with a variable degree of acute inflammatory cell infiltration.

Neuropathologic examination showed extensive, bilateral border zone infarcts involving the hemisphere regions between the anterior and middle cerebral artery distributions, the pa-

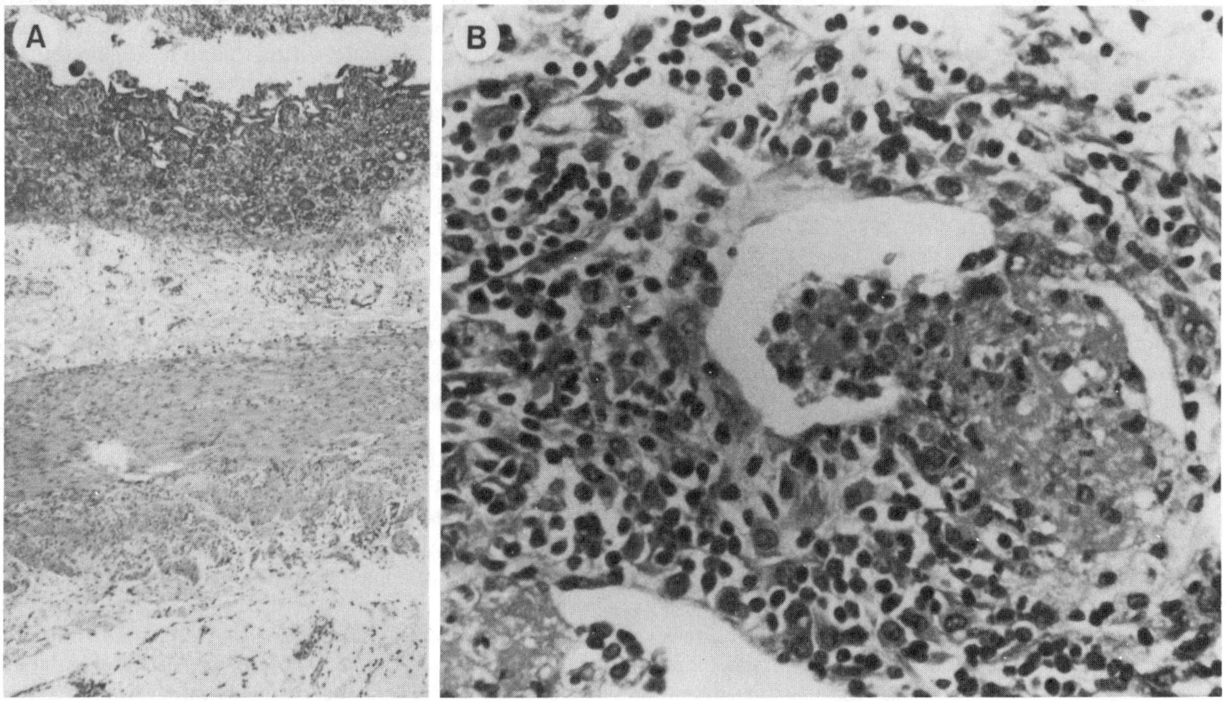

FIGURE 4. Micrographs of the removed intestinal allograft. A marked lymphocytic infiltrate is present in the lamina propria and extends into the muscular layer (A). Dense mesenteric infiltrate with recently thrombosed small vessel is shown (B). (H&E; ×20[A], ×200 [B]).

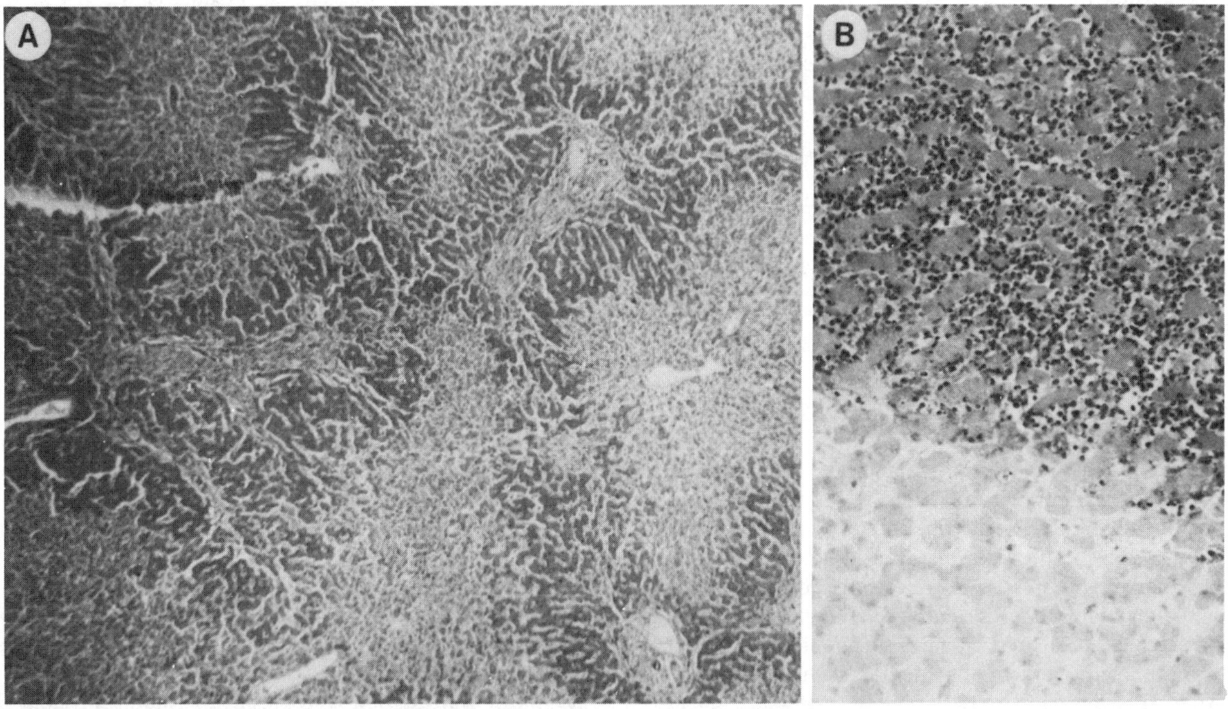

FIGURE 5. Micrographs of liver at postmortem examination. Multiple microinfarcts are present, mainly in zone 3(A). An advanced polymorphonuclear infiltrate is associated with many of the lesions (B). (H&E; ×20[A], ×80[B]).

rietooccipital region, and the thalami. Microscopy indicated widespread neuronal ischemic damage and recent infarction, consistent with the period of severe preterminal hypotension.

DISCUSSION

Monitors of rejection. The sequence of histologic changes seen in small bowel allograft rejection is well described in experimental canine models (*14*). The earliest signs are blunting of the villi, followed by increasing mononuclear infiltrates, and—ultimately—mucosal sloughing. Treatment with cyclosporine may delay (*14*) or abolish (*7*) these features. In a recent study (*15*) using CsA and prednisone immunosuppression in a canine model, 35-cm. segmental allografts were transplanted ectopically in the neck. Minimal or no cellular infiltration, and villi of normal appearance were seen in stomal biopsies.

The mild mononuclear cell infiltration seen in our patient's allograft biopsies during the first week (Fig. 2B) is of questionable significance. With the advent of fine-needle aspiration biopsy for routine monitoring of asymptomatic renal transplant recipients, several reports describe mononuclear infiltrates in a significant percentage of patients (*16–18*). These are neither diagnostic of, nor predictive of, graft rejection, and may be considered nonspecific and immunologically inactive. While these terms might be applied to the intestinal stoma biopsies during the first week posttransplant, it is apparent that a process of graft rejection was established by the 9th postoperative day, and was more advanced when the small bowel was removed on the 10th postoperative day (Figs. 2 and 4). The findings in the allograft itself correlate with the progressive changes in the daily biopsies, indicating that stomal biopsies can be used to monitor rejection in the clinical situation.

Peripheral blood procoagulant activity is a property of monocytes that may be induced by appropriate immunogenic stimuli including viruses, mitogens, and allogeneic cells. A membrane-bound prothrombinase results, leading to fibrin clot formation (*11*). The coagulation system is an important effector mechanism in organ transplant rejection, and studies of renal allograft rejection show correlation with radio-fibrinogen catabolism (*19*). Halloran (*20*) measured PCA in the peripheral blood of kidney transplant recipients and was able to correlate an increased activity with clinical rejection after the first 2 weeks. Recently, Cole (*10*) demonstrated impressive sensitivity of PCA in predicting incipient renal transplant rejection. A rise in PCA was associated with the clinical diagnosis of rejection in 20 of 21 episodes, and preceded it by 24 hr in 12 cases. However, the false-positive rate for the assay was 33%, indicating that some caution is required in interpretation.

Our own case represents the first use of a PCA assay in the monitoring of human small intestinal transplantation. Activity was absent during the period of relative histologic quiescence, rose on the 9th postoperative day coincident with increasing lymphocytic infiltrates in the intestinal graft biopsies, and was markedly elevated when more advanced rejection changes were identified in the removed graft. The importance of this potential serologic marker becomes apparent when one considers that functional, orthotopic bowel transplants may be relatively inaccessible for biopsy if no stoma is provided. In addition, to this date there is no early biochemical or immunologic marker of rejection following intestinal transplantation.

Assays of IL-1 and IL-2 activity may be useful as indicators of CsA efficacy of cellular immunosuppression. Current evidence suggests that CsA exerts its immunosuppressive effect primarily by altering macrophage and T lymphocyte immunologic responses. In vitro experimental studies have shown a reduction in IL-1 release from mitogen-stimulated macrophages exposed to CsA, as measured in a thymocyte proliferation assay (*21, 22*). Inducible lymphocyte IL-2 production is similarly decreased on exposure to CsA in vitro (*23, 24*). In our patient IL-1 and IL-2 activity were undetectable during the first postoperative week, suggesting that cellular immunosuppression was adequate during this time. (As prednisone has some IL-1-suppressive action it likely contributed to this result.) Spontaneous serum IL-1 and IL-2 measurements remained undetectable, however inducible levels were not measured on the last 3 days and no correlation can be drawn with the histological signs of rejection or the rise in PCA that occurred at that time.

Biliary excretion of cyclosporine. Dog experiments performed by Wagner (*25*) found that 76% of the radioactivity of an oral dose of labeled CsA was eliminated in the stool, with a similar amount after an intravenous dose. More than 50% of labeled CsA given intravenously to rats is recovered in the bile (*25*).

Seventeen CsA metabolites have been identified in urine and bile, and only 0.1% of the drug reaches the urine in unaltered form (*26, 27*). Recently, direct measurements of biliary concentrations of CsA and its crossreacting metabolites have confirmed the presence of very high levels of drug, primarily in metabolite form (*28*). It has been estimated that 43.8% of bioavailable drug appears in the bile within 12 hr of an oral dose (*28*).

Enterohepatic recirculation of CsA and its metabolites has been postulated on the basis of RIA-measured secondary serum peaks found in 36% of a series of renal transplant recipients. Serial CsA measurements in the serum and ileostomy output of a patient exhibited a pattern of sequential cycles, also suggesting recirculation (*29*).

Our measurements of serum and gastrostomy fluid CsA content permit several observations (Table 1). High CsA levels were present in the drainage as measured by RIA, reflecting high biliary excretion rates. The range of 4020–11,540 μg/L of CsA in gastrostomy fluid is lower than that reported for T-tube bile (9280–61,300) (*28*), and may represent the dilution effect of pancreatic and duodenal secretions, as well as differences in dosage and measurement regimens. The ratio of CsT to CsA, as reflected in the RIA:HPLC ratio, ranged from 11.5:1 to 19.9:1, indicating efficient hepatic metabolism with little parent compound being excreted. This again correlates with ratios found in bile measurements (18:1–36:1) (*28*). The low biliary concentration of parent CsA, as well as the very small net amounts present in collected bile (<1% over a dosage interval), make any significant enterohepatic recycling unlikely, as previously suggested (*28*). It is not known to what extent enterohepatic recirculation of CsA metabolites contributes to the serum levels of these substances, as measured by the difference in RIA and HPLC values. Another likely contributing mechanism is a process of metabolite back-diffusion into the blood from the hepatocytes and from tissue storage sites. In our patient, the maintenance of a normal proportion of crossreacting metabolites, despite the anatomic impossibility of enterohepatic recirculation appears to indicate the relative importance of this latter process.

Necropsy findings and cause of death. The interpretation of the histologic changes seen in the liver at postmortem examination is complex. The patient had been dependent on TPN for 2.5 years, and serum bilirubin and alkaline phosphatase levels had been in the abnormal range frequently in the months prior to transplantation. Therefore the cholestasis and hepatomegaly that were seen may have been attributable to TPN-related liver disease.

During the 36 hr following her clinical deterioration, the patient developed severe hypotension and was resuscitated from cardiac arrest. Foci of hepatocellular necrosis may be seen commonly in patients with prolonged hypotension, and may be considered a nonspecific reaction to a variety of insults (*30*). However, the polymorphonuclear infiltrates tend to place the time of genesis of these lesions prior to the period of clinical shock. As well, the chronology of serum bilirubin changes in relation to the liver pathology is obscured by the ongoing RBC hemolysis.

Other diagnostic possibilities to be considered in relation to the hepatic changes are acute graft-versus-host disease (GVHD) and cyclosporine hepatotoxicity. Although some investigators have reported periportal inflammation and hepatocellular necrosis in GVHD (*31, 32*), the classic hallmarks are small bile duct atypia and proliferation (*33, 34*). The other major target organs in GVHD, skin, and gastrointestinal tract, are almost invariably coaffected. The lack of bile duct changes, as well as normal skin and gastroduodenal histology, make GVHD an unlikely diagnosis.

CsA hepatotoxicity occurs not infrequently after organ transplantation. The diagnosis is usually made with the appearance of hyperbilirubinemia. It is associated with a higher dosage range (>17 mg/kg/day), and with CsA trough levels >400 μg/L (*35, 36*). The bilirubin falls upon lowering the dose and the trough levels. Biopsies are rarely done, and the histopathologic changes are not documented. Biopsy and necropsy reports have primarily come from bone marrow transplant patients, in whom GVHD, pretransplant chemotherapy and irradiation, and CsA toxicity present a multifactorial etiology for histological abnormalities in the liver (*34, 37*). Overall, the microscopic liver changes were probably the result of one or more of several contributing factors, among which were decreased perfusion related to hypotension, TPN-associated liver disease—and, possibly, cyclosporine toxicity.

The gross lower pole splenic infarction was almost certainly a result of the severe hypotension present during the last 36 hr. We can only speculate as to the cause of the splenic microinfarcts. An occult hypotensive episode or a previously unreported drug toxicity involving CsA or another of the several drugs in use are suspect.

Milder forms of neurologic toxicity, such as tremor and paresthesias, are seen in 10–39% of patients treated with CsA (*6*). As well, there have been reports of seizures associated with CsA. In some cases, hypertension, (*38*) high-dose steroids, (*39*) and hypomagnesemia (*40*) appear to be contributing factors.

Four recent reports have appeared describing severe CNS symptoms attributable to CsA. Atkinson (*41*) described 5 cases of CNS toxicity in bone marrow transplant recipients treated with CsA for the prophylaxis of GVHD. The symptom complex was characterized by motor spinal cord signs, a cerebellar-like syndrome, and mental confusion. Discontinuing the CsA produced rapid regression of symptoms. In 2 patients, later attempts to reintroduce the drug were associated with immediate recurrence of the symptoms. Pretransplant administration of cyclophosphamide and irradiation may have contributed to the morbidity. Wilczek (*42*) reported on a single renal transplant recipient given high-dose methylprednisolone in addition to CsA for a rejection episode. The patient gradually became somnolent, then comatose. When CsA was discontinued, there was rapid improvement. Later resumption of CsA at lower dosage again induced somnolence. Although anticytomegalovirus (CMV) antibodies were detected in the blood, the virus itself did not appear in the blood or the cerebrospinal fluid. Still an occult CMV encephalitis could not be completely ruled out. Berden (*43*) described a kidney recipient with elevated whole-blood CsA measurements of 600–1000 who developed a coma that persisted 44 days. CT scan was consistent with a leukoencephalopathy. Although the CsA was stopped at the onset, no other cause was identified for the coma, and the authors speculated that CsA was responsible. Finally, Beaman (*44*) reported 2 cases of patients, with high CsA levels after renal transplantation, who became encephalopathic and had grand mal seizures. The first patient's trough CsA level was 3992 μg/L. CsA was withheld, and recovery resulted within 36 hr. The second patient had a serum trough CsA level of 1583 μg/L, and symptoms similarly regressed soon after stopping the drug.

Of the 9 patients described, 8 demonstrate a close temporal relationship between withdrawal of the CsA and clearing of their encephalopathy. This relationship, as well as the absence of other positive diagnostic findings, tends to implicate CsA as the etiologic agent. A possible "permissive" factor is also present in the majority of cases (premarrow transplant conditioning, occult CMV infection, and hypertension), which may relate to similar observations in CsA-induced seizures.

Our patient's CsA trough levels were within the desired range, and none of the documented permissive factors were identified. In addition, there was no evidence of CsA-induced nephrotoxicity. Despite this, we speculate that the most likely explanation for her collapse remains CsA-induced central nervous system toxicity. The hypotension which followed secondarily was the cause of massive cerebral infarcts resulting in her death.

This case report represents the first human small intestinal transplantation in which cyclosporine and prednisone were used for immunosuppression. ABO incompatibility between the donor and the recipient resulted in a severe graft-versus-host type of hemolysis that was treated effectively by transfusing donor-compatible red blood cells. The large volume of lymphoid tissue present in the small intestine obviously predisposed to this complication, and we think that future small intestinal transplantation requires ABO compatibility or possibly allograft irradiation. Although the liver and spleen pathologic changes found at necropsy were somewhat obscure and probably multifactorial, the encephalopathy suffered by the patient adds to a growing volume of literature detailing CsA-associated severe central nervous system symptoms. There must be a high index of suspicion when neurologic deterioration develops in a patient treated with CsA, and it should be discontinued immediately.

The monitoring procedures undertaken in the patient verified that daily stomal biopsies are useful in identifying rejection within the intestinal graft, and that monocyte PCA may be a valuable serologic marker of rejection. One of the perceived problems at the outset of this allotransplant was an anticipated difficulty in monitoring CsA serum levels in the postoperative period. It was thought that the absence of an enterohepatic circuit for recycling CsA metabolites might lower the RIA/HPLC ratio in the serum. A therapeutically effective, safe range of trough values would be difficult to clearly identify in this situation. In fact, the normal ratio that was found indicated that enterohepatic recycling may not be an important mechanism in maintaining crossreactive metabolite levels in the serum, and that CsA monitoring in future small intestinal transplantation may be undertaken without significant regard for anatomic alterations in the recipient gastrointestinal tract.

Acknowledgments. We gratefully acknowledge the assistance of Dr. P.Y. Wong and Dr. P. Keown for performing the cyclosporine assays and sharing their knowledge and experience with us.

REFERENCES

1. Kirkman RL. Small bowel transplantation. Transplantation 1984; 37: 429.
2. Lillihei RC, Idezuki Y, Feemster JA, et al. Transplantation of stomach, intestine and pancreas: experimental and clinical observations. Surgery 1967; 62: 721.
3. Olivier CL, Rettori R, Olivier CH, Camilleri JP. Interruption of lymphatic vessels and its consequences in total homotransplantation of the small intestine and right side of the colon in man. Lymphology 1972; 5: 24.
4. Alican F, Hardy JD, Cayirli M, et al. Intestinal transplantation: laboratory experience and report of a clinical case. Am J Surg 1971; 121: 150.
5. Fortner JG, Sichuk G, Litwin SD, Beattie EJ. Immunological responses to an intestinal allograft with HLA-identical donor-recipient. Transplantation 1972; 14: 531.
6. Cohen D, Loertscher MD, Rubin M, Tilney N, Carpenter C, Strom T. Cyclosporine A: a new immunosuppressive agent for organ transplantation. Ann Intern Med 1984; 101: 667.
7. Craddock GN, Nordgren S, Reznick R, et al. Small intestinal transplantation in the dog using cyclosporine. Transplantation 1983; 35: 284.
8. Kirkman RL, Lear PA, Madara JL, Tilney NL. Small intestinal transplantation in the rat-immunology and function. Surgery 1984; 96: 280.
9. Ricour C, Revillon Y, Arnaud-Battandier F, et al. Successful small bowel in piglets using cyclosporine. Transplant Proc 1983; 15: 3019.
10. Cole E, Cardella CJ, Schulman J, Levy G. Monocyte procoagulant activity and plasminogen activator: role in human renal allograft rejection. Transplantation 1985; 40: 363.
11. Edgington TS, Helin H, Gregory S, Fair DS, Levy G, Schwartz BS. In Van Furthed R, ed. Cellular pathways and signals for the induction biosynthesis of initiators of the coagulation protease cascade and plasminogen activators mononuclear phagocytes. North Holland: Elsevier 1985; 687.
12. Mizel SB, Oppenheim JJ, Rosenstreich DL. Characterization of lymphocyte-activating factor (LAF) produced by the macrophage cell line, P388D1. I. Enhancement of LAF production by activated T lymphocytes. J Immunol 1978; 120: 1497.
13. Gillis S, Ferm MM, Ou W, Smith KA. T cell growth factor: parameters of production and a quantitative microassay for activity. J Immunol 1978; 120: 2027.
14. Lossing A, Nordgren S, Cohen Z, Cullen J, Craddock G, Langer B. Histologic monitoring of rejection in small intestinal transplantation. Transplant Proc 1982; 14: 643.
15. Raju S, Didlake R, Cayirli M, Turner MD, Grogan JB, Achord J. Experimental small bowel transplantation utilizing cyclosporine. Transplantation 1984; 38: 561.
16. Tufveson G, Backman U, Claesson K, Frodin L, Stenquist B, Wahlberg J. Renal transplant cytology: the impact of different immunosuppressive protocols and biopsy techniques. Transplant Proc 1985; 17: 2087.
17. O'Brian JP, Horsburgh T, Veitch P, Bell P. Experience with fine needle aspiration biopsies from renal transplant patients on different immunosuppressive regimens. Transplant Proc 1985; 17: 2089.
18. Egidi F, Tarantino A, De Vecchi A, Zubani R, Ponticelli C. Patterns of inflammation in fine needle aspiration biopsies in renal transplant patients treated with different immunosuppressive agents. Transplant Proc 1985; 17: 2091.
19. Wardle E, Uldall PR, Swinney JS. Radio-fibrinogen catabolism studies in human renal allograft recipients. Transplantation 1974; 18: 508.
20. Halloran P, Aprile M, Haddad G, Robinette M. The significance of elevated procoagulant activity in the monocytes of renal transplant recipients. Transplant Proc 1982; 14: 669.
21. Bunjes D, Hardt C, Rollinghof M, Wagner H. Cyclosporine A mediates immunosuppression of primary cytotoxic T cell responses by impairing the release of interleukin-1 and interleukin-2. Eur J Immunol 1981; 8: 657.
22. Uyemura K, Dixon JFP, Parker JW. CsA inhibits macrophage accessory cell function in mitogen-induced lymphocyte proliferation. Transplant Proc 1985; 17: 1374.
23. Ryffel B, Tammi K, Grieder A, Hess AD. Effect of CsA on human T cell activation. Transplant Proc 1985; 17: 1268.
24. Wagner H. Cyclosporin A mode of action. Transplant Proc 1983; 15: 523.
25. Beveridge T. Pharmacokinetics and metabolism of cyclosporin A. In: White DJ, ed. Cyclosporin A. Amsterdam: Elsevier, 1982: 36.
26. Abbott L, Pippenger CE. Cyclosporin: its clinical utility, methods of analysis, and TDM. Diagn Med 1985; (May): 36.
27. Wood AJ, Maurer G, Niederberger W, Beveridge T. Cyclosporine: pharmacokinetics, metabolism and drug interactions. Transplant Proc 1983; 15: 2409.
28. Venkataramanan R, Starzl TE, Yang S, et al. Biliary excretion of cyclosporin in liver transplant patients. Transplant Proc 1985; 17: 286.
29. Kahan BD, Reid M, Newburger J. Pharmacokinetics of cyclosporin in human renal transplantation. Transplant Proc 1983; 15: 446.
30. Hamilton DV, Evans DB, Thiru S. Toxicity of Cyclosporin in organ grafting. In: White DJ, ed. Cyclosporin A. Amsterdam: Elsevier, 1982: 393.
31. Lerner KG, Kao GF, Storb R, Buckner CD, Clift RA, Thomas ED. Histopathology of graft versus host reaction (GVHD) in human recipients of marrow from HL-A-matched sibling donors. Transplant Proc 1976; 6: 367.
32. Berk PD, Popper H, Kruges GRF, Decter J, Herzig G, Graw RG Jr. Veno-occlusive of the liver after allogeneic bone marrow transplantation. Ann Intern Med 1979; 90: 158.
33. Atkinson K, Biggs J, Dodds A, Concannon A. Cyclosporine-associated hepatotoxicity after allogeneic marrow transplantation in man: differentiation from other causes of post-transplant liver disease. Transplant Proc 1983; 15: 2761.
34. Sloane JP, Farthing MJ, Powles RL. Histopathological changes in the liver after allogeneic bone marrow transplantation. J Clin Pathol 1980; 33: 344.
35. Laupacis A, Keown PA, Ulan RA, et al. Hyperbilirubinemia and Cyclosporin A levels. Lancet 1981; 2: 1426.
36. Keown PA, Stiller CR, Sinclair NR, et al. The clinical relevance of cyclosporine blood levels as measured by radioimmunoassay. Transplant Proc 1983; 15: (suppl 1): 2438.
37. Powles RL, Clink H, Sloane J, Barrett AJ, Kay HE, McElwain TJ. Cyclosporin A for the treatment of graft vs. host disease in man. Lancet 1978; 2: 1327.
38. Joss DV, Barrett AJ, Kendra JR, Lucas CF, Desai S. Hypertension and convulsions in children receiving cyclosporin A. Lancet 1982; 1: 906.
39. Durrant S, Chipping PM, Palmer S, Gordon-Smith EL. Cyclosporin A, methylprednisolone, and convulsions. Lancet 1982; 2: 829.
40. Thompson CB, June CH, Sullivan KM, Thomas ED. Association between cyclosporine neurotoxicity and hypomagnesemia. Lan-

cet 1984; 2(8412): 1116.
41. Atkinson K, Biggs J, Darveniza P, Boland J Concannon A, Dodds A. Cyclosporine-associated central nervous system toxicity after allogeneic bone marrow transplantation. Transplantation 1984; 38: 34.
42. Wilczek H, Ringden O, Tyden G. Cyclosporin-associated central nervous system toxicity after renal transplantation. Transplantation 1985; 39: 110.
43. Berden JHM, Hoitsma AJ, Merx JL, Keyser A. Severe central nervous system toxicity associated with cyclosporin [Letter]. Lancet 1985; 1(8422): 219.
44. Beaman M, Parvin S, Veitch PS, Walls J. Convulsions associated with Cyclosporin A in renal transplant recipients. Brit Med J 1985; 290: 139.

Received 30 December 1985.
Accepted 26 February 1986.

0041-1337/86/4206-0621$02.00/0
TRANSPLANTATION

Vol. 42, No. 6
Printed in U.S.A.

EVIDENCE THAT SECONDARY MIXED LEUKOCYTE CULTURE SUPERNATANT MEDIATES CHANGES IN CELLULAR RECRUITMENT, BLOOD FLOW, AND VASCULAR PERMEABILITY[1]

DOUGLAS W. HANTO,[2] JOHN T. HARTY, ROSEMARY A. HOFFMAN, AND RICHARD L. SIMMONS

The Department of Surgery, University of Minnesota Health Sciences Center, Minneapolis, Minnesota 55455

Lymphokines produced as a result of allostimulation may play an important role in allograft rejection, mediating changes in cellular infiltration and migration, regional blood flow, and vascular permeability in a manner similar to that of delayed type hypersensitivity reactions. Changes in cellular recruitment (CR), regional blood flow (RBF), and vascular permeabilty (VP) were studied in paired healed subcutaneous urethane sponge grafts inoculated with secondary mixed leukocyte culture supernatant (2° MLC SN), a rich source of a variety of lymphokines secreted in response to allostimulation. Intravenous injection of Indium-111-labeled unsensitized lymphocytes (UL), Rubidium-86-chloride, and Iodine-125-labeled albumin were used to assess CR, RBF, and VP, respectively. An increase in CR (*$P<0.001$*), RBF (*$P<0.05$*), and VP (*$P<0.001$*) could be demonstrated at the site of injection of allogeneically restimulated 2° MLC SN compared with the syngeneically restimulated 2° MLC SN. The quantitative response and the kinetics of CR using 2°MLC SN were similar to previous studies in which specifically sensitized lymphocytes were injected with target cells bearing the sensitizing alloantigen, but the increase in RBF and VP were less. Injection of purified human interleukin 2, serotonin, histamine, and bradykinin had no significant effect on CR. Injection of purified human interleukin 1 resulted in a moderate increase in CR. These results are consistent with previous studies suggesting that the in vivo elaboration of lymphokines during allogeneic cellular interactions leads to an increase in CR, RBF, and VP. The small changes in RBF and VP in these experiments, however, do not account for the greater magnitude of the changes in CR. It is likely that other specific or nonspecific chemoattractants or inhibitors of cell migration also play a significant role in CR in vivo.

Allograft rejection is characterized by the accumulation at the graft site of alloantigen-specific helper and cytolytic T lymphocytes and nonspecific inflammatory cells, including unsensitized lymphocytes (UL), macrophages, neutrophils, and monocytes (*1*). The mechanisms which lead to the accumulation of these cells in the graft have been the focus of our studies. We have shown in a modified sponge matrix allograft model that the interaction between sensitized T cells and target cells bearing the sensitizing alloantigens results in an increase in the accumulation at the graft site of circulating unsensitized and sensitized lymphocytes regardless of their immunologic specificity (*2–6*). This increase in cellular recruitment (CR)* is accompanied by a parallel increase in regional blood flow (RBF) and vascular permeability (VP) (*4*). Using alloantigen-specific cloned T lymphocytes we have also shown that cytolytic, helper, and helper-independent cytolytic T cells are capable of mediating changes in CR when injected in combination with specific alloantigen bearing target cells (*6*). We have postulated that

[1] This work was supported by Grant AI 16869 from the National Institutes of Health.

[2] To whom requests for reprints should be addressed, at Washington University School of Medicine, Department of Surgery, 4989 Barnes Hospital Plaza, St. Louis, MO 63110.

* Abbreviations used: BALB, BALB/c; BFI, blood flow index; B6, C57BL/6; CO cardiac output; CR, cellular recruitment; DBA, DBA/2J; DTH, delayed-type hypersensitivity; IL-1, interleukin 1; IL-2, interleukin 2; MEM, minimal essential medium; MLC, mixed leukocyte culture; RBF, regional blood flow; RI, recruitment index; SN, supernatant; SSL, specifically sensitized lymphocytes; 2°, secondary; UL, unsensitized lymphocytes; VP, vascular permeability.

these changes in CR, RBF, and VP are the result of the secretion of one or more lymphokines by the responding specifically sensitized lymphocytes (SSL), resulting in the attraction of additional cells from the circulation, thereby expanding the pool of both specifically sensitized and nonspecific inflammatory cells at the graft site.

It is well established that allostimulation of sensitized lymphocytes results in the synthesis and release of a variety of lymphokines (*7*). No published in vivo studies, however, have directly addressed the possiblity that these soluble products of allostimulation can mediate inflammatory events. The present studies were designed to investigate the ability of various soluble mediators to increase the in vivo accumulation of circulating cells at the injection site and to test their ability to mediate changes in blood flow and vascular permeability as a more direct test of the hypothesis that allogeneic cellular interactions can generate soluble factors that can nonspecifically attract circulating lymphocytes similar to delayed-type hypersensitivity (DTH) reactions (*8*).

MATERIALS AND METHODS

Mice. Female BALB/c (BALB, H-2^d) and C57BL/6 (B6, H-2^b) mice were obtained from Charles River Breeding Laboratories, Wilmington, MA, and DBA/2J (DBA, H-2^d) mice were procured from The Jackson Laboratory, Bar Harbor, ME. They were housed in plastic cages, provided with purina rodent chow and tap water ad lib, and used at 8–12 weeks of age.

Experimental design. In the experiment described, BALB mice were used 13 days after implantation of two cell-free sterile urethane sponges on opposite sides of the lateral thorax. One sponge was injected with the experimental mediator and the opposite sponge with the appropriate control (see below). At 4 hr after sponge injection, indium-111-oxine–labeled unsensitized BALB spleen cells (UL), ^{86}RbCl, or ^{125}I-albumin were injected intravenously i.v. Sponges were removed and counted at intervals after i.v. injection of the respective isotopes to determine the relative accumulation of the labeled cells or isotopes in the two sponges. The percent of injected activity recovered in the sponges was calculated after correcting for the background count.

$$\% \text{ injected activity recovered in sponge} = \frac{\text{cpm in sponge} - \text{background cpm}}{\text{cpm injected} - \text{background cpm}}$$

The cellular recruitment index (RI) (^{111}In-oxine), blood flow index (BFI)(^{86}RbCl), and vascular permeability index (VPI) (^{125}I-albumin) were calculated by dividing the % injected activity in the test sponge by the % injected activity in the control sponge.

$$\text{RI, BFI, VPI} = \frac{\% \text{ injected activity in experimental sponge}}{\% \text{ injected activity in control sponge}}$$

The RI, BFI, and VPI will equal 1.00 if the injected label enters the sponges at random. Any value significantly greater than 1.00 indicates preferential localization of label in the experimental sponge matrix graft.

Sponge matrix. Urethane sponges were cut into 20×10×10-mm pieces weighing 31±1 mg. The sponges were thoroughly washed and autoclaved before use. Two cell-free sponges were implanted subcutaneously on opposite sides of the lateral thorax of BALB recipients and allowed to heal for 13 days. All surgical procedures were performed under aseptic conditions.

Generation of secondary mixed leukocyte culture supernatant (2° MLC SN). B6 and DBA spleens were removed aseptically and gently compressed with a glass stopper in minimal essential medium (MEM; Flow Laboratories, McLean, VA). The cell suspensions were centrifuged at 250×G for 5 min. The cells were resuspended in MEM and washed twice. The final cell pellet was resuspended in D-MEM (Gibco) supplemented with 2% fetal calf serum (Gibco) at a final concentration of 1 mM sodium pyruvate (M.A. Bioproducts), 100 units/ml penicillin (Gibco), 100 μg/ml streptomycin (Gibco), 1.4×10^{-2} mM folic acid (Gibco), 2.7×10^{-1} mM L-asparagine (Gibco), 1.5 mM L-glutamine (Gibco), 5.5×10^{-1} mM L-arginine HCl (Gibco), 5×10^{-2} mM 2-mercaptoethanol (Sigma), and 10 mM Hepes Buffer (Gibco). Responder spleen cells (B6, 5×10^7) were incubated with 10×10^7 irradiated (2000 rads)(^{137}Cs Mark 1, Shepard 806 R/min) DBA stimulator spleen cells in 40 ml of supplemented medium in tissue culture flasks (No. 3024; Falcon, Oxnard, CA) and placed horizontally. After 14 days at 37°C in a moist atmosphere of 10% CO_2 and air, cultures were harvested, washed once, and counted. Allogeneic or syngeneic restimulation was initiated by culturing 3×10^7 day-14 MLC cells with 12×10^7 fresh, irradiated DBA (allogeneic) spleen cells or 12×10^7 fresh irradiated B6 (syngeneic) spleen cells in 30 ml of supplemented D-MEM. Cultures were incubated 18–24 hr and the supernatant harvested. Supernatants were millipore-filtered (0.22-μ pore size) and stored at −20°C until use. Obvious changes in the pH of the culture media in allogeneic or syngeneic cultures over 24 hr were not observed.

Mediators. Serotonin (5-hydroxytryptamine creatine sulfate complex, M.W. 387.4 daltons), histamine (histamine dihydrochloride, M.W. 184 daltons), and bradykinin (bradykinin triacetate salt, M.W. 1240.5 dalton) were obtained from the Sigma Co., St. Louis, MO. Serotonin, histamine, and bradykinin were diluted to the appropriate concentrations in MEM immediately before sponge inoculation. Purified human interleukin 1 (IL-1) (activity>100 U/ml); specific activity = 8U/pg protein; T cell growth factor 1.0%; interferon 1 U/ml; endotoxin = nil) and interleukin 2 (IL-2) (activity 5000 half maximal units/ml 70 U/ug; Il-1, interferon, colony-stimulating factor, macrophage activating factor, PMA, PHA, and endotoxin = nil) (known to also react with mouse cells) were obtained from the Genzyme Co., Norwalk, CN, and diluted to the appropriate concentration with RPMI 1640 with 5% fetal calf serum.

IL-2 assay. 2° MLC supernatants were assayed for IL-2 activity by the method of Gillis et al. (*9*). Day-14 MLC cells (B6 anti-DBA_x, 2×10^4) were suspended in supplemented D-MEM, and plated in groups of 4 with serial dilutions of 2°MLC SN in flat-bottomed microtiter plates (No. 3596, Costar). Plates were incubated 48 hr at 37°C in 10% CO_2 and pulsed with 2 μCI ^{3}H-TdR per well for 6.5 hr. Plates were harvested onto glass fiber filter paper and the ^{3}H-TdR incorporation was determined by liquid scintillation spectrophotometry.

Labeling of unsensitized spleen cells with indium-111-oxine. Indium-111-oxine was obtained from Amersham, Arlington Heights, IL. Cells were labeled in a modified technique described by Frost et al. (*10*). BALB spleens were excised, compressed, filtered, and centrifuged as above. The pellet was resuspended in buffered ammonium chloride solution. After 10 min the suspension was diluted in MEM and washed once. The pellet was washed once and resuspended in buffered ammonium chloride solution. After 10 min the suspension was diluted in MEM and washed once. The pellet was washed once and resuspended in phosphate-buffered saline solution. 5.0×10^7 cells were incubated with 25 μCi of indium-111-oxine in 0.5 ml of phosphate buffered saline for 10 min at 37°C. Cells were then washed 3 times in phosphate-buffered saline and resuspended in MEM at 4×10^7 cells/ml. The viability of the labeled cells was checked by trypan blue exclusion, and in all experiments was essentially unchanged (85–95%) after the labeling procedure. Labeled cells in 0.5 ml (2×10^7) were injected via the lateral tail vein. An aliquot of the labeled cell suspension was counted along with the experimental samples in order to calculate the percentage of the total injected activity.

Measurement of regional blood flow (% cardiac output). Measurement of regional blood flow was assessed as a percentage of cardiac output (% CO) going to the sponge using a modification of the method described by Ottaway and Parrott (*11*), using ^{86}RbCl. ^{86}RbCl obtained from New England Nuclear was diluted to 80 μCi/ml in phosphate-buffered saline, and a 10-μl aliquot (0.8 μCi) was counted in order to calculate the percentage of total injected activity. At various intervals after sponge inoculation 0.5 ml of ^{86}RbCl (40 μCi) solution was administered i.v. into a lateral tail vein in awake mice. After 45 sec, the animal was sacrificed by injecting saturated KCL solution i.v. The abdomen was opened and the aorta and inferior vena cava were cut in order to exsanguinate the animal. The sponges were removed and counted in a Biogamma II (Beckman Instruments). The peak energy of emission for ^{86}Rb is 1.1 MeV (*11*). Background counts were measured. The percentage of the cardiac output going to each sponge was calculated according to the formula:

$$\%\text{CO} = \frac{\text{cpm in sponge} - \text{background cpm}}{\text{injected cpm} - \text{background cpm}} \text{ X } 100$$

The regional blood flow index was calculated as the ratio of the % CO in the experimental sponge divided by the % CO in the control sponge.

$$\text{BFI} = \frac{\%\text{CO (experimental sponge)}}{\%\text{CO (control sponge)}}$$

Measurement of local changes in vascular permeability. Measurement of local changes in vascular permeability in injected sponges were performed using ^{125}I-albumin. ^{125}I-albumin obtained from New England Nuclear was diluted to 8 μCi/ml in MEM and a 10-μl aliquot (0.08 μCi) was counted in order to calculate the percentage of total injected activity. At 4 hr after sponge inoculation, 0.5 ml (4 μCi) of the ^{125}I-albumin solution was injected into the lateral tail vein of awake mice. At various intervals thereafter, mice were sacrificed and the sponges removed and counted in a Biogamma II. The peak emission of ^{125}I is 0.035 MeV. Background counts were measured. The percentage of injected activity and the vascular permeability index were calculated as noted above.

Statistical analyses. Statistical significance was determined by the Wilcoxon two-tailed Student's *t* test. Values are expressed as mean ± SE ($\bar{X}$±SE). The *P* value of the RI, BFI, and VPI compared with 1.00 was calculated using the formula:

$$t = \frac{\text{RI, BFI, VPI} - 1.00}{\text{SE}} \text{ with } n - 1 \text{ degrees of freedom}$$

RESULTS

IL-2 activity of allogeneic and syngeneic 2° MLC SN. Allogeneic and syngeneic supernatant were generated in vitro by restimulation of D-14 B6 anti-DBA MLC cells with DBA or B6 irradiated spleen cells, respectively. These supernatants were tested for IL-2 activity using resting D-14 MLC cells as indicator cells in a proliferative assay as noted above. This assay tests for the presence of only one of many lymphokines produced by allogeneic restimulation of sensitized cells and is therefore only a general confirmation of the presence or absence of restimulation and lymphokine production. Figure 1 demonstrates the presence of strong IL-2 activity when D-14 MLC cells are restimulated with allogeneic cells and minimal activity when restimulated with syngeneic cells. Other lymphokines that are a byproduct of allostimulation in this system are presumably also present at low levels in the syngeneic SN compared with the allogeneic SN.

2°MLC SN-mediated cellular recruitment to the site of in vivo injection—dose response. Thirteen days after subcutaneous implantation, paired, healed subcutaneous sponges were injected with allogeneic 2° MLC SN on the experimental side and with syngeneic 2°MLC SN on the control side. Four hours later 20×10^6 ^{111}In-oxine-labeled unsensitized BALB spleen cells were injected i.v. Sponges were removed and counted 1 hr later and the recruitment index calculated. Table 1 demonstrates that when both sponges were injected with 0.4 cc syngeneic 2° MLC SN there was no preferential accumulation of intravenously injected labeled cells in either sponge (RI=1.14±0.06, *P* compared with 1.00 = NS). This is consistent with our previous

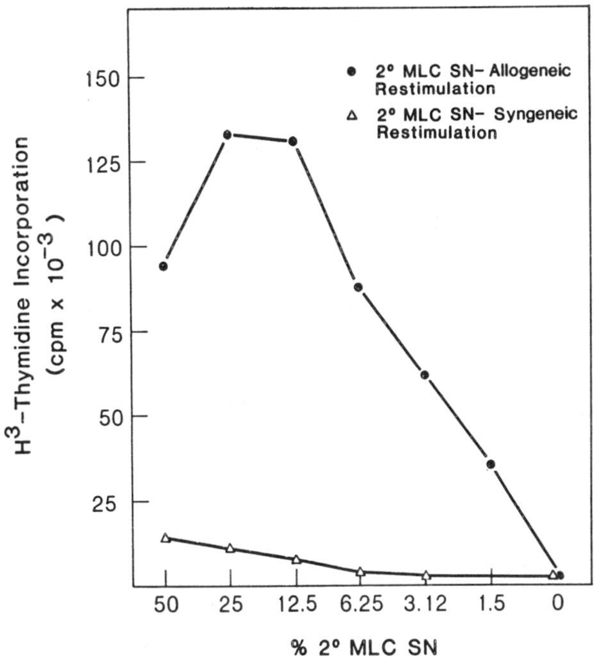

FIGURE 1. IL-2 activity of allogeneic and syngeneic supernatant. Allogeneic (●) and syngeneic (△) supernatant were generated in vitro by restimulation of D-14 B6 anti-DBA MLC cells (3×10^7) with DBA (12×10^7) or B6 (12×10^7) irradiated spleen cells, respectively, and harvested at 18 hr. The supernatants were tested for IL2 activity using D-14 MLC cells as indicator cells in a 6.5-hr proliferative assay (*9*). In the control syngeneic supernatant there is no significant IL-2 activity demonstrating the absence of restimulation.

studies demonstrating that anatomic variation or differences in healing or injection between the sponge grafts were not responsible for subsequently shown differences in RI. Table 1 shows that whenever one sponge was injected with 2° MLC SN and the other with syngeneic 2° MLC SN, there was a preferential increase in cellular recruitment to the sponge injected with allogeneic 2° MLC SN. When sponges were injected with differing volumes of 2° MLC SN, there was a dose-dependent increase in the preferential cellular recruitment to the site of allogeneic 2° MLC SN. Maximal preferential cellular recruitment was obtained with volumes equal to or greater than 0.6 ml.

2° MLC SN-mediated cellular recruitment—kinetics. Sponges were injected as before with 0.4 ml allogeneic 2° MLC SN or syngeneic 2° MLC SN. Then 4 hr later 20×10^6 ^{111}In-oxine-labeled unsensitized BALB spleen cells were injected i.v. Sponges were removed and counted at intervals after i.v. injection. Table 2 demonstrates that the preferential recruitment to the site of allogeneic 2° MLC SN injection, compared with the syngeneic SN, was demonstrable by 1 hr after i.v. injection (5 hr after sponge injection) and peaked by 4 hr after i.v. injection (8 hr after sponge injection) (see Fig. 2). From 4 hr to 24 hr there was only a slight decline in the RI from 2.07±0.07 to 1.81±0.09. This is in part due to an increase in nonspecific recruitment to the sponge injected with syngeneic supernatant, a phenomenon also observed in recruitment assays using sensitized cells and alloantigen (*3, 4*).

TABLE 1. Cellular recruitment properties of 2° MLC SN: dose response[a]

Volume of 2° MLC SN injected (ml)	% ($\bar{X}$ ± SE) of i.v. injected activity recovered in sponge		Recruitment index (RI) ($\bar{X}$ ± SE)	P[b] value
	Syngeneic SN:	Syngeneic SN:		
Control[c]	0.37±0.02	0.36±0.02	1.04±0.05	NS
	Allogeneic SN:	Syngeneic SN:		
0.2	0.57±0.04	0.41±0.04	1.45±0.08	<0.001
0.4	0.75±0.07	0.48±0.04	1.55±0.09	<0.001
0.6	0.82±0.06	0.51±0.05	1.71±0.11	<0.001
0.8	0.81±0.05	0.47±0.03	1.75±0.08	<0.001

[a] B6 anti-DBA SSL were generated in MLC; 2° MLC SN was generated by 24-hr allogeneic (DBA) or syngeneic (B6) restimulation with fresh irradiated DBA or B6 spleen cells, respectively. Allogeneic or syngeneic SN were then injected into plain sponge matrix grafts that had been implanted s.c. on opposite sides of the lateral thorax in BALB recipients 12 days earlier. Four hours later 20×10^6 ^{111}In-labeled fresh BALB spleen cells were injected i.v. Sponges were removed and counted 1 hr later.

[b] P value of RI compared with 1.00.

[c] In control animals both sponges were injected with syngeneic SN.

TABLE 2. Cellular recruitment properties of 2° MLC SN: kinetics[a]

Time (hours) of sponge removal after i.v. injection of ^{111}In-labeled cells	% ($\bar{X}$ ± SE) of i.v.-injected activity recovered in sponge: Allogeneic SN	Syngeneic SN	Recruitment index (RI) ($\bar{X}$ ± SE)	P value[b]
1	0.75±0.07	0.48±0.04	1.55±0.09	<0.001
2	0.98±0.03	0.51±0.02	1.96±0.11	<0.001
4	0.95±0.05	0.46±0.03	2.07±0.07	<0.001
8	0.89±0.03	0.44±0.01	2.03±0.09	<0.001
16	1.51±0.07	0.85±0.05	1.80±0.09	<0.001
24	1.56±0.07	0.87±0.03	1.81±0.09	<0.001

[a] Healed s.c. sponges were injected with allogeneic or syngeneic SN as before. Then 4 hr later 20×10^6 ^{111}In-labeled BALB spleen cells were injected i.v. Sponges were removed at intervals after i.v. injection and counted.

[b] P value of RI compared with 1.00.

2° MLC SN-mediated cellular recruitment—duration of effect. Sponges were injected as before, and at various intervals thereafter ^{111}In-labeled BALB spleen cells were injected i.v. Sponges were removed and counted 1 hr after i.v. injection, in contrast to the previous set of experiments where the time of i.v.injection was held constant and the interval to sponge removal was varied. Table 3 demonstrates a progressive increase in preferential cellular recruitment to the sponge injected with allogeneic SN up to 18 hr after injection. By 24 hr the effect of the 2° MLC SN at the graft site has begun to decrease.

Regional blood flow and vascular permeability at the site of in vivo injection of 2° MLC SN. Regional blood flow, expressed as percent of cardiac output, was examined in sponges injected with 0.4 ml of allogeneic or syngeneic 2° MLC SN. ^{86}RbCl (40 μCi) was injected i.v. at intervals following sponge injection, and animals were sacrificed and exsanguinated 45 sec after ^{86}RbCl injection as noted above. Sponges were removed and counted. Table 4 demonstrates there was a small but significant increase in blood flow at the site of allogeneic 2° MLC SN at

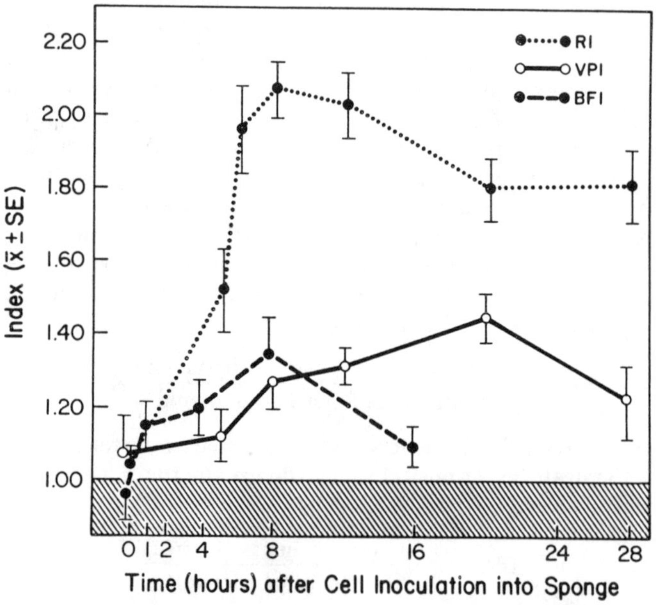

FIGURE 2. Effect of 2° MLC SN on the kinetics of lymphocytes recruitment, blood flow, and vascular permeability. The RI (● ··· ●), BFI (● --- ●), and VPI (O – O) (Tables 2, 4, and 5) have been plotted on the same time scale (i.e. hours after cell inoculation into sponge) for ease of comparison.

TABLE 3. Cellular recruitment properties of 2° MLC SN: duration of effect[a]

Time (hours) of i.v. injection of ^{111}In-labeled cells after sponge inoculation	% ($\bar{X}$ ± SE) of i.v.-injected activity recovered in sponge: Allogeneic SN	Syngeneic SN	Recruitment index (RI) ($\bar{X}$ ± SE)	P value[b]
2	0.50±0.04	0.42±0.02	1.18±0.05	<0.005
4	0.72±0.04	0.51±0.03	1.43±0.05	<0.001
6	0.85±0.09	0.53±0.05	1.55±0.06	<0.001
8	0.85±0.08	0.51±0.04	1.63±0.05	<0.001
18	1.24±0.04	0.61±0.04	2.08±0.08	<0.001
24	0.96±0.06	0.56±0.03	1.70±0.06	<0.001

[a] Healed s.c. sponges were injected as before. At intervals thereafter 20×10^6 ^{111}In-labeled BALB spleen cells were injected i.v. Sponges were removed and counted 1 hr after i.v. injection.

[b] P value compared with 1.00.

1, 4, and 8 hr, but not at 16 hr, after sponge injection (Fig. 2).

^{125}I-albumin (4 μCi) was injected i.v. 4 hr after sponge inoculation with 0.4 ml of allogeneic or syngeneic 2° MLC SN. Sponges were removed and counted at intervals after i.v. injection. Table 5 demonstrates that the VIP was elevated within 4 hours, peaked at 16 hr, and declined by 24 hr after i.v. injection (Fig. 2).

Effect of various mediators on cellular recruitment. The ability of human IL-1, IL-2, serotonin, histamine, and bradykinin to mediate cellular recruitment in vivo were compared with SSL + targets and 2°MLC SN as shown in Table 6. The data shown compared the maximal RI for each mediator, although each was tested over a range of time and dosage in several small pilot experiments. For example, IL-1, serotonin, histamine, and bradykinin were all tested for changes in CR at 0.25, 0.5, 1.0, 2.0, and 4.0 hr (data not shown). Serotonin was also tested at 1×10^{-2} M; IL-1, at 0.01, 0.1, 1.0, and 10.0 units; and IL-2 at 50, 100, and 200 half-maximal units. IL-2, serotonin, histamine, and bradykinin do not mediate a significant change in CR. In contrast IL-1 does mediate a slight increase in CR, but not as great as that mediated by SSL and targets or 2° MLC SN.

TABLE 4. Regional blood flow at the site of in vivo injection of 2° MLC SN[a]

Time (hours) of ^{86}RbCl injection after 2° MLC SN inoculation into sponge	% ($\bar{X}$ ± SE) cardiac output to sponges		Blood flow index (BFI) ($\bar{X}$ ± SE)	P value[b]
	Allogeneic SN	Syngeneic SN		
1	0.64±0.04	0.55±0.02	1.15±0.06	<0.05
4	0.61±0.04	0.52±0.04	1.20±0.07	<0.02
8	0.65±0.05	0.49±0.04	1.36±0.14	<0.05
16	0.51±0.03	0.47±0.02	1.10±0.05	NS (<0.10)

[a] Healed s.c. sponges were injected as before. At intervals thereafter 40 μCi ^{86}RbCl was injected i.v.; 45 sec later KCl was given, then animals were exsanguinated, and sponges were removed and counted. The blood flow to each sponge is expressed as a percentage of cardiac output.

[b] P value of BFI compared with 1.00.

TABLE 5. Vascular permeability at the site of injection of 2° MLC SN[a]

Time (hours) of sponge removal after i.v. injection of ^{125}I-albumin	% ($\bar{X}$ ± SE) of injected label recovered in sponge		Vascular permeability index (VPI) ($\bar{X}$ ± SE)	P value[b]
	Allogeneic SN	Syngeneic SN		
1	1.43±0.05	1.34±0.14	1.12±0.08	NS
4	2.78±0.09	2.24±0.15	1.27±0.07	<0.02
8	3.03±0.18	2.33±0.15	1.31±0.05	<0.01
16	3.13±0.21	2.19±0.13	1.44±0.07	<0.01
24	2.29±0.17	1.92±0.06	1.21±0.10	NS

[a] Healed s.c. sponges were injected as before. Then 4 hr later 4 μCi of ^{125}I-albumin was injected i.v. Sponges were removed at intervals after i.v. injection and counted.

[b] P value of VPI compared with 1.00.

TABLE 6. Comparison of the maximal cellular recruitment ability of various mediators[a]

Mediator	% ($\bar{X}$ ± SE) of injected activity recovered in sponge		Recruitment index (RI) ($\bar{X}$ ± SE)	P value[b]
	Experimental sponge	Control sponge		
B6 anti-DBA SSL + DBA or B6 Targets	0.76±0.05	0.38±0.03	2.04±0.23	<0.01
2° MLC SN (0.8 ml)	0.81±0.05	0.47±0.03	1.75±0.08	<0.001
IL-1 (1 unit)	0.59±0.03	0.46±0.02	1.31±0.05	<0.001
IL-2 (100 1/2 maximal units)	0.62±0.04	0.54±0.04	1.14±0.05	NS
Serotonin (4×10^{-4} M)	0.39±0.02	0.39±0.02	1.02±0.05	NS
Histamine (10^{-3} M)	0.39±0.04	0.35±0.02	1.07±0.07	NS
Bradykinin (40 μg)	0.36±0.01	0.39±0.02	0.93±0.04	NS

[a] Healed s.c. sponges were injected as before; 4 hr later 20×10^{6} ^{111}In-labeled BALB spleen cells were injected i.v. Sponges were removed 1 hr after i.v. injection and counted.

[b] P value of RI compared with 1.00.

DISCUSSION

Evidence is accumulating that both cytolytic and helper T lymphocytes play a major role in allograft rejection and that many of their effects may be mediated or enhanced by lymphokines produced as a result of allostimulation (*12–14*). Most in vivo studies have utilized adoptive transfer of bulk-sensitized lymphocytes that have been enriched for helper or cytolytic T cells on the basis of cell surface differentiation antigens. Some investigators have concluded that noncytotoxic Lyt-$1^{+}2^{-}$ cells in the mouse (*15–17*) or $OX8^{-}$, $W3/25^{+}$ cells in the rat (*18*) are primarily responsible for allograft rejection. These investigators argue that allograft destruction in these experiments is mediated by lymphokines and resembles a delayed-type hyersensitivity reaction. Other studies, utilizing adoptive transfer of cloned T lymphocytes, have demonstrated that cytolytic Lyt-2^{+} cells are capable of mediating the rejection of syngeneic and allogeneic tumors, leading to the conclusion that graft destruction is the result of direct cell mediated killing (*19–20*). It is possible, and in fact likely that both mechanisms are important in allograft rejection. A recent study in the T-cell-deprived rat demonstrated that a combination of cytotoxic $OX8^{+}$, $W3/25^{-}$ and noncytotoxic $OX8^{-}$, $W3/25^{+}$ lymphocytes was more effective than either cell population alone in mediating heart allograft rejection (*13*). Furthermore, recent evidence that most cytolytic T lymphocytes also produce lymphokines (*7*), including cytotoxic lymphokines (*21*), raises the possibility that even graft destruction mediated by these cells may involve lymphokines.

Lymphokines may play an important role in allograft rejection by mediating the accumulation of circulating allosensitized lymphocytes and other inflammatory cells at the graft site. The cellular infiltrate in rejecting allografts and in DTH reactions includes a few SSL—but UL, macrophages, neutrophils, and monocytes predominate (*1*). Although some studies have shown small amounts of specific migration of SSL to the sites of rejecting allografts and DTH reactions (*22–24*), most studies have shown lymphocytes accumulate randomly (*2, 25–31*). We have postulated that the chance encounter between a few circulating SSL (released from the lymphoid depots where initial allosensitization occurs) and graft alloantigen results in the release of lymphokines that mediate the nonspecific accumulation of additional SSL and other inflammatory cells, cause changes in local blood flow and vascular permeability, and mediate tissue injury. This would account for the heterogeneity and nonspecificity of the cellular infiltrate in rejecting allografts—and, since the circulating pool is enriched for SSL, nonspecific recruitment might serve as a specific amplification mechanism in rejection. This hypothesis is supported by our previous studies. We have demonstrated that the in vivo interaction between sensitized T cells and alloantigen-bearing target results in an increase in cellular recruitment, blood flow, and vascular permeability at the graft site (3, 4). SSL and UL accumulate equally and randomly (2, 3). We have also shown that alloantigen-specific cloned cytolytic, helper, and helper-cell-independent cytolytic T cells mediate an increase in cellular recruitment, confirming that any functional subclass of allosensitized T cell can mediate these changes, and that only target cell recognition, not cell killing, is required (6).

The present study was designed to determine whether soluble factors produced during allostimulation in vitro were capable of mediating changes in vivo in cellular recruitment, regional blood flow, and vascular permeablity. The ability of the supernatants obtained from restimulation of allosensitized lymphocytes to mediate such inflammatory events in vivo has not previously been examined. Using 2° MLC SN, a rich source of a variety of lymphokines synthesized and secreted by activated cells in response to allogeneic stimulation, a rapid, dose-related increase in cellular recruitment to the site of injection was demonstrated. The quantitative response and the kinetics of the accumulation of ^{111}In-labeled lymphocytes in response to 2° MLC SN were similar to previous studies in which SSL were injected with allogeneic targets (2, 4). These similarities emphasize the somewhat surprising rapidity with which the interation between SSL and alloantigen in these experiments led to the release of putative lymphokines capable of mediating changes in CR. The effect of 2° MLC SN on RBF and VP was also rapid, but quantitatively less than prior studies using SSL and alloantigen, and the VPI peaked later (4). Since CR was similar in the two studies, 2° MLC SN may contain other chemoattractants or migration inhibitory factors that are as important as changes in RBF and VP for CR.

Conventional inflammatory mediators such as serotonin, bradykinin, and histamine—which may participate in DTH reactions by increasing local blood flow, vascular permeability to protein, and cellular extravasation (32–34)—did not alter cellular recruitment in this model. Therefore, even though there are some similarities between these lymphokine mediated events in allograft rejection and DTH reactions, there are also clear differences. It is possible that the mediators required are in fact different, or changes in cellular recruitment may require the simultaneous action or interaction of several different factors. It is not surprising that IL-2 had no effect on cellular recruitment since we have shown before that CTL clones that do not secrete IL-2 are capable of mediating CR. IL-1, a product of activated macrophages that are present in large numbers in rejecting allografts, may be an important inflammatory mediator. More detailed investigations of its role in this model are in progress.

In conclusion, we have demonstrated that 2° MLC SN derived from in vitro restimulation of resting allosensitized T cells is capable of mediating in vivo changes in cellular recruitment, blood flow, and vascular permeability. There data are consistent with previous studies suggesting that the elaboration of lymphokines as a direct result of in vivo allogeneic cellular interactions results in the nonspecific attraction of circulating SSL and inflammatory cells to the graft site, which amplifies the host response. The small changes in RBF and VP in the present experiments do not account for the greater magnitude in CR. It is likely that other specific or nonspecific chemoattractants that are inhibitors of cell migration also play a significant role in CR in vivo.

REFERENCES

1. Ascher NL, Hoffman R, Hanto DW, Simmons RL. Cellular basis of allograft rejection. Immunol Rev 1984; 77: 217.
2. Hopt UT, Sullivan W, Hoffman R, Simmons RL. Migration and cell recruiting activity of specifically sensitized lymphocytes in sponge matrix allografts. Transplantation 1980; 30: 411.
3. Hanto DW, Hopt UT, Hoffman R, Simmons RL. The recruitment of unsensitized circulating lymphocytes to sites of allogeneic cellular interations. Transplantation 1982; 33: 541.
4. Hanto DW, Hopt UT, Hoffman R, Simmons RL. Lymphocyte recruitment, regional blood flow, and vascular permeability at sites of allogeneic cellular interactions. J Immunol 1982; 129: 2437.
5. Hanto DW, Harty JT, Simmons RL. Lymphocyte recruitment properties of regional lymph node or spleen cells during skin allograft rejection. Transplantation 1983; 36: 578.
6. Hanto DW, Widmer MB, Simmons RL. Functionally distinct T-cell clones mediate cellular recruitment in vivo. Transplantation 1986; 42: 168.
7. Prystowsky MB, Ely JM, Beller DI, et al. Alloreactive cloned T cell lines. VI. Multiple lymphokine activities secreted by helper and cytolytic cloned T lymphocytes. J Immunol 1982; 129: 2337.
8. Dvorak HF, Galli SJ, Dvorak AM. Expression of cell-mediated hypersensitivity in vivo—recent advances. Int Rev Exp Pathol 1980; 21: 119.
9. Gillis S, Ferm MM, Ou W, Smith KA. T cell growth factor: parameters of production and a quantitative microassay for activity. J Immunol 1978; 120: 2027.
10. Frost P, Smith J, Frost H. The radiolabelling of lymphocytes and tumor cells with ^{111}Indium. Proc Soc Exp Biol Med 1978; 157: 61.
11. Ottaway CA, Parrott DMV. Regional blood flow and its relationship to lymphocyte and lymphoblast traffic during a primary immune reaction. J Exp Med 1979; 150: 218.
12. Steinmuller D. Which T cells mediate allograft rejection. Transplantation 1985; 40: 229.
13. Heidecke CD, Kupiec-Weglinski JW, Lear PA, et al. Interactions between T lymphocyte subsets supported by interleukin 2-rich lymphokines produce acute rejection of vascularized cardiac allografts in T cell deprived rats. J Immunol 1984; 133: 582.
14. Kirkman RL, Barrett LV, Gaulton GN, Kelley VE, Ythier A, Strom TB. Administration of an anti-interleukin 2 receptor monoclonal antibody prolongs cardiac allograft survival in mice. J Exp Med 1985; 162: 358.
15. Loveland BE, Hogarth PM, Ceredig RH, McKenzie IFC. Cells mediating graft rejection in the mouse. I. Lyt-1 cells mediate skin graft rejection. J Exp Med 1981; 153: 1044.
16. Loveland BE, McKenzie IFC. Cells mediating graft rejection in the mouse. II. The Ly phenotypes of cells producing tumor allograft rejection. Transplantation 1982; 33: 174.
17. Loveland BE, McKenzie IFC. Cells mediating graft rejection in the mouse. III. Ly-1$^+$ precursor T cells generate skin graft rejection. Transplantation 1982; 33: 407.
18. Dallman MJ, Mason DW, Webb M. The roles of host and donor cells in the rejection of skin allografts by T cell deprived rats injected with syngeneic T cells. Eur J Immunol 1982; 12: 511.
19. Engers HD, Glasebrook AL, Sorenson GD. Allogeneic tumor rejection induced by the intravenous injection of Lyt-2$^+$ cytolytic T lymphocyte clones. J Exp Med 1982; 156: 1280.
20. Engers HD, Lahaye T, Sorenson GD, et al. Functional activity in vivo of effector T cell populations. II. Anti-tumor activity exhibited by syngeneic anti-Mo MULV-specific cytolytic T cell clones. J Immunol 1984; 133: 664.
21. Green LM, Stern ML, Haviland DL, Mills BJ, Ware CF. Cytotoxic lymphokines produced by cloned human cytotoxic T lymphocytes. I. Cytotoxins produced by antigen-specific and natural killer- like CTL are dissimilar to classical lymphotoxins. J Immunol 1985; 135: 4034.
22. Tilney NL, Notis-Mcconarty J, Strom TB. Specificity of cellular migration into cardiac allografts in rats. Transplantation 1978; 26: 181.
23. Emeson EE. Migratory behavior of lymphocytes with specific reactivity to alloantigens. II. Selective recruitment to lymphoid cell

allografts and their draining lymph nodes. J Exp Med 1978; 147: 13.
24. Chang AE, Sugarbaker PH. Preferential homin of passively transferred T cells into skin allografts of mice. Transplantation 1979; 28: 247.
25. Moore AR, Hall JG. Nonspecific entry of thoracic duct immunoblasts into intradermal foci of antigens. Cell Immunol 1973; 8: 112.
26. Allwood GG. The migratory behavior of T blasts to contact sensitivity reactions in actively and passively sensitized mice. Immunology 1975; 28: 681.
27. McCluskey RT, Benacerraf B, McCluskey JW. Studies on the specificity of the cellular infiltrate in delayed hypersensitivity reactions. J Immunol 1963; 90: 466.
28. Turk JL, Oort J. A histological study of the early stages of the development of the tuberculin reaction after passive transfer of cells labelled with ^{3}H Thymidine. Immunology 1963; 6: 140.
29. Prendergast RA. Cellular specificity in the homograft reaction. J Exp Med 1969; 119: 377.
30. Hall JG. Studies of the cells in the afferent and efferent lymph of lymph nodes draining the site of skin homografts. J Exp Med 1967; 125: 737.
31. Jungi TW, McGregor DD. Activated lymphocytes trigger lymphoblast extravasation. Cell Immunol 1978; 38: 76.
32. Rose ML, Parrott DMV. Vascular permeability and lymphoblast extravasation into inflamed skin are not related. Cell Immunol 1977; 33: 62.
33. Gershon RK, Askenase PW, Gershon MD. Requirement for vasoactive amines for production of delayed-type by hypersensitivity skin reactions. J Exp Med 1975; 142: 732.
34. Galli SJ, Hammel I. Unequivocal delayed hypersensitivity in mast cell-deficient and beige mice. Science 1984; 226: 710.

Received 4 February 1986.
Accepted 18 March 1986.

0041-1337/86/4206-0627$02.00/0
TRANSPLANTATION
Vol. 42, No. 6
Printed in U.S.A.

EVIDENCE OF A CYCLOSPORINE-BINDING PROTEIN IN HUMAN ERYTHROCYTES

RAGHUNATH P. AGARWAL, RICHARD A. MCPHERSON,[1] AND GREGORY A. THREATTE

Departments of Laboratory Medicine and Pathology, Georgetown University Medical Center, Washington, D.C. 20007

To investigate the phenomenon of different erythrocyte saturation capacities for cyclosporine (CsA) in the blood of different individuals, hemolysates of washed red cells were examined for the presence of a CsA-binding protein. Using gel filtration column chromatography of hemolysates from patients receiving CsA orally, the majority of erythrocyte-associated CsA eluted as a single peak with M_r 15,000–17,000, distinct from hemoglobin and carbonic anhydrase. [^{3}H]CsA added to a hemolysate in vitro eluted similarly. [^{125}I]CsA added to a hemolysate eluted much later in the same position as [^{3}H]CsA mixed with albumin and myoglobin (presumably as free unbound drug). These findings indicate that CsA normally binds to an intraerythrocytic protein similar in molecular size to calf thymus cyclophilin (M_r 15,000). By equilibrium dialysis, the purified erythrocyte proteins calmodulin (M_r 16,700) and cytochrome b_5 (M_r 15,000) failed to bind CsA. By equilibrium dialysis, [^{3}H] CsA did bind to column fractions containing the CsA-binding protein, but [^{125}I]CsA did not, suggesting that attachment to CsA occurs at or near a carbon-carbon double bond in an unusual nine-carbon amino acid of CsA. These results have important implications for CsA therapy with regard to distribution space, pharmacokinetics, and a possible protein-receptor mechanism of action.

Cyclosporine (CsA) * is an 11-amino acid cyclic peptide with immunosuppressive action on t lymphocytes (*1*), apparently at the level of inhibiting transcription from the gene for the lymphokine interleukin 2 (IL-2) (*2–4*). Clinical use of CsA for prevention of organ rejection requires therapeutic drug monitoring to reduce the risk of toxicity, particularly to the kidneys, liver, and central nervous system (*5–7*).

Due to its lipophilic nature, CsA distributes in body tissues largely according to organ fat content with extensive deposits in liver and kidney (*8–10*). Although the therapeutic target of CsA is t lymphocytes, there does not appear to be a surface membrane receptor for CsA on those cells (*11*). In the circulation, CsA binds preferentially to blood cells up to saturation of the cells (*9, 12*). Above that concentration, the fraction of CsA in plasma increases. The distribution between plasma and cells is influenced by temperature with more binding to cells at lower temperatures (*9, 13*). While CsA does bind to lipoproteins in plasma, the circulating levels of cholesterol and triglycerides apparently have little or no influence on whole-blood levels of CsA (*14, 15*).

Because of these influences on the distribution of CsA between cellular and plasma phases, therapeutic monitoring of the drug is commonly performed on whole blood for ease of sample preparation (*6, 16*). Hematocrit does influence the

[1] Address correspondence to: Richard A. McPherson, Department of Laboratory Medicine, Georgetown University Hospital, 3800 Reservoir Road, N.W., Washington, D.C. 20007.

* Abbreviations used: B, bound; CsA, cyclosporine; CsBP, cyclosporine-binding protein; EDTA, ethylenediaminotetraacetate; F, free; IL-2, interleukin-2; RBC, red blood cell; RIA, radioimmunoassay; SDS, sodium dodecyl sulphate.

distribution of CsA between cells and plasma in a predictable manner (*15*). However, we have previously found that patients demonstrate different saturation capacities in their red cells independent of hematocrit or hemoglobin content (*17*). Accordingly there appeared to be some component of red cells other than cell membrane lipids that selectively bound CsA.

The purpose of this investigation was to identify any proteins present in human erythrocytes that were able to bind CsA.

MATERIALS AND METHODS

Sephacryl S-200, Sephadex G-25, and Sephadex G-75 were obtained from Pharmacia Fine Chemicals, Piscataway, NJ. Tween 20, myoglobin, and calmodulin were from Sigma Chemical Co., St. Louis, MO. [^{3}H]CsA (label positions: 95% [Abu-^{3}H]-cyclosporine and 5 percent ([N-methyl-^{3}H]-Sar)cyclosporine) was generously supplied by Sandoz Ltd., Basel, Switzerland. [^{125}I]CsA (2.2 μCi/ml) was purchased from Immuno Nuclear Corporation, Stillwater, MN. Cytochrome b_5, isolated from bovine liver, was kindly supplied by Dr. Patrick Fleming, Department of Biochemistry, Georgetown University Medical Center, Washington, D.C. Polyacrylamide, N,N′-methylene-bis-acrylamide (Bis), TEMED, sodium dodecyl sulfate (SDS), and molecular weight standards were obtained from Bio-Rad, Richmond, CA. All other reagents were reagent grade and were used without further purification. Solutions from the Sephadex chromatography were concentrated by pressure dialysis using YM-2 membranes obtained from Amicon Corp., Lexington, MA.

Blood was collected by venipuncture into vacuum tubes containing ethylenediaminetetraacetic acid (EDTA) from kidney transplant recipients receiving CsA orally every twelve hours. All such blood specimens were obtained as trough levels for purposes of therapeutic drug monitoring. Blood samples were allowed to stand at 4°C for 24 hr for equilibration of the drug between various components and centrifuged at 2500×g for 10 min at 4°C. Plasma and buffy layer were removed, and red blood cells (RBC) were washed five times with buffer containing 150 mM NaCl and 10 mM Na phosphate (pH 7.4). The washed RBC were then lysed by freezing and thawing after the addition of four volumes of deionized water. RBC membranes were separated by centrifugation at 22,000 ×g for 1 hr in a refrigerated centrifuge (Sorvall RC2B). The upper layer was removed and chromatographed on Sephacryl or Sephadex columns operated with 10 mM Na phosphate (pH 6.8) at 4°C.

Protein concentrations in column eluates were monitored by absorbance at 280 nm (A_{280}), absorbance at 415 nm (A_{415}—i.e., spectral indicator of hemoglobin), and the difference in absorbances at 215 and 225 nm ($\Delta A = A_{215} - A_{225}$—i.e., predominantly peptide bonds). Absorbances were measured on a Beckman DU-8 spectrophotometer. Protein concentrations in the eluates were estimated from the values of ΔA (*18*). Carbonic anydrase activity was assayed by the colorimetric method of Wilburg and Anderson (*19, 20*). The assay mixture contained 2 ml of 0.025 M veronal buffer (pH 8.2) with 1 mg/100 ml of bromthymol blue, and 1 ml of the test sample appropriately diluted, to which was added 2 ml of saturated solution of cold carbon dioxide, all at 2°C. The time from injection of carbon dioxide until the indicator color changed from blue to yellow was recorded. Activity of the enzyme (U) was calculated from the following formula (*20*):

$$U = 10D([T_b/T_c] - 1)$$

where D is the dilution factor of the enzyme, Tb is the time of uncatalyzed reaction and Tc is the time of enzyme-catalyzed reaction.

The concentrations of CsA in the column eluates were measured by radioimmunoassay (RIA) using a kit supplied by Sandoz Ltd. In these measurements eluates from the Sephadex chromatography were used without further dilution. SDS-polyacrylamide gel electrophoresis was performed by the method of Weber and Osborn (*21*).

Equilibrium dialysis was performed on an apparatus made of rigid acrylic plastic, consisting of five separate pairs of chambers, which allowed for the performance of five simultaneous studies. Each chamber was separated into two compartments (1 ml capacity) by a semipermeable membrane (Spectrapor-1). At the top of each half-cell an opening for introducing or withdrawing solutions was provided. The [^{3}H] CsA solutions used in these studies were prepared by the dilution of 10 μl of the stock solution of the drug (58 μCi containing 6.8 μg CsA/ml) into 5 ml Tris buffer (0.05 M, pH 7.4) that contained 0.05% Tween 20. The [^{125}I] CsA solutions were prepared by the dilution of 0.1 ml stock solution (2.2 μCi/ml) into 2 ml of the same buffer containing 0.05% Tween 20. [^{3}H]CsA (or [^{125}I]CsA) solutions (0.8 ml) were introduced by a syringe into the half-cells (A_1-A_5) on one side of the dialysis apparatus and protein solutions (0.8 ml, 0.05% in Tween 20) were introduced into the opposite half-cells (B_1-B_5). The solutions were then equilibrated by agitating on an automatic shaker for 24 hr at room temperature. At the end of an experiment, 25-μl aliquots were withdrawn from each half-cell and counted (dpm) for tritium in a Beckman scintillation counter. In the case of [^{125}I]CsA, the radioactivity of 1-ml aliquots was measured in a Compac 120 Picker gamma counter. Recoveries of radiolabeled cyclosporine in solution (chamber A plus chamber B) after equilibrium dialysis were consistently greater than 90% (i.e., less than 10% loss by adsorption to chamber surfaces and membrane).

For the determination of binding constants, 0.2-ml aliquots of a hemolysate (diluted five-fold) prepared from washed erythrocytes of a normal individual were mixed with 0.4 ml of TT buffer (0.05 M trishydroxymethylaminomethane pH 7.4, 0.05% Tween 20). To each mixture 0.02 ml of [^{3}H]CsA (diluted 500-fold in ethanol from stock solution) was added and incubated at 4°C for 1 hr. Then 0.02 ml of unlabeled CsA was added in increasing concentrations and again incubated at 4°C for 1 hr. To adsorb the free CsA, 0.2 ml of a 1% charcoal suspension in TT buffer containing 0.2% bovine serum albumin was added, quickly vortexed, and incubated at 4°C for 10 min before centrifugation at 3000 rpm. Aliquots of 0.1 ml of the supernatants were counted for radioactivity with 5 ml of scintillation fluid. These counts represented bound [^{3}H]CsA. Nonspecific binding measured by using TT buffer in place of hemolysate was subtracted from the bound counts. To calculate free [^{3}H] CsA, corrected bound counts were subtracted from total counts. The ratio of bound-to-free was plotted versus bound. Binding constant and capacity were obtained by standard Scatchard analysis using least squares linear regression fit to a straight line of bound-to-free versus bound CsA.

RESULTS

Column fractionation of CsA in a hemolysate. The experimental strategy was to fractionate by gel filtration the proteins present in hemolysates prepared from erythrocytes of patients receiving CsA orally. The various fractions were then assessed for CsA content (by RIA) as well as for the presence of hemoglobin (as A_{415}), carbonic anhydrase activity, and total protein concentration (as A_{280}).

Fractionation of the hemolysate on a Sephacryl S-200 column (1.5×20-cm; effective resolution for M_r 5000 to 250,000 Da) operated with 10 mM Na phosphate (pH 6.8) at a flow rate of 30 ml/hr in 1.4-ml fractions showed that hemoglobin eluted in tubes 9–17 (peak in tube 12) while the CsA eluted in tubes 11-16 (peak in tube 14). This result showed that despite considerable overlap in the elution profiles of hemoglobin and CsA, the drug did elute in a position corresponding to a smaller size than human hemoglobin (M_r 64,500 Da).

By filtration through Sephadex G-25 (effective resolution for M_r 1000–5000 Da) using the same column parameters as above, both hemoglobin and CsA eluted in the void volume, indicating that the molecular size of the CsA-associated species was larger than 5,000 Da.

The hemolysate was next fractionated on a Sephadex G-75 column (2.5×100-cm; effective resolution for M_r 3000 to 80,000) operated with 10 mM Na phosphate (pH 6.8) as above. Under these conditions, there was virtually complete separation of hemoglobin (fractions 35–47, peak in 41) from CsA (fractions 52–65, peak in 57) and only partial overlap between carbonic anhydrase (CA; fractions 44–58, peak in 50) and CsA (Fig. 1). No CsA was detected in subsequent fractions out to tube 80, indicating that all the CsA in the hemolysate eluted in this single peak. The sum of CsA measured in fractions 52–65 accounted for 94% of the CsA from the original unfractionated hemolysate. The protein elution profile as assessed by A_{280} essentially paralleled that for hemoglobin (A_{415}). The values of A_{280} in the CsA-containing fractions (52–65) ranged from 0.43 to 0.03 with no distinct peak. Similarly the values of A_{415} in the same fractions ranged from 0.49 to 0.03, indicating only a minor trailing of hemoglobin perhaps as dissociated monomers. The total protein concentration in the peak CsA-containing fraction (tube 57) was 0.49 mg/ml as calculated from ΔA.

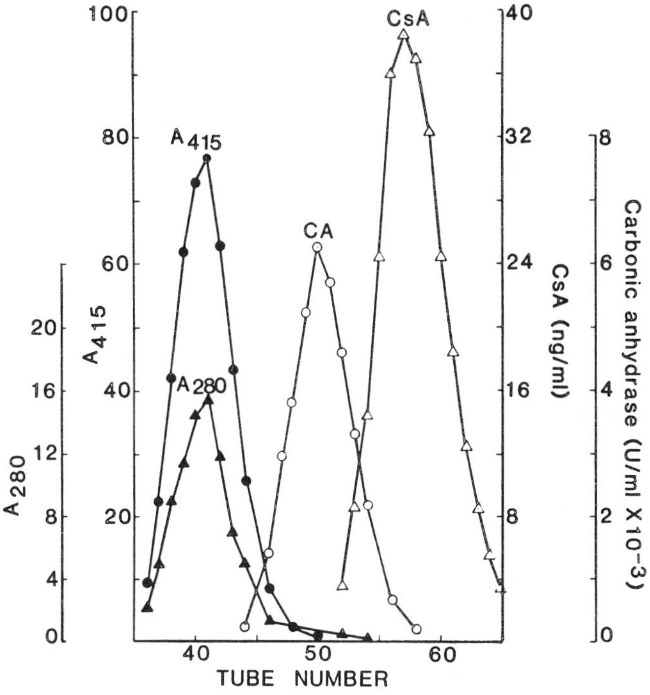

FIGURE 1. Gel filtration of a washed erythrocyte lysate from blood of a patient receiving CsA orally. A 5-ml sample was applied to a Sephadex G-75 column (2.5×100-cm) operated with 10 mM Na phosphate (pH 6.8). Fractions of 4.6 ml were collected at a flow rate of 30 ml/hr. Protein elution was monitored by measurement of absorbance at 415 nm (hemoglobin) and at 280 nm (total protein). Carbonic anhydrase (CA) was measured as enzyme activity; CsA was estimated by radioimmunoassay.

Erythrocytic uptake of radiolabeled CsA. The intraerythrocytic accumulation of CsA was analyzed directly by incubating blood from a normal individual with [^{3}H]CsA. In order to prevent any possible alteration of erythrocytes during the initial mixing with [^{3}H]CsA dissolved in alcohol, the [^{3}H]CsA was first mixed with plasma separated from EDTA-anticoagulated whole blood and then that plasma was added back to the remainder of the whole blood sample. In this manner, 0.05 ml of [^{3}H]CsA (29 μCi/3.4 μg) was added to 10 ml of whole blood and incubated for 3 hr at room temperature (22°C) with continuous gentle mixing by inversion. The sample was then centrifuged at 4°C, and the erythrocytes were washed and lysed. When the [^{3}H]CsA-containing hemolysate was fractionated on Sephadex G-75, the elution profile for hemoglobin and CsA was identical to that in Figure 1.

Attempts to incorporate [^{125}I]CsA into erythrocytes were unsuccessful. Accordingly [^{125}I]CsA was mixed with a hemolysate of normal erythrocytes, and this mixture was chromatographed on a Sephadex G-75 column under the same conditions described above. In this instance all of the ^{125}I radioactivity eluted in fractions 69–84 (peak in tube 76) (Fig. 2), which is far beyond the position where [^{3}H]CsA eluted (Fig. 1). Apparently unlabeled CsA and [^{3}H]CsA are both able to complex with a component of hemolysates, thereby eluting earlier on Sephadex G-75 than [^{125}I]CsA, which probably elutes as the free drug not complexed with other molecules. To confirm this interpretation, a mixture of dextran blue, equine myoglobin, and [^{3}H] CsA was fractionated under identical experimental conditions to determine how free CsA eluted in the absence of erythrocyte proteins. Dextran blue (void volume indicator) eluted in fractions 28–33 (peak in tube 30), myoglobin eluted in fractions 53–68 (peak in tube 59), and [^{3}H]CsA eluted in the same position as the [^{125}I]CsA in Figure 2. Thus CsA in the hemolysate appears to bind to a protein, but in the absence of that protein elutes as the smaller-molecular-sized free drug. By least squares linear regression analysis of logarithm of molecular weights for hemoglobin (64,500 Da), carbonic anhydrase (30,000 Da), and myoglobin (17,200 Da) versus elution volumes, the calculated relative molecular mass of the CsA-containing complex in erythrocytes was 17,300 Da. Since the M_r of CsA is 1203 Da, the actual size of the binding protein would be close to 16,100 Da, assuming an association ratio of one molecule of CsA to one molecule of the binding protein.

Attempts to resolve this protein by SDS polyacrylamide gel electrophoresis of CsA-containing fractions from the elution shown in Figure 1 were unsuccessful due to the presence of trace amounts of hemoglobin in all fractions. Hemoglobin, which was denaturated to its monomeric form in the treatment of the samples with SDS prior to electrophoresis, comigrated with the CsA binding protein, thereby obscuring its detection.

Equilibrium dialysis of CsA and proteins. In order to investigate whether some known purified proteins were able to bind CsA, radiolabeled CsA (in compartment A) was dialyzed against selected proteins (in compartment B). Since human erythro-

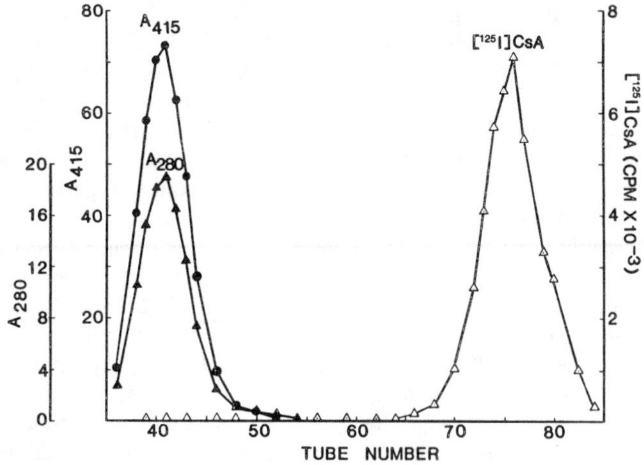

FIGURE 2. Fractionation of [^{125}I]CsA (0.3 ml) added to a hemolysate (5 ml) of erythrocytes from a normal individual on a Sephadex G-75 column with conditions as in Figure 1. The mixture of hemolysate and [^{125}I]CsA was incubated at room temperature for 1 hr before application to the column. The elution of [^{125}I]CsA was monitored by measurement of radioactivity in 1-ml aliquots of eluates in a gamma counter.

cytes contain appreciable amounts of calmodulin (M_r 16,700) (*22–24*) and cytochrome b_5 (M_r 15,000) (*25*), these proteins were assessed for CsA binding. After 24 hr of dialysis against [^{3}H]CsA, there were approximately equal amounts of radioactivity on each side of the membrane (Table 1), thus ruling out calmodulin and cytochrome b_5 as CsA-binding proteins (CsBP). Although the dpm of compartment A (radiolabeled CsA starting side) were slightly higher than those of compartment B (test protein side) at 24 hr, by 48 hr the dpm on each side were virtually identical. The same delay in achieving complete equilibrium distribution of [^{3}H]CsA was also observed when buffer with no protein was used in compartment B. The column fractions 41 (rich in hemoglobin) and 50 (rich in carbonic anhydrase) likewise showed no binding of [^{3}H]CsA by dialysis. Fraction 57, which originally was rich in CsA, did show a major binding of [^{3}H]CsA with the ratio of 1.925 between compartment B (protein) and compartment A (free drug), even in the presence of the CsA from in vivo administration. When [^{125}I] CsA was used in place of [^{3}H]CsA in dialysis against fraction 57 (rich in CsBP), there was no preferential accumulation in compartment B that confirmed the finding in Fig. 2 that [^{125}I] CsA did not bind to the erythrocyte CsBP. The structural feature of CsA that is recognized by CsBP, therefore, is likely to be close to or include the site of iodination on the CsA molecule that is the single carbon-carbon double bond in amino acid 1 (Fig. 3) (*26*).

Determination of binding constant. Addition of charcoal to a hemolysate mixed with [^{3}H]CsA and unlabeled CsA left an amount of [^{3}H]CsA in the supernatant that varied with concentration of CsA. This maneuver allowed for ready separation of free (F) CsA (charcoal adsorbed) from bound (B) CsA (in supernatant).

For total CsA concentrations of 60–800 picoM, Scatchard analysis of B/F versus B yielded a straight line with correlation coefficient of −0.969 (duplicate analysis with five data points each). Charcoal adsorption was adequate for these concentrations as judged by constant nonspecific binding (approximately 12%). The calculated dissociation constant (reciprocal negative slope) was 5×10^{-8} M, and the binding capacity (intercept on

TABLE 1. Dialysis of [^{3}H]CsA against proteins

Test protein	Radioactivity (dpm) after 24 h		
	Chamber A[a]	Chamber B[b]	DPM_B/DPM_A
Calmodulin (14 μg/ml)	17,893	17,373	0.971
Cytochrome b_5 (15 μg/ml)	17,358	16,706	0.962
Sephadex G-75 fractions:			
Tube 41 (hemoglobin)	17,560	16,901	0.962
Tube 50 (carbonic anhydrase)	17,251	16,749	0.973
Tube 57 (CsA-binding protein)	11,850	22,815	1.925
Tube 57 (CsA-binding protein)	8,380[c]	8,034[c]	0.959

[a] [^{3}H]CsA or [^{125}I]CsA was initially placed into chamber A.
[b] The test protein or fraction was placed into chamber B.
[c] [^{125}I]CsA was used in place of [^{3}H]CsA.

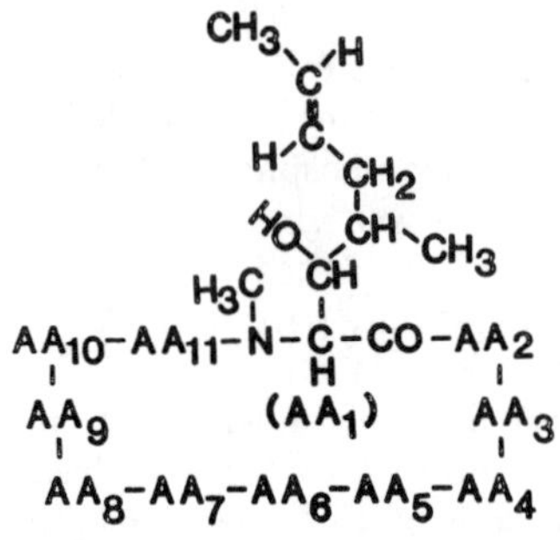

FIGURE 3. Structure of CsA showing the lone carbon-carbon double bond in amino acid 1 (AA_1). The other amino acids (AA_2-AA_{11}) are aminobutyric acid, sarcosine, methylleucine, valine, methylleucine, L-alanine, D-alanine, methylleucine, methylleucine, and methylvaline, respectively.

x-axis) was 2.0×10^{-7} M. This capacity in the test system corresponds to a binding capacity of 4 μM within erythrocytes. A mid-range therapeutic whole-blood level of CsA is about 0.4 μM (480 ng/ml). Thus the capacity of erythrocyte CsBP is more than sufficient to bind all the CsA associated with erythrocytes.

DISCUSSION

Therapeutic monitoring of CsA in blood is typically performed at trough levels in plasma or in whole blood that is frozen and thawed to release CsA contained in erythrocytes (*6, 13*). Because of the temperature-dependent binding of CsA to red cells (*16*), measurement of the drug in plasma requires very standardized incubation conditions of the whole-blood sample prior to centrifugation to avoid shifts of the drug into plasma from erythrocytes and vice versa. Alternatively, measurement of CsA in lysed whole blood does not require such precise conditions of equilibration prior to centrifugation. Accordingly, whole-blood CsA determinations are preferable for routine measurement in clinical laboratories. The draw back to whole-blood levels is that fluctuations in hematocrit can vastly affect CsA content of blood due to generally higher concentrations in erythrocytes than in plasma up to saturation of the erythrocytes (*9, 15*). Thus the therapeutic level of CsA (plus its metabolites) as measured by radioimmunoassay has a wide range in whole blood (250–800 ng/ml at the 24-hr trough according to the manufacturer, Sandoz, Ltd.).

In addition to this background, we have now provided evidence that there is a distinct protein in human erythrocytes that binds CsA in vivo—and, in fact, probably binds the majority of CsA in erythrocytes. This erythrocytic CsBP may differ in concentration between red cells of different patients, thus lending further variability to cellular binding pools of CsA. This erythrocyte CsBP is likely to play a major role in the general pharmacokinetics of CsA with regard to drug availability and distribution in tissues and organs of the body. In particular, it could substantially affect initial drug distribution following intravenous administration as opposed to oral administration.

A cyclosporine-binding protein designated *cyclophilin* has been demonstrated in the cytoplasmic fraction of bovine thymus (*27–29*). Cyclophilin has an apparent molecular weight of 15,000 Da, which is similar to that of the erythrocytic CsBP, which we have identified. Cyclophilin also has a similar dissociation constant for CsA to that of erythrocyte CsBP (e.g., 2×10^{-7} M versus 0.5×10^{-7} M). These independent observations indicate that proteins capable of binding CsA may have widespread distribution in many tissues of the body. It has generally been assumed that CsA distribution in different tissues depends on the fat content of each tissue due to the hydrophobic nature of CsA (*8–10*). However, a cellular-biniding protein might play a considerable role in determining specific tissue levels of CsA as well as availability of the drug to interact with target lymphocytes in transplanted organs.

Cyclophilin most likely interacts with CsA at the position of an aromatic amino acid residue in cyclophilin, since A_{280} of that protein is enhanced by addition of CsA (*29*). Our findings indicate that the region of CsA that interacts with the erythrocyte-binding protein includes the residue containing the only carbon-carbon double bond in CsA (*30*). It is noteworthy that cyclophilin can bind [^{3}H-dihydro]-H_2 cyclosporine (*27, 28*), in which that double bond is reduced, indicating that the double bond is not necessary for binding of CsA. Iodination of CsA also occurs across the double bond with reduction and tetrahydofuran formation in the side chain of amino acid 1 (*31*). The resulting diminished flexibility may fix the side chain into a conformation unfavorable for complex formation between CsA and erythrocyte CsBP. Assuming similarity between cyclophilin and the erythrocyte CsBP, it is reasonable to speculate that CsA may interact directly with an aromatic group in its binding protein. If such a hydrophobic attraction is the basis for binding, it should be diminished by higher temperatures, since erythrocytes demonstrate greater affinity and capacity for CsA at lower temperatures (*9*).

The motivation to search for a CsA binder in thymus was to identify a possible receptor on target cells by which CsA might act on t lymphocytes (*27–29*). Our findings that a CsBP exists in erythrocytes suggest two possibilities with regard to the functional nature of these binders. One is that major amounts of nonspecific CsA binders occur intracellularly and merely tie up CsA without mediating its pharmacologic activity in much the same way that serum albumin binds drugs and hormones in the circulation (*32*). The other more interesting possibility is that this CsBP or group of CsBPs directly mediates the action of CsA. Based on information that CsA probably acts by reversibly blocking transcription of IL-2 (*2–4*), we might postulate that the CsBP when complexed with CsA could then interact directly with the IL-2 gene to prevent transcription. This action would have physiologic significance only in t lymphocytes that normally produce IL-2. A better understanding of CsA's mechanism of action at the molecular level may be achieved by use of purified CsBP, such as that described in this study, added to in vitro transcription systems in the presence and absence of CsA.

REFERENCES

1. Borel JF, Feurer C, Magnee C, Stahelin H. Effects of the new antilymphocytic peptide cyclosporin A in animals. Immunology 1977; 32: 1017.
2. Kronke M, Leonard WJ, Depper JM, Arya SK, Wong-Staal F, Gallo RC, Waldmann TA, Greene WC. Cyclosporin A inhibits T-cell growth factor gene expression at the level of mRNA transcription. Proc Natl Acad Sci USA 1984; 81: 5214.
3. Hess AD. Effect of interleukin 2 on the immunosuppressive action of cyclosporin. Transplantation 1985; 39: 62.
4. Kermani-Arab V, Salehmoghaddam S, Danovitch G, Hirji K, Rezai A. Mediation of the antiproliferative effect of cyclosporine on human lymphocytes by blockade of interleukin 2 biosynthesis. Transplantation 1985; 39: 439.
5. Keown PA, Stiller CR, Sinclair NR, Carruthers G, et al. The clinical relevance of cyclosporin blood levels as measured by radioimmunoassay. Transplant Proc 1983; 15: 2438.
6. Bowers LD, Canafax DM. Cyclosporin: experience with therapeutic monitoring. Ther Drug Monit 1984; 6: 142.
7. Merion RM, White DJG, Thiru S, Evans DB, Calne RY. Cyclosporin: five years' experience in cadaveric renal transplantation. N Engl J Med 1984; 310: 148.
8. Von Willebrand E, Hayry P. Cyclosporin-A deposits in renal allografts. Lancet 1983; 2: 189.
9. Niederberger W, Lemaire M, Maurer G, Nussbaumer K, Wagner O. Distribution and binding of cyclosporin in blood and tissues. Transplant Proc 1983; 15: 2419.
10. Ried M, Gibbons S, Kowk D, Van Buren CT, Flechner S, Kahan BD. Cyclosporin levels in human tissues of patients treated for one week to one year. Transplant Proc 1983; 15: 2434.
11. LeGrue SJ, Friedman AW, Kahan BD. Lack of evidence for a cyclosporin receptor on human lymphocyte membranes. Transplant Proc 1983; 15: 2259.
12. Lemaire M, Tillement JP. Role of lipoproteins and erythrocytes in the in vivo binding and distribution of cyclosporin A in blood. J Pharm Pharmacol 1982; 34: 715.
13. Wenk M, Follath F, Abisch E. Temperature dependency of apparent cyclosporin A concentrations in plasma. Clin Chem 1983; 29: 1865.
14. Mraz W, Zink RA, Graf A, et al. Distribution and transfer of cyclosporine among the various human lipoprotein classes. Transplant Proc 1983; 15: 2426.
15. Rosano TB. Effect of hematocrit on cyclosporine (cyclosporin A) in whole blood and plasma of renal-transplant patients. Clin Chem 1985; 31: 410.
16. Yatscoff RW, Rush DN, Jeffery JR. Effects of sample preparation on concentrations of cyclosporin A measured in plasma. Clin Chem 1984; 30: 1812.
17. Agarwal RP, McPherson RA, Threatte GA. Assessment of cyclosporin A in whole blood and plasma in five patients with different hematocrits. Ther Drug Monit 1985; 7: 61.
18. Waddell WJ. A simple ultraviolet spectrophotometric method for the determination of protein. J Lab Clin Med 1956; 48: 311.
19. Wilbur KM, Anderson NG. Electrometric and colorimetric determination of carbonic anhydrase. J Biol Chem 1948; 176: 147.
20. Rickli EE, Ghazanfar SAS, Gibbons BH, Edsall JT. Carbonic anhydrase from human erythrocytes. J Biol Chem 1964; 239: 1065.
21. Weber K, Osborn M. The reliability of molecular weight determination by dodecyl sulfate-polyacrylamide gel electrophoresis. J Biol Chem 1969; 244: 4406.
22. Schreiber WE, Gentry R, Fischer EH. Calmodulin and cyclic

nucleotide phosphodiesterase activities in erythrocytes from normal and schizophrenic subjects. Biochem Biophys Res Commun 1981; 100: 1415.
23. Postnov YV, Orlov SLN, Reznikova MB, Rjazhsky GG, Pokudin NI. Calmodulin distribution and Ca^{2+} transport in the erythrocytes of patients with essential hypertension. Clin Sci 1984; 66: 459.
24. Klee CB, Crouch TH, Richman PG. Calmodulin. Ann Rev Biochem 1980; 49: 489.
25. Hultquist DE. Methemoglobin reduction system of erythrocytes. Methods Enzymol 1978; 52: 463.
26. Mahoney WC, Orf JW. Derivatives of cyclosporin compatible with antibody-based assay. I. The generation of [^{125}I]-labeled cyclosporin. Clin Chem 1985; 31: 459.
27. Merker M, Rice J, Schweitzer B, Handschumacher RE. Cyclosporin binding component in BW5147 lymphoblasts and normal lymphoid tissue. Transplant Proc 1983; 15: 2265.
28. Merker MM, Handschumacher RE. Uptake and nature of the intracellular binding of cyclosporin A in a murine thymoma cell line, BW 5147. J Immunol 1984; 132: 3064.
29. Handschumacher RE, Harding MW, Rice J, Drugge RJ. Cyclophilin: a specific cytosolic binding protein for cyclosporin A. Science 1984; 226: 544.
30. Wenger RM. Synthesis of cyclosporin. I. Synthesis of enantiomerically pure (2S,3R,4R,6E)-3-hydroxy-4-methyl-2-methylamino-6-octenoic acid, starting from tartaric acid. Helv Chim Acta 1983; 66: 2308.
31. Petcher TJ, Weber H-P, Ruegger A. Crystal and molecular structure of an iodo-derivative of the cyclic undecapeptide cyclosporin A. Helv Chim Acta 1976; 59: 1480.
32. Koch-Weser J, Sellers EM. Drug therapy. Binding of drugs to serum albumin. N Engl J Med 1976; part 1, 294: 311; part 2, 294: 526.

Received 26 November 1985.
Accepted 21 March 1986.

0041-1337/86/4206-0632$02.00/0
TRANSPLANTATION
Vol. 42, No. 6
Printed in U.S.A.

INDUCTION OF ANTIIDIOTYPIC ANTIBODIES BY BLOOD TRANSFUSIONS

CHARACTERIZATION OF T CELL ALLOANTIGEN-SPECIFIC RECEPTORS BY SERA FROM TRANSFUSED MICE[1]

D.P. SINGAL,[2] D. LUDWIN, S. JOSEPH, M.A. BLAJCHMAN, F.A. OFOSU, AND S-K. LIAO

Departments of Pathology and Medicine, McMaster University; and the Canadian Red Cross Blood Transfusion Service, Hamilton, Ontario, Canada

Balb/c (H-2^d) mice were transfused weekly with 0.1 ml of whole blood from C3H (H-2^k) mice. One week after 3 blood transfusions (BT), the mice were bled and the sera collected and pooled. The 3BT serum was absorbed twice with C3H lymphocytes and IgG isolated by ion-exchange chromatography. Balb/c anti-C3H, Balb/c anti-Balb/c, and Balb/c anti-SJL (H-2^s) lymphocytes were generated in the mixed lymphocyte cultures and metabolically labeled with ^{35}S-methionine. Cell lysates were prepared from labeled lymphocytes and precleared by absorption with normal mouse serum. Immunoprecipitation was carried out by 3BT-IgG and NMS-IgG. 3BT-IgG specifically precipitated 7 molecules (30K, 60K, 72K, 86K, 92K, 97K, 145K) from Balb/c anti-C3H lymphocytes. In contrast, 3BT-IgG did not precipitate these molecules from Balb/c anti-Balb/c or from Balb/c anti-SJL lymphocytes. The data suggest that BT induces antibodies directed against the blood donor alloantigen-specific receptors on recipient's T lymphocytes.

[1]This work was supported by research grants from the Kidney Foundation of Canada, the Canadian Red Cross Society, BTS, and the St. Joseph's Foundation, Hamilton.

[2]Address correspondence to: D. P. Singal, Ph.D., Department of Pathology, McMaster University, 1200 Main St. West, Hamilton, Ontario, Canada L8N 3Z5.

One of the most significant factors influencing clinical renal allograft survival is pretransplant blood transfusion (BT)* (*1, 2*). BT has also been shown to be effective in experimental transplantation in prolonging the survival of kidney, heart, and skin allografts in dogs, monkeys, rats, and mice (*2*). The beneficial effect of BT has been attributed to active immunologic unresponsiveness to donor's alloantigens. It is known that immunologic unresponsiveness can be induced by suppressor cells (*3–6*) or by antibodies directed against the T cell antigen-specific receptors—i.e., antiidiotypic antibodies (*5–12*). In our attempts to identify factors that may be responsible for the beneficial effect of BT, we have examined the possibility that BT may induce the production of antiidiotypic antibodies, which suppress the recipient's immune response to the allograft. In renal transplant patients, we have demonstrated that BT induces antibodies directed against the T cell antigen-specific receptors and have suggested that these antibodies may be an important factor in enhanced allograft survival (*7–9*). Using a systematic transfusion protocol in drug-unmodified mice, we have previously shown that sera from B6AF$_1$ mice

* Abbreviations used: BT, blood transfusion; CML, cell-mediated lympholysis; FBS, fetal bovine serum; GVHD, graft-versus-host disease; MEM, minimal essential medium; NMS, normal mouse serum; PBS, phosphate-buffered saline; SDS, sodium dodecyl sulphate.

transfused with DBA/2 blood can specifically inhibit responses of normal $B6AF_1$ mice against stimulator cells from the specific blood donor mice in MLC and in CML (*5, 10*). We have subsequently shown that Balb/c mice transfused with C3H blood develop antiidiotypic antibodies capable of inhibiting proliferative responses in MLC (*11*). The present study is a continuation of our work in the Balb/c-C3H combination and deals with the preliminary immunochemical characterization of the T cell alloantigen-specific receptors recognized by antibodies induced following BT.

MATERIALS AND METHODS

Mice. Adult male mice of Balb/c ($H\text{-}2^d$), C3H/HeJ (C3H) ($H\text{-}2^k$), and SJL ($H\text{-}2^s$) strains were purchased from the Jackson Laboratories, Bar Harbor, ME.

Blood Transfusions. Balb/c mice were transfused with 0.1 ml of fresh whole blood from C3H mice i.v. through the tail vein. BT were carried out at weekly intervals. Serum samples were collected and pooled under aseptic conditions one week after three BT (henceforth called 3BT serum). One ml of 3BT serum was absorbed twice, each time with 10^7 spleen cells from C3H mice, first at room temperature for 1 hr followed by 4°C for 1 hr.

IgG was prepared from 3BT serum and from normal mouse (Balb/c) serum (NMS) by ion-exchange chromatography on DEAE-Sephadex followed by binding and elution from a protein-A Sepharose (Pharmacia, Quebec) column.

Mixed lymphocyte culture (MLC), metabolic labeling of cells, and preparation of alloantigen-specific antigen. Cell suspensions were prepared aseptically from the spleens of mice. MLC was performed as described by us previously (*13*). Briefly 6×10^7 responder (Balb/c) spleen cells were cultured with an equal number of x-irradiated (1800 rads) stimulator (C3H or SJL) spleen cells in 60-ml volume in 75-cm^2 tissue culture flasks (Falcon Plastics). The medium consisted of alpha-minimum essential medium (MEM) supplemented with 10% fetal bovine serum (FBS), 20 mM Hepes, 1% sodium bicarbonate, 100 U/ml penicillin, 100 μg/ml streptomycin and 5×10^{-5} M 2-mercaptoethanol. The cultures were incubated at 37°C in a humidified 5% CO_2-in-air atmosphere for 5 days. Lymphocytes were collected from these cultures and washed twice with 30 ml of sterile phosphate-buffered saline (PBS), pH 7.4. Lymphocytes were metabolically labeled with 500 μCi of L-^{35}S-methionine (specific activity 1120 Ci/mM, New England Nuclear, Boston, MA) in 10 ml methionine-free MEM containing 10% FBS, 20 mM Hepes, 1% sodium bicarbonate, 100 U/ml penicillin, 100 μg/ml streptomycin and 5×10^{-5} M 2-mercaptoethanol for 18 hr.

Labeled lymphocytes were obtained from culture flasks, pelleted and washed 3 times with PBS, pH 7.4. The cell pellet was extracted with 1 ml of RIPA (50 mM Tris-HCl containing 0.15 M NaCl, 1% Triton, 1% sodium deoxycholate, 0.1% sodium dodecyl sulphate (SDS) and 0.1 mM phenylmethylsulfonyl fluoride) buffer (pH 7.2) and cellular debris was removed by centrifugation at 100,000 g for 1 hr.

Immunoprecipitation. The cell-lysate was precleared by absorption with 50 μl of NMS and 50 μl of packed protein-A Sepharose beads. Immunoprecipitation was carried out by mixing 50 μl of IgG (3BT serum or NMS) with 300 μl of cell-lysate at room temperature for 90 min. Then 30 μl of packed protein-A Sepharose beads was added. After additional mixing for 30 min at 4°C, beads were pelleted and washed 3 times with RIPA and 3 times with 100 mM Tris-HCl, pH 7.0, containing 0.2 M lithium chloride, to elute the immune complexes. Immune complexes were dissociated by heating beads at 100°C for 5 min in 50 μl of sample buffer (Tris-HCl (pH 6.8) 2 ml, glycerol 2 ml, 20% SDS 2.5 ml, 14.4 M 2-mercaptoethanol 0.7 ml, and 0.05% bromophenol blue 0.1 ml).

SDS-polyacrylamide Gel electrophoresis (SDS-PAGE). High resolution SDS-polyacrylamide slab gels (1.5-mm-thick) were prepared according to the method of Laemmli (*14*). Samples were anlayzed under reducing conditions by electrophoresis on SDS slab gels at a constant current of 150 mA per gel for 5 hr. After electrophoresis, gels were prepared for autoradiography and radiolabeled bands were detected on Kodak XAR-5 x-ray film. Molecular weights of the ^{35}S-methionine labeled proteins were estimated by reference to ^{14}C-labeled protein molecular weight markers (New England Nuclear, Boston, MA), which were included in each gel electrophoresis.

RESULTS

Experiments were performed by means of ^{35}S-methionine incorporation by lymphocytes for 18 hr followed by immunoprecipitation and SDS-PAGE under reducing conditions. In these experiments, the cell lysates were prepared from Balb/c anti-Balb/c, Balb/c anti-C3H, or Balb/c anti-SJL lymphocytes, and immunoprecipitation carried out with 3BT-IgG and NMS-IgG. Results from one such experiment are shown in Figure 1. It is evident that 3BT-IgG specifically precipitated 7 molecules with apparent molecular weights of 30K, 60K, 72K, 86K, 92K, 97K, and 145K on Balb/c anti-C3H lymphocytes. These molecules were not precipitable either by the NMS-IgG on Balb/c anti-C3H lymphocytes or by 3BT-IgG and NMS-IgG on Balb/c anti-Balb/c lymphocytes. Similarly, 3BT-IgG and NMS-IgG did not precipitate these molecules on Balb/c anti-SJL lymphcytes (results not shown). Similar results were obtained in six other experiments.

In these experiments, 3BT-IgG also precipitated two bands with apparent molecular weights of 41K and 81K, which were also precipitated by NMS-IgG (Fig. 1). In some experiments, additional molecules (for example, 47K and 49K molecules in Fig. 1) were detected by 3BT-IgG, but these molecules did not appear in all experiments. Therefore, 3BT-IgG specifically precipitated 7 molecules from Balb/c anti-C3H lymphocytes.

Under nonreducing conditions, only two distinct radioactive bands were visible after electrophoresis: the larger did not enter the stacking gel, and the second had an apparent molecular weight greater than 200K.

DISCUSSION

The results in the present study demonstrate that IgG prepared from sera obtained from Balb/c mice transfused with 3 weekly transfusions of C3H blood contained antibodies that specifically bind to the alloantigen-specific molecules on Balb/c anti-C3H lymphocytes. On the other hand, these antibodies did not bind to Balb/c anti-Balb/c lymphocytes or to Balb/c anti-SJL lymphocytes. The data suggest that BT may induce antibodies directed against the blood-donor-alloantigen–specific receptors on recipient's T lymphocytes.

The biochemical nature of the T cell antigen-specific receptor still remains obscure despite rather intensive study by numerous investigators. Binz et al. (*15*) showed that Lewis anti-DA T cell receptor molecules were able to bind strongly to DA Ag-

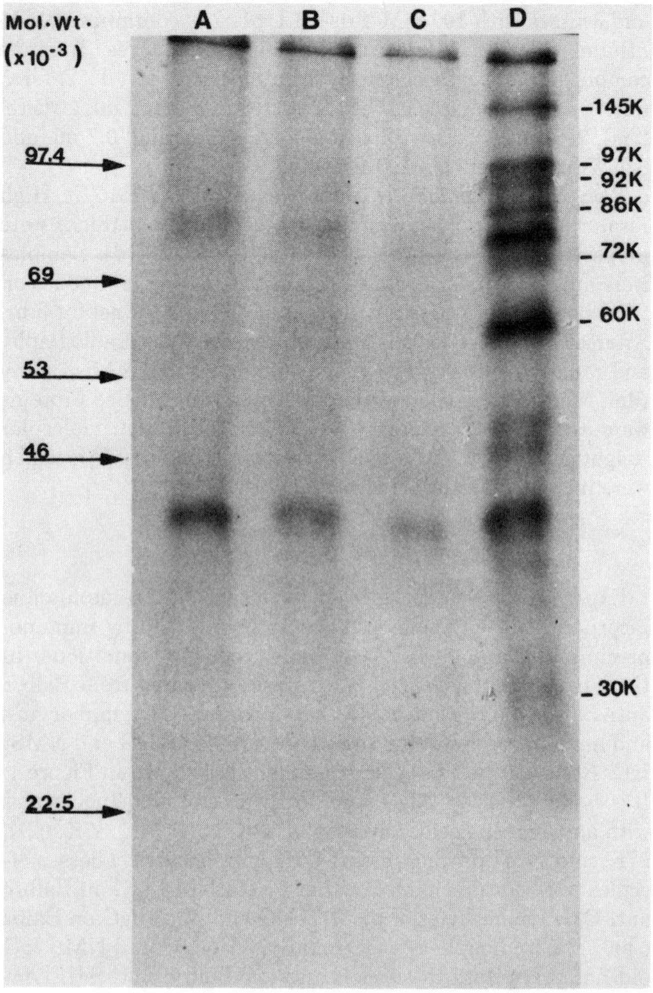

FIGURE 1. SDS-PAGE profiles of radiolabeled cell lysates precipitated by 3BT-IgG and NMS-IgG. Balb/c anti-Balb/c (lanes A,B) and Balb/c anti-C3H (lanes C,D) lymphocytes were metabolically labeled with ^{35}S-methionine and lysed with RIPA. The cell lysates were immunoprecipitated with NMS-IgG (lanes A,C) or with 3BT-IgG (lanes B,D) and analyzed on SDS-PAGE under reducing conditions. Molecular weight markers are indicated to the left of the figure. The positions of 7 molecules specifically precipitated by 3BT-IgG from Balb/c anti-C3H lymphocytes are indicated on the right of the figure.

B chain as well as the heavy DA Ia chain (27K, 33K, 44K). Bourgois et al. (*16*) utilized two antisera, an antiidiotypic serum and an anti-T-cell receptor serum, and described three T cell antigen-specific molecules (75K, 62K and 50K) present on B6 anti-CBA lymphoblasts. Morita et al. (*17*) described 4 major species of molecules with apparent molecular weights of 92K, 68-72K, 42K, and 14K, all associated with the T cell antigen receptors for haptens. In the present study, we detected 7 major molecules with approximate molecular weights of 30K, 60K, 72K, 86K, 92K, 97K, and 145K on Balb/c anti-C3H lymphoblasts with sera obtained from Balb/c mice transfused with C3H blood. The earlier data (*15–17*) together with the results in the present study support the concept that T cells are functionally complex and their complexity may be reflected in a chemical and genetic heterogeneity of their antigen-specific products (*18*). It is perhaps not surprising that we detect several molecules on Balb/c anti-C3H lymphocytes, since we are dealing with a mixed population of cells. Although results in the present investigation identify 7 alloantigen-specific molecules on Balb/c anti-C3H lymphocytes, no conclusions can be drawn about their functional significance. Further studies will be necessary to determine their biological role.

The conditions employed for the reduction of membrane proteins may not have resulted in complete reduction of disulfide bonds. This, however, is unlikely as these are the conditions generally used to reduce heterogenous mixtures of proteins. Since the 145K protein is significantly larger than those reported by other investigators (*15–17*), it is possible that this particular protein may be the one which interacts with but is not necessarily a part of the T cell alloantigen-specific receptor that is precipitated with the antiidiotypic antibody.

T lymphocytes reactive against alloantigens bear idiotypic determinants. Antiidiotypic antibodies raised against T cell idiotypes have been shown to suppress T cell functions, such as MLC, cell-mediated lympholysis (CML), and graft-versus-host disease (GVHD) reactions, as well as rejection of allografts (*19–22*). It is possible to induce antiidiotypic antibodies specific for allo-MHC reactive T cells by immunization with a number of reagents—including alloantibody molecules, purified T cell receptors, and selected heavy chains from specific IgG molecules—or with alloreactive T blasts generated in in vitro MLC cultures (*19*, *23*, *24*). In a functional assay, we have previously shown that antibodies directed against recognition sites on T lymphocytes can be induced by BT (*2*, *5–11*). In the present study, we have utilized sera obtained after 3BT to characterize the receptors generated on in vitro alloreactive T lymphocytes. Therefore, we have utilized polyclonal idiotype and antiidiotypes in our studies. The polyclonal idiotype preparation contains a mixture of antibody molecules directed against a variable number of antigen epitopes. It appears that antiidiotypic response following BT includes antibodies to several idiotypic determinants.

We have recently demonstrated that sera from Balb/c mice transfused with C3H blood can specifically inhibit proliferative responses of Balb/c cells to stimulator cells from the blood donor (C3H) mice in MLC (*11*). On the other hand, no inhibition was observed with stimulator cells from the third-party SJL mice. In addition, the inhibition in MLC was specific for the responder cells from the recipient Balb/c mice and for the stimulator lymphocytes from the blood donor C3H mice (*11*). The inhibition in MLC, therefore, was not due to alloreactive antibodies to the blood donor C3H cells. These results, together with data in the present study, suggest that BT may induce production of antibodies directed against the blood donor alloantigen-specific receptors on recipient's T lymphocytes—i.e., antiidiotypic antibodies—which suppress the host's immune response to the blood donor alloantigens.

In renal transplant patients, we have observed that BT induces antibodies directed against the T cell antigen-specific receptors (*7–9*). Renal transplant recipients maintaining functional allografts were found to have antibodies that inhibited responses in MLC against alloantigens present in the kidney donor. These antibodies were not demonstrable in patients who had rejected their allografts. Since these initial observations, a number of investigators have demonstrated the presence of MLC-inhibiting antibodies in renal transplant patients following BT (*25–27*), and the presence of these antibodies has been correlated with enhanced allograft survival. These data on renal transplant patients, together with our results on BT in mice (*5*, *10*, *11*), suggest that BT may imbalance the host's immunoregulatory circuits triggering the production of antiidiotypic antibodies. These antibodies may in turn be responsible for modulating the recipient's immune responses to the donor's alloantigens, thereby enhancing allograft survival.

In the present study, serum from Balb/c mice transfused with C3H blood was utilized for immunochemical characterization of the alloantigen-specific receptor's on the recipient's T lymphocytes. We have previously shown that the sera from transfused mice caused significant inhibition of proliferative responses of the recipient Balb/c mice against stimulator cells from the specific blood donor mice in MLC (*11*). Using the serum transfer experiments, Nagata et al. (*28*) demonstrated that the serum from blood-conditioned animals significantly prolonged heart allograft survival in rats. Further studies, however, are required to determine the role of the specific molecules identified in the present study in allograft enhancement.

REFERENCES

1. Opelz G. Current relevance of the transfusion effect in renal transplantation. Transplant Proc 1985; 17: 1015.
2. Singal DP, Ludwin D, Blajchman MA. Blood transfusion and renal transplantation. Br J Hematol 1985; 61: 595.
3. Brent L, Horsburgh T, Wood PJ. Induction of suppressor cells and allograft tolerance. Transplant Proc 1980; 12: 464
4. Maki J, Okazaki H, Wood ML, Monaco AP. Suppressor cells in mice bearing intact skin allografts after blood transfusions. Transplantation 1981; 32: 463.
5. Nagarkatti PS, Singal DP. Blood-transfusion-induced suppression of cytotoxic T lymphocyte responses in mice. Transplantation 1983; 36: 520.
6. Singal DP, Joseph S, Ludwin D. Blood transfusions, suppressor cells, and antiidiotypic antibodies. Transplant Proc 1985; 17: 1104.
7. Singal DP, Jospeh S. Role of blood transfusions on the induction of antibodies against recognition sites on T lymphocytes in renal transplant patients. Hum Immunol 1982; 4: 93.
8. Singal DP, Joseph S, Szewczuk M. Possible mechanism of the beneficial effect of pretransplant blood transfusion on renal allograft survival in man. Transplant Proc 1982; 14: 316.
9. Fagnilli L, Singal DP. Blood transfusions may induce anti-T cell receptor antibodies in renal patients. Transplant Proc 1982; 14: 319.
10. Nagarkatti PS, Joseph S, Singal DP. Induction of antibodies by blood transfusions capable of inhibiting responses on MLC. Transplantation 1983; 36: 695.
11. Ludwin D, Joseph S, Singal DP. MLC inhibiting antibodies in mice after blood transfusions. Transplantation 1986; 41: 100.
12. Suciu-Foca N, Reemtsma K, King DW. The significance of the idiotypic anti-idiotypic networks in humans. Transplant Proc 1986; 18: 230.
13. Singal DP, deVera R. Generation of memory cells in one-way mixed lymphocyte culture. II. Responses of lymphocytes from renal transplant recipients and normal individuals to subsellular alloantigens in vitro. Transplant Proc 1977; 9: 211.
14. Laemmli UK. Cleavage of structural proteins during the assembly of the head of bacteriophage T4. Nature 1970; 227: 680.
15. Binz H, Frischknecht H, Mercolli C, Dunst S, Wigzell H. Binding of purified, soluble major histocompatibility complex polypeptide chain onto isolated T-cell receptor. J Exp Med 1979; 150: 1084.
16. Bourgois A, Kahn-Perles B, Rubin B. The T cell receptor heavy chain is coded for by loci linked to Ig-V_H and C_H loci, and it displays structural similarities with Ig heavy chains. In: Janeway C, Sercarz EE, Wigzell H, eds. Immunoglobulin idiotypes. New York: Academic, 1981: 449.
17. Morita CT, Scott DM, Goodman JW, Lewis GK. Characterization of molecules released by hapten immunized lymphocytes. In: Janeway C, Sercarz EE, Wigzell H, eds. Immunoglobulin idiotypes. New York: Academic, 1981: 407.
18. Janeway CA, Owen FL. Summary Workshop: the T cell receptors. In: Janeway C, Sercarz EE, Wigzell H, eds. Immunoglobulin idiotypes. New York: Academic, 1981: 509.
19. Binz H, Wigzell H. Idiotypic, alloantigen-reactive T lymphocyte receptors and their use to induce specific transplantation tolerance. Prog Allergy 1977; 23: 154.
20. Braun M, Saal F. The T-cell receptor and cytotoxicity. An anti-idiotype antiserum that inhibits a graft-versus-host reaction does not inhibit cell-mediated cytotoxicity. Cell Immunol 1977; 30: 254.
21. Krawinkel U, Cramer M, Melchers I, Imanishi-Kari T, Rajewski K. Isolated hapten-binding receptors of sensitized lymphocytes. III. Evidence for idiotypic restriction of T-cell receptors. J Exp Med 1978; 147: 1341.
22. Strong DM, Ahmed A, Leapman SB, et al. Induction of memory cells in vitro with an anti-idiotypic serum against the recognition structure specific for cells primed for histocompatibility determinants. Transplant Proc 1979; 11: 928.
23. Andersson LC, Binz H, Wigzell H. Specific unresponsiveness to transplantation antigens induced by auto-immunization with syngeneic, antigenspecific T lymphoblasts. Nature 1976; 264: 778.
24. Frischknecht H, Binz H, Wigzell H. Induction of specific transplantation immune reactions using anti-idiotypic antibodies. J Exp Med 1978; 147: 500.
25. Cheigh JS, Suthanthiran M, Kaplan M, et al. Induction of immune alterations and successful renal transplantation with a simplified method of donor-specific blood transfusion. Transplantation 1984; 38: 501.
26. Takeuchi H, Sakagami K, Seki Y, et al. Antiidiotypic antibodies and suppressor cells induced by donor-specific transfusion of potential kidney transplant recipients. Transplant Proc 1985; 17: 1059.
27. Sollinger HW, Burlingham WJ, Sparks EMF, Glass NR, Belzer FO. Donor-specific transfusions in unrelated and related HLA-mismatched donor-recipient combinations. Transplantation 1984; 38: 612.
28. Nagata M, Ochiai T, Asano T, et al. Role of Ia-positive cells in the beneficial effect of donor blood transfusion and induction of suppressor cells in cardiac allograft transplantation of rats. Transplantation 1984; 38: 522.

Received 4 October 1985.
Accepted 18 March 1986.

0041-1337/86/4206-0636$02.00/0
TRANSPLANTATION
Copyright © 1986 by The Williams & Wilkins Co.

Vol. 42, No. 6
Printed in U.S.A.

REJECTION OF SKIN GRAFTS AND GENERATION OF CYTOTOXIC T CELLS BY MICE DEPLETED OF L3T4+ CELLS[1]

JANET WOODCOCK, DAVID WOFSY, ERÉNE ERIKSSON, JANET H. SCOTT, AND WILLIAM E. SEAMAN[2]

Arthritis/Immunology Section, San Francisco VA Medical Center; and the University of California, San Francisco, California

In mice, "helper/inducer" T cells can be depleted by treatment with a rat monoclonal antibody to the cell surface antigen, L3T4, which is homologous to the human antigen T4 (CD4). In order to examine the contribution of "helper/inducer" T cells to cellular immunity, C57BL/6 (H-2^b) mice were treated weekly with 1 mg i.v. of a monoclonal antibody to L3T4. Three days after the first injection, the mice received skin grafts from BALB/c (H-2^d) mice. The mice were then examined for skin graft rejection and for the development of cytotoxic cells. Treatment with anti-L3T4 prolonged skin graft survival from 9 to 18 days. Graft rejection was associated with the development of cellular cytotoxicity against H-2^d targets. Cytotoxicity developed despite ≥90% depletion of splenic L3T4$^+$ cells. Allospecific cytotoxic T cells could also be generated in vitro from C57BL/6 spleen cells depleted of L3T4$^+$ cells, when these were exposed in a mixed leukocyte culture to irradiated, T-cell-depleted, BALB/c spleen cells. In a mixed leukocyte culture using responder spleen cells from untreated C57BL/6 mice, both proliferation and interleukin 2 production were inhibited in the presence of antibody to L3T4 and, to a lesser extent, by antibody to Lyt-2. Complete inhibition was achieved by the presence of both antibodies. In a mixed leukocyte culture using responder spleen cells from C57BL/6 mice that had been treated with anti-L3T4, both proliferation and interleukin 2 production were inhibited largely by antibody to Lyt-2, although the presence of both anti-Lyt-2 and anti-L3T4 was most inhibitory. These findings indicate that graft rejection and cellular cytotoxicity can be generated in mice depleted of L3T4$^+$ cells by methods that have previously been shown to abrogate humoral immunity. Cellular immunity appears to require few, if any, L3T4$^+$ cells. These findings have implications for the clinical use of antibodies to "helper/inducer" T cells.

Antilymphocyte or antithymocyte globulins have been in clinical use for over 20 years as a means of suppressing host immunity to organ grafts (*1, 2*). Despite evidence that these preparations are efficacious, it has been difficult to produce batches of globulin that have identical effects in vivo. Also, the repeated use of antithymocyte globulin frequently leads to serum sickness (*3, 4*). The development of monoclonal antibodies (MAb)* against lymphocyte surface antigens has provided a more specific means for deleting lymphocyte subsets in vivo (*5, 6*). A murine MAb to the T3 (CD3) antigen, on all human T cells, has been used successfully to reverse acute rejection of renal allografts (*6, 7*). However, like heterologous antibodies, these MAb provoke a host immune response that may preclude their use for chronic therapy (*8, 9*).

To examine the consequences of using xenogeneic MAb to deplete T cells, we have treated mice with rat MAbs to mouse T cell antigens. In mice, as in humans, extrathymic T lymphocytes can be divided into two mutually exclusive subsets on the basis of surface antigens that participate in the immune response (*10–12*). Mouse "helper/inducer" T cells express L3T4, which is homologous to the human antigen, T4 (CD4) (*13*). These T cells recognize class II major histocompatibility antigens (MHA II), and their ability to bind and respond to MHA II$^+$ cells is blocked by antibody to L3T4 (*14*). Mouse "suppressor/cytotoxic" T cells express Lyt-2, homologous to the human antigen T8 (CD8) (*15, 16*). These T cells recognize class I major histocompatibility antigens (MHA I), and their ability to bind and respond to MHA I$^+$ cells is blocked by antibody to Lyt-2 (*12*).

We and others have found that mice injected repeatedly with rat MAb to L3T4, in amounts sufficient to deplete L3T4$^+$ cells, make little or no antibody to the rat MAb (*17, 18*). This is in contrast to a brisk immune response that develops in mice treated with rat MAb to other mouse T cell antigens, including Lyt-2, Thy-1.2, or Ly-1 (unpublished observations). The lack of a host response to the anti-L3T4 MAb allows sustained depletion of L3T4$^+$ cells from the blood, spleen, lymph nodes, and Peyer's patches, which is accompanied by a profound suppression of humoral immunity (*18, 19*). In euthymic mice, L3T4$^+$ cells recover when treatment with anti-L3T4 is stopped, but in thymectomized mice, the L3T4$^+$ cells do not recover (*18*).

Cobbold et al., demonstrated that depletion of L3T4$^+$ cells from thymectomized mice prolonged the survival of allogeneic skin grafts, while depletion of Lyt-2$^+$ cells did not affect graft rejection (*18*). The immunosuppressive effects of anti-L3T4 were not absolute; grafts that differed at the major histocompatibility locus were rejected after 25 days, compared to 11 days in untreated mice (18). Similar results were obtained in euthymic mice treated daily with anti-L3T4 during the first 14 days of engraftment (*18*).

In the present studies, we demonstrate that cellular immunity can be suppressed in intact animals by MAb to L3T4, but suppression is not complete, even though L3T4$^+$ cells are profoundly depleted. Skin grafts still elicit allospecific cellular cytotoxicity, leading to graft rejection. In vitro studies support

[1] This work was supported by the Veterans Administration, by USPHS Grant AM33004, and by the University of California Task Force on AIDS.

[2] Send reprint requests to Dr. Seaman at VAMC 111R, 4150 Clement St., San Francisco, CA 94121.

* Abbreviations used: FACS, fluorescence-activated cell sorter; GVHR, graft-versus-host reaction IL-2, interleukin 2; MAb, monoclonal antibody; MHA I, class I major histocompatibility antigen(s); MHA II, class II major histocompatibility antigen(s); MLC, mixed lymphocyte culture; NK, natural killer.

the hypothesis that allospecific cytotoxic Lyt-2^+ cells can develop with little or no contribution from L3T4^+ cells.

MATERIALS AND METHODS

Mice. Female C57BL/6 and BALB/c mice were obtained from Simonsen Laboratories (Gilroy, CA).

Skin grafting. BALB/c (H-2^d) donor mice were sacrificed, and flank and abdominal skin was removed surgically. Full-thickness grafts, 1-cm^2, were transplanted to the flanks of (C57BL/6 [H-2^b]) recipient mice under anesthesia. Graft sites were covered with petrolatum-impregnated gauze and a plaster dressing for 6 days. Rejection, defined as total loss of viable epithelium of the graft surface, was assessed on a daily basis (by an observer blinded to treatment).

Monoclonal antibodies (MAbs). MAb to L3T4 (rat IgG2b) was produced by hybridoma GK1.5 (*20*), the kind gift of Dr. Frank Fitch (University of Chicago). The hybridoma was grown as ascites in irradiated (450R) BALB/c mice. Anti-Lyt-2 (hybridoma 53-6 [*21, 22*]) anti-Lyt-2.2 (hybridoma 2.43 [*23*]), anti-Thy 1.2 (hybridoma 30-H12 [*24*]) and anti-ThB (hybridoma 53-9 [*22, 24*]) were grown as ascites in athymic (*nu/nu*) BALB/c mice. MAbs were partially purified by ammonium sulfate precipitation, dialyzed against phosphate-buffered saline, and quantified by absorbance at 280 nm and by quantitative cellulose acetate electrophoresis. Nonimmune rat IgG was purchased from Jackson Immunoresearch Laboratories, Avondale, PA.

Skin graft treatment protocol. Graft recipients were treated with weekly i.v. injections of 1 mg anti-L3T4. The first injection was given 3 days prior to grafting. Controls are noted in the *Results* section.

Fluorescence analysis of mononuclear cells. Spleen cells and peripheral blood mononuclear cells were stained with fluorescein-conjugated MAbs as previously described (*25*). The MAbs identified T cells (anti-Thy-1.2), "helper-inducer" T cells (anti-L3T4), "suppressor/cytotoxic" T cells (anti-Lyt-2), and B cells (anti-ThB). In addition, cells were stained with mouse MAb to rat immunoglobulin kappa chain (hybridoma MAR 18.5 [*26*]) in order to quantify cells bearing the anti-L3T4 rat MAb used in treatment. A minimum of 2000 (usually 5000) cells was analyzed for each stain, by using a fluorescence-activated cell sorter (FACS II, Becton Dickinson, Sunnyvale, CA).

Medium. Cell cultures were performed in RPMI-1640 with 10% heat inactivated fetal bovine serum (Grand Island Biological Co, Grand Island, NY) with penicillin, streptomycin, and L-glutamine. For mixed leukocyte cultures, medium was further supplemented with 2×10^{-5} M 2-mercaptoethanol.

Mixed leukocyte culture (MLC). Spleen cells from C57BL/6 mice treated with anti-L3T4 or with saline were stimulated by irradiated (2000 rads) non-T spleen cells from BALB/c mice, depleted of T cells by treatment of donor mice with 1 mg anti-Thy-1.2 at 7 and 4 days prior to sacrifice. Responder spleen cells were obtained from C57BL/6 mice treated with 1 mg anti-L3T4 or with saline 7 days and 4 days prior to sacrifice.

Cell proliferation in the MLC was assayed in flat-bottomed 96-well microtiter plates (Corning) with 5×10^5 responder cells and 2.5×10^5 stimulator cells per well in 0.2 ml, with triplicates for each assay. To assess the inhibitory effect of MAb to L3T4 or Lyt-2, the MAb were added alone or in combination at a concentration of 2 μg/well, at least a 10-fold excess of the amount required for saturation binding of target antigens. During the last 6 hr of incubation, wells were pulsed with 1 μCi [^{3}H]-thymidine (Schwartz/Mann, Spring Valley, NY). Cellular radioactivity was determined by using a liquid scintillation spectrophotometer.

To examine the generation of IL-2 in the MLC, 5×10^6 responder and 2×10^6 stimulator cells were cultured in 24-well plates (Corning) in a volume of 2 ml/well. Supernatants were harvested after 48 hr for the quantification of IL-2, as described below. To assess the inhibitory effect of MAb to L3T4 or Lyt-2, the MAb were added alone or in combination at 10 μg/well.

To generate cytotoxic cells in the MLC, 25×10^6 responders and 12.5×10^6 stimulators were cultured in 10 ml in 25-cm^2 tissue culture flasks (Corning) for 6 days. Cells were washed and used directly in cytotoxicity assays.

IL-2 bioassay. The IL-2 content of MLC supernatants was assayed by using the IL-2-dependent T cell line CTLL-20 (*27*). CTLL-20 cells were washed thoroughly and then cultured at 3×10^3 cells/well in flat-bottomed microtiter plates containing serial dilutions of supernatants of a standard IL-2 preparation. All assays were run in triplicate. The cells were incubated overnight, pulsed with [^{3}H]-thymidine at 1 μCi/well for 6 hr, and then harvested. An IL-2 standard, produced by Con-A stimulation of spleen cells, was run with each assay. Results in cpm from experimental cultures were converted to equivalent concentrations of standard and are expressed as % standard (vol/vol) $\pm$ SEM.

Cytotoxicity assays. Spleen cells from grafted mice or from the MLC were tested for allospecific cytotoxicity against P815 (DBA/2 mastocytoma, H-2^d) and, as a control for nonspecific cytotoxicity, against EL-4 target cells (C57BL/6 T cell, H-2^b). Target cells were labeled with ^{51}Cr by incubation in $Na_2(^{51}Cr)O_4$ (New England Nuclear, Boston, MA), and 10^4 targets were incubated with effector cells at varying concentrations in V-bottomed 96-well microtiter plates (Flow Laboratories, Inc, McClean, VA) at 37°C in a 5% CO_2 atmosphere. Following the MLC, killing of P815 could be assessed in a 4-hr assay, while killing of P815 by spleen cells from grafted mice was significant only after 18 hr. After incubation for cytotoxicity, half the supernatant was harvested for determination of radioactivity. Spontaneous release was determined by incubation of labeled targets alone; maximum release was determined by incubation of cells in saponin and 0.1% EDTA. Percent cytotoxicity was calculated by:

$$\% \text{ cytotoxicity} = \left[\frac{cpm_{sample} - cpm_{spont}}{cpm_{max} - cpm_{spont}}\right] \times 100$$

Because spleen cells from grafted mice lacked allospecific T cell killing at 4 hr of incubation, it was possible also to assess natural killer (NK) cell activity against YAC-1 (A/J Maloney virus-induced T cell lymphoma, H-$2^{d/k}$) in a 4-hr assay, under the same conditions as above, without a contribution of T cell cytotoxicity.

Complement-mediated lysis. To examine the phenotype of cytotoxic cells, cytotoxicity was assessed after selective depletion of lymphocyte subsets by antilymphocyte MAbs and complement. Samples of 5×10^6 cells from each of triplicate cultures were incubated for 40 min at 4°C in 0.5 ml of phosphate buffered saline (pH 7.4) supplemented with 2% fetal bovine serum, containing 5 μg of MAb to Thy-1.2, L3T4, or Lyt-2.2. The cells were washed twice and incubated for 40 min at 37°C in 0.5 ml low-toxicity rabbit complement (Cedarlane) diluted 1:6 in saline. After 2 washes, all tubes were diluted to 1 ml and used in cytotoxicity assays on the basis of the initial cell concentrations.

Statistical analysis. The significance of differences in graft survival between treatment and control groups was determined by the Wilcoxon rank sum test. Differences in means among cytotoxicity assays and proliferation assays were analyzed by Student's *t* test.

RESULTS

Rejection of skin grafts by mice treated with anti-L3T4 is accompanied by the development of cytotoxic T cells. When C57BL/6 mice were grafted with BALB/c skin, graft survival was prolonged from 9.3±1.0 (SEM) days to 18.1±3.1 days by treating the recipients with 1 mg of MAb to L3T4 beginning 3 days before the graft and continuing weekly thereafter (Fig. 1). Despite treatment with anti-L3T4, however, both athymic and euthymic mice eventually reject skin grafts that differ at the major histocompatibility locus. As a first step toward examining the mechanism of rejection, grafted mice were tested for the presence of allospecific cytotoxic cells.

Thirty-two days after grafting, spleen cells from grafted mice were tested for cytotoxicity against the mastocytoma tumor line P815, which shares $H\text{-}2^d$ antigens with the BALB/c graft donors. Spleen cells from mice treated with anti-L3T4 were able to generate a significant allospecific response (Fig. 2), although they had less cytotoxicity against P815 than spleen cells from untreated control mice ($P<0.02$ at 100:1 effector:target ratio). Spleen cells from ungrafted mice did not kill P815. No cells were capable of lysing EL-4 ($H\text{-}2^b$) targets. These studies indicated that allospecific cytotoxic cells developed in grafted mice despite depletion of $L3T4^+$ cells.

Grafted mice treated with anti-L3T4, including cohorts sacrificed early in the course of therapy, were depleted of $L3T4^+$ cells in blood, spleen, and lymph nodes. Figure 3 presents the depletion of $L3T4^+$ cells at days 3, 7, and 35 of weekly treatment. After 3 days, $L3T4^+$ cells were depleted over 85% compared with control values and were depleted by >90% thereafter. The depletion of cells at days 7 and 35 was assessed one week after the previous treatment, indicating that weekly treatment with anti-L3T4 sufficed for target cell depletion. If the

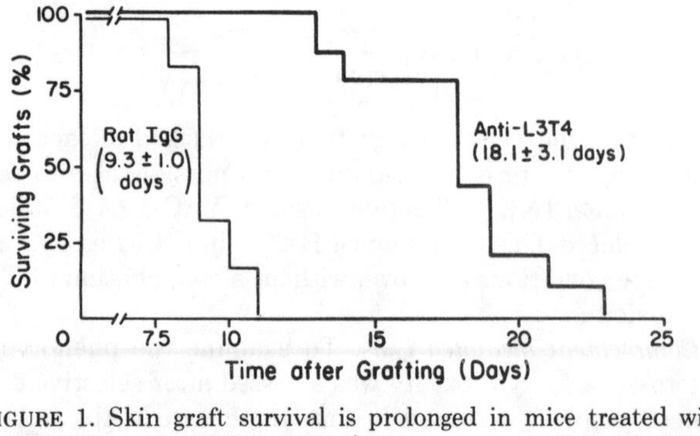

FIGURE 1. Skin graft survival is prolonged in mice treated with anti-L3T4. Recipient C57BL/6 ($H\text{-}2^b$) mice were treated weekly with 1 mg of MAb to L3T4, iv, beginning 3 days prior to transplantation of a 1-cm^2 graft from BALB/c ($H\text{-}2^d$) mice. Graft survival in control mice, treated with nonimmune rat IgG, was 9.3±1.0 (SEM) days (thin line, n=6) compared with 18.1±3.1 days in mice treated with anti-L3T4 (thick line, n=9). Values are the mean ± SEM.

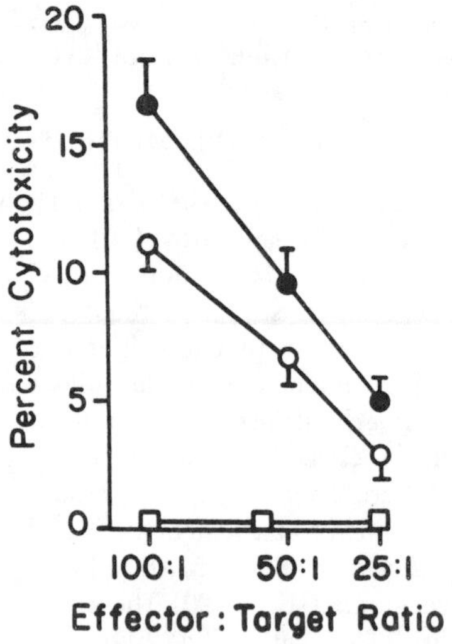

FIGURE 2. Cytotoxicity by spleen cells from C57BL/6 mice against P815 ($H\text{-}2^d$) targets. Spleen cells from mice that received BALB/c ($H\text{-}2^d$) skin grafts 32 days earlier had significant killing, whether treated with nonimmune rat IgG (controls, solid circles) or with anti-L3T4 (open circles). Cells from ungrafted mice had no cytotoxicity (squares).

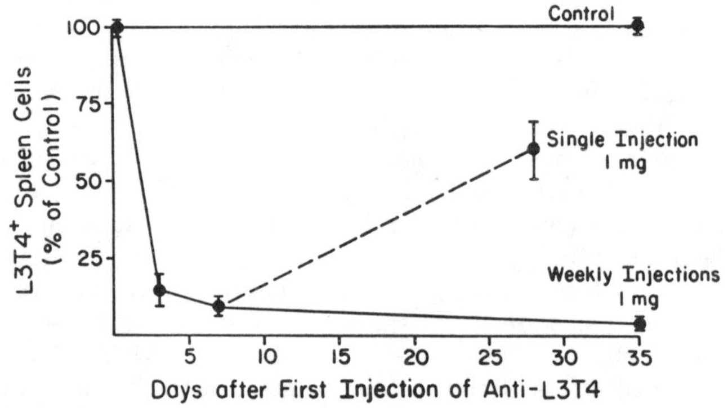

FIGURE 3. Weekly injection of MAb to L3T4 causes sustained depletion of $L3T4^+$ cells in the spleen. The number of $L3T4^+$ spleen cells are presented as a percentage of control mice. Three days after a single injection of 1 mg of anti-L3T4, when mice received skin grafts, $L3T4^+$ cells were reduced by over 85%; $L3T4^+$ cells continued to fall over the next 4 days, after which repeated weekly injections produced a sustained depletion of over 90% (solid line). If only a single injection was given, there was partial recovery of $L3T4^+$ cells after 4 weeks (dashed line).

first injection was not followed by weekly injections, however, $L3T4^+$ cells partially recovered over the ensuing month (Fig. 3). Cells from mice treated with anti-L3T4 were stained with a panel of antibodies to confirm that the loss of $L3T4^+$ cells from extrathymic organs was due to cell depletion. First, rat immunoglobulin was not detected on the surface of lymphocytes from treated mice, indicating that the MAb used in treatment was not blocking the antigen. Second, all of the T cells ($Thy\text{-}1.2^+$) were accounted for by cells expressing Lyt-2. Third, the ratio of T cells ($Thy\text{-}1.2^+$) to B cells (ThB^+) fell, indicating a partial depletion of T cells. Thus, within the limits of detection by these methods, the loss of $L3T4^+$ cells was not due to modulation of the L3T4 antigen from the surface of the cell (data not shown).

These studies demonstrate that cytotoxic T cells develop in grafted mice that are markedly depleted of $L3T4^+$ cells. However, treatment with anti-L3T4 does not rapidly eliminate L3T4⁺ cells from the thymus (unpublished observations), and there may be other areas where L3T4⁺ cells persist in vivo, contributing to the development of cytotoxic cells. We therefore examined the requirement for L3T4⁺ cells in the generation of allospecific cytotoxic T cells in vitro, where the elimination of L3T4⁺ cells could be documented.

Cytotoxic T cells are generated during an MLC by spleen cells depleted of L3T4⁺ cells. In order to assess the response of L3T4-depleted spleen cells in an MLC, spleen cells from C57BL/6 mice were obtained after two in vivo administrations of 1 mg of anti-L3T4 7 days and 4 days before mice were sacrificed. Fluorescence analysis documented that L3T4⁺ cells were below the level of detection both before and after the MLC. The stimulator cells were BALB/c spleen cells from which all T cells had been depleted by in vivo treatment with anti-Thy1.2, using the same protocol as for anti-L3T4. Preliminary studies indicated that this step was necessary in order to prevent stimulation of the responder cells by lymphokines released by the irradiated BALB/c stimulator cells. After a six day MLC, cells were tested for cytotoxicity against P815 and EL4 in a 4-hr ^{51}Cr release assay. No killing of EL4 was observed. In each of five experiments, cells from both untreated and treated mice were cytotoxic for P815. In 4 of 5 experiments, cytotoxicity by cells from mice that had been treated with anti-L3T4 was significantly lower than cytotoxicity by cells from control mice (range for the 5 experiments, 20–100% of control killing, on a per cell basis). Results from one of the 5 experiments are shown in Figure 4 which compares cytotoxicity generated by untreated spleen cells (Fig. 4a) to cytotoxicity generated by spleen cells depleted of L3T4⁺ cells (Fig. 4b). In both instances, the phenotype of the killer cells was shown to be Thy-1⁺, Lyt-2⁺, L3T4⁻ (Fig. 4). Thus, the cytotoxic T cells generated by L3T4-depleted spleen cells have the same phenotype as cytotoxic cells generated by intact spleen cells. Analysis of the cytotoxic cell population by microscopy or by light scatter on the cell sorter revealed that most of the live cells were blasts, indicating that the generation of cytotoxic T cells was accompanied by blast transformation. We therefore next examined directly whether L3T4-depleted spleen cells could be stimulated in an MLC to proliferate.

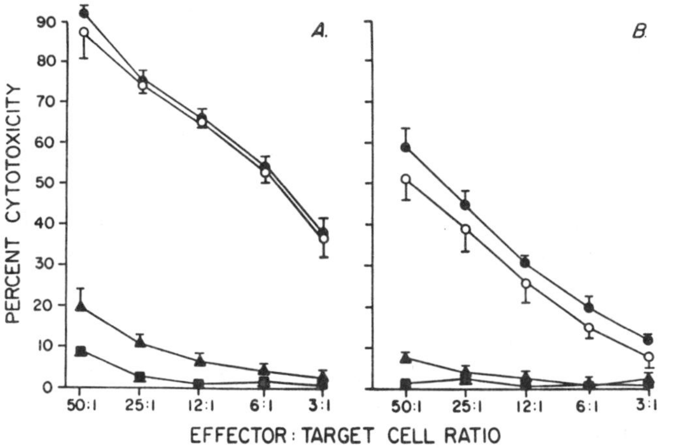

FIGURE 4. The generation of T cells cytotoxic for P815 during an MLC of C57BL/6 spleen cells against irradiated T cell-depleted BALB/c spleen cells. (A [left]) shows cytotoxicity by spleen cells from C57BL/6 mice treated with nonimmune rat IgG (controls). (B [right]) shows cytotoxicity by spleen cells from mice treated twice with MAb to L3T4. Following the MLC, the spleen cells were treated as follows: complement alone (controls, solid circles), anti-L3T4 plus complement (open circles), anti-Lyt-2.2 plus complement (solid triangles), or anti-Thy-1.2 plus complement (solid squares). For both intact and L3T4-depleted spleen cells, the phenotype of the killer cell is L3T4⁻, Lyt-2.2⁺, Thy-1.2⁺.

Proliferation and production of IL-2 in the MLC by spleen cells depleted of L3T4⁺ cells. The response of L3T4⁺ cells to alloantigens can be blocked by the presence of antibody to L3T4, and the response of Lyt-2⁺ cells can be blocked by antibody to Lyt-2. It was therefore possible to compare intact spleen cells with L3T4-depleted spleen cells not only with regard to proliferation in the MLC but also with regard to the inhibitory effects of antibody to L3T4 or to Lyt-2. To do so, these antibodies, alone or in combination, were included in the MLC from the onset.

Spleen cells depleted of L3T4⁺ cells responded in the MLC, but the response was reduced when compared with the response of control spleen cells (Fig. 5). Proliferation by spleen cells from untreated mice was significantly inhibited by both anti-L3T4 and anti-Lyt-2, but anti-L3T4 was more effective (Fig. 5). The combination of both antibodies completely prevented proliferation. Proliferation by spleen cells depleted of L3T4⁺ cells was inhibited 85% by anti-Lyt-2 ($P<0.01$) but only 35% by anti-L3T4 (not significant, $P>0.05$). The combination of both antibodies was more inhibitory than anti-Lyt-2 alone, indicating that there may be a contribution to proliferation by L3T4⁺ cells that cannot be detected by fluorescence analysis. If so, this contribution is clearly diminished when compared with spleen cells from untreated mice. A similar pattern of response and inhibition was seen when IL-2 was directly assessed by stimulation of the IL-2-dependent T cell line, CTLL-20 (Fig. 6). These findings suggest that Lyt-2⁺ cells are able to secrete IL-2 and trigger proliferation after an allogeneic stimulus in a manner that is independent of L3T4⁺ cells or requires very low numbers of L3T4⁺ cells.

DISCUSSION

Our studies demonstrate that the rejection of skin grafts by mice treated with anti-L3T4 is accompanied by the development of allospecific cytotoxic cells, despite a profound depletion of extrathymic L3T4⁺ T cells. Additionally, spleen cells from ungrafted mice treated with anti-L3T4 were able to proliferate, secrete IL-2, and generate cytotoxic Lyt-2⁺ T cells in response to allogenic challenge in an MLC. Blocking experiments performed during the MLC indicated that the phenotype of the responding cells in the treated group was primarily Lyt-2⁺, L3T4⁻.

Our demonstration that L3T4⁻ spleen cells can respond in an MLC is in contrast to the findings of Cobbold et al., who found little or no response by L3T4⁻ CBA spleen cells to BALB/c spleen cells (*19*). In our experiments, the response by L3T4⁻ spleen cells in the MLC was largely inhibited by anti-Lyt-2, but there was additional inhibition in the presence of anti-L3T4, indicating a possible contribution of L3T4 cells, even though these cells could not be detected by fluorescence analysis either before or after the MLC. It is possible that treatment with anti-L3T4 allows the survival of small numbers of L3T4⁺ cells that are sufficient to contribute to the proliferation of T cells and to the generation of cytotoxic T cells in vitro. If so, proliferation and IL-2 production are still predominantly dependent on the function of Lyt-2⁺ cells.

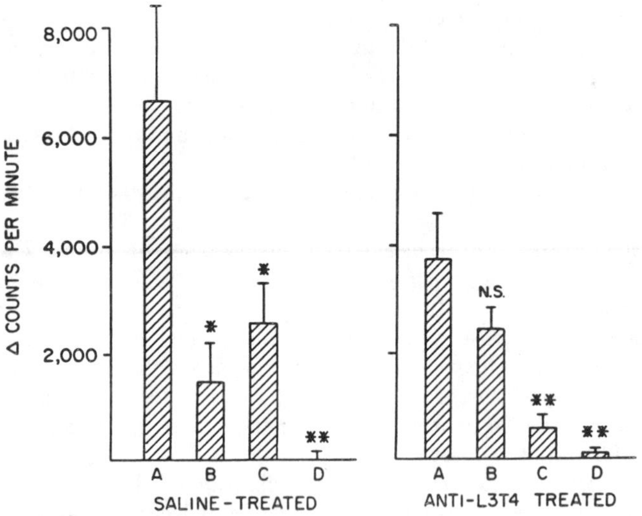

FIGURE 5. Proliferation of C57BL/6 spleen cells in an MLC with irradiated, T-cell-depleted BALB/c spleen cells. The left panel shows proliferation by spleen cells from C57BL/6 mice treated with nonimmune rat IgG (controls). The right panel shows proliferation by spleen cells from C57BL/6 mice treated twice with MAb to L3T4. In each panel, *A* is the proliferative response in the absence of MAb, *B* is the response in the presence of anti-L3T4, *C* is the response in the presence of anti-Lyt-2, and *D* is the response in the presence of both anti-L3T4 and anti-Lyt-2. ([*] $P<0.05$, [**] $P<0.01$ compared with A).

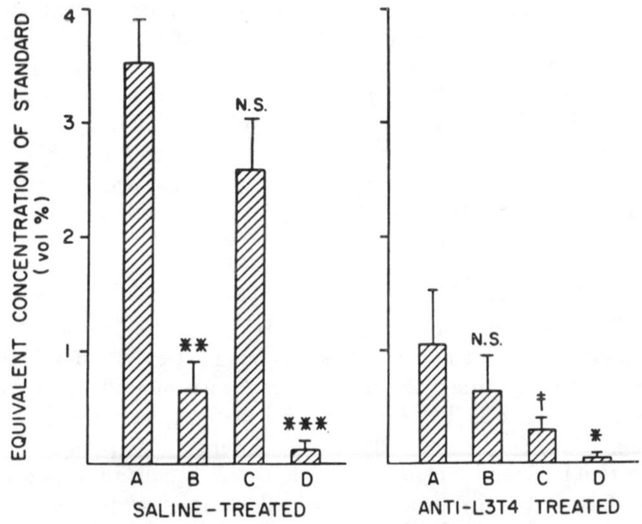

FIGURE 6. Production of IL-2 by C57BL/6 spleen cells in an MLC with irradiated, T-cell-depleted BALB/c spleen cells. The left panel shows IL-2 production by spleen cells from C57BL/6 mice treated with nonimmune rat IgG (controls). The right panels shows IL-2 production by spleen cells from C57BL/6 mice treated twice with MAb to L3T4. In each panel, *A* is the level of IL-2 produced in the absence of MAb, *B* is the level produced in the presence of anti-L3T4, *C* is the level produced in the presence of anti-Lyt-2, and *D* is the level produced in the presence of both. IL-2 was assessed by the ability to sustain proliferation of CTLL-20 as compared with serial dilutions of a standard. Results are expressed as a fraction of the standard. ([‡] P 0.10>0.05, [*] $P<0.05$, [**] $P<0.01$, [***] $P<0.005$.

In our in vivo experiments, the prolongation of graft survival by weekly treatment of euthymic mice was similar to the prolongation of graft survival seen by Cobbold et al., in thymectomized mice treated with anti-L3T4, in which L3T4$^+$ cells were permanently eliminated (*18*). Their findings and ours suggest that L3T4$^+$ cells may not be required for graft rejection. A lack of requirement for L3T4$^+$ cells in skin graft rejection is also supported by the recent findings of Holáň and Hašek (*28*). These authors found that treatment of B10.A mice with anti-Lyt-2.2, but not anti-L3T4, delayed rejection of skin grafts from B10.A(2R) or B10.A(4R) mice. Because these grafts differ from the recipient at MHA I but not at MHA II, the results suggest that L3T4$^+$ cells have little or no role in skin grafts that differ only at MHA I.

Studies in other experimental systems also support the contention that L3T4$^+$ cells may not be required at all for the development of cytotoxic T cells. Instead, IL-2 and other mediators of T cell "help" for the development of cytotoxic T cells may be generated by the Lyt-2$^+$, L3T4$^-$ T cell population. Prior to the description of the L3T4 antigen, treatment of mouse spleen cells with anti-Ly-1 was shown to remove their ability to generate IL-2 activity in response to MHA II, but not in response to MHA I, (*29*). Antibody to Ly-1 binds to all T cells but preferentially kills L3T4$^+$ T cells. More recently, Mizuochi et al., demonstrated that L3T4$^-$, Lyt-2$^+$ T cells produce IL-2 and generate cytotoxic T cells against allogeneic MHA I (*30*). Sprent and Schaefer have found that purified C57BL/6 Lyt-2$^+$ cells respond in an MLR to C57BL/6.C-H-2^{bm1} cells, which differ from C57BL/6 mice only in three amino acids in a class I major hisotcompatibility antigen (H-2K) (*31*). Other studies have indicated that this response relies on recognition of the H-2^{bm1} antigen in association with self-MHA II (*32, 33*), but the studies by Sprent and Schaefer support the finding that highly purified Lyt-2$^+$ cells respond to MHA I but not MHA II in an MLR, while highly purified L3T4$^+$ cells respond to MHA II but not MHA I (*31*). Interestingly, in these studies, MAb to L3T4 had no effect on the MLR by Lyt-2$^+$ cells, but the response was dependent on the expression of MHA II by the stimulator cells, not the responder cells, even though the stimulators and responders had identical MHA II (*31*).

In studies of the graft-versus-host reaction (GVHR), Korngold and Sprent demonstrated that a GVHR between cells that differ only at MHA I is prevented by pretreating the donor cells with anti-Lyt-2 (and complement) but not anti-L3T4 (*34*). GVHR between cells that differ only at MHA II is prevented by pretreating the donor cells with anti-L3T4, but not anti-Lyt-2. Piguet cloned allospecific cytolytic T cell lines from mice undergoing a GVHR against MHA I and found them all to be Lyt-2$^+$ but poorly proliferative and incapable of producing IL-2 (*35*). However, studies with cloned human T cells indicate that IL-2 is produced by about 15% of clones that express T8, the human homologue for Lyt-2 (*36*).

These studies of the response to allogeneic MHA suggest that the eventual rejection of grafts by mice treated with anti-L3T4 may be due to an independent response by Lyt-2 cells to MHA I. Alternatively, graft rejection may require relatively few L3T4$^+$ cells, and sufficient numbers persist after treatment with anti-L3T4. In either event our model demonstrates that even profound depletion of L3T4$^+$ cells in vivo is not sufficient to block graft rejection and the development of cytotoxic T cells. This is in contrast to the elimination of humoral immunity by the same therapy (*18, 19*). This suggests that the response of B cells in vivo to T-dependent antigens is either uniquely dependent on L3T4$^+$ cells or that, under the conditions that have been studied, more L3T4$^+$ cells are required for humoral immunity than are necessary for the development of cellular immunity.

The failure of anti-L3T4 to completely suppress cellular

immunity may have advantages in the treatment of autoimmunity. We have shown that MAb to L3T4 blocks the development of autoimmunity in NZB/NZW mice, which develop an illness resembling systemic lupus erythematosus (*17*). Treatment after the onset of autoimmunity also blocks disease and prolongs survival (Wofsy D. et al., unpublished observations). Treatment with anti-L3T4 blocks humoral immunity, so survival of animals may depend in part on the ability to generate cellular immunity.

Because treatment with anti-L3T4 delays, but does not prevent, skin graft rejection, treatment of humans with anti-T4 is not likely to sustain histoincompatible skin grafts. Skin, however, is an immunologically active organ with great immunogenicity. The role of T cell subsets in the rejection of visceral organ grafts may be different. Antibodies to T4 (CD4), the human homologue to L3T4, have been tested in monkeys. In one study, the antibodies prolonged the survival of kidney allografts from 9 to 11 days, in controls, to a maximum of 7 weeks in animals treated with anti-T4 (*37*). The antibodies tested were of isotypes that did not efficiently clear target cells; only a maximum of 80% of circulating target cells was removed. In a second study, a mixture of both IgG2a and IgG2b antibodies was used. There was variability in the depletion of target cells. Treatment suppressed acute graft rejection in graft recipients that had not previously received blood transfusions (*38*). In animals that had not previously been tranfused, the anti-T4 antibodies did not prolong graft survival more than treatment with azathioprine and prednisone. Further studies are warranted to assess the effects of anti-CD4 on immunity in primates.

Acknowledgments. We thank Denise Go for preparing the manuscript. Drs. Frank Fitch and Jeffrey Ledbetter kindly provided hybridomas for the production of the monoclonal antibodies used in these studies.

REFERENCES

1. Starzl TE. Heterologous antilymphocyte globulin. N Engl J Med 1968; 279: 700.
2. Heyworth MF. Clinical experience with antilymphocyte serum. Immunol Rev 1982; 65: 79.
3. Lawley IJ, Bielory L, Gascon P, Yencey KB, Young NS, Frank MM. A prospective clinical and immunologic analysis of patients with serum sickness. N Engl J Med 1984; 311: 1407.
4. Tatum AH, Bollinger RR, Sanfilippo F. Rapid serologic diagnosis of serum sickness from antithymocyte globulin therapy using enzyme immunoassay. Transplantation 1984; 38: 582.
5. Kohler G, Milstein C. Continuous cultures of fused cells secreting antibody of predefined specificity. Nature 1975; 256: 495.
6. Cosimi AB, Colvin RB, Burton RC, et al. Use of monoclonal antibodies to T cell subsets for immunologic monitoring and treatment in recipients of renal allografts. N Engl J Med 1981; 305: 308.
7. Ortho Multicenter Transplant Study Group. A randomized clinical trial of OKT3 monoclonal antibody for acute rejection of cadaveric renal transplants. N Engl J Med 1985; 313: 337.
8. Colvin RB, Cosimi AB, Burton RB. Anti-idiotype antibodies in patients treated with murine monoclonal antibody OKT3. Fed Proc 1982; 41: 363.
9. Burton RC, Cosimi AB, Colvin RB, et al. Monoclonal antibodies to human T cell subsets: use for immunological monitoring and immunosuppression in renal transplantation. J Clin Immunol 1982; 2(July suppl): 142S.
10. Reinherz EL, Schlossman SF. The differentiation and functions of human T lymphocytes. Cell 1980; 19: 821.
11. Engleman EG, Benike CJ, Grumet FC, Evans RL. Activation of human T lymphocyte subsets: helper and suppressor/cytotoxic T cells recognize and respond to distinct histocompatibility antigens. J Immunol 1981; 127: 2124.
12. Swain SL. T cell subsets and the recognition of MHC class. Immunol Rev 1983; 74: 129.
13. Dialynas DP, Quan ZS, Wall KA. Characterization of the murine T cell molecule, designated L3T4, identified by monoclonal antibody GK1.5: similarity of L3T4 to the human Leu-3/T4 molecule. J Immunol 1983; 131: 2445.
14. Wilde DB, Marrack P, Kappler J, Dialynas DP, Fitch FW. Evidence implicating L3T4 in class II MHC antigen reactivity: monoclonal antibody GK1.5 (anti-L3T4a) blocks class II MHC antigen-specific proliferation, release of lymphokines, and binding by cloned murine helper T lymphocyte lines. J Immunol 1983; 131: 2178.
15. Cantor H, Boyse EA. Functional subclasses of T lymphocytes bearing different Ly antigens. I. The generation of functionally distinct T cell subclasses is a differentiative process independent of antigen. J Exp Med 1975; 141: 1376.
16. Ledbetter JA, Evans RL, Lipinski M, Cunningham-Rundles C, Good RA, Herzenberg LA. Evolutionary conservation of surface molecules that distinguish T lymphocyte helper/inducer and cytotoxic/suppressor subpopulations in mouse and man. J Exp Med 1981; 153: 310.
17. Wofsy D, Seaman WE. Successful treatment of autoimmunity in NZB/NZW F_1 mice with monoclonal antibody to L3T4. J Exp Med 1985; 161: 378.
18. Cobbold SP, Jayesuriya A, Nash A, Prospeno TD, Waldmann H. Therapy with monoclonal antibodies by elimination of T-cell subsets in vivo. Nature 1984; 312: 548.
19. Wofsy D, Mayes DC, Woodcock J, Seaman WE. Inhibition of humoral immunity in vivo by monoclonal antibody to L3T4: studies with soluble antigens in intact mice. J Immunol 1985; 135: 1698.
20. Dialynas DP, Wilde DB, Marrack P, et al. Characterization of the murine antigenic determinant, designated L3T4a, recognized by monoclonal antibody GK1.5: expression of L3T4a by functional T cell clones appears to correlate primarily with class II MHC antigen-reactivity. Immunol Rev 1983; 74: 29.
21. Ledbetter JA, Rouse RV, Micklem HS, Herzenberg LA. T cell subsets defined by expression of Lyt-1,2,3 and Thy-1 antigens. Two parameter immunofluorescence and cytotoxicity analysis with monoclonal antibodies modifies current views. J Exp Med 1980; 152: 280.
22. Micklem HS, Ledbetter JA, Eckhardt LA, Herzenberg LA. Analysis of T lymphocyte subpopulations with monoclonal antibodies to Thy-1, Lyt-1, Lyt-2 and ThB antigens. In: Pernis B, Vogel HJ, eds. Regulatory T lymphocytes. New York: Academic, 1980: 119.
23. Sarmiento M, Glasebrook AL, Fitch FW. IgG or IgM monoclonal antibodies reactive with different determinants on the molecular complex bearing Lyt 2 antigen block T cell-mediated cytolysis in the absence of complement. J Immunol 1980; 125: 2665.
24. Ledbetter JA, Goding JW, Tokuhisa T, Herzenberg LA. Murine T-cell differentiation antigens detected by monoclonal antibodies. In: Kennett RH, McKearn TJ, Bechtol KB, eds. Monoclonal antibodies. New York: Plenum 1980: 235.
25. Seaman WE, Wofsy D, Greenspan JS, Ledbetter JA. Treatment of autoimmune MRL/1pr mice with a monoclonal antibody to Thy-1.2: a single injection has sustained effects on lymphoproliferation and renal disease. J Immunol 1983; 130: 1713.
26. Lanier LL, Gutman GA, Lewis DE, Griswold ST, Warner NL. Monoclonal antibodies against rat immunoglobulin kappa chains. Hybridoma 1982; 1: 125.
27. Clouse KA, Bach FH, Orosz CG. Detection of HSV-1 induced lymphokine production in human cells by a direct indicator cell addition assay. J Immunol 1984; 132: 2961.
28. Holáň V, Hašek M. Prolonged or permanent survival of skin allografts induced by monoclonal antibodies against lymphocyte subpopulations. Folia Biol (Praha) 1985; 31: 50.

29. Okada M, Henney CS. The differentiation of cytotoxic cells in vitro. II. Amplifying factor(s) produced in primary mixed lymphocyte cultures against K/D stimuli require the presence of Lyt-2+ cells but not Lyt-1+ cells. J Immunol 1980; 125: 300.
30. Mizuochi T, Golding H, Rosenberg AS, Glimcher LH, Malek TR, Singer A. Both L3T4+ and Lyt-2+ helper T cells initiate cytotoxic T lymphocyte responses against allogeneic major histocompatibility antigens but not against trinitrophenyl-modified self. J Exp Med 1985; 162: 427.
31. Sprent J, Schaefer M. Properties of purified T cell subsets. I. In vitro responses to class I vs class II H-2 alloantigens. J Exp Med 1986; 163: 998.
32. Rock K, Barnes MC, Germain RN, Benacerraf B. The role of Ia molecules in the activation of T lymphocytes. II. Ia-restricted recognition of allo K/D antigens is required for class I MHC-stimulated mixed lymphocyte responses. J Immunol 1983; 130: 457.
33. Weinberger O, Germain RN, Burakoff SJ. Responses to the H-2K^{ba} mutant involve recognition of syngeneic Ia molecules. Nature 1983; 302: 429.
34. Korngold R, Sprent J. Surface markers of T cells causing lethal graft-vs-host disease to class I vs class II H-2 differences. J Immunol 1985; 135: 3004.
35. Piguet PF. GVHR elicited by products of class I or class II loci of the MHC: analysis of the response of mouse T lymphocytes to products of class I and class II loci of the MHC in correlation with GVHR-induced mortality, medullary aplasia, and enteropathy. J Immunol 1985; 135: 1637.
36. Mingari MC, Moretta A, Maggi E, et al. Frequent coexpression of cytolytic activity and lymphokine production among human T lymphocytes. Production of B cell growth factor and interleukin 2 by T8+ and T4+ cytolytic clones. Eur J Immunol 1984; 14: 1066.
37. Cosimi AB, Colvin RB, Jaffers GJ, et al. Immunologic monitoring of monoclonal antibody therapy: comparison of five antibodies as immunosuppressants of renal allograft rejection. Transplant Proc 1984; 16: 1459.
38. Jonker M, Neuhaus P, Zurcher C, Fucello A, Goldstein G. OKT4 and OKT4A antibody treatment as immunosuppression for kidney transplantation in rhesus monkeys. Transplantation 1985; 39: 247.

Received 9 December 1985.
Accepted 18 March 1986.

0041-1337/86/4206-0642$02.00/0
TRANSPLANTATION

Vol. 42, No. 6
Printed in U.S.A.

THE REQUIREMENT FOR THE RENAL TRANSPLANT TO INDUCE ALLOGRAFT UNRESPONSIVENESS BY THE COMBINATION OF EXTRACTED HISTOCOMPATIBILITY ANTIGEN AND CYCLOSPORINE[1]

NORIO YOSHIMURA AND BARRY D. KAHAN

The Division of Immunology and Organ Transplantation, Department of Surgery, The University of Texas Medical School at Houston, Texas 77030

The impact of the presence of the allograft on the induction of unresponsiveness by the immunosuppressive combination of cyclosporine (CsA) and 3M KCl-extracted histocompatibility Antigen (Ag) was assessed by comparing the outcome of renal transplants when the regimen was used pretransplantation versus peri- and posttransplantation. WFu rat hosts, which had been pretreated with either one (−11, −10, −9) or three (−25, −24, −23, −18, −17, −16, −11, −10, −9) cycles of CsA and BUF Ag (−11 or −25, −18, −11) prior to implantation of BUF renal allografts, failed to display the prolonged graft survival achieved with this regimen administered in the peri- (−1, 0, +1) and immediate posttransplant (+7, 8, 9, 14, 15, 16) period. However, OX-8 positive, putative T-suppressor (T_s) cells in the spleens of pretreated hosts were able to transfer slightly prolonged BUF allograft survival to virgin, secondary syngeneic hosts. The OX-8-positive cells induced by pretreatment were apparently inhibited from prolonging BUF allografts in primary hosts by cellular elements vulnerable to splenectomy, total-body irradiation, or a three-day peritransplant course of CsA therapy. Therefore the presence of the renal graft at the time of peri- and immediate posttransplant administration of Ag-CsA facilitates the induction of unresponsiveness, possibly due to continued release of histocompatibility antigen to stimulate, and/or to providing an important peripheral environment promoting differentiation and maturation of, T_s cells.

The potent immunosuppressive effects of cyclosporine (CsA),* a hydrophobic, cyclic, fungal endecapeptide of novel chemical structure that has improved the outcome of human renal transplants (*1, 2*), exerts a relatively selective inhibition of T-helper functions, as documented in vivo (*3, 4*) and in vitro (*5, 6*), but not T-suppressor (T_s) activity (*7, 8*). The combination of donor histocompatibility antigen (Ag), which is extracted from spleen cells with 3M KCl and specifically stimulates T_s cells, with a three-day peritransplant course of CsA,

[1] This work was supported by Grant 1R01 AI 22664 from the National Institute of Allergy and Infectious Disease.

* Abbreviations used: BN, Brown Norway; BUF, Buffalo; CsA, cyclosporine; MST, median survival time (days); WFU, Wistar-Furth.

which dampens helper functions, causes synergistic immunosuppression. The mean survival of RT-1-incompatible Buffalo (BUF) rat renal allografts is prolonged in Wistar-Furth (WFu) recipients from 7 to 24 days (*9*). The unresponsive state induced by Ag-CsA is mediated by splenic and peripheral blood T_s cells, which are adherent neither to plastic nor nylon-wool, are OX-8-phenotype–positive, and cyclophosphamide-sensitive (*10, 11*). Moreover, adoptive transfer of purified T_s cells from Ag-CsA treated hosts prolongs the survival of donor BUF, but not third-party Brown-Norway (BN), grafts in secondary WFu hosts. T_s cells were also demonstrated to have infiltrated renal transplants that had enjoyed prolonged survival in primary hosts (*12*). In order to assess the significance of the allograft for the induction and maintenance of unresponsiveness mediated by T_s cells, the studies presented herein examined the efficacy of the Ag-CsA regimen administered to hosts in the absence of—namely, prior to—renal transplantation. Thus rather than imitiating the immunosuppressive regimen at the time of transplantation, these studies administered three cycles of the Ag-CsA regimen beginning 25 days prior to transplantation. If the Ag-CsA regimen by itself established an allounresponsive state, similar to that observed in 40% of hosts when therapy is commenced in the peri- and postoperative period, there would be no need for immunosuppressive therapy after implantation of the renal allograft.

MATERIALS AND METHODS

Animals. A bilateral recipient nephrectomy was combined with an orthotopic renal transplant, using a modified microsurgical technique (*13*). Inbred 150–300-g Buffalo (BUF, RT-1^b) male rats were used as donors to recipient Wistar-Furth (WFu, RT-1^u) male rats, which were maintained on ad libitum feedings of laboratory chow (Harlan Sprague-Dawley, Hasslett, MI). One group of animals underwent splenectomy concomitant with the nephrectomy and transplant. Since all hosts underwent the nephrectomy-transplant procedure, there was no necessity for a sham-operated control for the splenectomy group. The average total ischemic time for the renal transplant was less than 30 min. Renal graft function was assessed by recipient survival; death due to rejection was confirmed by histological examination.

Immunosuppressive regimens. CsA, which was donated by Sandoz (Basel, Switzerland) as a white powder, was dissolved in olive oil at a concentration of 20 mg/ml. Rats were administered three-day courses of oral CsA 10 mg/kg/day by gavage either as a single cycle on days −11, −10, −9 before transplantation, or as three cycles at intervals of seven days—namely, days −25, −24, −23; −18, −17, −16, and −11, −10, −9 before transplantation. This time sequence exploited the findings in previous experiments that CsA administered on days −1, 0, +1, with Ag on day −1 induced the generation of T_s cells in spleens harvested ten days after transplantation. Donor antigen was extracted from BUF spleen cells by the 3M KCl method (*14*). Protein concentrations in extracts were estimated by the Bradford method (*15*). Rats treated with one cycle of CsA on days −11, −10, −9 were i.v. with 5 mg antigen extract on day −11 or on days −11, −7, −4 and −1. Animals treated with three cycles of CsA received Ag on days −25, −18, and −11. On day 0 all WFu rats received a BUF kidney transplant.

In some experiments spleen cells were harvested on day 0 from WFu rats, pretreated with either one or three cycles of the Ag-CsA regimen. After separation of elements not adherent to plastic and nylon-wool, the cell population was depleted of W3/25-positive cells by a modification of the rosetting technique of Mason (*16*). This population, which was previously demonstrated to be enriched in OX-8 positive T cells (*10, 11*), was adoptively transferred i.v. into virgin, untreated, secondary, syngeneic WFu hosts (10^6 cells per recipient) on the day of BUF kidney transplantation.

RESULTS

Ag-CsA pretreatment to induce unresponsiveness. Table 1 shows that pretreatment of hosts with either one or three cycles of Ag-CsA did not prolong the survival of subsequent renal allografts. Untreated WFu hosts reject BUF kidney grafts at 7.2±0.6 days (group 1). Neither a single (group 2) nor three (group 3) cycles of Ag-CsA pretreatment affected the subsequent survival of challenge BUF allografts placed onto WFu hosts that did not receive posttransplant immunosuppression (MST 7.7± 0.5 and 7.4±0.5 days, respectively). However, secondary virgin WFu animals displayed significant prolongation of challenge BUF grafts after adoptive transfer of 1×10^6 T_s cells, which had been harvested on day 0 and purified from the spleens of WFu rats that were pretreated with either one (−11, −10, −9) or three (−25, −24, −23, −18, −17, −16, −11, −10, −9) cycles of the Ag-CsA regimen—namely, 12.4±4.2 (group 5) and 11.6±4.6 (group 6) days, respectively. However, the mean survival times of groups 5 and 6 were significantly shorter than that displayed by secondary, virgin WFu hosts receiving T_s cells harvested ten days after BUF kidney transplantation and perioperative treatment with a single cycle of the Ag-CsA regimen (group 7)—namely, CsA by gavage on days −1, 0, +1 and Ag i.v. on the day (−1) prior to transplantation (MST 17.5±8.0 days, $P < 0.05$). The Ag component of the regimen was critical: the OX-8-positive splenic population harvested and purified from hosts receiving three cycles of CsA pretreatment without antigen (group 8) failed to prolong graft survival (MST 7.3±0.5 days). In aggregate, these results suggest that suppressor cells generated in WFu rats during pretreatment with the Ag-CsA regimen prior to transplantation are less potent than the cells generated in hosts allografted at the time of induction of the immunosuppressive therapy. Thus, the presence of the graft reinforces the generation of suppressor cells.

In order to address the question whether the effect was solely due to the transplant releasing additional histocompatibility antigen that repetitively stimulates suppressor elements, donor extract was administered on days −11, −7, −4, and −1 in the interim between pretreatment with the one-cycle Ag-CsA regimen and transplantation (group 4). After multiple injections of donor Ag, graft survival time was not significantly prolonged (MST 12.1±8.4 days) compared with hosts receiving either one-cycle Ag-CsA or no pretreatment, due primarily to the large standard deviation from 2/8 hosts surviving more than 24 days.

Effect of splenectomy. The capacity of enriched OX-8-positive cells to confer prolonged allograft survival on virgin syngeneic hosts demonstrated the presence of T_s elements in the spleens of pretreated hosts. Since pretreated animals with intact spleens did not display allograft prolongation, it appeared likely that cells generating host resistance toward allografts predominated over the T_s elements in the spleen. In order to assess the immunologic activity of the nonsplenic lymphoid system after Ag-CsA pretreatment, splenectomy was performed at the time of transplantation (Table 2). A single cycle of Ag-CsA pretreatment (days −11, −10, −9) combined with splenectomy at the time of transplantation (day 0) significantly prolonged

TABLE 1. Effect of Pretreatment With Ag-CsA on BUF renal allograft survival in primary and in secondary WFu rats receiving adoptive transfer of T lymphocytes

Group	Treatment	n	Survival (days)	Mean (±SD)	P value[e]			
1	None	10	6, 7, 7, 7, 7, 7, 7, 8, 8, 8	7.2±0.6	NS (1 vs 2)	NS (1–3)		<0.05 (1–4)
2	1-Cycle Ag-CsA pretreatment[a]	7	7, 7, 8, 8, 8, 8, 8	7.7±0.5	NS (2 vs 3)		NS[f] (2–4)	
3	3-Cycle Ag-CsA pretreatment[b]	7	7, 7, 7, 7, 8, 8, 8	7.4±0.5	NS[f] (3 vs 4)			
4	1-Cycle Ag-CsA pretreatment Ag (−11, −7, −4, −1)	8	7, 7, 7, 7, 7, 9, 25, 28	12.1±8.4				
5	T_s cells from 1-cycle Ag-CsA pretreatment only[c]	10	8, 8, 9, 10, 11, 12, 13, 13, 19, 21	12.4±4.2	NS (5 vs 6)	<0.05 (5–7)		
6	T_s cells from 3-cycle Ag-CsA pretreatment	11	7, 8, 9, 9, 9, 10, 10, 13, 13, 16, 24	11.6±4.6	<0.05 (6 vs 7)		<0.01 (6–8)	
7	T_s cells from 1-cycle perioperative treatment[d]	11	8, 9, 10, 12, 13, 16, 18, 22, 23, 26, 35	17.5±8.0	<0.01 (7 vs 8)			
8	T_s cells from 3-cycle CsA only pretreatment	6	7, 7, 7, 7, 8, 8	7.3±0.5				

[a] The one-cycle pretreatment of WFu hosts included CsA (10 mg/kg/day) administered by gavage on days −11, −10, −9, and 3M-KCl-extracted donor antigen (5 mg) injected i.v. on day −11 prior to BUF kidney transplantation on day 0.

[b] The three-cycle pretreatment included CsA (10 mg/kg/day) administered on days −25, −24, −23, days −18, −17, −16, and days −11, −10, −9, and Ag injected on days −25, −18, −11 prior to BUF kidney transplantation on day 0.

[c] From splenic lymphoid cells harvested on day 0 from either one-cycle or three-cycle Ag-CsA-pretreated WFu rats, was prepared the OX-8 positive T cell subpopulation after dish separation, nylon-wool adherence, and rosetting using monoclonal antibodies, as previously described (*10*). T_s cells (1×10^6) were adoptively transferred into WFu rats on the day of BUF kidney transplantation.

[d] Lymphoid cells, harvested ten days after BUF kidney transplantation of WFu hosts that had received Ag (5 mg) on day −1 and CsA (10 mg/kg/day) on days −1, 0, +1. The OX-8-positive T cell subset, which had been fractionated by dish, nylon-wool and rosette techniques using monoclonal antibodies, were administered to virgin, secondary WFu hosts at a dose of 1×10^6 cells i.v. on the day of BUF kidney transplantation.

[e] Statistical significance assessed by the Kruskal-Wallis statistic.

[f] Statistical significance assessed toward one-cycle and three-cycle Ag-CsA-pretreated groups by Student's *t* test.

TABLE 2. Effect of splenectomy on BUF renal allograft survival in Ag-CsA-pretreated WFu hosts

Group	CsA pretreatment[a]	Ag	Splenectomy[b]	n	Survival (days)	Mean (±SD)	P value[c]		
1	1-Cycle	+	−	7	7, 7, 8, 8, 8, 8, 8	7.7± 0.5	<0.025 (1 vs 2)		
2	1-Cycle	+	+	6	7, 9, 16, 18, 29, 37	19.3±10.6			<0.01 (2–6)
3	3-Cycle	+	−	7	7, 7, 7, 7, 8, 8, 8	7.4± 0.5	<0.001 (3 vs 4)		
4	3-Cycle	+	+	7	10, 10, 17, 19, 30, 36, 48	24.3±13.2	<0.005 (4 vs 5)	<0.001 (4–6)	
5	3-Cycle	−	+	8	8, 8, 8, 8, 8, 9, 9, 10	8.5± 0.7	NS (5 vs 6)		
6	None	−	+	8	6, 7, 8, 9, 9, 9, 10, 11	8.6± 1.5			

[a] WFu rats received either one cycle of Ag-CsA pretreatment, including CsA (10 mg/kg/day) on days −11, −10, −9 and 3M KCl-extracted donor antigen (5 mg) on day −11, or three cycles of pretreatment including CsA (10 mg/kg/day) on days −25, −24, −23, −18, −17, −16, −11, −10, −9, and 5 mg donor antigen on days −25, −18, −11, followed by BUF kidney transplantation on day 0.

[b] Splenectomy was done at the time of transplantation in hosts denoted (+).

[c] Statistical significance between groups assessed by Newman-Keul's *Q* statistic.

BUF allograft survival to 19.3±10.6 days ($P < 0.025$), in spite of the fact that the animals did not receive any posttransplant immunosuppression. Further prolongation of BUF graft survival to 24.3±13.2 days ($P < 0.001$) was obtained when three cycles of Ag-CsA pretreatment were combined with splenectomy. Splenectomy combined with three cycles of pretreatment with CsA only (without extracted antigen) failed to prolong graft survival (MST 8.5±0.7 days) compared with control virgin WFu rats that had undergone only BUF transplantation and splenectomy without CsA therapy (MST 8.6±1.5 days, NS). These findings suggest that suppressor elements predominate in the nonsplenic lymphoid organs of Ag-CsA-pretreated hosts.

Effect of combined therapy with other immunosuppressants. Sublethal total-body irradiation (500 rads, day −1), or perioperative CsA treatment (10 mg/kg on days −1, 0, +1) was used for adjunctive therapy, in order to augment the immunosuppressive effect of Ag-CsA pretreatment upon WFu host resistance toward BUF allografts (Table 3). Hosts receiving irradiation on day −1 after three cycles of Ag-CsA pretreatment demonstrated slight, but significantly, prolonged BUF graft survival (MST 11.9±0.8 days) compared with the control group receiving only irradiation (MST 8.3±1.8 days, $P < 0.01$). Moreover, the combination of three cycles of Ag-CsA pretreatment with a fourth peritransplant three-day course of CsA adminis-

TABLE 3. Survival of BUF renal allografts in hosts receiving Ag-CsA pretreatment plus perioperative immunosuppression with CsA or with sublethal irradiation

Group	Ag-CsA pretreatment[a]	CsA perioperative treatment[b]	Irradiation[c]	n	Survival (days)	Mean (±SD)	P value[d]
1	None	−	−	10	6, 7, 7, 7, 7, 7, 7, 8, 8, 8	7.2±0.6	NS
2	3-Cycle	−	−	7	7, 7, 7, 7, 8, 8, 8	7.4±0.5	<0.01; <0.01
3	3-Cycle	+	−	7	9, 9, 11, 12, 15, 27, 28	15.9±7.6	<0.01
4	None	+	−	10	9, 10, 11, 11, 11,12, 12, 13, 16, 17	12.2±2.4	<0.01
5	3-Cycle	−	+	7	11, 11, 11, 12, 12, 13, 13	11.9±0.8	
6	None	−	+	6	6, 7, 7, 9, 10, 11	8.3±1.8	<0.01

[a] WFu rats pretreated with three cycles of Ag-CsA received CsA on days −25, −24, −23, −18, −17, −16, −11, −10, −9 and 3M KCl-extracted donor antigen (5 mg) on days −25, −18 and −11 in relation to BUF kidney transplantation on day 0.

[b] CsA (10 mg/kg/day) was administered perioperatively on days −1, 0, +1.

[c] WFu rats received 500 rads whole-body irradiation one day prior to BUF renal transplantation.

[d] Statistical significance assessed by the Kruskal-Wallis statistic.

tration yielded further prolongation (MST 15.9±7.6 days) compared with the control group, which only received perioperative CsA treatment (MST 12.2±2.4 days, $P < 0.01$). Thus immunosuppressive maneuvers in the peritransplant period augment the unresponsiveness induced by the pretransplant regimen.

DISCUSSION

The present experiments demonstrate that the presence of a transplant is important for the development and/or maturation of suppressor cell elements, and thereby the induction of unresponsiveness by combined Ag-CsA therapy. In contradistinction to the permanent unresponsiveness to donor tissue observed in 40% of hosts treated with three cycles of Ag-CsA in the peri- and immediate posttransplant period, animals given the regimen prior to allografting fail to show dampened resistance.

The presence of suppressor cells was only evident when an enriched population was selectively transferred to virgin animals, or when the pretreated, primary host underwent splenectomy, total-body irradiation, or CsA immunosuppression at the time of transplantation. The status of host resistance in pretreated animals was dissected by systemic adoptive transfer experiments. Previous experiments demonstrated that the peritransplant regimen of Ag-CsA-induced splenic T_s cells capable of adoptively transferring prolonged survival of BUF allografts to virgin, syngeneic WFu hosts (*10*). Adoptive transfer of T_s cells, obtained from animals pretreated with the Ag-CsA regimen in the absence of a graft and enriched by depletion of adherent and MAb W3/25 positive elements, prolonged graft survival, although to a lesser extent than T_s cells that had been obtained ten days after BUF kidney transplantation into a WFu host treated perioperatively with Ag-CsA.

The absence of a transplant during the inductive phase of Ag-CsA immunosuppression inhibited the maturation of splenic T_s cells, which thereby failed to gain dominance over cells favoring rejection. Thus challenge grafts placed 11 days after Ag-CsA pretreatment were not prolonged, suggesting that helper cell activity was stronger than the T_s stimulation. Therefore in an attempt to reduce helper activity, splenectomy, or a three-day perioperative course of CsA administration, or sublethal total-body irradiation was combined with the three-cycle Ag-CsA pretreatment regimen. One or three cycles of Ag-CsA pretreatment combined with splenectomy at the time of kidney transplantation prolonged graft survival time to 19.3 days and 24.3 days, respectively, compared with 8.6 days displayed by the group solely undergoing splenectomy. Splenectomy was performed on the day of transplantation rather than at the inception of the immunosuppressive regimen. Using a vascularized murine heart transplant model to dissect the effect of donor-specific transfusions, Shelby et al. (*17*) previously reported that T_s cell induction depended upon the presence of the spleen. Similar considerations may explain the controversy concerning pretransplant splenectomy for renal allograft recipients; restrospective analyses by some groups suggest a beneficial effect (*18, 19*), while others do not find a difference (*20, 21*). Moreover, some prolongation was obtained with a perioperative three-day course of CsA therapy or sublethal irradiation superimposed upon three cycles of Ag-CsA pretreatment. However this degree of allograft prolongation in the absence of the transplant was clearly inferior to that observed in hosts treated in the peri- and immediate posttransplant period, wherein 40% of animals were permanently unresponsive.

The presence of the allograft may facilitate the differentiation, maturation, and emergence of suppressor cells by two mechanisms: continuous release of antigen, and/or providing a relatively privileged site. Preliminary studies presented herein suggested that intermittent delivery of donor histocompatibility antigen extracted from lymphoid tissue on days −11, −7, −4, −1 tended to encourage the emergence of unresponsiveness. Although the phenomenon was not consistent, 2/8 WFu hosts pretreated with combined CsA and repeated exogenous BUF antigen displayed graft survival prolonged beyond 25 days. It is also possible that the effect of the allograft in prolonging survival is due to a unique aspect of its antigen compared with the extracted material. Whether this is purely due to cell-associated, histocompatibility antigen, as could be presented on irradiated lymphocytes, or to a unique aspect of kidney cell or associated dendritic elements is unclear. The argument that renal transplantation produces a special inductive stimulus for immunosuppression, reinforcing generation of T_s cells, is consistent with the observations of Salaman et al. (*22*) that AS_2

rats reject AS skin grafts unless they are conditioned by a previous successful AS renal transplant. Our previous studies (*12*), which demonstrated antigen-specific suppressor T cells in situ within renal allografts of hosts rendered unresponsive by perioperative administration of the Ag-CsA regimen, suggest that the allograft may provide a special maturation environment either for T_s cells differentiated in another organ, such as the spleen, and homing to the allograft, or for precursor T_s elements migrating directly into the kidney. However, Wood and Monaco (*23*) observed that skin grafts placed before or at, but not after, the time of bone marrow infusion in mice treated with antilymphocyte serum displayed prolonged survival. Since this model appears to be mediated by T_s cells (*24*), as does the Ag-CsA system, these findings suggest that intragraft events may apply to skin as well as to kidney, that continued graft antigen delivery is necessary for the induction of T_s-effected unresponsiveness, or that critical events or mediators of unresponsiveness dissipate early after the administration of the induction regimen. Thus understanding the role of the allograft in promoting the induction and/or maintenance of antigen-specific T_s cells may afford new insights into the establishment of transplantation unresponsiveness in adult animals.

REFERENCES

1. Starzl TE, Klintmalm GBG, Weil R, et al. Cyclosporin A and steroid therapy in 66 cadaver kidney recipients. Surg Gynecol Obstet 1981; 153: 486.
2. Kahan BD, Van Buren C, Flechner S, Payne WD, Boileau M, Kerman R. Cyclosporine immunosuppression mitigates immunological risk factors in renal transplantation. Transplant Proc 1983; 15: 2469.
3. Van Buren CT, Kerman RH, Agostino G, Payne W, Flechner S, Kahan BD. The cellular target of cyclosporin A action in humans. Surgery 1982; 92: 167.
4. Klaus GGB, Kunkl A. Dissociation of T helper cell function and helper cell priming by cyclosporin A. Transplant Proc 1983; 15: 2321.
5. Yoshimura N, Oka T, Ohmori Y, et al. Induction of suppressor T lymphocytes in mice treated with cyclosporine. Transplant Proc 1983; 15: 2334.
6. Orosz CG, Roofenian DC, Widmer MB, Bach FH. Analysis of cloned T cell function. II. Differential blockade of various cloned T cell functions by cyclosporine. Transplantation 1983; 36: 706.
7. Hess AD, Donneberg A, Tutschka PJ. Effect of cyclosporin on human lymphocyte responses in vitro. V. Analysis of responding T-lymphocyte subpopulations in primary MLR with monoclonal antibodies. J Immunol 1983; 130; 717.
8. Kupiec-Weglinski JW, Leak PA, Bordes-Aznar J, Heidecke CD, Strom TB, Tilney NL. Restoring immune responsiveness toward cardiac allografts in cyclosporin-A-treated rats. Transplant Proc 1983; 15: 1917.
9. Yasumura T, Kahan BD. Prolongation of allograft survival by repeated cycle of donor antigen and cyclosporine in rat kidney transplantation. Transplantation 1984; 38: 418.
10. Yoshimura N, Kahan BD. Nature of the suppressor cells mediating prolonged graft survival after administration of extracted histocompatibility antigen and cyclosporine. Transplantation 1985; 39: 162.
11. Yoshimura N, Kahan BD. The immunosuppressive action of suppressor cells from antigen-cyclosporine treated hosts on renal allograft survival. Transplantation 1985; 40: 384.
12. Yoshimura N, Kahan BD. Suppressor cell activity of cells infiltrating rat renal allografts prolonged by perioperative administration on extracted histocompatibility antigen and cyclosporine. Transplantation 1985; 40: 708.
13. Lee S. An improved technique of renal transplantation in the rat. Surgery 1967; 61: 771.
14. Reisfeld RA, Kahan BD. Biological and chemical characterization of human histocompatibility antigens. Fed Proc 1970; 29: 2034.
15. Bradford MM. A rapid and sensitive method for the quantitation of microgram quantities of protein utilizing the principles of protein-dye binding. Anal Biochem 1976; 72: 248.
16. Mason DW, Arthur RP, Dallman MJ, Green JR, Spickett GP, Thomas ML. Function of rat T-lymphocyte subsets isolated by means of monoclonal antibodies. Immunol Rev 1983; 74: 57.
17. Shelby J, Wakely E, Corry RJ. Splenectomy abrogates the improved graft survival achieved by donor-specific transfusion. Transplant Proc 1985; 17: 1083.
18. Stuart FP, Reckard CR, Kettle BL, Schulak JA. Effect of splenectomy on first cadaver kidney transplants. Ann Surg 1980; 192: 553.
19. Sutherland DER, Fryd DS, So SKS, et al. Long-term effect of splenectomy versus no splenectomy in renal transplant patients. Transplantation 1984; 38: 619.
20. Veith FJ, Luck RJ, Murray JE. The effects of splenectomy on immunosuppressive regimens in dog and man. Surg Gynecol Obstet 1965; 121: 1.
21. Opelz G, Terasaki P. Effect of splenectomy on human renal transplants. Transplantation 1973; 15: 605.
22. Salaman JR, Elves MW, Festenstein H. Factors contributing to survival of rats transplanted with kidneys mismatched at major locus. Transplant Proc 1971; 3: 577.
23. Wood ML, Monaco AP. The effect of timing of skin grafts on subsequent survival in ALS-treated, marrow-infused mice. Transplantation 1977; 23: 78.
24. Wood ML, Monaco AP. Suppressor cells in specific unresponsiveness to skin allografts in ALS-treated, marrow-injected mice. Transplantation 1980; 29: 196.

Received 19 December 1985.
Accepted 28 February 1986.

0041-1337/86/4206-0647$02.00/0
TRANSPLANTATION
Vol. 42, No. 6

Printed in U.S.A.

HUMAN CLASS II ANTIGENS

IMPLICATION OF CARBOHYDRATE IN THE DETERMINANTS RECOGNIZED BY SEVERAL ANTIHUMAN CLASS II MONOCLONAL ANTIBODIES[1]

ROSEMARY L. SPARROW, HILARY A. VAUGHAN, AND IAN F. C. MCKENZIE[2]

Research Centre for Cancer and Transplantation, Department of Pathology, University of Melbourne, Parkville, Victoria, 3052 Australia

Several monoclonal antibodies (McAbs) to human class II antigens are described; three of these recognize monomorphic epitopes, and two are polymorphic. The biochemical nature of the reactive epitopes was investigated by determining the binding ability of the McAbs to protease- or glycosidase-treated antigen preparations. Both of the polymorphic McAbs recognized protein-defined epitopes. However, for one of the antibodies F5C9, carbohydrate residues were also implicated. The extent of carbohydrate involvement varied with class II antigens of different DR specificity, suggesting that the proximity of the F5C9 epitope to carbohydrate side chains can vary. One of the three monomorphic McAbs recognized a protein-defined epitope, while the other two antibodies detected epitopes in which carbohydrates were involved. These results indicate that both protein and carbohydrate residues of the human class II antigens can influence the epitopes recognized by murine McAbs. This could explain some of the apparent complexities of the anti-human class II McAbs.

The human class II histocompatibility antigens are a group of heterodimeric glycoproteins encoded by three genetic subregions, HLA-DR, DQ, and DP (*1, 2*). Each subregion codes for multiple α and β chain gene products. It is not yet known however, whether these can all form functional class II antigens. These subregion-encoded class II antigens differ not only biochemically but also in their roles in various class II antigen dependent immune mechanisms (*3–5*) and tissue distribution (*6, 7*).

Much of this current knowledge has resulted from the use of McAbs recognizing a wide array of monomorphic and polymorphic class II epitopes. Although their contribution has been invaluable, conclusions drawn from the reactivity profiles of anti-class II McAbs are not always straightforward. For example, it is not clear whether subregion sharing of monomorphic epitopes occurs, although this is evident for some polymorphic epitopes (*8, 9*). In studies comparing the binding of several monoclonal antibodies (McAbs) to monomorphic class II epitopes, we and others have shown that the molecular populations recognized are not always superimposable (*10–13*). This would suggest that subregion sharing of some monomorphic epitopes does occur, or that some epitopes are not expressed or are inaccessible for antibody binding on subpopulations of class II antigens. Based on recent evidence, it would seem at least the latter situation is true. Shackelford et al. (*14*) have suggested that some McAbs recognize class II molecules at different stages of post-translational modification. Thus, two McAbs may recognize the same precursor molecule but the epitope for one of them may become unavailable following the addition of carbohydrate residues and subsequent conformational changes to the class II polypeptide. Furthermore, Beckman et al. (*15*) have demonstrated that the topographical distribution of some monomorphic epitopes on class II antigens varies with different HLA-DR specificities. Hence, two epitopes on a molecule of a particular DR specificity may be spatially distinct, whereas on a molecule of another DR specificity they may be spatially related.

In an allogeneic situation, it is apparent that polymorphism, and therefore immunogenicity, resides in the polypeptide chain rather than the carbohydrate groups (*16*). However, in a xenogeneic response, such as for the production of murine anti-human class II McAbs, where there are many more immunogeneic sites available, lack of carbohydrate involvement cannot be assumed. Several anti-class II McAbs are described here and the biochemical nature of the epitopes they recognize investigated.

MATERIALS AND METHODS

Anti-class II McAbs. The murine anti-human class II McAbs described herein were generated in three separate cell fusions. The fusion procedure was performed as described elsewhere (*17*) using mouse NS-1 myeloma cells. Details of the antibodies are given in Table 1. The polymorphic anti-class II McAb 26.1 has been described previously (*18*). Antibody-containing culture supernatants were used for all experiments except where indicated.

Cells. Peripheral blood lymphocytes (PBL) were isolated from heparinized whole blood by separation on Ficoll-Paque (Pharmacia, Uppsala, Sweden); B cells were enriched by separation of E-rosette-forming T cells; null cells were isolated by depletion of Ig^+ rosette-forming E^-B cells. PHA-activated cells were generated by incubating 3×10^7 cells/6 ml with 5 μg/ml leukoagglutinin (Pharmacia) in a 25-cm^2 culture flask for 3 days at 37°C in a 10% CO_2 atmosphere. Thymus specimens were obtained at operation and platelets from a pool of 60 platelet packs. Erythrocytes were prepared from whole blood by removal of buffy-coat cells following each of four washes in medium. Leukemic cells were obtained by direct donation from patients. Cultured cell lines were maintained in RPMI-1640 medium supplemented with 10% newborn calf serum (NCS).

Detection of cell-bound antibody. The sheep anti mouse im-

[1]This work was supported by the National Health and Medical Research Council (Australia) and the Anti-Cancer Council of Victoria.
[2] To whom correspondence should be addressed.

Abbreviations used: LCL, lymphoblastoid cell line; McAb, monoclonal antibody; Mr, apparent molecular weight; NCS, newborn calf serum; PBL, peripheral blood lymphocytes; PBS, phosphate-buffered saline; PMSF, phenylmethyl sulphonyl fluoride; SAMG, sheep anti-mouse immunoglobulin G; SDS, sodium dodecyl sulphate; SDS-PAGE, sodium dodecyl sulphate polyacrylamide gel electrophoresis.

TABLE 1. Murine antihuman class II monoclonal antibodies

Name	Immunization	Ig class	Binding[a] pA	Binding[a] C′	Reactivity on cell panel
B5.1	C3H anti-PBL + LCL	G2b	+	+	Monomorphic
1B10.1	Biozzi anti-Bashir LCL	G1	−	−	Monomorphic
3F1.1	Biozzi anti-Bashir LCL	G2a	+	+	Monomorphic
F5C9	CBA anti-B-CLL	G2a	+	+	Polymorphic
26.1[b]	CBA anti-Raji LCL	G2a	+	+	Polymorphic

[a] pA: protein A; C′: complement; +: binding; −: no binding.
[b] Described by Thompson et al. (*18*).

munoglobulin (SAMG)-rosetting assay (*19*) and the complement-dependent microcytotoxicity test (*20*) were used to detect the binding of monoclonal antibodies to target cells. For absorption studies with platelets and erythrocytes, equal volumes of packed cells were incubated with monoclonal antibodies (appropriate dilutions) for 30 min on ice. The supernatants were then collected and reincubated with fresh cells, after which the antibody activities of the supernatants were determined by the SAMG-rosetting assay.

Immunoprecipitation and electrophoretic analysis. LD-B cells, an HLA homozygous B-lymphoblastoid cell line (LCL) (HLA-A3, B7, DR2), were surface-labeled with ^{125}I using lactoperoxidase and solubilized with 0.5% NP-40 in 0.01 M tris, 0.15 M NaCl, 1 mM phenylmethyl sulphonyl fluoride (PMSF), pH 7.5. Aliquots of cell lysate were incubated with antibody for 2 hr on ice and the immune complexes precipitated with formalin-fixed *Staphylococcus aureus*. The immunoprecipitates were boiled in sodium dodecyl sulphate (SDS) buffer containing the reducing reagent dithiothreitol and the supernatants analyzed by SDS-polyacrylamide gel electrophoresis (SDS-PAGE) on a 13% polyacrylamide slab gel (*21*). Low molecular weight standards (Pharmacia) were also included. The gel was subsequently stained for protein, dried, and autoradiographed.

Enzyme treatment of cell lysates and inhibition assays. This procedure was performed as described elsewhere (*22, 23*). Briefly, cell lysates were prepared by solubilizing cells with NP-40 detergent (10^8 cells/ml 0.5% NP-40 in 0.01 M tris, 0.15 M NaCl, 1 mM PMSF, pH 7.5); excess detergent was subsequently removed by incubating with an equal volume of detergent-binding resin beads (Amberlite XAD-8; Rohm and Haas, Melbourne, Australia) for 15–20 min on ice. Aliquots (0.1 ml) of cell lysate were treated with one of the following enzymes: 1. 10 μg pronase (Calbiochem, San Diego, CA) diluted with phosphate-buffered saline (PBS); 2. 10 μg of papain (Sigma, St. Louis, MO) diluted with PBS, pH 6.2 containing 5 mM cysteine (final concentration); 3. 10 μg mixed glycosidases (from *Charonia lampas*) (Seikagaki Kogyu Co., Tokyo, Japan) diluted with 1 mM $Ca/MgCl_2$ in normal saline; 4. 2 U neuraminidase (influenza virus) (Calbiochem), pH 6.2; or 5. PBS as a control. Following a 4-hr incubation at 37°C, enzymatic cleavage was diverted by the addition of 50 μl of NCS. Periodate oxidation of carbohydrate residues was accomplished by incubating equal volumes (0.1 ml) of cell lysate with 0.2 mM potassium periodate in PBS. At this concentration of periodate, oxidation is restricted to the vicinyl hydroxyl groups of carbohydrate residue (*24*). The reaction was performed in the dark for 30 min at room temperature and was quenched by the addition of 50 μl 0.1 M glycerol in PBS. The treated cell lysates were then tested for their ability to compete with target cells for antibody binding in the rosette inhibition assay. In the wells of a 96-well microtiter plate, a constant amount of a predetermined dilution of antibody was incubated with titrations of the cell lysates

TABLE 2. Cell distribution of determinants recognized by anti-class-II monoclonal antibodies[a]

Positive cells	Negative cells
PBL (5–20%)[b]	Granulocytes
PHA-activated PBL (50%)	Null cells
	Thymocytes
	Platelets[c]
	Erythrocytes[c]
B-CLL	T-CLL, T-ALL
B-LCL	
Raji, Daudi, SY-15, LD-B, SM-7, UU, UW	T-LCL -MOLT 4, CEM
Bashir, Brooks, Bordin	Erythroleukemia, K562
	Histiocytic lymphoma, U937
Myeloma, RPMI 1788	

[a] Tested by SAMG-rosetting.
[b] Numbers in parentheses refer to % positive cells.
[c] Tested by absorption.

overnight at 4°C. Residual antibody activity was then determined by the degree of binding to target cells (the same cells used to prepare the cell lysate) in the SAMG-rosetting assay.

Endoglycosidase F treatment. A lysate of ^{125}I-surface-labeled Raji cells was prepared in Triton X-100 detergent, and then equilibrated by dialysis in 0.1 M sodium phosphate buffer, pH 6.1 containing 50 mM EDTA, 1% Tween-20, 1 mM PMSF. Excess Triton X-100 was removed by incubation with Bio-Beads SM2 (Bio-Rad, Richmond, CA). The lysate was then treated with 5 U endo-β-N-acetylglucosaminidase F (endoglycosidase F; New England Nuclear, Boston, MA), or with an equal volume of PBS as an untreated control. Digestion proceeded for 72 hr at 37°C with fresh additions of enzyme at 24 and 48 hr time points, after which the enzyme cleavage was inhibited by the addition of serum. Immunoprecipitation, using McAb ascites fluid, and SDS-PAGE were performed as described above.

RESULTS

Cell specificity. The specificities of the B5.1, 3F1.1, F5C9, and 1B10.1 McAbs were determined by their reactivities with a panel of different cell types (Table 2). Antibody binding was detected by the SAMG-rosetting assay. Each antibody reacted with a minor proportion (5–20%) of PBLs from normal donors. This proportion was increased to approximately 50% following PHA activation of PBLs, which is in agreement with previous findings that activated T cells express class II antigens (*25*). Other positive cell types included PBLs from B cell-CLL patients, B-LCLs and a myeloma cell line, RPMI 1788. Cells of the T lymphocyte lineage (thymocytes, peripheral T cells, leukemic T cells, and T cell lines) were unreactive, as were peripheral granulocytes, null cells, erythrocytes, platelets, the erythroleukemic cell line K562, and the histiocytic lymphoma line U937.

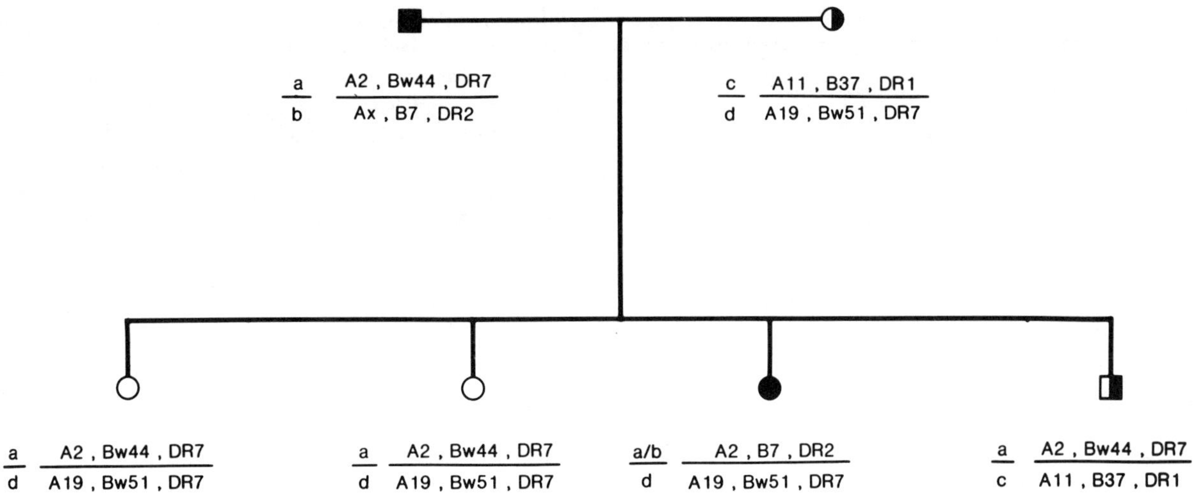

FIGURE 1. Segregation of F5C9 antibody reactivity in an HLA-typed family. Tested by the SAMG-rosetting and cytotoxicity assays using E⁻B cells. Open symbols: F5C9 unreactive; partially closed symbols: F5C9 weak positive (<50% F5C9 binding cells); and closed symbols: F5C9 strong positive (>80% F5C9-binding cells).

Population distribution. Panel testing on E⁻B cells indicated that the B5.1, 3F1.1, and 1B10.1 McAbs recognize invariant or monomorphic epitopes; only the F5C9 McAb displayed polymorphic binding.

Individuals who failed to bind the F5C9 antibody all expressed DR3 or DR7 specificities. This was not completely inclusive, however, as a minor proportion of DR3 or 7-positive individuals did react with the F5C9 antibody. Analysis of a family typed for HLA-A, B, DR showed that the F5C9-epitope segregated with HLA (Fig. 1). Reactivity was assessed on E⁻B cells in both the SAMG-rosetting and the complement-dependent cytotoxicity assays. The paternal *a* haplotype and the maternal *d* haplotype (both of which code for the HLA-DR7 specificity) did not code for the F5C9 reactivity; the maternal *c* haplotype (HLA-DR1) corresponded to weak reactivity (<50% of B cells bound F5C9 McAb), while strong reactivity (>80% of cells F5C9+ve) was associated with the paternal *b* haplotype (HLA-DR2). These reactivities segregated as expected in the offspring, demonstrating that the expression of the F5C9-epitope is linked to the HLA gene complex.

Additional information regarding these antibodies was gained from extensive workshop analysis. The B5.1, 26.1 and F5C9 McAbs were tested in the Second Asia-Oceanic Histocompatibility Workshop 1981, involving over 2000 individual typings. The results indicated, as expected, that the B5.1 McAb recognized a monomorphic determinant expressed by 100% of the population, while the 26.1 and F5C9 McAbs gave polymorphic reactions, with 30% and 85% of the populations being positive, respectively (*26*). Comprehensive analysis by serology, two-dimensional gels, and functional assays verified that the B5.1 and 3F1.1 McAbs each recognize monomorphic determinants on HLA-DR antigens, while the 26.1 recognizes a polymorphic HLA-DR determinant. The F5C9 McAb, however, recognizes a determinant on HLA-DQ antigens (personal communication, M. Steel, Coordinator, First International Workshop on Monoclonal Antibodies to Human MHC Class II Antigens, 1983).

Molecular identity. SDS-PAGE analysis of B5.1, F5C9, and 3F1.1 immunoprecipitates revealed bands of Mr 29K and 34K, characteristic of the class II antigens (Fig. 2). An additional band of 44K was also noted; this is thought to be actin, which

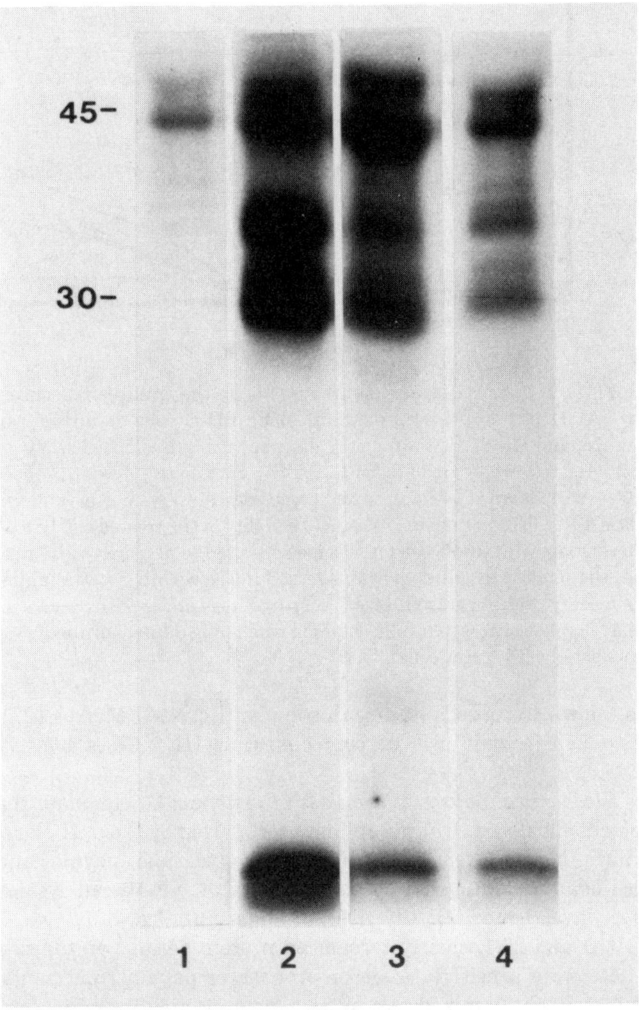

FIGURE 2. SDS-PAGE analysis under reducing conditions of immunoprecipitates obtained by incubating culture medium (lane 1), B5.1 (lane 2), F5C9 (lane 3), and 3F.1. (lane 4) with NP-40 lysates of ^{125}I-LD-B cells. The band at the bottom of the gel represents material running at the dye-front. Positions of molecular weight standards are indicated.

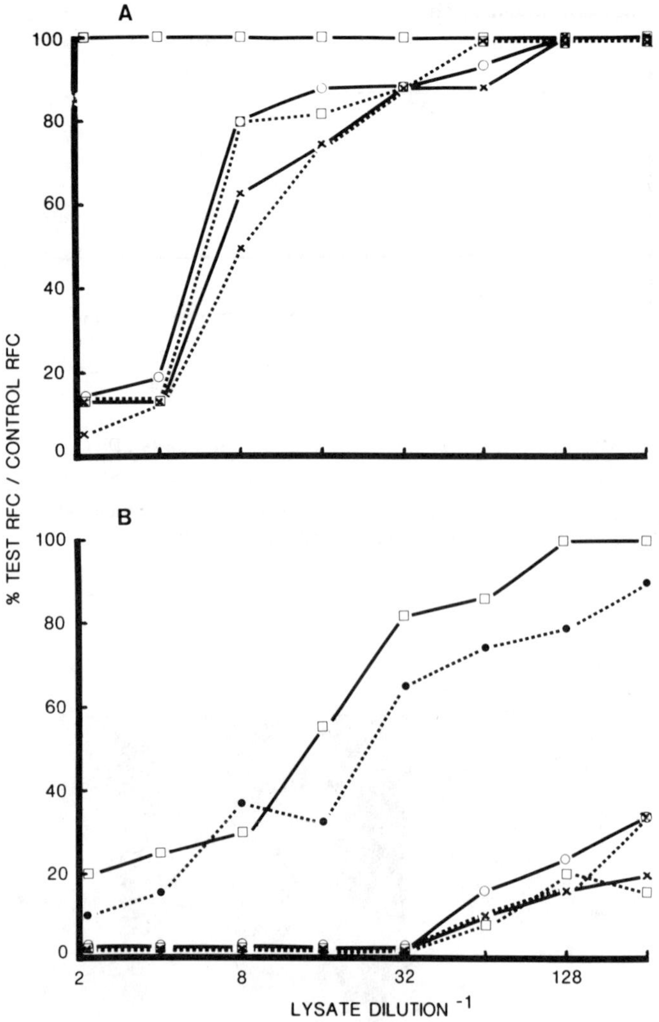

FIGURE 3. Effect of enzyme treatments on the epitopes recognized by (A) 1B10.1 McAb (1:8 dilution) using LD-B cells as an antigen source, and (B) 26.1 McAb (1:100 dilution) using Bashir cells. NP-40 cell lysates were treated with: PBS control (×——×); pronase (●----●); papain (□——□); mixed glycosidases (○——○); neuraminidase (□---□); or periodate (×---×). The ability of the treated cell lysates to compete with whole cells (the same cells used to prepare the lysates) for the binding of antibody was assessed in the SAMG-rosette inhibition assay. Results are expressed as a percentage of the positive control (i.e., number of rosetted cells obtained when only diluted antibody was incubated with target cells).

is known to coprecipitate with some anti-class-II McAbs (*27*), although it could also be coprecipitating HLA Class I heavy chain.

Biochemical nature of the class II epitopes. To elucidate the biochemical nature of the epitopes recognized by the anti-class-II McAbs, the effect of proteolytic and glycosidic enzymes and periodate oxidation on the antigenicity of NP-40 cell lysates was investigated. Of the five antibodies studied, only two, 1 BIO.1 and 26.1, clearly recognized protein-defined epitopes—these were sensitive to either pronase or papain treatments, but resistant to mixed glycosidases, neuraminidase, and periodate oxidation (Fig. 3). These results have been confirmed using lysates prepared from at least one other cell line (data not shown).

The epitopes recognized by two other antibodies, B5.1 and 3F1.1 (both monomorphic McAbs), appeared to involve carbohydrate residues (Fig. 4). The B5.1 epitope was sensitive to carbohydrate-specific cleavage by mixed glycosidases, neuraminidase, and periodate, whereas the 3F1.1 epitope was sensitive predominantly to neuraminidase treatment. Similar results were obtained using lysates of two other cell lines (data not shown). It was also noted that protease treatment increased the inhibitory capacity of the cell lysates for these two antibodies—a finding that supports the involvement of carbohydrate within the epitopes, as it is thought that proteolytic cleavage exposes additional carbohydrate antigenic sites (*28*).

Treatment of a radiolabeled cell lysate with endoglycosidase F followed by immunoprecipitation and analysis by SDS-PAGE confirmed these results (Fig. 5). The B5.1 McAb failed to precipitate any bands from the endoglycosidase-treated cell lysate (lane D). In contrast, the 26.1 McAb precipitated two bands (lane B), although it was evident that the endoclycosidase F-treatment had favored cleavage of the α chain.

The results obtained using the polymorphic F5C9 antibody indicated that both protein and carbohydrate groups formed the F5C9 epitope. However, the degree of involvement of carbohydrate varied with different sources of cell lysates. When LD-B cells (homozygous DR 2) were used as a source of antigen the F5C9-epitope was clearly protein-defined, being sensitive

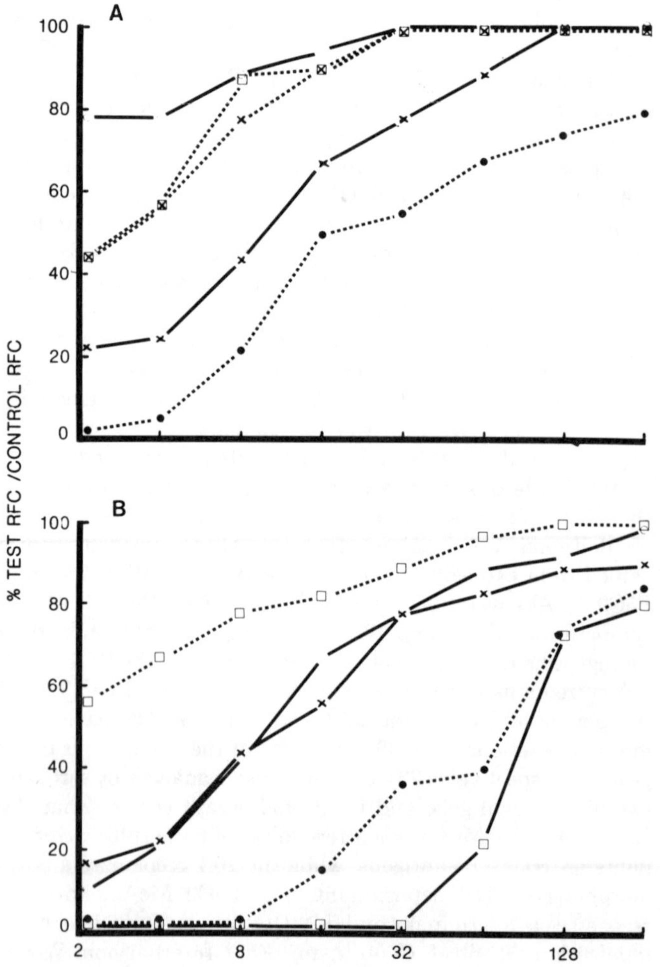

FIGURE 4. Effect of enzyme treatments on the epitopes recognized by (A) B5.1 McAb (1:50 dilution) using Raji cells as an antigen source, and (B) 3F1.1. McAb (1:50 dilution) using LD-B cells. (See legend to Figure 3 for further explanation.)

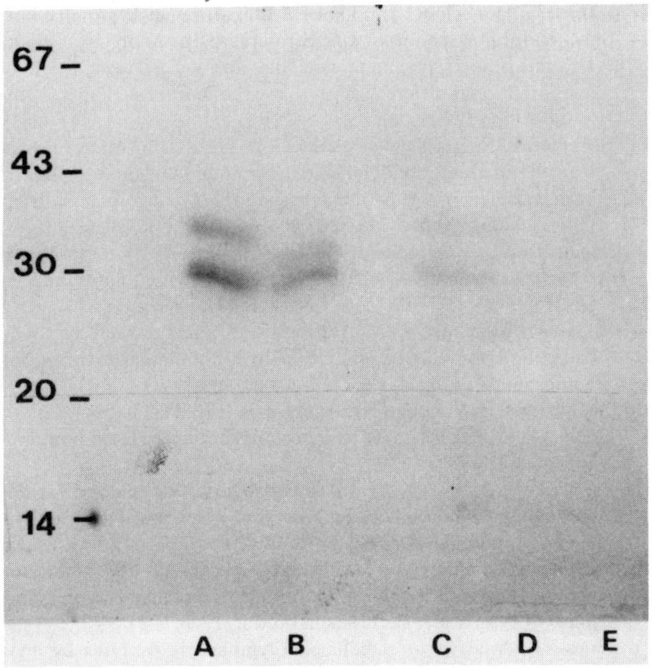

FIGURE 5. Effect of endoglycosidase F treatment of a ^{125}I-Raji cell lysate on the ability of the 26.1 and B5.1 McAbs to precipitate their reactive antigens, analyzed by SDS-PAGE on a 13% polyacrylamide gel under reducing conditions. Lane A: 26.1 and untreated lysate; Lane B: 26.1 and endoglycosidase F-treated lysate; Lane C: B5.1 and untreated lysate; Lane D: B5.1 and endoglycosidase F-treated lysate. Lane E: mouse ascites fluid control. Positions of molecular weight standards are indicated.

to pronase and papain treatments, but resistant to cleavage by mixed glycosidases or neuraminidase (Fig. 6A). Sensitivity of the F5C9-epitope to all enzyme treatments (proteolytic and glycosidic) when either Raji (DR 3/6) or Bashir cells (DR 5) were used suggested involvement of both protein and carbohydrate groups (Fig. 6B and 6C, respectively).

DISCUSSION

The four McAbs—B5.1, 3F1.1, 1B10.1, and F5C9-described in this paper recognize epitopes expressed on human class II antigens. This is evidenced by the restricted cell distribution of the epitopes, and immunochemical analysis of immunoprecipitates obtained with the McAbs. Three of the McAbs—B5.1, 3F1.1, and 1B10.1—recognize monomorphic epitopes, while the F5C9 McAb is polymorphic, recognizing an epitope expressed on HLA-DQ antigens. This latter antibody appears similar to two previously described anti-HLA-DQ McAbs (*29–31*).

We have investigated the molecular nature of the epitopes recognized by our group of anti-class II McAbs with the view to determine the involvement, if any, of the carbohydrate side chains. The two polymorphic anti-class II McAbs—F5C9 and 26.1 (*18*)—recognize protein-defined epitopes. This is consistent with previous findings that class II antigen polymorphism is attributed to variations in amino acid sequence rather than carbohydrate (*16*). The results for the F5C9 antibody were of particular interest, however. For some antigen specificities at least some carbohydrate involvement was indicated, whereas for other specificities there was none. Thus it would appear that the proximity of the protein-defined F5C9-epitope to carbohydrate side chains varies with class II antigens of different specificity. Heterogeneity in the topographical distribution of class II antigen epitopes in relation to different polymorphic specificities has recently been demonstrated by Beckman et al. (*15*).

Of significance was the finding that treatment of an antigen pool with glycosidic enzymes reduced the binding ability of two monomorphic anti-class II McAbs, B5.1 and 3F1.1. This was demonstrated both by the lysate-inhibition assay and by immunoprecipitation following endoglycosidase F treatment of the antigen pool. These results suggest that carbohydrate residues, either specifically or in combination with protein sequences, form the reactive epitopes. Alternatively, gylcosidic cleavage may induce considerable conformational changes such that protein-defined epitopes can no longer be recognized by the McAbs.

In a previous study we demonstrated that the 3F1.1 McAb recognizes a subpopulation of the molecules precipitated by the B5.1 McAb (*13*). Thus, it would seem that different monomorphic epitopes are recognized by these two antibodies—

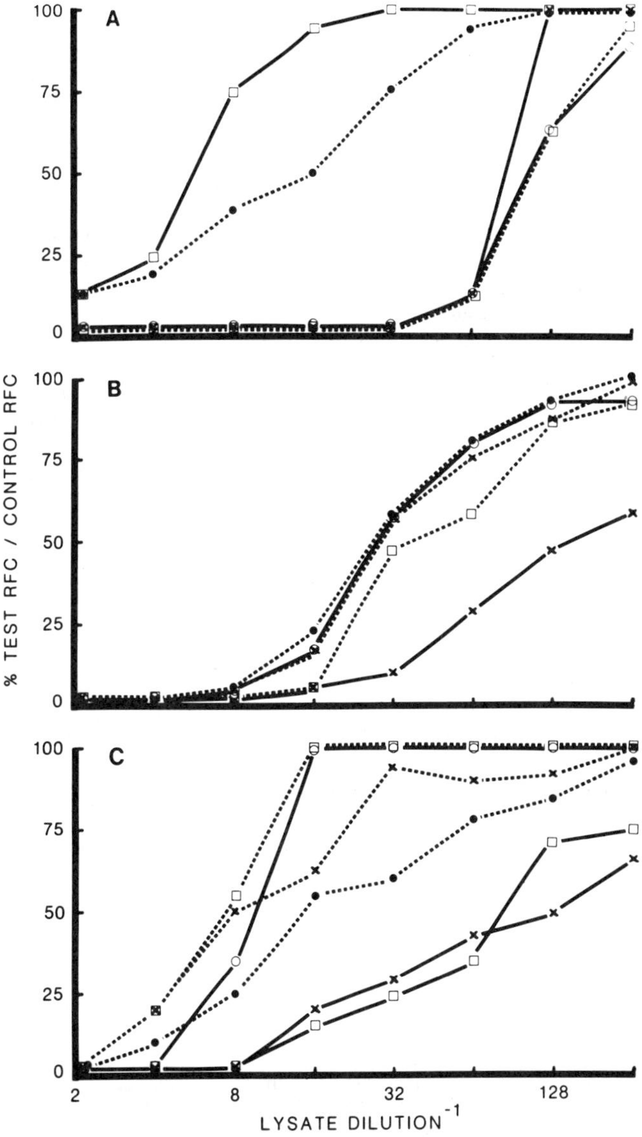

FIGURE 6. Effect of enzyme treatments on the epitopes recognized by the F5C9 McAb (1:80 dilution) when (A) LD-B cells, (B) Raji cells, and (C) Bashir cells were used as sources of antigen. (See legend to Figure 3 for further explanation.)

although, as shown here, both epitopes involved carbohydrate residues. Shackelford et al. (*14*) have suggested that some anti-class II McAbs distinguish antigens at various stages of post-translational modification. It is conceivable that such a relationship exists between the antigens recognized by the B5.1 and 3F1.1 McAbs.

A third monomorphic McAb 1 B10.1, described in this paper, recognized a protein-defined epitope. It is clear that both protein and carbohydrate, either separately or in combination, can form the epitopes defined by anti-class-II McAbs. Thus some of the apparent complexities of the class II antigens that have become evident since the use of McAbs, may well be explained by the molecular nature of the epitopes recognized. At this time the nature of the carbohydrate involved in the "carbohydrate defined" epitopes is not clear; neither is the functional significance, if any, of the difference between the two types of epitopes.

Acknowledgments. We thank Janet Cameron and Mimi Morgan for typing the manuscript.

REFERENCES

1. Kaufman JF, Auffray C, Korman AJ, Shackelford DA, Strominger JL. The class II molecules of the human and murine histocompatibility complex. Cell 1984; 36: 1.
2. Bodmer WF, Albert E, Bodmer JG, et al. Nomenclature for factors of the HLA system 1984. Immunogenetics 1984; 20: 593.
3. Corte G, Moretta A, Cosulich ME, Ramarli D, Bargellesi A. A monoclonal anti-DC1 antibody selectively inhibits the generation of effector T cells mediating specific cytolytic activity. J Exp Med 1982; 156: 1539.
4. Eckels DD, Lake P, Lamb JR, et al. SB-restricted presentation of influenza and herpes simplex virus to human T-lymphocyte clones. Nature 1983; 301: 716.
5. Navarrete C, Jaraquemada D, Fainboim L, et al. Genetic and functional relationship of the HLA-DR and HLA-DQ antigens. Immunogenetics 1985; 21: 97.
6. Natali PG, Segatto O, Ferrone S, Tosi R, Corte G. Differential tissue distribution and ontogeny of DC-1 and HLA-DR antigens. Immunogenetics 1984; 19: 109.
7. Neppert J, Nunez G, Stastny P. HLA-A, B, C, -DR, -MT, -MB and SB antigens on unstimulated human endothelial cells. Tissue Antigens 1984; 24: 40.
8. Hurley CK, Shaw S, Nadler L, Schlossman S, Capra JD. Alpha and beta chains on SB and DR antigens are structurally distinct. J Exp Med 1982; 156: 1557.
9. Karr RW, Kannapell CC, Zangara RJ, Goyert SM, Silver J, Schwartz BD. An HLA-DR5 homozygous cell line expresses two DS (I-A like) molecules. J Exp Med 1983; 158: 1374.
10. Lampson LA, Levy R. Two populations of Ia-like molecules on a human B cell line. J Immunol 1980; 125: 293.
11. Quaranta V, Pellegrino MA, Ferrone S. Serological and immunochemical characterization of the specificity of four monoclonal antibodies to distinct antigenic determinants expressed on subpopulations of human Ia-like antigens. J Immunol 1981; 126: 548.
12. Addis JBL, Tisch R, Falk JA, Letarte M. The analysis with monoclonal antibodies of the heterogeneity of Ia glycoproteins on chronic lymphocyte leukemia cells. J Immunol 1982; 129: 2033.
13. Sparrow RL, McKenzie IFC. Human 'Ia' antigen populations defined by monoclonal antibodies. J Immunogenet 1983; 10: 179.
14. Shackelford DA, Lampson LA, Strominger JL. Analysis of HLA-DR antigens by using monoclonal antibodies: recognition of conformational differences in biosynthetic intermediates. J Immunol 1981; 127: 1403.
15. Beckman IGR, Bradley J, Brooks D, Zola H. Delineation of serologically distinct monomorphic determinants of human class II antigens: evidence of heterogeneity in their topographical distribution. Mol Immunol 1984; 21: 205.
16. Shackelford DA, Strominger JL. Demonstration of structural polymorphism among HLA-DR light chains by two-dimensional gel electrophoresis. J Exp Med 1980; 151: 144.
17. Hogarth PM, Craig J, McKenzie IFC. A monoclonal antibody detecting the Ly-9.2 (Lgp 100) cell-membrane alloantigen. Immunogenetics 1980; 11: 65.
18. Thompson CH, Vaughan HA, McKenzie IFC. The definition of an MB related specificity by a monoclonal antibody. Hum Immunol 1983; 6: 133.
19. Parish CR, McKenzie IFC. A sensitive rosetting method for detecting subpopulations of lymphocytes which react with alloantisera. J Immunol Methods 1978; 20: 173.
20. Mittal KK, Mickey ME, Singal DP, Terasaki PI. Serotyping for homotransplantation. XXVIII. Refinement of microdroplet lymphocyte cytotoxic test. Transplantation 1968; 6: 913.
21. Jones PP. Analysis of radiolabeled lymphocyte proteins by one- and two-dimensional polyacrylamide gel electrophoresis. In: Mishell BB, Shiigi SM, eds. Selected methods in cellular immunology. San Francisco: WH Freeman, 1980: 398.
22. Sandrin MS, McKenzie IFC, Higgins TJ, Parish CR. Isolation and characterization of low molecular weight Ia antigens from normal human serum. Mol Immunol 1981; 18: 513.
23. Sparrow RL, McKenzie IFC. Hu Ly-m5: a unique antigen physically associated with HLA molecules. Hum Immunol 1983; 7: 1.
24. Marshall RD, Neuberger A. Structural analysis of the carbohydrate groups of glycoproteins. In: Gottschalk A, ed. Glycoproteins. Their composition, structure and function. Amsterdam: Elsevier, 1972: 322.
25. Reinherz EL, Kung PC, Pesando JM, Ritz J, Goldstein G, Schlossman SF. Ia determinants on human T-cell subsets defined by monoclonal antibody. Activation stimuli required for expression. J Exp Med 1979; 150: 1472.
26. Simons MJ, Tait BD. Proceedings of the Second Asia-oceania Histocompatibility Workshop Conference. Melbourne: Immunopublishing, 1983.
27. Allore RJ, Barber BH. Inter- and intra- molecular disulphide bonding among lymphocyte plasma membrane proteins and glycoproteins. Mol Immunol 1983; 20: 383.
28. Parish CR, Higgins TJ, McKenzie IFC. Carbohydrate Ia antigens in mouse and man. In: Ferrone S, David CS, Eds. Ia antigens. Vol I. Mice. Boca Raton: CRC Press, 1982: 143.
29. Marti GE, Kuo M-C, Shaw S, et al. A novel HLA-D/DR like antigen specific for human B lymphoid cells. Biochemical evidence for similarity to but non-identity with known HLA-D/DR antigens. J Exp Med 1983; 158: 1924.
30. Li X-M, Sogn JA, Coligan JE, et al. Specificity of the HLA class II reactive monoclonal antibody 33.1. Immunogenetics 1984; 20: 465
31. Chen Y-X, Evans RL, Pollack MS, et al. Characterization and expression of the HLA-DC antigens defined by anti-Leu 10. Hum Immunol 1984; 10: 221.

Received 10 December 1985.
Accepted 20 February 1986.

0041-1337/86/4206-0653$02.00/0
TRANSPLANTATION
Copyright © 1986 by The Williams & Wilkins Co.

Vol. 42, No. 6
Printed in U.S.A.

ULTRAVIOLET IRRADIATION OF CANINE DENDRITIC CELLS PREVENTS MITOGEN-INDUCED CLUSTER FORMATION AND LYMPHOCYTE PROLIFERATION[1]

JOSEPH APRILE[2], AND H. JOACHIM DEEG

The Fred Hutchinson Cancer Research Center, Division of Oncology; and the Department of Medicine, University of Washington School of Medicine, Seattle Washington 98104

The objectives of this study were to characterize canine peripheral blood dendritic cells (DC), to compare their functional role in lectin (Con-A) induced and oxidative ($NaIO_4$-induced) mitogenesis, and to investigate the effect of ultraviolet (UV) irradiation on DC function. We used, sequentially, Ficoll-Hypaque fractionation, discontinuous percoll gradients, rosette, sedimentation with human red blood cells, adherence to plastic and cytofluorometric sorting after labeling with an anti-Ia monoclonal antibody (7.2) to obtain cells of low buoyant density that were rosette-negative, plastic-nonadherent, Ia-positive, nonspecific-esterase-negative, and nonphagocytic. By transmission and scanning electron microscopy these cells had large irregular nuclei, numerous spherical mitochondria, elongated cytoplasmatic processes, and lacked phagosomes. These features clearly separate these cells from canine monocytes and characterize them as DC. These cells were capable of reconstituting the proliferative responses of accessory-cell-depleted autologous lymphocytes to both Con-A and $NaIO_4$. The responses to both mitogens showed a similar time course: an initial cluster formation of lymphocytes with DC was followed by lymphocyte blastogenesis (48–72 hr) and proliferation (72–96 hr). UV irradiation of DC before culture completely abrogated accessory activity for the response to both Con-A and $NaIO_4$, and neither cluster formation nor blast transformation or proliferation occurred. These data provide evidence that a UV-sensitive step of direct interaction of lymphocytes and DC is involved in the mechanism of T cell activation and proliferation.

Purified monocytes at various concentrations fail to function as accessory cells in the proliferative response of lymphocytes to Con-A in several species including the dog (*1*, *2*). On the other hand macrophage-depleted T cells from rat mesenteric lymph nodes proliferate in response to Con-A, especially at high cell density (*3*). Based mostly on work in rodents, it is clear that other low-density large mononuclear cells, first described by Steinman and Cohn (*4*) and termed *dendritic cells* (DC)* play a pivotal role in the process of antigen presentation and T cell activation (*5–9*). In the mouse and rat, loosely adherent low-buoyant-density Ia-positive DC provide accessory function in oxidative mitogenesis of T cells obtained from either lymph nodes or spleen (*10*, *11*). In the murine system these interactions involve the direct contact of DC with lymphocytes, which can be observed in the form of cell clusters (*8*, *12*).

In agreement with those studies, we observed in the dog that the most potent accessory function for T lymphocyte proliferation in response to Con-A resided in a low-buoyant-density fraction of plastic nonadherent, nonphagocytic, nonspecific esterase (NSE) negative cells with the morphological features of DC (*1*). In the present study we show that canine peripheral blood DC function as accessory cells both for lectin (Con-A)-induced, and oxidative ($NaIO_4$-induced) mitogenesis. Our data suggest that the mechanisms involved are similar. In both instances blast transformation and proliferation are preceded by cluster formation. Cluster formation is abrogated if DC are UV-exposed (*13*, *14*) before being assayed in add-back experiments to accessory-cell-depleted lymphocytes, and neither blast transformation nor proliferation occurs.

MATERIALS AND METHODS

Cells and Reagents

Canine cells. Heparinized whole blood was obtained by venipuncture from normal dogs, and peripheral blood mononuclear cells (PBMC) were separated on Ficoll-Hypaque discontinuous density gradients (1.074) as described (*15*).

Human red blood cells (HRBC). Heparinized whole blood obtained from healthy donors was separated over lymphocyte separation medium (LSM) (Litton Bionetics, Kensington, MD). The red cell pellet was washed three times with phosphate-buffered saline (PBS), and a 1:100 dilution (v/v) was made with PBS.

Preparation of Percoll. Percoll (Pharmacia, Uppsala, Sweden) was prepared as described (*1*) and concentrations of 64%, 56%, 54.3%, 52.7%, 51.1%, and 49.6% Percoll relative to the stock solution were used for gradients.

Nylon wool. Nylon wool columns were prepared as described (*16*). Briefly, nylon wool was soaked in normal saline, rinsed and soaked in distilled water, dried, packed in the barrel of a 10-ml sterile syringe and equilibrated with Hank's balanced salt solution (HBSS) with 10% (v/v) fetal calf serum (FCS) at 37°C in a humidified, 5% CO_2/air atmosphere for 1 hr prior to the addition of cells (*17*).

Monoclonal antibodies. Monoclonal antibody 7.2 (IgG2b) was a gift from Drs. J. Hansen and P. Martin. This antibody is specific for Ia-like antigens (DR and DQ) on human cells (*18*)

[1] This work was supported in part by PHS Grants HL 33859, CA 31787, CA 18221, and HL 36444 (formerly CA 30924), awarded by the National Cancer Institute and the National Heart, Lung, and Blood Institute, DHHS, and by contract DNA 001-83-C-0294, Defense Nuclear Agency.

[2] Address reprint requests to: Joseph Aprile, Fred Hutchinson Cancer Research Center, 1124 Columbia Street, Seattle, WA 98104.

* Abbreviations used 2-ME, 2-mercaptoethanol; Con-A, concanavalin-A; DC, dendritic cells; EM, electron microscopy; FCS, fetal calf serum; HBSS, Hank's balanced salt solution; HRBC, Human red blood cells; $HRFC^-$, cells not forming rosettes with HRBC; MLR, mixed leukocyte reaction; NDS, normal dog serum; NSE, nonspecific esterase; PBMC, peripheral blood mononuclear cells; PBS, phosphate-buffered saline.

and crossreactive with antigens of the same molecular size on canine cells (*19*).

Enrichment and Depletion of Cell Populations

Dendritic Cells (DC). Fractionation of cells on discontinuous Percoll gradients was carried out as described (*1*). Briefly, cells were suspended in 10.5 ml of the 64% Percoll solution, in a conical plastic centrifuge tube (Corning; Corning, NY), and 7 ml of the 56% Percoll solution followed by all subsequent concentrations and 3.5 ml PBS (Ca^{++} and Mg^{++}-free) were layered on top. This gradient was centrifuged at 800 g for 30 min at room temperature. The rotor was accelerated manually to speed, and following centrifugation was allowed to coast to a stop. Aliquots of 7 ml were removed stepwise, and labeled "fraction 1" through "fraction 7" accordingly. Fractions 1 and 2 were pooled and are referred to as the *low-buoyant-density fraction* F(1,2); fractions 5 through 7 were pooled and are referred to as the *lymphocyte-rich fraction* F(5–7).

Rosette fractionation with HRBCs. This method has been described previously (*17*). Briefly, cells from fraction F(1,2) were adjusted to 5×10^6 cells/ml, an equal volume of HRBCs (diluted 1:100 v/v) was added, and the mixture centrifuged at 200 g for 5 min at room temperature. The pellet was resuspended using a wide-bore Pasteur pipette to avoid disruption of rosetted cells. For use in further studies, these cells were layered over LSM in 15-ml plastic conical centrifuge tubes (Corning), and centrifuged at 390 g for 20 min at room temperature (*17*). Interface cells were collected, washed twice with medium, and designated as nonrosetting cells. For further purification nonrosetting cells were suspended in Waymouth's minimal medium containing 10% FCS (V/V) and incubated on plastic dishes (Falcon No. 3003, Oxnard, CA) overnight at 37°C, in a 5% CO_2/air atmosphere.

Cell sorting. F(1, 2) nonrosetting plastic nonadherent cells were incubated with antibody 7.2, for 30 min at 4°C, washed twice, and resuspended in PBS containing 1% (w/v) bovine serum albumin (BSA). These cells were subsequently sorted for 7.2 $(Ia)^+$ large cells on a fluorescence-activated cell sorter (FACS 440, Becton Dickinson) as previously described (*20*).

Accessory-cell-depleted lymphocytes. From 50 to 150 $\times10^6$ F(5–7) lymphocytes were suspended in 0.5 ml of HBSS containing 10% FCS (v/v) and passaged over a nylon wool column as described above. Nonadherent cells, termed F(5–7) NWNA, were collected.

UV irradiation. Cells suspended in Waymouth's medium in open plastic dishes (Falcon No. 3003, Oxnard, Ca), and placed on a shaker platform were exposed to a low-pressure mercury UV lamp with about 85% of radiant emission at 254 nm for a total of $10 mJ/cm^2$, as determined with a Black Ray electronic shortwave UV meter (Model J225, U.V. products) calibrated for measurement of shortwave radiant incidence from low-pressure mercury arc sources. Cells were then quantitatively removed from the plastic dishes, washed twice with Waymouth's medium, and resuspended at a concentration of 1.0×10^6 PBMC/ml in Waymouth's minimal medium containing 20% (v/v) heat-inactivated normal dog serum (NDS).

Gamma irradiation. When appropriate, cells were irradiated with a ^{137}Cs source (1380) rads before being used in in vitro assays as described previously (*1*).

Characterization of Cells

Cytochemical stains. Cell types by morphology were determined using Wright-stained cytocentrifuge preparations. Monocytes were further characterized by the presence of NSE activity. Viability was determined by trypan-blue exclusion and by acridine orange as a vital stain according to the method of Melamed et al. by (*21*).

Phagocytosis. For this study, 5×10^6 cells were suspended in 0.95 μl complete medium and 5 μl of a 5% solution of Latex beads (1.1-μ) (Sigma, St. Louis, MO), incubated for 1 hr at 37°C in a humidified 5% CO_2/air atmosphere, and excess beads were removed by a FCS gradient. Cells were Wright-stained, and examined for ingested beads.

Scanning electronmicroscopy (EM). Cells in suspension were fixed for 30 min in 0.1M cacodylate buffer containing 2.5% glutaraldehyde, washed in 0.1M cacodylate buffer (pH 7.4), spun onto polylysine-coated 18-mm circular coverslips, reintroduced to glutaraldehyde, dehydrated in graded alcohols (10, 20, 50, and 70%), subjected to critical drying, and coated with gold. Specimens were scanned with a Cambridge Stereoscan Mark II-A at a tilt of 25°.

Functional Assays

Lectin stimulation. Mitogen cultures were carried out as described (*15*). PBMC (1×10^5) were plated in triplicate in round-bottomed wells (No. B799, Costar, Cambridge, MA), and Con-A was added at the optimal concentration of 20 μg/ml. Cultures were incubated at 37°C in a humidified 5% CO_2/air atmosphere. After 72 hr, 1 μCi of ^3H-thymidine with a specific activity of 2.0 Ci/mmol (Amersham, Arlington Heights, IL) was added to each well, and cells were harvested 18–24 hr later. ^3H-activity was counted in a liquid scintillation counter (Beckman, Fullerton, CA). Results are expressed in cpm.

Oxidative mitogenesis. Cells were suspended at a concentration of 5×10^6 PBMC/ml in PBS containing 5 mM $NaIO_4$ (Sigma, St. Louis, MO), incubated for 15 min at 4°C, washed twice with Waymouth's minimal media, and resuspended at 1.0×10^6 PBMC/ml in Waymouth's media containing 20% NDS (v/v) and 1×10^{-5}M 2-mercaptoethanol (2-ME). Aliquots of 100 μl of each population were plated in triplicate. Cultures, ^3H labeling, harvesting, and counting were carried out as for Con-A, except that the culture period was 96 hr.

Cellular proliferation assay. $NaIO_4$-treated cells or cells to which Con-A was added, were placed in 1.0 ml aliquots in 24-well dishes (Corning No.25820, Corning, NY) at a concentration of 1.0×10^6 PBMC/ml. At 24, 48, 72, and 96 hr, respectively, the contents of different wells were removed, washed, and resuspended. Aliquots were removed for cell counts and viability, and 3×10^5 cells were cytospun and stained as described. On the cytospun preparations, clusters, lymphoblasts, and cells in mitotic phase were enumerated for each cell population.

Add-back experiments. In addition, we studied the effect of add-back of putative accessory cells (normal, UV- or gamma-irradiated) on accessory-cell-depleted lymphocytes (see above). For this purpose 5×10^3 DC-enriched cells were added to 10^5 lymphocytes for Con-A and $NaIO_4$ stimulation, and 5×10^4 DC-enriched cells were added to 10^6 lymphocytes for cellular proliferation assays. Assay conditions were as described above.

RESULTS

Characteristics of DC

Purification of DC. The scheme for purification of DC is illustrated in Figure 1 and results are summarized in Table 1. The frequency of DC in peripheral blood was always less than 1%. The Percoll low-buoyant-density fraction F(1,2) was en-

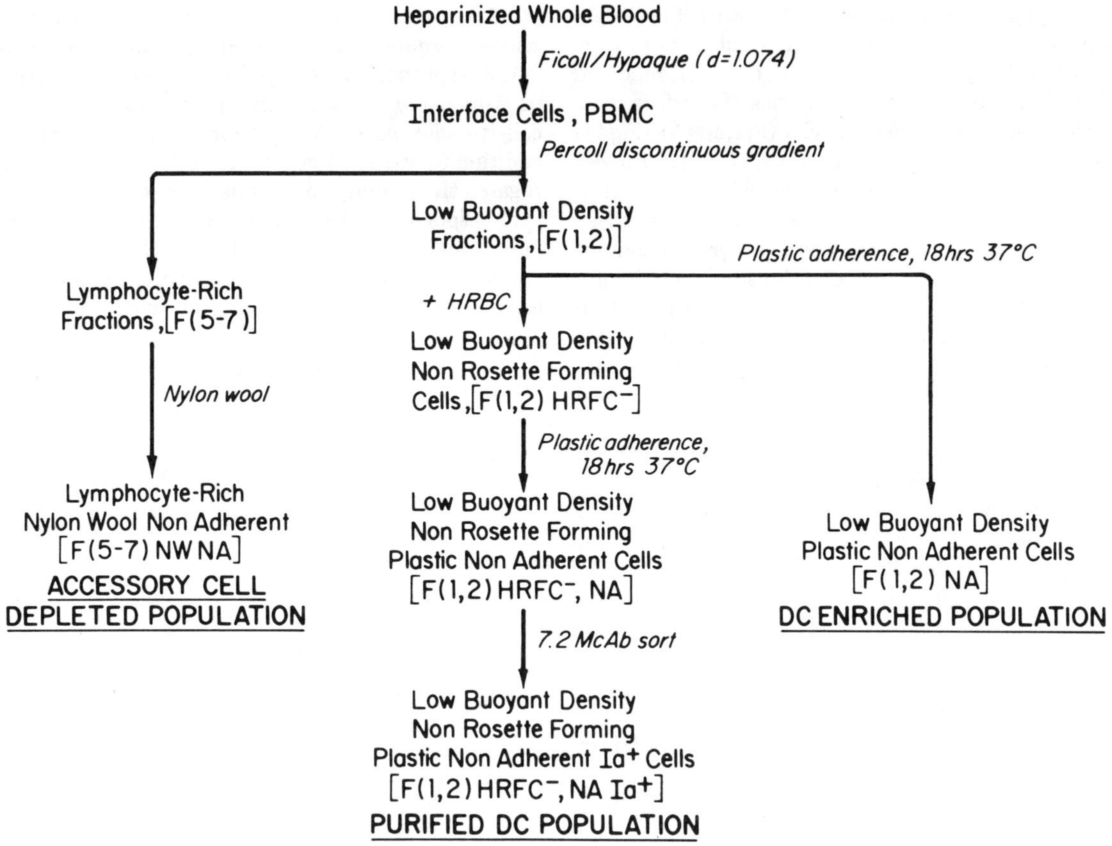

FIGURE 1. Scheme for the preparation of purified DC, enriched DC, and accessory-cell-depleted lymphocyte populations.

TABLE 1. Purification of canine peripheral blood dendritic cells[a]

Purification step	Number of cells ($\times10^6$)	Viability (%)	Differential count (%)			DC[b]	Total Cells (%)[d]	DC[e] Yield (%)
			Granulocytes	Lymphocytes	Monocytes			
1. Unfractionated cells: PBMC	96.5±23.0	97±2	16±6	76±6	7±1	<1	100	100
2. Percoll discontinuous gradient: low buoyant density fraction (F[1,2])	11.6±2.1	96±2	16±8	42±3	35±4	7±2	12.0±2.2	84.1±14.1
3. Rosetting with HRBC: low buoyant density nonrosetting cells (F[1,2] nonrosetting)	3.5±1.3	95±3	2±5	81±9	6±3	11±2	3.6±1.2	39.9±7.3
4. Plastic adherence: low buoyant density nonrosetting plastic nonadherent cells (F[1,2] nonrosetting, NA)	1.0±0.6	93±4	8±3	58±4	0	34±5	1.0±0.7	35.2±5.2
5. McAb[c] 7.2$^+$ sort: low buoyant density nonrosetting plastic nonadherent Ia$^+$ cells (F[1,2] nonrosetting, NA Ia$^+$)	0.3±0.02	89±2	ND[f]	ND	ND	92±5	0.3±0.1	28.6±1.6

[a] Shown is the mean (± 1 SD) of 8 experiments.
[b] DC were enumerated based on their unique morphological properties under phase-contrast microscopy and confirmed by electronmicroscopy.
[c] McAb: monoclonal antibody.
[d] % starting population.
[e] Yield of DC based upon a frequency of 1% in the unfractionated population.
[f] ND: not done.

riched for both DC (7±2%, mean±1 SD) and monocytes (35±4%). Rosette sedimentation with HRBC and plastic adherence of nonrosetting cells effectively removed monocytes and enriched DC to 34±5%. Further enrichment of DC (92±5%) was achieved by sorting for 7.2 (Ia)-positive cells. These DC-enriched populations reconstituted responsiveness of accessory-cell-depleted lymphocytes to Con-A in a dose-dependent fashion, as shown in detail below.

Scanning electron microscopy of purified low-buoyant-density nonrosetting plastic-nonadherent Ia$^+$ cells from peripheral blood showed elongated cytoplasmatic processes, and transmission EM revealed large irregularly shaped nuclei, many mitochrondria, and absence of phagosomes (not shown). These data reflect the histochemical, physical, and morphological properties of DC (*22*). The low yield of purified DC, however, rendered this method impractical for extensive studies. Therefore, low-buoyant-density plastic-nonadherent cells (F[1,2]NA) (Fig. 1) were used as the DC-enriched population (23±8%) for further functional studies. This population was devoid of monocytes, as ascertained by staining for NSE and absence of phagocytosis.

Accessory cell activity of DC. Con-A assays were carried out as described (*1, 15*). Optimal assay conditions for the stimulation of PBL by treatment with $NaIO_4$ were determined in preliminary studies. Maximum proliferation of lymphocytes occurred after pretreatment with 5 mM $NaIO_4$ for 15 min, followed by 4 days in culture. In all subsequent experiments 5 mM $NaIO_4$ and 4-day cultures were used.

Results of Con-A-induced mitogenesis are summarized in Figure 2A. Accessory-cell-depleted lymphocytes were unresponsive to Con-A. There was a dose-dependent reconstitution of lymphocyte proliferation by DC-enriched cells (F[1,2]NA, F(1,2) nonrosetting NA, or F(1,2) nonrosetting NA Ia^+). As shown in Figure 2B, with progressive enrichment of DC to 23, 34% and 92%, respectively, the number of DC required for a relative response (RR) of 1.0 were 5, 3.8, and 1.1×10^3, respectively. Extrapolation suggests that with an ideal purity of 100%, approximately 0.55×10^3 DC—i.e., a concentration of 0.5%, which closely corresponds to the actual concentration of DC in PBMC—would be required for an RR of 1.0.

The fact that low-buoyant-density cells that had not been further fractionated reconstituted lymphocyte proliferation only incompletely may have been due to the high concentration of monocytes (35±4%) that can result in suppression of lymphocyte proliferation, as shown previously (*23, 24*).

UV exposure of canine PBMC abolishes their ability to proliferate (*14*). As shown in Figure 3, exposure of DC-enriched cells to shortwave UV light for a total of 10 mJ/cm² prior to addition to accessory cell-depleted lymphocytes completely abrogated their ability to provide accessory function for lymphocyte responses to Con-A. Similar results were obtained with $NaIO_4$-induced mitogenesis (Fig. 4). The viability of UV-irradiated cells, when measured either by trypan blue exclusion or acridine orange uptake, was greater than 95% immediately after

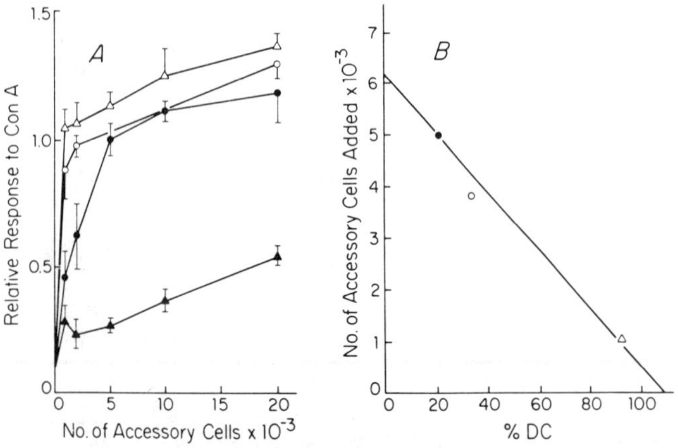

FIGURE 2. Assessment of accessory function of DC-enriched populations in Con-A-stimulated cultures. (A) 10^5 lymphocytes obtained from Percoll high-density fractions and nonadherent to nylon wool (F[5–7]NWNA) were used as responder cells in Con-A-stimulated assays. As accessory cells 1.0–20×10^3 cells from the populations F(1,2) (▲——▲), F(1,2)NA (●——●), F(1,2) nonrosetting-NA (○——○), or F(1,2) nonrosetting $NAIa^+$ (△——△), were added. Results each represent the mean ± 1 SD of four experiments, and are expressed as the relative response (RR) as compared with unfractionated PBMC that had shown a ^{3}H-thymidine uptake of 43,400±1400 cpm (mean ± 1 SD of four experiments always carried out in parallel) after stimulation with Con-A. (B) The number of cells from the F(1,2)NA, F(1,2) nonrosetting NA, and F(1,2) nonrosetting NA Ia^+ populations that were needed in add-back experiments to fully reconstitute (100%) the response of 1×10^5 F(5–7) NWNA cells to stimulation by Con-A is plotted against the purity (%) of DC in each of these populations.

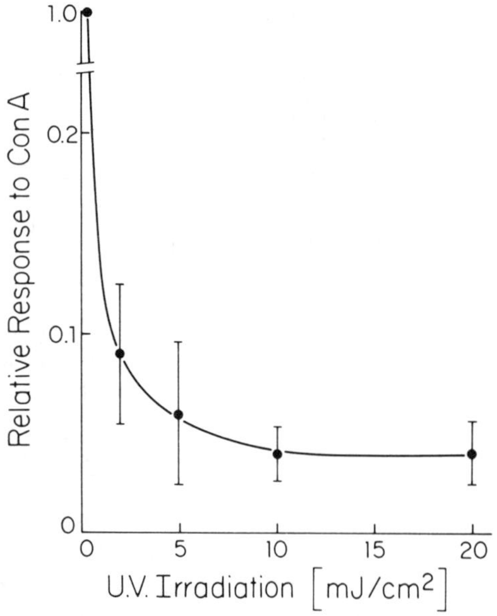

FIGURE 3. Effect of UV irradiation on accessory cell function: 1×10^5 accessory cell-depleted lymphocytes (F[5–7]NWNA) were cocultured with 5×10^3 DC-enriched (F[1,2]NA) cells, either untreated or exposed to 2–20 mJ/cm² of UV light prior to use. Results are expressed as relative response (RR) as compared with unfractionated PBMC.

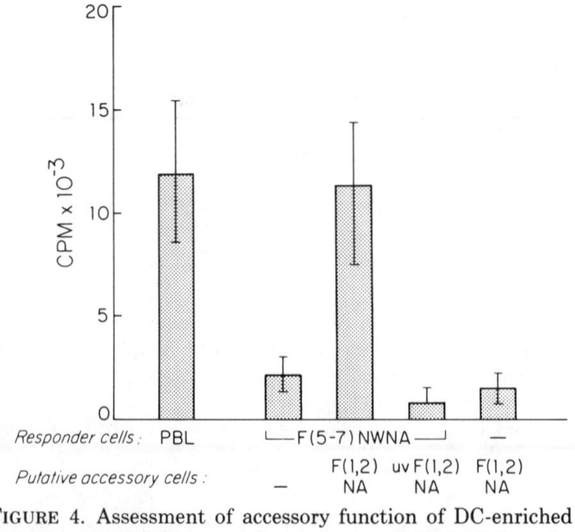

FIGURE 4. Assessment of accessory function of DC-enriched cells in $NaIO_4$-treated cultures: 10^5 accessory-cell-depleted lymphocytes (F[5–7]NWNA) served as responder cells and were cultured either alone or with the addition of untreated or UV-exposed (10 mJ/cm²) DC-enriched cells (F[1,2]NA). Results represent the mean ±1 SD of ^{3}H-thymidine uptake (cpm) of 5 experiments.

irradiation and 79±5%, 74±2%, and 58±4% following 24, 48, and 72 hr in culture, respectively.

Characteristics of Cluster Formation and Proliferation

The kinetics of cluster formation and responses of accessory-cell-depleted lymphocytes to which different populations of accessory cells were added is illustrated in Figure 5. At 24 hr

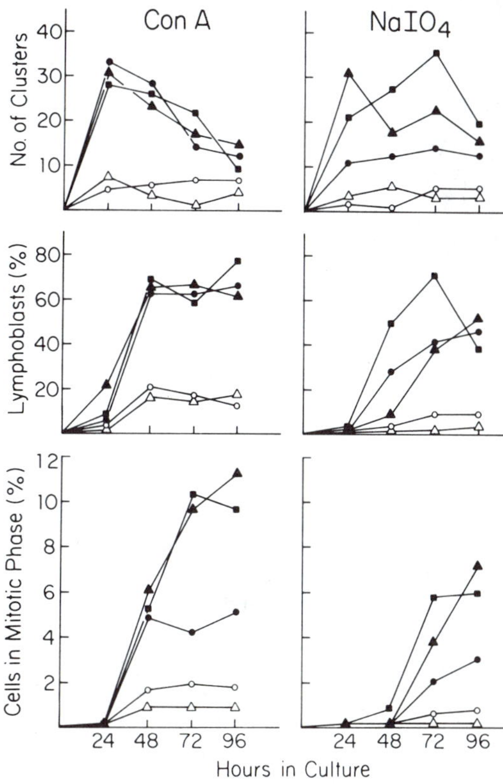

FIGURE 5. Cellular proliferation assay. Cytospun samples from cultures of 1×10[6] normal PBMC (■——■), accessory-cell-depleted lymphocytes (F[5–7]NWNA) (△——△), or F(5–7)NWNA cells, to which 5×10[4] DC-enriched cells (F[1,2]NA), untreated (▲——▲) or UV-exposed (○——○), or gamma-irradiated (●——●) were added. Cells were stimulated by either Con-A or $NaIO_4$ and cultured for 0, 24, 48, 72, and 96 hr, respectively. These samples were assayed for cluster formation, percent lymphoblasts, and percent cells in mitotic phase. Given is the mean (±SEM) or five experiments.

clustering of lymphocytes around DC was seen with normal PBMC. Only a few clusters were seen with accessory cell depleted lymphocytes. The addition of DC-enriched cells, untreated or gamma-irradiated, resulted in an increase in the number and size of clusters. When DC were UV-exposed the number of clusters did not differ from the background observed with lymphocytes alone. Cluster counts obtained from cytospun samples were in good agreement with counts obtained by counting directly in culture wells (using an inverted microscope), indicating that these clusters were tight and did not represent an artifact of sample preparation. The apparent decrease in the number of clusters by 96 hr was a result of confluence of adjoining clusters. The appearance of 24-hr clusters of F(1,2) NA cells by scanning EM is shown in Figure 6. The appearance of cultures with UV-exposed DC was identical to that of unstimulated PBL (data not shown).

At 48 hr, more than 50% of lymphocytes in the appropriate cluster-forming cultures had transformed into lymphoblasts. Only few lymphoblasts were observed in cultures with few or no clusters. The pattern was similar for Con-A-stimulated and $NaIO_4$ treated cultures.

Finally, an increase in the number of mitotic figures was observed in cluster-forming cultures, with a delay of 24–48 hr after blast transformation. These events are illustrated in Figure 7. The extent of blast transformation and mitosis was in good agreement with increased ^{3}H-thymidine uptake.

DISCUSSION

We have previously shown that purified canine peripheral blood monocytes fail to function as accessory cells in Con-A-induced mitogenesis. Rather, accessory cell function resided in a different low-buoyant-density plastic-nonadherent non-monocytic cell population (*1*). Preliminary morphologic analysis suggested that the functionally active fraction in that population consisted of DC. The present study expands those experiments and shows that these cells are NSE$^-$, Ia$^+$ and have the electron microscopic features of DC, as described in other species (*2, 5–9, 12*).

In addition, we have shown that monocyte-depleted cells enriched for DC function as potent accessory cells in both Con-A-induced and oxidative mitogenesis, whereas the low-buoyant-density fraction (F[1,2]), which was not further fractionated and contained substantial numbers of monocytes, exhibited less accessory potency. This finding is in agreement with the

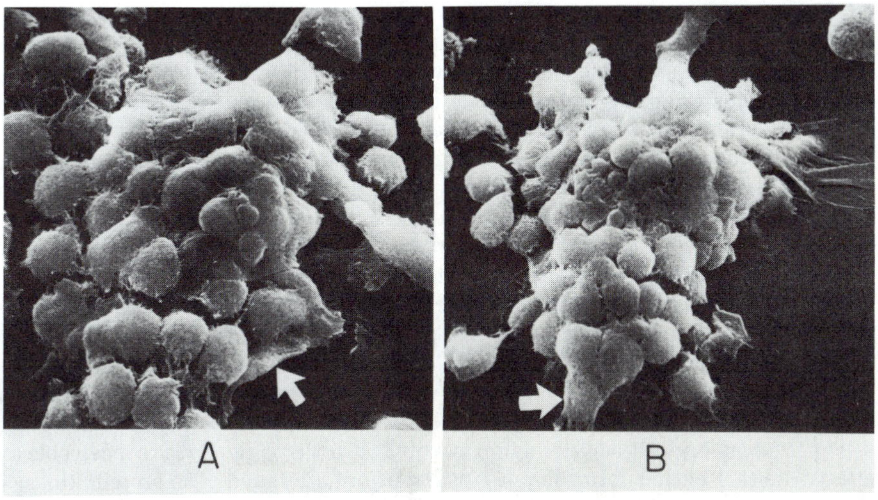

FIG. 6. Scanning electron micrographs of DC/lymphocyte clusters after 24-hr cultures of DC-enriched cells with Con-A (panel A, ×2270) or 24 hr after treatment with $NaIO_4$ (panel B, ×1050); lymphocytes are adhering to cytoplasmatic flaps (arrows) of DC.

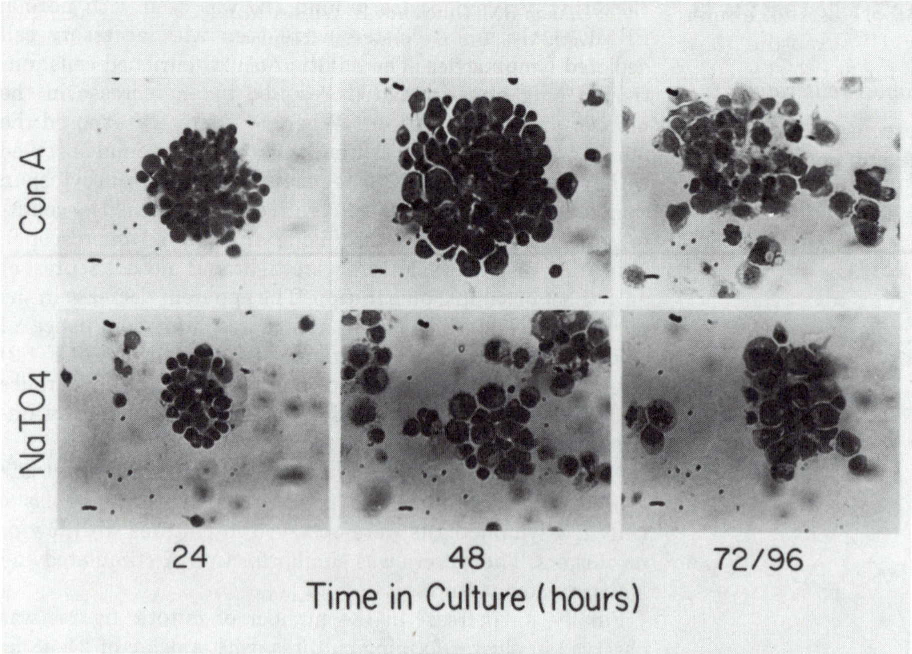

FIG. 7. Photomicrographs of DC/lymphocyte clusters from cytospun samples of PBMC following 24, 48, and 72 hr, respectively, in culture with Con-A (panel A, ×400) or 24, 48, and 96 hr, respectively, following treatment with $NaIO_4$ (panel B, ×400). At 24 hr only normal-appearing lymphocytes are visible; at 48 hr lymphocytes undergo blast transformation, and at 72 and 96 hr some lymphocytes have entered mitosis.

results of a study in rats showing that macrophages had no accessory activity in oxidative mitogenesis (*25*). Furthermore, monocytes have been found to have a suppressive effect on antigen-presenting capacity of DC in vitro (*23*). These data suggest, therefore, that the lesser ability of the low-buoyant-density cells to provide accessory function may have been related to an inhibitory effect of monocytes (*24*).

Common to both Con-A and $NaIO_4$-induced mitogenesis was a cluster formation of DC and lymphocytes occurring within 24 hr of initiation of culture. Cluster formation was consistently followed by lymphoblast transformation and proliferation, as indicated by the appearance of mitotic figures and a rise in thymidine uptake. Cluster formation has also been implicated in the mouse syngeneic mixed leukocyte reaction (*7*), in the rat mixed lymphocyte reaction (*26*), and in human autologous and mixed leukocyte reactions (*9*)—suggesting that the interaction between DC and lymphocytes represents a central step in the activation of lymphocytes. This is further supported by in situ observations in various lymphoid organs. In rat spleen DC have been shown to extend their processes between T lymphocytes (*27*), and it has been proposed that DC in human tonsils and adenoids form clusters with lymphocytes, thus generating centers of immunological activity (*28*). Similar interactions of a population of DC and lymphoid cells have been described in human thymus (*29*). The present study shows that not only DC from various lymphoid organs but also DC derived from peripheral blood interact with lymphocytes via cluster formation as a necessary first step of lymphocyte activation.

In agreement with studies in other species, UV irradiation of canine DC completely abrograted accessory function (*23*). Our data indicate that the loss of accessory function was related to the inability of UV irradiated DC to form clusters. This applied to both lectin-induced and oxidative mitogenesis. The lack of accessory function of DC was not due to a lack of viable DC since >90% of UV-exposed cells remained viable as determined by standard procedures. Gamma irradiation of DC before addition to accessory-cell-depleted lymphocytes had little or no effect on either cluster formation or blast transformation and proliferation. Similar observations have been made in a rat model (*25*).

The exact mechanism of action of UV irradiation is not known. It has been reported that UV exposure impairs interleukin production (*30*). There is also evidence that UV-induced inhibition of antigen presentation can be bypassed by interleukin 1 (*31*)—and, under certain conditions, with partially purified interleukin 2. (*31*). In agreement with this, we found that interleukin 2 can partially restore responsiveness of lymphocytes in the presence of UV-irradiated DC (unpublished observations). Moreover, gamma irradiation that does not immediately interrupt interleukin release (*30, 31*) does not prevent cluster formation. Alternatively, it has been suggested that the expression of Ia-like antigens decreases with time after UV exposure (*31*) thus interfering with the cell's antigen presenting function. In the present study, however, we did not find a change in Ia expression, as determined by monoclonal antibody 7.2, specific for a framework determinant on Ia-like antigens (*18*) (data not shown). One might speculate that different epitopes not recognized by this antibody were altered, or that functional capacity of Ia antigens was affected by UV exposure (*31*). However, the observation that the addition of exogenous IL 2 partially restored lymphocyte responsiveness argues against this explanation.

Activation of lymphocytes by Con-A has been found to require calcium ions (*32*). T cell activation can be abrogated by calcium-blocking agents such as verapamil and nifedipine (*33*). For these reasons calcium ions have been implicated as a transmembrane messenger in T cell activation. Preliminary studies in our laboratory show that Con-A-stimulated cells not only fail to proliferate in the presence of verapamil but also fail to form clusters with normal DC (unpublished observations). By analogy these results suggest that UV irradiation of DC may interfere with calcium influx into DC, thereby interfering with a calcium-dependent mechanism for interleukin production, as has been demonstrated in murine cell lines (*34*). It is also conceivable that other membrane-associated proteins, such as protein kinase C, are affected by UV exposure. In this case one might expect that the addition of phorbol esters to cultures would circumvent the block caused by UV exposure (*35*). Clearly, additional studies are required to further elucidate the mechanism of UV inactivation of DC.

Several in vivo experiments support the notion that DC play a central role in antigen presentation and immunogenicity, and that these functions can be altered by UV irradiation (*36*). Lechler and Batchelor have shown that rat kidney allografts depleted of DC can be transplanted successfully across major histocompatibility barriers, whereas grafts reconstituted with syngeneic DC are rejected (*37*). Lau et al. have observed prolonged survival of rat pancreatic islet cell allografts after prior UV irradiation of the graft (*38*), implying that UV-sensitive passenger leukocytes, presumably DC, provide the immunogenic signal for rejection. In a canine marrow transplant model we have shown that dogs transfused with normal whole blood from DLA-identical littermate donors uniformly become immunized (sensitized) as shown by the subsequent rejection of a marrow graft from the same donor (*39, 40*). If, however, the blood is exposed, prior to transfusion, to UV irradiation at doses sufficient to abolish the accessory capacity of DC as tested in vitro, transfusions apparently do not lead to sensitization, and dogs achieve sustained engraftment of marrow (*14*). If, instead, blood is exposed to gamma irradiation in vitro it maintains its ability to sensitize in vivo (*14*).

In conclusion, DC play a central role in antigen presentation and lymphocyte activation. In in vitro studies the direct interaction of DC from peripheral blood or lymphoid organs with lymphocytes in the form of cluster formation represents a general phenomenon involved in lymphocyte activation. Cluster formation is prevented by UV exposure of DC. This, in turn, results in an inability of normal lymphocytes to undergo transformation and mitosis, presumably due to a failure of UV exposed DC to provide the necessary signal, presumably interleukins.

Acknowledgments. We thank John Louton for his help with cell sorting experiments, Liz Caldwell for transmission electronmicroscopy, Arnold Schmidt for scanning electronmicroscopy pictures, and Susan Waisanen for preparing the manuscript.

REFERENCES

1. Aprile JA, Deeg HJ, Wulff JC, Raff RF. Purified canine monocytes fail to confer concanavalin-A responsiveness to accessory-cell-depleted lymphocytes. Exp Hematol 1984; 12: 45.
2. Tatsumi M, Imamura Y. Accessory cells distinct from macrophages in lymphocyte proliferation of cynomolgus monkeys. Immunology 1984; 52: 25.
3. Resch K, Heckmann B, Schober I, Barlin E, Gemsa D. The role of macrophages in the activation of T lymphocytes by Con-A. II. Macrophage-independent activation. Eur J Immunol 1981; 11: 120.
4. Steinman RM, Cohn ZA. Identification of a novel cell type in peripheral lymphoid organs of mice. I. Morphology, quantitatum, tissue distribution. J Exp Med 1973; 137: 1142.
5. Miyazaki H, Toshiaki O. Accessory functions and mutual cooperation of murine macrophages and dendritic cells. Eur J Immunol 1983; 13: 984.
6. Van Voorhuis W, Valensky J, Hoffman E, Lubon J, Hair LS, Steinman RM. Relative efficiency of human monocytes and dendritic cells as accessory cells for T cell replication. J Exp Med 1983; 158: 174.
7. Nussenzweig MC, Steinman RM. Contribution of dendritic cells to stimulation of the murine syngenic mixed leukocyte reaction. J Exp Med 1980; 151: 1196.
8. Steinman RM, Gutchinov B, Witmer MD, Nussenzweig MC. Dendritic cells are the principal stimulators of the primary mixed leukocyte reaction in mice. J Exp Med 1983; 157: 613.
9. Crow NK, Kunkel HG. Human dendritic cells: major stimulators of the autologous and allogeneic mixed leucocyte reactions. Clin Exp Immunol 1982; 49: 338.
10. Phillips LM, Parker JW, Jeffry AF, O'Brien RL. Characterization of responding cells in oxidative mitogen stimulation. II. Identification of an IA-bearing adherent accessory cell. J Immunol 1980; 124: 2700.
11. Klinkert WEF, LaBodie JH, O'Brien JP, Beyer CF, Bowers WE. Rat dendritic cells function as accessory cells and control the production of a soluble factor required for mitogenic responses of T lymphocytes. Proc Natl Acad Sci USA 1980; 77: 5414.
12. Inaba K, Witmer MD, Steinman RM. Clustering of dendritic cells, helper T lymphocytes and histocompatible B cells during primary antibody responses in vitro. J Exp Med 1984; 160: 858.
13. Lindahl-Kiessling K, Safwenberg J. Inability of UV irradiated lymphocytes to stimulate allogeneic cells in mixed lymphocyte culture. Int Arch Allergy Appl Immunol 1971; 41: 670.
14. Deeg HJ, Aprile J, Graham TC, Appelbaum FR, Storb R. Ultraviolet irradiation of blood prevent transfusion-induced sensitization and marrow graft rejection in dogs. Blood 1986; 67: 537.
15. Deeg HJ, Storb R, Gerhard-Miller L, Shulman HM, Weiden PL, Thomas ED. Cyclosporin A, a powerful immunosuppressant in vivo and in vitro in the dog, fails to induce tolerance. Transplantation 1980; 29: 230.
16. Julius MH, Simpson E, Herzenberg LA. A rapid method for the isolation of functional thymus-derived murine lymphocytes. Eur J Immunol 1973; 3: 645.
17. Atkinson K, Deeg HJ, Storb R, et al. Canine lymphocyte subpopulations. Exp Hematol 1980; 8: 821.
18. Hansen JA, Martin PJ, Nowinski RC. Monoclonal antibodies identifying a novel T-cell antigen and Ia antigens of human lymphocytes. Immunogenetics 1980; 10: 247.
19. Deeg HJ, Wulff JC, DeRose S, et al. Unusual distribution of Ia-like antigens on canine lymphocytes. Immunogenetics 1982; 16: 445.
20. Torok-Storb B, Deeg HJ, Storb R. Functional subsets of peripheral blood mononuclear cells in transfused dogs separated by size with fluorescence activated cell sorter. Exp Hematol 1980; 8: 906.
21. Melamed MR, Adams LR, Zimring A, Murnick JG, Mayer MA, Mayer K. Preliminary evaluation of acridine orange as a vital stain for automated differential leukocyte counts. Am J Clin Pathol 1972; 57: 95.
22. Steinman RM, Nussenzweig MC. Dendritic cells: features and functions. Immunol Rev 1980; 53: 127.
23. Bjercke S, Gaudernack G. Dendritic cells and monocytes as accessory cells in T-cell responses in man. II. Function as antigen-presenting cells. Scand J Immunol 1985; 21: 501.
24. Deeg HJ, Storb R. Functional dichotomy of canine thoracic duct lymphocytes: proliferation in mixed leukocyte culture and unresponsiveness to plant lectins. J Reticuloendothel Soc 1981; 29: 395.
25. Bowers WE, Berkowitz M, LaBadie JH, Klinkert WEF. Rat dendritic cells isolated from different tissues. Transplant Proc 1983; 15: 320.
26. Mason W, Pugh CW, Webb M. The rat mixed lymphocyte reaction: roles of a dendritic cell in intestinal lymph and T-cell subsets defined by monoclonal antibodies. Immunology 1981; 44: 75.
27. Dijkstia CD. Characterization of nonlymphoid cells in rat spleen, with special reference to strongly Ia-positive branched cells in T-cell areas. J Reticuloendothel Soc 1982; 32: 167.
28. Tilet-Leclercq C, Radoub D, Heiner E, et al. Isolation of follicular dendritic cells from human tonsils and adenoids. I. Procedure and morphological characterization. J Immunol Methods 1984; 66: 235.
29. Wekerle H, Ketelsen V-P. Thymic murine cells—Ia bearing epi-

thelium involved in T-lymphocyte differentiation? Nature 1980; 283: 402.
30. Lafferty KJ, Andrus L, Prowse SJ. Role of lymphokine and antigen in the control of specific T cell responses. Immunol Rev 1980; 51: 279.
31. Granstein RD, Tominaga A, Mizel SB, Parrish JA, Greene MI. Molecular signals in antigen presentation. II. Activation of cytolytic cells in vitro after ultraviolet radiation or combined gamma and ultraviolet radiation treatment of antigen-presenting cells. J Immunol 1984; 132: 2210.
32. Milner SM. Activation of lymphocytes by conconavalin A requires calcium ions. Cell Biol Int Rep 1979; 3: 35.
33. Birx DL, Berger M, Fleisher TA. The interference of T cell activation by calcium blocking agents. J Immunol 1984; 133: 2904.
34. Simon PL. Calcium mediates one of the signals required for interleukin 1 and 2 production by murine cell lines. Cell Immunol 1984; 87: 720.
35. Nishezuka Y. The role of protein kinase C in cell surface signal transduction and tumor promotion. Nature 1984; 308: 693.
36. Stingl G, Gazze-Stingl LA, Aberer W, Wolff K. Antigen presentation by murine epidermal Langerhans cells and its alteration by ultraviolet B light. J Immunol 1981; 127: 1707.
37. Lechler RI, Batchelor JR. Restoration of immunogenicity to passenger cell-depleted kidney allografts by the addition of donor strain dendritic cells. J Exp Med 1982; 155: 31.
38. Lau H, Reemtsma K, Hardy MA. Prolongation of rat islet allograft survival by direct ultraviolet irradiation of the graft. Science 1984; 223: 607.
39. Storb R, Weiden PL, Deeg HJ, et al. Rejection of marrow from DLA-identical canine littermates given transfusions before grafting: antigens involved are expressed on leukocytes and skin epithelial cells but not on platelets and red blood cells. Blood 1979; 54: 477.
40. Deeg HJ, Torok-Storb B, Storb R, et al. Rejection of DLA-identical canine littermate marrow after transfusion-induced sensitization: antigens involved are expressed on cotton-wool adherent but not on nonadherent mononuclear cells, granulocytes, or thoracic duct lymphocytes. Exp Hematol Today 1981; 27: 31.

Received 23 December 1985.
Accepted 24 February 1986.

0041-1337/86/4206-0660$02.00/0
TRANSPLANTATION

Vol. 42, No. 6
Printed in U.S.A.

INHIBITION OF RAT MIXED LYMPHOCYTE PANCREATIC ISLET CULTURES WITH ANTI-Ia IMMUNOTOXIN[1]

JUDITH A. SHIZURU, S. RAMAKRISHNAN,[2] THURMAN HUNT, RONALD C. MERRELL,[3,4] AND C. GARRISON FATHMAN

Division of Immunology, Department of Medicine and Department of Surgery, Stanford University Medical Center, Stanford, California, 94305

Studies reported here indicate that an anti-Ia immunotoxin can eliminate the allostimulatory subpopulation of cells present within the islets of Langerhans without damaging the hormone-secreting cells. Such studies made use of an in vitro correlate of transplantation rejection, the mixed lymphocyte islet cell (MLIC) reaction. Using the MLIC, it was demonstrated that an anti-Ia immunotoxin removed cells capable of stimulating the MLIC in a dose-dependent fashion without altering the hormone-secreting functions of the remaining cells when challenged with glucose and theophylline. These studies suggest the feasibility of using such anti-Ia immunotoxins in islet allograft transplantation models to circumvent problems inherent in complement-mediated cytotoxicity, a previously documented effective form of inducing islet allotransplantation tolerance.

[1]This work was supported by NIH grant AI 18716, the Juvenile Diabetes Foundation, and Cetus Corporation.
[2] Cetus Corporation, Emeryville, California, 94608
[3] Department of Surgery
[4] Present address: The Department of Surgery, University of Texas Health Science Center, Houston, Texas 77030.

The recent development of immunotoxins, a novel class of pharmacologic agents composed of highly toxic proteins, such as ricin or diphtheria toxin, covalently coupled to monoclonal antibodies, has offered a rational approach to selective cell killing (*1–8*). Exquisite target cell specificity is provided by the antibody portion of the molecule—and, once bound and internalized, the toxic moiety kills the cells by enzymatic inhibition of protein synthesis (*4*). One molecule of the bacterial exotoxin, diphtheria toxin, or of the plant toxins abrin or ricin may be sufficient to kill the cell it penetrates (*1*).

Thus far, application of these reagents has been limited to two fields: immunotoxins have been tested primarily as antineoplastic agents, the antibody portion being directed against target tumors (*3–6*); and pretreatment of donor bone marrow cells has been done with anti-T-lymphocyte antibody/toxin conjugates to specifically eliminate the cell-mediating graft-versus-host disease (*7, 8*). Results from both systems are encouraging. With respect to transplantation of organs other than bone marrow, the revival of the notion that a subset of nonparenchymal cells (passenger leukocytes) are responsible for initiation of graft rejection (*9–14*), and the discovery that these cells are distinguishable by the presence of MHC class II (Ia) antigens on their cell surface suggest that immunotoxin technology may additionally be applicable to the field of organ allograft tolerance induction.

The islets of Langerhans provide an ideal transplantation model for testing the efficacy of anti-Ia immunotoxins on allograft survival. Ia-bearing cells are only a small minority (2–3%) of the total islet population, the majority being the Ia-negative functional hormone-secreting cells (*15, 16*). Each islet is a tightly linked cellular community that possesses its own matrix of connective tissue and an extensive capillary endothelium (*17, 18*). Immunocytochemical staining studies have located Ia antigen on the lymphocytes, macrophages, dendritic cells, and capillary endothelium found within freshly isolated rat islets (*12, 19, 20*). Compared with other tissue allografts, untreated islets are particularly susceptible to rejection—however, successful abrogation of islet immunogenicity has been accomplished by a variety of regimens aimed at eliminating or altering the Ia-positive cells. These include long-term culturing of islets at low temperatures (*21*) or in an oxygen-rich atmosphere (*22*), restructuring of native islets into the so-called pseudoislets or neoislets (*23, 24*), and pretreatment of islets with heterogeneous anti-Ia antisera and complement (*25*).

Using a murine anti-Ia monoclonal antibody (13.4) conjugated to ricin A chain, we have recently demonstrated the suppression of the primary mixed lymphocyte reaction (MLR) stimulation (*26*). This assay is considered to be an *in vitro* correlate of graft rejection (*27*). Ia-positive cells are essential stimulator cells in the inductive phase of the primary MLR (*27, 28*).* In the present study, we extend the use of monoclonal 13.4 conjugated to whole ricin toxin to study the potential use of this reagent in the pretreatment of islets of Langerhans for allotransplantation. So that islet immunogenicity may be directly measured, a variant form of the MLR, the mixed lymphocyte/islet culture (MLIC), was utilized. Whole isolated islets, rather than lymphocytes, function as the stimulator population in this assay, which provides a method for titrating the activity of the immunotoxin.

MATERIALS AND METHODS

Antibodies. Monoclonal antibody 13.4 was generously provided by Dr. Gunter Hammerling (Heidelberg, Federal Republic of Germany) and purified via protein A column chromatography. This antibody, which has been described previously (*29*), binds to the mouse I-E^k molecule and has been associated with specificity Ia.7. Crossreactivity of anti-IE antibodies with rat splenocytes has been previously demonstrated (*26, 30*). Purified antibody from the MOPC 21 plasmacytoma line (*31, 32*) was selected as the appropriate irrelevant control antibody for specificity studies.

Immunotoxin preparation. Antibody 13.4 was derivatized with the heterobifunctional cross-linking reagent N-succinimidyl 3-(2-pyridyldithio) propionate (SPDP) and analyzed for the extent of derivatization as previously described (*33*). On the average, 4 mol of pyridyl-2-disulfide groups were introduced per mole of 13.4. To expose free sulfydryl groups, the SPDP-derivatized 13.4 was reduced with 5.0 mM dithiothreital (DTT) and desalted on a Sephadex G-25 column in phosphate buffered saline (PBS, pH 6.5).

Ricin, purified from the seed of *Ricinus communis* (*34*), was derivatized with m-maleimidobenzoyl-N-hydroxy-succinimide (MBS) using a method described by Youle and Neville (*8*). Incubation of ricin at 2 mg/ml with a 10-fold MBS molar excess was carried out for 30 min at 25°C followed by gel filtration on a G-25 column equilibrated in PBS (pH 6.5) to remove unreacted MBS. For conjugation, derivatized 13.4 thiolated at 3.1 μM was mixed with 9.8 μM ricin-MBS. The reaction was allowed to proceed for 1 hr at 25°C, then for 18 hr at 4°C. Purification of the 13.4 thioether-linked ricin toxin product (13.4×RT) was by HPLC gel permeation chromatography on a TSK-250 column as described elsewhere (*33*). The irrelevant immunotoxin MOPC 21×RT was prepared in a manner similar to that of 13.4×RT.

We also employed an alternate conjugation strategy in which the ricin toxin, rather than the antibody, was thiolated using SPDP derivatization (3 mol/L excess) and then reacted with MBS derivatized IgGs (3 mol/L excess). Immunotoxins prepared by either protocol had identical cytotoxic potencies (unpublished data).

The conjugates were analyzed by sodium dodecyl sulfate polyacrylamide gel electrophoresis (SDS-PAGE, 7.5%) and found to consist predominantly of a 1:1 molar ratio of ricin to antibody. The amount of free unconjugated antibody in the final preparation was less than 10% of the total mass. Free ricin toxin was not detected in the conjugate preparation.

Protein synthesis inhibition assay. The murine B cell lymphoma cell line, L10A2J, previously shown to express the I-E antigen (*35*), was used as target cells in a protein synthesis inhibition assay to assess immunotoxin activity. The cells were maintained in culture medium consisting of RPMI-1640 medium supplemented with 10% fetal bovine serum (FBS), 2.0 mM glutamine, and 50.0 μM β-mercaptoethanol. Then 1×10^5 target cells in a volume of 80.0 μl were mixed with 100.0 μl of 200 mM lactose in culture medium, and immunotoxin in an aliquot of 20.0 μl was added to triplicate cultures. Following 18 hr of incubation at 37°C, cells were centrifuged (500 ×G for 10 min) and resuspended in 0.2 ml of leucine-free RPMI-1640 substituted with 1.0 μCi ^{3}H-leucine. At the end of a 2-hr pulse period, the cultures were harvested on glass fiber filter discs (Gelman, 25-mm type A/E), precipitated with 5.0% trichloroacetic acid, and washed with cold ethanol. The extent of ^{3}H-leucine incorporation into protein was measured in a Packard Tri-Carb liquid scintillation counter following standard procedure.

Specificity index. The specificity index for the 13.4 immunotoxin was calculated by comparing the concentration of 13.4×RT required to yield 50% inhibition ($TCID_{50}$) in both the protein synthesis inhibition and MLR assays with the $TCID_{50}$ values for the control irrelevant immunotoxin, MOPC 21×RT.

Islet isolation. Pancreatic islets were isolated by collagenase digestion (Type IV, Cooper Biomedicals) and Ficoll gradient purification (*36*). Inbred male Lewis rats ($RT1^a$) 10–15 weeks of age, weighing 200–300 g (Charles River Company) were the islet source for mixed culture and function studies. The islets were maintained in tissue culture media (TCM) consisting of RPMI 1640 (GIBCO) supplemented with 10 mM $NaHCO_3$, 10 mM HEPES, 10% FBS, 1×10^{-3} M L-glutamine, 3×10^{-5} M 2-mercaptoethanol, nonessential amino acid, 100 units/ml peni-

* Abbreviations used: DTT, dithiothreital; FBS, fetal bovine serum; MBS, m-maleimidobenzoyl-N-hydroxy-succinimide; MLIC, mixed lymphocyte islet culture; MLR, mixed lymphocyte reaction; SPDP, N-succinimidyl 3-(2-pyridyldithio) propionate; TCM, tissue culture media.

cillin, and 100 μg/ml streptomycin (GIBCO) and glucose to a final concentration of 150 mg/dl. Intact purified islets were cultured 12–24 hr in a 37°C-humidified incubator (95% air/5% CO_2) prior to treatment with immunotoxin.

Lymphocyte preparation. For the MLIC studies, peripheral lymph node lymphocytes were obtained from male ACI rats (Laboratory Animal Supply) 12–18 weeks of age, weighing 200–300 g. Nodes were teased apart in TCM and passed through a nitex nylon mesh (Tetko Fabrics) giving a single cell suspension. Lymphocytes were then centrifuged at 1200 rpm for 10 min and washed twice in a similar manner.

For the MLR specificity studies, single-cell suspensions of spleen and lymph node cells obtained from adult male A/J (H-2^a) and C57BL/6 (H-2^b) mice, 6–8 weeks old (Jackson Laboratories) were prepared in a manner similar to that used for the rats.

Treatment of stimulator islets and spleen cells with immunotoxin. Following isolation and short-term culture, islets were hand-picked and divided into groups of 100–300. The groups were placed into 15-ml conical centrifuge tubes, washed twice, and pelleted at 1800 rpm for 1 min. Toxin conjugate 13.4×RT or MOPC21×RT was then added in a 0.1-ml volume with alpha lactose (final concentration 100 mM). Final volume in the tubes was 0.3 ml, and this suspension was incubated in 95% air/5% CO_2, 37°C for 15 min.

Allogeneic control islets were treated similarly by incubation in 100 mM lactose excluding the immunotoxin. Following incubation islets were washed two times in TCM supplemented with 100 mM lactose (1800 rpm, 1 min) and twice more with TCM alone.

Stimulator spleen cells for MLR studies were divided into groups of 2×10^7 in conical tubes and centrifuged at 1200 rpm for 10 min. Treatment with varying amounts of immunotoxin and alpha lactose was performed as described for islets above. Incubation was allowed for 15 min at 37°C followed by two washes with the 100 mM lactose TCM solution and two washes with TCM alone (1200 rpm, 10 min).

Mixed lymphocyte islet culture (MLIC). To prevent proliferation in the stimulator population, control and immunotoxin-treated islets were irradiated (2000 rads in a cesium irradiator). Following one wash with TCM, the groups were transferred in a volume of less than 0.3 ml into 96-well flat-bottomed microtiter plates (Falcon, No. 3072). The number of islets added per well varied depending upon the experiment. Wells were aspirated to 0.15 ml prior to addition of responder lymphocytes, and 2.5×10^5 ACI lymphocytes were added in a 0.1 ml volume to the islets, after which the plates were allowed to incubate in a 37°C humidified incubator (95% air/5% CO_2). On the fourth day of coculture, ^{3}H-thymidine (5 μCi, Research Products International Corporation) was added to each well with a mini-MASH (M.A. Bioproducts), and wells were harvested 16–18 hr later.

Mixed lymphocyte reaction (MLR). Viable splenic lymphocytes irradiated with 3300 rads were plated at a concentration of 1×10^6/well with 0.5×10^6 responder lymph node cells. The mixed cultures were incubated for 3 days at 37°C in a humidified atmosphere of 5% CO_2/95% air, labeled with tritiated thymidine (1 μCi/well), and incubated for 16–18 hr. Cells were harvested and thymidine incorporation determined as described for the MLIC above. These experiments were set up in triplicate.

Insulin secretion function studies. To assess the functional capacity of 13.4×RT-treated versus control islets, block stimulation studies were performed in parallel with the MLIC's 72 hr after immunotoxin exposure. For the duration of the study, 10–25 treated or untreated control islets were placed into conical centrifuge tubes and incubated at 37°C, 95% air/5% CO_2. Following two washes by centrifugation at room temperature (1 min, 1,800 rpm), a 30-min basal insulin secretion was established in Medium 199 (GIBCO) containing 5.6 mM glucose, 10 mM NaHCO3, 100 units/ml penicillin, 100 μg/ml streptomycin, and 0.5% bovine serum albumin (Fraction V, Sigma). Islets were then pelleted, and the supernatants collected, washed once, and resuspended in Medium 199 with stimulating concentrations of glucose (22 mM) and theophylline (10 mM) for an additional 30 min. At the end of the stimulation period, the tubes were centrifuged and the supernatants transferred to separate tubes. Supernatants were assayed for insulin by the method described below.

Insulin assay. Insulin was measured by double antibody radioimmunoassay as described by Morgan and Lazarow (*37*). Crystalline rat insulin was generously provided by the Eli Lilly Company. Guinea pig/antirat insulin antiserum (Linco, Lot No. ARI-02) was used as a first antibody, and was precipitated by a second goat/anti-guinea-pig antiserum (Linco, Lot No. 2011). ^{125}I-insulin (89 μCi/mg) was purchased from New England Nuclear. Before precipitation, 1 ml of 22.5% polyethylene glycol (molecular weight approximately 8,000, Sigma) was added to each tube to facilitate dilution and stabilization of the pellet.

RESULTS

Specificity and activity of Anti-Ia immunotoxin. In order to study the potential effects of anti-immunotoxins on inhibition of mixed lymphocyte islet cell cultures (MLIC), it was first necessary to demonstrate specific activity of the immunotoxin construct. Although the MLIC studies described below have been performed in rats, the most appropriate test of specificity of the immunotoxin is in a murine MLR. The antibody 13.4 has selective reactivity among mice for strains that bear products of the I-E subregion. As has been previously demonstrated, anti-I-E antibodies raised against murine MHC class II products crossreact with all Ia bearing rat lymphocytes tested (*30*). Thus, we took advantage of the fact that lymphocytes from C57BL/6 mice, which do not express I-E region products, could be assayed in conventional mixed lymphocyte reactions in reciprocal combination with lymphocytes from strain A/J, which do express I-E molecules. Data presented in Figure 1A demonstrate the selectivity of the 13.4×RT immunotoxin in the suppression of the murine MLR. Spleen cells from strain A/J mice, when treated with the anti-Ia immunotoxin, were inhibited in their ability to stimulate a response in C57BL/6 lymphocytes in a dose-dependent manner. Alternatively, treatment of C57BL/6 lymphocytes with immunotoxin 13.4×RT was no more efficient that treatment of the same lymphocytes with an irrelevant immunotoxin MOPC 21×RT. Parallel protein synthesis inhibition studies of the appropriate immunotoxin (13.4×RT) versus the MOPC 21×RT control on a murine target cell line, L10A2J, which expresses the I-E surface antigen, gave results similar to those demonstrated in Figure 1B. In both assays the observed cytotoxicity of the MOPC 21×RT conjugate at higher doses can be attributed to the nonspecific uptake of the immunotoxin by pinocytosis, in contrast to the specific internalization of 13.4×RT via receptor (Ia antigen)-

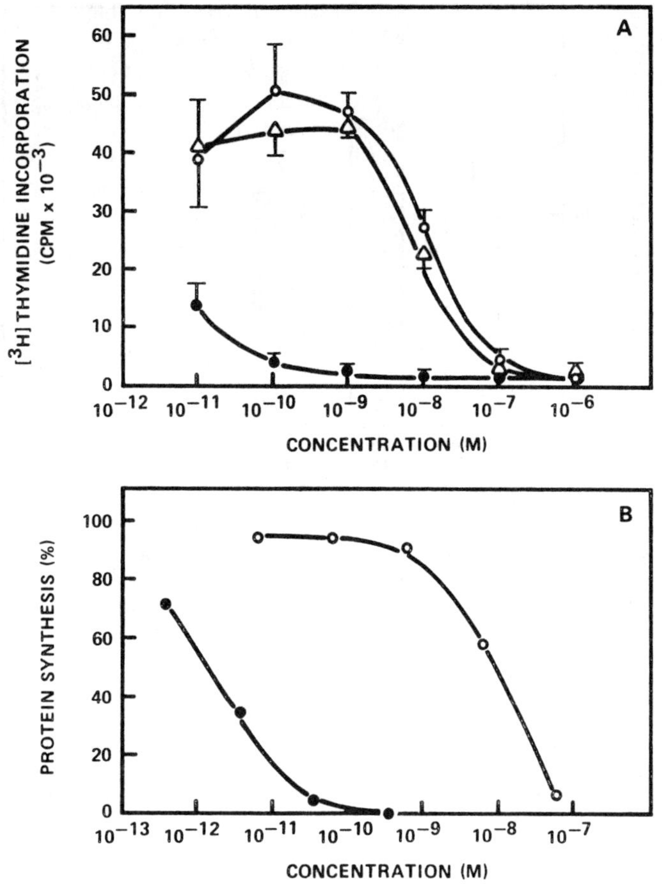

FIGURE 1. Specificity studies of 13.4×RT conjugate. (A) Murine MLR with pretreatment of stimulator cells at increasing concentrations of 13.4×RT and MOPC 21×RT. Treatment of 13.4×RT spleen cells from the strain A/J (●—●, C57BL/6 anti-A/J) demonstrate $TCID_{50}$ values of $<10^{-11}$M. Treatment of either the IE-negative C57BL/6 stimulator cells with 13.4×RT (O—O, A/J anti-C57BL/6) or of the A/J stimulators with the irrelevant immunotoxin MOPC 21×RT (Δ—Δ, C57BL/6 anti-A/J) yields $TCID_{50}$ values of approximately 10^{-8}M. Values are mean ± SD of triplicate wells. The specificity index of immunotoxin 13.4 as measured by this assay is greater than 5000-fold. (B) Dose-dependent cytotoxicity elicited by 13.4×RT (●—●) and the control immunotoxin prepared with MOPC 21 and ricin toxin (O—O). The IE-expressing murine cell line L10A2J was used as target cells and the percentage of protein synthesis taken as an index of cytotoxicity. Percent protein synthesis is expressed in relation to the level of H^3-leucine incorporation in control untreated cultures (100%). Each value is the mean of triplicate independent determinations.

mediated endocytosis. These data support the fact that the 13.4×RT conjugate is selectively cytotoxic, and has a specificity index in either the inhibition of the murine MLR or in protein synthesis inhibition of IE-positive murine target cells greater than 5000-fold.

Stimulatory capacity of islets In vitro: the MLIC. Earlier studies have shown that Ia-bearing cells are essential in the inductive phase of the primary MLR (*27, 28*). Thus, an analogous assay was developed to detect the presence of Ia-positive cells within rat islets. Irradiated Lewis islets were cultured in the presence of allogeneic responder ACI lymphocytes for several days, and the proliferative response measured by ^{3}H-thymidine incorporation. Data presented in Figure 2 demonstrated the kinetics of the MLIC for this rodent system. Increasing numbers of stimulator islets were plated with 2.5×10^5 allogeneic lymphocytes in microculture wells and harvested on sequential days. The proliferative response to 100 islets peaked on the fifth day of coculture. The dose-response curve is shown in Figure 3, in which ^{3}H-thymidine incorporation varies directly as a function of the number of islets in each well. Parallel studies, holding the number of stimulator islets constant (*20*) and titrating responder lymphocytes, demonstrated that 2.5 to 5×10^5 responder cells was optimal (data not shown).

Titration of immunotoxin 13.4×RT in MLIC. Immunotoxin 13.4×RT activity on rat islets was evaluated by titrating its ability to effectively eliminate the stimulatory response when compared with untreated allogeneic controls. Islets were exposed for 15 min to increasing concentrations of immunotoxins in the presence of lactose, and then plated with responder lymphocytes (MLIC) (Fig. 4). This incubation time was selected based on the murine experiments presented above and on studies with 13.4-RTA conjugate on spleen cells, which dem-

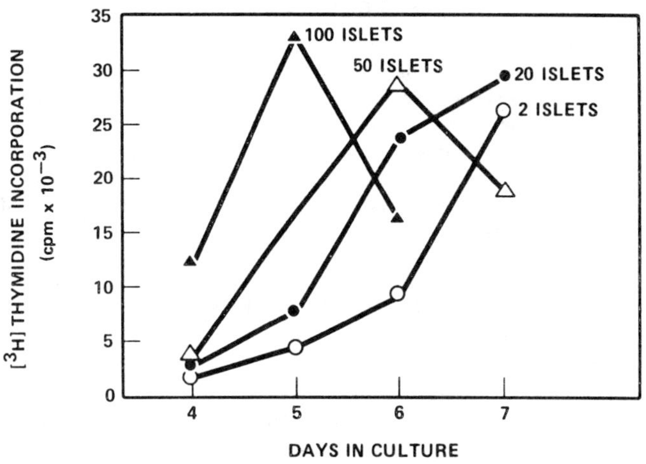

FIGURE 2. Kinetics of the MLIC proliferative response. ^{3}H-thymidine incorporation following a 16–18 hr pulse of 2.5×10^5 ACI ($RT1^a$) lymph node lymphocytes to varying numbers of x-irradiated (2000 rads) Lewis ($RT1^l$) islets in cultures harvested on consecutive days is presented as cpm. Data on the abscissa represent the incubation time in days; data on the ordinate show the mean value of three experiments, each triplicate cultures.

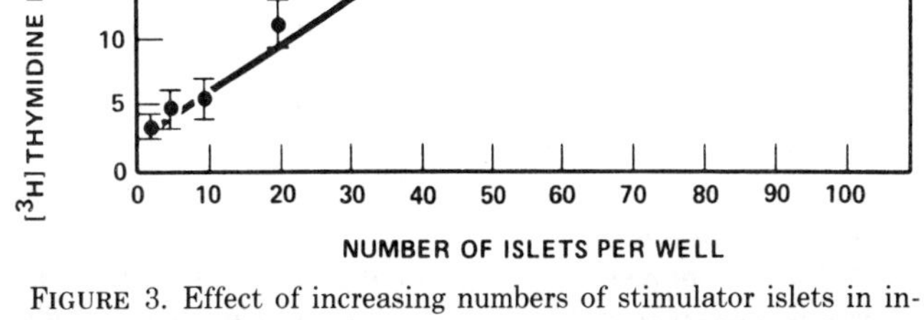

FIGURE 3. Effect of increasing numbers of stimulator islets in inducing an MLIC. ^{3}H-thymidine uptake of responder ACI lymphocytes (2.5×10^5 well) is measured in response to various doses of stimulator Lewis islets after five days in culture. Data on the ordinate represent the mean of two experiments set up in triplicate.

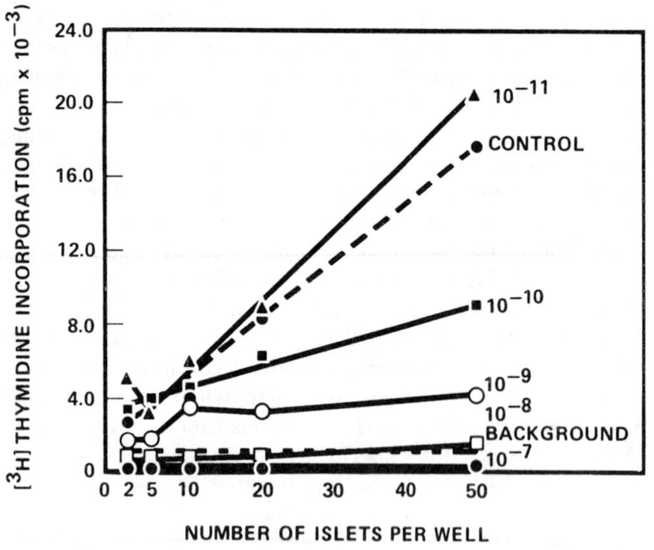

FIGURE 4. Titration of immunotoxin 13.4×RT. Potency of the anti-Ia immunotoxin in abolishing the MLIC proliferative response is demonstrated over a range of 4 logs of immunotoxin concentration. Number of islets versus ^{3}H-thymidine incorporation is plotted as a dose-response. Solid lines represent immunotoxin concentrations from 10^{-11} M to 10^{-7} M; dotted lines represent the allogeneic control and the lymphocyte background. Data plotted on the ordinate are the means of triplicate cultures.

onstrated that an incubation time of 4 hr was no more effective at suppressing an MLR than was 4 min (*26*). As shown in Figure 4, concentrations below 10^{-11}M were ineffective in reducing the stimulation potential of treated islets—however, above this concentration, stimulatory activity was inhibited over a range of 3 logs and complete abolishment of lymphocyte stimulation induction was achieved at $<10^{-8}$M. As control, MLICs were performed using unconjugated 13.4 antibody and the irrelevant immunotoxins MOPC 21×RT at 10^{-9}M. No inhibitory effect was demonstrated by either of these control reagents (Fig. 5).

Morphology and function of treated islets. We were concerned that the suppressive effects seen following immunotoxin treatment of islets in the MLIC might involve nonspecific killing of parenchymal cells, as well as the Ia-bearing cells. Therefore, 13.4×RT treated islets were cultured in the absence of lymphocytes and periodically examined under light microscopy and tested for insulin secretory function. The time required to kill target cells following immunotoxin treatment can vary widely depending on the number of immunotoxin molecules bound per cell and the antibody class (*1, 2*). Values ranging from 1.5 to 60 hr have been previously reported as the time necessary to decrease the rate of protein synthesis by one order of magnitude (*38*). Gross islet morphology was, therefore, examined immediately after treatment, and at 24, 48, and 72 hr following exposure to 13.4×RT. Treated islets viewed in suspension culture in the presence of the vital dye trypan blue showed no difference from untreated controls at any of the time points examined (data not included).

Functional competence of immunotoxin-treated versus untreated islets was tested at 72 hr by glucose stimulation studies (Fig. 6). Basal insulin secretion of treated islets at low glucose concentrations (5.6 mM), and the response of treated islets to high glucose concentrations (22.2 mM) plus theophylline (10

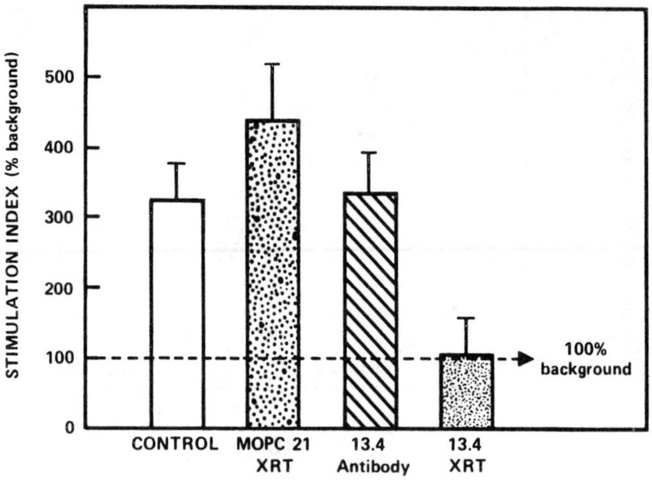

FIGURE 5. MLIC with unconjugated 13.4 antibody and irrelevant immunotoxin control. Comparative study of Lewis islets pretreated with 10^{-9} M 13.4×RT (□), 13.4 unconjugated antibody (▨), MOPC 21×RT (□), or media alone (□). Values were obtained from 3 independent experiments and expressed as a percentage of the lymphocyte background.

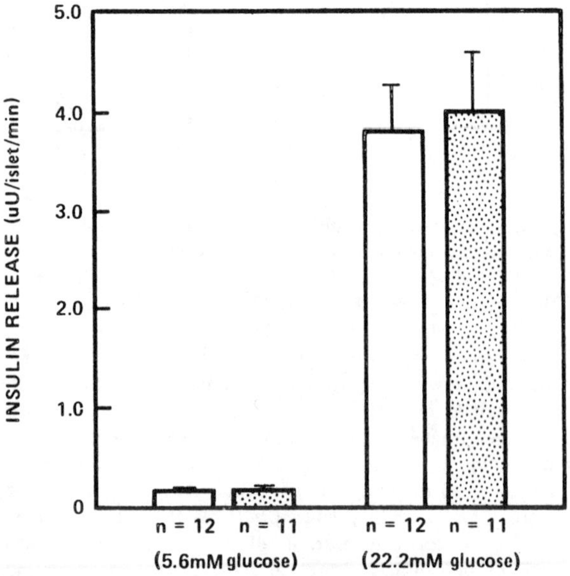

FIGURE 6. Insulin secretory response to glucose and theophylline from 13.4×RT-treated versus nontreated islets. At 72 hr following exposure to immunotoxin, 10–25 islets were equilibrated in a 5.6 mM glucose-containing medium for 30 min (basal insulin secretion). The groups were then washed and resuspended in 22 mM glucose plus 10 mM theophylline for a 30-min stimulation period. Insulin release was measured by radioimmunoassay, and is expressed here as microunits of insulin per islet per minute. Unshaded bars denote insulin release from untreated islets, stippled bars denote islets treated with 10^{-8} 13.4×RT.

mM), was comparable to that of untreated islets cultured under similar conditions. The results of these studies indicate that treatment of islets with immunotoxin leaves the hormone-secreting cells unimpaired.

DISCUSSION

The results of this study indicate that an anti-Ia immunotoxin can eliminate the allostimulatory subpopulation of cells present within the islets of Langerhans without damaging the hormone-secreting cells. Since cells bearing the Ia alloantigen are believed to initiate the immune rejection process (*9–12*), this method offers a potential approach to the prolongation of islet allografts. Thus far, use of anti-Ia antibodies for islet allograft tolerance induction has been dependent upon complement-mediated lysis as an effector mechanism for cell-specific killing (*4, 25*). The application of complement for this purpose is limited in a large-scale clinical setting, since nonspecific toxicity and difficulties in reproducibility from complement sources are a persistent problem. Additionally, using the same monoclonal antibody (13.4) we have previously demonstrated that toxin conjugates are more effective in suppressing the MLR than antibody-plus-complement (*26*). In this study we have substituted immunotoxin-mediated cytotoxicity as a means of correcting these apparent deficiencies in anti-Ia and complement-mediated tolerance induction. Although immunotoxin 13.4×RT demonstrates specific cytotoxic activity on Ia-positive cells within rat islets, it is useful to note that in shifting from the murine MLR to the rat MLIC system there was a decrease in the specific activity. Studies from our laboratory using a 13.4 ricin-A chain conjugate in rat MLR combinations similar to the MLIC responder/stimulator combinations presented here also exhibited a lower specific activity than seen in the murine MLR (*26*). The decrease in specific activity shown in the MLIC and in the rat MLR is presumably due to the lower affinity of the antibody for rat MHC class II antigens. Differences in antibody-binding affinity directly influence immunotoxin potency (*39, 40*) and should therefore be considered when evaluating activity of these agents. In our system, greater than 10 times more immunotoxin was needed for inhibition of the rat MLR (or MLIC), an increase that did not appreciably change its differential killing ability.

The relative vulnerability of transplanted pancreatic islets to destruction by host immune mechanisms compared with other organs has been thoroughly demonstrated by comparative allotransplantation studies in animals (*41–44*). The reasons for the differences in susceptibility of islet transplants are not clear. Other have speculated that the physical structure of islets may play a role—i.e., transplanted islets are dispersed throughout the host tissue (usually the liver) and are not protected by the usual stromal elements (*42, 43*). The mixed lymphocyte islet culture (MLIC) was used in these studies to assess the immunogenicity of islets. In an earlier MLIC study, Rabinovitch et al. observed both an allogeneic and an autologous lymphocyte response to collagenase-digested canine islets (*45*). Since neither collagenase-digested liver cells nor lymph node cells were autostimulatory, they concluded that the islets of Langerhans may contain tissue-specific antigens as well as alloantigens. Our results are in contrast to these findings. The response of lymphocytes to allogeneic islets was completely eliminated by treatment with an anti-Ia immunotoxin. These data strongly support our hypothesis that MHC Class II bearing cells (Ia-positive) are the source of allostimulation in MLIC, and that tissue-specific antigens, if present, will act like MHC Class I histocompatibility antigens and remain nonstimulatory in the absence of Ia induction of response.

Islets contain approximately 1–2×10^3 cells in toto; approximately 2–3% of these are Ia-positive (*19, 20*). Data presented here suggest that a very small number of Ia-bearing cells (i.e., 20–30) are sufficient to induce stimulation in an MLIC. Why islets are so efficient in stimulating an MLIC is an interesting but unanswered question. The suggestion that islets contain the immunogenic interstitial dendritic cell (*12–14, 42*) offers one explanation for their stimulatory properties. Whatever the mechanism of Ia-induced MLIC proliferation, it was our goal to design a convenient and quantitative method for evaluating immunotoxin effectiveness. Our data clearly demonstrate that anti-Ia immunotoxin treatment of islets specifically ablates MLIC stimulation. These results suggest that ricin toxin anti-Ia immunotoxin conjugates may be successfullly used in inducing islet allograft transplantation tolerance by removing the stimulatory Ia-bearing cells from the islet without interfering with the functional hormone-secreting cells. Preliminary unpublished results from our laboratory have suggested that such immunotoxin treatment of islets will allow successful islet transplantation across major histocompatibility barriers in a rodent model.

Acknowledgments. We thank Brian Fendly and Mike Bjorn (Cetus Corporation) for their expert technical assistance, and we offer special thanks to Robyn Kizer and Diane O'Neill for their careful and patient secretarial assistance in the preparation of the manuscript.

REFERENCES

1. Olsnes S, Pihl A. Chimeric toxins. Pharmacol Ther 1981; 15: 355.
2. Raso V. Antibody mediated delivery of toxic molecules to antigen bearing target cells. Immunol Rev 1982; 62: 93.
3. Krolick KA, Uhr JW, Vitetta ES. Selective killing of leukemia cells by antibody-toxin conjugates: implications for autologous bone marrow transplantation. Nature 1982; 295: 604.
4. Vitetta ES, Krolick KA, Miyama-Inaba M, Cushley W, Uhr JW. Immunotoxins: a new approach to cancer therapy. Science 1983; 219: 644.
5. Blythman HE, Casellas O, Gros P, et al. Immunotoxins: hybrid molecules of monoclonal antibodies and a toxin subunit specifically kill tumor cells. Nature 1981; 290: 145.
6. Thorpe PE, Mason DW, Brown ANF, et al. Selective killing of malignant cells in a leukemic rat bone marrow using an antibody-ricin conjugate. Nature 1982; 297: 594.
7. Vallera DA, Youle RJ, Neville, Jr. DM, Kersey JH. Bone marrow transplantation across major histocompatibility barriers. V. Protection of mice from lethal graft-vs-host disease by pretreatment of donor cells with monoclonal anti-Thy-1.2 coupled to the toxin ricin. J Exp Med 1982; 155: 949.
8. Youle RJ, Neville DM Jr. Anti-Thy 1.2 monoclonal antibody linked to ricin is a potent cell-type-specific toxin. Proc Natl Acad USA 1980; 77: 5483.
9. Steinmuller D. Passenger leukocytes and immunogenicity of skin allografts: a critical reevaluation. Transplant Proc 1982; 8: 1094.
10. Talmage DW, Dart G, Radovich J, Lafferty KJ. Activation of transplant immunity. Effect of donor leukocytes on thyroid allograft rejection. Science 1976; 191: 385.
11. Lacy PE, Davie JM, Finke ED. Induction of rejection of successful allografts or rat islets by donor peritoneal exudate cells. Transplantation 1979; 28: 415.
12. Faustman D, Lacy PE, Davie JM. Transplantation without immunosuppression. Diabetes 1982; 31(suppl 4): 11.
13. Lafferty KJ, Prowse SJ, Simeonovic CJ, Warren HS. Immunobiology of tissue transplantation: a return to the passenger leukocyte concept. Ann Rev Immunol 1983; 1: 143.
14. Lacy PE, Davie JM. Transplantation of pancreatic islets. Ann Rev Immunol 1984; 2: 183.
15. Faustman D, Hauptfeld V, Davie JM, Lacy PE, Shreffler D. Murine pancreatic B-cells expressed H-2K and H-2D but not Ia antigens. J Exp Med 1980; 151: 1563.
16. Baekkeskov S, Takahiro K, Klareskog L, et al. Expression of major histocompatibility antigens on pancreatic islet cells. Proc Natl

Acad Sci USA 1980; 78: 6456.
17. Lacy PE, Greider MH. Anatomy and ultrastructural organization of pancreatic islets. Endocrinology. New York: Grune & Stratton, 1979.
18. Unger RH, Dobbs RE, Orci L. Insulin, glucagon and somatostatin secretion in the regulation of metabolism. Ann Rev Physiol 1978; 40: 307.
19. Rabinovitch A, Rodolfo A, Noel J, Brunschig J, Ryan US. Tissue culture reduced Ia antigen-bearing cells in rat islets and prolongs allograft survival Diabetes 1982; 31(suppl 4): 48.
20. Hart DNJ, Newton MR, Reece-Smith H, Fabre JW, Morris PJ. Major histocompatibility complex antigens in the rat pancreas, isolated pancreatic islets, thyroid, and adrenal. Transplantation 1983; 36: 431.
21. Lacy PE, Davie JM, Finke EH. Prolongation of islet allograft survival following in vitro culture (24°C) with a single injection of ALS. Science 1978; 204: 312.
22. Lacy PE, Finke EH, Janney CG, Davie JM. Prolongation of islet xenograft survival by in vitro culture of rat megaislets in 95% O_2. Transplantation 1982; 33: 588.
23. Tze WJ, Tai J. Pseudoislet allotransplantation study in rats. Diabetes 1983; 31(suppl 1): 168A.
24. Shizuru JA, Trager D, Merrell RC. Structure, function and immune properties of reassociated islet cells. Diabetes 1985; 34: 898.
25. Faustman D, Hauptfeld V, Lacy P, Davie J. Prolongation of murine islet allograft survival by pretreatment of islets with antibody directed to Ia determinants. Proc Natl Acad Sci USA 1981; 78: 5156.
26. Nakahara K, Bjorn MJ, Kaplan D, Fathman CG. The effectiveness of anti-Ia immunotoxins in suppression of MLR. Transplantation 1985; 40: 62.
27. Minami M, Shreffler DC. Ia-positive stimulator cells are required in primary but not in secondary mixed leukocyte reactions against H-2K and H-2D differences. J Immunol 1981; 126: 1774.
28. Fathman CG, Handwerger BS, Sachs DH. Evidence for a role of Ir associated alloantigens in mixed lymphocyte culture stimulation. J Exp Med 1974; 140: 853.
29. Hammerling FJ, Hammerling U, Lemke H. Isolation of twelve monoclonal antibodies against Ia and H-2 antigens. Serological characterization and reactivity with B and T lymphocytes. Immunogenetics 1979; 8: 433.
30. Wettstein PJ, Frelinger JG, Hood L. Serological and biochemical characterization of rat (RT1) Class II molecules with restricted mouse anti-Ia sera. Immunogenetics 1981; 13: 93.
31. Svasti J, Milstein C. The complete amino acid sequence of a mouse kappa light chain. Biochemistry 1972; 128: 427.
32. Potter M. Antigen binding myeloma proteins of mice. Adv Immunol 1977; 25: 141.
33. Bjorn MJ, Ring D, Frankel A. Evaluation of monoclonal antibodies for the development of breast cancer immunotoxins. Cancer Res 1985; 45: 1214.
34. Nicolson GL, Blaustein J. The interaction of ricinus communis agglutinin with normal and tumor cell surfaces. Biochim Biophys Acta 1972; 266: 543.
35. McKean DJ, Infante AJ, Nilson A, et al. Major histocompatibility complex-restricted antigen presentation to antigen-reactive T cells by B lymphocyte tumor cells. J Exp Med 1981; 154: 1419.
36. Lernmark A, Nathans A, Steiner DF. Preparation and characterization of plasma membrane-enriched fractions from rat pancreatic islets. J Cell Bio 1976; 71: 606.
37. Morgan CR, Lazarow A. Immunoassay of insulin: two antibody system. Diabetes 1963; 12: 115.
38. Casellas P, Bourrie BJP, Gros P, Jansen FK. Kinetics of cytotoxicity induced by immunotoxins. J Biol Chem 1984; 259: 9359.
39. Neville DM Jr, Youle RJ. Monoclonal antibody-ricin or ricin A-chain hybrids: kinetic analysis of cell killing for tumor therapy. Immunol Rev 1982; 62: 75.
40. Ramakrishnan S, Houston LL. Prevention of growth of leukemia cells in mice by monoclonal antibodies directed against Thy 1.1 antigen disulfide linked to two ribosomal inhibitors: pokeweed antiviral protein or ricin A-chain. Cancer Res 1984; 44: 1398.
41. Reckard CR, Stuart FP, Schulak JA. Immunologic comparisons of isolated pancreatic islet and whole-organ allografts. Transplant Proc 1979; 11: 563.
42. Nash JR, Peters M, Bell PRF. Comparative survival of pancreatic islets, heart, kidney and skin allografts in rats with and without enhancement. Transplantation 1977; 24: 70.
43. Naji A, Barker CF, Silvers WK. Relative vulnerability of isolated pancreatic islets, parathyroid, and skin allografts to cellular and humoral immunity. Transplant Proc 1979; 11: 560.
44. Sutherland DER, Rynasiewicz JJ, Kawahara K, Gorecki P, Najarian JS. Rejection of islets versus immediately vascularized pancreatic allografts: a quantitative comparison. J Surg Res 1980; 29: 240.
45. Rabinovitch A, Fuller L, Mintz D, et al. Responses of canine lymphocytes to allogeneic and autologous islets of Langerhans in mixed cell cultures. J Clin Invest 1981; 67: 1507.
46. Gebel HM, Yasunami Y, Diekgraefe B, Davie JM, Lacy PE. Ia-bearing cells within isolated canine islets. Transplantation 1983; 36: 346.

Received 11 April 1985.
Accepted 12 February 1986.

0041-1337/86/4206-0667$02.00/0
TRANSPLANTATION
Vol. 42, No. 6

Printed in U.S.A.

THE ROLE OF RESIDENT ACCESSORY CELLS IN CORNEAL ALLOGRAFT REJECTION IN THE RABBIT[1]

K. A. WILLIAMS,[2] T. S. MANN, M. LEWIS, AND D. J. COSTER

Department of Ophthalmology, Flinders University of South Australia, Bedford Park, South Australia

Corneal grafts are more likely to be rejected when placed in a vascularized rather than in a normal host cornea. Using immunohistochemical techniques, normal rabbit cornea was found to contain measurable numbers of cells of hemopoietic origin, probably of either macrophage or dendritic lineage. After the deliberate induction of corneal inflammation and neovascularization, the number of these accessory cells was found to increase significantly. There was also a marked increase in the number of T cells present. Enzyme staining indicated a degree of heterogeneity in the infiltrate. The process of rejection of rabbit corneal grafts was found to occur earlier when additional infiltrating cells were present in either donor button or graft bed, and earlier still when the load of infiltrating cells was increased in both donor and recipient. We hypothesize that resident accessory cells of recipient origin may be implicated in graft rejection in vascularized, inflamed corneas.

Corneal grafts performed in patients with diseased but avascular, noninflamed corneas are generally successful and a clear graft is almost always achieved. In keratoconus, a dystrophic condition of the corneal stroma that results in thinning and subsequent distortion of the refracting surface of the cornea, the clear graft rate is better than 95% at one year. However, the results of transplantation into recipient eyes that show evidence of corneal neovascularization and inflammation are much less satisfactory; approximately half such grafts will fail, with the majority being lost to irreversible rejection (*1*). In practice, then, the so-called immunological privilege supposedly enjoyed by the cornea does not operate and the outcome of clinical corneal transplantation is determined very largely by the state of the graft bed into which the donor cornea is transferred (*2*). The reasons for the increased frequency of rejection in high-risk patients are unclear.

In humans, the principal difference between high-risk and normal corneas, or those excised from low-risk patients, is that they contain vascular endothelium, together with a large number of what are probably immune accessory cells (*3*). Such cells may be of monocyte/macrophage or dendritic lineage. Cells of both lineages bear the leukocyte-common antigen (a marker of hemopoietic derivation), together with class I and (depending on the species and the stage of differentiation/activation in the case of macrophages) class II major histocompatibility complex (MHC)* antigens, and may function as antigen-presenting cells (*4*). Small numbers of accessory-type cells are also present in normal central corneal stroma (*3*) and in epithelium (*5, 6*).

It has been suggested that the interstitial dendritic cell may be the predominant type of passenger leukocyte in transplanted tissue (*7*) and may provide the major immunogenic stimulus in a graft (*8*). The role of these cells in the recipient graft bed is unknown. In order to examine the importance of immune accessory cells in corneal transplantation, we have examined the cellular infiltrate in normal and deliberately vascularized, inflamed rabbit corneas by enzyme and immunoperoxidase staining, and have correlated the presence of accessory cells in both donor and recipient with subsequent corneal allograft survival.

MATERIALS AND METHODS

Experimental animals. Twelve-week-old virgin female rabbits of the New Zealand White strain were used as recipients of Colored strain donor corneas.

Corneal vascularization. Inflammation and vascularization were induced in some normal rabbit corneas by placing 8–0 braided silk sutures in each quadrant. Knots were left exposed. After 2–3 weeks, when vessels had grown into the cornea and anterior segment inflammation was evident, the sutures were removed and the animals grafted.

Corneal transplantation. Penetrating grafts 8 mm in diameter were performed as described elsewhere (*9*). Postoperatively, grafts were treated with one drop each of 1% atropine sulphate and 0.5% chloramphenicol daily for the first 12 days, after which the graft sutures were removed. No topical immunosuppression was administered. All animals were examined each day at the slit lamp, and the day of rejection was recorded. Rejection was defined as the first day when a rejection line was observed in a previously clear, thin graft, or the first day on which spreading edema was noted in the absence of such a line. Animals were killed once rejection was established, or at 100 days in the case of long-surviving grafts. All grafts were harvested for end-point histology. Survival data were analysed using the Mann-Whitney *U* test.

Enzyme and immunohistochemical staining. Cryostat-cut 6-μ sections of periodate-lysin-paraformaldehyde–fixed, snap-frozen material were examined (*3*). Both normal and vascularized, inflamed corneas were stained. Published methods were employed for ATP-ase (*10*) abnd β-glucuronidase (*11*) staining. Immunoperoxidase staining was performed using mouse anti-rabbit monoclonal antibodies together with a Vectastain ABC kit (Vector Laboratories) (*12*). Dual staining for immunoperoxidase and β-glucuronidase was performed on some sections.

Monoclonal antibodies. Antibody 2C4 (detecting class II MHC antigens) was the gift of Dr K. Knight (*13*). Antibodies M109 (detecting a leukocyte-common antigen); M107 (detecting an antigen present on 98% of a T cell line, on a majority of

[1] This work was supported by grants from the NH & MRC (No. 840518) and the O.R.I.A. K.A. Williams is supported by the Wellcome Trust.

[2] Address correspondence to: Dr. K. A. Williams, Dept. Ophthalmology, Flinders Medical Centre, Bedford Park S.A. 5042, Australia.

* Abbreviations used: IL-1, interleukin-1; MHC, major histocompatibility complex.

peripheral T cells, on a small subpopulation of thymocytes (<30%), and on less than 10% of B cells); M108 (detecting an antigen present on T cell blasts, on a majority of peripheral T cells, on less than 10% of B cells, and on a minor subpopulation of monocytes); and M110 (detecting an antigen present on 60–80% of thymocytes and on a small subpopulation of peripheral T cells, but absent from B cells and from a T cell line) were obtained from UCB-Bioproducts, Belgium (*14*). Antibody L 11/135 (American Type Culture Collection) detects an antigen present on all peripheral T cells (*15*). The characterization of LION 3A will be described elsewhere; however, the antibody reacts with approximately 60% of thymocytes and 50% of peripheral lymphocytes; is unreactive with monocytes, polymorphonuclear granulocytes, and platelets; and stains mononuclear cells in the T-dependent areas of lymph node and spleen. The negative control was culture supernatant from the mouse myeloma cell line P3653, used as fusion parent in the production of LION 3A.

Scoring of cells in corneal sections. Central and limbal areas of cornea were assessed separately. Counts of immunoperoxidase-positive cells were performed as described elsewhere (*3*). Briefly, however, cell counts were made over three randomly-selected fields of known area, in each of at least two duplicate corneal sections, using a microscope eyepiece grid; the number of immunoperoxidase-positive cells per square millimeter was then calculated.

RESULTS

Immunohistochemical staining. Immunoperoxidase staining of normal rabbit corneas demonstrated the presence of small numbers of cells bearing the leukocyte-common antigen in the central stroma and of increased numbers of such cells in the limbal stroma (Table 1). These cells were predominantly elongated, with large nuclei. The pattern of class II MHC antigen–positive cells was similar, with many cells exhibiting streaming, dendritic-like cytoplasmic processes. No class II antigen was observed on epithelial cells, keratocytes, or corneal endothelium. There were few cells with the nuclear morphology of neutrophils within either central or limbal stroma, and few cells positive for T cell markers.

Immunoperoxidase staining of vascularized and inflamed corneas (Table 1) demonstrated the presence, in the central stroma, of significantly increased numbers of M109-positive (anti-leukocyte-common antigen–positive) cells ($P<0.002$, 1-tailed t test), 2C4-positive (anti-MHC-class-II antigen–positive) cells ($P<0.001$, 1-tailed), LION 3A-positive (anti-T-cell-subset–positive) cells ($P<0.02$, 1-tailed), and L11/135-positive (anti-peripheral-T-cell–positive) cells ($P<0.002$, 1-tailed). There was no change in the number of M107, M108, or M110-positive (anti–T-cell-subset) cells in the vascularized, as compared with the normal, corneas. Vascular endothelial cells were identifiable morphologically, but were negative for all markers examined, including 2C4 (anti–MHC-class-II antigen), irrespective of whether the vessels were located in limbal or central cornea.

Enzyme staining. Enzyme staining of normal and prevascularized, inflamed rabbit corneas showed a significant increase in the number of cells positive for ATP-ase ($P<0.01$) in the central stroma of the vascularized corneas (Table 2), with numbers increasing towards the limbus. The increase in the number of β-glucuronidase-positive cells in the vascularized corneas did not reach significance at the 5% level. Cells positive for ATP-ase had a characteristic morphological appearance, with long processes streaming into the stroma. Those positive for β-glucuronidase were more heterogeneous and included some keratocytes (weakly positive), some cells with the nuclear morphology of polymorphonuclear granulocytes, some mononuclear cells, and some cells with long dendritic processes. Double staining indicated the presence of a population of β-glucuronidase-positive and leukocyte-common antigen-positive cells, as well as a population positive for the latter only.

Corneal graft experiments. Four contemporaneous groups were set up: group 1, normal avascular donor corneas transplanted into normal recipient beds; group 2, prevascularized donor corneas transplanted into normal recipient beds; group 3, normal donor corneas transplanted into prevascularized recipient beds; and group 4, prevascularized donor corneas transplanted into prevascularized recipient beds. Graft survival data are presented in Table 3. The median day to rejection differed significantly when group 1 was compared with groups 2 and 3 ($P<0.05$), and with group 4 ($P<0.002$). Groups 2 and 3 did not differ significantly from each other but did differ significantly from group 4 ($P<0.05$). End-point histology performed on all grafts confirmed that graft failure was consistent with rejection in every case.

DISCUSSION

The essential findings from this study were that cells with a morphological appearance and surface phenotype consistent with those of accessory cells were found in small numbers in normal central stroma of rabbit cornea, and in increased numbers in vascularized, inflamed corneas. The latter also showed an influx of T cells. Furthermore, the presence of accessory cells and T cells in either host or donor cornea was found to prejudice corneal allograft survival. The major phenotypic

TABLE 1. Immunoperoxidase staining of normal and vascularized, inflamed rabbit corneas

Monoclonal antibody	Type of cornea	Number	Number of positive cells/mm² (mean ± SD)	
			Central cornea	Limbal cornea
Negative control	Normal	10	0.0±0.0	0.2±0.5
	Vascularized	6	1.4±3.6	0.0±0.0
M109	Normal	10	2.7±2.1	170.1±101.4
	Vascularized	5	75.5±56.0	391.4±157.0
2C4	Normal	10	6.3±2.5	134.9±44.7
	Vascularized	6	48.0±18.7	237.2±52.3
LION 3A	Normal	10	0.9±1.4	11.3±9.0
	Vascularized	6	5.4±4.5	26.7±22.2
M107	Normal	5	0.8±1.3	2.3±2.3
	Vascularized	4	0.2±0.4	5.4±5.2
M108	Normal	6	1.0±1.6	2.3±2.3
	Vascularized	4	0.7±1.5	10.1±8.9
M110	Normal	6	0.6±1.2	1.5±2.1
	Vascularized	4	0.4±0.8	1.3±1.5
L11/135	Normal	6	0.7±1.2	33.4±17.8
	Vascularized	4	38.6±19.7	121.6±51.7

TABLE 2. Enzyme staining of normal and vascularized, inflamed corneas

Enzyme stain	Area of cornea	Number	Number of positive cells/mm² (mean ± SD)	
			Central cornea	Limbal cornea
ATP-ase	Normal	9	17.1±7.6	24.2±14.6
	Vascularized	3	40.3±6.6	23.3±3.4
β-glucuronidase	Normal	4	173.8±45.7	635.5±53.6
	Vascularized	4	413.8±53.7	914.8±161.5

TABLE 3. Effect of donor and recipient corneal prevascularization on penetrating corneal graft outcome

Donor cornea	Recipient cornea	Number	Day to rejection	Median day to rejection
Avascular, noninflamed	Avascular, noninflamed	8	22, 28, 62, 98,[a] 100, 100, 100, 100	100
Vascularized, inflamed	Avascular, noninflamed	9	12, 13, 17, 18, 20, 21, 21, 28, 100	20
Avascular, noninflamed	Vascularized, inflamed	14	15, 17, 18, 18, 21, 21, 21, 21, 42, 100, 100, 100, 100, 100	21
Vascularized, inflamed	Vascularized, inflamed	13	10, 12, 12, 12, 13, 13, 13, 14, 14, 15, 18, 18, 19	13

[a] Destroyed because of a damaged foot; graft in perfect condition.

markers of accessory cells in man, rat, and mouse include the leukocyte-common antigen and class II MHC antigens; there is general consensus that the presence of class II antigens is a requirement for effective antigen presentation (*16–22*). The distribution of class II MHC antigens on various accessory cells of the rabbit has recently been shown to be similar to that in the mouse (*23*).

Normal central corneal stroma in the rabbit was found to contain measurable numbers of cells bearing the leukocyte-common antigen. Approximately the same number of class II MHC antigen–positive cells were found, and, in view of their similarity in morphological appearance and anatomical distribution, it seemed likely that the one population was involved, although double staining was not performed. Most of these infiltrating cells had large, irregular-shaped oval nuclei and elongated cytoplasmic processes. They did not react with antibodies detecting various T cell markers. They were distinct from keratocytes which were smaller, slimmer, did not have stellate dendritic processes, and were negative for both leukocyte-common and class II MHC antigen markers. Staining and morphological characteristics were thus consistent with these cells being accessory cells, probably of the macrophage or dendritic lineage, scattered within the corneal stroma and epithelium. Precisely the same observations have been made in normal human cornea (*3, 24*).

Vascularized, inflamed corneas contained considerably more of these accessory-like cells, but the infiltrate was heterogeneous. There was a significant increase in the number of L11/135-positive cells in the absence of any increase in the number of cells positive for the T cell markers LION 3A, M107, M108, or M110. The L11/135 antigen is a marker of virtually all peripheral T cells (*15*) but has also been reported to react with some macrophages and neutrophils (*25*). Expression of some T lineage differentiation markers on accessory cells has been reported previously (*26, 27*). Cells bearing the L11/135 antigen in vascularized rabbit corneas comprised two distinct cell types—one population with the morphological appearance of accessory cells and the majority with the appearance of mononuclear cell blasts, presumably T blasts.

Further evidence for the heterogeneity of the infiltrate in vascularized, inflamed corneas came from investigation of the enzyme markers. The enzyme ATP-ase is a useful marker of the mouse epidermal Langerhans cell, but is not present in all murine dendritic cells (*28*). Cells positive for ATP-ase in rabbit cornea, all bore the morphological characteristics of accessory cells. Lysosomal β-glucuronidase is predominantly a marker of epidermal Langerhans cells (*29*), monocytes, macrophages, and reticuloendothelial cells (*30, 31*). Normal rabbit keratocytes were found to be weakly positive for β-glucuronidase, but occasional very strongly positive cells with accessory-cell-like morphology were also observed. Vascularized corneas contained both positive accessory cells and mononuclear cells.

The transplantation experiments reflect graft outcome under circumstances of varying infiltrating cell load in both donor button and graft bed. The median day to rejection among a group of normal rabbits grafted with normal donor tissue was greater than 100 days, with the majority of animals going on to bear long-surviving grafts, whereas the median day to rejection in a group in which the recipient bed had been prevascularized and inflamed prior to transplantation was 21 days. These two groups correspond to the clinical low-risk and high-risk groups respectively, and the results are similar to those reported by others (*32*). By contrast, in the contrived experimental situation in which a vascularized, inflamed cornea was transplanted into a normal graft bed, rejection occurred at the same tempo as it did when a normal button was grafted into a vascularized bed. This finding strongly implicates wandering cells—that is, nonstructural cells present in th cornea—as being of preeminent importance in corneal graft rejection. Deliberately vascularized cornea contains vascular endothelial cells (MHC class II antigen–negative) and more infiltrating leukocytes than does normal cornea; both of these cell types might be expected to affect graft survival simply by contributing to the total load of foreign histocompatibility antigen in the cornea.

Lafferty and colleagues have argued persuasively that two signals, specifically foreign antigen and the cytokine interleukin-1 (IL-1), are required for effective T cell activation. Activation generally occurs when antigen is presented to an antigen-reactive cell on the surface of an accessory cell (bearing autologous class II MHC antigens) that is capable of delivering the second signal, IL-1 (*33*). The allogeneic reaction is considered to reflect a special case in which donor-type cells bearing foreign MHC antigens and capable of producing IL-1, stimulate recipient T cells directly. Experimental evidence for this proposition has come from studies in which depletion of donor-type accessory cells from the graft by ultraviolet light (*34*), culture in oxygen (*35*), or pretreatment of donors with cyclophosphamide and x-irradiation (*36, 37*), has reduced the incidence of subsequent graft rejection. Furthermore, addition of donor-type accessory cells to an animal bearing a long-surviving allograft has been found to result in graft rejection (*8*). Probably both class I and II MHC antigens can stimulate allogeneic responses directly, provided they are present on a cell capable of making 1L-1, but class II antigens are the more effective.

In the context of the cornea, then, it might be expected that the accessory-like cells present, even in a normal cornea, could well be potent immunogens, and that increasing their numbers would affect rejection. This was indeed found to be the case. In the rabbit, donor-type accessory cells are more likely to be the strong stimulator cells than are vascular endothelial cells, as the latter were found not to carry class II antigens. Our results may provide an experimental foundation for the observations of the Dutch group, which has reported a greater incidence in rejection in large, compared with small, clinical grafts (*38*): the smaller and more central the donor button, the fewer the number of accessory cells likely to be transferred in the graft. However, patients requiring large corneal grafts are also likely to have more anterior segment disease—for example, glaucoma and aphakia.

The finding that inflammation and vascularization of the graft bed influence corneal graft survival is more difficult to explain. However, recent evidence has indicated that immune induction in allogeneic interactions can also take place through the classic pathway by which foreign class I and II antigens can be presented to alloreactive T cells by host accessory cells (*39*). We have suggested that recipient accessory cells contiguous with the graft margin may pick up, process, and present foreign histocompatibility antigens shed from the corneal graft to nearby T cells, thereby inducing host sensitization. In other words, the influx of immunologically competent cells that accompanies inflammation and vascularization renders the recipient bed a hostile place.

In the final experimental situation considered, in which both recipient and donor corneas were vascularized and inflamed, rejection consistently occurred early and within a narrow time span, considering the outbred nature of the model (median day 13, range 10–19 days), and there were no long-term survivors. Thus, immunogenicity of donor button and the presence of lymphocytes and accessory cells of hematological origin in proximity to the graft both determine the rate of initial sensitization, and together compound the inevitability of final graft destruction.

Acknowledgments. We thank S. Erikson and L. Noack for technical assistance, E. Andrea for preparing the manuscript, and W. Laffer for editorial assistance.

REFERENCES

1. Coster DJ. Factors affecting the outcome of corneal transplantation. Ann R Coll Surg Engl 1981; 63: 91.
2. Silverstein AM, Khodadoust AA. Transplantation immunobiology of the cornea. In: Porter R, Knight J, eds. Corneal graft failure. Ciba Foundation Symposium 15. Amsterdam: Elsevier, Excerpta Medica, North-Holland, 1973; 105.
3. Williams KA, Ash JK, Coster DJ. Histocompatibility antigen and passenger cell content of normal and diseased human cornea. Transplantation 1985; 39: 265.
4. Stingl G, Katz SI, Shevach EM, Rosenthal AS, Green I. Analogous functions of macrophages and Langerhans cells in the initiation of the immune response. J Invest Dermatol 1978; 71: 59.
5. Rodrigues MM, Rowden G, Hackett J, Bakos I. Langerhans cells in the normal conjunctiva and peripheral cornea of selected species. Invest Ophthalmol Vis Sci 1981; 21: 759.
6. Gillette TE, Chandler JW, Greiner JV. Langerhans cells of the ocular surface. Ophthalmology (Rochester) 1982; 89: 700.
7. Hart DNJ, Fabre JW. Demonstration and characterization of Ia-positive dendritic cells in the interstitial connective tissue of rat heart and other tissues, but not brain. J Exp Med 1981; 154: 347.
8. Lechler RI, Batchelor JR. Restoration of immunogenicity to passenger leucocyte-depleted kidney allografts by the addition of donor strain dendritic cells. J Exp Med 1982; 155: 31.
9. Williams KA, Grutzmacher RD, Roussel TJ, Coster DJ. A comparison of the effects of topical cyclosporin A and topical steroid on rabbit corneal allograft rejection. Transplantation 1985; 39: 242.
10. Juhlin L, Shelley WB. New staining techniques for the Langerhans cell. Acta Dermatov 1977; 57: 289.
11. Hayashi M, Nakajima Y, Fishman WH. The cytologic demonstration of β-glucuronidase employing naphthol AS-BI glucuronide and hexazonium pararosanilin; a preliminary report. J Histochem Cytochem 1964; 12: 293.
12. Hsu S-M, Raine L, Fanger H. Use of avidin-biotin-peroxidase complex (ABC) in immunoperoxidase techniques: a comparison between ABC and unlabeled antibody (PAP) procedures. J Histochem Cytochem 1981; 29: 577.
13. Lobel SA, Knight KL. The role of rabbit Ia molecules in immune functions as determined with the use of an anti Ia monoclonal antibody. Immunology 1984; 51: 35.
14. De Smet W, Brys L, Vaeck M, Hamers R. Monoclonal antibodies defining rabbit lymphocyte subpopulations. Protides Biol Fluids 1981; 29: 687.
15. Jackson S, Chused TM, Wilkinson JM, Leiserson WM, Kindt TJ. Differentiation antigens identify subpopulations of rabbit T and B lymphocytes. Definition by flow cytometry. J Exp Med 1983; 157: 34.
16. Van Voorhis WC, Hair LS, Steinman RM, Kaplan G. Human dendritic cells. Enrichment and characterization from peripheral blood. J Exp Med 1982; 155: 1172.
17. Pugh CW, MacPherson GG, Steer HW. Characterization of non-lymphoid cells derived from rat peripheral lymph. J Exp Med 1983; 157: 1758.
18. Steinman RM, Nussenzweig MC. Dendritic cells: features and functions. Immunol Rev 1980; 53: 127.
19. Van Voorhis WC, Valinsky J, Hoffman E, Luban J, Hair LS, Steinman RM. Relative efficacy of human monocytes and dendritic cells as accessory cells for T cell replication. J Exp Med 1983; 158: 174.
20. Klinkert WEF, LaBadie JM, Bowers WE. Accessory and stimulating properties of dendritic cells and macrophages isolated from various rat tissues. J Exp Med 1982; 156: 1.
21. Cowing C, Schwartz BD, Dickler HB. Macrophage Ia antigens. I. Macrophage populations differ in their expression of Ia antigens. J Immunol 1978; 120: 378.
22. Unanue ER, Beller DI, Lu CY, Allen PM. Antigen presentation: comments on its regulation and mechanism. J Immunol 1984; 132: 1.
23. Kapsenberg ML, Stiekema F, Leene W. Differential requirements for rabbit dendritic cells and macrophages in T lymphocyte proliferation induced by various mitogens. Immunology 1985; 55: 301.
24. Mayer DJ, Daar AS, Casey TA, Fabre JW. Localization of HLA-A,B,C and HLA-DR antigens in the human cornea: practical significance for grafting technique and HLA typing. Transplant Proc 1983; 15: 126.
25. Chen Z, Metzger DW, Adler FL. Characterization of a monoclonal antibody reactive with rabbit T lymphocytes and neutrophils. Cellular Immunol 1984; 85: 297.
26. Fithian E, Kung P, Goldstein G, Rubenfeld M, Fenoglio C, Edelson R. Reactivity of Langerhans cells with hybridoma antibody. Proc

Natl Acad Sci USA 1981; 78: 2541.
27. Wood GS, Warner NL, Warnke RA. Anti-leu-3/T4 antibodies react with cells of monocyte/macrophage and Langerhans lineage. J Immunol 1983; 131: 212.
28. Steinman RM. Dendritic cells. Transplantation 1981; 31: 151.
29. Mackenzie IC, Bickenbach JR, Rittman BR. Reactivity of epidermal Langerhans cells to a histochemical method for demonstration of β-glucuronidase. J Invest Dermatol 1982; 78: 239.
30. Hayashi M. Distribution of β-glucuronidase activity in rat tissues employing the naphthol AS-BI glucuronidase hexazonium pararosanilin method. J Histochem Cytochem 1964; 12: 659.
31. Lorbacher P, Yam LT, Mitus WJ. Cytochemical demonstration of β-glucuronidase activity in blood and bone marrow cells. J Histochem Cytochem 1967; 15: 680.
32. Khodadoust AA, Silverstein AM. Studies on the nature of the privilege enjoyed by corneal allografts. Invest Ophthalmol 1972; 11: 137.
33. Lafferty KJ, Andrus L, Prowse SJ. Role of lymphokine and antigen in the control of specific T cell responses. Immunol Rev 1980; 51: 279.
34. Lau H, Reemtsma K, Hardy MA. Prolongation of rat islet allograft survival by direct ultraviolet irradiation of the graft. Science 1984; 223: 607.
35. Lafferty KJ, Bootes A, Dart G, Talmage DW. Effect of organ culture on the survival of thyroid allografts in mice. Transplantation 1976; 22: 138.
36. McKenzie JL, Beard MEJ, Hart DNJ. Depletion of donor kidney dendritic cells prolongs graft survival. Transplant Proc 1984; 16: 948.
37. McKenzie JL, Beard MEJ, Hart DNJ. The effect of donor pretreatment on interstitial dendritic cell content and rat cardiac allograft survival. Transplantation 1984; 38: 371.
38. Volker-Dieben HJM. The effect of immunological and non-immunological factors on corneal graft survival. Doc Ophthalmol 1984; 57(1–2): 1.
39. Dutta D, Meeusen E, Boyle W. Indirect presentation of allogeneic major histocompatibility complex antigens by syngeneic macrophages. Transplant Proc 1985; 17: 1661.

Received 24 November 1985.
Accepted 13 February 1986.

0041-1337/86/4206-0671$02.00/0
TRANSPLANTATION
Vol. 42, No. 6
Printed in U.S.A.

EXPRESSION OF HLA ANTIGENS ON RENAL TUBULAR CELLS IN CULTURE

I. EVIDENCE THAT MIXED LYMPHOCYTE CULTURE SUPERNATANTS AND GAMMA INTERFERON INCREASE BOTH CLASS I AND CLASS II HLA ANTIGENS[1]

G. ALEX BISHOP, BRUCE M. HALL, MICHAEL G. SURANYI, DAVID J. TILLER, JOHN S. HORVATH, AND GEOFFREY G. DUGGIN

Department of Renal Medicine, Royal Prince Alfred Hospital, Missenden Road, Camperdown 2050 NSW, Australia

The altered expression of HLA antigens on tissues during rejection is of potential importance to both the initiation and effector arms of the alloimmune response. Associated with rejection episodes, renal tubular cell expression of HLA DR (class II) antigens has been observed to be markedly increased. In this study an in vitro assay using cultured renal tubular cells from normal human kidneys was developed. Monoclonal antibodies to detect HLA DR and HLA A,B,C (class I) molecules were used to identify these antigens on cultured tubular cells either by indirect immunofluorescence stains and flow cytometric analysis or by immunoperoxidase stains with cytological analysis. With these techniques normal cultured cells had little membrane or cytoplasmic HLA DR but did have membrane HLA A,B,C. Culture of renal tubular cells with either supernatants from mixed lymphocyte cultures or purified gamma interferon induced expression of HLA DR, with maximum expression occuring between day 4 and day 6. Increased HLA A,B,C expression was also observed. This increased expression of HLA antigens was shown not to be dependent upon increased cell division of the cultured cells, and removal of gamma interferon from the cultures resulted in a decay in both HLA DR and A,B,C expression within days. HLA expression was inhibited by addition of protein synthesis inhibitor cycloheximide, but not by the addition of puromycin, mitomycin C, or actinomycin D—which suggested that tubular cells had transcribed m RNA for both HLA DR and A,B,C antigens. Expression of HLA antigens was not inhibited by cyclosporine, corticosteroids, or azathioprine.

These studies demonstrate that the increased expression of HLA antigens seen in renal allografts at the time of rejection episodes can be explained by the release of lymphokines, especially gamma interferon, by infiltrating cells, and that reduced HLA DR expression of transplanted kidneys in patients treated with cyclosporine is

[1] This work was supported by grants from The National Health and Medical Research Council of Australia, The Australian Kidney Foundation, and the Lions Clubs of District 102N2.

not due to the drug directly inhibiting HLA expression by graft cells.

It is well established that there is a difference in the expression of class I (HLA A,B,C) and class II (HLA DR) HLA antigens on normal tissue (*1, 2*). HLA A,B,C antigens can be identified on the surface of nearly all nucleated cells, but HLA DR are only found on B cells, monocytes, macrophages, dendritic cells, Langerhans cells—and, in some species, on vascular endothelium. Although epithelial cells in normal tissue usually do not express HLA DR, they have been observed to do so in tissue with inflammatory changes (*3–5*).

In normal human kidneys there is some uncertainity as to the expression of HLA DR antigen on renal tubular cells. Initial reports could not demonstrate HLA DR on tubular cells (*2, 3*), although later studies using sensitive immunostaining techniques observed HLA DR on proximal tubular cells of many normal kidneys, particularly in the cytoplasm of these cells (*6–8*). In human renal allografts biopsies from allografts with minimal or no evidence of cellular rejection showed little or no expression of tubular cell HLA DR antigen, whereas biopsies from allografts with evidence of severe cellular rejection showed strong expression of HLA DR antigens (*3, 9, 10*). Kidneys from patients treated with cyclosporine tend to have less expression of HLA-DR antigens than those from azathioprine-treated patients (*10*). Similar expression of class II antigens on graft tissue has been shown in animal models of organ graft rejection (*11, 12*). These results parallel those in other immune-mediated diseases, such as thyroiditis (*4*) or graft-versus-host disease (*5*), in which tissues that are normally HLA DR-negative express HLA DR, and this expression is associated with a cellular infiltrate. In vivo it is not known whether the altered expression of HLA antigens is a direct result of immune effector mechanisms or a nonspecific response to tissue damage. However, it has been known for some time that activated T lymphocytes (*13*) and NK cells (*14*) can produce gamma interferon in vitro and that gamma interferon can induce HLA DR antigens on a variety of different cultured cell lines (*15–17*).

This study investigated whether expression of HLA DR antigen by tubular cells in rejecting human renal allografts is due to cell-mediated immune reactions associated with rejection, in particular lymphokines released from activated T cells. This report describes an in vitro model in which cultured human kidney cells can be induced to express HLA DR and increased amounts of HLA A,B,C antigen by filtered supernatants from mixed lymphocyte culture or purified gamma interferon. The kinetics of this increased expression of HLA antigens were examined, as were the effects of various metabolic inhibitors and immunosuppressive drugs on its induction. A preliminary report of part of this work has been published (*18*).

MATERIALS AND METHODS

Cell Cultures

Human kidney cell cultures. Human kidneys, some obtained at nephrectomy because of renal tumor and some donated for transplantation but unsuitable for use, were dissected aseptically to separate cortex. Diced cortical tissue was trypsinized at 37°C in a solution consisting of 0.25% trypsin and 0.05% EDTA in trypsin diluent, with 3 changes of solution over a period of 90 min. Trypsin diluent consisted of NaCl, 8.0 g/L; K Cl, 0.4 g/L; Na_2HPO_4, 0.06 g/L; KH_2PO_4, 0.06 g/L and $NaHCO_3$, 0.5 g/L. Trypsinized cells were centrifuged for 5 min at 300 ×g, and the cell pellet was resuspended in medium 199 (Flow Laboratories, North Ryde, N.S.W. Australia), supplemented with 2 mM glutamine, 15 mM HEPES, 50 U/ml Penicillin. 50 μg/ml Streptomycin and 20% heat-inactivated fetal calf serum (FCS)* (Flow Labs). Cells in medium 199 were cultured in 75-cm^2 plastic tissue culture bottles (Corning Glass Works, Corning, NY) or stored frozen in liquid nitrogen.

Cells were subcultured by washing with 0.05% EDTA in trypsin diluent and incubated with 0.25% trypsin plus 0.05% EDTA in trypsin diluent at 37°C for approximately 1 min, then gently washing the cells off the substrate. FCS was added to cells in suspension to a final concentration of 10%; then the suspension was centrifuged for 5 min at 300 ×g. The cell pellet was resuspended in medium 199 at a 1:3 split ratio.

For experiments to test induction of HLA DR antigens, cells from subculture were inoculated into 96-well flat-bottomed tissue culture trays (Falcon, Oxnard, CA).

Mixed lymphocyte culture. Peripheral blood was collected from healthy volunteers into ammonium heparin and diluted with an equal volume of mixed lymphocyte culture (MLC) medium. MLC medium consisted of RPMI 1640 medium (Flow Labs) plus L-glutamine, 2 mM; penicillin 50 U/ml; streptomycin 50 μg/ml; heparin 4 U/ml and HEPES buffer 20 mM. Diluted blood was layered over Ficoll/Hypaque (Pharmacia, N. Ryde, NSW, Australia) and centrifuged at 600 ×g for 20 min. The lymphocyte layer was collected and washed twice by suspension in MLC medium, followed by centrifugation at 300 ×g for 5 min. Lymphocytes were made to 1×10^6/ml with MLC medium plus 20% FCS, and stimulator lymphocytes were irradiated with 2500 rads. Stimulator and responder lymphocytes were cultured in bulk in 25-cm^2 plastic culture bottles; 5 ml of each was added on day 0, and 1 ml aliquots of the supernatant were removed daily and replaced with fresh medium. Aliquots were filtered through a 0.22-μ filter (Millipore) to remove cellular material, and stored at −70°C.

Culture of other cells. Human diploid fibroblasts (MRC 5, passage 32) and human epithelial cell cultures (Hep 2 unknown passage), a kind gift of Dr. M. Cloonan, Virology Dept., Prince Henry Hospital, Little Bay, Australia, were cultured as for renal epithelial cells.

Human vascular endothelial cells were prepared in primary culture by the method of Gimbrone (*19*).

Monoclonal Antibodies

The monoclonal antibodies used and their specificity were; HLA-D M1 (HLA DR), HLA A,B,C M1 (HLA A,B,C), F8 (factor VIII) (Australian Monoclonal Development Pty Ltd. Artarmon, N.S.W. Australia); I_2 (HLA DR), B_1 (B lymphocytes) (Coulter Electronics, Hialeah, FL); OKIal (HLA-DR), OKM_1 (monocytes), OKT_3 (T lymphocytes) (Ortho Pharmaceuticals, Raritan, NJ) and EMA (epithelial membrane antigen) (Dako, Copenhagen, Denmark).

Immunofluorescence stains of cultured cells. Cultured cells were trypsinized and washed in phosphate-buffered saline (PBS). Washed cells were resuspended in medium 199 plus 10% human A serum, and 50-μl aliquots were incubated with 5 μl of mouse monoclonal antibody. After 30 min on ice, cells were washed twice by addition of 2 ml PBS followed by cen-

* Abbreviations used: FCS, fetal calf serum; MLC, mixed lymphocyte culture; PBS, phosphate-buffered saline.

trifugation and aspiration of the supernatant. To the washed cell pellet was added 50 μl of a sheep-antimouse FITC conjugate (Silenus Laboratories, Dandenong, Victoria, Australia) and 20 μl of A serum. After 30 min on ice, cells were washed once in PBS and resuspended in PBS and analyzed by flow cytometry, with a Spectrum III flow cytometer (Ortho Diagnostics, Westwood, MA).

Immunoperoxidase stains of cultured cells. Cultured cells were trypsinized and washed in PBS, then resuspended in medium 199. Aliquots were cytocentrifuged onto microscope slides, fixed in buffered formal acetone, and stained by a four-step immunoperoxidase staining technique that has been described previously (*20*). Monoclonal antibodies were used at dilutions that had been previously shown to give reproducible staining (*3*).

Human interferon. Human gamma interferon purified from supernatant of PHA activated blasts was purchased from Cellular Products (Buffalo NY) and was free of PHA-P, and T cell and B cell growth factor. It had an initial specific activity of 1×10^6 IU/mg. Unless otherwise stated, the concentration of gamma interferon in these experiments was 20 IU/ml as assayed with a radioimmunoassay kit (Centocor Malvern, PA).

Metabolic inhibitor experiments. Actinomycin D, mitomycin C, and puromycin (Sigma) were added to cultures for 1 hr at concentrations within their range of biological activity (*21, 22*) or in separate experiments throughout the culture period. The cultures were then washed in the medium and exposed to gamma interferon for 4 days before expression of HLA DR antigens was assayed. Cycloheximide (Sigma), azathioprine (Wellcome, Cabarita NSW Australia), cyclosporine (a gift of Sandoz Australia, North Ryde, NSW Australia) and methylprednisolone (Upjohn, Rydalmere NSW Australia) were added at concentrations in the range that have been shown to have suppressive effect in vivo and vitro (*23, 24*). These chemicals were added with gamma interferon for the 4-day period of the culture.

RESULTS

Characterization of cultured human kidney cells. Human kidney cells could be subcultured at least 10 times but the results reported here are with cells at passage 4 or less. The identity of the low-passage-cultured cells was established as predominantly epithelial on the following criteria. The predominant cell in culture was cuboid, with morphology of epithelial cells. Colonies of small clusters of cells appeared attached to the culture flask within 24 hr and these grew to coalesce and produce a confluent monolayer by day 5 of culture. Electron microscopy of cultured kidney cells showed most cells had tight intercellular junctions, a feature unique to epithelial cells. Immunofluorescent or immunoperoxidase stains of cultured cells with EMA showed a variable proportion (35–70%) of the cultured human kidney cells stained, indicating that at least half the cultured cells were of tubular cell origin (Table 1). However EMA stains underestimate the proportion of tubular cells, as in immunoperoxidase stains of normal kidneys not all tubular cells were seen to react with EMA. In particular proximal tubular cells do not stain with EMA. Antibody to factor VIII, which reacts with cytoplasmic factor VIII in vascular endothelial cells did not stain cultured human kidney cells, but did stain control cultures of vascular endothelial cells in immunoperoxidase stains. This indicated that there were no cells of vascular endothelial origin in the cultured human kidney cells. Stains with lymphocyte-specific monoclonal antibodies OKT3, B_1, and monocyte-specific, OKMI, always stained less than 10% of cells in culture (Table 1). Early cultures morphologically had few or no fibroblast cells on light microscopy, but passage 4 cultures and later did have some fibroblast overgrowth. Thus the majority of other cells that were not positively identified by EMA were probably either renal tubular cells not expressing EMA or fibroblasts.

TABLE 1. Staining of cultured human kidney cells with a panel of monoclonal antibodies: comparison of cells prior to and after culture with human gamma interferon

Monoclonal antibody specificity	Name	After culture	Before culture
HLA DR	I2	51.3	4.3
HLA ABC	AMD ABC	98.2	95.9
Epithelial membrane antigen	EMA	57.8	46.6
Factor VIII	F8	4.8	3.9
Monocytes	OKM1	5.4	2.7
T lymphocytes	OKT3	5.8	3.2
B lymphocytes	BI	7.8	2.6
Antiinfluenza neuramidise	Control	5.7	3.2

Cultured human kidney cells were stained with monoclonal antibodies and analyzed by flow cytometry. Figures show percentage of cells labeled with each monoclonal antibody before culture and after culture for 4 days with human gamma interferon.

HLA antigen expression on human kidney cells after culture with MLC supernatant or gamma interferon. In all the cultures from 5 kidneys only a small proportion (<10%) of normal cultured human kidney cells stained positively for HLA DR, but all stained for HLA, A,B,C antigen. After culture with MLC supernatant or with gamma-interferon for 4 days, a large proportion (35–90%) of cells expressed HLA DR antigen when assayed either by immunofluorescence (Table 1) or immunoperoxidase staining (Fig. 1). HLA A,B,C intensity of expression was measured by mean channel of fluorescence on a cytofluorograph, and increased expression of HLA A,B,C antigens was also demonstrated. Human kidney cells from 5 different kidneys were assayed and all showed a similar pattern of induction of HLA antigens. Figure 2 shows a representative experiment that used day 6 MLC supernatant to induce HLA antigens; there were increased numbers of cells with HLA DR by day 2 of culture and this increased up to at least day 4. HLA A,B,C antigens increased slightly more rapidly. In 5 experiments similar results were obtained, with HLA A,B,C antigen expression always appearing before HLA DR. Similar results were obtained with gamma interferon.

Supernatants from day 1 through day 6 of MLC were taken to examine the time of appearance of the capacity of MLC supernatants to induce HLA expression of cultured kidney cells. Significant activity did not appear in the supernatant until day 3 of MLC, peaked at day 5, and persisted to day 6 (Fig. 3). In subsequent experiments day 5 or 6 MLC supernatants were used for induction of HLA antigens.

The increase in HLA antigen expression induced by gamma interferon or MLC supernatant was not accompanied by an increase in cell size as determined by light scattering properties on flow cytometry or on microscopic examination of the cultures. Thus the increased expression of HLA antigens appeared to be due to an increased density of HLA A,B,C and HLA DR molecules on the cell surface, and not due to an increase in the area of the cell membrane. In early cultures (passage 1–4) a greater proportion of cells (usually >60%) expressed HLA DR,

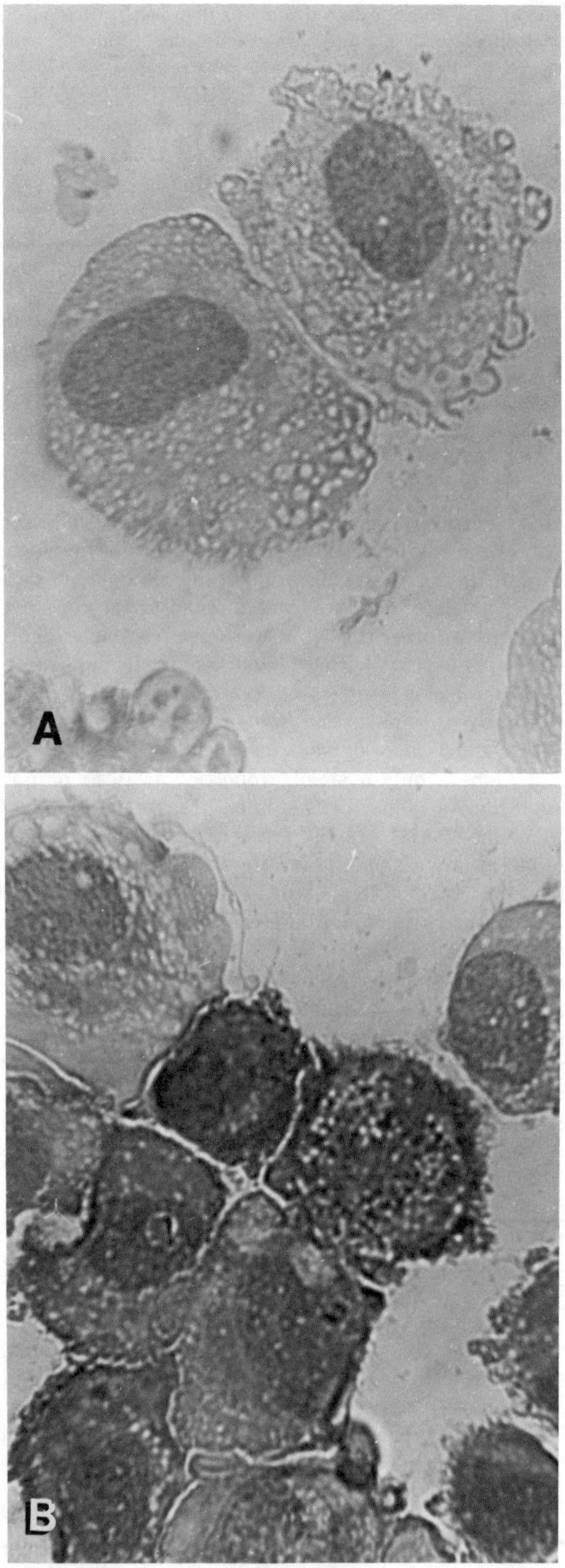

FIGURE 1. Immunoperoxidase stains of cultured human kidney cells stained to identify HLA DR antigen. Stained cells appear dark gray to black, while unstained cells appear light gray. (A) normal human kidney cells negative for HLA DR; (B) human kidney cells cultured for 4 days with MLC supernatant. Most cells express HLA DR antigen.

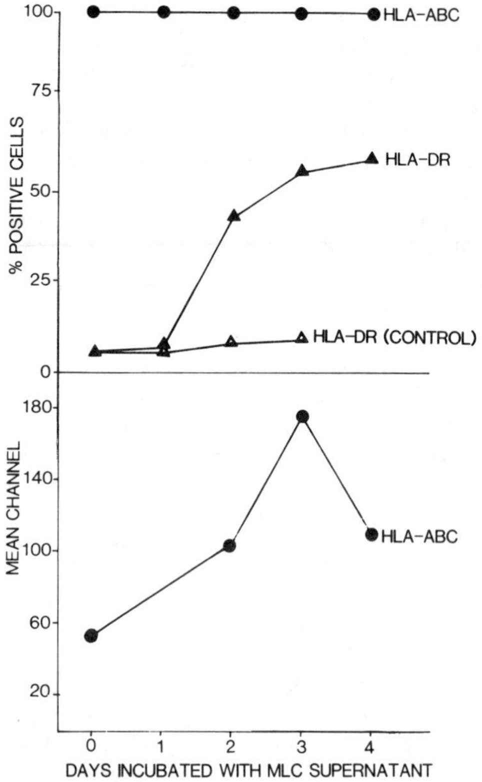

FIGURE 2. Time course of increase of HLA antigen expression by cultured human kidney cells after addition of mixed lymphocyte culture (MLC) supernatant. (●—●) cells stained to identify HLA A,B,C, antigens, (▲—▲) cells stained to identify HLA DR antigens. Cells were stained by an indirect immunofluorescence technique and analyzed by flow cytometry. Intensity of fluorescence of cells stained for HLA A,B,C, antigens was expressed as mean channel (lower panel) on a scale of increasing intensity from 0 to 225. Control cells were incubated without MLC supernatant.

compared with later passage cultures. This was probably due to the higher proportion of fibroblasts in late-passage cultures.

The possibility that gamma interferon affected the culture population to alter its constituent HLA-DR positive subpopulations was examined in three ways: by enumeration of the subpopulations of cells before and after exposure to lymphokine, by examination of the capacity of pure fibroblast cultures to express HLA antigens, and by examination of the effect of gamma interferon on cell proliferation.

Examination of the kidney cell culture subpopulations prior to and after exposure to gamma interferon. Cultured kidney cells were stained with a panel of monoclonal antibodies to identify cell populations prior to and after culture with gamma interferon (Table 1). There was little or no change in the proportion of cells defined by EMA or the markers for lymphocytes and monocytes counted on a cytofluorograph. After culture more than 50% of treated cells reacted with the EMA marker, which identifies some, but not all, renal tubular cells. Over 50% of all cells were HLA-DR-positive in treated cultures compared with 5% of cells in untreated cultures. The intensity of HLA ABC staining was also increased in the gamma-interferon-treated kidney cells. The cells remaining in culture had morphology similar to that of the pretreatment cultures, and no cells with cytoplasmic staining for factor VIII were identified in the

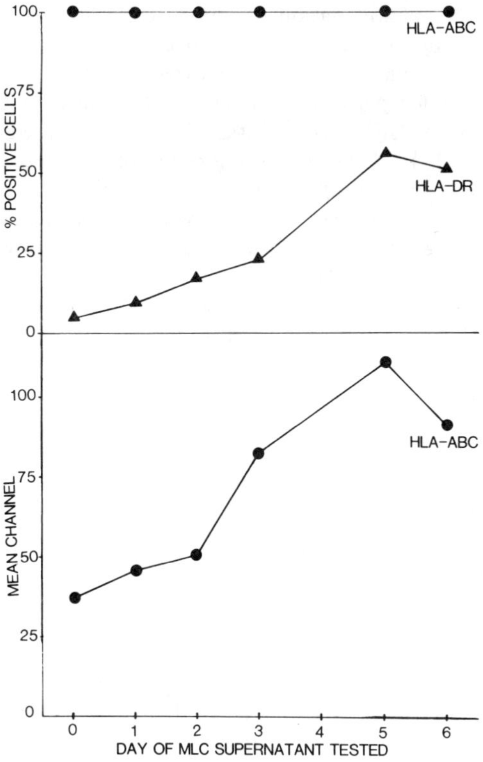

FIGURE 3. Time-course of development of the HLA antigen-inducing factor in mixed lymphocyte culture (MLC) supernatants. Human kidney cells were incubated for 4 days in the presence of MLC supernatant obtained from day 0 to day 6 of MLC. Treated cells were stained to identify HLA DR (▲—▲) and HLA A,B,C (●—●), and analyzed by flow cytometry. The percentage of HLA DR⁺ cells is shown in the top panel. Expression of HLA A,B,C is shown in the lower panel and is expressed as mean channel. Mean channel increases with increasing staining intensity on a scale from 0 to 255, which is a measure of intensity of staining recorded in the cytofluorograph. Significant HLA-antigen-inducing activity does not appear in MLC supernatants until days 2 or 3 of MLC, and peaks at day 5.

cultures either before or after gamma interferon treatment. These studies showed there was no change in the constituent cells in culture during treatment with gamma interferon and thus it was concluded that the cultured renal tubular cells treated with gamma interferon expressed HLA DR antigen.

Comparison of HLA antigen expression by cultured fibroblasts, epithelial cells, and kidney cells on exposure to gamma interferon. HLA-antigen expression by cultures of fibroblasts (MRC 5) and epithelial cells (Hep_2 carcinoma of larynx) induced with a range of concentrations of gamma interferon was compared with HLA antigen expression by human kidney cell cultures (Fig. 4). Fibroblasts had a moderate increase in intensity of expression of HLA A,B,C antigen that occurred at similar concentrations of gamma interferon to the increase in HLA A, B,C antigen of human kidney cell cultures. However, there was only a slight increase in HLA DR antigen expression by interferon-treated fibroblast cultures, in which about 25% of fibroblasts expressed HLA DR antigen at the maximum concentration of interferon. In contrast, approximately 90% of human kidney cells were HLA DR-positive at the highest concentration of gamma interferon. This result suggested that the increased HLA DR expression in renal tubular cell cultures was probably not due to the contaminating fibroblasts in the human kidney cell culture.

Hep_2 cultures showed a significant increase in HLA DR antigen with gamma interferon, and the percentage of cells expressing HLA DR antigen at maximum concentration of gamma-interferon was similar to that of human kidney cell cultures. Increased intensity of expression of HLA A,B,C antigen by Hep_2 cells was modest, with a maximum increase of approximately 80%, compared with approximately 200% for kidney cell cultures and approximately 100% for fibroblasts.

Increased HLA antigen expression was observed with concentrations of gamma interferon down to 0.5 units/ml, and nearly all cultured cells were induced to express increased HLA

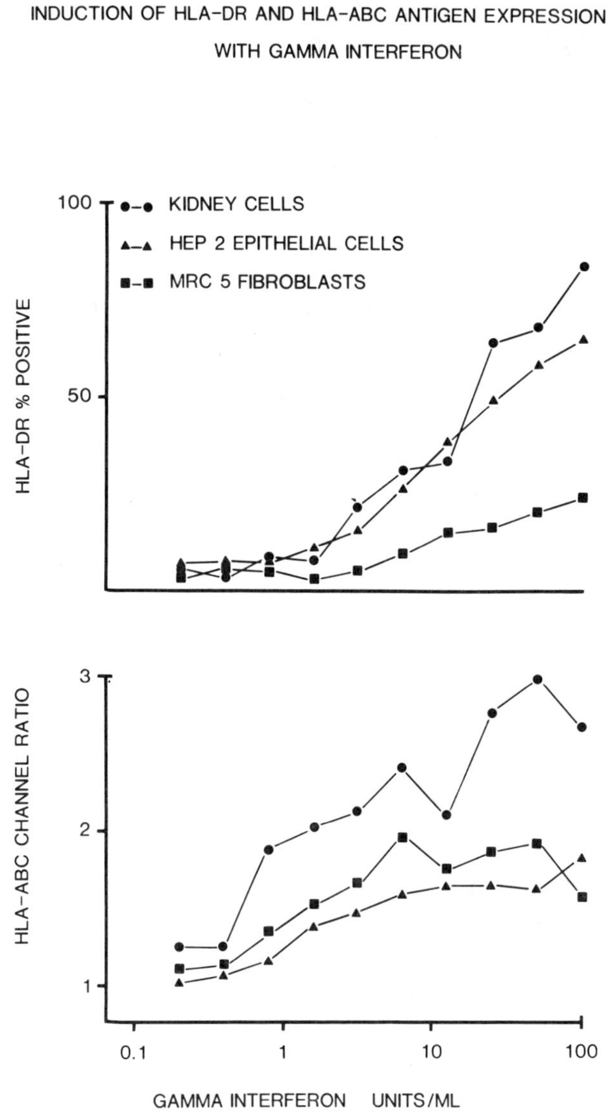

FIGURE 4. Induction of increased HLA antigen expression on three cultured human cell types by gamma interferon. Cells were incubated for four days with gamma interferon at a range of concentrations from 0.2 U/ml to 100 U/ml, then stained to identify HLA DR antigen (top panel) and HLA A,B,C antigen (lower panel). HLA A,B,C staining intensity is shown as channel ratio, which is calculated as a ratio of the mean channel of staining intensity of treated cells to the mean channel of staining intensity of untreated cells.

DR antigen at gamma interferon concentrations of about 20 U/ml. Half maximal stimulation for HLA DR was observed at a gamma-interferon concentration of approximately 10 U/ml and for HLA A,B,C at approximately 2 U/ml (Fig. 4).

Effect of gamma interferon on kidney cell replication. The possibility that HLA DR and HLA A,B,C antigen expression resulted from increased cell replication, induced by MLC supernatant or gamma interferon rather than a direct effect of gamma interferon on nondividing cells was examined. The incorporation of ^{3}H-thymidine, which is proportional to the rate of cell replication, and expression of HLA antigens of cultured kidney cells incubated with gamma interferon was examined at different time points (Fig. 5). There was a decreased incorporation of ^{3}H thymidine, after the addition of gamma interferon to cultured kidney cells, which suggested that gamma interferon does not increase HLA antigen expression by increasing cell division.

Time course induction and disappearance of HLA antigens. The rate of increase in expression of HLA A,B,C and DR antigens with time after addition of gamma interferon to kidney cell cultures is shown in Figure 5. No increase was observed in HLA DR antigen after one day, however there was a significant increase by day 2 and the amount of HLA DR expression peaked by days 4 or 5. Five experiments were performed to determine the time-course of induction of HLA A,B,C and HLA DR, and in each experiment HLA A,B,C always increased in intensity on day 1 before the appearance of HLA DR.

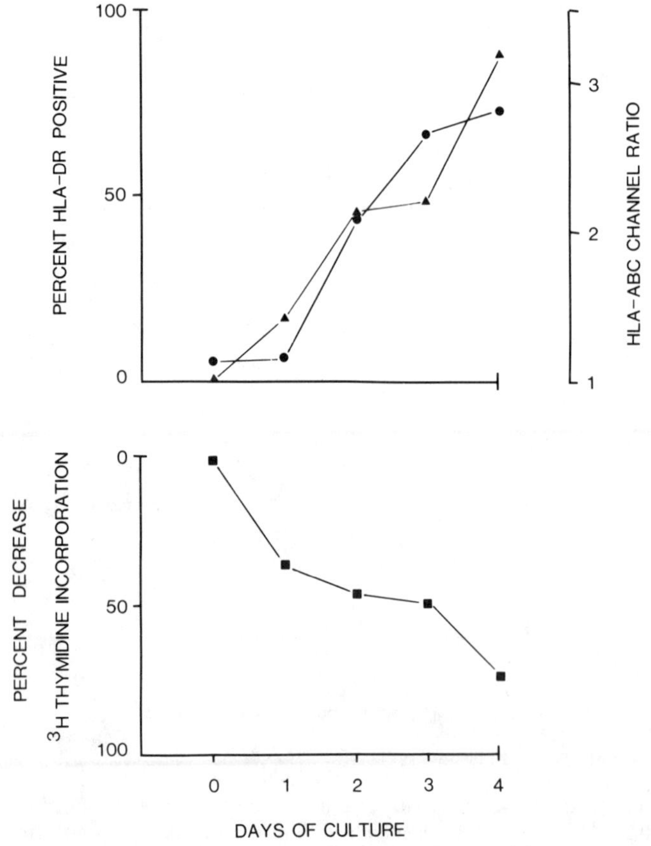

FIGURE 5. Comparison of the effects of gamma interferon treatment of human kidney cell cultures on HLA antigen expression (top panel), and cell replication as measured by ^{3}H thymidine incorporation (lower panel). Addition of gamma interferon causes a simultaneous increase in HLA antigen expression and a decrease in cell replication.

The effect of incubation of kidney cells for various times with MLC supernatants on the expression of HLA DR antigen is shown in Figure 6. Kidney cells were incubated with MLC supernatant for periods from 30 min to 6 days followed by removal of the MLC supernatant by repeated washing with medium 199. HLA DR antigen expression increased slightly with incubation periods as short as 30 min, and increased antigen expression was observed with increasing length of incubation period. Removal of the MLC supernatant resulted in a decrease of HLA DR antigen toward control values. Thus the expression of HLA DR antigens was dependent on the continued exposure of cells to MLC supernatant.

Attempts to inhibit gamma-interferon-induced expression of HLA DR antigens by cultured renal tubular cells. Metabolic inhibitors: Cultures were exposed to varing concentrations of actinomycin D, mitomycin C, puromycin, and cycloheximide (Table 2). Only cycloheximide significantly inhibited HLA DR antigen expression in concentrations that did not kill the cultured cells. Actinomycin D, mitomycin C and puromycin at concentrations low enough to allow continued cell viability did not inhibit HLA DR expression, and similar results were obtained whether they were removed after 1 hr or left in the culture. Cell survival was markedly reduced if inhibitors were left in the culture, however. Taken together these results suggest transcribed mRNA for HLA DR exists in renal tubular cells, and that increased expression of these antigens is only dependent upon increased protein synthesis.

Immunosuppressive drugs: Because kidney biopsies in patients treated with cyclosporine have less HLA DR expression

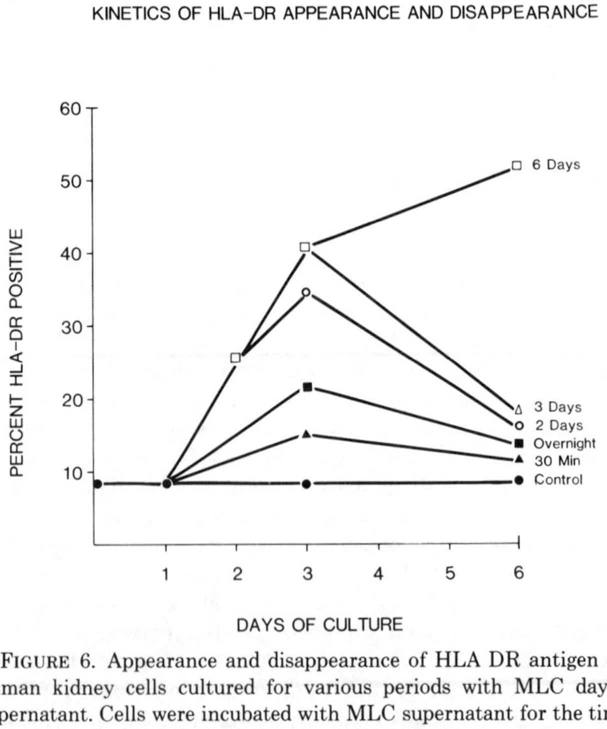

FIGURE 6. Appearance and disappearance of HLA DR antigen on human kidney cells cultured for various periods with MLC day 6 supernatant. Cells were incubated with MLC supernatant for the time shown, then washed thoroughly with medium 199 to remove the supernatant, then cultured in medium 199. Cells were stained to identify HLA DR antigen expression on day 3 and day 6 of culture. The percentage of cells expressing HLA DR antigen increased with time of incubation in MLC supernatant. Removal of supernatant resulted in a decrease of HLA DR antigen expression toward normal levels. Control cells were not treated with MLC supernatant.

TABLE 2. Effect of metabolic inhibitors on gamma-interferon-induced HLA antigen expression by human kidney cells[a]

	Concentration	Percentage of change in HLA antigen expression with metabolic inhibitor	
		Change in HLA DR[b]	Change in HLA A,B,C[c]
Actinomycin D	1 μg/ml	+2	+14
	0.5 μg/ml	+19	+46
	0.1 μg/ml	+16	+14
Mitomycin C	50 μg/ml	+15	+44
	5 μg/ml	−1	+119
	0.5 μg/ml	−11	+163
Puromycin	20 μg/ml	−11	+9
	2 μg/ml	−17	+5
	0.2 μg/ml	−12	+13
Cycloheximide	20 μg/ml	−99	−99
	2 μg/ml	−76	−91
	0.2 μg/ml	−46	−15
	0.02 μg/ml	+5	3

[a] Cultured human kidney cells were incubated with metabolic inhibitors and gamma interferon as described in the Materials and Methods section. The percentage of cells expressing HLA DR antigen and the intensity of expression of HLA A,B,C antigen as measured by mean channel of fluorescence intensity were determined by flow cytometry. Figures show % change of HLA antigen expression in cells treated with metabolic inhibitor and gamma interferon compared with a positive control of cells treated with gamma interferon alone.

[b] Change in percentage of cells stained for HLA DR.

[c] Change in the mean channel of fluorescence of cells stained for HLA A,B,C.

on renal tubular cells in mild-to-moderate rejection than occurs in azathioprine and corticosteroid-treated patients (*10*), the effects of these drugs on in vitro kidney cell expression of HLA DR was examined. Cyclosporine in the range 0.06–4 μg/ml or methylprednisolone in the range 1.56–100 μg/ml had no effect on the expression of HLA DR antigen. Azathioprine caused a moderate decrease in the percentage of cells expressing HLA DR antigen at the highest concentration tested (40 μg/ml) but had no effect at lower concentrations. Overall HLA DR antigen expression induced by gamma interferon in the presence of these agents was similar to that induced by gamma interferon alone.

DISCUSSION

In tissues that do not normally express HLA DR antigens it has been shown that during cell mediated immune attack such as allograft rejection these tissues can express these antigens. In this study we have demonstrated that human kidney cells in culture can be induced to express HLA DR by exposure to lymphokines released from alloactivated T cells, in particular gamma interferon.

There is some contention as to whether normal kidney tubular cells express HLA DR antigen or not (*1, 6–8, 25*). Flow cytometric analysis, a method that will only detect cell surface antigens showed that less than 10% of cultured kidney cells from all five cultured kidneys express HLA DR antigen. This low level of expression by a minority of cells may be due to their nonspecific staining due to the uptake of phenol red from the tissue culture medium (*26*) or a minority HLA DR$^+$ population. It thus appears that the human kidney tubular epithelial cells, which constitute the bulk of cells in primary culture, do not express cell membrane HLA DR antigens. Immunoperoxidase staining of normal kidney cultures using fixed cytological preparations, a method that can identify cytoplasmic HLA DR, also did not reveal any HLA DR antigen expression.

In contrast, cultured kidney cells that had been treated with MLC supernatant or purified gamma interferon showed strong HLA DR staining. Flow cytometry showed moderate-to-strong HLA DR staining of the treated cells, confirming that at least part of the HLA DR expression was confined to the plasma membrane. There was also an increase in HLA A,B,C (class I) antigen expression on the plasma membrane after treatment. A partially purified preparation of gamma interferon was as effective as MLC supernatant, which indicates that the effect of MLC supernatants in increasing kidney cell HLA expression is mediated at least in part by gamma interferon it contains. A cloned gamma interferon would provide absolute proof. These findings with human kidney cells are similar to those reported with a variety of other cultured cells—including human vascular endothelial cells (*27*), dermal fibroblasts (*28*), macrophages (*29, 30*), and melanoma (*15*) and carcinoma (*16*) cell lines on which gamma interferon has been shown to induce HLA DR and increased amounts of HLA A,B,C antigens.

In primary and low-passage cultures of kidney cortex cells there is a mixture of cell types, although there is a preponderance of tubular cells. We could not demonstrate an alteration in the basic population of cells in culture after MLC supernatant or gamma interferon treatment, with renal tubular cells the majority cell before and after treatment. Cell division per se, or an overgrowth of a minority population with high HLA expression did not account for this increase in HLA expression. The absence of a requirement for cell division was confirmed with the metabolic inhibitor studies, which suggest the expression of HLA DR in rejecting kidneys is not due to regeneration of damaged tubular cells but is probably a direct consequence of lymphokines released in the rejection process.

The course of expression of increased HLA antigens was similar when either MLC supernatant or gamma interferon were used for induction. It is also similar to that observed with tumor cell lines, melanoma (*31*), and other epithelial cell lines. In our experiments HLA A,B,C antigens increased slightly before HLA DR. Removal of gamma interferon resulted in a decrease of HLA antigen expression toward normal levels. This suggests the higher expression of HLA is dependent upon persistent exposure of the cell to gamma interferon. A similar reduction in renal tubular expression of HLA DR in vivo has been seen after the successful treatment of rejection (*20*). From these studies it could be concluded that appearance of HLA DR in kidney grafts may occur days after the appearance of the infiltrate of activated T cells that releases gamma interferon, and will also take days to subside after elimination of activated T cells on successful treatment of rejection.

Studies with metabolic inhibitors suggested that DNA transcription was not necessary and that renal tubular cells have preformed mRNA for both the HLA DR and HLA A,B,C antigens. The protein synthesis inhibitor cycloheximide blocked production of these antigens by renal tubular cells. These results are in contrast to those of Wong et al. (*17*) who were able to inhibit HLA DR antigen expression by brain cells with inhibitors of DNA transcription, and of Collins et al. (*28*) who detected de novo synthesis of mRNA in human endothelial cells and dermal fibroblasts with gamma interferon. The difference may be due to the fact that normal renal tubular cells have a low expression of HLA DR, particularly in the cytoplasm

(*6–8*), that is difficult to detect with indirect immunostaining techniques. If this is the case these cells would have the mRNA for HLA-DR and would only require protein synthesis to increase the expression of HLA DR. Other cells, such as brain and fibroblasts, which have no natural expression of HLA DR, would need to synthesize new mRNA. Taken together, these findings show that renal tubules have the mechanisms in place to produce HLA DR antigens, but that without lymphokine stimulation they do not always produce sufficient molecules for it to be detected, and that without continued stimulation the expression of HLA DR antigens wanes.

Neither cyclosporine nor methylprednisolone in concentrations known to suppress other immune functions in vitro or in vivo affected induction of HLA antigen expression on renal tubular cells by gamma interferon or MLC supernatants. This is similar to the findings of Groenewegen et al. (*26*) that cyclosporine could not inhibit MLC supernatant induced expression of HLA DR antigens on vascular endothelium, but if added to the MLC itself it can reduce the efficacy of the supernatant to induce HLA DR expression. Thus the observed lower frequency and intensity of HLA DR antigens on renal tubular cells of kidney allografts in patients treated with cyclosporine (*10*) compared with that in patients treated with azathioprine, cannot be attributed to a direct effect of cyclosporine on graft cells. However this effect may be due to cyclosporine inhibiting the release of gamma interferon from activated T cells (*26, 32*).

These findings in vitro correlate with the in vivo finding that, in T-cell-mediated inflammation, both HLA A,B,C and DR antigen expression is increased in tissue. This has been seen in renal allograft rejection in man (*3, 9*) and mice (*11*), in heart graft rejection in rats (*12*), in graft-versus-host disease (*5*), and in autoimmune diseases such as thyroiditis and primary biliary cirrhosis (*4*). After the T cell attack has subsided, the increased expression of HLA DR antigens persists for days to weeks, but in the absence of further cellular infiltrate will return to normal levels (*20*).

The relevance of the capacity of activated T cells to release gamma interferon that in turn induces increased expression of HLA antigens, has not been resolved. There are two potentially important consequences in terms of the immune response. First, HLA DR (class II) MHC expression may give cells the capacity to act as antigen-presenting cells and activate a greater immune response against the graft, as has been shown to happen with cultured vascular endothelial cells after induction of HLA DR (*33*). Second, and probably more important, is that the increased number of MHC antigens on graft cells increase the potential target molecules that effector T cells may recognize. Although the role of increased HLA expression in allograft rejection is yet to be established, it is unlikely that it will have beneficial consequences for the indefinite survival of the allograft.

Acknowledgments. We thank Jenny Waugh for her technical assistance and Karen Hynes for typing the manuscript.

REFERENCES

1. Koyama K, Fukunishi T, Barcos M, Tanigaki N, Pressman D. Human Ia-like antigens on non-lymphoid organs. Immunology 1979; 38: 333.
2. Hayry P, Von Willebrand E, Andersson LC. Expression of HLA-ABC and DR locus antigens on human kidney, endothelial, tubular and glomerular cells. Scan J Immunol 1980; 11: 303.
3. Hall BM, Bishop GA, Duggin GG, Horvath JS, Philips J, Tiller DJ. Increased expression of HLA DR antigens on renal tubular cells in renal transplants: relevance to the rejection response. Lancet 1984; 2: 247.
4. Hanafusa T, Pujol-Borrel R, Chiovato L, Russell RCG, Doniach D, Bottazzo GF. Aberrant expression of HLA DR antigen on thyrocytes in Graves' disease: relevance for autoimmunity. Lancet 1983; 2: 1111.
5. Lambert IA, Suitters AJ, Chisholm PM. Expression of Ia antigen on epidermal keratinocytes in graft-versus-host disease. Nature 1981; 293: 149.
6. Hancock WW, Kraft N, Atkins RC. The immunohistochemical demonstration of major histocompatibility antigens in the human kidney using monoclonal antibodies. Pathology 1982; 14: 409.
7. Fuggle SV, Errasti P, Daar AS, Fabre JW, Ting A, Morris PJ. Localization of major histocompatibility complex (HLA-ABC and DR) antigens in 46 kidneys. Transplantation 1983; 35: 385.
8. Daar AS, Fuggle SV, Fabre JW, Ting A, Morris PJ. The detailed distribution of MHC class II antigens in normal human organs. Transplantation 1984; 38: 293.
9. Hayry P, Von Willebrand E, Ahonen J, Eklund B. Do well-to-do and repeatedly rejecting renal allografts express the transplantation antigens similarly on their surface? Scand J Urol Nephrol 1981; 64 suppl: 52.
10. Bishop GA, Hall BM, Duggin GG, Horvath JS, Sheil AGR, Tiller DJ. Immunopathology of renal allograft rejection analysed with monoclonal antibodies to mononuclear cell markers. Kidney Int 1986; 29: 708.
11. Benson EM, Colvin RB, Russell PS. Induction of Ia antigens in murine renal transplants. J Immunol 1985; 134: 7.
12. Milton AD, Fabre JW. Massive induction of donor-type Class I and Class II major histocompatibility complex antigens in rejecting cardiac allografts in the rat. J Exp Med 1985; 161: 98.
13. Kasahara T, Hooks JJ, Dougherty SF, Oppenhein JJ. Interleukin 2- mediated immune interferon production by human T cells and T cell subsets. J Immunol 1983; 130: 1984.
14. Trinchieri B, Matsumoto-Kobayashi M, Clark SC, Seehra J, London L, Perussia B. Response of resting human peripheral blood natural killer cells to interleukin 2. J Exp Med 1984; 160: 1147.
15. Houghton AN, Thomson TM, Gross D, Oettgen HF, Old LJ. Surface antigens of melanoma and melanocytes. Specificity of induction of Ia antigens by human gamma-interferon. J Exp Med 1984; 160: 255.
16. Schwartz R, Momburg F, Moldenhauer G, Dorken B, Schirrmacher V. Induction of HLA class II antigen expression on human carcinoma cell lines by IFN-gamma. Int J Cancer 1985; 35: 245.
17. Wong GH, Bartlett PF, Clark-Lewis I, McKimm-Breschkin JL, Schrader JW. Interferon-gamma induces the expression of H-2 and Ia antigens on brain cells. J Neuroimmunology 1985; 7: 255.
18. Bishop GA, Suranyi MG, Hall BM, Duggin GG, Tiller DJ, Horvath JS. Induction of HLA-DR antigens on cultured human kidney cells. Transplant Proc 1986; 18: 290.
19. Gimbrone MA, Cotran RS, Folkman J. Human vascular endothelial cells in culture. Growth and DNA synthesis. J Cell Biol 1974; 60: 673.
20. Bishop GA, Hall BM, Philips J, et al. Expression of HLA DR antigens on renal tubular cells during rejection. Transplant Proc 1985; 17: 64.
21. Dianzani F, Zucca M, Scupham A, Georgiades JA. Immune and virus-induced interferons may activate cells by different derepressional mechanisms. Nature 1980; 283: 400.
22. Kuwata T, Fuse A, Morinaga N. Effects of cycloheximide and puromycin on the antiviral and anticellular activities of human interferon. J Gen Virol 1977; 37: 195.
23. Larsson EL. Cyclosporin A and Dexamethasone suppress T cell responses by selectively acting at distinct sites of the triggering process. J Immunol 1980; 124: 2828.
24. Dupont E, Wybran J, Toussaint C. Glucocorticosteroids and organ

transplantation 1984; 37: 331
25. Scott H, Brandtzaeg P, Hirschberg H, Solheim BG, Thorsby E. Vascular and renal distribution of HLA-DR like antigens. Tissue Antigens 1981; 18: 195.
26. Groenewegen B, Buurman WA, Jeunhomme GMAA, Van Der Linden CJ. Effect of Cyclosporine on MHC class II antigen expression on arterial and venous endothelium in vitro. Transplantation 1985; 40: 21.
27. Pober JS, Gimbrone MA, Cotran RS, et al. Ia expression by vascular endothelium is inducible by activated T cells and by human gamma-interferon. J Exp Med 1983; 157: 1339.
28. Collins T, Korman AJ, Wake CT, et al. Immune interferon activates multiple class II major histocompatibility complex genes and the associated invariant chain gene in human endothelial cells and dermal fibroblasts. Proc Nat Acad Sci USA 1984; 81: 4917.
29. Steeg PS, Moore RN, Johnson HM, Oppenheim JJ. Regulation of murine macrophage Ia antigen expression by a lymphokine with immune interferon activity. J Exp Med 1982; 156: 1780.
30. Becker S. Interferons as modulators of human monocyte-macrophage differentiation. I. Interferon-gamma increases HLA-DR expression and inhibits phagocytosis of zymosan. J Immunol 1984; 132: 1249.
31. Carrel S, Schmidt-Kessen A, Giuffre L. Recombinant interferon-gamma can induce the expression of HLA-DR and DC on DR negative melanoma cells and enhance the expression of HLA-ABC and tumor-associated antigens. Eur J Immumol 1985; 15: 118.
32. Palacios R, Martinez-Maza O, Deley M. Production of human interferon (HU IFN-gamma) studied at the single cell level. Origin, evidence for spontaneous secretion and effect of Cyclosporin A. Eur J Immunol 1983; 13: 221.
33. Wagner CR, Vetto RM, Burger DR. Subcultured human endothelial cells can function independently as fully competent antigen presenting cells. Hum Immunol 1985; 13: 33.

Received 10 December 1985.
Accepted 13 February 1986.

0041-1337/86/4206-0679$02.00/0
TRANSPLANTATION
Vol. 42, No. 6
Printed in U.S.A.

COMPARISON OF THE IMMUNOSUPPRESSIVE EFFECTS OF CYCLOSPORINE, LIPID-SOLUBLE ANESTHETICS, AND CALMODULIN ANTAGONISTS

RESPONSE TO EXOGENOUS INTERLEUKIN 2[1]

STEPHEN J. LEGRUE,[2] AND C. GWYNETH MUNN

The Department of Immunology, The University of Texas M. D. Anderson Hospital and Tumor Institute at Houston, Houston, TX 77030

The purpose of these investigations was to compare the immunosuppressive mechanism of cyclosporine (CsA) with those of lipid-soluble local anesthetics and calmodulin antagonists. Chlorpromazine (CPZ) and pentobarbital (PB) both inhibit lymphocyte activation by attenuating sodium and potassium ion potentials. CPZ and N-(6-aminohexyl)-5-chloro-1-naphthalene sulfonamide (W-7) can also block calcium-dependent activation processes by inhibition of calmodulin and protein kinase C. All four compounds were found to suppress human and murine lymphoproliferation to both alloantigen or mitogen in a dose-dependent and saturable manner. Exogenous interleukin-2 (IL-2) restored mitogenic responsiveness to cultures suppressed using W-7 and CsA, but not to lymphocytes suppressed with either CPZ or PB. Cytofluorographic analysis revealed that the degree of suppression in drug-treated lymphocytes was significantly correlated with the surface expression of receptors for transferrin and interleukin-2. Inhibition of IL-2 activation by PB was demonstrated to result from a blockade of the mitogenic growth factor signal using the IL-2-dependent cell line HT-2. Thus, the mechanism of action of cyclosporine can be differentiated from those of anesthetic immunosuppressants at the level of responsiveness to interleukin-2. The data support the hypothesis that cyclosporine may be an antagonist of calmodulin that selectively blocks early events in T lymphocyte activation leading to IL-2 synthesis, but does not inhibit the expression or function of the IL-2 receptor.

Cyclosporine (CsA)* is a cyclic endecapeptide of fungal origin that has proved extremely effective as an immunosuppressive

[1]This work was supported in part by the University of Texas Cancer Foundation.

[2]To whom correspondence should be addressed, at the Department of Immunology, The University of Texas M. D. Anderson Hospital and Tumor Institute, at Houston, 6723 Bertner Ave., Box 178, Houston, TX 77030.

*Abbreviations used: CsA, cyclosporine; CPZ, chlorpromazine; PB, pentobarbital; W-7, N-(6-aminohexyl)-5-chloro-1-naphthalene sulfonamide hydrochloride; IL-2, interleukin-2; Con-A, concanavalin-A; FBS, fetal bovine serum; HEPES, N-2 hydroxyethylpiperazine-N-2-ethane sulfonic acid; MLC, mixed lymphocyte culture; PBL, peripheral blood lymphocytes; IL-2R, interleukin-2 receptor; TfR, transferrin receptor; TPA, 12-O-tetradecanoylphorbol-13-acetate.

agent in organ transplantation (*1*). In vitro studies of CsA-induced immunosuppression have demonstrated that the drug inhibits the production and release of monokines and lymphokines (*2, 3*) by the specific blockage of messenger RNA transcription (*4–6*). The exact mechanism of this transcriptional blockade remains obscure, but recent evidence (*7*) suggests that binding of CsA to calmodulin may be involved (see *Note added in proof* below).

We have previously demonstrated that the hydrophobic CsA molecule does not associate with lymphocyte membranes via a specific receptor, but by partitioning into the lipid bilayer (*8*). Although others have postulated the involvement of specific plasma membrane or cytoplasmic receptors (*9–11*), we have hypothesized that CsA might exert its suppressive effects by disruption of membrane hyperpolarization and ion fluxes during the earliest stages of lymphocyte activation (*8, 12–15*). If this model is correct, CsA would be acting much like a lipid-soluble anesthetic (*16*). The purpose of this study was to test directly our hypothesis for a membrane involvement in the mechanism of CsA-induced unresponsiveness to alloantigens and to the polyclonal T cell mitogen Con-A.

There is ample evidence, both in vitro and in vivo, that lipid-soluble phenothiazines and barbiturates can be profoundly immunosuppressive at concentrations that also induce local anesthesia (*17–21*). Suppression by PB is thought to result primarily from the disruption of membrane hyperpolarization through the blockade of voltage-gated Na^+/K^+ and Ca^{2+} channels (*16, 19, 22, 23*). In addition to blocking voltage-gated ion channels, phenothiazines such as CPZ also bind to and inactivate calmodulin (*24, 25*). In contrast, immunosuppression mediated by the naphthalene sulfonamide derivative, W-7, is thought to result from its antagonistic effect on both calmodulin and protein kinase C activity (*26–29*). Thus, these compounds provide models to distinguish between a membrane-stabilizing, a calmodulin-antagonizing, and a protein kinase C-antagonizing mechanism of CsA-mediated immunosuppression.

MATERIALS AND METHODS

Lymphocytes. Murine splenocytes were harvested aseptically from specific-pathogen-free C57BL/6 (Animal Production Facility, Frederick, MD) and C3H/HeN (Charles River, Kingston, NY) mice using Lympholyte M (Accurate Chemical Co, Westbury, NY). Normal human peripheral blood mononuclear cells (PBL) from one author (S.J.L.) were isolated using Lymphoprep (Nyegaard, Oslo, Norway). The IL-2-dependent cell line, HT-2, was obtained from Dr. Susan Rich (Baylor College of Medicine, Houston, TX), and cultured as described by Watson (*30*).

Pharmaceuticals. Cyclosporine was a product of Sandoz (Basel, Switzerland) and was the kind gift of Dr. David Drath (The University of Texas Medical School at Houston, TX). A stock solution of 10^{-3} M CsA in ethanol was used to prepare dilutions for culture. Thus, a medium containing the highest concentration of CsA used in these studies (10^{-6} M) also contained 1% ethanol (*8*). Chlorpromazine-hydrochloride (25 mg/ml) was obtained as a sterile aqueous solution from Smith-Klein-Beckman (Philadelphia, PA), stabilized with 6 mg/ml NaCl, 2 mg/ml ascorbic acid, 1 mg/ml sodium bisulfite, and 1 mg/ml sodium sulfite. Sodium pentobarbital (50 mg/ml) was obtained as a sterile solution (40% propylene glycol, 10% ethanol) from Abbott Laboratories (North Chicago, IL). W-7 was obtained from Sigma (St. Louis, MO). Ethanol and 1-butanol were analytical grade reagents. Drugs and alcohols were diluted into serum-free RPMI-1640 medium (Gibco, Grand Island, NY) and stored at 4°C in the dark.

Rat IL-2 was purchased as a lyophilized, lectin-free preparation from Collaborative Research (Lexington, MA). It was reconstituted using RPMI-1640 medium supplemented with 2% serum to a final concentration of 200–250 units/ml.

Mixed lymphocyte culture (MLC). Isolated splenocytes from C57BL/6 and C3H/HeN mice were used for one-way MLC studies (*31*). C3H stimulator spleen cells were treated with mitomycin C (Sigma Chemical, St. Louis, MO), and 5×10^5 C3H cells in RPMI-1640 medium were seeded into 96-well flat-bottomed microtiter plates with 1×10^6 C57BL/6 responder cells in the presence of titered drug concentrations. Cultures were incubated for 96 hr in RPMI-1640 containing 2% fetal bovine serum (FBS). Cultures were pulsed with 1 μCi [^{3}H]-thymidine (33 Ci/mmol) for 18–24 hr and harvested onto glass-fiber filters prior to counting. The stimulation index of unsuppressed MLCs was always greater than 25.

Mitogen blastogenesis. Splenocytes from C57BL/6 mice or normal PBL were incubated with 1 μg/ml Con-A (Pharmacia, Piscataway, NJ) in RPMI-1640 medium containing 2 mM L-glutamine, 20 mM HEPES buffer pH 7.2, 50 μM 2-mercaptoethanol, and 2% heat-inactivated serum. Murine cells were incubated with FBS, whereas human cells received pooled human A/B serum. Titered concentrations of drug and IL-2 were added in a constant volume. Controls were incubated with Con-A alone or without mitogen. For proliferation studies, 5×10^5 cells were grown in flat-bottomed microtiter wells. After 3 days of incubation, cultures received 0.5 μCi [^{3}H]-thymidine for 6–8 hr prior to harvest onto glass-fiber filters. During 14 separate experiments using both human and murine lymphocytes, Con-A-stimulated lymphoblasts incorporated (mean ± SE) 160,440±28,762 cpm of [^{3}H]-thymidine, and unstimulated cells incorporated 2635±574 cpm of [^{3}H]-thymidine, yielding a median stimulation index of 80.3 (range: 46.7–151.5). The percent suppression attributable to the presence of drug was calculated using the formula: % suppression = 1 − (cpm drug − cpm spont.)/(cpm control − cpm spont.) × 100. Statistical significance was determined using Students' *t* test on the individual percentage values of replicate assays, transformed to the arcsine to provide a normal distribution.

Flow cytometry. Human cells used for cytofluorographic analysis were cultured in 24-well Costar (Cambridge, MA) plates at a density of 5×10^6 cells/well in 2 ml RPMI-1640 medium. After 3 days of mitogen culture in the presence or absence of drugs, aliquots were removed and pulsed with [^{3}H]-thymidine to confirm the immune status of the cells. The remaining cells were pooled and stained with fluorescein-isothiocyanate-conjugated monoclonal antibodies specific for the IL-2 receptor (IL-2R) and for the transferrin receptor (TfR). These antibodies were kindly provided by Dr. Christopher Snow of the Becton Dickenson Co. (Sunnyvale, CA). The percentage of cells expressing these cellular activation markers was determined using an Ortho Spectrum III flow cytometer (Ortho, Westwood, NJ).

RESULTS

Anesthetic-induced immunosuppression. The immunosuppressive activities of several lipid-soluble local anesthetics and calmodulin antagonists were compared with that of CsA (Fig.

1). All six of the compounds examined yielded sigmoidal curves for the inhibition of lymphoproliferation, as measured by the incorporation of [^{3}H]-thymidine into macromolecular DNA. No significant differences were observed in the abilities of the compounds to block either human or murine allospecific or mitogen-driven lymphoproliferation. As previously reported (*17, 19*), the suppression was not due to cytotoxic effects of the drugs, since treated and untreated cultures displayed similar abilities to exclude trypan blue.

The concentration range of ethanol and butanol yielding 10% to 90% suppression of [^{3}H]-thymidine incorporation (Fig. 1) closely paralleled the concentrations reported to affect nerve function and plasma membrane fluidity (Table 1). PB induced suppression of lymphoproliferation at concentrations 10-fold below those reported to affect membrane structure (*16*). However, the observed suppression engendered by PB was in the concentration range reported to be effective in blocking voltage-gated Na^+ and Ca^{2+} channels (*22*). Interestingly, log-fold lower concentrations of PB ($\leq 2\times10^{-5}$ M) consistently enhanced mitogen-stimulated [^{3}H]-thymidine incorporation by 10% to 20% (data not shown). Together, these results (Table 1) suggest that simple alcohols act by virtue of their membrane stabilizing effects, while the suppressive activity of PB is attributable to inhibition of ion channel function.

CPZ was suppressive at concentrations (1–10 μM) that have been reported to inhibit calmodulin and protein kinase C activation (*32–34*), as well as inhibiting voltage-gated Ca^{2+} channels (*35*). The calmodulin antagonist W-7 was active at 10–100 μM concentrations, where it inhibits calmodulin-dependent cascades, but not those regulated by protein kinase-C or cyclic nucleotide-dependent kinases (Table 1). These latter kinases require 0.1–1 mM concentrations of W-7 to block their activity (*28*). The dose-response curve for CsA spanned two logs of concentration, from 1 to 100 nM (Fig. 1). CsA has been reported to block Ca^{2+}-dependent lymphocyte activation at the lower boundaries of this range, and to inhibit TPA activation at higher concentrations (Table 1).

Interleukin-2 rescue of drug-induced suppression. The known sensitivity of CsA-suppressed lymphocyte cultures to rescue by exogenous IL-2 (*2, 3, 36, 37*) suggested a method to compare the effects of CPZ, PB, and W-7 with that of CsA. Murine splenocytes were cultured with Con-A in the presence of high or intermediate doses of each drug, and with or without 4 units of rat IL-2 (Fig. 2). The presence of IL-2 throughout the culture

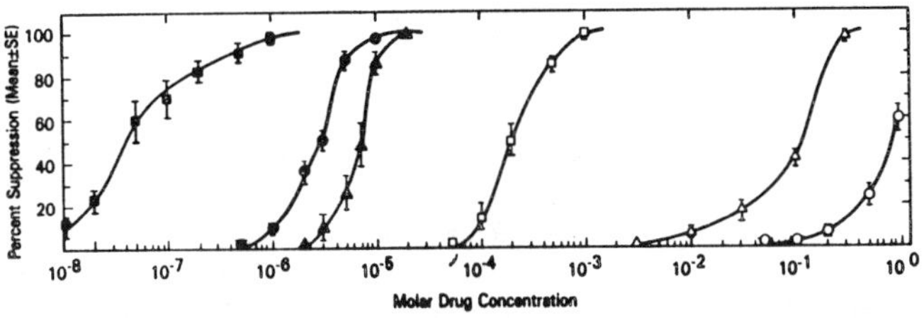

FIGURE 1. Titration of immunosuppressive lipid-soluble anesthetics, calmodulin antagonists, and cyclosporine. The percent suppression of alloantigen or mitogen-driven proliferation of human or murine lymphocytes engendered by titered doses of ethanol (○), butanol (△), pentobarbital (□), W-7 (▲), chlorpromazine (●), and cyclosporine (■) are presented. Values are the mean ± SE of three (ethanol and butanol) to eleven separate determinations for each compound.

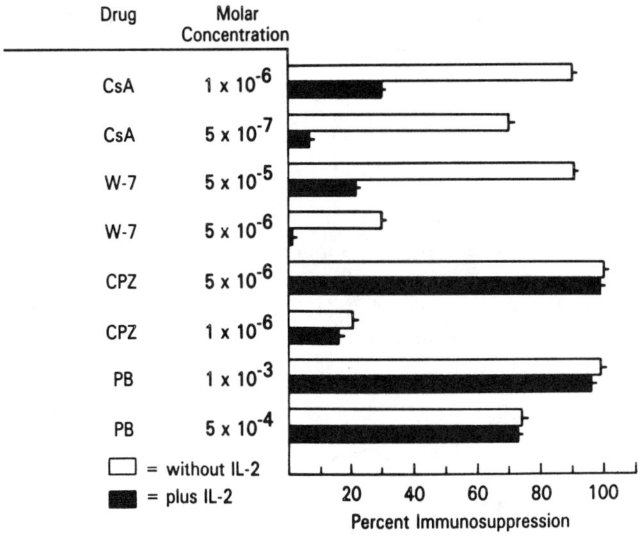

FIGURE 2. Effects of exogenous IL-2 on drug-mediated suppression of Con-A lymphoproliferation. Murine splenocytes were cultured for 3 days in the presence of the indicated drug concentrations, with or without 4 units of IL-2 added at time zero. The release from CsA- and W-7-induced suppression in the presence of IL-2 was statistically significant (*P*<0.01). Values are the means of three separate determinations.

TABLE 1. Anesthetic, immunosuppressive, and inhibitory activities of investigational drugs

Drug	C_{block}[a]	AH_{50}[b]	SD_{50}[c]	CaM[d]	PKC[e]	cXMP[f]	Channels[g]	References
Ethanol	5×10^{-1}	6×10^{-1}	7×10^{-1}	None	None	None	None	*16*
Butanol	7×10^{-2}	4×10^{-2}	8×10^{-2}	None	None	None	None	*16*
Pentobarbital	2×10^{-3}	2×10^{-3}	2×10^{-4}	ND[h]	ND	ND	3×10^{-4}	*16, 17, 19, 22*
Chlorpromazine	1×10^{-5}	1×10^{-5}	3×10^{-6}	1×10^{-5}	1×10^{-5}	None	1×10^{-5}	*16, 17, 24, 25, 32–35*
W-7	ND	ND	7×10^{-6}	1×10^{-5}	3×10^{-4}	2×10^{-4}	ND	*7, 28, 29*
Cyclosporine	ND	ND	5×10^{-8}	5×10^{-8}	1×10^{-6}	ND	ND	*2, 3, 6, 7, 40, 41, 43, 44*

[a] The molar concentration necessary to block frog sciatic nerve function.
[b] The molar concentration necessary to reduce hypotonic hemolysis by 50%.
[c] The molar concentration yielding a 50% reduction in lymphoproliferation (cf. Fig. 1).
[d] The molar concentration yielding a 50% reduction in calmodulin-dependent activation cascades or Ca^{2+} ionophore-mediated cellular activation.
[e] The molar concentration yielding a 50% reduction in protein kinase C-dependent activation cascades or phorbol-ester-mediated cellular activation.
[f] The molar concentration yielding a 50% reduction in cyclic nucleotide-dependent protein kinase activity.
[g] The molar concentration yielding a 50% reduction in voltage-gated ion flux.
[h] ND: not determined.

period significantly increased lymphoproliferation at both concentrations of W-7 and CsA. However, IL-2 had no effect on lymphocytes suppressed with either CPZ or PB. Titration of IL-2 concentrations from 0.2 to 4 units/culture effected a dose-dependent increase in lymphoproliferation of both W-7 and CsA-treated cells, but again had no significant effect on either CPZ or PB suppression (Fig. 3). When the degree of CsA- or W-7-induced suppression was 80%, 4 units of IL-2 completely restored the proliferative response to Con-A, as measured by incorporation of [^{3}H]-thymidine. At higher drug concentrations exogenous IL-2 could only effect a partial restoration of the proliferative response to lectin. Analogous results were obtained when drug-treated human PBL were incubated with exogenous IL-2 (data not shown).

Expression of IL-2R and TfR markers. The observed unresponsiveness of CPZ- and PB-treated lymphocytes to exogenous IL-2 might have been due either to a lack of IL-2 receptor expression or to an inability to transduce the proliferative stimulus following IL-2 binding. To test these possibilities, human PBL were stimulated with Con-A in the presence or absence of CsA, CPZ, W-7, or PB, and the membrane expression of the IL-2R and TfR lymphocyte activation markers was assessed by flow cytometry. For all four drugs, the percentage of cells binding anti-IL-2R and anti-TfR monoclonal antibodies showed a strong inverse correlation with the degree of drug-induced immunosuppression (Fig. 4). The coefficients of correlation (r) between percent suppression and the proportion of cells reacting with anti-IL-2R antibodies were as follows: CsA, r = −0.990; W-7, r = −0.995; CPZ, r = −0.977; PB, r = −0.964 (P<0.001 for each drug). When the data for all four compounds were pooled, r=−0.946 (P<0.001). Similarly, the coefficients of correlation between percent suppression and the proportion of cells reacting with the anti-TfR antibodies were: CsA, r = −0.963; W-7, r = −0.949; CPZ, r = −0.926; PB, r = −0.945 (P<0.001 for each drug). When the data for all four compounds were pooled (Fig. 4), the correlation between proliferation and TfR expression was −0.912 (P<0.001). Thus, the ability of drug-treated lymphocytes to proliferate in response to mitogen was strongly correlated with the expression of the cell surface T cell activation markers IL-2R and TfR.

The unresponsiveness of PB- and CPZ-treated cultures to exogenous IL-2 might also result from an inability of the lymphokine-receptor complex to transduce the mitogenic signal. To investigate this possibility, we employed the IL-2-dependent T lymphocyte cell line, HT-2 (Table 2). CsA affected IL-2-dependent growth only at the highest concentrations, where effects of the ethanol vehicle can also be documented (Table 1). Similarly, W-7 and CPZ were active only at high concentrations, and did not induce a significant reduction in

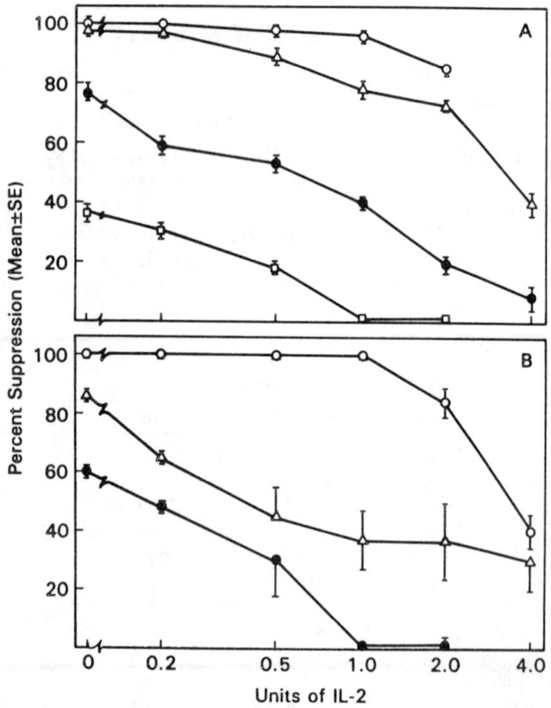

FIGURE 3. Titration of IL-2 activity. Murine spleen cells were cultured for three days with Con-A in the presence of CsA or W-7, with titered doses of rat IL-2. *A*: Splenocytes were stimulated in the presence of 5×10^{-7} M CsA (○), 2×10^{-7} M CsA (△), 5×10^{-8} M CsA (●), or 2×10^{-8} M CsA (□); *B*: Splenocytes were stimulated in the presence of 1×10^{-5} M W-7 (○), 7×10^{-6} M W-7 (△), or 5×10^{-6} M W-7 (●).

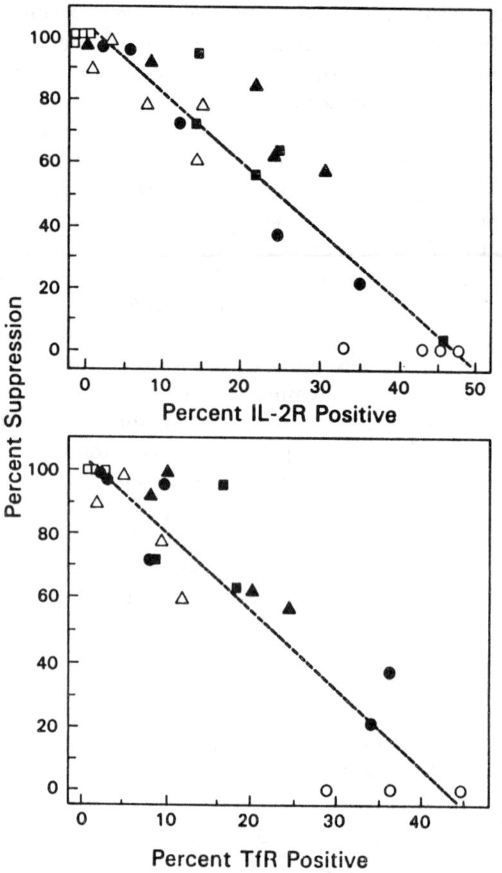

FIGURE 4. Correlation diagrams of percent suppression versus the expression of T cell activation markers. Human PBL were stimulated with Con-A in the presence of various concentrations of CsA (△), W-7 (●), CPZ (■) or PB (▲). Control cultures received Con-A alone (○) or no mitogen (□). After 3 days, aliquots were removed from each culture and pulsed with [^{3}H]-thymidine to determine the degree of immunosuppression. The remaining cells were analyzed by flow cytometry for expression of the IL-2 receptor (panel A), or for expression of the transferrin receptor (panel B). The coefficient of correlation (r) for IL-2R expression pooled from the data for all four drugs was −0.946 (P<0.001). The pooled coefficient of correlation for TfR expression was −0.912 (P<0.001).

TABLE 2. Effect of immunosuppressive drugs on IL-2 stimulation of HT-2 cells[a]

Drug concentration	cpm × 10^{-3} (mean ± SE)	Percent suppression	Level of significance
None	128.9±8.6		—
5×10^{-8}M CsA	126.4±9.6	2.7%	NS[b]
1×10^{-7}M CsA	120.4±2.7	9.2%	NS
1×10^{-6}M CsA	97.8±7.3	33.7%	NS
2×10^{-6}M W-7	121.1±4.9	8.4%	NS
5×10^{-6}M W-7	122.1±13.9	7.4%	NS
7×10^{-6}M W-7	117.3±6.5	12.6%	NS
1×10^{-5}M W-7	102.9±8.0	28.1%	NS
2×10^{-5}M W-7	56.0±4.0	78.7%	<0.005[c]
5×10^{-5}M PB	135.1±15.2	−6.6%	NS
1×10^{-4}M PB	86.1±9.7	45.7%	<0.05[c]
2×10^{-4}M PB	78.4±6.7	54.6%	<0.01[c]
5×10^{-4}M PB	52.0±3.7	83.0%	<0.005[c]
1×10^{-3}M PB	20.3±0.2	117.3%	<0.001[c]
5×10^{-7}M CPZ	124.6±0.3	4.7%	NS
1×10^{-6}M CPZ	130.4±10.1	−1.5%	NS
3×10^{-6}M CPZ	119.4±3.9	10.3%	NS
1×10^{-5}M CPZ	70.2±5.1	63.4%	<0.005[c]

[a] Triplicate microtiter cultures containing 5×10^{-4} HT-2 cells and 2.5 units/ml of rat IL-2 were incubated for 18 hr in the presence or absence of immunosuppressive drugs. Cultures were pulsed with [^{3}H]-thymidine and incubated for and additional 8 hr prior to harvest. Unstimulated cells incorporated 36.3±3.8. cpm ($\times10^{-3}$) of radiolabel.

[b] NS: not statistically significant.

[c] Statistically significantly different from controls receiving 2.5 units/ml of IL-2.

growth factor activity at concentrations that blocked mitogen-driven proliferation (Fig. 1). The ability of IL-2 to stimulate the proliferation of HT-2 cells, but not normal Con-A lymphoblasts in the presence of CPZ suggests that these models are not completely analogous, owing to the pleiotrophic activities of CPZ. PB inhibited IL-2-dependent growth of HT-2 cells (Table 2) at the same concentrations that blocked mitogen activation of normal lymphocytes (Fig. 1).

DISCUSSION

The extremely hydrophobic structure of CsA is consistent with a mechanism in which the drug enters the cell by partitioning into the phospholipid bilayer of the lymphocyte plasma membrane. We have previously demonstrated that the association of CsA with lymphocytes and phospholipid vesicles exhibits similar kinetics and affinity (*8*). We had hypothesized that CsA may exert its selective effects on lymphocyte function at the level of the plasma membrane, much like a lipid-soluble local anesthetic (*16*).

The binding of antigen or mitogen to receptors on the T lymphocyte plasma membrane initiates several metabolic cascades that eventually result in lymphokine production and blastogenesis through the elicitation of various second messengers. Activation systems may include voltage-gated or receptor-operated Na^+, K^+, or Ca^{2+} channels (*13, 22, 23*), cyclic nucleotide-dependent protein kinases, and protein kinases that are activated subsequent to the hydrolysis of phosphatidylinositol-4,5-bisphosphate to diacylglycerol and inositol trisphosphate (*38, 39*). The latter group of kinases include the Ca^{2+}/calmodulin-activated kinases and the Ca^{2+}/phospholipid-dependent protein kinase C. Lymphocyte activation can also be achieved using the protein kinase C activator TPA or the calcium ionophore A23187, either alone or together (*6, 29, 39, 40–43*).

The two alcohols and four drugs under investigation are all hydrophobic immunosuppressives that inhibited both mitogen- and alloantigen-driven lymphoproliferation of human and murine cells. Our results are in good agreement with previously published studies of these compounds (*2, 3, 8, 16–20, 26, 27, 36*). Alcohols, CPZ and PB are thought to act as local anesthetics by partitioning into the phospholipid phase of the plasma membrane, where they can uncouple the generation of action potentials (*16–19, 25, 29*). The significantly lower concentration of CPZ needed to suppress mitogen- or lymphokine-driven proliferation suggests that a simple membrane stabilizing mechanism is not responsible for the observed activity. PB and CPZ have also been reported to block K^+ and Ca^{2+} channels (*22, 25*) at concentrations that inhibited mitogen stimulation.

CPZ and W-7 can also interfere with both arms of the polyphosphoinositide-diacylglyceride activation cascade (Table 1). CPZ and W-7 block Ca^{2+}-dependent enzyme activation, at concentrations that inhibited mitogen-driven lymphoproliferation, by binding to hydrophobic enzyme interaction sites (*7, 24, 27, 34, 44, 45*). CPZ and W-7 can also inhibit protein kinase C activation by competitively inhibiting the binding of phospholipid (*28, 29, 32, 33*). We observed that mitogen stimulation was blocked using concentrations of W-7 that also inhibit calmodulin activity (*34*), but 10-fold below those required to inhibit protein kinase C and cyclic nucleotide-dependent kinases (*28*). However, CsA does not inhibit Ca^{2+} and phospholipid-dependent protein kinase C isolated from rat brain (Shenolakar S and LeGrue S., unpublished observations).

Recently, CsA has been reported to bind to and inactivate calmodulin by a Ca^{2+}-dependent mechanism (*7*). Furthermore, W-7 competitively inhibited the association CsA with calmodulin, suggesting a common binding site on the hydrophobic face of the protein exposed after Ca^{2+} binding. These workers did not investigate other activation cascades that are known to be sensitive to W-7. The available evidence is thus consistent with CsA, CPZ and W-7 sharing multiple sites of action on calmodulin, and possibly other target enzymes. The Ca^{2+}-dependent inactivation of calmodulin by CsA would explain the lack of evidence for an effect of CsA on intracellular Ca^{2+} concentrations during activation (*8, 12, 46*), because the drug would block activation at a site following Ca^{2+} mobilization (See *Note added in proof* below).

Transduction of the mitogenic signal following the association of IL-2 with its receptor has been reported to be either dependent (*47*) or independent (*48*) of changes in cytoplasmic free Ca^{2+}. Recent evidence suggests that IL-2 stimulation activates pathways distinct from those used during the initial stimulation by antigen or mitogen, because the combination of TPA and ionophore A23187 cannot substitute for the unique lymphokinetic signal provided by IL-2 (*49*). A calmodulin-independent mechanism for IL-2 stimulation is consistent with the reported calmodulin-binding properties of W-7 and CsA.

Suppression engendered by either W-7 or CsA could be partially or totally reversed, in a dose-dependent manner, by the addition of exogenous IL-2. Suppression of mitogen stimulation mediated by PB or CPZ was refractory to rescue by exogenous IL-2. The inability of lymphocytes to respond to IL-2 in the presence of PB was confirmed using the lymphokine-dependent cell line HT-2. Immunosuppressive concentrations of PB reduced the proliferative response of HT-2 cells to resting levels. Only the highest concentrations of CsA, CPZ, and W-7 could significantly reduce IL-2-dependent growth. The responsiveness of CPZ-treated HT-2 cells to IL-2 was in contrast to the results obtained using mitogen-stimulated murine splenocytes, and may be due to metabolic differences between the lymphokine-dependent cell line and normal murine lymphocytes, or to CPZ inhibition of metabolic processes in normal lymphocytes not directly related to IL-2 stimulation. Together, these results suggest a role for either protein kinase C or voltage-gated ion channels during IL-2 stimulation, independent of calmodulin activity.

Partial inhibition of lymphoproliferation by all four drugs was inversely correlated with an intermediate expression of the IL-2R and TfR T lymphocyte activation antigens. The responsiveness of CsA and W-7-treated splenocytes to exogenous IL-2, despite reduced expression of IL-2R, may reflect a lymphokine-dependant increase in receptor expression, or a preponderance of functional high affinity receptors in the remaining population (*50*).

Other investigators have also examined the effect of CsA on the expression of the T lymphocyte activation antigens IL-2R and TfR (*36, 51*). Miyawaki et al. (*36*) reported that, using an immunoperoxidase assay, the binding of anti-Tac antibody to mitogen-stimulated T lymphocytes was not affected by CsA concentrations up to 4×10^{-6} M, while reactivity with OKT9 anti-TfR antibodies was significantly reduced. Conversely, Lillehoj et al. (*51*) demonstrated by flow cytometry that 72 hr after addition of CsA to mitogen-stimulated murine splenocytes, the expression of IL-2 and transferrin receptors was significantly inhibited. Interestingly, after only 24 hr of mitogen activation in the presence of CsA, expression of both activation markers was normal. However, these authors were not able to rescue CsA-treated cultures using exogenous IL-2 (*51*). This observation is in sharp contrast to our results, and those reported by others (*2, 3, 36*). Our results do support those of Lillehoj et al. concerning the drug dose-dependent inhibition of IL-2 receptor expression 72 hr after initiation of culture (*51*). Furthermore, we have demonstrated a strict relationship for CsA and W-7 between the degree of drug-induced suppression of lymphoproliferation, the expression of the IL-2R activation marker, and responsiveness to exogenous IL-2.

The results presented here are consistent with a mechanism in which CsA exerts its suppressive action by mimicking lipid-soluble inhibitors of calmodulin. Furthermore, our evidence confirms that mitogen activation and IL-2 stimulation use different pathways. CPZ, W-7, and CsA enter the cell passively by partitioning into the lipid bilayer (*8, 16*), and probably inhibit key enzymes in the activation cascades by competitively binding to hydrophobic sites (*28, 29, 32, 33*). The differential sensitivity of PB- and CsA-suppressed lymphocytes to rescue by exogenous IL-2 argues against the hypothesized (*8*) direct effect of CsA on membrane hyperpolarization, although inhibition of voltage-gated K^+ channels or passive Ca^{2+} channels is consistent with the available evidence (*13, 23*). Further "drug-mapping" experiments should elucidate the pharmacologic mechanisms of these and other compounds in immune suppression.

Note added in proof. After submission of this manuscript, we directly evaluated the biological significance of CsA binding to calmodulin (LeGrue SJ, Turner R, Weisbrodt N., Dedman JR. Does the binding of cyclosporine to calmodulin result in immunosuppression? Science 1986; 234: 68.). Although we could document that CsA does bind to calmodulin in a Ca^{2+}-dependent manner, both active and inactive cyclosporine isomers were equipotent and could not inhibit calmodulin activity at immunopharmacologically relevant concentrations. Thus we do not favor calmodulin as a primary intracellular target for the action of CsA.

Acknowledgments. We are grateful to Sharon Pawlowski and Tasi-Ling Sheu for technical assistance, and to Alice Burnett for word processing.

REFERENCES

1. Borel JF. Cyclosporine: historical perspectives. Transplant Proc 1983; 15: 2219.
2. Larson E-L. Cyclosporin A and dexamethasone suppress T-cell responses by selectively acting at distinct sites of the triggering process. J Immunol 1980; 124: 2828.
3. Bunjes D, Hardt C, Rollinghoff M, Wagner H. Cyclosporin A mediates immunosuppression of primary cytotoxic T-cell responses by impairing the release of interleukin 1 and interleukin 2. Eur J Immunol 1981; 11: 657.
4. Kronke M, Leonard WJ, Depper JM, et al. Cyclosporin A inhibits T-cell growth factor gene expression at the level of mRNA transcription. Proc Natl Acad Sci USA 1984; 81: 5214.
5. Elliott JF, Lin Y, Mizel SB, Bleackly RC, Harnish DG, Paetkau V. Induction of interleukin 2 messenger RNA inhibited by cyclosporin A. Science 1984; 226: 1439.
6. Granelli-Piperno A, Inaba K, Steinman RM. Stimulation of lymphokine release from T-lymphoblasts: requirement for mRNA synthesis and inhibition by Cyclosporin-A. J Exp Med 1984; 160: 1792.
7. Colombani PM, Robb A, Hess AD. Cyclosporin A binding to calmodulin: a possible site of action on T lymphocytes. Science 1985; 228: 337.
8. LeGrue SJ, Friedman AW, Kahan BD. Binding of cyclosporin by human lymphocytes and phospholipid vesicles. J Immunol 1983; 131: 712.
9. Ryffel B, Donatsch P, Gotz U, Tschopp M. Cyclosporin receptor on mouse lymphocytes. Immunology 1980; 41: 913.
10. Ryffel B, Gotz U, Heuberger B. Cyclosporin receptors on human lymphocytes. J Immunol 1982; 129: 1978.
11. Handschumacher RE, Harding MW, Rice J, Drugge RJ, Speicher DW. Cyclophilin: a specific cytosolic binding protein for cyclosporin A. Science 1984; 226: 544.
12. Tsien RY, Pozzan T, Rink TJ. T-cell mitogens cause early changes in cytoplasmic free Ca^{2+} and membrane potential in lymphocytes. Nature 1982; 295: 68.
13. Birx DL, Berger M, Fleisher TA. The interference of T-cell activation by calcium channel blocking agents. J Immunol 1984; 133: 2904.
14. Weiss A, Imboden J, Shoback D, Stobo J. Role of T3 surface molecules in human T-cell activation: T3-dependent activation results in an increase in cytoplasmic free calcium. Proc Natl Acad Sci USA 1984; 81: 4169.
15. Weiss MJ, Daley JF, Hodgdon JC, Reinherz EL. Calcium dependency of antigen-specific (T3-Ti) and alternative (T11) pathways of human T-cell activation. Proc Natl Acad Sci USA 1984; 81: 6836.
16. Seeman P. The membrane actions of anesthetics and tranquilizers. Pharmacol Rev 1972; 24: 583.
17. Ferguson RM, Schmidtke JR, Simmons RL. Inhibition of mitogen-induced lymphocyte transformation by local anesthetics. J Immunol 1976; 116: 627.
18. Portoles A, Ojeda G, Portoles MP, Rojo JM. Effects of several neuroleptic compounds on the blastogenic response of spleen cells from mice. Int J Tissue React 1982; 4: 133.
19. Neuwelt EA, Kikuchi K, Hill SA, Lipsky P, Frenkel E. Barbiturate inhibition of lymphocyte function. J Neurosurg 1982; 56: 254.

20. Thomas J, Carver M, Haisch C, Thomas F, Welch J, Carchman R. Differential effects of intravenous anesthetic agents on cell-mediated immunity in the Rhesus monkey. Clin Exp Immunol 1982; 47: 457.
21. Stavitsky AB, Dasch JR, Astrachan L. Effects of Trifluoperazine, a calmodulin antagonist, on rabbit T- and B-cell responses to mitogens and antigen. Cell Immunol 1984; 87: 411.
22. Harris AR, Bruno P. Membrane disordering by anesthetic drugs: relationship to synaptosomal sodium and calcium fluxes. J Neurochem 1985; 44: 1274.
23. Chandy KG, DeCoursey TE, Cahalan MD, McLaughlin C, Gupta S. Voltage-gated potassium channels are required for human T-lymphocyte activation. J Exp Med 1984; 160: 369.
24. Marshak DR, Lukas TJ, Watterson DM. Drug-protein interactions: binding of chlorpromazine to calmodulin, calmodulin fragments, and related calcium-binding proteins. Biochemistry 1985; 24: 144.
25. Flaim SF, Brannan MD, Swigart SC, Gleason MM, Muschek LD. Neuroleptic drugs attenuate calcium influx and tension development in rabbit thoracic aorta: effects of pimozide, penfluridol, chlorpromazine and haloperidol. Proc Natl Acad Sci USA 1985; 82: 1237.
26. MacNeil S, Walker S, Brown B, Tomlinson S. Evidence that calmodulin may be involved in phytohaemagglutinin-stimulated lymphocyte division. Biosci Rep 1982; 2: 891.
27. Wolberg G, Zimmerman TP. Effects of calmodulin antagonists on immune mouse lymphocytes. Mol Pharmacol 1984; 26: 286.
28. Schatzman RC, Raynor RL, Kuo JF. N-(6-aminohexyl)-5-chloro-1-naphthalenesulfonamide (W-7) a calmodulin antagonist, also inhibits phospholipid-sensitive calcium dependent protein kinase. Biochim Biophys Acta 1983; 755: 144.
29. Sanchez A, Hallam TJ, Rink RJ. Trifluoperazine and chlorpromazine block secretion from human platelets evoked at basal cytoplasmic free calcium by activators of C-kinase. FEBS Lett 1983; 164: 43.
30. Watson J. Continuous proliferation of murine antigen-specific helper T-lymphocytes in culture. J Exp Med 1979; 150: 1510.
31. Meo T. The MLR test in the mouse. In: Lefkovits I, Pernis B. Immunological Methods, Vol I. New York: Academic 1979: 227.
32. Mori T, Takai Y, Minakuchi R, Yu B, Nishizuka Y. Inhibitory action of Chlorpromazine, Dibucaine and other phospholipid-interacting drugs on calcium-activated, phospholipid-dependent protein kinase. J Biol Chem 1985; 255: 8378.
33. Uratsuji Y, Nakamishi H, Takeyama T, Kishimoto A, Nishizuka Y. Activation by cellular protein kinase C and mode of inhibitory action of phospholipid-interacting compounds. Biochem Biophys Res Commun 1985; 130: 654.
34. Veigl ML, Vanaman TC, Sedwick WD. Calcium and calmodulin in cell growth and transformation. Biochim Biophys Acta 1984; 73: 21.
35. Schneider M, Shieh B, Pezzementi L, Schmidt J. Trifluorperazine receptor synthesis in cultured chick myotubes. J Neurochem 1984; 42: 1395.
36. Miyawaki T, Yackie A, Ohzeki S, Nagaoki T, Taniguchi N. Cyclosporin A does not prevent expression of Tac antigen, a probable TCGF receptor molecule, on mitogen-stimulated human T-cells. J Immunol 1983; 130: 2737.
37. Kaufmann Y, Chang AE, Robb RJ, Rosenberg SA. Mechanism of action of cyclosporin A: inhibition of lymphokine secretion studied with antigen-stimulated T-cell hybridomas. J Immunol 1984; 133: 3107.
38. Berridge MJ, Irvine RF. Inositol trisphosphate, a novel second messenger in cellular signal transduction. Nature 1984; 312: 315.
39. Ku Y, Kishimoto A, Takai Y, Ogawa Y, Kimura S, Nishizuka Y. A new possible regulatory system for protein phosphorylation in human peripheral blood lymphocytes. II. Possible relation to phosphatidylinositol turnover induced by mitogens. J Immunol 1981; 127: 1375.
40. Geshwendt M, Kittstein W, Horn F, Marks F. Cyclosporin-A inhibits biological effects of tumor promoting phorbol esters. Biochem Biophys Res Commun 1985; 126: 327.
41. Kay JE, Benzie CR, Borghetti AF. Effect of cyclosporin-A on lymphocyte activation by the calcium ionophore A23187. Immunology 1983; 50: 441.
42. Winkelstein A. The effects of cyclosporin and hydrocortisone on human T-lymphocyte colony formation. Cell Immunol 1984; 86: 413.
43. Edwards MC, Nouri AM, Gordon D, Evans JF. Tumor-promoting proinflammatory esters act as human lymphocyte mitogens with different sensitivities to inhibition by cyclosporin-A. Mol Pharmacol 1983; 23: 703.
44. Tanaka T, Ohmura T, Hidaka H. Hydrophobic interaction of the Ca^{2+} calmodulin complex with calmodulin antagonists: naphthalene-sulfonamide derivatives. Mol Pharmacol 1982; 22: 403.
45. Nishikawa M, Hidaka H. Role of calmodulin in platelet aggregation. Structure-activity relationship of calmodulin antagonists. J Clin Invest 1982; 69: 1348.
46. Metcalfe S. Cyclosporine does not prevent cytoplasmic calcium changes associated with lymphocyte activation. Transplantation 1984; 38: 161.
47. Gearing AJH, Wadhwa M, Perris AD. Interleukin 2 stimulates T-cell proliferation using a calcium flux. Immunol Lett 1985; 10: 297.
48. Mills GB, Cheung RK, Grinstein S, Gelfand EW. Interleukin-2-induced lymphocyte proliferation is independent of increases in cytosolic-free calcium concentrations. J Immunol 1985; 134: 2431.
49. Truneh A, Francoise A, Goldstein P, Schmitt-Verhurst AM. Early steps of lymphocyte activation bypassed by synergy between calcium ionophores and phorbol ester. Nature 1985; 313: 318.
50. Smith K. Interleukin-2. Ann Rev Immunol 1984; 2: 319.
51. Lillehoj HS, Malek TR, Shevach EM. Differential effect of Cyclosporin A on the expression of T and B lymphocyte activation antigens. J Immunol 1984; 133: 244.

Received 20 January 1986.
Accepted 7 April 1986.

0041-1337/86/4206-0686$02.00/0
TRANSPLANTATION

Vol. 42, No. 6
Printed in U.S.A.

Transplantation

BRIEF COMMUNICATIONS

THE EFFECT OF IRRADIATION OF THE DONOR SPLEEN ON REJECTION OF PORCINE PANCREATICODUODENOSPLENIC ALLOGRAFTS

Thrombosis of the pancreatic graft is responsible for the early loss of a significant proportion of pancreatic transplants (*1*). During the phase of acute pancreatitis following transplantation, it is thought taht low flow through the graft occurs and venous thrombosis may be precipitated. Attempts to prevent thrombosis have included the creation of a distal arteriovenous fistula (AVF)* between the splenic artery and vein (*2*). This approach raised concern about venous hypertension and/or a "steal" from the gland parenchyma to the venous circulation. In primates, such an AVF uniformly resulted in hemorrhagic pancreatitis (*3*). Starzl and colleagues proposed that the thrombosis problem could be avoided by the transplantation of a composite graft of whole pancreas, a segment of duodenum and the spleen (*4*). The inclusion of the spleen was purported to provide a physiological arteriovenous fistula maintaining vascular patency. The immunological consequences of including the spleen were uncertain. Based on islet cell transplantation work, the inclusion of a sensitizing cell mass such as the spleen in the transplant seems ill-advised (*5*). However, in small animal studies the transplantation of the spleen has been associated with an improvement of pancreas graft survival (*6*). Our studies in the porcine pancreaticoduodenal allograft (PDA) model clearly demonstrated the inclusion of the spleen (S) in the PDA (PDA+S) was detrimental to graft survival: increased graft loss in the PDA+S group was due to rejection (*7*). Furthermore, reports of graft-versus-host disease (GVHD) in human recipients of PDA+S discouraged continued use of this technique (*8, 9*).

If the immunocompetent cells in the graft spleen could be eradicated by irradition, for example, then the hemodynamic advantage of PDA+S might be preserved and the immunological disadvantages eliminated. Indeed, irradiation of the spleen of the PDA+S has been used to reverse signs of possible GVHD in the clinical setting (*9*). In this trial, we used our well-developed porcine PDA and PDA+S model to study the effect of pretransplantation irradiation of the spleen on graft function and survival.

Five pancreatectomized pigs received PDA+S grafts but, prior to transplantation, the graft spleen was exposed to 1000 rads (irradiated PDA+S). The techniques applied have been described thoroughly in a prior communication (*7*). Briefly, the graft consisted of the whole pancreas, a segment of duodenum and the spleen. The graft was transplanted intraperitoneally sewing the donor aortic cylinder (including the celiac axis and superior mesenteric artery) and portal vein to the recipient distal aorta and inferior vena cava. One end of the donor duodenal segment was oversewn and the other anastomosed to recipient small bowel. The irradiated PDA+S graft was immediately flushed with cold lactated Ringer's solution. The spleen of the graft was then irradiated; the remaining graft was excluded by lead shielding. Irradiation was given using a ^{60}Co machine with a source-to-graft distance of 65 cm. Dose rate was 102 rads/min and total treatment time was 6.96 min for 1000 rads calculated at a depth of 1 cm below the surface of the spleen. Total thickness of the spleen was 2 cm, thus there was a ±5% dose gradient over the entire volume of the spleen. The irradiated PDA+S grafts were transplanted after a mean cold ischemic time of 56±22 min (±SD) with a range of 30–90 min. The serum warm ischemic time (anastomosis time) was 26±6 min.

The immunosuppressive regimen was cyclosporine (Sandoz Co., East Hanover, NJ), 6 mg/kg i.v. and prednisolone, 1.5 mg/kg i.v. initially. The cyclosporine dose held constant at 6 mg/kg i.v. daily but the prednisolone dose was tapered to 0.5 mg/kg i.v. daily by the 7th day following transplantation and maintained. On the 28th day after transplantation cyclosporine was discontinued. Prednisolone was tapered and stopped within five days. Animals were fed once daily with pancreatic exocrine enzyme replacement. Cimetidine and perioperative antibiotic coverage were given as has been described (*7*).

Normoglycemia was established in irradiated PDA+S recipients for the 28 days of full immunosuppression (Table 1). This finding was similar to the experience we reported in 10 PDA recipients (*7*). There was no hyperglycemia (defined as blood glucose >150 mg/dl for three consecutive days) indicative of acute rejection in the 28 day posttransplantation period. On the other hand, 5 of 8 PDA+S recipients without irradiation of the graft spleen developed hyperglycemia an average of 13 days after transplantation ($P<0.05$ by the Fisher exact test). Intravenous glucose tolerance tests (ivGTT), .5 g/kg, were carried out on irradiated PDA+S recipients 28 days after transplantation. This data showed function comparable to PDA and surviving PDA+S grafts in previous studies. The K value, the slope of the linear regression of glucose on time calculated from ivGTT data, was −2.45 in irradiated PDA+S recipients (n = 5), −2.40 in PDA recipients (n = 10), and −2.24 n PDA+S recipients (n = 3). Hyperglycemia was associated with the reported characteristic histological findings of rejection—fibrosis, round cell infiltrate and loss of acinar cells—in every instance. The irradiated spleen was largely replaced with fibrosis. There were no signs of GVHD in any of the groups.

We found that the detrimental effect of inclusion of the spleen on graft survival in the porcine PDA model could be

TABLE 1. Mean daily blood glucose (mg/dl±SD)

	Experimental groups (n)		
	pda (10)	pda+s (8)	pda+s (5)
No rejection	95±8 (10)	95±13 (3)	92±23 (5)
Rejection	0/10	5/8	0/5

* Abbreviations used: AVF, arteriovenous fistula; GVHD, graft-versus-host disease; i.v. GTT, intravenous glucose tolerance test; PDA, pancreaticoduodenal allograft; S, spleen.

abrogated by irradiation of the spleen. Irradiation of the graft spleen prior to transplantation had no effect on the function of irradiated PDA+S grafts. In rats, when parental strain donor pancreaticosplenic grafts were transplanted into streptozotocin diabetic F_1 hybrids, resulting GVHD could be avoided by irradiation (250–1000 rads) of the graft without adversely affecting pancreatic graft function (Schulak JA, personal communication). In this study, 1000 rads to the graft spleen was chosen based on studies demonstrating this dose is lethal to splenocytes (*10*). A lesser dose might have selectively depleted radiosensitive suppressor cells, perhaps fostering a rejection episode. Histological examination of the irradiated graft spleen from normoglycemic reicpients showed extensive fibrosis, loss of germinal centers, dystrophic calcifications, giant cells, vacuolization, and proliferation of endothelial cells, sclerotic vessels and a round cell infiltrate. The splenic cellular infiltrate may be due to inflammation, host immunologic response—or, possibly, resident donor cells surviving irradiation. The delivery of antigen from the newly irradiated graft spleen and splenocyte destruction did not appear to have any effect (using rejection as an endpoint) in tolerizing or sensitizing the host.

Since the main impetus for including the spleen in the PDA graft is hemodynamic—that is, the avoidance of thrombosis—it would be important to determine differences in graft blood flow in groups that have received PDA, PDA+S and irradiated PDA+S grafts. This issue was not addressed in this trial. It could be reasoned that since the structural and vascular "skeleton" of the spleen remains following irradiation, it may provide the sought hemodynamic benefits. If hemodynamic studies of the irradiated PDA+S graft showed a beneficial effect on graft blood flow, then inclusion of the irradiated spleen in PDA transplantation could provide protection against thrombosis and become a tenable practice.

Donald C. Dafoe[1,2]
Darrell A. Campbell, Jr.[3]

[1] Department of Surgery.
[2] Address correspondence to: Donald C. Dafoe, M.D., 2926B Taubman Center, Box 0331, University of Michigan, Ann Arbor, MI 48109.
[3] Department of Radiation Therapy.

William H. Marks[3]
Anders Borgstrom[3]
Allen S. Lichter[1]
Jeremiah G. Turcotte[1]
The Departments of Surgery and Radiation Therapy
The University of Michigan Medical Center
Ann Arbor, Michigan 48109

REFERENCES

1. Sutherland DER, Chinn PL, Goetz FG, Elick BA, Najarian JS. Minnesota experience with 85 pancreas transplants between 1978 and 1983. World J Surg 1984, 8: 244.
2. Calne RY, McMaster P, Rolles K, Duffy TJ: Technical observations in sequential pancreas allografting: observations on pancreatic blood flow. Transplant Proc 1980; 12: 51.
3. DuToit DF, Heydenrych JJ, Louw G, et al. Intraperitoneal transplantation of vascularized segmental pancreatic autografts without duct ligation in the primate. Surgery 1983; 94: 471.
4. Starzl TE, Iwatsuki S, Shaw BW Jr, et al. Pancreaticoduodenal transplantation in humans. Surg Gynecol Obstet 1984; 159: 265.
5. Lacy PE. Experimental immuno-alteration. World J Surg 1984; 8: 198.
6. Bitter-Suermann H, Shevach EM. Induction of transplantation tolerance in guinea pigs by spleen allografts. I. Operative techniques and clinical results. Transplantation 1982; 33: 45.
7. Dafoe DC, Campbell DA Jr, Marks WH, Borgstrom A, Lloyd EV, Turcotte JG. Inclusion of the donor spleen in pancreaticoduodenal transplantation is associated with rejection. Transplantation 1985; 40: 579.
8. Sollinger HW, Kalayoglu M, Hoffman RM, Deierhoi, MH, Belzer FO. Experience with pnacreaticocystostomy in 24 consecutive pancreas transplants. Transplant Proc 1875; 17: 141.
9. Gonwa TA, Goeken NE, Schulak JA, Hghiam DD, Corry RJ. Failure of cyclosporine to prevent in vivo T cell priming in man: studies in allogeneic spleen transplantation. Transplantation 1985; 40: 299.
10. Thomas ED, Storb R, Buckner CD. Total-body irradiation in preparation for marrow engraftment. Transplant Proc 1976; 8: 591.

Received 18 February 1986.
Accepted 18 March 1986.

SUPPRESSION OF HOST-VERSUS-GRAFT RESPONSE IN EXPERIMENTAL BILIARY OBSTRUCTION

Despite the intensity of clinical and experimental investigation in hepatic transplantation in recent years, little remains known of the effect of cholestasis on cellular and humoral immune mechanisms, the mediators of allograft rejection. The data presented herein evaluate in vitro lymphoproliferative response to thymus-dependent and thymus independent mitogen and in vivo host-versus-graft reactivity in the cholestatic bile duct ligated rat model described by Lee. (*1*)

Female Sprague-Dawley (SD)* rats (Timco Laboratories, Houston, Texas) weighing 225–250 g were used in this study. Rats were assigned to three groups: bile duct ligation (BDL), sham operation (sham) or normal control (NC). Throughout the study rats were housed in metabolic cages, fed standard chow (Purina Formulab Chow 5008), and allowed water ad libitum. Sham animals were pair-fed with the BDL group to prevent a nutritional bias influencing lymphocytic function (*2*). Serum total bilirubin (Jendrassik Grof method) was determined at day 0 and at day 21 following operation. All sera from study animals were filtered and refrigerated at −70°C. Lymphoproliferative response to thymus-dependent and thymus independent mitogen, in vivo host versus graft reactivity to allogeneic F_{344} splenic lymphoid cells, and liver histology were performed on day 21.

Rat splenic lymphocyte proliferative response to T and B cell mitogens was tested using a modified method of Strong et al (*3*). Purified lymphoid cells were obtained in the following manner: rat spleens were harvested aseptically, cut into small pieces, and then teased through 100-mm stainless steel screens to make single cell suspensions in RPMI-1640 medium containing Pen Strep. The suspensions were spun at 1200 rpm for 10 min in a refrigerated centrifuge. Contaminating red blood cells were removed by treatment with tris ammonium chloride.

* Abbreviations used: BDL, bile duct ligation; FBS, fetal bovine serum; LPS, lipopolysaccharide; NC, normal control; PHA, phytohemagglutinin; SD, Sprague-Dawley.

The cell suspensions were further washed three times in RPMI-1640, and finally resuspended in complete RPMI containing 10% fetal bovine serum (FBS), pen strep, L glutamine, and 0.2 M Hepes. The cell suspensions were then enumerated and the cell concentration adjusted to 5×10^6 cells/ml in complete RPMI. The cells were dispersed in a microtiter well plate at 5×10^5 cells/well in 0.1 ml volume. Then 50 μl of the mitogen phytohemagglutinin (PHA) (Gibco) and lipopolysaccharide (LPS) (Calbiochem) were added in triplicate wells at 1:10, 1:25, and 1:50 dilutions of PHA stock solution and 1 mg/ml LPS solution. Volume per well was adjusted to 0.2 ml total by addition of the appropriate amount of complete RPMI. Microtiter plates were incubated for 48 hr at 37°C with a humidified 5% CO_2 air mixture. Following incubation cells were pulse-labeled with ^{3}H-thymidine (1 μCi/well, 6.7 Ci/mol; specific activity) for 16–18 hr. The cells were then harvested on a Mash II harvester. Disks were transferred to vials and 5 ml of scintillation cocktail was added. Incorporation of ^{3}H-thymidine was determined in a Beckman/LS-8000 liquid scintillation counter and results expressed as the difference in ^{3}H-thymidine uptake between mitogen stimulated and nonstimulated samples (Δ). Host versus graft reactivity to allogeneic F_{344} lymphoid cells was determined by the popliteal lymph node assay as described by Ford (*4*). Purified splenic F_{344} (allogeneic) and SD (syngeneic) lymphoid cells were obtained in the manner described above, and diluted in complete RPMI medium at a concentration of 250×10^6 cells/ml. BDL, Sham, and NC animals were subjected to ether anesthesia and 25×10^6 F_{344} cells injected into the right (allogeneic) footpad and 25×10^6 SD cells injected into the left (syngeneic) footpad. Seven days later animals were specified and popliteal lymph nodes dissected from right and left popliteal fossae and weighed. Host-versus-graft reactivity was exposed as the difference in weight between allogeneic and syngeneic stimulated nodes (Δ). All results were expressed as mean ± SEM and subjected to Student's unpaired *t* test.

At day 21 mean serum total bilirubin was elevated in BDL compared with sham and NC groups (9.8±0.7 vs. 0.3±0.2 and 0.1±0 mg/dl, respectively, $P<0.01$). Liver histology demonstrated bile duct proliferation, hepatocyte aptosis, early evidence of periportal fibrosis, and portal venous engorgement in BDL animals compared with sham and NC groups.

Lymphocytic responsiveness to PHA stimulation was depressed in BDL animals compared with Sham and NC rats at 1:10 (2331±941 vs. 50,146±2593 and 56,557±16,632 cpm, $P<0.001$), 1:25 (2352±738 vs. 38,622±1628 and 68,014±15,867 cpm $P<0.001$), and 1:50 (3761±420 vs. 26,120±2439 and 22,847±10,331 cpm $P<0.001$) dilutions of PHA stock solution (Table 1). Proliferative response to LPS demonstrated no difference among BDL, Sham, and NC animals at 1:10 (3691 vs. 4631±497 and 3177±546 cpm), 1:25 (4383±1062 vs. 2986±811 and 4244±1611 cpm), and 1:50 (3598±969 vs. 4233±7 and 6304±1202 cpm) dilutions of LPS stock solution (Table 1).

Host-versus-graft reactivity was markedly depressed in the BDL group compared with Sham and NC groups (Δ: −3.4±2.4 vs. 16.7±8.5 and 34.6±4.5 mg $P<0.04$ and 0.01, respectively) (Figs. 1 and 2).

To determine whether the observed suppression of BDL lymphoproliferative response to PHA and allogeneic F_{344} lymphoid cells was due to a serum related factor, the lymphoproliferative response of PHA-stimulated NC lymphocytes was determined as described previously following a 4-hr incubation of NC cells with 50 μl filtered BDL, Sham, and NC sera. Electrophoretic studies (cellulose acetate pH 8.6) were also performed on sera to determine concentrations of the immunoregulatory protein fraction α_2 macroglobulin in this model (*5*). Results failed to demonstrate suppressive activity in BDL sera (Table 1). In addition, no specific elevation in α_2 macroglobulin levels was apparent in BDL compared with Sham and

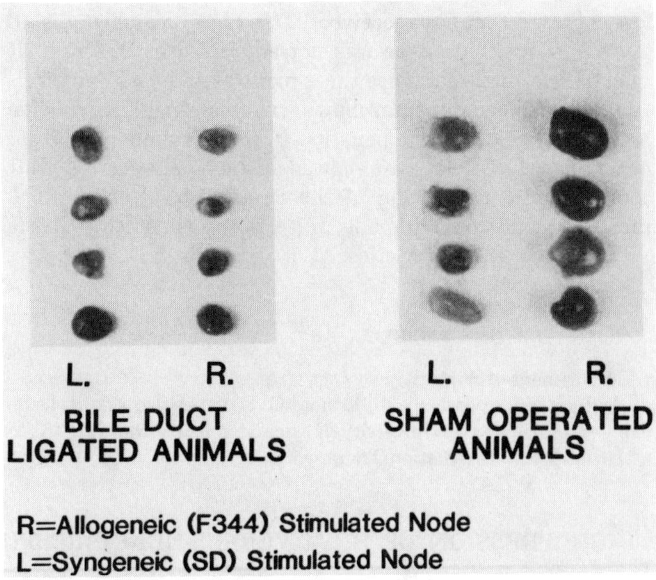

FIGURE 1. Popliteal lymph node assay in BDL and Sham animals (day 21).

TABLE 1. In vitro mitogen studies (day 21): uptake of ^{3}H thymidine (cpm [mean ± SEM])

	A. Lymphoproliferative response to PHA and LPS in BDL Sham, and NC groups						B. Lymphoproliferative response of NC cells preincubated with BDL, Sham, and NC sera	
	PHA (Δ)[a]			LPS (Δ)[a]				PHA (Δ)[a]
	1:10	1:25	1:50	1:10	1:25	1:50		1:10
BDL	2331[b]	2,352[b]	3,761[b]	3,691	4,631	3,177	NC cells + BDL serum	17714
(n = 4)	±941	±738	±420	±1,191	±497	±546	(n = 7)	±2834
Sham	50,146	38,622	26,120	4,383	2,986	4,244	NC cells + sham	17310
(n = 4)	±2,593	±1,628	±2,439	±1,062	±811	±1,611	serum (n = 7)	±2789
NC	56,557	68,014	22,847	3,598	4,233	6,304	NC cells + NC serum	17382
(n = 4)	±16,632	±15,867	±10,331	±969	±7	±1,202	(n = 7)	±2608

[a] Δ = cpm stimulated sample − cpm unstimulated sample.

[b] $P<0.001$ compared with sham and NC.

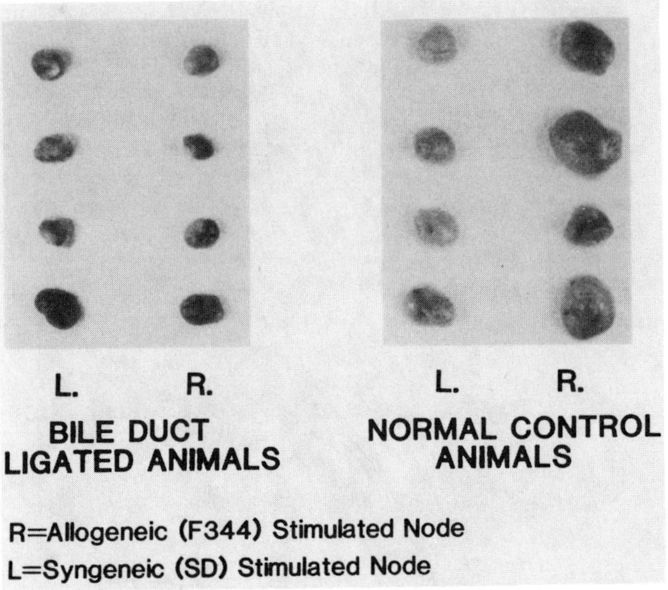

FIGURE 2. Popliteal lymph node assay in BDL and NC animals (day 21).

NC sera (0.51±0.09 vs. 0.54±0.02 and 0.29±0.08 mg/dl, respectively).

This study demonstrates that biliary obstruction results in impairment of lymphoproliferative response to T cell dependent, but not T cell independent mitogen in vitro. This suggests an impairment of cellular but not humoral immune mechanisms in this model. Suppression of cellular immune mechanisms, demonstrated as an impaired host-versus-graft response to allogeneic F_{344} lymphoid cells was apparent in BDL animals in vivo. This demonstrates an impaired effector response to histoincompatible tissue in the cholestatic host. In vitro mitogen studies failed to demonstrate lymphocytic suppressive activity in sera related from cholestatic animals or elevated levels of immunoregulatory α_2 globulin fractions in this model. Elucidation of the mechanism of suppressed T cell activity in biliary obstruction will require investigation of T cell subsets, T_HT_S function, accessory macrophage function, and in vivo lymphoinhibitory serum studies. Such studies will improve our understanding of the altered immunological status of the cholestatic host and have relevant implications in the science of transplantology.

P. T. ROUGHNEEN[1]
A. D. KULKARNI
D. J. GOUMA
W. C. FANSLOW
B. J. ROWLANDS
The University of Texas Medical School
Department of Surgery
Houston, Texas 77030

[1] Address correspondence to: P. T. Roughneen, M.B., Ch.B., Department of Surgery, Rm. 4.162, The University of Texas Medical School, 6431 Fannin, Houston, Texas 77030.

REFERENCES

1. Lee E. The effect of obstructive jaundice on migration of reticuloendothelial cells and fibroblasts into early experimental granulomata. Br J Surg 1972; 59: 875.
2. Kahan BD. Nutrition and host defence mechanisms. Surg Clin N Amer 1981; 61: 557.
3. Strong DM, Ahmed AA, Thurman GB, Sell KW. In vitro stimulation of murine spleen cells using a microculture system and a multiple automated sample harvester. J Immunol Methods 1973; 2: 279.
4. Ford WH, Burr W, Simonsen M. A lymph node weight assay for the graft versus host activity of rat lymphoid cells. Transplantation 1970; 10: 258.
5. Mowbray JF. Effect of large doses of an alpha 2 globulin fraction on the survival of rat skin homografts. Transplantation 1963; 1: 15.

Received 17 December 1985.
Accepted 3 March 1986.

ISOLATION OF RAT PANCREATIC ISLETS BY DUCTAL INJECTION OF COLLAGENASE[1]

The reversal of streptozotocin-induced diabetes in the rat by pancreatic islet transplantation became possible after Lacy and Kostianovsky developed the method of islet isolation first described by Moskalewski (*1–3*). Among the essential features of their technique are initial distension of the pancreas by a ductal injection of physiological saline, incubation of the minced pancreas in a collagenase solution, and subsequent centrifugation of the dispersed tissue on a Ficoll density gradient. This method, with minor variations, has become the standard technique for the preparation of rat islets in most laboratories (*4*, *5*). Depending on the site of islet transplantation, up to 6 donor pancreases must be processed in this way for a sufficient islet yield to consistently reverse streptozotocin-induced diabetes in one recipient (*6*). In our own laboratories over the past 10 years we have used pancreata from 4–6 donors to obtain approximately 1200 islets by this method, ensuring reliable reversal of streptozotocin-induced diabetes in each recipient (*7*, *8*). Unfortunately the technique has only limited application to other species, and has never been successfully applied to human islet transplantation for diabetes mellitus (*5*). More recently high yields of islets have been obtained from canine and human pancreases when collagenase is used in the initial pancreatic distention (*9*, *10*). We describe the application of this latter technique in the rat, and successful reversal of streptozotocin-induced diabetes with islets obtained from one donor.

Islet isolation. Anesthesia was induced in Dark Agouti and Lewis rats using an ether inhalation and maintained with 250 mg/kg of i.p. chloral. The lower end of the common bile duct of each donor was cannulated with a 2 FG cannula tied in place to prevent passage of collagenase solution into the duodenum. The right and left hepatic ducts were then ligated separately above the region of entry of the pancreatic ducts into the biliary tree. The donor was killed by exsanguination and 3 ml of Hank's solution (Flow Labs Ltd, Irvine, Ayrshire, Scotland) containing 7.5 mmol/L calcium chloride, 20 mmol/L HEPES buffer, and a varied amount of collagenase (1–6 mg/ml of type I, Sigma Chemical Co, St. Louis, MO) were injected through

[1] This work was supported by a grant from the medical research council and the British Diabetic Association.

the cannula to uniformly distend the pancreas. The pancreas was then excised and placed in a beaker on ice, prior to incubation in Hanks' solution containing 20 mmol/L HEPES buffer at 37°C. After various periods (13–29 min) the pancreas was removed from the incubation medium and placed into Hanks' solution containing 5 g/L bovine serum albumin and 20 mmol/L HEPES buffer at 4°C. This last solution was used in all subsequent steps of the isolation procedure. All the pancreatic tissue was then gently syringed through a 14 FG needle, suspended in further Hanks' solution, centrifuged at 50 g for 10 sec, and the supernatant discarded. The pellet of tissue was resuspended and gently syringed again. Another wash was done in the same way, after which the dispersed tissue was passed through a nylon mesh filter of 500-μ pore size (Henry Simon Ltd., Stockport, Cheshire, UK). The filtered tissue was centrifuged at 350 g for 5 sec, the supernatant discarded, and the tissue then suspended in 25% Ficoll made up in Hanks' solution with 20 mmol/L HEPES buffer, on which was layered a discontinuous density gradient of 23%, 20%, and 11% Ficoll solutions. The density gradient containing the tissue was spun at 750 g for 10 min at 4°C. The tissue obtained from the upper two interfaces was then washed three times in Hanks' solution as before, and viewed through a dissecting microscope for hand picking of the islets.

Islet identification. Hand picking of the islets was performed by selecting rounded, opaque islets from a Petri dish viewed through a dissecting microscope using slide illumination against a black background at a magnification of 15×. In each of the first 10 donor rats islets were stained during the isolation procedure prior to exsanguination by a 2-ml intraaortic injection of 1 in 1000 w/v neutral red in 0.9% saline, since this stain is selective for islet tissue and assists hand picking (*11*). Islet identification was confirmed by the use of the green light technique (*12*), and both light and electron microscopy (Fig. 1).

Development of the method. Initial experiments of rat islet isolation by this method were carried out with an incubation of 25 min. The mean number of islets obtained from 1 pancreas using 6 mg/ml collagenase was 647 (n=17, SD=135, range = 400–1010), whereas using 3 mg/ml it was 653 (n=42), SD=170, range = 334–1000); both mean yields were equivalent to approximately 1200 islets/g of pancreas. Using 3 mg/ml collagenase, the time of incubation was shortened to 17 min, with a similar mean islet yield of 659 (n=18, SD=88, range = 500–753), but after only 13 min incubation the mean yield of 273 (n=4, SD=152, range = 154–463) was significantly lower ($P<0.001$, t test). Poorer yields were also obtained using lower concentrations of collagenase and longer periods of incubation. There was no significant difference between the islet yields obtained from 52 Dark Agouti and 28 Lewis pancreases processed in these experiments.

Final method. A concentration of 3 mg/ml collagenase and an incubation period of 17 min was chosen on the basis of these results. Calcium chloride and HEPES buffer were added, as mentioned earlier, to ensure maximum collagenase activity at physiological pH. Further experiments refer to islets obtained by this technique. Acid alcohol insulin extraction assays were performed on 200–400 freshly isolated, hand picked islets from each of 5 donor pancreases, and a mean value of 0.34 mU/islet was obtained. From each of 10 further donor pancreases 200–400 freshly isolated, hand picked islets were implanted beneath the capsule of each of 10 kidneys in 6 normal syngeneic recipients. These kidneys were removed at laparotomy 2 weeks later and ground for insulin extraction; a mean of 138.7 mU insulin/kidney (0.47 mU/islet) was obtained. Both normal kidneys without an islet implant produced less than 1.5 mU insulin each.

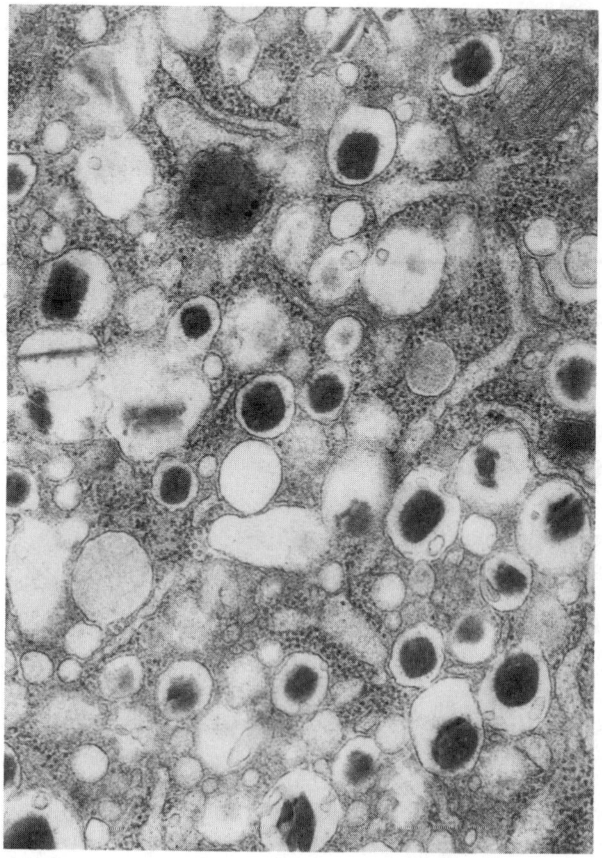

FIGURE 1. Electron micrograph showing well-preserved cytosol of a rat B cell with many typical granules, representative of hand picked islets obtained by ductal injection of collagenase (lead citrate and uranyl acetate; ×32,500).

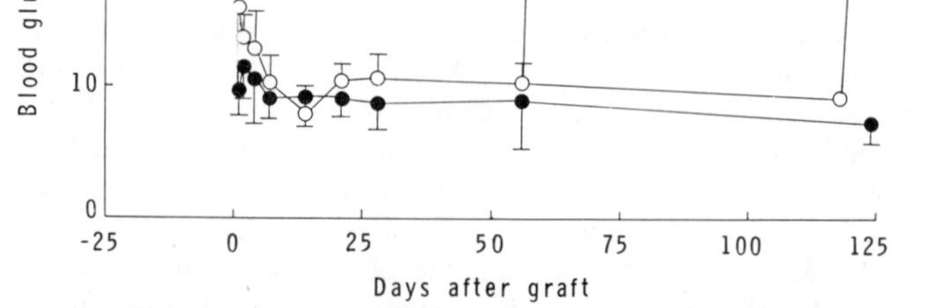

FIGURE 2. Blood sugar levels in 10 rats with streptozotocin-induced diabetes after each received an islet isograft obtained by ductal injection of collagenase; 5 intraportal grafts are represented by closed circles and 5 renal subcapsular grafts by open circles. Return of diabetes is demonstrated following the removal of renal subcapsular grafts from 2 recipients.

Reversal of streptozotocin-induced diabetes. Recipient rats were made diabetic 14 or more days before transplantation by a single i.v. injection of 65 mg/kg streptozotocin. The blood glucose of all recipients was over 22 mmol/L at the time of transplantation. At laparotomy freshly isolated islets from up to 3 donor pancreata were either slowly injected into the portal vein or implanted beneath the left renal capsule. The blood glucose of each recipient was monitored both before and after transplantation. In each of 5 recipients of islets from a single donor pancreas given into the portal vein normoglycemia was reestablished within 14 days, but for this to occur within 48 hr islets from at least 2 donor pancreases were required (Fig. 2). Subsequently the left kidneys of 2 renal subcapsular islet graft recipients were removed to confirm that the reversal of diabetes had dependend on the presence of the graft. Histology of these kidneys demonstrated viable islet grafts (not shown).

The isolation of 500–800 islets per adult rat pancreas is more than twice the number that can be obtained by the technique described earlier (*2–6*). A single donor-to-recipient ratio is desirable, and we have achieved this with the new method of isolation when the islets are grafted intraportally. The use of up to 3 donors has enabled us to confidently reverse streptozotocin-induced diabetes by renal subcapsular grafting, and has provided a method of ensuring the return of normoglycemia within 48 hr of intraportal islet transplantation in allogeneic recipients among whom graft failure can subsequently be attributed to rejection of an otherwise adequate graft. The method for islet isolation presented here was developed independently but bears great resemblance to a recently reported isolation method for mouse islets (*13*). Other groups are also using a similar, although unpublished, method based on intraductal collagenase injection (D. H. Mintz, M. Marshall, recent personal communication), and have obtained similar results. It would seem reasonable to propose that ductal collagenase injection with static incubation should not become the standard method for islet preparation from the rat pancreas.

Acknowledgments. We thank Dr. P. R. Millard of the Histopathology Department, John Radcliffe Hospital, for the electron micrograph.

Robert Sutton
Maureen Peters
Philip McShane
Derek W. R. Gray
Peter J. Morris
Nuffield Department of Surgery
University of Oxford
John Radcliffe Hospital
Headington, Oxford, United Kingdom OX3 9DU

REFERENCES

1. Moskalewski S. Isolation and culture of the islets of Langerhans of the guinea pig. Gen Comp Endocrinol 1965; 5: 342.
2. Lacy PE, Kostianovsky M. Method for the isolation of intact islets of Langerhans from the rat pancreas. Diabetes 1967; 16: 35.
3. Ballinger WF, Lacy PE. Transplantation of intact pancreatic islets in rats. Surgery 1972; 72: 175.
4. Scharp DW. Isolation and transplantation of islet tissue. World J Surg 1984; 8: 143.
5. Gray DWR, Morris PJ. Progress in pancreatic islet and fetal pancreas transplantation. In: Morris PJ, Tilney NL, eds. Progress in transplantation III. Edinburgh: Churchill Livingstone (in press).
6. Matas AJ, Sutherland DER, Steffes MW, Najarian JS. Islet transplantation. Surg Gynecol Obstet 1977; 145: 757.
7. Finch DR, Wise PH, Morris PJ. Successful intra-splenic transplantation of syngeneic and allogeneic isolated pancreatic islets. Diabetologia 1977; 13: 195.
8. Reece-Smith H, DuToit DF, McShane P, Morris PJ. Prolonged survival of pancreatic islet allografts transplanted beneath the renal capsule. Transplantation 1981; 31: 305.
9. Horaguchi A, Merrell RC. Preparation of viable islet cells from dogs by a new method. Diabetes 1981; 30: 455.
10. Gray DWR, McShane P, Grant A, Morris PJ. A method for isolation of islets of Langerhans from the human pancreas. Diabetes 1984; 33: 1055.
11. Gray DWR, Millard PR, McShane P, Morris PJ. The use of the dye neutral red as a specific, non-toxic, intra-vital stain of islets of Langerhans. Br J Exp Pathol 1983; 64: 553.
12. Finke EH, Lacy PE, Ono J. Use of reflected green light for specific identification of islets in vitro after collagenase digestion. Diabetes 1979; 28: 612.
13. Gotoh M, Maki T, Kiyoizumi T, Satomi S, Monaco AP. An improved method for isolation of mouse pancreatic islets. Transplantation 1985; 40: 437.

Received 6 February 1986.
Accepted 26 February 1986.

ENUMERATION OF TRANSFERRIN-RECEPTOR-EXPRESSING LYMPHOCYTES AS A POTENTIAL MARKER FOR REJECTION IN HUMAN CARDIAC TRANSPLANT RECIPIENTS[1]

With the tremendous increase in the number of cardiac transplantations in recent years, the necessity to accurately diagnose impending rejections by some means other than the use of invasive biopsy procedures has assumed increasing importance. Early diagnosis of cardiac rejections is very cumbersome as well as costly, and it is primarily based on histopathological diagnosis of endomyocardial biopsies taken serially after transplant operations. In this regard, even if a new method could only eliminate some routine biopsies, it would certainly reduce the risks, as well as the cost, of posttransplant care of the patients. Since monoclonal antibodies directed against transferrin receptors are available (*1, 2*) and it has been demonstrated that murine and human lymphocytes express transferrin receptors (TR)* during early stages of the cell cycle following antigenic stimulus (*3–7*), it seemed reasonable that enumerating the TR would assist in the early diagnosis of cardiac transplant rejection.

Nineteen cardiac transplant recipients were monitored serially for percentage of circulating lymphocytes expressing TR during their immediate posttransplant period ranging from 28 to 89 days (60.1±19.3). All patients were treated with cyclosporine and prednisone, and acute rejections were treated with a methylprednisone pulse for three days and/or rabbit antithymocyte globulin therapy. The diagnosis of acute rejection was done by the clinical service, independently of the laboratory performing TR enumeration, and was based upon the clinical symptoms, EKG changes, and histopathological diagnoses of

[1] This work was supported by NIH grant AM 32253. T. M. is a recipient of ACS FRA 246.

* Abbreviation used: TR, transferrin receptor.

endomyocardial biopsies; the results were kept blind. Time periods were arbitrarily set based on the first day of clinical diagnosis of rejection being defined as day 0, prerejection (day −14 to day −2), during rejection (day −1 to day +4), and after the treatment of rejection (day +5 to day +14). The percentage of TR-positive lymphocytes was determined using fluorescein-isothiocyanate-conjugated monoclonal antihuman TR (OKT9, Ortho Diagnostic Systems, Inc.) (*1*) and a fluorescence-activated flow cytometer (Ortho Spectrum III). The mean value of the %TR-positive cells in 15 healthy volunteers was 3.5±1.5, and the values above 8.0 (the mean + 3 SD) were considered significantly elevated. Statistical analysis was done using student's *t* test with Welch's solution or the chi square test with Yates' correction.

TR-positive circulating lymphocytes were monitored two to three times weekly and the average value was calculated. Our results of the analysis of TR on various clinical stages of cardiac transplant patients are given in Figure 1. The mean value of the percentage of TR-positive lymphocytes during the clinically stable period was 5.0±3.3, and only 8 of the 67 determinations exceeded the value of 8.0. During the prerejection and rejection periods, the mean values increased significantly ($P<0.001$) to 10.4±3.6 and 13.4±6.5, respectively. Eleven of the 15 determinations (73.3%) during the prerejection period, and 11 of the 12 determinations (91.7%) during the rejection period, were over the cut-off value of 8.0. After treatment of rejection, there was a significant decrease in the percentage of TR cells (5.3±2.7, $P<0.01$) and only 2 of 10 determinations remained above

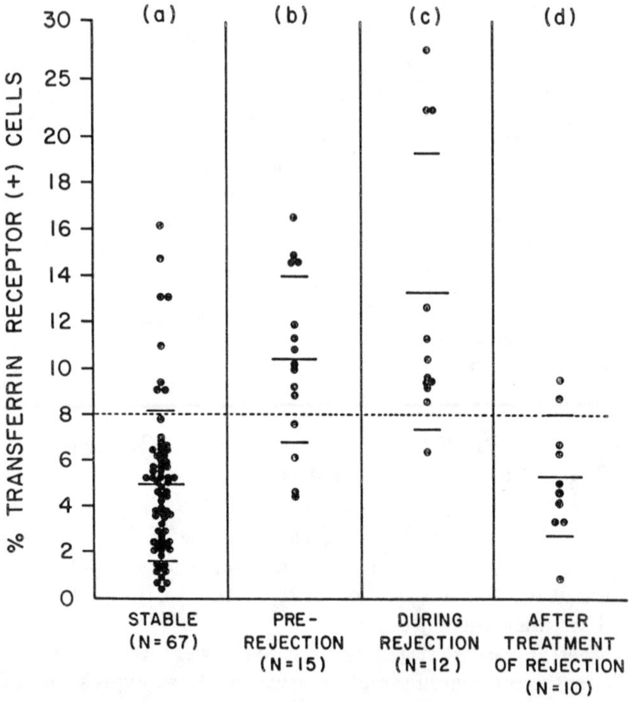

FIGURE 1. The values of circulating percentages of TR(+) lymphocytes in cardiac transplant recipients are presented in association with their clinical status. Each dot represents the average value of percentages of TR(+) cells in one week. Although the data were collected longitudinally in 19 patients, the number of determinations in each clinical classification were not equal, mainly due to the difference in periods in each classification. Statistical significances calculated using Student's *t* test with Welch's solution are as follows: a-b ($P<0.001$), a-c ($P<0.001$), b-d ($P<0.01$), and c-d ($P<0.01$).

TABLE 1. Association of impending rejections with circulating percentage of TR(+) lymphocytes during clinical quiescences of cardiac transplant recipients[a,c]

	Number of determinations	
	Rejection (−) within 2 weeks	Rejection (+) within 2 weeks
%TR(+) cells[a] ≥8.0[b]	8	11
%TR(+) cells <8.0	59	4

[a] Mean value of circulating %TR(+) cells in one week.

[b] Mean value plus 3 SD of circulating %TR(+) cells in 15 healthy volunteers.

[c] Statistical significance was calculated using the chi-square test with Yates' correction ($\chi^2 = 22.615$, $P < 0.001$).

TABLE 2. Association of recurrent rejections with circulating percentage of TR(+) lymphocytes after treatments of rejections in cardiac transplant recipients[a]

	Number of patients	
	Recurrent rejection (−)	Recurrent rejection (+)
%TR(+) cells[b] ≥8.0[c]	1[d]	4
%TR(+) cells <8.0	12	0

[a] Statistical significance was calculated using the chi-square test with Yates' correction ($\chi^2 = 8.501$, $P < 0.01$).

[b] Values of circulating %TR(+) cells between 7th and 10th days of rejection treatments.

[c] Mean value plus 3 SD of circulating %TR(+) cells in 15 healthy volunteers.

[d] This patient had a septicemia after the rejection treatment.

8.0. Thus, a significant correlation between elevated numbers of TR-positive cells in the circulation and clinical rejection episodes was noted. Moreover, the values of TR greater than 8.0% in clinically quiescent patients were highly associated with impending rejection episodes within two weeks ($P<0.001$) indicating the possible use of TR as an early predictor for allograft rejection or at least as a marker suggesting the need for a biopsy (Table 1). If the percentage of TR cells increased to values greater than 8.0, 11 of the 19 determinations (57.9%) were associated with acute rejections within 2 weeks. On the other hand, if the percentage of TR cells remained less than 8.0, only 4 of the 63 determinations (6.3%) had rejection episodes.

In order to determine whether the TR expression on lymphocytes could be used as an indicator for the efficacy of rejection treatments, the percentage of TR cells was enumerated before and after treatment of rejection episodes. Results presented in Table 2 demonstrate that if the percentage of TR-positive cells decreased and remained below 8.0 within 10 days posttreatment, none of the 12 patients had recurrent rejection episodes within the next 4 weeks. However, if the percentage of TR remained elevated above the value of 8.0, 4 of the 5 patients underwent rejection episodes requiring further treatment ($P<0.01$). The patient in whom the percentage of TR value did not decrease after treatment, although there was no clinically evident rejection, had a serious septicemia (Fig. 2a), thus suggesting that the percentage of TR elevation may also be an indicator of infections. This is further substantiated in Figure 2b, wherein the percentage of TR increased prior to a viral respiratory infection and the percentage of TR decreased below 8.0 with concurrent clearance of symptoms. In four of

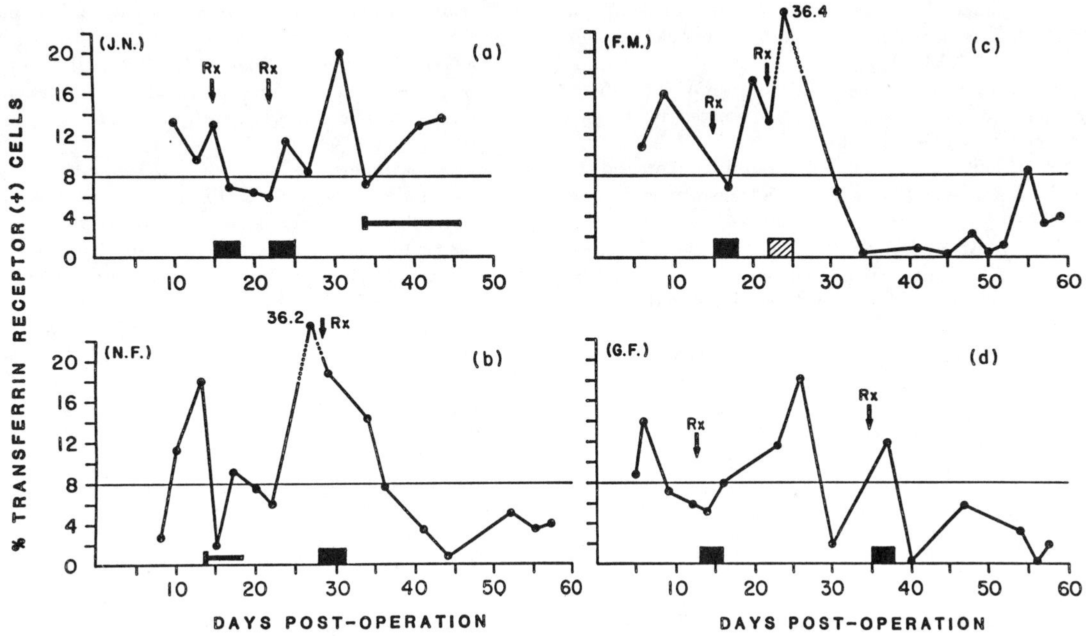

FIGURE 2. Representative patterns of circulating percentages of TR(+) lymphocytes and clinical courses of 4 cardiac transplant recipients: (↓) indicates the day of clinical diagnosis of rejection. Durations of rejection treatments using methylprednisolone (■) and rabbit ATG (▨) are also presented. Infectious complications are shown by horizontal bars (⊢).

five patients with infectious complications (two bacterial and two viral), although the percentage of TR was elevated above 8.0, the T4/T8 ratio was low (0.28–0.98). Thus, an increase in the percentage of TR with low T4/T8 ratios may be indicative of infections rather than rejections, but further analysis is needed to confirm this finding. Correlations between the increased percentage of TR and rejection episodes, as well as the potential use of percentage of TR in monitoring the rejection treatment can be seen in Figure 2, c and d. The percentage of TR values were greater than 8.0 prior to rejection episodes in both patients; these values continued to be high even after rejection treatments, which correlated well with the diagnosis of continuing rejections. Subsequent to a second course of rejection treatment, the percentage of TR decreased and the patients showed no recurrence of rejections. Thus, the data presented clearly indicate that monitoring for the number of TR expressing lymphocytes may serve as an indicator of impending rejections warranting the need for biopsies, as well as being a possible monitor of the efficacy of rejection treatment. Recent clinical studies have suggested the correlation between spontaneous lymphocyte blastogenesis and acute rejections in renal transplant recipients (*8, 9*). These results agree with our findings, since most human lymphoblasts (>90%) have been reported to have TR (*10*). It is also of significance to note that both bacterial and viral infections can increase the numbers of TR expressing lymphocytes in the circulation; however, this might be distinguished by analyzing the T4/T8 ratio simultaneously. Interestingly, recent studies in renal (*11, 12*) and cardiac transplantations (*13*) also reported the association of decreased T4/T8 ratio with cytomegalovirus infection or E-B virus infection. Our experience indicates that the percentage of TR should be monitored frequently, at least three times weekly, since TR is expressed on the surface of activated lymphocytes primarily during the early stages of the cell cycle (*3–7*). In summary, this study demonstrates the utility of enumerating transferrin receptors on circulating lymphocytes in cardiac transplant recipients as a simple means to forecast a possible rejection episode that may be further proved using endomyocardial biopsies before starting rejection treatment. Furthermore, preliminary data also suggest that a continued presence of elevated numbers of TR expressing cells even after treatment may be indicative of less-than-adequate treatment.

T. MOHANAKUMAR[2]
K. HOSHINAGA
N. L. WOOD
S. SZENTPETERY
R. R. LOWER
The Departments of Surgery and Microbiology
Medical College of Virginia
Virginia Commonwealth University
Richmond, Virginia

REFERENCES

1. Goding JW, Burns GF. Monoclonal antibody OKT-9 recognizes the receptor for transferrin on human acute lymphocytic cells. J Immunol 1981; 127: 1256.
2. Trowbridge IS, Lesley J, Schulte R. Murine cell surface transferrin receptor: studies with an anti-receptor monoclonal antibody. J Cell Physiol 1982; 112: 403.
3. Galbraith RM, Galbraith GMP. Expression of transferrin receptors on mitogen-stimulated human peripheral lymphocytes: relation to cellular activation and related metabolic events. Immunology 1981; 44: 703.
4. Frazier JL, Caskey JH, Yoffe M, Seligman PA. Studies of the transferrin receptor on both human reticulocytes and nucleated human cells in culture. J Clin Invest 1982; 69: 853.
5. Neckers LM, Cossman J. Transferrin receptor induction in mito-

[2] Address correspondence to: T. Mohanakumar, Ph.D., Medical College of Virginia, P.O. Box 5, MCV Station, Richmond, Virginia 23298-0001.

gen-stimulated human T lymphocytes is required for DNA synthesis and cell division and is regulated by interleukin 2. Proc Natl Acad Sci USA 1983; 80: 3494.

6. Salmon M, Bacon PA, Symmons DPM, Walton KW. Transferrin receptor expression by stimulated cells in mixed lymphocyte culture. Immunology 1985; 54: 559.
7. Hamilton TA. Regulation of transferrin receptor expression in concanavalin A stimulated and gross virus transformed rat lymphoblasts. J Cell Physiol 1982; 113: 40.
8. Kerman RH, Floyd M, Van Buren C, McConnell BJ, McConnell R, Kahan BD. Correlation of nonspecific immune monitoring with rejection or impaired function of renal allografts. Transplantation 1981; 32: 16.
9. Tanimura S, Taguchi Y, Kunori T, Satomi S, Kaneda I, Kasai M. Monitoring of in vivo blastogenic response in kidney transplant patients by flow cytometry. Transplant Proc 1985; 17: 652.
10. Hammarström ML, Axelsson B, Ivansen M, Hammarström S, Perlmann P. Transferrin receptors on mitogen-stimulated human thymus-derived lymphocytes. Scand J Immunol 1982; 16: 355.
11. Fiche M, Soulillou JP, Bignon JD, Billaudel S, Guenel J. T lymphocyte monitoring in kidney transplant recipients undergoing cytomegalovirus infection or rejection episodes. Transplantation 1984; 37: 421.
12. van Es A, Baldwin WM, Oljans PJ, Tanke HJ, Ploem JS, van Es LA. Expression of HLA-DR on T lymphocytes following renal transplantation, and association with graft-rejection episodes and cytomegalo-virus infection. Transplantation 1984; 37: 65.
13. Dummer JS, Ho M, Rabin B, Griffith BP, Hardesty RL, Bahnson HT. The effect of cytomegalovirus and Epstein-Barr virus infection on T lymphocyte subsets in cardiac transplant patients on cyclosporine. Transplantation 1984; 38: 433.

Received 5 December 1985.
Accepted 24 February 1986.

THE EFFECT OF REPEATED PREGNANCIES ON RENAL ALLOGRAFT FUNCTION

Approximately one of every 50 women of childbearing age with a functioning renal allograft becomes pregnant, and over 1200 cases of successful pregnancies in kidney transplant patients have already been reported (*1*). However, it was recently emphasized that most of these patients have had only one pregnancy; there is little information available regarding repeated pregnancies and the effects that they might have on the transplanted kidney (*2*). This has become an important issue in counseling these women about contraception, sterilization, and the safety of future pregnancies. We present a patient who has had six pregnancies since she received her renal allograft 15 years ago and whose renal function remains normal.

Case report. This 35-year-old gravida 6, para 5, abortus 1 patient was maintained on hemodialysis for chronic glomerulonephritis for two years until she underwent transplantation at age 21 of a four-antigen-match kidney from her brother. Following the operation her general condition improved, and her renal function remained normal while she continued to take azathioprine 75 mg and prednisone 5 mg daily. The patient's first pregnancy occurred five years after transplantation, and a 3300-g female infant was delivered by cesarean section because of failure to progress in labor and fetal distress. Her second pregnancy ended as a spontaneous abortion, but subsequent pregnancies (which have been followed with frequent antepartum visits, serial ultrasound examinations, and renal function tests) have been relatively uncomplicated. She has been delivered each time between 36 and 40 weeks gestation by repeat cesarean section, and birth weights of the two boys and three girls were 3300, 3420, 2600, 3050, and 2775 g. She was mildly hypertensive (diastolic blood pressures in the range of 80–90 mm Hg) toward the end of her first and sixth pregnancies, but there were no other signs or symptoms of preeclampsia. Asymptomatic bacteruria was treated at 24 weeks gestation during the fifth pregnancy, but she has never had albuminuria, glycosuria, or deterioration of renal function (Fig. 1). She experienced a moderate postpartum depression following her fifth pregnancy, which gradually resolved spontaneously, and tubal sterilization was performed at the time of the last cesarean section. Her health has remained good, and all of the children (ages 10, 6, 4, 3, and 1 year) are growing and developing normally and have had no unusual infections or immunologic problems.

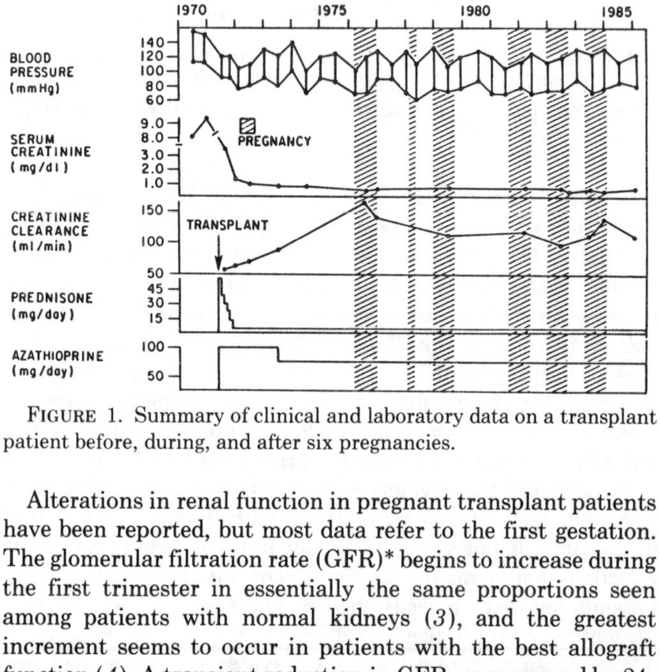

FIGURE 1. Summary of clinical and laboratory data on a transplant patient before, during, and after six pregnancies.

Alterations in renal function in pregnant transplant patients have been reported, but most data refer to the first gestation. The glomerular filtration rate (GFR)* begins to increase during the first trimester in essentially the same proportions seen among patients with normal kidneys (*3*), and the greatest increment seems to occur in patients with the best allograft function (*4*). A transient reduction in GFR, as measured by 24-hr creatinine clearance, sometimes occurs during the third trimester, but in most cases GFR has returned to prepregnancy levels by 8–12 weeks postpartum (*3*). The occurrence or worsening of proteinuria is present near term in 30–40% of patients, but this usually resolves postpartum—and, in the absence of other symptoms, requires no specific management (*4*). Permanent impairment of renal function following pregnancy has been seen in 7–15% of patients, but this is similar to the incidence of allograft deterioration in the nonpregnant renal transplant population (*5–7*). Because most cases of permanent graft impairment have occurred in patients with poor preconceptual renal function (plasma creatinine >2 mg/dl), even the first pregnancy should be avoided in those cases. Significant reduction of renal function in any transplant patient during pregnancy also remains as indication for pregnancy termination because of the risk that such damage may become permanent.

* Abbreviation used: GFR, glomerular filtration rate.

The effect of pregnancy in transplant patients has been found to be unrelated to prior rejection episodes or human leukocyte antigen types (*8*). Pregnancy outcome is correlated closely with renal function, and there is little evidence that the gestation has an adverse effect on the renal allograft. As with other chronic renal diseases, hypertension and azotemia at conception are associated with a higher risk to both mother and infant (1, 6, 9, 10). The ideal timing of pregnancy appears to be between two and five years after transplantation, when renal function has stabilized and immunosuppressive medication has been reduced to moderate dosages. When pregnancy occurs five or more years after transplantation, the postpartum renal function is not as good in some patients as it was before pregnancy and does not recover (*6*). However, adequate renal function rather than parity is the important factor in the success of the pregnancy, and long-term prognosis for the transplanted kidney. In patients with any type of chronic renal disease, pregnancy outcome has uniformly been good and deterioration of renal function has been unusual if the serum creatinine is less than 1.5 mg/dl (*1, 9, 10*). These clinical data now permit the clinician to distinguish transplant patients who are likely to experience difficulty from those in whom pregnancy can be undertaken with high expectation of success.

Our patient tolerated five term pregnancies and one spontaneous abortion with no deterioration of renal function. It is important to note that she has always remained in good health since her transplant with no rejection episodes, hypertension, or apparent contraindications to pregnancy. The greatest number of pregnancies reported in any other patient following renal transplantation is four (*11*). That patient also had no change in the functioning of her renal allograft during or after the pregnancies. Of the two patients who have had three pregnancies, one has done well. The other experienced severe preeclampsia during the third pregnancy, and postpartum renal deterioration eventually contributed to her death (*11, 12*). Therefore, it is clear that the success of one pregnancy in a particular patient does not always predict or guarantee the success of subsequent gestations. However, many transplant patients have achieved two successful pregnancies (*11, 17*), and others have been delivered of twins and triplets (*17, 18*). Our patient also shows that repeated pregnancies are not invariably contraindicated in renal transplant patients.

James R. Scott[1]
D. Ware Branch

[1] Address Reprint Requests to: James R. Scott, M.D., Department of Obstetrics and Gynecology, University of Utah Medical Center, Salt Lake City, Utah 84132.

Neil K. Kochenour
Ronald M. Larkin
Department of Obstetrics and Gynecology
University of Utah Medical Center,
Salt Lake City, Utah 84132

REFERENCES

1. Hou S. Pregnancy in women with chronic renal disease. N Engl J Med 1985; 312: 836.
2. Taylor ES. Editorial comment. Obstet Gynecol Surv 1985; 40: 627.
3. Davison JM. The effect of pregnancy on kidney function in renal allograft recipients. Kidney Int 1985; 27: 74.
4. Scott JR. Gynecologic and obstetric problems in renal allograft recipients. In: Buchsbaum HV, Schmidt J, eds. Gynecologic and obstetric urology. 2nd edition. Philadelphia: Saunders, 1982: 547.
5. Penn I, Makowski EL, Harris P. Parenthood following renal transplantation. Kidney Int 1980; 18: 221.
6. Davison JM, Lindheimer MD. Pregnancy in renal transplant recipients. J Reprod Med 1982; 27: 613.
7. Fine RN. Pregnancy in renal allograft recipients. Am J Nephrol 1982; 2: 117.
8. Lau RJ, Scott JR. Pregnancy following renal transplantation. Clin Obstet Gynecol 1985; 28: 339.
9. Bear RA. Pregnancy in patients with chronic renal disease. CMAJ 1978; 118: 663.
10. Shinichi A, Yasuhiro A, Konosuke K, et al. The influence of antecedent renal disease on pregnancy. Am J Obstet Gynecol 1985; 153: 508.
11. Makowski EL, Penn I. Parenthood following renal transplantation. In: de Alvarez R, ed. The kidney in pregnancy. New York: Wiley, 1976: 215.
12. Sciarra J, Toledo-Pereyra LH, Bendel RP, et al. Pregnancy following renal transplantation. Am J Obstet Gynecol 1975; 123: 411.
13. Golby M. Fertility after renal transplantation. Transplantation 1970; 10: 201.
14. Salant DJ, Marcus RG, Milne FJ, et al. Pregnancy in renal transplant recipients. S Afr Med J 1976; 50: 1288.
15. Waltzer WC, Coulam CB, Zincke H, et al. Pregnancy in renal transplantation. Transplant Proc 1980; 12: 221.
16. Whethem JCG, Cardella C, Harding M. Effect of pregnancy on graft survival in renal cadaver transplant patients. Am J Obstet Gynecol 1983; 145: 193.
17. Successful pregnancies in women treated by dialysis and kidney transplantation. Report from the Registration committee of the European Dialysis and Transplant Association). Br J Obstet Gynaecol 1980; 87: 839.
18. MacLean AB, Sharp F, Briggs JD, et al. Successful triplet pregnancy following renal transplantation. Scott Med J 1980; 25: 320.

Received 10 March 1986.
Accepted 7 April 1986.

ASSESSMENT OF FACTORS ASSOCIATED WITH DONOR-SPECIFIC SENSITIZATION IN PATIENTS GIVEN DONOR-SPECIFIC BLOOD TRANSFUSIONS

Recipient preparation for renal transplantation from mismatched living, related donors (LRD),* may include pretreatment with donor-specific blood transfusions (DST) (*1*). Even though the results of LRD renal transplantation have steadily improved during the past few years with the use of DST (*2*), this form of treatment adds a 30% risk of inducing donor-specific sensitization (*1, 2*). If low-dose azathioprine (AZA) is given throughout the transfusion period, the risk for patients developing antidonor T cell antibodies is decreased to 15% (*3*). Unfortunately, the majority of patients who become sensitized respond, not only against the mismatched HLA antigens of their donor, but also against many other HLA antigens—as is evidenced by a sharp increase in serum antibody titers directed

* Abbreviations used: AZA, azothioprine; DST, donor-specific transfusion; LRD, living-related donor; PRA, percentage of reactive antibody.

against a panel of lymphocytes. As a consequence sensitized patients may have to wait for a considerable period of time to receive a crossmatch-negative cadaveric kidney. We have reviewed factors known to be associated with the development of recipient sensitization and have identified some factors as highly predictive of future sensitization with DST.

Eighty-one potential recipients of mismatched LRD renal allografts were pretreated with DST between September 1981 and May 1985. All patients who received DST after January 1983 also received concomitant low-dose AZA throughout the transfusion period. Of the 81 patients, 2 had previously rejected a renal transplant; 11 had had previous pregnancies; and 5 had been previously transfused. All recipients received 200 ml of packed cells from their potential donor on three occasions at two-week intervals (*1*). Some received azathioprine (0.5 mg/kg/day) beginning 5 days before their first transfusion. The AZA was continued as tolerated, to keep the leukocyte count greater than 2000 cells/mm^3, until transfusion or until development of a positive crossmatch.

All patients and donors were tissue-typed by microcytotoxic techniques (*4*). Prior to beginning the DST protocol, and two weeks after each DST, the recipient's serum was crossmatched against the donor's T and B lymphocytes, which had been purified with nylon-wool, according to standard NIH techniques (*5*). T cell crossmatches were performed at room temperature, and B cell crossmatches were performed at 37°C and 4°C for both the donor and the recipient. A crossmatch was considered to be positive if cell death in the patient's serum was 10% greater than that found in a control of heat-inactivated fetal calf serum. A positive T cell crossmatch was considered to be an absolute contraindication for continued DSTs and for use of the potential LRD for renal transplantation. Alloreactivity studies, the percentage of reactive antibody titers (PRA), were derived from a panel of lymphocytes obtained from 25 selected individuals by standard complement-mediated cytotoxicity tests (*5*).

Prior to initiating DST, 13 patients had high (30%) PRA levels (median 54%: range 30%–99%) and 7 (54%) of them developed donor-specific sensitization (Table 1). Four patients (Nos. 1–4) underwent DST without AZA and 3 (75%) became sensitized. However, 4 (44%) of the remaining nine highly sensitized patients who received AZA during DST period also became sensitized (Nos. 5–8).

Of the 81 patients, 68 had PRA titers of less than 30%. The incidence of sensitization during DST with and without concomitant AZA treatment was also evaluated in these patients. A total of 34 patients were not immunosuppressed during the DST period, and 7 (21%) became sensitized. Another 34 low-PRA-titer patients received AZA during DST, and only 3 (9%) were sensitized to their donor.

Eleven multiparous women underwent DST. Five had high PRA titers and received DST from haploidentical siblings (Nos. 6, 8, 9, 11, 13). Two of the women (Nos. 6 and 8) also received random blood transfusions prior to initiating DST, and only these two women developed donor-specific sensitization. Six multiparous women had low PRA levels, yet all three women who received DST from offspring became sensitized. Two of these three sensitized women received concomitant AZA during DST.

Only two uremics with a previously rejected renal transplant entered the DST protocol. One patient received multiple random blood transfusions and had high PRA titer prior to DST, the other received no transfusions and had low PRA titer prior to DST—yet only the patient who received prior random transfusions developed donor-specific sensitivity.

Standard NIH crossmatch techniques have been shown to be less sensitive at detecting low levels of antidonor antibodies than either indirect immunofluorescence or flow cytometry techniques (6, 7). Perhaps either of these methods might have more accurately detected donor/recipient crossmatch positivity prior to beginning DST. Nevertheless, our data suggest that: 1. potential recipients with a high PRA titer prior to DST are extremely susceptible to donor-specific sensitization despite accompanying azathioprine treatment; 2. women with a high PRA titer and a history of previous pregnancies and random blood transfusions are at high risk to become sensitized to a DST donor; 3. multiparous women may be likely to become sensitized to offspring DST donors; and 4. prior recipients of rejected allografts who have received random transfusions may be susceptible to donor sensitization during DST.

We realize that the last two conclusions have been derived from a very small number of patients. The validity of these two conclusions need to be verified on a larger patient population.

In general, patients with high PRA titers seem more likely to develop donor-specific sensitization as a result of DST and probably should be offered cyclosporine for maintenance immunosuppression and rejection prophylaxis (*8*). The greatest benefit of DST with concomitant AZA is observed in patients with low PRA levels prior to DST, in whom sensitization is minimized and the full benefit of DST may be accrued.

Smita Vaidya[1]
Bruce G. Sommer
Eva Pagel
Maureen Koegel
Ronald M. Ferguson

TABLE 1. Results of concomitant azathioprine treatment during DST in patients with high PRA (30%)

Patient	Immunological history	PRA before DST (after DST)	Azathioprine treatment	Sensitization
1[a]	Random transfusion	54(90)	No	Yes
2[a]	Prior cadaveric transplant & rejection; Random transfusion	68(99)	No	Yes
3[a]	Random transfusion	30(ND)[b]	No	Yes
4[a]	Random transfusion	56(ND)	No	No
5	Noncontributory	34(79)	Yes	Yes[c]
6	Pregnancy; random transfusion	82(99)	Yes	Yes
7	Random transfusion	99(99)	Yes	Yes
8	Pregnancy; random transfusion	96(99)	Yes	Yes
9	Pregnancy	34(16)	Yes	No
10	Random transfusion	68(44)	Yes	No
11	Pregnancy	52(58)	Yes	No
12	Noncontributory	38(40)	Yes	No
13	Pregnancy	42(46)	Yes	No

[a] Received no immunosuppressive therapy during DST.
[b] ND: not determined.
[c] Azathioprine discontinued after third DST treatment.

[1] Current address: Pathology Department, University of Texas Medical Branch, Galveston, Texas 77550.

Division of Transplantation,
Department of Surgery,
The Ohio State University College of Medicine,
Columbus, Ohio 43210

REFERENCES

1. Salvatierra O, Vincenti F, Amend W, et al. Deliberate donor-specific blood transfusions prior to living related transplantation: a new approach. Ann Surg 1980; 192: 543.
2. Salvatierra O Jr, Iwaki Y, Vincenti F, et al. Incidence, characteristics and outcome of recipients sensitized after donor-specific blood transfusions. Transplantation 1981; 32: 528.
3. Anderson CB, Sicard GA, Ethredge EE. Pretreatment of renal allograft recipients with azathioprine and donor-specific blood products. Surgery 1982; 92: 315.
4. Terasaki PI, Bernoco D, Park MS, et al. Microdroplet testing for HLA-A, -B, -C, and -D antigens. Am J Clin Pathol 1978; 69: 103.
5. Amos BD. Cytotoxicity testing. In: Ray JG Jr, Hare BD, Penderson PD, Mullally DI, eds. NIAID manual of tissue typing techniques. Publication No. (NIH) 77-545. Washington, DC: US DHEW 1976: 25.
6. Sanfilippo F, Vaughn WK, Bollinger RR, Spees EK. Comparative effects of pregnancy, transfusion, and prior graft rejection on sensitization and renal transplant results. Transplantation 1982; 34: 360.
7. Garovoy MR, Rheinschmidt MA, Bigos M, et al. Flow cytometry analysis. Transplant Proc 1983; 15: 1939.
8. Sommer BG, Ferguson RM. Mismatched living related renal transplantation: a prospective randomized study. Surgery 1985; 98: 269.

Received 12 November 1985.
Accepted 24 February 1986.

CELL-MEDIATED LYMPHOLYSIS IN KAPOSI'S SARCOMA AFTER RENAL ALLOGRAFT

REPORT OF TWO CASES

Immunologic evaluation of patients with Kaposi's sarcoma (KS)* reveals defects in cell-mediated immunity but relatively intact humoral and neutrophil function (*1–4*). Thus, when peripheral lymphocytes are stimulated in vitro by mitogens or by allogeneic cells in mixed lymphocyte culture (MLC), they usually show marked depression in their ability to proliferate and incorporate ^{3}H-thymidine (*5, 6*).

The T lymphocyte competence can also be assessed in vitro by the measurement of certain effector functions (*1–10*), such as eliciting an allogeneic cytotoxic lymphocyte response against genetically related or unrelated subjects. To our knowledge no such type of study has been communicated so far in KS. The use of a cell-mediated lympholysis (CML) assay could also give insight into the type of cells involved in the deficient immune response described in this condition.

KS has been reported with increasing frequency in renal allograft recipients (*5, 11*). This report describes a de novo development of KS in two patients after renal allograft from living-related donors, in whom CML assay revealed an unspecific hyporesponsiveness.

Patient 1 (S.M.). On December 3, 1982, an 18-year-old man was transplanted with a renal allograft from his father.

Methylprednisone and azathioprine were instituted. Three episodes of acute rejection were treated with i.v. boluses of methylprednisone (total of 7 g) and 600 rads of local radiotherapy. On January 24, 1983, serum creatinine rose to 2.58 mg% and a total dose of 1240 mg methylprednisone was given. In December 1983, he noted a small purplish indurated nodule in the scrotum. A biopsy was performed and the diagnosis of KS was made. Histologically the lesion consisted of areas of spindle cells among which erythrocytes were enmeshed. There were numerous vascular lumina lined by endothelial cells. Mitotic figures were also present. Thereafter, similar lesions appeared on both legs, arms, head, mouth and nasopharynx. On February 4, 1984, a chest roentgenogram revealed nodular and interstitial infiltrates. Azathioprine was stopped and methylprednisone was tapered to 10 mg/day. On February 27, 1984, radiotherapy to the mouth and nasopharynx was begun, with a total of 3500 rads. In April 1984 the patient complained of increasing cough, mucopurulent discharge, and dyspnea. Serum creatinine was 2.42 mg%. Severe respiratory insufficiency developed and the patient died on May 6, 1984. At autopsy, multiple purplish indurated nodules were found in the lymph nodes, liver and left adrenal gland. A nodule, 1.5-cm in diameter was present in the duodenum; three similar lesions were located in the small intestine. The transplanted kidney showed histological signs of chronic rejection. It was free of sarcomatous lesions, in spite of heavy infiltration of perirenal tissues. The lungs showed multiple nodules, which were third of the whole parenchyma. Finally, two exofitic partially obstructing Kaposi's tumors were found in the trachea and in a main bronchus.

Patient 2 (M.M.). On October 26, 1977, a 20-year-old woman was tranplanted with a renal allograft from her father. Methylprednisone and azathioprine were instituted. An acute rejection was treated with a total dose of 4 g methylprednisone given by i.v. boluses. In May 1982 purplish indurated lesions appeared in the left thigh. A skin biopsy revealed KS, as described above. Azathioprine was discontinued and prednisone maintained at 30 mg/day, and the skin lesions gradually disappeared, azathioprine being reinstituted in October 1982. On March 9, 1984, fever, coma, and renal failure developed. Analysis of spinal fluid revealed *Cryptococcus neoformans* and *Streptococcus fecalis.* She was treated with amphotericin and vancomycin with good response. Renal function did not improve and a renal biopsy showed chronic rejection. In September 1984 she resumed chronic hemodialysis.

For cellular immune studies blood was collected from the recipients, donors, and unrelated healthy subjects. The lymphocytes were separated by Ficoll-hypaque gradient centrifugation.

Spontaneous sheep erythrocyte (E) and sheep erythrocyte coated with antibody and complement (EAC)-rosette-forming lymphocytes were considered to represent T and B populations, respectively (*12*); T cell subtypes were distinguished by complement-dependent cytotoxicity (CDC) using the monoclonal antibodies OKT3, OKT4, and OKT8 (Ortho Pharmaceuticals, Raritan, NJ).

*Abbreviations used: CDC, complement-dependent cytotoxicity; CML, cell-mediated lympholysis; Con A, concanavalin A; EAC, sheep erythrocyte, coated with antibody and complement; E, spontaneous sheep erythrocyte; KS, Kaposi's sarcoma; MLC, mixed lymphocyte culture; PHA, phytohemagglutinin; PWM, pokeweed mitogen.

The CML assay was performed according to the macromethod described by Lightbody (*13*). Briefly, the peripheral blood lymphocytes of the recipients were sensitized in vitro against the irradiated peripheral blood lymphocytes from both kidney donors and unrelated healthy subjects, in a one-way MLC. The effector cells (i.e., recipient antidonor, recipient anticontrol) were cultured for 6 days. Each combination was performed in triplicate. The percentages of donor-specific lysis and control cell lysis were determined in relation to phytohemagglutinin-stimulated blast cells, in a 4-hr ^{51}Cr assay, utilizing a ratio of effector/target cells of 100:1. The percentage of lysis (% CML) was calculated as follows:

$$\frac{\text{experimental mean cpm} - \text{spontaneous release mean cpm}}{\text{maximum release mean cpm} - \text{spontaneous release mean cpm}} \times 100$$

Values are expressed as $\bar{x} \pm$ ES.

The culture medium for both the MLC and CML assays was RPMI 1640 supplemented with 20% heat-inactivated pooled human AB serum from male donors, 25 nM HEPES (N-2-hydroxy-ethyl-piperazine-n′-2-ethane sulfonic acid), 20 mM L-glutamine, 100 UI penicillin/ml, and 100 μg of streptomycin/ml. Typing for HLA-A, B and C was performed as previously described (*14*).

Circulating lymphocytes were in the normal range in both patients. As shown in Table 1, the percentage of E and EAC-rosette-forming lymphocytes was normal in both patients. The percentage of T lymphocytes staining positively with the OKT3 was normal, the OKT4 population being only slightly depressed; the percentage of suppressor/cytotoxic T lymphocytes staining positively with the OKT8 monoclonal antibody was increased 1.76-fold. Thus the ratio of helper to suppressor/cytotoxic lymphocytes was decreased 2-fold. In vitro studies of PHA-induced lymphocyte proliferation showed a 4-fold to 1.8-fold decrease in ^{3}H-thymidine incorporation by lymphocytes from KS patients compared with lymphocytes from normal controls.

CML was 10% and 13% between recipient and donor, and 48% and 45% between recipient and unrelated healthy subjects' cells (Table 2). These figures are similar to those encountered in our laboratory between functioning renal allograft recipients without KS and their donors (13%±2.8), but lower than values found between functioning renal allograft recipients without KS and unrelated healthy subject cells (78.5%±4), and between unrelated controls as well (72.7%±3.9) (unpublished data).

Our finding of an unspecific CML hyporesponsiveness must be compared with CML responses in renal allograft recipients without KS. We have only found similar results in a patient without KS who discontinued immunosuppressive therapy after renal allograft and who showed normal renal function during a follow-up of 8 months (*15*). Otherwise, all of our immunosuppressed well-functioning allograft recipients without KS have shown an impaired CML response against their donor's lymphocytes (13%±2.8), with a normal CML response against unrelated healthy subjects' cells (78.5%±4). This last figure is similar to that found by us between unrelated healthy subjects (72.7%±3.9) (unpublished data). On the other hand, Goulmy et al. have reported that unspecific CML hyporesponsiveness can also be demonstrated in some well-functioning cadaveric renal allograft recipients (*16, 17*).

Thus the ability to mount a cytotoxic activity was unspecifically impaired in KS patients. The question of whether the immune alterations antedated the appearance of sarcomatous lesions cannot be answered here. The fact that renal allograft recipients without KS can also exhibit CML unspecific hyporesponsiveness (*16, 17*) would suggest that a low CML does not necessarily predispose to KS. Our data do not permit us to hypothesize about the mechanisms of the CML hyporesponsiveness.

Whether the diminished ratio of helper to suppressor/cytotoxic lymphocytes in the presence of a poor CML response was due to an increase in the number of suppressor cells is not conclusively answered in this study.

In summary, we have presented two renal allograft recipients with KS who showed an impaired CML response, both to their donors and to unrelated subjects. Further studies should clarify the mechanism of this hyporesponsiveness and its relation to KS.

TABLE 1. Cellular immune studies in renal allograft recipients with Kaposi's sarcoma

Cellular immune studies in peripheral blood (%)	Normal control subjects	Patient 1[a]	Patient 2[b]
E rosettes	65–85	71	69
EAC rosettes	20–35	26	28
OKT3 (pan-T) lymphocytes	85–90	95	90
OKT4 (T-helper/inducer) lymphocytes	65–75	50	47
OKT8 (T-suppressor/cytotoxic) lymphocytes	25–35	45	43
Ratio OKT4/OKT8 cells	2.1–2.6	1.1	1.1
Phytohemagglutinin-induced transformation	100	25	31

[a] On methylprednisone, 10 mg/day; no azathioprine; disseminated KS at the time of the study, 1–3 months after diagnosis.

[b] No prednisone, no azathioprine; KS in complete remission at the time of the study, 2 years after diagnosis.

TABLE 2. CML (%) in renal allografts with and without Kaposi's sarcoma and in controls

Combinations	Without KS	With KS	
		Patient 1[a]	Patient 2[a]
Functioning renal allograft recipient—donor	13±2.8 (n=7)	10	13
Functioning renal allograft recipient—control	78.5±4 (n=7)	48	45
Control—unrelated control	72.7±3.9 (n=3)	—	—

[a] See footnotes to Table 1.

Acknowledgments. We thank Dr. J.A. Barcat, Dr. L. Verruno, Dr. J. Abulafia, and Mrs. B. Castro for their cooperation in this study.

SUSANA GERTRUDIS RODRÍGUEZ[1]
RODOLFO SANTIAGO MARTÍN
HUGO ANTONIO ARAUJO
CLARISA LAURA ALVAREZ

[1]Address correspondence to: Dra. Susana G. Rodríguez, Instituto de Investigaciones Médicas Alfredo Lanari Donato Alvarez 3150, 1427 Buenos Aires, Argentina.

María del Carmen Samaniego
Instituto de Investigaciones Médicas Alfredo Lanari
Facultad de Medicina
Universidad de Buenos Aires
Argentina

REFERENCES

1. Mazzaferri ME, Penn GM. Kaposi's sarcoma associated with multiple myeloma. Arch Intern Med 1968; 122: 521.
2. Master SP, Taylor JF, Kyalwazi SK, Ziegler JL. Immunological studies in Kaposi's sarcoma in Uganda. Br Med J 1970; 1: 600.
3. Dobozy A, Husz S, Hunyadi J, Berkó G, Simon N. Immune deficiencies and Kaposi's sarcoma [Letter]. Lancet 1973; 1: 625.
4. Friedman-Kien AE, Laubenstein LJ, Rubinstein P, et al. Disseminated Kaposi's sarcoma in homosexual men. Ann Intern Med 1982; 96: 693.
5. Hardy MA, Goldfarb P, Levine S, et al. De novo Kaposi's sarcoma in renal transplantation. Cancer 1976; 38: 144.
6. Harwood AR, Osoba D, Hofstader SL, et al. Kaposi's sarcoma in recipients of renal transplants. Am J Med 1979; 67: 759.
7. Penn I. Kaposi's sarcoma in organ transplant recipients. Transplantation 1979; 27: 8.
8. Birkeland SA. Malignant tumors in renal transplant patients. The Scandia transplant material. Cancer 1983; 51: 1571.
9. Akhtar M, Bunuan H, Ali MA, Godwin JT. Kaposi's sarcoma in renal transplant recipients. Cancer 1984; 53: 258.
10. Luderschmidt C, Hillebrand G, Castro LA, Hammer C. Kutannoduläres Kaposi-Sarkom nach Nierentransplantation und Immunosuppression. Klin Wochenschr 1984; 62: 803.
11. Penn I. Cancer in immunosuppressed patients. Transplant Proc 1984; 16: 492.
12. Winchester RJ, Ross G. Methods for enumerating lymphocyte populations. In: Rose NR, Friedman H, eds. Manual of clinical immunology. Washington: American Society for Microbiology, 1976: 64.
13. Lightbody J. Use of the cell-mediated lympholysis test in transplantation immunity. In: Rose NR, Friedman H, eds. Manual of clinical immunology. Washington: American Society for Microbiology, 1976: 851.
14. Terasaki PI, McClelland JD. Microdroplet assay of human serum cytotoxins. Nature 1964; 204: 998.
15. Samaniego MC, Aguirre C, Martín R, Manni J. Unspecific CML hyporesponsiveness in a successful renal transplant patient after complete discontinuation of immuno-suppression [Abstract]. Fourth International Congress of Immunology, Paris, 1980: 8.3.22.
16. Goulmy E, Persijn G, Blokland E, D'amaro J, van Rood JJ. Cell-mediated lympholysis studies in renal allograft recipients. Transplantation 1981; 31: 210.
17. Goulmy E, Blokland E. Occurrence of posttransplant donor specific cell-mediated lympholysis nonreactivity in renal allograft recipients with perioperative transfusion only. Transplantation 1985; 39: 105.

Received 21 November 1985.
Accepted 24 February 1986.

IMMUNOFLUORESCENCE CAUSED BY CYCLOSPORINE IN URINARY EXFOLIATIVE CYTOLOGY IN RENAL TRANSPLANT RECIPIENTS

In spite of the efficacy of cyclosporine in preventing rejection of transplanted organs (*1, 2*), its main disadvantage is nephrotoxicity (*3*). Although it has been generally held that no morphologic damage of renal cells occurs (*4*), Cortesini (*5*) et al. have reported intracytoplasmic eosinophilic granulations in exfoliated proximal renal tubule cells of transplant patients on cyclosporine therapy. In an attempt to localize cyclosporine in exfoliated urinary tract cells, we examined urinary sediments for specific immunocytofluorescence due to cyclosporine in the first five patients treated with cyclosporine in our renal transplantation program. We also measured serum beta 2-microglobulin levels with the Phaedebas test (Pharmacia, Inc., Piscataway, NJ) to monitor nephrotoxicity and evaluated helper/suppressor (H/S) ratios by OKT4:OKT8 antiserum reactivity as an indicator of rejection. A two-year follow-up of renal graft function is presented.

Blood and urine specimens from five patients who had received kidneys from cadaver donors were tested at least weekly for five weeks (total specimens: 28). Patients received a preoperative dose of 5 mg/kg cyclosporine. Thereafter, patients were given oral doses of 12 mg/kg/day for five weeks unless blood levels indicated an adjustment of the dosage. Subsequently, conventional immunosuppression was substituted.

Twenty-four-hour urine specimens were collected on ice without preservative to correspond with blood specimens drawn for cyclosporine levels. A 50-ml aliquot was centrifuged, the sediment resuspended in a small amount of saline, and a cytospin preparation made. The slides were fixed in cold acetone for 10 min.

A drop of a 1:20 dilution of sheep anticyclosporine antiserum (Sandoz, East Hanover, NJ) in phosphate-buffered saline (PBS) was placed on each slide and incubated in a moist chamber at room temperature for 30 min. Slides were washed in PBS for 15 min. A drop of 1:20 dilution of PBS of rabbit antisheep antiserum (Kallestad, Austin, TX) was added to each slide and incubated at room temperature for 30 min and washed as before. Finally, a 1:20 dilution of fluoresceinated goat anti-rabbit antiserum (Tago, Inc., Burlingame, CA.) was added, incubated for 30 min at room temperature and washed as stated. The slides were coverslipped with mounting medium and examined under fluorescence microscopy. A clean-catch random urine from a normal person not on cyclosporine therapy was used as a negative control. Only squamous epithelial cells were seen in this normal sediment. Fluorescence was graded as weakly positive (0.5^+), positive (1^+) or strongly positive (2^+). In weakly positive specimens less than 10% of cells fluoresced, positive specimens showed fluorescence of 25–50% of cells and strongly positive specimens showed fluorescence of greater than 50% of cells. Both squamous and round epithelial cells were seen to fluoresce in positive specimens. In no specimen were cells absent from the sediment.

Of the 28 urinary sediments, 14 were negative for immunofluorescence and 14 were positive. One patient's urine remained negative for the entire five weeks.

Figure 1 is a photomicrograph of a urinary sediment preparation positive for immunofluorescence with cyclosporine antiserum.

The mechanism by which cyclosporine causes nephrotoxicity is not known. Damage may require time or cumulative effects of the drug, since no specimen was positive for fluorescence at

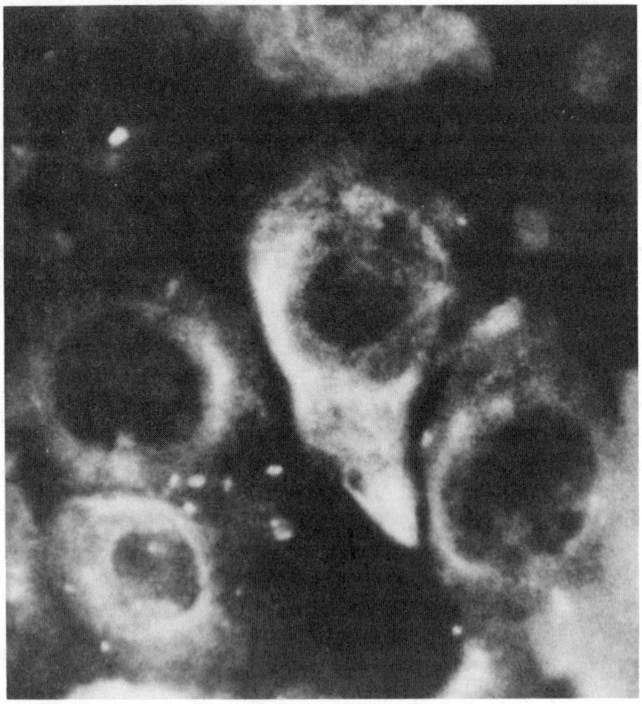

FIGURE 1. Cytospin preparation from a 24-hr urine specimen obtained from a renal transplant patient on cyclosporine therapy. The cells exhibit positive immunofluorescence after treatment with antiserum to cyclosporine.

less than seven days of cyclosporine therapy as shown in Figure 2. von Willebrand and Hayry (*6*) have reported finding cyclosporine deposits detectable by immunofluorescence in fine-needle biopsies of transplanted kidneys. These deposits were always present when nephrotoxicity was noted, and deposits tended to correlate with blood levels of cyclosporine. Using serum creatinine, cyclosporine deposits in the graft and presence or absence of inflammatory cells in the graft as guides, they used this technique to differentiate nephrotoxicity from rejection. Occasionally both processes occurred together as we believe happened in our patient No. 1.

If immunofluorescence of exfoliated urinary cells represents damage to renal tubular cells by cyclosporine, this technique may be used to confirm nephrotoxicity. However, as shown in Figure 3, the negative correlation between immunofluorescence and blood levels of cyclosporine suggests a time lag between high blood levels of the drug and appearance of positive cells in the urine. Therefore, immunofluorescence does not appear useful in predicting renal toxicity, but due to marked variation in individual response to the drug immunofluorescence may have value in adjusting dosages in difficult patients.

We also found a negative correlation between cyclosporine levels and serum beta 2-microglobulin levels, again attributing this observation to a time lag in appearance of beta 2-microglobulin in the serum. Beta 2-microglobulin is a single polypeptide chain with a molecular weight of 11,000 daltons synthesized by regenerating membranes. Several investigators have used beta 2-microglobulin as an index of aminoglycoside-induced necrosis of proximal renal tubular cells (*7, 8*). The normal value for serum Beta-2 microglobulin is 1.1-1.9 mg/L. Values in all of our transplant patients exceeded these normals, but by posttransplant (P-TX) day 30 all showed less than 3.5 mg/L except the one patient in whom rejection was suspected whose value rose from 6.8 mg/L on P-TX day 2 to 18.2 mg/L on P-TX day 33.

Parameters measured in our five patients are summarized in Table 1, and their clinical courses are discussed below.

Patient No. 1, a 22-year-old woman receiving her third

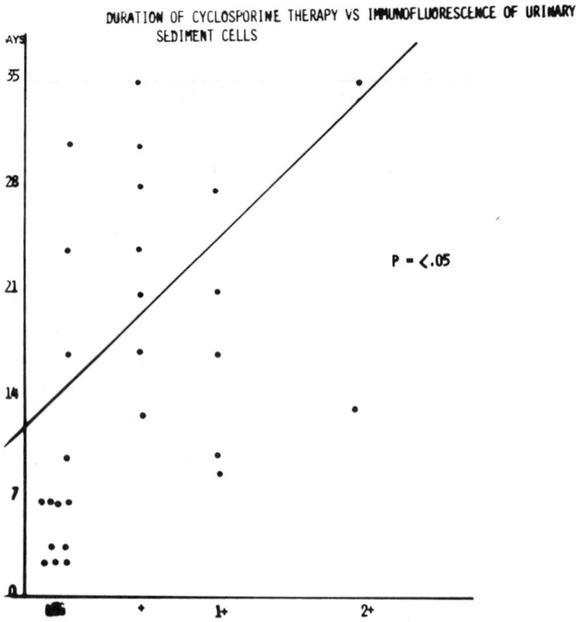

FIGURE 2. Comparison of the degree of immunofluorescence of urinary sediment cells and the duration of cyclosporine therapy.

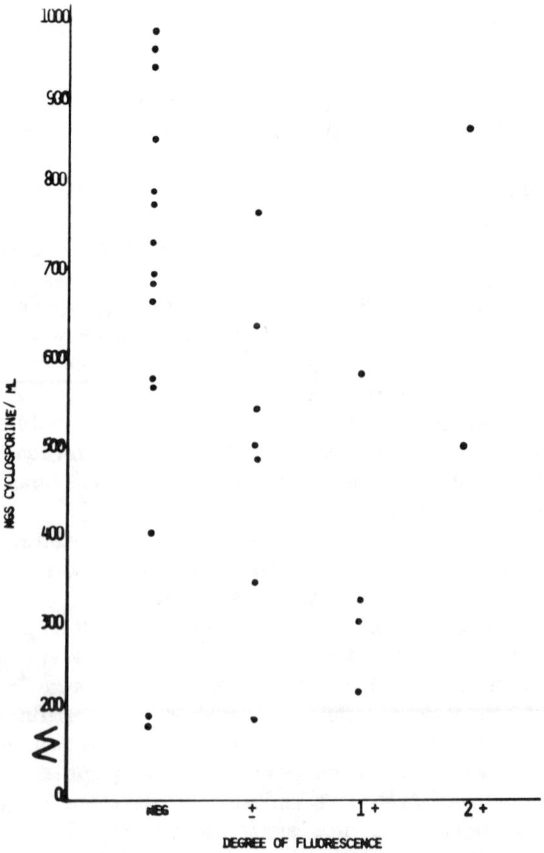

FIGURE 3. Correlation between the degree of immunofluorescence of urinary sediment cells and the concommitant blood levels of cyclosporine ($P = .001$).

TABLE 1. Summary of laboratory results obtained on five patients treated with cyclosporine after cadaveric renal transplantation[a]

P-TX Day	Fluorescence	Creatinine (mg/dl)	Serum-beta-2 microglobulin (mg/L)	H/S	Cyclosporine (ng/ml)
Normal:	Neg	0.5–1.5	1.1–1.9	0.9–1.5	250–800
Patient 1:					
2	Neg	1.4	6.8	1.1	—
5	1+	1.0	7.0	0.9	791
11	0.5+	1.8	16.9	0.9	507
19	0.5+	1.8	2.6	0.9	347
26	0.5+	1.9	17.6	0.9	187
33	0.5+	1.8	18.2	0.7	552
Patient 2:					
2	Neg	8.9	15.3	1.1	199
6	Neg	6.0	9.2	1.2	846
9	Neg	2.8	6.0	1.0	738
16	Neg	2.0	4.4	1.1	664
23	Neg	1.8	3.4	0.8	670
30	—	1.8	—	1.3	579
Patient 3:					
2	Neg	12.3	17.7	1.9	496
5	Neg	10.1	11.4	1.5	640
11	2+	2.1	3.8	1.4	514
19	1+	1.4	18.7	1.6	330
26	1+	1.8	2.7	1.7	309
33	2+	1.8	3.8	1.6	861
Patient 4:					
2	Neg	3.9	5.0	—	671
8	1+	2.6	7.3	1.3	575
16	1+	2.0	3.7	1.7	228
23	1+	2.1	3.0	1.6	844
30	Neg	2.0	3.0	1.4	410
Patient 5:					
2	Neg	6.8	7.7	1.2	199
6	Neg	3.6	4.9	1.0	965
9	1+	2.6	3.1	0.8	933
16	Neg	2.0	2.1	1.7	945
23	Neg	1.7	2.2	1.7	563
30	0.5+	1.8	3.5	1.3	769

cadaver transplant, consistently showed fluorescent cells in all urine specimens. Serum creatinine levels were essentially normal and cyclosporine blood levels were within the therapeutic range. However, creatinine clearance decreased progressively from 25 ml/min on P-TX day 9 to 14 ml/min on P-TX day 14, accompanied by a rise in serum beta 2-microglobulin from 7.0–16.9 mgs/L. From P-TX day 5, H/S ratios were 0.9. By P-TX day 33, the H/S ratio had fallen to 0.7, serum beta 2- microglobulin had risen to 18.2 mg/L and creatinine clearance was 24 ml/min. Rejection was diagnosed and azathioprine was added to cyclosporine therapy. At 24 months posttransplant, creatinine clearance was 63 ml/min, serum creatinine 0.9 mgs/dl and the patient is in good condition.

Patient No. 2, a 35-year-old man, was the only patient showing specimens consistently negative for fluorescence. Serum creatinine values became less than 2.0 mg/dl on P-TX day 13, and on P-TX day 25 creatinine clearance was 81 ml/min. On one occasion (day 6) cyclosporine levels were slightly increased (846 ng/ml) and on one occasion (P-TX day 23) the H/S ratio was slightly decreased (0.8). Beta 2-microglobulin levels fell consistently from 15.3 to 3.5 mg/L. At 24 months, serum creatinine was 1.8 mg/dl, creatinine clearance was 42 ml/min and the patient was in good condition.

Patient No. 3, a 30-year-old woman, showed the most intense cellular fluorescence of all patients. Specimens were positive on P-TX days 11, 19, 26, and 33, corresponding with serum creatinines of less than 2.1 mg/dl, normal H/S ratios and therapeutic blood levels of cyclosporine except on P-TX day 33 (861 ng/ml). However, serum beta 2-microglobulin rose from a previous 3.8 mg/L on day 11 to 18.7 mg/L on day 19, even though creatinine clearance increased during that time from 26 to 55 ml/min. On P-TX day 43 the patient became acutely ill, was found to be cytomegalovirus-positive, and remained febrile for 25 days. At six months posttransplant her creatinine clearance was 47 ml/min. She has moved out of the state and is lost to follow-up.

Patient No. 4, a 24-year-old man, showed fluorescent urinary cells on P-TX days 8, 16, and 23, corresponding with creatinine levels of less than 2.6 mg/dl and serum beta 2-microglobulin levels declining from 7.3 to 3.0 mgs/L. All H/S ratios were normal, and cyclosporine levels were elevated on only one occasion, P-TX day 23 (844 ng/ml). Creatinine clearances and serum creatinine levels were satisfactory for 16 months. The patient then developed cryptococcosis requiring amphotericin B therapy. At 24 months, serum creatinine is 6.5 mg/dl and creatinine clearance is 15 ml/min.

Patient No. 5, a 23-year-old man, showed fluorescent cells in his urine on P-TX days 9 and 30. The specimen from P-TX day 9 corresponded with both an increased cyclosporine blood level (933 ng/ml) and a depressed H/S ratio (0.8). Serum beta 2-microglobulin on day 9 was 3.1 mg/L, dropping to 2.2 and 2.1 mg/L on P-TX days 16 and 23 before rising to 3.5 mg/L on day 30 when urinary fluorescence again appeared. Cyclosporine blood levels were also elevated on days 6 and 16 (965 and 945 ng/ml) without a corresponding urinary fluorescence. At 60 days posttransplant this patient's creatinine clearance was 115 ml/min and his serum creatinine remained at less than 2.0 mg/dl for 12 months. At 24 months his serum creatinine was 3.3 mg/dl with a creatinine clearance of 26 ml/min.

From this limited series conclusions are not possible, but some inferences can be drawn. As seen in patient No. 1 rejection probably compounds the sensitivity to cyclosporine, as evidenced by fluorescence and markedly elevated beta 2-microglobulin in the face of decreasing H/S ratios. We also see fluorescence in a specimen from patient No. 5 when cyclosporine drug levels are slightly increased, and the H/S ratio is decreased (0.8). On the other hand, patient No. 2 failed to show fluorescent urinary cells with a depressed H/S (0.8) ratio when cyclosporine blood levels were in the therapeutic range. However, patient No. 4 showed fluorescent cells in spite of normal H/S ratios and declining beta 2-microglobulins, and only one elevated cyclosporine blood level.

Patient No. 3 remains enigmatic. Intense fluorescence of urinary cells with normal H/S ratios, therapeutic levels of cyclosporine and only one markedly elevated serum beta 2-microglobulin value, fails to fit into a pattern. Inasmuch as she developed cytomegalovirus infection on P-TX day 43, and the incubation period of this virus is prolonged, her kidney may have been more sensitive to cyclosporine due to viral injury.

In summary, 28 samples of blood and 24-hr urine collections were obtained from five patients for five weeks. The blood samples were analyzed for cyclosporine levels, beta 2-microglobulin levels and H/S ratios, and the sediments from urinary aliquots were examined for specific immunofluorescence to cyclosporine antiserum; 14 of the urine preparations were negative, and 14 were positive. No sample was positive before seven days of therapy. A time-lag was seen between high levels of cyclosporine in the blood and appearance of positive cells in the urine and/or increases in serum beta-2 microglobulin. Decreased H/S ratios in combination with increased beta-2-microglobulin and immunofluorescence suggested rejection in one patient.

If immunofluorescence correlates with nephrotoxicity, it may be useful in confirming renal damage, but will not have predictive value. However, in patients with atypical sensitivity to the standard drug dosage, examination of urinary sediment for cytofluorescence may assist in dosage adjustment.

Acknowledgments. We appreciate the technologists of the Tissue Typing and Special Chemistry Laboratories, and Mary Haven, M.S., Clinical Chemist, University of Nebraska Medical Center; as well as the Coordinators of the Transplant Office, Bishop Clarkson Memorial Hospital, Omaha, Nebraska for their cooperation in this project.

ARDEN E. LARSEN
Department of Pathology and Microbiology
University of Nebraska Medical Center
Omaha, Nebraska 68105

REFERENCES

1. Merion RM, White DJG, Thiru S, Evans DB, Calne RY. Cyclosporine: five years' experience in cadaveric renal transplantation. N Engl J Med 1984; 310: 148.
2. Beveridge T. Cyclosporin-A: an evaluation of clinical results. Transplant Proc 1983; 15: 433.
3. Flechner SM, van Buren CT, Kahan BD. The University of Texas Medical School, Houston, TX. First International Congress on Cyclosporin, 1983.
4. Calne RY. Cyclosporin. Nephron 1980; 26: 57.
5. Cortesini R, Stella F, Molajoni et al. Urinary exfoliative cytology in kidney allografts under cyclosporine therapy. Transplant Proc 1984; 16: 1200.
6. von Willebrand E, Hayry P. Cyclosporine-A deposits in renal allografts. Lancet 1983; 8343: 189.
7. Schentag JJ, Sutfin TA, Plaut ME, Jusko WJ. Early detection of aminoglycoside nephrotoxicity with urinary beta-2 microglobulin. J Med 1978; 9: 201.
8. Valsamis J, Brauman H, Yourassowsky E. Plasma beta-2 microglobulin as a means of predicting gentamicin serum concentration. Antimicrob Agents Chemother 1980; 17: 530.

Received 31 October 1985.
Accepted 27 February 1986.

STORED-BLOOD DONOR-SPECIFIC TRANSFUSIONS WITH CYCLOSPORINE IN DISTANTLY RELATED AND UNRELATED DONOR-RECIPIENT PAIRS

Donor-specific blood transfusions (DST)* improve kidney graft survival between one-haplotype-matched donor-recipient pairs with a reactive mixed lymphocyte culture (MLC) (*1*). Early experience with DST produced a sensitization rate of approximately 30%. However, by giving azathioprine concurrently with DST (*2,3*), or by giving stored donor blood (*4,5*), the sensitization rate has been reduced significantly while maintaining improved graft survival.

In patients in whom the only potential donor was outside the immediate family an attempt was made to see if the use of stored blood DST and concurrent use of CsA would result in minimal donor-specific sensitization and high graft survival.

Ten patients without potential donors within their immediate families were evaluated for renal transplantation at the King Faisal Specialist Hospital and Research Centre between 1/84 and 7/85. There were nine men and one woman with an average age of 31 years (range 20–42 years). Five distant cousins, one uncle, one nephew, and three wives were volunteer renal donors.

Tissue typing for the HLA-A, -B, and -DR antigens was done in all donor-recipient pairs. A standard MLC was done in seven pairs. A stimulation index over 10 and a relative response rate greater than 35% were considered reactive. Seven patients received a one unit DST that had been stored seven days while taking oral CsA 10 mg/kg/day. One patient received three 150 ml stored-blood DSTs while taking CsA, and two patients received a 200-ml booster stored-blood DST with CsA after three previous 150-ml stored-blood DSTs. T cell and warm B cell crossmatches were done two weeks after the last DST. Negative T cell and warm B cell crossmatches were required immediately prior to surgery. One recipient developed a positive warm B cell crossmatch to his wife following three 150-ml stored blood DSTs. This became negative after receiving CsA and a booster DST.

CsA was continued and the dose was adjusted to achieve a 24-hr trough RIA whole blood level of around 600 ng/ml. Methylprednisolone 10 mg/kg was given on days −1 and 0, and then tapered from 100 mg on day 1 to 30 mg by day 19. Acute rejection episodes were treated with methylprednisolone or prednisone, 5 mg/kg/day for five days with a rapid taper to maintenance levels, or with antithymocyte globulin (AtGam) 15 mg/kg/day for a maximum of ten days.

The life table analysis method was used in calculating actuarial survivals.

The donor-recipient pairs shared a mean of 1.5 (range 0–5) HLA-A, -B and -DR antigens. The MLC was reactive in the seven pairs tested. None of the 10 patients were prevented from receiving a kidney from their potential donor because of donor-specific sensitization.

The recipients were followed for 5–22 months (mean 14 months). The actuarial one-year patient and graft survivals were 100%. At the most recent follow-up, the mean serum creatinine level was 1.9 mg/dl, with a range of 1.3–2.9 mg/dl.

One patient returned to Yemen 22 months after transplantation with a graft that was functioning well and died shortly thereafter from unknown causes. Two patients were switched from CsA to azathioprine at 8 and 16 months due to the financial impossibility of continuing CsA in Sudan and concern about nephrotoxicity and CsA blood level monitoring.

A total of 12 rejection crises were treated in eight patients, and two patients had no rejection episodes. The CsA doses, at current follow-up, ranged from 2.2–5.3 mg/kg/day, with a mean of 4 mg/kg/day.

A number of factors led to the use of kidneys from distantly related and unrelated volunteer donors. These include the improved graft survival seen following DST, methods to reduce the sensitization rate of DST, improved immunosuppression

* Abbreviations used: AtGam, antithymocyte globulin; DST, donor-specific blood transfusions; MLC, mixed lymphocyte culture.

with CsA, and the shortage of living-related donor and cadaver donor kidneys. In Saudi Arabia the extended family is often quite large and the individual wishing to donate a kidney may not be a sibling, parent, or child of the recipient. In all cases there was an obvious emotional bond between the donor and the recipient.

Early reports of DST and unrelated donors were discouraging. Using fresh packed cells, Ruzany and associates reported sensitization in 5 of 7 patients and prompt rejection of the two transplanted kidneys (*6*). In another report, three fresh blood DSTs in unrelated donor recipient pairs caused a 31% donor-specific sensitization rate and the 20 transplanted kidneys did not have improved survival rates when compared with unrelated donor kidney transplants without DST (*7*).

Several other reports, however, have shown excellent results with 100% graft survival in 11, 2, and 20 distantly related or unrelated pairs following DST (*8–10*). In addition, sensitization was minimized using a DST-plus-azathioprine protocol (*8*).

Donor-specific sensitization has been eliminated by avoiding DSTs and using CsA in one-haplotype-matched pairs with an actuarial one-year graft survival of 91% (*11*). When applied to unrelated pairs, an 80% graft survival was obtained (*12*), which is similar to results in cadaver kidney transplants with CsA immunosuppression.

The results of the current series indicate that stored blood DSTs plus CsA can be given in distantly related and unrelated donor-recipient pairs with a low incidence of sensitization and an excellent graft survival rate. It is probable that not all of the measures utilized (i.e., DSTs, stored blood, 4–6 weeks of preoperative CsA) in the preparation of the recipients are necessary. However, DSTs seem to be a reasonable insurance against graft failure in this group, and storage of the blood was convenient and was used routinely in our living-related one-haplotype-matched pairs. CsA caused flushing and abdominal discomfort in some patients; however, this decreased with time and disappeared in all patients after transplantation. The dose required to obtain the desired blood level was low. Although the use of CsA increases the expense of the preoperative period, it was not associated with leukopenia, which may occur with azathioprine.

THOMAS R. HEFTY[1]
JOHN M. BARRY

The Division of Renal Transplantation
King Faisal Specialist Hospital and Research Centre
Riyadh, Kingdom of Saudi Arabia
The Division of Urology
Oregon Health Sciences University
Portland, Oregon

[1] Address requests for reprints to: Thomas R. Hefty, M.D., Oregon Health Sciences University, 3181 S.W. Sam Jackson Park Road, Portland, Oregon 97201.

REFERENCES

1. Salvatierra O, Vincenti F, Amend W, et al. Deliberate donor-specific blood transfusion prior to living related renal transplantation: a new approach. Ann Surg 1980; 192: 543.
2. Anderson CB, Sicard GA, Etheredge EE. Pretreatment of renal allograft recipients with azathioprine and donor-specific blood products. Surgery 1982; 92: 315.
3. Sollinger HW, Glass NR, Miller DT, Belzer FO. Comparison between DST and DST plus Imuran in HLA-nonidentical living-related transplants. Transplant Proc 1984; 16: 8.
4. Whelchel JD, Shaw JF, Curtis JF, Luke RG, Diethelm AG. Effect of pretransplant stored donor-specific blood transfusions on early renal allograft survival in one-haplotype living related transplants. Transplantation 1982; 34: 326.
5. Light JA, Metz S, Oddenino K, et al. Donor-specific transfusion with diminished sensitization. Transplantation 1982; 34: 352.
6. Ruzany F, Moraes, JRF, de Queiroz Faria L, de Moraes Souza ER, Iwaki Y. Unrelated donor-specific blood transfusions in human renal transplantation. Transplantation 1983; 35: 101.
7. Sabbaga E, Ianhez LE, Chocair PR, Azevedo LS, Sarturi PS, de Goes GM. Kidney transplants from living nonrelated donors: an analysis of 87 cases, including 20 cases with specific blood transfusions from the donor. Transplant Proc. 1985; 17: 1741.
8. Sollinger HW, Burlingham WJ, Sparks EMF, Glass NR, Belzer FO. Donor-specific transfusions in unrelated and related HLA-mismatched donor-recipient combinations. Transplantation 1984; 38: 612.
9. Barry JM, Hefty T, Fischer SM, Norman DJ. Donor specific blood transfusions and successful spousal kidney transplantation. J Urol 1985; 133: 1024.
10. Salvatierra O. Advantages of continued use of kidney transplantation from living donors. Transplant Proc 1985; 17: 18.
11. Flechner SM, Kerman RH, Van Buren CT, Epps L, Kahan BD. The use of cyclosporine in living-related renal transplantation. Transplantation 1984; 38: 685.
12. Berloco P, Alfani D, Famulari A, et al. Utilization of living donor organs for clinical transplantation. Transplant Proc 1985; 17: 13.

Received 22 January 1986.
Accepted 18 March 1986.

AUTHOR INDEX

Adinolfi, M., 271
Aebi, M., 567
Agarwal, R. P., 627
Agnes, S., 443
Ahonen, J., 364, 598
Albrechtsen, D., 35
Alvarez, C. L., 697
Amend, W., 511
Amos, D., 515
Amos, D. E., 602
Anderson, C. B., 267, 502
Andersson, A., 588
Appelbaum, F. R., 19, 515
Aprile, J., 653
Araneda, D., 191
Araujo, H. A., 697
Armstrong, L., 171
Ayalon, M., 118

Bachman, U., 511
Backman, L., 368
Baird, M. A., 1, 542
Baldwin, W. M., 479
Barker, C. F., 473
Barry, J. M., 437, 702
Bartus, S. A., 562
Bayle, C., 252
Beekhuis-Brusse, J. A. M., 93
Beining, P. R., 524
Benotti, P. N., 484
Bensinger, W., 19
Bentin, J., 317
Beyer, W. E. P., 376
Biava, C., 511
Bishop, G. A., 671
Bismuth, H., 330
Björkhem, I., 368
Bjorn, M., 205
Blajchman, M. A., 632
Blanchard, J. M., 528
Blazer, B. R., 222
Bogman, M. J. J. T., 178
Bolton, E. M., 352
Borgstrom, A., 686
Bortin, M. M., 229
Bosman, F., 307
Bothe, A., Jr., 484
Bow, L. M., 562
Bradley, B. A., 39, 46
Bradley, M. P., 1
Branch, D. W., 694
Braquet, P., 86
Breimer, M. E., 88
Brenner, M. K., 257
Brown, D., 315
Brown, S., 271
Brown, Z., 150
Buckner, C. D., 515
Bue, C. M., 14
Bull, R. W., 390
Burakoff, S. J., 380
Burdick, J. F., 67
Burke, J. F., 473
Burnstein, M., 613
Busuttil, R. W., 85, 561
Buszta, C., 23, 154
Buurman, W. A., 130

Callaway, C., 315
Calne, R., 308
Cameron, J. L., 333
Cameron, S., 494
Cameron, S. J., 150
Campbell, Jr., D. A., 686
Carlson, I. H., 372
Carpentier, N., 159
Carson, D. A., 317
Carter, N. P., 352
Castagneto, M., 443
Catto, G. R. D., 400
Cerilli, J., 262
Chandler, J. W., 403
Chapman, J. R., 91, 144, 352, 608
Charrier, K., 19
Chase, D., 271
Citterio, F., 443
Clow, L. W., 67
Cobbold, S., 239
Cobourn, C. S., 537
Cohen, Z., 613
Colonna, J. O., II
Colvin, R. B., 507
Coppage, M. L., 439
Cornelissen, I. M. H. A., 178
Cos, L. R., 453
Cosimi, A. B., 507
Costello, P., 484
Coster, D. J., 667
Cranston, D., 302
Crawford, D. H., 50
Crimmins, M., 380
Cross, D. E., 267
Cullen, J., 613
Cunningham, B. A., 602
Cunningham, C., 400
Cunningham, R. J., 154

Dafoe, D. C., 686
Darby, H., 325
David, C. S., 429
Davidson, R. J. L., 395
Davis, W. C., 14
Dean, M., 271
De Araujo, J. F., 107
Deeg, H. J., 19, 497, 571, 653
DeFazio, S. R., 593
Delmon, L., 252
deMacedo, A. R., 327
Demidem, A., 274
Denegri, J. F., 212
De Paula, F. J., 107
Deutsch, H. L., 200
DeVos, D., 372
De Waal, R. M. W., 178
Dharmasena, F., 228
Diamantstein, T., 191
Diener, E., 192
Doran, M. M., 439
Dorsch, S. E., 532
Doxiadis, I., 64
Draibe, S. A., 80
Dresdale, A. R., 98
Duggin, G. G., 671
Duncan, J. I., 395
Duncan, W. R., 406
Dzik, W. H., 484

Edington, H. D. J., 200
Ehninger, G., 558
Ekert, H., 58
Eliopoulos, G. M., 484
Ellis, W. M., 58
Emde, C., 64
Emerson, S., 380
Emeson, E. E., 466
Eriksson, E., 636

Fabian, I., 312
Fabre, J. W., 337
Fajaco, R., 568
Falk, J. A., 537
Falk, R. E., 537
Falkenstein, D., 80
Fan, J., 417
Fang, W., 315
Fanslow, W. C., 687
Farber, E., 537
Fathman, C. G., 205, 660
Faure, M., 274
Feduska, N., 511
Fefer, A., 515
Fehir, K. M., 315
Fensom, A. H., 271
Ferguson, R. M., 695
Fields, B. L., 372
Figueiredo, J. F., 80
Filipovich, A. H., 222
Findon, G., 463
Fish, J. C., 439
Flatmark, A., 35
Flechner, S. M., 311
Foegh, M. L., 86, 94
Fogleman, I., 494
Fontannaz, J., 159
Freed, B. M., 262
Fridd, C. W., 453
Friedrich, W., 312
Friend, P., 308
Fuccello, A. J., 507
Fuggle, S. V., 144
Fujimoto, H., 548
Fukao, K., 61
Fukuhara, T., 548

Gale, R. P., 54
Gedroyc, W., 494
Gelber, R., 73
Gellert, K., 122
Georgiou, G. M., 58
Giest, H., 84
Gifford, R. R. M., 439
Gilks, W. R., 39, 46
Gill, T. J., III, 235, 297
Gill T. J., III, 109, 217
Glicklich, D., 556
Goldstein, G., 507
Goldstein, L. I., 561
Gondo, H., 281
Gonwa, T. A., 423
Goormastic, M., 154
Gordon, M. J. V., 556
Gordon-Smith, E. C., 228
Gore, S. M., 39, 46
Gotoh, M., 387
Gouma, D. J., 687
Gozzo, J. J., 593
Graham, T. C., 19
Granfors, K., 197
Gray, D. W. R., 686
Greenberg, G. R., 613
Gregg, C. M., 453, 458
Grob, J. Ph., 257
Grosse-Wilde, H., 64
Grossman, R. A., 473
Gugenhiem, J., 330
Guttmann, R. D., 347

Hackman, R. C., 602
Hale, G., 307
Hall, B. M., 671
Hamaguchi, H., 61
Hammer, S. M., 484
Hanto, D., 621
Hanto, D. W., 168
Harada, M., 320
Harada, S., 222
Harder, F., 567
Hardy, M. A., 98
Harris, H. W., 109
Hartner, W. C., 593
Harty, J. T., 621
Hattori, K., 320
Hawkins, R., 50
Hayat, M., 252
Häyry, P., 358, 364
Hefty, T. R., 702
Heirwegh, K. P. M., 130
Hennige, M., 491
Henning, M. H., 322
Henny, F. C., 479
Henry, M., 125
Hercend, Th., 252
Heslop, B. F., 1, 542
Hiatt, J. R., 85, 561
Hill, R., 515
Himeno, K., 281, 417
Hirose, S., 429
Hodgson, H. J., 325
Hoffbrand, A. V., 257
Hoffman, R. A., 621
Hoffman, T., 524
Ho-Hsieh, H., 154
Hoitsma, A. J., 220
Horvath, J. S., 671
Hoshinaga, K., 691
Houssin, D., 330
Howden, B., 125
Hudson, J. L., 171
Hunt, T., 660

Ianhez, L. E., 107
Iliescu, V., 50
Imamura, M., 548
Ishiguro, K., 581
Itaya, T., 548
Iwasaki, Y., 61

Jablonski, P., 125
Jalkanen, S., 197
Jarowenko, M. V., 311
Jarrell, B. E., 473
Jeannet, M., 159
Jenkins, R. L., 434, 484
Jensen, W. A., 484
Joseph, S., 632

Kahan, B. D., 311, 642
Kamada, N., 7, 581
Kamholz, S. L., 466
Kaplan, D., 205
Karchmer, A. W., 434, 484
Kasai, M., 548
Kedar, E., 118
Kersey, J. H., 222
Khettry, U., 484
Khirabadi, B. S., 86, 94
Klein, J., 102
Klingemann, H., 412
Kochenour, N. K., 694
Koegel, M., 695
Koene, R. A. P., 178, 220
Köhler, C. O., 491
Kojima, Y., 588
Kondo, I., 61
Kootstra, G., 130, 307
Kootte, A. M. M., 93
Koyama, I., 333
Kramer, W. G., 311
Krowka, J. F., 162
Krumbacher, K., 64
Kuhlbäck, B., 598
Kulkarni, A. D., 687
Kunz, H. W., 217, 235, 297
Kupiec-Weglinski, J. W., 191
Kurlansky, P., 441
Kurlansky, P. A., 98

Lafuse, W. P., 429
Lai, M. K., 458
Lambert, R., 125
Langer, B., 613
Larkin, R. M., 694
Larsen, A. E., 699
Lau, H., 98
Laurent, G., 380
Lazda, V. A., 528
Lee, G., 537
Lee, M. D., 235
Lee, S., 327, 329
LeFor, W. M., 28
Legendre, C. M., 347
LeGrue, S. J., 679
Lehtonen, L., 184
Leibel, B. S., 96
Leivestad, T., 35
Lempert, N., 262
Lensmeyer, G. L., 372
Leshem, B., 118
Leunissen, K. M. L., 307
Levy, G. A., 613
Lewis, M., 667
Liao, S. K., 632
Lichter, A. S., 686
Lindbäck, B., 368
Linke, C. A., 453, 458
Lizzio, E. F., 524
Lloyd, D. A., 235
Lois, J. F., 85
London, W. T., 473
Lorber, M. I., 311
Lower, F. E., 212
Lower, R. R., 691
Ludwin, D., 632
Luger, A. M., 267
Lyons, P., 473

Magalini, S. C., 443
Magnuson, N. S., 14
Mahmoud, H. K., 64
Maisey, M., 494
Majoor, G. D., 292
Maki, T., 387, 593
Makowka, L., 537, 613
Mandour, W. A., 458
Mann, T. S., 667
Marboe, C., 98
Markees, T. G., 593
Marks, W. H., 686
Marsh, J., 271
Marshall, V., 125
Martin, G., 239
Martin, J. M., 96
Martín, R. S., 697
Mason, R. J., 400
Masurel, N., 376
Matas, A. J., 556
Matsuda, T., 320
Mauduit, G., 274
Maurer, D. H., 315
Mayumi, H., 281, 417
McColl, I., 271
McConnachie, P. R., 212
McConnell, D. B., 437
McCormick, J. F., 429
McCullough, C. M., 200
McDonald, G. B., 602
McElroy, J., 23
McIntyre, J. A., 212
McKenzie, I. F. C., 322, 647
McManus, R. P., 98
McPherson, R. A., 627
McShane, P., 689
McWhinnie, D. L., 144, 352
Melzer, J., 511
Merchant, B., 524
Merrell, R. C., 660
Meyers, J. D., 602
Michler, R. E., 98, 441
Miller, R. A., 380
Miller, T. E., 463
Milton, A. D., 337
Miyazaki, T., 548
Mizoguchi, H., 320
Mohanakumar, T., 691
Moingeon, P., 252
Monaco, A. P., 387, 434, 593
Morgan, J. S., 518
Mori, T., 320
Morris, P. J., 91, 144, 227, 302, 352, 608, 689
Mottironi, V. D., 14
Mowat, A. McI., 141
Mulholland, N., 50
Munn, C. G., 679

Nachreiner, R., 390
Nakahara, K., 205
Nanni, G., 443
Neild, G., 494
Neild, G. H., 150
Nissen, C., 159
Nomoto, K., 281, 417
Norin, A. J., 466
Norman, D. J., 507
Novick, A. C., 23, 154
Nowill, A., 252

Ochs, H. D., 14
Ofosu, F. A., 632
Oldfather, J. W., 267
Oljans, P. J., 479
Opelz, G., 224, 491
Orosz, C. G., 105
Otto, G., 84, 122

Padberg, W., 191
Pagel, E., 695
Pasternack, A., 598
Patterson, J., 257
Paul, L. C., 93, 479
Pawelec, G., 559
Pease, L. R., 102
Pecego, R., 515
Perera, M. I. R., 297
Perren, S. M., 567
Perryman, L. E., 14
Peters, M., 689
Pettersson, E., 364
Peugh, W. N., 227
Phelan, D. L., 267
Pico, J. L., 252
Pierson, R., 98
Pilarski, L., 162
Pinsker, K. L., 466
Pollack, M. S., 315
Pollak, R., 528
Porter, J., 387
Power, D. A., 400
Powles, R., 50
Prentice, H. G., 257
Purtilo, D. T., 222

Quinn, T., 556
Quinones-Baldrich, W., 561
Quinones-Baldrich, W. J., 85

Rae, D., 125
Ramakrishnan, S., 660
Ramming, K. P., 85, 561
Ramos, O. L., 80
Ramsay, N. K. C., 222
Ramwell, P. W., 86, 94
Ravis, W. R., 390
Ray, R. A., 561
Ray-Keil, L., 403
Reemstma, K., 441
Reemtsma, K., 98
Regazzoni, P., 567
Reichert, T., 380
Reisner, Y., 312
Reittie, J. E., 257
Rimm, A. A., 229
Ringdén, O., 368, 445
Risius, B., 23
Ritz, J., 73, 252
Robertson, D. M., 58
Rodey, G. E., 267
Rodriguez, S. G., 697
Rohatiner, A., 73
Rosano, T. G., 262
Rose, E. A., 98, 441
Rose, R. M., 484
Roughneen, P. T., 687
Rovelli, M. A., 562
Rowe, M. R., 235
Rowlands, B. J., 687
Rowles, J. R., 86, 94
Rozans, M. K., 380
Ruers, Th. J. M., 307
Ruth, J. A., 439

Sabbaga, E., 107
Sabbaga, J., 107
Sachs, H., 98
Sadeghi, A. M., 441
Sakurada, K., 548
Salvatierra, O., 511
Samaniego, M. D. C., 697
Samuelsson, B. E., 88
Sandler, S., 588
Sanfilippo, F., 28
Saraf, P., 453
Sasaki, T. M., 437
Satomi, S., 387
Schaefer, U. W., 64
Schafer, A., 224
Schaffner, W., 518
Schall, W. D., 390
Schlossman, S. F., 73
Schmidt, E., 497
Schmidt, H., 558
Schmidt-Weinmar, A., 64
Schneider, T. M., 191
Schüning, F., 64
Schweizer, R. T., 562
Scott, J. H., 636
Scott, J. R., 694
Scott, M., 327
Seaman, W. E., 636
Selawry, H., 568
Selden, C., 325
Sells, R. A., 136
Selwood, N. H., 39
Settaf, A., 330
Shaffer, D., 434
Shalit, M., 118
Shield, C. F. III, 507
Shinomiya, T., 7, 581
Shinozuka, H., 297
Shiobara, S., 320
Shiozawa, C., 162
Shizuru, J., 660
Shofer, F. S., 473
Shulman, H. M., 497
Sicard, G. A., 502
Sigulem, D., 80
Silverman, R. E., 613
Simmons, R. L., 168, 621
Simonian, S. J., 473
Simpson, J. G., 395
Singal, D. P., 632
Slavin, S., 118
Smith, B. R., 380
Smith, C. R., 441
Snider, M. E., 171
Soberman, R., 556
Sollinger, H. W., 372
Somia, N. V., 150
Sommer, B. G., 695
Sparrow, R. L., 647
Speck, B., 159
Spees, E. K., 28
Spencer, G. D., 602
Spencer, S. C., 337
Steinhilber, D., 23, 154
Steinmuller, D., 23, 154, 171
Stephens, S., 257
Stepkowski, S. M., 406
Stone, W. J., 518
Storb, R., 19, 412, 494, 571
Streem, S. B., 23, 154
Strom, T. B., 191
Sugarbaker, P. H., 200
Sullivan, K. M., 320
Superina, R. A., 227
Suranyi, M. G., 671
Sutton, R., 686
Szentpetery, S., 691

Tamaki, T., 581
Tanaka, K., 417
Tange, J., 125
Taniguchi, K., 281
Tanke, H. J., 479
Taube, D., 494

Tavanlis, G., 125
Taylor, C., 91
Taylor, C. J., 608
Taylor, H. M., 144, 352
Tellis, V. A., 556
Termeer, A., 220
Thick, M., 271
Thivolet, J., 274
Thomas, E. D., 494, 515, 602
Thomas, W. G., 98, 441
Thompson, J. F., 352
Thomson, A. W., 395, 400
Thorsby, E., 35
Threatte, G. A., 627
Tiedemann, K., 58
Tiller, D. J., 671
Tilney, N. L., 191
Ting, A., 91, 608
Toivanen, P., 184, 197
Tokuda, N., 281, 417
Toledo-Pereyra, L. H., 443
Torry, D. S., 212
Towpik, E., 191
Trey, C., 484
Tsoi, M., 412
Tsoukas, C. D., 317
Turcotte, J. G., 686
Tyler, J. D., 105, 502

Ueda, M., 320
Uerlings, I., 122
Ullrich, S. E., 287

Vaidya, S., 695
Vainio, O., 184
Van Bekkum, D. W., 248
Van Bockel, J. H., 93
Van Breda-Vriesman, P. J. C., 292
Van Buren, C. T., 311
Van der Linden, C. J., 130
Van Es, L. A., 479
Van Hooff, J. P., 307
Vaughan, H. A., 647
Vaughan, J. H., 317
Vaughn, W. K., 28
Veith, F. J., 466, 556
Vermeulen, A. N., 178
Veromaa, T., 197
Versluis, D. J., 376
Vetto, R. M., 437
Vincenti, F., 511
Visser, T. P., 248
Von Willebrand, E., 358, 364
Vroeman, J. P. A. M., 130

Wagemaker, G., 248
Waldmann, H., 239, 307
Walshaw, R., 390
Wassef, R., 613
Waters, K. D., 58
Weening, J. J., 479
Weimar, W., 376
Weiss, L., 118
Welsh, K., 271
Wenting, G. J., 376
Wernet, P., 558
White, J. V., 390
White, R., 556
Whiting, P. H., 395
Whittington, K., 568
Widmer, M. B., 168
Williams, K. A., 667
Williams, M., 333
Williamson, E. P. M., 136
Willoughby, J. J., 150
Wimperis, J. Z., 257
Winsett, O. E., 439
Witherspoon, R. P., 320
Wofsy, D., 636
Wolff, H., 84, 122
Wood, K. J., 227, 302
Wood, N. L., 691
Wood, R. F. M., 352
Woodcock, J., 636
Wotherspoon, J. S., 532
Wyatt, C. R., 14

Yancey, D., 329
Yeager, R. A., 437
Yee, G. C., 494
Yip, G. H., 347
Yoshida, T., 320
Yoshimura, N., 642
Ythier, A., 252
Yuzawa, K., 61

Zelkowtiz, L., 222
Zingg, W., 96
Zuidema, G. D., 333
Zwartendijk, J., 93

U.S. Postal Service

STATEMENT OF OWNERSHIP, MANAGEMENT AND CIRCULATION

Required by 39 U.S.C. 3685)

1A. TITLE OF PUBLICATION: TRANSPLANTATION

1B. PUBLICATION NO.: 0 0 4 1 1 3 3 7

2. DATE OF FILING: Oct. 1, 1986

3. FREQUENCY OF ISSUE: Monthly

3A. NO. OF ISSUES PUBLISHED ANNUALLY: 12

3B. ANNUAL SUBSCRIPTION PRICE: $105.00

4. COMPLETE MAILING ADDRESS OF KNOWN OFFICE OF PUBLICATION *(Street, City, County, State and ZIP+4 Code) (Not printers)*

428 East Preston Street, Baltimore, Maryland 21202

5. COMPLETE MAILING ADDRESS OF THE HEADQUARTERS OF GENERAL BUSINESS OFFICES OF THE PUBLISHER *(Not printer)*

428 East Preston Street, Baltimore, Maryland 21202

6. FULL NAMES AND COMPLETE MAILING ADDRESS OF PUBLISHER, EDITOR, AND MANAGING EDITOR *(This item MUST NOT be blank)*

PUBLISHER *(Name and Complete Mailing Address)*

Williams & Wilkins, 428 E. Preston St., Baltimore, MD 21202

EDITOR *(Name and Complete Mailing Address)*

Dr. A.P. Monaco, New England Deaconess Hospital, 185 Pilgrim Rd., Boston, MA 02215

MANAGING EDITOR *(Name and Complete Mailing Address)*

7. OWNER *(If owned by a corporation, its name and address must be stated and also immediately thereunder the names and addresses of stockholders owning or holding 1 percent or more of total amount of stock. If not owned by a corporation, the names and addresses of the individual owners must be given. If owned by a partnership or other unincorporated firm, its name and address, as well as that of each individual must be given. If the publication is published by a nonprofit organization, its name and address must be stated.) (Item must be completed.)*

FULL NAME	COMPLETE MAILING ADDRESS
Waverly Press, Inc.	Mt. Royal & Guilford Aves.
	Baltimore, MD 21202

8. KNOWN BONDHOLDERS, MORTGAGEES, AND OTHER SECURITY HOLDERS OWNING OR HOLDING 1 PERCENT OR MORE OF TOTAL AMOUNT OF BONDS, MORTGAGES OR OTHER SECURITIES *(If there are none, so state)*

FULL NAME	COMPLETE MAILING ADDRESS
NONE	

9. FOR COMPLETION BY NONPROFIT ORGANIZATIONS AUTHORIZED TO MAIL AT SPECIAL RATES *(Section 423.12 DMM only)*
The purpose, function, and nonprofit status of this organization and the exempt status for Federal income tax purposes *(Check one)*

(1) [X] HAS NOT CHANGED DURING PRECEDING 12 MONTHS
(2) [ ] HAS CHANGED DURING PRECEDING 12 MONTHS
(If changed, publisher must submit explanation of change with this statement.)

10. EXTENT AND NATURE OF CIRCULATION *(See instructions on reverse side)*	AVERAGE NO. COPIES EACH ISSUE DURING PRECEDING 12 MONTHS	ACTUAL NO. COPIES OF SINGLE ISSUE PUBLISHED NEAREST TO FILING DATE
A. TOTAL NO. COPIES *(Net Press Run)*	3370	3409
B. PAID AND/OR REQUESTED CIRCULATION 1. Sales through dealers and carriers, street vendors and counter sales — See line 11	107	106
2. Mail Subscription *(Paid and/or requested)*	2573	2668
C. TOTAL PAID AND/OR REQUESTED CIRCULATION *(Sum of 10B1 and 10B2)*	2680	2774
D. FREE DISTRIBUTION BY MAIL, CARRIER OR OTHER MEANS SAMPLES, COMPLIMENTARY, AND OTHER FREE COPIES	80	87
E. TOTAL DISTRIBUTION *(Sum of C and D)*	2760	2861
F. COPIES NOT DISTRIBUTED 1. Office use, left over, unaccounted, spoiled after printing	610	548
2. Return from News Agents	NONE	NONE
G. TOTAL *(Sum of E, F1 and 2—should equal net press run shown in A)*	3370	3409

11. I certify that the statements made by me above are correct and complete

SIGNATURE AND TITLE OF EDITOR, PUBLISHER, BUSINESS MANAGER, OR OWNER

Publisher Alma J. Wills

.Paid subs mailed Via Canada Post

PS Form 3526, Dec. 1985 *(See instruction on reverse)*

SUBJECT INDEX

Accessory cell, role in corneal allograft rejection (rabbit), 667
Adenocarcinoma, intestinal, induction by cyclosporine (rat), 297
Alloantibody, responses, in nonrejector combination (rat), 7
Alloantigen, -specific receptors, T cell (mouse), 632
Allograft. *See also* Graft
  bone, revascularized (dog) (Communication), 564
  cornea, role of accessory cells in rejection (rabbit), 667
  drug-induced tolerance to (mouse), 417
  epidermal, survival and tolerance of (human), 274
  heart
    development of suppressor lymphocytes during rejection (rat), 191
    effect of cyclosporine and iloprost on survival (rat) (Communication), 94
    effects of cyclosporine on induction of donor class I and class II major histocompatibility complex antigens in (rat), 337
    postoperative bone marrow injections with cyclosporine or antithymocyte globulin in (rat) (Communication), 441
    prolongation of survival using buffy coat pretransfusions (dog) (Communication), 98
    prolongation of survival with BN 52021 (rat) (Communication), 86
    rejection (mouse), 67
    survival following administration of heat-treated donor lymphocytes (rat), 1
    vascularized (mouse) (Communication), 226
  kidney
    analysis of cellular infiltration assessed by monoclonal antibody labeling in biopsy of (human), 352
    antiglobulin cytotoxicity crossmatch in recipients treated with cyclosporine (human) (Communication), 439
    cell-mediated lympholysis in Kaposi's sarcoma after transplantation (human) (Communication), 697
    cytomegalovirus infection, class II antigen expression, and rejection of (human), 364
    effect of cyclosporine on function after extended preservation (human), 154
    effect of repeated pregnancies on function (human) (Communication), 694
    effects of cyclosporine on induction of donor class I and class II major histocompatibility complex antigens in (rat), 337
    HLA class II antigen expression in (human), 144
    immunosuppressive effect of spleen cells on (rat), 302
    immunosuppressive metabolites of cyclosporine in blood of recipients (human), 262
    ^{99m}Tc diethylamine pentacetic acid scans in rejection (human), 494
    nephrotoxicity caused by use of gentamicin and cyclosporine in recipients (human) (Communication), 220
    rejection in the presence of anti-HLA-Cw5 antibody (human) (Communication), 91
    survival in antilymphocyte serum-treated animals (dog), 593
  lung, rejection during cyclosporine dose tapering (dog), 466
  pancreaticoduodenosplenic, effect of irradiation of the donor spleen on rejection of (pig) (Communication), 686
  rejecting, T cells cloned from (mouse), 171
  rejection, splenic microenvironment and self-recognition as factors in (rat), 528
  skin
    expression of major histocompatibility antigens on vascular endothelium of (mouse), 178
    prolonged survival through enhancement effects of donor tissue (mouse), 200
  unresponsiveness, requirement for the kidney transplant to induce (rat), 642
Alloreactivity, humoral and cellular, effect of cyclosporine on (rat), 400
Allotransplantation, pancreatic (dog), 333
Amyloidosis, kidney transplantation in patients with, 598
Anastomosis
  portoportal, in liver transplantation (human) (Communication), 85
  vena cava, method for (rat) (Communication), 330
Anemia
  aplastic
    autolymphocytotoxins in patients with, 159
    marrow graft rejection and venoocclusive disease of the liver in patients with, 497
Anesthetics, lipid-soluble, immunosuppressive effects (mouse), 679
Angiography, digital subtraction, for kidney donor evaluation (human), 23
Antibody
  anti-CD3 (T3), -induced activation of T cells by cyclosporine (human) (Communication), 317
  antidiotypic, induction by blood transfusions (mouse), 632
  anti-HLA-Cw5, rejection of kidney allograft in the presence (human) (Communication), 91
  anti-IL 2 receptor monoclonal, preservation of suppression by (rat), 191
  Campath-1, study of (human) (Communication), 308
  causing positive T cell crossmatches, immunoglobulin class and specificity of (human), 608
  class II monoclonal, recognition of (mouse, human), 647
  host, to OKT3 (human), 507
  monoclonal
    depletion of T cells from bone marrow using (human), 73
    for prevention of graft-versus-host disease and marrow graft rejection (mouse), 239
    labeling in sequential kidney allograft biopsies (human), 352
  monoclonal antidinitrophenyl, suppression of B cell immunity to dinitrophenyl by serotherapy with (mouse), 524
  OKT3 monoclonal, plasma levels during therapy (human), 507
  response to Pa antigen, genetic control of (rat), 217
  screening using lymphocytes frozen in microtest trays, pretransplant (human) (Communication), 224
  serum HLA, crossmatch outcome in dialysis patients based on identification of, 267
Antigen
  allogeneic, drug-induced tolerance to (mouse), 281
  class I, expression (mouse) (Overview), 109
  class I major histocompatibility complex, immunosuppressive role for (rat), 1
  class II, cytomegalovirus infection, and kidney allograft rejection (human), 364
  class II (mouse, human), 647
  glycolipid-based blood group A, in kidney (human) (Communication), 88
  histocompatibility
    requirement for the kidney transplant to induce allograft unresponsiveness by using (rat), 642
    suppression of immune response to (mouse), 287
  histocompatibility complex
    effects of cyclosporine on induction of donor class I and class II (rat), 337
    influence of pattern of inflammation and administration of steroids on (human), 358
  HLA, expression on kidney tubular cells in culture (human), 671
  HLA class II, expression in kidney allografts (human), 144
  HLA-DR, expression on peripheral blood T lymphocytes and kidneys graft tubular epithelial cells (human), 479
  Ia, hybrid (human), 423
  major and minor, roles (mouse), 67
  major histocompatibility, expression on vascular endothelium of skin allografts (mouse), 178
  Pa, genetic control of antibody response to (rat), 217
  -specific helper T cell molecules, functional activity of (mouse), 162
Antilymphocyte serum, -treated animals, kidney allograft survival in (dog), 593
Antithymocyte globulin, in heart allografts, postoperative bone marrow injections with (rat) (Communication), 441
Autolymphocytotoxin, in patients with aplastic anemia, 159

Autotransplantation, neck segmental pancreatic (dog) (Communication), 437
Azathioprine
immunosuppression, modulation of response to interleukin 2 in recipients of donor-specific transfusions under (human), 502
impairment of immune response to influenza vaccination in kidney transplant recipients by (human), 376

B cell
activation, contribution of granular lymphocytes to (human), 257
immunity to dinitrophenyl by serotherapy with monoclonal antidinitrophenyl antibodies, suppression of (mouse), 524
islet, effects of fast cooling on function (mouse), 588
mechanisms of transplantation tolerance in (chicken), 184
response, induction (mouse), 162
tolerance, induction by doses of erythrocytes (rat), 292
Bile
duct varices (human) (Communication), 85
obstruction, suppression of host-versus-graft response in (rat) (Communication), 687
Biopsy, kidney allograft, analysis of cellular infiltration assessed by monoclonal antibody labeling in (human), 352
Blood
flow, leukocyte culture supernatant mediates changes in (sponge), 621
immunosuppressive metabolites of cyclosporine in (human), 262
Blood, whole, interferences in the radioimmunoassay for cyclosporine (human), 372
Blood group A, antigens in kidney, distribution of glyclipid-based (human) (Communication), 88
Blood stem cell, transplantation, cure of malignant lymphoma with (dog), 19
Bone, allograft, revascularized (dog) (Communication), 564
Bone marrow
assessment of T cell depletion before transplantation (human), 380
chimeras, suppressor cell activity in the spleen of (mouse), 548
density gradient-fractionated donor, postoperative injection of (dog), 593
depletion of T cells from (human), 73
-derived cells, Ia^+ (mouse), 141
E rosette-depleted, for transplantation (human) (Communication), 312
function, reconstitution by fraction 3 of Percoll density gradient-separated cells (human), 58
graft
donor-recipient pairs (dog), 64
failure after total body irradiation (dog) (Overview), 571
monoclonal antibodies for prevention of rejection (mouse), 239
grafting, effect of fibronectin on lymphocytes after (human), 412
graft rejection in patients with aplastic anemia conditioned with cyclophosphamide and cyclosporine, 497
injections with cyclosporine or antithymocyte globulin in heart allografts, postoperative (rat) (Communication), 441
transplantation
contribution of granular lymphocytes to B cell activation and differentiation after T cell-depleted (human), 257
correction of severe combined immunodeficiency (horse), 14
cure of thalassemia by (mouse), 248
cyclosporine in (Overview), 445
development of bullous pemphigoid after (human) (Communication), 320
for X-linked lymphoproliferative syndrome (human) (Communication), 222
HLA-DP matching and graft-versus-host disease in (human) (Communication), 558
increasing utilization (human) (Overview), 229
interstitial pneumonitis following (human), 515
monitoring natural killer responses following (human), 252
transmission of malaria by (human) (Letter), 228
unexplained nausea and vomiting (human), 602
utilization of HLA-typed donor pool for (human), 54
with T cell-depleted grafts (mouse), 118
transplant recipients, Epstein-Barr virus infection and immunity in (human), 50
Bowel, small, transplantation across major histocompatibility complex and nonmajor histocompatibility complex disparities (rat), 235
Buffy coat, pretransfusions, prolongation of heart allograft survival using (dog) (Communication), 98
Bullous pemphigoid, development after bone marrow transplantation (human) (Communication), 320
Bursectomy, inability to produce specific antibodies after (chicken), 197

Calmodulin, antagonists, immunosuppressive effects (mouse), 679
Campath-1, antibody, study of (human) (Communication), 308
Capsule, kidney, islet cell transplantation under the (dog) (Letter), 443
Carbohydrate, involvement with antibodies (mouse, human), 647
Cell. *See also* specific type
-mediated cytotoxicity in bronchoalveolar lavage fluid, concanavalin A-dependent (dog), 466
-mediated lympholysis in Kaposi's sarcoma after kidney allograft transplantation (human) (Communication), 697
Cellular infiltration, assessed by monoclonal antibody labeling in sequential kidney allograft biopsies, analysis (human), 352
Chimera, bone marrow, suppressor cell activity in the spleen of (mouse), 548
Chimerism, establishment by spleen cell transplantation from donors made tolerant to H-2-identical recipients (mouse), 417
Chromatid, exchange, induction (human), 61
Cimetidine
-treated recipient (human) (Communication), 311
Clone
T cell
cytotoxic (human), 423
mediation of cellular recruitment by (mouse), 168
Cluster, mitogen-induced, use of ultraviolet irradiation of dendritic cells to prevent (dog, human), 653
Coagulation, intravascular, and kidney donation (human) (Communication), 307
Collagenase, isolation of pancreatic islets by ductal injection of (rat) (Communication), 689
Collins' solution, effect on function and structure of tubules from kidneys (rabbit), 80
Complement
-dependent lymphocytotoxicity assay, ^{51}Cr release (mouse), 212
depletion of T cells from bone marrow using (human), 73
monoclonal antibody that fixes (human) (Communication), 308
Concanavalin A, -dependent cell-mediated cytotoxicity in bronchoalveolar lavage fluid (dog), 466
Cornea
allograft, role of accessory cells in rejection (rabbit), 667
transplant, reduction in the incidence of rejection of (mouse), 403
Crigler-Najjar syndrome, liver transplantation in (human) (Communication), 84
Crossmatch
antiglobulin cytotoxicity, in kidney allograft recipients treated with cyclosporine (human) (Communication), 439
outcome in dialysis patients based on identification of serum HLA antibodies, 267
T cell, immunoglobulin class and specificity of antibodies causing positive (human), 608
Cryopreservation, of pancreatic islets (mouse), 588
Cuff technique, for liver transplantation (rat) (Communication), 330
Culture
expression of HLA antigens on kidney tubule cells in (human), 671
leukocyte, supernatant mediates changes in cellular recruitment, blood flow, and vascular permeability (sponge), 621
lymphocyte, supernatants increase class I and class II HLA antigens (human), 671
lymphocyte pancreatic islet, inhibition of (mouse, rat), 660
Cyclophosphamide, and cyclosporine, marrow graft rejection and venoocclusive disease of the liver in patients with aplastic anemia conditioned with, 497
Cyclosporine
anaphylactic reaction to first exposure to (human) (Letter), 443

and gentamicin, nephrotoxicity caused by use in kidney allograft recipients (human) (Communication), 220
and Nva^{2}-cyclosporine, comparative toxicological study (rat), 395
antiglobulin cytotoxicity crossmatch in kidney allograft recipients treated with (human) (Communication), 439
binding protein in erythrocytes (human), 627
cyclophosphamide and, marrow graft rejection and venoocclusive disease of the liver in patients with aplastic anemia conditioned with, 497
donor kidney and, role in modifying rejection (dog), 333
dose tapering, lung allograft rejection during (dog), 466
effect on function of kidney allografts following extended preservation (human), 154
effect on humoral and cellular alloreactivity to pregnancy (rat), 400
effect on islet xenograft survival (rat) (Communication), 568
effect on survival of heart allografts (rat) (Communication), 94
effects on induction of donor class I and class II major histocompatibility complex antigens in heart and kidney allografts (rat), 337
extracted histocompatibility antigen and, requirement for kidney transplant to induce allograft unresponsiveness by the combination of (rat), 642
immunofluorescence caused by, in urinary cytology in kidney transplant recipients (human) (Communication), 699
immunosuppression, hepatocyte transplantation in the spleen under (rat), 537
immunosuppression by, revascularized bone allografts with (dog) (Communication), 564
immunosuppressive effects (mouse), 679
immunosuppressive metabolites of (human), 262
impairment of the immune response to influenza vaccination, in kidney transplant recipients by (human), 376
in bone marrow transplantation (Overview), 445
-induced nephrotoxicity (human), 368
induction of intestinal adenocarcinomas by (rat), 297
inhibition of anti-CD3 (T3) antibody-induced activation of T cells by (human) (Communication), 317
modulation of host defenses to pyogenic microorganisms by, 463
mutagenicity (human), 61
nephrotoxicity
factor VIII as index of vascular injury in (human), 150
^{99m}Tc diethylamine pentacetic acid scans in (human), 494
or antithymocyte globulin in heart allografts, postoperative bone marrow injections with (rat) (Communication), 441
pharmacokinetics (dog), 390
pretreatment to minimize interferences from whole blood in the radioimmunoassay for (human), 372
small intestine transplantation using (human), 613
-treated hepatocellular implants, prolonged survival (rat) (Communication), 325
-treated recipient (human) (Communication), 311
use with donor-specific blood transfusion (human) (Communication), 702
Cytology
urinary, in kidney transplant recipients (human) (Communication), 699
urine, in relation to urinary tract malignancies in transplant patients (Communication), 93
Cytomegalovirus
infection, in kidney transplant recipients (human), 368
infection, class II antigen expression, and kidney allograft rejection (human), 364
Cytotoxicity
cell-mediated, in bronchoalveolar lavage fluid (dog), 466
crossmatch in kidney allograft recipients treated with cyclosporine, antiglobulin (human) (Communication), 439
of T cells cloned from rejecting allografts (mouse), 171

Dendritic cell, ultraviolet irradiation of (dog, human), 653
Density gradient
-fractionated donor bone marrow, postoperative injection of (dog), 593
-separated cells, Percoll (human), 58
Diabetes mellitus, pancreas transplantation in (rat) (Communication), 327
Dialysis, crossmatch outcome in patients using, 267
Diary of Forthcoming Events, T29x, 107, 332
Diethylamine pentacetic acid, ^{99m}Tc, scans in kidney allograft rejection and cyclosporine nephrotoxicity (human), 494
Dilution, culture methods, assessment of T cell depletion from bone marrow before transplantation using (human), 380
Dinitrophenyl, suppression of B cell immunity to, by serotherapy with antidinitrophenyl antibodies (mouse), 524
Drug
-induced tolerance to allogeneic antigens (mouse), 281
-induced tolerance to allografts (mouse), 417
Duct
parotid, segmental pancreatic neck autotransplantation with exocrine drainage to (dog) (Communication), 437
thorax, drainage (sheep), 136
varices, bile (human) (Communication), 85
Dye, exclusion (mouse), 212

Endothelium, vascular, expression of major histocompatibility antigens on (mouse), 178
Enzyme, deficiencies in patients with Hunter's or Hurler's disorders, transplantation of fetal fibroblasts and correction of, 271
Enzyme deficiency disease, hepatocyte transplantation for (rat), 130
Epithelial cell, kidney graft, expression of HLA-DR antigens on peripheral blood T lymphocytes and (human), 479
Epstein-Barr virus, infection and immunity in bone marrow transplant recipients (human), 50
E rosette, -depleted bone marrow for transplantation, preparation (human) (Communication), 312
Erratum, 332
Erythrocyte
cyclosporine binding protein in (human), 627
induction of B cell tolerance by doses of (rat), 292
Exocrine, drainage to the parotid duct, segmental pancreatic neck autotransplantation with (dog) (Communication), 437

Factor VIII, as index of vascular injury in cyclosporine nephrotoxicity (human), 150
Fibroblast, fetal, transplantation in patients with Hunter's or Hurler's disorders, 271
Fibronectin, effect on lymphocytes after marrow grafting (human), 412
Fistula, chyloesophageal (sheep), 136
Fluid, bronchoalveolar lavage, concanavalin A-dependent cell-mediated cytotoxicity in (dog), 466
Fraction 3, marrow function reconstitution by (human), 58

Gene, conversion, serological confirmation in Ia mutant B6.C-H-2^{bm12} of (mouse), 429
Gentamicin, and cyclosporine, nephrotoxicity caused by use in kidney allograft recipients (human) (Communication), 220
Globulin, antithymocyte, postoperative bone marrow injections with (rat) (Communication), 441
Glomerulus, function in autotransplanted kidneys preserved by hypothermic storage or machine perfusion, recovery (dog), 453
Glycolipid, -based blood group A antigens in kidney related to A_1/A_2, Lewis, and secretor status, distribution (human) (Communication), 88
Graft. *See also* Allograft
bone marrow
donor-recipient pairs (dog), 64
failure after total body irradiation (dog) (Overview), 571
monoclonal antibodies for prevention of rejection (mouse), 239
rejection in patients with aplastic anemia conditioned with cyclophosphamide and cyclosporine, 497
heart, enhancement (rat), 581
-infiltrating T cells, analysis (rat), 406
kidney, tubular epithelial cells, expression of HLA-DR antigens on peripheral blood T lymphocytes and (human), 479
pancreas islet, characteristics (mouse), 387

Graft—*Continued*
rejection, role of T_{DTH} and T_C populations in (rat), 406
serum, immunosuppressive activity of serum from (rat), 581
skin, rejection (mouse), 636
survival following removal of the regional lymph node, mechanism of (rat), 532
T cell-depleted, bone marrow transplantation with (mouse), 118
Grafting, bone marrow, effect of fibronectin on lymphocytes after (human), 412
Graft-versus-host disease
HLA-DP matching and, in bone marrow transplantation (human) (Communication), 558
monoclonal antibodies for prevention of (mouse), 239
Graft-versus-host reaction, Ia^+ bone marrow-derived cells are stimulus for intestinal phase of (mouse), 141

Heart
allograft
development of suppressor lymphocytes during rejection (rat), 191
effect of cyclosporine and iloprost on survival (rat) (Communication), 94
effects of cyclosporine on induction of donor class I and class II major histocompatibility complex antigens in (rat), 337
postoperative bone marrow injections with cyclosporine or antithymocyte globulin in (rat) (Communication), 441
prolongation of survival using buffy coat pretransfusions (dog) (Communication), 98
prolongation of survival with BN 52021 (rat) (Communication), 86
rejection (mouse), 67
survival following administration of heat-treated donor lymphocytes (rat), 1
vascularized (mouse) (Communication), 226
graft, enhancement (rat), 581
-lung transplantation, technique for (mouse) (Communication), 329
transplant recipients, marker for rejection in (human) (Communication), 691
Heat treatment, immunosuppressive effect of spleen cells on kidney allografts by (rat), 302
Henoch-Schönlein purpura, course following kidney transplantation (human), 511
Hepatocyte
transplantation, in the spleen under cyclosporine immunosuppression (rat), 537
transplantation for enzyme deficiency disease (rat), 130
Heroin, abuse, kidney transplantation in patients with a history of (Communication), 556
Histocompatibility
antigen
expression on vascular endothelium of skin allografts (mouse), 178
requirement for the kidney transplant to induce allograft unresponsiveness with (rat), 642
suppression of immune response to (mouse), 287
loci associated with lymphocyte alloantigenic loci (mouse) (Communication), 322
Histocompatibility complex
and non-major histocompatibility complex disparities, transplantation of the small bowel across (rat), 235
antigen, influence of pattern of inflammation and administration of steroids on (human), 358
antigens, effects of cyclosporine on induction of donor class I and class II (rat), 337
class I major, immunosuppressive role for (rat), 1
HLA typing, studies involving leukemia, use of phytohemagglutinin-stimulated mononuclear cell subpopulations for (human) (Communication), 315
Host-versus-graft response, in biliary obstruction, suppression (rat) (Communication), 687
Hunter's disorder, transplantation of fetal fibroblasts and correction of enzymatic deficiencies in patients with, 271
Hurler's disorder, transplantation of fetal fibroblasts and correction of enzymatic deficiencies in patients with, 271
Hybrid, Ia antigens (human), 423

Iloprost, effect on survival of heart allografts (rat) (Communication), 94
Immune response, to influenza vaccination in kidney transplant recipients, impairment by cyclosporine (human), 376
Immunity
B cell, to dinitrophenyl by serotherapy with monoclonal antidinitrophenyl antibodies (mouse), 524
Esptein-Barr virus, and infection in bone marrow transplant recipients (human), 50
Immunodeficiency, severe combined, correction by bone marrow transplantation (horse), 14
Immunofluorescence, caused by cyclosporine in urinary cytology in kidney transplant recipients (human) (Communication), 699
Immunogenetics, and clinical factors affecting kidney transplantation (human), 39
Immunoglobulin
class and specificity of antibodies causing positive T cell crossmatches (human), 608
subclasses, differences (human), 212
Immunosuppressant, use in organ transplantation (human) (Communication), 308
Immunosuppression
azathioprine, modulation of response to interleukin 2 in recipients of donor-specific transfusions under (human), 502
by cyclosporine, revascularized bone allografts with (dog) (Communication), 564
cyclosporine, hepatocyte transplantation in the spleen under (rat), 537
regimens, different (human), 35
Immunosuppressive activity, of serum from liver grafts (rat), 581
Immunosuppressive effect, of spleen cells on kidney allografts (rat), 302
Immunosuppressive effects, of cyclosporine, lipid-soluble anesthetics, and calmodulin antagonists (mouse), 679
Immunotoxin
anti-Ia
effectiveness in suppression of mixed lymphocyte reaction (mouse), 205
inhibition of lymphocyte pancreatic islet cultures with (mouse, rat), 660
Implant, hepatocellular, survival of cyclosporine-treated (rat) (Communication), 325
Indium 111, -labeled cells, study using (rat), 528
Infection
cytomegalovirus
class II antigen expression, and kidney allograft rejection (human), 364
in kidney transplant recipients (human), 368
Esptein-Barr virus, and immunity in bone marrow transplant recipients (human), 50
Inflammation, pattern, influence (human), 358
Influenza, vaccination in kidney transplant recipients, impairment of immune response by cyclosporine to (human), 376
Injection
bone marrow, with cyclosporine or antithymocyte globulin in heart allografts (rat) (Communication), 441
of collagenase, isolation of pancreatic islets by (rat) (Communication), 689
of density gradient-fractionated donor bone marrow, postoperative (dog), 593
Interferon, γ, increases class I and class II HLA antigens (human), 671
Interleukin 2
in recipients of donor-specific transfusions under azathioprine immunosuppression, modulation of response to (human), 502
use (mouse), 679
Intestine, small, transplantation using cyclosporine (human), 613
Irradiation
immunosuppressive effect of spleen cells on kidney allografts by (rat), 302
of the donor spleen, effect on rejection (pig) (Communication), 686
total body, failure of marrow grafts after (dog) (Overview), 571
ultraviolet, of dendritic cells to prevent mitogen-induced cluster formation and lymphocyte proliferation (dog, human), 653
Ischemia, damage, in autotransplanted kidneys preserved by hypothermic storage (dog), 458
Islet
B cell, effects of fast cooling on function (mouse), 588
graft, pancreatic (mouse), 387
pancreatic
cryopreservation of (mouse), 588
inhibition of culture (mouse, rat), 660
isolation by ductal injection of collagenase (rat) (Communication), 689
transplantation, outcome (mouse), 588

xenograft, effect of cyclosporine on survival (rat) (Communication), 568
Islet, pancreatic, transplants, tolerance to (rat) (Communication), 96
Islet cell, transplantation under the kidney capsule (dog) (Letter), 443

Kaposi's sarcoma, cell-mediated lympholysis in, after kidney allograft transplantation (human) (Communication), 697
Kidney
allograft
analysis of cellular infiltration assessed by monoclonal antibody labeling in biopsy of (human), 352
cell-mediated lympholysis in Kaposi's sarcoma after transplantation (human) (Communication), 697
cytomegalovirus infection, class II antigen expression, and rejection of (human), 364
effect of cyclosporine on function after extended preservation (human), 154
effect of repeated pregnancies on function (human) (Communication), 694
effects of cyclosporine on induction of donor class I and class II major histocompatibility complex antigens in (rat), 337
HLA class II antigen expression in (human), 144
immunosuppressive effect of spleen cells on (rat), 302
^{99m}Tc diethylamine pentacetic acid scans in rejection (human), 494
rejection in the presence of anti-HLA-Cw5 antibody (human) (Communication), 91
survival in antilymphocyte serum-treated animals (dog), 593
allograft recipients
antiglobulin cytotoxicity crossmatch in (human) (Communication), 439
immunosuppressive metabolites of cyclosporine in blood of (human), 262
natural killer cell subsets in (human), 347
nephrotoxicity caused by use of gentamicin and cyclosporine in (human) (Communication), 220
capsule, islet cell transplantation under the (dog) (Letter), 443
distribution of glycolipid-based blood group A antigens in (human) (Communication), 88
donation, intravascular coagulation and (human) (Communication), 307
donor, role in modifying rejection (dog), 333
donor evaluation, analysis of accuracy and cost-effectiveness of digital subtraction angiography for (human), 23
graft tubular epithelial cells, expression of HLA-DR antigens on peripheral blood T lymphocytes and (human), 479
preservation, glomerular damage after (rat), 125
preserved by hypothermic storage or machine perfusion, recovery of glomerular and tubular function in (dog), 453
preserved by hypothermic storage, warm ischemic damage in autotransplanted (dog), 458
transplant
analyzing survival data (human), 46
effect of splenectomy on survival of patients with more than one, 473
from HIA-haploidentical donors (human), 35
outcome (human), 608
prediction model of success rates (human), 491
requirement for inducing allograft unresponsiveness by combining extracted histocompatibility antigen and cyclosporine (rat), 642
transplantation
course of IgA nephropathy and Henoch-Schönlein purpura following (human), 511
immunogenetic and clinical factors affecting (human), 39
in patients with a history of heroin abuse (Communication), 556
in patients with amyloidosis, 598
multivariate analysis of risk factors in (human), 29
use of donor-specific transfusions for living-related (human) (Communication), 562
transplant patients, urine cytology in relation to urinary tract malignancies in (Communication), 93
transplant recipients
immunofluorescence caused by cyclosporine in urinary cytology in (human) (Communication), 699
impairment of the immune response to influenza vaccination by cyclosporine in (human), 376
serum β_2-microglobulin during rejection, cyclosporine-induced nephrotoxicity, and cytomegalovirus infection in (human), 368
strongyloidiasis in (human), 518
transplants, influence of pattern of inflammation and administration of steroids on class II major histocompatibility complex antigen expression in (human), 358
tubule cells, expression of HLA antigens on (human), 671
tubules from, effect of Collins' solution on function and structure (rabbit), 80

Lavage fluid, bronchoalveolar, concanavalin A-dependent cell-mediated cytotoxicity in (dog), 466
Letters to the Editor, 102
Leukemia, myelogenous, use of phytohemagglutinin-stimulated mononuclear cell subpopulations for HLA typing studies involving (human) (Communication), 315
Leukemia cell, anti-, characterization (human), 252
Leukocyte, culture supernatant mediates changes in cellular recruitment, blood flow, and vascular permeability (sponge), 621
Lipid, -soluble anesthetics, immunosuppressive effects (mouse), 679
Liver
graft, immunosuppressive activity of serum from (rat), 581
transplantation
cuff technique for (rat) (Communication), 330
for hepatobiliary malignancy (human) (Communication), 561
in Crigler-Najjar syndrome (human) (Communication), 84
portoportal anastomosis in (human) (Communication), 85
preservation damage in (pig), 122
pulmonary complications of (human), 484
serology of (rat), 7
toxic shock syndrome complicating (human) (Communication), 437
venoocclusive disease of, in patients with aplastic anemia conditioned with cyclophosphamide and cyclosporine, 497
L3T4$^+$ cell, depletion of (mouse), 636
Lung
allograft, rejection during cyclosporine dose tapering (dog), 466
heart transplantation, technique for (mouse) (Communication), 329
Lymph node, regional, mechanism of graft survival following removal (rat), 532
Lymphocyte
alloantigenic loci, histocompatibility loci associated with (mouse) (Communication), 322
culture, supernatants increase class I and class II HLA antigens (human), 671
effect of fibronectin on (human), 412
frozen, pretransplant antibody screening using (human) (Communication), 224
granular, contribution to B cell activation (human), 257
heat-treated, survival of heart allografts following administration of (rat), 1
pancreatic islet cultures, inhibition of (mouse, rat), 660
proliferation, use of ultraviolet irradiation of dendritic cells to prevent mitogen-induced cluster formation and (dog, human), 653
reaction, effectiveness of anti-Ia immunotoxins in suppression of (mouse), 205
suppressor, development during rejection of heart allografts (rat), 191
T
activity in transplant patients (Letter), 105
expression of HLA-DR antigens on (human), 479
transferrin receptor expressing (human) (Communication), 691
Lymphocytotoxicity, assay, ^{51}Cr release complement-dependent (mouse), 212
Lympholysis, cell-mediated, in Kaposi's sarcoma after kidney allograft transplantation (human) (Communication), 697
Lymphoma, malignant, cure (dog), 19
Lymphoproliferative syndrome, X-linked, bone marrow transplantation for (human) (Communication), 222

Malaria, transmission by bone marrow transplantation (human) (Letter), 228
Malignancy, hepatobiliary, liver transplantation for (human) (Communication), 561

Matching, HLA-DP, and graft-versus-host disease in bone marrow transplantation (human) (Communication), 558
Metabolite, immunosuppressive, of cyclosporine in the blood of kidney allograft recipients (human), 262
β_2-microglobulin, serum, during rejection (human), 368
Microorganism, pyogenic, modulation of host defenses by cyclosporine, 463
Microtest trays, pretransplant antibody screening using lymphocytes frozen in (human) (Communication), 224
Mitogen
-induced cluster formation and lymphocyte proliferation, use of ultraviolet irradiation of dendritic cells to prevent (dog, human), 653
Molecule, T cell, functional activity of antigen-specific helper (mouse), 162
Mononuclear cell, subpopulations, use of phytohemagglutinin-stimulated (human) (Communication), 315
^{99m}Tc, diethylamine pentacetic acid scans in kidney allograft rejection and cyclosporine nephrotoxicity (human), 494
Mutagenicity, of cyclosporine (human), 61
Mutant, B6.C-H-2^{bm12}, Ia, serological confirmation of gene conversion in (mouse), 429

Natural killer cell, subsets in kidney allograft recipients (human), 347
Nausea, unexplained, after marrow transplantation (human), 602
Nephropathy, IgA, course following kidney transplantation (human), 511
Nephrotoxicity
caused by use of gentamicin and cyclosporine in kidney allograft recipients (human) (Communication), 220
cyclosporine
factor VIII as index of vascular injury in (human), 150
^{99m}Tc diethylamine pentacetic acid scans in (human), 494
cyclosporine-induced (human), 368
N-methyl-*N*-nitrosourea, induction of intestinal adenocarcinomas by cyclosporine in animals given (rat), 297
Node, lymph, mechanism of graft survival following removal (rat), 532
Nva^2-cyclosporine, cyclosporine and, comparative toxicological study (rat), 395

OKT3 monoclonal antibody, plasma levels during therapy (human), 507

Pancreas
allotransplantation (dog), 333
islet grafts, characteristics (mouse), 387
transplantation, technique update (rat) (Communication), 327
Pancreatectomy, cyclosporine pharmacokinetics (dog), 390
Parotid, duct, segmental pancreatic neck autotransplantation with exocrine drainage to (dog) (Communication), 437
Percoll, density gradient-separated cells, marrow function reconstitution by fraction 3 of (human), 58
Perfusion, machine, recovery of glomerular and tubular function in autotransplanted kidneys preserved by (dog), 453
Pharmacokinetics, cyclosporine (dog), 390
Phytohemagglutinin, -stimulated mononuclear cell subpopulations, use for HLA typing studies involving leukemia (human) (Communication), 315
Plasma, levels during therapy, OKT3 monoclonal antibody (human), 507
Platelet
-activating factor (rat) (Communication), 86
Pneumonitis, interstitial, following bone marrow transplantation (human), 515
Pregnancy
effect of cyclosporine on humoral and cellular alloreactivity to (rat), 400
repeated, effect on kidney allograft function (mouse) (Communication), 694
Preservation
damage in liver transplantation (pig), 122
extended, effect of cyclosporine on function of kidney allografts after (human), 154
kidney, glomerular damage after (rat), 125
Protein, cyclosporine binding, in erythrocyte (human), 627
Pulmonary complications, of liver transplantation (human), 484
Purpura, Henoch-Schönlein, course following kidney transplantation (human), 511

Radiation
ultraviolet
reduction in the incidence of rejection of corneal transplants by pretreatment with (mouse), 403
suppression of immune response to histocompatibility antigens by (mouse), 287
Radioimmunoassay, for cyclosporine, pretreatment to minimize interferences from whole blood in (human), 372
Ranitidine
-treated recipient (human) (Communication), 311
Reaction
graft-versus-host, Ia$^+$ bone marrow-derived cells are stimulus for intestinal phase of (mouse), 141
lymphocyte, effectiveness of anti-Ia immunotoxins in suppression of (mouse), 205
to first exposure to cyclosporine, anaphylactic (human) (Letter), 443
Receptor
anti-IL 2, preservation of suppression by (rat), 191
T cell alloantigen-specific (mouse), 632
transferrin, expressing lymphocytes (human) (Communication), 691
Reconstitution, of immunohemopoietic functions (mouse), 118
Rejection
allograft, splenic microenvironment and self-recognition as factors in (rat), 528
bone marrow graft
in patients with aplastic anemia conditioned with cyclophosphamide and cyclosporine, 497
monoclonal antibodies for prevention of (mouse), 239
cornea allograft, role of accessory cells in (rabbit), 667
cornea transplants, reduction in the incidence by pretreatment with ultraviolet radiation (mouse), 403
effect of irradiation of the donor spleen on (pig) (Communication), 686
expression of HLA-DR antigens on peripheral blood T lymphocytes and kidney graft tubular epithelial cells in association with (human), 479
graft, role of T_{DTH} and T_C populations in (rat), 406
heart allograft, development of suppressor lymphocytes during (rat), 191
heart allografts (mouse), 67
in heart transplant recipients, marker for (human) (Communication), 691
kidney allograft
cytomegalovirus infection, class II antigen expression, and (human), 364
in the presence of anti-HLA-Cw5 antibody (human) (Communication), 91
^{99m}Tc diethylamine pentacetic acid scans in (human), 494
lung allograft, during cyclosporine dose tapering (dog), 466
role of donor kidney and cyclosporine in modifying (dog), 333
serum β_2-microglobulin during (human), 368
skin grafts (mouse), 636
Response
alloantibody, in nonrejector combination (rat), 7
antibody, to Pa antigen (rat), 217
host-versus-graft, in biliary obstruction (rat) (Communication), 687
immune
suppression (mouse), 287
to influenza vaccination in kidney transplant recipients (human), 376
natural killer, following bone marrow transplantation (human), 252
to interleukin 2 in recipients of donor-specific transfusions under azathioprine immunosuppression, modulation (human), 502

Sarcoma, Kaposi's, cell-mediated lympholysis in (human) (Communication), 697
Scans, ^{99m}Tc diethylamine pentacetic acid, in kidney allograft rejection and cyclosporine nephrotoxicity (human), 494
Sensitization, in patients given donor-specific blood transfusions ((Communication), 695
Serology, of liver transplantation (rat), 7
Serotherapy, suppression of B cell immunity to dinitrophenyl by (mouse), 524
Serum
antilymphocyte, kidney allograft survival in animals treated with (dog), 593
from liver grafts, immunosuppressive activity of (rat), 581
HLA antibodies, crossmatch outcome in dialysis patients based on identification of, 267
β_2-microglobulin during rejection, increased (human), 368
Skin
allograft
expression of major histocompatibility

antigens on vascular endothelium of (mouse), 178
prolonged survival through enhancement effects of donor tissue (mouse), 200
graft, rejection (mouse), 636
Spleen
donor, effect of irradiation on rejection (pig) (Communication), 686
hepatocyte transplantation in (rat), 537
microenvironment and self-recognition as factors in allograft rejection (rat), 528
of bone marrow chimeras, suppressor cell activity in (mouse), 548
Spleen cell
donor, immunosuppressive effect on kidney allografts (rat), 302
transplantation, establishment of chimerism by (mouse), 417
Splenectomy, effect on survival of patients with more than one kidney transplant, 473
Stem cell, cure of thalassemia by bone marrow transplantation without eradication of (mouse), 248
Steroid, influence of administration on class II major histocompatibility complex antigen expression in kidney transplants (human), 358
Storage
hypothermic
recovery of glomerular and tubular function in autotransplanted kidneys preserved by (dog), 453
warm ischemic damage in autotransplanted kidneys preserved by (dog), 458
Strongyloidiasis, in kidney transplant recipients (human), 518
Suppression
B cell immunity to dinitrophenyl by serotherapy with monoclonal anti-dinitrophenyl antibodies (mouse), 524
by anti-IL 2 receptor monoclonal antibody, preservation (rat), 191
mixed lymphocyte reaction, effectiveness of anti-Ia immunotoxins in (mouse), 205
of host-versus-graft response in biliary obstruction (rat) (Communication), 687
of immune response (mouse), 287
Suppressor cell, activity in the spleen of bone marrow chimeras (mouse), 548

T cell
alloantigen-specific receptors, characterization (mouse), 632
clone, mediation of cellular recruitment by (mouse), 168
cloned from rejecting allografts, cytotoxicity (mouse), 171
clones, cytotoxic (human), 423
crossmatch, immunoglobulin class and specificity of antibodies causing positive (human), 608
cytotoxic, generation (mouse), 636
-depleted bone marrow transplantation, contribution of granular lymphocytes to B cell activation and differentiation after (human), 257
-depleted grafts, bone marrow transplantation with (mouse), 118
depletion from bone marrow before transplantation, assessment (human), 380
depletion from bone marrow using monoclonal antibodies and complement (human), 73
graft-infiltrating, analysis (rat), 406
growth factor, impairment of tolerance by (chicken), 184
inhibition of anti-CD3 (T3) antibody-induced activation by cyclosporine (human) (Communication), 317
molecules, functional activity of antigen-specific helper (mouse), 162
response, induction (mouse), 162
subsets, depletion of (mouse), 239
Thalassemia, cure by bone marrow transplantation without eradication of stem cells (mouse), 248
Thorax, duct drainage (sheep), 136
Tissue, donor, prolonged skin allograft survival through enhancement effects on (mouse), 200
Tolerance
B cell, induction by doses of erythrocytes (rat), 292
in B cells (chicken), 184
induced, to pancreatic islet transplants (rat) (Communication), 96
in nonrejector combination (rat), 7
of epidermal allografts produced in culture, 274
systemic, induction (rat), 581
to allografts, drug-induced (mouse), 417
Toxic shock syndrome, complicating liver transplantation (human), 434
Transferrin, receptor expressing lymphocytes (human) (Communication), 691
Transfusion, blood
collapse curves (rat), 542
donor-specific
for living-related kidney transplantation (human) (Communication), 562
influence (human), 35
sensitization in patients given (Communication), 695
use of cyclosporine with (human) (Communication), 702
induction of antidiotypic antibodies by (mouse), 632
Transfusions, blood, donor-specific, modulation of response to interleukin 2 in recipients of (human), 502
Tubule
from kidney, effect of Collins' solution on function and structure (rabbit), 80
function in autotransplanted kidneys preseved by hypothermic storage or machine perfusion, recovery (dog), 453
Tubule cell, kidney, expression of HLA antigens on (human), 671

Ultraviolet
irradiation, of dendritic cells to prevent mitogen-induced cluster formation and lymphocyte proliferation (dog, human), 653
radiation
reduction in the incidence of rejection of corneal transplants by pretreatment with (mouse), 403
suppression of immune response to histocompatibility antigens by (mouse), 287
Urinary tract, malignancies in transplant patients, urine cytology in relation to (Communication), 93
Urine, cytology in relation to urinary tract malignancies in transplant patients (Communication), 93

Vaccination, influenza, impairment of the immune response to (human), 376
Varix, bile duct (human) (Communication), 85
Vena cava, anastomosis, method for (rat) (Communication), 330
Venoocclusive disease, of the liver in patients with aplastic anemia conditioned with cyclophosphamide and cyclosporine, 497
Virus, Epstein-Barr, infection and immunity in bone marrow transplant recipients (human), 50
Vomiting, after marrow transplantation (human), 602

Xenograft, islet, effect of cyclosporine on survival (rat) (Communication), 568

-42.